ARTHRITIS AND ALLIED CONDITIONS
A Textbook of Rheumatology

ARTHRITIS AND ALLIED CONDITIONS
A Textbook of Rheumatology

Daniel J. McCarty, M.D.

Will and Cava Ross Professor and Chairman
Department of Medicine
The Medical College of Wisconsin
Milwaukee, Wisconsin

Foreword By
Joseph Lee Hollander, M.D.

eleventh edition

Lea & Febiger

1989

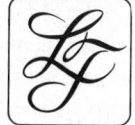

Philadelphia • London

Lea & Febiger
600 Washington Square
Philadelphia, PA   19106-4198
U.S.A.
(215) 922-1330

First Edition, 1940   Seventh Edition, 1966
Second Edition, 1941   Eighth Edition, 1972
Third Edition, 1944   Ninth Edition, 1979
Fourth Edition, 1949   Tenth Edition, 1985
Fifth Edition, 1953   Eleventh Edition, 1989
Sixth Edition, 1960

Library of Congress Cataloging in Publication Data

Arthritis and allied conditions.

  Includes bibliographies and index.
  1. Arthritis. 2. Rheumatism. 3. Rheumatology.
I. McCarty, Daniel J., 1928–   . [DNLM: 1. Arthritis.
WE 344 A7866]
RC933.A64   1988   616.7'22   88-4729
ISBN 0-8121-1123-0

Print Number 3   2   1

foreword

Fifty years have passed since Bernard I. Comroe started writing the first edition of ARTHRITIS AND ALLIED CONDITIONS—A TEXTBOOK OF RHEU-MATOLOGY. At that time the study of the rheumatic diseases was in its infancy. The American Rheumatism Association (ARA), now the largest national professional society for study of arthritis and related conditions, had only recently come into being. Only a few devoted pioneers were trying to study arthritis, eager to find some way to help the millions of sufferers and prevent the widespread crippling. Practically no funds were available for arthritis research, and only a small number of medical schools included in the faculty anyone even slightly interested in arthritis. It was in this barren environment that Dr. Comroe undertook to compose a textbook, organizing what little was known in a comprehensive and comprehensible form.

Dr. Comroe had obtained much of his data from the *Rheumatism Reviews*, started only a few years before by a small group of ARA members led by Dr. Philip Hench. The *Reviews* were a compendium of articles in the British and American literature on arthritis and related subjects. During the War years two more successful editions of ARTHRITIS appeared, but Dr. Comroe died in 1945.

When I took on the assignment of revising and rewriting ARTHRITIS AND ALLIED CONDITIONS in 1947 I realized that a single individual could not write or even collate the rapidly accumulating clinical research data in this expanding field, so I asked a group of colleagues to contribute. That fourth edition, coinciding with the discovery of cortisone in 1949 by Dr. Hench and his colleagues, was the first textbook to include an account of this epoch-making discovery. Truly, the discovery of the dramatic anti-inflammatory effect of cortisone started an explosive increase of interest in rheumatic diseases, and, indeed, in all types of inflammatory reactions, in the immune response, and in the physiology of lymphocytes, complement, and other mediators in the whole process of body reaction to infection and trauma. Even though, as the more optimistic had hoped, cortisone never proved to be a cure for rheumatoid arthritis, systemic lupus erythematosus, or the many other forms of inflammatory diseases of joints and other connective tissues, it truly was the catalyst of the "Renaissance of Rheumatology." Older rheumatologists may date themselves by stating they were rheumatologists "B.C." (before cortisone), acknowledging this turning point in their field.

Successive editions of ARTHRITIS—the 5th Edition of 1953, the 6th Edition of 1960, the 7th Edition of 1966, and the 8th Edition of 1972—have collated and interpreted the many advances in Rheumatology, both clinical and basic. By the eighth edition I was aware that the task of organizing, collating, and editing had become too much for me, even with the help of section editors. (The former young upstart was becoming the old downstop.) I therefore secured the assistance of Daniel J. McCarty for that task. He has ably carried on the tremendous work of organizing and editing the 9th Edition, in 1979, the 10th Edition, in 1985, and now the 11th Edition.

In previous editions I had written an introductory chapter that dealt with the history of Rheumatology, the classification of rheumatic diseases, and the development of organizations to cope with the problem. Because of the tremendous growth of scientific knowledge to be collated in this edition, and because all the material had been well documented in HISTORY OF RHEUMATOLOGY IN THE UNITED STATES, written by three former collaborating editors of ARTHRITIS AND ALLIED CONDITIONS, namely Charley J. Smyth, Richard H. Freyberg, and Currier McEwen, it was decided to eliminate that chapter. All interested readers are referred to this excellent book, published by the Arthritis Foundation in 1985.

Dr. McCarty did a splendid job editing the past two editions of ARTHRITIS and has improved on the standards set by Dr. Comroe and by me. This edition marks the continued coverage of the field of Rheumatology throughout a half century!

Joseph Lee Hollander, M.D.

preface

A comprehensive single-volume textbook of Rheumatology with a solitary editor has become the exception rather than the rule. The 11th Edition of ARTHRITIS AND ALLIED CONDITIONS—A TEXTBOOK OF RHEUMATOLOGY, a thoroughly revised and updated version of its venerable ancestors dating back to 1940, remains such a text.

New chapters have been devoted to mast cells and eosinophils, both of which have increasingly been implicated in the pathogenesis of rheumatic disorders. A separate new chapter is devoted to the anticardiolipin syndrome, an important, recently recognized subset of systemic lupus erythematosus that I have found to be common. Also, the signals controlling various lymphocyte populations in lupus are now sufficiently understood to warrant separate treatment. A new chapter discusses the arthritis associated with food allergy and the influence of diet. This subject was covered in the earlier editions and deleted in the past few volumes because of lack of data. Recent evidence now justifies its inclusion once again. Although the association is rare, the subject is raised by patients so frequently that clinicians need to have timely authoritative views.

New chapters are devoted to the pseudovasculitis syndromes that must be differentiated from true vasculitis; uveitis, a subject poorly understood by most rheumatologists; the nerve entrapment syndromes; and metabolic diseases of muscle, knowledge about which has been expanding rapidly. Diabetic stiff-hand syndrome has been added to the chapter on Duyputren's contracture and plantar fasciitis. Spinal stenosis has been highlighted as a separate chapter as it is both common and commonly overlooked. Finally, rapidly expanding knowledge about the particulate matter of synovial fluid justified a new chapter on the "other" crystals and particulates that may be associated with joint symptoms.

Space for all of these subjects was created by deletion of Harry K. Genant's classic chapter on radiology, which remains immortalized in past editions for ready reference. New chapters on magnetic resonance imaging and techniques for assessment of bone mineral have also been added. Certainly, the newer technologies are the cutting edge in the radiologic aspects of the rheumatic diseases.

In summary, all of the basic science advances that should be comprehended by the consultant-level rheumatologist are up to date. The individual rheumatic syndromes are discussed in both a theoretic and a practical manner by experts.

The advent of computer literature search capability and retrieval, together with the proliferation of new sources of original clinical observations and original research in arthritis and allied conditions, rapidly renders any textbook obsolete. This revision follows the 10th Edition by only 4 years, and I plan future revisions at not greater than 4-year intervals. As the medical community becomes more sophisticated and computer literate, all textbooks, including this one, may like the dinosaur become extinct. In the meanwhile, comprehensive, affordable, current texts like this one should serve as a useful source of reference and continuing education for those of us caring for patients suffering from arthritis and allied conditions.

Milwaukee, Wisconsin   Daniel J. McCarty, M.D.

In Memoriam

John J. Calabro, M.D.
Eliot A. Goldings, M.D.

contributors

Graciela S. Alarcón, M.D., M.P.H.
Associate Professor of Medicine
The University of Alabama at Birmingham
Birmingham, Alabama

Marlene A. Aldo-Benson, M.D.
Professor of Medicine, Microbiology, and Immunology
Indiana University School of Medicine
Indianapolis, Indiana

Roy D. Altman, M.D.
Professor of Medicine
University of Miami School of Medicine
Chief, Arthritis Section
Miami Veterans Administration Medical Center
Miami, Florida

Frank C. Arnett, M.D.
Professor of Medicine
Director, Rheumatology Division
University of Texas
Houston, Texas

Paul A. Bacon, M.D.
Professor of Rheumatology
Arthritis and Rheumatology Council
University of Birmingham Medical School
Birmingham, England

Gene V. Ball, M.D.
Professor of Medicine
University of Alabama at Birmingham
Birmingham, Alabama

John Baum, M.D.
Professor, Medicine and Pediatrics and
    Preventive Family and Rehabilitation Medicine
University of Rochester School of Medicine and
    Dentistry
Director, Clinical Immunology Unit
Monroe Community Hospital
Rochester, New York

Timothy W. Behrens, M.D.
Instructor in Medicine
Department of Medicine
Medical College of Wisconsin
Milwaukee, Wisconsin

Nicholas Bellamy, M.D.
Associate Professor of Medicine and Epidemiology
University of Western Ontario
London, Ontario

J. Claude Bennett, M.D.
Professor and Chairman
Department of Medicine
University of Alabama at Birmingham
Birmingham, Alabama

Robert M. Bennett, M.D.

Professor of Medicine
Head, Arthritis and Rheumatic Diseases Division
Oregon Health Sciences University
Portland, Oregon

Kenneth D. Brandt, M.D.

Professor of Medicine
Division of Rheumatology
Indiana University School of Medicine
Indianapolis, Indiana

W. Watson Buchanan, M.D.

Professor of Medicine
McMaster University
Hamilton, Ontario, Canada

John J. Calabro, M.D.*

Professor of Medicine and Pediatrics
University of Massachusetts School of Medicine
Director, Division of Rheumatology
St. Vincent Hospital
Worcester, Massachusetts

Grant W. Cannon, M.D.

Assistant Professor of Medicine
Division of Rheumatology
University of Utah and
    Veterans Administration Medical Center
Salt Lake City, Utah

Juan J. Canoso, M.D.

Professor of Medicine
Tufts University School of Medicine
Director of Clinical Rheumatology
New England Medical Center
Boston, Massachusetts

Guillermo F. Carrera, M.D.

Professor of Radiology
Medical College of Wisconsin
Milwaukee, Wisconsin

Dennis A. Carson, M.D.

Scripps Clinic and Research Foundation
La Jolla, California

C. William Castor, M.D.

Professor of Internal Medicine
Member, Rackham Arthritis Research Unit and
    Rheumatology Division
University of Michigan Medical School
Ann Arbor, Michigan

Mack L. Clayton, M.D.

Denver Orthopedic Clinic
Denver, Colorado

Alan S. Cohen, M.D.

Conrad Wesselhoeft Professor of Medicine
Chief of Medicine and Director, Thorndike Memorial
    Laboratory
Boston City Hospital
Boston University School of Medicine
Boston, Massachusetts

Mary E. Cronin, M.D.

Assistant Professor of Medicine
Loyola University Stritch School of Medicine
Maywood, Illinois

Bruce N. Cronstein, M.D.

Assistant Professor of Medicine
New York University Medical Center
New York, New York

Paul Dieppe, M.D.

ARC Professor of Rheumatology
Bristol Royal Infirmary
Bristol, England

Joseph Duffy, M.D.

Internal Medicine/Rheumatology
Mayo Clinic
Rochester, Minnesota

George E. Ehrlich, M.D.

Adjunct Professor of Clinical Medicine
New York University
New York, New York

Michael H. Ellman, M.D.

Associate Professor of Clinical Medicine
Director, Division of Rheumatology
Michael Reese Hospital and Medical Center
Pritzger School of Medicine
University of Chicago
Chicago, Illinois

Anthony S. Fauci, M.D.

Director, National Institutes of Allergy and Infectious
    Diseases
National Institutes of Health
Bethesda, Maryland

Douglas T. Fearon, M.D.

Professor of Medicine
Director, Division of Molecular and Clinical
    Rheumatology
Johns Hopkins University School of Medicine
Baltimore, Maryland

---

*Deceased

Adrian E. Flatt, M.D.

Professor and Chief, Department of Orthopedic
    Surgery
Baylor University Medical Center
Dallas, Texas

Denys K. Ford, M.D.

Professor of Medicine
Division of Rheumatology
Department of Medicine
University of British Columbia
Vancouver, B.C., Canada

Robert I. Fox, M.D., Ph.D.

Assistant Member
Scripps Clinic and Research Foundation
La Jolla, California

Daniel E. Furst, M.D.

Associate Professor of Medicine
Department of Medicine
University of Iowa
Iowa City, Iowa

Robert A. Gatter, M.D.

Associate Clinical Professor of Medicine
University of Pennsylvania School of Medicine
Philadelphia, Pennsylvania
Physician-in-Chief, Division of Rheumatology
Abington Memorial Hospital
Abington, Pennsylvania
Director, Center for Arthritis and Back Pain
Willow Grove, Pennsylvania

Harry K. Genant, M.D.

Professor, Departments of Radiology, Medicine, and
    Orthopaedic Surgery
University of California at San Francisco
San Francisco, California

Mark H. Ginsberg, M.D.

Associate Member
Division of Immunology and Rheumatology
Scripps Clinic and Research Foundation
La Jolla, California

Edward J. Goetzl, M.D.

Professor of Medicine
University of California at San Francisco
Moffitt Hospital
San Francisco, California

Don L. Goldenberg, M.D.

Clinical Program Director
Arthritis Section
Professor of Medicine
Boston University School of Medicine
Boston, Massachusetts

Eliot A. Goldings, M.D.*

Assistant Professor of Internal Medicine
University of Texas Southwestern Medical School
Dallas, Texas

Ira M. Goldstein, M.D.

Professor of Medicine
University of California at San Francisco
San Francisco General Hospital
San Francisco, California

James S. Goodwin, M.D.

Professor and Vice Chairman
Department of Medicine
Medical College of Wisconsin
Milwaukee, Wisconsin

John S. Gould, M.D.

Professor and Chairman
Department of Orthopedic Surgery
Medical College of Wisconsin
Milwaukee, Wisconsin

Barry L. Gruber, M.D.

Department of Medicine
State University of New York at Stony Brook
Health Science Center
Stony Brook, New York

Nortin M. Hadler, M.D.

Professor of Medicine and Microbiology/Immunology
Department of Medicine
University of North Carolina School of Medicine
Chapel Hill, North Carolina

Bevra H. Hahn, M.D.

Professor of Medicine and Director of Rheumatology
University of California at Los Angeles
Los Angeles, California

Paul B. Halverson, M.D.

Associate Professor of Medicine
Medical College of Wisconsin
St. Joseph's Hospital
Milwaukee, Wisconsin

E. Nigel Harris, M.D., D.M.

Deputy Director
Lupus Research Laboratory
The Rayne Institute
St. Thomas Hospital
Division of Rheumatology
University of Louisville
Louisville, Kentucky

*Deceased

Louis A. Healey, M.D.

The Mason Clinic
Seattle, Washington

George Ho, Jr., M.D.

Assistant Professor of Medicine
Department of Medicine
The Miriam Hospital
Brown University
Providence, Rhode Island

David A. Horwitz, M.D.

Professor of Medicine and Head, Rheumatology Section
Los Angeles County University of Southern California
    Medical Center
Los Angeles, California

Aubrey J. Hough, Jr., M.D.

Professor and Chairman
Department of Pathology
University of Arkansas for Medical Sciences
Little Rock, Arkansas

David S. Howell, M.D.

Professor of Medicine and Medical Investigator
Veterans Administration Medical Center
University of Miami School of Medicine
Miami, Florida

Graham R.V. Hughes, M.D.

Department of Rheumatology
St. Thomas Hospital
London, England

Allan E. Inglis, M.D.

Hospital for Special Surgery
New York, New York

John N. Insall, M.D.

Professor of Clinical Surgery
Cornell University Medical College
Department of Orthopedic Surgery
Hospital for Special Surgery
New York, New York

Israeli A. Jaffe, M.D.

Professor of Clinical Medicine
College of Physicians and Surgeons
Columbia University
New York, New York

Hugo E. Jasin, M.D.

Professor of Internal Medicine
University of Texas Southwestern Medical School
Dallas, Texas

Roger P. Johnson, M.S., M.D.

Clinical Professor of Orthopaedic Surgery
Medical Director, Musculo Skeletal Center
St. Francis Hospital
Milwaukee, Wisconsin

John P. Jones, Jr., M.D.

Medical Research Director
Diagnostic Osteonecrosis Center and Research
    Foundations
Kellseyville, California

Lawrence J. Kagen, M.D.

Professor of Medicine
Department of Medicine
Cornell University Medical Center
Hospital for Special Surgery
New York, New York

Allen P. Kaplan, M.D.

Chairman, Department of Medicine
State University of New York at Stony Brook
Health Sciences Center
Stony Brook, New York

Franklin Kozin, M.D.

Department of Rheumatology
Scripps Clinic and Research Foundation
La Jolla, California

Stephen M. Krane, M.D.

Professor of Medicine and Chief, Arthritis Institute
Massachusetts General Hospital
Boston, Massachusetts

Randi Y. Leavitt, M.D., Ph.D.

Senior Investigator
Laboratory of Immunoregulation
National Institute of Allergy and Infectious Diseases
National Institutes of Health
Bethesda, Maryland

David B. Levine, M.D.

Clinical Professor of Orthopaedic Surgery
Cornell University Medical College
Director, Department of Orthopaedic Surgery
Hospital for Special Surgery
Attending Orthopaedic Surgeon
New York Hospital
New York, New York

Dennis J. Levinson, M.D.

Associate Professor of Clinical Medicine
Department of Medicine
Michael Reese Hospital and Medical Center
Pritzker School of Medicine
University of Chicago
Chicago, Illinois

Robert W. Lightfoot, Jr., M.D.

Professor of Medicine
Director, Division of Rheumatology
University of Kentucky School of Medicine
Lexington, Kentucky

Martin Lotz, M.D.

Senior Research Associate
Department of Basic and Clinical Research
La Jolla, California

Daniel J. McCarty, M.D.

Will and Cava Ross Professor and Chairman
Department of Medicine
The Medical College of Wisconsin
Milwaukee, Wisconsin

Stephen E. Malawista, M.D.

Professor of Medicine
Chief, Section of Rheumatology
Department of Internal Medicine
Yale University School of Medicine
New Haven, Connecticut

Brian F. Mandell, M.D., Ph.D.

Assistant Professor of Medicine
University of Pennsylvania School of Medicine
Philadelphia, Pennsylvania

Henry J. Mankin, M.D.

Ashley Professor of Orthopedics and Surgery
Harvard Medical School
Massachusetts General Hospital
Boston, Massachusetts

Mart Mannik, M.D.

Professor of Medicine
Head, Division of Rheumatology
University of Washington
Seattle, Washington

Alfonse T. Masi, M.D., D.R.P.H.

Professor of Medicine
Department of Medicine
University of Illinois College of Medicine at Peoria
Peoria, Illinois

Thomas A. Medsger, Jr., M.D.

Professor of Medicine
Chief, Division of Rheumatology and
    Clinical Immunology
University of Pittsburgh
School of Medicine
Pittsburgh, Pennsylvania

Ronald P. Messner, M.D.

Professor of Medicine
Director, Section of Rheumatology
University of Minnesota School of Medicine
Minneapolis, Minnesota

Glenn A. Meyer, M.D.

Professor of Neurosurgery
Medical College of Wisconsin
Milwaukee, Wisconsin

Roland W. Moskowitz, M.D.

Professor of Medicine
Case Western Reserve University
Director, Division of Rheumatic Diseases
University Hospitals
Cleveland, Ohio

Gerald T. Nepom, M.D., Ph.D.

Director, Immunology Program
Virginia Mason Research Center
Seattle, Washington

J. Desmond O'Duffy, M.D.

Professor of Medicine
Department of Rheumatology
Mayo Clinic
Rochester, Minnesota

Richard S. Panush, M.D.

Professor and Chief
Division of Clinical Immunology, Rheumatology, and
    Allergy
Department of Medicine
College of Medicine
University of Florida and Veterans Administration
    Medical Center
Gainesville, Florida

Harold E. Paulus, M.D.

Professor of Medicine
University of California at Los Angeles
School of Medicine
Los Angeles, California

Paul E. Phillips, M.D.

Professor of Medicine and Pediatrics
Chief, Division of Clinical Immunology
State University of New York Health Science Center
Syracuse, New York

Janice Smith Pigg, R.N., B.S.N., M.S.

Manager and Nurse Consultant
Midwest Arthritis Treatment Center
Columbia Hospital
Milwaukee, Wisconsin

Taina Pihlajaniemi, M.D.

Department of Medical Chemistry
University of Oulu
Oulu, Finland

Marilyn C. Pike, M.D., Ph.D.

Assistant Professor, Department of Internal Medicine
Division of Rheumatology
The University of Michigan Medical Center
Ann Arbor, Michigan

Robert S. Pinals, M.D.

Professor and Acting Chairman
Department of Medicine
University of Medicine and Dentistry of New Jersey
Piscataway, New Jersey
Chairman, Department of Medicine
The Medical Center at Princeton
Princeton, New Jersey

Seth H. Pincus, M.D.

Laboratory of Microbial Structure and Function
Rocky Mountain Laboratory
National Institutes of Health
Hamilton, Montana

Darwin J. Prockop, M.D.

Professor and Chairman
Department of Biochemistry and Molecular Biology
Thomas Jefferson University
Philadelphia, Pennsylvania

Reed E. Pyeritz, M.D., Ph.D.

Associate Professor of Medicine and Pediatrics
Division of Medical Genetics
The Johns Hopkins Hospital
Baltimore, Maryland

Eric Radin, M.D.

Professor and Chairman
Orthopedic Surgery
West Virginia University Medical Center
Morgantown, West Virginia

Antonio J. Reginato, M.D.

Chief, Arthritis Section
Cooper Hospital
University Medical Center
Camden, New Jersey
Associate Professor of Medicine
University of Medicine and Dentistry of New Jersey
Piscataway, New Jersey
Clinical Associate Professor of Medicine
University of Pennsylvania
Philadelphia, Pennsylvania

Morris Reichlin, M.D.

Professor of Medicine
Chief of Immunology
Oklahoma Medical Research Foundation
Oklahoma City, Oklahoma

Juliet M. Rogers, M.D., Ch.B.

Lecturer, Paleopathology
Rheumatology Unit
Bristol Royal Infirmary
Bristol, England

Lawrence Rosenberg, M.D.

Professor of Orthopedic Surgery
Albert Einstein University
Orthopedic and Connective Tissue
    Research Laboratories
Montefiore Hospital and Medical Center
Bronx, New York

James T. Rosenbaum, M.D.

Associate Professor of Medicine, Ophthalmology, and
    Cell Biology
Department of Medicine
Oregon Health Sciences University
Portland, Oregon

Naomi F. Rothfield, M.D.

Professor of Medicine
Chief, Division of Rheumatic Diseases
University of Connecticut
Farmington, Connecticut

Bruce M. Rothschild, M.D.

Professor of Medicine
Northeast Ohio Universities
College of Medicine
Rootstown, Ohio
Director of Rheumatology
St. Elizabeth's Hospital
Youngtown, Ohio

Lorne A. Runge, M.D.

Assistant Professor of Medicine
Department of Rehabilitation Medicine
State University of New York Upstate Medical Center
Syracuse, New York

Doran E. Ryan, D.D.S., M.S.

Associate Professor and Chairman
Department of Oral and Maxillofacial Surgery
Medical College of Wisconsin
Milwaukee County Medical Complex
Milwaukee, Wisconsin

Lawrence M. Ryan, M.D.

Associate Professor of Medicine
Co-Chief, Rheumatology Division
Medical College of Wisconsin
Milwaukee, Wisconsin

Jane Green Schaller, M.D.

Professor and Chairman
Department of Pediatrics
Tufts University
Boston, Massachusetts

Frank R. Schmid, M.D.

Professor of Medicine
Chief, Arthritis Section
Northwestern University Medical School
Chicago, Illinois

H. Ralph Schumacher, Jr., M.D.

Professor of Medicine
University of Pennsylvania School of Medicine
Director, Arthritis Immunology Center
Veterans Administration Medical Center
Philadelphia, Pennsylvania

Edith R. Schwartz, Ph.D.

Professor of Orthopedic Surgery
Department of Orthopedic Surgery
Tufts University School of Medicine
Boston, Massachusetts

Gordon C. Sharp, M.D.

Professor of Medicine
University of Missouri at Columbia
Division of Immunology and Rheumatology
Columbia, Missouri

Wilmer L. Sibbitt, Jr., M.D.

Associate Professor of Medicine
University of New Mexico Medical School
Albuquerque, New Mexico

Leonard H. Sigal, M.D.

Assistant Professor of Medicine, Microbiology, and
    Immunology
Rheumatology/Medicine
Veterans Administration Medical Center at Syracuse
    University
Syracuse, New York

Peter A. Simkin, M.D.

Professor of Medicine
University of Washington
Seattle, Washington

Bernhard H. Singsen, M.D.

Chief, Division of Rheumatology
Alfred I. Dupont Institute
Wilmington, Delaware

John L. Skosey, M.D., Ph.D.

Professor of Medicine
Chief, Section of Rheumatology
University of Illinois College of Medicine
Chicago, Illinois

Hugh A. Smythe, M.D.

Wellesley Hospital
Toronto, Ontario, Canada

Ralph Snyderman, M.D.

Genetech, Inc.
San Francisco, California

Leon Sokoloff, M.D.

Professor of Pathology
State University of New York at Stony Brook
Stony Brook, New York

Isaias Spilberg, M.D.

Associate Professor of Medicine
Washington University School of Medicine
St. Louis, Missouri

Richard N. Stauffer, M.D.

Associate Professor of Orthopedic Surgery
Department of Orthopedic Surgery
Mayo Clinic
Rochester, Minnesota

Allen C. Steere, M.D.

Professor of Medicine
Tufts University School of Medicine
Chief, Rheumatology/Immunology
New England Medical Center
Boston, Massachusetts

John D. Stobo, M.D.

William Osler Professor of Medicine
Chairman, Department of Medicine
The Johns Hopkins Hospital
Baltimore, Maryland

James E. Stoll, M.D.

Assistant Professor of Orthopedics
Chief, Division of Spinal Surgery
Medical College of Wisconsin
Milwaukee, Wisconsin

David W. Stoller, M.D.

Assistant Professor, Department of Radiology
University of California School of Medicine at San
    Francisco
San Francisco, California

Robert L. Swezey, M.D.

Clinical Professor of Medicine
University of California School of Medicine at Los
    Angeles
Medical Director
The Arthritis and Back Pain Center
Swezey Institute
Santa Monica, California

Norman Talal, M.D.

Professor of Medicine
Department of Medicine
The University of Texas Health Science Center
Clinical Immunology Section
Audie L. Murphy Veterans Administration Hospital
San Antonio, Texas

Eng M. Tan, M.D.

Head, Autoimmune Disease Center
Scripps Clinic and Research Foundation
La Jolla, California

Angelo Taranta, M.D.

Professor of Medicine
New York Medical College
Director of Medicine,
   Cabrini Medical Center
New York, New York

Robert A. Terkeltaub, M.D.

Chief, Rheumatology Section
San Diego Veterans Administration Medical Center
Assistant Professor of Medicine in Residence
University of California at San Diego
School of Medicine
San Diego, California

David E. Trentham, M.D.

Assistant Professor of Medicine
Harvard Medical School
Chief, Division of Rheumatology
Beth Israel Hospital
Boston, Massachusetts

John R. Ward, M.D.

Professor of Medicine
Chief, Division of Rheumatology
University of Utah
Salt Lake City, Utah

Michael H. Weisman, M.D.

Associate Professor of Medicine
Department of Medicine
University of California at San Diego
San Diego, California

Gerald Weissmann, M.D.

Professor of Medicine
Director, Division of Rheumatology
New York University Medical Center
New York, New York

Peter F. Weller, M.D.

Associate Professor of Medicine
Harvard Medical School
Beth Israel Hospital
Boston, Massachusetts

Russell E. Windsor, M.D.

Hospital for Special Surgery
New York, New York

Robert L. Wortmann, M.D.

Associate Professor of Medicine
Co-Chief, Division of Rheumatology
Medical College of Wisconsin
Milwaukee, Wisconsin

Morris Ziff, Ph.D., M.D.

Ashbel Smith Professor Emeritus of Internal Medicine
Morris Ziff Professor Emeritus of Rheumatology
University of Texas Southwestern Medical Center
Attending Physician
Parkland Memorial Hospital
Dallas Veterans Administration Hospital
Dallas, Texas

Nathan J. Zvaifler, M.D.

Professor of Medicine
University of California at San Diego
San Diego, California

contents

*Deceased

| III. | **CLINICAL PHARMACOLOGY OF ANTIRHEUMATIC DRUGS** |

| IV. | **RHEUMATOID ARTHRITIS** |

*Due to unforeseen circumstances the manuscript for this chapter was delayed, preventing us from placing the material in its proper sequence. Chapter 44 appears immediately after Chapter 119 on page 1967.

The Publisher and Author regret any inconvenience this situation may cause the reader.

V.   OTHER INFLAMMATORY ARTHRITIC SYNDROMES

VI.   SYSTEMIC RHEUMATIC DISEASES

*Deceased

VII. MISCELLANEOUS RHEUMATIC DISEASES

VIII. REGIONAL DISORDERS OF JOINTS AND RELATED STRUCTURES

XI. INFECTIOUS ARTHRITIS

section   I

INTRODUCTION TO THE STUDY OF THE RHEUMATIC DISEASES

SKELETAL PALEOPATHOLOGY OF RHEUMATIC DISEASES: THE SUBPRIMATE CONNECTION

1

BRUCE M. ROTHSCHILD

Paleontology, like rheumatology, is a source of popular fascination and misconception. Even Thomas Jefferson's interest in the subject is documented.[1] In 1791, he published his description of "Certain bones of a quadruped of the clawed kind in the western parts of Virginia."[2] The antiquity of rheumatic disease, as represented in the paleontologic record, was discussed in an earlier edition of this book.[1] While referred to as osteoarthritis, the rheumatic disease actually represents spondylosis deformans.[1,3] Fossil specimens represent singular point observations in time often from a perspective dissimilar to that routinely encountered. Once recognized, an abnormality must be determined to be reflecting either reality or artifact. Reconciliation of representation with clinical significance often offers a challenge, regardless of whether one is dealing with a reconstruction or the actual specimen (see also Chapter 2).

OSTEOARTHRITIS

Identification of osteoarthritis (diarthrodial joint degeneration) in dinosaurs has proven elusive. Recently, the disease has been identified in the ankle (Fig. 1–1) of 2 of 39 Iguanodon in the famous herd on exhibit in Brussels. The normal articular surface in dinosaurs is scrotal in appearance. A thick cartilaginous cap would have been required to cover such a surface. The underlying bone appears to have been well protected from osteophyte development. Assessment of subchondral sclerosis or cysts awaits systematic population radiography, a process that has been applied thus far only to marine reptiles.[4] Preliminary radiologic study of sauropods (Camarosaurus, Apatosaurus, Diplodocus), Stegosaur, Allosaurus, Triceratops, and Hadrosaurs has demonstrated no subchondral erosions or cysts.

Physician interest in paleontology in general and in dinosaurs in particular dates to 1822, nineteen years prior to Sir Richard Owen's coining of the term dinosaur,[5] when Gideon Algernon Mantell, a family doctor from Sussex, England, initiated medical interest in dinosaur skeletons and Samuel Wendall Williston, founder and first Dean of the Kansas University School of Medicine, established the Kansas Museum of Natural History. Therefore, it is fitting that the first example of dinosauran osteoarthritis was noted in the group of dinosaurs that first attracted medical attention.[5]

Although dinosauran osteoarthritis appears to be an isolated phenomenon, population studies in Pleistocene mammals have been done. The frequency (26%) of osteoarthritis of the ankle in fossil marsupials is similar to that noted in the weight-bearing joints of contemporary humans.[6] The foothills of the little Big Horn have contributed more than their share to history and prehistory. A 120-foot-deep trap cave produced a diverse apparently unbiased sampling of animals (herds) that had crossed a Pleistocene game trail.[7] Examination of the excavated fossils revealed that only 6 of 21 genera showed osteophyte formation.[7] Further analysis of this cross section should

FIG. 1–1. Earliest example of osteoarthritis in an Iguanodon (dating back 125 million years). Note remodeling with osteophyte formation.

FIG. 1–2. Subchondral erosive metapodial arthritis in a 20,000-year-old bovid. Note marginal erosion of proximal metapodialia with undermining of subchondral bone.

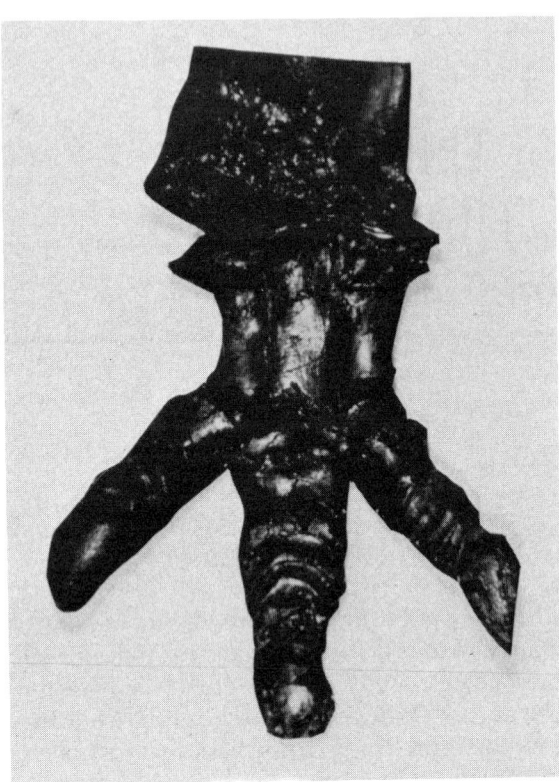

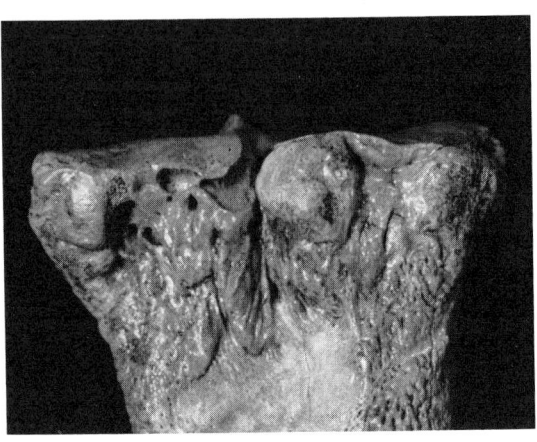

in bovids but not equids raises the question of species susceptibility or habitat exposure in determining occurrence of erosive disease. Because tuberculosis and brucellosis were endemic to American Indians,[8] it is conceivable that this portion of their food chain was responsible for transmitting the infecting agent.

Similar infections are natural to contemporary bison and can cause subchondral erosions characteristic of granulomatous disease.[9,10] Direct immunofluorescence microscopy with conjugated antisyphilitic antisera support the treponemal origin of a spiculated bone reaction recently described in a Pleistocene bear.[11] Application of scanning electron microscopy to a specimen of infected mosasaur spine has identified what appears to be the causative organism, Coccolithus.[12]

contribute to a better understanding of the relationship between bone structure and movement.

EROSIVE AND INFECTIOUS ARTHRITIS

Natural Trap Cave also provided an opportunity to study the population frequency of erosive joint disease. Among the species examined (representing bears, lions, cheetahs, wolves, wolverines, martens, marmots, voles, antelope, horses, camels, sheep, bison, musk oxen, mammoths, pika, lemmings, and rabbits), dated at 17,000 to 20,000 years, only three showed evidence of erosive disease.[7] Fifteen percent of Ovis (big horn sheep) and 50% of Bison and Bootherium (musk ox) had marginal subchondral erosions (Fig. 1–2), the distribution of which was limited to monoarticular involvement of the proximal portion of metacarpals in the big horn sheep and of metatarsals in the musk ox. Perierosive osteopenia was prominent, but reactive sclerosis was absent and periosteal reaction was minimal. An infectious etiology is suspected but confirmation of possible infectious organisms awaits further study. The occurrence of lesions

SPINAL FUSION

Fusion of the first three cervical vertebrae was found among a family of horned (Ceratopsian) dinosaurs: Monoclonius, Arrhinoceratops, Pachyrhinosaurus, Styracosaurus, Chasmosaurus, and Triceratops. The primitive ceratopsians, Protoceratops, Leptoceratops, and Montanoceratops, lack such fusion.[13] Smaller representatives (apparently juveniles) of more derived forms, Monoclonius and Triceratops, lack fusion, but the cervical vertebrae of adults are fully fused, suggesting an ontologically acquired phenomenon. Cervical fusion in dinosaurs may have occurred to facilitate support of the increasingly massive skull, which represented a significant portion of body weight. Such phylogenic development also suggests that fusion may have been a protective mechanism.

Syndromes of spine and spinal ligament calcification have been a source of controversy: Do they represent pathologic responses or protective phenomena? A recent controlled study of diffuse idiopathic skeletal hyperostosis (DISH) in humans revealed no correlation between ligamentous calcification and clinical musculoskeletal complaints.[14] This suggests that such calcification may be protective. Similar caudal bridging was documented in 50% of the Diplodocus and Apatosaurus specimens available for examination.[13] Bridging, when present, involved two to four contiguous vertebrae at one or two stressed points in each affected individual. Similar to DISH in humans, the zygapophyseal joints in dinosaurs were spared. Ligamentous calcifications frequently appear in dinosaurs.[15] Calcification of groups of spinal ligaments is present universally in ceratopsians (horned dinosaurs), hadrosaurs (duck-billed dinosaurs), and therasaurs (carnivorous tyrannosaur-like dinosaurs). Examples in the Paleolithic mammalian record include Mastodons, Teleoceras, and Menoceras (early rhinocera), Gigantocamelus, Michenia, and Protolabis (early camels), Smiledon (saber-toothed tigers), Equus sp. (an extinct early horse), Bison bison, Canis dirus, and fossil whales. Interestingly, a Mystocetan whale (Thinocetus), dated at 12 million years, was given the species name *arthritus* because of the mistaken idea that such bridging represented arthritis.[15] Such widespread evidence of DISH in the paleontologic record strengthens the concept that ligamentous calcification may not represent a disease after all, and may even have been useful to dinosaurs. Even though they had prominent tails, there is little evidence in the fossil record of tail drag marks.[16] The current

FIG. 1–3. Photograph of six vertebrae of the famous Lucy (4 million years old), the best preserved example of Australopithecus afarensis from the Hadar site in Ethiopia. Extensive bony proliferation anterior and lateral to the vertebral bodies (centra) superficially resembles the ankylosing hyperostosis of Forestier and Rotes-Querol. But this diagnosis was thought unlikely given the similarity in the superoinferior diameter of the centra and their bony extensions and lack of separation of the overgrowth from the vertebral body. If intravertebral bridging had been present and lost post mortem, a less regular distribution of bone in the anterior proliferative extensions would be expected. (Courtesy of C. Owen Lovejoy, Ph.D., Kent State University.)

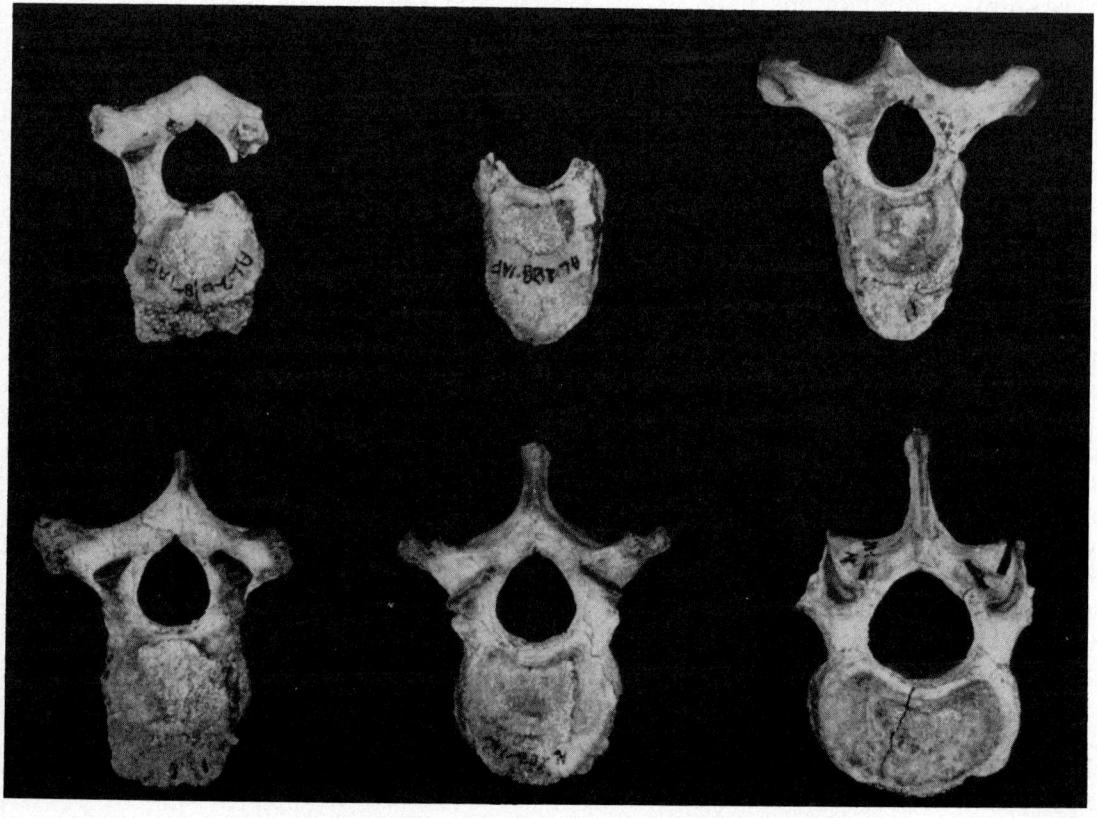

thinking is that dinosaurs kept their tails in the air (Gordon Edmund, personal communication). Occurrence of ligamentous calcification at mechanically stressed points might have aided this posture, it may also have facilitated use of the tail as an effective whip-like defensive weapon against predators and for intraspecies territorial or courting competition, as evidenced in the dinosaur track record.[15]

The vertebrae of the hominid Lucy are shown life-size in Figure 1–3. The massive bony proliferation anterior and lateral to the vertebral bodies cannot be diagnosed at present.[17] No facet joint osteoarthritis was present. While this bony proliferation may represent a pathologic state, it may also represent a protective vertebral response to loss of trabeculae (osteoporosis).[18]

AVASCULAR NECROSIS

The bone pathology of avascular necrosis was recently documented for the first time in early residents (exclusive of man) of what was to become Kansas.[4] The closest analogue in the veterinary literature is Legg-Calve-Perthe disease, slippage of the proximal femoral epiphysis.[19] This disorder was subsequently identified in specimens from Alabama and Belgium. Avascular necrosis was invariably present in Platecarpus, Tylosaur, Mosasaurus, Plioplatecarpus, Prognathodon, and Hainosaurus, and invariably absent from Clidastes, Ectenosaurus, and Halisaurus, independent of locale.[4,20] The frequency of occurrence within a given genera was also uniform, independent of locale. Occurrence of avascular necrosis was segregated according to diving habits, being uniformly present in deep divers and uniformly absent in shallow divers.[4,20,21] Although avascular necrosis in humans has a number of precipitating factors (see Chapter 98) only radiation, bismuth poisoning, and decompression syndrome could be potential etiologic factors in mosasaurs. Absence of radiation effects or variation in bismuth levels in affected versus unaffected vertebrae and species suggests decompression sickness as the etiologic factor.[22] Decompression sickness has been observed in humans subsequent to breath-holding dives.[22] Zoologic precedent is found in Berkson's report of seal death from decompression syndrome after forced surfacing from 300 m.[23]

SUMMARY

One of the problems of paleopathology is recognition of phenomena. Paleontologists, trained in systematics and anatomy rather than pathology, generally will recognize an abnormality but not necessarily its cause and pathogenesis. To physicians, the cause may seem obvious, but often it is not. As in all other branches of science, hypotheses must be subjected to critical evaluation. Fossil records have provided insight not only into characteristics but also into the evolution of species. This may also yield information about disease pathogenesis. The occurrence and presentation of such phenomena through the ages could even uncover clues to patterns of contemporary disease and disability.

REFERENCES

1. Bedini, S.A.: Thomas Jefferson and American Vertebrate Paleontology. Virginia Division of Mineral Resources Publication, *61*:1–26, 1985.
2. Jefferson, T.: A memoir on the discovery of certain bones of a quadruped of the clawed kind in the western parts of Virginia. Trans. Amer. Philos. Soc., *4(30)*:246–260, 1799.
3. Abrams, N.R.: Etiology and pathogenesis of degenerative joint disease. *In* Arthritis and Allied Conditions. 5th Ed. Edited by J.L. Hollander. Philadelphia, Lea & Febiger, 1953, p. 691.
4. Rothschild, B.M., and Martin, L.D.: Avascular necrosis: Occurrence in diving Cretaceous mosasaurs. Science, *236*:75–77, 1987.
5. Norman, D.: The Illustrated Encyclopedia of Dinosaurs. New York, Crescent Books, 1985.
6. Rothschild, B.M.: Osteoarthritis in fossil marsupial populations of Australia. Ann. Carnegie Museum (in press).
7. Rothschild, B.M., and Martin, L.D.: Erosive disease in the Pleistocene: A study of three populations. Quaternary Research (in press).
8. Enarson, D.A., Fujii, M., Nakielna, E.M., and Grzybowski, S.: Bone and joint tuberculosis: A continuing problem. Can. Med. Assoc. J., *120*:139–145, 1979.
9. Roux, J.: Epidemiologie et prevention de la brucellose. Bull WHO, *57*:179–195, 1979.
10. Jones, T.C., and Hunt, R.D.: Veterinary Pathology. Philadelphia, Lea & Febiger, 1983.
11. Rothschild, B.M., and Turnbull, W.: Treponemal infection in a Pleistocene bear. Nature, *329*:61–62, 1987.
12. Rothschild, B.M., and Martin, L.: Shark-induced infectious spondylitis: Evidence in the Cretaceous record. Paleogeogr., Paleoclimatol., and Paleoecol. (Submitted).
13. Rothschild, B.M.: Paleopathology of ankylosing spondylitis and diffuse idiopathic skeletal hyperostosis. Arthritis Rheum., *28*:595, 1985. (abstract)
14. Rothschild, B.M.: Diffuse idiopathic hyperostosis: Misconceptions and reality. Clin. Rheum., *4*:207–212, 1985.
15. Rothschild, B.M.: Diffuse idiopathic skeletal hyperostosis (DISH) as reflected in the paleontologic record: Dinosaurs and early mammals. Semin. Arthritis Rheum. (in press).
16. Thulborn, R.: Dinosaur trackways in the Winton formation (Mid-Cretaceous) of Queensland. Memoirs Queensland Museum., *21*:413–417, 1984.
17. Johanson, D.C., et al.: Morphology of the pliocene partial skeleton (AL. 288–1) from the Hadar formation. Ethiop. Amer. J. Phys. Anthropol., *57*:403–451, 1982.

18. Mosekilde, L., and Mosekilde, L.: Normal vertebral body size and compressive strength. Bone, *7*:207–212, 1986.

19. Innes, J.R.: "Inherited dysplasia" of the hip-joint in dogs and rabbits. Lab. Invest., *8*:1170–1178, 1959.

20. Rothschild, B.M.: Implications of paleopathology in the Belgium fossil record: Avascular necrosis in diving reptiles. Bull. Inst. Royal Sci. Naturelle (in press).

21. Rothschild, B.M.: Decompresson syndrome in turtles: Implications of the fossil record pathology, avascular necrosis. Ann. Carnegie Museum (in press).

22. Pauley, P.: Decompression sickness following repeated breath-hold dives. J. Appl. Physiol., *20*:1028–1030, 1965.

23. Berkson, H: Physiologic adjustments to deep diving in the Pacific green turtle (Chelonia mydas agassizii). Comp. Biochem. Physiol., *21*:507–524, 1967.

SKELETAL PALEOPATHOLOGY OF RHEUMATIC DISORDERS

2

PAUL DIEPPE and JULIET M. ROGERS

Paleopathology is the study of the antiquity of disease. Evidence comes from old medical manuscripts, traditional historical sources, literature, and art. In the case of bone and joint diseases, skeletons provide a particularly pertinent source of data.

Skeletal paleopathology of arthritic diseases has recently been explored by several groups interested in rheumatic disease epidemiology. It has the potential to provide evidence on the temporal and geographic origins of disorders such as rheumatoid arthritis. Careful study of skeletons may also provide insight into the way in which changes on and around the joint surface appear. Obviously, the best approach is multidisciplinary, with input from historians, anthropologists, radiologists, rheumatologists, and others.

SKELETAL PALEOPATHOLOGY AND THE ANTIQUITY OF RHEUMATIC DISEASES

Human joint disease is as old as man, as skeletons attest. Changes on and around joint surfaces have been seen in Australopithecus afarensis, an early hominid,[1] Neanderthal man,[2] Neolithic man,[3] and ancient mummies.[4,5] Archeologic excavations of material from all ages and from all areas of the world have always provided some evidence of joint disease, often extensive and serious.[6] Interpretation of the nature and significance of the changes seen remains difficult. Bones have often been examined without help from specialists in rheumatic diseases. Criteria to provide conformity in the description and interpretation of the findings have not been adequately developed.

Our present classification and understanding of rheumatic diseases are also relatively new. Many conditions now regarded as commonplace have only been recognized in the last few decades. It is therefore naive to expect older descriptions of skeletal remains to be easily interpreted in modern times. Skeletal data need to be interpreted in the light of the prevailing conditions and knowledge of both the period from which the skeleton comes and the time when it was excavated and examined.

HISTORICAL BACKGROUND

Physicians have always attempted to describe and to classify the disorders they saw. Hippocrates provided convincing descriptions of gout,[7] but other currently accepted rheumatic diseases or syndromes are not easily recognizable from early medical texts. Early art and literature also document that man was often in pain and disabled by musculoskeletal problems, but it is impossible to say whether specific disorders of the type seen today accounted for such morbidity.

The dark ages were a period in which art, literature, and medicine were stifled by blind belief. Progress followed the Reformation. Galenic theory was challenged. Clinicians correlated clinical observations with data from anatomic and postmortem studies. Examples from this period include the work of Sydenham (gout) and Connor (spondylitis).[8,9] Further

8

differentiation of rheumatic disorders came in the eighteenth and nineteenth centuries. The contributions of Charcot and Marie in France,[10,11] of Heberden and Scudamore in England,[12,13] and of others are well documented.[14] Their work led to the recognition of nodal osteoarthritis, rheumatic fever, neuropathic arthropathy, and ankylosing spondylitis. The rate of recognition of various rheumatic syndromes accelerated with the application of new technologies, beginning at the turn of this century, with the use of roentgen rays. It allowed arthritis to be classified, first as atrophic or hypertrophic,[15] and subsequently as rheumatoid or osteoarthritis, by Garrod,[16] as well as by others. Subsequent discoveries of rheumatoid and antinuclear factors, of crystals, and of disease-susceptibility genes have increased the sophistication of rheumatology, leading to the description of more discrete disease entities. The development of human skeletal paleopathology must be viewed against the concurrently developing background.

SKELETAL PALEOPATHOLOGY AS A SPECIFIC DISCIPLINE

Sir Marc Armand Ruffer, an important pioneer among skeletal paleopathologists, was working in Cairo as a bacteriologist when he became interested in the pathology of Egyptian mummies.[17] One of his findings was extensive spinal diseases, described by a variety of terms including spondylitis deformans. His work has since been reviewed by Zorab,[18] as well as by Rogers and colleagues,[19] and it seems clear that much of the spinal disease that he observed was due to ankylosing hyperostosis (Forestier's disease). This condition had not yet been described when Ruffer was working. Page May observed severe destructive joint disease in an early skeleton,[20] and he thought that this process might have been due to rheumatoid arthritis, despite extensive ankylosis and proliferative bony changes. A contemporary rheumatologist or paleopathologist might have interpreted the findings quite differently.

Other early contributors to the field include Wood-Jones,[21] Hrdlicka,[22] and Moodie.[23] After World War II, the work of Calvin Wells stimulated the field.[24] The publication of Brothwell and Sandison is a benchmark,[25] bringing order and more rigorous scientific approaches to the study of old bones. The careful academic studies of Steinbock,[26] Ortner and Putscher,[27] and others, using the modern multidisciplinary approach, have led to further advances.

MATERIALS AND METHODS

Single specimens, such as Egyptian mummies or corpses preserved in ice or peat, become available for study from time to time, but most workers rely on archeologic material. Such material is of two types: (1) that previously excavated and in a museum or private collection; and (2) skeletons recovered during current digs.

CONDITON OF THE MATERIAL

The condition of the material varies. Individual skeletons buried under favorable conditions may be beautifully preserved and may even be identifiable if coffin labels survive. Most burial grounds in Europe have been used for hundreds of years. Many of the earlier burials have been disturbed, so large numbers of disarticulated bones are all that survive. Excavations carried out under less-than-ideal conditions often result in the loss of the small bones of the hands and feet that are of great interest to the rheumatologist. Such incomplete skeletons are a frequent problem.

ANTEMORTEM VERSUS POSTMORTEM CHANGES

Making this distinction is another problem, especially for the inexperienced paleopathologist. Some soil, such as chalk, can abrade the bone surface, and mechanical damage during excavation is common. Antemortem changes usually show accompanying evidence of bony reaction or remodeling.

CARE IN HANDLING

Careful handling of specimens is essential. Ideally, a paleopathologist should be on site when material is recovered. Digs are organized by archeologists and may be of great interest to anthropologists and others as well as the paleopathologist. The different goals and interests of the various disciplines may produce conflicts in the way in which the material is excavated, cleaned, labeled, and measured, all essential steps in the process. Old, soil-damaged, osteoporotic bone may be fragile, and some potentially valuable findings may literally crumble away in the hands of colleagues.

METHODS

The methods used by all skeletal biologists are similar. When possible, a description of the in situ findings comes first. The site, time, and place of excavation and the posture of the skeleton in the ground should be recorded (Fig. 2–1). Photography on site is valuable. Excavation is followed by careful cleaning and labeling of specimens before they are transferred to the laboratory for further study. Thereafter, the techniques used are the same for all samples, irrespective of source. Each skeleton is carefully measured and described. A variety of standard indices are used to determine the age and sex of the specimen, although these determinations are often difficult. Gross pathologic features are then examined in more detail. Photographs and radiographs should be obtained before samples are handled extensively. Abnormalities are described carefully and are discussed with colleagues. Pathologic changes seen in a bone are not treated as isolated entities but are related to findings in the whole available skeleton. A variety of specialized techniques, such as slab radiography, bone histology, scanning electron microscopy, and extraction of material for biochemical analysis, may be useful.

MORPHOLOGIC CHANGES

These changes are described in two steps: (1) a detailed analysis of any abnormality seen on an indi-

FIG. 2–1. Medieval skeleton in situ. Note the flexed knees; this position was not a burial custom and suggests fixed flexion deformities antemortem. Subsequent examination showed an extensive, asymmetric sacroiliitis, spondylitis, and peripheral erosive arthropathy with bony proliferation. This picture is cautiously interpreted as a possible example of psoriatic or reactive spondyloarthropathy.

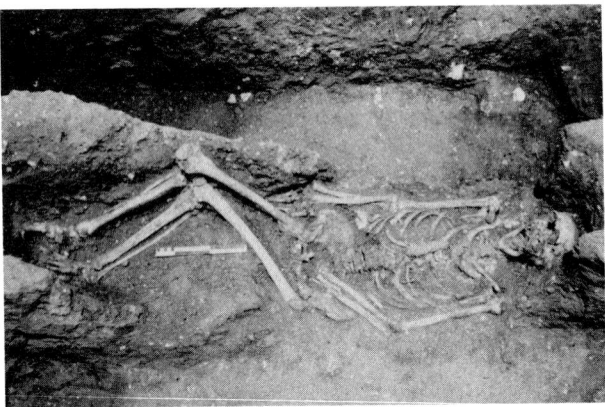

vidual bone; and (2) a chart of all abnormalities seen in the whole skeleton together with their distribution.

CHANGES AT A SINGLE JOINT SITE

Rheumatic disease can cause only a limited number of changes at bone ends, and each possibility must be carefully noted. The contour and texture of the joint surface may be abnormal, particularly in osteoarthritis (OA). The joint margin and periarticular bone shafts are common sites of change in all diseases. At each of these sites, only two basic types of pathologic features are observable: (1) bone loss through erosion or destruction; and (2) new bone formation. Although it is not always easy to distinguish between such changes, or to relate them to a precise anatomic area or structure, the attempt should always be made.

DISTRIBUTION OF CHANGES

Both the axial and the appendicular skeleton need to be considered. Obviously, the amount of skeleton recovered affects the apparent distribution of pathologic change; a note should always be made of the bones that are missing.[28]

Mistakes are easily made if the whole skeleton is not examined. For example, a peripheral erosive arthropathy may signify one thing if the spine is unavailable or has not been examined, but quite another if the sacroiliac joints are fused (Fig. 2–2).

INTERPRETATION OF FINDINGS

Interpretation is the biggest problem. Everyone feels pressure to find abnormalities and to explain them. Both archeologist and layman want to know how their ancestors fared: what diseases did they suffer from and why? It is always tempting to explain any skeletal abnormality in terms of occupation or physical activity.

Disease expression may alter with time and in different environments. Great care needs to be exercised before a definite diagnosis is made relative to a particular finding in an old specimen.

The literature of paleopathology reflects a gradual change in the level of sophistication in interpreting changes in old bones. It used to be said that any joint damage reflected wear and tear, indicative of some aspect of the individual's physical activity.[29] Osteophytes were then distinguished from other changes, but confusion over their interpretation remains. For

FIG. 2–2. Some of the patterns of distribution of joint disease described today. When skeletons are examined these patterns must be looked for, in addition to descriptions of individual changes at one joint site. RA = rheumatoid arthritis; OA = osteoarthritis; DISH = diffuse idiopathic skeletal hyperostosis; AS = ankylosing spondylitis.

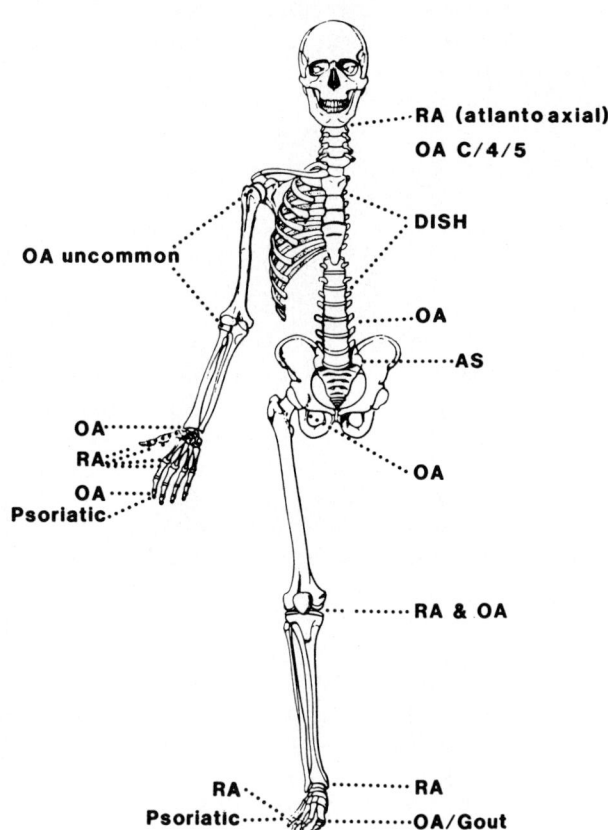

dral bone as well as of marginal osteophytes. The presence of these osteophytes may well be an aging phenomenon unrelated to OA.[32] This distinction has not always been recognized in the literature of paleopathology. Nevertheless, no doubt exists that true OA was common in our ancestors. Whether or not it was the same as the disease we see today is difficult to know. Many cases of hip and knee disease compatible with contemporary OA have been recorded (Fig. 2–3),[33] and severe OA is obvious in our oldest neolithic specimens.[3]

SPONDYLOSIS

Severe osteophytosis of vertebral bodies is another common finding in all skeletal samples examined. It is often accompanied by changes in the contours of the vertebrae and by apophyseal joint damage consistent with a diagnosis of severe lumbar or cervical spondylosis (Fig. 2–4).

GOUT

Given that clinical descriptions of gout appeared in the earliest medical writings, it is surprising that until

FIG. 2–3. Tibia of a Saxon skeleton showing extensive bony changes of the medial condyle. The signs include severe osteophytosis, sclerosis and disruption of the subchondral bone, and remodeling, suggestive of advanced osteoarthritis.

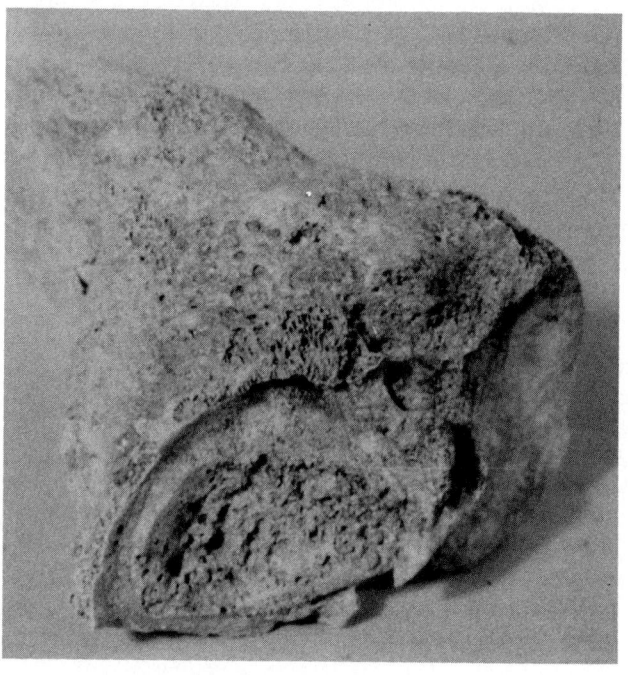

example, osteophytes are often used as an index of aging.[30] More recently, knowledge of erosive and other arthropathies has increased, but problems still arise from lack of medical consultation and the misinterpretation of findings such as joint ankylosis. The field is still in its infancy, and normality has yet to be defined.

RHEUMATIC DISEASES POSITIVELY IDENTIFIED IN ANCIENT SKELETONS

OSTEOARTHRITIS

Osteoarthritis (OA) is the commonest disease seen in ancient skeletons.[31] The problem of differentiating OA from osteophytosis itself, however, is important. In the absence of evidence of antemortem cartilage loss, OA should probably only be diagnosed if one has evidence of sclerosis or remodeling of subchon-

FIG. 2–4. Cervical vertebra from a Saxon skeleton showing eburnation and grooving of the facet joint. Note the osteophytosis of the vertebral body as well as the facet joints, indicating cervical spondylosis.

FIG. 2–5. *A,* Small bones of the hand and feet of a Saxon skeleton with large areas of juxta-articular erosion. *B,* Radiograph of the same specimens showing well-defined erosions with marginal hooks characteristic of gout.

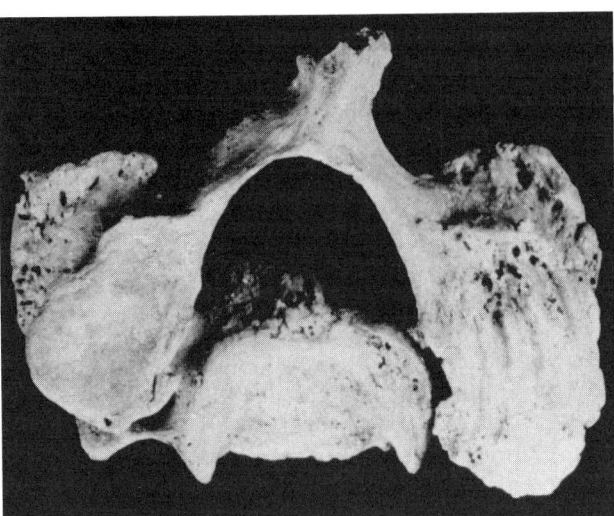

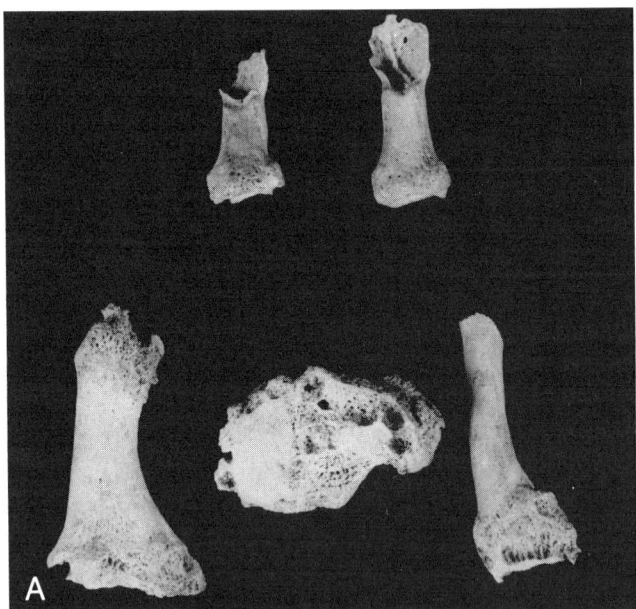

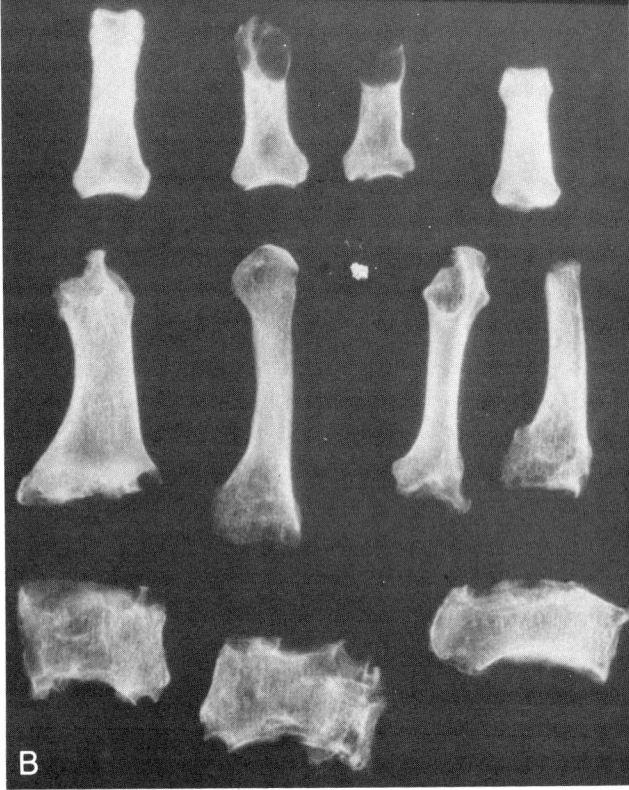

recently there were only two good descriptions of typical gouty erosions in old bones,[34,35] perhaps partly because paleopathologists and archeologists did not know what to look for and partly because such changes usually occur in the small bones of the feet and hands which are easily lost, damaged, or ignored in excavations. Gout is certainly apparent if you look for it. We have seen several cases of classic "punched out" erosions with sclerotic margins in the typical distribution that make any other interpretation difficult (Fig. 2–5). In one Egyptian skeleton, the tophi are still preserved, and the urate crystal deposits can be identified in the bony erosions.[36] That high levels of lead were detected in the bone suggests the diagnosis of saturnine gout.[37]

SACROILIITIS AND SPONDYLARTHROPATHIES

Ankylosing spondylitis (AS) has been overdiagnosed in the paleopathologic literature because of a tendency to label any fusing or erosive spondylarthritis as AS. A few cases, however, survive the closest scrutiny,[38] suggesting that it has existed for many hundreds of years. We and others have also seen a number of skeletons with an asymmetric sacroiliitis, some of which also have asymmetric fusion of the facet joints, vertebrae, or peripheral joints.[39] We have interpreted these changes as indications of either psoriatic arthropathy or Reiter's disease. In a few skeletons, unequivocal evidence of a peripheral erosive arthritis has accompanied the spinal changes. Proliferative bone growth occurs around the erosions, and both periostitis and "cup-and-pencil" deformities, suggestive of psoriatic spondylarthritis, have been seen (Fig. 2–6). Although it is difficult to distinguish among the different diseases within this group, numerous cases with some form of spondylarthropathy, with or without peripheral erosive disease, have been identified.

DIFFUSE IDIOPATHIC SKELETAL HYPEROSTOSIS

Diffuse idiopathic skeletal hyperostosis (DISH) is easy to identify because the characteristic right-sided, anterolateral, flowing osteophytes, bridging vertebrae, are so striking. Many extensive cases have been seen, some of which appear much less impressive on a radiograph than on visual inspection (Fig. 2–7). Several of our skeletons have also shown an extensive ossification of peripheral entheses that allows us to label them DISH, rather than simple ankylosing hy-

FIG. 2–6. *A,* Foot from a medieval skeleton showing fusion of midtarsal joints and erosive changes. Note the poor preservation of this specimen. Antemortem change, such as erosions in the interphalangeal joint of the great toe, could be clearly differentiated from the postmortem changes, however. *B,* This radiograph of the same specimen gives the proliferative erosive changes and fusion more clarity. This picture, which also shows evidence of sacroiliitis and spondylitis, is thought to be consistent with psoriatic spondylarthritis.

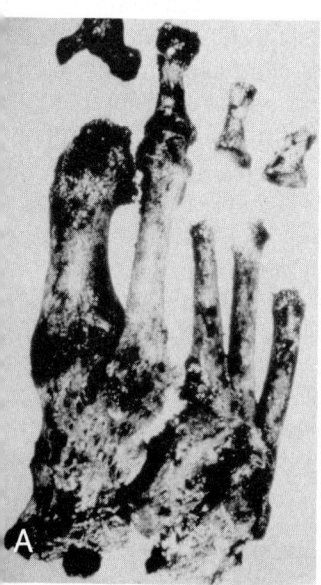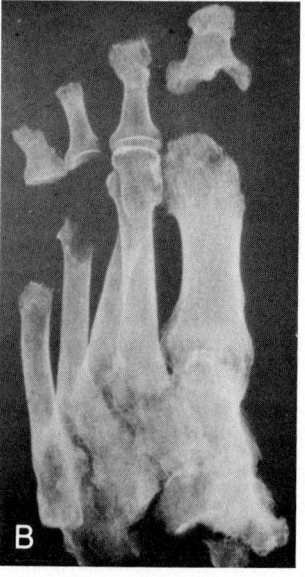

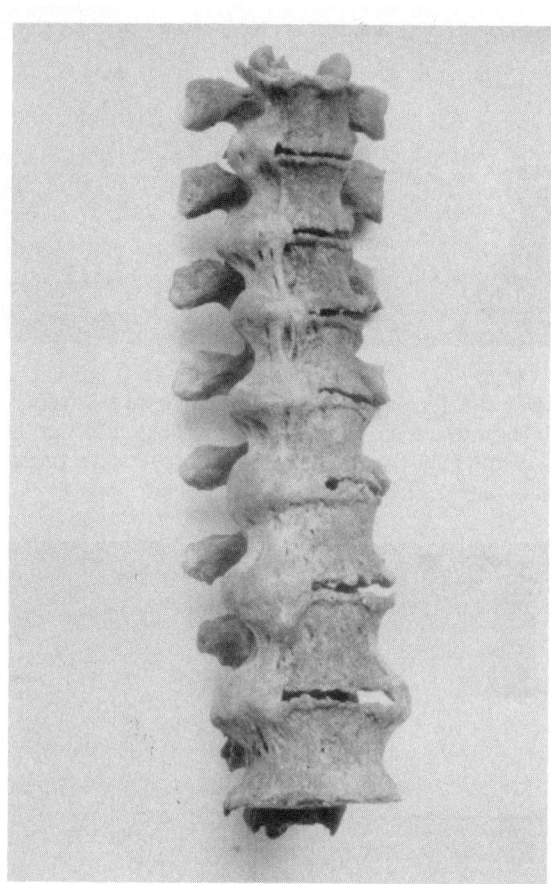

FIG. 2–7. Thoracic spine from a Saxon bishop showing right-sided anterolateral new bone, with fusion, typical of ankylosing hyperostosis (Forestier's disease). The changes are much less obvious on standard radiographic views.

perostosis of the spine.[39] The definitive description of this condition by Forestier and Rotes-Querol only appeared in 1950,[40] so it was unknown to early paleopathologists.

JOINT INFECTIONS

A few cases of severe joint damage with marked periosteal reaction compatible with a diagnosis of septic arthritis have been described (Fig. 2–8).[27] Spinal segments illustrated in Figure 2–9 show destruction and fusion of adjacent vertebrae with a "gibbus" angulation suggesting tuberculosis. Leprosy and syphilis can also leave characteristic marks on the skeleton.[41,42] Old osteomyelitis is even easier to identify with certainty, and some impressive cases have been described, indicating long survival after extensive bony infection.[26]

FIG. 2–8. The knee joints of a postmedieval specimen. The destructive changes, with periostitis and sinuses in bone, suggest septic arthritis.

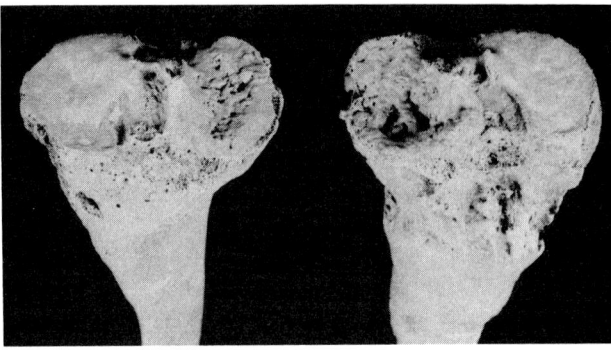

FIG. 2–9. A severely damaged hip joint from a Saxon skeleton. The bone loss, remodeling, and destruction on both sides of the joint suggest an indolent, destructive process, perhaps tuberculosis.

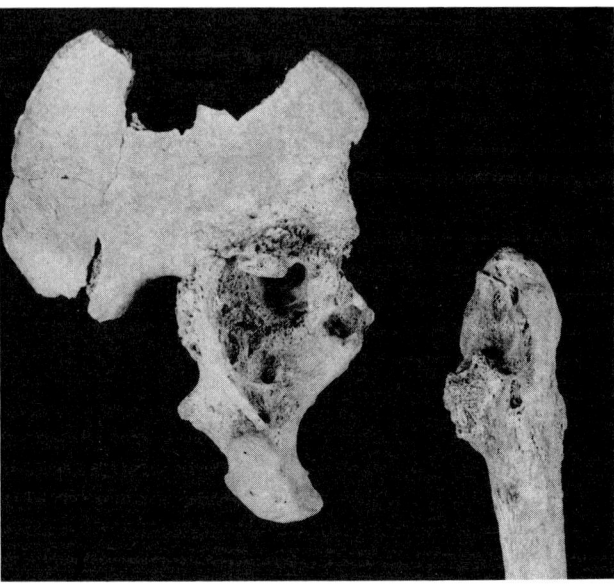

ANTIQUITY OF RHEUMATOID ARTHRITIS

Rheumatoid arthritis (RA) was not listed as one of the rheumatic diseases definitely identified in ancient skeletons. In addition to the foregoing findings, a number of singular joint changes are often observed. These changes include odd, isolated examples of joint destruction, fusion, erosion, or cyst formation, often in disarticulated bones or in one or a few joints of a poorly preserved skeleton; any attempt at diagnosis is virtually impossible. A few authors have described more widespread "erosive" changes suggesting pos-sible RA.[19,27,43,44] Careful scrutiny of most of these cases shows the presence of spondylarthritis, joint fusion, limited asymmetric changes, or isolated erosions in sites such as the feet. We have yet to be convinced that any of these skeletons show unequivocal RA of the type or severity common today.

The antiquity of RA has been questioned on other grounds.[45,46] The first convincing clinical descriptions of the disease are as recent as the early nineteenth century,[47] and unlike gout, for example, it cannot be clearly identified in any old art or literature. It may be a recent disease.[48] Paleopathology has a potential role in determining the likely time and place in which this disease first appeared. Most evidence suggests that RA of the severity seen today must have been uncommon, if present at all, in previous centuries. However, an alternative view has been advanced by rheumatologists in both the U.S. and Mexico. Pre-Columbian skeletons with erosive changes that may represent RA have been described. In view of the absence of such changes in European collections, it has been suggested that RA, like syphilis, could be a New World disease that was subsequently spread to Europe. This is an attractive idea, with far-reaching consequences concerning the etiology of RA. It will be interesting to follow this story as the skeletons are examined further and scrutinized by multidisciplinary experts. The antiquity of RA remains a tantalizing, but unsolved riddle.

TEMPORAL PERSPECTIVE

Paleopathology adds a temporal perspective to rheumatology. It highlights the antiquity of arthritis, shows that man has suffered pain and disability from joint disease through the ages, and reminds us that diseases and disease expression can change with time. Skeletal paleopathology is a rewarding, educational discipline of both historical and contemporary value.

REFERENCES

1. Cook, D.C., et al.: Vertebral pathology in Afar australopithecines. Am. J. Phys. Anthrop., *60*:83–101, 1983.
2. Straus, W.L., Jr., and Cave, A.J.E.: Pathology and posture of Neanderthal man. Q. Rev. Biol., *32*:348–363, 1957.
3. Rogers, J.M.: Report of skeletal remains from Hazelton Long Barrow. In preparation.
4. Torre, C., Giacobini, G., and Sicuro, A.: The skull and vertebral column pathology of ancient Egyptians: study of the Marro Collection. J. Hum. Evol., *9*:41–44, 1980.
5. Ruffer, M.A.: Arthritis deformans and spondylitis in ancient Egypt. J. Pathol. Bacteriol., *22*:152–196, 1918.

6. Bourke, J.B.: A review of palaeopathology of arthritic diseases. *In* Diseases in Antiquity. Edited by D. Brothwell and A.T. Sandison. Springfield, IL, Charles C Thomas, 1967, pp. 352–370.

7. Hormell, R.S.: Notes on the history of rheumatism and gout. N. Engl. J. Med., 223:754–759, 1940.

8. Sydenham, T.: The Works of Thomas Sydenham M.D. Translated by R.G. Latham. London, Sydenham Society, 1840.

9. Blumberg, B.S.: Bernard Connor's description of the pathology of ankylosing spondylitis. Arthritis Rheum., 1:553–563, 1958.

10. Charcot, J.M.: Clinical Lectures on the Diseases of Old Age. Translated by L.H. Hunt, New York, W. Wood, 1881.

11. Copeman, W.S.C.: A Short History of Gout and the Rheumatic Diseases. Berkeley, University of California Press, 1964.

12. Heberden, W.: Commentaries on the History and Cure of Diseases. London, T. Payne, 1802.

13. Scudamore, C.: A Treatise on the Nature and Cure of Gout and Gravel, 4th Ed. London, Longman, Hurst, Rees, Orme and Brown, 1823.

14. Benedek, T., and Rodnan, G.P.: A brief history of the rheumatic diseases. Bull. Rheum. Dis., 32:59–68, 1982.

15. Goldthwait, J.E.: The differential diagnosis and treatment of the so-called rheumatoid diseases. Boston Med. Surg. J., 151:529–534, 1904.

16. Garrod, A.B.: The great practical importance of separating rheumatoid arthritis from gout. Lancet, 2:1,033–1,037, 1892.

17. Ruffer, M.A., and Rietti, A.: On osseous lesions in ancient Egyptians. J. Pathol. Bacteriol., 16:439–447, 1912.

18. Zorab, P.A.: The historical and prehistorical background to ankylosing spondylitis. Proc. R. Soc. Med. 54:415–420, 1961.

19. Rogers, J., Watt, I., and Dieppe, P.: Palaeopathology of spinal osteophytosis, vertebral ankylosis, ankylosing spondylitis and vertebral hyperostosis. Ann. Rheum. Dis., 44:113–120, 1985.

20. Page May, W.: Rheumatoid arthritis (osteitis deformans) affecting bones 5,500 years old. Br. Med. J., 2:1,631–1,632, 1897.

21. Wood-Jones, F.: General pathology (including diseases of teeth). *In* Archaeological Survey of Nubia Report for 1907–1908, Vol II. Report on the Human Remains. Edited by G. Elliot-Smith and F. Wood-Jones. Cairo, National Printing Department, 1910, pp. 263–292.

22. Hrdlicka, A.: Special Notes on Some of the Pathological Conditions Shown by the Skeletal Material of the Ancient Peruvians. Smithsonian Misc. Coll., 93:1–100, 1914.

23. Moodie, R.L.: The Antiquity of Disease. Chicago, University of Chicago Science Series, 1923.

24. Wells, C.: Bones, Bodies and Disease. London, Thames and Hudson, 1964.

25. Brothwell, D., and Sandison, A.: Diseases in Antiquity. Springfield, IL, Charles C Thomas, 1967.

26. Steinbock, R.T.: Palaeopathological Diagnosis and Interpretation. Springfield, IL, Charles C Thomas, 1976.

27. Ortner, D.J., and Putscher, W.G.J.: Identification of Pathological Conditions in Human Skeletal Remains. Washington, Smithsonian Institution, 1981.

28. Rogers, J., Waldron, T., Dieppe, P., and Watt, I.: Arthropathies in paleopathology: the basis of classification according to most probable cause. J. Archeol. Sci., 14:179–193, 1987.

29. Wells, C.: The human burials. *In* Romano British Cemeteries at Cirencester. Edited by A. McWhirr, L. Viner, and C. Wells. Cirencester, England, Cirencester Excavation Committee, 1982, pp. 135–202.

30. Clarke, G.A., and Delmond, J.A.: Vertebral osteophytosis in Dickson Mound populations: a biochemical interpretation. *In* Arthritis: modern concepts and ancient evidence. Henry Ford Hosp. Med. J., 21:54–58, 1979.

31. Angel, J.L.: Osteoarthritis in prehistoric Turkey and Medieval Byzantium. *In* Arthritis: modern concepts and ancient evidence. Henry Ford Hosp. Med. J., 21:38–43, 1979.

32. Wood, P.H.N.: Osteoarthritis in the community. Clin. Rheum. Dis., 2:495–508, 1977.

33. Rogers, J., Watt, I., and Dieppe, P.: Arthritis in Saxon and mediaeval skeletons. Br. Med. J., 283:1,668–1,671, 1981.

34. Wells, C.: A palaeopathological rarity in a skeleton of Roman date. Med. Hist., 17:399–400, 1973.

35. Elliot Smith, G., and Dawson, W.R.: Egyptian Mummies. New York, Dial Press, 1924.

36. Rowling, J.T.: Pathological change in mummies. Proc. R. Soc. Med., 54:409–415, 1961.

37. Molleson, T.I.: The early Christian case of gout from Biga, NR Philae in the British Museum (Natural History), London. (Abstract.) Clin. Rheumatol., 5:15, 1986.

38. Kramar, C.: A case of ankylosing spondylitis in mediaeval Geneva. Ossa, 8:115–128, 1982.

39. Rogers, J., and Dieppe, P.: Lessons from paleopathology. Practitioner, 227:1,191–1,199, 1983.

40. Forestier, J., and Lagier, R.: Ankylosing hyperostosis of the spine. Clin. Orthop., 74:65–83, 1971.

41. Manchester, K.: A leprous skeleton of the 7th century from Eccles, Kent, and the present evidence of leprosy in early Britain. J. Archaeol. Sci., 8:205–209, 1981.

42. Hackett, C.J.: Diagnostic criteria of syphylis, yaws, and treponarid (treponaematoses) and of some other diseases in dry bones. *In* Sitzungsberichte der Heidelberger Akademie der Wissenschaften Mathematisch-Naturwissen-Schaftliche Klasse. Monograph 4. Berlin, Springer, 1976.

43. Klepinger, L.L.: Paleopathological evidence for the evolution of rheumatoid arthritis. Am. J. Phys. Anthropol., 50:119–122, 1979.

44. Karsh, R.S., and McCarty, J.D.: Archeology and arthritis. A.M.A. Arch. Intern. Med., 105:172–175, 1960.

45. Buchanan, W.W., and Murdoch, R.M.: Hypothesis: that rheumatoid arthritis will disappear. J. Rheumatol., 6:324–329, 1979.

46. Wood, P.H.N.: Is rheumatoid arthritis a recent disease? *In* Infection and Immunology in the Rheumatic Diseases. Edited by D.C. Dumonde. Oxford, Blackwell, 1976, pp. 619–622.

47. Parish, L.C.: An historical approach to the nomenclature of rheumatoid arthritis. Arthritis Rheum., 6:138–158, 1963.

48. Short, C.L.: The antiquity of rheumatoid arthritis. Arthritis Rheum., 17:193–205, 1974.

EPIDEMIOLOGY OF THE RHEUMATIC DISEASES

3

ALFONSE T. MASI and THOMAS A. MEDSGER, JR.

Epidemiology (*epi*, upon; *demos*, people; *logy*, science) is the study of the frequency and distribution of disease in populations and of factors determining or associated with disease occurrence. This discipline has made significant contributions to the understanding and control of many conditions, both infectious and noncommunicable. Epidemiology has a broad mission, and its methods affect other major disciplines, including clinical, public health, and laboratory sciences.

Depending on the level of understanding of a disease, epidemiologic investigations may be designed as descriptive, integrative, hypothesis-testing, experimental, or disease-control studies. Although studies of acute rheumatic fever have encompassed all levels, most rheumatic disease epidemiology has, thus far, focused on the more elementary descriptions of disease occurrence. The next stages are to infer concepts of disease by synthesizing such descriptive data and to generate testable etiologic hypotheses.

The descriptive epidemiology of the rheumatic diseases is voluminous, and important past contributions may be found in reviews, and proceedings of international conferences.[1–9] Accordingly, we have emphasized more recent studies illustrating epidemiologic concepts and principles and have selected the major disorders not associated with known infectious agents. Infection-related arthritis is covered in other chapters.

BASIC EPIDEMIOLOGIC CONCEPTS

CLASSIFICATION OF DISEASE

Because case frequencies reported in population surveys depend directly on disease definition, emphasis has been given to developing accurate, or at least reliable, criteria for the classification or diagnosis of rheumatic diseases, as described subsequently. No clear distinction exists between epidemiologic and clinical studies of disease classification, although epidemiologic investigations are usually based on defined populations, and clinical studies rely on data from one or more medical care institutions.

The purpose of criteria for *disease classification* is to allow comparison of groups of patients from diverse sources, such as from different institutions or countries. In contrast, *criteria for diagnosis* refer to decisions concerning the individual patient. It is thus appropriate that some patients with a definite clinical diagnosis may not satisfy a different set of classification criteria.

INCIDENCE AND PREVALENCE

Incidence is the rate of occurrence of new cases of disease (or its manifestations) during a given period in a defined population at risk.[10] It is estimated by determining the number of new cases that occur in a population over time. *Prevalence* is the percentage or proportion of cases, identified by interview or examination, in a population at a given point in time (point prevalence) or during a specified interval (interval or period prevalence). Point prevalence is determined in a single survey, whereas interval prevalence is determined in one or more surveys.

A numeric relationship exists between incidence (I) and prevalence (P) during stable periods of occurrence of a disease; that is, incidence times average duration of disease (D) equals prevalence (I $\times$ D = P). Because disease duration, including likelihood of remission or mortality, may vary with factors such as onset age, sex, race, and socioeconomic status, prevalence reflects both the risk of acquiring a disease and those factors that influence its duration. Hence, incidence is a more sensitive and specific indicator of disease acquisition risk than is prevalence and is thus superior for inferring mechanisms of etiology or host predisposition to onset. Studies of incidence are generally more demanding than prevalence studies because larger populations are required to derive a suitable number of new cases, and definition of disease at onset or first diagnosis may be difficult.

SENSITIVITY AND SPECIFICITY

These terms refer to the comparison of a true classification of a population with a classification based on a test or criterion result, as illustrated in a two-by-two table (Table 3–1). Sensitivity of a test or criterion is the proportion of persons who truly have a condition and whose results are positive on the test or criterion. Specificity of a test or criterion is the proportion of persons who truly do not have the condition and whose results are negative on the test or criterion.

MULTIFACTORIAL CONTRIBUTIONS TO ETIOLOGY

Most chronic acquired diseases are now believed to result from the interaction of multiple factors related to the host, environment, and at times, infecting agents (Fig. 3–1). Multifactorial mechanisms of disease often obscure recognition of the primary determining factor(s) by virtue of complex interactions and sequences of events. Epidemiology helps one to develop a holistic perspective of disease and a conceptual synthesis that can clarify such interrelationships and lead to promising directions for future studies. This goal may be accomplished by identifying a broader or narrower spectrum of a disease in the population or by recognizing characteristic disease course patterns that correlate closely with specific host, environmental, and other factors. Comprehensive approaches combining epidemiologic, clinical, and laboratory methods offer hope in unraveling the currently obscure primary interactions in these complex disorders.

RHEUMATOID ARTHRITIS

The epidemiology of rheumatoid arthritis (RA), including juvenile rheumatoid arthritis (JRA),[11] and the relationship between seropositive and seronegative RA have been reviewed.[12–14]

CLASSIFICATION OF DISEASE

RA illustrates the dilemma that lack of accurate definition poses to investigators seeking to determine the frequency or natural course of a disease. Thus, differences in reported incidence and prevalence may result mainly from differences in definition or severity, rather than actual disease occurrence. Although classic advanced RA can be more reliably diagnosed, it represents a minority of the total disease spectrum, and conclusions based on such narrow subsets must be properly qualified and not overgeneralized. Unfortunately, recognition and definition of RA during its earliest stages are difficult because the disease may follow a variable, nonspecific pattern for months or years before becoming "typical."

CRITERIA

A committee of the American Rheumatism Association (ARA) proposed criteria based on a set of 11 symptoms, signs, and laboratory features of RA as well as specific exclusions that increase the specificity[15] (Table 3–2). Five or more criteria (definite RA) yielded a sensitivity of 70% for rheumatologist-diagnosed definite RA and a specificity of 91%. Three

Table 3–1.   Sensitivity and Specificity Measures

Test or Criteria	True or Standard Classification		
	Yes	No	Total
Positive	a	b	a + b
Negative	c	d	c + d
Total	a + c	b + d	Total

Sensitivity equals a/a + c
Specificity equals d/b + d

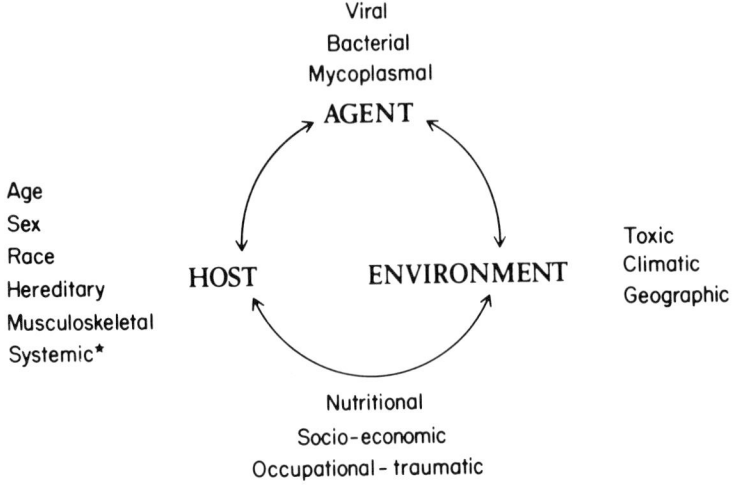

FIG. 3–1. Factors contributing to arthritis: holistic model of disease.

*e.g., circulatory, endocrinologic, immunologic, metabolic, neurologic, psychologic

or more criteria (probable RA) had a sensitivity of 88% for clinically probable or definite disease and specificity of 77%. Definite and probable categories were recommended for study or reporting purposes on the features, course, or treatment of RA, but not for establishing a diagnosis in an individual patient.[16] A less rigid classification of "possible" RA was also proposed to include early and atypical cases and patients with other disorders.[15,16] The duration of articular manifestations required to satisfy clinical criteria was purposely set at 6 weeks to eliminate inclusion of the more acute forms of arthritis caused by infection, trauma, or rheumatic fever.

At the Second International Symposium on Population Studies in the Rheumatic Diseases held in Rome in 1961, these criteria were modified to make them more suitable for epidemiologic studies. Synovial fluid analysis, synovial histology, and microscopic confirmation of subcutaneous nodules, which could not be expected to be routinely ascertained, were eliminated.[17] Deficiencies in the criteria included the difficulty in quantitating morning stiffness and its low reliability, the low frequency of subcutaneous nodules, and marked variation in use of different serologic tests for rheumatoid factor and grading of radiographs.[11]

Table 3–2. Rheumatoid Arthritis Diagnostic Criteria (ARA 1958 Revision)

1. Morning stiffness.
2. Pain on motion or tenderness in at least one joint.*
3. Swelling (soft tissue thickening or fluid, not bony overgrowth alone) in at least one joint.*
4. Swelling of at least one other joint.*†
5. Symmetric joint swelling with simultaneous involvement of the same joint on both sides of the body.*†
   Terminal phalangeal joint involvement does not satisfy the criterion.
6. Subcutaneous nodules over bony prominences, on extensor surfaces or in juxta-articular regions.*
7. Roentgenographic changes typical of rheumatoid arthritis (which must include at least bony decalcification localized
   to or greatest around the involved joints and not just degenerative changes).†
8. Positive agglutination (anti-gamma globulin) test.†
9. Poor mucin precipitate from synovial fluid (with shreds and cloudy solution).
10. Characteristic histologic changes in synovial membrane.†
11. Characteristic histologic changes in nodules.†

Categories†	Number of Criteria Required	Minimum Duration of Continuous Symptoms	Exclusion‡
Classic	7 of 11	6 weeks (nos. 1–5)	any of listed
Definite	5 of 11	6 weeks (nos. 1–5)	any of listed
Probable	3 of 11	3 weeks (one of nos. 1–5)	any of listed

*Observed by a physician.
†Refer to original references for further specification.
‡Refer to original references for listing of exclusions.
(Data from Ropes, M.W., Bennett, G.A., and Cobb, S.: 1958 Revision of diagnostic criteria for rheumatoid arthritis. Arthritis Rheum., 2:16–20, 1959; and Ropes, M.W., et al.: Proposed diagnostic criteria for rheumatoid arthritis. Ann. Rheum. Dis., 16:118–125, 1957.)

Another set of RA criteria proposed mainly for population studies[18] was derived from the Third International Symposium held in New York in 1966[7] (Table 3-3). The roentgenographic and serologic components of the Rome criteria were retained, but the New York criteria included different clinical items. They emphasized the pattern of affected joints, requiring involvement of a distal extremity joint (hand, wrist, or foot) and symmetry of an acceptable joint pair. These criteria list no exclusions or required duration of joint manifestations.

Both sets of criteria have been compared in the same populations: the Sudbury, Massachusetts study of 4552 adults and a comparative criteria study among 1748 Pima Indians over 14 years of age.[19,20] In the Massachusetts study, 118 persons initially met Rome criteria for probable or definite RA, as opposed to only 17 who satisfied the more selective physical examination item of the New York criteria.[19] After a 3- to 5-year followup, only 15% of those who initially satisfied probable Rome criteria remained so classified, whereas 65% of persons who initially satisfied New York criteria continued to do so. These studies suggest that some individuals with transient, nondeforming RA were included. It is likely that different criteria measure different stages in the evolution of RA or identify other conditions that mimic it. For example, females with bilateral knee involvement who have osteoarthritis may be considered to have RA by satisfying the second New York criterion.[20] Another obvious source of false positive results is the patient with polymyalgia rheumatica and peripheral joint involvement, who is not excluded from the Rome criteria and can satisfy both Rome and New York criteria.[21]

Revised criteria for the classification of RA were recently proposed[22] (Table 3-4). The presence of 4 or more of the 7 criteria defines "rheumatoid arthritis," and no further qualifications (classic, definite, probable) or lists of exclusions are required. In addition, a "classification tree" schema performs equally well as the traditional (4+ of 7) format. The new criteria has a 91 to 94% sensitivity and an 89% specificity for RA when compared to control subjects with non-RA rheumatic disease.[22]

Criteria developed for clinical remission in RA include: morning stiffness absent or less than 15 minutes in duration, no fatigue, no joint pain by history, no joint or tendon sheath swelling, and a normal erythrocyte sedimentation rate.[23] In the study sample of 344 RA patients, 5 or more of these criteria present in an individual patient indicated clinical remission, with 72% sensitivity and 100% specificity. Under the terms of the ARA remission criteria in a series of 458 RA patients, 18% had at least one remission (median length 10 months) during a mean followup of 2.5 years. The criteria were 80% sensitive and 96% specific against the investigators' assessment.[24]

AGE AND SEX DISTRIBUTION

It is generally agreed that the prevalence of "definite" RA increases with age for both males and females and approaches 2% and 5%, respectively, over age 55; these studies have been comprehensively reviewed.[11] The overall sex ratio of almost 3 females to 1 male is also a consistent finding; however, the sex ratio is 5:1 or more with onset under age 60, but approximately 2:1 or less when onset is at an older age.[11,25-27] The last ratio may be related to an abrupt increase in RA among older males.[26] Sex ratio data in younger adult RA subjects are limited, but they indicate a relative infrequency in males.[12,28,29] More recently, a peculiarly high predisposition to RA in younger adult females was found in studies of Yakima Indians,[29] with a tendency to more progressive disease.[30]

Analysis of 5-year average annual incidence rates for RA in Rochester, Minnesota showed a dramatic decrease among females from 92.3 per 100,000 from 1960 to 1964 to 39.7 per 100,000 from 1970 to 1974.[31] These investigators suggested a temporal relationship between the decline in incidence and the concomitant increase in the use of oral contraceptives. This concept was supported by a previous Royal College of General Practitioners study that indicated a reduction in incidence of RA associated with oral contraceptives.[32] The Rochester, Minnesota followup case-control study of the current or prior use of estrogens in

---

Table 3–3.   Rheumatoid Arthritis Population Survey Criteria (New York, 1966)*

1. History, past or present, of any episode of joint pain involving three or more limb joints without stipulation as to duration. The joints on either side shall count separately, but joints that occur in groups (e.g., the PIP or MCP joints) on one side shall count only as a single joint.

2. Swelling, limitation, subluxation, or ankylosis of at least three limb joints, including one hand, wrist, or foot with symmetry of at least one joint pair. (Joints excluded from criteria are the DIP, the fifth PIP, the first CMC joints, the hips, and the first MTP. Subluxation of the lateral MTP must be irreducible.)

3. X-ray features of grade 2 or more erosive arthritis in the hands, wrists, or feet.

4. Positive serologic reaction for rheumatoid (anti-gamma globulin) factor.

*Recommendations for summation of the criteria were not made. (Data from Bennett, P.H., and Burch, T.A.: New York symposium on population studies in the rheumatic diseases: new diagnostic criteria. Bull. Rheum. Dis., *17*:458, 1967.)

Table 3–4. 1987 Revised Criteria for Classification of Rheumatoid Arthritis (RA)*

Criterion	Definition
1. Morning stiffness	Morning stiffness in and around the joints lasting at least an hour before maximal improvement.
2. Arthritis of three or more joint areas	At least 3 joint areas with simultaneous soft-tissue swelling or fluid (not bony overgrowth alone) observed by a physician. The 14 possible joint areas are right or left PIP, MCP, wrist, elbow, knee, ankle, and MTP joints.
3. Arthritis of hand joints	At least one joint area swollen as above in a wrist, MCP, or PIP.
4. Symmetric arthritis	Simultaneous involvement of the same joint areas (as in 2) on both sides of the body (bilateral involvement of PIP, MCP, or MTP is acceptable without absolute symmetry).
5. Rheumatoid nodules	Subcutaneous nodules over bony prominences, or extensor surfaces, or in juxta-articular regions, observed by a physician.
6. Serum rheumatoid factor	Demonstration of abnormal amounts of serum "rheumatoid factor" by any method that has been positive in fewer than 5% of normal control subjects.
7. Radiographic changes	Radiographic changes typical of RA on posteroanterior wrist radiographs, including erosions or unequivocal bony decalcification localized to or most marked adjacent to the involved joints (osteoarthritic changes alone do not qualify).

*For classification purposes, a patient shall be said to have RA if he has satisfied at least 4 of the above 7 criteria. Criteria 1 to 4 must have been present for at least 6 weeks. Patients with two clinical diagnoses are not excluded. Designation as "classic," "definite," or "probable" RA is *not* to be made.
(Data from Arnett, F.C., et al.: The 1987 revised American Rheumatism Association criteria for classification of rheumatoid arthritis. Arthritis Rheum. (in press).)

women with and without RA showed no differences.[33] The question is unsettled because a Dutch report claims that oral contraceptives have a preventive effect on RA,[34] whereas another American study in a large cohort of nurses showed no protective effect.[35]

Sex-related host factors seem to play an important role in determining the onset and severity of RA. This concept is consistent with recognized pregnancy-induced remission and postpartum exacerbation or new onset of RA.[36] Males may have a protective factor that may be lost at older ages.

Urinary excretion[37] and plasma levels[38] of adrenal androgens are decreased in female RA patients as compared with control subjects. Steroid sex hormones may alter either microvascular or immunologic function, thereby influencing predisposition to RA and related disorders.[37,39–41]

ETHNIC AND GEOGRAPHIC DISTRIBUTION

All races seem capable of developing RA. Although differences in case definition make prevalence rates from various sources difficult to compare, estimates for definite RA are remarkably constant at 1.0% in white populations.[11] The prevalence of RA was similar for whites and blacks in the United States.[42] When ARA criteria for definite disease have been used, the

prevalence in major reported surveys for the average adult (age 15 and older) has ranged from a low of 0.1% in a rural black South African community[43] to 3.0% among Finnish whites.[44] The high prevalence of RA-like disease in young adult Yakima females was not associated with either HLA-Dw4 or HLA-DR4, in contrast to most other populations.[29,30] A Chippewa band was reported with a minimal prevalence of RA of 5.3% and a significant correlation of HLA-DR4 with RA, paralleling the high prevalence (68%) of HLA-DR4 in this closed population.[45] Climate itself does not seem to be a factor. Although most population studies of RA do not permit the calculation of incidence, annual estimates vary from 1 to 3/1000 persons at risk.[11,26]

Despite general similarity, reported population frequency differences seem real. Emphasis in future field studies should be directed at critically evaluating criteria, incidence, and course of RA in populations that offer particular logistic advantages or suggest unusually high or low frequencies. Additionally, further emphasis should be placed on controlled analysis of personal, historical, and environmental factors with which the disease may be associated in order to gain clues to etiology or pathogenesis.

ENVIRONMENTAL FACTORS

An increased prevalence of RA has been noted in single and divorced women,[46] as well as in association with lower income and lower educational achievement.[42,47] The marked increase in prevalence of definite RA in genetically close, related South African black urban populations, compared with rural populations, implicates sociologic and environmental factors in disease occurrence.[43,48]

Lack of association of RA in marital partners and failure to demonstrate evidence of an infectious agent do not support this mechanism of transmission.[49] An association between Epstein-Barr (EB) virus and RA has been suggested. Defective cytotoxic T-cell response to EB virus in RA has been reported, but it appears to be related to disease activity and occurs also in other inflammatory arthritides.[50] A parvovirus-like agent (RA-1 virus), unrelated to human B19 parvovirus, has been found in RA synovial membrane.[51] Further studies are required to elucidate this relationship (see Chapter 31). Surgical removal of lymphoid tissue has been reported to increase the risk of subsequent development of RA, with a risk associated with the quantity of lymphoid tissue excised.[52,53] This relationship has been disputed, however.[54,55] Failure to find disease similarity in sibling pairs with RA suggests that various environmental factors contribute to heterogeneity in RA.[56]

GENETIC INFLUENCES

The incidence of adult-onset RA (probable, definite, and classic) was studied in 496 first-degree relatives, 120 parents, 218 siblings, and 158 children, of 78 probands, and the incidence was compared to that in general population of Rochester, Minnesota.[57] The ratio of age- and sex-adjusted rates in first-degree relatives was 1.7 (95% confidence interval of 1.0 to 2.9). Although only 15 first-degree relatives developed RA in the study interval of 1945 to 1981, the major excess incidence was concentrated in the 16- to 39-year risk group (5 cases observed versus 1 expected). Moreover, a significant excess was only found among first-degree relatives of probands who had a diagnosis of RA made under 40 years of age, suggesting heterogeneity in the inheritance pattern. The conclusion is that, overall, the familial aggregation of RA is weak, and a putative susceptibility gene must have a low penetrance.[57]

Twin and family studies confined to probands with erosive seropositive arthritis showed a 6-fold increase in RA prevalence among siblings or dizygotic twins versus control subjects.[58] In monozygotic twins, the association was over 30 times that expected among controls. The data were most consistent with a polygenic pattern of inheritance.[58] A recent nationwide

Finnish twin cohort study indicated a relative risk of RA of 8.6 for monozygotic pairs and 3.4 for dizygotic pairs.[59] These figures are lower than those previously observed in family studies, but they are consistent with the sampling differences and severity of disease of probands. Family studies reported in a recent symposium showed that factors at or near the HLA locus confer increased risk for the development of RA.[59a]

Rapid advances are being made in the immunogenetic associations with RA, both positive (seropositive) and negative (seronegative) for serum IgM rheumatoid factor.[14] Essentially, all studies show a significant association between HLA-DR4 and seropositive RA, but only about half show such association with seronegative RA.[60] A summary of those results shows a relative risk of 4.7 for seropositive RA and 2.4 for seronegative RA in the presence of HLA-DR4 versus normal control subjects (Table 3–5). Subsets of DR4 have now been identified, some of which are associated with increased risk for the development of RA.[61] HLA-DR1 also associates with seropositive (relative risk 2.1) and seronegative (relative risk 2.9) RA, especially with HLA-DR4-negative, seronegative RA.[62] These data suggest that both seropositive and seronegative RA have a common, overlapping genetic predisposition.[14] Other genetic factors at or near the HLA locus may also be important in the expression of RA,[63] including an epitope related to 109d6 and MC1.[64,64a] The heterogeneity of RA is illustrated by a population study in the Netherlands in which overall frequency of DR4 was similar in cases and control subjects, and was increased only in the subset of RA patients with either erosions or rheumatoid factor or both.[65] Combined family and immunogenetic studies in RA deserve high priority.

COURSE OF DISEASE

The natural history of RA is variable. Three major patterns of articular involvement have been documented in its early course in younger adults, as illustrated in Figure 3–2.[66] Most reviews of outcome in RA have dealt with patients having well-established disease and thus may not represent the total spectrum. Essentially all studies, however, concur that serum rheumatoid factor and bony erosions indicate a poor prognosis.[11] Other early features found by multivariate analysis to be associated with worse disease on followup include female sex, white race, two or more swollen upper-extremity joints, Raynaud-like phenomena, and malaise or weakness.[12,67,68]

Because of the systemic nature of RA, it is not surprising that total mortality is reported to be greater

Table 3–5. Percentage of HLA-DR4 in Rheumatoid Factor-Positive and -Negative Rheumatoid Arthritis (RA): Summary Results (RF+ and RF−) (From 14 Published Reports)

Reported HLA-DR4 Associations		Percentage of Positive HLA-DR4		
		RF+ RA	RF− RA	Normal Subjects
RF+ only	(6 reports)	60	28	20
RF+ and RF−	(8 reports)	56	52	24
Total	(14 reports)	57	40	22
Number of RA patients		(887)	(329)	—

(Data from Gran, J.T., and Husby, G.: Seronegative rheumatoid arthritis and HLA DR4: proposal for criteria (Editorial). J. Rheumatol., *14*:1079–1082, 1987.)

than expected.[69] First evaluation findings that predict premature death include ARA functional class, rheumatoid factor titer, and number of involved joints; that is, variables that reflect the severity of disease and not its therapy.[70–72] A disproportionately frequent cause of death is infection, mainly of the respiratory tract and upper gastrointestinal tract disease, and bleeding attributed to therapy.[70,72] Cardiac deaths occur at an expected or increased rate, with no apparent relation to medications used. Considering the increased use of immunosuppressive drugs for severe RA, the frequency of cancer of the hematopoietic system could be excessive, although not malignant neoplasms in total.[73] In one controlled study, cyclophosphamide-treated patients had a 4-fold increase in occurrence of new cancers and a 15-fold increase in hematologic and lymphoreticular cancers.[74] Another controlled study of 119 cyclophosphamide-treated RA patients showed an excess in cases versus control subjects of urinary bladder (6 vs. 0), skin (8 vs. 0), and hematologic (5 vs. 1) cancers.[75]

In long-term followup studies, disease stage and duration adversely affect work capability, as do female sex, increased age at onset, initial functional class, and development of functional impairment early in the course of disease.[76,77] Control over the

FIG. 3–2. Schema of articular course patterns over five years in early diagnosed young adult rheumatoid arthritis patients. (From Masi, A.T., Feigenbaum, S.L., and Kaplan, S.B. Articular patterns in the early course of rheumatoid arthritis. Am. J. Med., *75* (Suppl.):16–26, 1983.)

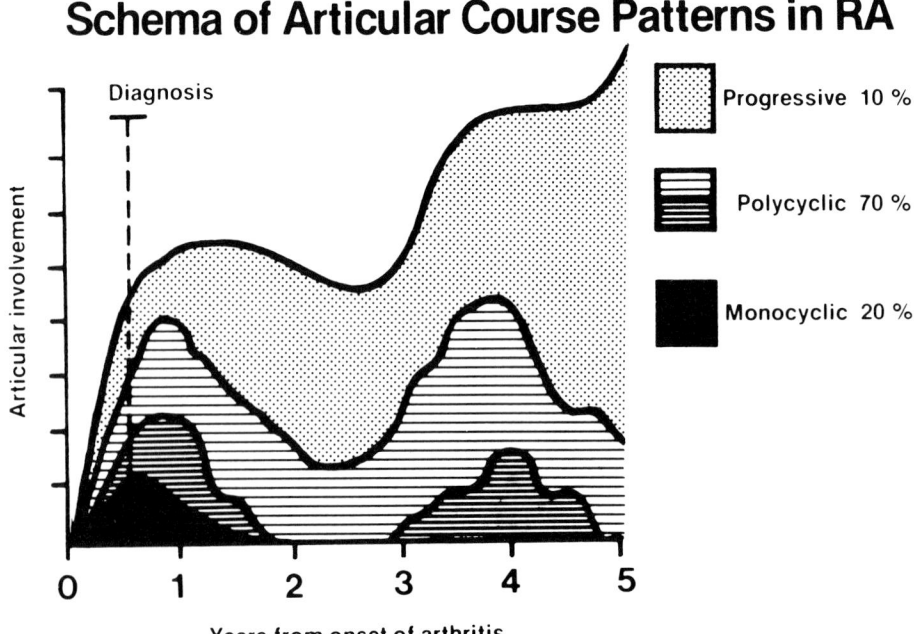

pace and activities of work and self-employment status most influenced continued employment.[78] Annual inpatient and overall costs attributable to RA were determined in multicenter studies and paralleled disease severity and disability.[79-81] Total annual medical costs averaged over $2500, and lifetime economic costs were estimated to approximate those of stroke and coronary heart disease.[81,82]

JUVENILE ARTHRITIS

DEFINITION OF DISEASE

Chronic forms of juvenile-onset arthritis include JRA, juvenile ankylosing spondylitis and related HLA-B27-associated disorders, numerous specific rheumatic and nonrheumatic conditions manifesting arthritis, and a residual group of unclassified arthritides. In England, the term juvenile chronic polyarthritis is often used for idiopathic, chronic juvenile-onset arthritis, with "JRA" limited to the 10 to 15% of children with positive tests for serum rheumatoid factor. Although arbitrary, the upper age limit for juvenile onset is usually considered to be the sixteenth birthday.

An ARA subcommittee reviewed and validated the 1977 classification criteria for JRA using a computerized data base of 250 children with prolonged followup.[83] The criteria include disease manifestations present during the first six months after onset, that is, polyarticular (5 or more joints) onset (manifestations most closely resembling those of adult seropositive RA), pauciarticular onset, and systemic onset. Rheumatoid rash was a good discriminator for the systemic-onset type. In a comparison study, Soviet and American patients were remarkably similar in the frequency of subtype onset, in sex and onset age within subtype, and in the distribution by subtype after followup.[84] No population survey criteria for chronic juvenile-onset arthritis have been proposed.

JRA POPULATION FREQUENCY

Figures derived from referral hospitals or specialty clinics undoubtedly underestimate the occurrence of JRA and are subject to selection biases. A summary of existing prevalence estimates suggests a figure of 0.2 to 1.0 cases per 1000 individuals.[85] One community-based epidemiologic study (Rochester, Minnesota, 1960 to 1980) has been published using 1977 ARA criteria for juvenile arthritis.[86] A comparable prevalence rate of 0.96 to 1.13 per 1000 was reported. The overall incidence was 13.9 per 100,000 population, with patterns indicating a female predominance before age 5. A greater proportion of the patients (74%) was classified as having pauciarticular onset in this community study than in referral medical center series. Using the criteria of the European League Against Rheumatism (EULAR) for juvenile chronic polyarthritis (JCP),[87] a population survey in western Sweden in 1983 yielded an annual incidence of 12 per 100,000 and a prevalence of 56 per 100,000. Prevalence decreased with age and the girl-to-boy ratio was 3:2.[88] Using ARA criteria for JRA, an incidence survey in urban Finnish children yielded a rate of 19.6 per 100,000 annually, with 76% having pauciarticular disease.[89] Other reported juvenile arthritis incidence rates are lower, ranging from 2.2 to 9.2 per 100,000 children at risk.[11]

AGE AND SEX DISTRIBUTION

Age and sex variations occur according to the previously mentioned onset patterns.[88] The sex ratio in the systemic onset (Still's) type is approximately equal, with the majority (over 80%) having onset under 10 years of age.[90] Numerous similar cases have been reported with onset in late adolescence and adulthood. Polyarticular onset usually begins later, and females predominate,[88,90] as in young adult–onset RA.

In the pauciarticular category, further subdivisions can be made. Young girls with serum antinuclear antibodies and chronic iridocyclitis have an average onset age of under 5 years.[83] Boys with HLA-B27 and one or another of the associated arthritis variants usually have onset at age 10 or older. One followup study showed that 15 individuals who had progressed to either clear-cut spondylitis or sacroiliitis were nearly all male and B27-positive with a mean onset age of 10.6 years.[91]

RACIAL AND ETHNIC DISTRIBUTIONS

Adequate data on racial and ethnic frequencies of JRA are lacking.[11] A clinical survey of JCP in black and Indian South African children revealed a high relative frequency of polyarticular onset and rheumatoid factor positivity, equal sex ratio, and absence of a specific subgroup with pauciarticular onset and positive antinuclear antibodies.[92] Bias of sampling more severe disease may have contributed to such findings. Further epidemiologic studies are needed in this area.

FAMILIAL OCCURRENCE

Within each of three families, pairs of first-degree relatives manifested the same onset subtype and strikingly similar clinical features.[93] As anticipated, a higher-than-expected frequency of clinical ankylosing spondylitis and radiographic sacroiliitis has been found among male relatives, especially of those probands with sacroiliitis and HLA-B27. The presence of this antigen also enables one to identify a group of young girls with dominant peripheral arthritis and cervical spondylitis, which may closely mimic RA.[93]

Early-onset (under nine years of age) pauciarticular arthritis with antinuclear antibody and iritis was associated with HLA-DRW5 in one study and with DRW8 and an antigen "Tmo," related to DW7 and DW11, in others.[94,95] The mode of inheritance in a study of 158 British JCP patients favors the existence of at least two DR-linked "disease" genes with the combination of DR5 and DRw8 enhancing susceptibility to early onset pauciarticular disease.[96] As in adult RA, polyarticular disease is associated with DW4. Four genetic markers, BW35, B8, DR4, and DW7, have been reported to have increased frequency in systemic onset juvenile arthritis,[95,97,98] with differences observed between childhood and adult types of Still's disease.[98] These studies support the clinical subgrouping and suggest genetic predisposition to their development, but a great deal of heterogeneity with respect to these markers is obvious.

OTHER FACTORS

In a study of juvenile patients not further subclassified, those whose arthritis was preceded by an emotionally stressful event had higher antiviral antibody titers than those without such events.[99] The possible role of microbial agents in the occurrence and precipitation of chronic rheumatic disease in children has been reviewed, with emphasis on diseases that typify several different mechanisms of microbe-host interaction.[100]

NATURAL HISTORY

Although the overall prognosis in juvenile arthritis is better than in adult RA,[101,102] about half in one series had active disease at some time between the fifth and fifteenth years after onset, and functional class III or IV disability was present in 34 of 123 (28%).[101] Most (11 of 18) systemic-onset versus only 11 of 101 pauciarticular-onset patients had developed polyarticular involvement after 5 years.[84] In a European followup study of 433 hospitalized patients followed an average of 15 years (range 10 to 22), the mortality rate in the systemic group was 13.8% (mainly from amyloidosis), versus 1% in the nonsystemic polyarticular and none in the pauciarticular-onset group.[103] Eight of 9 deaths in one English series of 100 patients were in children with systemic onset.[104] In another followup study of 100 patients, the worst prognosis at 15 years was associated with polyarticular onset or persistent polyarthritis; all 3 deaths and 13 instances of "severe disability" derived from this group.[105] Long-term mortality ranges from 1 to 3% in U.S. series to nearly 10% in England and Europe, with differences possibly due to definition of disease and the increased frequency of secondary amyloidosis in Europe.[106] Interestingly, the sex ratio of fatal cases is equal.

JRA AND RA: A CONTINUUM OR SEPARATE DISEASES?

Clinical and epidemiologic differences between the onset types of juvenile arthritis suggest that a variety of syndromes overlap age limits, such as adult-onset Still's disease,[107] and that the age distinction between adult and juvenile cases is artificial. As indicated by tissue typing associations with certain juvenile-onset arthritis syndromes, separate host predispositions to disease are suggested for different onset types, supporting concepts of disease not restricted to age limits.[11,98] Additional genetic studies are needed for more definitive conclusions.[95]

ARTHRITIS SYNDROMES RELATED TO HLA-B27

Prior to the HLA-B27 discoveries, a genetic predisposition was suspected in several overlapping spinal and peripheral arthritis syndromes, including cases diagnosed as juvenile and adult ankylosing spondylitis, sacroiliitis, and Reiter's syndrome. These typically rheumatoid factor-negative (seronegative) conditions are now grouped into a family of spondyloarthritis syndromes and also include yersinia-reactive arthritis, spondylitis associated with chronic inflammatory bowel disease or psoriasis, and certain forms of oligoarticular peripheral arthritis in juveniles or younger adults.[108] The population prevalence of these disorders varies and is correlated with the occurrence of B27 in the described populations.[109,110,111] These conditions may occur in the absence of B27, however, and they may appear identical in terms of clinical features and severity except for the association of acute anterior uveitis with B27 positivity.[112,113] In family studies, homozygosity for HLA-B27 does not seem to influence the severity or the occurrence of ankylosing spondylitis.[114] B27 may serve as a marker for as yet undetermined genetic determinants of disease, as has been suggested by restriction fragment length polymorphism analysis.[115] Alternately, a common host predisposition might be conditioned by exogenous factors that determine the clinical manifestations. HLA-D locus typing has not usually shown significant associations with ankylosing spondylitis or Reiter's syndrome, although one study of ankylosing spondylitis showed a positive linkage disequilibrium between DR1 and B27 and a linkage of DR7 with erosive peripheral arthritis.[116]

Activation of ankylosing spondylitis in HLA-B27-positive persons by virtue of antigenic cross-reactivity with certain microorganisms, specifically enteric carriage of Klebsiella pneumoniae has been proposed,[117] but is difficult to interpret.[118] Although various gram-negative enteric infections can precipitate Reiter's syndrome and similar reactive arthritis disorders, as previously mentioned, no such mechanism has yet been documented for ankylosing spondylitis or psoriatic arthritis. The epidemiology of the spondyloarthritis syndromes and concepts of etiology have been reviewed.[119]

ANKYLOSING SPONDYLITIS

Because of its variable severity, the reported frequency of ankylosing spondylitis depends on disease definition.[120] Prevalence varies in different populations, ranging from a virtual absence in Australian aborigines or black Africans to a 4.2% diagnosed frequency in adult male Haida Indians.[109,110,121] The usual reported prevalence of "definite" ankylosing spondylitis is 1 per 1000 population, based on hospital or clinical survey techniques with a sex ratio of 3 males to 1 female.[122,123] Among HLA-B27-positive "healthy" males and females, a 20% frequency of "definite" and "possible" ankylosing spondylitis has been reported, but most subjects had radiographic sacroiliitis, rather than ankylosing spondylitis.[124] Lower prevalences of spondylitis among B27-positive individuals have been observed, including 11% in males and 1.5% in females in Tromso, Norway,[125] 3% in males and 0.6% in females in Hungary,[125a] 1.6% in the Busselton population study in Australia,[126] and 1.3% in persons aged 45 or older in the Netherlands.[127]

CRITERIA

Criteria for population study of ankylosing spondylitis were proposed at the 1961 Rome symposium,[2] and a revised set was introduced in New York in 1966.[7] They are compared in Table 3–6. The Rome criteria permit a diagnosis of ankylosing spondylitis without bilateral sacroiliitis on roentgenographs, whereas the New York criteria allow a "probable" diagnosis based solely on roentgenographic evidence of sacroiliitis without clinical disease. Certainly, the second syndrome is not synonymous with clinical ankylosing spondylitis, although both may be associated with HLA-B27 and may belong to the spectrum of spondyloarthropathy. Future criteria studies should further define differences between clinically manifest ankylosing spondylitis and more limited radiographic syndromes.[128]

Considerable variability may be expected in the determination and interpretation of symptoms of pain and stiffness in the dorsal and lumbar spine.[129] A high degree of variability has also been found in the interpretation of radiographic sacroiliitis,[11,130] especially unilateral and milder bilateral changes and in films of persons aged 50 or younger.[130] In one study, the pain item in the New York criteria had a specificity of only 4.9% and thus must be considered a nonspecific criterion as it was defined.[129] Certain manifestations of back pain may be more characteristic of spondylitis than of degenerative disease, however, such as onset before 40 years of age, insidious development, persistence longer than 3 months, morning stiffness, and relief with mild exercise.[131] In a psoriatic arthritis study, the physical findings of limited back movement in all directions and limited chest expansion had high specificity (over 95%) for roentgenographic disease, but a low sensitivity (less than 15%).[129] It has been suggested that the New York pain criterion for ankylosing spondylitis be modified by substituting the Rome pain criterion (low-back pain for more than 3 months), for greater specificity.[132]

AGE AND SEX DISTRIBUTION

Ankylosing spondylitis is typically diagnosed in young adult males, with the usual age of onset between 15 and 35 years. Females tend to have milder disease,[133] although not in a case-control study, which indicated more neck, shoulder, and hip arthropathy in women, as well as higher proportions with anemia, uveitis, and relatives with spondyloarthropathy.[134] Nevertheless, ankylosing spondylitis is clinically diagnosed predominantly in males. Although marked

Table 3–6. Ankylosing Spondylitis Population Survey Criteria

Rome, 1961[2]	New York, 1966[7]
CLINICAL CRITERIA	
1. Low back pain and stiffness for more than 3 months that is not relieved by rest.	Pain at the dorsolumbar junction or in the lumbar spine by history or at present.
2. Pain and stiffness in the thoracic region.	
3. Limited motion in the lumbar spine.	Limitation of motion of the lumbar spine in all three planes: anterior flexion, lateral flexion, and extension.
4. Limited chest expansion.	Limitation of chest expansion to 1 inch (2.5 cm) or less, measured at the level of the fourth intercostal space.
5. Iritis or its sequelae (history or evidence).	
RADIOGRAPHIC CRITERIA	
Bilateral sacroiliac changes characteristic of ankylosing spondylitis	Grade 3 to 4 bilateral sacroiliitis.
DEFINITE ANKYLOSING SPONDYLITIS	
Positive roentgenogram and 1 or more clinical criteria, or Four of the five clinical criteria.	Grade 3 to 4 bilateral sacroiliitis and 1 or more clinical criteria, or Grade 3 or 4 unilateral or grade 2 bilateral sacroiliitis either with limitation of back movement in all planes, or with both other clinical criteria.
PROBABLE ANKYLOSING SPONDYLITIS	
	Grade 3 to 4 bilateral sacroiliitis with no clinical criteria.

male preponderance of about 10 to 1 was reported previously, later studies noted a lower ratio,[119,122] about 3 or 4 to 1, probably reflecting a greater proportion of women with milder disease. Radiographic sacroiliitis occurs in nearly equal proportions of B27-positive males and females, with or without peripheral arthritis.[131,135] These findings suggest important age- and sex-related factors contributing to the disease expression.

ETHNIC AND GENETIC DISTRIBUTION

Ankylosing spondylitis is unusual in blacks. Over 90% of unrelated white males and females with ankylosing spondylitis have B27, versus only about half the blacks.[112] Family studies indicate that genetic susceptibility to ankylosing spondylitis closely associates with HLA-B27,[127] but may occur sporadically in its absence.[136] Histocompatibility antigens B7, BW22, B40, and BW42 and the "public" antigen have been found to associate with spondyloarthritis syndromes in B27-negative white and black Americans, however.[137,138] Furthermore, restriction fragment length polymorphism analysis of genetic material has shown a 9.2 kilobase fragment in B27-positive individuals with ankylosing spondylitis more often than in B27-positive persons who do not have this disease (relative risk 297).[115] These findings imply a more direct role of the B27-related antigens in pathogenesis. This concept is supported by family studies showing close

segregation of the disorder with HLA-B27.[127,139,140] HLA-B27 subtypes of this antigen can now be defined, and of the seven so far identified, ankylosing spondylitis does not seem to be correlated with any type.[141] Homozygosity for B27 may have some influence on severity, but not on risk of development, of this disease.[142] Epidemiologic data suggest the possibility of a relation to hormonal factors as well. Diagnostically, HLA-B27 determination is most useful when the pretest likelihood of ankylosing spondylitis or Reiter's syndrome is clinically neither low nor high, but in the middle ranges of probability where the test result can influence decision.[143] The coexistence of ankylosing spondylitis and RA in the same patient appears to occur by chance, and each disorder is associated with its respective HLA marker.[144]

NATURAL HISTORY

Prognosis varies with the severity of the disorder and its treatment, but it is generally favorable because the disease is often mild or self-limited. Among 836 patients with ankylosing spondylitis diagnosed between 1935 and 1957 and not given radiation therapy in the United Kingdom, an increased mortality rate in males only from arthritis-related causes was reported.[145] In a United States clinical series of 56 cases (49 males) diagnosed between 1934 and 1960, reduced survival was detected only by 20 years after diagnosis or after approximately 30 years of symptomatic disease.[146] Only 4 of these individuals had received radiotherapy. A population sample of 102 patients with ankylosing spondylitis from Rochester, Minnesota diagnosed from 1935 through 1973, including 73 males and 29 females, had decreased survival for the females only, beginning about 10 years after diagnosis and not attributable to irradiation, but the number of deaths was small.[122] The prognosis for functional capacity and occupational performance was good in ankylosing spondylitis after a mean duration of 38 years of disease.[147]

OTHER SERONEGATIVE SPONDYLOARTHRITIS SYNDROMES

REITER'S DISEASE

Reiter's disease has been reported in epidemic occurrences, such as following bacillary dysentery,[148,149] and as an endemic or sporadic event following venereal urethritis.[150] An ARA subcommittee has proposed criteria for Reiter's syndrome based on analysis of 83 Reiter's syndrome, 53 ankylosing spondylitis, 33 seronegative RA, 53 psoriatic arthritis, and 27 gonococcal arthritis patients submitted from 7 centers.[151] Clinically acceptable Reiter's syndrome consists of peripheral arthritis of more than 1 month's duration in association with urethritis or cervicitis. These criteria had 84% sensitivity at the initial episode and 97.6% when subsequent episodes were included. Specificity against the comparison groups varied from 96 to 100%.

Although once considered to be rare, Reiter's disease is now recognized commonly in young adult males and is perhaps the leading cause of admissions to military hospitals for noninfectious arthritis.[28] The venereal acquisition of this disorder by women is unusual.[152] Postvenereal Reiter's syndrome is endemic in certain indigenous (Eskimo) populations of Greenland, with a high B27 frequency (circa 27%) and a high incidence of venereal disease. The estimated annual incidence in males was 0.3% for 1970 to 1983.[152] Following a bacillary dysentery epidemic in Finland in the summer of 1944, 0.2% of the enteritis victims developed Reiter's syndrome.[148] Interestingly, 10% of the enteric-acquired cases occurred in women, suggesting that the epidemic rather than endemic form of Reiter's syndrome is more common in women.[150,152] In an epidemic in June 1962, aboard an American naval vessel, 10 of 602 (1.5%) men with shigella dysentery subsequently acquired Reiter's syndrome within several weeks.[149] In a more recent cruise ship outbreak of Shigella flexneri 2a enteritis, 5 (2.5%) of

205 passengers studied had probable Reiter's syndrome or reactive arthritis.[153] In both these instances, HLA-B27 was identified in 4 of 5 patients subsequently tested.[153,154] In a large community outbreak of Shigella sonnei in Puerto Rico, however, no case of Reiter's syndrome was disclosed among 1970 patients surveyed.[155] Sporadic cases of Reiter's syndrome have been reported after enteric infection with Yersinia enterocolitica, Salmonella enteritidis, and Campylobacter fetus.

A survey of Reiter's disease in venereal clinics in the United Kingdom between 1960 and 1964 yielded 1 female and 100 male cases; 35 males residing in a particular area were examined along with their relatives and spouses.[150] Radiographic evidence of sacroiliitis was found in 23% of the probands, and its frequency increased with duration of symptoms. Clinical spondylitis and radiographic changes (Rome criteria) were 2 to 8 times as frequent among relatives as in a population control sample, and none of the spouses had spondylitis. An even wider spectrum of disease is suggested by studies of probands in Finland, indicating an association with acute peripheral polyarthritis among first-degree relatives.[156] The description of "incomplete" Reiter's syndrome also favors a broader disease spectrum.[28]

Following the HLA-B27 discovery, numerous clinical series of sporadic Reiter's syndrome were reported, with striking B27 associations of 63 to 96% among adult white patients, highest in those individuals with clinical or roentgenographic evidence of sacroiliitis.[120] HLA-B27 shows a lower association, approximately 40%, among American blacks with Reiter's syndrome,[157] but a complementary association with B7 CREG antigens may occur.[137] Among childhood cases of Reiter's syndrome, at least 12 of 13 reported had B27.[158] In addition, the epidemic form has been associated with B27,[153,154,159] with an estimated Reiter's syndrome attack frequency of one sixth to one third in B27-positive young adult males infected with shigella.[154] In a comparative familial study, aggregation of Reiter's syndrome was 10%, similar to the 14% found in ankylosing spondylitis, and the 2 diseases seemed to "breed true" within families.[160] The natural history of Reiter's syndrome was recently reported and reviewed.[161]

Followup of an American series of 122 patients with Reiter's syndrome showed that 16% had to change jobs and 11% were unemployable over a mean interval of 5.6 years of disease.[162] No specific entry factors correlated with outcome.

REACTIVE ARTHRITIS

A large series of Scandinavian Reiter's disease and yersinia-reactive arthritis patients was reported with special reference to HLA-B27.[163] The male-to-female ratio was nearly 20:1 in Reiter's syndrome, but 1:1 in yersinia arthritis, with a similar mean age of 30 and 31 and HLA-B27 positivity of 81 and 73%, respectively. Chronic back pain and joint symptoms were frequent in all the groups over the average 5-year followup, but most patients were able to lead normal lives. In 16% of patients with Reiter's syndrome, the acute disease progressed to a chronic destructive peripheral arthritis.

In addition, B27-positive individuals are also prone to arthritis following gastroenteritis caused by the gram-negative organisms salmonella[164] and Campylobacter jejuni.[165] HLA Bw62 was more frequent in patients with B27-negative reactive arthritis (48%) and ankylosing spondylitis (25%) than in healthy blood donors (7.2%).[166] Moreover, Bw62 was more frequent in patients with Crohn's disease (27%) and spondyloarthropathy with chronic gut inflammation (30%).

These observations indicate that a genetically susceptible host (HLA-B27-positive) may encounter an environmental inciting or infective agent that precipitates disease, possibly through circulating immune complex mechanisms.[167] Moreover, in patients with reactive arthritis and ankylosing spondylitis with peripheral arthritis, a strong relationship was found between clinical articular inflammation and inflammatory gut lesions found on biopsy specimens from the ileum.[168]

INFLAMMATORY BOWEL DISEASE ARTHRITIS

Although only a small proportion of patients with ulcerative colitis or regional enteritis develop spondylitis, their risk is estimated to be 30 times greater than in the general population, and approximately 50% are HLA-B27-positive;[169] however, neither asymptomatic roentgenographic sacroiliitis nor peripheral arthritis alone, occurring during the course of chronic inflammatory bowel disease, is associated with B27.[120,170] Population frequency, family studies, and HLA-B27 associations of the arthropathy of inflammatory bowel disease have been reviewed.[119]

PSORIATIC ARTHRITIS

Spondylitis occurs in approximately 2% of individuals with psoriasis, and 35 to over 70% of these spondylitis patients are HLA-B27 positive.[119] Among patients with psoriasis and only peripheral arthritis without sacroiliitis, a slightly increased frequency of

B27 has been observed in some series.[119,169] A proportion of these B27-positive patients may eventually develop spondylitis.

In comparison to normal subjects, patients with psoriasis and peripheral arthritis more often had HLA-BW38 (38% vs. 6%), as well as HLA-DRW4 (54% vs. 32%).[171] Another study, instead, found a higher frequency of DR7 in patients with peripheral arthritis only (52%) than in those with spinal involvement (35%) or blood donor control subjects (23%).[172] Patients with severe peripheral arthritis had the highest frequency of DR7 (71%). HLA-DR4 was found in higher frequency in patients with bone erosions (46%) than in those without (18%) or in control subjects (29%). These and other studies suggest that multiple factors, controlled by genes in the major histocompatibility complex, appear to contribute to psoriasis and psoriatic arthritis.[173] The association of HLA-DR4 is interesting because it is also associated with more advanced RA, whether seropositive or seronegative.[13,14]

Psoriatic arthritis in childhood has clinical features similar to those of the adult disease.[174] A sex ratio of 17 girls to 7 boys was found in one series, consistent with the female predominance of 2:1 in childhood-onset psoriasis. Arthropathy antedated skin changes in 14 (58%) of the 24 patients, and clinical evidence of tendinitis (36%) was also more common than in the adult disease. A larger series of 60 juvenile patients also showed a female predominance (3.2:1), a family history of psoriasis in almost half, and presentation with arthritis alone in 26 (43%).[175]

Peripheral arthritis is generally believed to occur in about 5% of psoriasis patients, but in one Italian survey, this proportion was over 25%.[175a] Arthritis is presumably frequent in those with more advanced skin involvement,[176] and occurs after psoriasis in the majority of cases.[175a] Psoriatic arthritis patients more frequently had sibs with this condition than did psoriasis patients without arthritis (4 versus 0.3%), but no difference was noted in the family history of psoriasis itself (both 7%).[176] Microvascular changes similar to those seen in RA have been identified in psoriatic synovium and implicated in pathogenesis.[171] Autoimmunity to collagen and association with HLA-DR4 are also shared features of psoriatic arthritis and RA.[171,173,177] Furthermore, the native collagen mouse model of arthritis shows histologic and radiographic similarities to both psoriatic arthritis and RA.[178] Thus, host predisposition as evidenced by certain HLA genotypes, immunologic reactivity to collagen, and microvasculopathy may contribute to the pathogenesis of both psoriatic arthritis and RA.

HOST PREDISPOSITION TO PERIPHERAL AND SPINAL ARTHRITIS SYNDROMES

Accumulating evidence indicates significant correlations between host factors, such as onset age, sex, and race, with various arthritis syndromes, some having recognized genetic or immunologic markers. For example, the onset age of spondyloarthritis syndromes is usually earlier than in RA, and males are favored. Among newly diagnosed younger peripheral arthritis patients with clinical diagnoses of RA, unclassified arthritis, and spondyloarthritis syndromes, but without evidence of classic ankylosing spondylitis,[12] HLA-B27 correlated with maleness and younger adult onset age (15 to 29 years). In contrast, rheumatoid factor positivity was found predominantly in females, particularly in those with older onset age (30 to 44 years), as seen in Table 3–7. These data emphasize powerful host-factor effects on the type of rheumatic disease syndrome manifested.[12,13] The largest group of newly diagnosed peripheral arthritis patients had neither rheumatoid factor nor B27. Their total frequency was equal in each age group studied, but a significant sex ratio reversal occurred between the juvenile and young adult ages.

Overlapping relationships among these largely undefined syndromes are schematized in Figure 3–3. Their further characterization provides an important challenge for future integrated epidemiologic, clinical, and laboratory research.[13]

CONNECTIVE TISSUE DISORDERS (ACQUIRED)

SYSTEMIC LUPUS ERYTHEMATOSUS

A review of the epidemiology of systemic lupus erythematosus (SLE) has been published.[179]

Criteria for Classification

The use, evaluations, and criticisms of the 1971 preliminary criteria for the classification of SLE were reviewed in 299 articles published in 3 rheumatology journals and 4 general medical journals.[180,181] The main criticism of these criteria was the failure to incorporate new immunologic knowledge. This problem was addressed in the 1982 revised criteria report with lupus and control patient data obtained from 18 institutions.[182] Antinuclear, anti-DNA, and anti-Sm antibodies were added, whereas Raynaud's phenomenon and alopecia were dropped (Table 3–8). If any 4 or more of the 11 criteria were present, serially or simultaneously, during any interval of observation, SLE could be diagnosed with 96% sensitivity and 96% specificity. The control group consisted predominantly of patients with RA, although the revised criteria performed well in an independent sample of 172 SLE patients and against a combined group of 299 patients with systemic sclerosis and 119 patients with polymyositis-dermatomyositis from the Scleroderma Criteria Cooperative Study (83% sensitivity, 89% specificity).[182,183]

Incidence and Prevalence

Reports of the occurrence of SLE in populations have been summarized in Table 3–9. The first population studies were performed using mainly hospital discharge record indexes, supplemented by clinic, laboratory, or pathology records.[184,185] In New York City, the 1965 estimated annual SLE incidence was over 3.0 new cases per 100,000 population.[185] During 1965 to 1973, the incidence was calculated as 7.4 per 100,000 in 120,000 San Francisco city and county residents belonging to a group health plan.[187] In the California study, the prevalence was 1 case in 700 white women aged 15 to 64 years, and 1 in 245 black women of this age.

Reports from areas with a variety of racial types throughout the world suggest that SLE is common.[179] The age-adjusted prevalence rates for Chinese, Filipinos, and Japanese living on Oahu Island, Hawaii

---

Table 3–7.   Distribution of Early Diagnosed Peripheral Arthritis Patients by Onset Age, Sex, Rheumatoid Factor (RF), and HLA-B27 Status*

Onset Age	RF + B27 −			RF − B27 −			RF − B27 +			Total		
	F	M	T	F	M	T	F	M	T	F	M	T
<15	1	1	2	10	20	30	2	5	7	13	26	39
15–29	9	0	9	23	12	35	4	15	19	36	27	63
30–44	15	2	17	31	8	39	4	2	6	50	12	62
<45	25	3	28	64	40	104	10	22	32	99	65	164

*Three B27 patients excluded with associated rheumatoid factor positivity.
(Data from the Memphis and Shelby County Arthritis Research Program: Masi, A.T., et al.: Prospective study of the early course of rheumatoid arthritis in young adults: comparison of patients with and without rheumatoid factor positivity at entry and identification of variables correlating with outcome. Semin. Arthritis Rheum., 5:299–326, 1976.)

FIG. 3–3. Schematic relationship between spondylitis, peripheral arthritis, HLA-B27, and rheumatoid factor (RF).

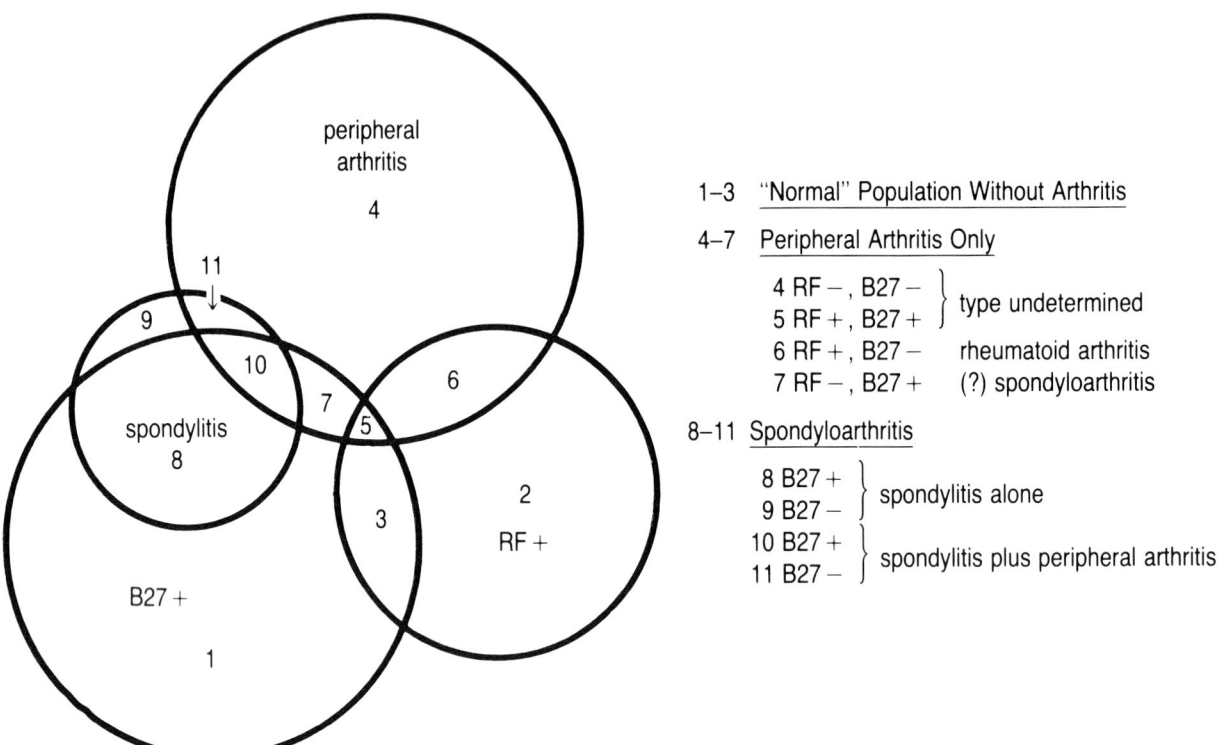

1–3   "Normal" Population Without Arthritis

4–7   Peripheral Arthritis Only

    4 RF −, B27 − ⎫
    5 RF +, B27 + ⎭ type undetermined
    6 RF +, B27 −   rheumatoid arthritis
    7 RF −, B27 +   (?) spondyloarthritis

8–11   Spondyloarthritis

    8 B27 + ⎫
    9 B27 − ⎭ spondylitis alone
    10 B27 + ⎫
    11 B27 − ⎭ spondylitis plus peripheral arthritis

were 3 to 4 times greater than those for whites.[189] Polynesians also had a severalfold higher incidence and mortality than whites in Auckland, New Zealand.[190] The Crow, Arapahoe, and Sioux tribes of North American Indians had annual incidence in excess of 10 per 100,000 population, using the 1971 ARA classification criteria.[192] The estimated annual incidence of SLE was 31.3 per 100,000 for full-blooded Sioux, but these rates were based on small numbers of cases.

It is not known whether the increasing incidence with time reflects heightened awareness by physicians of lupus or a true increase in frequency. The worldwide distribution of lupus suggests a multifactorial origin and pathogenesis.

Age, Race, and Sex Distribution

Females, particularly young women, have a striking susceptibility to SLE, as observed in virtually all epidemiologic studies. This dramatic incidence increases early in the second decade, peaks in the third, remains high during the childbearing years, decreases during the 45- to 64-year period, and declines further thereafter.[185] Conversely, males showed no impressive incidence variation with age in the small number of cases reported in the New York City study.[185] Over

all ages, females exceed males in clinical series in a ratio of at least 5:1, and to a greater extent during the childbearing years.[194,195]

Under age 12, the female-to-male ratio of new SLE cases is low (2 to 3:1).[196] Similarly, this ratio approaches equality after age 65.[185,197] Moreover, SLE may begin or may be exacerbated during pregnancy or the postpartum period,[198] when marked hormonal changes occur. The female preponderance in SLE may thus be associated more with sexual maturation or hormonal factors than with the female genotype itself.[195]

A role for endocrine factors in the pathogenesis of SLE is also suggested by its reported association with Klinefelter's syndrome and metabolic data showing prolonged estrogenic stimulation in such cases.[195,199] Additional support comes from low levels of plasma androgens in women with SLE and the protective effects of androgen (testosterone) administration in the murine lupus model.[200,201] Clinical and experimental data from a variety of sources suggest heightened humoral immunity and depressed cellular immunity in females, compared with males; these differences appear to be mediated by sex hormones.[202]

An incidence ratio of black to white females of about

Table 3–8. 1982 Revised Criteria for the Classification of Systemic Lupus Erythematosus*

Disorder	Signs
1. Malar rash	Fixed erythema, flat or raised, over the malar eminences, tending to spare the nasolabial folds
2. Discoid rash	Erythematous raised patches with adherent keratotic scaling and follicular plugging; atrophic scarring may occur in older lesions
3. Photosensitivity	Skin rash as a result of unusual reaction to sunlight, by patient's history or observation by a physician
4. Oral ulcers	Oral or nasopharyngeal ulceration, usually painless, observed by a physician
5. Arthritis	Nonerosive arthritis involving two or more peripheral joints, characterized by tenderness, swelling, or effusion
6. Serositis	a. Pleuritis—convincing history of pleuritic pain or rub heard by a physician or evidence of pleural effusion; OR b. Pericarditis—documented by electrocardiogram or rub or evidence of pericardial effusion
7. Renal disorder	a. Persistent proteinuria greater than 0.5 g/day or greater than 3+ if quantitation not performed; OR b. Cellular casts—may be red cell, hemoglobin, granular, tubular, or mixed
8. Neurologic disorder	a. Seizures—in the absence of offending drugs or known metabolic derangements, such as uremia, ketoacidosis, or electrolyte imbalance; OR b. Psychosis—in the absence of offending drugs or known metabolic derangements, such as uremia, ketoacidosis, or electrolyte imbalance
9. Hematologic disorder	a. Hemolytic anemia—with reticulocytosis; OR b. Leukopenia—less than 4,000/mm³ total on 2 or more occasions; OR c. Lymphopenia—less than 1,500/mm³ on 2 or more occasions; OR d. Thrombocytopenia—less than 100,000/mm³ in the absence of offending drugs
10. Immunologic disorder	a. Positive LE cell preparation: OR b. Anti-DNA: antibody to native DNA in abnormal titer; OR c. Anti-Sm: presence of antibody to Sm nuclear antigen: OR d. False-positive serologic test for syphilis known to be positive for at least 6 months and confirmed by Treponema pallidum immobilization or fluorescent treponemal antibody absorption test
11. Antinuclear antibody	An abnormal titer of antinuclear antibody by immunofluorescence or an equivalent assay at any time and in the absence of drugs known to be associated with "drug-induced lupus" syndrome

*The proposed classification is based on 11 criteria. For the purpose of identifying patients in clinical studies, a person shall be said to have systemic lupus erythematosus if any 4 or more of the 11 criteria are present, serially or simultaneously, during any interval of observation. (Data from Tan, E.M., et al.: The 1982 revised criteria for the classification of systemic lupus erythematosus. Arthritis Rheum., 25:1271–1272, 1982.)

3:1 was first reported in New York City based on small numbers.[184] This conclusion has now been amply supported in larger case series,[187,203] and mortality analyses confirm the findings.[204] Whether the incidence is increased in black over white males is not known because community population data are limited.

Genetic Factors

Although familial SLE has been described frequently, one cannot prove familial aggregation without a population denominator and a known frequency of disease in the population at risk;[179] however, the impressive number of reports, including males,[205] suggests a familial occurrence that is greater than chance.[179,206] Such aggregation appears to operate generally at a low level whether environmental, genetic, or infectious agent factors may contribute.[207,208] HLA-DR2 and DR3 were reported with greater frequency than in control populations, and in those subsets with precipitating antibodies to RNA-nucleoprotein antigens (anti-Ro/SSA or La/SSB), DR3 was increased.[209] The sharing of HLA haplotypes by 38 affected SLE sib pairs is no greater than expected by chance

alone.[206] The previous studies and immunologic characterization of identical twins clinically discordant for SLE argue that SLE susceptibility is not linked to the HLA-DR locus or that the primary mechanism is an inherited deficiency of immune function[206,209,210] (see also Chapter 69).

The healthy relatives of SLE patients have increased frequency of both serum lymphocytotoxic antibodies[208] and impaired suppressor cell function,[211] but these abnormalities have not been correlated.[211] Thus, although these findings represent defects in immunoregulation, they may not necessarily lead to disease.

Another association is that of congenital complete heart block with maternal SLE.[212,213] Many other cardiac abnormalities have also been noted in these infants. In at least half the cases, the women had few or no findings of lupus prior to the delivery. A striking proportion (over 80%) of the mothers had serum SS-A Ro antibodies in these retrospective studies.[214,215]

Environmental and Socioeconomic Associations

Studies of housing quality and crowding in New York City SLE cases and control subjects have shown

Table 3–9. Prevalence and Average Annual Incidence of Systemic Lupus Erythematosus (Frequency per 100,000 Population)

Source	Location of Study Population	Survey Period	Type of Survey	Prevalence		Incidence
Leonhardt[179]#	Scania*	1955–1961	Hospital	2.3		0.5
	Malmö	1955–1961		6.0		1.0
Siegel, et al.[184,185]	New York City	1954–1956	Multi-institutional	4.0		1.5
		1960–1962		10.0		1.5
		<u>1964–1966</u>		<u>15.0</u>		<u>3.5</u>
		1956–1965		14.6		2.0
Michet, et al.[186]	Rochester, Minnesota	1950–1979	Multiclinic	40.0		1.8
Fessel[187]	San Francisco	1965–1973	Health plan	50.8		7.4
Hochberg[188]	Baltimore	1970–1977	Hospital	—		4.6
Serdula and Rhoads[189]	Oahu, Hawaii	1970–1975	General hospital	5.8	(white)	
				24.1	(Chinese)	
				19.9	(Filipino)	
				20.4	(part-Hawaiian)	
				18.2	(Japanese)	
Hart, et al.[190]	Auckland, New Zealand	1975–1980	Hospital	14.6	(white)	
				50.6	(Polynesian)	
				19.1	(other)	
Helve[191]	Finland	Dec. 1978	Hospital	28		
Morton, et al.[192]	Crow Indians	1971–1975	Hospital index	—		27.1
	Arapahoe Indians			—		24.3
	Sioux Indians			67.0†		16.6
	Other Indian tribes			—		5.0‡
Chantler et al.[179]#	Southern Nevada	15 years	Isolated community	—		16.0
Nived, et al.[193]	Southern Sweden	1973–1982	Hospital and clinic	39.0§		4.8§

*Except Malmö.
†Period prevalence (20 cases in 30,210 population).
‡Median of other tribes.
§Age 15 or older.
#Cited in Reference 179.

no significant associations.[216] Antinuclear antibodies have been found in the serum of consanguineous female relatives of SLE patients, irrespective of household contact with the proband.[208] In addition, lymphocytotoxic antibodies have been noted in laboratory personnel who have studied lupus sera.[217] Neither SLE nor autoantibodies were more frequent in human household contacts of dogs with SLE.[218,219]

The etiologic role of type C viruses in human lupus remains controversial. In several reports, extensive studies failed to identify type C oncornavirus or its p30-related antigens.[220,221] High-titer (1:20 or greater) serum antibodies to Rickettsia haemobartonella, Anaplasmataceae, were found in all 22 SLE patients, compared with only 13 of 102 controls.[222] Free haemobartonella antigen was demonstrated in the glomeruli of one of these antibody-positive patients with lupus nephritis. The specificity and primary nature of this finding are not known.

Course of Disease and Survival

Reported survival rates from the time of first diagnosis have improved over the years, from the ear-lier hospital-based studies indicating a 4-year 51% survival rate,[223] to more recent, clinic-based results suggesting a 10-year 70 to 90% survival rate.[187,224] Interpretations of such marked differences are complex and are still unresolved. Clinical series have shown a more favorable prognosis in older individuals,[225] in patients with a longer interval from onset to diagnosis, and in those without renal or central nervous system involvement or superimposed bacterial infections.[194,224,226] In patients with lupus nephritis, a bimodal mortality pattern has been observed, with an excess of early deaths (within 2 years from onset to death) due to active lupus and sepsis and later deaths attributable to vascular events, such as atherosclerosis plus active SLE that may persist or reappear.[227] It was reported earlier that juvenile-onset patients had a poorer prognosis than expected, but more recent studies indicate that survival is at least comparable to that in adults.[228] Racial differences in prognosis were not detected in the New York City study.[229]

The role of corticosteroids in survival is unclear in

retrospective series, primarily because patients could not be matched for disease severity and other prognostically important organ system involvement. In one study, patients were stratified using a prognostic index that included scoring of disease severity according to clinical and laboratory evidence of intensity of involvement and number of organs affected.[230] Corticosteroid use was associated with improved survival only among high-risk patients who were identified by having at least 2 of the following clinical features defined by the investigators: 4+ severity at any time, total average severity of 2+ or greater, and nephritis.

Drug-Activated SLE-Like Syndromes

The relationship of drug-induced disease to idiopathic SLE is not clear. A hospital study of 258 SLE patients showed that 12 (4.7%) had received a possible inducing drug for at least 2 months preceding onset.[231] During 1957 to 1966, 59 cases of drug-induced SLE were detected in a New York City hospital survey.[232] The frequency increased with age, and females predominated over males, notwithstanding differences in drug exposure. No racial predisposition was observed, unlike in idiopathic SLE. In Rochester, Minnesota, drug-induced disease had an annual incidence of 0.8 per 100,000, compared with 1.8 for the natural disease.[186] In one series, hydralazine-induced lupus developed only in "slow acetylators" of the drug,[233] suggesting host metabolic predisposition to this syndrome, unlike in idiopathic SLE.[234]

SYSTEMIC SCLEROSIS (SCLERODERMA)

The term scleroderma encompasses a variety of disorders associated with hardening of the skin, whereas "systemic sclerosis" implies a multisystemic disorder affecting both skin and internal organs. The spectrum of systemic sclerosis ranges from classic disease with diffuse cutaneous involvement to limited cutaneous disease (the CREST syndrome), in which one sees prominent calcinosis, Raynaud's phenomenon, esophageal involvement, sclerodactyly, and telangiectasia.[235] Systemic sclerosis may also be encountered in the setting of "overlap" syndromes, such as "mixed connective tissue disease,"[236] and it may coexist with RA. Important clinical and natural history differences between these systemic sclerosis variants suggest that they represent distinct subsets of the disease.[237] The specificity of serum anti-Scl 70 and anticentromere antibody for these subsets supports this concept.[238,239]

Classification Criteria

Recent reviews of the epidemiology and classification of systemic sclerosis have been reported.[240,241]

Criteria for classification of definite systemic sclerosis have been proposed by a subcommittee of the ARA based on a multicenter longitudinal evaluation of 264 systemic sclerosis patients and 413 patients with other connective tissue disease (Table 3–10).[183] One major criterion, i.e. proximal scleroderma (scleroderma proximal to the digits), or at least 2 of 3 minor criteria (including sclerodactyly, digital pitting scars, and bilateral basilar pulmonary fibrosis on chest roentgenogram) served to identify 256 systemic sclerosis patients (97% sensitivity), but only 10 comparison patients (98% specificity). These criteria for definite disease were accurate in an external validation completed as part of the study. Assessment of the criteria made on 50 patients with systemic sclerosis and 199 patients with other connective tissue disease from New Zealand showed a 100% specificity and an anticipated lower sensitivity of 79%.[242] The lower sensitivity is attributable to a higher proportion of patients with limited scleroderma and early, mild disease in this population-based study. Definition of early, mild, and limited scleroderma should be addressed in subsequent ARA criteria studies.

Age, Race, and Sex-Specific Incidence and Mortality

Community and national epidemiologic surveys of systemic sclerosis incidence or mortality have been performed in the United States, based on hospital or death certificate records (Table 3–11). The estimated annual incidence has varied, but is believed to be 5 to 10 new cases per million population at risk. An incidence of 6.3 new patients per million per year was found from 1970 to 1979 in Auckland, with no significant difference between Caucasians and Polyne-

---

Table 3–10. ARA Scleroderma Criteria Cooperative Study (SCCS): Preliminary Clinical Criteria for Systemic Sclerosis*[183]

1. Proximal scleroderma is the single major criterion; sensitivity was 91% and specificity was over 99%.

2. Sclerodactyly, digital pitting scars of fingertips or loss of substance of the distal finger pad, and bibasilar pulmonary fibrosis contributed further as minor criteria in the absence of proximal scleroderma.

3. One major or two or more minor criteria were found in 97% of definite systemic sclerosis patients, but only in 2% of the comparison patients with systemic lupus erythematosus, polymyositis/dermatomyositis, or Raynaud's phenomenon.

*Excludes localized scleroderma and pseudosclerodermatous disorders.
(From Masi, A.T., et al.: Preliminary criteria for the classification of systemic sclerosis (scleroderma). Arthritis Rheum., 23:581–590, 1980.)

Table 3–11. Average Annual Incidence of Systemic Sclerosis Per Million Population

First Author	(Year)	Population Area	Study Period	Type of Survey	Incidence
Medsger	(1971)	Shelby County, TN	1947–1952	Multihospital	0.6
			1953–1957		1.5
			1958–1962		4.1
			1963–1968		4.5
Wigley	(1980)	South Island, NZ	1950–1973	Public hospital	2.3
Kurland	(1969)	Rochester, MN	1951–1967	Multi-institutional	12
Michet	(1985)	Rochester, MN	1950–1979	Multi-institutional	10
Bosmansky	(1971)	Piešt'any, Czech (dist. of 100,000)	1961–1969	Multi-institutional	7
Medsger	(1978)	US male veterans	1963–1968	Veterans hospital	2.3
Medsger	(1985)	Allegheny County, PA	1963–1972	Multi-institutional	10
Eason	(1981)	Auckland, NZ	1970–1979	Hospital and specialty practice	6.3

(From Masi, A.T.: Clinical-epidemiologic perspective of systemic sclerosis (scleroderma). *In* Systemic Sclerosis-Scleroderma. Edited by M.I.V. Jayson and C.M. Black. Sussex, England, John Wiley and Sons Ltd., 1988, pp 7–31.)

sians.[243] The female-to-male ratio is almost 3:1 in Anglo-Saxon populations,[240] but is exaggerated during the childbearing years of 15 to 44 or in populations with younger median ages of onset (circa 35 years or less).[240,244] The first convincing case of systemic sclerosis in a patient with Klinefelter's syndrome was reported.[245] Childhood or adolescent onset is unusual,[246] and incidence appears to increase steadily with age, especially in females.[244] Some excess is present in blacks, especially among females, but this tendency is small compared with findings in SLE.[247]

Geographic, Occupational, and Environmental Factors

Systemic sclerosis occurs throughout the world.[240,247] In the United States, no geographic concentration of cases has been recognized.[1,248] It has been suggested that the disease is more common among underground coal and gold miners and others occupationally exposed to silica dust.[240,247] Scleroderma-like cutaneous lesions, Raynaud's phenomenon, nail fold capillary changes, and osteolysis of the distal phalanges have been described in workers exposed to vinyl chloride monomer used in the manufacture of plastics.[249] The relationship of this syndrome to systemic sclerosis is unsettled; in a series of 44 cases tested, none had anti-Scl 70 or anticentromere antibodies.[250] Japanese workmen exposed to the vapor of epoxy resin developed cutaneous sclerosis.[251] In Japan, silicone or paraffin implantation for breast augmentation has been followed after many years by a scleroderma-like illness.[252] An acute multisystem disease with eosinophilia, culminating in fibrosis of the skin and subcutis, reached epidemic proportions in Spain and has been attributed to the ingestion of denatured rapeseed oil.[253] A vasculopathy with pronounced intimal proliferation is found in later stages of this syndrome and may be responsible for multiorgan dysfunction.[254]

Familial Occurrence

Although citations of the familial occurrence of systemic sclerosis remain limited, at least 17 such reports indicate that first-degree relatives are affected.[240,255] HLA testing of six families showed common types among the affected first-degree relatives within five of the families, but not among the families.[240] HLA-A, B, and DR typing has been unrewarding in identifying a genetic link.[256,257]

Natural History

The course of systemic sclerosis is variable, but survival studies have almost identical results.[240,247,248,258,259] The overall 5-year cumulative survival rates from diagnosis ranged from 34 to 73%. Recent advances in the treatment of "scleroderma renal crisis," including renal dialysis and the use of potent antihypertensive agents, should improve survival during the next few years.[247]

Outcome and survival are clearly influenced by the type of organ system involvement attributable to systemic sclerosis (see Chapter 73). Within the first one or two years of disease, the extent of skin involvement also correlates with prognosis as well as serologic reactivity,[259,260] adding validity to such subgrouping, such as sclerodactyly, acrosclerotic (intermediate) cutaneous disease, and diffuse cutaneous disease.[241,259,260] Anticentromere antibody is almost exclusively found in patients with limited cutaneous disease, such as sclerodactyly, and these patients have the lowest frequency of Scl 70 antibody (antibody to DNA topoisomerase-1 degradation products).[261,262] To the contrary, anticentromere antibody is rarely found in early diffuse (truncal) cutaneous disease, which has a high frequency of anti-Scl 70, as does the intermediate cutaneous subgroup. The frequency of antinucleolar antibody increases with the extent of early cutaneous involvement.[241,259,260] Future studies should analyze in a multivariate fashion the cutaneous classification of systemic sclerosis as well as serologic, organ involvement, and demographic features, both at an early stage and during followup, for better understanding of the natural history.

The coexistence of cancer and systemic sclerosis has been the subject of several reports and two epidemiologic studies.[263-265] An increased relative risk for lung cancer was observed, especially in scleroderma of prolonged duration with pulmonary interstitial fibrosis and independent of smoking,[264,265] and a subset of women was identified with breast cancer diagnosed at or near the time of onset of systemic sclerosis.[264]

Disease Models

Several potential models of systemic sclerosis have been described. Long-term survivors of bone marrow transplantation have developed multisystem involvement resembling systemic sclerosis.[266] The chemotherapeutic agent bleomycin is capable of inducing scleroderma.[267] In addition, "scleroderma chicken" and "tight-skinned mouse" models have been reported.[268,269] Although these conditions differ in a number of ways from systemic sclerosis, they may lead to important insights into the pathogenesis of tissue fibrosis. No animal model of microvascular occlusive disease is yet available for research.

POLYMYOSITIS AND DERMATOMYOSITIS

Because no clear-cut distinction exists,[270,271] polymyositis is the preferred term. In childhood, polymyositis is less well recognized than the more acute dermatomyositis, but critical comparison of these two juvenile disorders has shown similarities also favoring a common disease spectrum.[272]

Classification

Because of the variability in clinical and laboratory features, the problem of disease classification has been handled differently by various authors. One generally accepted system includes the following subgroups: adult polymyositis, adult dermatomyositis, inflammatory myositis associated with cancer,

childhood myositis, and myositis associated with other connective tissue diseases (overlap syndromes).[270]

No official criteria have as yet been proposed for polymyositis; however, for epidemiologic purposes, the classification criteria of Medsger and associates and the diagnostic criteria of Bohan and Peter are most frequently used.[271,273] They require various combinations of findings, including objective proximal muscle weakness, abnormal muscle biopsy, electromyographic features, serum muscle enzyme elevations, increased urine creatine excretion, and evidence of corticoid responsiveness, with exclusion of patients having a primary diagnosis of another connective tissue disease or other cause of primary myopathy (Table 3–12).

Age, Sex, and Race Incidence

A hospital-based epidemiologic survey of polymyositis (including dermatomyositis) in Memphis and Shelby County, Tennessee from 1947 to 1968 showed an average annual incidence of 5.0 cases per million population.[271] As with scleroderma, incidence increased during the study interval, reaching 8.4 during the period from 1963 to 1968; greater awareness of diagnosis and availability of serum muscle enzyme tests were believed to explain this trend. A bimodal age distribution was found, with the first incidence peak of 4.3 in the 10-to-14 age group, a nadir of 1.0 in the 15-to-24 age group, and a second peak of 10.2 in the 45-to-64 age group. Similar results were obtained in Israel, where the overall incidence was 2.2 new cases diagnosed annually per million population from 1960 to 1976, and childhood and adult incidence peaks were also observed.[274] Such patterns contrast with SLE in females, in whom the peak incidence occurs in the 15-to-44 age group and with lower incidence in the younger and older ages, especially in blacks.

In an expanded Memphis survey (1948 to 1972) of patients under age 20, the average annual incidence was 3.2 per million.[272] Under age 10, the incidence was identical in females and males (3.2F:3.1M) but in the second decade, a higher female-to-male ratio was noted (6.0F:0.7M). Thus, a female preponderance seems to emerge again in adolescence, as observed for RA, SLE, and systemic sclerosis, that suggests common factors related to sexual maturation as important in occurrence or precipitation of these conditions.

As with SLE, the incidence was 4 times greater in black than white females.[271] No overall sex difference was found in adult whites, but in blacks, females predominated twofold over males. In the Transvaal,

Table 3–12. Diagnostic Criteria for Polymyositis-Dermatomyositis

Manifestations

1. Typical skin rash of dermatomyositis
2. Symmetric proximal muscle weakness by history and physical examination
3. Elevation of one or more serum muscle enzymes
4. Myopathic changes on electromyogram
5. Typical polymyositis on muscle biopsy
6. Elevated urine creatine excretion
7. Objective improvement in muscle weakness on corticosteroid therapy

| | Bohan and Peter[273] | | Medsger and Masi[271] |
	Dermatomyositis	Polymyositis	Polymyositis
Definite	(1) + any 3 of (2), (3), (4) or (5)	all 4 of (2), (3), (4) and (5)	(2) and (5) *or* (2), (4) and either (3) or (6)
Probable	(1) + any 2 of (2), (3), (4) or (5)	any 3 of (2), (3), (4) or (5)	(2) and (4) *or* (2) and either (3) or (6)
Possible	(1) + any 1 of (2), (3), (4) or (5)	any 2 of (2), (3), (4) or (5)	(2) and (7)

the annual incidence of dermatomyositis among the Bantus was estimated to be not less than 2.1 cases per million, nearly 10 times that observed among whites in the same region.[275] The disease was twice as frequent as SLE in this population, it tended to occur in the "young adult" age group, and patients had some features suggesting overlap syndromes. The female-to-male sex ratio is usually greater in polymyositis patients whose manifestations overlap with those of other connective tissue diseases.[270]

Genetic Factors

Familial aggregation has rarely been reported, but studies of histocompatibility antigens have shown an increased frequency of HLA-B8 and DRW3 in both children and adults.[276,277] DRW3 correlated with the presence of Jo-1,[278] one of several antibody systems identified in the serum of polymyositis patients, especially those with fibrosing alveolitis.[279] This autoantibody is directed at the cellular enzyme histidyl-t RNA synthetase,[280] but its role in the pathogenesis of polymyositis and dermatomyositis is not yet clear.

Geographic and Socioeconomic Distribution

Polymyositis has been reported to occur in nearly all climates and geographic areas of the globe. No association with family income or household crowding and no evidence of temporal-spatial clustering of cases were found in Memphis.[271] In juveniles, a concentration of case onsets during colder months,[271] or with possible exposure to bacteriologically proved streptococcal diseases,[281] suggests upper respiratory infection as a precipitating factor. High Coxsackie B-2 complement-fixing and neutralizing antibody titers have been noted in childhood dermatomyositis in a case-controlled study.[282] Complementary DNA (cDNA) hybridization probes specific for Coxsackie B virus were used to detect viral RNA in muscle biopsies. Strong absolute binding was found in a five-year-

old boy with acute dermatomyositis.[283] The ratio of binding of the Coxsackie B virus cDNA to the control β-tubulin cDNA probe is difficult to interpret because of unknown factors that may affect the latter.

A new experimental model of Coxsackie virus-induced myositis has been described in mice,[284] and familial canine dermatomyositis has recently been identified in collie dogs, although no infectious agent has yet been incriminated in the latter model of juvenile dermatomyositis.[285] Complement-fixing antibodies to Toxoplasma gondii have been found in the serum of 7 of 20 (35%) of polymyositis patients, but rarely in individuals with dermatomyositis or in age-, race-, and sex-matched controls.[286] Patients with the highest titers had disease of more recent onset (mean less than 2 years) and more frequently had antitoxoplasma IgM antibodies, favoring recent infection.[287] Direct immunofluorescence has identified free toxoplasma tachyzoites in a child with dermatomyositis.[288] Identical twins were reported to develop childhood dermatomyositis 2 weeks apart following upper respiratory infections,[289] again indicating that some juvenile cases may be precipitated, but not necessarily caused, by infectious agents.

Natural History

Life-table analysis of 124 patients with polymyositis showed an overall 53% survival at 7 years, similar to that for systemic sclerosis.[290] Age over 50 years, black race, and the presence of marked muscle weakness, dysphagia, and aspiration pneumonia were signs of a poor prognosis if identified at the time of first hospital diagnosis. In a series from comparable years, dysphagia and severe proximal weakness at entry also were considered signs of a poor prognosis, and case fatality was 45%.[291] A lower overall fatality of 28%, increasing with age, was determined in 118 cases of polymyositis over a mean interval of 6 years.[292] Outcome and actuarial survival were recently reported from different continents, and each showed a worse prognosis with older age at onset.[293-295] As expected, patients who had more severe disease at onset and those who did not respond to initial therapy had worse outcomes.[293,294]

The increased mortality among older patients is not explained by associated cancer alone. Cardiac involvement was the most important factor associated with poor prognosis in one study and was additive to age.[295] The cardiac hazard was found in another large study of prognosis.[296]

Mortality data from a 1968 to 1978 United States study of nearly 2000 deaths attributed to polymyositis or dermatomyositis showed the highest mortality rates in nonwhite females.[297] It has been suggested that the prognosis in patients referred to large urban medical centers may be unrepresentative, and that milder disease with a higher remission rate is more characteristic.[298] Survival among patients with childhood polymyositis in 2 series is 90% or more after 6 years of followup.[290,299]

Although earlier studies suggested that many middle-aged or older adults with dermatomyositis had various associated cancers, larger, more representative surveys indicate a frequency of about 10%.[270,271,293-296] Reliable statistical data based on large epidemiologic surveys are not available to settle the question of magnitude or significance of association between adult dermatomyositis-polymyositis and malignant neoplasms.[300,301] A study from Mayo Clinic did not exclude an association between polymyositis-dermatomyositis and malignant disease, but concluded that a clinically significant relationship seems unlikely, and intensive clinical investigation to exclude "occult" underlying malignant disease was not cost effective.[302] A recent review of the literature suggests the possibility of an increased occurrence of malignancy within 2 years of the initial diagnosis of myositis.[302a]

VASCULITIS SYNDROMES

Disorders characterized by inflammation of arteries, capillaries, or veins may occur independently or in association with other rheumatic diseases. Nomenclature varies, depending on the frame of reference, whether clinical, etiologic, histologic, or immunologic[303,304] (see Chapter 74).

Polyarteritis Nodosa

Classic polyarteritis, originally termed "periarteritis nodosa," may be the end stage of a variety of necrotizing processes affecting muscular arteries. Infec-

tious agents have long been suspected as participants in the cause, but they have been difficult to demonstrate.

Concomitant infection with hepatitis B virus has been associated with 30 to 60% of cases of classic polyarteritis, and vasculitis has been reported in circumstances hyperendemic for hepatitis B.[305-308] Immune complexes containing hepatitis B surface antigen and antibody have been demonstrated in the circulation and blood vessel walls of some polyarteritis patients.[309] Use of certain intravenous drugs, particularly methamphetamines,[310] may lead to polyarteritis, presumably of toxic origin. Other associations reported include hyposensitization treatment for allergies,[311] serous otitis media,[312] and "hairy cell" leukemia.[313] No genetic factors have yet been identified in this disorder.

The population frequency of polyarteritis is not known, but middle-aged adults are mainly affected, with a male predominance in most series.[314,315] Mortality data from New York City showed 103 deaths attributed to polyarteritis nodosa from 1951 through 1959, during which time 340 deaths were attributed to SLE.[184] Similar mortality data were obtained from a sampling of United States death certificates.[1] Unfortunately, many types of vasculitis are probably included in these reports because subclassification on the basis of pathologic features was not popular at that time.

Childhood polyarteritis is unusual. Such patients may be classified within the multiple categories that compose the broad group of necrotizing vasculitis in adults.[316] Allergic granulomatous angiitis (Churg-Strauss syndrome) usually begins with asthma, followed by fever, eosinophilia, and a systemic necrotizing granulomatous vasculitis.[317] No favored host or environmental factor has been identified, although patients often have a strong personal history of allergy.

The prognosis in polyarteritis is poor regardless of whether it is associated with hepatitis B infection. The 5-year survival rate in one large series was 48% for patients treated with corticosteroids and 13% for untreated patients.[314] Renal involvement and associated hypertension at initial evaluation were the features most indicative of a poor prognosis.

Kawasaki Disease

Infantile polyarteritis, a rare condition with a particular affinity for the coronary arteries, affects children mainly under 1 year of age.[316] Kawasaki disease (mucocutaneous lymph node syndrome), presumably of infectious origin, has many similarities to infantile polyarteritis, but is a more varied systemic disorder.

It has been reported in increasing, epidemic proportions in Japan,[318] but is also described worldwide. This syndrome may be a final common pathway for a variety of infectious agents. Cases have been reported in association with Epstein-Barr virus[318a] and pseudomonas septicemia.[319] A retroviral cause has been suggested by a report of reverse transcriptase activity in blood samples of 8 of 18 recent-onset Kawasaki patients compared with only 1 of 18 control subjects.[320]

Hypersensitivity Vasculitis

Hypersensitivity implies an allergic or immune response to a foreign antigen and, indeed, illnesses such as serum sickness can be shown to result from the formation and tissue deposition of immune complexes containing the antigen. A specific offending antigen is found in only half of reported cases of small-vessel vasculitis, however, and thus the more uniform histologic finding of leukocytoclastic angiitis has been proposed as a better inclusive term. This pathologic change is also part of the spectrum of vessel damage seen in cases of hepatitis B infection. Henoch-Schönlein vasculitis, with skin, joint, gastrointestinal tract, and kidney target organ involvement, mainly affects children but may occur at all ages.[321] Various precipitating factors, such as viral or bacterial infections, drug exposures,[322] and other allergic mechanisms, have been implicated.[321]

Wegener's Granulomatosis

Wegener's granulomatosis, necrotizing granulomatous angiitis of the upper and lower respiratory tract associated with focal necrotizing glomerulonephritis, affects mainly adults of either sex with a slight (3:2) male predominance,[303,323] but cases have been reported in children.[324] Prognosis in this disease has been dramatically improved by the use of immunosuppressive drugs, especially cyclophosphamide.[303,323]

Giant Cell Arteritis

Arteritis characterized pathologically by giant cell formation may involve the aorta or any of its major branches (Takayasu's arteritis or pulseless disease), or may be restricted to the cranial vessels. The syndrome of polymyalgia rheumatica is associated with temporal arteritis in one third of cases; polymyalgia rheumatica primarily affects older adults, and familial aggregation is reported.[325] In both disorders, however, HLA associations have been controversial.[326,327] In contrast, Takayasu's arteritis affects mainly adolescent and younger adult females of many races,[328–330] but especially those of Oriental origin.[318] Excessive

estrogen secretion has been implicated in this disorder.[331]

Details of recent studies on the incidence of temporal arteritis and temporal arteritis or polymyalgia rheumatica are shown in Table 3–13. A 25-year experience in Olmstead County, Minnesota suggests steadily increasing incidence of temporal arteritis with age and an annual rate of 2.4 per 100,000 overall, and rising to 11.7 per 100,000 in individuals 50 and over.[332] Similar age-related incidence patterns have been reported from Scotland,[333] where the overall annual incidence rate, using only biopsy-proved cases, was 1.3 per 100,000 persons and 4.2 in persons aged 50 and over. In contrast, a United States southern urban location (Memphis and Shelby County, Tennessee) had a lower rate reported of 0.35 per 100,000, which increased to 1.6 for those over age 50.[334] Incidence was 7 times higher among women than men and among whites than blacks. Racial distribution does not account fully for differences between Minnesota and Tennessee. Additional studies are required to determine whether climate or other host or environmental factors are implicated. No confirmed environmental risk factors have been identified. In epidemiologic studies of temporal arteritis (giant cell arteritis) or polymyalgia rheumatica, the reported incidence rates were higher,[335,336] as might be expected. The incidence in Göteborg, Sweden was 9.3 overall and 28.6 per 100,000 persons age 50 or older.[335] In this study, the incidence of patients with histologic evidence of arteritis by temporal artery biopsy was 5.5 per 100,000 in all ages, and 16.8 in those 50 or older.[335] In the most recent prospective study from a Danish county, the respective annual incidences were 21.5 and 76.6.[336] In Olmstead County, Minnesota the incidence of polymyalgia rheumatica, including temporal arteritis, was 11.1 overall and 53.7 per 100,000 persons age 50 or older.[337] The prevalence of active and remitted polymyalgia rheumatica in persons over age 50 was estimated at 0.5%.[337]

Criteria have been proposed for classification of polymyalgia rheumatica based on 236 unequivocal cases and 253 comparison patients from 11 rheumatic disease centers in Great Britain.[338] Three or more of the 7 criteria were considered to identify cases. They had 92% sensitivity and 80% specificity when applied to the original study group. As expected, the criteria were less accurate (80% sensitivity) in a population chosen for external validation.

Behçet's Syndrome

Behçet's syndrome is also a cause of vasculitis, especially phlebitis, and is best known for the triad of oral and genital ulceration and ocular inflammation.

Table 3–13. Annual Incidence of Temporal Arteritis per 100,000 Population and of Temporal Arteritis or Polymyalgia Rheumatica (PMR)

Author(s), Reference	Year	Population Area	Study Period	Type of Survey	Annual Incidence*
Huston, et al.[332]	1978	Olmstead County, Minnesota	1950–1974	Temporal arteritis	2.4 11.7 (50+)
Jonasson, et al.[333]	1979	Lothian Region, Scotland	1964–1977	Biopsy-proved temporal arteritis	1.3 4.2 (50+)
Smith, et al.[334]	1983	Memphis and Shelby County, Tennessee	1971–1980	Temporal arteritis	0.35 1.6 (50+)
Bengtsson, and Malmvall[335]	1981	Göteborg, Sweden	1973–1975	Temporal arteritis or PMR	9.3 28.6 (50+)
				Biopsy-proved temporal arteritis	5.5 16.8 (50+)
Chuang, et al.[337]	1982	Olmstead County, Minnesota	1970–1979	PMR (including temporal arteritis)	11.1 53.7 (50+)
Boesen, and Freisleben Sorensen[336]	1987	Ribe County, Denmark	1982–1985	Temporal arteritis or PMR	21.5 76.6 (50+)

*Annual incidence of all ages (upper figure) and from age 50 or older (lower figure).

Several sets of diagnostic criteria have been proposed.[339,340] The disease is especially frequent in Japan and the Middle East; in Japan, its prevalence has been estimated at 1 per 10,000 population.[341] For unknown reasons, the marked male predominance (approximately 5 to 1) noted in reports from eastern Mediterranean countries is not found in smaller series from the United States.[303] Familial aggregation has been reported, but genetic analysis of 15 families from the United Kingdom and 9 from Turkey showed data incompatible with simple autosomal recessive inheritance.[343] An excess of like-sex sibling pairs for both sexes has been reported for Behçet's disease, implying effects of environmental exposures that like-sex siblings are more apt to share than unlike-sex siblings.[344] An increased frequency of HLA-B5 has been noted in Japan[345] and several countries in Europe, and B51 in Turkey.[345,345–347]

CONCEPTUAL DEVELOPMENTS

The connective tissue diseases, including RA, share several features:

1. Host and genetic predisposition.[58,95,348] The impressive body of epidemiologic data described here and reports of familial occurrence indicate important underlying host predisposing factors in disease expression. Similarities in the demographic patterns of these diseases reflect such host influences, such as female preponderance and increased incidence with development of sexual maturation, especially in blacks.
2. Overlapping clinical features.[236,270] Clinical and laboratory similarities among the diseases, and difficulty in classification of individual patients at any one time, or over a period of time, have led authors to consider them a family of "collagen vascular diseases" or "connective tissue diseases." More specifically, authors now use such terms as "sclerodermatomyositis," "lupoderma," and the "mixed connective tissue disease syndrome" (Fig. 3–4).
3. Blood vessels as an important target organ.[39,254,318,349,350] Vascular alterations are particularly frequent in these conditions and may affect arteries, capillaries, or veins of any size, including a spectrum of changes from noninflammatory intimal proliferative responses to acute necrotizing lesions.
4. Immunologic correlates.[277,305,351] Immune alterations often appear to be correlated with organ injury as a primary or secondary mechanism, as indicated by the presence of circulating and tissue-localized immunoglobulins, immune complexes, complement components, and changes in cell-mediated immunity.

Clinical epidemiologic data suggest that these disorders share important pathogenetic mechanisms, but vary in manifestations, perhaps by virtue of different combinations of predisposing and precipitating factors operating on the major target tissues. Vasculature seems to be vitally involved in these diseases, with increasing recognition of the pathophysiologic contributions and interrelationships of the immune and endocrine systems.[37,40,199,200,202]

HYPERURICEMIA AND PRIMARY GOUT

Gouty arthritis, recognized since antiquity, affects mainly men, in contrast to RA, SLE, and most other

FIG. 3–4. Schematic representation of interrelationships among the connective tissue diseases. To show other recognized "overlaps" would require a three-dimensional model. RA = Rheumatoid arthritis; PAN = polyarteritis nodosa; SS = systemic sclerosis; SLE = systemic lupus erythematosus; PM/DM = polymyositis/dermatomyositis.

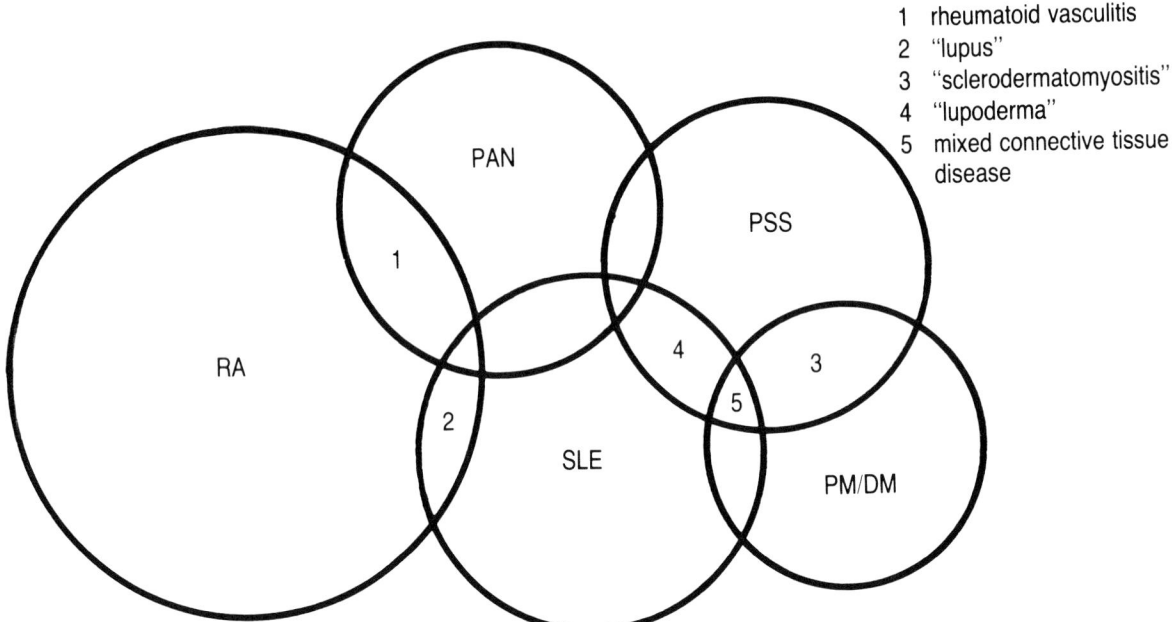

1 rheumatoid vasculitis
2 "lupus"
3 "sclerodermatomyositis"
4 "lupoderma"
5 mixed connective tissue
  disease

connective tissue diseases. Gout and RA rarely co-exist, but the reasons for this dissociation are unknown.[352–353]

Hyperuricemia predisposes one to crystal formation, and the presence of monosodium urate crystals in intra- and periarticular tissue spaces precipitates acute gouty inflammation. A close correlation exists between factors that influence hyperuricemia and those that contribute to gout. The risk of developing hyperuricemia and primary gout depends on a complex interaction of multiple factors, such as diet, environment, age, sex, and heredity.[354–356]

SERUM URIC ACID VALUES

The influence of heredity on serum uric acid level has been debated; a polygenic hypothesis appears most tenable.[357] First-degree relatives have serum uric acid levels closer to one another than do spouses, even after height and weight are considered.[358] In Japanese, black Africans, and the mixed populations of the United States and most European countries, the normal mean level for males is about 5 mg/dl.[355,359–361] In contrast, surveys in the South Pacific have shown similar mean levels ranging from 6.1 to 7.3 mg/dl, when one uses nonautoanalyzer assay methods,[356,362,363] and a recent epidemiologic study from

this area confirmed these levels in several population groups.[356] In native Filipinos, the mean serum uric acid level was normal (5.2 mg/dl), with a low frequency of gout, whereas hyperuricemia and increased frequency of gout were noted in Filipinos living in the northeastern United States, Alaska, and Hawaii.[364,365] Differences in dietary habits between the native and westernized cultures have been implicated, as well as a more frequent inability in Filipinos to increase renal urate excretion to compensate for a purine load.[364] A renal mechanism is also suggested by the finding that normouricemic New Zealand Maori men have a reduced fractional urate clearance.[365a] The role of obesity in these findings needs further study.

Several population surveys in the United States have indicated that the distribution of serum uric acid values is a continuous unimodal curve for both sexes.[355,359,366,367] The mean levels rise during childhood, irrespective of sex, but starting at 15 to 19 years of age, the average male values are higher, with maximum difference of almost 1.5 mg/dl in the 20-to-24 age group. The mean female values gradually increase from age 40, reaching about 0.5 mg/dl of the male values after the menopause. Levels in males remain essentially constant throughout adulthood, as do those in females from about age 50 and older.[368] These age and sex relationships suggest hormonal influ ences, but how such factors may be operating has not been demonstrated.[362]

Serum uric acid appears to be associated with alcohol intake and with hypertension,[369,370] but not independently with ischemic heart disease or with diabetes mellitus.[360,371] Cross-sectional studies have also identified correlations with physical (such as weight) and biochemical (such as hyperlipidemia) factors.[355,370]

CRITERIA

Criteria for population studies of gout, independent of hyperuricemia, were recommended at the 1966 New York symposium.[18] They included either (1) the presence of monosodium urate crystals in synovial fluid or in the tissues, demonstrated by chemical or microscopic examination; or (2) the presence of two or more of the following:

a. History or observation of at least two typical gouty arthritis attacks.
b. A clear history or observation of podagra.
c. The presence of a tophus.
d. A clear history or observation of a good response to colchicine.

An ARA subcommittee proposed the following preliminary criteria for the classification of the acute arthritis of primary gout:[372]

1. The presence of characteristic urate crystals in the joint fluid (item 12 in Table 3–14), or
2. A tophus proved to contain urate crystals by chemical or polarized light microscopic means, or
3. The presence of 6 out of 12 clinical, laboratory, and radiographic features (excluding items 1 and 2 in Table 3–14).

The combined criteria were sensitive (98%) and specific (98% against RA of greater than 2 years' duration and 89% against pseudogout and septic arthritis). This set of criteria was modified for epidemiologic survey purposes. The information to be ascertained during a single visit, by history, or by review of clinic records had a sensitivity for gout of 85% and a specificity of 93% or greater. The reliability of these preliminary criteria must be tested against independent clinical and population samples of gout and control arthritis patients.

AGE, SEX, AND RACE DISTRIBUTION

In Great Britain, the annual incidence of diagnosis of gout was determined to be 25 to 35 new cases per 100,000 population.[373] As expected, the prevalence and incidence of gout correlate closely with levels of

Table 3–14.   Proposed Criteria for Acute Arthritis of Primary Gout

1. More than one attack of acute arthritis
2. Maximum inflammation developed within one day
3. Monoarthritis attack
4. Redness observed over joints
5. First metatarsophalangeal joint painful or swollen
6. Unilateral first metatarsophalangeal joint attack
7. Unilateral tarsal joint attack
8. Tophus (proved or suspected)
9. Hyperuricemia
10. Asymmetric swelling within a joint on radiograph*
11. Subcortical cysts without erosions on radiograph
12. Monosodium urate monohydrate microcrystals in joint fluid during attack
13. Joint fluid culture negative for organisms during attack

*This swelling could logically be found on examination as well as on radiograph; however, the protocol did not request this information in regard to examination.
(From Wallace, S.L., et al.: Preliminary criteria for the classification of the acute arthritis of primary gout. Arthritis Rheum., *20:*895–900, 1977.)

serum uric acid in the population,[354,366,367,370,374] but gout seems to be increased also in relatives of patients, whether such individuals were initially determined to be hyperuricemic or normouricemic.[375] Prevalence figures as high as 15 per thousand have been estimated, with a 6:1 male-to-female ratio.[366] The prevalence of gouty arthritis in the elderly was 1.3% overall and similar for men and women in a population sample from Göteborg, Sweden.[376] Family history of gouty arthritis is especially correlated with early age of onset of gout and its occurrence in premenopausal women;[377] in one study, over half these women had such a history.[377,378] The relative protection from gout in women appears to be due to their prolonged lower mean serum uric acid levels, but other influences, particularly hormonal, are possible.

Primary gout was believed to be rare among native races living in their original habitat.[379,380] With changing life styles at present, however, gout is frequently seen in Orientals, Filipinos, Polynesians, and United States blacks.[362,363,365,381] In one large study of United States blacks, the male-to-female ratio was only 2:1.[381]

FAMILIAL OCCURRENCE

Gout has been recognized as a familial disorder since antiquity. The reported frequency of familial occurrence ranges from 6% to as high as 80%.[382] In 1964, the Lesch-Nyhan syndrome, a rare complete deficiency of the enzyme hypoxanthine-guanine phosphoribosyltransferase, was reported. Patients with this X-linked condition develop severe hyperuricemia, gout, and profound neurologic complications.

Since that time, a number of inborn errors of uric acid metabolism have been described,[382] some of which are associated with clinical gout and others with hypouricemia.[383,384] Although partial enzyme deficiency states were predicted to account for a considerable portion of the hyperuricemic population, such is not the case. In fact, only rarely is an enzymatic defect in purine metabolism identified in gouty individuals.

OSTEOARTHRITIS

Osteoarthritis (OA) is considered the most frequent articular disorder among white populations. Its prevalence is based on the presence of symptomatic and nonsymptomatic roentgenographic degenerative articular changes, the latter considered to be the most reliable criterion available.[385] Standardization of roentgenographic criteria has been developed in the form of the *Atlas of Standard Radiographs,* which has been used in several population studies.[386] The problem of interobserver variation remains, along with its effect on cross-cultural comparisons. It has been estimated that about 30% of persons with radiographic evidence of degenerative joint changes complain of pain at such sites. The ARA has proposed criteria for the classification of OA of the knee by means of data derived from clinical examination, laboratory testing, and radiographs.[387]

At present, factors contributing to OA can only be incompletely listed, with little understanding of their interaction. It is likely that each type and anatomic location of OA must be studied separately with regard to etiologic factors because cartilage degeneration may be a final common pathway of many pathophysiologic processes.[388]

PREVALENCE BY AGE, SEX, AND RACE

Age appears to be the most consistent factor in the occurrence of OA.[388,389] A nationwide sample of 6672 adults 18 to 79 years of age was studied for evidence of OA, including radiographs of the hands and feet, in the 1960 to 1962 United States Health Examination Survey.[390] All degrees of radiographic osteoarthrosis of the extremities increased steadily with age from 4% in persons 18 to 24 years of age to 85% among individuals 75 to 79 years of age, with an average of 37% in both males and females. Males appear to be affected more commonly than females before 45 to 54 years of age, but the sex ratio is reversed thereafter.[3] Moderate or severe involvement (9% overall) was almost twice as prevalent in females (11%) as males (6%), adjusted for age.[390] No racial or urban-rural difference was found. Subjects (4225 individuals) from the National Health and Nutrition Examination Survey (HANES) had an association of obesity with OA of the knee, in males, females, whites, and nonwhites, an association that was strongest among females.[391]

Roentgenographic surveys of other populations have shown a number of different patterns. American Indians have an increased prevalence of osteoarthrosis, with age-adjusted prevalence of all degrees of OA being 74% for males and 61% for females.[390] Moderate and severe grades of OA were highest among the Indian men, about 4 times the United States male prevalence. In contrast, Eskimos showed a lower incidence of OA than found in United States males and females.[392] Multiple osteoarthrosis and Heberden's nodes showed a low prevalence in a rural African community, with a similar prevalence in males and females, in contrast to white surveys.[393] Endemic OA of the hip is common in the black population around Mseleni in northern Kwa Zulu, South Africa, affecting some 7.4% of females and 3.0% of males in 1981.[394] The cause may be related to both environmental and congenital hip dysplasia mechanisms.

Several host and environmental factors, particularly those involving patterns and frequency of joint usage, have been postulated to explain these differences. Hypothesis-testing prevalence studies are needed to clarify these geographic and cultural differences.

PREVALENCE BY OCCUPATION AND BODY MEASUREMENTS

Theories of the etiology of OA have included mechanical factors, such as wear and tear, prolonged immobilization, continuous pressure, impact loading, anatomic abnormalities, previous inflammatory joint injury, and others.[388,389] In general, epidemiologic surveys confirm such associations.[3] Patterns of stereotyped, repetitive usage of hands in industry was associated with roentgenographic changes in particular joints;[395] however, no association has been found between long-distance running and clinical evidence of OA in lower extremities,[396,397] although female runners had more sclerosis and spur formation on knee roentgenograms.[397] That coxarthrosis was equally frequent in shipyard laborers and white-collar workers suggests no difference between heavy manual and sedentary work.[398] Clerical and sales workers had a lower-than-expected frequency of hand involvement, but higher-than-expected foot involvement.[399] The opposite was true of craftsmen, foremen, and similar workers. Finance, insurance, and real estate industry employees had lower-than-expected hand involvement. Other studies have suggested that occupation is important in determining the distribution and severity of OA,[1,4,400] but caution should be used in interpreting such data.[401] For example, competitive sports, such as running or football, were not found to predispose persons to OA of the hips or ankles, respectively.[402,403] More could be done to identify the work specifics, such as lifting, bending, twisting, and bumping, which predispose persons to OA in certain occupations.

A positive association has been noted between a number of body measurements and osteoarthrosis in both sexes.[404] The relationship is stronger for measurements reflecting body and limb girth and breadth rather than length. These trends are stronger in women than in men and apply to osteoarthrosis of both hands and feet. In one investigation of risk factors, 100 patients with severe OA who were hospitalized for total hip replacement were compared with an age-, sex-, and race-matched control group.[405] Matched pair analysis showed osteoarthritis to be more strongly associated with increased body weight, amount of education, and a family history of arthritis, but not with tobacco or alcohol consumption or athletic activity. Cause and effect in the relationship between OA and obesity have not been clearly identified, however. Anthropometric comparison of 25 women with generalized OA and 27 with symptomatic osteoporosis showed that those with OA were more obese and had greater muscle mass and strength despite comparable age and skeletal size.[406]

FAMILIAL ASSOCIATION

Primary coxarthrosis in sibs of patients treated by total hip replacement was 8%, as compared to 3.8% in control subjects, suggesting a hereditary factor, although OA of the knees did not differ.[407] An influence of heredity is most conspicuous in distal interphalangeal joint involvement (Heberden's nodes), with suspected dominant transmission in women and recessive transmission in men.[407a] The prevalence of radiographic evidence of generalized osteoarthrosis (involvement of three or more joint groups) is increased in families and twins of index cases, indicating an influence of genetic factors.[4] An excess of generalized osteoarthrosis has been noted in male and female siblings of affected probands, and a greater concordance has been reported in monozygotic than dizygotic twins. The increased frequencies do not fit simple mendelian inheritance patterns and may be determined by multiple genes.

NONARTICULAR RHEUMATISM AND FIBROMYALGIA SYNDROMES

The primary forms of these conditions are not associated with arthritis or connective tissue diseases or other rheumatic disorders having an immunologic, infectious, metabolic or systemic mechanism. They are included in the ARA classification of the rheumatic diseases under category IX, nonarticular rheumatism.[408] Some of these common disorders are regional, including sports-related and occupational soft tissue rheumatism problems, whereas others are generalized, such as fibromyalgia syndrome (see Chapter 80).[409–413] The literature on nonarticular rheumatism was summarized in the Twenty-fifth Rheumatism Review of the ARA.[414]

FREQUENCY

Almost everyone experiences transient symptoms or signs of soft-tissue rheumatism due to periodic excesses of normal living. When symptoms become acute or persistent, however, they usually result from injuries, strains of muscles or tendons, or overloading and fatigue of such tissues. Chronic complaints attributed to nonarticular rheumatism and miscellaneous back disorders were estimated to occur in about 3% of the adult (18 to 70 years) United States population in the 1976 National Health Interview Survey.[415] This frequency compared to about 3% of symptoms attributed to RA and 8% to degenerative joint disease. Among younger and middle-aged adults, problems caused by soft tissue rheumatism collectively may be expected to be the most common rheumatic disorders, possibly the major cause of absenteeism and decreased productivity. Proper epidemiologic studies of these disorders, except low-back pain, have not yet been conducted.

DIAGNOSIS AND CLASSIFICATION

A major dilemma with nonarticular rheumatism is the nature of the illness and its diagnosis. These conditions may be considered tissue reactions to multifactorial stresses rather than actual diseases, which connote distinct, recognizable pathologic entities with presumably uniform causation and precise therapy. At least for generalized fibromyalgia syndrome, consistent and accurate clinical diagnosis can be made, which is helpful in professional communications and management of patients.[409-413,416] Multicenter, cooperative criteria studies of fibromyalgia have been initiated and promise to standardize its classification.

AGE AND SEX DISTRIBUTION OF PRIMARY FIBROMYALGIA

This subset of patients has a homogeneous clinical pattern among the various age and sex groups.[409] For unknown reasons, the disorder is rare under the age of 10 years, increases in frequency during teen and young adult ages, and may decrease in older ages. Overall, females are predominantly affected, by a ratio of at least 5:1.[409,412] Under age 50, this disorder is probably the most common condition among females who consult rheumatologists, but its true incidence is not known. Little information is available on ethnic, socioeconomic, racial, or genetic predisposition.

COURSE OF DISEASE

Because the biologic gradients of severity of nonarticular rheumatism and fibromyalgia syndromes are vast, ranging from incidental minor symptoms to incapacitating disability, one cannot generalize on their course or outcome. Regarding primary fibromyalgia, initial clinical studies suggest persistent symptoms and manifestations in the majority of patients.[411] Hospitalization rates for various manifestations decrease after diagnosis and management.[412] Considerable clinical-epidemiologic research needs to be done on the functional, psychologic, and social influences of these disorders, to understand determinants of their course and outcome.

PERSPECTIVES

Gout illustrates a metabolically determined form of arthritis with important interactions of genetic, dietary, other host factors, and the environment in pathogenesis. OA, perhaps more than other forms of arthritis, demonstrates important local and biomechanical factors influencing joint involvement, although systemic and genetic factors also participate. To what extent degenerative and mechanical processes contribute to articular manifestations in other forms of chronic arthritis, such as gout and RA, is difficult to quantitate, but is nevertheless believed to

be important. Similarly, the significance of genetic and other host characteristics in many arthritic conditions is increasingly recognized. Thus, interrelated factors contribute to each arthritis syndrome, which may be classified by clinical, radiologic, or laboratory markers of greater or lesser accuracy. Classification of disease, identification of risk and other associated factors, and definition of its course are important challenges for future research, especially for clinical epidemiology.

Broad perspectives of disease and of pathogenetic mechanisms can provide valuable biologic insights and new directions to profitable lines of investigation and, ultimately, to improved care of patients. Integrated multidisciplinary studies, including longitudinal observations, cost time, effort, and money, but they are essential to a proper understanding of these multifactorial diseases. Regrettably, support for such efforts has not kept pace with perceived needs.[417] Detailed clinical-laboratory descriptive surveys should be performed, to define more clearly the diagnostic ranges and boundaries of the major arthritis syndromes. Although advanced "typical" stages of rheumatic disorders are readily recognized, studies of the mildest or earliest detectable diseases are vital to search for factors associated with onset, predisposition, and subsequent outcome. In addition, multidisciplinary analytic studies must be designed to refine and to test specific hypotheses in populations.

REFERENCES

1. Cobb, S.: The Frequency of the Rheumatic Diseases. American Public Health Association Monograph. Cambridge, Harvard University Press, 1971.
2. Kellgren, J.H., Jeffrey, M.R., and Ball, J.: The Epidemiology of Chronic Rheumatism. Oxford, Blackwell Scientific Publications, 1963.
3. Kelsey, J.L.: Epidemiology of Musculoskeletal Diseases. New York, Oxford University Press, 1982.
4. Lawrence, J.S.: Rheumatism in Populations. London, William Heinemann Medical Books, 1977.
5. Medsger, T.A., Jr., and Masi, A.T.: Epidemiology of the rheumatic diseases. *In* Arthritis and Allied Conditions. 10th Ed. Edited by D.J. McCarty. Philadelphia, Lea & Febiger, 1985, pp. 9–39.
6. Mikkelsen, W.M.: *In* Arthritis and Allied Conditions, 8th Ed. Edited by J.L. Hollander and D.J. McCarty. Philadelphia, Lea & Febiger, 1972, p. 211.
7. Bennett, P.H., and Wood, P.H.: Proceedings of the Third International Symposium on Population Studies of the Rheumatic Diseases. Amsterdam, Excerpta Medica, 1968.
8. Engleman, E., Bombardier, C., and Hochberg, M.C. (Eds.): Conference on Epidemiology of Rheumatic Diseases: specific needs of developing and developed countries. J. Rheumatol., 10:1–107, 1983.
9. Lawrence, R.C., and Shulman, L.E. (Eds.): Epidemiology of

the Rheumatic Diseases: Proceedings of the Fourth International Conference, National Institutes of Health. New York, Gower Medical Publishing, 1984.

10. Dorn, H.F.: Methods of measuring incidence and prevalence of disease. Am. J. Public Health, 41:271–278, 1951.

11. Hochberg, M.C.: Adult and juvenile rheumatoid arthritis: Current epidemiologic concepts. Epidemiol. Rev., 3:27–44, 1981.

12. Masi, A.T., et al.: Prospective study of the early course of rheumatoid arthritis in young adults: comparison of patients with and without rheumatoid factor positivity at entry and identification of variables correlating with outcome. Semin. Arthritis Rheum., 5:299–326, 1976.

13. Masi, A.T., and Feigenbaum, S.: Seronegative rheumatoid arthritis: fact or fiction? Arch. Intern. Med., 143:2167–2172, 1983.

14. Masi, A.T.: Rheumatoid factor negative (seronegative) RA: evolving clinical classification and immunopathogenetic associations. (Editorial.) J. Rheumatol., 15:4–6, 1988.

15. Ropes, M.W., Bennett, G.A., and Cobb, S.: 1958 Revision of diagnostic criteria for rheumatoid arthritis. Arthritis Rheum., 2:16–20, 1959.

16. Ropes, M.W., et al.: Proposed diagnostic criteria for rheumatoid arthritis. Ann. Rheum. Dis., 16:118–125, 1957.

17. Kellgren, J.H., Jeffrey, M.R., and Ball, J.: Proposed diagnostic criteria for use of population studies: active rheumatoid arthritis. In The Epidemiology of Chronic Rheumatism. Oxford, Blackwell Scientific Publications, 1963, pp. 324–327.

18. Bennett, P.H., and Burch, T.A.: New York symposium on population studies in the rheumatic diseases: new diagnostic criteria. Bull. Rheum. Dis., 17:458, 1967.

19. O'Sullivan, J.B., and Cathcart, E.S.: The prevalence of rheumatoid arthritis: follow-up evaluation of the effect of criteria on rates in Sudbury, Massachusetts. Ann. Intern. Med., 76:573–577, 1972.

20. Henrard, J., Bennett, P.H., and Burch, T.A.: Rheumatoid arthritis in the Pima Indians of Arizona: an assessment of the clinical components of the New York criteria. Int. J. Epidemiol., 4:119–126, 1975.

21. Healey, L.A.: Polymyalgia rheumatica and the American Rheumatism Association criteria for rheumatoid arthritis. Arthritis Rheum., 26:1417–1418, 1983.

22. Arnett, F.C., et al.: The 1987 revised American Rheumatism Association criteria for classification of rheumatoid arthritis. Arthritis Rheum. (in press).

23. Pinals, R.S., Masi, A.T., and Larsen, R.A.: Preliminary criteria for clinical remission in rheumatoid arthritis. Arthritis Rheum., 24:1308–1315, 1981.

24. Wolfe, F., and Hawley, D.J.: Remission in rheumatoid arthritis. J. Rheumatol., 12:245–252, 1985.

25. Josipovic, D.B., and Masi, A.T.: Marked female preponderance in rheumatoid arthritis patients with younger adult onset and positive rheumatoid factor (RF). (Abstract.) Proceedings of the Fourteenth International Congress of Rheumatology, 1977, p. 249.

26. Kato, H., et al.: Rheumatoid arthritis and gout in Hiroshima and Nagasaki, Japan: a prevalence and incidence study. J. Chronic Dis., 23:659–679, 1971.

27. Terkeltaub, R., et al.: A clinical study of older age rheumatoid arthritis with comparison to a younger onset group. J. Rheumatol., 10:418–424, 1983.

28. Arnett, F.C., et al.: Incomplete Reiter's syndrome: discriminating features and HL-A W27 in diagnosis. Ann. Intern. Med., 84:8–12, 1976.

29. Willkens, R.F., et al.: HLA antigens in Yakima Indians with rheumatoid arthritis: lack of association with HLA-Dw4 and HLA-DR4. Arthritis Rheum., 25:1435–1439, 1982.

30. Willkens, R.F., et al.: Studies of rheumatoid arthritis among a tribe of Northwest Indians. J. Rheumatol., 3:9–14, 1976.

31. Linos, A., et al.: The epidemiology of rheumatoid arthritis in Rochester, Minnesota: a study of incidence, prevalence, and mortality. Am. J. Epidemiol., 111:87–98, 1980.

32. Wingrave, S.J., and Kay, S.R.: Reduction in incidence of rheumatoid arthritis associated with oral contraceptives. Lancet, 1:569–570, 1978.

33. Del Junco, D.J., et al.: Do oral contraceptives prevent rheumatoid arthritis? JAMA, 254:1938–1941, 1985.

34. Vandenbroucke, J.P., et al.: Noncontraceptive hormones and rheumatoid arthritis in perimenopausal and postmenopausal women. JAMA, 255:1299–1303, 1986.

35. Liang, M.H., et al.: Oestrogen-use, menopausal status, and relationship to rheumatoid arthritis. Ann. Rheum. Dis., 43:115–116, 1984.

36. Persellin, R.H.: The effect of pregnancy on rheumatoid arthritis. Bull. Rheum. Dis., 27:922–927, 1976–1977.

37. Masi, A.T., Josipovic, D.B., and Jefferson, W.E.: Decreased 11-deoxy-17-ketosteroid excretion in women with rheumatoid arthritis (RA): Gas liquid chromatographic (GLC) studies of RA patients and matched controls implicating a deficiency of androgenic-anabolic steroids in RA. Semin. Arthritis Rheum., 14:1–23, 1984.

38. Feher, K.G., and Feher, T.: Plasma dehydroepiandrosterone, dehydroepiandrosterone sulfate and androsterone sulfate levels and their interaction with plasma proteins in rheumatoid arthritis. Exp. Clin. Endocrinol., 84:197–202, 1984.

39. Rothschild, B.M., and Masi, A.T.: Pathogenesis of rheumatoid arthritis: a vascular hypothesis. Semin. Arthritis Rheum., 12:11–31, 1982.

40. Ahlqvist, J.: Endocrine influences on lymphatic organs, immune responses, inflammation and autoimmunity: Acta Endocrinol., 83(Suppl. 206):1–136, 1976.

41. Lahita, R.G.: Sex steroids and the rheumatic diseases. Arthritis Rheum., 28:121–126, 1985.

42. National Center for Health Statistics. Public Health Service Publication No. 1000, Series 11, No. 17. Washington, United States Government Printing Office, 1966.

43. Beighton, P., Solomon, L., and Valkenburg, H.A.: Rheumatoid arthritis in a rural South African Negro population. Ann. Rheum. Dis., 34:136–141, 1975.

44. Laine, V.A.I.: Rheumatic complaints in an urban population in Finland. Acta Rheum. Scand., 8:81–88, 1962.

45. Harvey, J., et al.: Rheumatoid arthritis in a Chippewa band. II. Field study with clinical serologic and HLA-D correlations. J. Rheumatol., 10:28–32, 1983.

46. Medsger, A.R., and Robinson, H.: Comparative study of divorce in rheumatoid arthritis and other rheumatic diseases. J. Chronic Dis., 25:269–275, 1972.

47. Pincus, T., and Callahan, L.F.: Taking mortality in rheumatoid arthritis seriously—predictive markers, socioeconomic status and comorbidity. J. Rheumatol., 13:841–845, 1986.

48. Solomon, L., Robin, G., and Valkenburg, H.A.: Rheumatoid arthritis in an urban South African Negro population. Ann. Rheum. Dis., 34:128–135, 1975.

49. Hellgren, L.: Rheumatoid arthritis in both marital partners. Acta Rheum. Scand., 15:135–138, 1969.

50. Gaston, J.S.H., Rickinson, A.B., Yao, Q.Y., and Epstein, M.A.: The abnormal cytotoxic T cell response to Epstein-Barr virus in rheumatoid arthritis is correlated with disease activity

and occurs in other arthropathies. Ann. Rheum. Dis., 45:932–936, 1986.

51. Stierle, G., et al.: Parvovirus associated antigen in the synovial membrane of patients with rheumatoid arthritis. Ann. Rheum. Dis., 46:219–223, 1987.

52. Gottlieb, N.L., et al.: Antecedent tonsillectomy and appendectomy in rheumatic arthritis. J. Rheumatol., 6:316–323, 1979.

53. Fernandez-Madrid, F., Reed, A.H., Karvonen, R.L., and Granda, J.L.: Influence of antecedent lymphoid surgery on the odds of acquiring rheumatoid arthritis. J. Rheumatol., 12:43–48, 1985.

54. Wolfe, F., and Young, D.Y.: Rheumatoid arthritis and antecedent tonsillectomy. J. Rheumatol., 10:309–312, 1983.

55. Patel, S.B., and Eastmond, C.J.: Preceding tonsillectomy and appendicectomy in rheumatoid and degenerative arthritis. J. Rheumatol., 10:313–315, 1983.

56. Silman, A.J., Ollier, W.E.R., and Currey, H.L.F.: Failure to find disease similarity in sibling pairs with rheumatoid arthritis. Ann. Rheum. Dis., 46:135–138, 1987.

57. Del Junco, D.J., et al.: The familial aggregation of rheumatoid arthritis and its relationship to the HLA-DR 4 association. Am. J. Epidemiol., 119:813–829, 1984.

58. Lawrence, J.S.: Heberden Oration, 1969. Rheumoid arthritis—nature or nurture? Ann. Rheum. Dis., 29:357–379, 1970.

59. Aho, K., Koskenvuo, M., Tuominen, J., and Kaprio, J.: Occurrence of rheumatoid arthritis in a nationwide series of twins. J. Rheumatol., 13:899–902, 1986.

59a. Ollier, W., Festenstein, H., Filman, A., and Turry, H.T.L.F.: Workshop on immunogenetics and rheumatoid arthritis. Dis. Markers, 4:1–200, 1986.

60. Gran, J.T., and Husby, G.: Seronegative rheumatoid arthritis and HLA DR4: proposal for criteria (Editorial). J. Rheumatol., 14:1079–1082, 1987.

61. Nepom, G.T., Hansen, J.A., and Nepom, B.S.: The molecular basis for HLA class II associations with rheumatoid arthritis. J. Clin. Immunol., 7:1–7, 1987.

62. Stastny, P., et al.: HLA-DR4 and other genetic markers in rheumatoid arthritis. Br. J. Rheum. (in press).

63. Ollier, W., et al.: HLA antigen associations with extra-articular rheumatoid arthritis. Tissue Antigens, 24:279–291, 1984.

64. Lee, S.H., et al.: Strong associations of rheumatoid arthritis with the presence of a polymorphic Ia epitope defined by a monoclonal antibody: comparison with the allodeterminant DR4. Rheumatol. Int., 4(Suppl.):17–23, 1984.

64a. Duquesnoy, R.J., Marrari, M., Hackbarth, S., and Zeevi, A.: Serological and cellular definition of a new HLA-DR associated determinant, MCl, and its association with rheumatoid arthritis. Hum. Immunol., 10:165–176, 1984.

65. DeJongh, B.M., et al.: Epidemiological study of HLA and GM in rheumatoid arthritis and related symptoms in an open Dutch population. Ann. Rheum. Dis., 43:613–619, 1984.

66. Masi, A.T., Feigenbaum, S.L., and Kaplan, S.B.: Articular patterns in the early course of rheumatoid arthritis. Am. J. Med., 75:(Suppl.):16–26, 1983.

67. Feigenbaum, S.L., Masi, A.T., and Kaplan, S.B.: Prognosis in rheumatoid arthritis: a longitudinal study of newly diagnosed younger adult patients. Am. J. Med., 66:377–384, 1979.

68. Josipovic, D.: Prognostic indicators in early rheumatoid arthritis. (Abstract.) Clin. Exp. Rheumatol., 5(Suppl 2):26, 1987.

69. Abruzzo, J.L.: Rheumatoid arthritis and mortality. Arthritis Rheum., 25:1020–1023, 1982.

70. Mitchell, D.M., et al.: Survival, prognosis and causes of death in rheumatoid arthritis. Arthritis Rheum., 29:106–113, 1986.

71. Allebeck, P., Rodvall, Y., and Allander, E.: Mortality in rheumatoid arthritis, particularly as regards drug use. Scand. J. Rheumatol., 14:102–108, 1985.

72. Vandenbroucke, J.P., Hazevoet, H.M., and Cats, A.: Survival and cause of death in rheumatoid arthritis: a 25-year prospective follow-up. J. Rheumatol., 11:158–161, 1984.

73. Laakso, M., Mutru, O., Isomaki, H., and Koota, K.: Cancer mortality in patients with rheumatoid arthritis. J. Rheumatol., 13:522–526, 1986.

74. Baltus, J.A.M., et al.: The occurrence of malignancies in patients with rheumatoid arthritis treated with cyclophosphamide: a controlled retrospective follow-up. Ann. Rheum. Dis., 42:368–373, 1983.

75. Baker, G.L., et al.: Malignancy following treatment of rheumatoid arthritis with cyclophosphamide: long-term case-control follow-up study. Am. J. Med., 83:1–9, 1987.

76. Rasker, J.J., and Cosh, J.A.: The natural history of rheumatoid arthritis: a fifteen year follow-up study. The prognostic significance of features noted in the first year. Clin. Rheumatol., 3:11–20, 1984.

77. Sherrer, Y.S., et al.: The development of disability in rheumatoid arthritis. Arthritis Rheum., 29:494–500, 1986.

78. Yelin, E., et al.: Work disability in rheumatoid arthritis: effects of disease, social, and work factors. Ann. Intern. Med., 93:551–556, 1980.

79. Wolfe, F., et al.: A multicenter study of hospitalization in rheumatoid arthritis: effect of health care system, severity, and regional difference. J. Rheumatol., 13:277–284, 1986.

80. Lubeck, D.P., et al.: A multicenter study of annual health service utilization and costs in rheumatoid arthritis. Arthritis Rheum., 29:488–493, 1986.

81. Liang, M.H., et al.: Costs and outcomes in rheumatoid arthritis and osteoarthritis. Arthritis Rheum., 27:522–529, 1984.

82. Stone, C.E.: The lifetime economic costs of rheumatoid arthritis. J. Rheumatol., 11:819–827, 1984.

83. Cassidy, J.T., et al.: A study of classification criteria for children with juvenile rheumatoid arthritis. Arthritis Rheum., 29:274–281, 1986.

84. Baum, J., et al.: Juvenile rheumatoid arthritis: a comparison of patients from the USSR and USA. Arthritis Rheum., 23:977–984, 1980.

85. Gewanter, H.L., Roghmann, K.J., and Baum, J.: The prevalence of juvenile arthritis. Arthritis Rheum., 26:599–603, 1983.

86. Towner, S.R., et al.: The epidemiology of juvenile arthritis in Rochester, Minnesota 1960–1979. Arthritis Rheum., 26:1208–1213, 1983.

87. Wood, P.H.: Nomenclature and classification of arthritis in children. In The Care of Rheumatic Children. Edited by E. Munthe. Basel, EULAR, 1978, p. 47.

88. Andersson, G.B., et al.: Incidence and prevalence of juvenile chronic arthritis: a population survey. Ann. Rheum. Dis., 46:277–281, 1987.

89. Kunnamo, I., Kallio, P., and Pelkonen, P.: Incidence of arthritis in urban Finnish children: a prospective study. Arthritis Rheum., 29:1232–1238, 1986.

90. Stillman, J.S., and Barry, P.E.: Juvenile rheumatoid arthritis: Series 2. Arthritis Rheum., 20:171–175, 1977.

91. Edmonds, J., et al.: Follow-up study of juvenile chronic polyarthritis with particular reference to histocompatibility antigen W 27. Ann. Rheum. Dis., 33:289–292, 1974.

92. Haffejee, I.E., Raga, J., and Coovadia, H.M.: Juvenile chronic arthritis in black and Indian South African children. S. Afr. Med. J., 65:510–514, 1984.

93. Rosenberg, A.M., and Petty, R.E.: Similar patterns of juvenile

rheumatoid arthritis within families. Arthritis Rheum., 23:951–953, 1980.

94. Glass, D., et al.: Early-onset pauciarticular juvenile rheumatoid arthritis associated with human leukocyte antigen-DRW5, iritis, and antinuclear antibody. J. Clin. Invest., 66:426–429, 1980.

95. Rossen, R.D., et al.: Familial rheumatoid arthritis: a kindred identified through a proband with seronegative juvenile arthritis includes members with seropositive, adult onset disease. Hum. Immunol., 4:183–196, 1982.

96. Hall, P.J., et al.: Genetic susceptibility to early onset pauciarticular juvenile chronic arthritis: a study of HLA and complement markers in 158 British patients. Ann. Rheum. Dis., 45:464–474, 1986.

97. Glass, D.N., and Litvin, D.A.: Heterogeneity of HLA associations in systemic onset juvenile rheumatoid arthritis. Arthritis Rheum., 23:796–799, 1980.

98. Miller, M.L., et al.: HLA gene frequencies in children and adults with systemic onset juvenile rheumatic arthritis. Arthritis Rheum., 28:146–150, 1985.

99. Rimon, R., Viukari, M., and Halonen, P.: Relationship between life stress factors and viral antibody levels in patients with juvenile rheumatoid arthritis. Scand. J. Rheumatol., 8:62–64, 1979.

100. Phillips, P.E.: Infection and chronic rheumatic disease in children. Semin. Arthritis Rheum., 10:92–99, 1980.

101. Hanson, V., et al.: Prognosis of juvenile rheumatoid arthritis. Arthritis Rheum., 20:279–284, 1977.

102. Laaksonen, A.L.: A prognostic study of rheumatoid arthritis. Acta Paediatr. Scand. (Suppl. 166):1–79, 1966.

103. Stoeber, E.: Prognosis in juvenile chronic arthritis: follow-up of 433 chronic rheumatic children. Eur. J. Pediatr., 135:225–228, 1981.

104. Goel, K.M., and Shanks, R.A.: Follow-up study of 100 cases of juvenile rheumatoid arthritis. Ann. Rheum. Dis., 33:25–31, 1974.

105. Calabro, J.J., et al.: Juvenile rheumatoid arthritis: a general review and report of 100 patients observed for years. Semin. Arthritis Rheum., 5:257–298, 1976.

106. Baum, J., and Gutowska, G.: Death in juvenile rheumatoid arthritis. Arthritis Rheum., 20:253–255, 1977.

107. Cush, J.J., et al.: Adult-onset Still's disease: clinical course and outcome. Arthritis Rheum., 30:186–194, 1987.

108. Wright, V., and Moll, J.M.H.: Seronegative Polyarthritis. New York, Elsevier/North-Holland Biomedical Press, 1976.

109. Cleland, L.G., Hay, J.A.R., and Milazzo, S.C.: Absence of HL-A 27 and of ankylosing spondylitis in central Australian aboriginals. (Abstract.) Scand. J. Rheumatol., 8:30, 1975.

110. Gofton, J.P., et al.: HL-A 27 and ankylosing spondylitis in B.C. Indians. J. Rheumatol., 2:314–318, 1975.

111. Woodrow, J.C.: Histocompatibility antigens and rheumatic diseases. Semin. Arthritis Rheum., 6:257–276, 1977.

112. Khan, M.A., et al.: HLA B27 in ankylosing spondylitis: differences in frequency and relative risk in American blacks and Caucasians. J. Rheumatol., 4 (Suppl 3):39–43, 1977.

113. Khan, M.A., Kushner, I., and Bran, W.E.: Comparison of clinical features in HLA-B27 positive and negative patients with ankylosing spondylitis. Arthritis Rheum., 20:909–912, 1977.

114. Spencer, D.G., Dick, H.M., and Dick, W.C.: Ankylosing spondylitis—the role of HLA-B27 homozygosity. Tissue Antigens, 14:379–384, 1974.

115. McDaniel, D.O., et al.: Polymorphism with ankylosing spondylitis. Arthritis Rheum., 30:894–900, 1987.

116. Sanmarti, R., et al.: HLA class II antigens (DR, DQ loci) and peripheral arthritis in ankylosing spondylitis. Ann. Rheum. Dis., 46:497–500, 1987.

117. Ebringer, R.W., et al.: Sequential studies in ankylosing spondylitis: association of Klebsiella pneumoniae with active disease. Ann. Rheum. Dis., 37:146–151, 1978.

118. Geczy, A.F., et al.: HLA-B27, molecular mimicry and ankylosing spondylitis: popular misconceptions. Ann. Rheum. Dis., 46:171–172, 1987.

119. Masi, A.T., and Medsger, T.A.: A new look at the epidemiology of ankylosing spondylitis and related syndromes. Clin. Orthop., 143:15–29, 1979.

120. Brewerton, D.A.: Joseph J. Bunim Memorial Lecture: HLA-B27 and the inheritance of susceptibility to rheumatic disease. Arthritis Rheum., 19:656–668, 1976.

121. Solomon, L., et al.: Rheumatic disorders in the South African Negro. Part I. Rheumatoid arthritis and ankylosing spondylitis. S. Afr. Med. J., 49:1292–1296, 1975.

122. Carter, E.T., et al.: Epidemiology of ankylosing spondylitis in Rochester, Minnesota: 1935–1973. Arthritis Rheum., 22:365–370, 1979.

123. Masi, A.T.: Epidemiology of B-27 associated diseases. Ann. Rheum. Dis., 38:131–134, 1979.

124. Calin, A., and Fries, J.: Striking prevalence of ankylosing spondylitis in "healthy" W27 positive males and females: a controlled study. N. Engl. J. Med., 293:835–839, 1975.

125. Gran, J.T., Husby, G. and Hordvik, A.M.: Prevalence of ankylosing spondylitis in males and females in a young middle-aged population of Tromso, Northern Norway. Ann. Rheum. Dis., 44:359–367, 1985.

125a.Gömor, B., Gyodi, E., and Bakos, L.: Distribution of HLA B27 and ankylosing spondylitis in the Hungarian population. J. Rheumatol., 4(Suppl. 3):33–35, 1977.

126. Dawkins, R.L., et al.: Prevalence of ankylosing spondylitis and radiological abnormalities of the sacroiliac joints in HLA-B27 positive individuals. (Letter.) J. Rheumatol., 8:1025, 1981.

127. Van der Linden, S.M., et al.: The risk of developing ankylosing spondylitis in HLA-B27 positive individuals: a comparison of relatives of spondylitis patients with the general population. Arthritis Rheum., 27:241–249, 1984.

128. Gran, J.T., and Husby, G.: Ankylosing spondylitis: a comparative study of patients in an epidemiological survey, and those admitted to a department of rheumatology. J. Rheumatol., 11:788–793, 1984.

129. Moll, J.M.B., and Wright, V.: New York clinical criteria for ankylosing spondylitis: a statistical evaluation. Ann. Rheum. Dis., 32:354–363, 1973.

130. Hollingsworth, P.N., et al.: Observer variation in grading sacroiliac radiographs in HLA-B27 positive individuals. J. Rheumatol., 10:247–254, 1983.

131. Calin, A., et al.: Clinical history as a screening test for ankylosing spondylitis. JAMA, 237:2613–2614, 1977.

132. van der Linden, S., Valkenburg, H.A., and Cats, A.: Evaluation of diagnostic criteria for ankylosing spondylitis: A proposal for modification of the New York criteria. Arthritis Rheum., 27:361–368, 1984.

133. McBryde, A.M. Jr., and McCollum, D.E.: Ankylosing spondylitis in women. The disease and its prognosis. N.C. Med. J., 34:34–37, 1973.

134. Marks, S.H., Barnett, M., and Calin, A.: Ankylosing spondylitis in women and men: a case-control study. J. Rheumatol., 10:624–628, 1983.

135. Nasrallah, N.S., et al.: HLA-B27 antigen and rheumatoid factor negative (seronegative) peripheral arthritis: studies in

early-diagnosed younger patients. Am. J. Med., *63*:379–386, 1977.

136. Bensen, W.G., and Singal, D.P.: Is HLA-B27 the ankylosing spondylitis susceptibility gene? J. Rheumatol., *12*:949–952, 1985.

137. Arnett, F.C., Hochberg, M.C., and Bias, W.B.: Cross-reactive HLA antigens in B27-negative Reiter's syndrome and sacroiliitis. Johns Hopkins Med. J., *141*:193–197, 1977.

138. Schwartz, B.D., Luehrman, L.R., and Rodey, G.E.: Public antigenic determinant on a family of HLA-B molecules: basis for cross-reactivity and a possible link with disease predisposition. J. Clin. Invest., *64*:938–947, 1979.

139. Hammoudeh, M., and Khan, M.: Genetics of HLA associated disease: ankylosing spondylitis. J. Rheumatol., *10*:301–304, 1983.

140. Lockhead, J.A., et al.: HLA-B27 haplotypes in family studies of ankylosing spondylitis. Arthritis Rheum., *26*:1011–1016, 1983.

141. Breur-Vriesendorp, B.S., Dekker-Saeys, A.J., and Ivanyi, P.: Distribution of HLA-B27 subtypes in patients with ankylosing spondylitis: the disease is associated with a common determinant of the various B27 molecules. Ann. Rheum. Dis., *46*:353–356, 1987.

142. Suarez-Almazor, M.E., and Russell, A.S.: B27 homozygosity and ankylosing spondylitis. J. Rheumatol., *14*:302–304, 1987.

143. Khan, M.A., and Khan, M.K.: Diagnostic value of HLA-B27 testing in ankylosing spondylitis and Reiter's syndrome. Ann. Intern. Med., *96*:70–76, 1982.

144. Fallet, G.H., et al.: Coexisting rheumatoid arthritis and ankylosing spondylitis. J. Rheumatol., *14*:1135–1138, 1987.

145. Radford, E.P., Doll, R., and Smith, P.G.: Mortality among patients with ankylosing spondylitis not given x-ray therapy. N. Engl. J. Med., *297*:572–576, 1977.

146. Khan, M.A. Khan, M.K., and Kushner, I.: Survival among patients with ankylosing spondylitis: a life table analysis. J. Rheumatol., *8*:86–90, 1981.

147. Carette, S., et al.: The natural disease course of ankylosing spondylitis. Arthritis Rheum., *26*:186–190, 1985.

148. Paronen, I.: Reiter's disease: a study of 344 cases observed in Finland. Acta Med. Scand., *131* (Suppl. 212):7–114, 1948.

149. Noer, H.R.: An "experimental" epidemic of Reiter's syndrome. JAMA, *198*:693–698, 1966.

150. Lawrence, J.S.: Family survey of Reiter's disease. Br. J. Vener. Dis., *50*:140–145, 1974.

151. Willkens, R.F., et al.: Reiter's syndrome: evaluation of preliminary criteria for definite disease. Arthritis Rheum., *24*:844–849, 1981.

152. Bardin, T., Enel, C., Lathrop, M., and Becker-Christensen, F.: Reiter's syndrome in Greenland: a clinical and epidemiological study of two communities. Scand. J. Rheumatol., *14*:369–374, 1985.

153. Finch, M., Rodey, G., Lawrence, D., and Blake, P.: Epidemic Reiter's syndrome following an outbreak of shigellosis. Eur. J. Epidemiol., *2*:26–30, 1986.

154. Calin, A., and Fries, J.F.: An "experimental" epidemic of Reiter's syndrome revisited: follow-up evidence of genetic and environmental factors. Ann. Intern. Med., *84*:564–566, 1976.

155. Kaslow, R.A., Ryder, R.W., and Calin, A.: Search for Reiter's syndrome after an outbreak of *Shigella sonnei* dysentery. J. Rheumatol., *6*:562–566, 1979.

156. Kousa, M., et al.: Family study of Reiter's disease and HLA B27 distribution. J. Rheumatol., *4*:95–102, 1977.

157. Khan, M.A., et al.: Low association of HLA-B27 with Reiter's syndrome in blacks. Ann. Intern. Med., *90*:202–203, 1979.

158. Rosenberg, A.M., and Petty, R.E.: Reiter's disease in children. Am. J. Dis. Child., *133*:394–398, 1979.

159. Sairanen, E., and Tillikainen, A.: HL-A 27 in Reiter's disease following shigellosis. (Abstract) Scand. J. Rheumatol., *4* (Suppl. 8):30, 1975.

160. Calin, A., Marder, A., Marks, S., and Burns, T.: Familial aggregation of Reiter's syndrome and ankylosing spondylitis: a comparative study. J. Rheumatol., *11*:672–677, 1984.

161. Marks, J.S., and Holt, P.J.L.: The natural history of Reiter's disease—21 years of observations. Q. J. Med., *231*:685–697, 1986.

162. Fox, R., et al.: The chronicity of symptoms and disability in Reiter's syndrome. Ann. Intern. Med., *91*:190–193, 1979.

163. Leirisalo, M., et al.: Followup study on patients with Reiter's disease and reactive arthritis, with special reference to HLA-B27. Arthritis Rheum., *25*:249–259, 1982.

164. Aho, K., Leirisalo, R.M., and Repo, H.: Reactive arthritis. Clin. Rheum. Dis., *11*:11–40, 1985.

165. Bekassy, A.N., Enell, H., and Schalen, C.: Severe polyarthritis following Campylobacter enteritis in a 12-year old boy. Acta Paediatr. Scand., *69*:269–271, 1980.

166. Mielants, H., et al.: HLA antigens in seronegative spondyloarthropathies. Reactive arthritis and arthritis in ankylosing spondylitis: relation to gut inflammation. J. Rheumatol., *14*:466–471, 1987.

167. Lahesmaa-Rantala, R., Granfors, K., Kekomaki, R., and Toivanen, A.: Circulating yersinia specific immune complexes after acute yersiniosis: a follow-up study of patients with and without reactive arthritis. Ann. Rheum. Dis., *46*:121–126, 1987.

168. Mielants, H., et al.: Repeat ileocolonoscopy in reactive arthritis. J. Rheumatol., *14*:456–458, 1987.

169. Brewerton, D.A., and James, D.C.: The histocompatibility antigen (HLA 27) and disease. Semin. Arthritis Rheum., *4*:191–207, 1975.

170. Hyla, J.F., Franck, W.A., and Davis, J.S.: Lack of association of HLA B27 with radiographic sacroiliitis in inflammatory bowel disease. J. Rheumatol., *3*:196–200, 1976.

171. Espinoza, L.R., et al.: Histocompatibility typing in the seronegative spondyloarthropathies: a survey. Semin. Arthritis Rheum., *11*:375–381, 1982.

172. McHugh, N.J., et al.: Psoriatic arthritis: clinical subgroups and histocompatibility antigens. Ann. Rheum. Dis., *46*:184–188, 1987.

173. Murray, C., et al.: Histocompatibility alloantigens in psoriasis and psoriatic arthritis: Evidence for the influence of multiple genes in the major histocompatibility complex. J. Clin. Invest., *66*:670–674, 1980.

174. Sills, E.M.: Psoriatic arthritis in childhood. Johns Hopkins Med. J., *146*:49–53, 1980.

175. Shore, A., and Ansell, B.M.: Juvenile psoriatic arthritis—an analysis of 60 cases. J. Pediatr., *100*:529–535, 1982.

175a. Taylor, R., and Ford, G.: The chief scientist reports. Arthritis/rheumatism in an elderly population: prevalence and service use. Health Bull. (Edinb.), *42*:274–281, 1984.

176. Stern, R.S.: The epidemiology of joint complaints in patients with psoriasis. J. Rheumatol., *12*:315–320, 1985.

177. Trentham, D.E., et al.: Autoimmunity to collagen: shared feature of psoriatic and rheumatoid arthritis. Arthritis Rheum., *24*:1363–1369, 1981.

178. Trentham, D.E.: Collagen arthritis as a relevant model of rheumatoid arthritis: evidence pro and con. Arthritis Rheum., *25*:911–916, 1982.

179. Masi, A.T.: Clinical epidemiologic perspective of systemic lu-

pus erythematosus. *In* Epidemiology of the Rheumatic Diseases. Proceedings of the Fourth International Conference. National Institutes of Health. New York, Gower Medical Publishing, 1984, pp. 145–163.

180. Cohen, A.S., et al.: Preliminary criteria for the classification of systemic lupus erythematosus. Bull. Rheum. Dis., *21*:643–648, 1971.

181. Canoso, J.J., and Cohen, A.S.: A review of the evaluations, and criticisms of the preliminary criteria for the classification of systemic lupus erythematosus. Arthritis Rheum., *22*:917–921, 1979.

182. Tan, E.M., et al.: The 1982 revised criteria for the classification of systemic lupus erythematosus. Arthritis Rheum., *25*:1271–1277, 1982.

183. Masi, A.T., et al.: Preliminary criteria for the classification of systemic sclerosis (scleroderma). Arthritis Rheum., *23*:581–590, 1980.

184. Siegel, M., et al.: The epidemiology of systemic lupus erythematosus: preliminary results in New York City. J. Chronic Dis., *15*:131–140, 1962.

185. Siegel, M., and Lee, S.L.: The epidemiology of systemic lupus erythematosus. Semin. Arthritis Rheum., *3*:1–53, 1973.

186. Michet, C.J., et al.: Epidemiology of systemic lupus erythematosus and other connective tissue diseases in Rochester, Minnesota, 1950–1979. Mayo Clin. Proc., *60*:105–113, 1985.

187. Fessel, W.J.: Systemic lupus erythematosus in the community: incidence, prevalence, outcome, and first symptoms, the high prevalence in black women. Arch. Intern. Med., *134*:1027–1035, 1974.

188. Hochberg, M.C.: The incidence of systemic lupus erythematosus in Baltimore, Maryland, 1970–1977. Arthritis Rheum., *28*:80–86, 1985.

189. Serdula, M.K., and Rhoads, G.G.: Frequency of systemic lupus erythematosus in different ethnic groups in Hawaii. Arthritis Rheum., *2*:328–333, 1979.

190. Hart, H.H., Grigor, R.R., and Caughey, D.E.: Ethnic difference in the prevalence of systemic lupus erythematosus. Ann. Rheum. Dis., *42*:529–532, 1983.

191. Helve, T.: Prevalence and mortality rates of systemic lupus erythematosus and causes of death in SLE patients in Finland. Scand. J. Rheumatol., *14*:43–46, 1985.

192. Morton, R.O., et al.: The incidence of systemic lupus erythematosus in North American Indians. J. Rheumatol., *3*:186–190, 1976.

193. Nived, D., Sturfelt, G., and Wollheim, F.: Systemic lupus erythematosus in an adult population in southern Sweden: incidence, prevalence and validity of ARA revised classification criteria. Br. J. Rheumatol., *24*:147–154, 1985.

194. Estes, D., and Christian, C.L.: The natural history of systemic lupus erythematosus by prospective analysis. Medicine, *50*:85–95, 1971.

195. Masi, A.T., and Kaslow, R.A.: Sex effects in systemic lupus erythematosus: a clue to pathogenesis. Arthritis Rheum., *21*:480–484, 1978.

196. King, K.K., et al.: The clinical spectrum of systemic lupus erythematosus in childhood. Arthritis Rheum., *20*:287–294, 1977.

197. Maddock, R.K.: Incidence of systemic lupus erythematosus by age and sex. JAMA, *191*:137–138, 1965.

198. Dubois, E.L.: The clinical picture of systemic lupus erythematosus. *In* Lupus Erythematosus. Los Angeles, University of Southern California Press, 1974, pp. 232–379.

199. Lahita, R.G., and Bradlow, H.L.: Klinefelter's syndrome: hormone metabolism in hypogonadal males with systemic lupus erythematosus. J. Rheumatol., *14*(Suppl. 13):154–157, 1987.

200. Lahita, R.G., et al.: Low plasma androgens in women with systemic lupus erythematosus. Arthritis Rheum., *30*:241–248, 1987.

201. Roubinian, J.R., et al.: Delayed androgen treatment prolongs survival in murine lupus. J. Clin. Invest., *63*:902–911, 1979.

202. Inman, R.D.: Immunologic sex differences and the female predominance in systemic lupus erythematosus. Arthritis Rheum., *21*:849–852, 1978.

203. Siegel, M., Holley, H.L., and Lee, S.L.: Epidemiologic studies on systemic lupus erythematosus: comparative data for New York City and Jefferson County, Alabama, 1956–1965. Arthritis Rheum., *13*:802–811, 1970.

204. Kaslow, R.L., and Masi, A.T.: Age, sex, and race effects on mortality due to systemic lupus erythematosus in the United States. Arthritis Rheum., *21*:473–479, 1978.

205. Lahita, R.G., et al.: Familial systemic lupus erythematosus in males. Arthritis Rheum., *26*:39–44, 1983.

206. Arnett, F.C., et al.: Systemic lupus erythematosus: current state of the genetic hypothesis. Semin. Arthritis Rheum., *14*:24–35, 1984.

207. Block, S.R., et al.: Studies of twins with systemic lupus erythematosus: a review of the literature and presentation of 12 additional sets. Am. J. Med., *59*:533–552, 1975.

208. Messner, R.P., DeHoratius, R., and Ferrone, S.: Lymphocytotoxic antibodies in systemic lupus erythematosus patients and their relatives: reactivity with the HLA antigenic molecular complex. Arthritis Rheum., *23*:265–272, 1980.

209. Smolen, J.S., et al.: HLA-DR antigens in systemic lupus erythematosus: association with specificity of autoantibody responses to nuclear antigens. Ann. Rheum. Dis., *46*:457–462, 1987.

210. Soppi, E., Eskola, J., and Lehtonen, A.: Evidence against HLA and immunological dependence of disease outbreak in SLE: immunological characterisation of identical twins clinically discordant for SLE. Ann. Rheum. Dis., *44*:45–49, 1985.

211. Miller, K.B., and Schwartz, R.S.: Familial abnormalities of suppressor-cell function in systemic lupus erythematosus. N. Engl. J. Med., *301*:803–809, 1979.

212. Esscher, E., and Scott, J.S.: Congenital heart block and maternal systemic lupus erythematosus. Br. Med. J., *1*:1235–1238, 1979.

213. Hardy, J.D., et al.: Congenital complete heart block in the newborn associated with maternal systemic lupus erythematosus and other connective tissue disorders. Arch. Dis. Child., *54*:7–13, 1979.

214. Scott, J.S., et al.: Connective-tissue disease, antibodies to ribonucleoprotein and congenital heart block. N. Engl. J. Med., *309*:209–212, 1983.

215. Watson, R.M., et al.: Neonatal lupus erythematosus: a clinical, serological and immunogenetic study with review of the literature. Medicine, *63*:362–378, 1984.

216. Siegel, M., and Seelenfreund, M.: Racial and social factors in systemic lupus erythematosus. JAMA, *191*:77–80, 1965.

217. Lowenstein, M.B., and Rothfield, N.F.: Family study of systemic lupus erythematosus: analysis of the clinical history, skin immunofluorescence and serologic parameters. Arthritis Rheum., *20*:1293–1303, 1977.

218. Clair, D., et al.: Autoantibodies in human contacts of SLE dogs. Arthritis Rheum., *23*:251–253, 1980.

219. Reinertsen, J.L., et al.: An epidemiologic study of households exposed to canine systemic lupus erythematosus. Arthritis Rheum., *23*:564–567, 1980.

220. Hicks, J.T., et al.: Search for Epstein-Barr and type C oncornaviruses in systemic lupus erythematosus. Arthritis Rheum., 22:845–857, 1979.

221. Kimura, M., Andon, T., and Kai, K.: Failure to detect type-C virus p30-related antigen in systemic lupus erythematosus: false-positive reaction due to protease activity. Arthritis Rheum., 23:111–113, 1980.

222. Kallick, C.A., Thadhani, K.C., and Rice, T.W.: Identification of anaplasmataceae (Haemobartonella) antigen and antibodies in systemic lupus erythematosus. Arthritis Rheum., 23:197–205, 1980.

223. Merrell, M., and Shulman, L.E.: Determination of prognosis in chronic disease illustrated by systemic lupus erythematosus. J. Chronic Dis., 1:12–32, 1955.

224. Ginzler, E.M., et al.: A multicenter study of outcome in systemic lupus erythematosus. I. Entry variables as predictors of prognosis. Arthritis Rheum., 25:601–611, 1982.

225. Dimant, J., et al.: Systemic lupus erythematosus in the older age group: computer analysis. J. Am. Geriatr. Soc., 27:58–61, 1979.

226. Lee, P., et al.: Systemic lupus erythematosus: a review of 110 cases with reference to nephritis, the nervous system, infections, aseptic necrosis and prognosis. Q. J. Med., 181:1–32, 1977.

227. Rubin, L.A., Urowitz, M.B., and Gladman, D.D.: Mortality in systemic lupus erythematosus: the bimodal pattern revisited. Q. J. Med., 216:87–98, 1985.

228. Abeles, M., et al.: Systemic lupus erythematosus in the younger patient: survival studies. J. Rheumatol., 7:515–522, 1980.

229. Siegel, M., et al.: Survivorship in systemic lupus erythematosus: relationship to race and pregnancy. Arthritis Rheum., 12:117–125, 1969.

230. Albert, D.A., Hadler, H.M., and Ropes, M.W.: Does corticosteroid therapy affect the survival of patients with systemic lupus erythematosus? Arthritis Rheum., 22:945–953, 1979.

231. Lee, S.L., Rivero, I., and Siegel, M.: Activation of systemic lupus erythematosus by drugs. Arch. Intern. Med., 117:620–626, 1966.

232. Siegel, M., Lee, S.L., and Persee, N.S.: The epidemiology of drug-induced systemic lupus erythematosus. Arthritis Rheum., 10:407–415, 1967.

233. Perry, H.M., et al.: Relationship of acetyl transferase activity to antinuclear antibodies and toxic symptoms in hypertensive patients treated with hydralazine. J. Lab. Clin. Med., 76:114–125, 1970.

234. Baer, A.N., Woosley, R.L., and Pincus, T.: Further evidence for the lack of association between acetylator phenotype and systemic lupus erythematosus. Arthritis Rheum., 29:508–514, 1986.

235. Rodman, G.P., Jablonska, S., and Medsger, T.A., Jr.: Classification and nomenclature of progressive systemic sclerosis (scleroderma). Clin. Rheum. Dis., 5:5–13, 1979.

236. Sharp, G.C., et al.: Mixed connective tissue disease—an apparently distinct rheumatic disease syndrome associated with a specific antibody to an extractable nuclear antigen (ENA). Am. J. Med., 52:148–159, 1972.

237. Medsger, T.A., Jr.: Progressive systemic sclerosis and associated disorders. In Principles of Rheumatic Diseases. Edited by R.S. Panush. New York, John Wiley and Sons, 1981, pp. 331–350.

238. Tan, E.M., et al.: Diversity of antinuclear antibodies in progressive systemic sclerosis (scleroderma): Anticentromere antibody and its relationship to CREST syndrome. Arthritis Rheum., 23:617–625, 1980.

239. Steen, V.D., Powell, D.L., and Medsger, T.A., Jr.: Clinical correlations and prognosis based on serum autoantibodies in systemic sclerosis. Arthritis Rheum. (in press).

240. Masi, A.T.: Clinical-epidemiologic perspective of systemic sclerosis (scleroderma). In Systemic Sclerosis-Scleroderma. Edited by M.I.V. Jayson and C.M. Black. Sussex, England, John Wiley and Sons Ltd., 1988, pp. 7–31.

241. Masi, A.T.: Epidemiology and classification of systemic sclerosis. Connect. Tissue Dis. (in press).

242. Tan, P.L.J., Wigley, R.D., and Borman, C.B.: Clinical criteria for systemic sclerosis. Arthritis Rheum., 24:1589–1590, 1981.

243. Eason, R.J., Tan, P.L., and Gow, P.J.: Progressive systemic sclerosis in Auckland: a ten year review with emphasis on prognostic features. Aust. N.Z. J. Med., 11:657–662, 1981.

244. Medsger, T.A., Jr., and Masi, A.T.: Epidemiology of systemic sclerosis (scleroderma). Ann. Intern. Med., 74:714–721, 1971.

245. O'Donoghue, D.J.: Klinefelter's syndrome associated with systemic sclerosis. Postgrad. Med. J., 58:575–576, 1982.

246. Tuffanelli, D.L., and Winkelmann, R.K.: Systemic scleroderma: a clinical study of 727 cases. Arch. Dermatol., 84:359–371, 1961.

247. Medsger, T.A., Jr.: Epidemiology of progressive systemic sclerosis. In Systemic Sclerosis (Scleroderma). Edited by C.M. Black and A.R. Myers. New York, Gower Medical Publishing, 1985, pp. 53–60.

248. Medsger, T.A., and Masi, A.T.: The epidemiology of systemic sclerosis (scleroderma) among male U.S. veterans. J. Chronic Dis., 31:73–85, 1978.

249. Maricq, H.R., et al.: Capillary abnormalities in polyvinyl chloride production workers: examination by in vivo microscopy. JAMA, 236:1368–1371, 1976.

250. Black, C., et al.: Genetic susceptibility to scleroderma-like syndrome in symptomatic and asymptomatic workers exposed to vinyl chloride. J. Rheumatol., 13:1059–1062, 1986.

251. Yamakage, A., et al.: Occupational scleroderma-like disorder occurring in men engaged in the polymerization of epoxy resins. Dermatologica, 161:33–44, 1980.

252. Kumagai, Y., et al.: Clinical spectrum of connective tissue disease after cosmetic surgery (human adjuvant disease): observations in eighteen patients and a review of the Japanese literature. Arthritis Rheum., 26:1–12, 1984.

253. Kilbourne, E.M., et al.: Clinical epidemiology of toxic-oil syndrome: manifestations of a new illness. N. Engl. J. Med., 309:1408–1414, 1983.

254. Alonso-Ruiz, A., et al.: Toxic oil syndrome: a syndrome with features overlapping those of various forms of scleroderma. Semin. Arthritis Rheum., 15:200–212, 1986.

255. Medsger, T.A., Jr., and Masi, A.T.: Epidemiology of progressive systemic sclerosis. Clin. Rheum. Dis., 5:15–25, 1979.

256. Lynch, C.J., et al.: Histocompatibility antigens in progressive systemic sclerosis (PSS, scleroderma). J. Clin. Immunol., 2:314–318, 1982.

257. Whiteside, T.L., Medsger, T.A., Jr., and Rodnan, G.P.: HLA-DR antigens in progressive systemic sclerosis (scleroderma). J. Rheumatol., 10:128–131, 1983.

258. Medsger, T.A., Jr., et al.: Survival with systemic sclerosis (scleredema). Ann. Intern. Med., 75:369–376, 1971.

259. Giordano, M., et al.: Different antibody patterns and different prognoses in patients with scleroderma with various extent of skin sclerosis. J. Rheumatol., 13:911–916, 1986.

260. Barnett, A., Miller, M., and Littlejohn, G.: A survival study of scleroderma patients diagnosed over 30 years (1953–1983):

The value of a simple cutaneous classification in the early stages of this disease. J. Rheumatol. (in press).

261. Moroi, Y., et al.: Autoantibody to centromere (kinetochore) in scleroderma sera. Proc. Natl. Acad. Sci. U.S.A., 77:1627–1631, 1980.

262. Sherd, J.H., Bordwell, B., Rothfield, N.F., and Earnshaw, W.C.: High titers of autoantibodies to topoisomerase I (Scl-70) in sera from scleroderma patients. Science, 231:737–740, 1986.

263. Black, K.A., et al.: Cancer in connective tissue disease. Arthritis Rheum., 25:1130–1133, 1982.

264. Roumm, A.D., and Medsger, T.A., Jr.: Cancer and systemic sclerosis: an epidemiologic study. Arthritis Rheum., 28:344–360, 1985.

265. Peters-Golden, M., et al.: Incidence of lung cancer in systemic sclerosis. J. Rheumatol., 12:1136–1139, 1985.

266. Furst, D.E., et al.: A syndrome resembling progressive systemic sclerosis after bone marrow transplantation: model for scleroderma? Arthritis Rheum., 22:904–910, 1979.

267. Finch, W.R., et al.: Bleomycin induced scleroderma. J. Rheumatol., 7:651–659, 1980.

268. Gershwin, M.E., et al.: Characterization of a spontaneous disease of White Leghorn chickens resembling progressive systemic sclerosis (scleroderma). J. Exp. Med., 153:1640–1659, 1981.

269. Green, M.C., Sweet, H.O., and Bunker, L.E.: Tight-skin, a new mutation of the mouse causing excessive growth of connective tissue and skeleton. Am. J. Pathol., 82:493–507, 1976.

270. Bohan, A., et al.: A computer-assisted analysis of 153 patients with polymyositis and dermatomyositis. Medicine, 56:255–286, 1977.

271. Medsger, T.A., Jr., Dawson, W.N., Jr., and Masi, A.T.: The epidemiology of polymyositis. Am. J. Med., 48:715–723, 1970.

272. Hanissian, A.S., et al.: Comparison of childhood polymyositis and dermatomyositis: An epidemiologic and clinical comparative analysis. J. Rheumatol., 9:390–394, 1982.

273. Bohan, A., and Peter, J.B.: Polymyositis and dermatomyositis. N. Engl. J. Med., 292:344–347, 403–407, 1975.

274. Benbassat, J., Geffel, D., and Zlotnick, A.: Epidemiology of polymyositis-dermatomyositis in Israel, 1960–1976. Isr. J. Med. Sci., 16:197–200, 1980.

275. Findlay, G.H., Whiting, D.A., and Simson, I.W.: Dermatomyositis in the Transvaal and its occurrence in the Bantu. S. Afr. Med. J., 43:694–697, 1969.

276. Friedman, J.M., et al.: Immunogenetic studies of juvenile dermatomyositis: HLA-DR antigen frequencies. Arthritis Rheum., 26:214–216, 1983.

277. Behan, W.M.H., and Behan, P.O.: Immunological features of polymyositis/dermatomyositis. Springer Semin. Immunopathol., 8:267–293, 1985.

278. Arnett, F.C., et al.: The Jo-1 antibody system in myositis: relationships to clinical features and HLA. J. Rheumatol., 8:925–930, 1981.

279. Bernstein, R.M., et al.: Anti-Jo-1 antibody: a marker for myositis with interstitial lung disease. Br. Med. J., 289:151–152, 1984.

280. Mathews, M.B., and Bernstein, R.M.: Myositis antibody inhibits histidyl-t RNA synthetase: a model for autoimmunity. Nature, 304:177–179, 1983.

281. Koch, M.J., Brody, J.A., and Gillespie, M.M.: Childhood polymyositis: a case-control study. Am. J. Epidemiol., 104:627–631, 1976.

282. Christensen, M.L., et al.: Prevalence of Coxsackie B virus antibodies in patients with juvenile dermatomyositis. Arthritis Rheum., 29:1365–1370, 1986.

283. Bowles, N.E., Dubowitz, V., Sewry, C.A., and Archard, L.C.: Dermatomyositis, polymyositis, and Coxsackie-B-virus infection. Lancet, 1:1004–1007, 1987.

284. Strongwater, S.L., et al.: A murine model of polymyositis induced by Coxsackievirus B1 (Tucson strain). Arthritis Rheum., 27:433–442, 1984.

285. Hargis, A.M., et al.: Familial canine dermatomyositis: initial characterization of the cutaneous and muscular lesions. Am. J. Pathol., 116:234–244, 1984.

286. Phillips, P.E., Kassan, S.S., and Kagen, L.J.: Increased toxoplasma antibodies in idiopathic inflammatory muscle disease: a case-controlled study. Arthritis Rheum., 22:209–214, 1979.

287. Magid, S.K., and Kagen, L.J.: Serologic evidence for acute toxoplasmosis in polymyositis-dermatomyositis: increased frequency of specific anti-Toxoplasma IgM antibodies. Am. J. Med., 75:313–320, 1983.

288. Hendricks, G.F.M., et al.: Dermatomyositis and toxoplasmosis. Ann. Neurol., 5:393–395, 1979.

289. Harati, Y., Niakan, E., and Bergman, E.W.: Childhood dermatomyositis in monozygotic twins. Neurology, 36:721–723, 1986.

290. Medsger, T.A., Jr., Robinson, H., and Masi, A.T.: Factors affecting survivorship in polymyositis: a life-table study of 124 patients. Arthritis Rheum., 14:249–258, 1971.

291. Carpenter, J.R., et al.: Survival in polymyositis: corticosteroids and risk factors. J. Rheumatol., 4:207–214, 1977.

292. DeVere, R., and Bradley, W.G.: Polymyositis: its presentation, morbidity and mortality. Brain, 98:637–666, 1975.

293. Tymms, K.E., and Webb, J.: Dermatopolymyositis and other connective tissue diseases: a review of 105 cases. J. Rheumatol., 12:1140–1148, 1985.

294. Benbassat, J., et al.: Prognostic factors in polymyositis/dermatomyositis: a computer-assisted analysis of ninety-two cases. Arthritis Rheum., 28:249–255, 1985.

295. Hochberg, M.C., Feldman, D., and Stevens, M.B.: Adult onset polymyositis/dermatomyositis: an analysis of clinical and laboratory features and survival in 76 patients with a review of the literature. Semin. Arthritis Rheum., 15:168–178, 1986.

296. Henrikkson, K.G., and Sandstedt, P.: Polymyositis-treatment and prognosis: a study of 107 patients. Acta Neurol. Scand., 65:280–300, 1982.

297. Hochberg, M.C., Lopez-Acuna, D., and Gittelsohn, A.M.: Mortality from polymyositis and dermatomyositis in the United States, 1968–1978. Arthritis Rheum., 26:1465–1471, 1983.

298. Hoffman, G.S., et al.: Presentation, treatment, and prognosis of idiopathic inflammatory muscle disease in a rural hospital. Am. J. Med., 75:433–438, 1983.

299. Sullivan, D.B., Cassidy, J.T., and Petty, R.E.: Dermatomyositis in the pediatric patient. Arthritis Rheum., 20:327–331, 1977.

300. Barnes, B.E., and Mawr, B.: Dermatomyositis and malignancy: a review of the literature. Ann. Intern. Med., 84:68–76, 1976.

301. Talbott, J.H.: Acute dermatomyositis-polymyositis and malignancy. Semin. Arthritis Rheum., 6:305–360, 1977.

302. Lakhanpal, S., Bunch, T.W., Ilstrup, D.M., and Melton, L.J.: Polymyositis-dermatomyositis and malignant lesions: does an association exist? Mayo Clin. Proc., 61:645–653, 1986.

302a. Masi, A.T., and Hochberg, M.C.: Temporal association of polymyositis-dermatomyositis with malignancy: methodological and clinical considerations. Mt. Sinai J. Med. (in press).

303. Cupps, T.R., and Fauci, A.S.: Classification of the vasculitides. Major Probl. Intern. Med., 21:1–5, 1981.

304. Fauci, A.S., Haynes, B.F., and Katz, P.: The spectrum of vasculitis: clinical, pathologic, immunologic and therapeutic considerations. Ann. Intern. Med., 89:660–676, 1978.

305. Gocke, D.J., et al.: Association between polyarteritis and Australia antigen. Lancet, 2:1149–1153, 1970.

306. Trepo, C.G., et al.: The role of circulating hepatitis B antigen-antibody complexes in the pathogenesis of vascular and hepatic manifestations in polyarteritis nodosa. J. Clin. Pathol., 27:863–868, 1974.

307. Drueke, T., et al.: Hepatitis B antigen-associated periarteritis nodosa in patients undergoing long-term hemodialysis. Am. J. Med., 68:86–90, 1980.

308. McMahon, B.J., et al.: Vasculitis in Eskimos living in an area hyperendemic for hepatitis B. JAMA, 244:2180–2182, 1980.

309. Michalik, T.: Immune complexes of hepatitis B surface antigen in the pathogenesis of polyarteritis nodosa. Am. J. Pathol., 90:619–628, 1978.

310. Citron, B.F., et al.: Necrotizing angiitis associated with drug abuse. N. Engl. J. Med., 283:1003–1011, 1970.

311. Phanupnak, P., and Kohler, P.F.: Onset of polyarteritis nodosa during allergic hyposensitization treatment. Am. J. Med., 68:479–485, 1980.

312. Sergent, J.S., and Christian, C.C.: Necrotizing vasculitis after acute serous otitis media. Ann. Intern. Med., 81:195–199, 1974.

313. Elkon, K.B., et al.: Hairy-cell leukaemia with polyarteritis nodosa. Lancet, 2:280–282, 1979.

314. Frohnert, P.P., and Sheps, S.G.: Long-term follow-up study of periarteritis nodosa. Am. J. Med., 43:8–14, 1967.

315. Moskowitz, R.W., Baggenstoss, A.H., and Slocum, C.H.: Histopathologic classification of periarteritis nodosa: a study of 56 cases confirmed at necropsy. Mayo Clin. Proc., 38:345–357, 1963.

316. Fink, C.W.: Polyarteritis and other diseases with necrotizing vasculitis in childhood. Arthritis Rheum., 20:378–384, 1977.

317. Chumbley, L.C., Harrison, E.G., and DeRemee, R.A.: Allergic granulomatosis and angiitis (Churg-Strauss syndrome): report and analysis of 30 cases. Mayo Clin. Proc., 52:477–484, 1977.

318. Shiokawa, Y.: Vascular Lesions of Collagen Diseases and Related Conditions. Baltimore, University Park Press, 1977.

318a. Barbour, A.G., et al.: Kawasaki-like disease in a young adult: association with primary Epstein-Barr virus infection. JAMA, 241:397–398, 1979.

319. Keren, G., et al.: Kawasaki's disease and infantile polyarteritis nodosa: is pseudomonas infection responsible? Report of a case. Isr. J. Med. Sci., 15:592–600, 1979.

320. Shulman, S.T., and Rowley, A.H.: Does Kawasaki disease have a retroviral etiology? Lancet, 2:545–546, 1986.

321. Cream, J.J., Gumpel, J.M., and Peachey, R.D.G.: Schonlein-Henoch purpura in the adult: a study of 77 adults with anaphylactoid or Schonlein-Henoch purpura. Q. J. Med., 39:461–484, 1970.

322. Mullick, F.G., et al.: Drug related vasculitis. Clinicopathologic correlations in 30 patients. Hum. Pathol., 10:313–325, 1979.

323. Fauci, A.S., Haynes, B.F., Katz, P., and Wolff, S.M.: Wegener's granulomatosis: prospective clinical and therapeutic experience with 85 patients for 21 years. Ann. Intern. Med., 98:76–85, 1983.

324. Orlowski, J.P., Clough, J.D., and Dyment, P.G.: Wegener's granulomatosis in the pediatric age group. Pediatrics, 61:83–90, 1978.

325. Liang, G.C., et al.: Familial aggregation of polymyalgia rheumatica and giant cell arteritis. Arthritis Rheum., 17:19–24, 1974.

326. Hunder, G.G., et al.: HLA antigens in patients with giant cell arteritis and polymyalgia rheumatica. J. Rheumatol., 4:321–323, 1977.

327. Malmvall, B.E., Bengtsson, B.A., and Rydberg, L.: HLA antigens in patients with giant cell arteritis, compared with two control groups of different ages. Scand. J. Rheumatol., 9:65–68, 1980.

328. Fraga, A., et al.: Takayasu's arteritis: frequency of systemic manifestations (study of 22 patients) and favorable response to maintenance steroid therapy with adrenocorticosteroids (12 patients). Arthritis Rheum., 15:617–624, 1972.

329. Warshaw, J.B., and Spach, M.S.: Takayasu's disease (primary aortitis) in childhood: case report with review of literature. Pediatrics, 35:626–630, 1965.

330. Waern, A.V., Andersson, P., and Hemmingsson, A.: Takayasu's arteritis: a hospital region based study on occurrence, treatment and prognosis. Angiology, 34:311–320, 1983.

331. Numano, F., and Shimamoto, T.: Hypersecretion of estrogen in Takayasu's disease. Am. Heart J., 81:591–596, 1971.

332. Huston, K.A., et al.: Temporal arteritis: A 25-year epidemiologic, clinical and pathologic study. Ann. Intern. Med., 88:162–167, 1978.

333. Jonasson, F., Cullen, J.F., and Elton, R.A.: Temporal arteritis: a 14-year epidemiological, clinical and prognostic study. Scott. Med. J., 24:111–117, 1979.

334. Smith, C.A., Fidler, W.J., and Pinals, R.S.: The epidemiology of giant cell arteritis: report of a ten-year study in Shelby County, Tennessee. Arthritis Rheum., 26:1214–1219, 1983.

335. Bengtsson, B.A., and Malmvall, B.E.: The epidemiology of giant cell arteritis including temporal arteritis and polymyalgia rheumatica: incidences of different clinical presentations and eye complications. Arthritis Rheum., 24:899–904, 1981.

336. Boesen, P., and Freisleben Sorensen, S.: Giant cell arteritis, temporal arteritis, and polymyalgia rheumatica in a Danish county: a prospective investigation, 1982–1985. Arthritis Rheum., 30:294–299, 1987.

337. Chuang, T.-Y., Hunder, G.G., Ilstrup, D.M., and Kurland, L.T.: Polymyalgia rheumatica: a 10-year epidemiologic and clinical study. Ann. Intern. Med., 97:672–680, 1982.

338. Bird, H.A., et al.: An evaluation of criteria for polymyalgia rheumatica. Ann. Rheum. Dis., 38:434–439, 1979.

339. Behçet's Disease Research Committee of Japan: Behçet's disease: guide to diagnosis of Behçet disease. Jpn. J. Ophthalmol., 18:291–294, 1974.

340. Mason, R.M., and Barnes, C.C.: Behçet's syndrome with arthritis. Ann. Rheum. Dis., 28:95–103, 1969.

341. Aoki, K., Fujioka, K., and Katsumata, H.: Epidemiological studies in Behçet's disease in the Hokkaido district. Jpn. J. Clin. Ophthalmol., 25:2239–2243, 1971.

342. Berman, L., Trappler, B., and Jenkins, T.: Behçet's syndrome: a family, study and the elucidation of a genetic role. Ann. Rheum. Dis., 38:118–121, 1979.

343. Bird Stewart, J.A.: Genetic analysis of families of patients with Behçet's syndrome: data incompatible with autosomal recessive inheritance. Ann. Rheum. Dis., 45:265–268, 1986.

344. Grufferman, S., Barton, J.W., III, and Eby, N.L.: Increased sex concordance of sibling pairs with Behçet's disease, Hodgkin's disease, multiple sclerosis, and sarcoidosis. Am. J. Epidemiol., 126:365–369, 1987.

345. Ohno, S., et al.: Specific histocompatibility antigens associated with Behçet disease. Am. J. Ophthalmol., *80*:636–641, 1975.

346. Adorno, D., et al.: HLA-B5 and Behçet disease. Tissue Antigens, *14*:444–448, 1979.

347. Rosselet, E., Saudan, Y., and Jeannet, M.: Recherche antigens HLA dans la maladie de Behçet. Ophthalmologica, *172*:116–119, 1976.

348. Block, S.R., et al.: Immunologic observations on 9 sets of twins either concordant or discordant for SLE. Arthritis Rheum., *19*:545–554, 1976.

349. Banker, B.Q., and Victor, M.: Dermatomyositis (systemic angiopathy) of childhood. Medicine, *45*:261–289, 1966.

350. Campbell, P.M., and LeRoy, E.C.: Pathogenesis of systemic sclerosis: a vascular hypothesis. Semin. Arthritis Rheum., *4*:351–368, 1975.

351. Winkelstein, A., and Rabin, B.S.: Theories of autoimmunity. Bull. Rheum. Dis., *26*:842–847, 1975.

352. McCarty, D.J.: Coexistent gout and rheumatoid arthritis. J. Rheumatol., *8*:253–254, 1981.

353. Wallace, D.J., et al.: Coexistent gout in rheumatoid arthritis. Arthritis Rheum., *22*:81–86, 1979.

354. Acheson, R.M.: Epidemiology of serum uric acid and gout: an example of the complexities of multifactorial causation. Proc. R. Soc. Med., *63*:193–197, 1970.

355. Yano, K., Rhoads, G.G., and Kagan, A.: Epidemiology of serum uric acid among 8000 Japanese-American men in Hawaii. J. Chronic Dis., *30*:171–184, 1977.

356. Prior, I.: Epidemiology of rheumatic disorders in the Pacific with particular emphasis on hyperuricemia and gout. Semin. Arthritis Rheum., *11*:213–229, 1981.

357. Morton, N.E.: Genetics of hyperuricemia in families with gout. Am. J. Med. Genet., *4*:103–106, 1979.

358. Ahern, F.M., Johnson, R.C., and Ashton, G.C.: Family resemblances in serum uric acid level. Behav. Genet., *10*:303–307, 1980.

359. Dodge, H.J., and Mikkelsen, W.M.: Observations on the distribution of serum uric acid levels in participants of the Tecumseh, Michigan, community health studies. J. Chronic Dis., *23*:161–172, 1970.

360. Okada, M., et al.: Factors influencing the serum uric acid level: a study based on a population survey in Hisayamatown, Kyushu, Japan. J. Chronic Dis., *33*:607–612, 1980.

361. Akizuki, S.: A population study of hyperuricaemia and gout in Japan—analysis of sex, age and occupational differences in thirty-four thousand people living in Nagano prefecture. Ryumachi, *22*:201–208, 1982.

362. Healey, L.A.: Epidemiology of hyperuricemia. Arthritis Rheum., *18*:709–712, 1975.

363. Rose, B.S.: Gout in Maoris. Semin. Arthritis Rheum., *5*:121–145, 1975.

364. Healey, L.A., and Bayani-Sioson, P.S.: A defect in the renal excretion of uric acid in Filipinos. Arthritis Rheum., *14*:721–726, 1971.

365. Torralba, T.P., and Bayani-Sioson, P.S.: The Filipino and gout. Semin. Arthritis Rheum., *4*:307–320, 1975.

365a.Gibson, T., et al.: Hyperuricaemia, gout and kidney function in New Zealand Maori men. Br. J. Rheumatol., *23*:276–282, 1984.

366. Hall, A.P., et al.: Epidemiology of gout and hyperuricemia: a long-term population study. Am. J. Med., *47*:27–37, 1967.

367. O'Sullivan, J.B.: The incidence of gout and related uric acid levels in Sudbury, Massachusetts. In Population Studies of the Rheumatic Diseases. Amsterdam, Excerpta Medica Foundation, 1968, pp. 371–376.

368. Stewart, R.B., et al.: Epidemiology of hyperuricemia in an ambulatory elderly population. J. Am. Geriatr. Soc., *27*:552–554, 1979.

369. Ramsay, L.E.: Hyperuricaemia in hypertension: role of alcohol. Br. Med. J., *1*:653–654, 1979.

370. Campion, E.W., Glynn, R.J., and DeLabry, L.O.: Asymptomatic hyperuricemia: risks and consequences in the normative aging study. Am. J. Med., *82*:421–426, 1987.

371. Persky, V.M., et al.: Uric acid: a risk factor for coronary heart disease. Circulation, *59*:969–977, 1979.

372. Wallace, S.L., et al.: Preliminary criteria for the classification of the acute arthritis of primary gout. Arthritis Rheum., *20*:895–900, 1977.

373. Currie, W.J.C.: Prevalence and incidence of the diagnosis of gout in Great Britain. Ann. Rheum. Dis., *38*:101–106, 1979.

374. DeMuckadell, O.B., and Gyntelberg, G.: Occurrence of gout in Copenhagen males aged 40–59. Int. J. Epidemiol., *5*:153–158, 1976.

375. Rakic, M.T., et al.: Observations on the natural history of hyperuricemia and gout. I. An eighteen year follow-up of nineteen gouty families. Am. J. Med., *37*:862–871, 1964.

376. Bergström, G., et al.: Prevalence of rheumatoid arthritis, osteoarthritis, chondrocalcinosis and gouty arthritis at age 79. J. Rheumatol., *13*:527–534, 1986.

377. Yu, T.F.: Some unusual features of gouty arthritis in females. Semin. Arthritis Rheum., *6*:247–255, 1977.

378. Yu, T.-F.: Diversity of clinical features in gouty arthritis. Semin. Arthritis Rheum., *13*:360–368, 1984.

379. Beighton, P., et al.: Serum uric acid concentrations in an urbanized South African Negro population. Ann. Rheum. Dis., *33*:442–445, 1974.

380. Mody, G.M., and Naidoo, P.D.: Gout in South African blacks. Ann. Rheum. Dis., *43*:394–397, 1984.

381. Talbott, J.H., et al.: Gouty arthritis in the black. Semin. Arthritis Rheum., *4*:209–239, 1975.

382. Kelley, W.N.: Inborn errors of purine metabolism—1977. Arthritis Rheum., *20*:S221–S227, 1977.

383. Wyngaarden, J.B., and Kelley, W.N.: Hereditary xanthinuria. In Gout and Hyperuricemia. New York, Grune and Stratton, 1976, pp. 397–410.

384. Wyngaarden, J.B., and Kelley, W.N.: Miscellaneous forms of hypouricemia. In Gout and Hyperuricemia. New York, Grune and Stratton, 1976, pp. 411–418.

385. Laine, V.A.: International standardization of the diagnosis of rheumatoid arthritis and osteoarthritis, clinical aspects. Milbank Mem. Fund Q., *43*:133–141, 1964.

386. Symposium on the Epidemiology of Chronic Rheumatism, Volume II. Atlas of Standard Radiographs. Oxford, Blackwell Scientific Publications, 1963.

387. ARA Diagnostic Subcommittee for OA: Development of criteria for the classification and reporting of osteoarthritis: classification of osteoarthritis of the knee. Arthritis Rheum., *29*:1039–1049, 1986.

388. Peyron, J.G.: Osteoarthritis: the epidemiologic viewpoint. Clin. Orthop., *213*:13–19, 1986.

389. Acheson, R.M.: Heberden Oration 1981: epidemiology and the arthritides. Ann. Rheum. Dis., *41*:325–334, 1982.

390. National Center for Health Statistics. Public Health Service, Publication No. 1000, Series 11, No. 15, Washington, U.S. Government Printing Office, 1966.

391. Hartz, A.J., et al.: The association of obesity with joint pain

and osteoarthritis in the HANES data. J. Chronic Dis., *39*:311–319, 1986.

392. Andersen, S.: The epidemiology of primary osteoarthrosis of the knee in Greenland. Scand. J. Rheumatol., *7*:109–112, 1978.

393. Brighton, S.W.: The prevalence of osteoarthrosis in a rural African community. Br. J. Rheumatol., *24*:321–325, 1985.

394. Yach, D., and Botha, J.L.: Mseleni joint disease in 1981: decreased prevalence rates, wider geographical location than before, and socioeconomic impact of an endemic osteoarthrosis in an underdeveloped community in South Africa. Int. J. Epidemiol., *14*:276–284, 1985.

395. Hadler, N.M., et al.: Hand structure and function in an industrial setting: the influence of three patterns of stereotype, repetitive usage. Arthritis Rheum., *21*:210–220, 1978.

396. Panush, R.S., et al.: Is running associated with degenerative joint disease? JAMA, *225*:1152–1154, 1986.

397. Lane, N.E., et al.: Long-distance running, bone density, and osteoarthritis. JAMA, *255*:1147–1151, 1986.

398. Lindberg, H., and Danielsson, L.G.: The relation between labor and coxarthrosis. Clin. Orthop., *191*:159–161, 1984.

399. National Center for Health Statistics. Public Health Service, Publication No. 1000, Series 11, No. 20. Washington, U.S. Government Printing Office, 1966.

400. Kellgren, J.H., and Lawrence, J.S.: Rheumatism in miners. II. X-ray study. Br. J. Ind. Med., *9*:197–207, 1952.

401. Hadler, N.M.: Industrial rheumatology: clinical investigations into influence of pattern of usage on the pattern of regional musculoskeletal disease. Arthritis Rheum., *20*:1019–1025, 1977.

402. Puranen, J., et al.: Running and primary osteoarthritis of the hip. Br. Med. J., *2*:424–425, 1975.

403. Adams, I.D.: Osteoarthrosis and sport. J. R. Soc. Med., *72*:185–187, 1979.

404. National Center for Health Statistics. Public Health Service, Publication No. 1000, Series 11, No. 29. Washington, U.S. Government Printing Office, 1968.

405. Kraus, J.F., et al.: Epidemiological study of severe osteoarthritis. Orthopedics, *1*:37–42, 1978.

406. Dequeker, J., Goris, P., and Uytterhoeven, R.: Osteoporosis and osteoarthritis (osteoarthrosis): anthropometric distinctions. JAMA, *249*:1448–1451, 1983.

407. Lindberg, H.: Prevalence of primary coxarthrosis in siblings of patients with primary coxarthrosis. Clin. Orthop., *203*:273–275, 1986.

407a. Peyron, J.G.: Epidemiologic and etiologic approach to osteoarthritis. Semin. Arthritis Rheum., *8*:288–306, 1979.

408. Rodnan, G.P, Schumacher, H.R., and Zvaifler, N.J. (Eds.): Primer on the Rheumatic Diseases, 8th Ed. Atlanta, Arthritis Foundation, 1983, p. 36.

409. Yunus, M., et al.: Primary fibromyalgia (fibrositis): clinical study of 50 patients with matched normal controls. Semin. Arthritis Rheum., *11*:151–171, 1981.

410. Champbell, S.M., et al.: Clinical characteristics of fibrositis. I. A "blinded," controlled study of symptoms and tender points. Arthritis Rheum., *26*:817–824, 1983.

411. Felson, D.T., and Goldenberg, D.L.: Natural history of fibromyalgia. Arthritis Rheum., *29*:1522–1526, 1986.

412. Bennett, R.M. (Ed.): The fibrositis/fibromyalgia syndrome: current issues and perspectives. Am. J. Med., *81*:1–115, 1986.

413. Bengtsson, A.: Primary Fibromyalgia: A Clinical Laboratory Study. Linköping, Sweden, Linköping University medical disseration 1986 (No. 224), pp. 1–59.

414. Medsger, T.A., Jr., et al.: Nonarticular rheumatism. Arthritis Rheum., *26*:35–40, 1983.

415. National Center for Health Statistics (1976). Public Health Service, Publication No. 79–1552, Series 10, No. 124. Washington, D.C., U.S. Government Printing Office, 1976.

416. Yunus, M.B., Masi, A.T., and Aldag, J.C.: Criteria studies of primary fibromyalgia syndrome (PFS). (Abstract.) Arthritis Rheum., *30*:S21, 1987.

417. Allander, E., et al.: Rheumatology in perspective. The epidemiological view. Scand. J. Rheumatol., *46*(Suppl.):5–49, 1982.

DIFFERENTIAL DIAGNOSIS OF ARTHRITIS: ANALYSIS OF SIGNS AND SYMPTOMS

4

DANIEL J. McCARTY

Rational prognosis and therapy require precise diagnosis, and diagnosis depends primarily on skillful history taking and physical examination with subsequent help from the laboratory, the radiology department, or the surgical staff when indicated. I have assumed that the reader has acquired general clinical skills and will concentrate, therefore, on the interpretation of those aspects of the clinical history (symptoms) and the physical examination (signs) that relate to the differential diagnosis of arthritis and allied conditions (Table 4–1).

The purpose of the history and physical examination is to classify a patient's problem into one of four broad categories: inflammatory, degenerative-metabolic, functional (neurotic), or of unknown origin. These categories represent the primary nature of the diseases listed in Table 4–2. This classification does not deny the existence of an inflammatory component in osteoarthritis or a degenerative component of inflammatory arthritides such as rheumatoid arthritis (RA) or psoriatic arthritis. There may be an organic component even in those syndromes listed as "psychogenic," an organic peg on which is hung a psychoneurotic hat. Conversely, there is often a functional component to most organic illnesses. The "unknown" category is important because of the tendency by many clinicians to "force" a given patient's musculoskeletal complaints into a diagnostic pigeonhole. New syndromes and subsets of old ones are constantly being recognized. At least 10% of patients with musculoskeletal complaints that I have seen through the years cannot be given a diagnosis

with certainty. In the remainder, however, a reasonable differential diagnosis can be formulated after the initial examination.

HISTORY

CHIEF COMPLAINT

Patients consult physicians only for pain (or pain equivalent) or anxiety. Pain equivalents include subpainful unpleasantries such as itching, aching, stiffness, and nausea. Almost all other complaints are not presented to the doctor unless the patient, or a relative with some degree of control over the patient, is concerned (anxious) about their presence. Thus, treatment depends on relief of the pain or other unpleasant sensation, an explanation of the pertinent pathophysiology to the patient in lay terms, and a brief explanation of how the prescribed regimen is expected to correct the problem. The history should include detailed inquiry about the patient's motivation in coming to the doctor, especially in the *absence* of pain or pain equivalent. Why the anxiety? Could the older notion that RA is a psychosomatic illness have come from those extra office visits by anxious patients with mild disease while their stoic counterparts were at the movies? Could the patients with "fibrositis," making up 28% of new patients in private rheumatologic practice,[1] represent the anxious protruding tip of the mountain of individuals with tense neck and shoulder muscles? Are patients in a rheu-

55

Table 4–1. Signs and Symptoms Useful in Differential Diagnosis of Arthritis

Symptoms	Degenerative	Inflammatory	Psychogenic
Stiffness (duration)	Few minutes; "gelling" after prolonged rest	Hours (often); most pronounced after rest	Little or no variation in intensity with rest or activity
Pain	Follows activity; relieved by rest	Even at rest; nocturnal pain may interfere with sleep	Little or no variation in intensity with rest or activity
Weakness	Present, usually localized and not severe	Often pronounced	Often a complaint; "neurasthenia"
Fatigue	Not usual	Often severe with onset in afternoon	Often in A.M. on arising
Emotional depression and lability	Not usual	Common, coincides with fatigue; often disappears if disease remits	Often present
Signs			
Tenderness localized over afflicted joint	Usually present	Almost always; the most sensitive indication of inflammation	Tender "all over;" "touch-me-not attitude;" tendency to push away or to grasp the examining hand
Swelling	Effusion common; little synovial reaction	Effusion common; often synovial proliferation and thickening	None
Heat and erythema (skin)	Unusual but may occur	More common	None
Crepitus	Coarse to medium	Medium to fine	None, except with coexistent osteoarthritis
Bony spurs	Common	Sometimes found, usually with antecedent osteoarthritis	None, except with coexistent osteoarthritis

matic disease practice more likely to come to the office with a shopping list of questions written on a slip of paper (*petit morceau de papier* syndrome)? Find out precisely why the patient consulted you, with particular attention to the reason for the anxiety underlying all chief complaints.

HISTORY OF PRESENT ILLNESS

In general, one attempts to determine whether the patient has a systemic disease or a purely local condition. A localized condition may affect multiple sites, of course. What joints or other structures are involved?*

What was the pattern of involvement? In what order did joint involvement occur? How fast did it occur? At what time of the day did it start? If joint involvement is painful, severity can be estimated by whether it interfered with function of the affected extremity or with sleep or work. Was involvement self-limited, migratory, or additive (progressive)? If limited, how long was the episode? *Migratory* means that the process subsided completely in an affected

---

*"Joint" will be used hereafter, although tendon sheaths and bursae are often involved as well.

joint while cropping up in an erstwhile normal joint. *Progressive* or addictive means that the first joint stays afflicted while additional joints are involved by the pathologic process. Was treatment sought? What and how much was given and for how long? What was its effect on the disease? Side effects of therapy should be recorded.

Certain symptoms can be analyzed almost objectively, producing reliable data that deserve much weight diagnostically. The *duration of morning stiffness* is such a measurement and also serves as a convenient clinical yardstick to measure inflammatory activity (see Chapter 9). Patients are often emotional about the magnitude of morning stiffness, but not about its duration. Two questions suffice: what time do you get out of bed (not awake) and about when are you as "loose" as you are going to get? The physician then determines the duration of stiffness by subtraction. If a single question is asked, "How long are you stiff after getting up in the morning?" the patient will provide an answer. This answer will nearly always be different (shorter) than that obtained with the two-question technique.

The duration of morning stiffness is directly proportional to the severity of an inflammatory process in an extremity, whether this be arthritis, myositis,

Table 4–2.   Examples of Diseases in Various Categories

Noninflammatory†	Inflammatory	Psychogenic
Erosive osteoarthritis	*Tenosynovitis { calcific (BCP) / other }	*Primary fibrositis (tension rheumatism)
*Primary generalized osteoarthritis (OA)	*Rheumatoid arthritis	*Restless leg syndrome
*Isolated OA, e.g., hip, knee, first CMC	Seronegative polyarthritis	*Hysteria
*Cervical syndrome	*Systemic lupus erythematosus	
*Traumatic arthritis	Mixed connective tissue disease	
Aseptic (osteo)necrosis	Polyarteritis nodosa	
Amyloid arthropathy	Polymyositis	
*Pseudogout (some types)	Dermatomyositis	
Metabolic arthropathy	Rheumatic fever	
Hemachromatosis	*Reiter's syndrome ("reactive" arthritis)	
Acromegaly	*Psoriatic arthritis	
Hypothyroidism	*Ankylosing spondylitis	
Hyperparathyroidism	*Juvenile rheumatoid arthritis	
Ochronosis	Inflammatory bowel disease arthritis	
Neuroarthropathy (Charcot)	*Crystal synovitis	
*Enthesopathy	Gout (MSU)	
Tumors	Pseudogout (CPPD)	
Pigmented villonodular Synovitis	Other (BCP, postcorticosteroid injection flare)	
Synovial cell sarcoma	*Polymyalgia rheumatica	
*Mechanical abnormalities, e.g., torn menisci, tibial torsion	*Palindromic rheumatism	
*Reflex sympathetic dystrophies, e.g., shoulder-hand	Viral arthritis (e.g., rubella, mumps, hepatitis B)	
*Periarthritis of shoulder	Infectious arthritis	
*Tendonitis	Bacterial	
Blood dyscrasias, e.g., hemophilia	Tuberculous	
	Fungal	
	Immune complex arthritis, e.g., cryoglobulinemia, bacterial endocarditis, infected ventriculoatrial shunt	

*Common conditions encountered by every clinician.
†An inflammatory component may be present intermittently in some of these conditions.

bursitis, or sunburn. It signifies, nonspecifically, *inflammation*. Variations in its duration can be used to quantify inflammation and its response to treatment. Indeed, it is one of the best ways to follow inflammation clinically, and in this modern world of complex testing, it is both free of charge and immediately available. It is more precise than the erythrocyte sedimentation rate in following rheumatoid inflammation. True stiffness should be differentiated from the "articular gelling" of osteoarthritis, which lasts only for a few minutes or even seconds. The hesitant stiff first few steps of an elderly person crossing the room to switch channels on a TV set are a familiar example of the "gelling" phenomenon.

The sunburned limb becomes flexible sooner with each passing day, a faithful reflection of the resolution of the thermal injury and the accompanying inflammatory response. The protracted morning stiffness characteristic of polymyalgia rheumatica vanishes completely when low doses of prednisone are given. The average untreated patient with RA is stiff for about 4 hours after arising in the morning. The mechanism of stiffness after immobilization of an inflamed part is unclear, but it may be the subjective perception of increased resistance to motion that has been measured objectively,[2] which in turn is probably related to localized tissue edema and accumulation of the metabolic products of the inflammatory process. Motion activates the milking action of the muscles on both lymphatic flow and venous return. Increased stiffness of an inflamed part occurs not only after sleeping, but after any prolonged immobility, such as watching television or movies or catnapping.

If a structure is severely inflamed, it is *painful* on motion, just as sunburned skin over a joint is painful on motion. Overt pain at rest is found only in intense inflammation. Pain is difficult to describe, much less to quantify or localize. If trauma, including the microtrauma of motion, is pathogenetically important, then pain occurs on motion and subsides with rest. If there is no pattern of pain at all, a psychogenic factor might be involved. In patients with musculo-skeletal diseases, pain may arise from stimulation of synovial, capsular, periosteal, ligamentous, or ten-dinous nerve endings by mechanical irritation or by inflammation; from pressure on entrapped nerves, such as the median in the carpal tunnel at the wrist, the suprascapular in the shoulder, or from nerve roots in the cervical foramina; or from muscle spasm, either directly or, with increased muscle tone, on nerves coursing through the tightened muscle. Pain does not arise from cartilage. Electromyographers report little or no evidence of increased muscular contraction (spasm) about inflamed joints at rest, and to differ-entiate pathologically increased from normally in-creased electrical activity in contracting muscles is dif-ficult. If a patient complains of parietal pain and has no increased stiffness after prolonged immobility, di-rect nerve irritation or a psychologic problem is im-mediately suspected. Elicited pain *(tenderness)* is much more important clinically and can be localized accu-rately.

Systemic *fatigue,* like stiffness, is a subjective phe-nomenon and is not disease-specific. The time of on-set of fatigue after arising from bed is inversely pro-portional to the severity of the inflammatory process. This time is determined by subtracting the point of "bone tiredness" from the time of arising. The av-erage untreated rheumatoid patient has about 3.5 hours before fatigue sets in. The cause of such path-ologic fatigue is unknown. Perhaps the products of inflammation, milked from the involved sites by mus-cular activity, as already outlined, produce tissue ef-fects that subjectively represent fatigue. When asked about fatigue, patients often state that tiredness is present on arising. In the absence of insomnia, ane-mia, or metabolic disease, such fatigue is of neurotic origin, a desire perhaps to remain in the womb. This sensation usually disappears soon after the patient is up and about. Most of us have had this experience occasionally.

WEAKNESS

Disuse atrophy occurs rapidly, often in a few days, in muscles that move painful joints. In the diffuse systemic rheumatic diseases, direct muscle involve-ment often occurs as well. With upper-extremity in-volvement, "clumsiness" or weakness of grip may be the complaint, whereas difficulty in arising from a chair or in going up or down stairs may be experi-enced in lower-extremity involvement. This subjec-tive complaint can be verified and measured by meas-urement of grip strength or by timing a set task using lower-extremity muscles.[3]

DEPRESSION, HYSTERIA, AND EMOTIONAL LABILITY

Depresson may be the most common symptom of the twentieth century and is often noted in rheu-matologic practice. It is nearly always present in pa-tients with "fibrositis" (see Chapter 80), and, usually in reactive form, in patients with systemic rheumatic diseases. In RA, it often corresponds to the time of onset of pathologic fatigue, when emotional lability (crying, temper tantrums, or withdrawal) also occurs. These symptoms may disappear as the disease remits. Hysteria is less common and is usually dramatic. A patient cannot write clearly and has pain in the fingers (writer's cramp), cannot bend over or straighten up (camptocormia), or cannot straighten a bent extrem-ity. *Restless legs syndrome* is common and appears to be an hysterical condition or a depressive equivalent. Such patients are inordinately open to suggestion. Almost any medication that is prescribed with con-viction will work miraculously, but is certain to pro-duce unpleasant side effects; these patients are no-torious "placebo reactors" (see Chapter 80).

SYSTEMIC REVIEW

This is part of the routine history and should be done in all cases.

PAST HISTORY

A previous account of musculoskeletal or systemic disease may shed light on the current problem. Cho-rea or "growing pains" in childhood may aid in dif-ferentiating rheumatic fever or juvenile rheumatoid arthritis in an adult patient. A recent history of ex-posure to ticks or viral illness may clarify an otherwise obscure arthritis. Even more important is a history of sexual deviance or promiscuity in a patient suspected of having gonorrheal arthritis or Reiter's syndrome.

FAMILY HISTORY

A history of diabetes mellitus, hypertension or heart disease can often be obtained accurately. Diabetes is associated with adhesive capsulitis of the shoulders. Dupuytren's contracture, and osteoarthritis. A family history of arthritis may be obtained in patients with gout, pseudogout, ankylosing spondylitis, and RA, to name a few. I have often found it difficult to be sure of the diagnosis of arthritis from the family history, let alone what type of arthritis was actually present. This aspect of history taking may become more important with recent advances in immunogenetics (see Chapters 28, 29).

SOCIAL HISTORY

Stability of family life and the stability and type of job are important points to establish because much of the treatment program in arthritis involves them. Avocations should also be recorded because these, too, must often be dealt with in designing a treatment program. Current drug intake should be listed here, including alcohol and tobacco. Some idea of the patient's ability to perceive reality and of emotional maturity should be obtained at this point.

PHYSICAL EXAMINATION

An "arthralgia" is often an arthritis without a physical examination.

PALPATION

The rheumatologist's fingers are his stethoscope. Although various devices are useful to quantify tenderness, joint swelling, and skin temperature, none supplant the fingers in the physical examination. A working knowledge of topographic anatomy is essential. The examiner must know what structure(s) lies under his hand. This is particularly true when eliciting *tenderness*, which is the most sensitive sign available, albeit not specific. The neophyte uses too little force when pressing even on superficial structures. I exert sufficient force to blanch my thumbnail,[4,5] about 74 pounds per square inch, when examining areas that are not obviously inflamed. Obviously, one could reduce return office visits sharply by pressing this hard on red, swollen joints. Common sense must prevail. I use tenderness primarily to *exclude* disease. If none is present at 74 pounds per square inch, underlying inflammation, in the absence of congenital or acquired insensitivity to pain, is ruled out. If tenderness is present, then either a low pain threshold or pathologic change may be

responsible. Fortunately, most tenderness due to an organic cause is accompanied by more specific findings, such as swelling, crepitus, and increased local heat. Tenderness of joints is best elicited by pressure over the areas of synovial reflexion, whereas tendons should be stretched gently and then subjected to pressure. Direct pressure should be exerted on "fibrositic" areas in every patient. These areas include the lateral neck strap muscles, the belly of the trapezius, the epicondylar area, the medial knee over the collateral ligament and anserine bursa, and the lateral thigh over the tensor fasciae latae (see Chapter 80).

Areas of tenderness can be "controlled" by similar pressure over other nearby areas. A neurotic patient may be tender everywhere on the body. Such patients grasp the examiner's hand or draw the part away from the examiner's grasp—the "touch-me-not" sign. It is important to distinguish tender bones from tender soft tissues. For example, the anterior tibia is tender in most elderly subjects for reasons unknown to me. Bone tenderness is present in severe osteoporosis and other forms of systemic bone disease. In reflex sympathetic dystrophies, the entire hand (or foot) is tender. Even allowing for periarticular accentuation of tenderness, tenderness between the joints, over both bone and soft tissue, often suggests this condition rather than a true synovitis (see Chapter 97).

Deep-seated joints, such as the hips, spine and sacroiliac joints, require even more pressure to elicit tenderness because the intervening "pad" of soft tissue attenuates the applied force. Here, I exert pressure with the weight of my body against the flat of my hand held over the hip or over my thumb in the case of spine or sacroiliac joints. It is helpful to drape the patient over the examining table with the legs hanging down and the feet touching the floor, but not bearing weight (Fig. 4–1). The lumbar lordotic curve is flattened in this position. The sacroiliac joints lie between the roof of the sciatic notch and the posterior-inferior iliac spine, both of which can be identified easily. Inflammation of the sacroiliac joint is faithfully reflected by localized tenderness. Pressure can be exerted over each vertebral spine separately. The "skip areas" of spinal involvement so common in Reiter's syndrome, a septic discitis, or the precise level of lumbar degenerative disc disease, can often be mapped out readily with this technique.

A skilled examiner can lay hands on every peripheral joint in the body and can record the presence of tenderness on an appropriate form in about three minutes. Examination of the spine requires an additional three minutes.

FIG. 4–1. Optimal position for examination of sacroiliac joints and lumbar spine is shown. The posterior aspect of the sacroiliac joints lies between the sciatic notch and the posterior-inferior iliac spine (insert—arrows).

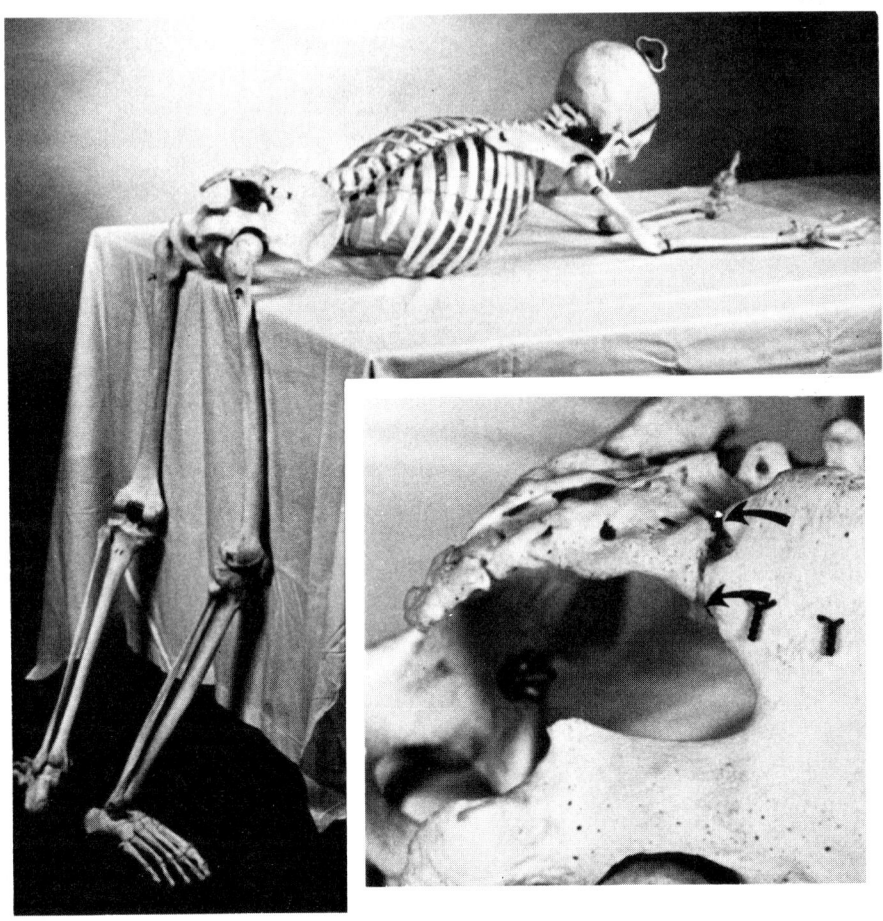

RANGE OF MOTION

Passive motion of a joint is an ancillary method of eliciting pain and is also necessary to check for contractures or limitation of motion. When pain is present on passive motion, it is often impossible to determine its origin without further examination. For example, pain on attempting to straighten the elbow to 0° or beyond can arise from intrinsic joint disease such as synovitis, or it may be due to extrinsic causes such as biceps tendonitis. Pain on motion of a hip or shoulder joint is often due to abnormalities in the joint capsule, bursae, or surrounding tendons. It is my practice to examine the anatomic structures about any joint that is painful on passive motion to determine exactly what is and what is not tender. Thus, the absence of pain on passive motion rules out pathologic abnormalities of many structures, but its presence demands further palpatory dissection of the local anatomy in search of its cause.

The *range of motion* of all joints should be determined while one attempts to elicit tenderness and pain on passive motion (Fig. 4–2). Loss of normal motion can be due to articular changes such as subluxation (partial dislocation), luxation (complete dislocation), capsular contraction, intra-articular adhesion, fibrous ankylosis, a tense effusion, extremely thickened synovium, or an intra-articular loose body. Bony ankylosis occurs commonly in some conditions such as JRA, ankylosing spondylitis, psoriatic arthritis, Reiter's disease, and, rarely, in gout, pseudogout, RA and osteoarthritis. Extra-articular causes such as ruptured or dislocated tendons, muscle spasm, tendon inflammation or shortening, or subchondral bony fractures are perhaps even more common causes of loss of motion.

Abnormal motion of joints should also be noted. The subchondral bony collapse of the medial tibial plateau, so common in osteoarthritis of the knee, produces a genu varus deformity and an abnormal lateral

FIG. 4–2. Normal range of motion of all joints is shown graphically. MCP = Metacarpophalangeal; PIP = proximal interphalangeal; DIP = distal interphalangeal; IP = interphalangeal. (Chart designed by Dr. J. Kenneth Herd in 1965 at Buffalo Children's Hospital and S.U.N.Y. at Buffalo.)

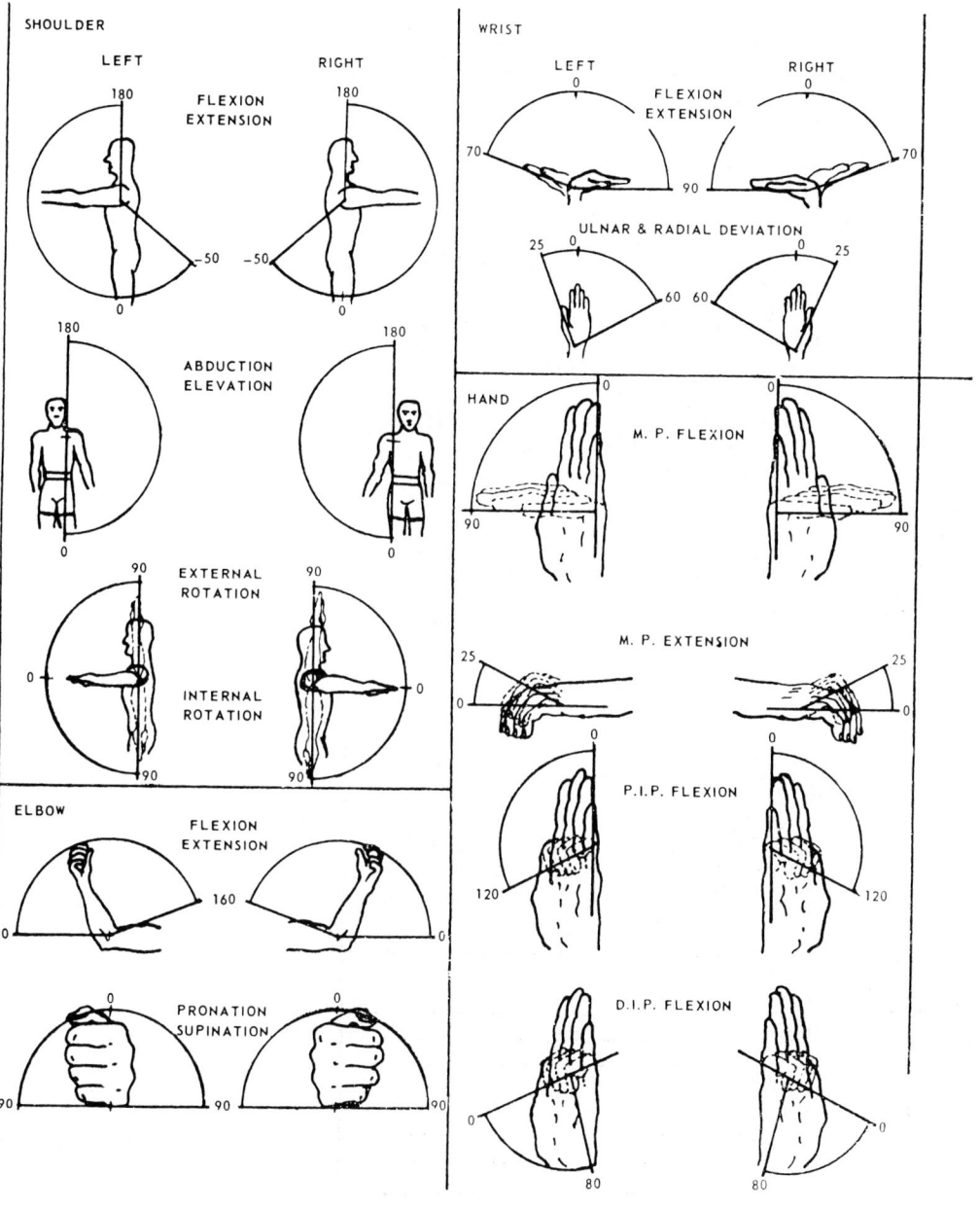

FIG. 4–2 (continued).

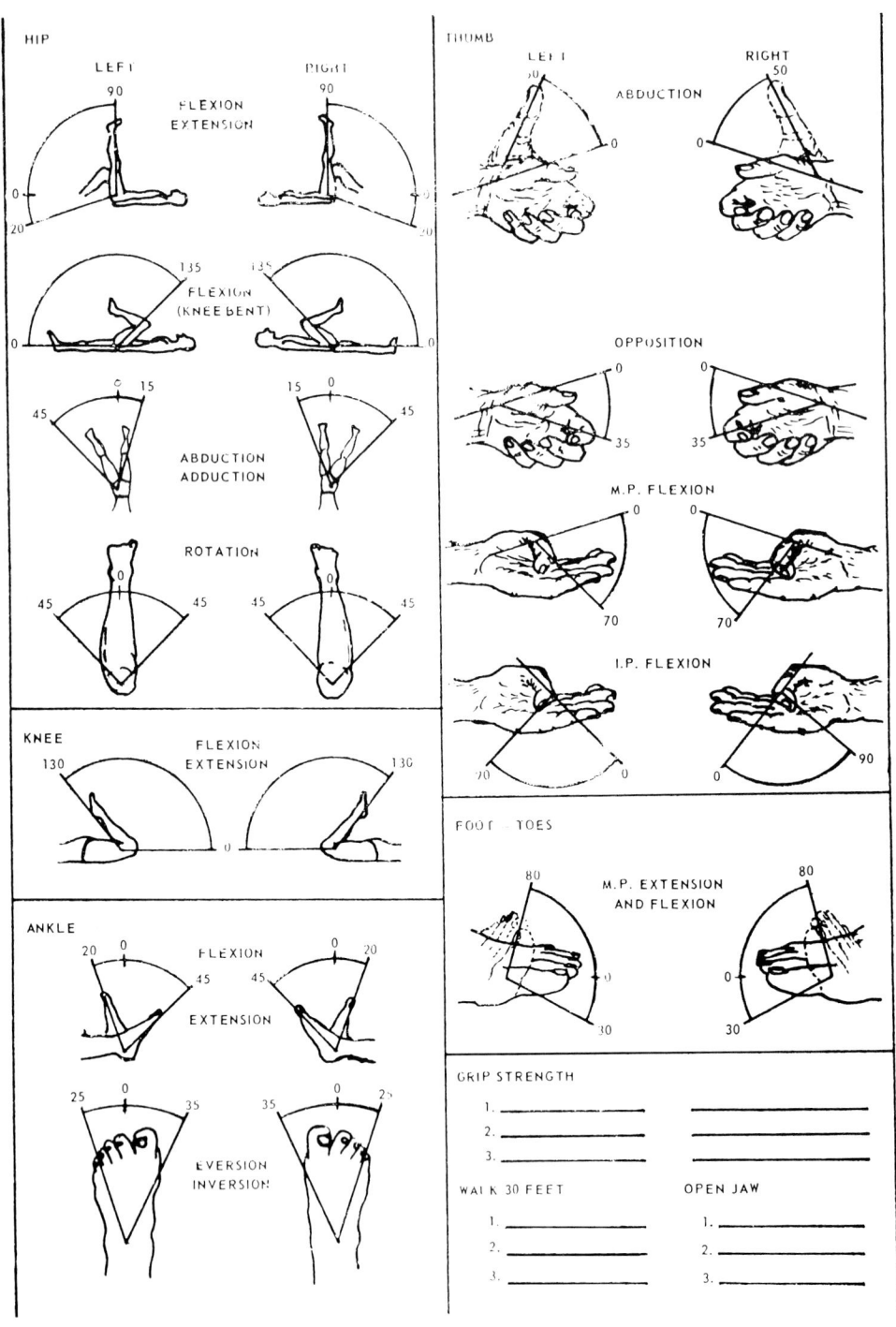

motion of the unstable knee owing to the slack in the medial collateral ligament. Early loss of lateral stability of the knee should be determined while the knee is flexed to about 25°. Except in carpal or tarsal joints, RA is apt to result in unstable, not fused, joints. Three common examples are the valgus and flexion deformities of laterally unstable knees, sliding atlantoaxial joints, and abnormal lateral motion of the second metacarpophalangeal (MCP) joint owing to erosion and rupture of its medial collateral ligament. These deformities should be looked for with the joint flexed to 90°, which stretches the collateral ligaments to tautness. Occasionally, in osteoarthritis, one knee develops a varus, and the other a valgus, deformity, resulting in a "windswept" appearance.

SWELLING

Swelling of joints, bursae, and tendons is an important sign that is always abnormal. Unlike tenderness, swelling specifically indicates organic disease. Swelling is most often due to underlying inflammation and can be due to synovial thickening, increased volume of joint fluid, or local edema. Detection of synovial thickening requires a knowledge of the anatomic synovial reflexions. Joints that lie just under the skin such as the knee, elbow, wrist, MCP, proximal and distal interphalangeal (PIP and DIP), and metatarsophalangeal (MTP) joints, are particularly suitable. If a "pad" of thickened tissue is felt, particularly in multiple areas, synovium is probably thickened owing either to inflammatory proliferation or to storage of abnormal material such as amyloid. The synovia of tendons frequently share in the proliferative process, leading to detectable swelling in the hand with bulging of palmar fat between the tendons (Fig. 4–3). Swelling of the synovium of the MTP joints

FIG. 4–3. Thickening of the synovium of the flexor digitorum tendons can be felt easily. Displaced tissues produce abnormal bulging between the tendons in the palm.

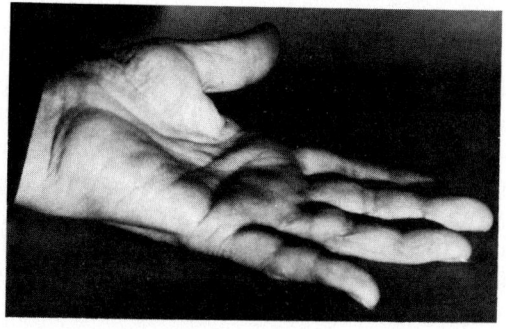

FIG. 4–4. Synovial thickening of the metatarsophalangeal joints spreads the forefoot, separating the toes, and producing the "window sign."

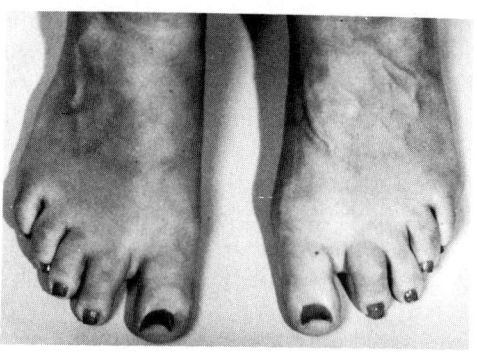

leads to abnormal separation of the toes—the "window" sign (Fig. 4–4). Synovial thickening in a tendon sheath, common in Reiter's syndrome or psoriatic arthritis, produces a "sausage finger" or "sausage toe" appearance. In general synovial swelling is most pronounced on extensor surfaces of joints where the capsule is more distensible.

Effusions are particularly common in large weight-bearing joints with distensible communicating bursae. Thus, fluid is often found in the knee, is less common in hip or ankle with their tighter joint capsules, and is much less common in upper-extremity joints, where the presence of detectable fluid is related directly to joint size. Fluid is often present in shoulder joints of patients with RA, but these joints are involved in relatively few patients. The wrist has a tight capsule, and fluid rarely is obtained unless the joint is intensely inflamed. Fluid is rarely, if ever, obtained from small hand joints. The importance of detecting fluid lies in its great diagnostic value. (See Chapters 5 and 39 for the techniques of arthrocentesis and synovianalysis.)

Osteophytes also produce a swollen appearance and are easily palpable along the margins of joints or parts of joints that lie just under the skin, such as the MTP, knee, PIP, and DIP joints. These are hard to the touch and may be tender. They are often more striking on clinical than on radiologic examination.

Nodular swellings felt over joints or areas exposed to repeated trauma—such as the olecranon, back of the head or heel, the ischial tuberosity, the external ear, and bridge of the nose in persons wearing eyeglasses—may be due to rheumatoid nodules, gouty tophi, or (rarely) xanthomata or amyloid masses. Clinically, a nodule is only a nodule until its contents are examined microscopically. Most "nodules" over rheumatoid finger joints turn out to be synovium herniated through defects in the joint capsule. Such herniae are usually reducible. Tendon nodules often occur in RA, systemic lupus, and rheumatic fever.

Skin Temperature. Increased warmth of skin overlying an inflamed deeper structure, sometimes accompanied by erythema in those individuals with relatively little skin pigment, is common and nonspecific. Differences between the temperature of the skin over an inflamed part and the surrounding skin can be estimated to within ±0.5°C using the *back* of the fingers. This determination is most helpful over large joints for obvious reasons. Unlike tenderness, which is a sensitive parameter because normal structures have none, increased warmth is inherently insensitive because normal parts are normally warm. It is more difficult to be certain of an increase of 0.5° C on a background temperature of 32°C than it is to feel secure that a PIP joint is tender when other PIP joints in the same hand are not.

Crepitus. Crepitus (noise) may be hard or, more often, felt as the joints are put through a range of motion. The coarse crackle in the joints of some individuals is of no pathologic significance. This noise is due to tendons snapping over bony prominences or perhaps to the "cracking" phenomenon (see Chapter 11). Generally, the finer the crepitus, the more significant it is clinically. Crepitus can be felt frequently, even when no noise is heard, as a fine vibratory sensation. Crepitus can arise from the grating of roughened cartilages against one another, or from bone rubbing against bone, as in advanced osteoarthritis.

A peculiar, fine crepitus can often be felt or heard when a chronically involved rheumatoid joint is moved, especially when loaded, such as in knees or hips on weight-bearing. This crepitus is presumably due to friction between destroyed articular cartilages. It always occurs in joints showing severe generalized cartilage loss radiographically and has been likened to the rubbing together of two sheets of old parchment. Extensive fibrin deposition in certain kinds of trauma or inflammation often gives rise to tendon crepitus. Thus, the patient with scleroderma may generate much noise while on the stairs, and the Achilles tendons of the weekend golfing enthusiast may audibly rebel on Monday. Typically, the latter types of crepitus are prominent after rest and diminish with repetitive movement. They are detected easily by the first, but not the last, student to examine the patient. Some idea of the integrity of the articular cartilages can be obtained by rubbing the distal part of a joint against the firmly anchored proximal part. The patella can be rubbed up and down in its groove as the patient lies supine with the quadriceps muscle relaxed.

The humeral head can be grated against the glenoid with the scapula held firmly by the examiner's other hand. The MTP, PIP, and first carpometacarpal (CMC) joint surfaces can be rubbed together at the same time that stability, range of motion, and tenderness are checked. Thus, the examiner can determine the extent of inflammation that is present and its long-term sequelae: deformity, instability, and cartilage damage.

The mechanism of knuckle cracking has been examined.[6] This phenomenon is due to mechanical subluxation of the joint, with gas formation in the joint due to the accompanying great decrease in intra-articular pressure. The subsequent vaporization of joint fluid releases enough free energy to produce an audible "crack." Once cracked, a knuckle cannot be cracked again until the gas has been absorbed and the increased space between the bone returns to normal. This process takes about 30 minutes.

WEAKNESS

Atrophy of muscle, especially the extensors, occurs rapidly about an inflamed or injured joint. Such a joint is almost always flexed to midposition, the position of maximum comfort. Muscle strength can be quantified readily by measuring grip with an appropriately rolled blood pressure cuff and by timing a repetitive action involving lower-extremity muscles.[3] It is often helpful to measure the circumference of the limb at a measured distance above or below a fixed point, such as the olecranon process or patella. Serial measurement provides a method to monitor an exercise program designed to restore missing muscle bulk.

SPECIFIC RHEUMATOLOGIC EXAMINATION

Each clinician should develop a standard, disciplined routine examination of the musculoskeletal system just as for the abdominal or chest examination. The approach may differ among individual physicians, but it should be the same for a given clinician each time he lays hands on a patient. This routine can easily be integrated into the general examination, reference to which is omitted for the sake of brevity in the following description. Particular attention is given to sites about which the patient specifically complains or those having abnormalities of which the patient is often unaware.

I start at the top with the temporomandibular joints, commonly involved in RA, but almost never in gout. Press over the joint, which lies just below the zygomatic arch in front of the ear. The joint can also be felt by placing a finger in the external auditory canal. Ask the patient to open wide and then bite. The space between the front teeth should accommodate two to three fingers. Next the range of motion of the cervical spine is examined. Have the patient touch the chin to both shoulders (rotation). Then, with the patient's nose kept in the midline, have him attempt to touch first one shoulder and then the other with his ear (lateral flexion). He should then place the chin to the chest, and then extend the neck as far as possible. The inion process of the occiput should come within three finger-breadths of the spinous process of C7. The usual "fibrositic" areas in the neck are pressed at the same time. Arthritic conditions generally produce limitation of rotation or lateral flexion before limitation of flexion or extension occurs. If these last motions are disproportionately restricted, or if they are more painful than attempted lateral flexion or rotation, a lesion affecting the spinal cord itself, rather than the cervical nerve roots, should be suspected.

Next, apply pressure with the thumb over the acromioclavicular (AC) and sternoclavicular (SC) joints, which are also examined for synovial thickening. Both are commonly affected by RA, and the AC joints often develop osteoarthritic changes. The sternomanubrial cleft and the costal cartilages are next compressed, and the chest expansion measured as an index of costovertebral motion. The lateral motion of the spine is determined as the patient sits. The shoulder joints are then put through a full range of motion, always testing abduction by holding the scapula down with one hand.

The cartilages of the humeral head and glenoid are rubbed together, the fibrous capsule is felt, and the supraspinatus and bicipital tendons are compressed. The last can be "twanged" like a bowstring as it lies in the bicipital groove. The extension of the elbows is next examined, and these joints are examined for synovial thickening. The olecranon and proximal ulna are palpated for bursal enlargement and for lumps that might suggest tophi, rheumatoid nodules, xanthoma, or amyloid deposits.

The wrist is put through a range of motion and examined for synovial thickening and extensor tenosynovitis or deQuervain's tenosynovitis (extensor tendons of thumb). The radiocarpal joint, the carpal joints and the ulnar bursa (distal radioulnar joint and contiguous bursa over the distal ulna) are each pressed separately for tenderness. The integrity of the distal radioulnar joint, often eroded by RA with dorsal displacement of the ulna, is assessed. The abnormal vertical motion of the distal ulna has been likened to that of a piano key—thus the "piano key" sign. The MCP joints are pressed together laterally and are then checked separately if any tenderness is elicited. Synovial thickening, range of motion, instability, and cartilage integrity are checked. Tenderness, swelling, and range of motion of all PIP and DIP joints, and of the IP, MCP, and first carpometacarpal joints of the

---

Table 4–3. Differential Diagnosis of Inflammatory Monarthritis

A. *Crystal-induced*

   1. Gout—man, lower extremity, previous attack, nocturnal onset, precipitated by medical illness or surgical procedures, response to colchicine, hyperuricemia, sodium urate crystals in joint fluid with neutrophils predominating, and WBC 10,000 to 60,000/mm³.

   2. Pseudogout—elderly patient, knee or other large joint, previous attack, precipitated by medical illness or surgical procedure, flexion contractures, chondrocalcinosis on radiography, calcium pyrophosphate dihydrate crystals in joint fluid with neutrophils predominating, and WBC 5,000 to 60,000/mm³.

   3. Calcific tendonitis or equivalent—extra-articular, tendon or capsule of larger joints, previous attack same or other area, calcification on radiography, chalky or milky material aspirated from area, neutrophils with phagocytosed ovoid bodies microscopically.

B. *Palindromic rheumatism*

   Middle-aged or elderly man, sudden onset, little systemic reaction, previous attacks, may be positive rheumatoid factors, little or no residual chronic joint inflammation, olecranon bursal enlargement.

C. *Infectious arthritis*

   1. Septic—severe inflammation, primary septic focus, drug or alcohol abuse, joint fluid with neutrophils predominating, WBC 50,000 to 300,000/mm³ (pus), infectious agents identified on smear and culture, or bacterial antigens identified in joint fluid.

   2. Tubercular—primary focus elsewhere, drug or alcohol abuse, marked joint swelling for long period, joint fluid with neutrophils predominating, acid-fast organisms on smear and culture.

   3. Fungal—similar to tuberculosis.

   4. Viral—antecedent or concomitant systemic viral illness, joint fluid can be of inflammatory or noninflammatory type, either mononuclear cells or neutrophils may predominate.

D. *Other*

   1. Tendonitis—as in A.3, but without radiologic calcification, antecedent trauma including repetitive motion.

   2. Bursitis—as above, but inflamed area is more diffuse, antecedent trauma.

   3. Juvenile rheumatoid arthritis—one or both knees swollen in preteen or teenager without systemic reaction, no erosions, mildly inflammatory joint fluid with some neutrophils, and no depression in synovial fluid $C'H_{50}$ levels.

Table 4–4.   Differential Diagnosis of Inflammatory Polyarthritis

A. *Rheumatoid arthritis* (RA)

    1. Seropositive—female patient, symmetrical joint and tendon involvement, synovial thickening, joint inflammation "in phase," nodules, weakness, systemic reaction, erosions on radiogram, rheumatoid factor present, $C'H_{50}$ level depressed in joint fluid that has 5,000 to 30,000 WBC/mm³, about 50 to 80% neutrophils; possible occurrence in children.

    2. Seronegative—either sex, symmetrical joint and tendon involvement, joint inflammation "in phase," more bony reaction radiographically (sclerosis, osteophytes, fusion, periostitis), rheumatoid factor absent, $C'H_{50}$ not depressed in joint fluid that has 3,000 to 20,000 WBC/mm³, about 20 to 60% neutrophils; more asymmetric than in seropositive cases; some cases probably are adult JRA.

B. *Collagen-vascular disease*

    1. Systemic lupus erythematosus—female patient, symmetric joint distribution identical to RA, hair loss, mucosal lesions, rash, systemic reaction, visceral organ or brain involvement, leukopenia, positive STS, no erosions radiographically, noninflammatory joint fluid with good viscosity and mucin clot and 1,000 to 2,000 WBC/mm³, mostly small lymphocytes; serum $C'H_{50}$ often depressed, antinuclear antibody (ANA) titer elevated, antinative human DNA antibody titer increased, anti-Sm antibody increased; anti SSA (Ro) subset (subacute cutaneous lupus).

    2. Scleroderma—tight skin, Raynaud's, resorption of digits, dysphagia, constipation, lung, heart or kidney involvement, symmetric tendon contractures, little or no synovial thickening, radiographic calcinosis circumscripta, positive ANA with speckled or nucleolar pattern, anti SCL-70 (systemic) and anti-centromere antibodies (CREST syndrome).

    3. Polymyositis (dermatomyositis)—proximal muscle weakness in pelvic and pectoral girdles, tender muscles, rash, typical nailbed and knuckle pad erythema, symmetric joint involvement, EMG showing combined myopathic and denervation pattern, muscle biopsy abnormal, elevated serum creatinine phosphokinase.

    4. Mixed connective tissue disease—swollen hands, Raynaud's, tight skin, symmetric joint and tendon involvement, possible evidence of joint erosions radiographically, positive ANA speckled pattern, anti-RNP antibody increased, strong response to corticosteroid therapy in anti-inflammatory doses.

    5. Polyarteritis nodosa—symmetric involvement, diverse clinical picture of systemic disease, histologic or angiographic diagnosis.

C. *Rheumatic fever*

    Young (2 to 40 yrs patient), sore throat, Gp A streptococci, migratory arthritis, rash, pancarditis or pericardial involvement, elevated ASO titers, joint inflammation responds dramatically to aspirin treatment, often no cardiac findings in adults.

D. *Juvenile rheumatoid arthritis*

    Symmetric joint involvement, rash, fever, absence of rheumatoid factor, radiographic periostitis, erosions late, possibly beginning or recurring in an adult. ANA-positive pauciarticular girls may develop iridocyclitis; B27-positive boys with possible fusion of sacroiliac and spinal joints.

E. *Psoriatic arthritis*

    Asymmetric boggy joint and tendon swelling, skin or nail lesions not always prominent or may follow arthritis, DIP joints may be prominently involved, radiologic periostitis or erosions, no rheumatoid factor, $C'H_{50}$ usually not depressed in inflammatory joint fluid with neutrophilic predominance.

F. *Reiter's syndrome* (reactive arthritis)

    Male patient, sexually deviant or promiscuous, urethritis, iritis, conjunctivitis, asymmetric joints, lower extremity, nonpainful mucous membrane ulcerative lesion, balanitis circinata, keratodermia blenorrhagica, weight loss, $C'H_{50}$ increased in serum and in joint fluid with 5,000 to 30,000 WBC/mm³; macrophages in joint fluid with 3 to 5 phagocytosed neutrophils ("Reiter's" cell); possible sequela of enteric infections or urethritis; syndrome may be incomplete and may affect females.

G. *Gonorrheal arthritis*

    Migratory arthritis or tenosynovitis finally settling in one or more joints or tendons, either sex, primary focus urethra, female genitourinary tract, rectum or oropharynx, skin lesions, vesicles, gram-negative diplococci on smear but not on culture of vesicular fluid, positive culture at primary site, blood, or joint fluid.

H. *Polymyalgia rheumatica*

    Elderly patient (>50 yrs), symmetric pelvic or pectoral girdle complaints without loss of strength, morning stiffness of long duration, prominent fatigue, weight loss, possible joint involvement, especially of shoulders, sternoclavicular joint, knees; sedimentation rate elevated, fibrinogen and alpha 2 and gamma globulin elevation, anemia, complete response to low doses (10 to 20 mg) prednisone, serum CPK normal, elevated alkaline phosphatase (liver).

I. *Crystal-induced*

    1. Monosodium urate (MSU) crystals (gout)—symmetric arthritis, flexion contractures, prior history of acute attacks, tophi, out-of-phase joint inflammation, systemic corticosteroid treatment for "RA," hyperuricemia, MSU crystals in joint fluid.

    2. Calcium pyrophosphate dihydrate (CPPD) crystals (pseudogout)—symmetric arthritis, MCP flexion contractures, as well as of wrist, elbow, shoulder, hips, knees, and ankles, prior acute attacks (sometimes), out-of-phase joint inflammation, CPPD crystals in joint fluid.

    3. Basic calcium phosphate (BCP) crystals (Milwaukee shoulder).

J. *Other*

    Amyloid arthropathy, peripheral arthritis of inflammatory bowel disease, tuberculosis, SBE, viral or spirochetal arthritis.

Table 4–5. Differential Diagnosis of Inflammatory Spondyloarthropathy*

A. *Ankylosing spondylitis*—male patient, symmetric sacroiliitis clinically and radiologically, limitation of spinal motion, uveitis, smooth symmetric spinal ligamentous calcification, ankylosis (often complete), absence of skip areas, family history, HLA-B27 antigen usually present, good response to nonsteroidal anti-inflammatory drugs (NSAIDs).

B. *Reiter's syndrome*—sexually promiscuous or deviant man with urethritis, skin-eye-heel, asymmetric peripheral joint involvement, sacroiliitis often asymmetric and "skip" areas of involvement in spine, coarse asymmetric syndesmophytes in spine, incomplete and asymmetric ankylosis, HLA-B27 often present, equivocal response to NSAIDs.

C. *Psoriatic spondylitis*—skin or peripheral joint involvement, asymmetric sacroiliitis, skip areas, possible ankylosis, HLA-B27 often present.

D. *Inflammatory bowel disease*—sacroiliitis, often symmetric, ankylosis, possibly silent bowel disease, spinal inflammation: unlike peripheral arthritis, does not vary with and is not responsive to treatment directed at bowel inflammation; HLA-B27 often present.

E. *Other*—infection (bacterial, tuberculous, fungal), osteochondritis, multiple epiphysitis in young adult.

*JRA spondyloarthropathy occurs almost entirely in HLA-B27-positive boys and is regarded as juvenile ankylosing spondylitis.

thumb are assessed. The hand is turned over and is examined for palmar erythema, palmar thickening, and Dupuytren's contracture. Each tendon is compressed and is felt for thickening when the finger has been fully extended. The flexor carpi radialis and flexor carpi ulnaris tendons are next compressed.

With the patient supine, each hip is flexed, abducted, and externally rotated (Patrick's maneuver). If a flexion contraction is suspected, the opposite hip is held in full flexion to flatten fully the lumbar lordosis, and the hip in question is fully extended. This maneuver prevents disguise of the flexion deformity by an increased lumbar lordosis. The hip joint is compressed from above, and then the tensor fasciae latae and trochanteric bursa are compressed from the side.

The range of motion of the knee is determined. The condition of the quadriceps, presence of synovial thickening, foreign bodies, fluid, warmth, osteophytes, stability, and cartilage integrity, especially of the patellofemoral compartment, are determined. Popliteal cysts are sought, and the fat pads under the patellar tendons are compressed. The ankles and subtalar joints are examined separately, as are the posterior and anterior tibialis and peroneal tendons. Synovial thickening at the ankle is often difficult to determine because of the normal increase in the periarticular tissues here in middle age and beyond, especially in women.

The tarsal joints are compressed as a group. The MTP joints are squeezed together laterally and are examined separately if any tenderness ensues. The first MTP joint is felt for osteophytes, range of motion, and cartilage integrity. The bunion bursa and sesamoids in the flexor hallucis tendon are examined. The latter is an extremely common site of symptomatic osteoarthritis, perhaps even more common than the patellofemoral compartment. The position of the metatarsal fat pad, nature's metatarsal support, is checked. This pad often slides forward under the toes in RA and leaves the swollen metatarsal heads just under the skin. The toes are next examined for ankylosis, and for "cock-up" or hammer deformities.

Table 4–6. Differential Diagnosis of Degenerative or Metabolic Arthropathy

A. *Primary generalized "nodal" osteoarthritis*
Heberden's nodes DIP joints, Bouchard's nodes PIP joints, arthritis of first CMC, knee, first MTP joints, symmetric, familial, no systemic reaction, Gp 1 joint fluid.
Variants
1. Erosive osteoarthritis—same but with more inflammatory features; possible bony ankylosis.
2. Localized osteoarthritis of DIP, first CMC, first MTP, other joints.

B. *"Non-nodal" osteoarthritis*
1. Osteoarthritis localized to one or (usually) both knees—flexion and varus deformities in middle-aged or elderly patient, Gp 1 joint fluid, subchondral microfractures with collapse of the medial tibial plateau; predominant involvement of medial tibiofemoral compartment.
2. Primary osteoarthritis of hip—(a) unilateral—superior joint space narrowing, long leg on ipsilateral side; (b) bilateral—medial joint space narrowing with medial migration of femoral heads, equal leg lengths.
3. Secondary osteoarthritis—any joint, traumatic origin, slipped epiphysis, mechanical problem, congenital malformation, another antecedent arthritis.
4. Osteoarthritis associated with CPPD or BCP crystals. Symmetric involvement, elderly patient, flexion contractures of joints listed in Table 4–4, prior acute attacks, associated metabolic diseases, familial incidence; lateral tibiofemoral and patellofemoral compartments often predominant.

C. *Metabolic*
Diffuse or localized musculoskeletal complaints in patient with endocrine or metabolic disease.

Foot deformities such as pes cavus or pes planus are noted with the patient standing. The spine is examined as already described.

Each of these areas can be examined in greater detail if necessary, with abnormalities pinpointed to specific ligaments, bursae, and tendons. The reader is referred to the excellent monograph by Polley and Hunder for further details on the clinical examination.[7]

DATA SYNTHESIS AND DIFFERENTIAL DIAGNOSIS

The mind of the clinician stores data in much the same way as a computer, but it also does more. It weighs each datum and weighs each datum differently in each individual. When one is writing about this process, generalizations must be made, but in full recognition of the more subtle analysis actually made in real life. The relative weights of the various signs and symptoms have been indicated in a general way in the foregoing descriptions.

The general category within which a patient's problem falls is usually obvious from the history and physical examination. To pinpoint the diagnosis, however, laboratory examination, including gross and microscopic joint fluid analysis, radiologic study, specialized tests and, occasionally, biopsy for ordinary or special microscopy, are indicated.

If the process is inflammatory, the diagnostic possibilities differ according to whether it is confined to one joint or is polyarticular and whether it affects the axial (spine, shoulders, hips) or the appendicular (peripheral) joints. The differential diagnosis of some representative common inflammatory conditions is given in Table 4–3 for monarthritis, Table 4–4 for polyarthritis, Table 4–5 for inflammatory spondyloarthropathy, and Table 4–6 for degenerative arthropathy. Such brief vignettes of findings are necessarily superficial and incomplete and are offered here with some diffidence. These tables may be of use to medical students and house staff in their earliest encounters with arthritic patients.

REFERENCES

1. A.R.A. Committee on Rheumatologic Practice: A description of rheumatology practice. Arthritis Rheum., 20:1278–1281, 1977.
2. Wright, V., and Johns, R.J.: Observations on the measurement of joint stiffness. Arthritis Rheum., 3:328–340, 1960.
3. Csuka, M.E., and McCarty, D.J.: A rapid method for measurement of lower extremity muscle strength. Am. J. Med., 78:77–81, 1985.
4. McCarty, D.J., Gatter, R.A., and Phelps, P.: A dolorimeter for quantification of articular tenderness. Arthritis Rheum., 8:551–559, 1965.
5. McCarty, D.J., Gatter, R.A., and Steele, A.D.: A twenty pound dolorimeter for quantification of articular tenderness. Arthritis Rheum., 11:696–698, 1968.
6. Unsworth, A., Dowson, D., and Wright, V.: "Cracking joints." Ann. Rheum. Dis., 30:348–358, 1971.
7. Polley, H.F., and Hunder, G.G.: Rheumatologic Interviewing and Physical Examination of the Joints, 2nd Ed. Philadelphia, W.B. Saunders, 1978.

5

SYNOVIAL FLUID

DANIEL J. McCARTY

Paracelsus called joint fluid *synovia* (like egg).[1] "Synovial fluid" is an often used redundancy for this clear, sticky liquid reminiscent of egg white. The *synovium* is the tissue lining the joint space containing synovia. It terminates at the margin of the articular cartilage and is supported by a dense fibrous joint capsule, much as the pia mater and arachnoid are supported by the fibrous dura mater about the brain. It is richly supplied with both blood vessels and lymphatics. Synovia is a dialysate of blood plasma into which hyaluronate, a glycosaminoglycan of high molecular weight, is secreted by the synoviocytes (synovial lining cells). These are normally arranged in a layer only 1 to 3 cells thick, embedded in ground substance but with no basement membrane. The synovium is not a true membrane, but a modified tissue space.[2]

Synovia may be obtained readily from the larger joints by arthrocentesis, described in detail in Chapter 39. Even with strict aseptic technique, probably some bacteria are introduced into the joint with every needle thrust through the skin. Leukocyte accumulation in canine joint fluid was greatly reduced if the skin was first cut and the needle thrust through sterile subcutaneous tissues exposed by spreading the wound.[3] A critical number of bacteria had to be inoculated before rabbit joints could be infected experimentally.[4] This probably also applies to human joints.

It is also impossible to thrust a needle through the vascular synovium, especially an inflamed synovium, without rupturing at least a few capillaries with subsequent micro-bleeding into the joint fluid. Thus, at least a few erythrocytes are seen in every aspirated joint fluid. Some may have entered the joint fluid by diapedesis through synovial capillaries secondary to the underlying disease, but some almost certainly are due to the needling itself. The greatest danger of joint infection from arthrocentesis lies in the inoculation of bacteria from the blood during bacteremia (see Chapter 39).

Information about various arthritic diseases and systemic rheumatic diseases with prominent joint involvement has been gained by gross, microscopic, and laboratory analyses of the synovia. Most of this information is pertinent to the contemporary practice of rheumatology and is the primary focus of this chapter. Other data, of only theoretical interest at this time, will be discussed briefly. A practical handbook of joint fluid analysis is available.[5]

Samples of the synovium may be obtained by the use of needles adapted to hollow organ biopsy, such as the Cope, or needles specifically designed for joints, such as the Parker-Pearson, the Williamson-Holt, or the Polley-Bickel. I have used all three, but the Polley-Bickel has proved most satisfactory because larger samples of tissue and a full-thickness specimen, including the articular capsule, are obtained. Synovial biopsy is of less practical value than aspiration of synovia (actually a "liquid biopsy") but may be helpful in the diagnosis of granulomatous diseases, tumors, and in clinical research.

Biopsy of synovium or articular cartilage in large joints such as the knee and shoulder by direct vision through an arthroscope has been performed in many centers. Technical improvements may extend the range of this procedure to smaller joints, gradually supplanting the need for open surgical biopsy.

The structure and function of the synovium, including joint lubrication by the synovia, are covered in Chapters 10 and 11.

SYNOVIANALYSIS

The term synovianalysis was originally coined to indicate an analogy with urinalysis.[6] Tests on synovia are at least as important in the differential diagnosis of joint disease as are those on the urine in urinary tract disease. The types of routine and special tests that may be useful are listed in Table 5–1.

GROSS ANALYSIS

The gross analysis of joint fluid is an office or bedside procedure. Its purpose is to divide a given fluid into one of five groups: normal, noninflammatory (group I of Ropes and Bauer),[2] inflammatory (group II), purulent, or hemorrhagic. A specific diagnosis is rarely made from gross analysis alone. Table 5–2 provides normal joint fluid values for selected items. Normal fluid is often difficult to obtain; it is scant and viscous. The normal knee joint—the body's largest—contains only a few drops to a maximum of 4 ml. Although normal, postmortem, and traumatic fluids

Table 5–1. Synovianalysis: Types of Studies

A. *Routine*
  1. Gross analysis
    a. Amount
    b. Color
    c. Clarity
    d. Viscosity
    e. "Mucin" clot
  2. Microscopic
    a. Leukocyte concentration
    b. Differential leukocyte count
    c. Wet smear inspection by polarized and phase contrast microscopy
B. *Special*
  1. Microbiologic
    a. Culture for bacteria, fungi, viruses, or tubercle bacilli
    b. Countercurrent immunoelectrophoresis for microbial antigens
  2. Serologic
    a. Hemolytic complement titration ($C'H_{50}$)
    b. Complement components (C_3 and C_4) by immunodiffusion
  3. Chemical
    a. Glucose
    b. Protein
    c. Enzymes

Table 5–2. Normal Synovial Fluid Values*

	Range	Mean
pH	7.3–7.43	7.38
WBC/cmm	13–180	63
Differential WBC (%)		
polymorphonuclear	0–25	7
lymphocytes	0–78	24
monocytes	0–71	48
clasmatocytes	0–26	10
synovial lining cells	0–12	4
Total protein g/dl	1.2–3.0	1.8
albumin (%)	56 –63	60
globulin (%)	37 –44	40
Hyaluronate g/dl		0.3

*Values represent combined data from various reports; references summarized in 7b.

are somewhat similar, protein concentrations are sufficiently increased in the latter two that they cannot be studied as substitutes for normal fluid. A partial list of the diseases producing fluids of the various groups is in Table 5–3. The noninflammatory or only mild inflammatory character of fluid from joints affected with very early rheumatoid arthritis is surprising and important.[7] Some bacterial arthritis presents group II rather than frankly purulent effusions, although I have listed them here only in the latter group. The range of values found for the various tests in each group is given in Table 5–4.

Normal fluid in increased amounts is found in the knee in myxedema, congestive heart failure, anasarca, or other conditions causing tissue edema. Fluid transudation into the joint space occurs as into any other tissue space. Transient, asymptomatic, noninflammatory synovial effusions may accompany high-dose corticosteroid therapy.[7a] Such effusions generally have cell counts within the normal range.

Although it is often possible to obtain a large volume of joint fluid, only a few drops are needed for the most useful tests. Only one drop or less (about 0.05 ml) is needed for bacteriologic culture, for a total leukocyte count, for Wright's staining, and for a wet preparation to look for crystals and other particulates. If phase-contrast microscopy is available, the predominant type of leukocyte may be determined, their concentration and morphology estimated, and particulates studied all with one drop of fluid! Almost any joint that is inflamed and anatomically accessible will yield a drop of fluid after skillful puncture.

Clot Formation. Normal synovial fluid does not clot because it lacks fibrinogen as well as prothrombin, factors V and VII, tissue thromboplastin, and antithrombin.[8] Most pathologic fluids do clot, however, and the rapidity of clotting and the size of the clot are roughly proportional to the severity of inflam-

Table 5–3. Examples of Diseases Producing Fluids of Different Groups

Noninflammatory (Group I)	Inflammatory† (Group II)	Purulent†† (Group III)	Hemorrhagic (Group IV)
Osteoarthritis	Rheumatoid arthritis	Bacterial infections	Trauma, especially fracture
Early rheumatoid arthritis	Reiter's syndrome	Tuberculosis	Neuroarthropathy (Charcot joint)
Trauma	Crystal synovitis, acute (gout,		Blood dyscrasia (e.g., hemophilia)
Osteochondritis dissecans	pseudogout, other)		Tumor, especially pigmented
Osteonecrosis	Psoriatic arthritis		villonodular synovitis or
Osteochondromatosis	Arthritis of inflammatory bowel		hemangioma
Crystal synovitis; chronic or	disease		Chondrocalcinosis
subsiding acute (gout and	Viral arthritis		Anticoagulant therapy
pseudogout)	Rheumatic fever		Joint prostheses
*Systemic lupus erythematosus	Behçet's syndrome		Thrombocytosis
*Polyarteritis nodosa	Fat droplet synovitis		Sickle cell trait or disease
Scleroderma			Myeloproliferative disease
Amyloidosis (articular)			
Polymyalgia rheumatica			
High-dose corticosteroid therapy			

*May occasionally be inflammatory.

†As a disease in these groups remits, the exudate (fluid) passes through a group I phase before returning to normal.

mation. All fluids should be transferred immediately from the syringe used for aspiration into a tube containing heparin, 50 units per milliliter of joint fluid. Oxalated tubes should not be used because calcium oxalate crystals will form and, in the presence of leukocytes, will be phagocytosed, often leading to confusion.[9]

Color. Truly normal fluid is colorless, like water. It is likely that the diapedesis of red cells, accompanying even mild inflammation, and their subsequent breakdown release hemoglobin, the heme moiety of which is metabolized locally to bilirubin, giving a yellow (xanthochromic) color to the fluid. Cerebrospinal fluid becomes similarly xanthochromic after subarachnoid hemorrhage. The leukocytes render the fluid white, and the degree of whiteness is proportional to their concentration. Pus, containing 150,000 to 300,000 leukocytes/cmm, is characteristically cream-colored, the "off-white" being due to heme pigments or to chromogen from the invading bacteria. For example, *Staphylococcus aureus* adds some golden pigment and the saprophytic *Serratia marcescens*, a reddish hue. Gray synovial fluid containing 2,550 µg of lead/dl was ob-

tained from a hip joint of a patient with retained bullet fragments.[10]

A grossly bloody fluid may be due to a traumatic arthrocentesis, which is usually evident during the procedure when the fluid entering the syringe shows an uneven distribution of blood. Bleeding owing to trauma may decrease as aspiration continues or, more commonly, blood may appear for the first time in the syringe near the end of the procedure. A hematocrit reading should always be obtained on a truly bloody effusion to determine whether it is blood per se, or whether it is blood admixed with joint fluid. Even 5 to 10% admixture makes joint fluid look like whole blood. A truly bloody effusion, unlike that caused by a "bloody tap," often fails to clot.

The differential diagnosis of a bloody effusion is given in Table 5–3. If a joint swells *immediately* after trauma, aspiration reveals frank blood with a hematocrit and leukocyte count approaching, or even identical to, that of whole blood from the same patient. In the absence of an underlying bleeding disorder, such as hemophilia, a fracture into the joint must be assumed to be present, and appropriate radiographic

Table 5–4. Gross Analysis of Joint Fluid

Criteria	Normal	Noninflammatory (Group I)	Inflammatory (Group II)	Purulent (Group III)
1. Volume (ml) (knee)	<4	often >4	often >4	often >4
2. Color	clear to pale yellow	xanthochromic	xanthochromic to white	white
3. Clarity	transparent	transparent	translucent to opaque	opaque
4. Viscosity	very high	high	low	very low, may be high with coagulase-positive staphylococcus
5. Mucin clot*	good	fair to good	fair to poor	poor
6. Spontaneous clot	none	often	often	often

*Recent effusions do not give firm clot because of serum admixture.

views should be obtained. Recurrent bleeding into a knee joint that appears normal on physical and radiologic examination between episodes is almost diagnostic of a hemangioma.[11]

Trauma, neuroarthropathy, bleeding disorders, and tumors are the most common causes of hemarthrosis, but chondrocalcinosis,[12,13] anticoagulant therapy,[14,15,16] joint prostheses,[17] thrombocytosis,[18] sickle cell trait,[19] and sickle cell disease[20] all have been described as rarer causes. Bone marrow in joint fluid, either fat droplets or blood-forming elements, is suggestive of a fracture into the joint, although fat droplets both free and within synovial fluid leukoyctes have been found in large number even in the absence of trauma.[21] Most fluids showing fat droplets have been obtained from traumatized joints.[22–24]

Patients with hemophilia and other coagulation defects are particularly prone to hemarthrosis (see Chapter 84), even after minor trauma.

Clarity. Normal joint fluids and those from joints affected with diseases that are fundamentally noninflammatory, such as osteoarthritis, are transparent. Ordinary newsprint can be read through a tube containing such fluid (Fig. 5–1A). Fluids with higher leukocyte counts from inflamed joints are opaque, and the degree of opacity is proportional to the leukocyte count.

Rarely, erythrocytes are present in sufficient number to given a cloudy, but not pink, fluid. These cells settle rapidly. Leukocytes also settle in joint fluid in vivo just as they do in a tube after aspiration.[25] Thus, both tube and joint must be inverted to mix their contents uniformly before samples are taken for counting cells. This important point has been ignored by many clinicians, and serious errors have occurred as a result. Fluids otherwise classified as group I may be opaque because of large numbers of monosodium urate (MSU), calcium pyrophosphate dihydrate (CPPD), basic calcium phosphate (BCP), cholesterol crystals, or fat droplets.

Viscosity. Normal and group I fluids are viscous owing to the high concentration of hyaluronate. Hyaluronate is degraded in some types of inflammatory joint disease (e.g., RA), and the viscosity is reduced appreciably. An approximation of viscosity, satisfactory for clinical purposes, can be obtained by watching the fall of a drop of fluid during transfer from aspirating syringe to glass tube. Viscous fluid "strings out" like molasses, often to a length of 10 cm or more (Fig. 5–1B). It strings out ("spinbarkheit") when a drop is compressed between thumb and index finger, which are then pulled apart suddenly (Fig. 5–1C). Fluids with reduced viscosity form a shorter string or even fall in discrete drops like water. More precise data can be obtained by using a viscometer[2] or by adapting an ordinary white blood cell diluting pipette,[26] but this is not necessary in everyday practice.

Mucin Clot. Although synovial fluid hyaluronic acid can be measured by several different techniques[27] the qualitative "mucin clot" test is the most practical. It estimates the degree of polymerization of hyaluronate sufficiently to classify clots as "good," "fair," or "poor." The supernatant from a *centrifuged* specimen is transferred to a clean glass tube. A few drops of

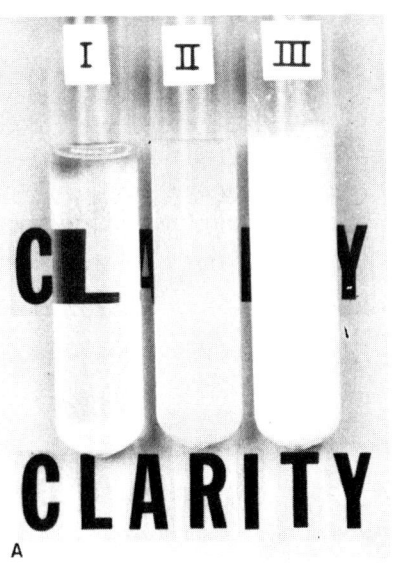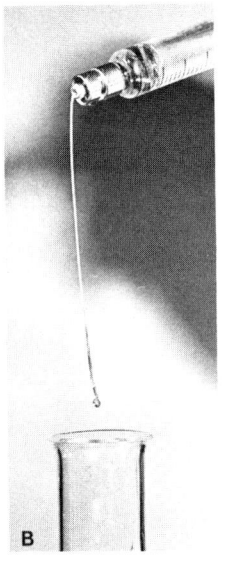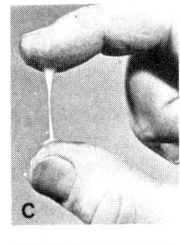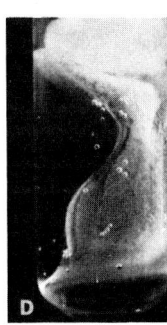

FIG. 5–1. *A,* Noninflammatory (group I), inflammatory (group II), and purulent (group III) joint fluids have been transferred to glass tubes. Group I fluids typically contain few leukocytes and are transparent, whereas fluids in groups II and III are opaque. *B,* Viscosity of a fluid can be judged by the length of "stringing" of a falling drop. This "string" is nearly 8 cm long and illustrates the relatively high viscosity of fluid from an osteoarthritic knee joint. *C,* Viscosity of joint fluid can also be tested like motor oil. The "stringing" of a drop as thumb and forefinger are separated is proportional to its viscosity. *D,* The dense white precipitate of protein hyaluronate developed after a few drops of glacial acetic acid were added to a tube containing nearly normal joint fluid. This "mucin clot" remained intact even after the tube was shaken (note bubbles), leading to its designation as "good."

glacial acetic acid are placed on the surface of the fluid. The heavier acid settles to the bottom of the tube, leaving a dense white precipitate of *protein hyaluronate* in its wake (Fig. 5–1D). This white clump of a "good" clot remains intact even when the tube is shaken.

An alternative method of producing a mucin clot, especially useful when the amount of fluid is limited, involves the addition of one part of whole joint fluid to four parts of 2% acetic acid (usually 1 to 4 ml). Fair and poor clots are shown in Figure 5–2. Prior use of hyaluronidase prevents the formation of even a poor clot.

The mechanism for the failure of most fluids from inflamed joints to form good mucin clots is not well understood. The higher than normal protein concentration, the presence in the protein-hyaluronate complex of inter-alpha trypsin inhibitor, and the lower degree of polymerization of the hyaluronate caused by its catabolism or by differences in its synthesis by the synoviocytes have all been invoked to explain it.[27]

Occasionally it is useful to reduce the viscosity of joint fluid to prepare a fluid for other tests. We have found that 1 mg (about 400 units) of testicular hyaluronidase* per milliliter of joint fluid reduces the viscosity approximately to that of serum after 30 minutes of incubation at 37° C.[28]

Analysis of Data. From the amount, color, and viscosity of the fluid and the mucin clot produced by acetic acid, a fluid can usually be classified into one of the five categories already described. No single gross measurement is of great significance or of di-

FIG. 5–2. "Mucin" clots can also be produced by adding one part of whole joint fluid to four parts of 2% acetic acid. A "fair" clot is seen on the left and a "poor" clot, composed of poorly formed shreds in a turbid solution, is in the middle. Treatment of the fluid shown in Figure 5–1D with hyaluronidase abolished mucin clot formation completely *(right)*.

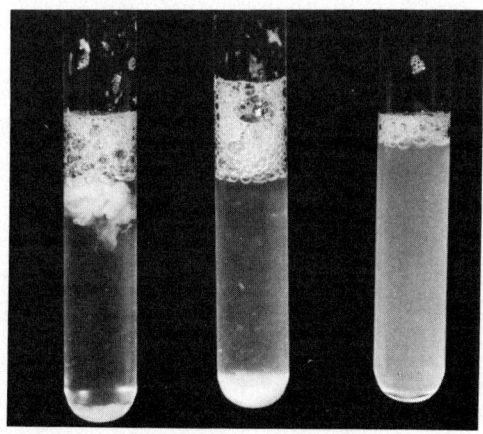

*Worthington Biochem.

agnostic importance per se. Septic, normal, and hemorrhagic fluids are easily distinguished. Most confusion arises in differentiating group I from group II. We sometimes speak of "group 1½." A pale-yellow, clear, highly viscous fluid producing a good mucin clot from a patient with symmetric polyarthritis is suggestive of lupus erythematosus rather than rheumatoid arthritis, for example.

Rheumatic fever is an example of a condition producing a group II fluid with good preservation of viscosity and mucin clot.[2] Group I effusions of recent onset can show reduced viscosity and mucin clot owing to serum admixture. As with all tests, joint fluid findings must be interpreted in light of the clinical picture.

MICROSCOPIC SYNOVIANALYSIS

Microscopic synovianalysis is also easily done in an office or outpatient clinic setting and requires an ordinary light microscope with oil immersion optics and a polarizing microscope equipped with a first-order red plate compensator.

Routine Cytology. A total leukocyte count is obtained on all group II or III fluids, just as for blood, except that care must be taken to thoroughly mix the contents of the tube before sampling to uniformly resuspend the cells. Cells also sediment in vivo. This finding is particularly evident in the presence of severe inflammation when the patient is supine for an extended period because of pain. The joint contents should be mixed by barbotage before a sample is taken for analysis. Some of the unexpected divergent synovial fluid leukocyte counts that have attracted attention might also be due to this phenomenon.[29] Normal saline (0.9 g/dl) must be used instead of acetic acid, or the bulk of the leukocytes will be entrapped in a mini-mucin clot. Erythrocytes will be lysed preferentially if hypotonic saline (0.3 g/dl) is used as diluent. This facilitates enumeration of leukocytes, which should be done at ×400 magnification.

A thin smear for leukocyte differential counting can be prepared on either a coverslip or a glass slide. For sharp detail, as one might wish for photography, it is best to treat the fluid with hyaluronidase before making the slide. It is rarely necessary to obtain total or differential leukocyte counts on group I fluids. If these are needed, the fluid can be centrifuged and the pellet resuspended in a smaller volume before smearing. Here again, pretreatment with hyaluronidase and the use of a cytocentrifuge are helpful.[30]

A summary of the findings in normal fluids and in those of groups I, II, and III appears in Table 5–5.

Table 5–5. Cytology of Joint Fluid

	Normal	*Gp I	Gp II	Gp III
Leukocytes cmm⁻¹	<150	<3,000	3,000–50,000	50,000–300,000
Polymorphonuclears (%)	<25	<25	>70	>90

*Group designations of Ropes and Bauer.[2]

Although total and differential leukocyte counts are nonspecific, they are useful in differential diagnosis between groups. If a fluid is grossly opaque, yellow-white, of reduced viscosity, and gives a poor mucin clot test, generally it shows, as expected, a high total leukocyte count with polymorphonuclear cell predominance. In general, small lymphocytes, monocytes, and macrophages (or synovial lining cells) make up the remainder of the leukocytes, and some of each can be found in most joint fluids. Normal human or bovine synovial fluid contains only a few leukocytes, and polymorphonuclear cells are difficult or even impossible to find (see Table 5–2),[2] but normal canine fluid contains a higher leukocyte count and polymorph percentage.[3]

Occasionally, an eosinophilic predominance is found in the differential leukocyte counts.[31–36] The differential diagnosis of synovial fluid eosinophilia is given in Table 5–6. The association with acute or chronic urticaria is of particular interest in that Charcot-Leyden crystals have been noted,[31,34,36] some of which were intracellular.

Radioimmunoassay for a specific eosinophil-derived protein showed that most synovial fluids containing neutrophils also evidence eosinophil degranulation.[37] The dissociation between the appearance of eosinophil products but not intact eosinophils has been related to the known tendency for these cells to accumulate in the *periphery* of inflammatory foci.

Monocytosis is another unusual finding occurring with acute, self-limited arthritis associated with viral disease. Chronic monocytosis has been found in a patient with ANA-negative, Ro (SSA)-positive lupus, however.[38]

Special Qualitative Cytologic Findings. Qualitatively peculiar cells found in joint fluid are listed in Table 5–6. "Inclusion body cells" or "ragocytes" (raisin cells)[39] originally called "RA cells,"[40] are often seen in fluids of the inflammatory type (Fig. 5–3A–C). The polymorphonuclear leukocytes in rheumatoid arthritis contain much phagocytosed material, including immunoglobulins G and M, rheumatoid factors, fibrin, antinuclear factors, immune complexes, and DNA particles. The significance of these inclusions is discussed in Chapter 40. Polymorphs in inflammatory joint fluids from other diseases, however, also contain inclusion bodies with similar contents. Inclusion bod-

ies are best seen in a "wet" preparation of joint fluid prepared as described subsequently. They appear as vacuoles (phagosomes) by phase contrast microscopy (Fig. 5–3A,B). By ordinary light they appear as round or raisin-shaped dark granules (Fig. 5–3C), usually located at the periphery of the phagocyte, even during locomotion (Fig. 5–4A). Such cells show vacuolization in Wright's stained smears.

Classic LE cells, described as an in vivo phenomenon, are seen in Wright's stained smears.[41,42] These cells must be differentiated from "tart" cells, polymorphonuclear leukocytes that have phagocytosed nuclear debris. The LE cell test is obsolete. The chance identification of LE cells in joint fluid is rarely critical

Table 5–6. Cellular Peculiarities in Synovial Fluid

I. Quantitatively Peculiar	References
A. *Monocytosis*	38,46
1. Acute, self-limited	
Viral arthritis	
Serum sickness	
Idiopathic	
2. Chronic	
Ro (SSA) positive SLE	38
Undifferentiated connective tissue disease	47
B. *Eosinophilia*	33
1. Rheumatoid arthritis	48
2. Rheumatic fever	48
3. Parasitic infections	48
4. Metastatic adenocarcinoma	48
5. Arthrography	32,48
Air	
Dye	
6. Therapeutic x-irradiation	49
7. Urticaria	
Acute	33,34
Chronic	31,36,48
8. Idiopathic	35

II. Qualitatively Peculiar	References
A. *Nonspecific*	
1. Ragocytes (PMN with large peripheral granules)	40
2. LE cells	41,42
3. Reiter's cells (macrophages containing PMNs)	43,45
4. Bone marrow cells	49
B. *Specific*	
1. Sickled erythrocytes	19,20,50
2. Gaucher cells	
3. Tumor cells	

FIG. 5–3. *A,* Inclusion bodies are seen as well-defined vacuoles in a motile polymorpho-nuclear leukocyte (phase contrast, ×1000). *B,* The vacuoles are typically located in the periphery of the leukocyte, and often contain an eccentrically placed dark body when viewed by phase contrast microscopy under oil immersion (×1250). *C,* By ordinary light microscopy, the inclusion bodies appear as dark, dense granules (×1250). *D,* Crystals of triamcinolone hexacetonide, a corticosteroid ester, are similar to monosodium urate or calcium pyro-phosphate crystals in size and shape (phase contrast, ×1000). These are rapidly ingested by joint fluid leukocytes and are often seen lying within phagosomes (*insert*: phase contrast, ×800, reduced by two-thirds). *E,* A large triclinic crystal of calcium pyrophosphate dihydrate within a polymorphonuclear leukocyte phagosome (phase contrast, ×1000). *F,* A phago-cytosed monosodium urate crystal appears to lie free in the cytoplasm of a joint fluid polymorphonuclear leukocyte (polarized light, ×1000). *G,* A phagocyte is about to ingest a calcium pyrophosphate crystal (phase contrast, ×1000).

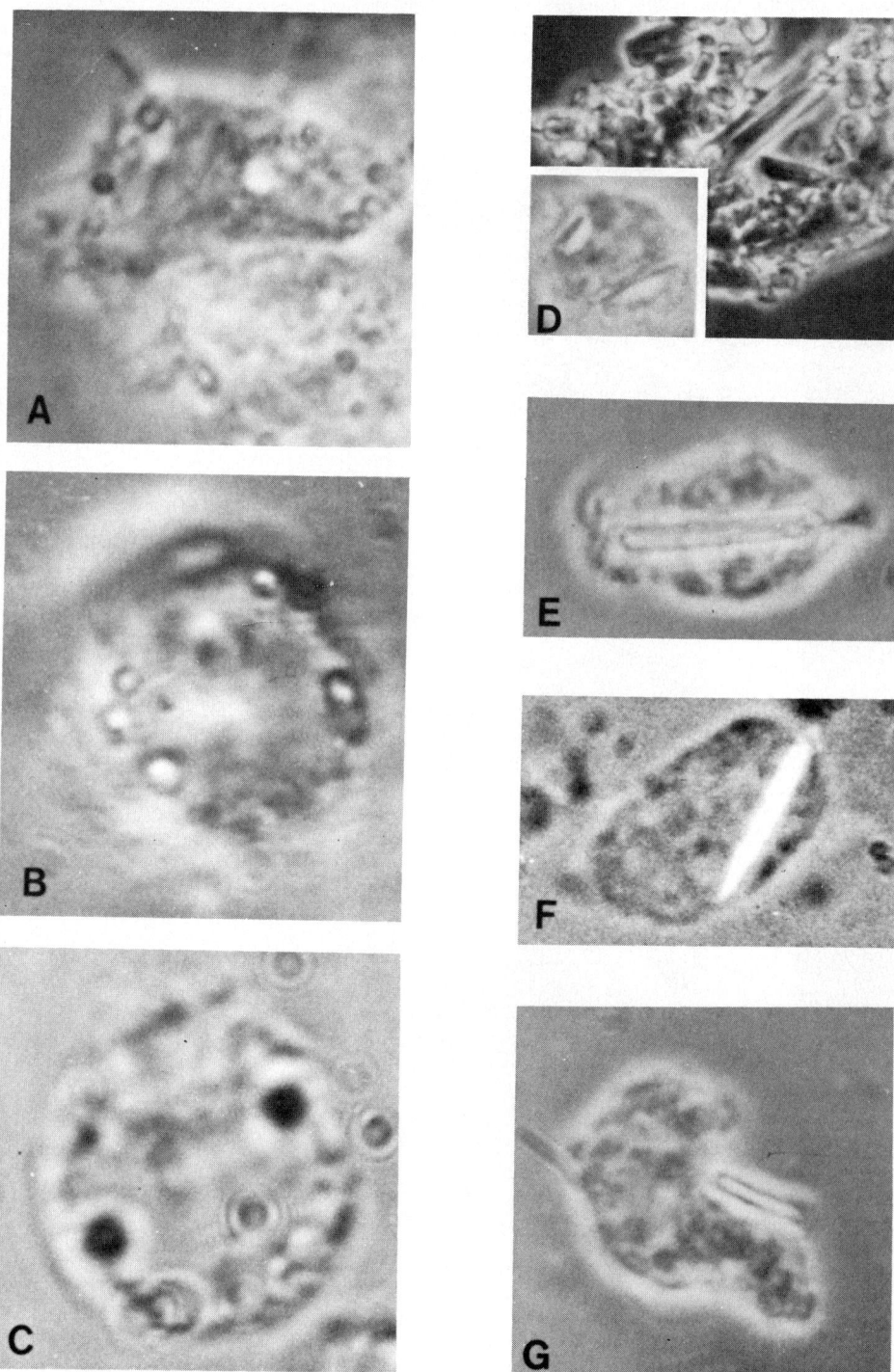

FIG. 5–4. *A,* A centrifuged pellet of fluid from an osteoarthritic knee joint showing collagen fibers (electron micrograph ×40,000). *B,* Homogenized normal cartilage produces some debris that appears fibrillar by light microscopy (phase contrast, ×1200). Other debris is birefringent and must be differentiated from microcrystals. The fibrils cannot be distinguished from fibrin by light microscopy. *C,* An electron micrograph of the fibrils reveals typical collagen periodicity (×100,000). *D,* A macrophage with at least three phagocytosed polymorphonuclear leukocytes is seen in a Wright's stained smear of synovial fluid from a patient with psoriatic arthritis (×1000 reduced by 50%). *E,* Wright's stained smear showing phagocytosed MSU crystals in a polymorphonuclear leukocyte (polarized light, ×1200). The nucleus of the cell on the right has become denser and the internuclear bridges, characteristic of the healthy polymorph, are lost. *F,* Wright's stained smear showing phagocytosis of MSU crystals by a monocyte.

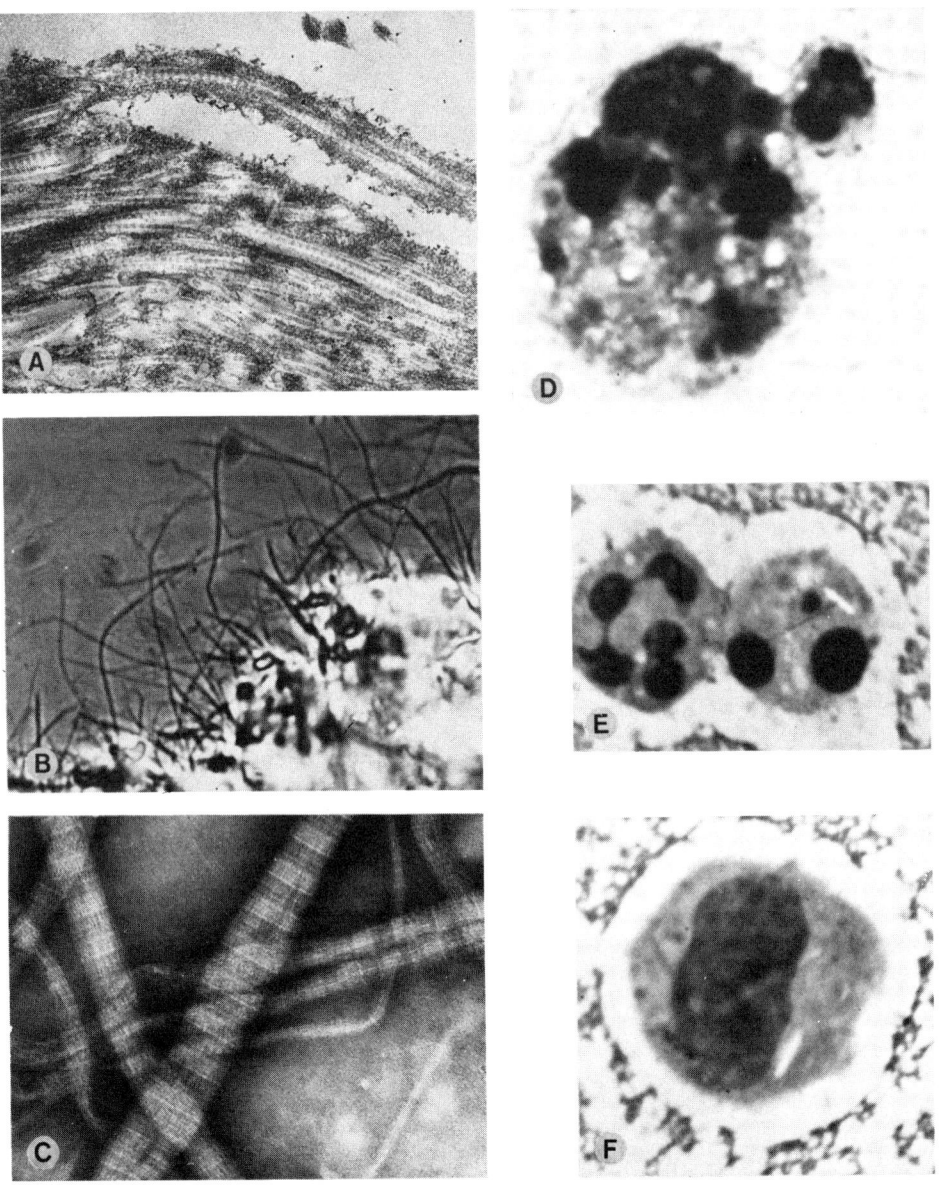

or even helpful in differential diagnosis, and is no reason for resurrection of the test.

Dead, degranulated polymorphonuclear leukocytes may disintegrate completely or may be phagocytosed relatively intact by scavenger cells such as monocytes or macrophages. Macrophages can ingest 3 to 5 polymorph "cadavers" (Fig. 5–4D), whereas the smaller monocytes cannot ingest more than one. Macrophages with ingested polymorphs may constitute up to 2% of the joint fluid leukocyte population in acute Reiter's syndrome, and were originally described as the "Reiter's cell," a misnomer implying disease specificity.[43] These cells have also been described in Reiter's synovium by electron microsopy[44] and in the Schwartzman reaction produced experimentally by bacterial endotoxin. These cells are an inconstant feature of Reiter's syndrome, and phagocytosis of polymorphs by mononuclear cells has been found in many inflammatory joint fluids.[45] The phenomenon is common in fluids from patients with juvenile rheumatoid arthritis. The finding of a single polymorph in a monocyte is also common, especially in fluids from gouty joints.

Many immunologic and cytologic studies have attempted to define subpopulations of mononucleated cells or their products, but none have been accepted as useful diagnostic or prognostic indicators.[30,51,52,53,54,54a,54b]

Phagocytosis of "hydroxyapatite" crystal aggregates by polymorphonuclear leukocytes (Fig. 5–5C) has been described in wet smears by light microscopy,[55,56] and by electron microscopy.[57,58,59] These particles, microspheroidal by scanning electron microscopy, are composed of aggregates of hydroxyapatite, largely carbonate substituted, and octacalcium phosphate or tricalcium phosphate.[60] Because these crystals are all *basic calcium phosphates*, the term *"BCP crystal deposition disease"* is preferred (see Chap. 108). Cytoplasmic inclusions in joint fluid polymorphs, staining a dark purple with Wright's stain, may represent clumps of BCP crystals.[59] This finding is nonspecific, since similar inclusions have been found in cells from effusions without demonstrable apatite crystals, and they were found in only 9 of 12 fluids showing "apatite" crystals by electron microscopy.

Sickled erythrocytes have been found in fluid from patients with either sickle cell disease or trait.[19,20,50] Gaucher cells and tumor cells have also been identified in synovial fluids.

Platelets also gain access to joint fluid. They have been enumerated directly in RA, JRA, and OA.[60a,61,62] In studies of RA fluids, they correlated with the leu-

FIG. 5–5. *A,* A focus of calcification in the periarticular tissues of a knee is shown by the von Kossa's stain (×80). The granular nature of the lesion is evident. An x-ray diffraction pattern revealed only hydroxyapatite. *B,* An inspissated chalk-like deposit removed from a shoulder joint capsule showed preservation of the sphere-like masses, some of which now contain birefringent crystals *(arrow)* (polarized light ×1250). *C,* Small spherical or disc-shaped particles containing eccentric or concentric striations were seen by phase contrast microscopy (×1250). These were phagocytosed by polymorphonuclear leukocytes *(insert).* (*B* and *C* from McCarty and Gatter.[56])

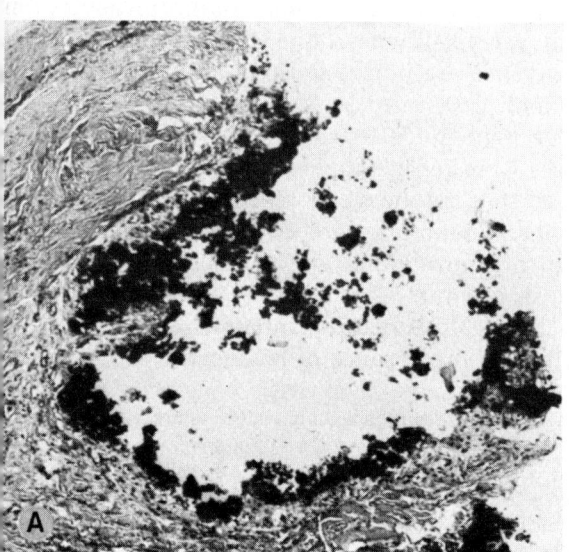
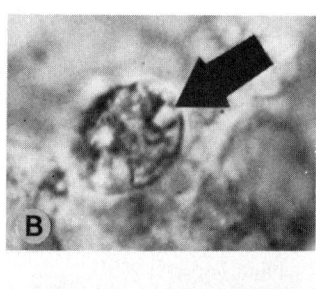
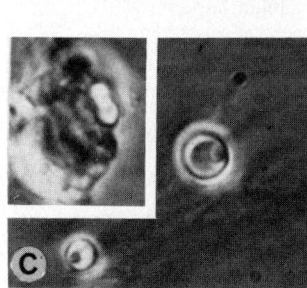

kocyte count, and clumps were noted with platelets adherent to synovial fluid lymphocytes.[60a] Moreover, platelet products such as beta thromboglobulin and connective tissue activating peptide III were detected in synovial fluids. Levels were higher in RA fluids, although neutrophilic leukocytes consume these proteins.[63]

Histamine levels in joint fluid were higher than in plasma from the same patient and were higher in samples from inflamed joints.[64]

Mast cells have been identified in synovial fluid[65,66] and in synovium;[67,68] mast cell number in joint fluids correlated with histamine levels. These data, obtained with more specific contemporary techniques, have revived interest in these cells and in histamine as agents of tissue damage in arthritis. Histamine is rapidly destroyed by histaminase in vivo, so its mere presence does not implicate it pathogenetically.

IDENTIFICATION OF CRYSTALS

The pathogenesis of crystal-induced inflammation is discussed in Chapter 106. Microcrystalline substances found in joint fluid are listed in Table 5–7. Here, the techniques useful or potentially useful in routine clinical work and in current clinical research will be discussed.

"Wet Smear" Preparation. Both the glass slide and

Table 5–7.   Particulate Matter of Synovial Fluid

I. *Crystals*
  A. Monosodium urate monohydrate (MSU)
    1. Ultramicroscopic
    2. Spherulites
  B. Calcium pyrophosphate dehydrate (CPPD)
    1. Ultramicroscopic
  C. Basic calcium phosphate (BCP)
    1. Carbonate-substituted hydroxyapatite (HA)
    2. Octacalcium phosphate (OCP)
    3. Tricalcium phosphate (TCP) (Whitlockite)
  D. Dicalcium phosphate dehydrate (DCPD) (Brushite)
  E. Calcium oxalate
  F. Cholesterol
  G. Lipid
  H. Aluminum phosphate
  I. Charcot-Leyden
  J. Artifactual—corticosteroid esters, lithium heparin, MSU, DCPD, calcium oxalate

II. *Other Particulates*
  A. Collagens
  B. "Wear" particles
    1. Cartilage fragments
    2. Prosthesis fragments
  C. "Rice" bodies (collagen types I, III, and V, enriched with fibrin)
  D. Fibrin
  E. Amyloid

coverslip must be free of dust and scratches. Dust particles are positively birefringent. One drop (about 0.05 ml) of freshly obtained joint fluid is placed on the slide and covered with a coverslip, the edges of which are sealed immediately with clear fingernail polish. This measure retards, but does not prevent, evaporation at the edges. Crystalline material may form at the junction of the fingernail polish and joint fluid if these touch. Such particles should be ignored. As the slide dries out, microcrystals of various types form at the edges of the fluid, but should also be ignored. To avoid confusion, the wet preparation should be examined immediately.

Sodium heparin should be used as anticoagulant. Lithium heparin may persist in crystalline form.[69a] These and calcium oxalate crystals from the use of oxalate anticoagulant[9] can prove confounding. Silicon-containing particles found by electron microscopy and x-ray energy dispersive analysis were thought to represent artifacts generated from glassware.[69*]

Light Microscopy. Monosodium urate monohydrate (MSU) crystals are strongly birefringent and are easily seen, even by ordinary light microscopy, as needle-shaped rods.[70] MSU crystals are usually 5 to 20 μ long, but crystals as short as 1 to 2 μ may be the only ones found, especially in persistent asymptomatic effusions after an acute attack. Some patients form only small crystals, and with every acute attack, only these are found. It is important to examine a wet smear as soon as possible after aspiration, using oil immersion and, preferably, compensated polarized light microscopy. In acute gout, many intraleukocytic crystals are found (Fig. 5–3F). They may be present for weeks after all clinical signs of inflammation have subsided.

Fluid obtained from a hyperuricemic patient and stored in a refrigerator for some hours after aspiration may show crystals when none were present initially.[71] Such crystals are unusually long and appear to nucleate and grow in or around leukocytes. Fifty consecutive joint fluids from patients with a variety of diseases were refrigerated for 24 hours and failed to show crystals if none were present in the fresh fluid.[72] This phenomenon is rare and inconstant and, although not now interpretable, does not justify the diagnosis of gout.

MSU crystals and acute inflammation have been described in the absence of leukocytes[73] and inflam-

---

*R. Gatter and I found silicon dioxide crystals, whose identity we confirmed by x ray diffraction, in a number of synovial fluids processed together on a Monday morning some years ago. The crystals were found to be contaminants from sand particles from under the fingernails of the technician, who had spent the weekend at the beach!

matory joint fluids have been seen from putative gout in the absence of MSU crystals.[74] In the former instance, a focus of neutrophil accumulation might occur in a contiguous synovial or extrasynovial compartment, and the obtained fluid may represent a "sympathetic" effusion in a joint near another compartment where crystal-induced inflammation is actually occurring. The *settling phenomenon* already discussed[25] could account for some of these cases. Moreover, small MSU and CPPD crystals have been found only by electron microscopy in several instances.[75,76] Light microscopic examination alone cannot definitely exclude the presence of crystals in joint fluid. The presence of "sphere urates" may explain some of these cases.[77] Alternatively, the clinical inflammation is due to causes other than gout. In my own experience over 28 years, I rarely have been perplexed by either phenomenon. Repeated clinical examination during several days, as inflammation subsides and becomes more precisely localizable, invariably disclosed the primary focus of inflammation.

Specific identification of MSU crystals is easiest with a quality polarizing microscope. Every arthritis center should invest in one. Some have advocated adapting an ordinary microscope with polarizing filters and a makeshift compensator using cellophane tape on a glass slide.[78,79] Although this may be better than no polarized light at all, the results using this technique or even an inexpensive polarizing microscope are inferior.

The depth of field with polarized light optics is flat, tending to minimize cellular detail, so that nonrefractile crystals and intracellular details are difficult to see. The addition of phase contrast is therefore helpful. We use a polarizing microscope equipped with a rotating stage; a built-in polarizer, analyzer, and first-order red plate compensator; a phase-contrast condenser, and ×10, ×40, and ×100 phase objectives; and a ×10 or ×12.5 eyepiece.

The wet preparaton is first scanned under the ×10 objective to localize suspicious objects. These objects are then observed under oil immersion (×100).

The *morphology* of a putative microcrystal is noted, as is whether it is birefringent. The *strength* and *sign* of birefringence and the *extinction angle* are then noted. Thus, four different descriptive items are obtained for an observed crystal. Birefringence is a property of many substances ordered in three dimensions. Not all birefringent objects are truly crystalline, for example, house dust, collagen, and pieces of cartilage. Not all crystals are birefringent, for example, in NaCl, a cuboidal crystal, the velocity of light passing through the crystal is identical in all directions. Bi-

refringence is caused by an observable difference in the velocity of light passing through an ordered structure in different directions, analogous to the velocity of an axe being driven into a log in different directions with the same applied force. In most logs, the velocity of the axe is greatest when its blade is parallel to the grain and slowest when it is across the grain. The blade penetrates deeper in the first instance. If the difference in the depth of penetration is great, the log is said to be "grainy." If the light is passing through a grainy crystal, strong birefringence is seen, whereas a nongrainy crystal may appear weakly birefringent or even nonbirefringent (isotropic).

Another variable is the mass of ordered material being examined. The amount of light being slowed must be sufficient to be appreciated visually. If a grainy log is thin, the axe might penetrate it completely regardless of the direction of the blow, and no difference in penetrability is noted. A thin crystal or a small collagen mass may appear nonrefractile by polarized light, whereas a larger mass of the same substance shows birefringence.

MSU crystals show strong birefringence, which disappears when their long axis is parallel to that of the crossed polarizer or analyzer (Fig. 5–6A; see also Fig. 5–8). This is called the position of *extinction* and is analogous to the axe striking the log obliquely, at a 45° angle to the cross grain, from either side. The difference in depth of penetration is now zero. MSU crystals extinguish when their long axis is parallel to the axis of the polarizer or analyzer; this is called *parallel* or *axial* extinction. Calcium pyrophosphate dihydrate (CPPD) crystals that show any birefringence extinguish when their long axis is oblique to the axis of the polarizer or analyzer; this is called *oblique* or *inclined* extinction (Fig. 5–6B). The angle between the axis of the polarizer or analyzer and the extinct crystal is called the *extinction angle;* in the case of CPPD crystals, this angle is between 20 and 30°.

The findings by plane-polarized light are augmented by the use of a first-order red quartz retardation plate, or "compensator." This plate slows the red component of white light by one-quarter wavelength so that the background now appears red rather than black. Now a MSU crystal appears red in the four positions of extinction shown in Figure 5–6A, and, instead of the four positions of brightness where it appeared white, it shows its optical sign of birefringence. When its long axis is perpendicular to the direction of slow vibration of the light in the compensator, it appears blue, and when its long axis is parallel to this direction, it appears yellow (Fig. 5–7A). Red is called the "sensitive tint," since it is relatively easy to shift from it to a slower (blue) or

FIG. 5–6. *A,* The typical properties under plane-polarized light of the strongly birefringent MSU crystal are illustrated *(top).* The crystal becomes nonrefractile when its long axis lies parallel to that of the polarizer or analyzer—the position of extinction. It is maximally bright when its long axis is in a position 45° oblique to these axes—the position of maximal brightness. This property is called axial or parallel extinction. *B,* The typical properties under plane-polarized light of the weakly birefringent CPPD crystal are illustrated *(bottom).* Extinction occurs when the long axis of the crystal is at an oblique angle to the axis of the polarizer or analyzer. This is called oblique or inclined extinction.

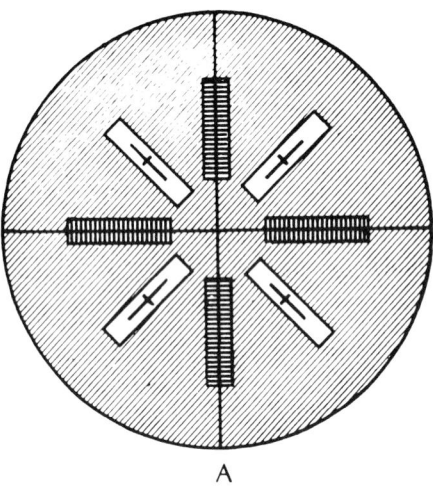

A

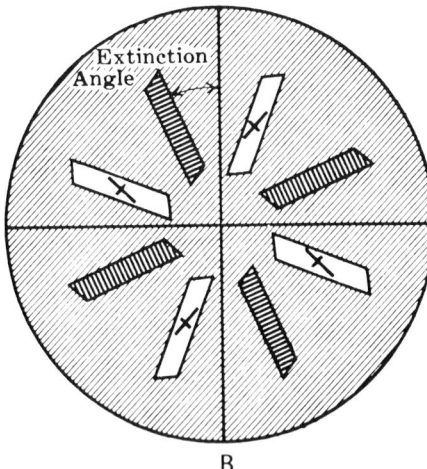

B

faster (yellow) wavelength of the visible spectrum, as shown in Figure 5–7B. First-order yellow and second-order blue are equidistant from first-order red. MSU crystals in blue or yellow positions of brightness or in positions of extinction are shown in Figure 5–8A.

The sign of birefringence is a characteristic of biaxial crystals like MSU and CPPD. Such crystals have two optic axes (biaxial), which means that two directions

permit light to pass through the lattice without being refracted at all. Our hypothetical axe would pass through the log from one end to the other without meeting any resistance at all in two directions.

The slow and fast rays of biaxial crystals bisect the angles formed by the optic axes. A crystal is optically (+) if its slow ray bisects the acute angles and optically (−) if its fast ray bisects the acute angles (Fig. 5–7C). As the fast ray of MSU crystals bisects the angle acutely in the morphologically long dimension of the crystal, it adds velocity to the light coming from the compensator and shifts the color to a higher wavelength—second-order blue (Fig. 5–7B). In crystallographic jargon, this phenomenon is known as (−) elongation. MSU crystals are thus analogous to a "grainy" log. When the morphologically long axis of CPPD crystal is at right angles to the direction of slow vibration of light in the compensator, its slow wave bisects the acute optic axis angle, slowing the velocity of the light even further and shifting the light to first-order yellow (Fig. 5–7B). CPPD crystals are like a log, the modest grain of which lies at right angles to its long dimension.

Fiechtner and Simkin have described "sphere-urates" in gouty synovial fluid[77] (Fig. 5–8B). In a few instances these were the only MSU crystalline phase present.

A high-quality polarizing light microscope with a compensator provides multiple parameters: morphology, strength of birefringence, the optical sign of birefringence (elongation), and the extinction angle. Excellent descriptions of this method have been published since compensated polarized light microscopy was first used to characterize MSU[80] and CPPD[12] microcrystals, and should be consulted for further details.[5,81,82]

Other Methods. X-ray diffraction "powder patterns" were used initially to classify pathologic calcifications in the 1960s.[83,84] Satisfactory patterns were obtained on as little as 50 μg of crystals. Specific digestion with uricase was used initially to substantiate the identity of MSU crystals,[80] but this is not necessary in routine work. The initial identification of both CPPD and dicalcium phosphate dehydrate (DCPD) was accomplished by infrared spectroscopy of crystals compressed into a sodium bromide disc.[84,85] This is a good method for identifying phosphate groups. The calcium moiety was identified in both crystals by routine chemical methods after crystal dissolution.

BCP but not CPPD or MSU crystals bind (^{14}C) diphosphonate (EHDP), and this is a useful, rapid, semiquantitative screening test.[28] Alizarin red staining, also used for this purpose,[86] is more sensitive but less specific. We examine the pellets of fluids that bind

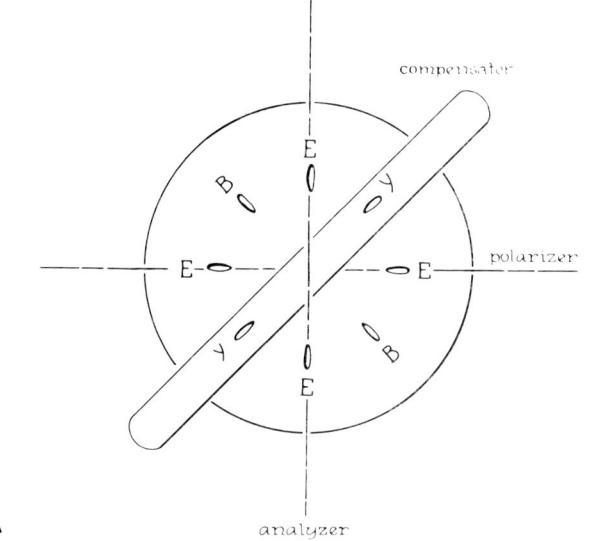

A

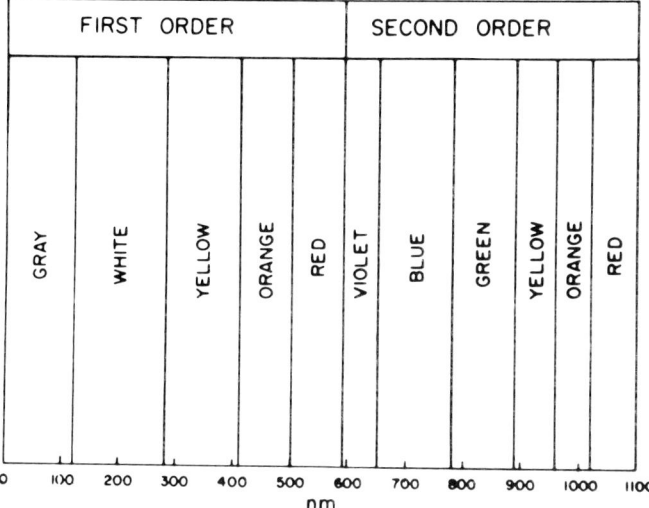

B

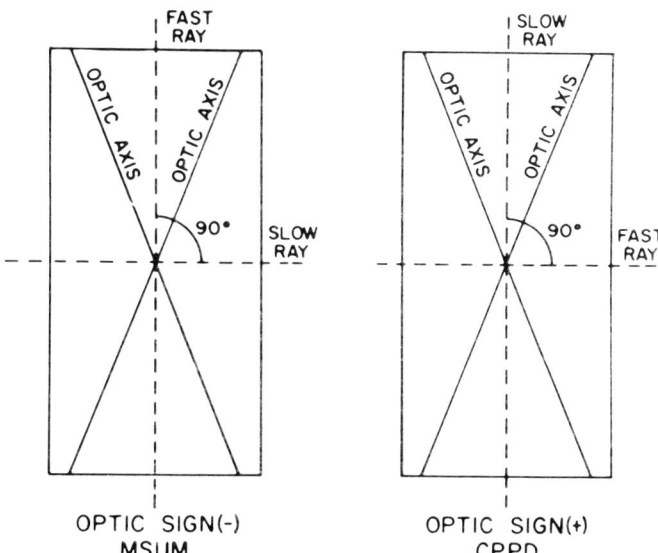

C

FIG. 5–7. *A,* The plane of slow vibration of light in the compensator is indicated by the wedge in the diagram, inserted at a 45° angle to the crossed polarizer and analyzer. A single MSU crystal rotated under the objective appears maximally blue (B) when its long axis is perpendicular to the plane of slow vibration of light in the compensator, and maximally yellow (Y) when it is parallel. The position of extinction (E) occurs when it lies parallel to the plane of the polarizer or analyzer. (From McCarty, D.J., and Hollander, J.L.[80]) *B,* First and second orders of colors produced from polarized white light are shown. (From Gatter, R.A.[82]) *C,* Optical sign determination in biaxial crystals; a crystal is (+) when the slow ray from the compensator besects the optic axes acutely and (−) when the fast ray from the compensator bisects the optic axes acutely. (From Gatter, R.A.[82])

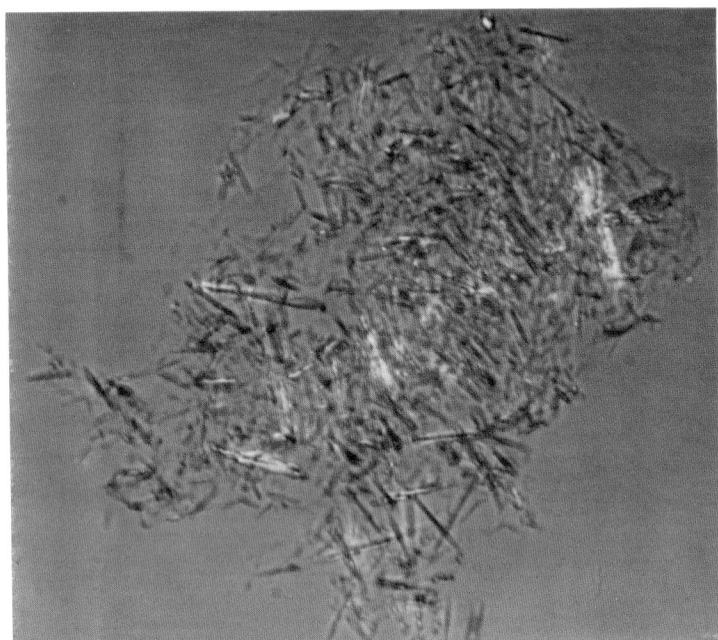

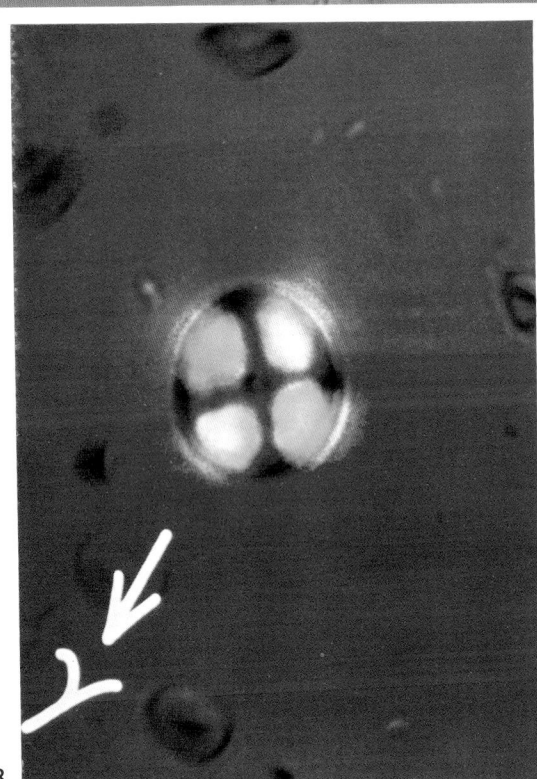

FIG. 5–8. *A,* MSU crystals in a drop of joint fluid from an 80-year-old dentist with chronic tophaceous gout. Viewed by compensated polarized light microscopy (×500). *B,* Negatively birefringent spherulite in synovial fluid of a patient with gouty arthritis. These spherulites may be (rarely) present as the only MSU crystalline phase or may be accompanied by the typical needle-shaped crystals (×1000). (From Fiechtner, J.J., and Simkin, P.A.[77]).

(^{14}C) EHDP by scanning electron microscopy (SEM).[87] Others have used rapid transmission electron microscopy (TEM), which is more sensitive and provides better definition of crystal morphology and location, e.g., intracellular versus extracellular.[88] Particulates found can be characterized further by x-ray energy dispersive analysis, which provides the ratio of calcium to phosphorus atoms.[87]

Fourier transform infrared (FTIR) spectrophotometry has been used to characterize calcium phosphate crystal aggregates.[60] These contained particulate collagen, hydroxyapatite partially substituted with carbonate and either octacalcium phosphate (OCP) or tricalcium phosphate (TCP). Chapter 108 provides more detail relative to identification of calcium-containing crystals.

Dicalcium Phosphate Dihydrate (DCPD). These orthophosphate crystals, a dimorph of brushite (Ca$HPO_4 \cdot 2H_2O$), were initially identified in cadaver cartilage[85,89] by infrared spectroscopy and x ray diffraction. They show strong (+) birefringence. They are more soluble than CPPD crystals—K_{sp}, about 10^{-7} versus 10^{-15}. They have been identified in articular cartilage in a patient with a destructive arthropathy.[90] Identification was made by scanning electron microscopy (see Fig. 106–2) and by x ray diffraction.

Basic Calcium Phosphate (BCP) Crystals. These crystals have been listed previously. The individual crystals are too small to be seen by optical microscopy. The largest are only 1 μm long. By TEM they appear as needles or plates. They are invariably aggregated and by phase contrast appear as "shiny coins" as shown in Figure 5–5B, or as microspheroidal "snowballs" by SEM as shown in Figure 108–3A. Particulate collagens are a constant feature of these fluids.[60,87] If many crystals are oriented with respect to their long axis they may appear birefringent (Fig. 5–5B).[90a]

Other Crystals (see also Chapter 109). These crystals are listed in Table 5–7. Cholesterol crystals, usually occurring as flat rhomboid plates with notched corners, have been described in joint fluids and in inflammatory and degenerative types of joint disease, usually in long-standing effusions.[91–95] These crystals are usually large, often more than 100 μm. They are thin plates, and although strongly birefringent, the mass refracting light in a single crystal may be insufficient to demonstrate this. When stacked like poker chips, however, their strong birefringence is evident.

Needle-shaped cholesterol crystals, as well as rhomboid plates, have been described in both joint fluid and pericardial fluid.[91,92,94] Both forms have an identical x-ray diffraction powder pattern resembling that of anhydrous cholesterol rather than cholesterol monohydrate.[94] Such cholesterol crystals were not pure, but contained small to moderate amounts of cholesterol ester, triglyceride, phospholipids, and small quantities of protein. These components absorbed to pure cholesterol crystals added to the supernatant effusion fluid. Conversion of rhomboid cholesterol crystals to needle-shaped crystals occurred with time. These needles were large and negatively birefringent. They were readily soluble in ether, which distinguished them immediately from the smaller MSU. Small cholesterol (5- to 10-μm) crystals have been described in osteoarthritic joint fluids.[92] More important, cholesterol crystals are never phagocytosed. They may be sufficiently numerous to render an effusion milky, but they have no known pathogenetic or phlogistic role.

Calcium oxalate crystals form readily if joint fluid is placed in an oxalated tube. Such crystals are cuboidal or rhomboid, about 2 to 10 μ across, and are phagocytosed by viable neutrophils in the joint fluid.[9] They have been found in patients on maintenance dialysis who have hyperoxalemia (see Chapter 109).[96,97] These may be intracellular.[98,99]

Crystals of corticosteroid esters are prepared as an injectable suspension by the drug companies by the grinding of larger crystals in a colloid mill and are often irregular in size and shape as a result. They are brightly birefringent. Most preparations are optically (+), but some are (−). They are usually 1 to 20 μ long and are avidly phagocytized by joint fluid leukocytes.[70] They may be present in joint fluid for as long as one month after injection. Storage, different crystal lots, and amount of shaking before injection may alter crystal appearance.

Lithium, but not sodium, heparin anticoagulant has been reported to produce crystals in joint fluid resembling CPPD.[69a] Such crystals are 2 to 5 μ long with varied shape. Calcium phosphorus mineral can precipitate artifactually from joint fluids exposed to air since the pH rises to >8 coincident with CO_2 loss.[28] As mentioned already, birefringent fat droplets resembling a Maltese cross have been seen both free and phagocytized, usually, but not always, associated with trauma.[21–24,47,100]

Aluminum phosphates have been found in French patients with renal disease who were taking aluminum-containing gels to control blood phosphorus.[101]

Metal fragments have been described in joint fluid from a joint that had had a metal prosthesis inserted.[17]

Amyloid fragments have been identified in synovial fluid by polarized light microscopic examination of pellets stained with Congo red.[102,103]

Cartilage Fragments. Normal articular cartilage ground in a tissue homogenizer showed many non-birefringent fibrils by ordinary light or phase contrast microscopy (Fig. 5–4B), and also birefringent chunks of cartilage.[104] The fibrils showed the typical periodicity of collagen by electron microscopy (Fig. 5–4C). Similar fibrils were seen in joint fluid pellets by both light and electron microscopy (Fig. 5–4A), and these same pellets contained hydroxyproline.[104] Collagen is a highly ordered molecule and is birefringent if enough is present to refract sufficient light. Collagen in parallel array with the highly ordered glycosaminoglycans arranged neatly between fibers is strongly (+) birefringent. Small birefringent, irregular-shaped particles are seen frequently in joint fluid and are thought to represent pieces of articular cartilage. Such fragments have been well characterized by histochemical methods in synovium, where they had become embedded after desquamation.[105]

Particulate collagens have been further identified by type.[106] Types I and III characteristic of synovial membrane, are found in patients with RA, whereas fluids from patients with osteoarthritis contain type II, the predominant collagen type in hyaline articular cartilage.

Wear particles have been characterized ferrographically.[107] In addition to the potential diagnostic importance of this technique, the wear particles themselves are capable of provoking collagenase and prostaglandin release from synovial cells. An excellent correlation was found between the number and microscopic features of cartilage fragments obtained by filtering synovial lavage fluid and the arthroscopic appearance of the cartilaginous surface.[108] Both of these techniques have great potential for diagnosis and prognosis of selected types of arthritis.

Rice Bodies. Bits of tissue resembling polished white rice are seen in many fluids from the affected joints of patients with rheumatoid arthritis, systemic lupus, or septic arthritis. Some of these contain a core of collagen with a mantle of fibrin, whereas others contain only fibrin.[109] On analysis, it is clear that the collagen is types I, III, and V in a proportion (40-40-20) identical to that of synovial membrane.[110] Whether these rice bodies represent infarcted ischemic synovium[111] or newly synthesized collagen by synovial cells that become entwined in particulate fibrin[109] is unclear.

CLINICAL LABORATORY STUDIES

Proteins. The total protein of normal synovial fluid averages about 1.8 g/dl (see Table 5–2). In general, the smaller protein molecules such as albumin are present in greater concentrations than larger molecules such as globulins. As discussed fully in Chapter 11, the entry and egress of small molecules are explained by diffusion between synovial lining cells, whereas the factor limiting protein entry is probably the number and size of the fenestrations in subsynovial capillaries. With diseases producing inflammation and increased synovial blood flow, protein entry may often increase out of proportion to the entry of small molecules. Therefore, virtually all protein molecules found in plasma enter the joint. With increasing inflammation, their concentration in synovia approaches the concentration of the patient's plasma. Protein egress from both normal and diseased joints is by lymphatic drainage. There is nearly a 1:1 ratio between lymphatics and capillaries in normal synovium.

That molecular size is not the only factor limiting protein entry into normal joints is obvious from the virtual absence of prothrombin (MW 63,000)[8] and the low levels of haptoglobin (MW 85,000)[112] and fibrinogen.

The concentration of lysosomal enzymes and other leukocyte-derived proteins, such as the antimicrobial substance lactoferrin,[113,114] also increase with the degrees of inflammation.

The presence of fibrin strands was alluded to in the discussion of particulate matter in synovia. Fibrin degradation products of high molecular weight, often in aggregates quite different from those found in blood owing to plasmin digestion of fibrin, have been found in inflammatory synovial fluids.[115] Antiplasmins were presumed to be responsible for this phenomenon. Even osteoarthritic fluids contained small amounts of these peculiar fibrin degradation products. Fibrin is chemotactic for and is phagocytized by synovial fluid leukocytes. It composes the bulk of the rice body. Small fragments of plasminogen, thought to be generated by the action of neutrophil elastase, have been identified in fluid from inflamed but not degenerative joints.[116] These fragments are not inhibited by the plasmin inhibitor and have been postulated to play a role in joint destruction, by acting either directly or as a procollagenase activator. Plasminogen activator levels were elevated in rheumatoid but not osteoarthritis joint fluid.[117]

Many studies have been performed on various other enzymes in joint fluid.[2,27] Leukocyte elastase and free collagenase activity correlated with polymorphonuclear leukocyte levels in joint fluid.[118]

Total Hemolytic Complement ($C'H_{50}$). The measurement of $C'H_{50}$, which measures the functional activity of all complement component proteins in synovial fluid, is sometimes helpful diagnostically. Normal synovial fluids show, as expected, low levels of $C'H_{50}$. Whether this is due to low levels of all or selected components is not known. In diseased synovia, the $C'H_{50}$ level is proportional to the total protein in the same fluid and to serum $C'H_{50}$, unless there is local consumption during the inflammatory process.[119–122] Generally, synovial $C'H_{50}$ is one third to one half of the patient's serum in the absence of local consumption. Table 5–8 summarizes the reported data. The serum $C'H_{50}$ is often low in systemic lupus erythematosus and high in Reiter's syndrome, psoriatic arthritis, and gonococcal arthritis and correspondingly low or high in fluids obtained from joints affected with these diseases; this situation simply reflects the serum levels of the component proteins.

Significant depression of joint fluid complement occurs most predictably in seropositive RA, when sepsis and the crystal deposition diseases are excluded. Exclusion is relatively easy in both instances by the specific features of these conditions, i.e., crystals or bacteria. The depression of $C'H_{50}$ in joint fluid is a reflection of the local Arthus-like immune complex disease that is an integral feature of RA (see Chapter 40). C3 levels corrected for synovial fluid globulin levels, can be substituted for $C'H_{50}$ and protein levels.[123] Activation of C2 and factor B was found in synovial fluids from a variety of inflammatory types of arthritis but not osteoarthritis.[124] A correlation existed between the amount of conversion and the synovial fluid polymorphonuclear leukocyte count. Such correlation was also noted in fluid from joints of patients with JRA;[125] complement activation correlated also with C-reactive protein but not with clinical disease activity.

Other Serologic Tests. Rheumatoid factors have been measured in synovial fluid.[126,127] In most instances, their titer is identical to or slightly lower than that in the patient's serum. In a few instances, they were found in the fluid and not in the serum or vice versa. Antigamma globulins are also found in joint fluids from other inflammatory types of arthritis and from osteoarthritic joints.[128] Assays for rheumatoid factors in either cells or synovia have not been shown to be helpful, for either diagnosis or prognosis.

Both antinuclear antibodies and DNA[129,130] have been found in synovial fluid, but no disease specificity has been found for either. DNA may be derived nonspecifically from the breakdown of cells during the inflammatory process.

Cryoproteins have been found in both rheumatoid and nonrheumatoid fluids.[131,132] These occurred in virtually all RA fluids and contained mixed immunoglobulins and bound complement, DNA, and rheumatoid factors. Those in non-RA fluids contained mostly fibrinogen and did not fix complement. Fibrin and fibronectin are present in synovial fluid in soluble and precipitated form in RA, although levels of the latter are normal in the serum.[133]

Small Molecules. The synovial transport of small molecules is discussed in Chapter 11. Most small molecules diffuse into synovia from the blood; some (such as lactate, CO_2, and inorganic pyrophosphate) are produced by joint tissues and may achieve higher concentrations in synovia as compared with plasma. Antimicrobial and antirheumatic drug molecules diffuse into synovia readily (see Chapter 114).

Concentrations of free drug in synovial fluid approximated those in plasma except in rheumatoid and infectious arthritis, which may have important therapeutic implications.[134] Immunoreactive vasoactive "gastrointestinal" peptide levels were higher in inflammatory synovial fluid than in the corresponding serum, suggesting its local production.[135]

Glucose. This vital molecule enters the synovia from plasma by facilitated diffusion, and its measurement in both compartments is sometimes diagnostically helpful. True glucose (Somogyi-Nelson), not total reducing substances, must be measured. The patient must be fasting to permit measurement of a stable serum level and the attainment of equilibrium between it and the joint fluid.[2] Table 5–9 summarizes the data of Cohen and associates relative to mean glucose serum-synovia differences in various joint diseases.[27] Differences greater than 40 mg/dl were seen regularly only in cases of bacterial or tubercular

Table 5–8.   Synovial Fluid Hemolytic Complement Levels (references summarized in ref 7b)

Disease	Serum $C'H_{50}$†	Synovial Fluid $C'H_{50}$
Rheumatoid arthritis		
seropositive	N or I	N or D (usually)
seronegative	N or I	N
Juvenile RA*		N
seronegative	N or I	
Systemic lupus erythematosus	N or D (usually)	N or D (usually)
Crystal deposition disease (gout and pseudogout)	N or I	N or D (often)
Reiter's syndrome	N or I (usually)	N
Ankylosing spondylitis	N or I	N
Psoriatic arthritis	N or I	N
Septic arthritis	N or I (usually)	N or D (often)
Other diffuse connective tissue diseases		
drug LE	N	inadequate data
polyarteritis	N, I, or D	inadequate data
scleroderma	N	inadequate data
polymyositis	N	inadequate data
Mixed cryoglobulinemia	D	inadequate data

N = normal; I = increased; D = decreased. (N, I, or D in synovial fluid is given with respect to that predicted from serum $C'H_{50}$ and joint fluid protein.)
*Seropositive children show findings as in adult seropositive RA.
†May be decreased with systemic vasculitis, so-called hypocomplementemic RA.

Table 5–9.   Serum-Synovial Fluid Glucose Differences in Joint Diseases

Disease	N	OA,Tr	LE	RF	Reiter's	Gout	RA	Tb	Bact
mean Δ glucose (mg/dl)	0	5	22	6	9	11	30	70	91
number of fluids	29	79	16	12	16	86	80	27	21

From data of Cohen et al.[25]
N = normal; OA = osteoarthritis; Tr = trauma; LE = lupus erythematosus; RF = rheumatic fever; RA = rheumatoid arthritis; Tb = tuberculosis;
Bact = bacterial arthritis.

infection, but overlap in values between septic and nonseptic inflammatory conditions often occurred, which limits the reliability of this test.

Hyaluronate. The molecular weight distribution of hyaluronate in RA synovial fluid showed that the average was similar to that from other joint diseases and moderately lower than that in normal fluid.[136] The total amount of hyaluronate was actually increased, however. Pathologic fluids are therefore characterized not by lack of high molecular weight hyaluronate, but rather by its dilution (see mucin clot test above).

Lipids. Normal fluid contains little lipid despite the large amount of fat in normal synovium. With inflammation, the content of lipid in synovia increases; cholesterol, phospholipids, neutral fat, and triglycerides all rise.[93,137–139] Cholesterol crystals may be found. Lipids of synovia may be synthesized by joint tissues or may derive from the lipid-rich membrane constituents of inflammatory cells. No specific diagnostic inflammation can be obtained from lipid analysis of synovia, except for (possibly) elevated free fatty acids in the pancreatitis-arthritis syndrome.[140] Injection of free fatty acids into rabbit joints induced an inflammatory response, including intracellular fat globules within neutrophils as found in patients. The possible phlogistic potential of fat droplets is discussed above under Particulate Matter and in Chapter 109.

An excellent review of synovial fluid lipid abnormalities has appeared.[141] A number of different mechanisms have been proposed to account for the release or formation of lipid droplets in synovia. These are sudanophilic, they may or may not be birefringent (Maltese-cross), and they may appear free in the fluid and within mononuclear or polymorphonuclear phagocytes. Fluids containing them may be either group I, group II,[2] bloody or chylous, with formation of a supernatant lipid layer on standing or centrifugation. Experimental hemarthrosis produced by injection of autologous blood induced mild inflammation associated with intracellular "Maltese-cross" birefringent spherulites.[142]

The weight of descriptive evidence favors the idea that some particulate lipids are biologically active, although the mechanism of such activity remains obscure.

Microbiologic Study. Like serum, joint fluid is an excellent culture medium. Data have been presented suggesting that synovial fluid inhibits the in vitro killing of Staphylococcus aureus by neutrophils.[143] Moreover, neutrophils from rheumatoid joint fluid were thought to be relatively effete.[144] However, more recent work has shown that rheumatoid synovial fluid supports the phagocytosis of S. aureus as well as serum does, that neutrophils from RA synovial fluid engulf organisms more efficiently than patient or donor cells do, and that RA synovial fluid neutrophils are as active in killing the organisms as cells from healthy donors are.[144a] Considering the ability of the synovium to trap circulating organisms (see Chapter 114) and the frequency of bacteremia, it is surprising a priori that septic arthritis is not more common. An increased incidence of joint sepsis in the presence of pre-existing joint disease and in patients whose defenses are compromised by drugs or systemic diseases such as cancer or cirrhosis is easy to comprehend.

Infection must be ruled out whenever joint inflammation accompanies a septic process elsewhere in a patient (e.g., heart valve, pneumonia, urinary tract, or skin). A joint fluid leukocyte count greater than 50,000/cmm should heighten the suspicion of infection. Arthrocentesis is again indispensable, with the caveat that infectious organisms may be introduced into the joint from the infected blood owing to the bleeding that invariably accompanies this procedure. The unsolved problem is how to make a rapid diagnosis. Antimicrobials are usually given empirically while the results of culture are awaited. Several new techniques for rapid microbiologic diagnosis have been advocated. These techniques are reviewed elsewhere.[145]

Even more promising is the use of gas-liquid chromatographic (GLC) analysis of synovial fluid.[146] Lactic acid levels aid in detecting infection, but only when above 250 mg/dl and when no antimicrobials have been given. In one study, succinic acid measured by GLC separated all septic fluids caused by gram-positive or gram-negative bacteria, including N. gonorrhoeae, in patients not given antibiotics, from fluids obtained from joints with sterile inflammatory types of arthritis.[147] Only 5 of 39 of the latter group had detectable succinic acid levels by GLC analysis. Moreover, succinic acid was detected in joint fluids in all 8 instances in which antibiotics had already been given. The combination of WBC count >50,000, synovial fluid glucose <40 mg/dl, and succinic acid level was nearly 100% accurate in diagnosing septic arthritis. These data need confirmation and extension but appear promising.

The examination of synovia is an excellent, rapid adjunct to clinical examination in differential diagnosis of arthritis. Culture for microbes and identification of crystals and other particulates provides specific clues, whereas gross parameters of analysis and selected laboratory procedures, such as total and differential leukocyte counts, total protein and hemolytic complement assay, and serum-synovial fluid differential glucose concentrations, provide ancillary data. Future studies of joint fluid will almost certainly yield additional information of both practical and theoretic importance in the rheumatic diseases. Magnetic resonance imaging, for example, is highly sensitive for joint fluid; 84% of normal hips contained detectable fluid by this method.[147] The usefulness of joint fluid analysis is being scrutinized along with other diagnostic tests,[148] and efforts at standardizaiton have begun.[149]

REFERENCES

1. Rodnan, G.P., Benedek, T.G., and Panetta, W.C.: The early history of synovial (joint) fluid. Ann. Intern. Med., 65:821–842, 1966.
2. Ropes, M.W., and Bauer, W.: Synovial Fluid Changes in Joint Diseases. Boston, Harvard University Press, 1953.
3. McCarty, D.J., Phelps, P., and Pyenson, P.: Crystal induced inflammation in canine joints. I. An experimental model with quantification of the host response. J. Exp. Med., 124:99–114, 1966.
4. Nagel, D.A., Albright, J.A., and Hollingsworth, J.W.: Studies on the pathophysiology and some host defense factors in staphylococcal arthritis in the rabbit and on the relationship of aseptic inflammation to infection rate. Yale J. Biol. Med., 39:119–128, 1966.
5. Gatter, R.A.: A Practical Handbook of Joint Fluid Analysis. Philadelphia, Lea & Febiger, 1984.
6. Hollander, J.L., Jessar, R.A., and McCarty, D.J.: Synovianalysis. Bull. Rheum. Dis., 12:263–264, 1961.
7. Schumacher, H.R., and Kitridou, R.C.: Synovitis of recent onset. Arthritis Rheum., 15:465–485, 1972.
7a. Lally, E.V.: High-dose corticosteroid therapy: Association with noninflammatory synovial effusions. Arthritis Rheum., 26:1283–1287, 1983.
7b. McCarty, D.J.: Synovial fluid. In Arthritis and Allied Conditions: A Textbook of Rheumatology, 10th Ed. Edited by D.J. McCarty, Lea & Febiger, Philadelphia, 1985.
8. Cho, N.H., and Neuhaus, O.W.: Absence of blood clotting substances from synovial fluid. Thrombosis et Diathesis Haemorrhagica, 5:108–111, 1960.
9. Schumacher, H.R.: Intracellular crystals in synovial fluid anticoagulated with oxalate. N. Engl. J. Med., 274:1372–1373, 1966.
10. Roberts, R.D., Wong, S.W., and Thiel, G.B.: An unusual case of lead nephropathy. Arthritis Rheum., 26:1048–1051, 1983.
11. Stevens, J., et al.: Synovial hemangioma of the knee. Arthritis Rheum., 12:647, 1969.
12. McCarty, D.J., Kohn, N.N., and Faires, J.S.: The significance of calcium phosphate crystals in the synovial fluid of arthritis patients: The "pseudogout syndrome." I. Clinical Aspects. Ann. Intern. Med., 56:711–737, 1962.
13. Stevens, L.W., and Spiera, H.: Hemarthrosis in chondrocalcinosis (pseudogout). Arthritis Rheum., 16:651–653, 1972.
14. Wild, J.H., and Zvaifler, N.J.: Hemarthrosis associated with sodium warfarin therapy. Arthritis Rheum., 19:98–102, 1976.
15. McLaughlin, G.E., McCarty, D.J., and Segal, B.L.: Hemarthrosis complicating anticoagulant therapy: Report of three cases. JAMA, 196:1020–1021, 1966.
16. Jaffer, A.M., and Schmid, F.R.: Hemarthrosis associated with sodium warfarin. J. Rheumatol., 4:215–217, 1977.
17. Kitridou, R.C., et al.: Recurrent hemarthrosis after prosthetic knee arthroplasty: Identification of metal particles in the synovial fluid. Arthritis Rheum., 12:520–528, 1969.
18. Harris, B.K., and Ross, H.A.: Hemarthrosis as the presenting manifestation of myeloproliferative disease. Arthritis Rheum., 17:969–970, 1974.
19. Casey, D.J., and Cathcart, E.S.: Hemarthrosis and sickle cell trait. Arthritis Rheum., 13:882–886, 1970.
20. Espinoza, L.K., Spilberg, I., and Osterland, C.K.: Joint manifestations of sickle cell disease. Medicine, 53:295–305, 1974.
21. Weinstein, J.: Synovial fluid leukocytosis associated with intracellular lipid inclusions. Arch. Intern. Med., 140:560–561, 1980.
22. Graham, J., and Goldman, J.H.: Fat droplets and synovial fluid leukocytes in traumatic arthritis. Arthritis Rheum., 21:76–80, 1978.
23. White, R.E., Wise, C.M., and Agudelo, C.A.: Post traumatic chylous joint effusion. Arthritis Rheum., 28:1303–1306, 1985.
24. Reginato, A.J., Feldman, E., and Rabinowitz, J.L.: Traumatic chylous knee effusion. Ann. Rheum. Dis., 44:793–797, 1985.
25. Hasselbacher, P., Passero, F.C., and Ludvico, C.L.: Sedimentation of leukocytes within the joint space. Pa. Med., 8:L54–55, 1978.
26. Hasselbacher, P.: Measuring synovial fluid viscosity with a white blood cell diluting pipette. Arthritis Rheum., 19:1358–1363, 1976.
27. Cohen, A.S., and Goldenberg, D.: Synovial fluid. In Laboratory Diagnostic Procedures in the Rheumatic Diseases. Edited by A.S. Cohen. 3rd Ed. Grune & Stratton, 1985.
28. Halverson, P.B., and McCarty, D.J.: Identification of hydroxyapatite crystals in synovial fluid. Arthritis Rheum., 22:389–395, 1979.
29. Krey, R.P., and Bailen, D.A.: Synovial fluid leukocytosis: A study of extremes. Am. J. Med., 67:436–442, 1979.
30. Poulter, L.W., et al.: Immunocytology of synovial fluid cells may be of diagnostic and prognostic value in arthritis. Ann. Rheum. Dis., 45:584–590, 1986.
31. Dougados, M., et al.: Charcot-Leyden crystals in synovial fluid. Arthritis Rheum., 26:1416, 1983.
32. Hasselbacher, P.: Synovial fluid eosinophilia following arthrography. J. Rheumatol., 5:173–176, 1978.
33. Lugar, M.J., and Friedman, B.M.: Acute synovial fluid eosinophilia. J. Rheumatol., 9:961–962, 1982.

34. Menard, H.A., et al.: Charcot-Leyden crystals in synovial fluid (letter). Arthritis Rheum., 24:1591–1593, 1981.
35. Podell, T.E., et al.: Synovial fluid eosinophilia. Arthritis Rheum., 23:1060–1061, 1980.
36. Brown, J.P., et al.: Eosinophilic synovitis: Clinical observations on a newly recognized subset of patients with dermatographism. Arthritis Rheum., 29:1147–1451, 1986.
37. Hallgren, R., Bjelle, A., and Venge, P.: Eosinophilic cationic protein in inflammatory synovial effusions as evidence of eosinophil involvement. Ann. Rheum. Dis., 43:556–562, 1984.
38. George, D., et al.: Chronic monocytic arthritis. Arthritis Rheum., 26:674–677, 1983.
39. Delbarre, F., Kahan, A., and Amor, B.: Le ragocyte synovial. Presse Med., 72:2129–2132, 1964.
40. Hollander, J.L., et al.: Studies on the pathogenesis of rheumatoid joint inflammation. I. The "RA cell" and a working hypothesis. Ann. Intern. Med., 62:271–280, 1965.
41. Hollander, J.L., Reginato, A., and Torralba, T.P.: Examination of synovial fluid as a diagnostic aid in arthritis. Med. Clin. North Am., 50:1281–1293, 1966.
42. Hunder, G.C., and Pierre, R.V.: In vivo LE cell formation in synovial fluid. Arthritis Rheum., 13:448–454, 1970.
43. Pekin, T.J., Malinin, T.I., and Zvaifler, M.J.: Unusual synovial fluid findings in Reiter's syndrome. Ann. Intern. Med., 66:677–684, 1967.
44. Norton, W.L., Lewis, D., and Ziff, M.: Light and electron microscopic observations on the synovitis of Reiter's disease. Arthritis Rheum., 9:747–757, 1966.
45. Takasugi, K., and Hollingsworth, J.W.: Morphologic studies of mononuclear cells of human synovial fluid. Arthritis Rheum., 10:495–501, 1967.
46. Yurdakul, S., et al.: The arthritis of Behçet's disease: A prospective study. Ann. Rheum. Dis., 42:505–515, 1983.
47. Schlesigner, P.A., Stillman, M.T., and Peterson, L.: Polyarthritis with birefringent lipid within synovial fluid macrophages: Case report and ultrastructural study. Arthritis Rheum., 25:1365–1368, 1982.
48. Klofkorn, R.W., and Lehman, T.J.: Eosinophilic synovial effusions complicating chronic urticaria and angioedema. Arthritis Rheum., 25:708–709, 1982.
49. Hasselbacher, P., and Schumacher, H.R.: Bilateral protrusia acetabuli following pelvic irradiation. J. Rheumatol., 4:189–196, 1977.
50. Hasselbacher, P.: Sickled erythrocytes in synovial fluid. Arthritis Rheum., 23:127–128, 1980.
51. Traycoff, R.B., Pascual, E., and Schumacher, H.R.: Mononuclear cells in human synovial fluid. Arthritis Rheum., 19:743–748, 1976.
52. Kinsella, T.D., Baum, J., and Ziff, M.: Studies of isolated synovial lining cells of rheumatoid and non-rheumatoid synovial membranes. Arthritis Rheum., 13:734–753, 1970.
53. Kinsella, T.D.: Transformation of human lymphocytes in vitro by autologous and allogenic rheumatoid synovial fluid. Ann. Rheum. Dis., 35:8–13, 1976.
54. Stastny, P., et al.: Lymphokines in the rheumatoid joint. Arthritis Rheum., 18:237–243, 1975.
54a. Nordstrom, D., et al.: Synovial fluid cells in Reiter's syndrome. Ann. Rheum. Dis., 44:852–856, 1985.
54b. Harding, B., and Knight, S.C.: The distribution of dendritic cells in the synovial fluid of patients with arthritis. Clin. Exp. Immunol., 63:594–600, 1986.
55. Brandt, K.D., and Krey, P.R.: Chalky joint effusion. Arthritis Rheum., 20:792–796, 1977.
56. McCarty, D.J., and Gatter, R.A.: Recurrent acute inflammation associated with focal apatite deposition. Arthritis Rheum., 9:804–819, 1966.
57. Dieppe, P.A., et al.: Apatite deposition disease. Lancet, 1:266–270, 1976.
58. Crocker, P.R. et al.: The identification of particulate matter in biological tissues and fluids. J. Pathol., 121:37–40, 1977.
59. Schumacher, H.R., et al.: Arthritis associated with apatite crystals. Ann. Intern. Med., 87:411–416, 1977.
60. McCarty, D.J., Lehr, J.R., and Halverson, P.B.: Crystal populations in human synovial fluid: Identification of apatite, octacalcium phosphate and beta tricalcium phosphate. Arthritis Rheum., 26:1220–1224, 1983.
60a. Endresen, G.K.M.: Investigation of blood platelets in synovial fluid from patients with rheumatoid arthritis. Scand. J. Rheumatol., 10:204–208, 1981.
61. Farr, M., et al.: Platelets in the synovial fluid of patients with rheumatoid arthritis. Rheumatol. Int., 4:13–18, 1984.
62. Yaron, M., and Djaldetti, M.: Platelets in synovial fluid (letter). Arthritis Rheum., 21:607–608, 1978.
63. Hallgren, R., Bjelle, A., and Venge, P.: Beta thromboglobulin in inflammatory synovial fluid. Inflammation, 7:311–319, 1983.
64. Frewin, D.B., et al.: Histamine levels in rheumatoid synovial fluid. J. Rheumatol., 13:13–14, 1986.
65. Malone, D.G.: Mast cell numbers and histamine levels in synovial fluid from patients with diverse arthritides. Arthritis Rheum., 29:956–963, 1986.
66. Fremont, A.J., and Denton, J.: Disease distribution of synovial fluid mast cells and cytophagic mononuclear cells in inflammatory arthritis. Ann. Rheum. Dis., 44:312–315, 1985.
67. Crisp, A.J., et al.: Articular mastocytosis in rheumatoid arthritis. Arthritis Rheum., 27:845–851, 1984.
68. Godfrey, H.P., et al.: Quantitation of human synovial mast cells in rheumatoid arthritis and other rheumatic diseases. Arthritis Rheum., 27:852–856, 1984.
69. Bardin, T., et al.: Transmission electron microscopic identification of silicon-containing particles in synovial fluid: Potential confusion with calcium pyrophosphate dihydrate and apatite crystals. Ann. Rheum. Dis., 43:624–627, 1984.
69a. Tnaphaichitr, K., Spilberg, I., and Hahn, B.: Lithium heparin crystals simulating CPPD crystals. Arthritis Rheum., 19:966–968, 1976.
70. McCarty, D.J., and Hogan, J.M.: Inflammatory reaction after intrasynovial injection of microcrystalline adrenocorticosteroid esters. Arthritis Rheum., 7:359–367, 1964.
71. Bluhm, G.B., Riddle, J.M., and Barnhardt, M.I.: Crystal dynamics in gout and pseudogout. Med. Times, 97:135–144, 1969.
72. Bible, M.W., and Pinals, R.S.: Late precipitation of monosodium urate crystals. J. Rheumatol., 9:480, 1982.
73. Ortel, R.W., and Newcombe, D.S.: Acute gouty arthritis and response to colchicine in the virtual absence of synovial fluid leukocytes. N. Engl. J. Med., 290:1363–1364, 1974.
74. Schumacher, H.R., et al.: Acute gouty arthritis without urate crystals identified on initial examination of synovial fluid. Arthritis Rheum., 18:603–612, 1975.
75. Bjelle, A., Crocker, P., and Willoughby, D.: Ultramicrocrystals in pyrophosphate arthropathy. Acta Med. Scand., 207:89–92, 1980.
76. Honig, S., et al.: Crystal deposition disease. Am. J. Med., 63:161–164, 1979.
77. Giechtner, J.J., and Simkin, P.A.: Urate spherulites in gouty synovia. JAMA, 245:1533–1536, 1981.
78. Fagan, T.J., and Lidsky, M.D.: Compensated polarized light

microscopy using cellophane adhesive tape. Arthritis Rheum., 17:256–262, 1974.

79. Owen, D.S.: A cheap and useful compensated polarizing microscope. N. Engl. J. Med., 285:1152, 1971.

80. McCarty, D.J., and Hollander, J.L.: Identification of urate crystals in gouty synovial fluid. Ann. Intern. Med., 54:452–460, 1961.

81. Gatter, R.A.: Use of the compensated polarizing microscope. Clin. Rheum. Dis., 3:91–103, 1977.

82. Gatter, R.A.: The compensated polarized light microscope in clinical rheumatology. Arthritis Rheum., 17:253–255, 1974.

83. Gatter, R.A., and McCarty, D.J.: Pathological tissue calcifications in man. Arch. Pathol., 84:346–353, 1967.

84. Kohn, N.N., et al.: The significance of calcium phosphate crystals in the synovial fluid of arthritis patients: The "pseudogout syndrome." II. Identification of crystals. Ann. Intern. Med., 56:738–745, 1962.

85. McCarty, D.J., and Gatter, R.A.: Identification of calcium hydrogen phosphate dihydrate crystals in human fibrocartilage. Nature, 201:391–392, 1963.

86. Paul, H., Reginato, A.J., and Schumacher, H.R.: Alizarin red staining as a screening test to detect calcium compounds in synovial fluid. Arthritis Rheum., 26:191–200, 1983.

87. Halverson, P.B., et al.: "Milwaukee shoulder": Association of microspheroids containing hydroxyapatite crystals, active collagenase and neutral protease with rotator cuff defects. II. Synovial fluid studies. Arthritis Rheum., 24:474–483, 1981.

88. Cherian, P.V., and Schumacher, H.R.: Diagnostic potential of rapid electron microscopic analysis of joint effusions. Arthritis Rheum., 25:98–100, 1982.

89. McCarty, D.J., et al.: Studies on pathological calcifications in human cartilage. I. Prevalence and types of crystal deposits in the menisci of two hundred fifteen cadavera. J. Bone Joint Surg., 48:309–325, 1966.

90. Gaucher, A., et al.: Identification des Cristaux observes dans les arthropathies destructrices de la chondrocalcinosis. Rev. Rhum. Mal. Osteoartic., 44:407–414, 1977.

90a. Schumacher, H.R., and Rothfuss, S.: Unusual laminated birefringent arrays of apatite crystals in inflammatory arthritis. Arthritis Rheum., 30:5106, 1987.

91. Ettlinger, R.E., and Hunder, G.C.: Synovial effusions containing cholesterol crystals. Mayo Clin. Proc., 54:366–374, 1979.

92. Fam, A.G., et al.: Cholesterol crystals in osteoarthritis joint effusions. J. Rheumatol., 8:273–280, 1981.

93. Newcombe, D.S., and Cohen, A.S.: Chylous synovial effusion in rheumatoid arthritis. Am. J. Med., 38:156–163, 1965.

94. Nye, W.H.R., Terry, R., and Rosenbaum, D.L.: Two forms of crystalline lipid in "cholesterol" effusions. Am. J. Clin. Pathol., 49:718–728, 1968.

95. Zuchner, J., Uddin, J., and Gantner, G.E.: Cholesterol crystals in synovial fluid. Ann. Intern. Med., 60:436–446, 1964.

96. Hoffman, G.S., et al.: Calcium oxalate microcrystalline-associated arthritis in end stage renal disease. Ann. Intern. Med., 97:36–42, 1982.

97. Reginato, A.J., et al.: Arthropathy and cutaneous calcinosis in hemodialysis oxalosis. Arthritis Rheum., 29:1387–1396, 1986.

98. Rosenthal, A., Ryan, L.M., and McCarty, D.J.: Intracellular calcium oxalate crystals in a patient receiving peritoneal dialysis. (submitted)

99. Schumacher, H.R., Reginato, A.J., and Pullman, S.: Synovial fluid oxalate deposition complicating rheumatoid arthritis

with amyloidosis and renal failure: Demonstration of intracellular oxalate crystals. J. Rheumatol., 14:361–366, 1987.

100. Gregg, J.R., Nixon, J.E., and Distefona, V.: Neutral fat globules in traumatized knees. Clin. Orthop., 132:219–224, 1978.

101. Netter, P., et al.: Inflammatory effect of aluminum phosphate. Ann. Rheum. Dis., 42:114, 1983.

102. Gordon, D.A., Pruzanski, W., and Ogryzlo, M.A.: Synovial fluid examination for the diagnosis of amyloidosis. Ann. Rheum. Dis., 32:328–430, 1973.

103. Munoz-Gomez, J., et al.: Synovial fluid examination for the diagnosis of synovial amyloidosis in patients with chronic renal failure undergoing hemodialysis. Ann. Rheum. Dis., 324:3–26, 1987.

104. Kitridou, R., et al.: Identification of collagen in synovial fluid. Arthritis Rheum., 12:580–588, 1969.

105. Hulten, O., and Gillerstedt, N.: Uber abnutzungsproduke in Gelenken und thu resorption unter dem bilde synovits detritca. Acta Chir. Scand., 84:1–29, 1940.

106. Cheung, H.S., et al.: Identification of collagen subtypes in synovial fluid from arthritis patients. Am. J. Med., 68:73–79, 1980.

107. Evans, C.H., Mears, D.C., and McKnight, J.: A preliminary ferrographic survey of the wear particles in human synovial fluid. Arthritis Rheum., 24:912–918, 1981.

108. Hotchkiss, R.N., Tew, W.P., and Hungerford, D.S.: Cartilaginous debris in the injured human knee. Clin. Orthop., 168:144–156, 1982.

109. Popert, A.G. et al.: Frequency of occurrence mode of development and significance of rice bodies in rheumatoid joints. Ann. Rheum. Dis., 41:109–117, 1982.

110. Cheung, H.S., et al.: Synovial origins of rice bodies in joint fluid. Arthritis Rheum., 23:72–76, 1980.

111. McCarty, D.J., and Cheung, H.S.: Origin and significance of rice bodies in synovial fluid. Lancet, 2:715–716, 1982.

112. Niedermeier, W., Cretitz, E.E., and Holley, H.L.: Trace metal composition of synovial fluid from patients with rheumatoid arthritis. Arthritis Rheum., 5:439–444, 1962.

113. Bennett, R.M., and Skosey, J.L.: Lactoferrin and lysozyme levels in synovial fluid. Arthritis Rheum., 20:84–90, 1977.

114. Decoteau, E.: Lactoferrin in synovial fluid of patients with inflammatory arthritis. Arthritis Rheum., 15:324–325, 1972.

115. Gormsen, J., Andersen, R.B., and Feddersen, C.: Fibrinogen-fibrin breakdown products in pathologic synovial fluids. Arthritis Rheum., 14:503–512, 1971.

116. Moroz, L.A., Wing, S., and Liote, F.: Mini-plasminogen-like fragments of plasminogen in synovial fluid in acute inflammatory arthritis. Thromb. Res., 43:417–424, 1986.

117. Mochan, E., and Uhl, J.: Elevations in synovial fluid plasminogen activator in patients with rheumatoid arthritis. J. Rheumatol., 11:123–128, 1984.

118. Cohen, G., Fehr, K., and Wagenhauser, F.J.: Leukocyte elastase and free collagenase activity in synovial effusions: Relation to numbers of polymorphonuclear leukocytes. Rheumatol. Int., 3:89–95, 1983.

119. Hedberg, H.: The depressed synovial complement activity in adult and juvenile rheumatoid arthritis. Acta Rheum. Scand., 10:109–127, 1964.

120. Kim, H.J., et al.: Clinical significance of synovial fluid total hemolytic complement activity. J. Rheumatol., 7:143–152, 1980.

121. Townes, A.S., and Sowa, J.M.: Complement in synovial fluid. Johns Hopkins Med. J., 127:23–37, 1970.

122. Pekin, T.J., and Zvaifler, N.J.: Hemolyic complement in synovial fluid. J. Clin. Invest., 43:1372–1382, 1964.

123. Hasselbacher, P.: Immunoelectrophoretic assay for synovial fluid C3 with correction for synovial fluid globulin. Arthritis Rheum., 22:243–250, 1979.

124. Hunder, G.C., McDuffie, F.C., and Mullen, B.J.: Activation of complement components C2 and B in synovial fluids. J. Lab. Clin. Med., 89:161–171, 1977.

125. Mollnes, E.T., and Paus, A.: Complement activation in synovial fluid and tissue from patients with juvenile rheumatoid arthritis. Arthritis Rheum., 27:1359–1364, 1986.

126. Bland, J.H., and Clark, L.: Rheumatoid factors in serum and joint fluid. Ann. Intern. Med., 58:829–836, 1963.

127. Rodnan, G.P., Eisenbeis, C.H., and Creighton, A.S.: The occurrence of rheumatoid factor in synovial fluid. Am. J. Med., 35:182–188, 1963.

128. Parker, L.P., Seward, C.W., and Osterland, C.K.: Occurrence of antigammaglobulins in effusion fluids of diverse etiology. Ann. Rheum. Dis., 33:262–267, 1974.

129. Hughes, G.R.V., et al.: The release of DNA into serum and synovial fluid. Arthritis Rheum., 14:259–266, 1971.

130. Leon, S.A., et al.: DNA in synovial fluid and the circulation of patients with arthritis. Arthritis Rheum., 24:1142–1150, 1981.

131. Marcus, R.L., and Townes, A.S.: The occurrence of cryoproteins in synovial fluid: The association of a complement fixing activity in rheumatoid synovial fluid with cold precipitable protein. J. Clin. Invest., 50:282–293, 1971.

132. Cracchiolo, A., Goldberg, L.S., and Barnett, A.V.: Studies of cryoprecipitate from synovial fluid of rheumatoid patients. Immunology, 20:1067–1077, 1971.

133. Clemmersen, I., Holund, B., and Andersen, R.B.: Fibrin and fibronectin in rheumatoid synovial membrane and rheumatoid synovial fluid. Arthritis Rheum., 26:479–485, 1983.

134. Wallis, W.J., and Simkin, P.A.: Anti-rheumatic drug concentrations in human synovial fluid and synovial tissue: Observations on extravascular pharmacokinetics. Clin. Pharmacokinet., 8:496–522, 1983.

135. Lygren, I., et al.: Gastrointestinal peptides in serum and synovial fluid from patients with inflammatory joint disease. Ann. Rheum. Dis., 45:637–640, 1986.

136. Dahl, L.B., et al.: Concentration and molecular weight of sodium hyduronate in synovial fluid from patients with rheumatoid arthritis and other arthropathies. Ann. Rheum. Dis., 44:817–822, 1985.

137. Bole, G.G.: Synovial fluid lipids in normal individuals and patients with rheumatoid arthritis. Arthritis Rheum., 5:589–601, 1962.

138. Chung, A.C., Shanahan, J.R., and Brown, E.M.: Synovial fluid lipids in rheumatoid and osteoarthritis. Arthritis Rheum., 5:176–183, 1962.

139. Small, D.M., Cohen, A.S., and Schmid, K.: Lipoproteins of synovial fluid as studied by analytical ultracentrifugation. J. Clin. Invest., 43:2070–2079, 1964.

140. Simkin, P.A., et al.: Free fatty acids in the pancreatic arthritis syndrome. Arthritis Rheum., 26:127–132, 1983.

141. Wise, C.M., White, R.E., and Agudelo, C.A.: Synovial fluid lipid abnormalities in various disease states: review and classification. Semin. Arthritis Rheum., 16:222–230, 1987.

142. Choi, S.J., Schumacher, H.R., and Clayburne, G.: Experimental hemarthrosis produces mild inflammation associated with intracellular Maltese crosses. Ann. Rheum. Dis., 45:1025–1028, 1986.

143. Simon, G.L., Niller, H., and Borenstein, D.G.: Synovial fluid inhibits killing of Staphylococcus aureus by neutrophils. Infect. Immun., 40:1004–1010, 1983.

144. Bodel, P.T., and Hollingsworth, J.W.: Comparative morphology, respiration and phagocytic function of leukocytes from blood and joint fluid in rheumatoid arthritis. J. Clin. Invest., 45:580–589, 1966.

144a. Breedveld, F.C., et al.: Phagocytosis and intracellular killing of staphylococcus aureus by polymorphonuclear cells from synovial fluid of patients with rheumatoid arthritis. Arthritis Rheum., 29:166–173, 1986.

145. Rytel, M.W.: Rapid Diagnosis of Infectious Disease. Edited by M.W. Rytel. CRC Press, 1979, pp. 7–16.

146. Borenstein, D.G., Gibbs, C.A., and Jacobs, R.P.: Gas liquid chromatographic analysis of synovial fluid: Succinic acid and lactic acid as markers for septic arthritis. Arthritis Rheum., 25:947–953, 1982.

147. Mitchell, D.G., et al.: MRI of joint fluid in the normal and ischemic hip. Am. J. Roentgenol., 146:1215–1218, 1986.

148. Eisenberg, J.M., et al.: Usefulness of synovial fluid analysis in the evaluation of joint effusions: Use of threshold analysis and likelihood ratios to assess a diagnostic test. Arch. Intern. Med., 144:715–719, 1984.

149. Schumacher, H.R., et al.: Reproductivity of synovial fluid analyses. Arthritis Rheum., 29:770–774, 1986.

MAGNETIC RESONANCE IMAGING OF THE JOINTS

6

DAVID W. STOLLER and HARRY K. GENANT

Therapeutic and rehabilitative advances in the management of arthritis have necessitated earlier and more-precise noninvasive radiologic assessments. Magnetic resonance imaging (MRI), with its ability to generate detailed high-contrast and high-resolution images of articular joints, supporting muscles, ligaments, cartilage, and synovia, has a unique role in the radiologic assessment of arthritis.[1] MRI provides direct multiplanar imaging of complex articulations in nonorthogonal planes with off-axis fields of view and can differentiate fat, fluid, muscle, cartilage, and cortical bone in both normal and pathologic states. The ability to noninvasively image and characterize early changes in marrow, subchondral bone, and cartilage allows more-precise evaluation in patients presenting with inflammatory or degenerative arthritis of both the axial and appendicular skeletons. In comparison, plain film radiography, although important in patient assessment, may not be an accurate predictor of the initial and subsequent alterations in joint function and structure. Computed tomography (CT) complements MRI and provides good surface cortical bone detail in infection, inflammation, and trauma (see Chapter 8).

TECHNICAL CONSIDERATONS

PHYSICAL PRINCIPLES UNDERLYING MRI

MRI is the presently accepted term describing a form of imaging based on the phenomenon of nuclear magnetic resonance (NMR). NMR was discovered in 1946 and had initial applications in the fields of chemistry and physics as a spectroscopy tool.[2,3] In 1973, Lauterbur proposed the use of NMR signals as the basis of a diagnostic imaging modality that has evolved into MRI as we know it today.

MRI is a function of the behavior of specified nuclei in a magnetic field.[4,5] Nuclei with an odd number of protons or neutrons develop magnetic moments or small magnetic fields. When a hydrogen proton is placed in a uniform magnetic field, it aligns its field in the direction of the external magnetic field. Because the proton also has spin, it precesses around the axis of the applied magnetic field lines in a fashion similar to a spinning top wobbling in the earth's gravitational field. This precession, or *resonance*, occurs at a fixed frequency called the *Lamour frequency*, which is directly proportional to the strength of the magnetic field. Groups of protons, precessing in phase relative to one another, generate a net magnetic moment that is parallel to the external magnetic field.

The application of a radio frequency pulse at the Lamour frequency causes the net magnetic moment to tilt away from its alignment with the external field. The amount of tilt depends on the strength and duration of the applied radio frequency pulse. Because the tilted protons continue to precess, the net magnetic moment also precesses. This precession, or *magnetic resonance*, produces the radio frequency signal, which, when detected and suitably recorded, provides the basis for MRI.

Water molecules, which are free (unattached) or

bound to larger macromolecules, provide the main source of protons (hydrogen nuclei) that are imaged and that characterize the MRI signal. The intensity of the emitted MRI radio frequency signal from any point in the patient depends on several factors, including hydrogen density, flow (laminar and pulsatile), and unique tissue contrast determinants called T1 and T2. *T1 time*, or *spin-lattice relaxation time*, represents the time required to re-establish longitudinal magnetization (the component parallel to the external magnetic field) subsequent to a 90° radio frequency pulse. T1 relaxation is a function of proton thermal interactions with the surrounding lattice or environment of resonating protons. *T2 time*, or *spin-spin relaxation time*, represents the loss of phase coherence of resonating protons after a 90° radio frequency pulse. This loss of phase coherence is a result of local spin interactions between neighboring protons. Free and bound water molecules influence molecular motion and tissue relaxation times.

T1 and T2 tissue contrast can be selectively emphasized by designating *TR (pulse repetition)* and *TE (echo delay)* times. A short TR and TE sequence will generate a T1-weighted image, whereas prolonged TR and TE settings will favor a T2-weighted image. Generally, a T1-weighted image provides superior tissue contrast and anatomic detail, whereas T2-weighted images are more sensitive to tissues with longer T1 and T2 values, such as tumors.

Fluid, edema, and inflamed tissues are characterized by prolonged T2 values and therefore demonstrate increased signal intensity on T2-weighted images. Compact bone (cortex) generates low signal intensity on all pulse sequences because of limited proton motion within its rigid hydrogen lattice. Yellow (fatty) marrow, however, will generate a high signal intensity on short TR, or T1-weighted, acquisitions. Ligaments and tendons, which are of low-spin density, image with low signal intensity, and adjacent muscle or hyaline articular cartilage demonstrates an intermediate signal intensity.

ADVANTAGES OF MRI

The principles and physics of MRI are completely different from CT, which relies on ionizing radiation. In MRI the generation of the imaging signal is based on events occurring at the molecular level, thus offering the potential to provide *physiologic and biochemical*, as well as anatomic, information about tissues. MRI further offers the unique capability of obtaining direct multiplanar acquisitions with off axis, oblique, cine, and vascular imaging modes, without the constraints of rigid imaging (plane of section and reconstruction) and without ionizing radiation. The ability to directly acquire multiplanar and oblique imaging at small centimeter fields of view is advantageous in studying small and complex musculoskeletal articulations. Thin slice sections (less than 3 mm) and high spatial resolution (less than 6 mm) produce images that approach the highest-quality CT images.

MRI TECHNIQUES

Unlike CT, MRI requires specialized protocols and specific technical parameters tailored to individual patients and to specific pathologic processes. Optimal imaging results require the creative selection of appropriate parameters—TR and TE, field of view, matrix, number of signal excitations (NEX), slice thickness, plane, and axis designations. Separate acquisitions are performed for each plane of section or type of tissue contrast required. Although multiple reconstructions are not generated from a signal data base, as they are with CT, developments in three-dimensional MRI acquisitions do allow for volumetric data acquisition.

The use of extremity and axial spine surface coils, positioned near the anatomic region of interest, will optimize signal-to-noise ratios, especially when imaging with higher-resolution acquisitions at smaller fields of view.

Conventional spin echo imaging techniques use a 90 to 180° radio frequency pulse pair to generate T1- or T2-weighted images based on selected TR and TE parameters. Although the selection of a heavily T2-weighted sequence (long TR and TE) produces increased signal-to-noise ratios, this improvement is offset by the disadvantages of prolonged acquisition times. Shorter TR sequences, which reduce imaging time, emphasize T1-weighting and are subject to greater noise. With the advent of new *gradient echo techniques* using pulse sequences with flip angles of less than 90° (fast-scan imaging), effective T2-weighted contrast can be generated in a fraction of the time required for traditional spin echo sequences. *Chemical-shift imaging*, using a chemical-shift artifact at fat-water interfaces, can be used to subtract relative contributions of fat and water to distinguish better a variety of pathologic processes.

Volumetric acquisition techniques and gradient echo imaging can be employed to change the low-intensity signal of flowing blood on conventional spin echo imaging to create an MRI angiogram effect, with enhancement of arterial and venous flow. In three-dimensional MRI, acquisitions are resolved with a *sec-*

ond phase encoding gradient, in addition to the standard decoding phase and frequency gradients used in processing received radio frequency signals.

CLINICAL APPLICATIONS OF MR IMAGING OF THE JOINTS

MRI OF THE KNEE

As a noninvasive imaging modality, allowing anatomic and pathologic definition of osseous, soft-tissue, ligamentous, cartilaginous, and marrow elements of the knee, MRI is rapidly replacing arthrography and CT for evaluation of inflammatory disorders of this joint.[6-8] In addition to the detection and subsequent followup of early inflammatory arthropathies, MRI has potential for use in the characterization of synovial- and cartilage-based disorders as well. The ability to visualize hyaline articular cartilage directly with MRI has been instrumental in characterizing synovial-based and cartilage-based disorders.

Imaging Protocol for the Knee. In a routine knee protocol, axial, sagittal, and coronal T1-weighted images are acquired in less than 10 min of imaging time. The patellofemoral joint and cartilage are best evaluated in the axial plane. The collateral ligaments are demonstrated on coronal images, and the menisci and cruciate ligaments are defined in the sagittal imaging plane.

Meniscal Pathology. Although the intact meniscus is of low signal intensity, meniscal degeneration is imaged with increased signal intensity in a spectrum pattern. An MRI grading system, rating the structure of the increased signal intensity (in relation to an articular surface), has been developed and correlated with a pathologic model. MRI is sensitive to changes in the menisci ranging from mucinous degeneration (grades 1 and 2) to frank tear (grade 3) (Figs. 6–1 and 6–2).[9,10] The increased signal intensity, observed on both T1- and T2-weighted images, results from increased local proton density and a shortening of T1 relaxation time, caused by synovial fluid absorbed into degenerative or torn meniscal surfaces. With MRI studies, histologic alterations in the fibrocartilaginous meniscus can thus be assessed *prior to the appearance of the surface changes* seen on arthrographic or arthroscopic examinations.

Complex meniscal tears, degenerative fibrillation, and meniscal capsular separations can all be visualized in MRI in the coronal and sagittal planes. *Hypoplastic menisci* have been observed in patients with juvenile rheumatoid (chronic) arthritis. (Hypoplastic

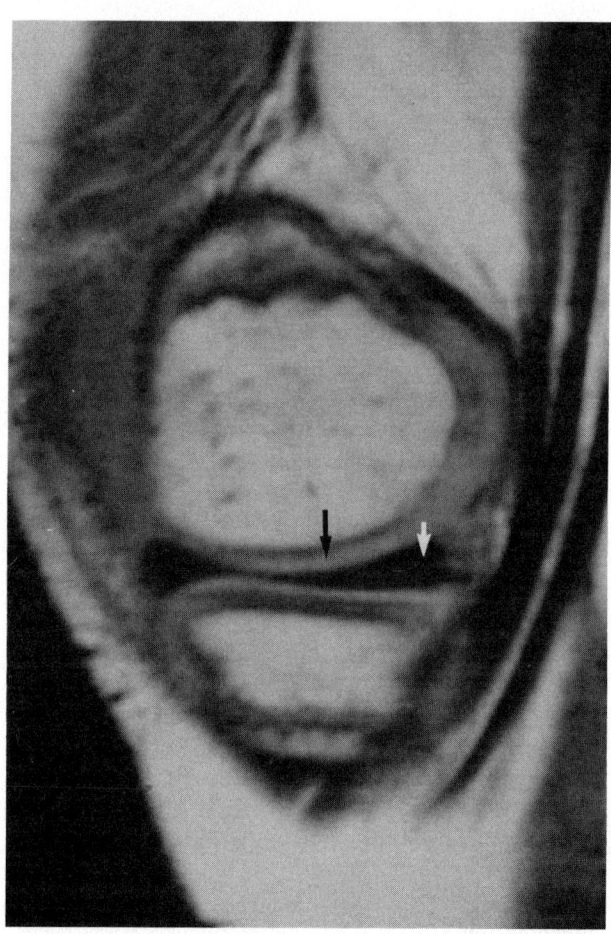

FIG. 6–1. MRI showing grade 2 signal intensity (white arrow) in meniscal degeneration. Hyaline articular cartilage is of intermediate signal intensity (black arrow). (T1-weighted sagittal image; TR = 800 msec, TE = 25 msec)

FIG. 6–2.   Grade 3 signal intensity extending to the inferior articular surface in a tear of the posterior horn of the medial meniscus (arrow). (T1-weighted sagittal image; TR = 800 msec, TE = 25 msec)

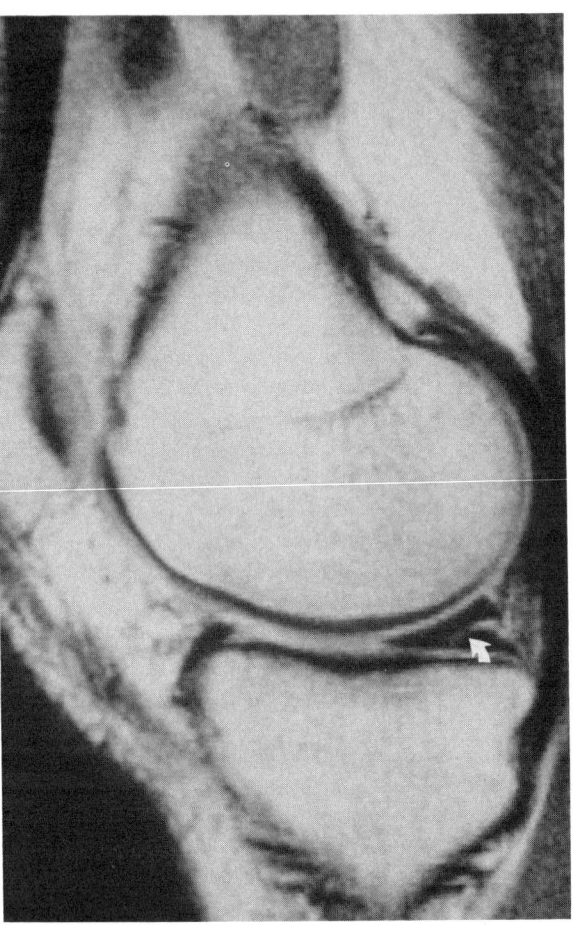

menisci might represent an impairment in synovial nutrition that affects normal fibrocartilage development.) On sagittal images, *dysplastic (discoid) menisci,* which are associated with an increased frequency of meniscal cysts and tears, appear as a continuous band, without separating into anterior and posterior horn segments. On coronal images, a discoid meniscus may extend toward the intercondylar notch.

Chondrocalcinosis has not yet been imaged in pathologically proved specimens, probably because both calcium crystals and fibrocartilage generate similar low-intensity signals.

Cruciate Ligament Pathology. Tears, avulsions, and edema in the cruciate ligaments can be imaged in both the coronal and sagittal planes (Figs. 6–3, 6–4, and 6–5). In acute and chronic injuries, disruptions of both the medial and lateral collateral ligaments are visualized on T1- and T2-weighted coronal images (Figs. 6–6 and 6–7). Complete tears or avulsions of the medial collateral or anterior cruciate ligaments are frequently associated with large hemorrhagic joint effusions.

Articular Cartilage Pathology. Patellar, femoral, and tibial hyaline articular cartilage image with a signal of intermediate intensity on both T1- and T2-weighted sequences (Fig. 6–8). On fast-scan MR images, using partial flip angles of less than 90°, hyaline articular cartilage will increase in signal intensity and appear bright (Fig. 6–9). On fast-scan gradient echo refocused images, *cartilage-fluid interfaces* can be defined even in the presence of large joint effusions. This allows a more accurate determination of cartilage thickness in erosive and degenerative arthropathies. In children, the hyaline articular cartilage on the surface of the distal femur and proximal tibia is thicker and more abundant, allowing earlier detection of erosions (Fig. 6–10).

In patients with juvenile rheumatoid arthritis, hemophilia, or osteoarthritis, attenuated cartilage and focal erosions, which may be underestimated on conventional radiographs, can be detected on MRI. Subchondral sclerosis, frequently seen in association with cartilage loss and joint space narrowing, images with low signal intensity on both T1- and T2-weighted sequences. Subarticular cysts containing fluid or mucinous material generate low signal intensity on T1-weighted images and uniformly generate high signal intensity on T2-weighted sequences.

Early identification of chondromalacia is often possible by visualizing a characteristic area of lower signal intensity within the patella representing bony softening, which *precedes* the loss of posterior facet hyaline cartilage.

Synovial Disorders. Although MRI cannot directly

FIG. 6–3. Intact anterior cruciate ligament (long solid arrow), femoral condylar hyaline articular cartilage (short solid arrow), and joint fluid of high signal intensity (open arrow). (T2-weighted sagittal image; TR = 2000 msec, TE = 40 msec)

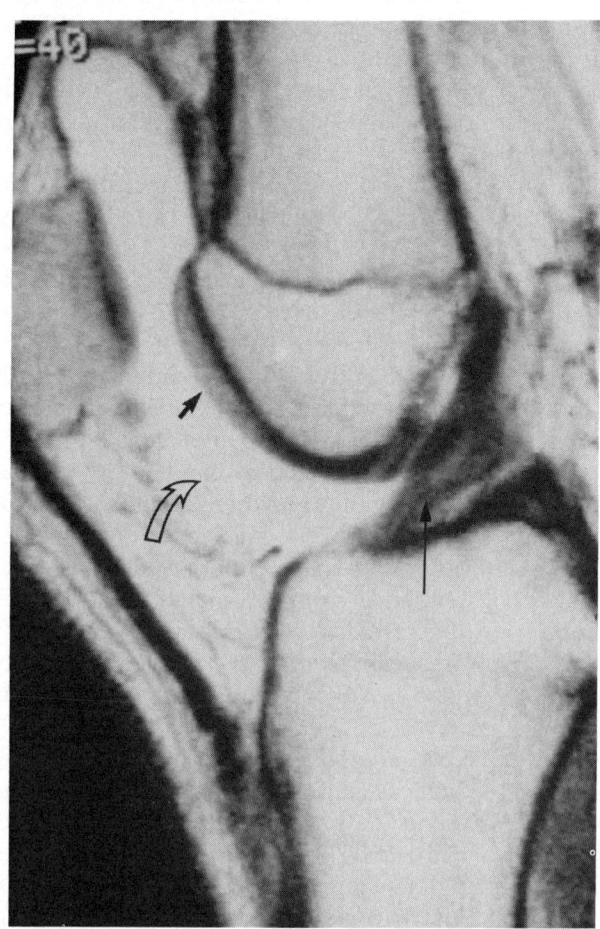

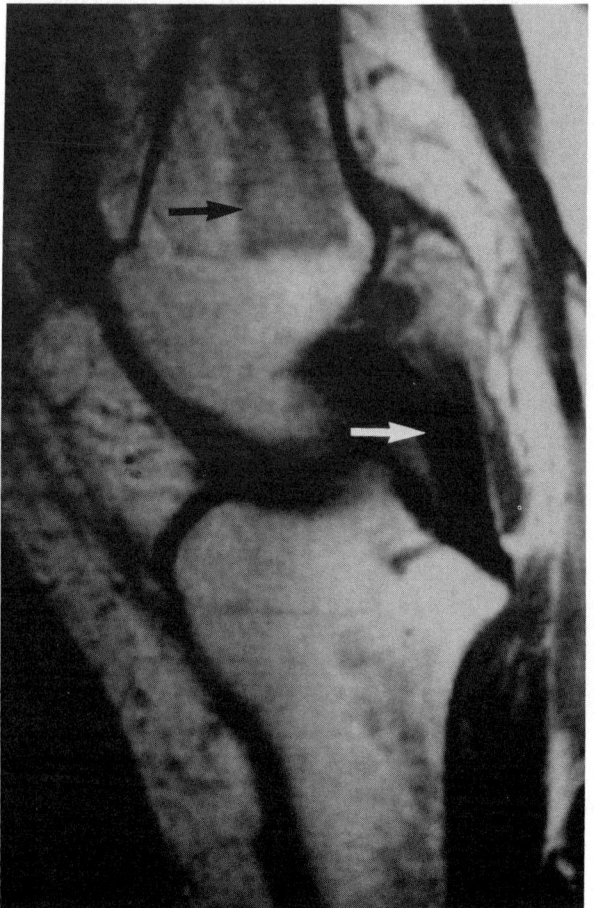

FIG. 6–4. Intact posterior cruciate ligament visualizes with low signal intensity (white arrow). Inhomogeneity of signal is seen in normal marrow in diametaphyseal region (black arrow). (T1-weighted sagittal image; TR = 800 msec, TE = 25 msec)

FIG. 6–5. Midsubstance tear in posterior cruciate ligament (arrow). (T1-weighted sagittal image; TR = 800 msec, TE = 25 msec)

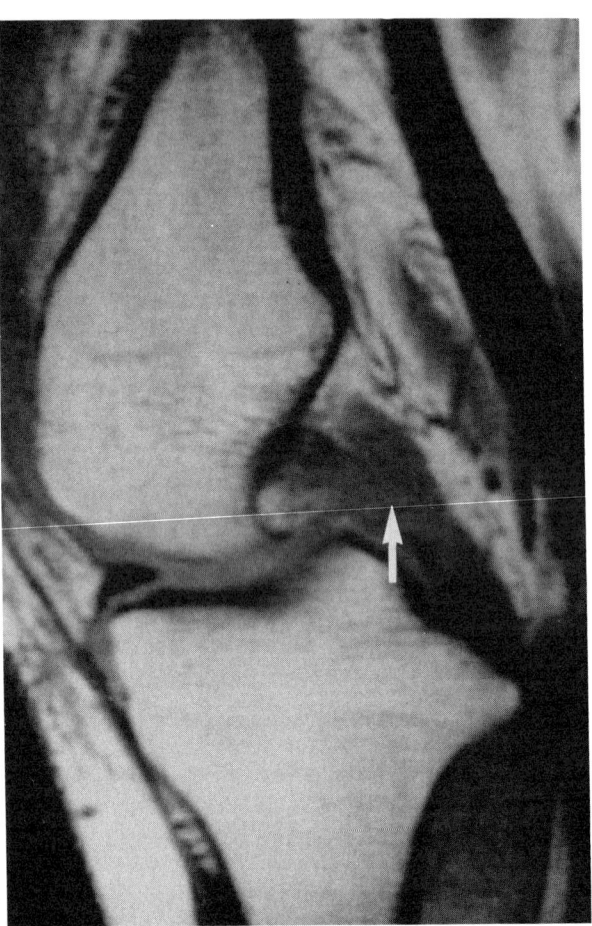

image intact synovia, early synovial irritations can be identified by the corrugated appearance of the normally concave free edge of Hoffa's infrapatellar fat pad (Fig. 6–11A,B). This pattern of early synovitis has been observed in patients with juvenile rheumatoid arthritis, hemophilia, Lyme disease, and hemorrhagic traumatic synovitis (Fig. 6–12). Hemosiderin deposits, which accumulate along this synovial reflection, and hypertrophied synovial masses have been documented in pigmented villonodular synovitis and in hemophilia (Figs. 6–13 and 6–14).

Pannus formation in inflammatory arthritis can be visualized with low to intermediate signal intensity on both T1- and T2-weighted images. This visualization is in contrast to associated joint effusions, which brighten to high signal intensity on T2-weighted sequences. Synovium-lined meniscal cysts, traceable to the joint line, image with high signal intensity on T2-weighted images. Medial patellar and suprapatellar plica (embryologic synovial remnants of the knee joint compartments) are visualized as bands of low signal intensity, which may thicken when inflamed and subsequently interfere with the quadriceps mechanism.

Fragments in synovial osteochondromatosis are visualized with either low or high signal intensity, depending on the presence of metaplastic cartilage or fatty marrow, respectively (Fig. 6–15). Nonuniformity of fragment size favors a secondary cause such as trauma.

Joint effusions generate high signal intensity on T2-weighted sequences (Figs. 6–16 and 6–17). With the patient in the supine position, effusions imaged in the coronal plane layer into a "saddlebag" distribution, with fluid tracking into medial and lateral suprapatellar bursal extensions. In trauma and in arthritis, fluid is reflected over the meniscal surfaces, posterior capsule, and cruciate ligaments without interfering with diagnostic interpretation. In suprapatellar effusions, fat-fluid, fluid-fluid, and air-fluid levels can be differentiated. Although inflammatory effusions can not yet be differentiated from noninflammatory effusions, inferences can be made from the presence of detritus, synovial hypertrophy, and inhomogeneity of marrow signal intensity on T1- and T2-weighted images. Further developments in MRI spectroscopy may more clearly differentiate inflammatory from noninflammatory joint effusions.

Popliteal Cysts. Popliteal cysts of the gastrocnemius-semimembranosus bursa are common. Popliteal cysts containing synovial fluid visualize with low signal intensity on T1-weighted images and high signal intensity on T2-weighted images (Fig. 6–18). Although frequently located posteromedial and deep to the gastrocnemius muscle, atypical presentations of

FIG. 6–6. *A,* Thickened medial collateral ligament in a partial tear images with low signal intensity (arrow). (T1-weighted coronal image; TR = 800 msec, TE = 20 msec). *B,* Corresponding T2-weighted gradient echo acquisition shows disruption and edema within the medial collateral ligament (arrow). (TR = 400 msec, TE = 30 msec, θ = 30°)

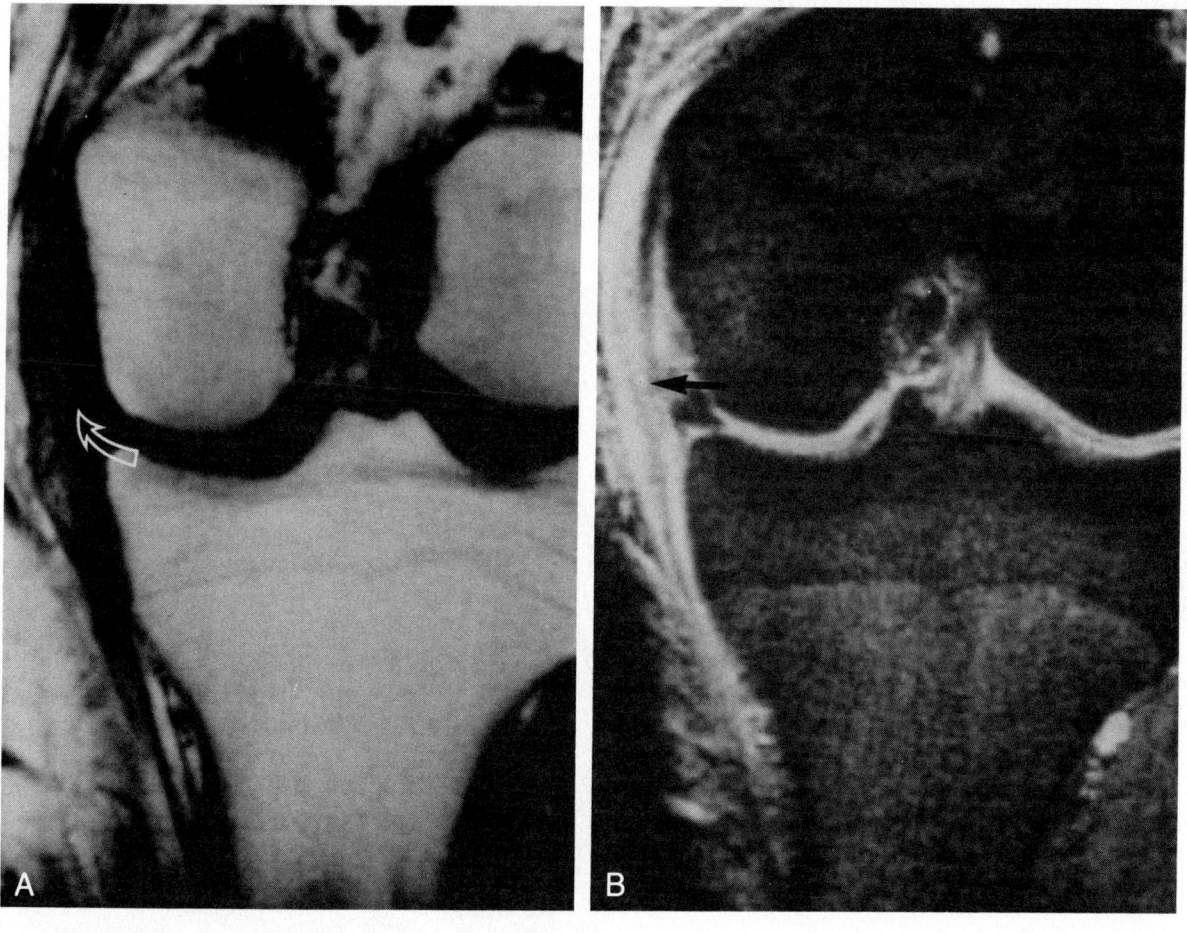

FIG. 6–7. Complete avulsion of the medial collateral ligament from its femoral epicondylar attachment (arrow). High-intensity signal represents subacute hemorrhage. (T1-weighted coronal image; TR = 1000 msec, TE = 40 msec)

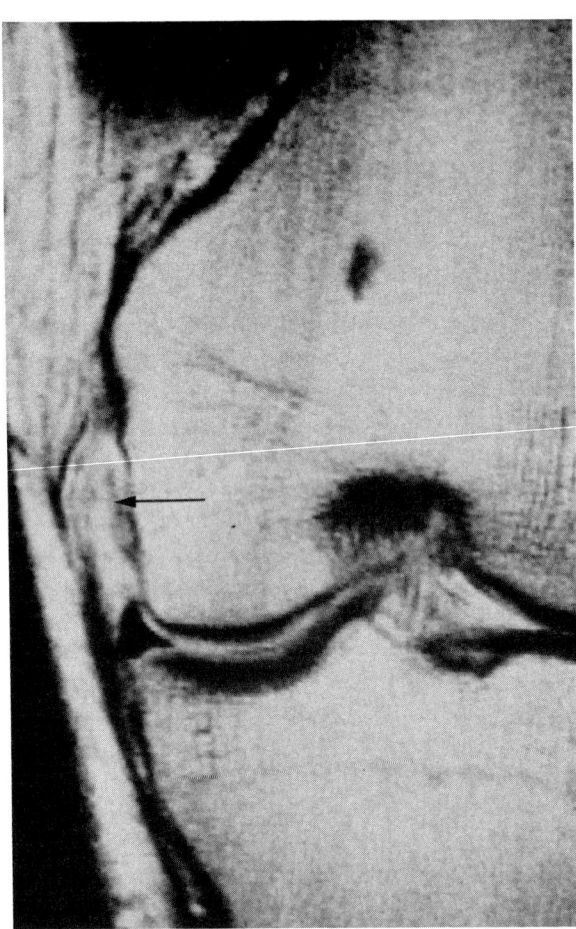

FIG. 6–8. Intact medial retinacular patellar attachments (solid black arrows) and posterior patellar hyaline articular cartilage of normal thickness (open arrow). (T1-weighted axial image; TR = 1000 msec, TE = 40 msec)

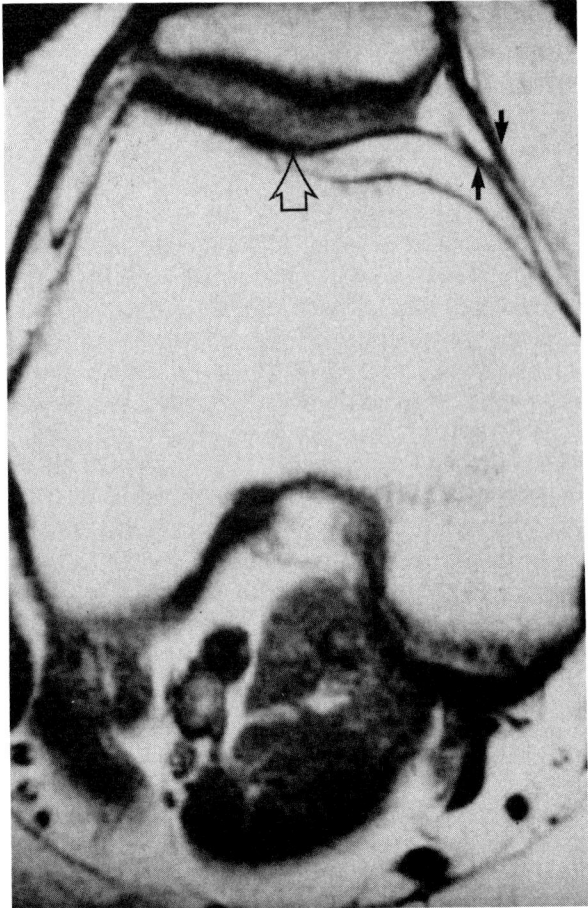

FIG. 6–9. Cartilage (straight arrow)-fluid (arrowhead) interface can be differentiated from the brighter signal intensity of the fluid in the suprapatellar bursa and the high signal intensity of the distal femoral hyaline articular cartilage. A subacute tear of the posterior cruciate ligament can also be seen (curved arrow) with increased intrasubstance signal intensity. (T2-weighted sagittal gradient recall image; TR = 600 msec, TE = 30 msec, flip angle of 15°)

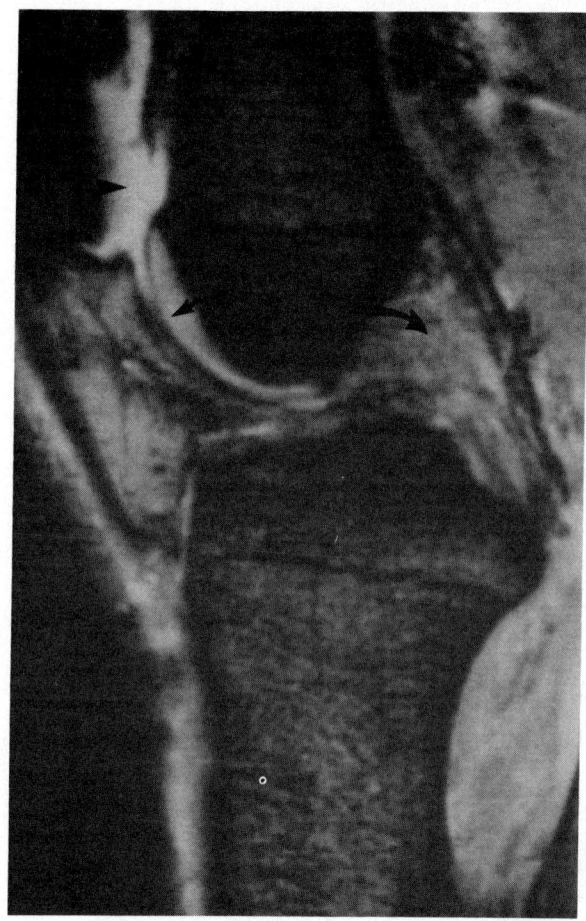

FIG. 6–10. Irregular, thick hyaline articular cartilage surface of intermediate signal intensity (black arrow) in a child with hemophilia. Hemosiderin deposits of low signal intensity are distributed in irritated synovial reflection (white arrow). (T1-weighted sagittal image; TR = 800 msec, TE = 25 msec)

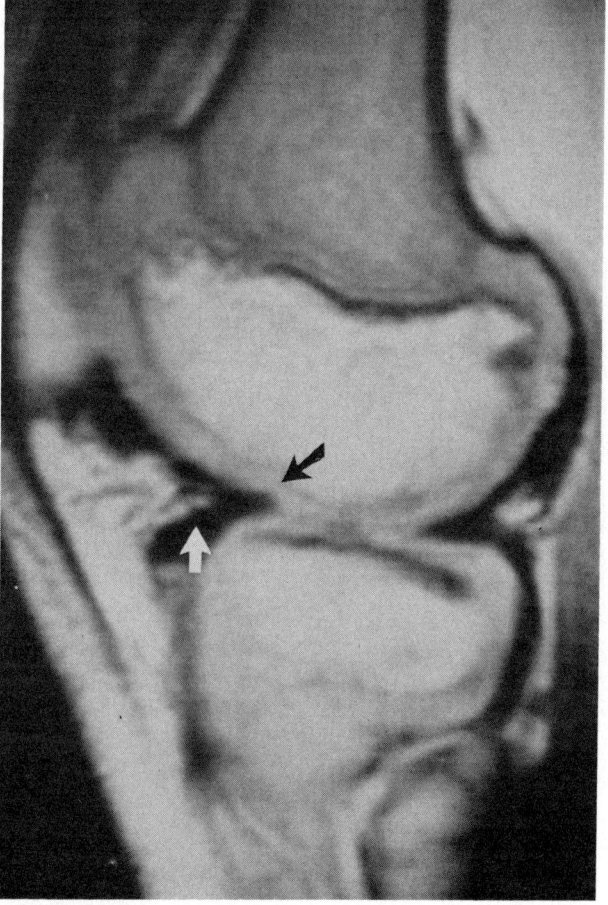

FIG. 6–11. *A,* Asymptomatic knee in a patient with Lyme disease showing normal concave appearance of Hoffa's infrapatellar fat pad (arrow). *B,* Synovial irritation in the knee of a patient with Lyme disease showing corrugated appearance of Hoffa's infrapatellar fat pad (white arrows) and joint effusion. (T1-weighted sagittal image; TR = 800 msec, TE = 25 msec)

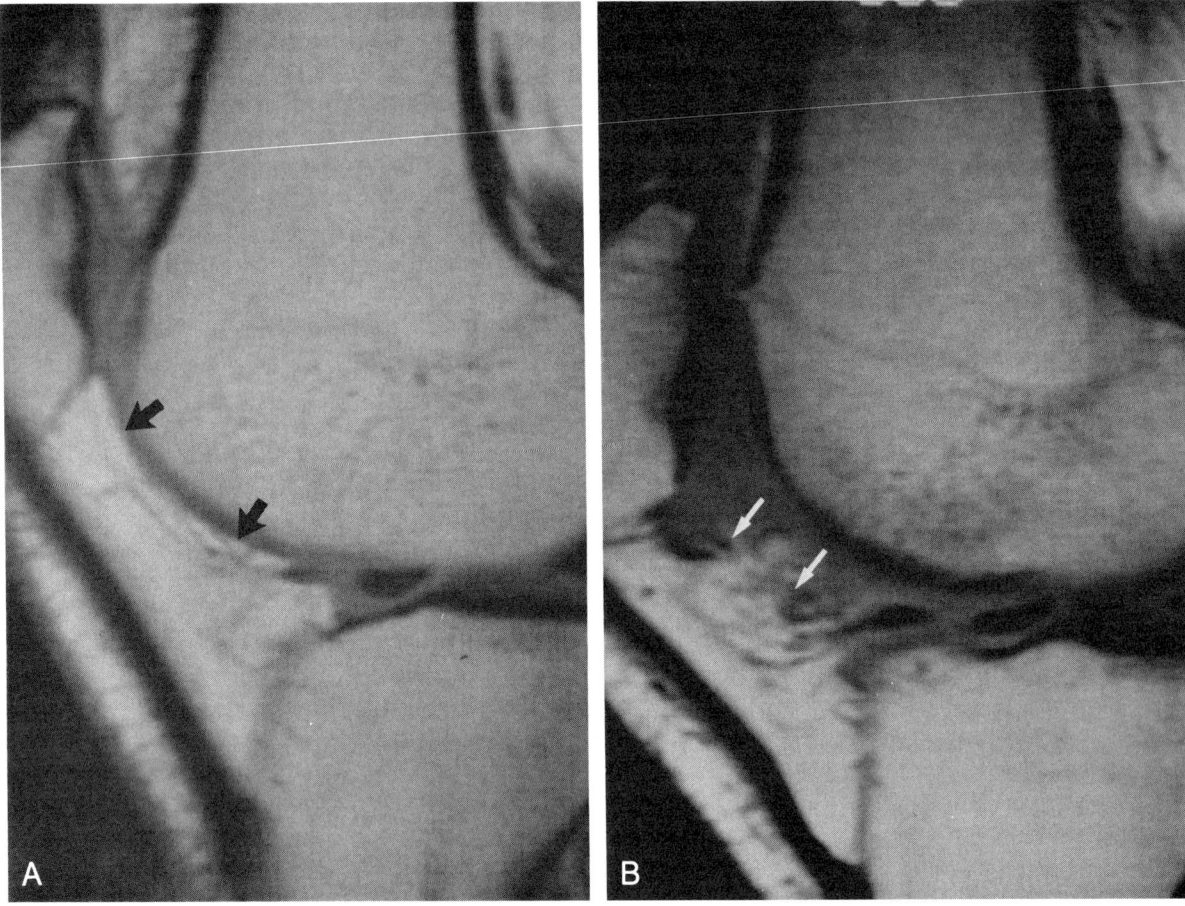

FIG. 6–12. Glanzman thrombocytopenia with hemorrhagic effusion and irregular synovial interface with the free edge of Hoffa's infrapatellar fat pad (arrow). (T2-weighted sagittal image; TR = 2000 msec, TE = 40 msec)

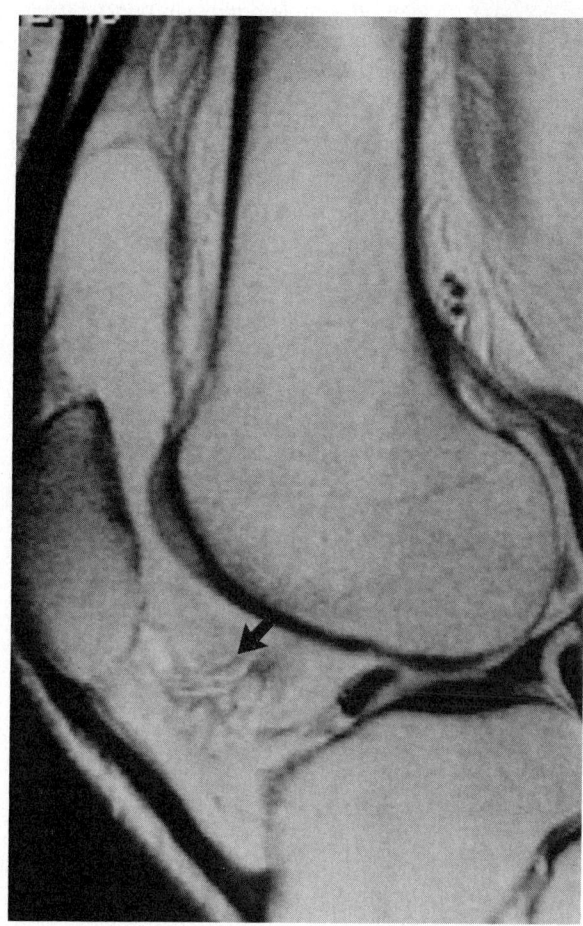

FIG. 6–13. Synovial hypertrophy in diffuse pigmented villonodular synovitis. Hemosiderin-laden masses image with low signal intensity (arrows). (Relative or intermediate T1-weighted sagittal image; TR = 1500 msec, TE = 40 msec)

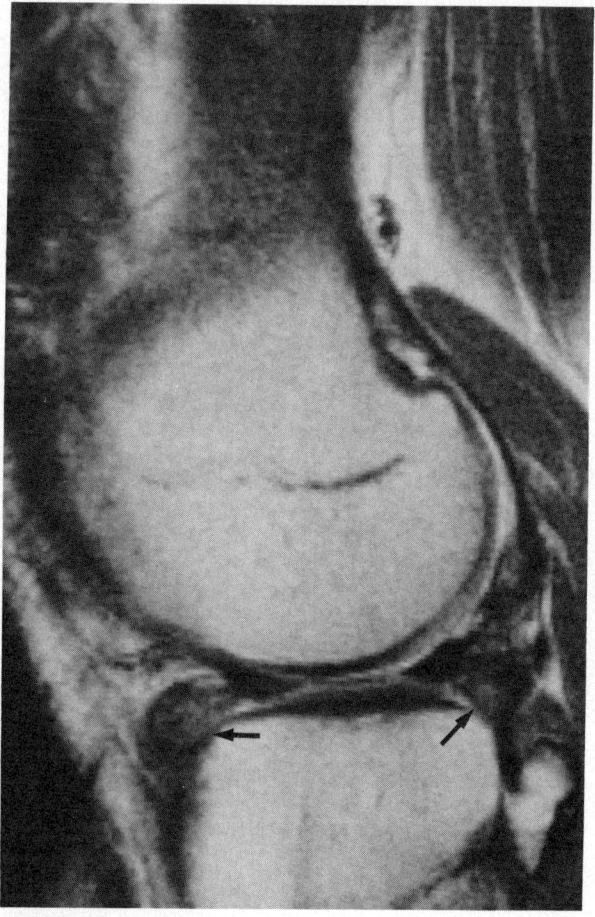

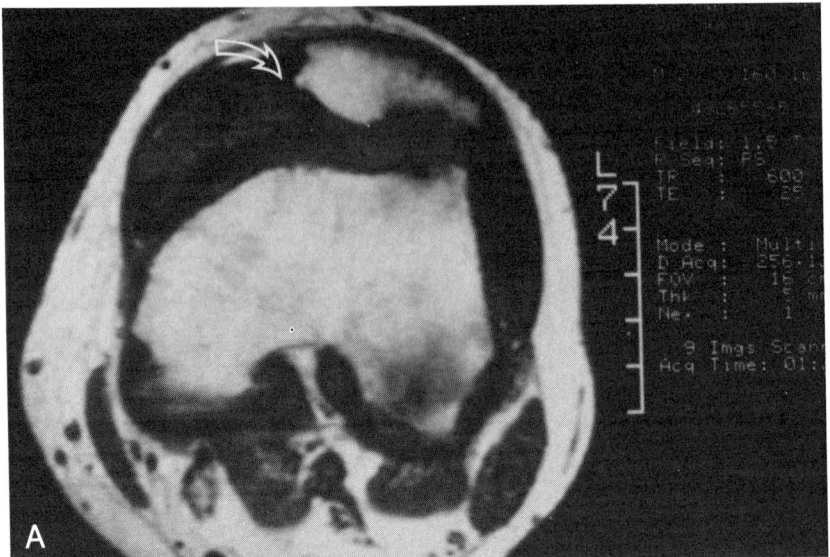

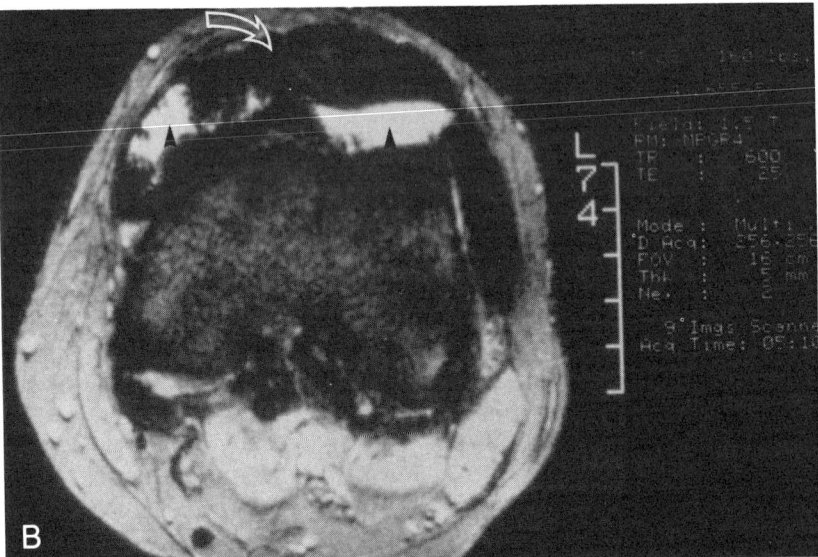

FIG. 6–14. Synovial hemosiderin deposits and adjacent joint effusion in knee joint of a hemophiliac patient. *A,* With conventional T1-weighting, the hemosiderin deposits (open arrow) appear low in signal intensity, whereas the adjacent joint effusion (arrowheads) is of intermediate signal intensity. (TR = 600 msec; TE = 25 msec) *B,* On gradient echo–acquired images, the joint effusion images with bright signal intensity (T2-weighted axial image; TR = 600 msec, TE = 25 msec, flip angle of 15°)

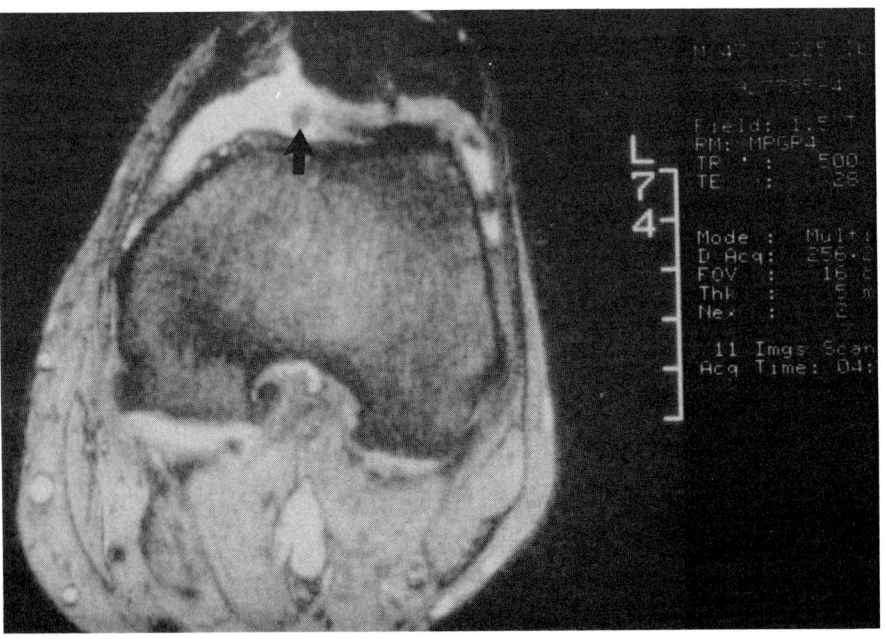

FIG. 6–15. Synovial-based nodules (arrow) in osteochondromatosis of the knee image with low signal intensity (arrow). The high signal intensity of synovial fluid creates an "arthrographic" effect. (T2-weighted axial gradient recall echo image; TR = 500 msec, TE = 28 msec, flip angle of 15°)

FIG. 6–16. High signal intensity of synovial fluid (arrow) on surface of hyaline articular cartilage. (T2-weighted sagittal image; TR = 2000 msec, TE = 60 msec)

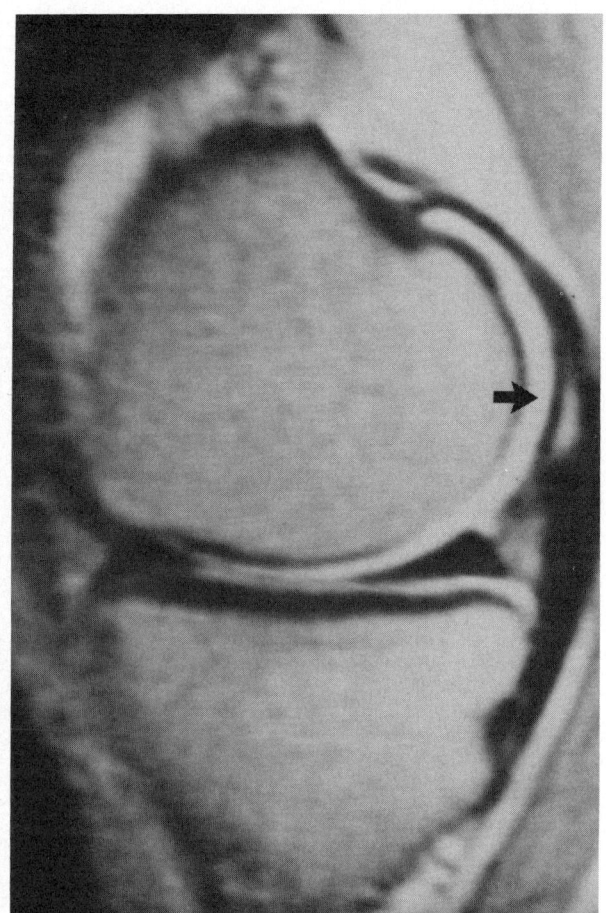

FIG. 6–17. Torn retinacular attachments (long arrow) and associated chondral fragment (short arrow) can be differentiated from adjacent suprapatellar effusion (curved arrows). (T2-weighted axial image; TR = 2000 msec, TE = 80 msec)

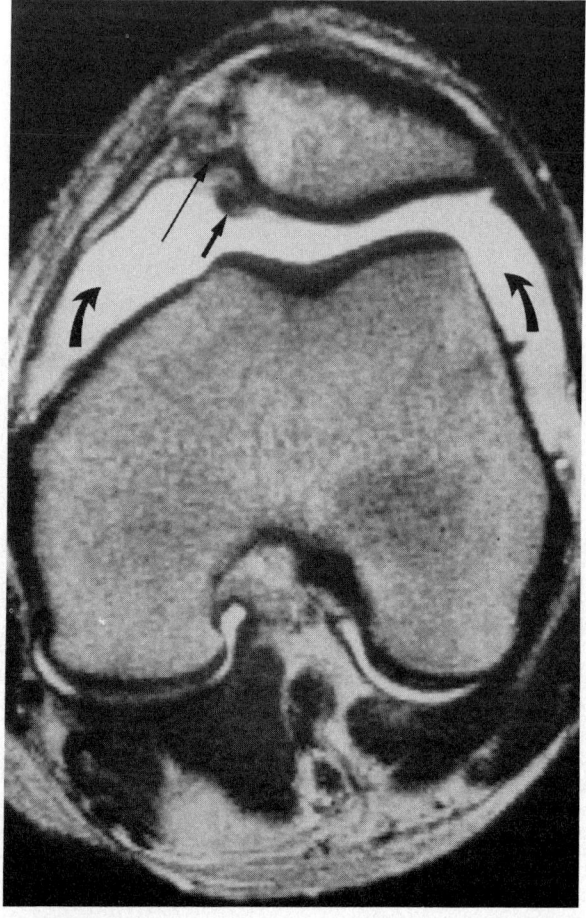

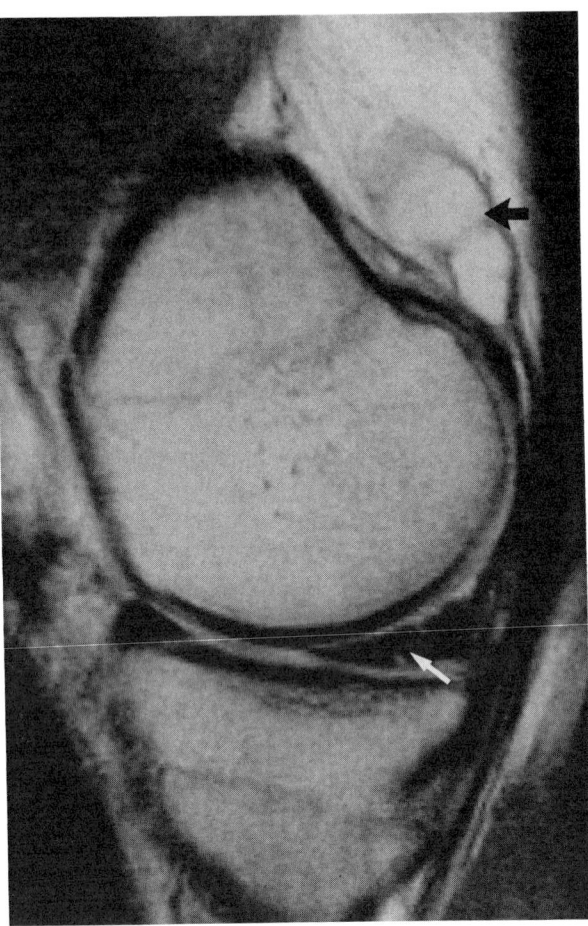

FIG. 6–18.   Popliteal cyst (black arrow) of high signal intensity in association with vertical tear (white arrow) in posterior horn segment of medial meniscus. (T2-weighted sagittal image; TR = 2000 msec, TE = 40 msec)

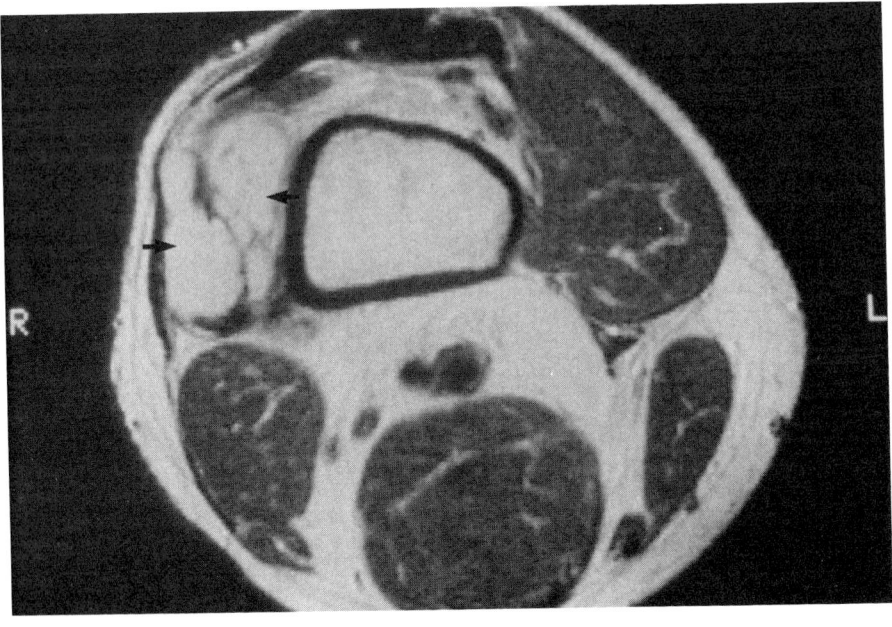

FIG. 6–19.   Atypical presentation of popliteal cyst tracking along the distal lateral femur (arrows). Intermediate weighting produces high signal intensity. (TR = 2000 msec, TE = 40 msec)

popliteal cysts have been observed with proximal or distal dissection relative to the joint (Fig. 6–19). In adults, intra-articular pathology, particularly meniscal tears, are often seen in association with popliteal cyst fluid collections.

Degenerative and Traumatic Disorders. Osteoarthritis is characterized by subchondral sclerosis (loss of signal intensity), attenuated hyaline cartilage, osteophytosis, and subchondral cysts (Fig. 6–20). With T2-weighting, degenerative cysts containing mucinous or synovial fluid generate increased signal intensity.

Spontaneous osteonecrosis and osteochondritis dissecans of the medial femoral condyle visualize with low signal intensity (Fig. 6–21). This visualization represents the area of devitalized bone. The overlying hyaline cartilage can then be examined for surface defects.[11]

MRI is also sensitive for detection of compression fractures of the tibial plateau (Fig. 6–22). These injuries can result in secondary osteoarthritis and are often associated with collateral or cruciate ligament injuries. Using MRI, fractures can be detected even in the absence of findings on initial plain radiography. Acute fractures have associated marrow edema and demonstrate increased signal intensity on T2-weighted images (Fig. 6–23). It is important not to mistake the epiphyseal scar for a fracture in an adult patient.

Neoplastic Disease. Preoperative assessment of primary neoplasms, commonly found about the knee joint, can be performed with T1-weighted sagittal or coronal images and T2-weighted axial planar images (Fig. 6–24). Initial diagnostic imaging should be performed before biopsy, because a subsequent inflammatory response may produce peritumoral edema, which images with high signal intensity and may simulate neoplastic spread. Candidates for limb salvage protocols who are receiving chemotherapy can be monitored with MRI.[12] Tumor recurrence can be distinguished from postoperative fibrosis even in the presence of metallic hardware or joint arthroplasties (Fig. 6–25). The size of the orthopedic hardware does not always indicate the degree of metallic artifact; *small screws and needles can produce large signal artifacts* (Fig. 6–26).

MRI OF THE HIP

MRI has the potential to directly image the hip in coronal, sagittal, and axial planes. Acetabular and femoral cartilage, as well as capsular structures, can be visualized with small fields of view using a high-

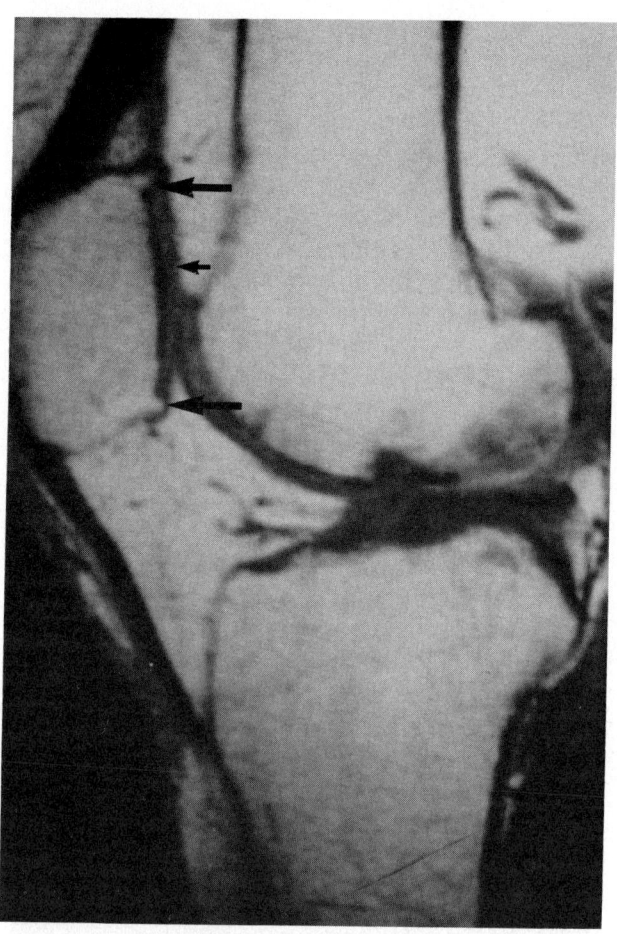

FIG. 6–20. Patella with attenuated patellar facet cartilage (short arrow) and osteophytosis (large arrows) in patient with chondromalacia. (T1-weighted sagittal image; TR = 800 msec, TE = 25 msec)

FIG. 6–21. Focus of spontaneous osteonecrosis (arrow) in medial femoral condyle. (T1-weighted sagittal image; TR = 800 msec, TE = 25 msec)

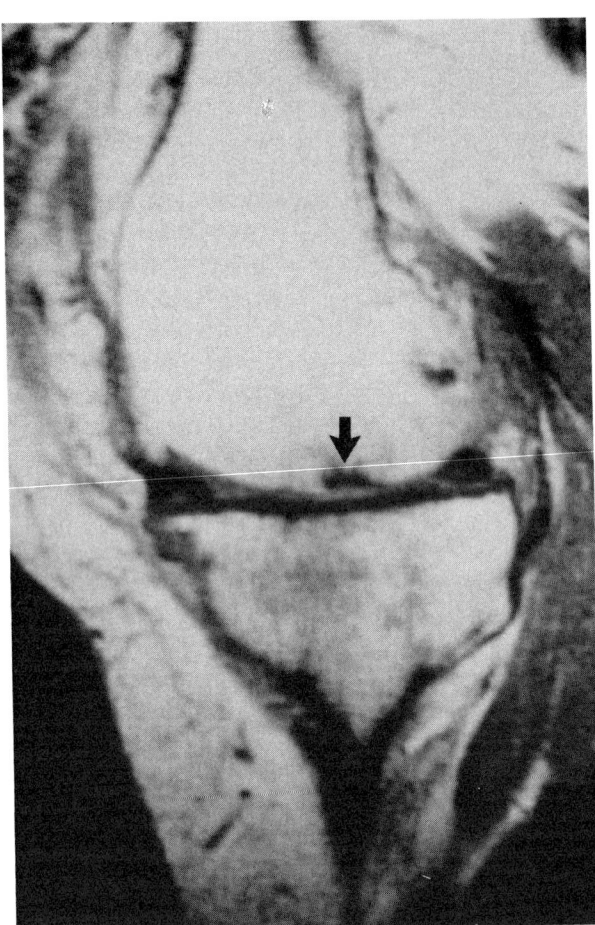

FIG. 6–22. Lateral tibial plateau fracture with ingrowth of granulation tissue (arrow) and disrupted articular surface. (Relative T1-weighted sagittal image; TR = 1500 msec, TE = 40 msec)

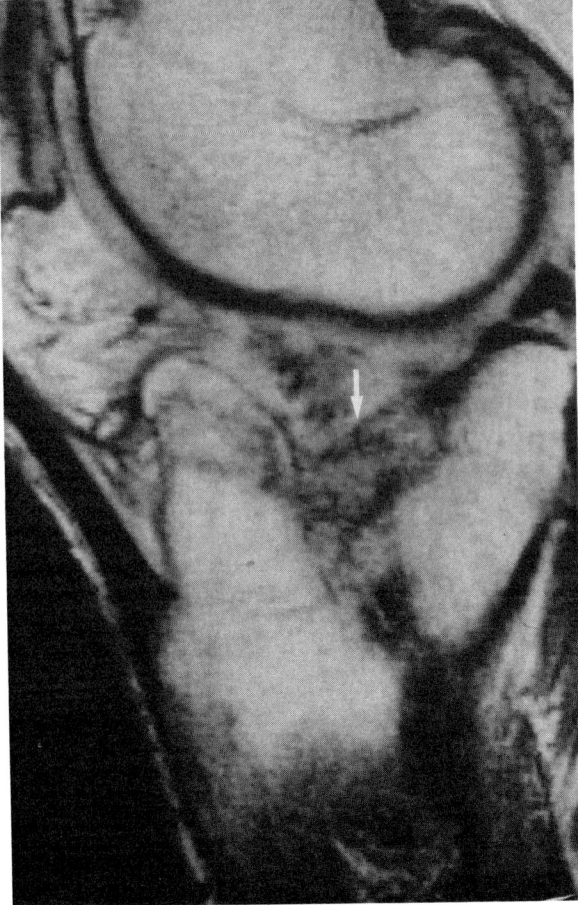

FIG. 6–23. Marrow edema in lateral facet patellar fracture (arrow) images with high signal intensity. (T2-weighted axial image: TR = 2000 msec, TE = 40 msec)

FIG. 6–24. Low signal intensity of blastic osteogenic sarcoma (white arrow) of the tibia with adjacent popliteus muscle edema (black arrow). (T2-weighted image; TR = 2000 msec, TE = 40 msec)

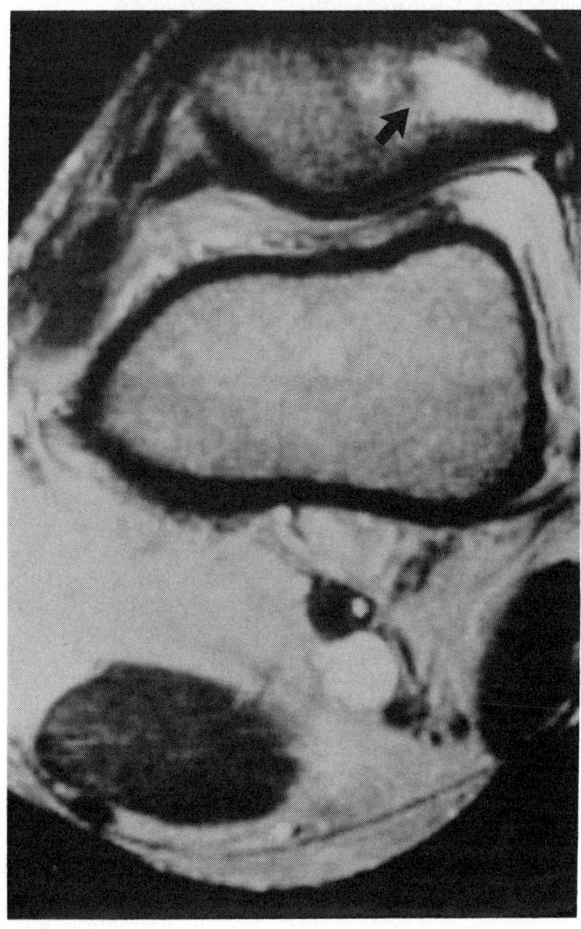

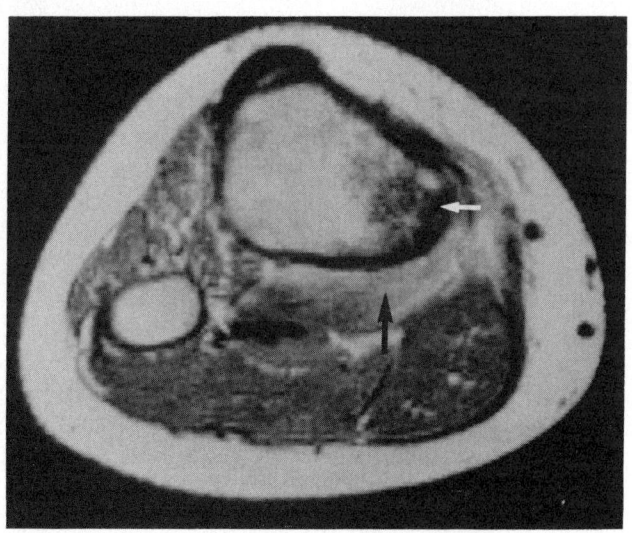

FIG. 6–25. Local metallic artifact (white arrow) does not obscure visualization of postoperative fibrosis (black arrow) in a patient with a limb salvage procedure for osteosarcoma. (Relative T1-weighted image; TR = 1500 msec, TE = 40 msec)

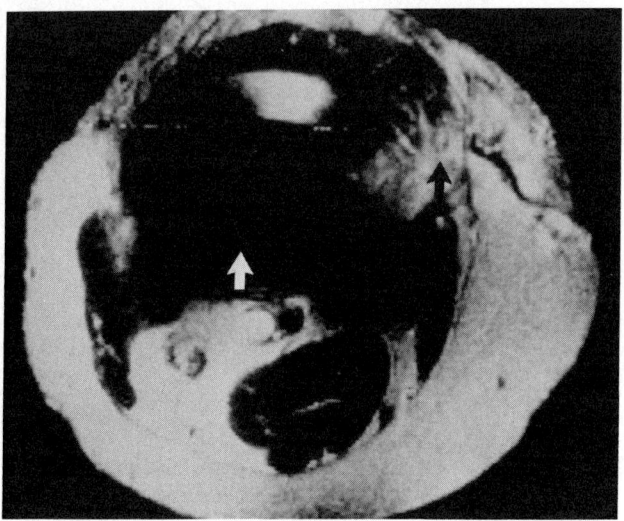

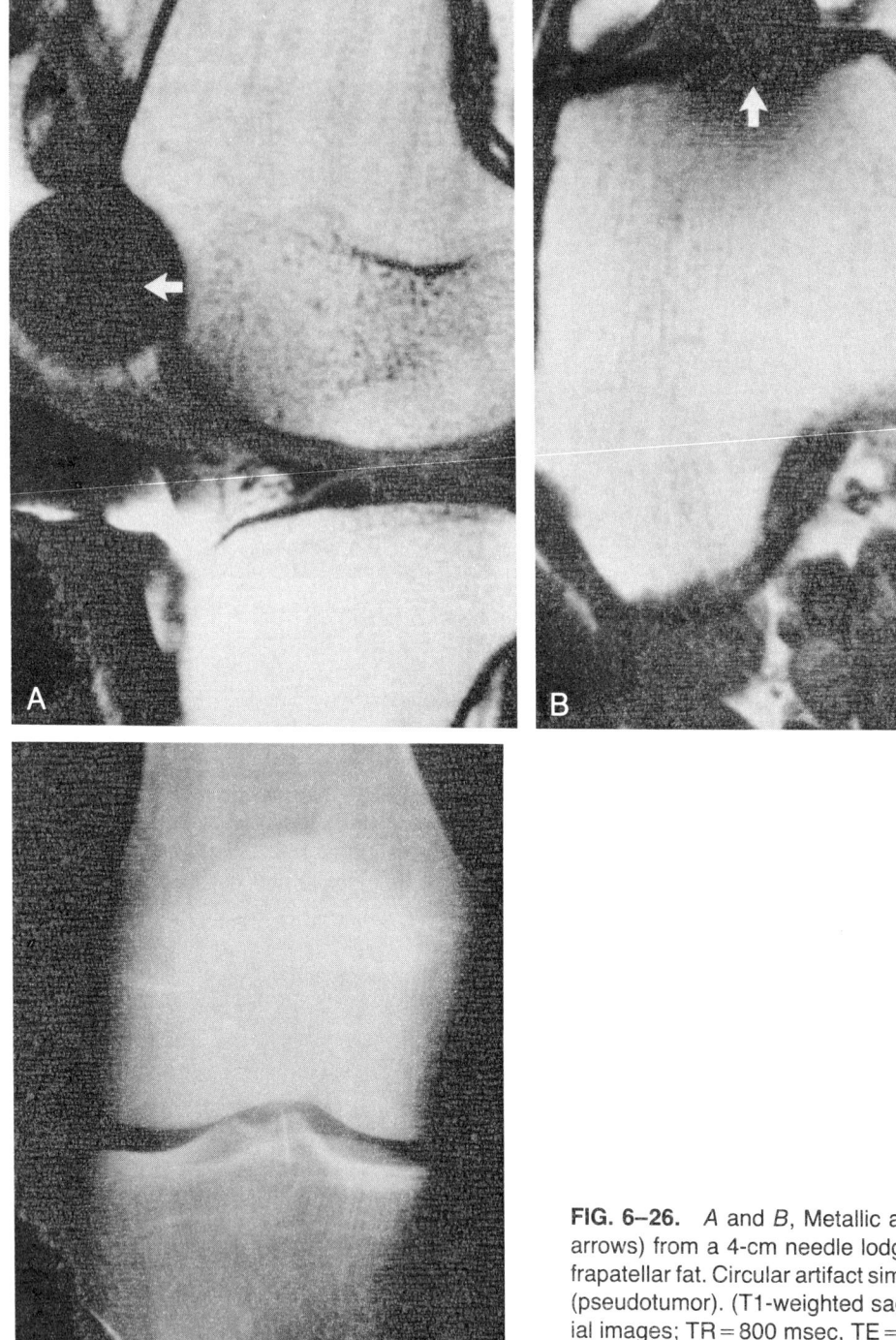

FIG. 6–26. *A* and *B*, Metallic artifact (white arrows) from a 4-cm needle lodged in the infrapatellar fat. Circular artifact simulates a cyst (pseudotumor). (T1-weighted sagittal and axial images; TR = 800 msec, TE = 25 msec) *C*, Corresponding plain radiograph showing needle fragment lodged in soft tissues (fat pad) within the knee joint.

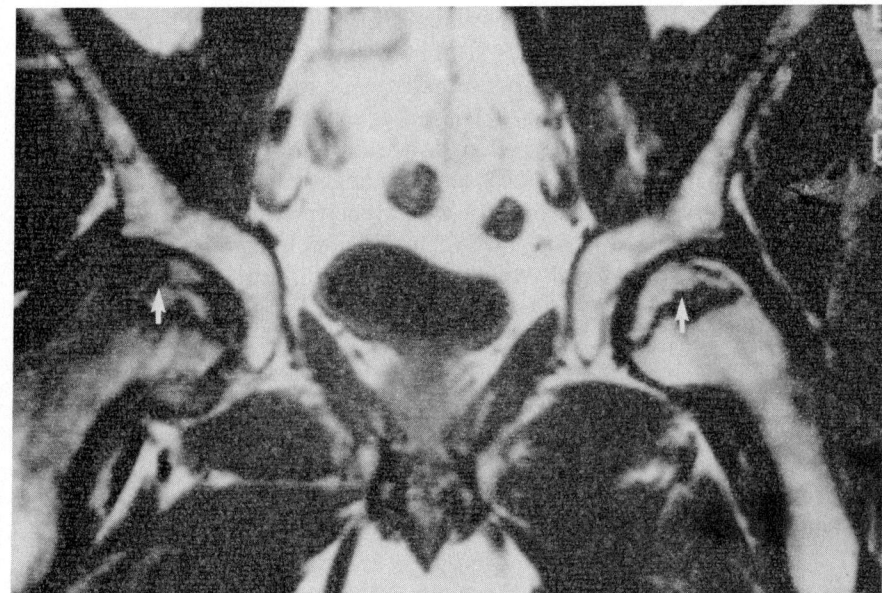

FIG. 6–27. Bilateral foci of avascular necrosis of the femoral head. The periphery images with low signal intensity, and the central portion images with higher signal intensity (arrows). (T1-weighted coronal image; TR = 800 msec, TE = 20 msec)

resolution matrix. Hip effusions of high signal intensity can be clearly identified on T2-weighted images.

Avascular Necrosis. One of the earliest, and still most useful, applications of MRI to the hip has been in the detection and staging of avascular necrosis (AVN) of the femoral head.[13,14] (See also Chapter 98.) Early identification of AVN is important, because treatment with rotational osteotomies or core decompression achieves best results during the initial stages of the disease. By the time subchondral sclerosis and collapse are detected with conventional radiography or CT, pathology is often advanced. Nuclear scintigraphy, with ^{99m}Tc-MDP and sulfur colloid bone agents, can be nonspecific, particularly when sulfur colloid agents are used in patients with decreased or abnormal marrow stores. In cases of trauma, scintigraphic flow studies might be necessary to identify ischemia.

A central area of altered signal intensity seen in association with the focus of AVN has been characterized and staged in T1- and T2-weighted images (Figs. 6–27 and 6–28). In the early stages of AVN, fat and blood constituents contribute to intermediate to high signal intensity on T1- and T2-weighted images, respectively. In the chronic phase of fibrous replacement, however, low signal intensity is observed on both T1- and T2-weighted images. A characteristic finding, called the *double line sign*, is seen with pro-

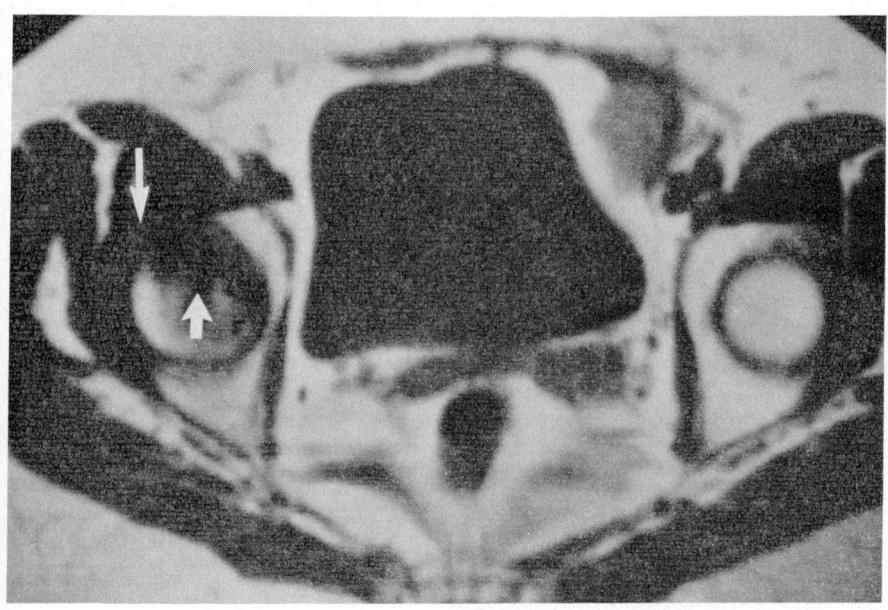

FIG. 6–28. Area of low signal intensity avascular necrosis (short arrow) with associated effusion (long arrow). The inferior pole of the transplanted kidney can also be seen. (T1-weighted axial image; TR = 600 msec, TE = 25 msec)

longed TR and TE settings. This finding is attributed to a hyperemic or inflammatory interface (high signal intensity) adjacent to a peripheral sclerotic rim (low signal intensity). The double line sign has been associated with AVN in 80% of cases studied. On T1-weighted images, a separate pattern of low signal intensity in marrow (probably representing hypervascularity) can be seen extending distally into the femoral neck. This signal demonstrates isointensity with marrow on T2-weighted images. On T2-weighted images, hip effusions associated with AVN are visualized with high signal intensity. The prognostic significance of presence or absence of fluid in AVN is uncertain.

In *Legg-Calvé-Perthes disease*, both the viability of epiphyseal marrow (necessary for surgical staging and osteotomy) and the presence of contralateral hip involvement can be evaluated with MRI studies (Fig. 6–29). MRI also will document the position of the nonossified femoral head in congenital hip dislocations (Fig. 6–30). Acetabular remodeling and interposed soft tissue or muscle, preventing anatomic reduction, can be demonstrated with coronal and axial MRI. Abduction cast therapy can be serially monitored with MRI studies, without the artifact or ionizing radiation that complicates CT.

Trauma. In traumatic hip dislocations, MRI can be used to detect *marrow edema* associated with acetabular or femoral head compression fractures. On T1-weighted images, loose bodies with marrow image generate high signal intensity, whereas chondral fragments might not generate signal intensity on either T1- or T2-weighted images.

Labral cartilage tears can be identified on coronal and sagittal images with small fields of view. Thin section axial images have also been useful in detecting the small nidus seen in *osteoid osteoma* lesions (Fig. 6–31).

The superior marrow contrast provided by MRI enables the detection of acetabular and femoral stress fractures when bone scintigraphy is positive but plain films or CT scans are negative (Figs. 6–32 and 6–33). In the presence of extensive reactive marrow edema, thin section (1.5 to 3 mm) CT frequently assists in identifying subtle cortical disruptions.

Arthritis. On T2-weighted images, degenerative subchondral cysts demonstrate enhanced signal intensity and can be differentiated from overlying cartilage. In juvenile rheumatoid arthritis, early articular erosions have been identified prior to detection of changes on conventional radiographs. MRI is especially sensitive in detecting AVN, synovial hypertrophy, and capsular effusions in these patients. Infiltrative disorders of marrow and juxta-articular soft-tissue masses (e.g., amyloid) can also be identified on T1- and T2-weighted images (Fig. 6–34).

Neoplastic Disease. Metastatic disease affecting the hip will image with high signal intensity on T2-weighted images. Peritumoral edema or postbiopsy tissue inflammation can mask the true extent of neoplastic involvement, however. Axial images are useful in detecting small lesions that require high-resolution and thin section capability. The longitudinal extent of marrow involvement is displayed on both coronal and sagittal images.

MRI OF THE ANKLE

With the use of a dedicated extremity coil, direct coronal, sagittal, axial, and oblique MRI images can

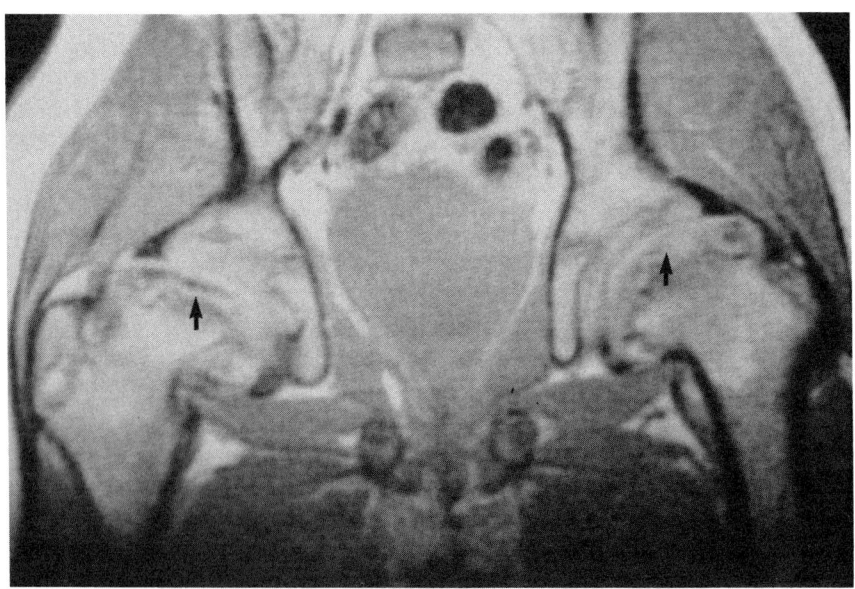

FIG. 6–29. Bilateral ischemic necrosis and subchondral collapse (arrows) of femoral epiphyseal centers in patient with Legg-Calvé-Perthes disease. Absence of signal from epiphyseal yellow marrow indicates loss of vascular viability (T1-weighted coronal image; TR = 1000 msec, TE = 20 msec)

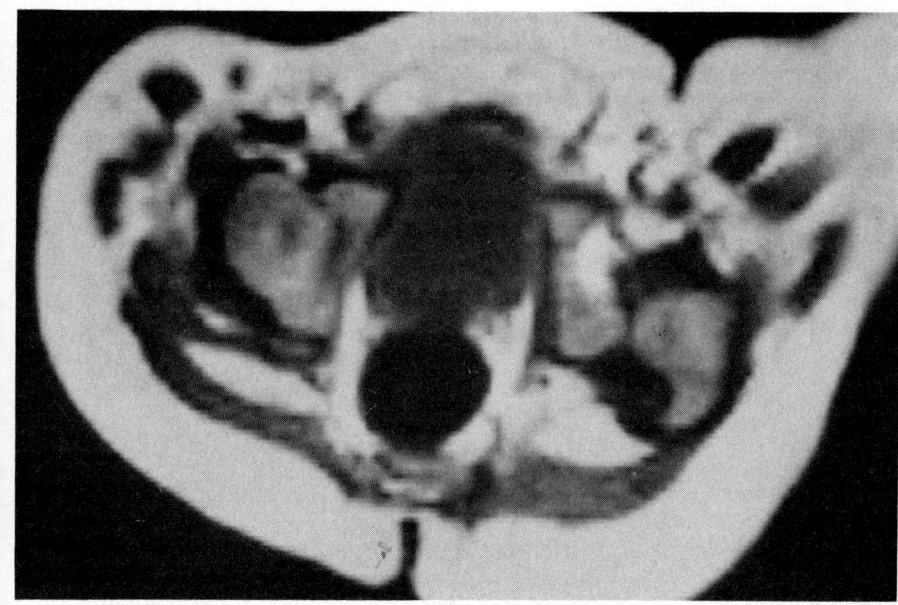

FIG. 6–30. Posterior displaced left hip relative to the acetabulum in congenital hip dislocation. (T1-weighted axial image; TR = 800 msec, TE = 20 msec)

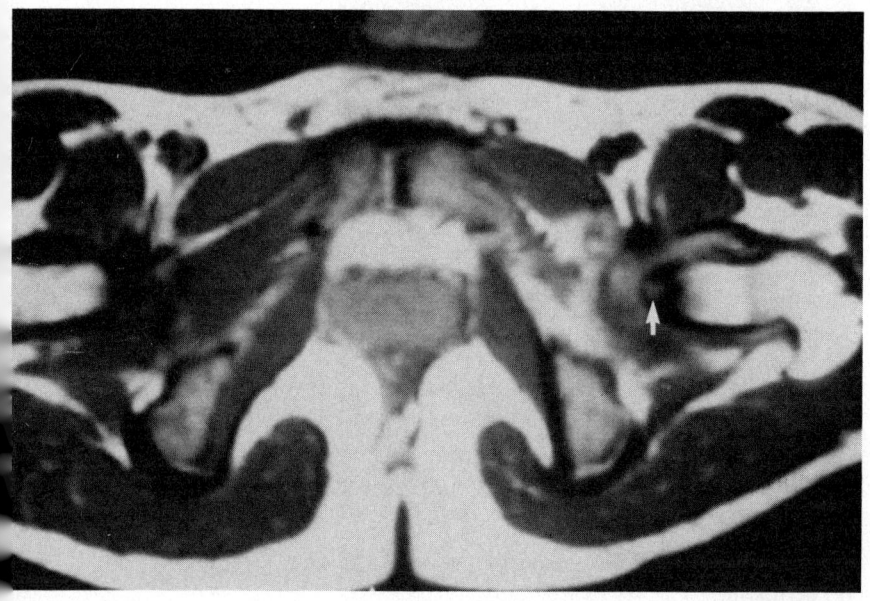

FIG. 6–31. Osteoid osteoma in thickened left femoral cortex. Central nidus is seen with intermediate signal intensity (arrow). (T1-weighted axial image through the hips; TR = 800 msec, TE = 20 msec)

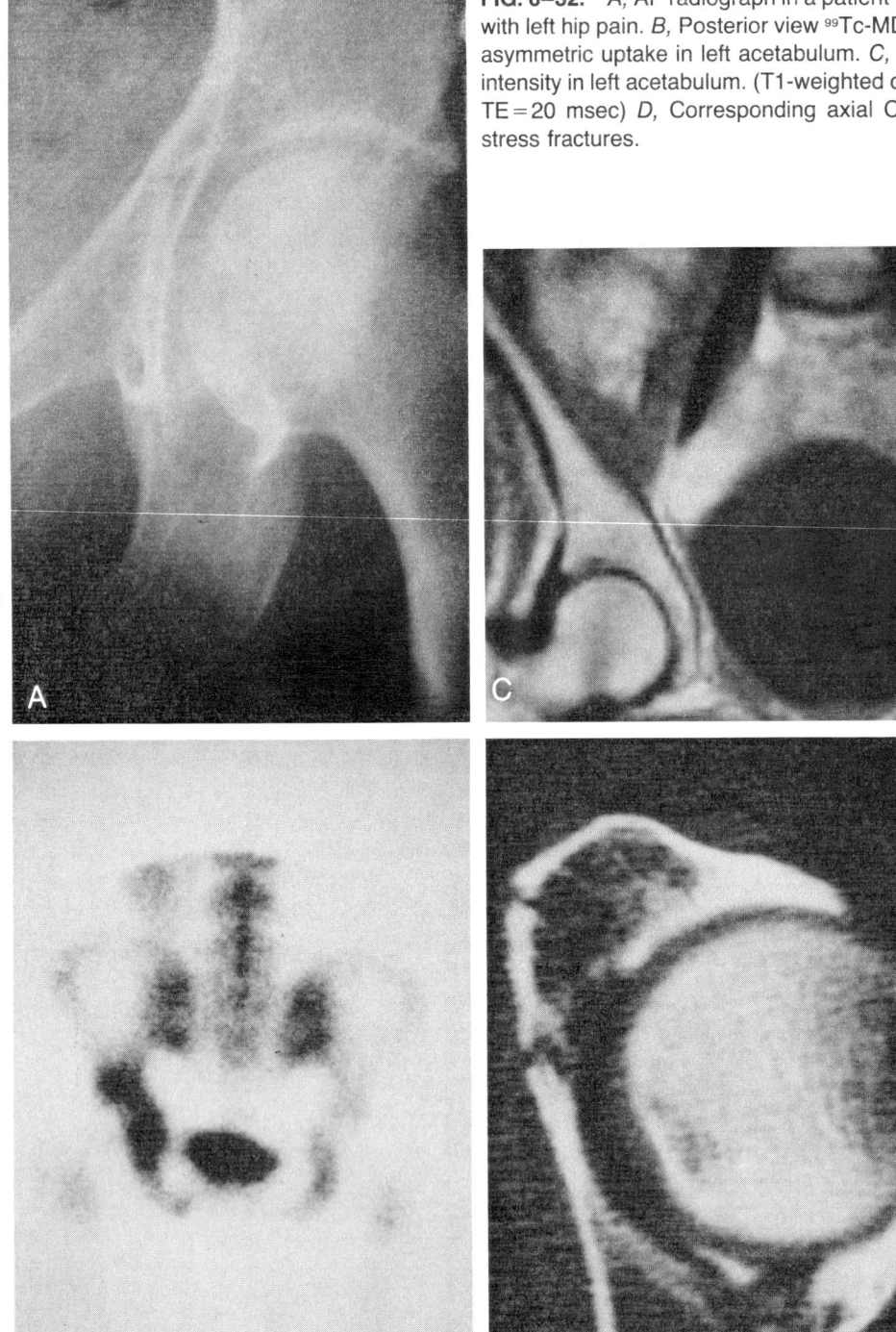

FIG. 6–32. *A,* AP radiograph in a patient with biliary cirrhosis presenting with left hip pain. *B,* Posterior view ^{99}Tc-MDP nuclear scintigram showing asymmetric uptake in left acetabulum. *C,* MRI demonstrating low signal intensity in left acetabulum. (T1-weighted coronal image; TR = 800 msec, TE = 20 msec) *D,* Corresponding axial CT scan identifying acetabular stress fractures.

FIG. 6–33. *A,* AP radiograph showing thickened femoral shaft cortex (arrow) in a patient presenting with pain in the thigh. *B,* MRI showing decreased signal intensity in marrow (arrow) adjacent to hypertrophied cortex. (T1-weighted coronal image; TR = 1000 msec, TE = 40 msec) *C,* Stress fracture adjacent to thickened cortex is revealed on axial CT scan (arrow).

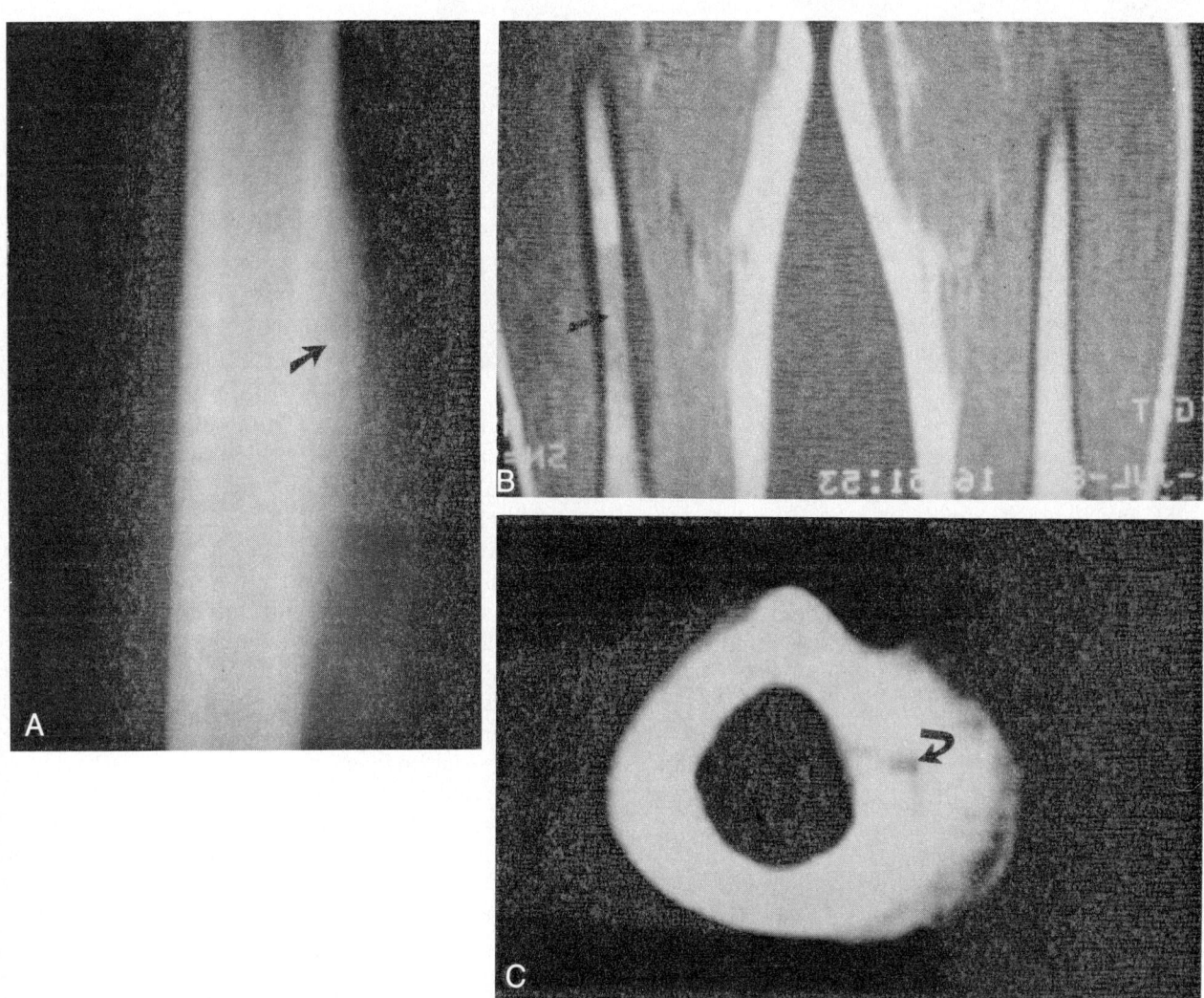

be obtained with high resolution at small fields of view.[15] On routine T1-weighted images, cortex, ligaments, and tendons are visualized with low signal intensity, and hyaline articular cartilage generates intermediate signal intensity. Axial images display the tendons around the ankle in cross section, whereas long-axis tendon anatomy is demonstrated in the sagittal imaging plane. The flexor and extensor tendon groups are shown in images through the tibiotalar joint and posterior facet of the subtalar joint. The pre-Achilles fat pad, of high signal intensity, is seen anterior to the Achilles tendon, which images with uniformly low signal intensity.

T2-weighted images are used to highlight capsular fluid, synovial inflammation, joint debris (detritus), and neoplasia. Ligamentous and tendinous disruptions can also be visualized on MRI of the ankle. MRI capability in detecting *ruptures of the Achilles tendon* is superior to other imaging modalities, because both the proximal and distal fibers can be identified. MRI can also be used to follow tendinous and ligamentous disruptions and interval healing of soft tissue. In addition, postoperative ankle reconstructions can be evaluated for points of ligamentous fixation and surgical complications such as infection or fracture.

Juxta-articular and subcortical cysts containing synovial fluid or mucinous substances are visualized with low signal intensity on T1-weighted images and with

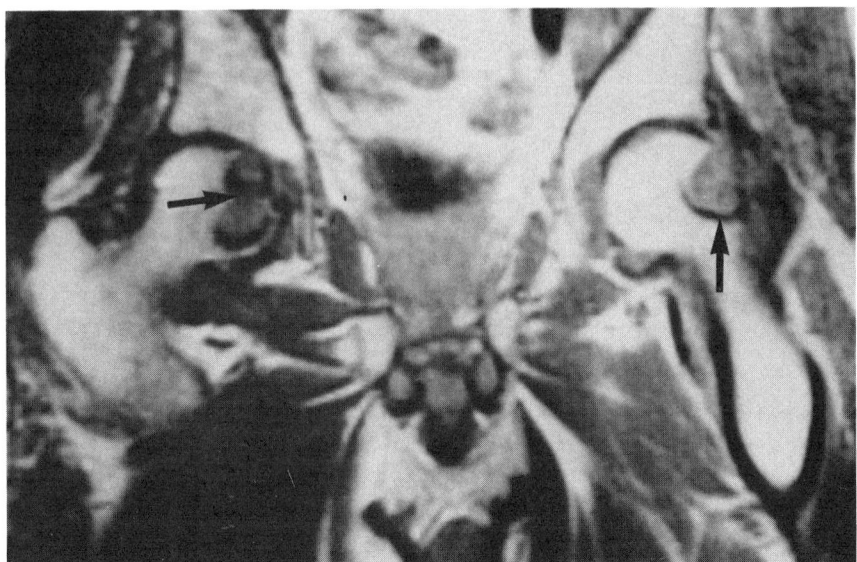

FIG. 6–34. Cystic erosions of amyloid (arrows) in femoral head and neck regions in a patient on chronic renal dialysis. (T1-weighted image; TR = 1000 msec, TE = 20 msec)

high signal intensity on T2-weighted images (Figs. 6–35A–C and 6–36). Detailed anatomy of the plafond and talar domes is best seen on T1-weighted images. In evaluating osteochondritis dissecans and transchondral fractures, MRI studies can be used to assess the congruity and thickness of articular cartilage (Fig. 6–37). On heavily T2-weighted images, which simulate arthrography, loose bodies (secondary to trauma, osteonecrosis, or arthritis) are outlined by the high-intensity signal of joint fluid (Fig. 6–38).

In the staging of neoplasms, axial images demonstrate separate fascial compartments. Infiltration along tendon sheaths, with adjacent cortical extension, has been documented in *synovial sarcomas* and other tumors around the ankle joint (Fig. 6–39).

In degenerative arthritis, early subchondral sclerosis images with low signal intensity. Denuded hyaline cartilage can be measured in both the tibiotalar and subtalar joints. Osteophytes and fractures can also be observed in ankle arthrosis.

MRI OF THE SHOULDER

Off-center field of viewing is required to evaluate the glenohumeral joint because the shoulder cannot be easily positioned within the center of the magnetic field. The supporting muscles of the shoulder image with intermediate signal intensity, whereas the rotator cuff tendons, glenoid labrum, and bony cortex generate low-intensity signals.[16] The "critical zone" of the supraspinatus tendon portion of the rotator cuff is seen on images in either the coronal (frontal) or sagittal plane (Fig. 6–40). The inherent nonuniformity of signal intensity within the musculotendinous ro-

tator cuff decreases the sensitivity of MRI in identifying *partial tears* somewhat. Sensitivity for detection of tears can be increased by T2-weighting, however, which highlights the fluid in torn rotator cuff fibers and can show the extension of synovial fluid between the glenohumeral joint and the subacromio-subdeltoid bursa overlying the cuff. Air contrast arthrography, followed by CT, is still more accurate in demonstrating labral and capsular deficiencies.* *Bicipital tendinitis* with irritation of the surrounding synovial sheath images with high signal intensity of T2-weighted axial images.

Osteomyelitis of the humerus, with various degrees of soft tissue inflammation, sequestra, and infectious tracking, has also been characterized on MRI studies. Defects in hyaline articular cartilage can be imaged early in the course of degenerative or inflammatory arthritis.

Evaluation of shoulder neoplasms is optimally performed with T1-weighted coronal and T2-weighted axial images. This method allows differentiation of invasion of marrow, bone cortex, and muscle (Fig. 6–41). The proximal and distal extent of disease is demonstrated on either coronal or sagittal acquisitions.

MRI OF THE HAND, WRIST, AND ELBOW

Smaller, saddle-shaped or circular surface coils are used for optimal field of viewing in coronal, axial, and sagittal planes (Fig. 6–42).[17,18] Flexor and extensor ten-

Editor's note. Ultrasonography is an excellent noninvasive means for evaluation of the integrity of the rotator cuff (see also Chapter 97).

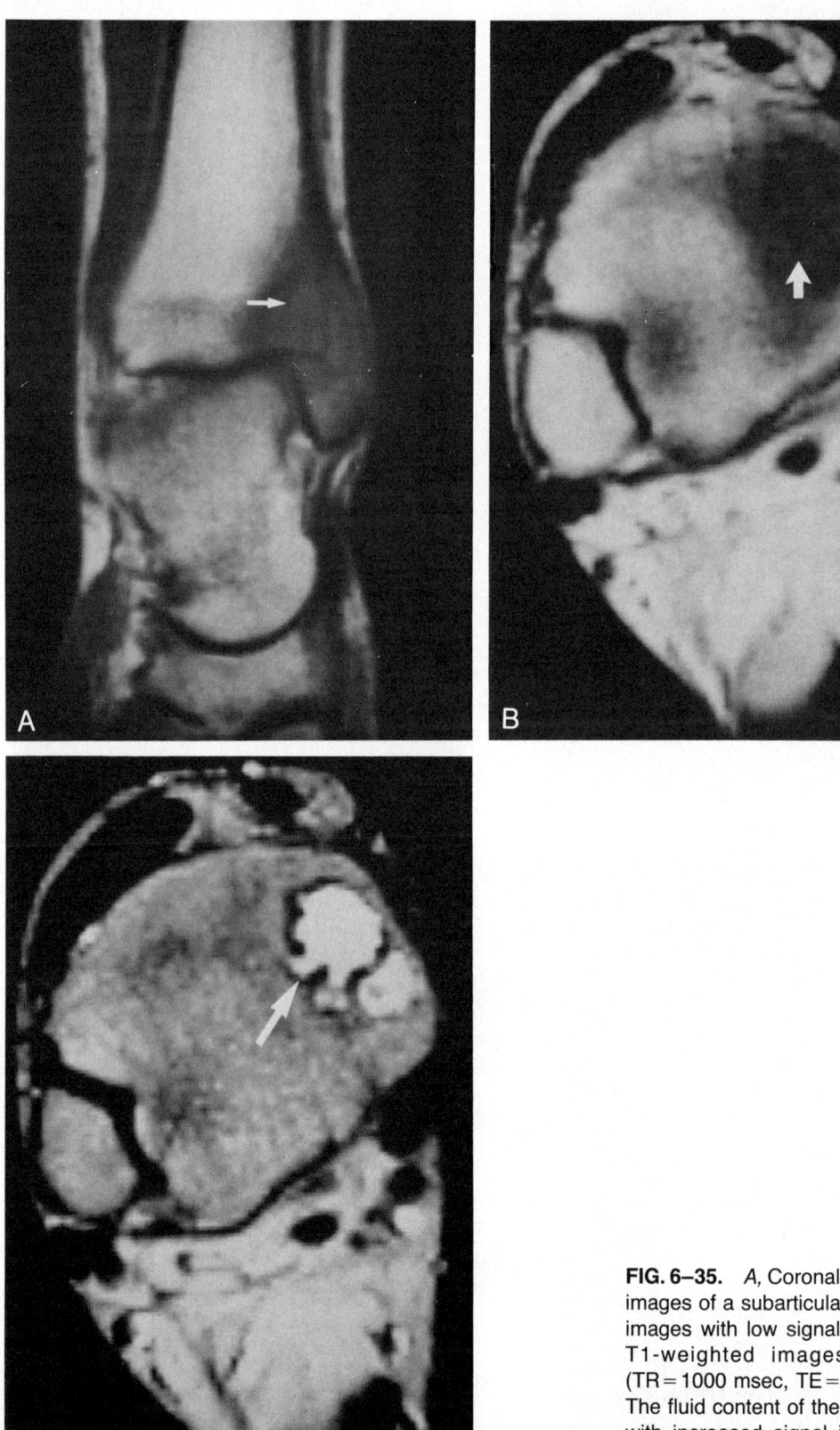

FIG. 6–35. *A,* Coronal and, *B,* axial images of a subarticular cyst, which images with low signal intensity on T1-weighted images (arrows). (TR = 1000 msec, TE = 40 msec) *C,* The fluid content of the cyst images with increased signal intensity (arrow) on T2-weighted axial image. (TR = 2000 msec, TE = 40 msec)

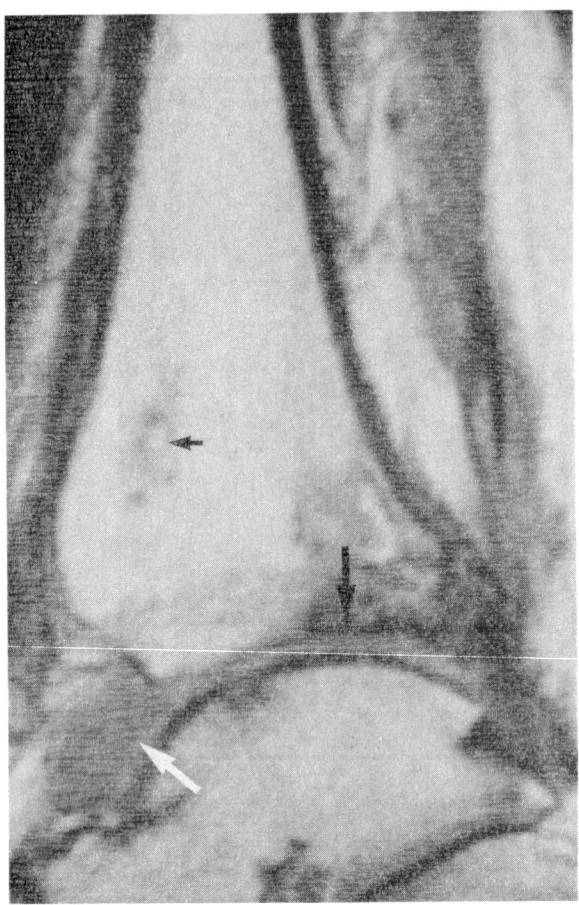

FIG. 6–36.   A sagittal image through the ankle joint shows low signal intensity of joint effusion and capsular distension (white arrow), subarticular cyst of distal tibia (large black arrow), and metaphyseal bone infarct (small black arrow) in a case of old trauma. (T1-weighted image; TR = 1800 msec, TE = 20 msec)

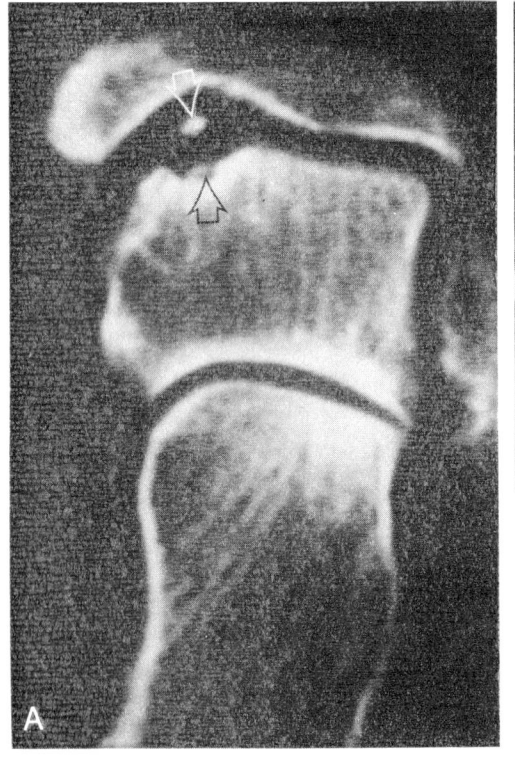

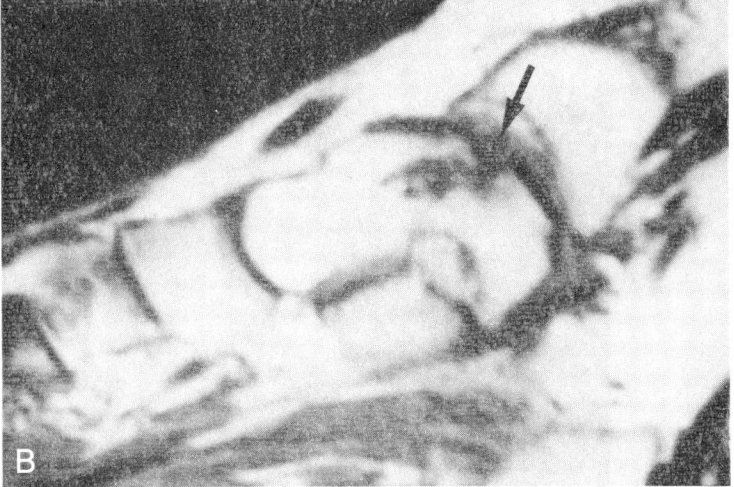

FIG. 6–37.   *A,* Axial CT scan through the ankle joint shows area of osteochondritis dissecans (black arrow). Detached osteochondral fragment indicated (white arrow). *B,* On corresponding sagittal MR image focus of osteochondritis with cortical defect (arrow) images with low signal intensity. (T1-weighted image; TR = 800 msec, TE = 20 msec)

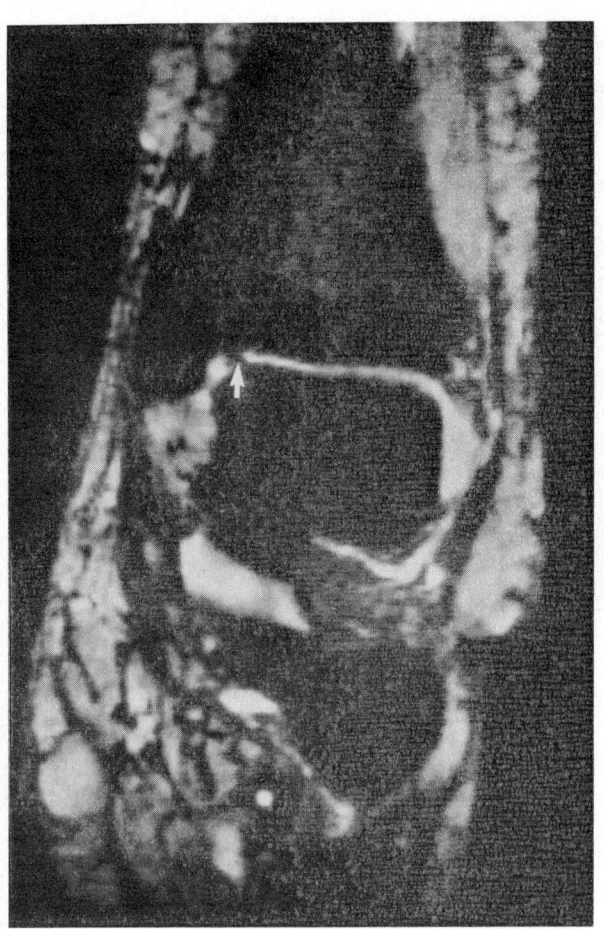

FIG. 6–38. Free fragment in tibiotalar joint (arrow) images with low signal intensity. (T2-weighted gradient echo coronal image; TR = 400 msec, TE = 30 msec, flip angle of 30°)

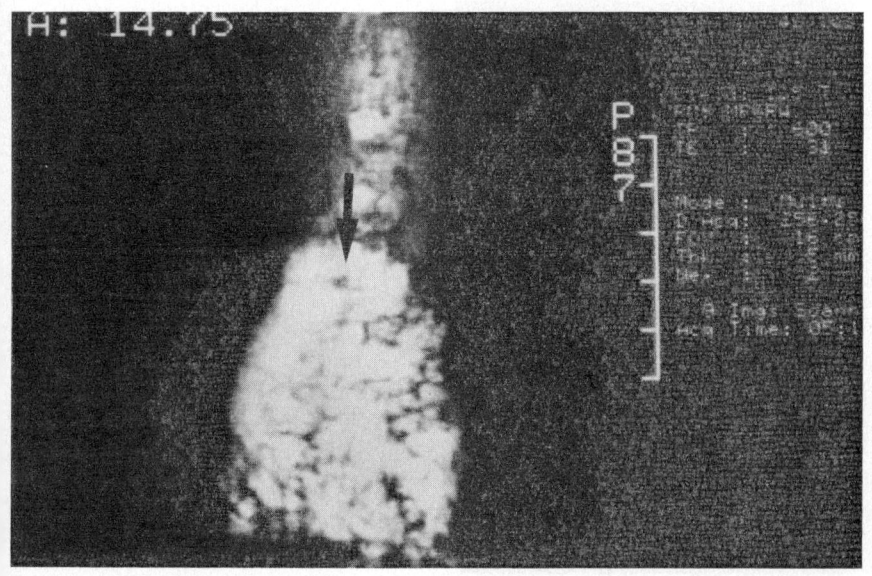

FIG. 6–39. Large, soft-tissue neurofibroma projects from the lateral aspect of the angle. (T2-weighted gradient echo image; TR = 600 msec, TE = 30 msec, flip angle of 15°)

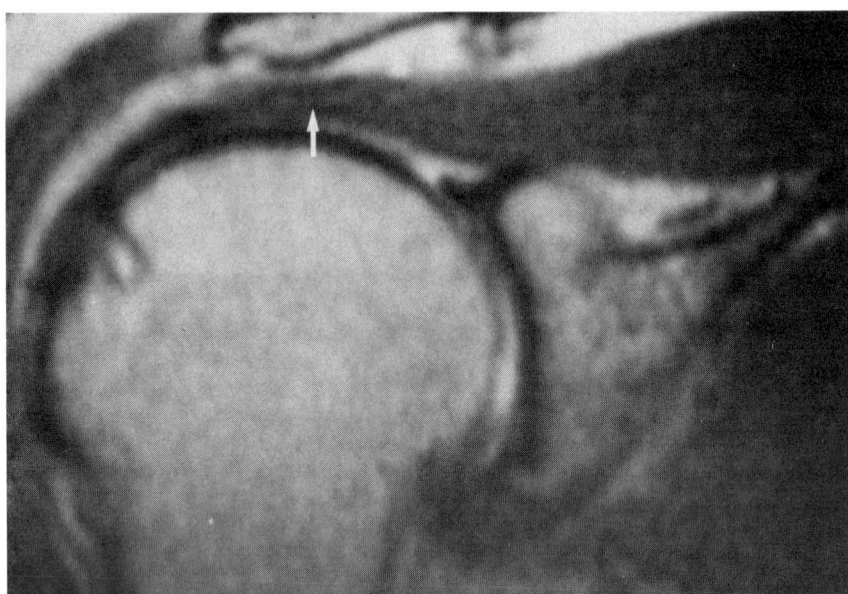

FIG. 6–40. Intact rotator cuff supraspinatus tendon (arrow). (T1-weighted coronal image through the shoulder; TR = 800 msec, TE = 20 msec)

dons are imaged in profile in the sagittal plane and seen en face on coronal images.

Osteonecrosis of the scaphoid and lunate *(Kienböck's disease)* can be evaluated by MRI early in the course of disease (Fig. 6–43).[19] Decreased signal intensity on T1-weighted images corresponds to loss of marrow viability, the detection of which can influence the treatment decision of whether to graft or to excise bone.

The triangular fibrocartilage complex separating the radiocarpal and inferior radioulnar joints is outlined on coronal images and generates a uniform, low-intensity signal. Partial fibrocartilage tears and intercompartmental fluid communication, including extension into the inferior radioulnar joint, are demonstrated on T2-weighted acquisitions. On partial flip angle fast-scan images, articular cartilage will generate high signal intensity.

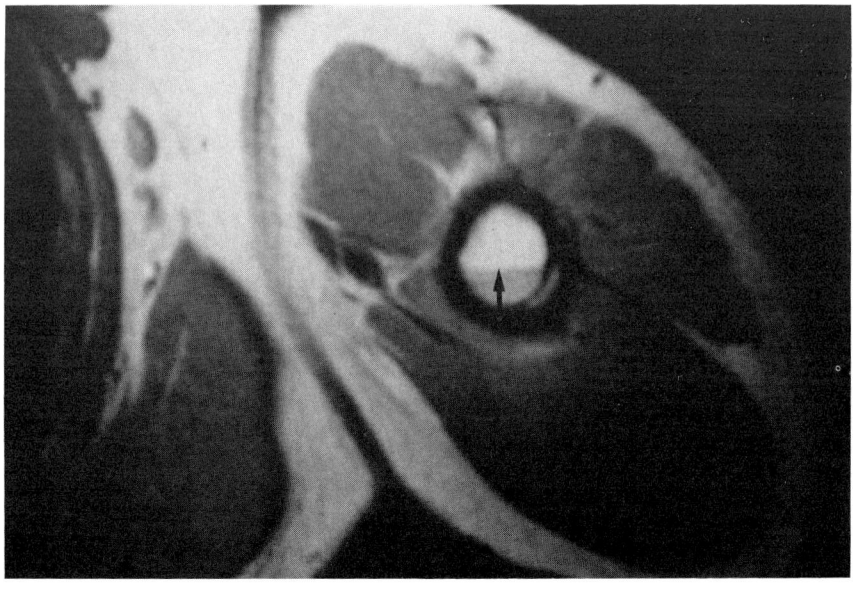

FIG. 6–41. Necrotic marrow fluid-fluid level (arrow) in a patient with dedifferentiated osteosarcoma. (TR = 2000 msec, TE = 20 msec)

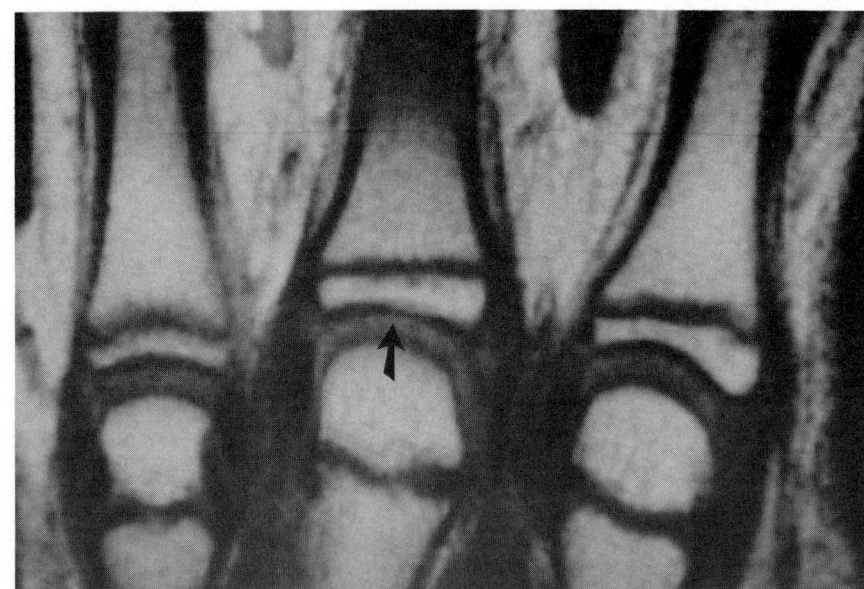

FIG. 6–42. Intact metacarpophalangeal hyaline articular cartilage (arrow) in a child. (T1-weighted coronal image; TR = 800 msec, TE = 20 msec)

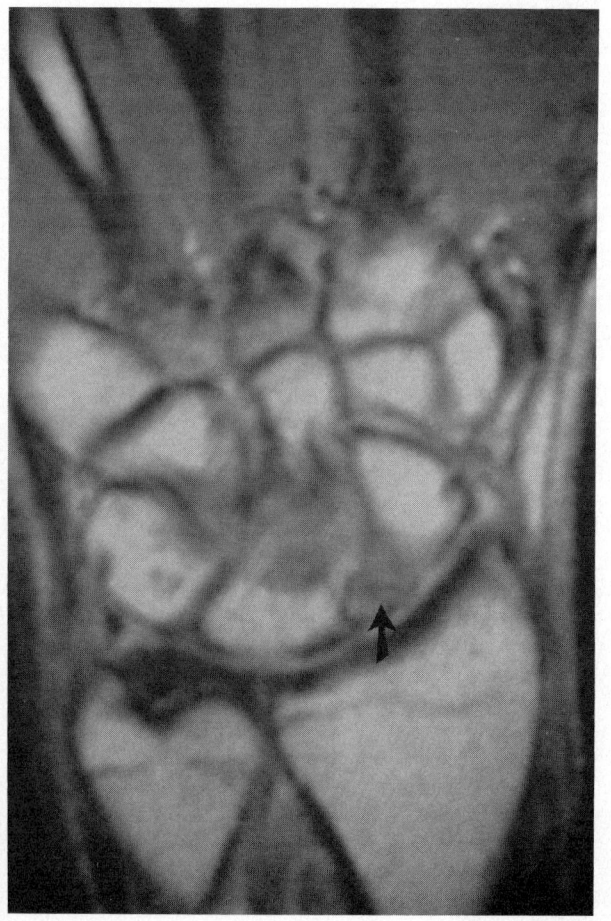

FIG. 6–43. Area of low signal intensity (arrow) represents avascular necrosis involving the proximal pole of the scaphoid. (T1-weighted image; TR = 800 msec, TE = 25 msec)

Carpal tunnel anatomy and pathology are shown on axial T1- and T2-weighted images. Inflammation and infiltration of the median nerve and surrounding tendon sheaths are visualized with long TR and TE settings on T2-weighted sequences (Fig. 6–44). With T1- and T2-weighting, lipomas, ganglions, sarcomas, hemangiomas, and arteriovenous malformations can be differentiated by the strength and homogeneity of signal intensity (Fig. 6–45). As discussed already, in gradient echo imaging, flow is enhanced in arterial and venous structures creating a peripheral MR "angiogram" effect (Fig. 6–46). T2-weighted images show the distribution of radiocarpal or intercarpal joint effusions (Fig. 6–47).

Axial images best illustrate the complex anatomy of the elbow joint, clearly demonstrating the relationship between the superior radioulnar joint and the elbow (ulnohumeral) joint proper. T2-weighting scanning techniques and thin-section (3 to 5 mm) capability are needed to image juxta-articular cysts, free fragments, and neoplasms (Figs. 6–48, 6–49A,B). Even when conventional plain-film radiographs are negative, osteochondroses and post-traumatic subarticular cysts can be seen on MRI study.

MRI OF THE SPINE

MRI of the spine has assumed an important role in the evaluation of degenerative diseases, infection,

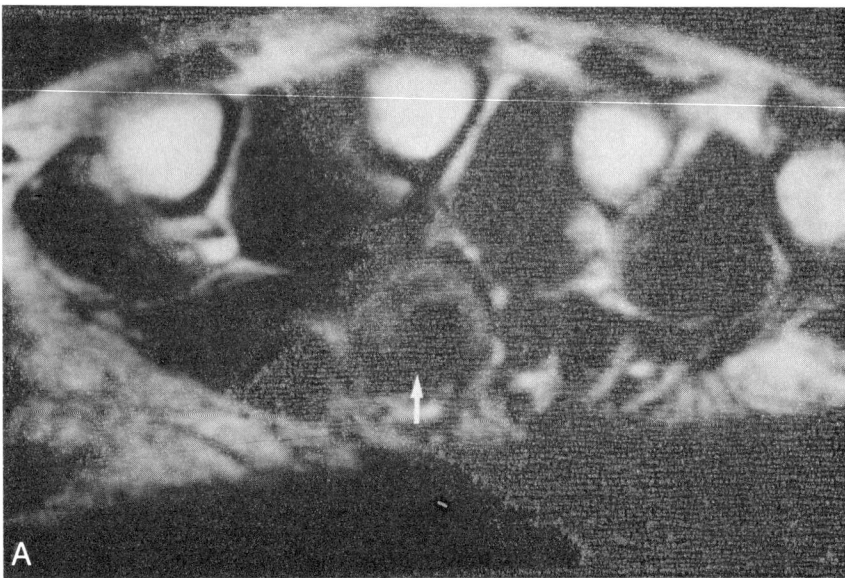

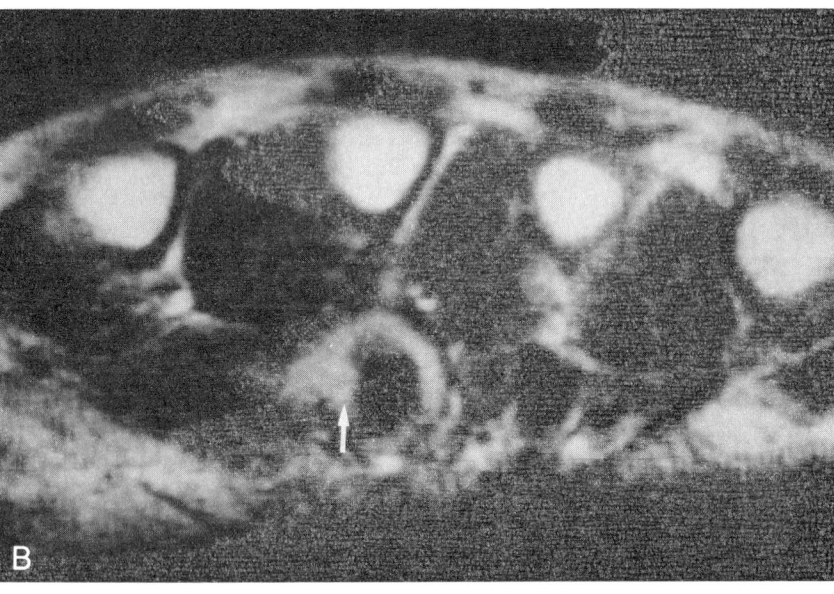

FIG. 6–44. Peritendinous edema in tenosynovitis of flexor tendon images. *A,* Low signal intensity on T1-weighted axial images (arrow). (TR = 1000 msec, TE = 20 msec) *B,* High signal intensity on T2-weighted axial images. (TR = 1500 msec, TE = 60 msec)

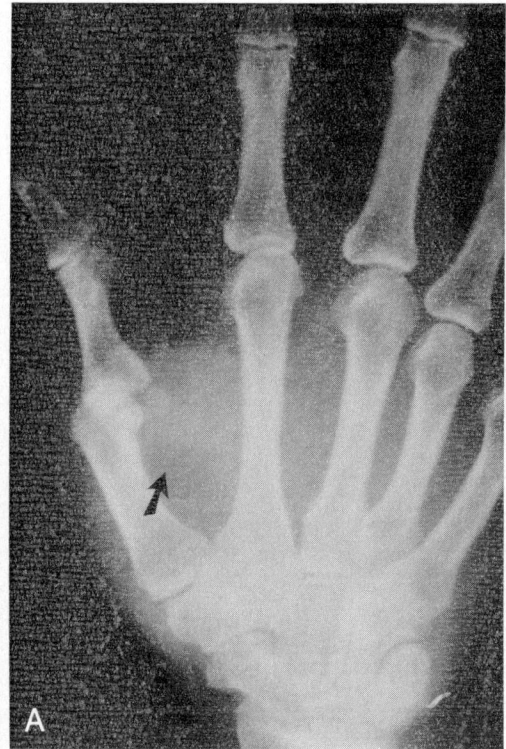

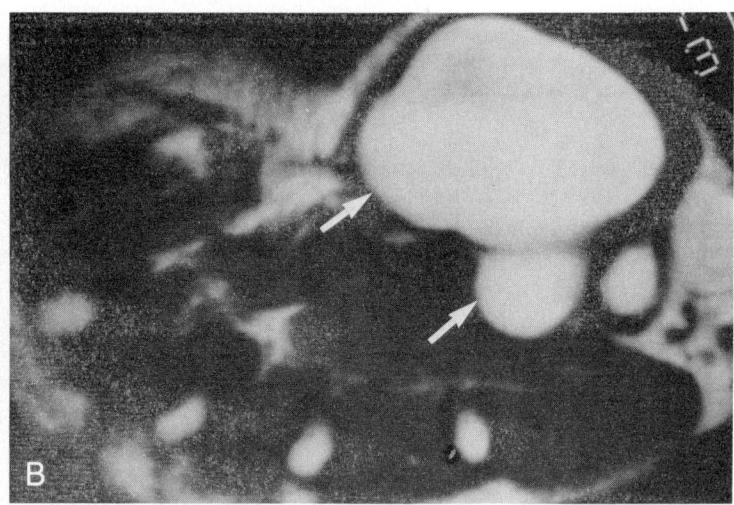

FIG. 6–45. *A,* AP radiograph of low-density soft-tissue mass involving the thenar eminence (arrow). *B,* Corresponding MRI image showing multilobulated lipoma imaging with subcutaneous fat high signal intensity (arrows). (T1-weighted axial image; TR = 800 msec, TE = 20 msec)

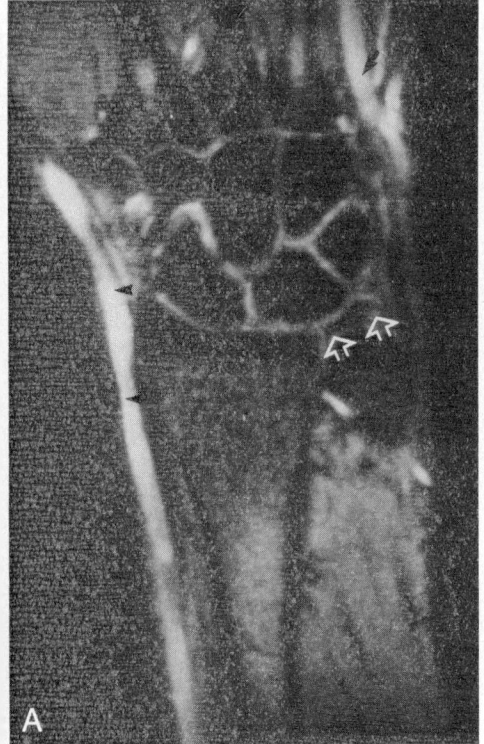

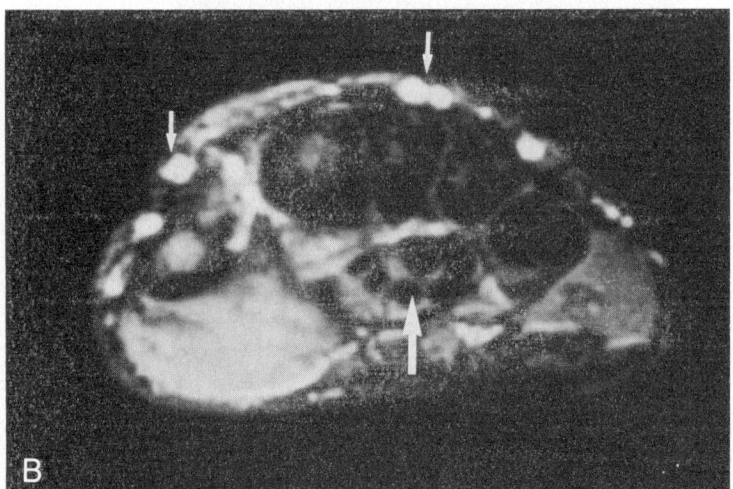

FIG. 6–46. T2-weighting provides vascular enhancement (arrowheads) in gradient echo coronal image in *A.* White arrows outline intact triangular fibrocartilage. Flexor tendons in the carpal tunnel can be differentiated by their low signal intensity (large arrow) in *B.* (T2-weighted gradient echo axial image through the wrist) (TR = 400 msec, TE = 30 msec, θ = 30°)

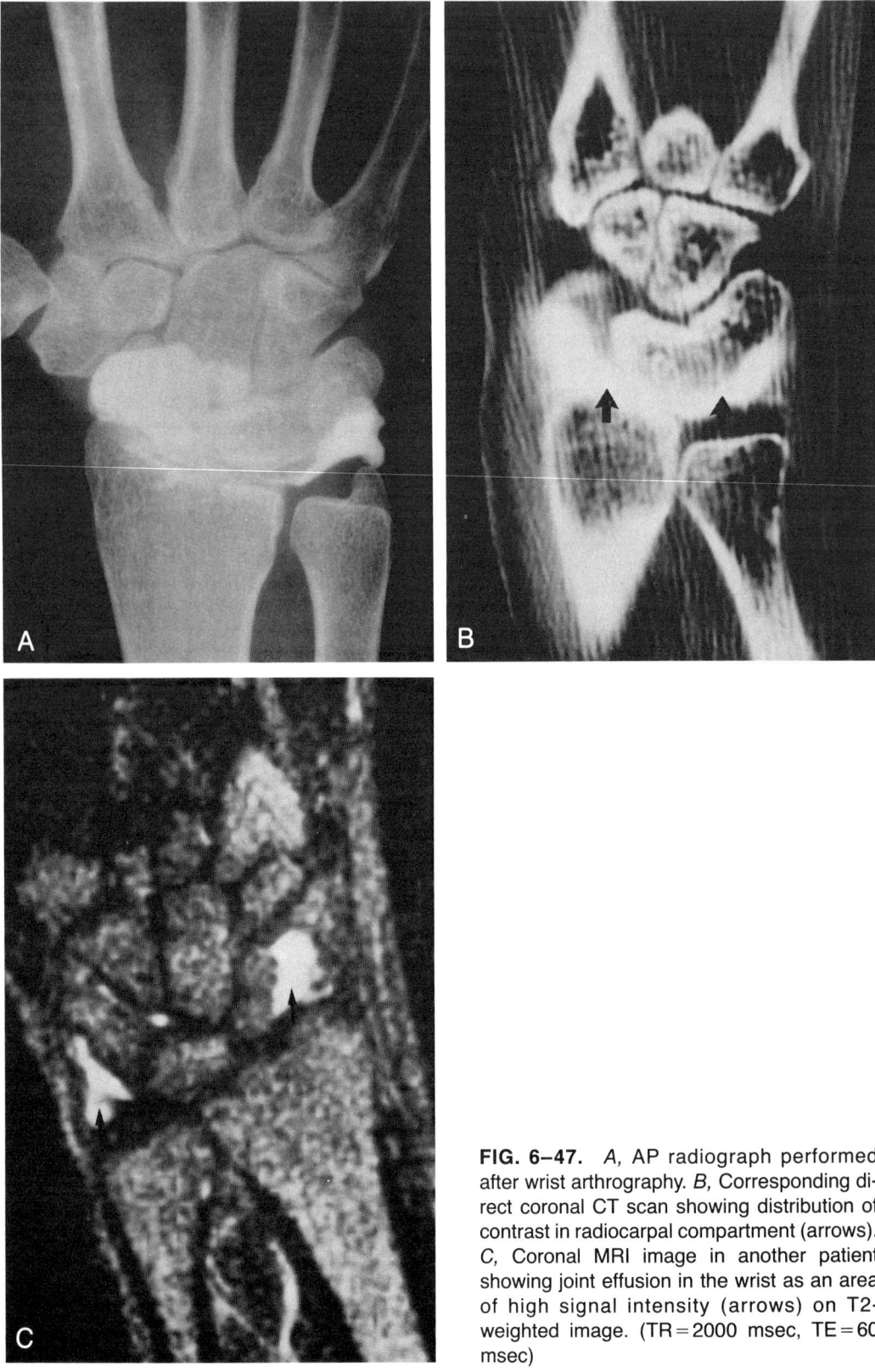

FIG. 6–47. *A,* AP radiograph performed after wrist arthrography. *B,* Corresponding direct coronal CT scan showing distribution of contrast in radiocarpal compartment (arrows). *C,* Coronal MRI image in another patient showing joint effusion in the wrist as an area of high signal intensity (arrows) on T2-weighted image. (TR = 2000 msec, TE = 60 msec)

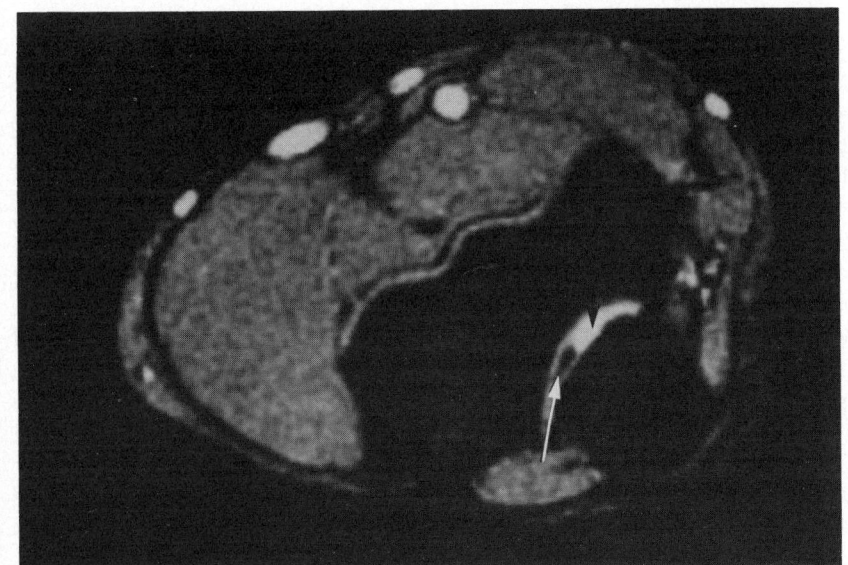

FIG. 6–48. Free fragment in elbow joint (long arrow) images with low signal intensity in contrast to adjacent synovial fluid (arrowhead), which images with high signal intensity. (T2-weighted gradient echo image) (TR = 400 msec, TE = 30 msec, θ = 30°)

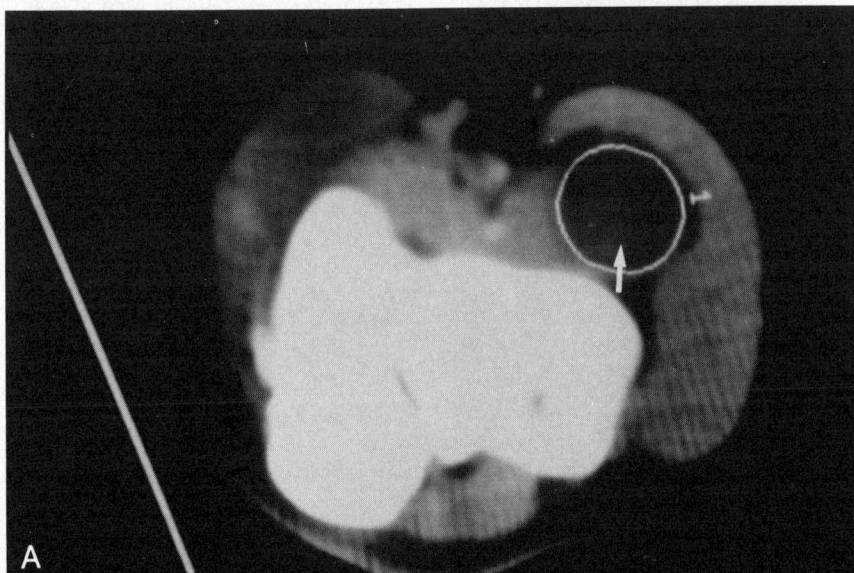
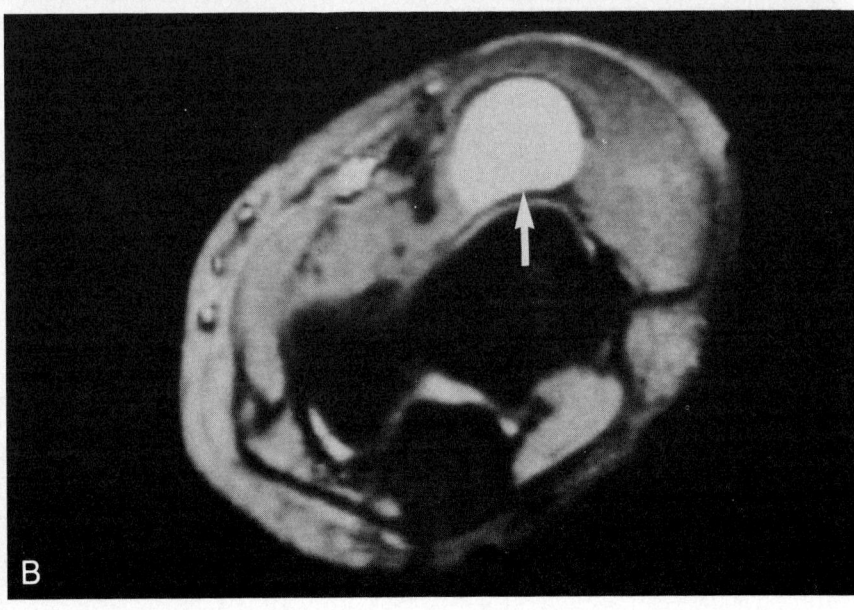

FIG. 6–49. *A,* Axial CT scan identifying low density mass deep to the brachioradialis muscle group (arrow). *B,* Corresponding MRI image showing high-intensity signal of synovial fluid (arrow) within surgically proven juxta-articular ganglion of the elbow joint. (T2-weighted gradient echo image) (TR = 400 msec, TE = 30 msec, θ = 30°)

trauma, and neoplasia.[20-24] In patients without history of fusion or laminectomy, MRI is frequently used as the examination of choice in the cervical, thoracic, and lumbar regions. CT is useful in providing detailed osseous anatomy in complicated postoperative and failed back patients, in whom stability and pseudoarthrosis are in question. Unlike CT, however, MRI can provide direct imaging in the sagittal, axial, and oblique planes without requiring reconstructions. With advances in spine surface coils and software, routine spine examinations have undergone significant reduction in imaging times.

The lumbar spine is studied with T1- and T2-weighting in both sagittal and axial imaging planes (Figs. 6–50 and 6–51). Cerebrospinal fluid (CSF) and discs image with low signal intensity on T1-weighted

images. With progressively greater T2-weighting, a sagittal myelographic effect (CSF of high signal intensity) is achieved. In the absence of desiccation and degeneration, the hydrated nucleus pulposus also generates a high-intensity signal on T2-weighting (Fig. 6–52). Neural foramina are best seen on T1-weighted sagittal or axial images, where exiting nerve roots can be visualized in contrast with epidural fat of high signal intensity (Fig. 6–53). On T2-weighted images the disc-thecal sac interface is separated.

Stenosis, facet pathology, and intrinsic cord abnormalities are displayed on either axial or sagittal images. The status of fractures, infection (osteomyelitis), or metastases can be assessed with the use of T1- and T2-weighting (Fig. 6–54). Infection produces regions of high signal intensity crossing the disco-

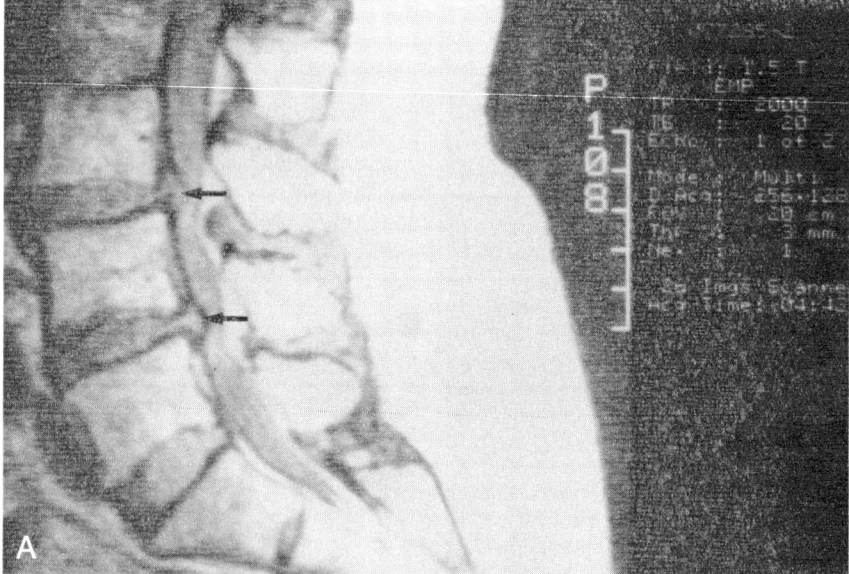

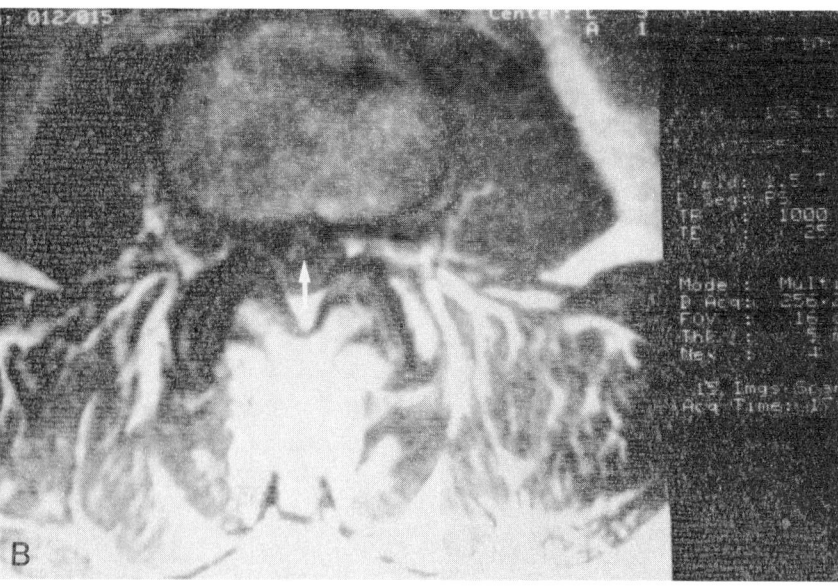

FIG. 6–50. *A*, Sagittal MRI image of the lumbar spine showing herniated discs (arrows) at levels L3-4 and L4-5. (Intermediate-weighted image; TR = 2000, TE = 20 msec) *B*, Corresponding axial image showing herniated nuclear material (arrow) and resultant central canal stenosis. (T1-weighted image; TR = 1000 msec, TE = 20 msec)

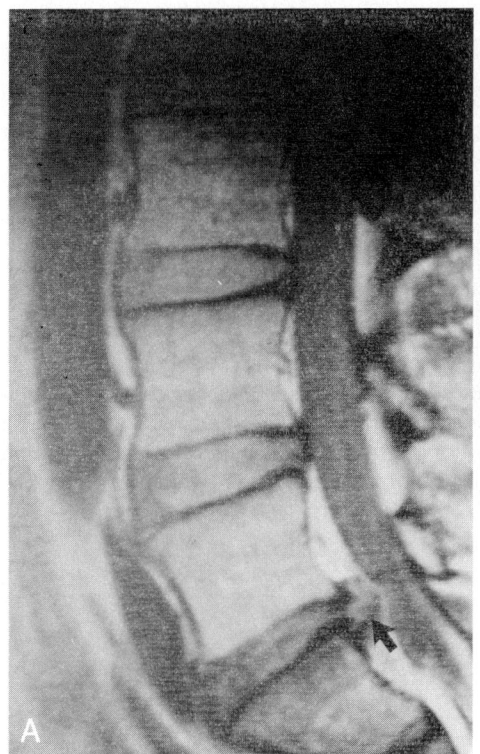

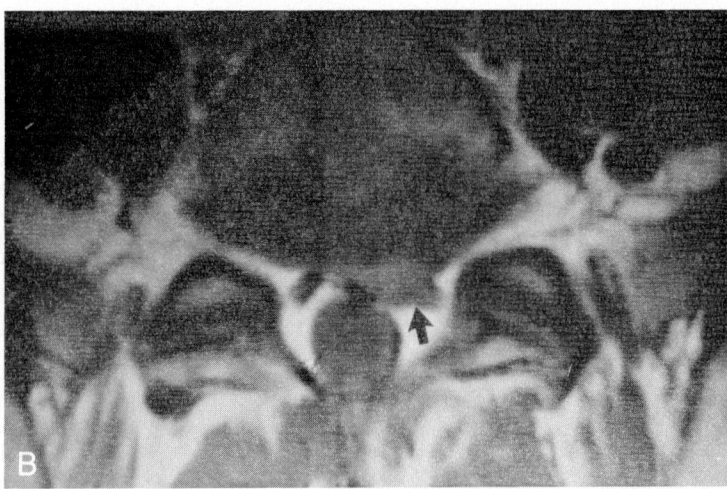

FIG. 6–51. *A,* T1-weighted sagittal image showing severe disk herniation at L5-S1 level (arrow). (TR = 1000 msec, TE = 20 msec) *B,* On axial image, effacement of left S1 nerve root by herniated nuclear material (arrow) is demonstrated (T1-weighted image; TR = 1000 msec, TE = 20 msec)

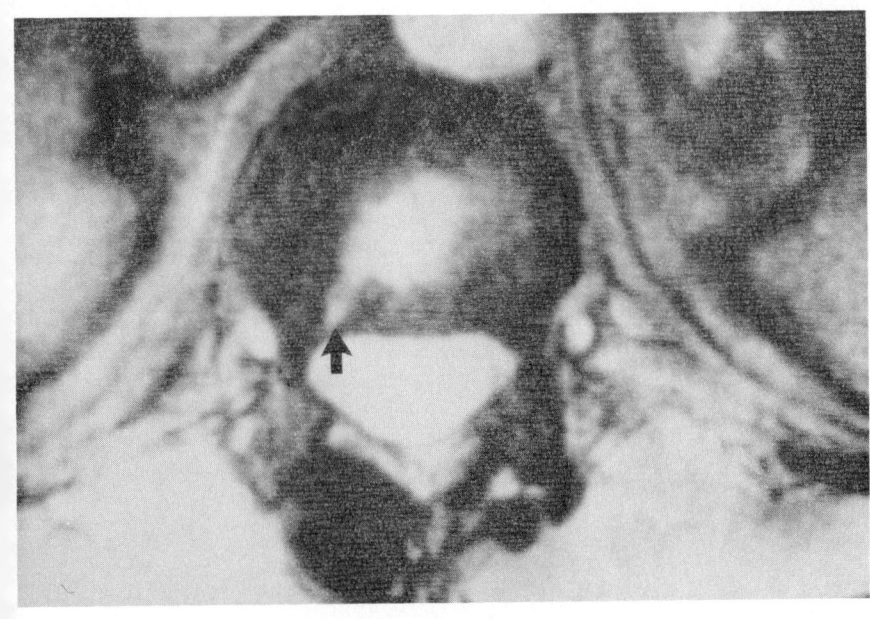

FIG. 6–52. Right posterolateral path of herniated nuclear material (arrow). (T2-weighted gradient echo axial image, TR = 400 msec, TE 30 msec, θ = 30°)

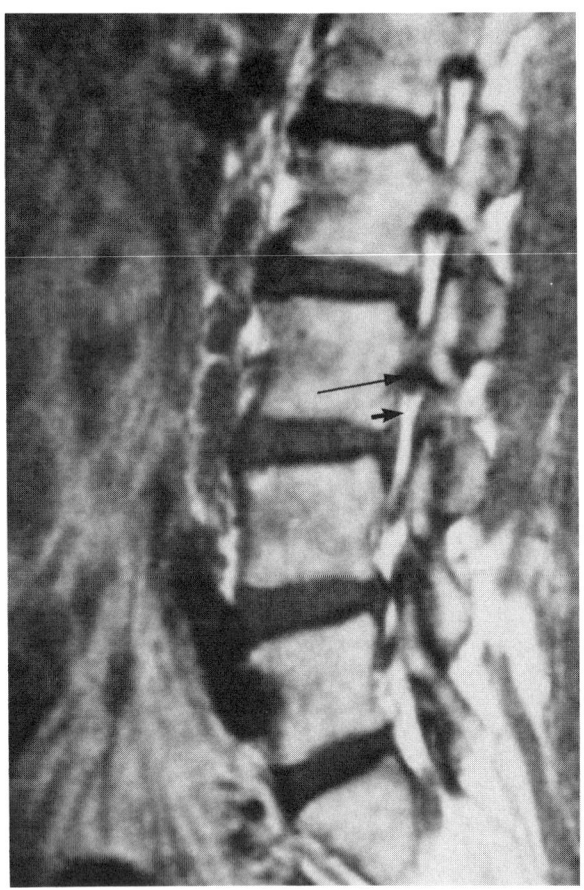

FIG. 6–53. Peripheral sagittal image demonstrating normal anatomy of neural foramen. Nerve root images with low signal intensity (long arrow) in contrast to high signal intensity of foraminal fat (short arrow). (T1-weighted image; TR = 1000 msec, TE = 20 msec)

FIG. 6–54.   *A,* Vertebral osteomyelitis with low signal intensity crossing the L4 and L5 vertebral bodies (arrows). (TR = 600 msec, TR = 20 msec) *B,* On T2-weighted images signal intensity is enhanced (arrows) with extension across the discovertebral junction. (TR = 2000 msec, TE = 60 msec)

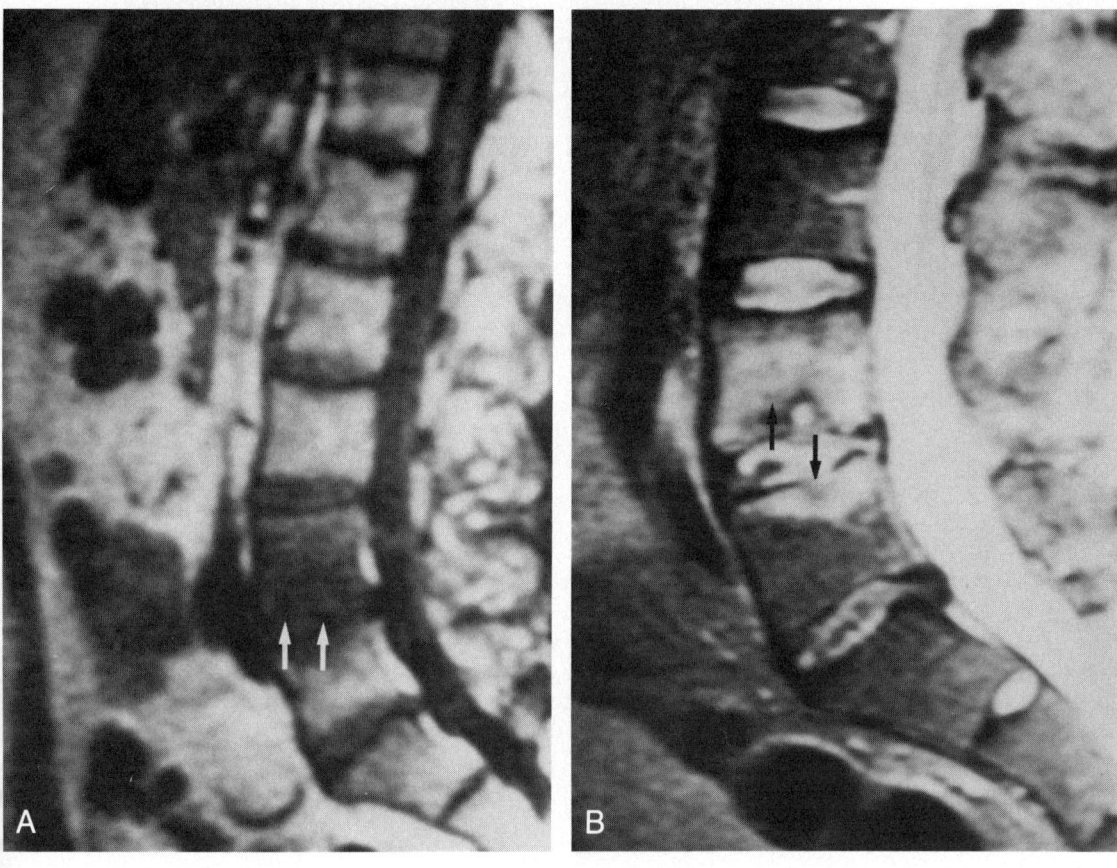

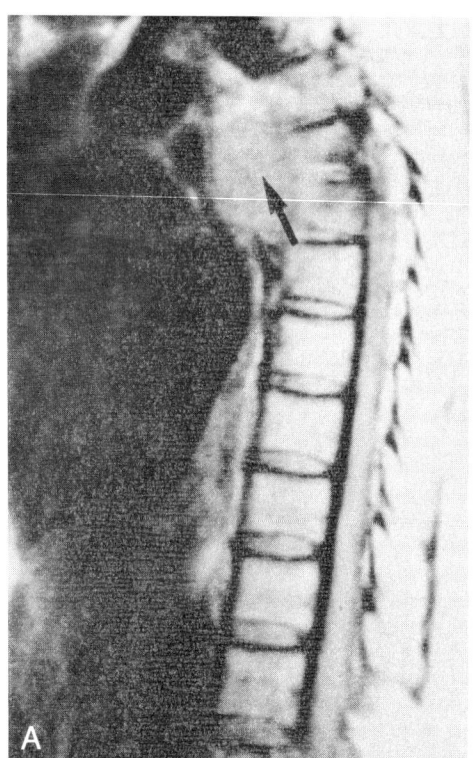

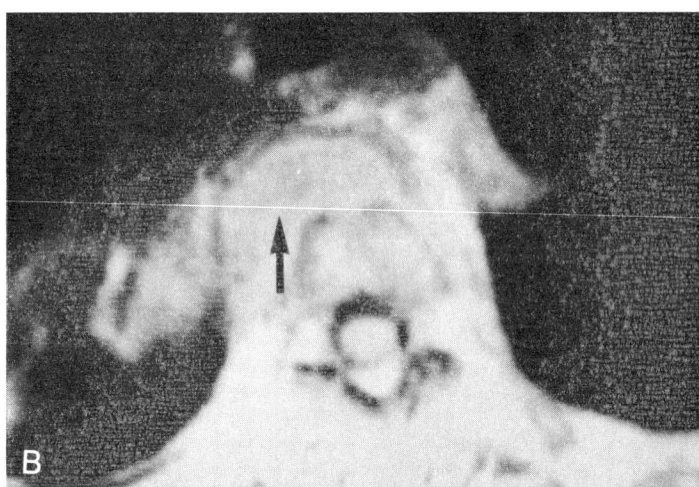

FIG. 6–55. *A,* Sagittal and, *B,* axial MRI images through the thoracic spine in a patient with spinal tuberculosis. Soft-tissue mass and adjacent vertebral body destruction (arrows) can be seen. (T1-weighted image; TR = 1000 msec, TE = 20 msec)

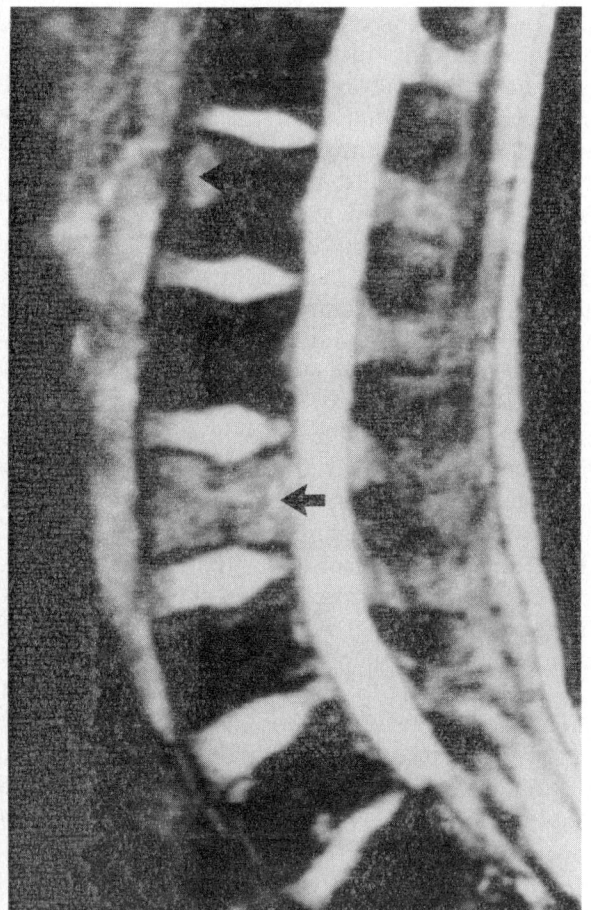

FIG. 6–56. Metastatic deposits in L1 and L3 vertebral bodies (arrows) in a patient with Ewing sarcoma. With T2-weighted gradient echo acquisition the tumor images with high signal intensity. (TR = 400 msec, TE = 30 msec, θ = 30°)

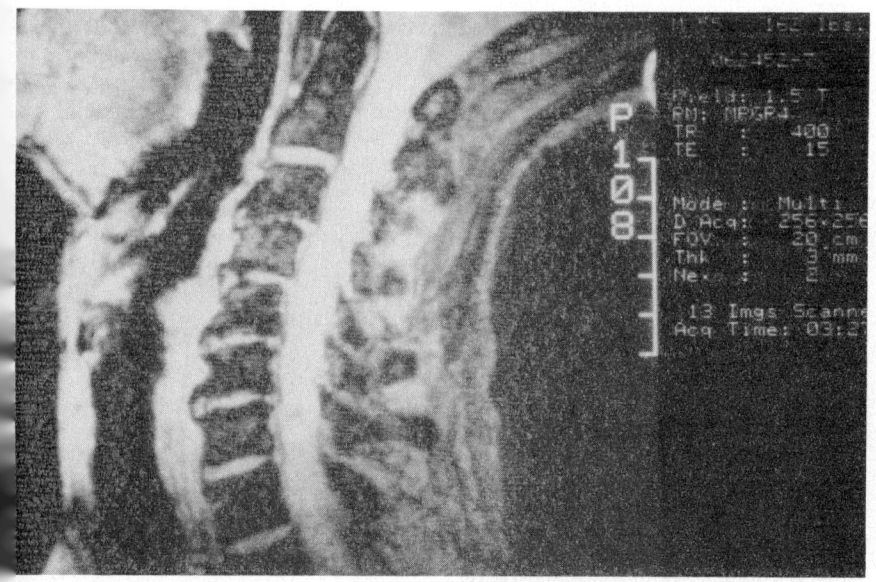

FIG. 6–57. Degenerative osteoarthritis of the cervical spine with disc space narrowing and anterior osteophytosis. (T2-weighted gradient echo image; TR = 400 msec, TE = 30 msec, θ = 30°)

vertebral junction, whereas metastases remain limited to the vertebral bodies or posterior elements (Figs. 6–55 and 6–56).

The cervicothoracic regions require fast scanning techniques to minimize artifacts from pulsatile CSF flow (Fig. 6–57). Using sagittal and axial images, cervical disc herniations, osteophytes, and cord tumors can be adequately studied. Functional imaging and changing the patient's positioning (flexion and extension) can be used to assess *atlantoaxial instabilities*. Oblique or angled sections are needed to delineate the course of exiting cervical nerve roots. MRI has also shown potential in demonstrating bilateral disc herniations that may be overlooked on CT.

MRI OF THE TEMPOROMANDIBULAR JOINT (see also Chapter 91)

The temporomandibular joint (TMJ) is subject to derangements of its fibrous disc and may be a target for both degenerative and inflammatory arthropathies. Patients with ankylosing spondylitis and rheumatoid arthritis are often subject to TMJ dysfunction, which needs to be distinguished from internal disc derangements. MRI offers a distinct advantage over CT in its ability to directly characterize meniscal structure. TMJ arthrography is still used to document disc perforations, however, and in the absence of anterior displacement, conservative treatment is indicated.

Disorders of the TMJ are best imaged in the sagittal plane using small (3 in.) surface coils and T1-weighted sequences.[25] Functional imaging, in closemouthed and openmouthed positions, is performed routinely in bilateral joint evaluations.

The TMJ meniscus represents a fibrous condensation composed of a thick posterior band, a thin intermediate zone, and an anterior band. The lateral pterygoid muscle is attached to the anterior band. The posterior band is continuous with a bilaminar-retrodiscal tissue complex. Spasm of the lateral pterygoid muscle can initiate or exacerbate discal displacements. The TMJ meniscus most commonly displaces in an anteromedial direction, as determined by condylar anatomy and pterygoid muscle pull. Upper and lower synovial joint spaces are divided by the TMJ meniscus. When the meniscus is anteriorly displaced, the posterior band is positioned anterior to the condylar head of the mandible. Anterior displacement may stretch the meniscus and retrodiscal attachments. In the intact meniscus, the posterior band occupies a 12 o'clock orientation with respect to the condylar head, and the intermediate zone is situated midway between the opposing structures of the articular eminence and the condylar head. In less than 5 min. of imaging time, complete medial to lateral joint coverage is possible with 3-mm sections. T2-weighted sequences can be used to differentiate joint fluid from a displaced meniscus or fibrous adhesions (Fig. 6–58). Joint fluid anterior to the condylar head can outline a displaced meniscus that is otherwise difficult to identify.

Degenerative and erosive arthritis of the TMJ visualize as narrowing and flattening of the condylar head and/or undercutting of the articular eminence. Lower marrow signal intensity and cortical thinning can be demonstrated on T1-weighted images. Fracture and free fragments (as can be found in synovial osteochondromatosis) are visualized in direct sagittal plane images.

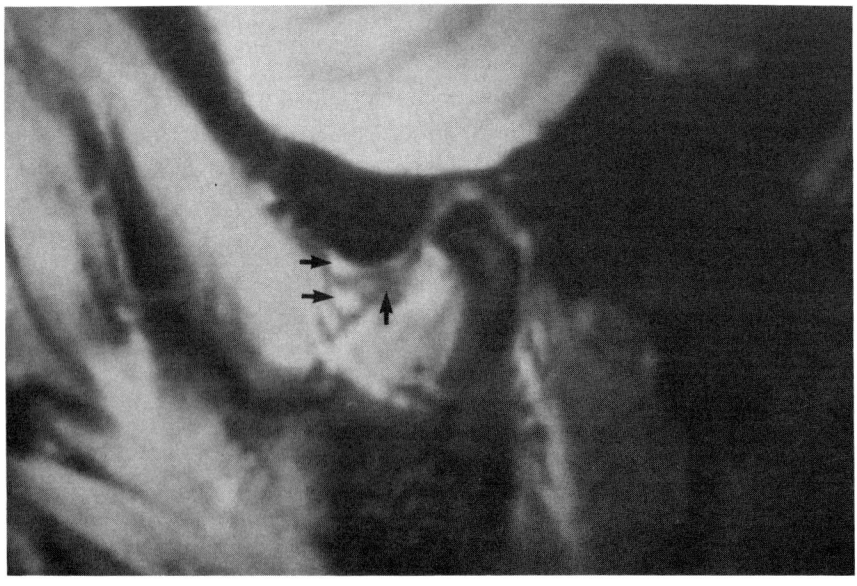

FIG. 6–58. Fluid in upper and lower TMJ compartments (horizontal arrows) and anteriorly displaced meniscus (vertical arrow). (T2-weighted sagittal gradient echo image; TR = 400 msec TE = 30 msec, θ = 30°)

SUMMARY AND CONCLUSIONS

MRI offers a unique contribution in musculoskeletal imaging. As a noninvasive modality able to produce high-contrast and high-resolution images without exposure to ionizing radiation, MRI is now the procedure of choice in the evaluation of many musculoskeletal disorders. Because the generation of the imaging signal in MRI is based on events occurring at the molecular level, MRI offers the potential to provide biochemical and physiologic information, as well as anatomic visualization. Tissue characterization in MRI is superior, and early changes in marrow, subchondral bone, and cartilage can be evaluated in patients presenting with either inflammatory or degenerative arthritis.

REFERENCES

1. Moon, K.L., Jr., et al.: Musculoskeletal applications of nuclear resonance. Radiology, 147:161–171, 1983.
2. Bloch, F., Hansen, W.W., and Parkard, M.E.: Nuclear induction. Phys. Rev., 69:127, 1946.
3. Purcell, E.M., Torrey, H.C., and Pound, R.V.: Resonance absorption by nuclear magnetic moments in solid. Physiol. Rev., 69:37, 1946.
4. Margulis, A.R., et al., eds.: Clinical Magnetic Resonance Imaging. San Francisco, Radiology Research and Education Foundation, University of California, 1983.
5. Moon, K.L., Jr., et al.: Nuclear magnetic resonance imaging in orthopaedics: Principles and applications. J. Orthop. Res., 1:101–114, 1983.
6. Reicher, M.A., et al.: Meniscal injuries: Detection using MR imaging. Radiology, 159:753–757, 1986.
7. Li, D.K.B., Adams, M.E., and McConkey, S.: Magnetic resonance imaging of the ligaments and menisci of the knee. Radiol. Clin. North Am., 24:209–228, 1986.
8. Kean, D.M., et al.: NMR imaging of the knee: Example of normal anatomy and pathology. Br. J. Radiol., 56:355–364, 1984.
9. Stoller, D.W., et al.: MRI-pathologic correlation of meniscal tears. Proceedings of the Fifth Annual Meeting of the Society of Magnetic Resonance in Medicine, 2:279, 1986.
10. Stoller, D.W., et al.: MRI-pathologic correlation of meniscal tears. Radiology, 163:731–735, 1987.
11. Pollack, M.S., Dalinka, M.K., Kressel, H.Y., and Spritzer, C.E.: MRI in the evaluation of osteonecrosis of the knee. In Proceedings of the Fifth Annual Meeting of the Society of Magnetic Resonance in Medicine, 4:1187–1188, 1986.
12. Sundaram, M., et al.: Magnetic resonance imaging in planning limb-salvage surgery for primary malignant tumors of bone. J. Bone Joint Surg., 68(A):809–819, 1986.
13. Mitchell, R.G., et al.: Femoral head avascular necrosis: Correlation of MR imaging, radiographic staging, radionuclide imaging, and clinical findings. Radiology, 162:709–715, 1987.
14. Mitchell, M.D., et al.: Avascular necrosis of the hip: Comparison of MR, CT and scintigraphy. A.J.R., 147:67–71, 1986.
15. Beltran, J., et al.: Ankle: Surface coil MR imaging at 1.5 T. Radiology, 161:203–209, 1986.
16. Kieft, G.J., et al.: Normal shoulder: MR imaging. Radiology, 159:741–745, 1986.
17. Koenig, H., Lucas, D., and Meissner, R.: The wrist: A preliminary report on high-resolution MR imaging. Radiology, 160:463–467, 1986.
18. Weiss, K.L., et al.: High-field MR surface-coil imaging of the hand and wrist. Part I. Radiology, 160:143–146, 1986.
19. Reinus, W.R., et al.: Carpal avascular necrosis: MR imaging. Radiology, 160:689–693, 1986.
20. Flannigan, B.D., et al.: MR imaging of the cervical spine: Neurovascular anatomy. A.J.R., 148:785–790, 1987.
21. Beltran, J., Noto, A.M., Chakeres, D.W., and Christoforedis, A.J.: Tumor of the osseous spine: Staging with MR imaging versus CT. Radiology, 162:565–569, 1987.
22. Burnett, K.R., Levine, J.B., and Sieger, L.: MRI evaluation of the cervical spine at high field strength. Appl. Radiol., 14(6):47–50, 1985.
23. Modic, M.T., et al.: Vertebral osteomyelitis: Assessment using MR. Radiology, 157:157–166, 1985.
24. Stoller, D.W., and Genant, H.K.: Fast imaging in the spine. In Spine Update. Edited by H.K. Genant. Berkeley, Ca., Radiology Research & Education Foundation, Univ. Press, 1987.
25. Harms, S.E., et al.: The temporomandibular joint: Magnetic resonance imaging using surface coils. Radiology, 157:133–136, 1985.

OSTEOPOROSIS AND BONE MINERAL ASSESSMENT

7

HARRY K. GENANT

Osteoporosis, a common disorder affecting large numbers of adults, results in considerable morbidity, mortality, and public-health expenditure.[1,2] Each year, hundreds of thousands of elderly people, particularly women, are disabled by broken bones, with the spine being the earliest and most common site of involvement. Osteoporosis is believed to precipitate 250,000 hip fractures annually, primarily in elderly women, and is the major cause of physical disability in old age.[3] Of elderly people who experience fractured hips, 10 to 20% die within 6 months of their injury. The sex-related difference in osteoporosis is especially significant because women in the 65-and-older age group are the fastest-growing segment of the U.S. population. It is expected that by the year 2035, the number of women and men over the age of 65 will increase by more than 200%.[4] This staggering growth rate will most likely result in a concomitant increase in the incidence of osteoporotic fractures of all kinds.

Recently the media has been informing women of the "silent epidemic" of osteoporosis, which results in an insidious loss of bone mass primarily evident through crush fractures of the vertebrae and fractures of the wrist and hip. Public consciousness of osteoporosis has also been heightened by the toll in health-care dollars measuring approximately 4 billion dollars annually, by the recent U.S. Congressional Action designating one week in May as the Annual National Osteoporosis Week, and by the convening of a National Institutes of Health Consensus Conference on this subject in the spring of 1984. The consensus panel recommended that studies be undertaken to develop accurate, safe, and inexpensive methods for determining the level of risk for osteoporosis, early diagnosis of the condition, and assessment of the clinical course of the disease.[1] Clinical aspects of osteopenia are discussed in Chapter 112.

QUANTITATIVE BONE MINERAL ANALYSIS

Considerable effort has been expended in the development of methods for quantitatively assessing the skeleton to detect osteoporosis early, and to monitor its progression and response to therapy. Consensus has not yet been reached on which methods are most efficacious for diagnosing and monitoring of the individual patient or for mass screening of large populations. In this regard, the selection of anatomic sites and of methods for quantifying skeletal mass is of considerable current importance.

The skeleton is composed of about 80% cortical or compact bone and 20% trabecular or cancellous bone (Table 7–1). The appendicular skeleton is composed predominantly of cortical bone, while the spine is composed of a combination of cancellous bone mostly in the vertebral bodies, and compact bone mostly in the dense end-plates and posterior elements. Trabecular bone has a high turnover rate, about eight times that of compact bone, partly as a result of its high surface-to-volume ratio. This high turnover rate makes trabecular bone a measuring site highly re-

Table 7–1. Comparison of Cortical and Trabecular Bone

Bone Tissue	Relative Amounts		
	Total Volume	Surface-to-Volume Ratio	Bone-Turnover Rate
Cortical-compact	4	1	1
Trabecular-cancellous	1	4	8

sponsive to metabolic stimuli. Osteoporotic fractures occur first in the vertebral bodies or distal radius, areas of predominantly trabecular bone.

Numerous methods have been used for quantitative assessment of the skeleton in osteoporosis with variable *precision, accuracy,* and *sensitivity,* precision here meaning longitudinal reproducibility in serial studies, accuracy meaning reliability that the measured value reflects true mineral content, and sensitivity meaning capacity to readily separate an abnormal patient from a normal population or to readily detect changes with time in a patient or in a population. The requirements for a clinically useful measurement of bone mineral differ, depending on the specific clinical problem under investigation. For serial determination in a given patient, precision and sensitivity are critical. On the other hand, as a diagnostic procedure to separate a patient from a normal population, accuracy and sensitivity are required. The various techniques available strive to accomplish one or all of these major goals.

The pattern and rate of bone loss in the peripheral versus the axial skeleton or in compact versus cancellous bone may vary appreciably in different disease states. Therefore, the variations in sensitivity observed for different types of measurements made at different anatomic sites are not only a function of systematic errors found with each technique but are also complicated by the physiologic variation occurring naturally at different regions of the body. Additionally, a comparison of the sensitivity of techniques is complicated by the problem of clinically defining "normal" and "diseased" populations.

For example, by all methods of measurement of age-related bone loss, it is apparent that overlap exists between osteoporotic patients and age-matched controls, and, in general, the difference between the two groups is on the order of one standard deviation.[5] Osteoporotic patients in this setting are generally defined as those individuals sustaining vertebral fractures, the so-called *vertebral crush syndrome.* But it is clear that some osteoporotic patients do not suffer fractures of the spine, whereas others with relatively minor osteopenia may do so, and patients with femoral neck fractures may differ in some respects from those with vertebral fractures, although both patients are frequently osteoporotic. Thus, these biologic discrepancies in combination with technical errors lessen the discrimination capability or diagnostic potential of any given technique.

The first quantitative bone mineral methods to be developed were radiogrammetry,[6] photodensitometry,[7,8] and photon absorptiometry,[9,10] which measure primarily cortical bone of the peripheral appendicular skeleton. Later-developed techniques can quantify bone mineral content in the spine, the site of early osteoporosis. Dual photon absorptiometry (DPA)[11–14] measures an integral of compact and cancellous bone of the axial skeleton or entire skeleton, while quantitative computed tomography (QCT)[15–30] provides a measure of purely trabecular bone of the vertebral spongiosum, or at other sites.

APPENDICULAR CORTICAL BONE MEASUREMENTS

Measurements of peripheral appendicular mineral content are relatively easy to perform and the techniques are generally available. They have provided important population-based information on skeletal mass (e.g., whites have less bone than blacks at all ages; in all ethnic groups men have more bone than women; both sexes lose bone with aging; and accelerated bone loss follows the menopause). These peripheral cortical bone measurements may be of limited diagnostic usefulness in the individual osteoporotic patient, however, because they overlap considerably with measurements in control populations; and peripheral cortical measurements do not necessarily correlate with spinal measurements, the site of early bone loss and fractures.[13,20,22,26]

RADIOGRAMMETRY

Cortical thickness is easy to measure with a caliper, or with a hand lens having a reticle. It is reproducible within 5% depending on the site measured, and is backed by a large body of normative data.[31–33] Simple cortical measurements may be represented in several ways: the summation of both cortices as an index of bone mass; the combined cortical thickness divided by total bone width as a measure of density; or a circular cross section of bone may be assumed with the bone width and cortical thickness measurements converted to cortical areas, which more closely parallel actual physical mass (Fig. 7–1).

Radiogrammetry is insensitive and has limited clinical application because of the failure to measure intracortical resorption or porosity and irregular endosteal scalloping or erosion. Intracortical resorption and trabecular bone resorption are important determinants of high bone turnover states and are not measured by this technique.[34–40]

PHOTODENSITOMETRY

Photodensitometry (radiodensitometry)[7,8,39,41] employs an x ray source, radiographic film, and a known standard wedge. It has proved reproducible in experienced hands and is possibly more sensitive than simple cortical measurement.

The photographic density on a film is roughly proportional to the mass of bone in the beam. However, relatively large changes in bone mineral (25 to 50%) must occur before differences can be determined by visual examination of radiographs. In an effort to quantitate bone mass, certain investigators[42–48] have measured the optical density of radiographs that have been exposed with the anatomic part and a reference wedge simultaneously. Multiple technical problems arise, including nonuniformity of the x ray intensity, beam hardening resulting from the polychromatic radiation source, and variation in film sensitivity related to processing. Although the precision and accuracy of photodensitometry generally are on the order of

5% for the peripheral skeleton, some centers have reported better results.[7,31,41,49]

Population studies using photodensitometry have documented the fundamental sexual dimorphism in cortical bone mass. The pioneering study of Meema[39] shows that, at all ages, women have less cortical bone than men and that age-related bone loss starts earlier, proceeds more rapidly, and results in a much greater depletion of the skeleton in women than in men (Fig. 7–2). Men first show significant loss of peripheral cortex, measured here in the radius, at age 60 to 70. By this time, in women the hydroxyapatite content of the radius, measured by radiodensitometry, has decreased from 700 mg per cm² to 350 mg per cm².

SINGLE PHOTON ABSORPTIOMETRY

Photon absorptiometry requires a gamma ray source, a detector, and intervening electronics to measure the beam attenuation through bone and express the result in some convenient form. The Norland-Cameron absorptiometer,[9,50] currently the most widely accepted and clinically applied device of this type (Fig. 7–3), measures the radial shaft by use of a ^{125}I source and a sodium iodide scintillation detector. The forearm is surrounded by a water bag or water bath so that the path thickness for the beam is kept constant, and a baseline measurement is obtained in

FIG. 7–2. Hydroxyapatite (mg/cm²) of radius by radiodensitometry in 305 normal white men and 308 normal white women. Bars indicate SE of mean. (From Meema, S., and Meema, H.E.: Menopausal bone loss and estrogen replacement. Israel J. Med. Sci., *12*:601–606, 1976.)

FIG. 7–1. Schematic representation of a cross-section of a tubular bone, showing several parameters determined by radiogrammetry.

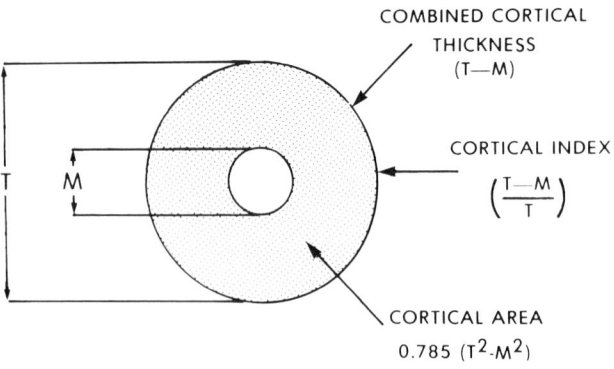

COMBINED CORTICAL
THICKNESS
(T—M)

CORTICAL INDEX

$$\left(\frac{T-M}{T}\right)$$

CORTICAL AREA
$0.785\ (T^2 - M^2)$

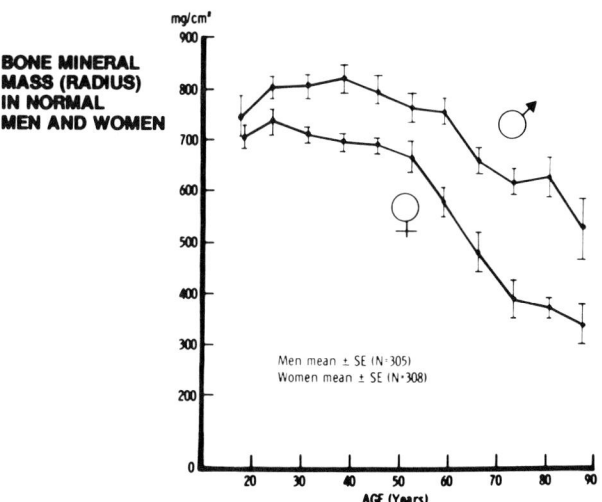

BONE MINERAL
MASS (RADIUS)
IN NORMAL
MEN AND WOMEN

Men mean ± SE (N·305)
Women mean ± SE (N·308)

AGE (Years)

FIG. 7–3. The commercially available Norland-Cameron densitometer.

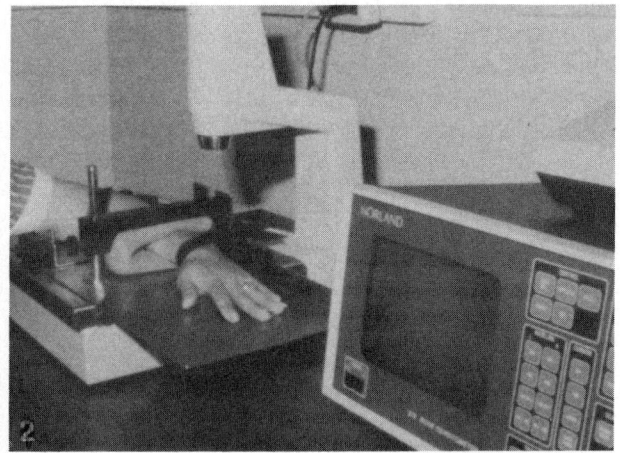

FIG. 7–4. Sexual dimorphism is shown for radial bone mineral by single photon absorptiometry (SPA) as a function of age.

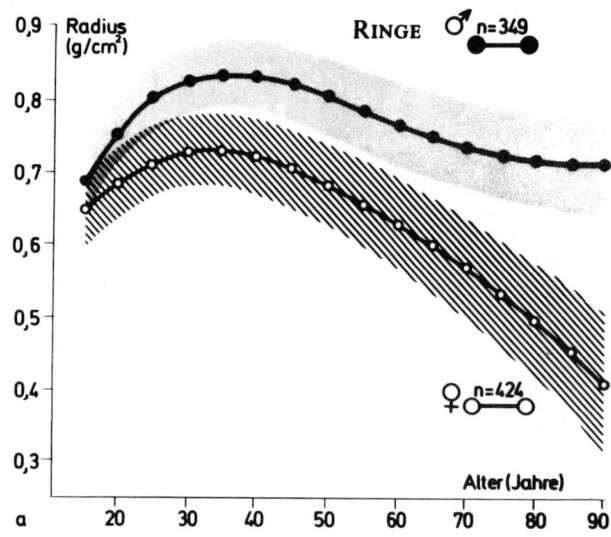

the region of the interosseous membrane. The gamma ray source and detector are then translated across the forearm, and changes in beam intensity are measured. The electronics in the device use these measurements to calculate the average attenuation of the ^{125}I beam caused by the bone interference and then compare this result with a standard curve derived from K_2HPO_4 (dipotassium hydrogen phosphate) and stored electrically. In the Norland-Cameron device, the number of grams of bone mineral contained in a 1-cm-wide path through the radius are read out in units of grams per centimeter. Bone width is also automatically determined, and the amount of bone mineral per area scanned is also calculated (g/cm²). Two sites are commonly measured in the radius: the mid-diaphysis, which consists of nearly 100% cortical bone, and the distal radial metaphysis, which contains about 75% cortical bone and 25% trabecular bone.[51]

Photon absorptiometry overcomes some of the technical problems of photodensitometry. Considerable normative data are available, and many clinical studies have supported its usefulness in population studies (Fig. 7–4). The precision of this technique is about 2% and the accuracy is about 6%.[50] Radiation exposure for this technique is low (less than 10 mrem).

The measurements obtained by photon absorptiometry correlate with weight of bone, mass at other scan sites, weight of other long bones, total skeletal weight, and total body calcium.[5] Wilson has shown measurements of the radius and ulnar shafts that are highly correlated ($r = 0.85$) with bone mineral content (BMC) of the femoral neck and less highly correlated ($r = 0.7$) with bone mineral content in the spine.[54] Others have found generally lower correlations.[26,55,56]

Studies of radial BMC in normal and osteoporotic persons show that people with osteoporosis fall about one standard deviation (15%) below levels of age-matched controls and two standard deviations (30%) below levels of young adults.[10,37,57–59] These results indicate considerable overlap between osteoporotic patients and controls, but they are similar to those obtained by iliac crest biopsy and trabecular bone volume determination.[5]

Photon absorptiometry has provided important population-based information on the central role of estrogen in the evolution of postmenopausal osteoporosis. Lindsay and co-workers studied 120 women who had just undergone hysterectomy with bilateral oophorectomy.[60] Bone mass was measured in two metacarpals by photon absorptiometry (Fig. 7–5). Sixty-three of these women received 20 µg of mestranol daily, a small dose found in low-dose contraceptive tablets. Fifty-seven women received a placebo, and these women lost bone throughout the 5 years, while the mestranol-treated women actually gained a small amount of bone mass. This study, which continued for 10 years, showed that the women taking the placebo continued to lose bone and had lost an average 1.5 cm in height, and radiographs of their lumbar spines showed beginning wedging of the vertebrae.[61] The 38 women who continued estrogen replacement for 10 years lost no bone and no height, and their vertebrae showed no evidence of wedging.

A major limitation of the *standard* photon absorptiometry techniques is that they reflect the status of peripheral tubular bones and measure primarily the

FIG. 7–5. Mean metacarpal mineral content during the 5-year follow-up of a group observed from 3 years after bilateral oophorectomy (zero time). (From Lindsay, R., et al.: Long-term prevention of post-menopausal osteoporosis by oestrogen. Lancet, *1*:1038, 1976.)

FIG. 7–6. The linear attenuation coefficient of phalangeal bone is shown for hyperparathyroid patients prior to parathyroidectomy and 1 to 3 years postoperatively. Most patients show remineralization following parathyroidectomy. (From Genant, H.K., et al.: Primary hyperparathyroidism. A comprehensive study of clinical, biochemical and radiographic manifestations. Radiology, *109*:513, 1973.)

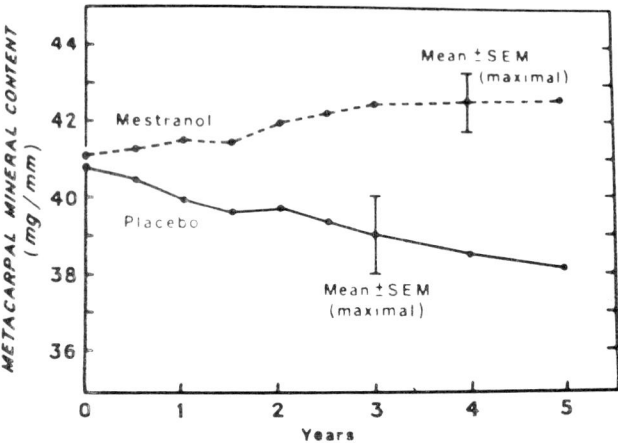

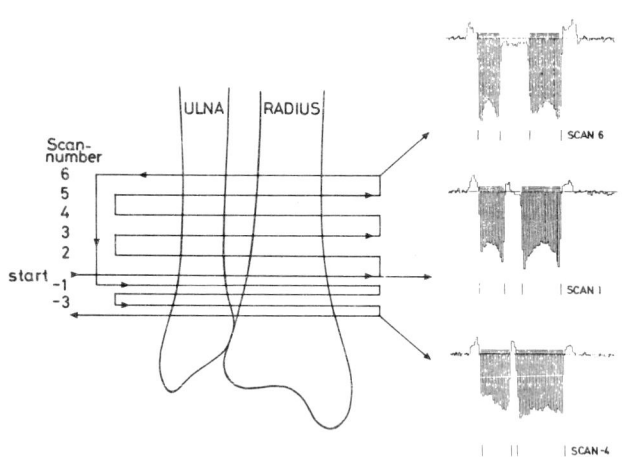

cortex. These measurements may not reflect the overall skeletal status for an individual patient in many metabolic diseases and, therefore, may be of restricted diagnostic value.[13,26] Evidence suggests that metabolic processes occur more rapidly in cancellous bone.[20,31,38,62,63] Recent modifications have been introduced in photon absorptiometry to provide raster or rectilinear scanning of the more distal radius[56,64,65] or of the calcaneus[66–69] and provide higher precision than previously achievable. These advances in instrumentation have been reviewed recently.[68] Two groups have reported their experiences using single-photon absorptiometry to study the radius at the site where the percentage of trabecular bone is similar to that found in the lumbar spine, a site referred to as the "ultradistal" radius.[56,64] The major difficulty in studying the ultradistal radius is the large change in bone mineral content over a short distance along the radial metaphysis. Methods that depend on palpation of bony landmarks such as the ulnar styloid process do not permit accurate relocation of the scanning site. Nilas and co-workers[56] scanned the radius and ulna and then used a computer-based edge detection program to determine the site at which the radius-ulna gap was 8 mm (Fig. 7–6). From this point, four scans were made at 2-mm increments distally. Awbrey and co-workers also used the radius-ulna gap to permit accurate repositioning but they made only one scan, where the radius-ulna was 5 mm.[64]

Nilas reported a correlation coefficient of 0.56 between bone density of the ultradistal radius and that of the lumbar spine.[56] From measurements made at the "5-mm" site in normal women, Grubb found a correlation coefficient of 0.52 with the spine.[70] These correlation coefficients, while significant, are inadequate to predict lumbar spine density from ultradistal radius density for an individual and are similar to results obtained when predicting lumbar spine density from age alone.[68]

The rectilinear, area-scanning approach has been applied also to measurement of the calcaneus as a convenient appendicular site containing purely trabecular bone. The single photon absorptiometry (SPA) technique used for the calcaneus is similar to that used in the study of bone loss during the Apollo and Skylab space missions.[67,71] It consists of a mechanical rectilinear scanner capable of scanning in either a horizontal or vertical plane. The os calcis scan encompasses a 2.5-cm section through the central portion which corresponds to the area of least mineral content as well as the area of greatest mineral loss during bed rest studies.[67] The ability to obtain a permanent record of the bone profiles ensures comparable sampling sites at each examination, essential for high precision. Population studies show that measurements at the os calcis are closely related to body weight and exercise, and that they discriminate spinal fractures comparably to measurements at the radius. Preliminary studies suggest that calcaneus measurement may discriminate appendicular fractures better than other techniques.[72] Additional studies are needed to determine the relative merit of photon absorptiometry of the calcaneus compared to direc spinal measurements, either for screening purposes or for monitoring disease progression and response to therapy.

DUAL PHOTON ABSORPTIOMETRY

Dual photon absorptiometry (DPA) has been studied extensively as a technique to measure spinal mineral as well as that of the hip and total body.[11–14,71,73,74] A high-purity, high-activity gadolinium source, which has photons of predominantly 44 keV and 100 keV, is used as the transmission source, and the scans are performed on a rectilinear scanner usually covering L2 to L4 (Fig. 7–7). The bone mineral content quantified is expressed in grams per cm², an area rather than density measurement.[75] This measurement assesses the sum or integral of all mineral within the scan path, which includes not only the predominantly trabecular bone of the vertebral bodies but also

FIG. 7–7. *A,* The Norland DPA system measuring the lumbar spine. *B,* Video display showing normal lumbar spine measured by DPA.

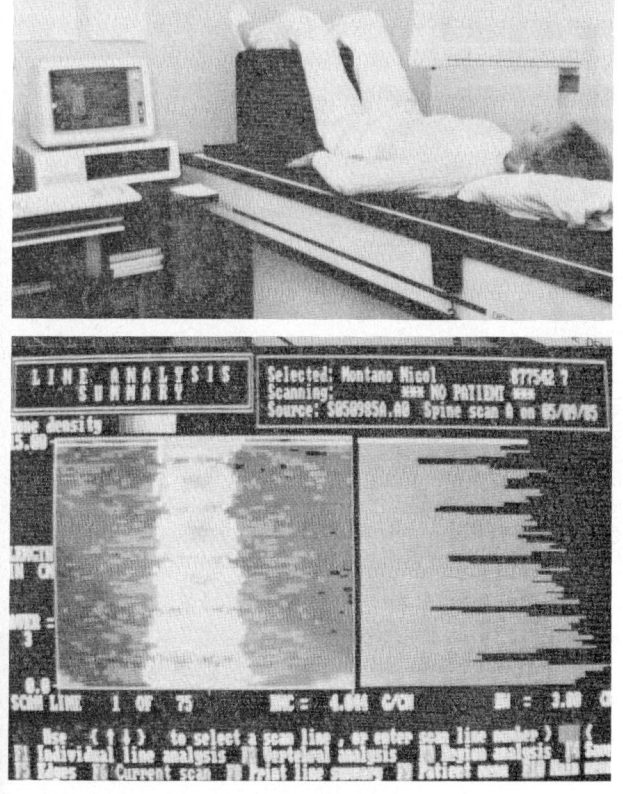

the vertebral end-plates and posterior elements with their greater percentage of compact bone. Vertebral compression fractures with callus formation, kyphoscoliosis, articular facet hypertrophy, discogenc sclerosis, marginal osteophytosis, and extraosseous calcification (aorta) are also included in the integral measurement and may result in inaccurate and poorly reproducible vertebral measurements.[76,77] Unfortunately, all of these findings are common in elderly subjects. In healthy subjects, the precision is on the order of 2% to 3%. The accuracy in phantom scanning is about 1% to 2%, and in vertebral specimens it is 4% to 10%[73,78,79] (Table 7–2).

The usual radiation dose with DPA is about 15 to 20 mrem, although conventional anteroposterior radiography, which often accompanies dual energy photon absorptiometry (DPA) for localization purposes, raises the dose to 200 to 300 mrem. DPA is also used to determine total body mineral content and is a useful replacement for calcium balance methods or total body neutron activation analysis for research purposes. DPA measurement of the hip is a potentially important application because of the magnitude of the problem of hip fractures. DPA measurement of the hip is superior to measurement of the spine for prediction of hip fracture risk, but it remains to be determined whether this site will be suitable for monitoring disease.

Extensive normative data and clinical results have been reported for DPA spinal measurement. A comprehensive analysis of DPA and SPA examined the patterns of bone loss in the axial and the appendicular skeleton in 187 normal volunteers (105 women and 82 men; age range, 20 to 89 years [Fig. 7–8]) and in 76 women and 9 men with vertebral fractures resulting from osteoporosis.[13] Bone mineral density was measured at the lumbar spine by dual photon absorptiometry and at both the midradius and distal radius by single photon absorptiometry. In normal women, bone diminution from the vertebrae began in young adulthood and was linear (Fig. 7–8A). In the appendicular skeleton, bone diminution did not occur until age 50 years, accelerated from age 51 to 65 years, and then decelerated somewhat after age 65 (Fig. 7–9A). Overall bone diminution throughout life was 47% for the vertebrae, 30% for the midradius, and 39% for the distal radius. In normal men, vertebral and appendicular bone diminution with aging was minimal or insignificant (Fig. 7–8B and Fig. 7–9B). Mean bone mineral density was lower in patients with osteoporosis than in age- and sex-matched normal subjects at all three sites, although spinal measurements discriminated best (Fig. 7–9A,B); however, considerable overlap occurred. By age 65, half

Table 7–2. Comparison Between Spinal QCT and DPA

Measurement	QCT Trabecular	DPA Integral
Sensitivity	3×	1×
Precision	1.5%–5%	2%–4%
Accuracy	5%–15%	5%–?
Radiation	100–500 mrem	10–20 mrem
Time	10–15 min.	30–45 min.

of the normal women (and by age 85, virtually all of them) had vertebral bone mineral density values below the 90th percentile of women with vertebral fractures and, thus, might be considered to have asymptomatic osteoporosis. For men, the degree of overlap was less. Disproportionate loss of trabecular bone from the axial skeleton appeared to be a distinguishing characteristic of spinal osteoporosis.

NEUTRON ACTIVATION ANALYSIS

Neutron activation analysis (NAA) in vivo has been under investigation at several centers for the past decade.[80-83] Neutrons bombard a small fraction of the total ^{48}Ca in the body, producing ^{49}Ca (half-life of 8.8 minutes), which is then counted externally. The neutrons (with energies of 1 to 15 MeV) are derived from accelerators, reactors, or alpha neutron sources. The technique provides an estimate of bone mineral content because, at least in the skeleton, calcium makes up a constant fraction (0.395) of the mineral. Radiation doses for such measures range from 200 to 3000 mrem, depending on the neutron energy and the detector efficiency. Precision and accuracy are on the order of 2% to 5%.[84]

A total body calcium measurement by NAA reflects primarily compact bone, which constitutes approximately 80% of the total skeletal mass and, therefore, correlates closely with other measurements of cortical bone.[5] Total body calcium measurements by neutron activation have been compared with results obtained by peripheral photon absorptiometry, and correlation coefficients on the order of 0.9 were obtained.[57,85,86] Processes occurring initially or predominantly in cancellous bone may not be as readily detected with this technique. For example, in osteoporotic patients, the correlation between peripheral measurements by photon absorptiometry and total body neutron activation is not ideal. Heterotopic calcification, such as vascular and costochondral calcification, or heterotopic ossification, such as osteophytosis and myositis ossificans, causes inaccuracies in the estimation of skeletal calcium by NAA.

FIG. 7–8. DPA spinal bone mineral for scattergram of normal females *(A)* and males *(B)* as a function of age. A linear relationship is shown for both sexes by DPA.

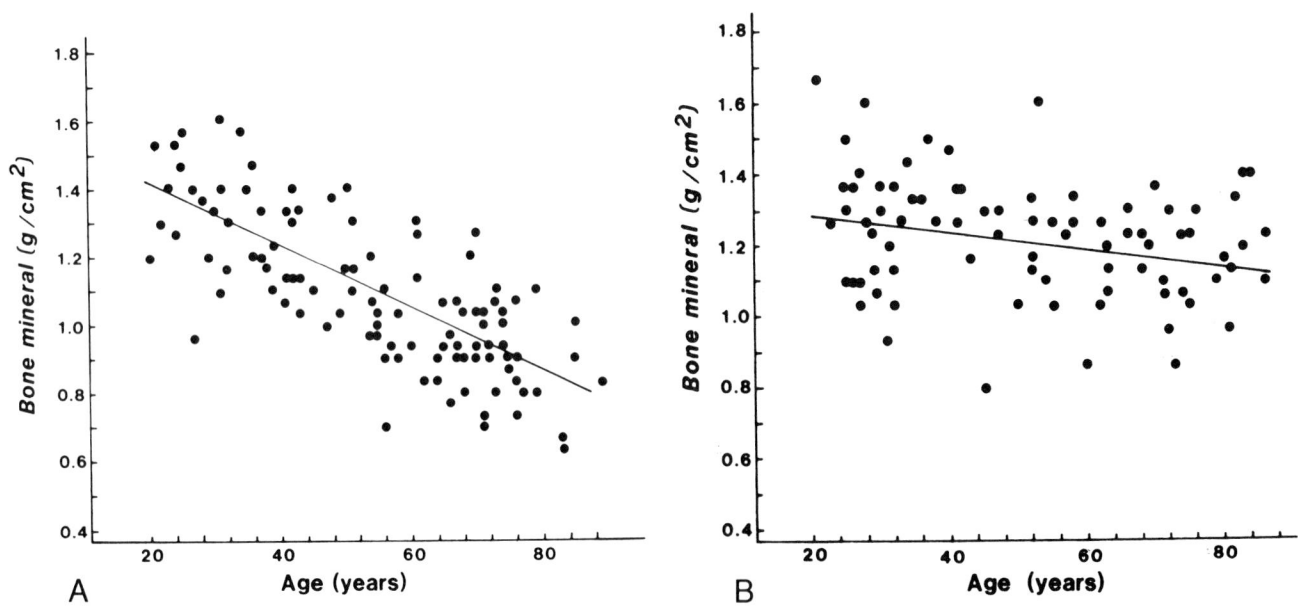

FIG. 7–9. *A*, SPA radial diaphyseal bone mineral content for normal females as a function of age. The 90% intervals are shown and contrasted with the plotted osteoporotic women. *B*, DPA spinal bone mineral content for normal females with 90% intervals shown. Osteoporotic females are plotted showing modest discrimination.

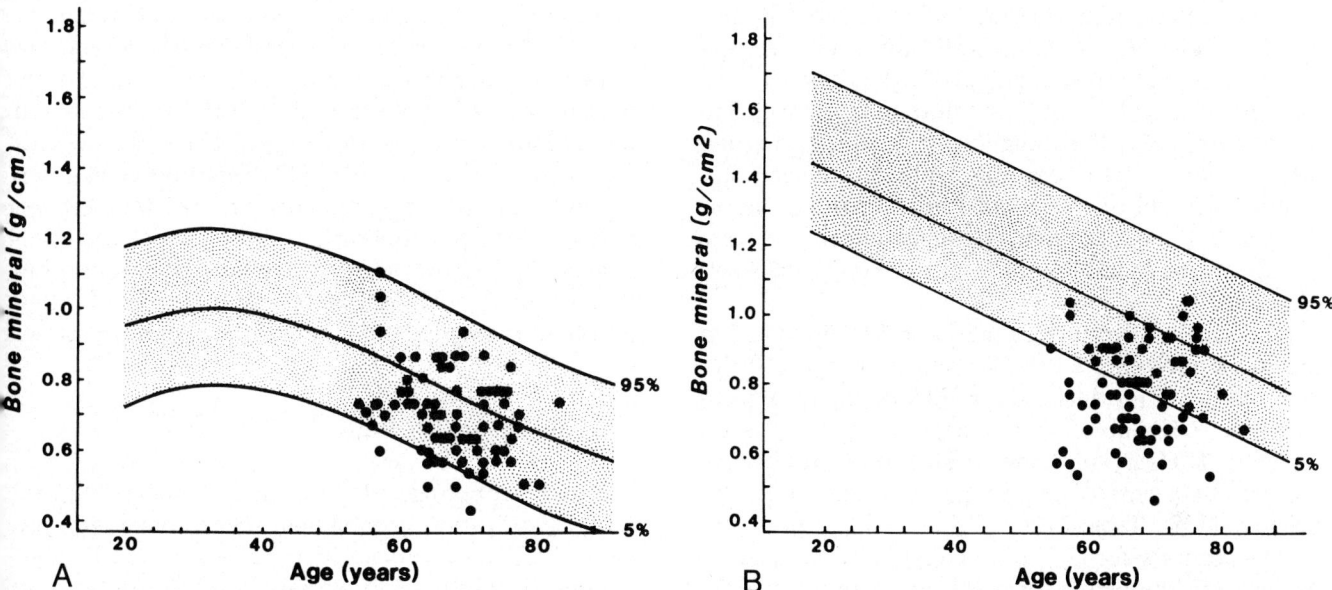

Complicated technical requirements and the expensive equipment used confine the availability of this technique to several large research centers. The dual energy photon absorptiometry technique would appear to give similar information to that of partial body activation at a substantially lower (several orders of magnitude less) level of radiation exposure[87] and it uses less expensive and far more readily available equipment.[5,87]

COMPUTED TOMOGRAPHY FOR BONE MINERAL ANALYSIS

Computed tomography (CT) has been widely investigated in recent years as a means of noninvasive quantitative bone mineral determination.[15–30] The usefulness of CT for measuring bone mineral lies in its ability to provide a quantitative image and, thereby, measure trabecular, cortical, or integral bone, centrally or peripherally. For measuring the spine, the potential advantages of quantitative computed tomography (QCT)[20,21,26] over DPA are its capability for precise three-dimensional anatomic localization providing a direct density measurement, and its capability for spatial separation of highly responsive cancellous bone from less responsive cortical bone. The lumbar vertebrae contain substantial amounts of compact bone, with only part of the spinal minerals

being high-turnover trabecular bone. The sensitivity of a technique measuring an integral of compact and cancellous bone (such as area projection with DPA) may be low compared to QCT because of inclusion of low-turnover compact bone and extraosseous mineral such as osteophytes or aortic calcification. The selective localization and the direct density measurement provided by QCT permit exclusion of these causes of low sensitivity or error and inclusion of purely trabecular bone.

QCT measures changes in trabecular mineral content in the spine and in the radius and tibia with great sensitivity and precision.[15–30] Conventional CT scanners are used, but the extraction of quantitative information from the CT image requires sophisticated calibration and positioning techniques and careful technical monitoring. Specifically designed, small-scale CT scanners using isotope or x ray sources have also been developed and applied, principally for measurement of the peripheral and trabecular and cortical skeleton as a research tool.[23,28]

TECHNICAL CONSIDERATIONS FOR VERTEBRAL QCT

QCT measurements using techniques developed at University of California, San Francisco (UCSF)[16,19,20] are made with commercially available CT scanners using a mineral reference standard for simultaneous calibration, a computed radiograph (scout view) for localization, and either single- or dual-energy techniques[16,17,19,24] (Fig. 7–10). Representative volumes (approximately 4 cm³) of purely trabecular bone at the midplane of two to four lumbar vertebral bodies are quantified and averaged, and the results are expressed in mineral equivalents of K_2HPO_4 in mg/cm³ (a density measurement). The examination takes 5 to 10 minutes, and the radiation exposure is approximately 100 to 200 mrem (one-tenth the dosage of a routine CT study). The radiation exposure can be higher on some CT systems if the manufacturers have restricted the capability for reducing kvp or mAs settings.

The precision (reproducibility) of vertebral QCT in normal subjects is 1% to 3% for single-energy (80 kVp) and 3% to 5% for dual-energy (80 kVp/120 kVp) techniques.[20,21] The accuracy of single-energy QCT is 1% to 2% for K_2HPO_4 solutions, and 5% to 15% for human vertebral specimens spanning a wide age-range[22,26,27] (Fig. 7–11, A, Table 7–1).

The accuracy for QCT (and DPA), however, can be reduced in the elderly osteoporotic population.[19,22,24] In QCT, the sources of error are different but are par-

tially correctable. The density of yellow marrow is less than that of red marrow because of the presence of fat, which falsely reduces the measured spinal mineral value (by about 7 mg per 10% fat by volume at 80 kVp), and can result in inaccuracies of 20 to 30% in an elderly osteoporotic population.[88] Dual-energy QCT,[17,19,24] now offered by several manufacturers, can reduce the magnitude of this fat error in the elderly to approximately 5% but with reduced precision and higher radiation exposure (Fig. 7–11B). *It is considered unnecessary for most clinical applications;* however, when highly accurate measurements are needed, for example in research applications, both single- and dual-energy QCT can be performed initially at baseline and then single-energy QCT alone can be applied for longitudinal followup, thus maintaining high precision.

CLINICAL AVAILABILITY OF QCT

Rapid technologic advances in CT, especially in external localization capabilities, mean that many advanced CT scanners can be modified for QCT measurements relatively inexpensively. Reductions in scanning time and radiation exposure make this an

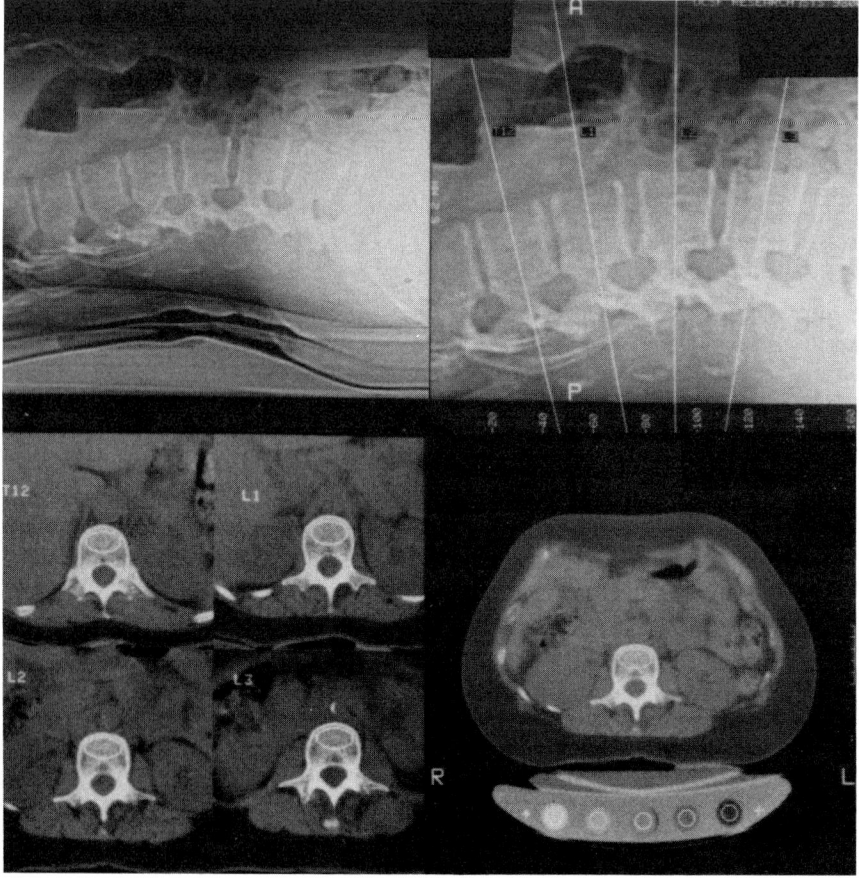

FIG. 7–10. Quantitative CT using the GE 9800 CT scanner. Lateral scout view provides rapid and simple localization approach in which the midplane of four vertebral bodies are defined on the video monitor and a single 10-mm-thick section is obtained at each level. An oval region of interest, centered in the midvertebral body, is used to determine cancellous bone mineral content (g/cm³), while circular regions of interest are used to quantify the K_2HPO_4 solutions in the calibration phantom.

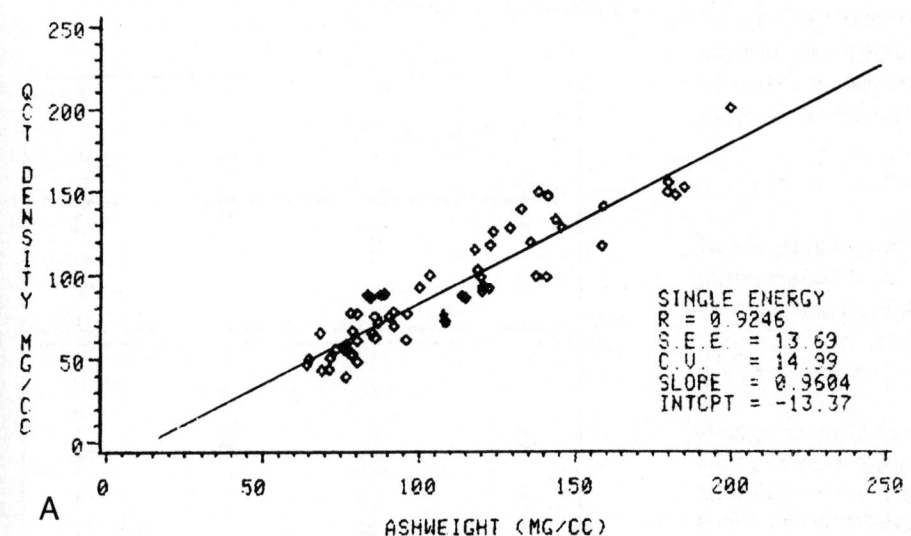

FIG. 7–11. The accuracy of single energy QCT *(A)* is shown for fresh vertebral specimen (derived from 62 samples) from 28 cadavers (20 males and 8 females with a mean age of 60). The predictive error of 13 mg/cc is acceptable diagnostically because of the large decrements observed cross-sectionally from health to disease, typically 30 to 100 mg/cc. Accuracy is improved with dual energy QCT *(B)* but at a cost of higher dose and lower precision.

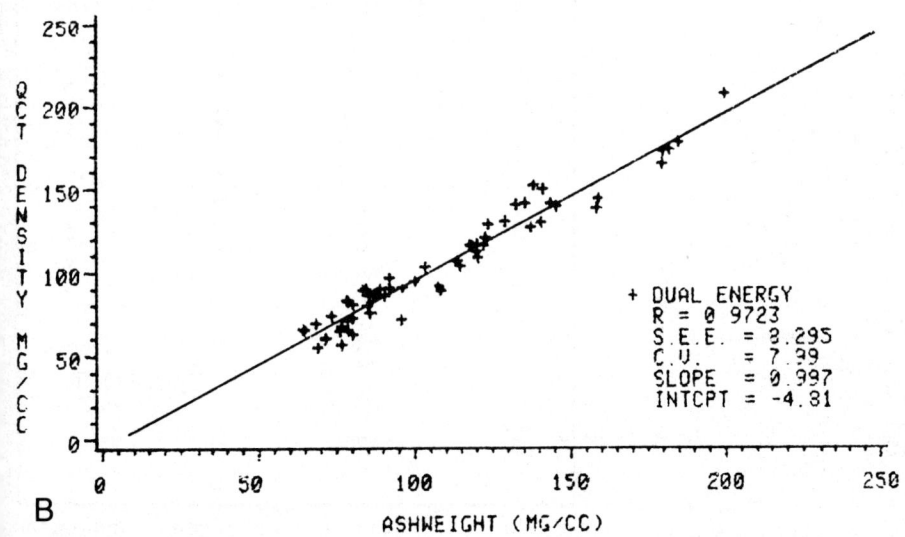

attractive technique for noninvasive bone mass measurement. We have assessed[21,22] the scanner independence of vertebral QCT measurement by determining the interscanner variability on four separate CT scanners using these techniques. A coefficient of variation between scanners of 3 to 4% was found, indicating that, with careful cross-calibration, normative data and clinical results obtained on a scanner at one site may be extrapolated to those obtained at different sites. Currently, QCT vertebral mineral determination by this approach has been implemented at over 1000 sites encompassing a wide geographic distribution and a wide array of commercial scanners. With a worldwide distribution of approximately 8000 advanced CT body scanners, the capability exists for widespread application of vertebral bone mineral determination by quantitative computed tomography.

CLINICAL APPLICATIONS OF QCT

QCT techniques for vertebral mineral determination have been used to study skeletal changes in osteoporosis and other metabolic bone diseases. Longitudinal and cross-sectional bone mass measurements have been obtained at UCSF in over 3000 patients seen clinically or on research protocols. The results presented here illustrate the use of QCT spinal mineral measurement in the delineation of normal age-related bone loss, in the evaluation of estrogen effects on bone, and in the assessment of fracture threshold and risk.

Age-Related Bone Loss

Normal ranges of vertebral mineral and age-related bone losses were determined from cross-sectional studies of 120 normal males and 203 normal females aged 20 to 80[17,22] (Fig. 7–12A, B). The normal mean value for young males and females is approximately

FIG. 7–12. *A,* Normal female values for vertebral cancellous mineral content by QCT, using a cubic regression with 95% confidence intervals; an accelerated loss is observed after menopause. *B,* Normal male values for vertebral cancellous mineral content by QCT, using a linear regression with 95% confidence intervals.

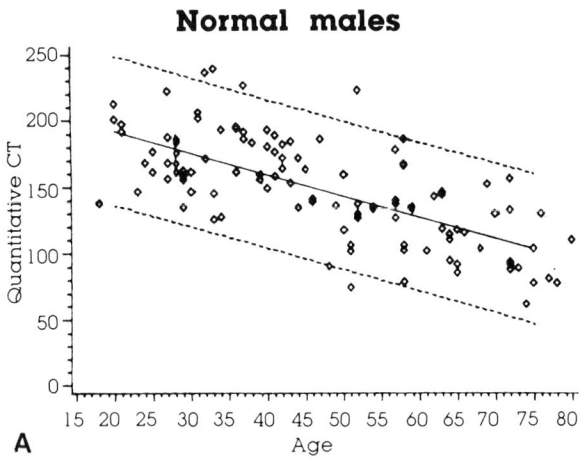

Normal males

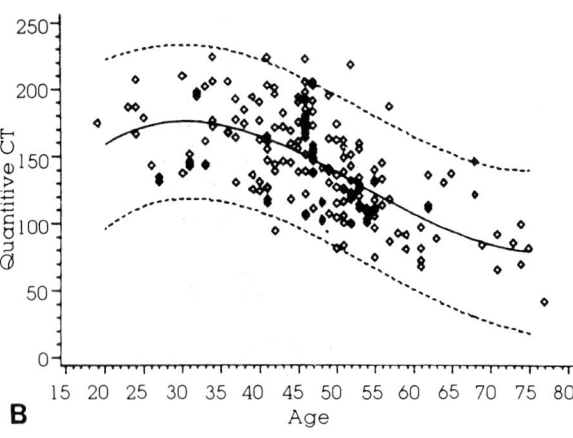

Normal females

FIG. 7–13. Vertebral trabecular bone loss in 83 climacteric women following natural menopause. Changes in spinal QCT, metacarpal cortical thickness, and radial photon absorptiometry over 24 months (three-point data per patient) are shown as a function of treatment.

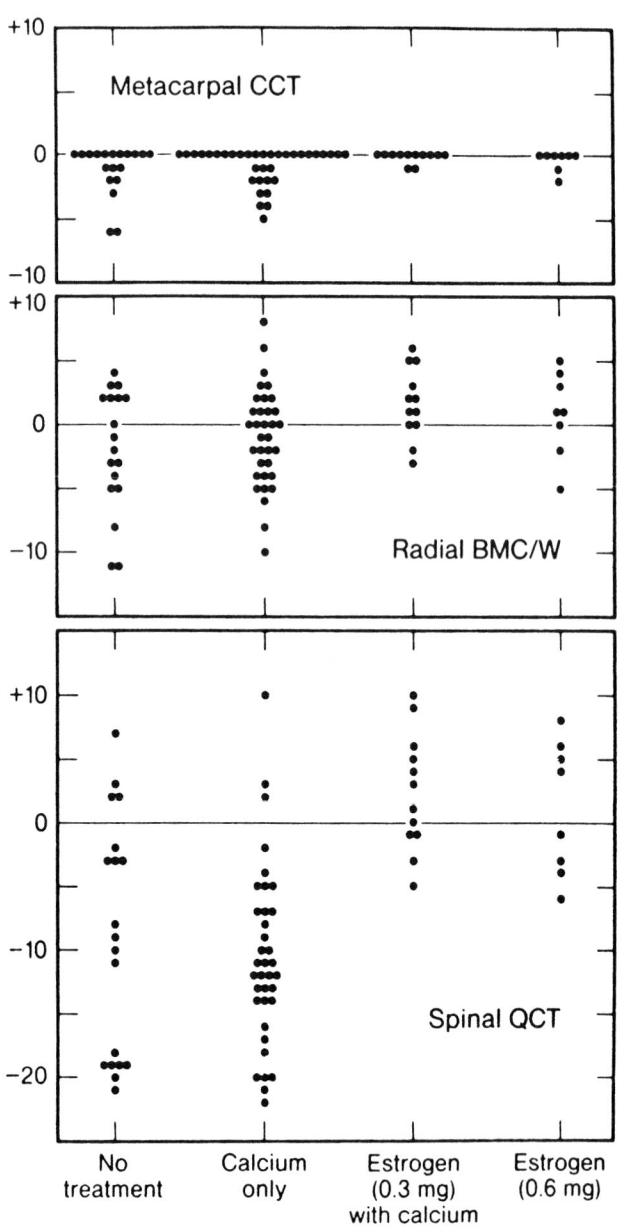

175 mg/cm³. Males, by linear regression, lose an average 0.94%/year so that by age 75, the mineral content is reduced by 40% to approximately 110 mg/cm³. Females, by cubic regression, lose an average 1.24%/year, which rate is accelerated at menopause, and by age 75, mineral content is reduced by 50% to approximately 90 mg/cm³. Correcting for age-related marrow fat alters the observed rates of loss by only

about 10% (e.g., in females, 1.08%/year versus 1.2%/year).[17,21] These rates of spinal trabecular bone loss are greater than those observed in DPA of the spine[13] due to the latter's inclusion of compact and extraneous bone in the integral measurements.

Influence of Estrogen on Skeletal Integrity in Women

The importance of estrogen in maintaining skeletal mass in women has now been shown convincingly[60] and is supported by recent studies using spinal QCT. Furthermore, the natural rates of postmenopausal bone loss and the dose response for estrogen replacement therapy are being established by noninvasive measurement techniques. Longitudinal studies performed over 24 months in 75 climacteric women (within 3 years of menopause) show an alarming average cumulative vertebral mineral loss of 9% while a minimal loss of 1 to 2% is observed in the appendicular skeleton over 2 years[89] (Fig. 7–13). Furthermore, spinal QCT shows that treatment with 1500 mg calcium per day is ineffective (10% cumulative loss), while calcium plus 0.3 mg conjugated estrogen daily is effective (+1.8%) and 0.625 mg conjugated estrogen alone is similarly effective (+1.6%).

The rate of spinal trabecular loss is even more extreme with abrupt cessation of ovarian function following surgical menopause. Longitudinal studies in women following oophorectomy show an average 9% annual vertebral cancellous loss[20] (Fig. 7–14), while integral vertebral loss (as with DPA) is only 4% and peripheral cortical bone loss is 2% to 3%. By QCT, the minimum protective dose of conjugated estrogen for preventing spinal bone loss following oophorectomy (as with natural menopause) is 0.625 mg/daily.

Ample evidence exists, then, that estrogen replacement therapy begun soon after spontaneous menopause or oophorectomy prevents bone loss. The *long-*

FIG. 7–14. Cumulative bone loss observed over a period of 24 months in 37 women as a function of quantitative technique and therapy with conjugated estrogen.

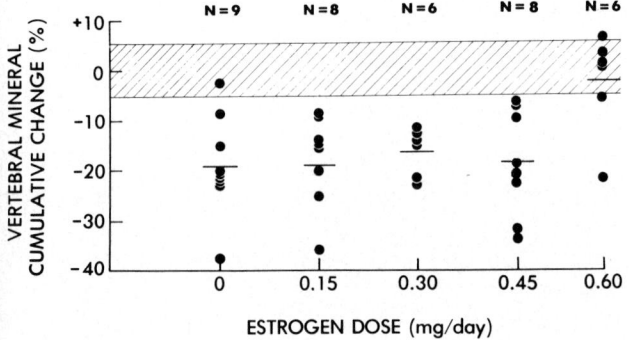

FIG. 7–15. Vertebral mineral content in the subset of 18 long-term estrogen-treated women contrasted with 17 age-matched controls.

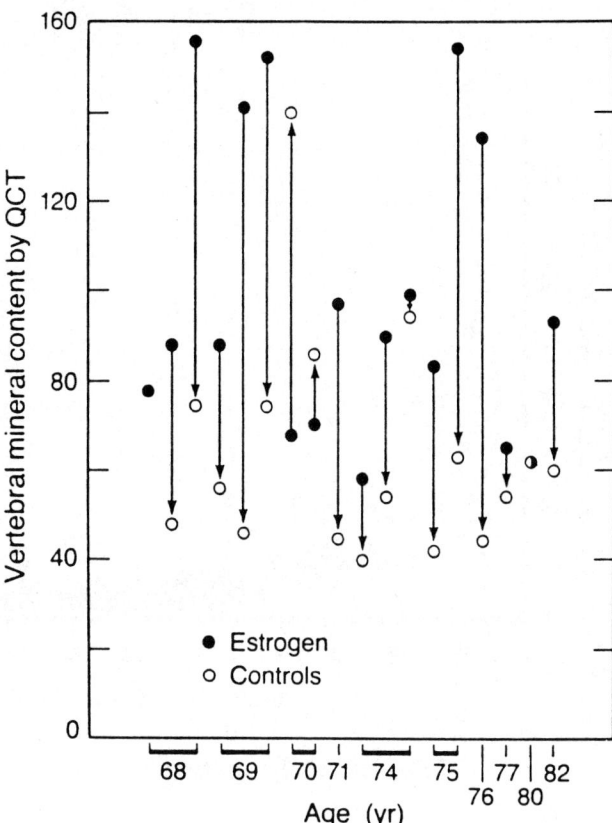

term benefits of estrogen use on skeletal mass and integrity, however, are not well established. To quantify the degree to which estrogen replacement therapy prevents postmenopausal osteoporosis, we performed a retrospective study comparing the occurrence of fractures in 245 long-term estrogen users and 245 case-matched controls, followed for an average of 17.6 years.[90] Quantitative bone mineral assessments were obtained from 18 women using estrogen replacement therapy and their controls (average age, 73 years) (Fig 7–15). Osteoporotic fracture incidence in estrogen users was 50% as great as in the controls ($p < 0.01$). Estrogen users showed significantly greater bone mineral: 54.2% greater spinal mineral ($p < 0.0002$), 19.4% greater forearm mineral ($p < 0.0005$), and 15.6% greater metacarpal cortical thickness ($p < 0.0005$). The results of this study strongly suggest that long-term estrogen replacement therapy confers significant protection against bone loss and fracture.

FIG. 7–16.   Scatter plot of spinal fracture index versus quantitative CT. Moderate correlation is observed between these two measurements.

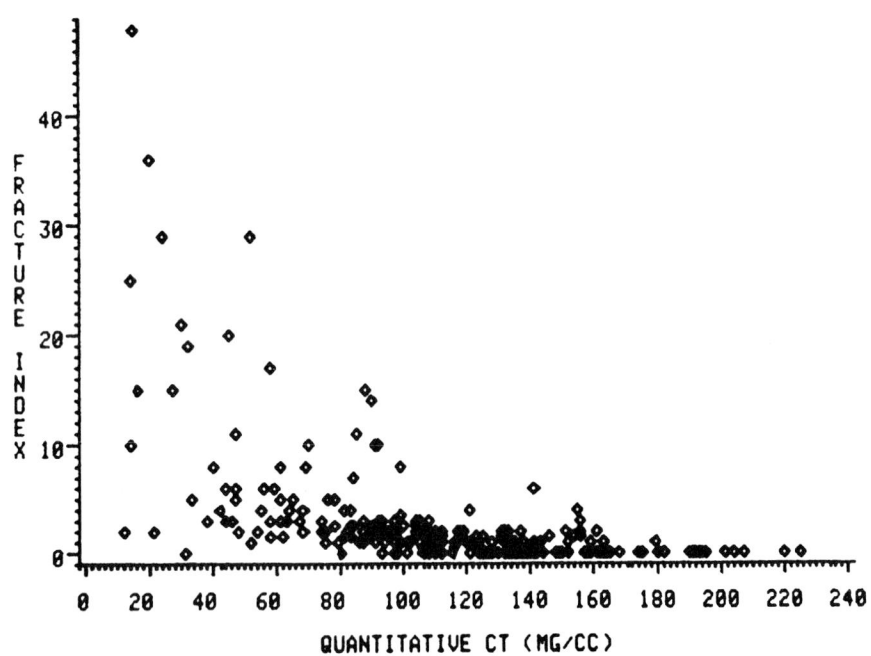

FRACTURE INDEX VS. QCT
R = −0.74

Osteoporotic males

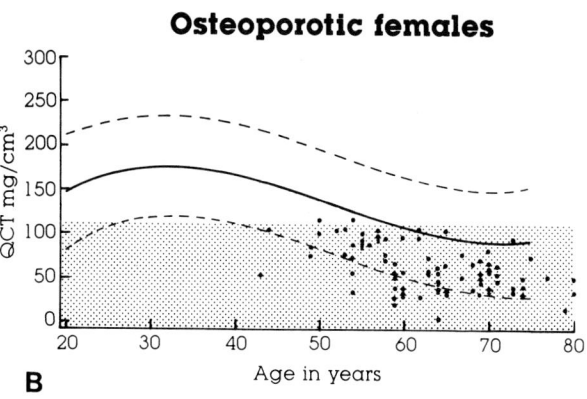

A

Osteoporotic females

B

FIG. 7–17.   A, Males with idiopathic osteoporosis and vertebral fractures are plotted as closed circles against the normal curve drawn with 95% confidence intervals. B, Females with postmenopausal osteoporosis and crushed or wedged vertebrae are plotted against the normal curve. For both males and females a fracture threshold or permissive level is observed below approximately 110 mg/cm³ (cross-hatched area).

Fracture Threshold and QCT

The relationship between fracture and vertebral mineral density has been examined. Vertebral QCT measurements in both males and females correlate well with the severity of vertebral fracture[26] (Fig. 7–16) and provide an index of fracture risk by revealing a permissive level at approximately 110 mg/cm^3, above which fractures are rare and below which fractures may occur (Fig. 7–17).[17,21] Substantial overlap exists, however, particularly in older women, between the osteoporotic group, as defined by atraumatic vertebral fracture, and the normal population; this overlap reduces the prediction value of spinal QCT, as with all other measurements of bone mass, for the individual patient, and also underscores the potential importance of other risk factors such as quality of bone tissue or propensity for falls. Nevertheless, all studies that have compared QCT and DPA in the same patients have found a better separation of osteoporotics from normals or a better correlation with fracture for spinal trabecular measurement by QCT than for spinal integral measurement by DPA.[55,91–96]

REFERENCES

1. Osteoporosis: Consensus Conference. JAMA, *252*:799–802, 1984.
2. Whedon, G.S.: Osteoporosis. N. Engl. J. Med., *305*:397–399, 1981.
3. National Institutes of Health: Special Report on Aging: 1979. National Institute on Aging, NIH Publication No. 79–1907, Bethesda, MD, Sept. 1979.
4. Butler, R.N.: The old woman: Continuities and discontinuities. Report from the National Institute on Aging and the National Institute on Mental Health Workshop. Bethesda, MD, Sept. 14–16, 1978.
5. Mazess, R.B.: Non-invasive measurement of bone. *In* Osteoporosis, Vol. II. Edited by U.S. Barzel. New York, Grune & Stratton, 1979, p. 5–26.
6. Garn, S.M.: Earlier gain and the later loss of cortical bone. *In* Nutritional Perspective. Edited by S.M. Garn. Springfield, IL, Charles C Thomas, 1970, p. 146.
7. Colbert, C., Mazess, R.B., and Schmidt, P.B.: Bone mineral determination in vitro by radiographic photodensitometry and direct photon absorptiometry. Invest. Radiol., *5*:336–340, 1970.
8. Doyle, F.H.: Some quantitative radiological observations in primary and secondary hyperparathyroidism. Br. J. Radiol., *39*:161, 1966.
9. Cameron, J.R., and Sorenson, J.A.: Measurement of bone mineral in vivo: An improved method. Science, *142*:230–232, 1963.
10. Smith, D.M., Khairi, M.R.A., and Johnston, C., Jr.: The loss of bone mineral with aging and its relationship to risk of fracture. J. Clin. Invest., *56*:311–318, 1975.
11. Krølner, B., and Nielsen, P.S.: Measurement of bone mineral content (BMC) of the lumbar spine. I. Theory and application of a new two-dimensional dual-photon attenuation method. Scand. J. Clin. Lab. Invest., *40*:485–487, 1980.
12. Peppler, W.W., and Mazess, R.B.: Total body bone mineral and lean body mass by dual photon absorptiometry. I. Theory and measurement procedure. Calcif. Tissue Int., *33*:353–359, 1981.
13. Riggs, B.L., et al.: Differential changes in bone mineral density of the appendicular and axial skeleton with aging. J. Clin. Invest., *67*:328–335, 1981.
14. Roos, B., Rosengren, B., and Skoldborn, H.: Determination of bone mineral content in lumbar vertebrae by a double gamma-ray technique. *In* Proceedings of the Bone Measurement Conference: USAEC Conf-700515. Edited by J.R. Cameron. Springfield, VA, Clearinghouse for Federal Scientific and Technical Information, National Bureau of Standards, U.S. Dept. of Commerce, 1970, pp. 243–254.
15. Adams, J.E., et al.: Dual energy computed tomography (CT) and the estimation of bone mass (abstract). J. Comput. Assist. Tomogr., *6*:204, 1982.
16. Cann, C.E., and Genant, H.K.: Precise measurement of vertebral mineral content using computed tomography. J. Comput. Assist. Tomogr., *4*:493–500, 1980.
17. Cann, C.E., and Genant, H.K.: Single versus dual-energy CT for vertebral mineral quantification. J. Comput. Assist. Tomogr., *7(3)*:551, 1983.
18. Cann, C.E., Genant, H.K., Kolb, F.O., and Ettinger, B.: Quantitative computed tomography for prediction of vertebral fracture risk. Bone, *6*:1–7, 1985.
19. Genant, H.K., and Boyd, D.P.: Quantitative bone mineral analysis using dual energy computed tomography. Invest. Radiol., *12*:545–551, 1977.
20. Genant, H.K., Cann, C.E., Ettinger, B., and Gordan, G.S.: Quantitative computed tomography of vertebral spondiosa: A sensitive method for detecting early bone loss after oophorectomy. Ann. Intern. Med., *97*:699–705, 1982.
21. Genant, H.K., et al.: Quantitative computed tomography for vertebral mineral determination. *In* Clinical Disorders of Bone and Mineral Metabolism. Edited by B. Frame and J.T. Potts. New York, Excerpta Medica, 1983, pp. 40–47.
22. Genant, H.K., et al.: Quantitative computed tomography for spinal mineral assessment: Current status. J. Comput. Assist. Tomogr., *9(3)*:602–604, 1985.
23. Hangartner, T.N., and Overton, T.R.: The Alberta gamma CT system. J. Comput. Assist. Tomogr., *6*:1156, 1983.
24. Laval-Jeantet, A.M., Cann, C.E., Roger, B.M., and Dallant, P.: A post-processing dual energy technique for vertebral CT densitometry. J. Comput. Assist. Tomogr., *9*:1164–1167, 1984.
25. Orphanoudakis, S.C., et al.: Bone mineral analysis using single energy computed tomography. Invest. Radiol., *14*:122–130, 1979.
26. Richardson, M.L., et al.: Assessment of metabolic bone disease by quantitative computed tomography. Clin. Orthop., *195*:224–238, 1985.
27. Rohloff, R., Hitzler, H., Arndt, W., and Frey, W.: Vergleichende Messungen des Kalksalzgehaltes spongioser Knochen mittels Computertomographie und J-125-Photonen-Absorptionsmethode. *In* CT '82. Edited by J. Lissner and J.L. Doppman. Konstanz, Germany, Schnetztor-Verlag, 1983, pp. 126–130.
28. Roos, B.: Dual Photon Absorptiometry in Lumbar Vertebrae. Goteborg, Sweden, Akademisk Avahling, 1974, p. 264–290.
29. Stebler, B., and Ruegsegger, P.: Special-purpose CT-system for quantitative bone evaluation in the appendicular skeleton. Biomed. Tech. (Berlin), *28*:196–205, 1983.
30. Weissberger, M.A., Zamenhof, R.G., Aronow, S., and Neer, R.M.: Computed tomography for the measurement of bone mineral in the human spine. J. Comput. Assist. Tomogr., *2*:253–262, 1978.

31. Dequeker, J.: Bone and aging: occasional surgery. Ann. Rheum. Dis., *34*:100–115, 1975.

32. Garn, S.M., Poznanski, A.K., and Nagy, J.M.: Bone measurement in the differential diagnosis of osteopenia and osteoporosis. Radiology, *100*:509–518, 1971.

33. Virtama, P., and Helela, T.: Radiographic measurements of cortical bone. Acta. Radiol. (Suppl) (Stockholm), *293*:268, 1969.

34. Duncan, H.: Cortical porosis: A morphological evaluation. *In* Proceedings of the First Workshop on Bone Morphometry. Edited by Z.F.G. Jaworski. Ottawa, Ontario, University of Ottawa Press, 1976, p. 78–83.

35. Genant, H.K., et al.: Primary hyperparathyroidism. A comprehensive study of clinical, biochemical and radiographic manifestations. Radiology, *109*:513–524, 1973.

36. Genant, H.K., et al.: The reflex sympathetic dystrophy syndrome. A comprehensive analysis using fine-detail radiography, photon absorptiometry, and bone and joint scintigraphy. Radiology, *117*:21–32, 1975.

37. Goldsmith, N.F., et al.: Bone mineral estimation in normal and osteoporotic women. J. Bone Joint Surg., *53A*:83, 1971.

38. Gordan, G.S., and Vaughan, C.: Clinical Management of the Osteoporoses. Acton, MA, Publishing Sciences Group, Inc., 1976.

39. Meema, H.E., and Meema, S.: Comparison of microradioscopic and morphometric findings in the hand bones with densitometric findings in the proximal radius in thyrotoxicosis and in renal osteodystrophy. Invest. Radiol., *7*:88–96, 1972.

40. Steinbach, H.L.: The roentgen appearance of osteoporosis. Radiol. Clin. North Am., *2*:191, 1964.

41. Mack, P.B.: Radiographic bone densitometry. Washington, DC, National Aeronautics and Space Administration, March 25, 1965, p. 31–46.

42. Anderson, J.B., Simmins, J., and Smith, D.A.: A new technique for measurement of metacarpal density. Br. J. Radiol., *39*:443, 1966.

43. Baylink, D.J., Vose, G.P., Doller, W.E., Hurxthal, L.M.: Two new methods for the study of osteoporosis and other metabolic bone diseases. II. Vertebral bone densitometry. Lahey Clin. Bull., *13*:217, 1964.

44. Mack, P.B., O'Brien, A.T., Smith, J.M., and Bauman, A.W.: A method of estimating the degree of mineralization of bones from tracings of roentgenograms. Science, *89*:467, 1939.

45. Mack, P.B., Brown, W.N., and Trapp, H.D.: The quantitative evaluation of bone density. AJR, *61*:808, 1949.

46. Meema, H.E., Bunker, M.L., and Meema, S.: Loss of compact bone due to menopause. Obstet. Gynecol., *26*:333, 1965.

47. Pridie, R.B.: The diagnosis of senile osteoporosis using a new bone density index. Br. J. Radiol., *40*:251–255, 1967.

48. Schraer, H., Schraer, R., Trostle, H.G., and D'Alfonso, A.: The validity of measuring bone density from roentgenograms by means of a bone density computing apparatus. Arch. Biochem. Biophys., *83*:486, 1959.

49. Meema, H.E., and Meema, S.: Cortical bone mineral density versus cortical thickness in the diagnosis of osteoporosis: A roentgenologic-densitometric study. J. Am. Geriatr. Soc., *17*:120, 1969.

50. Cameron, J.R., Mazess, R.B., and Sorenson, J.A.: Precision and accuracy of bone mineral determination by the direct photon absorptiometric method. Invest. Radiol., *3*:141–150, 1968.

51. Schlenker, R.A., and Von Seggen, W.W.: The distribution of cortical and trabecular bone mass along the lengths of the radius and ulna and the implications for in vivo bone measurements. Calcif. Tissue Res., *20*:41–52, 1976.

52. Hahn, I.J., Boisseau, V.C., and Aloia, L.V.: Effect of chronic corticosteroid administration on diaphyseal and metaphyseal bone mass. J. Clin. Endocrinol. Metab., *39*:274, 1974.

53. Smith, D.M., Johnston, C. Jr., and Yu, P.-L.: In vivo measurement of bone mass. JAMA, *219*:325–329, 1972.

54. Wilson, C.R.: Prediction of femoral neck and spine bone mineral content from the BMC of the radius or ulna and the relationship between bone strength and BMC. *In* Proceedings of the International Conference on Bone Mineral Measurement. Edited by R.B. Mazess. Washington, DC, National Institute of Arthritis, Metabolism, and Digestive Diseases, 1974, p. 51–59.

55. Genant, H.K., et al.: Comparison of methods for in vivo spinal bone mineral measurement. *In* Osteoporosis. Edited by C. Christiansen. Aalborg Stiftsborgtrykkeri, Denmark, 1984, p. 97.

56. Nilas, L., et al.: Comparison of single and dual photon absorptiometry in postmenopausal bone mineral loss. J. Nucl. Med., *26*:1257–1262, 1985.

57. Cohn, S.H., et al.: Absolute and relative deficit in total-skeletal calcium and radial bone mineral in osteoporosis. J. Nucl. Med., *15*:428–435, 1974.

58. Shapiro, J.R., et al.: Osteoporosis: Evaluation of diagnosis and therapy. Arch. Intern. Med., *135*:563, 1975.

59. Wahner, H., Riggs, B.L., and Beaubout, J.W.: Diagnosis of osteoporosis: Usefulness of photon absorptiometry at the radius. J. Nucl. Med., *18*:432–437, 1977.

60. Lindsay, R., et al.: Prevention of spinal osteoporosis in oophorectomized women. Lancet, *2*:1151–1154, 1980.

61. Lindsay, R., et al.: Long-term prevention of post-menopausal osteoporosis by oestrogen. Lancet, *1*:1038–1041, 1976.

62. Madsen, M., Peppler, W., and Mazess, R.B.: Vertebral and total body bone mineral content by dual photon absorptiometry. Invest. Radiol., *12*:185–188, 1977.

63. Posner, I., and Griffiths, H.J.: Comparison of CT scanning with photon absorptiometric measurement of bone mineral content in the appendicular skeleton. Invest. Radiol., *12*:524–544, 1977.

64. Awbrey, B.J., et al.: Bone density in women: A modified procedure for measurement of distal radial density. J. Orthop. Res., *2*:314–321, 1984.

65. Ruegsegger, P., et al.: Bone loss in premenopausal and postmenopausal women. J. Bone Joint Surg., *66A*:1015, 1984.

66. Vogel, J.M., Anderson, J.T.: Rectilinear transmission scanning of irregular bones for quantification of mineral content. J. Nucl. Med., *13*:13–18, 1972.

67. Vogel, J.M.: Bone mineral measurement: Skylab experiment M-078. Acta Astronautica, *2*:129–139, 1975.

68. Wahner, H.W., Eastell, R., Riggs, B.L.: Bone mineral density of the radius: Where do we stand? J. Nucl. Med., *26*:1339, 1985.

69. Yano, K., Wasnich, R.D., Vogel, J.M., Heilbrun, L.K.: Bone mineral measurement among middle-aged and elderly Japanese residents in Hawaii. Am. J. Epidemiol., *119*:751–764, 1984.

70. Grubb, S.A., et al.: Comparison of single and dual photon absorptiometry in postmenopausal bone mineral loss. J. Nucl. Med., *26*:1257, 1984.

71. Vogel, J.M., et al.: Microcomputer based dual energy photon absorptiometric bone mineral analyzer (VCH). IEEE Trans. Nucl. Sci., *26*:576–582, 1979.

72. Wasnich, R.D., Ross, P.D., Heilbrun, L.K., Vogel, J.: Prediction of postmenopausal fracture risk with bone mineral measurements. Am. J. Obstet. Gynecol., *153*:745, 1985.

73. Dunn, W., Wahner, H.W., and Riggs, B.L.: Measurement of bone mineral content in human vertebrae and hip by dual photon absorptiometry. Radiology, *136*:485–487, 1980.

74. Wahner, H., et al.: Dual-photon Gd-153 absorptiometry of bone. Radiology, *156*:203–206, 1985.

75. Riggs, B.L., et al.: Differential changes in bone mineral density

of the appendicular and axial skeleton with aging. J. Clin. Invest., *67*:328–335, 1981.

76. Cann, C.E., Rutt, B.K., and Genant, H.K.: Effect of extra-osseous calcification on vertebral mineral measurement (Abstract). *In* Proceedings of the Fifth Annual Meeting of the American Society of Bone Mineral Research. Calcif. Tissue Int., *35*:647, 1983.

77. Genant, HK., Gordan, G.S., and Hoffman, P.G., Jr.: Osteoporosis: Part I. Advanced radiologic assessment using quantitative computed tomography. West. J. Med., *139*:75–84, 1983.

78. Marhard, L., et al.: Abstract presented at the Symposium on Clinical Disorders of Bone and Mineral Metabolism. Detroit, MI, 1983.

79. Mazess, R.B.: The noninvasive measurement of skeletal mass. *In* Bone and Mineral Research—Annual 1. Edited by W.A. Peck. Amsterdam, Excerpta Medica, 1983, p. 223–279.

80. Chamberlain, M.R., Fremlin, J.H., Holloway, I., and Peters, D.K.: Use of the cyclotron for whole body neutron activation analysis: Theoretical and practical considerations. Int. J. Appl. Radiat. Isot., *21*:725, 1970.

81. Cohn, S.H., Dombrowski, C.S., and Fairchild, R.G.: In vivo neutron activation analysis of calcium in man. Int. J. Appl. Radiat. Isot., *21*:127, 1970.

82. Cohn, S.H., Shukla, K.K., Dombrowski, C.S., and Fairchild, R.G.: Design and calibration of a "broad-beam" ^{238}Pu, Be neutron source for total-body neutron activation analysis. J. Nucl. Med., *13*:487–492, 1972.

83. Palmer, H.E., Nelp, W.B., Murano, R., and Rich, C.: The feasibility of in vivo neutron activation analysis of total body calcium and other elements of body composition. Phys. Med. Biol., *13*:269–279, 1968.

84. Williams, E.D., Boddy, K., Harvey, I., and Haywood, J.K.: Calibration and evaluation of a system for total body in vivo activation analysis using 14 MeV neutrons. Phys. Med. Biol., *23*:405–415, 1978.

85. Aloia, J.R., et al.: Radiographic morphometry and osteopenia and spinal osteoporosis. J. Nucl. Med., *18*:425–431, 1977.

86. Manzke, E., et al.: Relationship between local and total bone mass in osteoporosis. Metabolism, *24*:605–615, 1975.

87. Wilson, C.R., and Madsen, N.: Dichromatic absorptiometry of vertebral bone mineral content. Invest. Radiol., *12*:180–184, 1977.

88. Sorenson, J.A., and Mazess, R.B.: Effects of fat on bone mineral measurements. *In* Proceedings of the Bone Measurement Conference. Edited by J.R. Cameron. USAEC Conf. 700515, Springfield, VA, Clearinghouse for Federal Scientific and Technical Information, 1970, pp. 255–262.

89. Ettinger, B., Genant, H.K., Cann, C.E.: Menopausal bone loss can be prevented by low dose estrogen with calcium supplements. J. Comput. Assist. Tomogr., *9*:633, 1985.

90. Ettinger, B., Genant, H.K., Cann, C.E.: Long-term estrogen replacement therapy prevents bone loss and fracture. Ann. Intern. Med., *102*:319–324, 1985.

91. Gallagher, C., Golgar, D., Mahoney, P., and McGill, J.: Measurement of spine density in normal and osteoporotic subjects using computed tomography: Relationship of spine density to fracture threshold and fracture index. J. Comput. Assist. Tomogr., *9*:634–635, 1985.

92. Mack, L.A., et al.: Correlation between fracture index and bone densitometry by CT and dual photon absorptiometry. J. Comput. Assist. Tomogr., *9*:635–636, 1985.

93. Powell, M.R., et al.: Comparison of dual photon absorptiometry and quantitative computed tomography of the lumbar spine in the same subjects. *In* Clinical Disorders of Bone and Mineral Metabolism. Edited by B. Frame and J.T. Potts. Amsterdam, Excerpta Medica, 1983, pp. 58–61.

94. Raymakers, J.A., et al.: Osteoporotic fracture prevalence and bone mineral mass measured with CT and DPA. Skeletal Radiol., *15*:191–197, 1986.

95. Reinbold, W.D., et al.: Measurement of bone mineral content in early postmenopausal and postmenopausal osteoporotic women. A comparison of methods. Radiology, *160*:469–478, 1986.

96. Sambrook, P.N., et al.: Measurement of lumbar spine bone mineral: A comparison of dual photon absorptiometry and computed tomography. Br. J. Radiol., *58*:621–624, 1985.

COMPUTED TOMOGRAPHY OF THE LUMBAR SPINE, CERVICAL SPINE, AND SACROILIAC JOINT

8

GUILLERMO F. CARRERA

Low-back pain is a common complaint. The lumbar spine and sacroiliac joint are affected by many conditions that can result in localized or radiating back pain, sometimes accompanied by evidence of neural dysfunction. Radiographic evaluation of the lumbar spine and sacroiliac joints is complicated by numerous factors. In the peripheral skeleton, relatively thin osteoarticular structures surrounded by uniform soft tissues are the rule. Conventional high-resolution radiography can provide exquisite demonstration of peripheral skeletal structure and abnormality. The lumbar spine and sacroiliac joints, in contrast, are anatomically complex structures. The presence of overlying abdominal visceral contents, the thickness of the trunk, and the importance of demonstrating neural structures render conventional radiographic techniques disappointingly insensitive in the evaluation of early or subtle abnormalities.

High-resolution computed tomography (CT) has become accepted as the best technique for evaluating the anatomy of the spine and spinal canal in the lumbar area, as well as for demonstrating the complex anatomy of the sacroiliac joints. Subtle abnormalities of the intervertebral discs, lumbar facet joints, and neural arches can now be properly evaluated using CT, and myelography can be avoided in most cases of mechanical backache. Radiographic findings diagnostic of sacroiliitis can in many cases be shown better using high-resolution CT than with conventional radiography. CT, therefore, offers a rapid, accurate, noninvasive technique for detecting pathologic anatomy in a wide spectrum of patients being

evaluated for low-back, pelvic, and radiating leg or hip pain.

CT has been applied also to the diagnosis of cervical disc disease and foraminal stenosis, but with somewhat less success and enthusiasm than for lumbar disease. Specific problems have limited application of CT in the cervical spine, particularly when extremely fine resolution is necessary, as in the evaluation of degenerative disc disease. Artifact from dental fillings can limit the plane of section available in the upper and midcervical areas. Artifact from the thickness of the shoulder girdle is a substantial limiting factor in evaluating the lower cervical spine. Despite these limitations, CT has found a place in evaluating cervical disc and foraminal disease and is embraced enthusiastically by some practitioners.[1,2]

CT OF THE LUMBAR SPINE

Radiographic evaluation of patients with low-back and sciatic pain requires demonstration of the vertebral bodies and neural arches, and also good delineation of the soft-tissue structures in the spinal canal. The diagnosis and discrimination of such conditions as herniated nucleus pulposus, spinal canal and neural foraminal stenosis, spondylolysis, and lumbar facet arthritis constitute the most important reasons for radiographic evaluation of patients with chronic backache. Systemic disorders such as metastatic disease to the vertebral column and noninfectious spondylitis are generally diagnosed prior to detailed radiographic evaluation of the vertebral segments for low-back or radiating leg pain. CT, using techniques that allow a high degree of spatial resolution and contrast resolution adequate for discriminating soft tissues in the spinal canal, can effectively diagnose most anatomically demonstrable lesions causing low-back pain and can obviate the need for complex and invasive tests such as contrast myelography, gas myelography, epidural venography, and discography.[3–10]

CT TECHNIQUES

A variety of instruments for performing high-resolution CT have become available in the past several years. The techniques for obtaining adequate CT images of the lumbar spinal canal and intervertebral discs vary from instrument to instrument. The CT study of the lumbar spine as performed at the Milwaukee Regional Medical Center furnishes an example of satisfactory technique.[5]

A General Electric CT/T 9800 scanner with a tilting gantry and large patient aperture is used to examine the lumbar spine. The patients are supine to minimize motion. Factors including 20-cm field of view, 3-second scan time, 5-mm contiguous slices, 600 mAS, and 120 kvp allow CT imaging with contrast resolution less than 0.5%, spatial resolution of 0.75 mm, and 4-rad radiation dose to the skin per examination. A preliminary lateral localizer image (computed radiograph) is obtained prior to transaxial examination to select the gantry level and angle for producing opti-

FIG. 8–1. Lateral computed radiograph shows the gantry angle and level chosen to produce an image in the midplane of the L4-L5 intervertebral disc and lumbar facet joints (dotted line). (From Carrera, G.F., et al.[3])

mal images in (or near) the plane of the intervertebral disc and perpendicular to the plane of the lumbar facet joints (Fig. 8–1).

NORMAL ANATOMY

CT images should be obtained at both "bone" and "soft tissue" image settings for full evaluation of the spine and spinal canal. Contiguous images covering the entire neural foramen from pedicle to pedicle allow complete assessment of the neural arch at each segment. The intervertebral discs, lumbar facet joints, bony structures of the neural arch, thecal sac, and nerve root sheaths can be clearly demonstrated. Epidural fat surrounds many important structures in the lumbar spine canal and allows easy discrimination of the thecal anatomy (Figs. 8–2, 8–3, and 8–4).

HERNIATED INTERVERTEBRAL DISC

Because of the differential density of intervertebral disc material and epidural fat, the abnormal contour of a herniated intervertebral disc can be clearly demonstrated using CT. Asymmetric protrusion of the intervertebral disc, either centrally or posterolaterally, can be readily appreciated, as can the effects of the intervertebral disc on adjacent nerve-root sheaths (Figs. 8–5 and 8–6). Unusual lesions such as lateral disc herniations and extruded fragments can be

FIG. 8–2. CT image through a normal L4-L5 intervertebral disc shows a smooth, slightly convex posterior interface with the spinal canal. The disc margin is congruent with a small area of density representing vertebral endplate (arrowhead). The spinal canal, thecal sac, nerve roots, and ligamenta flava are easily identified.

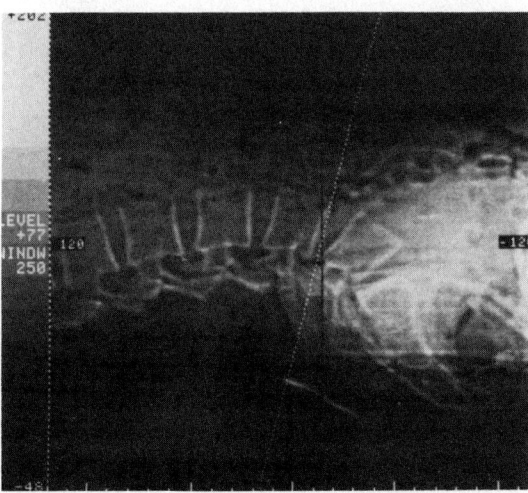

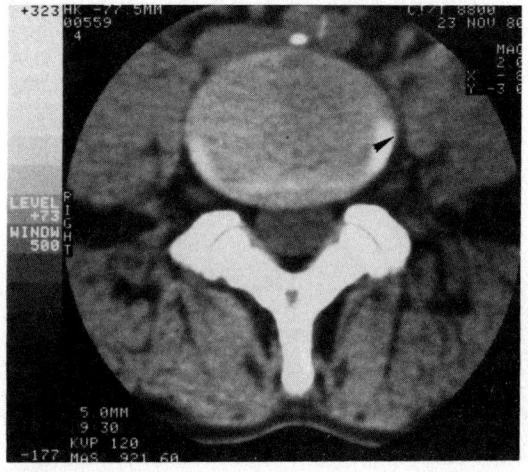

FIG. 8–3. CT scan at the L5-S1 level shows normal lumbar facet joints. The articular surfaces are straight and parallel, and normal osseous structure, including a corticomedullary discrimination (arrows), is apparent.

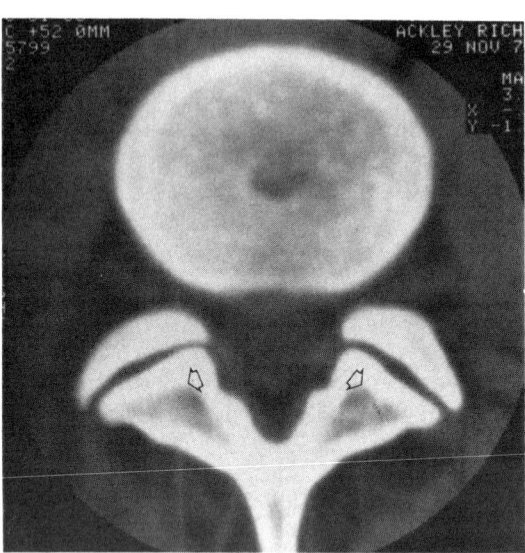

clearly identified, often better than with myelography.[10,11]

BULGING ANULUS

The myelographic discrimination between a diffusely bulging anulus fibrosus and a focal disc protrusion can be complex. CT can clearly demonstrate the symmetric bulge of a degenerated anulus fibrosus and allows discrimination from focal protrusion or herniation of intervertebral disc material[6,7,11] (Fig. 8–7).

LUMBAR FACET ARTHROPATHY

Subtle anatomic abnormalities of the lumbar facet joints can be easily demonstrated. Adequate CT images readily show such findings as joint space narrowing, osteophytes, reactive sclerosis, and erosions.

FIG. 8–5. CT image through the L5-S1 interspace shows as asymmetric posterior protrusion of intervertebral disc (open arrows). The left S1 root sheath (solid arrow) is easily identified. The right S1 root sheath has been displaced and obscured by the herniated intervertebral sac. (From Eldevik, O.P., et al.: Radiology, *145*:85, 1982.)

FIG. 8–4. CT scan through the L4-L5 interspace demonstrates use of a computer program to measure the right L4-L5 lumbar facet joint. In a series of normal volunteers, joint widths of 2.0 to 3.5 mm were measured. Joint narrowing should be diagnosed when a width less than 2 mm is encountered. (From Carrera, G.F., et al.[3])

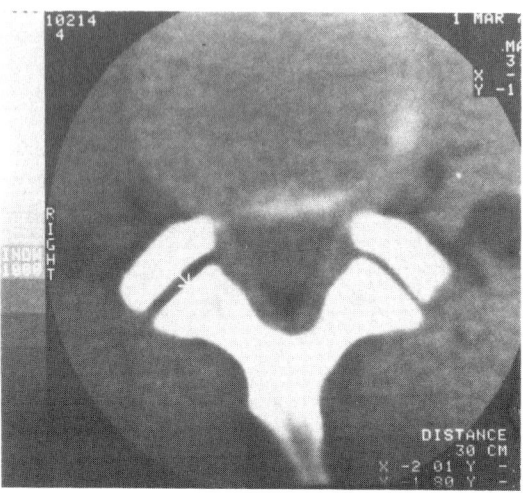

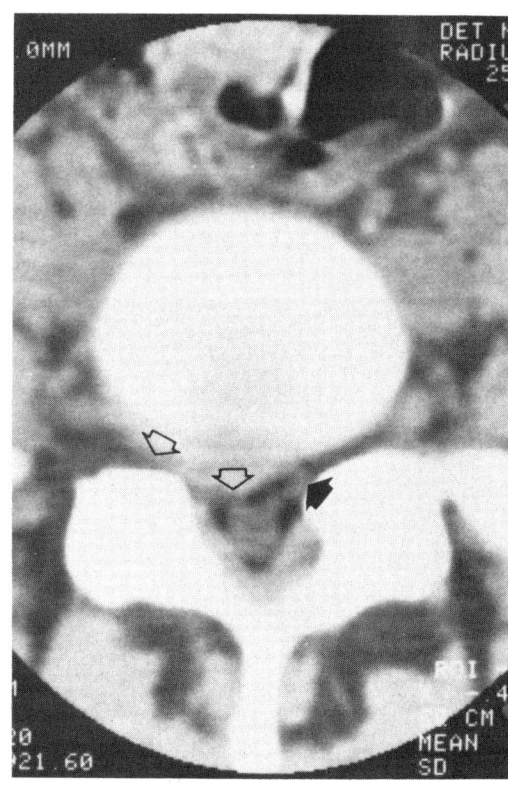

FIG. 8–6. CT image at the L5-S1 level shows a large central herniation of a relatively high-density intervertebral disc. The dural sac is posteriorly compressed and deformed by this central herniated nucleus pulposus.

FIG. 8–8. Extensive degenerative disease of the right L4-L5 facet joint. There is asymmetric narrowing of the joint, subchondral sclerosis involving both superior and inferior articular facets, posterior osteophyte formation, and a small amount of gas within the facet joint (vacuum phenomenon). (From Carrera, G.F., et al.[3])

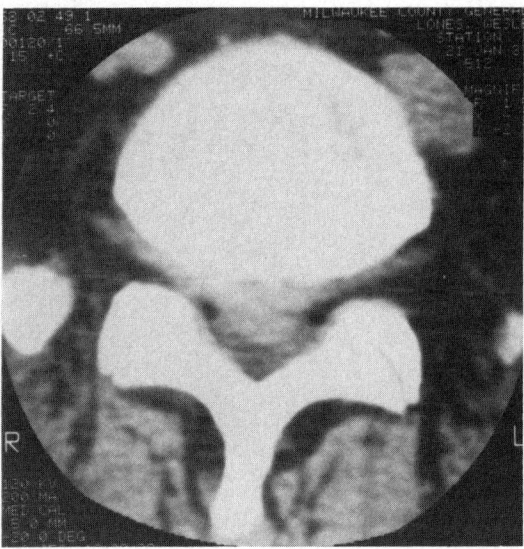

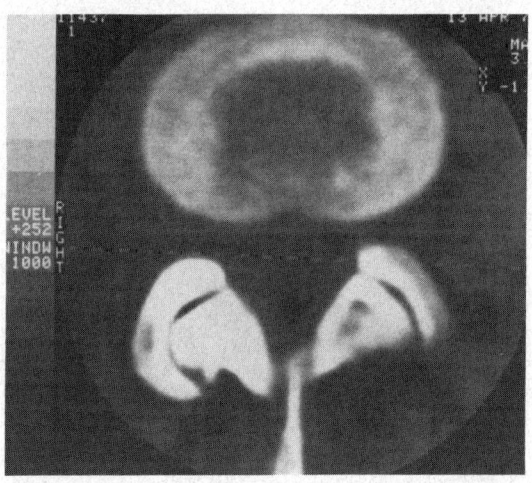

Unusual findings, such as facet capsular calcifications, can be seen[3,12] (Figs. 8–8, 8–9, 8–10).

SPINAL STENOSIS (See Chapter 93)

Spinal stenosis, either central canal stenosis or neural foraminal stenosis, remains largely a clinical diagnosis. The role of CT in establishing the anatomic

FIG. 8–7. CT image demonstrates symmetric circumferential bulge of the anulus, projecting beyond the vertebral endplate.

level of potential stenosis is still not clearly defined, but CT images demonstrating severe constriction of the spinal canal or narrowing of the lateral recess of the neural foramen can be valuable in surgical planning for patients with the clinical diagnosis of spinal stenosis.[3,8,11,13] Myelography is still needed to localize all lesions prior to surgery (see Chapter 93).

FIG. 8–9. Extensive facet arthritis in a patient who has had a laminectomy. Prominent subchondral erosions (arrows) as well as subchondral sclerosis are present. A small drop of residual myelographic contrast material is seen adjacent to the left facet joint. (From Carrera, G.F.., et al.[3])

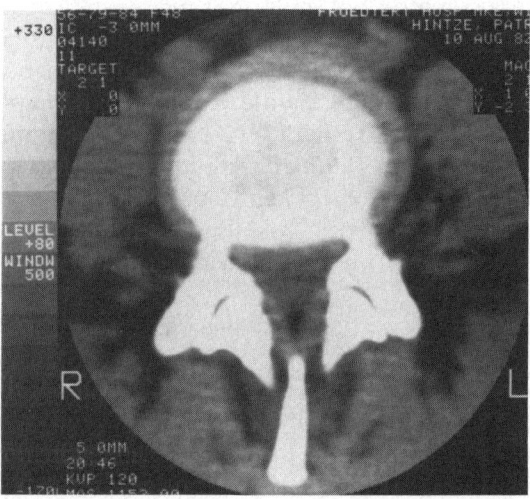

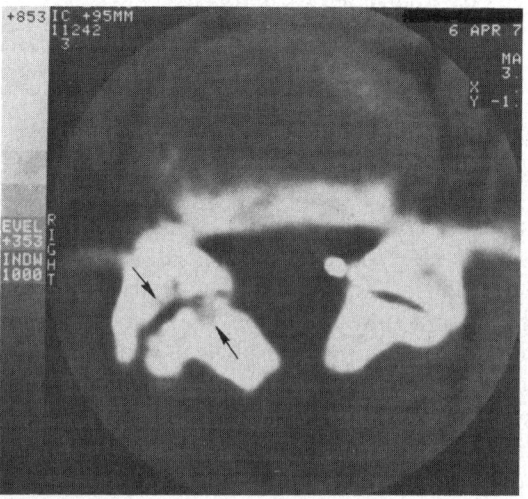

FIG. 8–10. Bilaminar calcification of the anterior capsular structures of the left L5-S1 lumbar facet joint. The innermost calcification (arrow) is in the ligamentum flavum. The calcification adjacent to the joint itself is in the anterior joint capsule. (From Carrera, G.F., et al.[3])

FIG. 8–11. CT image through the neural arch of L5 reveals irregular and sclerotic defects through the pars interarticularis (arrows). A dysmorphic pars and lamina are seen on the right. A deformed and elongated spinal canal is also apparent. These findings are characteristic of bilateral spondylolysis.

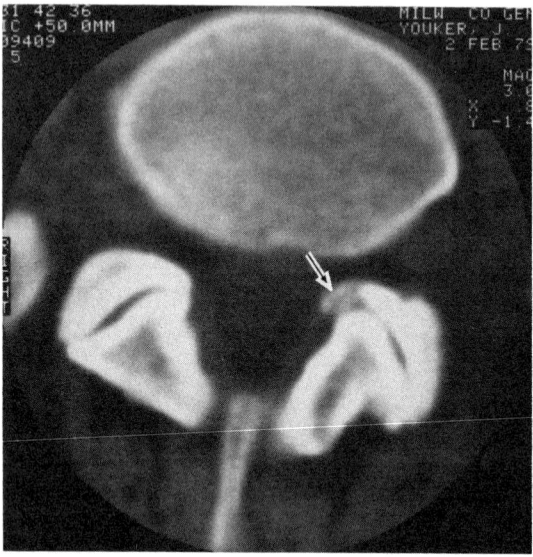

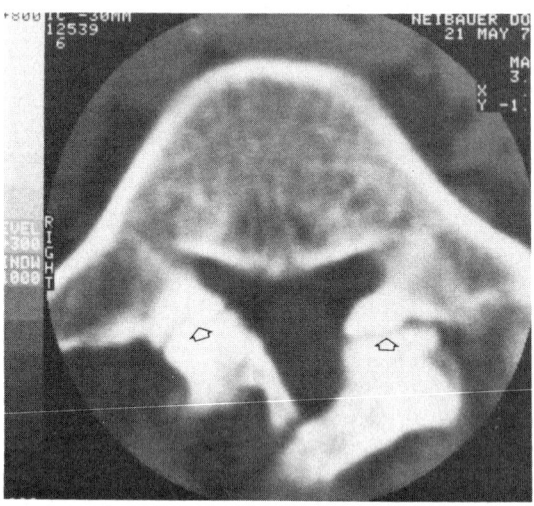

SPONDYLOLYSIS

Defects in the pars interarticularis can be difficult to diagnose using conventional films. If contiguous CT images are obtained from pedicle to pedicle in each vertebral segment under study, the entire neural arch is demonstrated, and defects in the pars interarticularis, degenerative changes, or evidence of maldevelopment of the pars interarticularis can be clearly seen[14] (Fig. 8–11).

IMPLICATIONS OF CT EXAMINATION OF THE LUMBAR SPINE

Conventional radiographic evaluation of the lumbar spine in patients with chronic low-back and/or sciatic pain as a major or exclusive complaint is relatively insensitive for the diagnosis of herniated disc, spinal stenosis, and lumbar facet arthropathy, and these are the anatomically demonstrable, treatable causes of mechanical low-back pain. Conventional radiographic examination of the lumbar spine is most useful in screening for a variety of focal or multifocal disorders such as metastases to the spine, infectious lesions, osteoporosis with compression fracture, trauma, and Paget's disease. High-resolution CT has been found to be more reliable than myelography in the diagnosis of intervertebral disc herniation, which

is the major surgically approachable lesion in patients with chronic low-back pain and sciatica.[11] CT diagnosis of lumbar facet arthropathy in patients with localized radiating back pain has proved to be an effective guide to diagnostic and therapeutic lumbar facet joint injection.[12,15]

COMPUTED TOMOGRAPHY OF SACROILIAC (SI) JOINTS

Sacroiliitis is an important feature of the seronegative spondyloarthropathies, such as psoriatic arthritis. Reiter's syndrome, ankylosing spondylitis, and enteropathic spondyloarthritis. Infectious sacroiliitis is a less common but important diagnostic consideration in patients with inflammatory low-back pain. Their complex anatomy and location in the pelvis, surrounded by a thick mantle of abdominal and pelvic contents, make radiographic evaluation of the SI joints using conventional techniques such as plain radiography difficult. Evidence of sacroiliitis, such as joint space narrowing, osteoporosis, subchondral sclerosis, erosion, and ankylosis, can be difficult to define.[16]

CT produces sectional images of the SI joints with high-spatial resolution, free of the confusing shadows caused by overlying soft-tissue structures. The natural irregularities of these joints are easily resolved by the tomographic nature of CT images. CT has been shown to be an effective and accurate method for SI joint evaluation.[16-18] Combined with careful clinical evaluation, screening conventional radiography, and (on occasion) radioisotope studies, CT contributes greatly to the diagnosis of sacroiliac disorders.[19]

CT TECHNIQUE

As in the evaluation of the lumbar spine, regardless of the CT instrument and protocol chosen, certain essential features must be addressed to produce adequate images. Essential elements of a successful CT examination include adequate spatial resolution and slice orientation in the axis of the sacrum to allow discrimination and evaluation of both ligamentous and diarthrodial compartments of the joint.

We use the General Electric CT/T 9800 scanner. A lateral localizer image is obtained first to select the best gantry level and angle for the CT cuts (Figs. 8–12, 8–13). Five-mm-thick contiguous sections through the sacroiliac joints are then performed using either a small field of view or target reconstruction algorithm. The scans are displayed with a window width of 1000 Hounsfield units (HU) and an image level of +250 to +350 Hounsfield units. This protocol allows discrimination of both compartments of the SI joint and produces high-resolution, high-contrast images clearly showing the normal subchondral cortex, medullary space, and all other anatomic landmarks.[20]

NORMAL ANATOMY

The SI joint consists of two anatomic compartments. The entire dorsal surface as well as superior aspect of the joint (approximately 25 to 30% of the total craniocaudal length) is ligamentous (syndesmosis). The strong sacroiliac ligaments are surrounded by fat and traversing muscles and insert into a series of ligamentous "pits" on the sacrum. This compartment is sharply oblique when compared to the diarthrodial (synovial) compartment. The oval-shaped diarthrodial compartment occupies the anterior and inferior portions of the sacroiliac joint and is oriented in, or near, the sagittal anatomic plane[2,19,20] (Figs. 8–14 and 8–15).

FIG. 8–12. Lateral computed radiography of the gantry level and angle required to produce contiguous images through the sacroiliac joint in the plane of the sacrum (dotted line).

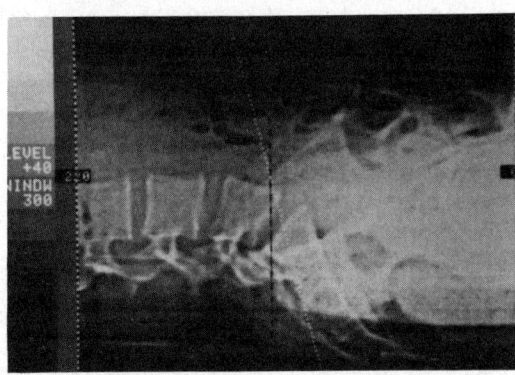

FIG. 8–13. Lateral computed radiograph displays the CT scan sequence used to image the sacroiliac joints. (From Carrera, G.F., et al.[17])

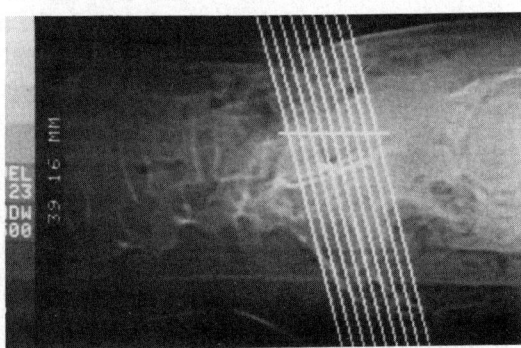

FIG. 8–14. Diagrammatic representation of a disarticulated sacroiliac joint viewed from the lateral aspect. Plane B represents the steeply oblique ligamentous portion of the joint, which lies dorsal and cephalad to the oval more sagittally oriented diarthrodial compartment of the joint (plane A). (From Carrera, G.F., et al.[17])

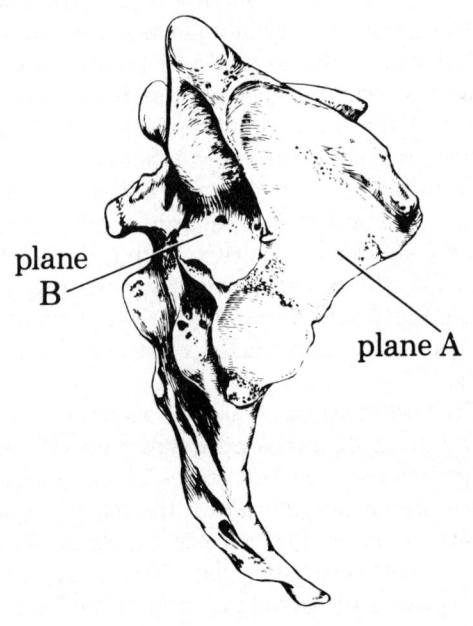

plane B

plane A

FIG. 8–15. CT scan through the diarthrodial compartment of the normal sacroiliac joints shows smooth, parallel articular surfaces. A sharp subchondral demarcation is seen on the sacral side of the joint. A somewhat broader zone of increased density is seen on the iliac side of both joints. This is a normal finding and should not be confused with subchondral reactive sclerosis. (From Carrera, G.F., et al.[17])

FIG. 8–16. CT scan through the diarthrodial compartment of the sacroiliac joints in a patient with ankylosing spondylitis shows advanced bilateral sacroiliitis. There is severe joint narrowing and irregularity. Small erosions (open arrows) are seen in both joints. Reactive sclerosis, present as a band of increased density separated from the subchondral plate by a lucent zone, is particularly apparent in the right joint (arrowheads). (From Carrera, G.F., et al.[17])

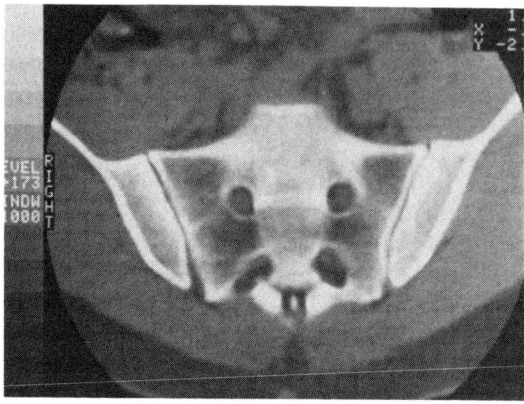

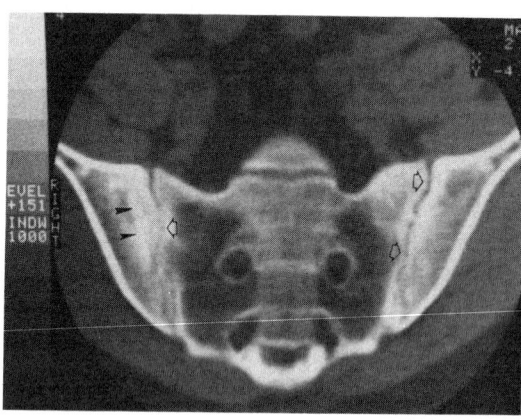

SACROILIITIS

The findings of sacroiliitis are similar to those found on conventional films. Early synovitis and hyperemia cause osteoporosis in a juxta-articular distribution. CT shows well-defined areas of decreased absorption (decreased density of mineral) near the articular cortex, frequently separated from the subchondral bone by a band of adjacent sclerosis. As an isolated finding, this zone of decreased absorption can be difficult to interpret even on CT images. Continued inflammatory disease leads to narrowing of the articular cartilage. In a series of normal volunteers, we found the normal SI joint width to be 2.5 to 4.0 mm. We therefore diagnose narrowing when the diarthrodial compartment of the joint measures less than 2 mm by computer program. Continued inflammatory disease causes erosions of the subchondral bone, evidenced on CT by indistinct cortical margins and/or interruptions of the subchondral cortex. With progressive erosive disease, these cortical interruptions progress to frank osteodestructive lesions and deep, irregular erosions, frequently surrounded by a zone of reactive sclerosis.

Reactive sclerosis in an area of sacroiliitis is manifested by areas of increased density on CT images. Although sclerosis on both sides of the joint is frequently stated as a criterion for the reactive sclerosis of sacroiliitis, *the predominant sclerosis almost always occurs on the iliac side of the joint.* This is true even in advanced cases of sacroiliitis, and should not deter

one from diagnosing reactive sclerosis caused by sacroiliitis.

Ankylosis appears on CT scans, as on plain films, as mature bone bridging the sacroiliac space[17,19] (Figs. 8–16, 8–17, 8–18).

IMPLICATIONS OF CT IN SACROILIITIS

The SI joint can participate in many inflammatory and mechanical conditions, resulting in findings suggesting sacroiliitis, Indistinct articular margins, osteoporosis, and cortical erosion are nonspecific changes that do not discriminate infectious, spondyloarthritic, or mechanical etiologies. Careful correlation of the radiographic findings (including CT) with the clinical findings is necessary to properly diagnose suspected sacroiliitis.

Bilateral sacroiliitis, particularly if spondylitis or peripheral arthritis is present, is essentially diagnostic of one of the seronegative spondyloarthritic syndromes. Although symmetric bilateral sacroiliitis is most characteristic of ankylosing spondylitis, and asymmetric bilateral sacroiliitis is most common in psoriatic arthritis or Reiter's syndrome, the findings in the SI joints alone frequently do not serve to discriminate these conditions. Although bilateral asymmetric sacroiliitis is somewhat more common in the latter two conditions than in ankylosing spondylitis, extensive bilateral changes are frequently found.

Pure unilateral sacroiliitis, although occasionally

FIG. 8–17. CT scan through the diarthrodial compartment of the sacroiliac joints shows asymmetric erosive sacroiliitis. There is mild irregularity and narrowing of the left sacroiliac joint, with erosions and subchondral sclerosis. Severe subchondral sclerosis is present in the right sacroiliac joint. Large erosions (arrows) are seen in the more involved right sacroiliac joint. (From Carrera, G.F., et al.[17])

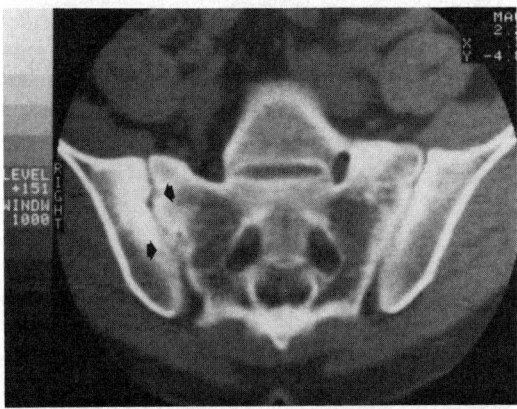

FIG. 8–18. CT scan in a patient with ankylosing spondylitis shows bilateral joint narrowing, sclerosis, and erosions. Focal ankylosis, seen as solid bars of bone traversing the joint, is present in both joints. (From Carrera, G.F., et al.[17])

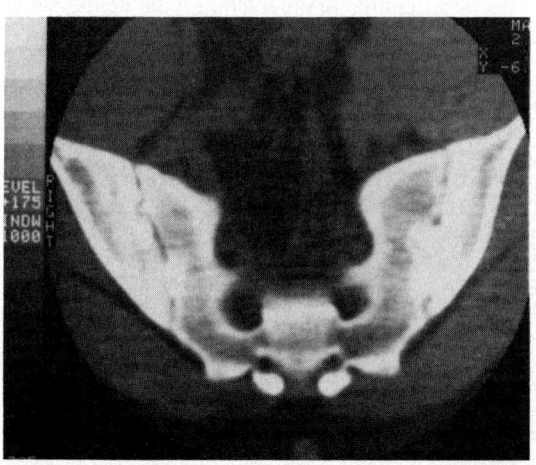

seen in seronegative spondyloarthritis, is more suggestive of joint infection. In the absence of strong clinical evidence for one of the seronegative spondyloarthritic syndromes, unilateral sacroiliitis suggests a presumptive diagnosis of infectious arthritis and should prompt vigorous attempts to isolate an organism.

Other etiologies for destructive SI joint disease, such as mechanical or neoplastic disorders, are generally accompanied by a history and clinical findings suggesting the primary condition. Osseous destruc-

tion on one side of the SI joint suggests metastasis, particularly if no systemic evidence of inflammatory disease is present[19] (Fig. 8–19).

CT, therefore, can play a significant role in the diagnosis and evaluation of patients with suspected sacroiliitis. When plain films are negative or equivocal, and clinical suspicion of sacroiliitis is high, CT is indicated. It is the most sensitive and accurate anatomic method now available for evaluation of the SI joints.

CT OF THE CERVICAL SPINE

The basic principles of CT examination of the cervical spine are similar to those used in studying the lumbar spine. Fractures of the cervical spine, a subject beyond the scope of this chapter, are easily studied using both axial- and sagittal-reformation CT. Because the resolution requirements are less for evaluating fractures than for evaluating spinal canal encroachment by herniated disc or osteophyte, rapid scanning, using contiguous 0.5-mm sections with relatively low radiation loads, is possible. The thinness of the intervertebral disc in the cervical area, the small size of the neural foramen, and the *absence of an epidural fat sleeve around the thecal sac* mandate extremely meticulous technique when CT examination for disc or foraminal disease is performed. Contrast enhancement of the thecal sac is often necessary to allow confident diagnosis of herniated cervical disc.[14] CT is still an adjunct to cervical myelography. It is likely that magnetic resonance imaging (MRI) will become the dominant technique in evaluating the cervical spine, particularly because direct sagittal and coronal plane

FIG. 8–19. CT scan in a patient with prostatic carcinoma shows a normal left sacroiliac joint. The right joint is irregular, but most of the irregularity is on the iliac side of the joint. A dense, sclerotic metastatic lesion is seen occupying the ilium adjacent to the right sacroiliac joint. (From Carrera, G.F.[19])

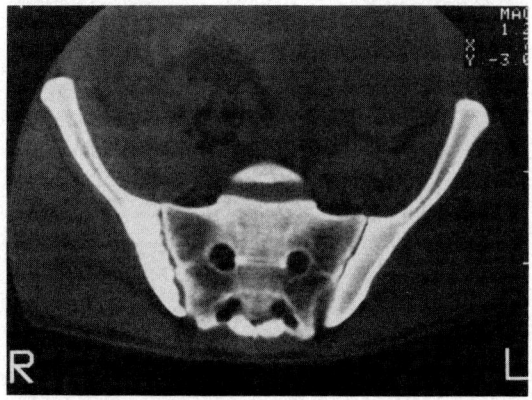

images at high resolution are easily available using this modality (see Chapter 6).

CT TECHNIQUES

As in the lumbar spine, many instruments using a variety of imaging protocols are available for studying the cervical spine. Our protocol serves as an example of an adequate technique for examining this complex region. A General Electric CT/T 9800 scanner with tilting gantry is used. The patient is examined supine with the position of the jaw determined following lateral preliminary computed radiography. Examining the localizer image prior to axial scanning allows both selection of optimal images in (or near) the plane of the intervertebral disc and proper patient positioning to avoid (as much as possible) the confusing effects of dental fillings in the plane of section. Technical factors include a 13-cm field of view (medium body calibration) which can be changed to a 10-cm field of view after preliminary localization. The smaller field of view improves resolution significantly. The technique employed requires 200 mAS, 3-second scan time, and 120 kvp. Seven contiguous 1.5-mm scans are obtained, with the center slice through the intervertebral disc. Higher scans might be needed for evaluating adjacent bony disease.

FIG. 8–20. CT scan through normal apophyseal joints at C4-C5, using bone windows. The articular surfaces are parallel with no evidence of osteophyte, erosion, or subchondral sclerosis. (Courtesy David L. Daniels, M.D.)

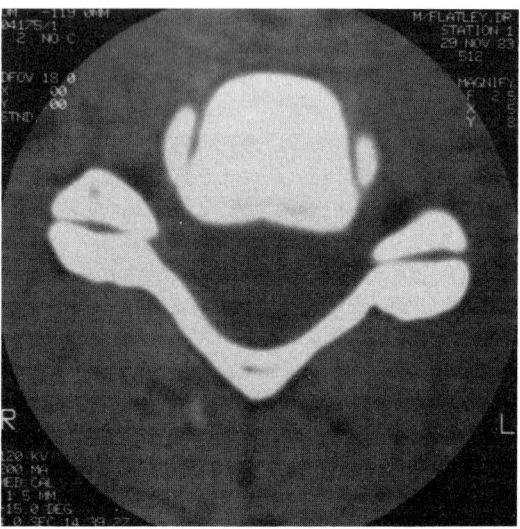

FIG. 8–21. CT scan through a normal C5-C6 intervertebral disc with thecal enhancement using metrizamide. Spinal cord is seen as a low-density structure within the contrast-enhanced thecal sac. Axillary pouches can be identified in the neural foramina (arrows). (Courtesy David L. Daniels, M.D.)

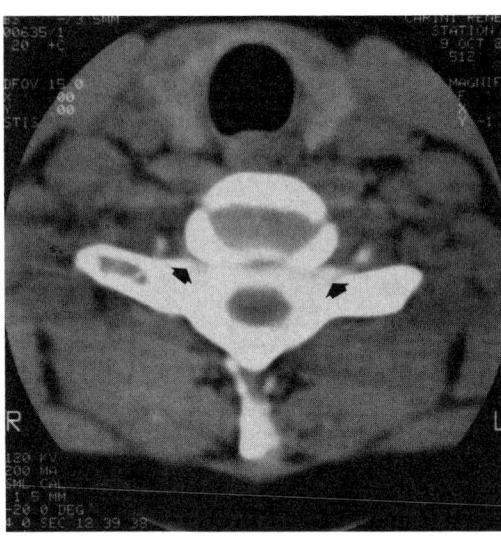

FIG. 8–22. CT scan at C5-C6 shows a posterolateral herniated intervertebral disc (arrows). The contrast-enhanced thecal sac is displaced by a soft-tissue mass representing herniated disc material encroaching on the spinal canal and vertebral foramen. (Courtesy David L. Daniels, M.D.)

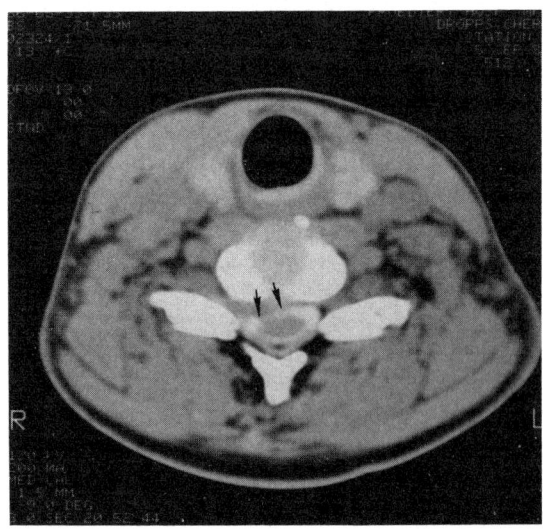

ANATOMY AND DISC PATHOLOGY

CT images should be obtained at both "bone" and "soft tissue" image windows to evaluate all of the structures in or near the cervical discs. The spinal cord can frequently be resolved within the cerebrospinal fluid-filled thecal sac, but details of cord structure are

FIG. 8–23. CT image through C4-C5 shows osteophytes from the uncinate joints narrowing the vertebral foramen (arrows). (Courtesy David L. Daniels, M.D.)

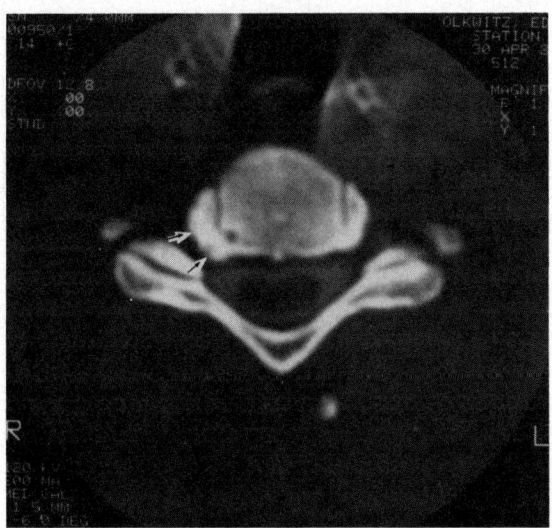

only variably resolved. The absence of epidural fat makes diagnosis of subtle herniated disc difficult.

The uncinate processes from the vertebral body below the level of the disc selected are apparent laterally. Minor asymmetry can result from positioning or developmental differences from side to side. The neural foramina similarly lie posteriorly and laterally to the uncinate (lateral interbody) joints and should be symmetric and free of encroachment[2] (Fig. 8–20).

Full evaluation for cervical disc disease often requires intrathecal contrast enhancement. We use a water-soluble contrast material such as metrizamide, or iopamidol (Fig. 8–21). Because contrast-enhanced studies imply invasion of the thecal sac, CT is often used as an adjunct to cervical myelography. Herniated intervertebral disc looks the same in the cervical spine as it does in the lumbar spine on CT images, except that distortion of the cerebrospinal fluid-filled, or contrast-enhanced thecal sac, rather than intrusion of disc material into the epidural fat spaces is seen (Fig. 8–22). Osteophytic encroachment on neural foramina (Fig. 8–23) can be seen at both bone and soft-tissue windows. Bone windows are useful to assess the exact size of the osteophyte, whereas soft-tissue windows are helpful in evaluating the neural structures traversing the foramen. Posterior transverse bars, or posterior osteophytes, are also readily apparent on CT images.

REFERENCES

1. Coin, C.G., and Coin, J.T.: Technical note. Computed tomography of cervical disk disease. Technical considerations with representative case reports. J. Comput. Assist. Tomogr., 5:275–280, 1981.
2. Simeone, F.A., and Rothman, R.H.: Cervical disc disease. In The Spine. Edited by R.H. Rothman, and F.A. Simeone. Philadelphia, WB Saunders, 1974.
3. Carrera G.F., et al.: Computed tomography of the lumbar facet joints. Radiology, 134:145, 1980.
4. Carrera, G.F., Williams, A.L., and Haughton, V.M.: Computed tomography in sciatica. Radiology, 137:433, 1980.
5. Hammerschlag, S.B., Wolpert, S.M., and Carter, B.L.: Computed tomography of the spinal canal. Radiology, 121:361, 1976.
6. Haughton, V.M., Syvertsen, A., and Williams, A.L.: Soft tissue anatomy within the spinal canal as seen on CT. Radiology, 134:649, 1980.
7. Haughton, V.M., and Williams, A.L.: CT anatomy of the spine. CRC Crit. Rev. Diagn. Imaging, 15:173–192, 1981.
8. Lee, B.C.V., Kazam, E., and Newman, A.D.: Computed tomography of the spine and spinal cord. Radiology, 128:95, 1978.
9. Sheldon, J.J., Sersland, T., and LeBorgne, J.: Computed tomography of the lower lumbar vertebral column. Radiology, 124:113, 1977.
10. Williams, A.L., Haughton, V.M., and Syvertsen, A.: Computed tomography in the diagnosis of herniated nucleus pulposus. Radiology, 135:95, 1980.
11. Haughton, V.M., et al.: A prospective comparison of computed tomography and myelography in the diagnosis of herniated lumbar disk. Radiology, 142:103, 1982.
12. Carrera, G.F.: Lumbar facet arthropathy. In Computed Tomography of the Spine. Edited by V.M. Haughton. New York, Churchill Livingstone, 1983.
13. Brown, H.A.: Enlargement of the ligamentum flavum—a cause of low-back pain with sciatic radiation. J. Bone Joint Surg., 20:325, 1938.
14. Grogan, J.P., et al.: Spondylosis studies with computed tomography. Radiology, 145:737, 1982.
15. Carrera, G.F.: Lumbar facet joint injection in low back pain and sciatica (I) and (II). Radiology, 136:661–667, 1980.
16. Ryan, L.M., et al.: The radiographic diagnosis of sacroiliitis: A comparison of different views with computed tomograms of the sacroiliac joint. Arthritis Rheum., 26(6):760–763, 1983.
17. Carrera, G.F., et al.: Computed tomography of sacroiliitis. AJR, 136:41–46, 1981.
18. Kozin, F., et al.: Computed tomography in the diagnosis of sacroiliitis. Arthritis Rheum., 24:1479–1485, 1981.
19. Carrera, G.F.: Current concepts in the evaluation of sacroiliitis. Postgr. Rad., 3:97, 1983.
20. Lawson, T.L., et al.: The sacroiliac joints; anatomic, plain roentgenographic, and computed tomographic analysis. J. Comput. Assist. Tomogr., 6:307–314, 1982.

CLINICAL EVALUATION IN RHEUMATIC DISEASES

NICHOLAS BELLAMY and W. WATSON BUCHANAN

. . . I took twelve patients in the scurvy . . . Their cases were as similar as I could have made them. They lay together in one place . . . and had one diet common to all . . . Two of these were ordered each a quart of cyder a-day. Two others took twenty-five gutts of *elixir vitriol* three times a day . . . Two others took two spoonfuls of vinegar three times a day . . . Two of the worst patients . . . were put on a course of sea-water . . . Two others had each two oranges and one lemon given them every day.

The consequence was, that the most sudden and visible good effects were perceived from the use of the oranges and lemons; one of those who had taken them, being at the end of six days fit for duty.

James Lind, 1753[1]

Since the dawn of time, doctors have tried out their pills and potions and, even more serious, their surgery on countless thousands of suffering patients. Conclusions about the efficacy of treatment were often based on a single or, at most, a few observations. This method worked well, and many of the major drugs in modern medicine were introduced in this way, including morphine, digitalis, penicillin, salicylates, gold, and cortisone, for which a clinical rheumatologist, the late Dr. Philip S. Hench, shared a Nobel Prize in Medicine. Indeed, there are relatively few examples of great modern therapeutic advances that have arisen from the sheer intellectualism of the discoverer's planning his research with a certain objective in view.[2] The experiments that led to the eradication of smallpox by Edward Jenner were unethical by today's standards and statistically uncontrolled.[3] James Lind is credited as the first to perform a prop-

erly controlled therapeutic trial,[1] although some 42 years were to elapse before the Lords of the Admiralty put his precepts into practice and made scurvy obsolete in the Royal Navy, thereby causing British seamen to be known by the sobriquet of limeys. The era of controlled clinical therapeutic trials began only after the Second World War, however, and it is gratifying that clinical rheumatologists were among the first to try out their drugs in this manner. The late Thomas N. Fraser of Glasgow, Scotland, was probably the first to report a double-blinded, controlled trial in rheumatic diseases when he compared injectable gold to placebo in patients with rheumatoid arthritis.[4] In the 1950s, several well-designed controlled trials were performed of salicylates and corticosteroids in rheumatic fever[5] and rheumatoid arthritis,[6–10] chrysotherapy in rheumatoid arthritis,[11,12] and radiotherapy in ankylosing spondylitis.[13] Concurrently, the statistical basis of clinical evaluation of therapeutic agents was established.[14–17]

With the ever-increasing number of new antirheumatic drugs being produced by the pharmaceutical industry, there is no substitute for properly designed and controlled trials to test their efficacy. Clinical impressions can be misleading; for example, two thirds of patients with rheumatoid arthritis "improved" after tonsillectomy,[18] and even "cures" were claimed.[19] The controlled clinical trial, although the most powerful design for assessing effectiveness of therapy,[20–28] needs to be critically assessed before one accepts its conclusions, and it needs to be placed in the appropriate clinical context.[29–38]

Because the quality of many clinical therapeutic trials of antirheumatic drugs leaves little ground for complacency,[39-41] an outline of the design and statistical interpretation is appropriate.

DESIGN AND INTERPRETATION OF CLINICAL TRIALS

Much has been written assessing the clinical trial literature. Although some authors have focused on specific areas of deficiency,[42,43] others have developed criteria for evaluating the quality of clinical studies that are applicable to both designers and assessors of clinical research protocols and publications.[44-51] Irrespective of the criteria used, there are nine basic components to a clinical trial, namely (1) research objective; (2) trial design; (3) patient selection; (4) randomization and stratification; (5) sample size calculation; (6) intervention, cointervention, contamination, and compliance; (7) outcome assessment; (8) statistical analysis; and (9) interpretation.

RESEARCH OBJECTIVE

Clear definition of the research objective is the major determinant of appropriate trial design selection and successful hypothesis testing. Although there is a great temptation a priori to probe multiple objectives and even greater temptation post hoc to "dredge" the data set, such hypothesis-generating activities should be clearly differentiated from those activities testing the principal hypothesis. Because different objectives generally require different and often very specific methodologic elements, *testing should be restricted to one or, at most, two major hypotheses.* At the completion of the trial design, the investigator should reflect on the adequacy of the selected methodology not only to *reject* the null hypothesis if false but also to *accept* it if true within conventional levels of statistical significance and respecting the *clinical importance* of the differences sought.

TRIAL DESIGN

One of five types are generally used in the evaluation of antirheumatic drugs: randomized parallel; randomized crossover; sequential; nonrandomized comparative groups; and one-group noncomparative open designs. While parallel designs offer operational simplicity, they potentially require larger sample sizes than comparable crossover designs and are unable to address issues of preference or within-patient response differences.[52] Crossover and factorial designs, however, are operationally more complex. Drug interactions and carry-over effects may occur, and the statistical and conceptual advantages of the design are frequently outweighed. A recent variation on this theme is the N-of-1 trial design described by Guyatt et al.,[53] which has potential application in the evaluation of individual patient responses to short-acting antirheumatic drugs. Nonrandomized comparative group designs, and one-group noncomparative open designs, lack the necessary rigor essential to assess the relative and absolute efficacy and tolerability of antirheumatic compounds.[54] In early trials, where the absolute response to a drug is unknown, it is appropriate to use a placebo control group. In later trials, when the superiority of the compound over placebo has already been demonstrated, it is more appropriate, from both scientific and ethical standpoints, to compare the response to the new compound against one or more standard therapies.

PATIENT SELECTION

"Selection" implies that certain patients will be excluded from study, and therefore trial results are only generalized to patients with characteristics similar to those actually studied. Great caution must be exercised in generalizing beyond such obvious limits, because beneficial and adverse responses can vary significantly in other subgroups. In general, selection criteria attempt to exclude patients in whom the probability of response is decreased and the probability of an adverse reaction is increased. For this reason, very young patients, elderly patients, pregnant patients, those with concurrent illness, or patients receiving other drug therapy are often excluded from early studies of new compounds.

The statistical efficiency of studying a relatively homogeneous group of compliant patients with very active and potentially responsive disease needs to be weighed against the more limited generalizability of the study result. Finally, it should be noted that patients who volunteer or consent for clinical studies may differ prognostically from those who refuse to participate.[55,56]

RANDOMIZATION AND STRATIFICATION

In a parallel trial design, the relative effectiveness of two antirheumatic compounds can be determined from the resultant response data only if the two treatment groups are known to have been prognostically similar. Group comparability can be guaranteed with respect to certain defined variables of potential prognostic importance by the process of *stratification*.[57] In contrast, the process of *randomization* gives no such guarantees, but is merely an attempt to increase the probability that undefined variables of potential prognostic importance are evenly distributed between the treatment groups.[58,59]

Although it is customary to assess group comparability and, therefore, the apparent success of the allocation process by statistical analysis, it is recognized that just as type II errors (see below) can occur in the analysis of outcome variables, so can they occur in the analysis of randomization variables. Thus, in spite of randomization and stratification, important prognostic differences can escape detection on statistical testing. The major variable in determining the response to antirheumatic drugs is the amount of pain or inflammation present at baseline.[60] This fact was first noted by Maclagan, over a century ago, in his paper on the use of salicin in acute rheumatoid fever.[61] Two alternative methods of assigning patients to treatment groups are minimization[63] and self-adjusting randomization[64] procedures, which attempt to enhance comparability by dynamically minimizing between-group differences during the allocation process.

SAMPLE SIZE CALCULATION

The number of patients required for a clinical trial is a function of several factors including trial design, the magnitude of the type I and type II errors, the size of the difference sought, and the variability in the underlying data set.[65,66] The expected differences sought are a function of the potency of the treatment, the responsiveness of the study subjects, and the sensitivity of the measuring instruments. Likewise, the variability is a function of the heterogeneity of the study population and the reliability of the outcome measures utilized.

Sample size requirements may be calculated from a number of standard formulas (Table 9–1). The type I (α) error is traditionally set at .05, i.e., when <.05, then the probability that the difference detected has risen entirely by chance is 1 in 20 or less. There is no such clearly defined level for the type II (β) error, but <.10 is usually regarded as acceptable. At this level the investigator accepts a 1 in 10 or less probability that a true difference at a specified level has been overlooked. The power of the study is expressed by

the formula $1 - \beta$. Thus, when β is set at .1, the study has a 90% probability of detecting a postulated difference if one truly exists. In designing a clinical trial, therefore, sufficient patients must be included to allow a reasonable probability that the smallest clinically important difference achieves statistical significance. Many clinical trials have relatively small sample sizes and are at risk of producing false negative results. As shown in Table 9–2, sample size requirements for detecting even a 25% risk reduction are substantial if the event rate in the control group is .05. The detection of smaller effects requires even larger sample sizes. Most clinical trials use a variety of outcome measures to capture the multidimensionality of the response.[41] The more outcomes that are assessed, the more likely that one will achieve a p value of <.05 because of chance alone. Statistical adjustment for multiple comparisons, however, further constrains the upper limit for significance and decreases the likelihood of demonstration of a true difference on any single variable. The probability of a type I error can be avoided by defining a priori one or two principal outcome measures, relegating the remainder to minor outcome measure status, and apportioning differential type I errors to them.[67] Sample size requirements, therefore, are clearly speculative, and although α and β may be conveniently fixed, the magnitude of the response may be smaller, and the variance larger, than projected.

INTERVENTION, COINTERVENTION, CONTAMINATION, AND COMPLIANCE

Intervention. Intervention is the term applied to the use of a specific treatment in a study. The agent tested may be given in a fixed dose or titrated according to a predetermined schedule or to the patient's requirements. Although clinical practice is best simulated by the titration strategy, because it commits patients to neither excessive nor inadequate therapy and thereby minimizes response failures because of either inefficacy or adverse reactions, it renders dose-based comparative analyses difficult owing to the small residual sample sizes at each dose level.[68] A fixed dose strategy allows conclusion about the efficacy and tolerability of a single specified dose, but fails to address the issue of optimal therapy in routine clinical practice.

In either strategy, drug administration may be preceded, punctuated, or followed by a "washout" period. Such periods may be anti-inflammatory drug free or totally drug free depending on the disease, the objective, and the class of anti-inflammatory drug under consideration. It may be single-blinded, dou-

Table 9–1. Standard Formulas for Calculating Sample Size

Comparison of two related means (crossover design)*
  Number of pairs = $[\sigma_d(Z\alpha + Z\beta)/\Delta]^2$

Comparison of two independent means (parallel design)
  Number per group = $2\,[\sigma(Z\alpha + Z\beta)/\Delta]^2$

Comparison of two related proportions (crossover design)†
  Number of pairs =
    $\{Z\alpha[\pi_0(1 - \pi_0)]^{1/2} + Z\beta[\pi_1(1 - \pi_1)]^{1/2}\}^2/(\pi_1 - \pi_0)$

Comparison of two independent proportions (parallel design)‡
  Number per group =
    $2\{(Z\alpha + Z\beta)/[2\,\sin^{-1}(\pi_1)^{1/2}] - [2\,\sin^{-1}(\pi_2)^{1/2}]\}^2$

---

*$Z\alpha$ = the magnitude of the type I error; this value expresses the risk the test designer is willing to take that the null hypothesis would be erroneously rejected, $Z\beta$ = the magnitude of the type II error; this value expresses the risk that the null hypothesis would be accepted erroneously, Δ = the magnitude of the change in the principle outcome measure, σ = estimate of the expected variance of the principal outcome measure.

†π_0 and π_1 (in crossover design) = refer to proportion of patients preferring some new treatment under null and alternate hypothesis, respectively. Usually $\pi_0 = 0.5$ and $\pi_1 > 0.5$.

‡π_1 and π_2 (in parallel design) = true proportions for a specified outcome in both treatment groups.

---

ble-blinded, triple-blinded, or unblinded. For practical and ethical reasons, analgesia with acetaminophen is usually allowed during washout periods. A sudden cessation of systemic corticosteroid therapy, however, is both inappropriate and hazardous, and the suspension of disease-modifying drugs impractical, the effects being inapparent for several weeks or months. Washout periods are generally restricted, therefore, to the withdrawal of nonsteroidal anti-inflammatory compounds. Because this withdrawal may be poorly tolerated by patients with active joint inflammation, a provision is usually made to advance such patients prematurely ("trap door" provision) to the active treatment phase. In spite of these problems, washout periods are advantageous in that they allow assessment of the baseline status of study patients, and they amplify any subsequent response to active drug therapy, thereby minimizing sample size requirements for detecting statistically significant improvements. Also, they facilitate assessment of patient responsiveness and absolute magnitude of the change, minimize carry-over effects from prior treatments, allow clinical baselines to be re-established in crossover studies, and, when performed at the end of a trial, serve to redefine group comparability and the persistence of patient responsiveness.

Cointervention. Cointervention refers to the administration of another potentially efficacious treatment at the same time as the intervention treatment. It can take many forms including concomitant analgesia, corticosteroids, or disease-modifying antirheumatic drugs, hospitalization, physiotherapy, and surgery. Because these often have a major biasing effect, confounding interpretation of trial results, cointervention should be minimized, monitored, and taken into account in formulating any conclusions.[69] As pain relief is the principal measurement of outcome in most antirheumatic drug trials, such caution is particularly relevant for concomitant analgesics because their use is ubiquitous whether they are officially permitted or not. Thus, unrecognized differential analgesic consumption rates can minimize between-group differences in pain control and lead incorrectly to the assumption that no difference exists. Analgesic consumption is, in fact, a surrogate measure of pain control for most patients and therefore is itself an important end point. With respect to other classes of antirheumatic compounds, patients taking corticosteroids should be on a stable dosage for at least one month prior to entry and during the study, whereas those on slow-acting disease-modifying agents should have been maintained at a constant dose level for at least the preceding 3 months.

Contamination. Contamination is rarely a problem in well-structured clinical trials of antirheumatic drugs. It occurs when an individual, instead of receiving the intended medication, receives a drug specifically designated for individuals in one of the other treatment groups. Its biasing effects are obvious, and if the effects are unrecognized, patients will be analyzed according to the drug that they were scheduled to receive, rather than that which they truly received.

Compliance. Compliance is a measure of the extent to which a patient adheres to the protocol, in general, and to drug ingestion, in particular. It can be measured in four ways: by direct observation, patient report (verbal or diary), pill counting, and plasma drug level monitoring. Each method has its limitations, so that noncompliant patients can appear compliant and vice versa. Even when the monitoring procedure is satisfactory, there is no standard definition for any level of compliance below which the therapeutic re-

Table 9–2. Sample Size Requirements

Rate of Events in the Control Group	Number of Trial Patients Required per Treatment Group to Show Clinically Significant Differences (Risk Reductions) of:*		
	10%	25%	50%
.01	116,213	17,121	3,587
.02	57,967	8,485	1,780
.03	37,994	5,606	1,178
.04	28,217	4,167	877
.05	22,350	3,304	696
.06	18,439	2,728	576
.07	15,646	2,317	490
.08	13,474	2,008	425
.09	11,921	1,768	375
.10	10,617	1,576	335
.12	8,662	1,289	274
.14	7,265	1,083	231
.16	6,217	929	199
.18	5,403	809	174
.20	4,751	713	154
.22	4,218	634	138
.24	3,773	569	124
.26	3,397	513	112
.28	3,075	466	102
.30	2,795	425	94
.35	2,237	343	76
.40	1,818	281	63
.45	1,492	233	53
.50	1,231	194	45
.55	1,018	163	39
.60	840	136	33
.65	689	114	28
.70	561	95	24
.75	449	78	21
.80	354	63	17
.85	265	50	14
.90	188	38	12
.95	119	27	9
.9999	58	12	5

*One-tailed $\alpha = .05$, $\beta = .2$

sponse is significantly compromised.[70] As enrollment is entirely voluntary, and as patients are in constant pain and under close supervision, we believe that compliance levels are reasonably high, and patient report (by diary) and pill counting are entirely adequate.[71] Indeed, the level of compliance can be a surrogate measure of efficacy and tolerance because if the drug is efficacious and produces no side effects it will usually be continued (although the converse is not always true).

OUTCOME ASSESSMENT

The timing and nature of outcome assessments should respect both the potential adverse and the potential beneficial effects of test compounds. Thus, although adverse reactions to both nonsteroidal and disease-modifying antirheumatic drugs can occur at any time after administration, the induction-response interval for nonsteroidal anti-inflammatory drugs (NSAIDs) is much shorter than that for slow-acting disease-modifying medications. Even with respect to adverse reactions to slow-acting agents, certain toxic effects (thrombocytopenia) can become more rapidly apparent than others (anemia) because of physiologic variability in the target cells. For both safety and scientific rigor, patients should be appropriately monitored for both clinical and laboratory intolerance in accordance with the known pharmacokinetics and pharmacodynamics of the drug under study. Some assessment points may be required to assess toxicity, others for efficacy, and still others may meet both requirements.

Clinical tolerance can be monitored by spontaneous patient report or open-ended or close-ended questioning. In general, the more rigorous the probe, the greater the incidence of intolerance and the more difficult the task of ascribing it to the studied drug. Even in a healthy population there is a background level of transient symptoms such as headache, diarrhea, and dyspepsia.

Outcome measures used to assess drug efficacy should be able to detect the smallest *clinically important* change and, at the same time, be both reliable and valid with respect to capturing the dimensionality of the clinical and pathophysiologic responses.[50,72] To avoid bias, both patients and assessors should not know who is receiving what treatment (double-blinded study). Usually, the test treatments are given in an identical format, either as indistinguishable compounds or using the "double-dummy" technique. When only a *single-blinded* technique is used, either the patient, or, more usually, the assessor can be compromised by an expectation bias that may either enhance or abrogate the clinical result. In a *triple-blinded* format, not only the patient and assessor are blind, but also a third party who has responsibility for administering certain aspects of the trial, e.g., termination of the study on ethical grounds if adverse reactions or response failures are unexpectedly high in one or other treatment group. In a triple-blinded scheme, such decisions can be made without prejudice.

STATISTICAL ANALYSIS

The results should be analyzed and presented in a way that demonstrates both their clinical importance and their statistical significance.[73] If composite indices have been used, they should be reported so that interpretation by physicians in general is possible. The vagaries of the type I and type II errors have already been discussed and are exceeded only by difficulty in defining levels of clinical importance for changes on outcome variables. It may be preferable to define a clinically important change as that discernible by the patient. Improvement or deterioration in variables such as pain and physical disability are, after all, most important to the patient. Although this dictum may be applied readily to subjective variables, it is much harder to define for a semiobjective variable such as grip strength, or for an objective variable such as erythrocyte sedimentation rate (ESR), because important changes in clinical status can occur at different levels of sphygmomanometric or ESR change in different individuals.

Two types of analytic philosophy are commonly used: *explicative*, or per protocol, and *management*, or intention to treat.[74] In the explicative approach, all patients failing to complete the study exactly according to protocol are excluded from analysis. In a management trial all patients entered into the trial are included in the analysis. Although the former strategy is operationally simple, it runs the risk of producing a biased result, usually by eroding wholly or partly any true differences in drug efficacy or tolerability. In the management strategy, dropouts, who often represent important drug-dependent events, are included in the analysis. Management is currently the preferred method for analysis in most studies. We recommend that if an explicative strategy is used, the analysis be duplicated using a management approach to establish the stability of the result and the integrity of the conclusions.[11]

Although randomization attempts to achieve group comparability, this does not guarantee a balance of potential confounding variables. If an imbalance is recognized in factors such as disease severity or duration, response potential, and (possibly) age or sex, the analysis should adjust for it.

INTERPRETATION

Caution is necessary in extrapolating the results of a study and in generalizing them to other patient groups that may differ in their response potential to both beneficial and adverse effects. Such groups include the elderly, the young, the pregnant, those with comorbid disease, and those who received concurrent drug therapy.[75–78] The results of a trial should be viewed, therefore, in the appropriate clinical context.[29–35,37,38,77] Furthermore, they should be interpreted with respect to other relevant data obtained from both open studies and clinical practice, as well as from other randomized controlled trials.[14,34,35,37,38,78–80] Although trial subjects are highly selected and closely observed and can derive certain benefits from study participation, the toxicity of NSAIDs reported in clinical trials actually corresponds fairly well to that found in the general population.[81]

Considering the large number of reported clinical trials, the many potential sources of bias, and the need to carefully appraise the quality and value of new data, the Ad Hoc Committee on Critical Appraisal of the Medical Literature has proposed a novel system for summarizing essential methodologic information in the abstracts of scientific papers.[82]

METHODS OF ASSESSMENT

Inflammation has long been recognized as notoriously difficult to measure both in clinical practice and in the laboratory.[83] The methods most commonly used are essentially based on quantitation of its cardinal features: dolor, tumor, calor, et rubor (Celsus 53 BC to AD 7), functio laesa (Galen c129 to c200), and et rigor.[84] The methods are, at best, indirect and have been aptly described by Lansbury[85] as being "analogous to estimating the size and heat of an underground fire by the amount of smoke, flame and heat detected above ground." Laboratory tests play a relatively small part in assessment, because a drug that only reduces the ESR without relieving joint pain is clearly of no interest to either patient or physician. Antirheumatic drugs available at present are relatively weak agents, and differences between NSAIDs and placebo in short-term trials are relatively small[86] (Table 9–3). At present, no single ideal method is capable of accurately reflecting disease activity in arthritis. As a result, some authors have suggested aggregation of end points into a composite index.[85,87–100]

COMPOSITE INDICES

Composite indices are constructed by statistical or judgmental procedures that allow aggregation of scores assigned to different end points.[100] Such end points may be on the same dimension (e.g., Ritchie Articular Index[90] and Lansbury Articular Index[87]) or different dimensions (Pooled Index[95]). Composite indices have two advantages over multiple end points. First, they provide a basis for combining all relevant end points into a single value. Second, they increase

Table 9–3. Mean Differences in Clinical and Laboratory Parameters Between Placebo and Salicylate, Indomethacin, Ibuprofen, and Prednisolone in 37 Patients with Rheumatoid Arthritis‡

Clinical and Laboratory Parameters	Salicylate	Indomethacin	Ibuprofen	Prednisolone
Pain index	−6	−10	−6	−7
Articular index	−6	−10	−6	−7
Grip strength (mm Hg)				
right	+12.3†	+14.5†	+17.5†	+16.5
left	+10.6	+11.1	+12.7	+11.3
Digital joint circumference (mm)				
right	−1	−4	0	−4
left	−3	−3	−3	−1
^{99m}Tc Knee joint uptake (percent $\times$ 10^{-2})				
right	−9.3	−12.0†	−8.3	−11.7†
left	−7.5	−10.9†	−10.9†	−12.1

*Oral daily dosage: Sodium salicylate 1 g four times a day, indomethacin 25 mg four times a day, ibuprofen 400 mg three times a day, and prednisolone 5 mg three times a day. Each preparation was given in double-blinded, crossover fashion, for one week.
†Statistically significant at the 5% level.
‡(From Deodhar, S.D., et al.: Measurement of clinical response to anti-inflammatory drug therapy in rheumatoid arthritis. Q. J. Med., 42:387–401, 1973.)

the statistical efficiency of clinical trials by avoiding the issue of p value adjustment for multiple comparisons, thereby reducing sample size requirements. Enthusiasm for such neo-Pythagorean numerology must be tempered by recognition that the derivation of a single-number value from a complex phenomenon does not necessarily imply any greater knowledge about that phenomenon than before. For this reason, composite indices require extensive and elaborate validation prior to general utilization.

Despite rigorous validation, many such indices use different weighting systems for the individual components of the index, and the preferred method of weighting remains controversial.[99] Thus, the Ritchie Articular Index weighs selected joints or groups of joints according to a four-point tenderness scale, whereas the Lansbury Articular Index uses joint size as the basis for such weighting. Such judgmental preferences have recently been supplanted by weighting systems based on statistical techniques such as derived units,[95] discriminate analysis,[91] and generalizability coefficient analysis.[98] When applied to multidimensional indices (particularly those that measure a wide spectrum of dimensions, e.g., pain, ESR, grip strength, and physical function), the purely statistical weighting techniques are at risk of producing relative weights for the individual components differing substantially from their relative clinical importance. With such techniques, for example, the ESR can make a much greater contribution to the final index score than more clinically relevant variables such as pain and physical function. To circumvent these problems, attempts have been made to combine the advantages of the statistical techniques with the relative clinical importance of each component.[101] Conceptually, however, it is relatively easy to cope with aggregating items on a single dimension (e.g., physical function), more difficult to aggregate across related dimensions (e.g., physical, social, and emotional function), and extremely difficult to combine scores across widely differing dimensions (e.g., pain, sedimentation rate, and grip strength).

MEASUREMENT OF ERROR

Sir Thomas Lewis, the acknowledged father of clinical science in the United Kingdom, remarked, "It is crucial in measuring to know the error of the method; to have but an inaccurate measure may be regrettable, but to have it and not to know it is deplorable."[102] Surprisingly, few authors reporting clinical therapeutic trials of antirheumatic drugs provide any information on the error of their methods.[103] This failure can lead to misinterpretation of the clinical significance of results. For example, the intraobserver error of digital joint circumference by the Geigy spring apparatus is approximately 2 mm.[104] In a trial of ketoprofen compared to placebo in rheumatoid arthritis, the reported reduction in digital joint circumference using this instrument was small and less than the error of the method.[105] Systematic errors not reflected by the standard deviation can also occur in clinical therapeutic trials. One example of this is assessment of joint tenderness at different times of the day, which has been shown to vary.[106] Only good trial design can eliminate this type of error.[107]

OBJECTIVE VERSUS SUBJECTIVE OUTCOME MEASURES

Naturally, objective measurements are needed in clinical therapeutic trials of antirheumatic drugs. Clin ical trials in rheumatology are only as good as their end points. In a comprehensive review of the literature on clinical trials of indomethacin, O'Brien showed that in those studies using objective measurements, only 25% of patients had "good" or "excellent" responses, whereas in those studies primarily based on subjective indices, the average "good" or "excellent" response was 60%.[39] These differences might also be explained by the quality of the trial designs, because those employing objective measures were better controlled than those using patients' subjective responses. The point is not that objective measures are not necessarily better than subjective ones, but that sensitive measures are better than insensitive ones.[108] The most sensitive parameter to change with antirheumatic drug therapy in rheumatoid arthritis is the patient's subjective assessment of pain relief.[86] The objective measurement of radionuclide joint uptake, on the other hand, is sometimes unable to discriminate between active drugs and placebo.[109] The "softer" subjective responses ranked high in importance to a panel of clinical rheumatologists.[99]

CHOICE OF END POINTS

The choice of end points is a choice of what to measure and how to measure it.[100] The decision can be made by a number of processes and use a variety of different individuals (i.e., patients, physicians in general, key informants, or a statistical lottery). Whatever the process, the measures selected should reflect the nature of the disease, the study population, the pharmacodynamics of the test compounds, and the research hypothesis. Different measures may be required for rheumatoid arthritis patients as opposed to osteoarthritis patients, for children as opposed to adults, and for slow-acting as opposed to fast-acting antirheumatic drugs. Irrespective of the specific protocol, the criteria we consider important for evaluative indices for clinical trials are illustrated in Table 9–4 and discussed below.[100]

1. The index should be designed for a specific purpose: Thus, measures such as ESR and Ritchie Articular Index used in rheumatoid arthritis trials may be inappropriate for osteoarthritis patients either because of a lack of expected change or fundamental differences in target joint involvement. Likewise, adults may be able to complete a self-administered questionnaire regarding physical function that is completely beyond the capability of a child with juvenile rheumatoid arthritis. Temporal factors may also be relevant. Thus, although progression of radiographic erosion might be a useful indicator of response to a

Table 9–4. Criteria for Evaluative Indices for Musculoskeletal Clinical Trials*

1. The index should be designed for a specific purpose.
2. The index should have been validated on individuals or populations having similar characteristics to future study populations.
3. Reliability should be adequate for achieving measurement objectives.
4. Validity (face, content, criterion, and construct) should be adequate for achieving measurement objectives.
5. The index must be responsive, i.e., able to detect significant change in the underlying variable.
6. Index performance should have been maintained in subsequent applications under similar study conditions.
7. The method of deriving scores, particularly in composite indices, should be both credible and comprehensible.
8. The feasibility of data collection and instrument application should not be constrained by time or cost.
9. The measurement process must be ethical.
10. Utilization of the index should have been adopted by other clinical investigators.

*(From Bellamy, N., and Buchanan, W.W.: A preliminary evaluation of the dimensionality and clinical importance of pain and disability in osteoarthritis of the hip and knee. Clin. Rheumatol., 5:231–241, 1986.)

slow-acting disease-modifying agent in rheumatoid arthritis, it is an inappropriate measure for a short-term study, particularly if it involves an NSAID. Furthermore, although some indices may be applicable to the study of pathologic aspects of disease[110,111] or to the radiographic appearance of the articulations,[112] other equally specific and sophisticated instruments may be needed to assess the clinical progress of patients with chronic arthritis.[100] Finally, the different research objectives of description, prediction, and evaluation should be kept clearly separated because each requires a different type of instrumentation.[113]

2. The index should have been validated on individuals or groups of patients having characteristics similar to the proposed study population: Validation studies were infrequently reported for earlier indices but are now a necessary requirement for new measuring instruments. Although borrowing an index from the rheumatoid arthritis literature and applying it in osteoarthritis trials may be convenient, the borrowed index's applicability must be demonstrated rather than just assumed. For this reason, the target joints for the Ritchie[90] and Doyle[114] indices differ, each respecting the differing patterns of joint involvement peculiar to the two forms of arthritis. Furthermore, while an index may be responsive in one setting (e.g., joint replacement surgery), it may be too insensitive to detect smaller responses accompanied by greater variability in another setting (e.g., NSAID therapy). The instrument selected for a clinical trial, therefore,

should be of demonstrated *reliability, validity,* and *responsiveness* in the *relevant* clinical setting.

3. Reliability should be adequate for achieving measurement objectives: Reliability is a synonym for consistency, or agreement, and is the extent to which a measurement procedure yields the same result on repeated applications when there has been no change in the underlying phenomenon. Because repeated measures rarely equal one another exactly, some degree of inconsistency is invariable. This form of measurement error is referred to as *noise,* or *random error.* Low levels of reliability are reflected in the magnitude of the standard deviation and result in increased sample size requirements for clinical trials employing such instruments (Table 9–1). In contrast to systematic error, i.e., bias, random error can be minimized by increasing the sample size. Although there is no absolute level for acceptable reliability in general, reliability coefficients should exceed .8.

Although a number of methods can be used to assess reliability, the two most commonly used are test-retest reliability,[72] and internal consistency.[115] The former, an expression of stability, requires two separate administrations of the test at appropriate intervals. In contrast, internal consistency is determined on a single administration of the test and estimates interitem correlation. In the special case when the measuring instruments are human observers, interobserver and intraobserver variability can be expressed to take into account the level of agreement beyond that expected as a result of chance alone using Cohen's kappa statistic.[116]

The major sources of measurement error can be divided among the patient, the observer, and the instrument. Patient variability often arises from circadian variation in symptoms, or from fatigue, poor memory, or inattention. Observers are liable to experience fatigue, particularly if the assessment task is lengthy or complex, or requires judgments based on visual or tactile perception.[117] Instruments may also vary as a function of some mechanic component of the instrument, e.g., cuff size in a sphygmomanometer or compliance in a dynamometer. Whatever the source of variability, it should be quantitated and, if unacceptably high, be minimized by design modification of the instruments, training of the assessors, or modification of the measurement process to improve patient performance. Such training procedures may have a profound impact on the sample size requirements for a clinical trial.[118]

4. Validity should be adequate for achieving measurement objectives. There are four types of validity: face, content, criterion, and construct.[72,119–121]

Face Validity. A measure has face validity if informed individuals (investigators and clinicians) judge that it measures part or all of the defined phenomenon. In many instances (e.g., hemoglobin, weight), this decision is self-evident, whereas in others, particularly in subjective measures for functional status, face validity alone may be insufficient, and other forms of validity must also be demonstrated.

Content Validity. An instrument can have face validity but fail to capture the dimension of interest in its entirety. A measure, therefore, has content validity if it is comprehensive, i.e., it encompasses all relevant aspects of the defined attributes. Like face validity, content validity is also subjective but can be conferred either by a single individual or by a group of individuals using one of several consensus-development techniques. The decision about which measure should be included in an instrument and which excluded is critical because it defines the nature of the instrument, and both guides and constrains the instrument's subsequent applicability. Any subsequent addition or deletion of measures creates, in essence, a new instrument requiring revalidation.

Some instruments use only objective measures, others only subjective measures, and still others a combination of both. In general, evaluative instruments for clinical trials should include some measures that comprehensively probe symptoms that occur frequently and are clinically important to patients. The definition of importance can be decided by groups of patients polled to assess the dimensions of their symptoms,[101] by clinical investigators whose decision is based on their perception of the patient's symptoms, or by the results of validation studies probing instrument performance.

An alternative measurement strategy that is devoid of content validity individualizes the measurement process using a signal strategy.[122,123] Here, each patient identifies a symptom or anatomic area of importance that subsequently becomes the principal, or possibly the only, measurement target. This method usually results in measuring different end points in different patients—a concept presently not totally accepted by either clinicians or biostatisticians. Our own experience with signal strategies suggests that they may be useful if subjects can be appropriately counseled into setting relevant and realistic goals, but that they lack the predictability, the comprehendibility, and, in some instances, the credibility of more traditional approaches.

Criterion Validity. Criterion validity is assessed statistically by comparing the new instrument against a current independent criterion or standard (concurrent criterion validity) or against a future standard (predictive criterion validity). It is, therefore, an estimate of the extent to which a measure agrees with the true value of an independent measure of health status, either present or future. The attainment of concurrent criterion validity is usually frustrated by the lack of any available standard whereas predictive criterion validity is not immediately relevant to evaluative objectives.

Construct Validity. Construct validity is of two types: convergent and discriminant. Both represent statistical attempts to demonstrate adherence between instrument values and a theoretical manifestation (construct), or consequence of the attribute. Convergent construct validity testing assesses the correlation between scores on a single health component as measured by two different instruments. If the coefficient is positive and appreciably above zero, the new measure is said to have *convergent* construct validity. In contrast, *discriminant* construct validity testing compares the correlation between scores on the same health component as measured by two different instruments (e.g., measures of physical function) and between scores on that health component and each of several other health components (e.g., measures of social and emotional function). A measure has discriminant construct validity if the proposed measure correlates better with a second measure accepted as more closely related to the construct than it does with a third, more distantly related measure.[120] Validity, like reliability, has no absolute level, and its adequacy depends on the measurement objective.

To circumvent some of the judgmental requirements of validity testing, several of the more recent multidimensional indices have used multivariant analytic techniques to select items for inclusion and also to evaluate index performance. While model building should supplement, rather than replace, judgmental activities, these advanced statistical techniques can nevertheless provide additional useful information regarding validity. In contrast to random error, systematic error (bias) produces invalid results that are not reflected in the standard deviation and cannot be negated by simply increasing sample size.

5. An evaluative index must be responsive to change, i.e., capable of detecting differential change in health status occurring in two or more groups of individuals exposed to competing interventions: This is an absolute prerequisite for an evaluative instrument and requires careful documentation. Not only should the instrument be responsive in general, but it also should be specifically responsive in the clinical setting in which it is to be applied. A number of factors can influence instrument sensitivity, one of the most important being *scaling*. With the exception of the Guttman/cumulative scaling techniques, dichoto-

mous scales generally lack the sensitivity required because of the restricted response options they offer. In contrast, 10-cm horizontal visual analogue scales[124] (Fig. 9–1) and 5-point Likert adjectival scales[125] offer adequate response options. The relative sensitivity of these two scales remains controversial, but the visual analogue scale may be more sensitive.[126]

6. Index performance should have been maintained in subsequent applications under similar study conditions: The repeated observation of expected relationships between intergroup differences and differential index scores when the instrument has been used under similar study conditions provides evidence for consistent performance. Such consistency has been observed, for example, in the measurement of osteoarthritis pain by visual analogue and Likert-type scales.[127]

7. The method of deriving index scores, particularly in composite indices, should be credible and comprehendible: Although clinical investigators and the biostatisticians with whom they associate may understand the construction of index scores, the methods may not be readily appreciated by physicians in general, who will be the appliers of any new knowledge. *The responsibility of the investigators to convey the methods used in score derivation cannot be overemphasized.* This is particularly true for composite indices for which analytic techniques integrate the magnitude and variability of any change occurring on each of several different dimensions but may disregard the relative clinical importance of the contribution of each of the components.

8. The feasibility of data collection should not be constrained by time or cost: Measurement procedures that are complex and excessively lengthy run the risk of patient and assessor fatigue, with a resultant decline in data quality. Similarly, measurement methods that are prohibitively expensive lack general applicability, although for certain projects cost may not be an overriding consideration.

9. The measurement process must be ethical: Measurement procedures that are painful, embarrassing, or hazardous to the study's subjects raise ethical issues. Such issues must be fully disclosed to participants, and, if possible, less invasive procedures sought. The necessity for data collection must be carefully weighed against the risks, and the final procedures reviewed by an independent committee versed in judging ethical issues in medical research protocols. Fortunately, safety issues are rarely encountered in the application of musculoskeletal indices.

10. Use of the index should have been adopted by other clinical investigators: This is a retrospective judgment and a relative one, because poor indices

may be repeatedly used, possibly because they are familiar, whereas high-performance indices may be neglected because they are either novel or use innovative, but incomprehendible, statistical techniques.

The current diversity of opinion regarding outcome measurement in osteoarthritis trials can be appreciated by comparing the FDA guidelines for 1977,[128] Altman and Hochberg's recommendations,[128] and a review of outcome measures used in 63 clinical trials of NSAIDs from 1962 to 1982[127] (Table 9–5). Pain and physician and patient global assessments are uniformly recommended by these authors, although the exact methods of measuring these dimensions are far from standardized. The 50-foot walking time, while recommended by the FDA and Altman and Hochberg,[128] has in fact displayed poor performance characteristics in differentiating active drugs from placebo in several NSAID studies. In contrast, the assessment of functional disability (the second most important symptom of osteoarthritis) is absent from both sets of guidelines and has been frequently omitted from NSAID trials, but is a measurable dimension containing responsive end points.

Although the Doyle[114] and Lequesne[129] indices were developed to assess osteoarthritis patients, they have been rarely applied in clinical trials. Furthermore, supposedly multipurpose instruments developed for the assessment of rheumatoid arthritis patients have not to date made an appreciable impact on outcome measurement in osteoarthritis trials. In spite of these criticisms, *clinical metrology* is a rapidly evolving discipline in which several recent instruments have shown high-performance characteristics on multiple dimensions. Although we remain less enthusiastic regarding multipurpose indices (i.e., indices to evaluate several different types of arthritis) because of substantial disease-dependent differences, formal comparisons of multipurpose- and purpose-built instruments remain to be conducted.

PAIN

Because pain is the major complaint of the rheumatic sufferer, measurement of pain relief becomes extremely important in assessing clinical response to antirheumatic drug medication. "Pain is known to us by experience and described by illustrations," wrote Sir Thomas Lewis, and the absence of a more precise definition highlights the difficulty in recognizing and grading the pain response.[102] Pain is an entirely subjective phenomenon and can be measured only by the patient who experiences it. Keele proposed a pain chart on which the patient recorded his pain on the adjectival scale: slight, moderate, severe, and agonizing.[130] In practice, few patients recorded their pain as "agonizing"; most tended to select "moderate." On other scales, however, the "moderate" score often corresponds to either "slight" or "severe."[131] The adjectival scale is controversial because the number of descriptions is insufficient for patients to regularly rank them.[132] Numeric values can be given to the adjectival scale as follows: 0 = no pain, 1 = slight pain, 2 = moderate pain, 3 = severe pain, and 4 = ex-

Table 9–5. Outcome Measures for Clinical Trials in Osteoarthritis

FDA Guidelines (1977)*	Altman and Hochberg[128]	Bellamy and Buchanan[127]	Out of 63 Trials
1. Joint swelling	1. Pain (using visual analogue scales)	1. Pain	58
2. Joint redness	2. Tenderness on pressure/motion	2. Patient global assessment	51
3. Tenderness on pressure	3. Clinician's global assessment of current status and degree of change in status	3. Range of movement	45
4. Pain at rest or on motion	4. Patient's global assessment of current status and degree of change in status	4. Physician global assessment	42
5. Range of motion	5. 50-foot walking time (for patients with hip and/or knee involvement)	5. Joint stiffness	35
6. 50-foot walking time	6. Grip strength (for patients with hand involvement)	6. Qualitative aspects of sleep	28
7. Clinician's global assessment		7. Walking time	23
8. Patient's global assessment		8. Activities of daily living	22
		9. Joint tenderness	19
		10. Analgesic compound	15
		11. Joint swelling	15
		12. Signal joints	10
		13. Ascent time	3
		14. Muscle power	3
		15. Hand function	3
		16. Radiology	2
		17. Joint temperature	1

*Source: Altman and Hochberg.[128]

tremely severe, or agonizing pain. Such a scale is capable of discriminating between use of nonsteroidal anti-inflammatory analgesics and placebo in short-term clinical trials.[133] Reading[134] found a poor correlation between the McGill pain questionnaire[135–137] and adjectival assessment, although Burckhardt[138] has claimed the former to be useful in arthritis.

Currently, the most popular method of recording pain is with the *visual analogue scale*.[124,139–143] This is merely a line taken to represent the continuum of pain, the ends defining the extremes of the experience, i.e., "no pain" and "as severe as it could be" (Fig. 9–1). The patient marks the line at a point corresponding to his estimate of pain, and the distance from zero is taken to represent the severity of pain. Scott and Huskisson have shown that the performance of a visual analogue scale is profoundly affected by its design.[145] Thus, for example, descriptions of pain at intervals along the line result in a clustering of points opposite the descriptions, converting the visual analogue scale into a graphic rating scale, resulting in loss of sensitivity[124] (Fig. 9–2). A good correlation has been found between horizontal and vertical scales.[146]

In one study, the descriptions were evenly spread along the line, the results were uniformly distributed, and the aforementioned problem with clustering was avoided.[144] There is excellent agreement between repeated measurements of pain using the visual analogue scale.[143,144] One of the problems of a visual analogue scale is that patients may have difficulty in understanding the concept, at least initially.[147,148] About 5% of patients in our experience have initial difficulty in understanding the concept of a visual analogue scale, and time taken for careful explanation is well-spent. The line should have stops at either end to limit the distribution of results.[149] The conventional length of the line is 10 cm, and it is important to note that this will change with photocopying.[150] Normal subjects asked to remember the position of a mark on the line perform less well than patients with pain.[151] The method has shown a good correlation with verbal rating scales,[152,153] has proved sensitive to change,[154] and has been found applicable to patients regardless

FIG. 9–1. Visual analogue pain scale. This scale may be either vertical or horizontal.[144] The ends of the line should be marked; otherwise, some patients will record their pain beyond the end of the line.

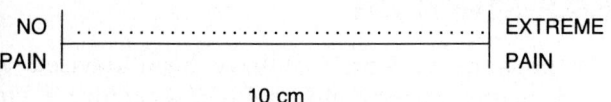

10 cm

FIG. 9–2. *A*, The use of descriptive terms along a visual analogue scale converts it to a graphic rating scale so that sensitivity is lost. *B*, The scale, however, is satisfactory if the descriptive terms are spread out evenly along the line.

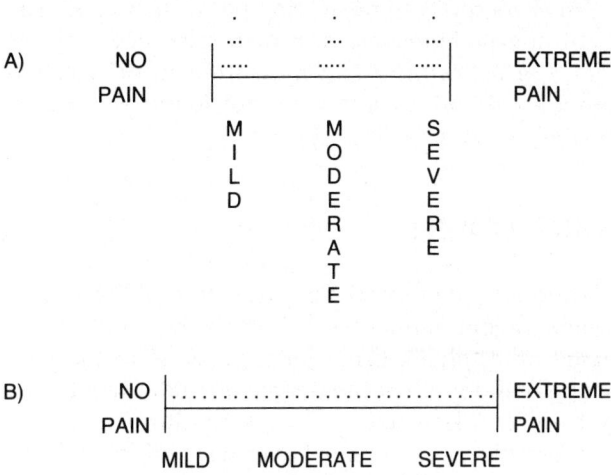

of ethnic background and even to children under 5 years of age.[155]

Beecher aptly stated that "Pain is measured in terms of its relief."[83] Huskisson made a plea to measure pain relief rather than pain directly.[131] Grossi and colleagues[156] modified the standard visual analogue scale with a chromatic addition and claimed increase in sensitivity. The relief variant of the visual analogue pain scale has the advantage that all patients start at the same baseline, but has the disadvantage that all patients do not start with the same degree of pain, and there is no opportunity to get worse.[124,131] Jacobsen contends that patients should not have access to previous scores when measuring subjective states such as pain.[157] Scott and Huskisson[145] and Carlsson[158] observed that as time goes on, patients tend to overestimate pain severity, but quickly correct their scores when shown their starting point. This observation is clearly important in long-term studies, and in rheumatic disease trials, it is now our practice to provide the patient with his previous scores. Pain varies at different times of the day, and it is therefore wise to standardize the timing of measurements.[131] Dequeker and Wuestenraed[159] also showed that weather conditions affect patients' pain, an obviously important consideration in long-term clinical trials.

The visual analogue scale for assessing pain has been criticized on the basis that it is nonlinear and prone to bias,[153,160] and is poorly comprehended by the patient.[147,148] Sriwatanakul et al.[161] have suggested that interindividual variations may be minimized if patients mark words used as descriptive terms on a visual analogue scale, then assign these terms the values obtained for individual subjects, instead of using arbitrary values of 1, 2, and 3 of the ordinal scale. This innovative method needs further testing in rheumatic diseases.

Other methods of measuring pain, such as assessment of pain threshold and pain tolerance,[84] observation of behavior,[162] and measurement of catecholamine excretion rates,[130] have not found acceptance in clinical trial practice.

JOINT COUNT

Various methods have been used to evolve a scoring system of joint tenderness.[87–90,164–170] These indices are based on applying firm digital pressure to the joint margins and grading the degree of tenderness by the patient's response. The articular index of Lansbury[89,167] was designed to provide information on the extent of articular involvement. An estimate of disease activity was based on joint size, as determined by the area of the articular surface, but the degree of joint inflammation was not taken into account. It should be noted that there are no data on the area of the articular surface in joints of the human body. Lansbury's Articular Index has a close correlation with the systemic index described by the same author,[87] and both have proved useful in charting the individual patient's progress, although most workers found that they take considerable time to perform.

The Cooperating Clinics Committee of the American Rheumatism Association employs a simple count of clinically active joints, as determined by pain on passive motion, tenderness on pressure, or inflammatory joint swelling.[168,169] This index has been widely used for the assessment of antirheumatic drugs, in both short- and long-term trials. Ward and his colleagues have provided evidence that scoring a few selected "signal" joints gives a better assessment of drug effect than a total joint count, but only one trial in which signal joints were used has been reported.[122] If signal joints become accepted, then the instruments variously described as "dolorimeters" or "palpameters,"[171–176] may come back into vogue, because, at present, they cannot generally be applied to all the joints. McCarty and colleagues[176] developed and standardized their dolorimeter against the Lansbury indices with the idea of making precise measurements of "one slice of the inflammatory pie." The reproducability of this instrument is very high; the interobserver and intraobserver errors are identical.

The articular index devised by Ritchie and colleagues is based on the summation of joint responses after firm digital pressure. The responses are recorded

as 0 = the patient has no tenderness, +1 = the patient says it is tender, +2 = the patient says it is tender and winces, and +3 = the patient says it is tender, winces, and withdraws the limb. Tenderness of the cervical spine, hip joints, and talocalcaneal and midtarsal joints is elicited by passive movement. Some joints are treated as single units: temporomandibular, sternoclavicular, acromioclavicular, metacarpophalangeal, metatarsophalangeal, and proximal interphalangeal joints of the hands. The sum of the Ritchie Articular Index is 78; it has been shown to reflect exacerbations of disease and improvement induced by antirheumatic drugs.

The Ritchie index correlates well (r = 0.89) with the articular index of the Cooperating Clinics Committee of the American Rheumatism Association (ARA).[90] Both indices show clear differences in short-term clinical therapeutic trials of antirheumatic drugs compared with placebo. The articular index of the Cooperating Clinics Committee of the ARA gives lower mean differences between active drugs and placebo, but this finding is offset by its smaller variability. Both articular indices are satisfactory for clinical trial purposes. The intraobserver error with the Ritchie index when performed within 30 min is highly acceptable (mean difference between 1 and 2 units). The interobserver error is high, and it has been calculated that differences less than 20 between two observers in an individual patient cannot be interpreted as significant.

This finding once again emphasizes the need for a single observer to make the measurements in a clinical therapeutic trial. Hart et al.[177,178] demonstrated that the interobserver error could be significantly reduced if only a single count of tender joints were used rather than grading the response, but this has the potential disadvantage of reduced sensitivity.[179] The Ritchie Articular Index of joint tenderness correlates with the patient's assessment of pain,[86] in the upper limbs with grip strength, and in the lower limbs with the time to walk 50 feet.[90] The Ritchie Articular Index of joint tenderness has the advantage that it can be performed by nonmedical personnel with an amanuensis in 2½ min.[90] It is the method chosen by the European League Against Rheumatism Standing Committee on International Clinical Studies,[129] but others[180] have not found it as satisfactory. As with pain scales, the Ritchie Articular Index of joint tenderness may be influenced by the weather.[159]

GRIP STRENGTH

Various instruments[181–183] have been devised to measure grip strength during the past century,[184] but they have failed to provide any advantage over the Davis bag[185] or sphygmomanometer cuff.[164,166,172] The intraobserver error with the Davis bag is up to 10 mm Hg; the interobserver error is 20 mm Hg.[186] Day-to-day and week-to-week variations in patients with stable disease gave no greater difference than that observed in intraobserver studies.[186] A circadian rhythm has been noted in one study in normal subjects[187] and in patients with rheumatoid arthritis,[97] but not in another study.[186] *It seems prudent to standardize the time of measurement of grip strength, as with other indices, in clinical therapeutic trials.* The determinants of grip strength are the strength of the muscles in the forearm and hand, and the pain and degree of joint destruction in the wrist, hand, and finger joints: grip strength, as previously noted, correlates with the Ritchie Articular Index of joint tenderness in the upper limbs, and also with a functional index[188,189] in the upper limbs. Grip strength is not particularly sensitive to change with antirheumatic drug therapy,[86,186] and its continued use in clinical trials rests largely on its simplicity and rapidity.

Myers and colleagues have described the use of an electronic apparatus that measures pressure-time recordings as well as maximum grip.[190]* This method requires more study to determine its value as an outcome measure in clinical trials.[191] Downie et al. found a poor correlation between measured grip strength and that assessed using a visual analogue scale.[192]

DIGITAL JOINT CIRCUMFERENCE

Jeweler's rings were first used by Boardman and Hart to measure the circumference of the proximal interphalangeal joints and the interphalangeal joint of the thumb.[193] These measurements correlate well with those obtained with the Geigy plastic spring gauge apparatus.[193] Webb et al. found a relatively small intraobserver error with the Geigy plastic spring gauge (approximately 2 mm) but a large interobserver error (approximately 10 mm).[104] The results of digital joint circumference measurement in patients with rheumatoid arthritis are reproducible from day to day and week to week in stable disease.[104] No correlation has been found with radionuclide (^{99m}Tc) joint uptakes,[194] and Rhind et al.[195] found no correlation with other clinical measurements. A diurnal rhythm in digital joint circumference has been found by some,[195,196]

Editor's note. This method is very impressive as values greater than 300 mm Hg can be measured. Not only do rheumatoid patients show weak grips, but the time required to peak grip is prolonged. The "area under the curve" is much more sensitive to circadian, drug, and other effects.

but not all,[104] investigators. Reduction in joint circumference can occur only in patients who have soft-tissue inflammatory joint swelling; in this instance, signal joints have proved to be of value.[104] Wilkens et al. have introduced an arthrocircameter with a fully flexed polyethylene loop that more readily adapts to irregular shapes than the Geigy spring gauge,[197] but there is still no proof of its superiority.

The circumference of the knee joint has been shown to decrease with NSAIDs, but this measurement has not been frequently employed in clinical therapeutic trials of antirheumatic drugs.

MORNING STIFFNESS, LIMBERING-UP TIME, TIME OF ONSET OF FATIGUE, AND SLEEP

Huskisson emphasized that rigor is an important component of joint inflammation, and few clinicians or patients would disagree.[84] The problem of measuring morning stiffness, "limbering-up" time, and time of onset of fatigue results essentially from lack of precise definition and inadequate methods of quantitation.[84,198–202] Many patients have difficulty in separating pain from stiffness, although in our experience this difficulty can be resolved with careful explanation. The duration of morning stiffness does correlate reasonably well with other clinical and laboratory parameters,[194] although some researchers disagree.[202] Morning stiffness, limbering-up time, and time of onset of fatigue do change with antirheumatic drug medication. Huskisson has pointed out that the morning stops at noon, and that assessment of morning stiffness should have an adjustment for time of first getting out of bed.[84] Laboratory methods of objectively quantitating joint stiffness[202–206] are applicable to only a few joints and have not, as yet, been used in clinical therapeutic trials. Morning stiffness can also be measured from diurnal changes in grip.[190,191,207] Although morning stiffness is probably due to accumulation of fluid in and around joints as a result of fluid retention during sleep,[203,208] it is not relieved by a diuretic.[209] Climatic conditions do, however, influence morning stiffness.[210]

One of the functions that is most disturbed in rheumatoid arthritis is sleep. Only one study has been reported on the nocturnal effects of an NSAID in rheumatoid arthritis.[211] It showed that somatic movements monitored overnight by a video recorder were not significantly different, but the quality of sleep was improved with NSAIDs.

RANGE OF JOINT AND SPINAL MOVEMENT

The range of motion of peripheral joints in normal subjects has been determined by the American Academy of Orthopedic Surgeons,[212] and the subject reviewed in detail by Wright.[213] Range of movement of the knee by a goniometer is highly reproducible,[214,215] but of limited value in assessing drug therapy.

Much effort has been put into defining spinal movement and chest expansion in assessing progress in ankylosing spondylitis. Normal range of spinal movement for different ages in both sexes has been established.[216] Spinal movement has been measured by several methods, including the Dunham spondylometer,[217–222] skin distraction,[216,223–226] an inclinometer,[227,228] and now-abandoned radiologic procedures.[229–231] Reynolds has compared the three modern clinical techniques for measuring spinal mobility.[232] The spondylometer was found to be the quickest method but applicable to certain movements only; the goniometer, the most versatile and of accepted accuracy; and the skin distraction method, inaccurate and complicated.

How does measurement of fingertip to floor, occiput to wall, range of spinal movement, and chest expansion perform in clinical trials? In a review of 22 reports in the literature, we found that only 8 showed differences (and these were extremely small) in spinal movement and only 6 in chest expansion as a result of NSAID therapy, although other parameters suggested that these drugs were efficacious. At present, we doubt the value of these time-consuming measurements in clinical therapeutic trials in ankylosing spondylitis.*

FUNCTIONAL INDICES

Disability is a major feature of rheumatic disease, but its measurement has proved difficult. Nevertheless, as previously mentioned, improvement in function was the principal measurement in the first controlled clinical therapeutic trial in rheumatic diseases.[4] Early descriptive methods based on four- or five-point scales can detect only major changes in functional ability and are too insensitive to detect differences with antirheumatic drug medication.[233,234] More elaborate scoring systems in common use in rehabilitation centers use as many as 100 or more separate "activities of daily living" and are either too complex and time-

*Editor's note. I have found them very useful in following patients' response to antirheumatic agents and use all three measurements routinely in clinical practice.

consuming or often not sufficiently sensitive to detect change with antirheumatic drug therapy.[188,235–240] Other more recent scoring systems, however, have shown greater promise.[241–244]

Timing of certain movements or set maneuvers related to activities of daily living, such as tying knots, picking up pins, hopping on one foot, standing on toes, flailing arms, walking a certain distance, and climbing and descending stairs, are now seldom used, with the exception of time to walk 50 feet.[166,174,188,240,245] An unresolved problem with functional assessment, whether global or limited to a particular movement, is that it does not differentiate reversible disability as a result of joint inflammation from the irreversible form that is associated with joint destruction and ligamentous laxity. More elaborate questionnaires have been designed to test the quality of life, health status, and sickness impact, as well as helplessness, impairment of social activity, economic consequences of loss of working time, and functional impairment in patients with rheumatoid arthritis,[188,242,246–263] but their value in short- and long-term trials remains to be established. An important point in such assessments is whether the questionnaire should be self-administered. Spiegel et al.[264] have shown that patients are more likely to report difficulties by such rather than to an interviewer. Although difficult to determine, an overall assessment of a patient's progress[265–271] has been found to be a valuable measure outcome. A "signal function" approach analogous to the signal joint approach of Ward[122] (discussed previously in the section Joint Count), which involves the identification of "specific responsive functional disabilities" important to the patient, can detect clinically significant changes in function.

THERMOGRAPHY

Increase in warmth of overlying skin is a cardinal feature of inflammation and, in joint disease, can be measured in various ways.[272] Skin temperature, as determined by thermography, correlates with the intra-articular temperature, albeit some 4 to 5° C higher, and with other clinical features of inflammation[273] with synovial perfusion as determined by xenon joint clearance,[274] pertechnetate joint uptake,[109] plethysmography, and synovial fluid cell count, protein concentration, and volume.[272] The thermographic pattern also correlates with the anatomic site of synovial hyperemia[275] and release of cathepsin-D.[36]

Most thermographic equipment is designed around an indium antimonide detector that is sensitive to infrared energy in the wavelengths of 2 to 5 μ. Infrared quantitative thermography, when carefully conducted with attention to methodologic requirements, especially control of ambient temperature, is capable of demonstrating reproducible changes in disease activity and shows significant changes following treatment with nonsteroidal anti-inflammatory analgesics,[274,276–278] intra-articular corticosteroids,[272,279,280] D-penicillamine,[281] and cyclophosphamide.[282] A thermographic index has been described and validated.[205]

Thermography provides a noninvasive, reproducible, sensitive, and quantifiable method of assessing improvement in joint inflammation and is not subject to circadian variation.[283–284] The initial cost of equipment is high, and the procedure must be carried out with strict attention to ambient temperature. As a result, thermography has not been widely used in clinical therapeutic trials of antirheumatic drugs. A study by Paterson and associates comparing clinical indices, radioisotope uptake, and thermography in assessing knee joint inflammation revealed differences in the time course of the rate of change of the various methods, emphasizing the need to interpret the results of each separately.[285] A differential thermometer may provide an alternative to thermography, but more work is needed to evaluate its usefulness.[286] Clinical evaluation of temperature changes over joints has rarely been used in clinical trials of antirheumatic drugs,[287] and changes in skin color have never been used, because generally only skin over septic or acute gouty joints becomes red. Fraser et al.[288] found a good correlation between microwave thermography and clinical features of joint inflammation.

ROUTINE LABORATORY TESTS

Certain laboratory tests reflect to some extent the severity of joint inflammation. The most frequently used test is the ESR. Nonsteroidal anti-inflammatory analgesics do not reduce the ESR,[169,289–291] although, peculiarly, fenclofenac does,[292] and oral corticosteroids cause only a temporary reduction lasting approximately 1 week. Few clinical trials take into consideration patients' smoking habits; smoking reduces the ESR.[293] The chief value of determining the ESR or other acute-phase reactants, such as C-reactive protein, haptoglobin, fibrinogen, α-2 macroglobulin, and plasma viscosity, is in trials of slow-acting "remission-inducing" drugs such as gold, chloroquine, and D-penicillamine.[294–310] Improvement in the albumin/globulin ratio and level of serum gammaglobulin also may be used to monitor slow-acting drugs, such as gold,[311–316] D-penicillamine,[317] cyclophosphamide,[318]

and levamisole treatment.[319] NSAIDs have no effect on the titer of IgM rheumatoid factor or of immune complexes, which has been variously noted to fall with gold, chloroquine, D-penicillamine, and cytotoxic agents,[308,311–332] but not with low-dose oral corticosteroids. No correlation has been found between immunologic parameters and clinical effects in patients treated with azathioprine or cyclophosphamide.[333,334] Laurent and Panayi concluded that on present evidence, rheumatoid factor titers are not a reliable measure of patient response to antirheumatic drug treatment.[273] Tests of lymphocyte function are relevant only to drugs that might exert their action by this means (e.g., levamisole).[333–336]

A normocytic, normochromic anemia is common in rheumatoid arthritis[337–338] and responds to drugs such as gold, D-penicillamine, and orgotein,[322,337–339] although it correlates poorly with disease activity.[340] A low serum iron concentration,[310] eosinophilia,[341] and thrombocytosis,[342,343] are found in active disease, but have not as yet been used as outcome measures.

The essential amino acid L-tryptophan is displaced from serum albumin by nonsteroidal anti-inflammatory analgesics and other drugs such as gold, D-penicillamine, and chloroquine.[344] In rheumatoid arthritis there is an increase in the protein-bound fraction and a corresponding fall in free plasma tryptophan that correlates with disease activity.[296,344,345] The significance, if any, of changes in tryptophan in clinical therapeutic trials remains to be determined.

Serum concentrations of sulfhydryl groups are reduced in rheumatoid arthritis[346] paralleling disease activity.[347,348] There is evidence that both nonsteroidal anti-inflammatory analgesics and drugs such as gold, D-penicillamine, and levamisole may increase sulfhydryl group reactivity,[349–353] but the value of this laboratory parameter in clinical therapeutic trials remains to be explored.

Serum copper concentrations are elevated in rheumatoid arthritis and correlate with ceruloplasmin levels and disease activity.[354,355] Whether serum copper estimations would be of use in clinical trials also remains to be determined.

Serum propeptide levels are higher in patients with active diseases and may prove useful as a prognostic marker for joint erosions.[356,357]

Synovial fluid analysis seems relevant only in clinical trials of intra-articular drugs,[358] and synovial biopsies are worthless because of the marked differences in synovial lesions in different regions of the same joint.[359]

In a critical appraisal of outcome measures in the assessment of antirheumatic drugs, Dixon and Wright[360] draw a distinction between the results of laboratory tests, which they called process measures, and the true outcome of therapy, i.e., whether the patient's health has improved or not.

RADIOLOGY

Of all the outcome measures in therapeutic trials of antirheumatic drugs, the most controversial is radiologic assessment of disease progression. Some contend that there is currently no treatment that can stop radiologic evidence of progressive joint damage in rheumatoid arthritis;[361,362] others maintain that corticosteroids, oral and parenteral chrysotherapy, D-penicillamine, and cyclophosphamide do.[8,9,12,318,363-371] A third group feels that the evidence is inconclusive.[372-374] Gofton[375] pointed out that in only three long-term clinical therapeutic trials in rheumatoid arthritis did the radiologic improvement reach statistical significance.[10,318,364] Hernandez et al.[376] reported healing of rheumatoid juxta-articular erosions with first-line drugs. Dawes et al.[377] found they were unable to predict outcome of radiologic changes, but, interestingly, observed that those drugs that reduced the C-reactive protein, but not the ESR, led to radiologic improvement.[378]

Various methods have been used to score radiologic changes in rheumatoid arthritis.[233,379-403] Most authors, with the exception of Mewa et al.[396] and others,[369,397] have found acceptable reproducibility both in counting erosions and assessing joint space narrowing.[383,388-393,398-403] A case has been made for counting erosions and cartilage loss separately,[404] and Jacoby et al.[405] have pointed out that changes in the small joints of the hand do not necessarily correlate with those in large joints. Only weak correlations have been observed between clinical and laboratory parameters, such as the C-reactive protein and ESR, and radiologic changes;[370,373,378,384,399,400,402,406-413] Luukainen et al.[411] suggest that only 50% of radiologic changes can be explained in terms of clinical and laboratory variables.

Gofton et al.[371] found the metacarpophalangeal joints best for recording radiological change, whereas others[401,410] have argued for a combination of different joints, using 17 to 23 joints for counting erosions and 16 to 18 for assessing joint space narrowing. Clearly, many problems still exist in assessing radiologic change in rheumatoid arthritis:[375,414] new techniques, such as microfocal radiography[415] and image analysis,[416] may prove useful. It has not been possible to assess the amount of joint inflammation by nuclear magnetic resonance imaging.[417]

Important disagreement in interpreting radiologic changes in joints of the hands in osteoarthritis,[418] in the sacroiliac joints in ankylosing spondylitis,[419-421] and in the lumbar spine[422] have been recorded.

RADIONUCLIDES

Various radionuclides have been used to quantify joint inflammation.[423-425] These may be administered intra-articularly and the rate of clearance from the joint determined or, alternatively, they may be administered intravenously and the rate of accumulation over a joint (or joints) measured. The clearance of radioactive xenon (^{133}Xe) after intra-articular injection provides an indirect measurement of synovial blood flow[426,427] and has been used to investigate physiologic and pharmacologic control of the synovial microcirculation.[428-433] The ^{133}Xe clearance method correlates with clinical assessment of joint inflammation,[426,433,434] but has shown poor discrimination between antirheumatic drug medication and placebo compared to standard methods in clinical therapeutic trials.[433,435]

The accumulation of radionuclide in joints after intravenous injection can be measured as a quantitative determination of peak count rate or monitored by a display scintiscan.[426,436-442] None of the various methods for quantifying synovitis using radionuclides has proved entirely satisfactory,[425] but measurement of the absolute uptake per unit joint area seems to give the best separation between normal joints and joints affected with rheumatoid arthritis.[438] The optimum time to scan after intravenous injection of the isotope remains undecided. Some workers find 15 min adequate, whereas others argue for a longer time.[423,424,436,437,442,443] Technetium 99^m given as the pertechnetate (^{99m}TcO$_4$) has been found superior to radioiodinated (I^{125}) human fibrinogen.[439] Technetium pyrophosphate or diphosphonate compounds absorb to juxta-articular bone and are consequently somewhat less useful than ^{99m}TcO$_4$ itself.[444] It should be noted that increased uptake of Tc pyrophosphate or diphosphonate compounds also occurs in bone in rheumatoid arthritis.[445]

These problems notwithstanding, isotopic joint uptake has an acceptable reproducibility and correlates reasonably well with clinical assessments of joint inflammation and the rate of clearance of intra-articularly injected radioactive xenon.[426,434,436,437,445] Polyarticular isotope indices have been described.[439,440,446,447] Radionuclide joint uptakes in both large and small joints are reduced with nonsteroidal anti-inflammatory analgesics, therapy with corticosteroids, gold or D-penicillamine,[86,447-449] and synovectomy.[450]

At a conference on outcome measures in rheumatologic clinical trials in inflammatory peripheral joint disease, a pessimistic view was expressed regarding the use of radionuclide joint scans,[109] the limiting factors being the initial capital cost of equipment, the lack of portability, and the time required for each individual measurement. Nevertheless, radionuclide measurements have a role in clinical therapeutic trials of antirheumatic drugs, provided due attention is directed to methods and interpretation, especially because these techniques provide an *objective* measurement of articular inflammation.

In ankylosing spondylitis, the sacroiliac joint/sacral ratio of radionuclide uptake shows considerable overlap between patients and controls, thus reducing its diagnostic value.[451,452] Significant reduction in such ratios occurred, however, after as little as three weeks of treatment with NSAIDs.[453–456] Further study is required to evaluate this method in clinical therapeutic trials in ankylosing spondylitis.

ETHICAL ISSUES

It is appropriate to conclude with a comment on some of the ethical issues relevant to clinical trials. In some respects the randomized clinical trial is an extremely artificial milieu in which to determine the success or failure of a new therapeutic agent. A variety of factors can motivate investigators and patients to participate in such studies, and both groups can vary significantly from those who will subsequently prescribe and receive the new treatment once it is approved. The clinical investigator, in particular, places himself in a morally ambiguous position.[457] As the patient's personal physician, he is committed exclusively to the patient; as an investigator, he is committed to the acquisition of scientific knowledge. The potential conflict of obligation is obvious and can be substantial. If, however, such a conflict arises and can be identified, it is our contention that the investigators' obligation must be primarily to the patient rather than to the project. A number of mechanisms exist to reduce the risk of such conflicts:

1. The trial should employ a valid design and should be efficient in its use of both patients and resources, such that generalizations can be made with respect to the data generated,[458] i.e., "fulfill the ethics of design."
2. The project should comply with the ethical standards of the declaration of Helsinki.[459]
3. The project should comply with the standards of an impartial, independently appointed, and appropriately constituted committee on biomedical ethics.
4. The trial should be monitored by an independent agency charged with responsibility for aborting the trial if therapeutic failures or adverse reactions exceed predetermined boundaries.
5. The patient should be viewed as a partner in the research enterprise rather than merely test material. Relevant information must be shared. Informed consent must be obtained.

The issue of informed consent remains contentious. Although it is the investigators' moral obligation to inform the patient of the nature of the investigation and of any potential benefits and risks anticipated, it remains unclear whether patients as a whole fully comprehend what they are told, and, therefore, whether the consent they give is adequately informed.[460] It has been argued that informed consent is only obtainable from medically trained individuals, whereas that obtained from lay people may constitute only partially informed or uninformed consent.[461] Elderly individuals, in particular, show significantly poorer comprehension of consent information.[462] Two recent randomized trials have indicated that the informed consent process in itself may influence the execution,[463] and possibly the outcome,[464] of clinical trials. Thus, total disclosure of all information may result in a better understanding of treatment and adverse reactions, but less willingness to agree to randomization and increased patient anxiety.[463] Given the continued evolution of medicolegal and moral philosophy and a general increase in health awareness and educational standards, it is inevitable that informed consent procedures will undergo further development and subsequent revision.

Our own position has been well summarized by the legendary French physiologist Claude Bernard (1813–1979).[465]

Among the experiments that may be tried on man, those that can only harm are forbidden; those that are innocent are permissible; and those that may do good are obligatory.

REFERENCES

1. Lind, J.: Diagnostics of the scurvy. *In* A Treatise of the Scurvy. London, Sands, Murray, and Cochran, 1753.
2. Lasagna, L.: *In* Drugs in Our Society. Edited by P. Talalay. Baltimore, Johns Hopkins Press, 1964.
3. Jenner, E.: An Enquiry into the Causes and Effects of the Variolae Vaccinae (1798). Denver, The Range Press, 1949.
4. Fraser, T.N.: Gold therapy in rheumatoid arthritis. Ann. Rheum. Dis., 4:71–75, 1945.
5. Combined Rheumatic Fever Study Group: A comparison of prednisone and acetylsalicyclic acid on the incidence of rheumatic heart disease. N. Engl. J. Med., 262:895–902, 1960.

6. Bywater, E.G.L., Dixon, A., St. J., and Wild, J.B.: Deoxycortone and ascorbic acid in the treatment of rheumatoid arthritis. Lancet, 1:951–953, 1950.

7. Medical Research Council: A comparison of cortisone and aspirin in the treatment of early cases of rheumatoid arthritis. Br. Med. J., 1:1223–1227, 1954.

8. Empire Rheumatism Council: Multicentre controlled trial comparing cortisone acetate and acetylsalicylic acid in long-term treatment of rheumatoid arthritis. Ann. Rheum. Dis., 14:353–370, 1950.

9. Empire Rheumatism Council: Multicentre controlled trial comparing cortisone acetate and acetylcalicylic acid in long-term treatment of rheumatoid arthritis. Ann. Rheum. Dis., 16:277–289, 1957.

10. Medical Research Council: A comparison of cortisone and aspirin in the treatment of early cases of rheumatoid arthritis. Br. Med. J., 1:847–850, 1957.

11. Empire Rheumatism Council: Gold therapy in rheumatoid arthritis: Report of a multicentre controlled trial. Ann. Rheum. Dis., 19:95–119, 1960.

12. Empire Rheumatism Council: Gold therapy in rheumatoid arthritis: Final report of a multicentre controlled trial. Ann. Rheum. Dis., 20:315–334, 1961.

13. Desmaris, M.H.L.: Radiotherapy in arthritis. Ann. Rheum. Dis., 12:25–28, 1953.

14. Hill, A.B.: The clinical trial. Br. Med. Bull., 1:278–282, 1951.

15. Hill, A.B.: The clinical trial. N. Engl. J. Med., 247:113–119, 1952.

16. Greenberg, B.G.: Conduct of cooperative field and clinical trials. Am. Stat., 13:13–28, 1959.

17. Hill, A.B.: Statistical Methods of Clinical and Preventive Medicine. New York, Oxford University Press, 1962.

18. Stainsby, W.J., and Nicholls, E.: Results of treatment in rheumatoid arthritis with reference to foci of infection and streptococcus vaccine. J. Lab. Clin. Med., 18:881–890, 1933.

19. Miltner, L.J., and Kulowski, J.: The effect of treatment and eradication of foci and infection in chronic arthritis (focal infection). J. Bone Joint Surg., 15A:383–393, 1973.

20. Savage, O.: Criteria for measurement in chronic diseases. Report on a Symposium on Clinical Trials. Pfizer, Kent, England, 32, 1958.

21. Witts, L.J., ed.: Medical Surveys and Clinical Trials, 2nd ed. London, Oxford University Press, 1964.

22. Bridgman, J.F., et al.: Irradiation of the synovium in the treatment of rheumatoid arthritis. Q. J. Med., New Series, 42:357–367, 1973.

23. Sartwell, P.E.: Retrospective studies—A review for the clinician. Ann. Intern. Med., 81:381–386, 1974.

24. Chambers, T.C., Block, J.B., and Lee, S.: Controlled studies in clinical cancer research. N. Engl. J. Med., 287:75–78, 1972.

25. Juhl, E., Christensen, E., and Tygstrup, N.: The epidemiology of the gastrointestinal randomized clinical trial. N. Engl. J. Med., 296:20–22, 1977.

26. Byar, D.P., et al.: Randomized clinical trials—Perspectives on some recent ideas. N. Engl. J. Med., 295:74–80, 1976.

27. Carbone, P.P.: The case for clinical trials. C. A., 30:53–54, 1980.

28. Friedman, L.M., Furberg, D.L., and DeMets, D.L.: Fundamentals of Clinical Trials, 2nd Ed. Massachusetts, Littlejohn, PSG Publishing Co., 1985.

29. Gehan, E.A., and Freireich, E.J.: Non-randomized controls in cancer clinical trials. N. Engl. J. Med., 290:198–203, 1974.

30. Pocock, S.J.: The combination of randomized and historical controls in clinical trials. J. Chronic Dis., 29:175–188, 1976.

31. Burkhardt, R., and Kienle, G.: Controlled clinical trials and medical ethics. Lancet, 2:1356–1359, 1978.

32. White, K.L.: Improved medical care: Statistics and the health services system. Public Health Rep., 82:847–854, 1967.

33. Leading article: Controlled trials: Planned deceptions? Lancet, 1:534–535, 1979.

34. Feinstein, A.R.: On steroids for publication of therapeutic research. J. Chronic Dis., 33:65–66, 1980.

35. Feinstein, A.R.: Should placebo-controlled trials be abolished? Eur. J. Clin. Pharmacol., 17:1–4, 1980.

36. Poole, A.R., et al.: Extracellular release of cathepsin-D from cells in human normal and rheumatoid synovial membranes. Ann. Rheum. Dis., 33:405–408, 1974.

37. Horwitz, R.E., and Feinstein, A.R.: The application of therapeutic-trial principles to improve the design of epidemiologic research: A case-control study suggesting that anticoagulants reduce mortality in patients with myocardial infarction. J. Chronic Dis., 34:575–583, 1981.

38. Horwitz, R.I., and Feinstein, A.R.: Improved observational method for studying therapeutic efficacy. Suggestive evidence that lidocaine prophylaxis prevents death in acute myocardial infarction. JAMA, 246:2455–2459, 1981.

39. O'Brien, W.M.: Indomethacin: A survey of clinical trials. Clin. Pharmacol. Ther., 9:94–107, 1968.

40. Sturrock, R., et al.: Eine Bewertung der Phenylalkanoinsaure—Derivate in der Behandlung rheumatischer Erkrankungen sowie einige Erlauterungen zur lehre der klinischen Versuchsmethoden. Z. Rheumatforsch., 34:55–67, 1975.

41. Rosenbloom, D., Brooks, P., Bellamy, N., and Buchanan, W.: Clinical Trials in the Rheumatic Diseases. A Selected Critical Review. New York, Praeger, 1985.

42. Reiffenstein, R.J., Schiltroth, A.J., and Todd, D.M.: Current standards in reported drug trials. Can. Med. Assoc. J., 9:1134–1135, 1968.

43. Frieman, J.A., Chalmers, T.C., Smith, H.G., and Kuebler, R.R.: The importance of beta, the type II error and sample size in the design and interpretation of the randomized control trial. N. Engl. J. Med., 25:761–764, 1978.

44. Chilton, M.W., and Barbano, J.P.: Guidelines for reporting clinical trials. J. Periodont. Res., 9(Suppl. 14):207–208, 1974.

45. O'Fallon, J.R., et al.: Should there be statistical guidelines for medical research papers? Biometrics, 34:687–695, 1978.

46. Mosteller, F.: Problems of omission in communications. Clin. Pharmacol. Ther., 25:761–764, 1979.

47. Mosteller, F., Gilbert, J.P., and McPeek, B.: Reporting standards in research strategies for controlled trials. Controlled Clin. Trials, 1:37–58, 1980.

48. Chalmers, T.C., et al.: Method for assessing the quality of a randomized control trial. Controlled Clin. Trials, 2:31–39, 1981.

49. DerSimonian, R., Charette, J., McPeek, P., and Mosteller, F.: Reporting on methods of clinical trials. N. Engl. J. Med., 306:1332–1337, 1982.

50. Tugwell, P., and Bombardier, C.A.: A methodologic framework for developing and selecting endpoints in clinical trials. J. Rheumatol., 9:758–762, 1982.

51. Bellamy, N., and Buchanan, W.W.: The codification of clinical trial methodology. Eur. League Against Rheum. Bull., 13:16, 1984.

52. Paulus, H.E.: The crossover study design is not dead. In Symposia Medica Hoechst 16. Controversies in the Clinical Evaluation of Analgesic Anti-Inflammatory Anti-Rheumatic Drugs. Edited by H.E. Paulus, G.E. Ehrlich, and E. Lindenlaub. Stuttgart, Schattauer-Verlag, 1981.

53. Guyatt, G., et al.: Determining optimal therapy-randomized trials in individual patients. N. Engl. J. Med., 314(Suppl. 14):889–892, 1986.

54. Cook, T.D., and Campbell, D.T.: Quasiexperimentation: Design and Analysis Issues for Field Settings. Boston, Houghton Mifflin, 1979.

55. Shapiro, S., Strax, P., and Venet, L.: Periodic breast cancer screening in reducing mortality from breast cancer. JAMA, 215:1777–1783, 1971.

56. Wilhelmsen, L., Ljungberg, S., Wedel, H., and Werko, L.: A comparison between participants and non-participants in a primary preventive trial. J. Chronic Dis., 29:331–339, 1976.

57. Zelin, M.: The randomization and stratification of patients to clinical trials. J. Chronic Dis., 27:365–375, 1974.

58. Feinstein, A.R.: Clinical biostatistics XXIV—The role of randomization in sampling, testing, allocation, and credulous idolating (conclusion). Clin. Pharmacol. Ther., 14:1035–1051, 1973.

59. Gore, S.M.: Assessing clinical trials—Simple randomization. Br. Med. J., 282:2036–2039, 1981.

60. Lee, P., Webb, J., Anderson, J.A., and Buchanan, W.W.: A method for assessing the therapeutic potential of anti-inflammatory, antirheumatic drugs in rheumatoid arthritis. Br. Med. J., 2:685–688, 1973.

61. Maclagan, T.J.: The treatment of acute rheumatism by salicin. Lancet, 1:342–343, 1876.

62. Buchanan, W.W., and Smythe, H.A.: Can clinicians and statisticians be friends? J. Rheumatol., 9:653–654, 1982.

63. Taves, D.R.: Minimization: A new method of assigning patients to treatment and control groups. Clin. Pharmacol. Ther., 15:443–453, 1974.

64. Nordle, O., and Brantmark, B.: A self-adjusting randomization plan for allocation of patients into two treatment groups. Clin. Pharmacol. Ther., 22:825–830, 1977.

65. Colton, T.: Inferences on means. Statistics in Medicine. Boston, Little Brown, 1974.

66. Colton, T.: Inferences on proportions. Statistics in Medicine. Boston, Little Brown, 1974.

67. Chaput de Saintonge, D.M., and Charman, V.L.: Bizepam or nitrazepam? A question of cost. Br. J. Clin. Pharmacol., 4:422–444, 1977.

68. Cromie, B.W.: The feet of clay of the double-blind trial. Lancet, 2:994–997, 1963.

69. Feinstein, A.R.: Clinical biostatistics: III. The architecture of clinical research. Clin. Pharmacol. Ther., 11:432–441, 1970.

70. Gordis, L.: Conceptual and methodologic problems in measuring patient compliance. In Compliance in Health Care. Edited by R.B. Haynes, D.W. Taylor, and D.L. Sackett. Baltimore, Johns Hopkins University Press, 1979.

71. Deyo, R.A., Inui, T.S., and Sullivan, B.: Non-compliance with arthritis drugs: Magnitude, correlates and clinical implications. J. Rheumatol., 8:931–936, 1981.

72. Carmines, E.G., and Zeller, R.A.: Reliability and Validity Assessment. Beverly Hills, Sage Publications, 1979.

73. Bellamy, N., and Buchanan, W.W.: Interpreting clinical trials of anti-rheumatic drug therapy. Bull. Rheum. Dis., 36:1–10, 1986.

74. Sackett, D.L., and Gent, M.: Controversy in counting and attributing events in clinical trials. N. Engl. J. Med., 301:1410–1412, 1979.

75. Lacher, M.J.: Physicians and patients as obstacles to a randomized trial. Clin. Res., 26:375–379, 1978.

76. Lasagna, L.: Placebo and controlled trials under attack. Eur. J. Clin. Pharmacol., 15:373–374, 1979.

77. Ritter, J.M.: Placebo-controlled, double-blind clinical trials can impede medical progress. Lancet, 1:1126–1127, 1980.

78. Sheiner, L.B.: Clinical trials and the illusion of objectivity. In Drug Therapeutic—Concepts for Physicians. Edited by K.L. Melman. New York, Elsevier-North Holland, 1979.

79. Ingelfinger, F.J.: The randomized clinical trial. N. Engl. J. Med., 287:100–101, 1972.

80. Gilbert, J.P.: Randomization of human subjects. N. Engl. J. Med., 291:1303–1306, 1974.

81. Coles, L.S., Fries, J.F., Kraines, R.G., and Roth, S.H.: From experiment to experience: Side effects of nonsteroidal anti-inflammatory drugs. Am. J. Med., 74:820–828, 1983.

82. Ad Hoc Working Group for Critical Appraisal of the Medical Literature: A proposal for more informative abstracts of clinical articles. Ann. Intern. Med., 106:598–604, 1987.

83. Beecher, H.K.: Measurement of Subjective Responses. Oxford, Oxford University Press, 1959, p. viii.

84. Huskisson, E.C.: Assessment in clinical trials. Clin. Rheum. Dis., 2:37–49, 1976.

85. Lansbury, J.: Methods for evaluating rheumatoid arthritis. In Arthritis and Allied Conditions, 6th ed. Edited by J.L. Hollander. Philadelphia, Lea & Febiger, 1960, p. 134.

86. Deodhar, S.D., et al.: Measurement of clinical response to anti-inflammatory drug therapy in rheumatoid arthritis. Q,. J. Med., New Series, XLII, No. 166, 42:387–401, 1973.

87. Lansbury, J.: Report of a three-year study on the systemic and articular indexes in rheumatoid arthritis. Arthritis Rheum., 1:505–522, 1958.

88. Mainland, D.: The estimation of inflammatory activity in rheumatoid arthritis. Role of composition indices. Arthritis Rheum., 10:71–77, 1967.

89. Lansbury, J.: Clinical appraisal of the activity index as a measure of rheumatoid activity. Arthritis Rheum., 11:599–605, 1968.

90. Ritchie, D.M., et al.: Clinical studies with an articular index for the assessment of joint tenderness in patients with rheumatoid arthritis. Q. J. Med., New Series, XXXVII, 147, 37:393–406, 1968.

91. McQuire, R.J., and Wright, V.: Statistical approach to indices of disease activity in rheumatoid arthritis. Ann. Rheum. Dis., 30:574–580, 1971.

92. Oka, M., Rekonen, A., and Ruotsi, A.: ^{99m}Tc in the study of systemic inflammatory activity in rheumatoid arthritis. Acta Rheumatol. Scand., 17:27–30, 1971.

93. Keitel, W., et al.: Ermittlung der prozentualen, Funkionsminderung der Gelenke durch einen Bewegungsfunktionstest in der Rheumatologie. Dtsch. Gesundheitsw., 26:1901–1903, 1971.

94. Fellinger, K., et al.: Computer Dokumentation einer Rheumastation. Z. Rheumatol., 32:257–271, 1973.

95. Smythe, H.A., Helewa, A., and Goldsmith, C.H.: "Independent assessor" and "pooled index" as techniques for measuring treatment effects in rheumatoid arthritis. J. Rheumatol., 4:114–152, 1977.

96. Lewi, P.J., and Symeons, J.: Levamisole in rheumatoid arthritis—A multivariate analysis of multicentre study. J. Rheumatol., 5(Suppl. 4):17–25, 1978.

97. Kotzin, B.L., et al.: Treatment of intractable rheumatoid arthritis with total lymphoid irradiation. N. Engl. J. Med., 305:969–976, 1981.

98. Eberl, R.: Are morning stiffness and time to onset of fatigue really measurable? Is measurement of ranges of motion useful? How much change is clinically significant? In Symposia Medica Hoechst 16. Controversies in the Clinical Evaluation

of Analgesic Anti-Inflammatory-Antirheumatic Drugs. Edited by H.E. Paulus, G.E. Ehrlich, and E. Lindenlaub. Stuttgart, Schattauer Verlag, 1981.

99. Bombardier, C., Tugwell, P., and Sinclair, A.: Preference for endpoint measures in clinical trials: Results of structured workshops. J. Rheumatol., 9:797–800, 1982.

100. Bellamy, N.: The clinical evaluation of osteoarthritis in the elderly. Clin. Rheum. Dis., 12:131–153, 1986.

101. Bellamy, N., and Buchanan, W.W.: A preliminary evaluation of the dimensionality and clinical importance of pain and disability in osteoarthritis of the hip and knee. Clin. Rheumatol., 5:231–241, 1986.

102. Lewis, T.: Pain. New York, Macmillan Publishing Co., 1942, p. 43.

103. Eberl, D.R., et al.: Repeatability and objectivity of various measurements in rheumatoid arthritis. A comparative study. Arthritis Rheum., 19:1278–1286, 1976.

104. Webb, J., et al.: Evaluation of digital joint circumference measurements in rheumatoid arthritis. Scand. J. Rheumatol., 2:127–131, 1973.

105. Mills, S.B., Bloch, M., and Bruckner, F.E.: Double-blind cross-over study of ketoprofen and ibuprofen in management of rheumatoid arthritis. Br. Med. J., 4:82–84, 1973.

106. Harkness, J.A.L., et al.: Circadian variation in disease activity in rheumatoid arthritis. Br. Med. J., 284:551–554, 1982.

107. Hart, F.D., and Huskisson, E.C.: Measurement in rheumatoid arthritis. Lancet, 1:28–30, 1972.

108. Joyce, C.R.B.: Patient cooperation and the sensitivity of drug trials. J. Chronic Dis., 15:1025–1036, 1962.

109. Lee, P.: Isotopes in the measurement of joint inflammation. J. Rheumatol., 9:767, 1982.

110. Outerbridge, R.E.: The aetiology of chondromalacia patellae. J. Bone Joint Surg., 43B:752–757, 1961.

111. Mankin, H.J., and Lippiello, L.: Biochemical and metabolic abnormalities in articular cartilage for osteoarthritic human hips. J. Bone Joint Surg., 52A:424–433.

112. Kellgren, L.H., and Lawrence, J.S.: Radiological assessment of osteoarthritis. Ann. Rheum. Dis., 16:494–501, 1957.

113. Kirshner, B., and Gyuatt, G.: A methodological framework for assessing health indices. J. Chron. Dis., 38:27–36, 1985.

114. Doyle, D.V., et al.: An articular index for the assessment of osteoarthritis. Ann. Rheum. Dis., 40:75–78, 1981.

115. Cronbach, L.J.: Coefficient alpha and internal structure of tests. Psychometrika, 16:297–334, 1951.

116. Cohen, J.: A coefficient of agreement for normal scales. Educ. Psych. Measurement, 20:27–47, 1960.

117. Sackett, D.L.: Clinical disagreement: 1. How often it occurs and why. Can. Med. Assoc. J., 123:499–504, 1980.

118. Klinkhoff, A., et al.: An experiment in reducing interobserver variability in joint count. J. Rheumatol. (in press).

119. Reliability and Validity in Standards for Educational and Psychological Tests. Washington, D.C., American Psychological Association, 1974, pp. 25–55.

120. Kaplan, R.M., Bush, J.W., and Berry, C.C.: Health status: Types of validity for an index of well-being. Health Serv. Res., 11:478–507, 1976.

121. Parkerson, G.R., et al.: The Duke-UNC Health Profile: An adult health status instrument for primary care. Med. Care, 19:806–828, 1981.

122. Ward, J.R., Niethammer, T.A., and Egger, M.J.: Can we just measure signal joints? Should ring size and walking time be analyzed only in selected patients? In Symposia Medica Hoechst 16. Controversies in the Clinical Evaluation of Analgesic Anti-inflammatory Antirheumatic Drugs. Edited by H.E. Paulus, G.E. Ehrlich, and E. Lindenlaub. Stuttgart, Schattauer Verlag, 1981.

123. Egger, M.J., et al.: Reduced joint count indices in the evaluation of rheumatoid arthritis. Arthritis Rheum., 28:613–619, 1985.

124. Huskisson, E.C.: Measurement of pain. Lancet, 2:1127–1131, 1974.

125. Likert, R.: A technique for the measurement of attitudes. Arch. Psychol., 140:44–60, 1932.

126. Huskisson, E.C.: Measurement of pain. Lancet, 2:1127–1131, 1974.

127. Bellamy, N., and Buchanan, W.W.: Outcome measurement in osteoarthritis clinical trials: The case for standardization. Clin. Rheumatol., 3:293–305, 1984.

128. Altman, R.D., and Hochberg, M.C.: Degenerative joint disease. Clin. Rheum. Dis., 9:681–693, 1983.

129. Lequesne, M.: European guidelines for clinical trials of new antirheumatic drugs. EULAR Bull., 9(Suppl.):171–175, 1980.

130. Keele, K.D.: Pain chart. Lancet, 255:6–8, 1948.

131. Huskisson, E.C.: Measurement of pain. J. Rheumatol., 9:768–769, 1982.

132. Wagstaff, S., Smith, O.V., and Wood, P.H.N.: Verbal pain, descriptions used by patients with arthritis. Ann. Rheum. Dis., 44:262–265, 1985.

133. Lee, P.: Evaluation of analgesic action and efficacy of antirheumatic drugs. J. Rheumatol., 3:283–294, 1976.

134. Reading, A.E.: The McGill pain questionnaire: An appraisal. In Pain Measurement and Assessment. Edited by R. Melzack, New York, Raven, 1984.

135. Melzack, R., and Torgerson, W.S.: On the language of pain. Anesthesiology, 34:50–59, 1971.

136. Melzack, R.: The McGill pain questionnaire: Major properties and scoring methods. Pain, 1:277–299, 1975.

137. Gracely, R.H., McGrath, P., and Dubner, R.: Validity and sensitivity of ratio scales of sensory and affective verbal pain descriptions: Manipulation of affect by diazepam. Pain, 5:19–29, 1978.

138. Burckhardt, C.S.: The use of the McGill pain questionnaire in assessing arthritis pain. Pain, 19:305–314, 1984.

139. Joyce, C.R.B., Zutshi, D.W., Hrubes, V., and Itasom, R.M.: Comparison of fixed interval and visual analogue scale for rating pain. Eur. J. Clin. Pharmacol., 8:415, 1975.

140. Revill, S.I., et al.: The reliability of a linear analysis for evaluating pain. Anaesthesia, 31:1191–1198, 1976.

141. Downie, W.W., et al.: Studies with pain rating scales. Ann. Rheum. Dis., 37:378–381, 1978.

142. Dixon, J.S., et al.: Discriminatory indices of response of patients with rheumatoid arthritis treated with D-penicillamine. Ann. Rheum. Dis., 39:301–311, 1980.

143. Sriwatanakul, K., et al.: Studies with different types of visual analog scales for measurement of pain. Clin. Pharmacol. Ther., 34:234–239, 1983.

144. Scott, J.T., and Huskisson, E.C.: Graphic representation of pain. Pain, 2:175–184, 1976.

145. Scott, J., and Huskisson, E.C.: Accuracy of subjective measurements made with or without previous scores: An important source of error in serial measurement of subjective states. Ann. Rheum. Dis., 38:558–559, 1979.

146. Dixon, J.S.: Agreement between horizontal and vertical visual analogue scales. Letter to the Editor. Br. J. Rheumatol., 25:415–416, 1986.

147. Maxwell, C.: Sensitivity and accuracy of the visual analogue scale: A psycho-physical classroom experiment. Br. J. Clin. Pharmacol., 6:15–24, 1978.

148. Stubbs, D.F.: Visual analogue scales. Br. J. Clin. Pharmacol., 7:124, 1979.
149. Huskisson, E.C., and Scott, P.J.: Flectafenine: A new analgesic for use in rheumatic diseases. Rheumatol. Rehabil., 16:54–57, 1977.
150. Bloomfield, S.S., and Hanks, G.W.: The visual analogue scale. Br. J. Clin.Pharmacol., 11:98, 1981.
151. Dickson, J.S., and Bird, H.A.: Reproducibility along a 10 cm vertical visual analogue scale. Ann. Rheum. Dis., 40:87–89, 1981.
152. Woodforde, J.M., and Merskey, H.: Some relationships between subjective measures of pain. J. Psychosom. Res., 16:173–178, 1972.
153. Revill, S.I., Robinson, J.O., Rosen, M., and Hogg, M.I.J.: The reliability of a linear analogue for evaluating pain. Anaesthesia, 31:1191–1198, 1976.
154. Ohnhaus, E.E., and Adler, R.: Methodological problems in the measurement of pain: A comparison between the verbal rating scale and the visual analogue scale. Pain, 1:379–384, 1975.
155. Scott, P.J., Ansell, B.M., and Huskisson, E.C.: Measurement of pain in juvenile chronic polyarthritis. Arthritis Rheum., 14:54–57, 1977.
156. Grossi, E., et al.: Analogue chromatic continuous scale (ACCS): A new method for pain assessment. Clin. Exp. Rheumatol., 1:337–340, 1983.
157. Jacobsen, M.: The use of rating scales in clinical research. Br. J. Psychiatry, 111:545–546, 1965.
158. Carlsson, A.M.: Assessment of chronic pain: I: Aspects of the reliability and validity of the visual analogue scale. Pain, 16:87–101, 1983.
159. Dequeker, J., and Wuestenraed, L.: The effect of biometerological factors on Ritchie articular index and pain in rheumatoid arthritis. Scand. J. Rheumatol., 15:280–284, 1986.
160. Langley, G.B., and Sheppard, H.: The visual analogue scale: Its use in pain measurement. Rheumatol. Int., 5:145–148, 1985.
161. Sriwatanakul, K., Kelvie, W., and Lasagna, L.: The quantitative of pain: An analysis of words used to describe pain and analgesia in clinical trials. Clin. Pharmacol. and Ther., 32:143–148, 1982.
162. Anderson, K.O., et al.: The assessment of pain in rheumatoid arthritis. Validity of a behavioral observation method. Arthritis Rheum., 30:36–43, 1987.
163. Huskisson, E.C.: Catecholamine excretion and pain. Br. J. Clin. Pharmacol., 1:80–82, 1974.
164. Copeman, W.S.C., et al.: A study of cortisone and other steroids in rheumatoid arthritis. Br. Med. J., 2:849–855, 1950.
165. Hench, P.S., et al.: Effects of cortisone acetate and pituitary ACTH on rheumatoid arthritis, rheumatic fever and certain other conditions: Study in clinical physiology. Arch. Intern. Med., 85:545–666, 1950.
166. Quin, C.E., Mason, R.M., and Knoweldon, J.: Clinical assessment of rapidly acting agents in rheumatoid arthritis. Br. Med. J., 2:810–813, 1950.
167. Lansbury, J., and Haut, D.D.: Quantitation of the manifestations of rheumatoid arthritis. 4. Area of joint surfaces as an index of total joint inflammation and deformity. Am. J. Med. Sci., 232:15–155, 1956.
168. Cooperating Clinics Committee of the American Rheumatism Association: A seven-day variability study of 499 patients with peripheral rheumatoid arthritis. Arthritis Rheum., 8:302–334, 1965.
169. Cooperating Clinics Committee of the American Rheumatism Association: A three-month trial of indomethacin in rheumatoid arthritis with special reference to analysis and inference. Clin. Pharmacol. Ther., 8:11–38, 1967.
170. Camp, A.V.: An articular index for the assessment of rheumatoid arthritis. Orthopedics, 4:39–45, 1971.
171. Steinbrocker, O.: A simple pressure gauge for measured palpation in physical diagnosis and therapy. Arch. Phys. Med., 30:289–290, 1949.
172. Duthie, J.J.R.: Clinical trials of ACTH: Preliminary report. Edinb. Med. J., 57:341–364, 1950.
173. Jonus, O.: Objective assessment in rheumatoid arthritis. Br. Med. J., 2:1244–1249, 1950.
174. Mandel, L.: Assessment of therapeutic agents in rheumatoid arthritis. Can. Med. Assoc. J., 74:515–521, 1956.
175. Hollander, J.L., and Young, D.C.: The palpameter, an instrument of quantification of joint tenderness. Arthritis Rheum., 6:277, 1963.
176. McCarty, D.J., Gatter, R.A., and Phelps, P.: A dolorimeter for quantification of articular tenderness. Arthritis Rheum., 8:551–559, 1965.
177. Hart, L.E., et al.: Grading of tenderness as a source of interrater error in the Ritchie articular index. J. Rheumatol., 12:716–717, 1985.
178. Hart, L.E., Tugwell, P., and Buchanan, W.W.: Observer variation and the Ritchie articular index. Letter to the Editor. J. Rheumatol., 13:836–837, 1986.
179. Thompson, P.W., and Kirwan, J.R.: Observer variation and the Ritchie articular index. Letter to the Editor. J. Rheumatol., 13:836, 1986.
180. Scott, D.L.: Clinical measurements in rheumatology. Editorial Br. J. Rheumatol., 26:81–83, 1987.
181. Dresher, E., Pugh, L.G.C., and Wild, J.B.: ACTH in rheumatoid arthritis compared with intramuscular adrenaline and with deoxycortone and ascorbic acid. Lancet, 1:1149–1153, 1950.
182. Cousins, G.R.: Effect of trained and untrained testers upon the administration of grip strength tests. Res. Q., 26:273–276, 1955.
183. DeChoisy, J.: A new method of assessing grip strength and wrist and arm movement in the arthritic patients. Rheumatol. Rehabil., 12(Suppl.):81–84, 1973.
184. Hunsicker, R.A., and Donnelly, R.V.: Instruments to measure strength. Res. Q., 26:408–419, 1955.
185. Savage, O.: Criteria for measurement in chronic diseases. Proc. R. Soc. Med., 51(Suppl. 59):85–88, 1958.
186. Lee, P., et al.: An assessment of grip strength measurement in rheumatoid arthritis. Scand. J. Rheumatol., 3:17–23, 1974.
187. Wright, V.: Some observations on diurnal variation on grip strength. Clin. Sci., 18:17–23, 1959.
188. Lee, P., et al.: The evaluation of a functional index in rheumatoid arthritis. Scand. J. Rheumatol., 2:71–77, 1973.
189. Spiegel, J.S., et al.: What are we measuring? An examination of walk time and grip strength. J. Rheumatol., 14:80–86, 1987.
190. Myers, D.B., Grennan, D.M., and Plamer, D.G.: Hand grip function in patients with rheumatoid arthritis. Arch. Phys. Med. Rehabil., 61:369–373, 1980.
191. Buchanan, W.W., et al.: Rheumatoid hand weakness characterising indices and clinical data acquisition. Eng. Med., 13:115–120, 1984.
192. Downie, W.W., Leatham, P.A., and Rhind, V.M.: The visual analogue scale in the assessment of grip strength. Ann. Rheum. Dis., 37:382–384, 1978.
193. Boardman, P.L., and Hart, F.D.: Clinical measurement of the

anti-inflammatory effects of salicylates in rheumatoid arthritis. Br. Med. J., *4*:264–268, 1967.

194. Collins, K.E., et al.: Radioactive technetium (^{99m}Tc) uptake in the proximal interphalangeal joints and the effects of oral corticosteroids. Ann. Rheum. Dis., *30*:401–405, 1971.

195. Rhind, V.M., Bird, W.A., and Wright, V.: A comparison of clinical assessments of disease activity in rheumatoid arthritis. Ann. Rheum. Dis., *39*:35–137, 1980.

196. Fremont-Smith, F., Harter, J.G., and Halberg, F.: Circadian rhythmicity of proximal interphalangeal (PIP) joint circumference in patients with rheumatoid arthritis. Arthritis Rheum., *12*:294, 1969.

197. Wilkens, R.F., Gleichert, J.E., and Gade, E.T.: Proximal interphalangeal joint measurement by arthrocircameter. Ann. Rheum. Dis., *32*:585–586, 1973.

198. Goetzl, E.J., et al.: A physical approach to the assessment of disease activity in rheumatoid arthritis. J. Clin. Invest., *50*:1167–1180, 1971.

199. Lee, P., et al.: The evaluation of antirheumatic drugs. Curr. Med. Res. Opin., *1*:427–443, 1973.

200. Steinberg, A.D.: On morning stiffness. J. Rheumatol., *5*:3–6, 1978.

201. Buchanan, W.W., and Tugwell, P.: Traditional assessment of articular diseases. Clin. Rheum. Dis., *9*:515–529, 1983.

202. Jobbins, B., Bird, H.A., and Wright, V.: A finger arthrography for the quantification of joint stiffness. Eng. Med., *10*:85–88, 1981.

203. Wright, V., and Johns, R.J.: Physical factors concerned with the stiffness of normal diseased joints. Johns Hopkins Hosp. Bull., *106*:215–231, 1960.

204. Backlund, L., and Tiselius, P.: Objective measurement of joint stiffness in rheumatoid arthritis. Acta Rheumatol. Scand., *13*:175–288, 1967.

205. Ingpen, M.L.: The quantitative measurement of joint changes in rheumatoid arthritis. Ann. Phys. Med., *9*:322–327, 1968.

206. Howe, A., Thompson, D., and Wright, V.: Reference values for metacarpo-phalangeal joint stiffness in normals. Ann. Rheum. Dis., *44*:469–476, 1985.

207. Pearson, R., et al.: Diurnal and sequential grip function in normal subjects and effects of temperature change and exercise of the forearm on grip function in patients with rheumatoid arthritis and in normal controls. Scand. J. Rheumatol., *11*:113–118, 1982.

208. Scott, J.T.: Morning stiffness in rheumatoid arthritis. Ann. Rheum. Dis., *19*:361–368, 1960.

209. Magder, R., Baxter, M.L., and Kassam, Y.B.: Does a diuretic improve morning stiffness? Letter to the Editor. Br. J. Rheumatol., *25*:318–319, 1986.

210. Rasker, J.J., Peters, H.J.G., and Boon, K.L.: Influence of weather on stiffness and force in patients with rheumatoid arthritis. Scand. J. Rheumatol., *15*:27–36, 1986.

211. Khong, T.K., et al.: Sleep disturbance due to arthritis: The efficacy of piroxicam in rheumatoid arthritis. New York, Academic Professional Information Service, 1982.

212. American Academy of Orthopaedic Surgeons: Joint Motion: Method of Measuring and Recording. Edinburgh, Churchill Livingstone, 1966.

213. Wright, V.: Measurement of Joint Movement. Philadelphia, W.B. Saunders Co., 1982.

214. Mitchell, W.S., Miller, J., and Sturrock, R.: An evaluation of goniometry as an objective parameter for measuring joint motion. Scott. Med. J., *20*:57–59, 1975.

215. Johnson, F.: The knee. Clin. Rheum. Dis., *8*:677–702, 1092.

216. Moll, J.M.H., and Wright, V.: Normal range of spinal mobility. Ann. Rheum. Dis., *30*:381–386, 1971.

217. Dunham, W.F.: Ankylosing spondylitis—Measurement of hip and spine movement. Br. J. Phys. Med., *12*:126–129, 1949.

218. Hart, F.D., and MacLagan, N.F.: Ankylosing spondylitis. A review of 184 cases. Ann. Rheum. Dis., *14*:77–89, 1955.

219. Goff, B., and Rose, G.K.: The use of a modified spondylometer in the treatment of ankylosing spondylitis. Rheumatism, *20*:63–66, 1964.

220. Sturrock, R.D., Wojtulewski, J., and Hart, F.D.: Spondylometry in a normal population and in ankylosing spondylitis. Rheumatol. Rehabil., *12*:135–142, 1973.

221. Hart, F.D., Strickland, D., and Cliffe, P.: Measurement of spinal mobility. Ann. Rheum. Dis., *33*:136–139, 1974.

222. Anderson, J.A.D.: The thoraco-lumbar spine. *In* Measurement of Joint Movement. Edited by V. Wright. Clin. Rheum. Dis., *8*:631–653, 1982.

223. Schober, P.: Tendenwirbelsaule und Kreuzschmerzen. Munch. Med. Wschr., *84*:336–338, 1937.

224. Macrae, J.F., and Wright, V.: Measurement of back movement. Ann. Rheum. Dis., *28*:548–589, 1969.

225. Moll, J.M.H., Liyanage, S.P., and Wright, V.: An objective clinical method to measure lateral spinal flexion. Rheum. Phys. Med., *11*:225–239, 1972.

226. Moll, J.M.H., Liyanage, S.P., and Wright, V.: An objective clinical method to measure spinal extension. Rheum. Phys. Med., *11*:293–312, 1972.

227. Loebl, W.Y.: Measurement of spinal posture and range of spinal movement. Ann. Phys. Med., *9*:103–110, 1967.

228. Domjan, L., and Balint, G.: A new goniometer for measuring spinal and peripheral joint mobility. Hung. Rheum., *28*(Suppl.):71–76, 1987.

229. Wiles, P.: Movement of the lumbar vertebrae during flexion and extension. Proc. R. Soc. Med., *26*:647–651, 1935.

230. Tanz, S.S.: Motion of the lumbar spine: A roentgenologic study. Am. J. Roentgenol., *69*:399–412, 1953.

231. Jonck, L.M., and van Niekerk, J.M.: A roentgenological study of the motion of the lumbar spine in the Bantu. S. Afr. J. Lab. Clin. Med., *7*:67–71, 1961.

232. Reynolds, P.M.G.: Measurement of spinal mobility: A comparison of three methods. Rheumatol. Rehabil., *14*:180–185, 1975.

233. Steinbrocker, O., Traeger, C.H., and Batterman, R.C.: Therapeutic criteria in rheumatoid arthritis. JAMA, *140*:659–662, 1949.

234. Lee, P., and Dick, W.C.: The assessment of disease activity and drug evaluation in rheumatoid arthritis. *In* Recent Advances in Rheumatology I. Part 2. Edited by W.W. Buchanan, and W.C. Dick. New York, Churchill Livingstone, 1976.

235. Lowman, E.W.: Rehabilitation of the rheumatoid cripple: A five-year study. Arthritis Rheum., *1*:38–43, 1958.

236. Mahoney, F.I., and Barthel, D.W.: Functional evaluation: The Barthel index. Md State Med. J., *14*:61–65, 1965.

237. Mason, R.M., et al.: Assessment of drugs in outpatients with rheumatoid arthritis. Ann. Rheum. Dis., *26*:373–388, 1967.

238. McEwen, C.: Evaluation of the patient as a whole and evaluation of the individual functional units of the musculoskeletal system. *In* The Surgical Management of Rheumatoid Arthritis. Edited by L. Preston and C. McEwen. Philadelphia, W.B. Saunders Co., 1968.

239. Convery, F.R., et al.: Polyarticular disability: A functional assessment. Arch. Phys. Med. Rehabil., *58*:494–499, 1977.

240. Savage, O.: Criteria for measurement in chronic diseases. Re-

port on a Symposium on Clinical Trials. Pfizer, Kent, England, 32, 1958.

241. Liang, M.H., and Jette, A.M.: Measuring functional ability in chronic arthritis. Arthritis Rheum., 24:80–86, 1981.

242. Helewa, A., Goldsmith, C.H., and Smythe, H.A.: Independent measurement of functional capacity in rheumatoid arthritis. J. Rheumatol., 9:793–796, 1982.

243. Jette, A.M.: Functional capacity evaluation: An empirical approach. Arch. Phys. Med. Rehabil., 61:85–89, 1980.

244. Tugwell, P., et al.: The ability of MACTAR Disability Questionnaire to detect sensitivity to change in rheumatoid arthritis. Clin. Res., 31:129A, 1983.

245. Grace, E.M., Gerecz, E.M., Kassam, Y.B., and Buchanan, W.W.: Fifty-foot walking time: An inappropriate outcome measure in clinical therapeutic trials of anti-rheumatic drugs. Br. J. Rheumatol., (in press).

246. Bergner, M., et al.: The sickness impact profile: Validation of a health status measure. Med. Care, 14:57–67, 1976.

247. Kaplan, R.M., Bush, J.W., and Berry, C.C.: Health status: Types of validity for an index of well-being. Health Serv. Res., 11:478–507, 1976.

248. Meenan, R.F., Gertman, P.M., and Mason, J.H.: Measuring health status in arthritis: The arthritis impact measurement scales. Arthritis Rheum., 23:146–152, 1980.

249. Fries, J.F., et al.: Measurement of patient outcome in arthritis. Arthritis Rheum., 23:137–145, 1980.

250. Chambers, L.W., et al.: The McMaster Health Index Questionnaire as a measure of quality of life for patients with rheumatoid disease. J. Rheumatol., 9:780–784, 1982.

251. Liang, M.H., Cullen, K., and Larson, M.: In search of a more perfect mousetrap (health status or quality of life instrument). J. Rheumatol., 9:775–779, 1982.

252. Schipper, H.: Editorial. Why measure quality of life? Can. Med. Assoc. J., 128:1367–1370, 1983.

253. Liang, M.H., et al.: Cost and outcomes in rheumatoid arthritis and osteoarthritis. Arthritis Rheum., 27:522–529, 1984.

254. Meenan, R.F., et al.: Outcome assessment in clinical trials. Evidence for the sensitivity of a health status measure. Arthritis Rheum., 27:1344–1352, 1984.

255. Nevitt, M.C., Epstein, W.V., Masem, M., and Murray, W.R.: Work disability before and after total hip arthroplasty. Arthritis Rheum., 27:410–421, 1984.

256. Durham, J., et al.: The M.D.R. index of function in rheumatoid arthritis. Clin. Exp. Rheumatol., 3:297–302, 1985.

257. Liang, M.H., Larson, M.G., Cullen, K.E., and Schwartz, J.A.: Comparative measurement efficiency and sensitivity of five health status instruments for arthritis research. Arthritis Rheum., 28:542–547, 1985.

258. Nicassio, P.M., et al.: The measurement of helplessness in rheumatoid arthritis. The development of the arthritis helplessness index. J. Rheumatol., 12:462–467, 1985.

259. Fries, J.F., et al.: Impact of specific therapy upon rheumatoid arthritis. Arthritis Rheum., 29:620–627, 1986.

260. Guyatt, G.H., Bombardier, C., and Tugwell, P.: Measuring disease-specific quality of life in clinical trials. Can. Med. Assoc. J., 134:889–895, 1986.

261. Kirwan, J.R., and Reeback, J.S.: Standard Health Assessment Questionnaire modified to assess disability in British patients with rheumatoid arthritis. Br. J. Rheumatol., 25:206–209, 1986.

262. Yelin, E.H., Henke, C.J., and Epstein, W.W.: Work disability among persons with musculoskeletal conditions. Arthritis Rheum., 29:1322–1333, 1986.

263. Sullivan, M., Ahlmen, M., Archenholtz, B., and Svensson, G.: Measuring health in rheumatic disorders by means of a Swedish version of the sickness impact profile. Scand. J. Rheumatol., 15:193–200, 1986.

264. Spiegel, J.S., Hirshfield, M.S., and Spiegel, T.M.: Evaluating self-care activities: Comparison of a self-reported questionnaire with an occupational therapist interview. Br. J. Rheumatol., 24:357–361, 1985.

265. Kirwan, J.R., et al.: An international comparison of judgment in rheumatoid arthritis. J. Rheumatol., 10:901–905, 1983.

266. Kirwan, J.R., Chaput de Saintonge, D.M., Joyce, C.R.B., and Currey, H.L.F.: Clinical judgment in rheumatoid arthritis I. Rheumatologists' opinions and the development of "paper patients." Ann. Rheum. Dis., 42:644–647, 1983.

267. Kirwan, J.R., Chaput de Saintonge, D.M., Joyce, C.R.B., and Currey, M.L.F.: Clinical judgment in rheumatoid arthritis II. Judging current disease activity in clinical practice. Ann. Rheum. Dis., 42:648–651, 1983.

268. Kirwan, J.R., Chaput de Saintonge, D.M., Joyce, C.R.B., and Currey, H.L.F.: Clinical judgment of rheumatoid arthritis III. British rheumatologists' judgments of "change in response to therapy." Ann. Rheum. Dis., 43:686–694, 1984.

269. Kirwan, J.R., and Currey, H.L.F.: Clinical judgment in rheumatoid arthritis IV. Rheumatologists' assessments of disease remain stable over long periods. Ann. Rheum. Dis., 43:695–697, 1984.

270. Williams, H.J., et al.: Comparison of low-dose oral pulse methotrexate and placebo in the treatment of rheumatoid arthritis. A controlled clinical trial. Arthritis Rheum., 28:721–730, 1985.

271. Potts, M.K., and Brandt, K.D.: Evidence of the validity of the arthritis impact measurement scales. Arthritis Rheum., 30:93–96, 1987.

272. Bacon, P.A., et al.: Thermography in the assessment of inflammatory arthritis. Clin. Rheum. Dis., 2:51–65, 1976.

273. Laurent, M.R., and Panayi, G.S.: Biochemical parameters in the assessment of anti-inflammatory drugs. A review. Agents Actions, 7(Suppl.):310–317, 1980.

274. Huskisson, E.C., and Scott, P.J.: Flectafenine: A new analgesic for use in rheumatic diseases. Rheumatol. Rehabil., 16:54–57, 1977.

275. Davidson, J.W., and Thomson, J.G.: Thermographic survey in chronic rheumatic diseases. Med. Thermography, 1978, pp. 267–271.

276. Haberman, J.A., et al.: Thermography in arthritis. Arthritis Rheum., 14:387, 1971.

277. Ring, E.F.J., et al.: Quantitation of thermography in arthritis using multi-isothermal analysis II. Effect of nonsteroidal anti-inflammatory therapy on the thermographic plus index. Ann. Rheum. Dis., 33:353–356, 1974.

278. Bacon, P.A., Collins, A.J., and Cosh, J.A.: Thermographic assessment of the anti-inflammatory effect of flurbiprofen in rheumatoid arthritis. Scand. J. Rheumatol., 4(Suppl. 8):11–17, 1975.

279. Bird, H.A., et al.: Comparison of intra-articular methotrexate with intra-articular triamcinolone hexacetonide by thermography. Curr. Med. Res. Opin., 5:141–146, 1977.

280. Bird, H.A., Ring, E.F.J., and Bacon, P.A.: A thermographic and clinical comparison of the intra-articular steroid preparations in rheumatoid arthritis. Ann. Rheum. Dis., 38:36–39, 1979.

281. Bucknall, R.C., et al.: A thermographic assessment of the anti-inflammatory effect of D-pencillamine in rheumatoid arthritis. Scand. J. Rheumatol., 4(Suppl. 8):21–29, 1975.

282. Hall, N.D., et al.: A combined clinical and immunological

assessment of four cyclophosphamide regimes in rheumatoid arthritis. Agents Actions, *9*:97–102, 1979.

283. Devereaux, M.D., Parr, G.R., Page Thomas, D.P., and Hazleman, B.L.: Disease activity indexes in rheumatoid arthritis; a prospective, comparative study with thermography. Ann. Rheum. Dis., *44*:434–437, 1985.

284. DeSilva, M., et al.: Assessment of inflammation in the rheumatoid knee joint: Correlation between clinical radioisotopic, and thermographic methods. Ann. Rheum. Dis., *45*:277–280, 1986.

285. Paterson, J., et al.: The assessment of rheumatoid inflammation in the knee. Ann. Rheum. Dis., *37*:48–52, 1978.

286. Thomas, D., et al.: Knee-joint temperature measurement using a differential thermistor thermometer. Rheumatol. Rehabil., *19*:8–13, 1980.

287. Levinson, J.E., et al.: Comparison of tolmetin sodium and aspirin in the treatment of juvenile rheumatoid arthritis. J. Pediatr., *91*:799–904, 1977.

288. Fraser, S., Land, D., and Sturrock, R.D.: Microwave thermography—An index in inflammatory joint disease. Br. J. Rheumatol., *26*:37–39, 1987.

289. Mowat, A.G.: Hematological abnormalities in rheumatoid arthritis. Semin. Arthritis Rheum., *1*:195–198, 1971.

290. Wright, V., et al.: Erythrocyte sedimentation rate (ESR) *In* Symposia Medica Hoechst 16. Controversies in the Clinical Evaluation of Analgesic Anti-inflammatory-Antirheumatic Drugs. Edited by H.E. Paulus, G.E. Ehrlich, and E. Lindenlaub. Stuttgart, Schattauer Verlag, 1981.

291. Grindulis, K.A., et al.: A comparison between clinical and laboratory tests in rheumatoid arthritis. Scand. J. Rheumatol., *12*:285–288, 1983.

292. Berry, H., et al.: Antirheumatic activity of fenclofenac. Ann. Rheum. Dis., *39*:473–475, 1980.

293. Larkin, J.G., Lowe, G.D.O., Sturrock, R.D., and Forbes, C.D.: The relationship of plasma and serum viscosity to disease activity and smoking habit in rheumatoid arthritis. Br. J. Rheumatol., *23*:15–19, 1984.

294. McConkey, B., et al.: The effects of some anti-inflammatory drugs on the acute phase reactants in rheumatoid arthritis. A study based on measurements of serum acute phase reactants. Q. J. Med., New Series, *41*:115–125, 1972.

295. McConkey, B., et al.: The effects of some anti-inflammatory drugs on the acute phase reactants in rheumatoid arthritis. Q. J. Med., New Series, *42*:785–791, 1973.

296. Alyward, M., et al.: A study of the influence of various antirheumatic drug regimens on serum acute phase proteins, plasma tryptophan and erythrocyte sedimentation rate in rheumatoid arthritis. Rheumatol. Rehabil., *14*:101–114, 1975.

297. Constable, T.J., Crockson, R.A., Crockson, A.P., and McConkey, B.: Drug treatment of rheumatoid arthritis. Lancet, *1*:1176–1179, 1975.

298. McConkey, B., et al.: Dapsone in rheumatoid arthritis. Rheumatol. Rehabil., *15*:230, 1976.

299. Amos, R.S., et al.: Rheumatoid arthritis: A relation of serum C-reactive protein and erythrocyte sedimentation rate to radiographic changes. Br. Med. J., *1*:195–197, 1977.

300. Runge, L.A., et al.: Treatment of rheumatoid arthritis with levamisole. A controlled trial. Arthritis Rheum., *20*:1445–1448, 1977.

301. Amos, R.S., et al.: Rheumatoid arthritis: Relation of CRP and ESR to radiographic changes. Br. Med. J., *1*:195, 1977.

302. McConkey, B., et al.: Effects of gold, dapsone and prednisolone and C-reactive protein and serum haptoglobin and erythrocyte sedimentation rate in rheumatoid arthritis. Ann. Rheum. Dis., *38*:141–144, 1979.

303. Walsh, L., Davies, P., and McConkey, B.: Relationship between erythrocyte sedimentation rate and C-reactive protein in rheumatoid arthritis. Ann. Rheum. Dis., *38*:362–363, 1979.

304. Crook, L., et al.: Erythrocyte sedimentation, viscosity and plasma proteins in disease detection. Ann. Clin. Lab. Sci., *10*:368–376, 1980.

305. Dixon, J.S., et al.: C-reactive protein in the serial assessment of disease activity in rheumatoid arthritis. Scand. J. Rheumatol., *13*:39–44, 1984.

306. Dixon, J.S.: Relationship between plasma viscosity on ESR and the Ritchie articular index. Letter to the Editor. Br. J. Rheumatol., *23*:232–236, 1984.

307. Larkin, J.: Relationship between plasma viscosity or ESR and the Ritchie articular index. Letter to the Editor. Br. J. Rheumatol., *23*:235, 1984.

308. Mielke, H., and Deicher, H.: Correlation of inflammatory RA disease activity with laboratory parameters. Scand. J. Rheumatol., *16*:22–24, 1985.

309. Dawes, P.J., et al.: Rheumatoid arthritis: Treatment which controls the C-reactive protein and erythrocyte sedimentation rate reduces radiological progression. Br. J. Rheumatol., *25*:44–49, 1986.

310. Cockel, R., et al.: Serum biochemical values in rheumatoid disease. Ann. Rheum. Dis., *30*:166–170, 1971.

311. Gotlieb, N.L., Kiem, I.M., Penneys, N.S., and Schultz, D.R.: The influence of chrysotherapy on serum protein and immunoglobulin levels, rheumatoid factor and anti-epithelial antibody titres. J. Lab. Clin. Med., *86*:962–972, 1975.

312. Lorber, A., et al.: Chrysotherapy: Suppression of immunoglobulin synthesis. Arthritis Rheum., *21*:785–791, 1978.

313. Alarcon, G.S., Koopman, W.J., and Schrohenloher, R.E.: In-vitro IgM and IgM rheumatoid factor production and response to remittive agents in rheumatoid arthritis. Letter to the Editor. Arthritis Rheum., *28*:356–357, 1985.

314. Pope, R.M., Lessard, J., and Nunnery, E.: Differential effects of therapeutic regimens on specific classes of rheumatoid factor. Ann. Rheum. Dis., *45*:183–189, 1986.

315. Robbins, D.L., et al.: Complement activation by 19S rheumatoid factor: Relationship to disease activity in rheumatoid arthritis. J. Rheumatol., *13*:33–39, 1986.

316. Robbins, D.L., Feigal, D.W. Jr., and Leek, J.C.: Relationship of serum IgG rheumatoid factor to IgM rheumatoid factor and disease activity in rheumatoid arthritis. J. Rheumatol., *13*:259–262, 1986.

317. Bluestone, R., and Goldberg, L.S.: Effects of D-penicillamine on serum immunoglobulins and rheumatoid factor. Ann. Rheum. Dis., *32*:50–52, 1973.

318. Cooperating Clinics Committee of the American Rheumatism Association: Controlled trial of cyclophosphamide in rheumatoid arthritis. N. Engl. J. Med., *283*:883–889, 1970.

319. Szpilman, H., et al.: Levamisole, cell-mediated immunity and serum immunoglobulins in rheumatoid arthritis. Lancet, *2*:208–209, 1976.

320. Popert, A.J., et al.: Chloroquine diphosphate in rheumatoid arthritis. Ann. Rheum. Dis., *20*:18–33, 1961.

321. Klinefelter, H.F., and Achurra, A.: Effect of gold salts and antimalarials on the rheumatoid factor titre in rheumatoid arthritis. Scand. J. Rheumatol., *2*:177–182, 1973.

322. Multicentre Trial Group: Controlled trials of D(−) penicillamine in severe rheumatoid arthritis. Lancet, *2*:75–280, 1973.

323. Day, A.T.: Penicillamine in rheumatoid disease: A long term study. Br. Med. J., *1*:180–183, 1974.

324. De Seze, S., and Kahn, M.F.: Immunosuppressive drugs in rheumatoid arthritis: Clinical results. Adv. Clin. Pharmacol., 6:89, 1974.

325. Mouridsen, H.T., Baerentsen, O., and Rossing, N.: Lack of effective gold therapy on abnormal IgG and IgM metabolism in rheumatoid arthritis. Arthritis Rheum., 17:391–396, 1974.

326. Berry, H., et al.: Azathioprine and penicillamine in treatment of rheumatoid arthritis: A controlled trial. Br. Med. J., 1:1052–1054, 1976.

327. Lorber, A., et al.: Chrysotherapy: Suppression of immunoglobulin synthesis. Arthritis Rheum., 21:785–791, 1978.

328. Amor, B., and Mery, C.: Chlorambucil in rheumatoid arthritis. Clin. Rheum. Dis., 6:567–584, 1980.

329. McKenzie, A.H., and Scherbel, A.L.: Chloroquine and hydroxychloroquine in rheumatological therapy. Clin. Rheum. Dis., 6:545–566, 1980.

330. Reeback, J.S., et al.: Circulating immune complexes and rheumatoid arthritis: A comparison of different assay methods and their early predictive value for disease activity and outcome. Ann. Rheum. Dis., 44:79–82, 1986.

331. Segal-Eiras, A., et al.: Effect of antimalarial treatment in circulating immune complexes in rheumatoid arthritis. J. Rheumatol., 12:87–89, 1985.

332. Reynolds, W.J., et al.: Circulating immune complexes in rheumatoid arthritis: A prospective study using five immunoassays. J. Rheumatol., 13:700–706, 1986.

333. Alepa, F.P., Zvaifler, N.J., and Sliwinski, A.J.: Immunologic effects of cyclophosphamide treatment in rheumatoid arthritis. Arthritis Rheum., 13:754–760, 1970.

334. Swanson, M.A., and Schwartz, R.S.: Immunosuppressure therapy: The relations between clinical response and immunology competence. N. Engl. J. Med., 277:163–170, 1967.

335. Multicentre Study Group: Levamisole in rheumatoid arthritis: A randomized double-blind study comparing two dosage regimens of levamisole with placebo. Lancet, 2:1007–1012, 1978.

336. Mille, B., et al.: Double-blind placebo controlled crossover evaluation of levamisole in rheumatoid arthritis. Arthritis Rheum., 23:172–182, 1980.

337. Mowat, A.G., Hothersall, T.E., and Aitchison, W.R.C.: Nature of anaemia in rheumatoid arthritis. Ann. Rheum. Dis., 28:303–309, 1969.

338. Harvey, A.R., et al.: Anemia associated with rheumatoid disease. Arthritis Rheum., 26:28–34, 1983.

339. Menander-Huber, K.B.: Orogotein in the treatment of rheumatoid arthritis. In International Workshop New Aspects of Therapy for Inflammation. Eur. J. Rheum. Inflamm., 4(Suppl.):201–211, 1981.

340. Grennan, D.M., et al.: Relationship between hemoglobin and other clinical and laboratory parameters in rheumatoid arthritis. Curr. Med. Res. Opin., 3:104–108, 1975.

341. Winchester, R.J., et al.: Observation on the eosinophilia of certain patients with rheumatoid arthritis. Arthritis Rheum., 14:650–655, 1971.

342. Hernandez, L.A., et al.: Thrombocytosis in rheumatoid arthritis: A clinical study of 200 patients. Rhumatologie, 5:635–640, 1975.

343. Hutchinson, R.M., Davis, P., and Jayson, M.I.V.: Thrombocytosis in rheumatoid arthritis. Ann. Rheum. Dis., 35:138–142, 1976.

344. Aylward, M., and Maddock, J.: Total and free tryptophan concentrations in rheumatic disease. J. Pharm. Pharmacol., 25:570–572, 1973.

345. McArthur, J.N., Dawkins, P.D., and Smith, M.J.H.: The displacement of L-tryptophan and dipeptides from bovine albumin in vitro and from human plasma in vivo by antirheumatic drugs. J. Pharm. Pharmacol., 23:393–398, 1971.

346. Lorber, A., et al.: Serum sulphydryl determinations and their significance in connective tissue diseases. Ann. Intern. Med., 61:423–434, 1964.

347. Lorber, A., Bovy, R.A., and Chang, C.C.: Sulphydryl deficiency in connective tissue disorders. Correlation with disease activity and protein alterations. Metabolism, 20:446–455, 1971.

348. Haataja, M., Nissila, M., and Ruutsalo, H.K.: Serum sulphydryl levels in rheumatoid patients treated with gold thiomalate and penicillamine. Scand. J. Rheumatol., 7:212–214, 1978.

349. Dixon, J.S., et al.: Discriminating indices of response of patients with rheumatoid arthritis treated with D-penicillamine. Ann. Rheum. Dis., 39:301–381, 1980.

350. Conference Proceedings: Do drugs alter the course of rheumatoid arthritis? Ann. Rheum. Dis., 41:549–550, 1982.

351. Grimaldi, M.G.: Serum sulfhydryl levels in rheumatoid patients treated with cyclophosphamide. Scand. J. Rheumatol., 9:237–240, 1980.

352. Ambanelli, U., Spisni, A., and Ferraccioli, G.F.: Serum antioxidant activity and related variables in rheumatoid arthritis. Scand. J. Rheumatol., 11:203–207, 1982.

353. Rae, K.J., et al.: Early and late changes in sulphydryl group and copper protein concentrations and activities during drug treatment with aurothiomalate and auranofin. Ann. Rheum. Dis., 45:839–846, 1986.

354. White, A.G., et al.: Copper—An index of erosive activity. Rheumatol. Rehabil., 17:3–5, 1978.

355. Brown, D.H., et al.: Serum copper and its relationship to clinical symptoms in rheumatoid arthritis. Ann. Rheum. Dis., 38:174–176, 1979.

356. Halberg, P., et al.: Double-blind trial of levamisole, penicillamine and azathioprine in rheumatoid arthritis. Danish Med. Bull., 31:403–409, 1984.

357. Horslev-Petersen, K., Bentsen, K.D., Junker, P., and Lorenzen, I.: Serum amino-terminal type III procollagen peptide in rheumatoid arthritis. Relationship to disease activity, treatment, and development of joint erosions. Arthritis Rheum., 29:592–599, 1986.

358. Hall, S.H., et al.: Intra-articular methotrexate clinical and laboratory study in rheumatoid and psoriatic arthritis. Ann. Rheum. Dis., 37:351–356, 1978.

359. Cruickshank, B.: Interpretation of multiple biopsies of synovial tissue in rheumatic diseases. Ann. Rheum. Dis., 11:137–143, 1952.

360. Dixon, J.S., Wright, V.: Outcome measure and anti-rheumatoid drugs: A critical appraisal. Editorial. Clin. Exp. Rheumatol., 4:1–2, 1986.

361. Pullar, T., Hunter, J.A., and Capell, H.A.: Does second-line therapy affect the radiological progression of rheumatoid arthritis? Ann. Rheum. Dis., 43:18–23, 1983.

362. Pullar, T., and Capell, H.A.: Can treatment really influence the radiological progression of rheumatoid arthritis? Editorial. Br. J. Rheumatol., 25:2–6, 1986.

363. Lidsky, M.D., Sharp, J.T., and Billings, S.: Double-blind study of cyclophosphamide in rheumatoid arthritis. Arthritis Rheum., 16:148–153, 1973.

364. Sigler, J.W., Bluhm, G.B., and Duncan, H.: Gold salts in the treatment of RA. A double-blind study. Ann. Intern. Med., 80:21–26, 1974.

365. Gibson, T., et al.: Evidence that D-penicillamine alters the course of rheumatoid arthritis. Rheumatol. Rehabil., 15:211–215, 1976.

366. Luukkainen, R., Isomaki, H., and Kajander, A.: Effect of gold

treatment on the progression of erosions in R.A. patients. Scand. J. Rheumatol., 6:123–127, 1977.

367. Luukkainen, R., Kajander, A., and Isomaki, H.: Effect of gold in progression of erosions in rheumatoid arthritis. Better results with early treatment. Scand. J. Rheumatol., 6:189–192, 1977.

368. Wright, V., and Amos, R.: Do drugs change the course of rheumatoid arthritis? Br. Med. J., 280:964–966, 1980.

369. Gofton, J.P., and O'Brien, W.M.: Effects of auranofin on the radiological progression of joint erosion in rheumatoid arthritis. J. Rheumatol., 9(Suppl. 8):169–172, 1982.

370. Sharp, J.T., Lidsky, M.D., and Duffy, J.: Clinical responses during gold therapy for rheumatoid arthritis. Arthritis Rheum., 25:540–549, 1982.

371. Gofton, J.P., and O'Brien, W.M.: Radiographic evaluation of erosion in rheumatoid arthritis: Double blind study of auranofin vs placebo. J. Rheumatol., 11:768–771, 1984.

372. Iannauzzi, L., Dawson, N., Zein, N., and Kushner, I.: Does any therapy slow radiographic deterioration in rheumatoid arthritis? N. Engl. J. Med., 309:1023–1028, 1983.

373. Ingeman-Nielwn, M., et al.: Clinical synovitis and radiological lesions in rheumatoid arthritis. Scand. J. Rheumatol., 12:237–240, 1983.

374. Kirwan, J.R., and Currey, H.L.F.: Rheumatoid arthritis—Disease modifying anti-rheumatic drugs. Clin. Rheum. Dis., 9:581–600, 1983.

375. Gofton, J.P.: Problems associated with measurement of radiological progression of disease in rheumatoid arthritis. J. Rheumatol., 10:177–179, 1983.

376. Hernandez, L.A., et al.: Rheumatoid juxta-articular erosions: Healing with first line drugs. Rheumatology, 7:41–45, 1978.

377. Dawes, P.T., et al.: Prediction of progressive joint damage in patients with rheumatoid arthritis receiving gold or D-penicillamine therapy. Ann. Rheum. Dis., 45:945–949, 1986.

378. Dawes, P.T., et al.: Rheumatoid arthritis: Treatment which controls the C-reactive protein and erythrocyte sedimentation rate reduces radiological progression. Br. J. Rheumatol., 25:44–49, 1986.

379. Kellgren, J.H., Jeffrey, M.R., and Ball, J.: Atlas of Standard Radiograph of Arthritis. Blackwell Scientific Publications, Oxford, 1963.

380. Norgaard, F.: Earliest roentgenological changes in polyarthritis of the rheumatoid type: Rheumatoid arthritis. Radiology, 85:325–239, 1965.

381. Brewerton, D.A.: Instrumental and technical roles. A tangential radiographic projection for demonstrating involvement of the metacarpal heads in R.A. Br. J. Radiol., 40:233–234, 1967.

382. Sharp, J.T., et al.: Methods of scoring the progression of radiological changes in rheumatoid arthritis. Arthritis Rheum., 14:706–720, 1971.

383. Larsen, A.: Radiological grading of rheumatoid arthritis: An inter-observer study. Scand. J. Rheumatol., 2:136–138, 1973.

384. Amos, R.S., et al.: Rheumatoid arthritis: Relation of serum C-reaction protein and erythrocyte sedimentation rates to radiographic changes. Br. Med. J., 1:195–197, 1985.

385. Larsen, A., Dale, K., and Eek, M.: Radiographic evaluation of rheumatoid arthritis and related conditions by standard reference films. Acta Radiol. Diagnosis, 18:481–491, 1977.

386. Larsen, A., et al.: Interobserver variation in the evaluation of radiologic changes of rheumatoid arthritis. Scand. J. Rheumatol., 8:109–112, 1979.

387. De Carvalho, A., and Graudal, H.: Radiographic progression of rheumatoid arthritis related to some clinical and laboratory parameters. Acta Radiol. Diagnosis, 21:551–555, 1980.

388. DeCarvalho, A., Graudal, H., and Jrgensen, B.: Radiologic evaluation of the progression of rheumatoid arthritis. Acta Radiol. Diagnosis, 21:115–121, 1980.

389. DeCarvalho, A.: Discriminative power of Larsen's grading system for assessing the course of rheumatoid arthritis. Acta Radiol. Diagnosis, 22:77–80, 1981.

390. Buckland-Wright, J.C.: X-ray assessment of activity in rheumatoid disease. Br. J. Rheumatol., 22:3–10, 1981.

391. Buckland-Wright, J.C.: Advances in the radiological assessment of rheumatoid arthritis. Br. J. Rheumatol., 22(Suppl. 1):34–43, 1983.

392. Genant, H.K.: Methods of assessing radiographic change in rheumatoid arthritis. Am. J. Med., 74:35–47, 1983.

393. Grindulis, K.A., Scott, D.L., and Struthers, G.R.: The assessment of radiographical progression in the hands and wrists in rheumatoid arthritis. Rheumatol. Int., 3:39–42, 1983.

394. Larsen, A., Horton, J., and Osborne, C.: Auranofin compared with intramuscular gold in the long term treatment of rheumatoid arthritis: An x-ray analysis. In Auranofin. Edited by H.A. Capell, D.S. Cole, K.K. Manghani and R.W. Morris. Amsterdam, Excerpta Medica, 1983.

395. Sharp, J.T.: Radiographic evaluation of the course of articular disease. Clin. Rheum. Dis., 9:541–548, 1983.

396. Mewa, A.A.M., et al.: Observer differences in detecting erosions in radiographs of rheumatoid arthritis. A comparison of posteroanterior, Norgaard and Brewerton views. J. Rheumatol., 12:216–221, 1983.

397. Bland, J.H., et al.: A study of inter- and intra-observer error in reading plain roentgenograms of the hands. Am. J. Roentgenol., 105:853, 1969.

398. Smith, D.W., and Bluhm, G.B.: Rater reliability in reading PA films of hand for bone and cartilage changes in rheumatoid arthritis. Eur. J. Rheumatol. Inflamm., 5:198–225, 1982.

399. Luukkainen, R., Isomaki, H., and Kajander, A.: Prognostic value of the type of onset of rheumatoid arthritis. Ann. Rheum. Dis., 42:274–275, 1983.

400. Scott, D.L., Coulton, B.L., Bacon, P.A., and Popert, A.J.: Methods of x-ray assessment in rheumatoid arthritis: a reevaluation. Br. J. Rheum., 24:31–39, 1985.

401. Scott, D.L., et al.: Anti-rheumatic drugs and joint damage in rheumatoid arthritis. Q. J. Med., 54:49–59, 1985.

402. Sjoblom, K.G., Saxne, T., Pettersson, H., and Wollheim, F.A.: Factors related to the progression of joint destruction in rheumatoid arthritis. Scand. J. Rheumatol., 1:21–27, 1984.

403. Sharp, J.T., et al.: Reproducibility of multiple-observer scoring of radiological abnormalities in the hands and wrists of patients with rheumatoid arthritis. Arthritis Rheum., 28:16–24, 1985.

404. Burns, T.M., and Calin, A.: The hand radiograph as a diagnostic discriminant between seropositive and seronegative "rheumatoid arthritis": A controlled study. Ann. Rheum. Dis., 42:605–612, 1983.

405. Jacoby, R.K., Jayson, M.I.V., and Cosh, J.A.: Onset, early stages, and prognosis in rheumatoid arthritis: A clinical study of 100 patients with 11 year follow-up. Br. Med. J., 2:96–100, 1973.

406. Brook, A., Fleming, A., and Corbett, M.: Relationship of radiological change to clinical outcome in rheumatoid arthritis. Ann. Rheum. Dis., 36:274–275, 1977.

407. Young, A., Corbett, M., and Brook, A.: The clinical assessment of joint inflammatory activity in rheumatoid arthritis related to radiological progression. Rheumatol. Rehabil., 19:14–19, 1980.

408. Bjelle, A., Bjornham, A., Larsen, A., and Mjorndal, T.: Chlor-

oquine in long-term treatment of rheumatoid arthritis. Clin. Rheumatol., 2:393–399, 1983.

409. Bluhm, G.B., Smith, D.W., and Mikulashek, W.M.: A radiologic method of assessment of bone and joint destruction in rheumatoid arthritis. Henry Ford Hosp. Med. J., 31:152–161, 1983.

410. Luukkainen, R., Isomaki, H., and Kajander, A.: Prognostic value of the type of onset of rheumatoid arthritis. Ann. Rheum. Dis., 42:274–275, 1983.

411. Luukkainen, R., et al.: The prediction of radiological destruction during the early stages of rheumatoid arthritis. Clin. Exp. Rheumatol., 1:295–298, 1983.

412. Scott, D.L., et al.: The long-term effects of treating rheumatoid arthritis. J. R. Coll. Physicians (London), 17:79–85, 1983.

413. Scott, D.L., et al.: Progression of radiological changes in rheumatoid arthritis. Ann. Rheum. Dis., 43:8–17, 1984.

414. Edwards, J.C.W., Edwards, S.E., and Huskisson, E.C.: The value of radiography in the management of rheumatoid arthritis. Clin. Radiol., 34:413–416, 1983.

415. Buckland-Wright, J.C.: Microfocal radiographic examinations of erosions in the wrist and hand of patients with rheumatoid arthritis. Ann. Rheum. Dis., 43:160–171, 1984.

416. Gaydecki, P.A., Browne, M., Mamtora, H., and Grennan, D.M.: Measurement of radiographic changes occurring in rheumatoid arthritis by image analysis techniques. Ann. Rheum. Dis., 46:396–401, 1987.

417. Baker, D.G., Schumacher, H.R., and Wolf, G.L.: Nuclear magnetic resonance evaluation of synovial fluid and articular disease. J. Rheumatol., 12:1062–1065, 1985.

418. Wright, E.C., and Acheson, R.M.: New Haven survey of joint diseases XI. Observer variability in the assessment of x-rays for osteoarthritis of the hands. Am. J. Epidemiol., 91:378–392, 1970.

419. Koran, L.M.: The reliability of clinical methods, data, and judgments. N. Engl. J. Med., 293:642–646, 1975.

420. Hollingsworth, P.N., et al.: Observer variation in grading sacroiliac radiographs in HLA-B27 positive individuals. J. Rheumatol., 10:247–254, 1983.

421. Bellamy, N., et al.: Perception—A problem in the grading of sacroiliac joint radiographs. Scand. J. Rheumatol., 13:113–120, 1984.

422. Deyo, R.A., McNiesh, L.M., and Cone, R.O., III.: Observer variability in the interpretation of lumbar spine radiographs. Arthritis Rheum., 28:1066–1070, 1985.

423. Dick, W.C.: The use of radioisotopes in normal and diseased joints. Semin. Arthritis Rheum., 1:301–325, 1972.

424. Dick, W.C., and Grennan, D.M.: Radioisotopes in the study of normal and inflamed joints. Clin. Rheum. Dis., 2:67–76, 1976.

425. Wallace, D.J., Brachman, M., and Klinenberg, J.R.: Joint scanning in rheumatoid arthritis. A literature review. Semin. Arthritis Rheum., 11:172–176, 1981.

426. Dick, W.C., et al.: Isotope studies in normal and diseased knee joints: ^{99m}Tc uptake related to clinical assessment and to synovial perfusion measured by the ^{133}Xe clearance technique. Clin. Sci., 40:327–336, 1971.

427. Dick, W.C., et al.: Derivation of knee joint synovial perfusion using the xenon (^{133}Xe) clearance technique. Ann. Rheum. Dis., 29:131–134, 1970.

428. Dick, W.C., et al.: The effect of thymoxamine on peripheral blood vessels as monitored by the ^{133}Xe clearance technique. J. Pharm. Pharmacol., 23:204–208, 1971.

429. Dick, W.C., et al.: Studies on the sympathetic control of normal and diseased synovial blood vessels: The effect of A and B receptor stimulation and inhibition, monitored by the ^{133}xenon clearance technique. Clin. Sci., 40:197–209, 1971.

430. St. Onge, R.A., et al.: The effect of external heat and exercise on the ^{133}xenon clearance rate in normal and diseased human joints, and of injection volume, methacholine, and atropine on the ^{133}xenon clearance rate in the normal canine joint. Rev. Rhum., 38:87–101, 1971.

431. Grennan, D.M., et al.: Histamine receptors in the synovial microcirculation. Eur. J. Clin. Invest., 5:75–82, 1975.

432. Grennan, D.M., Zeitlin, I.J., and Dick, W.C.: Effects of inflammatory mediators on synovial blood flow. Prostaglandins, 9:799–816, 1975.

433. Dick, W.C., et al.: Clinical studies on inflammation in human knee joints: Xenon (^{133}Xe) clearances correlated with clinical assessment in various arthritides and studies on the effect of intra-articularly administered hydrocortisone in rheumatoid arthritis. Clin. Sci., 38:123–133, 1970.

434. Dick, W.C., et al.: Indices of inflammatory activity. Relationship between isotope studies and clinical methods. Ann. Rheum. Dis., 29:643–648, 1970.

435. Dick, W.C., et al.: Effects of anti-inflammatory drug therapy on clearance of ^{133}Xe from knee joints on patients with rheumatoid arthritis. Br. Med. J., 3:278–280, 1969.

436. McCarty, D.J., et al.: ^{99m}technetium scintiphotography in arthritis. I. Technic and interpretation. Arthritis Rheum., 13:11–21, 1970.

437. McCarty, D.J., Polcyn, R.E., and Collins, P.A.: ^{99m}technetium scintiphotography in arthritis. II. Its nonspecific and clinical and roentgenographic correlations in rheumatoid arthritis. Arthritis Rheum., 13:21–32, 1970.

438. Rosenspire, K.C., et al.: Comparison of four methods of analysis of ^{99}Tc pyrophosphate uptake in RA joints. J. Rheumatol., 7:461–468, 1980.

439. Lee, P., et al.: The technetium radioiodinated human fibrinogen and clinical indices in the assessment of disease activity in rheumatoid arthritis. J. Rheumatol., 1:432–440, 1974.

440. Huskisson, E.C., Scott, J., and Balme, H.W.: Objective measurement of R.A. using technetium index. Ann. Rheum. Dis., 35:81–82, 1976.

441. Berry, H., et al.: Radioisotope scanning using a gamma camera. Ann. Rheum. Dis., 37:76–77, 1978.

442. Boerbooms, A.M., and Buys, W.C.: Rapid assessment of ^{99m}Tc pertechnetate uptake in the knee joint as a parameter of inflammatory activity. Arthritis Rheum., 21:348–352, 1978.

443. Hays, M.T., and Green, F.A.: The pertechnetate joint scan. Ann. Rheum. Dis., 31:272–277, 1972.

444. Hoffer, P.B., and Genant, H.K.: Radionuclide joint imaging. Semin. Nucl. Med., 6:168–184, 1976.

445. Rosenspire, K.C., et al.: Investigation of the metabolic activity of bone in rheumatoid arthritis. J. Rheumatol., 7:469–473, 1980.

446. Oka, M., et al.: Measurement of systemic inflammatory activity in rheumatoid arthritis by the ^{99m}Tc method. Scand. J. Rheumatol., 2:101–107, 1973.

447. Rekonen, A., Juikka, J., and Oka, M.: Measurement of joint inflammation. Scand. J. Rheumatol., 3:75–78, 1974.

448. Collins, K.E., et al.: Radioisotope study of small joint inflammation in rheumatoid arthritis. Radioactive technetium (^{99m}Tc) uptake in the proximal interphalangeal joints and the effects of oral corticosteroids. Ann. Rheum. Dis., 30:401–405, 1971.

449. Sturrock, R.D., Nicholson, R., and Wojtulewski, J.: Technetium counting in rheumatoid arthritis: Evaluation in the small joints of the hands. Arthritis Rheum., 17:417–420, 1974.

450. Dick, W.C., et al.: Effect of synovectomy on the clearance of

radioactive xenon (^{133}Xe) from the knee joint of patients with rheumatoid arthritis. J. Bone Joint Surg., *5213*:70–76, 1970.

451. Chalmers, I.M., et al.: Sacroiliitis detected by bone scintiscanning: A clinical, radiological and scintigraphic follow-up study. Ann. Rheum. Dis., *38*:112, 1979.

452. Spencer, D.G., et al.: Scintiscanning in ankylosing spondylitis: A clinical, radiological and quantitative radioisotopic study. J. Rheumatol., *6*:426–431, 1979.

453. Russell, A.S., Lentle, B.C., and Percy, J.S.: Investigation of sacroiliac disease. J. Rheumatol., *2*:45–51, 1974.

454. Russell, A.S., Lentle, B.C., and Percy, J.S.: Investigation of sacroiliac disease. J. Rheumatol., *2*:45–51, 1985.

455. Namey, T.C., McIntyre, J., and Dune, M.: Nucleoradiographic studies of axial spondyloarthropathies. Arthritis Rheum., *20*:1058, 1977.

456. Ho, G., Jr., et al.: Quantitative sacroiliac scintigraphy. A critical assessment. Arthritis Rheum., *22*:837–844, 1979.

457. Shafer, A.: The ethics of the randomized clinical trial. N. Engl. J. Med., *307*:719–724, 1982.

458. Sackett, D.L.: The competing objectives of randomized trials. N. Engl. J. Med., *303*:1059–1060, 1980.

459. World Medical Association: Human experimentation, code of ethics of the World Medical Association. Declaration of Helsinski. Br. Med. J., *2*:177, 1964.

460. Meisel, A., and Roth, L.H.: What we do or do not know about informed consent. JAMA, *246*:2473–2477, 1981.

461. Garnham, J.C.: Some observations on informed consent in non-therapeutic research. J. Med. Ethics, *1*:138–145, 1975.

462. Stanley, B., Guido, J., Stanley, M., and Shortell, D.: The elderly patient and informed consent. JAMA, *252*:1302–1306, 1982.

463. Simes, R.J., et al.: Randomized comparison of procedures for obtaining informed consent in clinical trials of treatment for cancer. Br. Med. J., *293*:1065–1068, 1986.

464. Daham, R., et al.: Does informed consent influence therapeutic outcome? A clinical trial of the hypnotic activity of placebo in patients admitted to hospital. Br. Med. J., *293*:363–364, 1986.

465. Bernard, C.: An introduction to the study of experimental medicine. Translated by H.C. Greene, New York, Collier Books, 1961, p. 130.

SCIENTIFIC BASIS FOR THE STUDY OF THE RHEUMATIC DISEASES

STRUCTURE AND FUNCTION OF JOINTS

10

HENRY J. MANKIN and ERIC RADIN

The rigidity of structure and segmental stability of the human frame are provided by the bony skeleton. Interruptions in the rigid framework, the *joints*, allow controlled and almost frictionless movement. The bones and joints provide structural support and protection to vital parts, yet allow sufficient directed movement for the functions of locomotion and prehension. The purpose of this chapter is to discuss, in detail, the structure and function of the joint. Although all joints will be considered, synovial joints and the intervertebral disc will be emphasized, because they constitute most joints and are the most often involved by the disease processes discussed in this volume.

CLASSIFICATION OF JOINTS

Joints are most often classified according to the type of motion that occurs. Three groups are recognized: the immovable joints (synarthroses); slightly movable joints (amphiarthroses); and movable joints (diarthroses).[1] Another less commonly used classification is based on the nature of the specialized forms of connective tissue that are present.[1] The two classifications are interrelated in that the constituent bones of the immovable joints or slightly movable joints are connected by fibrous or cartilaginous membranes (syndesmoses or synchondroses), whereas the component bony parts of the movable joints, although covered by hyaline cartilage, are completely separated and contain between them a joint cavity lined by a synovial membrane (synovial joints).[1,2]

Synarthroses are generally found in the skull. The contributing bony plates that compose the joints are held firmly to each other by fibrous or cartilaginous elements. *Amphiarthroses* are characterized by the presence of broad, flattened discs of fibrocartilage connecting the articulating surfaces. The bony portions of the joint are usually covered by hyaline cartilage, and the entire structure is invested by a fibrous capsule. Such joints are those between the vertebrae, the distal tibiofibular articulation, and the pubic symphysis. *Diarthroses* include most of the joints of the extremities. The joint space articular cartilages and synovial membrane allow the wide ranges of motion necessary for the functions of locomotion and prehension.[1,2]

SYNOVIAL JOINTS

GENERAL STRUCTURE

The synovial (diarthrodial) joints comprise most of the body's articulations and are characterized by wide ranges of almost frictionless movement. The articulating bony surfaces have at their ends a thin plate of dense cortical bone, known as the articular end-plate. Beneath this lies the cancellous bone often containing red (hematopoietic) marrow, and tightly adherent to the bony end-plate is the hyaline articular cartilage, a specialized form of connective tissue that serves as the bearing and gliding surface. The joint cavity is a tissue space, containing only a few milliliters of synovial fluid (Fig. 10–1).

The movement of the cartilaginous surfaces on one another provides the joint with the almost frictionless *mobility* essential to function; by definition, joints must also have *stability* to prevent movement in abnormal planes or excessive slipping under load. Stability is provided by the bony configuration of the joint, the ligamentous and capsular support systems, and the muscles controlling the joint. Each joint has a unique configuration that dictates not only the range but the degree of control of that range exerted by the various factors. For example, the hip is a ball and socket; the knee is a rounded, condylar, cam-shaped, four-bar linkage that allows not only flexion and extension but a surprising amount of rotation; the ankle is a complexly shaped mortised hinge; each intervertebral facet joint is a slightly convex-concave flat on a slightly convex flat; the shoulder is a ball on a disc. The configuration of each individual joint provides the maximum contact area for the usual positions of loading, with a range of motion and sufficient stability to allow high-efficiency performance.[3] Each joint has somewhat different load and positional requirements, reflected appropriately in its individual design. Uniaxial, biaxial, or polyaxial motion occurs, depending on the fit of the component parts at the various ranges. Thus, the bony structure of the ankle joint (a hinge joint) is the primary factor that dictates that motion will occur mainly in the sagittal plane

through an axis running transverse to the long axis of the limb and through the body of the talus. The medial malleolus, anterior lip, and posterior margin of the tibia and the fibular malleolus prevent abnormal movement by bony impingement on the talus and provide the stability necessary for normal dorsi- and plantar flexion under heavy load. On the other hand, the ball-and-shallow-socket bony configuration of the shoulder joint contributes almost nothing to its stability, which is provided almost entirely by a surprisingly loose capsule, ligaments, and of course by the major factor, the heavy and closely applied controlling musculature.[4]

Accessory structures that aid in maintaining the integrity of the joint are the fibrous capsules and ligaments.[4-6] The fibrous capsule for most joints is a firm structure consisting of dense connective tissue that invests the entire joint and inserts into the bones usually close to the articulating surfaces. Within the capsule are thick bands or condensations of parallel collagen fibers known as ligaments. These, too, insert on the bony parts and vary in their tightness from anatomic site to site, depending considerably on the position in which the joint is placed.

Within the joint capsule and defining the interarticular space is a specialized layer of connective tissue cells, the synoviocytes, which secrete the synovial fluid.[7,8] Deep to this layer are varying amounts of highly vascular adipose, fibrous or areolar tissue supporting the synoviocytes and allowing the sac to be appropriately loose in certain ranges of motion, with-

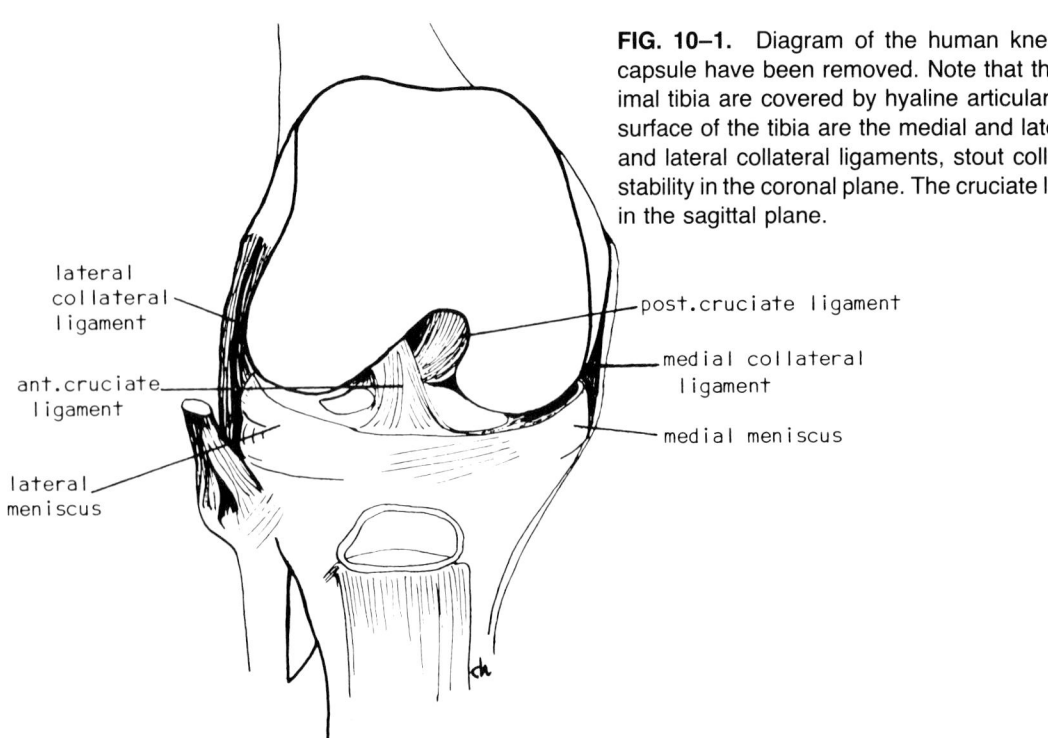

lateral collateral ligament

ant.cruciate ligament

lateral meniscus

post.cruciate ligament

medial collateral ligament

medial meniscus

FIG. 10–1. Diagram of the human knee joint. The patella and capsule have been removed. Note that the distal femur and proximal tibia are covered by hyaline articular cartilage. Affixed to the surface of the tibia are the medial and lateral menisci. The medial and lateral collateral ligaments, stout collagenous bands, provide stability in the coronal plane. The cruciate ligaments control stability in the sagittal plane.

out allowing the synovial folds to become entrapped between the joint surfaces during movement.[9,10] The synovial sac is "incomplete" in that, although it faithfully replicates the inner surface of the capsule, is reflected at the capsular insertion into the bone, and then extends along the bone to the margin of the articular cartilage, it does not cover the cartilage surfaces.[9] The synovial tissue is endowed with a rich blood supply necessary not only to support the synoviocytes but to serve as the source of the synovial fluid. It also has numerous nerve endings[8] that along with those in the capsule and spindles in the muscles, ligaments, and tendons, are responsible for the keen proprioceptive sense and deep pain perception that protect the joints.[11–13]

Certain of the body's joints have within their cavities complete or, more often, incomplete fibrocartilaginous discoid partitions known as menisci. The menisci are inconstant in some areas (e.g., acromioclavicular joint) and highly developed and well defined in others (e.g., knee, temporomandibular joint, and sternoclavicular joints).[1] Synovium does not cover the avascular, aneural fibrocartilaginous menisci, which are firmly fixed to the joint margin by attachment to bone and to ligaments or capsule, preventing abnormal movement or intra-articular displacement during joint function. The function of the menisci varies from site to site, but most authorities feel they contribute to joint stability.

EMBRYOLOGY AND DEVELOPMENT

Shortly after the limb buds appear in the human embryo (26 to 28 days; crown-rump [C-R] length 3 to 6 mm), an axial condensation or blastema develops within them.[14] The arm bud appears first (in 26 days), and within 2 days the leg bud is noted. At approximately 5 postovulatory weeks, the blastema becomes chondrified in the region of future bones; the chondrification proceeds in a proximodistal sequence.[14] The precartilage so formed undergoes an orderly sequence of maturation that proceeds in a fashion approximating epiphyseal cartilage maturation. The bony segments differentiate and become surrounded by a two-layered perichondrium.[15,16] The joint ends of the rudimentary bones are surrounded by concentric rings of flattened cells, and the site of the future joint is the intersection (known as the interzone) of the arcs of cells from one bony rudiment with those of the adjacent one.[17]

Early development of the large joints of the limbs involves two critical phases: the formation and differentiation of the interzones, and the appearance of cavities. The cells of the interzone at first appear identical but soon develop into three layers: a central loosely arranged layer and two denser layers on both sides, which subsequently become the articular cartilages.[14,17] The mesenchyme that surrounds the joints (synovial mesenchyme) becomes vascularized, and the capsule and the peri- and intra-articular structures (ligaments, menisci, and synovial membrane) differentiate from it.[15,16] By 8 postovulatory weeks, the components of the developing joint resemble the adult joint, except that the joint space has not yet appeared.[16–18]

At the end of the embryonic period or early in the fetal period (47 to 60 days), minute spaces appear in the undifferentiated interzone synovial mesenchyme of the larger joints. These spaces result from autolysis and liquefaction of the cells and are thought to be mediated by locally synthesized enzymes.[14] Lysosomal bodies are noted in embryonic cells early in their differentiation, and the enzymes contained within the sacs are believed to be released in response to an alteration in pH or oxygen tension.[14,19] The enzymes destroy the matrix and cells, forming minute cavities, which subsequently coalesce to form the joint cavity. The joint space is lined by rudimentary articular cartilage centrally, but peripherally by a single layer of flattened cells, which becomes the synovial membrane. Early in fetal life the synovial membrane is a relatively smooth, two-cell-layered lining with a subjacent vascular network. Subsequently, convolutions and villiform irregularities appear.

To illustrate this point, as Sledge[14] has pointed out for the shoulder joint, chondrification occurs at a C-R length of 11 mm; external features, such as condyles and tuberosities, and a visible interzone can be noted at C-R length of 17 mm. By 18 mm, the fibrous capsule and synovial mesenchyme are evident, and by 20 mm, the glenoid labra can be noted. By 30 mm of C-R length, the interzone begins to liquefy, and by 34 mm, the joint cavity is clearly evident. By 40 mm, the articular surfaces are well separated.

In terms of congenital abnormalities of joints, there is a critical period in the life of the developing fetus when an alteration in physiologic balance resulting from a genetic error or an intrauterine insult could lead to a major disturbance in joint structure. The upper limb buds appear at 26 days and the lower at 28, and the cavitation to form the joint does not occur until approximately 40 to 60 days.[17] It is reasonable to suppose that the joints are in maximum danger of maldevelopment as a result of insult occurring between the third and sixth week after conception. Insults before this time may include joint and limb abnormalities but will probably be considerably more extensive (somitic in distribution), and those that occur after complete development of the joint (80 days) are unlikely to have a significant effect on the structure of the joint.[14]

STRUCTURE AND CHEMISTRY OF COMPONENT PARTS

Ligaments and Capsule. Ligaments and capsular structures vary considerably in thickness and position, depending on the joint studied and the site within that joint.[1] Structures range from the thin, redundant articular capsule of the shoulder joint[4] to the thick, dense collagenous collateral and cruciate ligaments of the knee.[5,20–22] In some, the ligaments are condensations within the capsule, and in others they are discrete and separated from the capsule by an areolar layer. Capsular redundancy is an important aspect of joint function, particularly in relation to the range of motion. The inferior medial portion of the capsule of the shoulder joint is a loose, redundant sac, which does not become tense until the shoulder is fully abducted or flexed.[4] The posterior capsule of the knee is quite loose in flexion, but so tight in extension that it becomes an important stabilizer.[5]

Although some variation exists depending on the site studied, the periarticular ligaments and capsule are fairly uniform in histologic appearance, chemical composition, and tissue organization. The structures consist principally of parallel bundles or fascicles of collagen, sparsely populated with fibrocytes.[6,23] Blood vessels traverse a tortuous course between the fascicles, and an occasional nerve fiber is noted, most frequently perivascular, but occasionally free in the ligament or capsule. The collagen fibers range from 150 to 1500 nm in diameter, and an occasional elastic fiber is interspersed.[6,20,24] Together the fibrous proteins (collagen and elastin) account for over 90% of the dry weight of the tissue.[24–26] The collagen of ligaments and capsule is mostly type I $(2\alpha_1{}^1,1\alpha_2)$, similar but not identical in biochemical composition, glycosylation, and cross-linking to that found in dermis and bone.[24]

Mammalian ligaments and capsule are hyperhydrated with estimates of water ranging up to approximately 70%.[25] Most of the remaining inorganic solids consists of collagen (and elastin), although a small but important fraction is in the form of proteoglycans.[25] The glycosaminoglycan chains associated with these macromolecules differ somewhat from those found in cartilage in that approximately 35% consists of hyaluronic acid, with chondroitin sulfate (40%) and dermatan sulfate (20%) comprising the remainder.[24,25]

The insertions of ligaments and capsule into the adjacent bones demonstrate a zonal organization. Parallel bundles of collagen first become invested with a fibrocartilaginous stroma and, as they near the bone, become calcified.[1] The collagen fibers, continuous with the ligament, then enter the cortical osseous tissue in a manner analogous to Sharpey's fibers[27] (Fig. 10–2). The gradual transition of ligaments to mineralized fibrocartilage and then to bone enhances the ability of the insertions to distribute forces evenly and decreases the likelihood of a pull-out failure.[27]

Articular Cartilage. The articular cartilages are the principal "working" components of the diarthrodial joint and, in large measure, they and the synovial fluid are responsible for the almost frictionless movement of the articulating surfaces on each other[28] (Fig. 10–3). These specialized connective tissue components are firmly attached to the underlying bones and measure less than 5 mm in thickness in human joints,[1] with considerable variation depending on joint and site within the joint.[29,30] Articular cartilage is dense and white on gross inspection tending to become somewhat yellow with age.[31] Despite the high water content (estimated at over 70%, even for adults), cartilage feels semisolid. Contrary to expectations, the surface is not smooth, and a number of studies using the scanning electron microscope have demonstrated gentle undulations and irregular depressions that appear to correspond to the location and shape of cells lying just beneath the surface.[32] These depressions

FIG. 10–2. Photomicrograph showing the insertion of a collateral ligament of an interphalangeal ligament into the cortex of the phalanx. Note the parallel bundles of collagen that comprise the ligament, becoming first fibrocartilaginous, then calcified, prior to entering the substance of the cortical bone in a fashion similar to Sharpey's fibers (hematoxylin and eosin stain ×50).

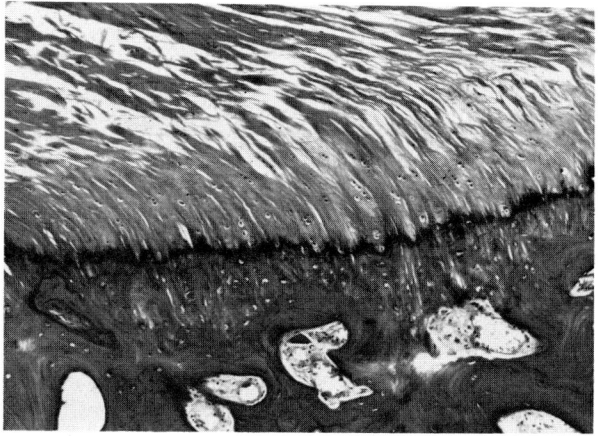

FIG. 10–3. Low-power photomicrograph of adult articular cartilage. Note the zonal distribution of the cells, the calcified layer separated from the radial zone by the "tidemark," and the cortical bone of the underlying bony end-plate. Articular cartilage is sparsely cellular, and the bulk of the tissue consists of extracellular matrix (hematoxylin and eosin stain ×40).

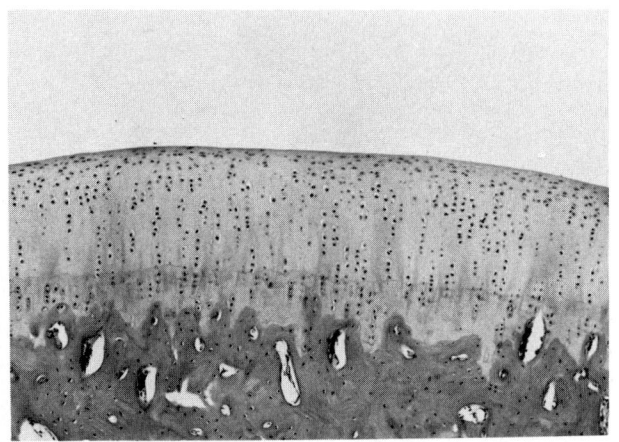

FIG. 10–4. Scanning electron micrograph of the surface of articular cartilage demonstrating irregularly placed rounded or ovoid depressions averaging 20 to 40 μm in diameter. (×440) (Courtesy of Dr. Ian Clark.)

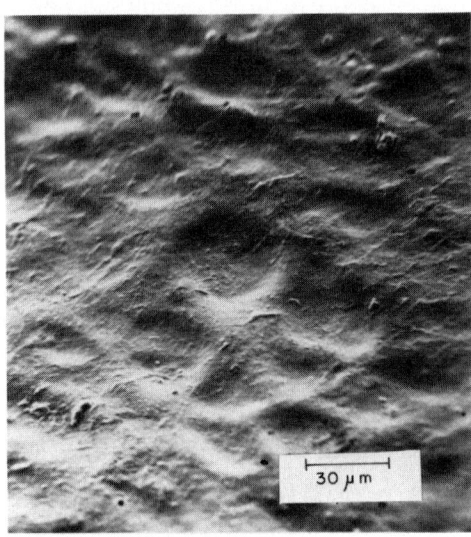

average 20 to 40 μm in diameter and occur with a frequency of 430/mm² (Fig. 10–4).[33,34]

The articular cartilages are aneural, avascular, and alymphatic. Thus, at least in adult humans, they derive their nutrition by a double diffusion system.[9,35] Because the blood vessels in synovium are situated along the (outer) capsular surface,[36] the articulating (inner) surface is relatively avascular, and nutrients must first diffuse across the synovial membrane into the synovial fluid and then through the dense matrix of the cartilage to reach the chondrocyte (see Chapter 16).[9,37,38] Because there are no nerves in articular cartilage, the bearing surfaces of the joint depend on nerve endings in the capsule, synovium, muscles, and subchondral bone for appreciation of pain and proprioception.[11–13,15]

Histologic and ultrastructural examination of the cartilage demonstrates a preponderance of extracellular matrix and only sparse cellularity[35,39] (see Fig. 10–3). The distribution of cells is not random, and four more or less distinct zones have been described:[39] a *tangential or gliding zone* in which the cells are elongated with their long axes parallel to surface; a *transitional zone* in which the cells are rounded and appear randomly distributed; a *radial zone* in which the cells appear to line up in short irregular columns; and a calcified zone, the matrix and cells of which are heavily encrusted with hydroxyapatite. The *calcified zone* is separated from the radial zone superficial to it by a wavy, irregular bluish line (on hematoxylin and eosin staining) called the "tidemark,"[40,41] and on its deep surface merges with the end-plate of the underlying bone[42] (Fig. 10–5). The tidemark is similar in appearance and composition to the cement lines in bone and may act as a limit to calcification[42,43] or, as has been suggested by Redler and co-workers,[41] may represent a variation in the structure of the collagen fibers to increase the resistance to shearing forces.

The biochemical composition of articular cartilage is quite different from that of other connective tissues involved in the joint. As indicated above, water content ranges up to almost 80%.[44] The water of articular cartilage is freely exchangeable with synovial fluid and appears to be held in the form of proteoglycan-collagen gel.[44] The movement of water and, more specifically, "weeping" of the cartilage may be essential features of a boundary lubrication system.[35,45] Collagen is the most prevalent organic constituent, accounting for over 50% of the remaining material.[35,46] The most superficial collagen fibers are arranged in bundles and sheets parallel to the surface of the cartilage forming a "skin," but distribution is more random in the deeper layers[46,47] (Fig. 10–6). Collagen of cartilage (type II) is of a different genetic species from that of skin or bone (type I) and consists of three identical α_1^{11} chains in a helical form. The chains differ from those of type I collagen principally in the increased concentration of hydroxylysine and excessive glycosylation (see Chapter 12).[48–50] Minor collagens, types IX and X, can also play an important role in the structure of the cartilage,[48,51] as do such protein constituents as anchorin[52,53] and chondronectin.[54–56] The

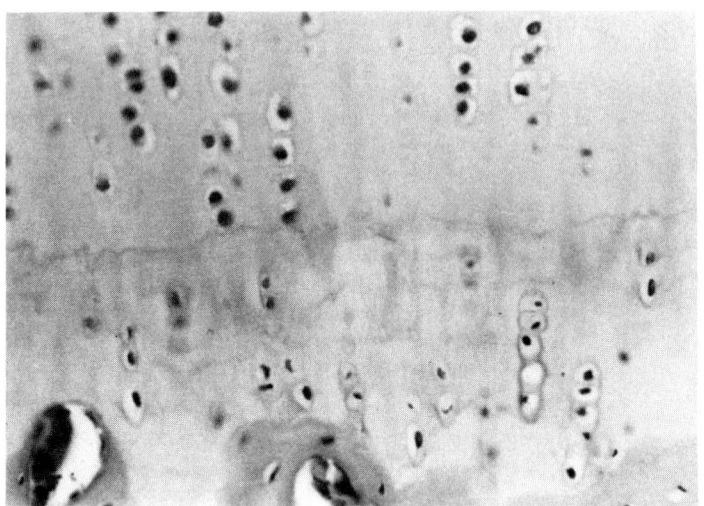

FIG. 10–5. Photomicrograph of mature articular cartilage showing the "tidemark," a wavy bluish line (or series of lines) separating the calcified zone below from the radial zone above. The matrix and cells of the calcified zone are heavily encrusted with apatitic salts (hematoxylin and eosin stain ×250).

FIG. 10–6. Diagram of the fibrous architecture of human articular cartilage according to a scheme proposed by Lane and Weiss. The lamina splendens (LS) is a layer several micra deep, composed of the fine fibers that cover the articular surface. Beneath this lies the tangential zone (TAN), which consists of tightly packed bundles of individual collagen fibers arranged parallel to the articular surface, often at right angles to each other. The collagen fibers in the transitional zone (TRANS) are randomly arranged. Collagen fibers of the radial zone (RAD) are also randomly arranged, but are of larger diameter, while those of the calcified zone (CAL) are arranged perpendicular to the articular surface. (From Lane, J.M., and Weiss, C.: Current comment: Review of articular cartilage collagen research. Arthritis Rheum., *18*:558, 1975).

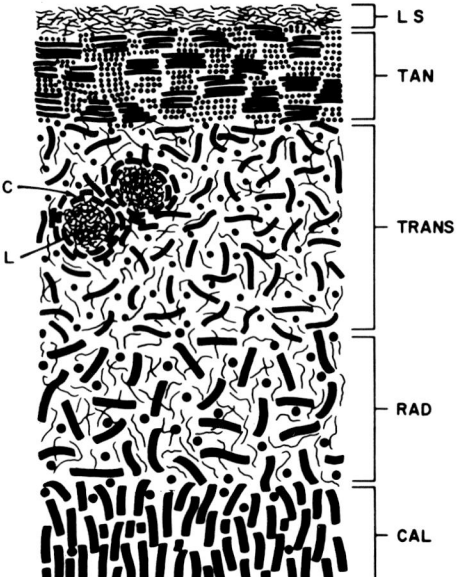

remainder of the organic solids are mostly proteoglycans,[35] macromolecules consisting in their simplest form (subunit) of a linear protein core approximately 180 to 210 nm in length, to which are attached glycosaminoglycans of three species: chondroitin 6-sulfate; chondroitin 4-sulfate; and keratan sulfate in varying numbers depending on the age of the individuals and site.[57–59] The molecular weight of the subunit is about 2 million Daltons, with as many as 50 glycosaminoglycan chains extended at right angles from the core protein.[59,60] Because the three polysaccharides are markedly anionic, the molecule exerts an enormous electronegative domain, causing it to remain stiffly extended in space (see Chapter 13).[35] This factor is probably crucial in maintenance of the resiliency of the tissue. The component glycosaminoglycans vary with age, with chondroitin 4-sulfate and chondroitin 6-sulfate being the principal constituents in immature animals, whereas in adults chondroitin 4-sulfate is diminished to less than 5% and keratan sulfate accounts for up to approximately 50%.[35,59,61] It is unlikely that the 2 million Dalton subunit exists as such in the natural state, and most of the proteoglycan is in the form of highly ordered, sometimes enormously large aggregates.[58,59] Aggregation of the subunits has been shown to occur along a thin filament of hyaluronic acid, which accounts for less than 1% of the total glycosaminoglycan present within the tissue,[58] but is obviously of critical importance in maintaining the physical properties,[59] and for the interaction with collagen.[62,63] Low-molecular-weight proteins, known as link proteins, play a role in aggregation.[64,65]

Articular cartilage also contains other materials in small quantities. Approximately 5 to 6% of the tissue is in the form of inorganic constituents, mostly calcium salts.[35] Lipids[66] account for less than 1% of the dry weight, and studies have suggested the presence of a glycoprotein or "matrix protein," constituting up to 15% of the total dry weight.[67]

Studies of the metabolism of articular cartilage contradict the inert appearance of the tissue, demonstrating a surprising rate of synthesis and degradation of the component matrix materials.[68] Specifically, radiotracer studies have demonstrated that the articular chondrocytes are responsible for the synthesis of the proteoglycan[68] and that at least a small portion of it turns over at a rapid rate.[68] Collagen is also synthesized by the cartilage cells, but is considerably more stable than the proteoglycan.[69] The rapid turnover of at least a small portion of the proteoglycan suggests the presence of an internal remodeling system, and evidence has accumulated that this system is based on the release of lysosomal enzymes from the chondrocytes, which have as their principal substrate the proteoglycan.[70–72] Although no hyaluronidase is identifiable in chondrocytes, a hyaluronidase-like material clearly operates in normal and especially osteoarthritic articular cartilage. As to the core protein, numerous investigators have implicated the acid cathepsins[35,70,72] and neutral protease.[71–73] Collagenase clearly evident in osteoarthritic articular cartilage is probably present in normal tissue, but tightly bound to inhibitors.[35,74]

Of considerable importance in the metabolism of articular cartilage are numerous factors altering the rates of synthesis or degradation of the cartilage by the cells. These include *humoral factors* such as insulin, somatomedin and cortisol; drugs such as nonsteroidal anti-inflammatory agents; mechanical forces acting on the cartilage, and electrical or magnetic fields.[35,75] Of perhaps greater influence on the cartilage are synovial factors, including a series of low-molecular-weight mediators such as interleukin-1 and the synovial prostaglandins.[76–79] Chondrocytes are also capable of responding to local factors such as chondrocyte-synthesized prostaglandins, collagenase-activating protein, altered pH, concentration of calcium, or other materials such as heat-shock proteins.[75,80,81]

Synovial Membrane and Synovial Fluid of Diarthrodial Joints. The synovial fluid and synovial membrane are discussed in Chapters 5 and 11, respectively, and hence are reviewed only briefly here. The synovial membrane is a vascular connective tissue lining the inner surface of the capsule but not covering the articular cartilage. As indicated, there is considerable anatomic difference between the lining cells (synoviocytes) and the subsynovial tissues, which consist of an avascular connective tissue framework with varying amounts of fibrous, areolar, and fatty tissues with elements of the reticuloendothelial system and, more specifically, lymphocytes interspersed[7,82] (Fig.

10–7). The synoviocytes themselves are the unique feature of this tissue and, as will be discussed, have been divided according to ultrastructural and cytochemical characteristics into types A and B,[8,83] which vary in their functions (fibrogenesis, phagocytosis, synthesis of hyaluronate, and synthesis of low-molecular-weight mediators—IL-1, prostaglandins, and proteases—all of which can affect the cartilage).[7,8,82] Ultrastructural studies have shown that the surface or lining cells form a discontinuous layer, lacking a basement membrane, and that cell processes (which may interdigitate) project from the cells toward the surface.[8,82] Thin branching filaments, probably of reticular origin, appear to serve as a supportive membrane for the cells, rather than collagen fibers, which are usually absent.[8]

The synovial membrane is endowed with a rich plexus of blood vessels in the subsynovial layers, which is thought to be responsible for the transfer of blood constituents into the synovial cavity and the formation of synovial fluid.[36,84] Filtration may be variable depending on the constituent studied, and it is apparent that there is a selective element to the transudative and especially the exudative processes. Excellent evidence demonstrates that the synovial cells

FIG. 10–7. Photomicrograph of normal synovium showing the surface layers of synovial cells and the presence of areolar and fatty synovial tissue (hematoxylin and eosin stain ×225).

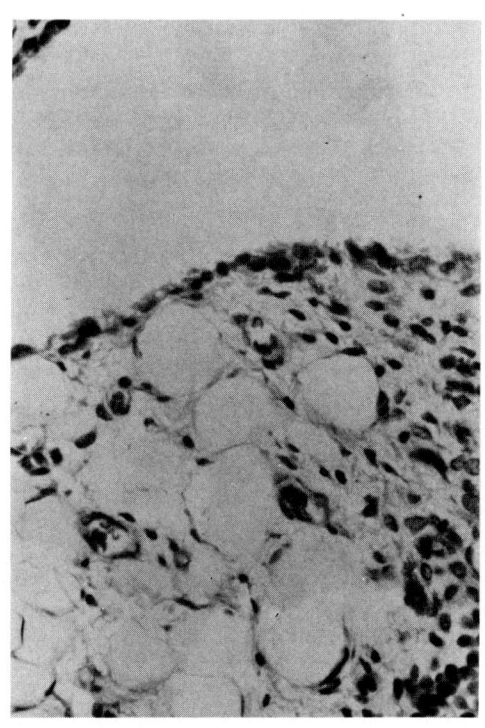

synthesize and secrete hyaluronate, an "additive" to the plasma constituents that forms the synovial fluid and an important aspect in lubrication mechanisms.[7,84] Equally important are some not as yet fully described protein materials that may be responsible in part for the lubrication system,[85–87] and the previously mentioned IL-1 (formerly known as catabolin).[76,80,88,89]

Normal synovial fluid is clear, pale yellow, and viscous. It is normally present in very small amounts. One to four milliliters is found in the human knee, and less in smaller joints. The viscosity of the fluid is due to the presence of the hyaluronate and proteinaceous materials, which have considerable importance in lubrication.[85–87]

Menisci of Diarthrodial Joints. As already stated, menisci normally occur only in the knee and temporomandibular, sternoclavicular, distal radioulnar, and acromioclavicular joints. They consist of complete or incomplete flattened, triangular, or somewhat irregularly shaped fibrocartilaginous discs, firmly attached to the fibrous capsules and often to one of the adjacent bones[1,2] (Fig. 10–8A,B).

The menisci, like articular cartilages, are for the most part avascular, but at the site of bony attachment they usually display a vascular arcade. No nerves or lymphatics have been identified in the meniscal tissues. They presumably derive their nutrition from synovial fluid, but also by diffusion from vascular plexuses, which are present in the soft tissues adjacent to their attachment to bone or fibrous capsule. Examination of the menisci of the knee under polarized or light microscopy has shown that the collagen fibers are arranged circumferentially, presumably to withstand the tension of load bearing[90] (Fig. 10–8B).

The fibrocartilage of the meniscus has a biochemical composition considerably different from that of articular cartilage.[91,92] The water content ranges between 70 and 78%. Inorganic ash accounts for approximately 3% of the wet weight. The remainder of the material, the inorganic solids, are principally collagen with type I ($2\alpha_1^1, 1\alpha_2$) predominating.[46] Collagen accounts for 60 to 90% of the organic solids.[91,93,94] Elastin is present in low concentration (<1%). Proteoglycans constitute less than 10% of the dry weight, and the constituent glycosaminoglycans are principally chondroitin sulfates and dermatan sulfate with keratan sulfate representing only a minor component.[92] Meniscal fibrocartilage appears to have a much more sluggish metabolism than hyaline articular cartilage has. Unlike hyaline articular cartilage, however, when meniscal fibrocartilage is injured, it can undergo repair. Such repair is almost invariably located in the vascular

FIG. 10–8. *A,* Photograph of a normal human medial meniscus. Note the semilunar shape with a thin free edge and considerably thickened marginal attachment site. Menisci increase the stability of the joint and serve as weight-bearing structures in the knee. *B,* Low-power photomicrograph of a fibrocartilaginous human medial meniscus. Note the presence of large numbers of parallel bundles of collagen and the sparse cellularity (hematoxylin and eosin stain ×40).

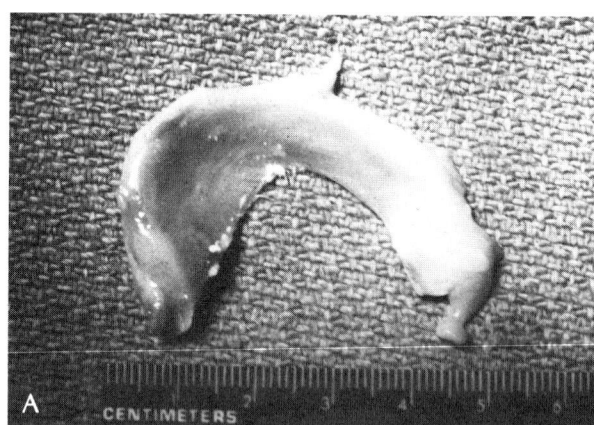

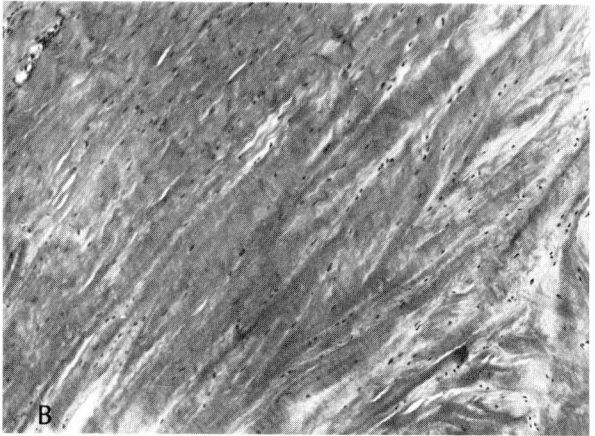

zone adjacent to the bony attachment site and is probably fibroblastic, rather than chondrocytic, in origin.

Subchondral Bone. Although at the ultrastructural and biochemical levels the bone making up the subchondral cortex and the cancellous bone that supports it are indistinguishable from bone from other sites, the organization of the subchondral bone is specific. The subchondral plate on which the calcified cartilage lies is thinner than cortical bone in most areas and can contain variable numbers of mature haversian systems. The distribution of these systems has been well established, but they appear to run parallel to the joint rather than parallel to the long axis of the bone (Fig. 10–9). The sheets and interconnecting struts of cancellous bone that support the plate and fill the epiphyseal end of the bone differ considerably

FIG. 10–9. Photomicrograph of distal femur of an adult rabbit showing the subchondral bone. Note the relationship of the bone to the cartilage and the compact nature of the subchondral plate. The haversian canals appear to be parallel to the joint surface (Masson trichrome ×50).

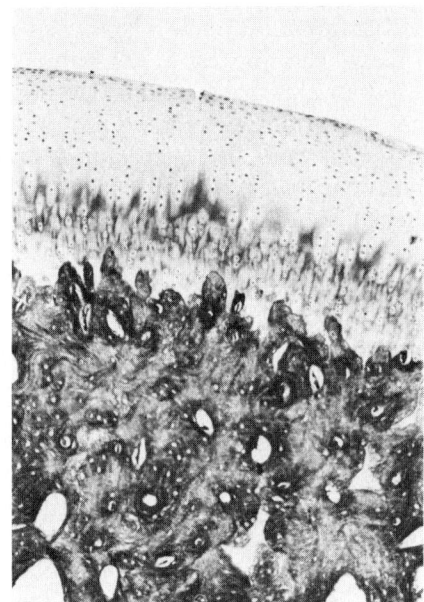

from joint to joint, but are highly ordered and characteristic for any one joint. The major plates are arranged at right angles to the predominating stresses and, together with the subchondral bony end-plate, are approximately 10 times more deformable than is the cortical bony shaft.[95] Stiffening of the subchondral bone, a change that occurs with osteoarthritis, is considered deleterious to the function of the joint and the "health" of the articular cartilages.[96]

Calcified Cartilage. A thin layer of calcified cartilage separates the articular cartilage from its bony subchondral bed. The junction between these tissues undulates, making it more difficult for the articular cartilage to be peeled off.[97,98]

The chondrocytes in the calcified cartilage are alive but metabolically they are relatively inactive.[99] The junction between the hyaline articular cartilage and the calcified cartilage stains deeply with basophilic dyes and is called the *tidemark*. In pathologic situations, such as osteoarthrosis, vessels penetrate the subchondral plate and the calcified cartilage.[39,100] The calcified cartilage can then act as a source of enchondral calcification, remodeling the subchondral plate and creating a new tidemark.[42] After substantial remodeling the tidemark can even be duplicated.[101]

FUNCTION

The compressive stress under which diarthrodial joints function is considerably greater than that associated with support of body weight. Muscles have poor mechanical advantage compared to body weight, which works through relatively long lever arms. Because muscular contraction balances the body over these joints and stabilizes them, the major joints of the lower extremity—the knee, the hip, and the ankle—usually function under loads approximately 2½ to 10 times that of body weight.[102] Similar compressive stresses (about 150 to 300 psi) are not uncommon in the joints of the upper extremity. Further, the load on joints is not constant, because activities are intermittent and often create high peak dynamic loads.[103] Joint motion is characterized by frequent rapid starts and equally rapid stops, both of which, but especially the starts, are associated with high compressive loads. It is remarkable that under such potentially punishing mechanical conditions most joints function throughout the life of the individual without evidence of destruction of their major load-bearing areas.

Role of Ligaments, Joint Capsule, and Surrounding Muscles. The ligaments, joint capsule, and surrounding muscles provide stability to joints. The role of muscles in this regard cannot be over-emphasized. Even though all periarticular structures are intact, complete paralysis of muscle abolishes the stability of a joint, and partial paralysis creates significant functional limitations. Muscles are most important in stabilizing the large proximal joints—the shoulder and the hip—which are of ball-and-socket design and thus have the least configurational stability. Energy conservation requires that the diameter of the extremities become smaller as one moves farther from the center of the body, so that bulky musculature can only exist close to the trunk. The wrist and foot cannot be totally surrounded by muscles as are the more centrally placed joints. Although muscles remain important in the stabilization of small joints, the configuration of the bone and the dense ligamentous interconnections of the wrist and foot play the major role in their stability.

The contribution of the joint capsule to joint stability has already been discussed. The capsular volume of joints varies considerably from joint to joint and also with position of the joint. Variations in intra-articular pressure (IAP) with joint position have been studied extensively.[104,105] The range of IAP in the knee varies from 5 cm of water at 15 to 60° of flexion to 60 cm of water at full extension and full flexion. These authors have also found that each joint has a position

SCIENTIFIC BASIS FOR THE STUDY OF THE RHEUMATIC DISEASES

in which the intracapsular volume is potentially largest (for example, at 30° of knee flexion).[104] Joints with significant effusions are maintained in this position to maximize intracapsular volume and minimize IAP.

Ligamentous structures prevent the joint from subluxation or dislocation and act to constrain and guide joint motion.[5,22] Ligaments are variable in their architecture and are complicated not only in structure but in relationship to adjacent tissues. In the fingers, ligaments are closely approximated to tendinous insertions. The collateral ligaments of the knee are constructed so that some portion of their fibers is under tension in all degrees of flexion. In combination with the cruciate ligaments, the collateral ligaments of the knee guide the complicated rolling and gliding motion of the distal femur of the proximal tibia (Fig. 10–1).[5,22] Many of the small joints of the hands and feet have thickened volar capsules forming a plate. These structures greatly add to the stability of those joints.

Role of Articular Cartilage. Articular cartilage represents the bearing surface of the joint and is structured to resist the repetitive rubbing and considerable deformation this surface is subjected to over years. The cartilage matrix, for the most part, is composed of a systematically oriented fibrous network of collagen and highly charged proteoglycan molecules. The collagen fibers at the surface run parallel to the surface and act as a membrane holding the matrix together. The collagen fibers in the basilar region of the articular cartilage run vertically and actually connect the articular cartilage with its underlying calcified bone, preventing shear failure during joint motion. The fibers in the mid-zone of the cartilage appear to be randomly oriented, but when the cartilage is subjected to axial compression, the fibers tend to line up perpendicular to the compressive force (Fig. 10–10),[106] the most advantageous arrangement in resisting a compressive load.

The lack of vessels in articular cartilage would appear to be of significant functional advantage. Under physiologic conditions, articular cartilage can be compressed to as much as 20% of its original height; if blood vessels traversed it, they would be rendered useless. On the basis of the diffusion rates in the tissue and the metabolic requirement of the cells, Maroudas calculated that the maximal thickness of the cartilage assuring chondrocyte viability is 6 mm.[107] Patellar cartilage, the thickest in the human body, is under 6 mm thick. Mechanical considerations clearly indicate that such thin layers have little meaningful role as shock absorbers. The appearance of articular cartilage may belie its mechanical integrity. One must judge cartilage biochemically or mechanically in order not to be misled.[108,109]

The function of articular cartilage is that of a bearing and contact surface. If the articular cartilage is removed, the subchondral bony plates of the joint will not fit well. It is the relatively deformable articular cartilage that provides the largest possible surface contact area when force is applied to a joint.[110] Simon and colleagues have shown that cartilage thickness is related to the degree of underlying bony incongruity.[111] Cartilage thickness is maximal in joints that fit less well and thinnest in joints that are most congruous. Cartilage thickness appears to depend on physiologic and mechanical factors.[112] Articular cartilage acts to transmit load to the underlying bony bed, but does little to distribute that load.[113] In fact, it is the subchondral bone that deforms under physiologic load.[114] Joints must be slightly incongruous in the unloaded state[115] (Fig. 10–11), so that when they deform under load they will become congruous. Deformation of subchondral bone is important in achieving an effective distribution of stress within a joint. This deformation of the subchondral bone results in a low-frequency, physiologically occurring, trabecular microfracture.[116] It has been suggested that microfractures of the interconnected plates of subchondral

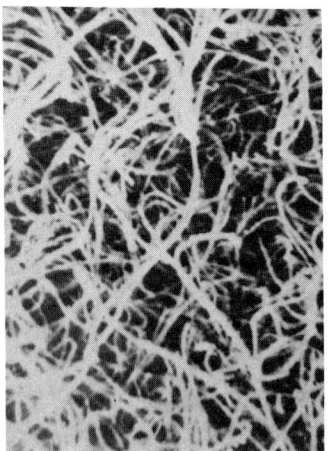 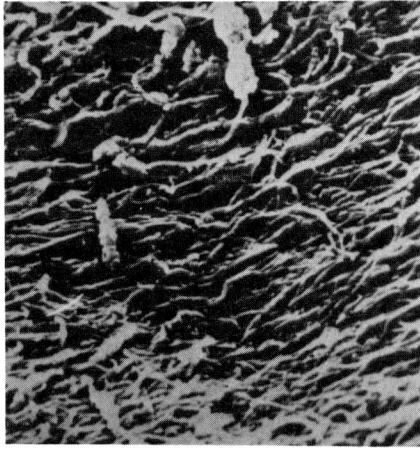

FIG. 10–10. On the left a scanning electron micrograph of the mid-zone collagen fibers of articular cartilage in the unloaded state. Note the essentially random orientation. The picture on the right is the same area of the cartilage with compressive load applied. Note how the fibers line up perpendicular to the load. (From McCall, J.[106])

FIG. 10–11. Normally unloaded joints are not completely congruous; under load they become so. It is deformation of the articular cartilage and subchondral bone that allows maximal contact under load. The larger the contact under load the lower the force per unit area and the stress on these tissues. (From Radin, E.L., et al.: The mechanics of joints as it relates to their degeneration. *In* American Academy of Orthopaedic Surgeons: Symposium on Osteoarthritis. St. Louis, The C.V. Mosby Co., 1976, p. 41.)

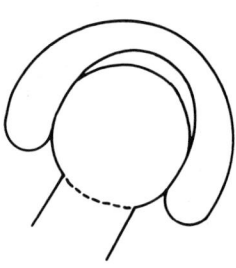

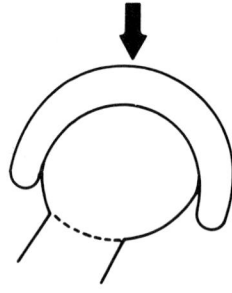

FIG. 10–12. Radiogram of an osteoarthritic hip that is beginning to sublux laterally. Note the condensation of bone at the lateral rim of the acetabulum and directly across from that area in the femoral head. Where stress is increased above normal, bone becomes sclerotic. If the stress is even greater, case cysts will form. Unloaded bone becomes relatively osteopenic.

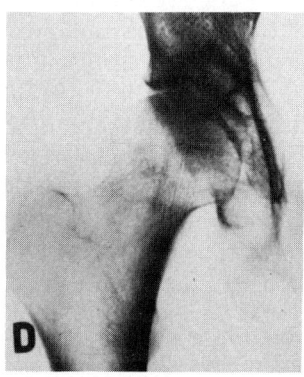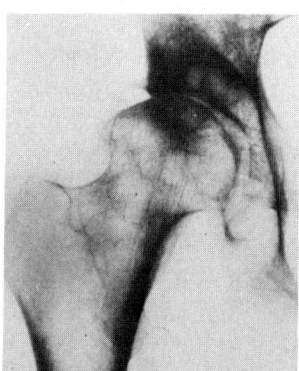

bone and the subsequent healing and remodeling results in structural patterns that provide maximum strength.[117] The subchondral bone pattern accurately reflects the stress distribution within the joint. From the overall orientation of the trabecular pattern of a joint radiogram one can determine whether this pattern of stresses is normal or abnormal.[36] In cases of localization of stress, subchondral bone becomes sclerotic and dense (Fig. 10–12).

Role of Menisci. The sites of intra-articular fibrocartilages or menisci have already been mentioned. Analyses of the types of joint that contain menisci show that they are basically hinge joints that also rotate. To achieve this type of motion, the edges to the hinge are rounded off, and it is the menisci that fill the gap (Fig. 10–13).[118] Without these "washers," such joints would have fairly small central articular cartilage contact areas and would be less stable. The menisci bear load[119] and also act as shock absorbers by squeezing outward.[120]

Joint Lubrication. The joint is lubricated by synovial fluid that contains hyaluronate, a large glycoprotein molecule whose average molecular weight is in excess of 1 million. It is this giant molecule that is responsible for the *"thixotropic"* flow characteristics of the synovial fluid (the more slowly it flows the more viscous it becomes). Based on the observations regarding the thixotropic character of the fluid, scientists originally concluded that joints were lubricated by a hydrodynamic system in which the fluid is held between the bearing surfaces by the continuing rotation of one part of the bearing. Joints are poorly suited to this form of lubrication, however, because they oscillate rather than rotate.[28] The finding that the coefficient of friction remains unchanged in joints lubricated with hyaluronidase-treated synovial fluid negated this hydrodynamic theory.[121]

The frictional resistance of animal joints lubricated with synovial fluid has been measured to be as low

FIG. 10–13. The knee is a hinge with rounded off corners to allow rotation as well as flexion in extension. "Washers" are needed in such a design to maintain stability, particularly in full extension. (From Radin, E.L.[118])

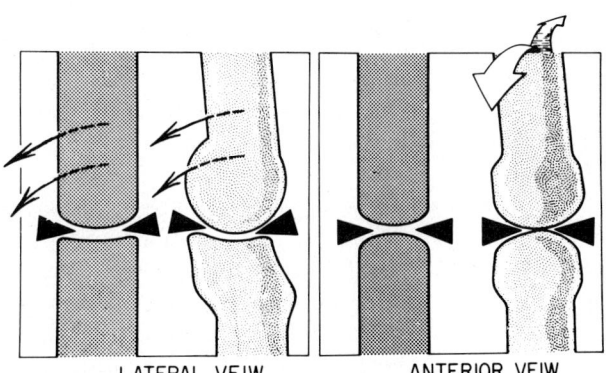

LATERAL VEIW　　　　ANTERIOR VEIW

as 0.002, which is twice as low as that of rubber on steel and one tenth that of an ice skate on ice.[122] Two hydrated cartilage surfaces under load are separated by a thin film of fluid under physiologic circumstances, and there is ample evidence that this fluid is water "squeezed" from the hyperhydrated cartilage.[123] Although the major part of water in cartilage is in the form of a proteoglycan-collagen gel,[44] it is freely exchangeable with synovial fluid, and a significant portion can be liberated by pressure on the cartilage.[124] Because in the adult there is little or no traverse of water through the subchondral plate or flow through the substance of the cartilage, the water displaced by cartilage compression is expressed onto the surface of the cartilage, preferentially peripheral to the zone of impending contact. Mow and Mansour have concluded that, under the most usual circumstances of joint motion, water tends to be pushed out just in front of the contact area.[125] When the compression is released, the matrix within the cartilage contains enough of a fixed charge to osmotically attract the water and small solutes back into the matrix, and the cartilage regains its original height.[126] Thus, the fluid film that exists between moving cartilage layers is made up of the cartilaginous interstitial fluid, which is squeezed onto the surface as the cartilage compresses the synovial fluid already trapped in the contact zone. The mechanism of lubrication is referred to as *hydrostatic*.

The hydrostatic mechanism obviously functions best under substantial loads, because under small loads there would be little cartilage compression and little weeping of fluid onto the surface. Physiologically, however, joints frequently move under relatively light load. Under such circumstances a hydrostatic mechanism would not generate a substantial fluid film, particularly just at the moment motion begins. Thus, it would be advantageous to have a second lubrication mechanism function primarily under these conditions. Such a mechanism exists, and it involves the binding of a special glycoprotein found in synovial fluid, *the lubricating glycoprotein*,[87] which is affixed to the cartilage surfaces and keeps them from touching, a mechanism referred to as *boundary lubrication*. Joints are thus lubricated by two complementary systems: a hydrostatic system, which functions primarily at high loads, and a boundary system, most effective at low loads.

Hyaluronate appears to have no place in cartilage-on-cartilage lubrication, but does play an important role as the boundary lubricant for synovial tissue.[86] Because the friction of cartilage rubbing on cartilage is so low, the preponderance of frictional resistance in joint movement is in the periarticular soft tissues,

which also in most joints make up the bulk of the articulating area within the joint capsule (Fig. 10–14). Hyaluronate serves as a boundary lubricant in this system.[86]

INTERVERTEBRAL DISCS

GENERAL STRUCTURE

Intervertebral discs are fibrocartilaginous complexes that form the articulation between the bodies of two adjacent vertebrae. Motion between any two vertebral segments is limited to a few degrees in any plane by the configuration of the discal tissue and intervertebral facets, but the sum of the motion in the joints of the entire column provides the range necessary for the extraordinary mobility of the human spine. Discs from various regions of the spine (cervical, thoracic, and lumbar) vary in size and shape, but are basically identical in their organization.[127] Each consists of three components: the outer fibrous restraining band, the annulus fibrosus; the central semifluid mass, the nucleus pulposus; and the restraining superior and inferior surfaces, the vertebral cartilaginous plates (Fig. 10–15A,B).

The annulus fibrosus consists of a ring of fibrous lamellae that encases the nucleus and unites the vertebral bodies by creating contiguity of the fibrous structure with the margin of vertebral segment and with the investing anterior and posterior longitudinal

FIG. 10–14. In most joints the surface area of synovium that rubs on itself and on articular cartilage is far greater than the area of the cartilage that rubs on cartilage. The synovium is redundant so that it will not interfere with joint motion.

JOINTS CONTAIN TWO

SYSTEMS WHICH REQUIRE

LUBRICATION

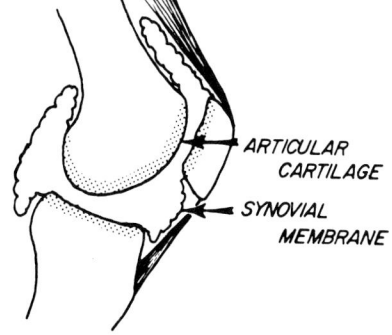

ARTICULAR CARTILAGE

SYNOVIAL MEMBRANE

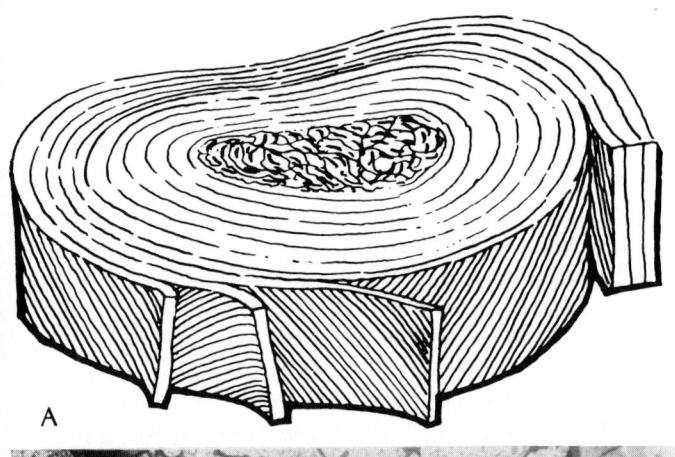

A

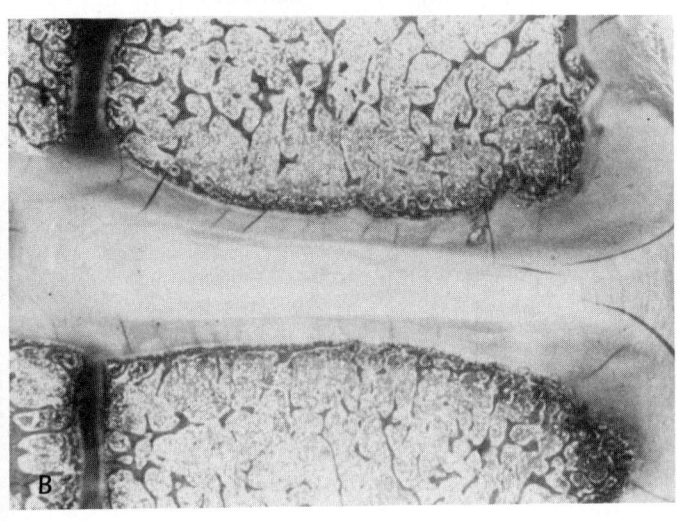

B

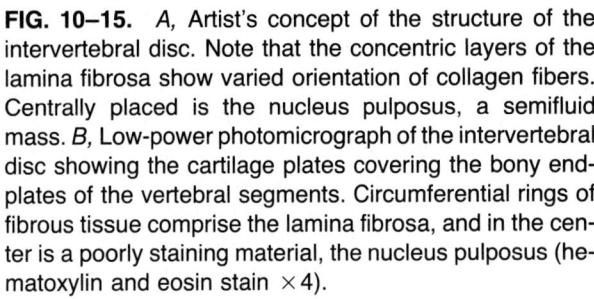

FIG. 10–15. *A*, Artist's concept of the structure of the intervertebral disc. Note that the concentric layers of the lamina fibrosa show varied orientation of collagen fibers. Centrally placed is the nucleus pulposus, a semifluid mass. *B*, Low-power photomicrograph of the intervertebral disc showing the cartilage plates covering the bony end-plates of the vertebral segments. Circumferential rings of fibrous tissue comprise the lamina fibrosa, and in the center is a poorly staining material, the nucleus pulposus (hematoxylin and eosin stain ×4).

ligaments.[1,127] The fibrous layers of the annulus are approximately 20 μm thick and, on polarized microscopic examination, show an organization such that alternating sheets of collagen are set at an angle to each other.[128–130] Flexibility is achieved by random arrangement of the fibers (0.1 to 0.2 μm in diameter) within the substance of the plates of collagen and by a relatively high proportion of proteoglycan and interstitial fluid in the annulus as compared with the more rigid tendons or ligaments.[102,131] The annulus is not uniformly thick throughout the substance. The plates in the anterior third of the disc are stoutest and most distinct; those in the posterior aspect are more closely packed and somewhat thinner.[132]

The second component of the disc is the nucleus pulposus, which occupies the central portion of the disc and is surrounded by the annulus. Actually, the nucleus is not centrally placed within the confines of the annulus, but usually lies closer to the posterior margin of the disc.[132] The nature of this material and its function in the joint are most evident when, on transverse or sagittal sectioning of the disc, it is found to bulge prominently beyond the plane of the section. The nucleus consists of a viscid fluid structure, which histologically is sparsely cellular and consists princi-

pally of loose delicate fibrous strands embedded in a gelatinous matrix.[5] In the central portion of the nucleus, the fibers appear randomly distributed, but as they approach the superior and inferior cartilage plates they assume an oblique angular orientation to become embedded in the cartilage at the peripheral attachment of the nucleus.[102,128,132] The structural interspace between the nucleus and the annulus is difficult to appreciate, and in many older subjects the two tissues blend imperceptibly.[127,128]

The disc is contained superiorly and inferiorly by cartilaginous plates, which are firmly fixed to the bony end-plates of the adjacent vertebral segments and differ little in structure from the hyaline articular cartilage seen in diarthrodial joints, except that they have no collagenous "skin," or indeed any discrete superficial surface.[127,132] Instead, the cartilage serves as an anchor for the fine filamented fibers of the nucleus pulposus in its central portion and the coarse fibrous plates of the annulus fibrosus peripherally.

EMBRYOLOGY AND DEVELOPMENT

The development of the intervertebral disc in humans occurs early in fetal life. Following formation of the morula, the mass of primitive cells becomes the blastocyst, which rapidly undergoes proliferation and differentiation into ectoderm and endoderm, which in turn combine to form the embryonic disc.[133] A primitive streak develops at the caudal end of the dorsum of the embryonic disc. The groove deepens, and at the most caudal portion, the primitive node develops. At this site, cells arising from the mesoderm give rise to the notochord, which thickens and rolls up into the neural folds to form the neural tube.[134,135] The mesodermal tissues on each side of the notochord form the primitive somites, and at approximately the third week of gestation, distinct spinal segments can be identified. The central portions of the somite on either side of the notochord form the vertebral column, mesodermal cells from each side joining to form the vertebral bony elements, including not only the cartilaginous end-plates but the annulus fibrosus and the peripheral portions of the nucleus pulposus.[133] The notochord, which originally lies centrally placed in the vertebral body and disc, is compressed as chondrification of the vertebra progresses and within a short time is destroyed.[135] No notochordal remnants can be found in the vertebral body in the mature fetus or adult (except in an occasional patient who develops a chordoma). That portion of the notochord that lies in the intervertebral disc area, however, becomes the major central portion of the nucleus pulposus.[135] The annulus develops early in embryonic life from the densely aggregated cells about each pole of the somitic segment and eventually surrounds the notochord completely. Ossification begins in the vertebral body at the 50- to 60-mm stage (third month) as vessels invade the cartilaginous precursors, but the endplates remain cartilaginous and serve as the attachment site for the adult nucleus pulposus and annulus fibrosus.[136]

BIOCHEMISTRY

The anulus fibrosus is principally collagenous but is relatively hyperhydrated compared with other fibrous tissues, with water estimates ranging between 65 and 70%.[129,131] Collagen accounts for approximately 50 to 55% of the dry weight. The remainder of the material consists of proteoglycan, the principal glycosaminoglycans, including chondroitin sulfate and keratan sulfate.[137,138] A small amount of glycoprotein is present.[139]

The nucleus has a much higher water content than the anulus, with estimates for immature animals ranging up to 88%. The value falls to about 65% in aged individuals.[129] Collagen is also present in the nucleus

(mostly type II), but accounts for a considerably smaller percentage of the dry weight (20 to 30%) than in other joint connective tissues.[43,86,129,137,140] Most of the material within the nucleus consists of proteoglycan[137] and other as yet poorly defined proteinaceous materials.[139] The distribution of glycosaminoglycans varies considerably, depending on the age of the patient and the amount of degeneration that has occurred, but chondroitin 6-sulfate (approximately 40%), chondroitin 4-sulfate (5%), keratan sulfate (approximately 50%), and hyaluronic acid (<2%) have all been reported.[137,138] Pearson and co-workers have described the presence of other proteins, probably glycoproteins, which are believed to be important in maintaining the physical properties of the material.[139] Lysosomal enzymes have been described that presumably play a role in the normal turnover of the proteoglycans.[130] Synthetic activity takes place in the outer ring of cells of the nucleus.[141]

FUNCTION

Over the last several years, several investigations by physicians and engineers have attempted to define the functional behavior of the intervertebral disc.[142-144] It is evident that the unit serves as a load-bearing structure, and that the resistance to axial loading (compression) is mediated through the compressibility of the hyperhydrated nucleus, which, with its surrounding envelope of anulus, resists and modifies pressures by "barrelling" (losing height while gaining in width).[142,144,145] The application of compressive force to the disc compresses the nucleus pulposus, which tends to push on the anulus fibrosus containing the nucleus. The anulus is designed to absorb most of the barrelling of the disc by stretching its collagen network. The disc thus mainly acts as a shock absorber.

Integrity and congruence of the intervertebral facet joints require the maintenance of the intervertebral disc space. Loss of disc height from rupture and extravasation of disc material, digestion of the nuclear proteoglycans, or surgical excision of the disc will lead to intervertebral space collapse and settling of the intervertebral facet joints, resulting in articular incongruity with diminution of their contact areas.[146,147] The disc should not be considered a separate unit, however, but an integral part of the intervertebral joint that includes the facet joints and the anterior and posterior longitudinal ligaments. All components acting together maintain the axial resistance to compression and stability of the spine.[143,148]

REFERENCES

1. Gray, H.: Anatomy of the Human Body, 29th ed. Edited by C.M. Goss. Philadelphia, Lea & Febiger, 1973.
2. Gardner, E.: The physiology of joints. J. Bone Joint Surg., 45A:1061–1066, 1963.
3. Inman, V.T.: Functional aspects of the abductor muscles of the hip. J. Bone Joint Surg., 29:607–619, 1947.
4. Rothman, R.H., Marvel, J.P., Jr., and Heppenstall, R.B.: Anatomic considerations in the glenohumeral joint. Orthop. Clin. North Am., 6:341–352, 1975.
5. Brantigan, O.C., and Voshell, A.F.: Mechanics of ligaments and menisci of the knee joint. J. Bone Joint Surg., 23A:44–66, 1941.
6. Kennedy, J.C., Weinberg, H.W., and Wilson, A.S.: The anatomy and function of the anterior cruciate ligament. J. Bone Joint Surg., 56A:223–235, 1974.
7. Hamerman, D., Rosenberg, L.D., and Schubert, M.: Diarthrodial joints revisited. J. Bone Joint Surg., 52A:725–774, 1970.
8. Lever, J.D., and Ford, E.H.R.: Histological, histochemical and electron microscopic observations on synovial membrane. Anat. Rec., 132:525–539, 1958.
9. Barnett, C.H., Davies, D.V., and MacConnail, M.A.: Synovial Joints: Their Structure and Mechanics. Springfield, IL, Charles C Thomas, 1961.
10. Redler, I., and Zimny, M.L.: Scanning electron microscopy of normal and abnormal articular cartilage and synovium. J. Bone Joint Surg., 52A:1395–1404, 1970.
11. Peterson, H.A., Winkelmann, R.K., and Coventry, M.B.: Nerve endings in the hip joint of the cat: Their morphology, distribution and density. J. Bone Joint Surg., 54A:333–343, 1972.
12. Ralston, H.J., III, Miller, M.R., and Kasahara, M.: Nerve endings in human fasciae, tendons, ligaments, periosteum, and joint synovial membrane. Anat. Rec., 136:137–147, 1960.
13. Gardner, E.: Innervation of the knee joint. Anat. Rec., 101:109–130, 1948.
14. Sledge, C.B.: Developmental anatomy of joints. In Diagnosis of Bone and Joint Disorders. Edited by D. Resnick and M.A.G. Niwagama. Philadelphia, W.B. Saunders, 1981, pp 1–20.
15. Gardner, E.: Physiology of movable joints. Physiol. Rev., 30:127–176, 1950.
16. Gardner, E., and O'Rahilly, R.: The early development of the knee joint in staged human embryos. J. Anat., 102:289–299, 1968.
17. Haines, R.W.: The development of joints. J. Anat., 81:33–55, 1947.
18. O'Rahilly, R., and Gardner, E.: The development of the knee joint of the chick and its correlation with embryonic staging. J. Morphol., 98:49–88, 1956.
19. Sledge, C.B., and Dingle, J.T.: Activation of lysosomes by oxygen. Nature, 205:140–141, 1965.
20. Arnoscky, S.P.: Anatomy of the anterior cruciate ligament. Clin. Orthop., 172:19–25, 1983.
21. Ellison, A.E.: Embryology, anatomy, and function of the anterior cruciate ligament. Orthop. Clin. North Am., 16:3–14, 1985.
22. Girges, F.G., Marshall, J.L., and Monajem, A.: The cruciate ligaments of the knee joint. Clin. Orthop., 106:216–231, 1975.
23. Venn, G., Mehta, M.H., and Mason, R.M.: Characterization of collagen from normal and scoliotic human spinal ligament. Biochim. Biophys. Acta, 757:259–267, 1983.
24. Amiel, D. et al.: Tendons and ligaments: A morphological and biochemical comparison. J. Orthop. Res., 1:257–265, 1984.
25. Akeson, W.H., Amiel, D., and LaViolette, D.: The connective tissue response to immobility: A study of chondroitin 4- and 6-sulfate and dermatan sulfate changes in periarticular connective tissue of control and immobilized knees of dogs. Clin. Orthop., 51:183–197, 1967.
26. Enneking, W.F., and Horowitz, M.: The intraarticular effects of immobilization on the human knee. J. Bone Joint Surg., 54A:973–985, 1972.
27. Noyes, F.R. et al.: Biomechanics of ligament failure. J. Bone Joint Surg., 56A:1406–1418, 1974.
28. Charnley, J.: Symposium on Biomechanics. London, Institute of Mechanical Engineering, 1969.
29. Meachim, G.: Effect of age on the thickness of adult articular cartilage at the shoulder joint. Ann. Rheum. Dis., 30:43–46, 1971.
30. Simon, W.H.: Scale effects in animal joints. I. Articular cartilage thickness and compressive stress. Arthritis Rheum., 13:244–256, 1970.
31. Van Der Korst, J.K., Sokoloff, L., and Miller, E.J.: Senescent pigmentation of cartilage and degenerative joint disease. Arch. Pathol., 86:40–46, 1968.
32. Ghadially, F.N.: Fine structure of joints. In The Joints and Synovial Fluid, Vol. 1. Edited by L. Sokoloff. New York, Academic Press, 1978, pp 105–168.
33. Clark, I.C.: Human articular surface contours and related surface depression frequency studies. Ann. Rheum. Dis., 20:15–23, 1971.
34. Clark, I.C.: Surface characteristics of human articular cartilage—A scanning electron microscope study. J. Anat., 108:23–30, 1971.
35. Mankin, H.J.: The articular cartilage, cartilage healing, and osteoarthrosis. In Adult Orthopedics. Edited by R.L. Cruess and W.R.J. Renme. New York, Churchill-Livingstone, 1984, pp 163–270.
36. Davies, D.V., and Edwards, D.A.W.: Blood supply of synovial membrane and intra-articular structures. Ann. Coll. Surg. Engl., 2:142–156, 1948.
37. Brower, T.D., Akahoski, Y., and Orlic, P.L.: Diffusion of dyes through articular cartilage in vivo. J. Bone Joint Surg., 44A:456–463, 1962.
38. McKibben, B., and Holdsworth, F.S.: The nutrition of immature joint cartilage in the lamb. J. Bone Joint Surg., 48B:793–803, 1966.
39. Stockwell, R.A.: Biology of Cartilage Cells. Cambridge, Cambridge University Press, 1979.
40. Fawns, H.T., and Landells, I.W.: Histological studies of rheumatic conditions. I. Observations on the fine structure of the matrix of normal bone and cartilage. Ann. Rheum. Dis., 12:105–113, 1953.
41. Redler, I. et al.: The ultrastructure and biochemical significance of the tidemark of articular cartilage. Clin. Orthop., 112:357–362, 1975.
42. Green, W.T., Jr. et al.: Microradiographic study of the calcified layer of articular cartilage. Arch. Pathol., 90:151–158, 1970.
43. Thompson, A.M., and Stockwell, R.A.: An ultrastructural study of the marginal transitional zone in the rabbit knee koint. J. Anat., 136:701–713, 1983.
44. Mankin, H.J., and Thrasher, A.Z.: Water content and binding in normal and osteoarthritic human cartilage. J. Bone Joint Surg., 57A:76–80, 1975.
45. Torzilli, P.A.: Influence of cartilage conformation on its equilibrium water partition. J. Orthop. Res., 3:473–483, 1985.
46. Lane, J.M., and Weiss, C.: Current comment: Review of ar-

ticular cartilage collagen research. Arthritis Rheum., 18:553–562, 1975.

47. Weiss, C., Rosenberg, L., and Helfet, A.J.: An ultrastructural study of normal young adult human articular cartilage. J. Bone Joint Surg., 50A:663–674, 1968.

48. Miller, E.J.: The collagen of joints. In The Joints and Synovial Fluid, Vol. 1. Edited by L. Sokoloff. New York, Academic Press, 1978, p. 205–236.

49. Goldwasser, M. et al.: Analysis of the type of collagen present in osteoarthritic human cartilage. Clin. Orthop., 167:296–302, 1982.

50. Hui-chou, C.S., and Lust, G.: The type of collagen made by the articular cartilage in joints of dogs with degenerative joint disease. Coll. Relat. Res., 2:245–256, 1982.

51. Nemeth-Csoka, M., and Meszaros, T.: Minor collagens in arthrotic human cartilage. Change in content of 1 alpha, 2 alpha, 3 alpha, and M-collagen with age and in osteoarthrosis. Acta Orthop. Scand., 54:613–619, 1983.

52. Mollenhauer, J., Bee, J.A., Lizarbe, M.A., and von der Mark, K.: Role of anchorin CII, a 31,000 mol. wt. membrane protein, in the interaction of chondrocytes with type II collagen. J. Cell. Biol., 98:1572–1579, 1984.

53. von der Mark, K., Mollenhauer, J., Muller, P.K., and Pfaffle, M.: Anchorin CII, a type II collagen-binding glycoprotein from chondrocyte membranes. Ann. N.Y. Acad. Sci., 460:214–232, 1985.

54. Varner, H.H., Horn, V.J., Martin, G.R., and Hewitt, A.T.: Chondronectin interactions with proteoglycan. Arch. Biochem. Biophys., 244:824–830, 1986.

55. Hewitt, A.T., Varner, H.H., Silver, M.H., and Martin, G.R.: The role of chondronectin and cartilage proteoglycan in the attachment of chondrocytes to collagen. Prog. Clin. Biol. Res., 110B:25–33, 1982.

56. Hewitt, A.T. et al.: The isolation and partial characterization of chondronectin, an attachment factor for chondrocytes. J. Biol. Chem., 257:2330–2334, 1982.

57. Bayliss, M.T. et al.: Structure of proteoglycans from different layers of human articular cartilage. Biochem. J., 209:387–400, 1983.

58. Muir, H., and Hardingham, I.E.: Structures of proteoglycans. In MPP International Review of Science, Biochemistry Series One, Vol. 5: Biochemistry of Carbohydrates. Edited by W.J. Whelan. Baltimore, University Park Press, 1975, pp. 153–222.

59. Hardingham, T.E. et al.: Cartilage proteoglycans. CIBA Found. Symp., 124:30–46, 1986.

60. Rosenberg, L., Hellman, W., and Kleinschmidt, A.K.: Electron microscopic studies of proteoglycan aggregates from bovine articular cartilage. J. Biol. Chem., 250:1877–1883, 1975.

61. Elliott, R.J., and Gardner, D.L.: Changes with age in the glycosaminoglycans of human articular cartilage. Ann. Rheum. Dis., 38:371–377, 1979.

62. Poole, A.R., Pidoux, I., Reiner, A., and Rosenberg, L.: An immunoelectron microscope study of the organization of proteoglycan monomer, link protein, and collagen in the matrix of articular cartilage. J. Cell. Biol., 93:921–937, 1982.

63. Broom, N.D., and Poole, C.A.: Articular cartilage collagen and proteoglycans. Their functional interdependency. Arthritis Rheum., 26:1111–1119, 1983.

64. Ryu, J., Towle, C.A., and Treadwell, B.V.: Characterization of human articular cartilage link proteins from normal and osteoarthritic cartilage. Ann. Rheum. Dis., 41:164–167, 1982.

65. Melching, L.I., and Roughley, P.J.: The role of link protein in mediating the interaction between hyaluronic acid and

66. Bonner, W.M. et al.: Changes in the lipids of human articular cartilage with age. Arthritis Rheum., 18:461–473, 1975.

67. Paulsson, M., and Heinegard, D.: Noncollagenous cartilage proteins: Current status of an emerging research field. Coll. Relat. Res., 4:219–229, 1984.

68. Mankin, H.J., and Lippiello, L.: The turnover of adult rabbit articular cartilage. J. Bone Joint Surg., 51A:1591–1600, 1969.

69. Lippiello, L., Hall, D., and Mankin, N.J.: Collagen synthesis in normal and osteoarthritic human cartilage. J. Clin. Invest., 59:593–600, 1977.

70. Azzo, W., and Woessner, J.F., Jr.: Purification and characterization of an acid metalloproteinase from human articular cartilage. J. Biol. Chem., 261:5434–5441, 1986.

71. Sapolsky, A.I., and Howell, D.S.: Further characterization of a neutral metalloprotease isolated from human articular cartilage. Arthritis Rheum., 25:981–988, 1982.

72. Ehrlich, M.G.: Degradative enzyme systems in osteoarthritic cartilage. J. Orthop. Res., 3:170–184, 1985.

73. Morales, T.I., and Kuettner, K.: The properties of the neutral proteinase released by primary chondrocyte cultures and its action on proteoglycan aggregate. Biochim. Biophys. Acta, 705:92–101, 1982.

74. Ehrlich, M.G. et al.: Collagenase inhibitors in osteoarthritic and normal cartilage. J. Clin. Invest., 59:226–233, 1977.

75. Treadwell, B.V., and Mankin, H.J.: The synthetic processes of articular cartilage. Clin. Orthop., 213:50–61, 1986.

76. Dingle, J.T.: The effect of synovial catabolin on cartilage synthetic activity. Connect. Tissue Res., 12:277–286, 1984.

77. Treadwell, B.V. et al.: Purification and characterization of collagenase activator protein synthesized by articular cartilage. Arch. Biochem. Biophys., 251:715–723, 1986.

78. Fulkerson, J.P., and Damiamo, P.: Effect of prostaglandin E2 on adult pig articular cartilage slices in culture. Clin. Orthop., 179:266–269, 1983.

79. Mitrovic, D. et al.: Anti-inflammatory drugs, prostanoid and proteoglycan production by cultured bovine articular chondrocytes. Prostaglandins, 28:417–434, 1984.

80. Ollivierre, F. et al.: Expression of IL-1 genes in human and bovine chondrocytes: A mechanism for autocrine control of cartilage matrix degradation. Biochem. Biophys. Res. Commun., 141:904–911, 1986.

81. Treadwell, B.V. et al.: Stimulation of the synthesis of collagenase activator protein in cartilage by a factor present in synovial conditioned medium. Arch. Biochem. Biophys., 251:724–731, 1986.

82. Ghadially, F.N., and Roy, S.: Ultrastructure of Synovial Joints in Health and Disease. London, Butterworth, 1969.

83. Barland, P., Novikoff, A.B., and Hamerman, D.: Electron microscopy of the human synovial membrane. J. Cell Biol., 14:207–220, 1962.

84. Adkins, E.W.O., and Davies, D.V.: Absorption from the joint cavity. Q. J. Exp. Physiol., 30:147–154, 1940.

85. Radin, E.L., Swann, D.A., and Weisser, P.: Separation of a hyaluronate free lubricating fraction from synovial fluid. Nature, 288:377–378, 1970.

86. Swann, D.A. et al.: Role of hyaluronic acid in joint lubrication. Ann. Rheum. Dis., 33:318–326, 1974.

87. Swann, D.A., and Radin, E.L.: The molecular basis of articular lubrication. I. Purification and properties of a lubricating fraction from bovine synovial fluid. J. Biol. Chem., 274:8069–8073, 1972.

88. Dingle, J.T.: Catabolin—A cartilage catabolic factor from synovium. Clin. Orthop., *156*:219–231, 1980.
89. Jubb, R.W., and Fell, H.B.: The effect of synovial tissue on the synthesis of proteoglycan by the articular cartilage of young pigs. Arthritis Rheum., 23:545–555, 1980.
90. Bullough, P.G. et al.: The strength of the menisci of the knee as it relates to their fine structure. J. Bone Joint Surg., *52B*:564–570, 1970.
91. Peters, T.J., and Smillie, I.S.: Studies on the chemical composition of the menisci of the knee joint with special reference to the horizontal cleavage lesion. Clin. Orthop., *86*:245–252, 1972.
92. Solheim, K.: The glycosaminoglycans of human semilunar cartilage. J. Oslo City Hosp., *15*:127–132, 1965.
93. Eyre, D.R., and Wu, J.J.: Collagen of fibrocartilage: A distinctive molecular phenotype in bovine meniscus. FEBS Lett., *158*:265–270, 1983.
94. Aspden, R.M., Yarker, Y.E., and Hukins, D.W.: Collagen orientations in the meniscus of the knee joint. J. Anat., *140* (3):371–380, 1985.
95. Radin, E.L., Paul, I.L., and Lowy, M.: A comparison of the dynamic force transmitting properties of subchondral bone and articular cartilage. J. Bone Joint Surg., *52A*:444–456, 1970.
96. Radin, E.L. et al.: Effect of prolonged walking on concrete on the knees of sheep. J. Biomech., *15*:487–492, 1982.
97. Radin, E.L., and Rose, R.M.: Role of subchondral bone in the initiation and progression of cartilage damage. Clin. Orthop., *213*:34–40, 1986.
98. Redler, I., Mow, V.C., Zimny, A.L., and Mansell, J.: The ultrastructure and biomechanical significance of the tidemark of articular cartilage. Clin. Orthop., *112*:357–362, 1975.
99. Kenzora, J.E., Yosipovitch, Z., and Glimcher, M.J.: The calcified cartilage zone of adult articular cartilage: A viable functional entity. Orthop. Trans., *2*:120, 1978.
100. Bullough, P.G., and Jagannath, A.: The morphology of the calcification front in articular cartilage. Its significance in joint function. J. Bone Joint Surg., *65B*:72–78, 1983.
101. Johnson, L.C.: Kinetics of osteoarthritis. Lab. Invest., *8*:1223, 1959.
102. Inoue, H., and Tetsuaki, T.: Three dimensional observation of collagen framework of lumbar intervertebral discs. Acta Orthop. Scand., *46*:949–956, 1975.
103. Simon, S.R. et al: Peak dynamic force in human gait. J. Biomech., *14*:817–822, 1981.
104. Eyring, E.J., and Murray, W.R.: The effect of joint position on the pressure of intra-articular effusion. J. Bone Joint Surg., *46A*:1235–1241, 1964.
105. Myers, D.B., and Palmer, D.G.: Capsular compliance and pressure-volume relationships in normal and arthritic knees. J. Bone Joint Surg., *54B*:710–716, 1972.
106. McCall, J.: Load deformation response of the microstructure of articular cartilage. *In* Lubrication and Wear in Joints. Edited by V. Wright. London, Sector Publ. Ltd., 1969, pp. 39–48.
107. Maroudas, A.: Distribution and diffusion of solutes in articular cartilage. Biophys. J., *10*:365–379, 1970.
108. Armstrong, C.B., and Mow, V.C.: Variations in the intrinsic mechanical properties of human articular cartilage with age, degeneration, and water content. J. Bone Joint Surg., *64A*:88–94, 1982.
109. Donohue, J.M. et al.: The effects of indirect blunt trauma on adult canine articular cartilage. J. Bone Joint Surg., *65A*:948–957, 1983.
110. Hayes, W.C., and Mockros, L.F.: Viscoelastic properties of human articular cartilage. J. Appl. Physiol., *31*:462–568, 1971.
111. Simon, W.H., Friedenberg, S., and Richardson, S.: Joint congruence. A correlation of joint congruence and thickness of articular cartilage in dogs. J. Bone Joint Surg., *55A*:1614–1620, 1973.
112. Armstrong, C.G., and Gardner, D.L.: Thickness and distribution of human femoral head articular cartilage. Ann. Rheum. Dis., *36*:407–412, 1977.
113. Radin, E.L., and Paul, I.L.: Does cartilage compliance reduce skeletal inpact loads? The relative force—attenuating properties of articular cartilages, synovial fluid, periarticular soft tissues and bone. Arthritis Rheum., *13*:139–144, 1970.
114. Mital, M.A.: Human Hip Joints. M.S. Thesis. Glasgow University Strathclyde, 1970.
115. Bullough, P., Goodfellow, J., and O'Connor, J.: The relationship between degenerative changes and load-bearing in the human hip. J. Bone Joint Surg., *55*:746–758, 1973.
116. Radin, E.L., et al.: Response of joints to impact loading. III. Relationship between trabecular microfractures and cartilage degeneration. J. Biomech., *6*:51–57, 1973.
117. Pugh, J.W., Rose, R.M., and Radin, E.L.: A possible mechanism of Wolff's law: Trabecular microfractures. Arch. Int. Physiol. Biochim., *81*:27–40, 1973.
118. Radin, E.L.: Biomechanics of the knee joint. Orthop. Clin. North Am., *4*:539–546, 1973.
119. Fairbank, T.J.: Knee joint changes after meniscectomy. J. Bone Joint Surg., *30B*:664–670, 1948.
120. Shrive, N.G., O'Connor, J.J., and Goodfellow, J.W.: Load-bearing in the knee joint. Clin. Orthop., *131*:279–287, 1978.
121. Linn, F.C., and Radin, E.L.: Lubrication of animal joints. III. The effect of certain chemical alterations of the cartilage and lubricant. Arthritis Rheum., *11*:674–682, 1968.
122. Radin, E.L., and Paul, I.L.: Response of joints to impact loading. I. In vitro wear. Arthritis Rheum., *14*:356–362, 1971.
123. McCutchen, C.W.: Mechanism of animal joints. Nature, *184*:1284–1285, 1959.
124. Edwards, J.: Lubrication and Wear in Living and Artificial Human Joints. London, Institute of Mechanical Engineering, 1967.
125. Mow, V.C., and Mansour, J.M.: The nonlinear interaction between cartilage deformation and interstitial fluid flow. J. Biomech., *10*:31–39, 1977.
126. Linn, F.C., and Sokoloff, L.: Movement and composition of interstitial fluid of cartilage. Arthritis Rheum., *8*:481–493, 1965.
127. Coventry, M.B.: Anatomy of the invertebral disc. Clin. Orthop., *67*:9–15, 1969.
128. Happey, F.: Studies of the structure of the human intervertebral disc in relation to its functional and aging processes. *In* The Joints and Synovial Fluid, Vol. 2. Edited by L. Sokoloff. New York, Academic Press, 1980, pp 95–136.
129. Naylor, A.: The biochemical changes in the human intervertebral disc in degeneration and nuclear prolapse. Orthop. Clin. North Am., *2*:343–358, 1971.
130. Naylor, A. et al.: Enzymatic and immunological activity in the invertebral disc. Orthop. Clin. North Am., *6*:51–58, 1975.
131. Urban, J.P., and McMullin, J.F.: Swelling pressure of the intervertebral disc: Influence of proteoglycan and collagen contents. Biorheology, *22*:145–157, 1985.
132. Parke, W.W., and Schiff, D.C.M.: The applied anatomy of the invertebral disc. Orthop. Clin. North Am., *2*:309–324, 1971.
133. Sherk, H.H., and Nicholson, J.T.: Comparative anatomy and embryology of the cervical spine. Orthop. Clin. North Am., *2*:325–341, 1971.

134. Willis, T.A.: The phylogeny of the intervertebral disk: A pictorial review. Clin. Orthop., *54*:215–233, 1967.

135. Wolfe, H.J., Putschar, W.G.J., and Vickery, A.L.: Role of the notochord in human intervertebral disk. I. Fetus and infant. Clin. Orthop., *39*:205–212, 1965.

136. Gardner, E.: The development and growth of bones. J. Bone Joint Surg., *45A*:856–862, 1963.

137. Gower, W.E., and Pedrini, F.: Age related variations in protein polysaccharides from human nucleus pulposus, annulus fibrosus, and costal cartilage. J. Bone Joint Surg., *51A*:1154–1162, 1969.

138. Oegema, T.R., Jr., Bradford, D.S., Cooper, K.M., and Hunter, R.E.: Comparison of the biochemistry of proteoglycans isolated from normal, idiopathic scoliotic, and cerebral palsy spines. Spine, *8*:378–384, 1983.

139. Pearson, C.H. et al.: The non-collagenous proteins of the human intervertebral disc. Gerontologie, *15*:189–202, 1969.

140. Brickley-Parsons, D., and Glimcher, M.J.: Is the chemistry of collagen in intervertebral discs an expression of Wolff's law? A study of the human lumbar spine. Spine, *9*:148–163, 1984.

141. Souter, W., and Taylor, T.K.F.: Sulphated acid mucopolysaccharide metabolism in the rabbit intervertebral disc. J. Bone Joint Surg., *52B*:371–384, 1970.

142. Hirsch, C., and Nachemson, A.: New observations on mechanical behavior of lumbar discs. Acta Orthop. Scand., *23*:254–283, 1954.

143. Markolf, K.L.: Deformation of the thoracolumbar intervertebral joints in response to external loads. J. Bone Joint Surg., *54A*:511–533, 1972.

144. Nachemson, A., and Morris, J.M.: In vivo measurements of intradiscal pressure. J. Bone Joint Surg., *46A*:1077–1092, 1964.

145. Broberg, K.B.: On the mechanical behavior of the intervertebral discs. Spine, *8*:151–165, 1983.

146. Dunlop, R.B., Adams, M.A., and Hutton, W.C.: Disc space narrowing and the facet joints. J. Bone Joint Surg., *66B*:706–710, 1984.

147. Gotfried, Y., Bradford, D.S., and Oegema, T.R.: Facet joint changes after chemonucleolysis-induced disc space narrowing. Spine, *11*:944–950, 1986.

148. White, A.A., III, and Gordon, S.L.: Synopsis: Workshop on idiopathic low-back pain. Spine, *7*:141–149, 1982.

11

SYNOVIAL PHYSIOLOGY

PETER A. SIMKIN

Synovial joints are the bearings through which the human machine accomplishes its work. Surrounding tissues help to maintain, support, and renew these complex living bearings throughout the lifetime of the individual. Principal among these tissues is the synovium, which supports the normal joint in at least three important physiologic ways: (1) it provides an unobtrusive, low-friction lining; (2) it transports needed nutrients into the joint space while it removes metabolic wastes, and (3) it plays an important role in maintaining joint stability. These physiologic functions in health and their alterations in disease are reviewed here. A fourth important role, the provision of biologic lubricants, is discussed in Chapter 10.

SYNOVIAL LINING

Because motion is the business of joints, the synovial lining must be able to adapt to the full range of positions permitted by the surrounding tendons, ligaments, and joint capsule. As a finger flexes, for instance, the palmar synovium of each interphalangeal joint contracts while the dorsal synovium expands. As the finger re-extends, the roles are reversed (Fig. 11–1). This expansion and contraction of synovium appear more consistent with an accordion-like process of folding and unfolding than with an elastic stretching of the tissue.

Most expansion and contraction of the synovium takes place over unopposed surfaces of articular cartilage. For any joint to flex or extend, there must be a disparity in the surface areas of opposing cartilages. When the joint moves, the smaller area glides across or around the larger. Cartilage not in contact with opposing cartilage is temporarily covered by synovium as, for example, are the knuckles of a clenched fist. As the cartilage surfaces move on each other to return to their initial position, an effective lubrication system must prevent pinching of the adjacent, vascular synovial tissue. Were this system to fail, repeated hemarthroses would prove rapidly incapacitating. This lubrication problem has not received the attention devoted to that of cartilage on cartilage. Swann and associates have suggested, however, that the hyaluronate molecules that render synovial fluid viscous may find their major physiologic role in lubricating the synovium.[1]

The well-lubricated synovium must expand and contract within the confines of the joint capsule. The process is easier when the volume of synovial tissue is at a minimum and is impeded when the volume is excessive. The cellular infiltration, hyperplasia, and edema of active synovitis may thus limit joint motion when the synovium gathers as a mass lesion. This problem seems likely to be most acute in full flexion, because the capsule of "hinge" joints is normally thicker on the flexor surface, and compression of extracapsular soft tissue further compromises the available space. In addition to its effect on range of motion, this process may also contribute to the stiffness of many arthritic patients.

Studies of relaxed metacarpophalangeal joints undergoing passive manipulation have found that in-

FIG. 11–1. Lateral views of an interphalangeal joint in extension (A) and in flexion (B). The greater surface area of proximal articular cartilage permits the distal bone to move around the proximal. Redundant synovium (shown schematically) gathers above the superior margin in extension and below the inferior margin during flexion.

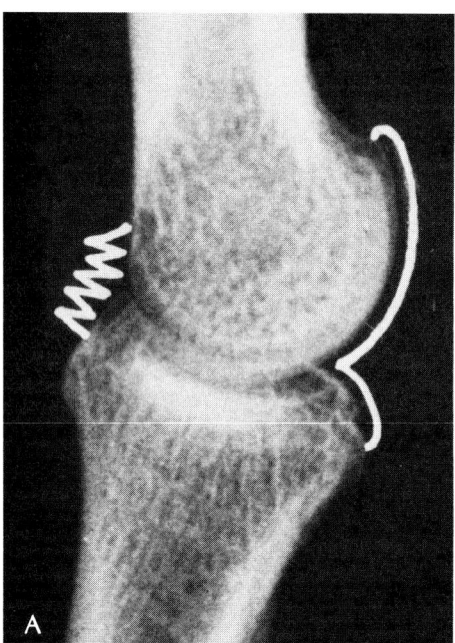

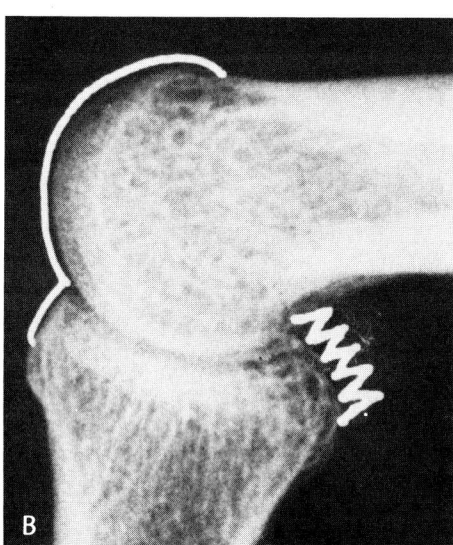

creased stiffness is readily demonstrable in the hands of patients with rheumatoid arthritis (RA) and this stiffness is greater in flexion than in extension.[2,3] Stiffness in normal joints is a complex phenomenon influenced by the time of day, varying inversely with grip strength and temperature, increasing progressively with age, occurring to a greater degree in men than in women, and affected by muscles, tendons,

and other periarticular structures, as well as by the capsule and synovium.[4] In the more severe stiffness characteristic of RA, the typical morning pattern suggests that tissue edema develops during periods of rest and then partially resolves with activity. The sensation of stiffness presumably results when redundant, edematous tissue interferes with free use of the joint.

SYNOVIAL TRANSPORT

In their classic studies of synovial effusions, Ropes and Bauer likened the synovial fluid to a dialysate of plasma.[5] They found a wide assortment of electrolytes and small molecules in the effusions at concentrations equivalent to those of plasma. The dialysate concept adequately explained the relative exclusion of most proteins in the presence of full equilibration of smaller molecules. Only hyaluronate, which is locally synthesized by synovial cells, departed from this pattern to a significant degree.

This model, however, is too simple to reflect the problem of synovial permeability fairly. The synovium is not a single inert membrane, but a complex living tissue (Fig. 11–2). As Bauer and colleagues also noted, transfer across the synovium "necessitates passage through an endothelial wall as well as diffusion through the intercellular spaces of the synovial membrane."[6] They were thus well aware that synovial permeability includes and implies both these barriers, but they were unable to dissect the individual contributions of the endothelium and interstitium.

The importance of considering these barriers separately may be illustrated by the "increased vascular permeability," regarded as a hallmark of inflammation. In this phenomenon, the inflamed endothelium is thought to leak an excessive amount of protein into the interstitium. If this excess is not cleared by a comparable increase in the rate of lymphatic clearance, the extravascular concentration of protein will rise toward the plasma level. The necessary result is a progressive diminution in the colloid osmotic pressure gradient between the two spaces. Because this pressure gradient drives venular reabsorption of water, increased vascular permeabiilty leads to edema in tissues and to effusions in joints. These principles reflect the Starling-Landis hypothesis of microvascular function and underscore the importance of the endothelium in retaining plasma proteins.[7]

It would be wrong, however, to infer that increased microvascular permeability to proteins necessarily means a significant increase in synovial permeability to smaller molecules as well. Small solutes normally

Joint space

Synovial lining cells

Interstitial space

Fenestrated endothelium

Blood

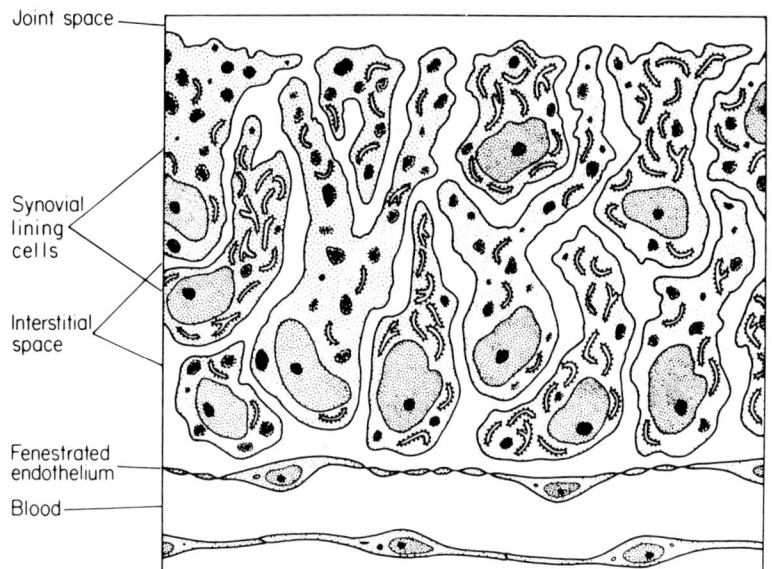

FIG. 11–2. The synovium. Molecules entering or leaving the joint space must traverse both the microvascular endothelium and the interstitial space between synovial cells. The endothelium provides the principal barrier limiting synovial permeability to proteins. The permeability of smaller molecules appears to be limited chiefly by their diffusibility across the synovial interstitium.

cross the endothelium not only through the "large pores" available to proteins, but also through a more abundant and highly permeable "small pore" system that excludes all large molecules. After leaving the microvessels, all molecules large and small must still traverse the synovial interstitium before they enter the synovial fluid. This tissue space, rather than the endothelium, appears to be the most important limiting factor in the overall transynovial exchange of small molecules. This functional duality (proteins limited by endothelium–small solutes limited by interstitium) permits independent changes in synovial permeability to large and to small solutes.

SMALL MOLECULES

Small physiologic molecules (those under 10,000 daltons in molecular weight) are usually in full equilibration between plasma and synovial fluid. To study the mechanism of their transynovial exchange, one must disturb this equilibrium and then measure and interpret the kinetics of the reequilibration process. This may be done in a number of ways.

A series of experiments in normal human knees provided the best evidence of the normal process of transynovial exchange and supported the critical importance of interstitial diffusion.[8] In this model, the knee was injected with saline solution containing trace amounts of tritiated water, benzyl alcohol, and ^{14}carbon (^{14}C)-labeled urea, urate, glucose, or sucrose. Serial samples of intrasynovial saline solution were then removed and were assayed for those exogenous tracer compounds as well as for endogenous urea, urate, glucose, creatinine, and total protein moving

from plasma into the saline solution. Over the course of the experiment, the concentration of endogenous molecules progressively rose toward full equilibration with plasma levels, whereas the concentration of exogenous molecules fell toward zero as they were cleared from the joint space. In a kinetic analysis of these data, the Fick diffusion equation permitted calculation of permeability values for each solute at the midpoint of every experiment. These experimental values, analogous to renal clearances, may be considered as the volume of intrasynovial saline solution equilibrating with plasma per unit time (ml/min).

For most compounds, synovial permeability is inversely related to the dimensions of the molecule. Thus, a plot of observed synovial permeability versus diffusion coefficient (which reflects configuration as well as size) yields a rather linear function (Fig. 11–3). This proportionality suggests that most small molecules cross the synovium by a process of free diffusion. Further analysis indicates that the limiting diffusion path is relatively long and narrow. These dimensions seem most consistent with those of the narrow channels between synovial lining cells. It thus appears that synovial permeability to most small molecules is determined by a process of free diffusion, limited mainly by the intercellular spaces of the synovium (see Fig. 11–2).

Additional evidence supporting this concept has been found in a high correlation between permeability and intrasynovial volume. Distention of the joint space accelerates the transynovial exchange of small molecules. This relationship is best explained by the probability that distention increases intercellular distances, thus facilitating the diffusion process. The positive correlation between volume and permeability

FIG. 11–3. Synovial permeability in normal, resting knees. The permeability is plotted against the diffusion coefficient. Egress and ingress are with respect to the joint space. Most data points are the mean values from 25 studies, but egress values for sucrose, glucose, urate, and urea are based on 7, 6, 6, and 6 studies, respectively. Benzyl alcohol leaving and glucose entering the joint space move rapidly because of diffusion into cells and specific transport, respectively. Protein enters slowly because of endothelial pore size limitation. Tritiated water leaves more slowly than predicted by its diffusion coefficient, probably because its egress is limited by effective synovial blood flow. All other small molecules (sucrose, urea, urate, creatinine, and glucose leaving the joint) cross the synovium at rates inversely proportional to their size as predicted by diffusion kinetics.

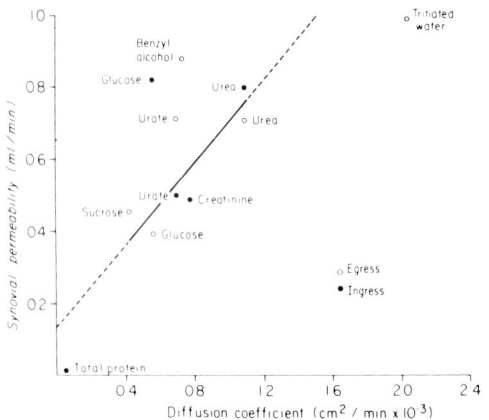

provides an interesting teleologic explanation for synovial effusions because the presence of an effusion enhances the delivery of nutrients to and the removal of wastes from the perturbed joint. In addition, these observations indicate that the intrasynovial volume should be known and considered in any comparative study of synovial permeabilities.

More recent evaluations of these and other data used a different analysis to reach the same interpretation of the synovium as a double barrier between plasma and synovial fluid. Once again, the microvascular endothelium was believed to be most critical for proteins, and the synovial interstitium was considered to be more important in determining the exchange of small solutes.[9,10]

In the aforementioned studies, the bidirectional permeability of urate ions was symmetric and consistent with simple diffusion kinetics. Dick and his associates have evidence, however, that egress of other anions from the joint space may be facilitated by a specific transport system. In their experiments, potassium perchlorate inhibited clearance of [99m]technetium (^{99m}Tc) and [131]iodine (^{131}I) from dog stifle joints and ^{99m}Tc from human knees.[11,12] These observations are of interest because effective active export of halide ions would be followed passively by sodium ions and by water. Such a system would thus be a "pump" capable of moving water out of the joint space.

Several other investigators have also studied the removal of ionic sodium and iodine from human knees.[13] The radioactive ions [24]sodium ([24]Na) and ^{131}I emit gamma rays that readily pass through human soft tissues. A counter placed over the joint is thus able continuously to monitor the disappearance of these isotopes after their intra-articular injection. These tracings characteristically follow a simple exponential pattern, which may be usefully expressed as either a half-life value or a clearance constant. In different series of normal knees, mean clearance constants for [24]Na have ranged from 0.022 to 0.051 min[-1], whereas similar determinations for ^{131}I have been from 0.022 to 0.055 min[-1]. These isotopes are thought to leave the knee by way of the blood, an interpretation supported by the work of Scholer and associates, who injected knees with heavy water (D_2O) and either [22]Na or [24]Na, followed the appearance of these isotopes in serial samples of arterial blood, and from these data calculated clearance constants in the same range as those obtained by external counting over the joint.[14] In addition, clearance of [24]Na from the knee was reduced when Harris and Millard inflated a tourniquet around the thigh to 60 mm Hg and was eliminated when they raised the pressure to 200 mm Hg.[15] These findings demonstrate that isotopic clearance depends on an effective circulation and diffusion into adjacent tissues plays no meaningful role.

The same isotopic clearance technique has been applied to the study of patients with joint diseases. Both in degenerative joint disease and in RA one sees a variable but consistently significant (up to threefold) increase above normal rates for the disappearance of both [24]Na and [131]I. The intrasynovial volume was not determined in these experiments, but clinical impressions suggested a positive correlation between effusion size and isotopic clearance rate. Intra-articular steroids caused a diminished clearance in a few individuals. In short, these investigators found that isotopic clearance correlated well with clinical signs of synovial inflammation. They attributed this finding to an enhanced synovial blood flow in active synovitis.

Clinical physiologists have long been interested in accurate determinations of the synovial blood flow. The vascular supply, however, is provided by many small vessels and is in part shared by the joint capsule, epiphyseal bone, and other perisynovial structures.[16] Thus, it is not possible to isolate and measure that

FIG. 11–4. Synovial permeability values of tritiated water from the resting knees of normal individuals, patients with rheumatoid arthritis, and subjects with other forms of arthritis. Under these experimental conditions, the effective synovial blood flow is not enhanced and may, indeed, be diminished in some of the patients with rheumatoid arthritis.

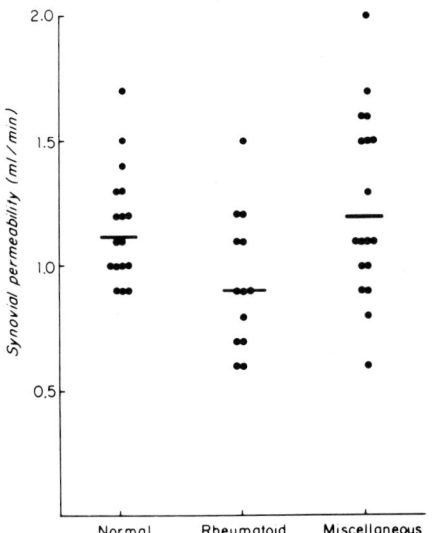

portion of the blood supply specifically destined for synovium, but the synovial blood flow may be indirectly approached by examining the clearance of small marker molecules from the joint space. In the event of full equilibration between synovial fluid and perfusing plasma, the clearance of such a marker would be equal to the synovial blood flow. Because it is unlikely that such equilibration is ever complete, all experimental values must be qualified with the adjective "effective." Using tritiated water as the marker, we found a mean effective synovial blood flow of 1 ml/min in normal knees.[8] When the same test system was used in inflamed arthritic knees, many with rheumatoid arthritis had diminished effective synovial blood flow, whereas those with other forms of joint disease had a wide range of values (Fig. 11–4). Unlike the studies of free ^{24}Na and ^{131}I, these experiments were conducted with equivalent intra-articular volumes and in the presence of a mild irritant (0.9% benzyl alcohol). The low rates found in many patients with RA suggest that they have an impaired capacity to respond to additional stimuli, as reflected by the data in Figure 11–4.

The effective blood flow has been re-examined using a new experimental method in 11 patients with rheumatoid arthritis and 9 people with osteoarthritis.[17,18] In this work, trace amounts of both free ^{123}I and ^{131}I-labeled human serum albumin were injected into existing knee effusions and were followed simultaneously by external counting. The apparent distribution volume was assessed by isotope dilution of the labeled albumin in a synovial fluid specimen aspirated after 24 hours. From the product of the rate constant for removal of free iodide (min^{-1}) and the volume (ml), one can determine a clearance value in ml/min (Table 11–1).

The clearance of free iodide (like that of tritiated water in the previous work), may be taken as an indicator of effective synovial blood flow. The values are comparable to those found with tritiated water but are higher, presumably because of the larger volumes that include the interstitial water of the synovial tissue as well as the recoverable effusion. Once again, the mean effective blood flow was lower in the rheumatoid patients, and 6 of the lowest 7 values were found in this disease. Within the rheumatoid group, the clearance of free iodine correlated with synovial fluid pH (r = 0.74), lactate (r = −0.77), synovial fluid/serum ratio of glucose (r = 0.81), and temperature (r = 0.88). The high correlation between apparent blood flow and these indices of circulatory metabolic imbalance suggests that the rheumatoid synovium is often hypoperfused and ischemic. Apparently, microvascular impairment may prevent an adequate circulatory response to the rheumatoid process.

The problems associated with studies of synovial blood flow must not be underestimated. Potential problems include inadequate mixing of injected solutes within the joint space, partial equilibration of the isotopic marker between plasma and interstitial fluid, experimental distortion of intrasynovial volume, pressure, or temperature, and varying levels of physical activity. No study has yet controlled most, let alone all, of these variables, and the problem of synovial blood flow thus remains an important area for further investigation.

GLUCOSE

Glucose is carried in plasma, is delivered by synovial transport, and is one of the most important nutrients required by chondrocytes. Because glucose concentration is easily measured in synovial fluid and is often low with severe synovitis, physicians have long been interested in its transynovial exchange.[19] Ropes, Muller, and Bauer were the first systematically to study normal mechanisms of glucose transport into joints.[20] They found that the concentration of glucose in synovial fluid usually was close to that of plasma. Between 3 and 4 hours after meals, however, levels were regularly higher within the joint space than they were in the perfusing blood. After a series of infusion

Table 11–1. Iodide Clearance from Rheumatoid and Osteoarthritic Knees

	n	Vol (ml)	Rate constant (min⁻¹)	Clearance (ml/min)
Rheumatoid arthritis	11	106 ± 23	0.018 ± 0.007	1.92 ± 0.98
Osteoarthritis	9	109 ± 105	0.028 ± 0.017	2.40 ± 1.44

experiments in man and in cattle, these investigators suggested that a specific transport system might facilitate the transfer of glucose from plasma to synovial fluid.

We used a different experimental approach (described previously) to confirm the presence of asymmetric glucose transport.[8] These studies used serial concentration changes within an injectate of saline solution to compare the egress of ^{14}C-labeled compounds with the ingress of physiologic "cold" molecules in normal human knees. Most small molecules, exemplified by urea in Figure 11–5, move freely in both directions between plasma and synovial fluid in accord with simple diffusion kinetics. In these studies, however, the finding that glucose entered the joint space more rapidly than would be expected from its size alone implicates a specific glucose transport system, a system that accelerates the entrance of glucose into the joint space, but does not affect its rate

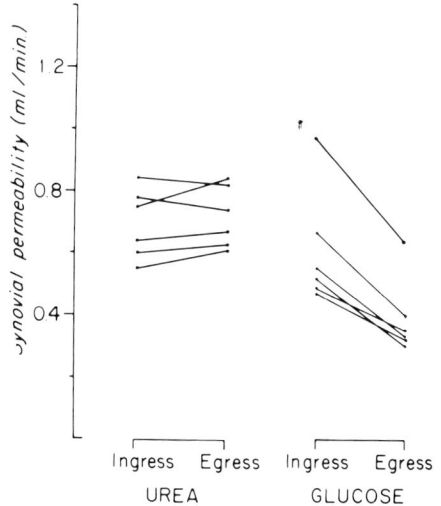

FIG. 11–5. Ingress of endogenous urea and glucose is compared with egress of the labeled molecules from resting normal knees. The synovium is symmetrically permeable to urea (mean ingress/egress = 0.97). Glucose, however, enters the joint at a rate faster than it leaves (mean ingress/egress = 1.59). These data are most consistent with a unidirectional transport system moving glucose into the joint. (From Simkin, P.A., and Pizzorno, J.E: Transynovial exchange of small molecules in normal human subjects. J. Appl. Physiol., 36:581–587, 1974.)

of return to the plasma. These studies do not establish whether the specific glucose transport occurs by active (energy requiring) transport or by facilitated diffusion, although the second mechanism appears more likely.

The synovial fluid glucose level in inflamed joints may be lower than plasma levels. Although most characteristic of sepsis, this finding is often present in rheumatoid disease (where levels may be undetectably low) and has occasionally been observed in gout, trauma, and other joint afflictions.[5] A low level thus offers no diagnostic specificity. Low glucose values may, however, offer valuable insight into the effectiveness of the synovial microcirculation. Specifically, any low value must indicate that the intrasynovial demand for glucose exceeds the supply and suggests that this circulatory-metabolic imbalance may apply for other nutrients as well. For instance, Falchuk, Goetzl, and Kulka found a low glucose concentration in 3 of 15 rheumatoid synovial fluids, and all 3 had remarkably low P_{O_2}, high P_{CO_2}, high lactate, and low pH.[21] Both increased consumption and impaired delivery reasonably may be implicated in this disruption of the normal equilibration between synovial fluid and plasma.

The white blood cells of synovial fluid consume little glucose in vitro and cannot be the most important factor in intrasynovial hypoglycemia.[20] Additional experiments in vitro suggest that hyperplastic synovium is the major user of glucose in rheumatoid joints, and presumably active synovitis of other origins may be similarly implicated.[22] Clearly, synovial consumption must be an important variable. Otherwise, even a marginal microcirculation would be able to maintain equilibration between synovial fluid and plasma.

Conversely, a microcirculation of maximal effectiveness should be able to supply an increased demand for glucose. Low glucose values indicate that the demand has not been met and suggest impaired microvascular function. The overall importance of vascular impairment is supported by the significant ($p < 0.005$) correlations we found between effective synovial blood flow (^{123}I clearance) and synovial fluid pH, lactate, glucose, and temperature in 11 rheumatoid synovial effusions. Obliteration of terminal blood vessels is a well-recognized histologic manifestation of rheumatoid synovitis. This direct vascular loss could well explain local synovial ischemia. The finding that "rice bodies" in a synovial fluid from patients with RA contain collagen types I, III, and V in a proportion of 40/40/20, identical to that of synovial membrane, strongly suggests that such local ischemia is accompanied by microinfarction and detachment of the infarcted tisssue to form the core of the "rice body."[23] In addition, as data of Ropes and Bauer suggest,[5] the high intrasynovial pressure of some rheumatoid effusions may further compromise the synovial microvessels by tamponade. Experimental support for this concept comes from the finding that a tense effusion markedly inhibited clearance of [133]xenon (^{133}Xe) from inflamed joints.[24]

In summary, a specific transport system accelerates the entrance of glucose into normal joints. Low levels of glucose often occur in the synovial effusions of intra-articular sepsis or rheumatoid arthritis. The precise mechanism of this intrasynovial hypoglycemia is unclear, but it appears to be caused both by increased local use and by impaired delivery of glucose into the joint space.

FAT-SOLUBLE SOLUTES

Because fat-soluble solutes can diffuse through, as well as between, cell membranes, they do not face the same synovial surface area restrictions as do hydrophilic molecules. The entire surface area of the synovium is available to lipophilic molecules diffusing in or out of the joint space. In our studies of normal knees, this phenomenon was seen with benzyl alcohol, a fat-soluble molecule that left the joint space faster than hydrophilic molecules of equivalent size.[8]

Physiologically, the most important fat-soluble molecules are the respiratory gases: oxygen and carbon dioxide. Since 1970, several investigators have studied the synovial fluid content of these crucial metabolites.[13,21,25] These studies show that many patients with RA (as well as a smaller number of patients with other joint diseases) have low P_{O_2} values, and this finding correlates with increased P_{CO_2}, decreased pH, and increased lactate (Fig. 11–6). Despite the high diffusibility of oxygen, its supply is unable to meet synovial demand in such joints. The resultant hypoxia makes synovial cells use the metabolically expensive glycolytic pathway with a consequent increase in consumption of glucose and production of lactic acid. Lactic acid, together with the carbonic acid produced by oxidative metabolism, leads to an intra-articular acidosis with synovial fluid pH values as low as 6.8.[25,26] All these changes reflect a severe circulatory-metabolic imbalance within the inflamed synovium, with the microvasculature unable either to supply sufficient metabolic fuels or to clear the products of their combustion adequately. As yet, little is known about the consequences to the bearer of such compromised joints. We do not know how well the cartilage withstands local hypoxia, hypoglycemia, and acidosis. It seems likely, however, that these factors may be important in the pathogenesis of rheumatoid lesions. Circulatory-metabolic imbalance in the synovium will require more investigation before the clinician will be able to recognize the problem readily and appropriately interpret its implications.

Lipophilic molecules (those having a high oil:water partition coefficient) pose a special problem because they accumulate in fatty tisues and are eluted slowly by the surrounding interstitial water. Recognition of this fact has led investigators to abandon ^{133}Xe clearance as a technique for the study of synovial blood flow. When ^{133}Xe was injected into a joint, its exponential clearance could be followed by external counting using the same techniques as described for [24]Na and [131]I. For example, the clearance constant from

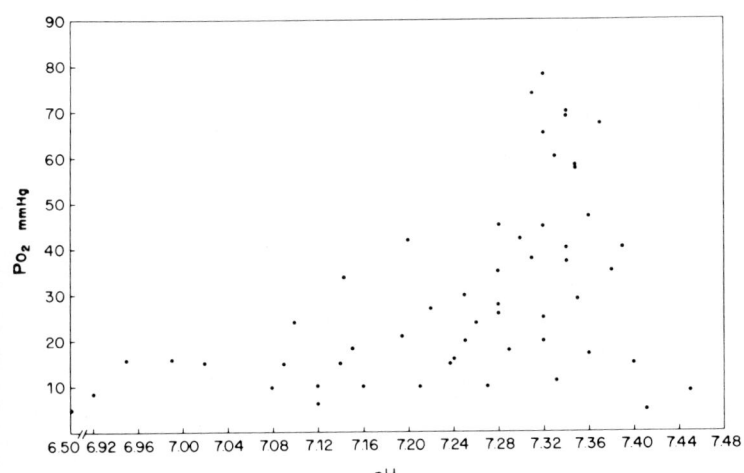

FIG. 11–6. Correlation of oxygen tension (P_{O_2}) with pH in synovial effusion of patients with various joint diseases. The pH varies little with modest local hypoxia, but usually becomes acidotic when the P_{O_2} falls below 30 mm Hg. (Courtesy of Dr. D.J. McCarty.)

normal knees was 0.0028, an order of magnitude less than that found for sodium or iodide.[27] Unfortunately, as Phelps, Steele, and McCarty demonstrated, the recorded clearance was from perisynovial fat rather than from the joint space.[24] The technique is therefore of little value in assessing synovial blood flow.

DRUGS

Physicians treating any form of arthritis are engaged in a battle against synovial inflammation. The principal weapons in this war are drugs intended to eliminate the cause or to ameliorate the effects of the inflammatory process, but how well do these agents reach their target? This question has been asked primarily by examining drug levels in synovial fluid and contrasting them with concurrent concentrations in plasma. Available data, obtained under a wide variety of clinical circumstances, indicate that drugs readily cross the double barrier of microvascular endothelium and synovial interstitium to appear in the synovial fluid.

We have reviewed an expanding literature on anti-inflammatory drug levels in synovial fluids and tissue.[28] For any orally administered drug, plasma levels reflect the sequential but overlapping processes of absorption, distribution, and elimination. Peak levels are usually reached within 1 or 2 hours, and the plasma concentration subsequently falls at rates reflecting first the distribution of the drug throughout the various tissue compartments and then the metabolism or elimination of that specific agent. The levels in synovial fluid lag behind those of plasma, reach a later and lower peak, and then begin their own descent. At some point, the downward slopes of both curves characteristically cross, and synovial fluid levels are subsequently higher than those of plasma (Fig. 11–7). After this time, the concentration gradient leads to diffusion of the agent from the tissues back into blood. The time required to reach this crossing or equilibration point appears to be a function primarily of the half-life of the drug. Short-lived agents such as aspirin have the earliest equilibration time, whereas long-lived drugs such as phenylbutazone have the latest, with intermediate agents falling in between (Fig. 11–8). This pattern may vary with the protein content of each effusion, the degree of protein binding of the agent, and the effective blood flow. Nevertheless, the available data indicate that synovial fluid levels exceed those of plasma by a passive, nonspecific process that is most readily observed in the case of short-lived therapeutic agents. On balance,

FIG. 11–7. Mean concentrations in serial samples of plasma and synovial fluid after a single oral dose of a therapeutic agent. Plasma levels rise rapidly with gastrointestinal absorption, fall as the drug is distributed throughout body compartments, and then decline steadily as a result of continuing metabolism and excretion. Synovial fluid levels initially lag behind those in plasma, but then cross over the plasma concentration (at the equilibration point) and eventually decline at a rate comparable to that in plasma. After equilibration, the drug diffuses down the concentration gradient from synovial fluid back into plasma. (Modified from indomethacin data of Emori, H.W., Champion, G.D., Bluestone, R., and Paulus, H.E.: Simultaneous pharmacokinetics of indomethacin in serum and synovial fluid. Ann. Rheum. Dis., 32:433–435, 1973.)

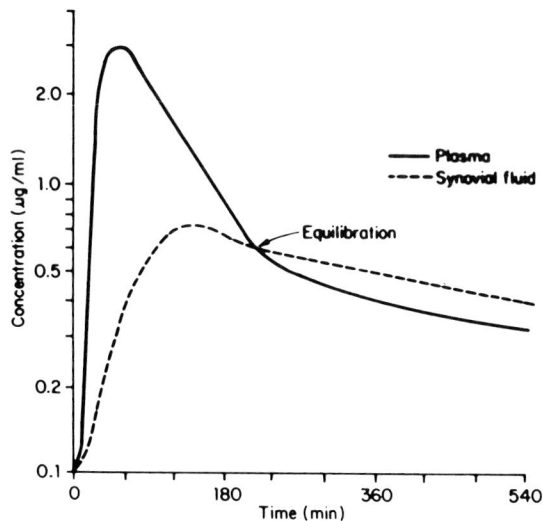

such drugs possess no apparent advantage over longer-lived agents.

Antibiotics constitute a second major class of drugs that has been studied in a similar way. Rapp and colleagues in patients with traumatic synovitis, Nelson in children, and Parker and Schmid in adults with acute septic arthritis have examined intrasynovial antibiotic concentrations.[29–31] They found that such levels lag behind peak plasma concentrations, with some suggestion that the lag is greater for antibiotics of larger molecular weight, such as erythromycin. In all cases, however, effective antibiotic levels were achieved within these repeatedly aspirated joints. It remains possible, and perhaps likely, however, that antibiotic access may be limited in tense, undrained effusions. Such conditions, analogous to any other abscess, would be most likely to occur in smaller or less accessible joints in which high-pressure effusions may be most easily overlooked. Therefore, *it remains unwise to assume that adequate antibiotic levels are present*

FIG. 11–8. Biological half-life versus equilibration time for nonsteroidal anti-inflammatory drugs. The linear relationship indicates that equilibration occurs early in the case of those agents that are rapidly cleared from plasma and late in those with a long biologic half-life. With usual dosage schedules, short-lived agents are often found with synovial fluid concentrations exceeding the concurrent levels in plasma. (From Wallis, W. J., and Simkin, P. A.: Antirheumatic drug levels in human synovial fluid and synovial tissue: observations on extravascular pharmacokinetics. Clin. Pharmacokinet., 8:496–522, 1983.)

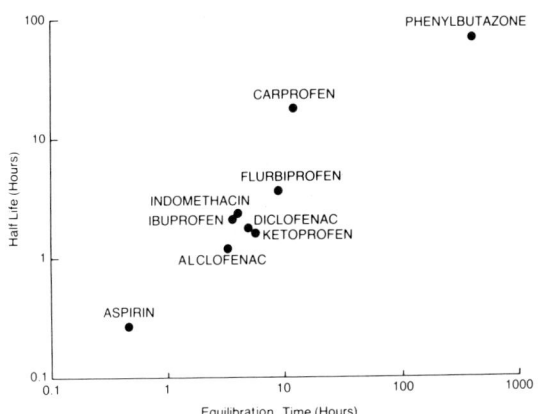

in any septic joint unless it is regularly aspirated or surgically drained.

PROTEIN

The proteins of synovial fluid are qualitatively the same as those of plasma, but there are major quantitative differences.[5,32] Normal synovial fluid from the human knee contains 1.3 g of total protein per 100 ml, and most of that protein is albumin.[33] The larger molecules such as fibrinogen, large globulins, and certain complement components are largely excluded. In "noninflammatory" effusions, found primarily in the knees of edematous patients, the same relative distribution holds, but with higher total protein concentrations. Because its small volumes make it inaccessible to investigators, there are few observations of truly normal human synovial fluid and essentially none from any joint other than the knee.

With active synovitis, proteins gain more ready access to the joint space. The fluid clots after aspiration, the complement activity increases (unless ongoing consumption is present), and the concentration of each protein approaches that of plasma. The rate of total protein ingress into normal and diseased joints was examined in our studies using serial sampling of "artificial effusions" comprised of comparable volumes of physiologic saline containing 0.9% benzyl alcohol (Table 11–2.)[34] The rate of protein entry was higher than normal (p <0.001) both in rheumatoid arthritis and in a diverse "miscellaneous synovitis" group including patients with osteoarthritis, septic arthritis, gout, and psoriasis. This increase in permeability to proteins was clearly not shared by smaller molecules exemplified by tritiated water $(^3H)H_2O$ in Figure 11–4. This important differential effect of inflammation is entirely consistent with the double-barrier model of synovial permeability. Active synovitis lowers the endothelial barrier to proteins but does not affect, or may even increase, the interstitial barrier that is the limiting factor in transynovial exchange of smaller molecules.

Both in normal and in diseased joints, one sees continuing turnover of synovial fluid proteins. Proteins entering the joint space do so at rates inversely proportional to their molecular size. In contrast, proteins of quite different dimensions have been found to leave the joint at essentially identical rates.[35,36] The presumed basis for this difference is that entering proteins primarily arrive by the size-selective process of diffusion, whereas all proteins leave the joint by the bulk flow of lymphatic drainage. In any stable effusion, these opposing processes are in balance, and the net flux into the joint (mg/min) is equaled by the net flux out. This net efflux of any protein may be obtained from the product of its concentration in synovial fluid (mg/ml) and the effective rate of lymphatic flow (ml/min).

We have determined the effective lymphatic flow in a series of patients with rheumatoid and osteoarthritis.[18] As in the case of effective blood flow, the lymphatic flow is assessed by the product of intracapsular volume (ml) and the rate constant for removal of a labeled marker (min^{-1}). These experiments used ^{131}I-labeled human serum albumin as the reference protein. The clearance rate of labeled albumin (interpreted as the effective synovial lymph flow) was

Table 11–2. Mean Synovial Permeability to Tritiated Water (THO) and Total Protein

	n	THO (ml/min)	Protein (ml/min)
Normal	17	1.11 ± 0.05	0.008 ± 0.001
Rheumatoid	13	0.90 ± 0.07	0.021 ± 0.002
Miscellaneous	18	1.11 ± 0.05	0.024 ± 0.003

0.071 ± 0.028 (SD) ml/min in 11 patients with RA and 0.039 ± 0.030 ml/min in patients with osteoarthritis. The difference between the 2 groups was significant, thus providing evidence for an accelerated rate of lymphatic flow in patients with rheumatoid disease.

The principal advantage of such information is the opportunity it provides for a kinetic interpretation of synovial fluid protein concentrations. A considerable body of evidence is now on hand regarding synovial fluid levels and synovial fluid:serum (SF/S) concentration ratios of specific plasma proteins.[33] Figure 11–9, for instance, gives data on SF/S for orosomucoid, transferrin, albumin, ceruloplasmin, and α_2-macroglobulin in fluid from patients with rheumatoid arthritis and osteoarthritis. The SF/S of these reference proteins bears a clear inverse relationship to their molecular size consistent with passive diffusion from plasma to synovial fluid. Similar plots have been useful to several other authors in qualitatively assessing whether immunoglobulins are locally produced in the synovium.[32,37] Values of SF/S above the passive regression line suggest local IgG synthesis in rheumatoid synovium, for instance, whereas an SF/S appropriate for the size of IgG makes local production unlikely in osteoarthritis. Although such assessments have been useful, these static observations provide no quantitative information regarding either synovial perme-

ability or local production of specific proteins. In fact, SF/S reflects the point of equilibrium between the opposing rates of permeability (in) and clearance (out).[9] Without appropriate kinetic information, one cannot determine whether a high SF/S, for instance, reflects increased permeability, decreased lymphatic flow, or a combination of the two.

An example of such a kinetic analysis is the measurement of protein flux through the articular cavity. Because the lymphatic egress of proteins is not size selective, the clearance rate of albumin can be assumed to reflect the clearance of all other passively

FIG. 11–9. Mean synovial fluid:serum ratios (SF/S) as a function of molecular radius for five plasma proteins (transferrin, orosomucoid, albumin, ceruloplasmin, and α_2 macroglobulin) in patients with rheumatoid arthritis and osteoarthritis. The concentration ratios differ by a degree that is not statistically significant. (From Wallis, W.J., Simkin, P.A., and Nelp, W.B.: Protein traffic in human synovial effusions. Arthritis Rheum., *30*:57–63, 1987.)

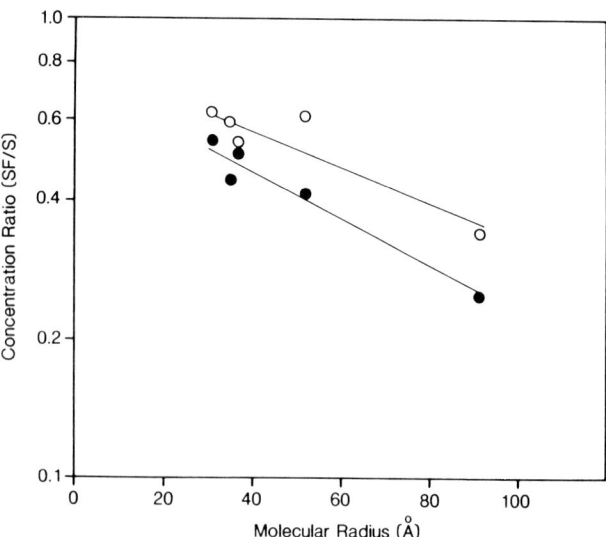

FIG. 11–10. Flux rates, in mg/min, for orosomucoid (Oroso), transferrin (Trans), albumin (Alb), ceruloplasmin (cerul), α_2 macroglobulin (Macro), and total protein in knee effusions of patients with osteoarthritis and rheumatoid arthritis. Albumin is the predominant protein traversing the joint space in both diseases. (From Wallis, W.J., Simkin, P.A., and Nelp, W.B.: Protein traffic in human synovial effusions. Arthritis Rheum., *30*:57–63, 1987.)

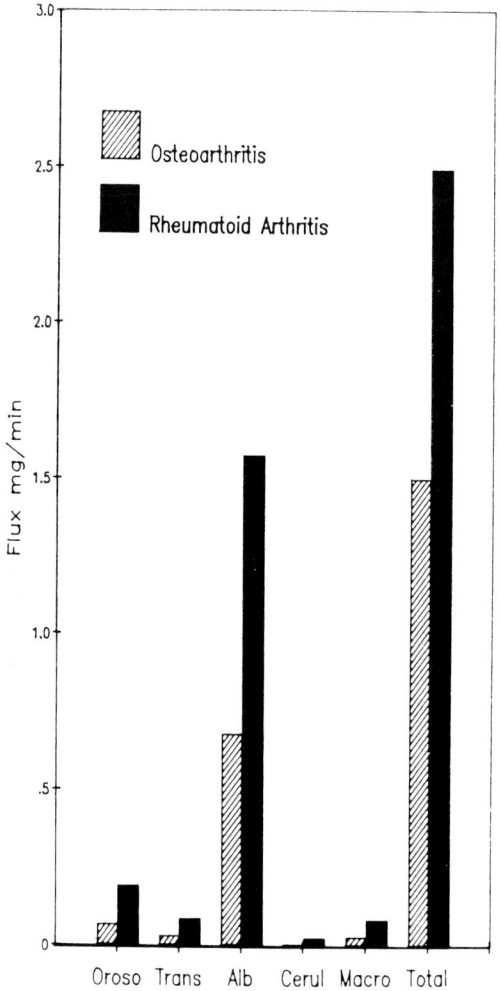

transported plasma proteins. The product of this value (ml/min) and the synovial fluid concentration (mg/ml) gives the removal rate of that protein in mg/min. When effusions are studied under steady-state conditions, this removal rate is the same as the rate of entry into the joint. These values express the articular flux rates of individual plasma proteins. They can be calculated readily in studies of stable effusions as illustrated in Figure 11–10. Not surprisingly, the predominant plasma protein, albumin, is also the principal protein traversing the joint space. Less prevalent proteins such as ceruloplasmin and α_2-macroglobulin have much slower flux rates. For each protein studied, the flux rate is much greater through rheumatoid effusions than through those of patients with osteoarthritis. These interdisease differences are much greater than those suggested by concentration ratios because their calculations include the finding that protein *clearance* is more rapid from rheumatoid than from osteoarthritic effusions.

Flux rate is a valuable means of evaluating protein traffic in synovial effusions. It is not, however, a measure of microvascular permeability. To address this important question, we evaluated the extraction of individual proteins from plasma into synovial fluid during a single passage through the articular microvasculature. As already described, the articular flux rate quantifies the egress of a given protein into the joint space. The delivery of that protein to synovial vessels may be similarly calculated in mg/min from the product of the plasma concentration (mg/ml) and the effective blood flow (ml/min). The ratio of the articular flux divided by the plasma delivery determines the fraction of a given protein that leaves the plasma, crosses the synovium, and enters synovial fluid during each passage through the synovial microvasculature. We have termed this value the *synovial permeance* and, in Figure 11–11, have recalculated and replotted the SF/S data as permeance values. By this assessment, it becomes apparent that the rheumatoid synovium is more permeable to protein than is the synovium in osteoarthritis. This prominent difference is not apparent from examination of SF/S ratios alone. Further development of this method should make it possible to quantify in vivo the synovial permeability to plasma proteins in individual patients and to calculate the net intra-articular production or consumption rates for specific proteins of interest. This ability may prove valuable, for instance, in assessing net local synthesis of rheumatoid factor, consumption of complement components, and release of enzymes.

INTRASYNOVIAL PRESSURE

The humeral head sits snugly in the glenoid fossa, regardless of whether the arm is supported. The hip

FIG. 11–11. Protein permeance in knee effusions of patients with arthritis. The microvascular escape of each of the five reference proteins is more than twice as great in rheumatoid arthritis as it is in osteoarthritis. (From Wallis, W.J., Simkin, P.A., and Nelp, W.B.: Protein traffic in human synovial effusions. Arthritis Rheum., *30*:57–63, 1987.)

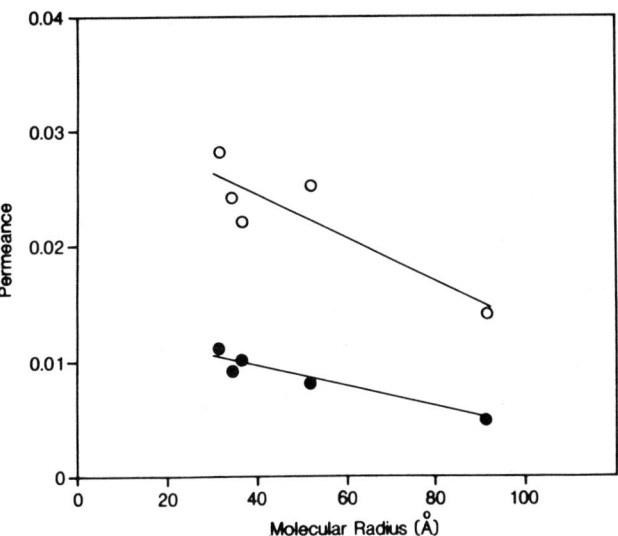

does not sublux during the swing-through phase of gait. Both at work and at rest, the opposing surfaces of articular cartilage remain in close approximation. This consistent apposition of articulating surfaces reflects a critical stabilizing capacity in normal joint function. Present data indicate that atmospheric pressure is one of the factors that sustain this apposition.

PRESSURES IN NORMAL JOINTS

Only a film of synovial fluid separates the moving surfaces in normal joints. Unlike the distended structure so often depicted in schematic drawings, the intra-articular cavity is primarily a potential space containing so little free fluid that none can be recovered by needle aspiration. Similarly, a microscopic layer of fluid fulfills the mission of lubrication in normal bursae and tendon sheaths. Each of these spaces, then, resembles a collapsed balloon with a wet, slippery inner surface. The state of collapse is apparently maintained by a subatmospheric intracavitary pressure. This concept was introduced by Müller, who found pressures of -8, -8, and -12 cm H_2O in 3 human knees without effusions and values from -4 to -6 cm H_2O in 4 additional knees with small effusions.[38] Müller also found that intra-articular pressures were negative (subatmospheric) in anesthetized dogs and in amputated limbs. This finding implies that subatmospheric pressures are generated neither by contraction of skeletal muscles nor by the active "pumping" of lymphatic vessels. These observations have been confirmed repeatedly in the normal, resting knees of several mammalian species.[39] A pressure differential of this magnitude is sufficient to explain the close apposition of synovium on cartilage, sheath on tendon, and bursal lining on itself, but how could these organs maintain such a differential without a specific pumping system and a continuous energy cost?

The exact mechanism of subatmospheric pressures remains controversial, but one reasonable explanation may be drawn from animal experiments using rigid perforated subcutaneous capsules.[39] The pressure in such capsules is consistently subatmospheric by as much as 7 mm Hg. In this model, an equal and opposite colloid osmotic pressure may maintain the negative hydrostatic pressure within the capsule (Fig. 11–12). This balance of forces requires fixation of glycosaminoglycans in the gel-like interstitial space of surrounding tissues. The high osmotic pressure of this fixed pericapsular gel may "draw" water from the capsule with a force sufficient to generate a negative pressure within the capsule. Infusions of either hyaluronidase or collagenase through the capsules disrupt the investing interstitial gel and cause equalization of pressures without and within the capsule.[40] This model indicates, then, both that an organized

matrix of high colloid osmotic pressure may maintain a negative hydrostatic pressure within an enclosed tissue space and that enzymatic disruption of interstitial matrix destroys the normal pressure relationships. Because the colloid osmotic pressure of normal, human synovial fluid approximates 10 mm Hg, that of the synovial interstitium would be predicted to be 14 mm Hg to maintain a resting intra-articular pressure at −4 mm Hg by this mechanism.

ROLE IN JOINT STABILITY

However achieved, a pressure differential of this magnitude may play a significant role in stabilizing joints. In concert with the action of tendons and ligaments, the "suction" of this phenomenon draws articulating surfaces into the best possible fit with each other and helps to guide the surface contacts as the joint moves through its range of motion. The magnitude of these forces was indicated by Jayson and Dixon's studies of 9 normal human knees.[41] With simple isometric exercise of the quadriceps, they found the mean intra-articular pressure to be −107 mm Hg. With severe distractive forces, the baseline pressure is driven farther downward and may ultimately go so low that dissolved gases come out of solution. This released gas appears coincident with sudden distraction of the joint surfaces and the well-known audible "knuckle crack." Both the bubble of gas and the distraction of the joint are readily demonstrated by serial radiographs.[42] This cavitation or "vacuum" phenomenon has generally been regarded as interesting, but of little practical value.

The observations are most instructive when assessed from the standpoint of joint stability, as illustrated in the finger. Normally, the extended middle finger may readily be moved throughout a lateral arc of approximately 40°, thus demonstrating laxity in the collateral ligaments of the metacarpophalangeal joint. On applying progressive increments of pull to relaxed third fingers, Unsworth and associates found that a force of 10 kg was required to "crack" the average knuckle (Fig. 11–13).[42] Only at this point did significant distraction occur and did the collateral ligaments accept a significant fraction of the force operating across the joint. At this force, then, an important stabilizing factor has been overcome. A metacarpophalangeal joint surface area is too small for atmospheric pressure alone to explain this 10-kg approximating force. The most likely explanation for the additional increment is the ability of synovial fluid to function as an adhesive as well as a lubricant. The effective lubrication of normal joints results principally from a

FIG. 11–12. Perforated subcutaneous capsule employed in physiologic studies of interstitial fluid. After implantation, the capsule is invested by granulation tissue. The colloid osmotic pressure of this tissue may exceed that of the fluid by an average value of 7 mm Hg, thus generating a subatmospheric pressure within the capsule. A similar discrepancy between colloid osmotic pressures of synovium and synovial fluid would explain the subatmospheric pressures reported in resting normal joints. (From Guyton, A.C.: A concept of negative interstitial pressure based on pressures in implanted perforated capsules. Circ. Res., *12*:399–414, 1963.)

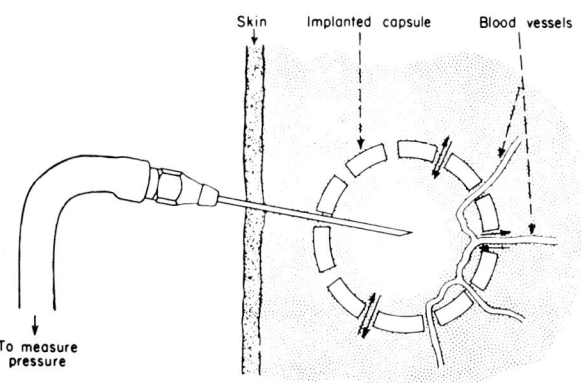

FIG. 11–13. "Cracking" of the third metacarpophalangeal joint. Despite progressive increments of pull up to 10 kg (lower curve with Xs), little separation is seen until the joint "cracks" with formation of a gas bubble within the joint space. When this happens, the adhesive properties of synovial fluid are overcome, and the load is transferred to the collateral ligaments of the joint. As long as the bubble remains, loading (open circles) and unloading (closed triangles) of the joint follow the upper curves. (From Unsworth, A., Dowson, D., and Wright, V.: "Cracking joints": a bioengineerng study of cavitation in the metacarpophalangeal joint. Ann. Rheum. Dis., *30*:348–358, 1971.)

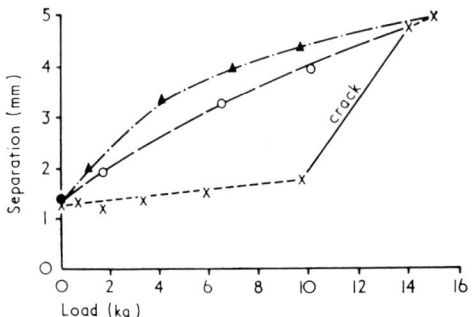

"boundary layer" mechanism. This term means that a layer of water adheres to each cartilaginous surface, an adherence mediated by the glycoprotein, lubricin.[43] Such a boundary layer reduces friction by reducing or eliminating the areas where one articular cartilage actually rubs against its mate. The same adherent layers should also bond the opposing surfaces to each other. Such an adhesive bond has been well recognized in other examples of boundary-layer lubrication.[44] Here, the cohesion of the solvent (water), perhaps enhanced by a principal solute (hyaluronate), serves to "glue" the opposing surfaces together. The functional advantage of such a water bond lies in that it has a high tensile strength and little or no shear strength. Thus, such a system enables opposing surfaces to slide freely across each other but limits their distraction.

When the metacarpophalangeal joint "cracks," the 10 kg of pull has overcome these adhesive properties. Here, as in other joints, the resultant bubble of intra-articular gas may then be used as a contrast agent for radiographic imaging of articular cartilage and other soft tissues within the joint. Radiologists have found this phenomenon to be useful in evaluating the knees, hips, and shoulders of infants and young children, although bubbles can be induced only rarely after the age of 2 years. Presumably, the surface area of these joints is sufficiently large in older children and adults to render the average radiologist unable or unwilling

to apply sufficient force to make the system fail. A simple comparison of the contact area of metacarpophalangeal joints with that of shoulders, elbows, and knees suggests that forces many times greater than 10 kg would be necessary to distract these joints. Simple atmospheric pressure, aided by adhesive properties of synovial fluid, must thus be able to contribute to the stabilization and congruent articulation of large joints. This is especially true in the polyaxial shoulder and hip joints, where ligaments can play only a limited role in maintaining joint stability.

EFFECT OF EFFUSIONS

In the presence of effusions, the resting intra-articular pressure usually becomes positive. The degree of positivity varies widely. Pressures between 10 and 20 mm Hg are common, and values as high as 80 mm Hg have been recorded in tense rheumatoid joints.[45] Although the degree of tension is often disregarded by clinicians, the consequences of elevated intra-articular pressure may be profound. Effusions of significant volume deprive the joint of the stabilizing effects of subatmospheric pressure and substitute instead a distending force that increases the stress on the ligaments and joint capsule (Fig. 11–14). In con-

FIG. 11–14. Isometric quadriceps contraction in normal knee containing 0, 10, and 20 ml added saline. With no injection, the intra-articular pressure is subatmospheric. This is no longer seen with 10 ml saline, and the pressure becomes positive with a simulated 20-ml effusion. (From Jayson, M.I.V., and Dixon, A.St.J.: Intra-articular pressure and rheumatoid geodes (bone "cysts"). Ann. Rheum. Dis., 29:496–502, 1970.)

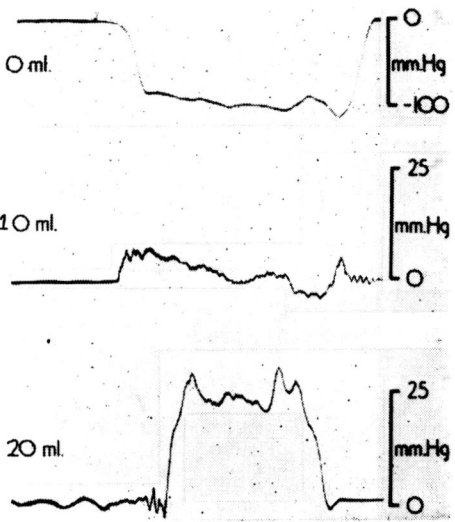

trast to normal joints, the pressures of effusions are greatest in full flexion and full extension, with lowest intra-articular pressures occurring at 30° of flexion. The thickened tissues of chronic synovitis are also less compliant than normal. This means that full flexion or extension may lead to high pressures in many inflamed joints. With passive knee flexion, for instance, Jayson and Dixon observed a mean pressure of 802 mm Hg in 3 rheumatoid patients injected with 100 ml intra-articular fluid.[41] These high pressures cause discomfort in chronically effused joints and thus limit the effective range of joint motion. They may also cause herniation through the capsule, progressive distention, or even rupture of the joint so often illustrated by "Baker's cysts" in the popliteal fossa. Such pressures also have been implicated in the pathogenesis of the subchondral cysts or "geodes" found in many kinds of joint diseases. As already mentioned, it seems likely that they may cause tamponade of the synovial microvasculature, thus contributing to the circulatory-metabolic imbalance of severe chronic synovitis. For all these reasons, the high-pressure effusion remains an important problem for investigation and a potentially critical reason for therapeutic intervention.

OPPORTUNITIES IN SYNOVIAL PHYSIOLOGY

Accurate diagnosis and appropriate therapy lie at the heart of good clinical rheumatology. The diagnostic criteria for most rheumatic diseases are broad, resting primarily on clinical observations supported by nonspecific laboratory findings. Within any diagnostic category, as illustrated for RA by Figures 11–4 and 11–6, is wide variation in pathophysiologic findings. As yet, however, the implications of this variation have rarely been explored. In which joints is the synovitis most likely to respond to intra-articular corticosteroids? Would the hydrostatic pressure, the pH, the oxygen tension, or some combination of physiologic parameters accurately predict joint destruction? Can such data serve as useful guides in therapeutic decision making? How well do antibiotics and other medications enter tense effusions? Does the "internal milieu" of the synovium or of cartilage predispose joints to infection by certain microorganisms? Do unique features of the synovial microvasculature lead to preferred deposition of circulating immune complexes? Do physiologic differences between joints explain characteristic patterns of rheumatic disease, such as the relative sparing by RA of the distal interphalangeal joints that are preferentially involved by

osteoarthritis? Does the subchondral bone share, to some extent, the subatmospheric pressure encountered in working joints? If so, do fluctuations in intraosseous pressure contribute to the lesions of decompression sickness and of other causes of aseptic necrosis? These and many other critical questions remain virtually unexplored. Answers will come only through a new commitment to the problems of articular physiology.

REFERENCES

1. Swann, D.A., et al.: Role of hyaluronic acid in joint lubrication. Ann. Rheum. Dis., 33:318–326, 1974.
2. Bäcklund, L., and Tiselius, P.: Objective measurement of joint stiffness in rheumatoid arthritis. Acta Rheumatol. Scand., 13:275–288, 1967.
3. Wright, V., and Johns, R.J.: Quantitative and qualitative analysis of joint stiffness in normal subjects and in patients with connective tissue diseases. Ann. Rheum. Dis., 20:36–45, 1961.
4. Such, C.H., Unsworth, A., Wright, V., and Dowson, D.: Quantitative study of stiffness in the knee joint. Ann. Rheum. Dis., 34:286–291, 1975.
5. Ropes, M.W., and Bauer, W.: Synovial fluid changes in joint disease. Cambridge, Harvard University Press, 1953.
6. Bauer, W., Ropes, M.W., and Waine, H.: The physiology of articular structures. Physiol. Rev., 20:272–312, 1940.
7. Levick, J.R.: Synovial fluid dynamics: the regulation of volume and pressure. In Studies in Joint Disease. Volume 2. Edited by E. Holborow and A. Maroudas. New York, Pitman, 1983, pp. 153–240.
8. Simkin, P.A., and Pizzorno, J.E.: Transynovial exchange of small molecules in normal human subjects. J. Appl. Physiol., 36:581–587, 1974.
9. Levick, J.R.: Permeability of rheumatoid and normal human synovium to specific plasma proteins. Arthritis Rheum., 24:1550–1560, 1981.
10. Levick, J.R.: Blood flow and mass transport in synovial joints. In Handbook of Physiology. Vol. IV. Microcirculation, Part 2. Edited by E.M. Renkin and C.C. Michel. Bethesda, MD, American Physiological Society, 1984, pp. 917–947.
11. Deodhar, S.D., O'Boyle, P.J., and Dick, W.C.: Anion transport from the canine synovial cavity. Nature, 231:61–63, 1971.
12. Kremer, D., Deodhar, S.D., and Dick, W.C.: A function of synovial membrane of normal and diseased humans in relation to the movement of small-molecular weight ions. Clin. Sci. Mol. Med., 44:611–615, 1973.
13. Simkin, P.A., and Nilson, K.L.: Trans-synovial exchange of large and small molecules. Clin. Rheum. Dis., 7:99–129, 1981.
14. Scholer, J.F., Lee, P.R., and Polley, H.F.: The absorption of heavy water and radioactive sodium from the knee joint of normal persons and patients with rheumatoid arthritis. Arthritis Rheum., 2:426–432, 1959.
15. Harris, R., and Millard, J.B.: Clearance of radioactive sodium from knee joint. Clin. Sci. Mol. Med., 15:9–15, 1956.
16. Liew, M., and Dick, W.C.: The anatomy and physiology of blood flow in a diarthrodial joint. Clin. Rheum. Dis., 7:131–148, 1981.
17. Wallis, W.J., Simkin, P.A., Nelp, W.B., and Foster, D.M.: Intra-articular volume and clearance in human synovial effusions. Arthritis Rheum., 28:441–449, 1985.

18. Wallis, W.J., Simkin, P.A., and Nelp, W.B.: Protein traffic in human synovial effusions. Arthritis Rheum., *30*:57–63, 1987.

19. Taylor, T.: Glucose metabolism and respiration. Clin. Rheum. Dis., *7*:167–175, 1981.

20. Ropes, M.W., Muller, A.F., and Bauer, W.: The entrance of glucose and other sugars into joints. Arthritis Rheum., *3*:496–513, 1960.

21. Falchuk, K.H., Goetzl, E.J., and Kulka, J.P.: Respiratory gases of synovial fluids: an approach to synovial tissue circulatory-metabolic imbalance in rheumatoid arthritis. Am. J. Med., *49*:223–231, 1970.

22. Roberts, J.E., McLees, B.D., and Kerby, G.P.: Pathways of glucose metabolism in rheumatoid and non-rheumatoid synovial membrane. J. Lab. Clin. Med., *70*:503–511, 1967.

23. Cheung, H.S., et al.: Synovial origin of rice bodies. Arthritis Rheum., *23*:72–76, 1980.

24. Phelps, P., Steele, A.D., and McCarty, D.J.: Significance of Xenon-133 clearance rate from canine and human joints. Arthritis Rheum., *15*:360–369, 1977.

25. McCarty, D.J.: Physiology of the normal synovium. *In* The Joints and Synovial Fluid. Edited by L. Sokoloff. New York, Academic Press, 1980.

26. Goetzl, E.J., et al.: A physiological approach to the assessment of disease activity in rheumatoid arthritis. J. Clin. Invest., *50*:1,167–1,180, 1971.

27. Dick, W.C., et al.: Clinical studies on inflammation in human knee joints. Clin. Sci., *38*:123–133, 1970.

28. Wallis, W.J., and Simkin, P.A.: Antirheumatic drug levels in human synovial fluid and synovial tissue: observations on extravascular pharmacokinetics. Clin. Pharmacokinet., *8*:496–522, 1983.

29. Rapp, G.F., Griffith, R.S., and Hebble, W.M.: The permeability of traumatically inflamed synovial membrane to commonly used antibiotics. J. Bone Joint Surg., *48A*:1,534–1,539, 1946.

30. Nelson, J.D.: Antibiotic concentrations in septic joint effusions. N. Engl. J. Med., *284*:349–353, 1971.

31. Parker, R.H., and Schmid, F.R.: Antibacterial activity of synovial fluid during therapy of septic arthritis. Arthritis Rheum., *14*:96–104, 1971.

32. Kusher, I., and Somerville, J.A.: Permeability of human synovial membrane to plasma proteins: relationship to molecular size and inflammation. Arthritis Rheum., *14*:560–570, 1971.

33. Balazs, E.A., Watson, D., Duff, I.F., and Roseman, S.: Hyaluronic acid in synovial fluid. Arthritis Rheum., *10*:357–376, 1967.

34. Simkin, P.A.: Synovial permeability in rheumatoid arthritis. Arthritis Rheum., *22*:689–696, 1979.

35. Brown, D., Cooper, A., and Bluestone, R.: Exchange of IgM and albumin between plasma and synovial fluid in rheumatoid arthritis. Ann. Rheum. Dis., *29*:644–651, 1969.

36. Rodnan, G.P., and MacLachlan, M.J.: The absorption of serum albumin and gamma globulin from the knee joint of man and rabbit. Arthritis Rheum., *3*:152–157, 1960.

37. Cecere, F., Lessard, J., McDuffy, S., and Pope, R.M.: Evidence for the local production and utilization of immune reactants in rheumatoid arthritis. Arthritis Rheum., *25*:1,307–1,315, 1982.

38. Müller, W.: Über den negativen Luftdruck im Gelenkraum. Dtsch. Z. Chir., *217*:395–401, 1929.

39. Levick, J.R.: Joint pressure-volume studies: their importance, design and interpretation. J. Rheumatol., *10*:353–357, 1983.

40. Stromberg, D.D., and Wiederhielm, C.A.: Effects of oncotic gradients and enzymes on negative pressures in implanted capsules. Am. J. Physiol., *219*:928–932, 1970.

41. Jayson, M.I.V., and Dixon, A.St.J.: Intra-articular pressure in rheumatoid arthritis of the knee. Ann. Rheum. Dis., *29*:401–408, 1970.

42. Unsworth, A., Dowson, D., and Wright, V.: "Cracking joints": a bioengineering study of cavitation in the metacarpophalangeal joint. Ann. Rheum. Dis., *30*:348–358, 1971.

43. Swann, D.A., et al.: The molecular structure and lubricating activity of lubricin isolated from bovine and human synovial fluids. Biochem. J., *225*:195–201, 1985.

44. Salomon, G.: The adhesion of liquids to solids. *In* Adhesion and Adhesives. Vol. 1. Edited by S. Houwink. New York, Elsevier Publishing, 1965, pp. 25–51.

45. Palmer, D.G., and Myers, D.B.: Some observations of joint effusions. Arthritis Rheum., *11*:745–755, 1968.

COLLAGEN IN NORMAL AND DISEASED CONNECTIVE TISSUE

12

DARWIN J. PROCKOP and TAINA PIHLAJANIEMI

Collagen is the major macromolecule of most connective tissues, and it is probably the most abundant protein in the human body. The other major macromolecules characteristic of connective tissues are elastin, a related fibrous protein, and a class of sugar-rich polymers known as proteoglycans (see Chapter 13). The amounts of collagen in tissues vary. Soft organs such as the liver contain little of the protein, whereas, in tissues such as skin and tendon, collagen accounts for over 70% of the dry weight (Table 12–1). Because collagen constitutes the bulk of most connective tissues, it makes a major contribution to their properties. Recent information about the biochemistry and chemistry of collagen (1) explains how the protein performs its important physiologic functions; (2) provides a molecular explanation for a number of genetic diseases of connective tissue; and (3) offers the promise of providing a basis for understanding the more common diseases of connective tissue that involve both genetic and environmental components.

FORMATION OF COLLAGEN FIBERS AND RELATED COLLAGEN STRUCTURES

Early in evolution nature had to solve the problem, how cells can be held together to constitute a multicellular organism. A major solution was the formation of extracellular collagen fibrils and fibers.

Collagen fibrils have approximately the same tensile strength as steel wires, and they act in most com-

plex organisms to hold together the cells of various tissues. The assembly of extracellular collagen fibrils is based on two relatively simple principles. The first principle is *"self-assembly,"* whereby a protein monomer of relatively small size aggregates with itself in a precise manner to form a much larger biologic structure.[2-4] Large connective tissue structures, such as ligaments and tendons, are composed of small bundles of collagen fibrils. The fibrils themselves are formed by the self-assembly of the collagen monomer (Fig 12–1). The collagen monomer permits such self-assembly because it is relatively long and rigid, it has the correct distribution of charge and hydrophobic amino acid side chains along its surface, and it has the correct length.

The second principle in the formation of collagen fibrils is that most collagens are first synthesized as precursors known as *procollagens* (Figs. 12–1, 12–2).[2-4] The procollagens contain additional amino acid sequences at both the N- and C-terminal ends of the monomers. These additional amino acid sequences constitute as much as one third of the mass of the procollagens. They have several important biologic functions, one of which is preventing the protein from self-assembling into fibrils and fibers prematurely.

At least 10 different kinds of collagen have now been identified in human connective tissues; these collagens can be considered a family of proteins (Table 12–2). The major subclassifications of the collagens is into the "fibrillar" and the "nonfibrillar" types. The fibrillar types form distinctive fibrils that are readily identified by their cross-striations, and they provide

Table 12–1.   Collagen, Elastin, and Proteoglycan Contents of Some Tissues*

Tissue	Collagen† (g/100 g dry wt)	Elastin‡ (g/100 g dry wt)	Proteoglycans§ (g/100 g dry wt)
Liver	4	0.2	
Lung	10	5	
Aorta	18	30	6
Ligamentum nuchae	17	75	
Cartilage	55		29
Cornea	68		5
Skin	72	0.6	
Tendon (Achilles)	86	4	0.5
Bone (mineral-free, cortical)	88		0.8

*Values are averages from references cited by Grant and Prockop.[1]

†Values for ligamentum nuchae, cartilage, and bone from bovine tissues; remainder from human tissue.

‡Values for ligamentum nuchae and Achilles tendon from bovine tissues; values for liver and skin from rat tissues; and remainder from human tissues.

§Value for aorta from rabbit tissues; value for cornea from human tissues; and remainder from bovine tissues.

FIG. 12–1.   Schematic representation of how a fibroblast assembles collagen fibrils. *A,* Intracellular post-translational modifications of proα chains, association of C-propeptide domains, and folding into triple-helical conformation. *B,* Enzymic cleavage of procollagen to collagen, self-assembly of collagen monomers into fibrils, and cross linking of fibrils. (From Prockop, D.J., and Kivirikko, K.I.[4] Reprinted by permission of the New England Journal of Medicine.)

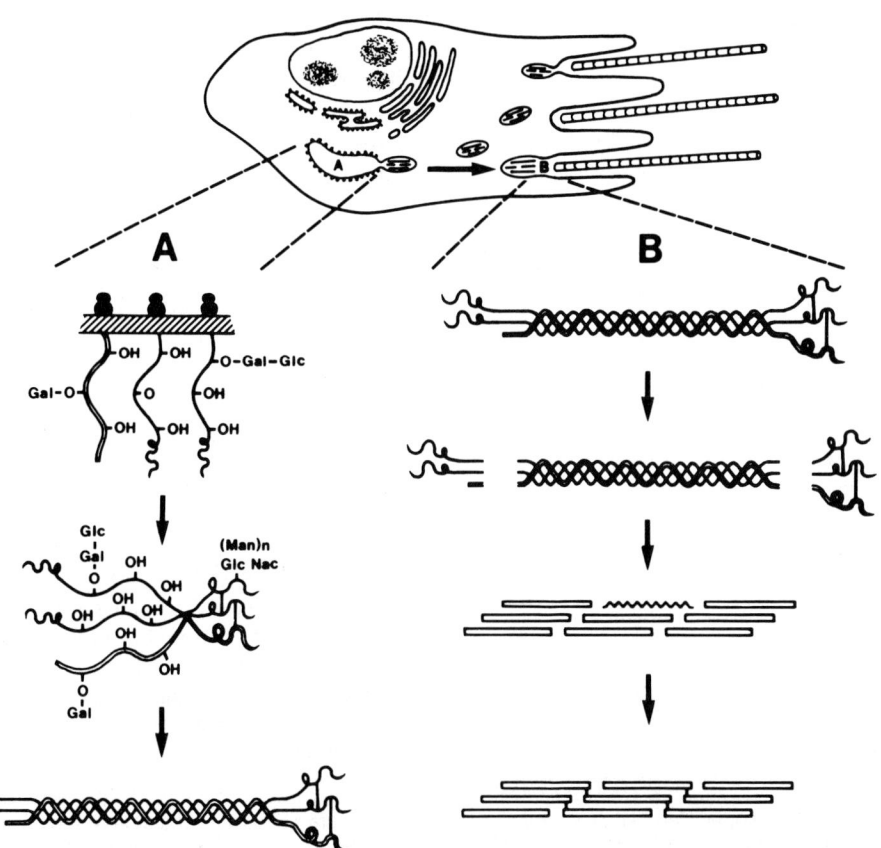

FIG. 12–2. Structure of a type I procollagen molecule. The molecule consists of two proα1(I) and one proα2(I) chains. It has the three distinct domains indicated. The C-propeptides of both kinds of proα chains contain a mannose-rich oligosaccharide. (From Prockop, D.J., and Kivirikko, K.I.[4] Reprinted by permission of the New England Journal of Medicine.)

PROCOLLAGEN MOLECULE

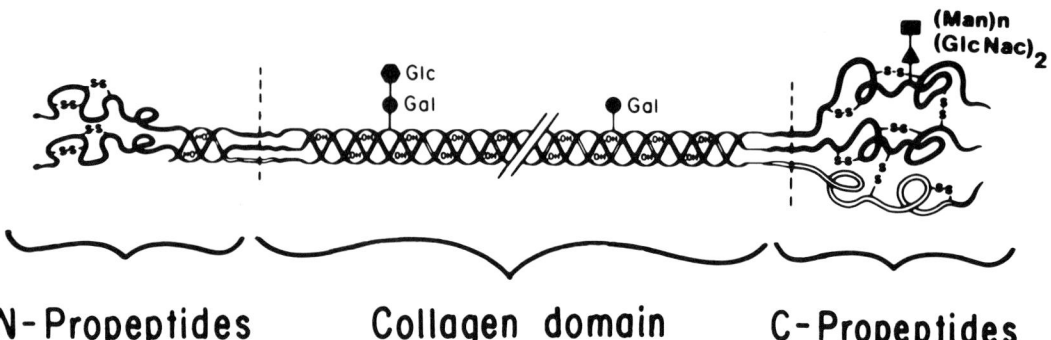

N-Propeptides   Collagen domain   C-Propeptides

the tensile strength required to hold tissues together. The small differences in their amino acid sequences are probably a major determinant in producing the kinds of fibrils that fibrillar collagens form in vivo (Fig. 12–3). The nonfibrillar collagens form network-like structures that serve as a scaffold for the binding of epithelial and endothelial cells. They also serve as filtration barriers in tissues such as the kidney. The most important difference between nonfibrillar collagens and fibrillar collagens is that the monomers of the nonfibrillar collagens contain large globular domains in addition to collagen domains. The presence of the globular domains means that the monomers self-assemble into structures that are more complex than the orderly array of fibrils seen in the structures formed only by fibrillar collagens.

Types I, II, and III collagen are the major fibrillar collagens.[2–4] Type I collagen is found ubiquitously in most connective tissues, including skin, bone, tendons, and ligaments. Type II collagen is the major collagen of hyaline cartilage. Type III collagen is less abundant than type I or type II collagen, but small amounts are found in most tissues that contain type I. The aorta and synovial membranes, however, are particularly rich in type III collagen; bone contains type I without any accompanying type III collagen.

Type IV collagen is the major nonfibrillar collagen of the body and is the major constituent of most basement membranes.[2–4,12] Type V collagen is found in a variety of tissues, particularly in blood vessels and smooth muscle cells. Type VI collagen and a family of other minor collagens are found in small amounts in various tissues.[7–10,12]

Types I and III collagen are the best studied and

Table 12–2.   Structurally and Genetically Distinct Collagens*

Type	Tissue Distribution	Polypeptide Chains	Chemical Characteristics
I	Bone, tendon, skin, dentin, ligament, fascia, arteries, and uterus	$[\alpha1(I)]_2\alpha2$	Hybrid composed of two kinds of chains. Low content of hydroxylysine and glycosylated hydroxylysine.
II	Hyaline cartilage	$[\alpha1(II)]_3$	Relatively high content of hydroxylysine and glycosylated hydroxylysine.
III	Skin, arteries, and uterus	$[\alpha1(III)]_3$	High content of hydroxyproline and low hydroxylysine. Contains interchain disulfide bonds.
IV	Basement membranes	$\alpha1(IV),\alpha2(IV)$	High content of cysteine, hydroxylysine, and glycosylated hydroxylysine. Contains large globular regions.
V	Blood vessels, other tissues	$\alpha1(V),\alpha2(V),\alpha3(V)$	

*Type VI and five or more additional types have been identified, but these are less abundant and are not as well characterized as types I, II, III, IV, and V. For more complete descriptions of these collagens see Bachinger et al.,[5] Bornstein and Sage,[6] Gibson et al.,[7] Mayne et al.,[8] Odermatt et al.,[9] Schmid and Conrad,[10] and Timpl et al.[11]

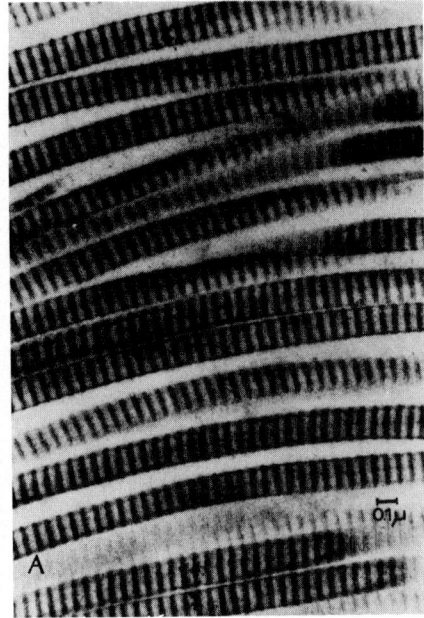 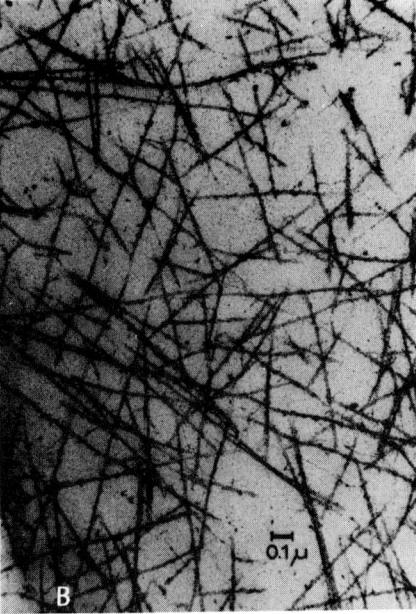

FIG. 12–3. *A,* Type I collagen fibrils in tendon and *B,* type II collagen fibrils in hyaline cartilage. Most current evidence suggests that the differences in fibril morphology as shown here are due to small differences in the genetically determined amino acid sequences. Morphology is probably also influenced by the presence of other connective tissue components, such as proteoglycans. (From Prockop, D.J., et al.[2] Reprinted by permission of the New England Journal of Medicine.)

have been most closely linked to human diseases. This discussion will focus primarily on these types.

The monomer of type I procollagen contains two proα1(I) chains and a slightly different proα2(I) chain (see Fig. 12–2). In contrast, the monomer of type III procollagen contains three identical proα1(III) chains that differ slightly in their structure from type I proα chains. Both type I and type III procollagen contain an N-propeptide domain, a collagen domain, and a C-propeptide domain.[2-4,6] Although the propeptides are, in general, globular structures similar to other globular proteins, the N-propeptide contains a short triple-helical subdomain similar to the collagen domain of the same protein. The C-propeptides are entirely globular, and they contain a mannose-rich oligosaccharide.

In the collagen domains of the proteins, each of the three chains is coiled into a left-handed helix with about three amino acids per turn. The three helical chains then twist around each other into a right-handed super-helix to form a rigid structure similar to a long and thin segment of rope. Each α chain contains about 1000 amino acid residues and, with the exception of short sequences at the ends of the chains, every third amino acid is glycine. Therefore, the molecular formula of an α chain can be represented as $(Gly-X-Y)_{333}$ where X and Y are amino acids other than glycine. Glycine, the smallest amino acid, must be present in every third position because the amino acid residue in this position occupies a restricted space in which the three helical chains come together in the center of the triple helix. The X and Y positions are frequently occupied by proline and 4-hydroxyproline, respectively. Because proline and hydroxyproline are ring amino acids, they provide rigidity to the structure. Other amino acids in the X and Y positions appear in clusters of charged hydrophobic amino acids whose side groups point away from the center of the triple helix. The pattern in which these clustered hydrophobic and charged amino acids appear on the surface of the monomer determines the precise manner in which the protein self-assembles (see Fig. 12–1B).

The genes for type I and type III procollagen have several unusual features.[13-21] One is that the protein coding sequences, or the exons of the genes, are divided by about 50 intervening sequences (Fig. 12–4). Most of the exons coding for the α chain domains are either 54 or 108 bases in length, and each of these exons begins with the codon for glycine and ends with the codon for a Y-position amino acid. These unexpected features of the genes have been interpreted as evidence that the procollagen gene originally arose as a 54-base primitive exon that was duplicated extensively at some stage during evolution.[13,18] However, it is also possible that the 54-base pattern of the exons arose through mechanisms designed to protect the gene from unequal crossover mutations. The exon pattern is similar in the proα1(I) and the proα2(I) genes, but the intervening sequences in the proα2(I) genes are longer. Therefore, the proα1(I) gene is 18,000 bases,[19] whereas the proα2(I) gene is 38,000 bases.[15-18] The same exon pattern has been seen in type II procollagen genes of chick embryos[20] and in type III procollagen genes from the same species.[21]

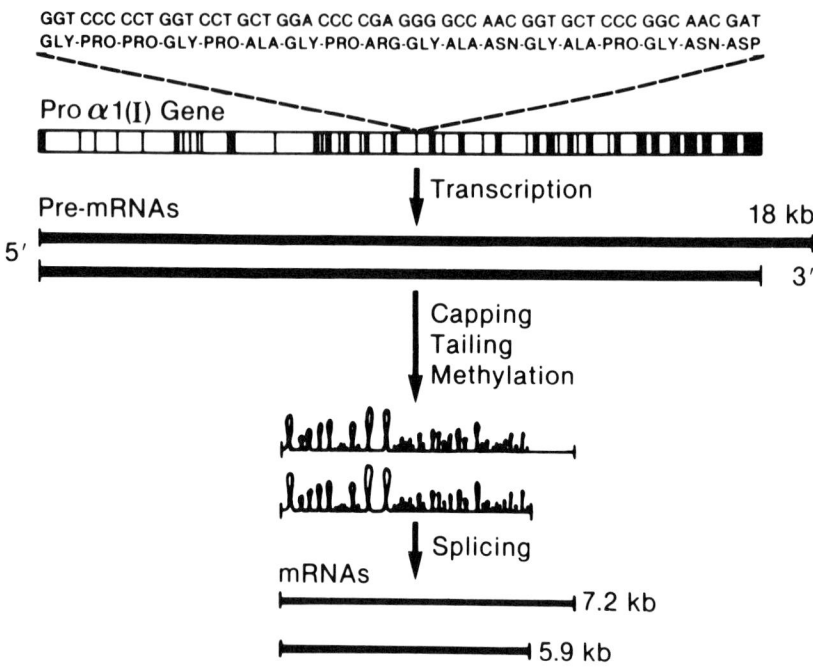

GGT CCC CCT GGT CCT GCT GGA CCC CGA GGG GCC AAC GGT GCT CCC GGC AAC GAT
GLY·PRO·PRO·GLY·PRO·ALA·GLY·PRO·ARG·GLY·ALA·ASN·GLY·ALA·PRO·GLY·ASN·ASP

FIG. 12–4. Schematic representation of the structure and of transcription of the proα1(I) gene. The top portion shows a typical 54-base pair exon encoding for a sequence of (Gly-X-Y)$_6$. The pattern of exons and introns in the proα1(I) gene is schematically represented on the basis of the similar pattern of the chick proα2(I) gene.[17] The gene is transcribed into two different pre-mRNAs, apparently because the first signal for polyadenylation is not entirely efficient. The initial RNA transcripts are about 18,000 bases (kilobases or kb) in length. Splicing out the intervening sequences reduces them to mRNAs of about 7.2 and 5.9 kb. The processing of the initial RNA transcripts also includes addition of a "cap" of the unusual base 7-methylguanylate at the 5'-end, addition of a "tail" of polyadenylate at the 3'-end, and methylation of a few bases. The two mRNAs with 3'-noncoding ends of different length are both used to synthesize proα1(I) chains with the same primary structure on polysomes. (From Prockop, D.J., and Kivirikko, K.I.[4] Reprinted by permission of the New England Journal of Medicine.)

The globular C-propeptides of types I, II, and III procollagen are coded for by relatively large exons.

The collagen genes are widely scattered on the human genome. The gene for the proα1(I) chain is on human chromosome 17, whereas the gene for the proα2(I) chain is on human chromosome 7.[22] The gene for the proα1(II) chain of type II procollagen is on chromosome 12 and the gene for the proα1(III) chain of type III procollagen is on chromosome 2. The gene for the α1 chain of type IV procollagen is located near the tip of chromosome 13.[23]

A variety of mRNAs of differing length for proα1(I) and proα2(I) chains have been found in fibroblasts synthesizing type I procollagen. The explanation for these mRNAs of different length is probably that the signals for the termination of transcription and for polyadenylation at the 3' end of RNA transcripts are relatively inefficient. As a result, two mRNAs of different length are synthesized from the proα1(I) gene and at least three mRNAs of different size from the proα2(I) gene.[24] Both genes appear to be present as single copies per haploid genome.[25] However, the steady-state levels of the mRNA for proα1(I) and proα2(I) chains are 2:1.[26] There appear to be major differences, therefore, in the rates at which the two genes are transcribed or the initial RNA transcripts of the genes are processed. However, the two kinds of proα chains are synthesized in a ratio of 2:1. It is apparent, then, that the mRNAs for proα1(I) and proα2(I) are translated at the same rate.[26]

POST-TRANSLATIONAL MODIFICATIONS

The intracellular assembly of the procollagen molecule is a complex process that requires at least eight specific enzymes and several nonspecific enzymes (see Fig. 12–1).[4,27–32] In the course of the intracellular processing of the polypeptide chains, over 100 amino acids in each proα chain are modified. After the procollagen molecule is secreted, one third of the mass is cleaved from the protein in the course of this conversion to the collagen monomer.

The complex processing that occurs both cotranslationally and post-translationally in fibroblasts includes the following steps (Table 12–3): (1) cleavage of "signal" peptides at the N-terminals of the chains; (2) hydroxylation of Y-position proline and lysine residues to 4-hydroxyproline and to hydroxylysine; (3) hydroxylation of a few Y-position proline residues to 3-hydroxyproline; (4) addition of galactose or both galactose and glucose to some of the hydroxylysine residues; (5) addition of a mannose-rich oligosaccharide to the C-propeptide; (6) association of the C-

Table 12–3. Stages in Collagen Metabolism

Process	Biologic Significance
Intracellular	
1. Transcription and translation	Determination of primary structure
2. Hydroxylation of prolyl residues	Stabilization of triple helix
3. Hydroxylation of lysyl residues	Site of attachment of galactose and glucose
	Needed for most stable cross-links
4. Galactosylation of hydroxylysyl residues	
5. Glycosylation of galactosyl-hydroxylysyl residues	
6. Glycosylation of procollagen propeptides	
7. Chain association, disulfide bonding, and helix formation	Helix required for normal rate of procollagen secretion
8. Translocation and secretion of complete procollagen molecule	
Extracellular Steps	
1. Conversion of procollagen to collagen	Fibril formation
2. Aggregation of collagen molecules	Fibril formation
3. Oxidation of lysyl and hydroxylysyl residues and subsequent cross-linking	Stabilization of fibrils
4. Degradation by collagenase(s)	Fibril turnover

terminal propeptides through a process directed by the structure of the C-terminal propeptide; and (7) formation of both intrachain and interchain disulfide bonds in the propeptides.

After the procollagen molecules are assembled and secreted from fibroblasts, the N-propeptides are cleaved by a procollagen N-proteinase, and the C-propeptides are cleaved by separate procollagen C-proteinase. The collagen then self-assembles into fibrils. After the fibrils are formed, a lysyl oxidase oxidizes lysine and hydroxylysine residues to aldehyde derivatives that form cross links with similar residues in adjacent molecules (Fig. 12–1B).

Specific functions can be assigned to several of these enzymatic modifications. The conversion of proline residues to 4-hydroxyproline is necessary for the α chain domains to fold ino a triple-helical conformation at body temperature. The hydroxylation of lysine residues to hydroxylysines is required for addition of sugar residues to hydroxylysine residues. This process is also required to form the most stable kinds of cross-links found in collagen fibrils. The disulfide bonds found between C-propeptides are probably required as a first step in the formation of the triple helix. To form collagen fibrils, however, the C-propeptides must be cleaved from procollagen. Fibrils can form without cleavage of the N-propeptide, but the protein containing the N-propeptides forms fibrils that are thin and irregular in their morphology. Stabilizing the fibril structure clearly requires lysyl oxidase reaction.[30] Without the formation of cross links initiated by lysyl oxidase, the fibrils do not achieve their maximal tensile strength.

Studies on the post-translational enzymes have demonstrated an unusual relationship between the conformation of the protein being processed and the enzymatic reactions themselves. In particular, the proα chains must be nonhelical to be substrates for some of the enzymes, but they must be triple-helical in order to be substrates for the others. Specifically, proα chains must be nonhelical in order to be substrates for 3-prolylhydroxylase, 4-prolylhydroxylase, lysylhydroxylase, and the two transferases that add sugars to hydroxylysine residues. Modification by these enzymes ceases once the protein folds into a triple-helical conformation. In addition, extensive work has demonstrated that after the protein has folded, it is rapidly secreted from fibroblasts. Conversely, if folding of the protein is delayed by circumstances, such as agents that inhibit the hydroxylation of prolyl residues, the time required for secretion is greatly increased. In contrast to the hydroxylating and glycosylating enzymes, the enzyme procollagen N-proteinase has the striking property of requiring that the protein be triple-helical in order to be cleaved by the enzyme.[29] In addition, lysyl oxidase will not oxidize lysine or hydroxylysine residues unless the protein has self-assembled into collagen fibrils.

One additional feature of interest about the post-translational modifications is that ascorbic acid is required by the prolylhydroxylases and lysylhydroxylases. Therefore, absence of ascorbic acid probably explains the failure of wounds to heal in scurvy. The hydroxylases also require oxygen, and limitations of oxygen may explain the failure of tissue repair in vascular insufficiency.[2,3]

GENETIC DISEASES SHOWN TO INVOLVE COLLAGEN

Within recent years, researchers have found definitive evidence for the involvement of collagen in a spectrum of genetic diseases (see also Chapter 85). The list of such genetic diseases of collagen now includes several specific forms of osteogenesis imperfecta (OI), and Marfan syndrome (MS), Ehlers-Danlos syndrome (EDS), and several related disorders (Table 12–4). Each of these conditions has proved to be highly heterogeneous at the molecular level. Many of them, however, can now be understood in terms of the basic information available about the biosynthesis of collagen. Although these diseases are relatively rare, they clearly provide paradigms for understanding more common diseases of connective tissue.

MOLECULAR DEFECTS IN OSTEOGENESIS IMPERFECTA

Although brittle bones are the most characteristic feature of OI, the disease is now recognized as involving most other tissues rich in type I collagen, such as ligaments, tendons, fasciae, sclerae, and teeth.[4,33–40]

Several different schemes for the classification of OI have been presented, each of which has considerable merit. The most commonly referred to classification, however, is the scheme of four major types as proposed by Sillence (Table 12–5).[39,40] In this classification, the type I form of OI is characterized by mildly brittle bones, blue sclerae, and an autosomal dominant mode of inheritance. This type is further subclassified as type IA if teeth are normal and type IB if opalescent teeth are present. Type II is the most severe form. The connective tissues are so fragile that the disease is usually lethal at birth. Type III is a moderately severe form with a recessive mode of inheritance but highly variable manifestations. Type IV is also a highly variable form characterized by a dominant mode of inheritance and normal sclerae.

The current information of molecular defects in OI demonstrates that the disease is even more heterogeneous than the clinical manifestations suggest. Unfortunately, definitive data are available on only a few patients, and it is difficult to present many generalizations on the kinds of molecular defects found in

each clinical phenotype (Table 12–6). Therefore, the information is best considered on a case-by-case basis as examples of specific variants of the disease.

The Lethal Variant Proα1(I)[s]. The most thoroughly studied variant of OI occurred in a patient who died at birth with connective tissues so weak that the head separated from the trunk during delivery.[41–44] The defect in this variant has been defined at the gene level and shown to be a deletion near the center of one allele for the proα1(I) gene (Fig. 12–5). Because of the deletion of the gene, fibroblasts from the patient synthesized both normal-length mRNAs for proα1(I) chains and mRNAs for proα1(I) chains that were shortened. The deletion in the proα1(I) gene was "in register" in the sense that the coding sequences on both sides of the deletion were in the correct phase to be translated into polypeptide chains. Therefore, the shortened mRNAs were translated into shortened proα1(I) chains.[41,44] Because the structure of the shortened chains was normal beyond the deletion, these chains became disulfide-linked to the normal proα1(I) and proα2(I) chains synthesized by the same fibroblast.[44] As a result, three fourths of the procollagen trimers assembled by the fibroblasts contained either one or two shortened proα1(I) chains (Fig. 12–6). The stability of procollagen trimers is directly related to the length of the α chain domain of the protein. In the case of the proα1(I) variant, the shortening in the proα1(I) chains was so great that the presence of even one shortened chain in a procollagen molecule prevented it from folding into a stable triple helix. Such molecules, therefore, were rapidly degraded either intracellularly or after secretion from the cells. As a consequence, a mutation that altered half the proα1(I) chains inactivated half the normal proα1(I) and three fourths of the normal proα2(I) chains synthesized by the fibroblasts (Fig. 12–6).

This inactivation of normal proα chains by shortened proα1(I) chains can be regarded as "protein self-inactivation" or "protein suicide" by analogy with "suicide inhibitors" of enzymes that bind irreversibly and inactivate enzymes. The phenomenon may be general and may help to explain how many hetero-

Table 12–4.   Genetic Diseases in Which Collagen Defects Have Been Demonstrated

Disease	Major Manifestations	Tissues Involved in Most Variants
Osteogenesis imperfecta (OI)	Brittle bones	Bone, skin, ligaments, tendons, fasciae, sclerae, ears, teeth
Marfan syndrome (MS)	Long, thin extremities	Skeleton, eye, aorta, ligaments
Ehlers-Danlos syndrome (EDS)	Skin changes and joint laxity	Skin, ligaments, tendons, fasciae, great vessels, bowel, and bones in some types
Menkes steely-hair syndrome	Cerebral degeneration	Brain, hair, arteries, bone, and bladder
Epidermolysis bullosa	Blistering of skin	Skin

Table 12–5.   Classification of Osteogenesis Imperfecta (OI) based on Clinical Manifestations and Mode of Inheritance as Proposed by Sillence et al.[39,40]

	Bone Fragility	Blue Sclerae	Dentinogenesis Imperfecta	Presenile Hearing Loss	Inheritance*
I	Mild	Present	Absent in IA† Present in IB‡	Present in some	AD
II	Extreme	Present	Present in some	Unknown	AR or S
III	Severe	Bluish at birth	Present or absent	Low incidence	AR
IV	Variable	Normal	Absent in IVA† Present in IVB‡	Low incidence	AD

*AD = autosomal dominant; AR = autosomal recessive; S = sporadic.
†A = normal teeth.
‡B = opalescent teeth.

Table 12–6.   Molecular Defects Identified in Osteogenesis Imperfecta (OI) and the Marfan Syndrome (MS)

Disease*	Molecular Defect†	Secondary Events
OI-I	Proα1(I)° Proα2(I)^S Other unidentified	Resistance to procollagen N-proteinase
OI-II	Proα1(I)^S Proα2(I)^S + Proα2(I)° Proα1(I)^{cys} Other unidentified	Unstable 3-helix; increased synthesis of proα1(III) Increased synthesis of proα1(IV) and proα2(IV) Unstable 3-helix; perhaps abnormal fibrils
OI-III	Proα2(I)^{cx} Proα1(I)^{cx} or Proα2(I)^{cx} Other unidentified	Synthesis of proα1(I) trimers Increased mannose in C-propeptide
MS	Decreased cross linking of elastin Other unidentified	

*OI-I, OI-II, and OI-III refer to the different types of OI as classified by Sillence (see Table 12–5).
†The molecular defects in most patients with OI and MS are still unknown. The statements here generally apply to single patients or to families with each type of disease in which the molecular defect has been defined.

FIG. 12–5.   Illustration of the molecular defect in one lethal variant of OI.[41–44] One allele for proα1(I) chains contains a deletion of about 0.5 kb in the middle of the gene. As a result, the mRNAs transcribed from the gene are shortened by 0.25 kb and about 80 amino acid residues. (From Prockop, D.J., and Kivirikko, K.I.[4] Reprinted by permission of the New England Journal of Medicine.)

FIG. 12–6.   Illustration of the phenomenon of "protein suicide" in a lethal variant of OI described in Figure 12–5. Because the deletion in the middle of the proα1(I) chain is in phase, the shortened proα1(I) chains associate with proα1(I) chains of normal length. The resulting trimers cannot fold into a stable triple helix at body temperature and are rapidly degraded. (From Prockop, D.J., and Kivirikko, K.I.[4] Reprinted by permission of the New England Journal of Medicine.)

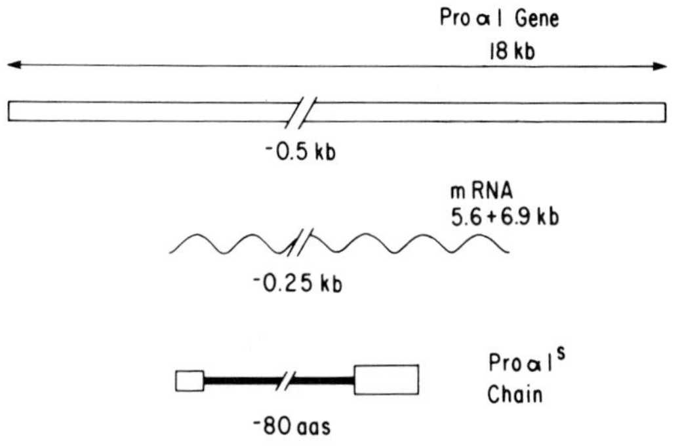

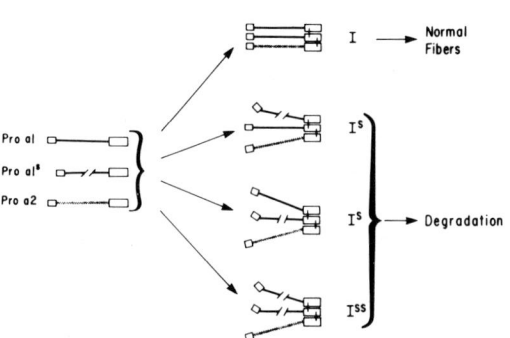

zygous gene defects, which reduce the amount of normal gene product by only one half, can produce a dominantly inherited disease. In the case of the variant called proα1(I)[s], the phenomenon of protein inactivation (or protein suicide) reduced the biologically useful procollagen synthesized by the fibroblasts to one quarter of the normal amount. This level of synthesis of type I procollagen was apparently insufficient to produce connective tissues with adequate tensile strength. Because the parents of the proband were phenotypically normal, the deletion in the proα1(I) chain apparently was a new, sporadic mutation. The same phenomenon of protein suicide has been seen in other lethal variants of OI caused by single base mutations that convert a glycine codon to a codon for arginine or cysteine (see below).

Three Variants of Proα2(I)[s]. Three OI variants have been shown to synthesize shortened proα2(I) chains of type I procollagen. Two involve deletions of amino acids from the N-terminal region of the proα2(I) chain.[45,46] The third involves a similar deletion from near the middle of the proα2(1) chain.[47]

The two variants with deletions near the N-terminal region of the proα2(I) chain were similar in that 20 to 30 amino acids were missing from the chain, and the deletions were located between amino acid residue number 7 and number 347 of the α2(I) chain. In one of these variants, half the proα2(I) chains synthesized by fibroblasts are shortened, whereas the other half are normal.[46] A similar situation was apparently present in the second variant,[45] but the clinical presentations differed. In one, the disease was apparently a sporadic one produced by a new mutation.[45] The proband was a middle-aged woman with multiple fractures and blue sclerae. In the second, the proband had extremely loose joints, blue sclerae, and roentgenographic evidence of wormian bones but no fractures.[46] His mother, who had the same molecular defect, was short and had blue sclerae but no other findings. Several affected members of the same family had a history of blue sclerae and fractures. This family is probably best considered as having an atypical variant of OI with a high degree of incomplete penetrance. The major clinical manifestations in some members of the family, however, were those of EDS.

The reasons for the differences in the clinical manifestations of these two variants with similar deletions in about the same region of the proα2(I) chains are not apparent. They may be explained by the possibility that one of the deletions is closer to the N-terminal of the proα2(I) chains and involves different amino acids.

In the second variant, the consequences of the deletion on the properties of procollagen were exam-

ined.[46] Two effects were found: (1) the deletion made procollagen molecules containing the shortened proα2(I) chain resistant to procollagen N-proteinase, apparently because the shortening altered the conformation of the cleavage site, and (2) procollagen trimers containing the shortened proα2(I) chains formed a triple-helical structure that was less stable than the triple-helical structure formed by normal type I procollagen. The data did not clearly resolve which of these two effects was the more important in vivo. The simplest explanation for the observations was that the shortening of the proα2(I) chains created a partial unfolding of the N-terminal region of the procollagen molecule. As a consequence, the N-propeptides were incompletely cleaved by procollagen N-proteinase. The persistence of the partially processed procollagen molecules in tissues probably explained the clinical manifestations of loose joints and fractures in some members of the family who inherited the defect.

The third variant that synthesized shortened proα2(I) chains was a lethal disease.[47] Two unrelated mutations were found, one in each of the two alleles for proα2(I) chains. The mutations in one allele produced a shortened chain, and the mutation in the second allele made it nonfunctional. The consequences of these two mutations were a decreased rate of synthesis of proα2(I) chains and shortening of all the proα2(I) chains synthesized by the patient's fibroblasts. The deletion of amino acids was again an "in-register" deletion so that the amino acid sequences of either side were normal. Therefore, the shortened chains were incorporated in the triple-helical trimers of procollagen. These trimers, however, apparently were not processed and not assembled into normal collagen fibrils. In addition, because there was a relative overproduction of proα1(I) chains compared with proα2(I) chains, the patient's fibroblasts probably synthesized trimers of proα1(I) chains, which do not have the same functional properties as normal trimers of type I procollagen. One additional observation on this variant was of interest. The father of the proband had one normal and one nonfunctioning allele for proα2(I). However, he was phenotypically normal, an observation that demonstrated that a nonfunctioning allele for the proα2(I) chain may be of no consequence. The mother of the proband had two normal proα2(I) alleles. Apparently, the allele that the proband had inherited from his mother underwent a sporadic mutation that generated the shortened proα2(I) chains.

The Variants Proα1(I)[cx] and Proα2(I)[cx]. Two variants of OI have mutations that change the structure of the C-propeptides of type I procollagen.[48–53] Both appear to cause a progressively deforming disease best classified as type III OI (see Table 12–5). The molecular defect in one of these variants has been only partially characterized, but a more precise characterization has been obtained for the second.

In the first variant, the patient's fibroblasts synthesized and secreted a type I procollagen that was less soluble than normal.[53] Examination of the structure of the C-propeptides of the type I procollagen demonstrated that it contained increased amounts of mannose. It was not established whether the excess mannose was in the proα1(I) or the proα2(I) chain. In addition, it was not established that the defect specifically involved a change in the amino acid sequence of the C-propeptides. The most likely explanation for the data, however, is that the mutation altered the amino acid sequence of the C-propeptide of one chain and that this change in amino acid sequence decreased the solubility of the procollagen and probably produced inappropriate aggregation of the protein in tissues. The increased mannose content may have directly contributed to the altered solubility of the protein, but it may also have been a secondary and less important phenomenon.

In the second variant with altered C-propeptides, the defect was precisely located to a change in amino acid sequence of the C-propeptide of the proα2(I) chain.[48–50] The dramatic finding in this patient was that none of the type I collagen in his skin, and presumably other tissues, contained any proα2(I) chains.[50] Since type I collagen had existed as a heterotrimer of two α1(I) and one α2(I) chains for about 800 million years of evolution,[51,52] it was generally assumed that the α2(I) chain is essential for life. This patient, however, had a form of OI that is only moderately debilitating. Examination of his fibroblasts demonstrated that the cells contained normal levels of mRNA for proα2(I) chains and that proα2(I) chains were synthesized by the fibroblasts.[48] However, none of the proα2(I) chains associated with proα1(I) chains. Therefore, the only procollagen trimer assembled and secreted by the fibroblasts consisted of three proα1(I) chains. Because the structure of the C-propeptide is critical for chain association, the results strongly suggested the molecular defect was an alteration of the structure of the C-propeptides of the proα2(I) chains. This suggestion has been confirmed by examination of both DNA and RNA from the patient's and his parents' fibroblasts.[49] The rate of proα2(I) synthesis by the patient's fibroblasts was less than that seen in control fibroblasts, apparently as a secondary consequence of the mutation in the coding sequences for the C-propeptide.[48] A similar molecular defect was probably present in an OI variant studied earlier.[54]

Single Base Substitutions in the Proα1(I) Chain in Lethal and Nonlethal Forms of OI. A series of single base mutations that change a single amino acid in the proα1(I) chain have been found.[55–61] Four of these mutations are lethal, but two produce only moderately severe forms of OI.

The four lethal variants all involve a single base mutation that converted a glycine codon in the proα1(I) chain to a codon for another amino acid.[58–61] In three of the variants the glycine codon was converted to cysteine[56–60] and in the fourth the glycine codon was converted to an arginine residue.[61] Although some of the data for the four variants is incomplete, the results suggest that all four were new mutations whereby a change of a single base and a single amino acid produced a lethal phenotype. Therefore these four variants constitute a dramatic example of how a change of just 1 of the 3 billion base pairs in the human genome can produce a lethal event. The probable explanation for the devastating effects of the mutations is that glycine, the smallest amino acid, must occupy every third amino acid position in a collagen α chain in order for the α chain to form a stable triple helix.[3] If a larger amino acid, such as cysteine or arginine, is inserted, the whole triple helix unfolds at body temperature and the protein is degraded before being used to form collagen fibrils.

The two nonlethal variants involving a change of a single amino acid have been less well characterized.[55,56] The mutations introduce a new cysteine residue into the α1(I) chain, but the amino acid replaced by cysteine was not defined. The current hypothesis is that the cysteine replaced an amino acid that is less essential than glycine for the stability of the triple helix.

Less Well-Defined Mutations in OI. An extensive study of patients with the type I form of OI demonstrated that cultured fibroblasts from three patients synthesized proα1(I) chains at a decreased rate as reflected by a decrease in the ratio of newly synthesized proα1(I) to proα2(I) chains.[62] Such defects may prove to be common in type I OI.

Fibroblasts from two patients with a lethal variant synthesized proα1(I) chains that migrated more slowly in polyacrylamide gels than normal chains.[63] The observations suggested that the fibroblasts were synthesizing lengthened proα1(I) chains, but this conclusion has not yet been definitely substantiated. In one of these variants, the ratio of mRNAs for proα1(I) to proα2(I) chains was 1:1 instead of the normal ratio of 2:1. Therefore, this patient appears to have one allele for a structurally altered proα1(I) chain and a second allele for proα1(I) that was not transcribed into mRNA.

In other variants, abnormalities in the migration of both α1(I) and α2(I) chains were found.[64,65] In still other variants, some of which may be the same as those studied by other investigators, changes in the ratio of α1(I) to α2(I) chains in pepsin digests of skin were observed.[66] The data suggested a mutation in one or more genes for type I procollagen, but the precise nature of the molecular defects is unclear.

Other Observations in OI. A frequent finding in OI is that the type I procollagen is overmodified, that is, it has an increased content of hydroxylysine and glycosylated hydroxylysine.[38,67,68] The most probable explanation for this observation is that the proα chains have changes in their structure that delay the time at which the chains fold into the triple helix. Any condition that delays helix formation will in itself produce an overmodification, because folding into the triple helix normally terminates and limits the extent of the post-translational modifications.

Another common observation in OI is a decrease in the ratio of type I to type III collagen in skin extracts, or a decrease in the ratio of the amounts of type I and type III procollagen secreted by cultured fibroblasts.[38,43] Some of these observations probably reflect either a decreased rate of synthesis of type I procollagen or the synthesis of a structurally abnormal type I procollagen, which is rapidly degraded in vivo. Some patients with OI, however, have type III collagen in bone, a tissue that normally does not contain this protein.[69,70] In these variants, therefore, the decrease in the ratio may represent an increased synthesis of type III collagen because of "gene switching."

Some observations point to mutations that change the expression of genes for other components of extracellular matrix. In fibroblasts from three patients with type II OI, an increased rate of synthesis of type IV collagen was observed.[47] Fibroblasts from several patients synthesized increased amounts of hyaluronic acid.[71] These effects may or may not be secondary to mutations in genes for type I procollagen.

MOLECULAR DEFECTS IN MARFAN SYNDROME

Marfan syndrome (MS) (see Table 12–4) is characterized by long, thin extremities, redundant ligaments and joint capsules, ectopia lentis, and dilation and rupture of the aorta.[33,35,37,72,73] As in OI, most of the affected tissues are rich in type I collagen. In addition, many of the characteristics of MS can be produced in young animals by inhibiting the cross linking of collagen either by severe copper deficiency or by admin-

istration of nitriles, which inhibit lysyl oxidase. Therefore, several investigators have suggested the MS is produced by mutations in the synthesis or structures of type I procollagen. Evidence for this suggestion has, however, been developed in only a few patients.[74–77]

In one patient, the rate of synthesis of type I procollagen in explants of aorta was decreased.[74] In several independent studies, about one third of the patients had increased excretion of peptide-bound hydroxyproline in the urine, an observation suggesting an increased rate of collagen turnover.[75] In some patients, skin collagen was more extractable than normal.[3,33,76] This observation and related findings suggest a defect in the cross linking of collagen. A deficiency in stable cross links of collagen was, in fact, observed in four patients.[77] However, extensive searches for a deficiency of lysyl oxidase, the critical enzyme for synthesis cross links, have proved to be negative.[78,79]

Some observations suggest defects in noncollagen genes. Aortas from six patients had a decreased content of elastin.[79,80] In addition, fibroblasts from some patients showed increased synthesis of hyaluronic acid.[81]

MOLECULAR DEFECTS IN EHLERS-DANLOS SYNDROME, THE MENKES STEELY-HAIR SYNDROME, AND RELATED DISEASES

EDS produces joint hypermobility and skin changes, such as thinness, extensibility, and fragility (see Table 12–4).[33,35,37,72,82–84] EDS has been classified into nine different types based primarily on the clinical manifestations (Table 12–7). As with OI, the precise molecular defects have been defined in only a few variants of EDS (Table 12–8), but these variants are instructive for understanding the others. Some forms are caused by mutations in genes for type I or type III procollagen, others by defects in enzymes required for the processing of type I procollagen. The defects in the processing enzymes mean that, at the molecular level, many forms of EDS resemble the Menkes syndrome and several related disorders.

Defects of Type III Procollagen in Ehlers-Danlos Syndrome Type IV. Type IV EDS is a rare but severe form of the syndrome. It frequently produces rupture of large arteries and hollow organs. All the patients apparently have a defect in type III procollagen.

One group of variants has a decreased rate of synthesis of proα1(III) chains by cultured fibroblasts.[85–88] In another group, proα1(III) chains are synthesized

Table 12–7.   Classification of EDS Based on Clinical Manifestations and Mode of Inheritance

Type	Joint Hypermobility	Skin Extensibility	Fragility	Bruising	Other Manifestations	Inheritance
I	Marked	Marked	Marked	Marked	Hernias, premature rupture of fetal membranes	AD*
II	Moderate	Moderate	Absent	Moderate		AD
III	Marked	Minimal	Minimal	Minimal		AD
IV	Limited to small joints	Minimal	Marked	Marked	Ruptures of large arteries and bowel; thin skin with prominent venous network; characteristic facies in some	AD or AR
V	Minimal	Moderate	Moderate	Moderate		XR
VI	Moderate	Moderate	Mild	Moderate	Ocular rupture; blue sclerae and other ocular abnormalities; scoliosis in some	AR
VII	Marked	Moderate	Moderate	Moderate	Multiple dislocations	AR or AD
VIII	Moderate	Moderate	Moderate	Moderate	Advanced periodontitis	AD
IX	Mild	Mild	Absent	Absent	Bladder diverticuli with spontaneous ruptures; hernias and skeletal abnormalities; skin laxity	XR or AR

*AD = autosomal dominant; AR = autosomal recessive; XR = X-linked recessive.

at about a normal rate but the secretion of type III procollagen is decreased.[89,90] By analogy with the defects seen in OI (discussed previously), these variants probably involve changes in the primary structure of proα1(III) chains that either prevent or delay folding of the chains into the triple helix and therefore interfere with normal secretion. This conclusion is supported by the observation that fibroblasts from some patients have greatly distended cisternae of the rough endoplasmic reticulum.[86,91] In another variant, fibroblasts secrete normal amounts of type III procollagen, but the protein contains both normal proα(III) chains and proα(III) chains with a slower electrophoretic mobility because of an alteration of amino acid sequence in the chain.[92] The type III procollagen containing the abnormal chains is unusually sensitive to digestion by proteinases and therefore may be rapidly degraded in vivo.

Hydroxylysine Deficiency in Ehlers-Danlos Syndrome Type VI. The characteristic of the type VI form of EDS is ocular changes, which frequently produce rupture of the eye. Severe skeletal deformities are also common. In the first family studied, there was both a deficiency of lysyl hydroxylase and a significant decrease in the hydroxylysine content of type I collagen in skin and other tissues.[93] The low hydroxylysine content probably explains the clinical symptoms because hydroxylysine is necessary for the synthesis of the most stable cross-links of collagen.[3]

Several families similar to the first have been identified,[94,95] but there are at least two other variants. In the second variant, assays of cultured fibroblasts show a deficiency of lysyl hydroxylase, but the hydroxylysine content of collagen extracted from tissues is essentially normal.[94,96] The third variant has the

Table 12–8.   Molecular Defects Identified in Ehlers-Danlos Syndromes (EDS)

EDS-IV	Proα(III)°	Decreased synthesis of type III procollagen
	Proα1(III)ᴸ	Unstable 3-helix of type III procollagen
	Proα1(III)ˣ	Decreased secretion rate of type III procollagen
	Other unidentified	
EDS-VI	Lysyl hydroxylase deficiency	Hydroxylysine-deficient collagen and defective cross-linking
	Other unidentified	
EDS-VII	Procollagen N-proteinase deficiency	Persistence of pNcollagen
	Proα2(I)ˣ	Resistance to procollagen N-proteinase and persistence of pNcollagen
	Other unidentified	
EDS-IX	Defect in Cu metabolism	Lysyl oxidase deficiency and defective cross-linking

same clinical picture, but there is no evidence of either a deficiency of lysyl hydroxylase or a decrease in the hydroxylysine content of collagen.[97] The molecular basis for this variant, therefore, is unclear.

Impaired Cleavage of N-Propeptides in Ehlers-Danlos Syndrome Type VII. The type VII form of EDS is characterized by laxity of joints severe enough to produce dislocations of the knees and unreducible dislocations of the hips. Two variants involve impaired removal of the N-propeptides from procollagen, but they are caused by distinctly different mutations.

In the type VIIA form, N-propeptides are incompletely removed from type I procollagen because of a deficiency of procollagen N-proteinase.[98] Partially processed proα1(I) and proα2(I) chains are found in tissue extracts, and the disease closely resembles dermatosparaxis, a recessively inherited disease found in cattle, sheep, dogs, and cats.[84,99,100] Examination of tissues from these animals, as well as studies on the self-assembly of the purified protein in vitro, has indicated that the partially processed procollagen that contains N-propeptides (pNcollagen) will form fibrils, but the fibrils are thin and irregular in outline. The failure of the fibrils to become thicker and more rounded probably explains the joint laxity in these individuals.

In the type VIIB form of EDS, the molecular defect is a structural alteration of the proα2(I) chain, which prevents cleavage by procollagen N-proteinase.[101] The consequence of the defect is again persistence of partially processed collagen containing the N-propeptide of the proα2(I) chain.

Altered Copper Metabolism and Deficient Lysyl Oxidase Activity in Ehlers-Danlos Syndrome Type IX, Menkes Syndrome, and Related Diseases. A variety of diseases of copper metabolism have been found to be associated with changes in collagen. These disorders include diseases previously classified as EDS type IX,[102,103] the Menkes syndrome,[104] and X-linked cutis laxa.[103] Because of similarities at the molecular level, it has been suggested that all these diseases be classifed as EDS type IX.[103,105] Under this classification, one variant of type IX is characterized by bladder diverticula with spontaneous rupture, inguinal hernias, mild skin changes, and skeletal abnormalities. The variant previously called the Menkes syndrome includes many of these changes together with arterial disease and deterioration of the central nervous system so severe that the condition is lethal.

The variants of EDS type IX are all characterized by low levels of copper and ceruloplasmin in serum, but high levels of copper in most cells.[103,104,106–109] The mutant cells also have increased amounts of the cation-binding protein metallothionein.[103,104] The change in metallothionein may be a primary alteration or it may be secondary to undefined alterations in copper metabolism. The low extracellular levels of copper probably decrease the cross linking of collagen because the critical enzyme in the cross linking of collagen (lysyl oxidase) requires copper.[110] Because all the disorders are X-linked, it is likely that the essential genes involved in copper metabolism are closely linked on the X-chromosome. The variability in the clinical manifestations, however, suggests that several different genes are involved.

Other Observations in Ehlers-Danlos Syndrome. The type V form of EDS is a moderately severe disorder in which a deficiency of lysyl oxidase has been reported in a few patients.[4] However, other families have not revealed any deficiencies of this enzyme,[111] and the initial observations of the deficiency probably need to be confirmed.

Alterations in the morphology of collagen fibers have been observed in almost every type of EDS and in animals with related disorders, but it has not yet been possible to relate the morphologic changes to specific molecular defects.[84,105,112]

CONCLUSIONS

This new information about genetic diseases of collagen has important implications for a broad range of common diseases. In addition, at least three surprises have been encountered.

One of the surprises has been the phenomenon called "protein suicide" discussed previously (see Fig. 12–6). A second surprise has been the broad range of different clinical manifestations produced by different mutations that change the structure of type I procollagen. The results demonstrate that a structural change in one part of the molecule produces a disease that primarily affects skin and ligaments (Fig. 12–7), but a similar change in another part of the same protein produces a disease that primarily affects bone. In effect, these diseases demonstrate that some parts of the type I procollagen molecule are critical for normal bone formation, whereas other parts are critical for the normal function of other connective tissues. A third surprise is the apparently high frequency of mutations in genes for type I procollagen in patients with genetic diseases of bone and related tissues. Although correct assembly and maintenance of bone requires the correct expression of a large number of genes, many of which must be bone specific, as many as one fourth of patients with OI and related heritable disorders of connective tissue have now been found to have mutations in either the proα1(I) or proα2(I) gene

FIG. 12–7. Approximate locations of mutations in the structure of type I procollagen. OI = osteogenesis imperfecta; EDS = Ehlers-Danlos syndrome.

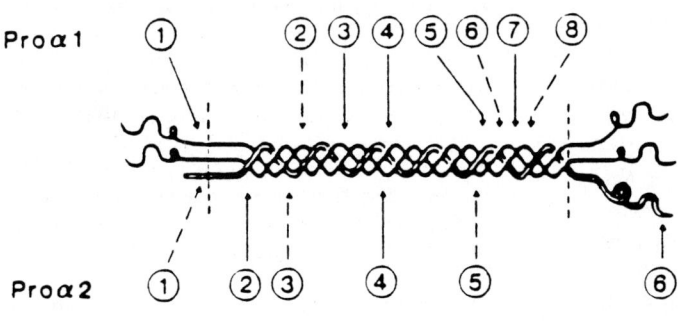

Proα1

①	Deletion 24 aas (Exon 6)	EDS VII
②	? → Cys	OI
③	Gly^{391} → Arg^{391}	Lethal OI
④	Deletion Exons 24–26 (–88 aas)	Lethal OI
⑤	Gly^{748} → Cys^{748}	Lethal OI
⑥	Gly^{904} → Cys^{904}	Lethal OI
⑦	Gly^{988} → Cys^{988}	Lethal OI
⑧	? → Cys	OI

Proα2

①	Deletion 18 aas (Exon 6)	EDS VII
②	Splice/Deletion Exon 11 (–18 aas)	EDS/OI
③	Deletion ~20 aas	OI
④	Splice Exon 28 (–18 aas)	Lethal OI
⑤	Deletion Exons 33 to 40 (–180 aas)	Lethal OI
⑥	Frameshift Deletion 4 bp	OI

for type I procollagen.[113] There are several explanations for this situation. One is that because collagen is a structural protein, a mutation that changes its structure is more likely to have a dominant effect than a mutation in a gene for an enzyme. Another reason is that the protein as a whole has a highly repetitive structure in which many of the amino acids must be preserved in order for it to function normally. As illustrated by the single base mutations in the proα1(I) chain (see above), a mutation that converts any one of the 338 glycine residues in the α1(I) chain is likely to have dramatic effects on destabilizing the protein and causing its rapid degradation. These features appear to make the genes for collagens particularly vulnerable to mutations that disturb the functional properties of connective tissues and produce disease syndromes.

The variants of OI and related diseases discussed here represent mutations in single genes of the collagen family that have overwhelming effects on the individual. The information about these diseases, however, makes it possible, perhaps for the first time, to think concretely about more common diseases that are multifactorial and that involve both genetic and environmental components.

There are, in fact, several reasons why mutations in collagen genes may be involved, as contributing factors, in relatively common diseases of midlife and beyond. One is a general consideration of the kinds of mutations one can expect to find in examining human collagen genes more thoroughly than has been done to date. From the example of a few patients with lethal OI (see Figs. 12–5, 12–6, Table 12–6), it is apparent that, at one extreme, there are mutations in type I procollagen genes that are incompatible with life. At the other extreme, it is likely that a detailed examination of genes from different individuals will reveal "neutral mutations," that is, changes in the genes that change the amino acid sequence of the protein but have no effect on its normal function. Between these two extremes, however, it is likely that mutations will be encountered that have subtle effects and require a long time to manifest themselves. Such subtle mutations may be particularly important in considering collagen. Collagen is a remarkably stable protein, and most of the collagen a person acquires during the growth spurt of adolescence remains with him the rest of his life. A broad time scale must therefore be considered in examining the biologic consequences of mutation in procollagen genes. One can readily imagine mutations that have no apparent consequence during childhood or early adult life. The same mutations, however, might produce change in the size or in other features of collagen fibrils to make connective tissues less fit than normal to withstand the stresses of 30 or 40 years of confrontation with the environment. These mutations may predispose a person to a slow manifestation of chronic diseases such as osteoporosis or osteoarthritis. The work on genetic diseases of collagen is clearly providing the experimental tools and the basic information necessary to examine such subtle mutations in collagen genes. Examining the medical consequences of the subtle mutations is likely to move the study of genetic diseases from the special realm of rare maladies to diseases of a broader population. In effect, it may be possible in the future to provide specific, molecular definitions of what physicians have long recognized as the genetic predisposition of many families and individuals to a variety of common chronic diseases.

REFERENCES

1. Grant, M.A., and Prockop, D.J.: The biosynthesis of collagen. N. Engl. J. Med., *286*:194, 242, 291, 1972.
2. Bornstein, P., and Traub, W.: The chemistry and biology of collagen. *In* The Proteins. Vol. 4. Edited by H. Neurath and R.L. Hill. New York, Academic Press, 1979, pp. 411–632.
3. Prockop, D.J., et al.: The biosynthesis of collagen and its disorders. N. Engl. J. Med., *301*:13–23, 77–85, 1979.
4. Prockop, D.J., and Kivirikko, K.I.: Heritable disorders of collagen. The lessons of rare maladies provide a basis for understanding common diseases. N. Engl. J. Med., *311*:376–386, 1984.
5. Bachinger, H.P., et al.: Structural implications from an electron microscopic comparison of procollagen V with procollagen I, pC-collagen I, procollagen IV, and a Drosophila procollagen. J. Biol. Chem., *257*:24590–24592, 1982.
6. Bornstein, P., and Sage, H.: Structurally distinct collagen types. Annu. Rev. Biochem., *49*:957–1003, 1980.
7. Gibson, G.J., Schor, S.L., and Grant, M.E.: Effect of matrix macromolecules on chondrocyte gene expression: Synthesis of a low molecular weight collagen species by cells cultured within collagen gels. J. Cell Biol., *93*:767–774, 1982.
8. Mayne, R., Reese, C.A., and Wiedemann, H.: New collagenous molecules from chicken hyaline cartilage. *In* New Trends in Basement Membrane Research. Edited by K. Kuhn, H.-H. Schoene, and R. Timpl. New York, Raven Press, 1982, pp. 121–126.
9. Odermatt, E., et al.: Structural diversity and domain composition of a unique collagenous fragment (intima collagen) obtained from human placenta. Biochem. J., *211*:295–302, 1983.
10. Schmid, T., and Conrad, H.E.: A unique low molecular weight collagen secreted by cultured chick embryo chondrocytes. J. Biol. Chem., *257*:12444–12450, 1982.
11. Timpl, R., et al.: A network model for the organization of type IV collagen molecules in basement membranes. Eur. J. Biochem., *120*:203–211, 1981.
12. Sage, H.: Collagens of basement membranes. J. Invest. Dermatol., *79*:51s–59s, 1982.
13. de Crombrugghe, B., and Pastan, I.: Structure and regulation of a collagen gene. Trends Biochem. Sci., 11–23, 1982.
14. Monson, J.M., and McCarthy, B.J.: Identification of a Balb/c mouse proα1(I) procollagen gene: Evidence for insertions or deletions in gene coding sequences. DNA, *1*:59–69, 1981.
15. Myers, J.C., et al.: Analysis of the 3' end of the human proα2(I) collagen gene: Utilization of multiple polyadenylation sites in cultured fibroblasts. J. Biol. Chem., *258*:10128–10135, 1983.
16. Tolstoshev, P., and Crystal, R.: The collagen alpha-2 chain gene. J. Invest. Dermatol., *79*:60S–64S, 1982.
17. Wozney, J., et al.: Structure of the proα2(I) collagen gene. Nature, *294*:129–135, 1981.
18. Yamada, Y., et al.: The collagen gene: Evidence for its evolutionary assembly by amplification of a DNA segment containing an exon of 54 bp. Cell *22*:887–892, 1980.
19. Chu, M.-L., et al.: Characterization of the human proα1(I) collagen gene. Fed. Proc., *42*:1758, 1983.
20. Sandell, L.J., et al.: Identification of the gene coding for type II procollagen. J. Biol. Chem., *258*:11617–11621, 1984.
21. Yamada, Y., et al.: Isolation and characterization of a genomic clone encoding chick αI and type III collagen. J. Biol. Chem., *258*:2758–2761, 1983.
22. Huerre, C., et al.: Human type I procollagen genes are located on different chromosomes. Proc. Natl. Acad. Sci. USA, *79*:6627–6630, 1982.
23. Boyd, C.D., et al.: The single copy gene coding for human α1(IV) procollagen is located at the terminal end of the long arm of chromosome 13. Hum. Genet., *74*:121–125, 1986.
24. Myers, L.C., et al.: Cloning a cDNA for the proα2 chain of human type I collagen. Proc. Natl. Acad. Sci. USA, *78*:3516–3520, 1981.
25. Dagleish, R., et al.: Copy number of a human type I α2 collagen gene. J. Biol. Chem., *257*:13816–13822, 1982.
26. de Wet, W.J., Chu, M.-L., and Prockop, D.J.: The mRNAs for the proα1(I) and proα2(I) chains of type I procollagen are translated at the same rate in normal human fibroblasts and in fibroblasts from two variants of osteogenesis imperfecta

with altered steady-state ratios of the two mRNAs. J. Biol. Chem., *258*:14385–14389, 1983.

27. Heathcote, J.C., and Grant, M.E.: Extracellular modification of connective tissue proteins. *In* The Enzymology of Post-translational Modifications of Proteins. Edited by R.B. Freedman and H.C. Hawkins. London, Academic Press, 1980, pp. 457–605.

28. Kivirikko, K.I., and Myllyla, R.: Biosynthesis of collagens. *In* Connective Tissue Biochemistry. Edited by K.A. Piez and A.H. Reddi. New York, Elsevier/North-Holland, 1984, pp. 83–158.

29. Tuderman, L., and Prockop, D.J.: Procollagen N-proteinase: Properties of the enzyme purified from chick embryo tendons. Eur. J. Biochem., *125*:545–549, 1982.

30. Siegel, R.C.: Lysyl oxidase. Int. Rev. Connect. Tissue Res., *8*:73–118, 1979.

31. Kivirikko, K.I., and Myllyla, R.: Post-translational modifications. *In* Collagen in Health and Disease. Edited by J.B. Weiss and M.I.V. Jayson. New York, Churchill Livingstone, 1982, pp. 101–120.

32. Kivirikko, K.I., and Myllyla, R.: Collagen glycosyltransferases. Int. Rev. Connect. Tissue Res., *8*:23–72, 1979.

33. Bornstein, P., and Byers, P.H.: Disorders of collagen metabolism. *In* Metabolic Control and Disease. Edited by P.K. Bondy and L.E. Rosenberg. Philadelphia, W.B. Saunders Co., 1980, pp. 1089–1153.

34. Hollister, D.W., Byers, P.H., and Holbrook, K.A.: Genetic disorders of collagen metabolism. Adv. Hum. Genet., *12*:1–87, 1982.

35. McKusick, V.A.: Heritable Disorders of Connective Tissue. Saint Louis, The C.V. Mosby Co., 1972.

36. Minor, R.R.: Collagen metabolism: A comparison of diseases of collagen and diseases affecting collagen. Am. J. Pathol., *98*:227–278, 1980.

37. Pinnell, S.R., and Murad, S.: Disorders of collagen. *In* The Metabolic Basis of Inherited Disease. Edited by J.B. Stanbury, et al. New York, McGraw-Hill Book Co., 1983, pp. 1425–1449.

38. Smith, R., Francis, M.J.O., and Houghton, G.R.: The Brittle Bone Syndrome: Osteogenesis Imperfecta. London, Butterworths, 1983.

39. Sillence, D.O.: Osteogenesis imperfecta: An expanding panorama of variants. Clin. Orthop. Rel. Res., *159*:11–25, 1981.

40. Sillence, D.O., Senn, A., and Danks, D.M.: Genetic heterogeneity in osteogenesis imperfecta. J. Med. Genet., *16*:101–116, 1979.

41. Barsh, G.S., and Byers, P.H.: Reduced secretion of structurally abnormal type I procollagen in a form of osteogenesis imperfecta. Proc. Natl. Acad. Sci. USA, *78*:5142–5146, 1981.

42. Chu, M.-L., et al.: Internal deletion in a collagen gene in a perinatal lethal form of osteogenesis imperfecta. Nature, *304*:78–80, 1983.

43. Penttinen, R.P., et al.: Abnormal collagen metabolism in cultured cells in osteogenesis imperfecta. Proc. Natl. Acad. Sci. USA, *72*:586–589, 1975.

44. Williams, C.J., and Prockop, D.J.: Synthesis and processing of a type I procollagen containing shortened proα1(I) chains by fibroblasts from a patient with osteogenesis imperfecta. J. Biol. Chem., *258*:5915–5921, 1983.

45. Byers, P.H., et al.: Abnormal α2-chain in type I collagen from a patient with a form of osteogenesis imperfecta. J. Clin. Invest., *71*:689–697, 1983.

46. Sippola, M., and Prockop, D.J.: A shortened proα2(I) chain in a mild variant of osteogenesis imperfecta. The altered structure makes type I procollagen resistant to procollagen N-proteinase. J. Cell Biol., *97*:229a, 1984.

47. de Wet, W.J., et al.: Synthesis of a shortened proα2(I) chain and decreased synthesis of proα2(I) chains in a proband with osteogenesis imperfecta. J. Biol. Chem., *258*:7721–7728, 1983.

48. Deak, S., et al.: The molecular defect in a non-lethal variant of osteogenesis imperfecta: Synthesis of proα2(I) chains which are not incorporated into trimers of type I procollagen. J. Biol. Chem., *258*:15192–15197, 1983.

49. Dickson, L., et al.: Nuclease S1 mapping of a homozygous mutation in the carboxy-propeptide coding region of the proα2(I) collagen gene in a patient with osteogenesis imperfecta. Proc. Natl. Acad. Sci. USA, *81*:4524–4528, 1984.

50. Nicholls, A.C., Pope, F.M., and Schloon, H.: Biochemical heterogeneity of osteogenesis imperfecta: New variant. Lancet, *1*:1193, 1979.

51. Bernard, M.P., et al.: Structure of a cDNA for the proα2 chain of human type I procollagen. Comparison with chick cDNA identifies structurally conserved features of the protein and gene. Biochemistry *22*:1139–1145, 1983.

52. Bernard, M.P., et al.: Nucleotide sequences of cDNAs for the proα1 chain of human type I procollagen. Statistical evaluation of structures which are conserved during evolution. Biochemistry, *22*:5213–5223, 1983.

53. Peltonen, L., Palotie, A., and Prockop, D.J.: A defect in the structure of type I procollagen in a patient who had osteogenesis imperfecta: Excess mannose in the COOH-terminal propeptide. Proc. Natl. Acad. Sci. USA, *77*:6179–6183, 1980.

54. Meigel, W.N., et al.: A constitutional disorder of connective tissue suggesting a defect in collagen biosynthesis. Klin. Wochenschr., *52*:906–912, 1974.

55. de Vries, W.N., and de Wet, W.J.: The molecular defect in an autosomal dominant form of osteogenesis imperfecta: Synthesis of type I procollagen containing cysteine in the triple-helical domain of proα1(I) chains. J. Biol. Chem., *261*:9056–9064, 1986.

56. Steinmann, B., Nicholls, A., and Pope, F.M.: Clinical variability of osteogenesis imperfecta reflecting molecular heterogeneity: Cysteine substitutions in the α1(I) collagen chain producing lethal and mild forms. J. Biol. Chem., *261*:8958–8964, 1986.

57. Steinmann, B., et al.: Cysteine in the triple-helical domain of one allele product of the α1(I) gene of type I collagen produces a lethal form of osteogenesis imperfecta. J. Biol. Chem., *259*:11129–11138, 1984.

58. Cohn, D.H., et al.: Lethal osteogenesis imperfecta resulting from a single nucleotide change in one human proα1(I) collagen allele. Proc. Natl. Acad. Sci. USA, *83*:6045–6047, 1986.

59. Vogel, B.E., et al.: A point mutation in a type I procollagen gene converts glycine 748 of the α1 chain to cysteine and destabilizes the triple helix in a lethal variant of osteogenesis imperfecta. J. Biol. Chem. In press, 1987.

60. Constantinou, C.D., Nielsen, K.B., and Prockop, D.J.: The molecular defect in a lethal variant of osteogenesis imperfecta is a single base mutation that substitutes cysteine for glycine 904 of the α1(I) chain of type I procollagen. (Submitted for publication.)

61. Bateman, J.F.: Lethal perinatal osteogenesis imperfecta due to the substitution of arginine for glycine at residue 391 of the α1(I)-chain of type I collagen. J. Biol. Chem., *262*:7021–7027, 1987.

62. Barsh, G.S., David, K.E., and Byers, P.H.: Type I osteogenesis imperfecta: A nonfunctional allele for proα2(I) chains of type I procollagen. Proc. Natl. Acad. Sci. USA, *79*:3838–3942, 1982.

63. Uitto, J., et al.: Synthesis of lengthened proα1(I) chains of type I procollagen by skin fibroblasts from two patients with lethal osteogenesis imperfecta. Clin. Res., 31:468A, 1983.

64. Bateman, J.F., et al.: Structural defects of type I procollagen in lethal perinatal osteogenesis imperfecta. Connect. Tissue Res., 9:203, 1982a.

65. Bateman, J.F., et al.: Defective type I procollagen secretion in lethal perinatal osteogenesis imperfecta. Connect. Tissue Res., 9:203, 1982.

66. Francis, M.J.O., et al.: The relative amounts of the collagen chains α1(I), α2 and α1(III) in the skin of 31 patients with osteogenesis imperfecta. Clin. Sci., 60:617a–623, 1981.

67. Kirsch, E., et al.: Disorder of collagen metabolism in a patient with osteogenesis imperfecta (Lethal type): Increased degree of hydroxylation of lysine in collagen types I and III. Eur. J. Clin. Invest., 11:30–47, 1981.

68. Trelstad, R.L., Rubin, D., and Gross, J.: Osteogenesis imperfecta congenita. Evidence for a generalized molecular disorder of collagen. Lab Invest., 36:501–508, 1977.

69. Müller, P.K., et al.: Presence of type III collagen in bone from a patient with osteogenesis imperfecta. Eur. J. Pediatr., 125:29–37, 1977.

70. Pope, F.M., et al.: Osteogenesis imperfecta (lethal) bones contain types III and V collagens. J. Clin. Pathol., 33:53408, 1980.

71. Turakainen, H., et al.: Synthesis of hyaluronic acid and collagen in skin fibroblasts cultured from patients with osteogenesis imperfecta. Biochim. Biophys. Acta, 628:388–397, 1980.

72. Nimmi, M.E.: Collagen: Structure, function, and metabolism in normal and fibrotic tissues. Semin. Arthritis Rheum., 13:1–86, 1983.

73. Pyeritz, R.E., and McKusick, V.A.: The Marfan syndrome: Diagnosis and management. N. Engl. J. Med., 300:772–777, 1979.

74. Halbritter, R., et al.: Case report and study of collagen metabolism in Marfan's syndrome. Klin. Wochenschr., 59:83–90, 1981.

75. Kivirikko, K.J.: Urinary excretion of hydroxyproline in health and disease. Int. Rev. Connect. Tissue Res., 5:93–163, 1970.

76. Byers, P.H., et al.: Marfan syndrome: Abnormal α2-chain in type I collagen. Proc. Natl. Acad. Sci. USA, 78:7745–7749, 1981.

77. Boucek, R.J., et al.: The Marfan syndrome: A deficiency in chemically stable collagen cross-links. N. Engl. J. Med., 305:988–991, 1981.

78. Royce, P.M., and Danks, D.M.: Normal lysyl oxidase activity in skin fibroblasts from patients with Marfan's syndrome. IRCS Med. Sci., 10:41, 1982.

79. Abraham, P.A., et al.: Marfan syndrome: Demonstration of abnormal elastin in aorta. J. Clin. Invest., 7:1245–1252, 1982.

80. Halme, T., et al.: Desmosines in aneurysms of the ascending aorta (annuloaortic ectasia). Biochim. Biophys. Acta, 717:105–110, 1982.

81. Appel, A., Horwitz, A.L., and Dorfman, A.: Cell-free synthesis of hyaluronic acid in Marfan syndrome. J. Biol. Chem., 254:12199–12203, 1979.

82. Pinnell, S.R., et al.: A heritable disorder of connective tissue. Hydroxylysine-deficient collagen disease. N. Engl. J. Med., 286:1013–1020, 1972.

83. Krieg, T., et al.: Molecular defects of collagen metabolism in the Ehlers-Danlos syndrome. Int. J. Dermatol., 20:415–425, 1981.

84. Minor, R.R., et al.: Defects in collagen fibrillogenesis causing hyperextensible, fragile skin in dogs. J. Am. Vet. Med. Assoc., 182:142–148, 1983.

85. Aumailley, M., et al.: Biochemical and immunological studies of fibroblasts derived from a patient with Ehlers-Danlos syndrome type IV demonstrate reduced type III collagen synthesis. Arch. Dermatol. Res., 269:169–177, 1980.

86. Byers, P.H., Barsh, G.S., and Holbrook, K.A.: Molecular mechanisms of connective tissue abnormalities in the Ehlers-Danlos syndrome. Coll. Rel. Res., 1:475–489, 1981.

87. Pope, F.M., et al.: EDS IV (acrogeria): New autosomal dominant and recessive types. J.R. Soc. Med., 73:180–186, 1980.

88. Pope, F.M., et al.: Patients with Ehlers-Danlos syndrome type IV lack type III collagen. Proc. Natl. Acad. Sci. USA, 72:1314–1316, 1975.

89. Byers, P.H., et al.: Altered secretion of type III procollagen in the form of type IV Ehlers-Danlos syndrome. Biochemical studies in cultured fibroblasts. Lab. Invest., 44:336–341, 1981.

90. Clark, J.G., et al.: Lung collagen in type IV Ehlers-Danlos syndrome: Ultrastructural and biochemical studies. Am. Rev. Respir. Dis., 122:971–978, 1980.

91. Uitto, J., et al.: The Ehlers-Danlos syndrome type IV: Clinical, genetic, and biochemical studies of a family. In American Academy of Orthopaedic Surgeons Symposium on Heritable Disorders of Connective Tissue. Edited by W.J. Akeson, P. Bornstein, and M.J. Glimcher. Saint Louis, The C.V. Mosby Co., 1982, pp. 82–95.

92. Stolle, C.A., et al.: Synthesis of an altered type III procollagen in a patient with type IV Ehlers-Danlos syndrome. A structural change in the α1(III) chain which makes the protein more susceptible to proteinases. J. Biol. Chem., 260:1937–1944, 1985.

93. Krane, S.M., Pinnell, S.R., and Erbe, R.W.: Lysyl-protocollagen hydroxylase deficiency in fibroblasts from siblings with hydroxylysine-deficient collagen. Proc. Natl. Acad. Sci. USA, 69:2899–2903, 1972.

94. Ihme, A., et al.: Biochemical characterization of variants of the Ehlers-Danlos syndrome type VI. Eur. J. Clin. Invest., 13:357–362, 1983.

95. Krane, S.M.: Hydroxylysine-deficient collagen disease: A form of Ehlers-Danlos syndrome type VI. In American Academy of Orthopaedic Surgeons Symposium on Heritable Disorders of Connective Tissue. Edited by W.H. Akeson, P. Bornstein, and M.J. Glimsincher. Saint Louis, The C.V. Mosby Co., 1982, pp. 61–75.

96. Steinmann, B., et al.: Ehlers-Danlos syndrome in two siblings with deficient lysyl hydroxylase activity in cultured skin fibroblasts but only mild hydroxylysine deficit in skin. Helv. Paediatr. Acta, 30:255–274, 1975.

97. Judisch, F.G., Waziri, M., and Krachmer, J.H.: Ocular Ehlers-Danlos syndrome with normal lysyl hydroxylase activity. Arch. Ophthalmol., 94:1489–1491, 1976.

98. Lichtenstein, J.R., et al.: Defect in conversion of procollagen to collagen in a form of Ehlers-Danlos syndrome. Science, 182:298–300, 1973.

99. Holbrook, K.A., et al.: Dermatosparaxis in a Himalayan cat: II. Ultrastructural studies of dermal collagen. J. Invest. Dermatol., 74:100–104, 1980.

100. Kohn, L.D., et al.: Calf tendon procollagen peptidase. Its purification and endopeptidase mode of action. Proc. Natl. Acad. Sci. USA, 71:40–44, 1974.

101. Steinmann, B., et al.: Evidence for a structural mutation of procollagen type I in a patient with the Ehlers-Danlos syndrome type VII. J. Biol. Chem., 255:8887–8893, 1980.

102. Byers, P.H., et al.: X-linked cutis laxa. Defective cross-link

formation in collagen due to decreased lysyl oxidase activity. N. Engl. J. Med., *303*:61–65, 1980.

103. Peltonen, L., et al.: Alterations in copper and collagen metabolism in the Menkes syndrome and a new subtype of the Ehlers-Danlos syndrome. Biochemistry, *22*:6156–6163, 1983.

104. Danks, D.M.: Hereditary disorders of copper metabolism in Wilson's disease and Menkes' disease. *In* The Metabolic Basis of Inherited Disease, 5th ed. Edited by J.B. Stanbury, et al. New York, McGraw-Hill Book Co., 1983, pp. 1251–1268.

105. Cupo, I.N., et al.: Ehlers-Danlos syndrome with abnormal collagen fibrils, sinus of valsalva aneurysms, myocardial infarction, panacinar emphysema and cerebral heterotopias. Am. J. Med., *71*:1051–1058, 1981.

106. Kivirikko, K.I., and Peltonen, L.: Abnormalities in copper metabolism and disturbances in the synthesis of collagen and elastin. Med. Biol., *60*:45–48, 1982.

107. Kuivaniemi, H., et al.: Abnormal copper metabolism and deficient lysyl oxidase activity in a heritable connective tissue disorder. J. Clin. Invest., *69*:730–733, 1982.

108. Rowe, D.W., et al.: Decreased lysyl oxidase activity in the aneurysm-prone mottled mouse. J. Biol. Chem., *252*:939–942, 1977.

109. Starcher, B., et al.: Abnormal cellular copper metabolism in the blotchy mouse. J. Nutr., *108*:1229–1233, 1978.

110. Siegel, R.C., Black, C.M., and Bailey, A.J.: Cross-linking of collagen in the X-linked Ehlers-Danlos type V. Biochem. Biophys. Res. Commun., *88*:281–287, 1979.

111. Siegel, R.C.: Lysyl oxidase. Int. Rev. Connect. Tissue Res., *8*:73–118, 1979.

112. Holbrook, K.A., and Byers, P.H.: Structural abnormalities in the dermal collagen and elastic matrix from the skin of patients with inherited connective tissue disorders. J. Invest. Dermatol., *79*:7s–16s, 1982.

113. Prockop, D.J.: A family with osteogenesis imperfecta as a model for genetic causes of osteoporosis and perhaps several other common diseases of connective tissue. Arthritis Rheum. In press, 1987.

STRUCTURE AND FUNCTION OF PROTEOGLYCANS

13

LAWRENCE ROSENBERG

Articular cartilage and nucleus pulposus are specialized connective tissues composed of few cells distributed throughout an abundant extracellular matrix. The extracellular matrix gives each tissue unusual mechanical properties essential for normal joint function. Articular cartilage provides a smooth covering for the osseous components of diarthrodial joints and contributes to the almost frictionless gliding of apposing joint surfaces. Articular cartilage is a hard, yet elastic tissue. Nucleus pulposus is softer, is more compressible and deformable, and has the capacity to undergo substantial changes in shape and volume with motion of the intervertebral joint. Both tissues transmit load, absorb impact, and sustain shearing forces, yet resist wear to a surprising degree.

The remarkable mechanical properties of these connective tissues are directly related to the structure and properties of the extracellular matrix, which is composed mainly of collagen, proteoglycans, and water. Collagen is an insoluble fibrous protein with tensile strength. Proteoglycans are elastic molecules that expand in solution and resist compression into a smaller volume of solution. The mechanical properties of normal articular cartilage and nucleus pulposus result from the structure and properties of the fibrous composite formed when proteoglycans at high concentration are entangled and constrained in a dense network of collagen fibers. Our understanding of the mechanical properties of normal articular cartilage and nucleus pulposus must be based on knowledge of the structures and physicochemical properties of proteoglycans and collagen and their interactions.

Current interest in the structure and properties of the molecular species comprising the intercellular substance of cartilage is based on other, more compelling considerations. Degradation of proteoglycans is a central event in osteoarthritis and rheumatoid arthritis that results in both a loss of the capacity of articular cartilage to resist wear and an acceleration of the destructive process. Each of these forms of arthritis may be viewed as a series of biochemical processes in which connective tissue macromolecules of elaborate structure are shattered in a characteristic fashion by specific enzymes. The clinical effect of the cartilage destruction is pain, limitation of motion of the affected joint, and increasing functional disability. A comprehensive view of the pathogenesis of a particular form of arthritis should include knowledge of the sequence of events at the cellular level in cartilage destruction and of the biochemical mechanisms underlying each event. The first section of this chapter describes the cartilage proteoglycans that are degraded in diseases such as osteoarthritis and rheumatoid arthritis.

CARTILAGE PROTEOGLYCANS

In the formation of both collagen and proteoglycans, a basic structural unit of low molecular weight is first formed. Many basic units then assemble into an ordered aggregate form of much higher molecular weight. The aggregate form exhibits the specific functional properties of the biochemical species, whereas

240

he basic structural unit does not, at least to the same degree. Such a process is frequently encountered in biochemistry.

The basic structural unit of cartilage ground substance is the proteoglycan monomer. A diagrammatic model of the structure of a cartilage proteoglycan monomer is shown in Figure 13–1. It consists of a protein core from which arise many chondroitin sulfate and keratan sulfate side chains. Chondroitin sulfate and keratan sulfate are covalently attached mainly to serine and threonine residues within the protein core. Proteoglycan monomers from different cartilages and nucleus pulposus vary in molecular weight and chemical composition, particularly the relative amounts of chondroitin sulfate and keratan sulfate. Indeed, proteoglycan monomers from the same cartilage are polydisperse and vary in size and composition; however, an average representative proteoglycan monomer would have a protein core of approximately M.W. 200,000 daltons, measuring about 300 nm long. To this protein core would be attached approximately 100 chondroitin sulfate side chains, each M.W. 20,000 to 30,000 daltons and approximately 50 to 60 nm long. Keratan sulfate chains, M.W. 5,000 to 10,000 daltons and 10 to 20 nm in length, would also be attached to the protein core. The entire proteoglycan monomer would be approximately M.W. 2 to 3 million daltons.

Chondroitin sulfate and keratan sulfate are linear polymers composed of sugar residues. They are members of the group of polysaccharides called glycosaminoglycans or mucopolysaccharides found in the ground substance of various connective tissues. The glycosaminoglycans are composed of two different sugar residues that alternate regularly in the polysaccharide chain. One sugar residue is an amino sugar, formed when the hydroxyl group of the number two carbon of glucose or galactose is replaced by an amino group, which is acetylated. Therefore, in the glycosaminoglycans, one sugar residue is the hexosamine N-acetylglycosamine or N-acetylgalactosamine. The other sugar residue is usually glucuronic acid, in which the number six carbon of glucose carries a carboxyl group. Each glycosaminoglycan is described in terms of the sugar residues that comprise its disaccharide repeating unit. The structures of the glycosaminoglycans and their linkage regions to protein core are shown in Figure 13–2.

The structure of the disaccharide repeating unit of chondroitin 6-sulfate is shown on the left of Figure 13–3. Chondroitin 6-sulfate chains are composed of approximately 40 to 60 repeating units consisting of glucuronic acid alternating with N-acetylgalactosamine. N-acetylgalactosamine carries an ester sulfate group on carbon number 6. The chondroitin sulfate chains are covalently bound to serine residues within the protein core by the neutral sugar trisaccharide galactose-galactose-xylose, shown on the right of Figure 13–3.[1–3] The structure of the keratan sulfate repeating unit is shown on the left of Figure 13–4. Keratan sulfate consists of galactose residues alternating regularly with N-acetylglucosamine residues. Keratan sulfate carries an ester sulfate group on the number 6 carbon of N-acetylglucosamine, and some or most of the galactose residues of keratan sulfate may be sulfated. Keratan sulfate chains consist of approximately 10 to 20 repeating units covalently bound mainly to threonine or serine residues of the protein core by N-acetylgalactosamine. As shown on the right of Figure 13–4, N-acetylneuraminic acid (sialic acid) and galactose residues are attached to the N-acetylgalactosamine residue lining each keratan sulfate chain to protein.[4,5]

The most important feature of the chemical structure of chondroitin sulfate and keratan sulfate is that the repeating units of the glycosaminoglycans carry closely spaced negatively charged groups. Glycosaminoglycan repeating units are approximately M.W. 450 to 500 daltons and 1 nm in length. Chondroitin 6-sulfate carries an ester sulfate group attached to carbon number 6 of N-acetylgalactosamine and the negatively charged carboxyl group of glucuronic acid. Thus, chondroitin 6-sulfate carries negatively charged groups at approximately 0.5-nm intervals. Keratan sulfate carries an ester sulfate group on carbon number 6 of N-acetylglucosamine, and some or most of the galactose residues may be sulfated, so keratan sulfate carries negatively charged groups at 0.5- to

FIG. 13–1. Diagrammatic model of the structure of the cartilage proteoglycan monomer.

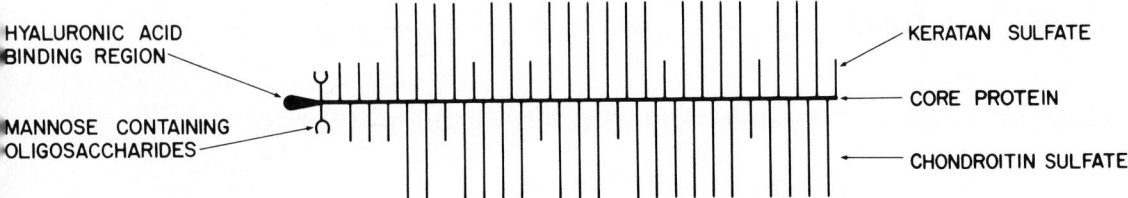

FIG. 13–2. Structures of the glycosaminoglycans and their linkage regions to protein. GlcUA = glucuronic acid; IdUA = iduronic acid; GlcNAc = N-acetylglucosamine; GalNAc = N-acetylgalacto-samine; Gal = galactose; Xyl = xylose; NeuAc = N-acetylneuraminic acid; Ser = serine; Thr = threonine; OSO₃⁻ = ester sulfate; GlcNSO₃⁻ = N-sulfo-D-glucosamine. Two disaccharide repeating units are shown to emphasize the microheterogeneity that exists in some cases. Heparan sulfate and heparin show many structural similarities; however, heparan sulfate contains more GlcNAc(α1→4)GlcUA repeating units, fewer glucosamine residues are N-sulfated, and fewer iduronic acid residues are sulfated at C2.

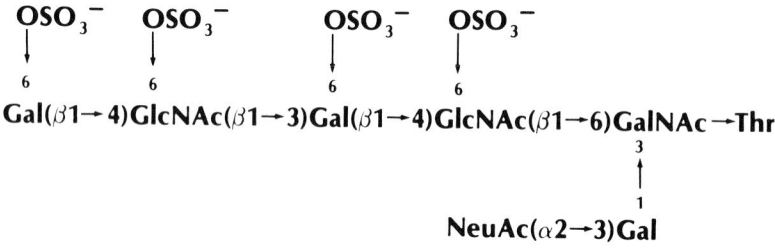

OSO₃⁻ ... OSO₃⁻

GalNAc(β1→4)GlcUA(β1→3)GalNAc(β1→4)GlcUA(β1→3)Gal(β1→3)Gal(β1→4)Xyl→Ser

CHONDROITIN 4-SULFATE

OSO₃⁻ OSO₃⁻ OSO₃⁻ OSO₃⁻

Gal(β1→4)GlcNAc(β1→3)Gal(β1→4)GlcNAc(β1→6)GalNAc→Thr
NeuAc(α2→3)Gal

KERATAN SULFATE

GlcNAc(β1→4)GlcUA(β1→3)GlcNAc(β1→4)GlcUA(β1→3)Gal(β1→3)Gal(β1→4)Xyl→Ser

HYALURONATE

OSO₃⁻ ... OSO₃⁻

GalNAc(β1→4)IdUA(α1→3)GalNAc(β1→4)GlcUA(β1→3)Gal(β1→3)Gal(β1→4)Xyl→Ser

DERMATAN SULFATE

OSO₃⁻ OSO₃⁻

GlcNAc(α1→4)IdUA(α1→4)GlcNAc(α1→4)GlcUA(β1→3)Gal(β1→3)Gal(β1→4)Xyl→Ser

HEPARAN SULFATE

OSO₃⁻ OSO₃⁻ OSO₃⁻

GlcNSO₃⁻(α1→4)IdUA(α1→4)GlcNAc(α1→4)GlcUA(β1→3)Gal(β1→3)Gal(β1→4)Xyl→Ser

HEPARIN

FIG. 13–3. Structure of chondroitin 6-sulfate and of its linkage region to protein. The disaccharide repeating unit of chondroitin 6-sulfate consists of glucuronic acid and N-acetylgalactosamine 6-sulfate. The chondroitin sulfate chain is covalently bound to serine by the trisaccharide containing galactose and xylose.

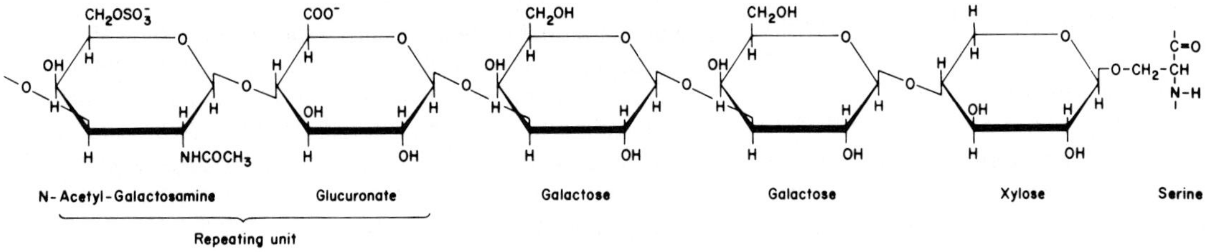

1-nm intervals. Because of the repelling forces of the closely spaced negatively charged groups, the glycosaminoglycan chains arising from proteoglycan monomer core protein are maintained in a stiffly extended conformation. The chondroitin sulfate and keratan sulfate chains stick out from core protein like the bristles on a brush, as shown in Figure 13–1. The proteoglycan monomer assumes an extended conformation and spreads out into a large volume of solution. The stiffness of the glycosaminoglycan chains makes the molecule resistant to compression into a

smaller volume of solution. This property is partially responsible for the elasticity of cartilage.

In addition to chondroitin sulfate and keratan sulfate, proteoglycan monomers contain two types of oligosaccharides.[6,7] The first type consists of oligosaccharides that resemble the linkage region of keratan sulfate to core protein and that are linked through N-acetylgalactosamine by O-glycosidic bonds to the hydroxyl groups of threonine or serine residues or core protein.

These oligosaccharides are located mainly in the

FIG. 13–4. Structure of keratan sulfate and its linkage region to protein. The disaccharide repeating unit of keratan sulfate consists of galactose and N-acetylglucosamine 6-sulfate. The keratan sulfate chain is covalently bound mainly to threonine by N-acetylgalactosamine.

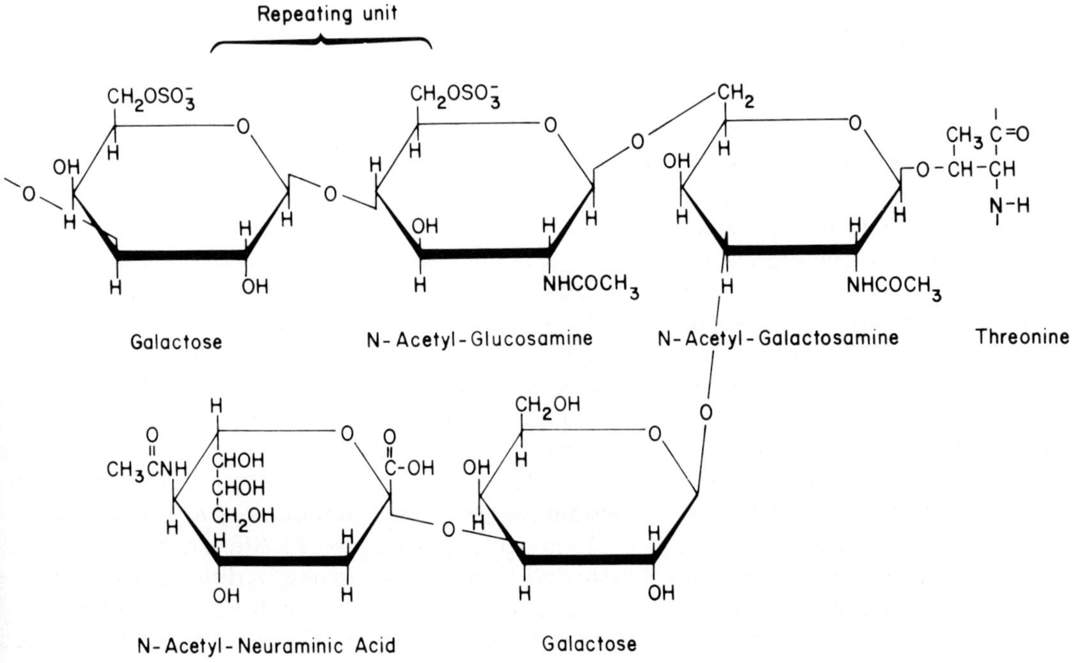

chondroitin sulfate-rich region of core protein. In developing (fetal) hyaline cartilages, the proportion of keratan-sulfate-linkage-region-like oligosaccharides is high, and the proportion of keratan sulfate chains in the chondroitin-sulfate-rich region is low. In mature hyaline cartilages, the proportion of keratan sulfate chains is high, and the proportion of keratan-sulfate-linkage-region-like oligosaccharides is low.

The second type of oligosaccharide is mannose-containing oligosaccharide, probably linked by N-glycosylamine bonds to asparagine residues in core protein. Although the structures of the mannose-containing oligosaccharides are only now being elucidated, they are probably similar to those of the mannose-rich oligosaccharides linked by N-glycosidic bonds to asparagine. These oligosaccharides are present in many glycoproteins. In proteoglycan monomers, the mannose-containing oligosaccharides are located near the hyaluronic acid-binding region, as shown in Figure 13–1.

STRUCTURE OF CARTILAGE PROTEOGLYCAN AGGREGATES

In native cartilage, most proteoglycan exists in the form of aggregates of high molecular weight.[8–28] The molecular architecture of a proteoglycan aggregate is shown in Figure 13–5. Hyaluronic acid forms the filamentous backbone of the aggregate.[10–13,15,26] The aggregate is formed by the noncovalent association of many proteoglycan monomers with hyaluronate. Proteoglycan monomers of varying size arise laterally at regular intervals from the opposite sides of the hyaluronic acid chain. A low-molecular-weight "link" protein is also a component of the aggregate. Link protein appears to stabilize or to strengthen the bond between proteoglycan monomer and hyaluronate.

A closer examination of the model shown in Figure 13–5 indicates that proteoglycan monomer core protein consists of 3 distinct regions that differ in structure and function. One end of the proteoglycan monomer core protein contains little or no chondroitin sulfate or keratan sulfate, and consists of a region of core protein of approximately M.W. 60,000 daltons with a globular conformation. This region contains the hyaluronic acid binding of proteoglycan monomer core protein.[18,23,29] Extending toward the other end of the molecule is a region of the protein core to which essentially all the chondroitin sulfate chains and some of the keratan sulfate chains are attached. It is called the chondroitin-sulfate-rich region. Between the hyaluronic acid-binding region and the chondroitin-sulfate-rich region is located a third region consisting of

FIG. 13–5. Diagrammatic model of the cartilage proteoglycan aggregate. The filamentous backbone of the aggregate is hyaluronic acid. Proteoglycan monomers of varying size arise at regular intervals from the opposite sides of the hyaluronic acid chain. One end of the proteoglycan monomer core protein has a globular conformation and contains the hyaluronic acid-binding region of the core protein. The other end of the core protein has an extended conformation and contains the attachment sites for chondroitin sulfate and keratan sulfate chains. The polydispersity in size and composition of proteoglycan monomers from mature cartilages results from the variable length of the chondroitin sulfate-rich region of proteoglycan monomer core protein. (From Rosenberg. L.: Structure of cartilage proteoglycans. *In* Dynamics of Connective Tissue Macromolecules. Edited by P.M.C. Burleigh and A.R. Poole. New York, Elsevier-North Holland, 1973, pp. 103–128.)

PROTEOGLYCAN AGGREGATE

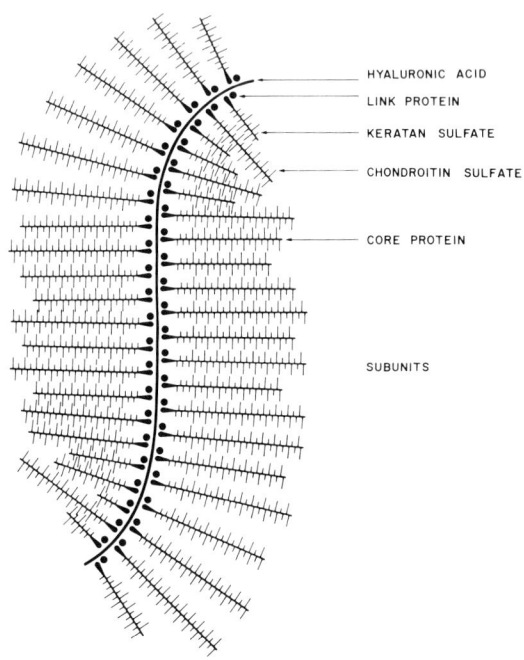

HYALURONIC ACID
LINK PROTEIN
KERATAN SULFATE
CHONDROITIN SULFATE

CORE PROTEIN

SUBUNITS

a short peptide to which are attached mainly keratan sulfate chains.[21,29] This region is called the keratan-sulfate-rich region.[21] In the proteoglycan aggregate, the link proteins are centrally located in the region where proteoglycan monomer binds to hyaluronate. The link proteins bind simultaneously to the hyaluronic acid-binding region of proteoglycan monomer core protein, and to hyaluronate, and stabilize the binding of proteoglycan monomer to hyaluronate.

Proteoglycan aggregates in different tissues vary in size and composition, owing to differences in hyaluronic acid chain lengths and in the size, chemical composition, and numbers of proteoglycan monomers noncovalently bound to hyaluronic acid in the proteoglycan aggregates. The mechanical properties of different tissues are related to these variations in the size and composition of proteoglycan aggregates. Even proteoglycan aggregates isolated from a particular cartilage are polydisperse. They consist of a population of molecules in which individual members vary in molecular weight, owing mainly to differences in the length of hyaluronic acid chain that forms the filamentous backbone of the proteoglycan aggregate. A representative proteoglycan aggregate from articular cartilage, however, would consist of over 100 proteoglycan monomers (each M.W. 2 million daltons) noncovalently bound together with link protein to a hyaluronic acid chain 4,000 nm in length. Such an aggregate would have a molecular weight of over 200 million daltons.

Because of the repelling forces of the thousands of negatively charged groups, these huge proteoglycan aggregates spread out into an enormous domain of solution. The volume of solution occupied by proteoglycan aggregates in vitro is far greater than that available to them in native cartilage, where the aggregates expand until they are constrained by the surrounding network of collagen fibers. The aggregates in native cartilage have elastic forces that are balanced by the tensile forces of collagen fibers. When articular cartilage is subjected to a compressive force, the aggregates are temporarily compressed into a smaller domain, and water is simultaneously extruded from the cartilage. When the compressive force is relieved, the aggregates expand, the articular cartilage simultaneously imbibes water, and the volume of the cartilage increases until further increases in volume are prevented by the collagen fibers. This kind of interaction is the basis for the elastic properties of articular cartilage.

The aforementioned structural concepts have been derived from studies of the chemical composition and physical properties of proteoglycan monomers and aggregates from different cartilages and from chemical binding studies between proteoglycan monomers, hyaluronate, and link protein. These studies required that proteoglycan monomers and proteoglycan aggregates first be isolated from cartilage. The procedure now generally used for the isolation of proteoglycan aggregates and monomers from cartilage involves four steps: (1) dissociative extraction; (2) reassociation; (3) equilibrium density gradient centrifugation under associative conditions; and (4) equilibrium density gradient centrifugation under dissociative conditions.

The purpose of step 1, dissociative extraction, is to bring proteoglycans into solution and to separate them from the insoluble network of collagen fibers. In native cartilage, most of the proteoglycan exists in the form of huge proteoglycan aggregates that are intricately entangled with, enmeshed in, and constrained by the dense network of collagen fibers. Little proteoglycan diffuses out of fresh, wet cartilage when it is stirred in the cold in isotonic solvents at neutral pH. The dissociative extraction method for extracting proteoglycans depends on one of the fundamental properties of the proteoglycan aggregate.

The noncovalent bonds between proteoglycan monomers, hyaluronate, and link protein are broken in concentrated solutions of guanidine hydrochloride (GuHCl) or divalent cations.[25,30,31] When fresh, wet cartilage is slowly stirred at 4° in 4 M GuHCl, pH 5.8 to 6.3, proteoglycan monomers, hyaluronate, and link proteins diffuse out of the insoluble collagen network at a rapid rate into the extraction solvent. The extract is separated from the insoluble collagenous cartilage residue by filtration. The filtered extract also contains a variety of noncollagenous matrix proteins that must be separated from the proteoglycans. To accomplish this goal, proteoglycan monomer, hyaluronate, and link proteins are first reassembled into proteoglycan aggregates by dialyzing off the guanidine hydrochloride. This is step 2: reassociation.

In step 3, matrix proteins are separated from the proteoglycan aggregates by equilibrium density gradient centrifugation under associative conditions. Cesium chloride (CsCl) is added to the reassociated extract, and the solution is centrifuged to equilibrium in a preparative ultracentrifuge. A gradient is established in which the concentration of CsCl and the density of the solution increase with distance from the top to the bottom of the solution. The gradient is divided into six equal fractions. The fractions from the bottom to the top of this associative gradient are called A1 through A6.[19,29] Proteoglycan aggregates are of high buoyant density and distribute in fraction A1 in the bottom sixth ($\rho \approx 1.6$ g/ml) of the gradient. The matrix proteins are of low buoyant density and distribute in fraction A6 ($\rho \approx 1.4$ g/ml) at the top of the gradient. Fraction A1 is the preparation used for the physical characterization of proteoglycan aggregates by sedimentation velocity experiments and by electron microscopy.[25,26]

In step 4, equilibrium density gradient centrifugation under dissociative conditions, the proteoglycan aggregate is separated into its component species. Fraction A1 from the associative gradient, which contains proteoglycan aggregate, is dissolved in 4 M GuHCl. The aggregate is dissociated into proteoglycan monomer, hyaluronate, and link protein. Cesium chloride is added. The solution is centrifuged to equi-

FIG. 13–6. Diagrammatic representation of the structural basis for the polydispersity of cartilage proteoglycan monomer. The polydispersity of the proteoglycan monomer is determined mainly by the variable length of the chondroitin-sulfate-rich region of the protein core. The ratio chondroitin sulfate to protein, buoyant density, and molecular weight of an individual proteoglycan monomer molecule are directly related to the length of the chondroitin-sulfate-rich region of core protein.

DISSOCIATIVE CONDITIONS   ASSOCIATIVE CONDITIONS

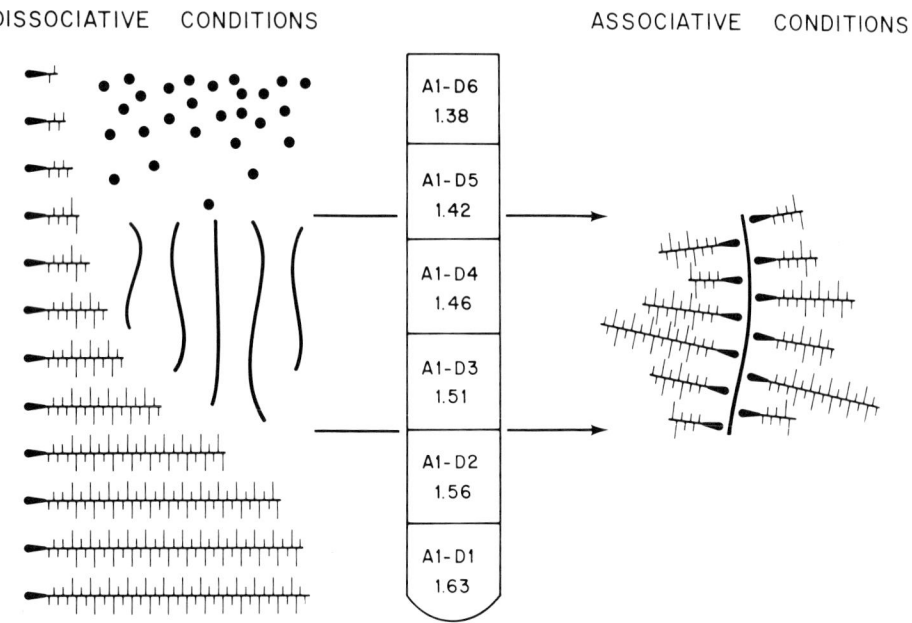

librium in a preparative ultracentrifuge. Six fractions called A1–D1 (bottom) through A1–D6 (top) are taken from this dissociative gradient. The effects of the dissociative gradient are shown diagrammatically in Figure 13–6.[29] Link protein is separated into the top of the gradient. Hyaluronic acid distributes in the middle of the 4 *M* GuHCl–3 *M* CsCl dissociative gradient. Proteoglycan monomers from mature hyaline cartilages distribute throughout the dissociative gradient. Individual members of the polydisperse population of proteoglycan monomers from mature hyaline cartilages band at buoyant densities determined mainly by their ratios of chondroitin sulfate and keratan sulfate to protein.

Figure 13–6 also expresses diagrammatically the structural basis for the polydispersity of proteoglycan monomers from a particular mature hyaline cartilage. The polydispersity of proteoglycan monomers appears to be determined mainly by the variable length of the chondroitin-sulfate-rich region of proteoglycan monomer core protein. Proteoglycan monomer core protein contains a hyaluronic acid-bonding region of constant size and composition, located in the region where the monomer binds to hyaluronate. Proteoglycan monomer core protein also contains a chondroitin-sulfate-rich region of variable length (composed

of variable numbers of possible homologous peptides providing attachment sites for chondroitin sulfate chains), which extends toward the other terminus. The ratio of chondroitin sulfate to protein, buoyant density, and molecular weight of an individual proteoglycan monomer are determined mainly by the length of the chondroitin-sulfate-rich region of the core protein.

This concept for the structural basis of the polydispersity of proteoglycan monomer is based on the results of several studies. In the first series of studies, the variable length of the chondroitin-sulfate-rich region has been deduced indirectly from the chemical composition and physical properties of individual members of the polydisperse population of proteoglycan monomers. For example, Table 13–1 shows the chemical composition and physical properties of eight monodisperse proteoglycan monomer fractions separated from the polydisperse population of proteoglycan monomers from bovine articular cartilage.[29] As shown in Table 13–1, the chondroitin sulfate content of each fraction, as indicated by the values for uronate or galactosamine, increases as the sedimentation coefficient of the proteoglycan monomer increases from 5.7 S to 14 S. These data indicate that the molecular weight of a proteoglycan monomer increases in pro-

Table 13–1. Chemical Composition and Physical Properties of Eight Proteoglycan Monomer Fractions Isolated from Bovine Articular Cartilage

Column	1	2	3	4	5	6	7	8
Yield, g/g	.019	.039	.036	.045	.074	.053	.209	.451
Uronate, %	9.7	10.3	11.5	15.3	16.1	17.1	19.0	20.1
Galactosamine	6.6	8.1	12.7	14.3	15.4	14.8	17.5	18.7
Hexose	12.5	13.5	12.9	14.3	13.3	11.7	11.8	12.2
Glucosamine	10.4	11.1	10.0	9.1	8.6	5.6	6.5	6.0
Sialate	3.0	3.1	2.9	2.4	2.8	1.8	1.8	1.4
Protein	30.7	23.9	17.3	13.0	14.9	10.3	11.1	9.9
s⁰⁄₀₀, subunit	5.7	7.8	8.8	9.7	10.3	10.8	12.7	14.3
s⁰⁄₀₀, aggregate		18.8	32.1					
Amino Acid Composition Residues/1000								
Aspartic acid	96	92	71	68	70	62	65	60
Threonine	61	65	68	63	65	62	62	61
Serine	69	77	90	105	103	115	123	125
Glutamic acid	139	138	149	147	141	150	146	150
Proline	84	96	101	111	110	104	105	101
Glycine	81	87	93	102	102	117	114	118
Alanine	75	76	77	74	76	71	73	70
Cysteine	20	21	17	14	17	12	13	12
Valine	60	56	56	59	56	59	59	57
Methionine	12	10	10	6	8	6	7	5
Isoleucine	35	34	33	32	31	32	33	40
Leucine	81	78	74	73	74	74	78	78
Tyrosine	42	27	33	29	20	27	25	24
Phenylalanine	40	45	41	43	41	39	38	38
Lysine	32	28	24	19	19	15	15	13
Histidine	14	17	12	11	11	12	13	13
Arginine	58	55	51	44	47	42	41	37

portion to its chondroitin sulfate content. The ratio of chondroitin sulfate to protein of the fractions also increases and is largely responsible for the differences in the buoyant densities of the fractions. One possible structural basis for this pattern of polydispersity might be that all proteoglycan monomer contains the same core protein, that is, polypeptide chains identical in molecular weight and composition in which chondroitin sulfate chains of different lengths are attached. The amino acid composition of proteoglycan monomers of different molecular weight is not constant, however. As shown in Table 13–1, the amino acid composition varies characteristically with molecular weight. The molecules of lowest weight are highest in cysteine, methionine, and aspartic acid and are lowest in serine and glycine. As the molecular weight increases, serine and glycine increase, and cysteine, methionine, and aspartic acid decrease.

What is the structural basis for this change in amino acid composition with molecular weight? The hyaluronic acid-binding region of proteoglycan monomer core protein has been isolated.[23] It is characterized by its high cysteine, methionine, and aspartic acid contents and by its low serine and glycine contents. The chondroitin-sulfate-rich region of proteoglycan monomer core protein is composed of variable numbers

of possibly homologous peptides each containing serine and glycine within a region, with the primary structure and conformation required for the initiation of the synthesis of a chondroitin sulfate chain.[32,33] The changes in the amino acid composition of proteoglycan monomer with molecular weight reflect the changes in the proportions of these two major domains of core protein. Proteoglycan monomers of the lowest molecular weight consist mainly of the hyaluronic acid-binding region. As the molecular weight of a proteoglycan monomer increases, the size of the chondroitin-sulfate-rich region increases, as indicated by the increase in serine and glycine contents. Thus, the polydispersity of proteoglycan monomers results mainly from the variable length of the chondroitin-sulfate-rich region of proteoglycan monomer core protein.

Direct evidence for the variable length of the chondroitin-sulfate-rich region has been presented in our electron microscopic study of the dimensions of cartilage proteoglycans.[34] A polydisperse population of proteoglycan monomers from bovine nasal cartilage was separated into a series of monodisperse fractions with sedimentation coefficients ranging from 8.3 S to 21.1 S. That no difference was noted in the lengths of the chondroitin sulfate chains or in the spacing between chains in the different proteoglycan monomer fractions indicates that neither increased chondroitin sulfate chain length nor decreased spacing between chains contributed to increases in monomer molecular weight. The length of the proteoglycan monomer core protein and the numbers of chondroitin sulfate chains per monomer increased as the sedimentation coefficients of the monomers increased, however, an indication that the length of the chondroitin-sulfate-rich region increases as the molecular weight of the monomer increases.

Electron microscopic measurements were also made of the chondroitin-sulfate-rich region in proteoglycan monomers bound to hyaluronate in proteoglycan aggregates.[34] Figure 13–7 shows the molecular architecture of a cartilage proteoglycan aggregate on nitrocellulose films. On these films, proteoglycan monomers bound to hyaluronic acid in proteoglycan aggregates consist of two distinct segments: a peripheral thick segment corresponding to the chondroitin-sulfate-rich region, and a central thin segment

that can be traced directly to the hyaluronic acid central filament.[35] This segment contains the hyaluronic acid-binding region. Direct measurements of these domains demonstrated that the size of a proteoglycan monomer is determined mainly by the length of the chondroitin-sulfate-rich region. The same methods might be used to investigate the structural changes in proteoglycans that occur in osteoarthritis.

STRUCTURE AND FUNCTION OF LINK PROTEINS

Cartilage proteoglycan aggregates contain 2 link proteins with molecular weights of approximately 44,000 and 48,000 daltons, based on sodium dodecyl sulfate-polyacrylamide gel electrophoresis.[36] Evidence suggests that: (1) the link proteins are components of native proteoglycan aggregates in vivo; and (2) the isolation of link proteins in association with proteoglycan aggregates is not an artifact re-

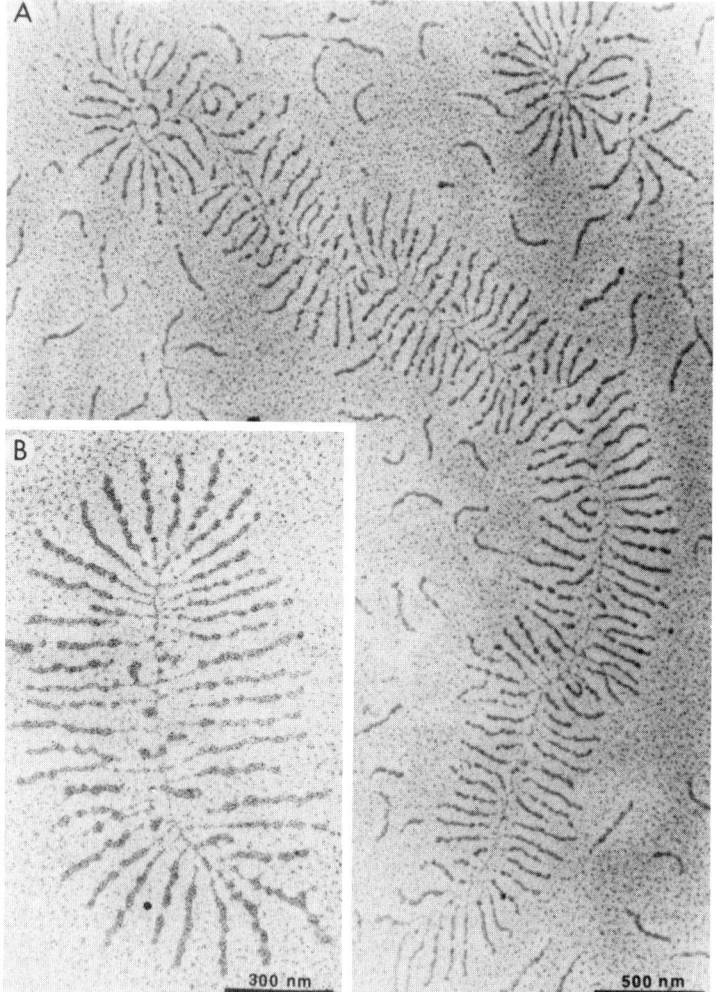

FIG. 13–7. *A* and *B*, Electron micrographs of proteoglycan aggregates from bovine fetal epiphyseal cartilage. The size of an individual proteoglycan aggregate is determined mainly by the length of the hyaluronic acid central filament. Proteoglycan aggregates isolated from a particular tissue vary in size over a broad range, owing to variations in: (1) the length of the hyaluronic acid central filament; (2) the numbers of proteoglycan monomers present in individual aggregates; (3) the spacing between monomers; and (4) the lengths of the proteoglycan monomers. On nitrocellulose films, chondroitin sulfate chains condense along the protein core, so the chondroitin-sulfate-rich region appears as a homogeneous, dense, widened area (thick segment). The centrally located thin segment is devoid of chondroitin sulfate chains and contains the hyaluronic acid-binding region. (From Buckwalter, J.A., and Rosenberg, L.C.: Structural changes during development in bovine fetal epiphyseal cartilage. II. Electron microscopic studies of proteoglycan monomers and aggregates. Coll. Relat. Res., *3*:489–504, 1983.)

sulting from the dissociative extraction and reassociation procedures commonly used to prepare proteoglycan aggregates.[37] Link protein has been isolated to homogeneity.[36] As indicated in Figure 13–6, fractions of low buoyant density (D5, D6) from the top of dissociative density gradients contain link protein mixed with small amounts of proteoglycan monomer. Link protein has been isolated from these fractions by gel chromatography on Sephacryl S-200 in 4 M GuHCl and has been characterized. Baker and Caterson have separated the 2 forms of link protein by preparative electrophoresis.[38] The link proteins differ in their carbohydrate composition; the link protein of higher molecular weight contains about 9% carbohydrate and more mannose and N-acetyglucosamine, whereas the link protein of lower molecular weight contains about 3% carbohydrate. The 2 forms of link protein are essentially identical in amino acid composition and in their peptide maps. The studies of Baker and Caterson suggest that these forms of link protein are identical in the primary structure of their polypeptide chains, but differ in their oligosaccharide components.[38]

In the proteoglycan aggregate, the two link proteins are centrally located in the region where proteoglycan monomer binds to hyaluronate, as indicated by the following observations (Fig. 13–8): In proteoglycan aggregates, the chondroitin-sulfate-rich region of proteoglycan monomer core protein is readily cleaved by trypsin or clostripain.[23,39] When proteoglycan aggregate is digested with trypsin or clostripain, the chondroitin-sulfate-rich region is shattered into small fragments. The central portion of the proteoglycan aggregate, however, which consists of link protein, the hyaluronic acid-binding region of core protein, and hyaluronic acid, is resistant to degradation by trypsin or clostripain. After digestion of proteoglycan aggregate with trypsin or clostripain, a complex consisting of link protein, hyaluronic acid-binding region, and hyaluronate may be isolated, as shown in Figure 13–8. These observations indicate that the link proteins are centrally located in the proteoglycan aggregate in the region where proteoglycan monomer binds to hyaluronate.

Link protein stabilizes proteoglycan aggregates against dissociation, apparently in binding simultaneously to proteoglycan monomer and hyaluronic acid, as shown in Figure 13–5.[8,36] The capacity of link protein to stabilize proteoglycan aggregates against dissociation has been demonstrated in sedimentation velocity experiments in the analytic ultracentrifuge.[36] If a prepared solution contains proteoglycan monomer and hyaluronate, a link-free aggregate will be formed that is stable at pH 7 and can be demonstrated in the analytic ultracentrifuge (Fig. 13–9). The link-free aggregate is unstable at low pH, so the amount of aggregate decreases at pH 5. The link-free aggregate is completely dissociated at pH 4; however, if link protein is added to the solution and a link protein-containing aggregate is formed, a greater amount of aggregate will be present at pH 7, and the aggregate will be stabilized against dissociation at pH 5.

FIG. 13–8. Demonstration of the central location of link protein in proteoglycan aggregate. The chondroitin-sulfate-rich region of proteoglycan monomers in aggregates is selectively cleaved by trypsin or clostripain, whereas the hyaluronic acid-binding region and link protein are not. Following digestion with trypsin or clostripain, a complex that contains link protein can be isolated: the hyaluronic acid-binding region and hyaluronate.

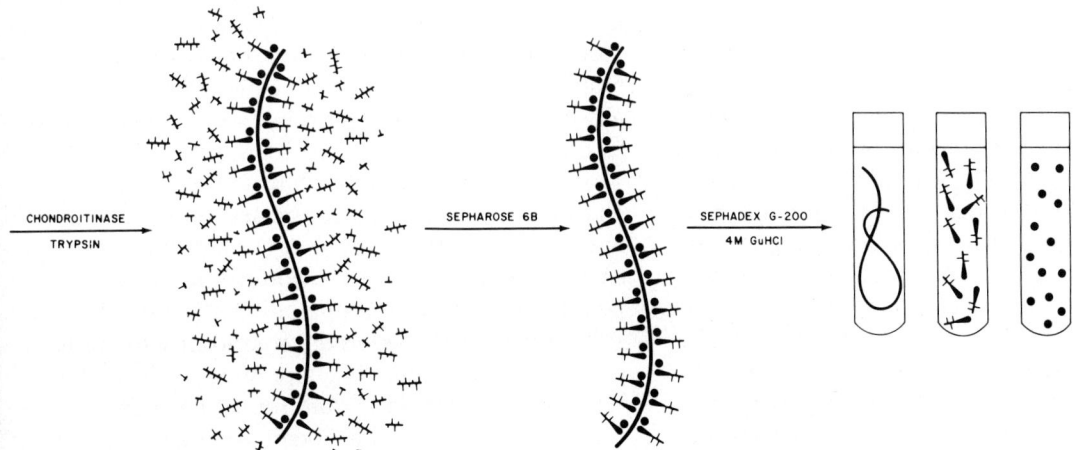

FIG. 13–9. Demonstration of the capacity of link protein to stabilize the proteoglycan aggregates against dissociation. On the left, a link-free aggregate has been prepared by mixing proteoglycan monomer and hyaluronate. The schlieren patterns show that the link-free aggregate is stable at pH 7, but largely dissociated at pH 5. On the right, a link-stabilized aggregate has been prepared by mixing proteoglycan monomer, link protein, and hyaluronate. More aggregate is present at pH 7, and the aggregate is not dissociated at pH 5. (From Tang, et al.: Proteoglycans from bovine nasal cartilage: properties of a soluble form of link protein. J. Biol. Chem., *254*: 10,523–10,531, 1979.)

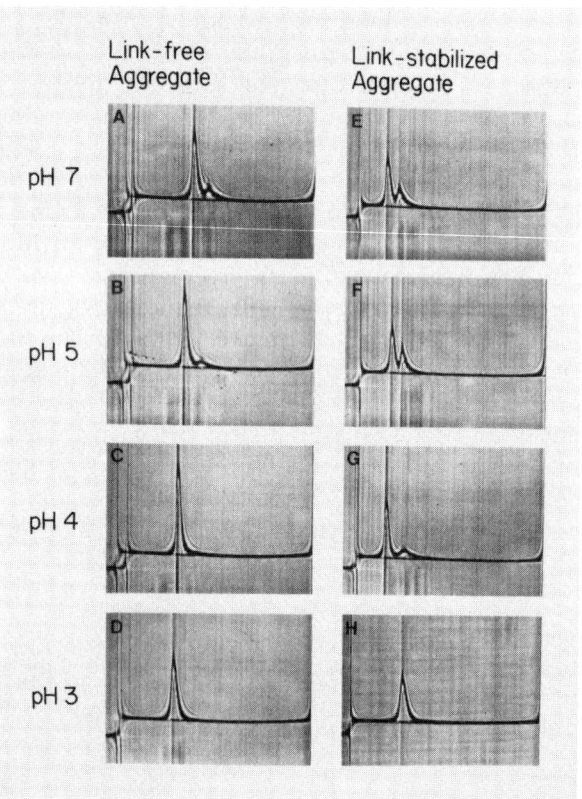

Taken together, the aforementioned observations indicate that the two forms of link protein probably represent two identical multifunctional subunits, each of which contains binding sites for both proteoglycan monomer and hyaluronate, fused into single and identical polypeptide chains. Rigorous proof of this concept requires that the two forms of link protein be separated from one another and the functional capacity of each form of link protein to bind to hyaluronate, to bind to proteoglycan monomer, and to stabilize proteoglycan aggregate against dissociation be examined.

DERMATAN SULFATE PROTEOGLYCANS

Dermatan sulfate proteoglycans are widely distributed in the extracellular matrix of undifferentiated mesenchymal tissue, fibrous connective tissues, blood vessel wall, skin, sclera, and lung. Compared with cartilage proteoglycan monomers, dermatan sulfate proteoglycan monomers are usually much smaller and do not bind with link protein to hyaluronate to form large, stable aggregates, but rather self-associate to form small, unstable aggregates. Systematic studies of the properties of dermatan sulfate proteoglycans have been initiated only recently, and detailed information on their structure and function is only now becoming available. Nonetheless, this class of proteoglycans will be important in understanding not only the properties of tissues, such as blood vessel wall where the proteoglycan is an essential structural component of normal extracellular matrix, but also the alterations in the structure and properties of articular cartilage that occur during aging and in response to injury. For example, the dermatan sulfate proteoglycan present in the extracellular matrix of undifferentiated fetal limb bud mesenchyme is largely replaced by cartilage proteoglycan after chondrogenesis, but reappears in increased concentration in some aging articular cartilages. The substitution during aging of a small dermatan sulfate proteoglycan with feeble elastic properties for the large cartilage proteoglyan aggregate with potent elastic properties may have deleterious effects on the elasticity of articular cartilage.

The structure of the glycosaminoglycan dermatan sulfate is shown in Figure 13–10. The disaccharide repeating unit of dermatan sulfate, shown on the left of Figure 13–10, consists of L-iduronic acid and N-acetylgalactosamine. L-iduronic acid is the C-5 epimer of D-glucuronic acid, in which the carboxyl group is in an axial rather than an equatorial position. The N-acetylgalactosamine residue of the dermatan sulfate repeating unit carries an ester sulfate group usually on carbon number four, but sometimes on carbon number six.[40] As indicated in the middle of Figure 13–10, dermatan sulfate chains also contain disaccharide repeating units composed of glucuronic acid and N-acetylgalactosamine.[40–46] The N-acetylgalactosamine residues in these chondroitin sulfate-like repeating units may be 4- or 6-sulfated. Thus, dermatan sulfate may be considered a hybrid in which the glycosaminoglycan chain is a copolymer of dermatan sulfate and chondroitin sulfate repeating units.

Dermatan sulfate has been isolated from skin,[47] heart valves,[48] blood vessels,[49–53] lung,[54] kidney,[55] nu-

FIG. 13–10. Structure of dermatan sulfate. The repeating unit of dermatan sulfate, shown on the left, consists of L-iduronic acid and N-acetylgalactosamine 4- or 6-sulfate. Dermatan sulfate chains also contain some disaccharide-repeating units consisting of glucuronic acid and N-acetylgalactosamine 4- or 6-sulfate. Dermatan sulfate is therefore a hybrid glycosaminoglycan. Dermatan sulfate chains are covalently bound to serine by the same linkage region as chondroitin sulfate; the first galactose of this linkage region is shown on the right.

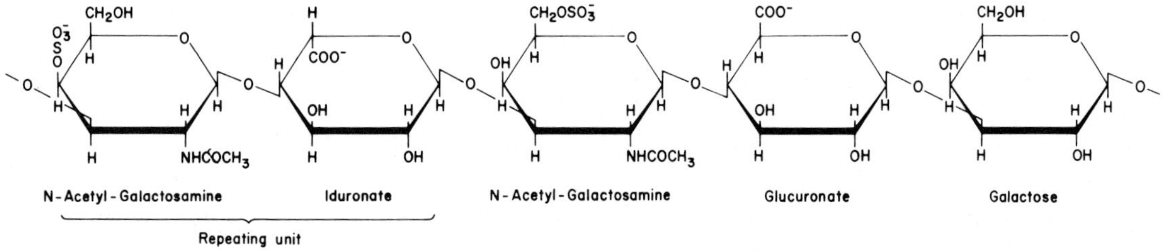

cleus pulposus.[56-58] and umbilical cord.[43] Dermatan sulfate accounts for much of the glycosaminoglycan present in lung and in the blood vessels of nonhuman primates frequently used in the studies of the pathogenesis of vascular diseases.[54,59,60] In these tissues, dermatan sulfate is covalently bound to a core protein in the form of a proteoglycan monomer. The linkage region of dermatan sulfate to protein is identical to that of chondroitin sulfate, shown in Figure 13–2.[41,61]

Proteoglycans containing dermatan sulfate are distributed in the extracellular matrix, where they interconnect collagen fibers, elastin, and cells. Wight and Ross studied the ultrastructural localization of proteoglycans in the intima of nonhuman primate arteries.[59,60] Numerous polygonal granules 20 to 50 nm in diameter with a marked affinity for ruthenium red were distributed throughout the extracellular matrix. The granules possessed filamentous projections 3 to 6 nm thick that appeared to interconnect adjacent granules. The granules and their filaments interconnected collagen fibers at regular intervals in register with the periodicity of the collagen fibers and elastic fibers and appeared to form connections between the plasma membranes of smooth-muscle cells and intercellular fibers. Most of the intercellular granules and filaments were removed with chondroitinase ABC. Wight and Ross also found that 60 to 80% of the glycosaminoglycan synthesized and secreted into the medium by arterial smooth muscle cells in culture was dermatan sulfate, whereas only 10 to 20% was chondroitin 4- or 6-sulfate.[60] Taken together, the results indicate that most of the extracellular matrix granules are dermatan sulfate proteoglycans. Wight and Ross suggested that the dermatan sulfate proteoglycan might function to hold collagen fibers, elastin, and cells together, and at the same time maintain tissue turgor as a result of their elastic properties. They suggested that the proteoglycans might function

as a type of plastic interstitial substance, important in absorbing or dissipating stress. Dermatan sulfate proteoglycans in the interstitium of lung parenchyma may possess similar functions.

Bovine sclera is a rich source of dermatan sulfate proteoglycans, which may be isolated in amounts sufficient for its detailed characterization and for studies of its unusual properties. Dermatan sulfate proteoglycans have been extensively studied by Fransson, Coster, and their co-workers.[62-69] The dermatan sulfate proteoglycans were extracted from bovine sclera with 4 M GuHCl in the presence of protease inhibitors. They were purified by ion-exchange chromatography on DEAE-cellulose in 6 M urea, by equilibrium density gradient centrifugation, and by gel chromatography on Sepharose CL-2B in 4 M GuHCl. Two proteoglycan monomers of different size, called proteoglycans I and II, were separated by gel chromatography on Sepharose CL-2B in 4 M GuHCl. Under associative conditions on gel chromatography, the large proteoglycan monomer (I) self-associated into aggregates, whereas the smaller proteoglycan monomer (II) did not. That the sizes of proteoglycans I and II under associative conditions were not increased by the addition of hyaluronic acid indicates that the dermatan sulfate proteoglycan monomers did not react with, or bind to, hyaluronate to form proteoglycan aggregates of the kind formed by cartilage proteoglycans.

The molecular weights of the scleral proteoglycan monomers were determined by sedimentation-velocity, diffusion, and sedimentation-equilibrium experiments in 6 M GuHCl. In 6 M GuHCl, the molecular weights of proteoglycan monomers I and II were 160,000, to 200,000 and 70,000 to 100,000 daltons, respectively. The molecular weight of the dermatan sulfate side chain was 24,000 daltons. Proteoglycan monomer I contained 45% protein, and proteoglycan monomer II contained 60% protein. Thus, the molecular weights of the protein cores of monomers I and II are approximately 85,000 and 46,000 daltons, respectively. This finding indicates that proteoglycan monomer II contains 1 or 2 dermatan sulfate chains bound to a core protein of approximately M.W. 46,000 daltons, whereas proteoglycan monomer I contains 4 or 5 dermatan sulfate chains bound to a core protein of M.W. 85,000 daltons.

Sedimentation-equilibrium and light-scattering studies under associative conditions in 0.15 M NaCl, pH 7.4, showed that proteoglycan monomers I and II self-associated to form aggregates of higher molecular weight. Moreover, the propensity to form aggregates and the size of the aggregates formed varied under different conditions and were dramatically increased under the conditions prevailing in the light-scattering experiments. Proteoglycan monomer I self-associated into aggregates of M.W. 500,000 to 800,000 daltons in sedimentation-equilibrium experiments in 0.15 M NaCl, whereas proteoglycan monomer II showed little tendency to self-associate and gave molecular weights of 90,000 to 110,000 daltons. In light-scattering experiments, both proteoglycan monomers I and II exhibited an enhanced propensity for self-association. Under associative conditions in 0.15 M NaCl, proteoglycan monomers I and II had molecular weights of 3.1×10^6 and 3.4×10^6, respectively. Thus, dermatan sulfate proteoglycans, even in a maximally aggregated state, have molecular weights that are approximately the same as those of cartilage proteoglycan monomers, and 20 to 100 times less than those of cartilage proteoglycan aggregates.

One of the most interesting properties of the dermatan sulfate proteoglycan is its capacity to undergo different degrees of self-association, depending on the experimental conditions. Thus, in light-scattering experiments, in which the macromolecules are not subjected to shearing forces or pressure, the highest degree of self-association into aggregates of large size readily occurs. In sedimentation-equilibrium experiments, in which the macromolecules are subjected to pressure, the degree of self-association is less. In gel-chromatography experiments, the large dermatan sulfate proteoglycan (proteoglycan I) self-associates to form small aggregates, whereas the smaller dermatan sulfate-containing proteoglycan (proteoglycan II) does not. The possibility exists that the proteoglycan aggregates formed by the self-association of dermatan sulfate proteoglycans are reversibly dissociated by shearing forces or pressure. Because of the small size of dermatan sulfate proteoglycan monomers and the instability of the small aggregates formed by the self-association of these proteoglycans, the substitution of

dermatan sulfate proteoglycans for cartilage proteoglycans in aging articular cartilage, or in the reparative tissue-filling cartilage defects, would have deleterious effects on the biomechanical properties of the articular cartilage.

MODULATION OF PROPORTIONS OF DERMATAN SULFATE PROTEOGLYCANS AND CARTILAGE PROTEOGLYCANS IN DEVELOPING AND AGING CARTILAGES

Prior to chondrogenesis, the developing limb bud consists of a core of mesenchyme covered by ectoderm. The mesenchymal cells are closely spaced and are separated by small amounts of extracellular matrix. Before chondrogenesis, the extracellular matrix of the mesenchyme contains mainly type I collagen and a dermatan sulfate proteoglycan, as well as much smaller amounts of cartilage proteoglycan. With the advent of chondrogenesis synthesis of the cartilage proteoglycan suddenly increases, and synthesis of the dermatan sulfate proteoglycan decreases. Goetinck and his co-workers have extensively studied the biosynthesis of the dermatan sulfate proteoglycan and the cartilage proteoglycan during chondrogenesis in limb bud development.[70-75]

Heretofore, it was assumed that the small dermatan sulfate proteoglycan that is a major component of the extracellular matrix of undifferentiated mesenchymal tissue would eventually be completely replaced by cartilage proteoglycan after chondrogenesis during fetal development. More recent studies have shown, however, that the dermatan sulfate proteoglycan is present in low concentrations in epiphyseal cartilage throughout fetal development.[76] Moreover, in some aging cartilages, the dermatan sulfate proteoglycan appears in increased concentration, in amounts over 10 times greater than those present in fetal epiphyseal cartilages. The dermatan sulfate proteoglycan isolated from bovine fetal epiphyseal cartilage and from aging bovine articular cartilage is polydisperse. Its molecular weight ranges from 80,000 to 140,000 daltons. Antisera have been prepared against the dermatan sulfate proteoglycan monomer and against the cartilage proteoglycan monomer from the same cartilage. The antiserum to the cartilage proteoglycan monomer does not react with the dermatan sulfate proteoglycan monomer, and the antiserum to the dermatan sulfate proteoglycan monomer does not react with the cartilage monomer. Thus, these proteoglycan monomers possess different protein cores.

The substitution of dermatan sulfate proteoglycan

for cartilage proteoglycan in the articular cartilage of some aging individuals, or in the reparative tissue-filling cartilage defects, would have profound effects on the biochemical properties of the articular cartilage. Cartilage proteoglycan aggregates, formed by the noncovalent association of proteoglycan monomers, link protein, and hyaluronate, and are stabilized against dissociation by link protein. There is no indication that they dissociate when subjected to shearing forces or pressure. On the other hand, aggregates formed by dermatan sulfate proteoglycans are smaller than the cartilage proteoglycan aggregates. They may dissociate into small dermatan sulfate proteoglycan monomers when subjected to shearing forces or to pressure similar to that to which articular cartilage is exposed. The small dermatan sulfate proteoglycans would be less effectively enmeshed with and constrained by the surrounding network of collagen fibers. In the next several years, research should indicate the effects of partial substitution of dermatan sulfate proteoglycans with feeble elastic properties for cartilage-specific proteoglycans with potent elastic properties on the biomechanical properties of articular cartilage.

REFERENCES

1. Lindahl, U., and Roden, L.: The chondroitin-4 sulfate-protein linkage. J. Biol. Chem., *241*:2,113–2,119, 1966.
2. Roden, L., and Armand, G.: Structure of the chondroitin 4-sulfate-protein linkage region: isolation and characterization of the disaccharide 3-O-β-D-glucuronosyl-D-galactose. J. Biol. Chem., *241*:65–70, 1966.
3. Roden, L., and Smith, R.: Structure of the neutral trisaccharide of the chondroitin-4 sulfate-protein linkage region. J. Biol. Chem., *241*:5,949–5,954, 1966.
4. Hopwood, J.J., and Robinson, H.C.: The alkali labile linkage region between keratan sulphate and protein. Biochem. J., *141*:57–69, 1974.
5. Hopwood, J.J., and Robinson, H.C.: The structure and composition of cartilage keratan sulphate. Biochem. J., *141*:517–526, 1974.
6. De Luca, S., et al.: Proteoglycans from chick limb bud chondrocyte cultures: keratan sulfate and oligosaccharides which contain mannose and sialic acid. J. Biol. Chem., *255*:6,077–6,083, 1980.
7. Lohmander, L.S., et al.: Oligosaccharides on proteoglycans from the Swarm rat chondrosarcoma. J. Biol. Chem., *255*:6,084–6,091, 1980.
8. Hardingham, T.E.: The role of link-protein in the structure of cartilage proteoglycan aggregates. Biochem. J., *177*:237–247, 1979.
9. Hardingham, T.E., Ewins, R.J.F., and Muir, H.: Cartilage proteoglycans. Structure and heterogeneity of the protein core and effects of specific protein modifications on the binding and hyaluronate. Biochem. J., *157*:127–143, 1976.
10. Hardingham, T.E., and Muir, H.: The specific interaction of hyaluronic acid with cartilage proteoglycans. Biochim. Biophys. Acta, *279*:401–405, 1972.
11. Hardingham, T.E., and Muir, H.: Hyaluronic acid in cartilage. Biochem. Soc. Trans. (Dublin), *1*:282–284, 1973.
12. Hardingham, T.E., and Muir, H.: Binding of oligosaccharides of hyaluronic acid to proteoglycans. Biochem. J., *135*:905–908, 1973.
13. Hardingham, T.E., and Muir, H.: Hyaluronic acid in cartilage and proteoglycan aggregation. Biochem. J., *139*:905–908, 1973.
14. Hascall, V.C., and Heinegard, D.: Aggregation of cartilage proteoglycans. I. The role of hyaluronic acid. J. Biol. Chem., *249*:4,232–4,241, 1974.
15. Hascall, V.C., and Heinegard, D.: Aggregation of cartilage proteoglycans. II. Oligosaccharide competitors of the proteoglycan-hyaluronic acid interaction. J. Biol. Chem., *249*:4,242–4,249, 1974.
16. Hascall, V.C., and Sajdera, S.W.: Physical properties and polydispersity of proteoglycan from bovine nasal cartilage. J. Biol. Chem., *245*:4,920–4,930, 1970.
17. Hascall, V.C., and Sajdera, S.W.: Protein polysaccharide complex from bovine nasal cartilage. The function of glycoprotein in the formation of aggregates. J. Biol. Chem., *244*:2,384–2,396, 1969.
18. Heinegard, D.: Polydispersity of cartilage proteoglycans: structural variations with size and buoyant density of the molecules. J. Biol. Chem., *252*:1,980–1,989, 1977.
19. Heinegard, D.: Extraction, fractionation and characterization of proteoglycans from bovine tracheal cartilage. Biochim. Biophys. Acta, *285*:181–192, 1972.
20. Heinegard, D.: Hyaluronidase digestion and alkaline treatment of bovine tracheal cartilage proteoglycans: isolation and characterization of different keratan sulfate proteins. Biochim. Biophys. Acta, *285*:193–297, 1972.
21. Heinegard, D., and Axelsson, I.: Distribution of keratan sulfate in cartilage proteoglycans. J. Biol. Chem., *252*:1,971–1,979, 1977.
22. Heinegard, D., and Hascall, V.C.: Characterization of chondroitin sulfate isolated from trypsin-chymotrypsin digest of cartilage proteoglycans. Arch. Biochem. Biophys., *165*:427–441, 1974.
23. Heinegard, D., and Hascall, V.C.: Aggregation of cartilage proteoglycans. III. Characteristics of the proteins isolated from trypsin digests of aggregates. J. Biol. Chem., *249*:4,250–4,256, 1974.
24. Rosenberg, L.: Structure of cartilage proteoglycans. In Dynamics of Connective Tissue Macromolecules. Edited by P.M.C. Burleigh and A.R. Poole. New York, Elsevier-North Holland., 1973, pp. 105–128.
25. Rosenberg, L., et al.: A comparison of proteinpolysaccharides of bovine nasal cartilage isolated and fractionated by different methods. J. Biol. Chem., *245*:4,112–4,122, 1970.
26. Rosenberg, L., Hellman, W., and Kleinschmidt, A.: Electron microscopic studies of proteoglycan aggregates from bovine articular cartilage. J. Biol. Chem., *250*:1,877–1,883, 1975.
27. Rosenberg, L., Pal, S., and Beale, R.: Proteoglycans from bovine proximal humeral articular cartilage. J. Biol. Chem., *248*:3,681–3,690, 1973.
28. Rosenberg, L., Schubert, M., and Sandson, J.: The protein-polysaccharides of bovine nucleus pulposus. J. Biol. Chem., *242*:4,691–4,701, 1967.
29. Rosenberg, L., et al.: Proteoglycans from bovine proximal humeral articular cartilage: structural basis for the polydispersity of proteoglycan subunit. J. Biol. Chem., *251*:6,439–6,444, 1976.
30. Mason, R.M., and Mayes, R.W.: Extraction of cartilage protein-

polysaccharides with inorganic salt solutions. Biochem. J., 131:535–540, 1973.

31. Sajdera, S.W., and Hascall, V.C.: Protein polysaccharide complex from bovine nasal cartilage: a comparison of low and high shear extraction procedures. J. Biol. Chem., 244:77–87, 1969.

32. Baker, J.R., Roden L., and Stoolmiller, A.C.: Biosynthesis of chondroitin sulfate proteoglycan: xylosyl transfer to Smith-degraded proteoglycan and other exogenous acceptors. J. Biol. Chem., 247:3,838–3,847, 1972.

33. Baker, J.R., Roden, L., and Yamagata, S.: Smith-degraded cartilage proteoglycan as an acceptor for xylosyl transfer. Biochem. J., 125:93P, 1971.

34. Buckwalter, J.A., and Rosenberg, L.C.: Electron microscopic studies of cartilage proteoglycans: direct evidence for the variable length of the chondroitin sulfate-rich region of proteoglycan subunit core protein. J. Biol. Chem., 257:9,830–9,839, 1982.

35. Buckwalter, J.A., and Rosenberg, L.C.: Structural changes during development in bovine fetal epiphyseal cartilage. II. Electron microscopic studies of proteoglycan monomers and aggregates. Coll. Relat. Res., 3:489–504, 1983.

36. Tang, L.H., et al.: Proteoglycans from bovine nasal cartilage: properties of a soluble form of link protein. J. Biol. Chem., 254:10,523–10,531, 1979.

37. Faltz, L.L., et al.: Characteristics of proteoglycans extracted from the Swarm rat chondrosarcoma with associative solvents. J. Biol. Chem., 54:1,375–1,380, 1979.

38. Baker, J.R., and Caterson, B.: The isolation and characterization of the link proteins from proteoglycan aggregates of bovine nasal cartilage. J. Biol. Chem., 254:2,387–2,393, 1979.

39. Caputo, C.B., et al.: Characterization of fragments produced by clostripain digestion of proteoglycans from the Swarm rat chondrosarcoma. Arch. Biochem. Biophys., 204:220–233, 1980.

40. Fransson, L.A.: Structure of dermatan sulfate. III. The hybrid structure of dermatan sulfate from umbilical cord. J. Biol. Chem., 243:1,504–1,510, 1968.

41. Fransson, L.A.: In Chemistry and Molecular Biology of the Intercellular Matrix. Edited by E.A. Balazs. New York, Academic Press, 1970, p. 823.

42. Fransson, L.A.: Structure of dermatan sulfate. 5. Hybrid structure of dermatan sulfate from hog intestinal mucosa. Arkiv. Kemi, 29:95–99, 1968.

43. Fransson, L.A.: Structure of dermatan sulfate. IV. Glycopeptides from the carbohydrate-protein linkage region of pig skin dermatan sulfate. Biochim. Biophys. Acta, 156:311–316, 1968.

44. Fransson, L.A., and Roden, L.: Structure of dermatan sulfate I. Degradation by testicular hyaluronidase. J. Biol. Chem., 242:4,161–4,169, 1967.

45. Fransson, L.A., and Roden, L.: Structure of dermatan sulfate. II. Characterization of products obtained by hyaluronidase digestion of dermatan sulfate. J. Biol. Chem., 242:4,170–4,175, 1967.

46. Malmstrom, A., et al.: The copolymeric structure of dermatan sulphate produced by cultured human fibroblasts: different distribution of iduronic acid- and glucuronic acid-containing units in soluble and cell-associated glycans. Biochem. J., 151:477–489, 1975.

47. Meyer, K., and Chaffee, E.: Mucopolysaccharides of skin. J. Biol. Chem., 138:491–499, 1941.

48. Deiss, W.P., and Leon, A.S.: Mucopolysaccharides of heart valve; mucoprotein. J. Biol. Chem., 215:685–689, 1955.

49. Berenson, G.S.: A study of acid mucopolysaccharides of bovine aorta with the aid of a chromatographic procedure for separating sulfated mucopolysaccharides. Biochim. Biophys. Acta, 28:176–183, 1958.

50. Engel, U.R.: Glycosaminoglycans in the aorta of six animal species. A chemical and morphological comparison of their topographic distribution. Atherosclerosis, 13:45–60, 1971.

51. Kumar, V., et al.: Acid mucopolysaccharides of human aorta. 1. Variations with maturation. J. Atheroscler. Res., 7:573–581, 1967.

52. Kumar, V., et al.: Acid mucopolysaccharides of human aorta. 2. Variation with atherosclerotic involvement. J. Atheroscler. Res., 7:583–590, 1967.

53. Murata, K., Nakazawa, K., and Hamai, A.: Distribution of acidic glycosaminoglycans in the intima, media and adventitia of bovine aorta and their anticoagulant properties. Atherosclerosis, 21:93–103, 1975.

54. Wusteman, F.S.: Glycosaminoglycans of bovine lung parenchyma and pleura. Experientia, 28:887–888, 1972.

55. Murata, K.: Polydisperse distribution of acidic glycosaminoglycans in bovine kidney tissue. Connect. Tissue Res., 4:131–140, 1976.

56. Butler, W.F., and Wels, C.M.: Glycosaminoglycans of cat intervertebral disc. Biochem. J., 122:647–652, 1971.

57. Davidson, E.A., and Woodhall, B.: Biochemical alterations in herniated intervertebral discs. J. Biol. Chem., 234:2,951–2,954, 1959.

58. Lyons, H., et al.: Changes in the protein polysaccharide fractions of nucleus pulposus from human intervertebral disc with age and disc herniation. J. Lab. Clin. Med., 68:930–939, 1966.

59. Wight, T., and Ross, R.: Proteoglycans in primate arteries. I. Ultrastructural localization and distribution in the intima. J. Cell Biol., 67:660–674, 1975.

60. Wight, T., and Ross, R.: Proteoglycans in primate arteries. II. Synthesis and secretion of glycosaminoglycans by arterial smooth muscle cells in culture. J. Cell Biol., 67:675–686, 1975.

61. Bella, A., Jr., and Danishefsky, I.: The dermatan sulfate-protein linkage region. J. Biol. Chem., 243:2,660–2,664, 1968.

62. Carlstedt, I., Coster, L., and Malmstrom, A.: Isolation and characterization of dermatan sulphate and heparan sulphate proteoglycans from fibroblast cultures. Biochem. J., 197:217–225, 1981.

63. Coster, L., et al.: Self-association of dermatan sulphate proteoglycans from bovine sclera. Biochem. J., 197:483–490, 1981.

64. Coster, L., et al.: The co-polymeric structure of pig skin dermatan sulphate: distribution of L-iduronic acid sulphate residues in co-polymeric chains. Biochem. J., 145:379–389, 1975.

65. Coster, L., and Fransson, L.A.: Isolation and characterization of dermatan sulphate proteoglycans from bovine sclera. Biochem. J., 193:143–153, 1981.

66. Fransson, L.A.: Interaction between dermatan sulphate chains. I. Affinity chromatography of copolymeric galactosaminoglycans on dermatan sulfate substituted agarose. Biochim. Biophys. Acta, 437:106–115, 1976.

67. Fransson, L.A., et al.: Self-association of scleral proteodermatan sulfate side chains. J. Biol. Chem., 257:6,333–6,338, 1982.

68. Fransson, L.A., et al.: Interactions between dermatan sulfate chains. III. Light-scattering and viscometry studies of self-association. Biochem. Biophys. Acta, 586:179–188, 1979.

69. Fransson, L.A., and Coster, L.: Interaction between dermatan sulphate chain. II. Structural studies on aggregating glycan chains and oligosaccharides with affinity for dermatan sulphate-substituted agarose. Biochim. Biophys. Acta, 582:132–144, 1979.

70. Goetinck, P.F., and Pennypacker, J.P.: Controls in the acquisition and maintenance of chondrogenic expression. In Ver-

tebrate Limb and Somite Morphogenesis. Edited by I.A. Ede, J.F. Hinchliffe, and M. Balls. Cambridge, Cambridge University Press, 1977.

71. Goetinck, P.F., Pennypacker, J.P., and Royal, P.D.: Proteochondroitin sulfate synthesis and chondrogenic expression. Exp. Cell Res., 87:241–248, 1974.

72. McKeown, P.J., and Goetinck, P.F.: A comparison of the proteoglycans synthesized in Meckel's and sternal cartilage from normal and nanomelic chick embryos. Dev. Biol., 71:203–215, 1979.

73. Pennypacker, J.P., and Goetnick, P.: Biochemical and ultrastructural studies of collagen and proteoglychondroitin sulfate in normal and nanomelic cartilage. Dev. Biol., 50:35–47, 1976.

74. Royal, P.D., and Goryinck, P.F.: *In vitro* chondrogenesis in mouse limb mesenchymal cells: changes in ultrastructure and proteoglycan. J. Embryol. Exp. Morphol., 39:79–95, 1977.

75. Royal, P.D., Sparks, K.J., and Goetinck, P.F.: Physical and immunochemical characterization of proteoglycans synthesized during chondrogenesis in the chick embryo. J. Biol. Chem., 255:9,870–9,878, 1980.

76. Rosenberg, L., et al.: Isolation, characterization and immunofluorescent localization of a dermatan sulfate-containing proteoglycan from bovine fetal epiphyseal cartilage. *In* Limb Development and Regeneration, Part B. Edited by R.O. Kelley, P.F. Goetinck, and J.A. MacCabe. New York, Alan R. Liss, 1983, pp. 67–84.

REGULATION OF CONNECTIVE TISSUE METABOLISM

14

C. WILLIAM CASTOR

The several connective tissues of mammals comprise a large and metabolically active portion of the body mass; they are no longer considered an inert fabric serving merely to support and bind together the parenchymal and neural structures. Mesenchymal derivatives account for 75% of the human body mass, and collagen alone constitutes one-third of total body protein. That the family of proteoglycans and glycosaminoglycans in the connective tissue ground substance probably amounts to less than 100 g per person emphasizes the enormous importance of these hydrophilic polyanions in regulating the movement of water and solutes in the extracellular matrix and in influencing its mechanical and lubricating properties.

Embryonic mesodermal cells differentiate to form different connective tissues, including fibroelastic, reticular, adipose, and elastic connective tissue, as well as bone, cartilage, synovial membrane, and the vascular system. A "connective tissue" consists of cellular and intercellular (matrix) components; the intracellular category is subdivided into fibrillar (collagen, elastin) and ground-substance materials including glycosaminoglycans, proteoglycans, glycoproteins, water, electrolytes, and other solutes. The proportion of these constituents varies with anatomic location and functional requirements. Thus, tendon and fascia have a disproportionate fibrillar component, whereas Wharton's jelly of the umbilical cord is predominantly ground substance; a greater cellular content is found in cartilage and synovial membrane. The vascular endowment of connective tissues ranges from the relative avascularity of cartilage to the profusion of interconnecting loops of fenestrated capillaries found in synovial membrane.

Mechanical support and protection are among the important functions performed by connective tissues. Bone protects viscera from mechanical injury, preserves intricate pressure relationships necessary for the life of the organism, and serves as a lever system through which tendons and fascia transmit mechanical energy derived from muscle contraction. The smooth transmission of mechanical energy to move the organism or its parts is facilitated by lubrication from ground-substance components located in the gliding planes of tendon sheaths, bursae, and joints. Because connective tissue matrix is everywhere interposed between the vascular system and epithelial structures, it functions as an organ of transport, conveying nutrients to the periphery and returning metabolic wastes. Energy reserves in the form of neutral fat are stored in, and released from, adipose connective tissue in response to direct hormonal influence, but the role of other metabolically active constituents, such as the glycoproteins of the ground substance, is less obvious.

No summary of the general functions of connective tissue would be complete without mention of its reparative potential. When injury disrupts the anatomic continuity of an organism, connective tissue rapidly bridges the defect. The cellular components effectively neutralize or destroy noxious agents, remove debris, and produce a framework of fibers and ground substance that restores anatomic continuity and, usually functional capacity to the injured part.

CONNECTIVE TISSUE METABOLISM

An analysis of connective tissue metabolism is concerned with the chemical and physical processes in the formation of the connective tissues and their maintenance in a functional state, as well as those processes involved in their degradation and remodeling. The anabolic aspect of connective tissue formation includes the formation of new cells, fibrillar proteins, and ground-substance components; catabolic events are concerned with the degradation and removal of these materials.

A plethora of factors with potential importance for the regulation of metabolism in diverse connective tissues is now being recorded and includes a growing list of autacoids ("growth factors," protein mediators of intercellular matrix formation, complex lipids, nucleotides, peptides, and biogenic amines), in addition to hormones and vitamins. In contrast to conventional hormones, many autacoid mediators are formed within the tissue they influence and have a limited radius of action, and their operational concentrations may not be accurately reflected in the plasma.

FACTORS REGULATING BOTH CELL REPLICATION AND GLYCOSAMINOGLYCAN FORMATION

The actions of many substances with regulatory potential have been studied only in vitro and have yet to be shown important in vivo or in man. Evaluation of signal molecules important in cell-to-cell communication continues to be fraught with difficulties. Most growth-promoting "factors" begin life as one element of a complex biologic mixture, declaring their presence by some measurable action in a bioassay system. Obscuring the significance of many autacoid factors is the peculiar array of assay systems, which often feature the effect of a protein isolated from one species on a narrow range of biochemical functions of cells or tissues from yet another species. Fortunately, several autacoid factors have now been sufficiently purified to permit amino acid sequence and other structural studies. Availability of nearly homogeneous proteins has not only permitted structural studies and assignment of biologic activities to specific molecules, but also has made possible the development of immunologic and receptor-binding assays to assist in detection and measurement of these regulatory proteins. Although these techniques have their own problems, they do offer an approach to measuring growth-regulatory factors in man. Major emphasis in this section is placed on materials and mechanisms

that appear to have importance in man for the regulation of connective tissue cell proliferation and the formation and breakdown of intercellular matrix materials in both basal and perturbed states. Characteristics of several mediators that stimulate connective tissue growth are recorded in Table 14–1.

EPIDERMAL GROWTH FACTOR (UROGASTRONE)

Epidermal growth factor (EGF) was first described in the mouse submaxillary gland and was later isolated from human urine as "urogastrone."[1] Excellent reviews summarize historical aspects of the discovery, isolation, and mechanism of action of EGF.[2,3] EGF isolated from mouse submaxillary gland and human urine has been sequenced and shown to be a heat-stable acidic polypeptide chain with 53 amino acid residues and 3 intramolecular disulfide bonds. Mouse EGF is synthesized and stored in the submandibular gland, where it is found in granular form in convoluted tubules. Localization of EGF in human platelet α granules was suggested by receptor binding and radioimmunoassay studies.[4] In both man and rat, immunohistochemical methods localize EGF in renal tubular cells, the serous glands of the nasal cavity, the submandibular glands, Brunner's glands, and the Paneth cells of the small intestine.[5] Alpha-adrenergic agents have been shown to stimulate secretion of EGF from the submandibular gland in both rat and mouse.[6] In the mouse, EGF is also known to be regulated by androgens; other evidence indicates that thyroid hormones and adrenocortical hormones regulate EGF in this species.[7] In senescent mice, the submandibular glands contain decreased amounts of EGF.[8]

In vitro actions of EGF include stimulation of cell proliferation in epithelial and fibroblastic cells of many types. EGF induces increased synthesis of DNA, RNA, cyclic nucleotides, and enhanced transport of nutritional precursors. In the appropriate cell types, EGF stimulates synthesis and secretion of specialized proteins (such as prolactin or collagen) and complex carbohydrates (such as hyaluronic acid). EGF-stimulated prolactin synthesis in rat pituitary cells was thought to depend on an increased transcription rate of the prolactin gene.[9] Nanogram amounts of EGF cause selective dose-dependent synthesis of collagen fibers by epithelial cells derived from rat liver.[10] Mouse EGF has little effect on collagen formation in cultures of rat liver fibroblasts, however,[11] and EGF actually reduces collagen synthesis in mouse osteoblastic cultures.[12] These data underline

Table 14–1. Growth Factors that Stimulate Connective Tissue Cell Replication and Extracellular Matrix Synthesis

Factor	Source	Characterization Status	Molecular Weight (daltons)	Possible Clinical Significance
Epidermal growth factor (EGF)	Platelets	Sequenced	6,045	Wound healing, neurofibromatosis
Connective tissue activating peptide-III (CTAP-III)	Platelets	Sequenced	9,278	Inflammation, wound healing, atherosclerosis, neoplasia
Platelet-derived growth factor (PDGF)	Platelets	Sequenced	31,000	Inflammation, wound healing, atherosclerosis, neoplasia
Insulin-like growth factor-I (IGF-I)	Plasma	Sequenced	7,649	Leprechaunism, mediation of human growth hormone (hGH) action
Insulin-like growth factor-II (IGF-II)	Plasma	Sequenced	7,471	Mediation of hGH action
Nerve growth factor (NGF)	Uncertain in man	Active subunit sequenced	13,259	Maintenance of sympathetic nervous system, neural neoplasms, Alzheimer's disease
Interleukin-1 (IL-1)	Human monocytes	Sequenced	17,500	Mediation of immune responses, connective tissue growth, and wound healing; an endogenous pyrogen
Connective tissue activating peptide-V (CTAP-V)	Connective tissue	Partially sequenced	16,000 and 28,000	Wound healing, inflammation, neoplasia
Connective tissue activating peptide-PMN (CTAP-PMN)	Human polymorphonuclear leukocytes	Highly purified, nonhomogeneous	12,000–16,000	Wound healing, inflammation

growth factor bioassay ambiguities that may arise from the species or tissue type of the target system.

In vivo, EGF stimulates cell proliferation, keratinization, and premature eruption of incisors, inhibits gastric acid secretion, and promotes healing or corneal ulcers. Intravenous infusion of EGF into merino sheep leads to temporary cessation of follicular activity and to the appearance of an abnormal wool protein.[13] Recent studies in rabbits suggest that both systemic and oral EGF may regulate the growth and postnatal maturation of the gastrointestinal tract.[14]

Fibroblasts have specific receptors for EGF, and binding of the peptide is said to be nearly irreversible. The gene for the human EGF receptor is believed to reside on chromosome 7.[15] Binding sites for EGF in skin fibroblasts from patients with neurofibromatosis are diminished when compared with age- and passage-matched normal strains.[16] Monoclonal antibodies against the EGF receptor induce some of the effects of EGF itself, including stimulation of thymidine incorporation into DNA. This observation supports the idea that information in the EGF-membrane receptor system resides primarily in the membrane receptor itself.[17] The binding characteristics of human placental membrane EGF receptor have been characterized[18]; studies leading to solubilization and isolation of the receptor suggest an apparent molecular weight of

160,000 to 180,000 daltons.[19] EGF binding to cellular receptors is followed by phosphorylation of the receptors, internalization, and proteolytic processing in lysosomes. "Remodeled" receptor fragments may serve as intracellular signals for the multiple specific activities attributed to EGF.[20]

PLATELET FACTORS

Nondialyzable factors in monkey serum promote proliferation of monkey arterial muscle cells in vitro; dialyzed serum prepared from recalcified platelet-poor plasma is much less mitogenic. Addition of platelets and calcium to platelet-poor plasma restores mitogenic activity. Furthermore, addition of a supernatant prepared from thrombin-aggregated platelets to platelet-poor plasma also stimulates proliferation of smooth muscle cells. These observations support the conclusion that much of the growth-promoting activity of dialyzed serum derives from platelets. This finding may be important in understanding the response of arteries to localized injury and may partially explain the source of serum factors that promote cell proliferation in vitro.[21]

It is clear that human platelets contain both cationic and anionic growth factors; one laboratory reported three different forms.[22] Current interest centers on three classes of defined entities: (1) cationic proteins such as connective tissue activating peptide-III (CTAP-III); (2) several molecular forms of "platelet-derived growth factors" (PDGF); and (3) the anionic platelet-derived growth factors which include CTAP-IV, transforming growth factor-β(TGFβ), and an endothelial cell growth factor (ECGF).[23-26]

CTAP-III, a thrombin-releasable growth-promoting factor in human platelets, has been isolated and studied in detail.[27-29] Isolated from fresh or outdated human platelets, CTAP-III is a 9,278-dalton single-chain protein with a mean isoelectric point of 8.5. Amino acid sequence and immunologic studies showed CTAP-III to differ from β-thromboglobulin (β-TG) only by the addition of an amino terminal tetrapeptide.[30,31] Proteolytic removal of the amino terminal tetrapeptide degrades CTAP-III to β-TG and obliterates growth factor activity. Growth factor activity, as measured by enhanced DNA or glycosaminoglycan synthesis in human fibroblast cultures, also depends on the intact status of one or both of the two intrachain disulfide bonds. Depending on the characteristics of the preparation, nanogram to microgram quantities of CTAP-III stimulate synthesis of DNA, hyaluronic acid, sulfated glycosaminoglycan chains, proteoglycan monomer, and proteoglycan core protein in human fibroblast cultures. CTAP-III also stimulates glucose transport, formation of prostaglandin E_2 (PGE$_2$), hyaluronic acid synthetase activity, and the synthesis and secretion of plasminogen activator.

Isoelectric point-related microheterogeneity was demonstrated in CTAP-III isolated both from outdated platelets and small samples processed rapidly from single individuals.[32] These findings are partially explained by variable lysine-linked glycosylation of the growth factor. The more basic variants of CTAP-III have higher specific activity in growth factor assays. That both CTAP-III antigen and biologic activity have been found in platelets of children deficient in growth hormone indicates that CTAP-III is not human growth-hormone dependent.[33] Specific antisera directed against CTAP-III ablate its mitogenic activity. Elevated plasma levels of CTAP-III antigen have been found by immunoassay in rheumatoid arthritis, in systemic lupus erythematosus, and in progressive systemic sclerosis and other forms of vasculitis. Because plasma CTAP-III levels appear to parallel clinical disease activity, a possible pathogenetic role is suggested.[34,35]

Immunoassay of CTAP-III in human serum shows concentrations ranging from 7000 to 25,000 ng/ml; such levels stimulate DNA and glycosaminoglycans synthesis in vitro and may approach the amounts seen by connective tissue cells in the microenvironments where platelet α-granule release occurs. Although CTAP-III has been studied primarily in relation to human connective tissue cells, it is a potent agonist in vitro for mouse and rat fibroblast and epithelial cell types and even, to a limited extent, for human epithelial neoplastic cell strains.

CTAP-IV is an anionic, platelet-derived growth factor that is a potent mitogen for synovial, cartilage, lung, and skin fibroblasts in cell culture; it is also a promoter of hyaluronate and sulfated proteoglycan synthesis. Unlike CTAP-III and PDGF, CTAP-IV has an acidic pI (4.5 to 5.0) with an apparent M_r of 24,000 to 25,000 daltons.[23] Amino acid composition of the isolated CTAP-IV protein includes 2 methionine and 4 tyrosine residues per mole and marked predominance of dicarboxylic over basic amino acid residues. TGFβ from platelets and other tissues resembles CTAP-IV in molecular weight, apparent subunit composition, and overall amino acid makeup; however, the CTAP-IV amino terminal sequence is unlike TFGβ.

Data concerning preparations of PDGF have suggested a molecule with 2 disulfide-linked chains, each with a molecular weight of 14,000 to 16,000 daltons.[36] PDGF is generally believed to exist in 2 forms, PDGF-1 and II, whose molecular weights are, respectively, 31,000 and 28,000 daltons.[37] Differences in glycosylation led some workers to postulate 4 molecular forms of PDGF.[38] Sequence studies of PDGF show little resemblance to CTAP-III.[39] Of considerable interest are reports that suggest that a transforming protein from simian sarcoma virus and PDGF are so closely related that they may be derived from the same or similar genes.[40,41]

PDGF has induced tyrosine-specific phosphorylation in human fibroblast membranes,[42] and it has stimulated synthesis of as many as five species of intracellular proteins.[43] Partially purified PDGF modified lipid metabolism by enhancing cholesterol synthesis and the number of LDL receptors in monkey aortic muscle cells.[44] The action of PDGF in promoting polyamine transport in arterial smooth muscle cells may relate to its role in cell division.[45] It now appears that PDGF is capable of stimulating cell division without the need for "progression factors" in plasma.[46] Other effects of PDGF include evidence that it is chemotactic for fibroblasts and vascular smooth muscle cells.[47] A related study showed that three platelet α-granule proteins, platelet factor 4, β-TG, and PDGF, each had chemotactic activity for human skin fibroblasts.[48] By radioreceptor assay, PDGF was not detectable in human plasma and [125]Iodine-PDGF injected intravenously into baboons was cleaved, with a half-life of

2 min; this evidence suggests a role for PDGF primarily at local sites of platelet α-granule release.[49] The significance of PDGE-like molecules synthesized by several other cell types, including macrophages, is uncertain.[50]

Studies of PDGF interactions with fibroblast receptors have suggested that PDGF and EGF are not processed by a common pathway, although PDGF and its receptor also may be internalized and degraded.[51-53] Phylogenetic surveys using a radioreceptor assay indicate that a PDGF-type protein is restricted to chordate members of the animal kingdom.[54]

INSULIN-LIKE GROWTH FACTORS AND SOMATOMEDINS

Cell replication in connective tissue occurs not only in response to acute or chronic injury, but also as a maintenance process. Although it is not certain that "replacement cell replication" depends on omnipresent plasma signals, several interesting materials in plasma are known to stimulate DNA synthesis. The advent of a radioimmunoassay that specifically recognized insulin proved that only 7% of the "insulin-like activity" of serum was actually insulin (and consequently suppressible by anti-insulin serum); the remainder was originally designated as nonsuppressible insulin-like activity (NSILA). The NSILA materials are themselves growth-hormone-dependent, and in turn have growth-promoting activity in chick embryo fibroblast cultures and in several other systems. NSILA has now been resolved into 2 entities, insulin-like growth factors I and II (IGF-I, IGF-II) whose covalent structures are known.[55,56] IGF-I is a single chain containing 70 residues (7,649 daltons) with 3 disulfide bonds and marked homology with proinsulin. IGF-II is a 7,471-dalton protein with 3 intrachain disulfide bonds; it shows substantial homology with IGF-1 and with proinsulin. Radioimmunoassay and radioreceptor assays indicate that IGF-I closely resembles somatomedin C.[57] Sequence analysis now confirms their identity.[58-60]

Growth hormone affects cartilage by inducing the formation of secondary substances, *somatomedins* ("sulfation factors"), which in turn interact with chondrocytes to modify their metabolism. Somatomedins in serum stimulate $^{35}SO_4$ uptake by cartilage from rats that have undergone hypophysectomy; serum from these rats is less stimulatory than that from normal rats, and administration of growth hormone restores stimulatory activity to serum of such animals.[61] Bioassay of somatomedins in human serum discloses high levels in acromegaly and low levels after hypophy-

sectomy and in patients with pituitary dwarfism. Administration of human growth hormone (hGF) to hypophysectomized patients or pituitary dwarfs restores human somatomedin levels to the normal range. At least 3 somatomedins (A, B, C) are present in human plasma. Somatomedin A isolated from human plasma was reported to have a molecular weight of approximately 7,000 daltons, with asparagine at its N-terminus. Somatomedin A stimulates incorporation of $^{35}SO_4$ into glycosaminoglycans in chick cartilage and DNA synthesis in both chick embryo and human fibroblasts.[62] IGF-I, IGF-II, and insulin induce marked "membrane ruffling" in KB cells, an effect thought to reflect rapid reorganization of the microfilament components of cytoskeletal structures.[63] Both insulin and IGF-I act through their own receptors; in rat hepatoma cells, metabolic responses to IGF-II were shown to be mediated by the insulin receptors.[64]

IGF-I and II are equally potent in stimulating DNA synthesis in chick embryonic tissue and $^{35}SO_4$ uptake in rat costal cartilage.[65] Both IGF species enhance mitosis in rabbit lens epithelial cells.[66] IGF stimulates 2-deoxyglucose uptake in skeletal muscle, fat, and heart cells, presumably not acting through the insulin receptor. Although IGF is 50 to 100 times more potent than insulin on growth parameters, it is ony one-sixtieth as potent as insulin with respect to 2-deoxyglucose uptake by fat cells.[67]

Skin fibroblasts have been shown by radioimmunoassay to secrete material resembling somatomedin C. Secretion is blocked by cycloheximide and stimulated by hGH, PDGF, and fibroblast growth factors (FGF), but not by EGF, thyroxine, or cortisol.[68]

Radioimmunoassay of IGF-I and II shows IGF-I levels to be elevated in acromegaly and depressed in hGH deficiency. Oversecretion of IGF-II in acromegaly is not seen; however, the low values in hGH deficiency support the idea that both factors are growth-hormone dependent. Extra pancreatic tumors associated with hypoglycemia are not associated with increased levels of IGF-I and II.[69]

Leprechaunism, a syndrome characterized by growth retardation, poor muscle development, and absence of fat, may result from deficiency of IGF activity. Some patients with this syndrome are reported to be deficient in cellular receptors for IGF-1.[70]

NERVE GROWTH FACTOR

Nerve growth factor (NGF) is present in many tissues, but is found in unusually high concentrations in some snake venoms and in the male mouse submaxillary gland.[71] It elicits overgrowth of sympathetic chain ganglia in vivo, generates a halo-like outgrowth of nerve fibers from embryonic sympathetic ganglia cultured in vitro, and is believed to be important in the regulation of neural cell growth and differentiation. NGF regulates the survival of peripheral sympathetic and spinal sensory neurons.

NGF isolated from the mouse submaxillary gland is a hexameric 140,000-dalton protein complex composed of α, β, and γ subunits. The α subunit subserves a regulatory function, the γ subunit is an arginine esteropeptidase, and the biologic activity resides in the β subunit.[72] The β subunit of NGF (BNGF) has been sequenced, and has a primary peptide with a molecular weight of 13,259 daltons that associates in 2 subunits with a molecular weight of 26,518 daltons. BNGF has 3 disulfide bonds with many acidic residues present in amide form, accounting for its basic nature. The biologic activity of BNGF is inhibited in the hexameric complex, which in turn protects the active components from proteolysis.

Antibodies to NGF cause total destruction of the sympathetic nervous system. NGF may be viewed as a protein hormone that exerts positive pleiotropic stimulation on developing nerve tissue and is required in small amounts to maintain the mature sympathetic nervous system. NGF activity immunologically identical to that of submaxillary glands has been found in blood and other peripheral organs.

The lack of data confirming the presence of NGF in human tissues is puzzling. One review emphasizes the possible role of NGF in neoplasms, including sarcoma, neuroblastoma, and gliomas.[73] Human melanoma cells in culture have been shown by indirect immunofluorescence to possess surface NGF; NGF receptors were thought to be present on the basis of both immunofluorescence and ^{125}I-NGF binding.[74] Highly purified receptor for NGF has also been prepared from membranes of a human melanoma cell line by affinity chromatography.[75] NGF has been shown to shorten the duration of action potential of dorsal root ganglia perikarya, mediated by an inward calcium ion current.[76] Such NGF regulation of calcium-dependent action potentials may provide a mechanism for altering the excitability of not only dorsal root ganglia perikarya, but also their associated terminals. In rats with electrolytic lesions of the medial septum, injection of NGF into the hippocampus actually impaired behavioral recovery.[77] Chromaffin cells exposed to NGF show an increased transport capacity for adenosine and a reduction in the transporter affinity for this purine.[78] The similarity of the physiologic deficits in Alzheimer's disease and the functions subserved by NGF has led to speculation that Alzheimer's disease may be caused either by a deficiency of NGF or by decreased responsiveness of cholinergic neurons to NGF.[79]

INTERLEUKIN 1

Interleukin I (IL-1), the first well-defined human "monokine," was originally known as lymphocyte activating factor (LAF). This potent thymocyte mitogen has been identified as an endogenous pyrogen and likely is an important mediator of inflammation in man.[80,81] IL-1 is secreted by activated macrophages of both man and mouse; synthesis of IL-1 also may be initiated by a cell-contact-dependent process involving activated lymphocytes and promoted by endotoxins and phagocytosis. IL-1 stimulates helper T-cell release of IL-2, a T-cell growth factor. IL-1 not only has a role in promoting T-cell proliferation, but also modifies in vitro immune responses and induces PGE_2 and collagenase synthesis and secretion by human synovial cells.[82-84] Both the murine and human forms of IL-1 have been purified to homogeneity, and the amino acid sequences have been deduced from the nucleotide sequence of their genes.[85-88] The mouse protein is active at concentrations of 10^{-11} to 10^{-10} M; it may be secreted as a 33,000-dalton molecule and subsequently enzymatically converted to a 17,500-dalton form. Two distinct human genes encoding proteins with IL-1 activity have been sequenced; the proteins IL-1α (pI = 5.0) and IL-lβ (pI = 7.0) exhibit distant homology but possess similar biologic activity. The 2 IL-1 proteins have similar affinity for a common class of receptors.[89] Recent work indicates that IL-1 stimulates DNA synthesis in normal human connective tissue cells and promotes formation of important extracellular matrix components, including glycosaminoglycans, but collagen synthesis by human dermal fibroblasts is suppressed.[90]

FIBROBLAST GROWTH FACTOR

Protein fractions from bovine brain and pituitary gland are "fibroblast growth factors" (FGF) in the sense that they stimulate DNA synthesis in one or more tissue culture systems, including mouse fibroblasts, chick myoblasts, and ovarian cell strains. At least one form is present as a contaminant of preparations of bovine thyroid-stimulating and luteinizing hormones and stimulates DNA synthesis in rabbit chondrocytes.

Both the basic FGF (bFGF) from bovine pituitary and acidic FGF (aFGF) from bovine brain have now been sequenced.[91,92] These substances are 53% homologous; both are potent mitogens for many cell types, including capillary endothelial and vascular smooth muscle cells. The FGF and IL-1 cytokines are approximately 25% homologous.

Although receptor-mediated hydrolysis of polyphosphoinositides is a commonly accepted pathway for transmembrane signaling for many agents, it apparently is not operative in the case of FGF because the FGF-induced rise in cytoplasmic free calcium (Ca^{2+}) is entirely dependent on the presence of extracellular Ca^{2+}, and protein kinase C is not activated by FGF.[93] Experiments in which FGF was used to treat the amputated limb stumps of adult frogs suggest that the peptide is active on parenchymal cells in vivo.[94] Both the acidic and basic forms of FGF have induced the growth of nontransformed cell lines in soft agar, a finding interpreted as supporting the notion that FGF plays a significant role in the in vivo growth of some types of tumors.[95]

ANGIOGENIC FACTORS

Regulation of angiogenesis in normal embryonic and adult tissues is an understudied subject. Information concerning the control of vascular proliferation in neoplasia indicates that a tumor angiogenesis factor (TAF) from some tumor cells diffuses over distances of 2 to 5 mm, causing migration of host capillaries to vascularize clusters of neoplastic cells. Extracts of lymph nodes and other tissues occasionally show traces of TAF activity. Early purification studies suggested that the molecular weight of the angiogenesis-promoting substance is approximately 100,000 daltons.[96] Partially purified TAF bioassayed on chick chorioallantoic membrane (CAM) stimulates new vessel formation with minimal evidence of lymphocyte accumulation. TAF increases cell growth of capillary, but not aortic, endothelial cells grown on a collagen substrate.[97]

Recently, a substance termed "angiogenin" was isolated from a serum-free medium that had supported the growth of an established human colonic adenocarcinoma cell strain.[98] Nanogram amounts of this small (M.W.~14,400 daltons) single-chain cationic (Ip>9.5) protein have stimulated angiogenesis in the CAM and rabbit corneal assays. Amino acid sequence determination showed the molecule to consist of 123 amino acids with 3 disulfide bonds; angiogenin was surprisingly homologous to pancreatic ribonuclease.[99]

Human platelets are also thought to contain endothelial cell growth factors (ENDO-GF); these materials have apparent molecular weights of 65,000 and 135,000 daltons, are heat labile, and are more active in stimulating DNA synthesis in endothelial cells than in fibroblasts.[25] Other researchers have reported platelet-derived proteins that stimulate proliferation of vascular endothelium (VEPF); although a 60,000-dalton species has been detected, the major bioactive protein has an apparent molecular weight of 20,000 daltons with an isoelectric point between 4.0 and 4.8. Like ENDO-GF, VEPF is heat labile and has greater mitogenic activity against endothelial cells than normal rat kidney fibroblasts.[26]

An *endothelial cell growth factor* (ECGF) isolated from bovine hypothalamus stimulates proliferation of quiescent populations of human umbilical vein endothelial cells.[100] ECGF is anionic and is found in high (70,000-dalton) and low (20,000- to 25,000-dalton) molecular-weight forms. This material stimulates DNA synthesis in mouse fibroblasts and human umbilical vein endothelial cells at 10 and 100 ng/ml, respectively. ECGF has a structural affinity for heparin, a glycosaminoglycan known to potentiate the biologic activity of this mitogen.[101] A recent review notes that most polypeptides mitogenic for endothelial cells bind to heparin.[102] These include cationic pituitary FGF, acidic brain FGF, basic brain FGF, brain endothelial cell growth factor (ECGF), retina-derived growth factor (RDGF), eye-derived growth factor (EDGF), and cartilage-derived growth factor (CDGF). Many of these entities appear to be closely related; their effects include not only mitogenesis, but also chemotaxis, protease induction, and lymphokine formation.

Tumor-induced angiogenesis can be inhibited by a diffusible factor present in cartilage.[103] Heat inactivation of cartilage destroys the antiangiogenesis activity of this notably avascular tissue. A cationic protease isolated from cartilage is believed to act by inhibiting the abilty of endothelial cells to penetrate and to vascularize cartilage. Such factors may be influential in the resistance of some tissues to invasion by blood vessels, reparative processes, and neoplasms.[104]

NEWLY DESCRIBED FACTORS

Transforming growth factors (TGF) are acidic, heat-stable proteins secreted by certain human tumor cell lines in culture that confer a transformed phenotype on untransformed fibroblasts.[105] Binding assays suggest that some TGFα are related to EGF. Some are potentiated by EGF. Production of TGFα by transformed cells and the response of normal cells to TGFα raise the possibility that cells may release factors that then bind to their own cell surface, thus stimulating their own growth.[106]

TGFβ has been found in human platelets, kidney, placenta, and tumors. It is a homodimer with an M_r of 25,000 daltons that binds to a receptor distinct from the EGF receptor. The amino acid sequence of TGFβ determined by protein sequencing and cDNA cloning shows this agonist to consist of 112 amino acids.[107] Important biologic actions attributed to TGFβ include stimulation of fibronectin and collagen synthesis and enhanced chemotactic migration of fibroblasts.[108] CDGF has been purified by heparin affinity chromatography; the isolated protein has an M_r of 19,000 daltons, and growth-factor activity was determined by tritiated thymidine incorporation in 3T3 cells.[109] This cationic protein also stimulates proliferation of chondrocytes and endothelial cells and synthesis of collagen and hyaluronic acid.[110,111]

CTAP-PMN is a human granulocyte-derived factor that stimulates DNA and glycosaminoglycan synthesis by human fibroblasts; it is heat stable, sensitive to thiols, and has a molecular weight between 12,700 and 15,700 daltons. Such a factor may play a role in chronic proliferative synovitis or in other settings where exudative inflammation is accompanied by connective tissue growth.[112]

CTAP-V is a growth factor in the urine of normal individuals that stimulates monolayer cultures of human synovial, cartilage, and dermal fibroblasts to synthesize incremental amounts of hyaluronic acid, proteoglycans, and DNA.[113,114] Immunohistochemical and immunobinding studies have detected the protein in normal human synovial, dermal, and cartilage fibroblasts and in endothelial cells. CTAP-V is a monomeric anionic polypeptide with 2 molecular size forms (M_r 28,000 and 16,000 daltons). Immunodiffusion or dot-blot analyses showed a CTAP-V-like material in the plasma or serum of 10 mammalian species including man; it was undetectable in 2 avian species. S-carboxymethylation or removal of sialic acid residues have failed to modify CTAP-V biologic activity. Rabbit antibodies raised against each of the purified CTAP-V proteins react with both antigens and neutralize their mitogenic activity. That amino-terminal amino acid sequence studies of the CTAP-V proteins were identical further confirms their structural similarity. The carbohydrate content of 28,000-and 16,000 dalton CTAP-V is 27 and 25% respectively, differing by additional N-acetylglucosamine and neuraminic acid residues present in the 28,000-dalton form. CTAP-V does not cross-react in a radioreceptor assay for insulin, basic somatomedin, or EGF-urogastrone. No homology exists with any known sequenced protein, including those proposed for both IL-1 forms.

CTAP-V may have significance in relation to autocrine mechanisms for growth regulation of conective tissue cells.

FACTORS REGULATING GLYCOSAMINOGLYCAN FORMATION

Structural characteristics of complex glycosaminoglycans are determined by the specificity of glycosyl transferases that in turn are determined by structural genes. Processes essential for synthesis of glycosaminoglycans include: (1) synthesis of sugar nucleotide precursors, (2) formation of sugar nucleotide transferases, and (3) synthesis of a specific protein core that can be appropriately xylosylated. Clearly, one may interfere with glycosaminoglycan synthesis at many levels. For example, selective inhibition of proteoglycan core protein formation with 5-bromodeoxyuridine reduces the synthesis of chondroitin sulfate.[115]

Molecular mechanisms directing the qualitative and quantitative makeup of ground substance glycosaminoglycans are poorly understood at best. Factors modifying the function of uridine diphosphate (UDP)-glucose dehydrogenase and UDP-glucose 4'-epimerase may play a significant role because in circumstances where the dehydrogenase shows greater affinity for UDP-glucose than the competing epimerase enzyme, chondroitin sulfate synthesis would be favored over keratan sulfate.[116] Similarly, UDP-xylose, an inhibitor of UDP-glucose dehydrogenase activity, does not inhibit UDP-glucose 4'-epimerase activity; thus, the concentration of UDP-xylose could direct UDP-glucose toward the synthesis of either chondroitin sulfate or keratan sulfate.

HORMONES AND VITAMINS

Knowledge of hormonal regulation of glycosaminoglycan metabolism is fragmentary, but the evidence indicates that normal levels of synthesis of these substances are supported by *insulin* and depressed by *glucocorticoids*. On the other hand, excess *thyroid hormone* modifies the milieu by retarding synthesis of sulfated glycosaminoglycans and increasing the rate of hyaluronate degradation. *Triiodothyronine* at physiologic concentration, has inhibited formation of glycosaminoglycans, primarily hyaluronic acid, by human skin fibroblasts.[117] *Parathyroid hormone* stimulates rodent bone in organ culture to form increased amounts of hyaluronate and to release calcium.[118] This effect has been seen with nanogram amounts of hormone and has been blocked by even smaller amounts of calcitonin. A direct relationship between the increased formation of hyaluronate and the removal of calcium during parathormone induced bone resorption is not clearly established.

In human synovial cultures, high medium concentrations of *ascorbic acid* result in accumulation of increased amounts of hyaluronic acid.[119] Guinea pigs, given large doses of ascorbic acid, develop minor increases in aortic sulfated glycosaminoglycans and hepatic aminotransferase activity.[120] *Retinoic acid*, a natural metabolite of vitamin A, inhibits sulfate fixation into glycosaminoglycan by chondrocytes in vitro at 10^{-9} M.[121] This is not a general phenomenon, however, because the relative proportion of N-sulfated glycosaminoglycan (heparan or heparin) increases as chondroitin-4 sulfate decreases.

PROSTAGLANDINS AND CYCLIC NUCLEOTIDES

Prostaglandins, particularly those of the E series, stimulate the formation of hyaluronic acid both in vitro and in vivo at pharmacologic concentrations; however, physiologic concentrations of prostaglandins potentiate glycosaminoglycan synthesis induced by CTAP-I and III.[122] In addition, E series prostaglandins stimulate incorporation of $^{35}SO_4^=$ into glycosaminoglycans synthesized by human dermal fibroblasts in cell culture. *Cyclic 3'5'adenosine monophosphate* (cAMP) in pharmacologic concentrations also enhances glycosaminoglycan synthesis, particularly hyaluronic acid, by human synovial and dermal fibroblasts; in lesser concentrations, cAMP potentiates the actions of CTAP-I and III.[123] Exposure of 3T3 mouse fibroblasts and their SV40 transformed counterparts to pharmacologic concentrations of cAMP modestly increases synthesis and secretion of chondroitin-4/6 sulfate, as well as dermatan sulfate.[124] These actions of cAMP may represent specific examples of cyclic nucleotide regulation of differentiated cell function.

PROTEIN FACTORS

CTAP-I from human lymphocytes is a low-molecular-weight protein (approximately 11,000 daltons) characterized by an essential sulfhydryl residue and low aromatic amino acid content.[125] Although CTAP-I is released by human lymphocytes in cultures, the process is not mediated by conventional lymphocyte mitogens. Major effects of CTAP-I on cultured synovial cells include release of E series prostaglandins into the medium, delayed accumulation of intracellular cAMP and, subsequently, accelerated glycolysis and glycosaminoglycan synthesis by activated synovial cells. Synovial cells are stimulated by CTAP-I to increase hyaluronate synthesis 4- to 50-fold; 2 to 4 times as much sulfated glycosaminoglycan is formed. Augmented hyaluronate synthesis by synovial cells in response to CTAP-I requires synthesis of RNA and protein, but not DNA. One can visualize how CTAP-I might enhance differentiated functions of connective tissue cells during perturbed states such as inflammation, but it is uncertain whether it has an important effect on the basal synthesis of connective tissue glycosaminoglycans. *CTAP-II* isolated from cultures of human laryngeal carcinoma cells is similar to CTAP-I in its isolation characteristics, electrophoretic mobility, and molecular weight, but it is much different in amino acid composition.[27] This peptide also has a biologically essential sulfhydryl residue and, like CTAP-I, the tumor-cell factor stimulates glycolysis and glycosaminoglycan synthesis by human synovial cells. CTAP-II may be an example of a tumor-related factor responsible for the generation of a connective tissue matrix suitable for an expanding tumor cell mass.

REGULATION OF COLLAGEN METABOLISM

Formation of the several known types of mature collagen fibrils is a multistep process, and many loci in the pathway are sensitive to regulatory action. Intracellular events leading to the formation of the collagen molecule include: (1) synthesis of mRNA specific for collagen; (2) formation of polyribosomal clusters; (3) association of polyribosomes and endoplasmic reticulum; (4) formation of an alignment segment of the polypeptide chains (registration peptide); (5) hydroxylation of specific proline and lysine residues; (6) glycosylation of selected hydroxylysine residues; and (7) conversion of procollagen to collagen by the action of procollagen peptidase and extrusion of tropocollagen into the extracellular milieu.[126]

Extracellular events include: (1) formation of peptide-bound aldehydes at specific lysine and hydroxylysine residues; (2) formation of intramolecular cross-links by an aldol condensation reaction; (3) formation of intermolecular cross-links peptide-bound aldehydes and unmodified amino groups of lysine or hydroxylysine residues as Schiff bases; and (4) aggregation of collagen fibers in the extracellular matrix to reflect specific structural characteristics in a given tissue.[126]

STIMULATION OF COLLAGEN FORMATION BY LOW-MOLECULAR-WEIGHT AGENTS

A notable gap in our understanding of connective tissue metabolism concerns *factors responsible for initiating or terminating collagen synthesis* in response to specific biologic requirements. A useful review has covered circumstances that modulate and regulate collagen synthesis in vitro, including cell density, aging, ascorbate, cell-to-cell interaction, and serum factors.[127] Although it is well known that *molecular oxygen, ferrous iron, α-ketoglutarate,* and *ascorbic acid* are required for collagen synthesis in man, little evidence suggests that these factors play a major regulatory role, except in deficiency states. *Ascorbic acid* promotes aggregation of ribosomes in the endoplasmic reticulum to facilitate collagen synthesis. Hydroxylation of lysine and proline in vivo can be inhibited by ascorbic acid deficiency or by chelation of ferrous iron by agents such as α,α'-dipyridyl. Human synovial cells incubated with pharmacologic concentrations of ascorbic acid form increased amounts of both soluble and fibrillar collagen.[119] Embryonic human lung fibroblasts depend on ascorbic acid for full hydroxylation of collagen, but not for maximal rate of synthesis.[128] Excess *vitamin A* modestly stimulates collagen accumulation[128] and may reverse the retarding effect of glucocorticoids on collagen formation. Although lysosomal labilizing compounds such as vitamin A, digitonin, testosterone, and papain are reported to stimulate collagen synthesis and repair, vitamin E reduces tensile strength and collagen accumulation in healing wounds and does not alter glucocorticoid inhibition of this process.[129]

Collagen synthesis is selectively increased by *bleomycin* in human fetal lung fibroblast cultures; prolyhydroxylase activity is also increased, as are collagen degradation processes.[130] *Uroporphyrin I* also stimulates collagen biosynthesis in human skin fibroblast cultures,[131] whereas modest increments of collagen are seen in sponge granulation tissue incubated with serotonin, bradykinin, histamine, and vasopressin.[132] Similarly, modest stimulation of proline and lysine hydroxylation occurs following exposure of chick embryo tissue to high concentrations of PGE_1 and $F_{1\alpha}$.[133] Collagen accumulation in female rat skin is promoted by estradiol, which apparently retards degradation rather than stimulating synthesis.[134]

PROTEIN FACTORS PROMOTING COLLAGEN ACCUMULATION

Although autacoid mediators may play a role in regulating collagen metabolism, few have been described, and none have been chemically characterized. "Lymphokine"-rich supernates (possibly IL-1) generated by phytohemagglutinin stimulation of human blood mononuclear cells modestly enhance collagen accumulation by WI-38 embryonic lung fibroblasts.[135] *Lymphokines* from human lymphocytes have been shown to stimulate synovial cell proliferation in culture as well as collagen synthesis, effects that are enhanced if the lymphocytes are lectin-activated.[136]

A *coupling factor* thought to mediate coupling of bone formation to bone resorption has been described.[137] This protein, extracted from human bone matrix, has been substantially purified and shown to stimulate bone growth by assays measuring bone cell DNA synthesis and incorporation of labeled proline into collagen. Coupling factor apparently is released during the course of bone resorption. It increases the growth rate of embryonic bone in culture and apparently is specific for bone and cartilage, but does not affect skin, kidney, muscle, or liver. Another *bone-derived growth factor* (BDGF) has been isolated from the conditioned medium used to nourish the calvaria of 21-day fetal rats. Two forms are found, one with a molecular weight of approximately 20,000 to 30,000 daltons, the other with a molecular weight between 6,000 and 13,000 daltons. Both fractions stimulate DNA, RNA, and proteoglycan synthesis in rabbit chondrocyte cultures. Others have shown that protein extracted from rat bone stimulates proliferation of both human and rat fibroblasts.[138]

TGFβ from human platelets stimulates collagen formation by human fibroblasts, an effect that appears to be antagonized by EGF.[24]

A *basic protein* secreted by rat macrophages stimulates formation of soluble collagen by rat fibroblasts in a cellulose sponge granuloma while depressing the formation of noncollagen proteins.[139] In experiments with fetal rat calvaria, *insulin* stimulates formation of type I collagen, an activity not shared with parathyroid hormone (PTH), EGF, or 1,25-dihydroxyvitamin D_3.[140]

AGENTS DEPRESSING COLLAGEN SYNTHESIS

Because collagen synthesis may require a membrane-bound mRNA-ribosome complex, it is possible that any agent that modifies membrane integrity may depress collagen biosynthesis. Cutaneous application of adrenal *glucocorticoids* decreases the thickness of rat dermis and its collagen content.[141] Direct suppression of collagen accumulation by hydrocortisone has also been shown in human fibroblast cultures.[119] Pharmacologic concentrations of natural and synthetic glucocorticoids inhibit incorporation of ^{14}C-proline into nondialyzable hydroxyproline in short-term tissue-slice experiments.[142] In mechanically damaged aortic tissue, prednisone modifies the repair process and especially inhibits the biosynthesis of collagen.[143] In uninjured aortic tissue, prednisone acts mainly antianabolically on the metabolism of collagen, as part of a general inhibition of protein synthesis.[144] Depression of collagen biosynthesis by adrenocortical hormones may reflect changes in the mRNA-tRNA complex because steroids cause a reduction in the amount of particulate RNA.

PTH-treated cultures of fetal rat calvaria show slow reversible inhibition of bone collagen synthesis, which is not opposed by calcitonin, an effect that may be mediated by cAMP.[145] This phenomenon may be specific for bone collagen because one sees little change in noncollagen protein or cartilage collagen. Both *osteoclast-activating factor* (OAF) from human lymphocytes and PTH inhibit collagen synthesis in fetal rat calvaria at concentrations that stimulate bone resorption. OAF-stimulated bone resorption is effectively inhibited by cortisol.[146] Because OAF, PTH, and PGE$_2$ are potential mediators of neoplastic and inflammatory bone loss, their interactions have been studied. The biologic actions of these agents are additive only at low concentrations. Human peripheral blood mononuclear cells, particularly B lymphocytes, may release soluble factors that preferentially inhibit collagen synthesis by normal human dermal fibroblasts.[147]

Lysyl oxidase activity is inhibited by β-amino proprionitrile, ethylenediamine tetra-acetic acid (EDTA), isonicotinic acid hydrazide, and D-penicillamine. Low doses of penicillamine act primarily by blocking aldehyde residues; higher levels are required to affect the activity of lysyl oxidase. The consequences of acutely inhibiting lysyl oxidase in healing wounds have been noted in rats treated by β-aminoproprionitrile, where transient lysyl oxidase inhibition in metabolically active wounds is associated with reduced wound strength.[148]

Chelating agents alter the incorporation and hydroxylation of proline and lysine, and the glycosylation of hydroxylysine.[149] For example, α,α'-dipyridyl and 8-hydroxyquinoline inhibit hydroxylation of proline and lysine as well as glycosylation of lysine derivatives, but EDTA, chlorpromazine, tetracycline,

hydralyzine, and procainamide inhibit hydroxylation and glycosylation in excess of their effect on the incorporation of ^{14}C-proline and ^{14}C-lysine. Penicillamine-type drugs affect incorporation of proline and lysine only at high concentrations. In a related vein, zinc deficiency may reduce collagen biosynthesis and depress the cross-linking process.[150]

PHYSICAL FACTORS REGULATING CONNECTIVE TISSUE METABOLISM

Clinicians have long known that *temperature* affects the musculoskeletal system, providing relief from pain and reducing stiffness and resistance to motion in articulation and fascial planes. Although the molecular basis for these effects is not understood, increased temperature reduces resistance to flow of viscous hyaluronate solutions, and collagen also undergoes temperature-related changes in physical state. Mammalian collagenase is four times as active at the higher temperatures within rheumatoid knee joints (36° C) than at normal joint temperature (33° C).[151] In a similar vein, small increases in joint temperature are associated with a marked increase in the responsiveness of synovial cells to CTAP-I-induced acceleration of glycolysis and hyaluronate formation.[152] *Shortwave diathermy*, a heat-inducing technique, increases uptake of ^{35}SO$_4$ and glycosaminoglycan concentration in rabbit articular tissues.[153] *Ionizing radiation* directed at normal and rheumatoid synovial cells in vitro stimulates hyaluronate formation and glucose use, an effect that requires both RNA and protein synthesis and is inhibited by hydrocortisone.[154]

Mechanical factors may influence organization of the extracellular matrix and the metabolic activity of the resident cells. The collagen fibers themselves may act as electrochemical transducers, transmitting information (force) to initiate changes in cellular metabolism important to the maintenance of the appropriate glycosaminoglycans and collagen matrix. Release of the normal *distractive forces* from rabbit Achilles tendons by tenotomy has resulted in increased accumulation of a glycosaminoglycan thought to be hyaluronic acid. The type and proportion of proteoglycan in *tension-* and *pressure*-bearing segments of rabbit tendons relate directly to the functional needs of the tissue.[120] Tendon segments subjected to substantial tension show thick collagen fibers of high tensional strength associated with a small amount of dermatan sulfate. Pressure-bearing segments contain chondroitin-4/6 sulfate with its greater water inclusion properties. Continuous mechanical pressure applied to cartilage appears to reduce both proteoglycan synthesis and breakdown. Further evidence for the importance of the *mechanical stimulation* to cell metabolism comes from in vitro experiments in which arterial smooth muscle cells were subjected either to stretching stimuli or to agitation without stretching. Repeated stretching and relaxation of rabbit aortic medial cells stimulate the synthesis of types I and III collagen, hyaluronate, and chondroitin-6 sulfate, but do not affect the rate of synthesis of chondroitin-4 sulfate or dermatan sulfate.[155]

ELECTRICAL FIELD EFFECTS

Current interest in electrical-field stimulation of fracture healing stems from work on piezoelectric effects in bone.[156] The known tissue interactions with nonionizing electromagnetic fields have been carefully reviewed.[157] Methods of applying electric current in the management of nonunited fractures include constant direct current, pulsing direct current, alternating current, and induced current; these techniques are introduced to patients by either invasive or noninvasive methods.[158] Most reports indicate that the various modes of electrical stimulation result in healing of 65 to 75% of fractures classified as nonunions.

Studies of mechanisms in electrical modulation of bone healing have focused attention on the idea that mechanically induced electrical polarization of biologic systems, resulting from the deformation of crystalline biopolymers (as collagen), may have major physiologic importance. An important observation was the demonstration that cartilage is electrically polarized on mechanical deformation with generation of electric potentials ranging from 0.5 to 2.0 mV. The joint face of articular cartilage becomes positively charged in a cyclical fashion in the face of intermittent loading.[159] Cells subjected to electrical fields in vitro show increased *protein synthesis* as well as *sulfate uptake* into presumptive glycosaminoglycans.[160] In addition, mouse fibroblasts subjected to an interrupted DC field show modest stimulation of DNA and collagen synthesis.[161] Other studies show that DNA synthesis in cartilage cells may be stimulated by oscillating electric fields, an effect said not to occur with skin fibroblasts.[162] Verapamil or tetrodotoxin blocks this electrical field effect, supporting the hypothesis that altered sodium (Na^+) and Ca^{2+} fluxes are important in triggering DNA synthesis in these cells. Epiphyseal cartilage shows changes in cAMP produced by electrical and mechanical perturbation. In an animal model of disuse osteoporosis, pulsed electromagnetic fields increased the rate of synthesis of proteoglycan

and collagen and diminished bone resorption.[163] In another study, electromagnetic fields inhibited bone cell responsiveness to parathyroid hormone in vitro.[164]

The accumulated data suggest that mechanical and electrical coupling in living organisms, at least in selected tissues, results in polarization of cells and other tissue components, with subsequent alterations in ion fluxes and cell membrane function. These translate into biologic responses important to growth, repair, and remodeling of tissues.

FACTORS RELATED TO CONNECTIVE TISSUE MATRIX DEGRADATION

Rheumatoid synovial tissue incubated in vitro elaborates collagenase as free enzyme or trypsin-releasable proenzyme. Collagenase secreted by synovial cells may complex with native collagen fibrils at physiologic temperatures and may subsequently be activated by plasmin generated from plasminogen by a plasminogen activator. Synthesis of both latent collagenase and plasminogen activator by synovial cells in inhibited by as little as 10^{-9} M dexamethasone or by larger amounts of other glucocorticoids, whereas progesterone has no inhibitory effect.[165] Indomethacin increases collagenase synthesis in cell culture while inhibiting the formation of PGE_2. Thus, it is unlikely that PGE_2 is a required antecedent of collagenase synthesis.[166] Collagenase production has been stimulated in macrophages by endotoxin and by lymphocyte products,[167,168] in tadpole explants by cAMP, and in bone cell cultures by heparin.[169] IL-1 derived from macrophages appears to be important in activating connective tissue cells and in causing enhanced collagenase synthesis and secretion in disease states.[36]

Because the action of mammalian collagenase on bone presupposes previous demineralization of the matrix, the action of agents promoting calcium loss is of considerable importance. Prostaglandin stimulation of bone resorption is greatest with PGE_2. Stimulation increases linearly over a range of 10^{-9} M through 10^{-3} M, when measured by release of ^{45}calcium from prelabeled fetal bone. The flat dose-response curve of PGE_2 differentiates it from other bone-resorption agents such as PTH, vitamin D_3, and OAF, all of which show steeper dose-response curves and cause more rapid bone resorption than do prostaglandins. The mechanism of action of prostaglandins in this phenomenon is not well understood.[170] Evidence suggests that rheumatoid synovial tissue in organ culture synthesizes primarily PGE_2 and $PGF_{2\alpha}$; it is possible that the PGE_2 produced by rheumatoid synovium may contribute to the tissue destruction of juxta-articular bone in rheumatoid arthritis.[171]

CTAP-III, a chemically defined factor, is known to stimulate synthesis and secretion of plasminogen activator by human synovial cells in culture.[172] Factors in the medium from lectin-stimulated human monocytes also stimulate plasminogen activator synthesis and secretion by human synovial fibrolast cultures.[173]

CONCLUSION

The foregoing summary hardly suggests that connective tissue metabolism is regulated by a dominant central control mechanism. Rather, connective tissue cells function as a community of diverse interacting cell types exerting a high degree of mutual local control over neighboring cells. In perturbed states, as in injury, those metabolic phenomena with survival value stand out, and their major thrust is repair. Metabolic functions of cells during the repair process are genetically programmed activities largely regulated by autacoid mediators, feedback control mechanisms, and environmental factors converging on the cell to yield an appropriate metabolic response. The polypeptide effector substances of connective tissue may be analogous to peptides such as the endorphins, which act in the local endocrine control of nervous system function. In the era ahead, present tentative speculations about roles of "growth factors" and their receptors in disease processes are likely to gel, become organized, and provide new avenues on which to approach refractory biologic problems, including those characterized by degenerative and inflammatory change in connective tissue, such as the various forms of arthritis.

REFERENCES

1. Gregory, H., and Preston, B.M.: The primary structure of human urogastrone. Int. J. Pept. Protein Res., 9:107–118, 1977.
2. Cohen, S.: The epidermal growth factor (EGF). Cancer, 51:1787–1791, 1983.
3. Hollenberg, M.D.: Epidermal growth factor—urogastrone, a polypeptide acquiring hormonal status. Vitam. Horm., 37:69–110, 1979.
4. Oka, Y., and Orth, D.N.: Human plasma epidermal growth factor/β-urogastrone is associated with blood platelets. J. Clin. Invest., 72:249–259, 1983.
5. Poulsen, S.S., et al.: Immunohistochemical localization of epidermal growth factor in rat and man. Histochemistry, 85:389–394, 1986.
6. Olsen, P.S., Kirkegaard, P., Poulsen, S.S., and Nexo, E.: Adrenergic effects on exocrine secretion of rat submandibular epidermal growth factor. Gut, 25:1234–1240, 1984.
7. Gresik, E.W., et al.: Hormonal regulation of epidermal growth factor and protease in the submandibular gland of the adult mouse. Endocrinology, 109:924–929, 1981.
8. Gresik, E.W., Brennan, M., and Azmitia, E.: Age-related changes in EGF and protease in submandibular glands of C57BL/6J Mice. Exp. Aging Res., 8:87–90, 1982.
9. Murdoch, G.H., et al.: Epidermal growth factor rapidly stimulates prolactin gene transcription. Nature, 300:192–194, 1982.
10. Kumegawa, M., et al.: Epidermal growth factor stimulates collagen synthesis in liver-derived epithelial clone cells. Biochim. Biophys. Acta, 675:305–308, 1983.
11. Kumegawa, M., et al.: Effect of epidermal growth factor on collagen formation in liver-derived epithelial clone cells. Endocrinology, 110:607–612, 1982.
12. Hiramatsu, M., et al.: Effect of epidermal growth factor on collagen synthesis in osteoblastic cells derived from newborn mouse calvaria. Endocrinology, 111:1810–1816, 1982.
13. Gillespie, J.M., et al: Changes in the proteins of wool following treatment of sheep with epidermal growth factor. J. Invest. Dermatol., 79:197–200, 1982.
14. O'Loughlin, E.V, et al.: Effect of epidermal growth factor on ontogeny of the gastrointestinal tract. Am. J. Physiol., 249:G674–G678, 1985.
15. Davies, R.L., et al.: Genetic analysis of epidermal growth factor action: assignment of human epidermal growth factor receptor gene to chromosome 7. Proc. Natl. Acad. Sci. U.S.A., 77:4188–4192, 1980.
16. Zelkowitz, M.: Neurofibromatosis fibroblasts: abnormal growth and binding to epidermal growth factor. Adv. Neurol., 29:173–188, 1981.
17. Schreiber, A.B., et al.: Monoclonal antibodies against receptor for epidermal growth factor induce early and delayed effects of epidermal growth factor. Proc. Natl. Acad. Sci. U.S.A., 78:7535–7539, 1981.
18. Hock, R.A., and Hollenberg, N.D.: Characterization of the receptor for epidermal growth factor-urogastrone in human placenta membranes. J. Biol. Chem., 255:10,731–10,736, 1980.
19. Hock, R.A., Nexo, E., and Hollenberg, M.D.: Solubilization and isolation of the human placenta receptor for epidermal growth factor-urogastrone. J. Biol. Chem., 255:10,737–10,743, 1980.
20. Fox, C.F., Linsley, P.S., and Wrann, M.: Receptor remodeling and regulation in the action of epidermal growth factor. Fed. Proc., 41:2988–2995, 1982.
21. Ross, R., et al.: A platelet-dependent serum factor that stimulates the proliferation of arterial smooth muscle cells in vitro. Proc. Natl. Acad. Sci. U.S.A., 71:1207–1210, 1974.
22. Heldin, C.H., Wasteson, A., and Westermark, B.: Partial purification and characterization of platelet factors stimulating the multiplication of normal human glial cells. Exp. Cell Res., 109:429–437, 1977.
23. Castor, C.W., et al.: Growth factors as mediators of extracellular matrix synthesis and degradation in man. In Protides of the Biological Fluids. Vol. 34. Edited by H. Peters. Oxford, Pergamon Press, 1986, pp. 247–250.
24. Roberts, A.B., et al.: Transforming growth factor type β: rapid induction of fibrosis and angiogenesis in vivo and stimulation of collagen formation in vitro. Proc. Natl. Acad. Sci. U.S.A., 83:4167–4171, 1986.
25. King, G.L., and Buchwald, S.: Characterization and partial purification of an endothelial cell growth factor from human platelets. J. Clin. Invest., 73:392–396, 1984.
26. Miyazono, KI., et al.: A platelet factor stimulating the prolif-

eration of vascular endothelial cells. Exp. Cell Res., 159:487–494, 1985.

27. Castor, C.W., et al.: Connective tissue activation. XIV. Composition and actions of a human platelet autacoid mediator. Arthritis Rheum., 22:260–272, 1979.
28. Castor, C.W., et al.: Connective tissue activation. XI. Stimulation of glycosaminoglycan and DNA formation by a platelet factor. Arthritis Rheum., 20:859–868, 1977.
29. Castor, C.W., et al.: Connective tissue activation: stimulation of DNA and glycosaminoglycan synthesis by a platelet factor. (Abstract.) Arthritis Rheum., 20:110, 1977.
30. Begg, G.S., et al.: Complete covalent structure of human beta-thromboglobulin. Biochemistry, 17:1739–1744, 1978.
31. Castor, C.W., Miller, J.W., and Waltz, D.A.: Structural and biological characteristics of connective tissue activating peptide (CTAP-III), a major human platelet-derived growth factor. Proc. Natl. Acad. Sci. U.S.A., 80:765–769, 1983.
32. Green, M.S. Hossler, P.A., and Castor, C.W.: Connective tissue activation. XXX. Isoelectric point microheterogeneity of CTAP-III, a human platelet derived growth factor. Proc. Soc. Exp. Biol. Med., 181:555–559, 1986.
33. Castor, C.W., et al.: Connective tissue activating peptide-III. XXII. A platelet growth factor in human growth hormone deficient patients. J. Clin. Endocrinol. Metab., 52:128–132, 1981.
34. MacCarter, D.K., Hossler, P.A., and Castor, C.W.: Connective tissue activation. XXIII. Increased plasma levels of a platelet growth factor (CTAP-III) in patients with rheumatic diseases. Clin. Chim. Acta, 115:125–134, 1981.
35. Myers, S.L., Hossler, P.A., and Castor, C.W.: Connective tissue activation. XIX. Plasma levels of the CTAP-III platelet antigen in rheumatoid arthritis. J. Rheumatol., 7:814–819, 1980.
36. Johnsson, A., et al.: Platelet-derived growth factor: identification of constituent polypeptide chains. Biochem. Biophys. Res. Commun., 104:66–74, 1982.
37. Deuel, T.F., et al.: Human platelet-derived growth factor. Purification and resolution into two active protein fractions. J. Biol. Chem., 256:8896–8899, 1981.
38. Raines, E.W., and Ross, R.: Platelet-derived growth factor: high yield purification and evidence for multiple forms. J. Biol. Chem., 257:5154–5160, 1982.
39. Antoniades, H.N., and Hunkapillar, M.W.: Human platelet-derived growth factor (PDGF): amino-terminal amino acid sequence. Science, 220:963–965, 1983.
40. Doolittle, R.F., et al.: Simian sarcoma virus onc gene, v-sis, is derived from the gene (or genes) encoding a platelet-derived growth factor. Science, 221:275–276, 1983.
41. Waterfield, M.D., et al.: Platelet derived growth factor is structurally related to the putative transforming protein P[28sis] of simian sarcoma virus. Nature, 304:35–39, 1983.
42. Ek, B., and Heldin, C.H.: Characterization of a tyrosine-specific kinase activity in human fibroblast membranes stimulated by platelet-derived growth factor. J. Biol. Chem., 257:10,486–10,492, 1982.
43. Pledger, W.J., et al.: Platelet-derived growth factor-modulated proteins: constitutive synthesis by a transformed cell line. Proc. Natl. Acad. Sci. U.S.A., 78:4358–4362, 1981.
44. Chait, A., et al.: Platelet-derived growth factor stimulates activity of low density lipoprotein receptors. Proc. Natl. Acad. Sci. U.S.A., 77:4084–4088, 1980.
45. Subbaiah, P.V., and Bagdale, J.D.: Polyamines and atherosclerosis: platelet releasate and other mitogens stimulate pu-

46. Heldin, C.H., Wasteson, A., and Westermark, B.: Growth of normal human glial cells in a defined medium containing platelet-derived growth factor. Proc. Natl. Acad. Sci. U.S.A., 77:6611–6615, 1980.
47. Grotendorst, G.R., et al.: Platelet-derived growth factor in chemoattractant for vascular smooth muscle cells. J. Cell. Physiol., 113:261–266, 1982.
48. Senior, R.M., et al.: Chemotactic activity of platelet alpha granule proteins for fibroblasts. J. Cell Biol., 96:382–385, 1983.
49. Bowen-Pope, D.F., Malpass, T.W., Foster, D.M., and Ross, R.: Platelet-derived growth factor in vivo: levels, activity, and rate of clearance. Blood, 64:458–469, 1984.
50. Shimakado, K., et al.: A significant part of macrophage-derived growth factor consists of at least two forms of PDGF. Cell, 43:277–286, 1985.
51. Bowen-Pope, D.F., and Ross, R.: Platelet-derived growth factor: specific binding to cultured cells. J. Biol. Chem., 257:5161–5171, 1982.
52. Heldin, C.H., Wasteson, A., and Westermark, B.: Interaction of platelet-derived growth factor with its fibroblast receptor. J. Biol. Chem., 257:4216–4221, 1982.
53. Huang, J.S., et al.: Platelet-derived growth factor: specific binding to target cells. J. Biol. Chem., 257:8130–8136, 1982.
54. Singh, J.P., Chaikin, M.A., and Stiles, C.D.: Phylogenetic analysis of platelet-derived growth factor by radioreceptor assay. J. Cell Biol., 95:667–671, 1982.
55. Rinderknecht, E., and Humbel, R.E.: The amino acid sequence of human insulin-like growth factor I and its structural homology with proinsulin. J. Biol. Chem., 253:2769–2776, 1978.
56. Rinderknecht, E., and Humbel, R.E.: Primary structure of human insulin-like growth factor II. FEBS Lett., 89:283–286, 1978.
57. Van Wyk, J.J., Svoboda, M.E., and Underwood, L.E.: Evidence from radio-ligand assays that somatomedin-C and insulin-like growth factor-I are similar to each other or different from other somatomedins. J. Clin. Endocrinol. Metab., 50:206–208, 1980.
58. Bala, R.M., and Bhaumick, B.: Purification of a basic somatomedin, from human plasma Cohn fraction IV-1, with physiochemical and radioimmuno-assay similarity to somatomedin-C and insulin-like growth factor. Can. J. Biochem., 57:1289–1298, 1979.
59. Klapper, D.G., Svoboda, M.E., and Van Wyk, J.J.: Sequence analysis of somatomedin-C: confirmation of identity with insulin-like growth factor I. Endocrinology, 112:2215–2217, 1983.
60. Svoboda, M.E., et al.: Purifcation of somatomedin-C from human plasma: chemical and biological properties, partial sequence analysis, and relationship to other somatomedins. Biochemistry, 19:790–797, 1980.
61. Salmon, W.D., Jr., and Daughaday, W.H.: A hormonally controlled serum factor which stimulates sulfate incorporation by cartilage in vitro. J. Lab. Clin. Med., 49:825–836, 1957.
62. Rechler, M.M., et al.: Purified human somatomedin A and rat multiplication stimulating activity: mitogens for cultured fibroblasts that cross-react with the same growth peptide receptors. Eur. J. Biochem., 82:5–12, 1978.
63. Kadowaki, T., et al.: Insulin-like growth factors, insulin, and epidermal growth factor cause rapid cytoskeletal reorganization in KB cells. J. Biol. Chem., 261:16,141–16,147, 1986.
64. Krett, N.L., Heaton, J.H., and Gelehrter, T.D.: Mediation of

insulin-like growth factor actions by the insulin receptor in H-35 rat hepatoma cells. Endocrinology, 120:401–408, 1987.

65. Zapf, J., Schoenle, E., and Froesch, E.R.: Insulin-like growth factors I and II: some biological actions and receptor binding characteristics of two purified constituents of nonsuppressible insulin-like activity of human serum. Eur. J. Biochem., 87:285–296, 1978.

66. Reddan, J.R., and Dziedzic, D.C.: Insulin-like growth factors, IGF-1, IGF-2 and somatomedin C trigger cell proliferation in mammalian epithelial cells cultured in a serum-free medium. Exp. Cell Res., 142:293–300, 1982.

67. Poggi, C., et al.: Effects and binding of insulin-like growth factor I in the isolated soleus muscle of lean and obese mice: comparison with insulin. Endocrinology, 105:723–730, 1979.

68. Clemmons, D.R., Underwood, L.E., and Van Wyk, J.J.: Hormonal control of immunoreactive somatomedin production by cultured human fibroblasts. J. Clin. Invest., 67:10–19, 1981.

69. Zapf, J., Walter, H., and Froesch, E.R.: Radioimmunological determination of insulin-like growth factors I and II in normal subjects and in patients with growth disorders and extrapancreatic tumor hypoglycemia. J. Clin. Invest., 68:1321–1330, 1981.

70. Van Obberghen-Schilling, E.E., et al.: Receptors for insulin-like growth factor I are defective in fibroblasts cultured from a patient with leprechaunism. J. Clin. Invest., 68:1356–1365, 1981.

71. Angeletti, R.H., and Bradshaw, R.A.: Nerve growth factor from mouse submaxillary gland: amino acid sequence. Proc. Natl. Acad. Sci. U.S.A., 68:2417–2420, 1971.

72. Harper, G.P., and Thoenen, H.: Nerve growth factor: biological significance, measurement, and distribution. J. Neurochem., 34:5–16, 1980.

73. Vinores, S.A., and Perez-Polo, J.R.: Nerve growth factor and neural oncology. J Neurosci. Res., 9:81–100, 1983.

74. Sherwin, S.A., Sliski, A.H., and Todaro, G.J.: Human melanoma cells have both nerve growth factor and nerve growth factor-specific receptors on their cell surfaces. Proc. Natl. Acad. Sci. U.S.A., 76:1288–1292, 1979.

75. Puma, P., et al.: Purification of the receptor for nerve growth factor from A875 melanoma cells by affinity chromatography. J. Biol. Chem., 258:3370–3375, 1983.

76. Chalazonitis, A., Peterson, E.R., and Crain, S.M.: Nerve growth factor regulates the action potential duration of mature sensory neurons. Proc. Natl. Acad. Sci. U.S.A., 84:289–293, 1987.

77. Pallage, V., Toniolo, G., Will, B., and Hefti, F.: Long-term effects of nerve growth factor and neural transplants on behavior of rats with medial septal lesions. Brain Res., 386:197–208, 1986.

78. Torres, M., Bader, M.F., Aunis, D., and Miras-Portugal, M.T.: Nerve growth factor effect on adenosine transport in cultured chromaffin cells. J. Neurochem., 48:233–235, 1987.

79. Hefti, F.: Is Alzheimer disease caused by lack of nerve growth factor? Ann. Neurol., 13:109–110, 1983.

80. Gery, I., Gershon, R.K., and Waksman, B.H.: Potentiation of the T-lymphocyte response to mitogens. I. The responding cell. J. Exp. Med., 136:128–142, 1972.

81. Lachman, L.B.: Human interleukin 1: purification and properties. Fed. Proc., 42:121–127, 1983.

82. Mizel, S.B. et al.: Stimulation of rheumatoid synovial cell collagenase and prostaglandin production by partially purified lymphocyte-activating factor (interleukin 1). Proc. Natl. Acad. Sci. U.S.A., 78:2474–2477, 1981.

83. Oppenheim, J.J., and Gery, I.: Interleukin 1 is more than an interleukin. Immunol. Today, 3:113–119, 1982.

84. Postlethwaite, A.E., et al.: Interleukin 1 stimulation of collagenase production by cultured fibroblasts. J. Exp. Med., 157:801–806, 1983.

85. Mizel, S.B., and Mizel, D.: Purification to apparent homogeneity of murine interleukin 1. J. Immunol., 126:834–837, 1981.

86. Schmidt, J.A.: Purification and partial biochemical characterization of normal human interleukin 1. J. Exp. Med., 160:772–787, 1984.

87. Lomedica, P.T., et al.: Cloning and expression of murine interleukin-1 cDNA in Escherichia coli. Nature, 312:458–462, 1984.

88. March, C.J., et al.: Cloning, sequence and expression of two distinct human interleukin-1 complementary DNAs. Nature, 315:641–647, 1985.

89. Bird, T.A., and Saklatvala, J.: Identification of a common class of high affinity receptors for both types of porcine interleukin-1 on connective tissue cells. Nature, 324:263–266, 1986.

90. Bhatnagar, R., et al.: Interleukin-1 inhibits the synthesis of collagen by fibroblasts. Biochem. Int., 13:709–720, 1986.

91. Esch, F., et al.: Primary structure of bovine pituitary basic fibroblast growth factor (FGF) and comparison with the amino-terminal sequence of bovine brain acidic FGF. Proc. Natl. Acad. Sci. U.S.A., 82:6507–6511, 1985.

92. Esch, F., et al.: Primary structure of bovine brain acidic fibroblast growth factor (FGF). Biochem. Biophys. Res. Commun., 133:554–562, 1985.

93. Magnaldo, I., et al.: The mitogenic signaling pathway of fibroblast growth factor is not mediated through polyphosphoinositide hydrolysis and protein kinase C activation in hamster fibroblasts. J. Biol. Chem., 261:16,916–16,922, 1986.

94. Gospodarowicz, D., et al.: Fibroblast growth factor: its localization, purification, mode of action, and physiological significance. In Advances in Metabolic Disorders. Vol. 8. Edited by R. Luft and K. Hall. New York, Academic Press, 1975, pp. 301–335.

95. Rizzino, A., and Ruff, E.: Fibroblast growth factor induces the soft agar growth of two non-transformed cell lines. In Vitro Cell. Dev. Biol., 22:749–755, 1986.

96. Folkman, J., and Cotran, R.: Relation of vascular proliferation to tumor growth. Int. Rev. Exp. Pathol., 16:207–248, 1976.

97. Keegan, A., et al.: Purified tumour angiogenesis factor enhances proliferation of capillary, but not aortic, endothelial cells in vitro. J. Cell Sci., 55:261–276, 1982.

98. Fett, J.W., et al.: Isolation and characterization of angiogenin, an angiogenic protein from human carcinoma cells. Biochemistry, 24:5480–5486, 1985.

99. Strydom, D.J., et al.: Amino acid sequence of human tumor derived angiogenin. Biochemistry, 24:5486–5494, 1985.

100. Maciag, T., Hoover, G.A., and Weinstein, R.: High and low molecular weight forms of endothelial cell growth factor. J. Biol. Chem., 257:5333–5336, 1982.

101. Maciag, T., Mehlman, T., and Friesel, R.: Heparin binds endothelial cell growth factor, the principal endothelial cell mitogen in bovine brain. Science, 225:932–935, 1984.

102. Lobb, R.R., Harper, J.W., and Fett, J.W.: Purification of heparin-binding growth factors. Anal. Biochem., 154:1–14, 1986.

103. Brem, H., Arensman, R., and Folkman, J.: Inhibition of tumor angiogenesis by a diffusible factor from cartilage. In Extracellular Matrix Influences on Gene Expression. Edited by H.C. Slavkin and R.C. Greulich. New York, Academic Press, 1975, pp. 767–772.

104. Kuettner, K.E., et al.: Regulation of epiphyseal cartilage maturation. *In* Extracellular Matrix Influences on Gene Expression. Edited by H.C. Slavkin and R.C. Greulich. New York, Academic Press, 1975, pp. 435–440.

105. Todaro, G.J., Fryling, C., and DeLarco, J.E.: Transforming growth factors produced by certain human tumor cells: polypeptides that interact with epidermal growth factor receptors. Proc. Natl. Acad. Sci. U.S.A., 77:5258–5262, 1980.

106. Todaro, G.J., et al.: Transforming growth factors (TGFs): properties and possible mechanisms of action. J. Supramol. Struct., 15:287–301, 1981.

107. Derynck, R., et al.: Human transforming growth factor-β complementary DNA sequence and expression in normal and transformed cells. Nature, 316:701–705, 1985.

108. Postlethwaite, A.E., Keski-Oja, J., Moses, H.S., and Kang, A.H.: Stimulation of the chemotactic migration of human fibroblasts by transforming growth factor β. J. Exp. Med., 165:251–256, 1987.

109. Sullivan, R., and Klagsbrun, M.: Purification of cartilage-derived growth factor by heparin affinity chromatography. J. Biol. Chem., 260:2399–2403, 1985.

110. Davidson, J.M., et al.: Accelerated wound repair, cell proliferation, and collagen accumulation are produced by a cartilage-derived growth factor. J. Cell Biol., 100:1219–1227, 1985.

111. Hammerman, D., Sasse, J., and Klagsbrun, M.: A cartilage-derived growth factor enhances hyaluronate synthesis and diminishes sulfated glycosaminoglycan synthesis in chondrocytes. J. Cell. Physiol., 127:317–322, 1986.

112. Myers, S.L., and Castor, C.W.: Connective tissue activation. XV. Stimulation of glycosaminoglycan and DNA synthesis by a polymorphonuclear leucocyte factor. Arthritis Rheum., 23:556–563, 1980.

113. Cabral, A.R., and Castor, C.W.: Connective tissue activation. XXXI. Identification of two molecular forms of a mesenchymal cell-derived growth factor, connective tissue activating peptide-V (CTAP-V). Arthritis Rheum., 30:1382–1392, 1987.

114. Cabral, A.R., Cole, L.A., Walz, D.A., and Castor, C.W.: Connective tissue activation. XXXII. Structural and biological characteristics of mesenchymal-derived connective tissue activating peptide-V (CTAP-V). Arthritis Rheum., 30:1393–1400, 1987.

115. Dorfman, A.: Adventures in viscous solutions. Mol. Cell. Biochem., 4:45–74, 1974.

116. DeLuca, G., Rindi, S., and Speziale, P.: Proceedings: regulatory mechanisms of glycosaminoglycan biosynthesis at the level of nucleotide-sugars precursors. Ital. J. Biochem., 25:179–181, 1976.

117. Smith, T.J., et al.: Regulation of glycosaminoglycan synthesis by thyroid hormone *in vitro*. J. Clin. Invest., 70:1066–1073, 1982.

118. Luben, R.A., and Cohn, D.V.: Effects of parathormone and calcitonin on citrate and hyalurate metabolism in cultured bone. Endocrinology, 98:413–419, 1976.

119. Castor, C.W.: Regulation of collagen and hyaluronate formation in human synovial fibroblast cultures. J. Lab. Clin. Med., 75:798–810, 1970.

120. Gillard, G.C., et al.: The proteoglycan content and the axial periodicity of collagen in tendon. Biochem. J., 163:145–151, 1977.

121. Shapiro, S.S., and Poon, J.P.: Effect of retinoic acid on chondrocyte glycosaminoglycan biosynthesis. Arch. Biochem. Biophys., 174:74–81, 1976.

122. Castor, C.W.: Connective tissue activation. VII. Evidence supporting a role for prostaglandin and cyclic nucleotides. J. Lab Clin. Med., 85:392–404, 1975.

123. Castor, C.W.: Connective tissue activation. VI. The effects of cyclic nucleotides on human synovial cells *in vitro*. J. Lab. Clin. Med., 83:46–66, 1974.

124. Goggins, J.F., Johnson, G.S., and Pastan, I.: The effect of dibutyryl cyclic adenosine monophosphate on synthesis of sulfated acid mucopolysaccharides by transformed fibroblasts. J. Biol. Chem., 247:5759–5764, 1972.

125. Castor, C.W.: Synovial cell activation induced by a polypeptide mediator. Ann. N.Y. Acad. Sci., 256:304–317, 1975.

126. Nimni, M.E.: Collagen: its structure and function in normal and pathological connective tissues. Semin. Arthritis Rheum., 4:95–150, 1974.

127. Muller, P.K., et al.: Some aspects of the modulations and regulation of collagen synthesis *in vitro*. Mol. Cell. Biochem., 34:73–85, 1981.

128. Paz, M.A., and Gallop, P.M.: Collagen synthesized and modified by aging fibroblasts in culture. In Vitro, 11:302–312, 1975.

129. Ehrlich, H.P., Tarver, H., and Hunt, T.K.: Inhibitory effects of vitamin E on collagen synthesis and wound repair. Ann. Surg., 175:235–240, 1972.

130. Sterling, K.M., Jr., et al.: Bleomycin-induced increase of collagen turnover in IMR-90 fibroblasts: an *in vitro* model of connective tissue restructuring during lung fibrosis. Cancer Res., 42:3502–3506, 1982.

131. Varigos, G., Schiltz, J.R., and Bickers, D.R.: Uroporphyrin I stimulation of collagen biosynthesis in human skin fibroblasts. J. Clin. Invest., 69:129–135, 1982.

132. Aalto, M., and Kulonen, E.: Effects of serotonin, indomethacin and other antirheumatic drugs on the synthesis of collagen and other proteins in granulation tissue slices. Biochem. Pharmacol., 21:2835–2840, 1972.

133. Blumenkrantz, N., and Sondergaard, J.: Effect of prostaglandin E1 and F1 on biosynthesis of collagen. Nature (New Biol.), 239:246, 1972.

134. Skosey, J.L., and Damgaard, E.: Effect of estradiol benzoate on the degradation of insoluble collagen of rat skin. Endocrinology, 93:311–315, 1973.

135. Johnson, R.L., and Ziff, M.: Lymphokine stimulation of collagen accumulation. J. Clin. Invest., 58:240–252, 1976.

136. Parrott, D.P., et al.: The effect of lymphokines on proliferation and collagen synthesis of cultured human synovial cells. Eur. J. Clin. Invest., 12:407–415, 1982.

137. Farley, J.R., and Baylink, D.J.: Isolation and partial purification of a putative coupling factor from human bone. Trans. Assoc. Am. Physicians, 94:80–87, 1981.

138. Sampath, T.K., DeSimone, D.P., and Reddi, A.H.: Extracellular bone matrix-derived growth factor. Exp. Cell Res., 142:460–464, 1982.

139. Jalkanen, M., and Penttinen, R.: Enhanced fibroblast collagen production by a macrophage-derived factor (CEMF). Biochem. Biophys. Res. Commun., 108:447–453, 1982.

140. Canalis, E.: Effect of hormones and growth factors on alkaline phosphatase activity and collagen synthesis in cultured rat calvariae. Metabolism, 32:14–20, 1983.

141. Castor, C.W., and Baker, B.L.: The local action of adrenocortical steroids on epidermis and connective tissue of the skin. Endocrinology, 47:234–241, 1950.

142. Uitto, J., Teir, H., and Mustakallio, K.K.: Corticosteroid-induced inhibition of the biosynthesis of human skin collagen. Biochem. Pharmacol., 21:2161–2167, 1972.

143. Manthorpe, R., Garbasch, C., and Lorenzen, I.: Glucocorticoid effect on repair processes in vascular connective tissue:

morphological examination and biochemical studies on collagen RNA and DNA in rabbit aorta. Acta Endocrinol., *80*:380–397, 1975.

144. Manthorpe, R., et al.: Effects of glucocorticoid on connective tissue of aorta and skin in rabbits: biochemical studies on collagen, glycosaminoglycans, DNA and RNA. Acta Endocrinol., *77*:310–324, 1974.

145. Dietrich, J.W., et al.: Hormonal control of bone collagen synthesis *in vitro:* effects of parathyroid hormone and calcitonin. Endocrinology, *98*:943–949, 1976.

146. Raisz, I.G., et al.: Effect of osteoclast activating factor from human leukocytes on bone metabolism. J. Clin. Invest., *56*:408–413, 1975.

147. McArthur, W., et al.: Immune modulation of connective tissue functions: studies on the production of collagen synthesis inhibitory factor by populations of human peripheral blood mononuclear cells. Cell. Immunol., *74*:126–139, 1982.

148. Arem, A.J., et al.: Effect of lysyl oxidase inhibition on healing wounds. Surg. Forum, *26*:67–69, 1975.

149. Blumenkrantz, N., and Asboe-Hansen, G.: Effect of chelating agents on the biosynthesis of collagen. Acta Derm. Venereol. (Stockh.), *53*:94–98, 1973.

150. McClain, P.E., et al.: Influence of zinc deficiency on synthesis and cross-linking of rat skin collagen. Biochim. Biophys. Acta, *304*:457–465, 1973.

151. Harris, E.D., Jr., and McCroskery, P.A.: The influence of temperature and fibril stability on degradation of cartilage collagen by rheumatoid synovial collagenase. N. Engl. J. Med., *290*:1–6, 1974.

152. Castor, C.W., and Yaron, M.: Connective tissue activation. VIII. The effects of temperature studies *in vitro*. Arch. Phys. Med. Rehabil., *57*:5–9, 1976.

153. Vanharanta, H., Eronen, I., and Videman, T.: Shortwave diathermy effects on ^{35}S-sulfate uptake and glycosaminoglycan concentration in rabbit knee tissue. Arch. Phys. Med. Rehabil., *63*:25–28, 1982.

154. Yaron, M., et al.: Hyaluronic acid production by irradiated human synovial fibroblasts. Arthritis Rheum., *20*:702–708, 1977.

155. Leung, D.Y., Glagov, S., and Mathews, M.B.: Cyclic stretching stimulates synthesis of matrix components by arterial smooth muscle cells *in vitro*. Science, *191*:475–477, 1976.

156. Fukada, F., and Yasuda, I.: On the piezoeffect of bone. J. Physiol. Soc. Jpn., *12*:1158, 1957.

157. Adey, W.R.: Tissue interactions with nonionizing electromagnetic fields. Physiol. Rev., *62*:435–514, 1981.

158. Lechner, F., Ascherl, R., and Uraus, W.: Treatment of pseudarthroses with electrodynamic potentials of low frequency range. Clin. Orthop., *161*:71–81, 1981.

159. Bassett, C.A.L., and Pawluk, R.J.: Electrical behavior of cartilage during loading. Science, *178*:982–983, 1972.

160. Transactions of the First Annual Meeting of the Bioelectrical Repair and Growth Society. Vol. I. Philadelphia, 1981.

161. Baserga, R., and Sasaki, T.: Protein synthesis in the prereplicative phase of isoproterenol-stimulated DNA synthesis. J. Cell Biol., *39*:9a, 1968.

162. Rodan, G.A., Bourret, L.A., and Norton, L.A.: DNA synthesis in cartilage cells is stimulated by oscillating electric fields. Science, *199*:690–692, 1978.

163. Cruess, R.L., Kan, K., and Bassett, C.A.L.: The effect of pulsing electromagnetic fields on bone metabolism in experimental disuse osteoporosis. Clin. Orthop., *173*:245–250, 1983.

164. Luben, R.A., et al.: Effects of electromagnetic stimuli on bone and bone cells *in vitro:* inhibition of responses to parathyroid hormone by low-energy low-frequency fields. Proc. Natl. Acad. Sci. U.S.A., *79*:4180–4184, 1982.

165. Werb, Z., et al.: Endogenous activation of latent collagenase by rheumatoid synovial cells: evidence for a role of plasminogen activator. N. Engl. J. Med., *296*:1017–1023, 1977.

166. Dayer, J.M., et al.: Production of collagenase and prostaglandins by isolated adherent rheumatoid synovial cells. Proc. Natl. Acad. Sci. U.S.A., *73*:945–949, 1976.

167. Wahl, L.M., et al.: Collagenase production by lymphokine-activated macrophages. Science, *187*:261–263, 1975.

168. Wahl, L.M., et al.: Collagenase production by endotoxin-activated macrophages. Proc. Natl. Acad. Sci. U.S.A., *71*:3598–3601, 1974.

169. Harris, E.D., Jr.: Recent insights into the pathogenesis of the proliferative lesion in rheumatoid arthritis. Arthritis Rheum., *19*:68–72, 1976.

170. Dietrich, J.W., Goodson, J.M., and Raisz, L.G.: Stimulation of bone resorption by various prostaglandins in organ culture. Prostaglandins, *10*:231–240, 1975.

171. Robinson, D.R., et al.: Prostaglandin synthesis by rheumatoid synovium and its stimulation of colchicine. Prostaglandins, *10*:67–85, 1975.

172. Ragsdale, C.G., et al.: Connective tissue activation: stimulation of plasminogen activator by CTAP-III. Arthritis Rheum., *25*:S100, 1982.

173. Hamilton, J.A., and Slywka, J.: Stimulation of human synovial fibroblast plasminogen activator production by mononuclear cell supernatants. J. Immunol., *126*:851–855, 1981.

15

STRUCTURE AND FUNCTION OF SYNOVIOCYTES

ROBERT I. FOX, MARTIN LOTZ, and DENNIS A. CARSON

The synovial membrane is the thin layer of tissue that lines the inner surfaces of joints, bursae, and tendon sheaths, with the exception of hyaline cartilage. The synoviocyte layer is located between the joint cavity and underlying fibroblasts or adipose tissue (the subsynovium) and is normally one to three cells thick (Fig. 15–1A). In arthritic joints, the precise identification of the synovial cell layer is difficult because of its increased thickness, the lack of a basement membrane demarcating it, and the often imperceptible blending of synovial cell layer into the subsynovium (see Fig. 15–1B,C). The cellular composition of the synovial layer is heterogeneous in normal and disease states, consisting of fibroblastoid, macrophage-like, and dendritic cells.

The synovial fibroblasts help form and modify the synovial fluid and extracellular matrix. Compared with typical connective tissue fibroblasts, the synovial fibroblasts have more secretory granules, and probably synthesize more hyaluronic acid and less collagen. The synovial macrophages keep the joint fluid free of debris by phagocytosing and degrading particulate material. The synovial dendritic cells may assist in this latter function by releasing collagenase into the joint fluid. No single property distinguishes the synovial lining macrophages from other connective tissue histiocytes.[1]

Changes in the structure and function of the synovial lining cells associated with repeated trauma, infection, metabolic imbalance, or deposition of immune complexes may contribute to the development of degenerative and inflammatory joint disease. For these reasons, an adequate comprehension of the specialized properties of synoviocytes is a major goal of rheumatologic research, although progress in this area has been hampered. It is difficult to obtain a pure cell population from a heterogeneous synovial lining only a few cells thick. Moreover, isolated synoviocytes seldom maintain a stable, differentiated phenotype during repeated passages in vitro. Indeed, if synoviocytes represent the reversible adaptation of connective tissue macrophages and fibroblasts to the particular environment of the joint, experiments with long-term cell lines may have limited applicability. Instead, the elucidation of properties that truly differentiate synovial lining cells from other fibroblasts and tissue histiocytes may depend on histochemical analyses conducted with short-term, nondividing, explant cultures.

Wherever possible, this chapter emphasizes those aspects of cell structure, metabolism, and function that distinguish the synovial lining cells from the other types.

STRUCTURE OF THE NORMAL SYNOVIAL MEMBRANE

On gross inspection, the normal human synovial membrane is smooth and shiny. Its minute folds, or microvilli, can be seen easily under a light microscope. The folds permit the expansion of the synovial membrane in response to joint movement or changes in intra-articular pressure.

273

FIG. 15–1. Histology of the synovial membrane in normal and rheumatoid arthritis joints. *A,* The normal synovial lining layer is one to three cells thick. The subsynovial tissue consists of fibrocytes, blood vessels, and a few histiocytes, all between collagen bundles. *B,* A biopsy of rheumatoid arthritis synovial membrane has hyperplasia and lymphocytic infiltration. *C,* A synovial biopsy from a different rheumatoid arthritis patient shows thickening of the synovial membrane associated with fibroblastic proliferation, but with few infiltrating lymphocytes.

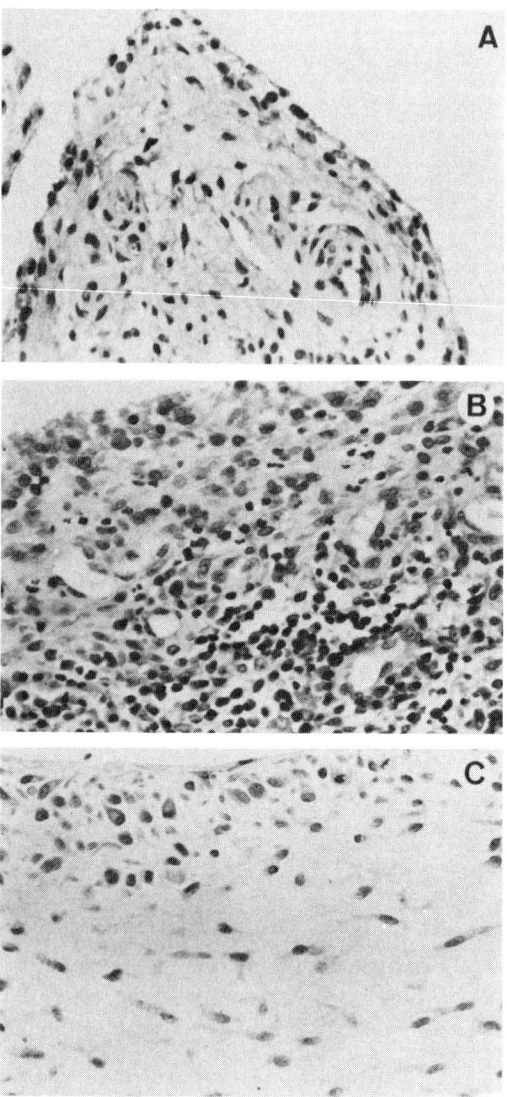

blood vessels and lymphatics penetrate the subsynovial tissue, they do not reach the synovial lining.

The ultrastructure of the synovial lining reveals two structurally distinct types of cells, originally termed A and B cells by Barland.[3] Type A synovial lining cells resemble tissue macrophages.[2,3] They possess a dense and heterochromatin-rich nucleus, abundant cytoplasmic vacuoles, and a poorly developed rough endoplasmic reticulum (Fig. 15–2). These cells possess finger-like extensions, filopodia, which protrude into and surround particles of extracellular matrix. Type B synovial cells have ultrastructural characteristics of connective tissue fibroblasts.[4,5] They have a pale nucleus, relatively few vacuoles and filopodia, a well-developed Golgi apparatus, and a prominent rough endoplasmic reticulum (Fig. 15–3). Approximately 70 to 80% of the normal synovial lining cells have fibroblast (type B cell) characteristics. The remaining 20 to 30% resemble macrophages (type A cells)[3,4] (Table

FIG. 15–2. Electron micrograph ($\times$14,000) of a type A rat synovial macrophage after intra-articular injection of horseradish peroxidase. Numerous small vessels and large vacuoles contain the ingested peroxidase reaction product, as indicated by the arrows. Other large vacuoles (V) are partly filled with a moderate electron-dense material. (From Graabeck, P.M.: Ultrastructural evidence for two distinct types of synoviocytes in rat synovial membrane. J. Ultrastruct. Res., *78*:321–339, 1982.)

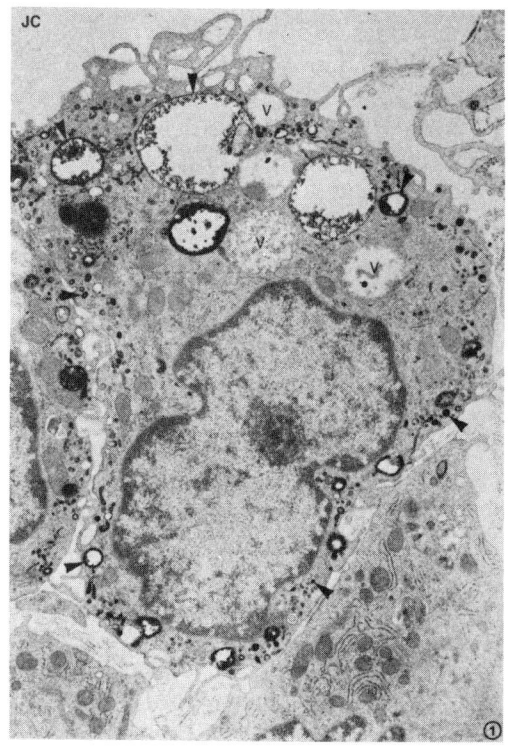

The synovial lining comprises an ill-defined layer, one to three cells deep, overlying a subsynovial layer composed of fibroblasts, adipocytes, unclassified cells, collagen fibers, and proteoglycans.[2] No basement membrane separates the synovial intima from the underlying connective tissue. Although abundant

FIG. 15–3. Electron micrograph ($\times$ 14,000) of a type B rat synovial fibroblast after intra-articular injection of horseradish peroxidase. The peroxidase reaction product has not been ingested. The prominent Golgi region (G) and rough endoplasmic reticulum (RER) are visible. Note the adjacent horseradish peroxidase positive synovial cell, which is the same as that shown in Figure 15–2. (From Graabaek, P.M.: Ultrastructural evidence for two distinct types of synoviocytes in rat synovial membrane. J. Ultrastruct. Res., 78:321–339, 1982.)

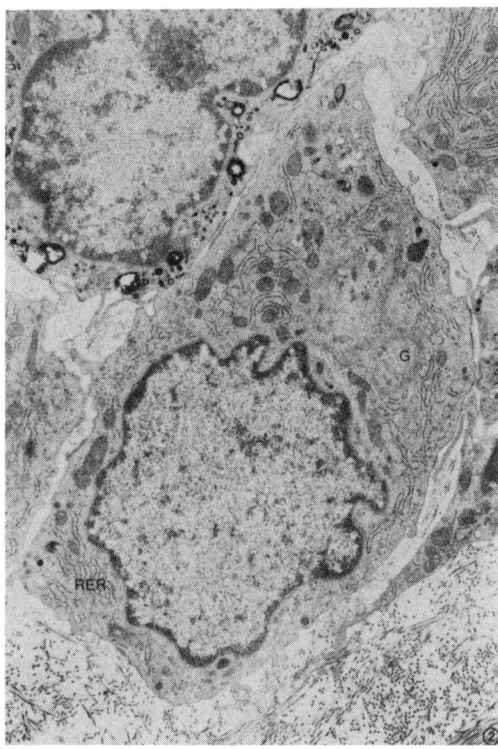

15–1). Cells with ultrastructural characteristics intermediate between fibroblasts and macrophages, the intermediate or type C cells, have also been described.[2,6]

Vascular endothelial cells are important in maintaining nutrition in the normal synovium and proliferate in rheumatoid arthritis (RA). Specialized postcapillary venules, referred to as high endothelial venules (HEVs), provide a site for lymphocytes to exit from the blood and migrate into the synovium.[7,8] HEVs can be identified by their characteristic cuboidal structure, ultrastructure, and histochemistry.[9] An example of HEVs in RA synovium is shown in Figure 15–4A.

Ultrastructurally, a basement membrane (BM) separates the endothelial cells from the underlying connective tissue. This BM consists of two layers: a moderately electron dense (lamina densa) layer located on the connective tissue side of the BM, and a translucent layer (lamina rara) that separates cells from the lamina densa. The BM has several components including type 4 collagen, laminin, and heparan sulfate proteoglycan.[10a] In RA, the BM is thickened and disrupted,[11] leading to possible functional alterations in the blood-tissue barrier.

The synovium and joint capsule are innervated by mechanoreceptors, nerve plexus, and free endings of unmyelinated nerves. The latter are linked to primary afferent neurons that provide sensory innervation and contain a neuropeptide called *Substance P* (SP).[12] The involvement of the nervous system in the pathogenesis of RA has been suggested by the symmetry of synovitis and by the observation that hemiplegic joints are generally spared from the inflammatory process. In adjuvant arthritis, sectioning of the peripheral nerve reduced the severity of arthritis in the denervated joint,[13] and nondenervated joints with the highest density of primary sensory neurons developed the most severe arthritis.[14]

SYNOVIAL LINING CELLS

EMBRYOLOGY

Certain aspects of the embryology of joints are important in understanding the structure and function of the synovial lining cells. In the fourth to sixth week of gestation, the synovial mesenchyme arises from a cellular aggregate or blastema associated with early limb-bud formation.[15] The primitive synovial mesenchyme is the progenitor of the secretory lining cells, the subsynovial fibroblasts, and the cells of the joint capsule.

The exact origin of the synovial cells is controversial.[4,16] Some workers feel that both type A and type B cells derive from a unique precursor, such as the "intermediate" cell that has features of primitive fibroblasts.[10a] However, experimental data now indicate that some type A synovial phagocytes arise from the circulating bone marrow-derived monocyte pool. Macrophages do not appear in the developing synovial membrane until the subsynovial tissue becomes vascularized.[6] Furthermore, if adult mice of one strain are lethally irradiated and reconstituted with bone marrow from a genetically distinct strain, the synovial macrophages are gradually replaced by cells with the genetic markers of the bone marrow donor.[17,18] In contrast, the secretory synovial fibroblasts display the genetic markers of the recipient strain of mice for at least 60 days following transplantation. One cannot exclude the possibility that during the period of ob-

Table 15–1. Properties of Synovial Lining Cells

	Cell Type		
	Macrophage (Type A Cell)	Fibroblast (Type B Cell)	Dendritic Cell
Cytoplasm and Organelles			
Vacuoles	+		
Filopodia	+		
Endoplasmic reticulum		+	
Lysosomes	+		
Prostaglandins			+
Collagenase			+
Hyaluronic acid		+	
Chondroitin sulfate		+	
Fibronectin		+	
Mononuclear cell factors	+		
Plasminogen activator		+	
Plasma Membrane			
HLA-DR	+		+
Fc receptor	+		−
C3 receptor	+		−
Function			
Phagocytosis	+		
Interaction with T-lymphocytes	+		+
Glycosaminoglycan and proteoglycan synthesis		+	

FIG. 15–4. Endothelial cells in synovium. *A,* At low power, a spectrum of vessels is revealed after endothelial cells in synovial frozen sections are stained with antibody to factor VIII. *B,* Higher power, showing several venules lined by high endothelium. *C,* Specific binding of peripheral blood lymphocytes (PBL) (dark, round cells) to synovial HEV in the in vitro binding assay. (From Jalkenen, S., Steere, A.C., Fox, R.I., and Butcher, E.C.: A distinct endothelial cell recognition system that controls lymphocyte traffic into inflamed synovium. Science, *233:*556–558, 1986. Copyright 1986 by the AAAS.[10])

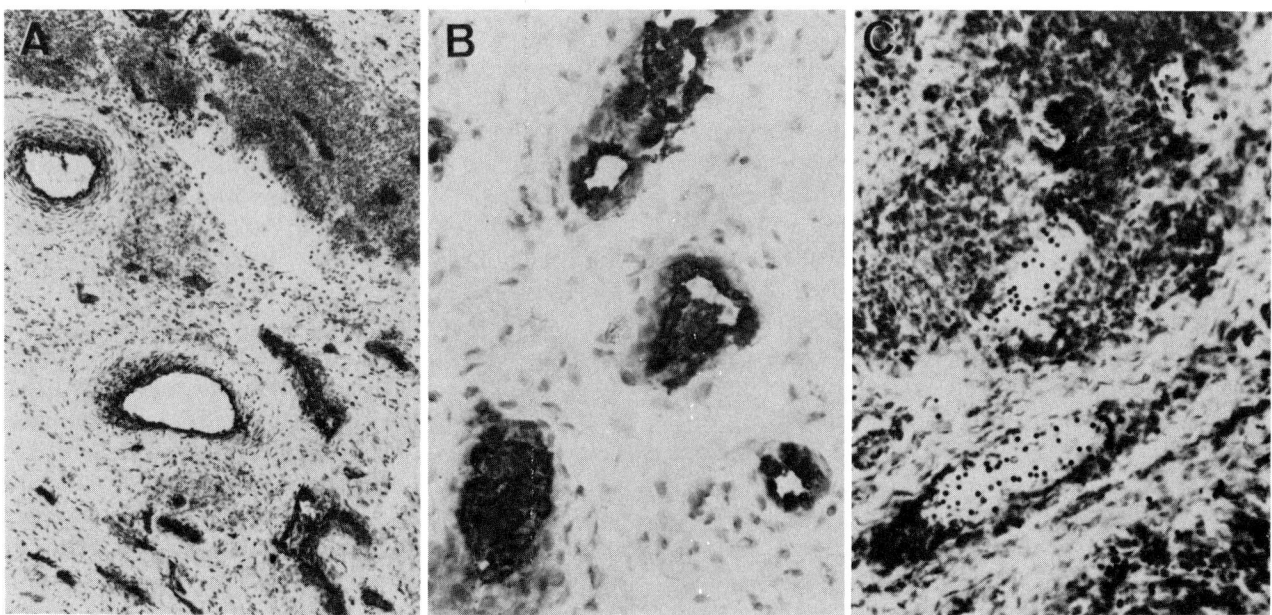

servation the repopulation of the synovial fibroblasts had not yet occurred. Nevertheless, a reasonable interpretation of the data is that most synovial macrophages arise from bone marrow-derived precursors, whereas most synovial fibroblasts develop from the primitive mesenchyme of the limb-bud.

Several types of synovial "dendritic" cells have been identified from immunohistologic studies, electron microscopy, and in vitro culture of cells eluted from synovial membrane by enzymatic digestion (Fig. 15-5). In synovial tissue sections, some dendritic cells interdigitate with immune T-lymphocytes[19] and express ATPase and HLA-class II antigens.[18,20,21] These synovial dendritic cells may be similar to the "interfollicular" dendritic cells found in the T-cell zones of normal cells of lymph nodes[18,22] and the Langerhan's cell found in skin.[23] The "dendritic" cells in synovial fluid described by Zvaifler and co-workers[24] appear similar to this type of synovial dendritic cell and to the "veiled" dendritic cell found in low frequency in blood and thoracic lymph.[25] An additional dendritic cell type, derived from synovial membrane digested with enzymes and cultured in vitro, is deficient in lysosome and lacks significant phagocytic activity.[20,21,26] Their "dendritic" structure in tissue culture is reversible, and time-lapse videomicroscopy has shown their ability to assume a fibroblast-like structure. They can, however, be reinduced to express a dendritic morphology by treatment with interleukin-1, prostaglandin E2, and cyclic AMP analogues.[28-30] Such "dendritic" cells appear to represent a differentiated fibroblast rather than a lineage from monocytes. The term "dendritic" is nonspecific, and cau-

tion must be used when identifying populations based on structure alone.

Even though fibroblasts belong to a different cell lineage than the macrophages, they may undergo phenotypic conversion when a selective pressure is applied. In one study, murine fibroblast cells were induced in vitro to express macrophage markers such as Ia antigen, phagocytosis, lysozyme, and nonspecific esterase.[10a,31] In another study, rabbit synoviocytes with the morphologic appearance of fibroblasts phagocytosed latex particles and released collagenase after maintenance in tissue culture.[32] Perhaps a fraction of the synovial fibroblasts are primitive mesenchymal cells that can reversibly differentiate into macrophages.

The stimuli that cause connective tissue fibroblasts and macrophages to assume the structure and function of synovial lining cells have not been defined precisely. The formation of the joint cavity during embryogenesis is preceded by the appearance of small clefts in the primitive synovial mesenchyme with accompanying cell and matrix lysis.[15,33] The clefts gradually enlarge and eventually coalesce to form the complete joint cavity, surrounded by a synovial lining. In one experimental model, injection of air into the subcutaneous tissues of rats induced the formation 10 to 14 days later of a cavity with a lining resembling synovium.[34] The lining was composed of macrophages and fibroblasts in a laminar arrangement, overlying a collagenous subintima and a zone of high vascularity. However, the composition of the fluid in the cavity was not analyzed. These results suggest, but do not prove, that tissue cavitation can stimulate fi-

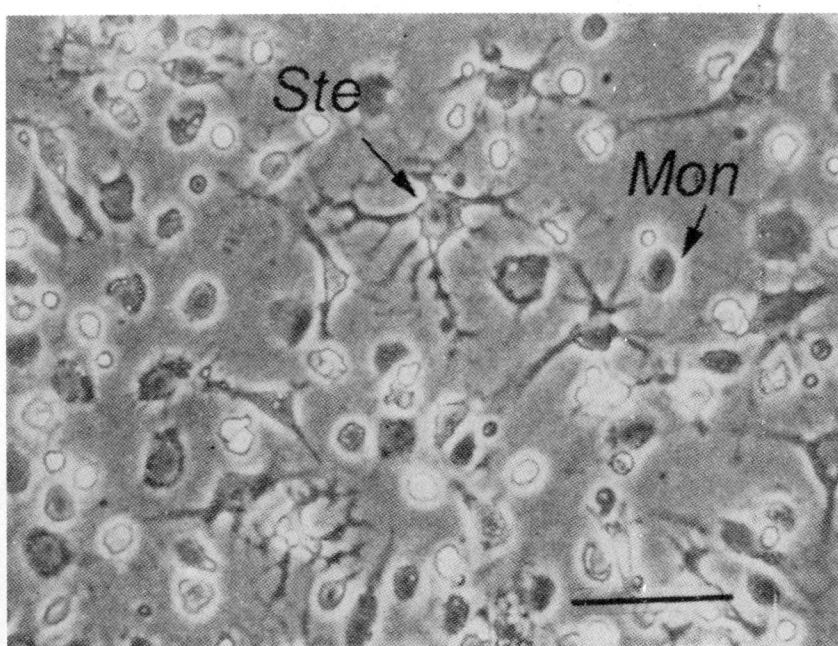

FIG. 15-5. Photomicrograph using phase contrast optics of a primary culture of rheumatoid synovium. Stellate cells (Ste) and probable monocytes (Mon) are designated by the arrows. (From Krane, S.M.[26])

broblasts and macrophages to develop into synovial lining cells. Apparently, the conversion is not irreversible. The structure and biochemical properties of normal synovial fibroblasts propagated in tissue culture do not differ reproducibly from fibroblasts obtained from other anatomic sites.[35] Presumably, a continuous interaction among the synovial lining cells, the synovial fluid, and the extracellular matrix is necessary to maintain their differentiated state.

LIFE SPAN

Under physiologic conditions, synovial lining cells proliferate slowly and have a prolonged life span.[36–38] Fewer than 1% of normal superficial lining cells in explanted synovium incorporated tritiated thymidine into DNA during a brief incubation (Fig. 15–6). The frequency of dividing synovial cells in patients with RA is considerably higher, although never exceeding a few percent of the total.[37,38]

The slow turnover of synovial cells may partly explain the prolonged retention of foreign materials deposited on the synovial membrane.[39] In RA, synovial phagocytes may harbor gold particles long after chrysotherapy has been discontinued.

Despite their intrinsically slow proliferation rate in vivo, synovial fibroblasts from normal adults retain the potential for rapid cell division. Following synovectomy or joint injury, the synovial lining can regenerate completely. The fibroblasts in the new lining layer probably derive from the mitosis of residual synoviocytes as well as of fibroblasts in the subsynovial tissue. The synovial macrophages, like other specialized tissue histiocytes, probably have a limited capacity for cell division. After injury or synovectomy, the synovial macrophages probably are replaced by precursor monocytes from the systemic circulation and subsynovial space rather than from direct cell division. A constant migration of monocytes from the circulation may be required for the persistence of chronic inflammatory synovitis. Whether synovial lin-

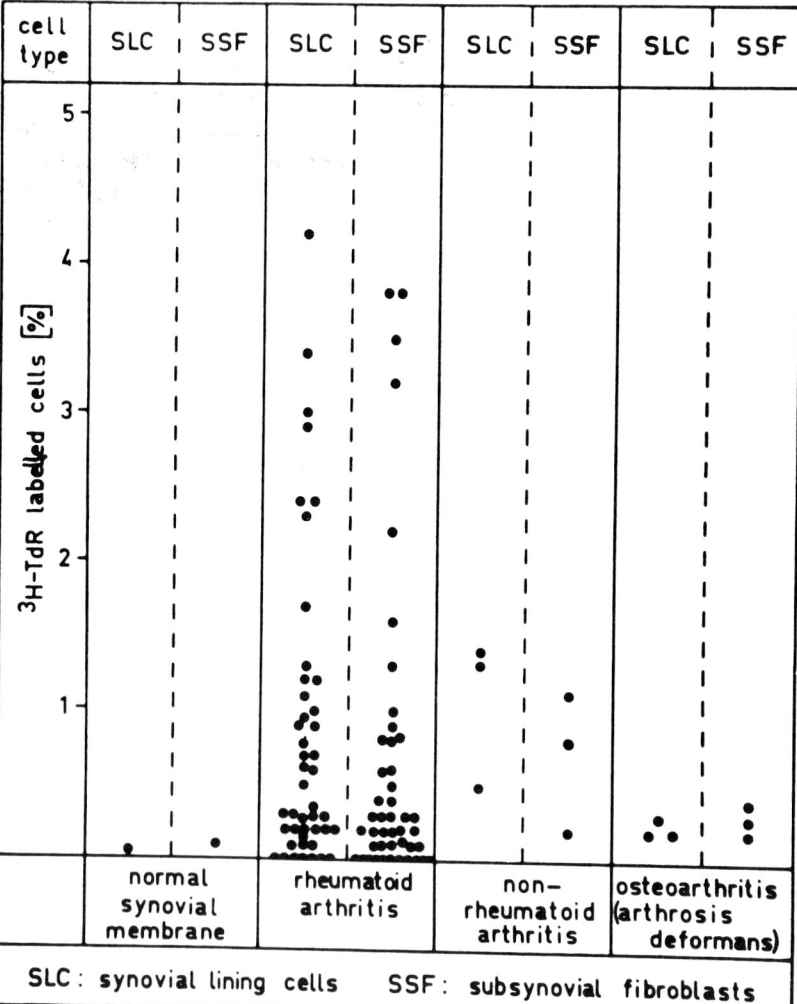

FIG. 15–6. Tritiated thymidine [³H]-TdR, labeling indices of synovial lining cells (SLC) and subsynovial fibroblasts (SSF) in various conditions. (From Mohr, W., Beneke, G. and Amohing, W.: Proliferation of synovial lining cells and fibroblasts. Ann. Rheum. Dis., *34:*219–224, 1975.)

ing cells ever actively migrate into the subsynovial tissue or into the systemic circulation is not known.

COMPOSITION AND BIOCHEMISTRY

Because synovial lining cells are difficult to obtain in quantity, knowledge of their composition and biochemistry has come from quantitative histochemical studies of carefully sectioned tissues,[2,35,40] and from metabolic analysis of dispersed cells maintained in short-term tissue culture.[26,41–45]

Nucleotide Metabolism. The DNA content of synoviocytes should be similar to that of other human diploid cells (i.e., about 8×10^{-12} g/cell). The RNA content in the secretory fibroblast is greater than in the phagocytic macrophage, reflecting the well-developed rough endoplasmic reticulum of the former cell type.[2,4,5] Explanted synovial fibroblasts synthesize RNA and DNA in a medium lacking exogenous purines and pyrimidines.[38] Hence, they presumably retain the capacity for de novo purine and pyrimidine biosynthesis. It seems likely that synovial macrophages, like other cells of the monocyte-macrophage series, should contain xanthine oxidase.

The endogenous production of pyrophosphate and hypoxanthine increases when cells proliferate. As shown in Figure 15–5, synovial cell turnover is accelerated in osteoarthritic and rheumatoid synovium. The potential contribution of endogenously generated pyrophosphate and uric acid to the pathogenesis of calcium pyrophosphate and monosodium urate deposition disease has not been fully evaluated.

Lysosomes. The abundant lysosomes of synovial lining macrophages have been studied in detail because of their potential role in the production of joint inflammation.[1,21,29,35] The organelles typically contain tartrate-inhibitable acid phosphatase(s) (Fig. 15–7), β-N-acetylglucosaminidase, cathepsin D, and nonspecific esterase.[27] The lysosomes lack significant amounts of alkaline phosphatase, peroxidase, and chloroacetate-reactive esterase.[29]

Lysosomes are less prominent in the synovial cells that assume a stellate or dendritic appearance in tissue culture.[26,35,46–48] However, the cytoplasmic processes of the dendritic cells do have numerous granules that contain immunoreactive collagenase in a latent form.[49]

Prostaglandins. The synovial membrane contains freely available unsaturated phospholipids, as detected by the acid hematin reaction.[35] Increased amounts of unsaturated phospholipids have been observed in rheumatoid synovial cells. The elevation may be related to an accelerated rate of prostaglandin synthesis. With immunofluorescent and immuno-electron-microscopic techniques, prostaglandin E has been detected in intracytoplasmic granules, presumably lysosomes, of synovial macrophages.[50] The prostaglandins are probably synthesized endogenously, because microsomal preparations from rheumatoid synovial lining contain enzymes capable of generating PGF_2 and $PGF_2\alpha$. Similarly, isolated adherent rheumatoid synovial cells produce prostaglandins in tissue culture.[52–54] Neither the enzymes mediating prostaglandin synthesis nor the prostaglandin molecules themselves have been detected within synovial fibroblasts. The leukotriene content and synthetic capacity of normal and rheumatoid synoviocytes are topics of current research.

Carbohydrates. Human synovial cells consume glucose and oxygen and generate lactic acid in vivo.[55] They contain an active glycolytic pathway, tricarboxycylic acid cycle, and hexose monophosphate shunt.[35] Cytochemical assays have also yielded evidence for mitochondrial oxidative activity. The quantitative importance of nonoxidative and oxidative glucose metabolism for the generation of ATP by synovial cells under various conditions has not been determined precisely.

FIG. 15–7. Cryostat section of a normal *(A)* and a rheumatoid synovium *(B* and *C)* stained for acid phosphatase. Note the intense staining at the lining areas. (From Theofilopoulos, A.N. et al.: Evidence for presence of receptors for C3 and IgG on human synovial cells. Arthritis Rheum., 23:6, 1980.[27])

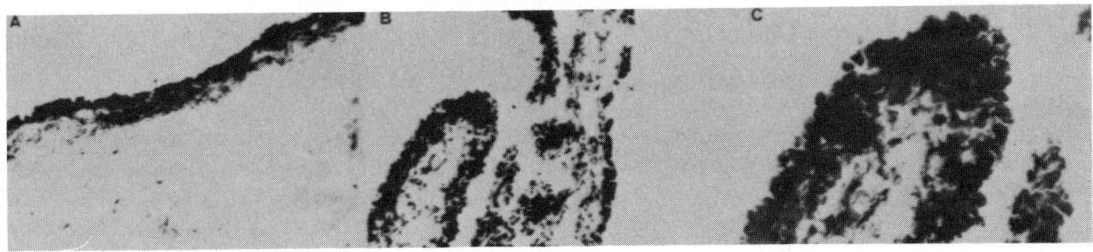

In chronic synovitis, synovial cells consume increased amounts of oxygen and generate more lactic acid. These changes undoubtedly reflect the enhanced proliferative and protein synthetic activity of the cells, as well as the entry into the joints of inflammatory cells from the circulation. The increased metabolic activity can cause a substantial fall in synovial fluid glucose, pH, and oxygen tension.[55] These changes may ultimately limit the energy-generating capacity of the synovial lining cells and adjacent chondrocytes, with resultant exacerbation of joint destruction.

Glycosaminoglycans. A basic physiologic function of the synovial lining fibroblasts is the synthesis and secretion of hyaluronic acid. This acidic glycosaminoglycan is a major component of the joint fluid and forms part of the extracellular matrix that surrounds the synovial lining cells. The hexuronic acid moiety of hyaluronic acid derives from UDP-glucuronic acid, which is formed by the action of UDP-glucose dehydrogenase.[56] Specific glycosyltransferases represent the rate-limiting step in hyaluronate formation.[45] Both UDP-glucose dehydrogenase and hyaluronic acid synthase activity are present in normal synovial lining fibroblasts propagated in vitro.

Human synovial lining fibroblasts incorporate radioactive sulfate into chondroitin sulfate and dermatan sulfate.[57] The two glycosaminoglycans, in association with proteoglycan core proteins, are part of the extracellular synovial lining matrix. They are also detectable in joint fluid. In accordance with the need to modify continually the joint fluid and extracellular matrix, the synovial lining fibroblasts probably synthesize and secrete proteoglycans constitutively. However, several distinct polypeptide hormones can affect the rate of production.[41] When the synovium is injured, the synovial macrophages, and other inflammatory cells, release specific connective tissue activating factors that enhance proteoglycan synthesis by the adjacent fibroblasts. The newly formed extracellular matrix coats the synovial lining and protects it from further injury. The control of connective tissue activation is discussed in detail in Chapter 14.

Collagen. Synovial fibroblast cells in culture synthesize types 1 and 3 collagen; this synthesis is augmented by interleukin-1[58] and inhibited by interferon-gamma.[59] Thus, synoviocytes may respond to functional signals derived from T-lymphocytes and macrophages. Although the synovial fibroblasts synthesize collagen in vitro, their doing so may represent an adaptation to tissue culture because collagen is not a significant component of normal synovial fluid, and collagen fibers are notably sparse in the superficial synovial layers. Normal rabbit synovial slices incorporated less proline (a collagen precursor) than glycine, tryptophan, or histidine into protein, suggesting that collagen was only a minor fraction of synovial protein synthesis in vivo.[44]

Collagenase and Plasminogen Activator. The non-phagocytic synovial dendritic cells contain collagenase in granules associated with the stellate processes.[49] When exposed to interleukin-1 produced by activated adjacent synovial macrophages, collagenase is released in a latent form into the extracellular space.[60] In a parallel fashion, normal synovial fibroblasts have been reported to release the proteolytic enzyme plasminogen activator, after exposure to supernatants of mononuclear phagocytes.[26,32,60] Plasminogen activator converts the latent collagenase to an active form. It also degrades fibrinogen directly, thereby preventing fibrin formation. The collagenase and plasminogen activator work with the phagocytic mechanism to prevent the accumulation of particulate material in the joint fluid.

Fibronectin. Fibronectin is a large extracellular glycoprotein that forms part of the extracellular matrix in both normal and RA synovial membranes.[61] This molecule is synthesized by different cell types, including synovial lining cells and vascular endothelial cells. Although there is only a single fibronectin gene, different tissues produce distinct fibronectin molecules by alternative methods of splicing the mRNA from this gene.[62–64] The concentration of fibronectin in RA synovial fluid is more than twice as high as in plasma from the same patients, suggesting that it is produced within the synovium.[65] High concentrations of fibronectin have been detected by immunohistology in areas of synovial lining cell proliferation, particularly at the margin of the pannus-invading cartilage.[65,66]

Fibroblasts and osteosarcoma cells have specific cell surface receptors for fibronectin.[66a] Specific amino acid sequences in fibronectin, including peptides containing arginine-glycine-asparagine (termed RGD based on the standard nomenclature for naming amino acids), are recognized by these receptors.[62,66a] The RGD receptor for fibronectin appears to be a member of a larger family of receptors for other cell adhesion molecules, including vitronectin, von Willebrand's factor, and fibrinogen.[66a] Thus, fibronectin and other related cell adhesion molecules help define the architecture of both normal and diseased synovium. Interruption of the interaction of cells with adhesive proteins provides a potential target for modulation of the arthritic process.

CHANGES IN SYNOVIOCYTES IN RHEUMATOID ARTHRITIS

In RA, the synovial lining becomes hyperemic and thickened with extensive growth and folding into villi.[67] The proliferation of synovial cells is an early event in pathogenesis and precedes the appearance of plasma cells.[68] The synovial layer may increase in thickness to 10 or more cells (see Fig. 15–1B and C). Individual synovial cells hypertrophy to double in size, predominantly owing to increased cytoplasm.[69] During the first months of disease, there may be significant variation in the degree of synovial hypertrophy and hyperplasia in different regions of the same joint,[70] but significant regional variations are less frequent in cases of long duration. In some patients, synovial giant cells are present (Table 15–2); such cells have 2 to 12 nuclei and resemble hypertrophied synoviocytes. Their location and features are distinct from "foreign body" giant cells and Langerhans' giant cells,[69,71,72] but they are not specific for RA because they are found in other types of arthritis also (see Table 15–2).

Both macrophage (type A) and fibroblast (type B) cells are increased in number in most RA patients, although some patients have a more pronounced increase in type B and intermediate cell types.[3] At the electron microscopic level, numerous differences are apparent between the type A cells in RA patients and those of normal individuals. The size and number of lysosomes are increased. The Golgi apparatus is smaller, and fewer filopodia are present. The mitochondria are frequently swollen and contain fewer cristae. The type B cells show increased rough endoplasmic reticulum and intermediate-sized filamentous fibers of the vimentin type.[3,73] The matrix of RA joints contains periodically banded collagen fibers as well as "fibrinoid" material that does not show cross-striation.[74] The fibroblasts in the subsynovium of RA joints do not show the changes noted in type A or type B cells and appear similar to fibroblasts in skin or normal joints.[2] At the junction of pannus and articular cartilage, both fibroblasts and type A cells are present, with the type A cells forming the cells actually invading the cartilage.[75,76]

Quantitative cytochemical measurements have revealed that synoviocytes from RA patients contain higher levels of various enzymes than normal synoviocytes; examples include elevated amounts of glucose 6-phosphatase, cathepsin D, enzymes of the glycolytic pathway, and prostaglandin synthetase.[35,41] Enzymes commonly found in monocytes, such as nonspecific esterase and lysozyme, are present in most of the synovial lining cells.[47,77] The intense staining of tissue sections for acid phosphatase (see Fig. 15–6) is due to the increased thickness of the synovium and to the increased lysozyme content per synoviocyte. Henderson has reviewed many additional studies performed on tissue slices and cells eluted from synovial membrane.[35] The relationship of these activities to those expressed by synoviocytes in situ remains a topic of intense research interest.

Studies have used monoclonal antibodies to further characterize antigens expressed by synovial cells.[20,46–48,78,79] Frozen tissue sections can be stained with particular monoclonal antibodies produced from mice immunized with human antigens. Synovial cells binding the monoclonal antibody are then detected with fluorescent or peroxidase conjugated anti-mouse IgG antiserum. Most rheumatoid synovial lining cells

Table 15–2. Percentage Incidence of Histopathologic Parameters in 10 Diagnostic Categories*

	Clinical Diagnoses (Number of Accessions in Percentages)						
	Definite or Classic Rheumatoid Arthritis (127)	Juvenile Rheumatoid Arthritis (23)	Psoriatic Arthropathy (13)	Reiter's Syndrome (9)	Ankylosing Spondylitis (17)	Enterocolitic Arthropathy (7)	Osteoarthritis (74)
1. Hypertrophy of synoviocytes	82.7	73.9	84.6	77.8	35.3	85.7	68.9
2. Hyperplasia of synoviocytes	63.0	69.6	76.9	77.8	47.1	57.1	63.5
3. Synovial giant cells	18.1	8.7	30.8	0	17.6	0	10.8
Synovial giant cells, superficial	15.7	4.3	23.1	0	17.6	0	6.8
Synovial giant cells in subsynoviocyte tissue	7.9	4.3	15.4	0	5.9	0	5.4
4. Ulceration of synovial surface	26.0	13.0	15.4	0	11.8	0	5.4
5. Fresh fibrin on synovial surface	32.5	21.7	38.5	0	23.5	28.6	24.3
6. Organizing fibrin on synovial surface	50.4	39.1	53.8	11.1	17.6	14.3	13.5
7. Fibrin in subsynoviocyte tissue	7.1	0	0	0	0	0	1.4
8. Proliferating fibroblasts	68.5	26.1	84.6	33.3	11.8	14.3	14.9

*Data from Cooper, N. et al.: Diagnostic specificity of synovial lesions. Hum. Pathol., 12:314–328, 1981.

express Ia antigen, the gene product of the HLA-DR locus (Fig. 15–8A and B). Synovial lining cells also express OKM-1 (Fig. 15–7C) and T200 (Fig. 15–7D) antigens; these markers are found on monocytes but not on fibroblasts.[40,79–81] They correspond to the receptors for complement-derived component iC3b and the common leukocyte antigen, respectively.[79,80] These results suggest that synovial proliferation in rheumatoid arthritis is due to bone marrow-derived cells. However, it remains possible that primitive mesenchymal cells can be induced to express these markers. Immunohistologic techniques can also be used to demonstrate that most mononuclear cells infiltrating the rheumatoid synovium are T cells (Fig. 15–9A), although some B cells (Fig. 15–9B) are also present. In contrast to rheumatoid synovium, normal joints have a smaller proportion of synovial cells reactive with anti-Ia antibody (Fig. 15–10A), OKM-1 (Fig. 15–10B), and T200 (Fig. 15–10C) antibodies. These results emphasize the increased number of macrophage-dendritic cells found in the rheumatoid joint.[20,21,46]

Several different patterns of lymphocyte infiltration have been noted in the synovium of different RA patients.[79,82,83] In some patients, synovial membrane biopsies contain germinal centers with immunohistologic characteristics similar to reactive lymph nodes.[46,79] Other RA patients have synovial lining cell proliferation with few infiltrating T- or B-lymphocytes.[79,84] It has been suggested that patterns of synovial histology may predict clinical outcome or response to particular medications,[82,83,85] but larger numbers of patients with long-term followup will be required to assess their predictive value. Synovial cells are also able to bind immune complexes, presumably through their receptors for the Fc portion of IgG or for complement components[27] (Fig. 15–11) Thus, synovial cells are able to concentrate particular antigens and present them in an immunogenic form to lymphocytes.

FIG. 15–8. Immunohistologic characterization of rheumatoid synovial membrane. Frozen tissue sections were reacted with monoclonal antibodies and peroxidase-coupled goat anti-mouse IgG. The presence of a positive reaction is shown by dark staining. *A,* Reaction with monoclonal anti-Ia antibody to detect the gene product of the HLA-DR gene locus. *B,* A higher magnification (×400) demonstrates that virtually all lining cells express Ia-antigen. *C,* Staining of the synovial lining cells with antibody OKM-1 which detects an antigen on monocytes. *D,* Reaction with the T200 antigen, a marker found on hematopoietic cells but not with normal fibroblasts.

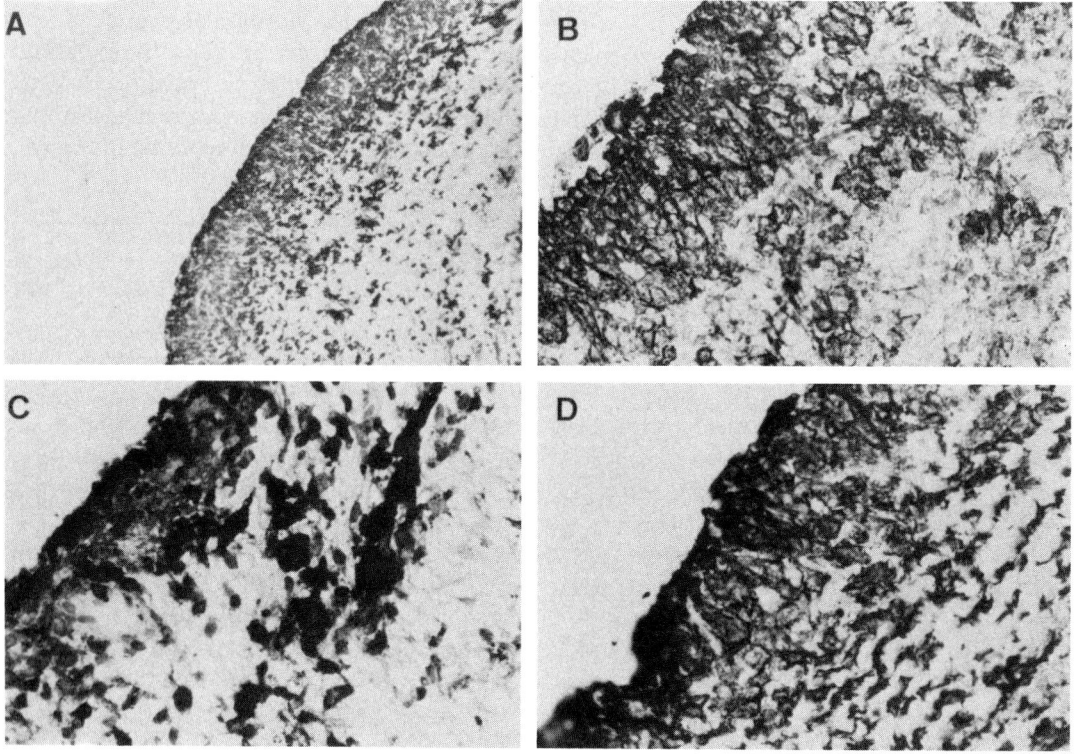

FIG. 15–9. Most mononuclear cells in the rheumatoid synovium are T cells based on staining with monoclonal antibody Leu 4 *(A)*; examples of the positively stained cell membranes are shown by arrows. Scattered B cells, detected by anti-kappa/lambda antibody *(B)*, are also present; an example of the cytoplasmic and membrane staining is shown by the arrow.

FIG. 15–10. Normal synovial membrane tissue sections stained with anti-Ia *(A)*, OKM-1 *(B)*, and T200 *(C)* monoclonal antibodies. Examples of positively stained cells are shown by the arrows.

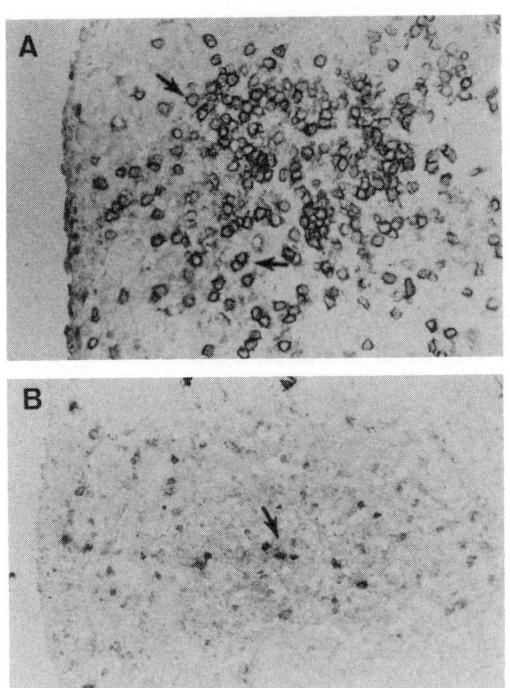

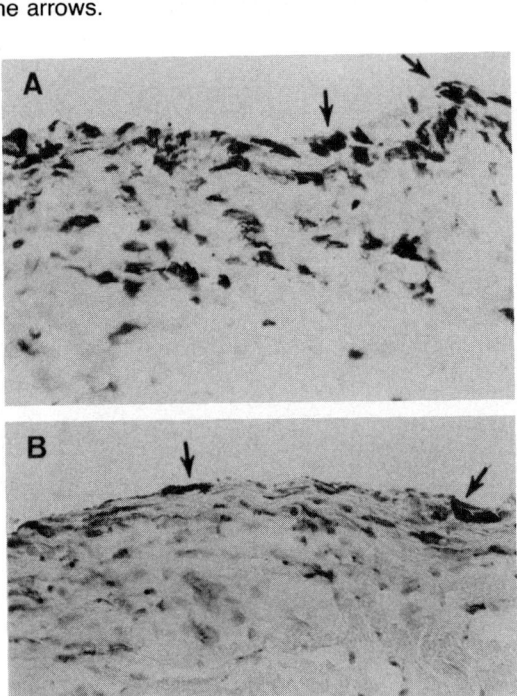

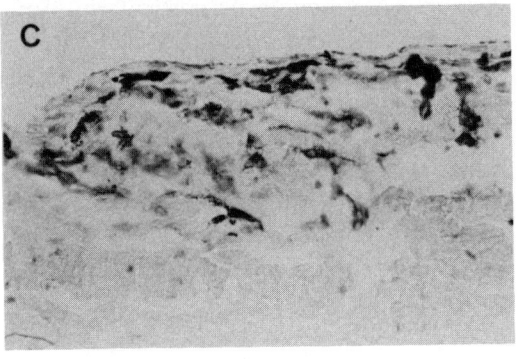

FUNCTIONAL PROPERTIES OF CELLS IN THE RA SYNOVIUM

The RA synovial membrane is infiltrated by a variety of cells including type A and type B synoviocytes, vascular endothelial cells, dendritic macrophage-like cells, and lymphocytes; their functional interactions partly depend on intimate cell-to-cell contact. Studies on cells eluted from the synovial membrane have characterized potentially important interactions, which can be divided into two categories: (1) the production of soluble factors from synoviocytes influencing the growth and differentiation of adjacent mesenchymal and lymphoid cells, and (2) synoviocyte or endothelial cell response to signals from lymphocytes or macrophages.

Synovial type A (macrophage-like) cells release interleukin-1,[86,87] which can (1) induce fibroblasts to produce procoagulants, which promote fibrin deposition, and to stimulate collagenase secretion;[58–60] (2) stimulate cultured endothelial cells to assume high endothelial venule (HEV) structure;[8] and (3) increase immune responsiveness among T-lymphocytes. Synoviocytes also produce a B cell stimulatory factor (BSF2) closely related to interferon β2.[88] The release of these factors by hyperplastic RA synovial cells provides a novel mechanism for perpetuation of a local immune response as they may be partly responsible for recruiting activated lymphocytes that produce antibody.

Synoviocytes may influence neighboring lymphocytes by expressing cell membrane molecules that influence immune responses. For example, synovial cells in normal or osteoarthritic joints express little histocompatibility antigen (HLA-DR). However, high

FIG. 15–11. Cryostat section of a normal synovium with attachment of the lining areas of fluorescinated gram-negative bacteria that had fixed complement as viewed by fluorescence *(A)* and phase *(B)* microscopy. (From Theofilopoulos, A.N. et al.: Evidence for presence of receptors for C3 and IgG Fc on human synovial cells. Arthritis Rheum., 23:6, 1980.)

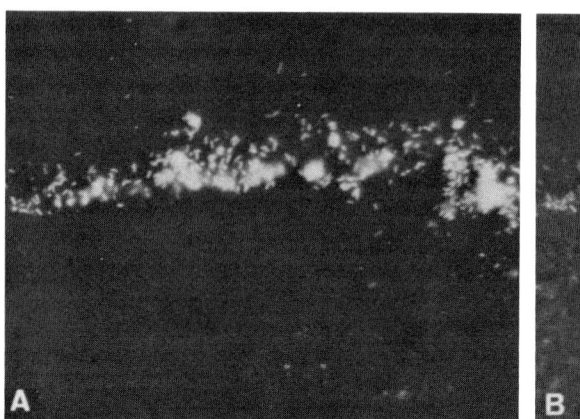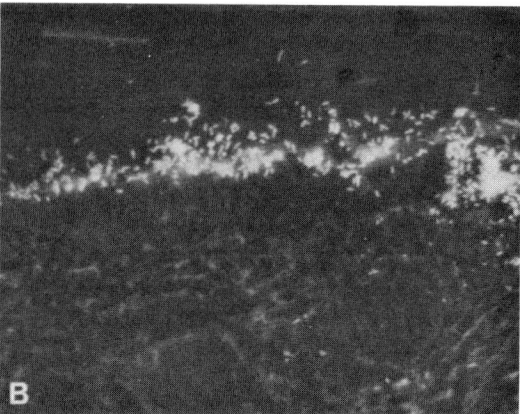

levels of HLA-DR are expressed on RA synovial lining cells (Figure 15–8A). HLA antigens allow synovial lining cells to directly stimulate lymphocyte proliferation and serve as a target for cytotoxic lymphocyte responses.[89] The induction of HLA-DR on the "target" cells in RA synovium is particularly intriguing in view of the close link with HLA-DR4.[90]

Finally, synovial lining cells may influence the immune response by presenting other targets for the immune lymphocytes. In rheumatic fever, immune responses are directed against synovial antigens sharing a cross-reactive antigen with certain strains of streptococcus,[91] a pathophysiologic process termed "molecular mimicry." Agents capable of eliciting molecular mimicry have been actively sought in RA research studies. One candidate is the Epstein-Barr virus (EBV), because RA patients have elevated titers of antibodies against nuclear antigens (e.g., EBNA-1) induced by this ubiquitous agent.[92–95] The stimulus for these increased antibody titers remains unclear but may result from difficulties in effectively regulating EBV-infected B-lymphocytes.[96] RA synovial membrane lining cells do contain at least one protein that is cross-reactive with the EBNA-1 antigen.[95] Because EBV DNA was not detected in the RA synovium,[97] it is unlikely that immune responses are directed against EBV-infected synovial cells. If immune responses against EBV play a role in pathogenesis, a process such as molecular mimicry may be responsible. Other candidates for molecular mimicry include cartilage antigens sharing cross-reactivity with

mycoplasma[98] and synovial antigens sharing cross-reactivity with parvoviruses.[99]

Synovial cells in vitro proliferate or differentiate in response to factors released from lymphocytes, monocytes, and platelets. Because many of these factors were initially defined by their ability to influence fibroblast growth, they were originally termed "connective tissue-activating peptides" (CTAPs) (see Chapter 14). CTAPs are identical to certain growth factors important in cancer cells, including epidermal, insulin-like, and platelet-derived growth factors. Additional factors released by mononuclear cells (i.e., lymphokines and monokines), such as interleukin-1, also augment synovial cell growth and collagen production.[41,58] The similarity of "growth" factors in RA and cancer is intriguing because both conditions involve unregulated growth and invasion of neighboring tissues. Information about molecular mechanism of carcinogenesis may provide further insight into synoviocyte proliferation and new treatment for arthritis.

Synovial cells in vitro also respond to neuropeptides such as Substance P (SP).[100] Because SP can be released into tissues from peripheral nerve endings of primary sensory neurons[101] and SP-like activity has been detected in synovial fluids,[102] the stimulation of RA synoviocytes by SP is likely to occur in vivo. Moreover, SP can enhance cellular synthesis of collagenase and prostaglandin E, molecules that may participate in cartilage destruction and perpetuation of the immune response. SP is a potent vasodilator that may allow extravasation of plasma and is able to activate

T-lymphocytes,[103] monocytes,[104] and neutrophils.[105] Thus, neuropeptides, as well as lymphokines and factors encoded by oncogenes, may participate in the pathogenesis of RA.

Harris and Brinkerhoff have pointed out the similarity between the destructive process in rheumatoid synovium and localized cancer.[51] They found that suspensions of synovial cells could survive after transplantation into nude (athymic) mice. These cells become organized into a pannus-like structure with fibroblasts, multinucleated giant cells, and collagen fibers. In comparison, normal human skin fibroblasts or normal rabbit synovial cells cannot be recovered from the injection site of nude mice.

In sum, the synovial lining cells have a notable capacity to (1) bind antigen-antibody complexes, (2) present antigen to T-lymphocytes, (3) produce cytokines that promote the activation and proliferation of T-lymphocytes, and (4) respond to signals from mononuclear cells. Hence, it is not surprising that the persistence of antigenic material in the synovium, or the intermittent deposition of immune complexes from the circulation, induces the infiltration of lymphocytes and plasma cells, and the disruption of the normal synovial architecture. Indeed, in some patients with RA, the synovial membrane eventually transforms into a lymphoid tissue that produces abundant immunoglobulin and lymphokines in situ, serving to remind us that the specialized structure and function of the synovial lining represent an adaptation to the milieu of the joint space and adjacent subsynovial tissue. When the external environment is altered, the character of the synovial lining changes accordingly.

PHARMACOLOGIC APPROACHES TO MODIFYING THE FUNCTION OF SYNOVIOCYTES

To varying degrees, all forms of chronic inflammatory synovitis are associated with hyperplasia of synovial fibroblasts, metabolic activation of synovial macrophages and dendritic cells, infiltration of leukocytes from the subsynovial space, and matrix disorganization. Not surprisingly, therefore, pharmacologic agents that block lysosomal enzyme release, prostaglandin synthesis, free radical formation, or cellular proliferation favorably alter the course of joint inflammation.[106] If such drugs could be administered in a form that localized preferentially to the synovial macrophages, and persisted for long periods, a more specific antiarthritic effect could be obtained. An objective for future research will be to develop antiarthritic substances that (1) impede the homing of monocytes to the synovial membrane, (2) block the synthesis of interleukin-1 and related lymphokines, (3) impair the ability of dendritic cells to present antigen to T-lymphocytes, and (4) interfere with the binding of polypeptide growth factors to specific receptors on synovial fibroblasts and dendritic cells. Agents with these properties could block the reciprocal interactions between synovial macrophages, dendritic cells, fibroblasts, and subsynovial lymphocytes necessary for sustained joint inflammation.

REFERENCES

1. Hermanns, W., and Schulz, L.C.: Enzyme histochemical studies of the homogeneity of the mononuclear phagocyte system with special reference to the synovium. Agents Actions, 11:117–129, 1982.
2. Gadially, F.N.: Fine structure of joints. In The Joints and Synovial Fluid. Edited by L. Sokoloff. New York, Academic Press, 1978, pp. 110–120.
3. Barland, P., Novikoff, A.B., and Hamerman, D.: Electron microscopy of the human synovial membrane. J. Cell Biol., 14:207–214, 1962.
4. Graabaek, P.M.: Ultrastructural evidence for two distinct types of synoviocytes in rat synovial membrane. J. Ultrastruct. Res., 78:321–339, 1982.
5. Okada, Y., Nakanishi, I., and Kajikawa, K.: Ultrastructure of the mouse synovial membrane. Arthritis Rheum., 24:835–843, 1981.
6. Krey, P.R. et al.: The human fetal synovium. Histology, fine structure and changes in organ culture. Arthritis Rheum., 14:319–325, 1971.
7. Freemont, A. et al.: Changes in vascular endothelium related to lymphocyte collections in diseased synovium. Arthritis Rheum., 26:1427–1433, 1983.
8. Cavender, D. et al.: Pathways to chronic inflammation in rheumatoid arthritis. Fed. Proc., 46:116–118, 1987.
9. Freemont, A., and Jones, C.: Light microscopic histochemical and ultrastructural studies of human lymph node paracortical venules. J. Anat., 136:349–362, 1983.
10. Jalkenen, S., Steere, A., Fox, R.I., and Butcher, E.C.: A distinct endothelial cell recognition system that controls lymphocyte traffic into inflamed synovium. Science 233:556–558, 1986.
10a.Krawisz, B., Florine, D., and Scott, R.: Differentiation of fibroblast-like cell into macrophages. Cancer Res., 41:2891–2899, 1981.
11. Matsuboru, T., and Ziff, M.: Basement membrane thickening of post capillary venules and capillaries in rheumatoid synovium. Arthritis Rheum., 30:18–29, 1987.
12. Pernow, B.: Substance P. Pharmacol. Rev., 35:85–141, 1983.
13. Courtright, L.J., and Kuzell, K.C.: Sparing effect of neurological deficit and trauma on the course of adjuvant arthritis in the rat. Ann. Rheum. Dis., 24:360–368, 1965.
14. Levine, J.D. et al.: Intraneuronal substance P contributes to the severity of experimental arthritis. Science, 226:547–549, 1984.
15. O'Rahilly, R., and Gardner, E.: The embryology of movable joints. In The Joints and Synovial Fluid. Edited by L. Sokoloff. New York, Academic Press, 1978, pp. 48–97.
16. Davies, D., and Palfray, A.: Studies on the Anatomy and Function of Bones and Joints. Pathology of Rheumatoid Arthritis. Edited by F. Evans. Berlin, Springer-Verlag, 1966, pp 130–143.
17. Edwards, J.C.W., and Willoughby, D.A.: Demonstration of bone marrow-derived cells in synovial lining by means of giant

intracellular granules as genetic markers. Ann. Rheum. Dis., *41*:177–182, 1982.

18. Klareskog, L. et al.: Immune functions of human synovial cells. Phenotypic and T-cell regulatory properties of macrophage-like cells that express HLA-DR. Arthritis Rheum., *25*:488–501, 1982.

19. Iguchi, T., Kurosaka, M., and Ziff, M.: Electron microscopic study of HLA-DR and monocyte/macrophage staining cells in rheumatoid synovial membrane. Arthritis Rheum., *29*:600–613, 1986.

20. Poulter, L.W. et al.: The involvement of interdigitating (antigen-presenting) cells in the pathogenesis of rheumatoid arthritis. Clin. Exp. Immunol., *51*:247–254, 1983.

21. Poulter, L.W. et al.: Histochemical discrimination of HLA-DR positive cell populations in the normal and arthritic synovial lining. Clin. Exp. Immunol., *48*:381–388, 1982.

22. Katz, S.I., Tamaki, K., and Sax, D.H.: Epidermal Langerhans cells are derived from cells originating in bone marrow. Nature, *282*:324–326, 1979.

23. Steinman, R.M.: Identification of a novel cell type in peripheral lymphoid organs of mice. V. Purification of spleen dendritic cells. New surface markers and maintenance in vitro. J. Exp. Med., *149*:1–8, 1979.

24. Zvaifler, N.J. et al.: Identification of immunostimulatory dendritic cells in the synovial effusions of patients with rheumatoid arthritis. J. Clin. Invest., *76*:789–800, 1985.

25. Fox, R., Fong, S., Tsoukas, C., and Vaughan, J.H.: Characterization of recirculating lymphocytes in rheumatoid arthritis patients. J. Immunol., *132*:2883–2887, 1984.

26. Krane, S.M.: Aspects of the cell biology of the rheumatoid synovial lesion. Ann. Rheum. Dis., *40*:433–448, 1981.

27. Theofilopoulos, A.N. et al.: Evidence for presence of receptors for C3 and IgG Fc on human synovial cells. Arthritis Rheum., *23*:1–9, 1980.

28. Hendler, P.L. et al.: Human synovial dendritic cells. Direct observation of transition to fibroblasts. J. Rheumatol., *12*:660–664, 1985.

29. Fraser, J.R.E., Clarris, B.J., and Baxter, E.: Patterns of induced variation in the morphology, hyaluronic acid secretion, and lysosomal enzyme activity of cultured human synovial cells. Ann. Rheum. Dis., *38*:287–294, 1979.

30. Baker, D.G. et al.: Rheumatoid synovial cell morphologic changes induced by a mononuclear cell factor in culture. Arthritis Rheum., *26*:8–14, 1983.

31. Reference deleted.

32. Werb, Z., and Reynolds, J.J.: Stimulation by endocytosis of the secretion of collagenase and neutral proteinase from rabbit synovial fibroblasts. J. Exp. Med., *140*:1482–1490, 1976.

33. Rajah, K.T., and Merker, H.J.: Joint formation in culture. Arthritis Rheum., *34*:200–205, 1975.

34. Edwards, J.C.W., Sedgwick, A.D., and Willoughby, D.A.: The formation of a structure with the essential features of synovial lining by subcutaneous injection of air. J. Pathol., *134*:147–156, 1981.

35. Henderson, J.A. et al.: The biochemistry of the human synovial lining with special reference to alterations in metabolism in rheumatoid arthritis. Pathol. Res. Pract., *172*:1–24, 1981.

36. Henderson, B., Glynn, L.E., and Chayen, J.: Cell division in the synovial lining in experimental allergic arthritis: Proliferation of cells during the development of chronic arthritis. Ann. Rheum. Dis., *41*:275–281, 1982.

37. Mohr, W., Beneke, G., and Amohing, W.: Proliferation of synovial lining cells and fibroblasts. Ann. Rheum. Dis., *34*:219–224, 1975.

38. Nykanen, T. et al.: Characterization of the DNA-synthesizing cells in rheumatoid synovial tissue. Scand. J. Rheumatol., *7*:118–122, 1978.

39. Webb, F.W., Ford, P.M., and Glynn, L.E.: Persistence of antigen in rabbit synovial membrane. Br. J. Exp. Pathol., *52*:31–41, 1971.

40. Reference deleted.

41. Amento, E.P. et al.: Modulation of synovial cell products by a factor from a human cell line: T lymphocyte induction of a mononuclear cell factor. Proc. Natl. Acad. Sci. USA, *79*:5307–5311, 1982.

42. Hamilton, J.A. et al.: Streptococcal cell walls and synovial cell activation. J. Exp. Med., *155*:1702–1717, 1982.

43. Kinsella, T.D., Baum, J., and Ziff, M.: Studies of isolated synovial lining cells of rheumatoid and nonrheumatoid synovial membranes. Arthritis Rheum., *13*:734–753, 1970.

44. Kitlowski, N.P. et al.: Protein synthesis in articular cartilage and synovium of the rabbit. Arthritis Rheum., *8*:456–458, 1965.

45. Sisson, J.C., Castor, C.W., and Klavons, J.A.: Connective tissue activation XVIII. Stimulation of hyaluronic acid synthetase activity. J. Lab. Clin. Med., *96*:189–197, 1980.

46. Reference deleted.

47. Reference deleted.

48. Reference deleted.

49. Woolley, D.E., Harris, E.D., and Brinckerhoff, C.E.: Collagenase immunolocation in cultures of rheumatoid synovial cells. Science, *200*:773–775, 1978.

50. Shiozawa, S., Williams, R.C., Jr., and Ziff, M.: Immunoelectron/microscopic demonstration of prostaglandin E in rheumatoid synovium. Arthritis Rheum., *25*:685–693, 1982.

51. Brinkerhoff, C., and Harris, E.: Survival of rheumatoid synovium implanted in nude mice. Am. J. Path., *103*:411–418, 1981.

52. Cheung, H.S., Halverson, P.D., and McCarty, D.J.: Release of collagenase, neutral protease, and prostaglandins from cultured mammalian synovial cells by hydroxyapatite and calcium pyrophosphate dihydrate crystals. Arthritis Rheum., *24*:1338–1344, 1981.

53. Collins, A.J.: Prostaglandin synthetase activity in synovial tissue from patients with rheumatoid arthritis after therapy with aspirin-like drugs. *In* Prostaglandins and Inflammation. Edited by G.P. Lewis. Vienna, Hans Huber, 1976, pp. 27–63.

54. McGuire, M.K.B. et al.: Messenger function of prostaglandins in cell-to-cell interactions and control of proteinase activity in the rheumatoid joint. Int. J. Immunopharmacol., *4*:91–102, 1982.

55. Goetzl, E.J. et al.: Physiological approach to the assessment of disease activity in rheumatoid arthritis. J. Clin. Invest., *50*:1167–1173, 1971.

56. Ross, G.T., Marsh, J.M., and Roback, D.W.: Uridine diphosphate glucose dehydrogenase in rheumatoid synovial cells in culture. J. Rheumatol., *8*:710–715, 1981.

57. Marsh, J.M. et al.: Synthesis of sulfated proteoglycans by rheumatoid and normal synovial tissue in culture. Ann. Rheum. Dis., *38*:166–170, 1979.

58. Krane, S.M. et al.: Mononuclear cell conditioned medium containing mononuclear cell factor (MCF) homologous with interleukin-1 stimulates collagen and fibronectin synthesis by adherent rheumatoid synovial cells: Effects of prostaglandin E2 and indomethacin. Coll. Relat. Res., *5*:99–117, 1985.

59. Amento, E.P. et al.: Influences of gamma interferon on synovial fibroblast like cells. Ia induction and inhibition of collagen synthesis. J. Clin. Invest., *76*:837–848, 1985.

60. Reference deleted.
61. Scott, C.L. et al.: Significance of fibronectin in rheumatoid arthritis and osteoarthrosis. Ann. Rheum. Dis., 40:142–153, 1981.
62. Oldberg, A., and Ruoslahti, E.: Evolution of the fibronectin gene. Exon structure of cell attachment domain. J. Biol. Chem., 261:2113–2116, 1986.
63. Kornblihtt, A.R. et al.: Primary structure of human fibronectin: Differential splicing may generate at least 10 polypeptides from a single gene. EMBO J., 4:1755–1759, 1985.
64. Schwarzbauer, J.E. et al.: Three different fibronectin mRNAs arise by alternative splicing within the coding region. Cell, 35:421–431, 1983.
65. Scott, D.L., and Walton, W.: The significance of fibronectin in rheumatoid arthritis. Semin. Arthritis Rheum., 13:244–254, 1984.
66. Scott, D., Delamere, J., and Walton, K.: The distribution of fibronectin in the pannus of rheumatoid arthritis. Br. J. Exp. Pathol., 62:362–365, 1981.
66a. Ruoslahti, E., and Pierschbachler, M.: Arg-Gly-Asp: A versatile cell recognition signal. Cell, 44:517–518, 1986.
67. Wyllie, J., Haust, M., and More, R.: The fine structure of synovial lining cells in rheumatoid arthritis. Lab. Invest., 15:519–529, 1966.
68. Schumacher, H.R., Jr.: Synovial membrane and fluid morphologic alterations in early rheumatoid arthritis: Microvascular injury and virus-like particles. Ann. N.Y. Acad. Sci., 256:39–64, 1975.
69. Fassbender, H.: Pathology of Rheumatic Diseases. New York, Springer-Verlag, 1980, pp. 2–94.
70. Cruickshank, B.: Interpretation of multiple biopsies of synovial tissue in rheumatic diseases. Ann. Rheum. Dis., 11:137–145, 1952.
71. Cooper, N., et al.: Diagnostic specificity of synovial lesions. Hum. Pathol., 12:314–328, 1981.
72. Soren, A., and Waugh, T.: The giant cells in synovial membrane. Ann. Rheum. Dis., 40:496–500, 1981.
73. Osung, O., Chandra, M., and Holborrow, E.: Intermediate filaments in synovial lining cells in rheumatoid arthritis are of the vimentin type. Ann. Rheum. Dis., 41:74–77, 1982.
74. Norton, W., and Ziff, M.: Electron microscopic observations on rheumatoid synovial membranes. Arthritis Rheum., 9:589, 1966.
75. Shiozawa, S., Jasin, H., and Ziff, M.: Absence of immunoglobulins in rheumatoid cartilage-pannus junctions. Arthritis Rheum., 23:816–821, 1980.
76. Shiozawa, S., Shiozawa, K., and Futita, T.: Morphologic observations in the early phase of the cartilage-pannus junction. Arthritis Rheum., 26:472–477, 1983.
77. Klareskog, L., Forsum, U., and Wigzell. H.: Murine synovial intima contains Ia,Ie/c positive bone marrow-derived cells. Scand. J. Immunol., 15:509–514, 1982.
78. Konttinen, Y. et al.: Characterization of the immunocompetent cells of rheumatoid synovium from tissue sections and eluates. Arthritis Rheum., 24:71–79, 1981.
79. Young, C.L. et al.: Immunohistologic characterization of synovial membrane lymphocytes in rheumatoid arthritis. Arthritis Rheum., 27:32–39, 1984.
80. Trowbridge, I.S., Omary, N.B., and Battifora, H.: Human analogue of murine T200 glycoprotein. J. Exp. Med., 152:842–852, 1980.
81. Kung, P.C. et al.: Strategies for generating monoclonal antibodies defining human T-lymphocyte differentiation antigens. Transplant. Proc., 12:141–146, 1980.
82. Malone, D.G. et al.: Immune function in severe, active rheumatoid arthritis. A relationship between peripheral blood mononuclear cell proliferation to soluble antigens and synovial tissue immunohistologic characteristics. J. Clin. Invest., 74:1173–1185, 1984.
83. Decker, J.L. et al.: NIH conference. Rheumatoid arthritis: Evolving concepts of pathogenesis and treatment. Ann. Intern. Med., 101:810–824, 1984.
84. Wilder, R.L. et al.: The pathogenesis of group A streptococcal cell wall-induced polyarthritis in the rat. Arthritis Rheum., 26:1442–1451, 1983.
85. Wahl, S.M. et al.: Leukapheresis in rheumatoid arthritis. Association of clinical improvement with reversal of anergy. Arthritis Rheum., 26:1076–1084, 1983.
86. Mizel, S.B.: Interleukin-1 and T cell activation. Immunol. Rev., 63:51–72, 1982.
87. Wood, D., Ihrie, E., and Hamerman, D.: Release of interleukin-1 from human synovial tissue in vitro. Arthritis Rheum., 28:853–860, 1985.
88. Muraguchi, A., et al.: The essential role of B cell stimulatory factor 2 (BSF2) for terminal differentiation of B-cells. J. Exp. Med., (in press), 1987.
89. Klareskog, L. et al.: Evidence in support of a self perpetuating HLA-DR dependent delayed type cell reaction in rheumatoid arthritis. Proc. Natl. Acad. Sci. USA, 79:3632–3636, 1982.
90. Stastny, P.: Rheumatoid arthritis: Relationship with HLA-D. Am. J. Med., 75:9–15, 1983.
91. Zabriske, J.B., and Freimer, E.H.: An immunological relationship between group A streptococcus and mammalian muscle. J. Exp. Med., 124:661–680, 1966.
92. Rhodes, G. et al.: Human immune responses to synthetic peptides from the Epstein-Barr nuclear antigen. J. Immunol., 134:221–216, 1985.
93. Alspaugh, M.A. et al.: Elevated levels of antibodies to Epstein-Barr virus antigens in sera and synovial fluids of patients with rheumatoid arthritis. J. Clin. Invest., 67:1134–1140, 1981.
94. Fox, R.I. et al.: Epstein-Barr virus in rheumatoid arthritis. Clin. Rheum. Dis., 11:665–688, 1985.
95. Fox, R.I. et al.: Rheumatoid arthritis synovial membrane contains a 62 Kd protein that shares an antigenic epitope with the Epstein-Barr virus encoded EBNA-1 antigen. J. Clin. Invest., 77:1539–1547, 1986.
96. Tosato, G., Steinberg, A.D., and Blaese, R.M.: Defective EBV-specific suppressor T-cell function in rheumatoid arthritis. N. Engl. J. Med., 305:1238–1243, 1981.
97. Fox, R.I. et al.: Lack of reactivity of rheumatoid arthritis synovial membrane with cloned Epstein Barr virus DNA probes. J. Immunol., 137:498–501, 1986.
98. Holoshitz, J. et al.: T-lymphocytes of rheumatoid arthritis patients show augmented reactivity to a fraction of any bacteria cross reactive with cartilage. Lancet, 2:305–309, 1986.
99. Simpson, R.W. et al.: Association of parvoviruses with rheumatoid arthritis of humans. Science, 223:1425–1428, 1984.
100. Lotz, M., Carson, D.A., and Vaughan, J.H.: Substance P activation of rheumatoid synoviocytes: Neural pathway in the pathogenesis of arthritis. Science, 235:893–895, 1987.
101. Lembeck, F., and Holzer, P.: Substance P as neurogenic mediator of antidromic vasodilation and neurogenic plasma extravasation. Naunyn Schmiedebergs Arch. Pharmacol., 310:175–183, 1979.
102. Inman, R.D., Chin, B., and Marshall, K.W.: Substance P and arthritis: Analysis of plasma and synovial fluid levels. Arthritis Rheum., 29:S9, 1986.

103. Payan, D.G. et al.: Substance P recognition by a subset of human T lymphocytes. J. Clin. Invest., *74*:1537–1539, 1984.

104. Hartung, H.P., Wolters, K., and Toyka, K.V.: Substance P: Binding properties and studies on cellular responses in guinea pig macrophages. J. Immunol.,*136*:3856–3863, 1986.

105. Bar-Shavit, Z. et al.: Enhancement of phagocytosis: A newly found activity of substance P residing in its N-terminal tetrapeptide sequence. Biochem. Biophys. Res. Commun., *94*:1445–1451, 1980.

106. Davies, P.: The effect of anti-rheumatic agents on macrophage function. Int. J. Immunopharmacol., *4*:111–118, 1982.

16

CHONDROCYTE STRUCTURE AND FUNCTION

EDITH R. SCHWARTZ

Articular cartilage is a unique tissue in that it is aneural, avascular, and alymphatic. It is also unusual in the relative sparsity of cells distributed throughout the preponderance of extracellular matrix. The shape, size, and arrangement of these cells, known as chondrocytes, vary according to their location within the articular cartilage.

On the basis of light microscopy, articular cartilage is divided into three zones: a tangential zone, a transitional zone, and a deep or radial zone. Chondrocytes in the superficial layer are small, are regularly aligned parallel to the articulating surface, and have a spindle shape. In the next zone descending from the articulating surface, the transitional zone, the chondrocytes are larger, round or ovoid in shape, and more heterogeneous in distribution. In the deep or radial zone, the chondrocytes are larger yet and are stacked in groups of four or five perpendicular to the articulating surface. In the deepest region of the radial zone, the calcified zone, the chondrocytes' shape is modified by events associated with mineralization.[1]

Chondrocytes have the full complement of subcellular components. Within the cell, the nucleus, surrounded by a nuclear envelope, is situated eccentrically inside the cytoplasm. Smooth and rough-surfaced endoplasmic reticulum, Golgi apparatus, mitochondria, and lysosomes are contained within the cytoplasm.[2]

Bones grow in length by the process of interstitial growth within cartilage followed by endochondral ossification. In long bones, the two sites for cartilaginous growth are articular cartilage and epiphyseal-plate or growth-plate cartilage. Whereas in long bones the articular cartilage is the growth plate for the epiphysis, the epiphyseal plate provides growth in length of the metaphysis and diaphysis. By convention, the epiphyseal-plate cartilage has been divided into four zones: the zones of resting cartilage, proliferative cartilage, maturing cartilage, and calcifying cartilage. The chondrocytes in the calcifying zone were formerly believed to be inactive or actually to have died as a result of calcification of the matrix.[3]

Improved techniques in prefixation and fixation of cartilage have given new insight into the changes associated with normal maturation of proliferating chondrocytes into hypertrophic cells in growth-plate cartilage. The hypertrophic zone in growth-plate cartilage extends from the lower limit of the proliferative zone to the region of vascular invasion (Figs. 16–1 and 16–2). Hypertrophic chondrocytes have now been shown to be differentiated and metabolically active cells with intact subcellular constituents. The metabolic products that they synthesize and secrete, as well as the ultrastructure of these cells, are distinct from those of chondrocytes that reside in the proliferative zone, however (Fig. 16–3).[4]

Thus, in contrast to the previous concept of chondrocytes as dormant cells, it now appears that chondrocytes are multipotential cells capable of carrying out all the functions necessary to synthesize and degrade the constituents of the extracellular matrix that surrounds them. Further, in addition to the presence of membrane receptors for systemically transported

289

FIG. 16–1. Frontal section through part of the proximal area of the tibia of the rat, illustrating the epiphyseal bone (E), growth-plate cartilage (G), zone of vascular invasion (V), and metaphysis (M) (toluidine blue O, ×10).

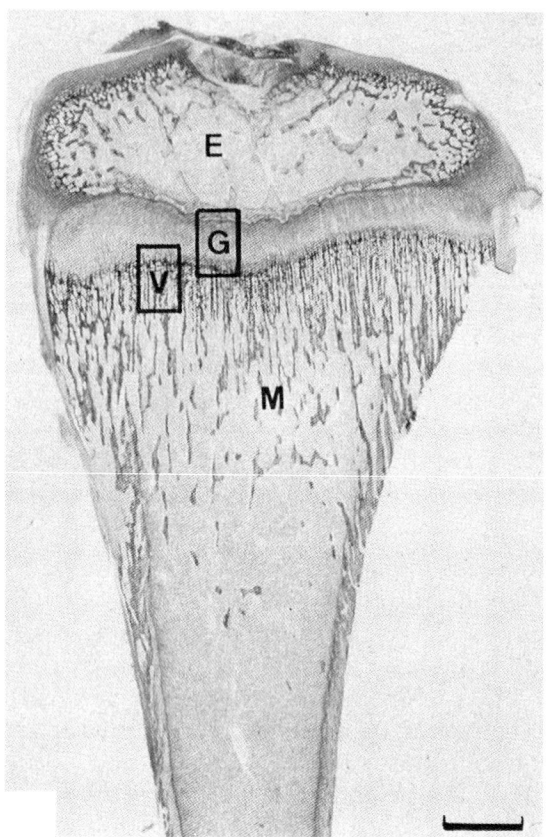

FIG. 16–2. High-magnification photomicrograph of the growth plate (inset G in Fig. 16–1), fixed in glutaraldehyde containing ruthenium hexamine trichloride and toluidine blue (×170). The proliferating zone (PZ) is characterized by flat cells with similar heights, arranged in distinct columns. The hypertrophic zone (HZ) consisting of a lower and upper half based on geometric considerations, extends from the lower limit of the proliferating zone to the region of vascular invasion (IZ).

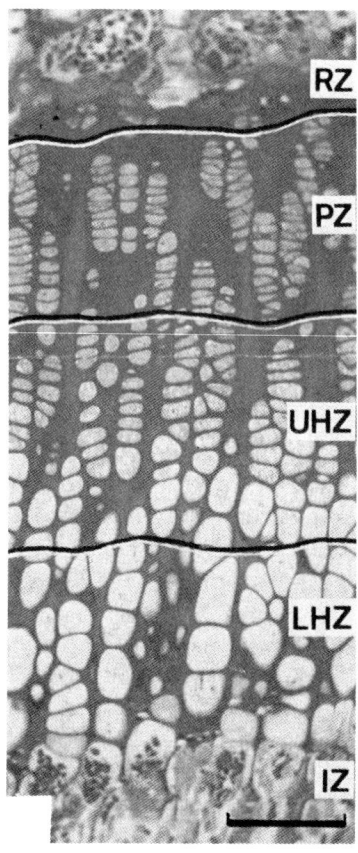

metabolic modulators, the cells themselves produce multiple factors necessary to regulate their milieu.

PRODUCTS OF CHONDROCYTE SYNTHESIS

Normal cartilage is about 70% hydrated.[5] In addition to water, the extracellular matrix constituents surrounding the chondrocytes include collagen, proteoglycans, and other simple and complex proteins, lipids, and carbohydrates.

Collagen is the largest component of articular cartilage by dry weight. Type II collagen, specific for cartilage and the most prevalent genetic type in cartilage, consists of three identical chains of 100,000 daltons each. The arrangement of collagen fibers varies and is site dependent, similar to the site dependency of the cells. The fibers along the articulating surface are thin, are regularly aligned, and lie parallel to this surface. Although the fibers are more randomly distributed in the transitional zone, they have prescribed geometric features with relation to the cells of this region. With the use of scanning electron microscopy, it has been shown that the collagen fibers form a "woven nest" about each chondrocyte. In the radial zone, the fibers are thick and are perpendicular to the articulating surface.[6]

Several other genetic types of collagen are synthesized in cartilage, albeit to a lesser extent. These include type IX, type X, and 1-α, 2-α, and 3-α chains (type XI). Type IX collagen has both a collagen and a proteoglycan domain. It consists of 3 chains of 68,000, 84,000, and 115,000 daltons. Chondroitin sulfate chains are attached exclusively to the largest component.[7] Type X collagen appears to be synthesized exclusively by chondrocytes in the lower hypertrophic

FIG. 16–3. Electron micrographs of a proliferating (top) and a hypertrophic (bottom) chondrocyte (fixation with ruthenium hexamine trichloride; top ×4300 and bottom ×2200). N = nucleus; M = mitochondria; E = rough endoplasmic reticulum; G = Golgi area; V = vacuoles; and P = pericellular matrix.

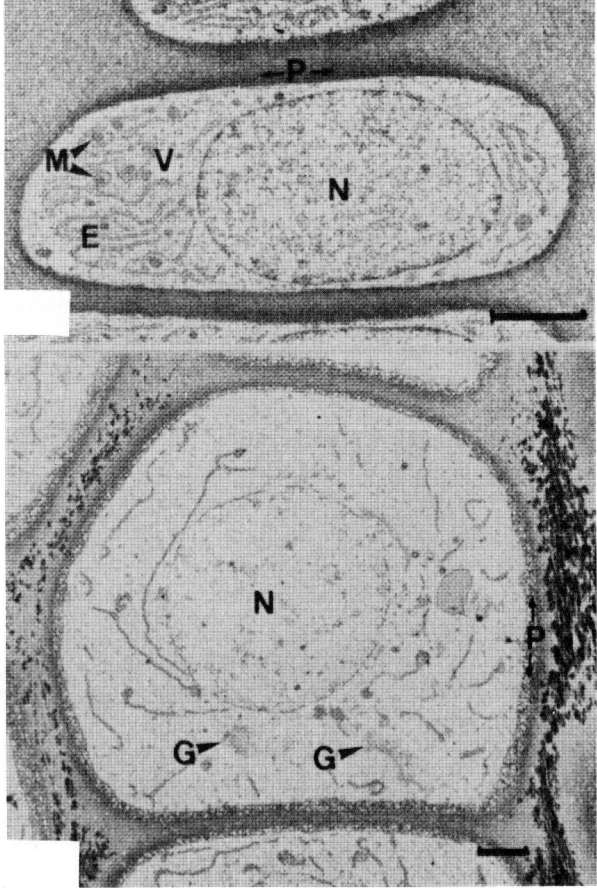

FIG. 16–4. Electrophoretic patterns of collagen purified from normal (N) and osteoarthritic (OA) cartilage derived from the knees of guinea pigs showing mild-to-severe osteoarthritic changes. The disease had been induced surgically in the right hind knee joint of the animals by severance of the anterior cruciate and medial collateral ligaments combined with partial meniscectomy. The normal cartilage was obtained from the contralateral nonoperated left knee joint. Starting from the left, lanes 1 and 2, lanes 3 and 4, and lanes 5 and 6 represent animals with mild, moderate, and severe osteoarthritic lesions, respectively. The characteristic pattern of type II collagen is evident. Type I collagen, purified from guinea pig skin, is shown for comparison purposes in the far-right lane.

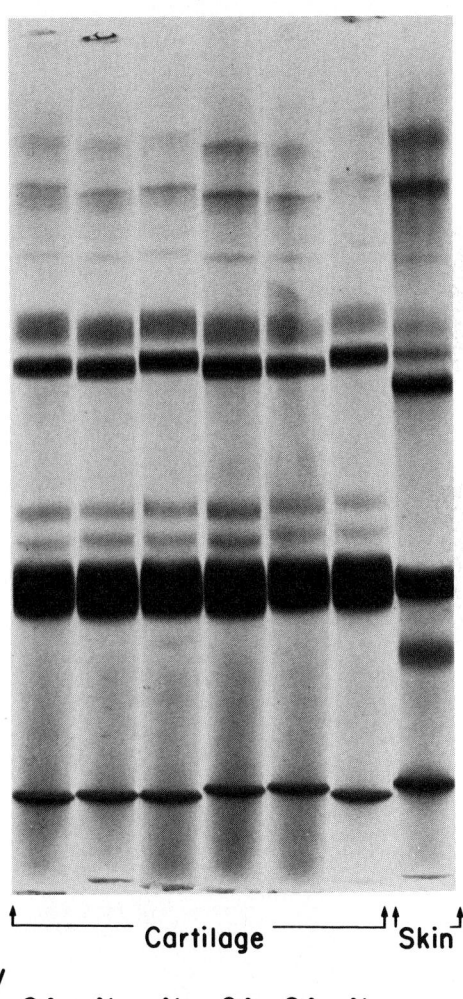

zone.[8] Comparison of collagen contained in normal and osteoarthritic articular cartilage derived from a guinea pig model of osteoarthritis, in which the disease was surgically induced, showed no quantitative changes in the composition of either type II or type XI collagen. The turnover rates of both collagens were higher in the diseased tissue, however[9] (Figs. 16–4 and 16–5). In contrast to a previous report, no conversion in the synthesis of type II to type I collagen was observed in organ cultures of osteoarthritic human articular cartilage.[10,11]

Proteoglycans, the other major component of the extracellular matrix, are complex macromolecules composed of protein and both sulfated and nonsulfated glycosaminoglycans. The suprastructure formed by proteoglycans in conjunction with collagen is responsible for the strength and resilience of articular cartilage. The basic proteoglycan structure, known as the proteoglycan subunit, consists of a protein core to which keratan sulfate, chondroitin sulfate, oligosaccharides, and phosphate moieties are attached covalently. These subunits, in turn, form aggregates through noncovalent interaction with hyalu-

FIG. 16–5. Lanes 1 and 2 (left to right) depict the electrophoretic patterns of type XI collagen from normal and osteoarthritic guinea pig articular cartilage, respectively, after separation from other collagens by fractional precipitation. The electrophoretic pattern of the purified total collagen is shown in lane 3 for normal and lane 4 for osteoarthritic guinea pig cartilage. The disease had been surgically induced in the right hind knee joint of the animal, as described in the legend to Figure 16–4.

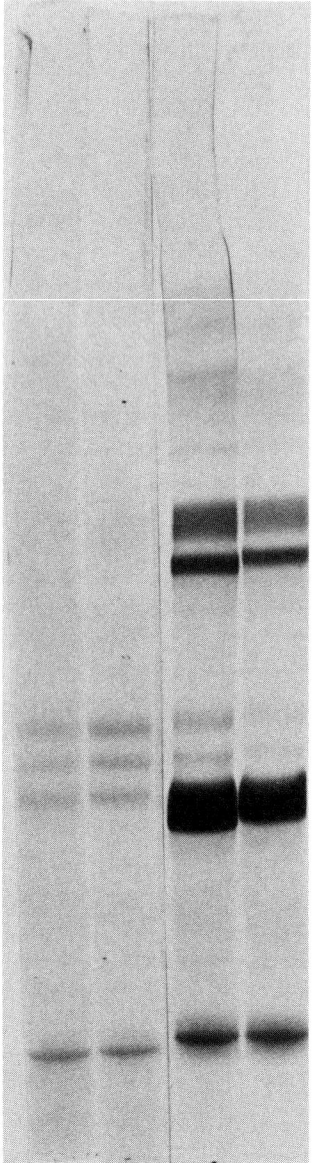

ronic acid. The stability of the aggregates is increased by glycoproteins known as link proteins, which bind both to hyaluronic acid and to proteoglycan.[12–14]

MECHANISMS OF SYNTHESIS AND METABOLISM BY CHONDROCYTES

Much of the present-day knowledge of proteoglycan structure and metabolism has come from studies of chondrocyte culture systems. With the use of appropriate media, it has been possible to simulate in vivo properties of cartilage in these cultures. For example, the higher metabolic turnover rate of proteoglycans that characterizes human osteoarthritic articular cartilage was reflected when this parameter was compared in cultures of chondrocytes derived from normal and osteoarthritic human articular cartilage. The increased metabolic activity of osteoarthritic chondrocytes was further enhanced when fetal calf serum was replaced by human serum in the culture medium. This finding suggests that circulating factors act synergistically with factors produced by chondrocytes to regulate proteoglycan metabolism.[15]

That chondrocytes reflect their in vivo activities with regard to proteoglycan metabolism was further demonstrated recently when chondrocytes isolated and cultured from different zones of cartilage were compared. Keratan sulfate predominates in the deeper zone of articular cartilage. When monolayer cultures were established from chondrocytes isolated from the more superficial and deeper zones of cartilage, cells with high keratan sulfate production came from the lower region of the articular cartilage. Those from the superficial zone were negative for keratan sulfate production.[16] Thus, although the chondrocyte is the unique cell type in cartilage, the structure of newly synthesized proteoglycans is controlled by the chondrocyte's location within the tissue. These specific properties are retained under proper culture conditions.

Studies of proteoglycan synthesis conducted in chondrocyte cultures have shown that the rate-limiting step is the synthesis of the protein core that occurs in the cisternae of the rough endoplasmic reticulum.[17] Subsequently, the core protein is phosphorylated, followed by the addition of oligosaccharides and glycosaminoglycans in the Golgi apparatus.[18,19] Specifically, chondroitin sulfate synthesis on the protein core occurs in the medial trans-Golgi compartment.[20] Although proteoglycan and link proteins have been shown to co-localize within Golgi vesicles of chondrocytes, hyaluronic acid appears to be synthesized elsewhere.[21,22] Proteoglycan aggregate formation, therefore, occurs only after the components have been secreted from the cell. Proteoglycan aggregate formation is regulated, in part, by the extent of phosphorylation of the core protein.[23]

In addition to these two major constituents, chondrocytes synthesize the other structural macromolecules, regulatory factors, and enzymes necessary for development and maintenance of cartilage. As with other cells, chondrocytes possess the machinery to process, if necessary, the newly synthesized molecules into active forms.

As previously indicated, much of our knowledge of the properties of chondrocytes comes from studies in cell culture. It has been important to verify that properties of chondrocytes in culture duplicate their behavior in all respects with those in situ. This duplication has been demonstrated in several laboratories. For example, my co-workers and I have shown that, under culture conditions, chondrocytes derived from osteoarthritic cartilage express hypermetabolic activity when compared with those derived from age-matched normal cartilage. This result is analogous to what is found in the tissue of origin. Even after cell passage, the chondrocytes from osteoarthritic cartilage express higher levels of degradative enzyme activities, such as arylsulfatase B and acid phosphatase. Thus, the information for this alteration is inherent in the chondrocyte and is retained on cell division.[24]

Chondrocytes can remain viable and continue to undergo metabolic turnover for several months when they are maintained in cell culture in the absence of growth factors. Under these long-term culture conditions, cell numbers remain static, however. Thus, although serum factors contribute to cell attachment, cell growth, and regulation of chondrocyte metabolism, the information necessary for basal levels of chondrocyte function is inherent in the cell.[25]

REGULATION OF METABOLIC ACTIVITIES OF CHONDROCYTES

Recently, clinicians and scientists have focused on factors that regulate the metabolic activities of chondrocytes and thus control cartilage development, normal turnover, and alterations associated with disease states. The earliest interest focused on "sulfation factor," a compound recognized to enhance sulfated proteoglycan synthesis in cartilage.[26] As the amino acid sequence of this polypeptide became known, it was recognized to be a member of a group of factors called somatomedins, specifically *somatomedin C*.[27] This compound was found to be synthesized by the liver in response to growth-hormone influence. In addition

to its action on liver cells, however, growth hormone has now been found to stimulate chondrocytes to synthesize and to secrete somatomedin C directly. This finding has suggested that the growth-promoting effect of growth hormone on cartilage in vivo is partly mediated by local production of somatomedin C.[28]

Results from binding studies, as well as the elucidation of the amino acid sequence, have shown significant homology between somatomedin C and insulin and have prompted the renaming of somatomedin C to *insulin-like growth factor 1* (IGF-1). Recent evidence has suggested a "dual-effector theory," which defines an essential metabolic role for IGF-1 in concert with growth hormone. It was proposed that growth hormone first causes cell differentiation, after which IGF-1 serves as a mitogenic signal to cause mitosis of newly differentiated chondrocytes.[29]

Trippel and co-workers have studied the effects of somatomedin C or IGF-1 on chondrocytes isolated from the epiphyseal growth plate, the tissue directly responsible for skeletal growth. Although chondrocytes of all the epiphyseal zones bind somatomedin C, the greatest binding was by the cells in the proliferative zone. Binding occurred through specific receptor interaction followed by internalization of somatomedin C by the cell.[30]

In addition to IGF-1, cartilage also produces *cartilage-derived growth factor* (CDGF), a peptide that causes proliferation of chondrocytes. In one study, proliferation was accompanied by an increase in hyaluronic acid synthesis and a decrease in sulfated glycosaminoglycan synthesis.[31] Furthermore, CDGF stimulated the proliferation of and was chemotactic for endothelial cells.[32] In the murine model, chondrocytes from the hypertrophic region synthesize a factor that is also chemotactic for endothelial cells. Although it is not known whether this factor is identical to CDGF, its secretion into the extracellular matrix by hypertrophic chondrocytes appears to induce capillaries to grow into the cartilaginous epiphysis toward the hypertrophic chondrocyte. It is postulated that these processes induce mineralization and endochondral bone formation.[33]

ROLE IN DISEASE

Chondrocytes are in a uniquely isolated environment in cartilage; yet they respond to local and systemic changes as do cells of other tissues. Chondrocytes play an active role in endochondral ossification and in the formation of primary and secondary centers of ossification. Furthermore, under normal conditions, they maintain a balanced extracellular matrix throughout their life. Disequilibrium of this homeostasis occurs frequently, however, and diseases of cartilage result, particularly in the various arthritides in which erosion of the articular cartilage characterizes disease progression. To understand the mechanisms that regulate cartilage breakdown, as well as the role of the chondrocyte in mediating these processes, local and systemic effectors that enter the cartilage by way of diffusion and modulate these processes need to be identified.

Several years ago, Dingle and co-workers described *catabolin*, a factor derived from synovium that stimulated chondrocytes to release degradative enzymes capable of causing cartilage breakdown.[34] Thereafter, Krane and co-workers reported the isolation of a monocyte-derived factor with similiar properties that also caused inflammation.[35] Both factors have now been identified as *interleukin-1* (IL-1), a mediator of numerous physiologic effects including fever production, bone resorption, and inflammation. With the use of rabbit articular chondrocytes in vitro, IL-1 enhanced the production and secretion of latent metalloproteinases and prostaglandin E_2 (PGE_2) and reduced the activity of plasminogen activator in a dose-dependent manner.[36]

Previous studies in vivo had shown that injection of recombinant IL-1 into the knees of rabbits resulted in the loss of proteoglycans from articular cartilage. In contrast to the in vitro studies, the pathologic response could not be attributed to an increased production of PGE_2, but rather appeared to result from stimulation of degradative enzymes.[37]

Other in vitro studies using rabbit articular chondrocytes showed that IL-1 also stimulated proteoglycanase production. This enzyme, a metalloproteinase that degrades proteoglycans, requires cobalt and calcium for activation.[38] The enhancement of phospholipase A_2 activity in rabbit articular chondrocytes by IL-1 was recently described by Chang and co-workers; it was proposed that this was the first step in the cascade of events by which the inflammatory action of IL-1 is manifested.[39] It is therefore clear that IL-1 has multiple effects on chondrocytes.

Other effectors have also been shown to mediate cartilage metabolism. Both *epidermal growth factor* and *transforming growth factor β* have inhibited collagen and glycosaminoglycan synthesis by rabbit articular chondrocytes. Together, these factors have been mitogenic.[40] Tumor necrosis factor, which shares some activities with IL-1, has stimulated the release of metalloproteinases from chondrocytes.[36]

In contrast to previous thinking, which attributed only a passive role to chondrocytes, these cells are now recognized to be active participants in the maintenance of intact cartilage under normal conditions as well as when challenged by disease. Chondrocytes are multipotential cells that respond to immunogenic challenges. Whereas normal human chondrocytes are negative for I_a antigens both in situ and in cell culture, these cell-surface antigens are readily inducible when chondrocytes are stimulated with recombinant γ-interferon.[41] These data further support the premise that chondrocytes play an active role in the destruction of cartilage in inflammatory joint diseases such as rheumatoid arthritis.

Chondrocytes also have receptors for numerous pharmacokinetic agents, including histamine. An initial observation detailed the dose-dependent increases in cyclic adenosine monophosphate (cAMP) and PGE_2 production when chondrocytes were exposed to histamine. The cells were shown to have histamine$_2$ (H_2) receptors. The PGE_2 production was further stimulated by pre-exposing the chondrocytes to factors released by the synovium. It appears that histamine-induced PGE_2 production by chondrocytes is mediated both by activation of H_1 and H_2 receptors and subsequent liberation of arachidonic acid.[42]

Despite its unique setting within a tissue that has neither lymphatic system nor blood supply, and has no nerve endings, the chondrocyte has exquisite sensitivity to alterations in the physiologic state of other parts of the body. This sensitivity is made possible through the processes of active and passive diffusion into the cartilage of multiple effectors that can bring and communicate appropriate signals to the chondrocyte through receptor interactions.

REFERENCES

1. Stockwell, R.A., and Meachim, G.: The chondrocytes. *In* Adult Articular Cartilage, 2nd Ed. Edited by M.A.R. Freeman. New York, Grune and Stratton, 1979, pp. 69–145.
2. Weiss, C., Rosenberg, L., and Helfet, A.J.: An ultrastructural study of normal young adult human articular cartilage. J. Bone Joint Surg. (Am.), *50*:664–674, 1968.
3. Salter, R.B.: Textbook of Disorders and Injuries of the Musculoskeletal System. Baltimore, Williams & Wilkins, 1983, p. 8.
4. Hunziker, E.B., Schenk, R.K., and Cruz-Orive, L.M.: Quantitation of chondrocyte performance in growth-plate cartilage during longitudinal bone growth. J. Bone Joint Surg. (Am.), *69*:162–173, 1987.
5. Mankin, H.J., and Thrasher, A.Z.: Water content and binding in normal and osteoarthritic cartilage. J. Bone Joint Surg. (Am.), *57*:76–80, 1975.
6. McDevitt, C.A.: Biochemistry of articular cartilage: nature of proteoglycans and collagen of articular cartilage and their role in aging and in osteoarthritis. Ann. Rheum. Dis., *32*:364–378, 1978.

7. Vaughn, L., Winterhalter, K.H., and Bruckner, P.: Proteoglycans Lt from chicken embryo sternum identified as type IX collagen. J. Biol. Chem., *260*:4758–4763, 1985.

8. Keilty, C.M., et al.: Type X collagen, a product of hypertrophic chondrocytes. Biochem. J., *227*:545–554, 1985.

9. Schwartz, E.R.: Surgically induced osteoarthritis in guinea pigs: studies of proteoglycans, collagen, and non-collagen proteins. *In* Osteoarthritis: Current Clinical and Fundamental Problems. Edited by J.G. Peyton. Paris, Ciba-Geigy, 1985, pp. 273–288.

10. Nimni, M., and Deshmukh, K.: Differences in collagen metabolism between normal and osteoarthritic human articular cartilage. Science, *181*:751–752, 1973.

11. Fukae, M.G., Mechanic, G., Adamy, L., and Schwartz, E.R.: Chromatographically different type II collagens from human normal and osteoarthritic cartilage. Biochem. Biophys. Res. Commun., *67*:1575–1580, 1975.

12. Heinegard, D., and Paulsson, M.: Structure and metabolism of proteoglycans. *In* Extracellular Matrix Biochemistry. Edited by K. Piez and H. Reddi. New York, Elsevier, pp. 277–328.

13. Tang, L.H., Rosenberg, L., Reiner, A., and Poole, A.: Proteoglycans from bovine nasal cartilage. J. Biochem., *254*:10,523–10,531, 1979.

14. Hardingham, T.E.: The role of link-protein in the structure of cartilage proteoglycan aggregates. Biochem. J., *177*:237–247, 1979.

15. Schwartz, E.R., Kirkpatrick, P.R., and Thompson, R.C.: Sulfate metabolism in human chondrocyte cultures. J. Clin. Invest., *54*:1056–1064, 1974.

16. Zanetti, M., Ratcliffe, A., and Watt, F.M.: Two subpopulations of differentiated chondrocytes identified with a monoclonal antibody to keratan sulfate. J. Cell Biol., *101*:53–59, 1985.

17. Kimura, J., Lohmander, S., and Hascall, V.C.: Studies on the biosynthesis of cartilage proteoglycans in a model system of cultured chondrocytes from the swarm rat chondrosarcoma. J. Cell Biochem., *26*:261–278, 1984.

18. Schwartz, E.R.: Phosphorylation of proteoglycans and link proteins in human cartilage. Orthop. Trans., *10*:437–438, 1986.

19. Kimura, J.H., Caputo, C.B., and Hascall, V.C.: The effects of cycloheximide on synthesis of proteoglycans by cultured chondrocytes from the swarm rat chondrosarcoma. J. Biol. Chem., *256*:4268–4376, 1984.

20. Ratcliffe, A., Fryer, P., and Hardingham, T.E.: Proteoglycan biosynthesis in chondrocytes: protein A-gold localization of proteoglycan protein core and chondroitin sulfate within Golgi subcompartments. J. Cell Biol., *101*:2355–2365, 1985.

21. Kimura, J.H., Hardingham, T.E., Hascall, V.C., and Solursh, M.: Biosynthesis of proteoglycans and their assembly into aggregates in cultures of chondrocytes from the swarm rat chondrosarcoma. J. Biol. Chem., *254*:2600–2609, 1979.

22. Philipson, L., and Schwartz, N.: Subcellular location of hyaluronate synthetase in oligodendroglioma cells. J. Biol. Chem., *259*:5017–5023, 1984.

23. Anderson, R.S., and Schwartz, E.R.: The effect of phosphorylation/dephosphorylation of human proteoglycan subunits on aggregate formation. Orthop. Trans., *9*:340–341, 1985.

24. Colofiore, J.R., and Schwartz, E.R.: Monensin stimulation of arylsulfatase B activity in human chondrocytes. J. Orthop. Res., *4*:273–280, 1986.

25. Schwartz, E.R., and Sugumaran, G.: Proliferation and maintenance of human chondrocyte cultures in defined medium. In Vitro, *18*:254–260, 1982.

26. Sledge, C.B.: Structure, development and function of joints. Orthop. Clin. North Am., *6*:619–628, 1975.

27. Van Wyck, J.J., Svoboda, M.E., and Underwood, L.E.: Evidence from radioligand assay that somatomedin-C and insulin-like growth factor-1 are similar to each other and different from other somatomedins. J. Clin. Endocrinol. Metab., *50*:206–208, 1980.

28. Schlechter, N.L., Russell, S.M., Spencer, E.M., Nicoll, C.S.: Evidence suggesting that the direct growth-promoting effect of growth hormone on cartilage in vivo is mediated by local production of somatomedin. Proc. Natl. Acad. Sci. U.S.A., *83*:7932–7934, 1986.

29. Nilsson, A., et al.: Regulation by growth hormone of number of chondrocytes containing IGF-1 in rat growth plate. Science, *233*:571–574, 1986.

30. Trippel, S., Van Wyk, J.J., and Mankin, H.J.: Localization of somatomedin C binding to bovine growth-plate chondrocytes in situ. J. Bone Joint Surg., *68*:897–903, 1986.

31. Hamerman, D., Sasse, J., and Klagsbrun, M.: A cartilage derived growth factor enhances hyaluronate synthesis and diminishes sulfated glycosaminoglycan synthesis in chondrocytes. J. Cell Physiol., *127*:317–322, 1986.

32. Lobb, R., et al.: Purification and characterization of heparin-binding endothelial cell growth factors. J. Biol. Chem., *261*:1924–1928, 1986.

33. Floyd, W.E., et al.: Vascular events associated with the appearance of the secondary center of ossification in the murine distal femoral epiphysis. J. Bone Joint Surg., *69*:185–190, 1987.

34. Dingle, J.T., et al.: A cartilage factor from synovium. Biochem. J., *184*:177–180, 1979.

35. Krane, S.M., Dayer, J.M., Simon, L.S., and Byrne, S.: Mononuclear cell-conditioned medium containing mononuclear cell factor (MCF), homologues with interleukin-1, stimulates collagen and fibronectin synthesis by adherent rheumatoid synovial cells: effects of prostaglandin E$_2$ and indomethacin. Collagen Relat. Res., *5*:99–117, 1985.

36. Schnyder, H.J.G., Payne, T., and Dinarello, C.: Human monocyte or recombinant interleukin 1's are specific for the secretion of a metalloproteinase from chondrocytes. J. Immunol., *138*:469–503, 1987.

37. Pettipher, E.R., Higgs, G.A., and Henderson, B.: Interleukin 1 induces leukocyte infiltration and cartilage proteoglycan degradation in the synovial joint. Proc. Natl. Acad. Sci. U.S.A., *83*:8749–8753, 1986.

38. Shimmei, M., Miyazaki, K., Kituchi, T., and Shimomura, Y.: An assay for proteoglycanase and its application to articular chondrocyte cultures. Agents Actions *18* (Suppl.):103–108, 1986.

39. Chang, J., Gilman, S.C., and Lewis, A.J.: Interleukin 1 activates phospholipase A$_2$ in rabbit chondrocytes: a possible signal for IL 1 action. J. Immunol., *136*:1283–1287, 1986.

40. Skantze, K.A., Brinckerhoff, C.E., and Collier, J.P.: Use of agarose culture to measure the effect of transforming growth factor beta and epidermal growth factor on rabbit articular chondrocytes. Cancer Res., *45*:4416–4421, 1985.

41. Jahn, B., et al.: Changes in cell surface antigen expression on human articular chondrocytes induced by gamma-interferon. Arthritis Rheum., *30*:64–74, 1987.

42. Taylor, D.J., Yoffe, J., Brown, D.M., and Wooley, D.E.: Histamine H$_2$ receptors on chondrocytes derived from human, canine, and bovine articular cartilage. Biochem. J., *225*:315–319, 1985.

17

IMMUNOGLOBULINS AND THEIR GENES

J. CLAUDE BENNETT

Immunoglobulin molecules are responsible for two major biologic functions: (1) the recognition of foreign substances (receptor function); and (2) the elimination or destruction of these foreign substances (effector function). The functions require that the immune system have the potential to interact with an almost limitless number of antigens. To react with these substances in highly specific ways, the immune system must generate an enormous degree of molecular diversity. Among immunoglobulin molecules, by far the most complex heterogeneity is found at the level of structural differences that relate to the specificity of an antibody binding site and define the idiotype. The specificity of all antibodies is determined by the primary structure of the combining region, variation in which is the main source of heterogeneity of immunoglobulins. In addition, other structural differences define the isotypes, recognized classes of immunoglobulins, whose existence has been demonstrated in all members of the species. Both serologic and amino acid sequencing studies have shown the existence of a limited number of these classes and subclasses of antibodies, which differ from each other in specific structural ways, although they are invariably related. They also each seem to have unique biologic properties. Finally, as one would expect, there are subtle yet specific genetic polymorphisms of immunoglobulins, as have been identified for many other families of protein molecules (allotype).

Several general features of the immunoglobulins deserve mention here in the context of our understanding of this system in relation to rheumatologic diseases. First, the various classes and subclasses of immunoglobulins seem to have special functions that relate to immunologic defense mechanisms. For example, IgA, the major class of immunoglobulin present in all external secretions, is responsible for protecting the mucosal surfaces from the primary attack of exogenous substances. A second general consideration is that, either as a result of cross reactivities or alteration of antigens that are presented to the immune system of the host or as a result of unique genetic rearrangements of immunoglobulin genes, certain sets of clones of cells may produce antibodies that are reactive with self-constituents.[1] Such aberrations in the immune response are most often encountered in rheumatoid arthritis, in systemic lupus erythematosus, and in related disorders. One would assume, as discussed in other chapters of this text, that these immunologic reactions play a significant role in the pathogenesis of some of the manifestations of these diseases.[2]

STRUCTURE OF AN ANTIBODY MOLECULE

The basic structure of all immunoglobulins is the same. Immunoglobulins are made of 2 types of polypeptide chains (Fig. 17–1). The larger is called the heavy (H) chain. The other, because it is smaller, is known as the light (L) chain. Each immunoglobulin subunit consists of 2 identical H and 2 identical L chains, which are generally held together by disulfide

FIG. 17–1.   Basic model of the immunoglobulin molecule structure. See text for description.

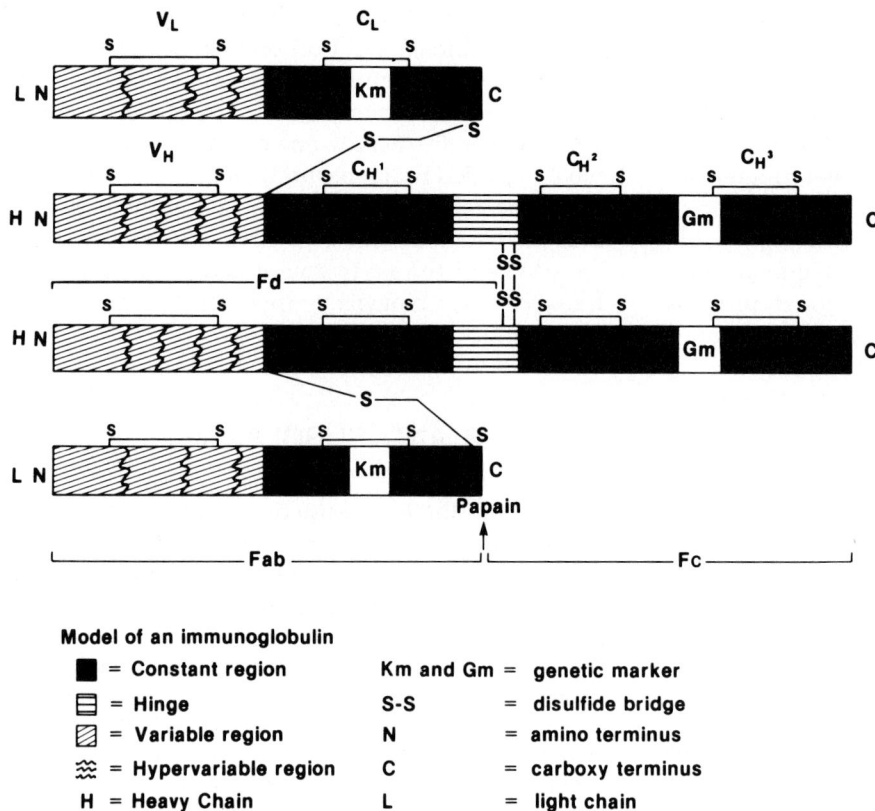

Model of an immunoglobulin

■ = Constant region	Km and Gm = genetic marker
▤ = Hinge	S-S = disulfide bridge
▨ = Variable region	N = amino terminus
≋ = Hypervariable region	C = carboxy terminus
H = Heavy Chain	L = light chain

bonds, and hence the molecular formula is H_2L_2.[3] The disulfide bonds joining the H and L chains connect the carboxy termini of the light chains to the heavy chains. The interheavy chain disulfide bridges vary in number from 1 to 11 for the different classes and subclasses and are generally located in the center of the H chain in a region known as the "hinge," which is unusually rich in cysteine and proline. The molecular weight of the light chain is about 25,000; that of the heavy chain varies between 25,000 and 65,000 daltons. The differences in size are related to differences in the structure of the "hinge," that is, in the γ3 subclass of IgG, or to the presence of an extra domain in the μ and ε heavy chains. Each polypeptide chain can be divided into a series of globular subunits or domains, each of which is about 110 residues in length and is characterized by a highly conserved intrachain disulfide bridge, which spans about 60 residues and makes the domain compact. The domains are separated by more extended regions known as the interdomain stretches. Based on amino acid sequence studies showing a high degree of homology between different domains, it would appear that they are the result of a series of gene duplications. In those classes, and in subclasses in which functional localization of

various biologic properties has been achieved, it seems that the several domains may have evolved to serve different biologic functions.[4]

Comparison of the amino acid sequences of a large number of homogeneous immunoglobulins has documented that each of the chains can be divided structurally and functionally into two major regions. One of these, the amino terminal (110–120 residues), is known as the variable (V) region because of the amino acid sequence variation among different myeloma proteins and antibodies belonging to a given class. The remaining half of the L chain and three-quarters of the H chain are known as the constant regions (C) because their structure is virtually the same for all molecules belonging to a single immunoglobulin class or subclass.

Abundant structural, functional, and x-ray diffraction evidence now supports the concept that the variable regions are directly involved in the antigen-binding sites of the molecule and that the sites are composed of one or more "hypervariable regions," which in the three-dimensional structure of the molecules are in close proximity and thus are able to react with the antigen.[5] The three hypervariable regions in the light chains and four in the heavy chains, though far separated in the linear sequence, are in close proximity in the fully folded molecule. It would appear from immunologic analyses that the hypervariable regions are intimately involved in the idiotypic determinants of the antibody, and antibodies with the same specificity commonly have similar if not identical hypervariable regions. Spanning the remainder of the variable segments are the so-called framework regions, which show less variability among different molecules and contribute to the variable region subclass specificity. Numerous amino acid sequence studies of myeloma proteins and Bence Jones proteins have shown the existence of subclasses of V regions for λ and κ chains, and at least three H chain variable region subclasses, which are found in all general classes and subclasses of heavy chains. The antigen-binding sites (one per H-L pair) are located at the tip of the molecule and consist of both H and L chains; however, in most antibodies studied to date, the H chain plays a greater role in determining the specificity of the antibody than the L chain.[5]

The constant region consists of either three or four domains and, in most classes, it also contains the interdomain or hinge region in the center of the molecule. Comparison of the structure of the constant regions of different classes and subclasses of H chains shows striking homologies among many of them. In the case of the four subclasses of IgG, this homology is greater than 95%. The structural features of the C regions seem to determine those biologic functions that distinguish different classes and subclasses of immunoglobulins from each other and to influence the localization and sites of action of all immunoglobulins. Thus, the C_H2 domain seems to be important in most subclasses in complement fixation and in regulating the catabolic properties of an antibody, whereas the C_H3 domain is important in the interaction of immunoglobulins with receptors on many cells, including monocytes, neutrophils, lymphocytes, and endothelial cells. Obviously, these interactions with a variety of cells are important in initiating the process of phagocytosis, in allowing certain subclasses to traverse the placenta, and in influencing many of the biologic functions of lymphocytes, platelets, and other cells. The antigenic determinants reactive with rheumatoid factors seem to be located in more than one domain.[6]

Although the H and L chains are the true structural subunits of immunoglobulins, a simple way of obtaining biologically active fragments with differing biologic properties is by proteolytic digestion, which occurs preferentially at the hinge region.[7] The products obtained differ for different enzymes. Thus, papain yields an Fc and two Fab fragments, whereas pepsin degrades the Fc fragment and yields the two Fab fragments still joined by a disulfide bridge—(Fab')2. Other enzymes, or these enzymes under different conditions, yield different types of fragments that are equally useful in dissecting the biologic functions of the molecule. These proteolytic fragments, which generally include one or more intact domains, have provided much useful biologic information, because the Fab fragments composed of the light chain and Fd fragment (see Fig. 17–1) can combine with antigen, and the Fc fragment can be used to study the secondary biologic properties of immunoglobulins.

CLASSES AND SUBCLASSES

Although the basic structure of all antibody molecules is similar, all species of animals studied to date have a series of immunoglobulin classes and subclasses (Fig. 17–2). They appear to have evolved from

FIG. 17–2. Basic subunit diagrams of the various immunoglobulin classes depicting their disulfide bonding patterns and, in the case of IgA$_1$, IgA$_2$, and IgM, indicating that they may exist as polymeric structures. See text for further description. (Redrawn from Hilschmann, N., et al.: Naturwissenschaften, *65*:617, 1978.)

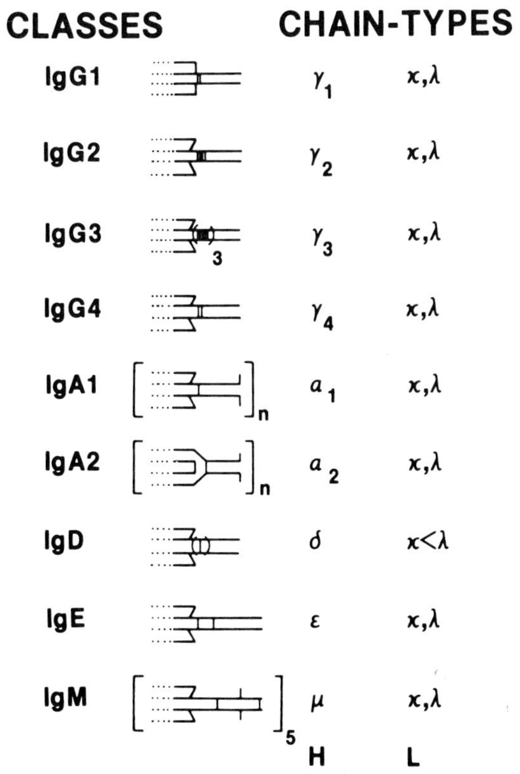

CLASSES		CHAIN-TYPES	
IgG1		γ_1	κ, λ
IgG2		γ_2	κ, λ
IgG3		γ_3	κ, λ
IgG4		γ_4	κ, λ
IgA1		a_1	κ, λ
IgA2		a_2	κ, λ
IgD		δ	$\kappa < \lambda$
IgE		ε	κ, λ
IgM		μ	κ, λ
		H	L

each other, but differ in the structure and, consequently, the function of the constant domains of the heavy chains. These are all under control of a series of closely linked genes,[8] as discussed later. In a broad sense, one can regard the classes and subclasses in a similar manner. For example, $IgG_{1,2,3,4}$ all have the same basic structural design and differ only in the primary sequence of their constant regions and the location of their interchain disulfide bonds. The H chain in each of these subclasses is referred to as γ_1, γ_2, and so forth. The L chain may be of either the κ or the λ type. IgA exists as two subclasses, with H chain designations as α_1 and α_2, respectively, and again the light chains may either be of the κ or λ type. IgD and IgE have H chains designated δ and ϵ, respectively, and in the case of IgM, which exists as a pentamer, the H chain is termed μ. Again, in all classes, the L chain may either be κ or λ. Furthermore, in additional polypeptide chains in those classes, molecules exist as polymers. One such chain, the J chain, is present in both IgA and IgM when they are in the polymeric state.[9] This 15,000-dalton molecule appears to be important in initiating the disulfide bonded polymer formation. In the case of IgA, a 70,000-dalton secretory component binds to the molecule and is present only in the external secretions. It seems to be important in playing a receptor-like role for IgA as it transits the secretory epithelial cells, as well as in allowing secretion. In addition, the secretory component may protect the polymers against proteolysis.[10] Table 17–1 lists the five major classes of immunoglobulins in man and describes some of their physical and chemical features. Table 17–2 compares the four subclasses of IgG, the two of IgA, and the classes of IgM, IgD, and IgE from the standpoint of their biologic function.

IgG

IgG, the major immunoglobulin class, provides the bulk of antibody activity in response to most antigens. Most IgG molecules are avid in reacting with complement and in initiating the enzymatic cascade consequent to complement fixation; however, IgG_1 and IgG_3 are most effective. IgG_4 does not fix complement effectively in the native state, but has been reported to do so after proteolytic cleavage. Studies with various types of fragments suggest that complement fixation is a property of the C_H2 domain. There are some differences in the ability of different subclasses to interact with receptors on the surface of neutrophils, monocytes, and lymphocytes. As a consequence, IgG_1 and IgG_3 are most active in opsonization by neutrophils and monocytes and participate most effectively in the phenomenon of antibody-mediated cytotoxicity. The Fc fragments of all four subclasses of IgG can interact with rheumatoid factors. IgG_1 and IgG_3 do so more effectively, however. The structural and genetic studies[11] suggest that the subclasses of IgG are under separate genetic control.

IgM

The biologic and clinical significance of this class of immunoglobulin was initially appreciated when it was recognized that rheumatoid factors present in serum are generally macroglobulins with antibody activity to IgG. In the last 20 years, however, its significance in many other areas of the immune response has been fully established. IgM exists in two forms. One is the basic subunit, the 8S 180,000-dalton IgM with a molecular formula μ_2L_2. This fraction is minor in serum, but appears to be the major component in lymphocyte surfaces.[12] The other and major form is the 19S, 900,000-dalton pentameric IgM $(\mu_2L_2)5J$, in which five subunits are disulfide bridged and generally contain one molecule of J chain, which joins two of the subunits by a disulfide bridge.[13] IgM is the predominant immunoglobulin in many primary immune responses and can, at times, as in the case of rheumatoid factors, cold agglutinins, and isoagglu-

Table 17–1.   Selected Properties of Immunoglobulin Classes

	IgG	IgA	IgM	IgD	IgE
Molecular weight	160,000	170,000 or polymer	900,000	160,000	180,000
Sedimentation constant	7S	7S (9, 11, 13)	19S	7S	8S
Approx. concentration serum (mg/dl)	1,000–1,500	250–300	100–150	.3–30	.0015–.2
Valence	2	2 (monomer)	10	2	2
Molecular formula	γ_2L_2	$(\alpha_2L_2)_n$	$(\mu_2L_2)_5$	δ_2L_2	ϵ_2L_2
Half-life (days)	23	6	5	3	2.5
Special property	Placental passage	Secretory Ig	Primary response Lymphocyte surface	Lymphocyte surface	Reagin

Table 17–2. Selected Biologic Properties of Classes and Subclasses of Immunoglobulins

	IgG				IgA		IgM	IgD	IgE
	1	2	3	4	1	2			
Percentage of total (%)	65	20	10	5	90	10			
Major genetic factors	Gm a, f, z	n	b, g	4 a, b	A_1m	A_2m			
Complement fixation	+ +	+	+ +	−	−	−	+ +	−	−
Complement fixation (alternative)					+	+		±	±
Placental passage	+	+	+	+	−	−	−	−	−
Fixing to mast cells or basophils	−	−	−	−	−	−	−	−	+
Binding to:									
—Macrophages	+	±	+	±	−	−	−	−	−
—Neutrophils	+	+	+	+	+	+	−	−	−
—Platelets	+	+	+	+	−	−	−	−	−
—Lymphocytes	+	+	+	+	−	−	+	−	−
Reaction with Staphylococcus A	+	+	−	+	−	−	−	−	−
Half-life (days)	23	23	8–9	23	6	6	5	3	2.5
Synthesis mg/kg/day	25	?	3.5	?	24	?	7	.4	.02

tinins, remain the major or sole antibody for long periods of time. It differs from most other immunoglobulins in having a heavy chain that is larger owing to the presence of an extra domain. IgM is avid in complement fixation, and studies suggest that this property resides in the $C\mu4$ domain.[14] As is the case for all immunoglobulins, the valence of the μ_2L_2 subunit is two. Because it consists of five subunits, IgM has ten combining sites for small antigens, but because of steric factors, half the sites appear to be blocked when IgM reacts with large protein antigens. As a consequence, the valence for large antigens is five, and rheumatoid factor exists in serum in the form of a 22S complex $(\mu_2L_2)5$-$(IgG)5$.

IgA

Second in concentration to IgG in serum is the IgA fraction, which generally exists in the form of a monomer (α_2L_2), but on occasion, especially in patients with myeloma, as a polymer $(\alpha_2L_2)2,3$-J. Although in serum there appears to be no particular function for IgA, it plays a major role in the so-called secretory immune system. The secretory IgA has several unique features. First, it is synthesized largely by plasma cells located in, or originating from, the lymphoid tissues in the intestinal tract. In the secretions, the molecule usually exists in the form of a polymer linked to another molecule, the 70,000-dalton secretory component (SC), which is synthesized by the epithelial cells lining the gut. The function of the SC remains uncertain. It appears to serve as a receptor for IgA[15] and thus may play a role in attracting IgA-bearing lymphocytes to the gut and other organs of secretion. It

may also attract circulating IgA to the surface of the epithelial cells within which the molecule combines to the secretory component. A second function may be to make the secretory IgA complex more resistant to proteolytic digestion; several in vitro studies have shown that the complex is more resistant to degradation than the IgA without secretory component.[16] The observation that several bacterial enzymes digest IgA_1 and not IgA_2 in the hinge region may explain why IgA_2 is more abundant in external secretions than in the serum, where it makes up a minor fraction of IgA.[17]

The importance of this immune system in the host defense cannot be overestimated. Most infectious agents enter through the gastrointestinal and respiratory tracts and initiate a local immune response involving, primarily, the IgA fraction. Consequently, as demonstrated in the polio vaccination program, oral vaccinations in general may prove to be more effective than those by the systemic route. It seems likely that this local immune system plays a major role also in the genitourinary, lacrimal, salivary, and respiratory systems and that it may be the primary defense against a variety of environmental pathogens, even though IgA is less able to activate the complement system or to initiate phagocytosis.

IgD

IgD is a minor immunoglobulin and, even though some serum antibodies have been identified in this class in man, it appears to serve no unusual function and is absent from the serum of mice and primates. Its primary role in man and all these species appears to be to function as one of the two major surface receptors on B lymphocytes together with monomeric IgM. Although it seems likely that the interaction of these surface molecules with antigen is necessary to trigger and perhaps also to suppress lymphoid function, no data are available to define a distinct biologic function in this regard for either of these two surface antigen recognition units. Free IgD differs from the other immunoglobulins in its unusual susceptibility to digestion by a variety of proteolytic enzymes.[18]

IgE

The distribution of IgE is largely extravascular, and its turnover is rapid, with a half-time of about 2 days. The major type of antibody associated with IgE is the reaginic antibody that plays a role in a variety of allergic conditions. Through their interaction with receptors on mast cells and basophils, the IgE reaginic antibodies, in the presence of antigens, cause the release of histamine and various other vasoactive substances, which are responsible for clinical manifestations of various allergic states. IgE antibodies may play a protective role in numerous parasitic infections, perhaps by increasing vascular permeability, thus permitting other types of antibodies to be active.

IMMUNOGLOBULIN GENE ORGANIZATION

As discussed in earlier sections of this chapter, pairs of light and heavy chains fold into discrete structural V region domains that bind the antigens. These domains consist of approximately 107 amino acids from a light chain and approximately 125 amino acids from a heavy chain. Within the V region domain, 3 short polypeptide loops (hypervariable regions) from each of the heavy and the light chains form the antigen-binding sites. This extraordinary degree of variability defined within the V regions also gives rise to the idiotypic determinants.

Extensive amino acid sequence determination on various myeloma proteins, both from man and from mouse, led to an appreciation that the heavy chains and the 2 types of light chains κ and λ, are each encoded by a separate multigene family. The variability of the V region of a single immunoglobulin polypeptide chain, in conjunction with a nearly invariant constant region, gave rise to the concept that the functionally distinct V and C regions of these polypeptides are encoded by independent genetic elements within each gene family.[19,20] That is, more than one gene is required to encode a single polypeptide chain.

The development of the technology for recombinant DNA led to the ability to clone immunoglobulin genes and to develop extensive libraries of gene fragments that could be used to determine the molecular organization of immunoglobulin genes.[21–25] The initial studies of the light chains confirmed the prediction and showed a large separation between the V and C regions. As shown in Figure 17–3, embryonic DNA contained gene elements coding for the leader sequence, a V region gene separated by over 3 kb from a C region gene, and an interspersed J region gene, which accounted for residues 98 through 110. In the process of message formation, the V and J regions were linked together through a deletion of the intervening sequence. In the case of a myeloma cell, there was already some juxtaposition in which the V-J joining had occurred, but the C sequences were still at some distance. This was faithfully transcribed in the primary RNA, and additional splicing occurred before a mature messenger was produced. This finding agreed with the 2 gene/1 polypeptide hypothesis; V and C sequences are encoded separately in the germ line and are rearranged to form an active V-C gene in antibody-producing cells.[19,20] The coding regions are referred to as *exons* and the intervening sequences as *introns*.

In the case of the V_κ sequences, which have a minimum of perhaps 300 different groups, it seems that a library of possible V_κ genes exists from which selected sequences undergo combination with one of the four J_κ regions. This would provide a mechanism for the generation of considerable diversity because J_κ segments are not restricted to any one V_κ group. Such V-J joining might occur through a mechanism of inverted palindrome reading. It is also evident from the way in which the joining occurs that sequence variation may be seen at the point of a junction. This would explain the exceptional variability at position 96 that has been observed in the mouse κ chains.[26,27]

The heavy chain genes are developed in a similar way, with the provisions for the immunoglobulin class switching that occurs during ontogeny.[28] In this situation, the various constant region areas related to each class or subclass can be spliced to a given V region through a switching recognition point. This event is shown in its simplest form in Figure 17–4. The actual picture, relative to the constant regions, is more complex. From what we know about the globular domains of the immunoglobulin C regions, and from what we have already learned about genes existing in fragments, we should not be surprised to see that the C genes exist with the C_H1 domain separated

FIG. 17–3. Genetic events involved in gene segment organization and messenger RNA (mRNA) splicing during the development of an immunoglobulin-secreting cell line. (L = leader sequence; V = variable region; J = joining region; C = constant region of the genome.) See text for further description.

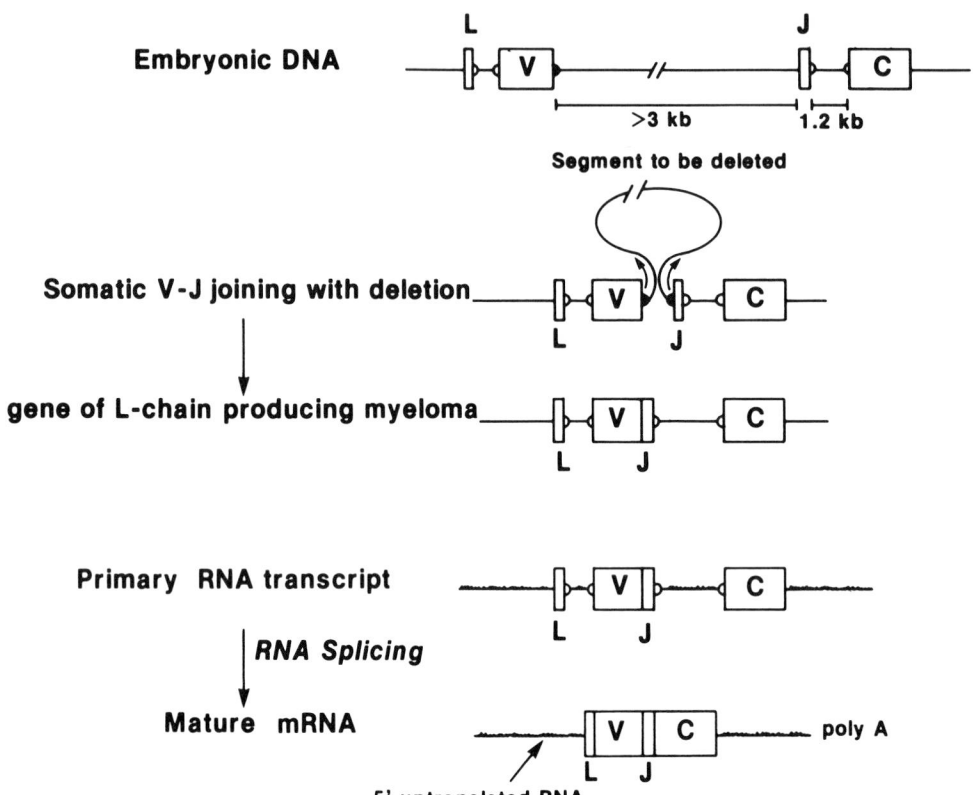

from the hinge region domain, separated from a C_H2 domain, separated from a C_H3 domain[29] as shown in Figure 17–5. Such a separation of the domains, requiring splicing before the final message is read, explains how certain of the heavy-chain diseases may develop.

Furthermore, the total variable region is more complex for the heavy chains, involving the splicing together of three segments (V, D, and J) rather than two, as in the light chain. The new area in heavy chain genes is called D because it may be viewed as a diversity-generating segment[23] (Fig. 17–6).

As can be seen in this joining scheme, a single V_H region is drawn from the V library, a single D is drawn from the D library, and a single J from the J library, all of which are then spliced together. Perhaps through a recognition mechanism, suggested by consistent intervening sequences, appropriate joining takes place. Thus, the whole pattern for differentiation of immunoglobulin heavy chains involves the joining of V, D, and J segments, as well as the nec-

essary switching of S segments that are homologous to each other and that identify recognition sets for splicing in the various C genes. This process seems to be enhanced by transcription.[30] If the heavy-chain gene family had 200 V, 12 D, and 4 J gene segments, 9.6×10^3 V_H genes ($200 \times 12 \times 4$) could be generated by combinatorial joining.[31] Similarly, class-specific switching may allow a single V_H gene to be associated with 8 different C_H genes, permitting distinct effector functions to be used. Six sources for the generation of somatic diversity may be seen: (1) combinatorial diversity, by combining the various gene segments; (2) junctional site diversity at the V_L-J_L, V_H-D, and D-J_H junctions, because of imprecise joining; (3) junctional insertion diversity where several nucleotides are inserted without template direction; (4) somatic mutational events;[32] especially near the junctional areas; (5) upstream exchange of rearranged V_H segments;[33] and (6) combinatorial association of heavy and light chains. Obviously, mechanisms 2, 3, 4, and 6 amplify the potential diversity implied in the combinatorial calculations.

FIG. 17–4. Immunoglobulin H chain class switching in the mouse. The molecular events involved in switching from expression of one class of immunoglobulin to another are depicted, showing first the gene organization during μ chain synthesis. In the second situation is shown a switch region recombination event resulting in a deletion of all the DNA up to the α gene necessary for ultimate expression of the α polypeptide chain. The S loci indicate switch-specific codons. (Adapted from Honjo, H.: Annu. Rev. Immunol., *1*:515, 1983.)

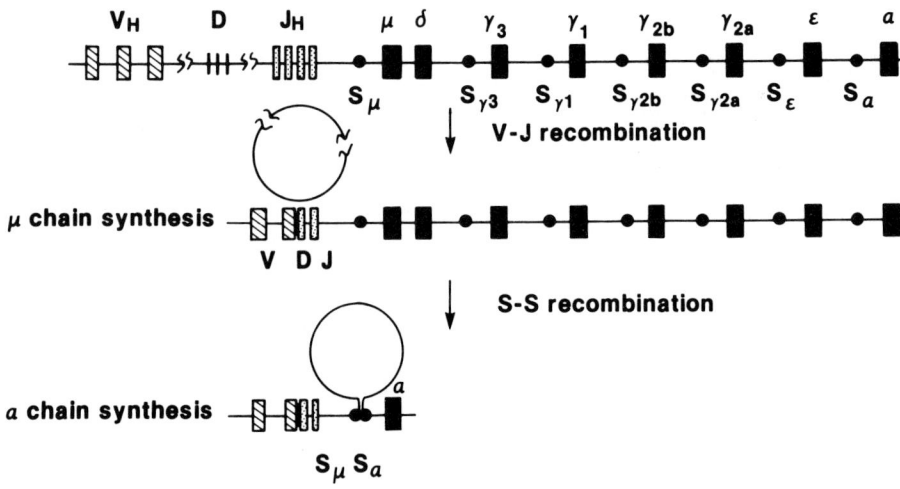

CLINICAL SIGNIFICANCE

Although one must be careful not to overuse and overemphasize technical assays in clinical situations, one must not overlook the importance of the immune system in analyzing the clinical status of the patients with rheumatic diseases. Clearly, evaluation of auto-antibodies, and particularly the clonal repertoire of response in disease states, is likely to be of increasing importance at not only the fundamental level but also the applied clinical level as well. The real significance of immunoglobulins as they relate to rheumatic diseases, however, stems from the knowledge they have given us of the immune system, its regulation, its genetic organization, as well as from the new avenues of approach provided us for defining ways in which perturbations of this system take place.[2] Only through these new approaches can we ever hope to modify such perturbations in a predetermined and clinically effective way. Additionally, studies of immunoglobulin genes have provided an exciting new avenue for the study of somatic cell differentiation and molecular

FIG. 17–5. Molecular events involved in gene segment splicing for the constant region domains of the heavy chain. See text for further description.

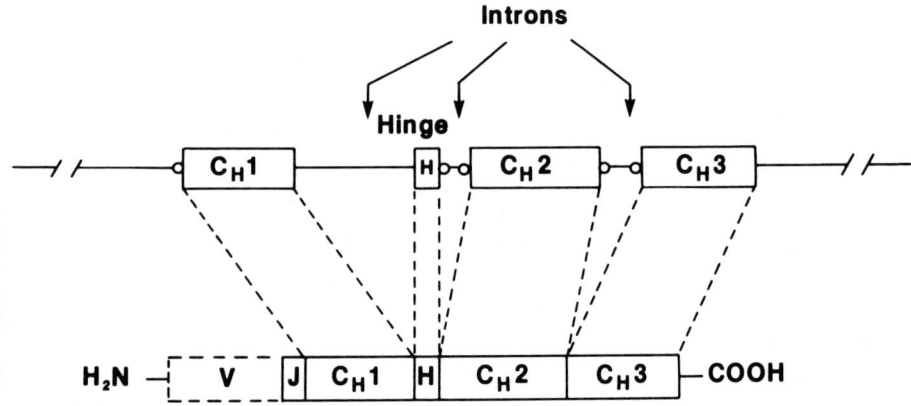

FIG. 17–6. Gene segment joining mechanisms generate diversity within the V region of the heavy chains. Shown is a combination of events selecting out V, D, and J regions of the heavy chain.

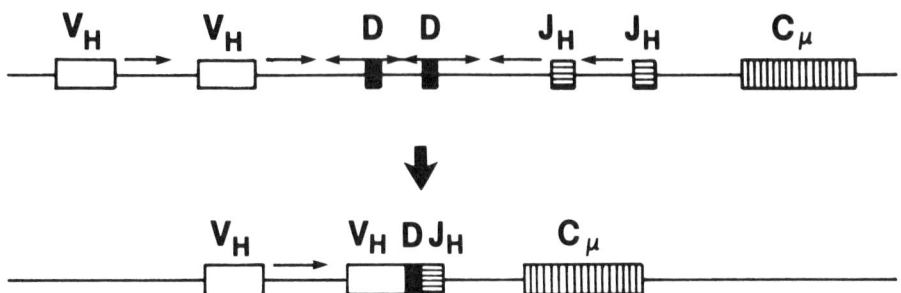

diversity in general.[34,35] As we come to understand the ways in which all these mechanisms are regulated at the molecular level, we should be able to apply the appropriate knowledge to reverse pathologic alterations in the immune system.

REFERENCES

1. Milstein, C.: From antibody structure to immunological diversification of immune response. Science, 231:1,261–1,268, 1986.
2. Arant, S.E., Griffin, J.A., and Koopman, W.J.: V$_H$ gene expression is restricted in anti-IgG antibodies from MRL autoimmune mice. J. Exp. Med., 164:1,284–1,300, 1986.
3. Edelman, G.M.: Antibody structure and molecular immunology. Science, 180:830–840, 1973.
4. Yasmeen, D., et al.: The structure and function of immunoglobulin domains. IV. The distribution of some effector functions among the Cγ2 and Cγ3 homology regions of human immunoglobulin G^1. J. Immunol., 116:518–526, 1976.
5. Davie, D.R., and Metzger, H.: Structural basis of antibody function. Annu. Rev. Immunol., 1:87–117, 1983.
6. Turner, M.W., et al.: Genetic (Gm) antigens associated with subfragments from the Fc fragment of human immunoglobulin G. Nature 221:1,166–1,169, 1969.
7. Franklin, E.C., and Frangione, B.: Structural variants of human immunoglobulin. In Contemporary Topics in Molecular Immunology. Edited by F.P. Inman, and W.J. Mandy. New York, Plenum Publishing, 1975, pp. 89–126.
8. Calame, K.L.: Mechanisms that regulate immunoglobulin gene expression. Annu. Rev. Immunol., 3:159–195, 1985.
9. Koshland, M.E.: The coming of age of the immunoglobulin J. chain. Annu. Rev. Immunol., 3:425–453, 1985.
10. Underdown, B.J., and Dorrington, K.J.: Studies on the structural and conformational basis for the relative resistance of serum and secretory immunoglobulin A to proteolysis. J. Immunol., 112:949–959, 1974.
11. Natvig, J.B., and Kunkel, H.G.: Human immunoglobulins: classes, subclasses, genetic variants, and idiotypes. Adv. Immunol., 16:1–59, 1973.
12. Marchalonis, J.J., Cone, R.E., and Atwell, J.L.: Isolation and partial characterization of lymphocyte surface immunoglobulins. J. Exp. Med., 135:956–971, 1972.
13. Zikan, J., et al.: Secondary structure of the immunoglobulin J chain. Proc. Natl. Acad. Sci. U.S.A., 82:5,905–5,909, 1985.
14. Hurst, M., et al.: The structural basis for binding of complement by immunoglobulin M. J. Exp. Med., 140:1,117–1,121, 1974.
15. Crago, S.S., et al.: Secretory component on epithelial cells is a surface receptor for polymeric immunoglobulin. J. Exp. Med., 147:1,832–1,837, 1978.
16. Brown, W.R., Newcomb, R.W., and Ishizaka, K.: Proteolytic degradation of exocrine and serum immunoglobulins. J. Clin. Invest., 49:1,374–1,380, 1970.
17. Plaut, A.G., et al.: Neisseria gonorrhoeae and Neisseria meningitidis: extracellular enzyme cleaves human immunoglobulin A. Science, 190:1,103–1,105, 1975.
18. Takahashi, Y., et al.: Complete covalent structure of a human immunoglobulin D: sequence of the λ light chain. Proc. Natl. Acad. Sci. U.S.A., 80:3,686–3,690, 1983.
19. Dreyer, W.J., and Bennett, J.C.: The molecular basis of antibody formation: a paradox. Proc. Natl. Acad. Sci. U.S.A., 54:864–869, 1965.
20. Seidman, J.G., and Leder, P.: The arrangement and rearrangement of antibody genes. Nature, 276:790–795, 1978.
21. Leder, P.: Mechanisms of gene evolution. JAMA, 248:1,582–1,591, 1982.
22. Perlmutter, R.M., et al.: Diversity in the germline antibody repertoire: Molecular evolution of the T15 V$_H$ gene family. J. Exp. Med., 162:1,998–2,016, 1985.
23. Sabano, H., et al.: Identification and nucleotide sequence of a diversity DNA segment (D) of immunoglobulin heavy-chain genes. Nature, 290:562–570, 1981.
24. Takahashi, N., et al.: Structure of human immunoglobulin gamma genes: Implications for evolution of a gene family. Cell, 29:671–679, 1982.
25. Waldmann, T.A., et al.: Molecular genetic analysis of human lymphoid neoplasms. Ann. Intern. Med., 102:497–510, 1985.
26. Leder, P.: The genetics of antibody diversity. Sci. Am., 246:102–115, 1982.
27. Max, E.E., Seidman, J.B., and Leder, P.: Sequences of five potential recombination sites enclosed close to an immunoglobulin κ constant region. Proc. Natl. Acad. Sci. U.S.A., 76:3,450–3,454, 1979.
28. Kataoka, T., Miyata, T., and Honjo, T.: Repetitive sequences in class-switch recombination regions of immunoglobulin heavy chain genes. Cell, 23:357–368, 1981.
29. Adams, J.M., et al.: Organization and expression of murine immunoglobulin genes. Immunol. Rev., 59:5–14, 1981.

30. Blackwell, T.K., et al.: Recombination between immunoglobulin variable region gene segments is enhanced by transcription. Nature 324:585–589, 1986.

31. Tonegawa, S.: Somatic generation of antibody diversity. Nature, 302:575–581, 1983.

32. Wysocki, L., Manser, T., and Gefter, M.L.: Somatic evolution of variable region structures during an immune response. Proc. Natl. Acad. Sci. U.S.A., 83:1,847–1,851, 1986.

33. Reth, M., et al.: A novel V_H to $V_H DJ_H$ joining mechanism in heavy-chain-negative (null) pre-B cells results in heavy-chain production. Nature, 322:840–842, 1986.

34. Staudt, L.M., et al.: A lymphoid-specific protein binding to the octamer motif of immunoglobulin genes. Nature, 323:640–643, 1986.

35. Yancopoulos, G.D., and Alt, F.W.: Developmentally controlled and tissue-specific expression of unrearranged V_H gene segments. Cell, 40:271–281, 1985.

STRUCTURE AND FUNCTION OF MONOCYTES AND MACROPHAGES

18

RALPH SNYDERMAN and MARILYN C. PIKE

The human immune system has evolved the capability of performing a number of vital protective functions, including defense against microbes, resistance to the development of neoplasms, and removal of denatured substances and nonvital tissues. Efficiency in the elimination of substances by the immune system depends on its ability to identify what is to be destroyed and to eliminate the identified agent rapidly. The immune system has unique features that permit the surveillance and removal of "unwanted" materials. In addition to fixed structures, such as the thymus, spleen, lymph nodes, and bone marrow, the immune system is comprised of motile cells that are able to localize rapidly at virtually any site within the host. For example, billions of leukocytes accumulate at sites of bacterial invasion within hours of their penetration into tissues. The immune system is also the only tissue with the potential to destroy other components of the host. The destructive potential of the immune system is necessary for its host-protective function, but it is also responsible for the tissue damage common to most rheumatic disorders.

Conceptually, the immune system can be divided into three functional units that mediate recognition, recruitment (amplification), and effector functions. The interaction of foreign or denatured substances with either nonspecific or specific recognition components of the immune system results in the generation of inflammatory mediators that then recruit and activate effector cells. Amplification systems are the source of mediators, termed "phlogistic" agents, which alter vascular permeability, enhance local blood flow, and stimulate the egress, chemoattraction, and activation of effector cells that destroy the inciting agent.[1]

The macrophage is central to the recognition, amplification, and effector functions of the immune system. Since the seminal observations of Elie Metchnikoff in the late nineteenth century, the phagocytic nature of macrophages has been recognized as an important component of host defense against infection.[2-5] Macrophages are wandering phagocytes that contain a broad repertoire of intracellular degradative and oxidative enzymes. Both polymorphonuclear leukocytes and macrophages have chemotactic, phagocytic, antibacterial, and secretory capabilities, but unlike polymorphonuclear leukocytes, macrophages play a crucial role in immunoregulation, have the ability to differentiate further (become activated), and often are the first components of the immune system to encounter an antigen. The nature of the interaction of macrophages with an antigen may subsequently determine the immunogenicity of the antigen or its ability to induce tolerance.[6,7] Processing of antigen by macrophages as well as its presentation in the context of mixed histocompatibility (MHC) loci is obligate for most subsequent lymphocyte responses. Lymphocytes and their secretory products, called *lymphokines*, may augment macrophage egress to inflammatory sites, enhance effector functions, or regulate macrophage functions in other ways. In turn, macrophages produce cytokines, termed *monokines*, which affect many other cell types (paracrine secretory products) and, as part of their comprehensive secretory capa-

306

bilities, may modulate their own function (autocrine secretory products) in inflammatory foci.

Macrophages are thus essential for the initiation and execution of nearly all immune processes. Macrophage differentiation and its roles as an effector, immune accessory, and secretory cell are reviewed here, with emphasis on relevance to the rheumatic diseases.

STRUCTURE AND DEVELOPMENT OF THE MONONUCLEAR PHAGOCYTE SYSTEM

The mononuclear phagocyte system consists of a group of cells, located in different tissues throughout the body, that share a common stem cell origin in the bone marrow, as well as certain functional and cytochemical characteristics.[5,8] In the blood, the cells are termed *monocytes*, whereas once they have migrated into tissues, they are called *macrophages*. The term mononuclear phagocyte includes all cells in this lineage. The mononuclear phagocyte system is a vital component of the immune system because it is the source of fixed tissue macrophages of the reticuloendothelial system as well as wandering phagocytic cells. The single most important characteristic of the mononuclear phagocyte is its ability to phagocytize and digest other substances, particularly substances coated (opsonized) by antibody. Mononuclear phagocytes are also capable of differentiating into cells with altered functional properties, depending on the environmental stimuli. As such, the mononuclear phagocyte system is admirably suited to its role as the primary effector in numerous host-defensive situations.

GENERAL CHARACTERISTICS

Cells of the mononuclear phagocyte system share several important characteristics despite tremendous biochemical and functional diversity, depending on tissue locus.[9,10] Morphologic features, such as low nuclear-to-cytoplasmic ratios, bilobed nuclei, and membrane ruffling, are evident at the light- and electron-microscopic level. Enzymatic features of macrophages demonstrated cytochemically or enzymatically include the presence of nonspecific esterase, peroxidase (depending on the state of differentiation), lysozyme, 5'nucleotidase, and aminopeptidase.[11–13] Membrane characteristics of macrophages include the presence of Ia antigens, receptors for chemotactic factors, Fc, C3b, certain sugars, and advanced glycosylation end

products. Moreover, a variety of specific antigenic determinants exist on the surface of macrophages (see the section on macrophage surface antigens in this chapter). The morphologic features of cells in the mononuclear phagocyte system are variable and are determined by the state of maturation, degree of differentiation, or content of ingested material. All macrophages share the ability to phagocytize particles and to adhere to charged surfaces. The cytotoxic and microbicidal capacities of macrophages are variable and relate to their state of activation[14] (see the section of this chapter on macrophage activation).

In different tissues, macrophages acquire certain distinct structural and metabolic properties. For examples, alveolar macrophages develop a high oxidative metabolic capacity, whereas splenic and peritoneal macrophages remain primarily dependent on anaerobic glycolysis.[15] Structurally, the macrophages that egress into tissues or into inflammatory sites as single cells may form granulomas and may develop into sheets of epithelioid cells, they may fuse to become multinucleated giant cells, or they may differentiate into osteoclasts.[16] Most data regarding the development of the mononuclear phagocyte system have been derived from the study of mice, guinea pigs, rats, or humans. The macrophages studied have been blood monocytes, resident peritoneal or alveolar macrophages, or macrophages called to an inflammatory site by phlogistic agents (elicited macrophages). The development of continuous cell lines with macrophage characteristics has allowed the further study of macrophage origins, differentiation, and functional development.[17–21]

ORIGIN

The earliest components of the mononuclear phagocyte system can be identified in the bone marrow. Primitive stem cells are called colony-forming units (CFU), and those committed to the granulocyte-monocyte line are termed GM-CFU. Dividing cells resident in the bone marrow include the CFU, GM-CFU, monoblasts, and promonocytes, whereas monocytes, the next level of cell maturity, are generally nondividing cells that first circulate in the blood and then egress into tissues, where they are called macrophages. Once in tissue or sites of granulomatous inflammation, macrophages may be long lived. Although monocytes are considered to be stem cells, a subpopulation appears capable of dividing at local tissue sites.[4,5] Macrophages enter various tissues and populate serous cavities (resident peritoneal macrophages), the lungs (alveolar macrophages), hepatic and splenic sinusoids (Kupffer's and sinusoidal cells), the brain (microglial elements), and bone (osteoclasts). The type A synovial lining cell is also an important part of the mononuclear phagocyte system (Fig. 18–1).

BONE MARROW MACROPHAGE PROGENITORS

Progression from the multipotential stem cell to the circulating monocyte is observed as macrophages develop.[11,12,22] The GM-CFU are the distinct progenitor cells for this lineage and can be induced to express Fc receptors.[23] Erythrocytes and lymphocytes have separate progenitors. Human GM-CFU proliferation is regulated by several diffusible factors, as are GM-CFU in other species. Among these are colony-stimulating factors (CSF), a term used to describe substances stimulating individual hemapoietic precursor

cells to divide and differentiate. CSF acting specifically on macrophage differentiation stimulate the oxidative burst and lysosomal enzyme release, besides enhancing differentiation.[24] CSF for GM-CFU are contained in supernatants of certain cell cultures (conditioned medium) such as stimulated lymphocytes, fibroblasts, and cell cultures of some tumor cell lines. CSF are acidic glycoproteins with a molecular weight in the range of 40,000 to 70,000 daltons.[25–27] The genes for 2 CSF molecules have been cloned thus far. Multi-CSF or interleukin-3 (IL-3) stimulates the proliferation of T cells, B cells, and mast cells, as well as granulocytes and macrophages.[28] Human GM-CSF has also been cloned, and it appears that one gene product of 14,000 daltons contains both CSF-α (macrophage, neutrophil and eosinophil stimulating activity) and CSF-β (exclusive stimulation of macrophages and neutrophils).[29]

That CSF for macrophages bind to cells of this lin-

FIG. 18–1. Mononuclear phagocyte system.

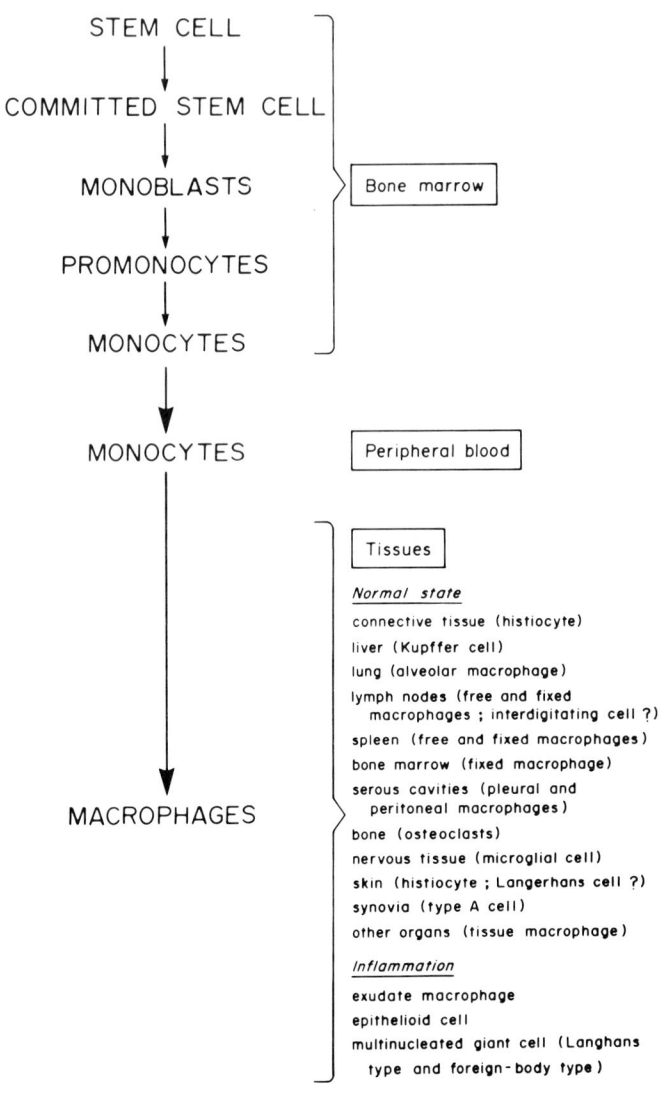

eage with high affinity suggests the presence of specific receptors. Indeed, a mouse mononuclear phagocyte growth factor, CSF-1, binds specifically to the c-fms proto-oncogene product,[30] suggesting that this transmembrane glycoprotein with its associated tyrosine kinase activity may represent the cell surface receptor for CSF-1. In contrast to the stimulatory effects of CSF, the combination of prostaglandins (PGE$_1$ and PGE$_2$) and acidic isoferritin activities (AIA) depresses macrophage differentiation.[31,32] Prostaglandins apparently play a role in the regulation of monocytopoiesis through their inhibitory effects on the GM-CFU cycle, thus providing a negative feedback loop. Because macrophages can synthesize prodigious amounts of PGE,[33,34] they may have the capacity to autoregulate their own progenitor cells.[35] Macrophages also appear to be the source of AIA, which are 21,000-dalton subunits of ferritin and are major components of this protein. AIA, in conjunction with prostaglandins, inhibit the stimulatory effects of CSF. Another cell-derived inhibitory factor acting on stem cells is lactoferrin.

In normal bone marrow, some cells produce a factor that suppresses the development of GM-CFU.[36] The cells producing this factor have Fc gamma receptors and do not require activation by mitogens for elaboration of the factor. Another factor regulating growth of macrophage precursors has been called synergistic activity (SA). When added with CSF to normal murine bone marrow cultures, SA results in the selection of a subset of macrophage progenitors with a high proliferative potential.[37] Activity such as this could induce a rapid turnover of macrophages when needed during an inflammatory response.

DIFFERENTIATION

The first level of differentiation from the stem cell is the monoblast, a round cell about 12 μ in diameter, that can be grown in culture from murine, but not as yet from human, bone marrow.[4,5,10,22,38,39] Monoblasts, which are characterized by a small amount of basophilic cytoplasm and a ruffled membrane, are esterase positive; they are also adherent phagocytes wth Fc receptors and apparently divide only once, into 2 promonocytes. Promonocytes are larger cells with an indented nucleus and more cytoplasm than monoblasts and are also peroxidase positive. The cell cycle time for promonocytes is longer than that for the monoblasts (about 12 hours versus 16 hours).[40,41] The promonocyte pool, twice as large as the monoblast pool, matures in the bone marrow for about 60 hours, then becomes part of the circulating or marginal pool for

approximately 9 hours. Inflammatory stimuli increase proliferation of promonocytes, enhance release of immature monocytes from bone marrow, and thus accelerate entry into the circulating-marginal pool.[41] Monocytes constitute a minority (less than 8%) of nucleated circulating blood elements,[42] but they are a readily available source of tissue macrophages.

Because marrow reserves of preformed monocytes are smaller than those of polymorphonuclear leukocytes, and the proliferative capacity of monocytes is limited, the participation of macrophages in host defense depends on the continued expansion of this small pool in response to various inflammatory stimuli. In mice, the circulation half-time is approximately 22 hours and ranges from 10 to over 70 hours in man.[4,9] The marginating monocyte pool is approximately 4 times the circulating pool. The extravascular pool, represented by the monocytes that have egressed into tissues, is large. Once out of the circulating pool, these cells, now termed macrophages, do not return. The kinetics of monocyte maturation are similar in mice and in humans.

In general, three mechanisms are known whereby monocyte levels are modulated by inflammatory stimuli: (1) earlier release of premature monocytes that would normally have been retained in the marrow; (2) temporary shortening of the cell cycle time, resulting in an increased output of younger monocytes; and (3) a sustained enlargement of the precursor pool as accomplished by an increase in the proportion of promonocytes.[42] Several possibilities for the regulation of monocytopoiesis during acute inflammation have been proposed.[39,43] In the normal steady state, monoblast production is controlled by bone marrow regulators of monocytopoiesis (local production of CSF). When an inflammatory stimulus develops, however, local macrophages may, after phagocytosis of an antigen, release a substance that has been called factor-increasing monocytopoiesis (FIM). This agent circulates to the bone marrow and stimulates increased monoblast production. This factor has been characterized as a protein of 18,000 to 24,000 daltons and elicits a rapid monocytopoiesis when injected into normal mice.[43]

TISSUE MACROPHAGES

Although most tissue macrophages arise from emigration from the circulating-marginating pool, precursor cells have some mitotic potential at local tissue sites.[44] Data concerning the fate of macrophages that have emigrated into tissues derive primarily from studies of experimentally induced granulomatous inflammation.[22,45] A hematogenous origin is currently held for peritoneal, alveolar, hepatic, and neural tissue macrophages, but in chronic granulomatous foci, evidence suggests local replication as well.[9,22,44,46] A small portion of circulating blood monocytes may be capable of dividing once at local tissue sites.[4] Depending on the particulate nature and digestibility of the antigenic stimulus, macrophages may become long-lived, immobile, nondividing cells, which fuse to become giant cells that do not divide, or they may become epithelioid macrophages.

In certain tissue sites, the macrophages may dramatically affect the regulation of the local environment. Two examples are the interactions among the synovial phagocytic cell and its neighboring plasma cells and lymphoblasts in the synovial membrane and the potential of alveolar macrophages to produce soluble factors affecting proliferation of lymphocytes to antigens and mitogens.[47]

The ability of blood monocytes to become resident cells in specific tissues is thought to be a random process and one in which further differentiation at the specific tissue is a consequence of local trophic influences. As more is learned about the development of macrophages and their heterogeneity, however, it would not be surprising to find that specific bone marrow precursors or subclasses of monocytes possess a unique capacity for differentiation and thus for eventual selection of their specific final tissue destination.

MACROPHAGES AS EFFECTOR CELLS

MECHANISMS OF MACROPHAGE ACCUMULATION

The accumulation of macrophages at local tissue sites is the result of a complex process that involves adherence to the vascular endothelium, migration through gaps between the endothelial cells, penetration of the basement membrane, and then locomotion through tissue spaces to the inflammatory site. The initial binding of blood monocytes to endothelial cells is likely to involve fibronectin, a complex high-molecular-weight molecule found in plasma, which is capable of binding to monocytes as well as to endothelial cells and a family of adhesion proteins termed Mac-1, lymphocyte function-associated-1 (LFA-1), and p 150, 95 (see the discussion of these proteins later in this chapter).[48–52] The passage of monocytes through vascular basement membrane may depend on the ability of these cells to secrete collagenase.[53,54] The actual migration of the cells to the

inflammatory site appears to be mediated by chemotaxis.[55]

Chemotactic factors are molecules that cause the directed migration of cells along a concentration gradient. Several different types of chemotactic factors are produced at sites of inflammation, depending on the stimulus to inflammation. Monocytes and macrophages have cell-surface receptors for chemotactic factors.[56–59] The binding of chemoattractants to the surface of resting blood monocytes leads to a change in the shape of the round cells to their motile triangular configuration.[60] Associated with this change are several metabolic events apparently required for chemotaxis to occur as discussed later in this chapter. These processes lead to a rapid change in the cytoskeleton of the cells and allow reorientation of actin filaments to the front of the cell with rearrangement of cytoskeletal elements, providing front-to-back polarization. The net effect of the chemoattractants is cellular migration along a gradient toward the site of inflammation (Fig. 18–2). Several chemotactic factors associated with macrophage accumulation in vivo have been described.

COMPLEMENT-DERIVED CHEMOTACTIC FACTORS

The fifth component of complement, C5, is composed of two chains, termed the α chain and the β chain.[61] Activation of C5 by the earlier-acting complement components (see Chapter 25) or a cleavage of C5 by proteases leads to the release of a fragmentation product termed C5a.[62,63] C5a is chemotactic for both polymorphonuclear leukocytes and monocyte-macrophages.[63–66] It also has anaphylatoxin activity in that it increases vascular permeability, contracts vascular smooth muscle, degranulates mast cells, and, on occasion, causes hypotension.[62,63]

C5a is a protein consisting of 74 amino acids, the carboxy-terminal constituent being arginine.[61,67] At higher concentrations, C5a can also lead to secretion of lysosomal enzymes by macrophages and stimulation of the respiratory burst with production of superoxide anion. C5a has been identified at inflammatory sites in vivo and has also been detected in synovial effusions from patients with rheumatoid arthritis.[68,69] C5a in the circulation in rapidly degraded to C5a-des-arg through the action of a carboxypeptidase.[61] This molecule retains chemotactic activity for mononuclear phagocytes, although it is less potent than C5a itself. C5a and C5a-des-arg are important chemoattractants in inflammatory conditions initiated by immune complexes,[70] bacterial endotoxins or non-

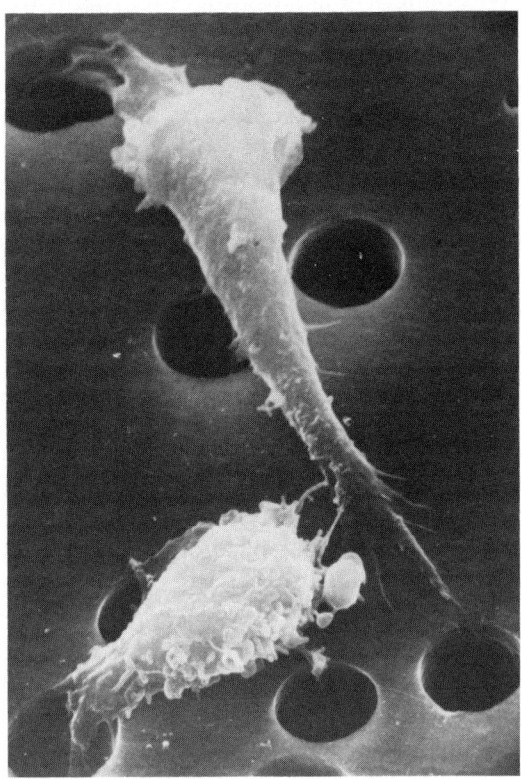

FIG. 18–2. Scanning electron micrograph of two human blood monocytes migrating through 5.0-μm pores of a polycarbonate filter in response to a chemotactic lymphokine (×4,000). The cell at the top has completely emerged through a pore and has advanced diagonally across the filter's surface. On the lower left another cell has begun to emerge through the filter. (From Snyderman, R., and Mergenhagen. S.E.[205])

specific tissue trauma that releases tissue proteases.[71] The production of C5a in patients undergoing renal dialysis, cardiopulmonary bypass, and nylon-fiber filtration leukapheresis is thought to be responsible for the immediate neutropenia and pulmonary-vascular leukostasis associated with these procedures.[72–74]

CELL-DERIVED CHEMOTACTIC FACTORS

Stimulation of lymphocytes by specific antigen or mitogens results in the synthesis and release of biologically active agents termed lymphokines. One particular lymphokine, lymphocyte-derived chemotactic factor (LDCF), is a chemoattractant for monocyte-macrophages.[65,75] This material has a molecular weight of approximately 12,000 daltons and has been isolated from supernatants of stimulated lymphocyte cultures as well as from delayed hypersensitivity reactions in vivo.[76]

OTHER CHEMOTACTIC FACTORS FOR MACROPHAGES

Several other chemotactic factors for monocyte-macrophages have been described. One well-defined group comprises the synthetic N-formylated oligopeptides thought to be analogous to chemotactic factors produced by rapidly dividing bacteria.[77] Certain N-formyl methionyl peptides, such as N-formyl-methionyl-leucyl-phenylalanine (f-met-leu-phe), are potent chemoattractants for monocyte-macrophages, which have specific membrane receptors for them.[58,59,78,79] By recognizing these peptides, mononuclear phagocytes may be able to accumulate at sites of bacterial growth.

Collagen (type I), as well as its degradation products are also chemoattractants for monocytes.[80] Kallikrein, proteins released by tumor cells, and a product released by fibroblasts also have monocyte-macrophage chemotactic activity.[53,81,83] Another potential source of chemoattractants for macrophages are the metabolites of arachidonic acid.[53,84] Certain phlogistic agents, such as C5a, interact with inflammatory cells, activating cellular phospholipase, which cleaves arachidonic acid from membrane phospholipids.[85] Metabolism of arachidonic acid by macrophages can result in the production of leukotriene B_4 (5'12 dihydroxyeicosatetraenoic acid or LTB_4).[86,87] LTB_4 is a chemoattractant for neutrophils and macrophages and has been detected in rheumatoid synovial effusions.[88,89] High-affinity receptors for LTB_4 have been identified on the surface of leukocytes.[90–92]

Another lipid-derived chemoattractant produced by monocytes and macrophages is a phospholipid derivative called platelet-activating factor (PAF). PAF is also secreted by polymorphonuclear leukocytes and basophils.[93,94] Phagocytic stimuli, as well as soluble activators, induce its secretion. The structure of this molecule is 1-0-alkyl 2-0-acetyl-5n-glycerol-3-phosphoryl choline.[95] In addition to possessing chemotactic activity for macrophages and polymorphonuclear leukocytes, PAF induces platelet aggregation and degranulation.

MECHANISMS OF MACROPHAGE CHEMOTAXIS

The precise biochemical mechanisms of macrophage chemotaxis are not fully understood. N-formylmethionyl peptides, such as (N-f-met-leu-phe) have provided an important tool for the study of chemotaxis because they are structurally defined and potent and because monocytes and macrophages have specific receptors for them.[56,58,59] The equilibrium dissociation constant (K_D) for f-met-leu-phe binding to human blood monocytes is 30 nM, and there are approximately 65,000 receptors per cell.[56] The receptor is a glycoprotein (M.W.~ 62,000 daltons) composed of approximately 50% carbohydrate.[18,96,97] In macrophage membranes, the receptor exists in a high- and low-affinity form with the 2 affinities in part interconvertible and regulated by guanine di- and trinucleotides. A nucleotide regulatory protein may be involved in regulating the biologic activity of the chemotactic factor receptor.[57] Similar regulation has been suggested for certain neurotransmitter receptors.[98]

The binding of chemoattractants to their receptor on human monocytes leads to the activation of phospholipase C and the degradation of phosphoinositides.[85,99–102] Activation of this enzyme leads to the formation of important second messenger molecules contained within the structure of the polyphosphoinositides, phosphatidylinositol-4-phosphate (PIP) and phosphatidylinositol 4,5-bisphosphate (PIP_2).[103–106] These include inositol-1,4,5-trisphosphate (IP_3), which releases calcium from intracellular stores, and diacylglycerol, which, together with calcium, activates protein kinase C and translocates this cytosolic enzyme activity to particulate membrane fractions.[107–112] Diacylglycerol is further metabolized to arachidonate, which serves as a precursor for the leukotrienes, thromboxanes, and prostaglandins, important mediators of the inflammatory response.[41,113–118] In addition, IP_3 is converted into inositol-1,3,4,5-tetrakisphosphate (IP_4), which causes influx of calcium into cells from extracellular stores.[119]

Phospholipase C activation in leukocytes by chemoattractants requires coupling to a guanine nucleotide regulatory protein (G protein) with subsequent hydrolysis of guanosine triphosphate.[100,120,121] This activity can be demonstrated in isolated plasma membranes.[100] The G protein used by human leukocytes during chemoattractant receptor-induced activation appears to be distinct from the G_s, G_o, G_i, and transducin described for the adrenergic receptor systems, as well as the muscarinic-cholinergic and rhodopsin receptors.[122] This G protein, termed G_c, M.W. about 40,000 daltons, is adenosine disphosphate (ADP)-ribosylated by both cholera toxin and pertussis toxin.[122]

In addition to coupling with a G protein, chemoattractant-mediated responses in macrophages and monocytes require transmethylation reactions mediated by S-adenosylmethionine.[123,124] Inhibition of methylation in intact macrophages reduces the affinity of the oligopeptide chemoattractant receptor.[125] In addition, phosphatidylinositol metabolism, presumably by phospholipase C, is inhibited by conditions that inhibit methylation in human monocytes.[85] The precise methylation reaction is unknown, although it has been shown that chemoattractants inhibit the methylation of phosphatidylethanolamine to form phosphatidylcholine,[126] which, in turn, inhibits phospholipase C that metabolizes the phosphoinositides.[105] Thus, by curtailing the synthesis of phosphatidylcholine, chemoattractants may activate this enzyme.

As mentioned previously, protein kinase C activation results from stimulation of the phosphoinositide pathway.[106] It has been postulated that activation of this enzyme by phorbol ester tumor promoters, 1,2 diacylglycerols, and chemoattractants is necessary for generation of superoxide anion.[110,111] Phorbol esters and diacylglycerol bind directly to protein kinase C,[127] and phorbol esters lead to the translocation of this enzyme from cytosolic to membrane fractions in human monocytes.[109] Chemoattractant substances produce the same effect in human leukocytes.

Leukocyte activation by single doses of chemoattractants is rapid and transient, and induced functional responses, such as rapid perpendicular light scattering, superoxide anion production, and lysosomal enzyme release, do not persist beyond 2 to 5 min.[128,129] This suggests activation of autoregulatory termination mechanisms.[122] It has been known for years that agents that increase cyclic adenosine-5′-monophosphate (cAMP) levels in monocytes and macrophages inhibit functional responses.[130,131] Chemoattractants, however, have been shown to cause a transient increase in cAMP in these cells.[132,133] Based on these data, it has been postulated that increases in cAMP produced by chemoattractants serve as a termination signal for leukocyte functional responses.[122,132,133] Increased intracellular cAMP decreases calcium mobilization from extracellular medium and, to a lesser degree, PIP_2 hydrolysis. These observations suggest that cAMP-dependent protein kinases may inhibit the formation of cation channels after PIP_2 hydrolysis.

Protein kinase C may also be involved in the termination of phagocyte activation by chemoattractants. Although activation of protein kinase C stimulates superoxide production,[109–111] high concentrations of phorbol esters, which directly activate this enzyme, inhibit the coupling of the activated G protein to phospholipase C.[134,135] The result is inhibition of PIP_2 hydrolysis by chemoattractants.[135]

MACROPHAGE RECEPTORS

Receptors trigger cells to respond appropriately to environmental stimuli. Considering the broad range of macrophage functions, it is not surprising that their plasma membranes are well endowed with receptors that selectively initiate various physiologic functions.[34,136] Biochemically, receptors are discrete cellular structures that bind specific ligands with high affinity and limited capacity. Functionally, the binding of a receptor with its ligand triggers a discrete biologic response by the cell.

Fc RECEPTORS

Clearance of immune complexes and endocytosis of opsonized particles is an important function of macrophages, which contain surface receptors for the Fc portion of immunoglobulin.[113,137–142] Cross-linkage of such receptors stimulates endocytosis. Fc receptors for distinct immunoglobulin subclasses are present on both human monocytes and murine macrophages. Studies in macrophages from guinea pig, rat, mouse, and man have all shown Fc receptor specificity for individual subclasses of immunoglobulin G (IgG), for example, mouse macrophages have distinct receptors for IgG2a, IgG2b-IgG1, and IgG3,[143–146] termed $FcR_{\gamma 2a}$, $FcR_{\gamma 2b-\gamma 1}$, and $FcR_{\gamma 3}$, respectively. Some evidence suggests that the signals generated by the binding of IgG to the different classes of Fc receptors in murine macrophages may stimulate different biologic activities, such as phagocytosis or cytotoxicity.[147] The murine Fc receptors themselves have differential susceptibility to proteases and phospholipases and cap independently.[142–148] In murine macrophages, all classes of Fc receptors appear to be single-chain glycoproteins of approximately 50,000 daltons. The mechanisms by which the binding of IgG to its receptor initiate cellular function are largely unknown, but in the case of the $FcR_{\gamma 2b-\gamma 1}$ receptor, a ligand-dependent channel initiating ion influx is operative.[149]

Fc receptors appear to react differently with respect to their ability to bind monomers and aggregates of immunoglobulins. Receptors for monomeric IgG are thought to bind cytophilic antibody of the human IgG1 and IgG3 subclasses. The function of such receptors may be to couple antibody to monocytes so they are better able to recognize specific antigens. Receptors for monomeric IgG are protease sensitive and do not lead to endocytosis of antigen unless they are subsequently cross-linked by other antibodies to the antigen. Some Fc receptors bind only aggregates of IgG or antigen-antibody complexes. Such binding results in antigen internalization. It is estimated that macrophages contain approximately 500,000 such receptors per cell.[150] Specific Fc receptors for IgE and IgM have been reported on mononuclear phagocytes and cell lines from several species, but their functional role is unclear.[114,151]

COMPLEMENT RECEPTORS

That monocytes and macrophages respond chemotactically to low doses of C5a implies the presence of a specific receptor.[66] Indeed, a common receptor for C5a and C5a des arg has been demonstrated on human polymorphonuclear leukocytes.[114] The C5a receptor initiates lysosomal enzyme secretion and activation of the respiratory burst enzyme in mononuclear phagocytes. Macrophages also contain receptors for fragments of the fourth and third component of complement. Complement receptor 1 (CR1) binds C3b as well as C4b.[152] Complement receptor 3 (CR3) binds C3bi,[153–155] a degradation product of C3b produced by the action of C3b inactivator, and further degradation products termed α2D or C3d,g. A monoclonal antibody that recognizes an antigen termed Mac-1 also binds to CR3; this finding indicates that Mac-1 and CR3 are identical surface molecules.[156] Monoclonal antibodies to the monocyte-granulocyte membrane glycoprotein Mo-1 also inhibit C3bi binding and thereby indicate an interaction with CR3.[157] The type 2 (CR2) complement receptor interacts with C3d and is present on lymphocytes, but not mononuclear or polymorphonuclear phagocytes.[155,158] The receptors for C3b and C3bi are antigenically distinct and are independently mobile in the plane of the membrane when activated. Moreover, the C3bi receptor requires Ca^{+2} and Mg^{+2} for optimal activity, whereas the C3b receptor does not.[159] Structurally, the C3b receptor is a 205,000-dalton single-chain membrane glycoprotein,[153] whereas the C3bi receptor is composed of 2-membrane glycoprotein chains of M.W. 180,000 and 100,000 daltons, respectively.[160,161] Binding of antigens to macrophages by complement receptors does not initiate endocytosis unless the macrophage is further stimulated by Fc receptors or other phlogistic stimuli.[160–162] The primary function of complement receptors appears to be the attachment of complement-bearing antigens to the macrophage surface. In the presence of low levels of IgG, complement receptor stimulation does enhance phagocytosis, however.

RECEPTORS FOR GLYCOPROTEINS

Clearance of serum proteins such as enzymes, as well as bacteria, may be mediated by receptors for specific sugars or glycoproteins on macrophages. A mannosyl-glucosyl receptor on macrophages mediates clearance on mannosyl, glucosyl, and acetyl-glucosamine terminal glycoproteins from the circulation. The clearance of lysosomal hydrolases appears to be through the mannosyl-glucosyl receptor on Kupffer's cells and alveolar macrophages.[163,164] A mouse macrophage-recognition system involving lectin-like receptors has been described and can bind the cell-wall sugars of certain microorganisms.[165] Receptors that bind sugars may be important in removing denatured proteins, effete cells, or bacteria from the circulation. Indeed, proteins modified by long-term exposure to glucose accumulate *advanced glycosylation end* products (AGE) as a function of protein age.[166] These proteins are recognized by specific receptors on macrophages that are distinct from the mannose-fucose receptor. The affinity of the AGE receptor on macrophages is 1.75×10^{-11} *M*. It has been postulated that incomplete removal of AGE proteins by macrophages could give rise to some of the physiologic changes that occur with normal aging.[166]

RECEPTOR FOR LIPOPROTEINS

Macrophages are important in the clearance of lipids from the circulation, and accumulation of fatty substances within macrophages may be involved in the pathogenesis of atherosclerosis. Human monocytes and macrophages contain receptors that bind low-density lipoproteins (LDL) containing lysine residues modified by acetylation, auto acetylation, or malondialdehyde treatment.[167–169] This receptor internalizes bound, chemically modified LDL and causes monocytes and macrophages to accumulate large amounts of cholesterol esters.[167,168] Accumulation of such lipid-laden "foam cells" in the subendothelial space is one of the early events in atherogenesis.[100,170] Arterial smooth muscle cells and endothelial cells have been shown to modify LDL chemically to the forms that react with the macrophage acetyl LDL receptor.[171,172] One mediator of this modification is superoxide anion, produced by arterial smooth muscle cells.[171] A secretory product derived from thrombin-activated platelets has been shown to interfere with the accumulation of cholesterol esters by macrophages.[173] Thus, complex interactions appear to exist among macrophage LDL receptors, endothelial cells, arterial smooth muscle cells, and platelets in the formation of foam cells.

HORMONE RECEPTORS ON MACROPHAGES

Macrophages contain receptors for several hormones that likely play a role in the regulation of mac-

rophage function.[34] Many classes of hormone receptors have been demonstrated, indirectly or directly, on macrophages, including receptors for polypeptide hormones, steroid hormones, and catecholamines. Direct binding studies have shown that macrophages contain adrenergic, insulin, glucagon, and thyrotropin receptors, as well as receptors for somatomedin, prostaglandins, and dexamethasone.[34] Rheumatoid synovial adherent macrophages have a steroid receptor.[174] Indirect evidence suggests that macrophages also have receptors for histamine, serotonin, parathyroid hormone, calcitonin, vitamin D, estrogen, and progesterone. Beta-adrenergic agonists inhibit chemotaxis as well as secretion and superoxide anion production, whereas alpha-adrenergic receptors, serotonin receptors, and muscarinic-cholinergic receptors appear to enhance chemoattractant-mediated functions.[138,175,176]

OTHER RECEPTORS ON MACROPHAGES

Functional evidence suggests that macrophages have receptors for many agents that may affect their biologic activity. CSF binds to monocytes and macrophages. The binding site for CSF may be involved in the differentiation of these cells.[27] α-2-Macroglobulin-protease complexes are rapidly endocytized by macrophages and may provide an important mechanism for the clearance of proteolytic enzymes. Macrophages appear to have a membrane-binding site for α-2-macroglobulin-protease complex, but not for native α-2-macroglobulins.[177]

Macrophage-activating factor (MAF) has been shown to be identical or closely related to γ-interferon.[178,179] The potency of this material for activating macrophages suggest the presence of a receptor for γ–interferon. Similarly, macrophage migration-inhibitory factor (MIF) probably binds to a receptor on macrophages because its activity is blocked by sugars such as 1-fucose, as well as by pretreating the cells with fucosidase.[180–182] The receptor for MIF-MAF on guinea pig macrophages has been identified as a glycolipid.[183] Clearance of iron could be mediated by a lactoferrin receptor that has been described on murine macrophages.[184] Lactoferrin released from neutrophil-specific granules could be internalized by macrophages, thereby sequestering iron in the reticuloendothelial system.[184]

ENDOCYTOSIS

A central feature of macrophage function, enabling them to perform their many roles in host defense, is their ability avidly to ingest many different materials. *Endocytosis* is the generalized term for internalization of extracellular substances by invagination of the plasma membrane. Subsequent membrane fusion results in the formation of membrane-bound vesicles within the cell. The term *pinocytosis* is used to describe the internalization of fluids and solutes, whereas *phagocytosis* refers to the ingestion of particulate materials.

PINOCYTOSIS

Murine macrophages internalize twice their cell surface area per hour in pinocytic vesicles that deliver their contents to secondary lysozymes.[185] Recycling of the membrane from the lysosomal compartment back to the plasma membrane is continuous because the size of the vacuolar system and membrane remains constant. Thus, pinocytosis is a process that provides a means for the rapid recycling of plasma membrane to lysosomal compartments and back.[186]

PHAGOCYTOSIS

The ingestion of particles by macrophages requires two processes: (1) the binding of the particle to the macrophage plasma membrane; and (2) the actual ingestion of the particulate material.[187,188] Binding of particles to macrophages is enhanced by serum factors termed opsonins (agents that enhance phagocytosis), but the cells are capable of binding and ingesting nonopsonized material as well. In such a case, lectin-like receptors or carbohydrate receptors may be involved in stimulating the phagocytic process. The metabolic requirements for phagocytosis of nonopsonized particles differ in that ingestion of nonopsonized particles is blocked by 2-deoxyglucose.[118,189] Contact with opsonized particles results in their attachment to the macrophage plasma membrane, followed by the elaboration of pseudopods at the location of the particle. The responses by the macrophage to bound particles are segmental in that they occur only in the proximity of the material to be phagocytized.[190] Bystander particles, not containing opsonins, may be ignored while adjacent opsonized particles are phagocytized. The development of the pseudopods is dependent on the polymerization of actin filaments directly beneath the particle to be ingested,[191] and phagocytosis is blocked by cytochalasin B, an agent that inhibits actin polymerization (Fig. 18–3).

Energy for the movement of the macrophage membrane around an opsonized particle is likely to derive from adenosine triphosphate (ATP) and occurs in a "zipper"-like fashion.[192] That is, the movement of the membrane around an opsonized particle proceeds sequentially by interaction of receptors on the membrane with ligands on the particle. If macrophages confront particles only partially covered with opsonin, the pseudopods advance only as far as the opsonins are present and do not form a complete phagosome. When the bound particle is circumferentially opsonized, the macrophage membrane covers its entire surface and fuses, so the particle is inside the cell surrounded by what had been the macrophage plasma membrane. The internalized structure is termed a "phagosome."

Concomitant with the formation of the phagosome is the migration of lysosomal granules toward it. The membranes of these granules fuse with the membrane of the forming phagosome and discharge their contents into it.[193] The fusion of membrane of lysosomal granules with that of the phagosome causes the formation of a structure called a "phagolysosome." In addition to exposing the opsonized particle to the enzyme contents of lysosomal granules, the binding process leads to activation of the "respiratory burst enzyme," nicotinamide-adenine dinucleotide phosphate (NADPH) oxidase, which is associated with the plasma membrane.[194] Activation of this enzyme leads to the production of *superoxide anion*, which is further metabolized into several toxic oxygen products, including *hydrogen peroxide, hydroxyl radical, hypochlorous ion,* and *singlet oxygen,*[195–197] which are toxic to most microbes. The combination of toxic oxygen products with the contents of lysosomal granules makes it unlikely that all but the most resistant microorganisms survive phagocytosis by macrophages (see Fig. 18–3). During the process of phagocytosis, incomplete fusion of phagosomes prior to discharge of lysosomal contents, "regurgitation while feeding," can cause the release of toxic oxygen products and lysosomal contents into the extracellular environment.

Both Fc and C3 receptors promote phagocytosis, but the differences in their ability to do so are striking. Cross-linking of Fc receptors triggers phagocytosis whether or not the macrophages have been stimulated by inflammatory agents. In contrast, macrophages isolated from noninflammatory environments (resident peritoneal macrophages) bind, but do not internalize, particles coated with either C3b or C3bi alone. If the cells are stimulated with phorbol-myristate-acetate, a tumor promoter that initiates the respiratory burst as well as lysosomal enzyme secretion, the macrophages will then ingest both C3b- and C3bi-coated particles.[160,161] For C3b or C3bi receptors to stimulate ingestion, a second signal is needed, and

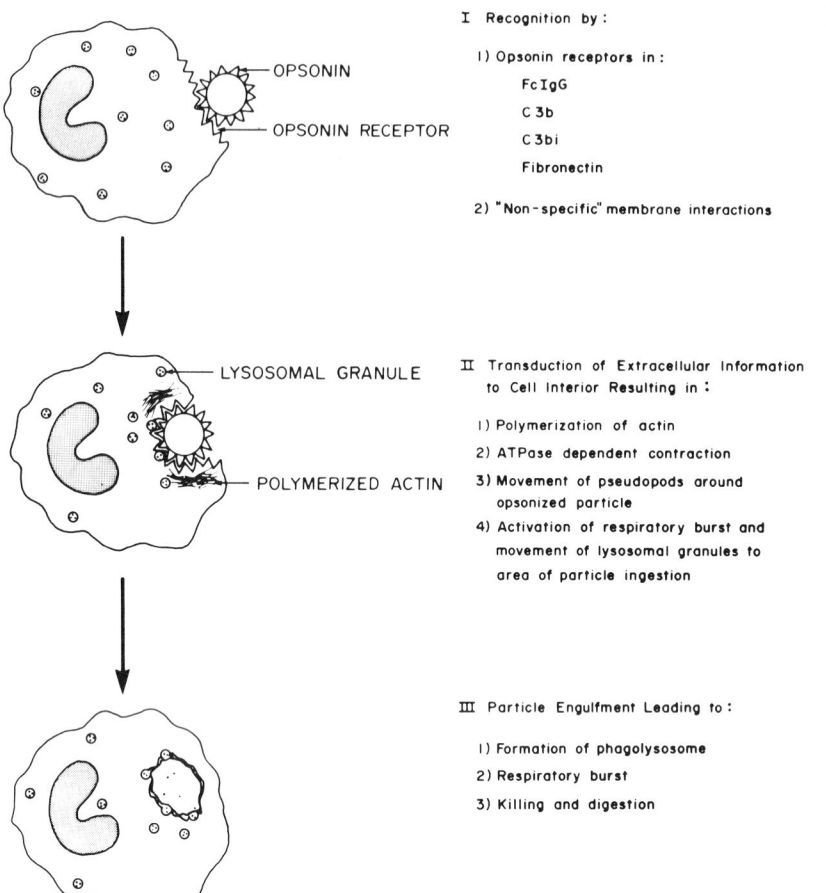

I Recognition by :

1) Opsonin receptors in :
    FcIgG
    C3b
    C3bi
    Fibronectin

2) "Non-specific" membrane interactions

II Transduction of Extracellular Information
    to Cell Interior Resulting in :

1) Polymerization of actin
2) ATPase dependent contraction
3) Movement of pseudopods around
    opsonized particle
4) Activation of respiratory burst and
    movement of lysosomal granules to
    area of particle ingestion

III Particle Engulfment Leading to :

1) Formation of phagolysosome
2) Respiratory burst
3) Killing and digestion

FIG. 18–3. Mechanisms of phagocytosis.

this can be provided by phlogistic stimuli. Macrophages, but not polymorphonuclear leukocytes, secrete complement-alternative pathway components able to opsonize particles locally.[198] C3b and C3bi have been eluted from zymosan particles incubated with human monocytes in the absence of serum components.[199] In addition to Fc receptors, CR3 receptors also promote phagocytosis. CR3 receptors are normally activated in the macrophage membrane and do not promote phagocytosis unless they are freely mobile within the lipid bilayer.[107] A lymphokine derived from human T cells activates C3-mediated phagocytosis by freeing the anchored receptors and allowing them to diffuse within the cells' plasma membrane.[200]

In addition to phagocytizing opsonized particles, macrophages readily ingest immune complexes or aggregated immunoglobulins. These agents, like opsonized particles, stimulate the respiratory burst and secretory events by macrophages. Immune complexes and cryoglobulins can also interfere with the phagocytosis of particles by monocytes, however, perhaps by blocking Fc receptors. Although little is known about regulation of phagocytosis in rheumatic diseases, it has been postulated that immune complexes

in the synovial fluid can prevent effective phagocytosis and elimination of particulate antigens.[201] In patients with rheumatoid arthritis, immune clearance is decreased, perhaps owing to the blocking of reticuloendothelial cell clearance mechanisms by intermittent exposure to immune complexes.[202] Moreover, patients with rheumatoid arthritis and vasculitis, who have circulating immune complexes, show defects of monocyte phagocytosis of yeast particles, a complement-dependent opsonic function. Patients with circulating immune complexes and cutaneous vasculitis, but without rheumatoid arthritis, also display an impairment of complement-mediated monocyte phagocytosis.[203] Stimulation of phagocytosis depends on membrane phenomena and is inhibited when macrophages are treated with antibodies to their membrane components.[204]

MACROPHAGES AS SECRETORY CELLS

Macrophages secrete products affecting many different host functions. The vast array of such products is just now being recognized, and secretion may be as important a macrophage function as endocytosis. Secretion occurs in several different patterns, one of which is triggered by chemoattractants or opsonized particles,[205] but other types of secretion are constitutive, not requiring exogenous stimulation.[115] Although many products of macrophage secretion are stored within lysosomal compartments, others are synthesized just before release.

ACID HYDROLASES

Abundant amounts of acid hydrolases are stored in macrophage lysosomes,[206] and after exposure to inflammatory substances, such as chemoattractants or opsonized particles, these are rapidly secreted by exocytosis. In general, substances capable of inducing chronic inflammation in vivo induce macrophage secretion of acid hydrolases in vitro,[33] for example, peptidoglycans of streptococcal cell walls.[207,208] That lysosomal discharge stimulated by chemoattractants occurs at doses generally 10 times higher than those required to initiate chemotaxis implies that secretion may not occur until macrophages reach the inflammatory site where such chemoattractants are in highest concentration.[209] Acid hydrolases may contribute to tissue destruction at inflammatory sites if the pH is sufficiently low. Hydrolases may also amplify inflammatory reactions by cleaving C5 or other proinflammatory molecules and may thereby produce additional biologically active cleavage products.[71] Other substrates for acid hydrolases may include collagen, proteoglycans, and the basement membrane of blood vessels.[210]

PLASMINOGEN ACTIVATOR

This neutral protease converts plasminogen to plasmin.[211,212] Plasmin degrades fibrin and can activate C1, cleave C3, and convert Hageman factor into prekallikrein activator.[213] Plasminogen activator is secreted at low levels by nonactivated macrophages or monocytes, but its secretion is enhanced by phlogistic stimuli.[214] In inflammatory macrophages, plasminogen activator exists in 2 active forms, a cell-associated enzyme and a soluble form released into the extracellular medium.[152,215] The cell-associated form is an ectoenzyme in the cell membrane, inhibitable by sodium chloride, with a K_M for plasminogen 20-fold lower than its soluble form.[152] This soluble form in macrophage cell lysates is difficult to measure because of the presence of endogenous inhibitors.[152,216] The

soluble form has a K_M of 16nM, has a high molecular weight, and is unstable.[216] The fibrinolytic inhibitor in mouse and human macrophages (M.W. 45,000 to 50,00 daltons) binds to the heavy chain of urokinase. The secretion of this inhibitor is not constitutive and requires prior cellular activation.[216] The secretion of plasminogen activators by macrophages may allow migration through fibrin clots to arrive at inflammatory sites. The ability of plasminogen activator to cleave Hageman factor and to activate complement at sites of inflammation may also generate additional phlogistic agents. Plasminogen activator can also activate collagenase from its proenzyme form, stimulating the destruction of collagen.[217]

COLLAGENASE

Collagenase is a neutral protease secreted in small amounts by unstimulated macrophages, but phagocytosis or endotoxin enhance secretion.[218,219] Lymphokines also induce macrophages to produce collagenase.[220] Degradation of collagen in chronic inflammatory sites, such as the rheumatoid synovium, could be caused, at least in part, by collagenases secreted by macrophages.[221] Macrophage-derived factors such as IL-1 stimulate collagenase and prostaglandin formation from rheumatoid tissues containing stellate cells.[222]

ELASTASE

Secretion of this neutral protease is stimulated by phagocytic stimuli as well as by inflammatory mediators.[223] Human monocytes secrete elastase when they are exposed to immune complexes.[224] Release of elastase at inflammatory sites can lead to irreversible tissue damage by destroying vascular structures.

LYSOZYME

This important component of macrophage secretions is capable of degrading the cell walls of bacteria. Lysozyme is a cationic protein that hydrolyzes n-actylmuramic-β1-4-n-acetyl, glucose linkages in bacterial cell walls.[225] Lysozyme has been found in human osteoarthritic cartilage.[117] Lysozyme is a constitutive secretion product of macrophages in that it is not stimulated by phagocytosis or by phlogistic agents.[206] Lysozyme is secreted at high levels by macrophages in culture, irrespective of their degree of activation.[193,226] Other enzymes secreted by macrophages are angiotensin-converting enzyme, arginase, and nonspecific esterases.[117,226]

ANTIPROTEASES

Regulation of proteolytic enzyme activity is important in limiting tissue destruction accompanying protease release into extracellular tissue sites; macrophages contain α-2-macroglobulin and α-1-antiprotease.[227,228] Proteases bound by macroglobulin include kallikrein, thrombin, elastase, collagenase, plasmin, and plasminogen activator. After binding a protease, α-2-macroglobulin is modified, internalized, and destroyed by macrophages, providing an important regulatory mechanism for limiting the damage from secretion of proteases by inflammatory cells. Human monocytes secrete α-2-macroglobulin in culture, but mechanisms regulating such secretion have not been elucidated.[229]

α-1-Antiprotease potently inhibits serine proteinases, such as elastase, by forming enzyme-inhibitor complexes. Low levels of α-1-antiprotease have been associated with emphysema and with adult respiratory distress syndrome, in which α-1-antiprotease levels in alveolar secretions are low because of the release of toxic neutrophil products.[230] Antiprotease-protease complexes are taken up by synovial inflammatory macrophages.[231] Abnormalities of antiproteases in rheumatic diseases have not been extensively evaluated; this area should be important for future research.

PROCOAGULANTS

Besides stimulating fibrinolysis by secretion of plasminogen activator, macrophages and monocytes have procoagulant activity stimulated by interaction with endotoxin, immune complexes, and C3b or by phagocytosis of bacteria.[232] Procoagulant activities produced by human monocytes include tissue factor, factor X activator, prothrombin activator and the vitamin-K-dependent clotting factors, II, VII, IX, and X.[233,234] Procoagulant activity released by monocytes has been implicated in the pathophysiology of allograft rejection.[28] Monocytes from patients with rheumatic disease appear to have higher procoagulant-generating activity than do normal monocytes. When phlogistic stimuli are introduced, however, monocytes from normal individuals make more procoagulant than monocytes from rheumatoid patients. Microvascular thromboses and fibrin deposition in chronic inflammatory states could be related to the release of procoagulant from macrophages.[235]

COMPLEMENT COMPONENTS

Macrophages synthesize a number of complement components and provide a source for opsonins and mediators of inflammation directly at local tissue sites.[190,236] C1, C4, C2, C3, C5, factor B, factor D, and properdin are all made by macrophages. Because the cleavage products of C3b and factor B of the alternate pathway are potent macrophage activators,[237,238] release of complement components at sites of inflammation could play an important role in macrophage activation.[239] Monocytes from patients with rheumatoid arthritis make more C2 than do those patients with osteoarthritis.[240]

ARACHIDONIC ACID METABOLITES

Stimulation of macrophages or monocytes by phlogistic agents activates cellular phospholipases that degrade membrane phospholipids,[158] with resulting release of arachidonic acid.[194,241-244] Arachidonic acid can be further metabolized into prostaglandins, thromboxanes, or leukotrienes by the action of either cyclooxygenase or lipoxygenase (see Chapter 26). PGE_2, the predominant prostaglandin synthesized by macrophages,[86,87] is secreted by unstimulated peritoneal macrophages, but secretion is increased after exposure to phlogistic stimuli. PGE_2 causes hyperalgesia and fever when it is injected into animal brains.[245]

Macrophages also synthesize leukotrienes and thromboxanes. The most predominant leukotrienes are of the 5-hydroxyeicosatetraenoic acid series.[246]

Leukotrienes C and D (slow-reactive substances of anaphylaxis or SRS-A) are also released by stimulated macrophages. Alveolar macrophages produce 12-hydroxyeicosatetraenoic acid (12-HETE), LTB_4, PGF_2, thromboxane A_2, and PAF.[84,169,247,248] PGE_2 stimulates the production of cAMP in macrophages as in other cells with PGE_2 receptors;[54] cAMP inhibits many cellular reactions, including chemotaxis, phagocytosis, the respiratory burst, lymphocyte mitogenesis, and lymphocyte-mediated cytotoxicity. Prostaglandins stimulate osteoclast activation, thereby enhancing bone resorption.[15] Thromboxanes are vasoconstrictors and LTB_4 is chemotactic for both neutrophils and macrophages.[53] Leukotrienes C and D stimulate smooth muscle contraction and bronchoconstriction. Macrophage-induced suppressor activity,[249] described in numerous inflammatory conditions including rheumatoid arthritis, may be mediated by the release of prostaglandins and leukotrienes.[56,250–252]

GROWTH-PROMOTING FACTORS

Macrophages produce a number of growth factors. The best defined of these is interleukin-1 (IL-1), previously termed lymphocyte-activating factor (LAF).[253,254] IL-1 is more than one protein, a fact appreciated after its genes were cloned.[255,256] Human IL-1α and IL-1β, synthesized by lipopolysaccharide-treated macrophages, are translated as approximately 30,000-M.W. precursors, which are apparently cleaved to M.W. 17,500. These molecules mediate many biologic activities including thymocyte proliferation by induction of IL-2 synthesis, fibroblast growth-factor activity, and prostaglandin and collagenase release from synovial cells.[115,253,254,257] IL-1 also causes acute-phase protein synthesis by hepatocytes and appears to be identical to endogenous pyrogen. Moreover, IL-1 enhances eosinophil oxidative metabolism induced by phorbol esters.[258]

IL-1 is produced in macrophages on stimulation with a variety of agents including silica, lipopolysaccharide, muramyldipeptide, and immune complexes.[253,254,257] IL-1 is either secreted or accumulates intracellularly, depending on the stimulus. This factor is also expressed on the surface of macrophages and can act as a cell contact dependent signal.[259] The production of IL-1 is inhibited by hydrocortisone, PGE$_2$, aging, and ultraviolet radiation.[260,261] T -cell-induced production of IL-1 is curtailed by the immunosuppressive drug cyclosporin.[262] IL-1 also has direct effects on connective tissue cells. The rate of cell division and prostaglandin and collagenase production by fibroblasts is accelerated by IL-1.[263] This substance promotes bone resorption by osteoblasts as well as the release of glycosaminoglycans from cartilage.[264] Exposure of rheumatoid synovial cells to IL-1 in vitro increases production of inflammatory products. IL-1 may also be identical to mononuclear cell factor (MCF) shown to stimulate synovial stellate cells to produce collagenase.[265]

Macrophages produce other less well defined growth factors. Colony-stimulating activity, which causes hematopoietic progenitor cells to form colonies in vitro, is released after the addition of endotoxin to macrophage cultures. Macrophages also release activities that stimulate fibroblast proliferation,[266] but the nature of these activities is still poorly defined.[267] Macrophages also synthesize low levels of α-interferon whereas γ-interferon may act as a differentiation

signal to macrophages by enhancing their expression of surface membrane components.[268,269]

TUMOR-NECROSIS FACTOR

Tumor-necrosis factor (TNF) is a potent biologic material produced and secreted by macrophages exposed to endotoxin.[270,271] The discovery of TNF dates to the late 1800s when Coley described dramatic antitumor responses in patients treated with extracts of pyogenic bacteria.[272] TNF was first isolated from the serum of animals treated with endotoxin. Injection of such sera resulted in necrosis of animal tumors, as well as other biologic activities including extreme cachexia (originally termed cachectin by some investigators),[273] lipemia secondary to complete suppression of lipoprotein lipase, hypotension, fever, and disseminated intravascular coagulation. TNF effects in different tissues are mediated by high-affinity receptors, the occupancy of which results in the suppression of specific messenger RNA expression.[270] TNF from several animal species has been cloned; is a highly conserved molecule suggesting that its in vivo biologic activity is important for survival.[270,274] The mature human gene product is composed of 157 amino acids with a molecular weight of 45,000 daltons by gel filtration and 17,000 daltons by sodium dodecyl sulfate gel electrophoresis.[270,274]

TNF may be important in the pathogenesis of certain rheumatic diseases in that many inflammatory disorders are characterized by mononuclear inflammatory infiltrates in the affected tissues. Indeed, TNF stimulates collagenase and PGE$_2$ production by human synovial cells and dermal fibroblasts,[275] and stimulates bone resorption, and inhibits synthesis of proteoglycans in cartilage.[276]

REACTIVE OXYGEN PRODUCTS

Release of reactive oxygen species is an important mechanism by which macrophages kill microbial agents and tumor cells.[195,277] Phagocytosis or exposure to agents such as chemoattractants initiates a "respiratory burst," a phenomenon associated with increased cellular oxygen consumption and the activation of a membrane-associated enzyme, NADPH oxidase.[194,278] This enzyme converts molecular oxygen into superoxide anion (O_2^-) as follows:

$$NADPH \times H^+ + 2O_2 = NADP^+ + 2H^+ 2O_2^-$$

Further metabolism of superoxide leads to the formation of hydrogen peroxide through the enzyme superoxide dismutase. Hydrogen peroxide and O_2, in the presence of iron, react to form singlet oxygen ($\cdot O_2$) and hydroxyl radical ($\cdot OH$). The enzyme myeloperoxidase and a halide such as chloride ion then convert singlet oxygen to hypochlorous ion.[279] Hydrogen peroxide, singlet oxygen, hydroxyl radical, and hypochlorous ion are potent oxidizing agents and inactivate the sulfhydryl groups of vital enzymes or proteins. Their release is affected by their state of macrophage activation. Macrophages activated to kill intracellular parasites or tumor cells can secrete large amounts of hydrogen peroxide.[121,195] Resident peritoneal macrophages or inflammatory macrophages, not stimulated with agents such as bacille Calmette Guérin (BCG), are far less capable of producing hydrogen peroxide. An interesting activity of oxidizing agents is their ability to inactivate biologically active products, such as chemoattractants or antiproteases, through oxidation of methionine residues to sulfoxides.[230,280] Oxidizing agents thus play additional roles in inflammation other than through direct cytotoxicity. For example, production of superoxide anion decreases the viscosity of synovial fluid through depolymerization of hyaluronate.[281]

FIBRONECTIN

This macromolecular glycoprotein mediates the adherence of cells such as fibroblasts to substrata; it is synthesized and released by activated macrophages. Because fibronectin is chemotactic for fibroblasts, activated macrophages can provide a stimulus for fibrogenesis at inflammatory sites.[282–285]

FACTORS AFFECTING LIPID METABOLISM

Apolipoprotein E is a 34,000- to 37,000-dalton glycoprotein that regulates lipoprotein and cholesterol metabolism. Peritoneal macrophages secrete large amounts of apolipoprotein E after they have been loaded with cholesterol.[168] Apolipoprotein E and cholesterol are secreted independently, but later associate with high-density lipoproteins (HDL), forming particles that deliver cholesterol to the liver.[286] Liver cells contain receptors for apolipoprotein E that stimulate the uptake of apolipoprotein E-associated lipids. The magnitude of apolipoprotein E secretion by cholesterol-laden macrophages suggests an important role for mononuclear phagocytes in atherogenesis.[287–289] That release of apolipoprotein E by macrophages is inhibited by endotoxin suggests a mechanism for the hyperlipidemia associated with endotoxemia.[289] Moreover, very low-density lipoproteins (VLDL) induce triglyceride synthesis by macrophages.[290] These findings indicate a potentially important role for macrophages in regulating lipid metabolism.

Monocytes display a much greater capacity for cholesterol synthesis from its precursors, acetate and mevalonate, than other leukocytes.[167,291] Lipid synthesis may be required for some inflammatory functions of monocyte-macrophages because inhibitors of such synthesis depress their chemotaxis, a process reversed by exogenous LDL.[292] Serial ultrastructural studies of vascular endothelium from animals fed high-cholesterol diets show that formation of atherosclerotic lesions is preceded by intimal penetration of blood-borne mononuclear cells that subsequently undergo transformation into "foam" cells in fatty streak lesions.[100,170–172] The interaction of arterial proteoglycans and LDL has been postulated to be an important factor in extracellular cholesterol accumulation in the arterial wall.[293] The cholesterol ester content of macrophages incubated with insoluble LDL-proteoglycan complexes was 20 times that observed in cells incubated with LDL alone;[293] these findings suggest that components of extracellular matrix, such as proteoglycans, can modify cellular catabolism of LDL.

NEUROPEPTIDES

Investigators have become increasingly aware of a bidirectional interplay between the immune and neuroendocrine systems. Several neuropeptides synthesized in the pituitary gland are also produced and secreted by macrophages and monocytes. The proopiomelanocortin-derived hormones, adrenocorticotropin (ACTH), and the endorphins are synthesized constitutively in the absence of cell stimulation.[294–296] These peptides signal the adrenal gland to release corticosteroids and have direct effects on immune functions. ACTH inhibits γ-interferon production by lymphocytes, for example,[297] and the endorphins augment both macrophage superoxide anion release and chemotaxis.[298,299]

The neuropeptide bombesin is also secreted by macrophages.[300] Its biologic effects include stimulation of hormone and enzyme secretion from endocrine and exocrine glands and mitogenic activity for fibroblasts, normal bronchial epithelial cells, and small-cell lung-cancer cells.[301–303] Bombesin is also chemotactic for human monocytes, but the significance of this finding is still obscure.[304]

Monocytes and macrophages also are stimulated to

produce superoxide anion by another neuropeptide, substance P, an undecapeptide secreted by unmyelinated C-type nerve terminals.[305,306] High-affinity receptors for substance P have been detected on macrophage surfaces.[305] Substance P has been implicated as a mediator of joint inflammation in an animal model of rheumatoid arthritis.[307,308]

Other Factors

Alveolar macrophages, isolated by bronchial lavage and placed in culture, make soluble factors that suppresss the proliferative response of peripheral blood lymphocytes to antigens and mitogens. These factors suppress T cells to a greater extent than B cells. Thus, the alveolar macrophage, formerly thought to have only nonspecific defensive functions, may have the capacity to adjust its own microenvironment.[47] A nonspecific immune-suppressor factor has been isolated from macrophages treated with soluble immune-response suppressor factor (SIRS).[45]

MICROBICIDAL ACTIVITY

When phagocytized by macrophages, microbial agents are exposed to hydrolases, toxic oxygen products, lysozyme and other antibacterial proteins. Such antimicrobial activity is one of the most important macrophage functions.[166] Some infectious agents, predominantly intracellular pathogens, escape destruction, however. These include certain viruses, and mycobacterial, chlamydial, rickettsial, and listerial organisms. Parasites such as trypanosoma, leishmania, and toxoplasma can even replicate in macrophages, whereas fungal organisms, including cryptococcus and aspergillus, and bacteria such as corynebacterium, salmonella, brucella, pasteurella, and nocardia can also survive macrophage phagocytosis. The ability to escape destruction by macrophages is far from complete, however; macrophages in the "activated" state, such as those treated with γ-interferon, kill the aforementioned organisms far more readily than do nonactivated cells. Macrophage activation is important in host defense, especially antimicrobial and tumoricidal activity.[309]

MACROPHAGE ACTIVATION

Macrophages and granulocytes have functions in common; however, some striking differences exist, one of the most important of which is the ability of macrophages to alter their functional activity in response to environmental stimuli. When isolated from blood or from noninflammatory tissue sites such as the peritoneal cavity, macrophages show chemotactic, phagocytic, and antimicrobial activity, but all these functions, as well as the magnitude of the respiratory burst, are enhanced during activation. Products synthesized by stimulated lymphocytes such as lymphokines or by small doses of endotoxins lead to macrophage activation.[108,310,311] The activated macrophage has enhanced ability to kill intracellular parasites as well as tumor cells in the absence of antitumor antibody.[50,312] Microbicidal activity for trypanosomes can be induced in human monocyte-derived macrophages if the cells are first exposed to soluble factors produced by lymphocytes.[313,314] Soluble factors from spleen cells enhance macrophage antimicrobial functions for chlamydia by enhancing hydroxyl-radical production.[315] Metabolites of the cyclo-oxygenase and lipoxygenase pathways are increased by treatment of macrophages with γ-interferon or BCG.[316] Macrophages can also use peroxidase enzymes released by other cells at inflammatory sites to augment their own killing potential.[317]

Macrophage activation can be divided into several distinct steps,[12,312,318] shown experimentally with murine peritoneal macrophages: resident macrophages have the lowest lysosomal enzyme content and low microbicidal and tumoricidal activity; macrophages elicited with nonimmune inflammatory agents such as proteose peptone contain more lysosomes and are more phagocytic, but are still unable to kill intracellular parasites or tumor cells; however, cells elicited using BCG are fully activated and kill intracellular organisms and tumor cells. Intermediate between inflammatory and activated macrophages are "primed" macrophages obtained from animals injected with the complex polysaccharide *pyran*. These cells become fully activated in vitro after treatment with MAF and small doses of endotoxin.[312,319] The enhancement of protein kinase C activity and the phosphorylation of several as yet unidentified proteins accompany macrophage activation.[320] Expression of mRNA for the proto-oncogenes c-fos and c-myc is also increased.[320] Chemoattractants, on the other hand, selectively increase expression of c-fos levels in human blood monocytes, apparently mediated by the release of 1,2-diacylglycerol.[321]

TUMOR CYTOTOXICITY

The development of direct tumor-cell cytotoxicity by macrophages is associated with selective binding to tumor, as opposed to nontumor, cells (Fig. 18–4).[312,322] As previously discussed, activated mac-

FIG. 18–4. Scanning electron micrograph of macrophages binding multiple tumor cells (×3,800). M = macrophage; T = tumor cell. (Courtesy of Dr. Dolph O. Adams, Duke University Medical Center.)

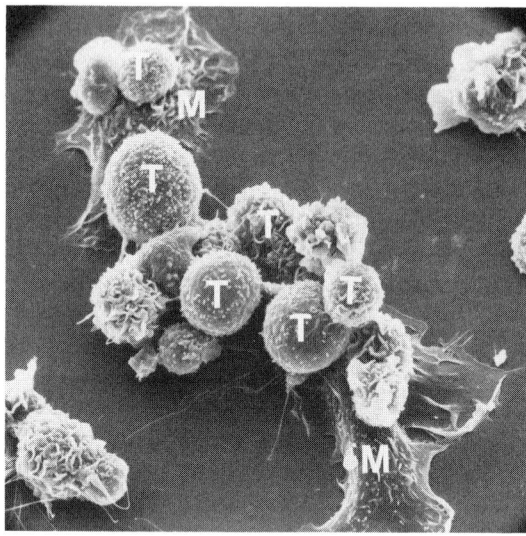

rophages have increased lysosomal hydrolase activity and a greater potential to produce hydrogen peroxide. In the presence of tumor cells, activated macrophages secrete a novel serine protease (M. W. approximately 40,000 daltons) not found in unactivated macrophages.[46] This protease and the production of hydrogen peroxide, TNF, and IL-1 by activated macrophages seem responsible for tumor cell killing,[323] although human blood monocytes are capable of lysing tumor cells by oxygen-independent mechanisms under some circumstances.[91] Macrophages can also kill tumor cells in the presence of antibody, a phenomenon termed antibody-dependent cell-mediated cytotoxicity; this process does not require activated macrophages. Although the biochemical correlates of activation are still unknown, functional changes include enhanced tumor cell binding activity and enhanced secretion of cytolytic protease.[324,325] Cell surface changes include decreased 5' nucleotidase activity and decreased numbers of mannose receptors.[64,326] Transmethylation, mediated by S-adenosyl-methionine, is required for direct tumor cell lysis.[327]

How then do clinically apparent tumors survive macrophage-mediated destruction? Tumor cells can produce factors that depress both macrophage accumulation at sites of inflammation in vivo and macrophage and monocyte chemotactic responsiveness in vitro.[99,328–331] A chemotactic defect has been noted in monocytes obtained from cancer patients, and such a defect is reversed by tumor removal.[332] The inhibi-

tion of chemotaxis associated with neoplasms may be due to the synthesis by tumor cells of a protein with similarities to the P15E structural component of oncogenic retroviruses.[333,334] Cancer cells thus may protect themselves from macrophage-mediated immune destruction.

MACROPHAGES AS IMMUNOREGULATORY CELLS

The importance of macrophages as effector cells has been recognized for over a century, but we now know that they are also essential in the afferent limb of the immune response. Macrophages are required, at some point, in almost all immunologic reactions because they regulate the function of both B and T lymphocytes.[6,7,335,336] Immune reactions begin with the antigen binding to the macrophage. The degree to which antigen is phagocytized and digested is important because it affects the quantity that will ultimately react with other immunocompetent cells. Most antigen given in vivo is destroyed by macrophages, with the fate of the remainder determined in part by its site of administration; antigen penetrating the circulation accumulates in splenic macrophages, whereas antigen administered in local tissue sites localizes in macrophages within draining lymphoid follicles.[337,338] Bound antigen is taken up by an active metabolic process involving micropinocytosis and becomes associated with Ia gene products. Limited regions of antigen molecules act as determinants (epitopes) for the stimulation of specific clones of T cells in the generation of helper cells for antibody production. "Antigen presentation" is the phenomenon whereby macrophages alter antigen in such a way that subsequent macrophage-lymphocyte interactions lead to the initiation of an immune response (see also Chapter 19).

Immune responses proceed only if Ia compatibility between macrophages and lymphocytes exists.[339] A physical interaction between macrophages and lymphocytes appears to be necessary for subsequent immunologic responses. Activation of T-helper cells requires antigen to be associated with class II MHC structures on macrophages, whereas activation of T-suppressor cells requires antigen to be associated with class I MHC structures. Some exceptions to the rule exist. Complex lipopolysaccharides and polysaccharides, such as endotoxins, appear to interact directly with B cells.

Besides specific antigen presentation, macrophages also affect immune responses through the secretion of nonantigen-specific factors such as interleukin-1 (IL-1) and tumor necrosis factor (TNF).[340,341] IL-1 is required for lymphocyte blastogenesis initiated by antigen or nonspecific mitogens, whereas TNF synergizes with IL-1 for most functions. Macrophages can also inhibit immune responses by the secretion of prostaglandins.[252,342–344]

MACROPHAGE ADHESION PROTEINS

A family of adhesion proteins present on the surface of monocytes and macrophages is needed for many cellular functions, including adherence, chemotaxis, endocytosis, and tumor cell lysis.[52] These molecules include LFA-1, Mac-1, and p150,95.[50–52] These high-molecular-weight surface glycoproteins contain an α and β subunit noncovalently associated in an $\alpha_1\beta_1$ structure. The β subunits have an M.W. of 95,000 daltons and are identical in the 3 molecules. The distinguishing characteristics of the molecules reside in the α subunit, which have different isoelectric points, molecular weights, and cell distributions and are immunologically noncross-reactive. The relative molecular weight of the Mac-1, LFA-1, and p150,95 α subunits are 165,000, 177,000, and 150,000 daltons, respectively.[50,51]

The LFA-1 and Mac-1 molecules contribute to a variety of adhesion-related functions of monocytes, granulocytes, and lymphocytes. LFA-1, whose expression on the cell surface is independent of cellular activation,[52] is expressed on lymphocytes, monocytes, granulocytes, and large granular lymphocytes. Monoclonal antibodies to LFA-1 inhibit cytolytic T-lymphocyte-mediated killing and T-helper cell responses, natural-killer activity, antibody-dependent cellular cytotoxicity, and phorbol ester-stimulated lymphocyte aggregation.[52] Presumably, this molecule mediates adhesion of monocytes to cell surfaces and may be important for antigen-presenting activity. Mac-1 was first detected by a monoclonal antibody recognizing a differentiation antigen present on myeloid, but not lymphoid, cells.[51,345] Later, it was found to be identical to CR3, which binds the inactivated segment (C3bi) of the third component of complement.[160] Mac-1 therefore mediates adherence and phagocytosis of C3bi-coated particles by granulocytes and monocytes. The expression of both Mac-1 and p150,95 on monocytes and granulocytes is enhanced by treatment with activators such as chemoattractants, phorbol esters, and calcium;[52] p150,95 is found on the surfaces of macrophages, monocytes, and granulocytes, but its specific function remains unknown.

An autosomal recessive disorder has been described in which the Mac-1, LFA-1, and p150,95 glycoproteins are deficient.[51] These patients have recurrent, life-threatening bacterial infections, lack of pus formation, and persistent granulocytosis. Each of the three α subunits and the common β subunit are deficient on the surface of all cells. Two phenotypes have been defined, severe deficiency and moderate deficiency, with surface expression of <0.2% and 5%, respectively, of the normal amounts of the three glycoproteins. In both phenotypes, the underlying defect is in the common β subunit.[51,52] In normal cells, α and β subunit precursors are synthesized and are noncovalently associated before transport to the Golgi complex, where carbohydrate processing and a slight increase in relative molecular mass occur. The mature molecules are then transported to the cell surface or to intracellular storage sites.[52] Cells from these patients lack β subunit synthesis. Because α and β association is required prior to transport to the cell surface, both subunits are absent on patient cells. The recurrent soft tissue infections appear to be due to the inability of granulocytes and monocytes to migrate to inflammatory sites.

DENDRITIC CELLS

A newly described nonlymphoid cell called "dendritic" because of its strikingly stellate appearance, appears to be an important component of immune responses.[176,346] These cells have potent antigen-presentation functions and are Ia positive. They are adherent to surfaces, but do not express Fc receptors and are nonphagocytic. Although not "officially" recognized as macrophages, dendritic cells stimulate allogeneic, syngeneic, and soluble antigen responses. They may be equivalent to the "interdigitating cell" in the T-cell nodal region of the lymph node where antigen is known to localize, but marker studies have not yet proved this concept conclusively.[343]

An elongated cell in human rheumatoid synovial tissue has also been called "dendritic." It is also Ia positive and nonphagocytic;[347] a potent source of collagenase, it is best referred to as a "stellate" cell[348,349] (see also Chapter 15).

DRUG EFFECTS ON MACROPHAGE FUNCTION

CORTICOSTEROIDS

Mononuclear phagocytes contain glucocorticoid receptors,[350] and glucocorticoids have a profound effect on macrophage function both in vivo and in vitro.

Hydrocortisone given intravenously in humans induces a monocytopenia within 4 hours, associated with depressed monocyte accumulation at inflammatory sites. Alternate-day administration of prednisone has less effect on monocyte function than does daily administration.[351] Corticosteroids also depress the release of monocytes from the bone marrow and decrease GM-CFU formation from bone marrow cells in vitro.[352] Monocytes from individuals taking prednisone show depressed bactericidal activity ex vivo while retaining normal chemotactic and phagocytic function.[353] Treatment of human monocytes with corticosteroids in vitro, however, depresses their chemotaxis,[131] and incubation of monocytes with hydrocortisone depresses their ability to bind opsonized erythrocytes.[354] Other functions of monocytes depressed by glucocorticoids include the secretion of collagenase, elastase, and plasminogen activator,[214,352] production of superoxide anion,[355] and differentiation to macrophages in vitro.[356] In contrast, spontaneous human monocyte-mediated cytotoxicity in vitro is enhanced by hydrocortisone.[357]

GOLD COMPOUNDS

Gold sodium thiomalate inhibits mixed leukocyte reactions of mononuclear cell preparations at concentrations compatible with those obtained therapeutically and is associated with the development of large intracytoplasmic vacuoles, diminished pinocytosis, and less phagocytosis of IgG-opsonized erythrocytes.[116,358] The phagocytic activity of macrophages isolated from synovium of gold-treated patients is similarly decreased.[228] Oral gold preparations are thought to have similar effects. This effect of gold may be selective because suppression of phagocytosis is greater in monocytes from patients with rheumatoid disease than in cells from normal persons.[359]

CYTOTOXIC AGENTS

These agents frequently decrease circulating monocyte levels, probably by affecting the development of monocytes in the bone marrow.[360,361] High doses of cyclophosphamide or methotrexate may also affect the accumulation of macrophages at inflammatory sites.[89,360] Vincristine similarly depresses the ability of macrophages to accumulate at sites of infection.[362]

PENICILLAMINE

In experimental animals, administration of D-penicillamine has a stimulatory effect on reticuloendothe-lial function, accompanied by an increased uptake of radiolabeled aggregated human gamma globulin by rat peritoneal macrophages.[363]

LEVAMISOLE

This immunostimulatory drug, initially developed as an antiparasitic agent, enhances monocyte chemotaxis in vitro and reverses defects of monocyte function associated with certain viral infections such as influenza.[364,365]

CYCLOSPORIN A

This immunosuppressive drug has profound effects on T-lymphocyte function and alters macrophage function when given to rats in vivo. Prostaglandin and thromboxane B_2 release by macrophages from animals treated intramuscularly with cyclosporin A was reduced.[366] That concentrations of these substances were reduced at sites of skin grafts in animals treated with cyclosporin suggests inhibition of macrophage accumulation at these sites.

L-LEUCINE METHYL ESTER

When human macrophages are incubated with L-leucine methyl ester, a metabolite is generated, L-leucyl-L-leucine methyl ester, which selectively inhibits cellular suppressive or cytolytic activities,[367] including OKT8+ suppressor T cells, MLC-activated and spontaneous natural-killer cells, and macrophages. A variety of other nonlymphoid and lymphoid cells remain unaffected by this material. These findings potentially provide a model of selective immunosuppressive therapy for certain rheumatic diseases.

MACROPHAGES IN RHEUMATIC DISEASES

The human immune system has evolved complex mechanisms designed to recognize specific epitopes on a variety of antigens. Nonetheless, the phagocytic cell is still central to the recognition and elimination of antigen, whether it be by fixed-tissue macrophages as components of the reticuloendothelial system or by wandering macrophages at tissue sites throughout the body. Macrophages participate in virtually all aspects of immunity. The properties that allow mac-

FIG. 18–5. Model for the pathogenesis of articular inflammation in rheumatoid arthritis. IL 1 = interleukin 1; LAF = lymphocyte activating factor; LDCG = lymphocyte-derived chemotactic factor; MAF = macrophage activating factor: RF = rheumatoid factor.

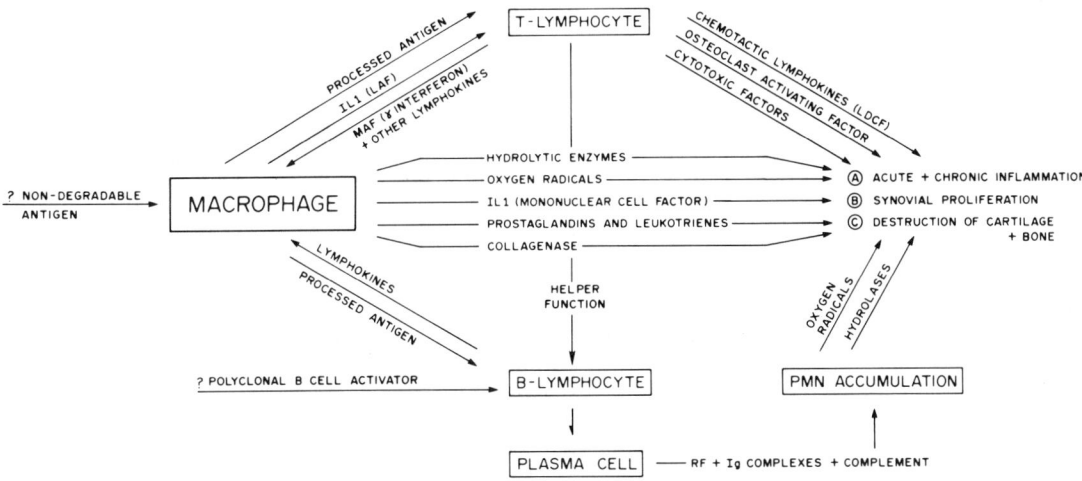

rophages to be so efficient in destroying nonself render them capable of being major participants in the tissue destruction associated with inflammatory diseases. In rheumatoid arthritis, polymorphonuclear leukocytes are the predominant phagocytic cells in the synovial fluid, but macrophages predominate in the synovium.[368] Although the stimulus initiating the inflammatory event in rheumatoid arthritis is unknown, synovial macrophages clearly produce copious amounts of prostaglandins, release enzymes such as collagenase, elastase, and plasminogen activator, and secrete IL-1 and TNF. The cartilage-degrading enzymes, collagenase and elastase, are derived from macrophages in the synovial pannus that invades the surrounding hard tissues. Cartilage-specific collagen may activate both macrophages and the alternative pathway of the complement cascade, thus interrelating two facets of the immunopathology of rheumatoid arthritis.[369]

Proteases aid in superficial cartilage destruction by uncross-linking collagen fibers and thereby making them more susceptible to proteolytic destruction. Stellate synovial cells are stimulated by IL-1 to produce abundant amounts of collagenase (see Chapter 42). Early in the development of rheumatoid arthritis, cartilage loss with decreased protoglycan content is manifested. Lysosomal proteases degrade aggregates of proteoglycans, which, when released from cartilage as solubilized components, are then sensitive to further enzymatic attack. IL-1 from macrophages also stimulates lymphocytes to produce lymphokines, at least one of which, termed *osteoclast-activating factor*, may stimulate bony demineralization. Prostaglan-

dins, leukotrienes, and other arachidonic acid metabolites may be responsible for long-term leaching of mineral from bony matrix. The net effect of an acute and chronic inflammatory response in the synovium is continued cellular influx, proliferation, and invasion of synovium into the surrounding joint structures (Fig. 18–5).

REFERENCES

1. Snyderman, R.: Mechanisms of inflammation and tissue destruction in the rheumatic diseases. *In* Cecil Textbook of Medicine, 16th Ed. Edited by L.H. Smith and J.B. Wyngaarden. Philadelphia, W.B. Saunders, 1982.
2. Normann, S.I., and Sorkin, F.: Macrophages and natural killer cells: regulation and function. Adv. Exp. Med. Biol., *155*:1–21, 1982.
3. Snyderman, R., and Goetzl, E.J.: Molecular and cellular mechanisms of leukocyte chemotaxis. Science, *213*:830–835, 1981.
4. Van Furth, R.: Mononuclear Phagocytes: Functional Aspects. The Hague, Martinus Nijhoff, 1980.
5. Van Furth, R.: Origin and kinetics of mononuclear phagocytes. Ann. N.Y. Acad. Sci., *278*:161–169, 1976.
6. Rosenthal, A.L, and Shevach, E.M.: The function of macrophages in T-lymphocyte antigen recognition. *In* Contemporary Topics in Immunobiology. Edited by W.O. Weigle. New York, Plenum Publishing, 1976.
7. Russell, I.J., and Tomasi, T.B.: Mechanism and abnormalities of immune regulation. Pathobiol. Ann., *8*:1–33, 1978.
8. Van Furth, R.: An approach to the characterization of mononuclear phagocytes involved in pathologic processes. Agents Actions, *6*:91–96, 1976.
9. Van Furth, R.: Mononuclear Phagocytes in Immunity, Infection and Pathology. Oxford, Blackwell Scientific Publications, 1975.
10. Van Furth, R., et al.: The mononuclear phagocyte system: a

new classification of macrophages, monocytes and their precursor cells. Bull. W.H.O., *46*:845–867, 1972.

11. Karnovsky, M.L.: Biochemical characteristics of activated macrophages. Ann. N.Y. Acad. Sci., *256*:266–270, 1975.

12. Karnovsky, M.L., and Lazdins, J.K.: Biochemical criteria for activated macrophages. J. Immunol., *121*:809–814, 1978.

13. Monohan, R.A., Dvorak, H.F., and Dvorak, A.M.: Ultrastructural localization of nonspecific esterase activity in guinea pig and human monocytes, macrophages, and lymphocytes. Blood, *58*:1089–1099, 1981.

14. North, R.J.: The concept of the activated macrophage. J. Immunol., *121*:806–810, 1978.

15. Byvoet, O.L., et al.: ADP in Paget's disease of bone: role of the mononuclear phagocyte system. Arthritis Rheum., *23*:1193, 1199, 1980.

16. Griffin, F.M., and Silverstein, S.: Segmental response of the macrophage plasma membrane to a phagocytic stimulus. J. Exp. Med., *139*:323–340, 1974.

17. Abboud, C.N., et al.: Hydrophobic adsorption chromatography of colony-stimulating activities and erythroid-enhancing activity from the human monocyte-like cell line, G.C.T. Blood, *58*–62:1148, 1981.

18. Kay, G.E., Laner, B.C., and Snyderman, R.: Induction of selective biological responses to chemoattractants in a human monocyte-like cell line. Infect. Immun., *41*–45:1166, 1983.

19. Koren, H.S., Handwerger, B.S., and Wunderlich, J.R.: Identification of macrophage-like characteristics in a cultured murine tumor line. J. Immunol., *114*:894–905, 1975.

20. Ralph, P.: Functions of macrophage cell lines. *In* Mononuclear Phagocytes: Functional Aspects. Edited by R. van Furth. The Hague, Martinus Nijhoff, 1980.

21. Rhodes, J.: Altered expression of human monocyte Fc receptors in malignant disease. Nature, *265*:253–270, 1977.

22. Spector, W.G.: The macrophage: its origin and role in pathology. Pathobiol. Ann., *4*:33–64, 1974.

23. Calcagno, M., et al.: Evidence of the existence of a factor that induces Fc receptors on bone marrow cells. Blood, *59*–69:756, 1982.

24. Wing, E.J., Ampel, N.M., Wahecd, A., and Shadduck, R.K.: Macrophage colony stimulating factor enhances the capacity of murine macrophages to secrete oxygen reduction products. J. Immunol., *135*:2052–2057, 1985.

25. North, R.J., and Mackaness, G.B.: Immunological control of macrophage proliferation in vitro. Infect. Immun., *8*:68–75, 1973.

26. Stanley, E.R., et al.: Colony stimulating factor and the regulation of granulopoiesis and macrophage production. Fed. Proc., *34*:2272–2278, 1976.

27. Stanley, E.R., and Gilbert, L.J.: Regulation of macrophage production by a colony-stimulating factor. *In* Mononuclear Phagocytes: Functional Aspects. Edited by R. van Furth. The Hague, Martinus Nijhoff, 1980.

28. Van Dingle, C.J.W., and van Agan, W.B.: Generation of tissue thromboplastin by human monocytes. *In* Mononuclear Phagocytes: Functional Aspects. Edited by R. van Furth. The Hague, Martinus Nijhoff, 1980.

29. Lee, F., et al.: Isolation of cDNA for a human granulocyte-macrophage colony-stimulating factor by functional expression in mammalian cells. Proc. Natl. Acad. Sci. U.S.A., *82*:4360–4365, 1985.

30. Sacca, R., Stanley, E.R., Sherr, C.J. and Rettenmier, C.W.: Specific binding of the mononuclear phagocyte colony-stimulating factor CSF-1 to the product of the v-fms oncogene. Proc. Natl. Acad. Sci. U.S.A., *83*:3331–3336, 1986.

31. Broxmeyer, H.E., et al.: Monocyte-macrophage-derived acidic isoferritins: normal feedback regulators of granulocyte-macrophage progenitor cells in vitro. Blood, *60*:595–604, 1982.

32. Pleus, L.M., Broxmeyer, H.G., and Moore, M.A.: Regulation of human myelopoiesis by prostaglandin E and lactoferrin. Cell Tissue Kinet., *14*:515–522, 1981.

33. Weissmann, G.: Lysosomal mechanisms of tissue injury in arthritis. N. Engl. J. Med., *286*:141–147, 1972.

34. Werb, Z.: Hormone receptors and hormonal regulation of macrophage physiological functions. *In* Mononuclear Phagocytes: Functional Aspects. Edited by R. van Furth. The Hague, Martinus Nijhoff, 1980.

35. Pelus, L.M.: Association between CFU-GM expression of HLA-DR antigen and control for granulocyte and macrophage production: a new role for prostaglandin E1. J. Clin. Invest., *70*:568–578, 1982.

36. Spitzer, G., and Verma, D.S.: Cells with Fc gamma receptors from normal donors suppress granulocytic macrophage colony formation. Blood, *60*:758–762, 1982.

37. Kriegler, A.B., et al.: Partial purification and characterization of a growth factor for macrophage progenitor cells with high proliferative potential in mouse bone marrow. Blood, *60*:503–510, 1982.

38. Goud, J.L.M., Schotte, C., and van Furth, R.: Identification and characterization of the monoblast in mononuclear phagocyte colonies grown in vitro. J. Exp. Med., *142*:1180–1189, 1975.

39. van Furth, R., et al.: The regulation of the participation of the mononuclear phagocyte system in inflammatory responses. *In* Experimental Models of Chronic Inflammatory Disease. Va Bayer Symposium. Edited by L.E. Glynn and H.D. Schlumberger. Berlin, Germany, Gross Leder, 1977.

40. Goud, J.L.M., and van Furth, R.: Proliferative characteristics of monoblasts grown in vitro. J. Exp. Med., *142*:1200–1208, 1975.

41. Meuret, G., Batara, E., and Furste, H.O.: Monocytopoiesis in normal man: pool size, proliferation activity and DNA synthesis time of promonocytes. Acta Haematol., *54*:261–270, 1975.

42. Volkman, A.: Monocyte kinetics and their changes in infection. *In* Immunobiology of the Macrophage. Edited by D.S. Nelson. New York, Academic Press, 1976.

43. van Waarde, D., Hulsing-Hessilink, E., and van Furth, R.: Properties of a factor increasing monocytopoiesis (FIM) occurring in serum during the early phase of an inflammatory reaction. Blood, *50*:727–734, 1977.

44. Volkman, A.: Disparity in origin of mononuclear phagocyte populations. J. Reticuloendothel. Soc., *19*:249–255, 1976

45. Aune, T.M., and Pierce, C.W.: Identification and initial characterization of a nonspecific suppressor factor (macrophage-SF) produced by soluble immune response suppressor (SIRS)-treated macrophages. J. Immunol., *127*:1828–1837, 1981.

46. Adams, D.O.: The granulomatous inflammatory responses. Am. J. Pathol., *84*:163–191, 1976.

47. McCombs, C.C., et al.: Human alveolar macrophages suppress the proliferative response of peripheral blood lymphocytes. Chest, *82*:266–274, 1982.

48. Czop, J.K., McGowan, S.E., and Center, D.M.: Opsonin-independent phagocytosis by human alveolar macrophages; augmentation by human plasma fibronectin. Am. Rev. Respir. Dis., *125*:607–617, 1982.

49. Perri, R.T., et al.: Fibronectin enhances in vitro monocyte-macrophage-mediated tumoricidal activity. Blood, *60*:430–438, 1982.

50. Sanchez-Madrid, F., et al.: A human leukocyte differentiation antigen family with distinct α-subunits and a common β-subunit. J. Exp. Med., *158–162*:1785, 1983.

51. Springer, T.A., et al.: Inherited deficiency of the Mac-1, LFA-1, p150,95 glycoprotein family and its molecular basis. J. Exp. Med., *160*:1901–1916, 1984.

52. Springer, T.A, and Anderson, D.C.: The importance of the Mac-1, LFA-1 glycoprotein family in monocyte and granulocyte adherence, chemotaxis and migration into inflammatory sites: insights from an experiment in nature. Ciba Found. Symp., *118*:102–140, 1986.

53. Valone, F.H.: Regulation of human leukocyte function by lipoxygenase products of arachidonic acid. *In* Contemporary Topics in Immunobiology: Regulation of Leukocyte Function. Edited by R. Snyderman. New York, Plenum Publishing, 1984.

54. Verghese, M.W., and Snyderman, R.: Hormonal activation of adenylate cyclase in macrophage membranes is regulated by guanine nucleotides. J. Immunol., *130*:869–878, 1983.

55. Snyderman, R., and Mergenhagen, S.E.: Chemotaxis of macrophages. *In* Immunobiology of the Macrophage. Edited by D.S. Nelson. New York, Academic Press, 1976.

56. Benyunes, M.C., and Snyderman, R.: Characterization of an oligopeptide chemoattractant receptor on human blood monocytes using a new radioligand. Blood, *63*:588–694, 1984.

57. Snyderman, R., et al.: A chemoattractant receptor on macrophages exists in two affinity states regulated by guanine nucleotides. J. Cell Biol., *98*:444–450, 1984.

58. Snyderman, R., and Fudman, E.J.: Demonstration of a chemotactic factor receptor on macrophages. J. Immunol., *124*:2754–2762, 1980.

59. Weinberg, J.B., Muscato, J.J., and Niedel, J.: Monocyte chemotactic peptide receptor. J. Clin. Invest., *68*:621–630, 1981.

60. Cianciolo, G.J., and Snyderman, R.: Monocyte responsiveness to chemotactic stimuli is a property of a sub-population of cells that can respond to multiple chemoattractants. J. Clin. Invest., *67*:60–69, 1981.

61. Hugli, T.E.: The structural basis for anaphylatoxin and chemotactic functions of C3a, C4a, and C5a. CRC Crit. Rev. Immunol., *4*:321–366, 1981.

62. Jensen, J., Snyderman, R., and Mergenhagen, S.E.: Chemotactic activity: a property of guinea pig, C5 anaphylatoxin. *In* Cellular and Humoral Mechanisms in Anaphylaxis and Allergy. Proceedings of the Third International Congress on Allergy and Anaphylaxis. S. Karger, Basel, 1969.

63. Shin, H.S., et al.: Chemotactic and anaphylatoxic fragment cleaved from the fifth component of guinea pig complement. Science, *162*:136–140, 1968.

64. Imber, M.J., et al.: Selective reduction of mannose specific binding on activated vs. inflammatory macrophage monolayers. J. Biol. Chem., *257*:129–136, 1982.

65. Snyderman, R., et al.: Human mononuclear leukocyte chemotaxis: Quantitative assay for mediators of humoral and cellular chemotactic factors. J. Immunol., *108*:857–863, 1972.

66. Snyderman, R., Shin, H.S., and Hausman, M.S.: A chemotactic factor for mononuclear leukocytes. Proc. Soc. Exp. Biol. Med., *138*:387–392, 1971.

67. Hugli, T.E., and Muller-Eberhard, H.J.: Anaphylatoxins: C3a and C5a. Adv. Immunol., *26*:1–38, 1978.

68. Snyderman, R., Phillips, J.K., and Mergenhagen, S.E.: Biological activity of complement in vivo: role for C5 in the accumulation of polymorphonuclear leukocytes in inflammatory exudates. J. Exp. Med., *134*:1131–1140, 1971.

69. Ward, P.A., and Zvaifler, N.: Complement-derived chemotactic factors in inflammatory fluids of humans. J. Clin. Invest., *50–62*:606, 1971.

70. Snyderman, R., Phillips, J.K., and Mergenhagen, S.E.: Polymorphonuclear leukocyte chemotactic activity in rabbit serum and guinea pig serum treated with immune complexes: evidence for C5a as the major chemotactic factor. Infec. Immun., *1*:521–532, 1970.

71. Snyderman, R., Shin, H.S., and Dannenberg, A.M., Jr.: Macrophage proteinase and inflammation: the production of chemotactic activity from the fifth component of complement by macrophage proteinase. J. Immunol., *109*:896–905, 1972.

72. Chenoweth, D.E., et al.: Complement activation during cardiopulmonary bypass: evidence for generation of C3a and C5a anaphylatoxins. N. Engl. J. Med., *304*:497–507, 1981.

73. Craddock, P.R., et al.: Complement and leukocyte-mediated pulmonary dysfunction in hemodialysis. N. Engl. J. Med., *296*:769–778, 1977.

74. Hammerschmidt, D.E., et al.: Complement activation and pulmonary leukostasis during nylon fiber filtration leukapheresis. Blood, *51*:721–730, 1978.

75. Altman, L.C., et al.: A human mononuclear leukocyte chemotactic factor: characterization, specificity, and kinetics of production by homologous leukocytes. J. Immunol., *110*:801–809, 1973.

76. Postlethwaite, A.E., and Snyderman, R.: Characterization of a cell mediated reaction in the guinea pig. J. Immunol., *114*:274–280, 1975.

77. Schiffmann, E., Corcoran, B., and Wahl, S.: N-formylmethionyl peptides as chemoattractants for leukocytes. Proc. Natl. Acad. Sci. U.S.A., *72*:1059–1064, 1975.

78. Auron, P.E., et al.: Nucleotide sequence of human monocyte interleukin-1 precursor cDNA. Proc. Natl. Acad. Sci. U.S.A., *81*:7907–7914, 1984.

79. Chang, J., Liu, M.C., and Newcombe, D.S.: Identification of two monohydroxyeicosatetraenoic acids synthesized by human pulmonary macrophages. Am. Rev. Respir. Dis., *126*:457–462, 1982.

80. Postlethwaite, A.E., and Kang, A.: Collagen and collagen peptide-induced chemotaxis of human monocytes. J. Exp. Med., *143*:1299–1310, 1976.

81. Gallin, J.I., and Kaplan, A.P.: Mononuclear cell chemotactic activity of kallikrein and plasminogen activator and its inhibition by C1 inhibitor and α2-macroglobulin. J. Immunol., *113*:1928–1936, 1974.

82. Katz, A.B., Papper, D.S., and Ewart, M.R.: Generation of chemotactic activity for leukocytes by the action of thrombin on human fibrinogen. Nature, *24*:56–60, 1973.

83. Meltzer, M.S., Stevenson, M.D., and Leonard, E.J.: Characterization of macrophage chemotaxins in tumor cell cultures and comparison with lymphocyte-derived chemotactic factors. Cancer Res., *37*:721–729, 1977.

84. Arnou, B., et al.: Release of platelet activating factor and arachidonic acid metabolites form alveolar macrophages. Agents Actions, *11*:555–565, 1981.

85. Pike, M.C., and Snyderman, R.: Transmethylation reactions are required for initial morphologic and biochemical responses of human monocytes to chemoattractants. J. Immunol., *127*:1444–1450, 1981.

86. Scott, W.A., et al.: Regulation of arachidonic acid metabolism by macrophage activation. J. Exp. Med., *155*:1148–1155, 1982.

87. Scott, W.A., et al.: Resting macrophages produce metabolites from exogenous arachidonic acid. J. Exp. Med., *155*:535–546, 1982.

88. Ford-Hutchinson, A.W., et al.: Leukotriene B, a potent chemokinetic and aggregating substance released form polymorphonuclear leukocytes. Nature, 286:264–268, 1980.

89. Gadeberg, O.V., Rhodes, J.M., and Larsen, S.: The effect of various immunosuppressive agents on mouse peritoneal macrophages and on the in vitro phagocytosis of Escherichia coli O5:K3:H5 and degradation of ^{125}I labelled HSA-antibody complexes by the cells. Immunology, 28:59–67, 1975.

90. Goldman, D.W., and Goetzl, E.J.: Specific binding of leukotriene B_4 to receptors on human polymorphonuclear leukocytes. J. Immunol., 129:1600–1606, 1982.

91. Kleinerman, E.S., et al.: Lysis of tumor cells by human blood monocytes by a mechanism independent of activation of the oxidative burst. Cancer Res., 45:2058–2065, 1985.

92. Kreisle, R.A., and Parker, C.W.: Specific binding of leukotriene B_4 to a receptor on human polymorphonuclear leukocytes. J. Exp. Med., 157:628–639, 1983.

93. Camussi, G.M., et al.: Release of platelet activating factor and histamine. II. The cellular origin of human PAF monocytes, polymorphonuclear leukocytes and basophils. Immunology, 42:191–198, 1981.

94. Mencia-Huerta, J.M., and Benveniste, J.: Platelet activating factor and macrophages. I. Evidence for the release from rat and mouse peritoneal macrophages and not from mastocytes. Eur. J. Immunol., 9:409–414, 1979.

95. Demopoulos, C.A., Pinkard, R.N., and Hanahan, D.J.: Platelet activating factor. J. Biol. Chem., 254:9355–9362, 1979.

96. Heiman, D.F., Gardner, J.T., Apferdorf, W.J., and Malech, H.L.: Effects of tunicamycin on the expression and function of formyl peptide chemotactic receptors of differentiated HL-60 cells. J. Immunol., 136:4623–4629, 1986.

97. Malech, H.L., Gardner, J.P., Heiman, D.F., and Rosensweig, S.A.: Asparagine-linked oligosaccharides on formyl peptide chemotactic receptors of human phagocytic cells. J. Biol. Chem., 260:2509–2514, 1985.

98. Stadel, J.M., DeLean, A., and Lefkowitz, R.J.: Molecular mechanisms of coupling in hormone receptor-adenylate cyclase systems. Adv. Enzymol., 53:1–32, 1982.

99. Normann, S.J., and Sorkin, F.: Inhibition of macrophage chemotaxis by neoplastic and other rapidly proliferating cells in vitro. Cancer Res., 37:705–715, 1977.

100. Schwartz, C.J., et al.: Monocyte-macrophage participation in atherogenesis: inflammatory components of pathogenesis. Semin. Thrombosis Hemostasis, 12:79–101, 1986.

101. Verghese, M.W., Smith, C.D., and Snyderman, R.: Potential role for a guanine nucleotide regulatory protein in chemoattractant receptor mediated polyphosphoinositide metabolism, calcium mobilization and cellular responses by leukocytes. Biochem. Biophys. Res. Commun., 127:450–454, 1985.

102. Volpi, M., et al.: Pertussis toxin inhibits fMet-Leu-Phe but not phorpol ester-stimulated changes in rabbit neutrophils: role of G proteins in excitation response coupling. Proc. Natl. Acad. Sci. U.S.A., 82:2708–2713, 1985.

103. Berridge, M.J.: Inositol trisphosphate and diacylglycerol as second messengers. Biochem. J., 220:345–349, 1984.

104. Farese, R.V.: Phospholipids as intermediates in hormone action. Mol. Cell. Endocrinol., 35:1–21, 1984.

105. Majerus, P.W., et al.: The metabolism of phosphoinositide-derived messenger molecules. Science, 234:1519–1522, 1986.

106. Nishizuka, Y.: The role of protein kinase C in cell surface signal transduction and tumor promotion. Nature, 308:693–699, 1984.

107. Griffin, F.M., Luben, R.A., and Golde, D.W.: A human lymphokine activates macrophage C3 receptors for phagocytosis: studies using monoclonal anti-lymphocyte antibodies. J. Leukocyte Biol., 36:95–106, 1984.

108. Mackaness, G.B.: Influence of immunologically committed lymphocytes on macrophage activity in vivo. J. Exp. Med., 129:973–987, 1969.

109. Myers, M.A., McPhail, L.C., and Snyderman, R.: Redistribution of protein kinase C activity in human monocytes: correlation with activation of the respiratory burst. J. Immunol., 135:3411–3418, 1985.

110. Nishihira, J., McPhail, L.C., and O'Flaherty, J.T.: Stimulus-dependent mobilization of protein kinase C. Biochem. Biophys. Res. Commun., 134:587–592, 1986.

111. Pike, M.C., Jakoi, L., McPhail, L.C., and Snyderman, R.: Chemoattractant-mediated stimulation of the respiratory burst in human polymorphonuclear leukocytes may require appearance of protein kinase activity in the cell's particulate fraction. Blood, 67:909–916, 1986.

112. Streb, H., Irvine, R.F., Berridge, M.J., and Schulz, I.: Release of calcium from a nonmitochondrial intracellular store in pancreatic acinar cells by inositol-1, 4,5-trisphosphate. Nature, 306:67–70, 1983.

113. Arend, W.P., and Mannik, M.: The macrophage receptor for IgG: number and affinity of binding sites. J. Immunol., 110:1455–1462, 1973.

114. Boltz-Nitulescu, G., Plummer, J.M., and Spiegelberg, H.L.: Fc receptors for IgE on mouse macrophages and macrophage-like cell lines. J. Immunol., 128:2265–2272, 1982.

115. Gordon, S., Todd, J., and Cohn, Z.A.: In vitro synthesis and secretion of lysozyme by mononuclear phagocytes. J. Exp. Med., 139:1228–1239, 1974.

116. Harth, M., and Stiller, C.R.: Inhibitory effects of gold and other drugs on mononuclear cell responses: a comparison. J. Rheumatol., 5 (Suppl.):112–118, 1979.

117. Howell, D.S., et al.: Presence and role of lysozyme in human osteoarthritic cartilage. J. Rheumatol., 1:31–39, 1974.

118. Michl, J., Ohlbaum, D.J., and Silverstein, S.C.: 2-Deoxyglucose selectively inhibits Fc and complement receptor-mediated phagocytosis in mouse peritoneal macrophages. I. Description of the inhibitory effect. J. Exp. Med., 144:1465–1472, 1976.

119. Irvine, R.F., et al.: The inositol tris/tetrakisphosphate pathway-demonstration of $Ins(1,4,5)P_3$ 3-kinase activity in animal tissue. Nature, 320:631–634, 1986.

120. Koo, C., Lefkowitz, R.J., and Snyderman, R.: Guanine nucleotides modulate the binding affinity of the oligopeptide chemoattractant receptor on human polymorphonuclear leukocytes. J. Clin. Invest., 72:748–755, 1983.

121. Nathan, C.F., et al.: Extracellular cytolysis by activated macrophages and granulocytes. II. Hydrogen peroxide as a mediator of cytotoxicity. J. Exp. Med., 149:100–114, 1979.

122. Snyderman, R., Smith, C.D., and Verghese, M.W.: Model for leukocyte regulation by chemoattractant receptors: roles of a guanine nucleotide regulatory protein and polyphosphoinositide metabolism. J. Leukocyte Biol., 1987. In press.

123. Pike, M.C., Kredich, N.M., and Snyderman, R.: Requirement of S-adenosylmethionine-mediated methylation for human monocyte chemotaxis. Proc. Natl. Acad. Sci. U.S.A., 75:3928–3934, 1978.

124. Pike, M.C., and Snyderman, R.: Requirements of transmethylation reactions for eukaryotic cell chemotaxis. In Covalent and Noncovalent Modification of Protein Function. Edited by D. Atkinson, and C.F. Fox, New York, Academic Press, 1980, p. 285–295.

125. Pike, M.C., and Snyderman, R.: Transmethylation reactions

regulate affinity and functional activity of chemotactic factor receptors on macrophages. Cell, 28:107–117, 1982.

126. Pike, M.C., Kredich, N.M., and Snyderman, R.: Phospholipid methylation in macrophages is inhibited by chemotactic factors. Proc. Natl. Acad. Sci. U.S.A., 76:2922–2927, 1979.

127. Niedel, J.E., Kuhn, L.J., and Vandenbark, G.R.: Phorbol diester receptor copurifies with protein kinase C. Proc. Natl. Acad. Sci. U.S.A., 80:36–41, 1983.

128. Painter, R.G., et al.: Activation of neutrophils by N-formyl chemotactic peptides. Fed. Proc., 43:2737–2742, 1984.

129. Sklar, L.A., and Oades, Z.G.: Signal transduction and ligand receptor dynamics in the neutrophil. J. Biol. Chem., 260:11,468–11,475, 1985.

130. Gallin, J.I., et al.: Agents that increase cyclic AMP inhibit accumulation of cGMP and depress human monocyte locomotion. J. Immunol., 120:492–499, 1978.

131. Stephens, C.G., and Snyderman, R.: Cyclic nucleotides regulate the morphologic alterations required for chemotaxis in monocytes. J. Immunol., 128:1192–1205, 1982.

132. Simchowitz, L., et al.: Induction of a transient elevation in intracellular levels of cAMP by chemotactic factors: an early event in human neutrophil activation. J. Immunol., 124:1482–1491, 1980.

133. Verghese, M.W., Smith, C.D., and Snyderman, R.: Role for a guanine nucleotide regulatory protein in chemoattractant mediated calcium mobilizaiton and cAMP formation in human neutrophils (PMNs). Clin. Res., 33:566A, 1985.

134. Naccache, P.H., et al.: Phorbol esters inhibit the fMet-Leu-Phe and leukotriene B4 stimulated calcium mobilization and enzyme secretion in rabbit neutrophils. J. Biol. Chem., 260:2125–2132, 1985.

135. Smith, C.D., Uhing, R.J., and Snyderman, R.: Nucleotide regulatory protein-mediated activation of phospholipase C in human polymorphonuclear leukocytes is disrupted by phorbol esters. J. Biol. Chem., 1987. In press.

136. Loor, F., and Roelants, G.E.: The dynamic state of the macrophage plasma membrane: attachment and fate of immunoglobulin, antigen and lectins. Eur. J. Immunol., 4:649–655, 1974.

137. Grey, H.M., and Anderson, C.L.: Structural characteristics of Fc receptors on macrophages. In Mononuclear Phagocytes: Functional Aspects. Edited by R. van Furth, The Hague, Martinus Nijhoff, 1980.

138. Heusser, C.H., Anderson, C.L., and Grey, H.M.: Receptors for IgG: subclass specificity of receptors on different mouse cell types and the definition of two distinct receptors on a macrophage cell line. J. Exp. Med., 145:131–140, 1977.

139. Huber, H., et al: Human monocytes: distinct receptor sites for the third component of complement and for immunoglobulin G. Science, 162:1281–1285, 1968.

140. Silverstein, S.C., Steinman, R.M., and Cohn, Z.A.: Endocytosis. Annu. Rev. Biochem., 46:669–695, 1977.

141. Unkeless, J.C.: Fc receptors of mouse macrophages. In Mononuclear Phagocytes: Functional Aspects. Edited by R. van Furth. The Hague, Martinus Nijhoff, 1980.

142. Unkeless, J.C., and Eisen, H.: Binding of monomeric immunoglobulins to Fc receptors of mouse macrophages. J. Exp. Med., 142:1520–1532, 1975.

143. Diamond, B., Bloom, B.R., and Scharff, M.D.: The Fc receptors of primary and cultured phagocytic cells studied with homogeneous antibodies. J. Immunol., 121:1978–1983, 1978.

144. Diamond, B., and Scharff, M.D.: IgG1 and IgG2b share the Fc receptor on mouse macrophages. J. Immunol., 125:631–640, 1980.

145. Diamond, B., and Yelton, D.E.: A new Fc receptor on mouse macrophages binding IgG3. J. Exp. Med., 153:514–520, 1981.

146. Walker, W.S.: Separate Fc receptors for immunoglobulins IgG2a and IgG2b on an established cell line of mouse macrophages. J. Immunol., 116:911–917, 1976.

147. Walker, W.S.: Mediation of macrophage cytolytic and phagocytic activities by antibodies of different classes and class-specific Fc receptors. J. Immunol., 119:367–373, 1977.

148. Anderson, C.L., and Grey, H.M.: Physiochemical separation of two distinct Fc receptors on murine macrophage-like cell lines. J. Immunol., 121:648–656, 1978.

149. Young, J.D.E., et al.: Macrophage membrane potential changes associated with γ2b/γ1 Fc receptor-ligand binding. Proc. Natl. Acad. Sci. U.S.A., 80:1357–1362, 1983.

150. Unkeless, J.C.: The presence of two Fc receptors on mouse macrophages: evidence from a variant cell line and differential trypsin sensitivity. J. Exp. Med., 145:931–943, 1977.

151. Finbloom, D.S., and Metzger, J.: Binding of immunoglobulin E to the receptor on rat periotoneal macrophages. J. Immunol., 129:2004–2009, 1982.

152. Lemaire, G., Draper, J.C., and Petit, J.F.: Importance, localization and functional properties of the cell-associated form of plasminogen activator in mouse peritoneal macrophages. Biochim. Biophys. Acta, 755:332–346, 1983.

153. Fearon, D.T.: Identifcation of the membrane glycoprotein that is the C3b receptor of the human erythrocyte, polymorphonuclear leukocyte, and monocyte. J.Exp. Med., 152:20–32, 1980.

154. Rabellino, E.M., Ross, G.D., and Polley, M.J.: Membrane receptors of mouse leukocytes. I. Two types of complement receptors for different regions of C3. J. Immunol., 120:879–883, 1978.

155. Ross, G.D.: Analysis of the different types of leukocyte membrane complement receptors and their interaction with the complement system. J. Immunol. Methods, 37:197–205, 1980.

156. Beller, D.I., Springer, T.A., and Schreiber, R.D.: Anti-MAC-1 selectively inhibits the mouse and human type three complement receptor. J. Exp. Med., 156:1000–1012, 1982.

157. Arnoult, M.J., et al.: Inhibition of phagocytosis of complement C3- or immunoglobulin C-coated particles and of C3bi binding monoclonal antibodies to a monocyte-granulocyte membrane glycoprotein. J. Clin. Invest., 71:171–184, 1983.

158. Lambris, J.D., Dobson, N.J., and Ross, G.D.: Isolation of lymphocyte membrane complement receptor type two (the C3d receptor) and preparation of receptor specific antibody. Proc. Natl. Acad. Sci. U.S.A., 78:1828–1833, 1981.

159. Wright, S.D., and Silverstein, S.C.: Phagocytosing macrophages exclude soluble macromolecules from the zone of contact with ligand-coated targets. Cell Biol., 95:433a, 1982.

160. Wright, S.,D., et al.: Identification of the C3bi receptor of human monocytes and macrophages with monoclonal antibodies. Proc. Natl. Acad. Sci. U.S.A., 80:5699–5704, 1983.

161. Wright,. S.D., Van Voorhis, W.C., and Silverstein, S.C.: Identification of the C3b receptor on human leukocytes using a monoclonal antibody. Fed. Proc., 42:1079–1088, 1983.

162. Bianco, C., Griffin, F.M., Jr., and Silverstein, S.C.: Studies of the macrophage complement receptor: alteration of receptor function upon macrophage activation. J. Exp. Med., 141:1278–1289, 1975.

163. Stahl, P., et al.: Evidence for receptor-mediated binding of glycoproteins, glycoconjugates, and lysosomal glycosidases by alveolar macrophages. Proc. Natl. Acad. Sci. U.S.A., 75:1399–1404, 1978.

164. Stahl, P., et al.: In vivo and in vitro evidence for a lysosomal

enzyme uptake system in macrophages. *In* Mononuclear Phagocytes: Functional Aspects. Edited by R. van Furth. The Hague, Martinus Nijhoff, 1980.

165. Weir, D.M., and Ogmundsdottir, H.M.: Cellular recognition by phagocytes: role of lectin-like receptor(s). *In* Mononuclear Phagocytes: Functional Aspects. Edited by R. van Furth. The Hague, Martinus Nijhoff, 1980.

166. Rodley, G.E., et al.: Defective bactericidal activity of monocytes in fatal granulomatous disease. Blood, 33:813–820, 1969.

167. Fogelman, A.M., et al.: Cholesterol biosynthesis in human lymphocytes, monocytes and granulocytes. Biochem. Biophys. Res. Commun., 76:167–171, 1977.

168. Goldstein, J.L., et al.: Binding site on macrophages that mediates uptake and degradation of acetylated low density lipoprotein, producing massive cholesterol depositon. Proc. Natl. Acad. Sci. U.S.A., 76:333–338, 1979.

169. Martin, T.R., et al.: Leukotriene B_4 production by the human alveolar macrophage: a potential mechanism for amplifying inflammation in the lung. Am. Rev. Respir. Dis., 129:106–124, 1984.

170. Sevitt, S.: Platelets and foam cells in the evolution of atherosclerosis: histological and immunohistological studies of human lesions. Atherosclerosis, 61:107–118, 1986.

171. Heinecke, J.W., et al.: Superoxide-mediated modification of low density lipoprotein by arterial smooth muscle. J. Clin. Invest., 77:757–769, 1986.

172. Small, D.M.: Physiocochemical and histical changes in the arterial wall of nonhuman primates during progression and regression of atherosclerosis. J. Clin. Invest., 73:1590–1602, 1984.

173. Phillips, D.R., Arnold, K., and Innerarity, T.L.: Platelet secretory products inhibit lipoprotein metabolism in macrophages. Nature, 316:746–750, 1985.

174. Braidman, L.P., et al.: Evidence for a steroid receptor in rheumatoid synovial tissue cells. Agents Actions, 7(Suppl.):233–240, 1980.

175. Sandler, J.A., et al.: The effect of serotonin (5-hydroxytryptamine) and derivatives on guanosine 3′,5′-monophosphate on human monocytes. J. Clin. Invest., 55:431–445, 1975.

176. Steinman, R.M., et al.: Dendritic cells and macrophages— current knowledge of their distinctive properties and functions. *In* Mononuclear Phagocytes: Functional Aspects. Edited by R. van Furth. The Hague, Martinus Nijhoff, 1980.

177. Debanne, M.T., Bell, R., and Dolovich, J.: Uptake of proteinase-macroglobulin complexes by macrophages. Biochim. Biophys. Acta, 411:295–305, 1975.

178. Nathan, C.F., et al.: Identification of interferon-γ as the lymphokine that activates human macrophage oxidative metabolism and antimicrobial activity. J. Exp. Med., 158:670–683, 1983.

179. Schreiber, R.D., et al.: Macrophage-activating factor produced by a T cell hybridoma: physicochemical and biosynthetic resemblance to interferon. J. Immunol., 131:826–834, 1983.

180. Higgins, T.J., et al.: Possible role of macrophage glycolipids as receptors for migration inhibitory factor (MIF). J. Immunol., 121:880–888, 1978.

181. Remold, H.G.: Requirement for α-L-fucose on the macrophage membrane receptor for MIF. J. Exp. Med., 138:1065–1072, 1973.

182. Rocklin, R.E.: Role of monosaccharides in the interaction of two lymphocyte mediators with their target cells. J. Immunol., 116:816–822, 1976.

183. David, J.R., et al.: MIF/MAF-macrophage interactions: biochemical characterization of a putative glycolipid receptor for MIF and the existence and properties of two distinct MIFs. *In* Mononuclear Phagocytes: Functional Aspects. Edited by R. van Furth. The Hague, Martinus Nijhoff, 1980.

184. Van Snick, J.L., and Masson, P.L.: Binding of human lactoferrin to mouse peritoneal cells. J. Exp. Med., 144:1568–1580, 1976.

185. Tulkens, P., Schneider, Y.J., and Trouet, A.: Membrane recycling (shuttle?) in endocytosis. *In* Mononuclear Phagocytes: Functional Aspects. Edited by R. van Furth. The Hague, Martinus Nijhoff, 1980.

186. Muller, W.A., Steinman, R.M., and Cohn, Z.A.: Membrane flow during endocytosis. *In* Mononuclear Phagocytes: Functional Aspects. Edited by R. van Furth. The Hague, Martinus Nijhoff, 1980.

187. Silverstein, S.C., and Loike, J.D.: Phagocytosis. *In* Mononuclear Phagocytes: Functional Aspects. Edited by R. van Furth. The Hague, Martinus Nijhoff, 1980.

188. Stossel, T.P.: Phagocytosis: recognition and ingestion. Semin. Hematol., 12:83–98, 1975.

189. Michl, J., Ohlbaum, D.J., and Silverstein, S.C.: 2-Deoxyglucose selectively inhibits Fc and complement receptor-mediated phagocytosis in mouse peritoneal macrophages. II. Dissociation of the inhibitory effect of 2-deoxyglucose on phagocytosis and ATP generation. J. Exp. Med., 144:1484–1500, 1976.

190. Einstein, L.P., Schneeberger, E.E., and Colten, H.R.: Synthesis of the second component of complement by long-term primary cultures of human monocytes. J. Exp. Med., 43:114–121, 1976.

191. Yin, H.L., and Stossel, T.P.: Control of cytoplasmic actin gelsol transformation by gelsolin, a calcium-dependent regulatory protein. Nature, 281:583–586, 1979.

192. Griffin, F.M., Jr., et al.: Studies on the mechanism of phagocytosis. I. Requirements for circumferential attachments of particle-bound ligands to specific receptors on the macrophage plasma membrane. J. Exp. Med., 142:1263–1274, 1975.

193. Schnyder, J., and Baggiolini, M.: Secretion of lysosomal enzymes by macrophages. *In* Mononuclear Phagocytes: Functional Aspects. Edited by R. van Furth. The Hague, Martinus Nijhoff, 1980.

194. McPhail, L.C., and Snyderman, R.: Oxygen-dependent microbicidal activity of leukocytes. Contemp. Top. Immunobiol., 14:247–281, 1984.

195. Johnston, R.B., Jr.: Oxygen metabolism and the microbicidal activity of macrophages. Fed. Proc., 39:93–100, 1978.

196. Klebanoff, S.J.: Oxygen intermediates and the microbicidal event. *In* Mononuclear Phagocytes: Functional Aspects. Edited by R. van Furth. The Hague, Martinus Nijhoff, 1980.

197. Nathan, C.F.: The release of hydrogen peroxide from mononuclear phagocytes and its role in extracellular cytolysis. *In* Mononuclear Phagocytes: Functional Aspects. Edited by R. van Furth. The Hague, Martinus Nijhoff, 1980.

198. Ezekowitz, R.A.B., et al.: Local opsonization by secreted macrophage complement components: role of receptors for complement in uptake of zymosan. J. Exp. Med., 159:244–255, 1984.

199. Ezekowitz, R.A.B., et al.: Interaction of human monocytes, macrophages, and polymorphonuclear leukocytes with zymosan in vitro. J. Clin. Invest., 76:2368–2378, 1985.

200. Griffin, F.M., Jr., and Mullinax, P.J.: Augmentation of macrophage complement receptor function in vitro. III. C3b receptors that promote phagocytosis migrate within the plane of the macrophage plasma membrane. J. Exp. Med., 154:291–302, 1981.

201. Svensson, B.O., Norberg, R., and Torshensson, R.: Effects of cytoglobulins and aggregated IgG on in vitro monocyte phagocytosis. Scand. J. Rheumatol., *31 (Suppl.)*:57–62, 1980.

202. Lawley, T.J.: Immune complexes and RES function in human diseases. J. Invest. Dermatol., *74*:339–348, 1980.

203. Hurst, N.P., and Nuki, G.: Evidence for defect of C-mediated phagocytes by monocytes from patients with RA and cutaneous vasculitis. Br. Med. J., *282*:2081–2095, 1980.

204. Holland, P., Holland, N.H., and Cohn, Z.A.: The selective inhibition of macrophage phagocytic receptors by antimembrane antibodies. J. Exp. Med., *135*:458–469, 1982.

205. Schnyder, J., and Baggiolini, M.: Secretion of lysosomal hydrolases by stimulated and nonstimulated macrophages. J. Exp. Med., *148*:435, 1978.

206. Davies, P., and Allison, A.C.: The macrophage as a secretory cell in chronic inflammation. Agents Actions, *6*:60–68, 1976.

207. Allison, A.C., Cardella, D., and Davies, P.: Immune complexes and induced release of lysosomal enzymes from mononuclear phagocytes in the pathogenesis of rheumatoid arthritis. In Immunological Aspects of Rheumatoid Arthritis: Rheumatology. Vol. 6. Edited by J. Clot and J. Sany. Basel, S. Karger, 1975.

208. Smialowicz, R.J., and Schwab, J.H.: Processing of streptococcal cell walls by rat macrophages and human monocytes, in vitro. Infect. Immun., *17*:591–600, 1977.

209. Snyderman, R., and Pike, M.C.: Transductional mechanisms of chemoattractant receptors on leukocytes. Comtemp. Top. Immunobiol., *14*:1–28, 1984.

210. Ziff, M.: Phagocytes and substrates in the joint. Scand. J. Rheumatol., *40 (Suppl.)*:10–32, 1981.

211. Gordon, S.: Macrophage neutral proteinase and chronic inflammation. Ann. N.Y. Acad. Sci., *278*:176–190, 1976.

212. Unkeless, J.C., Gordon, S., and Reich, E.: Secretion of plasminogen activator by stimulated macrophages. J. Exp. Med., *139*:834–938, 1974.

213. Kaplan, A.P.: The Hageman factor dependent pathways of human plasma. Microvasc. Res., *8*:92–101, 1974.

214. Vassalli, J.D., Hamilton, J., and Reich, E.: Macrophage plasminogen activator: modulation of enzyme production by anti-inflammatory steroids, mitotic inhibitors and cyclic nucleotides. Cell, *8*:271–276, 1976.

215. Solomon, J.A., et al.: Evidence for membrane association of plasminogen activator activity in mouse macrophages. Biochem. Biophys. Res. Commun., *94*:480–486, 1980.

216. Chapman, H.A., and Stone, O.L.: Characterization of macrophage-derived plasminogen-activator inhibitor. Biochem. J., *230*:109–117, 1985.

217. Evans, C., Mgars, D., and Cosgrove, C.: Release of neutral proteinase from mononuclear phagocytes and synovial cells in response to cartilaginous wear particles in vitro. Biochem. Biophys. Acta, *677*:287–298, 1981.

218. Wahl, L.J., et al.: Collagenase production by endotoxin activated macrophages. Proc. Natl. Acad. Sci. U.S.A., *71*:3598–3603, 1974.

219. Werb, Z., and Gordon, S.: Secretion of a specific collagenase by stimulated macrophages. J. Exp. Med., *142*:345–360, 1975.

220. Wahl, L.M., et al.: Collagenase production by lymphokine-activated macrophages. Science, *187*:261–264, 1975.

221. Dayer, J.M., et al.: Production of collagenase and prostaglandins by isolated adherent rheumatoid synovial cells. Proc. Natl. Acad. Sci. U.S.A., *73*:945–950, 1976.

222. Dayer, J.M., et al.: Purification of a factor from human blood monocyte which stimulates production of collagenase and

223. Werb, Z., and Gordon, S.: Elastase secretion by stimulated macrophages. J. Exp. Med., *142*:361–376, 1975.

224. Ragsdale, C.G., and Arend, W.P.: Neutral protease secretion by human monocytes: effect of surface-bound immune complexes. J. Exp. Med., *149*:954–968, 1979.

225. Spitznagel, J.K.: Non-oxidative antimicrobial reactions of leukocytes. Contemp. Immunobiol., *14*:283–344, 1984.

226. Gordon, S.: Lysozyme and plasminogen activator: constitutive and induced secretory products of mononuclear phagocytes. In Mononuclear Phagocytes: Functional Aspects. Edited by R. van Furth. The Hague, Martinus Nijhoff, 1980.

227. Hovi, T., Mosher, D., and Vaheri, A.: Cultured human monocytes synthesize and secrete α2-macroglobulin. J. Exp. Med., *145*:1580–1596, 1978.

228. Jessop, J.D., and Wilkins, M.: The effect of gold salts on the phagocytic activity of synovial macrophages in organ culture. J. Rheumatol., *5 (Suppl.)*:137–148, 1979.

229. Boldt, D.H., Chan, S.K., and Keaton, K.: Cell surface alpha 1-protease inhibitor on human peripheral mononuclear cells in culture. J. Immunol., *129*:1830–1838, 1982.

230. Cochrane, C., Spragg, R., and Revak, S.: Studies on the pathogenesis of the adult respiratory distress syndrome: evidence of oxidant activity in bronchoalveolar lavage fluid. J. Clin. Invest., *71*:754–769, 1983.

231. Vischer, T.L, Flory, E., and Muirden, K.: Proteinase complexes are taken up by synovial macrophages during joint inflammation. Adv. Exp. Med. Biol., *135*:635–642, 1982.

232. Geczy, C.L., and Meyer, P.A.: Leukocyte procoagulant activity in man: an in vitro correlate of delayed-type hypersensitivity. J. Immunol., *128*:331–340, 1982.

233. Edwards, R.L., and Rickles, F.R.: Macrophage procoagulants. Prog. Hemost. Thromb., *7*:183, 1984.

234. Shands, J.W.: Macrophage Procoagulants. Hemostasis, *14*:373–380, 1984.

235. Lyberg, T., et al.: Effect of immune-complex containing sera from patients with rheumatic diseases on thromboplastin activity of monocytes. Thromb. Res., *25*:193–200, 1982.

236. Brade, V., and Bentley, C.: Synthesis and release of complement components by macrophages. In Mononuclear Phagocytes: Functional Aspects. Edited by R. van Furth. The Hague, Martinus Nijhoff, 1980.

237. Bianco, C., Eden, A., and Cohn, Z.A.: The induction of macrophage spreading: role of coagulation factors and the complement system. J. Exp. Med., *144*:1531–1544, 1976.

238. Gotz, O., et al.: The stimulation of mononuclear phagocytes by components of the classical and the alternative pathways of complement activation. In Mononuclear Phagocytes: Functional Aspects. Edited by R. van Furth. The Hague, Martinus Nijhoff, 1980.

239. De Ceulaer, C., Papagoglau, S., and Whaley, K.: Increased biosynthesis of C components by cultured monocytes, synovial fluid macrophages and synovial membrane cells from plasma. J. Immunol., *41*:37–44, 1980.

240. Littman, B.H., and Ruddy, S.: Accelerated synthesis of second complement component (C2) by mononuclear cells from synovial fluid. Clin. Res., *25*:485A, 1977.

241. Davies, P., et al.: Synthesis of arachidonic acid oxygenation products by various mononuclear phagocyte populations. In Mononuclear Phagocytes: Functional Aspects. Edited by R. van Furth. The Hague, Martinus Nijhoff, 1980.

242. Kennerly, D.A., et al.: Diacylglycerol metabolism in mast cells:

a potential role in membrane fusion and arachidonic acid release. J. Exp. Med., *150*:1039–1049, 1979.

243. Lapetina, E.G., and Cuatrecasas, P.: Stimulation of phosphatidic acid production in platelets precedes the formation of arachidonate and parallels the release of serotonin. Biochim. Biophys. Acta, *573*:394–403, 1979.

244. Rittenhouse-Simmons, S.: Production of diglyceride from phosphatidylinositol in activated human platelets. J. Clin. Invest., *63*:580–594, 1979.

245. Feldberg, W., and Gupta, K.P.: Pyrogen fever and prostaglandin-like activity in cerebrospinal fluid. J. Physiol., *228*:41–55, 1973.

246. Claeys, M., et al.: 15-HETE formation by rabbit peritoneal tissue. Agents Actions, *11*:589–598, 1981.

247. Blusse van, O., Abbas, A., and van Furth, R.: Origin, kinetics, and characteristics of pulmonary macrophages in the normal steady state. J. Exp. Med., *149*:1504–1518, 1979.

248. Kaltreider, H.B.: Alveolar macrophages: enhancers or suppressors of pulmonary imune reactivity? (Editorial.) Chest, *82*:261–269, 1982.

249. Smolen, J.S., et al.: The human autologous mixed lymphocyte reaction. I. Suppression by macrophages and T-cells. J. Immunol., *127*:1987–1995, 1981.

250. Shibata, Y., Tamura, K., and Ishida, N.: In vivo analysis of the suppressive effects of immunosuppressive acidic protein, a type of z1-acid glycoprotein, in connection with its high level in tumor-bearing mice. Cancer Res., *43*:2889–2897, 1983.

251. Walinsky, S.I., et al.: Role of prostaglandins in the development of depressed cell mediated immune response in rheumatoid arthritis. Cell. Immunol. Immunopathol., *17*:3–9, 1980.

252. Webb, D.R., and Nowowiejski, I.: Control of suppressor cell activation via endogenous prostaglandin synthesis: the role of T cells and macrophages. Cell. Immunol., *63*:321–329, 1981.

253. Oppenheim, J.J., and Cohen, S. (Eds.): Interleukins, Lymphokines and Cytokines. Proceedings of the Third International Lymphokine Workshop. New York, Academic Press, 1983.

254. Pick, E. (Ed.): Lymphokines. New York, Academic Press, 1984.

255. Lomedico, P.T., et al.: Cloning and expression of murine interleukin-1 cDNA in E. coli. Nature, *312*:458–461, 1984.

256. March, C.J., et al.: Cloning, sequence and expression of two distinct human interleukin-1 complementary DNAs. Nature, *315*:641, 1985.

257. Dinarello, C.A., et al.: The influence of lipoxygenase inhibitors on the in vitro production of human leukocytic pyrogen and lymphocyte activating factor (interleukin 1). Int. J. Immunopharmacol., *6*:43–52, 1984.

258. Pincus, S.H., Whitcomb, E.A., and Dinarello, C.A.: Interaction of IL-1 and TPA in modulation of eosinophil function. J. Immunol., *137*:3509–3517, 1986.

259. Kurt-Jones, E.A., et al.: Identification of a membrane associated interleukin-1 in macrophages. Proc. Natl. Acad. Sci. U.S.A., *82–87*:1204, 1985.

260. Dinarello, C.A.: Interleukin-1. Rev. Infect. Dis., *6*:51–83, 1984.

261. Snyder, D.S., and Unanue, E.R.: Corticosteroids inhibit murine Ia expression and interleukin 1. J. Immunol., *129*:1803–1809, 1982.

262. Bunjes, D., et al.: Cyclosporin A mediates immunosuppression of primary cytotoxic T cell responses by impairing the release of interleukin 1 and interleukin 2. Eur. J. Immunol., *11*:657–669, 1981.

263. Schmidt, J.A., et al.: Silica-stimulated monocytes release fibroblast proliferation factors identical to interleukin 1: potential role for interleukin 1 in the pathogenesis of silicosis. J. Clin. Invest., *73*:1462–1474, 1984.

264. Gowne, M., et al.: An IL-1 like factor stimulates bone resorption in vitro. Nature, *306*:378–382, 1983.

265. Dayer, J.M., et al.: Participation of monocyte-macrophages and lymphocytes in the production of a factor which stimulates collagenase and prostaglandin release by rheumatoid synovial cells. J. Clin. Invest., *64*:1392–1399, 1979.

266. Bitterman, P.B., et al.: Human alveolar macrophage growth factor for fibroblasts: regulation and partial characterization. J. Clin. Invest., *70*:806–819, 1982.

267. Wharton, W., Walker, E., and Stewart, C.C.: Growth regulation by macrophages. *In* Macrophages and Natural Killer Cells: Regulation and Function. Edited by S.J. Normann and E. Sorkin. New York, Plenum Publishing, 1982.

268. Roberts, N.H., Jr., et al.: Virus-induced interferon production by human macrophages. J. Immunol., *123*:365–373, 1979.

269. Vogel, S.N., et al.: Correction of defective macrophage differentiation in C3H/HeJ mice by an interferon-like molecule. J. Immunol., *128*:380–388, 1982.

270. Old, I.J.: Tumor necrosis factor. Science, *230*:630–636, 1985.

271. Shalaby, M.R., Pennica, D., and Palladino, M.A., Jr.: An overview of the history and biologic properties of tumor necrosis factors. Springer Semin. Immunopathol., *9*:33–55, 1986.

272. Coley, W.B.: Contributions to the knowledge of sarcoma. Ann. Surg., *14*:199–221, 1891.

273. Beutler, K.B., and Cerami, A.: Cachectin and tumor necrosis factor as two sides of the same biological coin. Nature, *320*:584–587, 1986.

274. Pennica, D., et al.: Cloning and expression in Escherichia coli of the cDNA for murine tumor necrosis factor. Proc. Natl. Acad. Sci. U.S.A., *82*:6060–6065, 1985.

275. Dayer, J.M., Beutler, B., and Cerami, A.: Cachectin/tumor necrosis factor stimulates collagenase and prostaglandin E2 production by human synovial fibroblasts. J. Exp. Med., *162*:2163–2177, 1985.

276. Saklatvala, J.: Tumor necrosis factor α stimulates resorption and inhibits synthesis of proteoglycan in cartilage. Nature, *322*:547–550, 1986.

277. Babior, B.M.: Oxygen-dependent microbial killing by phagocytes. N. Engl. J. Med., *298*:659–665, 1978.

278. Johnston, R.B., Jr., Chadwick, D.A., and Pabst, M.J.: Release of superoxide anion by macrophages: effect of in vivo or in vitro priming. *In* Mononuclear Phagocytes: Functional Aspects. Edited by R. van Furth. The Hague, Martinus Nijhoff, 1980.

279. Klebanoff, S.J.: A peroxidase-mediated antimicrobial system in leukocytes. J. Clin. Invest., *46*:1078–1090, 1967.

280. Clark, R.A., and Szot, S.: Chemotactic factor inactivation by stimulated human neutrophils mediated by myeloperoxidase-catalyzed methionine oxidation. J. Immunol., *128*:1507–1514, 1982.

281. McCord, J.M.: Free radical and inflammation: protection of synovial fluid by superoxide dismutase. Science, *185*:529–533, 1974.

282. Alitalo, K., Hovi, T., and Vaheri, A.: Fibronectin is produced by human macrophages. J. Exp. Med., *151*:601–614, 1980.

283. Postlethwaite, A.E., et al.: Induction of fibroblast chemotaxis by fibronectin: localization of the chemotactic region to a 140K nongelatin binding fragment. J. Exp. Med., *153*:494–503, 1981.

284. Tsukamoto, Y., Helsel, W.E., and Wahl, S.M.: Macrophage production of fibronectin, a chemoattractant for fibroblasts. J. Immunol., *127*:673–681, 1981.

285. Wyler, D., and Postlethwaite, A.E.: Fibroblast stimulation in schistosomiasis. IV. Isolated egg granulomas elaborate a fibroblast chemoattractant in vitro. J. Immunol., 130:1371–1379, 1983.

286. Basu, S.K., Goldstein, J.L., and Brown, M.S.: Independent pathways for secretion of cholesterol and apolipoprotein E by macrophages. Science, 219:871–874, 1983.

287. Basu, S.K., et al.: Biochemical and genetic studies of the apoprotein E secreted by mouse macrophages and human monocytes. J. Biol. Chem., 257:9788–9796, 1982.

288. Basu, S.K., et al.: Mouse macrophages synthesize and secrete a protein resembling apolipoprotein E. Proc. Natl. Acad. Sci. U.S.A., 78:7545–7550, 1981.

289. Werb, Z., and Chin, J.R.: Endotoxin suppresses expression of apoprotein E by mouse macrophages in vivo and in culture. J. Biol. Chem., 258:10,642–10,649, 1983.

290. Gianturco, N., et al.: Hypertriglyceridemic very low density lipoproteins induce triglyceride synthesis and accumulation in mouse peritoneal macrophages. J. Clin. Invest., 70:168–176, 1982.

291. Yachnin, S., Toub, D.B., and Mannickarottu, V.: Divergence in cholesterol biosynthetic rates and 3-hydroxy-3-methyglutaryl-CoA reductase activity as a consequence of granulocyte versus monocyte-macrophage differentiation in HL-60 cells. Proc. Natl. Acad. Sci. U.S.A., 81:894–899, 1984.

292. Pike, M.C., and Snyderman, R.: Lipid requirements for leukocyte chemotaxis: effects of inhibitors of phospholipid and cholesterol synthesis. J. Immunol., 124:1963–1972, 1980.

293. Salisbury, B.G.J., Falcone, D.J., and Minick, C.R.: Insoluble low-density lipoprotein-proteoglycan complexes enhance cholesterol ester accumulation in macrophages. Am. J. Pathol., 120:6–14, 1985.

294. Blalock, J.F., Bost, K.L., and Smith, E.M.: Neuroendocrine peptide hormones and their receptors in the immune system. J. Neuroimmunol., 10:31–42, 1985.

295. Lolait, S.J., et al.: Immunoreactive β-endorphin in a subpopulation of mouse spleen macrophages. J. Clin. Invest., 73:277–290, 1984.

296. Smith, E.M., and Blalock, J.E.: Human lymphocyte production of corticotropin and endorphin-like substances: association with leukocyte interferon. Proc. Natl. Acad. Sci. U.S.A., 78:7530–7535, 1981.

297. Johnson, H.M., et al.: Regulation of lymphokine (γ-interferon) production by corticotropin. J. Immunol., 132:246–252, 1984.

298. Sharp, R.M., et al.: Opiod peptides rapidly stimulate superoxide production by human polymorphonuclear leukocytes. Endocrinology, 117:793–808, 1985.

299. Van Epps, D.F., and Saland, L.: B-endorphin and met-enkephalin stimulate human peripheral blood mononuclear cell chemotaxis. J. Immunol., 132:3046–3052, 1984.

300. Wiedermann, C.J., et al.: Bombesin in human and guinea pig alveolar macrophages. J. Immunol., 137:3928–3936, 1986.

301. Cuttitta, F., et al.: Bombesin-like peptides can function as autocrine growth factors in human small-cell lung cancer. Nature, 316:823–826, 1985.

302. Rosengurt, E., and Sinnett-Smith, J.: Bombesin stimulation of DNA synthesis and cell division in cultures of Swiss 3T3 cells. Proc. Natl. Acad. Sci. U.S.A., 80:2936–2941, 1983.

303. Willey, J.C., Lechner, J.F., and Harris, C.C.: Bombesin and the C-terminal tetradecapeptide of gastrin-releasing peptide are growth factors for normal human bronchial epithelial cells. Exp. Cell. Res., 153:245–255, 1984.

304. Ruff, M., et al.: Neuropeptides are chemoattractants for human monocytes: a possible mechanism for metastasis. Clin. Immunol. Immunopathol., 37:387–395, 1985.

305. Hartung, H.P., Wolters, K., and Toyka, K.V.: Substance P: binding properties and studies on cellular responses in guinea pig macrophages. J. Immunol., 136:3856–3864, 1986.

306. Hartung, H.P., and Toyka, K.V.: Activation of macrophages by substance P: induction of oxidative burst and thromboxane release. Eur. J. Pharmacol., 89:301, 1983.

307. Levine, J.D., et al.: Intraneuronal substance P contributes to the severity of experimental arthritis. Science, 226:547, 1984.

308. Levine, J.D., Moskowitz, M.A., and Basbaum, A.I.: The contribution of neurogenic inflammation in experimental arthritis. J. Immunol., 135:843s–849, 1985.

309. Cohn, Z.A.: The activation of mononuclear phagocytes: fact, fancy, and future. J. Immunol., 121:813–821, 1978.

310. David, J.R.: Macrophage activation by lymphocyte mediators. In Infection and Immunity in the Rheumatic Diseases. Edited by D.C. Dumonde. London, Blackwell Scientific, 1974.

311. Nakagawara, A., et al.: Lymphokines enhance the capacity of human monocytes to secrete reactive oxygen intermediates. J. Clin. Invest., 70:1042–1058, 1982.

312. Adams, D.O., Johnson, W.J., and Marino, P.A.: Mechanisms of target recognition and destruction in macrophage-mediated tumor cytotoxicity. Fed. Proc., 41:2212–2218, 1982.

313. Nogueira, N., et al.: Trypanosoma cruzi: induction of microbicidal activity in human mononuclear phagocytes. J. Immunol., 128:2142–2150, 1982.

314. Nogueira, N., and Cohn, Z.A.: Trypanosoma cruzi: mechanisms of entry and intracellular fate in mammalian cells. J. Exp. Med., 143–148:1402, 1976.

315. Bryne, G.I., and Faubian, C.L.: Lymphokine-mediated microbiostatic mechanisms restrict Chlamydia psittaci growth in macrophages. J. Immunol., 128:469–475, 1982.

316. Boraschi, D., et al.: Regulation of arachidonic acid metabolism in macrophages by immune and nonimmune interferons. J. Immunol., 135:502–510, 1985.

317. Lockley, R.M., Wilson, C.B., and Klebanoff, S.J.: Role of endogenous and acquired peroxidase in the toxoplasmacidal activity of murine and human mononuclear phagocytes. J. Clin. Invest., 69:1099–1110, 1982.

318. Meltzer, M.S., et al.: Macrophage activation for tumor cytotoxicity: analysis of intermediary reactions. J. Reticuloendothel. Soc., 26:403–412, 1979.

319. Ruco, L.P., and Meltzer, M.S.: Macrophage activation for tumor cytotoxicity: induction of tumoricidal macrophages by PPD in BCG immune mice. Cell. Immunol., 32:203–214, 1977.

320. Adams, D.O., and Hamilton, T.A.: The cell biology of macrophage activation. Annu. Rev. Immunol., 2:283–330, 1984.

321. Ho, Y., Lee, M.F., and Snyderman, R.: Chemoattractant-induced activation of c-fos gene expression in human monocytes. J. Exp. Med. In press.

322. Piessens, W.F.: Increased binding of tumor cells by macrophages activated in vitro with lymphocyte mediators. Cell. Immunol., 35:303–314, 1978.

323. Nathan, C.F., and Cohn, Z.A.: Role of oxygen dependent mechanisms in antibody-induced lysis of tumor cells by activated macrophages. J. Exp. Med., 152:198–212, 1980.

324. Johnston, W.J., Whisnant, C.C., and Adams, D.O.: The binding of BCG-activated macrophages to tumor targets stimulates secretion of cytolytic factor. J. Immunol., 127:1787–1798, 1981.

325. Marino, P.A., and Adams, D.O.: Interaction of Bacillus Calmette-Guerin-activated macrophages and neoplastic cells in vitro. Cell Immunol., 54:11–24, 1980.

326. Edelson, P.J.: Macrophage ecto-enzymes: their identification,

metabolism, and control. *In* Mononuclear Phagocytes: Functional Aspects. Edited by R. van Furth. The Hague, Martinus Nijhoff, 1980.

327. Admas, D.O., Pike, M.C., and Snyderman, R.: The role of transmethylation reactions in regulating the binding of BCG-activated murine macrophages to neoplastic target cells. J. Immunol., 127:225–232, 1981.

328. Nelson, M., and Nelson, D.S.: Macrophages and resistance to tumors. I. Inhibition of delayed-type hypersensitivity reactions by tumor cells and by soluble products affecting macrophages. Immunology, 34:277–285, 1978.

329. Snyderman, R., et al.: Effects of neoplasms on inflammation: depression of macrophage accumulation after tumor implantation. J. Immunol., 116:585–596, 1976.

330. Snyderman, R., and Pike, M.C.: A Inhibitor of macrophage chemotaxis produced by neoplasms. Science, 192:370–373, 1976.

331. Stevenson, M.M., and Meltzer, M.S.: Depressed chemotactic responses in vitro of peritoneal macrophages from tumor-bearing mice. J. Natl. Cancer Inst., 57:847–857, 1976.

332. Snyderman, R., et al.: Abnormal monocyte chemotaxis in patients with breast cancer: evidence for a tumor-mediated effect. J. Natl. Cancer Inst., 60:737–748, 1978.

333. Cianciolo, G.J., et al.: Murine malignant cells synthesize a 19,000 dalton protein which is physiochemically and antigenically related to the immunosuppressive retroviral protein, P15E. J. Exp. Med., 158:885–898, 1983.

334. Cianciolo, G.J., et al.: Inhibitors of monocyte responses to chemotaxins are present in human cancerous effusions and react with monoclonal antibodies to the P15E structural protein of retroviruses. J. Clin. Invest., 68:831–843, 1981.

335. Lipsky, P.E., and Rosenthal, A.S.: Macrophage-lymphocyte interaction I. Characteristics of the antigen-independent binding of guinea pig thymocytes to syngeneic macrophages. J. Exp. Med., 138:900–914, 1973.

336. Panayi, G.S., Corregall, V., and Youlden, L.F.: Immunoregulation in the rheumatic diseases. Scand. J. Rheumatol., 38 (Suppl.):9–920, 1982.

337. Unanue, E.R., et al.: Regulation of immunity and inflammation by mediators from macrophages. Am. J. Pathol., 85:465–476, 1976.

338. Unanue, E.R., and Calderon, J.: Evaluation of the role of macrophages in immune induction. Fed. Proc., 34:1737–1748, 1975.

339. Ziegler, K., and Unanue, E.R.: Identification of a macrophage antigen-processing agent required for I-region-restricted antigen presentation to T-lymphocytes. J. Immunol., 127:1869–1875, 1981.

340. Mizel, S.B., and Mizel, D.: Purification to apparent homogeneity of murine interleukin-1. J. Immunol., 126:834–842, 1981.

341. Moller, G.: Interleukins and lymphocyte activation. Immunol. Rev., 63:1–42, 1982.

342. Allison, A.C. Mechanisms by which activated macrophages inhibit lymphocyte responses. Immunol. Rev., 40:3–27, 1978.

343. Katz, D.R., et al.: A comparative study of accessory cells derived from the peritoneum and from solid tissues. Adv. Exp. Med., Biol., 155:421–438, 1982.

344. Morley, J.: Anti-inflammatory effects of prostaglandins. *In* Rheumatoid Arthritis. Edited by J.L. Gordon, and B. Hazelman. Amsterdam, Elsevier, 1977.

345. Ault, K.A., and Springer, T.A.: Cross reaction of a rat anti-mouse phagocyte specific monoclonal antibody (anti-Mac-1)

346. Hoefsand, E.C.M.: Macrophages, Langerhans' cells, interdigitating and dendrite accessory cells: a summary. Adv. Exp. Med. Biol., 155:463–472, 1982.

347. Winchester, R.J., and Burmester, G.R.: Demonstration of Ia antigens on certain dendrite cells and on a novel elongate cell found in human synovial tissue. Scand. J. Immunol., 14:439–450, 1981.

348. Dayer, J.M., and Drane, S.M.: The interaction of immunocompetent cells and chronic inflammation as exemplified by rheumatoid arthritis. Clin. Rheum. Dis., 4:517–545, 1978.

349. Wooley, D.E., et al.: Collagenase immunolocalization in cultures of rheumatoid synovial cells. Science, 200:773–776, 1978.

350. Werb, Z., Foley, R., and Munck, A.: Interaction of glucocorticoids with macrophages: identification of glucocorticoid receptors in monocytes and macrophages. J. Exp. Med., 147:1684–1698, 1978.

351. Dale, D.C., Fauci, A.S., and Wolff, S.M.: Alternate-day prednisone: leukocyte kinetics and susceptibility to infections. N. Engl. J. Med., 291:1154–1160, 1974.

352. Werb, Z.: Biochemical actions of glucocorticoids on macrophages in culture: specific inhibition of elastase, collagenase, and plasminogen activator secretion and effects on other metabolic functions. J. Exp. Med., 147:1695–1709, 1978.

353. Rinehart, J.J., et al.: Effects of corticosteroid therapy on human monocyte function. N. Engl. J. Med., 292:236–244, 1975.

354. Schrieber, A.D., et al.: Effect of corticosteroids on the human monocyte IgG and complement receptors. J. Clin. Invest., 56:1189–1201, 1975.

355. Lehmeyer, J.E., and Johnston, R.B., Jr.: Effect of anti-inflammatory drugs and agents that elevate intracellular cyclic AMP on the release of toxic oxygen metabolites by phagocytes: Studies in a model of tissue-bound IgG. Clin. Immunol. Immunopathol., 9:482–498, 1978.

356. Rinehart, J.J., Wuest, D., and Ackerman, G.A.: Corticosteroid alteration of human monocyte to macrophage differentiation J. Immunol., 129:1436–1445, 1982.

357. Kleinerman, E.S., et al.: Pharmacology of human spontaneous monocyte-mediated cytotoxicity: I. Enhancement by salicylates and steroids. Arthritis Rheum., 24:774–782, 1981.

358. Lipsky, P.E., Ugai, K., and Ziff, M.: Alterations in human monocyte structure and function induced by incubation with gold sodium thiomalate. J. Rheumatol., 5 (Suppl.):130–138, 1979.

359. Davis, P., Miller, C.L., and Johnston, C.A.: Effect of gold salts on adherent mononuclear cells in tissue culture. J. Rheumatol., 5 (Suppl.): 98–104, 1979.

360. Buhles, W.C., Jr., and Shifrine, M.: Effects of cyclosphosphamide on macrophage numbers, functions and progenitor cells. J. Reticuloendothel. Soc., 21:285–298, 1977.

361. Van Furth, R., et al.: The effect of azathioprine (Imuran) on the cell cycle of promonocytes and the production of monocytes in the bone marrow. J. Exp. Med., 141:531–548, 1975.

362. North, R.J.: Suppression of cell-mediated immunity to infection by an antimitotic drug: further evidence that migrant macrophages express immunity. J. Exp. Med., 132:535–549, 1970.

363. Binderup, L., Bramm, E., and Arrigoni-Martelli, E.: Effect of D-penicillamine in vitro and in vivo on macrophage phagocytosis. Biochem. Pharmacol., 29:2273–2284, 1980.

364. Pike, M.C., Daniels, C.A., and Snyderman, R.: Influenza induced depression of monocyte chemotaxis: reversal by levamisole. Cell. Immunol., 32:234–242, 1977.

365. Pike, M.C., and Snyderman, R.: Augmentation of human monocyte chemotaxis response by levamisole. Nature, *261*:136–139, 1976.

366. Fan, T.P.D., and Lewis, G.P.: Effect of cyclosporin A and inhibitors of arachidonic acid metabolism on blood flow and cyclo-oxygenase products in rat skin allografts. Br. J. Pharmacol., *81*:361–373, 1984.

367. Thiele, D.L., and Lipsky, P.E.: The immunosuppressive activity of L-leucyl-L-leucine methyl ester: selective ablation of cytotoxic lymphocytes and monocytes. J. Immunol., *136*:1038–1049, 1986.

368. Greenberg, P., and Zvaifler, N.J.: Immunobiology of rheumatoid arthritis. Pathobiol. Annu., *6*:279–297, 1976.

369. Hanauskeok-Abel, H.M., Pointz, B.F., and Schorlemmer, H.U.: Cartilage-specific collagen activates macrophages and the alternative pathway of C: Evidence for an immunopathogenic concept of RA. Ann. Rheum. Dis., *41*:168–182, 1982.

SUGGESTED READING

Chenoweth, D.E., and Hugli, T.E.: Demonstration of specific C5a receptor on intact human polymorphonuclear leukocytes. Proc. Natl. Acad. Sci. U.S.A., *75*:3943–3948, 1978.

Daniele, R.P., Diamond, M.S., and Holian, A.: Demonstration of a formyl peptide receptor on lung macrophages: correlation of binding properties with chemotaxis and release of superoxide anion. Am. Rev. Respir. Dis., *126*:274–279, 1982.

Dey, P.K., et al.: Fruther studies on the role of prostaglandins in fever. J. Physiol., *241*:629–638, 1974.

Ericsson, J.L.E.: Origin and structure of the osteoclast. *In* Mononuclear Phagocytes: Functional Aspects. Edited by R. van Furth. The Hague, Martinus Nijhoff, 1980.

Fauci, A.S., and Dale, D.C.: The effect of in vivo hydrocortisone on subpopulations of human lymphocytes. J. Clin. Invest., *52*:240–255, 1974.

Fogelman, A.M., et al.: Malondialdehyde alteration of low density lipoproteins leads to cholesterol ester accumulation in human monocytes-macrophages. Proc. Natl. Acad. Sci. U.S.A., *77*:2214–2219, 1980.

Goetzl, E.J., and Pickett, W.C.: The human PMN leukocyte chemotactic activity of complex hydroxy-eicosatetraenoic acids (HETEs). J. Immunol., *125*:1789–1974, 1980.

Hamilton, J., Vassalli, J.D., and Reich, E.: Macrophage plasminogen activator: induction by asbestos is blocked by anti-inflammatory steroids. J. Exp. Med., *144*:1689–1699, 1976.

Ho, M.K., and Springer, T.A.: Mac-1 antigen: quantitative expression in macrophage population and tissues, and immunofluorescent localization in spleen. J. Immunol., *128*:2281–2291, 1982.

Hseuh, W., Sun, F.F., and Henderson, S.: The biosynthesis of leukotriene B$_4$, the predominant lipoxygenase product in rabbit alveolar macrophages, is enhanced during immune activation. Biochim. Biophys. Acta, *835*:92–99, 1985.

Issacson, P., et al.: Alpha-1-antitrypsin in human macrophages. J. Clin. Pathol., *34*:982–1001, 1981.

Kay, M.B.: Mechanism of removal of senescent cells by human macrophages in situ. Proc. Natl. Acad. Sci. U.S.A., *72*:3521–3526, 1975.

Lohr, K., and Snyderman, R.: Amphotericin B alters the affinity and functional activity of the oligopeptide chemotactic factor receptor on human polymorphonuclear leukocytes. J. Immunol., *129*:1594–1603, 1982.

Mahley, R.W., et al.: Altered metabolism (in vivo and in vitro) of plasma lipoproteins after selective modification of lysine residues of the apoproteins. J. Clin. Invest., *64*:743–760, 1979.

Maino, V.C., Hayman, M.J., and Crumpton, M.J.: Relationship between enhanced turnover of phosphatidylinositol and lymphocyte activation by mitogens. Biochem. J., *146*:247–260, 1975.

Mizel, S.B., et al.: Stimulation of rheumatoid synovial cells: collagenase and prostaglandin production by partially purified lymphocyte activating factor (IL-1). Proc. Natl. Acad. Sci. U.S.A., *78*:2474–2479, 1981.

Pike, M.C., and Snyderman, R.: Leukocyte Chemoattractant Receptors. *In* The Receptors. Vol. 1. Edited by P.M. Conn. New York, Academic Press, 1984.

Rennick, D.M., et al.: A cloned MCGF cDNA encodes a multilineage hematopoietic growth factor: multiple activities of Interleukin 3. J. Immunol., *134*:910–918, 1985.

Serhan, C.N., et al.: LTB$_4$ and phosphatidic acid are calcium ionophores. J. Biol. Chem., *257*:4746–4754, 1982.

Smith, C.D., et al.: Chemoattractant receptor induced hydrolysis of phosphatidylinositol 4,5 bisphosphate in human polymorphonuclear leukocyte membranes. J. Biol. Chem., *260*:5875–5883, 1985.

Springer, T.A., and Anderson, D.C.: Functional and structural interrelationships among the Mac-1, LFA-1, family of leukocyte adhesion glycoproteins, and their deficiency in a novel, heritable disease. *In* Hybridoma Technology in the Biosciences and Medicine. Edited by T.A. Springer. New York, Plenum Publishing, p. 191, 1976.

Thompson, J., and van Furth, R.: The effect of glucorticosteroids on the proliferation and kinetics of promonocytes and monocytes of the bone marrow. J. Exp. Med., *137*:10–22, 1973.

Todd, R.F., III, and Schlossman, S.F.: Analysis of antigenic determinants on human monocytes and macrophage. Blood, *59*:775–782, 1982.

Vlassara, H., Brownlee, M., and Cerami, A.: High affinity receptor mediated uptake and degradation of glucose-modified proteins: a potential mechanism for removal of senescent macromolecules. Proc. Natl. Acad. Sci. U.S.A., *82*:5588–5593, 1985.

LYMPHOCYTES: STRUCTURE AND FUNCTION

19

JOHN D. STOBO

The last 40 years have witnessed an exponential increase in our understanding of the immune system. The most important events are summarized chronologically. Experiments in the 1950s clearly indicated that lymphocytes involved in the immune response could be divided into two broad populations. One population, requiring the thymus for normal differentiation, was termed thymus-derived lymphocytes (T cells). The other population, initially differentiated, at least in adult life, in the bone marrow, was called bone marrow-derived lymphocytes (B cells). T cells function as effector cells for cell-mediated reactions, such as delayed hypersensitivity, and also help B cells differentiate into antibody secreting plasma cells. Both T cells and B cells are required for full antibody responses to most antigens.

Experiments in the 1960s demonstrated that the immune response is controlled by genes in the major histocompatibility complex (MHC). Subsequently, it was demonstrated that products of these immune response genes are molecules expressed on the surface of antigen presenting cells such as macrophages. These immune-response associated, or Ia, molecules control both cell-mediated and humoral immunity by determining whether antigen is appropriately presented to effector and helper T cells.

Studies in the 1970s demonstrated that functionally distinct subpopulations of T and B cells could be distinguished by differences in cell surface molecules. In the 1980s, the advances of molecular biology and recombinant DNA technology allowed the delineation of the nature of the T-cell receptor for antigen and

allowed study of the molecular and biochemical events involved in the activation of both T cells and B cells.

This chapter will summarize and expand these advances.

MOLECULES PRESENT ON THE SURFACE OF T CELLS

Several molecules located on the T-cell surface play an important role in their differentiation and function. It will be helpful in discussing T-cell ontogeny and function to briefly review the most important. Although these molecules were initially designated by the monoclonal antibodies with which they react, recent internationally accepted terminology designates them as clusters of differentiation (CD). The CD determination refers to the whole molecule and not simply an epitope detected by a specific antibody.

CD2

CD2, a glycoprotein with a molecular weight of 50,000, is present on 95% of thymocytes and all peripheral T cells.[1] This molecule is the receptor by which T cells bind to sheep red blood cells and is responsible for the initial observation that human T cells can be quantitated by their ability to form rosettes with sheep red blood cells. The CD2 molecule appears

336

to play an important role in modulating T-cell reactivity.

Two groups of observations support this theory. First, monoclonal antibodies against the CD2 molecule can either inhibit or induce T-cell activation. Some CD2 monoclonal antibodies inhibit T-cell activation induced by mitogens or calcium ionophores. Other antibodies initiate activation. Monoclonal antibodies can detect three distinct epitopes in the CD2 molecule, $CD2_1$, $CD2_2$, and $CD2_3$. The $CD2_1$ and the $CD2_2$ epitopes are expressed on resting thymocytes and resting peripheral blood T cells, but the $CD2_3$ epitope is expressed only when T cells are activated. Addition of $CD2_2$ antibodies can induce expression of the $CD2_3$ epitope. Addition of either $CD2_1$ or $CD2_2$ antibodies to resting T cells does not induce their activation. However, simultaneous addition of $CD2_2$ and $CD2_3$ antibody induces T-cell proliferation, suggesting that the molecule can transmit activating signals. The mitogen phytohemagglutinin (PHA) may activate T cells via the CD2 molecule. PHA binds to the $CD2_2$ epitope, induces expression of $CD2_3$, and then binds to this epitope, inducing T-cell activation.

A second observation supporting a role for the CD2 molecule in T-cell activation is the demonstration of a natural ligand for CD2 called lymphocyte function associate 3 (LFA-3), molecular weight (MW) of 55,000 to 70,000. This molecule is expressed on the surface of a variety of cells including endothelial cells, epithelial cells, stromal cells of most organs, and human red blood cells. Solubilized LFA-3 binds to CD2. Antibodies against LFA-3 inhibit conjugate formation between the cytotoxic T cell and its target and therefore inhibit T-cell killing of target cells. Thymic epithelial cells display LFA-3, and thymocyte adherence to these epithelial cells is mediated by interactions between CD2 and LFA-3. LFA-3 antibodies inhibit the ability of thymic epithelial cells to function as accessory cells for mitogen-induced activation of thymocytes. CD2-LFA-3 binding may play an important role in thymocyte activation but requires further definition.

CD3

CD3 refers to three distinct molecules linked noncovalently on the surface on approximately 90% of thymocytes and all peripheral T cells. The three distinct molecules in the CD3 complex are referred to as CD3 γ, a 25,000-MW glycoprotein; CD3 δ, a 20,000 MW glycoprotein; and CD3 ε, a 20,000-MW nonglycosylated protein. The CD3 complex is linked noncovalently to the T-cell antigen receptor, both to the "classic" α/β heterodimer as well as to the recently described γ/δ heterodimer. Antibodies to the CD3 complex can serve as one signal required for T-cell activation. This linking of the CD3 complex with the T-cell antigen receptor may be important either in transducing activating signals or in stabilizing the antigen receptor heterodimer in the cell membrane. The finding that CD3 antibodies can substitute for antigen and serve as one signal required for T-cell activation supports a role for this molecule in T-cell activation. Cells that have been mutagenized so that they no longer express the α/β heterodimer also fail to express the CD3 complex, supporting a role for the CD3 molecules in allowing or stabilizing expression of the α/β heterodimer.

CD4

The CD4 molecule is a single polypeptide chain of 55,000 MW displayed by approximately 90% of thymocytes and 60% of peripheral blood T cells. This molecule marks cells whose activation depends on the recognition of class II MHC gene products, i.e., CD4-positive T cells recognize antigen in conjunction with class II MHC gene products. It has been hypothesized that CD4 binds to class II MHC molecules, enhancing avidity of binding between the reactive T cell and antigen presenting cell. This function would be most important when there is low avidity interaction between the antigen receptor and antigen presenting cell. This hypothesis is based on the inverse correlation observed between the amount of CD4 antibody necessary to block T-cell activation and the amount of antigen required for activation. Whether the CD4 molecule can transduce an activating signal is controversial. The CD4 molecule also serves as a receptor by which human immunodeficiency virus (HIV) can infect T cells and other cells.

CD8

The CD8 molecule is expressed on approximately 90% of thymocytes and 30% of peripheral blood T cells. On human thymocytes the CD8 molecule (33,000 MW) forms a heterodimer by complexing with a 45,000 MW molecule, CD1. CD1 is the human equivalent of the mouse class I MHC molecule, TL. On peripheral blood T cells, the CD8 molecule forms disulfide-linked homodimers and homomultimers, and it marks T cells whose activation requires recognition of antigen in conjunction with class I MHC gene products. Just as CD4 may act as an adhesion molecule required to increase the avidity with which CD4 positive cells react with antigen presenting cells, the CD8 may bind directly to class I MHC molecules and increase the interaction between CD8 positive cells and their target. CD8 antibodies block interactions between cytotoxic T cells and the target cell.

THE T-CELL RECEPTOR (TCR) FOR ANTIGEN

Experiments performed in the 1960s clearly demonstrated that T cells can manifest antigen specificity. Thus, immunization of animals with an antigen led to the generation of T cells capable of manifesting a secondary response specific to that antigen, implying that the T cell must have an antigen receptor. Because the receptor for antigen on the surface of B cells resembled immunoglobulin, it was assumed that the T-cell receptor would similarly resemble circulating immunoglobulins. However, this turned out not to be the case.[2] Instead, the first T-cell receptor for antigen was demonstrated to be a heterodimer linked by a disulfide bond made up of an acidic α chain of approximately 50,000 MW and a basic β chain of approximately 42,000 MW. Although this antigen receptor heterodimer is not actually immunoglobulin, it is similar to immunoglobulin in terms of both its general structure and the genetic mechanisms leading to its expression (Fig. 19–1). Like immunoglobulin, it can be divided into variable and constant regions. The variable region interacts with antigen; the function of

the constant region is still unknown. Isolation of the T-cell receptor from T-cell clones, each of which has specificity for distinct antigens, demonstrates a region in the amino terminal end of the α and β chains distinct for each T-cell clone. In contrast, the sequence of regions in the carboxy terminus of the α and β chains is relatively constant from clone to clone.

The T-cell repertoire must be capable of distinguishing among the approximately 1,000,000 different antigens to which it will be exposed. There is not sufficient room in the human genome for the existence of 1,000,000 genes, each encoding an antigen receptor with distinct specificity. Therefore, there must be a mechanism conserving genetic information and still providing the tremendous antigenic diversity required among the T-cell repertoire. This mechanism involves genetic rearrangements similar to those accounting for the diverse specificity among immunoglobulins (Chapter 17) (Fig. 19–1). Genes coding for the α chain exist on the fourteenth human chromosome and can be divided into three broad regions represented by variable (V), joining (J), and constant (C). Genes coding for the β chain are present on the seventh human chromosome and are similarly divided into V, J, and C regions. There is also a diversity (D) region between the V and J regions. The V, D, J, and C regions actually represent gene families, not single genes. For example, there are 60 V-region genes and 40 J-region genes present in α-chain genes. Similarly, there are multiple V-, D-, and J-region genes encoding the β chain.

Antigenic diversity is accounted for by three different mechanisms (Table 19–1). First, each different V-region gene can code for an α or a β chain with a different antigen specificity. There are approximately 60 different specificities encoded by the V region of the α chain and approximately 30 different specificities encoded by the V region of the β chain. Clearly, these specificities are not sufficient to account for 1 × 10⁶ different receptors.

Second, junctional diversity is created when a single V region is joined to a different D or J region. For example, interaction of a single V-region gene of the β chain with two different D regions results in two β

FIG. 19–1. The T-cell receptor for antigen. The T-cell receptor for antigen is a disulfide-linked heterodimer. Both the α and β chains can be divided into a variable region, which binds to antigen, and a constant region. The genetic mechanism which allows for antigenic diversity is recombinations among variable (V), diversity (D), joining (J), and constant (C) region genes.

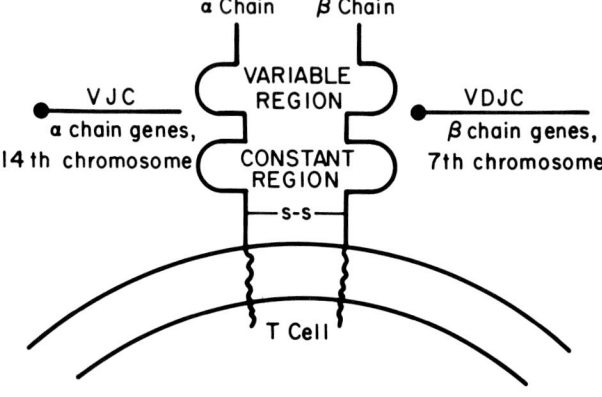

Table 19–1. Mechanisms which Contribute to T-cell Diversity

I.	Multiple V-region genes:
	α chain = 60
	β chain = 30
II.	Combinatorial, i.e., VDJ joining:
	α chain = 60V × 40J = 2400
	β chain = 30V × 2D × 12J = 720
III.	Differential α/β pairing:
	2400 α × 720 β = 1.7 × 10⁶

chains with different antigen specificities. Therefore, the specificity encoded for by the α and β chains is represented by the total number of V regions × D-region genes × J-region genes. Therefore, the total diversity represented by α-chain genes is 60 × 40, or 2400. In the case of the β chain, 30 different V regions can combine with any of the 2 different D regions and any of the 12 different J regions leading to a total diversity of 30 × 2 × 12, or 720.

But the antigen diversity in the T-cell repertoire is far greater than either 2400 or 720. Therefore, there must be other mechanisms that can create antigen receptors of different specificities up to approximately 1,000,000, and this is represented by the third mechanism leading to diversity, interactions between distinct α and β chains. It is clear that the antigen specificity of the receptor does not simply reside in the primary amino acid sequence of either the α or β chain, but seems to be dependent on interactions between the two chains. For example, a single α chain interacting with many β chains leads to a receptor with multiple antigen specificities, and a single β chain interacting with several different α chains leads to receptors with several different antigen specificities. Therefore, the total diversity present in the T-cell repertoire is represented by a multiple of the diversities inherent in each of the α and the β chains (720 × 2400), leading to a total diversity in excess of 1,000,000. Such gene rearrangements accounting for multiple specificities is very similar to the gene rearrangements accounting for multiple specificities among immunoglobulin molecules as described in Chapter 17.

Recently, another heterodimer noncovalently linked to the CD3 complex has been demonstrated on a small number of thymocytes and peripheral T cells. It is made up of two chains termed γ and δ, which are distinct from the α and β chains. The γ/δ heterodimer is expressed on approximately 5% of thymocytes and peripheral T cells. In both cases, it is present on cells lacking both CD4 and CD8. γ/δ antibodies can serve as one signal required for T-cell activation, suggesting that the γ/δ heterodimer may play a role in T-cell activation. In animals lacking a thymus, there are circulating T cells displaying the γ/δ heterodimer, but not the α/β heterodimer, suggesting that thymic maturation is necessary for expression of α/β but not for γ/δ. Multiple V-, J-, and C-region chain genes encode for the γ chain, and these undergo rearrangements similar to that demonstrated for the α and β chains, so that the γ/δ heterodimer is also capable of antigenic diversity. Exactly what role this receptor plays in T-cell differentiation or activation is still un-

clear. The molecules and receptors involved in T-cell activation are represented in Figure 19–2.

T-CELL DIFFERENTIATION

The differentiation of T cells proceeds as follows. Step cells migrate from the bone marrow to the thymic cortex and traverse the thymus as they move from

FIG. 19–2. Molecules and receptors involved in the activation of T4 positive and T8 positive T cells. For both T4 and T8 positive T cells, the receptor that recognized antigen in conjunction with MHC molecules is the α/β heterodimer shown in Figure 19–1. The receptor recognizes antigen plus class II MHC molecules in the case of T4 cells, and antigen plus class I MHC molecules in the case of T8 cells. The CD4 molecule on T4 positive cells binds to class II MHC molecules, whereas the CD8 molecules on T8 positive cells binds to class I MHC molecules. Interactions between CD2 and LFA-3 may be important in the activation of both cell types.

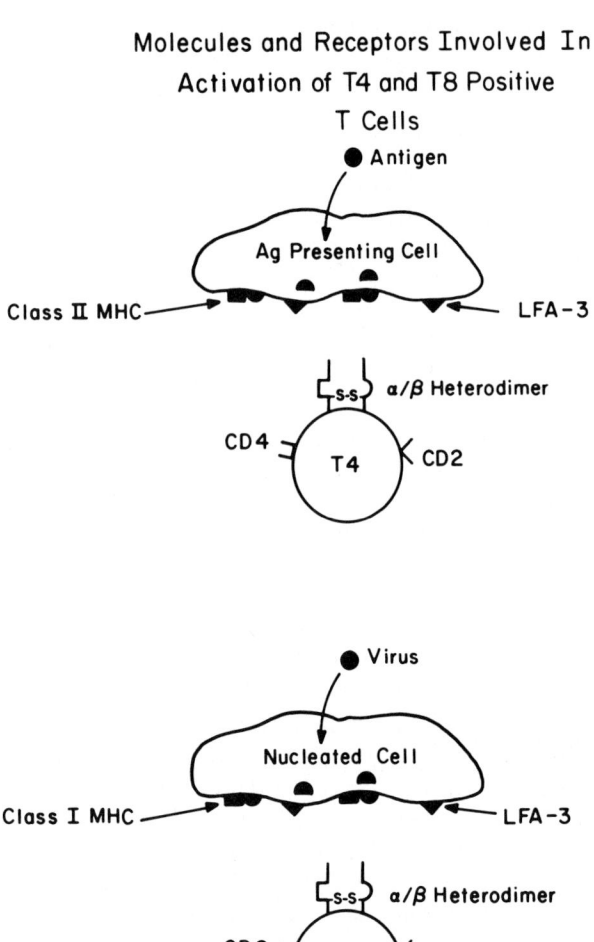

Molecules and Receptors Involved In Activation of T4 and T8 Positive T Cells

the cortex to the medulla, which takes approximately 3 days. During this migration, they develop functional maturity mirrored by changes in their expression of cell surface molecules. The first T-cell marker expressed on thymocytes is CD2, followed by CD3. When the thymocytes are first CD3 positive, they express CD3 in conjunction with the γ/δ heterodimer. At this stage, T cells do not express either CD4 or CD8. Next, the α/β heterodimer is expressed in conjunction with CD3. At this stage, the cells are both CD4 and CD8 positive. Once in the medulla, thymocytes divide into two distinct lineages: 65% of the T cells are CD4 positive and CD8 negative, while the remaining 35% are CD4 negative and CD8 positive. Both populations express CD2 and CD3 in conjunction with the α/β heterodimer. The cells then migrate to the periphery as two populations, distinguishable by their expression of CD4 or CD8.

Whether the small population of cells expressing the γ/δ heterodimer represents a distinct thymocyte population or a precursor to cells eventually destined to express the α/β heterodimer is unclear. No T cells have been found expressing both γ/δ and α/β, and culturing of γ/δ thymocytes fails to generate cells displaying α/β, supporting the concept that they represent distinct lineages. Because γ/δ positive heterodimer cells can be demonstrated in the periphery of athymic mice, it is not clear whether they necessarily derive from the thymus at all.

Development of functional maturity is one important event occurring during thymic differentiation. Another is the development of antigenic diversity. As will be discussed, activation of T cells by antigen requires that the T cells "see" antigen in conjunction with either class I or class II MHC gene products. It is during their maturation within the thymus that T cells express receptors with the capability of recognizing antigen in conjunction with *self* class I or *self* class II MHC gene products, as illustrated by the following observations:

Rodent T cells recognize antigen in conjunction with the animal's own class I or class II MHC gene products. If the thymus of that animal is replaced with the thymus of another strain of animal, however, then the T cells that differentiate in the thymus and pass to the periphery recognize antigen in conjunction with the class I or class II MHC determinants displayed on the *transplanted* thymic epithelium. Therefore, during thymic differentiation, T cells recognizing antigen in conjunction with MHC gene products expressed on thymic tissue are somehow selected. In the intact individual, this would involve recognition of self-MHC. T cells that recognize self-MHC gene products alone would presumably be autoreactive

and therefore be deleted during thymic development. The thymic epithelial cells appear to play an important role in determining MHC restriction. It is possible to demonstrate thymic epithelial cells that have engulfed large numbers (10 to 100) of thymus thymocytes. These thymic "nurse cells" display both class I and class II MHC molecules and may nurture MHC restriction. As discussed, interactions between CD2 on thymocytes and LFA-3 on thymic epithelium presumably play a role in such thymocyte-epithelial cell interactions. Exactly how this physical interaction is translated into the genetic rearrangements leading to T-cell receptor diversity is not known.

Immunocompetent T cells leave the thymus through postcapillary venules in the medulla, entering the bloodstream. They subsequently move to the thymic-dependent region of lymph nodes, periarterial sheaths of the spleen, or intranodular areas of Peyer's patches. In less than 24 hours, the T cells leave by efferent lymphatics, enter the large lymphatics, and return to the bloodstream via the thoracic duct. The movement of T cells from the circulation into lymphoid organs occurs through specialized areas in the blood vessels called *postcapillary, high-endothelial venules* (HEV). T cells bind to HEV by means of specific receptors, and specific receptors and specific ligands exist for different lymphoid organs. For example, if peripheral lymph node cells are injected back into an animal from which they are removed, they preferentially localize to the peripheral lymph nodes and not to the spleen or the Peyer's patches. Similarly, cells residing in Peyer's patches preferentially return to Peyer's patches. This specific homing depends on the expression of specific cell-surface molecules. If lymphocytes are treated with proteolytic enzymes that remove cell surface molecules, their homing becomes random. One molecule involved in directing T-cell migration to peripheral lymph nodes, as opposed to Peyer's patches, has been isolated. It has a molecular weight of 80,000 MW and can be detected by monoclonal antibody MEL-14. This antibody can inhibit the migration of T cells into the lymph node but does not affect their migration into Peyer's patches. Other molecules involved in directing lymphocyte "traffic" remain to be isolated.

T-CELL ACTIVATION

Clearly, T cells can manifest antigen specificity, and the α/β heterodimer is the major receptor by which they recognize antigen. It is equally clear that the T-cell receptor does not recognize antigen alone. Antigen alone does not bind to specific T cells, and antigen added to purified populations of T cells fails to induce activation. Instead, antigen must be first *processed* and then *presented* to T cells. The α/β heterodimer recognizes the processed antigen presented in conjunction with either class I or class II MHC gene products.

As mentioned previously, experiments in the 1960s clearly indicated that the immune response is under genetic control. Genes controlling this immune reactivity are localized to the MHC. Genes in the MHC regulating immune reactivity are termed class I or class II MHC genes (Fig. 19–3). The product of class I MHC genes is a 45,000 MW molecule expressed on the surface of all nucleated cells in conjunction with a smaller molecule, β-2 microglobulin (13,000 MW). (Genes coding for β-2 microglobulin are not located within the MHC.) Products of class II MHC genes are represented by an α/β heterodimer (distinct from the T-cell α/β heterodimer) whose expression is limited to antigen presenting cells such as monocytes/mac-

FIG. 19–3. MHC gene products. Genes in the MHC code for two classes of molecules important in T-cell activation. The product of class I genes is a 45,000-MW molecule which is associated with B$_2$ microglobulins on all nucleated cells. The product of class II genes is a noncovalently associated heterodimer displayed on the surface of antigen presenting cells such as monocytes/macrophages, B cells, and dendritic cells.

MHC GENE PRODUCTS

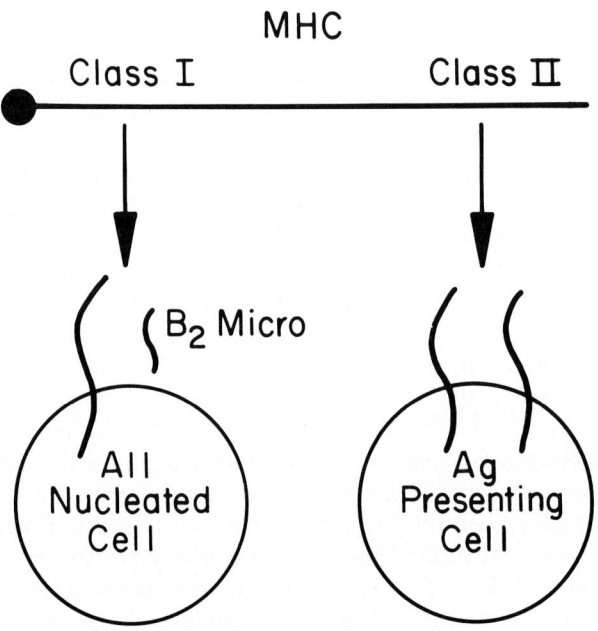

rophages, B-lymphocytes, activated T cells, dendritic cells, and in some cases, endothelial cells. Class II MHC genes and their products regulate immune reactivity to soluble, nonreplicating antigen, whereas class I MHC gene products are involved in determining immune reactivity to organisms such as viruses that can replicate intracellularly.

A physical association between some antigens and class II MHC gene products and some viruses and class I MHC gene products has been demonstrated. Therefore, it appears that these molecules control immune reactivity by serving as a type of receptor capable of interacting with soluble or replicating antigens. In a situation in which immune responsiveness to an antigen exists, interaction between the class I or class II MHC molecule and the antigen is such that the antigen can be appropriately viewed by the T-cell receptor. In a situation in which there is genetically determined unresponsiveness, the appropriate interaction between the class I or class II MHC molecule and antigen does not occur. The antigen-MHC complex cannot be appropriately viewed by the T-cell receptor, and T-cell activation does not occur.

The first step in T-cell activation by antigen is the appropriate processing of the antigen by the antigen presenting cell. Soluble antigens are physically taken up by antigen presenting cells such as monocytes or macrophages and are degraded. This process is energy dependent and can be inhibited by the drug chloroquine. A portion of the degraded antigen is then expressed on the cell surface in conjunction with the appropriate MHC gene product. The metabolic processes involved in the expression of replicating antigens such as viruses appear to be somewhat different. The process is not inhibited by chloroquine. Much remains to be learned about the process of antigen uptake, degradation, and expression.

For some soluble antigens, a physical association between the antigen and the class II MHC gene product has been shown, and for a limited number of viral antigens, it is possible to demonstrate an interaction between the virus and class I MHC gene products. Therefore, it is assumed that it is this physical interaction between antigen and MHC gene product that is seen by the α/β heterodimer. Because the T-cell receptor for antigen consists of two chains, it might be concluded that one chain recognizes the antigen and the other the MHC gene product, but this does not appear to be the case. Instead, the α/β heterodimer appears to recognize an associated determinant generated by interactions between antigen plus MHC of the product. Structure function relationship is similar to the interaction between specific antibody and antigen. The combination of the light and heavy chains best binds antigen.

Recognition of antigen in conjunction with class I or class II MHC gene products by the T-cell antigen receptor constitutes one signal required for activation (other signals involved will be discussed subsequently). The metabolic events involved in transmembrane signaling through the antigen receptor heterodimer can be summarized by the following (Fig. 19–4). A signal is transmitted either directly to the antigen receptor heterodimer or indirectly through the CD3 complex, activating a phosphodiesterase called *phospholipase C* that cleaves an important metabolite of membrane inositol, phosphotidylinositol-bisphosphate (PIP$_2$), into two crucial products.[3] The first is 1,4,5 *inositol trisphosphate* (1,4,5)P$_3$, which binds to receptors present on the endoplasmic reticulum of the cell and mobilizes calcium from bound intracellular stores, thereby increasing intracellular free calcium. A rise in cytoplasmic free calcium is one crucial intracellular signal necessary for activation. Although some of the increase in cytoplasmic free calcium seen

FIG. 19–4. Two stimuli and three signals are required for T-cell activation. Recognition of antigen plus MHC by the antigen receptor heterodimer–CD3 complex causes hydrolysis of PIP$_2$ into IP$_3$ and diacylglycerol. IP$_3$ increases intracellular calcium by mobilizing calcium from bound intracellular stores. Diacylglycerol activates protein kinase C (PKC). A second stimulus required for activation can be mediated by IL-1. Biochemical events involved in this pathway are unknown.

Two Stimuli and Three Signals are Required for T-Cell Activation

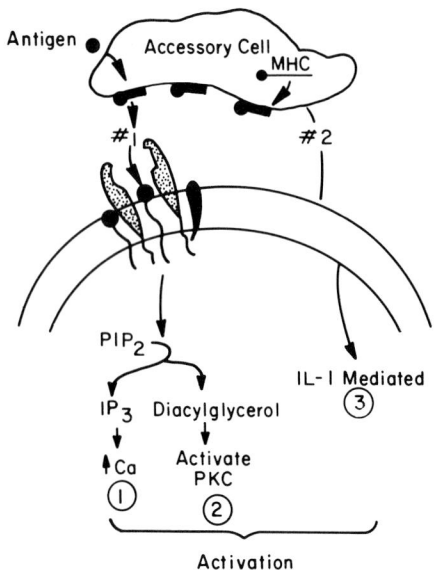

during T-cell activation represents calcium mobilized from bound intracellular stores, migration of calcium from the outside to the inside of the cell also contributes to the increased cytoplasmic free calcium observed. Exactly how this occurs is not known. In some systems there exists a kinase that generates IP$_4$ from (1,4,5)P$_3$. Possibly, IP$_4$ opens calcium channels in the cell membrane, allowing an influx of extracellular calcium. It has not been possible to demonstrate the classic, voltage-dependent calcium channels in lymphocytes.

The second major product generated from PIP$_2$ is *diacylglycerol (DG)* (Fig. 19–4), the physiologic activator of another intracellular enzyme called *protein kinase C* (PKC). Activation of this kinase constitutes a second crucial signal for T-cell activation. PKC presumably phosphorylates some other intracellular protein, which then transmits an important activating signal. Activation of PKC is accompanied by a fall in intracellular hydrogen ion concentration, reflected by an increase in intracellular pH by 0.1 to 0.15 units. Hydrogen ions are exported to the outside of the cell through a sodium-proton exchanger. Phosphorylation of this sodium-proton exchanger by the activated PKC may induce its action. The two signals (1,4,5)P$_3$ and DG generated through the T-cell antigen receptor can be reproduced using calcium ionophores, which directly increase cytoplasmic free calcium and phorbol esters that directly bind to and activate PKC. The combination of calcium ionophores and phorbol esters can substitute for antigen/MHC gene product to activate T cells.

Still another signal besides increased cytoplasmic free calcium and activation of PKC is necessary to activate resting T cells. In some systems, this signal can be represented by a soluble material called *interleukin-1* (IL-1), a lymphokine released by accessory cells. The biochemical events initiated by IL-1 involved in T-cell activation are unknown.

In summary, recognition of antigen plus MHC gene product by the T-cell antigen receptor/T3 complex results in two signals required for activation; i.e., an increased intracellular free calcium and activation of PKC. These two signals alone are not sufficient for the activation of resting T cells. A third signal that can be induced by IL-1 is required (Fig. 19–4).

T-cell activation can be represented by several events, including the synthesis of molecules that are secreted, expression of new molecules on the cell surface, and proliferation. Gamma-interferon is an example of a molecule synthesized and secreted after T-cell activation. This molecule plays an important role in host defense against viral infections. Another molecule that is secreted and appears to be very important in T-cell growth and differentiation is a lymphokine called *interleukin-2* (IL-2). With T-cell activation there is increased expression of the receptor for IL-2 on the activated T cell.[4] Therefore, IL-2 made by an activated T cell feeds back on the cell as an autocoid (see Chapter 14) enhancing its growth and differentiation. Subsequently, there is down regulation of the receptor for IL-2 so that uncontrolled, autonomous proliferation does not proceed.

T-CELL FUNCTION

T cells function in two ways, as effector cells for cell-mediated reactions and as regulatory cells that can regulate both cell-mediated and humoral immunity. Cell-mediated reactions for which T cells exist as effector cells include *delayed hypersensitivity and cytotoxicity*. Regulatory functions are represented by T cells required to amplify both cell-mediated reactivity and the differentiation of B cells into immunoglobulin-secreting plasma cells.

Clearly the proportion of circulating T cells specific for a given antigen is very small. Therefore, the number of antigen-specific T cells reacting to a foreign antigen consisting of 10 different antigenic determinants would be too small to constitute substantial host defense. T cells have, therefore, devised a means by which they can magnify their reactivity. They do this by secreting *lymphokines* that act on other cells such as lymphocytes and monocytes/macrophages in an antigen-nonspecific fashion to recruit them into host defense. Perhaps this process can be best exemplified by detailing the events that occur in a T-cell response to a viral infection.

A circulating virus cannot react with T cells because the replicating virus must be seen in conjunction with class I MHC gene products. Infection of any nucleated cell (remember, all nucleated cells express class I MHC, but only some express class II MHC molecules) results in the expression of the viral antigens in conjunction with class I MHC products on the cell surface. This complex is then recognized by the T-cell α/β heterodimer, and if the appropriate signals are generated, activation can ensue. As part of activation, molecules such as interferon that directly inhibit viral growth and replication are secreted and molecules such as *migration inhibition factor* (MIF) are released, resulting in a local accumulation of monocytes. Other molecules, macrophage-activating factors, are released and activate these cells to kill virus. IL-2 is secreted and increased expression of IL-2 receptors occurs, resulting in proliferation and expansion of the clone of T cells initially activated, accounting for the

amnestic or *secondary* response when the antigen is again introduced.

B-CELL DIFFERENTIATION

B cells constitute the effector cells for humoral immunity as they differentiate into the immunoglobulin secreting plasma cell. During fetal life, B-cell differentiation occurs in the liver. In adult life, stem cells undergo differentiation into B cells within the marrow and then pass to peripheral lymphoid tissue.

The hallmark of cells of the B-cell system is immunoglobulin. Immunoglobulin present on the surface of the B cell serves as the receptor for antigen and is involved in transmitting at least one signal necessary for its proliferation and differentiation. Plasma cells secrete immunoglobulin of the same specificity as the surface immunoglobulin displayed by the precursor B cell. As noted for T cells, B cells must be capable of distinguishing approximately 1,000,000 different antigens. The conserved genetic mechanisms leading to this diversity involve gene rearrangements similar to those described for the T-cell receptor (see Chapter 17). Like the genes for the T-cell receptor, immunoglobulin genes consist of multiple gene families termed V, D, J, and C genes. (Light-chain genes consist of V, J, and C genes.) Genes encoding the C region of the heavy chain consist of C_μ, C_δ, C_γ, C_ϵ, and C_α, representing genes encoding for the C region of IgM, IgD, IgG, IgE, and IgA respectively. During the differentiation of B cells, there is an orderly, sequential rearrangement in light- and heavy-chain genes that gives rise to polypeptides (light and heavy chains) that subsequently join to form an intact immunoglobulin molecule. The early stages of B-cell differentiation (pre-B cell through plasma cell) are mirrored by crucial rearrangements occurring among immunoglobulin genes (Fig. 19–5). A *pre-B cell* is a cell that has immunoglobulin in the cytoplasm but not on the cell surface. A *B cell* is a cell that has surface immunoglobulin but does not secrete large amounts of immunoglobulin. *Plasma cells* do not have surface immunoglobulin, but do secrete large amounts of immunoglobulin.

PRE-B CELL

The first event in B-cell differentiation is reflected by rearrangements among heavy-chain genes. First there is a DJ rearrangement, and then the DJ genes join to a V-region gene. Next, the VDJ gene complex assciates with a C_μ gene. An intact heavy chain is

FIG. 19–5. Events involved in the differentiation of B cells. The scheme traces the differentiation of B cells. The black line to the left indicates the presence of rearranged heavy to light chains.

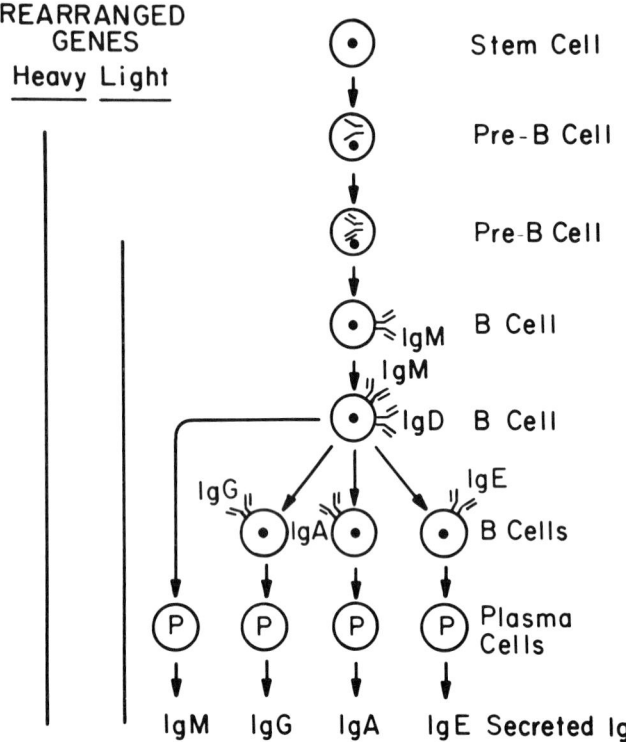

synthesized and appears in the cytoplasm. Next, rearrangements occur among the light-chain genes. The first rearrangements occur on one allele of the κ light chain. If this results in an effective VJC complex, an intact κ light chain is synthesized. If an effective rearrangement does not occur, then rearrangement switches to the other allele of the κ gene. If an effective VJC complex results, κ light chain synthesis ensues. If not, rearrangements switch first to one allele and, if unsuccessful, to the other allele of the λ genes. If no effective light-chain gene rearrangement occurs, then normal B-cell development does not proceed.

Once an effective light-chain gene rearrangement ensues, light chains are synthesized, appear in the cytoplasm, and become associated with heavy chains.

B CELL

The switch from pre-B cell to B cell is characterized by the appearance of membrane immunoglobulin. The B cell first expresses only IgM (monomeric, 7S IgM), and next synthesizes and expresses both IgM and IgD. At the gene level, this dual expression is represented by the association of a single VDJ complex and both C_μ and C_δ genes. Because VDJ genes code for the portions of Ig molecules that dictate their antigen specificity, and C genes code for portions that determine immunoglobulin class, it is easy to see how a single cell can synthesize two different classes of immunoglobulin, each of which has the same antigenic specificity. The display of both IgM and IgD appears to be an important event in B-cell activation. B cells displaying only surface IgM are difficult to activate and, in some models, appear particularly susceptible to the induction of tolerance. In contrast, the appearance of surface IgD provides a receptor that allows appropriate signals to push B-cell differentiation forward. At the next stage of B-cell development, the B cells express only IgD. From this point, they differentiate into cells that display only IgG, IgE, or IgA.

PLASMA CELL

At the plasma cell stage, all gene rearrangements have been completed and the cell is engaged in secreting large amounts of immunoglobulin of a single antigenic specificity and immunoglobulin class. In general, it can be assumed that B cells displaying a specific immunoglobulin class give rise to plasma cells secreting Ig of that same class. For example, IgG-bearing B cells generate IgG-secreting plasma cells, IgA-bearing B cells give rise to IgA-secreting plasma cells, and IgE-bearing B cells generate IgE-secreting plasma cells.

This ordered sequence of immunoglobulin class expression that occurs during B-cell differentiation is mirrored by the ontogeny of B cells and immunoglobulin production. In human fetuses, synthesis of IgM begins at 10 to 11 weeks of age, IgG at 12 weeks, and IgA after 30 weeks. Adult levels of IgM occur by 1 year of age, IgG by 5 years, and IgA by the early teens.

B-CELL ACTIVATION

The mechanisms involved in the activation of B cells by antigen are similar, but not identical, to those involved in the activation of T cells by antigen. One major difference is that surface immunoglobulin on B cells (the B-cell antigen receptor) is capable of recognizing antigen alone and does not need to have antigen processed or to "see" antigen in conjunction with MHC gene products. Interactions between the antigen and surface immunoglobulin on B cells produce intracellular biochemical events identical to those seen after activation of T cells.[5-7] Phosphotidylinositol-bisphosphate is cleaved into two important metabolites by phospholipase C, namely $(1,4,5)P_3$ and DG. The resultant rise in intracellular free calcium and protein kinase C activation stimulates the B cell to enter the G-I phase of the cell cycle. Further progression through the cell cycle does not occur unless the B cell comes into contact with a soluble factor or factors secreted by T cells. One of these factors, *B-cell stimulating factor*, or BSF-I, has three important effects: it increases the expression of MHC molecules on the surface of the B cell, it acts as a competence factor in preparing the cell to enter S phase, and it promotes

the secretion of both IgE and IgG_1 by B cells/plasma cells.

The ability of BSF-I to increase MHC gene expression by B cells may be important in allowing these cells to be effective presenters of antigen. For example, it is possible that within the microenvironment, antigen binds to the surface immunoglobulin receptor of B cells and is then processed and presented to T cells in conjunction with MHC gene products on the B-cell surface. B cells can serve as antigen presenting cells. As a result of the interaction between T cells, antigen, and MHC gene products on B cells, the T cells may be stimulated to produce BSF-I. The secreted lymphokine then enhances MHC gene expression by the B cell, allowing it to become a more effective antigen presenter and, in conjunction with antigen, allows further B-cell differentiation and proliferation (Fig. 19–6).

In vivo experiments looking at the effects of BSF-I on IgE antibody responses are intriguing. BSF-I increases IgE synthesized in response to parasitic infections. Therefore, it may have an important role in allergic responses.

Many factors have been demonstrated to modulate, in vitro, B-cell differentiation and proliferation. Which of these factors are important in vivo and which are different from BSF-I remains to be determined.

FIG. 19–6. T-B cell interactions in the antigen induced differentiation of B cells. Antigen binds to immunoglobulin receptors on B cells, is processed, and presented to T cells in conjunction with MHC molecules. Antigen-specific T cells are activated and release the lymphokine, BSF-1. BSF-1 increases MHC expression by the B cell allowing more efficient presentation of antigen, and then, in conjunction with the stimulus provided by antigen, allows the B cell to differentiate into antibody secreting plasma cells. Other factors released by T cells and macrophages are most likely required for B cell differentiation.

T–B Cell Interactions in the Antigen Induced Differentiation of B Cells

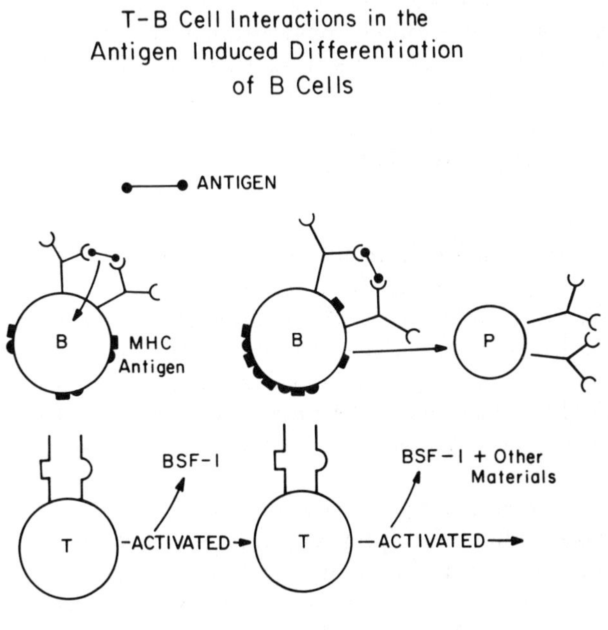

REFERENCES

1. Springer, T.A., Dustin, M.L., Kishimoto, T.K., and Marlin, S.D.: The lymphocyte function-associated LFA-1, CD2, and LFA-3 molecules: Cell adhesion receptors of the immune system. Annu. Rev. Immunol., 5:223–252, 1987.
2. Toyonaga, B., and Mak, T.: Genes of the T-cell antigen receptor in normal and malignant T cells. Annu. Rev. Immunol., 5:585–620.
3. Weiss, A., et al.: The role of the T3/antigen receptor complex in T-cell activation. Annu. Rev. Immunol., 4:593–620, 1986.
4. Greene, W.C., and Leonard, W.J.: The human interleukin-2-receptor. Annu. Rev. Immunol., 4:69–96, 1986.
5. Schrader, J.W.: The panspecific hemopoietin of activated T lymphocytes (Interleukin-3). Annu. Rev. Immunol., 4:205–230, 1986.
6. Hamaoka, T., and Ono, S.: Regulation of B-cell differentiation: Interactions of factors and corresponding receptors. Annu. Rev. Immunol., 4:167–204, 1986.
7. Cambier, J.C., and Ransom, J.T.: Molecular mechanisms of transmembrane signaling in B lymphocytes. Annu. Rev. Immunol., 5:175–199, 1987.

20

NEUTROPHIL STRUCTURE AND FUNCTION

BRUCE N. CRONSTEIN and GERALD WEISSMANN

The polymorphonuclear leukocytes (PMNs) are highly specialized cells whose primary function is the phagocytosis and destruction of microorganisms and other noxious agents. In addition to their role in host defense, PMNs are commonly present at sites of immunologically mediated tissue injury. PMNs mediate many of the events that occur at foci of acute inflammation.

Metchnikoff proposed, in the closing years of the nineteenth century, that leukocytes may liberate substances that are capable of damaging adjacent tissues.[1] It remained until the middle years of the twentieth century for the demonstration of the crucial role of PMNs in a variety of experimental immunologically induced inflammatory reactions. The first reaction shown to be neutrophil dependent was the Arthus reaction. The depletion of PMNs by either nitrogen mustard or heterologous antineutrophil antisera inhibited the Arthus reaction in several species.[1a] Despite deposition of antigen, antibody, and complement components in the vessels of antiserum-treated animals, no microscopic evidence of vascular injury could be found.[2-6] Other experimental models of immunologic injury have a similar dependence on the neutrophil for tissue damage. These models include the necrotizing arteritis of experimental serum sickness in rabbits,[7] the proteinuria associated with acute nephrotoxic vasculitis in rats and rabbits,[8] and arthritis in rabbits induced by an intra-articular reversed passive Arthus reaction.[9] In the last of these experimental systems, intra-articular injections of purified

suspensions of PMNs reconstituted the immunologic lesions in neutrophil-depleted rabbits.

These studies show that PMNs play an important role in mediating immunologically induced tissue injury by generating toxic metabolites and releasing various inflammatory molecules, especially those stored in cytoplasmic granules or lysosomes. These lysosomal substances cause tissue damage directly and interact with components of the complement and kinin systems to generate still other mediators of inflammation and tissue damage.

GENERAL DESCRIPTION OF THE PMNS

Mature PMNs are easily distinguished from other circulating cells. The diameter ranges from 8 to 15 μM and they have a multilobed nucleus (Fig. 20–1). Wright's stained blood smears show three types of granulocyte, namely neutrophils, eosinophils, and basophils.

The most common PMN type in blood and other tissues is the neutrophil, which is probably the most important for the mediation of tissue injury and for host defense. The neutrophil nucleus has from two to five lobes. There is plentiful cytoplasm and multiple granules that appear pink on Wright's stain. Electron microscopy demonstrates few mitochondria and sparse endoplasmic reticulum (Fig. 20–1).

Eosinophils, comprising 1 to 3% of the total leukocyte population in the peripheral blood of normal individuals, have large cytoplasmic granules that

FIG. 20–1. *A,* A transmission electron photomicrograph of a resting neutrophil (× 11,700). N = nucleus; GA = Golgi apparatus; G = granules; C = centrioles; M = mitochondrion. *B,* A higher power of this neutrophil demonstrating radiation of microtubules (MT) from centrioles (C) (× 44,100). *C,* The electron photomicrograph shows a neutrophil that has ingested monosodium urate crystals (MSU) (× 7,600). Marker indicates 1 μm. (Photomicrographs courtesy of Dr. Abby Rich.)

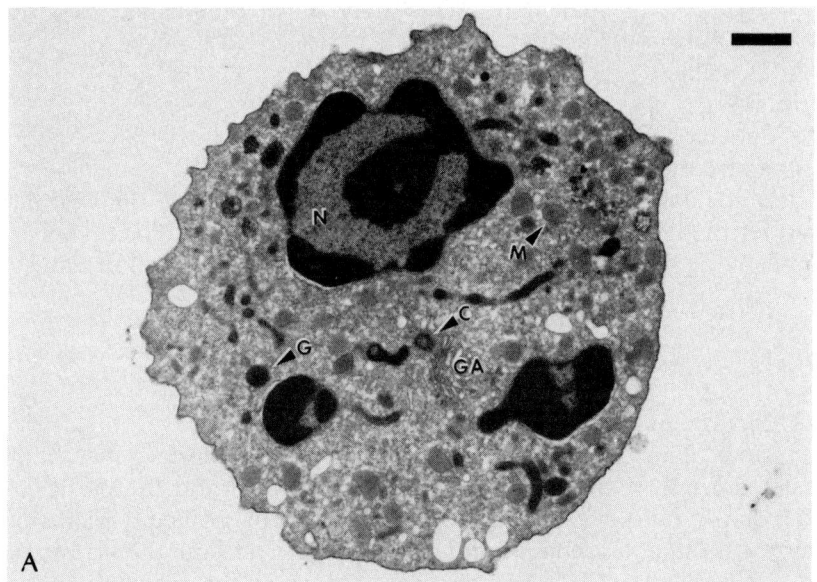

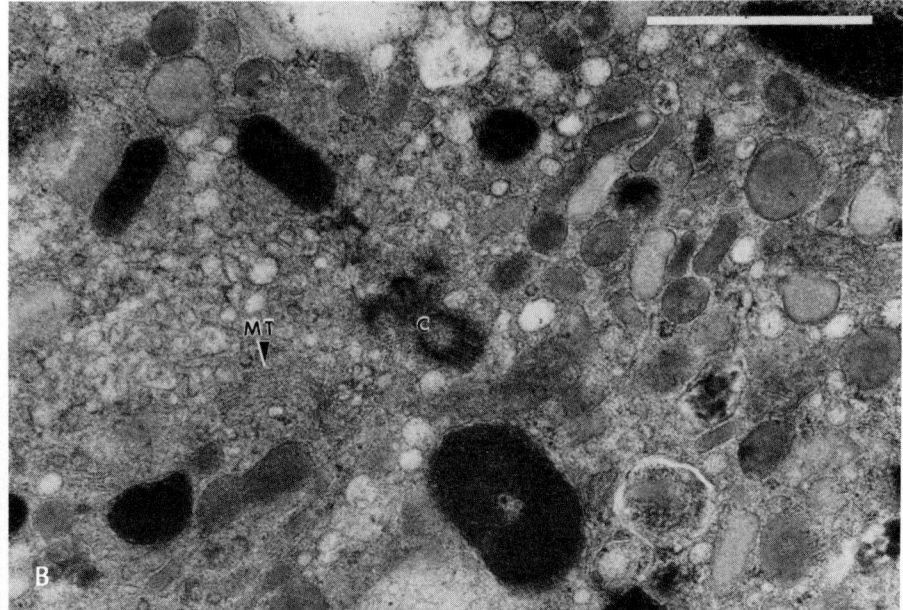

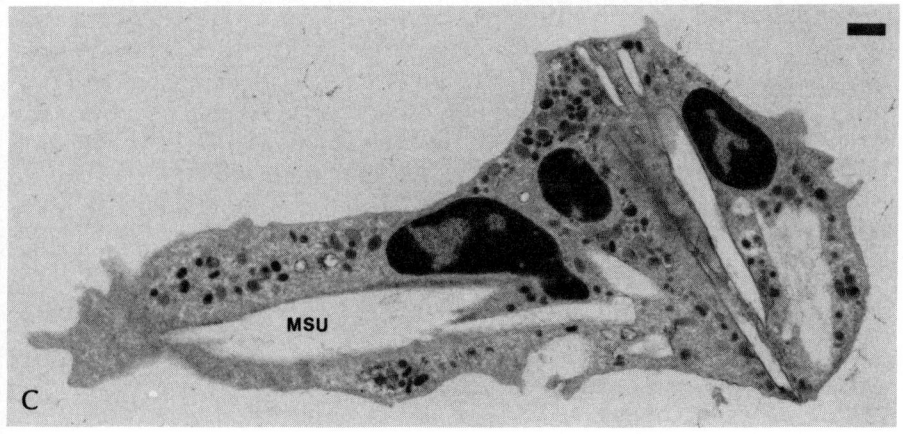

stain red. These cells are involved in the host response to parasites, although their function and role in host defense and response to injury are currently under intense study (see Chapter 21).

The basophil can be distinguished by large bluish-black cytoplasmic granules seen in Wright's stained smears that contain histamine and heparin. Basophils constitute less than 1% of the leukocyte population in the peripheral blood of normal persons and mediate immediate hypersensitivity (type I immunologic reactions). The discussion in the remainder of this chapter will refer exclusively to neutrophils.

PRODUCTION OF NEUTROPHILS

Neutrophils have an extremely rapid rate of turnover[10] and circulate for very short periods. The half-life of the mature neutrophil in the blood is only 6 to 7 hours. Because several days are required for the neutrophil to mature in the bone marrow, a large pool of marrow precursors is necessary for maintenance of circulating cells. The factors responsible for stimulation of neutrophil production, such as granulocyte-monocyte colony stimulating factor (GM-CSF), are being isolated and cloned for possible therapeutic use.[11–13]

In the bone marrow, neutrophil maturation proceeds through several histologically characteristic stages. The neutrophil precursors (myelocytes and promyelocytes) synthesize lysosomes in the Golgi apparatus.[14] Two granule types are morphologically evident. The first granule to appear during the maturation process is called the *primary* (azurophil) granule (because of its staining characteristics on Wright-Giemsa stain). These granules are relatively large and contain a number of hydrolytic enzymes and bactericidal molecules discussed in greater detail later. *Secondary* (specific) granules appear only after the full cellular complement of primary granules has been synthesized. These are smaller than primary granules and contain a different group of enzymes and bactericidal molecules. There are more secondary than primary granules in the mature neutrophil despite their later appearance during cellular maturation. Certain evidence suggests other subcellular storage sites for "granular" enzymes.[15] These enzymes can be released on appropriate stimulation.

Besides the morphologic changes, cellular metabolism also undergoes a transition during maturation. Neutrophil precursors contain many mitochondria and appear to use oxidative metabolism for protein synthesis. With maturation there is a shift to anaerobic glycolysis, presumably in preparation for function in hypoxic tissues.[16,17] Mobility, plasticity, and the capacity to ingest particles also accompany maturation. Immature neutrophils, released into the circulation prematurely, have diminished bactericidal activity.[18]

NEUTROPHIL FUNCTION

In host defense PMNs must leave the vasculature and migrate to infected or inflamed loci, where they ingest their targets for further intracellular digestion and destruction.

PHAGOCYTOSIS

Neutrophils invaginate their surface membrane at the point of contact and surround the particle. The resulting intracellular vacuole, called a *phagosome* or phagocytic vesicle, pinches off from the surface of the cell and becomes completely internalized within the cell cytoplasm.[19–21] After phagocytosis the cells become rounded and have less available surface membrane. Resting neutrophils, not exposed to particles, have a large surface area, seen in the form of surface pseudopods and blebs (Fig. 20–2). Despite its relatively large surface area, the plasma membrane's extent is finite, and limitations in availability of surface membrane may limit the number of particles that can be ingested by a single cell. Fusion of granule membranes with those of the phagosome begins the process of digestion of the phagocytosed particles. The lysosomal granules discharge their contents into the phagosome in a process known as *degranulation*.[22,23] The phagosome, now called a *phagolysosome*, contains a wide array of microbicidal proteins and degradative enzymes.

GRANULES AND THEIR CONTENTS

Neutrophils are well-adapted to their role as microbicidal and scavenging cells as their granules contain an assortment of microbicidal enzymes and proteases necessary to meet the challenge of many different types of bacteria, as well as for scavenging damaged tissues. Many of these enzymes are capable of damaging viable host tissues, but because they are usually sequestered within the granule and phagolysosome, they do not present a threat to the host. Generally, a minimal amount of granule contents is released by the cell during the phagocytic process, but under certain conditions massive release of gran-

FIG. 20–2. *A,* A scanning electron micrograph of two resting neutrophils. Note the ruffled edges, irregular shape, and large number of pseudopods extending from the cell surface. *B,* Neutrophils adherent to a surface coated with IgG. Note the flattened, rounded shape and loss of pseudopods as the neutrophils spread out and attempt to ingest the antibody coated surface. (Photomicrographs courtesy of Dr. Abby Rich.)

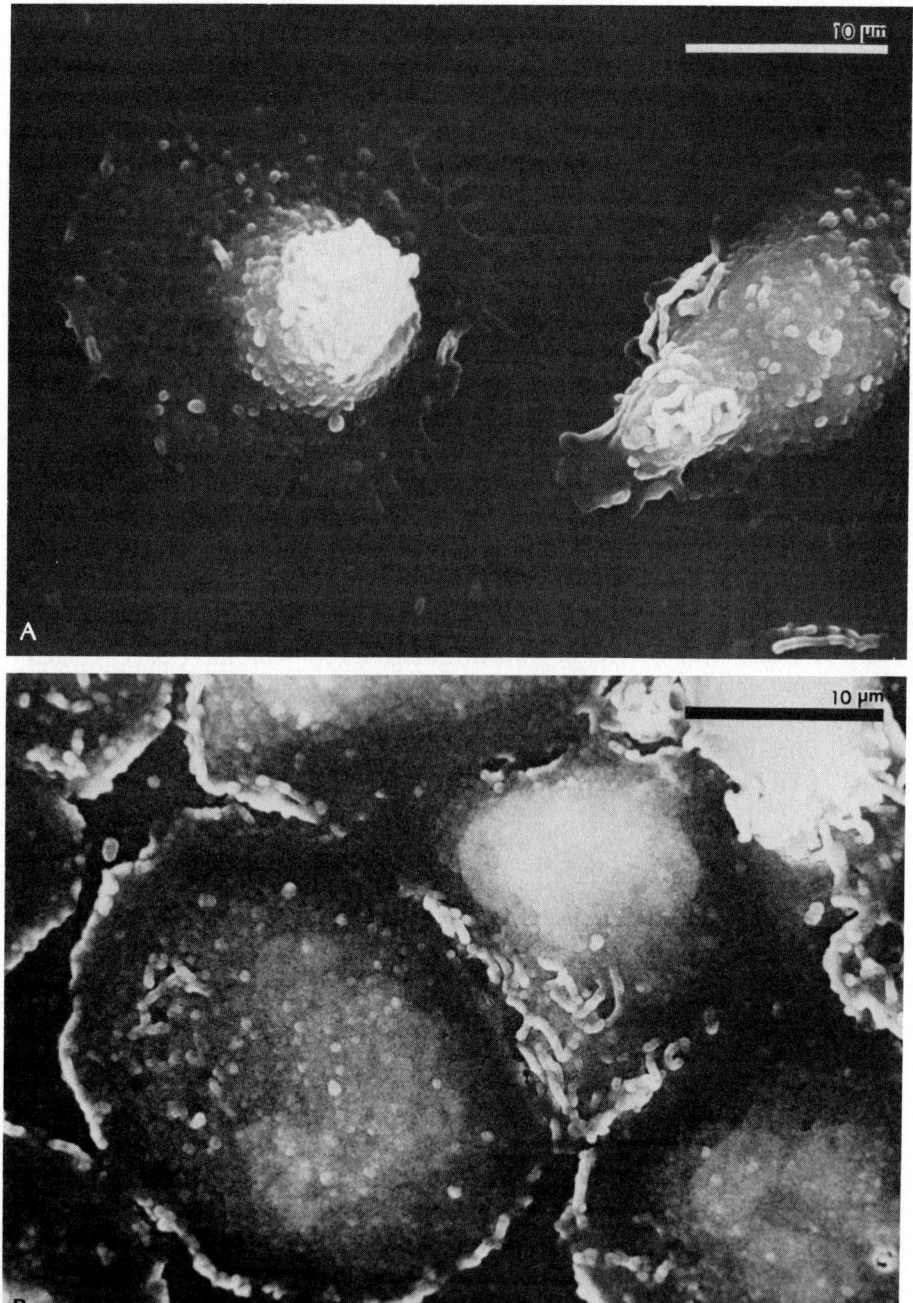

ule contents can promote tissue injury, leading to further inflammation. Extracellular release of granule contents occurs by several mechanisms, discussed later.

Granule Contents

Neutrophil granules contain many different types of compounds including microbicidal enzymes, proteases, and proteins with nonenzymatic microbicidal properties. *Lysozyme* is a bactericidal enzyme, found in both specific and azurophil granules, which hydrolyzes cell-wall peptidoglycans of many species of bacteria.[24,25] Specific granules also contain nonenzymatic molecules including lactoferrin,[25] a bacteriostatic protein, and vitamin B_{12}-binding protein.[26] Collagenase[27] and alkaline phosphatase[24] are neutral hydrolases also found in specific granules.[24a]

Azurophil granules also contain lysozyme,[10,25] but in contrast to the specific granules, the azurophil granules also contain myeloperoxidase, low-molecular-weight bactericidal proteins,[28–30] chondroitin sulfate, and the neutral and acid hydrolases.[19,25,31] Myeloperoxidase, together with hydrogen peroxide (H_2O_2) and a halide, constitute an important killing mechanism.[32,33] The low-molecular-weight bactericidal cationic proteins are a heterogenous group of molecules most active at acid pH and with different bactericidal specificities for gram-positive and gram-negative bacteria.[34] These proteins can also cause increased vascular permeability or histamine release when they escape into the extracellular environment. The neutral and acid hydrolases have digestive or scavenging functions as well as antibacterial proper-

ties. A representative group of granule contents is listed in Table 20–1.

The granule contents with the greatest potential for causing tissue damage are the proteases, which as a group have a broad substrate specificity. The neutral serine proteases, elastase and cathepsin G, and the metalloenzyme collagenase, though not the only proteolytic enzymes found in neutrophils, probably account for most of the damage to extracellular structures induced by lysosomal enzymes and thus will be described in more detail.

Cathepsin G. Human neutrophil "chymotrypsin-like" enzyme was recognized by its ability to hydrolyze phenylalanine esters.[35,36] It has a molecular weight of 26,000 daltons and is localized to azurophil granules.[37] It is immunologically distinct from neutrophil elastase and needs different conditions for its isolation from granules. Its substrate specificity is very broad; it has been reported to hydrolyze hemoglobin,[36] fibrinogen,[36] casein,[35] cryocasein,[38] insoluble collagen,[39] and cartilage proteoglycans.[38] It is inhibited by human plasma α-1-antitrypsin, α-2-macroglobulin, and, most effectively, α-1-antichymotrypsin.

Collagenase. This neutral protease has been localized to the azurophil granule by some investigators[23] and to the specific granule by others.[27] It is a metalloenzyme with an apparent molecular weight of approximately 76,000 daltons[40,41] that hydrolyzes *solubilized* native collagen but cannot cleave collagen fibrils without the participation of an additional neutral protease.[40] The preferred substrate for this enzyme is type I collagen, the predominant type of bone and tendon.[42] Like other metalloproteases, it is inhib-

Table 20–1. Neutrophil Granules and Their Contents

Substance	Azurophil Granules (Primary)	Specific Granules (Secondary)
Microbicidal enzymes	Myeloperoxidase Lysozyme	Lysozyme
Neutral proteases	Elastase Cathepsin C Cathepsin G Collagenase	Alkaline phosphatase Collagenase
Acid proteases	β-glucuronidase Acid β-glycerophosphatase N-acetyl β-glucosaminidase α-mannosidase Arylsulphatase β-galactosidase α-fucosidase Cathepsin B Cathepsin D	
Nonenzymatic	Cationic proteins Chondroitin sulfate Defensins	Lactoferrin Vitamin B_{12}-binding protein

ited by EDTA and cysteine, but unlike the other neutral proteases, neutrophil cytosol does not inhibit collagenase activity. Inhibitors of collagenase in plasma include α-1-antitrypsin and α-2-macroglobulin, which must first undergo proteolytic cleavage by collagenase as part of its mechanism of action.[41]

Elastase. Elastase is a neutral protease localized to the azurophil granule.[43] It is a basic glycoprotein with a molecular weight of approximately 30,000 to 34,000 daltons.[43] Together with collagenase it constitutes 5% of the dry weight of the neutrophil. The substrate specificity of elastase is broad; the enzyme has been reported to hydrolyze elastin from tendon, lung, basement membrane, native collagen, fibril, proteoglycan, cryocasein, hemoglobin, fibrinogen, and, in concert with collagenase, histone.[38,44] Elastase digests elastic arteries in vitro and provokes vascular injury when injected in vivo. PMN cytosol, α-1-antitrypsin, α-2-macroglobulin, and neutrophil cytosol are all effective inhibitors of elastase. Of the enzymes discussed here, elastase is probably the most important because of its abundance and broad substrate specificity.

Taken together, these enzymes have a remarkably broad substrate specificity, although of greater importance to the rheumatologist is the degradation of the two major components of articular cartilage, collagen and proteoglycans. The neutral proteases may also contribute to the inflammatory response by generating chemotactic factors from C5[45] and by cleaving plasma kininogen[46] and leukokininogen to kinins.[39] The existence of multiple plasma and cytosolic inhibitors for these proteolytic enzymes testifies to their potential for destruction when not confined to the granule.

CYTOSKELETAL STRUCTURES

Microtubules and microfilaments are the major constituents of the neutrophil cytoskeleton. These structures are not only involved in degranulation, cell motility,[47,48] and maintenance of the internal cellular organization, but also may mediate information transfer between the plasma membrane and the cell interior.

Microtubules are polymers of tubulin, a 55,000 dalton protein. The centrioles, located between the Golgi apparatus and nucleus, have an electron-dense organizing center from which almost all of the microtubules associated with these structures originate. The microtubules then radiate outward, passing very close to and appearing to graze membrane-bound organelles such as granules[49] (Fig. 20–1C).

The "assembly" and "disassembly" of microtubules are controlled in a variety of ways both in vitro and in vivo. Calcium ions promote dissolution of polymerized tubulin, as do decreased pH or medium osmolality.[30] Cyclic GMP and agents that elevate its intracellular levels such as phorbol myristate acetate and carbamylcholine promote assembly of tubulin, whereas cAMP and agents that elevate its intracellular levels such as PGE_1 and isoproterenol promote disassembly. The redox state of the cells may also regulate assembly of microtubule proteins.[51] Micromolar concentrations of the plant alkaloids colchicine and vinblastine induce reversible dissolution of microtubules. Studies done with the aid of these agents, especially colchicine, have made it possible to identify the function of these structures. There are separate binding sites in tubulin dimers for colchicine and vinblastine.

Microtubules are of particular importance in neutrophil function. Degranulation during phagocytosis is affected by agents influencing the state of assembly of microtubules.[52–56] Cyclic nucleotide–modulated increments and decrements in degranulation correlate with increments and decrements in microtubule numbers.[57] Cyclic GMP can induce assembly of microtubules in the absence of a stimulus but is itself incapable of stimulating degranulation.

Current evidence suggests that translocation of phagosomes rather than fusion is modulated by microtubules. Correlations between tubule assembly and disassembly and the degree of degranulation probably reflect earlier events in the degranulation sequence.

Assembly may enhance, or disassembly diminish, the chances for contact between neutrophil granule and stimulated areas of the plasma membrane. Other structures, perhaps contractile proteins, might play a more direct role in fusion between granules and the phagosome.

Microfilaments are 6 nm in diameter and constitute the cells' contractile system. They have been identified as actin polymers and are prominent in areas of the cell involved in adhesion and particle ingestion.[48] The neutrophil contractile system bears a striking resemblance to that of skeletal muscle. Actin, myosin (with actin-activated Mg^{2+}ATPase activity), actin-binding protein, and a cofactor that allows actin to activate the Mg^{2+}ATPase have all been isolated from phagocytic cells.[2] During normal phagocytosis, contractions occur in two directions. Contraction occurs under the particle to form an invagination that is directed along microtubule-defined tracks toward the cytocenter. Filaments are seen associated with the phagocytic vacuole, but granules fuse with vacuoles in the cytocenter, and microfilaments are not usually seen near sites of active fusion.

The second type of movement involves a filamentous web at the cell surface, containing actin and myosin. Contraction of this web that interacts with actin-binding protein results in a lateral movement of the plasma membrane which serves to close the phagocytic vacuole like a purse string. The microfilament system can be inhibited by interference with production of metabolic energy or by chelation of calcium, providing one possible mechanism for the modulation of degranulation by this ion. More specific disruption of the contractile system can be achieved using the fungal metabolite cytochalasin B, which interferes with the function of actin-binding protein.[58] Cytochalasin B inhibits the purse string contraction either by preventing the formation of actin-binding gels or by solubilizing them, thus preventing sol to gel transformation of cytoplasmic extracts.[58,59] Cytochalasin B is a powerful inhibitor of neutrophil migration and phagocytosis. In conjunction with the ultrastructure data, this suggests a vital role for microfilaments in these active processes.[47]

STIMULUS-RESPONSE COUPLING IN NEUTROPHILS

In response to an appropriate stimulus such as bacteria, foreign peptides, or certain soluble agents, neutrophils will aggregate, migrate toward the source of chemoattractants, ingest appropriately coated particles, degranulate, and generate toxic oxygen metabolites. The nature of this interaction between stimuli and neutrophils is now becoming clearer and can serve as a paradigm of cellular activation.

Opsonins and Their Receptors

The ability and speed with which neutrophils ingest a given particle depends at least partly on the surface characteristics of the particle. Surface charge and hydrophobicity profoundly influence ingestion, although the optimal surface characteristics for phagocytosis are still not completely understood. Certainly one explanation for the ability of some bacteria to evade phagocytic attack is a subtle alteration of their surface that makes them less appetizing.

Host humoral factors greatly facilitate phagocytosis. Particles exposed to fresh serum are ingested much more readily than are untreated particles. Those humoral factors coating particles in preparation for ingestion are known as *opsonins,* from the Greek "to prepare victuals." Opsonins have traditionally been divided into heat stable and heat labile factors. Im-

munoglobulins, in particular IgG (specifically subclasses IgG1 and IgG3), which are resistant to the effects of heating, comprise the heat-stable opsonins. The immunoglobulin molecule must be intact to promote phagocytosis. By proteolytic digestion of immunoglobulin molecules, two functional portions can be distinguished: the Fab portion of the antibody molecule, which binds to specific antigenic sites on the particle, and the Fc portion, which binds to a specific receptor on the neutrophil membrane. This receptor has been isolated and partially characterized as a protein with a molecular weight of 53,000 to 66,000 daltons. By using either a specific monoclonal antibody or labeled immune complexes, it can be calculated that there are 112,000 to 135,000 Fc-receptor sites per cell.[60]

Serum complement can also act as an opsonin and is characteristically heat labile. The most active opsonic agent generated from serum complement is C3b, generated by proteolytic cleavage of C3 resulting from activation of either the classic pathway of complement or the properdin system (alternative pathway). A receptor for C3b isolated from human erythrocytes has been shown to be identical to that found on neutrophils. The isolated receptor is a protein with a molecular weight of approximately 205,000 daltons. Use of a specific, labeled receptor antibody has shown that there are about 60,000 receptors per cell for C3b.[61]

Tuftsin is a tetrapeptide fragment of IgG that acts as a nonspecific stimulus for phagocytosis.[62]

The Activation Process

Once the neutrophil has engaged an appropriately opsonized particle a number of cellular responses occur. After stimulus of an appropriate receptor, there is a lag period before a measurable physiologic response, such as granule release or aggregation, occurs.[63,64] This lag period is stimulus specific and represents the time required for transmission of an excitatory signal and translation into an appropriate cellular response.

A family of guanine triphosphate (GTP) binding proteins appear to act as transmitters for activation by agents acting at the cell surface. These proteins have been termed G_i or G_s, depending on whether they inhibit (G_i) or stimulate (G_s) adenyl cyclase. The G_i protein also has the characteristic property that it is inactivated by pertussis toxin, whereas the G_s protein is irreversibly activated by cholera toxin. Occupancy of chemoattractant receptors in neutrophils leads to activation (GTP binding) of a G_i-like protein that then generates other intracellular messengers, e.g., active phospholipid intermediates (such as diacylglycerol and inositol trisphosphate) and calcium movements.[65–75]

One of the cellular alterations that is classically found as a first step in stimulus-response coupling is a change in the plasmalemmal transmembrane potential. Rapid hyperpolarization followed by depolarization has been found after appropiate stimulation.[76]

In addition to changes in membrane potential, calcium has been proposed as a second messenger for neutrophil activation. Four criteria for such second messenger status have been met. Translocation of extracellular calcium by the ionophore A23187 activates neutrophils, whereas removal of calcium from the extracellular environment markedly reduces cellular responses to a variety of stimuli.[77–79] Activated neutrophils take up labeled extracellular calcium and, after a variable period, actively extrude it. Cytoplasmic free calcium levels increase rapidly after stimulation; this probably represents mobilization of intracellular stores.[80–83] Calcium has been localized to several areas within neutrophils by cytochemical and ultrastructural techniques. There are discrete deposits along the plasmalemma in resting cells, in the heterochromatic region of the nucleus, in the azurophil granules, and associated with glycogen. Membrane-associated calcium is released very soon after neutrophil stimulation and may be the source of the rise in cytosolic free calcium.[84–86]

Cyclic nucleotides are classic second messengers in a number of secretory cells. Rapid transient rises in cAMP occur after activation of neutrophils with some, but not all, stimuli.[79,87,89] Increased cAMP concentrations are not necessary for neutrophil responses because inhibition of its formation has no effect on responses to stimuli that increase cAMP levels.[89] Agents raising intracellular cAMP levels, such as isoproterenol and theophylline, tend to diminish neutrophil responses,[56] suggesting that cyclic nucleotides play a role as a modulator but not as a signal for cell function.

Metabolic Response to Activation

After contact with appropriately opsonized particles, a number of metabolic changes occur. These include increased oxygen consumption ("the respiratory burst"),[90,91] and increases in hexose monophosphate shunt activity,[92] hydrogen peroxide[93] and superoxide anion generation,[94] phospholipid turnover,[95] and protein phosphorylation.[96] Protein phosphorylation is involved in the regulation of intracellular activities of many cell types. Both cAMP-sensitive and phospholipid-sensitive protein kinase activities have been found in activated neutrophils.[97,98] Phorbol esters, potent neutrophil activators, bind directly to a protein kinase C and thus appear to bypass the usual activation sequence.[99] Stimulation of human neutrophils leads to enhanced phosphorylation of four proteins and dephosphorylation of one.[96]

Stimulation of neutrophils also enhances turnover of the phosphatidylinositol/phosphatidic acid cycle, which may play a role in regulation of intracellular free calcium levels.[100] Additionally, breakdown of phosphatidylinositol or its diphosphorylated and triphosphorylated derivatives by phospholipase C could lead to generation of diacylglycerol, a known activator of protein kinase C. Phospholipid turnover can also provide free arachidonic acid leading to generation of products of the cyclo-oxygenase and lipoxygenase pathways, as discussed below.

The rapid consumption of oxygen by stimulated neutrophils leads, almost stoichiometrically, to production of hydrogen peroxide, superoxide anion radicals, singlet oxygen, and hydroxyl radicals. A critical first step in these events appears to be the reduction of molecular oxygen to superoxide anion by a plasma membrane bound NADPH-dependent oxidase. Consumption of NADPH by this oxidase leads to enhanced glucose metabolism by the hexose monophosphate shunt. Superoxide anion is enzymatically (by superoxide dismutase) or spontaneously converted to hydrogen peroxide, which can react with additional superoxide anion to form hydroxyl radicals. All of these oxygen species are highly reactive and possess varying degrees of bactericidal and cytocidal activity.[101,101a]

Evidence from granule free and nucleus free subcellular particles derived from human neutrophils strongly suggests that superoxide anion is generated by enzymes in the plasma membrane.[102] This localization of the superoxide anion generating system leads to a concentration of toxic microbicidal agents around ingested organisms once the phagosome is formed by the cell membrane, minimizing release of toxic oxygen species into the cell cytoplasm or the extracellular space.

RELEASE OF PROSTAGLANDINS, THROMBOXANES, AND LEUKOTRIENES

Neutrophils release activated products of arachidonate when exposed to phagocytic stimuli. These include products of the cyclo-oxygenase pathway, prostaglandins (PGs) and thromboxanes, and products of the lipoxygenase pathway, the leukotrienes. The exact role and interaction of these compounds with each other and other mediators of inflammation is not completely understood. In addition, these compounds appear to have both anti- and pro-inflammatory effects (see Chaper 26).

On stimulation, arachidonic acid is released from membrane phospholipids via the enzyme phospholipase C. This step is inhibited by anti-inflammatory corticosteroids. These C20 polyunsaturated fatty acids then interact with the active oxygen species generated during the respiratory burst.[103] Two enzyme systems may be operative at this point, cyclo-oxygenase to produce prostaglandins and thromboxanes, or the lipoxygenases to produce leukotrienes.

Cyclo-oxygenase, also called prostaglandin synthetase, is inhibited by aspirin and other nonsteroidal anti-inflammatory drugs (NSAIDs). The fatty acid endoperoxides thus formed (the PGG and PGH series) are weak potentiators of edema caused by bradykinin and histamine,[104] but more importantly serve as intermediates in the formation of other prostaglandins and thromboxanes via isomerization of the more stable PGs. Of these, PGE_2 and PGI_2 appear to be the primary mediators of inflammation because they cause vasodilatation and inflammation when injected, their injection into the midbrain of experimental animals causes fever, they act synergistically with mediators such as bradykinin and histamine to cause edema and vasodilatation, and they sensitize tissues to painful stimuli by other agents. These compounds are present in elevated concentrations in inflammatory exudates and their synthesis is inhibited by most anti-inflammatory drugs.[105] There is also some evidence that PGs are anti-inflammatory. The PGE series can stimulate cAMP production and thereby suppress immediate hypersensitivity reactions and reactions associated with cellular immunity such as lectin-induced T-cell mitogenesis[106] and neutrophil degranulation.[107]

The products of the lipoxygenase pathway have been elucidated, and their role in inflammation is becoming increasingly evident. The predominating pathway of leukotriene (LT) metabolism depends on the cell type: the 12-lipoxygenase in platelets, the 15-lipoxygenase in T-lymphocytes, and the 5-lipoxygenase in neutrophils. Arachidonic acid metabolism via the 5-lipoxygenase pathway is depicted in Figure 20–3. Lipoxygenase is not inhibited by the NSAIDs, except for benoxaprofen,[108] but is inhibited by ETYI. The lipoxygenase together with activated oxygen species forms 5-HETE, which is converted to the unstable epoxide LTA4,[109] which then is either enzymatically hydrolyzed to LTB4 or acted on via glutathione-5-transferase to LTC4. The latter can be further modified by glutamyl transpeptidase to form LTD4 and LTE4.[110,111]

LTB4 is released on activation of neutrophils,[112] and in nanomolar or smaller amounts causes leukocyte chemotaxis[113–116] and adhesion to endothelial cells.[117] At higher concentrations in the presence of neutrophils, LTB4 elicits extravasation of plasma from vessel wall.[118] LTB4 also activates neutrophils. Within seconds after addition to neutrophil suspensions, it causes aggregation, degranulation, generation of superoxide anion, and mobilization of membrane-associated calcium.[119,120]

Monosodium urate crystals (MSU) stimulate the formation of arachidonate metabolites by neutrophils and platelets. Neutrophils exposed to nonlytic quantities of MSU crystals generate 5-HETE, LTB4 (and its nonenzymatically formed isomers 6-*trans*-LTB4, 12-*epi*-6-*trans*-LTB4), and 20-COOH-LTB4 via the 5-lipoxygenase pathway. Neutrophils treated with colchicine are unable to form LTA4 from 5-HETE after addition of MSU crystals and thus do not form LTB4 and its isomers. This shifts metabolism of arachidonate to other metabolites such as 5S,12S-DiHETE, which antagonize the action of LTB4. Thus LTB4 and other products of arachidonate produced by platelets appear to be important mediators of inflammation in gouty arthritis. Colchicine may specifically affect the biosynthesis of these substances[121] (see Chapter 106).

The cysteine-containing leukotrienes (LTC4, LTD4, and LTE4), produced by macrophages and basophils, constitute the immunologically mediated "slow reactive substance of anaphylaxis" (SRS-A). They have diverse biologic effects. The discussion here will be confined to their influence on the inflammatory response. SRS-A, in nanomolar concentrations, causes an intense dose-dependent vascular contraction, most marked in the terminal arterioles. Although the vasoconstriction is short-lived, it is followed by a dose-dependent, reversible leakage of macromolecules at the postcapillary venules.[118] Thus, together with PGE_2 and PGI_2, SRS-A contributes to edema formation. These actions appear to be via a direct action on vessel walls because they occur rapidly and do not require PGs, histamine, or neutrophils.

The pro-inflammatory effects of the various products of arachidonic acid are summarized in Table 20–2.

DEGRANULATION

Neutrophil degranulation normally accompanies phagocytosis, suggesting common or similar triggering mechanisms.[122,122a] These have been discussed in the section describing stimulus-response coupling. After binding of a particle, a localized contraction occurs just underneath the point of contact and at right angles to the plasma membrane, resulting in a cup-

FIG. 20–3. Scheme of arachidonic acid metabolism via 5-lipoxygenase.

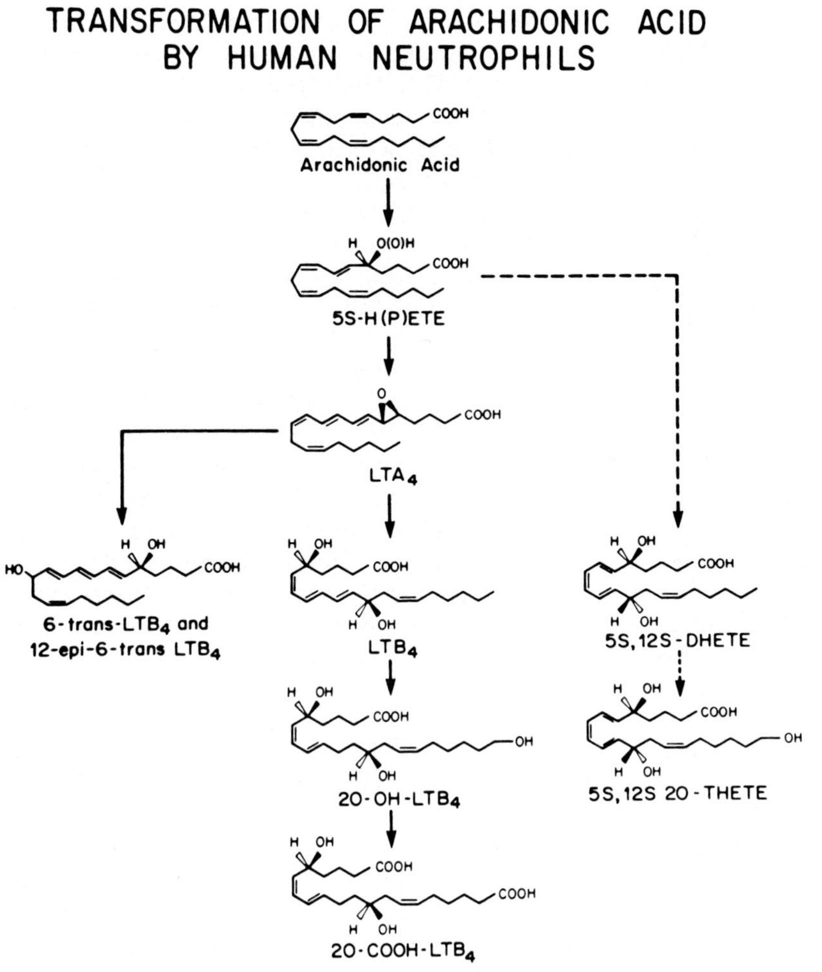

TRANSFORMATION OF ARACHIDONIC ACID
BY HUMAN NEUTROPHILS

Table 20–2. Inflammatory Effects of Arachidonate Metabolites

	Products of Cyclo-oxygenase	Products of Lipoxygenase
Vasodilatation	PGE$_2$ PGF$_2$	Not demonstrated
Pain, hyperalgesia	PGE$_2$ PGF$_2$ (PGG, PGH weak with bradykinin and histamine)	LTC$_4$
Fever	PGE$_2$ PGI$_2$	Not demonstrated
Neutrophil migration and adhesion	PGE$_2$ PGE$_2$, PGF$_2$, PGI$_2$ (inhibit)	Not demonstrated LTB$_4$
Released by neutrophil in response to monosodium urate	not demonstrated	LTB$_4$ and isomer, 5S, 12S DHETE

shaped depression into which the particle fits. The margins of the depression move inward to enclose the particle in a phagocytic vacuole or phagosome. This movement is inhibited by cytochalasin B, which interferes with microfilaments, and thus measurement of degranulation is possible. Azurophil and specific granules (lysosomes) join this newly formed vacuole at its internal border and discharge their contents, a process called degranulation. The fusion of the granule and plasma membranes is inhibited by corticosteroids. Usually the vacuole closes, preventing extracellular loss of enzymes; however, if there is too much to digest, the vacuole may remain open and some enzymes may be secreted extracellularly and attack host tissues. This mechanism of host injury will be discussed in detail below.

Degranulation takes place during phagocytosis but also occurs when neutrophils are exposed to sufficient concentrations of secretogogues, chemoattractants, lectins, tumor promotors, and calcium ionophores. The extracellular release of granule contents can be readily induced in vitro by exposing neutrophils to secretogogues in the presence of cytochalasin B. This technique has allowed kinetic studies of the stimulus-secretion coupling response. Continuous monitoring of secretion from cytochalasin B-treated cells revealed a distinct lag period between exposure to stimulant and lysosomal enzyme release. This period is stimulant-dependent varying from 15 seconds for the chemotactic peptide FMLP[123] to 60 seconds for calcium ionophore A23187.[129] These times were comparable to those seen for O_2^- generation using the same stimuli. In general, the lag periods for specific granule discharge are slightly less than those for azurophil granules.[107,123]

Possible explanations for the lag period include the time required to assemble or to disassemble cytoskeletal structures, to piece together a multicomponent oxidase system, or to transport secretory granules through the cytoplasm. The theory that has received most attention is that the lag period reflects the time required to accumulate a crucial second messenger as already discussed.

BACTERICIDAL MECHANISMS

Neutrophils play a major role in host defense against bacteria and fungi. Destruction of invading bacteria by neutrophils is most efficiently accomplished within phagosomes where the granule contents are concentrated around the invading organism yet remain isolated from the cytoplasm and from the extracellular tissues. The phagosome is well-adapted

for this function with an internal pH of 3.5 to 4.0, optimal for the acid hydrolases delivered by azurophil granules and for the conversion of superoxide anion produced during the respiratory burst to hydrogen peroxide (H_2O_2). Hydrogen peroxide has a bactericidal effect, but its potency is augmented by the myeloperoxidase present in the azurophil granules. This enzyme catalyzes the oxidation of halide ions (most likely Cl- in vivo)[77] with resultant halogenation of bacteria.[32] Myeloperoxidase may also directly degrade amino acid constituents of the bacterial wall.

The respiratory burst also gives rise to other active oxygen species with bactericidal activity, including hydroxyl radical and singlet oxygen. Which of the active oxygen species is most responsible for destruction of microbes is unclear, but it is likely that some combination of the above processes is responsible for microbial destruction in vivo. The large number of killing mechanisms provides neutrophils with an armory of sufficient redundancy and "overkill" to deal with a broad spectrum of microorganisms and constitutes a fail-safe system in the event that one component of active oxygen species is inoperative.

EXTRUSION OF NEUTROPHIL GRANULE ENZYMES IN TISSUE INJURY

Having presented evidence that neutrophil leukocytes have the potential to provide immune tissue injury, we will discuss the mechanisms whereby proteases and other lysosomal constituents are secreted and gain access to their specific substrates.

Cell Death

One mechanism is simply cell death (Fig. 20–4A). When neutrophils are exposed to toxins (for example, phospholipases in snake venom or materials that could be encountered in some forms of septic arthritis), injury to the plasma membrane is an early consequence, and all intracellular materials are released pari passu from the injured cell, including those ordinarily sequestered within lysosomes. Biologic detergents, such as the amphipath melitti, act in this manner to cause primary lysis of the cell membrane and, only subsequently, disruption of lysosomes.[125] Under these circumstances, cytoplasmic enzymes, potassium, and other cellular constituents, in addition to lysosomal hydrolases, are directly released into the surrounding tissues.

Perforation From Within

Another mechanism conforms to the "suicide sac" hypothesis of deDuve. Under some circumstances,

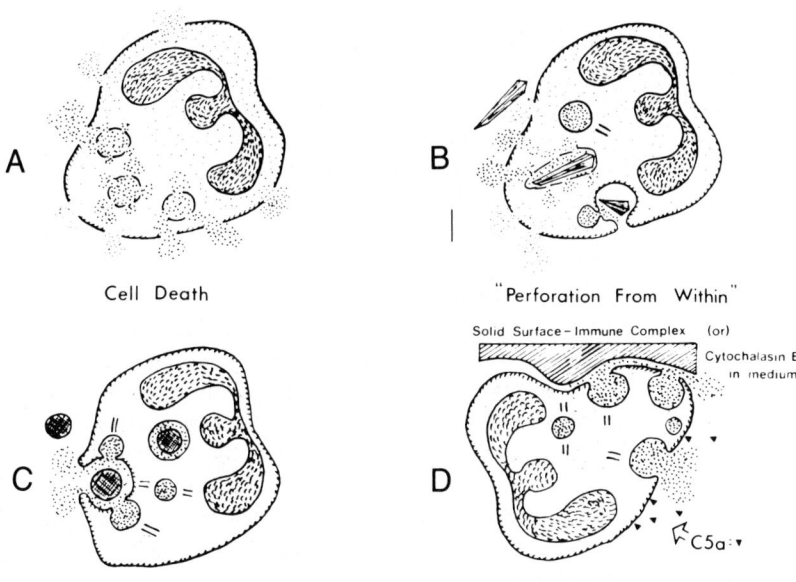

A. Cell Death

B. "Perforation From Within"

Solid Surface – Immune Complex (or)
Cytochalasin B in medium

C. "Regurgitation During Feeding"

D. "Reverse Endocytosis"

C5a

FIG. 20–4. Mechanisms of lysosomal enzyme release causing tissue injury.

materials gain access to the interior of the cells' vacuole system, wherein they cause rupture of lysosomal membranes from within (Fig. 20–4B). Damage to the organelles leads to the release of lysosomal enzymes concomitantly with the release of cytoplasmic enzymes and other intracellular constituents as the cell dies by perforation from within of its vacuolar system. Crystalline substances, such as monosodium urate and silica, act on phagocytic cells in this fashion.[48] Hence, this form of lysosomal enzyme release is a primary promoter of inflammation in gout.

Using neutroplasts (neutrophil fragments that lack granules but that retain the ability to phagocytize crystals), we have demonstrated that phagocytosis alone is not sufficient. Lysis from within requires the release of granule contents from the phagolysosome.[126]

Whereas these first two mechanisms of lysosomal enzyme release may account for tissue injury in some instances, two additional mechanisms involving intact, viable neutrophils have also been recognized. Both are relevant to the pathogenesis of immune tissue injury and often have been proven amenable to modification by a number of pharmacologic agents, particularly those that affect the state of assembly of cytoplasmic microtubules or the level of cyclic nucleotides within cells.

Regurgitation During Feeding

One mechanism of lysosomal enzyme release from intact, viable PMNs has been termed regurgitation during feeding (Fig. 20–4C). Under some circumstances, e.g., following the ingestion by these cells of insoluble immune complexes, as encountered in synovial fluid in rheumatoid arthritis, or of other particulates, a phagosome is formed that merges at its internal border with primary lysosomes. Because of either incomplete fusion of the vacuolar membrane or the persistence of endocytic channels, regurgitation of lysosomal hydrolases occurs and inflammatory materials are released into the surrounding tissues without associated phagocytic cell death or release of cytoplasmic enzymes.[127] Biochemical and morphologic evidence for this mechanism, called regurgitation during feeding, has been presented for a variety of systems involving particle ingestion by phagocytic cells. The cell remains viable but releases its lysosomal contents, which are free to act upon surrounding tissues. This is a common mechanism of tissue injury in a variety of disease states. Ohlsson has shown that the neutral proteases, elastase and collagenase, are regurgitated by this mechanism.[41]

Harlan et al.,[128] using human neutrophils activated with serum-treated zymosan, demonstrated endothelial cell detachment caused by neutral protease digestion of endothelial cell surface proteins, including fibronectin.

Reverse Endocytosis

Another mechanism of selective lysosomal enzyme extrusion from neutrophil has been termed reverse endocytosis, or frustrated phagocytosis (Fig. 20–4D). In this process, material previously stored within lysosomes is exported to the external milieu. For example, cells that encounter immune complexes (both soluble and insoluble) or aggregated immunoglobulins deposited on solid surfaces, such as millipore filters or collagen membranes, adhere to these surfaces and selectively release their lysosomal constituents.[129] Enzyme release then occurs by reverse endocytosis. Merging of granules with the plasma membrane results in discharge of lysosomal enzymes directly to the outside of the cell as though into a phagocytic vacuole. Phagocytosis per se does not occur, and the viability of the adherent cells is not altered. This mechanism of enzyme release seems pertinent to the pathogenesis of tissue injury when immune complexes are deposited on cell surfaces or extracellular structures, such as vascular basement membranes. For example, the nephritis of systemic lupus erythematosus could be generated by this form of granule enzyme release, stimulated by the surface deposition of immune complexes (DNA, anti-DNA IgG, and complement components).

Neutrophil surface recognition of, and stimulation by, three distinct ligands can provoke granule translocation, membrane fusion, and selective extracellular release of granule contents. These ligands include Fc regions of IgG molecules that have undergone a conformational change either as a result of combining with antigen or as a result of heat aggregation (Fc-receptor stimulus), fragments of the third component of complement (C3b-receptor stimulus), and the soluble, low-molecular-weight complement component C5a. For example, immune complexes prepared by heat-aggregated human IgG reacting with rheumatoid factor or heat-aggregated IgG per se, either in suspension or deposited on nonphagocytizable surfaces, are capable of provoking the selective discharge of lysosomal constituents from human neutrophils by reverse endocytosis.[56,125,127,130,131] Neutrophils exposed to fragments of C3 fixed on nonphagocytizable surfaces respond in a similar manner (in the presence of IgG). C5a, generated by activation of either the classic or alternative complement pathways, can interact with neutrophils in the absence of particles (or immunoglobulins) to stimulate membrane fusion between lysosomal granules and between these organelles and the plasma membrane.[130] In cytochalasin B-treated neutrophils[130] and in neutrophils adherent to nonphagocytizable surfaces,[131] this leads to selective extracellular release of lysosomal enzymes by reverse endocytosis.

Such degranulation following cell surface stimulation by immune reactants involves both major classes of neutrophil granules, azurophil and specific. Consequently, acid hydrolases such as β-glucuronidase (from azurophil granules) as well as lysozyme (from specific granules) can be detected in the medium surrounding such stimulated cells.[56,125,127,130,131] In contrast, some nonimmune stimuli appear to provoke selective discharge (by exocytosis) of only specific granule constituents (e.g., lysozyme). Such stimuli include the tumor promotor, phorbol myristate acetate,[57] concanavalin A,[132] and ionized calcium,[133] in either the presence or the absence of the divalent cation ionophore A23187. These observations, together with reported sequential degranulation during phagocytosis,[134] indicate that somewhat different mechanisms are responsible for discharge of the two types of granules.

Oxygen metabolites have also been implicated in extracellular cytolysis of host cells. Because the generation of oxygen metabolites occurs along with phagocytic uptake, these metabolites come in contact with surrounding tissues in one of the four methods outlined above. It is likely that these oxygen metabolites cause the same degree of tissue damage in autoimmune diseases once tissue-free radical scavengers that inhibit oxygen-metabolite-mediated cytolysis are exhausted.[135]

PHARMACOLOGIC CONTROL OF NEUTROPHIL FUNCTION

Because lysosomal enzyme release and generation of toxic oxygen metabolites may contribute to the pathogenesis of tissue injury during inflammation as well as propagation of the inflammatory reaction, it is likely that a reduction in their extracellular release could be beneficial in disease states characterized by aberrant inflammation. Much attention has been given to pharmacologic inhibition of enzyme release and superoxide anion generation. As expected, no inhibitors alter enzyme release found after cell death or after perforation from within. In general, two major types of compounds have been studied for their effect on granular enzyme release: those that affect the state or formation of cytoplasmic microtubules directly, and those that influence the intracellular level of cyclic nucleotides, cAMP and cGMP. Exogenous cAMP (plus theophylline) as well as agents that elevate intracellular levels of cAMP (e.g., PGE_1, isoproterenol) reduce enzyme release.[56] Exogenous cGMP and agents that elevate levels of cGMP (e.g., serotonin, carbamylcholine) enhance lysosomal enzyme release.[56] Similarly, agents that promote disassembly of cytoplasmic microtubules (e.g., colchicine and vinblastine) reduce, and agents that promote microtubule assembly (e.g., deuterium oxide) enhance, lysosomal enzyme release. For some of these agents, such as colchicine, which specifically inhibits leukotriene generation by neutrophils, alternative mechanisms of action may exist.[121]

The NSAIDs which, as a group, share the ability to block prostaglandin synthesis, appear to have a variety of effects on neutrophils. Aspirin and piroxicam inhibit neutrophil degranulation, aggregation, and superoxide anion generation. Ibuprofen inhibits only aggregation and degranulation, and indomethacin inhibits only aggregation.[136]

Our work suggests a potent endogenous modulator of neutrophil function, namely adenosine. This purine engages receptors on the neutrophil surface that selectively inhibit generation of superoxide anion and other toxic oxygen metabolites while still permitting degranulation. Surprisingly, adenosine and its analogues modulate neutrophil function in response to some (e.g., C5a, FMLP, opsonized zymosan particles) but not other stimuli (immune complexes). More surprisingly, engagement of adenosine receptors promotes chemotaxis by neutrophils.[137-143] Thus, adenosine, released from damaged tissue, may promote migration of neutrophils to sites of infection or tissue damage while preventing the activated neutrophils from damaging healthy tissues along the way.

Some of the anti-inflammatory effects of glucocorticosteroids can be attributed to inhibition of neutrophil locomotion, phagocytosis, and degranulation. One interesting explanation of this inhibition is that these drugs stabilize membranes, thus inhibiting fusion between membrane surfaces on which both phagocytosis and degranulation depend.[144]

Neutrophils, through their ability to release potentially toxic enzymes and oxygen metabolites, play a crucial role in the pathology of arthritis and other inflammatory conditions. Successful therapy of these conditions may be achieved by use of drugs directed at inhibition of neutrophil responses to inflammatory stimuli.

HERITABLE DISORDERS

Neutrophil function is regulated by a multitude of extrinsic and intrinsic factors, disruption of any one of which can lead to malfunction. At least 15 primary (probably inheritable) defects of neutrophil function with resultant recurrent infections have been identified, and at least twice as many conditions (including systemic lupus erythematosus and rheumatoid arthritis) secondarily resulting in decreased neutrophil function have been reported.[145] The defects identified include perturbations of neutrophil interactions with external stimulatory factors such as activated complement components, causing impaired chemotaxis and ingestion or impaired phagocytosis because of opsonin or tuftsin deficiency.

Abnormalities of neutrophil function can be classified in terms of their major responses to inflammatory stimuli. Intrinsic inherited defects can be classified in terms of defects of chemotaxis, ingestion, degranulation, receptor coupling, adherence, or bactericidal mechanisms. Studies of such rare defects have provided great insight into normal neutrophil function.

One of the most intriguing is the rare autosomal recessive disorder Chediak-Higashi syndrome, characterized clinically by a propensity to skin and subcutaneous infections and partial albinism. Neutrophils and monocytes from patients with this disorder contain large azurophil granules that do not fuse with phagosomes,[146] and degranulation is delayed. The respiratory burst is normal. Neutrophils from patients with this syndrome have increased levels of cAMP.[147] The basic cause of this syndrome is inadequate tubulin polymerization resulting in nonfunctional microtubules, and impaired chemotaxis and degranulation.[148,148a] Indeed, cells from patients with this disorder exhibit functional abnormalities like those of normal cells treated with colchicine, a microtubule-disrupting drug.[149,150] Agents increasing intracellular cAMP, such as carbachol and bethanacol, and ascorbic acid, which decreases cAMP, promote microtubule assembly and ameliorate cell dysfunction in vitro.[141,148]

An actin abnormality has been reported in a single patient with recurrent infections whose neutrophils failed to ingest particles and to respond to chemotactic stimuli.[151] Neutrophilic cytoplasm was deficient in microfilaments and the in vitro polymerization of isolated actin was poor. These neutrophils exhibited hyperactive degranulation.

Granulocytes from several patients with recurrent bacterial infections had a deficiency of a membrane glycoprotein (gp150).[152] This membrane glycoprotein is a member of a family of glycoproteins present in the plasma membranes of different types of leukocytes. Deficiency of gp150 results in a defect in receptor-coupled superoxide anion generation and degranulation stimulated by C3 and Fc receptors. The membrane glycoprotein gp150 is distinct from the receptors for opsonized particles but appears to be important for neutrophil adherence to particles or surfaces.

Lactoferrin deficiency was associated with altered granulocyte function in a single patient with recurrent bacterial infections.[153] Neutrophils from this patient had bilobed nuclei, a deficit of specific granules with abnormal membranes, less than 8% of the specific granules proteins lactoferrin, and vitamin B_{12}-transport protein, and impaired phagolysosome fusion, demonstrated by the presence of an increased number of primary granules and their products. Adherence, aggregation, the ability to decrease the cell surface charge in response to n-formyl-metrional-leucyl-phenylalanine (FMLP) stimulation, and hydroxyl radical production in response to phagocytosis, were all impaired. Addition of lactoferrin to in vitro suspensions of these cells normalized adherence and aggregation. These abnormalities suggest that specific granule products such as lactoferrin play a part in modulating granulocyte function.

Increasing interest has focused on heritable intrinsic disorders of the bactericidal respiratory burst mechanisms. The importance of the microbicidal system described by Klebanoff,[154] consisting of myeloperoxidase, hydrogen peroxide, and halide ions, is brought to light by some of these conditions. Chronic granulomatous disease (CGD) now appears to be a group of inheritable disorders characterized by recurrent bacterial and fungal infections. The respiratory burst normally accompanying phagocytosis by neutrophils and monocytes is completely defective and microbial killing is diminished.[155] In a multicenter European study,[156] two distinct inheritance patterns were demonstrated; the previously recognized X-linked inheritance pattern and a newly identified autosomal recessive inheritance. Two distinct abnormalities of the cellular machinery involved in the respiratory burst were identified. In autosomal recessive disease, neutrophils had normal cytochome b-245 which was not reduced in response to PMA. In this subset, disease seemed to result from an abnormality of an activation system, or an absence or malfunction of a proximal electron donor in the electron-transport chain. Absence of cytochrome b-245 was documented in males with the X-linked disease by the European group, but the gene for the deficient protein of CGD neutrophils has recently been isolated and does not appear to code for cytochrome b-245.[12,157,157a] Another report described a patient with an X-linked disorder similar to, but not as severe as, CGD.[158] This patient was believed to have a defect in oxidase enzyme activity with a decreased affinity for NADPH.

Neutrophils from patients with CGD can kill some bacteria, namely those that generate sufficient hydrogen peroxide to facilitate the oxidase system, thereby providing the means of their own destruction. However, some peroxide-generating bacteria also produce catalase (e.g., Staphylococcus aureus and Escherichia coli), thus destroying the small amounts of peroxide and once again leaving the killing system without a substrate. It is to such catalase-positive aerobic bacteria that CGD patients most often succumb.

Glucose-6-phosphate dehydrogenase deficiency causes a defect in hydrogen peroxide production that is rarely of clinical significance. The defect results in inability to maintain adequate levels of NADPH. Neutrophils from patients with this deficiency usually have normal or only slightly reduced bactericidal activity, unless the enzyme activity is entirely absent, in which case the syndrome closely resembles CGD.

Myeloperoxidase (azurophil granules) deficiency also disrupts the Klebanoff system. This autosomal recessive trait is usually of no clinical consequence, and in fact neutrophils from these patients often accumulate more hydrogen peroxide than do normal cells.[159] Some impairment of bactericidal activity is found in neutrophils of patients lacking lysozyme[25] and secondary granules.[160] One family has been reported with a deficiency of glutathione reductase, inherited as an autosomal recessive disorder. Glutathione (GSH) protects cells against oxidative damage by the highly reactive compounds produced during the respiratory burst and is oxidized to its dimer GSSG. GSH reductase catalyzes the reconversion of GSSH to GSH. Neutrophils from the affected family members appear to function normally in the presence of small numbers of bacteria, but with greater numbers of bacteria, hydrogen peroxide generation is increased with a concomitant shortening in the duration of the respiratory burst.[161,162]

Other inherited neutrophil disorders include a familial defect in chemotaxis[163] and the lazy leukocyte syndrome.[164]

REFERENCES

1. Metchnikoff, E.: Sur la lutte des cellules de l'organisme contre l'invasion des microbes. Ann. Inst. Pasteur, 1:321, 1887.
1a. Cochrane, C.G., Weigle, W.O., and Dixon, F.J.: The role of polymorphonuclear leukocytes in the initiation and cessation of the Arthus vasculitis. J. Exp. Med., 110:481–494, 1959.
2. Boxer, L.A., and Stossel, T.P.: Interactions of actin, myosin, and an actin-binding protein of chronic myelogenous leukemia leukocytes. J. Clin. Invest., 57:964–976, 1976.
3. DeShazo, C.V., et al.: The effect of complement depletion on neutrophil migration in acute immunologic arthritis. J. Immunol., 108:1414–1419, 1972.
4. Humphrey, J.H.: The mechanism of Arthus reactions. I. The role of polymorphonuclear leucocytes and other factors in reversed passive Arthus reactions in rabbits. Br. J. Exp. Pathol., 36:268–282, 1955.
5. Parish, W.E.: Effects of neutrophils on tissues. Experiments on the Arthus reaction, the flare phenomenon, and post-phagocytic release of lysosomal enzymes. Br. J. Dermatol., 81:28–35, 1969.
6. Stetson, C.A.: Similarities in the mechanisms determining the Arthus and Shwartzman phenomena. J. Exp. Med., 94:347–358, 1951.
7. Kniker, W.T., and Cochrane, C.G.: Pathogenic factors in vascular lesions of experimental serum sickness. J. Exp. Med., 122:83–98, 1965.
8. Cochrane, C.G., Unanue, E.R., and Dixon, F.J.: A role of polymorphonuclear leukocytes and complement in nephrotoxic nephritis. J. Exp. Med., 122:99–116, 1965.

9. DeShazo, C.V., Henson, P.M., and Cochrane, C.G.: Acute immunologic arthritis in rabbits. J. Clin. Invest., 51:50–57, 1972.
10. Cartwright, G.E., Athens, J.W., and Wintrobe, M.M.: The kinetics of granulopoiesis in normal man. Blood, 24:780–803, 1964.
11. Cohen, A.M., et al.: In vivo stimulation of granulopoiesis by recombinant human granulocyte colony-stimulating factor. Proc. Natl. Acad. Sci. USA, 84:2484–2488, 1987.
12. Kaushansky, K., et al.: Genomic cloning, characterization, and multilineage growth-promoting activity of human granulocyte-macrophage colony-stimulating factor. Proc. Natl. Acad. Sci. USA, 83:3101–3105, 1986.
13. Kohsaki, M., et al.: In vivo stimulation of murine granulopoiesis by human urinary extract from patients with aplastic anemia. Proc. Natl. Acad. Sci. USA, 80:3802–3806, 1983.
14. Fedorko, M.E., and Hirsch, J.G.: Cytoplasmic granule formation in myelocytes: An electron microscope radioautographic study on the mechanism of formation of cytoplasmic granules in rabbit heterophilic myelocytes. J. Cell Biol., 29:307–316, 1966.
15. Murphy, G., Bretz, U., Baggiolini, M., and Reynolds, J.J.: The latent collagenase and gelatinase of human polymorphonuclear neutrophil leucocytes. Biochem. J., 192:517–525, 1980.
16. Beck, W.S.: The control of leukocyte glycosis. J. Biol. Chem., 232:251–270, 1958.
17. Scott, R.E., and Horn, R.G.: Ultrastructural aspects of neutrophil granulocyte development in humans. Lab. Invest., 23:202–215, 1970.
18. Messner, R.R., et al.: A transient defect in leukocytic bactericidal capacity. Clin. Immunol. Immunopathol., 1:523–532, 1973.
19. Korn, E.D., and Weisman, R.A.: Phagocytosis of latex beads by Acanthamoeba II. Electron microscopic study of the initial events. J. Cell Biol., 34:219–227, 1969.
20. Mudd, J., McCutcheon, M., and Lucke, B.: Phagocytosis. Physiol. Rev., 14:210–275, 1934.
21. Zucker-Franklin, D., and Hirsch, J.G.: Electron microscope studies on the degranulation of rabbit peritoneal leukocytes during phagocytosis. J. Exp. Med., 120:569–576, 1964.
22. Cohn, Z.A., and Hirsch, J.G.: The influence of phagocytosis on the intracellular distribution of granule-associated components of polymorphonuclear leucocytes. J. Exp. Med., 112:1015–1022, 1960.
23. Ohlsson, K., Olsson, I., and Spitznagel, J.K.: Localization of chymotrypsin-like cationic protein, collagenase, and elastase in azurophil granules of human neutrophilic polymorphonuclear leukocytes. Hoppe Seylers Z. Physiol. Chem., 358:361–366, 1977.
24. Bretz, U., and Baggiolini, M.: Biochemical and morphological characterization of azurophil and specific granules of human neutrophilic polymorphonuclear leukocytes. J. Cell Biol., 63:251–269, 1974.
24a.Bretz, U., and Baggiolini, M.: Association of the alkaline phosphatase of rabbit polymorphonuclear leukocytes with the membrane of the specific granules. J. Cell Biol., 59:696–707, 1973.
25. Spitznagel, J.K., et al.: Selective deficiency of granules associated with lysozyme and lactoferrin in human polymorphs (PMN) with reduced microbicidal capacity. J. Clin. Invest., 51:93a, 1972.
26. Kane, S.P., and Peters, T.J.: Analytical subcellular fractionation of human granulocytes with reference to the localization

of vitamin B_{12}-binding proteins. Clin. Sci. Mol. Med., 49:171, 1975.
27. Murphy, G., Reynolds, J.J., Bretz, U., and Baggiolini, M.: Collagenase is a component of the specific granules of human neutrophil leucocytes. Biochem. J., 162:195–197, 1977.
28. Ganz, T.: Extracellular release of antimicrobial defensins by human polymorphonuclear leukocytes. Infect. Immun., 55:568–571, 1987.
29. Ganz, T., et al.: Defensins: Natural peptide antibiotics of human neutrophils. J. Clin. Invest., 76:1427–1435, 1987.
30a.Zeya, H.I., and Spitznagel, J.K.: Cationic protein bearing granules of polymorphonuclear leukocytes: Separation from enzyme-rich granules. Science, 163:1069–1071, 1969.
30b.Michell, R.H., Karnovsky, M.J., and Karnovsky, M.L.: The distribution of some granule-associated enzymes in guinea-pig polymorphonuclear leucocytes. Biochem. J., 116:207–216, 1970.
30c.Spitznagel, J.K., et al.: Character of azurophil and specific granules purified from human polymorphonuclear leukocytes. Lab. Invest., 30:774–787, 1984.
31. Olsson, I., and Venge, P.: Cationic proteins of human granulocytes I. Isolation of the cationic proteins from the granules of leukaemic myeloid cells. Scand. J. Haematol., 9:204–214, 1972.
32. Klebanoff, S.J.: Iodination of bacteria: A bactericidal mechanism. J. Exp. Med., 126:1063–1078, 1967.
33. Klebanoff, S.J.: Myeloperoxidase: Contribution to the microbicidal activity of intact leukocytes. Science, 169:1095–1097, 1970.
34. Zeya, H.I., and Spitznagel, J.K.: Arginine-rich proteins of polymorphonuclear leukocyte lysosomes. Antimicrobial specificity and biochemical heterogeneity. J. Exp. Med., 127:927–941, 1968.
35. Rindler-Ludwig, R., and Braunsteiner, H.: Cationic proteins from human neutrophil granulocytes: Evidence for their chymotrypsin-like properties. Biochim. Biophys. Acta, 379:606, 1975.
36. Schmidt, W., and Havemann, K.: Isolation of elastase-like and chymotrypsin-like neutral proteases from human granulocytes. Hoppe Seylers Z. Physiol. Chem., 355:1077–1082, 1974.
37. Feinstein, G., and Janoff, A.: A rapid method for purification of human granulocyte cationic neutral proteases: Purification and characterization of human granulocyte chymotrypsin-like enzyme. Biochim. Biophys. Acta, 403:477–492, 1975.
38. Starkey, P.M., and Barrett, A.J.: Neutral proteinases of human spleen. Biochem. J., 155:255–263, 1976.
39. Johnston, M., and Greenbaum, L.M.: Leukokinin-forming system in the ascitic fluid of a murine mastocytoma. Biochem Pharmacol., 22:1386–1389, 1973.
40. Lazarus, G.S., et al.: Role of granulocyte collagenase in collagen degradation. Am. J. Pathol., 68:565–576, 1972.
41. Ohlsson, K.: Granulocyte collagenase and elastase and their interactions with alpha 1-antitrypsin and alpha 2-macroglobulin. In Proteases and Biological Control. Edited by D.B. Reich and E. Shaw. New York, Cold Spring Harbor Lab., 1975.
42. Horwitz, A.J., Hance, A.J., and Crystal, R.G.: Granulocyte collagenase: Selective digestion of type I relative to type III collagen. Proc. Natl. Acad. Sci. USA, 74:897–901, 1977.
43. Dewald, B., et al.: Subcellular localization and heterogeneity of neutral proteases in neutrophilic polymorphonuclear leukocytes. J. Exp. Med., 141:709–723, 1975.
44. Janoff, A., et al.: Human neutrophil elastase: In vitro effects on natural substrates suggest important physiological and pathological actions. In Proteases and Biological Control. Ed-

ited by E. Reich, D.B. Rifkin, and E. Shaw. New York, Cold Spring Harbor Lab., 1975.

45. Ward, P.A., and Hill, J.H.: C5 chemotactic fragments produced by an enzyme in lysosomal granules of neutrophils. J. Immunol., *104*:535–536, 1970.

46. Movat, H.Z., Habal, F.M., and MacMoline, D.R.L.: Neutral proteases of human PMN leukocytes with kininogenase activity. Int. Arch. Allergy Appl. Immunol., *50*:257–281, 1976.

47. Allison, A.C., Davies, P., and DePetris, S.: Role of contractile microfilaments in macrophage movement and endocytosis. Nature [New Biol.], *232*:153–155, 1971.

48. Reaven, E.P., and Axline, S.G.: Subplasmalemmal microfilaments and microtubules in resting and phagocytizing cultivated macrophages. J. Cell Biol., *59*:12–27, 1976.

49. Weissmann, G., Smolen, J., Hoffstein, S., and Korchak, H.: The secretory code of the neutrophil. *In* Cellular Interactions. Edited by J.T. Dingle and J.L. Gordon. New York, Elsevier/North Holland Biomedical Press, 1981.

50. Rich, A.M., and Hoffstein, S.: Inverse correlation between neutrophil microtubule numbers and enhanced random migration. J. Cell Sci., *48*:181–191, 1981.

51. Mellon, M.G., and Rebhun, L.I.: Sulfhydryls and the in vitro polymerization of tubulin. J. Cell Biol., *70*:226–238, 1976.

52. Malawista, S.E.: Vinblastine can inhibit lysosomal degranulation without suppressing phagocytosis in human blood leukocytes. *In* Immunopathology of Inflammation. Edited by B.K. Forscher and J.C. Houck. Amsterdam, Excerpta Medica, 1971.

53. Weissmann, G., et al.: A general method, employing arsenazo III in liposomes, for study of calcium ionophores: Results with A23187 and prostaglandins. Proc. Natl. Acad. Sci. USA, *77*:1506–1510, 1980.

54. Weissmann, G., Smolen, J.E., and Korchak, H.M.: Release of inflammatory mediators from stimulated neutrophils. N. Engl. J. Med., *303*:27–34, 1980.

55. Wright, D.G., and Malawista, S.E.: Mobilization and extracellular release of granular enzymes from human leukocytes during phagocytosis: Inhibition by colchicine and cortisol but not by salicylate. Arthritis Rheum., *16*:749–758, 1973.

56. Zurier, R.B., et al.: Mechanisms of lysosomal enzyme release from human leukocytes. II. Effects of cAMP and cGMP, autonomic agonists, and agents which affect microtubule function. J. Clin. Invest., *53*:297–309, 1974.

57. Goldstein, I.M., Hoffstein, S., and Weissmann, G.: Mechanisms of lysosomal enzyme release from human polymorphonuclear leukocytes. J. Cell Biol., *66*:647–652, 1975.

58. Stossel, T.P., and Hartwig, J.H.: Interactions of actin, myosin, and a new actin-binding protein of rabbit pulmonary macrophages. II. Role in cytoplasmic movement and phagocytosis. J. Cell Biol., *68*:602–619, 1976.

59. Wehring, R.R.: Cytochalasin B inhibits actin-related gelation of HeLa cell extracts. J. Cell Biol., *71*:303–307, 1976.

60. Fleit, H.B., Wright, S.D., and Unkeless, J.C.: Human neutrophil Fc receptor distribution and structure. Proc. Natl. Acad. Sci. USA, *79*:3275–3279, 1982.

61. Fearon, D.J.: Identification of the membrane glycoprotein that is the C3b receptor of the human erythrocyte, polymorphonuclear leukocyte, B lymphocyte, and monocyte. J. Exp. Med., *152*:20–30, 1980.

62. Najjar, V.A., and Nishioka, K.: Tuftsin: A natural phagocytosis stimulating peptide. Nature, *228*:672–673, 1970.

63. Kaplan, H.B., Edelson, H.S., Friedman, R., and Weissmann, G.: The roles of degranulation and superoxide anion gener-

ation in neutrophil aggregation. Biochim. Biophys. Acta, *721*:55–63, 1982.

64. Sklar, L.A., et al.: A continuous, spectroscopic analysis of the kinetics of elastase secretion by neutrophils. J. Biol. Chem., *257*:5471–5475, 1982.

65. Becker, E.L., et al.: The inhibition of neutrophil granule enzyme secretion and chemotaxis by pertussis toxin. J. Cell Biol., *100*:1641–1646, 1985.

66. Bokoch, G.M., and Gilman, A.G.: Inhibition of receptor-mediated release of arachidonic acid by pertussis toxin. Cell, *39*:301–308, 1984.

67. Goldman, D.W., et al.: Pertussis toxin inhibition of chemotactic factor-induced calcium mobilization and function in human polymorphonuclear leukocytes. J. Exp. Med., *162*:145–156, 1985.

68. Krause, K.H., et al.: Chemotactic peptide activation of human neutrophils and HL-60 cells. Pertussis toxin reveals correlation between inositol trisphosphate generation, calcium ion transients and cellular activation. J. Clin. Invest., *76*:1348–1354, 1985.

69. Lad, P.M., Olson, C.V., and Smiley, P.A.: Association of the N-formyl-met-leu-phe receptor in human neutrophils with a GTP-binding protein sensitive to pertussis toxin. Proc. Natl. Acad. Sci. USA, *82*:869–873, 1985.

70. Ohta, H., Okajima, F., and Ui, M.: Inhibition by islet-activating protein of a chemotactic peptide-induced early breakdown of inositol phospholipids and Ca^{2+} mobilization in guinea pig neutrophils. J. Cell Biol., *260*:15771–15780.

71. Okajima, F., Katada, T., and Ui, M.: Coupling of the guanine nucleotide regulatory protein to chemotactic peptide receptors in neutrophil membranes and its uncoupling by islet-activating protein, pertussis toxin. J. Biol. Chem., *260*:6761–6768, 1985.

72. Okajima, F., and Ui, M.: ADP-ribosylation of the specific membrane protein by islet-activating protein, pertussis toxin, associated with inhibition of a chemotactic peptide-induced arachidonate release in neutrophils. J. Biol. Chem., *259*:13863–13871, 1985.

73. Smith, C.D., et al.: Chemoattractant receptor-induced hydrolysis of phosphatidylinositol 4,5-bisphosphate in human polymorphonuclear leukocyte membranes. Requirement for a guanine nucleotide regulating protein. J. Biol. Chem., *260*:5875–5878, 1985.

74. Verghese, M.W., Smith, C.D., and Snyderman, R.: Potential role for a guanine nucleotide regulatory protein in chemoattractant receptor mediated polyphosphoinositide metabolism, Ca^{++} mobilization and cellular responses by leukocytes. Biochem. Biophys. Res. Commun., *127*:450–457, 1985.

75a. Volpi, M., et al.: Pertussis toxin inhibits fmet-leu-phe but not phorbol ester-stimulated changes in rabbit neutrophils: Role of G proteins in excitation response coupling. Proc. Natl. Acad. Sci. USA, *82*:2708–2712, 1985.

75b. Lad, P.M., Olson, C.V., Grewal, I.S., and Scott, S.J.: A pertussis toxin-sensitive GTP-binding protein in the human neutrophil regulates multiple receptors, calcium mobilization, and lectin-induced capping. Proc. Natl. Acad. Sci. USA, *82*:8643–8647, 1985.

75c. Spiegel, A.M., Gierschik, P., Levine, M.A., and Downs, R.W., Jr.: Clinical implications of guanine nucleotide-binding proteins as receptor-effector couplers. N. Engl. J. Med., *312*:26–33, 1985.

76. Korchak, H.M., and Weissmann, G.: Changes in membrane potential of human granulocytes antecede the metabolic re-

sponses to surface stimulation. Proc. Natl. Acad. Sci. USA, 75:3818–3822, 1978.

77. Goldstein, I.M., Horn, J.K., Kaplan, H.B., and Weissmann, G.: Calcium-induced lysozyme secretion from human polymorphonuclear leukocytes. Biochem. Biophys. Res. Commun., 60:807–812, 1974.

78. O'Flaherty, J.T., Showell, H.J., Becker, E.L., and Ward, P.A.: Substances which aggregate neutrophils. Am. J. Pathol., 92:155–166, 1978.

79. Smolen, J.E., and Weissmann, G.: Stimuli which provoke secretion of azurophil enzymes from human neutrophils induced increments in adenosine cyclic 3′,5′-monophosphate. Biochim. Biophys. Acta, 672:197–206, 1981.

80. Korchak, H.M., Hoffstein, S.T., and Weissmann, G.: The neutrophil granule. In The Secretory Granule. Edited by A.M. Poisner and J.M. Trifaro. New York, Elsevier Medical Press, 1982.

81. Naccache, P.H., Showell, H.J., Becker, E.L., and Sha'afi, R.I.: Changes in ionic movements across rabbit polymorphonuclear leukocyte membranes during lysosomal enzyme release. Possible ionic basis for lysosomal enzyme release. J. Cell Biol., 75:635–649, 1977.

82. Pozzan, T., Lew, P.D., Wollheim, C.B., and Tsien, R.Y.: Monitoring cytoplasmic free calcium concentration, (Ca^{++}) in living polymorphonuclear leukocytes. Clin. Res., 31:320–329, 1983.

83. Serhan, C., et al.: Changes in phosphatidylinositol and phosphatidic acid in stimulated human neutrophils: Relationship to calcium mobilization, aggregation, and superoxide radical generation. Biochim. Biophys. Acta, 762:420–428, 1983.

84. Hoffstein, S.T.: Ultrastructural demonstration of calcium loss from local regions of the plasma membrane of surface-stimulated human granulocytes. J. Immunol., 123:1395–1402, 1979.

85. Naccache, P.H., Showell, H.J., Becker, E.L., and Sha'afi, R.I.: Involvement of membrane calcium in the response of rabbit neutrophils to chemotactic factors as evidenced by the fluorescence of chlorotetracycline. J. Cell Biol., 83:179–186, 1979.

86. Smolen, J.E., and Weissmann, G.: The fluorescence response of chlorotetracycline-loaded human polymorphonuclear leukocytes. I. The effect of various stimuli and calcium antagonists. Biochim. Biophys. Acta, 720:172–180, 1982.

87. Henson, P.M.: Mechanisms of mediator release from inflammatory cells. In Mediators of Inflammation. Edited by G. Weissmann. New York, Plenum Publishing, 1974.

88. Jackowski, S., and Sha'afi, R.I.: Response of adenosine cyclic 3′,5′-monophosphate level in rabbit neutrophils to the chemotactic peptide FMLP. Mol. Pharmacol., 16:473–481, 1979.

89. Simchowitz, L., Spilberg, I., and Atkinson, J.P.: Evidence that the functional responses of human neutrophils occur independently of transient elevations in cAMP levels. Fed. Proc., 42:1080, 1983.

90. Baldridge, C.W., and Gerard, R.W.: The extra respiration of phagocytosis. Am. J. Physiol., 103:235–236, 1933.

91. Sbarra, A.J., and Karnovsky, M.L.: The biochemical basis of phagocytosis I. Metabolic changes during the ingestion of particles by polymorphonuclear leukocytes. J. Biol. Chem., 234:1355–1362, 1959.

92. Evans, W.H., and Karnovsky, M.L.: The biochemical basis of phagocytosis. IV. Some aspects of carbohydrate metabolism during phagocytosis. Biochemistry, 1:159–166, 1962.

93. Iyer, G.Y.N., Islam, D.F.M., and Quastel, J.H.: Biochemical aspects of phagocytosis. Nature, 192:535–541, 1971.

94. Babior, B.M., Kipnes, R.S., and Curnutte, J.T.: Biological de-

fense mechanisms: The production by leukocytes of superoxide, a potential bacterial agent. J. Clin. Invest., 52:741–744, 1973.

95. Karnovsky, M.L., and Wallach, D.F.H.: The metabolic basis of phagocytosis III. Incorporation of inorganic phosphate into various classes of phosphatides during phagocytosis. J. Biol. Chem., 236:1895–1901, 1961.

96. Andrews, P.C., and Babior, B.M.: Endogenous protein phosphorylation by resting and activated human neutrophils. Blood, 61:333–340, 1983.

97. Huang, C-K., et al.: Effects of chemotactic factors on the protein phosphorylation of rabbit peritoneal neutrophils. Fed. Proc., 42:1080, 1983.

98. Tsung, P.K., Sakamoto, T., and Weissmann, G.: Protein kinase and phosphatases from human polymorphonuclear leukocytes. Biochem. J., 145:437–438, 1975.

99. Niedel, J.E., Kohn, I.J., and Vandenback, G.R.: Phorbol diester receptor copurifies with protein kinase C. Proc. Natl. Acad. Sci. USA, 80:36–40, 1983.

100. Serhan, C., et al.: Phosphatidate and oxidized fatty acids are calcium ionophores. Studies employing arsenazo III in liposomes. J. Biol. Chem., 256:2736–2741, 1981.

101. Fantone, J.C., and Ward, P.A.: Role of oxygen-derived free radicals and metabolites in leukocyte-dependent inflammatory reactions. Am. J. Pathol., 107:397–418, 1982.

101a. Babior, B.M.: Oxygen-dependent microbial killing by phagocytes. N. Engl. J. Med., 298:659–668, 1978.

102. Korchak, H.M., et al.: Granulocytes without degranulation: Neutrophil function in granule-depleted cytoplasts. Proc. Natl. Acad. Sci. USA, 80:4968–4972, 1983.

103. Perez, H.D., Weksler, B., and Goldstein, I.: A new mechanism for the generation of biologically active products from arachidonic acid. Clin. Res., 27:464a, 1979.

104. Kuehl, E.A.A., et al.: Role of prostaglandin endoperoxide PGG2 in inflammatory processes. Nature, 265:170–172, 1977.

105. Robinson, D.R., Curran, D.P., and Hamer, P.J.: Prostaglandins and related compounds in inflammatory rheumatic diseases. In Adv. in Inflammation Research. Edited by M. Ziff, G. Velo, and S. Gorini. New York, Raven Press, 1982.

106. Goodwin, J.S., Bankhurst, A.D., and Messner, R.P.: Suppression of human T-cell mitogenesis by prostaglandin: Existence of a prostaglandin-producing suppressor cell. J. Exp. Med., 146:1719–1734, 1977.

107. Smolen, J.E., Korchak, H.M., and Weissmann, G.: Increased levels of cyclic adenosine 3′,5′-monophosphate in human polymorphonuclear leukocytes after surface stimulation. J. Clin. Invest., 65:1077–1085, 1980.

108. Dawson, W., Boot, J.R., Harvey, J., and Walker, J.R.: The pharmacology of benoxaprofen with particular attention to effects on lipoxygenase product formation. Eur. J. Rheumatol. Inflamm., 5:61–68, 1982.

109. Radmark, O., et al.: Leukotriene A.: Stereochemistry and enzymatic conversion to leukotriene B. Biochem. Biophys. Res. Commun., 92:954–961, 1980.

110. Hammarstrom, S.: Metabolism of leukotriene C3 in the guinea pig. Identification of metabolites formed by lung, liver, and kidney. J. Biol. Chem., 256:9573–9578, 1981.

111. Hammarstrom, S., et al.: Rapid in vivo metabolism of LTB C3 in the monkey, Macaca irus. Biochem. Biophys. Res. Commun., 101:1109–1115, 1981.

112. Jubiz, W., et al.: A novel leukotriene produced by stimulation of leukocytes with formylmethionylleucylphenylalanine. J. Biol. Chem., 257:6106–6110, 1982.

113. Goetzl, E.J., and Pickett, W.C.: The human polymorpho-

nuclear leukocyte chemotactic activity of complex hydroxy-eicosatetraenoic acids (HETEs) 1. J. Immunol., 125:1789–1791, 1980.

114. Malmstein, C., Svensson, J., Hamberg, M., and Samuelsson, B.: The role of prostaglandin endoperoxides and thromboxanes in platelet aggregation. In Advances in Prostaglandin and Thromboxane Research, Vol. 1. Edited by B. Samuelsson and R. Paoletti. New York, Raven Press, 1976.

115. Palmer, R.M., Stepney, R.J., Higgs, G.A., and Eakins, K.E.: Chemokinetic activity of arachidonic and lipoxygenase products on leukocytes of different species. Prostaglandins, 20:411–418, 1980.

116. Smith, M.J., Ford-Hutchinson, A.W., and Bray, M.A.: Leukotriene B: A potential mediator of inflammation. J. Pharm. Pharmacol., 32:517–518, 1980.

117. Dahlen, S.-E., Hedqvist, P., Hammarstrom, S., and Samuelsson, B.: Leukotrienes are potent constrictors of human bronchi. Nature (London), 288:484–486, 1980.

118. Samuelsson, B.: Leukotrienes: Mediators of immediate hypersensitivity reactions and inflammation. Science, 220:568–575, 1983.

119. Feinmark, S.J., et al.: Stimulation of human leukocyte degranulation by leukotriene B4 and its omega-oxidized metabolites. FEBS Lett., 136:141–144, 1981.

120. Serhan, C.N., et al.: Leukotriene B4 and phosphatidic acid are calcium ionophores: Studies employing arsenazo III in liposomes. J. Biol. Chem., 257:4746, 1982.

121. Serhan, C.N., Lundberg, U., Weissmann, G., and Samuelsson, B.: Formation of leukotrienes and hydroxy acids by human neutrophils and platelets exposed to monosodium urate. J. Exp. Med. (In press).

122. Mandell, G.L.: Intraphagosomal pH of human polymorphonuclear neutrophils. Proc. Soc. Exp. Biol. Med., 134:447–449, 1970.

122a. Hirsch, J.G., and Cohn, Z.A.: Degranulation of polymorphonuclear leucocytes following phagocytosis of microorganisms. J. Exp. Med., 112:1005–1014, 1960.

123. Smolen, J.E., Korchak, H.M., and Weissmann, G.: Initial kinetics of lysosomal enzyme release and superoxide anion generation in human polymorphonuclear leukocytes. Inflammation, 4:145, 1980.

124. Weissmann, G., et al.: The secretory code of the neutrophil. J. Reticuloendothel Soc., 26:687–700, 1979.

125. Malmstein, C.L., et al.: Leukotriene B4: A highly potent and stereospecific factor stimulating migration of polymorphonuclear leukocytes. Acta Physiol. Scand., 110:449–451, 1980.

126. Rich, A.M., Giedd, K.N., Cristello, P., and Weissmann, G.: Granules are necessary for death of neutrophils after phagocytosis of crystalline monosodium urate, (in preparation).

127. Zurier, R.B., Hoffstein, S., and Weissmann, G.: Mechanisms of lysosomal enzyme release from human leukocytes. J. Cell Biol., 58:27–48, 1973.

128. Harlan, J.M., et al.: Neutrophil-mediated endothelial injury in vitro. Mechanisms of cell detachment. J. Clin. Invest., 68:1394–1403, 1981.

129. Herlin, T., Petersen, C.S., and Esmann, V.: The role of calcium and cyclic adenosine 3′,5′-monophosphate in the regulation of glycogen metabolism in phagocytozing human polymorphonuclear leukocytes. Biochim. Biophys. Acta, 542:63–76, 1978.

130. Goldstein, I., et al.: Mechanisms of lysosomal enzyme release from human leukocytes: Microtubule assembly and membrane fusion induced by a component of complement. Proc. Natl. Acad. Sci. USA, 70:2916–2920, 1973.

131. Zurier, R.B., Hoffstein, S., and Weissmann, G.: Cytochalasin B: Effect on lysosomal enzyme release from human leukocytes. Proc. Natl. Acad. Sci. USA, 70:844–848, 1973.

132. Hoffstein, S., et al.: Concanavalin A induces microtubule assembly and specific granule discharge in human polymorphonuclear leukocytes. J. Cell Biol., 68:781–787, 1976.

133. Goldstein, I.M., Hoffstein, S., and Weissmann, G.: Influence of divalent cations upon complement-mediated enzyme release from human polymorphonuclear leukocytes. J. Immunol., 115:665–670, 1975.

134. Bainton, D.F.: Sequential degranulation of the two types of polymorphonuclear leukocyte granules during phagocytosis of microorganisms. J. Cell Biol., 58:249–264, 1973.

135. Sacks, T., et al.: Oxygen radicals mediate endothelial cell damage by complement-stimulated granulocytes. J. Clin. Invest., 61:1161–1167, 1978.

136. Kaplan, H.B., et al.: Effects of non-steroidal anti-inflammatory agents on human neutrophil functions in vitro and in vivo. Biochem. Pharmacol. (In press).

137. Cronstein, B.N., et al.: Adenosine: A physiological modulator of superoxide anion generation by human neutrophils. II. Adenosine acts via an A2 receptor on human neutrophils. J. Immunol., 135:1366–1371, 1985.

138. Cronstein, B.N., et al.: Adenosine: An endogenous inhibitor of neutrophil mediated injury to endothelial cells. J. Clin. Invest., 78:760–770, 1986.

139. Cronstein, B.N., Kubersky, S.M., Weissmann, G., and Hirschhorn, R.: Engagement of adenosine receptors inhibits H2O2 release by activated human neutrophils. Clin. Immunol. Immunopathol., 42:76–85, 1987.

140. Cronstein, B.N., et al.: Engagement of adenosine receptors raises cAMP alone and in synergy with engagement of the FMLP receptor and inhibits membrane depolarization but does not affect stimulated Ca++ fluxes, 1987, (submitted).

141. Rose, F.R., Hirschhorn, R., Weissmann, G., and Cronstein, B.J.: Adenosine promotes chemotaxis. J. Exp. Med. (In Press)

142. Cronstein, B.N., et al.: Engagement of adenosine receptors inhibits neutrophil adherence to endothelial cells. (Submitted)

143. Cronstein, B.N., Kramer, S.B., Weissmann, G., and Hirschhorn, R.: Adenosine: A physiological modulator of superoxide anion generation by human neutrophils. J. Exp. Med., 153:1160–1177, 1983.

144. Dunham, P. et al.: Membrane fusion: Studies with a calcium-sensitive dye, arsenazo III, in liposomes. Proc. Natl. Acad. Sci. USA, 74:1580–1584, 1977.

145. Johnston, R.B., Jr.: Defects of neutrophil function. N. Engl. J. Med., 307:434–436, 1982.

146. Root, R.K., Rosenthal, A.S., and Balestra, D.J.: Abnormal bactericidal, metabolic, and lysosomal functions of Chediak-Higashi syndrome leukocytes. J. Clin. Invest., 51:649–665, 1972.

147. Boxer, L.A., et al.: Correction of leukocyte function in Chediak-Higashi syndrome by ascorbate. N. Engl. J. Med., 295:1041–1045, 1976.

148. Oliver, J.M., and Zurier, R.B.: Correction of characteristic abnormalities of microtubule function and granule morphology in Chediak-Higashi syndrome with cholinergic agonists. Studies in vitro in man and in vivo in the beige mouse. J. Clin. Invest., 57:1239–1247, 1976.

148a. Clark, R.A., and Kimball, H.R.: Defective granulocyte chemotaxis in the Chediak-Higashi syndrome. J. Clin. Invest., 50:2645–2652, 1971.

149. Gallin, J.I.: Abnormal phagocyte chemotaxis: Pathophysiol-

ogy, clinical manifestations, and management of patients. Rev. Infect. Dis., 3:1196–1220, 1981.

150. Johnson, R.B., Jr.: Biochemical defects of polymorphonuclear and mononuclear phagocytes associated with disease. *In* The Reticuloendothelial System. Edited by A.J. Sbarra and R.R. Strauss. New York; Plenum, 1980.

151. Boxer, L.A., Hedley-White, E.T., and Stossel, T.P.: Neutrophil actin dysfunction and abnormal neutrophil behavior. N. Engl. J. Med., 291:1093–1099, 1974.

152. Arnaout, M.A., et al.: Deficiency of a granulocyte-membrane glycoprotein (gp150) in a boy with recurrent bacterial infections. N. Engl. J. Med., 306:693–699, 1982.

153. Boxer, L.A., et al.: Lactoferrin deficiency associated with altered granulocyte function. N. Engl. J. Med., 307:404–410, 1982.

154. Klebanoff, S.J., and Hamon, C.B.: Role of myeloperoxidase-mediated antimicrobial systems in intact leukocytes. J. Reticuloendothel. Soc., 12:170–196, 1972.

155. Karnovsky, M.L.: Steps toward an understanding of chronic granulomatous disease. N. Engl. J. Med., 308:274–275, 1983.

156. Segal, A.L., et al.: Absence of cytochrome b-245 in chronic granulomatous disease. N. Engl. J. Med., 308:245–251, 1983.

157. Baehner, R.L., et al.: DNA linkage analysis of X chromosome-linked chronic granulomatous disease. Proc. Natl. Acad. Sci. USA, 83:3398–3401, 1986.

157a. Royer-Porkora, B., et al.: Cloning the gene for an inherited human disorder—chronic granulomatous disease—on the basis of its chromosomal location. Nature, 322:32–38, 1986.

158. Lew, P.D., et al.: A variant of chronic granulomatous disease: Deficient oxidative metabolism due to a low-affinity NADPH oxidase. N. Engl. J. Med., 305:1329–1333, 1981.

159. Salmon, S.E., Cline, M.J., Schultz, J., and Lehrer, R.I.: Myeloperoxidase deficiency. Immunologic study of a genetic leukocyte defect. N. Engl. J. Med., 282:250–253, 1970.

160. Strauss, R.G., et al.: An anomaly of neutrophil morphology with impaired function. N. Engl. J. Med., 290:478–484, 1974.

161. Loos, H., Roos, D., Weening, R., and Hourwerzyil, J.: Familial deficiency of glutathione reductase in human blood cells. Blood, 48:53–62, 1976.

162. Roos, D., et al.: Protection of phagocytic leukocytes by endogenous glutathione: Studies in a family with glutathione deficiency. Blood, 53:851–866, 1979.

163. Miller, M.E., et al.: A new familial defect of neutrophil movement. J. Lab. Clin. Med., 82:1–8, 1975.

164. Miller, M.E., Oski, F.A., and Harris, M.B.: Lazy-leucocyte syndrome. A new disorder of neutrophil function. Lancet, 1:665–669, 1971.

EOSINOPHIL STRUCTURE AND FUNCTION

21

PETER F. WELLER

The eosinophil, like the neutrophil and the basophil, is a bone marrow-derived polymorphonuclear leukocyte. Tinctorially, the eosinophil is readily differentiated from other leukocytes based on the affinity of the eosinophil's cytoplasmic granules for acidic dyes, such as eosin. Clinically, differences between eosinophils and neutrophils are indicated by the different diseases and immunologic responses with which the two classes of leukocytes are associated. Neutrophils function in host defense against bacteria and some other types of microbial organisms by phagocytizing and killing them. In contrast, eosinophils play no significant role in defense against traditional pyogenic organisms. The eosinophils' role in antimicrobial immunity is predominantly against stages of metazoan parasites, large and noningestible worms. Eosinophils usually constitute less than 5% of circulating blood leukocytes, but increased blood or tissue eosinophils occur not only with the metazoan parasitic infections but also with allergic diseases and a variety of other, often idiopathic conditions.[1,2]

Although the eosinophil has been studied less extensively than the quantitatively more predominant neutrophil, the eosinophil clearly differs from other polymorphonuclear leukocytes in its morphology, in some of its major constituent proteins and elaborated products, and in the diseases with which it is involved. While much remains to be learned about the participatory roles of eosinophils in many types of inflammatory responses, increasingly the structure and functional capabilities of eosinophilic leukocytes are being defined.[3]

PRODUCTION AND DISTRIBUTION OF EOSINOPHILS

After forming and maturing within the bone marrow, eosinophils are released into the blood where they circulate with a half-life of about 3 to 8 hours. Eosinophils leave the circulation to localize in tissues, especially those that interface with the outside world, such as the respiratory and gastrointestinal tracts. Eosinophils live longer than neutrophils and persist in tissues for at least several days. Although the pool of peripheral blood eosinophils is the only one accessible for enumeration, eosinophils are principally tissue-dwelling cells. Studies in animals indicate that for every eosinophil present in the circulation there are 300 to 500 in the tissues.[2]

Considerable evidence documents that the control of eosinophilopoiesis, in response to experimental stimuli for eosinophil production, is a T-lymphocyte-dependent process,[4,5] although the identity of the eosinophilopoietic factor(s) has not been ascertained. But athymic mice are not totally deficient in eosinophils,[6] indicating that other factors may help maintain a basal production of eosinophils. Experimentally, eosinophil development can be promoted by agents acting predominantly on other cell lines. Hence, granulocyte/macrophage colony-stimulating factor (GM-CSF) in elevated concentrations can stimulate eosinophil formation.[7] A stimulus that is specific, or preferential, for eosinophil formation, however, is likely to account for the heightened production of eosinophils encountered in some clinical and experimental conditions. Recently, a murine eosinophil-differentiating factor has been identified which acts as a specific eosinophil colony-stimulating factor and promotes the maturation of eosinophil development.[8] Undoubtedly, greater insights will be forthcoming in identifying the humoral factors and their cooperative interactions which result in the increased formation and release of mature eosinophils.

Eosinophils are motile cells and exhibit enhanced migration in response to specific stimuli. A number of compounds have been recognized as chemoattractant for eosinophils. Many of these substances are released by mast cells, including histamine in a limited concentration range,[9] a metabolite of histamine,[10] and two tetrapeptides, termed ECF-A (eosinophil chemotactic factor of anaphylaxis).[11] In addition, platelet-activating factor (PAF) has recently been identified as a chemotactic and chemokinetic factor for eosinophils. PAF is both more potent than the previously identified human eosinophil chemoattractant compounds and more specific for eosinophils than neutrophils.[12,13] Other immunologically generated moieties, chemotactic for both eosinophils and neutrophils, include the complement-derived components, C5a, the trimolecular complex $C_{\overline{567}}$ and leukotriene B_4.[12] Lymphokines that act specifically to augment eosinophil migration have also been recognized.[14,15] These chemoattractant substances provide a means whereby eosinophils can be recruited to sites of immunologic reactions and can also

serve to stimulate the functions of eosinophils in these local sites.

MORPHOLOGY OF EOSINOPHILS

The human eosinophil, which measures 12 to 17 μ in diameter, is only slightly larger than the neutrophil but, unlike the neutrophil, usually has a bilobed nucleus (Fig. 21–1). The most notable morphologic feature of the eosinophil is its content of large, distinctive intracytoplasmic granules. These *specific granules* are morphologically unique because within each of them is located one or more crystalloid cores. This crystalloid core, present only in the specific granules of eosinophils, is recognizable by transmission electron microscopy and usually appears electron dense (Fig. 21–1). Both the core and the surrounding matrix of these granules contain a number of cationic, positively charged, proteins which provide the basis for their staining with eosin.

Analogous to the situation in neutrophils (see Chapter 20), a second population of cytoplasmic granules, the *primary granules*, arises early in eosinophil maturation. These are clearly present in eosinophilic promyelocytes and may persist in lesser numbers in mature eosinophils.[16] Another distinct population of smaller cytoplasmic granules has been delineated morphologically using cytochemical identification of acid phosphatase and arylsulfatase B within these granules.[17] The cytoplasm of eosinophils participating

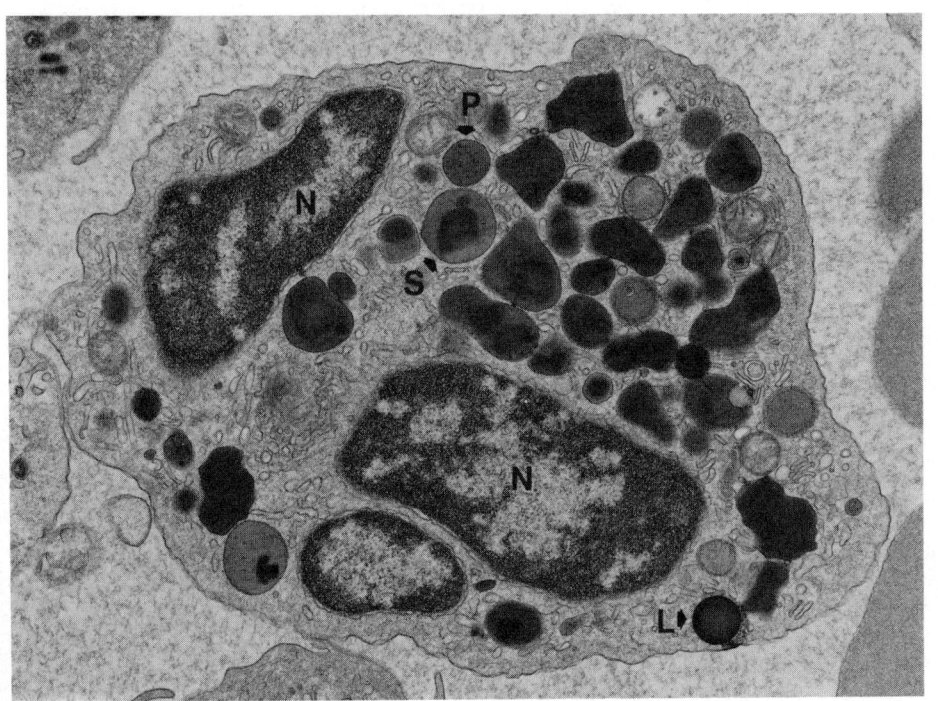

FIG. 21–1. Transmission electron micrograph of a human peripheral blood eosinophil. As is usual, the eosinophil has a bilobed nucleus (N). Cytoplasmic granules include the primary granule (P) and the large specific granule (S), many of which contain characteristic electron-dense crystalline cores. In addition, an osmiophilic, nonmembrane-bound lipid body (L) is seen within the cytoplasm. ($\times$ 12,600) (Courtesy of Ann. M. Dvorak, M.D., Beth Israel Hospital, Harvard Medical School, Boston)

in inflammatory reactions in tissues has increased numbers of these granules.[18] A fourth population of small morphologically distinct granules has also been recognized in human eosinophils.[19] In contrast to the cytoplasmic granule populations of the neutrophil, the only granule of the eosinophil isolated by subcellular fractionation is the specific granule. Hence, the definition of these other types of eosinophil cytoplasmic granules still rests on morphologic and cytochemical observations.

A cytoplasmic structure, sometimes confused with granules but distinct from them, is the lipid body (Fig. 21–1).[20] Lipid bodies are roughly globular in shape and range in size from minute to the size of large cytoplasmic granules. By electron microscopy they appear dark with osmium fixation due to their lipid content and can be shown to lack a delimiting membrane. Lipid bodies are also found in neutrophils. These organelles can serve as repositories of esterified arachidonic acid.[20]

CONSTITUENTS OF EOSINOPHILS

The large, specific granule of the eosinophil contains a variety of acid and neutral hydrolases analogous to the hydrolytic enzymes found in neutrophil granules.[21] Because of a paucity of studies of isolated cytoplasmic granules of eosinophils, the full content of enzymes present within the granules has not been defined, and many of them have not yet been characterized. The localization of some lysosomal enzymes to this granule population has been assumed but not proven. Eosinophils contain collagenase,[22,23] and cathepsins[24] but not elastase or neutral protease.[24] One enzyme of neutrophil-specific granules apparently absent from eosinophils is lysozyme.[21] A series of cationic proteins are recognized as distinctive to eosinophil specific granules (Table 21–1). *Major basic protein* (MBP) has been named because it is quantitatively predominant within the granule and has an isoelectric point in excess of 10.[25,26] MBP forms the crystalloid core of the granule.[27,28] It has a molecular weight of about 10,000 to 15,000,[26,29] and is also found in basophils.[30] Although to date MBP has no recognized enzymatic activity, it is potent biologically. A second granule protein is *eosinophil peroxidase*, an enzyme distinct physicochemically and biochemically from the myeloperoxidase of the neutrophil and monocyte.[31–33] *Eosinophil peroxidase*, like another basic granular constituent termed *eosinophil cationic protein* (ECP), is present in the matrix of the granule surrounding the crystalloid core.[28] A fourth cationic protein, *eosinophil-derived neurotoxin* (EDN), when injected intracerebrally into test animals, elicits a characteristic neuropathologic response, termed the "Gordon phenomenon," identical to that initially elicited by the injection of tissues containing human eosinophils.[34] Recently, both ECP and EDN have been found to share sequence homology with RNase, and both ECP and EDN have RNase activity.[35,36] ECP also may mediate potentially cytolytic, channel-forming activity by inducing the formation of pores across artificial and cellular membranes.[37]

Another protein of human eosinophils has long been associated with eosinophil-related diseases because of its propensity to crystallize in vivo, forming Charcot-Leyden crystals[2] (Fig. 21–2). The bipyramidal, elongated structures may be found in human tissues and fluids, including sputum, feces, pleural fluid, and synovial fluid (Chapter 5),[38] in association with a diversity of allergic, parasitic, and other eosinophil-related diseases.[2] These crystals are composed of a single 17,000 molecular weight protein, immunochemically and biochemically identical to an eosinophil-derived protein exhibiting lysophospholipase activity.[39–41] Unlike the other distinctive eosinophil proteins, this protein constitutes about 5% of cell protein. It is not found within the cytoplasmic granule but is associated with membranes and other intracellular structures.[41] The same protein exists in human basophils but not in other leukocytes.[42]

CELL SURFACE RECEPTORS

Eosinophils express plasma membrane receptors for complement components, including CR1, the C3b/C4b receptor, CR3, and receptors for C1q, C3a, and C5a.[43–46] Receptors for immunoglobulin include an Fc receptor for IgG, although the eosinophil receptor may differ structurally from the Fc gamma receptor present on neutrophils.[47] Unlike neutrophils, eosinophils can express a cell membrane receptor for IgE. This eosinophil IgE receptor has a lower affinity for

Table 21–1. Composition of Eosinophil Cytoplasmic Granules

Specific Granules—Contain unique crystalloid core
  Neutral and acidic lysosomal hydrolases

Cationic proteins:	Mol. Wt.	Location	Enzyme Activity
MBP—Major basic protein	10–15,000	core	none known
ECP—Eosinophil cationic protein	18,000	matrix	RNase
EDN—Eosinophil derived neurotoxin	20,000	matrix	RNase
EPO—Eosinophil peroxidase	75,000	matrix	peroxidase

Primary Granules—Predominant during eosinophil maturation
  Peroxidase, arylsulfatase, acid phosphatase
Small Granules
  Arylsulfatase, acid phosphatase

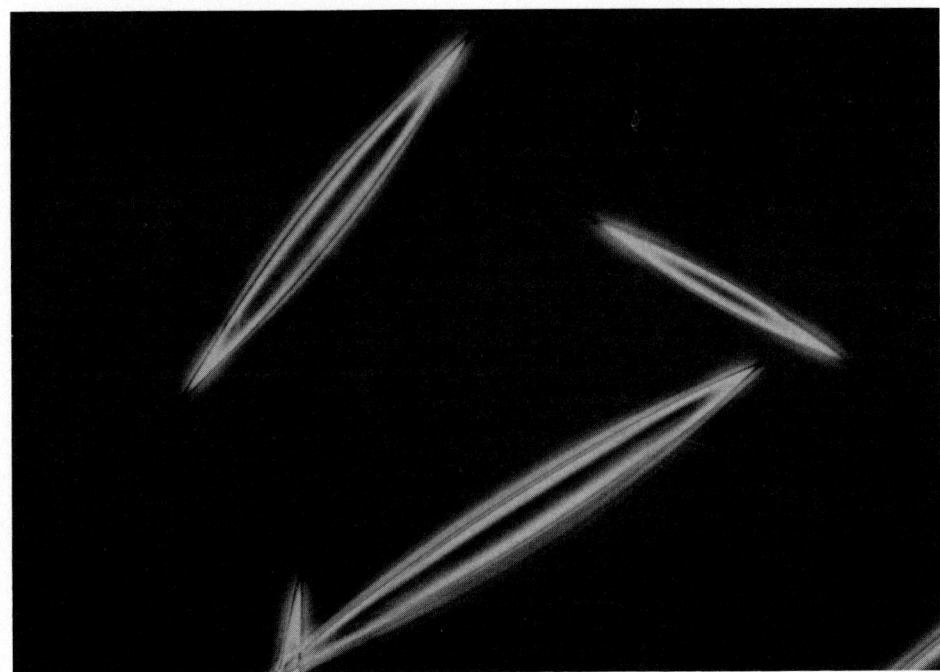

FIG. 21–2. Phase contrast micrograph of Charcot-Leyden crystals demonstrating their characteristic bipyramidal morphology. (×1,000) (Courtesy of Steven J. Ackerman, Ph.D., Beth Israel Hospital, Harvard Medical School, Boston)

its ligand than IgE receptors present on basophils and mast cells.[48]

LIPID PRODUCTS OF THE EOSINOPHIL

Eosinophils have the capacity to form and release biologically active lipids. The oxidative metabolism of arachidonic acid by the 5-lipoxygenase pathway in these cells leads to the intracellular production and subsequent release of leukotriene C_4 (LTC$_4$).[49,50] The elaboration of this eicosanoid by eosinophils differs from the predominant formation of leukotriene B_4 from neutrophils identically stimulated with the calcium ionophore A23187. Neutrophils contain an epoxide hydrolase that forms LTB$_4$ from LTA$_4$, but eosinophils possess a specific leukotriene C_4 synthetase which transfers a glutathione to the intermediate LTA$_4$ to produce LTC$_4$. LTC$_4$ mediates smooth muscle contractile, mucous secretory, and vasoconstrictive activities as opposed to LTB$_4$ which is an agonist of neutrophil and mononuclear cell functions. Eosinophils can also produce derivatives from the 15-lipoxygenase pathway of arachidonic acid metabolism, although the biologic activities of these compounds are not defined.[50]

Eosinophils can synthesize and release PAF, 1-0-alkyl-2-acetyl-3-phosphocholine, a potent inflammatory mediator with a wide range of biologic activities.[51]

ACTIVATED EOSINOPHILS

A variety of morphologic, biochemical, and functional data indicate both that eosinophils may become "activated" and that at least some blood eosinophils circulating in diseases associated with hypereosinophilia have been "activated" in vivo (Table 21–2). Morphologically, these cells may contain cytoplasmic vacuolizations with diminished numbers or size of large cytoplasmic granules.[52,53] Numbers of lipid bodies and small cytoplasmic granules increase as eosinophils engage in immunologic reactions.[20] Electron microscopy of such cells has shown that the electron-dense crystalloid cores of the granules have lost their normal electron density, suggesting that MBP within the core has been released.[54] "Activated" circulating blood eosinophils are metabolically more active than are unstimulated cells, with increased hexose monophosphate shunt activity and increased superoxide anion production in vitro.[53,55,56] Activated eosinophils, centrifuged and separated over density gradient media are less dense than normal eosinophils.[53] In-

Table 21–2. The "Activated" Eosinophil

Differences observed in eosinophils from patients with eosinophilia in comparison with normal eosinophils:
1. Morphology—Alteration in granule matrix/core, diminished granule numbers and size, vacuolization
2. Diminished cell density—Hypodense
3. Surface receptors—Increased receptors for IgE, IgG, and C3b
4. Parasite killing—Augmented ability
5. Enhanced leukotriene C_4 production
6. Increased metabolic activity

creased numbers of such circulating "hypodense" eosinophils have been associated with a number of diseases, including asthma.[57,58] Cells obtained from the blood of patients with eosinophilia may express increased numbers of cell surface receptors for IgG and complement components.[53] Hypodense eosinophils, in comparison with eosinophils of normal density, predominantly express IgE and CR3 receptors,[44,59] and show greater activity in parasite killing assays.[59,60] Whether all of these morphologic, biochemical, and functional attributes of "activated" eosinophils have the same underlying mechanism remains to be defined. Although cytokines, including lymphocyte and monocyte products, can experimentally induce some of these same alterations in eosinophils (reviewed in Ref. 3), the stimuli for eosinophil activation in vivo have not been ascertained. Additional knowledge of the mechanisms and consequences of eosinophil activation will undoubtedly promote a greater understanding of the contributions eosinophils make to those diseases with which they are associated.

FUNCTIONS OF EOSINOPHILS

Over the years, a number of functions have been hypothesized for the eosinophil. Currently, two major roles have been identified for this cell.

ROLES IN HOST DEFENSE

Experimentally eosinophils can phagocytize bacteria, mycoplasma, and other ingestible microorganisms, but they are less efficient than neutrophils in the phagocytosis of pathogens subject to intracellular killing.[61] With most bacterial and viral infections, eosinopenia develops, not eosinophilia. Specific factors mediate this eosinopenic response independent of adrenal corticosteroids, which also mediate eosinopenia.[62] Clinically, eosinophils do not have a major function as effector cells in the response to infection with unicellular microorganisms.[61]

The parasitic infections that stimulate blood or tissue eosinophilia are those involving multicellular metazoan (helminthic) parasites but not unicellular protozoans.[2] In such infections, which are often associated with augmented IgE antibody formation, eosinophils have a role in killing helminthic parasites, especially during their larval stages.[63] Examples of parasites that may be killed by eosinophils include Trichinella, schistosomes, schistosome eggs, and filaria, all of which are too large to be phagocytized.

The cells initially adhere to the worms; this may be effected by several classes of opsonins. The initial binding of eosinophils to the surface of the parasite may be mediated by eosinophil CR1 binding to C3b deposited on the surface of the worm, by Fc gamma-mediated binding with antiparasite IgG, or by Fc epsilon-mediated binding with antiparasite IgE.[59,63] Deposition of eosinophil cytoplasmic granule contents onto the surface of the parasite then occurs, accompanied by a tighter binding of the cell to the parasite. Cell products that can contribute to the death of the parasite include the cationic granule proteins, MBP, ECP, EDN, and eosinophil peroxidase which can catalyze the formation of highly reactive oxygen species (see Chapter 20). Other oxidative products, such as hydrogen peroxide, may also contribute to parasite cytotoxicity.[63]

Although other cell types are also important in the host defense against multicellular parasites, the role of eosinophils in containing helminthic infections has been clearly shown by the increased worm burdens in infected animals depleted of eosinophils by antieosinophil antiserum.[63]

ROLE IN DISEASE PATHOGENESIS

As with helminthic infections, the notable association of eosinophils with a variety of diseases of apparent allergic or uncertain etiologies has long prompted efforts to delineate the functions of eosinophils in these diseases. While increased blood and tissue eosinophils may imply their role in the immunopathogenesis of the associated disease, the absence of recognizable eosinophils in a disease does not obviate a possible role for these cells. An example of a disease *not* characteristically associated with eosinophilia is chronic urticaria. Using antisera specific for eosinophil granule MBP, the intralesional deposition of MBP has been demonstrated,[64] even in lesions not associated with dermal or blood eosinophilia. Therefore eosinophils may have participated in the immunopathogenesis of the disease despite absence of morphologic evidence of their presence. The finding of released eosinophil-specific granule proteins or of eosinophil-derived Charcot-Leyden crystals suggests the antecedent presence of eosinophils. In some circumstances eosinophils appear to lyse. Both cutaneous and pulmonary biopsies of eosinophil-associated diseases contain free, extracellular, but still membrane-bound, crystalloid-containing eosinophil granules.[65] The mechanism of cytolysis in such reactions is undefined but may occur more commonly than heretofore recognized. Thus, eosinophils may be involved even without lesional eosinophilia.*

In most diseases associated with eosinophils, their contribution to pathogenesis remains ill-defined. From their known functional capabilities and the mechanisms of their effector role in host defense against parasites, possible ways in which eosinophils may be involved can be inferred. For example, they may liberate compounds such as newly formed lipids or stored granule proteins, which could contribute to disease immunopathogenesis.

Release of Inflammatory Mediators

As noted above, eosinophils form two classes of biologically active lipids. And like other cells, they may liberate PAF.[51] The potent, diverse activities of PAF can be mediated directly or by stimulating other cells to release leukotrienes, prostaglandins, and complement peptides. Stimulated eosinophils also release LTC_4.[49,50] LTD_4 and LTF_4 are formed from LTC_4 by the sequential enzymatic removal of glutamic acid and glycine from its tripeptide glutathione side chain. LTC_4, and especially LTD_4, have bronchoconstrictor activity, constrict terminal arterioles, dilate venules, and stimulate airway mucous secretion.[66] Intracutaneous injection of these sulfidopeptide leukotrienes induces a wheal-and-flare response in humans.[66] Eosinophils stimulated with calcium ionophore or IgG-bearing zymosan particles[67] synthesize and release LTC_4. Thus, eosinophils are potential sources of two types of mediator lipids, the sulfidopeptide leukotrienes and the phospholipid analogue, PAF.

Release of mediators of inflammation from other cell types may also follow stimulation by eosinophil granule cationic proteins. The extracellular release of MBP and ECP from eosinophils has been documented in many conditions. Indirect immunofluorescence has demonstrated MBP in tissues from patients with eczema, urticaria, sinusitis, asthma, and dermatitis due to onchocerciasis. Radioimmunoassays have shown increased levels of MBP in blood.[2] Elevated levels of MBP have been found in the sputum of patients with asthma,[68] and increases in ECP have been documented in inflammatory synovial effusions.[69] MBP, which induces a wheal-and-flare reaction when injected intradermally, activates purified human basophils and rat mast cells to release histamine.[70] Although MBP is cytotoxic for parasites, the MBP-induced effect on mast cells occurs by a noncytotoxic, calcium- and energy-dependent mechanism.[70] Eosinophil peroxidase, by an enzymatic mechanism re-

quiring H_2O_2 and halide ion, also stimulates mediator release from mast cells.[71]

Release of Granule Proteins

Granule proteins may also contribute directly to the immunopathogenesis of eosinophil-related diseases by causing tissue dysfunction or destruction. Gleich and colleagues have provided evidence that one of these cationic proteins, MBP, may mediate cytotoxic as well as noncytotoxic activity on mammalian cells analogous to its action on parasites. Purified MBP applied to isolated guinea pig trachea in concentrations found in the sputum of asthmatics elicited dose-dependent effects on ciliated epithelial cells.[72-74] With lower concentrations of MBP, ciliary beating was impaired, whereas higher concentrations caused death and shedding of epithelial cells and pneumocytes. Airways of patients dying of asthma show similar shedding and desquamation of the bronchial epithelium down to the lamina propria and have extensive extracellular MBP deposits.[75] Thus, the eosinophil and its products may contribute to the pathologic changes accompaning asthma.[76] The possible role of eosinophil MBP in other diseases remains to be studied.

While MBP affects host cellular functioning by mechanisms that are uncertain except for its marked cationic charge, other granule constituents have enzymatic activities. As noted above, both EDN and ECP have RNase activity,[36] but whether their toxic effects are a consequence of this activity is unknown. ECP, unlike other eosinophil cationic proteins, can cause potentially lytic transmembrane pore formation.[37] Another cationic granule enzyme, eosinophil peroxidase, acting with cell-generated H_2O_2 and halide ion, can mediate toxic effects on host tissues and cells.[77]

Eosinophil granule collagenase cleaves collagen types I and III, and its release could damage connective tissue.[22,23,78] Eosinophils can also stimulate fibroblast proliferation.[79]

Although a beneficial role for the eosinophil as a helminthotoxic effector cell in the diverse immune response to parasitic infections appears certain, its role in other diseases is still unclear. Analogous to its role in killing parasites, the eosinophil may well be an effector cell contributing to their pathogenesis.

REFERENCES

1. Cohen, S.G., and Ottesen, E.A.: The eosinophil, eosinophilia, and eosinophil-related disorders. *In* Allergy Principles and Practice. 2nd Ed. Edited by E. Middleton, Jr., C.E. Reed, and E.F. Ellis. St. Louis, C.V. Mosby, 1983, pp. 701–769.

Editor's note. This is undoubtedly the case in synovial fluid, as discussed in Chapter 5.

2. Beeson, P.B., and Bass, D.A.: The Eosinophil. Philadelphia, W.B. Saunders, 1977.
3. Gleich, G.J., and Adolphson, C.R.: The eosinophilic leukocyte: Structure and function. Adv. Immunol., 39:177–253, 1986.
4. Basten, A., and Beeson, P.B.: Mechanism of eosinophilia. II. Role of the lymphocyte. J. Exp. Med., 131:1288–1305, 1970.
5. McGarry, M.P., Speirs, R.S., Jenkins, V.K., and Trentin, J.J.: Lymphoid cell dependence of eosinophil response to antigen. J. Exp. Med., 134:801–814, 1971.
6. Phillips, S.M., DiConza, J.J., Gold, J.A., and Reid, W.A.: Schistosomiasis in the congenitally athymic (nude) mouse. I. Thymic dependency of eosinophilia, granuloma formation, and host morbidity. J. Immunol., 118:594–599, 1977.
7. Metcalf, D.C., et al.: Biologic properties in vitro of a recombinant human granulocyte-macrophage colony-stimulating factor. Blood, 67:37–45, 1986.
8. Lopez, A.F., et al.: Murine eosinophil differentiation factor. An eosinophil-specific colony-stimulating factor with activity for human cells. J. Exp. Med., 163:1085–1099, 1986.
9. Clark, R.A.F., Gallin, J.I., and Kaplan, A.P.: The selective eosinophil chemotactic activity of histamine. J. Exp. Med., 142:1462–1476, 1975.
10. Goetzl, E.J., and Austen, K.F.: Purification and synthesis of eosinophilotactic tetrapeptides of human lung tissue. Identification as eosinophil chemotactic factor of anaphylaxis. Proc. Natl. Acad. Sci. U.S.A., 72:4123–4127, 1975.
11. Turnbull, L.W., and Kay, A.B.: Eosinophils and mediators of anaphylaxis. Histamine and imidazole acetic acid as chemotactic agents for human eosinophil leukocytes. Immunology, 31:797–802, 1976.
12. Wardlaw, A.J., Moqbel, R., Cromwell, O., and Kay, A.B.: Platelet-activating factor. A potent chemotactic and chemokinetic factor for human eosinophils. J. Clin. Invest., 78:1701–1706, 1986.
13. Sigal, C.E., Valone, F.H., Holtzman, M.J., and Goetzl, E.J.: Preferential human eosinophil chemotactic activity of the platelet-activating factor (PAF) 1-0-hexadecyl-2-acetyl-sn-glyceryl-3-phosphocholine (AGEPC). J. Clin. Immunol., 7:179–184, 1987.
14. Weller, P.F., Dvorak, J.A., and Whitehouse, W.C.: Human eosinophil stimulation promoter lymphokine: Production by antigen stimulated lymphocytes and assay with a new electro-optical technique. Cell. Immunol., 40:91–102, 1978.
15. Colley, D.G.: Lympholine-related eosinophil responses. Lymphokine Rep., 1:133–154, 1980.
16. Bainton, D.F., and Farquhar, M.G.: Segregation and packaging of granule enzymes in eosinophilic leukocytes. J. Cell. Biol., 45:54–73, 1970.
17. Parmley, R.T., and Spicer, S.S.: Cytochemical and ultrastructural identification of a small type granule in human late eosinophils. Lab. Invest., 30:557–567, 1974.
18. Parmley, R.T., and Spicer, S.S.: Altered tissue eosinophils in Hodgkin's disease. Exp. Mol. Pathol., 23:70–82, 1975.
19. Schaefer, H.E., Hubner, G., and Fischer, R.: Spezifische mikrogranula in eosinopilen. Acta Haematol. (Basel), 50:92–104, 1973.
20. Weller, P.F., and Dvorak, A.M.: Arachidonic acid incorporation by cytoplasmic lipid bodies of human eosinophils. Blood, 65:1269–1274, 1985.
21. West, B.C., Gelb, N.A., and Rosenthal, A.S.: Isolation and partial characterization of human eosinophil granules. Am. J. Pathol., 81:575–585, 1975.
22. Hibbs, M.S., Mainardi, C.L., and Kang, A.H.: Type-specific collagen degradation by eosinophils. Biochem. J., 207:621–624, 1982.
23. Davis, W.B., et al.: Eosinophil-mediated injury to lung parenchymal cells and interstitial matrix. J. Clin. Invest., 74:269–278, 1984.
24. Archer, G.T., and Hirsch, J.G.: Isolation of granules from eosinophil leucocytes and study of their enzyme content. J. Exp. Med., 118:277–284, 1963.
25. Gleich, G.J., et al.: Physicochemical and biological properties of the major basic protein in guinea pig eosinophil granules. J. Exp. Med., 140:313–332, 1974.
26. Gleich, G.J., et al.: Comparative properties of the Charcot-Leyden crystal protein and the major basic protein from human eosinophils. J. Clin. Invest., 57:633–640, 1976.
27. Lewis, D.M., Lewis, J.C., Loegering, D.A., and Gleich, G.J.: Localization of the guinea pig eosinophil major basic protein to the core of the granule. J. Cell. Biol., 77:702–713, 1978.
28. Peters, M.S., Rodriquez, M., and Gleich, G.J.: Localization of human eosinophil granule major basic protein, eosinophil cationic protein, and eosinophil-derived neurotoxin by immunoelectron microscopy. Lab. Invest., 54:656–662, 1986.
29. Weller, P.F., Ackerman, S.J., and Smith, J.A.: Eosinophil granule cationic proteins: Major basic protein is distinct from the smaller subunit of eosinophil peroxidase. J. Leukocyte Biol. (in press), 1988.
30. Ackerman, S.J., et al.: Localization of eosinophil granule major basic protein in human basophils. J. Exp. Med., 158:946–961, 1983.
31. Wever, R., Plat, H., and Hamers, M.N.: Human eosinophil peroxidase: A novel isolation procedure, spectral properties and chlorinating activity. FEBS Lett., 123:327–331, 1981.
32. Olsen, R.L., and Little, C.: Purification and some properties of myeloperoxidase and eosinophil peroxidase from human blood. Biochem J., 209:781–787, 1983.
33. Weiss, S.J., et al.: Brominating oxidants generated by human eosinophils. Science, 234:200–203, 1986.
34. Durack, D.T., Ackerman, S.J., Loegering, D.A., and Gleich, G.J.: Purification of human eosinophil-derived neurotoxin. Proc. Natl. Acad. Sci. U.S.A., 78:5165–5169, 1981.
35. Gleich, G.J., et al.: Biochemical and functional similarities between human eosinophil-derived neurotoxin and eosinophil cationic protein: Homology with ribonuclease. Proc. Natl. Acad. Sci. U.S.A., 83:3146–3150, 1986.
36. Slifman, N.R., Loegering, D.A., McKean, D.J., and Gleich, G.J.: Ribonuclease activity associated with human eosinophil-derived neurotoxin and eosinophil cationic protein. J. Immunol., 137:2913–2917, 1986.
37. Young, J. D-E., Peterson, C.G.B., Venge, P., and Cohn, Z.A.: Mechanism of membrane damage mediated by human eosinophil cationic protein. Nature, 321:613–616, 1986.
38. Brown, J.P., Rola-Pleszczynski, M., and Menard, H.-A.: Eosinophilic synovitis: Clinical observations on a newly recognized subset of patients with dermatographism. Arthritis Rheum., 29:1147–1151, 1986.
39. Weller, P.F., Goetzl, E.J., and Austen, K.F.: Identification of human eosinophil lysophospholipase as the constituent of Charcot-Leyden crystals. Proc. Natl. Acad. Sci. U.S.A., 77:7440–7443, 1980.
40. Weller, P.F., Bach, D., and Austen, K.F.: Human eosinophil lysophospholipase: The sole protein component of Charcot-Leyden crystals. J. Immunol., 128:1346–1349, 1982.
41. Weller, P.F., Bach, D.S., and Austen, K.F.: Biochemical characterization of human eosinophil Charcot-Leyden crystal protein (lysophospholipase). J. Biol. Chem., 259:15100–15104, 1984.
42. Ackerman, S.J., Weil, G.J., and Gleich, G.J.: Formation of Char-

cot-Leyden crystals by human basophils. J. Exp. Med., 155:1597–1609, 1982.

43. Changelian, P.S., and Fearon, D.T.: Tissue-specific phosphorylation of complement receptors CR1 and CR2. J. Exp. Med., 163:101–115, 1986.

44. Capron, M., et al.: Functional role of the α-chain of complement receptor type 3 in human eosinophil-dependent antibody-mediated cytotoxicity against schistosomes. J. Immunol., 139:2059–2065, 1987.

45. Hamada, A., and Greene, B.M.: C1q enhancement of IgG-dependent eosinophil-mediated killing of schistosomula in vitro. J. Immunol., 138:1240–1245, 1987.

46. Goers, J.W., et al.: Studies on C3a$_{hu}$ binding to human eosinophils: Characterization of binding. Int. Arch. Allergy Appl. Immunol., 74:147–151, 1984.

47. Kulczycki, A., Jr.: Human neutrophils and eosinophils have structurally distinct Fc gamma receptors. J. Immunol., 133:849–854, 1984.

48. Capron, M., et al.: Cytophilic IgE on human blood and tissue eosinophils: Detection by flow microfluorometry. J. Immunol., 134:3013–3018, 1985.

49. Weller, P.F., et al.: Generation and metabolism of 5-lipoxygenase pathway leukotrienes by human eosinophils: Predominant production of leukotriene C$_4$. Proc. Natl. Acad. Sci. U.S.A., 80:7626–7630, 1983.

50. Henderson, W.R., Harley, J.B., and Fauci, A.S.: Arachidonic acid metabolism in normal and hypereosinophilic syndrome human eosinophils: Generation of leukotrienes B$_4$, C$_4$, D$_4$ and 15-lipoxygenase products. Immunology, 51:679–686, 1984.

51. Lee, T., et al.: Increased biosynthesis of platelet-activating factor in activated human eosinophils. J. Biol. Chem., 259:5526–5530, 1984.

52. Spry, C.J.F., and Tai, P.C.: Studies on blood eosinophils. II. Patients with Loffler's cardiomyopathy. Clin. Exp. Immunol., 24:423–434, 1976.

53. Windqvist, I., et al.: Altered density, metabolism and surface receptors of eosinophils in eosinophilia. Immunology, 47:531–539, 1982.

54. Dvorak, A.M.: Ultrastructural evidence for release of major basic protein-containing crystalline cores of eosinophil granules in vivo: Cytotoxic potential in Crohn's disease. J. Immunol., 125:460–462, 1980.

55. Bass, D.A., et al.: Comparison of human eosinophils from normals and patients with eosinophilia. J. Clin. Invest., 66:1265–1273, 1980.

56. Pincus, S.H., Schooley, W.R., DiNapoli, A.M., and Broder, S.: Metabolic heterogeneity of eosinophils from normal and hypereosinophilic patients. Blood, 58:1175–1181, 1981.

57. Fukuda, T., et al.: Increased numbers of hypodense eosinophils in the blood of patients with bronchial asthma. Am. Rev. Respir. Dis., 132:981–985, 1985.

58. Prin, L., et al.: Heterogeneity of human peripheral blood eosinophils: Variability in cell density and cytotoxic ability in relation to the level and the origin of hypereosinophilia. Int. Arch. Allergy Appl. Immunol., 72:336–346, 1983.

59. Capron, M., et al.: Role of IgE receptors in effector function of human eosinophils. J. Immunol., 132:462–468, 1984.

60. David, J.R., et al.: Enhanced helminthotoxic capacity of eosinophils from patients with eosinophilia. N. Engl. J. Med., 303:1147–1152, 1980.

61. Kay, A.B.: The eosinophil in infectious disease. J. Infect. Dis., 129:606–613, 1974.

62. Bass, D.A., et al.: Eosinopenia of acute infection. Production of eosinopenia by chemotactic factors of acute inflammation. J. Clin. Invest., 65:1265–1271, 1980.

63. Butterworth, A.E.: Cell-mediated damage to helminths. Adv. Parasitol., 23:143–235, 1984.

64. Peters, M.S., Schroeter, A.L., Kephart, G.M. and Gleich, G.J.: Localization of eosinophil granule major basic protein in chronic urticaria. J. Invest. Dermatol., 81:39–43, 1983.

65. Gonzalez, E.B., et al.: Ultrastructural and immunohistochemical evidence for release of eosinophilic granules in vivo: Cytotoxic potential in chronic eosinophilic pneumonia. J. Allergy Clin. Immunol., 79:755–762, 1986.

66. Lewis, R.A., and Austen, K.F.: The biologically active leukotrienes. Biosynthesis, metabolism, receptors, functions, and pharmacology. J. Clin. Invest., 73:889–897, 1984.

67. Shaw, R.J., et al.: Activated human eosinophils generate SRS-A leukotrienes following IgG-dependent stimulation. Nature, 316:150–152, 1985.

68. Frigas, E., et al.: Elevated levels of the eosinophil granule major basic protein in the sputum of patients with bronchial asthma. Mayo Clin. Proc., 56:345–353, 1981.

69. Hallgren, R., Bjelle, A., and Venge, P.: Eosinophil cationic protein in inflammatory synovial effusions as evidence of eosinophil inolvement. Ann. Rheum. Dis., 43:556–562, 1984.

70. O'Donnell, M.C., Ackerman, S.J., Gleich, G.J., and Thomas, L.L.: Activation of basophil and mast cell histamine release by eosinophil granule major basic protein. J. Exp. Med., 157:1981–1991, 1983.

71. Henderson, W.R., Chi, E.Y., and Klebanoff, S.J.: Eosinophil peroxidase-induced mast cell secretion. J. Exp. Med., 152:265–279, 1980.

72. Frigas, E., Loegering, D.A., and Gleich, G.J.: Cytotoxic effects of the guinea pig eosinophil major basic protein on tracheal epithelium. Lab. Invest., 42:35–43, 1980.

73. Hastie, A.T., Loegering, D.A., Gleich, G.J., and Kueppers, F.: The effect of purified human eosinophil major basic protein on mammalian ciliary activity. Am. Rev. Respir. Dis., 135:848–853, 1987.

74. Ayars, G.H., et al.: Eosinophil- and eosinophil-granule mediated pneumocyte injury. J. Allergy Clin. Immunol., 76:595–604, 1985.

75. Filley, W.V., Holley, K.E., Kephart, G.M., and Gleich, G.J.: Identification by immunofluorescence of eosinophil granule major basic protein in lung tissues of patients with bronchial asthma. Lancet, 2:11–15, 1982.

76. Frigas, E., and Gleich, G.J.: The eosinophil and the pathophysiology of asthma. J. Allergy Clin. Immunol., 77:527–537, 1986.

77. Agosti, J.M., et al.: The injurious effect of eosinophil peroxidase, hydrogen peroxide, and halides on pneumocytes in vitro. J. Allergy Clin. Immunol., 790:496–504, 1987.

78. Bassett, E.G.: Eosinophils and connective tissue catabolism. Biochem. J., 213:769–770, 1983.

79. Pincus, S.H., Ramesch, K.S., and Wyler, D.J.: Eosinophils stimulate fibroblast DNA synthesis. Blood, 70:572–574, 1987.

THE MAST CELL IN RHEUMATIC DISEASES

22

BARRY L. GRUBER and ALLEN P. KAPLAN

The human mast cell is prominent beneath mucosal surfaces and is one of the critical cells responsible for allergic reactions. It possesses high-affinity surface receptors for immunoglobulin E (IgE) antibody. Interaction of bound IgE with allergens causes cell activation and degranulation, initiating the symptoms associated with immediate hypersensitivity. Human mast cells are also found throughout connective tissues, particularly around small blood vessels. Although in many pathologic conditions the number of these cells is increased, their precise contribution to the inflammatory reaction and to tissue injury remains unclear. Considerable evidence supports the idea that mast cells have the capability to modulate homeostasis in connective tissue, with obvious implications for our understanding of the complex events leading to articular destruction in the rheumatic disorders.

MORPHOLOGIC CHARACTERISTICS

Mast cells are large (12.6 μm in diameter); dense cytoplasmic granules occupy a sizable portion of the cell volume. These granules are 0.2 to 0.4 μm in diameter, and their contents react strongly with metachromatic dyes such as toluidine blue, azure A, methylene blue, or Giemsa stain. Nonmetachromatic stains, such as the chloracetate esters that react with granule-bound proteases, can also be used to identify mast cells.[1-3] Morphologists have further been able to identify mast cells in connective tissues by using flu-

orescence with berberine dyes or by allowing unconjugated avidin to react with the cytoplasmic granules.[4,5] Both these reactions depend on the granule core proteoglycan (heparin). Several cytoplasmic proteases are cell-specific, and monospecific antisera provide still another way to define mast cells in situ (Fig. 22–1).[6,7]

With better ability to recognize mast cells there has been a growing appreciation of the abundance of these cells in certain disease states. Some examples in humans include the tissue involved with advancing tumors, inflammatory synovium, senile osteoporosis, scleroderma, keloids, pulmonary fibrosis, chronic obstructive lung disease, inflammatory bowel disease, acute hepatitis, chronic urticaria, Behçet's disease, and chronic allograft rejection.[8-26] The significance of the increased numbers of mast cells in these disparate conditions is as yet unknown. A recurrent theme is their proximity to chronic inflammatory lesions leading to connective tissue alterations. Whether the mast cell population arises by proliferation in situ or by migration, (or both) is not known. That interleukin 4 (B-cell stimulating factor 1) causes proliferation of connective tissue mast cells favors the former possibility and indicates communication between mast cells and T lymphocytes.[27]

MEDIATORS

Considerable information exists about the secretory products derived from mast cells.[3,28,29] These products

374

FIG. 22–1. Mast cells in rheumatoid synovium visualized using immunoperoxidase techniques with monoclonal antibodies directed to the cytoplasmic protease tryptase. This enzyme is unique to mast cells and highlights these cells in the subsynovial layers of this tissue. ($\times$625). (Courtesy of Dr. L.B. Schwartz.)

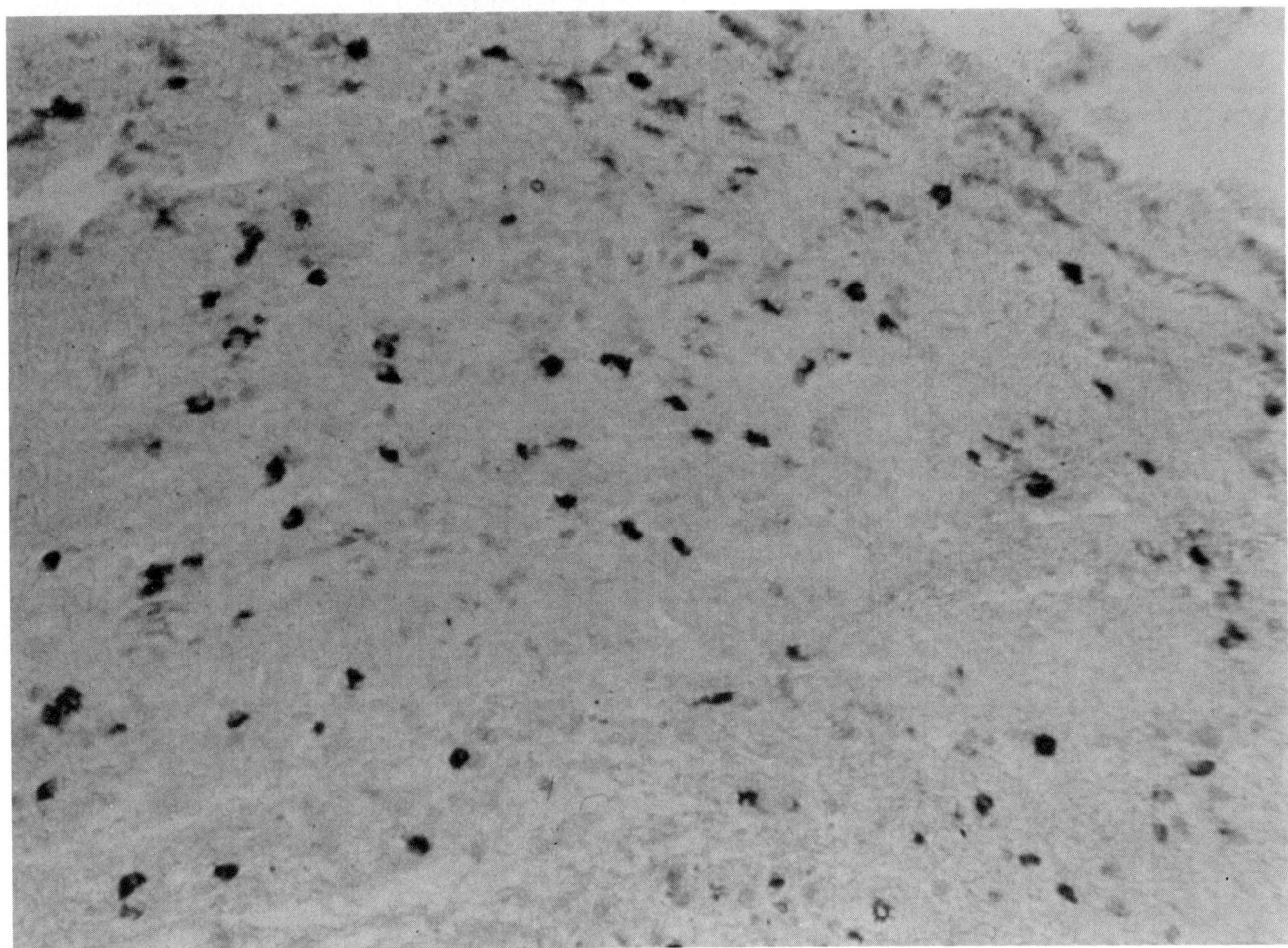

have been classified into (1) preformed; (2) newly synthesized; and (3) granule-associated (Table 22–1). Each of these compounds has diverse biologic effects (Table 22–2). Only a few compounds are unique and therefore specific markers of mast cell secretion. These include prostaglandin D_2, tryptase, and histamine; although histamine is also found in appreciable quantity in basophils. These markers can be quantitated in different diseases using radioenzymatic and immunoassays and reflect the degree of mast cell involvement. Although mast cells are also the major repository for heparin, sensitive and practical quantitative assays are still lacking.

SECRETION

The local release of granule constituents may follow a variety of stimuli. The sequence of biochemical events preceding release has been studied in detail.[30–32] The classic scheme for activation involves the cross linkage of at least two high-affinity IgE receptors on the cell membrane. This process may be initiated by aggregating membrane-bound specific IgE after antigen exposure. IgG_4 may also initiate degranulation through specific receptors, albeit less efficiently.[33] Many other compounds may activate these cells;[28,29] for example, basic anions such as compound 48/80, small basic peptides C3a and C5a derived from complement activation, bivalent concanavalin A, calcium ionophores A23187 and X537A, staphylococcal protein A, hyperosmolar mannitol, ionomycin, certain peptidases and lipases, thrombin, and substance P.[34–40] Moreover, other types of cells may secrete substances that then activate mast cells and basophils. Investigation of this secretion has begun to turn at-

Table 22–1. Human Mast Cell Mediators

Preformed and eluted
  Histamine
  Eosinophil chemotactic factors
  Neutrophil chemotactic factors
  Superoxide
  Arylsulfatase A
  Elastase
  β-Hexosaminidase
  β-Glucosonidase
  β-Galactosidase
  Kallikrein-like enzyme
Preformed and granule associated
  Heparin/chondroitin sulfate E
  Tryptase
  Chymotrypsin-like protease
  Superoxide dismutase, catalase (rodents)
  Arylsulfatase B
Newly generated
  Leukotrienes (LTC$_4$, LTD$_4$, LTE$_4$)
  Platelet-activating factor
  Prostaglandins (PGD$_2$)

tention from specific IgE-coupled activation to cytokine-mediated mast cell activation in chronic inflammatory disorders. Products secreted by monocytes, lymphocytes, neutrophils, and platelets have been shown to have histamine-releasing activity.[41-46] In vitro experiments with purified recombinant interleukin 1 and gamma interferon also suggest that these substances can either initiate or augment basophil (and perhaps mast cell) degranulation independently of the aforementioned "histamine releasing factors."[47,48] Preliminary data suggest that certain growth factors, such as interleukins 3, 4, and 5, may stimulate

the proliferation of mast cells,[49] but whether they also cause secretion is unclear.

Certain characteristic morphologic changes concomitant with mast cell activation can be seen by electron microscopy (Fig. 22–2). At the earliest stages, mast cell granules have highly organized crystalline-like structures containing scrolls, gratings, and lattice formation. These structures become swollen with reduced electron density coinciding with solubilization of the matrix. Individual granules then fuse, forming interconnecting channels that progressively expand and merge with the plasma membrane. Mediators and granule components are then extruded through small openings in these newly formed "degranulation sacs." This sequence is in contrast to that seen in human basophils, in which individual granules fuse with the plasma membrane.[50]

The cascade of biochemical events that accompany these morphologic events is complex. It appears that the process is initiated with the activation of a serine esterase, followed immediately by adenyl cyclase activation and methylation of membrane phospholipids (Fig. 22–3). The control and precise characteristics of the initial IgE-dependent esterase reaction remain unclear at present. The evidence for this enzyme stems from the observations that certain proteases in the presence of calcium may themselves initiate degranulation, and serine esterase inhibitors may modulate histamine release.[55,56]

Within seconds after aggregation of IgE receptors, intracellular cAMP levels rise,[57] and cAMP-dependent protein kinases are activated.[58] The adenyl cyclase activation appears to be regulated by the methylation

Table 22–2. Actions of Mast Cell Products

Selected Mediators	Actions
Histamine	Triple response of Lewis (vasodilatation, endothelial cell contraction and increased vascular permeability, axon reflex) (H$_1$), pruritus (H$_1$), gastric acid secretion (H$_2$), lymphocyte suppression (H$_2$), chondrocyte activation (H$_2$), regulation of synovial microcirculation (H$_2$), chemoattraction (eosinophils)
Heparin	Anticoagulation, anticomplementary (C1q binding, C$_4$, C$_2$, C$_3$ activation, C3bBb convertase), stimulation of angiogenesis, enhancement of elastase activity, modulation of parathyroid hormone-calcitonin to induce osteoporosis, stimulation of collagenase synthesis, inhibition of activated collagenase, stabilization of tryptase, potentiation of fibronectin binding to collagen
Tryptase	Cleavage of trypsin substrates, inactivation of fibrinogen and high molecular weight kininogen, generation of C3$_a$ from C$_3$, activation of latent synovial collagenase
Chymotrypsin-like protease	Cleavage of chymotrypsin substrates, cleavage by protease of fibronectin, laminin, conversion of angiotensin I to II, cleavage of dermal-epidermal junction
Prostaglandins (PGD$_2$)	Bronchoconstriction, chemoattraction, inhibition of platelet aggregation, vasodilatation, potentiation of LTC$_4$ on vasculature
Leukotrienes (LTC$_4$, LTD$_4$, LTE$_4$)	Slow-reacting substances of anaphylaxis, smooth muscle contraction, vasodilatation
Platelet-activating factor	Activation of neutrophils, platelets, smooth muscle contraction vasopermeability, chemotaxis for eosinophils and neutrophils
Kallikrein-like enzyme	Generation of bradykinin

FIG. 22–2. Ultrastructural analysis of human mast cells at rest (A) and 20 min. after exposure of antibody to IgE (B). Note that after activation the mast cell develops numerous degranulation channels containing altered granule matrix material. (A), ×9,000; (B), ×8,000. (From Dvorak, A.M., et al.: Basophil and mast cell degranulation: ultrastructural analysis of mechanisms of mediator release. Fed. Proc., 42:2,510–2,515, 1983.)

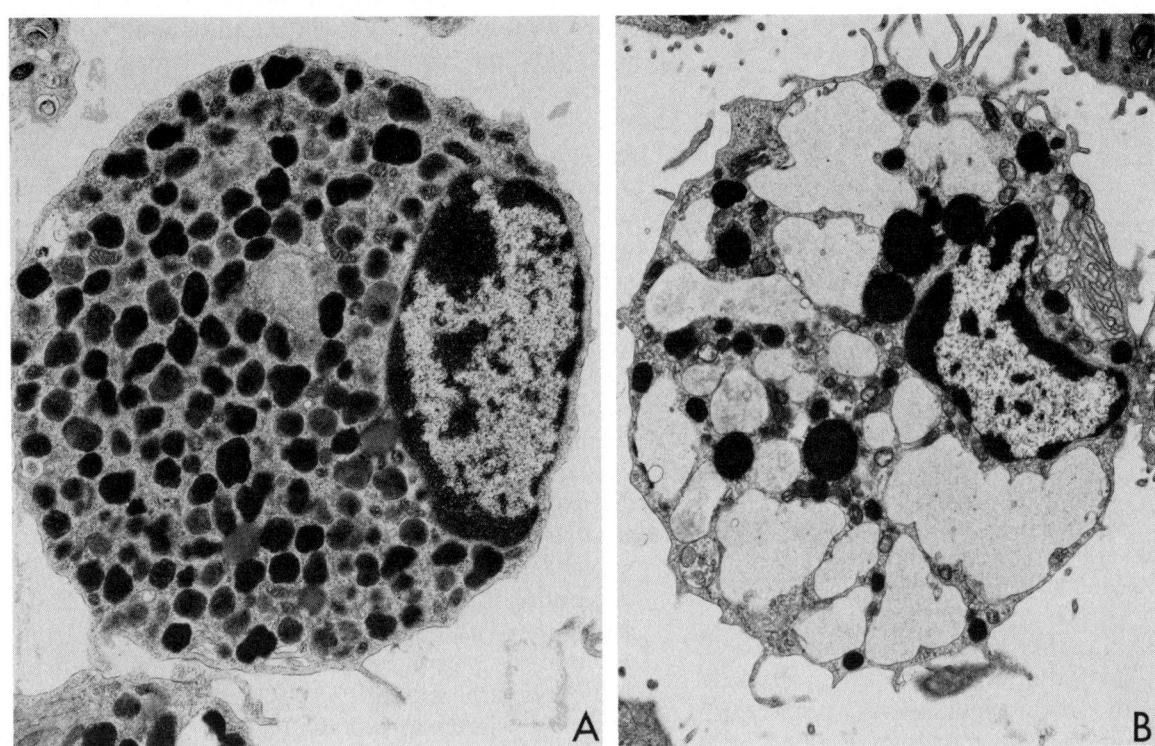

of membrane phospholipids because inhibition of the methyl transferase abrogates the rise in cAMP. In fact, the metabolism of the membrane phospholipids is critical for IgE-mediated histamine release.[59–61] The formation of phosphatidylethanolamine from phosphatidylserine and then donation of methyl groups to yield phosphatidylcholine appears requisite for the uptake of extracellular calcium necessary for degranulation. This turnover of phospholipids also provides substrates for endogenous-activated phospholipases A_2 and C to generate arachidonic acid and the fusogen, diacylglycerol. The liberated arachidonic acid is further metabolized to a variety of products, including prostaglandins, leukotrienes, and platelet-activating factor. These products, together with cyclic adenosine monophosphate (cAMP), appear to have a feedback role in the internal regulation of the activation process.[62]

HETEROGENEITY

Rodent mast cells studied displayed heterogeneity from one organ system to another, giving rise to the concept of *typical* and *atypical* mast cells, or *connective-tissue* and *mucosal-type* mast cells, respectively.[63–66] Differences in morphology, histochemistry, granule content, response to certain agonists and antagonists of histamine release, and growth requirements were recorded. The interest of immunologists was aroused by the discovery that the growth of mucosal or bone marrow-derived mast cells was dependent on factor(s) released from T lymphocytes, termed interleukin 3.[65–67] Recent work shows that differentiation into distinct cellular subsets is controlled by still undefined factors in the local tissue microenvironment. Differentiated mast cells take up residence in the appropriate organ system and show the expected phenotypic characteristics after they are injected into mast-cell deficient mice.[68,69]

Difficulties in extrapolating the rodent studies to the human system have led to considerable controversy. The lymphocyte-dependent mucosal or bone marrow-derived mast cell has not been clearly isolated in man. Nonetheless, mast cells isolated from human skin, nasal mucosa, lung parenchyma, or gastrointestinal mucosa behave differently in vitro.[70] Such dif-

FIG. 22–3. The cascade of membrane events following activation of IgE receptors, leading to degranulation. Stimuli that may be relevant in rheumatic disease to initiate degranulation are listed.

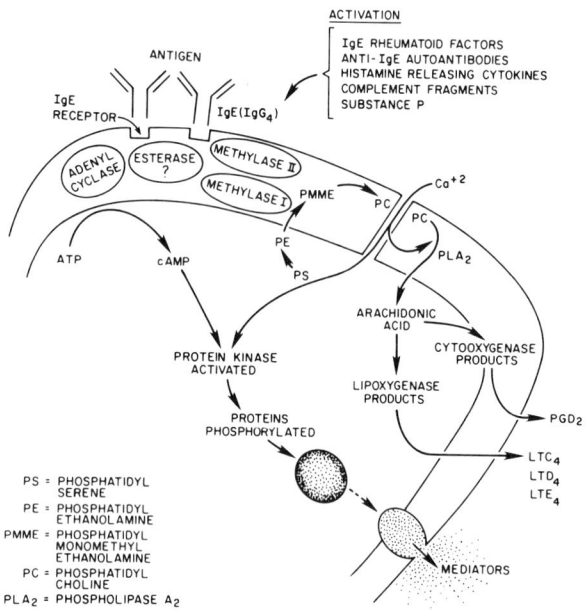

ferences include the profile of arachidonate metabolites, quantity of histamine, type of granule proteoglycan, and the expression of specific proteases. The responsiveness to certain secretagogues and the ability to inhibit degranulation by specific compounds also differ in cells obtained from different tissues.

Although the importance of cellular heterogeneity is not immediately evident, such differences may be useful when one attempts to manipulate mast cells in a given disease. Two separate types of mast cells can be identified in normal human intestinal mucosa by their protease content, but that only one type is observed in patients with acquired immunodeficiency suggests possible interplay between lymphocytes and distinct subsets of mast cells.[71] The relevance of this observation to mast cells arising in a lymphocyte-rich synovium or in the dermis of a patient with early scleroderma remains to be determined.

CONNECTIVE TISSUE DISORDERS

Mast cell numbers are increased in the synovium of patients with rheumatoid arthritis, juvenile arthritis, psoriatic arthritis, ankylosing spondylitis, Lyme arthritis, and rat adjuvant arthritis.[10–15,72–79] This increase is likely a non-specific finding. The degree of

local mast cell hyperplasia seems related to the extent of mononuclear cell infiltrate.[14] Mast cells in the rheumatoid synovium have been partially characterized and can be activated in vitro by both IgE-dependent mechanisms and mononuclear cell products.[10,80] Immunoperoxidase labeling techniques show mast cell-specific protease (tryptase) throughout the rheumatoid synovium (see Fig. 22–1). Different mast cell subsets, as defined by the specific granule-associated proteases, are scattered throughout the rheumatoid synovium.[81]

Initial speculations on the contribution of the mast cell to the pathogenesis of the rheumatoid lesion have focused on the release of mediators regulating the synovial inflammatory response. These mediators include compounds that have chemotactic and chemokinetic activity leading to the recruitment of inflammatory cells into the tissue while simultaneously enhancing vasopermeability. The synovial microcirculation contains specific H_2 receptors for histamine.[82] In addition, many of the low-molecular-weight mediators, such as histamine and the leukotrienes, are capable of modulating cellular immune responses.[83]

Perhaps the most intriguing observations are those implicating mast cells in matrix degradation and bone resorption. Accumulations of mast cells have been noted at the periphery of invasive adenocarcinomas and other tumors with morphologic evidence of degranulation in the area of matrix dissolution.[84–85] Similar findings have been noted in chronic periodontal disease, with ultrastructural evidence of fraying of collagen fibers near the site of mast cell degranulation.[86] Furthermore, drugs inhibiting mast cell degranulation in a canine model of periodontal disease diminished the degree of associated bone resorption.[87] Hence, the finding of mast cell clusters at the site of cartilage erosion near the pannus junction and along the resorbing subchondral bone in rheumatoid joints is of interest.[13,88] These observations have prompted studies suggesting that mast cell products may stimulate synoviocytes and chondrocytes to release collagenase and prostaglandin E_2.[89–91] Mast cell proteinases can activate latent collagenase and promote collagenolysis.[84,86,92–94] Tryptase may be important in this regard because it lacks any apparent natural serum inhibitors. Mast cell proteases may also play a role in digesting matrix glycoproteins and minor collagens; type IV collagen, fibronectin, and proteoglycans are all substrates for rodent mast cell proteases.[95–97]

Intercellular interactions involving mast cells may lead indirectly to connective tissue degradation. Fibroblasts ingest mast cell granules in vitro and respond by releasing collagenase and prostaglandin

E_2.[98] Chondrocytes are capable of responding to histamine by way of H_2 receptors with a rise in intracellular cAMP.[99] Another granule constituent, heparin, has potent skeletal effects. Long-term administration of heparin induces osteoporosis.[100–102] This effect may be secondary to complex interactions between parathyroid hormone, calcitonin, and heparin or perhaps mediated through procollagenase stimulation.[103–106] Whatever the mechanism, the association between osteopenia and mast cells is also seen in patients with systemic mastocytosis. Areas of both localized osteopenia and osteosclerosis are often manifested in the same patient.[107] Several reports have drawn attention to increased skeletal mast cells in idiopathic senile osteoporosis.[108,109]

An additional potential effect of heparin released from synovial mast cells is its ability to sustain angiogenesis. Proliferation of new blood vessels is an integral feature of rheumatoid pannus. In vitro, heparin has the ability to bind and stimulate migration of endothelial cells.[110–112]

Although most evidence supports a role for mast cells in degradative processes, mast cells may also participate in the growth and repair of connective tissues.[113] That the number of mast cells decreases in the vicinity of incisional wounds in rats suggests degranulation.[114,115] Others have noted increased mast cells at the site of experimentally induced bone fracture.[116] Certain conditions involving excessive synthesis of connective tissue elements have been associated with mast cells, such as keloids and pulmonary fibrosis.[117,119] Mast cell hyperplasia has been noted in the involved skin of patients with early scleroderma.[120] The significance of this finding is under scrutiny using a model of chronic graft-versus-host disease, where serial skin biopsies show progressive fibrosis associated with mast cell depletion, implying degranulation.[121] Another model for idiopathic scleroderma in humans is the toxic oil syndrome, where changes in the dermis include fibrosis and a marked mast cell infiltrate.[122]

ACTIVATION

Although considerable speculation and some supportive data indicate the potential for mast cells to modulate connective tissue metabolism, what stimulates mast cell secretion in these diseases? Histamine-releasing factors secreted from activated mononuclear cells may play an important role, and IgE antiglobulins in rheumatoid arthritis may allow binding to aggregates of IgG and subsequent degranulation.[123–125] Autoantibodies directed against IgE itself have been reported in systemic lupus erythematosus and rheumatoid arthritis.[126,127] Anaphylatoxins generated during complement activation may also act locally to activate mast cells. Neuropeptides, such as substance P, have been identified in rheumatoid joint fluid and can degranulate mast cells.[39,128]

Mast cells are potentially important in connective tissue homeostasis. They are gaining recognition as consistent components of the connective tissue disorders. Although much of the evidence for their pathogenetic role is indirect, advances are being made which should provide a conceptual framework regarding their contribution to the degradative or proliferative lesions in disease states.

REFERENCES

1. Benditt, E.P., and Lagunoff, D.: The mast cell: its structure and function. Prog. Allergy, *8*:195, 1964.
2. Kramer, H., and Windrum, G.M.: The metachromatic staining reaction. J. Histochem. Cytochem., *3*:227, 1955.
3. Metcalfe, D.D., Kaliner, M., and Donlon, M.A.: The mast cell. Crit. Rev. Immunol., *3*:23, 1981.
4. Enerback, L.: Berberine sulfate binding to mast cell polyanions: a cytofluorometric method for quantitation of heparin. Histochemistry, *42*:301–313, 1974.
5. Bergstresser, P.R., Tigelaar, R.E., and Thorp, M.D.: Conjugated avidin identified cutaneous rodent and human mast cells. J. Invest. Derm., *83*:214–218, 1984.
6. Schwartz, L.B., Foley, J.V., and Austen, K.F.: Localization of tryptase to human cutaneous mast cells and keratinocytes by immunofluorescence and immunoperoxidase cytochemistry with monoclonal anti-tryptase antibody. J. Allergy Clin. Immunol., *76*:182–190, 1985.
7. Schecter, N.M., et al.: Human skin mast cells contain high concentration of two serine proteinases with different specificities. (abstract.) J. Invest. Dermatol., *86*:505, 1986.
8. Dvorak, H.F., et al.: Human breast carcinoma: fibrin deposits and desmoplasia: inflammatory cell type and distribution. J. Natl. Cancer Inst., *67*:335–345, 1981.
9. Hartveit, F., Thoresen, S., Tangen, M., and Maartman-Moe, H.: Mast cell changes and tumor dissemination in human breast carcinoma. Invasion Metastasis, *4*:146–156, 1984.
10. Gruber, B., et al.: Characterization and functional studies of rheumatoid synovial mast cells: activation by secretagogues, anti-IgE and a histamine-releasing lymphokine. Arthritis Rheum., *29*:944–955, 1986.
11. Crisp, A.J., et al.: Articular mastocytosis in rheumatoid arthritis. Arthritis Rheum., *27*:845–855, 1984.
12. Godfrey, H.P., Ilardi, C.F., Engber, W., and Graziano, F.M.: Quantitation of human synovial mast cells in rheumatoid arthritis and other rheumatic diseases. Arthritis Rheum., *27*:852–856, 1984.
13. Bromley, M., Fischer, W.D., and Wooley, D.E.: Mast cells at site of cartilage erosion in the rheumatoid joint. Ann. Rheum. Dis., *43*:76–79, 1984.
14. Malone, D.G., Wilder, R.C., Saavedra-Delgado, A.M., and Metcalfe, D.D.: Mast cell numbers in rheumatoid synovial tissues: correlation with quantitative measures of lymphocytic

infiltration and modulation by anti-inflammatory therapy. Arthritis Rheum., *30*:130–138, 1987.

15. Freemont, A.J., and Denton, J.: Disease distribution of synovial fluid mast cells and cytophagocytic mononuclear cells in inflammatory arthritis. Ann. Rheum. Dis., *44*:312–315, 1985.

16. Cohen, I.K., Beaven, M.A., Horakova, Z., and Keiser, H.R.: Histamine and collagen synthesis in keloid and hypertrophic scars. Surg. Forum, 23:509–510, 1972.

17. Groto, T., Befus, D., Low, R., and Bienenstock, J.: Mast cell heterogeneity and hyperplasia in bleomycin-induced pulmonary fibrosis in rats. Am. Rev. Respir. Dis., *130*:797–802, 1984.

18. Kay, A. B., et al.: The mast cell and chronic bronchitis. *In* The Mast Cell—Its Role in Health and Disease. Edited by J. Pepys and A.M. Gordon. Kent, England, Pittman Medicine, 1979, pp. 236–248.

19. Lamb, D., and Lumden, A.: Intraepithelial mast cells in human airway epithelium: evidence for smoking induced changes in their frequency. Thorax, *37*:334–342, 1982.

20. McAuley, R.C., and Sommers, S.C.: Mast cells in nonspecific ulcerative colitis. Am. J. Dig. Dis., *6*:233–236, 1961.

21. Dvorak, A.M., Monahan, R.A., Osage, J.E., and Dickerson, G.R.: Mast cell degranulation in Crohn's disease. Lancet, *1*:498, 1978.

22. Bardadin, K.A., and Scheuer, P.J.: Mast cells in acute hepatitis. J. Pathol., *149*:315–325, 1986.

23. Natbony, S.F., Philips, M., Elias, J.M. and Kaplan, A.P.: Histologic studies of chronic idiopathic urticaria. J. Allergy Clin. Immunol., *71*:177, 1983.

24. Lichtig, L., Harohn, S., Hammel, I., and Friedman-Birnbaum, R.: The quantification and significance of mast cells in lesions of Behçet's disease. Br. J. Dermatol., *102*:255–259, 1980.

25. Colvin, R.B., and Dvorak, H.F.: Basophils and mast cells in renal allograft rejection. Lancet, *1*:212–214, 1974.

26. Moore, T.C., Thompson, D.P., and Glassock, R.J.: Elevation of urinary and blood histamine following clinical renal transplantation. Ann. Surg., *173*:381–388, 1971.

27. Mosmann, T.R., Bond, M.O., and Coffman, R.L.: T cells and mast cell lines respond to B cell stimulatory factor-1. Proc. Natl. Acad. Sci. U.S.A., *83*:5,654–5,658, 1986.

28. Schwartz, L.B.: The mast cells. *In* Allergy. Edited by A.P. Kaplan. New York, Churchill Livingstone, 1985, pp. 53–92.

29. Gershwin, M.E. (Ed.): The mast cell. Clin. Rev. Allergy, *1*:343–417, 1983.

30. Ishizaka, T.: Analysis of triggering events in mast cells for immunoglobulin E-mediated histamine release. J. Allergy Clin. Immunol., *167*:90–98, 1986.

31. Ishizaka, T., et al.: Bridging of IgE receptors activates phospholipid methylation and adenylate cyclase in mast cell plasma membranes. Proc. Natl. Acad. Sci. U.S.A., *78*:6,812–6,815, 1986.

32. Kennerly, D.A., Sullivan, T.J., and Parker, C.W.: Activation of phospholipid metabolism during mediator release from stimulated rat mast cells. J. Immunol., *122*:152–157, 1979.

33. Perelmutter, L.: IgG4 and the immune system. Clin. Rev. Allergy, *1*:269–281, 1983.

34. Foreman, J.C., Mongar, B.D., and Gomperts, B.D.: Calcium ionophores and movement of calcium ions following the physiological stimulus to a secretory process. Nature, *245*:249–251, 1973.

35. Siraganian, R.P.: Basophil activation by concanavalin A. *In* The Role of Mitogens in Immunology. Edited by J.J. Oppen-

heim, and D.L. Rosenstrich. New York, Academic Press, 1976, p. 69.

36. Hugli, T.E., and Muller-Eberhard, H.J.: Anaphylatoxins: C3a and C5a. Adv. Immunol., *26*:1–43, 1978.

37. Findlay, S.R., Dvorak, A.M., and Lichtenstein, L.M.: Hyperosmolar triggering of basophil histamine release. J. Allergy Clin. Immunol., *65*:170–176, 1980.

38. Marx, G., Barnes, D., and Razin, E.: Thrombin selective activation of mast cells. Fed. Proc., *45*:1,324, 1985.

39. Webber, S.E., and Foreman, J.C.: The effect of substance P and related peptides on the guinea pig lung strip. Agents Actions, *14*:425–428, 1984.

40. Foreman, J.C.: Peptides and histamine release. J. Allergy Clin. Imunol., *74*:127, 1984.

41. Thueson, D.O., Speck, L.S., Lett-Brown, M.A., and Grant, J.A.: Histamine-releasing activity (HRA) I. Production by mitogen or antigen-stimulated human mononuclear cells. J. Immunol., *123*:626–632, 1979.

42. Sedgwick, J.D., Hoit, P.G., and Turner, K.J.: Production of a histamine releasing lymphokine by antigen or mitogen-stimulated human peripheral T cells. Clin. Exp. Immunol., *45*:409–415, 1981.

43. Kaplan, A.P., Halbert, E., Fauci, A., and Dinarello, C.: A histamine releasing factor from activated human mononuclear cells. J. Immunol., *135*:2,027–2,032, 1985.

44. Schulman, E.S., et al.: Human lung macrophages induce histamine release from basophil and mast cells. Am. Rev. Respir. Dis., *131*:230–235, 1985.

45. White, M.V., Kaliner, M.A., and Baer, H.: Stimulated neutrophils release a histamine releasing factor. (Abstract.) J. Allergy Clin. Immunol., *77*:132, 1986.

46. Fisher, R.H., et al.: Platelet-basophil interactions: Clinical correlates. (abstract) J. Allergy Clin. Immunol., *79*:196, 1987.

47. Haak-Frendscho, M., et al.: Recombinant IL-1 causes histamine release from human basophils. (abstract.) J. Allergy Clin. Immunol., *77*:230, 1986.

48. Ida, S., et al.: Enhancement of IgE-mediated histamine release from human basophils by viruses: role of interferon. J. Exp. Med., *145*:892–900, 1977.

49. Hamaguchi, Y., et al.: Interleukin 4 as an essential growth factor for in vitro clonal growth of murine connective tissue-type mast cells. J. Exp. Med., *165*:268–273, 1987.

50. Dvorak, A.M., et al.: Basophil and mast cell degranulation: ultrastructural analysis of mechanisms of mediator release. Fed. Proc., *42*:2,510–2,515, 1983.

51. Ishizaka, T., Conrad, D.H., and Schulman, E.S.: Biochemical analysis of initial triggering events of IgE-mediated histamine release from human lung mast cells. J. Immunol., *130*:2,357–2,361, 1983.

52. Ishizaka, T., Hirata, F., and Sterk, A.R.: Bridging of IgE receptors activates phospholipid methylation and adenylate cyclase in mast cell plasma membranes. Proc. Natl. Acad. Sci. U.S.A., *78*:6,812–6,815, 1981.

53. Kaliner, M., and Austen, K.F.: A sequence of biochemical events in the antigen-induced release of chemical mediators from sensitized human lung tissue. J. Exp. Med., *138*:1,077–1,094, 1974.

54. Siraganian, R.P.: Biochemical events in basophil/mast cell activation and mediator secretion. *In* Allergy. Edited by A.P. Kaplan. New York, Churchill Livingstone, 1985, pp. 31–52.

55. Meier, H.L., et al.: Histamine release by esterase inhibitors. Int. Arch. Allergy Appl. Immunol., *77*:218–221, 1985.

56. Ishizaka, T.: Analysis of triggering events in mast cells for

immunoglobulin E-mediated histamine release. J. Allergy Clin. Immunol., 167:90–96, 1981.

57. Winslow, C.M., Lewis, R.A., and Austen, K.F.: Mast cell mediator release as a function of cyclic-AMP-dependent protein kinase activation. J. Exp. Med., 154:1,125–1,136, 1981.

58. Holgate, S.T., Lewis, R.A., and Austen, K.F.: Rat serosal mast cell 3′–5′ cyclic adenosine monophosphate-dependent protein kinase and its immunologic activation. J. Immunol., 124:2,093,–2,099, 1980.

59. McGivney, A., et al.: Rat basophilic leukemia cell lines defective in phospholipid methyltransferase enzymes, Ca^{2+} influx, and histamine release: reconstitution by hybridization. Proc. Natl. Acad. Sci. U.S.A., 78:6,176–6,179, 1981.

60. Ishizaka, T., et al.: IgE-mediated triggering signals for mediator release from human mast cells and basophils. Fed. Proc., 43:2,840–2,845, 1984.

61. Morita, Y., Chiang, P.K., and Siraganian, R.P.: Effect of inhibitors of transmethylation on histamine release from human basophils. Biochem. Pharm., 30:785–790, 1981.

62. Urata, C., and Siraganian, R.P.: Pharmacologic modulation of Ca^{2+} influx, phospholipase activation and histamine release in rat basophilic leukemic cells. Fed. Proc., 42:1,342–1,347, 1983.

63. Beinenstock, T., et al.: Comparative aspects of mast cell heterogeneity in different species and sites. Int. Arch. Allergy Appl. Immunol., 77:126–129, 1985.

64. Enerback, L.: Mast cells in rat gastrointestinal mucosa. I. Effects of fixation. Acta Pathol. Microbiol. Scand., 66:289–302, 1966.

65. Razin, E., et al.: Culture from mouse bone marrow of a subclass of mast cells possessing a distinct chondroitin sulfate proteoglycan with glycosaminoglycan rich in N-acetyl-galactosamine-4-6-disulfate. J. Biol. Chem., 257:7,229–7,236, 1982.

66. Haig, D.M., McKee, T.H., and Jarret, E.E.R.: Generation of mucosal mast cells is stimulated in vitro by factors derived from T cells of helminth-infected rats. Nature, 300:188–191, 1982.

67. Ihle, J.N., et al.: Biological properties of homogenous interleukin 3. I. Demonstration of WEH1-3 growth factor activity, mast cell growth activity, P-cell stimulatory activity, colony stimulating factor activity and histamine-producing cell-stimulating factor activity. J. Immunol., 130:282–286, 1983.

68. Otou, K., et al.: Phenotypic changes of bone marrow-derived mast cells after peritoneal transfer into w/w^2 mice that are genetically deficient in mast cells. J. Exp. Med., 165:615–628, 1987.

69. Nakano, T., et al.: Fate of bone marrow-derived cultured mast cells after intracutaneous, intraperitoneal, and intravenous transfer into genetically mast cell deficient $w/w^{/2}$ mice: evidence that cultured mast cells can give rise to both connective tissue type and mucosal mast cells. J. Exp. Med., 162:1,025–1,032, 1985.

70. Barrett, K.E., and Metcalfe, D.D.: Mast cell heterogeneity: evidence and implications. J. Clin. Immunol., 4:253–261, 1984.

71. Irani, A.A., et al.: Selective depletion of tryptase mast cells in intestinal mucosa of patients with defective T-lymphocyte function. (Abstract.) J. Allergy Clin. Immunol., 79:179, 1987.

72. Sajveiya, K.: Synovial mast cells. Indian J. Pathol. Microbiol., 26:111–115, 1983.

73. Okada, J.: The mast cell in synovial membrane of patients with joint diseases. Jpn. J. Orthop. Surg., 47:657–674, 1973.

74. Crisp, A.J.: Mast cells in rheumatoid arthritis. J. R. Soc. Med., 77:450–451, 1984.

75. Malone, D.A., Irani, A.M., and Schwartz, L.B.: Mast cell numbers and histamine levels in synovial fluids from patients with diverse arthritides. Arthritis Rheum., 29:956–963, 1986.

76. Athreya, B.H., Moser, G., and Schumacher, H.R.: Role of basophils and mast cells in juvenile rheumatoid arthritis. In The Mast Cell: Its Role in Health and Disease. Edited by J. Pepys and A.M. Edwards. London, Pittman Medicine, 1979, pp. 127–136.

77. Shichikawa, K., Tsujimoto, M., and Nishioka, T.: Histopathology of early sacroiliitis and enthesitis in ankylosing spondylitis. Adv. Inflamm. Res., 9:15–24, 1985.

78. Johnson, Y.E., et al.: Lyme arthritis spirochetes found in synovial microangiopathic lesions. Am. J. Pathol., 118:26–34, 1985.

79. Gryfe, A., Sanders, P.M., and Gardner, D.L.: The mast cell in early rat adjuvant arthritis. Ann. Rheum. Dis., 30:24–30, 1971.

80. Gruber, B.L., Haak-Frendscho, M., and Kaplan, A.P.: Mononuclear cell factor induces secretion of synovial mast cells. (Abstract.) Arthritis Rheum., 28:570, 1985.

81. Irani, A.M., Golzar, N., Deblois, G., and Gruber, B.L.: Distribution of mast cell subsets in rheumatoid arthritis and osteoarthritis synovia. (Abstract.) Arthritis Rheum., 30:566, 1987.

82. Grennan, D.M., Rooney, P.J., and Onge, P.M.: Histamine receptors in the synovial microcirculation. European J. Clin. Invest., 55:75–82, 1975.

83. Beer, D.T., and Rocklin, R.E.: Histamine-induced suppressor cell activity. J. Allergy Clin. Immunol., 73:332–334, 1984.

84. Dabbous, M.K., et al.: Mast cells and matrix degradation at sites of tumour invasion in rat mammary adenocarcinoma. Br. J. Cancer, 54:459–465, 1986.

85. Farnoush, A., and McKenzie, I.C.: Sequential histological changes and mast cell response in skin during chemically-induced carcinogenesis. J. Pathol., 12:300–311, 1983.

86. Dabbous, M.K., Tipton, D.A., and Haney, L.: Mast cell-mediated stimulation of collagen degradation by gingival fibroblasts. (Abstract.) J. Dent. Res., 66:2,005, 1987.

87. Jeffcoat, M.K., Williams, R.C., and Johnson, H.G.: Treatment of periodontal disease in beagles with iodoxamide ethyl, an inhibitor of mast cell release. J. Periodont. Res., 20:532–541, 1985.

88. Bromley, M., and Wooley, D.E.: Histopathology of the rheumatoid lesion: identification of cell types at sites of cartilage erosion. Arthritis Rheum., 27:857–863, 1984.

89. Yoffe, J., Taylor, D.J., and Wooley, D.E.: Mast cell products stimulate collagenase and prostaglandin E production by cultures of adherent rheumatoid synovial cells. Biochem. Biophys. Res. Commun., 122:270–276, 1984.

90. Yoffe, J.R., Taylor, D.T., and Wooley, D.E.: Mast cell products and heparin stimulate the production of mononuclear-cell factor by cultured human monocyte/macrophage. Biochem. J., 230:83–90, 1985.

91. Taylor, D.J., Yoffe, J.R., and Brown, D.M.: Histamine stimulates prostaglandin E production by rheumatoid synovial cells and human articular chondrocytes in culture. Arthritis Rheum., 29:160–166, 1986.

92. Hausen, H.B., Lobb, C.M., and Taylor, R.E.: Activation of fibroblast procollagenase by mast cell proteases. Biochim. Biophys. Acta, 438:273–286, 1976.

93. Gruber, B.L., Marchese, M.J., and Schwartz, L.B.: Regulation of synovial collagenase activation by mast cell proteases. (Abstract.) Arthritis Rheum., 30:S7, 1987.

94. Gruber, B.L., Marchese, M.J., and Zucker, S.: Interactions of human mast cell tryptase with latent collagenase: divergent

results dependent upon cellular source. (Abstract.) Fed. Proc., *46*:734, 1987.

95. Seppa, H., Vaananen, K., and Korhonen, K.: Effects of mast cell chymase of rat skin on intercellular matrix a histochemical study. Acta Histochem., *64*:64–71, 1979.

96. Sage, H., Woodbury, R.G., and Bornstein, P.: Structural studies on human type IV collagen. J. Biol. Chem., *254*:9,893–9,899, 1979.

97. Vartio, T., Seppa, H., and Vaheri, A.: Susceptibility of soluble and matrix fibronectins to degradation by tissue proteinases, mast cell chymase, and cathepsin G. J. Biol. Chem., *256*:471–478, 1981.

98. Subba Rao, R.V., Friedman, M.M., and Atkins, F.M.: Phagocytosis of mast cell granules by cultured fibroblasts. J. Immunol., *130*:341–349, 1983.

99. Taylor, D.J. Yoffe, J.R., Brown, D.M., and Woolley, D.E.: Histamine H₂ receptors on chondrocytes from human, canine and bovine articular cartilage. Biochem. J., *225*:315–319, 1985.

100. Griffith, G.C, Nichols, G., Asher, J.D., and Hanagan, B.: Heparin osteoporosis. JAMA, *193*:91–94, 1965.

101. Avioli, L.V.: Heparin-induced osteopenia: an appraisal. Adv. Exp. Med. Biol., *52*:375–387, 1975.

102. Squires, J.W.: Heparin induced spinal fractures. JAMA, *241*:2,417–2,420, 1979.

103. Crisp, A.J., Wright, J.K., and Hazelman, B.L.: Effects of heparin, histamine and salmon calcitonin on mouse calvarial bone resorption. Ann. Rheum. Dis., *45*:422–427, 1986.

104. Crisp, A.J., Roelke, M.S., Goldring, S.R., and Krane, S.M.: Heparin modulates intracellular c-AMP in human trabecular bone cells and adherent rheumatoid synovial cells. Ann. Rheum. Dis., *43*:628–634, 1984.

105. Goldhaber, P.: Heparin enhancement of factors stimulating bone resorption in tissue culture. Science, *147*:407–412, 1965.

106. Lanaers-Clays, G., and Vaes, G.: Collagenase, procollagenase and bone resorption: effects of heparin, parathyroid hormone and calcitonin. Biochim. Biophys. Acta, *438*:273–280, 1976.

107. Stark, E., Van Buskirk, F.W., and Daily, J.: Radiologic and pathologic bone changes associated with urticaria pigmentosa. Arch. Pathol., *62*:143–150, 1956.

108. Fallon, M.D., Whyte, M.P., Craig, Jr., R.B., and Teitelbaum, S.L.: Mast cell proliferation in post-menopausal osteoporosis. Calcif. Tissue Int., *35*:29–31, 1983.

109. Frame, B., and Nixon, R.K.: Bone marrow mast cells in osteoporosis of aging. N. Engl. J. Med., *279*:626–630, 1968.

110. Glimelius, B., Busch, C., and Hook, M.: Binding of heparin on the surface of cultured human endothelial cells. Thromb. Res., *12*:773–782, 1978.

111. Kessler, D.A., Langer, R.S., Pless, N.A., Folkman J.: Mast cells and tumor angiogenesis. Int. J. Cancer, *18*:703–709, 1976.

112. Azizkhan, R.G., Azizkhan, J.C., Zetter, B.R., and Folkman, J.: Mast cell heparin stimulates migration of capillary endothelial cells in vitro. J. Exp. Med., *152*:931–944, 1980.

113. Boyd, J.F., and Smith, A.N.: The effect of histamine and histamine-releasing agent (compound 48/80) on wound healing. J. Pathol. Bacteriol., *78*:379–388, 1959.

114. Persinger, M.A., Lepage, P., Simard, J.P., and Parker, G.H.: Mast cell numbers in incisional wounds in rat skin as a function of distance, time and treatment. Br. J. Dermatol., *108*:179–187, 1983.

115. Wichmann, B.E.: The mast cell count during the process of wound healing. Acta Pathol. Microbiol. Scand., *108*(Suppl.):5–35, 1955.

116. Severson, A.R.: Mast cells in areas of experimental bone resorption and remodelling. Br. J. Exp. Pathol., *50*:17–21, 1969.

117. Lykke, A.W.J., Schonell, M.E., and Stewart, B.W.: Atypical mast cell degranulation and focal hydropic degeneration of venular endothelium in diffuse fibrosing alveolitis. Experientia, *35*:1,492–1,496, 1979.

118. Watanabe, S., et al.: Mast cells in the rat alveolar septa undergoing fibrosis after ionizing radiation: ultrastructural and histochemical studies. Lab. Invest., *31*:555–567, 1974.

119. Kawanami, O., Ferrans, W.J., Fulmer, J.D., and Crystal, R.G.: Ultrastructure of pulmonary mast cells in patients with fibrotic lung disorders. Lab. Invest., *40*:717–734, 1979.

120. Hawkins, R.A., Claman, H.N., Clark, R.A., and Steigerwald, J.C.: Increased dermal mast cell populations in progressive systemic sclerosis: a link in chronic fibrosis? Ann. Intern. Med., *102*:182–186, 1985.

121. Claman, H.N.: Mast cell depletion in murine chronic graft-versus-host disease. J. Invest. Dermatol., *84*:246–248, 1985.

122. Fonseca, E., and Solis, J.: Mast cells in the skin: progressive systemic sclerosis and the toxic oil syndrome. (Letter.) Ann. Intern. Med., *102*:864–865, 1985.

123. Zurow, B.L., et al.: Immunoglobulin E-rheumatoid factor in the serum of patients with rheumatoid arthritis, asthma and other diseases. J. Clin. Invest., *68*:1,610–1,613, 1981.

124. Chatpar, P.C., Muller, D., and Gruber, B.: Prevalence of IgE rheumatoid factor in mixed cryoglobulinemia and rheumatoid arthritis. Clin. Exp. Rheum., *4*:106–111, 1986.

125. Permin, H., and Egeskold, E.M.: IgE anti IgG antibodies in patients with juvenile and adult rheumatoid arthritis including Felty's syndrome. Allergy, *37*:421–428, 1982.

126. Gruber, B.L., Kaufman, L., and Baeza, M.: Anti-IgE autoantibodies detection in connective tissue disease and ability to activate circulating basophils. (Abstract.) Arthritis Rheum. *29*:521, 1986.

127. DeClerck, L.S., Gigase, P.L., and Bridts, L.H.: Anti-IgE antibodies in rheumatoid arthritis in relation to clinical and laboratory findings. J. Allergy Clin. Immunol., *79*:220, 1987.

128. Lotz, M., Carson, D.A., and Vaughan, J.H.: Substance P activation of rheumatoid synoviocytes: neural pathway in pathogeneis of arthritis. Science, *235*:893–895, 1987.

23

GRANULOCYTE CHEMOTAXIS

ISAIAS SPILBERG and BRIAN F. MANDELL

The recruitment of granulocytes at the site of tissue injury is the histopathologic hallmark of acute inflammation. A great deal of information exists suggesting that the responding cells follow a common pathway to arrive at the exact location of tissue damage, independent of whether the potentially injurious substance is a bacterium, an immune complex, or a urate crystal. The local accumulation of cells is an active phenomenon. Loss of vascular integrity is not required for the cells to emigrate from the circulation. Microscopic studies indicate that neutrophils coursing through the microvasculature adjacent to an inflamed area are sidetracked from their normal pattern of flow. They clump together, adhere to the endothelial wall, crawl between endothelial cells, and traverse the interstitial matrix to arrive at the site of tissue injury. Once there, the neutrophil in all likelihood releases additional mediators, thereby amplifying the inflammatory process until the triggering stimulus for inflammation is removed. The critical role that granulocyte chemotaxis plays in normal host defense is dramatically underscored by the clinical and laboratory descriptions of several potentially lethal immunodeficiency states in which the defined alteration of host defense is depressed neutrophil migration. The reverse is observed in primary inflammatory disorders, in which the chronic stimulation of inflammatory cells leads to organ damage and dysfunction. In some clinical conditions excessive chemotactic factor elaboration and depressed neutrophil function coexist in the same patient as a manifestation of loss of immunoregulatory controls.

DEFINITION AND METHODOLOGY

Chemotaxis is the directed migration of cells along a chemical gradient. This must be distinguished from *chemokinesis*, in which cells are chemically stimulated to move faster, but not necessarily along a gradient.[1] The key distinction is that during chemotaxis the cells orient and maintain the same orientation during locomotion. The two processes can be differentiated experimentally by exposing the cells to a series of gradients obtained by varying the concentration of the test substance. Substances that are truly chemotactic produce the greatest enhancement of vectorial movement when they are spatially separated from the responding cells so that a diffusion gradient results. Studies on individual cells reveal that, on exposure to a concentration gradient of chemotactic factor, the initial pseudopod extension is directed toward the gradient peak.[1,2] Neutrophils thus are capable of sensing the strength of the gradient across their bodies. Migration following this extension is in a vector toward the maximal chemotactic factor concentration; continuous sensing of the gradient occurs, and alterations in the gradient rapidly change the direction of migration. In contrast, cells responding chemokinetically show increased movement, but no net vector of migration. This response can be correlated with absolute mediator concentration, as opposed to the strength of the gradient.[3,4] Characteristically, chemotactic factors, when incubated with cells in the absence of a gradient, are also chemokinetic. The relative contribution of chemokinesis and chemotaxis to

383

the local accumulation of inflammatory cells in vivo is not known.

Current methods used to study granulocyte movement in vitro fall into two general categories: (1) observation of the motion of individual cells, and (2) measurement of the migration of a cell population. In the first method, locomotion is analyzed by time-lapse cinematography of individual cells on a warmed glass slide.[2] The use of this technique has permitted the detailed description of the morphology of granulocytes in motion, but has been used less frequently to study various clinical states and drug effects. Study of the locomotion of individual cells is not suitable for evaluating potential clinical defects in cellular mobility, because of problems in quantifying the cellular events, because of technical difficulties in establishing stable concentration gradients, and because of problems in surveying the effects of a large number of agents on granulocyte motion. These difficulties are partially avoided by assessing the migration of cell populations using variations of the Boyden chamber and the "under agarose" assays.

In the Boyden chamber method, granulocytes are added to the upper, and the potential chemoattractant to the lower, of two compartments that are separated by a micropore filter.[5] After suitable incubation, migration is quantified microscopically by counting the stained granulocytes that have migrated through the filter, or by determining the actual distance traveled into the filter by the "leading front" of cells.[5] Filter pore sizes used in these experiments have ranged from 0.65 to 5 μm, too small to enable the cells to passively traverse the filter. The adaptation of computer-assisted image analyzers to the "leading front" technique allows for more rapid and extensive data collection as well as elimination of human counting error.[5a] A modification of the Boyden chamber assay[6] that also eliminates human counting error uses two micropore filters and radiolabeled leukocytes. Migration is quantified by counting the radioactivity in cells that has passed completely through the first filter and into the second. Highly purified cell populations are required in order to equate radioactivity with the migration of a given granulocyte class. The limitations of these techniques include filter lot variability, inability to study isolated cells, and the artificial constraint imposed by inflexible pores.

The "under agarose" method, also limited by the inability to study individual cells, uses visual evaluation of cells moving between agarose gel and the underlying petri dish.[7] The chemotactic and chemokinetic effects of an attractant can be assessed, but this method is less sensitive than the filter techniques. Population techniques do not allow for identification

of neutrophil subsets with varied migratory capabilities. All methods require controls for endogenous random granulocyte motility and for chemokinesis.

In vivo assessment of human neutrophil motility provides information that is difficult to quantify. One method uses a superficial skin abrasion made with a sterile scalpel blade, the "skin window" first described by Rebuck. The abrasion is covered with a coverslip that can be removed and stained at suitable times to count migrating cells.[8]

Another assay for in vivo chemotactic activity involves the implantation into the skin of a small patch of Dacron fabric coupled with a disk of ethylene vinyl acetate copolymer. Such polymers can release biologically active substances at a constant rate for several days. On removal from the host, the fabric patches are sectioned and stained to reveal the attracted cells.[8a]

The in vivo methods provide useful clinical estimates of total cell migration, but cannot distinguish between chemotaxis and chemokinesis.

White cell motility in vitro is influenced by the concentration of protein, partial pressure of oxygen, pH, temperature, and tonicity of the suspending medium.[1] It is unclear, however, whether the extremes required to change leukocyte function actually occur in vivo.

CHEMOTACTIC FACTORS

Substances reportedly chemotactic for granulocytes vary greatly in size and chemical composition as well as in the extent to which they have been studied. The initial interaction between a cell and chemotactic factor molecules is mediated by specific cell surface receptors. Such receptors have been described for the synthetic formylated peptides on both neutrophils[9,10] and macrophages.[11,12] These chemotactic factors, active at 10^{-10} M, may actually play a role in the attraction of neutrophils to metabolically active bacteria since similar materials have been isolated from the filtrates of E. coli growing in broth.[12a] The neurotransmitter *substance P,* a compound thought to play a potential role in rheumatoid arthritis, also binds to the N-formyl-methionine-leucine-phenylalanine (FMLP) receptor.[13] The availability of the formylated peptides has facilitated the study of the mechanism by which receptor binding is translated into chemotaxis. The biologic significance of chemotactic factor-receptor interaction is evidenced by the striking correlation between binding affinities and chemotactic activities observed in a large number of formylated peptides of a varying amino acid sequence.[30] Specific receptors have also been described for crystal-induced chemotactic factor (CCF),[14] complement component C5a,[15] leukotriene B_4 (LTB$_4$),[16] and the eosinophilic chemotactic factor of anaphylaxis.[23,25]

The chemotactic activity of complement is due to C5a and C5a-des-arg.[17] The latter is the residual C5a molecule after serum carboxypeptidase(s) cleaves the terminal arginine residue, and is probably the major circulating form of C5a. C5a-des-arg differs from C5a in that it has no anaphylatoxin activity, has roughly 10% of the chemotactic activity of native C5a, and probably requires a serum protein "helper factor" for such activity.[18] C5a is active at a concentration of 10^{-9}M. Patients deficient in C5 are at risk of developing disseminated infection.[41] C5-derived chemotactic activity has been suggested to be primarily responsible for PMN accumulation in experimental bacterial meningitis.[19] It seems likely that C5a-des-arg is the major initial chemotactic factor involved in inflammation caused by immune complex deposition and other reactions involving complement activation such as sepsis. The structure of the cellular receptor for C5a and other chemotactic factors remains largely unknown.

The phagocytosis of monosodium urate or calcium pyrophosphate crystals by neutrophils leads to the generation and secretion of a protein (CCF) first described by Phelps, which is chemotactically active at concentrations of less than 10^{-7} M for neutrophils and monocytes.[20] The production of this chemotactic factor is exquisitely sensitive to suppression by low doses of colchicine. This suppression has been proposed as the primary mechanism by which the drug acts in acute gout and pseudogout.[20] The intra-articular injection of CCF into rabbit joints induced an acute synovitis without a significant increase in vascular permeability; colchicine effectively suppressed monosodium urate crystal-induced arthritis in this model without affecting the inflammatory response to the intra-articular injection of CCF.[21]

The clinical success of nonsteroidal anti-inflammatory drugs, which share the ability to inhibit arachidonate-derived prostaglandins, has prompted an intense search among the metabolites of arachidonic acid for a pivotal mediator of inflammation. The most potent natural chemotactic factor described to date is a product of the lipoxygenase pathway.[22] Leukotriene B_4 or 5(S), 12(R)-hydroxy-eicosa-6,14-CIS 8,10-trans-tetraenoic acid (LTB$_4$) is chemotactically active for neutrophils at concentrations of less than 10^{-10} M. Other leukotriene derivatives are active, but less potent, chemotactic factors. Because their production is stimulated by exposure of neutrophils to other chemotactic factors, they may function in vivo to modulate the inflammatory process. Aspirin-like drugs do not dramatically suppress LTB$_4$ generation.

Type I allergic reactions are characterized by tissue infiltration with eosinophils and neutrophils and are mediated by the specific interaction of antigen with IgE on the surface of mast cells and basophils. Exposure in vitro or in vivo of sensitized mast-cell–rich tissues to a stimulating antigen results in the release of chemotactic factors for both eosinophils[23] and neutrophils.[24] The eosinophil chemotactic factor of anaphylaxis (ECF-A) is composed of at least two tetrapeptides: val-gly-ser-glu and ala-gly-ser-glu.[23] These peptides exist preformed in granules of mast cells and basophils and their release is apparently under the same control as histamine secretion. ECF-A exhibits peak activity at approximately 5×10^{-8} M and is capable of inducing chemotaxis and enzyme release from eosinophils, but not from neutrophils. The receptor for ECF-A exhibits marked conformational specificity toward related tetrapeptides.[25] The less studied basophil can also respond chemotactically to C5a and to an as yet unidentified product of lymphocyte culture.[26] Several other chemotactic factors have been described, some of which are listed in Table 23–1.

Chemotactic factors have multiple effects on granulocytes. Exposure of cells to relatively high concentrations of chemotactic factors in vitro causes prompt reversible aggregation. Intravenous infusion of the chemotactic factors FMLP or C5a-des-arg into animals elicits a transient thrombocytopenia, neutropenia, and pulmonary sequestration of granulocytes with an accompanying decrease in the PO$_2$ and increase in the alveolar-arterial oxygen gradient.[33] These effects may be analogous to those occurring in vivo with the initiation of hemodialysis, a procedure that activates C5, resulting in intravascular neutrophil aggregation, leukopenia, and transient hypoxia.[34] Incubation of neutrophils in vitro with most, but not all,[35] chemotactic factors induces lysosomal enzyme release and superoxide production. Factors vary in their potency, and fairly stringent incubation conditions are sometimes necessary to demonstrate this activity. Although exocytosis has been proposed as one mechanism by which cells regulate their own chemotactic response by way of chemotactic factor destruction and receptor recycling, the in vivo significance is unclear. The secreted neutrophil granule contents are also capable of generating additional chemotactic factors from their action(s) on complement, coagulation proteins, collagen, and other neutrophils.

Incubation of cells with high concentrations of chemotactic factors in the absence of a gradient leads to a reversible state of chemotactic unresponsiveness

Table 23–1. Granulocyte Chemotactic Factors

Chemotactic Factor	Characteristics	Comments
C5a[15,17]	Glycoprotein, MW 11,200	Specific receptor. Formed during hemodialysis.
C5a-des-arg[18]		Needs helper factor.
Crystal-induced CF[20]	Glycoprotein, MW 11,500	Specific receptor. Synthesis inhibited by colchicine.
Arachidonate metabolites[22]	LTB$_4$ product of lipoxygenase pathway, MW 330	Specific receptor. Most potent natural chemotactic factor described.
Hepatocyte derived lipid[27]	Non-polar byproduct of ethanol metabolism.	Perhaps active in ethanol hepatitis.
Nerve growth factor[28]	Protein, MW 100,000	Serine protease activity.
Interleukin 1[29]	Polypeptide(s)	Product of PMNs, monocytes, synovial cells. Endogenous pyrogen activity.
ECF-A[23]	Val-gly-ser-glu and other tetrapeptides, 300–500 MW	Specific receptor. From mast cells.
Ragweed antigen induced neutrophil chemotactic factor[24]	Protein, MW 150,000	Probably from mast cells.
Formylated peptides[9]	FMLP, MW 440, and related peptides	Specific receptor on neutrophils, macrophages.
Glycyl-L-histidyl-glycine[35]	MW 269	Does not induce exocytosis
Bacterial products[30]	MW 150–1500	From E. coli culture filtrate.
Platelet factor 4[31]	MW 7,800	From platelets
Denatured proteins[32]	Various proteins including albumin and hemoglobin	No specific receptor identified

(without decreased chemokinesis) termed *deactivation*. This state has been shown to be, in part, agent nonspecific and, therefore, unlikely to occur simply as a result of receptor binding or "down regulation" of receptors.[36] In vivo deactivation can be demonstrated in humans and may contribute to the accumulation of cells in an inflammatory focus by limiting the egress of cells initially attracted by a chemotactic gradient.[37] Several extracellular modulators of neutrophil chemotaxis have also been described, including a normal human serum component that irreversibly inactivates the C5 chemotactic peptide. This chemotactic factor inactivator can inhibit Arthus reactions and immune-complex–induced pulmonary damage.[38]

CELLULAR EFFECTS OF CHEMOTACTIC FACTORS

Leukocytes migrating in a chemotactic gradient exhibit a polarized structure.[1,39] A leading pseudopod generally free of organelles adheres to a substrate and is followed by the cell body containing the nucleus and a tail that may contain organelles. The position of the centriole is usually maintained between the leading pseudopod and the bulk of the nucleus; this arrangement has been used as a marker for orientation. The tail is not necessarily adherent to the substratum, although at times it may have extensions (retraction fibers) that are rich in microfilaments. Direct observation of migrating cells has shown that they crawl along a substrate, changing direction by a series of turns, each less than 90° from the previous direction. Actin-containing microfilaments are necessary for any migration to take place, and microtubules are probably required for accurate maintenance of orientation.[39] Assembly of both microfilaments and microtubules is stimulated by chemotactic factors. Patients with frequent infections and altered granulocyte migration that accompanies defects in microfilament assembly[40] and microtubule polymerization[41] have been described.

The biochemical steps by which receptor binding is translated into chemotaxis are still unclear. Chemotactic factor binding to neutrophils stimulates several rapid and transient metabolic events, including activation of Na$^+$K$^+$ ATPase, transmembrane potential changes, increased intracellular calcium, phosphoinositol turnover, decreased lipid methylation, tyrosinolation of tubulin, increased glucose and oxygen consumption and changes in cyclic nucleotide levels and arachidonic acid metabolism.[30,42–48] Stimulation of these metabolic processes by a chemotactic factor, however, does not necessarily indicate that the stimulation contributes directly to chemotaxis, nor that the events are even interdependent. For instance, chemotactic factors normally elicit a rapid increase in neutrophil transmembrane potential. Cells from patients with chronic granulomatous disease, a disorder marked by the inability of neutrophils to undergo a normal respiratory burst of increased oxygen consumption and superoxide production, do not respond to chemotactic factors with membrane hyperpolarization[42]; nevertheless, their chemotactic response is still 60% of normal. Microtubule polymerization occurs during both chemotaxis and exocytosis, although the two processes can be separated by altering membrane fluidity,[46] or by using the chemotactic factor gly-his-gly, an agent that polymerizes microtubules, but does not stimulate exocytosis.[35] The observed increases in cyclic nucleotides levels induced by chemotactic factors may not be required for chemotaxis;[48] extracellular calcium, however, appears to be required for unimpaired adhesion and migration.[44] Incubation of granulocytes with FMLP or phorbol esters results in an initial cytosolic acidification followed by a more sustained alkalinization.[49,50] These intracellular changes may influence PMN function to a degree yet to be determined; PMN from patients with chronic granulomatous disease do not undergo intracellular pH changes when challenged, yet their chemotactic response is still appreciable (although not normal).

Exposure of neutrophils to chemotactic factors leads to decreased methylation of phospholipids. This correlates with a rapid increase in the availability of arachidonate and its subsequent metabolism by way of cleavage from phospholipids by phospholipase A_2, an enzyme reportedly inhibited by high-dose glucocorticoids. This inhibition is produced by steroid-induced synthesis of a specific protein that inhibits both phospholipase A_2 and chemotaxis.[51] The activity of the endogenous inhibitor is suppressed by the increase in intracellular calcium evoked by chemotactic factors. Not all investigators have demonstrated glucocorticoid inhibition of chemotaxis, however. Products of both the cyclo-oxygenase and lipoxygenase pathways increase in response to heightened arachidonate mobilization. The various ratios of resultant prostaglandins and leukotrienes depend on cell type. Several of the lipoxygenase products, primarily LTB_4, have been shown to be chemotactic themselves. Since LTB_4 increases intracellular-free calcium, which is in turn capable of activating the actin system and modulating cell migration, it may act *in vivo* as an amplifier of the chemotactic response initiated by other chemoattractants.

The mechanism by which transduction of the binding signal to intracellular events occurs is still not clear. It has been shown that at least some chemotactic factor receptors (FMLP, LTB_4) exist in two kinetic forms in isolated membranes: high and low affinity. The high affinity form, the Km of which appears to correlate with the chemotactic response, can be converted to the low affinity form upon incubation of the membranes with guanine nucleotides.[52] Endogenous receptors seem, on interaction with their chemotactic factor, to reversibly associate with membrane proteins in a manner similar to that of the guanine nucleotide regulatory proteins described in catecholamine and other hormone-responsive adenyl-cyclase systems. This interaction can be altered by incubating cells with pertussis toxin, an agent that by ribosylating the regulatory protein breaks down the receptor-regulatory protein interaction.[53] Pertussis toxin inhibits several receptor-mediated metabolic processes, such as calcium flux, phosphoinositol turnover, and arachidonate metabolism, and suppresses both chemotaxis and exocytosis.[54]

CHEMOTAXIS AND THE RHEUMATIC DISEASES

Studies of cells from patients with various rheumatic diseases have reportedly demonstrated both reduced and enhanced chemotaxis.[41,55,55a] Clear-cut distinction between chemotaxis and chemokinesis have not always been provided, and interpretation of several of these studies is therefore limited. As a rule, peripheral blood granulocytes from most patients with rheumatic disorders behave normally, but the serum from some patients may be defective in its ability to induce chemotaxis. Peripheral blood neutrophils of some patients with rheumatoid arthritis, Felty's syndrome, and SLE have shown abnormal migration in vitro, and the extent of the defect has been correlated with disease activity.[41] Increased chemotaxis has been reported in vitro in neutrophils obtained from patients with Behçet's syndrome, HLA-positive ankylosing spondylitis and Yersinia arthritis, and familial Mediterranean fever (FMF).[55,55a,55b] A caveat to the interpretation of these data, however, lies in the fact that circulating neutrophils are not a homogeneous population,[41] so that studies on peripheral blood cells may actually reflect a subpopulation of cells that are not participating in the ongoing inflammatory process, either because of intrinsic cellular properties or secondary extracellular factors, such as in vivo deactivation. PMNs from HLA-27 positive healthy individuals have been reported to respond with increased chemotaxis to activated complement in vitro.[55a] The significance of this finding is presently unknown.

An inadequate capacity to generate chemotactic activity in serum has been described in some patients with SLE. The sera from these patients contain an inhibitor of the helper factor required by C5a-des-arg for full chemotactic activity. The inhibitor is antigenically related to the B6 fragment of human complement B.[18,18a]

A defect in the capacity to generate chemotactic activity from serum is frequently seen in a rheumatic disease-like syndrome associated with a genetic deficiency in early complement components. Patients with C1r, C4, or C2 deficiencies are prone to develop an SLE-like illness or, more rarely, a dermatomyositis-like syndrome or necrotizing vasculitis. Patients with C3 and C5 deficiencies have a more pronounced serum chemotactic defect and are prone to recurrent infections but, as a rule, do not develop a rheumatic-like syndrome.[41]

The recurring peritonitis and arthritis seen in FML have been linked to depressed levels of a C5a antagonist found in peritoneal and synovial fluids of these patients. The serum levels of this endogenous antagonist were reported to be normal. This may represent a specific defect in FMF, because synovial fluids from other arthritides were reported to have near-normal levels of the antagonist.[55b,56]

ANTI-INFLAMMATORY AGENTS AND CHEMOTAXIS

Anti-inflammatory drugs are generally thought to act on the PMN, limiting motility and/or cellular effector functions. There is, however, insufficient evidence documenting such effects on PMN chemotaxis. Corticosteroids are the most potent anti-inflammatory compounds available, and in vivo assays of cell motility reveal that hydrocortisone is capable of reducing neutrophil accumulation for up to 12 hours.[57] In vitro studies, however, have not demonstrated a primary defect on chemotaxis, suggesting that hydrocortisone may exert its effects through some in vivo mechanism, perhaps by interfering with neutrophil adhesion or endothelial cell interaction. A single intravenous dose of dexamethasone was shown not to alter neutrophil migration assessed in vitro even when the cells were obtained from volunteers at the peak of steroid-induced granulocytosis.[58] Colchicine, which depolymerizes microtubules, impairs chemotaxis in vitro when

assessed by the filter technique, but not by the agarose method, which does not require cells to penetrate the rigid channels of a filter.[59] Studies using an experimental rabbit model of crystal-induced arthritis showed that pharmacologic doses of intravenous colchicine impaired the ability of neutrophils to generate and secrete the crystal-induced chemotactic factor implicated in the pathogenesis of acute gout and pseudogout. The peripheral blood granulocytes of the colchicine-treated rabbits, however, retained their full ability to respond to a chemotactic challenge.[21] Normal chemotaxis has also been demonstrated testing peripheral blood neutrophils from colchicine-treated patients. Other drugs, including gold compounds, levamisol, and some nonsteroidal anti-inflammatory agents, have been shown to alter granulocyte chemotaxis in vitro.[41,60,61] Often such drugs have been tested in vitro at greater than their pharmacologic levels, and a clear distinction between chemotaxis and chemokinesis has not always been presented. Further studies are needed before conclusions can be drawn regarding the mechanism(s) of their in vivo effect. Interestingly, sulfasalazine, phenylbutazone, sulindac, and indomethacin have been shown to interfere in vitro with the binding of FMLP to its receptor.[61a]

Preliminary animal studies have shown that dietary enrichment with Borage oil, which contains precursors of PGE_1, instead of the usual arachidonate and PGE_2 precursors, dramatically suppresses both the in vivo neutrophil response to sodium urate crystals and adjuvant arthritis in rats.[62] Dietary supplementation with fish oils (eicosapentaenoic acids) decreases the human neutrophil response to LTB_4 as well as its generation.[63] Amelioration of the inflammatory response, including migration and tissue accumulation of neutrophils, may be possible through dietary supplementation with specific lipids.

In summary, leukocyte chemotaxis is the result of a complex series of intracellular events resulting in directional migration of potentially destructive cells into an inflammatory site. Rational manipulation of the inflammatory response will require a better understanding of the chemotactic process in order to hopefully suppress unwanted granulocyte-mediated tissue damage without unduly compromising normal host defense.

REFERENCES

1. Zigmond, S.H.: Chemotaxis of polymorphonuclear leukocytes. J. Cell Biol., 77:269–287, 1978.
2. Zigmond, S.H.: Mechanisms of sensing chemical gradients by polymorphonuclear leukocytes. Nature, 249:450–452, 1974.
3. Keller, H.U., et al.: A proposal for the definition of terms re-

lated to locomotion of leukocytes and other cells. Clin. Exp. Immunol., *27*:377–380, 1980.

4. Becker, E.L.: Chemotaxis. J. All. Clin. Immunol., *66*:97–105, 1980.

5. Zigmond, S.H., and Hirsh, J.G.: Leukocyte locomotion and chemotaxis: New methods for evaluation and demonstration of a cell-derived chemotactic factor. J. Exp. Med., *137*:387–410, 1973.

5a.Shore, B.L., Daughaday, C.C., and Spilberg, I.: Benign asbestos pleurisy in the rabbit. A model for the study of pathogenesis. Am. Rev. Resp. Dis., *128*:481–485, 1983.

6. Gallin, J.I., Clark, R.A., and Goetzl, E.J.: Radio-assay of leukocyte locomotion: A sensitive technique for clinical studies. *In* Leukocyte Chemotaxis: Methods, Physiology and Clinical Implications. Edited by J.I. Gallin and P.G. Quie. New York, Raven Press, 1978.

7. Nelson, R.D., Quie, P.G., and Simmons, R.L.: Chemotaxis under agarose: a new and simple method for measuring chemotaxis and spontaneous migration of human polymorphonuclear leukocytes and monocytes. J. Immunol., *115*:1650–1656, 1975.

8. Miller, M.E.: Cell movement and host defenses. Ann. Intern. Med., *78*:601–603, 1973.

8a.Zetter, B.R., Rasmussen, N., and Brown, L.: Methods in laboratory investigation. An in vivo assay for chemoattractant activity. Lab. Invest., *53*:362–368, 1985.

9. Aswanikumar, S., Corcoran, B., and Schiffmann, E.: Demonstration of a receptor on rabbit neutrophils for chemotactic peptides. Biochem. Biophys. Res. Commun., *4*:810–817, 1977.

10. Williams, L.T., Snyderman, R., Pike, M.C., and Lefkowitz, R.J.: Specific receptor sites for chemotactic peptides on human polymorphonuclear leukocytes. Proc. Natl. Acad. Sci. USA, *74*:1204–1206, 1977.

11. Snyderman, R., and Fudman, E.J.: Demonstration of a chemotactic factor receptor on macrophages. J. Immunol., *124*:2754–2757, 1980.

12. Spilberg, I., Mehta, J., Daughaday, C., and Simchowitz, L.: Determination of a specific receptor for formyl-methionyl-leucyl-phenylalanine on the pulmonary alveolar macrophage and its relationship to chemotaxis and superoxide production. J. Lab. Clin. Med., *97*:602–609, 1981.

12a.Marasco, W.A., et al.: Purification and identification of formyl-methionyl-leucyl-phenylalanine as the major peptide neutrophil chemotactic factor produced by *Escherichia coli.* J. Biol. Chem., *279*:5430–5439, 1984.

13. Marasco, W.A., Showell, H.J., and Becker, E.L.: Substance P binds to the formylpeptide chemotaxis receptor on the rabbit neutrophil. Biochem. Biophys. Res. Commun., *99*:1065–1072, 1981.

14. Spilberg, I., and Mehta, J.: Demonstration of a specific neutrophil receptor for a cell-derived chemotactic factor. J. Clin. Invest., *63*:85–88, 1979.

15. Chenoweth, D.E., and Hugli, T.E.: Demonstration of specific C5a receptor on intact human polymorphonuclear leukocytes. Proc. Natl. Acad. Sci. USA, *75*:3943–3947, 1978.

16. Goldman, D.W., and Goetzl, E.J.: Specific binding of leukotriene B$_4$ to receptors on human polymorphonuclear leukocytes. J. Immunol., *129*:1600–1604, 1982.

17. Shin, H.S., et al.: Chemotactic and anaphylatoxic fragment cleaved from the fifth component of guinea pig complement. Science, *162*:361–363, 1968.

18. Perez, H.D., Chenoweth, D.E., and Goldstein, I.M.: Attachment of human C5a-des-arg to its cochemotaxin is required for maximum expression of chemotactic activity. J. Clin. Invest., *78*:1589–1595, 1986.

18a.Perez, H.D., Hooper, C., Volanakis, J., and Veda, A.: Specific inhibitor of complement (C5)-derived chemotactic activity in systemic lupus erythematosus related antigenically to the Bb fragment of human factor B. J. Immunol., *139*:484–489, 1987.

19. Ernst, J.D., Hartiala, K.T., Goldstein, I.M., and Sande, M.A.: Complement (C5)-derived chemotactic activity accounts for accumulation of polymorphonuclear leukocytes in cerebrospinal fluid of rabbits with pneumococcal meningitis. Infect. Immun., *46*:81–86, 1984.

20. Spilberg, I., and Mandell, B.F.: Crystal-induced chemotactic factor. *In* Advances in Inflammation Research, Vol. 5. Edited by G. Weissmann. New York, Raven Press, 1983. pp. 57–65.

21. Spilberg, I., Mandell, B.F., Simchowitz, L., and Rosenberg, D.: Mechanism of action of colchicine in acute urate crystal-induced arthritis. J. Clin. Invest., *64*:775–780, 1979.

22. Goetzl, E.J.: Oxygenation products of arachidonic acid as mediators of hypersensitivity and inflammation. Med. Clin. N. Am., *65*:809–829, 1981.

23. Goetzl, E.J., and Austen, K.F.: Purification and synthesis of eosinophilic tetrapeptides of human lung tissue: Identification as eosinophil chemotactic factor of anaphylaxis. Proc. Natl. Acad. Sci. USA, *72*:4123–4127, 1975.

24. Atkins, P.C., Norman, M., Zweiman, B., and Rosenblum, F.: Further characterization and biologic activity of ragweed-antigen-induced-neutrophil chemotactic activity in man. J. All. Clin. Immunol., *64*:251–258, 1979.

25. Boswell, R.N., Austen, K.F., and Goetzl, E.: A chemotactic receptor for Val-Gly-Ser-Glu on human eosinophil polymorphonuclear leukocytes. Immunol. Comm., *5*:469–479, 1976.

26. Boetcher, D.A., and Leonard, E.J.: Basophil chemotaxis: Augmentation by a factor from stimulated lymphocyte cultures. Immunol. Comm., *2*:421–428, 1973.

27. Roll, F.J., Bissell, D.M., and Perez, H.D.: Human hepatocytes metabolizing ethanol generate a non-polar chemotactic factor for human neutrophils. Biochem. Biophys. Res. Commun., *137*:688–694, 1986.

28. Gee, A.P., et al.: Nerve growth factor: Stimulation of polymorphonuclear leukocyte chemotaxis in vitro. Proc. Natl. Acad. Sci. USA, *80*:7215–7217, 1983.

29. Sauder, D.N., et. al.: Chemotactic cytokines: the role of leukocytic pyrogen and epidermal cell thymocyte-activating factor in neutrophil chemotaxis. J. Immunol., *132*:828–832, 1984.

30. Schiffmann, E.: Leukocyte chemotaxis. Ann. Rev. Physiol., *44*:553–568, 1982.

31. Duel, T.F., et al.: Platelet factor 4 is chemotactic for neutrophils and monocytes. Proc. Natl. Acad. Sci. USA, *78*:4584–4587, 1981.

32. Wilkinson, P.C., and Allan, R.B.: Binding of protein chemotactic factors to the surface of neutrophil leukocytes and its modifications with lipid bacterial toxins. Mol. Cell Biochem., *20*:25–40, 1978.

33. Issekutz, A.C., and Ripley, M.: The effect of intravascular chemotactic factors on blood neutrophil and platelet kinetics. Am. J. Hematol., *21*:157–171, 1986.

34. Craddock, P.R., et al.: Complement (C5a)-induced granulocyte aggregation in vitro. A possible mechanism of complement-mediated leukostasis and leukopenia. J. Clin. Invest., *60*:260–264, 1977.

35. Spilberg, I., et al.: Dissociation of the neutrophil functions of exocytosis and chemotaxis. J. Lab. Clin. Med., *92*297–302, 1978.

36. Spilberg, I., Mandell, B.F., and Hoffstein, S.: A proposed

model for chemotactic factor deactivation: Evidence for micro-tubule modulation of polymorphonuclear leukocyte chemo-taxis. J. Lab. Clin. Med., *94*:361–369, 1979.

37. Center, D.M., Soter, N.A., Wasserman, S.I., and Austen, K.F.: Inhibition of neutrophil chemotaxis in association with exper-imental angioedema in patients with cold urticaria: A model of chemotactic deactivation in vivo.. Clin. Exp. Immunol., *35*:112–118, 1979.

38. Johnson, K.J., Anderson, T.P., and Ward, P.: Suppression of immune complex induced inflammation by the chemotactic factor inactivator. J. Clin. Invest., *59*:951–958, 1977.

39. Allan, R.B., and Wilkinson, P.C.: A visual analysis of chemo-tactic locomotion of human leukocytes: Use of a new chemo-tactic assay with Candida Albicans as a gradient source. Exp. Cell Res., *111*:191–198, 1978.

40. Boxer, L.A., Hedley-Whyte, E.T., and Stossel, T.P.: Neutrophil actin dysfunction and abnormal neutrophil behavior. New Engl. J. Med., *291*:1093–1099, 1974.

41. Gallin, J.: Abnormal phagocyte chemotaxis: Pathophysiology, clinical manifestations, and management of patients. Rev. In-fect. Dis., *3*:1196–1220, 1981.

42. Seligmann, B.E., and Gallin, J.I.: Use of lipophilic probes of membrane potentials to assess human neutrophil activation. J. Clin. Invest., *66*:493–503, 1980.

43. Bradford, P.G., and Rubin, R.P.: Characterization of formyl-methionyl-leucyl-phenylalanine. Stimulation of inositol tri-phosphate accumulation in rabbit neutrophils. Molec. Phar-macol., *27*:74–78, 1985.

44. Meshulam, T., Proto, P., Diamond, R.D., and Melnick, D.A.: Calcium modulation and chemotactic peptide receptor. J. Im-munol., *137*:1954–1960, 1986.

45. Naccache, P.H., Showell, H.S., Becker, E.L., and Shaafi, R.I.: Pharmacological differentiation between chemotactic factor in-duced calcium redistribution and transmembrane flux in rabbit neutrophils. Biochem. Biophys. Res. Commun., *89*:1224–1230, 1979.

46. Yuli, I., Tomonago, A., and Snyderman, R.: Chemoattractant receptor functions in human polymorphonuclear leukocytes are divergently altered by membrane fluidizers. Proc. Natl. Acad. Sci. USA, *79*:5906–5910, 1982.

47. Nath, J., Flavin, M., Corcoran, G., and Schiffmann, E.: Stim-ulation of tubulin tyrosylation in rabbit leukocytes evoked by the chemoattractant formyl-methionyl-leucyl-phenylalanine. J. Cell Biol., *91*:232–234, 1981.

48. Simchowitz, L., Spilberg, I., and Atkinson, J.P.: Evidence that the functional responses of human neutrophils occur inde-pendently of transient elevations in cyclic AMP levels. J.Cyc. Nucl. Prot. Phosph. Res., *16*:35–47, 1983.

49. Simchowitz, L., and Cragoe, E.J., Jr.: Regulation of human neutrophil chemotaxis by intracellular pH. J. Biol. Chem., *261*:6492–6500, 1986.

50. Grinstein, S., and Furuya, W.: Cytoplasmic pH regulation in phorbol ester-activated human neutrophils. Am. Physiol. Soc., *251*:C55–C65, 1986.

51. Hirata, F., et al.: A phospholipase A_2 inhibitory protein in rabbit neutrophils induced by glucocorticoids. Proc. Natl. Acad. Sci. USA, *77*:2533–2536, 1980.

52. Koo, C., Lefkowitz, R.J., and Snyderman, R.: Guanine nu-cleotides modulate the binding affinity of the oligopeptide chemo-attractant receptor on human polymorphonuclear leu-kocytes. J. Clin. Invest., *72*:748–753, 1983.

53. Okajima, F., Katada, T., and Ui, M.: Coupling of the guanine nucleotide regulatory protein to chemotactic peptide receptors in neutrophil membranes and its uncoupling by islet-activating protein, pertussis toxin. J. Biol. Chem., *260*:6761–6768, 1985.

54. Becker, E.L., et al.: The inhibition of neutrophil granule en-zyme secretion and chemotaxis by pertussis toxin. J. Cell Biol., *100*:1641–1646, 1985.

55. Pease, C.T., Fordam, J.N. and Currey, H.L.F.: Polymorpho-nuclear cell motility, ankylosing spondylitis, and HLA B27. Ann. Rheum. Dis., *43*:279–284, 1984.

55a. Leirisalo, et al.: Chemotaxis in yersinia arthritis. Arthritis Rheum., *23*:1036–1044, 1980.

55b. Matzner, Y., Partridge, R.E.H., Levy, M., and Babior, B.M.: Diminished activity of a chemotactic factor inhibitor in synovial fluids from patients with familial Mediterranean fever. Blood, *63*:629–633, 1984.

56. Matzner, Y., and Brzezinski, A.: C5a-inhibitor deficiency in peritoneal fluids from patients with familial Mediterranean fe-ver. New Engl. J. Med., *311*:287–290, 1984.

57. Boggs, D.R., Athens, J.W., and Cartwright, G.E.: The effect of adrenal glucocorticosteroids upon the cellular composition of inflammatory exudates. Am. J. Pathol., *44*:763–773, 1964.

58. Glasser, L., Huestic, D.W., and Jones, J.F.: Functional capa-bilities of steroid recruited neutrophils harvested for clinical transfusion. N. Engl. J. Med., *297*:1033–1036, 1979.

59. Daughaday, C.C., Bohrer, A.N., and Spilberg, I.: Lack of effect of colchicine on human neutrophil chemotaxis under agarose. Experientia, *37*:199–200, 1981.

60. Ho, P.P.K., Young, A.L., and Southard, G.L.: Methyl ester of N-formyl-methionyl-leucyl-phenylalanine. Chemotactic re-sponses of human blood monocytes and inhibition of gold compounds. Arthritis Rheum., *21*:133–136, 1978.

61. Meacock, S.C.R., and Kitchen, E.A.: Some effects of non-ster-oidal anti-inflammatory agents on leukocyte migration. Agents Actions, *6*:320–324, 1976.

61a. Stenson, W.F., Mehta, J., and Spilberg, I.: Sulfasalazine inhi-bition of binding of N-Formyl-Methionyl-Leucyl-Phenylalanine (FMLP) to its receptor on human neutrophils. Biochem. Pharm., *33*:407–412, 1984.

62. Tate, G., et al.: Suppression of experimental acute and chronic inflammation by diets enriched in gamma linolenic acid. (Ab-stract) Arthritis Rheum., *29*:S36, 1986.

63. Lee, T.H., et al.: Effect of dietary enrichment with eicosapen-taenoic and docosahexaenoic acids on in vitro neutrophil and monocyte leukotriene generation and neutrophil function. New Engl. J. Med., *312*:1217–1224, 1985.

24

PLATELETS IN RHEUMATIC DISEASE

ROBERT A. TERKELTAUB and MARK H. GINSBERG

The involvement of blood platelets in inflammatory processes has become recognized as an important aspect of their biology. Here we address the structure and function of platelets as they relate to a potential role in rheumatic disease. Evidence for platelet involvement in the pathogenesis of human rheumatic diseases and clinically significant events involving platelets in certain rheumatic diseases are also reviewed.

PLATELET STRUCTURE AND FUNCTION

Normal platelets are anucleate, discoid cell fragments, approximately 2 μm in diameter, which are derived from marrow megakaryocytes by budding from the peripheral cytoplasm as reviewed in detail elsewhere.[1] Platelets contain at least three types of storage organelles:[2,3] (1) alpha granules storing several platelet-specific proteins and adhesive glycoproteins; (2) dense bodies less numerous than the alpha granule, as the main storage site for biogenic amines, chiefly serotonin; and (3) lysosomes containing neutral and acid hydrolases. Virtually the entire blood content of serotonin is borne in platelet dense bodies. Adenine nucleotides, calcium, and inorganic pyrophosphate are also stored in the dense bodies.

The normal platelet life span in blood is 7 to 10 days, with removal either by the reticuleondothelial system when cells become senescent or by incorporation into hemostatic plugs. Platelets have little or no ability to synthesize proteins.

The main function of platelets is to initiate hemostasis by forming and helping to consolidate a cellular plug at sites of vascular injury.[4] Platelets are specialized for the functions of adhesion, aggregation, and secretion.[5] Adherence to exposed subendothelial collagen in blood vessels is followed by aggregation and release of mediators, which promote further aggregation and vasoconstriction to arrest hemorrhage. The mechanism of this "release action" is reviewed in detail elsewhere.[6] Aggregation and certain platelet adhesive reactions are mediated by the membrane glycoprotein heterodimer IIb/IIIa, which recognizes arginine-glycine-aspartic acid sequences in a variety of adhesive glycoproteins, including fibrinogen and fibronectin.[7] Platelet membrane glycoprotein IIb/IIa is therefore a member of a family of cytoadhesins.[7,8]

Because platelets possess receptors for IgG Fc, IgE, interferon-gamma, certain prostaglandins, and complement proteins, they can interact directly with a number of particulate inflammatory agents, including microorganisms, and may modulate clearance of some of these particles from the circulation. Platelets and their constituents also interact with other inflammatory cells (Table 24–1). Because platelets localize in areas of perturbation of vascular integrity, they participate in the earliest steps of coagulation, inflammation, and tissue repair.[9] They are believed to be critically important in wound healing and in atherogenesis.[4,10] Platelets are thought to participate in inflammation for the following reasons: (1) they release on activation and aggregation, a variety of inflammatory mediators; (2) they are stimulated by phlo-

391

Table 24–1. Platelet-Derived Mediators of Inflammation

Class		Mediator	Actions
I.	Cyclo-oxygenase-dependent	Thromboxanes A_2, B_2	Vasoconstriction, proaggregation, increased neutrophil adherence
		Prostaglandins D_2, E_2, $F_{2\alpha}$	Vasoactive, modulation of hemostasis and leukocyte function
		Hydroxyheptadecatrienoic acid	Chemotaxis
II.	Lipoxygenase-dependent	12-Hydroperoxyeicosatetraenoic acid	Vasoconstriction, cyclo-oxygenase inhibition, stimulation of leukocyte leukotreine B_4 synthesis
		12-Hydroxyeicosatetraenoic acid	Chemotaxis, stimulation of monocyte procoagulant activity
III.	Dense body contents	Serotonin	Vasoconstriction, increasesd vascular permeability, fibrogenesis
IV.	Alpha-granule contents	Thrombospondin, fibrinogen, fibronectin, von Willebrand factor	Adhesive glycoproteins, numerous functions
		Platelet factor 4 (PF4)	Proaggregation, chemotaxis, inhibition of neutral proteases
		Growth factors: platelet-derived (PDGF), transforming (TGF-beta), epidermal (EGF)	Growth and transforming factors
		High-molecular-weight kininogen, factor V	Coagulation proteins
V.	"Granule" contents	Cationic permeability factor	Stimulation of mast cell histamine release, chemotaxis
		Serum-activating enzymes	Generation of C5a in serum
		Cathepsins A, C, D, E	Acid proteinases
		Elastase, collagenase	Neutral proteinase
		α-1-Antitrypsin, α-2-macroglobulin, α-2-antiplasmin	Proteinase inhibition
		Heparitinase	Heparin sulfate-degrading endoglycosidase

gistic agents; (3) they participate in the pathogenesis of animal models of inflammatory disease; and (4) evidence suggests platelet localization and activation at sites of tissue injury in some human inflammatory diseases. Released "mediators" may be newly synthesized, as in the case of metabolites of arachidonic acid (see Chapter 26) or concentrated in storage organelles. The materials released from stimulated platelets may contribute to the inflammatory process by modulating hemostasis, vascular tone, and permeability, by attracting more inflammatory cells, by inducing tissue damage, and by initiating and modulating angiogenesis and matrix formation and repair by effects on connective tissue cells and constituents. Many of the platelet mediators capable of these functions are listed in Table 24–1. Four large adhesive glycoproteins released from alpha-granules (fibrinogen, von Willebrand factor, fibronectin, and thrombospondin) play a critical role in coagulation by forming contact interactions with platelet membrane proteins, vessel wall proteins, and one another.[7,9,11] Released constituents include important growth and transforming factors [platelet-derived growth factor

(PDGF),[10] transforming growth factor beta (TGF-beta),[12] and epidermal growth factor (EGF)[13]], as well as a heparan sulfate-degrading enzyme (heparitinase).[14]

POTENTIAL ACTIVATORS OF PLATELETS IN RHEUMATIC DISEASES

Platelets are activated at sites of vascular injury by hemostatic factors such as thrombin, adenosine diphosphate, arachidonate derivatives, and exposed subendothelial collagen. Other agents also stimulate platelets, several of which agents may be involved in the initiation or propagation of inflammatory responses. Examples of such agents are listed in Table 24–2. Evidence for platelet activation in certain immunologically mediated diseases such as asthma and cold urticaria,[15,16] and evidence for activation in vitro by IgE and interferon-gamma are discussed in detail in the references indicated.[17,18]

Table 24–2. Potential Activators of Platelets in Inflammatory Diseases

Types of Activation	Activator
Hemostatic	Thrombin
	Collagen
	Adenosine diphosphate
	Prostaglandins, thromboxanes
Immunologic	Platelet-activating factor (PAF)
	Immune aggregates
	IgG-coated surfaces
	Antibodies to certain drugs (e.g., quinidine)
	Antiplatelet antibodies
	IgE
	Complement
	Interferon-gamma
Nonimmunologic	Monosodium urate crystals
	Microorganisms
	Double-stranded DNA
Enhancers of activation	Complement
	Single-stranded DNA
	Certain bacterial lipopolysaccharides

PLATELET-ACTIVATING FACTOR

This well-characterized phospholipid mediator is released from stimulated human neutrophils, macrophages, and platelets,[19] aggregates platelets at subnanomolar concentrations, is leukotactic, and stimulates other cells, including neutrophils and vascular endothelial cells. Injection of platelet-activating factor (PAF) into animals induces thrombocytopenia, leukopenia, hypotension, and platelet-dependent bronchoconstriction. PAF generation and cell stimulation are not inhibited by nonsteroidal anti-inflammatory drugs in vitro.

IMMUNOGLOBULIN G-MEDIATED PLATELET ACTIVATION AND ANTIPLATELET ANTIBODIES

Immunoglobulin G (IgG) containing immune complexes, aggregated gamma globulin, and IgG-coated surfaces stimulate human platelets,[20] which possess a receptor for the Fc portion of IgG thought to be identical to membrane glycoprotein IIIa.[21] A 40,000 dalton single-chain platelet membrane protein, apparently identical to p40, a low-affinity receptor on U937 cells for monomeric IgG with the capacity to bind IgG aggregates or IgG-coated particles, has also been described, and monoclonal antibodies to p40 specifically block platelet aggregation induced by heat-aggregated IgG.[21a] Certain drug-induced thrombocytopenias are probably caused by immune complex-mediated platelet sequestration and lysis. Quin-

idine-induced purpura is the best studied reaction;[22] both immunologically specific and nonspecific adsorption of drug-antibody complexes to the platelet surface seem important in its pathogenesis. Such binding is mediated by the platelet Fc receptor and by Fab domain-mediated binding. Quinidine alone binds only weakly to platelets in the absence of drug-dependent antibody. Among antirheumatic drugs, aspirin, acetaminophen, phenylbutazone, and gold compounds have been implicated in some cases of immunologically mediated thrombocytopenias. Antibodies to antigens on the platelet surface may arise in autoimmune states, such as in systemic lupus erythematosus or idiopathic thrombocytopenic purpura, or as a result of isoimmunization after transfusion or pregnancy.[23] Antilymphocyte and antithymocyte globulins may possess antiplatelet activity. Antiplatelet antibodies may either stimulate platelets or inhibit their function, and thrombocytopenia may result from increased reticuloendothelial clearance. In the case of alloantibodies, anti-PlA1 has been clearly shown to react with a major cell surface glycoprotein,[24] whereas antilymphocyte globulins react in part with surface beta-2-microglobulin. In the case of autoantibodies, studies are just beginning to characterize these antigens. The membrane glycoproteins GPIIb/IIIa may be major antigens in some patients with chronic idiopathic thrombocytopenic purpura.[25,26]

MONOSODIUM URATE CRYSTAL-PLATELET INTERACTIONS

Platelets and monosodium urate (MSU) crystals, the causative agent of gouty inflammation, may interact at intravascular and extravascular sites. The study of platelet-crystal interaction has proved useful as a model system for cellular activation in gout and related microcrystalline diseases. MSU crystals induce a selective secretion of dense body constituents followed by platelet lysis in vitro.[27] Four platelet membrane glycoproteins (including GPIIb/IIIa) mediate such platelet stimulation. Removal of these proteins by chymotryptic digestion, or incubation of platelets with F(ab')2 fragments of an antibody directed against these proteins, specifically suppresses platelet secretory responses to MSU crystals.[28]

COMPLEMENT, DNA, LIPOPOLYSACCHARIDE, AND PLATELETS

Platelets interact with complement in a variety of ways.[20,29] First, complement-dependent sequelae to the binding of antiplatelet antibodies may modulate platelet lysis.[20,30] Second, platelets may activate complement by way of C5 cleavage by platelet-bound thrombin.[31] Third, platelets are directly activated by either classic or alternative-pathway complement activation in platelet-rich plasma. Platelet membrane assembly of C5b-9 results in increased binding of coagulation factors Va and Xa to the membrane and a dramatic increase in platelet prothrombinase activity. Thrombin-mediated platelet activation and conversion of arachidonate to thromboxanes are also enhanced in the presence of certain complement proteins. Complement proteins may modulate enhanced procoagulant activity in some diseases associated with complement activation, such as systemic lupus erythematosus. Prolonged bleeding times and impaired in vitro platelet aggregation occur in some individuals genetically deficient in one of the proteins necessary for C5b-9 formation.

Free DNA has been described in serum and plasma in several conditions associated with tissue injury, such as vasculitides and systemic lupus erythematosus. Single- and double-stranded (native) DNA both bind to platelets and the second induces in vitro serotonin release.[32] Single-stranded DNA, but not native DNA, enhances the platelet release reaction induced by heat-aggregated IgG.[32,33]

The bacterial lipopolysaccharide component of gram-negative bacteria may be responsible for a number of in vivo effects, including pyrogenicity, toxicity, and lethality.[34] Lipopolysaccharide may also have several important immunologic actions, in part mediated by effects in Fc receptor-bearing cells, such as macrophages and B cells. The lipid A region of lipopolysaccharide is responsible for many of these effects. Isolated lipid A and lipid A-rich lipopolysaccharide of certain strains have been found to enhance immune aggregate-induced platelet serotonin release approximately fifty-fold, and also enhances secretion of other platelet constituents.[35]

PLATELETS IN ANIMAL MODELS OF INFLAMMATORY DISEASES

Studies of animal models of human disease have assessed the effect of platelet depletion on tissue injury and have documented platelet localization at sites of inflammatory tissue damage.[36] Platelet deposition at sites of tissue injury has been detected quantitatively by the accumulation of [51]chromium (^{51}Cr)-labeled platelets or by ultrastructural pathologic features in such animal models as sponge implantation, reverse passive Arthus reaction in skin, and IgE-me-

diated anaphylaxis. Protective effects of platelet depletion have been reported in models such as IgE anaphylaxis, the Shwartzman reaction, the Arthus reaction in the joint, and serum sickness nephritis, in which released platelet permeability factors may influence the deposition of immune complexes in blood vessel walls. In the case of the Arthus reaction and IgE-dependent skin reactions in the rabbit, platelet depletion does not prevent the lesions, but may be associated with lessening of their severity. This finding exemplifies the inherent redundancy of the inflammatory response, but blocking platelet deposition is without effect in some other animal models. It is thus important to study platelets in human disease directly, rather than with animal models, because of the known functional differences between human and nonprimate platelets.

PLATELETS AS MEDIATORS IN HUMAN INFLAMMATORY DISEASE

Evidence for the role of platelets in human inflammation includes localization at sites of injury, activation in immunologic disease, and abnormalities in specific diseases.

LOCALIZATION AT SITES OF HUMAN TISSUE INJURY

Light-microscopic recognition of platelets in inflammatory lesions is difficult, but ultrastructural techniques have shown platelets in synovial fluids and platelet aggregation in glomerular capillaries.[37] The platelet-specific proteins platelet factor 4 and beta-thromboglobulin (B-TG) have been found in rheumatoid synovial fluids. Only suggestive evidence exists of platelet localization at sites of human immune injury. Use of immunolocalization techniques for platelet-specific antigens and [111]indium-labeled platelets with external imaging should settle this question.[38]

ACTIVATION IN HUMAN RHEUMATIC DISEASES

Measurement of platelet activation in disease has dual significance. First, it implicates platelets in the disease. Second, it may provide a means of monitoring drug effects on platelet activation and an opportunity to elucidate the relationship between disease activity and platelet activation.

Platelet turnover rate has been assessed in patients with immunologic disease, although this procedure is inconvenient and does not measure activation itself, but rather the increased turnover that presumably accompanies platelet activation. Assays of platelet activators in blood and tissue fluids of patients with immunologic disease have been used, but their presence is only an indirect indication of in vivo platelet activation. Assays for detection of in vivo secretion of platelet-specific proteins, however, provide a rapid, simple approach to assess platelet activation in human disease. Future clinical studies will probably use the known activation-dependent platelet expression of a specific protein derived from the alpha-granule membrane as a tissue probe.[38]

PROGRESSIVE SYSTEMIC SCLEROSIS (SCLERODERMA) AND RAYNAUD'S PHENOMENON

Platelet interaction with small-vessel subendothelium exposed by immune endothelial injury may be a factor in the early pathogenesis of scleroderma (see Chapter 73). Release of platelet mediators, including PDGF and a distinct endothelial cell growth factor,[39] would result in smooth muscle cell migration and intimal proliferation with luminal narrowing and eventual fibrosis. TGF-beta released from platelet alpha-granules during blood clotting, and also produced by activated T lymphocytes, promotes angiogenesis and is known to enhance collagen and fibronectin synthesis by fibroblasts.[12] This mechanism may contribute to the remarkable increase in deposition of these proteins in the dermis often seen in sclerodermal skin lesions. Serotonin may cause episodic vasoconstriction (Raynaud's phenomenon) and systemic fibrogenesis.[40,41] Platelets from patients with scleroderma contain decreased serotonin, compatible with an enhanced release of this moiety.[42] Other evidence of in vivo platelet participation in scleroderma includes elevated levels of circulating platelet aggregates and plasma concentrations of B-TG.[43]

Despite this evidence, the results of controlled and uncontrolled therapeutic trials of platelet inhibitors have been mixed. Nifedipine, a calcium-channel-blocking drug with vasodilatory activity, reduces the frequency of both primary and scleroderma-associated Raynaud's phenomenon and inhibits platelet aggregation in vitro.[44] In contrast, ketanserin, a selective antagonist of the platelet aggregating and vasoconstrictive actions of serotonin (binds to cellular S_2-serotonin receptors) may be more effective in relieving than in preventing cold-induced vasoconstriction in

primary Raynaud's phenomenon.[40] Platelet-inhibition therapy with dipyridamole and aspirin or use of dazoxiben, a selective thromboxane synthetase inhibitor that also may enhance prostacyclin synthesis, has not been beneficial.[45,46]

SYSTEMIC LUPUS ERYTHEMATOSUS AND GLOMERULONEPHRITIS

Defective platelet aggregation, independent of therapy with aspirin or nonsteroidal anti-inflammatory agents, occurs in some patients with systemic lupus erythematosus. That increased plasma levels of B-TG and an acquired deficiency of platelet-dense body contents (storage pool deficiency) have been found in patients with this defect suggests in vivo platelet activation as the cause.[47] Potential platelet activators in systemic lupus erythematosus include immune complexes, antiplatelet antibodies, exposed subendothelial collagen (vasculitis), and thrombin, by way of activation of the clotting cascade.[48] Increased plasma levels of free DNA are frequently observed in this disease. As already mentioned, single-stranded (ssDNA) and native DNA both bind to platelets and modulate platelet activation in vitro. Treatment of platelet-rich plasma in patients with this disease with deoxyribonuclease restores defective aggregation in response to collagen contact in platelets of some patients with an acquired storage pool deficiency; this finding suggests that this abnormality is mediated by DNA.[49]

Both acute and chronic thrombocytopenias are encountered in systemic lupus erythematosus, and the course of chronic thrombocytopenia may be similar to that of chronic idiopathic thrombocytopenic purpura.[23] In addition to antiplatelet antibodies, antibodies to platelet-bound ssDNA may play a pathogenetic role in this condition.[33]

Platelet involvment in proliferative glomerulonephritis, as well as other forms of glomerulonephritis, is recognized in patients with systemic lupus erythematosus.[50] A prospective, controlled clinical trial of platelet-inhibitor therapy (dipyridamole, 225 mg/day, and aspirin, 975 mg/day) in 40 patients with idiopathic type I membranoproliferative glomerulonephritis showed an inhibition of the rate of decline of renal function.[51]

RHEUMATOID ARTHRITIS

Sera and synovial fluids from patients with rheumatoid arthritis can activate normal platelets,[42] and increased plasma concentrations of B-TG have been found in some patients.[52] Increased amounts of platelet-activating material in sera and synovial fluids may be important because of the frequent occurrence of increased platelet production and net thrombocytosis in patients with this disease. The degree of thrombocytosis correlated directly with parameters of disease activity and inversely with the hematocrit.[53] Thrombocytosis is also related to the extra-articular manifestations of rheumatoid arthritis, particularly cutaneous vasculitis (see Chapter 44).

Degradation of articular cartilage is a consequence of synovial inflammation in rheumatoid arthritis. Proteolytic degradation of articular cartilage in vitro renders it active as an adhesion site and aggregating factor for platelets.[54] A possible role of platelets in cartilage damage and repair in human disease states remains to be determined.

OTHER VASCULAR INFLAMMATORY DISORDERS MEDIATED BY PLATELETS

A direct role of activated platelets in certain experimental vascular lesions is known.[4] Pathologic evidence now links primary platelet deposition and activation to the physiologic consequences of *erythromelalgia* and thrombotic thrombocytopenic purpura in humans. Platelets are also indirectly implicated in the pathogenesis of pre-eclampsia because early antiplatelet therapy may prevent this disorder.[55]

Platelet-Mediated Vascular Inflammation and Thrombosis in Myeloproliferative Disorders

A syndrome of burning pain and erythema in the extremities, known as erythromelalgia, has been seen in a primary form without underlying disease and in a secondary form associated with the thrombocytosis accompanying the myeloproliferative disorders polycythemia vera and primary thrombocythemia.[56]

The secondary syndrome is associated with histologic evidence of arteriolar inflammation and thrombotic occlusions in vessels from symptomatic areas. Abolition of symptoms follows low doses of aspirin or reduction of platelet counts to normal levels with cytotoxic drugs,[56] but inhibition of thromboxane synthesis with dazoxiben does not relieve symptoms or correct the increased platelet consumption associated with this condition. It has therefore been postulated that precursors of thromboxane A_2 mediate the pain and inflammation in this condition. Platelets from patients with myeloproliferative disorders, but not secondary thrombocytosis, are frequently deficient in lipoxygenase activity,[57] which could lead to increased

endoperoxide and stable prostaglandin production from arachidonic acid by way of cyclo-oxygenase.

Thrombotic Thrombocytopenic Purpura

This disorder, associated with heightened platelet deposition, is characterized by microangiopathic hemolytic anemia, thrombocytopenia, fever, renal dysfunction, and neurologic abnormalities. Sera from affected patients induce agglutination of normal platelets.[58] A 37-kilodalton protein isolated from the plasma of a patient with thrombotic thrombocytopenic purpura, but not from normal or other thrombocytopenic plasmas, possesses this activity.[59] Large multimers of plasma von Willebrand factor enhance the platelet-agglutinating activity of serum in patients with this disease.[58] That circulating large multimers of von Willebrand factor are increased in many patients with vascular inflammatory disorders such as giant cell arteritis and systemic lupus erythematosus,[60] may explain the reported association of thrombotic thrombocytopenic purpura and systemic lupus erythematosus.[61] The relative contributions of endothelial cells and platelets in the pathogenesis of thrombocytopenic purpura remain obscure.

PLATELET PHARMACOLOGY IN RHEUMATIC DISEASE

Many drugs with anti-inflammatory properties inhibit platelet function. Therapy with aspirin (or other nonsteroidal anti-inflammatory drugs, such as indomethacin), may affect platelet aggregation and release reactions.[62] Such drugs have been used successfully to reduce the frequency of thrombotic complications in the treatment of patients with atherosclerotic disease.[63]

Although antimalarial agents such as chloroquine also inhibit platelet function, their clinical significance is uncertain. Several other agents that inhibit platelets or platelet-derived mediators may be therapeutically helpful in inflammatory diseases, as already discussed. These include agents that antagonize serotonin, elevate platelet cyclic adenosine monophosphate, stabilize the cell membrane, and block certain membrane receptors.[64]

In summary, platelets are known to play an important role in thrombosis and thus contribute to the thrombotic complications of inflammation. Platelets are well equipped to function in inflammatory responses by releasing numerous mediators of inflammation.

Platelets may play a crucial early role in the genesis of the inflammatory lesions in some animal models, and growing evidence also suggests platelet localization at sites of tissue injury, platelet activation in the course of immunologic and inflammatory diseases, and direct mediation of vascular inflammation by platelets in humans.

REFERENCES

1. Penington, D.G.: Formation of platelets. *In* Platelets in Biology and Pathology. Vol. 2. Edited by J.L. Gordon. Amsterdam, Elsevier/North-Holland, 1981, pp. 19–42.

2. Da Prada, M., Richards, J.G., and Kettler, R.: Amine storage organelles in platelets. *In* Platelets in Biology and Pathology. Vol. 2. Edited by J.L. Gordon. Amsterdam, Elsevier/North-Holland, 1981, pp. 107–146.

3. Kaplan, K.L.: Platelet granule proteins: localization and secretion. *In* Platelets in Biology and Pathology. Vol. 2. Edited by J.L. Gordon. Amsterdam, Elsevier/North-Holland, 1981, pp. 77–90.

4. Packham, M.A., and Mustard, J.F.: The role of platelets in the development and complications of atherosclerosis. Semin. Hematol., 23:8–26, 1986.

5. De Clerck, F., Somers, Y., and van Gorp, L.: Platelet-vessel wall interactions in hemostasis: implications of 5-hydroxytryptamine. Agents Actions, 15:627–635, 1984.

6. Skaer, R.J.: Platelet degranulation. *In* Platelets in Biology and Pathology. Vol. 2. Edited by J.L. Gordon. Amsterdam, Elsevier/North-Holland, 1981, pp. 321–348.

7. Pytela, R., et al.: Platelet membrane glycoprotein IIb/IIIa: member of a family of Arg-Gly-Asp-specific adhesion receptors. Science, 231:1,559–1,562, 1986.

8. Plow, E.F., et al.: Immunologic relationship between platelet membrane glycoprotein Gp IIb/IIIa and cell surface molecules expressed by a variety of cells. Proc. Natl. Acad. Sci. U.S.A., 83:6,002–6,006, 1986.

9. Schmaier, A.H.: Platelet forms of plasma proteins: plasma cofactors, substrates, and inhibitors contained within platelets. Semin. Hematol., 22:187–202, 1985.

10. Ross, R., Raines, E.W., and Bowen-Pope, D.F.: The biology of platelet-derived growth factor. Cell, 46:155–169, 1986.

11. George, J.N., Nurden, A.T., and Phillips, D.R.: Molecular defects in interactions of platelets with the vessel wall. N. Engl. J. Med., 311:1,084–1,098, 1984.

12. Sporn, M.B., Roberts, A.B., Wakefield, L.M., and Assoian, R.K.: Transforming growth factor-beta: biological function and chemical structure. Science, 233:532–534, 1986.

13. Assoian, R.K., Grotendorst, G.R., Miller, D.M., and Sporn, M.B.: Cellular transformation by coordinated action of three peptide growth factors from human platelets. Nature, 309:804–806, 1984.

14. Castellot, J.J., Favreau, L.V., Karnovsky, M.J., and Rosenberg, R.D.: Inhibition of vascular smooth muscle cell growth by endothelial cell-derived heparin: possible role of a platelet endoglycosidase. J. Biol. Chem., 257:11,256–11,260, 1982.

15. Krauer, K.A.: Platelet activation during antigen-induced airway reactions in asthmatic subjects. N. Engl. J. Med., 304:1,404–1,406, 1981.

16. Grandel, K.E., et al.: Association of platelet activating factor with primary acquired cold urticaria. N. Engl. J. Med., 313:405–409, 1985.

17. Joseph, M., et al.: A new function for platelets: IgE-dependent killing of schistosomes. Nature, 303:810–812, 1983.

18. Molinas, F.C., Wietzerbin, J., and Falcoff, E.: Human platelets possess receptors for a lymphokine: demonstration of high specific receptors for Hu IFN-gamma. J. Immunol., 138:802–806, 1987.

19. O'Flaherty, J.T., et al.: Binding and metabolism of platelet-activating factor by human neutrophils. J. Clin. Invest., 78:381–388, 1986.

20. Henson, P.M., and Ginsberg, M.H.: Immunological reactions of platelets. *In* Platelets in Biology and Pathology. Vol. 2, Edited by J.L. Gordon. Amsterdam, Elsevier/North-Holland, 1981, pp. 265–308.

21. Steiner, M., and Luscher, E.: Identification of the immunoglobulin G receptor of human platelets. J. Biol. Chem., 261:73,230–73,235, 1986.

21a. Rosenfeld, S.I., et al.: Human platelet Fc receptor for immunoglobulin. J. Clin. Invest., 76:2,317–2,322, 1985.

22. Lerner, W., Caruso, R., Faig, D., and Karpatkin, S.: Drug-dependent and non-drug-dependent anti-platelet antibody in drug-induced immunologic thrombocytopenic purpura. Blood, 66:306–311, 1985.

23. McMillan, R.: Chronic idiopathic thrombocytopenic purpura. N. Engl. J. Med., 304:1,135–1,147, 1981.

24. Kunicki, T.J., and Aster, R.H.: Isolation and immunologic characterization of the human platelet alloantigen, PlAI. Mol. Immunol., 16:353–360, 1979.

25. Woods, V.L., Oh, E.H., Mason, D., and McMillan, R.: Autoantibodies against the platelet glycoprotein IIb/IIIa complex in patients with chronic ITP. Blood, 63:368–375, 1984.

26. Beardsley, D.S., et al.: Platelet membrane glycoprotein 111a contains target antigens that bind anti-platelet antibodies in immune thrombocytopenias. J. Clin. Invest., 74:1,701–1,707, 1985.

27. Ginsberg, M.H., Kozin, F., O'Malley, M., and McCarty, D.J.: Release of platelet constituents by monosodium urate crystals. J. Clin. Invest., 60:999–1,007, 1977.

28. Jaques, B.C., and Ginsberg, M.H.: The role of cell surface proteins in platelet stimulation by monosodium urate crystals. Arthritis Rheum., 25:508–521, 1982.

29. Wiedmer, T., Esmon, C.T., and Sims, P.J.: On the mechanism by which complement proteins C5b-9 increase platelet prothrombinase activity. Biol. Chem., 261:14,587–14,592, 1986.

30. Lehman, H.A., et al.: Complement-mediated autoimmune thrombocytopenia: monoclonal IgM antiplatelet antibody associated with lymphoreticular malignant disease. N. Engl. J. Med., 316:194–198, 1987.

31. Polley, M.J., and Nachman, R.L.: The human complement system in thrombin-mediated platelet function. *In* Platelets in Biology and Pathology. Vol. 2. Edited by J.L. Gordon. Amsterdam, Elsevier/North-Holland, 1981, pp. 309–319.

32. Dorsch, C.A., and Killmayer, J.: The effect of native- and single-stranded DNA on the platelet release reaction. Arthritis Rheum., 26:179–185, 1983.

33. Dorsch, C.A.: Enhancement of binding of single-strand DNA to human platelets by aggregated IgG and ADP. Arthritis Rheum., 23:666–667, 1980.

34. Mathison, J.C., and Ulevitch, R.J.: Mediators involved in the expression of endotoxic activity. Surv. Synth. Pathol. Res., 1:34–48, 1983.

35. Ginsberg, M.H., and Henson, P.M.: Enhancement of platelet response to immune complexes and IgG aggregates by lipid A-rich bacterial lipopolysaccharides. J. Exp. Med., 147:207–218, 1978.

36. Ginsberg, M.H.: Role of platelets in inflammation and rheumatic disease. Adv. Inflamm. Res., 2:53–71, 1986.

37. Duffy, J.L., Cinquez, T., Girishman, E., and Churg, J.: Intraglomerular fibrin, platelet aggregation, and subendothelial deposits in lipoid nephrosis. J. Clin. Invest., 49:251–258, 1970.

38. George, J.N., et al.: Platelet surface glycoproteins: studies on resting and activated platelets and platelet membrane microparticles in normal subjects, and observations in patients during adult respiratory distress syndrome and cardiac surgery. J. Clin. Invest., 78:340–348, 1986.

39. King, G.L., and Buchwald, S.: Characterization and partial purification of an endothelial cell growth factor from human platelets. J. Clin. Invest., 73:392–396, 1984.

40. Siebold, J.R., and Terregino, C.A.: Selective antagonism of S$_2$-serotonergic receptors relieves but does not prevent cold induced vasoconstriction in primary Raynaud's phenomenon. J. Rheumatol., 13:337–340, 1986.

41. Sternberg, E., et al.: Development of a scleroderma-like illness during therapy with L-5-hydroxytryptophan and carbidopa. N. Engl. J. Med., 303:782–787, 1980.

42. Zeller, J., et al.: Serotonin content of platelets in inflammatory rheumatic diseases. Arthritis Rheum., 26:532–540, 1983.

43. Kahaleh, M.B.,Osborn, I., and Leroy, E.C.: Elevated levels of circulating platelet aggregates and beta-thromboglobulin in scleroderma. Ann. Intern. Med., 96:610–613, 1982.

44. Han, P., Boatwright, D., and Ardlie, N.G.: Effect of the calcium-entry blocking agent nifedipine on activation of human platelets and comparison with verapamil. Thomb. Haemost., 50:513–517, 1983.

45. Beckett, U.L., et al.: Trial of platelet-inhibiting drug in scleroderma: double-blind study with dipyridamole and aspirin. Arthritis Rheum., 27:1,137–1,143, 1984.

46. Ettinger, W.H., Wise, R.A., Schaffhauser, D., and Wigley, F.M.: Controlled double-blind trial of dazoxiben and nifedipine in the treatment of Raynaud's phenomenon. Am. J. Med., 77:451–456, 1984.

47. Weiss, H.J., Rosove, M.H., Lages, B.A., and Kaplan, K.L.: Acquired storage pool deficiency with increased platelet-associated IgG. Am. J. Med., 69:711–717, 1980.

48. Hardin, J.A., et al.: Activation of blood clotting in patients with systemic lupus erythematosus. Am. J. Med., 65:430–436, 1978.

49. Dorsch, C.A., and Meyerhoff, J.: Elevated plasma beta-thromboglobulin levels in systemic lupus erythematosus. Thromb. Res., 20:617–622, 1980.

50. Partabni, A., Frampton, G., and Cameron, J.S.: Measurement of platelet release substances in glomerulonephritis. Thromb. Res., 19:177–189, 1980.

51. Donadio, J., et al.: Membranoproliferative glomerulonephritis: a prospective clinical trial of platelet-inhibitor therapy. N. Engl. J. Med., 310:1,421–1,426, 1984.

52. Myers, S.L., and Christie, T.A.: Measurement of beta-thromboglobulin connective tissue-activating peptide-III platelet antigen concentrations in pathologic synovial fluids. J. Rheumatol., 9:6–12, 1982.

53. Bennett, R.M.: Hematological changes in rheumatoid disease. Clin. Rheum. Dis., 3:433–465, 1977.

54. Zucker-Franklin, D., and Rosenberg, L.: Platelet interaction with modified articular cartilage. J. Clin. Invest., 59:641–651, 1977.

55. Beaufils, M., Uzan, S., Donsimoni, R., and Colau, J.C.: Prevention of pre-eclampsia by early antiplatelet therapy. Lancet, 1:840–842, 1985.

56. Michiels, J.J., et al.: Erythromelalgia caused by platelet-mediated arteriolar inflammation and thrombosis in thrombocythemia. Ann. Intern. Med., 102:466–471, 1985.

57. Schafer, A.I.: Deficiency of platelet lipoxygenase activity in myeloproliferative disorders. N. Engl. J. Med., 306:381–386, 1982.

58. Kelton, J.G., Moore, J., Santos, A., and Sheridan, D.: Detection of a platelet-agglutinating factor in thrombotic thrombocytopenic purpura. Ann. Intern. Med., 101:589–593, 1984.

59. Siddiqui, F.A., and Lian, E.: Novel platelet-agglutinating protein from a thrombotic thrombocytopenic purpura plasma. J. Clin. Invest., 76:1,330–1,337, 1985.

60. Nusinow, S., Federici, A.B., Zimmerman, T.S., and Curd, J.G.: Increased von Willebrand factor antigen in the plasma of patients with vasculitis. Arthritis Rheum., 27:1,405–1,410, 1984.

61. Amorosi, E.L., and Ultmann, J.E.: Thrombotic thrombocytopenic purpura. Medicine, 45:139–159, 1966.

62. Fuster, V., and Chesebro, J.H.: Antithrombotic therapy: role of platelet-inhibitor drugs. Mayo Clin. Proc., 56:102–112, 185–195, 265–273, 1981.

63. Cairns, J.A., et al.: Aspirin, sulfinpyrazone, or both in unstable angina. N. Engl. J. Med., 313:1,369–1,375, 1985.

64. Didisheim, P., and Fuster, V.: Actions and clinical status of platelet-suppressive agents. Semin. Hematol., 15:55–72, 1978.

25

COMPLEMENT MEDIATORS OF INFLAMMATION

DOUGLAS T. FEARON

Activation of the complement system leads to the generation of mediators that can induce an acute inflammatory response. This well-characterized function of the complement system normally serves to protect the individual from microbial infection by causing the accumulation of leukocytes and by modulating their function at sites of complement activation. However, these same functions of complement may be detrimental if activation is excessive or is triggered by host rather than foreign material, as may occur in the presence of large amounts of immune complexes comprised of autoantibodies. Accordingly, several experimental models of immunologically mediated diseases have emphasized the central position of the complement system in linking the humoral immune response to the recruitment of leukocytes to sites of immune complex deposition. Observations derived from these models have led to one view of the complement system as having only deleterious effects in rheumatic diseases. However, an opposing view, which is based on the frequent occurrence of autoimmune disease in individuals having inherited abnormalities of the complement system, suggests that this system may have beneficial or protective effects by regulating the biologic effects of immune complexes. This chapter presents the biochemistry and cell biology of the complement system which provide the foundation for hypotheses concerning the role of complement in rheumatic disease.

BIOCHEMISTRY OF THE COMPLEMENT SYSTEM

The complement system consists of 18 plasma proteins (Table 25–1) whose designations conform to two conventions. The classic components, which are the plasma proteins responsible for hemolysis of antibody-sensitized erythrocytes, are symbolized with a capital C and a number designating the component (e.g., C1, C4, C2, C3, and C5 through C9). The alternative pathway factors, so-called because they were discovered after the classic components, are denoted with a capital letter (e.g., B, D, and P [properdin]). A bar over a letter or number, as in $\overline{C1s}$, indicates the enzymatically active form of the protein, and cleavage fragments are suffixed with lower-case letters (e.g., C3a and C3b). The most critical step in the elaboration of the biologic functions of the complement system is generation of the major cleavage fragment of C3, C3b; all complement proteins may be grouped into functional divisions according to their interactions with C3 (Fig. 25–1). There are two pathways for initial cleavage of C3, the classic and the alternative; a single amplification mechanism comprised of alternative pathway proteins, which augments C3 cleavage once initial C3b has been generated; and a final common effector sequence that the initiating and amplifying pathways activate after C3b has been generated (Fig. 25–1).

Table 25–1. Physicochemical Characteristics of Proteins of the Complement System

	Approximate Molecular Weight (Daltons)	Serum Concentration (μg/ml)	Cleavage Fragments
Classic pathway of activation			
C1q	400,000	100	
C1r	95,000	50	
C1s	85,000	50	
C4	209,000	430	C4a, C4b, C4c, C4d
C2	117,000	30	C2a, C2b
Alternative pathway of activation and amplification			
Factor P (properdin)	160,000	25	
Factor D	25,000	2	
Factor B	93,000	240	Bb, Ba
C3	190,000	1300	C3a, C3b, iC3b, C3c, C3d,g
Attack sequence			
C5	206,000	75	C5a, C5b
C6	128,000	60	
C7	120,000	55	
C8	153,000	80	
C9	79,000	160	
Control proteins			
C$\overline{1}$INH	105,000	180	
Factor I (C3b/C4b inactivator)	93,000	50	
Factor H (β1H)	150,000	520	
C4bp	1.2×10^6	250	

CLASSIC PATHWAY OF ACTIVATION

The classic activating pathway[1-3] (Fig. 25–2) is comprised of five proteins, three of which—C1q, C1r, and C1s—are bound together in the presence of calcium to form C1 pentamolecular complex, C1qr$_2$s$_2$,[4] and C4 and C2. Initiation of the pathway follows binding of the C1q subcomponent of the Fc region of IgM or IgG1–3 that is present in antigen-antibody complexes. Activation of C1 requires the calcium-dependent intact C1 complex, and interaction of at least two of the six binding sites of C1q with immunoglobulin.[4] The latter requirement has been surmised from studies showing that while a single IgM molecule with its five Fc regions will suffice for conversion of C1 to C$\overline{1}$, at least two adjacent IgG molecules are necessary for this step to occur. Interaction of two C1q binding sites

FIG. 25–1. Relation of the classic and alternative pathways of complement activation to C3 and the effector sequence of complement. Antigen-antibody complexes AgAb initiate formation of the classic pathway C3 convertase, which can cleave C3 to generate C3b and activate C5 to C9. The alternative pathway amplification C3 convertase C3b,Bb is assembled when C3b that was initially generated by the priming C3 convertase C3,Bb or by C4b,2a is deposited on a surface with appropriate biochemical characteristics. This C3 convertase is termed "amplifying" because the product of C3 cleavage, C3b, is a subunit of the enzyme.

FIG. 25–2. The classic activating pathway. C$\overline{1}$, bound to and activated by antibody (Ab) within the antigen-antibody complex (AgAb) sequentially cleaves C4, whose major C4b fragment binds to AgAb and C2 to form the classic pathway C3 convertase, C4b,2a. The reaction is regulated by C$\overline{1}$IMH, which binds to and inhibits C$\overline{1}$, and by the combined effects of C4-bp and I, which result in cleavage of C4b into the inactive fragments, C4c and C4d.

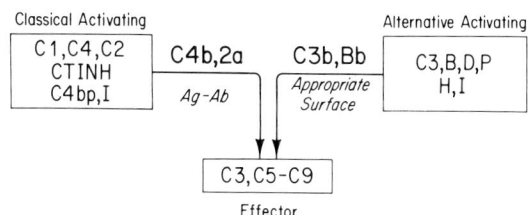

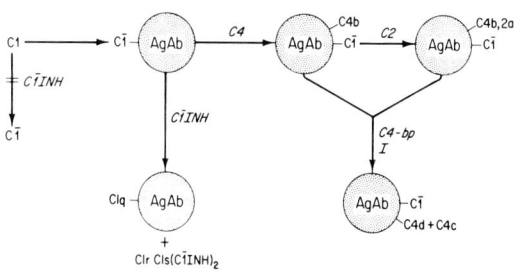

is thought to induce a steric change in the proenzyme C1r, thereby permitting autocatalytic activation to C̄1̄r. The serine protease-active site of C̄1̄r converts C1s to C̄1̄s by cleavage of a peptide bond to reveal its serine protease site. C̄1̄s sequentially acts on its two complement protein substrates, C4 and C2. C4 is cleaved into two fragments, the larger of which, C4b, continues the complement reaction, while the smaller fragment, C4a, has weak anaphylatoxic activity. Generation of C4b reveals a site that transiently has the capacity to bind covalently to membranes or immune complexes, thereby localizing the reaction to the initiating complex containing C̄1̄. This binding of C4b occurs by a transacylation reaction involving an internal thiolester present in the α-polypeptide of C4 and nucleophiles, such as amino or hydroxyl groups on the immune complex. Of the two C4 isotypes, C4A is better able to form amide linkages, whereas C4B forms ester linkages. The bound C4b then forms a reversible magnesium-dependent complex with C2, which is cleaved into its larger C2a and smaller C2b fragment by C̄1̄. The C2a cleavage fragment remains bound to C4b, and the complex is termed the classic C3 convertase because of its capacity to cleave C3. The enzymatic site for C3 cleavage resides on the C2a fragment, and irreversible decay-dissociation of C2a from C4b,2a releases C2i and abolishes C3 convertase activity. C4b is capable of reforming the convertase upon cleavage of additional native C2 and C̄1̄.

In addition to lability of the classic C3 convertase, activation of C3 by this pathway is limited by three control proteins: C̄1̄ inhibitor (C̄1̄INH), C4 binding protein (C4bp), and C3b/C4b inactivator (I). C̄1̄INH inhibits autoactivation of C1r, C̄1̄r activation of C1s, and C̄1̄s cleavage of C4 and C2. Irreversible C̄1̄r₂–C̄1̄INH₂ and C̄1̄s₂–C̄1̄INH₂ complexes are formed, which dissociate from C1q. C̄1̄INH also functions as a control protein for the Hageman factor-initiated pathways because it inhibits the capacity of activated Hageman factor to activate prekallikrein and factor XI of the clotting system and suppresses the kinin-generation of kallikrein. Inherited deficiency of this control protein results in the disease, hereditary angioedema, and is associated with chronically depressed serum levels of C4 and C2 because of their cleavage by uninhibited C1 that is spontaneously generated.

C4bp forms complexes with C4b, thereby blocking the binding of C2 and promoting the cleavage of C4b by I into the C4c and C4d fragments. The latter fragment remains bound to immune complexes and expresses either the Rogers or Chido antigen according to the C4 isotype.[5,6]

ALTERNATIVE AND AMPLIFYING PATHWAYS FOR GENERATION OF C3b

An alternative pathway for C3 cleavage was discovered when zymosan, an insoluble polysaccharide-containing derivative of yeast cell walls, was observed to inactivate C3 in serum without apparent utilization of C1, C4, C2, or specific antibody. Various substances are now known to activate this pathway and include: microbial polysaccharides, such as endotoxin; rabbit erythrocytes and lymphocytes; some human lymphoblastic and virus-infected cell lines; and large, insoluble immune complexes. Cleavage of C3 by the alternative pathway occurs in two distinct phases: continuous, low-grade generation of C3b and subsequent amplified cleavage of C3 by an enzyme that is initially formed with C3b derived from the low-grade reaction[3,7,8] (Fig. 25–3). This C3b-dependent C3 convertase is not only essential for expression of the alternative pathway, but it is inherently capable of amplifying C3 cleavage initiated by the classic pathway.

The constituent proteins of the amplification pathway are C3b, B, D, P, and two control proteins, I and H (see Table 25–1). Initial cleavage of C3 by the alternative pathway occurs continuously and in the absence of activators. C3 that possibly differs from the native form of the protein, in having acquired a C3b-like conformation by spontaneous hydrolysis of its thiolester, forms a fluid phase C3 convertase on interaction with B and D. Small amounts of C3 are cleaved by this enzyme, generating the larger C3b and smaller C3a fragments. As occurs following cleavage of C4, a thiolester within the α-polypeptide of C3b is capable of undergoing a transacylation reaction with amino or hydroxyl groups on nearby cell surfaces, leading to covalent attachment of C3b. This attachment may take place only in the immediate vicinity of C3b because of the short half-life of the thiolester in C3b, which otherwise reacts with H_2O. The bound C3b reversibly binds B in the presence of magnesium, thereby exposing a peptide bond in B that is susceptible to cleavage by D, a serine protease. The major cleavage fragment of B, Bb, remains bound to C3b to form the labile bimolecular complex, C3b,Bb, that is the amplification C3 convertase. The proteolytic site for C3 cleavage resides on the Bb fragment and can be expressed only as long as Bb is bound to C3b. Thus, the rapid irreversible decay-release of Bb, which becomes inactive Bbi, that occurs with a half-life of 4 min at 30° C results in loss of C3-cleaving activity. This intrinsic control of convertase function is overcome by P, which binds to C3b and retards decay-

FIG. 25–3. Competition between B and H for binding to membrane-associated C3b. C3b binds to both nonactivating (NA) and activating (A) cell surfaces, and discrimination between these surfaces by the alternative pathway occurs after this step. On a nonactivating cell, certain membrane constituents, such as sialic acid, promote the binding of H, which facilitates conversion of C3b to C3bi by I. On an activating cell, these membrane constituents are diminished or absent, and binding of B leads to formation of C3b,Bb, which can catalyze deposition of more C3b. Not shown is P, which enhances activation by binding to C3b and stabilizing the C3b,Bb complex.

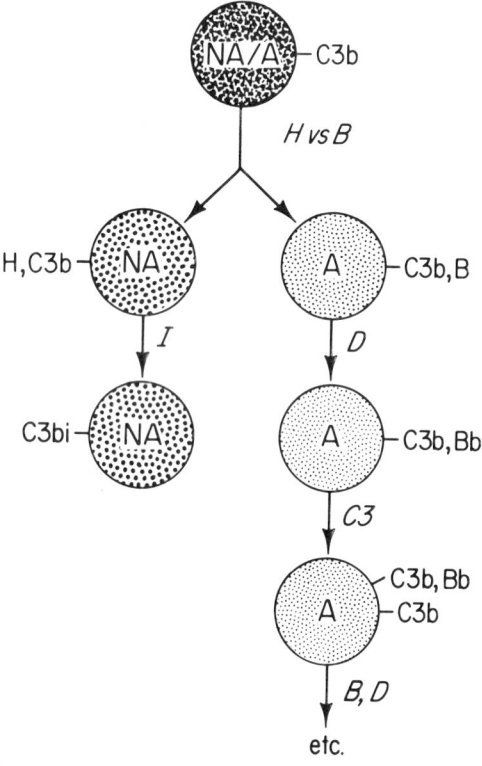

release of Bb from the complex, extending the half-life of C3b,Bb up to 40 min at 30° C.

Regulation of the amplification of C3 convertase is effected by H and I. H binds reversibly to C3b, inhibiting uptake of B or displacing B or Bb, which have already complexed with C3b. In addition, binding of H apparently induces an allosteric change in C3b so that I can cleave the α-polypeptide to generate inactive iC3b. The critical roles of these regulatory proteins are apparent in patients with homozygous deficiencies of H or I who have markedly depressed serum concentrations of C3 and B secondary to their hypercatabolism.

Whether a cell or particle activates the alternative pathway is determined by the relative affinity of bound C3b for B and for H, respectively. C3b that is fixed to the surface of a nonactivator binds H with almost a 100-fold greater affinity ($K_a = 1 \times 10^7$ M^{-1}) than that with which it binds B ($K_a = 1 \times 10^5$ M^{-1}) in the presence of 0.5 mM free Mg^{2+}. Fluid phase C3b also appears to complex with H more readily than it does with B. In contrast, C3b on the surface of a cell or particle that activates the alternative pathway binds both proteins with almost equal avidity. Its association constant for H decreases while that for B remains unchanged. With nonactivating surfaces, formation of the amplification C3 convertase is impaired because H effectively blocks uptake of B by C3b and promotes irreversible cleavage-inactivation of C3b by I. With activators, B can effectively compete with H for binding to C3b, and amplification of C3 cleavage occurs.

A cell surface constituent that regulates the affinity of membrane-associated C3b for H is sialic acid, which is present in some glycoproteins and glycolipids of cells. Naturally occurring activators of the human alternative pathway, such as zymosan or rabbit erythrocytes, have absent and diminished amounts of sialic acid on their surfaces, respectively. Enzymatic removal of sialic acid from sheep erythrocytes or chemical cleavage of its polyhydroxylated side chain converts this cell from a non-activator to an activator of the pathway by decreasing the affinity of membrane-bound C3b for H. The capacity of the alternative complement pathway to respond to cells that are relatively deficient in surface sialic acid may be relevant to its apparent role in natural resistance to infections. Most bacteria lack sialic acid. However, the bacterial species that have capsular sialic acid, such as type III, group B Streptococcus, groups B and C Neisseria meningitidis, and K1 Escherichia coli, are pathogenic for humans.

Specific antibody augments activation of the human alternative pathway by zymosan, rabbit erythrocytes, pneumococci, streptococci, and measles virus-infected HeLa cells, independent of any effects on the classic activating pathway. F(ab')$_2$ fragments are as active as intact IgG, Mg^{2+} but not Ca^{2+} is required, and the reactions can occur in C2-deficient human serum. Large, insoluble immune complexes also activate the alternative pathway with covalent attachment of C3b to the Fd region of IgG.

EFFECTOR COMPONENT REACTIONS

The C4b,2a and C3b,Bb enzymes are identical in their substrate specificities. They both cleave C3 at the Arg77-Ser78 bond of the α-polypeptide chain to generate C3a and C3b, and C5 at the Arg74-Ser75 bond of its α-polypeptide chain to generate C5a and

C5b fragments. The C3 convertases acquire C5 convertase activity only after C3b has attached to a site on the target that is adjacent to the enzyme, perhaps to C4b itself in the case of the classical convertase. This C3b functions by interacting with the substrate C5. The C5b fragment combines with C6 and C7, probably while it is still associated with the C5 convertase, and this trimolecular complex transfers from C3b to the membrane of the target. Uptake of C8 by membrane-associated C5b-7 apparently leads to further insertion of the complex into the bilayer, and binding of as many as five molecules of C9 to a single C5b-8 complex creates stable transmembrane channels by polymerization of C9.[9,10]

The C5b-9 complex can damage membranes by two means. The first is by formation of the transmembrane channel, which appears on electron microscopy as a hollow, thin-walled cylinder of approximately 10 nm height. This structure allows the passage of salt, water, and small proteins leading to net uptake of water by a cell, with consequent swelling and gross disruption of the membrane. The second means of membrane damage involves the disorganization of the lipid bilayer that occurs when large numbers of amphiphilic C5b-9 complexes are formed in target membranes. Membrane damage by this means may be important for lysis of viruses whose envelope membranes do not function as osmotic barriers.

BIOLOGY OF COMPLEMENT

Some of the cleavage fragments of complement proteins that are produced during activation of the system serve as ligands for specific receptors on certain cells, including polymorphonuclear leukocytes, eosinophils, monocytes and macrophages, mast cells, and lymphocytes. These ligand-receptor interactions account for many of the biologic effects of complement (Table 25–2).

The ligands generated during complement activation are of two general types: those that are bound to the target of complement activation, and those that are freely diffusible in the fluid phase. Examples of the former are C1q, C4b, and C3b, which directly promote the removal of microorganisms through endocytosis by leukocytes (opsonins). The diffusible ligands, which are low-molecular-weight cleavage peptides such as C3a and C5a, act as local hormones that cause receptor-mediated cellular responses of secretion, altered metabolism, and migration in the microenvironment. These ligand-receptor interactions also promote the clearance of complement-activating material by causing the accumulation of large numbers of phagocytic cells at sites of complement activation.

Table 25–2. Cell Types Bearing Complement Receptors

Receptor	Cell Type	Cellular Response
C1q	Neutrophil	Respiratory burst
	Monocyte	?
	Null cell	Enhanced ADCC
	B-lymphocyte	?
C4a, C3a	Mast cell	Secretion
CR1 (C3b)	Erythrocyte	Immune complex clearance, production of iC3b and C3d,g
	Neutrophil	Phagocytosis; adsorptive pinocytosis
	Monocyte/macrophage	Same as neutrophil
	Eosinophil	Enhanced phagocytosis
	B-lymphocyte	Enhanced differentation to plasma cell
	T-lymphocyte	?
	Glomerular podocyte	?
CR2 (C3dg)	B-lymphocyte	Synergistic interaction with sIg
CR3 (iC3b)	Neutrophil	Phagocytosis
	Monocyte	Phagocytosis
	Large granular lymphocyte	Enhanced ADCC
C3e	Neutrophil	Release from bone marrow
C5a	Mast cell	Secretion: leukotriene synthesis?
	Neutrophil	Chemotaxis; secretion; increased stickiness; increased C3b receptor expression
	Monocyte/macrophage	Chemotaxis; secretion; spreading; leukotriene synthesis?

BIOLOGIC REACTIONS INDUCED BY INTERACTION OF CELLULAR RECEPTORS WITH BOUND COMPLEMENT LIGANDS

Binding of C3a to specific receptors on mast cells and basophils causes the secretion of granule contents, including histamine, indicating a role for the peptide in altering vascular permeability.[11] C3a also suppresses the maturation of B lymphocytes induced by antigen and polyclonal activators. This has been attributed to inhibition of the production of T cell-derived helper factors, although the cell type that C3a interacts with in this reaction is not known. Removal of the C-terminal arginine by serum carboxypeptidase to generate C3a des Arg abolishes both biologic functions of the peptide.

C3e is a peptide of 10,000 molecular weight that is thought to be derived from the C3c fragment by unknown proteolytic enzymes. This peptide causes leukocytosis when injected into rabbits, and specific binding of C3e to neutrophils has been reported. This activity is also mediated by C3d-K, a kallikrein-derived fragment of C3.

C5a may be the most critical of the diffusible cleavage fragments of complement proteins. Receptors for this peptide exist on mast cells, basophils, neutrophils, and probably on eosinophils, monocytes, and macrophages.[11] Binding to mast cells and basophils induces secretion of histamine and other secretory granule constituents. Incubation of guinea pig lung strips with C5a causes production of slow-reacting substances of anaphylaxis, which are composed of the C-6 sulfidopeptide leukotrienes, but the cell type responding in this reaction to C5a has not been identified. Interaction of C5a with neutrophils causes a range of cellular responses: increased "stickness" that may promote adhesion to endothelial cells, chemotaxis along a concentration gradient of C5a, increased expression of CR1 and CR3 on the plasma membrane, increased oxygen consumption and superoxide generation, and secretion of specific granules. In general, these responses of the neutrophil promote its localization to a tissue site in which complement activation is occurring, and prepare it for endocytosis of the complement-activating material. C5a is also chemotactic for monocytes and induces slow secretion of glycolytic and proteolytic enzymes by this cell type. An interesting finding indicates that C5a causes production of interleukin-1 by macrophages and augments in vitro lymphocyte responses to antigen. In contrast to the effects of carboxypeptidase H on the activity of C3a, conversion of C5a to C5a des Arg by this enzyme does not abolish the biologic activities of

the peptide except, perhaps, that of inducing secretion of histamine by mast cells.

BIOLOGIC REACTIONS INDUCED BY INTERACTION OF CELLULAR RECEPTORS WITH BOUND COMPLEMENT LIGANDS

Three complement proteins attach to the target of complement activation—C1q, C3b and its further degradation fragments, and C4b—and have the capacity to interact with specific receptors present on leukocytes and certain other cell types. Therefore, these proteins mediate the uptake by certain cells of complement-activating complexes.[12]

The C1q subcomponent of activated $C\bar{1}$ becomes accessible for interacting with C1q receptors on leukocytes when $C\bar{1}INH$ binds to the $C\bar{1}r_2$ and $C\bar{1}s_2$ subcomponents, which causes them to dissociate from C1q. C1q receptors have been found on neutrophils, monocytes, B-lymphocytes, a small population of T cells, and some lymphocytes lacking B- and T-cell markers. These receptors probably mediate the attachment of C1q-coated particles and soluble immune complexes, but the consequences of these binding interactions by each cell type are incompletely understood. It has been shown that latex particles coated with C1q induce a respiratory burst by neutrophils, and that antibody-dependent cellular cytotoxicity mediated by lymphocytes is enhanced by the presence of C1q on target cells.

Three different receptors for fragments of C3 that are bound to complement-activating substances are thought to exist: CR1, CR2, and CR3.[13–17] CR1, which has also been termed the immune adherence receptor and the C3b/C4b receptor, binds C3b and C4b. This receptor, which is a 250,000 molecular weight glycoprotein, is found on erythrocytes, neutrophils, monocytes, macrophages, eosinophils, mast cells, all B-lymphocytes, 10% of T cells, and glomerular podocytes. The function of CR1 on erythrocytes may be to facilitate clearance of immune complexes bearing C3b from the blood. Because of its factor H-like activity, the erythrocyte CR1 also promotes the cleavage by factor I of immune complex-bound C3b to iC3b, and to the fragments C3d,g and C3c. CR1 on neutrophils and monocytes facilitates the phagocytosis of C3b-bearing particles and adsorptive pinocytosis of soluble C3b-bearing complexes. The functions of CR1 on B- and T-lymphocytes and glomerular podocytes are not yet understood. Although these receptors can mediate phagocytosis by mast cells of particles bearing C3b, endocytosis of particles would not seem to be a major role for this cell type.

CR2 binds the iC3b, C3dg, and C3d fragments of C3. It is a 145,000 MW glycoprotein that is present on all mature B-lymphocytes, follicular dendritic cells of the spleen, several T-lymphoblastoid cell lines, and pharyngeal epithelial cells. The function of the receptor is incompletely understood, but it has been shown recently to synergize with membrane IgM in the release of intracellular calcium when these two receptors are cross linked. In addition, monoclonal antibody to CR2 has been reported to induce T cell–dependent B cell proliferation. Polymeric human C3dg, perhaps by interaction with CR2, also caused proliferation of murine B cells that had been activated with lipopolysaccharide. Finally, CR2 is the B-cell receptor for the Epstein-Barr virus.

The C3 receptor termed CR3 is specific for iC3b. CR3 is a member of the Mac-1/LFA-1/p150,95 family of membrane proteins. It resides on large granular lymphocytes, macrophages, and neutrophils. This receptor is involved in the phagocytosis of iC3b-coated particles by neutrophils and monocytes, and enhances ADCC reactions of large granular lymphocytes.

INHERITED DEFICIENCIES OF COMPLEMENT PROTEINS

Individuals with an inherited deficiency of a complement component may present with a history of repeated bacterial infections, autoimmune disease, or angioedema, the syndrome being dependent on which component is absent (Table 25–3).

BACTERIAL INFECTIONS

Individuals with homozygous deficiency of C3 generally suffer repeated bacterial infections, making clear the central role of C3 in maintaining normal host defenses by opsonizing foreign organisms to promote their phagocytosis by neutrophils and macrophages. Interruption of complement activation at the C3 step also prevents the bactericidal reaction of the C5b-9 complex and the generation of C5a chemotactic factor, which would otherwise localize leukocytes to the infection site. When H or I is absent from the plasma, there is uncontrolled, spontaneous activation of the alternative pathway, hypercatabolism of C3 and B, and impaired host defense against bacterial infections.

Individuals with homozygous deficiencies of P, C5,

Table 25–3. Diseases Associated with Inherited Complement Component Deficiencies

Deficient Component	Associated Diseases
C1q	Systemic lupus erythematosus, chronic sepsis, skin disease
C1r	Systemic lupus erythematosus, chronic discoid lupus erythematosus
C1s	Systemic lupus erythematosus
C2	Systemic lupus erythematosus, chronic discoid lupus erythematosus, dermatomyositis, vasculitis and Schönlein-Henoch purpura, inflammatory bowel disease, glomerulonephritis, juvenile rheumatoid arthritis
C4	Systemic lupus erythematosus
C3	Recurrent bacterial infections, nephritis
C5	Recurrent Neisseria infections
C6	Recurrent Neisseria infections
C7	Recurrent Neisseria infections
C8	Recurrent Neisseria infections
C9	None
P	Recurrent Neisseria meningitis
C̄1INH	Hereditary angioedema, chronic discoid lupus erythematosus, systemic lupus erythematosus
I	Recurrent bacterial infections
H	Recurrent bacterial infections

C6, C7, or C8 appear to be unusually susceptible to systemic neisseria infections, suggesting that direct complement-mediated cytolysis by the C5b-9 complex may be an important factor in resistance to these organisms.

RHEUMATIC DISEASES

A newly appreciated role for the complement system in preventing autoimmune disease has become evident from analysis of its association with inherited deficiencies of components of the classic pathway of activation[18,19] (Table 25–3). Deficiency of even only one C4 isotype, C4A, predisposes to systemic lupus erythematosus, despite the presence of normal amounts of C4B.[20] The importance of these observations to the understanding of the pathogenesis of these diseases is indicated by the finding of a null allele for C4 and C2 in 80% of patients with SLE.

The molecular basis by which deficiencies of classic pathway components predispose to SLE is not known. Although the C4A, C4B, and C2 genes are located in the major histocompatibility complex, the association of their null alleles with autoimmune disease is secondary to the deficiency rather than being caused by linkage to a particular HLA haplotype. It has been suggested that these components, together with erythrocyte CR1, are important in the clearance of immune complexes.[20,21] The sequential activation of C1, C4, C2, and C3 maintains the solubility of complement-activating immune complexes and causes the covalent attachment of C3b to the complexes. The latter reaction prepares the complexes for a targeted clearance by cells expressing CR1 rather than nonspecific trapping in vascular organs such as the kidney (see also Chapter 27). A model for this type of complement-dependent handling of intravascular immune complexes has been provided by studies in nonhuman primates in which immune complexes infused intra-arterially are rapidly bound by erythrocytes, preventing their diffusion into tissues. Then, because CR1 also serves as a cofactor for the cleavage by factor I of C3b to iC3b and C3dg, the complexes eventually are released from the erythrocytes as these cells pass through the portal circulation, where they are perhaps taken up by Kupffer's cells for degradation. This mechanism for the handling of intravascular immune complexes is dependent not only on C1–C3, but also on the quantitative expression of CR1 by erythrocytes, a genetically regulated characteristic. The relative deficiency of CR1 on erythrocytes of patients with SLE, whether inherited or acquired, would also impair immune complexes clearance.[22-26] Other potential reactions of C1, C4, C2, and C3, such as the generation of ligands for interaction with CR2 on B cells, are less well understood but are certain to be involved in this most important function of the complement system, the regulation of the immune response in a manner that prevents autoimmune disease.

The complement system can prevent the formation of large, insoluble immune complexes and can disaggregate preformed insoluble antigen-antibody complexes in vitro (see Chapter 27). The former reaction appears to be dependent primarily on the classic activating pathway, whereas the latter, which is mediated by the binding of C3b to antibody within the immune complex, is principally dependent on activation of C3 by the alternative pathway. Thus, the absence of C1, C4, C2, or C3 may permit the formation in tissues of relatively larger aggregates of antigen-antibody classes which could induce an inflammatory reaction. Similarly, deficiencies of these components, or of CR1 on erythrocytes, may have the common consequence of impairing the clearance from the circulation of soluble immune complexes by decreasing their opsonization and cellular uptake. These complexes possibly may then deposit in sites other than the reticuloendothelial system where they could induce tissue damage.

The third possibility by which complement deficiencies may predispose to autoimmune disease relates to the recent findings that certain cleavage fragments of C3 may have down-regulatory effects on cellular immune responses. The absence of the components of the classic activating pathway or of C2 would prevent the generation of these fragments by immune complexes, thereby blocking this putative negative feedback role of the complement system. Although it is still not possible to choose among these various explanations, it is becoming more apparent that the complement system, and in particular the classic pathway, has an essential role in the homeostasis of the immune response and should no longer be considered as having only deleterious effects in inflammatory diseases.

ACQUIRED DEFICIENCIES OF COMPLEMENT PROTEINS

An acquired deficiency of a complement protein is caused by hypercatabolism alone or in combination with hyposynthesis. Hypercatabolism reflects complement activation, usually secondary to the presence of excessive amounts of immune complexes, and often correlates with the occurrence of clinical disease. Two unusual mechanisms of acquired hypercatabolism of C3 involve autoantibodies directed to the C3 convertase of the classic and alternative pathways. The former has been found in some patients with SLE and the latter, which has been termed C3 nephritic factor, occurs in some patients with membranoproliferative glomerulonephritis and partial lipodystrophy. These antibodies bind to and stabilize their respective C3 convertases thereby causing augmented C3 cleavage.

Relative functional depressions of C1, C4, C2, and C3 in synovial fluid of patients with seropositive rheumatoid arthritis are taken as evidence of intra-articular activation of the classic pathway, whereas depressions of these components in plasma are generally seen only in those patients having rheumatoid vasculitis. In patients with SLE, the plasma concentrations of C3 are frequently depressed in association with active renal disease, and response to therapy can sometimes be monitored by observing a return to normal plasma levels of the component, presumably indicating lower amounts of complement-activating immune complexes. Thus, acquired deficiencies of complement proteins usually indicate activation of the system by normal mechanisms and frequently indicate the presence of an immunologically mediated pathobiologic process.

CLINICAL ASSESSMENTS OF COMPLEMENT FUNCTION

Activation of a complement protein results in loss of its precursor, native activity, and in the generation of cleavage fragments that are usually more rapidly cleared from plasma than is the native form of the protein. If hypercatabolism is not compensated for by increased synthesis, the finding of a depressed concentration of a complement protein in plasma or other body fluids is evidence for activation of the system. Complement can be measured by assaying the function of its components by hemolytic assays that detect only native, unaltered proteins, or by measuring the protein on concentration of individual components and their cleavage fragments, usually by immuno-precipitation assays. The most frequently employed functional assay of complement activity is the determination of the amount of serum or other body fluid required to lyse 50% of a sample of sheep erythrocytes that have been sensitized with rabbit antibody, and is reported as CH_{50} units. The test measures the overall activity of C1–C9; is not influenced by the alternative pathway proteins B, D, or P; is relatively insensitive to a modest decrease in the activity of a single component; and requires that the sample be assayed immediately or promptly frozen at $-70°$ C. The CH_{50} is useful as an initial screen to detect marked consumption of complement proteins or homozygous deficiencies of individual components. Although specific functional assays for all components of both pathways have been developed, these require specialized reagents not available in most clinical laboratories, and individual components are usually measured by radial immunodiffusion assays.

For the evaluation of patients found to be hypo-complementemic, determination of the C4 and C3 protein concentrations is most informative. Low concentrations of C4 indicate that classic pathway activation has occurred, because C4 is extremely sensitive to C1. Depressed levels of C3 suggest that rather intense activation of either pathway is occurring and, if found to be associated with normal levels of C4, indicate that exclusive activation of the alternative pathway is occurring. A limitation of these assays is that they do not discriminate between native C4 and C3 and their high-molecular-weight cleavage fragments, C4c and C3c, respectively, because most of the antigenic determinants on the native proteins are also expressed by these degradation products. In compartments separated from the vascular system, such as synovial and pleural spaces, clearance of degradation fragments is slow, so that measurement of the protein concentrations will underestimate the extent of complement activation. Assays for C4a des Arg, C3a des Arg, and the C5b-9 complex[25] may be more informative because they provide direct evidence for complement activation. Finally, the involvement of complement in a pathologic process can be directly assessed by immunofluorescent staining of individual complement proteins in the involved tissue and by studies of the metabolism of radiolabeled complement proteins. The former is a useful diagnostic procedure, and the latter technique is useful in clinical investigative studies.

CONCLUDING COMMENTS

The complement system has two pathways for activation: the classic and alternative. The former, through its C1 component, is especially suitable for the recognition of immune complexes, and the latter, by its capacity to interact directly with bacterial cell surfaces in the absence or presence of specific antibody, may be critical for host defense. Activation of either pathway leads to the formation of C3 and C5 convertases which generate the soluble and target-bound cleavage fragments of C3 and C5 which may interact with specific cellular receptors to mediate most of the biologic effects of the complement system. Because many of these effects promote an inflammatory response, the primary role of complement in rheumatic diseases had generally been considered to be deleterious. However, the recognition of autoimmune diseases in a large proportion of individuals having inherited deficiencies of the components of the classic pathway, C1, C4, and C2, and of the C3b receptor, suggests that the complement system may also have a critical role in modulating the immune response. Understanding the molecular and cellular bases for the apparent predisposition of these individuals to rheumatic disease is essential for the definition of the pathobiologic and homeostatic functions of the complement system.

REFERENCES

1. Reid, K.B.M.: Activation and control of the complement system. Essays Biochem., *22*:27–68, 1986.
2. Reid, K.B.M., and Porter, R.R.: The proteolytic activation systems of complement. Annu. Rev. Biochem., *50*:433–464, 1981.
3. Porter, R.R.: The complement components coded in the major histocompatibility complexes and their biological activities. Immunol. Rev., *87*:7–17, 1985.
4. Colomb, M.G., Arlaud, G.J., and Villiers, C.L.: Activation of C1. Philos. Trans. R. Soc. Lond., *306*:283–292, 1984.
5. Yu, C.Y., et al.: Structural basis of the polymorphism of the complement components C4A and C4B: Gene size, reactivity and antigenicity. EMBO J., *5*:2873–2881, 1986.
6. Isenman, D.E., and Young, J.R.: The molecular basis for the difference in immune hemolysis activity of the Chido and Rogers isotypes of human complement C4. J. Immunol., *132*:3019–3027, 1984.

7. Fearon, D.T., and Austen, K.F.: The alternative pathway of complement: A system for host defense of microbial infection. N. Engl. J. Med., *303*:259–263, 1980.

8. Pangburn, M.K., and Muller-Eberhard, H.J.: The alternative pathway of complement. Springer Semin. Immunopathol., *7*:163–192, 1984.

9. Muller-Eberhard, H.J.: The membrane attack complex of complement. Annu. Rev. Immunol., *4*:503–528, 1986.

10. Podack, E.R.: Molecular mechanisms of cytolysis by complement and by cytolytic lymphocytes. J. Cell Biochem., *30*:133–170, 1986.

11. Huey, R., Fukuoka, Y., Hoeprich, P.D., Jr., and Hugli, T.E.: Cellular receptors to the anaphylatoxins C3a and C5a. Biochem. Soc. Symp., *51*:69–81, 1986.

12. Wong, W.W., and Fearon, D.T.: Complement-ligand receptor interactions that mediate biological responses. Annu. Rev. Immunol., *1*:243–271, 1983.

13. Fearon, D.T.: Cell and molecular biology of human complement receptors. *In* Progress in Immunology. Edited by B. Cinader and R.G. Miller. Orlando, Academic Press, pp. 291–298, 1986.

14. Ross, G.D., and Medof, M.E.: Membrane complement receptors specific for bound fragments of C3. Adv. Immunol., *37*:217–267, 1985.

15. Klichstein, L.B., et al.: Human C3b/C4b receptor (CR1): Demonstration of long homologous repeating domains that are composed of the short consensus repeats characteristic of C3/C4 binding proteins. J. Exp. Med., *165*:1095–1112, 1987.

16. Anderson, D.C., and Springer, T.A.: Leukocyte adhesion deficiency: An inherited defect in the Mac-1, LFA-1, p150,95 glycoproteins. Annu. Rev. Med., *38*:175–194, 1987.

17. Weis, J.J., et al.: Identification of a partial cDNA clone for the C3d/Epstein Barr virus receptor of human B lymphocytes: Homology with the receptor for fragments of C3b and C4b of the third and fourth components of complement. Proc. Natl. Acad. Sci. U.S.A., *83*:5639–5643, 1986.

18. Schifferli, J.A., Ng, Y.C., and Peters, D.K.: The role of complement in the elimination of immune complexes. N. Engl. J. Med., *315*:488–495, 1986.

19. Fries, L.F., O'Shea, J.J., and Frank, M.M.: Inherited deficiencies of complement and complement-related proteins. Clin. Immunol. Immunopathol., *40*:37–49, 1986.

20. Cornacoff, J.B., et al.: Primate erythrocyte-immune complex-clearing mechanism. J. Clin. Invest., *71*:236–247, 1983.

21. Cosio, F.G., et al.: Clearance of human antibody/DNA immune complexes and free DNA from the circulation of the nonhuman primate. Clin. Immunol. Immunopathol., *42*:1–9, 1987.

22. Iida, K., Mornaghi, R., and Nussenzweig, V.: Complement receptor deficiency in erythrocytes from patients with systemic lupus erythematosus. J. Exp. Med., *155*:1427–1438, 1982.

23. Wilson, J.G., Wong, W.W., Schur, P.H., and Fearon, D.T.: Mode of inheritance of decreased C3b receptors on erythrocytes of patients with systemic lupus erythematosus. N. Engl. J. Med., *307*:981–986, 1982.

24. Ross, G.D., et al.: Disease-associated loss of erythrocyte complement receptors (CR1, C3b receptors) in patients with systemic lupus erythematosus and other diseases involving autoantibodies and/or complement activation. J. Immunol., *135*:2005–2014, 1985.

25. Walport, M.J., et al.: Family studies of erythrocyte complement receptor type 1 levels: Reduced levels in patients with SLE are acquired, not inherited. Clin. Exp. Immunol., *59*:547–554, 1985.

26. Wilson, J.G., et al.: Deficiency of the C3b/C4b receptor (CR1) of erythrocytes in systemic lupus erythematosus: Analysis of the stability of the defect and of a restriction fragment length polymorphism of the CR1 gene. J. Immunol., *138*:2706–2710, 1987.

26

ARACHIDONIC ACID METABOLITES

EDWARD J. GOETZL and IRA M. GOLDSTEIN

The important roles of products of the oxygenation of arachidonic acid and other polyunsaturated fatty acids as mediators of inflammation and hypersensitivity have been delineated more clearly over the past decade.[1-6] In many different types of cells, arachidonic acid is released from membrane phospholipids in response to specific stimuli. The arachidonic acid is converted by the cyclo-oxygenase pathway to diverse prostaglandins and thromboxanes and by lipoxygenase pathways to hydroxyeicosatetraenoic acids (HETEs) and more complex polar metabolites. The cyclo-oxygenase and lipoxygenase pathways share a dependence on the availability of free arachidonic acid and oxygen and exhibit other common characteristics, such as a critical involvement of unstable epoxide and peroxide intermediates and the requirement for more than one type of cell for optimal generation of some products.

Most of the mediators derived from the oxygenation of arachidonic acid fulfill physiologic activities in normal organ function. For example, prostaglandins may participate in the regulation of ovulation, parturition, and vascular tone.[5] In some circumstances, deficient or excessive concentrations of the same products may initiate or modulate pathologic reactions. Such is the case for the contributions of prostaglandins to dysmenorrhea, anomalous central and peripheral vascular responses, and Bartter's syndrome.[5] The more recently characterized lipoxygenase products of arachidonic acid also appear to serve physiologic roles and have the capacity to evoke responses that are deleterious in some individuals. Lipoxygenase products are important mediators of inflammation and hypersensitivity and, in some instances, such as the constriction of pulmonary airways and stimulation of epithelial cell secretion, are 100 to 1000 times more potent than cyclo-oxygenase products.[2-6]

The purposes of this chapter are to describe the general features of the pathways of enzymatic and nonenzymatic oxygenation of arachidonic acid, the structural and biologic characteristics of the resultant mediators of inflammation, the possible roles of such mediators in rheumatic diseases, and the capacity to influence pharmacologically the generation and actions of the mediators.

MOBILIZATION AND OXYGENATION OF ARACHIDONIC ACID

The rate of metabolism of arachidonic acid by oxidative pathways in most types of cells is controlled primarily by the rate of release of arachidonic acid from phospholipids (Fig. 26–1). Although the events that initiate release of arachidonic acid are different for each type of cell, three general mechanisms have been implicated in the release process. In polymorphonuclear leukocytes and some mast cells, the primary mechanism is the degradation of phospholipase A_2, which releases arachidonic acid principally from phosphatidylcholine.[7] The second mechanism was suggested by the observations that phosphatidylinositol donates arachidonic acid at a signif-

409

icantly enhanced rate in stimulated leukocytes.[8-10] The action of a phosphatidylinositol-specific phospholipase C results in the generation of diacylglycerol, from which arachidonic acid is released by a diacylglycerol lipase. Phospholipase C also generates other potent mediators of cellular activation.[10,11] A third mechanism involves the conversion of phosphatidylethanolamine by sequential methylation to a phospholipase A_2-susceptible phosphatidylcholine, which serves as the source of arachidonic acid in some leukocytes.[12] The importance of the last pathway in mononuclear leukocytes and some mast cells was implied by the similar time-course of the degradation of phosphatidylethanolamine-derived phosphatidylcholine and the release of arachidonic acid, as well as by the capacity of phospholipase inhibitors and inhibitors of phospholipid methylation to block leukocyte functional responses.[12] The fate of free arachidonic acid is either reacylation into phospholipids or oxygenation to more polar compounds.

The cyclo-oxygenation of arachidonic acid consists of a sequence of complex molecular rearrangements and oxygenations that lead to the formation of 15-hydroperoxy-9-α, 11α-peroxidoprosta-5,13-dienoic acid, which is an endoperoxide designated PGG_2 (see Figure 26–1).[2,4] Reduction of the C-15 hydroperoxy-group of PGG_2 generates the more polar endoperoxide, PGH_2, which serves as the common precursor for prostaglandins, prostacyclin, and thromboxanes. PGH_2 is converted to PGE_2 by an isomerase and to $PGF_{2\alpha}$ by a reductase, while a distinct synthetase in the walls of blood vessels, mononuclear phagocytes, and some other cells transforms PGH_2 to prostacyclin, or PGI_2.[4,13,14]

PGH_2 is converted to thromboxane A_2 in platelets and some other types of cells.[3,15] Thromboxane A_2 and each of the prostaglandins have a unique profile of actions on blood vessels, smooth muscle, platelets, and other cells (Table 26–1). PGE_2 and PGI_2 decrease tone and increase the permeability of vessels in the microcirculation.[14-16] In contrast, thromboxane A_2 and $PGF_{2\alpha}$ increase microvascular tone, and $PGF_{2\alpha}$ decreases slightly the natural permeability of microvasculature as well as the increased permeability induced by other agonists.[3,14-16] Although less potent than some of the lipoxygenase products of arachidonic acid, $PGF_{2\alpha}$, PGI_2, and thromboxane A_2 constrict and PGE_2 dilates both large and small airways of the lungs.[5,14,16] The potent bidirectional effects of thromboxane A_2 and PGI_2 on platelet aggregation and other functions are intravascular activities critical to the control of hemostasis and the development of some atherosclerotic lesions.[5,17] Identical bidirectional effects of thromboxane A_2 and PGI_2 are expressed in relation to

the adherence of leukocytes to surfaces (see Table 26–1). Other direct and modulatory effects of prostaglandins on leukocyte functions are generally less pronounced than the corresponding activities of lipoxygenase products.[5,16] PGE_2 derived largely from macrophages suppresses the secretory and proliferative responses of subsets of T-lymphocytes to antigens and mitogenic lectins,[18-21] which appears to account for part of the suppressive function of macrophages and perhaps some T-lymphocytes.

The lipoxygenation of arachidonic acid by different pathways shares some features with the cyclo-oxygenation reactions and is equally complex (see Fig. 26–1). An unstable hydroperoxyeicosatetraenoic acid (HPETE) is the initial metabolite of each lipoxygenase pathway. The HPETE is either reduced to the more stable corresponding HETE or is transformed to an epoxide which serves as the precursor for more highly substituted and polar products.[2,4,5] The HPETEs and epoxides are analogous to the endoperoxides and to thromboxane A_2, respectively, in the cyclo-oxygenase pathway. Similarly, the HETEs and related derivatives are analogous to the prostaglandins. In both types of pathways, oxidation and hydrolysis are the predominant mechanisms for either conversion to less active mediators or degradation (see Fig. 26–1). HETEs and more complex products of the lipoxygenase pathways, such as leukotrienes, have the capacity to alter microvascular and smooth muscle function and to initiate and modify leukocyte activities, but have no consistent effects on platelets (see Table 26–1).[5,6,16]

Dioxygenation events are a more characteristic feature of the lipoxygenase pathways. The 5-lipoxygenation of 12-HETE by leukocytes and the 12-lipoxygenation of 5-HETE by platelets both generate isomers of 5,12-diHETE (Fig. 26–1). In addition, the 5-lipoxygenation of 15-HPETE or 15-HETE by leukocytes initiates a complex series of reactions that yields specific tri-HETEs, termed lipoxins,[22] capable of selectively stimulating some functions of PMN leukocytes and inhibiting the activity of human natural killer cells.[22,23]

Products of arachidonic acid are susceptible to precise quantification by both chromatographic and immunochemical techniques. The prostaglandins, HETEs, and other lipoxygenase products can be assayed directly, while thromboxane A_2 and PGI_2 are assessed in terms of their stable metabolites, thromboxane B_2 and 6-keto-$PGF_{1\alpha}$ respectively.

NONENZYMATIC PATHWAYS LEADING TO PRODUCTION OF BIOLOGICALLY ACTIVE ARACHIDONIC ACID METABOLITES

Because enzymatic conversion of arachidonic acid to biologically active hydroxy-derivatives proceeds

Table 26–1. Primary Inflammatory Effects of Arachidonic Acid Products

	LTB₄	LTC₄	LTD₄	TxA₂	PGF₂	PGI₂	PGE₂
Microvasculature	Increases permeability Decreases tone; may increase tone transiently	Increases permeability Decreases tone; may increase tone transiently	Increases permeability Decreases tone; may increase tone transiently	Increases tone	Decreases permeability Increases tone	Increases permeability Decreases tone	Increases permeability Decreases tone
Pulmonary airways	Constricts small > large LTD₄ > LTC₄ >> LTB₄	Constricts small > large	Constricts small > large	Constricts	Constricts small ≅ large	Constricts small ≅ large	Dilates
PMN leukocytes and macrophages	Stimulates chemotaxis; other specific functions			Increases adherence to surfaces		Enhances random migration Decreases adherence to surfaces	Enhances random migration
	Increases adherence to surfaces	Increases adherence to surfaces	Increases adherence to surfaces			Decreases some responses to other stimuli	Decreases some responses to other stimuli
T-lymphocytes	Inhibits transformation and secretion; induces suppressor cells						Inhibits transformation and secretion; induces suppressor cells
Platelets				Aggregates (through ADP)		Inhibits aggregation (through cAMP)	
Other actions	Stimulates pulmonary airway secretion of mucous glycoproteins LTC₄/D₄ > LTB₄	Stimulates pulmonary airway secretion of mucous glycoproteins LTC₄/D₄ > LTB₄	Stimulates pulmonary airway secretion of mucous glycoproteins LTC₄/D₄ > LTB₄			Induces hyperalgesia	

FIG. 26–1. Common characteristics of the cyclo-oxygenation and lipoxygenation of arachidonic acid. PG = prostaglandin; HETE = hydroxyeicosatetraenoic acid; DI-HETE = dihydroxyeicosatetraenoic acid; HPETE = hydroperoxyeicosatetraenoic acid; LT = leukotriene.

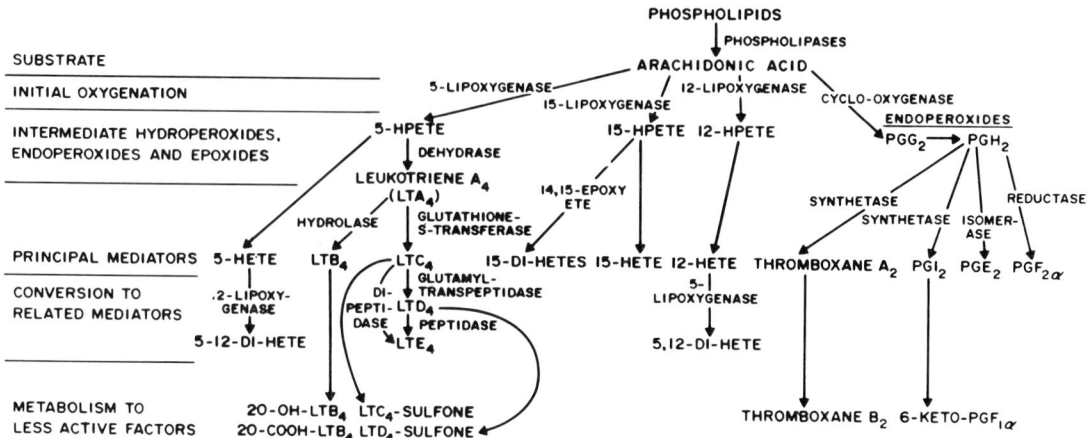

through the formation of hydroperoxides, it is not surprising that similar derivatives can be generated nonenzymatically by free radical-mediated reactions. Turner et al., for example, found that exposure of arachidonic acid either to air for 24 hours or to ultraviolet irradiation resulted in the generation of oxidized lipids that were chemotactic for human polymorphonuclear leukocytes.[24,25] The products generated in this fashion were identified as positional isomers of hydroxyeicosatetraenoic acids.

Perez et al. described another mechanism whereby arachidonic acid can be converted nonenzymatically to biologically active products.[26] Chemotactic activity for human polymorphonuclear leukocytes was generated upon exposure of arachidonic acid to a superoxide-generating system consisting of xanthine oxidase and acetaldehyde. Generation of chemotactic activity in this experimental system was time-dependent and could be inhibited significantly by scavengers of singlet oxygen, as well as by scavengers of superoxide, hydrogen peroxide, and hydroxyl radicals. Silica gel thin-layer radiochromatography demonstrated a product with chemotactic activity that was distinct from unaltered arachidonic acid and from 12-HETE. The isolated product was chemotactic for human polymorphonuclear leukocytes at a concentration (approximate) of 3.0 ng/ml and chemokinetic at concentrations of 0.75 to 1.5 ng/ml.

The precise identity of the chemotactic lipid formed from arachidonic acid by exposure to a superoxide-generating system was not determined. There is evidence, however, that hydroxyl radicals and singlet oxygen can convert arachidonic acid to several bio-

logically active products. Fridovich and Porter, for example, found that exposure to xanthine oxidase and acetaldehyde converted arachidonic acid to a series of conjugated diene hydroperoxides (i.e., HPETEs).[27] The 15-hydroperoxide and 5-substituted hydroperoxide were the major products formed. Co-oxidation of arachidonic acid by the xanthine oxidase-acetaldehyde system was inhibited by either superoxide dismutase or catalase and was stimulated by the addition of ferrous salts. These findings suggested that hydroxyl radicals, or similar reactive species generated by the iron-catalyzed interaction of superoxide with hydrogen peroxide, were responsible for the formation of hydroperoxy-acids from arachidonate. Porter et al. also found that arachidonic acid could be oxidized by exposure to either air or singlet oxygen (generated by photolysis) to yield a mixture of hydroperoxides, including 5-HPETE, 12-HPETE, and 15-HPETE.[28,29]

Phagocytic leukocytes (particularly polymorphonuclear leukocytes) are capable of generating abundant amounts of oxygen-derived free radicals and producing lipid peroxides.[30,31] Consequently, under conditions that exist at most foci of inflammation, it is possible for potent chemoattractants to be generated from arachidonic acid by mechanisms involving free radicals. Generation of chemotactic products from arachidonic acid may be important for amplifying inflammatory responses.

Another chemoattractant formed by the action of oxygen-derived free radicals was described by Petrone et al.[32] These investigators found that potent chemotactic activity for human polymorphonuclear leukocytes could be generated in vitro by exposing normal human plasma to a source of superoxide anion radicals (i.e., xanthine oxidase and sodium xanthine). Generation of chemotactic activity in this system was inhibited by superoxide dismutase, but not by catalase. When plasma that had been exposed to superoxide anion radicals was injected intradermally into rats, large numbers of polymorphonuclear leukocytes accumulated at the injection sites. Infiltration by these cells was evident as early as 30 minutes after injection and increased with time. A similar response was observed when rats were injected intradermally with xanthine oxidase and xanthine. No leukocyte infiltration was observed, however, if superoxide dismutase was injected simultaneously with the enzyme and substrate.

The chemotactic activity that was formed by exposing plasma to superoxide was heat-labile (56°C for 30 minutes), nondialyzable, and stable to lyophilization. The bulk of the activity was recovered after gel filtration and ion exchange chromatography of treated plasma in fractions containing albumin. Albumin per se, however, was not chemotactic. Rather, the chemotactic factor appeared to consist of a chloroform-extractable component (i.e., lipid) that was bound to albumin. Although the nature of the lipid was not determined, it is intriguing to speculate that it may be a hydroperoxy- or hydroxy-derivative of arachidonic acid.

Based on these findings, it has been proposed that (1) superoxide anion radicals produced by stimulated leukocytes interact with a plasma precursor to form a potent chemotactic factor that propagates and amplifies inflammatory reactions, and (2) superoxide dismutase ameliorates inflammation by preventing the formation of superoxide-dependent chemotactic activity.

PROINFLAMMATORY EFFECTS OF PROSTAGLANDINS

There is ample evidence that stable prostaglandins, thromboxanes, and prostacyclin are mediators of inflammation.[33-35] First, these compounds are capable of provoking many of the cardinal signs of inflammation (e.g., erythema, fever, pain, edema). Second, they are synthesized by phagocytic cells and are released in large amounts during inflammatory reactions. Finally, synthesis of stable prostaglandins, thromboxanes, and prostacyclin is inhibited by many anti-inflammatory drugs. Details concerning the proinflammatory effects of prostaglandins are summarized in the sections that follow.

Erythema and Fever. It has been demonstrated conclusively that products of the cyclo-oxygenase pathway of arachidonic acid metabolism contribute to the erythema, local increases in temperature, and fever associated with many forms of acute and chronic inflammation. PGI_2, PGE_1, PGE_2, PGD_2, and PGA_2, for example, have been found capable of provoking vasodilation.[14,36,37] The most potent of these compounds, PGI_2, markedly increases the diameter of precapillary arterioles.[38] In contrast, the cyclic endoperoxides (e.g., PGH_2) and thromboxane A_2 are potent vasoconstrictors.[14]

Prostaglandins of the E series, as well as arachidonic acid, produce fever in experimental animals when injected directly into the cerebral ventricles.[39] In addition, levels of prostaglandins are increased in the cerebrospinal fluid of animals rendered febrile by both endogenous and exogenous pyrogens.[40,41] These observations, together with the fact that almost all nonsteroidal anti-inflammatory agents also are antipyretic agents,[42] support the hypothesis that products of arachidonic acid formed by the cyclo-oxygenase pathway contribute to the development of hyperpyrexia.

Pain and Edema. The roles played by stable prostaglandins in provoking the pain and edema that accompany inflammation are more complex. For example, in a number of experimental models, stable prostaglandins (e.g., PGE compounds) have been found incapable of provoking pain directly.[43,44] They do, however, produce hyperalgesia and act synergistically with other mediators (e.g. histamine, bradykinin) to augment pain.[43,45] PGE_2, for example, when injected into human skin, causes a marked potentiation of the pain produced by intradermal injections of either histamine or bradykinin.[43] PGE_2 not only enhances the intensity of the pain provoked by these mediators, but prolongs the duration as well.

As in the case with pain, prostaglandins appear to be incapable of directly causing edema, but act synergistically with other mediators. Williams and Peck, for example, showed that intradermal injections of E-type prostaglandins in rabbits produce large increases in local blood flow with little, if any, plasma exudation.[37] Bradykinin and histamine, on the other hand, increased vascular permeability (resulting in plasma exudation) for 10 to 15 minutes after injection, but were far less potent with respect to their ability to increase blood flow. Prostaglandins potentiated the vascular permeability changes provoked by histamine and bradykinin. The ability of any individual prostaglandin to potentiate plasma exudation was directly related to its ability to enhance blood flow. It appears, therefore, that the edema of acute inflammation is not due directly to products of the cyclo-oxygenase pathway of arachidonic acid metabolism, but can be modulated by inhibitors of this pathway (e.g., nonsteroidal anti-inflammatory agents).

More recent evidence suggests that products of arachidonic acid play a role in provoking changes in vascular permeabilty mediated by complement and polymorphonuclear leukocytes. For example, purified rabbit and human C5a-des-arg (which lacks intrinsic anaphylatoxin activity) caused increased vascular permeability in rabbit skin only in the presence of added prostaglandins (e.g., PGE_1 and PGE_2) and only in animals with normal numbers of circulating polymorphonuclear leukocytes.[46,47] As indicated previously, prostaglandins probably enhance exudation of plasma across (or through) the endothelium by inducing vasodilatation and increased flow.

Other products of the cyclo-oxygenase pathway may promote vascular permeability changes. Prostacyclin (PGI_2), for example, dilates blood vessels and augments edema provoked by other mediators.[38,48] Thromboxane A_2 also may provoke some forms of vascular injury by enhancing adherence of polymorphonuclear leukocytes to endothelial surfaces.[49]

Tissue Injury (Resorption of Bone). Apart from their ability to influence vascular tone and permeability, prostaglandins show little evidence of directly causing tissue injury. It has been suggested, however, that at least some of the tissue damage that accompanies inflammation is produced indirectly by free radicals (e.g., hydroxyl radicals), which are generated during the enzymatic conversion of PGG_2 to PGH_2.[50] Inhibition of the formation of such free radicals or their elimination by scavengers may account for the potent anti-inflammatory effects of some drugs that do not inhibit the synthesis of stable prostaglandins.

Although prostaglandins generally are incapable of causing tissue injury, it has been demonstrated that PGE_2 stimulates bone resorption in vitro and in vivo.[51,52] PGE_2 produced by rheumatoid synovia promotes resorption of bone in the absence of other major products of the rheumatoid tissue. In addition, rheumatoid synovial tissue in culture produces approximately 10 times more PGE_2 than normal synovial tissue. It appears likely, therefore, that prostaglandins (particularly PGE_2) produced by hypertrophic and hyperplastic synovial tissue contribute to the destruction of juxta-articular bone in rheumatoid arthritis. Since PGE compounds also inhibit collagen biosynthesis in vitro,[53] enhanced production of prostaglandins by rheumatoid synovium may lead to additional detrimental effects in adjacent connective tissue.

Generation of Prostaglandins at Sites of Inflammation. Large amounts of stable prostaglandins have been detected at foci of inflammation, and these compounds are synthesized by phagocytic cells (i.e., polymorphonuclear leukocytes, monocytes, and macrophages).[54–56] Human polymorphonuclear leukocytes released prostaglandins of the E and F series to the surrounding medium when these cells were exposed to suitably opsonized zymosan particles.[56] Prostaglandin E was found in the highest concentration in the medium, and the prostaglandin E to prostaglandin F ratio was approximately 3:1. Prostaglandin release was not due to contamination of the reaction mixtures with platelets and was inhibited by indomethacin and aspirin. Stimulated human polymorphonuclear leukocytes also generated thromboxane A_2.[57,58] Finally, and perhaps most relevant to the types of inflammation observed in patients with rheumatoid disease, inflamed synovial tissue synthesized large amounts of PGE compounds (see the following section).

Inhibition of Prostaglandin Biosynthesis by Anti-Inflammatory Drugs. The most compelling evidence that stable prostaglandins are mediators of inflammation has come from studies of the effects of various drugs on the biosynthesis of these compounds. Most nonsteroidal anti-inflammatory agents and anti-inflammatory adrenal corticosteroids inhibit the biosynthesis of stable prostaglandins.

From the foregoing discussion, it might be concluded that stable prostaglandins are important mediators of inflammation and that many anti-inflammatory drugs produce their beneficial effects by inhibiting prostaglandin biosynthesis, but some observations suggest alternative conclusions.

INHIBITION OF LEUKOCYTE FUNCTIONS BY PROSTAGLANDINS

Abundant evidence has been accumulated during the past decade indicating that several functions of cells involved in acute and chronic inflammatory reactions (i.e., polymorphonuclear leukocytes, monocytes, macrophages, lymphocytes) can be modulated by cyclic nucleotides. For example, selective extracellular release of proinflammatory lysosomal constituents from stimulated human peripheal blood polymorphonuclear leukocytes in vitro, as well as release of mediators of inflammation from other cell types, can be inhibited either by cyclic 3′,5′-adenosine monophosphate (cAMP) directly or by pharmacologic agents that increase levels within cells of this cyclic nucleotide.[59–61] Therefore, consistent with their ability to increase cellular levels of cAMP, some prostaglandins (e.g., PGE_1, PGE_2) act as ''extracellular messengers" and inhibit release of mediators of inflammation from leukocytes.[62] Prostaglandins of the E series, as well as PGI_2, also inhibit leukocyte chemotaxis,[63,64] adherence to various substrates (including endothelium),[65,66] phagocytosis,[67] and generation of oxygen-derived free radicals.[68] Inhibitory effects on various functions of B- and T-lymphocytes have been reported as well. For example, PGE_1 and PGE_2 (with or without the phosphodiesterase inhibitor, theophylline) suppress proliferative responses of human lymphocytes to mitogen, lymphocyte-mediated cytotoxicity, and antibody production by B-lymphocytes.[20,69,70]

In contrast to the effects of cAMP, cyclic 3',5'-guanosine monophosphate (cGMP) and agents that elevate levels within cells of cGMP enhance some leukocyte functions. $PGF_{2\alpha}$, for example, increases levels of cGMP in polymorphonuclear leukocytes and enhances selective release from these cells of lysosomal constituents.[60–62] $PGF_{2\alpha}$ enhances other functions of polymorphonuclear leukocytes,[64] and augments certain functions of B and T lymphocytes.[69,70] It is not surprising, therefore, that considerable attention has been focused recently on the potential roles played by prostaglandins in regulating inflammatory reactions, as well as both humoral and cellular immune reactions. It has been suggested, for example, that by local, preferential biosynthesis of one or another of the prostaglandins, the very cells that release mediators of inflammation provide a mechanism for modulating inflammatory responses. PGF compounds may enhance inflammation, whereas PGE compounds, by acting as feedback, actually may provide a "shutoff" signal and reduce inflammation.

ANTI-INFLAMMATORY EFFECTS OF PROSTAGLANDINS IN EXPERIMENTAL ANIMALS

From the foregoing discussion, it seems possible that prostaglandins that inhibit leukocyte functions in vitro also may exhibit anti-inflammatory effects in vivo. Examples of some anti-inflammatory effects of prostaglandins in various forms of experimentally induced inflammation are discussed in the following sections.

Adjuvant Arthritis. Adjuvant disease in the rat includes a severe and persistent polyarthritis that appears 10 to 14 days after a single intradermal injection of complete Freund's adjuvant. PGE_2 significantly reduces tibiotarsal joint swelling in rats with adjuvant arthritis.[71] In subsequent studies,[72,73] it was observed that PGE_1 (500 µg administered intraperitoneally

twice daily) either prevented or suppressed adjuvant arthritis, while the same treatment with PGA_2 had no effect on the disease. Arthritis was prevented when rats were treated either from the day of adjuvant injection or from day seven. When treatment was begun on day 14, the typical explosive course of the arthritis was suppressed. Established inflammation was reduced significantly even when treatment was begun on day 21. Similar results were obtained with PGE_1 and PGE_2 in adrenalectomized rats.

Whereas treatment of rats with PGE compounds did not suppress delayed hypersensitivity reactions to mycobacterial antigens, anti-sheep red blood cell–antibody titers were reduced. Treatment with PGE compounds also reduced the numbers of circulating lymphocytes. Despite these and other observations relative to the effects of prostaglandins on humoral and cellular immune reactivity, the mechanisms whereby PGE compounds suppress adjuvant arthritis in rats is still unknown.

Carrageenan-Induced Inflammation. PGE_1 and PGE_2 also suppressed inflammation in rats injected with carrageenan.[72] Administration of PGE compounds into subcutaneous air blebs at the time of carrageenan injection reduced the number of polymorphonuclear leukocytes that entered the focus of inflammation. PGE_1 and PGE_2 also produced concentration-dependent reductions in exudate lysosomal enzyme (i.e., beta-glucuronidase) and cytoplasmic enzyme (i.e., lactate dehydrogenase) levels. Ultrastructural studies revealed that carrageenan was ingested by invading leukocytes and enclosed within phagocytic vacuoles, the membranes of which subsequently ruptured. More lysosomes apparently remained intact after carrageenan uptake by bleb leukocytes from PGE-treated rats than from control rats. There also was no loss of phagosomal membrane integrity in cells from treated rats.

Another carrageenan-induced lesion has been used to evaluate the effectiveness of anti-inflammatory drugs. Carrageenan-induced edema in the rat footpad is associated with three distinct phases of mediator-induced vascular permeability changes.[25] The initial phase probably results from the release of histamine and serotonin and is inhibited by antihistamines. The second phase has been attributed to the action of bradykinin. The third phase of persistent edema has been attributed to the local production of prostaglandins (particularly PGE_2) by inflammatory cells. Interestingly, treatment of rats systemically with either PGE_1 or the more stable derivative, 15-(S)-15 methyl PGE_1, significantly inhibits carrageenan-induced rat footpad edema.[74] Both the acute phase of edema formation and the later phases are reduced in a dose-dependent fashion by PGE_1 and PGE_2, but not by $PGF_{2\alpha}$.

The effects of PGE compounds on carrageenan-induced rat footpad edema coincide with the findings reported previously that PGE_1 and 15-(S)-15-methyl PGE_1 (but not PGA_2 or $PGF_{2\alpha}$) greatly reduce the increases in vascular permeability induced in rats by intradermal injections of histamine, serotonin, bradykinin, the complement-derived anaphylatoxin C3a, and compound 48/80.[75] Suppression by the PGE compounds of vascular permeability changes is associated ultrastructurally with preservation of tight junctions between endothelial cells. Interference with the local effects of vasopermeability mediators may account for the suppressive effects of PGE compounds on immune complex-induced inflammation and tissue injury in experimental animals.

Immune Complex–Induced Inflammation. Vascular permeability changes after induction of reversed passive Arthus reactions in rat skin were suppressed significantly by pretreatment with either PGE_1 or its stable derivative, 15-(S)-15-methyl PGE_1.[76] Suppression also was observed in animals treated with PGE_2 and PGD_2, but not $PGF_{2\alpha}$. Interestingly, the stable derivative of PGE_1 also was effective when administered orally. Diminished vascular permeability in treated animals was accompanied by markedly reduced exudation of polymorphonuclear leukocytes. For the most part, leukocytes remained within dermal venules and capillaries, despite the observations by transmission electron microscopy and/or by immunofluorescence microscopy that immune complexes and complement were deposited in the walls of these blood vessels. Ingestion of immune complexes by leukocytes also was reduced in treated animals. Polymorphononuclear leukocytes harvested from the blood of rats treated with PGE_1 exhibited depressed chemotactic responses in vitro as well as diminished lysosomal enzyme secretion after incubation with a chemotactic peptide.

Suppression of human polymorphonuclear leukocyte degranulation also has been observed following intravenous infusion of PGE_1 for the treatment of peripheral vascular disease.[77] A detailed study of this phenomenon[78] revealed evidence that administration systemically of 15-(S)-15-methyl PGE_1 reduces the binding affinity of the receptor on rat polymorphonuclear leukocytes for the synthetic chemotactic peptide. N-formyl-methionyl-leucyl-phenylalanine (FMLP). Whereas the dissociation constant (K_D) for FMLP binding was increased two- to three-fold, treatment with PGE_1 did not alter the total number of receptor sites per cell. Consistent with these findings, polymorphonuclear leukocytes from PGE_1-treated

rats exhibited significantly decreased responses to FMLP in vitro (i.e., degranulation and generation of superoxide anion radicals). These studies suggest that some of the anti-inflammatory effects observed after administration of PGE compounds may be mediated by altered functional responses of polymorphonuclear leukocytes to chemotactic peptides.

In addition to inhibiting immune complex-induced inflammation, 15-(S)-15-methyl PGE_1 has been found capable of suppressing inflammation caused by antitissue antibodies. The nephrotoxicity in rats caused by single intravenous injections of antibodies directed against glomerular basement membranes was suppressed significantly by treatment wtih PGE_1.[79] Treatment reduced glomerular hypercellularity and proteinuria, but did not affect binding of the antibodies to the glomerular basement membrane.

Murine Systemic Lupus Erythematosus. Female F_1 hybrids of New Zealand black (NZB) and white (NZW) mice spontaneously develop a disease that resembles systemic lupus erythematosus. The disease is associated with the appearance of circulating autoantibodies (e.g., anti-DNA antibodies) and progressive, immune complex-mediated glomerulonephritis. When female NZB/NZW F_1 hybrid mice were treated with PGE_1 (200 μm subcutaneously either once or twice daily) from 6 through 52 weeks of age, they not only were protected from the development of anemia and nephritis but also lived longer than untreated animals.[80] At 52 weeks, 18 of 19 treated mice were alive versus only 2 of 19 untreated controls. Survival of NZB/NZW mice also was prolonged when treatment with PGE_1 was begun at 24 weeks, at a time when these animals begin to develop nephritis. Interestingly, although treatment with PGE_1 did not prevent development of antibodies to nuclear antigens (including anti-DNA antibodies), it did prevent deposition of immunoglobulins and complement in glomeruli, as well as the development of proliferative nephritis. The milder disease observed in male NZB/NZW mice also was prevented by treatment with PGE_1.

In contrast to these as yet unexplained effects of pharmacologic amounts of PGE compounds on the course of murine lupus, evidence has appeared suggesting that inhibition of endogenous prostaglandin biosynthesis also may suppress this disease. Female NZB/NZW F_1 hybrid mice fed a diet rich in eicosapentaenoic acids (i.e., fatty acids containing five double-bonds) did not develop proteinuria and lived longer than similar mice fed a normal diet.[81] None of the animals fed the special diet died or exhibited proteinuria for the duration of the study (up to 13.5 months). Anti-double-stranded DNA antibodies were reduced by approximately 50% in treated animals. A diet rich in eicosapentaenoic acids also resulted in significant improvement in rates of mortality, proteinuria, and histologic evidence of glomerular injury when administered after the onset of renal disease.[82] Similar diets have reduced the severity of immune complex-mediated renal disease in other strains of mice and decreased the susceptibility of mice to Type II collagen-induced arthritis.[82,83] Because eicosapentaenoic acid inhibits conversion of arachidonic acid into thromboxanes and stable prostaglandins, it was concluded that arachidonic acid metabolites may play a role in the pathogenesis of murine lupus. Clearly, more work will be required to elucidate the mechanisms whereby prostaglandins modulate immune complex-mediated inflammation and tissue injury.

LEUKOTRIENES AS POTENT MEDIATORS OF INFLAMMATION AND HYPERSENSITIVITY

The 5-lipoxygenation of arachidonic acid in leukocytes generates 5-hydroperoxy-eicosatetraenoic acid (5-HPETE), which is the precursor for the production of a family of complex 5-hydroxyeicosatetraenoic acids (5-HETEs), termed leukotrienes, that contain additional polar substituents and three conjugated double bonds (see Fig. 26–1). The highly reactive 5,6-epoxy-eicosa-7,9,11,14-tetraenoic acid (leukotriene A_4 or LTA_4, where the subscript 4 indicates the total number of double bonds in the molecule) is derived from 5-HPETE.[84] LTA_4 is hydrated enzymatically to form 5(S),12(R)-dihydroxy-eicosa-6,14,cis-8,10, trans-tetraenoic acid (LTB_4),[85] a potent stimulus of chemotaxis and other functions of leukocytes in vitro and in vivo.[86–88] LTA_4 also combines enzymatically with glutathione to yield 5-hydroxy-6-sulfido-glutathionyl-7,9-trans-11, 14-cis-ETE (LTC_4), which is converted enzymatically to 5-hydroxy-6-sulfido-cysteinyl-glycine-ETE (LTD_4) and, subsequently, to 5-hydroxy-6-sulfido-cysteinyl-ETE (LTE_4).[4,5] A γ-glutamyltranspeptidase also transforms LTE_4 to a γ-glutamyl-LTE_4, designated LTF_4.[89] LTC_4, LTD_4, and LTE_4 are potent contractile and vasoactive factors, and represent the principal constituents of the slow-reacting substance of anaphylaxis (SRS-A) generated by immunologic stimulation of human lung and other tissues.[90] The conversion of HPETE to an epoxide, which reacts with one or more polar compounds, is a fundamental mechanism observed in each of the pathways. 15-HPETE similarly is transformed to an unstable 14,15-epoxide that is converted to two isomers of 14,15-diHETE and four of 8,15-diHETE. Although the

epoxide derived from 12-HPETE has not been characterized fully, the complex metabolites identified include an 11,12-diHETE and several trihydroxy-eicosatetraenoic acids. Although the biochemical and cellular characteristics of the generation of leukotrienes by leukocytes and other cells have not been defined fully, cell-to-cell interactions appear to be important for the achievement of maximal production rates of the mediators. The addition of platelets to polymorphonuclear (PMN) leukocytes in vitro enhances the rate of generation of 5,12-di-HETE isomers of LTB_4.

Fluid and tissue concentrations of the lipoxygenase products are regulated predominantly by the activities of the pathways of generation, as has been demonstrated by the greater than 80% suppression of the levels achieved with different classes of lipoxygenase inhibitors. In addition, further metabolism of leukotrienes may convert the primary principles either to mediators with different activities or to inactive products (see Fig. 26–1). The transformation of LTB_4 to 20-hydroxyl-LTB_4 and 20-carboxyl-LTB_4 reduces both the polymorphonuclear leukocyte chemotactic and aggregating potency and the smooth muscle contractile and microvascular activities in several in vitro systems.[91] The peroxidation of LTC_4 in human eosinophils rapidly yields sulfoxides and a sulfone of LTC_4, the latter of which retains smooth muscle and microvascular activities, and two 6-trans isomers of LTB_4, which exhibit leukocyte chemotactic activity that is not expressed by LTC_4.[92] The SRS-A activities of LTD_4 are diminished substantially by peptidolytic conversion to LTE_4,[93] and the activities of LTC_4, LTD_4, and LTE_4 are eliminated by 15-hydroxylation.[94] The quantitative importance and biologic significance of the secondary pathways of metabolism of the leukotrienes have not been established in vivo. The bulk of the radioactivity of [³H]-LTC_4 given systemically to rats accumulates in the liver and kidneys, which degrade and excrete the mediator in the bile and urine, respectively.[95,96] Other pathways for the metabolic inactivation of leukotrienes in distinct tissue compartments may contribute to their elimination after local reactions.

Although some of the smooth muscle and microvascular effects of LTB_4 may be attributable to stimulation by LTB_4 of the generation of thromboxanes and prostaglandins,[97] the activation of PMN leukocytes is initiated by the occupancy of receptors on the cell surface that selectively recognize LTB_4, as compared to other chemotactic factors. The dependence of the PMN leukocyte chemotacic activity on the structural integrity of several relatively polar domains of LTB_4 and the capacity of chemotactically less active derivatives and analogues of LTB_4 to inhibit the responses to LTB$_4$, but not to peptide chemotactic factors,[98] suggested that a subset of receptors was dedicated to LTB$_4$ and did not bind functionally similar stimuli of different structures. The application of direct binding assays has confirmed the presence on PMN leukocytes of a separate class of stereospecific receptors for LTB$_4$.[99] Human PMN leukocytes express approximately 5,000 receptors for LTB$_4$ with a Kd of 0.4 nM that transduce chemotactic responses to LTB$_4$, and 270,000 with a Kd of 60 nM that mediate degranulation and increases in generation of superoxide in response to high concentrations of LTB$_4$.[100] The receptors are composed of a 60 kD membrane protein with the combining site and a 41 kD guanine nucleotide-binding protein that interact in the presence of guanosine 5'-triphosphate to convert high-affinity to low-affinity binding.[101] The receptors for LTC$_4$ and LTD$_4$ on PMN leukocytes are of far lower affinity than those on smooth muscle cells and in lung tissues, but exhibit similar stereospecificity and transduce increases in adherence of the PMN leukocytes to surfaces. Unlike the receptors for LTB$_4$, those for LTC$_4$ and LTD$_4$ are not restricted to the plasma membrane, but are localized predominantly on lysosomal granules.[102,103]

The first functional classification of leukotrienes was based on the observations that the contractile and vasoactive factors, LTC$_4$ and LTD$_4$, lacked the capabilities of LTB$_4$ to stimulate leukocyte chemotaxis and other functions.[1,2] However, 3 to 300 nM LTC$_4$ and LTD$_4$ enhanced the adherence of PMN leukocytes to surfaces to the same extent as LTB$_4$ and peptide chemotactic factors.[104] Indomethacin inhibited the increase in PMN leukocyte adherence evoked by LTC$_4$ and LTD$_4$. Similar studies in animal models of the effects of indomethacin on the constriction of pulmonary airways by LTB$_4$ indicate that cyclo-oxygenase products of arachidonic acid are generated by the action of LTB$_4$ on lung tissues and contribute significantly to the contractile effects observed.[97] Thus, the involvement of cyclo-oxygenase metabolites in the biologic effects of lipoxygenase mediators may be a more general phenomenon.

Diverse metabolites of the 15-lipoxygenation and 5-lipoxygenation of arachidonic acid, including LTB$_4$, are generated in substantial quantities by human and murine T-lymphocytes.[105–107] 15-HETE, at concentrations attained in suspensions of stimulated lymphocytes, inhibits murine lymphocyte transformation[105] and human T-lymphocyte migration.[108] In contrast, LTB$_4$ and, to a lesser extent, 5-HETE enhance the migration of human T-lymphocytes in vitro.[108] A broader analysis of the direct effects of leukotrienes on other functions of purified human T-lymphocytes demon-

strated that 10^{-8}M–10^{-6}M LTB$_4$, but not LTC$_4$, LTD$_4$, or LTE$_4$, significantly inhibits proliferative and synthetic responses to mitogens and antigens.[109] In more complex interactions, LTB$_4$ also induced T-lymphocyte suppressor and cytotoxic activities. Enhancement by LTB$_4$ of T-lymphocyte cytotoxic activity required endogenous thromboxane production, while both adherent mononuclear leukocytes and endogenous prostaglandin production were essential for the suppressor activity exhibited by LTB$_4$-stimulated T-lymphocytes.[110,111]

The related symptoms of hyperalgesia or tenderness, aching, and stiffness in arthritis and other inflammatory diseases are attributable to the effects of specific mediators on the nociceptive pathways of the peripheral nervous system. LTB$_4$ and other leukotactic factors reduce the nociceptive threshold to a symptomatic level by a PMN leukocyte-dependent mechanism that is resistant to nonsteroidal anti-inflammatory drugs.[112] The primary mediator of hyperalgesia generated locally by the LTB$_4$-stimulated PMN leukocytes is the 8(R),15(S)-di-hydroxyeicosa-5 cis-9,11,13 trans-tetraenoic acid product of 15-lipoxygenation of arachidonic acid.[113] Another 8,15-diHETE isomer that antagonizes that hyperalgesia induced by the primary mediator also blocks LTB$_4$-evoked hyperalgesia.[113] Lipoxygenase inhibitors thus may provide more effective management of the sensory abnormalities of arthritis.

The results of the earliest comprehensive assays of arachidonic acid metabolites in human disease demonstrated highly significant increases in the concentrations of PGE$_2$, PGF$_{2\alpha}$, free arachidonic acid, and HETEs in psoriatic lesions as compared to uninvolved skin of the same patients.[114] Concurrent studies indicated that synovial fluid of patients with rheumatoid arthritis contains higher concentrations of PGE$_2$ and, to a lesser extent, PGF$_{2\alpha}$ and thromboxane B$_2$ than synovial fluid of subjects with noninflammatory arthropathies.[115,116] In addition, explants of synovial tissue and cultures of adherent synovial cells from patients with rheumatoid arthritis produced greater quantities of PGE$_2$ and some other cyclo-oxygenase products in vitro than did tissue from subjects with nonrheumatoid arthropathies.[117–120] The finding of significantly increased levels of LTB$_4$ in synovial fluid of patients with rhreumatoid arthritis or spondyloarthritis and of 5-HETE in rheumatoid synovial tissue was the first documentation of abnormal activity of the lipoxygenase pathway in human arthritis.[121] Interest in the pathophysiologic significance of the metabolism of arachidonic acid in human inflammatory states was enhanced by the detection of heightened tissue sensitivity to lipoxygenase products in psoriasis. The activity of soluble guanylate cyclase from psoriatic lesions and uninvolved skin of psoriasis patients was stimulated two- to three-fold by arachidonic acid or 12-L-HETE, whereas that from normal subjects was not altered, even though baseline levels were substantially lower than those of patient samples.[122] Although available data do not permit a meaningful integration of the abnormalities of arachidonic acid metabolism and of other systems in human inflammatory disease, a tentative model may be provided for rheumatoid arthritis. Macrophages and polymorphonuclear leukocytes that infiltrate the synovium in large numbers contribute to the elevated levels of PGE_2, thromboxanes, 5-HETE, and LTB_4. Synoviocytes also generate cyclo-oxygenase products, LTB_4, and 5-HETE. These products, along with complement-derived molecules, such as C5a, stimulate the local influx of more leukocytes. Other leukotrienes and, with a lower potency, LTB_4 might increase the permeability of regional microcirculatory beds.

Recent studies involving dietary supplements of alternative fatty acids, such as eicosapentaenoic acid (EPA), on human PMN leukocyte function have suggested an autacoid role for some metabolites of arachidonic acid. Normal subjects and patients with asthma who received gram quantities of EPA daily for 8 weeks showed increased leukocyte production of LTB_5, a chemotactic factor derived from EPA that is of far lower potency than LTB_4.[123] Moreover, leukocytes from EPA-supplemented subjects contained less arachidonic acid and generated less LTB_4 and PGE_2 in vitro.[124,125] Concurrently, the chemotactic responses of PMN leukocytes, but not monocytes, to multiple stimuli were suppressed significantly. EPA dietary supplements thus represent a new approach to anti-inflammatory therapy.

ANTI-INFLAMMATORY ACTIONS OF DRUGS THAT INHIBIT OXYGENATION OF ARACHIDONIC ACID

The pharmacologic characteristics of inhibitors of the oxygenation of arachidonic acid[126] and their clinical uses as anti-inflammatory drugs[42] have been reviewed comprehensively. Here we describe the properties of clinically relevant inhibitors of generation and antagonists of biologically active metabolites of arachidonic acid in relation to their mechanism of action and the consequent effect on inflammation (Table 26–2). Although numerous difficulties limit the applicability of information gained from in vitro analyses and studies of animal models, such information will be used to reinforce points that are not clearly established by clinical data.

Some of the inhibitors, most notably corticosteroids, suppress the release of arachidonic acid from phospholipids and thus may effectively inhibit the cyclo-oxygenase and lipoxygenase pathways. Other agents exhibit selectively either for or within one of the major pathways. For example, therapeutic doses of most nonsteroidal anti-inflammatory drugs inhibit cyclo-oxygenation, while sparing lipoxygenase activities. Phenylbutazone inhibits preferentially the formation of PGE_2, whereas gold has a similar effect on $PGE_{2\alpha}$ synthesis without influencing that of PGE_2.[127] Most commonly, the antirheumatic drugs have more than one type of effect on the reactions of oxygenation of arachidonic acid. Most nonsteroidal anti-inflammatory drugs and corticosteroids have other suppressive effects on inflammation, such as scavenging oxygen radicals, altering cyclic nucleotide metabolism, influencing the activities of various enzymes or transport systems, or blocking unrelated receptors. The capacity of the cyclo-oxygenase and lipoxygenase inhibitor eicosatetraynoic acid (ETYA) to suppress neutrophil chemotaxis to the synthetic peptide. N-formyl-methionyl-leucyl-phenylalanine (FMLP), for example, is attributable in part to inhibition of the FMLP to chemotactic receptors.[128] Indomethacin inhibits cyclic nucleotide phosphodiesterase activity, leading to elevated intracellular levels of cAMP, at concentrations that suppress cyclo-oxygenase activity.[129] Some actions of inhibitors of the oxygenation of arachidonic acid may attenuate their anti-inflammatory effects. Indomethacin and salicylates up-regulate some cellular receptors for prostaglandins,[130,131] which may augment or unmask the proinflammatory activities of prostaglandins.

ADRENAL CORTICOSTEROIDS

Since 1950, a staggering number of publications have appeared attesting to the ability of adrenal corticosteroids to suppress undesirable immune and inflammatory reactions (see also Chapter 37). Despite this, we still know relatively little about the precise mechanisms by which the anti-immunologic and anti-inflammatory benefits of these compounds are achieved. Evidence has appeared suggesting that adrenal corticosteroids may act to ameliorate inflammation by interfering with the metabolism of arachidonic acid. Several investigators have documented that corticosteroids inhibit production of PGE_2 and $PGF_{2\alpha}$ by inflamed synovial tissue.[118,119] It has also been reported that corticosteroids inhibit production

Table 26–2.   Inhibitors of Generation or Effects of Metabolites of Arachidonic Acid

Class	Agent	Action
Inhibitors of synthesis	Corticosteroids	Inhibit release of arachidonic acid
	Gold compounds	Block production of $PGF_{2\alpha}$
	Nonsteroidal anti-inflammatory drugs	Suppress generation of prostaglandins; retard conversion of HPETEs to HETEs
	Phenylbutazone	Blocks production of PGE_2
	Salicylazosulfapyridine	Inhibits lipoxygenase activity, with less effect on cyclo-oxygenase activity
	Tocopherols	Inhibit cyclo-oxygenase and lipoxygenase activities
	Ascorbic acid	Inhibits thromboxane synthesis, stimulates release of arachidonic acid; variable effect on prostaglandin synthesis
Inhibitors of effect	Colchicine, chloroquine, probenecid, methylxanthines, some nonsteroidal anti-inflammatory drugs	Suppress transport of prostaglandins into cells and/or the actions of prostaglandins

by stimulated leukocytes of thromboxane A_2 and stable prostaglandins, and that this inhibitory effect could be overcome by supplying the cells with exogenous arachidonic acid.[57,132] Several observations suggest that corticosteroids inhibit prostaglandin biosynthesis by binding to specific glucocorticoid receptors and by inducing synthesis and release of one or more cellular proteins that inhibit phospholipase activity.

Macrocortin. Three groups of investigators independently observed that inhibition by corticosteroids of prostaglandin production by rat renal papillae,[133] perfused guinea pig lungs,[134] and rat peritoneal leukocytes (a mixture of macrophages and polymorphonuclear leukocytes)[132,135] required prolonged incubations and could be prevented with agents that inhibit either DNA-directed RNA synthesis (e.g., actinomycin D) or protein synthesis (e.g., puromycin, cycloheximide). Incubation of rat peritoneal leukocytes with hydrocortisone for 90 minutes resulted in release into the medium surrounding these cells of a nondialyzable "factor" that inhibited production of prostaglandins by fresh leukocytes.[135] The steroid-induced inhibitor of prostaglandin biosynthesis was identified subsequently as a polypeptide, termed "macrocortin,"[136] which was partially purified from steroid-stimulated rat peritoneal leukocytes and was found to have an apparent molecular weight (MW) of 40,000.[137]

Lipomodulin. Preincubation of rabbit peritoneal leukocytes with adrenal corticosteroids for 16 hours resulted in inhibition of chemotactic factor induced release of [14C]-arachidonic acid previously incorporated into membrane phospholipids.[138] The inhibitory potency of various corticosteroids correlated well with their anti-inflammatory activity and with their ability to bind to glucocorticoid receptors. Evidence was presented that corticosteroids induced the synthesis of a

40,000 MW protein ("lipomodulin"), which directly inhibited the activity of porcine pancreatic phospholipase A_2. When human fibroblasts were stimulated with bradykinin in the presence of a monoclonal antibody directed against lipomodulin, the cells responded by releasing greater than normal amounts of previously incorporated [14C]-arachidonic acid.[139] This apparent enhancement of phospholipase activity was blocked by adding an excess of lipomodulin (partially purified from supernatants of rabbit polymorphonuclear leukocytes incubated for 16 hours with 1.0 μm fluocinolone acetonide). The activity of partially purified lipomodulin was decreased markedly after treatment with sera from patients with systemic lupus erythematosus, rheumatoid arthritis, and dermatomyositis, as well as with sera from NZB/NZW and MRL/1 mice. The decrease in phospholipase A_2-inhibitory activity paralleled the amount of [35S]-methionine-labeled lipomodulin that was precipitated by these sera. It was suggested that "autoantibodies" in patients with rheumatic diseases facilitate activation of phospholipase A_2 in vivo and play a role in the pathogenesis of immunologically-induced inflammation and tissue injury.

As attractive as this suggestion may be, no conclusive evidence exists that lipomodulin possesses anti-inflammatory activity. Lipomodulin and macrocortin appear to be identical with a 35 to 40 kilodalton (kD) protein found in the cytosol of a wide variety of mammalian cells (aptly named "lipocortin").[140] Lipocortin binds to phospholipids in the presence of calcium and thereby interferes with the action of phospholipase A_2.[141] It remains to be determined, however, whether lipocortin really mediates effects of anti-inflammatory corticosteroids on arachidonic acid metabolism by intact cells.

Whereas most nonsteroidal anti-inflammatory

agents effectively inhibit production by leukocytes of prostaglandins by inhibiting cyclo-oxygenase activity, these agents do not influence the formation of lipoxygenase products (e.g., hydroxy-acids, leukotrienes). It is unclear whether anti-inflammatory corticosteroids may act "proximally" to suppress phospholipase activity in vivo, thereby reducing the availability of arachidonic acid as a substrate and thus limiting production of inflammatory mediators by both the cyclo-oxygenase and lipoxygenase pathways.

NONSTEROIDAL ANTI-INFLAMMATORY DRUGS

The ability of most drugs to inhibit the generation of prostaglandins, thromboxanes, or HETEs has been assessed principally in vitro or in animal models (see also Chapter 32). However, indomethacin and related agents do block the production of prostaglandins by human synovial and cutaneous tissues and cells[120,142] and in human subjects[143,144] at clinically relevant concentrations. The specificity of drug action has not been established in most instances. This will be an important goal for future clinical trials in view of the observations that some nonsteroidal agents inhibit the conversion of HPETEs to HETEs.[145] Because HPETEs are potent inhibitors of some steps in the cyclo-oxygenation and further metabolism of arachidonic acid, the HPETEs that accumulate may contribute to the suppression of prostaglandin and thromboxane synthesis by some nonsteroidal agents.

Pronounced inhibition of the effects of prostaglandins on vascular tissue or smooth muscle and of their proinflammatory activities has suggested that some drugs block the transport and/or actions of prostaglandins (see Table 26–2). The competitive inhibition of the effects of prostaglandins was assessed in dog lung or rat intestinal blood vessels for chloroquine and methylxanthines; in uterine or intestinal muscle for indomethacin, naproxen, and cyproheptadine; and in a model of inflammation for colchicine.[146–149] Antagonism of the effects of an exogenous prostaglandin would seem to be an operationally specific test of mechanism. Few studies, however, have established direct antagonism by receptor analyses or have ruled out an involvement of secondary mediators that might have been the target of the inhibitors.

With respect to the lipoxygenase pathways, neither selective inhibitors of generation nor antagonists of the mediators have been developed for routine use in patients with inflammatory diseases. Although compounds such as sulfasalazine and colchicine have been found to be capable of inhibiting 5-lipoxygenase activity in human polymorphonuclear leukocytes in vitro,[150–152] it is not clear that such inhibition accounts for their beneficial actions in vivo. It remains to be determined whether other compounds that inhibit lipoxygenases will prove to be clinically useful as anti-inflammatory agents.[153,154]

REFERENCES

1. Goetzl, E.J.: Mediators of immediate hypersensitivity derived from arachidonic acid. N. Engl. J. Med., *303*:822–825, 1980.
2. Samuelsson, B.: Prostaglandins, thromboxanes, and leukotrienes: Formation and biological roles. The Harvey Lectures. Series 75. New York, Academic Press, 1981.
3. Halushka, P.V., and Lefer, A.M. (eds.): Thromboxane A$_2$ in health and disease. Fed. Proc., *46*:131–158, 1987.
4. Needleman, P., et al.: Arachidonic acid metabolism. In Annual Review of Biochemistry. 55. Edited by C.C. Richardson, P.D. Boyer, I.B. Dawid, and A. Meister. Palo Alto, CA, Annual Reviews, Inc., 1986, pp. 69–102.
5. Hayaishi, O., and Yamamoto, S. (eds.): Advances in Prostaglandin, Thromboxane, and Leukotriene Research. New York, Raven Press, 1985.
6. Goetzl, E.J., Burrall, B.A., and Koo, C.H.: Modulation of human leukocyte function in vitro and in vivo by leukotrienes and alternative fatty acids. Ann. N.Y. Acad. Sci., in press, 1988.
7. Irvine, R.F.: How is the level of free arachidonic acid controlled in mammalian cells? Biochem. J., *204*:3–16, 1982.
8. Rubin, R.P., Sink, L.E., and Freer, R.J.: Activation of (arachidonyl) phosphatidylinositol turnover in rabbit neutrophils by the calcium ionophore A23187. Biochem. J., *194*:497–505, 1981.
9. Walsh, C.E., et al.: Effect of phagocytosis and ionophores on release and metabolism of arachidonic acid from human neutrophils. Lipids, *16*:120–124, 1981.
10. Majerus, P.W., et al.: The metabolism of phosphoinositide-derived messenger molecules. Science, *234*:1519–1526, 1986.
11. Bell, R.M.: Protein kinase C activation by diacylglycerol second messengers. Cell, *45*:631–632, 1986.
12. Pike, M.C., Kredich, N.M., and Snyderman, R.: Phospholipid methylation in macrophages is inhibited by chemotactic factors. Proc. Natl. Acad. Sci. USA, *76*:2922–2926, 1979.
13. Johnson, R.A., et al.: The chemical structure of prostaglandin X (prostacyclin). Prostaglandins, *12*:915–928, 1976.
14. Moncada, S., and Vane, J.R.: Pharmacology and endogenous roles of prostaglandin endoperoxides, thromboxane A$_2$ and prostacyclin. Pharmacol. Rev., *30*:293–331, 1979.
15. Hamberg, M., Svensson, J., and Samuelsson, B.: Thromboxanes: A new group of biologically active compounds derived from prostaglandin endoperoxides. Proc. Natl. Acad. Sci. USA, *72*:2994–2998, 1975.
16. Davies, P., Bailey, P.J., Goldenberg, M.M., and Ford-Hutchinson, A.W.: The role of arachidonic acid oxygenation products in pain and inflammation. Ann. Rev. Immunol., *2*:335–357, 1984.
17. Kaley, G. (ed.): Control of coronary circulation and myocardial function by eicosanoids. Fed. Proc., *46*:46–88, 1987.
18. Goodwin, J.S., Kaszubowski, P.A., and Williams, R.C., Jr.: Cyclic AMP response to prostaglandin E on subpopulations of human lymphocytes. J. Exp. Med., *150*:1260–1264, 1979.
19. Webb, D.R., and Nowowiejski, I.: Mitogen-induced changes

in lymphocyte prostaglandin levels: A signal for the induction of suppressor cell activity. Cell. Immunol., *41*:72–85, 1978.

20. Webb, D.R., Rogers, T.J., and Nowowiejski, I.: Endogenous prostaglandin synthesis and the control of lymphocyte function. Ann. N.Y. Acad. Sci., *332*:262–270, 1980.

21. Fischer, A., LeDeist, F., Durandy, A., and Griscelli, C.: Separation of a population of human T-lymphocytes that bind prostaglandin E₂ and exert a suppressor activity. J. Immunol., *134*:815–819, 1985.

22. Serhan, C.N., Hamberg, M., and Samuelsson, B.: Lipoxins: Novel series of biologically active compounds formed from arachidonic acid in human leukocytes. Proc. Natl. Acad. Sci. USA, *81*:5335–5339, 1984.

23. Ramstedt, U., et al.: Inhibition of human natural killer cell activity by (14R,15S)-14,15-dihydroxy-5Z,8Z,10E,12E-icosatetraenoic acid. Proc. Natl. Acad. Sci. USA, *81*:6914–6918, 1984.

24. Turner, S.R., Campbell, J.A., and Lynn, W.S.: Polymorphonuclear leukocyte chemotaxis toward oxidized lipid components of cell membranes. J. Exp. Med., *141*:1437–1441, 1975.

25. Turner, S.R., Tainer, J.A., and Lynn, W.S.: Biogenesis of chemotactic molecules by the arachidonate lipoxygenase system of platelets. Nature (London), *257*:680–681, 1975.

26. Perez, H.D., Weksler, B.B., and Goldstein, I.M.: Generation of a chemotactic lipid from arachidonic acid by exposure to a superoxide-generating system. Inflammation, *4*:313–328, 1980.

27. Fridovich, S.E., and Porter, N.A.: Oxidation of arachidonic acid in micelles by superoxide and hydrogen peroxide. J. Biol. Chem., *256*:260–265, 1981.

28. Porter, N.A., Logan, J., and Kontoyiannidou, V.: Preparation and purification of arachidonic acid hydroperoxides of biological importance. J. Org. Chem., *44*:3177–3181, 1979.

29. Porter, N.A., Wolf, R.A., Yarbro, E.M., and Weenen, H.: The autoxidation of arachidonic acid: Formation of the proposed SRS-A intermediate. Biochem. Biophys. Res. Commun., *89*:1058–1064, 1979.

30. Goldstein, I.M., Roos, D., Kaplan, H.B., and Weissmann, G.: Complement and immunoglobulins stimulate superoxide production by human leukocytes independently of phagocytosis. J. Clin. Invest., *56*:1155–1163, 1975.

31. Stossel, T.P., Mason, R.J., and Smith, A.L.: Lipid peroxidation by human blood phagocytes. J. Clin. Invest., *54*:638–645, 1974.

32. Petrone, W.F., English, D.K., Wong, K., and McCord, J.M.: Free radicals and inflammation: Superoxide-dependent activation of a neutrophil chemotactic factor in plasma. Proc. Natl. Acad. Sci. USA, *77*:1159–1163, 1980.

33. Davies, P., et al.: The role of arachidonic acid oxygenation products in pain and inflammation. Annu. Rev. Immunol., *2*:335–357, 1984.

34. Goetzl, E.J.: Oxygenation products of arachidonic acid as mediators of hypersensitivity and inflammation. Med. Clin. North Am., *65*:809–828, 1981.

35. Kuehl, F.A., Jr., and Egan, R.W.: Prostaglandins, arachidonic acid, and inflammation. Science, *210*:978–984, 1980.

36. Williams, T.J.: Prostaglandin E₂, prostaglandin I₂, and the vascular changes of inflammation. Br. J. Pharmacol., *65*:517–524, 1979.

37. Williams, T.J., and Peck, M.J.: Role of prostaglandin-mediated vasodilation in inflammation. Nature (London), *270*:530–532, 1977.

38. Higgs, G.A., Cardinal, D.C., Moncada, S., and Vane, J.R.: Microcirculatory effects of prostacyclin (PGI₂) in the hamster cheek pouch. Microvasc. Res., *18*:245–254, 1979.

39. Cranston, W.I.: Central mechanisms of fever. Fed. Proc., *38*:49–51, 1979.

40. Dey, P.K., et al.: Further studies on the role of prostaglandin in fever. J. Physiol., *241*:629–646, 1974.

41. Ziel, R., and Krupp, P.: Influence of endogenous pyrogen on cerebral prostaglandin-synthetase system. Experienta, *32*:1451–1453, 1976.

42. Simon, L.S., and Mills, J.A.: Drug therapy: Nonsteroidal anti-inflammatory drugs (two parts), N. Engl. J. Med., *302*:1179–1185, 1237–1243, 1980.

43. Ferreira, S.H.: Prostaglandins, aspirin-like drugs and analgesia. Nature New Biol., *240*:200–203, 1972.

44. Ferreira, S.H., and Vane, J.R.: New aspects of the mode of action of nonsteroid anti-inflammatory drugs. Ann. Rev. Pharmacol., *14*:57–73, 1974.

45. Ferreira, S.H., Nakamura, M., and Castro, M.S.A.: The hyperalgesic effects of prostacyclin and prostglandin E₂. Prostaglandins, *16*:31–37, 1978.

46. Issekutz, A.C., and Movat, H.Z.: The effect of vasodilator prostaglandins on polymorphonuclear leukocyte infiltration and vascular injury. Am. J. Pathol., *107*:300–309, 1982.

47. Wedmore, C.V., and Williams, T.J.: Control of vascular permeability by polymorphonuclear leukocytes in inflammation. Nature (London), *289*:646–650, 1981.

48. Higgs, E.A., Moncada, S., and Vane, J.R.: Inflammatory effects of prostacyclin (PGI₂) and 6-oxo-PGF₁ in the rat paw. Prostaglandins, *16*:153–162, 1978.

49. Spagnuolo, P.J., Ellner, J.J., Hassid, A., and Dunn, M.J.: Thromboxane A₂ mediates augmented polymorphonuclear leukocyte adhesiveness. J. Clin. Invest., *66*:406–414, 1980.

50. Kuehl, F.A., Jr., et al.: Role of prostaglandin endoperoxide PGG₂ in inflammatory processes. Nature (London), *265*:170–173, 1977.

51. Klein, D.C., and Raisz, L.G.: Prostaglandins: Stimulation of bone resorption in tissue culture. Endocrinology, *86*:1436–1440, 1970.

52. Seyberth, H.W., et al.: Prostaglandins as mediators of hypercalcemia associated with certain types of cancer. N. Engl. J. Med., *293*:1278–1283, 1975.

53. Raisz, L.G., and Koolemans-Beynen, A.R.: Inhibition of bone collagen synthesis by prostaglandin E₂ in organ culture. Prostaglandins, *8*:377–385, 1974.

54. Goldyne, M.E., and Stobo, J.D.: Synthesis of prostaglandins by subpopulations of human peripheral blood monocytes. Prostaglandins, *18*:687–694, 1979.

55. Kurland, J.I., and Bockman, R.J.: Prostaglandin E production by human blood monocytes and mouse peritoneal macrophages. J. Exp. Med., *147*:952–957, 1978.

56. Zurier, R.B., and Sayadoff, D.M.: Release of prostaglandins from human polymorphonuclear leukocytes. Inflammation, *1*:93–101, 1975.

57. Goldstein, I.M., et al.: Thromboxane generation by human peripheral blood polymorphonuclear leukocytes. J. Exp. Med., *148*:787–792, 1978.

58. Goldstein, I.M., Malmsten, C.L., Samuelsson, B., and Weissmann, G.: Prostaglandins, thromboxanes, and polymorphonuclear leukocytes. Mediation and modulation of inflammation. Inflammation, *2*:309–317, 1977.

59. Bourne, H.R., et al.: Modulation of inflammation and immunity by cyclic AMP. Receptors for vasoactive hormones and mediators of inflammation regulate many leukocyte functions. Science, *184*:19–28, 1974.

60. Weissmann, G., et al.: Yin-yang modulation of lysosomal en-

zyme release from polymorphonuclear leukocytes by cyclic nucleotides. Ann. N.Y. Acad. Sci., 256:222–231, 1975.

61. Weissmann, G., Goldstein, I., Hoffstein, S., and Tsung, P.-K.: Reciprocal effects of cAMP and cGMP on microtubule-dependent release of lysosomal enzymes. Ann. N.Y. Acad. Sci., 253:750–762, 1975.

62. Zurier, R.B., et al.: Mechanisms of lysosomal enzyme release from human leukocytes. II. Effects of cAMP and cGMP, autonomic agonists, and agents which affect microtubule function. J. Clin. Invest., 53:297–309, 1974.

63. Gallin, J.I., et al.: Agents that increase cyclic AMP inhibit accumulation of cGMP and depress human monocyte locomotion. J. Immunol., 120:492–496, 1978.

64. Hatch, G.E., Nichols, W.K., and Hill, H.R.: Cyclic nucleotide changes in human neutrophils induced by chemo-attractants and chemotactic modulators. J. Immunol., 119:450–456, 1977.

65. Boxer, L.A., et al.: Inhibition of polymorphonuclear leukocyte adhesion by prostacyclin. J. Lab. Clin. Med., 95:672–678, 1980.

66. Bryant, R.E., and Sutcliffe, M.C.: The effect of 3′,5′-adenosine monophosphate on granulocyte adhesion. J. Clin. Invest., 54:1241–1244, 1974.

67. Cox, J.P., and Karnovsky, M.L.: The depression of phagocytosis by exogenous cyclic nucleotides, prostaglandins and theophylline. J. Cell Biol., 59:480–490, 1973.

68. Lehmeyer, J.E., and Johnston, R.B.: Effect of anti-inflammatory drugs and agents that elevate intracellular levels of cyclic AMP on the release of toxic oxygen metabolites by phagocytes: Studies in a model of tissue-bound IgG. Clin. Immunol. Immunopathol., 9:482–490, 1978.

69. Goldyne, M.E., and Stobo, J.D.: Immunoregulatory role of prostaglandins and related lipids. Crit. Rev. Immunol., 2:189–223, 1981.

70. Goodwin, J.S., and Webb, D.R.: Regulation of the immune response by prostaglandins. Clin. Immunol. Immunopathol., 15:106–122, 1980.

71. Aspinall, R.L., and Cammarata, P.S.: Effect of prostaglandin E_2 on adjuvant arthritis. Nature (London), 224:1320–1321, 1969.

72. Zurier, R.B., Hoffstein, S., and Weissmann, G.: Suppression of acute and chronic inflammation in adrenalectomized rats by pharmacologic amounts of prostaglandins. Arthritis Rheum., 16:606–618, 1973.

73. Zurier, R.B., and Quagliata, F.: Effect of prostaglandin E_1 on adjuvant arthritis. Nature (London), 234:304–305, 1971.

74. Fantone, J.C., Kunkel, S.L., and Weingarten, B.: Inhibition of carrageenan-induced rat footpad edema by systemic treatment with prostaglandins of the E series. Biochem. Pharmacol., 31:3126–3128, 1982.

75. Fantone, J.C., Kunkel, S.L., Ward, P.A., and Zurier, R.B.: Suppression by prostaglandin E_1 of vascular permeability induced by vasoactive inflammatory mediators. J. Immunol., 125:2591–2596, 1980.

76. Kunkel, S.L., et al.: Suppression of immune complex vasculitis in rats by prostaglandin. J. Clin. Invest., 64:1525–1529, 1979.

77. Fantone, J.C., Kunkel, S.L., and Ward, P.A.: Suppression of human polymorphonuclear function after intravenous infusion of prostaglandin E_1. Prostaglandins Med., 7:195–198, 1981.

78. Fantone, J.C., Marasco, W.A., Elgas, L.J., and Ward, P.A.: Anti-inflammatory effects of prostaglandin E_1: In vivo modulation of the formyl peptide chemotactic receptor on the rat neutrophil. J. Immunol., 130:1495–1497, 1983.

79. Kunkel, S.L., Zanetti, M., and Sapin, C.: Suppression of

80. Zurier, R.B., Damjanov, I., Miller, P.L., and Biewer, B.F.: Prostaglandin E treatment prevents progression of nephritis in murine lupus erythematosus. J. Clin. Lab. Immunol., 1:95–98, 1978.

81. Prickett, J.D., Robinson, D.R., and Steinberg, A.D.: Dietary enrichment with the polyunsaturated fatty acid eicosapentaenoic acid prevents proteinuria and prolongs survival in NZB × NZW F_1 mice. J. Clin. Invest., 68:556–559, 1981.

82. Robinson, D.R., et al.: Dietary fish oil reduces progression of established renal disease in (NZB × NZW) F_1 mice and delays renal disease in BXSB and MRL/1 strains. Arthritis Rheum., 29:539–546, 1986.

83. Leslie, C.A., et al.: Dietary fish oil modulates macrophage fatty acids and decreases arthritis susceptibility in mice. J. Exp. Med., 162:1336–1349, 1985.

84. Borgeat, P., and Samuelsson, B.: Arachidonic acid metabolism in polymorphonuclear leukocytes: Unstable intermediate in formation of dihydroxy acids. Proc. Natl. Acad. Sci. USA, 76:3213–3217, 1979.

85. Borgeat, P., and Samuelsson, B.: Metabolism of arachidonic acid in polymorphonuclear leukocytes. Structural analysis of novel hydroxylated compounds. J. Biol. Chem., 254:7865–7869, 1979.

86. Ford-Hutchinson, A.W., et al.: Leukotriene B_4, a potent chemotactic and aggregating substance released from polymorphonuclear leukocytes. Nature (London), 286:264–265, 1980.

87. Goetzl, E.J., and Pickett, W.C.: The human PMN leukocyte chemotactic activity of complex hydroxy-eicosatetraenoic acids (HETEs). J. Immunol., 125:1789–1791, 1980.

88. Lindblom, L., et al.: Leukotriene B_4 induces extravasation and migration of polymorphonuclear leukocytes in vivo. Acta Physiol. Scand., 116:105–108, 1982.

89. Bernström, K., and Hammarstrom, S.A.: A novel leukotriene formed by transpeptidation of leukotriene E. Biochem. Biophys. Res. Commun., 109:800–804, 1982.

90. Lewis, R.A., et al.: Slow reacting substances of anaphylaxis: Identification of leukotrienes C-1 and D from human and rat sources. Proc. Natl. Acad. Sci. USA, 77:3710–3714, 1979.

91. Hansson, G., et al.: Identification and biological activity of novel omega-oxidized metabolites of leukotriene B_4 from human leukocytes. F.E.B.S. Lett., 130:107–112, 1981.

92. Goetzl, E.J.: The conversion of leukotriene C_4 to isomers of leukotriene B_4 by human eosinophil peroxidase. Biochem. Biophys. Res. Commun., 106:270–275, 1982.

93. Lee, C.W., et al.: Conversion of leukotriene D_4 to leukotriene E_4 by a dipeptidase release from the specific granule of human polymorphonuclear leukocytes. Immunology, 48:27–35, 1983.

94. Morris, H.R., et al.: Slow reacting substances (SRSs). The structure identification of SRSs from rat basophil leukaemia (RBL-1) cells. Prostaglandins, 19:185–201, 1980.

95. Applegren, L.E., and Hammarstrom, S.A.: Distribution and metabolism of [3H]labeled leukotriene C_4 in the mouse. J. Biol. Chem., 257:531–535, 1982.

96. Ormstad, K., et al.: Uptake and metabolism of leukotriene C_4 by isolated rat organs and cells. Biochem. Biophys. Res. Commun., 104:1434–1440, 1982.

97. Sirois, P., et al.: In vivo effects of leukotriene B_4, C_4, and D_4. Evidence that changes in blood pressure are mediated by prostaglandins. Prostaglandins Med., 7:363–373, 1981.

98. Goetzl, E.J., and Pickett, W.C.: Novel structural determinants

of the human neutrophil chemotactic activity of leukotriene B. J. Exp. Med., *153*:482–487, 1981.

99. Goldman, D.W., and Goetzl, E.J.: Specific binding of leukotriene B₄ to receptors on human polymorphonuclear leukocytes. J. Immunol., *129*:1600–1604, 1982.

100. Goldman, D.W., and Goetzl, E.J.: Heterogeneity of human polymorphonuclear leukocyte receptors for leukotriene B₄. Identification of a subset of high affinity receptors that transduce the chemotactic response. J. Exp. Med., *159*:1027–1041, 1984.

101. Goldman, D.W., Gifford, L.A., Marotti, T., Koo, C.H., and Goetzl, E.J.: Molecular and cellular properties of human polymorphonuclear leukocyte receptors for leukotriene B₄. Fed. Proc., *46*:200–203, 1987.

102. Baud, L., Koo, C.H., and Goetzl, E.J.: Specificity and cellular distribution of human polymorphonuclear leukocyte receptors for leukotriene C₄. Immunology, in press, 1987.

103. Baud, L., et al.: Molecular and cellular diversity of the polymorphonuclear leukocyte receptors for leukotrienes. Advances in Prostaglandin, Thromboxane, and Leukotriene Research, vol. 17A. Edited by B. Samuelsson, P.W. Ramwell and R. Paoletti, New York, Raven Press, 1987, pp. 163–166.

104. Goetzl, E.J., Brindley, L.L., and Goldman, D.W.: Enhancement of human neutrophil adherence by synthetic leukotriene constituents of the slow-reacting substance of anaphylaxis. Immunology, *50*:35–41, 1983.

105. Bailey, J.M., et al.: Regulation of T-lymphocyte mitogene is by the leukocyte product 15-hydroxy-eicosatetraenoic acid (15-HETE). Cell. Immunol., *67*:112–120, 1982.

106. Kelly, J.P., and Parker, C.W.: Effects of arachidonic acid and other unsaturated fatty acids on mitogenesis in human lymphocytes. J. Immunol., *122*:1556–1562, 1979.

107. Goodwin, J.S., et al.: Mechanism of action of glucocorticosteroids: Inhibition of T-cell proliferation and interleukin-2 production by hydrocortisone is reversed by leukotriene B₄. J. Clin. Invest., *77*:1244–1250, 1986.

108. Payan, D.G., and Goetzl, E.J.: The dependence of human T-lymphocyte migration on the 5-lipoxygenation of endogenous arachidonic acid. J. Clin. Immunol., *1*:266–270, 1981.

109. Payan, D.G., and Goetzl, E.J.: Specific suppression of human T-lymphocyte function by leukotriene B₄. J. Immunol., *131*:551–553, 1983.

110. Rola-Pleszczynski, M., Borgeat, P., and Sirois, P.: Leukotriene B₄ induces human suppressor lymphocytes. Biochem. Biophys. Res. Commun., *108*:1531–1537, 1982.

111. Rola-Pleszczynski, M., Gagnon, L., and Sirois, P.: Leukotriene B₄ augments human natural cytotoxic cell activity. Biochem. Biophys. Res. Commun., *113*:531–537, 1983.

112. Levine, J.D., Lau, W., Kwait, G., and Goetzl, E.J.: Leukotriene B₄ produces hyperalgesia that is dependent on polymorphonuclear leukocytes. Science, *225*:743–745, 1984.

113. Levine, J.D., et al.: Hyperalgesic properties of 15-lipoxygenase products of arachidonic acid. Proc. Natl. Acad. Sci. USA, *83*:5331–5334, 1986.

114. Hammarstrom, S., et al.: Increased concentrations of non-esterified arachidonic acid, 12L-hydroxy-5,8,10,14-eicosatetraenoic acid, prostaglandin E₂, and prostaglandin F₂α in epidermis of psoriasis. Proc. Natl. Acad. Sci. USA, *72*:5130–5134, 1975.

115. Robinson, D.R., Dayer, J.M., and Krane, S.M.: Prostaglandins and their regulation in rheumatoid arthritis. Ann. N.Y. Acad. Sci., *332*:279–294, 1979.

116. Robinson, D.R., McGuire, M.B., and Levine, L.: Prostaglan-

dins in rheumatic diseases. Ann. N.Y. Acad. Sci., *256*:318–329, 1975.

117. Blotman, F., et al.: PGE₂, PGF₋₂α and TXB₂ biosynthesis by human rheumatoid synovia. *In* Advances in Prostaglandin and Thromboxane Research, Vol. 8. Edited by B. Samuelsson, P.W. Ramwell, and R. Paoletti. New York, Raven Press, 1980, pp. 1705–1708.

118. Floman, Y., Floman, N., and Zor, U.: Inhibition of prostaglandin E release by anti-inflammatory steroids. Prostaglandins, *11*:591–594, 1976.

119. Kantrowitz, F., et al.: Corticosteroids inhibit prostaglandin production by rheumatoid synovia. Nature (London), *258*:737–739, 1975.

120. Robinson, D.R., Tashjian, A.H., Jr., and Levine, L.: Prostaglandin-stimulated bone resorption by rheumatoid synovia. J. Clin. Invest., *56*:1181–1188, 1975.

121. Klickstein, L.B., Shapleigh, C., and Goetzl, E.J.: Lipoxygenation of arachidonic acid as a source of polymorphonuclear leukocyte chemotactic factors in synovial fluid and tissue in rheumatoid arthritis and spondyloarthritis. J. Clin. Invest., *66*:1166–1170, 1980.

122. Cantieri, J.S., Graff, G., and Goldberg, N.D.: Cyclic GMP metabolism in psoriasis: Activation of soluble epidermal guanylate cyclase by arachidonic acid and 12-hydroxy-5,8,10,14-eicosatetraenoic acid. J. Invest. Dermatol., *74*:234–237, 1980.

123. Goldman, D.W., Pickett, W.C., and Goetzl, E.J.: Human neutrophil chemotactic and degranulating activities of leukotriene B₅ (LTB₅) derived form eicosapentaenoic acid. Biochem. Biophys. Res. Commun., *117*:282–288, 1983.

124. Lee, T.H., et al.: Effect of dietary enrichment with eicosapentaenoic acid and docosahexaenoic acid on in vitro neutrophil and monocyte leukotriene generation and leukotriene function. N. Engl. J. Med., *312*:1217–1224, 1985.

125. Payan, D.G., et al.: Alterations in human leukocyte function induced by ingestion of eicosapentaenoic acid. J. Clin. Immunol., *6*:402–410, 1986.

126. Metz, S.A.: Anti-inflammatory agents as inhibitors of prostaglandin synthesis in man. Med. Clin. North Am., *65*:713–757, 1981.

127. Stone, K.J., Mather, S.J., and Gibson, P.P.: Selective inhibition of prostaglandin biosynthesis by gold salts and phenylbutazone. Prostaglandins, *10*:241–251, 1975.

128. Atkinson, J.P., Simchowitz, L., Mehta, J., and Stenson, W.: 5,8,11,14-eicosatetraynoic acid (ETYA) inhibits binding of N-formyl-methionyl-leucyl-phenylalanine (FMLP) to its receptor on human granulocytes. Immunopharmacology, *4*:1–9, 1982.

129. Stefanovich, V.: Inhibition of 3′,5′ cyclic AMP phosphodiesterase with anti-inflammatory agents. Res. Commun. Chem. Pathol. Pharmacol., *7*:573–582, 1974.

130. Metz, S.A., Robertson, R.P., and Fujimoto, W.Y.: Inhibition of prostaglandin E synthesis in cultured pancreas augments glucose-induced insulin secretion. Diabetes, *30*:551–557, 1981.

131. Rice, M.G., McRae, J.R., and Robertson, R.P.: The prostaglandin E receptor: Induction of density changes in rat liver membrane. Clin. Res., *28*:522A, 1980.

132. DiRosa, M., and Persico, P.: Mechanism of inhibition of prostaglandin biosynthesis by hydrocortisone in rat leukocytes. Br. J. Pharmacol., *66*:161–163, 1979.

133. Danon, A., and Assouline, G.: Inhibition of prostaglandin biosynthesis by corticosteroids requires RNA and protein synthesis. Nature (London), *273*:552–554, 1978.

134. Flower, R.J., and Blackwell, G.J.: Anti-inflammatory steroids induce biosynthesis of a phospholipase A₂ inhibitor which

prevents prostaglandin generation. Nature (London), 278:456–459, 1979.

135. Carnuccio, R., DiRosa, M., Flower, R.J., and Pinto, A.: The inhibition by hydrocortisone of prostaglandin biosynthesis in rat peritoneal leukocytes is correlated with intracellular macrocortin levels. Br. J. Pharmacol., 74:322–324, 1981.

136. Blackwell, G.J., et al.: Macrocortin: a polypeptide causing the anti-phospholipase effect of glucocorticoids. Nature (London), 287:147–149, 1980.

137. Blackwell, G.J., et al.: Glucocorticoids induce the formation and release of anti-inflammatory and anti-phospholipase proteins into the peritoneal cavity of the rat. Br. J. Pharmacol., 76:185–194, 1982.

138. Hirata, F., et al.: A phospholipase A_2 inhibitory protein in rabbit neutrophils induced by glucocorticoids. Proc. Natl. Acad. Sci. USA, 77:2533–2536, 1980.

139. Hirata, F., et al.: Presence of autoantibody for phospholipase inhibitory protein, lipomodulin, in patients with rheumatic diseases. Proc. Natl. Acad. Sci. USA, 78:3190–3194, 1981.

140. Wallner, B.P., et al.: Cloning and expression of human lipocortin, a phospholipase A_2 inhibitor with potential anti-inflammatory activity. Nature (London), 320:77–81, 1986.

141. Davidson, F.S., Dennis, E.A., Powell, M., and Glenney, J.R.: Inhibition of phospholipase A_2 by "lipocortins" and calpactins. An effect of binding to substrate phospholipids. J. Biol. Chem., 262:1698–1705, 1987.

142. Dayer, J.M., Robinson, D.R., and Krane, S.M.: Prostaglandin production by rheumatoid synovial cells. J. Exp. Med., 145:1399–1404, 1977.

143. Granstrom, E., and Kindahl, H.: Radioimmunoassay for urinary metabolites of prostaglandin F_2. Prostaglandins, 12:759–783, 1976.

144. Samuelsson, B.: Quantitative aspects of prostaglandin synthesis in man. Adv. Biosci., 9:7–12, 1973.

145. Siegel, M.I., et al.: Arachidonate metabolism via lipoxygenase and 12L-hydroperoxy-5,8,12,14-icosatetraenoic acid peroxidase sensitive to anti-inflammatory drugs. Proc. Natl. Acad. Sci. USA, 77:308–312, 1980.

146. Manku, M.S., and Horribin, D.F.: Chloroquine, quinine, procaine, quinidine and clomipramine are prostaglandin agonists and antagonists. Prostaglandins, 12:789–801, 1976.

147. Manku, M.S., and Horribin, D.F.: Chloroquine, quinine, procaine, quinidine, tricyclic antidepressants, and methylxanthines as prostaglandin agonists and antagonists. Lancet, 2:1115–1117, 1976.

148. Sanner, J.H.: Substances that inhibit the actions of prostaglandins. Arch. Intern. Med., 133:133–146, 1974.

149. Sanner, J.H., and Eakins, K.E.: Prostaglandin antagonists. In Prostaglandins. Chemical and Biochemical Aspects. Edited by S.M.M. Karim. Baltimore, University Park Press, 1976.

150. Stenson, W.F., and Lobos, E.: Sulfasalazine inhibits the synthesis of chemotactic lipids by neutrophils. J. Clin. Invest., 69:494–497, 1982.

151. Sircar, J.C., Schwender, C.F., and Carethers, M.E.: Inhibition of soybean lipoxygenase by sulfasalazine and 5-aminosalicylic acid: A possible mode of action in ulcerative colitis. Biochem. Pharmacol., 32:170–172, 1983.

152. Reibman, J., et al.: Colchicine inhibits ionophore-induced formation of leukotriene B_4 by human neutrophils: The role of microtubules. J. Immunol., 136:1027–1032, 1986.

153. Bach, M.K.: Prospects for the inhibition of leukotriene synthesis. Biochem. Pharmacol., 33:515–521, 1984.

154. Strasser, T., Fischer, S., and Weber, P.C.: Inhibition of leukotriene B_4 formation in human neutrophils after oral nafazatrom (Bay G6575). Biochem. Pharmacol., 34:1891–1894, 1985.

CHARACTERISTICS OF IMMUNE COMPLEXES AND PRINCIPLES OF IMMUNE COMPLEX DISEASES

27

MART MANNIK

Immunologic mechanisms of tissue injury include: (1) IgE-mediated anaphylaxis; (2) complement-induced cell lysis; (3) immune complex-mediated injury; (4) cell-mediated immune injury involving specifically sensitized lymphocytes or antibody-dependent cellular cytotoxity; and (5) antibody-mediated neutralization of biologically active molecules. In a given disease more than one mechanism may be operative to cause the clinical manifestations. This chapter will focus on injury mediated by immune complexes.

Tissue injury in immune complex-mediated diseases results from the presence of antigen-antibody complexes in tissues. The basement membranes of blood vessels, glomeruli, choroid plexus, and other organs are common locations for deposits of immune complexes. The antigen-antibody deposits may arise from deposition in tissues of circulating immune complexes or from local formation. The diseases mediated by immune complexes share common pathogenic mechanisms, but the underlying causes vary owing to the different origins of the antigens in immune complexes. Since the immune complex diseases have common pathologic mechanisms their clinical manifestations include common features such as glomerulonephritis, vasculitis, arthritis, skin eruptions, pleuritis, and pericarditis. Such multiple organ involvement is frequent in disorders that result from deposition of immune complexes from circulation. Diseases resulting from local immune complex formation, on the other hand, usually are associated with involvement of a single organ such as the kidney or thyroid gland. In disorders associated with circulating immune complexes, considerable variations occur in the extent of the manifestations among patients and even in a given patient during the course of the disease. The reasons for such variations are still not known. Differences in the nature of the immune complexes, differences in the involved antigens, or alterations in the mechanisms for disposal of circulating immune complexes may account for variations in the disease expression.

A disease can be categorized as an immune complex disease with certainty when the specific antibodies and antigens that participate in the disease process are identified. Specific antibodies and antigens have been identified in some of the currently established immune complex disorders by elution from one or more target organs, followed by immunochemical identification of the recovered materials. In other disorders the specific antigens in the lesions have been identified by immunofluorescence microscopy, using specific antibodies to the suspected antigens. The currently known human immune complex diseases can be categorized according to the source of antigen, i.e., administered antigens, antigens released from microorganisms, antigens originating from endogenous tissues, and antigens released from tumors. The chronicity of many immune complex diseases results from the continued or recurrent presence of the antigen. Table 27–1 provides several examples of established human immune complex diseases. The list of suspected immune complex diseases is long, and appropriate reviews should be consulted for further detail.[1-3] The clinical manifestations of these

Table 27–1. Examples of Established Human Immune Complex Diseases*†

1. *Due to administered antigens*
   Serum sickness (animal antitoxins and antiserums, other animal proteins and hormones, drugs)
2. *Due to microbial antigens*
   Post-Streptococcal glomerulonephritis (plasma membrane antigens of beta-hemolytic Streptococci)
   Glomerulonephritis of bacterial endocarditis (bacterial antigens)
   Glomerulonephritis of infected ventriculoatrial shunts (*Staphylococcus epidermidis* antigen)
   Glomerulonephritis of syphilis (treponemal antigen)
   Glomerulonephritis of typhoid fever (*Salmonella* Vi antigen)
   Immune complex disease of hepatitis B infection (hepatitis B antigen)
   Glomerulonephritis of toxoplasmosis (*Toxoplasma* antigen)
   Glomerulonephritis of quartan malaria (*Plasmodium malariae* antigen)
   Glomerulonephritis of schistosomiasis (*Schistosoma mansoni* antigen)
3. *Due to autologous antigens*
   Systemic lupus erythematosus (DNA, nucleoprotein)
   Rheumatoid arthritis (IgG as antigen for rheumatoid factors)
   Mixed cryoglobulinemia (IgG as antigen)
   Glomerulonephritis due to renal tubular antigen (renal tubular antigen)
   Thyroiditis with thyroid carcinoma (thyroglobulin)
   Nephropathy of autoerythrocyte-sensitization (red cell stroma)
4. *Due to tumor antigens*
   Colonic carcinoma with nephritis (specific tumor antigen, carcinoembryonic antigen)
   Bronchogenic carcinoma with nephritis (specific tumor antigen)
   Clear cell renal carcinoma with nephritis (proximal tubule brush border antigen)

*The identified antigens are indicated in parentheses.
†Selected references identifying the involved antigens were provided in a previous edition.[4]

"suspected" disorders resemble the findings in established immune complex diseases. Immunoglobulins and complement components exist in glomeruli, blood vessels, and other organs characteristic of immune complex diseases, but the specific antigens and antibodies are still not identified.

NATURE OF IMMUNE COMPLEXES

The essential constituents of all antigen-antibody complexes are antigens and antibodies. In any given immune complex, the number of antigen and antibody molecules may vary, depending on the characteristics of each of the reactants and the features of the antigen-antibody union. The biologic properties of immune complexes are related to the nature of the molecules forming the complexes, as well as the number of reactants in each complex.

ANTIGENS

Antigens are defined as substances that interact specifically with available antibodies or sensitized lymphocytes. The term *immunogen* is reserved for a substance that upon administration to a suitable host will elicit an immune response. This distinction is made because all substances that react with antibodies or with sensitized lymphocytes do not necessarily induce an immune response. Antigens may be proteins, polysaccharides, nucleic acids, lipoproteins, or other chemicals. The actual portion of an antigen molecule that interacts with the antibody-combining site or with a specific receptor of a sensitized lymphocyte is defined as an *antigenic determinant*. The number of antigenic determinants on a molecule defines its valence for the interaction with specific antibodies. Five to six amino acids or six to seven monosaccharide units form the optimal size of an antigenic determinant for the interaction with a specific antibody-combining site. Small molecules with a single antigenic determinant are called haptens. Macromolecules, on the other hand, may be multivalent with several distinct antigenic determinants. Most macromolecular proteins fall into the latter category of antigenic molecules, whereas molecules like DNA with a repeating sequence are more likely to have repeating single antigenic determinants. The number of antigenic determinants of a molecule profoundly influences the kinds of antigen-antibody complexes that may form with the specific antibodies. Clearly, the molecular complexity of antigens increases as one considers microorganisms, cells, or tissues as antigens. For detailed discussions of antigens and antigenic determinants, the reader should consult immunochemical texts.[5,6]

Chemical features of the antigen may influence the biologic properties of immune complexes. A few examples serve to emphasize this point. For instance, exposed galactose residues in a glycoprotein may hasten the removal from circulation of small-latticed immune complexes by interaction with galactose receptors on hepatocytes.[7] Large molecular weight DNA is removed quickly from circulation by the liver and, as a consequence, immune complexes containing such DNA are also quickly removed from circulation.[8] Finally, cationic (positively charged) antigens can interact with fixed negative charges in tissues and then contribute to local immune complex formation, including the kidney, as will be emphasized later.

ANTIBODIES

Antibodies are the other essential constituents of antigen-antibody complexes; they may belong to the IgG, IgA, IgM, IgD, or IgE classes of immunoglobulins (for detailed discussion of antibody structure see Chapter 16). IgG, monomeric IgA, IgD, and IgE have a valence of two. Dimeric IgA and trimeric IgA molecules have a valence of four and six, respectively. IgM molecules exhibit a valence of ten or five, depending on the nature of the antigen. Interestingly, when bivalent IgG molecules interact with a polyvalent antigen with appropriately spaced, repeating antigenic determinants, then both antibody-binding sites preferentially react with the same antigenic molecule, giving an apparent valence of one to the antibody molecule. This type of reaction is termed a monogamous bivalent reaction and does not favor the formation of immune complexes with many antigen and many antibody molecules.[9] Antibodies to DNA, for example, may bind with monogamous bivalent interactions to DNA of sufficient size and, in this interaction, cross-linking of DNA strands by antibodies is not favored.[10]

LATTICE OF IMMUNE COMPLEXES

When antigen-antibody union takes place, various immune complexes may form, ranging from a union of one antigen molecule and one antibody molecule to unions of many molecules of each reactant. The *lattice of immune complexes* is defined as the number of antigen molecules and the number of antibody molecules in a given immune complex. Examples of various lattice formations are schematically depicted in Figure 27–1.

The lattice formation of immune complexes influences their biologic properties. Several variables alter the lattice formation of immune complexes. The valence of most antibody molecules is two, as pointed out previously. Polymeric IgA molecules and IgM molecules might form different lattice structures. The valence of antigen molecules profoundly alters the lattice of formed complexes. A monovalent antigen can only form Ag_2Ab_1 complexes; larger lattices and immune precipitates cannot be formed. Bivalent antigens, depending on the distance between the antigenic determinants, may form Ag_1Ab_1, Ag_2Ab_2, circular Ag_3Ab_3, or larger open or closed complexes. Only multivalent antigens form immune complexes with high degrees of lattice and undergo immune precipitation.

The molar ratio of antigen to antibody influences

FIG. 27–1. Schematic representation of immune complexes (AgAb) with varying degrees of lattice formation. In A the interaction of two small monovalent antigen molecules (haptens) with one antibody molecule is depicted. Diagram B shows a small-latticed (Ag_2Ab_2) immune complex formed by multivalent antigen and IgG molecules. Diagram C depicts the monogamous bivalent interaction formed by an antigenic molecule with repeating antigenic determinants. A large-latticed (Ag_4Ab_4) immune complex is depicted in D, formed with antibodies of two different specificities and an antigen with two different antigenic determinants.

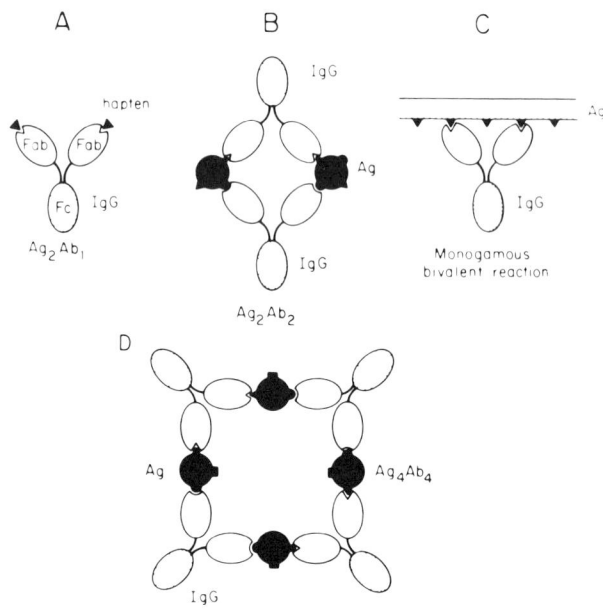

the degree of lattice formation, as illustrated by the classic precipitation curves. When an increasing amount of antigen is added to a constant amount of antibody, then an increasing amount of precipitate is formed in the antibody excess zone. At the point of equivalence, maxiumum amount of precipitate is formed, and free antigen and free antibody are not detectable in the supernatant. Addition of antigen beyond the point of equivalence results in soluble immune complexes, and the amount of formed precipitate decreases. With increasing antigen excess, the lattice formation of soluble immune complexes decreases. When a large excess of antigen is used, small soluble immune complexes are formed, consisting of Ag_1Ab_1, Ag_2Ab_2, or Ag_2Ab_1 complexes. In addition, the absolute concentrations of antigen and antibody influence the lattice formation independent of the antigen-antibody molar ratio. At a given degree of antigen excess, more small-latticed immune complexes (Ag_1Ab_1 and Ag_2Ab_2) are formed at microgram concentrations of reactants than at the same antigen-antibody ratio at milligram concentrations.

The association constant between the antigen and antibody influences the lattice formation of immune complexes. Low-affinity antibodies form smaller immune complexes than high-affinity antibodies with all other variables constant. The principles of determining association constants for monovalent antigens are well established. The principles and methods of measuring association constants for large, multivalent antigens and antibodies are complicated and may lead to errors, depending on the assumed simplifications. The reader interested in further study of the association constants and their measurement should consult texts on immunochemistry.[5,6]

The characteristics of immune complexes in human diseases have not yet been examined in sufficient detail to relate their features to the disease processes and disease outcome. The concepts established in experimental animals, however, have pointed to the need to develop this information.

BIOLOGIC PROPERTIES OF IMMUNE COMPLEXES

The key properties of antigen-antibody complexes with respect to immune complex diseases are activation of the complement systems, interaction with cell receptors, and deposition in tissues. These functions depend on the nature of antibodies in the complexes and the degree of lattice formation of the complexes. Other biologic properties of immune complexes, such as the influence on the immune response and alteration of the functions of lymphocytes, are less well understood at this time, but have been reviewed elsewhere.[1] Polyclonal B cell activation by immune complexes, however, is a biologic property of immune complexes that may have considerable importance in the concepts of autoimmune disorders. Studies in experimental animals have demonstrated that antigen-antibody complexes can lead to antigen independent B cell proliferation and to synthesis of specific antibodies not related to the constituents of immune complexes.[11]

COMPLEMENT FIXATION BY IMMUNE COMPLEXES

Complement fixation by immune complexes may proceed through the classic or the alternative pathways of complement activation (see Chapter 25 for discussion of the complement system).

Antibodies of the IgG and IgM class activate the complement system through the classic pathway,

provided sufficient lattice formation is present. Among the IgG class of antibodies, IgG1, IgG2, and IgG3 subclasses are efficient in complement activation, and the IgG4 subclass is inefficient. The initial step of complement activation through the classic pathway occurs by the binding of C1q to the immune complexes. The available evidence indicates that the complexes form a multivalent ligand to bind C1q, thereby activating the complement system, rather than by conformational changes induced by the antigen-antibody interaction. This view is consistent with the observations that even monomeric IgG molecules bind weakly to isolated C1q as examined by analytical ultracentrifugation, including all subclasses of IgG. With multiple IgG molecules, immune complexes are expected to form even firmer bonds with C1q, thus leading to complement activation. As a generalization, the greater the number of IgG molecules, the greater the effectiveness of immune complexes in binding to C1q and activating the complement system. Similarly, with heat-aggregated IgG, effective complement activation is achieved. The number of IgM molecules required in soluble immune complexes has not been carefully delineated, but on cell surface one IgM antibody molecule may suffice to activate the complement system. The other classes of antibodies in immune complexes do not fix complement.

The alternative complement pathway is activated by all immune complexes that trigger the classic complement pathway by generating C3b and thereby activating the C3b-dependent loop of the alternative pathway.

The complement system also significantly influences the nature of immune complexes by solubilizing already formed immune precipitates and by preventing immune precipitation. When immune precipitates are formed between antigen and antibody at equivalence, and fresh serum is added as a source of complement, the immune precipitates are converted to soluble, large-latticed immune complexes that contain covalently bound products of C3.[12] This binding of C3 breakdown products to antibody molecules is essential for dispersion of the immune precipitates and for the prevention of reformation of immune precipitates. These solubilized complexes are large. For example, when the system of bovine serum albumin and antibodies to bovine serum albumin is employed, the solublized complexes have sedimentation constants of 25 to 30 Svedberg units.

Furthermore, immune precipitation is prevented in a similar manner by the presence of complement. When precipitating antigens and antibodies are mixed in the presence of fresh serum as a source of complement, a precipitate is not formed, whereas the same reactants form a precipitate in a neutral buffer or in heated serum.[13] The immune complexes generated by either of these mechanisms remain soluble and contain C3b. The presence of C3b in these immune complexes mediates their interaction with the complement receptor CR1, which is present on phagocytic cells and primate erythrocytes. This receptor on red blood cells is now thought to play an important role in disposing of circulating C3b-containing immune complexes.[14]

INTERACTION OF IMMUNE COMPLEXES WITH CELL SURFACE RECEPTORS

The primary interaction of immune complexes with cells occurs through the Fc receptors on neutrophils, monocytes (including tissue macrophages throughout the body, as well as Kupffer's cells in the liver), platelets, and certain lymphocyte populations. These receptors are specific for IgG and do not interact with other classes of immunoglobulins. In addition to the Fc receptors, phagocytic cells and some lymphocytes also possess complement receptors. (For detailed discussion of receptors on lymphocytes, monocytes, and neutrophils, see Chapters 18, 19, and 20, respectively.)

The lattice structure of immune complexes influences significantly their interaction with the Fc receptors. Monomeric IgG molecules bind to these cell surface receptors weakly, but do not trigger the interiorization or engulfment of the attached molecules by the cell. Attachment of complexes with sufficient lattice, on the other hand, results in phagocytosis of the complexes. Small-latticed immune complexes, such as those prepared with divalent and monovalent antigens or prepared by high degrees of polyvalent antigen excess, are not phagocytized by neutrophils or by monocytes. Large-latticed immune complexes, defined as containing more than two antibody molecules, are attached to the Fc receptors and then apparently undergo further condensation or rearrangement to even larger lattices prior to phagocytosis.[15] This condensation to larger lattices was thought to result from the increased local concentration of the soluble immune complexes by interaction with Fc receptors on the monocyte surface. Monomeric IgG1 and IgG3 are effective in inhibiting the attachment of immune complexes to the Fc receptors of neutrophils and monocytes, but IgG2 and IgG4 are ineffective.

The interaction of immune complexes with monocyte receptors occurs via the Fc receptors and can lead to phagocytosis and degradation of the ingested immune complexes. If the immune complexes have reached a sufficient lattice to activate complement, then the C3b bound to immune complexes can facilitate their binding to and phagocytosis by monocytes through the interaction with C3b receptors on these cells. For example, if heat-aggregated IgG, as a surrogate for immune complexes, contains more than 16 IgG molecules, it is effective in complement activation, and phagocytosis of these large aggregates by monocytes is facilitated by the presence of complement.[16]

The principles of interactions of monocytes and immune complexes also apply to tissue macrophages, including Kupffer's cells in the liver. The interaction of immune complexes with Kupffer's cells is the basis for their removal from circulation.

As discussed in Chapter 20, during phagocytosis of large-latticed immune complexes, particularly when these materials are attached to a nonphagocytizable surface, lysosomal enzymes spill to the surrounding medium. This event is thought to be highly important in mediating tissue damage during immune complex deposition.

Human platelets interact with immune complexes without the presence of complement components, leading to platelet aggregation and release of platelet constituents that activate the clotting system (see Chapter 24). Platelet aggregation and release of platelet constituents require large-latticed immune complexes. During this release platelets are not lysed. Thus, through interactions with platelets, immune complexes can activate the clotting system, which then may contribute to the final pathways of tissue injury.

Human and other primate erythrocytes possess a receptor for C3b (CR1) that mediates the binding of immune complexes to the red cells. Erythrocytes from patients with active systemic lupus erythematosus (SLE) have a decrease in these receptors.[17] In one study, even the relatives of patients with SLE had decreased C3b receptors on erythrocytes, suggesting an inherited defect.[18] Available evidence, however, indicates that the reduced levels of CR1 on red blood cells of patients with SLE are acquired during active disease.[19,20] Furthermore, studies in monkeys have suggested that the C3b receptors on red cells contribute to the removal from circulation of very large immune complexes.[14]

FATE OF CIRCULATING IMMUNE COMPLEXES

Once immune complexes are formed in circulation, their subsequent fate and tissue deposition depend on several variables, including the lattice of immune complexes, the status of the mononuclear phagocyte system, the nature of antibodies in the complexes, and the nature of antigen molecules in the complexes. The principles involved in the removal of immune complexes from circulation have been studied in experimental animals.

When immune complexes with known degrees of lattice formation are injected into mice, rabbits, or monkeys, large-latticed immune complexes, composed of lattices larger than Ag_2Ab_2, are rapidly removed from the circulation by the mononuclear phagocyte system, predominantly by the Kupffer's cells of the liver. Small-latticed complexes, composed of Ag_2Ab_2 and Ag_1Ab_1 complexes, persist longer in circulation but are removed more quickly than the antibodies alone. Complement components are not required in this rapid uptake of large-latticed complexes since the depletion of complement with cobra venom factor or with aggregated IgG does not alter the kinetics or quantity of immune complexes cleared by the mononuclear phagocyte system. The mechanism of immune clearance by Kupffer's cells depends on Fc receptors of these cells. Furthermore, Kupffer's cells in hepatic sinusoids are not covered by endothelial cells and are thus directly exposed to the circulating complexes. The original data for these conclusions have been summarized in the literature.[21]

The mononuclear phagocyte system in the liver, previously called the reticuloendothelial system, is saturable with carbon particles or with other substances. Competitive uptake, and the inhibition of uptake of one substance by another, is an established phenomenon. The saturation of the mononuclear phagocyte system by large-latticed immune complexes was established by injecting increasing doses of immune complexes.[21] Saturation of this system leads to prolonged circulation of large-latticed immune complexes and thereby to increased risk of tissue deposition. This saturation was detected by using aggregated IgG as a probe for Kupffer's cell function in experimental animals as a surrogate of immune complexes. Small-latticed immune complexes in experimental animals do not alter the clearance kinetics or hepatic uptake of this probe.[22] Patients with systemic lupus erythematosus or other immune complex disease have decreased clearance of antibody-coated red cells in comparison to normal persons.[23] The antibody-coated red cells principally measure uptake by the spleen. Nevertheless, the clearance of these coated cells indicates a malfunction in patients with active SLE.

As pointed out, the class and subclass of antibody molecules influence the efficacy of their interactions with monocyte receptors in vitro. These observations suggest that large-latticed immune complexes, containing antibodies that are ineffective in interacting with monocyte receptors, would circulate longer than complexes containing antibodies that interact effectively with these receptors. For example, when the interchain disulfide bonds of the IgG class of antibodies are cleaved by reduction and alkylation, immune complexes made with such antibodies interact ineffectively with monocyte receptors in vitro. The clearance kinetics of such complexes are altered. The large-latticed complexes are removed slowly from the circulation of rabbits, monkeys, and mice owing to decreased hepatic uptake. Because of the prolonged circulation of these large-latticed immune complexes, deposition in renal glomeruli is enhanced.[21]

In experimental animals, immune complexes containing IgA class of antibodies are taken up rapidly by the liver when eight or more IgA antibodies are present in the immune complexes.[24] The critical number of eight antibody molecules is achieved either by eight monomeric IgA molecules or by four dimeric IgA molecules. The uptake of these large IgA complexes occurs by IgA receptors on Kupffer's cells.[25]

The nature of antigens in immune complexes can alter the fate of circulating immune complexes. For example, certain antigens are rapidly removed from circulation by the mononuclear phagocyte system without the presence of antibodies. Small-latticed immune complexes prepared with such antigens are also quickly removed from circulation. Specific examples of the role of antigens on the fate of immune complexes were already cited in the section on the nature of immune complexes.

TISSUE DEPOSITION OF IMMUNE COMPLEXES

As already pointed out, the presence of immune complexes in a variety of organs is associated with inflammation and tissue damage. Glomeruli, renal peritubular capillaries, renal tubular basement membranes, small and medium blood vessels in many organs, dermal-epidermal junction, choroid plexus, the basement membrane of thyroid follicles, interstitial spaces in synovial tissue, and articular cartilage are examples of the many sites where immune complexes have been identified. The presence of immune complexes at various sites may arise from deposition of circulating immune complexes or from local formation of antigen-antibody complexes at the site of their presence. The local formation of immune complexes can arise from interaction of antibodies with structural components of the tissue or from selective deposition or presence of an antigen at a given location, followed by specific immune complex formation. A clinical example of local immune complex formation with structural antigens in tissues occurs in Goodpasture's syndrome. In this disease, antibodies develop to the glomerular basement membrane antigens that also react with the alveolar basement membrane, leading to presence of antibodies uniformly deposited along the glomerular and alveolar basement membranes.

The Arthus reaction is the basic model of local immune complex disease, induced in actively or passively immunized animals by local injection of the antigen. Vasculitis at the site of antigen injection is caused by immune complexes in small vessels, leading to complement fixation and influx of polymorphonuclear leukocytes and later mononuclear cells.[26] Antigen-induced local immune complex disease can be generated experimentally in specific organs, such as joints, the pleural cavity, and lungs. Antigen-induced synovitis is an example of local antigen-induced disease, and the formation of immune complexes plays a significant part in the inflammatory process. In these experiments, the injected antigen in the form of immune complexes remains bound to the superficial layers of cartilage and ligaments for prolonged periods, thus prolonging the inflammation. As another example, once tolerance to an endogenous substance is broken, then the autologous tissues can serve as a continued source of antigen to maintain a chronic local inflammatory process. A well-studied example is the thyroiditis induced by injection of heterologous thyroglobulin. Tolerance is broken to thyroglobulin, antibodies are synthesized to thyroglobulin, and immune complexes form at the follicular basement membrane of thyroid follicles.[27] The key point in this disease model is that the follicular basement membrane is the site where the antigen and antibody union occurs, and the formed complexes remain largely localized in this area.

Information is not available to distinguish in human diseases the immune complexes that have arisen at a given location by deposition from circulation from those developed by local formation. The presence of circulating immune complexes in association with tissue deposition should not be considered as unequivocal evidence that the circulating immune complexes were deposited in the tissues. In recent years considerable progress has been made in understanding the development of immune complexes in glomeruli. Therefore, special emphasis will be given to the concepts that have evolved from studies in experimental animals.

In human glomerulonephritis, including the ne-

phritis of systemic lupus erythematosus, and in experimental models of glomerulonephritis, immune deposits are found in three locations. These locations are the mesangium, the subendothelial area, and the subepithelial area (Fig. 27–2). The glomerular mesangium, consisting of matrix and resident mesangial cells, is considered as glomerular interstitial tissue, surrounded by the glomerular capillary loops that are confined by the Bowman's capsule. The glomerular capillary wall is both a size and a charge barrier to macromolecules in circulation. Fixed negative charges are present in the glomerular basement membrane, both in the lamina rara interna (subendothelial area) and the lamina rara externa (subepithelial area). These fixed negative charges in the glomerular capillary wall significantly contribute to the mechanisms of immune complex formation and deposition in glomeruli. Experimental evidence indicates that some immune deposits in glomeruli arise from deposition of immune complexes from circulation and that other immune deposits in glomeruli develop by local formation of antigen-antibody complexes.

In chronic serum sickness models in experimental animals, the renal lesions contained mesangial, sub-

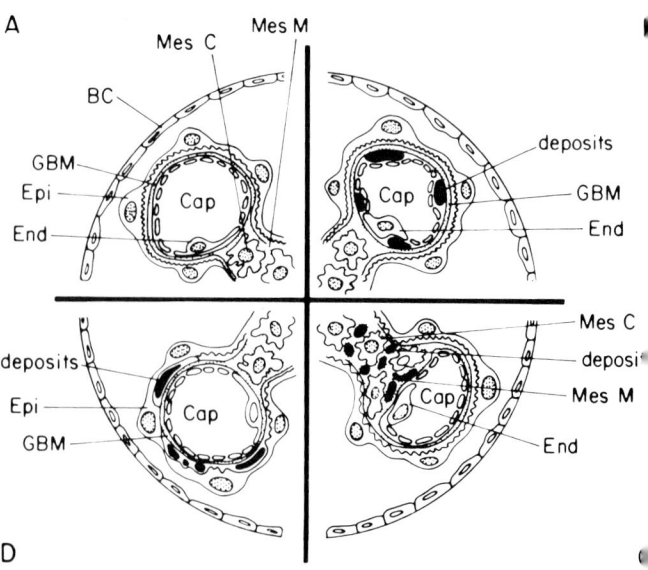

FIG. 27–2. Schematic representation of different localization of immune complexes within the glomerular capillaries. A, Normal capillary loop; B, pattern of subendothelial deposits; C, pattern of mesangial deposits; D, pattern of subepithelial deposits. BC = Bowman's capsule; US = urinary space; GBM = glomerular basement membrane; Cap = capillary lumen; Epi = epithelial cells with foot processes; End = endothelial cells with fenestrated cytoplasmic extensions covering the basement membrane; Mes C = mesangial cells; Mes M = mesangial matrix.

endothelial, and subepithelial immune deposits. Initially, all these deposits were thought to arise from deposition of circulating immune complexes. Experiments with injection of preformed immune complexes into unimmunized animals, however, showed that complexes in circulation deposit in the subendothelial area and in the mesangium. No deposits were found in the subepithelial area, using rabbit IgG antibodies to human serum albumin, bovine serum albumin, or to the dinitrophenyl antigenic determinants on bovine serum albumin as summarized in the literature.[28] Several lines of evidence indicate that the lattice of circulating immune complexes is highly important to their deposition in glomeruli. First, when mixtures of large-latticed (greater than Ag_2Ab_2) and small-latticed (Ag_2Ab_2 and Ag_1Ab_1) immune complexes in antigen excess are injected into mice, glomerular deposition of complexes progresses only while the large-latticed complexes remain in circulation. Second, the injection of small-latticed (Ab_2Ab_2, Ag_1Ab_1) immune complexes into mice causes no glomerular immune deposits. Third, when large-latticed immune complexes are deposited in glomeruli, the injection of a large excess of antigen results in complete removal of extracellular glomerular immune deposits, presumably by conversion of the immune deposits to small-latticed immune complexes.[28] Finally, immune complexes deposited from circulation into the subendothelial or mesangial areas must undergo condensation or rearrangement into even larger complexes or small precipitates to persist in glomeruli and to become visible as electron-dense deposits. Proof for this concept was obtained by injecting into mice large-latticed immune complexes that were covalently cross-linked so that these complexes could not rearrange or condense into precipitates. These complexes were only transiently deposited in glomeruli and did not evolve into electron-dense deposits. In contrast, when similar complexes without covalent bonds were administered to mice, the deposits that evolved then persisted and became visible as electron-dense deposits.[29]

These observations collectively indicate that large-latticed immune complexes containing more than two antibody molecules become locally concentrated in glomeruli, possibly as a result of transient interactions with glomerular structures. Then, as a consequence of this increased local concentration, they condense into even larger deposits, comparable to immune precipitates, that become visible as electron-dense deposits in the subendothelial or mesangial areas of the glomeruli. Immune deposits that do not undergo such rearrangement, such as nonprecipitating antigen-

antibody systems, persist in glomeruli only a relatively short time.

Electrostatic interactions constitute one mechanism for local increase in concentration of immune complexes in glomeruli. When chemically modified, cationic (positively charged) antibodies were used to prepare soluble immune complexes, the injection of these complexes caused extensive subendothelial deposits that persisted in this location much longer than complexes prepared with unaltered antibodies.[30] The lattice of the injected complexes is still important in that large-latticed complexes (containing more than two antibody molecules) result in deposits that persist for several days, whereas cationized antibodies or small-latticed immune complexes are present by immunofluorescence microscopy only for a few hours, owing to the interaction with the fixed negative charges in glomerular capillary walls. Since the glomerular capillary wall is partially permeable to cationic molecules of even 400,000 molecular weight, but not to cationic molecules of about 1×10^6 molecular weight,[31] the large-latticed complexes with more than two antibody molecules attach to the fixed negative charges in the lamina rara interna, achieve increased local concentration, and then condense to even larger deposits that persist and become visible as electron-dense deposits. Similar deposits evolve in the mesangial matrix. Other mechanisms must also be involved in the retention and condensation of immune complexes in the mesangial matrix, since even highly anionic (negatively charged) antibodies in large-latticed immune complexes result in mesangial deposits.[32]

The involvement of charge-charge interactions for the initial glomerular deposition of circulating, cationic immune complexes and subsequent condensation into large lattices was illustrated in mice with the following experiments. Cationic immune complexes were injected, leading to immediate deposits in glomeruli. These immune deposits were displaced from glomeruli by competing cationic molecules when injected 1 minute after the administration of immune complexes. If 1 hour elapsed between the injection of the same immune complexes and the competing cationic molecules, the immune deposits were not displaced.[33] As revealed by electron microscopy, the injected cationic molecules initially decorated the regularly spaced, fixed anionic sites in the laminae rarae, but with the passage of time, the electron-dense material condensed into larger deposits in the subendothelial or subepithelial area.[30] In rat kidneys pretreated with heparinase perfusion, cationic immune complexes did not cause immune deposits, indicating that heparan sulfate proteoglycans constitute the relevant fixed anionic sites for charge-charge interaction with immune complexes.[34]

Several experimental models exist for local immune complex formation in glomeruli due to antigens that become attached or planted in glomeruli, as reviewed in the literature.[35] Intravenously injected aggregated IgG or aggregated albumin becomes entrapped in the mesangial matrix, and when antibodies to these aggregated proteins are administered, immune deposits form and an acute inflammatory response ensues in the mesangial area of the glomeruli. Concanavalin A binds to the glomerular basement membrane, and when antibodies to Concanavalin A are administered, lumpy-bumpy immune deposits evolve.

Considerable evidence indicates that the subepithelial immune deposits, as seen in membranous glomerulonephritis, are locally formed rather than deposited from circulation.[35] Evidence for this was marshalled in rats with the $F \times 1A$ antigen derived from the brush border of proximal tubules, and with repeated perfusion of rat kidneys with bovine serum albumin and antibodies to bovine serum albumin. In these experiments the possible formation of immune complexes in the perfusate was excluded. In the first example, the $F \times 1A$ antigen is located in the subepithelial area, and the perfused antibodies combine with the antigen to form subepithelial immune deposits. In the second example, some of the perfused bovine serum albumin reaches the subepithelial area and is followed by antibody to form subepithelial immune complexes. The role of the charge on antigens has been extensively studied on glomerular localization. For example, cationized (positively charged) human IgG localizes in rat kidneys and persists there with a half-life of 4.2 hours due to interaction with the fixed negative charges in the glomeruli. When antibodies to IgG are injected after the antigen, subepithelial immune deposits form, and the antigen persists with a half-life of 12 days in rat glomeruli.[36] Furthermore, the chronic administration of cationic antigens results in extensive membranous glomerulonephritis with subepithelial deposits to a greater extent than achieved with neutral or anionic antigens.[37,38] For the persistence of immune deposits in the subepithelial area and the formation of electron-dense deposits, precipitating antigen-antibody systems are required. Nonprecipitating antigen-antibody systems form only transient deposits that do not become visible as electron-dense deposits.[39] It is also possible that positively charged antibodies become planted in the glomeruli first, followed by antigen, to form immune deposits in glomeruli.[40]

Relatively recent findings indicate that subepithelial immune deposits in glomeruli may arise from cell-surface antigens and antibodies directed to these molecules. When bivalent antibodies react with epithelial cell-surface antigens, capping and subsequent shedding of the antigen-antibody complexes from the epithelial cell membrane result in subepithelial granular immune deposits.[41,42]

Obviously, much work is required to identify and characterize the antigens involved in human glomerulonephritis, but the studies in experimental models have established principles that can be useful in this needed work.

When subepithelial deposits have formed, the glomerulus does not become hypercellular and monocytes do not accumulate; yet, proteinuria becomes prominent. The injury that leads to proteinuria is largely mediated by complement since extensive proteinuria did not evolve in C3-depleted rats with subepithelial deposits.[43]

EXPERIMENTAL MODELS OF IMMUNE COMPLEX DISEASES

The study of immune complex diseases in experimental animal models was first to establish many principles involved in these disorders. The experimental models can be classified as spontaneous disease models, diseases induced by administration of antigen (serum sickness), and abnormalities induced by injection of preformed immune complexes. In addition, the serum sickness models can be considered as acute or chronic abnormalities, depending on a single or multiple administration of antigen.

The best-known example of spontaneous immune complex disease is murine lupus in New Zealand and other strains of mice (see Chapter 30).

ACUTE IMMUNE COMPLEX DISEASES

The study of acute immune complex disease or serum sickness in rabbits has provided perhaps the greatest initial insight into the pathologic events in immune complex diseases. In this system, large quantities of an antigen are required for intravenous injection in unimmunized rabbits to produce significant disease. For example, 500 mg of bovine serum albumin (BSA) is used for a 2-kg rabbit.[44] When radiolabeled antigen is employed, the events of antigen disappearance can be easily followed (Fig. 27–3). Initially, the concentration of the injected antigen decreases rapidly as a result of intra- and extravascular equilibration. Thereafter, the concentration of the antigen declines gradually as a result of catabolism.

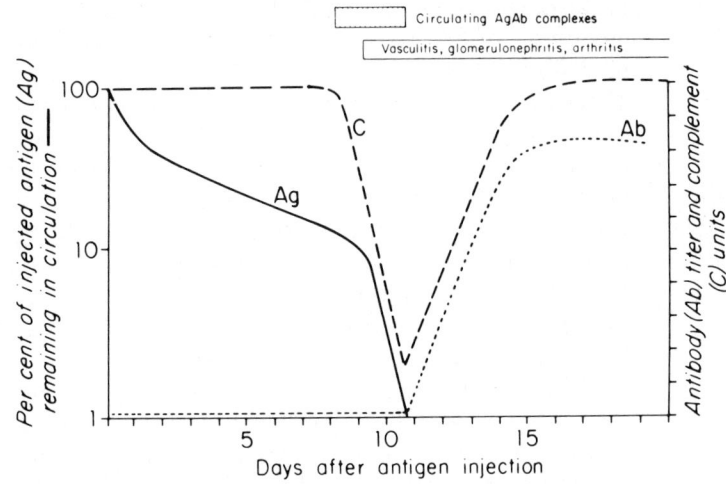

FIG. 27–3. Schematic representation of events in acute serum sickness. The percentage of injected antigen (Ag) in circulation initially declines rapidly as a result of intra- and extravascular equilibration, then decreases as a result of catabolism, and about nine days after injection undergoes immune clearance as a result of antibody synthesis. At the time of immune clearance, circulating immune complexes are detectable and complement (C) is consumed. Vasculitis, glomerulonephritis, and arthritis develop because of immune complex deposition. With the clearance of immune complexes by the mononuclear phagocyte system, the pathogenic process ceases, free antibody (Ab) becomes detectable, and the inflammatory lesions gradually subside.

When the immune response to the BSA develops after about eight days, the concentration of the antigen drops rapidly because of antigen-antibody complex formation, resulting in immune clearance of the foreign material. During the immune clearance phase and just prior to this event, circulating immune complexes are easily identified by the presence of a radiolabel on the injected BSA. At the time of immune clearance, the rabbit serum complement level decreases.

Coincident with the immune clearance of the injected BSA, resulting from the formation of large-latticed immune complexes, the rabbits develop glomerulonephritis, vasculitis of many organs, and synovitis. The injected antigen, rabbit IgG, and complement components are present in the glomerular and vascular lesions. This model does not distinguish whether the tissue deposits result from deposition of circulating complexes or from local formation. Vasculitis can be abrogated in this model when complement components (C3) are depleted with cobra venom factor prior to the onset of the immune clearance phase of the disease, thus preventing the development of complement-derived chemotactic factors. The vascular damage is also abrogated by neutropenia induced by nitrogen mustard.[45] Thus, the vascular damage is not caused per se by the deposition of immune complexes, but requires an influx of neutrophils. The development of glomerular lesions is more complex, since the depletion of complement components or neutrophils does not abrogate histologic lesions. On the other hand, a decrease in circulating monocytes decreases proteinuria, indicating that monocytes are involved in mediating the renal damage in this model.[46] The natural course of this acute illness in rabbits is self-limited and abates with return of complement to normal levels and gradual disappearance of the inflammatory lesions. The immune response in rabbits to BSA persists, but the pathogenic process ceases when the antigen is removed. Similarly, in human diseases when the presence of antigens ceases, the immune complex manifestations abate. The self-limited course of serum sickness from an injected foreign protein and the cessation of glomerulonephritis by appropriate antimicrobial treatment of infective endocarditis serve as excellent examples.

CHRONIC IMMUNE COMPLEX DISEASE

The acute serum sickness in rabbits is easily converted to a chronic disease model by injecting repeated doses of the same antigen. If the injected dose of BSA is varied according to the immune response in each rabbit, providing an antigen excess relative to the total amount of antibody, then the disease progresses, invariably leading to chronic glomerulonephritis and renal failure.[44] On the other hand, if a fixed dose of antigen is given (e.g., 12.5 mg. of BSA per injection), then the progression of disease varies according to the immune response of the rabbit.[47] Rabbits that mount a vigorous immune response develop no progressive disease, presumably owing to formation of large-latticed immune complexes that are effectively and promptly removed from the circulation. Rabbits that mount a relatively low immune response have demonstrable immune complexes in circulation, ranging from 500,000 to 700,000 daltons by sucrose density gradient ultracentrifugation; these persist in circulation up to 24 hours. These animals develop diffuse proliferative glomerulonephritis with deposits of immune complexes in capillary loops in the subepithelial area. As discussed previously under tissue deposition of immune complexes, current evidence indicates that these deposits may have arisen by the alternating presence of antigen and antibody. Rabbits that develop a moderate immune response have circulating complexes of about one million daltons that persist in circulation only for a few hours. These animals develop hypercellularity in glomeruli and mesangial deposits of immune complexes. In addition to glomerular pathology, chronic and frequent antigen administration to immunized animals also causes immune complex-mediated interstitial renal lesions.[48]

DISEASE INDUCED BY PREFORMED IMMUNE COMPLEXES

Vasculitis and glomerulonephritis are readily induced in mice by injecting large doses or repeated doses of soluble, preformed immune complexes. Similar experiments have not succeeded in rabbits, but this may have resulted from inadequate doses of injected complexes as compared to the doses required in mice.[1] Nevertheless, the observation that injected, preformed immune complexes can cause vasculitis and glomerulonephritis confirmed that circulating immune complexes cause lesions, and opened the way for further study of the physiology of circulating immune complexes and elucidation of mechanisms for their deposition in tissues as described previously. Glomerular deposition of preformed immune complexes has already been discussed in detail.

TESTS FOR DETECTING IMMUNE COMPLEXES AND CLINICAL APPLICATION OF THESE TESTS

The preceding sections pointed out the relevance of circulating immune complexes to the persistence and chronicity of immune complex–mediated disease processes in experimental animals. Therefore, it seems desirable to quantify and characterize the immune complexes in human diseases in order to predict disease outcome or even to identify the origin of involved antigens. Many methods have been proposed for the estimation of circulating immune complexes in human diseases. The presence of immune complexes has been demonstrated and claimed in many disorders.[2,3,49,50] No single assay, however, provides an accurate measure of all immune complexes. The most frequently used assays for immune complexes are listed in Table 27–2.

The physical methods for detection of immune complexes depend on separation of these materials from other serum components. Size separations by ultracentrifugation or gel filtration are insensitive and laborious. In addition, small complexes are difficult to distinguish from normal serum macromolecules. These methods alone or in combination with biologic methods remain tools for research laboratories. Addition to serum of low concentrations of polyethylene glycol can precipitate immune complexes, but some normal serum proteins are also precipitated with this quick technique. Cryoprecipitation is a property of some but not all immune complexes; certain myeloma proteins and Waldenström macroglobulins also have the same property.

The biologic methods for detection of immune complexes have been extensively employed. All these methods depend on one of several biologic properties of immune complexes already discussed earlier in this chapter. As pointed out, many of these properties depend on the lattice of immune complexes, on the class or subclass of antibodies in the complexes, and even on properties of the antigens. Therefore, these biologic tests detect various immune complexes with variable efficiency. Another problem is the lack of an ideal standard for the biologic assays for immune complexes. Aggregated human IgG is most commonly used as a surrogate standard for immune complexes, but the degree of aggregation is often not adequately standardized. The results are usually expressed as equivalents of µg or ng of aggregated human IgG. Some investigators prefer to express the results as standard deviations above the normal range, established with serums from normal persons.

The assays using C1q detect immune complexes that can bind this complement protein. A fluid-phase or a solid-phase assay is used. These methods detect immune complexes containing IgM or IgG that can interact with C1q. As a generalization, immune complexes with large lattices are detected more effectively than immune complexes with small lattices.[51] Thus, the same degree of positivity can arise from the presence of a relatively small amount of large-latticed immune complexes or a relatively large amount of small-latticed immune complexes. Monomeric IgG can interfere to some degree with these tests. Some patients have in serum materials sedimenting with normal IgG (6.6 Svedberg units) that bind to C1q in the solid-phase assay. Evidence suggests that this low molecular weight (6.6S) C1q-binding IgG may represent antibodies directed to C1q.[52] This low-molecular-weight C1q-binding material, as well as faster sedimenting immune complexes that bind to C1q, are present in serums of patients with proliferative forms of lupus glomerulonephritis.[53] Moreover, anionic molecules, including DNA, endotoxin, and heparin, can bind to C1q molecules and render the C1q insol-

Table 27-2. Selected Examples of Methods for Detecting Immune Complexes

Methods	Comments
1. *Physical methods*	
Analytical ultracentrifugation	Relatively insensitive
Sucrose density gradient ultracentrifugation and gel filtration	Can be combined with biologic assays to relate activity and size of complexes
Precipitation with polyethylene glycol	Immune complexes are less soluble in polyethylene glycol than other serum proteins
Cryoprecipitation	Some immune complexes, but also other proteins, are insoluble at 4°C
2. *Interaction with C1q*	
Precipitation of radiolabeled C1q with complexes in polyethylene glycol	Extensively used method, able to detect as little as 10 μg of aggregated IgG
C1q-coated polystyrene tubes	C1q-coated tubes bind complexes, detected with radiolabeled antibodies to IgG
3. *Interactions with rheumatoid factors (RF)*	
Solid-phase radioimmunoassay, RF bound to cellulose	Complexes inhibit binding of ^{125}I aggregated IgG by RF
Solid-phase radioimmunoassay, aggregated IgG bound to agarose	Complexes inhibit binding of RF to aggregated IgG conjugated to agarose
4. *Interactions with bovine conglutinin*	
Conglutinin-coated tubes	Coated tubes bind immune complexes that contain C3bi, detected with ^{125}I-antihuman-IgG
5. *Interaction with Fc and complement receptors on cells,*	
Raji cell assay	C3b and other complement receptors bind immune complexes, detected with ^{125}I-antihuman IgG
Interaction with macrophage receptors	Immune complexes inhibit uptake of aggregated IgG by macrophages

uble in polyethylene glycol in the fluid-phase assay. In a solid-phase C1q assay, these substances do not interfere with the test results, since binding to C1q is detected by antibodies to IgG or to IgM.

Rheumatoid factors bind to the Fc fragment of IgG and with higher efficiency when the IgG molecules are polymerized in immune complexes or nonspecifically aggregated. Thus, these assays only detect immune complexes containing IgG, and the presence of complement components is not required. Polyclonal rheumatoid factors from patients with rheumatoid arthritis or monoclonal rheumatoid factors from patients with B-cell tumors may be employed for these assays. Again, the assays with rheumatoid factors detect larger complexes more effectively than small complexes. In addition, high concentrations of monomeric IgG can cause false positive tests.

The conglutinin assay detects only immune complexes that have activated complement and contain C3bi. If C3b is present prior to inactivation by the C3b inactivator, the complexes are not detected. Once C3bi is cleaved into C3d and C3c, the immune complexes are no longer effectively detected by this assay. Other systems have taken advantage of specific antibodies to C3b or C3d, adsorbed on the surface of plastic tubes. The binding to the test tube of immune complexes with these complement components is then detected by antibodies to specific immunoglobulins. These systems also detect material in the size range of normal IgG. These species of molecules arise from covalent binding of C3b to IgG and subsequent cleavage of C3b to C3d, consisting of C3d bound to IgG without the presence of antigen molecules.[54]

The most commonly used assay employing cell receptors is the Raji cell assay. The Raji cells are lymphoblastoid B cells derived from a patient with Burkitt's lymphoma. These cells lack surface immunoglobulins, and have low-affinity receptors for IgG and high-affinity receptors for activated complement components. Hence, this assay detects immune complexes that have C3b and other complement components bound to them. The binding of immune complexes to the cells is detected with antibodies to IgG or other immunoglobulins. Therefore, the presence of lymphocytotoxic antibodies can lead to false positive results. Even antibodies to nuclear antigens may give false positive tests since these cells extrude or bind DNA at times.

Because all the assays for immune complexes mentioned are not antigen specific, these tests are not specific to a given disease and provide no assistance in reaching a specific diagnosis. The development of assays that identify specific antigens in systemic lupus erythematosus and other disorders may become useful in the future.[55] Several studies of rheumatic diseases and other disorders have reported a relationship between the concentration of circulating immune complexes and the severity of the disease. Positive correlations have been reported in patients with SLE, rheumatoid arthritis, certain leukemias, other cancers, Lyme arthritis, and other diseases.[2,49,50] Prospective studies demonstrating the usefulness of one or more tests for immune complexes in decisions concerning the clinical management of rheumatic or other diseases, however, have been lacking or inconclusive. Consequently, until more data become available from researchers, some groups have recommended only sparing and judicious use of tests for immune complexes in clinical diagnosis and management.[56] A clinician thoroughly familiar with the interpretation of these tests may find the assays for immune complexes useful as an adjunct to or in place of other tests (such as complement or complement component levels) in guiding therapeutic interventions. The indiscriminate use of these tests, however, should be discouraged.

REFERENCES

1. Haakenstad, A.O., and Mannik, M.: The biology of immune complexes. In Autoimmunity. Edited by N. Talal. New York, Academic Press, 1977, pp. 277–360.
2. Theofilopoulos, A.N., and Dixon, F.J.: The biology and detection of immune complexes. Adv. Immunol., 28:89–220, 1979.
3. Williams, R.C., Jr.: Immune Complexes in Clinical and Experimental Medicine. Cambridge, Harvard University Press, 1980.
4. Mannik, M.: Characteristics of immune complexes and principles of immune complex disease. In Arthritis and Allied Conditions, 9th Ed., Edited by D.J. McCarty. Philadelphia, Lea & Febiger, 1979, pp. 256–267.
5. Glynn, L.E., and Steward, M.W.: Immunochemistry: An Advanced Textbook. Chichester, John Wiley and Sons, 1977.
6. Atassi, M.Z., van Oss, C.J., and Absolom, D.R. (Eds.): Molecular Immunology. New York, Marcel Dekker, Inc., 1984.
7. Finbloom, D.S., et al.: The influence of antigen on immune complex behavior in mice. J. Clin. Invest., 68:214–224, 1981.
8. Emlen, W., and Mannik, M.: Clearance of circulating DNA-antiDNA immune complexes in mice. J. Exp. Med., 155:1210–1215, 1982.
9. Hornick, C.J., and Karush, F.: Antibody affinity. III. The role of multivalence. Immunochemistry, 9:325–340, 1972.
10. Papalian, M., et al.: Reaction of systemic lupus erythematosus antinative DNA antibodies with native DNA fragments from 20 to 1200 base pairs. J. Clin. Invest., 65:469–477, 1980.
11. Morgan, E.L., and Weigle, W.O.: Polyclonal activation of murine B lymphocytes by immune complexes. J. Immunol., 130:1066–1070, 1983.
12. Takahashi, M., et al.: Mechanisms of solubilization of immune aggregates by complement. Implication for immunopathology. Transplant Rev., 32:121–139, 1976
13. Schifferli, J.A., Woo, P., and Peters, D.K.: Complement-mediated inhibition of immune precipitation. I. Role of the classical and alternative pathways. Clin. Exp. Immunol., 47:555–562, 1982.
14. Schifferli, J.A., Ng, Y.C., and Peters, D.K.: The role of complement and its receptor in the elimination of immune complexes. N. Engl. J. Med., 315:488–495, 1986.
15. Dower, S.K., et al.: Mechanisms of binding of multivalent immune complexes to Fc receptors. 1. Equilibrium binding. Biochemistry, 20:6326–6334, 1981.
16. Kijlstra, A., van Es, L.A., and Daha, M.R.: The role of complement in the binding and degradation of immunoglobulin aggregates by macrophages. J. Immunol., 123:2488–2493, 1979.
17. Iida, K., Mornaghi, R., and Nussenzweig, V.: Complement receptor (CR₁) deficiency in erythrocytes from patients with systemic lupus erythematosus. J. Exp. Med., 155:1427–1438, 1982.
18. Wilson, J.G., et al.: Mode of inheritance of decreased C3b receptors on erythrocytes of patients with systemic lupus erythematosus. N. Engl. J. Med., 307:981–986, 1982.
19. Walport, M.J., et al.: Family studies of erythrocyte complement receptor type I levels: Reduced levels in patients with SLE are acquired, not inherited. Clin. Exp. Immunol., 59:547–554, 1985.
20. Yoshida, K., Yukiyama, Y., Hirose, S., and Miyamoto, T.: The change in C3b receptors on erythrocytes from patients with systemic lupus erythematosus. Clin. Exp. Immunol., 60:613–621, 1985.
21. Mannik, M.: Pathophysiology of circulating immune complexes. Arthritis Rheum., 25:783–787, 1982.
22. Jimenez, R.A.H., and Haakenstad, A.O., and Mannik, M.: Hepatic uptake of small-latticed immune complexes does not alter mononuclear phagocyte system function. Immunology, 48:205–210, 1983.
23. Kimberly, R.P., and Ralph, R.: Endocytosis by the mononuclear phagocyte system and autoimmune disease. Am. J. Med., 74:481–483, 1983.
24. Rifai, A., and Mannik, M.: Clearance kinetics and fate of mouse IgA immune complexes prepared with monomeric or dimeric IgA. J. Immunol., 130:1826–1832, 1983.
25. Rifai, A., and Mannik, M.: Clearance of circulating IgA immune complexes is mediated by a specific receptor on Kupffer cells in mice. J. Exp. Med., 160:125–137, 1984.
26. Crawford, J.P., Movat, H.Z., Ranadive, N.S., and Hay, J.B.: Pathways to inflammation induced by immune complexes: Development of the Arthus reaction. Fed. Proc., 41:2583–2587, 1982.
27. Claggett, J.A., Wilson, C.B., and Weigle, W.O.: Interstitial immune complex thyroiditis in mice. The role of autoantibody to thyroglobulin. J. Exp. Med., 140:1439–1456, 1974.
28. Mannik, M., and Gauthier, V.J.: Characteristics of circulating immune complexes that deposit in renal glomeruli. In Nephrology—Proceedings of the IXth International Congress of Nephrology. Edited by R.R. Robinson, et al. New York, Springer-Verlag, 1984, pp. 527–539.
29. Mannik, M., Agodoa, L.Y.C., and David, K.A.: Rearrangement of immune complexes in glomeruli leads to persistence and development of electron dense deposits. J. Exp. Med., 157:1516–1528, 1983.
30. Gauthier, V.J., Mannik, M., and Striker, G.E.: Effect of cationized antibodies in preformed immune complexes on deposition and persistence in renal glomeruli. J. Exp. Med., 156:766–777, 1982.
31. Vogt, A., et al.: Interaction of cationized antigen with rat glomerular basement membrane: In situ immune complex formation. Kidney Int., 22:27–35, 1982.
32. Gauthier, V.J., Striker, G.E., and Mannik, M.: Glomerular localization of immune complexes prepared with anionic antibodies or with cationic antigens. Lab. Invest., 50:636–644, 1984.
33. Gauthier, V.J., and Mannik, M.: Only the initial binding of cationic immune complexes to glomerular anionic sites is mediated by charge-charge interactions. J. Immunol., 136:3266–3271, 1986.

34. Kanwar, Y.S., Caulin-Glaser, T., Gallo, G.R., and Lamm, M.E.: Interaction of immune complexes with glomerular heparan sulfate-proteoglycans. Kidney Int., 30:842–851, 1986.

35. Couser, W.G., et al.: Mechanisms of immune complex formation and deposition in glomeruli. In Nephrology—Proceedings of the IXth International Congress of Nephrology. Edited by R.R. Robinson, et al. New York, Springer-Verlag, 1984, pp. 508–526.

36. Oite, T., et al.: Quantitative studies of in situ immune complex glomerulonephritis in the rat induced by planted, cationized antigen. J. Exp. Med., 155:460–474, 1982.

37. Border, W.A., et al.: Induction of membranous nephropathy in rabbits by administration of an exogenous cationic antigen: Demonstration of a pathogenic role for electrical charge. J. Clin. Invest., 69:451–461, 1982.

38. Gallo, G.R., et al.: Nephritogenicity and differential distribution of glomerular immune complexes related to immunogen charge. Lab. Invest., 48:353–362, 1983.

39. Agodoa, L.Y.C., Gauthier, V.J., and Mannik, M.: Precipitating antigen-antibody systems are required for the formation of subepithelial electron dense immune deposits in rat glomeruli. J. Exp. Med., 158:1259–1271, 1983.

40. Agodoa, L.Y.C., Gauthier, V.J., and Mannik, M.: Antibody localization in glomerular basement membrane may precede in situ immune deposit formation in rat glomeruli. J. Immunol., 134:880–884, 1985.

41. Camussi, G., et al.: Antibody-induced redistribution of Heymann antigen on the surface of cultured glomerular visceral epithelial cells: Possible role in the pathogenesis of Heymann glomerulonephritis. J. Immunol., 135:2409–2416, 1985.

42. Andres, G., et al.: Biology of disease: Formation of immune deposits and disease. Lab. Invest., 55:510–520, 1986.

43. Salant, D.J., et al.: A new role for complement in experimental membranous nephropathy in rats. J. Clin. Invest., 66:1339–1350, 1980.

44. Dixon, F.J., et al: Pathogenesis of serum sickness. A.M.A. Arch. Pathol., 65:18–28, 1958.

45. Cochrane, C.G.: Mediation of immunologic glomerular injury. Transplant. Proc., 1:949–958, 1969.

46. Holdsworth, S.R., Neale, T.J., and Wilson, C.B.: Abrogation of macrophage-dependent injury in experimental glomerulonephritis in the rabbit. Use of an antimacrophage serum. J. Clin. Invest., 68:686–698, 1981.

47. Germuth, F.G., Jr., and Rodriguez, E.: Immunopathology of the Renal Glomerulus. Boston, Little, Brown and Co., 1973.

48. Brentjens, J.R., et al.: Extra-glomerular lesions associated with deposition of circulating antigen-antibody complexes in kidneys of rabbits with chronic serum sickness. Clin. Immunol. Immunopathol., 3:112–126, 1974.

49. Zubler, R.H., and Lambert, P.H.: Detection of immune complexes in human diseases. Prog. Allergy, 24:1–48, 1978.

50. Agnello, V.: Immune complex assays in rheumatic diseases. Hum. Pathol., 14:343–349, 1983.

51. Wener, M.H., and Mannik, M.: Influence of immune complex lattice on the C1q solid phase assay as determined with covalently cross-linked immune complexes. Clin. Exp. Immunol., 52:543–550, 1983.

52. Uwatoko, S., et al.: Characterization of C1q-binding IgG complexes in systemic lupus erythematosus. Clin. Immunol. Immunopathol., 30:104–116, 1984.

53. Wener, M.H., Mannik, M., Schwartz, M.M. and Lewis, E.J.: Relationship between renal pathology and the size of circulating immune complexes in patients with systemic lupus erythematosus. Medicine, 66:85–97, 1987.

54. Pereira, A.B., Theofilopoulos, A.N., and Dixon, F.J.: Detection and partial characterization of circulating immune complexes with solid-phase anti-C3. J. Immunol., 125:763–770, 1980.

55. Maire, M.A., et al.: Identification of components of IC purified from human sera. I. Immune complexes purified from sera of patients with SLE. Clin. Exp. Immunol., 51:215–224, 1983.

56. Report of IUIS/WHO Working Group: Use and abuse of laboratory tests in clinical immunology: Critical considerations of eight widely used diagnostic procedures. Clin. Exp. Immunol., 46:662–674, 1981.

GENETIC STRUCTURE AND FUNCTIONS OF THE HUMAN MAJOR HISTO-COMPATIBILITY COMPLEX

28

GERALD T. NEPOM

The major histocompatibility complex (MHC) is a series of linked genes located on chromosome 6, which controls a number of key immunologic functions. Products of these genes elicit strong transplantation rejection reactions, which is the basis of the name "histocompatibility antigens." In addition, MHC gene products participate in the induction and regulation of immune responses. Known as the human leukocyte antigen (HLA) system, these MHC gene products play a fundamental role in immune recognition and response and are implicated in the genetic susceptibility of a number of rheumatoid diseases. HLA differences among different individuals lead to differing capacity for specific immune responses, so that the MHC gene complex contributes an important element of individual genetic variation.

An immune response is a complex process requiring multiple interactions and cellular events. The participation of MHC gene products is controlled by precise structural features of MHC genes themselves, and possibly also by mechanisms controlling their expression. The important structural and genetic features accounting for the genetic control of specific immune interactions are summarized here to illustrate how the structure and function of the MHC are inseparable. The high degree of variability among HLA genes is the hallmark of the MHC. Autoimmune and immune-mediated disease reactions depend on the same structural features of HLA genes and their products that interact in normal coordinated immune responses. The HLA system is "polymorphic" because many forms of distinct HLA genes and gene products

exist; these multiple forms have distinct functions in both histocompatibility and control of the immune response. Some of these polymorphisms directly account for individual variation in susceptibility to HLA-associated diseases.

The structure of human MHC genes and HLA molecules will be reviewed, emphasizing the diverse array of variable genes available for functional immune interactions. The mechanisms contributing to this structural polymorphism will be summarized and used to illustrate current methods to analyze the specific contribution of HLA genes to disease susceptibility.

THE GENE ORGANIZATION OF THE HUMAN MHC

The HLA system is located on the short arm of chromosome 6, approximately 15 centimorgans from the centromere. Genes of the HLA system cluster into three sets of structurally distinct regions: class I, class II, and class III (Fig. 28–1). These three regions are linked together within the HLA system, with the class II complex centromeric to the class I complex, and the class III complex juxtaposed between class I and class II genes. Each cluster contains numerous structurally and functionally interrelated genes. For clarity, we will consider each gene complex in order of its location on the chromosome.

FIG. 28–1. Genetic organization of the HLA complex. A portion of the short arm of chromosome 6 is illustrated, with the class II HLA genes (D region) and the class I HLA genes (HLA-A, B, C) flanking additional genes, encoding some complement components, known as the class III region. The DP region, most centromeric of the class II genes on chromosome 6, includes four loci. One of these loci encodes a functional β gene, known as DPβ; one encodes a functional α gene known as DPα. The dimer formed by the products of these two genes exists on the cell surface as the DP molecule. Other loci in the DP region encode β and α pseudogenes (i.e., apparently nonfunctional, vestigial, remnants of class II-related genes). Approximately 20,000 DNA nucleotides (20 kb, or kilobases) telomeric from the DP region lies the DZα gene. Little is known about the expression or function of DZα, and no class II protein product has been identified from this gene. Approximately 100 kb telomeric of DZα lies the DOβ gene. The DOβ gene has several structural characteristics distinguishing it from all other class II β genes, indicating that its origins probably represent some distant evolutionary event; its function is unknown. Approximately 20 kb telomeric of DOβ is the DQ region, consisting of four distinct loci. The DXβ and DXα loci are still mysterious as no known product of or function for these genes has yet been described. The DQβ gene locus is the structural gene for the DQβ polypeptide; the DQα locus encodes the structural gene for the DQα polypeptide. The HLA-DQ class II molecule on the cell surface consists of a dimer of the DQα and DQβ gene products. Approximately 40 kb telomeric of the DQ region is the DR region, which includes at least four loci. The DRβ$_1$ locus contains the structural gene for a DRβ polypeptide; the DRβ$_2$ locus appears to represent a pseudogene, in that it has lost much of the genetic material necessary to encode an intact protein. The DRβ$_3$ locus contains the structural gene for a second DRβ polypeptide, and the DRα locus contains the structural gene for the DRα polypeptide. The HLA-DR class II molecules expressed on cell surfaces consist of two types of dimer, in which the DRα polypeptide associates with either the DRβ$_1$ polypeptide or the DRβ$_3$ polypeptide.

Within the class I HLA region, the HLA-B, HLA-C, and HLA-A loci encode the structural proteins for the class I heavy chains which function as transplantation antigens. The class I molecules are expressed on the cell surface in association with β$_2$ microglobulin, a polypeptide encoded by a gene on another chromosome.

THE CLASS II GENE COMPLEX

The class II gene complex consists of at least 14 different genes. These genes exist as two distinct classes, called α (alpha) and β (beta), with six α and eight β genes currently recognized (see Fig. 28–1). The products of these genes form class II proteins (see below), which are cell surface dimers consisting of one α and one β chain noncovalently bound together. The genes of the class II complex are distributed in distinct clusters, with closely related genes within a cluster differing from genes in other clusters. These clusters are known by the designations DP, DQ, and DR, as established in 1984 by the World Health Organization (WHO) nomenclature committee on histocompatibility antigens. The DO and DZ genes represent distantly related class II genes which map outside the DP, DQ, or DR clusters.

HLA-DR molecules are expressed as dimers of products from a DRα and DRβ gene. In most individuals, two different DRβ genes on each chromosome are expressed, so that two types of αβ dimers can result. In addition, HLA-DQ molecules, derived from the DQα and DQβ genes, and HLA-DP molecules, from the DPα and DPβ genes, form two additional class II dimers. Other genes in the class II complex are of unknown function or are apparently not expressed (see Fig. 28–1).

THE CLASS III GENE COMPLEX

Genes of the class III complex are structurally unrelated to either the class I or class II genes but located within the HLA region. The class III complex consists of a rather heterogeneous set of genes, only some of which have been identified. The genes for complement factors C2, BF, C4A, and C4B are located within the class III complex. Structural genes for 21 hydroxylase are also located here, linked to the C4A and C4B genes. Recently, genes for tumor necrosis factor α and β have also been identified and provisionally mapped to the class III complex. Probably, additional analysis will identify many other genes in this region, but the significance of their location between HLA class II and HLA class I is unknown.

THE CLASS I GENE COMPLEX

As with the class II complex, HLA class I genes are arrayed in a complex set of interrelated regions. The total number of class I genes is not entirely known, and may vary among different ethnic lineages, but

The HLA Genetic Region
(Chromosome No.6)

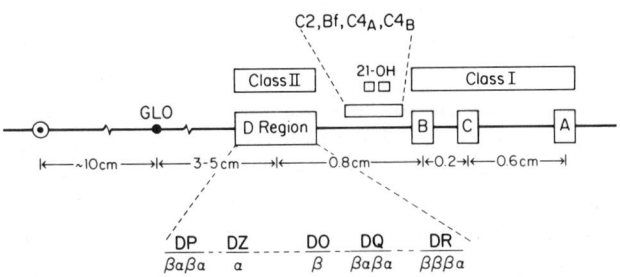

probably numbers around 20 or more. The HLA B, C, and A regions of the class I complex have been fairly well defined, with HLA B located closest to the class II and class III regions. Each of these three regions includes at least one functional locus encoding a class I polypeptide chain. The polypeptide class I product found on the cell surface is a dimer associated with a molecule called β_2 microglobulin, which is encoded by a gene found on a different chromosome.

The genetic structure of a single class I gene is compared to a single class II gene in Figure 28–2. The gene structure is marked by several characteristic features. A regulatory region precedes the structural gene itself. Specific DNA sequences within this regulatory region control the expression of the gene, regulating both basal levels and stimulated levels of transcription. The structural gene itself consists of a series of linked coding regions, called exons, separated by long stretches of noncoding DNA segments, called introns. The structural motif of similar repeating exons and introns in both class I and class II molecules is a feature shared not only by HLA molecules, but also by other molecules involved in immune recognition, including immunoglobulins and T-cell receptor genes. Class I genes contain one more "repeat unit" of an intron and an exon compared to the class II genes (see Fig. 28–2), which accounts for the larger size of class I proteins. The "tail" of each gene includes exons that encode the portion of the HLA molecule that spans the cell surface membrane and exons that encode the portion of the molecule anchored inside the cell (i.e., on the cytoplasmic side of the plasma membrane). Reported differences among different HLA genes in this "cytoplasmic tail" genetic region may be important for understanding the functional interaction of HLA molecules with specific cellular events.

STRUCTURE AND EXPRESSION OF HLA MOLECULES

CLASS II MOLECULES

Class II molecules, sometimes referred to as "Ia antigens," were first described in mice, where they were known as major histocompatibility complex I region associated or Ia antigens. The murine I region is homologous to the human class II region, hence the use of "Ia" as a synonym for class II molecules.

HLA class II molecules are glycoproteins composed of two chains, the α and β chains encoded by the class II α and β genes, respectively. Each chain consists of four "domains" with distinct functions; each domain is encoded by a specific exon (see Fig. 25–2). After translation, class II α and class II β molecules assort intracytoplasmically in concert with a third polypeptide called the *invariant chain*. During transport to the cell membrane of the $\alpha\beta$ dimer, the association with the invariant chain may be lost. The carboxy-terminal ends of both polypeptides remain intracytoplasmic, a hydrophobic portion of each passes through the plasma membrane, and the amino terminal ends including both extracellular domains are exposed to the environment, participating in recognition events and immune interactions.

Both the α and the β polypeptides are glycosylated. The β chain bears a single complex end-linked carbohydrate, attached to the protein at amino acid 19 in the first domain. Alpha (α) chains are also glycosylated, usually with two carbohydrates, one a complex N-linked sugar and one a high mannose structure. The role of the carbohydrate structures in immune recognition, if any, remains unclear.

Structural variation among the different class II gene products is the key to the functional differences in immune recognition which lead to histoincompatibility, immune recognition, and disease susceptibility. There are two types of structural variations. First, different class II regions are structurally dissimilar; thus, DP, DQ, and DR molecules, while related, diverge from each other by up to 30% in primary amino acid sequence. The second kind of structural variation is more subtle. Each of the class II genes exists in the population in different allelic forms (i.e., individual

FIG. 28–2. Structure of HLA genes and their polypeptide products. Schematic illustrations of the HLA genes are shown, emphasizing the similarities in overall structure of the class II β, class II α and class I genes. Each gene is composed of DNA with alternating exons (open boxes) separated by large intervening sequences (introns). Several of the exons encode the polypeptide structural domains of the HLA molecules themselves, as indicated by arrows. The structural domains of the HLA polypeptides, indicated by the loops, show considerable structural homology among the different members of these HLA molecular families.

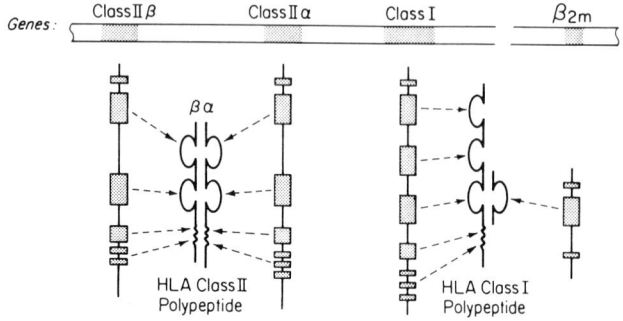

variation among particular class II genes is rampant in the outbred human population). The number of alleles at each of the expressed class II genes differs; there may be as few as two alleles for DRα, and as many as 50 to 80 alleles for DRβ, with allelic variation for DP and DQ somewhere in between.

Most of the variable sequences distinguishing one class II α gene from another, or one class II β gene from another, are clustered in the first domain of the polypeptide chain. As a consequence, the most polymorphic region is the most available for intercellular recognition. Specific "locus-specific" sequences characterize differences among DP, DQ, and DR molecules, and are located in both the first and second domains, as well as in some sequences around the carboxy-terminal. Sequences that differ among alleles of the same locus (e.g., among different DR molecules) cluster in three or four localized sites of variation within the first domain structure. By analogy with immunoglobulin structure, it appears that these regions of allelic "hypervariability" may be spatially oriented close to each other when the first domain folds into its native conformation. These sites of allelic variability probably create specific structural regions, or "epitopes," accounting for individual structural differences in immune recognition.

The class II molecules are expressed constitutively on B cells and monocytes. The levels of expression are inducible, being up-regulated by a number of mechanisms, including the lymphokine *gamma interferon*. Many other cell types, including T cells, melanoma cells, endothelial cells, and microglial cells, also are *inducible* for class II expression. The structural basis for this inducible quality appears to lie in the genetic control region located adjacent to each class II gene. Because each class II gene carries its own upstream regulatory region, different loci may be regulated differently. Support for this notion comes from the observation that interferon induces a greater increase in DQ than DR expression in monocytes. Also, many leukemic lines and possibly some normal cells express DR but not detectable levels of DQ, unless stimulated by an inducing agent. In addition to this locus-specific regulation of expression, there appears to be a more global class II regulation of expression (at least two case reports have been described in which individuals with immunodeficiency syndromes fail to express any class II molecules, even though class I expression is intact).

CLASS I MOLECULES

The class I gene products are glycoproteins located in the cell membrane noncovalently bound to a pep-

tide known as β_2 *microglobulin*. The HLA class I gene encodes a 44,000 mw glycoprotein heavy chain structure; the β_2 microglobulin gene encodes the 12,000 mw subunit on a separate chromosome.

The class I heavy chain structure consists of three extracellular domains, a transmembranous domain and a cytoplasmic domain. As with the class II molecule, each structural domain of the class I polypeptide is encoded in a specific exon (see Fig. 28–2). Allelic variation, accounting for differences in individual class I molecules, is concentrated in both the first and second domains. The roentgenographic crystallographic structure of a purified class I molecule has been reported. The amino acid residues of the first and second domains formed a series of parallel strands interconnected by short loops; these parallel strands appeared to form a "platform-like" structure presenting a broad surface available for potential extracellular interactions involved in immune recognition.

HLA POLYMORPHISMS

The structural variation among alleles for most of the class II loci is the mechanistic basis for the functional polymorphism of the MHC. This section will highlight three types of allelic variation to illustrate important mechanisms accounting for functional diversity attributed to specific HLA genes.

STRUCTURAL POLYMORPHISM DUE TO ALLELIC VARIATION

As mentioned above, the source of genetic diversity within the MHC is derived both from the multiple number of different HLA genes and from the high degree of allelic variability exhibited by most of these genes. There is a wide range of allelic differences among genes at the class II loci, such as $DR\beta_1$, from minimal changes, involving as few as one amino acid change, at one end of the spectrum, to very substantial changes, up to 25 to 30 amino acid differences, at the other. Although the exact number of alleles for the $DR\beta_1$ locus is not known, a reasonable estimate would be more than 50. In most cases described, these differences are sufficient to alter both allorecognition and immune reactivity. Of all the HLA class II loci, the $DR\beta_1$ locus exhibits the highest degree of this kind of allelic variation, attributable to localized amino acid variability. The number of recognized alleles at each of the class II loci will undoubtedly increase as analysis expands into diverse populations; currently the

DQα locus appears to encode at least seven alleles, the DQβ locus at least eight or nine alleles, and the DRβ₃ locus at least four alleles. The extent of allelic variation for the DP genes has not been well studied yet.

Allelic variation in class I genes is also primarily due to specific amino acid heterogeneity. The total number of alleles for the HLA, A, B, and C loci is not known; a reasonable estimate, however, would be that at least 40 or 50 alleles for HLA A and B exist as discrete structural and functional variants.

A second source of structural polymorphic variation, unique to the class II molecules, derives from the fact that the class II molecule is a dimer of an α gene product and a β gene product. *Recombination* events between the α gene and β gene rearrange the linkage between specific α and β alleles. Genetic rearrangement occurring between α and β genes generates novel genetic linkages resulting in new structural variants. For example, in Figure 28–3 three sets of alleles for the DQα and DQβ loci are shown. Line A illustrates the linkage between the DQβ 3.1 allele at the DQβ locus and the DQα .5+ DQα gene. This combination of α and β genes encodes a specific DQαβ dimer. Line B illustrates the linkage between a DQβ 3.2 gene and a DQα .5− DQα gene, a DQ gene pair frequently linked together resulting in the

expression of a different DQ dimer molecule. Recombination between the DQβ and DQα genes shown in Line A and Line B would result in a rearrangement of the linkage, such that the DQβ 3.1 allele could be found linked to the DQα .5− allele, as illustrated in Line C. This linkage does occur, resulting in the expression of a DQαβ dimer with structural and functional properties different from either of the dimers resulting from the genes illustrated in Lines A and B. Novel αβ dimers create new spatial conformations, or epitopes, consisting of structural portions contributed by both the α and the β chain. Thus, unique epitopes are formed by combinations of specific α and β genes. In this manner, recombination events generate new combinations of linked α and β genes, generating structural variation in expressed class II molecules.

A third type of structural diversity within the MHC, an intra-allelic recombination, generates polymorphic alleles. The best-studied example is the identification of three different related alleles of the HLA-A locus gene. Gene sequence analysis has identified a number of variable sequences in the A2 gene, which differ from the A28 gene. Sequence analysis of a third HLA-A allele, known as A69, indicates that this gene appears to be a hybrid allele, including a portion of the A2 gene with the remainder derived from the A28 gene. A probable explanation for the derivation of the A69 gene is that it represents an intragenic recombination event between two alleles, the A2 and A28 genes. This one example illustrates the extremely high degree of variability generated within genes of the MHC by recombination and mutation.

FIG. 28–3.   Recombination between linked class II genes generates diversity. The DQ genetic regions of three different haplotypes are illustrated. In the first haplotype, a linked DQβ and DQα gene generate a DQw3 positive DQ molecule, such as commonly found on haplotypes that type as DR5, DQw3. The second haplotype listed represents a different DQβ and a different DQα gene, commonly linked on haplotypes that type as DR4, DQw3. Although both DQ products type as DQw3, neither the β nor the α genes are the same in these two haplotypes. The third haplotype illustrated results from a recombination event between DQβ and DQα genes of the first two haplotypes. The resulting haplotype (3) carries a DQ3.1β gene linked to a DQα5⁻ gene, which results in a DQw3 positive molecule distinct from either of the first two haplotypes. This third haplotype is found in some individuals who type as DR4, DQw3.

EVOLUTION OF THE MHC

Allelic variation represents the genetic diversity produced by mutation and recombination, as described in the previous section. *Interlocus variation* represents additional genetic diversity which relies on another mechanism, namely gene duplication. Within a particular HLA region, such as HLA-DR, different β gene loci are more homologous to each other than they are to β gene loci in other regions. Thus, genes within a region appear to have duplicated, leading to the presence of multiple homologous loci within a single region. To trace the origins of the different regions within HLA, it is instructive to draw parallels with the evolution in other species. Interestingly, in mice, rats, rabbits, and humans, the basic organization of the MHC is remarkably similar. The basic pattern consists of multiple homologous class II genes clustered in discrete regions, separate from regions

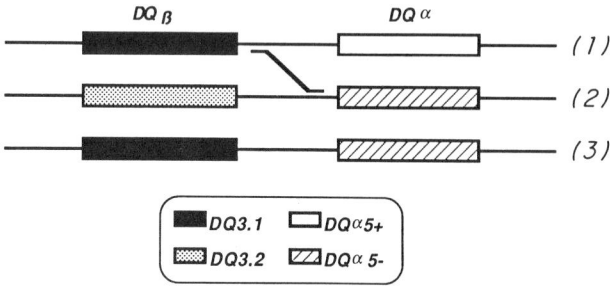

of class I genes. In some cases, such as the murine class I locus called H2K, the basic class I gene structure and function have remained intact, even though this gene has apparently moved on the chromosome centromeric of class II genes. The precise number of MHC genes varies among species, between 20 and 40 for the class I genes, for instance. Nevertheless, all class I genes studied appear to be related, indicating that an ancestral gene underwent a series of mutation, gene duplication, and recombination events. Viewed in this context, the process of selecting different functions for different MHC structural genes can be viewed as a process of *adaptive differentiation.* Although we know little about the selective pressures operating on MHC gene diversification, it is probable that the occurrence of "favorable" mutations and rearrangements led to the expression of the functional MHC genes whose gene products are an integral part of the immune response today. Conversely, nonessential MHC genes apparently accumulated mutations and rearrangements of no particular consequence and are recognizable in the genome as today's pseudogenes. In this context, the specific structural variation accounting for the function of a specific HLA gene can itself have diverse origins. In some cases, allelic variations resulting from mutation, and in other cases from gene recombination or rearrangements, directly correspond to the polymorphic features that determine HLA-associated immune function, HLA typing specificities, and HLA-associated disease susceptibility.

THE RELATIONSHIP BETWEEN STRUCTURE AND HLA TYPING

In 1984 the World Health Organization HLA nomenclature committee established a consensus nomenclature related to the known structural features of HLA genes and gene products and corresponding to the locus encoding a particular specificity. Thus, for instance, the HLA DR "types," such as DR1, DR2, DR3, . . . DRw14, represent specificities present on products of DR genes. Similarly, HLA-DQ specificities, DQw1, w2, and w3, are carried on products of DQ genes, and the same holds for HLA-DP, HLA-B, HLA-C, and HLA-A.

MULTIPLE ALLELES CARRY A SINGLE HLA TYPING SPECIFICITY

The serologically defined HLA specificities, HLA-A, B, C, DR, and DQ, correspond to epitopes, or

antibody recognition sites, on the HLA polypeptide chain itself. The structural basis for an HLA serologic typing reaction, then, is the presence of such a specific epitope on one of the HLA molecules being expressed.

In some cases, particular specificities have been mapped to specific loci. For instance, some of the HLA-DR specificities, such as HLA-DR3, HLA-DR4, and HLA-DR5, are carried on products of the DRβ_1 locus. HLA DQw3, similarly, is carried on products of the DQβ locus. In many cases, however, single locus assignments for HLA specificities are inadequate. For instance, the HLA DRw52 and w53 specificities appear to be encoded by the HLA DRβ_3 gene, but in some cases they may also occur on products of the HLA DRβ_1 gene. The HLA DQw1 specificity is another example which, although serologically allelic to DQw2 and w3, may actually require the expression of a particular DQα gene in order to type as DQw1.

A single typing specificity, such as DR2, DR4, or DR8, is found on multiple different HLA molecules. For instance, six different alleles at the DRβ_1 locus all encode different polypeptide chains sharing a DR4+ serologic epitope. *Thus, individuals carrying any of these six different genes all type as HLA-DR4.* Although there are over 50 alleles at DRβ_1, there are only 14 recognized DR typing specificities at this locus. The HLA serologic typing designation therefore is a *public serologic specificity* present on multiple different alleles.

An analogous situation exists for other HLA loci. The best-studied examples for class I genes relate to HLA-A2 and HLA-B27, which are both public serologic specificities present on multiple distinct allelic variants at the HLA-A and HLA-B loci, respectively. At least six different B27+ alleles and a similar number of A2+ alleles have been described, which differ from each other by scattered amino acid substitutions in the first and second domains. Different alleles with the same typing specificity are related by virtue of sharing the same epitope recognized by alloantisera, either anti-B27 or anti-A2 in these examples.

THE SEROLOGIC DEFINITION OF HLA SPECIFICITIES

HLA-A, HLA-B, HLA-C, HLA-DR, and HLA-DQ specificities are routinely typed by using maternal antisera. Leakage of fetal lymphocytes into the maternal circulation is sufficient to enable approximately 30% of women to develop a significant titer of anti-HLA antibodies in the weeks immediately following delivery. Thus, maternal antiserum may contain antibodies directed against specific HLA antigenic determinants present on fetal cells coming from the paternal haplotype. These antisera react with the lymphocytes of the fetus, of the father, and of anyone else in the population who shares these determinants. The maternal antisera, therefore, are used to identify the presence of these specificities in unrelated individuals. Extensive analysis over the last two decades has identified a number of consistent specificities frequently recognized by such maternal sera when tested on a large panel of normal donor lymphocytes. Specificities which segregate in the population in an allelic fashion have been assigned for each of the HLA loci. Twenty-three such specificities have been identified on products of the HLA-A locus; 49 on products of the HLA-B locus; 8 on products of the HLA-C locus; 14 on products of the $DR\beta_1$ locus; 2 on products of the $DR\beta_3$ locus; and 3 on products of the DQ loci. As emphasized above, these specificities represent antigenic epitopes on the HLA molecules which may occur on several different allelic products so that *there are actually far more structural alleles at each of these loci than the recognized specificities.* The serologically defined antigenic specificities have been assigned numbers as summarized in Table 28–1.

Because the recognized HLA serologic specificities are defined by maternal antisera, they represent the recognition of alloantigenic epitopes on HLA molecules. Recent advances in monoclonal antibody technology have expanded our understanding of epitope recognition on HLA molecules. Numerous monoclonal antibodies against HLA molecules have been produced, usually derived from mouse or rat species. Therefore, the epitopes recognized by such monoclonal antibodies represent xeno-epitopes, as opposed to the allo-epitopes defined by conventional typing antisera. HLA epitopes defined by monoclonal antibodies fall into three main clusters. First, some xeno-epitopes mimic allo-epitopes; that is, the specificity defined by a monoclonal antibody parallels the specificity defined by a multiparous antisera, and therefore matches a recognized HLA specificity. Second, some monoclonal antibodies recognize "private" epitopes which distinguish among different molecules sharing the same typing specificity; for instance, DQw3 is a public serologic specificity present on products of the $DQ\beta$ locus. At least three alleles at this locus carry the DQw3 allospecificity. Murine monoclonal antibodies have been described which recognize only one of these DQw3+ alleles. This serologic specficity is a xeno-epitope present on one of the DQw3+ alleles called DQw3.1, but not the others. Such a monoclonal antibody provides a serologic typing specificity more accurate for detailed HLA analysis than conventional maternal alloantisera. A third type of xeno-epitope is characterized by monoclonal antibodies to HLA molecules recognizing several different alleles which carry different allospecificities. For example, the $DQ\alpha5$ epitope is defined by a monoclonal antibody reacting with specific alleles of the $DQ\alpha$ locus. The product of this $DQ\alpha$ locus is expressed in a class II dimer in association with different $DQ\beta$ chains; some of these dimers carry the allospecificities recognized as DQw2, and others the specificities recognized as DQw3. Both types of DQ dimers, however, also carry the $DQ\alpha5$ xenospecificity. Monoclonal antibodies are therefore proving very useful as tools for the recognition of epitope variation not recognized by conventional HLA typing reagents.

THE CELLULAR DEFINITION OF HLA SPECIFICITIES

In addition to the HLA nomenclature defined by serologic reactivity described above, a useful nomenclature based on T-cell allorecognition has also been developed. The HLA class II complex is a primary stimulant for T-cell proliferation based on allorecognition. Differences in expressed class II molecules can be recognized by monitoring proliferation of lymphocytes from unrelated individuals mixed together in in vitro culture, called the *mixed lymphocyte reaction (MLR).*

The major stimulating epitopes in a primary MLR are found on the products of the $DR\beta_1$ locus. Therefore, when cells of unrelated individuals are mixed together and proliferation is measured, reactivity correlates with allelic differences at the $DR\beta_1$ locus. Because the serologic specificities carried on products of the $DR\beta_1$ locus are the DR specificities, the proliferative response, known by the name HLA-D, correlates reasonably well with the HLA-DR designations. There are 19 recognized primary stimulating specificities in MLR, known as the HLA-D antigenic series. The nomenclatures of the HLA-D specificities and the HLA-DR specificities is partially, although not wholly, analogous; thus, most DR1+ individuals type as Dw1, most DR3+ individuals type as Dw3, and so on. However, there are some important exceptions. For example, as described above, HLA-DR4 is a broad, public serologic specificity present on at least six different allelic products of the $DR\beta_1$ locus. Each of these different allelic variants, although identical for the DR serologic specificity DR4, differ in MLR reactivity, and therefore differ for HLA-D. Thus, the Dw4, Dw10, Dw13, Dw14, and Dw15 specificities all represent T-cell recognition allo-epitopes carried on different DR4+ alleles.

Table 28–1. The HLA Specificities

HLA A	B	C	[D]	DR	DQ	DP
A1	B5	Cw1	Dw1	DR1	DQw1	DPw1
A2	B7	Cw2	Dw2	DR2	DQw2	DPw2
A3	B8	Cw3	Dw3	DR3	DQw3	DPw3
A9	B12	Cw4	Dw4	DR4		DPw4
A10	B13	Cw5	Dw5	DR5		DPw5
A11	B14	Cw6	Dw6	DRw6		DPw6
Aw19	B15	Cw7	Dw7	DR7		
A23(9)	B16	Cw8	Dw8	DRw8		
A24(9)	B17		Dw9	DRw9		
A25(10)	B18		Dw10	DRw10		
A26(10)	B21		Dw11(w7)	DRw11(5)		
A28	Bw22		Dw12	DRw12(5)		
A29(w19)	B27		Dw13	DRw13(w6)		
A30(w19)	B35		Dw14	DRw14(w6)		
A31(w19)	B37		Dw15			
A32(w19)	B38(16)		Dw16	DRw52		
Aw33(w19)	B39(16)		Dw17(w7)	DRw53		
Aw34(10)	B40		Dw18(w6)			
Aw36	Bw41		Dw19(w6)			
Aw43	Bw42					
Aw66(10)	B44(12)					
Aw68(28)	B45(12)					
Aw69(28)	Bw46					
	Bw47					
	Bw48					
	B49(21)					
	Bw50(21)					
	B51(5)					
	Bw52(5)					
	Bw53					
	Bw54(w22)					
	Bw55(w22)					
	Bw56(w22)					
	Bw57(17)					
	Bw58(17)					
	Bw59					
	Bw60(40)					
	Bw61(40)					
	Bw62(15)					
	Bw63(15)					
	Bw64(14)					
	Bw65(14)					
	Bw67					
	Bw70					
	Bw71(w70)					
	Bw72(w70)					
	Bw73					
	Bw4					
	Bw6					

The definition of HLA-D specificities is not solely a function of the DRβ₁ locus. Differences at the HLA-DQ locus also contribute to allorecognition in MLR, especially between individuals with identical DRβ₁ alleles, but different DQ alleles. One example of this is illustrated by the MLR between cells that are DR7, DQw2, and cells that are DR7, DQw3. These two haplotypes are mutually alloreactive and distinguish the specificities whose D types are known as Dw11 and Dw17, although both carry the same DRβ₁ gene. *In effect, the HLA-D designations represent a separate nomenclature for a composite of HLA-DR and DQ allo-epitope recognition.* A schematic representation of the relationship among HLA-D, DR, and DQ is illustrated in Figure 28–4.

Another set of allo-epitopes recognized by T-cells

FIG. 28–4. The relationship between HLA-D and the HLA-DR and DQ class II specificities. Different linkages between DQ genes and DR genes result in the generation of distinct haplotypes. Five families of DQ specificities are listed, along with nine families of DR specificities. The HLA-D specificities are derived from a nomenclature based on stimulation of T-cell alloreactivity in mixed lymphocyte culture. The HLA-Dw1 through Dw19 specificities represent T-cell recognition patterns resulting from diverse class II molecule expression. This figure illustrates the usual DQ and DR specificities found associated with each of the major HLA-D types.

	DQw1	DQw2	DQw3.1	DQw3.2	DQ "X"
DR1	Dw1				
DR2	Dw2, Dw12				
DR3			Dw3		Dw "X"
DR4			Dw4	Dw4 Dw14 Dw10	Dw15
DR5(w11)			Dw5		
DR6(w13)	Dw18, 19				
DR6(w14)	Dw9		Dw16		
DR7		Dw17		Dw11	
DR8	Dw8.3		Dw8.2		Dw8.1
DR9				Dw "DB5"	

have been used to define a series of allelic specificities at the HLA-DP locus. Products of the HLA-DP genes are usually found in lower concentrations on lymphocyte cell surfaces compared to DR, and are much weaker in stimulating alloresponses in mixed lymphocyte culture. Nevertheless, secondary mixed lymphocyte cultures, in which sensitized T-cells are restimulated, generate a proliferative response sufficient to define a series of allo-epitopes encoded by DP genes. At least six such specificities have been described (see Table 28–1). Because the DP molecules are very weak stimulators of allorecognition, no consistent serologic characterization of these alleles has yet been described. As noted above, structural analysis indicates a multiplicity of alleles for the DP loci; therefore, it is probable that numerous other specificities for the DP products remain to be defined.

LINKAGE

The HLA complex is a series of linked genes, with each locus potentially found in many allelic forms in the population. One important feature of the complex is that particular alleles at one locus are frequently found linked to particular alleles at an adjacent locus.

For instance, DR5+ DRβ₁ genes are usually found on the same haplotype with DQw3.1+ DQβ genes. Similarly, HLA-B8 is found more often on the same haplotype with HLA-DR3 than it is with any of the other DR specificities. This phenomenon, termed *linkage disequilibrium,* indicates that the assortment of allelic specificities at different HLA loci is not random with respect to each other. This has important ramifications for population studies based on analysis of HLA genes. For instance, a disease associated with HLA-B8 in the population may actually be due to HLA-DR3, which is co-expressed and in linkage with B8, or to any other gene located between the HLA-B and the HLA-DR loci on the B8, DR3+ haplotype.

THE FUNCTION OF HLA MOLECULES

The structural features of HLA molecules directly relate to their function in immune response. In particular, the structural polymorphisms leading to allelic variation are responsible for the diversity of immune recognition within the population, different susceptibility to HLA-associated diseases, and to alloreactivity (transplantation rejection). The mechanism by which HLA molecules mediate these functions is triggered by recognition events designed to detect foreign molecules and result in immune recognition and activation.

REGULATION OF IMMUNE RESPONSE

Foreign antigens are recognized by the immune system in association with HLA molecules. This immune recognition, one of the earliest events in the induction of an immune response, is mediated by receptors on T cells which have a dual specificity. The T-cell receptor recognizes both the HLA molecule and the foreign antigen, apparently simultaneously and as part of a macromolecular complex involving not only the T-cell receptor molecule, the antigen, and the HLA molecule, but possibly other "accessory" molecules present on the T-cell surface. In this immune recognition event, the HLA molecule plays the role of a permissive signal, a "green light" in the pathway leading to T-cell activation, amplification, and effector function. In this early immune recognition process, the HLA molecules appear to physically associate with foreign antigens. Experimental data are most consistent with a model in which antigen-presenting cells in peripheral tissues, lymph nodes, spleen, and other lymphatics (macrophages, monocytes, and related cells) partially degrade and process foreign antigens, and "present" them to T cells. This antigen presentation function uses class II molecules to trigger and activate T cells with the appropriate specific receptor.

This recognition of HLA molecules together with antigen confers specificity, or "restriction," of immune responses for antigen in association with self-MHC products in early immune activation. Secondary immune recognition and effector responses by antigen-specific T cells are also MHC restricted. For example, cytotoxic or killer T-lymphocytes, which are responsible for direct cell-mediated cytotoxicity, recognize and kill their target only when the foreign antigen is expressed on cell surfaces in association with MHC products, usually class I molecules. Similarly, the activity of helper T-lymphocytes is restricted by the requirement for recognizing antigen only if it is present on a cell surface in association with the particular allelic specificity of the HLA molecule active in the initial immunization, usually a class II molecule. Thus, *MHC restriction of immune reactivity occurs both at the level of sensitization of cells against foreign antigens and at the level of cytotoxic T effector cells against viruses and chemical-modifying agents.*

The genetic control of this immune restriction function lies in the same structural features of the HLA molecules forming the basis for allelic variability. Thus, an individual's T cells sensitized in the context of one particular HLA allele can be restimulated and can function against that antigen subsequently only in the presence of the same specific allele. For example, virus-specific cytotoxic T-lymphocytes derived from an A2 + individual can lyse virus-infected cells from other A2 individuals with the same allele, but not lyse virus-infected cells from other individuals with different HLA-A alleles. Similarly, activation of T helper cells derived from an HLA-Dw14 individual, which proliferate in response to a bacterial antigen, can be stimulated by Dw14 + cells but not by the closely related Dw4 + cells. These types of studies indicate that the T-cell receptor is capable of extremely specific recognition, not only of the antigen but of the associated HLA molecule. *The epitope on the HLA molecule recognized by the T-cell receptor does not necessarily coincide with the allo-epitopes recognized by alloantisera used for HLA typing.* Thus, HLA restriction specificities do not necessarily parallel HLA typing specificities.

ALLOREACTIVITY

When tissues are transplanted between HLA-incompatible individuals, destruction of the transplanted tissue by the immune system generally oc-

curs. Graft rejection appears to be due to the same normal physiologic mechanisms the immune system musters to attack other foreign antigens. Sensitization of the immune system occurs as a result of recognition of foreign antigens on the graft tissue. Foreign HLA antigens are particularly potent sensitizers of immune recognition. Just as with antigen presentation, allogeneic HLA molecules are recognized by T-cell receptors from T helper and cytolytic T cells in a progressive response leading from initial antigen sensitization to amplification and effector response, including the formation of "memory" cells capable of rapidly rejecting a second transplant from a donor of the same histocompatibility type.

The mechanism for allorecognition by T cells is thought to parallel the recognition of nominal antigen in the context of self-HLA molecules. In other words, the precise structural features responsible for allelic variability between transplant donor and recipient are themselves viewed by the recipient T cells as if they represented a foreign antigen. In some cases, in fact, it has been possible to demonstrate that a single T-cell clone is capable of recognizing the combination of antigen with self-MHC as well as allo-MHC, using the same receptor. Both class I and class II allelic differences are sufficient to stimulate alloreactivity in transplant rejection reactions.

DISEASE SUSCEPTIBILITY

A number of rheumatic diseases are strongly associated with particular HLA specificities (see Chapter 29), for example with rheumatoid arthritis HLA-DR4 and with ankylosing spondylitis and Reiter's disease HLA-B27. Recent advances in understanding the structure and genetic organization of the HLA system, as summarized above, have provided new methods and approaches toward understanding the genetic basis of such disease susceptibility. Molecular techniques used to probe genetic susceptibility of the various forms of arthritis and allied rheumatic conditions are based on the concept that structural polymorphisms directly control and correlate with functional mechanisms of immune activation. Detailed analysis of structural variation in those HLA genes associated with particular diseases, therefore, revolves around the notion that immune activation in HLA-associated rheumatic diseases is triggered by specific recognition events involving HLA molecules.

The techniques used for analysis of HLA-associated diseases rely on an understanding of HLA genomic structure. Analysis of specific individual loci, and of specific allelic variants encoded in each loci, permits the detailed genetic mapping of disease susceptibility genes. For the reasons cited above, namely that typing specificities do not discriminate among subtle allelic polymorphisms, more structural approaches are now being used.

Specific allelic variation can be studied in terms of epitope expression, primary protein structure, and primary DNA structure. These approaches are illustrated by the analysis of the association between seropositive rheumatoid arthritis and the DR4 specificity. As described above, the DR4 specificity itself is a broad public serologic specificity recognizing an epitope shared by several different structural alleles of the DRβ₁ locus. Furthermore, the HLA-DR4 specificity is linked in Caucasian haplotypes to the DQw3 specificity carried on multiple different alleles of the DQβ₁ locus. Therefore, many different haplotypes, consisting of different arrays of linked DR and DQ genes, all represent different combinations of HLA genes indistinguishable by conventional HLA typing because all type as HLA-DR4 and DQw3. Several of these haplotypes are diagrammed in Table 28–2. Viewed in this context, it is clear that the association of HLA-DR4 with rheumatoid arthritis may, in fact, be due to any of these genes. Also, because other diseases, such as pemphigus vulgaris and type I diabetes (insulin-dependent diabetes mellitus) (IDDM) are also associated with HLA-DR4, it is apparent from Table 28–2 that different genes potentially account for the HLA predisposition in these diseases, even though each is associated with the DR4 specificity by conventional HLA typing.

Techniques designed to identify specific allelic variation distinguish among the genes and gene products expressed by the different DR4+ haplotypes. At the level of the expressed class II molecules, murine monoclonal antibodies can distinguish the DQ3.1 from the DQ3.2 DQβ molecules. Although no monoclonal antibodies have yet been described that can distinguish between the DRβ₁ alleles associated with DR4, T-cell clones have been derived that will recognize some, but not all, DR4+ DRβ₁ alleles. In addition to these

epitope-specific approaches, two direct structural approaches are currently in widespread use. First, the polypeptide gene products can be distinguished on the basis of electrophoretic mobility in isoelectric focusing. Therefore, two-dimensional gel electrophoresis analysis, supplemented by peptide mapping analysis, will distinguish specific allelic variants based on amino acid substitutions. Second, for direct genomic analysis, "Southern blotting" is used to distinguish between homologous genes with differing nucleotide sequences. *Southern blotting* involves the use of *specific restriction endonucleases,* enzymes that cleave DNA when characteristic DNA nucleotide sequences are recognized. When alleles differ in the region of these specific recognition sequences, they will differ also in their ability to be cut by a specific restriction endonuclease. These differences can be visualized by DNA gel electrophoresis, in which DNA fragments of various sizes are readily distinguished. A radioactive (or otherwise labeled) probe homologous to a particular HLA gene sequence is used to anneal to the test DNA to identify individual genes. An example of such hybridization analysis for the HLA-DQ genes is shown in Figure 28–5. The distinct DNA fragments carrying the HLA-DQ gene are evident, as are the different DNA fragment lengths for the DQ3.1 and DQ3.2 alleles after restriction endonuclease digestion. This *restriction fragment length polymorphism* (RFLP) is therefore a useful genomic marker to identify allelic variation among gene products that carry the same typing specificity, in this case DQw3.

The major limitation of RFLP is that DNA sequence variations distinguishing different alleles may not always correspond to differences recognized by a particular restriction enzyme. Therefore, this technique is not completely specific for identifying allelic variants. A more specific and accurate technique is the use of sequence-specific oligonucleotide probes to detect an individual gene of interest. Such probes are constructed based on the precise known DNA sequence which varies between closely related genes at the same locus. In some cases, these probes may differ by only a single nucleotide. Identification of individual HLA genes using such probes is based on manipulation of the hybridization conditions between the probe and the test DNA so that only an exact complementary base homology yields a positive hybridization signal. An example is shown in Figure 28–5,*B*, in which a sequence-specific oligonucleotide probe for the DQw3.2 gene has been used to precisely identify individual genes. The use of such probes takes advantage of the specific genetic information which, in functional terms, translates into the polymorphism contributing directly to immune recognition.

Table 28–2. Allelic Variation Among Some DR4+ Haplotypes Associated with Autoimmune Diseases

HLA-DQ		HLA-DR		Autoimmune
Gene	Specificity	Gene	Specificity	Disease Association*
DQ3.1	(DQw3)	Dw4	(DR4)	RA
DQ3.2	(DQw3)	Dw4	(DR4)	RA, IDDM
DQ3.2	(DQw3)	Dw14	(DR4)	RA, IDDM
DQ3.2	(DQw3)	Dw10	(DR4)	IDDM, PV

*RA, rheumatoid arthritis; IDDM, insulin-dependent diabetes mellitus; PV, pemphigus vulgaris

FIG. 28–5. The use of specific DNA probes to distinguish among HLA genes is illustrated. *A*, Genomic DNA from a variety of different individuals has been digested with a restriction endonuclease and electrophoresed in agar gels to separate DNA fragments based on size. Subsequently, a radioactive probe to the DQβ gene has been added. Hybridization between this probe and the DQβ gene results in a dark band, representing the DNA fragment containing the DQβ gene. Such hybridization analysis discriminates among different DQβ alleles. *B*, The same DNA samples have been hybridized to a different DNA probe which hybridizes only to the DQ3.2 sequence. Such methods provide a rapid and definitive identification of individual allelic variants.

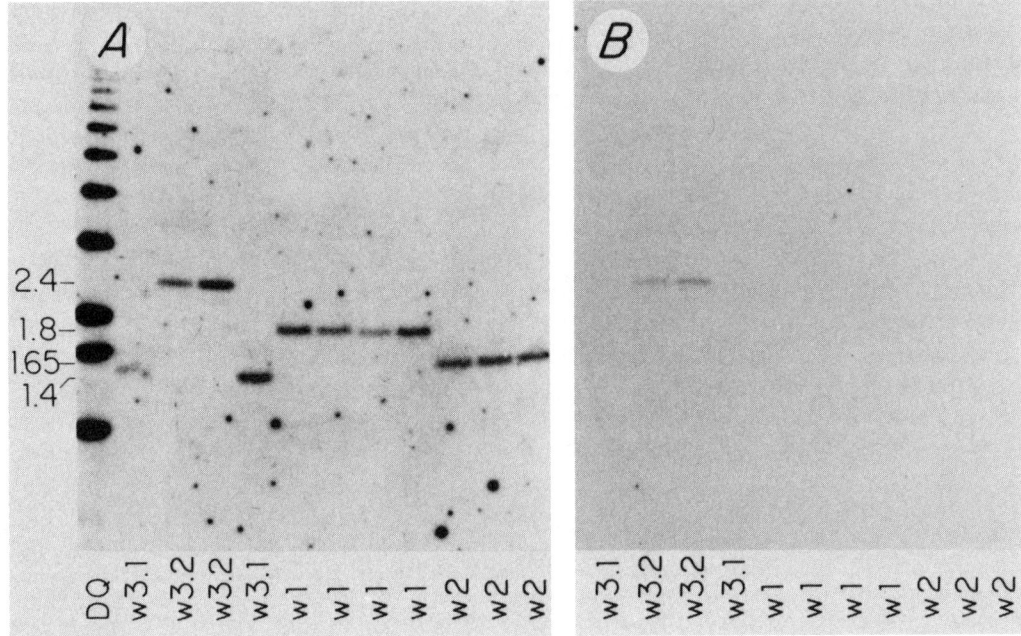

Recent studies have used such gene-specific probes, Southern blots, and two-dimensional gel analysis to clarify and identify precise associations between HLA genes and some diseases. In DR4-associated rheumatoid arthritis, the Dw4 and Dw14 alleles at the $DR\beta_1$ locus are highly associated with disease and appear to account for the association of the HLA DR4 specificity with this disease. In contrast, the DQw3.2 allele at the $DQ\beta_1$ locus appears to account for the association of HLA DR4 with type I diabetes. Thus, although both of these diseases are associated with the same HLA typing specificity, DR4, their genetic susceptibility is conferred by distinct genes (see Table 28–2). Some DR4+ haplotypes, such as those typing as Dw4, DQw3.1, are associated with rheumatoid arthritis but not with IDDM. Others, such as Dw4, DQw3.2, are associated with both rheumatoid arthritis and IDDM and probably account for sporadic reports of segregation of these two diseases together.

The identification of a specific HLA variant does not invariably predict disease outcome, although spe-cific genomic variants within HLA class II genes are highly correlated with disease expression (i.e., not all individuals with a particular susceptibility allele develop the disease). Two current models address this issue. On the one hand, it is possible that the identification of specific allelic variants highly associated with a particular disease merely reflects close genetic linkage with the actual genetic controlling element. In this model, the HLA allele is a marker gene, which may not have a direct role in the disease process. This model predicts that additional closely linked genes will be identified which more directly associate with disease. An alternative model postulates that the associated allelic variants are themselves the direct mechanistic link between HLA and the disease. But in this model other genetic or environmental factors are needed to "trigger" the required immune recognition events using the associated HLA gene product. In this scenario, the HLA susceptibility gene functions as a permissive element, not sufficient by itself for disease expression.

It is probable that examples of HLA-associated diseases that meet each of these alternative models will be identified. In most cases, resolution of the issue will require, for each particular disease, the precise genetic analysis of the associated allele and its flanking genes. In the examples cited above, in which the association of DR4 with rheumatoid arthritis maps to the $DR\beta_1$ locus, and the association of DR4 with IDDM maps to the $DQ\beta$ locus, some additional genomic analysis has been performed suggesting that specific allelic variants at these loci are themselves directly responsible for the HLA disease associations. Thus, in these two diseases, the function of the HLA gene itself appears to be as a permissive element in the aberrant immune response, accounting for the expression of the disease susceptibility trait.

GENERAL REFERENCES

1. Albert, E., Baur, M., and Mayr, W. (eds.): Histocompatibility Testing 1984. Berlin, Springer-Verlag, 1984.
2. Tiwari, J., and Terasaki, P.: HLA and Disease Associations. New York, Springer-Verlag, 1985.
3. Kaufman, J. et al.: The class II molecules of the human and murine major histocompatibility complex. Cell, 36:1–13, 1984.
4. Nepom, G.T.: Immunogenetics of HLA associated diseases. In Concepts in Immunopathology, Vol. 5. Edited by J. Cruse. Basel, Karger, 1987.

29

IMMUNOGENETICS AND RHEUMATIC DISEASES

FRANK C. ARNETT

A multitude of rheumatic diseases, particularly those believed to arise from disordered immunoregulation, have recently been associated with HLA antigens encoded by genes from within the major histocompatibility complex (MHC). Nosologic concepts of disease entitities and clusters, previously justified on clinical and serologic grounds, have been strengthened by commonalities and differences in HLA correlations. Equally important are the clues to pathogenesis underlying these rapidly evolving observations. Precise localization of the responsible genes and determination of their biologic functions in health and disease are currently areas of intense and fruitful investigation (see Chapter 28).

HLA AND THE SPONDYLITIC DISORDERS

Genetic predisposition to this family of diseases clusters around HLA-B, especially with the B27 antigen marker (Fig. 29–1). Each clinical disorder, however, demonstrates unique HLA correlations.

Ankylosing Spondylitis (AS). About 90% of Caucasian patients possess HLA-B27 compared to 6 to 8% of the general population in the United States and Europe (relative risk = 100 to 150).[1,2] Black Americans, whose B27 frequency is only 2 to 3%, develop the disease less often and also show a weaker B27 association of only 48 to 60%.[3] The prevalence of AS generally parallels the B27 antigen frequency in different populations, both being notably low in African blacks and Japanese and high in certain American Indians, especially the Haida, Pima, and Chippewa.[4] Among random B27-positive individuals and B27-positive relatives of normal probands with B27, the risk of AS is only 2%; however, B27-positive relatives of AS probands carry a 25% risk of disease.[5,6]

Multiple cases of AS in families almost invariably segregate with B27 unless there are members with psoriatic arthritis or inflammatory bowel disease.[2,7] Homozygosity for the antigen may promote more severe disease in terms of peripheral arthritis and uveitis.[8] HLA-B27-negative patients rarely have uveitis or cardiac involvement,[1,9] and B27 is less frequent (50 to 70%) in isolated sacroiliitis, perhaps a milder form of disease.[10,11] An excess of B7 cross-reacting antigens (the B7-Creg) and the psoriatic-associated specifici-

FIG. 29–1. HLA chromosomal region disease associations.

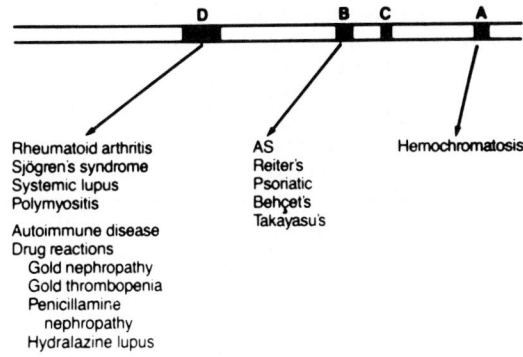

453

ties, Bw38 and Bw39, occur in B27-negative patients[9,10] (Table 29–1).

Reiter's Syndrome. HLA-B27 is found in 63 to 76% of patients with either postdysenteric or postvenereal Reiter's syndrome.[12,13] *Forme frustes*, such as incomplete Reiter's syndrome, isolated circinate balanitis, uveitis, heart block, keratodermia (pustular psoriasis), and dactylitis have also been associated with this antigen.[14] B27-negative patients rarely develop sacroiliitis or uveitis and generally pursue a milder course.[12–14]

A 20% disease risk for reactive arthritis has been calculated for B27-positive individuals who acquire one of the inciting enteric pathogens (*Shigella, Salmonella, or Yersinia*) or nongonococcal urethritis.[2,4,14] Family studies show that 10 to 12% of patients' relatives will also have arthritis, usually peripheral, which segregates with B27.[2,7] In fact, Reiter's syndrome and AS each tend to "breed true" within families and certain populations.[7,15] High prevalences have been found in Navajo Indians and the Inuit.[16,17]

Psoriatic Arthritis. Neither psoriasis vulgaris nor peripheral psoriatic arthritis is associated with HLA-B27.[2,4] Instead, psoriasis shows an excess of HLA-B17, B13, B37, Cw6, and DR7.[18,19] Psoriatic arthritis, moreover, is further associated with Bw38 and Bw39 (both formerly Bw16).[18,20,21] Disease susceptibility appears to lie closer to HLA-B or -C loci, especially Cw6,[19] than to DR. HLA-B27 is increased only in psoriatic spondylitis occurring in 40 to 50%.[4,18,20,21] HLA-Bw38 and Bw39 may also promote axial involvement.

Enteropathic Arthritis. The inflammatory bowel diseases (IBD), ulcerative colitis, and Crohn's disease, as well as their complicating peripheral arthritides, show no HLA correlations.[4] Enteropathic spondylitis, however, is associated with HLA-B27 in 30 to 50% of cases.[4,22] Family studies suggest than non-HLA linked genes that predispose to IBD may also confer suscep-

tibility to axial arthropathy even in the absence of expression of the bowel lesion.[22]

HLA-B27: PRIMARY OR LINKED GENE

It is unclear whether the B27 molecule itself confers disease susceptibility, serves as a marker for another closely linked gene, or does both. Evidence favoring a direct role for B27 includes the following: (1) the high relative risk (100 to 150) associated with B27;[1,2] (2) the fact that the correlation of B27 with spondyloarthropathies crosses geographic and ethnic barriers;[2,4] (3) the lack of stronger associations at HLA-A,C,D or the class III complement loci;[23] and (4) the apparent excess of B7 cross-reactive (CREG) antigens in B27-negative patients.[9,10] Moreover, the differential risks conferred by B27 haplotypes in relatives of AS patients (25%) versus random B27-positives (2%),[5,6] as well as the clinical differences between AS and Reiter's syndrome and their tendency to "breed true" in families,[7,15] suggest structural diversity in B27 molecules or additional tightly linked genes. Indeed, at least three variants of B27 have been defined by monoclonal antibodies,[24] cytotoxic T-cell responses,[25] and actual amino acid and/or nucleotide sequencing,[26,27] and six have been defined by isoelectric focusing.[28] None of these variants, however, has shown preferential segregation with disease. Recently, a 9.2 kilobase (kb) Pvu II restriction fragment-length polymorphism (RFLP) from the HLA-B locus (or closely adjacent) has been found in 73% of B27-positive AS patients but in only 23 to 27% of normal individuals, including normal B27 positives.[29] Alone, this RFLP confers a relative risk of only 7 for AS; however, when it occurs with B27, the relative risk approaches 300. It also appears to be increased in peripheral psoriatic arthritis (54%) but not in B27-negative AS, psoriatic

Table 29–1. HLA and the Spondyloarthropathies

	Frequency of HLA-B27	Other Associated HLA Antigens
Ankylosing spondylitis	85–90%	B7-Creg*; Bw16 (38 and 39)
with uveitis or carditis	95–100%	—
Acute anterior uveitis	50–56%	—
Reiter's syndrome	63–76%	B7-Creg*
with sacroiliitis, uveitis, carditis	90–100%	—
Inflammatory bowel diseases	Not increased	None
peripheral arthritis	Not increased	None
spondylitis	30–50%	None
Psoriasis vulgaris	Not increased	B13, B17, B37, Cw6, DR7
peripheral arthritis	Not increased	Bw38, Bw39
spondylitis	40–50%	Bw38, Bw39
Normal Caucasians	6–10%	—

*Includes B7, Bw22 (Bw 54, 55, 56), B40 (Bw 60, 61), Bw42 in addition to B27.

spondylitis, or Reiter's syndrome. In AS families, the 9.2 kb RFLP can be inherited from the B27 haplotype or from the alternative non-B27-bearing chromosome, suggesting gene complementation.[30] Thus, it appears that B27 and another B locus-linked gene are important.

Infectious agents as triggers or perpetuators for AS are strongly suspected, similar to those already known for Reiter's disease. Interactions between bacteria and B27 molecules are under active investigation. T-lymphocytes and serum antibodies from Americans with Reiter's syndrome recognize Yersinia enterocolitica (serotype 3), a bacterium that causes Reiter's disease in Europe.[31] Arthritogenic American strains of Shigella flexneri share a 92,000 MR outer membrane protein with the pathogenic Yersinia.[31] Monoclonal antibodies against both Yersinia and Klebsiella show cross-reactivity with B27. More recently, HLA-B27 has been found to share a sequence of six consecutive amino acids with Klebsiella pneumoniae nitrogenase, and both sequences are located in hydrophilic domains of their respective molecules. Antibodies to this synthesized peptide were found in the serum of 29% of AS patients, 53% of patients with Reiter's syndrome, and only 5% of normal B27-positive individuals. Thus, molecular mimicry between B27 and bacterial antigens has been proven, though whether this mechanism will explain disease remains to be proven.[32–33a] One laboratory has reported certain Klebsiella strains that modify the B27 molecule in AS patients by way of genomic insertion of a plasmid,[34,35] which elicited a cytotoxic T-cell response between two HLA-identical brothers (B27-positive), one with and one without AS.[35a]

HLA-B27: CLINICAL USES

Diagnosis of a spondyloarthropathy depends on careful clinical and radiographic assessment. Occasionally, testing for B27 may provide useful additional information. The following are examples of such situations. (1) A patient, usually young, whose chronic low back pain is inflammatory in character, may have sacroiliac roentgenograms that are normal or equivocal. A positive B27 does not establish a diagnosis of spondylitis, but it is supportive. The likelihood of a false-positive is only 8% (the normal population frequency), and a negative test makes spondylitis improbable since 90% of patients are positive. (2) Patients with incompletely expressed Reiter's syndrome and postvenereal or postdysenteric reactive arthritis are often diagnostic problems. A positive B27 test along with careful bacteriologic exclusion may prove

useful. (3) Finally, B27 positivity may help properly classify the child with seronegative juvenile arthritis. Although not absolutely predictive, it provides a high likelihood for a future spondylitic course.

RHEUMATOID ARTHRITIS

Rheumatoid arthritis, a disorder clinically, radiographically, and serologically distinctive from the spondyloarthropathies, shows important genetic differences as well. Susceptibility does not appear to arise from HLA-A, -B, or -C loci, but rather from the HLA-D region (see Fig. 29–1). Stastny first demonstrated a frequently occurring mixed lymphocyte response (MLR) in patients with rheumatoid arthritis, later defined by homozygous typing cells as HLA-Dw4.[36] This specificity occurred in 54% of Caucasian seropositive rheumatoids, but in only 16% of normal controls. With the advent of serologic typing for D-related (DR) B-cell alloantigens, HLA-DR4 was found to occur in even higher frequency in seropositive patients, 70% as compared to 25 to 28% of normal individuals (relative risk = 6).[36,37] Again, only rheumatoid factor-positive patients showed this association, and the frequency of DR4 was further increased in those with the highest serologic titers.[38] In fact, seronegative rheumatoid arthritis demonstrated no excess of DR4 or any other HLA antigen, suggesting that it develops on a different genetic background or is a separate disorder.[38]

Healthy women who were rheumatoid factor-positive also showed no excess of Dw4.[39] HLA-DR4 and Dw4 (coded by the DR beta 1 locus) also are tightly linked to DRw53 (DR β 3) and DQw3 (DQ α and β), both of which show similar relative risks for rheumatoid arthritis as DR4/Dw4.[40,41] Moreover, additional MLR specificities have been associated with DR4, including Dw10, Dw13, Dw14, and Dw15.[42] The DR4 association with seropositive rheumatoid arthritis is equally distributed between males and females and does not relate to age of disease onset.[38] On the other hand, although DR4 maintains a statistically significant correlation with the disease in most ethnic groups, including Japanese, Latin Americans, and Europeans, its frequency is highly variable.[38] Only 36 to 46% of American blacks with rheumatoid arthritis have the antigen, and its frequency is lower (10 to 14%) in normal blacks.[38,43,44] Studies in Ashkenazi Jews and Asian Indians show no association of disease with DR4, but rather an excess of HLA-DR1 in the former.[45] In fact, DR1 has now been found to occur in excess in DR4-negative Caucasians with rheumatoid arthritis.[45a] Two American Indian tribes, each with a high frequency of seropositive disease, show striking HLA contrasts. The Mille Lacs Chippewas show a high population frequency of DR4 (68%), which has been uniformly found in those with rheumatoid arthritis. The Yakimas, however, in whom DR4 normally occurs in 38%, show no DR or Dw associations with disease.[47]

Family studies also support a strong predisposition to rheumatoid arthritis carried on DR4-bearing haplotypes.[38] Multiple affected members usually share the same DR4 haplotype, but not uniformly. Furthermore, all DR4-positive family members do not express disease. Thus, a simple Mendelian dominant model with incomplete penetrance cannot be proposed currently for all families. In addition, it is unclear whether homozygosity for DR4 in adults increases disease risk or severity, although studies in juvenile rheumatoid arthritis (JRA) imply such an effect.[48,49] DR4 has been associated with radiographic erosions in adult RA.[49a]

Newer techniques are now better defining the DR4 haplotypes and "epitopes" most relevant to disease susceptibility (Table 29–2).[40,42,48–53] Certain "extended" DR4 haplotypes, including one with a rare C4B allele (C4B2.9), are more strongly associated with rheumatoid arthritis.[50,51] The molecular diversity of DR4 that accounts for the differing MLR responses (Dw4, Dw10, Dw13, Dw14, Dw15) is caused by relatively circumscribed amino acid differences around positions 70 and 86 in the DR4 beta 1 molecule.[42] The Dw4 and Dw14 specificities seem to predispose most strongly to rheumatoid arthritis in Caucasians,[48,49] while DQw3 beta RFLPs also show differential associations with these Dw types as well as rheumatoid disease and insulin-dependent diabetes mellitus (IDDM).[52] Sequence homology in the DR β third hypervariable region has been demonstrated between DR4 and DR1 molecules, and another (or the same)

disease-relevant epitope on other DR molecules in rheumatoid patients and families has been defined by a monoclonal antibody.[52a,52b] A DR β RFLP has been reported, which, along with DR4, increases the relative risk for rheumatoid arthritis to 50.[53]

IMMUNE RESPONSE TO COLLAGEN

A definite role for collagen autoimmunity in the initiation or perpetuation of rheumatoid arthritis has not yet been shown. Nevertheless, evidence from animal models and from in vitro human studies suggests that immune responses to collagen sub-types are controlled by the MHC and may be relevant to human disease. The induction of type II collagen arthritis in both rat and mouse models requires certain MHC-linked alleles.[54,55] Specifically, I region genes, the murine counterparts of HLA-D, are necessary for disease expression in mouse strains.[55] In humans, T-cell-dependent responses to denatured collagen as measured by leukocyte inhibitory factor release were correlated with DR4-positivity in both rheumatoid patients and normal individuals.[56] Furthermore, this "hyper-responsiveness" of the DR4-positive cell was related to an inherent lack of suppressor influence.[56]

SUSCEPTIBILITY TO DRUG TOXICITY

The risk of developing certain immunologically mediated adverse reactions to drugs used in the treatment of rheumatoid arthritis is increased in patients possessing certain HLA antigens. Gold-induced proteinuria/nephrotic syndrome, an immune complex nephropathy, occurs most commonly in DR3-positive individuals.[57] Of 24 rheumatoid patients who developed proteinuria on sodium aurothiomalate, 19 (80%)

Table 29–2. HLA-DR4 Haplotypes and Disease Susceptibility

HLA B	HLA C	Complement alleles*	HLA DR+	HLA D**	HLA DQ++	Disease associations		
						RA	JRA	IDDM
B15(62)	Cw3	S C 3 (2.9)	DR4	Dw4	DQw3.1	+	+	−
B12(44)	—	S C 3 0	DR4	Dw4	DQw3.2	+	+	+
B38	Cw7	—	DR4	Dw10	DQw3.2	−	−	+
B51	—	—	DR4	Dw13	—	?	?	?
B40(60)	Cw3	—	DR4	Dw14	DQw3.2	+	+	+
—	—	—	DR4	Dw15	DQwX	+	?	−

*Class III complement alleles for Bf, C2, C4A and C4B, respectively, defined electrophoretically.[50]
+ Defined by serologic HLA typing.
**Defined by mixed lymphocyte response and/or amino acid/nucleotide sequencing and/or DNA restriction enzyme analysis of DR beta 1 gene.[48,49]
++ Defined by DNA restriction enzyme analysis.[52]
Abbreviations: RA = rheumatoid arthritis; JRA = seropositive juvenile rheumatoid arthritis; IDDM = insulin-dependent diabetes mellitus.

possessed DR3 (relative risk = 32). Similarly, 69% of patients developing penicillamine-induced nephropathy had DR3.[57] Thus, a similar renal lesion induced by two different drugs has been associated with the same genetic marker, a phenomenon solidifying clinical observations that penicillamine proteinuria is more likely in patients having previous gold nephropathy. Ironically, studies suggest that good therapeutic response to gold is also associated with DR3.[58] Gold-induced thrombocytopenia, an immune-mediated peripheral destruction of platelets, also correlates with DR3 positivity.[59] Of 15 patients studied, 12 (80%) were positive for this tissue antigen (relative risk = 8.9). Notably, penicillamine-induced myasthenia appears to be more common (62%) in DR1-positive patients.[60] Additional HLA associations with adverse effects or favorable responses (DR3 reported for aurothioglucose)[61] from these and other therapeutic agents require further attention. Furthermore, it may soon become practical to determine DR status prior to initiation of drug therapy, with exclusion or more careful monitoring of patients at highest risk. The expected frequency of DR3 in a rheumatoid population, especially when DR4 is the dominant antigen, is approximately 10%.

JUVENILE CHRONIC ARTHRITIS (JCA)

Juvenile-onset chronic arthritis (JCA), often termed juvenile rheumatoid arthritis (JRA), is a heterogeneous group of rheumatic diseases beginning in childhood and often persisting into adulthood. Clinical

FIG. 29–2. Clinical/serologic subsets of juvenile arthritis and their HLA antigen associations. (Arnett, F.C., et al.: Juvenile rheumatoid arthritis. Johns Hopkins Med. J., *151*:313–317, 1982. Courtesy of the Johns Hopkins University Press.)

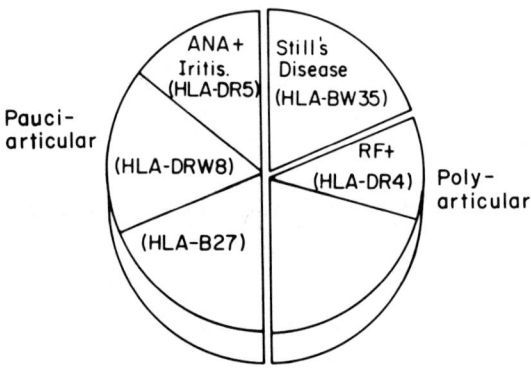

JUVENILE CHRONIC ARTHRITIS

subgroups have been established based on modes of presentation, numbers of affected joints, ocular disease, and serologic markers such as rheumatoid factor and antinuclear antibodies (ANA).[62] The application of HLA antigens has confirmed the rationale for establishing these subgroups and has provided impetus to more guided investigations into pathogenesis (Fig. 29–2).

Juvenile Spondylitis. Following the discovery of the strong association of HLA-B27 with ankylosing spondylitis and Reiter's disease, this antigen was also found in 26 to 42% of patients with juvenile chronic arthritis.[62,63] The majority are boys with late-onset pauciarticular involvement, usually affecting lower-extremity joints, who may later develop more typical symptoms and signs of spondylitis. Others, however, persist with a dominant peripheral arthritis. Girls may also be affected, and a deforming polyarthritis continuing into adulthood may ensue.[64] Cervical spine involvement with apophyseal joint fusion is a predominant finding in this unique B27-subset.[64]

Seropositive Polyarticular Onset (JRA). Only 10 to 15% of children with JCA have demonstrable IgM rheumatoid factor. This subset, in particular, clinically resembles adult rheumatoid disease because of the chronicity and severity of joint disease and the frequent appearance of subcutaneous nodules. HLA-DR4, especially its Dw4 (relative risk = 7) and Dw14 (relative risk = 11) subtypes, as in adult rheumatoid disease (Table 29–2), is significantly increased in such patients.[48] Moreover, homozygosity for Dw4 increases relative risk to 36, and the heterozygous combination of Dw4/Dw14 to 116.[48] Neither DR4 nor any other HLA antigen has been found in excess in seronegative patients with polyarticular onset.[63]

Pauciarticular Onset. This mode of onset, particularly at a young age in girls, is often accompanied by ANA positivity, which correlates strongly with the development of chronic iridocyclitis. HLA-Dw5, DR5 and extended DR5 haplotypes correlate with ANA and the ocular lesion.[63,65] HLA-Dw8, DRw8, DRw6 and DRw52 also associate with pauciarticular disease and may overlap with Dw5/DR5 in predisposing to eye disease. Notably, 10 concordant sib-pairs with pauciarticular JCA, the majority positive for DR5, were found to share two HLA haplotypes, thus implying recessive effects or *trans* gene complementation from the MHC.[66] HLA-DPw2 is also increased in this subset (53% vs 17% in controls; relative risk = 4.5), but is not in linkage disequilibrium with DR or DQ antigens because of a recombinational "hot spot".[67]

Acute Febrile Onset (Still's Disease). There may be

an association of Still's disease with HLA-Bw35 and DR4.[63]

SYSTEMIC LUPUS ERYTHEMATOSUS (SLE)

Systemic lupus erythematosus (SLE) is a multisystem inflammatory disorder characterized by multiple autoantibodies to plasma and cellular constituents and by immune complex formation resulting in immune-mediated tissue injury. Underlying genetic influences on its development and expression have long been suspected because of familial clustering of cases (10 to 12% of patients have another affected relative) and the 71% concordance of disease in monozygotic twins.[68] It is now clear that MHC-linked genes are exerting a profound effect on disease expression and are probably acting in concert with one or more non-HLA linked loci. Several class II antigens coded by the HLA-D region, as well as hereditary loss of function of nearby structural genes for the complement components C2 and C4, all show significant associations with SLE.[68,69]

Early studies of HLA-A and -B loci antigens in SLE patients suggested a weak link to B8 and, in retrospect, probably reflected linakge disequilibrium between B8 and DR3. It has now been well established that HLA-DR2 and HLA-DR3 occur in significantly increased frequencies in white patients (relative risk 2 to 3 for each).[37,68,70–73] Reports from different centers and geographic locations show great variability as to which DR specificity is more common, with some showing only an excess of DR2 and others DR3.[70–73] In most studies, DR2 and DR3 each occur in 40 to 60% of patients, with 75% possessing one or the other antigen. Both antigens also are common in normal Caucasians (DR2 in 22% and DR3 in 25%). Investigations in other racial groups are limited; black Americans show no HLA associations in some series and show elevated frequencies of DR2, DR3 and DR7 in others.[73] Moreover, the DR3 and DR2 associations in whites with SLE relate almost entirely to the Ro (SS-A) and La (SS-B) autoantibody subsets (see following).

The more recently recognized class II MHC antigens DQw1 (formerly MBI/MTI) and possibly DRw52 (formerly MT2) are also increased in SLE patients.[70,71,73] DQw1, previously defined by serum Ia-715,[70] is in tight linkage disequilibrium with DR1, 2, and w6 and occurs in approximately 69% of white SLE patients as compared to 55% of normal whites (relative risk 2 to 3). DRw52, previously defined by serum Ia-172[70] and a dominant antigen in Sjögren's

syndrome,[76] is strongly linked to DR3,5,w6, and w8 and occurs in excess in some SLE series. It remains unclear whether DR (β 1 or β 3) or DQ are the primary loci for disease predisposition.

Families containing more than one relative with SLE frequently have additional members with other immunologic disorders (e.g., thyroid disease, autoimmune hemolytic anemia, thrombocytopenic purpura) or serologic abnormalities (e.g., ANA, anti-ssDNA, false-positive tests for syphilis).[68,74] Studies of HLA haplotypes in such families show that neither affected SLE members nor relatives with other immune disorders or abnormal serologies share HLA haplotypes any more often than would be expected by chance alone.[68,74] In fact, formal genetic analyses using these disease/serologic abnormalities as "traits" show a Mendelian-dominant segregation pattern with no linkage to HLA.[75] On the other hand, the SLE relatives appear to have randomly inherited DR2- or DR3-bearing haplotypes, whereas their relatives with other diseases and serologic reactions have not. These observations raise the possibility that HLA may be acting only in a modifying role, since certain of its alleles are randomly superimposed on another dominant immunoregulatory gene common to many autoimmune disorders.[75] Theoretically, such HLA effects should be manifested as clinical or serologic phenomena highly characteristic for SLE.

Certain autoantibody responses, some distinctive of SLE, show strong associations with DR antigens.[68,69,71,77] Two Ro (SS-A) autoantibody genetic subsets of SLE have been defined in whites by ELISA assays (Fig. 29–3).[77] Anti-Ro (SS-A) accompanied by anti-La (SS-B) occurs in approximately 20% of SLE patients and correlates with DR3, older age of disease

FIG. 29–3. Circles represent major autoantibody systems in SLE and their respective HLA associations. Adjacent clinical features have been correlated with these antibodies. (From Alvarellos, A., et al.[69a])

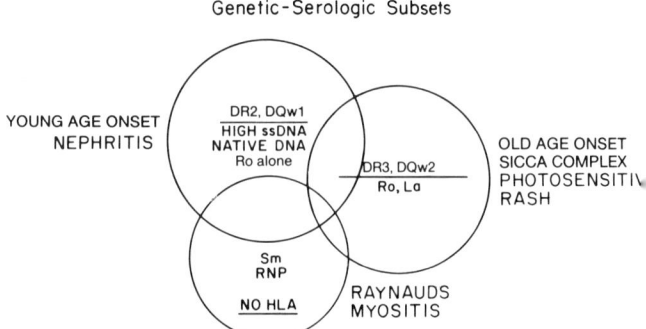

SYSTEMIC LUPUS ERYTHEMATOSUS
Genetic-Serologic Subsets

onset, sicca complex, and infrequent renal involvement. Anti-Ro (SS-A) without anti-La (SS-B) is found in another 26% and associates with DR2 and younger age of onset. Ro (SS-A) antibody levels are significantly lower in the Ro (SS-A) alone-DR2 subgroup compared to the Ro (SS-A) and La (SS-B)-DR3 subgroup, but both are often accompanied by IgM rheumatoid factor and hyperglobulinemia. Heterozygotes for DR2/DR3 show higher relative risks (7 to 15) for the presence of anti-Ro (SS-A) than non-heterozygotes. Also, a profound quantitative effect is apparent from DQ in that DQw1/DQw2 heterozygotes produce the highest levels of anti-Ro (SS-A). Whether this reflects the *trans* association of DQ alpha and beta chains with formation of "hybrid" DQ surface molecules, or the compound effect of the inheritance of two abnormal Ro (SS-A) immune responses (i.e., DQw1 is linked to DR2 and DQw2 is linked to DR3), remains unclear.

Anti-nDNA measured by Crithidia luciliae assay and high titers of anti-ssDNA show significant correlations with DR2.[69a] Anti-Sm and anti-nRNP show no positive HLA relationships (Fig. 29–3).[69a,77]

CLINICAL-SEROLOGIC-GENETIC LUPUS SUBSETS

Several newly recognized lupus subsets further support the role of HLA antigens in predisposing to autoantibody production, which in turn may prove to be pathogenic. An intimate link between Ro antibody, HLA-DR3, DR2, and cutaneous disease seems likely in these disorders.

Subacute Cutaneous Lupus Erythematosus (SCLE). A predominantly cutaneous disease, SCLE is marked by nonscarring, often photosensitive, annular, and/or papulosquamous lesions.[78] Serious systemic manifestations such as nephritis and nervous system involvement are unusual, and such patients are frequently ANA and anti-DNA negative. Anti-Ro(SS-A) has been found in 63% and anti-La(SS-B) in 25% of these patients. HLA-DR3 is strongly associated with SCLE, occurring in 77% of patients.[78]

Neonatal Lupus. Neonatal lupus is a syndrome characterized by photosensitive annular skin lesions and/or serious congenital heart block appearing shortly after birth.[79] Placentally transferred anti-Ro(SS-A) antibodies are uniformly found in these infants, and their anti-Ro–positive mothers are often asymptomatic. HLA-DR3 has been found in most mothers studied; however, the affected infants do not necessarily inherit DR3.[79] Thus, tissue injury in the neonate, whether by anti-Ro or other factors, does not require the presence of DR3. Moreover, anti-Ro–positive mothers who are DR2 positive do not usually produce infants with neonatal lupus.[79]

Lupus-Like Disease in Hereditary Complement Deficiencies. This disease has been recorded for nearly all components of the cascade.[69] Heterozygous C2 deficiency, the most common defect, occurs in 1 in 300 normal individuals, and the homozygous state in approximately 1 in 10,000. A lupus-like syndrome characterized by prominent cutaneous disease, including annular lesions, mild systemic features, and paucity of ANA and anti-DNA, occurs in approximately one third of homozygous C2 deficients.[69] Again, the anti-Ro(SS-A) antibody has been found to occur in 70% of such patients.[80] The "null" gene for C2 deficiency is linked to an A25,B18,Dw2/DR2-bearing haplotype. The prevalence of SLE in heterozygotes for C2 deficiency is unknown; however, the partially deficient C2 state has been found in approximately 6% of unselected SLE patients.[69]

Two structural genes for C4(C4A and C4B) also map between the HLA-B and -D loci. Homozygous C4 deficiency, requiring deletions or gene dysfunction of both C4A and C4B on both homologous chromosomes, is exceedingly rare but has been reported in a few patients with SLE.[81] Partial deficiency, however, resulting from "null" alleles at C4A or C4B are relatively common (22% for C4A and 28% for C4B). In fact, a C4A silent allele is in strong linkage disequilibrium with the HLA-A1,B8,Cw7 and DR3 haplotype, a gene cluster strongly associated with diseases of autoimmunity.[82,83] C4A "null" alleles are significantly increased in both white and black patients with SLE (relative risk = 3).[82,83] Homozygous C4A deficiency occurs in 11 to 13% of white SLE patients compared to less than 1% of normal patients, and confers a relative risk of 19.[83] Moreoever, the presence of both a C4A "null" allele and DR2 (which are not often linked on the same haplotype) results in a relative risk of 25 for SLE.[83] C4A null alleles and total C4 deficiency in SLE patients are heterogeneous at the gene level; some patients have deleted C4A genes while others have intact but noncoding DNA.[83a]

DRUG-INDUCED LUPUS

Hydralazine-induced lupus provides a model in which several genes are necessary after exposure to a sufficient quantity of drug.[72] The syndrome occurs primarily in slow acetylators of the drug. Female sex, another heritable factor, increases pre-disposition. Finally, HLA-DR4 has been found in 73% of such patients, occurring in 54% of affected females and 100%

of males. Thus, it appears that hydralazine does not promote the expression of a "lupus diathesis," since neither DR2 nor DR3 is the predisposing HLA type. Similarly, penicillamine-induced lupus has been reported in a small series of rheumatoid patients where the majority had A11, B15, DR4, and DRw8.[84]

SJÖGREN'S SYNDROME

Sjögren's syndrome (the sicca complex) is an autoimmune exocrinopathy characterized by unbridled B-cell proliferation, lymphocytic infiltration of multiple glandular and extraglandular organs, and myriad autoantibodies.[85] The disorder may occur alone (primary Sjögren's syndrome) or secondarily in the settings of rheumatoid arthritis, systemic lupus, and other connective tissue diseases.

Genetic predisposition to primary Sjögren's syndrome has been linked to HLA-B8 and more strongly to HLA-DR3.[86] In addition, early studies of B-cell reactivity to serum Ia-172, now known to be a DRw52 (MT2) defining reagent, had demonstrated that most primary and rheumatoid-associated Sjögren's patients were positive.[86] It now appears likely that DRw52, a class II MHC antigen (DR beta 3 gene) in linkage with DR3,5,w6, and w8, is the major HLA specificity associated with both primary and secondary forms of this disorder.[76] DRw52 is positive in approximately 90% of patients with primary Sjögren's syndrome and usually is carried on B8,DR3 haplotypes. DRw52 also is significantly associated with rheumatoid-Sjögren's and SLE-Sjögren's, as compared to both normal controls and rheumatoid and lupus controls without the sicca complex (Fig. 29–4). In these instances, DRw52 may be carried with DR3 but is more often allied with DR5, DRw6, or DRw8. Furthermore, because DRw52 is not linked to DR4 or DR2, the primary HLA associations for RA and SLE, respectively, this sicca-promoting factor usually is inherited on the alternate HLA haplotype.[76] DRw53 shows the strongest association with Sjögren's syndrome in Japanese patients.[87a]

Similar to the situation in SLE, the expression of the anti-Ro(SS-A)/anti-La(SS-B) antibody system appears to be intimately related to DR3 and DR2, and DQw1/DQw2 heterozygotes produce the highest levels of anti-Ro(SS-A).[72] In addition, anti-Ro associates strongly with hyperglobulinemia, rheumatoid factor, leukopenia, and vasculitis.[88] Thus, although susceptibility to disease seems intimately related to the DR beta-3 gene, the production of certain autoantibodies appears more closely allied to the DR beta-1 and DQ

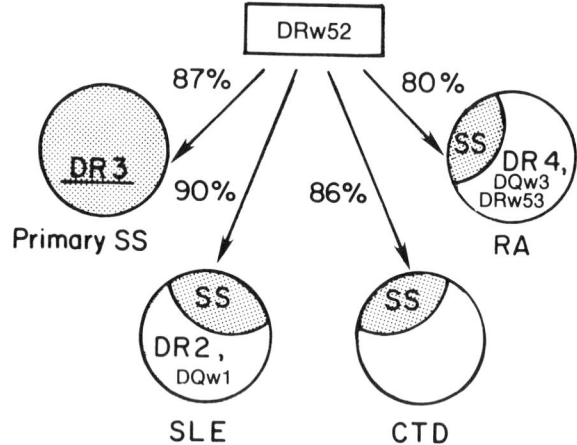

FIG. 29–4. Schematic representation of data presented in Wilson, R.W., et al.[76] showing the DRw52 specificity predisposing to Sjögren's syndrome in its primary and secondary settings. (From Wilson, R.W., et al.[76])

genes, suggesting close interaction between MHC linked loci.

POLYMYOSITIS/DERMATOMYOSITIS

Adult polymyositis in whites has been associated with HLA-DR3, whereas disease in blacks correlates with HLA-DRw6.[89] Supporting the possibility that dermatomyositis might be an immunogenetically different disorder, no HLA excesses have been found. Furthermore, a negative association of HLA-DR4 with all forms of myositis has been found, a phenomenon that suggests that DR4 may afford protection against the acquisition of inflammatory muscle disease.[89] Childhood dermatomyositis also shows a significant association with HLA-B8 and, more strongly, HLA-DR3.[90] The Jo-1 autoantibody (anti-histidyl tRNA synthetase), which is highly specific for polymyositis, has also been noted to correlate with HLA-DR3 and DRw6.[91]

PROGRESSIVE SYSTEMIC SCLEROSIS (SCLERODERMA)

Although progressive systemic sclerosis (PSS) shares many overlapping clinical and immunologic features with SLE and Sjögren's syndrome, evidence suggesting MHC influences on pathogenesis is weak.[92] An increased frequency of DR5 has been reported, as well as an excess of DR3, especially in the CREST variant. The B8/DR3 haplotype was also increased in a series of European patients and correlated with impaired cellular immunity. DR1 was found in 27.5% of 68 patients with diffuse scleroderma and 19.5% with CREST compared to 11.5% in normals.[92] Possibly of note was a significant correlation of DR1 (46%) with anticentromere antibodies.

OTHER AUTOIMMUNE DISORDERS

Multiple diseases resulting form aberrations in immune function have been associated with specific HLA types, the majority coded by the HLA-D region.[93] It is not uncommon to find may of these disorders occurring in patients with HLA-D related rheumatic disorders or in their family members.[68,74] In addition, several defects and disorders not believed to be of immune origin have also been linked to the MHC. A listing of these illnesses and HLA antigen correlations appears in Table 29–3.

BEHÇET'S DISEASE

Behçet's disease is strongly affiliated with HLA-B5 in Japanese, Turkish, Tunisian, Israeli, Greek, Italian,

French, and possibly Swiss and British patients.[94] For unclear reasons, no HLA-A or -B antigens, including B5, are increased in Americans with the disease. In Japan, the Middle East and Italy,[95] HLA-Bw51, a "split" of B5, appears to be the primary antigen. Other antigens that may be implicated include Aw31, DR5, DR7, and DRw52.[96]

TAKAYASU'S ARTERITIS

Takayasu's arteritis (aortic arch syndrome, pulseless disease of young women) has been strongly associated with HLA-B5 in Japanese patients.[97] More recently, Bw52, a "split" of B5, has been demonstrated to be the major specificity.[97] A weaker link exists for Dw12, an antigen in linkage with Bw52. No HLA-DR or DQ antigens have been implicated in Japanese. On the other hand, ten affected Americans showed no B locus association but, instead, high frequencies of HLA-DR4 (70%) and DQw3(MB3)(100%).[98]

OTHER VASCULITIDES

Giant cell arteritis and polymyalgia rheumatica have been weakly correlated with HLA-DR4 in French and American patients.[99] Similarly, an excess of HLA-DR2 was found in Wegener's granulomatosis, but no HLA-A,B,C, or DR associations have been found for polyarteritis or Churg-Strauss vasculitis.[100]

Table 29–3.   HLA and Nonrheumatic Diseases

Immunologic Disorders	HLA Associations
Graves' disease	B8, Dw3, DR3
Hashimoto's thyroiditis	Dw3
Addison's disease	B8, Dw3, DR3
Chronic active hepatitis	B8, Dw3, DR3
Celiac disease	B8, Dw3, DR3
Dermatitis herpetiformis	B8, Dw3, DR3
Myasthenia gravis	B8, Dw3, DR3
Juvenile diabetes	B8, Dw3, DR3 and B15, DR4
Multiple sclerosis	B7, Dw2, DR2
Optic neuritis	B7, Dw2
Goodpasture's syndrome	DR2
Pernicious anemia	B7, Dw2
Ragweed allergy (Ra 5)	B7, Dw2
Ragweed allergy (Rye I & II)	B8, Dw3
IgA deficiency	B8, DR3
Defective Fc receptors	B8, Dw3
Nonimmunologic Disorders	
21-hydroxylase deficiency	HLA-linked (Bw47)
Hemochromatosis	HLA-linked (A3)
Atrial septal defect (secundum)	HLA-linked
Spinocerebellar ataxia	HLA-linked
Narcolepsy	Dw2, DR2
Depressive disorders	HLA-linked
Longevity (>90 years in males)	A1, Cw7, B8, DR3

REFERENCES

1. Brewerton, D.A., et al.: Ankylosing spondylitis and HL-A27. Lancet, 1:904–907, 1973.
2. Woodrow, J.C.: Histocompatibility antigens and rheumatic diseases. Semin. Arthritis Rheum., 6:257–276, 1977.
3. Khan, M.A., et al.: HLA-B27 in ankylosing spondylitis: Differences in frequency and relative risk in American Blacks and Caucasians. J. Rheumatol. (Suppl. 3), 4:39–43, 1977.
4. Masi, A.T., and Medsger, T.A., Jr.: A new look at the epidemiology of ankylosing spondylitis and related syndromes. Clin. Orthop. Rel. Res., 143:15–29, 1979.
5. van der Linden, S.M., Valkenburg, H.A., and de Jongh, B.M.: The risk of developing ankylosing spondylitis in HLA-B27 positive individuals. Arthritis Rheum., 27:241–249, 1984.
6. Calin, A., Marder, A., Becks, E., and Burns, T.: Genetic differences between B27 positive patients with ankylosing spondylitis and B27 positive healthy controls. Arthritis Rheum., 26:1460–1464, 1983.
7. Hochberg, M.C., Bias, W.B., and Arnett, F.C.: Family studies of HLA-B27 associated arthritis. Medicine (Baltimore), 57:463–475, 1978.
8. Arnett, F.C., et al.: Homozygosity for HLA-B27. Impact on

rheumatic disease expression in two families. Arthritis Rheum., 20:797–804, 1977.

9. Khan, M.A., Kushner, I., and Braun, W.E.: Genetic heterogeneity in primary ankylosing spondylitis. J. Rheumatol., 7:383–386, 1980.

10. Arnett, F.C., Hochberg, M.C., and Bias, W.B.: Cross-reactive HLA antigens in B27-negative Reiter's syndrome and sacroiliitis. Johns Hopkins Med. J., 141:193–197, 1977.

11. Möller, E., and Olhagen, B.: Studies on the major histocompatibility system in patients with ankylosing spondylitis. Tissue Antigens, 6:237–246, 1975.

12. Brewerton, D.A., et al.: Reiter's disease and HL-A27. Lancet, 2:996–998, 1973.

13. McClusky, O.E., Lordon, R.E., and Arnett, F.C.: A genetic factor in disease susceptibility and expression. J. Rheumatol., 1:263–268, 1974.

14. Arnett, F.C.: The seronegative spondyloarthropathies. Bull. Rheum. Dis., (In press), 1987.

15. Calin, A., Marder, A., Marks, S., and Burns, T.: Familial aggregation of Reiter's syndrome and ankylosing spondylitis: A comparative study. J. Rheumatol., 11:672–677, 1984.

16. Morse, H.G., et al.: High frequency of HLA-B27 and Reiter's syndrome in Navajo Indians. J. Rheumatol., 7:900–902, 1980.

17. Oen, K., et al.: Rheumatic diseases in an Inuit population. Arthritis Rheum., 29:65–74, 1986.

18. Murry, C., et al.: Histocompatibility alloantigens in psoriasis and psoriatic arthritis. J. Clin. Invest., 66:670–675, 1980.

19. McMichael, A.J., et al.: HLA C and D antigens associated with psoriasis. Br. J. Dermatol., 98:287–292, 1978.

20. Espinoza, L.R., et al.: Histocompatiblity typing in the seronegative spondyloarthropathies. Semin. Arthritis Rheum., 11:375–381, 1982.

21. Bealieu, A.D., et al.: Psoriatic arthritis: Risk factors for patients with psoriasis—a study based on histocompatibility antigen frequencies. J. Rheumatol., 10:633–636, 1983.

22. Enlow, R.W., Bias, W.B., and Arnett, F.C.: The spondylitis of inflammatory bowel diseases. Evidence for a non-HLA linked axial arthropathy. Arthritis Rheum., 23:1359–1365, 1980.

23. Gran, J.T., et al.: HLA-B27 and allotypes of complement components in ankylosing spondylitis. J. Rheumatol., 11:324–326, 1984.

24. Turek, P.J., Grumet, F.C., and Engleman, E. G.: Molecular variants of the HLA-B27 antigen in healthy individuals and patients with spondyloarthropathies. Immunological Rev., 86:71–91, 1985.

25. Breuning, M.H., et al.: Anti-HLA-B27 cytotoxic T lymphocytes. Tissue Antigens, 22:267–282, 1983.

26. Rojo, S., et al.: HLA-B27 antigenicity: Antibodies against the chemically synthesized 68-84 peptide from HLA-B27.1 display alloantigenic specificity and discriminate among HLA-B27 subtypes. J. Immunol., 137:904–910, 1986.

27. Coppin, H.L., and McDevitt, H.O.: Absence of polymorphism between HLA-B27 genomic exon sequences isolated from normal donors and ankylosing spondylitis patients. J. Immunol., 137:2168–2172, 1986.

28. Choo, S.Y., et al.: Six variants of HLA-B27 identified by isoelectric focusing. Immunogenet.,23:24–29, 1986.

29. McDaniel, D.O., et al.: Association of a 9.2 kb Pvu II MHC class restriction fragment length polymorphism with ankylosing spondylitis. Arthritis Rheum., 30:894–900, 1987.

30. Reveille, J.D., et al.: Restriction fragment length polymorphism (RFLP) analysis in familial ankylosing spondylitis (AS): Independent segregation of a 9.2 kb Pvu II RFLP from B27 haplotypes. Arthritis Rheum., 30:S24, 1987. (Abstract)

31. Yu, D.T.Y., Ogasawara, M., Hill, J.L., and Kono, D.H.: Study of Reiter's syndrome, with special emphasis on Yersinia enterocolitica. Immunological Rev., 86:27–45, 1985.

32. Ogasawara, M., Kono, D.H., and Yu, D.T.Y.: Mimicry of human histocompatibility HLA-B27 antigens by Klebsiella pneumoniae. Infect. Immun., 51:901–908, 1986.

33. Kono, D.H., et al.: Ye-1, a monoclonal antibody that crossreacts with HLA-B27 lymphoblastoid cell lines and arthritis-causing bacteria. Clin. Exp. Immunol., 61:503–508, 1986.

33a. Schwimmbeck, P.L., et al.: Autoantibodies to HLA-B27 in the sera of HLA-B27 patients with ankylosing spondylitis and Reiter's syndrome. Molecular mimicry with Klebsiella pneumoniae as potential mechanism of autoimmune disease. J. Exp. Med., 166:173–181, 1987.

34. Geczy, A.F., Alexander, K., and Bashir, H.V.: A factor(s) in Klebsiella culture filtrate specifically modifies an HLA-B27 associated cell-surface component. Nature, 283:782–784, 1980.

35. Keat, A.: Is spondylitis caused by Klebsiella? Immunol. Today, 7:144–149, 1986.

35a. Geczy, A.F., et al.: Cytotoxic T lymphocytes against disease-associated determinant(s) in ankylosing spondylitis. J. Exp. Med., 164:932–937, 1986.

36. Stastny, P.: Association of the B-cell alloantigen DRw4 with rheumatoid arthritis. N. Engl. J. Med., 298:869–871, 1978.

37. Gibofsky, A., et al.: Contrasting patterns of newer histocompatibility determinants in patients with rheumatoid arthritis and systemic lupus erythematosus. Arthritis Rheum. (Suppl.), 21:S134–138, 1978.

38. Stastny, P.: Joint report: Rheumatoid arthritis. In Histocompatibility Testing 1980. Edited by P.I. Terasaki. Los Angeles, UCLA Tissue Typing Laboratory Press, 1980, pp. 681–686.

39. Engleman, E.G., et al.: Mixed lymphocyte reaction in healthy women with rheumatoid factor. Lack of association with Dw4. Arthritis Rheum., 21:690–693, 1978.

40. Duquesnoy, R.J., Marrari, M., Hackbarth, S., and Zeevi, A.: Serological and cellular definition of a new HLA-DR associated determinant, MCI, and its association with rheumatoid arthritis. Hum. Immunol., 10:165–176, 1984.

41. Lee, S.H., et al.: Strong associations of rheumatoid arthritis with the presence of a polymorphic Ia epitope defined by a monoclonal antibody: Comparison with the allodeterminant DR4. Rheumatol. Int., 4(Suppl):17–23, 1984.

42. Gregersen, P.K., et al.: Molecular diversity of HLA-DR4 haplotypes. Proc. Nat. Acad. Sci. USA, 83:2642–2646, 1986.

43. Alarif, L.I., et al.: HLA-DR antigens in blacks with rheumatoid arthritis and systemic lupus erythematosus. J. Rheumatol., 10:297–300, 1983.

44. Karr, R.W., et al.: Association of HLA-DRw4 with rheumatoid arthritis in black and white patients. Arthritis Rheum., 23:1241–1245, 1980.

45. Schiff, B., et al.: Association of Aw31 and HLA-DR1 with adult rheumatoid arthritis. Ann. Rheum. Dis., 41:403–404, 1982.

45a. Legrand, L., et al.: HLA-DR genotype risks in seropositive rheumatoid arthritis. Am. J. Hum. Genet., 36:690–699, 1984.

46. Harvey, J., et al.: Heterogeneity of HLA-DR4 in the rheumatoid arthritis of a Chippewa band. J. Rheumatol., 8:797–803, 1981.

47. Wilkens, R.F., et al.: HLA antigens in Yakima Indians with rheumatoid arthritis. Lack of association with HLA-Dw4 and HLA-DR4. Arthritis Rheum., 25:1435–1439, 1982.

48. Nepom, B.S., et al.: Specific HLA-DR4 associated histocompatibility molecules characterize patients with seropositive juvenile rheumatoid arthritis. J. Clin. Invest., 74:287–291, 1984.

49. Nepon, G.T., et al.: Identification of HLA-Dw14 genes in DR4 + rheumatoid arthritis. Lancet, 2:1002–1005, 1986.

49a. Gran, J.T., Husby, G., and Thorsby, E.: HLA antigens in palindromic rheumatism, nonerosive rheumatoid arthritis and classical rheumatoid arthritis. J. Rheumatol., 11:136–140, 1984.

50. Raum, D., et al.: Extended haplotypes of chromosome 6 in adult rheumatoid arthritis. Arthritis Rheum., 27:516–521, 1984.

51. O'Neill, G.J., et al.: Complement C4 is a marker for adult rheumatoid arthritis. Lancet, 2:214, 1982.

52. Nepom, B.S., et al.: Specific genomic markers for the HLA-DQ subregion discriminate between DR4+ insulin-dependent diabetes mellitus and DR4+ seropositive rheumatoid arthritis. J. Exp. Med., 164:345–350, 1986.

52a. Merryman, P., et al.: Nucleotide sequence of MHC class II region genes in a patient with DR4 negative rheumatoid arthritis (RA) from a multiplex family: simulation of a DR4 haplotype by trans complementation of the HVIII regions. Arthritis Rheum., 30:S31, 1987 (abstract).

52b. Lee, S.H., et al.: Ia antigens and susceptibility to rheumatoid arthritis. Clin. Rheum. Dis., 11:645–664, 1985.

53. McDaniel, D.O., et al.: Class II MHC restriction fragment length polymorphism (RFLP) and HLA-DR4 in rheumatoid arthritis (RA). Arthritis Rheum., 29:S11, 1986 (Abstract).

54. Griffiths, M.M., et al.: Immunogenetic control of experimental type II collagen-induced arthritis. I. Susceptiblity and resistance among inbred strains of rats. Arthritis Rheum., 24:781–789, 1981.

55. Wooley, P.H., et al.: Type II collagen-induced arthritis in mice:I. MHC (I region) linkage and antibody correlates. J. Exp. Med., 154:668–700, 1981.

56. Solinger, A.M., and Stobo, J.D.: Immune response gene control of collagen reactivity in man: Collagen unresponsiveness in HLA-DR4 negative nonresponders is due to the presence of T-dependent suppressive influences. J. Immunol., 129:1916–1920, 1982.

57. Wooley, P.H., et al: HLA-DR antigens and toxic reaction to sodium aurothiomalate and d-penicillamine in patients with rheumatoid arthritis. N. Engl. J. Med., 303:300–302, 1980.

58. Speerstra, F., et al.: The influence of HLA phenotypes on the response to parenteral gold in rheumatoid arthritis. Tissue Antigens, 28:1–7, 1986.

59. Coblyn, J.S., et al.: Gold-induced thrombocytopenia: A clinical and immunogenetic study of twenty-three patients. Ann. Intern. Med., 95:178–181, 1981.

60. Delamere, J.P., et al.: Penicillamine induced myasthenia in rheumatoid arthritis: Its clinical and genetic features. Ann. Rheum. Dis., 42:500–504, 1983.

61. van Riel, P.L.C.M., et al.: Association of HLA antigens, toxic reactions and therapeutic response to auroanofin and aurothioglucose in patients with rheumatoid arthritis. Tissue Antigens, 22:194–199, 1983.

62. Schaller, J.G.: Juvenile rheumatoid arthritis—series 1. Arthritis Rheum. (Suppl. 2), 20:165–170, 1977.

63. Miller, M.L., and Glass, D.N.: The major histocompatibility complex antigens in rheumatoid arthritis and juvenile arthritis. Bull. Rheum. Dis., 31:21–25, 1981.

64. Arnett, F.C., Bias, W.B., and Stevens, M.B.: Juvenile-onset chronic arthritis. Clinical and roentgenographic features of a unique HLA-B27 subset. Am. J. Med., 69:369–376, 1980.

65. Miller, M.L., et al.: Inherited predisposition to iridocyclitis with juvenile rheumatoid arthritis: Selectivity among HLA-DR5 haplotypes. Proc. Nat. Acad. Sci. USA, 81:3539–3542, 1984.

66. Clemens, L.E., Albert, E., and Ansell, B.M.: Sibling pairs affected by chronic arthritis of childhood: Evidence for a genetic predisposition. J. Rheumatol., 12:108–113, 1985.

67. Odum. N., et al.: Increased frequency of HLA-DPw2 in pauciarticular onset juvenile chronic arthritis. Tissue Antigens, 28:245–250, 1986.

68. Arnett, F.C., et al.: Systemic lupus erythematosus. Current state of the genetic hypothesis. Semin. Arthritis Rheum., 14:24–35, 1987.

69. Sehur, P.H.: Complement and lupus erythematosus. Arthritis Rheum., 25:793–798, 1982.

69a. Alvarellos, A., et al.: Relationships of HLA-DR and MT antigens to autoantibody expression in SLE. Arthritis Rheum., 26:1533–1535, 1983.

70. Reinersten, J.L., et al.: B lymphocyte alloantigens associated with systemic lupus erythematosus. N. Engl. J. Med., 299:515–518, 1978.

71. Ahearn, J.M., et al.: Interrelationships of HLA-DR, MB, and MT phenotypes, autoantibody expression, and clinical features in systemic lupus erythematosus. Arthritis Rheum., 25:1031–1040, 1982.

72. Batchelor, J.R., et al.: Hydralazine-induced systemic lupus erythematosus: Influence of HLA-DR and sex on susceptibility. Lancet, 2:1107–1109, 1980.

73. Hochberg, M.C., et al.: Systemic lupus erythematosus: A review of clinico-laboratory features and immunogenetic markers in 150 patients with emphasis on demographic subsets. Medicine, 64:285–295, 1985.

74. Reveille, J.D., et al.: Null alleles of the fourth component of complement and HLA haplotypes in familial systemic lupus erythematosus. Immunogenet., 21:299–311, 1985.

75. Bias, W.B., et al.: Evidence that autoimmunity in man is a Mendelian dominant trait. Amer. J. Hum. Genet., 39:584–602, 1986.

76. Wilson, R.W., et al.: Sjögren's syndrome: Influence of multiple HLA-D region specificities on clinical and serologic expression. Arthritis Rheum., 27:1245–1253, 1984.

77. Hamilton, R.G., et al.: Two Ro (SS-A) autoantibody responses in systemic lupus erythematosus. Arthritis Rheum. (In press)

78. Sontheimer, R.D., et al.: Serologic and HLA associations in subacute cutaneous lupus erythematosus. Ann. Intern. Med., 97:664–671, 1982.

79. Watson, R.M., et al.: Neonatal lupus erythematosus: A clinical, serological and immunogenetic study with review of the literature. Medicine, 63:362–378, 1984.

80. Provost, T.T., Arnett, F.C., and Reichlin, M.: C2 deficiency, lupus erythematosus and anticytoplasmic Ro(SS-A) antibodies. Arthritis Rheum., 26:1279–1282, 1983.

81. Tappeiner, G., et al.: Systemic lupus erythematosus in hereditary deficiency of the fourth component of complement. J. Am. Acad. Dermatol., 7:66–79, 1982.

82. Fielder, A.H.L., et al.: Family study of the major histocompatibility complex in patients with systemic lupus erythematosus: Importance of null genes of C4A and C4B in determining disease susceptibiltiy. Br. Med. J., 286:425–428, 1983.

83. Howard, P.F., et al.: Relationships between C4 null genes, HLA-D region antigens, and genetic susceptibility to systemic lupus erythematosus in Caucasian and Black Americans. Amer. J. Med., 81:187–295, 1985.

83a. Goldstein, R., et al.: Molecular heterogeneity of complement component C4 "null" and 21-hydroxylase genes in systemic lupus erythematosus. Arthritis Rheum. (In press.)

84. Chalmers, A., et al.: Systemic lupus erythematosus during penicillamine therapy for rheumatoid arthritis. Ann. Intern. Med., *97*:659–663, 1982.

85. Strand, V., and Talal, N.: Advances in the diagnosis and concept of Sjögren's syndrome (autoimmune exocrinopathy). Bull. Rheum. Dis., *30*:1046–1052, 1980.

86. Moutstopoulos, H.M., et al.: Genetic differences between primary and secondary sicca syndrome. N. Engl. J. Med., *301*:761–763, 1979.

87. Moriuchi, J., et al.: Association between HLA and Sjögren's Syndrome in Japanese patients. Arthritis Rheum., *29*:1518–1521, 1986.

87a. Harley, J.B., et al.: Gene interaction at HLA-DQ enhances autoantibody production in primary Sjögren's syndrome. Science, *232*:1145–1147, 1986.

88. Alexander, E.L., et al.: Sjögren's syndrome: Association of anti-Ro (SS-A) antibodies with vasculitis, hematologic abnormalities, and serologic reactivity. Ann. Intern. Med., *98*:155–159, 1983.

89. Hirsch, T.J., et al.: HLA-D related (DR) antigens in various kinds of myositis. Hum. Immunol., *3*:181–186, 1981.

90. Friedman, J.M., et al.: Immunogenetic studies of juvenile dermatomyositis: HLA-DR antigen frequencies. Arthritis Rheum., *26*:214–216, 1983.

91. Arnett, F.C., et al.: The Jo-1 antibody system in myositis: Relationships to clinical features and HLA. J. Rheumatol., *8*:925–930, 1981.

92. Whiteside, T.L., Medsger, T.A., Jr., and Rodnan, G.P.: HLA-DR antigens in progressive systemic sclerosis (scleroderma). J. Rheumatol., *10*:128–131, 1983.

93. Winchester, R.J.: The HLA system and susceptibility to diseases: An interpretation. Clin. Aspects Autoimmunity, *1*:9–24, 1986.

94. Ohno, S., et al.: Close association of HLA-Bw51 with Behçet's disease. Arch. Ophthalmol., *100*:1455–1458, 1982.

95. Baricordi, O.R., et al.: Behçet's disease associated with HLA-B51 and DRw52 antigens in Italians. Hum. Immunol., *17*:297–301, 1986.

96. O'Duffy, J.D., Lehner, T., and Barnes, C.G.: Summary of the Third International Conference on Behcet's Disease. J. Rheumatol., *10*:154–158, 1983.

97. Numano, F., et al: HLA-DR, MT and MB antigens in Takayasu disease. Tissue Antigens, *21*:208–212, 1983.

98. Volkman, D.J., Mann, D.L., and Fauci, A.: Association between Takayasu's arteritis and a B-cell alloantigen in North Americans. N. Engl. J. Med., *306*:464–465, 1982.

99. Barrier, J., et al.: Increased prevalence of HLA-DR4 in giant cell arteritis. (Letter.) N. Engl. J. Med., *305*:104–105, 1981.

100. Elkton, K.B., et al.: HLA antigen frequencies in systemic vasculitis: Increase in HLA-DR2 in Wegener's granulomatosis. Arthritis Rheum., *26*:102–105, 1983.

30

ARTHRITIS AND AUTOIMMUNITY IN ANIMALS

ELIOT A. GOLDINGS* and HUGO E. JASIN

Spontaneously occurring and experimental animal models of disease have traditionally provided important insights into mechanisms of human disease and have allowed for the development of effective therapeutic agents in many areas of human pathology. In the case of human rheumatoid arthritis (RA) and other autoimmune diseases, the sketchy knowledge available regarding causative factors and pathogenic mechanisms makes the task of selecting a pertinent animal model for any particular research endeavor extremely difficult. This difficulty is compounded by the absence of animal models that imitate closely the human diseases, and by the realization that more than one pathogenic mechanism can induce identical clinical and pathologic manifestations.

In most models of chronic arthritis, regardless of the inducing mechanisms used, the synovial inflammatory reaction tends to show a monotonous picture of lining cell layer hyperplasia, infiltration of the subsynovium with macrophages, lymphocytes, and plasma cells, and in severe lesions, the development of invasive pannus and cartilage destructive changes. The expression of autoimmunity may result from widely different genetic and regulatory abnormalities in the different strains under study. Thus, the studies carried out with animal models usually yield results and conclusions with limited applicability to the human counterpart. The fruitful transfer of knowledge derived from studies on animal models to human disease should result from a careful considera-

tion of the common features in both species. Overinterpretation must be avoided.

The list of animal models of arthritis and autoimmunity is long. An exhaustive description of all experimental and spontaneous models is clearly impossible. Models expressing a significant number of clinical, pathologic, and pathophysiologic features in common with the human counterparts have been selected for discussion here. A considerable amount of information is available on these animal models since they have attracted investigators precisely because of the features they share with human diseases.

ANIMAL MODELS OF ARTHRITIS

EXPERIMENTAL MODELS WITH IMMUNE PATHOGENESIS

Adjuvant Arthritis of Rats

Polyarthritis induced by a single injection of Freund's adjuvant containing bacterial components has been studied extensively. Its induction and severity are fairly predictable, leading to its widespread use by pharmacologists to study the potential value of immunosuppressive and anti-inflammatory drugs in the treatment of human chronic inflammatory arthritides. Adjuvant arthritis is species specific and can be produced only in rats. The development of adjuvant arthritis was first described by Stoerk et al.[1] in 1954 in rats injected with complete Freund's adjuvant (containing heat-killed acid-fast bacilli) and spleen homogenate. In 1956, Pearson[2] made similar observations using muscle homogenate instead of spleen

---

*Deceased

465

cells, and also showed that polyarthritis followed the use of complete Freund's adjuvant only, without addition of any tissue homogenate. Numerous studies have since dealt with multiple aspects of this model.[3]

Adjuvant arthritis is induced by intradermal injection of complete Freund's adjuvant into the back, tail, footpad, or directly into a lymph node. Not all breeds of rats are equally susceptible to the disease. Some strains such as Lewis and Sprague-Dawley develop arthritis with an incidence of over 90%, whereas the AVN, Buffalo, and other strains demonstrate significant resistance with an incidence of less than 10%. It has been shown that susceptibility to adjuvant arthritis is controlled in part by genes in or close to the rat major histocompatibility complex.[4]

After adjuvant injection, a latent period of about 10 to 12 days occurs prior to the appearance of polyarthritis, which consists of the abrupt onset of acute or subacute inflammation affecting the ankles, wrists, and tarsal and interphalangeal joints. Spine and tail structures are involved often concomitantly. Extra-articular manifestations such as tendonitis, keratitis, iridocyclytis, nodular lesions on exposed surfaces, skin rashes, urethritis, and diarrhea are common. The arthritis is usually self-limited. It increases in severity to a peak at 20 to 25 days after the adjuvant injection and then slowly involutes. In some animals, there is a tendency to spontaneous recurrences of a cyclic nature, usually at about 60 and 100 days after inoculation. In over 50% of the animals, the arthritis progresses to irreversible joint destruction and ankylosis as a result of the acute process.

The early synovial lesion consists of a perivascular mononuclear cell infiltrate and edema. Burstein and Waksman[5] showed that the earliest cells appearing in the affected tissues were proliferating mononuclear cells, probably macrophages derived from rapidly dividing bone-marrow precursors. Thus, the synovial lesions mimic in many ways the cellular events occurring at the site of a delayed hypersensitivity reaction in the skin. Soon after the onset of the synovial lesions, the inflammatory process becomes more intense. In addition to the increased cellular infiltration, there is fibrin deposition, joint effusion, and a concomitant proliferative response of fibroblasts and osteoblasts. Pannus invades the subchondral bone and occasionally the surface of the articular cartilage, leading to widespread joint destruction with fibrous and bony ankylosis.

Pathologically, the extra-articular lesions generally resemble the synovial inflammatory changes described previously.[6] The nodular lesions in the skin, eye, tendons, and genitalia are characterized by perivascular accumulation of mononuclear cells, predominantly histiocytes. There may be focal areas of fibrin deposition and occasional foci of necrosis. The proliferative aspects of the inflammatory synovitis are also seen in the extra-articular lesions with intense proliferative response of fibroblasts and osteoblasts. In the affected tendons, the fibroblast response leads to pannus formation contributing to fibrous ankylosis and further restriction of joint motion.

Several features strongly suggest that adjuvant disease is induced by a delayed hypersensitivity reaction to a disseminated antigen—the histologic picture, the induction of the disease by complete Freund's adjuvant, the latent period between inoculation and clinical expression of the inflammatory response, and the experimental studies to be described. The nature of the antigen(s) is not known, but there are compelling reasons suggesting that affected rats may develop an aberrant immune response to ubiquitous autoantigen(s). Early studies addressed the possibility that a latent infection was being activated as a result of the administration of adjuvant. However, multiple studies have failed to uncover an infectious agent, and the disease was not transferred by contact or by infusion of serum or joint tissue into an unaffected rat.[6] A viral etiology is still not ruled out because antiviral agents, including one that does not induce interferon synthesis, can ameliorate the expression of disease.[7] That adjuvant arthritis is due to a delayed hypersensitivity reaction to an unknown antigen was strongly suggested by passive transfer of sensitized T lymphocytes to naive recipients who then developed the disease.[8]

Although the nature of the sensitizing antigen(s) has not yet been elucidated, the finding that the arthritis can still be induced after replacing the mycobacterium in the Freund's adjuvant by apparently nonimmunogenic small-molecular-weight adjuvants[9] suggests that the antigen(s) involved may be endogenous. Indeed, as-yet-unconfirmed work suggests that helper T-cell lines reactive with Mycobacterium tuberculosis could transfer arthritis to irradiated naive recipients.[10] Moreover, arthritogenic clones selected from the original cell line react with a component of the proteoglycans of mammalian cartilage.[11,12] Pertinent to the pathogenesis of rheumatoid arthritis is the observation that lymphocytes obtained from rheumatoid peripheral blood and synovial fluid show augmented reactivity with M. tuberculosis antigen.[13] This observation may have a genetic basis because increased skin delayed hypersensitivity responses to M. tuberculosis antigens are associated with HLA-DR4 in a group of patients with leprosy.[14]

There are many reasons why rat adjuvant arthritis has been one of the most frequently used experimental models of inflammatory arthritis to study the mechanisms of action and therapeutic effects of various anti-inflammatory and immunomodulatory agents.[15,16] Its most attractive features include (1) similarities of its clinical and histopathologic picture to human rheumatoid arthritis and Reiter's syndrome; (2) the immunologic nature of its pathogenesis; (3) the ease and reproducibility of induction and clinical course in susceptible rat strains; and (4) the availability of reproducible objective quantitation of the severity of inflammatory joint involvement. Less attractive is its species specificity, and the tendency for soft tissue calcification, bony proliferation, and bony ankylosis, features found in Reiter's syndrome but almost never in rheumatoid arthritis.

Type II Collagen–Induced Arthritis

The arthritis induced in rats by immunization with homologous or heterologous type II collagen was first described by Trentham et al. in 1977.[17] This model is of particular interest because both cell-mediated and humoral immune responses to collagen have been described in patients with rheumatoid arthritis,[18,19] systemic lupus erythematosus,[20] progressive systemic sclerosis,[21] relapsing polychondritis,[22] and other inflammatory conditions.[19] The arthritis is induced in rats[17] or mice[23,24] by injection of native type II collagen in complete or incomplete Freund's adjuvant. The absolute requirement of homologous or heterologous *native* collagen II as the inducing antigen is of great interest. Immunization of rats or mice with denatured type II collagen or with type I or III collagen has been unsuccessful in generating arthritis. The ability of both incomplete and complete Freund's adjuvant to induce the arthritis is also significant. Because the disease has many clinical and histopathologic similarities to rat adjuvant arthritis, collagen II theoretically could act as an adjuvant in lieu of mycobacterium and give rise to adjuvant disease. Studies, however, have failed to show any evidence that type II collagen behaves as an adjuvant.[25] Although animals with either adjuvant disease or type II collagen–induced arthritis can develop cell-mediated and humoral immunity to collagen,[26] several features suggest that the two experimental models may have a different pathogenesis.[27]

In Wistar, Lewis, or Sprague-Dawley rats the incidence of clinically apparent arthritis is about 40 to 80%.[17] The onset of polyarthritis is usually abrupt, occurring 14 to 60 days after immunization, with a peak onset at 20 days. Although the joints of the hind limbs usually become involved, forepaw inflammation occurs only in about 10% of those rats developing arthritis. Involvement is predominantly distal, with

ankles and tarsal and interphalangeal joints most commonly affected. Inflammation reaches maximum severity within 4 or 5 days, and swelling usually persists from 5 to 8 weeks. The involved joints usually develop permanent deformity. In contrast to adjuvant arthritis, the spine is not involved and no extra-articular manifestations are observed. About 10% of the animals, however, develop erythema and nodular or diffuse induration of the ears, lesions clinically and histologically different from the ear lesions associated with adjuvant disease.

The disease in mice is induced by intradermal immunization of type II collagen in adjuvant followed by an intraperitoneal booster injection of collagen 21 days later. The onset of collagen-induced arthritis in mice is extremely variable, occurring 19 to 112 days after the initial immunizing injection, with a mean of 47 days. The incidence of arthritis is also variable, depending on the genetic susceptibility of the inbred strains used. In susceptible strains, the ankle joints are most often involved. Swelling and redness usually involve the entire foot, doubling the size of the dorsum of the foot and intermalleolar thicknesses. Spine involvement or extra-articular manifestations do not develop in mice either.

The earliest alterations include profuse fibrin deposition over the synovial and articular cartilage surfaces. Subsequently, the synovial lining cells become hyperplastic; the cells appear round with an increased number of filopodia. Fibrin deposition and hyperplasia may be seen in joints that do not develop cellular infiltrates. As arthritis progresses in about 20% of the animals, the subsynovium becomes infiltrated with mononuclear cells and polymorphonuclear leukocytes. The latter disappear about 6 or 7 weeks after immunization. The synovial proliferative changes lead to the formation of villi and of invasive pannus covering the articular surface of the cartilage. In the later stages, the synovium is hypertrophied and fibrotic. The articular cartilage and the subchondral bone covered by pannus show widespread erosive changes and periosteal new bone formation leading to joint ankylosis.[17] In mice, the histologic changes are similar.[23,24]

The histologic appearance of the auricular chondritis developing in about 10% of the immunized rats is of interest because it is similar to the picture seen in patients with relapsing polychondritis (see Chapter 78). The involved ears show focal cellular perichondrial infiltrates. The early lesions consist of polymorphonuclear leukocytes scattered over a mononuclear cell background with necrosis of chondrocytes and loss of matrix adjacent to the cell infiltrates. In later stages, the cartilage is surrounded by multinucleated giant cells and histiocytes. Occasionally, the inflammatory process leads to complete destruction of the normal auricular cartilage. The costal cartilage, tracheae, major bronchi, and aortic valves of the affected rats show no evidence of inflammation.[17,28]

Compelling evidence suggests that the arthritis in this model is mediated by a specific immune response to homologous or heterologous native type II collagen. The disease can be transferred passively with spleen and lymph node cells obtained from sensitized donor animals.[29] Helfgott et al.[30] have transferred the arthritis by intra-articular injection of T-cell supernatants from animals with collagen-induced arthritis. The exact pathogenic mechanisms responsible for the induction and maintenance of the chronic arthritis, however, are not completely understood, because the disease is associated with the development of high levels of both cell-mediated and humoral immunity. It is possible to passively transfer a transient arthritis in rats and mice[31-34] with serum containing anti–collagen II antibodies. Furthermore, the infused collagen antibodies have been shown to localize in the superficial areas of articular cartilage.[32,34] The importance of humoral mechanisms in the induction of inflammation is underscored by studies indicating that complement-fixing antibodies may be necessary for the generation of arthritis.[34,35] Studies of the immune response to different cyanogen bromide–cleaved peptides of type II collagen have shown that only a proportion of anti-collagen antibodies are arthritogenic, primarily those that react with a large peptide designated CD11.[36] It is likely that the arthritogenicity of these particular antibodies exists because this peptide contains the immunodominant epitopes of the native collagen molecules in terms of the magnitude or affinity of the antibody response elicited.

Immunogenetic studies using inbred mice have also emphasized the importance of humoral immunity in the induction of arthritis. Immunization of mice with type II collagen induces equally good skin-test reactivity to both native and denatured collagen, but humoral antibodies are more specific for the helical conformation of native collagen.[24,37] The antibody responses to collagen are under genetic control. Mice with H-2^b and H-2^s genotypes are high responders to type I collagen, whereas the H-2^q genotype determines high responses to type II collagen. With few exceptions, the mouse strains susceptible to the development of arthritis are also high responders to type II collagen. Although arthritis does not develop in the absence of an antibody response to type II collagen, the reverse is not always true. B10.S and B10.D2 mice are not susceptible to the development of arthritis but

their antibody responses to type II collagen reach high values. It has been argued that overt arthritis may depend on the development of a critical level of an antibody specific for a particular epitope on native type II collagen.[37] In B10 mice, the antibodies may have a different specificity, akin to those directed primarily against covalent structural determinants appearing after immunization with denatured collagens, although these cross-react with the native molecule.

The modulating role of collagen antibodies in chronic polyarthritis has been clearly demonstrated by Taurog et al.,[38] who showed that induction and passive transfer of adjuvant arthritis in the rat is facilitated, and the severity of arthritis greatly enhanced, by previous injection of the recipient animals with type II collagen antibodies. Additional studies with this model may contribute to a better delineation of the role of this autoimmune mechanism in human disease.

Antigen-Induced Arthritis

One of the major distinctive clinical features of RA is its chronic, relentless course. Both arthritis models just described may resemble human RA to some degree in their histologic picture, but both have a relatively short clinical course. It has been suggested that chronicity of RA may be due to a local immune response directed against a self-replicating infectious agent or to a renewable autoantigen (see Chapters 40 and 42). For these reasons, chronic infectious arthritis models or chronic arthritis induced by intra-articular injection of antigen into previously immunized animals may be better suited to study the mechanisms responsible for the long-term maintenance of chronic inflammation.

Experimental arthritis produced by intra-articular injection of antigen was first described over 70 years ago[39] but it attracted widespread attention only after Dumonde and Glynn[40] produced chronic arthritis in rabbits first sensitized to autologous or heterologous fibrin and subsequently injected intra-articularly with the insoluble antigen. The chronic synovitis that developed was postulated to be caused by a local delayed hypersensitivity reaction. Other soluble antigens such as ovalbumin,[41,42] bovine serum albumin,[42] ferritin,[43] or horseradish peroxidase[44] injected intra-articularly in rabbits previously immunized to the antigen in complete Freund's adjuvant also gave rise to a chronic arthritis, sometimes lasting more than 6 months. A chronic arthritis with the same features developed in mice[45] or rabbits immunized with the antigen in complete Freund's adjuvant. Several authors have emphasized the need to use complete adjuvant[40,50] because chronic arthritis did not develop in animals immunized with incomplete Freund's adjuvant. This suggests the need for a vigorous immune response to the injected antigen.

A few hours after the antigen injection, acute joint inflammation associated with severe swelling and exudation develops. The swelling then decreases slowly over 2 weeks to a variable plateau. About one third of the animals show a thickened synovium for 8 to 24 weeks. Inflammatory synovial fluid can be obtained from the joint in the first week after injection, but the chronic synovitis that follows is not associated with free exudate. Invasive pannus and cartilage erosions develop 4 to 6 weeks after the intra-articular injection, but the affected animals may not show any visible functional impairment.

Severe acute synovitis developing within a few hours after the intra-articular injection of antigen represents an Arthus reaction in animals with high titers of precipitating IgG antibodies.[46] Microscopically, 2 to 12 hours after injection there is widespread engorgement of many large and small vessels throughout the synovium. Tissue infiltration with large numbers of polymorphonuclear leukocytes (heterophils), hemorrhagic changes, vascular thrombosis, and tissue necrosis are seen in most specimens. In the initial 2 to 4 days the joint cavity is filled with an exudate loaded with erythrocytes and polymorphonuclear leukocytes. The synovial membrane and cartilage are often covered by a thick coat of fibrin. The articular cartilage shows widespread necrosis of the superficial chondrocytes and depletion of intracellular matrix. Three to six days after injection, the acute synovitis begins to subside. The heterophilic infiltrate becomes less prominent, and tissue macrophages and histiocytes appear in the subsynovium. The synovial cell lining layer shows active proliferation reaching a thickness of six to eight cells in many areas. The fibrinous exudate becomes infiltrated with round cells and fibroblasts and shows early evidence of organization. At this stage, the subsynovial cellular infiltrate is composed of heterophils and large mononuclear cells, but few lymphocytes and plasma cells.

By 3 to 4 weeks there is diffuse proliferation of synovial lining cells, scattered areas of fibrosis are seen in the deeper layers, and lymphocytes and plasma cells infiltrate the subsynovium. Moreover, at this stage of chronic synovitis, collections of lymphocytes resembling lymphoid follicles may occur, similar to those seen in established human rheumatoid synovitis. The articular cartilage shows small scattered erosions and, in some areas, early invasive pannus extends onto the articular surface. In later stages, 4 and 6 months after injection, about 30% of the animals still show evidence of active progressive chronic synovitis. Synovial proliferation, and subsynovial infiltration with foci of lymphocytes and plasma cells, are still prominent. The articular cartilage shows progressive damage with widespread erosions and replacement by fibrous tissue. In many areas, the chondrocytes appear dead and the remaining matrix is disrupted by amorphous deposits and fibrin. Electron microscopic studies confirm the light microscopic appearance, and the superficial areas of residual cartilage contain amorphous electron-dense deposits, identified as immune complexes.[47,48] The collagen network is disorganized and, in many areas, the fibers lose their typical banding.

The acute Arthus reaction[46] in the injected joints is not surprising, because its prerequisite high titers of precipitating IgG antigen-specific antibody are certainly present in most rabbits, but the mechanism maintaining long-term chronic synovitis is a matter of debate. Dumonde and Glynn[40] emphasized the use of complete adjuvant to establish a strong delayed hypersensitivity reaction to the antigen as a requirement for the development of the chronic stage of the disease. Support for this hypothesis was adduced as the development of chronic synovitis correlated better with the magnitude of cell-mediated immunity than with antibody titers in individual rabbits.[49,50] Alternatively, studies by Cooke et al.[42] suggested that humoral mechanisms may play an important part in the development of chronic synovitis. The inflamed synovial membranes synthesized immunoglobulins in vitro to the same extent as spleen or lymph nodes. Also, 30 to 40% of these immunoglobulins represented specific antibody to the antigen injected up to 8 weeks previously, suggesting that a sustained local antibody response was maintained by persisting antigen. Further study showed that the injected antigen was selectively retained in the joints of previously immunized animals and then released slowly.[47] Most of the retained antigen was localized to avascular collagenous tissues in the joint, that is, articular cartilage, menisci, and intra-articular ligaments, and was associated with specific antibody and complement components. Antigen retained within immune complexes may serve as the stimulus for prolonged local antibody synthesis in the synovium, providing a source of complement-fixing antigen-antibody complexes provoking a sustained inflammatory response. Local trapping of antigen depends on the presence of antibody in the extravascular compartment, because immune complex formation probably occurs within the articular collagen fiber network.[51,52] The exact role of the trapped immune complexes remains to be established, but when menisci containing immune complexes were surgically inserted into the suprapatellar pouches of previously immunized animals, a chronic inflammatory capsule developed around the donor tissue, reminiscent of the inflammatory pannus seen in rheumatoid cartilage.[53]

The chronic nature of this immune synovitis probably depends both on the presence of a critical number of antigen-specific circulating lymphocytes and on enough circulating antibody to retain sufficient antigen to establish a sustained local chronic inflammatory process. Local antibody synthesis may help maintain the sequestered complexes in antibody excess, ensuring their insolubility and slow release. In the mouse model of antigen-induced arthritis, chronic arthritis developed only after intra-articular injection of cationized antigen, which binds to cartilage by charge interactions with the acidic proteoglycan in much larger amounts than the native molecule.[54] The relevance of this model with regard to pathogenic mechanisms in human rheumatoid arthritis is strengthened by the observation that most pannus-free rheumatoid articular cartilage and meniscus specimens contained trapped immune complexes with the same localization shown for the rabbit model.[55]

Chronic arthritis might be due to the long-term retention of local antigen in the affected joints, because although the antigen is detectable for many weeks after injection, the arthritis may last more than 6 months in some animals. Although the number of retained antigen molecules needed to provoke arthritis is extremely small,[56] an inflammatory process of long duration may be due to the development of an immune reaction to autoantigen, probably a product of the inflammatory process itself.[57]

Streptococcal Cell Wall–Induced Arthritis

Attempts to induce chronic arthritis with streptococcal cell wall preparations arose from the observation that a single intradermal injection of sonically disrupted group A streptococci provoked a prolonged intermittent inflammatory lesion in rabbit skin.[58] This was related to the long-term persistence of the cell-wall material in macrophages.[59] Further work by the same group led to the development of models of chronic arthritis in rabbits[60] and rats[61] and a carditis resembling rheumatic fever in mice.[62]

In rabbits, a single intra-articular injection of isolated fragments of group A streptococcal cell walls induced an acute synovitis with maximal swelling 2 days after injection and subsidence in 4 to 5 days. Subsequent chronic synovitis may not be severe enough to be detectable clinically. A single intraperitoneal injection of large amounts of cell-wall sonicate induced acute polyarthritis in 100% of susceptible rat strains. By day 2 after injection, most animals showed

from 2 to 35 acutely inflamed joints, usually ankles, wrists, and interphalangeal, tarsophalangeal, carpophalangeal, tarsal, and carpal joints. About 50% of these animals had findings lasting 10 to 12 weeks, characterized by exacerbations and partial remissions. Many chronically involved joints showed gross deformities or ankylosis. The disease course was marked by at least two cycles of exacerbations and complete remissions in 40% of rats, peaking on weeks 5 and 10 after injection. Rats exhibiting this intermittent pattern of polyarthritis sometimes showed chronic deformities and ankylosis. This peculiar clinical course and the observation that the susceptibility to polyarthritis varied from strain to strain[61] suggest that this model may share pathogenic mechanisms with Freund's adjuvant-induced arthritis.

The early microscopic changes in the rabbit model consist of accumulation of a fibrinopurulent exudate, focal synovial necrosis, and intense infiltration with polymorphonuclear leukocytes within 2 or 3 weeks after the intra-articular injection, the exudative process is slowly replaced by hypertrophy of synovial villi, hyperplasia of the lining layer, and diffuse infiltration of the subsynovium by macrophages and giant cells. The macrophages are mostly replaced by focal accumulations of lymphocytes 4 to 6 weeks after injection. At the end of 9 weeks, inflammatory changes are minimal.

In susceptible rat strains, such as outbred Sprague-Dawleys, polyarthritis can be severely erosive. The initial acute inflammatory synovitis may be detectable as early as 5 hours after injection and is monotonously similar in all of the models discussed here. Acutely, synovitis is characterized by congestion, edema, profuse deposition of fibrin, lining cell layer hyperplasia, and intense infiltration with neutrophils and macrophages. The joint capsules and the periarticular and subcutaneous tissues are also involved acutely. This acute process is gradually replaced by a chronic erosive arthritis with proliferative synovitis and intense subsynovial infiltration with macrophages and lymphocytes. In severely involved joints, pannus invades cartilage and subchondral bone, replacing these tissues by vascular granulation tissue and disrupting their normal architecture. Chronic synovitis may subside without causing irreversible destructive changes in other joints. In most animals, synovitis is observed microscopically for 10 weeks after injection, but between 11 and 30 weeks only one third of the rats still showed active lesions.

The peptidoglycan portion of the streptococcal cell walls has been implicated in the genesis of the inflammatory changes. This macromolecule consists of a backbone of alternating N-acetylglucosamine and

N-acetyl-muramic acid units linked by β-1,4 bonds. In the streptococcus, the acetyl muramic acid residues are covalently linked to pentapeptide side chains composed of L-alanine, D-glutamine, L-lysine, and two D-alanine residues. The carbohydrate backbone is also linked to group-specific polysaccharide chains. The peptidoglycan moiety may be responsible for the toxic effects on the tissue, whereas the polysaccharide side chains protect the mucopeptide from digestion by intracellular lysozymes.[63] Such resistance to biodegradation leading to long-term persistence within macrophages correlates with prolonged inflammatory reactions.[60] In the rabbit arthritis model, the peptidoglycan persists in synovial macrophages for at least 5 weeks, and its presence within the joint correlates with the evolution of the inflammatory process.[60] Peptidoglycan could be detected within mononuclear cells up to 63 days after injection, and in spleen and liver throughout the 180 days of the study.[64]

Although the peptide and polysaccharide moieties of the cell wall fragments are both antigenic, specific immune mechanisms may play a secondary role in the development of arthritis. First, the acute inflammatory synovitis may be detected as early as 5 hours after intraperitoneal injection. Moreover, although many animals develop humoral[65] and cell-mediated immune responses[66] to the bacterial antigen, there is little or no correlation between these immune responses and the development or severity of arthritis. The early, acute phase of the disease appears to be complement dependent, because it is inhibited by cobra venom.[67] The late, chronic phase of the arthritis, which frequently results in widespread joint damage, may be thymus dependent.[68] In addition, the perivascular cell aggregates infiltrating the inflamed synovium are predominantly of T-helper/inducer phenotype.[68]

The pathogenic background of these four chronic arthritis models resides in the concept that an inflammatory process develops as a result of an immune response against a locally persisting foreign or autoantigen. Undigestible bacterial products persisting within cells may generate tissue injury through the same final common inflammatory pathway.

Experimental Production of Rheumatoid Factors

In human diseases characterized by intense and sustained antigenic stimulation, a significant proportion of patients develop positive tests for rheumatoid factor (see Chapter 46). Stimulation of autoantibody may be the result of nonspecific polyclonal activation of B-lymphocytes, containing a subpopulation of precursor cells programmed for rheumatoid factor synthesis. The experimental counterpart of this clinical finding has been reproduced in rabbits hyperimmunized with bacterial vaccines.[69] Repeated injections of streptococcal vaccines in susceptible rabbits induced the synthesis of large amounts of IgM and IgG rheumatoid factors,[70] which in some animals appeared homogeneous with common idiotypic determinants.[71] Rheumatoid factor production following hyperimmunization appears to be under genetic control since large quantitative differences have been observed between rabbit families. The development of rheumatoid factors caused by inordinate B-lymphocyte activation after hyperimmunization with foreign antigens may share common mechanisms with chronic graft versus host reactions in mice.

INFECTIOUS ARTHRITIS

Mycoplasma Arthritis

Mycoplasmas are small bacteria with fastidious growth requirements but without rigid cell walls; they are found in latent form in almost all species of laboratory animals. Many strains are arthritogenic, producing chronic arthritis either spontaneously or under experimental conditions. In swine, cattle, and rats, both epizootic and sporadic infections with Mycoplasma hyorhinis and M. arthritidis have been reported. Experimental arthritis has been described in pigs, rats, and rabbits.[72–75]

The clinical course of arthritis produced by M. arthritidis in rats or mice is somewhat different. In rats, the site of injection develops a well-capsulated abscess that soon resolves. The arthritis is relatively acute, developing a few days after injection, peaking at 7 to 14 days, and rapidly subsiding after 2 to 3 weeks.[76] In mice, the injection with viable organisms commonly produces severe and extensive abscesses, but the arthritis is less severe than in the rat and is characterized by gradual progression for as long as 9 months, with periods of remission and exacerbation.[73]

The acute suppurative synovitis in the rat frequently leads to irreversible, severe joint destruction. In mice, the synovium shows an initial acute phase with polymorphonuclear leukocyte infiltration and mild proliferative changes; the chronic phase is characterized by massive synovial proliferation, mononuclear cell infiltration, and erosions of articular cartilage, and bone associated with pannus formation.

Mycoplasmas can be recovered from the affected joints at all stages of the disease, although the number of microorganisms tends to be lower during the chronic inflammatory phase. The mechanisms of arthritogenesis of mycoplasma are not well understood, but several biologic characteristics may account for its ability to maintain chronic inflammation. Mycoplasmas can attach to and modify host cell membranes, mediate T- and B-lymphocyte activation, induce lymphocyte cytotoxicity, stimulate interferon production, and activate complement.[77] The role of the immune response to the injected agents in the development and maintenance of the synovitis has not been defined. Partial protection against the development of arthritis appears in animals previously infected or in mice injected with formalin-killed M. arthritidis.[72]

The rabbit model of mycoplasma arthritis developed at the University of Utah is of particular interest because it may represent an example of chronic "infectious" arthritis persisting in the apparent absence of the causative agent.[75] After intra-articular injection of viable M. arthritidis or M. pulmonis, an acute and chronic inflammatory reaction developed that may persist at least 1 year. The disease was characterized by an initial acute synovitis with heterophil infiltration during the first week, followed by a proliferative synovitis and subsynovial infiltration with lymphocytes and plasma cells, often organized around blood vessels and mimicking lymphoid follicles. Invasive pannus and articular cartilage erosions may develop in two thirds of the rabbits injected with M. arthritidis.

Despite the sustained synovitis persisting for many months, viable mycoplasmas or mycoplasma antigens cannot be found in joint tissues 7 weeks after injection. High antibody titers in synovial fluids persist for many weeks, however, suggesting a local immune response to the mycoplasma. Granular deposits containing IgG and complement in synovium and cartilage are detectable after the local disappearance of mycoplasma antigens.[78] It is possible to induce a chronic monoarthritis by intra-articular injection of nonviable mycoplasma in rabbits previously exposed to live M. arthritidis.[79] Here there is a strong correlation between synovial fluid antibody levels and the severity of the synovitis. In addition, immune complexes in cartilage and menisci are detected 7 weeks after the intra-articular injection. These observations suggest that immune mechanisms similar to those operative in antigen-induced arthritis may also play an important role both in this model and in the arthritis generated with live organisms. Alternatively, the failure to detect antigenic material in synovium or cartilage also suggests that the late chronic synovitis could be maintained by the development of immunity against an autoantigen present within the joint.

Erysipelothrix Insidiosa Arthritis

Spontaneous or experimental Erysipelothrix insidiosa (previously called E. rhusiopathiae) arthritis has been reported in swine, dogs, and rabbits.[80–82] This model has some features in common with mycoplasma arthritis. E. insidiosa arthritis is also characterized by an early acute stage followed by a prolonged chronic synovitis that may last several years and lead to severe destructive changes. The histologic changes are similar to the chronic synovitis induced by mycoplasma. The synovium shows hypertrophy and perivascular infiltration with lymphocytes, plasma cells, and macrophages. In severe cases, pannus formation and cartilage erosive changes are common.

This model shares other interesting characteristics with mycoplasma arthritis and also with human RA. Viable organisms can be recovered from the affected joints only in early disease. Using RNA-DNA hybridization, capable of detecting 1 organism per 50 mammalian cells, Steinman and Hsu[83] were unable to demonstrate E. insidiosa in synovial specimens from miniature pigs with chronic arthritis produced by intravenous injection of the organisms. Other studies, however, suggest that bacterial products may play a role in the induction of arthritis. Arthritis could be reproduced in rabbits by multiple intravenous injection of a cell-free extract of Erysipelothrix.[84] Bacterial products labeled with fluorescein localized in the inflamed synovium. In rabbits and dogs with experimental E. insidiosa arthritis,[80,81] serum rheumatoid factors were readily detected. Also, rheumatoid factor–like material was found in leukocyte inclusions obtained from rabbits with Erysipelothrix arthritis.[80]

The mechanisms responsible for chronicity in these infectious arthritis models have not been elucidated. Failure to detect bacterial products within the joint does not eliminate the possibility that these may still be directly or indirectly responsible for the maintenance of chronic inflammation. However, the alternative hypothesis that a second independent pathophysiologic process initiated by the infection may take over as the chronic stimulus is attractive, particularly in view of the current ideas on the pathogenetic mechanisms operative in RA (see Chapter 40).

Viral Arthritis

A spontaneous chronic viral arthritis in goats has been described.[85] A retrovirus with antigenic similarities to the visna virus has been shown to be responsible for the production of chronic progressive arthritis, tendonitis, and bursitis in adult animals and a demyelinating encephalomyelitis in kids. The arthritis is characterized by progressive mononuclear cell infiltration and lining cell hyperplasia, hypertrophy, and necrosis. Viral particles are present in lining layer cells up to 45 days after inoculation, and live virus has been isolated from inoculated goats up to 79 days after infection.

Two spontaneous forms of feline chronic progressive arthritis have been described. One is characterized by prominent periosteal bone formation around affected joints. The other resembles human RA and is associated with the development of subchondral marginal erosions and joint deformity. A feline syncytium-forming virus has been either isolated or detected serologically in all cats tested.[86]

A self-limiting chronic experimental arthritis has been induced in inoculated and contralateral rabbit knees by injection of herpesvirus of the hominis strain.[87] The arthritis persisted for 3 months, at which time no evidence of live virus could be detected. Histologically, subsynovial vessel formation, lymphocyte infiltration, and lining cell layer hyperplasia were seen. Some animals developed cartilage erosions and reactive periostitis.

ANIMAL MODELS OF AUTOIMMUNITY

Several well-characterized murine models for human systemic lupus erythematosus (SLE) are discussed in this chapter. Because the genetic background remains constant among different members of an inbred mouse strain, the sequence and spectrum of disease expression are rather homogeneous within that strain. The reproducibility of disease features within strains has permitted investigations of both the immunopathogenesis and therapy of SLE. For example, modification of the environment, diet, or hormonal status, or the administration of drugs, monoclonal antibodies, or certain forms of irradiation to mice of a given strain each has profoundly altered the expression of the autoimmune syndrome characteristic of that strain. Several strains in addition to New Zealand mice have been developed that express SLE-like autoimmunity. The clinical and immunopathologic manifestations of their illness have been described.[88] It has become painfully clear that pathogenic mechanisms or therapeutic success observed in one strain may not operate and fail in the others.[89,90] In recent years, therefore, investigators have performed experiments in several of the autoimmunity-prone strains before arriving at universal conclusions. Since the clinical manifestations of SLE in humans also exhibit considerable heterogeneity, this comparative approach in murine lupus research seems more likely to yield information regarding basic common mechanisms relevant to our understanding and treatment of lupus in humans.

NEW ZEALAND MICE

The prototype murine model of spontaneous autoimmunity is the New Zealand black (NZB) mouse. The immunopathology of this strain has been reviewed.[91] Virtually all NZB mice, male and female, develop a severe autoimmune hemolytic anemia associated with reticulocytosis and hepatosplenomegaly by 1 year of age. An indolent membranous glomerulonephritis often develops that terminally can acquire proliferative features. Approximately 12 to 20% of NZB mice develop a lymphoid cancer in their second year of life. Overall, untreated NZB mice live a life span equivalent to "middle age" in humans.

The immunologic abnormalities present in NZB mice are manifold, and their cellular basis is complex. Although the disease can be transferred with bone marrow cells,[92] defects of mature B- and T-lymphocytes and of macrophages have been documented in various experimental systems.[89,90] Consequently, considerable debate exists regarding the mechanism by which the activation of autoantibody-producing B cells occurs. It is clear that the immunopathology is a consequence of the overproduction of antibodies directed toward self-determinants. For example, accelerated maturation from the pre–B cell to the mature B cell occurs in the bone marrow of NZB mice at an early age.[93] Moreover, unusual Ly-1 positive B cells present in the spleens[94] can account for the spontaneous well-documented, polyclonal production of IgM, including IgM autoantibodies[95] in NZB mice.[96,97] Whether microenvironmental factors such as those exerted by cells of a monocyte/macrophage lineage, either in the bone marrow or spleen, might play a role of driving the differentiation of these B cells is not clear.[93] Functionally, the abnormality appears to reside within the B cells assayed in various systems, such as cloning in soft agar[98] or susceptibility to tolerance induction.[99–101] Theoretically, accelerated maturation of B cells could arise from defective thymic-derived lymphocyte regulation. Defects in T cells include abnormal responses to mitogens and in the autologous mixed lymphocyte reaction,[102] production of interleukin-2,[103] cytotoxic and suppressor T-cell generation, and susceptibility to tolerance induction.[90,104–106] Moreover, a defect in the generation of auto-anti-idiotypic antibodies to control the development of Coombs antibodies in NZB mice has been suggested.[107]

When NZB mice are mated with New Zealand white (NZW) mice, the F_1 offspring manifest an autoimmune syndrome distinct from that found in the parental NZB strain. NZB/W female mice develop an extensive membranoproliferative glomerulonephritis leading to death between 8 and 10 months of age. Male survival into the second year of life has been related to hormonal differences.[108] The glomerular lesions are associated with the deposition of DNA/anti-DNA immune complexes and complement.[109] Murine retroviral glycoprotein antigen, GP-70, and its specific antibody also have been eluted from glomerular lesions in NZB/W mice.[110,111] The relative nephritogenicity of these two antigen-antibody systems in murine lupus is still unclear.

Recent evidence has implicated an immunopathogenic role for T cells in NZB/W mice. Thus, treatment of NZB/W mice with a monoclonal anti-L3T4 antibody specific for helper-inducer T cells prevented the development of autoimmunity.[112] In addition, this treatment cured older mice with established autoimmune disease.[113] A requirement for NZB/W T cells has been shown as well for in vitro production of antihistone antibodies.[114] Moreover, production of pathogenic cationic anti-DNA antibodies with affinity for the glomerular basement membrane required both T cells and B cells from older animals.[115] Most recently, T cells were shown to augment the production of autoantibodies in vitro in the parental NZB strain.[116]

NZB/W mice may be a model for human Sjögren's syndrome because of mononuclear cell infiltration of lacrimal and salivary glands, and renal interstitium. NZB/W mice also develop lymphoid cancer, but to a lesser degree than in the NZB parent strain.[91,117] The Coombs-positive hemolytic anemia so characteristic of NZB mice is not clinically significant in the NZB/W F_1 hybrid. Similarly, overt central nervous system and skin disease are not apparent, but immune complex deposition in the choroid plexus[118] and at the dermal-epidermal junction[119] has been detected.

Because of the prominence of glomerulonephritis in female NZB/W mice, this model has been touted as an experimental analogue of lupus nephritis in man. The role of various drugs as well as diet and hormonal manipulations have been studied. Treatment with either corticosteroids or cyclophosphamide prolongs life, but greatly increases the incidence of neoplasm.[120,121] Prolonged survival also follows treatment with prostaglandin E_1,[122] essential fatty acid deprivation,[123] low-calorie diet,[124] zinc deprivation,[125] or total lymphoid irradiation,[126,127] or monoclonal antibodies to L3T4[112,113] or to Ia molecules.[128]

The genetics of autoimmunity expressed in New Zealand mice has been studied in detail and reviewed.[129] Sophisticated studies using recombinant inbred lines derived from F_2 generation matings between NZB and nonautoimmune mice have showed independent segregation of genes determining the various autoantibodies (antierythrocyte, natural thy-

mocytotoxic, and anti–single-strand DNA autoantibodies), those determining polyclonal B-cell activation, and those determining the expression of retroviruses.[130,131] Similarly, each of these genes segregates independently from other immunologic markers such as immunoglobulin heavy chain allotypes and the major histocompatibility locus. Therefore, mutiple genes are involved in the autoimmune disease of NZB mice. Moreover, interactions occur among various genes within the NZB mouse as well as with NZW genes in the NZB/W F_1 mouse hybrid.[129] For example, the production of IgG autoantibodies against DNA and histones has been linked to the major histocompatibility complex (H-2^z) of the NZW mice and not to the genes coding for the α- and β-chains of the T-cell receptors.[132]

Environmental factors impinging on this complex genetic background have been observed in a strain of NZB mice that expresses an X-linked immunodeficiency, primarily involving the lack of a B-cell population, designated Lyb5. Such congeneic NZB.CBA/N mice ordinarily do not manifest polyclonal B-cell activation or develop significant autoimmunity, but they do acquire the latter if continually stimulated by various polyclonal activators.[133] The NZB model of autoimmunity demonstrates well the complex interaction between multiple genes whose expression may be further modified by the unpredictable external environment.

MRL MICE

As noted already, genetic analyses of New Zealand mice have ruled out the concept of a single "autoimmunity" gene. In the late 1970s, additional models were developed in the Jackson Laboratory by Murphy and Roths. The MRL/Mp-*lpr/lpr* is a model for an accelerated membranoproliferative glomerulonephritis associated with anti-DNA production.[88] Both male and female members of this strain die between 5 and 7 months of age. A congeneic strain designated MRL/Mp−$^{+/+}$ develops a low-grade autoimmune syndrome, dying midway in the second year of life. Both strains develop antibody to the Sm antigen,[134] a specific marker for SLE in man. The MRL/Mp−$^{+/+}$ mouse, however, does not develop the impressive lymphoproliferative disorder present in the *lpr/lpr* counterpart. The MRL/Mp-*lpr/lpr* mouse is the only strain that develops a detectable synovitis in up to 75% of animals in addition to immune complex glomerulonephritis.[88,135] A high correlation between serum IgM rheumatoid factor and the development of erosive arthritis has been recorded.[135] This feature has been used to promote the MRL/Mp-*lpr/lpr* mouse as a natural occurring model of human RA. A necrotizing polyarteritis with dense infiltration by polymorphonuclear leukocytes and fibrinoid necrosis of medium-size arterial walls of kidneys, genital organs, and heart develops in 75% of this strain of mice.[88,136] Individual hybridomas derived from MRL/Mp-*lpr/lpr* mice have generated monoclonal antibodies with specificities. The antigenic determinant recognized was a phosphodiester linkage shared among several phospholipids.[137] Thus, a single monoclonal antibody derived from an unimmunized mouse produced a positive antinuclear antibody test, antibody reactions with DNA and other polynucleotides, antibody reactions with cardiolipin, and prolongation of the activated partial thromboplastin test characteristic of a lupus anticoagulant.[137]

The advantage of the MRL/Mp-*lpr/lpr* strain for drug and diet studies relates to the rapid pace of the autoimmune syndrome and the death of the mouse, both of which are markedly accelerated compared to the NZB/W female. The therapeutic efficacy of PGE$_1$,[138] total lymphoid irradiation[139] and cyclophosphamide,[140,141] and T-cell antibody[142] have been clearly shown in this model similar to their previously noted beneficial effects in NZB/W mice. The therapeutic effect of PGE$_1$ administration as well as low-calorie diet was more closely linked to the inhibition of formation of circulating endogenous retroviral envelope glycoprotein GP-70/anti-GP-70 immune complexes than to the inhibition of anti–native DNA autoantiodies.[124,138] The deposition of retroviral immune complexes in glomeruli may be highly pathogenic in MRL/Mp-*lpr/lpr* and NZB/W mice and critically important for the development of vasculitis in the former strain.[136]

The genetics of this model appears simpler than in the NZB mouse. The *lpr* gene is a single-locus autosomal recessive gene that merely functions as an accelerating factor interacting with MRL background genes present in the MRL/Mp − $^{+/+}$ mouse. The effect of the *lpr* gene by itself can be more clearly appreciated by the successful transfer of this gene to mice with no known autoimmune potential. Thus, C57BL/6-*lpr/lpr* and C3H/HeJ-*lpr/lpr* mice develop substantial lymphadenopathy and anti-DNA antibody,[143] and die at approximately 1 year of age. Rheumatoid factor production but not renal disease is characteristic.[144]

Clues to the mode of action of the *lpr* gene have been detected. In contrast to NZB, NZB/W, and BXSB/Mp strains in which neonatal thymectomy will dramatically accelerate the development of autoimmunity, such a maneuver abolishes its development in the MRL/MP-*lpr/lpr* mouse.[89] The T-cell dependence of MRL disease is further supported by the

observation of massive proliferation of T cells in the spleen and lymph nodes of the *lpr* mouse.[89] These have been shown to be rich in helper-cell activity with respect to antibody formation, and bear the unusual phenotype Ly1 + , Ly2 − , L3T4 − .[145] More recently, T-cell-derived lymphokines, designated B-cell differentiation factors, have been detected in the supernatants of cultured lymphoid cells from *lpr* mice whether on the MRL or C57BL/6 background.[146] It is probable that these factors play a role in the activation and maturation of nearby B cells and in their secretion of IgG autoantibodies. Mice with the *lpr* gene also exhibit defects in the production of interleukin-2 (T-cell growth factor) and in the production of receptors for interleukin-2.[147,148] The presence of such defects in all murine SLE strains suggests that these are not the primary expression of the *lpr* gene.[103] Similarly, increased Ia-positive peritoneal macrophages have been detected in MRL/MP-*lpr/lpr* and NZB mice in association with autoantibody formation, but their absence in *lpr* mice with the C57BL/6 and C3H/HeJ backgrounds indicates that this feature is not tightly linked to the expression of the *lpr* gene.[149]

BXSB MICE

Another strain developed by Murphy and Roths, the BXSB/Mp mouse, is unusual in that the males develop autoimmunity quite early, dying at 5 to 7 months of age, whereas the female BXSB/Mp mice develop an indolent autoimmune syndrome that does not lead to death until well into the second year of life. The BXSB/Mp male mice develop a Coombs-positive hemolytic anemia and, more importantly, a rapidly progressive immune complex membranoproliferative glomerulonephritis.[88] A striking monocytosis has been observed.[150]

In addition, a degenerative vascular disease involving the coronary arteries is noted in some mice of this strain,[88,136] but this is far more striking in the male offspring of a mating between BXSB/Mp males and NZW females.[151] Such coronary disease is observed in 100% of the (NZWxBXSB)F$_1$ males and is responsible for death at approximately 5 months of age. The pathologic findings reveal a paucity of cellular infiltrate in the coronary vessels. The pathogenesis of this lesion has been linked to sustained low levels of circulating immune complexes in contrast to the necrotizing polyarteritis of MRL/Mp-*lpr/lpr* mice, which is associated with high levels of circulating immune complexes that trigger an inflammatory reaction once deposited.[136] It is conceivable that vasospastic compounds such as thromboxanes may play a significant role in the pathogenesis of this lesion (see Chapter 26). Thus, this model may be ideally suited to examine the effect of thromboxane inhibitors, prostaglandin E_1, as well as diet modification, particularly with regard to lipid content, on the development of degenerative coronary vascular disease. As with MRL/Mp-*lpr/lpr* mice, the BXSB male and the (NZWxBXSB)F_1 male are ideal models for study of drug, diet, and other therapeutic modalities since their life span is significantly shortened and each has distinctive immunopathologic diseases.

Immunologic and genetic pathogenic factors in the SLE syndrome in BXSB/Mp male mice involve a Y-chromosome-linked factor that is *not* mediated by male hormones.[152,153] The abnormal B-cell function of BXSB/Mp male mice may be augmented by thymectomy.[154] Nevertheless, anti-T–cell antibodies retard lupus from developing in BXSB mice suggesting a role for helper T cells in this strain.[155] An enhanced response to normal T-cell–derived lymphokines by BXSB/Mp- and NZB-derived B cells, activated by either lipopolysaccharide or anti-immunoglobulin, has been demonstrated.[156] This observation, together with a defined defect in tolerance induction at the B-cell level,[157] indicates that the disease in the BXSB/Mp male, like that in the NZB mouse, involves an inherent B-cell abnormality in its pathogenesis.

PARENT TO F_1-INDUCED GRAFT VERSUS HOST REACTIONS

A model has been developed by Gleichmann and co-workers[158,159] that uses a chronic graft versus host reaction (GVHR) achieved by the transfer of parental helper T-cell–enriched, suppressor T-cell–depleted, spleen cells into nonirradiated F_1 hosts. Similarly, a chronic GVHR is achieved with certain strain combinations favoring the generation of T-cell help even with the transfer of unfractionated spleen cells (e.g., DBA/2→(C57BL/10xDBA/2)F_1, or combinations differing only at the I region locus). In both cases, the chronic GVHR triggers an SLE-like syndrome. Precedent for SLE-like autoimmunity and the development of scleroderma-like skin disease ensuing from a GVHR was first reported in rats[160] and later in mice.[161] The donor T cells recognize allogeneic F_1 major histocompatibility antigens, resulting in chronically augmented nonspecific T-cell helper function. These mice develop a whole series of autoantibodies characteristic of SLE,[159] including antinuclear antibodies, Coombs antibody, natural thymocytotoxic autoantibody, and anti-DNA antibody, with immuno-

pathologic consequences such as the development of immune complex glomerulonephritis.[162]

This murine model of SLE is created rather than inherited, offering the advantage of careful experimental manipulation and analysis. Gleichmann has proposed that F_1 host B cells are primed in vivo by autoantigens with multiple repeating antigenic determinants, rendering them responsive to abnormal T-cell help that is neither major histocompatibility complex restricted nor specific for the same autoantigens to which the B cells are committed. Such a novel mechanism could account for the development of various autoantibodies observed in human and murine SLE. Thus, helper T-cell activation generated by the acquisition of mutant major histocompatibility complex determinants (particularly of the I region in mice and D region in man), or the modification of I- or D-region antigens by viruses or drugs might trigger the onset of autoimmunity and the lupus syndrome. This process may ensue from appropriate T-cell recognition of autoantigens in the context of "new" I- or D-region antigens present on macrophages rather than from the generation of nonspecific T-cell help.[163] Pharmacologic, dietary, or other therapeutic approaches to the modification of the autoimmune disease produced in this model have not yet been reported.

CONCLUSION

All models discussed here, in addition to SLE-prone inbred Palmerston-North mice,[164] moth-eaten mice,[165] and the most recently described C3H/HeJ-*gld/gld* mice,[166] have in common the production of characteristic autoantibodies leading to immune complex mediated injury. The immunopathologic features of these various models are summarized in Table 30–1. In no model does there develop significant neurologic disorders, serositis, or skin involvement. Nevertheless, they provide models of glomerulonephritis, vasculitis, and synovitis that resemble the analogous manifestations of human SLE.

The immunoregulatory disorders associated with such pathology are varied. In certain instances, the induction of excess helper T lymphocyte activity, as in the cases of the chronic GVHR mice and the *lpr* mice, may in fact be the dominant mechanism. In the BXSB/Mp male and in the New Zealand mice, tissue injury may result from intrinsic abnormalities by B lymphocytes, although defective suppressor T-cell, and excessively active monocyte/macrophage and helper T-cell mechanisms may be operative as well. Cognizance of these heterogeneous models of SLE in

Table 30–1. Mouse Models of Systemic Lupus Erythematosus

Model	Immunopathology	Accelerating Factor	Mean Mortality Male; Female (months)	Helper-T-Cell Dependence	Primary B-Cell Abnormality	Autoantibodies
NZB	Autoimmune hemolytic anemia; membranous glomerulonephritis; lymphoid hyperplasia and cancer	Environment	15½; 14	+	Yes	Antierythrocyte Anti–single stranded DNA NTA*
(NZBxNZW)F₁	Membranoproliferative glomerulonephritis; Sjögren's syndrome	Estrogens	15; 9	+ +	Yes	Antinative DNA Anti-GP-70
MLR/Mp-*lpr/lpr*	Membranoproliferative glomerulonephritis; polyarteritis; erosive arthritis; lymphadenopathy	Autosomal recessive *lpr* gene	6; 5	+ + + +	No	Antinative DNA Anti-Sm Rheumatoid factor Anti-GP-70
BXSB/Mp	Proliferative glomerulonephritis; degenerative coronary disease	Y chromosome (not hormonal)	5; 20	+ +	Yes	Antinative DNA Antierythrocyte
Chronic GVHR†	Glomerulonephritis; arthritis; Sjögren's syndrome	—	>12	+ + + +	No	Anti-DNA Antierythrocyte NTA

*NTA = Natural thromocytotoxic autoantibody.
†GVHR = Graft versus host reaction.

mice should stimulate further clinical investigation of SLE and lead to a better understanding of the pathogenic mechanisms and to the development of more effective therapies.

REFERENCES

1. Stoerk, H.C., Bielinski, T.C., and Budzilovich, T.: Chronic polyarthritis in rats injected with spleen in adjuvants (Abstract.) Am. J. Pathol., 30:616, 1954.
2. Pearson, C.M.: Development of arthritis, periarthritis and periositis in rats given adjuvants. Proc. Soc. Exp. Biol. Med., 91:95–101, 1956.
3. Zahiri, H., et al.: Adjuvant experimental polyarthritis. Can. Med. Assoc. J., 101:269–278, 1969.
4. Battisto, J.R., et al.: Susceptibility to adjuvant arthritis in DA and F344 rats. A dominant trait controlled by an autosomal gene locus linked to the major histocompatibility complex. Arthritis Rheum., 25:1194–1200, 1982.
5. Burstein, N.A., and Waksman, B.H.: The pathogenesis of adjuvant disease in the rat. II. A radioautographic study of early lesions with the use of H³-thymidine. Yale J. Biol. Med., 37:195–203, 1964.
6. Pearson, C.M., Waksman, B.H., and Sharp, J.T.: Studies of arthritis and other lesions induced in rats by injection of mycobacterial adjuvant. V. Changes affecting the skin and mucous membranes. Comparison of the experimental process with human disease. J. Exp. Med., 113:485–510, 1961.
7. Kapusta, M.A., Young-Rodenchuk, M., and Kourounakis, L.: Restoration of diminished splenic responses to phytohemagglutinin and concanavalin A in adjuvant-induced disease by irrazole: Possible role of a virus and suppressor cells. J. Rheumatol., 6:507–518, 1979.
8. Taurog, J.D., Sandberg, G.P., and Mahowald, M.L.: The cellular basis of adjuvant arthritis. I. Enhancement of cell-mediated passive transfer by concanavalin A and by immuno- suppressive pretreatment of the recipient. Cell. Immunol., 75:271–282, 1983.
9. Chang, Y.-H., Pearson, C.M., and Chedid, L.: Adjuvant polyarthritis. V. Induction by N-acetylmuramyl L-alanyl-D-isoglutamine, the smallest peptide subunit of bacterial peptidoglycan. J. Exp. Med., 153:1021–1026, 1981.
10. Holoshitz, J., Naparstek, Y., Ben-Nun, A., and Cohen, I.R.: Lines of T lymphocytes induce or vaccinate against autoimmune arthritis. Science, 219:56–58, 1983.
11. Van-Eden, W., et al.: Arthritis induced by a T-lymphocyte clone that responds to Mycobacterium tuberculosis and to cartilage proteoglycans. Proc. Natl. Acad. Sci. USA, 82:5117–5120, 1985.
12. Cohen, I.R., Holoshitz, J., Van Eden, W., and Frenkel, A.: T lymphocyte clones illuminate pathogenesis and affect therapy of experimental arthritis. Arthritis Rheum., 28:841–845, 1985.
13. Holoshitz, J., et al.: T-lymphocytes of rheumatoid arthritis patients show augmented reactivity to a fraction of mycobacteria crossreactive with cartilage. Lancet, 2:305–309, 1986.
14. Ottenhoff, T.H., et al.: Evidence for an HLA-DR4-associated immune-response gene for Mycobacterium tuberculosis. Lancet, 2:310–313, 1986.
15. Rosenthale, M.E., and Nagra, C.L.: Comparative effects of some immunosuppressive and antiinflammatory drugs on allergic encephalomyelitis and adjuvant arthritis. Proc. Soc. Exp. Biol. Med., 125:149–153, 1967.
16. Swingle, K.F.: Evaluation of anti-inflammatory activity. In Anti-inflammatory Agents. Edited by R.A. Scherrer and M.W. Whitehouse. New York, Academic Press, 1974.
17. Trentham, D.E., Townes, A.S., and Kang, A.H.: Autoimmunity to type II collagen: An experimental model of arthritis. J. Exp. Med., 146:857–867, 1977.
18. Steffen, C.: Collagen as an autoantigen in rheumatoid arthritis. In Advances in Joint Disease. Edited by A. Maroudas and E.J. Holborow. Marshfield, MA, Pitman Publishing, 1981.
19. Stuart, J.M., et al.: Incidence and specificity of antibodies to types I, II, III, IV and V collagen in rheumatoid arthritis and other rheumatic diseases as measured by I¹²⁵-radioimmunoassay. Arthritis Rheum., 26:832–840, 1983.

20. Gioud, M., et al.: Antibodies to native type I and II collagens detected by an enzyme linked immunosorbent assay (ELISA) in rheumatoid arthritis and systemic lupus erythematosus. Coll. Relat. Res., 2:557–564, 1982.
21. Stuart, J.M., Postlethwaite, A.E., and Kang, A.H.: Evidence for cell-mediated immunity to collagen in progressive systemic sclerosis. J. Lab. Clin. Med., 88:601–607, 1976.
22. Foidart, J.M., et al.: Antibodies to type II collagen in relapsing polychondritis. N. Engl. J. Med., 299:1203–1207, 1978.
23. Courtenay, J.S., et al.: Immunization against heterologous type II collagen induces arthritis in mice. Nature, 283:666–668, 1980.
24. Wooley, P.H., et al.: Type II collagen-induced arthritis in mice. I. Major histocompatibility complex (I region) linkage and antibody correlates. J. Exp. Med., 154:688–700, 1981.
25. Cremer, M.A., Stuart J.M., and Townes, A.H.: A study of native type II collagen for adjuvant activity. J. Immunol., 124:2912–2918, 1980.
26. Trentham, D.E., et al.: Autoimmunity to collagen in adjuvant arthritis of rats. J. Clin. Invest., 66:1109–1118, 1980.
27. Iizuka, Y., and Chang, Y.-H.: Adjuvant polyarthritis. VII. The role of type II collagen in pathogenesis. Arthritis Rheum., 25:1325–1332, 1982.
28. Cremer, M.A., et al.: Auricular chondritis in rats. An experimental model of relapsing polychondritis induced with type II collagen. J. Exp. Med., 154:535–540, 1981.
29. Trentham, D.E., et al.: Passive transfer with cells of type II collagen-induced arthritis in rats. J. Clin. Invest., 62:359–366, 1978.
30. Helfgott, S.M., Dynesius-Trentham, R.A., Brahn, E., and Trentham, D.E.: An arthritogenic lymphokine in the rat. J. Exp. Med., 162:1531–1545, 1985.
31. Stuart, J.M., et al.: Type II collagen-induced arthritis in rats. Passive transfer with serum and evidence that IgG anti-collegen antibodies can cause arthritis. J. Exp. Med., 155:1–16, 1982.
32. Stuart, J.M., et al.: Serum transfer of collagen-induced arthritis. II. Identification and localization of autoantibody to type II collagen in donor and recipient rats. Arthritis Rheum., 26:1237–1244, 1983.
33. Stuart, J.M., and Dixon, F.J.: Serum transfer of collagen-induced arthritis in mice. J. Exp. Med., 158:378–392, 1983.
34. Kerwar, S.S., et al.: Type II collagen-induced arthritis: Studies with purified anticollagen immunoglobulin. Arthritis Rheum., 26:1120–1131, 1983.
35. Kerwar, S.S., et al.: Studies of type II collagen-induced polyarthritis: Effect of complement depletion. J. Immunopharmacol., 3:323–337, 1982.
36. Terato, K., et al.: Collagen-induced arthritis in mice. Localization of an arthritogenic determinant to a fragment of the type II collagen molecule. J. Exp. Med., 162:637–646, 1985.
37. Stuart, J.M., Townes, A.S., and Kang, A.H.: Nature and specificity of the immune response to collagen in type II collagen-induced arthritis in mice. J. Clin. Invest., 69:673–683, 1982.
38. Taurog, J.D., et al.: Synergy between adjuvant arthritis, and collagen-induced arthritis in rats. J. Exp. Med., 162:962–978, 1985.
39. Gardner, D.L.: The experimental production of arthritis. Ann. Rheum. Dis., 19:297–317, 1960.
40. Dumonde, D.C., and Gynn, L.E.: The production of arthritis in rabbits by an immunological reaction to fibrin. Br. J. Exp. Pathol., 43:373–383, 1962.
41. Consden, R., et al.: Production of a chronic arthritis with ovalbumin. Its retention in the rabbit knee joint. Ann. Rheum. Dis., 30:307–315, 1971.
42. Cooke, T.D., and Jasin, H.E.: The pathogenesis of chronic inflammation in experimental antigen-induced arthritis. I. The role of antigen on the local immune response. Arthritis Rheum., 15:327–337, 1972.
43. Tateishi, H., Jasin, H.E., and Ziff, M.: Electron microscopic study of synovial membrane and cartilage in a ferritin-induced arthritis. Arthritis Rheum., 16:133–134, 1973.
44. Graham, R.C., and Shannon, S.L.: Peroxidase arthritis. I. An immunologically mediated response with ultrastructural cytochemical localization of antigen and specific antibody. Am. J. Pathol., 67:69–82, 1972.
45. Brackertz, D., Mitchell, G.F., and Mackay, I.R.: Antigen-induced arthritis in mice. I. Induction of arthritis in various strains of mice. Arthritis Rheum., 20:841–850, 1977.
46. DeShazo, D.V., Henson, P., and Cochrane, C.G.: Acute immunologic arthritis in rabbits. J. Clin. Invest., 51:50–57, 1972.
47. Cooke, T.D., Hurd, E.R., Ziff, M., and Jasin, H.E.: The pathogenesis of chronic inflammation in experimental antigen-induced arthritis. II. Preferential localization of antigen-antibody complexes to collagenous tissues. J. Exp. Med., 135:323–328, 1972.
48. Ugai, K., Ziff, M., and Jasin, H.E.: Interaction of polymorphonuclear leukocytes with immune complexes trapped in joint collagenous tissues. Arthritis Rheum., 22:353–364, 1979.
49. Fox, A., and Glynn, L.E.: Persistence of antigen in non-arthritic joints. Ann. Rheum. Dis., 34:431–437, 1975.
50. Menard, H.A., and Denners, J.-C.: Use of a hapten-carrier system in experimental immune arthritis in the rabbit. Arthritis Rheum., 20:1402–1408, 1977.
51. Hollister, J.R., and Mannik, M.: Antigen retention in joint tissues in antigen-induced synovitis. Clin. Exp. Immunol., 16:615–627, 1974.
52. Jasin, H.E.: Mechanism of trapping of immune complexes in joint collagenous tissues. Clin. Exp. Immunol., 22:473–485, 1975.
53. Jasin, H.E., and Cooke, T.D.: The inflammatory role of immune complexes trapped in joint collagenous tissues. Clin. Exp. Immunol., 33:416–424, 1978.
54. van den Berg, W., et al.: Electrical charge of the antigen determines intraarticular antigen handling and chronicity of arthritis in mice. J. Clin. Invest., 74:1850–1859, 1984.
55. Cooke, T.D., et al.: Identification of immunoglobulins and complement in rheumatoid collagenous tissues. Arthritis Rheum., 18:541–551, 1975.
56. Webb, F.W., Ford, P.M., and Glynn, L.E.: Persistence of antigen in rabbit synovial membrane. Br. J. Exp. Pathol., 52:31–35, 1971.
57. Phillips, J.M., Kaklamanis, P., and Glynn, L.E.: Experimental arthritis associated with autoimmunization to inflammatory exudates. Ann. Rheum. Dis., 25:165–174, 1966.
58. Cromartie, W.J., Schwab, J.H., and Craddock, J.G.: The effect of a toxic cellular component of group A streptococci on connective tissue. Am. J. Pathol., 37:79–99, 1960.
59. Ohanian, S.H., and Schwab, J.H.: Persistence of group A streptococcal cell walls related to chronic inflammation of rabbit dermal connective tissue. J. Exp. Med., 125:1137–1148, 1967.
60. Schwab, J.H., et al.: Association of experimental chronic arthritis with the persistence of group A streptococcal cell walls in the articular tissue. J. Bacteriol., 94:1728–1735, 1967.
61. Cromartie, W.J., et al.: Arthritis in rats after systemic injection

of streptococcal cells or cell walls. J. Exp. Med., *146*:1585–1602, 1977.

62. Cromartie, W.J., and Craddock, J.G.: Rheumatic-like cardiac lesions in mice. Science, *154*:285–287, 1966.

63. Schwab, J.H., and Ohanian, S.H.: Degradation of streptococcal cell wall antigens in vivo. J. Bacteriol., *94*:1346–1352, 1967.

64. Dalldorf, F.G., et al.: The relation of experimental arthritis to the distribution of streptococcal cell wall fragments. Am. J. Pathol., *100*:383–402, 1980.

65. Greenblatt, J.J., Hunter, N., and Schwab, J.H.: Antibody response to streptococcal cell wall antigens associated with experimental arthritis in rats. Clin. Exp. Immunol., *42*:450–457, 1980.

66. Hunter, N., et al.: Cell-mediated immune response during experimental arthritis induced in rats with streptococcal cell walls. Clin. Exp. Immunol., *42*:441–449, 1980.

67. Schwab, J.H., et al.: Relationships of complement to experimental arthritis induced in rats with streptococcal cell walls. Immunology, *46*:83–88, 1982.

68. Allen, J.B., et al.: Role of the thymus in streptococcal cell wall–induced arthritis and hepatic granuloma formation. Comparative studies of pathology and cell wall distribution in athymic and euthymic mice. J. Clin. Invest., *76*:1042–1056, 1985.

69. Christian, C.L.: Rheumatoid factor properties of hyperimmune rabbit sera. J. Exp. Med., *118*:827–844, 1963.

70. Bokisch, V.A., Bernstein, D., and Krause, R.M.: Occurrence of 19S and 7S anti-IgG's during hyperimmunization of rabbits with streptococci. J. Exp. Med., *136*:799–815, 1972.

71. Bokisch, V.A., et al.: Isolation and immunochemical characterization of rabbit 7S anti-IgG with restricted heterogeneity. J. Exp. Med., *137*:1354–1368, 1973.

72. Cole, B.C., and Cassell, G.H.: Mycoplasma infections as models of chronic joint inflammation. Arthritis Rheum., *22*:1375–1381, 1979.

73. Cole, B.C., et al.: Chronic proliferative arthritis of mice induced by Mycoplasma arthritidis. I. Induction of disease and histopathological characteristics. Infect. Immun., *4*:344–355, 1971.

74. Sokoloff, L.: Animal model: Arthritis due to mycoplasma in rats and swine. Am. J. Pathol., *73*:261–264, 1973.

75. Washburn, L.R., et al.: Chronic arthritis of rabbits induced by mycoplasmas. I. Clinical microbiologic and histologic features. Arthritis Rheum., *23*:825–836, 1980.

76. Ward, J.R., and Jones, R.S.: The pathogenesis of mycoplasmal (PPLO) arthritis in rats. Arthritis Rheum., *5*:163–175, 1962.

77. Cole, B.C., et al.: Chronic proliferative arthritis of mice induced by Mycoplasma arthritidis. II. Serological responses of the host and effect of vaccines. Infect. Immun., *4*:431–440, 1971.

78. Washburn, L.R., Cole, B.C., and Ward, J.R.: Chronic arthritis of rabbits induced by mycoplasmas. II. Antibody response and the deposition of immune complexes. Arthritis Rheum., *23*:837–845, 1982.

79. Washburn, L.R., Cole, B.C., and Ward, J.R.: Chronic arthritis of rabbits induced by mycoplasmas. III. Induction with nonviable Mycoplasma arthritidis antigens. Arthritis Rheum., *25*:937–946, 1982.

80. Astorga, G.P.: Immunologic studies of an experiment chronic arthritis resembling rheumatoid arthritis. Arthritis Rheum., *12*:589–596, 1969.

81. Sikes, D., et al.: Electrophoretic and serologic changes of blood serum of arthritic (rheumatoid) dogs infected with Erysipelothrix insidiosa. Am. J. Vet. Res., *32*:1083–1087, 1971.

82. Sikes, D., Crimmins, L.T., and Fletcher, O.J.: Rheumatoid arthritis of swine: A comparative pathologic study of clinical spontaneous remissions and exacerbations. Am. J. Vet. Res., *30*:753–769, 1969.

83. Steinman, C.R., and Hsu, K.: Specific detection and semiquantitation of microorganisms in tissue by nucleic acid hybridization. II. Investigation of synovia from pigs with chronic Erysipelothrix arthritis. Arthritis Rheum., *19*:38–42, 1976.

84. White, T.G., Puls, J.L., and Mirikitani, F.K.: Rabbit arthritis induced by cell-free extracts of Erysipelothrix. Infect. Immun., *3*:715–722, 1971.

85. Crawford, T.B., Adams, D.S., and Cheevers, W.P.: Chronic arthritis in goats caused by a retrovirus. Science, *207*:997–999, 1980.

86. Pedersen, N.C., Pool, R.R., and O'Brien, T.: Feline chronic progressive polyarthritis. Am. J. Vet. Res., *41*:522–535, 1980.

87. Webb, F.W., et al.: Experimental viral arthritis induced with herpes simplex. Arthritis Rheum., *16*:241–250, 1973.

88. Andrews, B.A., et al.: Spontaneous murine lupus-like syndromes: Clinical and immunopathological manifestations in several strains. J. Exp. Med., *148*:1198–1215, 1978.

89. Theofilopoulos, A.N., and Dixon, F.J.: Murine models of systemic lupus erythematosus. Adv. Immunol., *37*:269–390, 1985.

90. Steinberg, A.D., et al.: The cellular and genetic basis of murine lupus. Immunol. Rev., *55*:121–154, 1981.

91. Milich, D.R., and Gershwin, M.E.: The pathogenesis of autoimmunity in New Zealand mice. Semin. Arthritis Rheum., *10*:111–147, 1980.

92. Morton, J.B., and Siegel, B.V.: Transplantation of autoimmune potential. I. Development of antinuclear antibodies in H-2 compatible recipients of NZB bone marrow. Proc. Natl. Acad. Sci. USA., *71*:2162–2165, 1974.

93. Jyonouchi, H., et al.: Age-dependent deficiency of B lymphocyte lineage precursors in NZB mice. J. Exp. Med., *155*:1665–1678, 1982.

94. Hayakawa, K., et al.: The "Ly-1 B" cell subpopulation in normal, immunodefective and autoimmune mice. J. Exp. Med., *157*:202–218, 1983.

95. Hayakawa, K., et al.: Functionally distinct lymphocytes that secrete IgM autoantibodies. Proc. Natl. Acad. Sci. USA., *81*:2494–2498, 1984.

96. Moutsopoulos, H.M., et al.: Demonstration of activation of B lymphocytes in New Zealand mice at birth by an immunoradiometric assay for murine IgM. J. Immunol., *119*:1639–1644, 1977.

97. Manny, N., Datta, S.K., and Schwartz, R.S.: Synthesis of IgM by cells of NZB and SWR mice and their crosses. J. Immunol., *122*:1220–1227, 1979.

98. Kincade, P.W., et al.: Abnormalities in clonable B lymphocytes and myeloid progenitors in autoimmune NZB mice. Proc. Natl. Acad. Sci. USA, *76*:3464–3468, 1979.

99. Goldings, E.A.: Defective B cell tolerance induction in New Zealand Black mice. I. Macrophage independence and comparison with other autoimmune strains. J. Immunol., *131*:2630–2634, 1983.

100. Brooks, M.S., and Aldo-Benson, M.: Defects in antigen-specific immune tolerance in continuous B cell lines from autoimmune mice. J. Clin. Invest., *78*:784–789, 1986.

101. Cowdery, J.S., Jacobi, S.M., Pitts, A.K., and Tyler, T.L.: Defective B cell clonal regulation and autoantibody production in New Zealand black mice. J. Immunol., *138*:760–764, 1987.

102. Glimcher, L.H., et al.: The autologous mixed lymphocyte re-

action in strains of mice with autoimmune disease. J. Immunol., 125:1832–1838, 1980.

103. Dauphinee, M.J., et al.: Interleukin 2 deficiency is a common feature of autoimmune mice. J. Immunol., 127:2483–2487, 1981.

104. Gerber, N.L., et al.: Loss with age in NZB/W mice of thymic suppressor cells in the graft-vs-host reaction. J. Immunol., 113:1618–1625, 1974.

105. Staples, P.J., and Talal, N.: Relative inability to induce tolerance in adult NZB and NZB/NZW F₁ mice. J. Exp. Med., 129:123–139, 1969.

106. Laskin, C.A., et al.: Studies of defective tolerance induction in NZB mice. Evidence for a marrow pre-T cell defect. J. Exp. Med., 155:1025–1036, 1982.

107. Cohen, P.L., and Eisenberg, R.A.: Anti-idiotypic antibodies to the Coombs antibody in NZB F₁ mice. J. Exp. Med., 156:173–180, 1982.

108. Roubinian, J.R., Papoian, R., and Talal, N.: Androgenic hormones modulate autoantibody responses and improve survival in murine lupus. J. Clin. Invest., 59:1066–1070, 1977.

109. Lambert, P.H., and Dixon, F.J.: Pathogenesis of glomerulonephritis of NZB/W mice. J. Exp. Med., 127:507–522, 1968.

110. Izui, S., et al.: Retroviral gp70 immune complexes in NZB × NZW F₂ mice with murine lupus nephritis. J. Exp. Med., 154:517–528, 1981.

111. Izui, S., et al.: Association of circulating retroviral gp70-anti-gp70 immune complexes with murine systemic lupus erythematosus. J. Exp. Med., 149:1099–1116, 1979.

112. Wofsy, D., and Seaman, W.E.: Successful treatment of autoimmunity in NZB/NZW F₁ mice with monoclonal antibody to L3T4. J. Exp. Med., 161:378–391, 1985.

113. Wofsy, D., and Seaman, W.E.: Reversal of advanced murine lupus in NZB/NZW F₁ mice by treatment with monoclonal antibody to L3T4. J. Immunol., 138:3247–3253, 1987.

114. O'Dell, J.R., and Kotzin, B.L.: In vitro production of antihistone antibodies by spleen cells from young autoantibody negative NZB/NZW mice. J. Immunol., 135:1101–1107, 1985.

115. Datta, S.K., Patel, H., and Berry, D.: Induction of a cationic shift in IgG anti-DNA autoantibodies: Role of helper cells with classical and novel phenotypes in three murine models of lupus nephritis. J. Exp. Med., 165:1252–1268, 1987.

116. Laskin, C.A., Haddad, G., and Soloninka, C.A.: Regulatory role of NZB T lymphocytes in the production of anti-DNA antibodies in vitro. J. Immunol., 137:1867–1873, 1986.

117. Talal, N., and Steinberg, A.D.: The pathogenesis of autoimmunity in NZB mice. In Current Topics in Microbiology and Immunology. Edited by W. Arber, et al. New York, Springer-Verlag, 1974, pp. 64–79.

118. Lampert, P.W., and Oldstone, M.: Host IgG and complement deposits in choroid plexus during spontaneous immune complex diseases. Science, 180:408–410, 1973.

119. Gilliam, J.N., Hurd, E.R., and Ziff, M.: Subepidermal deposition of immunoglobulin in NZB/NZW F₁ hybrid mice. J. Immunol., 114:133–137, 1975.

120. Walker, S.E., and Bole, G.G., Jr.: Augmented incidence of neoplasia in NZB/NZW mice treated with long-term cyclophosphamide. J. Lab. Clin. Med., 82:619–633, 1973.

121. Walker, S.E., et al.: Prolonged lifespan and high incidence of neoplasms in NZB/NZW mice treated with hydrocortisone sodium succinate. Kidney Int., 14:151–157, 1978.

122. Zurier, R.B., et al.: Prostaglandin E treatment prevents progression of nephritis in murine lupus erythematosus. J. Clin. Lab. Immunol., 1:95–98, 1978.

123. Hurd, E.R., et al.: Prevention of glomerulonephritis and prolonged survival in New Zealand black/New Zealand white F₁ hybrid mice fed an essential fatty acid–deficient diet. J. Clin. Invest., 67:476–485, 1981.

124. Izui, S., et al.: Low-calorie diet selectively reduces expression of retroviral envelope glycoprotein gp70 in sera of NZBxNZW F₁ hybrid mice. J. Exp. Med., 154:1116–1124, 1981.

125. Beach, R.S., Gershwin, M.E., and Hurley, L.S.: Nutritional factors and autoimmunity. II. Prolongation of survival in zinc-deprived NZB/W mice. J. Immunol., 128:308–313, 1982.

126. Kotzin, B.L., and Strober, S.: Reversal of NZB/NZW disease with total lymphoid irradiation. J. Exp. Med., 150:371–378, 1979.

127. Slavin, S.: Successful treatment of autoimmune disease in (NZB/NZW)F₁ female mice by using fractionated total lymphoid irradiation. Proc. Natl. Acad. Sci. USA, 76:5274–5276, 1979.

128. Adelman, N.E., Watling, D.L., and McDevitt, H.O.: Treatment of (NZBxNZW)F₁ disease with anti-Ia monoclonal antibodies. J. Exp. Med., 158:1350–1355, 1983.

129. Shirai, T.: The genetic basis of autoimmunity in murine lupus. Immunol. Today, 3:187–194, 1982.

130. Datta, S.K., et al.: Analysis of recombinant inbred lines derived from "autoimmune" (NZB) and "high leukemia" (C58) strains: Independent multigenic systems control B cell hyperactivity, retrovirus expression, and autoimmunity. J. Immunol., 129:1539–1544, 1982.

131. Raveche, E.S., et al.: Genetic studies in NZB mice. V. Recombinant inbred lines demonstrate that separate genes control autoimmune phenotype. J. Exp. Med., 153:1187–1197, 1981.

132. Kotzin, B.L., and Palmer, E.D.: The contribution of NZW genes to lupus-like disease in (NZBxNZW)F₁ mice. J. Exp. Med., 165:1237–1251, 1987.

133. Smathers, P.A., et al.: Effects of polyclonal immune stimulators upon NZB.xid congenic mice. J. Immunol., 128:1414–1419, 1982.

134. Eisenberg, R.A., Tan, E.M., and Dixon, F.J.: Presence of anti-Sm reactivity in autoimmune mouse strains. J. Exp. Med., 147:582–587, 1978.

135. Hang, L., Theofilopoulos, A.N., and Dixon, F.J.: A spontaneous rheumatoid arthritis–like disease in MRL/l mice. J. Exp. Med., 155:1690–1701, 1982.

136. Berden, J.J.M., Hang, L., McConahey, P.J., and Dixon, F.J.: Analysis of vascular lesions in murine SLE. I. Association with serologic abnormalities. J. Immunol., 130:1699–1705, 1983.

137. Lafer, E.M., et al.: Polyspecific monoclonal lupus-autoantibodies reactive with both polynucleotides and phospholipids. J. Exp. Med., 153:897–909, 1981.

138. Izui, S., et al.: Selective suppression of retroviral gp70-anti-gp70 immune complex formation by prostaglandin E₁ in murine systemic lupus erythematosus. J. Exp. Med., 152:1645–1658, 1980.

139. Theofilopoulos, A.N., et al.: Inhibition of T cell proliferation and SLE-like syndrome of MRL/l mice by whole body or total lymphoid irradiation. J. Immunol., 125:2137–2142, 1980.

140. Smith, H.R., Chused, T.M., and Steinberg, A.D.: Cyclophosphamide-induced changes in the MRL-lpr/lpr mouse: Effects upon cellular composition, immune function, and disease. Clin. Immunol. Immunopathol., 30:56–61, 1984.

141. Smith, H.R., et al.: Cyclophosphamide induced changes in the MRL-lpr/lpr mouse: Effects upon cellular composition, immune function, and disease. Arthritis Rheum., 26:S76, 1983.

142. Wofsy, D., Ledbetter, J.A., Hendler, P.L., and Seaman, W.E.:

Treatment of murine lupus with monoclonal anti-T cell antibody. J. Immunol., *134*:852–857, 1985.

143. Pisetsky, D.S., et al.: lpr gene control of the anti-DNA antibody response. J. Immunol., *128*:2322–2325, 1982.

144. Kelley, V.E., and Roths, J.B.: Interaction of mutant lpr gene with background strain influences renal disease. Clin. Immunol. Immunopathol., *37*:220–229, 1985.

145. Davidson, W.F., et al.: Phenotypic, functional and molecular genetic comparisons of the abnormal lymphoid cells of C3H-lpr/lpr and CD3-gld/gld mice. J. Immunol., *136*:4075–4084, 1986.

146. Prud'homme, G.J., et al.: Identification of a B cell differentiation factor(s) spontaneously produced by proliferating T cells in murine lupus strains of the lpr/lpr genotype. J. Exp. Med., *157*:730–742, 1983.

147. Altman, A., et al.: Analysis of T cell function in autoimmune murine strains. J. Exp. Med., *154*:791–808, 1981.

148. Wofsy, D., et al.: Deficient interleukin 2 activity in MRL/Mp and C57BL/6J mice bearing the lpr gene. J. Exp. Med., *154*:1671–1680, 1981.

149. Kelley, V.E., and Roths, J.B.: Increase in macrophage Ia expression in autoimmune mice: Role of the Lpr gene. J. Immunol., *129*:923–925, 1982.

150. Wofsy, D., Kerger, C.E., Seaman, W.E.: Monocytosis in the BXSB model for systemic lupus erythematosus. J. Exp. Med., *159*:629–634, 1984.

151. Hang, L.M., Izui, S., and Dixon, F.J.: (NZWxBXSB)F₁ hybrid, a model of acute lupus and coronary vascular disease with myocardial infarction. J. Exp. Med., *154*:216–221, 1981.

152. Eisenberg, R.A., and Dixon, F.J.: Effect of castration on male-determined acceleration of autoimmune disease in BXSB mice. J. Immunol., *125*:1959–1961, 1980.

153. Murphy, E., and Roths, J.B.: A Y chromosome associated factor in strain BXSB producing accelerated autoimmunity and lymphoproliferation. Arthritis Rheum., *22*:1188–1194, 1979.

154. Smith, H.R., et al.: Evidence for thymic regulation of autoimmunity in BXSB mice: Acceleration of disease by neonatal thymectomy. J. Immunol., *130*:1200–1204, 1983.

155. Wofsy, D.: Administration of monoclonal anti-T cell antibodies retards murine lupus in BXBS mice. J. Immunol., *36*:4544–4545, 1986.

156. Prud'homme, G.J., et al.: B cell dependence on and response to accessory signals in murine lupus strain. J. Exp. Med., *157*:1815–1827, 1983.

157. Hang, L., et al.: The cellular basis for resistance to induction of tolerance in BXSB systemic lupus erythematosus male mice. J. Immunol., *129*:787–789, 1982.

158. Elson, C.J.: Autoantibodies typical of SLE and graft-vs-host reactions. Immunol. Today, *3*:181–182, 1982.

159. Gleichmann, E., Van Elven, E.H., and VandenVeen, J.P.W.: A systemic lupus erythematosus (SLE)-like disease in mice induced by abnormal T-B cell cooperation. Preferential formation of autoantibodies characteristic of SLE. Eur. J. Immunol., *12*:152–159, 1982.

160. Stastny, P., Stembridge, V.A., and Ziff, M.: Homologous disease in the adult rat, a model for autoimmune disease. I. General features of cutaneous lesions. J. Exp. Med., *118*:635–648, 1963.

161. Jaffee, B.D., and Claman, H.H.: Chronic graft-versus-host disease (GVHD) as a model for scleroderma. I. Description of model systems. Cell. Immunol., *77*:1–12, 1983.

162. Rolink, A.G., Gleichmann, H., and Gleichmann, E.: Diseases caused by reactions of T lymphocytes to incompatible structures of the major histocompatibility complex. VII. Immune-complex glomerulonephritis. J. Immunol., *130*:209–215, 1983.

163. Eisenberg, R.A., and Cohen, P.L.: Class II major histocompatibility antigens and the etiology of systemic lupus erythematosus. Clin. Immunol. Immunopathol., *29*:1–6, 1983.

164. Walker, S.E., et al.: Palmerston-North mice, a new animal model for systemic lupus erythematosus. J. Lab. Clin. Med., *92*:932–945, 1978.

165. Davidson, W.F., et al.: Phenotypic and functional effects of the motheaten gene on murine T and B lymphocytes. J. Immunol., *122*:884, 891, 1978.

166. Roths, J.B., Murphy, E.D., and Eicher, E.M.: A new mutation, gld, that produces lymphoproliferation and autoimmunity in C3H/HeJ mice. J. Exp. Med., *159*:1–20, 1984.

INFECTIOUS AGENTS IN CHRONIC RHEUMATIC DISEASE

31

PAUL E. PHILLIPS

Genetic factors, immune responses, and inflammation are clearly involved in the pathogenesis of the systemic connective tissue diseases (CTDs). Histocompatibility antigen gene associations with specific CTDs have been defined; these genes probably affect immunoregulation, which seems to be disordered in most CTDs. Humoral and cellular immune responses to various antigens, many of host origin, apparently result in inflammation in various tissues.

The role of chronic infection in pathogenesis is less clear. Hypotheses are based on both animal models of disease and human arthritides in which the causal roles of microbial agents are explicit. The striking clinical and pathologic similarities between certain naturally occurring infectious diseases in animals and human diseases such as rheumatoid arthritis (RA), systemic lupus erythematosus (SLE), and vasculitis have stimulated a search for microbial etiologies of the human syndromes. With a few exceptions, such as hepatitis B–associated vasculitis and, more recently, Lyme disease, these efforts have been unsuccessful. However, as the few successes demonstrate, this generally negative experience is not definitive. For instance, successful microbial rescue may require as-yet-unrecognized experimental conditions: some clearly infectious agents, such as those in Whipple's disease and, until recently, Lyme disease, cannot be propagated in the laboratory under any known conditions. Furthermore, chronic arthritis initiated by infection in experimental animals may progress even when the microbial agent is no longer demonstrable. Even after a specific microorganism has been identi-

fied, its role must be defined: is it a nonspecific, perhaps even trivial, trigger, or is its persistence in some form essential to the recurring and chronic patterns of the CTD?

This chapter focuses on microbes as inciting or perpetuating factors in the pathogenesis of CTD. Known infections causing rheumatic disease in humans are used to illustrate the various microbe-host interactions that could lead to CTD, and the evidence for specific microbial involvement in each CTD is reviewed with emphasis on recent studies and controversial areas. Earlier work was discussed and referenced in previous editions of this book.[1]

MICROBE-HOST INTERACTION

It is difficult to test hypotheses for microbial roles in the CTD experimentally because the three principal factors in microbe-host interactions—host susceptibility, tropism of the microbe, and the host response—vary greatly.[1] The first two determine whether infection actually occurs. Host susceptibility can involve genetic factors that, for instance, can determine the presence of specific microbial receptors on cells. It is also affected by pre-existing immunity, including cross-reactivity toward other antigenically related microbes, and by the size and route of the microbial inoculum. Susceptibility can also influence the course and outcome of infection, but here microbial tropism and the host immune response are more important. Tropism refers not only to the species, but also to the cell type and tissues preferentially infected, and to whether infection is local or systemic. Local or distant damage may be caused by microbial replication or release of toxins. In the nonimmune host, the initial response can include interferon production, complement activation, local inflammation, and pyrogen or toxin release. Thereafter, the host develops specific immunity, and additional mechanisms for cell and tissue damage become operative. The importance of each immune mechanism in eliminating the infection varies with the specific microbe. Systemic spread is generally reduced or terminated by development of circulating antibody, but circulating or in situ immune complexes with microbial antigens may be formed, resulting in inflammation. Specific cellular immunity destroys intact bacteria and virus-infected cells. Residual or released microbes and their components are further degraded and eliminated by specific humoral and cellular recognition. The successful conclusion of these events is termination of infection and its symptoms, but if the microbe or its antigens persist or if reinfection occurs, recurrent or chronic inflammatory disease may result.[2] These results can also occur if the host responds immunologically to self-antigens, whether altered by inflammation or cross-reacting with microbial antigens. Rheumatic disease results if any of these mechanisms involves joint or other connective tissues and, depending on the specific microbe-host interaction, can vary in both severity and duration.

HUMAN MODELS FOR INFECTION IN THE CONNECTIVE TISSUE DISEASES

Animal models of chronic infection causing immunologically mediated disease are discussed in Chapter 30. The most significant recent development has concerned persistent infections with the lentivirus subfamily of retroviruses, particularly caprine arthritis-encephalitis, a model for RA, and equine infectious anemia, a model for SLE.[3] These important animal models have been overshadowed by the interest in Acquired Immune Deficiency Syndrome (AIDS), which is caused by another lentivirus, the human immunodeficiency virus (HIV).[4] As discussed below, the pathogenesis of SLE might mirror in reverse what happens in AIDS. Several other known infections causing rheumatic disease in humans are also useful as models, some for articular, and others for systemic CTD.

ARTICULAR CTD

The acute and subacute rheumatic systems occurring during certain recognized infections in humans are potential models for the pathogenesis of CTD primarily affecting joints, such as RA.[5] The pathogenesis of these models is not entirely understood, but a general classification can be made based on the relative importance of (1) presence of the microbe or its antigens in the local tissue, (2) the host immune response to the microbe, and (3) local presence of a host antigen cross-reactive with the microbe (Table 31-1). The causative microbes in most of these models are also candidate etiologic agents in the CTD themselves.

The arthritis occurring rarely after smallpox vaccination is an example of rheumatic disease resulting primarily from local presence of the microbe in the joint. The DNA poxvirus replicates there, causing cell necrosis and inflammation, perhaps by viral stimulation of synovial prostaglandin synthesis,[6] resulting in a monoarthritis lasting several weeks. The virus is then eliminated by the host immune response, inflammation resolves, and the arthritis does not recur. Arthritis thus results primarily from direct virus-induced cell damage; the major contribution of the immune response is to eliminate the virus. Unless a local host antigen was altered by the inflammation to become a perpetuating stimulus, this model for articular CTD is unlikely.

The arthritis occurring with acute hepatitis B (HB) virus infection is an example of rheumatic disease resulting from the immune response to the microbe or its antigens present somewhere other than the joint. Polyarthralgias, arthritis, and urticaria occur relatively early after infection with this DNA hepadnavirus, along with hypocomplementemia and HB antigenemia. The symptoms resolve with appearance of HB antibody and clinical hepatitis, disappearance of HB antigen, and normalization of serum complement. This serum sickness-like illness results from formation and deposition of circulating HB antigen-antibody immune complexes. Without any perpetuating antigen, this is also an unlikely model. The role of persistent HB infection in systemic vasculitis and other immunologically mediated diseases is discussed subsequently.

Rubella, an RNA togavirus, can be acquired either naturally or by immunization. It provides an example of rheumatic disease resulting from the immune response to the microbe or to its antigens present locally. Polyarthralgias and, less often, arthritis occur following viremia, coincident with or after antibody appearance. Virus has been found in the joint early in

Table 31–1.   Models for CTD Primarily Involving Joints: Human Arthritis with Known Infections

	Vaccinia Arthritis	Acute Hepatitis B Arthritis	Rubella Arthritis	Rheumatic Fever with Carditis	Lyme Disease
Local infection	+	0	+	0	+
Host immune response	0	+	+	+	+
Local cross-reactive host antigen	0	0	0	+	+

infection and possibly as late as 4 months after vaccination. Thus, although rubella replication generally does not destroy cells, it might cause joint disease directly early in infection. Most rheumatic symptoms occur later, probably from the immune response to virus or its antigens persisting locally for some weeks or months in joint tissues before being eliminated. An inflammation-altered host antigen might also contribute to perpetuation.

Rarely, rubella arthritis becomes chronic.[7] Studies on whether virus persistence is necessary for chronicity have generally been negative, but recently the virus was isolated from peripheral blood lymphocytes of 10 patients with chronic rubella arthritis up to 7 years after infection.[8] This discovery was somewhat surprising considering the previous difficulty of isolation even during the acute period. That previous failures may have been due to use of insensitive methods is illustrated by virus isolations from acute rubella arthritis synovial fluid requiring up to 11 blind cell culture passages in vitro, 3 being the routine.[9] The virus grew better in vitro at 32°C than at 37°C, as used in most previous studies.[10] In the chronic rubella arthritis study, serum antibody levels were normal, but lymphocyte proliferation in response to rubella antigen was increased compared to controls.[8] These studies suggest that the virus may persist in chronic rubella arthritis, stimulating a cellular immune response. The pathogenesis of antigen- and mycoplasma-induced arthritis in animals is probably similar. This model is applicable to articular CTD and has been a favorite hypothesis for several decades. Some direct evidence supports both the model, as discussed above, and as discussed later, rubella as a candidate etiologic agent in RA and juvenile RA (JRA).

Rheumatic fever, with carditis as the local target, is the best model for rheumatic disease caused by a cross-reactive immune response to local host antigen and a component of the microbial agent. Local presence of the microbe is not necessary. Following a distant streptococcal infection in the pharynx, the host antibody response to a streptococcal antigen cross-reacts with a host antigen present in the heart, resulting in local inflammation. The cycle is repeated or intensified with recurrent infections. Although the cross-reactive host antigen has been demonstrated,

its pathogenic role is less certain because it is not present in other affected tissues such as synovium. Thus, although the explanation outlined here seems best, others are possible. This model, postulating a host antigen in tissues cross-reactive with a microbial antigen, is also an attractive hypothesis for articular CTD. Some direct evidence exists for both the model and streptococcal infection as a candidate agent in RA and JRA.

Lyme disease is perhaps the best microbial model for RA, combining all three factors: local infection, the host immune response, and perhaps a local cross-reactive host antigen. The disease has a variety of acute and chronic manifestations, including proliferative arthritis, and is caused by infection with a spirochete, Borrelia burgdorferi.[11] Antigen-specific immune responses have been demonstrated in blood, cerebrospinal fluid, and the joint, where the microbe appears to persist.[12–14] Recent studies in Lyme neurologic disease suggest that the spirochete and neuronal cells share a cross-reactive antigen.[15] The microorganism can also alter immune responses in an antigen-nonspecific manner: an endotoxin-like substance with mitogenic properties[16] and interleukin-1 are produced,[17] and immunoglobulin production and cellular proliferation by unsensitized cells are increased.[18] Thus, it seems likely that both antigen-specific and nonspecific mechanisms are important in the pathogenesis of Lyme disease.

Taken together, the data from these human models and from the animal models discussed in Chapter 30 support a pathogenetic role both for microbial persistence with antigen-specific immune responses, and for antigen-nonspecific modulation of the immune response by microbial antigens leading to immunodysregulation (Table 31–2). All three factors listed in Table 31–1 could be important: a microbial infection, possibly in joint tissues, induces local inflammation either by an immune response to the microbial antigen, to an inflammation-altered host antigen, or to a cross-reactive host antigen present locally, or by directly inducing immunodysregulation. Local persistence of one or more of these processes then provides the perpetuating stimulus for recurrent or chronic arthritis, perhaps with microbial reinfections as an additional stimulus for exacerbations.

Table 31–2. Current Hypotheses for a Microbial Role in Articular CTD

Sequence: General Microbial Hypothesis
  Local microbial replication (bacteria/mycoplasma/virus)
  Microbe-specific immune response/nonspecific immunodysregulation
  Local antigen(s): microbial/cross-reactive/altered host
  Local inflammation
  Early arthritis
  Persistent local antigen(s): microbial/cross-reactive/altered host
  Persistent local inflammation
  Recurrent/chronic arthritis

Alternative Sequence: Bacterial Debris Hypothesis
  Endogenous gastrointestinal bacterial antigens
  Microbe-specific immune response
  Nonspecific immune response: rheumatoid factor
  Immune complex formation: local/systemic
  Recurrent/chronic arthritis

Alternative Sequence: Cross-Tolerance Hypothesis
  Endogenous/exogenous microbial infection
  Microbe-specific immune response
  Cross-reactive host antigen: HLA B27/other
  Local inflammation
  Recurrent/chronic arthritis

Many variations of this basic theme can be constructed to account for specific features of particular diseases. One is the bacterial debris hypothesis (Table 31–2) that endogenous gut bacteria provide microbial host antigen, and various immune complexes are formed by specific antibody, alteration of host IgG, and the induction of rheumatoid factor.[19] Formation of such complexes in joints results in articular CTD, whereas circulating complexes lead to systemic CTD. This mechanism could account for rheumatic disease after intestinal bypass surgery or inflammatory bowel disease. Alternatively, endogenous or exogenous microbial antigens can cross-react with host antigens, perhaps HLA-determined (Table 31–2).[20] Experimentally, monoclonal antibodies to many different viruses often cross-react with normal tissues.[21] Autoantibodies have also been postulated to be anti-idiotype antibodies to antiviral antibodies,[22] perhaps particularly involving viral and host cell Fc receptors.[23] Cellular oncogene activation, perhaps virus-induced, with the production of various specific cell growth factors could also be an important mechanism leading to immunodysregulation.[24]

SYSTEMIC CTD

Except for the bacterial debris hypothesis, the articular CTD models discussed above are not readily applicable to systemic CTD. The association of necrotizing vasculitis with hepatitis B (HB) virus infection was the first example of a CTD caused by chronic virus infection.[25] It is also an excellent model for other systemic CTD like SLE.

Although there may be some geographic variation, 30 to 50% of American and European patients with systemic vasculitis have evidence of chronic HB infection.[26,27] The clinical presentation of HB-positive patients may differ somewhat from the HB-negative group, but they are otherwise similar in the profound severity of their illness, their articular, central nervous system, renal, and other system involvement, their often poor response to treatment, and their generally poor prognosis.[28]

The frequency of vasculitis is low in chronic HB surface antigen (HBsAg) carriers—about 1% in a hemodialysis group.[29] Infection can be acquired parenterally or by contact, with vasculitis beginning 1.5 to 18 months later.[30] Clinical hepatitis occurs, if at all, 3 to 4 months before the vasculitis.[28] HBsAg is usually found in the blood using immunologic or ultrastructural methods. It is also present in vasculitic lesions by immunofluoresence, along with IgM and C3. The later appearance of specific antibody correlates with the recovery from acute illness. Antibody to core antigen is present in most patients, even those with persisting HBsAg.[27]

There is considerable evidence for a circulating immune complex pathogenesis of HB vasculitis. This includes the aggregated electron microscopic appearance of HB viral components from serum, suggesting they are complexed with antibody, the immunoreactants found in the lesions, the hypocomplementemia usually found during active disease, and the occasional presence of HBsAg and specific antibody simultaneously in blood.[25–27,31,32] However, direct demonstration of immune complexes has been difficult, with some types of tests negative and others positive, and the presence of complexes often does not correlate with clinical activity. In fact, both direct and indirect evidence of immune complexes is often present in other HB-associated diseases and even asymptomatic carriers.[33–37] In addition, the demonstration of specific antibody together with antigen in vascular lesions has been difficult,[28–32] although it has been done in serum.[33,37]

Thus, vasculitis probably results from the immune response to persistent systemic virus replication, with circulating immune complex formation and deposition. The clearance of such complexes can be impaired by defective Kupffer's cell function caused by viral damage or overload. Composition, size, complement-fixing ability, and timing of the complexes are factors affecting potential pathogenicity. In situ immune complex formation may also occur, and factors in addition to the humoral immune response are probably involved. For instance, at the subcellular level, host genetic control of virus and virus component production apparently leads to the vast excess of circulating HBsAg. The enhanced immunogenicity of the HB core antigen may reflect its ability to directly induce B-cell antibody production.[38] Still unrecognized virus strain variations or an abnormal cellular immune response might also be involved. Thus, HB infection can be viewed as the cause of a subset of necrotizing vasculitis, but only in concert with other equally critical host factors. An extraordinarily broad spectrum of immunopathology can occur during HB infections, ranging from the often fatal vasculitis or the acute arthritis discussed here, to both acute and chronic asymptomatic infections.[28,39] HB can also play a role in glomerulonephritis and essential mixed cryoglobulinemia,[40] as discussed later.

AIDS is another potential model for systemic CTD. Its cause, HIV, is one of a growing number of human retroviruses,[4] the first of which, the human T-lymphotropic virus type I (HTLV-I), causes adult T-cell leukemia.[41] Both HTLV-I and the related virus HTLV-II, which has been associated with hairy cell leukemia,[42] can transform human T cells in vitro,[43] while the less related HIV (formerly HTLV-III) is cytopathic for human T cells.[44] HTLV-IV and several related viruses were isolated recently in Africa; their disease associations are not yet known.

In vivo, these lentiviruses preferentially grow in macrophage/monocyte lineage cells in various organs or T cells. Thus, they can cause disordered immunoregulation in many ways. Using AIDS as an example, HIV binds to the T cell CD4 receptor,[45] infecting this helper/inducer subset preferentially and either interfering with their function or actually killing them.[44] Alternatively, dysfunction could be caused by idiotypic antibody and cytotoxic responses to the HIV envelope glycoprotein bound to CD4, which then cross-reacts with class II major histocompatibility antigens, interfering with the network regulation of the immune response.[46] This might also occur as a result of the widespread infection of macrophages in AIDS.[47,48] HIV can also act as a polyclonal B-cell activator,[49] which could result in the production of pathogenic autoantibodies. Another mechanism for inducing chronic inflammation may be stimulation of interferon production by HIV, leading to increased Ia antigen expression on macrophages and subsequent attraction of lymphocytes.[50]

In AIDS, these perturbations result in a multisystem disease with a number of similarities to SLE—arthralgias, thrombocytopenia, peripheral and central nervous system involvement, hypergammaglobulin-emia, lupus-type anticoagulant, and tubuloreticular inclusions, to name a few.[46,51,52] There are almost certainly other undiscovered retroviruses in humans; these might affect different immunologically active cell subsets, for instance, the T8 suppressor cell subset in SLE.[53] Thus, AIDS, with its profound immunodysregulation, is a good model for the CTD, particularly SLE.

A general hypothesis for microbial involvement in the systemic CTD can be constructed using HB vasculitis and AIDS as models (Table 31–3). This model differs from that for the articular CTD (Table 31–2) in the systemic distribution of both the microbial and host antigens, and in the immune interactions with them. Antigenic debris from endogenous gut bacteria or cross-reactive host antigens (Table 31–2) could also be involved here. Both hypotheses include various alternatives to account for the uncertain role of genetic factors, and the uncertain nature and location of the inciting and perpetuating microbial or host antigens. Other environmental agents (e.g., drugs or sunlight) can either mimic a microbial effect or unbalance a precarious host-microbe relationship in favor of disease. The microbe then might not be the prime immediate cause, but rather part of a multifactorial pathogenesis. These broad hypotheses also provide a framework for future experimentation, e.g., identification of an immune response to the antigens, whatever their origin, that should be present in joint tissues of at least some articular CTD patients.

EVIDENCE IMPLICATING INFECTIOUS AGENTS IN CTD

Many attempts at implicating different classes of microorganisms in most rheumatic syndromes have been made over the last 50 years. With the exception of HB vasculitis and Lyme disease, promising early findings have generally not been subsequently substantiated. Earlier enthusiasms, discussed in detail and referenced in previous editions,[1] are summarized

Table 31–3. Current Hypothesis for a Microbial Role in Systemic CTD

Sequence
Systemic microbial replication
Microbe-specific immune response/nonspecific immunodysregulation
Systemic antigen(s): microbial/cross-reactive/altered host
Immune complex formation: circulating/in situ
Systemic inflammation
Persistent systemic antigen(s)
Recurrent/chronic systemic inflammation

here. More recent efforts and controversial areas are discussed below.

ARTICULAR CTD

Rheumatoid Arthritis (RA). In part because of the ready availability of specimens from this common disease, extensive microbial isolation studies with an imposing array of methods have been done over the years. Attempts at isolating bacteria have not yielded consistent or reproducible results. Nevertheless, interest in the possible role of bacteria or their fragments has increased, largely because of their obvious role in reactive and enteropathic arthritis.[19] Immunologic evidence has been found for the presence of bacterial antigens in rheumatoid synovial fluids,[54] but a mass spectrometric study of synovial fluids and tissues was negative.[55] Regarding specific immunity to bacteria, both normal and high levels of antibodies to various streptococcal cell wall preparations have been found in RA and JRA compared to various controls,[56,57] and antibodies to proteus were higher in RA.[58] Immunoglobulin-secreting cell responses to bacterial peptidoglycan were markedly depressed in RA compared to other arthritides and normal controls.[59] Experimentally, antibodies to streptococcal peptidoglycan cross-reacted with human rheumatoid factor, suggesting an idiotypic complementarity between the two.[60] Cellular responses, but not serum antibodies, to a Mycobacterium tuberculosis fraction were higher in RA, particularly in early disease. Interestingly, antigenic cross-reactivity existed between this fraction and cartilage.[61] Thus, experimental studies provide some support for a link between bacterial infection and RA.

Interest in the role of mycoplasma persists mainly because of the chronic arthritis they cause in animals. Numerous earlier attempts to detect either the microorganisms or specific immunity to them have been generally negative, although antibiotic treatment has been claimed to help.[62] Neither the presence of an incompletely characterized transmissible agent in rheumatoid synovium nor the role of amebic infection in RA has been confirmed.

The enthusiasm for studying particular classes of microbes has been generated largely by available methods—thus the sequence from bacteria to mycoplasma and, during the last 20 years, to viruses. Earlier studies, both published and unpublished, were predominantly negative, including attempts at detecting both DNA and RNA viruses in RA tissues, and at transmitting the disease to baboons.[63]

The most credible current candidates are a parvovirus, Epstein-Barr virus (EBV), and rubella, with the human retroviruses (HTLV), cytomegalovirus (CMV), and others as less likely candidates. Synovial cellular immune responses suggested that CMV and mumps might be involved in RA,[64] and some RA patients had persistent synovial responses to CMV, but confirmatory evidence of CMV infection was not obtained.[65] Earlier, a single CMV isolation was reported from synovial cells.[66] CMV antibodies were not increased generally in RA,[67] but were elevated in some patients with early disease.[68]

Recent studies suggest some RA patients may have antibodies to HTLV-1 antigens,[69,70] but synovial lymphocyte cultures did not produce the viral enzyme reverse transcriptase.[71] Patients with large granular lymphocytic leukemia, which is frequently associated with RA and Felty's syndrome, had antibodies to HTLV-I core proteins, but controls with RA or Felty's alone did not.[72] Influenza, HB, adeno-, and other viruses have been mentioned recently in single reports.

Parvoviruses are small DNA viruses that can cause disease in many vertebrate species. The B19 strain causes erythema infectiosum, a rubella-like illness occurring mostly in children. This is often accompanied by a usually self-limited polyarthritis, particularly in adults.[73] A rare sequelae of B19 parvovirus infection is aplastic anemia. Another parvovirus, called RA-1, has been implicated in RA, initially by finding virus-like particles using electron microscopy, and subsequently by transmission in mice.[74] Further progress has been difficult because the virus cannot be grown in vitro, so that purified virus antigens and specific antisera have not been obtained. Unpublished studies seem to indicate the virus is distinct from other known parvoviruses, including B19. However, its actual human origin is still uncertain, and evidence of infection has been found in osteoarthritis specimens as well.[75] Such data, as have many earlier studies, suggest a possible etiologic role for CMV, HTLV, and parvoviruses, but can also represent isolation of an innocent passenger in vivo, acquisition of a laboratory contaminant in vitro, cross-reacting antibodies, or other problems.

EBV is a DNA herpesvirus that causes infectious mononucleosis. It has also been linked etiologically to Burkitt's lymphoma, nasopharyngeal carcinoma, and recently to a new clinical syndrome, chronic infectious mononucleosis. EBV causes a persistent infection of B-lymphocytes, both in vivo where proliferation is usually checked by T cells, and in vitro where it is not. It is also a polyclonal B-cell activator.[76] EBV was initially implicated in RA by the presence of anti-EBV antibodies in sera. The first observation was that most RA sera reacted with a nuclear antigen from an EBV-infected B-lymphoblastoid cell line.[77] Subsequent studies focusing on whether this RA-nuclear antigen (RANA) was an EBV-induced antigen showed that it resulted from EBV infection in vitro, that anti-RANA was found in vivo only after EBV infection, and that titers, but not prevalence, of anti-RANA and other EBV antibodies were generally increased in RA.[67,68,76,78]

More recent studies have shown that RA sera react with many EBV-specific polypeptides, but also with cellular components,[79] and that anti-RANA correlates best with antibody to the type 2 EBV nuclear antigen (EBNA-2).[80] RA sera also had high antibody titers to synthetic peptides derived from EBNA,[81] but SLE and scleroderma sera were also more reactive in these studies.[79,81] Such molecular biologic techniques have also been applied to defining the fine structure of EBV antigens and the precise specificities of the immune response to them in EBV-associated diseases,[82,83] but they have not yet defined specific abnormalities in RA. To date, genetic factors that explain the different EBV antibody responses in RA have not been identified.[84,85]

The second line of evidence regarding EBV was that RA blood lymphocytes behaved differently in vitro, in particular, transforming into lymphoblastoid cell lines more readily.[76,78,86] This transformation seemed to be due to defective EBV-specific suppressor T-cell function,[76,78] although this defect was variable in RA and also present to some extent in both normal and disease controls.[87] The specific defect might be failure of RA T cells to produce gamma interferon (IFNγ),[88] which in turn might be due to their enhanced sensitivity to the suppressive action of prostaglandins produced by the adherent cell population,[89] although this was not clearly confirmed in another study.[90] IFNγ did inhibit EBV-induced B-cell activation in vitro, although higher doses were required for RA cells.[91] The defect in T-cell suppression in RA patients correlated with increased EBV receptor expression on their lymphoblastoid cell lines.[92]

EBV-infected B cells were more frequent in RA blood,[76] but most studies did not find other evidence for increased virus expression in vivo.[78] Neither RANA nor other EBV antigens or genomes were found in RA tissues, including synovium, using various types of molecular probes.[93,94]

Overall, studies to date suggest that the increased antibody response to EBV antigens in RA could be due to increased viral expression in B cells in vivo, and that this and the abnormal behavior of RA lymphocytes in vitro is due to defective immunoregulation by T cells. The cause of the latter is unknown but is probably not EBV infection, which thus seems unlikely to be a prime cause of RA. The virus may

also act in an antigen-nonspecific manner as a polyclonal B-cell activator. Further studies are needed to determine whether increased expression of EBV in B cells, its effect on their function, or the immune response to it has a role in perpetuation of RA.

Rubella has been a perennial etiologic candidate in RA, but recent studies, like earlier ones, have yielded conflicting results. Repeated virus isolation was reported over a 2-year period from six patients with varying types of chronic arthritis including RA, but the specific identification of the isolates as rubella was not detailed,[95] and the report has been retracted.[96] Apparently rubella-specific immune responses have also been found; B cells secreting antibody to rubella, but only rarely to other viruses, were found in both peripheral blood and synovium of seven RA patients.[97] When indirect leukocyte migration inhibition was used, the cellular response of both rheumatoid synovial and blood lymphocytes to rubella antigen was somewhat more depressed than to other virus antigens,[98] but when proliferation was used, blood lymphocytes were generally hyporesponsive to virus antigens, including rubella.[99] In another study, the synovial lymphocytes of 1 of 10 RA patients proliferated somewhat specifically in response to rubella, and virus was isolated repeatedly from the same joint and from blood.[100,101] However, two careful studies failed to detect any evidence of rubella in RA joint or other tissues.[102,103] Further studies on the possible role of rubella need more rigorous classification of patients, better controls, and specific identification of any virus isolates. Studies relating rubella and JRA are discussed subsequently.

Both humoral and cellular immune responses to other viruses have been examined in RA. Antibodies in serum and synovial fluid to herpesviruses, measles, and other viruses were generally normal,[67,68,96] including in siblings discordant for RA.[104] B cells secreting antibody to various viruses were found rarely in blood and never in synovial tissue.[97] Measles antibodies were elevated in RA sera using immunofluorescence, but neither this nor elevation of any virus antibody other than EBV has been found generally.[1] RA synovial fluid differed from blood lymphocytes in being unable to support herpes simplex virus replication, apparently due to a cell-to-cell interaction, perhaps mediated by IFN.[105] As in SLE, high levels of both IFNα and IFNγ have been shown in RA blood and synovial fluid.[106] IFNα at least results from lymphocyte activation and does not indicate viral infection as directly as IFNγ may.

Earlier studies had not shown specific changes in the cellular response of blood lymphocytes to various viruses,[99] but recently Ford and co-workers reported that RA synovial lymphocytes do respond in a specific manner.[64,65] They had previously focused on Reiter's syndrome, finding that blood mononuclear cells seldom responded to microbial antigens, but that synovial fluid mononuclear cell responses were quite common. These were primarily to ureaplasma and chlamydia in venereally transmitted Reiter's syndrome, and to various enteric bacteria in the enteric form. However, responses were also seen to viral antigens, and unique responses to single microorganisms were seldom found, making their specificity less certain.[107] Concurrently, these workers examined synovial cell responses in RA finding that, in contrast to Reiter's syndrome, responses to the enteric and venereal microorganisms were generally much less, but that responses were usually found to several of the viruses tested, including rubella, mumps, adeno, respiratory syncytial, parainfluenza, reo, measles, and Coxsackie B4 and B5 viruses.[100,107,108] More recently, synovial lymphocyte responses to these antigens, plus CMV and varicella, were examined sequentially in four RA patients. Response patterns were variable, but in two, mumps and CMV, there appeared to be relatively consistent responses to single viruses, as discussed earlier. Substantial responses were also generally observed to one or more other viruses, however.[64,65] Several technical considerations limit the conclusions that can be drawn from these studies, but they indicate the importance of studying the local immune response and are a promising avenue for future investigations.[109]

With these generally inconclusive attempts at implicating specific viruses by different methods, various immunologic and other approaches have been used to detect an antigen unique to rheumatoid synovial cells, whether microbial in origin or not, so far with negative results.

Models for microbial involvement in JRA are similar to those in the adult disease. Earlier attempts at implicating specific agents both in JRA and in the other childhood rheumatic diseases were generally negative.[5] Several studies found increased serum antibodies to bacterial peptidoglycan in JRA, particularly the pauciarticular type with iridocyclitis,[56,57,110] and also in juvenile ankylosing spondylitis (AS).[110] In addition, inflammation of the gut was found endoscopically in 80% of pauciarticular JRA and juvenile AS.[111] The role of bacterial infection in JRA, as in RA, remains speculative.

Disease exacerbation in JRA was associated with preceding viral infections, but serum antiviral antibodies were similar to controls.[112] IFN was not found in JRA sera, but in vitro production was similar or increased compared to controls.[112] In contrast to adult RA, both blood and joint lymphocytes from JRA supported normal herpes simplex virus growth.[113]

Earlier studies of rubella in JRA had been conflicting,[5] and more recently, the claim of rubella isolation from one JRA patient[95] was retracted.[96] JRA blood lymphocytes had been found to be somewhat hyporesponsive to viral antigens including rubella,[98] but the most credible evidence for the association has come from Chantler and co-workers.[114] Rubella was isolated from synovial fluid and/or blood mononuclear cells from one of five systemic JRA, two polyarticular JRA, two of six pauciarticular, and two of six seronegative spondyloarthritis patients. Virus was isolated two or more times from four of the seven patients. Sixteen controls were negative. The virus isolates were specifically identified as rubella using both plaque reduction and immunoprecipitation followed by polyacrylamide gel electrophoresis.[114] The success of this group appears to depend principally on the discovery that lymphoreticular cells harbor the virus for long periods.[8,101]

In summary, there is little firm evidence implicating microbial agents in RA. The abnormalities observed with EBV most likely reflect an underlying immunoregulatory disturbance, the cause of which is still undetermined. Bacterial peptidoglycan, the RA-1 parvovirus, rubella, CMV, and retroviruses are other candidate etiologic agents. In JRA, the evidence implicating rubella is quite strong. These and other studies directly or indirectly implicating other microbes all require confirmation.

The Seronegative Spondyloarthropathies. These rheumatic syndromes share many clinical features such as spondylitis and peripheral arthritis, the absence of rheumatoid factor, and a high prevalence of the histocompatibility antigen gene HLA-B27 (Table 31-4). This gene strongly predisposes toward illness in most white populations, and is also associated with

Table 31-4.   Microorganisms Implicated in the Seronegative Spondyloarthropathies

Reactive Arthritis
   Enteric infection
      Reiter's: Shigella, Salmonella
        Reactive: Yersinia, Campylobacter, Brucella
   Venereal infection
      Reiter's: Chlamydia, Mycoplasma, Neisseria

Enteropathic Arthritis
   Inflammatory bowel disease: ? enteric flora
   Whipple's: Whipple's bacterium
   Intestinal-bypass: Escherichia coli, Bacteroides fragilis

Dermatopathic Arthritis
   Hidradenitis suppurativa/acne conglobata
   Psoriasis

Ankylosing spondylitis: ? Klebsiella

increased severity. Those lacking B27 might have immunologically cross-reactive antigens in the HLA-B7 group, but predisposing genes in nonwhite populations have not been identified.[115–118] Many of these syndromes are also associated with enteric or venereal infection.[116–119]

There is considerable clinical overlap between the various spondyloarthropathies, but particularly between Reiter's syndrome and reactive arthritis. When the distinctive extra-articular features of either disease are lacking, it is difficult to distinguish from seronegative RA. This difficulty has led to proposals that enteric infection is a major factor in RA,[19] and even in other CTDs.[120] Clinically and pathogenetically, Reiter's syndrome can be considered a form of reactive arthritis.[117] Both can follow enteric infection. In postdysenteric Reiter's syndrome, Shigella flexneri subtypes 1b and 2a were positively incriminated, but Shigella sonnei was not.[121] Reactive arthritis has been principally observed in Scandinavia following Yersinia enterocolitica bowel infections, but also after salmonella infections, and more recently Campylobacter jejuni and brucellosis.[116,122,123] The arthritis following yersinia infections occurs almost exclusively with serotypes 0:3 and 0:9, types prevalent in both Europe and Japan. Plasmids seem to determine enteropathogenicity,[124] but whether they are necessary for arthritogenicity is unknown.

Reactive arthritis patients with B27 not only usually have more severe disease, but also show several immunologic abnormalities. T-lymphocytopenia was found, along with decreased suppression of immunoglobulin synthesis in vitro.[125] Yersinia antibody titers were usually elevated, IgA antibodies being particularly associated with the arthritis.[126] The specific cellular response to Yersinia was higher than in seronegative RA patients lacking B27,[125] but lower than in patients with Yersinia infection without arthritis.[127] The latter study also found a depressed response to Escherichia coli, suggesting the enterobacterial common antigen may be involved in pathogenesis of the arthritis. Formation of circulating immune complexes, possibly with the bacteral antigens, may be responsible for the rheumatic symptoms.[128] Leukocyte chemotaxis and chemokinesis were higher in B27-positive subjects with or without Yersinia arthritis. Thus, B27 may predispose to more severe and prolonged symptoms by an enhanced inflammatory response.[129,130]

Reiter's syndrome more commonly follows venereal infection, but the responsible organisms continue to be debated. Candidates include Chlamydia trachomatis, various mycoplasma, and Neisseria gonorrhoeae.[131,132] Earlier studies on the role of chlamydia in sexually acquired reactive arthritis, including Rei-

ter's syndrome, were inconclusive.[132] More recent studies have again implicated these intracellular microorganisms by higher urethral isolation rates, increased antibody levels,[133] and immunologic evidence of chlamydia elementary bodies in joint materials.[134] Arthritis occurred more often in patients with B27, or with high IgG antibody to chlamydia.[133] Chlamydia were isolated from the joint in one case, and infection was definitely implicated even in B27-negative cases.[135] A clear pattern of specific cellular responses has not been reported, but more sensitive assays may yield definitive information.[136] Th exact chlamydia antigen involved is also unknown, but its major glycolipid shares both immunologic and physical characteristics with lipopolysaccharide from enteric bacteria.[137]

The synovial lymphocyte response in Reiter's syndrome to venereal (chlamydia, ureaplasma) or enteric microbial antigens (salmonella, shigella, yersinia, campylobacter) was often increased,[108] as discussed earlier. This increase distinguished between the venereal and enteric forms, and also helped to classify idiopathic knee arthritis.[100,108] The synovial lymphocyte response to the particular microbial antigen was far greater than the blood lymphocyte response in virtually all cases.[100,107,108] Except for the synovial response to ureaplasma, the earlier enthusiasm for mycoplasma in Reiter's syndrome has waned. However, these agents are definitely involved in nongonococcal urethritis, and new species continue to be isolated using more sensitive methods.[138] They continue, therefore, to be candidate etiologic agents. Virologic studies have been generally negative. One study suggested the cellular response to N. gonorrhoeae was increased in Reiter's syndrome.[139] The evidence for a pathogenetic role of cross-reactivity between HLA-B27 and klebsiella is discussed later.

In summary, many microorganisms, both enteric and venereally transmitted, can trigger Reiter's syndrome and reactive arthritis. Recognized agents are yersinia, certain species of shigella and salmonella, campylobacter, probably chlamydia, and possibly mycoplasma.

In enteropathic arthritis (Table 31–4),[119] both spondylitis and peripheral arthritis occur, but only the former is associated with B27. In inflammatory bowel disease, a previously reported transmissible agent was not confirmed. Whipple's disease is caused by an unculturable bacterium, which may invade joint tissues to cause symptoms. After intestinal bypass for morbid obesity, marked overgrowth of Escherichia coli and Bacteroides fragilis can occur in the resulting blind loop. Circulating immune complexes containing antibodies to these bacteria may then cause arthritis, which disappears when the bypass is taken down.[140,141]

"Dermatopathic" arthritis may also occur; severe chronic skin infections were associated with a reactive arthritis-like picture.[142] In psoriatic arthritis, high anti-DNAase B levels seemed to implicate streptococci, but the specificity of the antibody was not shown.[143] A retrovirus-like particle was isolated from a patient with psoriasis and although it has not been grown or fully characterized, possibly virus-related antigens may be expressed in psoriatic as well as other chronic arthritides.[144]

Studies of ankylosing spondylitis (AS), in which B27 is nearly always present, by two groups have implicated enteric bacteria.[20,118] Initially, Ebringer and co-workers found antigenic cross-reactivity between Klebsiella pneumoniae (formerly Aerobacter aerogenes) and the B27 antigen, and that klebsiella bowel infection was more prevalent in active AS.[20,145] Although the latter finding has not been generally confirmed,[146–148] active AS patients do have higher antibodies to klebsiella, and not to other bacteria like proteus.[58] Geczy and co-workers have presented considerable additional evidence for a cross-reactive antigen.[118] Lymphocytes from B27-positive AS proliferated less in response to klebsiella antigens than did those from B27-negative AS or B27-positive or -negative normal individuals. Antisera to certain klebsiella strains were cytotoxic to lymphocytes from 80% of B27-positive AS, 60% of B27-positive RS, and 20% of B27-positive uveitis patients, but not from B27-negative patients or B27-positive or -negative healthy controls.[118,149]

Geczy and co-workers also found that B27-positive but not B27-negative normal lymphocytes were lysed by the antisera after incubation either with a culture filtrate of the particular klebsiella strains,[150] or with a factor from lymphoblastoid cell lines derived from B27-positive AS patients.[151] The modifying factor in the culture filtrate was a 26,000 to 30,000-dalton bacterial outer membrane component. A number of compounds inhibited the modification process, implying a variety of different metabolic pathways were involved.[152] The factor has been partially purified and further characterized enzymatically.[153]

Approximately 8% of random klebsiella isolates had this cross-reactive antigen; they did not share particular capsular serotypes, bacteriophage types, or cultural characteristics.[118,154] Other kinds of bacteria with the cross-reactive antigen were found in all B27-positive AS patients, but only rarely in B27-positive normal persons.[155] T- and B-lymphocytes, platelets, fibroblasts, and lymphoblastoid cell lines from B27-positive AS patients, but not spermatozoa or

erythrocytes, carried the cross-reacting antigen. It persisted for many generations in cultured cells, but lymphocytes from HLA-identical normal siblings of B27-postive AS patients did not carry it.[118] Cytotoxic T-lymphocytes from a B27-positive normal donor were induced in vitro by either B27-positive AS or factor-modified autologous cells, which then specifically lysed B27-positive AS cells but not controls.[156] Antiserum to the factor from a B27-positive AS lymphoblastoid cell line also caused specific lysis.[157]

Geczy has summarized this work as showing that a cross-reactive determinant is present on both B27-positive AS lymphocytes and various strains of enteric bacteria particularly found in AS, which is transmissible between the two in some way, and suggesting that an interaction between the two may be an important early event in AS.[118] However, this area is controversial because of the difficulty other investigators have had in confirming the studies.[148,158,159] Some support has come from exchange of specimens and reagents, which provided confirmatory data.[159,160] Independent confirmation of cross-reactivity was shown between HLA B27-positive AS cells and chlamydia[161] and, using monoclonal antibodies, between HLA B27 and both klebsiella and yersinia.[162] A 6-amino acid homology was identified in HLA B27.1 and Klebsiella pneumoniae nitrogenase; 29% of B27-positive AS patients had serum antibody to the synthesized hexamer, and 46% to a 13-amino acid peptide containing the shared sequence from the klebsiella enzyme, compared to none of B27-positive healthy control individuals.[163] Similar results were obtained in Reiter's syndrome patients; 53% had antibody to the hexamer and 44% to the longer peptide.[163] Clinically, endoscopic evidence of gut inflammation was found in many patients with both adult and juvenile AS, as well as Reiter's syndrome.[111,164]

A number of apparently well-conducted studies, many using shared reagents from Ebringer and Geczy, have failed to confirm these studies.[118,148,158,159] Various assays including cytotoxicity failed to show any cross-reactivity between klebsiella and B27-positive AS cells. Two cell lines did show cross-reactivity, but further studies failed to show a specific antibody-antigen reaction.[165] Likewise, several other groups could not show lymphocytotoxicity of klebsiella antiserum for B27-positive AS cells.[166–168] AS cells did have a heightened lymphokine response to klebsiella in another study, but this was unrelated to the presence of B27, and was thought to be due to polyclonal B-cell activation.[169] Confirmation of a bacterial plasmid carrying the factor cross-reactive with B27 also was not obtained.[168] In Reiter's syndrome, cross-reactivity was not demonstrated between B27 and yersinia or chlamydia,[170] nor were serum antibodies to B27 found in yersinia-reactive arthritis patients or other patients following shigella and campylobacter infections.[171] The B27M2 epitope was not in itself sufficient to produce reactive arthritis after shigella infection.[172] Homology was not found between yersinia or chlamydia plasmids and 71 non-plasmid-carrying enteric bacteria strains associated with reactive arthritis, or with B27-positive DNA.[173] Earlier studies had also failed to provide confirmation, particularly regarding cytoxicity.[174–177]

In summary, the studies by Ebringer, Geczy, and co-workers show that a membrane antigen from particular klebsiella strains cross-reacts with a cell surface antigen determined by HLA-B27, or a closely associated gene, in AS and Reiter's syndrome. After in vitro exposure to klebsiella or B27-positive AS cell lines, normal B27-positive lymphocytes acquire the antigen. Thus, in vivo the cellular antigen seems to be acquired with disease and is not transmitted genetically, whereas in vitro it is transmissible both horizontally and vertically. One possible explanation might be a bacterial plasmid that can also infect human cells.[118] Confirmatory studies by other investigators have yielded conflicting results, but it seems clear that cross-reactivity between certain gut bacteria and HLA-B27 exists. However, similar cross-reactivities between host and environmental antigens (e.g., ABO blood group antigens and Escherichia coli, or DNA and klebsiella) are being described more often.[21,178] Thus, the critical question, still unanswered, is whether the B27-klebsiella cross-reactivity is pathogenetically important in AS.[148] Criticism of the Geczy work has also been directed at the appropriateness of control groups, the possible in vitro effects of in vivo drug treatment, and other technical variables.[179]

In other attempts at implicating microbes in the spondyloarthropathies, various bacteria, chlamydia, mycoplasma and viruses were similarly cytotoxic for B27-positive and -negative fibroblasts.[180] Serum antibodies to chlamydia and measles were not increased in AS.[181,182] Another finding indirectly suggesting a role for infection in B27-associated disease was the temporary T-lymphopenia found in patients with acute uveitis, their household contacts, and in quiescent AS patients, but not their contacts. This finding suggested horizontal transmission of an infective agent during attacks of uveitis.[183]

The clinical similarities of the spondyloarthropathies and their frequent association with both HLA-B27 and microbial infections suggest common pathogenetic mechanisms. The latter may include deposition of immune complexes containing bacterial antigens, or cross-reactivity of such antigens with host target tissue or responding cell antigens. Enteric bacteria, chlamydia, and mycoplasma are all candidate etiologic agents, but proof is difficult because (1) they are often found as normal flora, although only genetically susceptible individuals may acquire disease, and (2) many patients have been treated with antibiotics before they can be studied. Nonetheless, a role for endogenous bacteria in reactive arthritis at least seems certain, and should stimulate further investigation into similar pathogenetic mechanisms in other chronic arthritides.[19]

SYSTEMIC CTD

Systemic Lupus Erythematosus. Interest in the role of microbes, and particularly viruses, has declined both because of their secondary role in New Zealand mouse disease and because of the many negative studies over the past 20 years.[1,184] Earlier anaplasma and mycoplasma isolations from SLE patients and other transmissible effects have not been confirmed.[185] Regarding viruses, the tubuloreticular structures found by electron microscopy in many SLE patients are thought not to be viral, but rather a secondary manifestation of cellular injury. In vitro, they were induced by interferon (IFN),[186] levels of which were frequently high in sera from patients with active SLE.[186,187] This initially suggested an antiviral response, but elevated levels were also found in other CTD,[188] and the IFN is an unusual acid-labile α or leukocyte-derived type.[189,190] Antibodies to IFN have been found in SLE,[191] and it may also be deposited in the kidney.[192] Both the αIFN and the inclusions are also found in AIDS.[52] Interferons are a heterogenous group of substances, including various kinds of viral- and immune-induced compounds, which can alter many cellular, including lymphocyte, functions. It is not clear whether the elevated levels in CTD are a cause or a result of lymphocyte dysfunction,[188] but it seems more likely that they are a direct result of lymphocyte activation rather than of viral infection. Various other electron microscopic inclusions have been seen in SLE tissues, but none are convincingly viral.

During the mid-1970s, interest turned to type C or oncornaviruses, now called retroviruses. These RNA viruses have a unique enzyme, RNA-dependent DNA polymerase, and a characteristic electron microscopic appearance. They are found in many subhuman species and are sometimes oncogenic, but the first human retrovirus, HTLV-I, was isolated only recently.[41] It is one of a growing family of these viruses in humans.[4] Type C viruses were initially implicated in the autoimmune disease of New Zealand mice, but it now appears that any viral pathogenetic role is secondary.[184] Earlier studies of SLE, principally using immunofluorescence and radioimmunoassays with antiviral antisera, suggested that type C virus expression was enhanced,[1] and that virus-related antigens were present in renal glomeruli.[193,194] However, specificity was difficult to prove, especially because these viruses acquire envelopes as they bud from host cells, incorporating and adsorbing components from both the cell and the culture medium. Thus, the antiviral antisera invariably contained nonviral reactivities that often persisted even after extensive absorption.[184,195] Antibody binding to the carbohydrate moiety of viral glycoproteins was shown to be one source of false-positive reactions.[196]

A large number of other studies did not show increased type C virus expression in SLE.[1] Some, including the type C-like particles in placentas, their immunohistologic reactivity with viral antisera,[197,198] serum antibodies to type C viruses using cytotoxicity,[199] or viral enzyme inhibition, showed no difference between SLE patients and normal persons. One study did show baboon endogenous virus enzyme inhibition by 20% of SLE sera,[200] but most studies showed no evidence of viral expression.[201-204] Thus, a pathogenetic role for any of the subhuman type C viruses studied in the past seems unlikely.[1]

Recent studies have applied human retrovirus reagents to SLE. An increased prevalence of high IgM anti-HTLV-I antibodies was found using enzyme immunoassay and protein immunoblotting.[70] In contrast, IgG antibodies to HTLV-I were not elevated in this or several other studies.[70,205-209] Apparent antibody reactivity with both HTLV-I and HIV antigens was found in SLE sera and possible HTLV-I expression was found in cultured blood mononuclear cells.[210] Another study showed reactivity of unspecified autoimmune disease sera with murine retrovirus proteins using immunoblotting.[211] Antibodies to HTLV-2 and HIV have not been found in SLE sera.[70,208,209,212] Neither HTLV-I, HTLV-II, or HIV proviral sequences were found in SLE blood mononuclear cells,[209] but proto-oncogene expression was increased in both SLE and other autoimmune diseases.[213] The latter probably reflects lymphocyte activation, one cause of which can be retrovirus infection. The studies to date do not firmly implicate a retrovirus in SLE but rather, as in multiple sclerosis,[214] suggest that HTLV-I, or more likely, a related virus may be involved in pathogenesis.[70] Considering the recent isolation of the human retroviruses,[41] their T-cell tropism,[4] and their ability to cause immunoregulatory disturbances in both humans[46] and animals,[3]

these viruses remain major etiologic candidates in SLE.[53,215]

Other viruses, viral antigens, and viral genomes that have not been found more frequently, or at all, in SLE tissues include myxoviruses such as measles and influenza, hepatitis B, and papovaviruses. Measuring specific antibody levels has not provided any clues either. Serum antibody levels, particularly against measles and rubella, are often increased in SLE patients compared to controls, but this seems to be part of the general overproduction of antibodies so characteristic of SLE. As in the retrovirus studies, a major problem with these virus antibody tests is that they may also measure antibodies to nonviral antigens (medium, cellular components), which may also be increased in SLE.[216]

Recent studies have shown an increased prevalence in SLE of antibodies to the EBV early antigen,[79] but not to synthetic peptides derived from the EBV nuclear antigen.[81] Two thirds of SLE patients had IgG antibodies to herpes simplex type I, and one third to varicella-zoster. None had IgM antibodies, but controls were not included.[217] Mothers of babies with congenital heart block, who may have SLE, had a slightly increased prevalence of CMV antibodies, but not of EBV viral capsid antibodies, compared to normal controls.[218] One study showed the prevalence of HB antibody was increased in SLE, but not in RA, JRA, polymyalgia rheumatica, temporal arteritis, or other CTDs,[219] but no increase in HB antibody levels was found in another study.[220]

The response to immunization with both bacterial and viral antigens often seems to be blunted in SLE both in vivo and in vitro.[221-223] The nature of the defect is not clear, but theoretically it might reflect prior commitment to other antigens. The finding of antibodies to polynucleotides after viral illness was suggested as a possible mechanism for their occurrence in SLE and other CTD.[224] Cellular reactivity to viral antigens was generally reduced in SLE, probably owing to a generalized functional lymphocyte defect rather than to a failure of specific immune recognition.[225,226]

The La (SS-B), Ro (SS-A), and Smith (Sm) autoantibodies found in SLE and other CTD recognize protein antigens on intracellular ribonucleoprotein particles, including small nuclear RNAs complexed with protein (snRNPs).[227] The La antigen in particular appears to play a role in the functions of cellular mRNA, but also binds to viral mRNAs, including EBV, adeno, and vesicular stomatitis viruses.[228] In another study, antibodies to native DNA in SLE sera inhibited adenovirus DNA synthesis in vitro.[229] Thus, these autoantibodies react with cellular components that may also be involved in viral replication. Whether viruses are actually involved in induction of these autoantibodies is unknown, but these studies indicate a possible mechanism by which viruses could trigger autoimmune abnormalities.

Studies of antilymphocyte and other autoantibodies in family members of SLE patients, human contacts of canine SLE, and canine contacts of human SLE suggested possible horizontal transmission of an infectious agent.[230,231] Subsequent studies comparing microbial antibody titers in SLE patients and examining households with canine SLE have not supported this idea.[232,233] The origin of these autoantibodies is also heterogenous; they can result from viral infection, but they may simply reflect disordered immunoregulation in SLE.

In spite of the lack of evidence implicating infectious agents, it is still likely that SLE requires an initiating event, probably environmental and possibly infectious. In the setting of genetically determined perturbations of the immune system, an infectious trigger could be a trivial event clinically, and could be different in different patients. Once triggered, the immunologic abnormalities might be self-perpetuating so that the persistent infection and foreign antigens, as found in HB vasculitis, might not be needed in SLE. Current evidence has not implicated firmly any specific microbial agents, but on a theoretical basis, the human retroviruses are particularly attractive candidates.

Polymyositis and Dermatomyositis. The possible roles of Toxoplasma gondii and picornaviruses continue to be investigated.[234,235] Approximately 15% of polymyositis patients have high serum toxoplasma antibody levels, many with specific IgM antibodies suggesting current or recent infection.[234,236,237] Isolation attempts have been negative, and the clinical response to specific antimicrobial treatment has been equivocal.[234,236-238] The microorganism has occasionally been demonstrated in muscle using immunofluorescence.[239,240] The etiologic role of toxoplasmosis remains to be established, because latent infection is common and could be secondarily activated by the myositis.

Various possibly viral inclusions have been found in myositis using the electron microscope; the most convincing are the crystalline picornavirus-like arrays. One study found these inclusions could be digested with amylase, suggesting they were in fact glycogen.[241] Virus isolation attempts and antibody studies have not been revealing generally but in some patients have implicated coxsackieviruses, which belong to the picornavirus family. Recent studies, particularly in juvenile dermatomyositis, have shown a higher prevalence of Coxsackie B virus antibodies,[242] and the presence of viral RNA in muscle.[243] The myositis-specific Jo-1 and another autoantibody inhibited aminoacyl-tRNA synthetases, cellular enzymes that can be involved in the replication of RNA viruses like picornaviruses.[244,245] This work is analogous to that discussed above showing that La and other autoantibodies in SLE recognize cellular nucleic acid proteins that can also be involved in viral replication. Another point in favor of a role for coxsackieviruses is the excellent model of myositis in mice caused by the B1 virus.[246]

Influenza occasionally causes a severe acute myositis, but may also cause a syndrome called benign acute childhood myositis, which may be a mild form of polymyositis.[247] Polymyositis has occurred as an early manifestation of AIDS,[248] and has also been associated rarely with hepatitis B and BCG vaccination. Viruses have also been implicated occasionally in other forms of inflammatory muscle disease, such as inclusion body myositis.[249,250]

That such a variety of infectious agents has been implicated, but so rarely and in such a variety of myopathies, suggests again that the infectious triggers may be different in different patients. The underlying mechanisms may also be different, varying from direct invasion of muscle to various immunoregulatory disturbances. To date, toxoplasma and coxsackieviruses have been most firmly implicated in myositis, but only in some cases.

Other CTDs. Necrotizing vasculitis without evidence of HB infection presumably has other causes, possibly also infectious. Some adults presented with serous otitis media and episcleritis, suggesting infection, but virus antibody studies were inconclusive.[251] Streptococcal infection, rubella vaccination, CMV, and trichinosis have been implicated rarely in systemic vasculitis, but in most non-HB cases no agent can be identified. Herpes simplex and HTLV have been implicated in cutaneous vasculitis, as has varicella-zoster in central nervous system vasculitis.[252-254]

Infantile polyarteritis, the most severe form of Kawasaki disease, also called the mucocutaneous lymph node syndrome, has become a major epidemic disease in Japan.[255] Many cases seem to be linked to previous respiratory illnesses, but no specific agents have been identified.[256,257] Various etiologies have been proposed, inluding rickettsia,[258] rug shampoo's mobilizing house dust mites,[259] a variant strain of Propionibacterium acnes spread by mites,[260] a feline virus transmitted by fleas,[261] and retroviruses. The latter were implicated by transient viral reverse transcriptase production from cultured blood mononuclear cells,[262,263] which was also transmitted transiently to an established T-cell line.[263] Rare virus-like structures were also found in the mononuclear cells,[263] but no antibodies to HTLV-I or II, HIV, or simian immunodeficiency virus were found.[264] Overall, a retrovirus is the best current candidate agent in Kawasaki disease.

An infectious cause, particularly viral, has long been suspected in Behçet's disease. Most studies have been negative,[265,266] but several have suggested a possible viral role. As in RA synovial lymphocytes, herpes simplex virus replication was impaired in blood lymphocytes from patients with Behçet's disease, and chromosomal abnormalities were frequent.[267] Nucleic acid hybridization suggested the herpes genome persists in lymphocytes,[268] and blood mononuclear responses to both herpes and varicella-zoster were diminished.[269] As in SLE, IFN levels were also increased in Behçet's sera.[270] Thus, herpesviruses seem to be emerging as candidate agents in Behçet's disease.

Upper respiratory infections were frequently observed in Henoch-Schönlein vasculitis, but specific agents were not implicated.[271] No evidence was found to implicate HB infection in polymyalgia rheumatica and giant cell arteritis,[219,272,273] but possible horizontal transmission between spouses was reported.[274]

Goodpasture's syndrome may follow influenza rarely. Virus-like structures have been found with the electron microscope, but there has been no further evidence for an infectious origin. In children, a variety of antigens may be involved in glomerulonephritis.[275] Streptococcal infection has long been recognized as one of these, although the exact mechanism is still obscure.[276]

Elevated CMV antibodies, including IgM suggesting active infection, were found in Sjögren's syndrome,[277] although an earlier study was negative. EBV antigens and DNA were found in the salivary glands of patients with Sjögren's syndrome,[278] but antibodies to synthetic EBV peptides were not increased.[81] As in RA, these antibodies were significantly higher in scleroderma.[81] Evidence for HB infection was not found in scleroderma.[219]

CMV, as well as other viruses, has rarely been associated with both autoimmune hemolytic anemia and idiopathic thrombocytopenia. HB and other viral antigens were found frequently in the latter disease, but appropriate controls were lacking.[279] Herpesviruses were implicated in a syndrome consisting of arthralgias with acute urinary retention.[280] In Paget's disease, evidence for a chronic paramyxovirus infection continues to accumulate.[281,282] The rarity of most of these other CTD syndromes continues to be a major impediment to investigating their possible infectious etiologies.

Other Hepatitis B Syndromes. The spectrum of immunologic responses to HB infection is broad, ranging from the asymptomatic persistent virus carrier, through the acute arthritis-hepatitis syndrome, to fatal necrotizing vasculitis. Two other immunologically mediated diseases have been associated with HB infection: membranous glomerulonephritis and essential mixed cryoglobulinemia.[28] The former has been associated with HB infection predominantly in childhood; it appears to be the single most common cause.[275] Hepatitis is often present, but may be subclinical or overshadowed by the renal disease. Considerable evidence has been found for an immune complex pathogenesis, but the viral antigen involved is still unclear.

The association of essential mixed cryoglobulinemia with HB infection is more controversial. Initially, most patients were reported to have HB infection,[283] but this finding was not confirmed.[284,285] This was in part owing to differences in the number of patients with chronic liver disease, who had a higher HB prevalence and whom many would term secondary rather than essential cryoglobulinemia.[285] Nevertheless, it seems clear that HB infection, chronic liver disease, and cryoglobulinemia are associated, and that many of the clinical manifestations of the latter are due to immune complex-mediated vasculitis.

HB infection in humans continues to be unique because of the wide spectrum of associated immunologic disease. Recent reports indicate that hepatitis A can also be accompanied by arthralgias and rash acutely, and by arthritis, cutaneous vasculitis and cryoglobulinemia with relapsing infection.[286] Much is yet to be learned about both the viral and host factors involved in the pathogenesis of hepatitis virus infections.

PROBLEMS AND PROSPECTS

Many problems in studies of the role of infectious agents in rheumatic disease can be avoided by proper study design, but others will be recognized only by experimentation. Proper selection of patients, controls, and specimens is critical. Timing (early or late in the disease) may be crucial. Sensitivity of detection methods is also important, but must be balanced with the need for specificity. Culture procedures should include positive and negative controls to allow early recognition of both false-negatives and contaminants. Cross-reactivities of sera and antisera have been particularly troublesome, because there are so many other possible interpretations of a positive result besides specific antibody to the microbe being tested. These include recognition of culture components present on the microbial envelopes,[195,196,216] polyclonal B-cell activation in vivo by microbial agents,[76,287] and recognition of "true" cross-reacting determinants on microbes or microbe-induced host cell components, and host components themselves. This last category may or may not be of pathogenetic importance in the particular disease.[118,148,179,227–229,244,245] Using monoclonal antibodies instead of heteroantisera may help in this situation, but true microbe-host cross-reactions have been recognized increasingly with these reagents as well.[21,288]

Multiple factors, host and environmental, are probably involved in the pathogenesis of CTD. In addition, each of these diseases is really a syndrome, with different factors, and perhaps different environmental agents, involved in different subsets. Recognizable subsets include necrotizing vasculitis with hepatitis B infection, various enteric bacteria in reactive arthritis and Reiter's syndrome, and probably HB in cryoglobulinemia. Other subsets may emerge in the future from the circumstantial evidence now implicating various microbes as candidate etiologic agents. In RA, the abnormalities observed with EBV probably reflect an underlying immunoregulatory disturbance, the cause of which is still undetermined. Other candidates are rubella, which is even more strongly implicated in JRA, a parvovirus, and CMV. Bacterial peptidoglycan may be involved in both RA and JRA. In the spondyloarthropathies, a large body of controversial evidence implicates klebsiella and other enteric bacteria in both AS and Reiter's syndrome, with chlamydia and mycoplasma also implicated in the latter. The human retroviruses are strong candidates in SLE and Kawasaki disease, and perhaps in RA. Toxoplasma and Coxsackie B viruses have been implicated in myositis, herpes may have a role in Behçet's disease, and EBV may have a role in Sjögren's syndrome. These and the studies implicating other microbes, either directly or indirectly, require confirmation and so are necessary and potentially fruitful areas for further investigation.

Identification of other high potential research areas is more difficult. As in the past, much may depend on serendipitous observations. Serum antibody levels or lymphocyte responses to newly discovered agents, such as the human retroviruses, or in strictly defined populations (e.g., by genetic factors such as HLA-B27) may be helpful. Determination of the specificities of the local, as opposed to the systemic, immune response in chronic arthritis, and identification of the antigens and antibodies involved in immune com-

plexes in blood, synovial fluid, and tissues are more direct approaches. Recombinant DNA and monoclonal antibody technologies can determine the fine specificity of antibodies and the fine structure of antigens much better than past methods (e.g., as recently applied to EBV[79–82,288]). Longitudinal epidemiologic studies to elucidate transmission by contact or other vectors may also be worthwhile.

Microbial isolation and nucleic acid and antigen detection studies should use the most sensitive methods available. For instance, the expression of retroviruses is often very restricted, making it necessary to activate and grow the specific cell type in which they reside in order to isolate them.[3,4,41,44] They also show extensive antigenic variation, making immunologic detection methods less reliable. There are shared genomic sequences among all retroviruses, but there are also extensive differences even in the lentivirus subfamily. These differences, along with the potential rarity of infected cells in diseased tissues, make detection with cDNA probes and standard methods more difficult. The polymerase chain reaction method can increase sensitivity many orders of magnitude to overcome this.[289] This method combined with broadly specific oligonucleotide probes has great promise for detecting bacteria as well as other microbes.[290]

Another rewarding area of research should be further definition of the genetic loci involved in the CTD and their mechanisms of action. Genetically determined cell surface components probably act in combination with microbial antigens to allow immunologic recognition of the microbe as foreign. Any microbial antigen cross-reacting with cell surface components could then affect immune responses to other antigens, either up- or down-regulating them.

Initially, the disturbed host response might involve only the microbial agent or a host antigen, but with time, hyper-responsiveness to other host antigens might become established. Identifying specific responses, particularly locally in the tissues where they occur, and the antigens involved should clarify perpetuating mechanisms. Correlation of such responses with predisposing genetic factors might then allow prospective study of high-risk subjects so that microbial inciting events can be identified. Thus, it should be useful to explore disease-perpetuating, as well as disease-initiating, mechanisms in the host.

Antigen-nonspecific responses to microbial components may also be involved in the pathogenesis of CTD (e.g., polyclonal B cell activation by certain viruses[38,49,76]) or stimulation of IFN production. Microbial infection may also perturb normal cellular responses involving oncogene activation and specific cellular growth factor production.[24,213] Monoclonal antibody and recombinant DNA technologies provide the methods necessary to define strain differences in microorganisms from protozoans[291] down to bacterial plasmids,[292] and so should resolve the controversy about klebsiella and the spondyloarthropathies,[148] as well as being broadly applicable to microbial diagnosis.[293] Application of these techniques should eventually allow precise definition of the roles of genetic and microbial factors, and of disordered immunoregulation in the pathogenesis of the CTD.

REFERENCES

1. Phillips, P.E., and Christian, C.L.: Infectious agents in chronic rheumatic diseases. *In* Arthritis and Allied Conditions. Edited by D.J. McCarty. Philadelphia, Lea & Febiger; 9th Ed., 1979, pp. 320–328; 10th Ed., 1985, pp. 431–449.
2. Southern, P., and Oldstone, M.B.A.: Medical consequences of persistent viral infection. N. Engl. J. Med., *314*:359–367, 1986.
3. Haase, A.T.: Pathogenesis of lentivirus infections. Nature, *322*:130–136, 1986.
4. Wong-Staal, F., and Gallo, R.C.: Human T-lymphotropic retroviruses. Nature, *317*:395–403, 1985.
5. Phillips, P.E.: Infection and chronic rheumatic disease in children. Semin. Arthritis Rheum., *10*:92–99, 1980.
6. Yaron, M. et al.: RNA and DNA viral stimulation of prostaglandin E production by human synovial fibroblasts. Arthritis Rheum., *24*:1582–1586, 1981.
7. Polk, B.F., Modlin, J.F., White, J.A., and DeGirolami, P.C.: A controlled comparison of joint reactions among women receiving one of two rubella vaccines. Am. J. Epidemiol., *115*:19–25, 1982.
8. Tingle, A.J. et al.: Postpartum rubella immunization: Association with development of prolonged arthritis, neurological sequelae, and chronic rubella viremia. J. Infect. Dis., *152*:606–612, 1985.
9. Fraser, J.R.E. et al.: Rubella arthritis in adults. Isolation of virus, cytology and other aspects of the synovial reaction. Clin. Exp. Rheum., *1*:287–294, 1983.
10. Cunningham, A.L., and Fraser, J.R.: Persistent rubella virus infection of human synovial cells cultured in vitro. J. Infect. Dis., *151*:638–645, 1985.
11. Steere, A.C. et al.: The spirochetal etiology of Lyme disease. N. Engl. J. Med., *308*:733–740, 1983.
12. Sigal, L.H. et al.: Profliferative responses of mononuclear cells in Lyme disease: Concentration of *Borrelia burgdorferi*-reactive cells in joint fluid. Arthritis Rheum., *29*:761–769, 1986.
13. Pachner, A.R., Sigal, L.H., and Steere, A.C.: Antigen-specific proliferation of CSF lymphocytes in Lyme disease. Neurology, *35*:1642–1644, 1985.
14. Johnson, Y.E. et al.: Lyme arthritis: Spirochetes found in synovial microangiopathic lesions. Am. J. Pathol., *188*:26–34, 1985.
15. Sigal, L.H., and Tatum, A.H.: Molecular mimicry in Lyme neurologic disease: Cross-reactivity between *Borrelia burgdorferi* and neuronal antigens. (Submitted)
16. Beck, G. et al.: Chemical and biological characterization of a lipopolysaccharide extracted from the Lyme disease spirochete *(Borrelia burgdorferi)*. J. Infect. Dis., *152*:108–117, 1985.
17. Habicht, G.S. et al.: Lyme disease spirochetes induce human

18. Sigal, L.H., Steere, A.C., and Dwyer, J.M.: In vivo and in vitro evidence of B cell hyperactivity during Lyme disease. (Submitted)
19. Bennett, J.C.: The infectious etiology of RA: New considerations. Arthritis Rheum., *21*:531–538, 1978.
20. Young, C.R., Ebringer, A., and Archer, J.R.: Immune response inversion after hyperimmunization: Possible mechanism in the pathogenesis of HLA-linked diseases. Ann. Rheum. Dis., *37*:152–158, 1978.
21. Srinivasappa, J. et al.: Molecular mimicry: Frequency of reactivity of monoclonal antiviral antibodies with normal tissues. J. Virol., *57*:397–401, 1986.
22. Plotz, P.H.: Autoantibodies are anti-idiotype antibodies to antiviral antibodies. Lancet, *1*:824–826, 1983.
23. Mouritsen, S.: Rheumatoid factors are anti-idiotypic antibodies against virus-induced anti-Fc receptor antibodies: A hypothesis for the induction of some rheumatoid factors. Scand. J. Immunol., *24*:485–490, 1986.
24. Williams, R.C., Sibbitt, W.L., and Husby, G.: Oncogenes, viruses, or rheumogens? Am. J. Med., *80*:1011–1016, 1986.
25. Gocke, D.J. et al.: Association between polyarteritis and Australia antigen. Lancet, *2*:1149–1153, 1970.
26. Sergent, J.S., Lockshin, M.D., Christian, C.L., and Gocke, D.J.: Vasculitis with hepatitis B antigenemia: Long term observations in nine patients. Medicine, *55*:1–18, 1976.
27. Trepo, C.G., Zuckerman, A.J., Bird, R.C., and Prince, A.M.: The role of circulating hepatitis B antigen/antibody immune complexes in the pathogenesis of vascular and hepatic manifestations in polyarteritis. J. Clin. Pathol., *27*:863–868, 1974.
28. Inman, R.D.: Rheumatic manifestations of hepatitis B virus infection. Semin. Arthritis Rheum., *11*:406–420, 1982.
29. Drueke, T., et al.: Hepatitis B antigen-associated periarteritis nodosa in patients undergoing long-term hemodialysis. Am. J. Med., *68*:86–90, 1980.
30. McMahon, B.J., et al.: Vasculitis in Eskimos living in an area hyperendemic for hepatitis B. JAMA, *244*:2180–2182, 1980.
31. Gower, R.G., et al.: Small vessel vasculitis caused by hepatitis B virus immune complexes. J. Allergy Clin. Immunol., *62*:222–228, 1978.
32. Michalak, T.: Immune complexes of hepatitis B surface antigen in the pathogenesis of periarteritis nodosa. Am. J. Pathol., *90*:619–628, 1978.
33. Inman, R.D. et al.: Isolation and characterization of circulating immune complexes in patients with hepatitis B systemic vasculitis. Clin. Immunol. Immunopathol., *21*:364–374, 1981.
34. Lambert, P.H., et al.: Quantitation of immunoglobulin-associated HBs antigen in patients with acute and chronic hepatitis, in healthy carriers and in polyarteritis nodosa. J. Clin. Lab. Immunol., *3*:1–8, 1980.
35. Levo, Y. et al.: Laboratory stigmata of connective tissue disorders in asymptomatic carriers of hepatitis B virus. Am. J. Med. Sci., *282*:116–119, 1981.
36. Thomas, H.C. et al.: Metabolism of the third component of complement in acute type B hepatitis, HBs antigen positive glomerulonephritis, polyarteritis nodosum, and HBs antigen positive and negative chronic active liver disease. Gastroenterology, *76*:673–679, 1979.
37. Gupta, R.C., and Kohler, P.F.: Identification of HBsAg determinants in immune complexes from hepatitis B virus-associated vasculitis. J. Immunol., *132*:1223–1228, 1984.
38. Milich, D.R., and McLachlan, A.: The nucleocapsid of hep-

atitis B virus is both a T-cell-independent and a T-cell-dependent antigen. Science, 234:1398–1401, 1986.

39. Duffy, J. et al.: Polyarthritis, polyarteritis and hepatitis B. Medicine, 55:19–37, 1976.

40. Shusterman, N., and London, W.T.: Hepatitis B and immune-complex disease. N. Engl. J. Med., 310:43–46, 1984.

41. Poiesz, B.J. et al.: Detection and isolation of type C retrovirus particles from fresh and cultured lymphocytes of a patient with cutaneous T cell lymphoma. Proc. Natl. Acad. Sci. U.S.A., 77:7415–7419, 1980.

42. Rosenblatt, J.D. et al.: A second isolate of HTLV-II associated with atypical hairy-cell leukemia. N. Engl. J. Med., 315:372–377, 1986.

43. Merl, S. et al.: Efficient transformation of previously activated and dividing T-lymphocytes by HTLV. Blood, 64:967–974, 1985.

44. Broder, S., and Gallo, R.C.: A pathogenic retrovirus (HTLV-III) linked to AIDS. N. Engl. J. Med., 311:1292–1297, 1984.

45. McDougal, J.S. et al.: Binding of HTLV-III/LAV to T4+ T cells by a complex of the 100K viral protein and the T4 molecule. Science, 231:382–385, 1986.

46. Ziegler, J.L., and Stites, D.P.: Hypothesis: AIDS is an autoimmune disease directed at the immune system and triggered by a lymphotrophic retrovirus. Clin. Immunol. Immunopathol., 41:305–313, 1986.

47. Gartner, S. et al.: The role of mononuclear phagocytes in HTLV-III/LAV infection. Science, 233:215–219, 1986.

48. Koenig, S. et al.: Detection of AIDS virus in macrophages in brain tissue from AIDS patients with encephalopathy. Science, 233:1089–1093, 1986.

49. Schnittman, S.M. et al.: Direct polyclonal activation of human B lymphocytes by the acquired immune deficiency syndrome virus. Science, 233:1084–1086, 1986.

50. Kennedy, P.G.E. et al.: Persistent expression of Ia antigen and viral genome in visna-maedi virus-induced inflammatory cells. J. Exp. Med., 162:1970–1982, 1985.

51. Cohen, A.J., Philips, T.M., and Kessler, C.M.: Circulating coagulation inhibitors in the acquired immunodeficiency syndrome. Ann. Intern. Med., 104:175–180, 1986.

52. Kostianovsky, M., Orenstein, J.M., Schaff, Z., and Grimley, P.M.: Cytomembranous inclusions observed in acquired immunodeficiency syndrome. Arch. Pathol. Lab. Med., 111:218–222, 1987.

53. Phillips, P.E.: The virus hypothesis in systemic lupus erythematosus. Ann. Intern. Med., 83:709–715, 1975.

54. Bartholomew, L.E., and Bartholomew, F.N.: Antigenic bacterial polysaccharide in rheumatoid synovial effusion. Arthritis Rheum., 22:969–977, 1979.

55. Pritchard, D.G., Settine, R.L., and Bennett, J.C.: Sensitive mass spectrometric procedure for the detection of bacterial cell wall components in rheumatoid joints. Arthritis Rheum., 23:608–610, 1980.

56. Pope, R.M., Rutstein, J.E., and Straus, D.C.: Detection of antibodies to streptococcal mucopeptide in patients with rheumatic disorders and normal controls. Int. Arch. Allergy Appl. Immunol., 67:267–274, 1982.

57. Johnson, P.M. et al.: Antibody to streptococcal cell wall peptidoglycan-polysaccharide polymers in seropositive and seronegative rheumatic disease. Clin. Exp. Immunol., 55:115–124, 1984.

58. Ebringer, A. et al.: Antibodies to proteus in rheumatoid arthritis. Lancet, 2:305–307, 1985.

59. Pardo, I., Carafa, C., Dziarski, R., and Levinson, A.I.: Analysis of in vitro polyclonal B cell differentiation responses to bacterial peptidoglycan and pokeweed mitogen in rheumatoid arthritis. Clin. Exp. Immunol., 56:253–262, 1984.

60. Johnson, P.M., Phua, K.K., and Evans, H.B.: An idiotypic complementarity between rheumatoid factor and anti-peptidoglycan antibodies? Clin. Exp. Immunol., 61:373–378, 1985.

61. Holoshitz, J. et al.: T lymphocytes of rheumatoid arthritis patients show augmented reactivity to a fraction of mycobacteria cross-reactive with cartilage. Lancet, 2:305–309, 1986.

62. Brown, T. McP., Bailey, J.S., Iden, I.I., and Clark, H.W.: Antimycoplasma approach to the mechanism and the control of rheumatoid disease. In Inflammatory Diseases and Copper. Edited by J.R.J. Sorenson. Clifton, NJ, The Humana Press, 1982, pp. 391–407.

63. MacKay, J.M.K. et al.: Aetiology of rheumatoid arthritis: An attempt to transmit an infective agent from patients with rheumatoid arthritis to baboons. Ann. Rheum. Dis., 42:443–447, 1983.

64. Ford, D.K., and da Roza, D.M.: Further observations on the response of synovial lymphocytes to viral antigens in RA. J. Rheumatol., 13:113–117, 1986.

65. Ford, D.K. et al.: Persistent synovial lymphocyte responses to cytomegalovirus antigen in some patients with rheumatoid arthritis. Arthritis Rheum., 30:700–704, 1987.

66. Hamerman, D., Gresser, I., and Smith, C.: Isolation of cytomegalovirus from synovial cells of a patient with rheumatoid arthritis. J. Rheumatol., 9:658–664, 1982.

67. Catalano, M.A. et al.: Antibodies to EBV-determined antigens in normal subjects and in patients with seropositive RA. Proc. Natl. Acad. Sci. U.S.A., 76:5825–5828, 1979.

68. Male, D. et al.: Antibodies to EB virus- and cytomegalovirus-induced antigens in early rheumatoid disease. Clin. Exp. Immunol., 50:341–346, 1982.

69. Blomberg, J., Folsch, G., Nilsson, I., and Faldt, R.: Immunoglobulin G antibodies binding to a synthetic peptide deduced from the nucleotide sequence of the env gene of HTLV I in patients with leukemia and rheumatoid arthritis, HLA sensitized persons and blood donors. Leukemia Research, 9:1111–1116, 1985.

70. Phillips, P.E. et al.: High IgM antibody to human T-lymphotropic virus type I in systemic lupus erythematosus. J. Clin. Immunol., 6:234–241, 1986.

71. Galeazzi, M., Tuzi, T., Amici, C., and Benedetto, A.: Rheumatoid arthritis and human T cell lymphotrophic retroviruses. Arthritis Rheum., 29:1533–1534, 1986. (Letter)

72. Starkebaum, G. et al.: Serum reactivity to human T-cell leukaemia/lymphoma virus type I proteins in patients with large granular lymphocytic leukaemia. Lancet, 1:596–599, 1987.

73. Reid, D.M. et al.: Human parvovirus-associated arthritis: A clinical and laboratory description. Lancet, 1:422–425, 1985.

74. Simpson, R.W. et al.: Association of parvoviruses with rheumatoid arthritis of humans. Science, 223:1425–1428, 1984.

75. Smith, C.: Personal communication, 1987.

76. Tosato, G., and Blaese, R.M.: Epstein-Barr virus infection and immunoregulation in man. Adv. Immunol., 37:99–149, 1985.

77. Alspaugh, M.A., and Tan, E.M.: Serum antibody in RA reactive with a cell-associated antigen. Arthritis Rheum., 19:711–719, 1976.

78. Bluestein, H.G., and Hasler, F.: Epstein-Barr virus and rheumatoid arthritis. Surv. Immunol. Res., 3:70–77, 1984.

79. Sculley, D.G., Sculley, T.B., and Pope, J.H.: Reactions of sera from patients with rheumatoid arthritis, systemic lupus erythematosus and infectious mononucleosis to Epstein-Barr virus-induced polypeptides. J. Gen. Virol., 67:2253–2258, 1986.

80. Sculley, T.B., Pope, J.H., and Hazelton, R.A.: Correlation between the presence of antibodies to the Epstein-Barr virus nuclear antigen type 2 and antibodies to the rheumatoid arthritis nuclear antigen in patients with rheumatoid arthritis. Arthritis Rheum., *29*:964–970, 1986.

81. Rhodes, G. et al.: Human immune responses to synthetic peptides from the Epstein-Barr nuclear antigen. J. Immunol., *134*:211–216, 1985.

82. Miller, G. et al.: Antibody responses to two Epstein-Barr virus nuclear antigens defined by gene transfer. N. Engl. J. Med., *312*:750–755, 1985.

83. Halprin, J. et al.: Enzyme-linked immunosorbent assay of antibodies to Epstein-Barr virus nuclear and early antigens in patients with infectious mononucleosis and nasopharyngeal carcinoma. Ann. Intern. Med., *104*:331–337, 1986.

84. Bell, D.A., and Alspaugh, M.A.: Antibody to rheumatoid arthritis associated nuclear antigen (RANA) in familial rheumatoid arthritis. J. Rheumatol., *11*:277–281, 1984.

85. Cohen, J.H.M. et al.: HLA-DR antigens and the antibody response against Epstein-Barr virus. Tissue Antigens, *23*:156–162, 1984.

86. Slaughter, L. et al.: In vitro effects of EBV on peripheral blood monocytes from patients with rheumatoid arthritis and normal subjects. J. Exp. Med., *148*:1429–1434, 1978.

87. Kahan, A., Kahan, A., Amor, B., and Menkes, C.J.: Different defects of T cell regulation of Epstein-Barr virus-induced B cell activation in rheumatoid arthritis. Arthritis Rheum., *28*:961–970, 1985.

88. Hasler, F., Bluestein, H.G., Zvaifler, N.J., and Epstein, L.B.: Analysis of the defects responsible for the impaired regulation of Epstein-Barr virus-induced B cell proliferation by rheumatoid arthritis lymphocytes. I. Diminished gamma interferon production in response to autologous stimulation. J. Exp. Med., *157*:173–188, 1983.

89. Hasler, F., Bluestein, H.G., Zvaifler, N.J., and Epstein, L.B.: Analysis of the defects responsible for the impaired regulation of EBV-induced B cell proliferation by rheumatoid arthritis lymphocytes. II. Role of monocytes and the increased sensitivity of rheumatoid arthritis lymphocytes to prostaglandin E. J. Immunol., *131*:768–772, 1983.

90. Winrow, V.R. et al.: The effects of adherent cells on measurement of the hyper-responsiveness of rheumatoid B lymphocytes to Epstein-Barr virus. J. Immunol. Methods, *97*:221–227, 1987.

91. Lotz, M. et al.: Effects of recombinant human interferons on rheumatoid arthritis B lymphocytes activated by Epstein-Barr virus. J. Rheumatol., *14*:42–45, 1987.

92. Kahan, A. et al.: Increased expression of Epstein-Barr virus receptor of lymphoblastoid cell lines from subsets of patients with rheumatoid arthritis. J. Rheumatol., *13*:1024–1027, 1986.

93. Alspaugh, M.A., Shoji, H., and Nonoyama, M.: A search for rheumatoid arthritis-associated nuclear antigen and Epstein-Barr virus specific antigens or genomes in tissues and cells from patients with rheumatoid arthritis. Arthritis Rheum., *26*:712–720, 1983.

94. Fox, R.I., Chilton, T., Rhodes, G., and Vaughan, J.H.: Lack of reactivity of rheumatoid arthritis synovial membrane DNA with cloned Epstein-Barr virus DNA probes. J. Immunol., *137*:498–501, 1986.

95. Grahame, R. et al.: Chronic arthritis associated with the presence of intrasynovial rubella virus. Ann. Rheum. Dis., *42*:2–13, 1983.

96. Mims, C.A., Stokes, A., and Grahame, R.: Synthesis of an-

97. Chattopadhyay, H. et al.: Demonstration of anti-rubella antibody secreting cells in RA patients. Scand. J. Immunol., *10*:47–54, 1979.

98. Chattopadhyay, H., Chattopadhyay, C., and Natvig, J.B.: Hyporesponsiveness to virus antigens of rheumatoid synovial and blood lymphocytes using the indirect leucocyte migration inhibition test. Scand. J. Immunol., *10*:585–592, 1979.

99. Wolf, R.E.: Hyporesponsiveness of lymphocytes to virus antigens in RA. Arthritis Rheum., *21*:238–242, 1978.

100. Ford, D.K. et al.: Synovial mononuclear cell responses to rubella antigen in rheumatoid arthritis and unexplained persistent knee arthritis. J. Rheumatol., *9*:420–423, 1982.

101. Chantler, J.K. et al.: Sequential studies on synovial lymphocyte stimulation by rubella antigen, and rubella virus isolation in an adult with persistent arthritis. Ann. Rheum. Dis., *44*:564–568, 1985.

102. Hart, H., and Norval, M.: Search for viruses in rheumatoid macrophage-rich synovial cell populations. Ann. Rheum. Dis., *39*:159–163, 1980.

103. Norval, M., and Smth, C.: Search for viral nucleic acid sequences in rheumatoid cells. Ann. Rheum. Dis., *38*:456–462, 1979.

104. Walker, D.J., Griffiths, I.D., and Madeley, D.: Autoantibodies and antibodies to microorganisms in rheumatoid arthritis: Comparison of histocompatible siblings. J. Rheum., *14*:426–428, 1987.

105. Appleford, D.J.A., and Denman, A.M.: Fate of herpes simplex virus in lymphocytes from inflammatory joint effusions. I. Failure of the virus to grow in cultured lymphocytes. II. Mechanisms of non-permissiveness. Ann. Rheum. Dis., *38*:443–455, 1979.

106. Degre, M., Mellbye, O.J., and Clarke-Jenssen, O.: Immune interferon in serum and synovial fluid in rheumatoid arthritis and related disorders. Ann. Rheum. Dis., *42*:672–676, 1983.

107. Ford, D.K., da Roza, D.M., and Schulzer, M.: Lymphocytes from the site of disease but not blood lymphocytes indicate the cause of arthritis. Ann. Rheum. Dis., *44*:701–710, 1985.

108. Ford, D.K., and da Roza, D.M.: Observations on the responses of synovial lymphocytes to viral antigens in RA and Reiter's syndrome. J. Rheumatol., *10*:643–646, 1983.

109. Phillips, P.E.: Infectious agents in the pathogenesis of rheumatoid arthritis. Semin. Arthritis Rheum., *16*:1–10, 1986.

110. Burgos-Vargas, R., Howard, A., and Ansell, B.M.: Antibodies to peptidoglycan in juvenile onset ankylosing spondylitis and pauciarticular onset juvenile arthritis associated with chronic iridocyclitis. J. Rheumatol., *13*:760–762, 1986.

111. Mielants, H. et al.: Late onset pauciarticular juvenile chronic arthritis: Relation to gut inflammation. J. Rheumatol., *14*:459–465, 1987.

112. Devere-Tyndall, A. et al.: Infection and interferon production in systemic juvenile chronic arthritis: A prospective study. Ann. Rheum. Dis., *43*:1–7, 1984.

113. Hollingsworth, P. et al.: Fate of herpes simplex virus in lymphocytes from blood and joint effusions of systemic and pauciarticular juvenile chronic arthritis. Ann. Rheum. Dis., *42*:14–16, 1983.

114. Chantler, J.K., Tingle, A.J., and Petty, R.E.: Persistent rubella virus infection associated with chronic arthritis in children. N. Engl. J. Med., *313*:1117–1123, 1985.

115. Arnett, F.C., Hochberg, M.C., and Bias, W.B.: Cross-reactive HLA antigens in B27-negative Reiter's syndrome and sacroiliitis. Johns Hopkins Med. J., *141*:193–197, 1977.

116. Alarcon, G.S. et al.: Reactive arthritis associated with brucellosis: HLA studies. J. Rheumatol., 8:621–625, 1981.

117. Leirisalo, M. et al.: Followup study on patients with Reiter's disease and reactive arthritis, with special reference to HLA-B27. Arthritis Rheum., 25:249–259, 1982.

118. McGuigan, L.E., Geczy, A.F., and Edmonds, J.P.: The immunopathology of ankylosing spondylitis—A review. Semin. Arthritis Rheum., 15:81–105, 1985.

119. Inman, R.D.: Arthritis and enteritis—An interface of protean manifestations. J. Rheumatol., 14:406–410, 1987.

120. Larsen, J.H.: *Yersinia enterocolitica* infections and rheumatic disease. Scand. J. Rheumatol., 9:129–137, 1980.

121. Simon, D.G., et al.: Reiter's syndrome following epidemic shigellosis. J. Rheumatol., 8:969–973, 1981.

122. Kosunen, T.U., et al.: Arthritis associated with *Campylobacter jejuni* enteritis. Scand. J. Rheumatol., 10:77–80, 1981.

123. van de Putte, L.B.A. et al.: Reactive arthritis after *Campylobacter jejuni* enteritis. J. Rheumatol., 7:531–535, 1980.

124. Heesemann, J. et al.: Plasmids of human strains of *Yersinia enterocolitica*: Molecular relatedness and possible importance for pathogenesis. J. Infect. Dis., 147:107–115, 1983.

125. Goebel, K-M., Goebel, F-D., and Baier, R.: Impaired cell-mediated immunity among HLA-B27 related rheumatoid variants responding to yersinia antigen. J. Clin. Lab. Immunol., 8:75–81, 1982.

126. Granfors, K., Viljanen, M., Tiilikainen, A., and Toivanen, A.: Persistence of IgM, IgG, and IgA antibodies to yersinia in yersinia arthritis. J. Infect. Dis., 141:424–429, 1980.

127. Leino, R. et al.: Depressed lymphocyte transformation by yersinia and *Escherichia coli* in yersinia arthritis. Ann. Rheum. Dis., 42:176–181, 1983.

128. Manicourt, D.H., and Orloff, S.: Immune complexes in polyarthritis after salmonella gastroenteritis. J. Rheumatol., 8:613–620, 1981.

129. Leirisalo, M. et al.: Chemotaxis in yersinia arthritis. Arthritis Rheum., 23:1036–1044, 1980.

130. Repo, H., Leirisalo, M., Tiilikainen, A., and Laitinen, O.: Chemotaxis in yersinia arthritis. In vitro stimulation of neutrophil migration by HLA-B27 positive and negative sera. Arthritis Rheum., 25:655–661, 1982.

131. Goldenberg, D.L.: "Postinfectious" arthritis. New look at an old concept with particular attention to disseminated gonococcal infection. Am. J. Med., 74:925–928, 1983.

132. Kousa, M.: Evidence of chlamydial involvement in the development of arthritis. Scand. J. Infect. Dis., 32(Suppl):116–121, 1982.

133. Keat, A.C. et al.: Evidence of *Chlamydia trachomatis* infection in sexually acquired reactive arthritis. Ann. Rheum. Dis., 39:431–437, 1980.

134. Keat, A. et al.: *Chlamydia trachomatis* and reactive arthritis: The missing link. Lancet, 1:72–74, 1987.

135. Vilppula, A.H., Yli-Kerttula, U.I., Ahlroos, A.K., and Terho, P.E.: Chlamydial isolations and serology in Reiter's syndrome. Scand. J. Rheumatol., 10:181–185, 1981.

136. Brunham, R.C. et al.: Cellular immune response during uncomplicated genital infection with *Chlamydia trachomatis* in humans. Infect. Immun., 34:98–104, 1981.

137. Nurminen, M., Leinonen, M., Saikku, P., Makela, P.H.: The genus-specific antigen of chlamydia: Resemblance to the lipopolysaccharide of enteric bacteria. Science, 220:1279–1281, 1983.

138. Tully, J.G., Taylor-Robinson, D., Cole, R.M., and Rose, D.L.: A newly discovered mycoplasma in the human urogenital tract. Lancet, 1:1288–1291, 1981.

139. Rosenthal, L., and Danielsson, D.: Induction of DNA synthesis in lymphocytes in vitro by various bacteria, with special reference to *Neisseria gonorrhoeae*, in patients with uro-arthritis (Reiter's disease). Scand. J. Rheumatol., 7:101–108, 1978.

140. Wands, J.R., LaMont, J.T., Manne, E., and Isselbacher, K.J.: Arthritis associated with intestinal-bypass procedure for morbid obesity. N. Engl. J. Med., 294:121–124, 1976.

141. Leff, R.D., Aldo-Benson, M.A., and Madura, J.A.: The effect of revision of the intestinal bypass on post intestinal bypass arthritis. Arthritis Rheum., 26:678–681, 1983.

142. Rosner, I.A., et al.: Spondyloarthropathy associated with hidradenitis suppurativa and acne conglobata. Ann. Intern. Med., 97:520–525, 1982.

143. Vasey, F.B., et al.: Possible involvement of group A streptococci in the pathogenesis of psoriatic arthritis. J. Rheumatol., 9:719–722, 1982.

144. Rodahl, E., and Iversen, O.J.: Analysis of circulating immune complexes from patients with ankylosing spondylitis by gel electrophoresis and immunoblotting using antiserum against a psoriasis associated retrovirus-like particle. Ann. Rheum. Dis., 45:892–898, 1986.

145. Ebringer, R.W., Cawdell, D.R., Cowling, P., and Ebringer, A.: Sequential studies in ankylosing spondylitis: Association of *Klebsiella pneumoniae* with active disease. Ann. Rheum. Dis., 37:146–151, 1978.

146. Warren, R.E., and Brewerton, D.A.: Faecal carriage of klebsiella by patients with ankylosing spondylitis and rheumatoid arthritis. Ann. Rheum. Dis., 39:37–44, 1980.

147. Eastmond, C.J., et al.: A sequential study of the relationship between faecal *Klebsiella aerogenes* and the common clinical manifestations of ankylosing spondylitis. Ann. Rheum. Dis., 41:15–20, 1982.

148. Keat, A.: Is spondylitis caused by klebsiella? Immunology Today, 7:144–149, 1986.

149. Seager, K. et al.: Evidence for a specific B27-associated cell surface marker on lymphocytes of patients with ankylosing spondylitis. Nature, 277:68–70, 1979.

150. Geczy, A.F., Alexander, K., Bashir, H.V., Edmonds, J.P.: Characterization of a factor(s) present in klebsiella culture filtrates that specifically modifies an HLA-B27-associated cell-surface component. J. Exp. Med., 152:331s–340s, 1980.

151. Orban, P. et al.: A factor shed by lymphoblastoid cell lines of HLA-B27 positive patients with ankylosing spondylitis specifically modifies the cells of HLA-B27 positive normal individuals. Clin. Exp. Immunol., 53:10–16, 1983.

152. Sullivan, J.S., and Geczy, A.F.: The modification of HLA-B27-positive lymphocytes by the culture filtrate of *Klebsiella* K43 BTS 1 is a metabolically active process. Clin. Exp. Immunol., 62:672–677, 1985.

153. Upfold, L.I., Sullivan, J.S., and Geczy, A.F.: Biochemical studies on a factor isolated from *Klebsiella* K43-BTS1 that cross-reacts with cells from HLA-B27 positive patients with ankylosing spondylitis. Human Immunology, 17:224–238, 1986.

154. Pease, P.E. et al.: An investigation into the properties of klebsiella strains isolated from ankylosing spondylitis patients. J. Hyg. (Camb.), 89:119–123, 1982.

155. McGuigan, L.E. et al.: Significance of non-pathogenic cross reactive bowel flora in patients with ankylosing spondylitis. Ann. Rheum. Dis., 45:566–571, 1986.

156. Geczy, A.F., McGuigan, L.E., Sullivan, J.S., and Edmonds, J.P.: Cytotoxic T lymphocytes against disease-associated determinants(s) in ankylosing spondylitis. J. Exp. Med., 164:932–937, 1986.

157. Sullivan, J.S., and Geczy, A.F.: An antiserum to a disease-

associated factor from the cells of an HLA-B27 positive patient with ankylosing spondylitis specifically recognizes an HLA-B27 associated determinant. Arthritis Rheum., 30:439–442, 1987.

158. Terasaki, P.I., and Yu, D.T.Y.: Regarding the ankylosing spondylitis/klebsiella/HLA-B27 problem. Arthritis Rheum., 30:353–354, 1987.

159. Geczy, A.F., Sullivan, J.S., and McGuigan, L.E.: Response to the editorial by Terasaki and Yu. Arthritis Rheum., 30:714–715, 1987. (Letter)

160. Geczy, A.F. et al.: Blind confirmation in Leiden of Geczy factor on the cells of Dutch patients with ankylosing spondylitis. Human Immunol., 17:239–245, 1986.

161. Wakefield, D. et al.: Chlamydial antibody cross reactivity with peripheral blood mononuclear cells of patients with ankylosing spondylitis: The role of HLA B27. Clin. Exp. Immunol., 63:49–57, 1986.

162. Ogasawara, M., Kono, D.H., and Yu, D.T.Y.: Mimicry of human histocompatibility HLA-B27 antigens by Klebsiella pneumonia. Infect. Immun., 51:901–908, 1986.

163. Schwimmbeck, P.L., Yu, D.T.Y., and Oldstone, M.B.A.: Autoantibodies to HLA B27 in the sera of HLA B27 patients with ankylosing spondylitis and Reiter's syndrome. J. Exp. Med., 166:173–181, 1987.

164. Mielants, H. et al.: Repeat ileocolonoscopy in reactive arthritis. J. Rheumatol., 14:456–458, 1987.

165. Georgopoulos, K., Dick, W.C., Goodacre, J.A., and Pain, R.H.: A reinvestigation of the cross-reactivity between klebsiella and HLA-B27 in the aetiology of ankylosing spondylitis. Clin. Exp. Immunol., 62:662–671, 1985.

166. Kinsella, T.D., Fritzler, M.J., and Lewkonia, R.M.: Normal anti-klebsiella lymphocytotoxicity in ankylosing spondylitis. Arthritis Rheum., 29:358–362, 1986.

167. Cameron, F.H. et al.: Failure of Klebsiella pneumoniae antibodies to cross-react with peripheral blood mononuclear cells from patients with ankylosing spondylitis. Arthritis Rheum., 30:300–305, 1987.

168. Toubert, A., Philippon, A., and Amor, B.: HLA-B27, ankylosing spondylitis and Klebsiella pneumoniae: Toward a molecular approach. J. Rheumatol., 14:391–393, 1987. (Letter)

169. Gross, W.L., Ludemann, G., Schmidt, K., and Ullmann, U.: Lymphocyte response to klebsiella in ankylosing spondylitis. Eur. J. Clin. Invest., 16:338–346, 1986.

170. Inman, R.D., Chiu, B., Johnston, M.E.A., and Falk, J.: Molecular mimicry in Reiter's syndrome: Cytotoxicity and ELISA studies of HLA-microbial relationships. Immunology 58:501–506, 1986.

171. Cavender, D., and Ziff, M.: Anti-HLA-B27 antibodies in sera from patients with gram-negative bacterial infections. Arthritis Rheum., 29:352–357, 1986.

172. Van Bohemen, C.G. et al.: HLA-B27M1M2 and high immune responsiveness to Shigella flexneri in post-dysenteric arthritis. Immunol. Lett., 13:71–74, 1986.

173. Pulkkinen, L., Vuorio, E., Hyypia, T., and Toivanen, A.: Lack of DNA homology between arthritis triggering bacteria and plasmid of Yersinia enterocolitica or Chlamydia trachomatis. J. Rheumatol., 13:831–833, 1986. (Letter)

174. Archer, J.R.: Search for cross-reactivity between HLA-B27 and Klebsiella pneumoniae. Ann. Rheum. Dis., 40:400–403, 1981.

175. Shinebaum, R., Cooke, E.M., Siegerstetter, J., and Wright, V.: Effect of klebsiella capsular antisera on lymphocytes from patients with ankylosing spondylitis. J. Med. Microbiol., 14:451–456, 1981.

176. Enlow, R.W. et al.: Human lymphocyte response to selected infectious agents in Reiter's syndrome and ankylosing spondylitis. Rheumatol. Int., 1:171–175, 1982.

177. Beaulieu, A.D., Rousseau, F., Israel-Assayag, E., and Roy, R.: Klebsiella-related antigens in ankylosing spondylitis. J. Rheumatol., 10:102–105, 1983.

178. Naparstek, Y. et al.: Immunochemical similarities between monoclonal antibacterial Waldenstrom's macroglobulins and monoclonal anti-DNA lupus autoantibodies. J. Exp. Med., 161:1525–1538, 1985.

179. Kinsella, T.D., Fritzler, M.J., and McNeil, D.J.: Ankylosing spondylitis. A disease in search of microbes. J. Rheumatol., 10:2–4, 1983.

180. Dilley, D., Fan, P.G., and Bluestone, R.: Absence of cytotoxic effect of selected pathogens on HLA B27 positive fibroblasts. Proc. Soc. Exp. Biol. Med., 159:184–186, 1978.

181. Alcalay, M. et al.: Ankylosing spondylitis and chlamydial infection in apparently healthy HLA B27 blood donors. J. Rheumatol., 6:439–446, 1979.

182. Kalliomaki, J.L., Halonen, P., Arnadottir, T., and Voipio-Pulkki, L.M.: Antibodies to measles virus in ankylosing spondylitis. Scand. J. Rheumatol., 12:29–31, 1983.

183. Byrom, N.A. et al.: T and B lymphocytes in patients with acute anterior uveitis and AS, and in their household contacts. Lancet, 2:601–603, 1979.

184. Pincus, T.: Studies regarding a possible function for viruses in the pathogenesis of systemic lupus erythematosus. Arthritis Rheum., 25:847–856, 1982.

185. Kallick, C.A., Thadhani, K.C., and Rice, T.W.: Identification of Anaplasmataceae (haemobartonella) antigen and antibodies in SLE. Arthritis Rheum., 23:197–205, 1980.

186. Rich, S.A.: Human lupus inclusions and interferon. Science, 213:772–775, 1981.

187. Hooks, J.J., et al.: Immune interferon in the circulation of patients with autoimmune disease. N. Engl. J. Med., 301:5–8, 1979.

188. Moutsopoulos, H.M., and Hooks, J.J.: Interferon and autoimmunity. Clin. Exp. Rheum., 1:81–84, 1983.

189. Preble, O.T. et al.: Interferon-induced 2'-5' adenylate synthetase in vivo and interferon production in vitro by lymphocytes from systemic lupus erythematosus patients with and without circulating interferon. J. Exp. Med., 157:2140–2146, 1983.

190. Klippel, J.H. et al.: Serum alpha interferon and lymphocyte inclusions in systemic lupus erythematosus. Ann. Rheum. Dis., 44:104–108, 1985.

191. Suit, B.E. et al.: Detection of anti-interferon antibodies in systemic lupus erythematosus. Clin. Exp. Rheum., 1:133–135, 1983.

192. Panem, S., Ordonez, N., Vilcek, J.: Renal deposition of alpha interferon in systemic lupus erythematosus. Infect. Immun., 42:368–373, 1983.

193. Mellors, R.C., and Mellors, J.W.: Type C RNA virus-specific antibody in human SLE demonstrated by enzymoimmunoassay. Proc. Natl. Acad. Sci. U.S.A., 75:2463–2467, 1978.

194. Reynolds, J.T., and Panem, S.: Characterization of antibody to C-type virus antigens isolated from immune complexes in kidneys of patients with systemic lupus erythematosus. Lab. Invest., 44:410–419, 1981.

195. Pedersen, N.C. et al.: The causes of false-positives encountered during the screening of old-world primates for antibodies to human and simian retroviruses by ELISA. J. Virol. Methods, 14:213–228, 1986.

196. Markenson, J.A., and Snyder, H.W.: Reactivity of antisera to endogenous primate retrovirus with a human T cell mem-

brane protein: Recognition of a nonviral glycoprotein by antibodies directed only against carbohydrate components. J. Immunol., *132*:772–779, 1984.

197. Ueno, H., Imamura, M., and Kikuchi, K.: Frequency and antigenicity of type C retrovirus-like particles in human placentas. Virchows Arch. [A], *400*:31–41, 1983.

198. Maeda, S. et al.: Immunohistologic detection of antigen related to primate type C retrovirus p30 in normal human placentas. Am. J. Pathol., *112*:347–356, 1983.

199. Belkin, R.N., Anderson, K., and Phillips, P.E.: Lack of type C virus antibodies in systemic lupus erythematosus. J. Rheumatol., *9*:613–616, 1982.

200. Okamoto, T., Tamura, T., and Takano, T.: Evidence in patients with SLE of the presence of antibodies against RNA-dependent DNA polymerase of baboon endogenous virus. Clin. Exp. Immunol., *54*:747–755, 1983.

201. Kimura, M., Andoh, T., and Kai, K.: Failure to detect type C virus p30-related antigen in SLE: False positive reaction due to protease reactivity. Arthritis Rheum., *23*:111–113, 1980.

202. Aulakh, G.S., Hicks, J.T., Martin, W.J., and Phillips, P.E.: Search for type C oncornavirus-related genetic information in tissues from patients with systemic lupus erythematosus. Arthritis Rheum., *21*:880–884, 1978.

203. Phillips, P.E., Sellers, S.A., and Cotronei, S.L.: Type C oncornavirus isolation studies in systemic lupus erythematosus. III. Isolation of a putative retrovirus by triple cell fusion. Ann. Rheum. Dis., *37*:234–237, 1978.

204. Hicks, J.T. et al.: Search for Epstein-Barr and type C oncornaviruses in SLE. Arthritis Rheum., *22*:845–857, 1979.

205. Halbert, S.P. et al.: Quantitative estimation of HTLV-I antibodies by a standardized ELISA in adult T cell leukemia and AIDS. J. Clin. Microbiol., *23*:212–216, 1986.

206. Koike, T. et al.: Antibodies to human T cell leukemia virus are absent in patients with SLE. Arthritis Rheum., *28*:481–484, 1985.

207. Kurata, A. et al.: Production of a monoclonal antibody to a membrane antigen of human T-cell leukaemia virus (HTLV I/ATLV)-infected cell lines from a SLE patient; Serological analyses for HTLV I infections in SLE patients. Clin. Exp. Immunol., *62*:65–74, 1985.

208. McDougal, J.S., Kennedy, M.S., Kalyanaraman, V.S., and McDuffie, F.C.: Failure to demonstrate (cross-reacting) antibodies to human T lymphotropic viruses in patients with rheumatic diseases. Arthritis Rheum., *28*:1170–1174, 1985.

209. Boumpas, D.T. et al: Type C retroviruses of the human T cell leukemia family are not evident in patients with SLE. Arthritis Rheum., *29*:185–188, 1986.

210. Olsen, R.G. et al.: Serological and virological evidence of human T-lymphotropic virus in systemic lupus erythematosus. Med. Microbiol. Immunol., *176*:53–64, 1987.

211. Rucheton, M. et al.: Presence of circulating antibodies against gag-gene MuLV proteins in patients with autoimmune connective tissue disorders. Virology, *144*:468–480, 1985.

212. Kaminsky, L.S. et al.: High prevalence of antibodies to acquired immune deficiency syndrome (AIDS)-associated retrovirus (ARV) in AIDS and related conditions but not in other disease states. Proc. Natl. Acad. Sci. U.S.A., *82*:5535–5539, 1985.

213. Boumpas, D.T. et al.: Increased proto-oncogene expression in peripheral blood lymphocytes from patients with systemic lupus erythematosus and other autoimmune diseases. Arthritis Rheum., *29*:755–760, 1986.

214. Ohta, M. et al.: Sera from patients with multiple sclerosis react with human T cell lymphotropic virus-I gag proteins but not

env proteins—Western blotting analysis. J. Immunol., *137*:3440–3443, 1986.

215. Kapusta, M.A.: The virus-activated suppressor cell hypothesis in experimental and human rheumatic diseases. J. Rheumatol., *7*:309–315, 1980.

216. Pincus, T., Steinberg, A.D., Blacklow, N.R., and Decker, J.L.: Reactivities of SLE sera with cellular and virus antigen preparations. Arthritis Rheum., *21*:873–879, 1978.

217. Nagayama, Y., and Kazuyama, Y.: Serum anti-herpes virus antibody titre in patients with active systemic lupus erythematosus. Int. J. Immunotherapy, *3*:59–64, 1987.

218. Taylor, P.V. et al.: Maternal antibodies against fetal cardiac antigens in congenital complete heart block. N. Engl. J. Med., *315*:667–672, 1986.

219. Permin, H., Aldershvile, J., and Nielsen, J.O.: Hepatitis B virus infection in patients with rheumatic diseases. Ann. Rheum. Dis., *41*:479–482, 1982.

220. Bonafede, R.P., Van Staden, M., and Klemp, P.: Hepatitis B virus infection and liver function in patients with systemic lupus erythematosus. J. Rheumatol., *13*:1050–1052, 1986.

221. Jarrett, M.P., Schiffman, G., Barland, P., and Grayzel, A.I.: Impaired response to pneumococcal vaccine in systemic lupus erythematosus. Arthritis Rheum., *23*:1287–1293, 1980.

222. Nies, K., Boyer, R., Stevens, R., and Louie, J.: Antitetanus toxoid antibody synthesis after booster immunization in systemic lupus erythematosus. Arthritis Rheum., *23*:1343–1350, 1980.

223. Mitchell, D.M. et al.: Kinetics of specific anti-influenza antibody production by cultured lymphocytes from patients with systemic lupus erythematosus following influenza immunization. Clin. Exp. Immunol., *49*:290–296, 1982.

224. Spencer-Green, G. et al.: Polynucleotide antibodies in connective tissue disease: Viral markers or disease mediators? J. Lab. Clin. Med., *107*:159–165, 1986.

225. Wolf, R.E., and Ziff, M.: Lymphocyte response to virus antigens in SLE. Arthritis Rheum., *19*:1271–1277, 1976.

226. Pons, V.G., Reinertsen, J.L., Steinberg, A.D., and Dolin, R.: Decreased cell-mediated cytotoxicity against virus-infected cells in SLE. J. Med. Virol., *4*:15–23, 1979.

227. Lerner, E.A., et al.: Deciphering the mysteries of RNA-containing lupus antigens. Arthritis Rheum., *25*:761–766, 1982.

228. Francoeur, A.M., Chan, E.K.L., Garrels, J.I., and Mathews, M.B.: Characterization and purification of lupus antigen La, an RNA-binding protein. Mol. Cell. Biol., *5*:586–590, 1985.

229. Horwitz, M.S., Friefeld, B.R., and Keiser, H.D.: Inhibition of adenovirus DNA synthesis in vitro by sera from patients with systemic lupus erythematosus. Mol. Cell. Biol., *2*:1492–1500, 1982.

230. Allen, J.I., Searles, R.P., Messner, R.P., and Bankhurst, A.D.: Antilymphocyte antibodies in systemic lupus erythematosus patients and their relatives: Reactivity with nonhuman lymphocytes. Clin. Immunol. Immunopathol., *9*:371–378, 1978.

231. Folomeeva, O. et al.: Comparative studies of antilymphocyte, antipolynucleotide, and antiviral antibodies among families of patients with systemic lupus erythematosus. Arthritis Rheum., *21*:23–27, 1978.

232. Hazelton, R.A., Clark, S.O., Sturrock, R.D., and Sommerville, R.G.: Serologic titres to micro-organisms in systemic lupus erythematosus: A family study. Ann. Clin. Res., *15*:40–43, 1983.

233. Reinertsen, J.L. et al.: An epidemiologic study of households exposed to canine SLE. Arthritis Rheum., *23*:564–568, 1980.

234. Kagen, L.J.: Polymyositis and dermatomyositis. *In* Modern

Topics in Rheumatology. Edited by G.R.V. Hughes. London, Heineman, 1976, pp. 135–143.

235. Kallen, P.S., Louie, J.S., Nies, K.M., and Bayer, A.S.: Infectious myositis and related syndromes. Semin. Arthritis Rheum., 11:421–439, 1982.

236. Phillips, P.E., Kassan, S.S., and Kagen, L.J.: Increased toxoplasma antibodies in idiopathic inflammatory muscle disease: A case-control study. Arthritis Rheum., 22:209–214, 1979.

237. Magid, S.K., and Kagen, L.J.: Serologic evidence for acute toxoplasmosis in polymyositis-dermatomyositis. Increased frequency of specific antitoxoplasma IgM antibodies. Am. J. Med., 75:313–320, 1983.

238. Adams, E.M. et al.: The development of polymyositis in a patient with toxoplasmosis: Clinical and pathologic findings and review of literature. Clin. Exp. Rheumatol., 2:205–208, 1984.

239. Hendrickx, G.F.M., Verhage, J., Jennekens, F.G.I., and van Krapen, F.: Dermatomyositis and toxoplasmosis. Ann. Neurol., 5:393–395, 1978.

240. Quilis, M.R., and Damjanov, I.: Dermatomyositis as an immunologic complication of toxoplasmosis. Acta Neuropathol. (Berl.) 58:183–186, 1982.

241. Katsuragi, S., Miyayama, H., and Takeuchi, T.: Picornavirus-like inclusions in polymyositis—aggregation of glycogen particles of the same size. Neurology, 31:1476–1480, 1981.

242. Christensen, M.L. et al.: Prevalence of coxsackie B virus antibodies in patients with juvenile dermatomyositis. Arthritis Rheum., 29:1365–1370, 1986.

243. Bowles, N.E., Dubowitz, V., Sewry, C.A., and Archard, L.C.: Dermatomyositis, polymyositis, and coxsackie-B-virus infection. Lancet, 1:1004–1007, 1987.

244. Mathews, M.B., and Bernstein, R.M.: Myositis autoantibody inhibits histidyl-tRNA synthetase: A model for autoimmunity. Nature, 304:177–179, 1983.

245. Mathews, M.B., Reichlin, M., Hughes, G.R.V., and Bernstein, R.M.: Anti-threonyl-tRNA synthetase, a second myositis-related autoantibody. J. Exp. Med., 160:420–434, 1984.

246. Ytterberg, S.R.: Coxsackievirus B 1 induced murine polymyositis: Acute infection with active virus is required for myositis. J. Rheumatol., 14:12–18, 1987.

247. Ruff, R.L., and Secrist, D.: Viral studies in benign acute childhood myositis. Arch. Neurol., 39:261–263, 1982.

248. Dalakas, M.C., Pezeshkpour, G.H., Gravell, M., and Sever, J.L.: Polymyositis associated with AIDS retrovirus. JAMA, 256:2381–2383, 1986.

249. Calabrese, L.H., Mitsumoto, H., and Chou, S.M.: Inclusion body myositis presenting as treatment-resistant polymyositis. Arthritis Rheum., 30:397–403, 1987.

250. Mikol, J. et al.: Inclusion-body myositis: Clinicopathological studies and isolation of an adenovirus type 2 from muscle biopsy specimen. Ann. Neurol., 11:576–581, 1981.

251. Sergent, J.S., and Christian, C.L.: Necrotizing vasculitis after acute serous otitis media. Ann. Intern. Med., 81:195–199, 1974.

252. Kazmierowski, J.A., Peizner, D.S., and Wuepper, K.D.: Herpes simplex antigen in immune complexes of patients with erythema multiforme. JAMA, 247:2547–2550, 1982.

253. Haynes, B.F., et al.: Identification of human T cell leukemia virus in a Japanese patient with adult T cell leukemia and cutaneous lymphomatous vasculitis. Proc. Natl. Acad. Sci. U.S.A., 80:2054–2058, 1983.

254. MacKenzie, R.A., Forbes, G.S., and Karnes, W.E.: Angio-

graphic findings in herpes zoster arteritis. Ann. Neurol., 10:458–464, 1981.

255. Yanagawa, H., Nakamura, Y., Kawasaki, T., Shigematsu, I.: Nationwide epidemic of Kawasaki disease in Japan during winter of 1985–86. Lancet, 2:1138–1139, 1986.

256. Bell, D.M., et al.: Kawasaki syndrome: Description of two outbreaks in the United States. N. Engl. J. Med., 304:1568–1575, 1981.

257. Dean, A.G. et al.: An epidemic of Kawasaki syndrome in Hawaii. J. Pediatr., 100:552–557, 1982.

258. Tasaka, K., and Hamashima, Y.: Studies on rickettsia-like body in Kawasaki disease. Acta Pathol. Jpn., 28:235–245, 1978.

259. Patriarca, P.A. et al.: Kawasaki syndrome: Association with the application of rug shampoo. Lancet, 2:578–580, 1982.

260. Kato, H. et al.: Variant strain of *Propionibacterium acnes*: A clue to the aetiology of Kawasaki disease. Lancet, 2:1383–1388, 1983.

261. Moynahan, E.J.: Kawasaki disease: A novel feline virus transmitted by fleas? Lancet, 1:195, 1987.

262. Shulman, S.T., and Rowley, A.H.: Does Kawasaki disease have a retroviral aetiology? Lancet, 2:545–546, 1986.

263. Burns, J.C. et al.: Polymerase activity in lymphocyte culture supernatants from patients with Kawasaki disease. Nature, 323:814–816, 1986.

264. Rauch, A.M., Fultz, P.N., and Kalyanaraman, V.S.: Retrovirus serology and Kawasaki syndrome. Lancet, 1:1431, 1987. (Letter)

265. Martin, D.K., Nelms, D.C., Mackler, B.F., and Peavy, D.L.: Lymphoproliferative responses induced by streptococcal antigens in recurrent aphthous stomatitis and Behçet syndrome. Clin. Immunol. Immunopathol., 13:146–155, 1979.

266. O'Duffy, J.D., Lehner, T., and Barnes, C.G.: Summary of the Third International Conference on Behçet's disease. J. Rheumatol., 10:154–158, 1983.

267. Denman, A.M. et al.: Lymphocyte abnormalities in Behçet syndrome. Clin. Exp. Immunol., 42:175–185, 1980.

268. Eglin, R.P., Lehner, T., and Subak-Sharpe, J.H.: Detection of RNA complementary to herpes-simplex virus in mononuclear cells from patients with Behçet's syndrome and recurrent oral ulcers. Lancet, 2:1356–1361, 1982.

269. Efthimiou, J., Harikumar, M.K., Knight, R.A., and Snaith, M.L.: Inappropriate peripheral blood lymphocyte responses to herpes viruses in patients with Behçet syndrome. Immunol. Lett., 8:317–318, 1984.

270. Ohno, S. et al.: Detection of gamma interferon in the sera of patients with Behçet disease. Infect. Immun., 36:202–208, 1982.

271. Emery, H., Larter, W., and Schaller, J.G.: Henoch-Schönlein vasculitis. Arthritis Rheum., 20:385–388, 1977.

272. Bridgeford, P.H. et al.: Polymyalgia rheumatica and giant cell arteritis: Histocompatibility typing and HB infection studies. Arthritis Rheum., 23:516–518, 1980.

273. Elling, H., Skinhoj, P., and Elling, P.: Hepatitis B virus and polymyalgia rheumatica: A search for HBsAg, HBsAb, HBcAB, HBeAg, and HBeAb. Ann. Rheum. Dis., 39:511–513, 1980.

274. Hickstein, D.D., Gravelyn, T.R., and Wharton, M.: Giant cell arteritis and polymyalgia rheumatica in a conjugal pair. Arthritis Rheum., 24:1448–1450, 1981.

275. Kleinknecht, C., Levy, M., Gagnodoux, M.F., and Habib, R.: Membranous glomerulonephritis with extra-renal disorders in children. Medicine, 8:219–229, 1979.

276. Nissenson, A.R. (moderator): Poststreptococcal acute glo-

merulonephritis: Fact and controversy. Ann. Intern. Med., 91:76–86, 1979.

277. Shillitoe, E.J. et al.: Antibody to cytomegalovirus in patients with Sjögren's syndrome as determined by an enzyme-linked immunosorbent assay. Arthritis Rheum., 25:260–265, 1982.

278. Fox, R.I., Pearson, G., and Vaughan, J.H.: Detection of Epstein-Barr virus-associated antigens and DNA in salivary gland biopsies from patients with Sjögren's syndrome. J. Immunol., 137:3162–3168, 1986.

279. Lurhuma, A.Z., Riccomi, H., and Masson, P.L.: The occurrence of circulating immune complexes and viral antigens in idiopathic thrombocytopenic purpura. Clin. Exp. Immunol., 28:49–55, 1977.

280. Murphy, T.F., Senterfit, L.B., and Christian, C.L.: Arthralgia associated with acute urinary retention. A syndrome of probable viral etiology. Am. J. Med., 68:386–388, 1980.

281. Mills, B.G., and Singer, F.R.: Critical evaluation of viral antigen data in Paget's disease of bone. Clin. Orthop., 217:16–25, 1987.

282. Basle, M.F. et al.: On the trail of paramyxoviruses in Paget's disease of bone. Clin. Orthop., 217:9–15, 1987.

283. Levo, Y. et al.: Association between hepatitis B virus and essential mixed cryoglobulinemia. N. Engl. J. Med., 296:1501–1504, 1977.

284. Bombardieri, S. et al.: Liver involvement in essential mixed cryoglobulinemia. Ric. Clin. Lab., 9:361–368, 1979.

285. Popp, J.W., et al.: Essential mixed cryoglobulinemia without evidence for hepatitis B virus infection. Ann. Intern. Med., 92:379–383, 1980.

286. Gocke, D.J.: Hepatitis A revisited. Ann. Intern. Med., 105:960–961, 1986.

287. Cremer, N.E., Devlin, V.L., Riggs, J.L., and Hagens, S.J.: Anomalous antibody responses in viral infection: Specific stimulation or polyclonal activation? J. Clin. Microbiol., 20:468–472, 1984.

288. Luka, J. et al.: Identification and characterization of a cellular protein that cross-reacts with the Epstein-Barr virus nuclear antigen. J. Virol., 52:833–838, 1984.

289. Kwok, S. et al.: Identification of human immunodeficiency virus sequences by using in vitro enzymatic amplification and oligomer cleavage detection. J. Virol., 61:1690–1694, 1987.

290. Chen, K., Neimark, H., Steinman, C.: Characterization of a broadly specific oligonucleotide probe for detection of unknown eubacteria in putatively infected tissue. Arthritis Rheum., 30:S78, 1987 (Abstract).

291. Ware, P.L., and Kasper, L.H.: Strain-specific antigens of Toxoplasma gondii. Infect. Immun., 55:778–783, 1987.

292. Platt, D.J. et al.: Restriction enzyme fingerprinting of enterobacterial plasmids: A simple strategy with wide application. J. Hyg. (Camb.), 97:205–210, 1986.

293. Richman, D. et al.: Summary of a workshop on new and useful methods in rapid viral diagnosis. J. Infect. Dis., 150:941–951, 1984.

section | III |

CLINICAL PHARMACOLOGY OF ANTIRHEUMATIC DRUGS

ASPIRIN AND OTHER NONSTEROIDAL ANTI-INFLAMMATORY DRUGS

32

HAROLD E. PAULUS and DANIEL E. FURST

Many arthritic diseases are characterized by inflammation, causing tissue injury and loss of function. Therapy is therefore directed toward limiting the inflammatory process and its consequences. The several major categories of antirheumatic drugs differ substantially in their characteristics, mode of action, and clinical effects.

The nonsteroidal anti-inflammatory drugs (NSAIDs) reduce the signs and symptoms of established inflammation within the first few days of administration. Examples include aspirin, indomethacin, ibuprofen, fenoprofen, ketoprofen, naproxen, tolmetin, sulindac, meclofenamate, diflunisal, and piroxicam. They seem effective only while blood levels of drug are sustained; withdrawal of an NSAID is soon followed by recurrence of inflammation. Although moderated, chronic inflammatory arthritis is often not completely suppressed by NSAIDs, and damage to joints continues to occur during drug administration.

Slowly acting antirheumatic drugs (SAARDs), also called remission-inducing drugs (RIDs) or disease-modifying antirheumatic drugs (DMARDs), are diverse compounds sharing a common pattern of clinical response. Administration of one of these drugs has no immediate therapeutic benefit, but after weeks or months, the onset of clinical improvement may be detected. With continued administration, some or all disease manifestations may eventually be completely suppressed. If drug administration is discontinued, however, the manifestations of disease gradually recur. During a remission induced by SAARDs, damage to joints and other tissues probably stops, although it resumes when the drug is discontinued. Examples of SAARDs include the organic gold compounds, antimalarial drugs, antimetabolites, alkylating agents, D-penicillamine, and levamisole. All were developed for other indications and were then applied to the treatment of rheumatic diseases as an afterthought.

Corticosteroids share some characteristics with NSAIDs in that they rapidly moderate established inflammation and probably do not prevent the progression of joint damage. On the other hand, high doses of prednisone have prolonged effects on immunoglobulin synthesis, and the appearance of some drug effects may be delayed, as in treatment of vasculitis or nephritis.

The NSAIDs are discussed here. Although knowledge of their cellular and molecular effects on various aspects of the inflammatory process is increasing, their use in the rheumatic diseases remains empiric.

GENERAL CONSIDERATIONS

CHEMISTRY

Although they appear different from one another, the NSAIDs can be grouped by chemical structural similarities (Fig. 32–1).

A limited correlation exists between the pKa* of a

---

*pKa = pH at which a salt is half-ionized.

507

FIG. 32–1. Chemical structures of some nonsteroidal anti-inflammatory drugs.

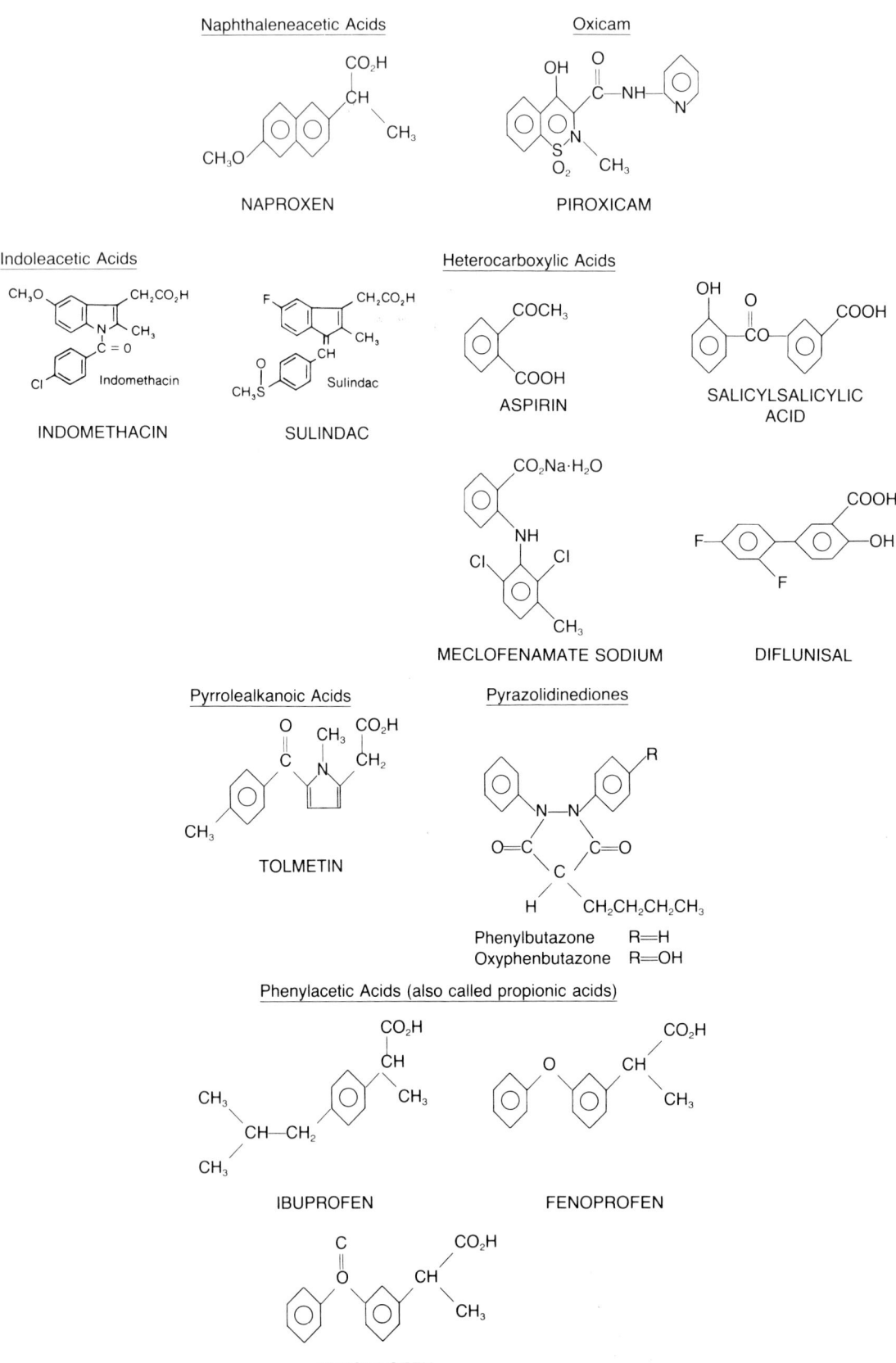

drug and both its plasma half-life* and its anti-inflammatory activity. Thus, as the pKa decreases, the plasma half-life decreases, probably owing to more rapid renal tubular excretion of the drug. A pKa of less than 3 diminishes anti-inflammatory activity and increases uricosuric activity.[1] Most NSAIDs have a pKa in the range of 3.5 to 5 and are not usually uricosuric.[1]

PHARMACOLOGIC ACTIVITIES

All NSAIDs have antipyretic and analgesic activities in animal models and anti-inflammatroy activity in various in vitro and in vivo tests. Because NSAIDs moderate established inflammation, they might be anticipated to affect numerous inflammatory processes.

Effects on Arachidonic Acid Metabolites

Arachidonic acid is a constituent of cell membrane phospholipids. This fatty acid is produced in response

*Plasma half-life (t 1/2) = the time necessary for the plasma concentration to decrease by half.

to inflammatory stimuli, and its synthesis is inhibited by glucocorticosteroids. Arachidonic acid is metabolized to form a remarkable array of biologically active substances (Fig. 32–2). The characterization and identification of these metabolites has focused attention on the mechanisms of acute and chronic inflammation (see Chapter 26). Chemotactic lipids may be produced by nonenzymatic oxidation of arachidonic acid, and various products result from its oxidation with the enzymes cyclo-oxygenase or lipoxygenase. NSAIDs block the conversion of arachidonic acid to the endoperoxides prostaglandins G_2 (PGG_2) and H_2 (PGH_2) by inhibiting the membrane-bound enzyme, cyclo-oxygenase (Fig. 32–2). In platelets, these endoperoxides are transformed into thromboxane A_2, whereas in inflamed tissue, PGE_2 is formed. The inhibition of endoperoxide formation by NSAIDs blocks the synthesis of both prostaglandins and thromboxanes.[2]

Vane has postulated that the antipyretic, anti-inflammatory, and analgesic properties of aspirin-like drugs are accounted for by their effect on prostaglandin synthetase (cyclo-oxygenase).[3] Prostaglandins have been demonstrated to cause inflammation in

FIG. 32–2. Arachidonic acid metabolism.

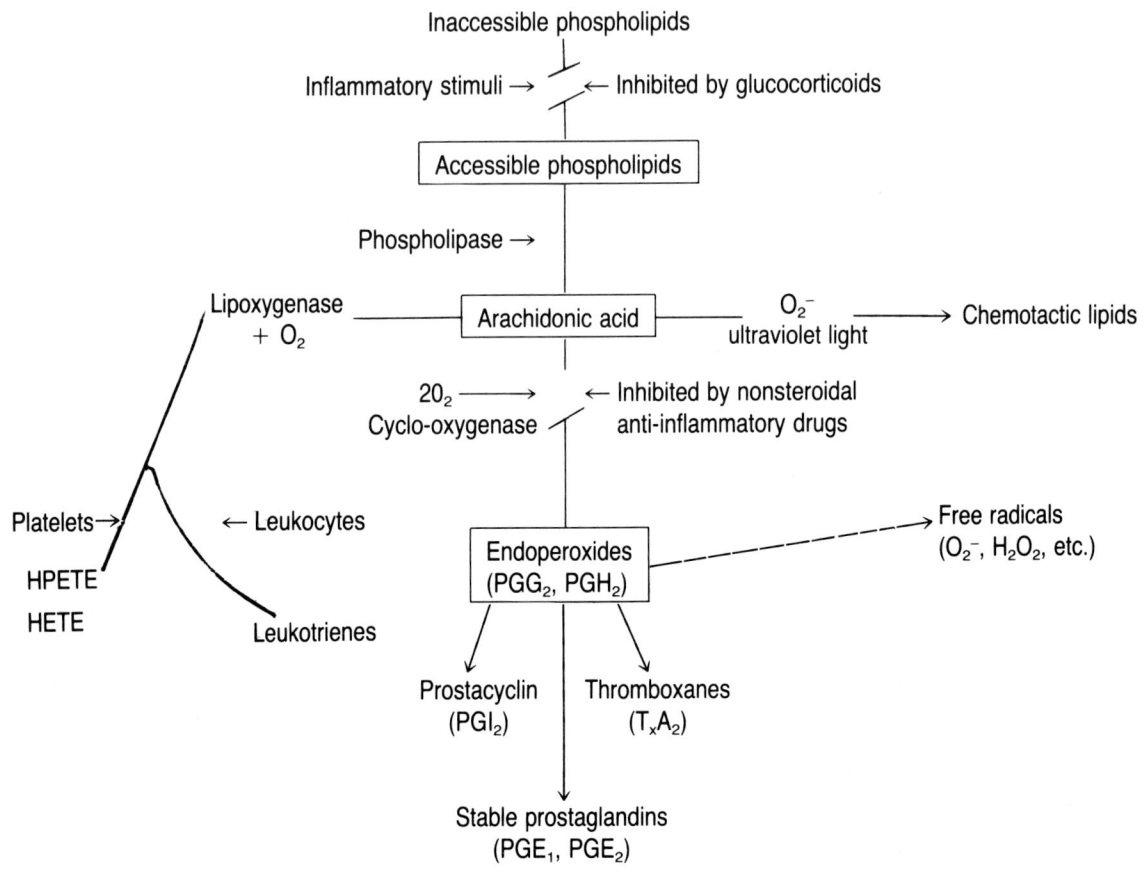

various experimental situations. PGE_1 is a potent pyrogen in animals,[4] and $PGF_{2\alpha}$ has caused fever in patients when given systemically to stimulate uterine contraction.[3] Edema, erythema, and some of the histologic changes of inflammation have been associated with prostaglandin administration to animals. Further, a variety of free radicals derived from molecular oxygen, including superoxide, hydroxyl, and perhydroxyl radicals, are involved in the biosynthesis of prostaglandins and can provoke cell injury themselves. These free radicals are produced by activated neutrophils and other elements of the inflammatory reaction. Many NSAIDs may act as free radical scavengers (antioxidants), in addition to inhibiting the formation of free radicals in the arachidonic acid pathway.

Arachidonic acid metabolites often have opposing effects on various mechanisms involved in inflammation. Vessel tone is increased by $PGF_{2\alpha}$ and T_xA_2 and decreased by PGE_2 and PGI_2, whereas vessel permeability is increased by PGE_2, PGI_2, and LTB_4, and decreased by $PGF_{2\alpha}$. Chemotaxis is stimulated by PGE_2 and LTB_4 and inhibited by PGI_2.

Thromboxane A_2 stimulates aggregation of platelets and increases neutrophil adherence. In the gastric mucosa, prostaglandins decrease acid production and increase gastric mucin secretion and gastroesophageal sphincter tone. In the kidney, vasodilatory prostaglandins help to regulate renal blood flow, glomerular filtration rate, and sodium and water excretion. Other specific effects of prostaglandins in various tissues include dilatation of the ductus arteriosus and contraction of uterine muscle fibers.

The inhibition of arachidonic acid metabolism by systemic administration of drugs has a variety of effects. Generally, NSAIDs inhibit cyclo-oxygenase; aspirin does so in an irreversible fashion, and the others reversibly in a concentration-related manner. Pain associated with arachidonic acid metabolites is reduced. Fever is moderated, and platelet aggregation is decreased. Gastric acid production increases, gastric mucin production decreases, and gastroesophageal sphincter tone may decrease, producing dyspepsia. Under certain circumstances, renal blood flow may decrease, causing a rise in creatinine levels, edema, hyperkalemia, and sometimes renal papillary necrosis. Uterine cramps may be suppressed, and a patent ductus arteriosus may be closed.

The order of potency* of cyclo-oxygenase inhibition by various NSAIDs correlates well with their potency in the carrageenan rat paw edema model of inflam-

---

*Potency = the relative quantity of drug required to produce a particular effect. Thus, one drug is more potent than another if less is required to produce a certain effect.

mation. Cyclo-oxygenases obtained from different tissues have different sensitivities to inhibition by NSAIDs, and their relative potencies vary according to the tissue preparations used to test them. For example, acetaminophen is reported to be as effective as aspirin in inhibition of cyclo-oxygenase obtained from the brain, but it has much less activity than aspirin on the enzyme obtained from the spleen; this finding may help to explain the effective antipyretic and analgesic activities of acetaminophen, and its lack of anti-inflammatory properties.[5] Aspirin, a potent inhibitor of cyclo-oxygenase, acts by acetylating the enzyme. The relative lack of activity of nonacetylated salicylate in cyclo-oxygenase inhibition assays is anomalous in that salicylate derived from nonacetylated sources suppresses inflammation as effectively as equivalent doses of aspirin in the treatment of patients with rheumatoid arthritis (RA).[6]

Additional evidence that suppression of cyclo-oxygenase activity does not completely explain the anti-inflammatory effects of NSAIDs is found in experiments with rats whose tissues have been made deficient in arachidonic acid by a diet deficient in a fatty acid essential to its production. When these rats that are deficient in arachidonic acid are injected with carrageenan, the expected paw edema is produced, but to a lesser degree than in normal rats. This finding suggests that the inability to produce metabolites of arachidonic acid indeed decreases the inflammatory response. But when such rats were given aspirin, paw edema further decreased. Quantitatively, the additional decrease in paw edema was similar to that produced by aspirin in the nondeficient rats, suggesting that the anti-inflammatory effects of NSAIDs are not completely explained by the suppression of cyclo-oxygenase.[7]

The foregoing observations have encouraged interest in the lipoxygenase pathway of arachidonic acid metabolism (Fig. 32–2). This pathway is active in both rabbit and human neutrophils.[2] Leukotriene B_4 (LTB_4) induces neutrophil aggregation, O_2^- generation, and degranulation.[8] It causes neutrophils to accumulate at local sites of inflammation by stimulating chemotaxis and enhancing leukocyte adherence to and diapedesis across postcapillary venule walls, and it also stimulates the production of guanylate and adenylate cyclase.[9] Piroxicam inhibited LTB_4-induced leukocyte aggregation,[9] but ibuprofen had no effect. Benoxaprofen was reported to be only a weak inhibitor of cyclo-oxygenase, but a more effective inhibitor of lipoxygenase, whereas indomethacin was a good inhibitor of cyclo-oxygenase and a poor inhibitor of lipoxygenase; ketoprofen was an effective inhibitor of both.[11] Differing effects on various aspects of arachidonic acid metabolism may be responsible for differences in clinical responses to specific NSAIDs, although such differences have not yet been clearly defined.

Effects on Other Soluble Factors

Bradykinin generation increases capillary permeability. Several NSAIDs inhibit bradykinin-induced edema at concentrations at the upper end of pharmacologic dosing regimens,[12] and these agents also inhibit serotonin release and the action of catecholamines in studies of platelet function in vitro and in turpentine-induced pleurisy. Yet the high concentrations needed make it unlikely that inhibition of kinin or amine release is a major mechanism of the clinical effect of NSAIDs. Enzymes involved in oxidative phosphorylation, transferases, RNA synthetases, and polymerases have been proposed as possible sites of action of NSAIDs, but effects on these enzyme systems are seen in isolated, unphysiologic preparations.[13] NSAIDs may scavenge free radicals directly, but high drug concentrations are required. Several NSAIDs have been demonstrated to inhibit intracellular influx of calcium and calcium-dependent cell aggregation.[14]

In concentrations within the therapeutic range, aspirin is an effective uncoupler of oxidative phosphorylation only in tissue isolates.[13,15] Further, some effective uncouplers of oxidative phosphorylation such as 2′, 4-dinitrophenol are devoid of anti-inflammatory activity.[16] Rat fetal tissue histidine decarboxylase, needed for histamine formation, is inhibited by 1 mM aspirin, and 4 g aspirin daily reduce histamine excretion by half in humans.[17]

Effects on Cellular Elements

Granulocyte and monocyte migration and phagocytosis can be inhibited in vitro by aspirin, phenylbutazone, indomethacin, and several other NSAIDs,[18,19] but the high concentrations required may produce general depression of cellular mechanisms. Aspirin and piroxicam inhibited neutrophil aggregation and degranulation when stimulated by N-formyl-methionyl-leucyl-phenylalanine (FMLP), but not when stimulated by phytohemagglutinin or concanavalin A. Lymphocyte transformation and DNA synthesis are suppressed by aspirin, phenylbutazone, oxyphenbutazone, indomethacin, and flufenamic acid.[20,21] Indomethacin, 10^{-1} and $10^{-5}M$, inhibits prostaglandin dehydrogenase and potentiates PGE_1-mediated cyclic adenosine monophosphate (cAMP) generation in human synoviocytes.[22] The actions of NSAIDs on cAMP phosphodiesterase are of particular interest because increased cAMP levels are associated with decreased lymphocyte and leukocyte responsiveness.[23] Caution must be exercised in interpreting these results because many factors may cause a rise or fall in cAMP, and the foregoing changes may have little to do with lymphocyte activity. Inhibition of neutrophil activation and lymphocyte immunoglobulin formation have been documented with therapeutic concentrations of indomethacin (1.5 to 10 μg/ml).[10,24] Indomethacin reversibly enhanced skin test reactivity in anergic patients with common variable immunodeficiency.[24]

Analgesia

Clinically, aspirin and other NSAIDs are effective analgesics. Based on cross-perfusion studies, the analgesic action of salicylates is generally considered to be peripheral,[15] in contrast to the central action of narcotics. When an isolated organ with nerves intact to the whole animal A, but with its circulation from animal B, is injected with minute amounts of bradykinin, pain is induced in animal A. Aspirin injected into the circulation of animal B blocks the bradykinin-invoked pain response in animal A; and aspirin injected into the circulation of animal A, in which it perfuses not the isolated organ, but the central nervous system of that animal, does not block the bradykinin-induced pain. Thus, salicylates and other NSAIDs can suppress chemically induced peripheral pain, but they do not block the transmission or perception of painful stimuli.[25]

Antipyresis

NSAIDs are effective antipyretics in humans, generally in short-term, placebo-controlled studies of patients with fevers of various causes. Little evidence suggests that any one drug has a better therapeutic ratio* than another.

Antirheumatic and Anti-Inflammatory Effects

The anti-inflammatory effects of the NSAIDs were noted centuries ago, with the use of salicylates by Pliny for gout.[26] Aspirin was shown conclusively to be effective in RA only in 1964.[27] These findings have been confirmed and extended by placebo-controlled studies using doses of at least 4.0 g/day.[28]

NSAIDs have been compared with placebo, with aspirin, and often with each other in the treatment of RA. The more recent trials have been double-blind and randomized with well-defined criteria for patient evaluation. Most trials of the newer NSAIDs suggest comparability to aspirin in anti-inflammatory doses

---

*Therapeutic ratio = beneficial effects/toxic effects.

with respect to efficacy, but with somewhat less toxicity.

The anti-inflammatory effects of NSAIDs have been documented best in RA, but such effects in other rheumatic diseases have been explored to some extent. Aspirin is probably efficacious against rheumatic fever. In juvenile RA (JRA), it is definitely the drug of first choice, presumably because of its combined analgesic, antipyretic, and anti-inflammatory activities.[29] Studies in Reiter's syndrome and psoriatic arthritis have been uncontrolled, but NSAIDs are widely used in these illnesses. A number of NSAIDs are clearly superior to placebo in treating ankylosing spondylitis, whereas aspirin is effective only occasionally.[30-32] Although aspirin is both anti-inflammatory and uricosuric in high doses, it is rarely used to treat gout.[33] Other NSAIDs are more effective than aspirin; indomethacin is one of the drugs of choice in the treatment of acute gout.[34-36] The use of aspirin and aspirin-like drugs in the treatment of osteoarthritis is appropriate and is nearly universal,[37] although it is not clear whether they are acting as analgesic or anti-inflammatory drugs in this situation. In vitro studies of NSAIDs' effects on cartilage metabolism and on various animal models of osteoarthritis have yielded variable and often contradictory results.

Effects on Platelet Function

Most NSAIDs decrease platelet aggregation induced by adenosine diphosphate, collagen, or epinephrine by inhibiting platelet cyclo-oxygenase.[38] For most NSAIDs, this effect is reversible and depends on the presence of adequate drug concentrations in the platelet, but aspirin irreversibly acetylates this enzyme.[39] Because platelets are unable to synthesize additional cyclo-oxygenase, this effect persists until the acetylated platelets are replaced by newly formed platelets from the bone marrow. As little as 300 mg aspirin may produce an antiaggregation effect that is still detectable 4 to 6 days later. Nonacetylated salicylates, which have minimal effect on prostaglandin synthesis, also have little or no effect on platelet aggregation and are a better choice for patients undergoing surgical procedures or at increased risk of bleeding.[7,40]

The antiplatelet aggregation effect of NSAIDs has been used in studies of aspirin for the prevention of cerebral and coronary artery occlusive events. It is thought that the production of thromboxane A_2 by platelets must be inhibited, whereas that of prostacyclin (PGI_2) by vascular endothelium must be maintained for most effective anticoagulation by aspirin.[41] Thromboxane A_2 promotes platelet aggregation, but PGI_2 prevents this aggregation and is also vasodila-

tory. Aspirin inhibits the production of both substances. Several approaches have been used to produce differential inhibition of thromboxane A_2 in platelets without inhibiting PGI_2 in vascular endothelium. Because platelets are unable to synthesize new cyclo-oxygenase to replace that which has been acetylated by aspirin, as can nucleated endothelial cells, the use of infrequent (once daily), low doses of aspirin should cause continual suppression of platelet cyclo-oxygenase, but only transient suppression of PGI_2 production by endothelial cells.[42] Another approach involves the use of slow-release aspirin or enteric-coated aspirin, which does not produce measurable aspirin (as opposed to salicylate) concentrations in the systemic circulation, presumably because of complete metabolism of the slowly absorbed aspirin on its first pass through the liver. In this situation, platelet cyclo-oxygenases are irreversibly acetylated during their brief exposure to aspirin in the portal circulation, but PGI_2 production is normal because the endothelial cells of the systemic circulation are not exposed to aspirin.[43]*

Other Effects

Induction of uterine muscle contraction was one of the earliest observed effects of prostaglandins. This effect can be suppressed by NSAIDs, and several of these agents have been recommended for treatment of menstrual cramps.[44] Indomethacin, used to assist in the closure of patent ductus arteriosus in infants, frequently averts the need for surgical intervention.[45]

SOME PHARMACOKINETIC DEFINITIONS

One-Compartment Open Model

This term is defined as the representation of the body as a single homogeneous unit. It assumes that a dose of drug is instantaneously mixed throughout the body, that plasma level changes reflect changes occurring at the tissue level, and that elimination from the body occurs in an exponential fashion. The word "open" refers to the presence of a way into and out of the body; that is, it is not a closed system (Fig. 32–3).

Two-Compartment Open Model

This term is defined as the representation of the body as two compartments. These compartments do not reflect specific anatomical or physiologic areas. They are generally viewed as a "central" compart-

---

*Editor's note. Bleeding times in patients receiving anti-inflammatory doses of aspirin (sufficient to provide a salicylate blood level of 20 to 30 mg/dL) are usually normal, as production of both T_xA_2 and PGI_2 is suppressed.

FIG. 32–3. Plasma level versus time curve for a one-compartment open model. IV = intravenous.

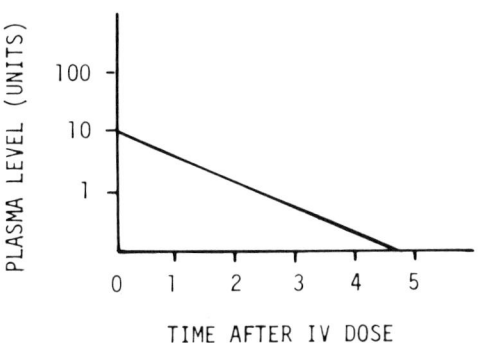

ment, representing highly perfused tissues, and a "peripheral" compartment, representing poorly perfused tissues. Any representation of the body as a two-compartment model results in a biexponential decline in plasma levels as a function of time after intravenous injection (Fig. 32–4).

Absorption Half-Life

This is the time required after administration of a drug for its concentration in blood or plasma to increase from a given level to twice that level.

Distribution Half-Life (t 1/2 α)

In a two-compartment open model, during the initial (distribution) phase of the biexponential curve, this half-life is the time required for the plasma drug level to decrease by half, after administration of an intravenous bolus. Conceptually, this term reflects the change in plasma drug level as the drug distributes from the central compartment into the peripheral compartment (Fig. 32–5).

FIG. 32–4. Plasma level versus time curve for a two-compartment open model. IV = intravenous.

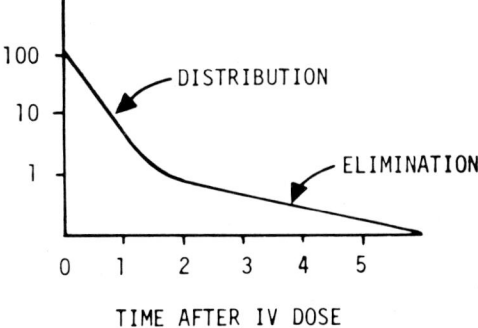

Elimination Half-Life (Beta Half-life, t 1/2 β)

In a two-compartment open model, during the final (elimination) phase of the biexponential curve, this half-life is the time required for the plasma drug level to decrease by half, after an intravenous bolus. Conceptually, this term reflects the change in plasma drug level in the central compartment, once distribution is complete, as the drug leaves the body (Fig. 32–5).

Area Under the Log Serum Concentration Versus Time Curve (AUC)

The AUC is the calculated area under the graphic representation of drug levels using a semilogarithmic plot of plasma drug level versus time. It is considered to represent the amount of drug that actually reaches the circulation (Fig. 32–5).

INTERACTIONS

Drug-Drug Interactions

Most NSAIDs are acidic compounds that bind tightly to serum albumin and therefore may displace, or may be displaced by, one another or by other drugs. NSAIDs may displace sulfonylurea oral hypoglycemic agents from albumin and may cause transient hypoglycemia.[46] In a patient treated with warfarin, phenylbutazone increased the prothrombin time by 85%.[47]

Concomitant use of salicylates and carbonic anhydrase inhibitors may induce metabolic acidosis.[48] Reversible acute renal failure or hyperkalemia may occur when NSAIDs and triamterene are combined.[49] Probenecid impairs the excretion of many NSAIDs. Brater has reviewed the evidence of many possible drug-drug and drug-disease interactions with NSAIDs.[50]

Drug-Patient Interactions

Cirrhosis may prolong phenylbutazone half-life.[51] Acute renal failure decreased renal drug excretion and also decreased protein binding of salicylate (40 mg/100 ml) and of phenylbutazone (50 mg/100 ml) by 26% and 20%, respectively.[52] Borga and co-workers found a decrease in the binding constants for salicylate in uremic patients.[53] Thus, uremia caused an increased unbound fraction* of salicylate, probably by decreasing the binding affinity of albumin. These effects may be true for other NSAIDs and must be considered in patients with renal impairment.

In 1982, benoxaprofen was withdrawn because of a number of deaths of elderly patients who developed hepatic or renal failure after weeks to months of ther-

---

*Unbound fraction = that fraction of drug in blood or plasma that is not bound to plasma protein or cells.

FIG. 32–5. Plasma level versus time curve for a two-compartment open model, following an oral dose. Absorption, distribution, and elimination phases and the area under the curve (AUC) are demonstrated.

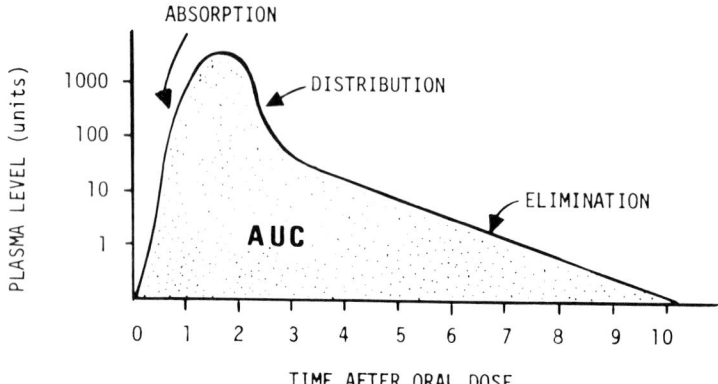

apy. The usual plasma half-life of benoxaprofen in persons with normal renal fuction is about 30 hours, but in persons with decreased creatinine clearance, the half-life may approach 150 hours, leading to excessive accumulation of the drug.[54]

Effect of Aging. Care must be taken when treating elderly patients with NSAIDs because toxicity may be increased by age-related aberrations in drug distribution, metabolism, or excretion. They have more illnesses and take more medications than younger patients, use more over-the-counter medications, and are more likely to self-medicate and to make errors in dosage and dosage schedules. Coexisting diseases may also affect drug metabolism in frail elderly patients, as differentiated from the increasing number of vigorous, healthy elderly persons.[55]

Total drug clearance by the liver and kidney may be reduced in the elderly, but for most of the currently available NSAIDs for which comparative studies have been done, the pharmacokinetics are not influenced significantly by age of the patient. Possible exceptions include ketoprofen, naproxen, and piroxicam.[50]

The serum half-life of phenylbutazone is often longer in elderly patients than in young adults (mean: 104.6 versus 81.2 hours)[56] and shorter in children (40.3 versus 75.8 hours).[57] For indomethacin, elderly and younger patients have equal serum half-lives and AUC, despite much lower renal clearance of the drug in older patients. Some workers postulate that a greater gastrointestinal elimination in the older group accounts for the lack of accumulation of drug.[58]

Various physiologic, pharmacokinetic, and pharmacodynamic changes may occur with increased age. Cardiac output decreases; flow to the heart, brain, and muscles is preserved, but flow to the liver and kidneys decreases by about 1 to 2% per year.[59] Hepatic

synthetic reactions such as conjugation and glucuronidation are probably less affected than preparative reactions such as oxidation and hydrolysis;[60] creatinine clearance and tubular maxima decrease. Little overall change occurs in drug absorption, although isolated examples exist of selective decreases in drug bioavailability in elderly patients (e.g., acetaminophen).[60,61]

With increased age, serum albumin concentration decreased from a mean of 3.9 to 3.0 g/dl.[62] Salicylate binding decreased from 92% in the young to 79% in the elderly, at total salicylate concentrations of 140 mg/L.[63] Thus, an increased unbound salicylate fraction can result in increased toxicity in the elderly. Drug distribution is altered by decreased total body water and lean body mass and increased body fat in the elderly.[64] Changes in drug receptors may occur with aging. Elderly rats have fewer glucocorticoid binding sites on fat cells than young rats, whereas binding affinity is comparable in all age groups.[65] Isoproterenol-stimulated, intracellular cAMP production is decreased in the lymphocytes of the elderly, as compared to young, normal, human volunteers—a finding suggesting a postreceptor defect.[66]

The net result is an increase in the incidence of adverse reactions with age. The most dramatic example was the occurrence of hepatorenal failure in elderly patients treated with benoxaprofen. SAARD may behave similarly. Penicillamine was equally effective in the treatment of young and old patients with RA, but the toxicity in elderly patients was doubled.[67]

Genetics. The metabolism of phenylbutazone and aspirin is under genetic control. Such control is polygenic for phenylbutazone and is also affected by environmental factors.[68,69]

Table 32–1. Adverse Effects of Nonsteroidal Anti-inflammatory Drugs

Drug	Gastro-intestinal Bleeding	Peptic Ulcer	Abdominal Pain, Heartburn, Dyspepsia	Rash	Headache	Tinnitus	Renal Failure	Blood Dyscrasia	Other
Placebo			+++		+				1, 3
Aspirin	[+]	[++]	++++	+++	++	++++	+		4(?), 5
Carprofen	?	[+]	+++	+++					5
Diflunisal (Dolobid)	[+]	[+]	+++	+++	+++	++			2(+++), 4
Fenoprofen (Nalfon)	[+]	[+]	+++	++		++	[+]	+	2(++), 3(++), 4(?)
Flurbiprofen	?		++++	?		?			
Ibuprofen (Motrin)	[+]	[+]	+++	+++		++	+	+	2(++), 3(+++), 5
Indomethacin (Indocin)	[+]	[+]	++++	+	[++++]	++		+	2(++), 3(++++), [5]
Ketoprofen	[+]	[+]	++++	+++	+++	++			2(+++)
Meclofenamate (Meclomen)	[+]	[++]	+++	+++	+++	++	+	+	[2(++++)], 3(+++), 4
Naproxen (Naprosyn)	[+]	[+]	+++	+++	+++	+++	+	+	3(+++)
Phenylbutazone (Butazolidin) and oxyphenbutazone	[+]	[+]	+++	++	+	+	+	[+]	[4] [5]
Piroxicam (Feldene)	[+]	[+]	+++	++	++	++		+	3(++)
Salicylate (nonacetylated)	?	?	+++	?		++++			
Sulindac (Clinoril)	[+]	[+]	+++	+++	+++	++		+	2(+++), 3(+++), [5]
Tolmetin (Tolectin)	[+]	[++]	+++	+	+++	++	+	+	3(+++)

? = insufficient data; incidence: + = <1%; ++ = 3%; +++ = 3%–9%; ++++ = > 10%; □ denotes important side-effects; 1 = drowsiness; 2 = diarrhea; 3 = dizziness; 4 = interaction with warfarin; 5 = hepatic toxicity.

ADVERSE EFFECTS

The side effects of NSAIDs are qualitatively similar, although the frequency of particular side effects varies with the compound. Table 32–1 lists the reported incidence and occurrence of side effects. Because true incidence figures are not available and because definitions of severity of side effects vary, this is an admittedly incomplete overview of toxic effects.

Gastrointestinal Effects

These side effects are common to all NSAIDs and may be considered a characteristic of this class of drugs. These effects may be related to common mechanisms of action. For example, PGE_1, PGE_2 and PGA inhibit gastric acid secretion in animals and humans. PGF_2 increases cardiac sphincter tone in humans, and PGE_1 and PGE_2 prevent ulcers.[70,71] Inhibition of these putative protective functions of prostaglandins by NSAIDs may explain some gastrointestinal toxicity. In addition, phenylbutazone, oxyphenbutazone, and indomethacin decrease gastric mucus production and increase shedding of cells from the gastric mucosa in animals and humans.[72] A number of NSAIDs increase acid secretion, cause local congestion and hemorrhage, and have other local effects such as precipitation of protective glycoprotein.[73,74] Some of these drugs have extensive enterohepatic recirculation.[75–78]

Such recirculation through the bowel correlates with the gastrointestinal toxicity of indomethacin and may be responsible for the similar toxicity of other NSAIDs.[76] Microscopic bleeding is usually less severe with most other NSAIDs than with aspirin.[55,79]

Hepatic Effects

Reversible hepatocellular toxicity with aspirin has been reported in patients with JRA and systemic lupus erythematosus (SLE) and has also been seen with other NSAIDs. In some cases, abnormal liver function tests return to normal even though the drug is continued, although in other cases, hepatic dysfunction may be severe enough to prolong prothrombin times.[80–82] A United States Food and Drug Administration (FDA) conference concluded that hepatic toxicity should be considered a class characteristic of these agents. During prospective clinical trials reported to the FDA, 67 of 1252 patients (5.4%) with RA treated with aspirin developed persistent elevations of one or more liver function tests such as serum glutamic-oxaloacetic transaminase (SGOT), serum glutamic-pyruvic transaminase (SGPT), lactic dehydrogenase (LDH), alkaline phosphatase, and total bilirubin. Elevation of SGOT or SGPT levels appears to be a reversible early warning, and it may be prudent to monitor these tests monthly during the first year of treatment. Advanced age, decreased renal function, multiple drug use, higher drug doses, increased duration of therapy, JRA, and SLE are likely to increase the risk of liver toxicity with NSAIDs.[83] Phenylbutazone may induce hepatocellular injury, cholestasis, and granulomatous hepatitis, which have resulted in a number of fatalities. Hepatotoxicity usually develops within the first 6 weeks of drug therapy and is more likely to develop in the elderly.[84]

Renal Effects

NSAIDs may decrease creatinine clearance and increase serum creatinine concentrations in patients predisposed by hypovolemia or impaired renal function, probably by impairing the compensatory vasodilatory function of renal prostaglandins. These changes often disappear spontaneously, even with continued use of the drug.[85,86] NSAIDs should be used with caution in patients with congestive heart failure, liver disease associated with ascites, hypertension, excessive diuresis, minimal renal arterial insufficiency, mild impairment of glomerular filtration, or multiple drug use.[87] Rarer renal complications include the following: acute renal failure with marked proteinuria and minimal change glomerulopathy, as reported with fenoprofen;[88] acute interstitial nephritis sometimes associated with eosinophilia or other signs

of a hypersensitivity reaction;[89] and papillary necrosis.[90] A review of the world literature between 1970 and 1985 revealed 274 cases of acute renal disease associated with NSAID use.[91] Renal toxicity is rare in prospective trials of NSAIDs in which carefully selected and closely monitored patients are studied, however, and a review of 46 patients treated with aspirin for an average of more than 20 years did not find any serious renal disease.[92] Nonetheless, older patients with borderline renal function may develop serious toxicity.[93]

SPECIFIC AGENTS

These include aspirin and other salicylate compounds, as well as other NSAIDs.

ASPIRIN AND OTHER SALICYLATE PREPARATIONS

The generic term "salicylate" is used here to include all salicylates, including aspirin, but not diflunisal. "Aspirin" refers only to acetylsalicylic acid.

Pharmacologic Properties

Absorption. Salicylate absorption is thought to be a passive process proportional to the concentration of the drug in the bowel, that is, a first-order process. The usual preparations of salicylates and aspirin are completely absorbed, with a peak plasma salicylate level occurring within 2 hours after a 975-mg dose.[94] Aspirin's plasma half-life is only 15 minutes because it is rapidly deacetylated to form salicylate; thus, little aspirin is found in the circulation.[95] Its metabolite, salicylic acid, is the substance usually measured.

Distribution. Salicylate is bound to albumin at two sites, and this binding varies nonlinearly with increasing concentrations of drug. Thus, at serum concentrations below 100 mg/L, it is approximately 92% bound, but at 300 mg/L, it is only 80% bound.[53] As higher concentrations of the drug are reached, more is unbound and thus is available to distribute into tissues.[96] Acid-base status also affects salicylate distribution because non-ionized drug diffuses through cell membranes more easily than ionized drug. Because salicylate has a pKa of 3.0, most is ionized at pH 7.4; a decrease in pH increases the proportion of nonionized drug. In rats, when arterial pH changed from 7.4 to 7.2, the amount of nonionized salicylate doubled, albeit only from 0.004 to 0.008%. This change was reflected by much wider tissue distribution of the drug, as demonstrated by autoradiography of ^{14}carbon (^{14}C)-labeled salicylic acid.[97] Thus, in severe salicylate poisoning, an early, rapid decrease in serum salicylate concentration may reflect increased distribution of salicylate into tissues because of acidosis and may indicate that both the clinical situation and the acidosis are growing worse, rather than better.

Metabolism and Elimination. Once aspirin is deacetylated, its metabolism is the same as all other salicylates. Five metabolites formed in the liver, and salicylic acid itself, are excreted in the urine.[98] Salicylic acid, gentisic acid, gentisuric acid, and salicylacylglucuronide, are eliminated by first-order kinetics;* as the plasma concentration of salicylic acid increases, the excretion rates of these compounds increase proportionately. Salicylurate and salicylphenylglucuronide are eliminated by capacity-limited (Michaelis-Menton) kinetics† because the enzymes that catalyze their formation become saturated. Thus, with salicylate concentrations greater than approximately 50 mg/L, salicylurate and salicylphenylglucuronide are formed at their maximum rates and, no matter how much the serum concentration of salicylic acid increases, their rate of production remains approximately the same.[98] At low doses, the predominant excretory form is salicylurate and the drug is eliminated rapidly, but as the dose increases, serum concentrations may build up more rapidly than expected. For example, with daily doses of 1 g aspirin, the body contains approximately 0.5 g salicylate when steady state‡ has been reached, but with 4 g daily, it contains about 5.6 g salicylate. The ratio is thereby changed from 0.5 to 1.4. With a single 650-mg dose of aspirin, the serum salicylate half-life is 3.5 to 4.5 hours; when given at a dose of 4.5 g daily, the average half-life is 15 to 20 hours.[98] Serum half-life correlates more closely with serum salicylate concentration than with dose and increases as serum concentrations increase.[7] At higher doses, it takes much longer to reach steady state and to excrete the drug. Thus, salicylates are

eliminated by parallel first-order and capacity-limited kinetics. Over the range of 100 to 300 mg/L, compensating mechanisms may render the relationship between dose and blood level more proportional.[96]

Salicylic acid excretion varies with urine pH. In four normal subjects, increasing the urine pH from 5.8 to 6.6 by administering sodium bicarbonate orally, decreased steady-state salicylate serum levels from 270 ± 79 mg/L to 150 ± 46 mg/L, by increasing salicylic acid excretion.[99]

Metabolism of salicylates may be induced by aspirin.[68,100]§

Variability of Dose Response. Equal doses in different individuals may elicit variable responses[101] (Fig. 32–6). *No evidence establishing a relationship between a given serum salicylate level and clinical efficacy has been published.* Salicylate metabolism in humans has a genetic influence.[68]

In summary, the handling of salicylate by the body is complex, influenced by the effects of systemic pH and nonlinear protein binding on distribution, by the effects of parallel first-order and capacity-limited metabolism, by the induction of salicylurate and salicylphenylglucuronide metabolism, and by the effects of urinary pH on excretion.

Acetylated Versus Nonacetylated Salicylates

Salicylates exist in many dosage forms. All the formulations, once metabolized to salicylate, are further metabolized and eliminated in a similar fashion. They may differ in their rates of disintegration, dissolution, and absorption, however.[7] Aspirin is a much more potent cyclo-oxygenase inhibitor in vitro than nonacetylated salicylates, although the efficacy of the two drugs is comparable in in vivo models of inflammation such as carrageenan-induced edema,[102] as well as in RA.[6,103,104]

In vitro tests of platelet aggregation and adhesiveness, and the availability of platelet factor 4, are inhibited for 72 hours after a single 300-mg aspirin dose, probably because of irreversible acetylation of platelet membranes. Nonacetylated salicylates, on the other hand, do not affect these in vitro tests of platelet aggregation.[40] This difference is important because it dictates different uses of acetylated and nonacetylated salicylates in circumstances in which one does, or does not, wish to influence platelet aggregation. Further, a relationship appears to exist between in vitro cyclo-oxygenase inhibition and the bronchospasm associated with the use of various NSAIDs.[7] Thus, some aspirin-sensitive asthmatic patients may still be able

---

*First-order kinetics = a process in which the amount of drug eliminated per unit of time is directly proportional to the amount of drug in the body at that time. Zero-order kinetics = a process in which the amount of drug eliminated per unit of time is independent of the amount of drug in the body; that is, despite increasing amounts of drug in the body, the amount eliminated per unit of time remains constant.

†Capacity-limited (Michaelis-Menton) kinetics = a combination of first-order and zero-order kinetics. When the body contains a small amount of drug, elimination approximates first order. When the amount in the body exceeds a threshold, it approaches zero order because of saturation of capacity-limited metabolic processes.

‡Steady state = that point during long-term drug therapy at which the rate of absorption of drug, usually equated with its rate of administration, equals its rate of elimination. During steady state, the amount of drug in the body remains the same.

§Induction of metabolism = an increased rate of drug metabolism, owing to an increase in the activity or amount of an enzyme that metabolizes it.

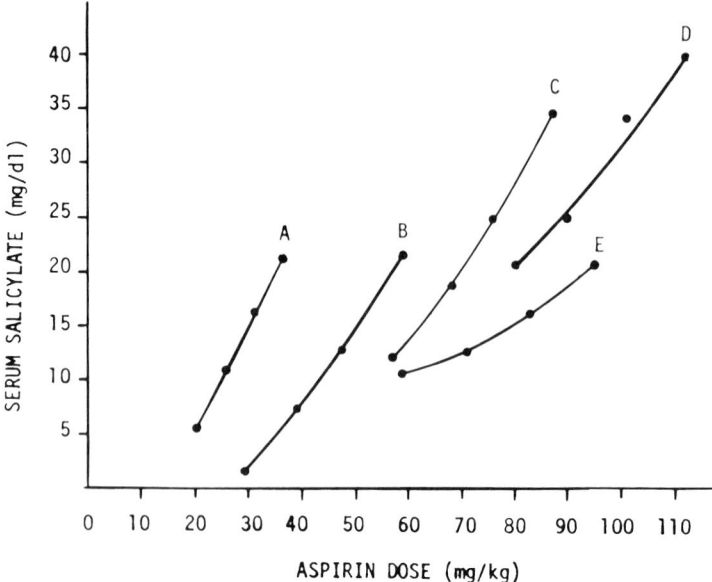

FIG. 32–6. Relationship of aspirin doses and serum salicylate concentrations in five patients (A, B, C, D, and E) with rheumatoid arthritis. Note the striking differences in serum levels attained by different patients taking similar aspirin doses.

to use a non-acetylated salicylate for anti-inflammatory therapy, although asthma has also been induced by nonacetylated salicylate in at least one patient.[105] Finally, it may be advantageous to use an anti-inflammatory drug that does not affect PGE_2 synthesis in patients with borderline or poor renal function.

Aspirin Formulations

Many forms of aspirin are available. The most desirable has rapid tablet disintegration, rapid dissolution and small particle size, to enhance rapid absorption, decrease contact time with the gastrointestinal mucosa, and lessen direct gastrointestinal irritation.[7] "Buffered" tablets are formulated with calcium and magnesium antacids that increase the pH in the microenvironment of the tablet, allowing rapid dissolution of aspirin in the high-pH dissolution layer. After diffusion into the acidic gastric juice, the aspirin probably reprecipitates as fine granules, allowing rapid absorption and less gastrointestinal irritation. Tablets containing sufficient antacid to raise the gastric pH above 5 may increase salicylate excretion by raising the urinary pH.[40]

Enteric dosage forms are designed to be insoluble below pH 3 and soluble above pH 5. Unfortunately, erratic, delayed, or even incomplete absorption may occur with some preparations or in patients with rapid gastrointestinal transit.[106] In addition, if gastric emptying is abnormal, large numbers of undissolved tablets rarely may accumulate in the stomach, with the potential to cause serious toxicity when they advance into the intestine.[107] In general, enteric-coated tablets result in later and lower peak concentrations, but in overall bioequivalence if disintegration and dissolution occur completely.[108]

Timed-release preparations use microencapsulated aspirin particles. The matrices in these tablets consist of waxes, resins, plastics, or polymers with different disintegration rates. This formulation results in different and delayed absorption rates with flattened plasma salicylate concentration versus time curves.[7] The advantage of these slow-releasing preparations is that the drug may be given less frequently; their disadvantage is the potential for incomplete absorption.

Rectal suppositories have been used in attempts to circumvent gastrointestinal irritation. The absorption half-life of suppositories is much longer (3 hours) than the absorption half-life of oral preparations (15 to 30 minutes), and the bioavailability of suppositories depends on retention time. For example, only 20 to 40% of the dose was absorbed in under 2 hours, whereas 60% was absorbed in 4 to 5 hours.[7] Generally, salicylate bioavailability from suppositories is less than that of oral salicylate preparations.[7]

Nonacetylated Salicylates

Sodium Salicylate. This compound is rapidly absorbed, and although it is a less potent analgesic than aspirin, it does appear to be an effective anti-inflammatory agent that causes less gastrointestinal bleeding.[7,109]

Choline Magnesium Trisalicylate. This compound provides 500 mg salicylic acid for each "500 mg" choline magnesium trisalicylate. It has been used to treat RA and osteoarthritis and it appears to cause less gastrointestinal blood loss than aspirin and to have fewer adverse gastrointestinal effects in general.[7,104,110] A liquid preparation providing 500 mg salicylate per 5 ml is also available.

Salicylsalicylic Acid. Although practically insoluble in the stomach, salicylsalicylic acid is soluble in the near-neutral pH of the small intestine. A 500-mg dose is equivalent to 698 mg salicylic acid. Only 77% of the possible salicylate in salicylsalicylic acid is found in the blood as salicylic acid, however, possibly because part of the salicylsalicylic acid is metabolized to its glucuronide and is excreted before it can be broken down to salicylate.[7] Like aspirin, this agent appears effective in the treatment of both osteoarthritis and RA.[111] It also causes less gastrointestinal blood loss than aspirin.[73,112]

Adverse Effects

Hypersensitivity to aspirin is estimated to occur in 0.2% of patients. The symptoms may be anaphylaxis with shock, asthma, urticaria, or angioedema. In a survey of 284 aspirin-intolerant individuals, 85% developed respiratory symptoms such as wheezing and asthma, 9.5% had urticaria or angioedema, and 6% has both skin and respiratory symptoms.[113] A triad of nasal polyposis, asthma, and aspirin sensitivity is influenced by both genetic and environmental factors.[113] Cyclo-oxygenase inhibition in these patients may reduce bronchodilating prostaglandins. In addition, diversion of arachidonic acid metabolism toward lipoxygenase products may augment the release of anaphylactic mediators, such as slow-reacting substance of anaphylaxis (SRSA). Patients exhibiting this reaction to aspirin generally are sensitive to all NSAIDs, and these drugs should be avoided.[114]

Hepatotoxicity. As discussed earlier, abnormal liver function tests have been reported in patients taking aspirin, particularly those with active SLE or JRA.[80,82]

Nephrotoxicity. The nephrotoxic potential of NSAIDs described earlier in this chapter is shared by aspirin.[85] Renal papillary necrosis has been reported in patients taking aspirin alone, as well as in patients taking aspirin-containing analgesic mixtures.[115] A survey of 908 patients in New Zealand, however, showed no association between aspirin ingestion and renal disease, even when large quantities of aspirin were ingested.[90]

Gastrointestinal Toxicity. Gastrointestinal irritation, with dyspepsia, nausea, and vomiting, is a common side-effect, but usually is not serious and is relieved if the drug is withheld. Gastrointestinal blood loss due to aspirin is well documented by studies using [51]chromium (^{51}Cr)-labeled red blood cells to monitor fecal blood loss.[116,117] In one study, during control periods, average blood loss was 0.5 ± 0.5 ml/day (SD), whereas after 2.6 g aspirin daily for 4 days, average blood loss was 3.0 ± 2.2 ml/day. No correlation was found between symptoms of gastric distress and occult gastrointestinal bleeding.[116] The clinical significance of this occult bleeding is uncertain; during 67 months of aspirin therapy, only 1.6% of 244 patients had a drop in hemoglobin greater than 20%.[118] Aspirin damages the gastric mucosa, probably at the tight junctions of the mucosal cells; thereafter, gastric acid passes through the damaged mucosa and injures capillaries and venules.[119] Thus, achlorhydria helps to prevent aspirin-induced occult gastrointestinal blood loss.[120]

In 15,000 patients without a predisposing cause, occasional aspirin use did not increase the incidence of major gastrointestinal bleeding, but use of aspirin for 4 or more days per week for at least 12 weeks was associated with diagnoses of benign gastric ulcers.[121]

In addition to the direct effects of aspirin on the gastric mucosa, its effects on platelets, bleeding time, and prothrombin time may place patients with pre-existing peptic ulcers or coagulation difficulties at a greater risk of major gastrointestinal bleeding. In such patients, aspirin should be avoided, or used with great caution. Nonacetylated salicylates, which do not affect the foregoing coagulation parameters, may be used, although caution must still be exercised.

Central Nervous System Effects. Reversible concentration-related tinnitus and hearing loss occur. Although most patients notice the onset of tinnitus at levels between 200 and 300 mg/L, it is not an accurate guide to dosage in patients with pre-existing hearing loss.

Salicylate Intoxication

Aspirin toxicity is less frequent with the widespread use of "child-proof" caps. Further, the possible pathogenetic role of aspirin in Reye's syndrome will probably lead to decreased use of aspirin in infants and small children, as will the availability of over-the-counter ibuprofen, in adults.[123,124] Nevertheless, aspirin remains an important cause of toxicity in children and adults.

General Metabolic Effects. Oxygen consumption increases rapidly after salicylate administration in either animals or humans.[16] An associated increase in P_{CO_2} helps to produce metabolic acidosis in infants and young children, but is overcompensated by hyperventilation in adults.[16] Particularly in children, high fevers may be encountered; marked sweating accompanies the fever, and serious dehydration can result.[16] Clinically important hyper- and hypoglycemia have been observed during aspirin intoxication.[16]

Central Nervous System Effects. The sensitivity of the respiratory center to changes in P_{CO_2} and pH is increased by aspirin. In dogs, the injection of low concentrations of salicylate into the cisterna magna caused a prompt increase in ventilatory volume and frequency, minutes before any changes occurred in PCO_2.[125] At high serum salicylate concentrations, respiratory depression occurs.[16]

Vomiting is thought to have both central and peripheral causes. Both intravenous and rectal salicylate doses cause vomiting, despite negligible gastric salicylate concentrations. A local effect is also considered likely because vomiting occurs at lower serum concentrations after oral than after intravenous salicylates (282 versus 392 mg/L) and because both vagal and spinal afferent pathways must be interrupted to afford complete protection against vomiting caused by oral salicylate.[16]

Other reported neurologic effects of aspirin toxicity include headache, hyperkineticity, excitement, hallucinations, delirium, convulsions, stupor, coma, and absent Babinski and deep-tendon reflexes.[16]

Acid-Base Disturbances. Acid-base changes during salicylate intoxication are related to the following: respiratory alkalosis due to stimulation of the respiratory center; loss of acids, salts, and fluids due to vomiting; fluid and salt losses due to profuse sweating; and metabolic acidosis due to uncoupling of oxidative phosphorylation and accumulation of organic acids. Children and infants are much more susceptible to metabolic acidosis than adults because the ability of children to increase alveolar ventilation is quickly overcome by accumulated acids.[16,126]

The combination of dehydration, salt and sodium losses caused by sweating and vomiting, and respiratory alkalosis can result in profound potassium depletion.[126] In this situation, respiratory alkalosis and urinary acidosis may coexist. Potassium and bicarbonate must be replaced, in addition to fluids and sodium. The net result of salicylate toxicity on the acid-base status of an individual patient depends on the relative contribution of each of the foregoing actions.

Treatment. Correlation of serum salicylate values with the severity of symptoms is difficult. Acidosis decreases salicylate ionization and increases membrane permeability, and the fraction of unbound salicylate increases with the total drug concentration. These effects increase diffusion of salicylates from blood into the tissues and lead to severe symptoms in the face of "relatively low" serum salicylate levels. Thus, in judging the severity of an overdose, the patient's history and symptoms, arterial blood pH, serum albumin concentration, and serum salicylate level all must be considered.

When a patient with a known aspirin overdose is first seen, induction of vomiting or gastric lavage should *always* be done because aspirin delays gastric emptying. One report states that 20.3 g salicylate were recovered by gastric lavage 9 hours after ingestion. If the patient is conscious, induced vomiting may empty the stomach more efficiently and more completely than lavage.[126,127]

Fluid and electrolyte therapy, with potassium supplements, replaces losses and induces diuresis. When potassium therapy is begun, alkalinization of the urine is recommended to increase the excretion of salicylates. Too-rapid alkalinization may be dangerous.[126] Careful monitoring of fluid and electrolyte balance is necessary to prevent overhydration, especially in elderly patients.

Respiratory depression, convulsions, and hyperpyrexia must be treated if they occur. If a patient has significant hemorrhage, an unusual complication of salicylate overdose, vitamin K should be administered, and routine treatment of gastrointestinal bleeding should be undertaken.[15,126]

More severe salicylate intoxication may be treated by peritoneal dialysis or hemodialysis. Hemodialysis is a rapid and efficient method for removing salicylates.[15,126] Schreiner and Teehan recommend consideration of hemodialysis with known acute absorption of 0.5 g/kg or blood levels above 800 mg/L.[128] Clinical judgment, however, rather than a single serum salicylate value, must guide one in deciding whether to undertake dialysis.

Dosage
Tablets containing 300 or 600 mg are available, as are enteric-coated tablets containing 300 to 1200 mg.
The dose of aspirin depends on the therapeutic goals. For anti-inflammatory effects, blood levels between 200 and 300 mg/L (20 and 30 mg/100 ml) are usually desired, requiring doses between 2 and 6 g daily. Because the doses needed to achieve therapeutic concentrations vary widely, the appropriate dose *must be individualized.* The maximum tolerated dose should be approached slowly because it may take as long as a week after each dosage change to achieve a new steady-state level.
For analgesia, doses in the range of 1.8 g daily usually suffice: the dosage may be increased to tolerance or effect, before changing to other analgesics.

PHENYLBUTAZONE

Pharmacology and Pharmacokinetics

Phenylbutazone (Butazolidin) has been available as an analgesic, antipyretic, and anti-inflammatory drug for more than 30 years. Although effective against RA, gout, ankylosing spondylitis, osteoarthritis, and various nonarticular musculoskeletal syndromes, phenylbutazone is no longer recommended as initial therapy for any indication because of its association with deaths caused by aplastic anemia and agranulocytosis, as well as rare severe hepatic reactions.[87] Oxyphenbutazone is no longer marketed by its original manufacturer.

Because of its diminishing importance, phenylbutazone will not be discussed in detail. Interested readers are referred to the tenth edition of this book for a more extensive discussion of this historically important NSAID.[129]

INDOMETHACIN

Indomethacin (Indocin) is an indole-acetic acid with anti-inflammatory, analgesic, and antipyretic properties.[1] Its potent inhibition of cyclo-oxygenase has resulted in its use in several unexpected areas of medicine.

Pharmacology and Pharmacokinetics

Indomethacin is completely and rapidly absorbed, reaching peak plasma levels of between 1 and 2 μg/ml in 1 to 3 hours after oral dosing. The plasma disappearance curve of indomethacin is biphasic, indicating that the kinetics fit a two-compartment model, with an elimination half-life of 2.2 to 11.2 hours in adults. Kinetic analysis indicates the presence of a nonsamplable "hypothetic organ" that causes a slower elimination of drug from the circulation than expected.[130] Completeness of absorption in humans has been shown. Only 2% of a 25-mg oral dose is excreted in the feces as unchanged indomethacin.[76] Both intravenous and oral indomethacin are about 65% excreted in the urine and 35% excreted in the feces. Whereas 16% of a dose appears as unchanged drug in the urine, the rest is inactive metabolites. Gastrointestinal toxicity was related to the amounts of indomethacin and its metabolites excreted in the bile in five animal species.[76] Because between 27 and 43% of the drug is excreted in the bile in humans, and much is reabsorbed, it is not surprising that indomethacin has significant gastrointestinal toxicity. Glucuronide metabolites of indomethacin are excreted in the bile and reabsorbed as indomethacin after hydrolysis in the bowel, increasing the terminal plasma half-life and the mean plasma indomethacin concentration.[131] Indomethacin is 99% bound to serum albumin; binding is not impaired in patients with chronic renal failure.[131]

A slow-release preparation (75-mg capsule) of indomethacin is available; its bioavailability and efficacy appear to be the same as formulations already available, but it may be taken twice a day.[131] Its absorption occurs predominantly within the first 8 hours after ingestion.[131] Indomethacin is also available as a completely bioavailable oral suspension (25 mg per 5 ml) and as 80 to 90% bioavailable rectal suppositories (50 mg per suppository). Vials containing 1 mg of lyophilized indomethacin for intravenous administration are also available for treatment of patent ductus arteriosus in premature infants.

Indomethacin elimination seems to be age dependent to some extent. The mean half-life in newborn infants whose mothers were taking indomethacin was 14.7 hours, although the half-life of the drug in the mothers was 2.2 hours.[132] Seven elderly patients (mean age 75.8 years) cleared 13% of a dose of indomethacin through their kidneys, whereas seven younger patients (mean age 33 years) cleared 30% by this route. Despite these findings, the serum half-lives and AUC were the same for both groups.[58,131] Thus, although renal elimination was decreased in the elderly, total elimination was the same, perhaps because of compensatory increased gastrointestinal elimination. Because of this characteristic, one would expect greater gastrointestinal toxicity from indomethacin in the elderly.

Similar to other NSAIDs, indomethacin may affect renal function, but 2 weeks of treatment with indomethacin, 150 mg daily, did not decrease renal function as measured by creatinine clearance, fractional sodium or potassium excretion, and free water reabsorption, in six normal subjects or in patients with previously normal renal function. Peripheral renin activity was decreased in all patients.[133] Life-threatening hyperkalemia has been reported, mostly in elderly patients receiving large doses for gouty arthritis.[93]

The interaction between aspirin and indomethacin is complex; the decreased indomethacin AUC after long-term administration of both drugs is due to a combination of reduced indomethacin absorption, increased biliary clearance, and decreased renal clearance.[134] Clinically, no difference in response was noted between aspirin and indomethacin given alone or in combination, although the incidence of side effects increased when the drugs were given together.[135]

Indomethacin causes sodium retention and decreases the natriuretic effect of furosemide, but this effect is easily overcome by increasing the dose of the diuretic.[136] Probenecid interferes with the excretion of indomethacin, probably by competing for a common tubular secretion mechanism.[137] The marked increase in indomethacin serum levels during concurrent probenecid administration was reported to increase the effect of indomethacin in 28 patients with RA who were given both drugs at bedtime;[138] this finding may be important when the drugs are used together to treat gout. Diflunisal caused a 210% increase in indomethacin AUC, from 0 to 12 hours, when the two drugs were given concomitantly.[139] Moreover, indomethacin increased lithium carbonate levels by 42% in seven subjects, probably because of decreased renal lithium clearance.[140] In normal subjects, indomethacin did not change the anticoagulant effect induced by warfarin.[141]

Uses

Despite some initial controversy, it is generally agreed that indomethacin is approximately as effective as aspirin in RA.[142,143] It may be more effective than aspirin in some patients and is a reasonable alternative in patients who are intolerant to aspirin.

Indomethacin is effective in acute gouty arthritis. Doses as high as 600 mg have been used for the first day, followed by 150 to 200 mg daily, continuing until 3 to 4 days after all pain has disappeared.[35] A daily dose of 100 mg is effective in patients with ankylosing spondylitis.[31] Its effect on osteoarthritis is documented in several short-term studies in which indomethacin, in doses of 75 to 225 mg/day, was compared with placebo,[144] as well as with other NSAIDs.[145] Doses greater than 100 mg daily are rarely indicated in this older population, however. Indomethacin has also been used in the following conditions: psoriatic arthritis, with about a 50% response rate; rheumatic fever, with an effectiveness equal to that of aspirin; Reiter's syndrome, with about a 75% response rate; and JRA, in which 12 of 13 children studied responded. Controlled trials are not available in any of these conditions.[142]

Indomethacin has also been used in other diseases as an anti-inflammatory drug or for its potent effect on prostaglandin synthesis. It has been reported to be effective in the nephrotic syndrome,[146] pericarditis,[147] pleuritic pain,[148] pancreatic cholera,[149] hypercalcemia related to some neoplasms,[150] premature labor,[151] treatment of patent ductus arteriosus in infants,[45] leprosy,[152] dysmenorrhea,[153] and uveitis.[154] Most of these uses of indomethacin are investigational, although the FDA has approved its use for the treatment of patent ductus arteriosus.*

Adverse Effects

In 1968, O'Brien reviewed published reports of toxicity to indomethacin.[142] In 15 studies, some undesirable reaction was reported in 35.6% of patients. Gas-

trointestinal side effects occurred in 12.5 to 44% of patients, and 2 to 5% developed ulcers with bleeding. Such ulcers may be gastric, duodenal, or jejunal and may be silent.[142,155] Gastrointestinal toxicity may be related to the amount of drug excreted in the bile. Local effects on gastric mucosa include inhibition of mucin secretion, increased acid secretion, and local congestion.[74]

Central nervous system effects, reported in 10 to 25% of patients,[142] include characteristic morning frontal headache, vertigo, feelings of dissociation or unreality, depression, and, rarely, hallucinations or psychosis. In a retrospective study, the occurrence of retinal abnormalities was the same in an indomethacin-treated group as in control subjects. Both groups showed changes consistent with age and arteriosclerosis.[156]

The International Agranulocytosis and Aplastic Anemia Study has reported that indomethacin use is associated with excess risks for both agranulocytosis (0.6 per million) and aplastic anemia (10.1 per million).[157] Because information from voluntary reporting systems and other studies[158] do not confirm these findings, however, warnings have not as yet been issued regarding increased bone marrow toxicity of indomethacin.

Other rarely reported toxicities include hepatitis, acute renal failure, angina pectoris, induction of antiplatelet antibodies, asthma, arthropathy of the hips, peripheral neuropathy, rashes, and two cases of pulmonary hypertension in infants of mothers given indomethacin to inhibit premature labor, perhaps related to early closure of the ductus arteriosus in utero.[142,159–163] Through secretion into breast milk, the drug may have caused convulsions in a 6-day-old breast-fed infant.[164] Oral indomethacin has a mild coronary artery vasoconstrictive effect, but this does not interfere substantially with the expected increase in myocardial blood flow during rapid atrial pacing, and does not alter the exercise threshold for angina pectoris.[165]†

Schaller reviewed the serious adverse experiences reported in children taking indomethacin and concluded that the drug should be given to children under age 14 only if lack of efficacy or toxicity associated with other NSAIDs warranted the risk; selected patients with JRA or juvenile ankylosing spondylitis may be treated with indomethacin for short periods, but the drug is not recommended for long-term use.[166]

---

*Editor's note. We have been impressed with the effects of indomethacin in treating the pleural and pericardial involvement in systemic lupus erythematosus.

†Editor's note. The sodium-retaining effects of indomethacin are weak, but we have noted recurrent edema in a patient with Addison's disease.

Dosage

Capsules containing 25 or 50 mg are available, as well as 75-mg timed release capsules, an oral suspension (25 mg/5 ml), and 50-mg rectal suppositories.

Indomethacin has a relatively short plasma elimination half-life; steady-state levels are reached within 1 to 2 days; dosing (25 mg) may be necessary every 4 or every 8 hours, depending on the half-life of the drug in individual patients. The slow-release (75-mg capsules) preparation may be used twice daily.

New uses for indomethacin may arise from its potent effects on prostaglandin synthesis. Gastrointestinal and central nervous system effects may be troublesome, and their incidence may increase with age.

IBUPROFEN

Ibuprofen (Motrin, Rufen, Advil, Nuprin, and others), a propionic acid with a pKa of 4.4, was first marketed in 1969 in Great Britain and in 1974 in the United States. Ibuprofen is more than 90% absorbed, and peak levels occur 45 to 90 minutes after tablet ingestion. Food delays absorption. The plasma-time concentration curves of the drug can be satisfactorily described by a one-compartment open model, with a half-life of approximately 2 hours. Increasing the dose linearly increases the AUC of unbound drug.[167] Despite its short half-life, pharmacologic effects continue for much longer. In a small pilot study, a fixed daily dose of ibuprofen was as effective when given every 12 hours as when given every 6 hours.[168] It is 98% protein bound and is cleared predominantly by the liver.[169] All metabolites are inactive, and induction of metabolism does not occur. In 13 subjects, most of the drug was either hydroxylated or carboxylated; only 12% was excreted by the kidney as the glucuronide, and only 1% appeared unchanged in the urine.[169] Despite strong protein binding, significant interaction between warfarin and ibuprofen does not occur in normal subjects.[170] Ibuprofen causes transient inhibition of platelet aggregation of shorter duration than that caused by aspirin.

Double-blind trials of ibuprofen (up to 1200 mg/day) versus placebo, aspirin (2.3 to 4.8 g/day), or other NSAIDs yielded equivocal results in RA, with definite analgesia, but questionable anti-inflammatory activity. At higher doses of 2100 to 2400 mg/day, the anti-inflammatory effect was more evident.[171] One study comparing doses of 2400 mg to 3200 mg ibuprofen daily in 61 patients with RA showed no difference between these dosing regimens.[172] Side effects were infrequent at lower doses but at the higher doses were equal to the side effects of other NSAIDs.[171]

Ibuprofen, at a daily dose of 1200 mg, is reported to be an effective analgesic in osteoarthritis. At 1800 mg daily, ibuprofen was as effective as 3.6 g aspirin in 437 osteoarthritis patients.[173] Success has also been shown in JRA, in comparison to aspirin;[174] in ankylosing spondylitis, although indomethacin is usually preferred;[175] and in gout.[175] In nonarticular rheumatism, indomethacin and ibuprofen are equally effective, although ibuprofen causes fewer side effects.[176] In addition, ibuprofen has been used successfully to inhibit uterine contraction and to treat dysmenorrhea.[177] Animal experiments indicate that ibuprofen limits the size of infarctions when given intravenously immediately after coronary artery occlusion. The mechanism of this effect is unknown.[178]

Adverse Reactions

Dyspepsia occurs in up to 16% of cases, and clinically significant gastrointestinal bleeding has been reported.[179] Although ibuprofen, like other NSAIDs, reversibly affects platelet aggregation, it has been given to hemophiliac patients with no greater effect than in normal subjects.[179] Occult gastrointestinal blood loss was less with ibuprofen than with aspirin, but greater than with placebo, and increased with increasing doses of ibuprofen. Headaches, drowsiness, tinnitus, vertigo, and rash occur, but are uncommon.[179] An unusual, idiosyncratic aseptic meningitis has been reported following ibuprofen administration in a few patients with SLE or mixed connective tissue disease.[180] As with other NSAIDs, ibuprofen has been associated with edema and precipitation of congestive heart failure in susceptible individuals, probably because of the effects of these drugs on renal homeostasis by cyclo-oxygenase inhibition. Ibuprofen has also been implicated in papillary necrosis, as well as in acute renal failure.[179] Other, rare, adverse reactions include asthma, agranulocytosis, and hepatic dysfunction.[114,181,182] However, no cases of acute liver or kidney disease or of other serious uncommon illnesses requiring hospitalization were found among 13,230 members of a group health cooperative who were prescribed ibuprofen as outpatients.[183]

Doses are given every 6 or 8 hours because of the short serum half-life of this drug, although one study compared 6- and 12-hour dosing intervals.[168] Because so little of it is cleared unchanged by the kidneys, the dose does not need to be modified in patients with renal failure. Although ibuprofen is predominantly cleared by the liver, alcoholic liver disease does not alter its kinetics.[184] Ibuprofen is tightly bound to albumin; nonetheless, no drug interactions of consequence have been reported.[169] This lack of interaction may be a significant advantage for patients taking warfarin anticoagulants.[179] Because ibuprofen is principally metabolized by oxidation, probenecid, which inhibits glucuronidation, does not raise ibuprofen serum concentrations.[185]

Overdose. Ibuprofen was released in 1984 for nonprescription sale to the general public as 200-mg tablets for use as an analgesic, with a maximum daily dose of 1200 mg. Increased availability as an alternative to aspirin and acetaminophen increases the potential for accidental or deliberate overdoses. Ibuprofen overdose has been rare, despite its extensive use as an NSAID. Only 75 cases of ibuprofen overdose were noted among 58,000 overdoses recorded in a 2-year survey by the British National Poisons Information Service.[186] Alleged overdoses ranged from 200 mg to 40 g; plasma concentrations as high as 704 mg/L were measured in asymptomatic patients. Only a single death was recorded. A 67-year-old woman died following vomiting, deafness, confusion, hyperventilation, coma, hypotension, and cardiac arrest after an overdose of both ibuprofen and salicylate.[186]

The Rocky Mountain Poison and Drug Center has reported 126 cases of ibuprofen overdose; 24 patients developed symptoms, all within 4 hours after drug ingestion, and one child died. Symptoms include CNS depression, seizures, apnea, nystagmus, blurred vision, diplopia, headache, tinnitus, bradycardia, hypotension, abdominal pain, nausea, vomiting, hematuria, and abnormal renal function.[187] Treatment generally included an emetic or gastric lavage, observation, and administration of fluids.

Dosage
The drug is available as 200-, 300-, 400-, 600-, or 800-mg tablets.
Because of its short plasma half-life, ibuprofen is usually given four times a day; 1200 to 1600 mg daily are adequate for analgesia, but 3000 to 3600 mg daily may be needed for an anti-inflammatory effect in RA. These higher doses are more likely to be associated with gastrointestinal side effects.

NAPROXEN

Naproxen (Naprosyn) is completely absorbed from tablet, capsule, or aqueous suspension. The absorption rate is increased by bicarbonate, is decreased by other antacids, and is slightly decreased by food. Naproxen contains only the active D(+) isomer; the L(−) isomer is inactive. A linear relationship exists between dose and serum concentration for doses up to 500 mg, but the relationship becomes nonlinear thereafter. A 50% increase of dose to 750 mg results in only a 25% increase in the AUC. This phenomenon is associated with increases in unbound fraction and renal excre-

tion, and indicates that protein-binding sites may be saturated at that level.[188,189] The drug is 97.6 to 99.5% protein bound at doses below 500 mg.[188] The plasma levels of naproxen fit a two-compartment open model with an elimination half-life of 12 to 15 hours. No difference is noted in half-life between adults and children.[188,189] From 77 to 100% is recovered in the urine, as conjugated drug (50 to 60%), or as metabolites (27 to 46%); only 0.5 to 2.5% appears in the feces.[188,189] In a study of patients taking 250 mg naproxen twice daily, mean synovial fluid concentrations were 50% of serum concentrations 3 to 4 hours after a dose and 74% of serum concentrations after 15 hours.[190]

The addition of aspirin decreased naproxen blood levels and decreased the AUC by 15%; however, when naproxen was given to subjects taking salicylates, the AUC of salicylate was decreased by only 2%.[188,191] An 8-week crossover study showed that a regimen of naproxen, 500 mg daily, added to aspirin, 1.3 to 5 g daily, was better than aspirin alone, with respect to patient preference, walking time, grip strength, and morning stiffness, but not with respect to inflamed joint count or joint swelling.[192] However, another study in RA patients showed that the efficacy of naproxen, 1500 mg daily, was not increased by adding sufficient choline magnesium salicylate to produce average plasma salicylate concentrations of 23.5 mg/dl.[103] No kinetic interactions have been found between naproxen and diflunisal,[193] but concomitant probenecid administration has increased steady-state naproxen concentrations by 50% and has increased plasma half-lives from 14 to 37 hours.[194]

Naproxen displaces warfarin from human serum albumin in vitro: a 14 to 17% increase in free warfarin concentration was found when therapeutic concentrations of naproxen were added.[195] In vivo studies show an increase in free warfarin concentrations in some subjects when these two drugs are used together, so patients treated with both warfarin and naproxen should be observed closely on initiation or change in therapy.[196] Unbound serum naproxen concentrations are increased in patients with renal insufficiency, but the half-life of the drug is unaltered.[197] Compared to normal individuals, 10 patients with alcoholic cirrhosis had a 60% reduction in clearance of unbound naproxen, but no difference in clearance of total drug or in volume of distribution. Therefore, it has been suggested that naproxen doses should be decreased by 50% or more in patients with alcoholic cirrhosis.[198]

In patients with RA, naproxen, at a dose of 400 to 750 mg daily, was more effective than placebo and was as effective as aspirin,[188] it was also roughly comparable to 150 mg indomethacin or to 2.4 g fenoprofen daily. Naproxen was also more effective than 2400 mg ibuprofen or 1500 mg flufenamic acid, although statistically significant differences were not found.[188] A dose-related increase in efficacy has been shown in 50 patients with RA treated with up to 1000 mg naproxen daily,[199] and a relationship of serum level to efficacy response was shown in 24 patients with RA given up to 1500 mg naproxen daily for 2 weeks.[200] In this study, trough naproxen concentrations, measured just before a dose, below 18 μg/ml were associated with no response, whereas 76% of patients with trough concentrations above 50 μg/ml responded.

Naproxen, 10 mg/kg/day, was as effective as aspirin, 75 mg/kg/day, in patients with JRA.[201] Naproxen, 250 mg twice daily, was more effective than placebo and was equal to indomethacin in osteoarthritis of large joints.[188] Many trials, using naproxen 500 to 750 mg versus other NSAIDs, such as proquazone, diclofenac, indomethacin, and flurbiprofen, did not show major differences between drugs in treating osteoarthritis.[188] Small numbers of patients with ankylosing spondylitis, acute gout, and "nonarticular rheumatism" have also been treated successfully with daily doses of 500 to 1000 mg naproxen.[32,36,188]

Side effects are similar to those of indomethacin and aspirin, but they are less frequent[188] (see Table 32–1).

Dosage

Tablets containing 250, 375, or 500 mg are available.

Because naproxen has a long elimination half-life, it can be given twice a day. Naproxen protein-binding sites become saturated at doses greater than 500 to 750 mg a day, and at higher doses, renal clearance increases. Despite this effect, increasing doses raise serum concentrations, and doses as high as 1500 mg daily have been used. Unchanged drug may be cleared to a modest extent, so some drug may accumulate in patients with renal impairment. Naproxen is tightly and extensively bound to serum protein, making drug-drug interactions more likely. In RA, the relationship between serum concentration and efficacy suggests that serum levels may be useful to adjust doses.

SULINDAC

Sulindac (Clinoril) is an indene-acetic acid derivative, chemically related to indomethacin, and may be considered as an isostere of indomethacin.[202] A sulfoxide, it is a prodrug because its sulfide metabolite is much more active than the parent drug in in vitro tests of anti-inflammatory activity and in animal studies of inflammation. For example, the sulfide is 500 times as active as the sulfoxide as a prostaglandin synthesis inhibitor. Sulindac is reversibly metabolized to the sulfide and is irreversibly metabolized to an inactive sulfone. In animal studies, the drug is transformed to the sulfide in all tissues. Except in lung and plasma, more sulfide is present than sulfoxide.[202] All forms of this drug undergo enterohepatic recirculation, with 5 to 30 times more sulindac than sulfide excreted in the bile. Sulindac is more than 88% bioavailable, although some may already be in the inactive sulfone form when absorbed. Peak plasma levels are achieved within an hour in fasted humans. The plasma half-life of sulindac itself is 7.8 hours, but the more active sulfide metabolite has a half-life of 16 to 18 hours. Both the sulfoxide and sulfide are tightly protein bound (93 to 98%); 45 to 50% of a single dose is excreted in the urine, whereas 25 to 30% is found in the feces. Although over 90% of the drug is recovered in the urine and feces, only 10% is recovered as sulfide, all in the feces.[75]

Two-hour postprandial blood glucose levels did not change when sulindac was given with tolbutamide for 7 days, although the fasting blood sugar levels of these patients did decrease from 120.5 to 112.9 mg/100 ml.[203] Sulindac had little effect on prothrombin time in volunteers taking warfarin, although those given warfarin without sulindac had a faster return of prothrombin times to normal than those taking warfarin and sulindac combined. This effect may indicate some inhibition of the excretion or metabolism of warfarin by sulindac; four patients developed hypothrombinemia in response to sulindac.[204] Aspirin did not change the peak plasma concentrations or AUC of sulindac, but it did decrease these parameters for the sulfide by 20 to 25%.[205] Unlike other NSAIDs, sulindac may not inhibit cyclo-oxygenase in the kidney because that organ can reoxidize the sulfide back to the inactive prodrug sulfoxide form.[206] It has been suggested that sulindac does not impair renal function or renal prostaglandin synthesis,[207] and it is sometimes preferred over other NSAIDs in patients at increased risk for NSAID renal toxicity. This renal sparing effect is not complete for all patients; reversible renal failure can be induced with sulindac and has been reported in suitably predisposed patients.[208,209]

Doses of 150 to 200 mg sulindac twice a day are more effective than placebo and are equivalent to 3.6 to 4.8 g aspirin in the treatment of both RA and osteoarthritis of the large joints.[210,211] Sulindac is more effective than ibuprofen, 1200 mg daily, in osteoarthritis of the hip.[210] A 1-year double-blind study of 387 patients with osteoarthritis compared 100 to 400 mg sulindac to 1.6 to 4.8 g aspirin daily; about 80% in both groups had an excellent or satisfactory response.[212] Sulindac, at a dose of 100 to 200 mg twice a day, may be as effective as indomethacin or phenylbutazone in ankylosing spondylitis, nonarticular shoulder pain, and gout.[210,213–215]

Adverse effects are less common with sulindac than with equieffective doses of aspirin. Of 864 patients with osteoarthritis or RA enrolled in controlled trials of sulindac versus aspirin, 10.4% of sulindac-treated patients discontinued the drug because of adverse effects, as compared to 17.3% of aspirin-treated patients.[212,216] As with other NSAIDs, gastrointestinal side effects were most common. In osteoarthritis patients, 1 ulcer was found in 387 patients; overall, the incidence of ulcer was 0.4% in 1865 patients.[212] Gastrointestinal blood loss while taking sulindac for a week was 2 ml daily, whereas blood loss while taking aspirin was 15 ml daily.[217]

Sulindac has the usual range of NSAID side effects, including rare reactions such as bone marrow aplasia, Stevens-Johnson syndrome, congestive heart failure, acute renal failure, aseptic meningitis, and severe hepatitis.[205,218–221]

Dosage

Tablets containing 150 or 200 mg are available.
Sulindac is given twice daily in doses of 300 to 400 mg/day. Gastrointestinal side effects may be decreased because the sulfide, which may be the active irritant, does not build up rapidly in the gastrointestinal tract. Because sulindac is tightly protein bound, drug-drug interactions are possible. May have advantages in some patients with renal insufficiency.

TOLMETIN

Tolmetin (Tolectin), a pyrrole derivative, is not chemically related to any of the previously described NSAIDs, although it shares their probable mechanism(s) of action and animal pharmacology.[222] Tolmetin is absorbed rapidly, with peak plasma concentrations in about 30 to 45 minutes. Plasma disposition curves have been fitted to one- and two-compartment open models, with elimination half-lives between 2.1 and 6.8 hours.[223–225] The longer half-life relates to the drug's elimination phase and makes up only a small portion of the drug's AUC; 99% of the drug is excreted in the urine. All metabolites are inactive; 10 to 17% unchanged tolmetin is recovered in urine, but may be an artifact because the glucuronide metabolite may spontaneously dissociate to tolmetin in the urine. Animal studies indicate that tolmetin does not have a significant enterohepatic circulation.[226]

Tolmetin is 99% protein bound,[224] but it did not influence warfarin-induced prolonged prothrombin times when added to an anticoagulant regimen for 3

weeks.[227] Magnesium-aluminum hydroxide (Maalox) did not decrease tolmetin's AUC.[223] In vitro, aspirin and salicylic acid substantially decreased tolmetin binding to albumin.[228] Tolmetin added to established aspirin therapy in RA patients for 10 weeks did not have any additional clinical effect.[229] The combined administration of tolmetin and aspirin for 18 days resulted in a fourfold increase in free tolmetin (from 1% to 3.8%), a 16% decrease in tolmetin AUC, and a 17% increase in tolmetin clearance.[225,230]

Tolmetin, at a dose of 1200 to 1500 mg daily, is better than placebo and is probably equal to 3.9 to 4.5 g aspirin, 100 to 150 mg indomethacin, 2400 mg ibuprofen, or 400 mg phenylbutazone per day in the treatment of RA and osteoarthritis.[222] In 107 children with JRA, tolmetin was equal to aspirin in effectiveness. In 10 gouty patients, it neither decreased serum uric acid levels nor suppressed acute gouty arthritis.[232] In an open study of 30 patients with ankylosing spondylitis, 90% had a satisfactory response.[233]

Gastrointestinal side effects severe enough to discontinue medication included ulcers in 3.6% of 420 patients; gastrointestinal bleeding occurred in 1% of 420 patients, and occasional nausea, pain, or diarrhea was noted.[234,235] In a review of 847 geriatric patients with osteoarthritis, 15.5% stopped tolmetin because of side effects, 3.2% developed peptic ulcers, and 1.3% developed gastrointestinal bleeding; in patients younger than 65 years in the same studies, ulcers developed in 1.9% and bleeding occurred in 0.4%.[236] The rare side effects of other NSAIDs can also occur in tolmetin-treated patients, despite the unique chemical structure of this agent. Thus, acute renal failure and interstitial nephritis, meningitis, anaphylactic reactions, and IgM-related allergic thrombocytopenic purpura have been documented.[89,237–239] An artifactual "pseudoproteinuria" may occur in patients taking tolmetin. When the sulfosalicylic acid test for urine protein is used, the acid precipitates the major metabolite of tolmetin, with an appearance resembling that of proteinuria. Use of tetrabromphenol blue (Albustix) or similar nonacidic or specific methods circumvents this laboratory artifact.[240]

Dosage

Tolmetin is given in doses of 600 to 1800 mg daily, divided into three or four doses; 200- and 400-mg tablets are available. Up to 2400 mg daily in RA and up to 1600 mg daily in osteoarthritis have been prescribed. Most of the drug is metabolized and then excreted in the urine. Because enterohepatic recirculation appears to be minimal, this drug is theoretically more useful in the elderly. No advantage exists to the simultaneous use of tolmetin and aspirin in RA. Tolmetin does not appear to be of use in gout, but it is an alternative to aspirin in the treatment of JRA, usually in divided doses of 15 to 35 mg/kg/day.

FENOPROFEN

Fenoprofen (Nalfon) is an arylpropionic acid with a pKa of 4.5. The (S)-fenoprofen enantiomer is 35 times more active than the (R)-isomer as an in vitro inhibitor of cyclo-oxygenase from human platelets. In vivo, the (R)-enantiomer is stereoselectively converted to the more active (S)-isomer.[241] Fenoprofen is 80% bioavailable, its disposition is well described by a two-compartment open model, and it has an enterohepatic circulation in humans. The elimination half-life of the drug is short (70 to 160 minutes); 90% of a single dose is excreted in the urine as glucuronides, and only 1 to 3% is eliminated as unchanged fenoprofen. The drug is 99% bound to serum proteins.[78,242,243]

Aspirin, at a daily dose of 3.9 g, decreased the area under the log plasma concentration–time curve of fenoprofen by 25 to 50% and decreased its serum half-life by 30% after multiple dosing in normal subjects. The mechanism of this effect was not clear because aspirin and fenoprofen bind at different sites on albumin, so drug displacement is not likely. It was postulated that aspirin might have induced increased metabolism of fenoprofen.[243] Absorption of fenoprofen is decreased by food, with a 20% decrease in AUC, as compared to the fasting state.[244] On the other hand, magnesium-aluminum hydroxide does not decrease absorption. No other significant drug-drug interactions with fenoprofen appear to exist, despite its high protein binding, although probenecid would be expected to increase fenoprofen serum concentrations.

Fenoprofen, at 1.2 to 3.2 g a day, is better than placebo and is generally comparable to a daily dose of aspirin of 3.6 g or more in the treatment of RA.[245] Similarly, fenoprofen, at 1.8 to 2.4 g a day, is effective in osteoarthritis.[246] It appeared to be effective in treating acute gout when a daily dose of 3.2 g was used in an open trial of 27 patients.[247] In a 2-week, double-blind, cross-over study of 19 patients with ankylosing spondylitis, 1800 mg fenoprofen daily was as effective as 150 mg indomethacin.[248]

Occult blood loss from the gastrointestinal tract in humans is less with short-term fenoprofen administration than with aspirin (2.25 versus 5 ml/day).[249] In a study of patients with RA, fewer gastrointestinal side effects and less tinnitus were noted with fenoprofen than with aspirin.[245] Like other NSAIDs, fenoprofen has been associated with rare hepatic dysfunction, agranulocytosis, and thrombocytopenia, as well as uncommon rashes, headaches, and drowsiness.[250] Of more concern is fenoprofen-induced renal failure. Fenoprofen appeared to be more nephrotoxic than other NSAIDs and its use sometimes resulted in multiple renal lesions within the same patient, according to a review of the world literature on NSAID-related renal complications.[91] Although oliguria may or may not be present, and the association with nephrotic syndrome is variable, interstitial nephritis and minimal-change glomerulonephritis are characteristic. Eosinophilia is seen in 30% of patients, and T-cell predominance and IgE-bearing B cells have been documented in renal tissue.[88]

Dosage

The drug is available as a 200- or 300-mg capsule or a 600-mg tablet. Usual doses are 1800 to 2400 mg daily, but doses as high as 3200 mg daily have been used in acute gout.

Fenoprofen should be given four times a day. It is an effective drug, but thus far accounts for a majority of NSAID-induced nephropathy, so it should be used cautiously.

MECLOFENAMATE SODIUM

Meclofenamate sodium (Meclomen) is the third generation of the fenamates. Flufenamic acid and mefenamic acid have also been marketed, but are used infrequently and are not discussed here. Meclofenamate sodium is a cyclo-oxygenase inhibitor that may inhibit phospholipase A_2 and may also impair prostaglandin activity at its receptor site.[251] It was more potent than benoxaprofen as an inhibitor of 5-lipoxygenase actvity in human neutrophils in vitro and thus can be considered a dual inhibitor of both 5-lipoxygenase and the cyclo-oxygenase pathways of arachidonic acid metabolism.[252] But no benefit occurred when it was used to treat the (possibly lipoxygenase-mediated) inflammation of psoriatic dermatitis.[253]

Meclofenamate is rapidly absorbed, with peak concentrations in 1 to 2 hours.[77] It is highly metabolized, and one of its metabolites, hydroxymethyl meclofenamic acid, has some anti-inflammatory activity.[77] From 50 to 70% of the drug is excreted in the urine, and 25 to 30% appears in the feces.[77] It probably undergoes enterohepatic recirculation. The elimination half-life of meclofenamic acid is 3.3 hours; no information is available on the half-life of the active metabolite.[77,254] Meclofenamic acid is 99.8% albumin bound, but is displaced from albumin by salicylate.[254]

Neither food nor magnesium-aluminum hydroxide (Maalox) affected its bioavailability, but sodium bicarbonate resulted in more rapid absorption and higher peak plasma levels.[254] Concomitant aspirin therapy decreased plasma meclofenamate concentrations; the AUC was 10% less when meclofenamate was given with aspirin.[255] Warfarin requirements were decreased by an average of 16% (range 0 to 25%) when given with meclofenamate sodium, but no interaction with propoxyphene or sulfinpyrazone appeared to be clinically significant.[255]

Meclofenamate sodium is effective in treating RA.[256] In 6- to 8-week trials, regimens of 200 mg and 300 mg daily were better than placebo; a daily dose of 300 mg was equivalent to 3.6 g aspirin or 150 mg indomethacin. In patients with osteoarthritis, 300 mg daily was better than placebo and was equivalent to phenylbutazone and naproxen regimens. With meclofenamate sodium, 76% of patients studied, versus 42% receiving placebo, felt overall improvement.[257] Meclofenamate appeared to be as effective as indomethacin in the treatment of ankylosing spondylitis or extra-articular conditions such as painful shoulder syndrome.[258,259] High doses, such as 800 mg the first day, followed by 300 mg/day for 6 days, were equivalent to 150 mg indomethacin daily in the treatment of acute gout.[260] A 4-week, open, uncontrolled study of 39 patients with JRA indicated that the drug was effective at daily doses of 3 to 7.5 mg/kg.[261] The 18% dropout rate in this study was higher than in previous similar studies of other NSAIDs by the same group (0 to 3%), however, and thus the usefulness of meclofenamate may be limited in children.[261]

Adverse Experiences

The types of adverse reactions with meclofenamate sodium are similar to those with other NSAIDs, but gastrointestinal problems seem to be more common. Among 2500 patients in controlled studies, dose-related diarrhea, the most common side effect, occurred in 11%, as compared to 2% of aspirin-treated patients.[262] Abdominal pain occurred in 7%, versus 1% with aspirin. Withdrawal of the drug for diarrhea occurred in only 2.2% of meclofenamate sodium-treated patients, however, as opposed to 1.8% of aspirin-treated patients.[262] The diarrhea was of small-bowel origin.[262] In long-term studies of 109 patients with RA in which 60% completed a year of treatment and 17% completed 2 years of treatment, gastrointestinal side effects were even more common and occurred in 30.6 to 43.3% of patients.[263] Therapy was discontinued in 29% because of these effects, which included abdominal pain in 8%, diarrhea in 7%, and peptic ulcers in 2.8%.[263] One of every six patients receiving meclofenamate sodium had a decrease in hemoglobin or hematocrit level, although no evidence of increased blood loss, bone marrow suppression, or hemolysis was found. Patients with osteoarthritis appeared to have fewer side effects than those with RA.[262,263]

Dosage
The drug is available in 50- and 100-mg capsules.
The daily dosing regimen recommended for meclofenamate sodium is 200 to 400 mg, given in four divided doses. Although effective, it may have greater incidence of gastrointestinal side-effects than other NSAIDs.

PIROXICAM

Piroxicam (Feldene), a carboxamide, was marketed in the United States in 1982. It is one of only three NSAIDs with a high pKa, of 6.32; phenylbutazone and oxyphenbutazone are the others.[264] In most other ways, piroxicam is similar to other NSAIDs. It is antipyretic, variably analgesic, and anti-inflammatory, and it reversibly inhibits platelet aggregation. Its principal mechanism of action is probably cyclo-oxygenase inhibition, but at high concentrations it also inhibits neutrophil migration, phagocytosis, and lysozymal enzyme release.[264] Piroxicam's long elimination half-life (mean 38 hours; range 14 to 158 hours) makes it suitable for administration once a day.[264] For the same reason, 7 to 21 days of therapy are required before steady-state plasma concentrations are achieved; thereafter plasma concentrations are relatively stable with once-daily drug administration. The presence of more than one peak in the plasma concentration curve suggests that piroxicam may undergo enterohepatic recycling.[265] It is well absorbed, highly metabolized, and renally excreted, although only 10% of a dose is excreted unchanged into the urine.[264] Its metabolites are clinically inactive.[264] The accumulation of this drug is linear, and it is 99% protein bound at a concentration between 5 and 50 μg/ml.[266] Synovial fluid concentrations are approximately 50% of serum concentrations.[264] Unlike many other NSAIDs, piroxicam is not displaced from albumin by aspirin, and drug-drug interactions are often insignificant; for example, no interaction was found with several antacids or digoxin.[264] Partial thromboplastin times, however, were prolonged when this drug was given with acenocoumarol.[264] Piroxicam levels are not elevated in patients with renal impairment because this drug is cleared from the plasma predominantly by hepatic metabolism.[267]

With piroxicam's long and variable half-life, there has been concern about possible piroxicam accumulation in elderly patients. One study reported an increased volume of distribution in older patients,[268] but this was not confirmed by another study.[269] However, the latter single-dose study of healthy subjects found that, compared with young women, elderly women had decreased clearances from the body, increased predicted steady-state plasma levels, and longer plasma half-lives of piroxicam; there were no differences in these measures between young and elderly men. A review of these and other single- and multiple-dose kinetic studies and therapeutic drug-level monitoring studies involving more than 1200 subjects concluded that there is an inconsistent tendency toward slightly increased steady-state piroxicam concentrations in elderly women, but that there is no evidence of an associated increased risk of adverse effects.[267]

Piroxicam has been studied in patients with RA, osteoarthritis, gout, ankylosing spondylitis, and acute musculoskeletal disorders.[264] In a 4-week double-blind cross-over study of 22 patients with RA, 20 mg piroxicam daily was better than placebo with respect to joint tenderness, joint swelling, morning stiffness, and global assessment. Seventy-nine patients with RA underwent a 12-week, parallel, double-blind comparison of aspirin, 3 g or more, and piroxicam, 20 mg daily. Stable prednisone and gold therapy were allowed. Patients in both drug groups improved equally with respect to pain, stiffness, joint pain and swelling, 50-foot walking time, and visual analogue scales. Grip strength improved more in patients taking aspirin, as did erythrocyte sedimentation rates.[270]

Piroxicam, at 20 mg daily, was comparable in efficacy to 100 to 200 mg indomethacin daily in 32 patients with RA. In osteoarthritis, piroxicam, 20 mg/day, was comparable to a daily dose of 2.6 to 3.9 g aspirin and was statistically superior in reducing the number of painful joints and in increasing lower-extremity range of motion.[271] In a 12-week, double-blind, randomized, parallel study of 2000 patients with osteoarthritis given 20 mg piroxicam or 750 mg naproxen daily, both drugs produced similar efficacy and toxicity.[272] For gout (40 mg/day piroxicam for 1 to 5 days) and ankylosing spondylitis (10 to 30 mg/day), only "positive-control" (versus indomethacin) or uncontrolled trials were done, but results indicated efficacy.[273,274]

Adverse Effects

Based on studies of over 3500 patients who have used the drug, the incidence and type of side effects from piroxicam are similar to those of other NSAIDs.[275] Gastrointestinal side effects occurred in 19% of patients studied and required discontinuance of the drug in 3.5%. One percent developed ulcers, as compared to 2.9% of those taking aspirin. Other gastrointestinal symptoms included dyspepsia, nausea, diarrhea, and cramping pain. Daily doses of piroxicam of 30 to 40 mg were associated with a higher incidence of ulcers than doses of 20 mg daily (up to 29% versus 1%). In one study, 4 of 10 patients taking

40 mg/day piroxicam and concurrent aspirin developed peptic ulcers.[276] Headaches and dizziness were unusual and occurred in about 3% of patients, as compared to 11 to 22% of those taking indomethacin. Other unusual side effects included rashes, liver dysfunction, allergic reactions, edema, and hematologic manifestations (0.9 to 2.4%).[275,276] Tinnitus occurred in 0.6% of patients. These findings were confirmed by an intensive review of the entire worldwide pre- and postmarketing experience with piroxicam in a data base of over 75,000 patients.[277] The FDA further reviewed the available data and concluded that there is no suggestion of an increased risk associated with piroxicam use as compared with other NSAIDs.

Dosage

The drug is available as 10- and 20-mg capsules.
Piroxicam has a half-life of 38 hours, so once-daily administration is sufficient. On the other hand, the drug has a narrow therapeutic range; 20 mg daily is the dose most frequently prescribed, a 10-mg dose is often ineffective, and a dose of 30 mg or more appears to be more toxic than the standard dose.

DIFLUNISAL

Diflunisal (Dolobid) is difluorophenyl salicylic acid.[278] It is not broken down into salicylic acid, although its metabolism is similar to that of salicylates. Like most NSAIDs, its principal mechanism of action is probably reversible cyclo-oxygenase inhibition.[278] Diflunisal may bind cyclo-oxygenase at a site close to, but not identical to, the aspirin and indomethacin binding site; it is also an effective free radical scavenger. Thus, the mechanism of action of this drug may differ from that of aspirin in some details, and it can inhibit the acetylation of cyclo-oxygenase by aspirin.[278] Diflunisal was first marketed in Great Britain in 1977 and marketed in the United States in 1982.[279]

Diflunisal is well absorbed. Like salicylates, it is subject to capacity-limited metabolism. Ninety percent is metabolized to two glucuronides, acyl and phenyl, that are excreted in the urine; 5% of a dose is excreted unchanged in the urine.[278] With 1000 mg daily doses, up to 30% may appear in the urine as diflunisal sulfate.[280] Protein binding is greater than 98%. Because the drug exhibits capacity-limited kinetics, plasma disappearance half-times increase with larger doses (8 to 10 hours with 500 mg daily; 15 hours with 1000 mg daily). With creatinine clearance of less than 30 ml/min, its half-life increases significantly; total body clearance decreases, but less than expected;

raised biliary clearance probably compensates for the lowered renal clearance.[278]

Concurrent naproxen and diflunisal administration decreases urinary naproxen excretion, but plasma naproxen profiles do not change; this finding implies compensatory biliary naproxen clearance. Diflunisal has decreased the renal clearance and increased plasma concentrations of indomethacin after their coadministration, however.[278] In one study, free warfarin concentrations increased minimally when diflunisal was given; similarly, diflunisal increased plasma concentrations of hydrochlorothiazide and acetaminophen. No interactions were detected when diflunisal was given with tolbutamide, furosemide, or magnesium hydroxide; however, aluminum hydroxide decreased diflunisal absorption by 40%.[278]

For postoperative oral surgical pain, 500- and 1000-mg doses of diflunisal were superior to placebo, and the effect generally lasted 12 hours. For peak analgesia, diflunisal doses of 500 and 1000 mg, were equivalent to each other, equal to 600 mg acetaminophen with 60 mg codeine, and better than 650 mg aspirin, 600 mg acetaminophen, 100 mg acetaminophen with 100 mg propoxyphene, and 100 mg propoxyphene napsylate. For overall analgesia, measured as pain intensity differences, 1000 mg diflunisal appeared superior to the comparison drugs at both 4 and 12 hours, whereas a 500-mg dose was superior only at 12 hours.[281]

In the treatment of osteoarthritis of the hips and knees, five studies included 1218 patients, of whom 657 were receiving diflunisal.[282] Daily doses of 500, 750 and 1000 mg were statistically better than placebo in all 10 disease activity criteria. When 791 patients were given aspirin, in daily doses of 2000 to 3000 mg, or diflunisal, in daily doses of 500 to 750 mg, in a 12-week, double-blind, parallel study, diflunisal was better than aspirin at 8 and 12 weeks for night pain, weight-bearing pain, stiffness, functional activity, and global response. Diflunisal, at 500 to 750 mg/day, was also better than 800- to 1200-mg doses of ibuprofen.[282]

Diflunisal 500 to 1000 mg daily has also been reported to be effective in rheumatoid arthritis[283,284] and ankylosing spondylitis.[285] Serum uric acid is moderately decreased by diflunisal, by a combination of uricosuria and competitive inhibition of xanthine oxidase.[286]

Adverse Effects

As expected for an NSAID, 25% of 657 patients had gastrointestinal effects: 0.5% had ulcers or hemorrhage; 17% had dyspepsia, pain, or cramps; and 9% had diarrhea or nausea. In addition, 0 to 5% had

rashes, dizziness, or drowsiness. In these studies, diflunisal was associated with fewer gastrointestinal effects than aspirin (47% for aspirin versus 25% for diflunisal), and tinnitus occurred in only 1%. Diflunisal caused less microscopic gastrointestinal bleeding than aspirin, as measured with (^{51}Cr)-labeled red cells; after 2 weeks, 8.8 ml/24 hours with aspirin, as compared with 2.1 ml/24 hours with diflunisal and 1.6 ml/24 hours with placebo.[287]

Dosage

The drug is supplied as 250- and 500-mg tablets.

Although it is a molecular modification of salicylic acid, diflunisal is not metabolized to salicylate and is not equivalent to the non-acetylated salicylates or aspirin in dose or mode of action.

Diflunisal has capacity-limited metabolism, and consequently, serum half-lives are raised by increasing doses. When one is using the usually recommended daily dose of 1000 mg, half-lives are about 12 hours and allow twice-daily administration. Although a dose of 1000 mg a day has no antiplatelet effects, a dose of 1500 mg daily reversibly inhibits platelet aggregation.

KETOPROFEN

Ketoprofen is a propionic acid derivative marketed in Europe since 1973, and in the United States since 1986. It is a potent inhibitor of prostaglandin synthesis,[288] and may also inhibit lipoxygenase.[10] Following a single oral dose, the drug is rapidly and completely absorbed, with peak concentrations 1 to 2 hours after the dose. The elimination half-life is approximately 2 hours in normal volunteers, although an observed multiexponential decline in serum concentrations limits the absolute accuracy of the terminal half-life.[289] It is 99% protein-bound, is extensively hydroxylated and glucuronidated, and is virtually completely excreted in the urine in the conjugated form.[290] Ketoprofen plasma clearance is decreased by 22 to 50% in the geriatric population.[291,292] Creatinine clearance and ketoprofen clearance are related, and dosing regimens may need to be altered in patients with renal disease.[293] Protein binding is decreased in cirrhotic patients, probably related to hypoalbuminemia. Despite the lack of significant change in total plasma clearance among cirrhotics, the amount of ketoprofen in the body was increased relative to normals (57.6 mg versus 102.2 mg after a single dose).[292] Therefore, patients with severely impaired liver function may require lower daily doses or less frequent administration.

Aspirin displaces ketoprofen from its albumin binding site and increases plasma clearance of unbound drug, but unbound concentrations do not change and ketoprofen efficacy is probably unaffected.[294] Probenecid raises both total and unbound ketoprofen plasma levels, prolongs plasma half-life, decreases protein binding, and lowers the rate of hepatic conjugation.[295]

Despite its half-life of approximately 2 hours, ketoprofen is sometimes given twice daily. Ketoprofen decreases synovial fluid prostaglandin E concentrations for more than 24 hours after a 100-mg ketoprofen dose.[292]

Efficacy and Toxicity

In Vavra's compendium of results from clinical studies of ketoprofen in RA, osteoarthritis, ankylosing spondylitis, and acute gout, ketoprofen in doses of 200 to 300 mg was more effective than placebo, and as effective as anti-inflammatory doses of aspirin, indomethacin, and ibuprofen.[292] Typically, 200 to 300 mg of ketoprofen improved joint tenderness by 45 to 49%, while joint tenderness improved by 23% in the placebo group. In longer trials, a 40% decrease in tenderness was noted in the ketoprofen and aspirin groups, although the swollen joint index improved only 11% for both. In acute gout, 92% improvement was noted within 24 hours in a ketoprofen group (compared with a 91% improvement in those receiving indomethacin). Ketoprofen was effective in an open trial of 34 JRA patients, as well as in small crossover studies of ankylosing spondylitis and Reiter's disease.[296–298]

Using pooled data from 978 ketoprofen-treated patients in double-blind trials, Vavra found that ketoprofen adhered to the usual NSAID profile of adverse reactions.[292] Dyspepsia occurred in 25.8% of patients and lower GI discomfort, including diarrhea and constipation, occurred in 15.3% of patients. CNS effects occurred in 3 to 9%, while rashes and edema occurred in 3 to 4% of patents. Tinnitus occurred in 7% of patients. All these findings were statistically less frequent than among aspirin-treated patients in aspirin-controlled trials. Thus far, no significant liver function abnormalities have been noted. Ketoprofen can produce increases in BUN, serum creatinine, and fluid retention, although these are usually transient and asymptomatic.

Dosage
Ketoprofen is available in 50- and 75-mg capsules. It is recommended for treatment of RA and osteoarthritis in three or four divided daily doses totaling 150 to 300 mg. Initial doses should be decreased 30 to 50% in the elderly and in patients with impaired renal function.

OTHER NONSTEROIDAL ANTI-INFLAMMATORY DRUGS

An efficient system has been developed for detecting chemicals with NSAID properties. Many such agents are being developed. Many await approval for marketing, and some have already been marketed in various parts of the world. Only a few examples are given here.

CARPROFEN

Carprofen, a carbazole-propionic acid derivative, is an inhibitor of cyclo-oxygenase, particularly as the more active carprofen (R)-isomer.[299] It may also inhibit neutrophil chemotaxis.[300] Like other NSAIDs, it inhibits the first wave of platelet aggregation and is active in the usual animal arthritis models (e.g., adjuvant arthritis), where its potency is approximately equivalent to indomethacin.[301]

Of ^{14}C-labeled carprofen, 75% appeared in the urine in humans, with 3 to 5% as intact carprofen and the rest as metabolites; 17 to 33% of the label appeared in the feces over 2 to 10 days. The drug probably undergoes enterohepatic recirculation in humans.[302] Administered as a racemic mixture, the in vitro ratio of S+ to R-isomer is always less than 2.[303] Its bioavailability relative to a solution is 88%, and its terminal half-life is 13 to 27 hours.[302] It is 99.4 to 99.9% protein bound. Because carprofen is an organic acid, it is excreted by glomerular filtration at low concentrations, reabsorbed at medium concentrations, and finally secreted into the urine at high concentrations.[304] Its concentration in synovial fluid varies between 30 and 103% of serum.[303]

The serum half-life of carprofen in the elderly is less than in the young (9.4 hours versus 15.7 hours), but the clearances for the two age groups are equal.[305] Hepatic cirrhosis has no effect on the pharmacokinetic profile of carprofen.[306]

Aspirin decreases the AUC of carprofen by 37%, possibly through increased biliary excretion of the carprofen.[307] Probenecid inhibits carprofen secretion, thereby increasing its total body retention. While effective in treating acute gout, carprofen is not uricosuric.[308] From a series of 242 RA patients culled from the literature, it appears that carprofen, at doses of 300 mg per day or more, is approximately equivalent to indomethacin and aspirin in the treatment of RA.[303] Carprofen is also equivalent to indomethacin in the treatment of osteoarthritis.[309]

In the above-mentioned 242 RA patients, carprofen was discontinued by 2% because of gastrointestinal toxicity; by 0.5% because of rash; and by 0.7% because of elevated liver function tests. In 1843 patients with various rheumatic conditions, there was a 2.1% incidence of blood in the stool, but no clinical peptic ulcers.[310] Photosensitive dermatitis has been reported.[311]

DICLOFENAC

Diclofenac is a phenylacetic acid (fenamate) derivative with a pKa of 4. It is a potent, reversible, inhibitor of cyclo-oxygenase in vitro and in vivo. It also decreases the availability of arachidonic acid by stimulating its uptake into triglycerides and inhibiting the release of intracellular arachidonic acid, thus also reducing formation of leukotrienes and 5-HETE.[312] Like all NSAIDs, it demonstrates anti-inflammatory, analgesic, and antipyretic activity in animals.[313]

The drug is completely absorbed in humans, is 99.7% bound to albumin, and has a terminal half-life of approximately 75 minutes.[314,315] Steady-state concentrations in synovial fluid are higher than those in plasma, and there is persistent suppression of PGE_2 for 8 to 12 hours after a dose.[316] Because the drug is more than 95% metabolized to inactive metabolites, renal functional impairment does not significantly influence the plasma clearance of active drug. The metabolites undergo enterohepatic recirculation.[317,318] Only 5% of the drug is recovered unchanged in the urine, while 50 to 60% is excreted as metabolites. Another 30 to 40% appears to be excreted in the bile.[315]

There is no change in diclofenac pharmacokinetics in the elderly compared to the young.[315] While in vitro studies of diclofenac reveal no serum-binding effects of salicylic acid, tolbutamide, prednisolone, or warfarin, aspirin decreased diclofenac's area under the curve in vivo.[319] In vivo aspirin increases diclofenac's biliary excretion and changes the distribution of the drug.[316]

In patients with RA, 75 to 150 mg daily diclofenac is superior to placebo and approximately equivalent to 3 to 5 g aspirin, 75 to 150 mg indomethacin, 500 mg naproxen, 1600 mg ibuprofen, or 300 mg phenylbutazone.[315] Double-blind investigations of JRA in Europe found that diclofenac (2 to 3 mg/kg/day) was superior to placebo and comparable to indomethacin (2 to 3 mg/kg/day) or aspirin (60 to 90 mg/kg/day).[316] Like other NSAIDs, it is effective in acute sprains and strains and in ankylosing spondylitis.[316] It also alleviates the symptoms of gout, where its intramuscular form is comparable to phenylbutazone.[315]

Summarizing over 422 publications, both controlled and open label, Catalano concluded that 21% of pa-

tients had gastrointestinal adverse reactions and 6.4% had central nervous system reactions. Adverse reactions were more frequent with the drug than with a placebo in comparative trials, less frequent than with aspirin, and approximately the same as those with ibuprofen and naproxen. In short-term trials in the United States, severe adverse reactions occurred in 4.6% of the patients taking 75 to 200 mg/day of diclofenac, compared with 4.5% for the placebo patients and 9.2% for the patients taking 2400 to 4800 mg/day of aspirin. Medically serious reactions in 1173 patients treated for up to 58 weeks were as follows: peptic ulcer disease (0.34%); gastrointestinal bleeding (0.17%); hepatitis (0.26%); thrombocytopenia (0.17%). No renal failure occurred.[320] No dose-related incidence of side effects occurred when comparing 75 and 150 mg daily doses of the drug. Doses higher than 200 mg daily may be associated with an increased incidence of adverse drug reactions.[321]

ETODOLAC

Etodolac, an indoleacetic acid derivative, is a cyclo-oxygenase inhibitor. Further, it probably "shunts" arachidonic acid metabolism into the lipoxygenase pathway as it inhibits cyclo-oxygenase.[322]

Etodolac is completely absorbed.[323] It has an elimination half-life of 6.1 hours, is greater than 99% bound to human serum proteins, is at least 95% metabolized, and is excreted in the urine (73%) and feces (14%). It has five metabolites, two of which may cause false-positive readings for bilirubin in the urine.[324] Etodolac is assumed though not proven to have an enterohepatic recirculation in humans.[323]

The kinetics of this drug were unchanged in elderly men, relative to young men. In renal disease, the AUC of etodolac is decreased by 50%, but because its free fraction is increased by a factor of 2, the AUC of the free drug is unchanged. Hemodialysis does not alter the drug's kinetics.[325] Aspirin decreased total etodolac concentrations by 51%, but also did not change free etodolac concentrations.[325]

Etodolac is effective in the treatment of RA, with increasing effectiveness as the dose of etodolac increases. The minimum effective dose is probably 200 mg per day in RA, and the highest dose used to date is 600 mg per day.[325,326] In a 1-year, aspirin-controlled, multicenter trial, serial joint roentgenograms suggested that etodolac slowed radiographic change,[326] although study design difficulties make this conclusion controversial. In osteoarthritis, 400 mg daily etodolac is equal to 4300 mg aspirin and better than placebo.[327]

Clinical toxicity was assessed in 739 etodolac-treated patients in ten double-blind, placebo-controlled trials. Gastrointestinal complaints were the most common. Indigestion occurred in 5.1% of patients on etodolac, 8.7% on aspirin, and 2.0% on placebo. Nausea, epigastric pain, heartburn, constipation, and dyspepsia were less frequent with etodolac than with aspirin. Tinnitus was less frequent with etodolac (1.3%) than with aspirin (18.3%). Headaches occurred in approximately 6% and rashes in approximately 2% with both drugs.[325]

Alkaline phosphatase was increased in 2.2% of patients treated with etodolac, but SGOT and SGPT were increased in less than 1%. A mild decrease in para-aminohippuric acid (PAH) clearance was noted in 30% of etodolac-treated patients with pre-existing renal impairment.[325] Overall, etodolac may have slightly less GI toxicity than other NSAIDs in clinical studies. This is supported by studies in rats, in which low doses of etodolac decreased gastric prostaglandin E_2 concentrations less than naproxen or piroxicam (25% decrease in PGE_2 with etodolac versus 60% decrease with the other two drugs). At higher doses, the three drugs affected PGE_2 equally.[328]

FENBUFEN

This phenylalkanoic acid derivative is a pro-drug. The inactive parent compound is metabolized to 4-biphenylacetic acid, a cyclo-oxygenase inhibitor. Six other metabolites are inactive in cyclo-oxygenase inhibition assays.[329]

Two hours after dosing, fenbufen is more than 78% absorbed; the active metabolite concentration peaks between 6 and 8 hours after administration.[330,331] Although the elimination half-life of the parent compound is 7 hours, the biphenylacetic acid metabolite remains present at significant concentrations for up to 72 hours after a single dose. Although no half-life of this metabolite has been published, it is safe to assume that its half-life is much longer than that of the parent compound and that once daily dosing is reasonable.[331] After administration of ^{14}C-labeled fenbufen, 66% of the label appears in the urine, 7.6% in the feces, and 11.7% in the expired air (when measured as ^{14}C). The urinary metabolites are excreted largely as conjugates.[331]

Fenbufen and its active metabolites are highly bound to serum proteins (98 to 99.9%) and are slightly displaced by salicylate. This slight displacement, however, may double the free fraction.[331] When warfarin and fenbufen are given together, a 14% increase in serum warfarin concentration and a slight increase in prothrombin time occur. This rases the possibility of an occasional clinically significant interaction.[329] Aspirin decreases the AUC of fenbufen by approximately 20%.[331] Trace amounts of fenbufen appear in breast milk. Additionally, fenbufen concentrations in synovial fluid are approximately one third those in serum.[329]

In 1981, Brogden summarized the published studies of fenbufen in osteoarthritis, RA, soft tissue rheumatism, and gout.[329] Fenbufen, 600 to 1000 mg daily is as effective as 3.6 to 4.8 g of aspirin in RA. It is also as effective as moderate doses of indomethacin or fenoprofen. Doses up to 1000 mg daily were effective in uncontrolled studies of gout.

In a German multicenter trial of over 7000 patients with rheumatic diseases treated for 8 weeks, the greatest proportion of adverse effects were gastrointestinal (12.8%), with 2% considered severe.[330] During the first 12 months of treatment, 8 of 1676 patients taking fenbufen, 5 of 326 patients taking aspirin, and 2 of 290 patients taking indomethacin developed ulcers.[330] Tinnitus was extremely rare while CNS effects occurred in 6% of patients on fenbufen (versus 20% on indomethacin).[332] Transient elevation of transaminases may occur after 3 to 6 weeks of fenbufen therapy.

FLURBIPROFEN

Flurbiprofen is a propionic acid derivative with a pKa of 4.2.[333] Like other NSAIDs, it is a potent inhibitor of cyclo-oxygenase and platelet aggregation.[334,335] It may inhibit enzyme release from neutrophils; it does not inhibit free radical generation nor does it affect the lipoxygenase pathway.[333]

Flurbiprofen's pharmacokinetics were reviewed by Kaiser and co-workers.[336] Although no formal absolute bioavailability studies have been published, flurbiprofen appears to have excellent relative bioavailability. It is greater than 99% bound to serum albumin, it is more than 94% excreted into the urine, and its hydroxylated metabolite is approximately 5% as active as the parent compound in anti-inflammatory tests.[333,336] Five to six percent of the drug is excreted unchanged and approximately 13% is excreted as its active metabolite. The rest of the drug is excreted as glucuronides and sulfate conjugates. An active enterohepatic recirculation occurs in baboons and probably also occurs in humans.

Although there is no significant interaction between phenprocoumon and flurbiprofen, aspirin decreases flurbiprofen area under the curve by 48%.[337] No formal studies of the effect of renal disease on flurbiprofen pharmacokinetics have been reported, but this drug should not require dosing changes in renal disease because it is metabolized to a large degree.

Flurbiprofen is more effective than placebo and as effective as aspirin, indomethacin, ibuprofen, sulindac, and mefenamic acid in 4- to 8-week trials in RA.[338] In these studies, the average flurbiprofen dosage was 50 mg four times a day. In a 52-week comparison study, flurbiprofen and aspirin were equal at year's end.[339] Interestingly, a 100-mg bid dose of flurbiprofen was equal to 50 mg qid in one study.[340] In addition, regimens using an evening dose were more effective than other regimens. A 50-mg bid or tid dose of flurbiprofen was equivalent to ibuprofen, naproxen, indomethacin, or acetaminophen in 4- to 6-week trials in osteoarthritis.[338] Flurbiprofen was equal to indomethacin and phenylbutazone in ankylosing spondylitis.[341,342] It was also used in short-term trials of acute shoulder syndrome and acute gout;[343,344] the starting dose was 300 to 400 mg daily for several days, after which the dose was reduced to 200 mg daily. Flurbiprofen equaled ibuprofen in the acute shoulder syndrome and indomethacin in treating acute gout.

The toxicity of flurbiprofen is exemplified by the results of a 52-week double-blind comparison of 200 mg flurbiprofen and 4000 mg aspirin in 822 RA patients;[339] 36% of flurbiprofen-treated patients and 63% of aspirin-treated patients reported side effects. As usual the principal side effect was digestive, with 27.4% in the flurbiprofen (F) group and 49.9% in the aspirin (A) group. CNS effects (F: 5.1% versus A: 10.5%), rashes (F: 5.2% versus A: 8.6%), hematologic (F: 1.7% versus A: 0.5%), and tinnitus/decreased hearing (F: 8.5% versus A: 28.8%) also occurred. Abnormal liver function tests or elevated serum creatinine values occurred very rarely.[345] Among 941 flurbiprofen-treated patients, alkaline phosphatase elevations occurred in 0.3% of patients, bilirubin tests were abnormal in 0.4%, and ASTs were elevated in 0.4%. Serum creatinine was elevated in only one patient.

CHOICE AND USE OF NONSTEROIDAL ANTI-INFLAMMATORY DRUGS

Of prime importance is the need to individualize dosage. In all kinetic studies of NSAIDs, one of the most striking findings is the great range of serum concentrations in individual patients. Such variability is best documented with aspirin, with which three- or fourfold differences in steady-state serum salicylate levels occur in small groups of patients taking the same weight-adjusted doses. Although the range of individual responses is obscured in many of the ki-

netic studies summarized here because mean values are used for clarity of presentation, substantial individual variability is actually present with respect to the pharmacology of these drugs.[346] Therefore, in treating any patient, it is essential to adjust the therapy to the patient's response, rather than to assume the appropriateness of an average recommended dose or dosage interval.

For aspirin and the nonacetylated salicylates, dosage can be most effectively individualized by monitoring serum salicylate concentrations; we aim for values between 10 and 30 mg/100 ml (100 to 300 μg/ml or 100 to 300 mg/L). These values overlap those at which symptoms of mild salicylism are seen. Thus, the development of tinnitus can be used as a general guide to adequate salicylate levels, although this observation is inconstant and is not valid in patients with pre-existing hearing loss.[347]

A relationship between naproxen serum levels and efficacy has been proposed;[200] if confirmed, recommendations for "therapeutic" naproxen serum levels may be useful as a guide for adjusting the dosage of this drug. Although easily measured, serum concentrations are not readily available for most NSAIDs. We recommend starting with the average recommended dose and then cautiously increasing stepwise to the maximum recommended dose until optimal therapeutic effects or minimal side effects develop. For some patients, the optimal dose may be low, whereas others may not achieve a satisfactory response even with the maximum recommended doses. With increasing clinical experience, the maximum doses of many of the newer NSAIDs have been raised.

Because aspirin has a long tradition in rheumatology, it has been customary to give it to nearly everyone and to add other medications to baseline aspirin therapy. With the proliferation of NSAIDs, it is now possible to give a single patient many NSAIDs simultaneously. We do not think that the data justify this practice. Studies in rat paw edema have not demonstrated additive anti-inflammatory effects with coadministration of more than one NSAID,[348] and rat adjuvant arthritis studies have shown decreased anti-inflammatory effect when a second drug was added to a background NSAID.[349] In one study, no increase in anti-inflammatory effect in RA patients was achieved by a combination of 100 mg indomethacin and 4 g aspirin daily, as compared to each drug given alone, and the toxicity of the combination was greater.[135] Similarly, when tolmetin was added to a background of aspirin therapy, no additive clinical effect was found,[229] and the addition of therapeutic serum salicylate levels to naproxen 1500 mg/day did not increase the efficacy of naproxen alone.[103]

The addition of aspirin has been demonstrated to decrease plasma levels of several NSAIDs,[350] and it may increase the risk of gastrointestinal bleeding with piroxicam.[276] The addition of 500 mg naproxen daily to aspirin, 1.3 to 5.2 g daily, however, was more effective than aspirin alone in RA,[192] but the patients receiving the larger aspirin doses showed the least improvement. This finding suggests that the combination was more effective only if the baseline therapy was suboptimal. The patients in this study may have been receiving all their benefit from the naproxen alone. Unless new data supporting specific combinations of NSAIDs become available, *we do not recommend concurrent administration of more than one NSAID.* Efficacy is unlikely to be increased, and toxicity may well be additive.

How should one choose an NSAID for a particular patient? Factors to consider include complicating illnesses and other drug intake. For example, if a patient is taking warfarin or has an ulcer, the effects of NSAIDs on coagulation must be weighed. In addition to individually variable dose-response relationships, some patients probably respond much better to one NSAID than they do to another, although the reasons for this phenomenon are unknown. In a number of well-designed cross-over studies, four or more NSAIDs were compared; the number of subjects per study ranged from 32 to 141.[351-356] In general, the preferences of the patient and the physician were the only measures useful in ranking the drugs. In five studies in RA, no first choice was noted in two, whereas naproxen ranked first in two and indomethacin first in one study. Indomethacin and naproxen were the most frequently preferred among six NSAIDs studied in ankylosing spondylitis,[356] and tolmetin was the first choice among four NSAIDs studied in osteoarthritis.[351] No study demonstrated an overwhelming preference for any single drug, however; each drug was strongly preferred by some patients. In all these comparative studies, aspirin was preferred by fewer patients, usually because it caused more side effects. It also appeared to be less effective against symptoms of ankylosing spondylitis.[31,356]

Because one cannot predict which NSAID will be most effective for an individual patient, treatment should be initiated with one drug, and the dose should be increased gradually until the optimal or maximum tolerated dose is reached. That dose should be continued for several weeks. If the patient has an inadequate therapeutic response, the first drug should be replaced with a second NSAID, and the process should be repeated. These individual therapeutic trials can be repeated with new drugs; one should persist for at least 2 weeks at the optimal tolerated dose, until the most effective drug for that particular patient has been found. Our prejudice against pyramiding NSAIDs does not apply to the appropriate addition of a slowly acting antirheumatic agent, such as a gold compound or D-penicillamine, to initial therapy with an NSAID.

REFERENCES

1. Scherrer, R.A.: Aryl- and hetero-arylcarboxylic acids. *In* Antiflammatory Agents. Vol. I. Edited by R.A. Scherrer and M.W. Whitehouse. New York, Academic Press, 1974, pp. 45–89.
2. Weissmann, G.: Prostaglandins in acute inflammation. *In* Current Concepts. Kalamazoo, MI, Upjohn, 1980, pp. 1–32.
3. Vane, J.R.: Inhibition of prostaglandin biosynthesis as the mechanism of action of aspirin-like drugs. *In* International Congress on Prostaglandins. Edited by S. Bergstrom and S. Bernhard. Oxford, Pergamon Press, 1973, pp. 395–411.
4. Melton, A.S., and Wendland, T.S.: A possible role for PGE, as a modulator for temperature regulation in the CNS of the cat. J. Physiol., *207*:76–77, 1970.
5. Flower, R.J., and Vane, J.R.: Inhibition of prostaglandin synthetase in brain explains the antipyretic activity of paracetamol (4 acetamidophenol). Nature, *240*:410–411, 1972.
6. Blechman, W.J., and Lechner, B.L.: Clinical comparative evaluation of choline magnesium trisalicylate and acetylsalicylic acid in rheumatoid arthritis. Rheumatol. Rehabil., *18*:119–124, 1979.
7. Dromgoole, S.H., Furst D.E., and Paulus, H.E.: Rational approaches to the use of salicylates in the treatment of rheumatoid arthritis. Semin. Arthritis Rheum., *11*:257–283, 1982.
8. Radin, A. et al.: Leukotriene B$_4$ (LTB$_4$) as a mediator of inflammation human neutrophil (PMN) activation and calcium (Ca) ionophoresis. Arthritis Rheum., *25(Suppl.)*:S-8, 1982.
9. Samuelsson, B.: Leukotrienes: a new class of mediators of immediate hypersensitivity reactions and inflammation. Adv. Prostaglandin Thromboxane Leukotriene Res., *11*:1–13, 1983.
10. Abramson, S. et al.: The neutrophil in rheumatoid arthritis: its role and the inhibition of its activation by nonsteroidal anti-inflammatory drugs. Semin. Arthritis Rheum., *13(Suppl. 1)*:148–153, 1983.
11. Dawson, W. et al.: The pharmacology of benoxaprofen with reference to effects on lipoxygenase product formation. Eur. J. Rheumatol. Inflamm., *5*:61–68, 1982.
12. Martelli, F.A.: Antagonism of inflammatory drugs on bradykinin induced increase of capillary permeability. J. Pharm. Pharmacol., *19*:617–620, 1967.
13. Smith, M.J.H., and Dawkins, P.D.: Salicylates and enzymes. J. Pharm. Pharmacol., *23*:729–744, 1971.
14. Weissmann, G. et al.: Marine sponge aggregation: A model for effects of NSAIDs on the calcium movements of cell aggregation. Semin. Arthritis Rheum., *15*:42–53, 1985.
15. Smith, M.J.H.: Toxicology. *In* The Salicylates. Edited by M.J.H. Smith and P.K. Smith. New York, John Wiley and Sons, 1966, pp. 233–306.
16. Smith, M.J.H.: The metabolic basis of the major symptoms in acute salicylate intoxication. Clin. Toxicol., *1*:387–407, 1968.
17. Liakakos, D., Vlachos, P., and Anoussakis, L.: Effect of acetylsalicylic acid (aspirin) on bone collagen in children. Clin. Chim. Acta, *44*:427–429, 1973.
18. Chang, Y.-H.: Studies on phagocytosis II. The effect of NSAID

on phagocytosis and on urate crystal-induced joint inflammation. J. Pharmacol. Exp. Ther., *183*:235–244, 1972.

19. DiRosa, M., Papadimitrion, J.M., and Willoughby, D.A.: A histopathological and pharmacological analysis of the mode of action of NSAID. J. Pathol., *105*:239–256, 1971.

20. Dewse, C.D.: Inhibition of DNA synthesis in cultured human lymphocytes by phenylbutazone and oxyphenbutazone.J. Pharm. Pharmacol., *28*:596–598, 1976.

21. Whitehouse, M.W.: Evaluation of potential antirheumatic drugs *in vitro* using lymphocytes and epithelial cells. The selective action of indoxole, methyl glyoxal and chloroquine. J. Pharm. Pharmacol., *19*:590–595, 1967.

22. Ciosek, C.P., Jr., et al.: Indomethacin potentiates PGE-stimulated C-AMP accumulation in human synoviocytes. Nature, *251*:145–150, 1974.

23. Weissmann, G.: Pathways of arachidonate oxidation to prostaglandins and leukotrienes. Semin. Arthritis Rheum., *13(Suppl. 1)*:123–129, 1983.

24. Goodwin, J.S., and Ceuppens, J.I.: Effect of nonsteroidal anti-inflammatory drugs on immune function. Semin. Arthritis Rheum., *13(Suppl. 1)*:134–143, 1983.

25. Lim, R.K.S.: Analgesia. *In* The Salicylates. Edited by M.J.H. Smith and P.K. Smith. New York, John Wiley and Sons, 1966, pp. 155–202.

26. Rodnan, G.P., and Benedek, T.G.: The early history of antirheumatic drugs. Arthritis Rheum., *13*:145–165, 1970.

27. Fremont-Smith, K., and Bayles, T.B.: Salicylate therapy in rheumatoid arthritis. JAMA, *192*:1133–1136, 1965.

28. Boardman. P.I., and Hart, F.D.: Clinical measurement of the anti-inflammatory effect of salicylates in rheumatoid arthritis. Br. Med. J., *4*:264–268, 1967.

29. Schaller, T.G.: Treatment of juvenile rheumatoid arthritis. *In* Arthritis and Allied Conditions. 10th Ed. Edited by D.J. McCarty. Philadelphia, Lea & Febiger, 1985, pp. 811–818.

30. Gibson, T., and Laurent, R.: Sulindac and indomethacin in treatment of ankylosing spondylitis: A double-blind crossover study. Rheumatol. Rehabil., *19*:189–192, 1980.

31. Godfrey, R.G. et al.: A double-blind crossover trial of aspirin, indomethacin and phenylbutazone in ankylosing spondylitis. Arthritis Rheum., *15*:110–111, 1972.

32. Hill, H.F.H., and Hill, A.G.S.: Ankylosing spondylitis: Open long-term and double-blind cross over studies with naproxen. J. Clin. Pharmacol., *15*:355–362, 1975.

33. Yu, T.F., and Gutman, A.B.: Study of the paradoxical effects of salicylates in low, intermediate and high dosage on the renal mechanism for excretion of urate in man. J. Clin. Invest., *38*:1298–1315, 1959.

34. Gall, E.P.: Hyperuricemia and gout: A modern approach to diagnosis and treatment. Postgrad. Med., *65*:163–171, 1979.

35. Smyth, C.J., and Percy, J.S.: Comparison of indomethacin and phenylbutazone in acute gout. Ann. Rheum. Dis., *32*:351–353, 1973.

36. Wilkens, R.F., Case, J.B., and Huix, F.J.: The treatment of acute gout with naproxen. J. Clin. Pharmacol., *15*:363–366, 1975.

37. Howell, D.S.: Osteoarthritis—etiology and pathogenesis. *In* Symposium on Osteoarthritis. St. Louis, C.V. Mosby. American Academy of Orthopedic Surgeon's Committee for Arthritis, 1976, pp. 44–47.

38. Moncada, S., and Vane, J.R.: Pharmacology and endogenous roles of prostaglandin endoperoxides, thromboxane A_2 and prostacyclin. Pharmacol. Rev., *30*:293–331, 1979.

39. Kocsis, J.J. et al.: Duration of inhibition of platelet prosta-

glandin aggregation by ingested aspirin or indomethacin. Prostaglandins, *3*:141–144, 1973.

40. Morris, H.G. et al.: Effects of salsalate (nonacetylated salicylate) and aspirin on serum prostaglandins in humans. Ther. Drug. Monit., *7*:435–438, 1985.

41. Massotti, G. et al.: Differential inhibition of prostaglandin production and platelet aggregation by aspirin. Lancet, *2*:1213–1217, 1979.

42. Weksler, B.B. et al.: Differential inhibition by aspirin of vascular and platelet prostaglandin synthesis in atherosclerotic patients. N. Engl. J. Med., *308*:800–805, 1983.

43. Siebert, D.J. et al.: Aspirin kinetics and platelet aggregation in man. Clin. Pharmacol. Ther., *33*:367–374, 1983.

44. Hanson, F.W.: Naproxen sodium, ibuprofen and placebo in dysmenorrhea. J. Reprod. Med., *27*:423–427, 1982.

45. Mahoney, I. et al.: Prophylactic indomethacin for patent ductus arteriosus. N. Engl. J. Med., *306*:506–510, 1982.

46. Hansten, P.D.: Drugs which may enhance the effects of diphenylhydantoin. *In* Drug Interactions. Edited by P.D. Hansten. Philadelphia, Lea & Febiger, 1973, pp. 54–69.

47. Aggeler, P.M. et al.: Potentiation of anticoagulant effect of warfarin by phenylbutazone. N. Engl. J. Med., *276*:496–501, 1967.

48. Cowan, R.A. et al.: Metabolic acidosis induced by carbonic anhydrase inhibitors and salicylates in patients with normal renal function. Br. Med. J., *289*:347–348, 1984.

49. Favre, L., Glasson, P., and Vallotton, M.B.: Reversible acute renal failure from combined triamterene and indomethacin. Ann. Intern. Med., *96*:317–320, 1986.

50. Brater, D.C.: Drug-drug and drug-disease interactions and nonsteroidal anti-inflammatory drugs. Am. J. Med., *80(Suppl. A)*:62–75, 1986.

51. Levi, A.J., Sherlock, S., and Walker, D.: Phenylbutazone and isoniazid in patients with liver disease in relation to previous drug therapy. Lancet, *1*:1275–1279, 1968.

52. Andreasen, F.: Protein binding of drugs in plasma from patients with acute renal failure. Acta Pharmacol. Toxicol., *12*:417–429, 1973.

53. Borga, O. et al.: Protein binding of salicylate in uremic and normal plasma. Clin. Pharmacol. Ther., *20*:464–475, 1976.

54. Hamdy, R.C. et al.: The pharmacokinetics of benoxaprofen in elderly subjects. Eur. J. Rheumatol. Rehabil., *5*:69–75, 1982.

55. Schlegel, S.I., and Paulus, H.E.: Nonsteroidal and analgesic therapy in the elderly. Clin. Rheum. Dis., *12*:245–273, 1986.

56. O'Malley, K. et al.: Effect of age and sex on human drug metabolism. Br. Med. J., *3*:607–609, 1971.

57. Alvares, A.P. et al.: Drug metabolism in normal children, lead poisoned children, and normal adults. Clin. Pharmacol. Ther., *17*:179–183, 1975.

58. Traeger, A. et al.: Pharmacokinetics of indomethacin in the aged. A. Alternesforsch., *27*:151–155, 1973.

59. Bender, A.D.: The effect of increasing age on the distribution of peripheral blood flow in man. J. Am. Geriatr. Soc., *13*:192–198, 1965.

60. Greenblatt, D.J., Sellers, F.M., and Shader, R.I.: Drug disposition in old age. N. Engl. J. Med., *306*:1081–1088, 1982.

61. Divoll, M. et al.: Effect of food on acetaminophen absorption in young and elderly subjects. J. Clin. Pharmacol., *22*:571–576, 1982.

62. Hayes, M.J., Langeman, M.J.S., and Short, A.H.: Changes in drug metabolism with increasing age: Warfarin binding and plasma proteins. Br. J. Clin. Pharmacol., *2*:69–72, 1975.

63. Lesko, L.J. et al.: Salicylate protein binding in young and

elderly serum as measured by diafiltration. (Abstract.) Clin. Pharmacol. Ther., 33:257, 1983.

64. Morgan, J., and Furst, D.E.: Implications of drug therapy in the elderly. Clin. Rheum. Dis., 12:227–244, 1986.

65. Roth, G.S., and Livingston, J.N.: Reductions in glucocorticoid inhibition of glucose oxidation and presumptive glucocorticoid receptor content in rat adipocytes during aging. Endocrinology, 99:831–839, 1976.

66. Dillon, N. et al.: Age and beta-adrenoceptor-mediated function. Clin. Pharmacol. Ther., 27:769–772, 1980.

67. Kean, W.F. et al.: Efficacy and toxicity of D-penicillamine for rheumatoid disease in the elderly. J. Am. Geriatr. Soc., 30:94–100, 1982.

68. Furst, D.E., Gupta, N., and Paulus, H.E.: Salicylate metabolism in twins. J. Clin. Invest., 60:32–38, 1977.

69. Vessell, E.S., and Page, J.G.: Genetic control of drug levels in man: Phenylbutazone. Science, 159:1479–1480, 1968.

70. Editorial. Lancet, 2:961–962, 1975.

71. Roberts, A. et al.: Gastric antisecretory and antiulcer properties of PGF$_2$, 15 Methyl PGE$_2$, and 16, 16-Dimethyl PGF$_2$. Gastroenterology, 70:359–370, 1976.

72. Max, M., and Menguy, R.: Influence of aspirin and phenylbutazone on the rate of turnover of gastric mucosal cells. Digestion, 2:67–72, 1969.

73. Lanza, P.L. et al.: A comparative endoscopic evaluation of the damaging effects of nonsteroidal anti-inflammatory agents in the gastric and duodenal mucosa. Am. J. Gastroenterol., 75:17–21, 1981.

74. Lin, T.M. et al.: Action of the anti-inflammatory agents, acetylsalicylic acid, indomethacin and fenoprofen on gastric mucosa of dogs. Res. Commun. Chem. Pathol. Pharmacol., 11:1–14, 1975.

75. Duggan, D.E. et al.: Disposition of sulindac. Clin. Pharmacol. Ther., 21:326–335, 1977.

76. Duggan, D.E. et al.: Enterohepatic circulation of indomethacin and intestinal irritation. Biochem. Pharmacol., 24:1749–1754, 1975.

77. Glazko, A.J. et al.: Metabolic disposition of meclofenamic acid (Meclomen) in laboratory animals and in man. Curr. Ther. Res., 23(Suppl.):22–41, 1978.

78. Rubin, A. et al.: Physiological disposition of fenoprofen in man. J. Pharm. Sci., 61:739–745, 1972.

79. Lussier, A., and Arsenault, A.: Gastrointestinal blood loss induced by ketoprofen, aspirin and placebo. Scand. J. Rheumatol., 5(Suppl. 14):73–76, 1976.

80. Athreya, B.H. et al.: Aspirin-induced hepatotoxicity in JRA. Arthritis Rheum., 18:347–352, 1975.

81. Rachelefsky, G.S. et al.: Serum enzyme abnormalities in juvenile rheumatoid arthritis. Pediatrics, 48:730–736, 1976.

82. Seaman, W.E., and Plotz, P.H.: Effect of aspirin on liver tests in patients with RA or SLE and in normal volunteers. Arthritis Rheum., 19:155–160, 1976.

83. Paulus, H.E.: Government affairs: FDA Arthritis Advisory Committee meeting. Arthritis Rheum., 25:1124–1125, 1982.

84. Benjamin, S.B. et al.: Phenylbutazone liver injury: A clinical pathologic survey of 23 cases and review of the literature. Hepatology, 1:255–268, 1981.

85. Kimberly, R.P., and Plotz, P.H.: Aspirin induced depression of renal function. N. Engl. J. Med., 296:418–423, 1977.

86. Levenson, D.J., Simmons, C.E., and Brenner, B.M.: Arachidonic acid metabolism, prostaglandins and kidney. Am. J. Med., 72:354–374, 1982.

87. Paulus, H.E.: Government affairs: FDA Arthritis Advisory Committee meeting. Phenylbutazone and oxyphenbutazone.

NSAID effects on renal function. Auranofin. Arthritis Rheum., 28:450–451, 1985.

88. Stachura, I., Jayakumar, S., and Bourke, E.: T and B lymphocyte subsets in fenoprofen nephropathy. Am. J. Med., 75:9–16, 1983.

89. Katz, S.N. et al.: Tolmetin association with reversible renal failure and acute interstitial nephritis. JAMA, 246:243–245, 1981.

90. New Zealand Rheumatism Association Study: Aspirin and the kidney. Br. Med. J., 1:593–596, 1974.

91. Carmichael, J., and Shankel, S.W.: Effects of nonsteroidal anti-inflammatory drugs on prostaglandins and renal function. Am. J. Med., 78:992–1000, 1985.

92. Emkey, R.D., and Mills, J.A.: Aspirin and analgesic nephropathy. JAMA, 247:55–57, 1982.

93. Findling, J.W. et al.: Indomethacin-induced hyperkalemia in three patients with gouty arthritis. JAMA, 244:1127–1128, 1980.

94. Levy, G., and Hollister, L.E.: Inter- and intrasubject variations in drug absorption kinetics. J. Pharm. Sci., 53:1446–1452, 1964.

95. Rowland, M., and Riegelman, S.: Absorption kinetics of aspirin in man following oral administration of an aqueous solution. J. Pharm. Sci., 61:379–395, 1972.

96. Furst, D.E., Tozer, T.N., and Melmon, K.L.: Salicylate clearance, the resultant of protein binding and metabolism. Clin. Pharmacol. Ther., 26:380–389, 1979.

97. Hill, J.B.: Salicylate intoxication. N. Engl. J. Med., 228:1110–1113, 1973.

98. Levy, G., and Tsuchiya, T.: Salicylate accumulation kinetics in man. N. Engl. J. Med., 287:430–432, 1972.

99. Levy, G., and Leonards, J.R.: Urine pH and salicylate therapy. JAMA, 217:81, 1971.

100. Miller, F.U., Hundt, H.K.L., and deKock, A.C.: Decreased steady-state salicylic acid plasma levels associated with chronic aspirin ingestion. Curr. Med. Res. Opin., 3:417–422, 1975.

101. Paulus, H.E. et al.: Variations of serum concentrations and 'half-life' of salicylate in patients with rheumatoid arthritis. Arthritis Rheum., 14:527–532, 1971.

102. Ferrera, S.H.: Prostaglandins and nonsteroidal anti-inflammatory drugs. In Prostaglandins and Thromboxanes. Edited by F. Berti, B. Samuelson, and G.P. Velvo. New York, Plenum Press, 1976, pp. 353–360.

103. Furst, D.E. et al.: A controlled study of concurrent therapy with a non-acetylated salicylate and naproxen in rheumatoid arthritis. Arthritis Rheum., 30:146–154, 1987.

104. Rothwell, K.G.: Efficacy and safety of a non-acetylated salicylate, choline magnesium trisalicylate, in the treatment of rheumatoid arthritis. J. Int. Med. Res., 11:343–348, 1983.

105. Chudwin, D.S. et al.: Sensitivity to non-acetylated salicylates in a patient with asthma, nasal polyps, and rheumatoid arthritis. Ann. Allergy, 57:133–134, 1986.

106. Briggs, D.F., Couts, R.T., and Walter, L.J.: A note on the bioavailability of five Canadian brands of acetylsalicylic acid tablets. Can. J. Pharm. Sci., 12:23–25, 1977.

107. Halla, J.T., Fallahi, S., and Hardin, J.G.: Acute and chronic salicylate intoxication in a patient with gastric outlet obstruction. Arthritis Rheum., 24:1205–1207, 1981.

108. Orozco-Alcola, J.J., and Baum, J.: Regular and enteric-coated aspirin: A re-evaluation. Arthritis Rheum., 22:1034–1037, 1979.

109. Leonards, J.R., and Levy, G.: Gastrointestinal blood loss from aspirin and sodium salicylate tablets in man. Clin. Pharmacol. Ther., 14:62–66, 1973.

110. Goldenberg, A., Rudnicki, R.D., and Koonce, M.L.: Clinical comparison of efficacy and safety of choline magnesium trisalicylate and indomethacin in treating osteoarthritis. Curr. Ther. Res., 24:245–260, 1978.

111. Liyange, S.P., and Tambar, P.K.: Comparative study of salsalate and aspirin in osteoarthrosis of the hip or knee. Curr. Med. Res. Opin., 5:450–453, 1978.

112. Deodhar, S.D. et al.: A short-term comparative trial of salsalate and indomethacin in rheumatoid arthritis. Curr. Med. Res., 5:185–188, 1977.

113. Samter, M.: Intolerance to aspirin. Hosp. Pract., 8:85–90, 1973.

114. Szczcklik, A.: Antipyretic analgesics and the allergic patient. Am. J. Med., 75:82–84, 1983.

115. Murray, T., and Goldberg, M.: Analgesic abuse and renal disease. Annu. Rev. Med., 26:537–550, 1975.

116. Holt, P.R.: Measurement of gastrointestinal blood loss in subjects taking aspirin. J. Lab. Clin. Invest., 56:717–729, 1960.

117. Ridolfo, A.S. et al.: Effect of fenoprofen and aspirin on gastrointestinal microbleeding in man. Clin. Pharmacol. Ther., 14:226–230, 1973.

118. Barager, F.D., and Duthie, J.J.R.: Importance of aspirin as a cause of anemia and peptic ulcer in rheumatoid arthritis. Br. Med. J., 1:1106–1108, 1960.

119. Davenport, H.W.: Salicylate damage to the gastric mucosa barrier. N. Engl. J. Med., 276:1307–1312, 1967.

120. Jabbari, M., and Vallberg, L.S.: Role of acid secretion in aspirin-induced gastric mucosal injury. Can. Med. Assoc. J., 102:178–182, 1970.

121. Levy, M.: Aspirin use in patients with major upper GI bleeding and peptic ulcer disease. N. Engl. J. Med., 290:1157–1162, 1974.

122. Mongan, E. et al.: Tinnitus as an indication of therapeutic serum salicylate levels. JAMA, 226:142–145, 1973.

123. Partin, J.S. et al.: Serum salicylate concentrations in Reye's disease. Lancet, 1:191–194, 1982.

124. Remington, P.L. et al.: Reye's syndrome and juvenile rheumatoid arthritis in Michigan. Am. J. Dis. Child., 139:870–872, 1985.

125. Tenney, S.M., and Miller, R.M.: The respiratory and circulatory actions of salicylates. Am. J. Med., 19:498–503, 1955.

126. Melmon, K.L., Rowland, M., and Morreli, H.: The clinical pharmacology of salicylates. Calif. Med., 110:410–422, 1969.

127. Matthew, H. et al.: Gastric aspiration and lavage in acute poisoning. Br. Med. J., 1:1333–1337, 1966.

128. Schreiner, G.E., and Techan, B.P.: Dialysis of poisons and drugs. Trans. Am. Soc. Artif. Intern. Organs, 18:563–599, 1972.

129. Paulus, H.E., and Furst, D.E.: Aspirin and other nonsteroidal anti-inflammatory drugs. In Arthritis and Allied Conditions, 10th Ed. Edited by D.J. McCarty. Philadelphia, Lea & Febiger, 1985, p. 467–468.

130. Kwan, K.C. et al.: Kinetics of indomethacin absorption, elimination and enterohepatic circulation in man. J. Pharmacokinet. Biopharm., 4:255–280, 1976.

131. Yeh, K.C.: Pharmacokinetic overview of indomethacin and sustained-release indomethacin. Am. J. Med., 79(Suppl. 4C):3–12, 1985.

132. Traeger, A., Noschel, H., and Zaumseil, J.: Pharmacokinetics of indomethacin in pregnant and parturient women and in their newborn infants. Zentralbl. Gynaekol., 95:635–641, 1973.

133. Williams, R.L., et al.: Effects of indomethacin and carprofen on renal homeostasis in rheumatoid arthritis patients and in healthy individuals. J. Clin. Pharmacol., 21:493–500, 1981.

134. Kwan, K.C. et al.: Effect of concomitant aspirin administration on the pharmacokinetics of indomethacin in man. J. Pharmacokinet. Biopharm., 6:451–475, 1978.

135. Brooks, P.M. et al.: Indomethacin-aspirin interactions: A clinical appraisal. Br. Med. J., 3:69–71, 1975.

136. Patak, R.V. et al.: Antagonism of the effects of furosemide by indomethacin in normal and hypertensive man. Prostaglandins, 10:649–659, 1975.

137. Baber, N. et al.: The interaction between indomethacin and probenecid. Clin. Pharmacol. Ther., 24:298–306, 1978.

138. Brooks, P.M. et al.: The clinical significance of indomethacin-probenecid interactions. Br. J. Clin. Pharmacol., 1:287–290, 1974.

139. Tjandramaga, T.B. et al.: Interaction of diflunisal with indomethacin. In World Conference on Clinical Pharmacology and Therapeutics. (Abstract 658.) London, August 3 to 9, 1980.

140. Hansten, P.D. (Ed.): Lithium and indomethacin. Drug Interaction Newsl., 1:47–48, 1981.

141. Vessell, E.S., Passananti, G.T., and Johnson, A.O.: Failure of indomethacin and warfarin to interact in normal human volunteers. J. Clin. Pharmacol., 15:486–495, 1975.

142. O'Brien, W.M.: Indomethacin: A survey of clinical trials. Clin. Pharmacol. Ther., 9:94–106, 1968.

143. Wright, V., Walker, W.C., and McGuire, R.J.: Indomethacin in the treatment of rheumatoid arthritis. Ann. Rheum. Dis., 28:157–162, 1969.

144. Wanka, J., and Dixon, A.S.J.: Treatment of osteoarthritis of the hip with indomethacin, a controlled clinical trial. Ann. Rheum. Dis., 23:288–294, 1964.

145. Desproges-Gotteron, R., Comte, B., and Leroy, V.: A double blind comparison of alclofenac and indomethacin in osteoarthritis of the hip. Curr. Ther. Res., 13:393–397, 1971.

146. Arisz, L. et al.: The effect of indomethacin on proteinuria and kidney function in the nephrotic syndrome. Acta Med. Scand., 199:121–125, 1976.

147. Minuth, A.N. et al.: Indomethacin treatment of pericarditis in chronic hemodialysis patients. Arch. Intern. Med., 135:807–810, 1975.

148. Sacks, P.V., and Kanarek, D.: Treatment of acute pleuritic pain. Comparison between indomethacin and a placebo. Am. Rev. Respir. Dis., 108:666–669, 1973.

149. Jaffe, H.N. et al.: Indomethacin responsive pancreatic cholera. N. Engl. J. Med., 97:817–820, 1977.

150. Ito, H. et al.: Indomethacin responsive hypercalcemia. N. Engl. J. Med., 293:558–559, 1975.

151. Zuckerman, H., Reiss, U., and Rubinstein, I.: Inhibition of human premature labor by indomethacin. Obstet. Gynecol., 44:787–792, 1974.

152. Karat, A.B., Thomas, G., and Rao, P.S.: Indomethacin in the management of erythema nodosum leprosum: A double blind controlled trial. Lepr. Rev., 40:153–158, 1969.

153. Ladipo, O.A.: Primary dysmenorrhea treated with indomethacin. Int. J. Gynecol. Obstet., 15:221–222, 1977.

154. Perkins, E.S., and MacFaul, P.A.: Indomethacin in the treatment of uveitis: A double blind trial. Trans. Ophthalmol. Soc. U.K., 85:53–58, 1965.

155. Somogyi, A., Kovacs, K., and Selye, H.: Jejunal ulcers produced by indomethacin. J. Pharm. Pharmacol., 21:122–123, 1969.

156. Carr, R.E., and Siegel, I.M.: Retinal function in patients treated with indomethacin. Am. J. Ophthalmol., 75:302–306, 1973.

157. International Agranulocytosis and Aplastic Anemia Study: Risks of agranulocytosis and aplastic anemia. A first report of

their relation to drug use with special reference to analgesics. JAMA, *256*:1749–1757, 1986.

158. Inman, W.H.: Study of fatal bone marrow depression with special reference to phenylbutazone and oxyphenbutazone. Br. Med. J., *1*:1500–1505, 1977.

159. Cuthbert, M.F.: Adverse reactions to nonsteroidal anti-inflammatory drugs. Curr. Med. Res. Opin., *2*:600–610, 1974.

160. Davidson, C., and Manohitharajah, S.M.: Drug-induced antiplatelet antibodies. Br. Med. J., *3*:545, 1973.

161. Eade, O.E. et al.: Peripheral neuropathy and indomethacin. Br. Med. J., *2*:66–67, 1975.

162. Kelsey, W.M., and Scharyj, M.: Fatal hepatitis probably due to indomethacin. JAMA, *199*:586–587, 1967.

163. Manchester, D., Margolis, H.S., and Sheldon, R.E.: Possible association between maternal indomethacin and primary pulmonary hypertension of the newborn. Am. J. Obstet. Gynecol., *126*:467–469, 1976.

164. Eeg-Olofsson, O. et al.: Convulsions in a breast fed infant after maternal indomethacin. Lancet, *2*:215, 1978.

165. Pacold, I. et al.: Effects of indomethacin on coronary hemodynamics, myocardial metabolism and anginal threshold in coronary artery disease. Am. J. Cardiol., *57*:912–915, 1986.

166. Schaller, J.G.: Report to the FDA Arthritis Advisory Committee, May 19–20, 1977.

167. Lockwood, G.F. et al.: Pharmacokinetics of ibuprofen in man. I. Free and total area/dose relationships. Clin. Pharmacol. Ther., *34*:97–103, 1983.

168. Brugueras, N.E., LeZotte, L.A., and Moxley, T.E.: Ibuprofen: A double-blind comparison of twice-a-day therapy with four-times-a-day therapy. Clin. Ther., *2*:13–21, 1978.

169. Albert, K.S., and Gernaat, C.M.: Pharmacokinetics of ibuprofen. Am. J. Med., *77*(Suppl. 1A):40–46, 1984.

170. Penner, J.A., and Albrecht, P.H.: Lack of interaction between ibuprofen and warfarin. Curr. Ther. Res., *18*:862–871, 1975.

171. Ward, J.R.: Update on ibuprofen for rheumatoid arthritis. Am. J. Med., *77*(Suppl. 1A):3–9, 1984.

172. Molnar, J.P., and Moxley, T.E.: Ibuprofen, a double-blind comparison of two dosages, 2400 mg and 3200 mg daily, for treating rheumatoid arthritis. Curr. Ther. Res., *26*:581–591, 1979.

173. Altman, R.D.: Review of ibuprofen for osteoarthritis. Am. J. Med., *77*(Suppl. 1A):10–18, 1984.

174. Brewer, E.J.: Non-steroidal anti-inflammatory agents. Arthritis Rheum., *20*:513–516, 1977.

175. Kantor, T.G.: Ibuprofen. Ann. Intern. Med., *91*:877–882, 1979.

176. Valtonen, E.J., and Busson, M.: A comparative study of ibuprofen and indomethacin in nonarticular rheumatism. Scand. J. Rheumatol., *7*:183–188, 1978.

177. Owen, P.R.: Prostaglandin synthetase inhibitors in the treatment of primary dysmenorrhea. Outcome trials reviewed. Am. J. Obstet. Gynecol., *148*:96–103, 1984.

178. Jugdutt, B.I. et al.: Salvage of ischemic myocardium by ibuprofen during infarction in the conscious dog. Am. J. Cardiol., *46*:74–82, 1980.

179. Royer, G.L., Seckman, C.E., and Welshman, I.R.: Safety profile: Fifteen years of clinical experience with ibuprofen. Am. J. Med., *77(Suppl. 1A)*:25–34, 1984.

180. Widener, H.L., and Littman, D.H.: Ibuprofen induced meningitis in systemic lupus erythematosus. JAMA, *239*:1062–1064, 1978.

181. Gryffe, C.I., and Rubenzahl, S.: Agranulocytosis and aplastic anemia possibly due to ibuprofen. Can. Med. Assoc. J., *114*:877–880, 1976.

182. Stempel, D.A., and Miller, J.J., III.: Lymphopenia and hepatic toxicity with ibuprofen. J. Pediatr., *90*:657–658, 1977.

183. Johnson, J.H. et al.: A followup study of ibuprofen users. J. Rheumatol., *12*:549–552, 1985.

184. Johl, R.P. et al.: Ibuprofen and sulindac kinetics in alcoholic liver disease. Clin. Pharmacol. Ther., *31*:104–109, 1983.

185. Graham, G.G. et al.: The pharmacokinetics of ibuprofen in healthy subjects and patients with rheumatoid arthritis. Personal communication, 1982.

186. Court, J., Streete, P., and Volans, G.: Acute poisoning with ibuprofen. Hum. Toxicol., *2*:381–384, 1983.

187. Hall, A.H. et al.: Ibupofen overdose: 126 cases. Ann. Emerg. Med., *15*:1308–1313, 1986.

188. Brogden, R.N. et al.: Naproxen up to date: A review of its pharmacological properties and therapeutic efficacy and use in rheumatic diseases and pain states. Drugs, *18*:241–277, 1979.

189. Runkel, R. et al.: Pharmacokinetics of naproxen overdoses. Clin. Pharmacol. Ther., *20*:269–277, 1976.

190. Jalava, S. et al.: Naproxen concentrations in serum, synovial fluid and synovium. Scand. J. Rheumatol., *6*:155–157, 1977.

191. Segre, F.J. et al.: Naproxen-aspirin interactions in man. Clin. Pharmacol. Ther., *15*:374–379, 1974.

192. Wilkens, R.F., and Segre, E.J.: Combination therapy with naproxen and aspirin in rheumatoid arthritis. Arthritis Rheum., *19*:677—682, 1976.

193. Dresse, A. et al.: Effect of diflunisal on the human plasma levels and on the urinary excretion of naproxen. Arch. Int. Pharmacodyn. Ther., *236*:276–284, 1978.

194. Runkel, R. et al.: Naproxen-probenecid interaction. Clin. Pharmacol. Ther., *24*:706–713, 1978.

195. Yacobi, A., and Levy, G.: Effect of naproxen on protein binding of warfarin. Res. Commun. Chem. Pathol. Pharmacol., *15*:369–372, 1976.

196. Jain, A. et al.: Effect of naproxen on the steady state serum concentration and anticoagulant activity of warfarin. Clin. Pharmacol. Ther., *25*:61–66, 1979.

197. Antilla, M., Haataja, M., and Kasanen, A.: Pharmacokinetics of naproxen in subjects with normal and impaired renal function. Eur. J. Clin. Pharmacol., *11*:263–268, 1980.

198. Williams, R.L. et al.: Naproxen disposition in patients with alcoholic cirrhosis. Eur. J. Clin. Pharmacol., *27*:291–296, 1984.

199. Luftschein, S. et al.: Increasing doses of naproxen in rheumatoid arthritis: use with and without corticosteroids. J. Rheumatol., *6*:397–404, 1979.

200. Day, R.O. et al.: Relationship of serum naproxen concentration to efficacy in rheumatoid arthritis. Clin. Pharmacol. Ther., *31*:733–740, 1982.

201. Kvien, T.K., Hoyeraal, H.M., and Sandstad, B.: Naproxen and acetylsalicylic acid in the treatment of pauciarticular and polyarticular juvenile rheumatoid arthritis. Assessment of tolerance and efficacy in a single-centre 24 week double-blind parallel study. Scand. J. Rheumatol., *13*:342–350, 1984.

202. Duggan, D.E.: Sulindac: Therapeutic implications of the prodrug/pharmacophore equilibrium. Drug. Metab. Rev., *12*:325–337, 1981.

203. Ryan, J.R. et al.: On the question of an interaction between sulindac and tolbutamide in the control of diabetes. Clin. Pharmacol. Ther., *21*:231–233, 1977.

204. Hansten, P.D. (Ed.): Sulindac and warfarin. Drug Interaction Newsl., *1*:26, 1981.

205. Drug Bulletin. November, 1979.

206. Miller, M.J.S., Bednar, M.M., and McGiff, J.C.: Renal metabolism of sulindac, a novel non-steroidal anti-inflammatory

agent. Adv. Prostaglandin Thromboxane Leukotriene Res., 11:487–491, 1983.

207. Ciabottoni, G. et al.: Effects of sulindac and ibuprofen in patients with chronic glomerular disease. N. Engl. J. Med., 310:279–283, 1984.

208. Blackshear, J.L., Davidman, M., and Stillman, M.T.: Identification of risk factors for renal insufficiency from nonsteroidal anti-inflammatory drugs. Arch. Intern. Med., 143:1130–1134, 1983.

209. Roberts, D.G. et al.: Sulindac is not renal sparing in man. Clin. Pharmacol. Ther., 38:258–265, 1985.

210. Brogden, R.N. et al.: Sulindac: a review of its pharmacological properties and therapeutic efficacy in rheumatic diseases. Drugs, 16:97–114, 1978.

211. Dieppe, P.A. et al.: Sulindac and osteoarthritis of the hip. Rheumatol. Rehabil., 15:112–115, 1976.

212. Andelman, S.Y.: Long-term double blind comparison of sulindac and aspirin in the treatment of osteoarthritis. Postgrad. Med. Comm., Special Report:21–32, 1979.

213. Diamond, H.S., and Bankhurst, A.D.: Double blind comparison of sulindac and phenylbutazone in acute gouty arthritis. Postgrad. Med. Comm., Special Report:75–80, 1979.

214. Gengos, D, Pingeon, R.A., and Andrew, A.: Double blind evaluation of sulindac and oxyphenbutazone in the treatment of acute pain of the shoulder. Postgrad. Med. Comm., Special Report:69–74, 1979.

215. Liebling, M.R.: Multi-clinic double blind trial of sulindac in ankylosing spondylitis. Postgrad. Med. Comm., Special Report:61–68, 1979.

216. Merck, Sharpe and Dohme. FDA presentation. May, 1977.

217. Richter, J.A., and Swader, J.: Comparison of fecal blood loss after use of aspirin and sulindac. Postgrad. Med. Comm., Special Report:81–85, 1979.

218. Ballas, Z.K., and Donta, S.T.: Sulindac induced aseptic meningitis. Arch. Intern. Med., 142:165–166, 1982.

219. Levitt, L., and Pearson, R.W.: Sulindac-induced Steven's-Johnson toxic epidermal necrolysis syndrome. JAMA, 243:1262–1263, 1980.

220. Miller, J.L.: Marrow aplasia and sulindac. (Letter.) Ann. Intern. Med., 92:129, 1979.

221. Park, G.D. et al.: Serious adverse reactions associated with sulindac. Arch. Intern. Med., 142:1292–1294, 1982.

222. Brogden, R.N. et al.: Tolmetin: a review of its pharmacological properties and therapeutic efficacy in rheumatic diseases. Drugs, 15:429–450, 1978.

223. Ayres, J.R. et al.: Linear and non-linear assessment of tolmetin pharmacokinetics. Res. Commun. Chem. Pathol. Pharmacol., 17:583–593, 1977.

224. Furst, D.E. et al.: Comparison of tolmetin kinetics in rheumatoid arthritis and matched healthy controls. J. Clin. Pharmacol., 23:329–335, 1983.

225. Hashimoto, M. et al.: Studies on disposition and metabolism of tolmetin, a new anti-inflammatory agent, in rats and mice. I and II. Drug Metab. Dispos., 7:14–23, 1979.

226. Selley, M.L. et al.: Pharmacokinetic studies of tolmetin in man. Clin. Pharmacol. Ther., 17:599–605, 1975.

227. Whitsett, T.L. et al: Tolmetin and warfarin: a clinical investigation to determine if an interaction exists. In Tolmetin. Edited by J.H. Ward. Princeton, Excerpta Medica, 1975, pp. 160–167.

228. Selley, M.L., Madsen, B.W., and Thomas, J.: Protein binding of tolmetin. Clin. Pharmacol. Ther., 24:694–705, 1978.

229. Robinson, H. et al.: Concomitant tolmetin and aspirin therapy

in rheumatoid arthritis. In Tolmetin. Edited by J. H. Ward. Princeton, Excerpta Medica, 1975, pp. 102–111.

230. Plostnicks, J. et al.: Human metabolism of tolmetin. In Tolmetin. Edited by J.H. Ward. Princeton, Excerpta Medica, 1975, pp. 23–33.

231. Levinson, J.E. et al.: Comparison of tolmetin sodium and aspirin in the treatment of juvenile rheumatoid arthritis. J. Pediatr., 91:799–804, 1977.

232. Jentsch, D.D.: Tolectin treatment for rheumatoid arthritis and gout. In Thirteenth International Congress of Rheumatology. Princeton, Excerpta Medica, 1975, p. 114.

233. Schattenkirchner, M., Schattenkirchner, U., and Muller-Fassbender, H.: Klinische erfahrungen mit Tolectin in der Langzeitbehandlung der Spondylitis ankylosans. Therapiewoche, 27:2298–2306, 1977.

234. Caldwell, J. et al.: Double blind comparison of the efficacy and side-effect liability of tolmetin and indomethacin. In Tolmetin. Edited by J.R. Ward. Princeton, Excerpta Medica, 1975, pp. 71–84.

235. Ehrlich, G.E., et al.: Long-term therapy with rheumatoid arthritis. In Tolmetin. Edited by J.R. Ward. Princeton, Excerpta Medica, 1975, pp. 85–101.

236. O'Brien, W.M.: Long-term efficacy and safety of tolmetin sodium in treatment of geriatric patients with rheumatoid arthritis and osteoarthritis: a retrospective study. J. Clin. Pharmacol., 23:309–329, 1983.

237. Restivo, C., and Paulus, H.E.: Anaphylaxis from tolmetin. JAMA, 240:246, 1978.

238. Ruppert, G.B., and Barth, W.F.: Tolmetin-induced aseptic meningitis. JAMA, 245:67–68, 1981.

239. Stefanini, M., and Nassif, R.I.: Acute thrombocytopenic purpura traced to tolmetin related antibody. Va. Med., 109:171–175, 1982.

240. Ehrlich, G.E., and Wortham, G.F.: Pseudo-proteinuria in tolmetin-treated patients. Clin. Pharmacol. Ther., 17:467–468, 1975.

241. Rubin, A., et al.: Stereoselective inversion of (R)-fenoprofen to (S)-fenoprofen in humans. J. Pharm. Sci., 74:82–84, 1985.

242. Gruber, C.M., Jr.: Clinical pharmacology of fenoprofen: A review. J. Rheumatol., 3(Suppl. 2):8–17, 1976.

243. Rubin, A. et al.: Interactions of aspirin with non-steroidal anti-inflammatory drugs in man. Arthritis Rheum., 16:635–645, 1973.

244. Chernish, S.M. et al.: The physiological disposition of fenoprofen in man. IV. J. Med. (Basel), 83:249–257, 1972.

245. Gum, O.B.: Fenoprofen in rheumatoid arthritis: A controlled multicentered study. J. Rheumatol., 3(Suppl. 2):26–31, 1976.

246. Brooke, J.W.: Fenoprofen therapy in large joint osteoarthritis: Double blind comparison with aspirin and long-term experience. J. Rheumatol., 3(Suppl. 2):71–75, 1976.

247. Wanasukapunt, S., Lertratanakul, Y., and Rubinstein, H.M.: Effect of fenoprofen calcium on acute gouty arthritis. Arthritis Rheum., 19:933–935, 1976.

248. Shipley, M., Berry, H., and Bloom, B.: A double blind cross over trial of indomethacin, fenoprofen and placebo in ankylosing spondylitis, with comments on patient assessment. Rheumatol. Rehabil., 19:122–125, 1980.

249. Loebl, D.H.T. et al.: Gastrointestinal blood loss. Effect of aspirin, fenoprofen, and acetaminophen in rheumatoid arthritis as determined by sequential gastroscopy and radioactive fecal markers. JAMA, 237:976–979, 1977.

250. Wendland, M.L., Wagoner, R.D., and Holley, K.E.: Renal failure associated with fenoprofen. Mayo Clin. Proc., 56:103–107, 1980.

251. McLean, J.R., and Gluckman, M.I.: On the mechanism of the pharmacologic activity of meclofenamate sodium. Arzneim. Forsch., 33:627–630, 1983.
252. Boctor, A.M., Eickholt, M., and Pugsley, T.A.: Meclofenamate sodium is an inhibitor of both the 5-lipoxygenase and cyclooxygenase pathways of the arachidonic acid cascade *in vitro*. Prostaglandins Leukotrienes Med., 23:229–233, 1986.
253. Ellis, C.N. et al.: Effects of oral meclofenamate therapy in psoriasis. J. Am. Acad. Dermatol., 14:49–52, 1986.
254. Smith, T.C.: Clinical pharmacology studies of sodium meclofenamate (Meclomen). Curr. Ther. Res., 23(Suppl.):42–50, 1978.
255. Barager, F.D., and Smith, T.C.: Drug interaction studies with sodium meclofenamate (Meclomen). Curr. Ther. Res., 23(Suppl.):51–59, 1978.
256. Petrick, T.J., and Black, M.E.: Double-blind multicenter studies with meclofenamate sodium in the treatment of rheumatoid arthritis in the United States and Canada. Arzneim. Forsch., 33:631–635, 1983.
257. Petrick, T.J., and Bovenkerk, W.E.: Multicenter studies in the United States and Canada of meclofenamate sodium in osteoarthritis of the hip and knee. Arzneim. Forsch., 33:644–648, 1983.
258. Bonssina, I., Gunthner, W., and Marti' Masso', R.: Double-blind multicenter study comparing meclofenamate sodium with indomethacin and placebo in the treatment of extra-articular rheumatic disease. Arzneim. Forsch., 33:649–652, 1983.
259. Ebner, W., Ballarin, J.M.P., and Bonssina, I.: Meclofenamate sodium in the treatment of ankylosing spondylitis. Arzneim. Forsch., 33:(Suppl. 4a):660–663, 1983.
260. Eberl, R., and Dunky, A.: Meclofenamate sodium in the treatment of acute gout. Arzneim. Forsch., 33(Suppl. 4a):641–643, 1983.
261. Brewer, E.J. et al.: Sodium meclofenemate (Meclomen) in the treatment of juvenile rheumatoid arthritis. J. Rheumatol., 9:129–134, 1982.
262. Preston, S.N.: Safety of meclofenamate sodium. Curr. Ther. Res., 23(Suppl.):107–112, 1978.
263. Eberl, R.: Long-term experience with meclofenamate sodium. Arzneim. Forsch., 33(Suppl. 4a):667–678, 1983.
264. Dahl, S.I., and Ward, J.R.: Pharmacology, clinical efficacy and adverse effects of piroxicam, a new nonsteroidal anti-inflammatory agent. Pharmacotherapy, 2:80–90, 1982.
265. Hobbs, D.C.: Pharmacokinetics of piroxicam in man. Eur. J. Rheumatol. Inflamm., 6:46–55, 1983.
266. Verbeek, R.K., Richardson, C.J., and Blocka, K.L.: Clinical pharmacokinetics of piroxicam. J. Rheumatol., 13:789–796, 1986.
267. Hobbs, D.C.: Piroxicam pharmacokinetics: Recent clinical results relating kinetics and plasma levels to age, sex and adverse effects. Am. J. Med. 81(Suppl. 5B):22–28, 1986.
268. Woolf, A.D. et al.: Pharmacokinetic observations on piroxicam in adult middle-aged and elderly patients. Br. J. Clin. Pharmacol., 16:433–437, 1983.
269. Richardson, C.J. et al.: Effect of age and sex on piroxicam disposition. Clin. Pharmacol. Therap., 37:13–18, 1985.
270. Wilkens, R.F. et al.: Double-blind study comparing piroxicam and aspirin in the treatment of rheumatoid arthritis. Am. J. Med., 72(Suppl 2A):23–26, 1982.
271. Abruzzo, J.L., Gordan, G.V., and Meyers, D.R.: Double-blind study comparing piroxicam and aspirin in the treatment of osteoarthritis. Am. J. Med., 72(Suppl. 2A):45–49, 1982.
272. Husby, G.: The Norwegian Multicenter Study. Am. J. Med., 81(Suppl. 5B):6–10, 1986.
273. Bluestone, R.: Safety and efficacy of piroxicam in the treatment of gout. Am. J. Med., 72(Suppl. 2A):66–69, 1982.
274. Romberg, O.: Comparison of piroxicam with indomethacin in ankylosing spondylitis. A double-blind cross over trial. Am. J. Med., 72(Suppl. 2A):58–62, 1982.
275. Pitts, N.E.: Efficacy and safety of piroxicam. Am. J. Med., 72(Suppl. 2A):77–87, 1982.
276. Benoxaprofen and piroxicam: Two new drugs for arthritis. Med. Lett. Drugs Ther., 24:63–66, 1982.
277. Piroxicam Symposium: Piroxicam: A clinical perspective. Am. J. Med., 82(Suppl. 5B):1–55, 1986.
278. Davies, R.O.: Review of the animal and clinical pharmacology of diflunisal. Pharmacotherapy, 3:23S–37S, 1983.
279. Diflunisal. Med. Lett. Drugs Ther., 24:76–78, 1982.
280. Lowen, G.R., McKay, G., and Verbeek, R.K.: Isolation and identification of a new major metabolite of diflunisal in man. The sulfate conjugate. Drug Metab. Dispos., 14:127–131, 1986.
281. Beaver, W.T., Forbes, J.A., and Shackleford, R.W.: A method for the 12 hour evaluation of analgesic efficacy in outpatients with postoperative oral surgery pain. Pharmacotherapy, 3:23S–37S, 1983.
282. Umbenhauer, E.R.: Diflunisal in the treatment of pain in osteoarthritis. Pharmacotherapy, 3:55S–60S, 1983.
283. Devereaux, M.D., and Douglas, W.A.: A double-blind comparative study of diflunisal and naproxen in the treatment of rheumatoid arthritis. Eur. J. Rheumatol. Inflamm., 6:274–278, 1983.
284. Turner, R.A., Whipple, J.P., and Shackleford, R.W.: Diflunisal 500–750 mg versus aspirin 2,600–3,900 mg in the treatment of rheumatoid arthritis. Pharmacotherapy, 4:151–157, 1984.
285. Franssen, M.J., Gribnau, F.W., and van de Putte, L.B.: A comparison of diflunisal and phenylbutazone in the treatment of ankylosing spondylitis. Clin. Rheumatol., 5:210–220, 1986.
286. Ferraccioli, G., Spiani, A., and Ambanelli, U.: Hypouricemic action of diflunisal in gouty patients: *in vitro* and *in vivo* studies. J. Rheumatol., 11:330–332, 1984.
287. Rider, J.A.: Comparison of fecal blood loss after use of aspirin and diflunisal. Pharmacotherapy, 3:61S–64S, 1983.
288. Matsuda, K. et al.: Decrease of urinary PGE_2 and $PGF_{2\alpha}$ excretion by non-steroidal anti-inflammatory drugs in rats. Biochem. Pharmacol., 32:1347–1352, 1983.
289. Upton, R.A. et al.: Ketoprofen pharmacokinetics and bioavailability based on an improved sensitive and specific assay. Eur. J. Clin. Pharmacol., 20:127–133, 1981.
290. Upton, R.A. et al.: Negligible excretion of unchanged ketoprofen, naproxen and probenecid in urine. J. Pharm. Sci., 69:1254–1257, 1980.
291. Advenier, C.A. et al.: Pharmacokinetics of ketoprofen in the elderly. Br. J. Clin. Pharmacol., 16:65–70, 1983.
292. Vavra, I.: Ketoprofen. *In* Newer Anti-inflammatory Agents: Clinical Implications. Edited by A.J. Lewis and D.E. Furst. New York, Marcel Dekker, Inc., 1987, pp. 419–437.
293. Stafanger, G. et al.: Pharmacokinetics of ketoprofen in patients with chronic renal failure. Scand. J. Rheumatol., 10:189–192, 1981.
294. Williams, R.L. et al.: Ketoprofen–aspirin interactions. Clin. Pharmacol. Ther., 30:226–231, 1981.
295. Upton, R.A. et al.: Effects of probenecid on ketoprofen kinetics. Clin. Pharmacol. Ther., 31:705–712, 1982.
296. Brewer, E.J. et al.: Ketoprofen in the treatment of juvenile rheumatoid arthritis. J. Rheumatol., 9:144–148, 1982.
297. Woggon, J., Charlot, F., and Villiaumey, J.: Comparative study of benoxaprofen and ketoprofen in ankylosing spondylitis. Eur. J. Clin. Pharmacol., 19:305–307, 1981.

298. Juvakoski, T., and Lassus, A.: A double-blind cross-over evaluation of ketoprofen and indomethacin in Reiter's disease. Scand. J. Rheumatol., 11:106–108, 1982.
299. Gaut, Z.N. et al.: Stereoisomeric relationships among anti-inflammatory activity, inhibition of platelet aggregation and inhibition of prostaglandin synthetase. Prostaglandins, 10:59–66, 1975.
300. Tursi, A. et al.: In vitro studies of anti-inflammatory activity of carprofen. Eur. J. Rheumatol. Inflamm., 5:488–491, 1982.
301. Randall, L.O., and Baruth, H.: Analgesic and anti-inflammatory activity of 6-chloro-α-methyl-carbazole-acetic acid (C-5720). Arch. Int. Pharmacodyn. Ther., 220:94–114, 1976.
302. Ray J.E., and Wade, D.N.: The pharmacokinetics and metabolism of ^{14}C-carprofen in man. Biopharm. Drug Dispos., 3:29–38, 1982.
303. Enthoven, D., Coffey, J.W., and Wyler-Plaut, R.: Carprofen. In Newer Anti-inflammatory Agents: Clinical Implications. Edited by A.J. Lewis and D.E. Furst. New York, Marcel Dekker, Inc., 1987, pp. 313–328.
304. Berkesky, I., and Colburn, W.A.: Renal clearance of carprofen in the isolated perfused rat kidney. Drug Metab. Dispos., 9:25–29, 1980.
305. Holazo, A.A. et al.: Pharmacokinetics of carprofen in man during tid administration (Abstract.) American Pharmacology Association (127th Annual Meeting), Washington, DC, April 1980, p. 88.
306. Holazo, A.A. et al.: The influence of liver dysfunction on the pharmacokinetics of carprofen. J. Clin. Pharmacol., 25:109–114, 1985.
307. Schneck, D.W. et al.: The effect of aspirin on the disposition of carprofen in humans. Pharmacology, 21:166, 1979.
308. Yu, T.F., and Perel, J.: Pharmacokinetics and clinical studies of carprofen in gout. J. Clin. Pharmacol., 20:347–351, 1980.
309. Dickey, R.A. et al.: Double-blind cross-over trial of carprofen in osteoarthritis (Abstract.) In Proceedings of the International Meeting on Inflammation, Verona, September 24 to 27, 1979, p. 75.
310. Furst, D.E.: Personal communication with Hoffman-LaRoche, 1987.
311. Goh, C.L., and Kwok, S.F.: Photosensitivity associated with carprofen (Imadyl). Dermatologica, 170:74–76, 1985.
312. Ku, E.C. et al.: Effect of diclofenac sodium on the arachidonic acid cascade. Am. J. Med., 80 (Suppl. 4B):18–23, 1986.
313. Scholer, D.W. et al.: Pharmacology of diclofenac sodium. Am. J. Med., 80(Suppl. 4B):34–38, 1986.
314. Reiss, W. et al.: Pharmacokinetics and metabolism of the anti-inflammatory agent, Voltaren. Scand. J. Rheumatol., 22(Suppl.):17–29, 1978.
315. Brogden, R.N. et al.: Diclofenac sodium: A review of its pharmacologic properties and therapeutic use in rheumatic diseases and pain of varying origin. Drugs,20:24–48, 1980.
316. Liauw, H.L., Moscaritola, J.D., and Burcher, J.: Diclofenac sodium (Voltaren). In Newer Anti-inflammatory Agents: Clinical Implications. Edited by A.J. Lewis and D.E. Furst. New York, Marcel Dekker, Inc., 1987, pp. 329–347.
317. Stierlin, H., and Faigle, J.W.: Biotransformation of diclofenac sodium in animals and in man: II. Quantitative determination of the unchanged drug and principal phenolic metabolites in urine and bile. Xenobiotica, 9:611–621, 1971.
318. Stierlin, H., Faigle, J.W., and Colombi, A.: Pharmacokinetics of diclofenac sodium (Voltaren) and metabolites in patients with impaired renal function. Scand. J. Rheumatol., 22:30–35, 1978.
319. Wagner, J., and Salc, M.: Binding of diclofenac sodium to serum proteins of different species and interactions with other drugs and protein binding. Aktuel Rheumatol., 4:153, 1979.
320. Catalano, M.A.: Worldwide safety experience with diclofenac. Am. J. Med., 80(Suppl. 4B):81–87, 1986.
321. Serra-Peralba, A.: A clinical trial of a new anti-rheumatic agent: Diclofenac sodium. Med. Clin., 67:418–423, 1976.
322. Sirois, P. et al.: Comparative effect of etodolac, indomethacin and benoxaprofen on eicosanoid biosynthesis. Inflammation, 8:353–364, 1984.
323. Sayen, M.N. et al.: The metabolic disposition of etodolac in rats, dogs and man. Drug Metabol. Rev., 12:339–362, 1981.
324. Ferdinandi, E.S. et al.: Disposition and biotransformation of C-14 etodolac in man. Xenobiotica, 16:153–166, 1986.
325. Sanda, M. et al.: Etodolac. In Newer Anti-inflammatory Agents: Clinical Implications. Edited by A.J. Lewis and D.E. Furst. New York, Marcel Dekker, Inc., 1987, pp. 349–370.
326. Jacob, G. et al.: A 52-week double-blind trial of etodolac vs aspirin in the treatment of rheumatoid arthritis. Adv. Ther., 2:82–89, 1985.
327. Andelman, S.Y.: Etodolac, aspirin, and placebo in patients with degenerative joint disease: A 12 week study. Clin. Therap., 52:651–661, 1983.
328. Lee, D., and Dvornik, D.: Etodolac: Effect on prostaglandin concentrations in gastric mucosa of rats. Life Sci., 36:1157–1162, 1985.
329. Brogden, R.N. et al.: Fenbufen: A review of its pharmacological properties and therapeutic use in rheumatic disease and acute pain. Drugs, 21:1–22, 1981.
330. Sloboda, A.E. et al.: Fenbufen. In Newer Anti-inflammatory Agents: Clinical Implications. Edited by A.J. Lewis and D.E. Furst. New York, Marcel Dekker, Inc., 1987, pp. 371–392.
331. Chiccarelli, F.S., Eisner, H.J., and Van Lear, G.E.: Metabolic and pharmacokinetic studies of fenbufen in man. Arzneim. Forsch., 4A:728–735, 1980.
332. Anderson, L.G., and Bina, P.R.C.: Double-blind cross-over trial comparing fenbufen and acetylsalicylic acid in rheumatoid arthritis. Arzneim. Forsch., 4A:735–739, 1980.
333. Smith, R.J., Lomen, P.L., and Kaiser, D.G.: Flurbiprofen. In Newer Anti-inflammatory Agents: Clinical Implications. Edited by A.J. Lewis and D.E. Furst. New York, Marcel Dekker, Inc., 1987, pp. 393–418.
334. Nishizawa, E.E. et al.: Flurbiprofen: A new potent inhibitor of platelet aggregation. Throm. Res., 3:577–588, 1973.
335. Tyers, M.B., and Haywood, H.: Effects of prostaglandins on peripheral nociceptors in acute inflammation. Agents Actions, 6(Suppl.):65–78, 1979.
336. Kaiser, D.G., Brooks, C.D., and Lomen, P.L.: Pharmacokinetics of flurbiprofen. Am. J. Med., 80(Suppl. 3A):10–15, 1986.
337. Brooks, P.M., and Khong, T.K.: Flurbiprofen-aspirin interaction: A double-blind cross-over study. Curr. Med. Res. Opin., 5:53–57, 1977.
338. Brogden, R.N. et al.: Flurbiprofen: A review of its pharmacological properties and therapeutic use in rheumatic diseases. Drugs, 18:417–438, 1979.
339. Lomen, P.L. et al.: Flurbiprofen in the treatment of arthritis: A comparison with aspirin. Am. J. Med., 80(Suppl. 3A):89–95, 1986.
340. Kowanko, J.C. et al.: Circadian variations in the signs and symptoms of rheumatoid arthritis and in the therapeutic effectiveness of flurbiprofen at different times of the day. Br. J. Clin. Pharmacol., 11:477–484, 1981.
341. Lomen, P.L. et al.: Flurbiprofen in the treatment of ankylosing spondylitis: A comparison with phenylbutazone. Am. J. Med., 80(Suppl. 3A):120–126, 1986.

342. Lomen, P.L. et al.: Flurbiprofen in the treatment of ankylosing spondylitis: A comparison with indomethacin. Am. J. Med., *80(Suppl. 3A)*:127–132, 1986.

343. Lomen, P.L. et al.: Flurbiprofen in the treatment of acute gout: A comparison with indomethacin. Am. J. Med., *80(Suppl. 3A)*:134–139, 1986.

344. Mena, H.R. et al.: Treatment of acute shoulder syndrome with flurbiprofen. Am. J. Med., *80(Suppl. 3A)*:141–144, 1986.

345. Lomen, P.L., Turner, L.F., and Lamborn, K.R.: Safety of flurbiprofen in the treatment of ankylosing spondylitis, osteoarthritis and rheumatoid arthritis. Am. J. Med., *80(Suppl. 3A)*:23–30, 1986.

346. Fries, J.F., and Britton, M.C.: Fenoprofen calcium in rheumatoid arthritis. Arthritis Rheum., *16*:629–634, 1973.

347. Tugwell, P. et al.: Controlled trial of the clinical utility of serum salicylate monitoring in rheumatoid arthritis. J. Rheumatol., *11*:457–461, 1984.

348. Mielens, Z.E. et al.: Interactions of aspirin with nonsteroidal anti-inflammatory drugs in rats. J. Pharm. Pharmacol., *20*:567–569, 1968.

349. Van Armen, C.G., Nuss, G.W., and Risley, E.A.: Interactions of aspirin, indomethacin, and other drugs in adjuvant-induced arthritis in the rat. J. Pharmacol. Exp. Ther., *187*:400–414, 1973.

350. Miller, D.R.: Combination use of nonsteroidal anti-inflammatory drugs. Drug. Intell. Clin. Pharm., *15*:3–7, 1981.

351. Caldwell, J.R. et al.: Four-way, multicenter, cross over trial of ibuprofen, fenoprofen calcium, naproxen and tolmetin sodium in osteoarthritis. South. Med. J., *76*:706–711, 1983.

352. Capell, H.A. et al.: Patent compliance: A novel method of testing nonsteroidal anti-inflammatory analgesics in rheumatoid arthritis. J. Rheumatol., *6*:584–593, 1979.

353. Gall, E.P. et al.: Clinical comparison of ibuprofen, fenoprofen calcium, naproxen, and tolmetin sodium in rheumatoid arthritis. J. Rheumatol., *9*:402–407, 1982.

354. Huskisson, E.C. et al.: Four new anti-inflammatory drugs: Responses and variations. Br. Med. J., *1*:1048–1049, 1976.

355. Scott, D.L. et al.: Variations in responses to nonsteroidal anti-inflammatory drugs. Br. J. Clin. Pharmacol., *14*:691–694, 1982.

356. Wasner, C. et al.: Nonsteroidal anti-inflammatory agents in rheumatoid arthritis and ankylosing spondylitis. JAMA, *246*:2168–2172, 1981.

33

GOLD COMPOUNDS

JOHN L. SKOSEY

Gold compounds have been used in therapeutics since medieval times. In the late nineteenth and early twentieth centuries, they were used primarily for the treatment of tuberculosis and other infections. By modern standards of evaluation, the responses obtained did not warrant the enthusiasm with which they were used.[1] Forestier is credited with having pioneered the use of these compounds in the treatment of rheumatoid arthritis (RA).[2,3] The first use of gold in RA, as Solganal, was recorded by Lande in 1927.[4] Because of excessive toxicity associated with the large doses initially used, the popularity of gold declined. Gold compounds have been the "second line" agent of first choice for the treatment of RA for nearly 60 years. They have become the standard against which many other drugs have been judged. Table 33–1 lists currently available compounds.

CHEMISTRY

Elemental gold was used in ancient times to treat pruritus of the palms. Gold leaf has been used as an adjunct in the therapy of cutaneous ulcers. Radioactive gold (^{198}Au) in colloidal form has been used to treat malignant pleural and peritoneal effusions and has been injected intra-articularly in patients with RA. With these minor exceptions, gold is used in compounds in which the metal in the monovalent aurous form (Au^+) is stabilized by attachment to a sulfur-containing ligand.[5] The most popular injectable gold preparations used in the United States include au-

Table 33–1. Nomenclature of Gold Compounds

Generic Name	Proprietary Name
Gold sodium thiomalate	Myochrysine
Aurothioglucose	Solganal
Gold thioglycoanilid	Lauron
Gold sodium thiosulfate (IV)	Sanochrysine, Crisalbine
Colloidal gold sulfide (oral, IV)	Aurol-sulfide
Calcium aurothioglycolate	Myoral
Sodium aurothiobenzimidazole carboxylic acid (IV)	Triphal
Methylglucamide of aurothiodiglycollic acid	Parmanil
Sodium auroallylthiourea benzoate (IV)	Lopion
Sodium aurothiopropanol sulfonate	Allochrysine
Sulfhydryl gold naphthyl trisulfocarbonium	Aurocein
Triethylphosphine gold thioglucosetetra-acetate (oral)	Auranofin

IV = Intravenous.
(Adapted from Gottlieb, N.L., and Gray, R.G.: Pharmacokinetics of gold in rheumatoid arthritis. Agents Actions, *8(Suppl.)*:529–538, 1981.)

rothioglucose (Solganal) and sodium aurothiomalate (Myochrysine). Each of these compounds is approximately 50% gold by weight. Sodium aurothiosulfate (Sanochrysine), aurothioglycoanilide (Boron), and sodium aurothiopropanol sulfonate (Allochrysine), also administered by intramuscular injection, are available in other parts of the world. Triethylphosphine gold thioglucosetetra-acetate (Auranofin), the only gold compound absorbed after oral ingestion, is widely available throughout the world.[6]

PHARMACOLOGIC ACTIONS

Gold compounds have a number of actions that may be of pharmacologic interest. The origin of RA and the related diseases for which these drugs are widely used is not known, and the relative importance of putative pathogenic influences remains uncertain. Similarly, the relative importance of the multiple pharmacologic effects of gold compounds in the treatment of RA is unclear.

ANTIMICROBIAL EFFECTS

Koch demonstrated that potassium aurocyanide [KAu(CN$_2$)] arrested the growth of Mycobacterium tuberculosis in vitro. Subsequently, gold compounds have been shown to arrest or to inhibit growth of, or to kill, various strains of bacteria, mycoplasma, and protozoa in vitro and to protect against viral infections. The early observations of the effects of gold compounds on tubercle bacilli led to their use in RA, a chronic disease considered to have characteristics in common with chronic infectious diseases such as tuberculosis.[2]

A number of arguments have challenged the thesis that antimicrobial effects represent an important therapeutic action of gold compounds in RA.[7] First, in spite of great interest in a possible infectious cause of RA, no infectious agent has been identified consistently in this disease. A virus is the most likely infectious agent in the pathogenesis of RA, and gold compounds do not affect viral growth. Moreover, no evidence suggests that treatment with gold compounds reduces the incidence of specific infectious diseases in patients with RA. Finally, unlike in experimental models of infectious arthritis, in which gold compounds must be administered early in the disease to be effective, these preparations are often beneficial in RA even when they are administered years after disease onset.

ALTERATION OF IMMUNE FUNCTION

Immunologic considerations include experimental disease and the effects of gold compounds on lymphocytes, monocytes and macrophages, and immune complexes.

Experimental Immunologically Mediated Disease

The effects of gold compounds on experimental inflammatory diseases with immunologic abnormalities reminiscent of RA have been studied. Gold has an inconsistent effect on adjuvant arthritis in rats.[7] In allergic encephalomyelitis, the onset of clinical signs of disease is delayed by treatment with gold compounds given in doses 50 times greater, on the basis of weight, than those used in human disease. Lymph node cells from animals treated with gold compounds are capable of transferring the disease. This finding suggests that the drug inhibits the effector process, that is, inflammation, rather than acting on a more basic immune process.

Lymphocytes

Lymphocytes tested in vitro from patients with RA have a decreased response to mitogens, in comparison with cells from control subjects. Responses of lymphocytes obtained from these patients after treatment with sodium aurothiomalate approach a normal range.[8] Paradoxically, lymphocytes from patients treated with the oral gold compound Auranofin show a further *decrease* in mitogen response.[9] This decrease may reflect differences in the distribution of elemental gold because a greater amount is found in cells after administration of the oral preparation. Sera from patients with active RA suppress lymphocyte responses to mitogens, probably due to their content of immune complexes. Following treatment with sodium aurothiomalate, immune complex levels fall, and the inhibitory effects of serum are diminished.[10] Both oral and injectable gold compounds added in vitro suppress lymphocyte responses to mitogens.[9] Given the conflicting effects of gold compounds on lymphocyte mitogenic responses, it is unlikely that the major therapeutic effect of these drugs is mediated through alteration of lymphocyte function as assessed by responses to mitogens. Low-density (activated) lymphocytes are present in increased numbers in the blood of patients with RA. Their numbers return to normal after treatment with gold compounds or with D-penicillamine.[11]

Treatment with gold compounds interferes with immunoglobulin-synthesizing cells. Serum levels of rheumatoid factor and other immunoglobulins decrease, in rare cases leading to hypogammaglobulinemia.[12] As noted previously, serum levels of immune complexes also fall in patients treated with these drugs.[8,10] The spontaneous synthesis of immunoglobulin M (IgM) rheumatoid factor by peripheral blood mononuclear cells correlates with disease activity in RA. Synthesis of IgM rheumatoid factor by cells from patients is diminished following treatment with either gold compounds or D-penicillamine.[13]

Monocytes and Macrophages

Gold compounds variably affect the function of monocytes and macrophages. *Aurosomes* develop in phagocytic cells of various tissues of patients treated with gold compounds.[14] These structures are lysosomal bodies with myelinoid membranes enclosing rod-like inclusions, presumably derived from the membranes, and electron-dense deposits of gold. Aurosomes are formed after administration to experimental animals of a variety of soluble gold salts, including the therapeutically inactive form, sodium chloroaurate ($NaAuCl_4$). Sodium thiomalate treatment induces the formation of a structure that lacks the characteristic dense (gold) deposit, but possesses the myelinoid membrane with rod-like inclusions. As already noted, sodium aurothiomalate also inhibits the proliferatve responses of lymphocytes to mitogens in vitro. Similar effects are observed with the auric compound, $NaAuCl_4$.[15,16] This inhibition is probably secondary to suppression of monocyte factors required for lymphocyte responses because it can be overcome by the addition of fresh monocytes not previously exposed to gold compounds. On the other hand, the response of splenic lymphocytes from rats with adjuvant arthritis is inhibited by adherent spleen cells, and this inhibition is overcome by treatment of the animals with gold sodium thiomalate.[17] It is not clear whether the enhancement by sodium aurothiomalate of mitogen responses of peripheral blood lymphocytes from patients with RA is similarly mediated through suppression of monocytes and macrophages. Thus, although it is difficult to reconcile the in vitro and in vivo effects of gold compounds on lymphocyte proliferation, it appears that, in each case, these effects are mediated through actions on cells of the monocyte-macrophage system.

Treatment of mice with large doses of sodium aurothiomalate increases the susceptibility of these animals to infection with a usually avirulent strain of Semliki forest virus. This increased susceptibility has been attributed to impairment of phagocytosis and degradation of virus by the mouse macrophages.[18] The increased phagocytosis of carbon particles by macrophages of patients with RA is also decreased and approaches normal levels with chrysotherapy. Gold compounds, in vitro and in vivo, inhibit chemotaxis by macrophages.[19] Thus, ample opportunity exists for the effects of gold compounds in RA to be mediated through alteration of macrophage function. Definition of the importance of these effects awaits clarification of the role of the monocyte-macrophage system in the pathogenesis of RA and related conditions.

Immune Complexes

Circulating immune complexes, measured by C1q binding activity, are often elevated in patients with RA and consist largely of IgM rheumatoid factor complexed to IgG. During treatment with gold compounds, immune complex levels often fall, but only when evidence of decreased joint inflammation is present. This sequence suggests that the effect on immune complexes reflects suppression of inflammation rather than an effect on a primary pathogenic process.[10]

ANTI-INFLAMMATORY EFFECTS

These effects include actions on acute-phase proteins and oxygen-derived free radicals.

Acute-Phase Proteins

Serum levels of acute-phase proteins such as C-reactive protein (CRP), fibrinogen, haptoglobin, ceruloplasmin, α_1-antitrypsin, and a α_1-acid glycoprotein rise nonspecifically in response to inflammation. High levels of CRP may correlate with severe arthritis and the development of erosive disease. Although evidence suggests a role for some of these proteins in the pathogenesis of inflammation, the significance of these observations is not yet clear. Treatment with gold results in a fall in the serum level of acute-phase proteins that parallels clinical improvement.[10,19]

Oxygen-Derived Free Radicals

Inflammatory mediator cells such as neutrophils and macrophages, when stimulated, produce metabolites of oxygen that possess a high degree of chemical reactivity. These metabolites include superoxide anion, hydrogen peroxide, hydroxyl radical, singlet oxygen, and hypochlorous acid. For convenience, they are referred to collectively as oxygen-derived free radicals, even though not all have the unpaired electron characteristic of free radicals. Gold compounds may protect against the oxidant properties of these free radicals. Levels of natural scavengers of free radicals, such as reduced glutathione in erythrocytes and serum free sulfhydryl moieties and ceruloplasmin, are diminished in active RA, possibly as a result of the action of free radicals produced during the inflammatory process.[10,20] These natural scavengers return to normal levels during treatment with gold compounds. In vitro, both sodium aurothiomalate and triethylphosphine gold thioglucosetetra-acetate inhibit leukocyte iodination, a function that requires free radical action.[21] Free radicals inactivate α_1-proteinase inhibitior, a polypeptide that can protect against damage from lysosomal enzymes released by inflammatory mediator cells. Gold compounds protect α_1-proteinase inhibitor from oxidative damage resulting from the action of free radicals in vitro. That this effect of the drugs is shared by their thiol ligands, thiomalate, thioglucose, and thioglucosetetra-acetate, emphasizes the potential role of the sulfhydryl moieties of these drugs in their biologic effects.[22,23]

ENZYME INHIBITION

Gold compounds directly inhibit a number of enzymes, probably because of the ability of the elemental gold monovalent cation to bind to sulfhydryl groups at critical sites of the enzyme.

A potential mechanism of action of gold compounds in the treatment of erosive synovitis is their inhibition of enzymes such as elastase, collagenase, and hyaluronidase, which are capable of degrading connective tissue components.[7,19] As previously noted, gold compounds and their sulfhydryl ligands may inhibit enzymes indirectly by protecting α_1-proteinase inhibitor from oxidative damage. Moreover, gold is concentrated within lysosomes, where it can combine with and possibly inhibit destructive enzymes. The activity of lysosomal enzymes extracted from cells exposed to gold compounds, or from animals treated with gold compounds, is diminished. Gold is also capable of inhibiting metabolic enzymes involved in such functions as macromolecular synthesis and oxidative phosphorylation.[7] The gold moiety of sodium aurothiomalate or of triethylphosphine gold thioglucosetetra-acetate inhibits a trypsin-like neutral protease on the surface of Ehrlich ascites tumor cells.[24] This enzyme is responsible for the activation of procollagenase, believed to be an important requirement for tumor invasiveness through connective tissue. A similar mechanism may contribute to the invasiveness of synovial pannus. Sodium aurothiomalate inhibits proliferation of, and collagen synthesis by, cultured human synovial cells.[25]

OTHER EFFECTS

The amino acid tryptophan has been postulated to have anti-inflammatory effects. Its plasma level increases when it is displaced from protein-binding sites by gold compounds.[7,19] Other amino acids or oligopeptides with potential anti-inflammatory effects may be similarly displaced. Gold binds with and irreversibly inactivates the first component of complement. The treatment of rats with gold sodium thiosulfate alters the electron-microscopic morphologic features of tail tendon collagen and changes the physicochemical measurements in a manner suggesting increased intermolecular cross-linking. Gold compounds protect albumin and γ globulin from the effects of a number of denaturing agents. Treatment of rats with gold sodium thiomalate results in a decrease in the numbers of unmyelinated, but not of myelinated, nerve fibers. This observation has led to the speculation that gold may produce an anti-inflammatory effect through a neurotoxic effect on the (unmyelinated) nociceptive afferent and sympathetic efferent fibers of the peripheral nervous system that contribute to the pathophysiology of inflammation.[26]

PHARMACOKINETICS

When patients are given weekly injections of 50 mg gold sodium thiomalate, the concentration of elemental gold in serum reaches a peak of approximately 700 µg/dl about 2 hours after injection. The level then declines to half this value over the next 7 days. Gold thioglucose, which is supplied in a sesame oil vehicle, is absorbed more slowly and produces a lower peak gold level. Serum levels a week after injection are comparable to those attained when gold sodium thiomalate is used, however. After 6 to 8 weeks of weekly injections, the serum gold level stabilizes at 300 to 400 µg/dl. Maintenance gold therapy of 50 mg every 3 to 4 weeks results in a steady-state serum gold level of 75 to 125 µg/dl. A small amount of injected gold is first found in the erythrocytes several days after administration and reaches a peak in these cells at about 7 days. It is bound primarily to hemoglobin and replaces hydrogen in the sulfhydryl groups. The finding that gold administered in injectable form is not present in erythrocytes for several days after injection suggests its incorporation into bone marrow precursors.[6]

Erythrocytes of smokers contain a much higher fraction of total blood gold than erythrocytes of nonsmokers, 18% as opposed to 3%. This difference has been attributed to the raised levels of cyanide and thiocyanate in the blood of smokers. These compounds can form complexes with gold that are then able to enter erythrocytes.[27] Ninety-two percent of intravascular gold is bound to serum proteins, primarily to albumin, with smaller amounts bound to complement and immunoglobulins. With higher doses and, consequently, higher blood levels of gold, albumin-binding sites become saturated, and the percentage bound to other serum proteins increases.[6]

Approximately 40% of the gold in sodium aurothiomalate given weekly is excreted. Of the excreted gold, approximately 70% is found in urine and 30% in feces.[6] The concentration in breast milk is low, but the serum gold level in newborns of mothers receiving chrysotherapy is over half that in maternal circulation.[28]

About 25% of gold from the oral gold preparation Auranofin is absorbed. The blood gold level is proportional to the dose of ingested gold, but it is lower than that with injectable gold. A whole blood gold level of approximately 90 μg/dl is achieved after continuous therapy with 9 mg per day. In contrast to the findings with injectable gold preparations, 25 to 50% of whole blood gold is in the cellular fraction. In the serum fraction, 82% is bound to albumin, and the remainder is bound primarily to globulins. The excretion of Auranofin is much more complete than that of injectable gold preparations; 95% is recovered in feces and 5% in urine. The greater fecal recovery probably reflects, in part, incomplete absorption.[6,29]

The amount of gold retained depends on the compound, the dose, and the frequency and route of administration. In patients receiving weekly injections, approximately 60% of gold is retained, whereas only 20% is retained when injections are given monthly. Less (30%) is retained from Auranofin. None is retained when a dose of 2 mg is given daily for a similar period. Gold is stored in highest concentration in organs with the highest content of reticuloendothelial tissue: lymph nodes, adrenal glands, liver, kidney, bone marrow, and spleen. Equilibrium is achieved rapidly between blood and synovial fluid, where the gold concentration is about half that of blood. Gold accumulates in synovial macrophages, more rapidly in inflamed than in uninflamed synovium. Low concentrations of gold are detected in skin and its appendages and in the cornea and lens of the eye.[6]

Interest has been increasing in the potential therapeutic role of the sulfhydryl ligands of the gold compounds, but few data are available on the pharmacokinetics of these moieties. When patients receive weekly injections of sodium aurothiomalate, the thiomalate portion of the drug disappears rapidly from plasma; about 60% is recovered in urine by the end of the first day after injection. In mice, thiomalate is retained primarily in the kidney, liver, spleen, lung, muscle, and skin.[30]

THERAPEUTIC USES

Gold compounds are used most commonly for the treatment of RA, although they have been used in the therapy of other inflammatory diseases as well.[31–33] Therapy with gold compounds produces benefits, as assessed by reductions in patients' dis-

ability and pain. Although these drugs induce remission in fewer than 10% of patients, they reduce the rate of progression of joint damage.[34–37]

The mode of administration has been dictated primarily by tradition. Typically, a small initial dose of 10 mg sodium aurothiomalate or aurothioglucose, designed to identify idiosyncratic reactions, is given intramuscularly. This dose is followed in a week by an injection of 25 or 50 mg; 50 mg is then given weekly until a total of 1 g drug (500 mg elemental gold) has been administered. Pain at the injection site can be reduced by the addition of a local anesthetic such as lidocaine to the syringe containing the drug.[38] It is then customary to continue "maintenance" therapy, 50 mg every 2 weeks for 4 to 8 injections, then every 3 weeks for 4 to 6 injections, then monthly. The frequency and dosage of maintenance therapy are altered according to the clinician's perception of therapeutic and toxic responses. Other regimens in which the dosage or frequency of injection is either increased or decreased have produced results that are sometimes better and sometimes worse than the traditional regimen, and the value of maintenance therapy has been questioned. Nonetheless, most practitioners currently follow the traditional method of administering gold compounds. Although maintenance therapy is often continued indefinitely, evidence suggests that patients who have received a total of 6 g gold compound receive no further benefit from the drug.[39] Further, patients in whom gold is discontinued when the disease is in remission are unlikely to respond to the drug a second time if the disease recurs.[40] Auranofin, which is 29% elemental gold by weight, is administered orally, at 6 to 9 mg daily (3 mg BID or TID).

It used to be common to withhold gold compounds until the patient had an inadequate response to an adequate trial of aspirin or another nonsteroidal anti-inflammatory drug. It also used to be customary to wait until the disease has been present for at least 1 year, to ensure that chrysotherapy would not be given unnecessarily to a patient who could experience a spontaneous remission. The current trend is toward a more aggressive approach to the treatment of RA and earlier use of gold compounds and other second-line drugs. Results of chrysotherapy are best when it is initiated earlier, rather than later, in the natural history of the disease, particularly, as would be expected, to retard joint erosion.[36,41,42] The development of juxta-articular erosions or persistent inflammation unresponsive to nonsteroidal agents dictates earlier institution of therapy with gold compounds. The rate of progression of joint damage, as assessed by radiography, is least in those patients who have a strong clinical response to the drug.[37]

Most contraindications for therapy with gold compounds are relative, rather than absolute. They include pre-existing proteinuria and dermatitis, which would be difficult to distinguish from toxic effects of the drug. Anemia and leukopenia are not absolute contraindications and may, when they are the result of the underlying disease process such as anemia of chronic inflammation or Felty's syndrome,[43] improve with treatment. As noted previously, gold crosses the placenta and can be recovered in the fetal circulation in signifcant quantities, but children born to mothers treated with gold compounds throughout pregnancy have not been reported to have abnormalities attributable to therapy.[28] Gold compounds are as efficacious in patients over 60 years of age as they are in younger individuals, and the incidence of toxicity is not notably different in the older group.[44]

Forestier, in an early report of his experience with the use of gold compounds in the treatment of RA and related diseases, stated that toxicity would require discontinuing the drug in 25% of patients, and 60% would be "greatly benefited."[2] Although individual reports vary in the relative frequencies of therapeutic success and toxicity, these figures are within the generally accepted range. It is often stated that beneficial effects are not observed for weeks or months after the institution of therapy. Some studies show, however, a gradual improvement in morning stiffness, pain, systemic symptoms, and other measures of inflammation that, by extrapolation, seems to have begun soon after the institution of therapy.[45] The effects on sedimentation rate and on other laboratory correlates of inflammation lag behind the clinical findings. Although the beneficial effects of gold compounds on the clinical manifestations of inflammation are important, the ability of these agents to retard the progression of articular damage is of even more significance. It is unusual for these drugs to arrest joint damage completely, but a number of studies have shown that treatment of patients with RA with gold compounds retards cartilage loss and the development of cysts and erosions. In some cases, mineralization, as assessed by serial radiographs, improves.[35]

Both oral and parenteral gold compounds are effective in patients with psoriatic arthritis with a rheumatoid pattern of involvement, as well as in the treatment of peripheral arthritis in patients with spondylitis.[46] Similar toxicity is also observed, but contrary to earlier teachings, cutaneous toxicity does not appear to be excessive or frequent when gold compounds are used in psoriatic arthritis, nor does chrysotherapy appear to benefit the skin of psoriatic patients.[47]

Gold compounds have been successful in the treatment of juvenile RA (JRA). The dose must be adjusted for the age and size of the child.

Chrysotherapy has been used for the treatment of palindromic rheumatism and of intermittent hydrarthrosis (see Chapter 64). It is said to be ineffective in the treatment of the axial joints in ankylosing spondylitis. It has been used successfully in the treatment of nonrheumatic disorders such as pemphigus vulgaris and asthma.[48–50]

TOXICITY

Unfortunately, the incidence of toxicity is high and frequently necessitates cessation of therapy (Fig. 33–1). During a standard course (20 injections of 50 mg) of therapy with gold compounds, approximately 35% of patients experience toxic side effects, and these effects are severe enough to require discontinuance of the drug in about 14% (Table 33–2). During continued maintenance therapy, the incidence of toxicity and treatment termination increases, so by 4 to 5 years, only 16 to 50% of patients still receive treatment (Fig. 33–1).[51] Dermatitis, nearly always pruritic, is by far the most common side effect; proteinuria, neutropenia, and thrombocytopenia occur much less frequently. Uncommon side effects include the nitritoid reaction (a cutaneous flush soon after injection), post-injection flares of joint inflammation, and gastrointestinal, pulmonary, neurologic, and muscular effects. The incidence of toxic effects is similar with both sodium aurothiomalate and aurothioglucose, but nitritoid reactions and postinjection flares are practically limited to patients receiving the former compound. The incidence of toxicity with the oral preparation is similar to that with the injectable compounds, but diarrhea is the most common side effect, and rash is less frequent. Results to date suggest that the overall toxicity of the oral gold preparation is less than that of parenteral gold compounds, although the parenteral drugs are usually more effective.[52–54] Concomitant administration of glucocorticoids does not alter the incidence or severity of toxic reactions to gold compounds.

Toxicity to gold may be mediated by immune mechanisms under genetic control. Antibodies of the IgE class directed toward sodium aurothiomalate have been associated with toxic reactions.[55] Eosinophilia may accompany gold toxicity, but because it may be observed in RA unrelated to therapy it is not a useful predictor of adverse reactions or of their severity.[56]

FIG. 33–1. Termination incidence for rash, for lack of benefit, for proteinuria for other reasons, and for total causes during gold therapy. (From Richter, J.A., et al.: Analysis of treatment terminations with gold and antimalarial compounds in rheumatoid arthritis. J. Rheumatol., 7:153–159, 1980.)

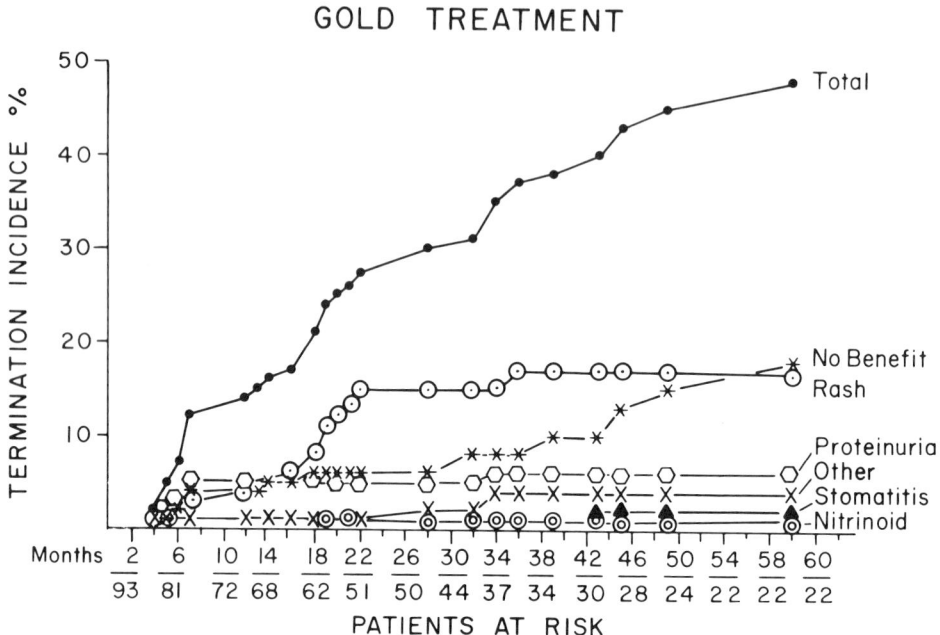

Immunologically mediated drug toxicity may be influenced by histocompatibility genes, which, in turn, may control cells concerned with immune responses. An increased incidence of toxicity, especially proteinuria, to gold compounds is seen in white patients with human leukocyte (HLA) antigen haplotypes A1, B8, Cw7, and DR3.[57] Other investigators have found an

Table 33–2. Toxicity of Gold Compounds

Mucocutaneous Effects
Pruritus
Rash
Mucous membrane ulcers
Bone Marrow Effects
Leukopenia
Thrombocytopenia
Renal Effects
Proteinuria
Acute renal failure (hypersensitivity reaction)
Gastrointestinal Effects
Diarrhea
Enterocolitis
Hepatocellular damage
Pulmonary Effects
Reduced pulmonary function
Neurologic Effects
Polyneuropathy
Chrysiasis
Nitritoid reaction
Postinjection inflammation flare

association of DR3 with skin eruptions as well as with proteinuria, and have found that the incidence of DR4 or DR7 antigen is decreased in patients who develop toxic reactions to either gold or penicillamine.[58,59] The conclusion that these HLA antigens afford a protective benefit must be entertained with caution, however, because an increase in the incidence of an HLA antigen found at any locus is necessarily associated with a decrease in the frequency of other antigens found at that locus. DR3 and B8 antigens are associated with the development of an immune-mediated peripheral destruction of platelets in patients treated with gold, but not with thrombocytopenia that appears to develop by nonimmune mechanisms.[60,61] B35 antigen has been associated with mucocutaneous toxic reactions.[62] That these associations are not found in American black RA patients, however, emphasizes that caution must be exercised in extrapolating these findings to other racial groups.[63]

MUCOCUTANEOUS EFFECTS

Rash, pruritus, and mucous membrane ulcers are among the most common side effects in patients treated with gold compounds. The rash is almost always pruritic, and pruritus can occur without the rash. A nonspecific dermatitis is usually seen, but the rash may be similar to lichen planus, pityriasis rosea, or various forms of eczema.[64] It typically is located in cutaneous folds such as around the neck, the armpits, the groin, or under the breasts. Usually, however, it has no distinguishing characteristics. Eosinophilia variably accompanies rash and, when present, may precede or appear simultaneously with it. Severe reactions such as exfoliative dermatitis or toxic epidermal necrolysis occur rarely. Although mucocutaneous reactions represent the side effects most commonly associated with therapy with gold compounds, they also occur frequently in control populations. The reported incidence of toxic reactions in control populations may be spuriously high, however, because in some studies, the control injection consisted of small doses of gold compound. These small doses, although ineffective therapeutically, may well have been capable of inducing hypersensitivity reactions.

BONE MARROW EFFECTS

Although rare, the complication of bone marrow suppression is serious. Approximately 5% of patients develop some degree of leukopenia or thrombocytopenia. Usually, these disorders are minor and are not associated with increased risk of infection, bleeding, or other serious complications. It is often possible to continue therapy with gold compounds in the face of mild to moderate chronic granulocytopenia.[65] Thrombocytopenia may be the result of drug-induced thrombocytopenia.[66] Aplastic anemia, although rare, has occurred in patients treated with gold compounds and it can be life-threatening.[34]

RENAL EFFECTS

Proteinuria is second only to rash in incidence as a manifestation of toxicity and occurs in up to 10% of patients treated with gold compounds. Gold therapy must be differentiated from other causes such as renal amyloidosis, a complication of RA still common in many parts of the world.[67] The renal damage is usually mild, especially if recognized early and if treated by drug withdrawal. Nephrotic syndrome and renal failure have occurred, however. Immune complexes have been found in glomerular basement membrane. The nature of the antigen has not been determined. Early studies suggested that the immune complexes contained elemental gold, but later studies have not borne out this finding. Aurosomes are present in proximal and distal renal tubule cells, and increased

urinary excretion of lysosomal enzymes occurs early in the development of nephrotoxicity. These findings have led to the suggestion that the initial injury is to renal tubules. It is postulated that released antigens then complex with autoantibodies and give rise to autoimmune membranous nephropathy.[68] Rarely, acute renal failure develops as a hypersensitivity reaction.

OTHER TOXIC REACTIONS

Less-common toxic reactions in patients treated with gold compounds involve the gastrointestinal tract, the lung, and the neuromuscular system. As noted previously, mild diarrhea is the most common side effect of treatment with the oral gold preparation. This may result from decreased absorption from the colonic lumen of Na^+ and fluid, subsequent to inhibition by Auranofin of a colonic mucosal (Na^+ + K^+)adenosine triphosphatase.[69] Life-threatening enterocolitis and ileitis have been reported as complications of parenteral therapy.[70–72] The gastrointestinal tract may be affected throughout its length, from the stomach to the colon, in which a clinical picture similar to toxic megacolon may develop.[73] Histologic examination of biopsies of colon in such cases shows ulceration, edema, hemorrhage, and dense mononuclear cell infiltration. Reversible liver damage has been reported, associated with various histologic abnormalities and sometimes with lymphadenopathy, pulmonary infiltrates, and rash.[74]

Acute pulmonary damage, characterized by symptoms of rapidly progressing dyspnea, cough (occasionally with sputum production), pleuritic chest pain, fever, and rash, has been reported. Roentgenograms show diffuse infiltrates with patchy consolidation involving both lungs ("gold lung") (Fig. 33–2). Pulmonary function tests show a restrictive lung defect, reduced lung volume, and marked reduction in diffusing capacity. Histologic examination of lung biopsies shows edema, interstitial fibrosis, and alveolar wall thickening with marked lymphocytic and plasma cell infiltration.[75] This complication is usually self-limited, but may be fatal.[76] A variety of neurologic complications occur rarely as a result of therapy with gold compounds, polyneuropathy being the most common.[77] Either a mixed sensory and motor neuropathy, which is predominantly distal, or an acute polyneuropathy of the Guillian-Barré type is seen. Axonal degeneration and segmental demyelination are seen in histologic examination of sural nerve biopsies.[78] Encephalopathy may occur rarely.[79] Gold compounds have been reported to exert toxic effects on

FIG. 33–2. Posteroanterior chest radiographs of a patient with "gold lung." *A,* On hospital admission. *B,* Three months later, after successful treatment. (From Cooke, N., and Bamji, A.: Gold lung. Rheumatol. Rehabil., *20:*129–135, 1981.)

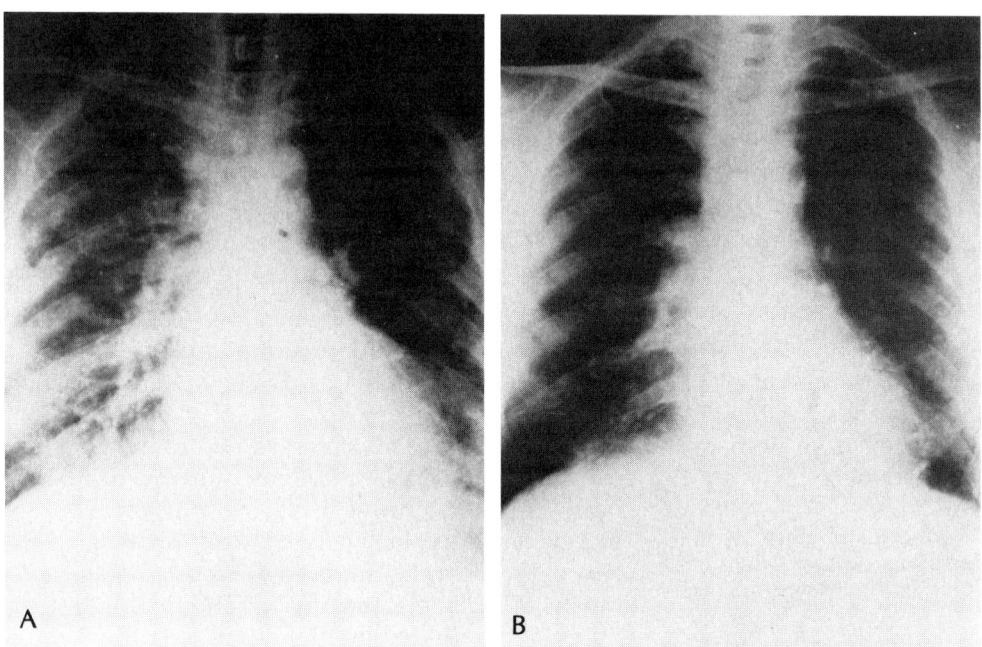

muscle that result in continuous muscle fiber activity.[80]

Corneal chrysiasis, or deposition of elemental gold in the cornea, detected by slit-lamp examination, occurs in almost all patients who have received as much as 1 g of gold compounds. About half have deposits of gold in the lens.[81] These deposits are of limited, if any, clinical significance. More extensive deposition of elemental gold in skin occurs rarely and may be mistaken for cyanosis.[82] Gold compounds may cause reactions similar to those caused by nitrites. These nitritoid reactions consist of facial flushing, nausea, dizziness, and sometimes, hypotension. Postinjection reactions of transient stiffness, arthralgia, myalgia, and constitutional symptoms accounted for only a few withdrawals from therapy in controlled series. They occur, however, in as many as 15% of patients and may result in unnecessary and premature cessation of therapy.[83] Both nitritoid and postinjection reactions are more common in patients receiving sodium aurothiomalate than in those treated with aurothioglucose. These reactions usually can be managed by substitution of aurothioglucose for aurothiomalate.

MANAGEMENT OF TOXIC REACTIONS

Most toxic side effects of therapy with gold compounds, if detected early, can be managed simply by discontinuing the drug. Nitritoid and postinjection reactions respond to a change in gold compound. Aurothioglucose can often be used to continue treatment of patients who have had moderate to severe adverse reactions to aurothiomalate.[84] More severe toxicity, such as nephrosis with significant proteinuria, exfoliative dermatitis or other severe skin toxicity, or marked leukopenia or thrombocytopenia, requires the use of glucocorticoids, the equivalent of 40 to 60 mg prednisone daily, in divided doses.[85] A combination of glucocorticoids and agents capable of chelating gold, such as British anti-Lewisite (BAL), has sometimes been used with apparent success. No clear-cut evidence suggests that chelating agents provide additional benefit, however. N-acetylcysteine (Mucomyst), which binds but does not chelate monovalent gold, has been used alone in doses of 2 to 9 g infused intravenously over 2 to 6 hours to treat hematologic reactions to gold. This agent lacks the toxicity of BAL and is apparently effective.*[86] Enterocolitis, when associated with eosinophilia, has been reported to respond to cromolyn sodium, 20 mg qid.[71]

Editor's note. We have successfully treated a patient with severe aplastic anemia with 10 g n-acetylcysteine given every 24 hours through a Hickman catheter and using an infusion pump. Treatment for 4 months was necessary to reverse gold toxicity and to stabilize the bone marrow output at normal levels. (Hansen, et al.: J. Rheumatol., *12:*794–797, 1985).

Monitoring Toxicity during Therapy

Before each injection, the patient should be questioned regarding symptoms of toxicity. Pruritus usually precedes other manifestations of rash. Traditionally, also prior to each injection, patients have a complete blood count, which includes a differential white count and either a platelet count or examination of the peripheral smear for platelet adequacy. A urinalysis is also done, in particular to assess the presence of proteinuria.* These laboratory tests should not be relied on completely to exclude toxic reactions. Leukopenia or thrombocytopenia can occur precipitously. The patient should be advised to contact the physician should fever, oral ulceration, purpura or other bleeding, or other sign of bone marrow suppression develop. Usually, however, a gradual decline in peripheral blood elements is observed and allows for reduction in dosage or cessation of treatment. Hematuria is an unlikely result of treatment with gold compounds.[87] If it occurs, another cause should be sought.[88]

Reinstitution of Therapy after Toxic Reactions

After severe reactions, such as marked thrombocytopenia or leukopenia, exfoliative dermatitis, nephrotic syndrome, colitis, or pulmonary reaction, therapy with gold compounds should not be reinstituted. After mild toxic reactions, however, it is often possible to resume therapy with gold compounds at a lower dose or at decreased frequency. Should a toxic reaction recur, another "remission-inducing" agent, such as penicillamine, azathioprine, or methotrexate, may be given. Most studies have shown that toxicity to gold compounds is not predictive of the probability or the type of potential toxic reaction to one of the other drugs.

REFERENCES

1. Keers, R.Y.: The gold rush 1925–35. Thorax, *35*:884–889, 1980.
2. Forestier, J.: Rheumatoid arthritis and its treatment by gold salts. J. Lab. Clin. Med., *20*:827–840, 1935.
3. Kean, W.F., et al.: The history of gold therapy in rheumatoid disease. Semin. Arthritis Rheum., *14*:180–186, 1985.
4. Lande, K.: Die gunstique Baunflussung Schleichender Dauerinfekte durch Solganal. MMW, *74*:1132–1134, 1927.
5. Sadler, P.J.: The biological chemistry of gold: a metallo-drug and heavy-atom label with variable valency. Struct. Bond., *29*:171–214, 1976.
6. Gottlieb, N.L., and Gray, R.G.: Pharmacokinetics of gold in rheumatoid arthritis. Agents Actions, *8 [Suppl.]*:529–538, 1981.
7. Leibfarth, J.H., and Persellin, R.H.: Mechanisms of action of gold. Agents Actions, *11*:458–472, 1981.

8. Highton, J., et al.: Changes in immune function in patients with rheumatoid arthritis following treatment with sodium aurothiomalate. Ann. Rheum. Dis., *40*:254–262, 1981.
9. Lorber, A., Jackson, W.H., and Simon, T.M.: Assessment of immune response during chrysotherapy: comparison of gold sodium thiomalate vs. auranofin. Scand. J. Rheumatol., *10*:129–137, 1981.
10. Laurent, M.R., and Panayi, G.S.: Biochemical parameters in the assessment of anti-inflammatory drugs—a review. Agents Actions, *7[Suppl.]*:310–317, 1980.
11. Alexander, G.J., et al.: Low density lymphocytes: their relationship to disease activity and to antirheumatic therapy. Br. J. Rheumatol., *23*:6–14, 1984.
12. So, A.K., Peskett, S.A., and Webster, A.D.: Hypogammaglobulinaemia associated with gold therapy. Ann. Rheum. Dis., *43*:581–582, 1984.
13. Olsen, N., Ziff, M., and Jasin, H.E.: Spontaneous synthesis of IgM rheumatoid factor by blood mononuclear cells from patients with rheumatoid arthritis: effect of treatment with gold salts or D-penicillamine. J. Rheumatol., *11*:17–21, 1984.
14. Ghadially, F.N., et al.: The morphology and atomic composition of aurosomes produced by sodium aurothiomalate in human monocytes. Ann. Pathol., *2*:117–125, 1982.
15. Lipsky, P.E., and Ziff, M.: Inhibition of antigen- and mitogen-induced human lymphocyte proliferation by gold compounds. J. Clin. Invest., *59*:455–466, 1977.
16. Lipsky, P.E., and Ziff, M.: The mechanisms of action of gold and D-penicillamine in rheumatoid arthritis. *In* Advances in Inflammation Research. Vol. III. Rheumatoid Arthritis. Edited by M. Ziff, G.P. Velo, and S. Gorini. New York, Raven Press, 1982, pp. 219–235.
17. Binderup, L., Bramm, E., and Arrigoni-Martelli, E.: The effect of some antirheumatic drugs *in vivo* on the response of spleen cells to concanavalin A in rats with chronic inflammation. Int. J. Immunopharmacol., *4*:57–66, 1982.
18. Oaten, S.W., Jagelman, S., and Webb, H.E.: Further studies of macrophages in relationship to avirulent Semlikki forest virus infections. Br. J. Exp. Pathol., *61*:150–155, 1980.
19. Vernon-Roberts, B.: Action of gold salts on the inflammatory response and inflammatory cell function. J. Rheumatol., *6[Suppl 5]*:120–129, 1979.
20. Munthe, E., Kass, E., and Jellum, E.: Evidence for enhanced radical scavenging prior to drug response in rheumatoid arthritis. *In* Advances in Inflammation Research. Vol. III. Rheumatoid Arthritis. Edited by M. Ziff, G.P. Velo, and S. Gorini. New York, Raven Press, 1982, pp. 211–218.
21. Sliwinski, A.J., and Guertin, M.A.: Gold suppression of human neutrophil function *in vitro*. Biochem. Pharmacol., *31*:671–676, 1982.
22. Skosey, J.L., and Chow, D.C.: Inactivation of serum elastase inhibitory capacity by products of stimulated neutrophils: protection by gold salts and D-penicillamine. *In* Advances in Inflammation Research. Vol. III. Rheumatoid Arthritis. Edited by M. Ziff, G.P. Velo, and S. Gorini. New York, Raven Press, 1982, pp. 245–253.
23. Skosey, J.L., et al.: Drug interference with inactivation of serum alpha-1-proteinase inhibitor by oxygen radicals. *In* Oxy Radicals and Their Scavenger Systems. Vol. II. Cellular and Medical Aspects. Edited by R.A. Greenwald and G. Cohen. New York, Elsevier Biomedical, 1983, pp. 264–267.
24. Short, A.K., et al.: β-Naphthylamidase activity of the cell surface of Ehrlich ascites cells: reversible control of enzyme activity by metal ions and thiols. Br. J. Cancer, *44*:709–716, 1981.
25. Goldberg, R.L., et al.: A mechanism of action of gold sodium

---

Editor's note. I generally have patients test their urine for protein every 2 weeks with Albustix.

thiomalate in diseases characterized by a proliferative synovitis: reversible changes in collagen production in cultured human synovial cells. J. Pharmacol. Exp. Ther., 218:395–403, 1981.

26. Levine, J.D., et al.: The neurotoxic effect of gold sodium thiomalate on the peripheral nerves of the rat: insights into the anti-inflammatory actions of gold therapy. Arthritis Rheum., 29:897–901, 1986.

27. Graham, G.G., et al.: The effect of smoking on the distribution of gold in blood. J. Rheumatol., 9:527–531, 1982.

28. Cohen, D.L., Orzel, J., and Taylor, A.: Infants of mothers receiving gold therapy. (Letter.) Arthritis Rheum., 24:104–105, 1981.

29. Gottlieb, N.L.: Comparison of the kinetics of parenteral and oral gold. Scand. J. Rheumatol., 51[Suppl]:10–14, 1983.

30. Jellum, E., and Munthe, E.: Fate of the thiomalate part after intramuscular administration of aurothiomalate in rheumatoid arthritis. Ann. Rheum. Dis., 41:431–432, 1982.

31. Cooperating Clinics Committee of the American Rheumatism Association: A controlled trial of gold salt therapy in rheumatoid arthritis. Arthritis Rheum., 16:353–358, 1973.

32. Empire Rheumatism Council: Gold therapy in rheumatoid arthritis: report of a multi-centre controlled trial. Ann. Rheum. Dis., 19:95–119, 1960.

33. Empire Rheumatism Council: Gold therapy in rheumatoid arthritis: final report of a multicentre controlled trial. Ann. Rheum. Dis., 20:315–352, 1961.

34. Lockie, L.M., and Smith, D.M.: Forty-seven years experience with gold therapy in 1,019 rheumatoid arthritis patients. Semin. Arthritis Rheum., 14:238–246, 1985.

35. Iannuzzi, L., et al.: Does drug therapy slow radiographic deterioration in rheumatoid arthritis? N. Engl. J. Med., 309:1023–1028, 1983.

36. Luukainen, R.: Chrysotherapy in rheumatoid arthritis: with particular emphasis on the effect of chrysotherapy on radiographical changes and on the optimal time of initiation of therapy. Scand. J. Rheumatol., 34[Suppl]:1–56, 1980.

37. Scott, D.L. and Farr, M.: Assessing the progression of joint damage in rheumatoid arthritis. Drugs, 32[Suppl 1]:63–70, 1986.

38. Kovalesky, A., Sherry, D.D., and Lehman, T.J.: The use of lidocaine to reduce the pain of myochrysine injections for children with juvenile rheumatoid arthritis. J. Rheumatol., 13:356–357, 1986.

39. Van der Leeden, H., et al.: A double-blind study on the effect of discontinuation of gold therapy in patients with rheumatoid arthritis. Clin. Rheumatol., 5:56–61, 1986.

40. Evers, A.E., and Sundstrom, W.R.: Second course gold therapy in the treatment of rheumatoid arthritis. Arthritis Rheum., 26:1071–1075, 1983.

41. Dawes, P.T., et al.: Prediction of progressive joint damage in patients with rheumatoid arthritis receiving gold or D-penicillamine therapy. Ann. Rheum. Dis., 45:945–949, 1986.

42. Sharp, J.T., Lidsky, M.D., and Duffy, J.: Clinical responses during gold therapy for rheumatoid arthritis: changes in synovitis, radiologically detectable erosive lesions, serum proteins, and serologic abnormalities. Arthritis Rheum., 25:540–549, 1982.

43. Dillon, A.M., et al.: Parenteral gold therapy in the Felty syndrome: experience with 20 patients. Medicine (Baltimore), 65:107–112, 1986.

44. Kean, W.F., Bellamy, N., and Brooks, P.M.: Gold therapy in the elderly rheumatoid arthritis patient. Arthritis Rheum., 26:705–711, 1983.

45. Schattenkirchner, M., et al.: Auranofin and sodium aurothio-

malate in the treatment of rheumatoid arthritis. J. Rheumatol., 9[Suppl. 8]:184–189, 1982.

46. Dequeker, J., et al.: Longterm experience with oral gold in rheumatoid arthritis and psoriatic arthritis. Clin. Rheumatol., 3[Suppl. 1]:67–74, 1984.

47. Richter, M.B., Kinsella, P., and Corbett, M.: Gold in psoriatic arthropathy. Ann. Rheum. Dis., 39:279–280, 1980.

48. Salomon, D., and Saurat, J.H.: Oral gold therapy (Auranofin) in pemphigus vulgaris. Dermatologica, 172:310–314, 1986.

49. Miyamoto, T.: Treatment of bronchial asthma in Japan. Chest., 90[Suppl. 5]:71S–73S, 1986.

50. Okatani, Y.: A few clinical statistical observations on the use of Solganal-B-oleosum in bronchial asthma. J. Asthma Res.,17:165–173, 1980.

51. Richter, J.A. et al.: Analysis of treatment terminations with gold and antimalarial compounds in rheumatoid arthritis. J. Rheumatol., 7:153–159, 1980.

52. Chaffman, M., et al.: Auranofin: a preliminary review of its pharmacological properties and therapeutic use in rheumatoid arthritis. Drugs, 27:378–424, 1984.

53. Davis, P., and Harth, M. (Eds.): Proceedings: Therapeutic innovation in rheumatoid arthritis: worldwide Auranofin symposium. J. Rheumatol., 9[Suppl. 8]:1–209, 1982.

54. Williams, H.J., et al.: Auranofin, gold sodium thiomalate, and placebo in the treatment of rheumatoid arthritis: cooperative systematic studies of rheumatic diseases. Clin. Rheumatol., 3[Suppl 1]:39–50, 1984.

55. Bretza, J., Wels, I. and Novey, H.S.: Association of IgE antibodies to sodium aurothiomalate and adverse reactions to chrysotherapy for rheumatoid arthritis. Am. J. Med., 74:945–950, 1983.

56. Dawes, P.T., Smith, D.H., and Scott, D.L.: Massive eosinophilia in rheumatoid arthritis: report of four cases. Clin. Rheumatol., 5:62–65, 1986.

57. Bardin, T., et al.: HLA system and side effects of gold salts and D-penicillamine treatment of rheumatoid arthritis. Ann. Rheum. Dis., 41:599–601, 1982.

58. Bensen, W.G., et al.: HLA antigens and toxic reactions to sodium aurothiomalate in patients with rheumatoid arthritis. J. Rheumatol., 11:358–361, 1984.

59. Perrier, P., et al.: HLA antigens and toxic reactions to sodium aurothiopropanol sulphonate and D-penicillamine in patients with rheumatoid arthritis. Ann. Rheum. Dis., 44:621–624, 1985.

60. Adachi, J.D., et al.: Gold induced thrombocytopenia: platelet associated IgG and HLA typing in three patients. J. Rheumatol., 11:355–357, 1984.

61. Madhok, R., et al.: Chrysotherapy and thrombocytopenia. Ann. Rheum. Dis., 44:589–591, 1985.

62. Nusslein, H.G., et al.: Association of HLA-Bw35 with mucocutaneous lesions in rheumatoid arthritis patients undergoing sodium aurothiomalate therapy. Arthritis Rheum., 27:833–836, 1984.

63. Alarcon, G.S., et al.: HLA antigens and gold toxicity in American blacks with rheumatoid arthritis. Rheumatol. Int., 6:13–17, 1986.

64. Hofmann, C., Burg, G., and Jung, C.: Kutane Nebenwirkungen der Goldtherapie: klinische und histologische Ergebnisse. Z. Rheumatol., 45:100–106, 1986.

65. Aaron, S., Davis, P., and Percy, J.: Neutropenia occurring during the course of chrysotherapy: a review of 25 cases. J. Rheumatol., 12:897–899, 1985.

66. Von dem Borne, A.E., et al.: Thrombocytopenia associated with gold therapy: a drug-induced autoimmune disease? Br. J. Haematol., 63:509–516, 1986.

67. Bourke, B.E., Woodrow, D.F., and Scott, J.T.: Proteinuria in rheumatoid arthritis—drug-induced or amyloid? Ann. Rheum. Dis., 40:240–244, 1981.

68. Ainsworth, S.K., et al.: Gold nephropathy: ultrastructural, fluorescent, and energy-dispersive x-ray microanalysis study. Arch. Pathol. Lab. Med., 105:373–378, 1981.

69. Hardcastle, J., et al.: The effect of auranofin on the colonic transport of Na$^+$ and fluid in the rat. J. Pharm. Pharmacol., 38:466–468, 1986.

70. Jackson, C.W., et al.: Gold induced enterocolitis. Gut, 27:452–456, 1986.

71. Martin, D.M., et al.: Gold-induced eosinophilic enterocolitis: response to oral cromolyn sodium. Gastroenterology, 80:1567–1570, 1981.

72. Geltner, D., et al.: Gold-induced ileitis. J. Clin. Gastroenterol., 8:184–186, 1986.

73. Benfield, G.F., Asquith, P., and Felix-Davies, D.D.: Widespread gastric ulceration during Auranofin therapy. [Letter.] J. Rheumatol., 13:228–229, 1986.

74. Lowthian, P.J., Cleland, L.G., and Vernon-Roberts, B.: Hepatotoxicity with aurothioglucose therapy. Arthritis Rheum., 27:230–232, 1984.

75. Cooke, N., and Bamji, A.: Gold lung. Rheumatol. Rehabil., 20:129–135, 1981.

76. Chatzigiannis, I., Schmidt, K.L., and Stambolis, C.: Todliche Lungenfibrose durch Goldtherapie? Z. Rheumatol., 43:49–58, 1984.

77. Fam, A.G., et al.: Neurologic complications associated with gold therapy for rheumatoid arthritis. J. Rheumatol., 11:700–706, 1984.

78. Katrak, S.M., et al.: Clinical and morphological features of gold neuropathy. Brain, 103:671–693, 1980.

79. Perry, R.P., and Jacobsen, E.S.: Gold induced encephalopathy: case report. J. Rheumatol., 11:233–234, 1984.

80. Grisold, W., and Mamoli, B.: The syndrome of continuous muscle fibre activity following gold therapy. J. Neurol., 231:244–249, 1984.

81. McCormick, S.A., et al.: Ocular chrysiasis. Ophthalmology, 92:1432–1435, 1985.

82. Beckett, V.L., et al.: Chrysiasis resulting from gold therapy in rheumatoid arthritis: identification of gold by x-ray microanalysis. Mayo Clin. Proc., 57:773–777, 1982.

83. Halla, J.T., Harden, J.G., and Linn, J.E.: Postinjection non-vasomotor reactions during chrysotherapy. Arthritis Rheum., 20:1188–1191, 1977.

84. McGirr, E.E., et al.: Aurothioglucose in rheumatoid arthritis: outcome of treatment in patients intolerant of sodium aurothiomalate. Med. J. Aust., 141:349–351, 1984.

85. Coblyn, J.S., et al.: Gold-induced thrombocytopenia. Ann. Intern. Med., 95:178–181, 1981.

86. Godfrey, N.F., et al.: IV N-acetyl-cysteine treatment of hematologic reactions to chrysotherapy. J. Rheumatol., 9:519–526, 1982.

87. White, E.G., Smith, D.H., and Zaphiropoulos, G.C.: Haematuria occurring during antirheumatoid therapy. Br. J. Rheumatol., 23:57–60, 1984.

88. Hordon, L.D., et al.: Haematuria in rheumatoid arthritis: an association with mesangial glomerulonephritis. Ann. Rheum. Dis., 43:440–443, 1984.

34

ANTIMALARIALS

LORNE A. RUNGE

Trial-and-error experimentation has shown that antimalarial drugs effectively treat rheumatoid arthritis (RA).[1-3] These drugs were enthusiastically tried for various conditions after World War II, with two reports appearing in 1951 describing suppression of lupus[4] and rheumatoid arthritis.[5] The initial incomplete knowledge of their pharmacology resulted in blindness in some patients. The mechanisms of such toxicity were unknown, and the first case of associated retinopathy attributed the lesion to systemic lupus erythematosus (SLE).[6]

Controlled and uncontrolled studies[7-31] of antimalarial compounds (Fig. 34–1) show that 30 to 90% of patients note some benefit, 10 to 50% are unchanged or worse, and 0 to 30% stop treatment within a few months because of the development of side effects. High doses of chloroquine are more effective but induce more side effects. The degree of response seen with currently recommended doses of hydroxychloroquine is comparable to that seen with gold (both intramuscular and oral), D-penicillamine, and azathioprine.

PHARMACOKINETICS

All synthetic antimalarial drugs are well absorbed orally within hours and become widely distributed in the body.[2] They are retained in tissues for prolonged periods, and the total dose is probably never completely excreted. Pigmented animals retain much more of the drug in melanized tissues than do albino animals.

These drugs can theoretically exert a pharmacologic effect in low doses because they are concentrated within important effector cells (e.g., leukocytes) and persist for long periods.

MOLECULAR INTERACTIONS

Ferriprotoporphyrin IX

Ferriprotoporphyrin IX is made when the malarial parasite (schizont) in the erythrocytic phase of the disease digests hemoglobin within its phagocytic vacuole. The remarkable effectiveness of the synthetic antimalarials is due to their strong affinity for ferriprotoporphyrin IX[32] and the marked toxicity of this combination for the schizont.

Melanin

Antimalarial drugs have an affinity for melanin nearly as great as that for ferriprotoporphyrin IX. Melanin protects the skin from ultraviolet irradiation damage,[33] acting as a biologic transducer so that ultraviolet light is more rapidly dissipated and unable to induce the formation of free radicals. Melanin in the eye might well have a similar function. Melanin within the inner ear may reduce sound damage by dissipating physical force in biologic structures.[34] The melanosomes in the skin are transferred to the keratinocytes and are lost with epithelial replacement; however, those in the eye and inner ear are normally

FIG. 34–1. Chemical structures, molecular formulas, and molecular weights for representative antimalarial compounds.

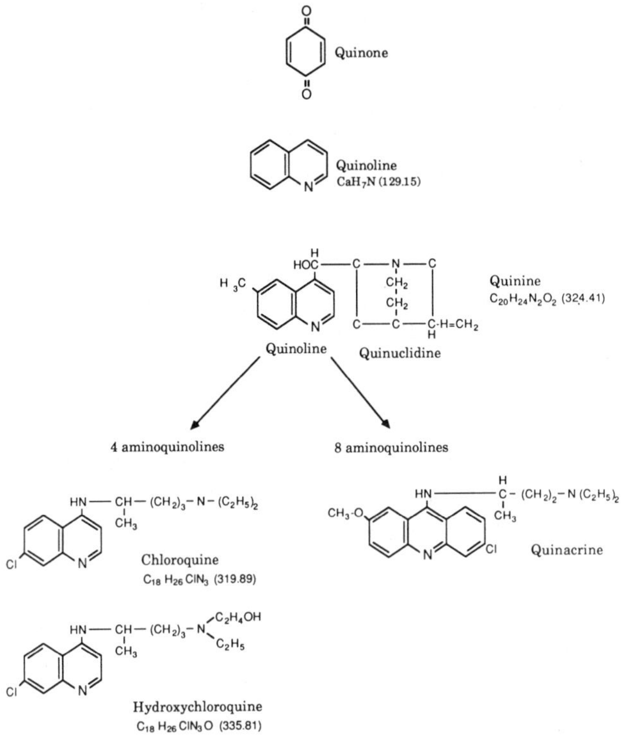

not released into surrounding cells, so bound drug remains indefinitely.

Lysosomes

Cell biologists use chloroquine because it concentrates within endocytic vacuoles and alters their function. Receptor-mediated phagocytosis is normally followed by activation of an adenosine triphosphate (ATP)-driven proton pump which lowers intralysosomal pH, which dissociates the receptor from its ligand. The receptor then migrates back to the cell surface, and the ingested material is subjected to enzymatic attack.[35–37] Antimalarials concentrate within the acidic vacuoles[38,39] due to the positive charges of their nitrogen atoms. They either poison the proton pump or become a proton sink, interfering with phagosomal acidification and with dissociation of the receptor-ligand complexes. Receptor recirculation is reduced as is their affinity for various molecular ligands,[40–45] including immunoglobulins on B lymphocytes,[40] antigen in antigen-processing cells,[41] lysosomal enzymes,[42] and asialo-glycoproteins.[37,43,44] Intralysosomal digestion is impaired.[45] Antimalarials also concentrate in the small vacuoles that bud from the Golgi apparatus and can interfere with glycosy-

lation of synthesized proteins. Ia antigens[46] and immunoglobulins[47] are affected by this mechanism. Chloroquine is also used to strip adsorbed human leukocyte antigens (HLA) from the surfaces of platelets.[48]

Older studies describing drug effects on isolated lysosomes[49] have proved difficult to interpret[35] but have stimulated much investigation of the adverse effects of lysosomal enzymes on joint tissue.[50,51]

DNA

Antimalarial drugs have a strong affinity for DNA and interfere with its function. DNA polymerase and RNA/DNA polymerase are inhibited by high concentrations of antimalarial drugs.[52,53] High concentrations also inhibit the development of the lupus erythematosus (LE) cell phenomenon.[54] Such inhibition is due to an effect on DNA itself rather than on antibody. The drug becomes intercalated into the DNA molecule.[55] These effects probably occur in vivo, because RA patients treated with chloroquine have more chromosomal damage in cultured lymphocytes than do control subjects.[56]

Protein

Antimalarial drugs bind to plasma proteins and inhibit their denaturation, probably by protection of sulfhydryl bonds.[57] This effect may account for the desludging action of the drug in RA treatment.[27]

ORGAN EFFECTS

Immune

Antibody production to human rabies vaccine is decreased due to brief chloroquine prophylaxis for malaria.[58] RA patients taking chloroquine show depressed lymphocyte responsiveness to both nonspecific mitogens and specific antigens.[59,60] The mechanism underlying this effect remains unclear. Lymphocyte lysosomes seem more sensitive to chloroquine inhibition than do neutrophil lysosomes in vitro.[61]

Bone

The osteoclastic bone resorption surface has lysosomal characteristics (i.e., it is a closed space with a low pH lined by a membrane containing a proton pump).[62] Antimalarial drugs accumulate in bones,[63] and if they concentrate at the osteoclast-bone interface they could interfere with resorption. One study of rheumatoid forefeet did show histologic evidence of decreased bony resorption in patients taking antimalarial drugs.[64] Additional studies along these lines would be of great interest.

Eye

The pigmented epithelial cells of the eye participate actively in many metabolic processes. Pigment in the rods and cones is normally transferred to and catabolized by the lysosomes of the pigmented epithelium. Melanosomes are very closely associated anatomically with such phagocytic activity.[65] Antimalarial drugs, therefore, have two reasons to become localized at the tip of the pigmented epithelium (lysosomes and melanin). This is surely an important first step in the development of antimalarial drug retinopathy.

SIDE EFFECTS

Eye

Retinopathy may develop during long-term antimalarial drug use.[65-71] A subtle mottling of the retinal pigment eventually progresses to a characteristic "bull's eye" appearance, due to pigment localization in a ring pattern around the fovea centralis. Concurrent with these physical changes, a visual field defect to red light develops and progresses to paracentral scotoma which can lead to permanent blindness. Patients first note the inability to read long words as their constricted visual fields permit recognition of only a few letters at a time.

Accumulated experience has resolved some of the issues relevant to retinopathy. Hydroxychloroquine doses above 6 mg/kg/day for prolonged periods (generally more than 1 year) may cause visual lesions.[68] Serum blood levels correlate well with both dosage and risk of eye changes.[72] Eye lesions may progress even after the drug is stopped, but this may occur only if excessve dosages have been used.[73] Scotoma alone, pigmented changes alone, and concurrent changes may develop. Chloroquine may be more toxic than hydroxychloroquine,[70] and age over 60 years may also be a significant risk factor.[74]

Other ocular effects include corneal deposits which cause haloes to appear around lights. These deposits are often linear-appearing below the pupil by slit lamp examination, occurring in the anterior third of the cornea.[75] Crystals in the fluid layer have been noted and are thought to be composed of the drug itself.[76] Corneal anesthesia may accompany corneal drug deposits.

In high doses, antimalarial drugs can impair visual accommodation due to dysfunction of the ciliary body. The problem is usually experienced as blurred vision or diplopia when looking up from fixation on a nearby object. Both corneal deposits and impaired accommodation correlate with high blood levels, resolve with reduced dosage, and do not result in permanent damage or dysfunction.

Ear

Tinnitus is a characteristic component of cinchonism noted when using various bark extracts to treat fever. Other drugs that interfere with hearing, such as the mycin antibiotics, also have an affinity for melanin thus leading to the suspicion that melanin binding underlies antimalarial ototoxicity.[34] The relative ototoxicity of these drugs correlates with their drug-melanin binding affinity.[77] This effect is rare when the drug is used in moderate doses.

Central Nervous System

Rarely, a patient may develop hypomanic behavior after taking antimalarials, with accompanying insomnia and increased motor activity reminiscent of corticosteroid effects.

Skin

Antimalarial drugs depress abnormal inflammatory reactions to ultraviolet-induced injury[78] and depress the tanning response. Fair-skinned patients should be warned about sun exposure when using these drugs.

Patients taking synthetic antimalarial drugs for prolonged periods may develop *skin mottling* with a grayish appearance. Patches of dark pigment may develop, particularly over the shins and hard palate.

Maculopapular rashes occur in 3% to 10% of patients treated for RA, probably due to hypersensitivity.

Muscle

Cells in tissue cultures become intensely vacuolated after addition of chloroquine to the media due to the development of giant lysosomes.[79] Muscle biopsies from patients developing weakness during the course of antimalarial treatment show similar changes.[80] This complication is probably rare; reported series contain no more than four patients each.[80-86] Muscular weakness develops slowly after months to years of treatment and is associated with depressed deep tendon reflexes, fatigue, and weakness. Peripheral striated muscle is generally involved, but two cases of biopsy-proven cardiomyopathy have been noted.[87] A repeated biopsy showed decreased vacuolization after stopping the drug in one of these patients. Understandably, no reported case has been rechallenged to confirm the suspicion that the antimalarial drug caused the problem.

Bone Marrow

Leukopenia and aplastic anemia have developed during antimalarial treatment. Only isolated case reports support the association without rechallenge.[88-90]

TREATMENT INDICATIONS IN RHEUMATIC DISEASE

RHEUMATOID ARTHRITIS

Appropriate treatment decisions are based on best estimates of efficiency and toxicity (therapeutic index) so that the patient knowingly accepts the unavoidable risks. Controlled trials show suppression of joint inflammation in 50 to 70% of patients treated with chloroquine[7,8,9,11,12,13,15] or hydroxychloroquine.[13,16,17,19,20] Similar results were noted in uncontrolled trials.[13,16,17,19,20,22,27–31] Side effects severe enough to warrant stopping the drug occur in only 3 to 8% of patients at doses currently used. Gastrointestinal toxicity is infrequent accounting for 4% of side effects. This problem almost always can be managed by giving the drug at bedtime. Skin rashes occur in 3% to 10% of patients but may be extensive and progress to exfoliative dermatitis. Ototoxicity is rare but should be suspected if vertigo or tinnitus develops during the course of long-term treatment.

Our previous studies using life table analysis to describe the outcome of treatment confirm the lower incidence of toxicity[27] of hydroxychloroquine, which, compared to intramuscular gold and D-penicillamine, are indeed very minimal. Toxicity increases with time, however; prolonged observation over years gives a more useful estimate of drug side effects. The minimal risk of adverse reactions is one of the major advantages for using hydroxychloroquine. Physicians who feel secure in using intramuscular gold or D-penicillamine should have no problem adjusting to the hazards of antimalarial drugs.

The problem of retinopathy has significantly inhibited their widespread use, and many different approaches have been advocated to avoid this complication without convincing documentation. Available evidence suggests that a daily dose of hydroxychloroquine less than 6 mg/kg is relatively safe when combined with ophthalmologic exams not less than every 6 months. Testing for paracentral scotoma (visual fields using a red target), a visual (Amsler) grid (Fig. 34–2), and ophthalmoscopy for detection of pigment mottling constitute a sufficient monitoring program during long-term treatment. In patients under age 60, ophthalmologic consultation should be sought after 1 year of therapy or 100 g cumulative dose and at yearly intervals thereafter, as there are no recorded cases of ocular toxicity at lower doses. In patients over 60 years old, a baseline eye examination is useful to determine whether senile macular degenerative changes or drusen is present. The Amsler grid is very sensitive and

FIG. 34–2. Amsler grid. The following instructions are given to patients:

Proper use of the Amsler grid will enable you to detect subtle changes in your vision due to even a small amount of fluid from under your retina.

To perform the test, wear the glasses that you normally use while reading. If you wear bifocals, use the bottom portion or reading portion of the glass. Attach the grid to a wall at eye level and stand 12 to 14 inches away from it. Cover one eye. With the other eye, look at the center dot.

While you are looking at the center dot, you should be able to see the four corners of the square. You should also be able to see that the large square is composed of many smaller squares.

The first day you observe the grid, mark with a pencil any areas of distortion, any gray or blurry spots, or any blank spots. This is your baseline pattern.

Each Monday morning thereafter, look at the center dot of the grid. If you notice new areas of distortion, wavy instead of straight lines, or enlargement of the blank spot, especially toward the center, please call me promptly.

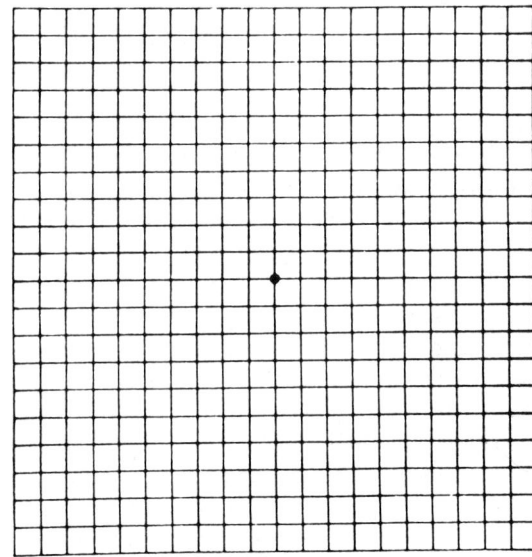

can be used by the office nurse to test each patient during the routine visit.

I consider using hydroxychloroquine in patients who have had RA for 6 months or more and an insufficient response to optimal treatment wth a nonsteroidal anti-inflammatory agent. A reliable patient less than 60 years old with persistent synovitis in multiple joints early in the course of disease is an ideal candidate.[91] Should initial fundoscopy show a pigment abnormality or if there is a history of significant visual problems, a complete ophthalmologic assessment is mandatory before treatment is begun. Senile macular degeneration resembles antimalarial damage and is a strong contraindication for use of these drugs. Therapy is started at 6 mg/kg/day or less (about 400 mg/day for the usual adult). Many women receive only 300 mg/day and a small thin woman may require only 200 mg/day. Regular ophthalmologic exams are begun after 4 to 6 months of therapy if it is decided that the beneficial effect has been worthwhile. The drug is discontinued if no benefit has occurred. Severe side effects usually occur within the first 6 months of treatment; patents doing well after 6 months are candidates for prolonged treatment. Useless ophthalmologic evaluations are avoided for those without prior visual problems or those who will not be taking prolonged treatment. The risk of blame for subsequent visual impairment is acceptably low.

More conservative approaches have included beginning with a small dose 3 days per week[23] and monitoring blood levels in addition to ophthalmologic examinations. This additional precaution is definitely worth considering in children.[73] Other suggestions have included using dark glasses to prevent retinal exposure to ultraviolet light* and stopping treatment for 1 month during early summer to reduce sunlight effects.

There are few drug interactions to worry about during hydroxychloroquine treatment. Acute intermittent porphyria can be provoked by this class of drugs. One well-designed trial indicated that the combination of D-penicillamine and hydroxychloroquine did worse than Dpenicillamine alone.[19] An uncontrolled trial combined hydroxychloroquine with low dose cyclophosphamide and azathioprine in patients with intractable disease.[92] This regimen showed little toxicity attributed to hydroxychloroquine.

The drugs should probably not be used during pregnancy due to possible ear and eye damage; however, the risk with usual doses may be minimal.[69]

Antimalarial drugs are widely used for discoid lupus,[93] systemic lupus erythematosus,[94] juvenile rheumatoid arthritis (JRA),[95] and psoriatic arthritis.[96] The only controlled trial in JRA failed to show significant improvement, except for decreased pain on motion.[95] Nevertheless, multiple uncontrolled series strongly suggest that at least the arthritic component of the above diseases is effectively suppressed.

The skin involvement of lupus erythematosus usually responds to antimalarial therapy. In both discoid lupus and subacute cutaneous (Ro positive) lupus, antimalarials are the initial drug of choice.

A well-understood therapeutic mechanism supports the use of synthetic antimalarial drugs in prophylaxis for chloroquine-sensitive malaria. Small doses (400 mg hydroxychloroquine once weekly) induce few side effects and are exceptionally effective. In rheumatic diseases the mechanism of action is less well understood. In doses needed for disease suppression the drug accumulates in the eye, skin, muscle, and inner ear, and in sufficient concentrations can cause tissue damage. The chronic ingestion of antimalarial drugs affects many tissues by binding to melanin and by interfering with lysosomal function. As with other slow-acting agents, their use in rheumatic diseases remains empiric, but their therapeutic index is relatively high compared to other available effective agents.

These drugs offer substantial relief, are generally well tolerated, and deserve consideration despite the threat of blindness. The patient must be reliable and have periodic ophthalmologic examinations. The daily dose of hydroxychloroquine should never exceed 6 mg/kg/day.

REFERENCES

1. Folfheinz, W., and Merkli, B.: Quinine and quinine analogues. *In* Handbook of Experimental Pharmacology. Antimalarial Drugs 11. Vol. 68. Edited by W. Peters and W.H.G. Richards. New York, Springer-Verlag, 1984.
2. McChesney W., and Merkli, B.: 4-aminoquinolines. *In* Handbook of Expermental Pharmacology. Antimalarial Drugs 11. Vol. 68. Edited by W. Peters and W.H.G. Richards. New York, Springer-Verlag, 1984.
3. Coatney, G.R.: Pitfalls in a discovery: The chronicle of chloroquine. Am. J. Trop. Med. Hyg., *12*:121, 1963.
4. Page, F.: Treatment of lupus erythematosus with mepacrine. Lancet, *2*:755, 1951.
5. Brennecke, F.E., et al.: A preliminary report on the effect of certain 8-aminoquinolines in the treatment of rheumatoid arthritis. J. Lab. Clin. Med., *38*:795, 1951.
6. Cambiaggi, A.: Unusual ocular lesions in a case of systemic lupus erythematosus. Arch. Ophthalmol., *57*:451, 1957.
7. Bagnall, A.W.: The value of chloroquine in rheumatoid disease; A four year study of continuous therapy. Can. Med. Assoc. J., *77*:182, 1957.
8. Cohen, A.S., and Calkins, E.: A controlled study of chloroquine as an antirheumatic agent. Arthritis Rheum., *1*:297, 1958.
9. Rinehart, R.E., Rosenbaum, E.E., and Hopkins, C.E.: Chloroquine therapy in rheumatoid arthritis. Northwest Med., *56*:703, 1957.
10. Bepler, C.R., et al.: A 15 month controlled study of the effects of amodiaquin in rheumatoid arthritis. Arthritis Rheum., *2*:403, 1959.
11. Freedman, A., and Steinberg, V.L.: Chloroquine in rheumatoid arthritis. A double blindfold trial of treatment for one year. Ann. Rheum. Dis., *19*:243, 1960.
12. Popert, A.J., Meijers, K.A.E., Sharp, J., Bier, F.: Chloroquine diphosphate in rheumatoid arthritis. Ann. Rheum. Dis., *20*:18, 1961.

Editor's note. The effect of dark glasses is at least partially abrogated by pupillary dilation. I have treated more than 500 patients with hydroxychloroquine over a 27-year period, some up to 20 years, without serious ocular toxicity.

13. Scull, E.: Chloroquine and hydroxychloroquine therapy in rheumatoid arthritis. Arthritis Rheum., *5*:30, 1962.

14. Bartholomew, L.E., and Duff, I.F.: Amopyroquin (propoquin) in rheumatoid arthritis. Arthritis Rheum., *6*:356, 1963.

15. Dwosh, L., et al.: Azathioprine in early rheumatoid arthritis. Arthritis Rheum., *20*:685, 1977.

16. Kersley, G.D., and Palin, A.G.: Amodiaquine and hydroxychloroquine in rheumatoid arthritis. Lancet, 2:886, 1959.

17. Mainland, D., and Sutcliffe, M.I.: Hydroxychloroquine sulfate in rheumatoid arthritis, a six month, double-blind trial. Bull. Rheum. Dis., *13*:287, 1962.

18. Hamilton, E.B.D., and Scott, J.T.: Hydroxychloroquine sulfate ("Plaquenil") in treatment of rheumatoid arthritis. Arthritis Rheum., *5*:502, 1962.

19. Bunch, T.W., et al.: Controlled trial of hydroxychloroquine and D-penicillamine in the treatment of rheumatoid arthritis. Arthritis Rheum., *27*:267, 1984.

20. Kvien, T.K., Hoyeraal, H.M., and Sandstad B.: Slow acting antirheumatic drugs in patients with juvenile rheumatoid arthritis evaluated in a randomized, parallel 50-week clinical trial. J. Rheumatol., *12*:533, 1985.

21. Haydu, G.G.: Rheumatoid arthritis therapy: A rationale and the use of chloroquine diphosphate. Am. J. Med. Sci., *225*:71, 1953.

22. Scherbel, A.L., Schuchter, S.L., and Harrison, J.W.: Comparison of effects of two antimalarial agents, hydroxychloroquine sulfate and chloroquine phosphate, in patients with rheumatoid arthritis. Cleve. Clin. Q., *24*:98, 1957.

23. Young, J.P.: Chloroquine phosphate (Aralen) in the long-term treatment of rheumatoid arthritis. Ann. Intern. Med., *51*:1159, 1959.

24. Cramer, Q.: Rheumatoid diseases antimalarials (chloroquine and hydroxychloroquine) as therapeutic aids. Mo. Med., *55*:1203, 1958.

25. Klinefelter, H.F., and Achurra, A.: Effect of gold salts and antimalarials on the rheumatoid factor in rheumatoid arthritis. Scand. J. Rheumatol., *2*:177, 1973.

26. Fowler, P.D., Shadforth, M.F., Crook, P.R., and Lawton, A.: Report on chloroquine and dapsone in the treatment of rheumatoid arthritis: A 6-month comparative study. Ann. Rheum. Dis., *43*:200, 1984.

27. Cecchi, E., and Ferraris, F.: Desludging action of hydroxychloroquine in rheumatoid arthritis. Acta Rheum. Scand., *8*:214, 1961.

28. Wollheim, F.A., Hanson, A., and Bertil Laurell, C.: Chloroquine treatment in rheumatoid arthritis. Scand. J. Rheumatol., *7*:171, 1978.

29. Husain, Z., and Runge, L.: Treatment complications of rheumatoid arthritis with gold, hydroxychloroquine, D-penicillamine, and levamisole. J. Rheumatol., *6*:825, 1980.

30. Dixon, J.S., et al.: Biochemical indices of response to hydroxychloroquine and sodium aurothiomalate in rheumatoid arthritis. Ann. Rheum. Dis., *40*:480, 1981.

31. Adams, E.M., Yocum, D.E., and Bell, C.L.: Hydroxychloroquine in the treatment of rheumatoid arthritis. Am. J. Med., *75*:321, 1983.

32. Chou, A.C., Chevli, R., and Fitch, C.D.: Ferriprotoporphyrin IX fulfills the criteria for identification as the chloroquine receptor of malaria parasites. Biochemistry, *19*:1543, 1980.

33. Quevedo, W.G., Fitzpatrick, T.B., Szabo G., and Jimbow, K.: Biology of melanocytes. *In* Dermatology in General Medicine, 3rd Ed. Edited by T.B. Fitzpatrick, et al. New York, McGraw-Hill, 1987.

34. Proctor, P., McGinnes, J., and Corry, P.: A hypothesis on the preferential destruction of melanized tissues. J Theor. Biol., *48*:19, 1974.

35. deDuve, C.: Lysosomes revisited. J. Biochem., *137*:391, 1983.

36. Marzella, L., and Glaumann, H.: Biogenesis, translocation, and function of lysosomal enzymes. Int. Rev. Exp. Pathol., *25*:278, 1983.

37. Breitfeld, P.P., et al.: Cell biology of the asialoglycoprotein receptor system: A model of receptor-mediated endocytosis. Int. Rev. Cytol., *97*:47, 1985.

38. Allison, A.C., and Young, M.R.: Uptake of dyes and drugs by living cells in culture. Life Sci., *3*:1407, 1964.

39. Dingle, J.T., and Barrett, A.J.: Uptake of biologically active substances by lysosomes. Proc. R. Soc. Lond. [Biol.], *173*:85, 1969.

40. Ramanadham, M., Gollapudi, S.V.S., and Kern, M.: Anti-immunoglobulin induced proliferation of B cells. Exp. Cell. Res., *148*:303, 1983.

41. Grey, H.M., and Chestnut, R.: Antigen processing and presentation to T cells. Immunology Today, *6*:101, 1985.

42. Gonzalez-Noriega, A., Grubb, J.H., Talkad, V., Sly, W.S.: Chloroquine inhibits lysosomal enzyme pinocytosis and enhances lysosomal enzyme secretion by impairing receptor recycling. J. Cell. Biol., *85*:839, 1980.

43. Hasilik, A., and Neufeld, E.F.: Biosynthesis of lysosomal enzymes in fibroblasts. J. Biol. Chem., *225*:4946, 1980.

44. Tolleshaug, H., and Berg, T.: Chloroquine reduces the number of asialoglycoprotein receptors in the hepatocytes plasma membrane. Biochem. Pharmacol., *28*:2919, 1979.

45. Wibo, M., and Poole, B.: Protein degradation in cultured cells. J. Cell. Biol., *63*:430, 1974.

46. Nowell, J., and Quaranta, V.: Chloroquine affects biosynthesis of Ia molecules by inhibiting dissociation of invariant (γ) chains from a-B dimers in B cells. J. Exp. Med., *162*:1371, 1985.

47. Thorens, B., and Vassalli, P.: Chloroquine and ammonium chloride prevent terminal glycosylation of immunoglobulins in plasma cells without affecting secretion. Nature, *321*:618, 1986.

48. Minchinton, R.M., and Waters, A.H.: Chloroquine stripping of HLA antigens from neutrophils without removal of neutrophil specific antigens. Br. J. Haematol., *57*:703, 1984.

49. Weissmann, G.: Labilization and stabilization of lysosomes. Fed. Proc., *23*:1038, 1964.

50. Weissmann, G., Spilberg, I., and Krakauer, K.: Arthritis induced in rabbits by lysates of granulocyte lysosomes. Arthritis Rheum., *12*:103, 1969.

51. Zvaiffler, N.J.: A speculation of the pathogenesis of joint inflammation in rheumatoid arthritis. Arthritis Rheum., *8*:289, 1965.

52. Cohen, S.N., and Yielding, K.L.: Inhibition of DNA and RNA polymerase reactions by chloroquine. Proc. Natl. Acad. Sci., U.S.A., *54*:521, 1965.

53. Stollar, D., and Levine, L.: Antibodies to denatured deoxyribonucleic acid in lupus erythematosus serum v. mechanism of DNA-anti-DNA inhibition by chloroquine. Arch. Biochem. Biophys., *101*:335, 1963.

54. Dubois, E.L.: Quinacrine (Atabrine) in treatment of systemic and discoid lupus erythematosus. Arch. Intern. Med., *94*:131, 1954.

55. Bolte, J., Demuynck, C., and Lhomme, J.: Synthetic models of deoxyribonucleic acid complexes with antimalarial compounds. J. Med. Chem., *20*:1607, 1977.

56. Neill, W.A.: Action of chloroquine phosphate in rheumatoid arthritis. Ann. Rheum. Dis., *32*:547, 1973.

57. Gerber, D.A.: Effect of chloroquine on the sulfhydryl group

and the denaturation of bovine serum albumin. Arthritis Rheum., 7:193, 1964.

58. Pappaioanou, M., et al.: Antibody response to preexposure human diploid-cell rabies vaccine given concurrently with chloroquine. N. Engl. J. Med., 314:280, 1986.

59. Hurvitz, D., and Hirschhorn, K.: Suppression of in vitro lymphocyte responses by chloroquine. N. Engl. J. Med., 273:23, 1965.

60. Panayi, G.S., Neill, W.A., Duthie, J.J.R., and McCormick, J.N.: Action of chloroquine phosphate in rheumatoid arthritis. Ann. Rheum. Dis., 32:316, 1973.

61. Jones, C.J.P., and Jayson, M.I.V.: Chloroquine: Its effect on leucocyte auto- and heterophagocytosis. Ann. Rheum. Dis., 43:205, 1984.

62. Baron, R., Neff, L., Louvard, D., and Courtoy, P.J.: Cell-mediated extracellular acidification and bone resorption: Evidence for a low pH in resorbing lacunae and localization of a 100-kD lysosome. J. Cell Biol., 101:2210, 1985.

63. Fischer, V.W., and Fitch, C.D.: Affinity of chloroquine for bone. J. Pharm. Pharmacol., 27:527, 1975.

64. Julkunen, H., Rokkanen, P., and Laine, H.: Chloroquine treatment and bone changes in rheumatoid arthritis. Scand. J. Rheumatol., 5:36, 1976.

65. Zinn, K.M., and Marmor, M.F.: The Retinal Pigment Epithelium. Cambridge, Harvard University Press, 1979.

66. Nylander, U.: Ocular damage in chloroquine therapy. Acta Ophthalmol., 44:335, 1966.

67. Bernstein, H.N., and Ginsberg, J.: The pathology of chloroquine retinopathy. Arch. Ophthalmol., 71:238, 1964.

68. Scherbel, A.L.: Chloroquine and hydroxychloroquine in rheumatological therapy. Clin. Rheum. Dis., 6:545, 1980.

69. Rynes, R.I., et al.: Ophthalmologic safety of long-term hydroxychloroquine treatment. Arthritis Rheum., 22:832, 1979.

70. Finbloom, D.S., Silver, K., Newsome, D.A., and Gunkel, R.: Comparison of hydroxychloroquine and chloroquine use and the development of retinal toxicity. J. Rheumatol., 12:692, 1985.

71. Voipio, H.: Incidence of chloroquine retinopathy. Acta Ophthalmol., 44:349, 1966.

72. Laaksonen, A., Kaskiahde, B., and Juva, K.: Dosage of antimalarial drugs for children with juvenile rheumatoid arthritis and systemic lupus erythematosus. Scand. J. Rheumatol., 3:103, 1974.

73. Maksymowych, W., and Russell, A.S.: Antimalarials in rheumatology: Efficacy and safety. Arthritis Rheum., 16:206, 1987.

74. Elman, A.: Chloroquine retinopathy in patients with rheumatoid arthritis. Scand. J. Rheumatol., 5:161, 1976.

75. Sandvig, K.: Chloroquine (Resochin) effects on the cornea. Acta Ophthalmol., 44:355, 1966.

76. Beebe, W.E., Abbott, R.L., and Fung, W.E.: Hydroxychloroquine crystals in tear film of a patient with rheumatoid arthritis. Am. J. Ophthalmol., 101:377, 1968.

77. Dencker, L., Lindquist, N.G., and Ullberg, S.: Mechanism of drug-induced chronic lesions. Role of drug accumulation on the melanin of the inner ear. Experientia, 29:1362, 1973.

78. Lester, R.S., Burnham, T.K., Fine, G., and Murry, K.: Immunologic concepts of light reactions in lupus erythematosus and polymorphous light eruptions. Arch. Dermatol., 96:1, 1967.

79. Fedorko, M.E., Hirsch, J.G., and Cohn, Z.A.: Autophagic vacuoles produced in vitro. J. Cell Biol., 38:377, 1968.

80. Whisnant, J.P., Espinosa, R.E., Kierland, R.R., and Lambert, E.H.: Chloroquine neuromyopathy. Mayo Clin. Proc., 23:502, 1963.

81. Loftus, L.R.: Peripheral neuropathy following chloroquine therapy. Can. Med. Assoc. J., 89:917, 1963.

82. Begg, T.B., and Simpson, J.A.: Chloroquine neuromyopathy. Br. Med. J., 1:770, 1964.

83. Millingen, K.S., and Suerth, E.: Peripheral neuromyopathy following chloroquine therapy. Med. J. Aust., 1:840, 1966.

84. Smith, B., O'Grady, F.: Experimental chloroquine myopathy. J. Neurol. Neurosurg. Psychiatry, 29:255, 1966.

85. Hughes, J.T., Esirie, M., Oxbury, J.M., and Whitty, C.W.M.: Chloroquine myopathy. Q.J. Med., 157:85, 1971.

86. Marks, J.S.: Motor polyneuropathy and nystagmus associated with chloroquine phosphate. Postgrad. Med. J., 55:569, 1979.

87. Ratliffe, N.B.: Diagnosis of chloroquine cardiomyopathy by endomyocardial biopsy. N. Engl. J. Med., 316:191, 1987.

88. McDuffie, F.C.: Bone marrow depression after drug therapy in patients with SLE and rheumatoid diseases. Ann. Rheum. Dis., 24:289, 1965.

89. Polano, M.K., Cats, A., and Van Olden, G.A.J.: Agranulocytosis following treatment with hydroxychloroquine sulphate. Lancet, 1:1275, 1965.

90. Propp, R.T., and Stillman, J.S.: Agranulocytosis and hydroxychloroquine. N. Engl. J. Med., 244:492, 1967.

91. Mackenzie A.: Antimalarial drugs for rheumatoid arthritis. Am. J. Med., 75:48, 1983.

92. Csuka, M.E., Carrera, G.F., and McCarty, D.J.: Treatment of intractable rheumatoid arthritis with combined cyclophosphamide, azathioprine, and hydroxychloroquine. JAMA, 255:2315, 1986.

93. Swanbeck, G.: Aminoquinolines. In Dermatology in General Medicine, 3rd Ed. Edited by T.B. Fitzpatrick, et al. New York, McGraw-Hill, 1987.

94. Rudnicki, R.D., Gresham, G.E., and Rothfield, N.F.: The efficacy of antimalarials in systemic lupus erythematosus. J. Rheumatol., 2:323, 1975.

95. Brewer, E.J., Giannini, E.H., Kuzmina, N., and Aleksew, L.: Penicillamine and hydroxychloroquine in the treatment of severe juvenile rheumatoid arthritis. N. Engl. J. Med., 314:1269, 1986.

96. Krammer, G.M., et al.: Psoriatic arthritis: A clinical, immunologic and HLA study of 100 patients. Semin. Arthritis Rheum. 9:75, 1979.

CYTOTOXIC DRUGS AND SULFASALAZINE

GRANT W. CANNON and JOHN R. WARD

This chapter deals with the use of cytotoxic agents and sulfasalazine in antirheumatic therapy. Although many of the applications of these drugs are still considered investigational, they are widely used. By including these agents in the same chapter, we do not mean to imply that their antirheumatic effects, mechanism of action, magnitude of effect, or toxicity are similar. Rather, these agents are presented to allow comparison of their differences and determine their proper role in the treatment of rheumatic diseases. Chapter 38 discusses additional agents that have been or are now being investigated for potential use in the rheumatic diseases.

THE CYTOTOXIC DRUGS

The cytotoxic drugs were initially used to treat malignancies and later were employed in the management of rheumatic diseases. Well-designed clinical trials have shown that these agents are highly effective, but that significant toxicity is associated with their use. Major emphasis is currently centered on the risk/benefit ratio of these agents to determine their ultimate role in the rheumatic diseases.

The agents discussed here have been referred to by various authors as "cytotoxic," "immunoregulatory," and even "anti-inflammatory" agents. The exact effect of these drugs may depend on the dose, the administration schedule, and the nature of the underlying disease process. The term *cytotoxic agent* is chosen because cytotoxicity is the primary effect of these

drugs. Proliferating cells are particularly sensitive to the toxic effects of these agents, hence their extensive use in treating neoplastic diseases. The target cells on which these agents exert their antirheumatic effect are not known but might include lymphocytes, hematopoietic precursors, synovial cells in rheumatoid arthritis (RA), or renal cells in the proliferative glomerulonephritis of systemic lupus erythematosus (SLE). The dosing schedules used for many of these drugs often do not correspond to the known cell cycle kinetics of potential target cells.

Occasionally, these drugs are termed "immunoregulatory" agents because of their potent and generally suppressive effects on the immune system. Because lymphocyte proliferation is such an integral part of the generation of an immune response, the immunoregulatory effect is likely to be mediated by toxicity to these proliferating cells. We refer to these compounds as "cytotoxic" rather than "immunoregulatory" drugs for two reasons. First, many agents other than the cytotoxic drugs may act as immunoregulatory agents (e.g., cytokines, antibodies, etc.), as discussed in Chapter 38. Second, it remains to be proven that the antirheumatic effects of these drugs are primarily based on their effect on the immune system.

Because of the toxicity associated with the use of these agents, a careful analysis of the expected benefits must be performed. Toxicities frequently encountered include bone marrow suppression, increased risk of infection, teratogenicity, infertility, and carcinogenicity. The frequency of these problems as well as unique toxicities are discussed in the section on each agent. After careful consideration of the risks versus the benefits, individual patients may be candidates for cytotoxic therapy.

AZATHIOPRINE

HISTORY

In the early 1960s, 6-mercaptopurine (6-MP) was reported effective in multiple "autoimmune diseases" including RA.[1,2] Efforts to protect 6-MP from rapid metabolism led to the development of azathioprine, which is metabolized in vivo to 6-MP.[3,4] Subsequent reports described benefit with azathioprine in the treatment of RA[5–9] and SLE.[5,6] Later, controlled trials were performed that documented the effectiveness of azathioprine in RA[10–12] with long-term followup studies confirming continued clinical efficacy.[13–16] The role of azathioprine in SLE,[17–26] inflammatory myopathy,[27–30] and psoriatic arthritis[10,14] remains debated.

PHARMACOLOGY

Pharmacokinetics

Azathioprine is 6-[(1-methyl-4-nitro-imidazol-5-yl)thio]purine (Fig. 35–1). Azathioprine is well absorbed,[4] and approximately 30% of circulating azathioprine is protein bound.[31] About 2 to 10% of the drug is excreted unchanged in the urine.[31,32] The plasma half-life of azathioprine is 3 hours in subjects with normal renal and hepatic function.[31]

Azathioprine itself is not an active compound but is metabolized to 6-MP by the liver and erythro-

FIG. 35–1.   Structure of azathioprine.

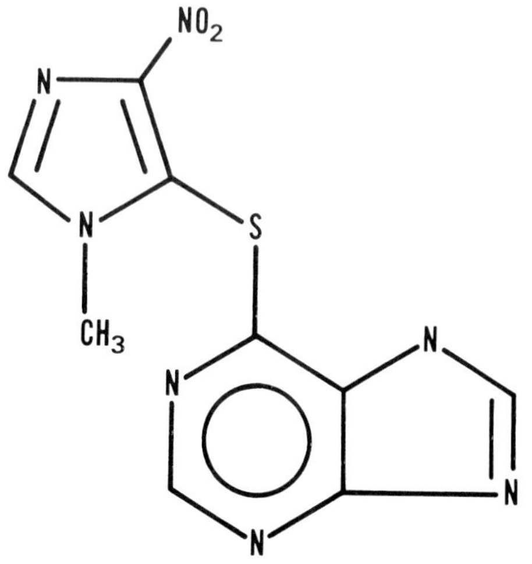

cytes.[33,34] Multiple metabolites of 6-MP have been identified including the cytotoxic compounds 6-thioinosinic acid and 6-thioguanylic acid.[3] Xanthine oxidase degrades azathioprine metabolites to 6-thiouric acid.[34]

Although hepatic metabolism is important, the clinical effects of liver disease on azathioprine metabolism are unclear. Some patients with liver disease have near normal azathioprine metabolism,[35] while other patients with chronic liver disease may be at higher risk for hematologic toxicity.[36] The half-life of azathioprine may increase in renal failure,[37] although this effect is often not clinically significant.[32]

Drug interactions with azathioprine are uncommon. Although the pharmacokinetics of 6-MP are not significantly altered by allopurinol in some patients,[38] the inhibition of azathioprine metabolism by allopurinol is potentially life-threatening if unrecognized. Azathioprine and 6-MP are eventually metabolized to 6-thiouric acid by xanthine oxidase. Allopurinol blocks this action and allows prolonged accumulation of azathioprine and its metabolites. *The simultaneous administration of these compounds should be avoided.* If azathioprine and allopurinol are to be used concurrently, the dose of azathioprine must be reduced by 75% and close monitoring performed to avoid toxicity.[34] Trimethoprim has been reported to increase the hematologic toxicity of azathioprine.[39]

Proposed Mechanisms of Action

The exact mechanism of action of azathioprine in rheumatic diseases remains unclear, although the drug's major effects result from its cleavage in vivo to 6-MP.[4] 6-Thioinosinic acid, formed by the action of hypoxanthine phosphoribosyl transferase on 6-MP, suppresses several steps in the synthesis of adenine and guanine by preventing interconversion of purine bases, especially inosinic and guanylic acid. 6-Thioinosinic acid also acts as a feedback inhibitor of inosinic acid production to inhibit de novo biosynthesis of purines.[34] 6-MP may also be incorporated into RNA and DNA as 6-thioguanine.[40] These effects lead to cell cytotoxicity, although the role of cell cytotoxicity remains unclear in the action of these agents in RA.

In addition to cytotoxic effects, azathioprine has been found to suppress natural killer cell activity,[41] antibody production,[4] antibody-dependent cellular cytotoxicity,[41] and cellular immune assays.[42] B cells may be selectively altered during treatment with azathioprine.[43] No change in adenosine deaminase is seen.[44] In general, the immunologic parameters of patients with rheumatic disease receiving azathioprine is not grossly altered.[10] Azathioprine has suppressed the production of autoantibodies in animal models of

SLE[45,46] and has been reported to lower rheumatoid factor[47,48] in RA patients, although this is not universally seen.[7,11,12,49,50] It is unknown if this alteration of antibody level is a primary or secondary drug effect.[45,46]

ADVERSE DRUG EFFECTS

From 19 to 32% of patients must discontinue azathioprine because of significant adverse reactions (Table 35–1).[49–51] In the majority of instances these events are rapidly reversible on discontinuing azathioprine. Studies comparing differing doses of azathioprine have suggested, but not proven, a dose-related increased incidence of adverse effects.[12,52] Often, patients experiencing mild toxicity can take the drug at a lower dose without difficulty.

Hematologic

Hematologic toxicity is encountered frequently. Leukopenia,[5,8–11,13,14,47–49,51–53] thrombocytopenia,[10,47,54] anemia,[9,14,53] pure red cell aplasia,[53] and pancytopenia[15] have all been reported in RA patients. Severe leukopenia may lead to serious infections.[14]

Table 35–1. Adverse Effects of Azathioprine

Hematologic
Leukopenia[5,8–11,13,14,47–49,51,52,53]*
Thrombocytopenia[10,47]*
Anemia[9,14]*
Pure red cell aplasia[53]
Pancytopenia[15]*
Gastrointestinal
Nausea/epigastric pain[5,8,11,13,14,47–55]*
Stomatitis[47]*
Gastrointestinal hemorrhage[9]*
Gastric ulcer[14]*
Diarrhea[47,54]*
Pancreatitis[56–58]
Hepatic
Elevated liver enzymes[52,55]*
Hepatitis[60]
Cholestasis[60–63]
Fibrosis[61,62]
Cirrhosis[59]
Pulmonary
Interstitial pneumonitis[64,65]
Diffuse alveolar damage[64]
Dermatologic
Maculopapular rash[8–10,14,47,49,51,52]*
Reproductive
Congenital deformities[68–70]
Chromosomal damage[13,70]
Miscellaneous
Herpes zoster[10,49]*
Proteinuria[49]*
Peripheral neuropathy[84]

*Reported during the treatment of rheumatic diseases.

Gastrointestinal

Nausea, vomiting, and epigastric pain are frequent complaints in patients receiving azathioprine.[5,8,11,13,14,47–52,54,55] Less frequently, stomatitis,[47,54] gastrointestinal hemorrhage,[9] gastric ulcer,[14] and diarrhea[47,54] are reported. Pancreatitis has been seen during azathioprine treatment of inflammatory bowel disease and renal transplantation[56–58] but not during the treatment of rheumatic diseases.

Hepatic

Liver toxicity from azathioprine is uncommon. Evaluation of liver disease in renal transplant patients receiving azathioprine suggests that azathioprine is an uncommon cause of hepatic injury in these patients, with infections the most common cause of liver disease.[36] The most common abnormality is mild elevation of liver enzymes,[52,55] which may not require that therapy be stopped. In the one report of fatal progressive liver failure and cirrhosis with azathioprine, elevated liver enzymes were noted 6 months before death.[59] It is unknown if the liver disease would have been reversible if the azathioprine had been discontinued. In some reports, hepatitis and abnormal liver enzymes have completely resolved with cessation of azathioprine,[60] and some cases of fibrosis have not progressed on serial biopsy during azathioprine treatment.[61,62] Hepatocellular injury with cholestasis has also been noted.[60–63]

Pulmonary

Pulmonary disease is rarely reported during azathioprine therapy and has never been reported during the treatment of rheumatic diseases. Interstitial pneumonitis[64,65] and diffuse alveolar damage[64] have occurred, with deaths seen in patients with severe respiratory failure.[64]

Dermatologic

Maculopapular rashes are reported in most series of azathioprine therapy in RA.[8–10,14,47,49,51,52] No major dermatologic complications have been reported in these patients. Psoriasis has often improved in patients with psoriatic arthritis receiving azathioprine.[8,10]

Reproductive

Azathioprine should not be used in pregnancy if possible. Azathioprine and its metabolites have been demonstrated to cross the placenta.[66] Successful pregnancies have occurred in patients receiving azathioprine during the first trimester and throughout pregnancy;[67] however, significant neonatal complications and chromosomal damage have occurred in the offspring of patients receiving azathioprine during pregnancy.[68–70]

Malignancy

Malignancies are increased in renal transplant patients receiving azathioprine and corticosteroids,[71] though perhaps these malignancies would have occurred independent of immunosuppressive therapy.[72] Azathioprine therapy has been associated with chromosomal abnormalities with long-term use.[13] The possibility of increased malignancies in nontransplant patients is still unresolved, but the evidence suggests that secondary malignancies after treatment of rheumatic diseases are unlikely. During the treatment of RA with azathioprine, leukemias,[73,74] lymphomas,[74] and solid tumors have occurred.[8,14,15,74] Epidemiologic studies of malignancies in nontransplant patients receiving azathioprine suggest an increase in malignancies as compared to the expected malignancy rates.[75] Complicating the evaluation of this literature are the conflicting reports of increased malignancies in RA patients independent of cytotoxic antirheumatic therapies.[76–78] To truly define the malignancy potential of cytotoxic agents, studies must include RA control patients who had no cytotoxic exposure. Studies comparing the incidence of malignancies in patients with RA receiving azathioprine to that in control RA patients have not shown a detectable malignancy risk.[79–82] One study did suggest that azathioprine may increase malignancy rates in RA patients, but many of these individuals had received alkylating agents, which are known definitely to induce malignancies.[83]

Miscellaneous

Infections may be increased in patients receiving azathioprine.[14] In particular, herpes zoster may develop during azathioprine treatment.[10,49] Although rarely seen, proteinuria[49] and peripheral neuropathy[84] are reported.

CLINICAL EXPERIENCE

Rheumatoid Arthritis

Multiple studies have demonstrated effectiveness of azathioprine in RA. The doses used range from 1.0 to 4.8 mg/kg/day,[14,15] with 1.25[12,51,52] and 2.5[9,11,12,47,49,50,52] mg/kg/day most frequently employed. Studies directly comparing 1.25 versus 2.5 mg/kg/day doses did not demonstrate statistically significant differences in clinical outcomes but did suggest that the higher doses may be more effective in controlling antirheumatic activity.[12,52] Adverse drug reactions may have been more common at the higher dose.[52] In a large multicenter trial of azathioprine (1.25 to 1.5 mg/

kg/day), 44% of patients experienced "important clinical improvement," defined as improvement in >30% of tender joints.[51] Comparisons of azathioprine with D-penicillamine,[47,50,51,54] gold,[48,49] cyclophosphamide,[49] chloroquine,[48] and levamisole,[54] have suggested that azathioprine is equally effective as these agents, in the study populations tested. Continued treatment with azathioprine is required to maintain the clinical improvement achieved.[13,15]

The disease-modifying effects of azathioprine in RA are unclear. Rheumatoid factor has fallen in some studies, but this effect is not universal.[11,12,55] Reports of progression[13,50] and improvement of bone erosions are reported.[54,55] One study comparing gold and azathioprine suggested that fewer erosions developed during azathioprine therapy than during gold therapy.[49] Rheumatoid vasculitis has improved during treatment with azathioprine.[14]

The recommended initial dose for azathioprine is 1 mg/kg, and this may be increased to a maximum dose of 2.5 mg/kg in severe cases. Because of the slow onset of action by azathioprine, a trial of at least 12 weeks and probably up to 24 weeks is required to ensure an adequate opportunity for a clinical response. Complete blood counts with platelet counts should be performed at the beginning and at least every 4 weeks throughout therapy. The measurement of liver function tests at baseline seems appropriate, with repeated evaluation at 1 month and then every 3 to 6 months thereafter. Clinical evaluations should include inquiries for gastrointestinal upset, stomatitis, and skin rash. The use of allopurinol should be avoided. If azathioprine and allopurinol are used concurrently, the dose of azathioprine must be reduced by 75%.[34]

Systemic Lupus Erythematosus

The role of azathioprine in SLE is not well defined. Azathioprine doses have ranged from 1.0 to 4.0 mg/kg/day[17,25] with adjustments for leukopenia. The greatest experience with cytotoxic drugs in SLE is at the National Institutes of Health (NIH), where a large cohort of SLE patients with renal disease was followed for several years in randomized protocols.[17–22] These studies have been complicated by a general trend toward improvement of SLE outcome over the last decades, which makes temporal comparison between the different protocols difficult.[85] In general, these protocols have shown that cytotoxic drugs retard the progression to end-stage renal disease when compared to prednisone used alone. The NIH results favor cyclophosphamide as the most effective agent, with azathioprine producing some intermediate benefit.[17] Other authors have suggested that azathioprine is much more effective than prednisone used alone in

SLE renal disease;[23,25] however, these studies did not compare azathioprine and cyclophosphamide. Discoid lupus has also been treated successfully with azathioprine.[26]

Inflammatory Muscle Disease

Reports of uncontrolled studies describe improvement of inflammatory myopathy with azathioprine.[28,29] A controlled trial evaluating azathioprine and prednisone versus prednisone alone showed no significant clinical differences after 3 months in the small groups of patients studied,[27] but at 6 months the group receiving both azathioprine and prednisone experienced greater functional improvement and possible steroid-sparing effects.[30]

Psoriatic Arthritis

No controlled trials are available for azathioprine in psoriatic arthritis; however reports of uncontrolled trials suggest improvement of clinical disease activity[8,10,14] and improvement of skin lesions.[8,14]

Miscellaneous

Uncontrolled studies have reported success with the use of azathioprine in several vasculitis syndromes. Alkylating agents are often used before azathioprine in severe vasculitides and appear to be more effective.[86] Benefit with azathioprine in Wegener's granulomatosis,[87,88] Takayasu's arteritis[89,90] and other necrotizing vasculitis syndrome, however, is reported.[91] Weber-Christian disease is also sometimes responsive to azathioprine.[92] Corticosteroids given in large doses are often administered with azathioprine in the preceding diseases.

SUMMARY

Azathioprine is clearly an effective agent in the treatment of RA wth similar efficacy to other approved slow-acting antirheumatic drugs. Regular monitoring for toxicity is required to prevent serious adverse drug effects. The question of carcinogenicity is still being evaluated. Currently available data, however, show that the drug has little carcinogenic potential in rheumatic disease patients. The role of azathioprine in SLE needs further definition; however, cyclophosphamide appears to be more effective than azathioprine in SLE nephritis.

METHOTREXATE

HISTORY

In 1951, Gubner et al.[93] first reported that methotrexate produced clinical improvement in RA. Later,

open-label trials reported similar effectiveness.[94–101] Controlled clinical trials have conclusively confirmed its efficacy in RA.[102–106] Improvement in psoriatic arthritis,[107–110] Reiter's syndrome,[111,112] and inflammatory muscle disease[113–116] has also been noted with methotrexate. Long-term followup studies now under way should more clearly define the role of this agent in the treatment of rheumatic diseases.[117–121]

PHARMACOLOGY

Pharmacokinetics

Methotrexate (Fig. 35–2) is a folic acid analogue that is absorbed by the gastrointestinal tract after oral ingestion but with significant variability, ranging from 23 to 95%.[122–125] In RA patients, the mean bioavailability is 67% of the ingested dose with a range from 40 to 100%.[126] Ingestion with food, particularly milk products, could in part explain the alterations seen in methotrexate absorption.[127] From 50 to 84% of methotrexate is bound by plasma proteins.[128,129] Intravenous or intramuscular dosing gives excellent bioavailability and equivalent serum levels.[130]

After absorption, methotrexate is transported into cells, metabolized to polyglutamates and 7-hydroxy-methotrexate,[131,132] and excreted. After initial redistribution, the terminal half-life with low doses of methotrexate is probably 7 to 10 hours.[126,130] Most uptake of methotrexate by cells involves an energy-dependent (active) transport, although passive transport also occurs with high extracellular methotrexate concentrations.[133,134] It is unlikely that such high concentrations are achieved with the relatively small doses used to treat rheumatic diseases. After 24 hours, the majority of intracellular methotrexate is polyglutamated.

Polyglutamates appear to remain in cells longer than unglutamated methotrexate does.[135–137] Polyglutamates are active[137] and may even have greater potency than unglutamated methotrexate.[138–140] Methotrexate is also metabolized to 7-hydroxy-methotrexate, which is also an active compound, although less potent than methotrexate.[136] Both 7-hydroxy-methotrexate and methotrexate circulate in the blood and are primarily eliminated by the kidney. Renal excretion involves filtration, and probably both active secretion[138] and tubular resorption.[138,141] Methotrexate may also undergo some enterohepatic circulation.[141,142] Compensatory increases in biliary excretion may occur if renal clearance of the drug decreases.[143]

Multiple drug interactions have been reported with methotrexate.[144] Although methotrexate toxicity precipitated by drug interactions has been reported,[145–146] the clinical significance of the majority of these rela-

FIG. 35–2. Structure of methotrexate.

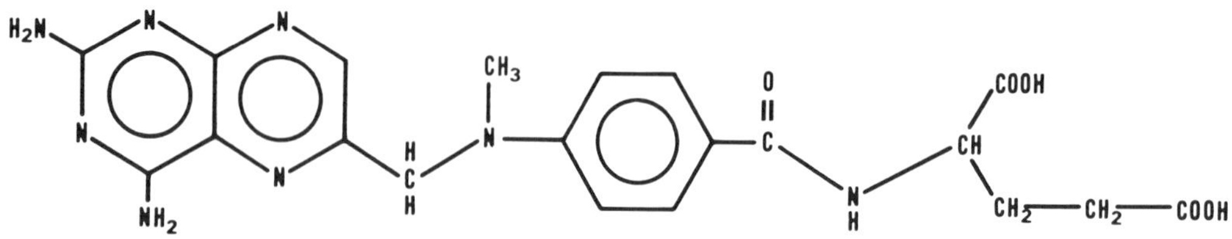

tionships remains unknown. Absorption,[147] protein binding,[128,148] intracellular transport, and renal excretion[129,149–151] of methotrexate may be altered by other agents.[144] Potentially significant interactions may occur with aspirin when there is some displacement of methotrexate from protein-binding sites[128,148] and decrease in renal excretion,[98,129] although clinically this interaction does not appear to cause significant problems in the majority of patients.[128,152] Nonsteroidal anti-inflammatory agents decrease tubular secretion of methotrexate in vitro,[150] and case reports of methotrexate toxicity precipitated by these agents have appeared.[145,146] Probenecid also appears to reduce both renal clearance and biliary elimination of methotrexate.[128,149,151]

Proposed Mechanisms of Action

Methotrexate inhibits dihydrofolate reductase, leading to a depletion of intracellular pools of reduced folate. Thymidylate synthesis is inhibited by depletion of $N^{5–10}$ methylene-FH_4,[153] and purine synthesis is inhibited by depletion of N^{10}-formyl-FH4.[154,155] The intracellular concentration of polyglutamated methotrexate may play an important role in these enzyme inhibitions.[156] Although these steps are important in the cytotoxic effects of methotrexate, the role of cell cytotoxicity in the antirheumatic properties of methotrexate remains unknown.[157] No significant lymphocyte depletion during the treatment of RA with methotrexate has been demonstrated, although there is a slight decrease in the number of circulating monocytes.[158]

In addition to having cytotoxic effects, it has been suggested that methotrexate is an immunomodulator. High doses of methotrexate alter antibody production and may alter cellular immunity, but whether these effects occur at the low doses of methotrexate used in rheumatic disease thereby remains unclear. Methotrexate treatment of RA may suppress delayed-type hypersensitivity reactions,[158] although this is not always seen. Acute inflammation is not affected.[158,159] Significant changes in immunologic function[103,106,158]— as determined by measurements of circulating immune complexes, lymphocyte cell-surface markers for

T-helper cells and T-suppressor/cytotoxic cells, or antibody production[159]—do not occur during short-term methotrexate therapy. Long-term methotrexate therapy may be associated with a decrease in T-suppressor cells.[160] In vitro IgM rheumatoid factor production by lymphocytes from RA patients receiving methotrexate may be reduced.[161] Circulating monocytes may decrease, and a decrease in spontaneous ³H-thymidine uptake by peripheral blood lymphocytes has accompanied methotrexate treatment.[159] In vitro tests show that methotrexate may depress neutrophil chemotaxis,[162,163] and granulocyte phagocytosis[164] and may augment natural killer cell function.[165] In summary, no conclusive evidence shows that methotrexate exerts immunomodulating effects during the treatment of RA.

Methotrexate decreases the severity of adjuvant-induced arthritis in rats,[166–169] which is associated with a return of mitogen-induced lymphocyte transformation assays to normal.[167] In most of these experiments, however, the doses used were significantly higher than those used in the treatment of RA. In one study an antirheumatic effect of methotrexate was observed at doses equivalent to those used in the treatment of human RA.[166]

In summary, the mechanism of action of methotrexate in RA remains unknown. Although cytotoxicity accompanies the use of high doses of methotrexate, this effect of methotrexate in the therapy of human RA is uncertain. The drug may have an immunomodulating activity, but these data are primarily based on in vitro experiments and not on in vivo drug effects.[103,106,158–165]

ADVERSE EFFECTS

Adverse reactions (Table 35–2) are the major limitations of both short-term and long-term use of methotrexate in RA. Adverse drug effects required methotrexate to be discontinued in 5 to 32%[104,106] in short-term trials and 5 to 31%[119,170] in long-term followup studies. Clinical and immunologic markers cannot consistently predict which patients are at an

Table 35–2.   Adverse Effects of Methotrexate

Hepatic
  Elevated liver enzymes/nonspecific
    hepatitis[97–99,101,104–106,117,118,173,174,178–180,184]*
  Fatty liver[173,174,178]*
  Fibrosis[94–117,173–180]*
  Cirrhosis[173,174,176]
Gastrointestinal
  Nausea/vomiting[97–99,102,104,106,107,118,184,186]*
  Stomatitis[97,99,102–104,109,117,118,184]*
  Diarrhea[106]*
  Gastric ulcer with bleeding[121]*
  Mucosal damage[121]
  Malabsorption[124,190]
Hematologic
  Leukopenia[98,102,104,118,121,191]*
  Thrombocytopenia[97,102,104,117,191]*
  Pancytopenia[103,104,121,191]*
Pulmonary
  Acute pneumonitis[118,121,184,192–196]*
  Fibrosis[192,205–206]*
Neurologic
  Headache[104,106,107,118,211]*
  Seizures[121,208]*
  Nerve palsy[207,209]
  Speech impediments[207,208]
  Hemiparesis[207,208]
  Emotional disturbances[208]
  Loss of consciousness[208]
  Status epilepticus[208]
  Rapidly progressive ascending neuromuscular paralysis[208,209]
  Mental status changes[208,209]
  Paraplegia[210]
Dermatologic
  Maculopapular rash[103,104,106,109,186]*
  Hair loss[107,186]*
  Skin ulcers[214]
  Erythema and desquamation[213]
Reproductive
  Congenital abnormalities[215,216]
  Oligospermia[220,221]
Miscellaneous
  Renal[228]
  Vasculitis[230,231]*
  Herpes zoster[97,98,102,117,232]*
  Pneumocystis[233]

*Reported during the treatment of rheumatic diseases.

increased risk for methotrexate toxicity, although increased methotrexate toxicity has been associated with older patients[119] and patients with malnutrition[171] or impaired renal function.[119] Methotrexate toxicity may occur less often in patients bearing HLA-DR 53.[172]

Hepatic

Liver injury has been a major concern during methotrexate treatment. Although methotrexate-induced liver disease involves a large spectrum of abnormalities, the greatest concern is the development of fibrosis[94,117,173–180] and cirrhosis.[173,174,176] Several liver biopsy grading scales have been developed to quan-

titate the severity of methotrexate-induced disease.[173,174;,176,180,181] These systems generally classify the disease as minimal change (fatty infiltration and mild lymphocytic infiltrates); nonspecific hepatitis (periportal round cell infiltration); fibrosis; and cirrhosis.[180,181] During the use of methotrexate in RA, up to 76% of patients showed histologic abnormalities on biopsy,[180] mostly fatty infiltration and mild, nonspecific hepatitis. Some RA patients had mild hepatic abnormalities without fibrosis on pretreatment liver biopsies.[118] Fibrosis is seen in up to 34% of RA patients after 2 years of treatment[180] and appears to be a definite sign of methotrexate-induced hepatic injury. In RA patients, serial biopsies have not shown a progression of hepatic abnormalities.[118,182] Although cirrhosis has been seen in patients receiving methotrexate for cancer and psoriasis[173,174,176] with a prevalence of up to 25.6% after 5 years,[176] cirrhosis has not yet been reported in RA patients. The experience in psoriasis patients suggests that cirrhosis developing during methotrexate treatment may be less severe than that seen from other causes.[176]

It is impossible to predict which patients are at risk for methotrexate-induced hepatotoxicity. Risk factors for methotrexate-induced liver disease include alcohol abuse,[174,176] increasing age,[174,175] obesity,[175] diabetes mellitus,[176] impaired renal function,[176] and previous arsenic,[176] or other hepatotoxin exposure.[174] Longer duration of treatment, greater total dose received, and higher frequency of administration are thought to increase the risk of liver damage with methotrexate.[173–176,183]

Efforts with noninvasive techniques to detect hepatic injury have been unsuccessful. Although low-serum albumin and sustained elevations of aminotransferase and/or alkaline phosphatase may be mild indicators of liver damage, these abnormalities are too nonspecific to be clinically useful.[176,180] ''Liver'' enzymes are elevated during methotrexate treatment in up to 76% of patients[97–99,101,104–106,117,118,173,174,178–180,184] but show little correlation with histologic changes.[118,180] During controlled clinical trials with methotrexate in RA, up to 19% of patients discontinued the drug because of liver enzyme abnormalities.[104] Bromsulphalein (BSP) testing[173] has not proven useful in detecting significant methotrexate-induced liver disease. Technetium-99 liver scans have not consistently detected methotrexate-induced liver damage later shown on biopsy.[177,185] Ultrasonography may have a role in screening for methotrexate-induced liver damage.[179] Liver biopsies therefore remain the gold standard for evaluating liver damage from methotrexate. Liver biopsies should probably be performed at least every 2 years during methotrexate treatment and at more frequent intervals in patients with underlying risk factors.

Gastrointestinal

Nausea, vomiting,[97–99,102,104,106,107,118,184,186] stomatitis,[97,99,102–104,109,117,118,184] and diarrhea[106] are common side effects during the use of methotrexate in RA patients and may be severe enough to require discontinuation of the drug. Gastric ulceration with bleeding has been reported.[121] Alteration of small-bowel histology has been seen after methotrexate use to treat malignancies, both when used as the single agent[187,188] or in combination chemotherapy.[189] These effects may induce malabsorption.[124,190] There was no correlation of such histologic changes with diarrhea or with gastrointestinal symptoms in these patients.[189]

Hematologic

Leukopenia,[98,102,104,118,121,191] thrombocytopenia,[97,102,104,117,191] and pancytopenia[103,104,121,191] have been reported during methotrexate therapy of RA. Impaired renal function,[103,191] pre-existing marrow injury,[191] and dosage errors[191] are reported risk factors. Age over 60 years, concurrent use of multiple medications, and hypoalbuminemia may also predispose to methotrexate-induced hematologic toxicity, although bone marrow toxicity certainly occurs in patients without these abnormalities. Leucovorin treatment has been used to reverse methotrexate-induced bone marrow injury, with marrow recovery in four of five patients with pancytopenia.[191] Severe infections may develop in patients with significant leukopenia.[121]

Pulmonary

Acute pneumonitis and interstitial fibrosis have been reported during treatment of RA with methotrexate.[118,121,184,192–196] The former presents as an acute or subacute respiratory disease characterized by dry nonproductive cough, shortness of breath, and fever.[192–204] Crackles are heard, often at the base of the lungs.[192] Hypoxemia accompanies interstitial and alveolar infiltrates, which are usually bilateral.[198] Histologic findings are typically those of a hypersensitivity pneumonitis with interstitial round-cell infiltration, bronchiolitis, and giant cells.[192,193] Steroids may reduce the severity of this reaction,[192] which appears to be idiosyncratic, without known predisposing factors.[192] Underlying pulmonary disease may predispose to the development of this problem.[196] Interstitial pulmonary fibrosis has also been reported during methotrexate therapy of both RA[192] and other diseases.[205,206]

Neurologic

Treatment with high doses of methotrexate has produced transient neurologic problems in cancer patients.[207–210] These include headache,[104,106,107,118,209] nerve palsy,[207–209] speech impediments,[207,208] hemiparesis,[207,208] emotional disturbances,[208] focal seizures,[121,208] generalized seizures with loss of consciousness,[208] status epilepticus,[208] rapidly progressive ascending neuromuscular paralysis,[208,209] and mental status changes.[208,209] Seizures have occurred in RA patients receiving methotrexate.[121] Intrathecal methotrexate has been associated with the development of paraplegia, which was almost totally reversible.[210] Psycho-organic changes appear to be very uncommon.[211] Studies of cerebrospinal fluid (CSF) methotrexate levels in patients with and without methotrexate-induced neurotoxicity suggest that these neurologic adverse drug effects are in part related to CSF methotrexate levels.[209] Electroencephalograms have not shown any changes during methotrexate therapy.[212]

Dermatologic

Maculopapular eruptions of drug hypersensitivity occur during methotrexate treatment of RA.[103,104,106,109,186] More serious toxic reactions include erythema and desquamation over the distal extremities[213] and skin ulcers.[214] Hair loss has accompanied treatment of RA with methotrexate.[107,186]

Reproductive

Methotrexate should not be administered to pregnant women or women who are not practicing effective contraception. Fetal abnormalities can occur, particularly when the drug is given during the first trimester. Congenital defects have included multiple skeletal abnormalities, hydrocephalus, ear anomalies, cleft palate, meningomyelocele, and anencephaly.[215,216] Offspring of women who have previously received methotrexate have had no clear-cut increase in congenital abnormalities,[217,218] though the possibility of a slight increase cannot be completely excluded.[219]

Oligospermia has been seen in some men during treatment of psoriasis with methotrexate, but this effect is often reversible after the drug is stopped.[220,221]

Malignancy Potential

Although some evidence suggests that methotrexate may have a mutagenic effect,[222] none suggests that its use predisposes to the development of malignancies.[223,224] Anecdotal reports have appeared.[225–227] A thymoma was noted in an RA patient receiving methotrexate.[225] Metastatic squamous cell carcinoma[226] and a nasopharyngeal carcinoma[227] have been reported in psoriatic patients receiving methotrexate. Careful epidemiologic analyses, however, have failed to show an increase in second tumors in patients receiving methotrexate for malignant diseases.[223,224] Long-term followup is needed to completely exclude the carcinogenic potential of methotrexate treatment in RA patients, but available data are encouraging.

Miscellaneous

High-dose methotrexate therapy in patients with malignancies can cause histologically evident damage to the renal tubular epithelium with a concurrent increase in blood urea nitrogen (BUN) and decrease in renal clearance of inulin and p-aminohippurate (PAH).[228] No histologic changes have been seen on renal biopsies in patients receiving methotrexate for psoriasis.[229] Underlying renal insufficiency may increase the risk of other drug-induced adverse reactions. Leukocytoclastic vasculitis has been reported after high-dose methotrexate therapy in osteogenic sarcoma[230] and during treatment of RA.[231] Herpes zoster[97,98,102,117,232] and Pneumocystis carinii pneumonia[233] occurred during treatment of RA with methotrexate.

CLINICAL EXPERIENCE

Rheumatoid Arthritis

Open-label[93,96–101] and controlled trials[102–106] have reported clinical improvement during treatment of RA with methotrexate. Such improvement has followed oral, intravenous,[99,223] and intramuscular drug use.[103] Intra-articular injections have generally been ineffective,[234,235] although success with this method has been reported.[236] Reported effective doses of methotrexate range from 5 to 25 mg/week. Greater than 50% improvement in the number of swollen joints occurred in 21 to 54% of patients during short-term trials[104,106] with remissions reported.[118,121] Improvement in erosions on serial radiographs were found in 7 of 11 patients receiving methotrexate during a long-term prospective trial without progression in any patient.[118] An increased mean number of erosions on hand roentgenograms over 1 year in 35 patients was found in another study, although 23 (65.7%) of patients showed no progression of erosions.[184] Improvement in rheumatoid vasculitis[237] and reduction of both the rheumatoid factor titer[238] and the number of rheumatoid nodules have also been reported.[104] Although the majority of these reports in RA show favorable effects of therapy, FitzGerald and co-workers reported "poor" long-term results.[186]

The most effective dose and route of administration of methotrexate is not yet completely defined. Most studies have used oral "pulse" doses, although single-dose weekly therapy also appears to be effective.[118] There was no detectable difference in clinical efficacy in one trial comparing methotrexate 10 versus 25 mg/week.[102] In a clinical trial allowing dose increases from 7.5 to 15.0 mg/week after 6 weeks of therapy in RA patients, the subset showing the greatest improvement experienced an early response with the lower dose.[239] Although some clinical improvement eventually occurred in patients given the 15-mg/week dose, it is unknown if improvement would have occurred on the lower dose. Some patients needed higher drug doses to maintain disease suppression in one long-term study.[118]

A dose of 7.5 mg/week is currently most widely used initially, with subsequent adjustments upward, depending on the observed clinical response and toxicity.* Doses of 15 mg/week may be required in some patients, but most patients showing a beneficial effect will do so at lower doses.

As with any drug therapy, the expected benefits should be discussed with the patient in terms of the possible risk, and the most common adverse reactions should be described. Monitoring for methotrexate toxicity should include screening for renal insufficiency (serum creatinine) before beginning therapy with repeat creatinine levels every 3 to 6 months during treatment. Patients with significant renal disease should not receive the drug. Patients with mild renal insufficiency may be treated with reduced doses. Complete blood counts including platelets and "liver" enzymes should be measured before beginning methotrexate therapy. Complete blood and platelet counts should be obtained at least monthly, and liver enzymes monitored every 2 months during therapy. A liver biopsy should be performed after 2 years of treatment and at more frequent intervals in patients with significant risk factors for liver disease. Patients should be alerted to the potential of pulmonary disease during methotrexate treatment and advised to seek medical attention if pulmonary symptoms develop.

Psoriatic Arthritis

The role of methotrexate in the treatment of psoriatic arthritis is unclear. Several authors report improvement of psoriatic arthritis during treatment with methotrexate.[107–110] A controlled trial by Willkens et al.[240] showed a significant improvement in physician assessment of disease severity but not in other pa-

*Editor's note. Many clinicians give 2.5 mg (one tablet) every 12 hours for three doses once a week. The 12-hour interval was derived from the rate of division of skin cells in psoriasis.

rameters of disease activity in 37 psoriatic arthritis patients enrolled in a placebo-controlled trial. A cross-over trial suggested improvement of psoriatic arthritis during treatment with relatively high dosages, up to 2 mg/kg every 10 days.[108]

Polymyositis/Dermatomyositis

There are no controlled trials of methotrexate in inflammatory muscle disease, although several reports have suggested that the agent may be effective in patients refractory to steroids.[113–116] Higher doses of methotrexate given intravenously were generally used in the treatment of inflammatory muscle disease. One group's initial report used between 5 and 100 mg/day (mean 50 mg/day) with subsequent maintenance doses of 30 to 75 mg/week (mean 42 mg/week) in combination with steroids,[114] with improvement noted in 77% of patients.[114] Another study reported improvement in only 5 of 16 patients, however.[116] Fisher et al.[113] used 1 mg/kg/week to successfully treat childhood dermatomyositis and polymyositis. The steroid-sparing effects of methotrexate are emphasized in all of these reports.[113–116]* The drug has no beneficial effect in inclusion-body myositis.

Reiter's Syndrome

Methotrexate has been used effectively in the treatment of Reiter's syndrome.[111,112] An improvement in 90% of skin lesions and in 75% of arthritis was recorded,[112] but no controlled trials are reported.

SUMMARY

Methotrexate is clearly effective in the treatment of many but not all RA patients.[93–106] Inconclusive data suggest that methotrexate may also be effective in the treatment of psoriatic arthritis,[107–110] inflammatory muscle disease,[113–116] and Reiter's syndrome.[111,112] Careful monitoring is required in following patients receiving this drug. Long-term studies should clarify the role of methotrexate in the treatment of these rheumatic diseases.

ALKYLATING AGENTS

HISTORY

The biologic activity of alkylating agents was first recognized in the late 1800s,[241] and they were used to

*Editor's note. In uncontrolled studies we have used intravenous methotrexate (UCLA protocol[114]) combined with azathioprine, 50 mg/day, with very encouraging results in corticosteroid-resistant disease.

FIG. 35–3. Structure of cyclophosphamide.

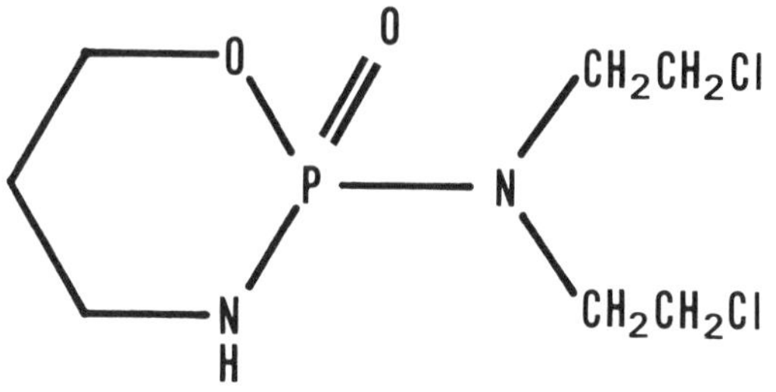

treat malignant diseases. Nitrogen mustard was first used in the treatment of refractory RA in 1951.[242] Subsequently, cyclophosphamide (Fig. 35–3) and chlorambucil (Fig. 35–4) became the principal alkylating agents used to treat rheumatic diseases. Cyclophosphamide was used predominantly by British and American investigators, while chlorambucil was used extensively in France. Initial reports involved their use in RA and SLE with extension to the vasculitides and other rheumatic conditions. Their role in rheumatic disease therapy is under re-evaluation. They have proven efficacy in several situations but uncertainty over their long-term toxicity, including the induction of malignancies, is a major concern.

PHARMACOLOGY

Pharmacokinetics

Cyclophosphamide is well absorbed after oral ingestion.[243] Twelve to 14% of the drug is bound to plasma proteins;[244] it is mostly metabolized by the liver, although there may be some metabolism by the lung and kidney.[241] Its plasma half-life is 2 to 10 hours. Less than 20% of cyclophosphamide is excreted unchanged in the urine over the first 24 hours.[241] Cyclophosphamide is an inactive compound that is activated by the cytochrome P-450 mixed-function oxidase system.[243] Cyclophosphamide is first metabolized to 4-hydroxycyclophosphamide, which is in a steady state with aldophosphamide. Additional oxidation leads to the inactive metabolites, 4-ketocyclophosphamide and carboxyphosphamide, and the active metabolites, phosphoramide mustard and acrolein.[243] The activity of the inducible hepatic mi-

FIG. 35–4. Structure of chlorambucil.

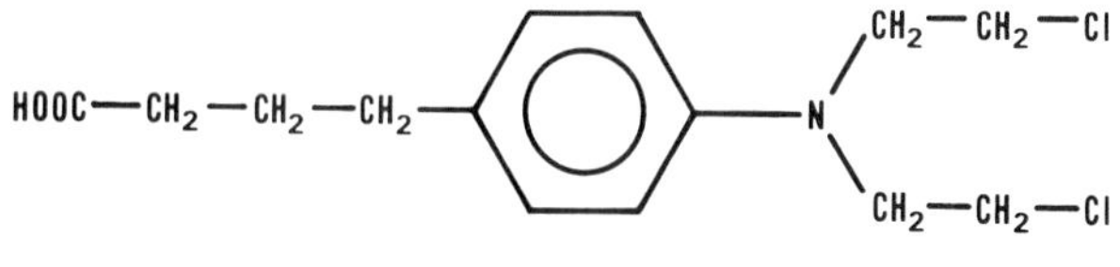

crosomal enzymes, and therefore the rate of cyclophosphamide metabolism, can be increased by prior exposure to various drugs[241] including previous cyclophosphamide therapy.[244]

Chlorambucil pharmacokinetics are not well defined.[241,245] It is rapidly and almost completely absorbed orally, with peak serum concentrations occurring after 30 to 70 minutes and metabolism to phenylacetic acid mustard and other metabolites with a serum half-life of 1.5 to 1.7 hours. Twenty to 70% of labeled chlorambucil is excreted in the urine in the form of various metabolites over the first 24 hours.

Drug interactions with cyclophosphamide and chlorambucil appear to be rare. Enhanced cyclophosphamide toxicity during concurrent allopurinol therapy has been reported, however,[246] perhaps secondary to inhibition of the hepatic P-450 enzymes.[247] In animal models, chloroquine may inhibit DNA repair enzymes and thus increase cyclophosphamide toxicity.[248,249] Agents that induce cytochrome P-450 enzymes may increase cyclophosphamide metabolism[244] but do not have a clinically significant effect on the antineoplastic effects of cyclophosphamide in animal models.[250–253] Steroids may inhibit cyclophosphamide metabolism.[254] Overall, most drug interactions with cyclophosphamide appear to have little clinical importance.

Proposed Mechanisms of Action

Cyclophosphamide metabolites and chlorambucil inhibit a wide variety of cellular processes and are cytotoxic through the alkylation of various cellular constituents. The alkylation of guanine in DNA can lead to miscoding, destruction of the purine ring, and blocked DNA replication through cross-linking.[241] These actions are nonspecific, but some cell populations may be protected from alkylating agents by greater content of thiols or oxidative enzyme activity.[241]

Alkylating agents may alter immune function, as evaluated by in vitro and in vivo studies in both humans and animals. In vitro evaluation of cyclophosphamide is difficult because the compound is itself inactive; therefore, the effects of its active metabolites must be evaluated.[255] The actions of alkylating agents on the immune system depend on the drug dose, the duration of therapy, and the temporal relationship of drug administration to an immunogen stimulus. The depletion of lymphoid tissues,[256–261] including both T cells and B cells,[256–259,262] can occur after cyclophosphamide and chlorambucil therapy. Differential cytotoxicity for various lymphoid cell populations is reported.[247,256,258,263–265] B cells may be more sensitive to cyclophosphamide than T cells.[256,258] Low-dose cyclo-

phosphamide therapy in children with minimal change nephropathy is associated with a decrease in helper T-cell subsets.[266] These values return to normal after 6 to 12 months.[266] Cellular immune function can be either enhanced[267–272] or suppressed[257,273–277] depending on the experimental system used. The enhancement of cellular immunity may result from inhibition of suppressor functions[271,272] rather than a direct enhancing property. Humoral immunity has generally been depressed,[276,278–285] though rare examples of enhancement have been reported.[286] Many immunologic assays may remain unaltered during cyclophosphamide treatment in humans.[287] In addition to immunologic effects, the alkylating agents exert anti-inflammatory actions.[288]

In summary, alkylating agents appear to act through cytotoxic effects on various components of the complex inflammatory and immune systems. The overall result appears to be both anti-inflammatory and immunosuppressive, with decrease in both cellular and humoral functions. However, the possibility of enhancement of the immune system may occur through inhibition of suppressor function.

ADVERSE DRUGS EFFECTS (Table 35–3)

Hematologic

Hematologic complications are the most common adverse reactions, requiring either dose adjustment or drug discontinuation in the treatment of rheumatic diseases. Leukopenia,[277,289–303] thrombocytopenia,[289,290,293,299,304,305] anemia,[290,298,300] pancytopenia,[298,300,306–308] and eosinophilia[290] are all reported. The exact incidence of these complications is unclear because many investigators have adjusted the drug dose to produce "mild leukopenia," generally in the range of 3000 cells per mm³.[297] Therefore, the reported cases often represent severe leukopenia that did not reverse on reducing the dose. Despite these reservations, Deshayes et al.[300] reported the overall incidence of hematologic complications to be 20% during chlorambucil treatment: leukopenia (14%), thrombocytopenia (8%), anemia (5%), and pancytopenia (3%). Others[296] have reported the incidence of leukopenia to be as high as 50%. Leukopenia during cyclophosphamide treatment of RA is probably dose dependent.[302] The hematologic abnormalities may persist for several months after the drug is stopped.[289] In pulse therapy with alkylating agents, the nadir for blood leukocyte and platelet levels usually occurs 8 to 12 days after dosing and returns to normal in 2 to 3 weeks.[309]

574 CLINICAL PHARMACOLOGY OF ANTIRHEUMATIC DRUGS

Table 35–3. Adverse Effects of Alkylating Agents

Hematologic
 Leukopenia[277,289–303]*
 Thrombocytopenia[289,290,293,299,304,305]*
 Anemia[290,298,300]*
 Pancytopenia[298,300,306–308]*
 Eosinophilia[290]*‡
Gastrointestinal
 Nausea/epigastric pain[293,295,300–303,310,311]*
 Stomatitis[302,310]*
 Diarrhea[302,305]*
 Hepatotoxicity with cholestasis[312]*
Infections
 Pneumonia[292,295,313]*
 Septic arthritis[307]*
 Sepsis[290,291,295,299,300,306]*
 Herpes zoster[17,290–293,297–299,305,306,307,310,311]*
Urologic†
 Hemorrhagic cystitis[17,301,302,305,310,311]*
 Chronic cystitis[314–316]
 Carcinoma of the bladder[317–319]
Pulmonary
 Pulmonary fibrosis[321]
 Pulmonary infiltrates[303]*
Dermatologic
 Maculopapular rash[290,292,293,295,300,311]*
 Hair loss[292–295,307,322]*
 Urticaria[323]
Reproductive
 Male infertility[324–328]*
 Ovarian failure[290,292,293,300,301,303,305,311]*
 Teratogenicity[332–335]
Potential for malignancies
 Leukemia[289,298,304,336–345]*
 Lymphomas[321,346–348]*
 Solid tumors[298,336,348]*
 Chromosomal damage[331,349]*
Miscellaneous
 Cardiotoxicity[309,352]
 Impaired water excretion[351]

*Reported during the treatment of rheumatic diseases.
†Reported only with cyclophosphamide.
‡Reported only with chlorambucil.

Gastrointestinal

Gastrointestinal upset,[293,295,300–303,310,311] stomatitis,[302,310] diarrhea,[302,305] and rare hepatotoxicity with cholestasis[312] have occurred during alkylating agent therapy.

Infections

Significant bacterial and opportunistic infections can occur during treatment with alkylating agents.[17,290,295,298,300,307,313] These infections include pneumonia,[292,295,313] septic arthritis,[307] and septicemia.[290,291,295,299,300,306] These events are often associated with leukopenia, but they can occur in the absence of peripheral blood abnormalities. Herpes zoster frequently accompanies treatment of rheumatic

disease with cyclophosphamide,[17,305,310,311] or chlorambucil.[290–293,297–299,306,307]

Urologic

Cyclophosphamide treatment is often complicated by hemorrhagic cystitis,[17,301,302,305,310,311] chronic cystitis,[314–316] and carcinoma of the bladder.[317–319] These complications are probably caused by renal excretion of the toxic metabolite acrolein. Efforts to reduce bladder exposure to this agent include vigorous hydration and the use of agents with sulfhydryl groups.[320] Urologic complications do not occur with chlorambucil therapy.

Pulmonary

Pulmonary fibrosis has been seen in patients receiving combination chemotherapy and attributed to cyclophosphamide.[321] Pulmonary reactions during cyclophosphamide therapy are rare. Those reported in patients with rheumatic disease may have been due to infection.[303]

Dermatologic

Maculopapular rash, often severe enough to require discontinuing cyclophosphamide[311] or chlorambucil,[290,292,293,295,300] have been described infrequently. Varying degrees of hair loss are also mentioned,[292–295,307,322] and urticaria is reported.[323]

Reproductive

Male infertility involves both toxicity to the germinal epithelium in the seminiferous tubules[324–326] and Leydig's cell dysfunction,[327,328] which may be prolonged.[324,325,328] Recovery of fertility is variable. Many patients became permanently sterile,[328] but others subsequently fathered normal children.[329,330] Ovarian failure and amenorrhea is a well-documented complication of both cyclophosphamide[301,303,305,311] and chlorambucil[290,292,293,300] treatment. The ovarian fibrosis and follicular destruction often leads to permanent infertility. The use of pulse cyclophosphamide may produce less ovarian failure than daily oral treatment.[17]

The teratogenic effects of cyclophosphamide and chlorambucil are ill-defined because pregnancies are generally avoided after alkylating agent treatment. Chromosomal damage occurs in RA patients receiving cyclophosphamide.[331] Fetal abnormalities have been reported after cyclophosphamide[332–334] and chlorambucil[335] treatment, although there are also reports of normal pregnancies after cyclophosphamide treatment.[218]

Potential for Malignancies

The potential for induction of malignancies is raised by frequent reports of leukemia,[289,298,304,336-345] lymphomas,[321,346-348] solid tumors,[298,336,348] and chromosomal damage[331,349] in patients receiving alkylating agents. Thirty-eight deaths with 15 malignancies (7 lymphomas and leukemias) were reported in one series of 131 RA patients receiving chlorambucil between 1965 and 1973.[298] The prevalence of leukemia in 1612 RA patients receiving chlorambucil has been estimated at 0.74%.[337] A controlled evaluation of the prevalence of malignancies in RA patients who had received cyclophosphamide were compared to a similar population who had not received this drug.[348] There was a four-fold increase of solid tumors in the patients who had received cyclophosphamide and a 16-fold increased incidence of lymphoreticular malignancy (compared to the general population). This is probably the most convincing study[348] of the neoplastic potential of alkylating agents in RA. The only other explanations for these data are that the most severely active rheumatoid disease patients received alkylating therapy and severe RA is per se accompanied by an increased risk of malignancy. Other reports have suggested increased malignancies following cyclophosphamide and chlorambucil therapy in RA.[289,350] *The data strongly suggest that cyclophosphamide and chlorambucil increase the risk of malignancy.* This potential risk should be discussed with all patients before they use alkylating agents.

Miscellaneous

Rare complications include water retention,[351] cardiotoxicity,[309,352] anaphylaxis with fever,[353] and acute oropharyngeal dysesthesias.[354]

CLINICAL EXPERIENCE

Cyclophosphamide and chlorambucil are approved by the Food and Drug Administration (FDA) only for the treatment of malignancies. *No alkylating agents are approved for the treatment of rheumatic disease.* All patients receiving these cytotoxic agents should give informed consent before their administration, and a thorough evaluation should be performed to ensure that the potential risks of this therapy are justified.

Rheumatoid Arthritis

Multiple uncontrolled[242,289,301,311] and controlled trials[302,305,310] have evaluated cyclophosphamide and chlorambucil therapy in RA patients. Clinical improvement occurred in 48 to 94% of patients.[289] The daily dose of cyclophosphamide used in RA is gen-

erally 1 to 2 mg/kg. One trial found no greater clinical benefit in patients treated with 75 mg/day compared with a group treated with 150 mg/day.[302] A trend toward increased toxicity was observed, however, in patients receiving the higher dose. Chlorambucil doses range from 0.03 to 0.3 mg/kg/day, with the dose frequently adjusted to maintain leukopenia.[289]

Reduction in erythrocyte sedimentation rate,[291,299,206,355] rheumatoid factor,[277,299,355] and healing of erosions[356] have been reported during alkylating agent therapy. Clinical monitoring during therapy with these agents should include complete blood counts at least monthly, and patients receiving cyclophosphamide should be instructed to maintain high urine flow. Periodic urinalysis is needed to detect hematuria suggesting possible cyclophosphamide bladder toxicity. Because of their carcinogenicity alkylating agents are now rarely used to treat RA.

Systemic Lupus Erythematosus

Both cyclophosphamide[17-22] and chlorambucil[357] have been used to treat patients with SLE, especially those with nephritis. NIH studies have shown that end-stage renal failure is prevented in patients receiving cytotoxic drugs in addition to corticosteroids as compared to patients receiving steroids alone.[17-22,85] Cyclophosphamide appears to be the most effective agent in these studies. "Pulse" cyclophosphamide, consisting of intravenous cyclophosphamide (0.5 to 1.0 g/m²),[17,85,358] given every 1 to 3 months with subsequent maintenance therapy, has been used most recently. Blood counts are obtained 8 to 12 days post injection to assess hematologic toxicity. In another report, the use of cyclophosphamide in SLE without concurrent steroids was ineffective.[303]

Vasculitis

Wegener's granulomatosis, a previously fatal disease, has been suppressed predictably with cyclophosphamide. Long-term remissions are often obtained, and survival is clearly superior to that obtained with prednisone therapy alone.[359] Cyclophosphamide treatment failures have been reported, however.[87,88]

Polyarteritis nodosa,[91] rheumatoid vasculitis,[360] Takayasu's arthritis,[361] Churg-Strauss syndrome,[90] and systemic necrotizing vasculitis[86] have all been effectively treated with cyclophosphamide, generally used in combination with high-dose corticosteroids.

Miscellaneous

Cyclophosphamide or chlorambucil have been used to treat juvenile RA,[341,362] inflammatory muscle disease,[303,363] essential mixed cryoglobulinemia,[364] Behçet's syndrome,[313,365,366] Goodpasture's syndrome,[367] Henoch-Schönlein purpura,[368] and scleroderma.[331,369] Data are insufficient to predict results in any of these conditions.

SUMMARY

Alkylating agents are often effective in suppressing disease activity in RA, SLE, vasculitis, and (possibly) other rheumatic conditions. Toxic reactions, while common and often dose-related, usually resolve after the drug is discontinued. The carcinogenicity of these agents is frightening and continues for years after treatment. This problem has dampened the original enthusiasm for their use in therapy of nonlethal disease. Wegener's granulomatosis, severe SLE, and aggressive necrotizing vasculitis represent diseases with such a grim prognosis that the potential benefit offered by alkylating agents still justifies their use.

CYTOTOXIC DRUGS IN COMBINATION

Combination chemotherapy has been used in oncology for many years. Combinations of "long-acting" agents have recently been employed to treat intractable RA. In these open trials, lower doses of drugs are used than when each is used individually. Cyclophosphamide, azathioprine, and hydroxychloroquine were used in combination in one study of 31 patients with intractable RA.[370,371] Doses of cyclophosphamide and azathioprine were adjusted to maintain a leukopenia of 2500 to 4000 or until a "definite clinical response was noted."[370] Maintenance doses of azathioprine were 25 to 200 mg/day (mean, 74 mg) and of cyclophosphamide were 6 to 100 mg/day (mean 30 mg). Thirty patients improved during combination treatment. Sixteen achieved complete remission, seven "near remission," and seven "partial response." But only six patients had no adverse effects. Four patients died of malignancies (erythroleukemia and colon, lung, and endometrial cancer). Other adverse effects included herpes zoster, infections, pruritus, epigastric distress, diarrhea, cystitis, stomatitis, alopecia, amenorrhea, thrombocytopenia,and vasculitic leg ulcers.[370,371]

Another group of 18 patients with intractable RA were randomized to receive either a combination of methotrexate, cyclophosphamide, and hydroxychloroquine; methotrexate alone; or "continuation of other remittive agents."[372,373] Improvement in patients receiving combination protocol exceeded that seen in the other two groups. The authors suggested that this program was "not only efficacious and associated with recortication of erosions, but was also relatively free of serious adverse effects."[372]

Still another uncontrolled study[373b] combined methotrexate, azathioprine, and hydroxychloroquine to treat patients with seropositive RA whose disease was resistant to either of the first two drugs used alone. Of 20 patients completing the study, 17 showed marked disease suppression with only minor toxicity.[373b*] A controlled trial using this combination has been organized (personal communication). Chlorambucil was combined with D-penicillamine (DPA) or with gold and compared with a gold–DPA combination.[374] There was improvement in all treatment groups, but the best results were noted in the patients receiving gold and DPA in combination.

Combination therapy with cytotoxic drugs or other slow-acting antirheumatic drugs is an interesting concept that will require controlled trials and long-term followup of adverse drug effects to determine its role in the treatment of RA and other rheumatic diseases.

SULFASALAZINE

HISTORY

Svartz[375] originally described the use of sulfasalazine in the treatment of RA and inflammatory bowel disease in 1942. Following a report of a large uncontrolled experience,[376] Sinclair and Duthie[377] performed an unblinded comparison of sulfasalazine, gold, and placebo in 60 RA patients as part of an intensive inpatient treatment program. All 3 groups of patients improved, but as no significant difference between the placebo and treatment groups was found, the authors concluded that sulfasalazine ". . . does not appear to be of any specific value in the treatment of this disease."[377] A possible type II statistical error was not considered. Although Kuzell and Gardner[378] also found sulfasalazine was effective in RA, the negative report by Sinclair and Duthie[377] discouraged further investigation of sulfasalazine in RA until the late 1970s, when McConkey et al.[379,380] reported its efficacy based on uncontrolled experience. Subsequently, several reports have suggested that sulfasalazine is an effective agent in treatment of RA[381–389] and other rheumatic diseases.[390–398]

---

*Editor's note. I have used this combination with similarly promising results in refractory RA.

FIG. 35–5. Structure of sulfasalazine.

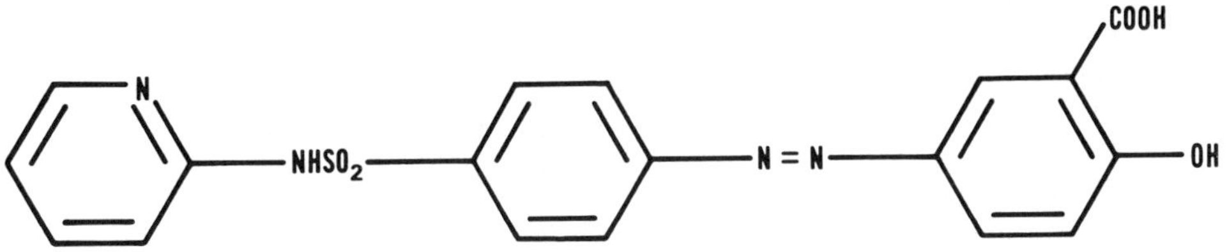

PHARMACOLOGY

Pharmacokinetics

Sulfasalazine has been referred to by several names including salicylazosulphapyridine, salazopyrin, and azopyrin. Sulfasalazine (Fig. 35–5) is a conjugate of 5-aminosalicylic acid (5-ASA), a salicylate, and sulfapyridine, a sulfonamide, linked by an azo bond. Little data are available concerning sulfasalazine pharmacology in RA patients, but this agent has been studied extensively in normal subjects and in patients with inflammatory bowel disease.[399–402] Absorption varies widely among individuals but does not exceed 10 to 33%[402,403] with less than 10% of the absorbed compound appearing unaltered in the urine.[403] The majority of sulfasalazine reaches the colon unaltered[404] where the azo bond is reduced by bacterial flora to release 5-ASA and sulfapyridine.[405] Some of the compound undergoes enterohepatic circulation before cleavage.[406]

Most 5-ASA is recovered unchanged in the feces, although up to 33% may be absorbed systemically.[403] The majority of the absorbed 5-ASA is acetylated to form acetyl-5-ASA, which is excreted in the urine. Some of the 5-ASA is excreted in the feces as acetyl-5-ASA, which may be partially the result of local as well as systemic acetylation.[407]

Sulfapyridine is almost completely absorbed.[403] Sulfapyridine is metabolized by acetylation, ring hydroxylation, and conjugation to glucuronic acid.[400] Subjects with slow acetylator phenotypes have higher sulfapyridine serum levels than patients with fast acetylator phenotypes.[403] This phenomenon may explain why patients with the slow acetylator phenotype have an increased incidence of toxic side effects.[383,387,388,408–410] It was suggested that RA patients who are fast acetylators may have less benefit with sulfasalazine,[388] but no difference in efficacy was found in RA patients of different acetylator phenotypes[387,388] or different drug blood levels.[386–388]

Mechanism of Action

The mechanism of action of sulfasalazine in treatment of RA remains uknown, but observations during therapy in inflammatory bowel disease patients and in vitro assay may have relevance to its action in RA. These postulated mechanisms of action include immunologic effects, potential changes in prostaglandin synthesis and folate metabolism, and changes in gut flora.

Immunologic studies have yielded conflicting results.[411–415] In ulcerative colitis patients receiving sulfasalazine, one study found no change in numbers of blood T- or B-lymphocytes, skin test reactivity, or complement receptors on lymphocytes.[411,412] Another study, however, found decreased mitogen-induced lymphocyte activation, decreased numbers of T-cells, and a return of monocyte phagocytosis to normal.[413] The in vitro addition of sulfasalazine had no effect on these immunologic parameters, leading to the postulate that the drug has an "indirect" effect on immune function so that disease control is followed by a return of immunologic function toward normal. In mice treatment with sulfasalazine increased susceptibility of the intestine to malignant ascites cells.[414] The drug effect could be transferred by spleen cells from treated animals to naive animals. Changes in natural killer activity with sulfasalazine have been reported.[415] There are no evaluations of immunologic function in RA patients treated with sulfasalazine.

Both sulfasalazine and 5-ASA inhibit in vitro prostaglandin synthesis,[416] but there is no evidence that this effect correlates with the effects of sulfasalazine in either RA or inflammatory bowel disease. Sulfasalazine inhibits platelet thromboxane synthetase,[417] random migration of polymorphonuclear leukocytes (PMNs), superoxide production by neutrophils, myeloperoxidase-mediated iodination,[418] and the production of leukotrienes and certain other hydroxy fatty acids.[419]

Folate malabsorption can occur in patients taking sulfasalazine for either inflammatory bowel disease[420–423] or RA.[380] Serum folate levels are reduced, and three enzymes involved in folate metabolism (dihydrofolate reductase, methylenetetrahydrofolate reductase, and serine transhydroxymethylase) are inhibited by the drug.[424] These effects appear to be due to the whole molecule rather than its components, 5-

ASA or sulfapyridine.[420] In view of the efficacy of methotrexate, a folic acid antagonist, in RA, this observation may be of some importance. The precise effects of sulfasalazine on folic acid metabolism in RA patients is not well defined, although megaloblastic anemia has been reported.[380,384,425–428]

Sulfasalazine changes the composition of the bowel flora when given to patients with inflammatory bowel disease.[429] The effects of sulfasalazine on the bowel flora in RA are unknown, although sulphamethoxazole, a somewhat similar sulfa antibiotic, is reportedly effective in RA.[430] Abnormal bowel permeability has been found in HLA-B27–associated arthritis and RA,[431] and abnormal mucosal histology accompanies ankylosing spondylitis.[432] Whether bowel flora changes occur in RA patients during treatment with sulfasalazine is unknown.

Studies have compared the effects of the separate administration of 5-ASA and sulfapyridine in both inflammatory bowel disease and RA. The active component of sulfasalazine in inflammatory bowel diseases appears to be 5-ASA,[433,434] whereas in RA patients the sulfapyridine moiety appears to provide the disease-suppressing activity.[435,436] Although the RA patients were randomly assigned to two treatment groups, these studies were not blinded, and the therapeutic efficacy of sulfasalazine was not compared with that of its two components.

ADVERSE EFFECTS

Complete reviews of sulfasalazine toxicity are available (Table 35–4).[425,437,438] Most data come from treatment of inflammatory bowel disease, although information on long-term therapy in RA is being collected.[425] No evidence suggests a difference in drug toxicity patterns in these two diseases. The doses reported to be effective in RA (2 to 3 g/day) are somewhat lower than those used in patients with inflammatory bowel disease. Because of the lower dose, sulfasalazine may be better tolerated in RA patients.

Long-term studies of sulfasalazine therapy in inflammatory bowel disease show that 30%[438] of patients discontinue the drug with many additional patients experiencing minor adverse affects not requiring cessation of therapy.[438] Adverse effects requiring permanent discontinuation of sulfasalazine in RA patients range from 26 to 33%.[384,425]

The side effects follow two patterns, one dose related and the second idiosyncratic. Most side effects are dose related, occurring more commonly in patients with the slow acetylator phenotype who have higher blood levels of the drug. These effects are most

Table 35–4. Adverse Effects of Sulfasalazine

Systemic
Fever[377,378,389,409,438]*
Headache[379,380,384,409,438]*
Gastrointestinal
Vomiting/nausea[377,378,380, 382,383,385,387,389,425,435]*
Abdominal discomfort[377,379,382,385,389,425,435]*
Mouth ulcers[383,425]*
Pancreatitis[439]
Diarrhea[440–442]
Pseudomembranous colitis[443]
Malabsorption[380,420,422,423,425,444]
Hepatic
Hepatitis[387,425,438,445–456]*
Hepatic necrosis[447–449]
Cholestasis[457,458]*
Hematologic
Neutropenia[379,383,384,387,389,409,425]*
Agranulocytosis[409,452,459–465]*
Thrombocytopenia[425,466]*
Megaloblastic anemia[380,384,426–428]*
Hemolytic anemia[409,467–472]
Red cell aplasia[473]
Methemoglobinemia[437]
Sulfhemoglobinemia[437]
Dermatologic
Maculopapular eruptions[382–385,387–389,409,437,445,456]*
Urticaria[425,438]*
Toxic epidermal necrolysis[478]*
Exfoliative dermatitis[448]*
Stevens-Johnson syndrome[449]*
"Cyanosis" without oxygen desaturation[375,409]*
Erythema multiforme[450]
Musculoskeletal
Drug-induced lupus[479–481]
Raynaud's phenomenon[482]
Pulmonary
Dyspnea[425,484]*
Hypersensitivity pneumonitis[483–485]*
Subacute fibrosis alveolitis[486]*
Reproductive
Male infertility[488,489]
Fetal wastage[490,491]
Neurologic
Paresthesias[425]*
Confusion[449]
Neck stiffness[449]
Seizures[449]
Ataxia[449]
Miscellaneous
Tachycardia[492]
Renal[450]
Anosmia[438]

*Reported during the treatment of rheumatic diseases.

marked in patients taking 4 g or more of sulfasalazine daily and include nausea, vomiting, headache, malaise, hemolytic anemia, reticulocytosis, and methemoglobinemia. Idiosyncratic drug reactions that have no relationship to acetylator phenotype or blood drug level tend to occur early in the course of therapy and are unpredictable.

Systemic

Fever[377–389,409,438] and headache[379,380,384,409,438] commonly occur early in the course of therapy and may be controlled by reducing the sulfasalazine dose.

Gastrointestinal

Nausea with or without vomiting[377,378,380,382,383,385,387,389,425,435] and abdominal discomfort[377,379,382,385,389,425,435] are among the most frequent gastrointestinal side effects of sulfasalazine. Mouth sores have occurred during treatment of RA.[383,425] Pancreatitis,[439] bloody diarrhea,[440–442] pseudomembranous colitis,[443] and malabsorption of folate[380,420,422,423,425] and digoxin[444] are described.

Hepatic

Sulfasalazine can induce several liver problems. Hepatitis can present with jaundice, fever, rash, lymphadenopathy, and hepatomegaly[387,425,438,445–456] associated with abnormal liver chemistries and biopsies showing focal necrosis with surrounding inflammatory infiltration, eosinophilia, and rare granulomas.[447–449] Cholestasis without jaundice or elevations of serum transaminases has been reported in RA patients receiving sulfasalazine.[457] A patient with "combined features of SLE, polymyositis and RA" developed fatal cholestasis and agranulocytosis.[458]

Hematologic

Hematologic abnormalities during treatment with sulfasalazine have included neutropenia,[379,383,384,387,389,409,425] agranulocytosis,[409,458–465] thrombocytopenia,[425,466] hemolytic anemia,[409,467–472] methemoglobinemia,[437] sulfhemoglobinemia,[437] megaloblastic anemia,[380,384,426–428] and red cell aplasia.[473] The hemolytic anemia has been associated with the slow acetylator phenotype[409] and glucose-6-phosphate dehydrogenase deficiency.[467] Agranulocytosis has proved fatal.[458] Multiple hematologic abnormalities may also appear.[474]

Dermatologic

Various cutaneous eruptions are associated with sulfasalazine therapy. Macular or papular eruptions, which usually occur early in the course of therapy, often within the first 24 hours,[382–385,387–389,409,435,437,445,456] and urticaria are the most common skin reactions.[425,438] Most of these rashes resolve spontaneously after the drug is stopped. Desensitization has been used successfully in some patients.[437,475–477] More serious dermatologic complications of sulfasalazine therapy include toxic epidermal necrolysis (Lyell's syndrome),[478] exfoliative dermatitis,[448] Stevens-John-

son syndrome,[449] and erythema multiforme.[450] "Cyanosis" without oxygen desaturation, methemoglobinemia, and sulfhemoglobinemia has been reported.[375,409]

Musculoskeletal

Drug-induced SLE has occurred in patients with ulcerative colitis[479,480] or Sjogren's syndrome treated with sulfasalazine.[481] Isolated Raynaud's phenomenon has accompanied sulfasalazine treatment.[482] In each of these cases symptoms resolved when therapy was stopped and returned on rechallenge in one case.[480]

Pulmonary

Pulmonary reactions to sulfasalazine are rare but include hypersensitivity pneumonitis,[483–485] subacute fibrosing alveolitis,[486] and tracheolaryngitis with bronchospasm.[437] Hypersensitivity pneumonitis often presents with fever,[483] rashes,[484] dyspnea,[425,484] eosinophilia,[484] and pulmonary infiltrates[483,484] on chest roentgenogram. With drug discontinuation, the symptoms and signs resolve. Reinstitution of sulfasalazine therapy has resulted in recurrent pulmonary disease.[484,485] Subacute fibrosing alveolitis has been fatal.[486] These reactions appear to be idiosyncratic. Pulmonary function tests in patients with inflammatory bowel disease showed no significant changes when patients were taking sulfasalazine.[487]

Reproductive

Reversible male infertility without associated hormonal abnormalities has been reported.[488,489] Specific abnormalities included decreased sperm mobility, disturbed morphology, and reduced density.[488] Although abnormal sperm morphology persisted for up to several months after withdrawal of sulfasalazine, whether or not permanent teratogenic effects occur is still unknown. Fertility can return after the drug is withdrawn.[488,489] Sulfasalazine does not alter fertility in women, but a slight increase in fetal loss without increased congenital abnormalities has been reported.[490,491] Despite these data the use of sulfasalazine should be avoided during pregnancy.

Neurologic

Neurotoxicity includes paresthesias,[425] confusion, neck stiffness, seizures, and ataxia.[455] These symptoms were all reversible on discontinuation of sulfasalazine.

Miscellaneous

Other adverse effects associated with sulfasalazine therapy include tachycardia,[492] glomerulonephritis,[456] and anosmia.[438]

Desensitization

Desensitization has been used in patients with adverse reactions to the drug,[437,475–477] mostly in patients with skin or systemic complaints. Reinstituting sulfasalazine in patients who have had severe side effects is not recommended. Desensitization involves use of initial low doses of sulfasalazine (1 to 125 mg/day) with slow, stepwise increases until therapeutic doses are achieved.

CLINICAL EXPERIENCE

Rheumatoid Arthritis

Suppression of disease activity has been documented in many studies.[375,376,378–389] The major difficulty in assessing these studies has been the failure to include appropriate control groups. In the first controlled trial, Sinclair and Duthie[377] compared patients receiving sulfasalazine to patients given gold or placebo during an intensive inpatient evaluation and therapy program. Although treatment was neither randomized nor blinded, the authors concluded that sulfasalazine was ineffective.[377] More recent trials comparing sulfasalazine to D-penicillamine[382,384,493] or gold[383,384] suggest that the antirheumatic activity of sulfasalazine is comparable to these more traditional agents. Placebo-controlled studies also show that sulfasalazine had greater effect than placebo.[383,389] Sulfasalazine definitely has antirheumatic activity in RA, but the degree of this activity needs better definition.

The optimal dose for use in rheumatic disease has not been defined. Studies in RA patients have generally used either 2 g/day[379,380,382,384–386,435] or 3 g/day,[381,383,387,389] although 4 g/day[378] and 6 g/day have been given.[377] The drug is usually given in three or four divided doses. Side effects increase with the increasing dose. In comparing doses of 1.5 and 3.0 g/day in RA patients stratified according to acetylator phenotype, Pullar et al.[387] found greater improvement in patients given the higher dose. This trial was not designed to test the efficacy of the two doses in all patients but rather to compare efficacy and toxicity relative to acetylator phenotype.

Monitoring sulfasalazine treatment of RA is still ill defined. Clearly, close clinical and laboratory followup is needed during the first 3 months of therapy, as the majority of toxic reactions occur during this period.[425] Rash and gastrointestinal side effects are easily detected clinically; monitoring for hematologic complications (primarily neutropenias) requires complete blood counts, including platelets and differential leukocyte counts at regular intervals. Suggested monitoring frequencies vary from every 2 to 4 weeks. Studies obtained every 2 weeks for the first 3 months and monthly thereafter appear prudent. Liver enzyme levels should be obtained at least quarterly.

Ankylosing Spondylitis

Placebo-controlled trials of 37[390] and 60[392] patients with ankylosing spondylitis reported significant improvement with added sulfasalazine compared to the use of the baseline nonsteroidal anti-inflammatory medication only. Assessment of drug effect in these studies primarily relied on subjective improvement of pain and stiffness.

Miscellaneous

Apart from the studies in RA and ankylosing spondylitis, there are few controlled trials of sulfasalazine in the treatment of other rheumatic diseases. Uncontrolled trials in reactive arthritis,[393,394] scleroderma,[395,396] and juvenile rheumatoid arthritis[398] have reported improvement. The improvement seen in patients with HLA-B27 related arthritis during sulfasalazine therapy may be related to treatment of subclinical inflammatory bowel disease.[432]

SUMMARY

Although not yet approved by the FDA for the treatment of any rheumatic disease, sulfasalazine holds promise as a potential agent for the treatment of RA and other rheumatic disorders. Tolerability appears similar to or better than that seen when it is used to treat inflammatory bowel disease, perhaps related to the use of lower doses. Additional studies should clarify its comparative efficacy and its role relative to the standard "second-line" agents now available for the treatment of RA.

REFERENCES

1. Dameshek, W., and Schwartz, R.: Treatment of certain "autoimmune" diseases with antimetabolites; a preliminary report. Trans. Assoc. Am. Physicians, 73:113–127, 1960.
2. Myles, A.B.: 6-Mercaptopurine (6 M.P.) in the treatment of rheumatoid arthritis and related conditions. Ann. Rheum. Dis., 24:179–180, 1965.
3. Elion, G.B.: Biochemistry and pharmacology of purine analogues. Fed. Proc., 26:898–904, 1967.
4. Elion, C.B., and Hitchings, G.H.: Azathioprine. In Antineoplastic and Immunosuppressive Agents. Part 2. Edited by C. Sartorelli and D.G. Johns. Berlin, Springer-Verlag, 1975.
5. Lorenzen, I., and Videbaek, A.: Treatment of collagen diseases with cytostatics. Lancet, 2:558–561, 1965.
6. Corley, C.C., Lessner, H.E., and Larsen, W.E.: Azathioprine therapy of "autoimmune" diseases. Am. J. Med., 41:404–412, 1966.

7. Philips, V.K., Bergen, W., and Rothermich, N.O.: Azathioprine therapy in twenty-five patients with rheumatoid arthritis. Arthritis Rheum., 10:305, 1967.

8. Mason, M., et al.: Azathioprine in rheumatoid arthritis. Br. Med. J., 1:420–422, 1969.

9. Harris, J., Jessop, J.D., and deSaintonge, D.M.C.: Further experience with azathioprine in rheumatoid arthritis. Br. Med. J., 4:463–464, 1971.

10. Levy, J., et al.: A double-blind controlled evaluation of azathioprine treatment in rheumatoid arthritis and psoriatic arthritis. Arthritis Rheum., 15:116–117, 1972.

11. Urowitz, M.B., et al.: Azathioprine in rheumatoid arthritis. A double-blind, cross-over study. Arthritis Rheum., 16:411–418, 1973.

12. Urowitz, M.B., et al.: Azathioprine in rheumatoid arthritis: A double-blind study comparing full dose to half dose. J. Rheumatol., 1:274–281, 1974.

13. Hunter, T., et al.: Azathioprine in rheumatoid arthritis. A long-term follow-up study. Arthritis Rheum., 18:15–20, 1975.

14. Pinals, R.S.: Azathioprine in the treatment of chronic polyarthritis: Longterm results and adverse effects in 25 patients. J. Rheumatol., 3:140–144, 1976.

15. DeSilva, M., and Hazleman, B.L.: Long-term azathioprine in rheumatoid arthritis: A double-blind study. Ann. Rheum. Dis., 40:560–563, 1981.

16. Thompson, P.W., Kirwan, J.R., and Barnes, C.G.: Practical results of treatment with disease-modifying antirheumatoid drugs. Br. J. Rheumatol., 24:167–175, 1985.

17. Austin, H.A., III: Therapy of lupus nephritis. Controlled trial of prednisone and cytotoxic drugs. N. Engl. J. Med., 314:614–619, 1986.

18. Steinberg, A.D., and Decker, J.L.: A double-blind controlled trial comparing cyclophosphamide, azathioprine and placebo in the treatment of lupus glomerulonephritis. Arthritis Rheum., 17:923–937, 1974.

19. Decker, J.L., et al.: Cyclophosphamide or azathioprine in lupus glomerulonephritis: A controlled trial: Results at 28 months. Ann. Intern. Med., 83:606–615, 1975.

20. Klippel, H.J.: Studies in the treatment of lupus nephritis. In Systemic lupus erythematosus: Evolving concepts. Moderated by J.L Decker. Ann. Intern. Med., 91:587–604, 1979.

21. Dinant, H.J., et al.: Alternative modes of cyclophosphamide and azathioprine therapy in lupus nephritis. Ann. Intern. Med., 96:728–736, 1982.

22. Carette, S., et al.: Controlled studies of oral immunosuppressive drugs in lupus nephritis: A long-term follow-up. Ann. Intern. Med., 99:1–8, 1983.

23. Sztejnbok, M., Stewart, A., Diamond, H., and Kaplan, D.: Azathioprine in the treatment of systemic lupus erythematosus. A controlled study. Arthritis Rheum., 14:639–645, 1971.

24. Gelfand, M.C., and Steinberg, A.D.: Therapeutic studies in NZB/W mice. II. Relative efficacy of azathioprine, cyclophosphamide and methylprednisolone. Arthritis Rheum., 15:247–252, 1972.

25. Cade, R., et al.: Comparison of azathioprine, prednisone, heparin alone or combined in treating lupus nephritis. Nephron, 10:37–56, 1963.

26. Tsokos, G.C., Caughman, S.W., and Klippel, J.H.: Successful treatment of generalized discoid skin lesions with azathioprine. Its use in a patient with systemic lupus erythematosus. Arch. Dermatol., 121:1323–1325, 1985.

27. Bunch, T.W., et al.: Azathioprine with prednisone for polymyositis. A controlled, clinical trial. Ann. Intern. Med., 92:365–369, 1980.

28. Benson, M.D., and Aldo, M.A.: Azathioprine therapy in polymyositis. Arch. Intern. Med., 132:547–551,1973.

29. McFarlin, D.E., and Griggs, R.C.: Treatment of inflammatory myopathies with azathioprine. Trans. Am. Neurol. Assoc., 93:244–246, 1968.

30. Bunch, T.W.: Prednisone and azathioprine for polymyositis. Long-term followup. Arthritis Rheum., 24:45–48, 1981.

31. Huskisson, E.C.: Azathioprine. Clin. Rheum. Dis., 10:325–332,1984.

32. Bach, J-F., and Dardenne, M.: The metabolism of azathioprine in renal failure. Transplantation, 12:253–259, 1971.

33. Clements, P.J., and Davis, J.: Cytotoxic drugs: Their clinical application to the rheumatic diseases. Semin. Arthritis Rheum., 15:231–254, 1986.

34. Bertino, J.R.: Chemical action and pharmacology of methotrexate, azathioprine and cyclophosphamide in man. Arthritis Rheum., 16:79–83, 1973.

35. Bach, J., and Dardenne, M.: Serum immunosuppressive activity of azathioprine in normal subjects and patients with liver diseases. Proc. R. Soc. Med., 65:260–263, 1972.

36. Ware, A.J., et al.: Etiology of liver disease in renal transplant patients. Ann. Intern. Med., 91:364–371, 1979.

37. Maddocks, J.L.: Clinical pharmacological observations on azathioprine in kidney transplant patients. Clin. Sci. Mol. Med., 55:20P, 1978.

38. Coffey, J.J., et al.: Effect of allopurinol on the pharmacokinetics of 6-mercaptopurine (NSC 755) in cancer patients. Cancer Res., 32:1283–1289, 1972.

39. Bailey, R.R.: Leukopenia due to a trimethoprim–azathioprine interaction. N.Z. Med. J., 97:739, 1984.

40. LePage, G.A.: Incorporation of 6-thioguanine into nucleic acids. Cancer Res., 20:403–408, 1960.

41. Prince, H.E., et al.: Azathioprine suppression of natural killer activity and antibody-dependent cellular cytotoxicity in renal transplant recipients. Transplant. Proc., 16:1475–1477, 1984.

42. Al-Safi, S.A., and Maddocks, J.L.: Strength of the human mixed lymphocyte reaction (MLR) and its suppression by azathioprine or 6-mercaptopurine. Br. J. Clin. Pharmacol., 19:105–107, 1985.

43. Abdou, N.I., Zweiman, B., and Casella, S.R.: Effects of azathioprine therapy on bone marrow-dependent and thymus-dependent cells in man. Clin. Exp. Immunol., 13:55–64, 1973.

44. Maddocks, H.L., and Al-Safi, S.A.: Lack of inhibition of purine nucleoside phosphorylase and adenosine deaminase in patients treated with azathioprine. Br. J. Clin. Pharmacol., 19:108–111, 1985.

45. Hahn, B.H., et al.: Comparison of therapeutic and immunosuppressive effects of azathioprine, prednisolone and combined therapy in NZP/NZW mice. Arthritis Rheum., 16:163–170, 1973.

46. Gelfand, M.C., et al.: Therapeutic studies in NZB/W mice. I. Synergy of azathioprine, cyclophosphamide and methylprednisolone in combination. Arthritis Rheum., 15:239–246, 1972.

47. Berry, H., et al.: Azathioprine and penicillamine in treatment of rheumatoid arthritis: A controlled trial. Br. Med. J., 1:1052–1054, 1976.

48. Dwosh, J.L., et al.: Azathioprine in early rheumatoid arthritis. Comparison with gold and chloroquine. Arthritis Rheum., 20:685–692, 1977.

49. Currey, H.L.F., et al.: Comparison of azathioprine, cyclophosphamide, and gold in treatment of rheumatoid arthritis. Br. Med. J., 3:763–766, 1974.

50. Berry, H., et al.: Trial comparing azathioprine and penicillam-

ine in treatment of rheumatoid arthritis. Ann. Rheum. Dis., **35**:542–543, 1976.

51. Paulus, H.E., et al.: Azathioprine versus D-penicillamine in rheumatoid arthritis patients who have been treated unsuccessfully with gold. Arthritis Rheum., *27*:721–727, 1984.

52. Woodland, J., et al.: Azathioprine in rheumatoid arthritis: Double-blind study of full versus half doses versus placebo. Ann. Rheum. Dis., *40*:355–359, 1981.

53. Old, C.W., et al.: Azathioprine-induced pure red blood cell aplasia. JAMA, *240*:552–554, 1978.

54. Halberg, P., et al.: Double-blind trial of levamisone, penicillamine and azathioprine in rheumatoid arthritis. Dan. Med. Bull., *31*:403–409, 1984.

55. Cade, R., et al.: Low dose, long-term treatment of rheumatoid arthritis with azathioprine. South. Med. J., *69*:388–392, 1976.

56. Guillaume, P., Grandjean, E., and Male, P.J.: Azathioprine-associated acute pancreatitis in the course of chronic active hepatitis. Dig. Dis. Sci., *29*:78–80, 1984.

57. Taft, P.M., Jones, A.C., Collins, G.M., and Halacz, N.A.: Acute pancreatitis following renal transplantation. A lethal complication. Am. J. Dig. Dis., *23*:541–544, 1978.

58. Kawanishi, H., Randolph, E., and Bull, F.E.: Azathioprine-induced acute pancreatitis. N. Engl. J. Med., *289*:357, 1973.

59. Zarday, Z., et al.: Irreversible liver damage after azathioprine. JAMA, *222*:690–691, 1972.

60. DePinho, R.A., Goldberg, C.S., and Lefkowitch, J.H.: Azathioprine and the liver. Evidence favoring idiosyncratic, mixed cholestatic-hepatocellular injury in humans. Gastroenterology, *86*:162–165, 1984.

61. DuVivier, A., Munro, D.D., and Verbov, J.: Treatment of psoriasis with azathioprine. Br. Med. J., *1*:49–51, 1974.

62. Munro, D.D.: Azathioprine in psoriasis. Proc. R. Soc. Med., *66*:747–748, 1973.

63. Sparberg, M., Simon, N., and Del Greco, F.: Intrahepatic cholestasis due to azathioprine. Gastroenterology, *57*:439–441, 1969.

64. Bedrossian, C.W.M., et al.: Azathioprine-associated interstitial pneumonitis. Am. J. Clin. Pathol., *82*:148–154, 1984.

65. Carmichael, D.J.S., et al.: Interstitial pneumonitis secondary to azathioprine in a renal transplant patient. Thorax, *38*:951–952, 1983.

66. Saarikoski, S., and Seppala, M.: Immunosuppression during pregnancy: Transmission of azathioprine and its metabolites from the mother to the fetus. Am. J. Obstet. Gynecol., *115*:1100–1106, 1973.

67. Sharon, E., et al.: Pregnancy and azathioprine in systemic lupus erythematosus. Am. J. Obstet. Gynecol., *118*:25–28, 1974.

68. DeWitte, D.B., et al.: Neonatal pancytopenia and severe combined immunodeficiency associated with antenatal administration of azathioprine and prednisone. J. Pediatr., *105*:625–628, 1984.

69. Cote, C.J., Meuwissen, H.J., and Pickering, R.J.: Effects on the neonate of prednisone and azathioprine administered to the mother during pregnancy. J. Pediatr., *85*:324–328, 1974.

70. Leb, D.W., Weisskopf, B., and Kanovitz, B.S.: Chromosome aberrations in the child of a kidney transplant recipient. Arch. Intern. Med., *128*:441–444, 1971.

71. Penn, I., Halgrimson, C.G., and Starzl, T.E.: De novo malignant tumors in organ transplant recipients. Transplant. Proc., *3*:773–778, 1971.

72. Hoover, R., and Fraument, J.R., Jr.: Risk of cancer in renal-transplant recipients. Lancet, *2*:55–57, 1973.

73. Seidenfeld, A.M., et al.: Acute leukemia in rheumatoid arthritis treated with cytotoxic agents. J. Rheumatol., *11*:586–587, 1984.

74. Tilson, H.H., and Whisnant, J.: Pharmaco-epidemiology—drugs, arthritis, and neoplasms: Industry contribution to the data. Am. J. Med., *78*(Suppl. 1A):69–76, 1985.

75. Kinlen, L.J., et al.: Collaborative United Kingdom–Australasian study of cancer in patients treated with immunosuppressive drugs. Br. Med. J., *2*:1461–1466, 1979.

76. Prior, P., et al.: Cancer morbidity in rheumatoid arthritis. Ann. Rheum. Dis., *43*:128–131, 1984.

77. Symmons, D.P.M.: Lymphoproliferative malignancy in rheumatoid arthritis: A study of 20 cases. Ann. Rheum. Dis., *43*:132–135, 1984.

78. Isomaki, H.A., Mutru, O., and Koota, K.: Death rate and causes of death in patients with rheumatoid arthritis. Scand. J. Rheumatol., *4*:205–208, 1975.

79. Prior, P.: Cancer and rheumatoid arthritis: Epidemiologic considerations. Am. J. Med., *78*(Suppl. 1A):15–21, 1985.

80. Symmons, D.P.M.: Neoplasms of the immune system in rheumatoid arthritis. Am. J. Med., *78*(Suppl. 1A):22–28, 1985.

81. Hazleman, B.: Incidence of neoplasms in patients with rheumatoid arthritis exposed to different treatment regimens. Am. J. Med., *78*(Suppl. 1A):39–43, 1985.

82. Kinlen, L.J.: Incidence of cancer in rheumatoid arthritis and other disorders after immunosuppressive treatment. Am. J. Med., *78*(Suppl. 1A):45–49, 1985.

83. Lewis, P., Hazleman, B.L., Hanka, R., and Roberts, S.: Cause of death in patients with rheumatoid arthritis with particular reference to azathioprine. Ann. Rheum. Dis., *39*:457–461, 1980.

84. Fathring, M.J.G., Coxon, A.Y., and Sheaff, P.C.: Polyneuritis associated with azathioprine sensitivity reaction. Br. Med. J., *280*:367, 1980.

85. Balow, J.E., et al.: Lupus nephritis. Ann. Intern. Med., *106*:79–94, 1987.

86. Fauci, A.S., et al.: Cyclophosphamide therapy of severe systemic necrotizing vasculitis. N. Engl. J. Med., *301*:235–238, 1979.

87. Brandwein, S., et al.: Wegener's granulomatosis. Clinical features and outcome in 13 patients. Arch. Intern. Med., *143*:476–479, 1983.

88. Weiner, S.R., and Paulus, S.R.: Treatment of Wegener's granulomatosis with cyclophosphamide: Outcome analysis. Arthritis Rheum., *26*:S65, 1983.

89. Hall, S., et al.: Takayasu arteritis. A study of 32 North American patients. Medicine, *64*:89–99, 1985.

90. Lanham, J.G., et al.: Systemic vasculitis with asthma and esoinophilia: A clinical approach to the Churg-Strauss syndrome. Medicine, *63*:65–81, 1984.

91. Leib, E.S., Restivo, C., and Paulus, H.E.: Immunosuppressive and corticosteroid therapy of polyarteritis nodosa. Am. J. Med., *67*:941–947, 1979.

92. Panush, R.S., et al.: Weber-Christian disease: Analysis of 15 cases and review of the literature. Medicine, *64*:181–191, 1985.

93. Gubner, R., August, S., and Ginsberg, V.: Therapeutic suppression of tissue reactivity. II. Effect of aminopterin in rheumatoid arthritis and psoriasis. Am. J. Med. Sci., *221*:176–182, 1951.

94. Hoffmeister, R.T.: Methotrexate in rheumatoid arthritis. Arthritis Rheum., *15*:114, 1972.

95. Wilke, W.S., Calabrese, L.H., and Scherbel, A.L.: Methotrexate in the treatment of rheumatoid arthritis. Pilot study. Cleve. Clin. Q., *47*:305–309, 1980.

96. Willkens, R.F., Watson, M.A., and Paxson, C.S.: Low dose

pulse methotrexate therapy in rheumatoid arthritis. J. Rheumatol., 7:501–505, 1980.

97. Steinsson, K., Weinstein, A., Korn, J., and Abeles, M.: Low dose methotrexate in rheumatoid arthritis. J. Rheumatol., 9:860–866, 1982.

98. Groff, G.D., Shenberger, K.N., Wilke, W.S., and Taylor, T.H.: Low dose oral methotrexate in rheumatoid arthritis: An uncontrolled trial and review of the literature. Semin. Arthritis Rheum., 12:333–347, 1983.

99. Michaels, R.M., et al.: Weekly intravenous methotrexate in the treatment of rheumatoid arthritis. Arthritis Rheum., 25:339–341, 1982.

100. Willkens, R.F., and Watson, M.A.: Methotrexate: A perspective of its use in the treatment of rheumatic diseases. J. Lab. Clin. Med., 100:314–321, 1982.

101. Hoffmeister, R.T.: Methotrexate therapy in rheumatoid arthritis: 15 years experience. Am. J. Med., 12(Suppl.):69–73, 1983.

102. Thompson, R.N., et al.: A controlled two-centre trial of parenteral methotrexate therapy for refractory rheumatoid arthritis. J. Rheumatol., 11:760–763, 1984.

103. Andersen, P.A., et al.: Weekly pulse methotrexate in rheumatoid arthritis. Clinical and immunologic effects in a randomized, double-blind study. Ann. Intern. Med., 103:489–496, 1985.

104. Williams, H.J., et al.: Comparison of low-dose oral pulse methotrexate and placebo in the treatment of rheumatoid arthritis. A controlled clinical trial. Arthritis Rheum., 28:721–730, 1985.

105. Wilke, W.S., et al.: 24 week double-blind crossover study of methotrexate in rheumatoid arthritis. (Abstract.) Clin. Res., 33:884A, 1985.

106. Weinblatt, M.E., et al.: Efficacy of low-dose methotrexate in rheumatoid arthritis. N. Engl. J. Med., 312:818–822, 1985.

107. Nyfors, A.: Benefits and adverse drug experiences during long-term methotrexate treatment of 248 psoriatics. Dan. Med. Bull., 25:208–211, 1978.

108. Black, R.L., et al.: Methotrexate therapy in psoriatic arthritis. Double-blind study on 21 patients. JAMA, 189:743–747, 1964.

109. Kersley, G.D.: Amethopterin (methotrexate) in connective tissue disease—Psoriasis and polyarthritis. Ann. Rheum. Dis., 27:64–66, 1968.

110. Gowans, J.D.C., et al.: Long term therapy of psoriatic and rheumatoid arthritis with oral methotrexate monitored by serial liver biopsies. (Abstract.) Arthritis Rheum., 22:615–616, 1979.

111. Owen, E.T., and Cohen, M.L.: Methotrexate in Reiter's disease. Ann. Rheum. Dis., 38:48–50, 1979.

112. Lally, E.V., and Ho, George, Jr.: A review of methotrexate therapy in Reiter syndrome. Semin. Arthritis Rheum., 15:139–145, 1985.

113. Fischer, T.J., et al.: Childhood dermatomyositis and polymyositis—Treatment with methotrexate and prednisone. Am. J. Dis. Child., 133:386–389, 1979.

114. Metzger, A.L., et al.: Polymyositis and dermatomyositis—Combined methotrexate and corticosteroid therapy. Ann. Intern. Med., 81:182–189, 1974.

115. Sokoloff, M.C., Goldberg, L.S., and Pearson, C.M.: Treatment of corticosteroid resistant polymyositis with methotrexate. Lancet, 1:14–16, 1971.

116. Arnett, F.C., et al.: Methotrexate therapy in polymyositis. Ann. Rheum. Dis., 32:536–546, 1973.

117. Weinstein, A., Marlowe, S., Korn, J., and Farouhar, F.: Low-

118. dose methotrexate treatment of rheumatoid arthritis. Long-term observations. Am. J. Med., 79:331–337, 1985.

118. Kremer, J.M., and Lee, J.K.: The safety and efficacy of the use of methotrexate in long-term therapy for rheumatoid arthritis. Arthritis Rheum., 29:822–831,1986.

119. Fehlauer, C.S., Carson, C.W., Cannon, G.W., and Ward, J.R.: Two year follow-up of efficacy and toxicity of methotrexate therapy in rheumatoid arthritis. Arthritis Rheum., 29(Suppl.):S76, 1986.

120. Weinblatt, M.E., et al.: Long term prospective study of methotrexate in rheumatoid arthritis. Arthritis Rheum., 29(Suppl.):S76, 1986.

121. Gispen, J.G., et al.: Toxicity to methotrexate in rheumatoid arthritis. J. Rheumatol., 14:74–79, 1987.

122. Jolivet, J., et al.: The pharmacology and clinical use of methotrexate. N. Engl. J. Med., 309:1094–1104, 1983.

123. Balis, F.M., Savitch, J.L., and Bleyer, W.A.: Pharmacokinetics of oral methotrexate in children. Cancer Res., 43:2342–2345, 1983.

124. Craft, A.W., Kay, H.E.M., Lawson, D.N., and McElwain, T.J.: Methotrexate-induced malabsorption in children with acute lymphoblastic leukaemia. Br. Med. J., 2:1511–1512, 1977.

125. Henderson, E.S., Adamson, R.H., and Oliverio, V.T.: The metabolic fate of tritiated methotrexate. II. Absorption and excretion in man. Cancer Res.,25:1018–1023, 1965.

126. Furst, D.E.: Clinical pharmacology of very low dose methotrexate for use in rheumatoid arthritis. J. Rheumatol., 12(Suppl. 12):11–14, 1985.

127. Pinkerton, C.R., Glasgow, J.F.T., Welshman, S.G., and Bridges, J.M.: Can food influence the absorption of methotrexate in children with acute lymphoblastic leukaemia? Lancet, 2:8197–8209, 1980.

128. Taylor, J.R., and Halprin, K.M.: Effect of sodium salicylate and indomethacin on methotrexate-serum albumin binding. Arch. Dermatol., 113:588–591, 1977.

129. Liegler, D.G., et al.: The effect of organic acids on renal clearance of methotrexate in man. Clin. Pharmacol. Ther., 10:849–857, 1969.

130. Edelman, M.B., Biggs, D.F., Jamali, F., and Russell, A.S.: Low-dose methotrexate kinetics in arthritis. Clin. Pharmacol. Ther., 35:382–386, 1984.

131. Goldman, I.D., and Matherly, L.H.: The cellular pharmacology of methotrexate. Pharmacol. Ther., 28:77–102, 1985.

132. Chan, K.K., Nayar, M.S.B., and Cohen, J.L.: Metabolism of methotrexate in man after high and conventional doses. Chem. Pathol. Pharmacol., 28:551–561, 1980.

133. Warren, R.D., Nichols, A.P., and Bender, R.A.: Membrane transport of methotrexate in human lymphoblastoid cells. Cancer Res., 38:668–671, 1978.

134. Hill, B.T., Bailey, B.D., White, J.C., and Goldman, I.D.: Characteristics of transport of 4-amino antifolates and folate compounds by two lines of L5178Y lymphoblasts, one with impaired transport of methotrexate. Cancer Res., 39:2440–2446, 1979.

135. Jolivet, J., Schilsky, R.L., Bailey, B.C., and Chabner, B.A.: The synthesis and retention of methotrexate polyglutamates in cultured human breast cancer cells. Ann. N.Y. Acad. Sci., 397:184–192, 1982.

136. Jolivet, J., and Chabner, B.A.: Intracellular pharmacokinetics of methotrexate polyglutamates in human breast cancer cells: Selective retention and less dissociable binding of 4-NH$_2$-10-CH$_5$PteGlu$_4$ and $_5$ to dihydrofolate reductase. J. Clin. Invest., 72:773–778, 1983.

137. Rosenblatt, D.S., et al.: Prolonged inhibition of DNA synthe-

sis associated with the accumulation of methotrexate poly-glutamates by cultured human cells. Mol. Pharmacol., 14:1143–1147, 1978.

138. Jacobs, S.A., et al.: Stoichiometric inhibition of mammalian dihydrofolate reductase by the gamma-glutamyl metabolite of methotrexate: 4-amino-4-deoxy-N10-methylpteroylglutamyl-gamma-glutamate. Biochem. Biophys. Res. Commun., 63:692–698, 1975.

139. McGuire, J.J., Hsieh, P., Coward, J.K., and Bertino, J.R.: Enzymatic synthesis of folylpolyglutamates: Characterization of the reaction and its products. J. Biol. Chem., 255:5776–5788, 1980.

140. McGuire, J.J., and Bertino, J.R.: Enzymatic synthesis and function of folylpolyglutamates. Mol. Cell Biochem., 38:19–48, 1981.

141. Calvert, A.H., Bondy, P.K., and Harrap, K.R.: Some observations on the human pharmacology of methotrexate. Cancer Treat. Rep., 61:1647–1656, 1977.

142. Hendel, J., and Brodthagen, H.: Enterohepatic cycling of methotrexate estimated by the use of the D-isomer as a reference marker. Eur. J. Clin. Pharmacol., 26:103–107, 1984.

143. Steinberg, S.E., et al.: Enterohepatic circulation of methotrexate in rats in vivo. Cancer Res.,42:1279–1282, 1982.

144. Evans, W.E., and Christensen, M.L.: Drug interactions with methotrexate. J. Rheumatol., 12(Suppl. 12):15–20, 1985.

145. Daly, H.M., Scott, G.L., Boyle, J., and Roberts, C.J.C.: Methotrexate toxicity precipitated by azapropazone. Br. J. Dermatol., 114:733–735, 1986.

146. Thyss, A., et al.: Clinical and pharmacokinetic evidence of a life-threatening interaction between methotrexate and ketoprofen. Lancet, 1:256–258, 1986.

147. Cohen, M.N., et al.: Effect of oral prophylactic broad spectrum nonabsorbable antibiotics on the gastrointestinal absorption of nutrients and methotrexate in small cell bronchogenic cancer. Cancer, 38:1556–1559, 1976.

148. Dixon, R.L., Henderson, E.S., and Rall, D.P.: Plasma protein binding of methotrexate and its displacement by various drugs. Fed. Proc., 24:454, 1965.

149. Bourke, R.S., et al.: Inhibition of renal tubular transport of methotrexate by probenecid. Cancer Res., 35:110–116, 1975.

150. Nierenberg, D.W.: Competitive inhibition of methotrexate accumulation in rabbit kidney slices by nonsteroidal anti-inflammatory drugs. J. Pharm. Exp. Ther., 226:1–6, 1983.

151. Kates, R.E., Tozer, T.N., and Sorby, D.L.: Increased methotrexate toxicity due to concurrent probenecid administration. Biochem. Pharmacol., 25:1485–1488, 1976.

152. Rooney, T.W., and Furst, D.E.: Comparison of toxicity in methotrexate (MTX) treated rheumatoid arthritis (RA) patients also taking aspirin or other NSAID. Arthritis Rheum., 29(Suppl.):S76, 1986.

153. Chabner, B.A., and Young, R.C.: Threshold methotrexate concentration for in vivo inhibition of DNA synthesis in normal and tumorous target issues. J. Clin. Invest., 52:1804–1811, 1973.

154. Smith, G.K., Benkovic, P.A., and Benkovic, S.J.: L(−)-10-formyltetra-hydrofolate is the cofactor for glycinamide ribonucleotide transformylase from chicken liver. Biochemistry, 20:4034–4036, 1981.

155. Zaharko, D.S., Fung, W.-P., and Yang, K.-H.: Relative biochemical aspects of low and high doses of methotrexate in mice. Cancer Res., 37:1602–1607, 1977.

156. Galivan, J.: Evidence for the cytotoxic activity of polyglutamate derivatives of methotrexate. Mol. Pharmacol., 17:105–110, 1980.

157. Sikes, D.H., et al.: Lack of inhibition of thymidylate synthetase activity with low dose oral methotrexate in rheumatoid arthritis. Arthritis Rheum., 29(Suppl.):S18, 1986.

158. O'Callaghan, J.W., Bretscher, P., and Russell, A.S.: The effect of low dose chronic intermittent parental methotrexate on delayed type hypersensitivity and acute inflammation in a mouse model. J. Rheumatol., 13:710–714, 1986.

159. Johnston, C.A., Russell, A.S., Kovithavongs, T., and Dasgupta, M.: Measures of immunologic and inflammatory responses in vitro in rheumatoid patients treated with methotrexate. J. Rheumatol., 13:294–296, 1986.

160. Kremer, J.M.: Lymphocyte subset analysis after long-term methotrexate therapy for rheumatoid arthritis. Arthritis Rheum., 29(Suppl.):S75, 1986.

161. Olsen, N., Baer, A., and Pincus, T.: Methotrexate induces early, specific decreases in IgM-rheumatoid factor synthesis in rheumatoid arthritis patients. Arthritis Rheum., 29(Suppl.):S75, 1986.

162. Cream, J.J., and Pole, D.S.: The effect of methotrexate and hydroxyurea on neutrophil chemotaxis. Br. J. Dermatol., 102:557–563, 1980.

163. Suarez, C.R., et al.: Effect of low dose methotrexate on neutrophil chemotaxis induced by leukotriene B4 and complement C5a. J. Rheumatol., 14:9–11, 1987.

164. Marhaugh, G., Bratlid, D., and Moe, P.J.: Effect of methotrexate on phagocytosis and killing of staphylococcus aureus and human granulocytes. Scand. J. Infect. Dis., 12:61–65, 1980.

165. Matheson, D.S., Green, B., and Hoar, D.I.: The influence of methotrexate and thymidine on the human natural killer cell function in vitro. J. Immunol., 131:1619–1621, 1983.

166. Welles, W.L., et al.: Studies on the effect of low dose methotrexate on rat adjuvant arthritis. J. Rheumatol., 12:904–906, 1985.

167. Kourounakis, L., and Kapusta, M.A.: Restoration of diminished T-cell function in adjuvant induced disease by methotrexate: Evidence for two populations of splenic T-cell suppressors. J. Rheumatol., 3:346–354, 1976.

168. Mizushima, Y., Tsukada, W., and Akimoto, T.: A modification of rat adjuvant arthritis for testing antirheumatic drugs. J. Pharm. Pharmacol., 24:781–785, 1972.

169. Ward, J.R., Cloud, R.S., Krawitt, E.L., and Jones, R.S.: Studies on adjuvant-induced polyarthritis in rats. III. The effect of "immunosuppressive agents" on arthritis and tuberculin hypersensitivity. Arthritis Rheum., 7:654–661, 1964.

170. Boh, L., et al.: Long term use of methotrexate (MTX) in inflammatory arthritis: Clinical and X-ray evaluation. Arthritis Rheum., 28(Suppl.):S46, 1985.

171. Mihranian, M.H., Wang, Y.M., and Daly, J.M.: Effects of nutritional depletion and repletion on plasma methotrexate pharmacokinetics. Cancer, 54:2268–2271, 1984.

172. Alarcón, G.S., et al.: Toxicity to methotrexate in rheumatoid arthritis: Clinical and HLA studies. (Abstract.) Arthritis Rheum., 28:S36, 1985.

173. Podurgiel, B.J., et al.: Liver injury associated with methotrexate therapy for psoriasis. Mayo Clin. Proc., 48:787–792, 1973.

174. Nyfors, A.: Liver biopsies from psoriatics related to methotrexate therapy. Acta Pathol. Microbiol. Scand. [A], 85:511–518, 1977.

175. Robinson, J.K., Baughman, R.D., Auerbach, R., and Cimis, R.J.: Methotrexate hepatotoxicity in psoriasis. Consideration of liver biopsies at regular intervals. Arch. Dermatol., 116:413–415, 1980.

176. Zachariae, H., Kragballe, K., and Sogaard, H.: Methotrexate induced liver cirrhosis. Br. J. Derm., *102*:407–412, 1980.

177. Geronemus, R.G., Auerbach, R., and Tobias, H.: Liver biopsies v liver scans in methotrexate-treated patients with psoriasis. Arch. Dermatol., *118*:649–651, 1982.

178. Lanse, S.B., Arnold, G.L., Gowans, J.D.C., and Kaplan, M.M.: Low incidence of hepatotoxicity associated with long-term, low-dose oral methotrexate in treatment of refractory psoriasis, psoriatic arthritis, and rheumatoid arthritis. An acceptable risk/benefit ratio. Dig. Dis. Sci., *30*:104–109, 1985.

179. Miller, J.A., et al: Ultrasound as a screening procedure for methotrexate-induced hepatic damage in severe psoriasis. Br. J. Dermatol., *113*:699–705, 1985.

180. Tolman, K.G., Clegg, D.O., Lee, R.G., and Ward, J.R.: Methotrexate and the liver. J. Rheumatol., *12*(Suppl. 12):29–34, 1985.

181. Roenigk, H.H., Jr., et al.: Methotrexate guidelines, revised. J. Am. Acad. Dermatol., *6*:145–155, 1982.

182. Rolf, R., and Karger, T.: Liver biopsy findings in patients with rheumatoid arthritis and psoriatic arthritis on long-term treatment with methotrexate. Arthritis Rheum., *29*(Suppl.):S76, 1986.

183. Dahl, M.G., Gregory, M.M., and Scheuer, P.J.: Methotrexate hepatotoxicity in psoriasis—Comparison of different dose regimens. Br. Med. J., *1*:644–656, 1972.

184. Boh, L.E., et al.: Low-dose weekly oral methotrexate therapy for inflammatory arthritis. Clin. Pharmacol., *5*:503–508, 1986.

185. Kersey, P., and Dahl, M.: Comparison of liver scans and liver biopsies in patients with psoriasis. Br. J. Dermatol., *103*(Suppl. 18):15–16, 1980.

186. FitzGerald, O., Hanly, J., Molony, J., and Bresnihan, B.: Poor long-term results from low-dose methotrexate therapy in rheumatoid arthritis. Letter to the Editor. Arthritis Rheum., *27*:599–600, 1984.

187. Trier, J.S.: Morphological alterations induced by methotrexate in the mucosa of human proximal intestine. Gastroenterology, *42*:295–305, 1962.

188. Gwavava, N.J.T., et al.: Small bowel enterocyte abnormalities caused by methotrexate treatment in acute lymphoblastic leukaemia of childhood. J. Clin. Pathol., *34*:790–795, 1981.

189. Cunningham, D., et al.: Functional and structural changes of the human proximal small intestine after cytotoxic therapy. J. Clin Pathol., *38*:265–270, 1985.

190. Craft, W.W., Rankin, A., Aherne, W.: Methotrexate absorption in children with acute lymphoblastic leukemia. Cancer Treat. Rep., *65*(Suppl. 1):77–81, 1981.

191. MacKinnon, S.K., Starkebaum, G., and Willkens, R.F.: Pancytopenia associated with low dose pulse methotrexate in the treatment of rheumatoid arthritis. Semin. Arthritis Rheum., *15*:119–126, 1985.

192. Carson, C.W., et al.: Pulmonary disease during the treatment of rheumatoid arthritis with low dose pulse methotrexate. Semin. Arthritis Rheum., *16*:186–195, 1987.

193. Cannon, G.W., et al.: Acute lung disease associated with low-dose pulse methotrexate therapy in patients with rheumatoid arthritis. Arthritis Rheum., *26*:1269–1274, 1983.

194. Engelbrecht, J.A., Calhoon, S.L., and Scherrer, J.J.: Methotrexate pneumonitis after low-dose therapy for rheumatoid arthritis. Arthritis Rheum., *26*:1275–1278, 1983.

195. St Clair, E.W., Rice, J.R., and Snyderman, R.: Pneumonitis complicating low-dose methotrexate therapy in rheumatoid arthritis. Arch. Intern. Med., *245*:2035–2038, 1985.

196. Bell, M.J., Geddie, W.R., Gordon, D.A., and Reynolds, W.J.: Pre-existing lung disease in patients with rheumatoid arthritis may predispose to methotrexate lung. Arthritis Rheum., *29*(Suppl.):S75, 1986.

197. Goldman, G.C., and Moschella, S.L.: Severe pneumonitis occurring during methotrexate therapy. Report of two cases. Arch. Dermatol., *103*:194–197, 1971.

198. Everts, C.S., Westcott, J.L., and Bragg, D.G.: Methotrexate therapy and pulmonary disease. Radiology, *107*:539–543, 1973.

199. Lascari, A.D., Strano, A.J., Johnson, W.W., and Collins, J.G.P.: Methotrexate-induced sudden fatal pulmonary reaction. Cancer, *40*:1393–1397, 1977.

200. Clarysse, A.M., Cathey, W.J., Cartwright, G.E., and Wintrobe, M.M.: Pulmonary disease complicating intermittent therapy with methotrexate. JAMA, *209*:1861–1864, 1969.

201. Acute Leukemia Group B Cooperative Study: Acute lymphocytic leukemia in children. Maintenance therapy with methotrexate administered intermittently. JAMA, *207*:923–928, 1969.

202. Filip, D.A., Logue, G.L., Harle, T.S., and Farrar, W.H.: Pulmonary and hepatic complications of methotrexate therapy of psoriasis. JAMA, *216*:881–882, 1971.

203. Sostman, H.D., Matthay, R.A., Putnam, C.E., and Smith, W.G.J.: Methotrexate-induced pneumonitis. Medicine, *55*:371–388, 1976.

204. Whitcomb, M.E., Schwarz, M.I., and Tormey, D.C.: Methotrexate pneumonitis: Case report and review of the literature. Thorax, *27*:636–639, 1972.

205. Kaplan, R.L., and Waite, D.H.: Progressive interstitial lung disease from prolonged methotrexate therapy. Arch. Dermatol., *114*:1800–1802, 1978.

206. Bedrossian, C.W.M., Miller, W.C., and Luna, M.A.: Methotrexate-induced diffuse interstitial pulmonary fibrosis. South. Med. J., *72*:313–318, 1979.

207. Martino, R.L., et al.: Transient neurologic dysfunction following moderate-dose methotrexate for undifferentiated lymphoma. Cancer, *54*:2003–2005, 1984.

208. Jaffe, N., Takaue, Y., Takashi, A., and Robertson, R.: Transient neurologic disturbances induced by high-dose methotrexate treatment. Cancer, *56*:1356–1360, 1985.

209. Bleyer, W.A., Drake, J.C., and Chabner, B.A.: Neurotoxicity and elevated cerebrospinal-fluid methotrexate concentration in meningeal leukemia. N. Engl. J. Med., *289*:770–773, 1973.

210. Gagliano, R.G., and Costanzi, J.J.: Paraplegia following intrathecal methotrexate. Cancer, *37*:1663–1668, 1976.

211. Duller, P., and van de Kerhof, P.C.M.: Impact of methotrexate on psycho-organic functioning. Letter to Editor. Br. J. Dermatol., *113*:503–504, 1985.

212. Ibsen, H.H.W.: Electroencephalographic examination in seven patients treated with methotrexate for psoriasis. Acta Pharmacol. Toxicol. (Copenh), *58*:303–304, 1986.

213. Doyle, L.A., Gerg, C., Bottino, G., and Chabner, B.: Erythema and desquamation after high-dose methotrexate. Ann. Intern. Med., *98*:611–612, 1983.

214. Lawrence, C.M., and Dahl, M.G.C.: Two patterns of skin ulceration induced by methotrexate in patients with psoriasis. J. Am. Acad. Dermatol., *11*:1059–1065, 1984.

215. Milunsky, A., Graef, J.W., and Gaynor, M.D.: Methotrexate-induced congenital malformations. J. Pediatr., *72*:790–795, 1968.

216. Warkany, J.: Aminopterin and methotrexate: Folic acid deficiency. Teratology, *17*:353–358, 1978.

217. Rustin, G.J.S., et al.: Pregnancy after cytotoxic chemotherapy for gestational trophoblastic tumours. Br. Med. J., *288*:103–106, 1984.

218. Blatt, J., et al.: Pregnancy outcome following cancer chemotherapy. Am. J. Med., 69:828–832, 1980.

219. Ross, G.T.: Congenital anomalies among children born of mothers receiving chemotherapy for gestational trophoblastic neoplasms. Cancer, 37:1043–1047, 1976.

220. El-Beheiry, A., El-Mansy, E., Kamel, N., and Salama, N.: Methotrexate and fertility in men. Arch. Androl., 3:177–179, 1979.

221. Sussman, A., and Leonard, J.M.: Psoriasis, methotrexate and oligospermia. Arch. Dermatol., 116:215–217, 1980.

222. Lindskov, R., Wulf, H.C., Wantzin, G.L., and Niebuhr, E.: Sister chromatid exchange in patients treated with methotrexate for psoriasis. J. Invest. Dermatol., 82:458–459, 1984.

223. Bailin, P.L., et al.: Is methotrexate therapy for psoriasis carcinogenic? A modified retrospective analysis. JAMA, 232:359–362, 1975.

224. Rustin, G.J.S., et al.: No increase in second tumors after cytotoxic chemotherapy for gestational trophoblastic tumors. N. Engl. J. Med., 308:473–476, 1983.

225. Colburn, K.K., and Cao, J.D.: Thymoma associated with rheumatoid arthritis in a patient taking methotrexate. J. Rheumatol., 13:437–439, 1986.

226. Harris, C.C.: Malignancy during methotrexate and steroid therapy for psoriasis. Arch. Dermatol., 103:501–504, 1971.

227. Craig, S.R., and Rosenberg, E.W.: Methotrexate-induced carcinoma? Arch. Dermatol., 103:505–506, 1971.

228. Condit, P.T., Chanes, R.E., and Joel, W.: Renal toxicity of methotrexate. Cancer, 23:126–131, 1967.

229. Zachariae, H., Grunnet, E., and Sogaard, H.: Accidental kidney biopsies in psoriasis. Br. J. Dermatol., 94:655–657, 1976.

230. Navarro, M., et al.: Leukocytoclastic vasculitis after high-dose methotrexate. Letter to the Editor. Ann. Intern. Med., 105:471–472, 1986.

231. Marks, C.A., Willkens, R.F., Wilske, K.R., and Brown, P.B.: Small-vessel vasculitis and methotrexate. Ann. Intern. Med., 100:916, 1984.

232. Bachman, D.M.: Pulsed intravenous methotrexate treatment in rheumatoid arthritis. Arthritis Rheum., 25(Suppl.):S65, 1982.

233. Perruquet, J.L., Harrington, T.M., and Davis, D.E.: *Pneumocystis carinii* pneumonia following methotrexate therapy for rheumatoid arthritis. Arthritis Rheum., 26:1291–1292, 1983.

234. Hall, G.G., et al.: Intra-articular methotrexate: Clinical and laboratory study in rheumatoid and psoriatic arthritis. Ann. Rheum. Dis., 37:351–356, 1978.

235. Wigginton, S.M., et al.: Methotrexate pharmacokinetics after intra-articular injection in patients with rheumatoid arthritis. Arthritis Rheum., 23:119–122, 1980.

236. Tiliakos, N.A., Lawrence, T.A.B., and Wilson, C.H.: Intra-articular methotrexate in intractable rheumatoid knees. Arthritis Rheum., 25(Suppl.):S65, 1982.

237. Tiliakos, N.: Pulse methotrexate therapy for intractable rheumatoid cutaneous ulcers. Arthritis Rheum., 28(Suppl.):S37, 1986.

238. Cannon, G.W., et al.: Association of clinical and laboratory parameters in rheumatoid arthritis during treatment with methotrexate. Arthritis Rheum., 29(Suppl.):S75, 1986.

239. Williams, H.J., et al.: Effect of increasing dose of methotrexate in patients with rheumatoid arthritis. Arthritis Rheum., 28(Suppl.):S87, 1986.

240. Willkens, R.F., et al.: Randomized, double-blind, placebo controlled trial of low-dose pulse methotrexate in psoriatic arthritis. Arthritis Rheum., 27:376–381, 1984.

241. Kovarsky, J.: Clinical pharmacology and toxicology of cyclophosphamide: Emphasis on use in rheumatic disease. Semin. Arthritis Rheum., 12:359–372, 1983.

242. Diaz, C.J., Garcia, E.L., and Mechante, A.: Treatment of rheumatoid arthritis with nitrogen mustard. Preliminary report. JAMA, 147:1418–1419, 1951.

243. Calabresi, P., and Parks, R.J., Jr.: Antiproliferative agents and drugs used for immunosuppression. *In* The Pharmacological Basis of Therapeutics. 7th Ed. Edited by A.G. Gilman, L.S. Goodman, T.W. Rall, and F. Murad. New York, Macmillan Publishing Co., 1985.

244. Bagley, C.M., Jr., Bostick, F.W., and DeVita, V.T., Jr.: Clinical pharmacology of cyclophosphamide. Cancer Res., 33:226–233, 1973.

245. McLean, A., Newell, D., and Baker, G.: The metabolism of chlorambucil. Biochem. Pharmacol., 25:2331–2335, 1976.

246. Boston Collaborative Drug Surveillance Program: Allopurinol and cytotoxic drugs. Interaction in relation to bone marrow depression. JAMA, 227:1036–1040, 1974.

247. Vesell, E.W., Passanati, G.T., and Greene, F.E.: Impairment of drug metabolism in man by allopurinol and nortriptyline. N. Engl. J. Med., 283:1484–1488, 1970.

248. Kovacs, K., and Steinberg, A.D.: Cyclophosphamide: Drug interactions and bone marrow transplantation. Transplantation, 13:316–321, 1972.

249. Gaudin, D., and Yielding, K.L.: Response of a "resistant" plasmocytoma to alkylating agents and x-ray in combination with the "exercision repair inhibitors" caffeine and chloroquine. Proc. Soc. Exp. Biol. Med., 131:1413–1416, 1969.

250. Alberts, D.S., and vanDaalen Wetters, T.: The effect of phenobarbital on cyclophosphamide anti-tumor activity. Cancer Res., 36:2785–2789, 1976.

251. Hart, L.G., and Adamson, R.H.: Effect of microsomal enzyme modifiers on toxicity and therapeutic activity of cyclophosphamide in mice. Arch. Int. Pharmacodyn., 180:391–401, 1969.

252. Field, R.B., et al.: The effect of phenobarbital or 2-diethylaminoethyl-2,2-diphenylvalerate on the activation of cyclophosphamide in vivo. J. Pharmacol. Exp. Ther., 180:475–483, 1972.

253. Sladek, N.E.: Therapeutic efficacy of cyclophosphamide as a function of its metabolism. Cancer Res., 32:535–542, 1972.

254. Kayakawa, T., et al.: Effect of steroid hormone on activation of endoxan (cyclophosphamide). Biochem. Pharmacol., 18:129–135, 1969.

255. Shand, F.L., and Howard, J.G.: Induction in vitro of reversible immunosuppression and inhibition of B cell receptor regeneration by defined metabolites of cyclophosphamide. Eur. J. Immunol., 9:17–21, 1979.

256. Turk, J.L., and Poulter, L.W.: Selective depletion of lymphoid tissue by cyclophosphamide. Clin. Exp. Immunol., 10:285–296, 1972.

257. Turk, J.L., and Poulter, L.W.: Effects of cyclophosphamide on lymphoid tissues labeled with 5-iodo-2-deoxyuridine-^{125}I and [51]Cr. Int. Arch. Allergy, 43:620–629, 1972.

258. Stockman, G.D., et al.: Differential effects of cyclophosphamide on the B and T cell compartments of adult mice. J. Immunol., 110:277–282, 1973.

259. Winkelstein, A.: Effect of immunosuppressive drugs on T and B lymphocytes in guinea pigs. Blood, 50:81–91, 1977.

260. Hurd, E.R., and Guiliano, V.J.: The effect of cyclophosphamide on B and T lymphocytes in patients with connective tissue diseases. Arthritis Rheum., 18:67–75, 1975.

261. Clements, P.J., et al.: Effects of cyclophosphamide on B- and

T-lymphocytes in rheumatoid arthritis. Arthritis Rheum., 17:347–353, 1974.

262. Dale, D.C., Fauci, A.S., and Wolff, S.M.: The effect of cyclophosphamide on leukocyte kinetics and susceptibility to infection in patients with Wegener's granulomatosis. Arthritis Rheum., 16:657–664, 1973.

263. Diamantstein, R., Willinger, E., and Reiman, J.: T-suppressor cells sensitive to cyclophosphamide and to its in vitro active derivative 4-hydroperoxycyclophosphamide control: The mitogenic response of murine splenic B cells to dextran sulfate. A direct proof for different sensitivities of lymphocyte subsets to cyclophosphamide. J. Exp. Med., 150:1571–1576, 1979.

264. Kaufman, S.H.E., Hahn, H., and Diamantstein, T.: Relative susceptibilities of T cell subsets involved in delayed-type hypersensitivity to sheep red blood cells to the in vitro action of 4-hydroperoxycyclophosphamide. J. Immunol., 125:1104–1108, 1980.

265. Ozer, H., et al.: In vitro effects of 4-hydroperoxycyclophosphamide on human immunoregulatory T subset function. I. Selective effects on lymphocyte function in T-B cell collaboration. J. Exp. Med., 155:276–290, 1982.

266. Feehally, J., et al.: Modulation of cellular immune function by cyclophosphamide in children with minimal-change nephropathy. N. Engl. J. Med., 310:415–420, 1984.

267. Maguire, H.D., and von Ettore, L.: Enhancement of dinitrochlorobenzene (DNCB) contact sensitization by cyclophosphamide in the guinea pig. J. Invest. Dermatol., 48:39–43, 1967.

268. Turk, J.L., Parker, D., and Poulter, L.W.: Functional aspects of the selective depletion of lymphoid tissue by cyclophosphamide. Immunology, 23:493–501, 1972.

269. Lagrange, P.H., MacKaness, G.B., and Miller, T.E.: Potentiation of T-cell-mediated immunity by selective suppression of antibody formation with cyclophosphamide. J. Exp. Med., 139:1529–1539, 1974.

270. Kerkhaert, J.A.M., Hofhuis, F.M.A., and Willers, J.M.N.: Influence of cyclophosphamide on delayed hypersensitivity and acquired cellular resistance to Listeria monocytogenes in the mouse. Immunology, 32:1027–1032, 1977.

271. Rollinghoff, M., et al.: Cyclophosphamide-sensitive T-lymphocytes suppress the in vivo generation of antigen-specific cytotoxic T-lymphocytes. J. Exp. Med., 45:455–459, 1977.

272. Ferguson, R.M., and Simmons, R.L.: Differential cyclophosphamide sensitivity of suppressor and cytotoxic cell precursors. Transplantation, 25:36–38, 1978.

273. Maguire, H.C.: Specific acquired immune unresponsiveness to contact allergens with cyclophosphamide in the mouse. Int. Arch. Allergy, 50:651–658, 1976.

274. Berenbaum, M.D., and Brown, I.N.: Prolongation of homograft survival in mice with single doses of cyclophosphamide. Nature, 200:84, 1963.

275. Owens, A.H., Jr., and Santos, G.W.: The effect of cytotoxic drugs on graft versus host disease in mice. Transplantation, 11:378–382, 1971.

276. Steinberg, A.D., Daley, G.G., and Talal, N.: Tolerance to polyinosine-polycytidylic acid in NZB/NZW mice. Science, 167:870–871, 1970.

277. Bontoux, D., et al.: Effect and mode of action of chlorambucil in rheumatoid disease. Value of the lymphoblast transformation test. Rev. Rheum. Mal. Osteoartic., 38:759–764, 1971.

278. Kahn, M., and de Seze, S.: Immunosuppression agents in rheumatology. Indications, results, and long-term adverse effects. Ann. Med. Interne (Paris), 125:449–506, 1974.

279. Alpea, F.P., Zvaifler, N.J., and Sliwinski, A.J.: Immunologic

280. Stevenson, H.D., and Fauci, A.S., Activation of human B lymphocytes. XII. Differential effects of in vitro cyclophosphamide on human lymphocyte subpopulations involved in B cell activation. Immunology, 39:391–397, 1980.

281. Santos, G.W., and Owen, A.H.:19S and 7S antibody production in the cyclophosphamide or methotrexate treated rat. Nature, 209:622–624, 1966.

282. Aisenberg, A.C.: Immunosuppression by alkylating agents—tolerance induction. Transplant. Proc., 5:1221–1226, 1973.

283. Kawaguchi, S.: Studies on the induction of immunological paralysis to bovine globulin in adult mice. II. The effect of cyclophosphamide. Immunology, 19:291–299, 1970.

284. Many, A., and Schwartz, R.S.: On the mechanism of immunological tolerance in cyclophosphamide-treated mice. Clin. Exp. Immunol., 6:87–99, 1970.

285. Turk, J.L., and Parker, D.: Further studies on B-lymphocyte suppression in delayed hypersensitivity, indicating a possible mechanism for Jones-Mote hypersensitivity. Immunology, 24:751–758, 1973.

286. Duclos, H., et al.: Enhancing effect of low dose cyclophosphamide on the in vitro antibody response. Eur. J. Immunol., 7:679–684, 1977.

287. Curtis, J.E., et al.: Immune response of patients with rheumatoid arthritis during cyclophosphamide treatment. Arthritis Rheum., 16:34–42, 1973.

288. Hersh, E.M., Wong, V.G., and Freireich, E.J.: Inhibition of the local inflammatory response in man by antimetabolites. Blood, 27:38–48, 1966.

289. Cannon, G.W., et al.: Chlorambucil therapy in rheumatoid arthritis: Clinical experience in 28 patients and literature review. Semin. Arthritis Rheum., 15:106–118, 1985.

290. Renier, J.C., et al.: Le traitement de la polyarthrite rhumatoide par le chlorambucil. Etude de 113 observations. Arch. Med. de l'Ouest, 1:47–58, 1971.

291. Vignon, G., and Bied, J.: Comparative study of the various immunosuppressive agents in rheumatoid arthritis. Rev. Rhum. Mal. Osteoartic., 38:785–795, 1971.

292. Cayla, J., and Rondier, J.: The treatment of 67 cases of rheumatoid arthritis with chlorambucil drugs. Rev. Rhum. Mal. Oseoartic., 38:765–770, 1971.

293. Arlet, J., Mole, J., and Debrock, J.: Our experience of the treatment of chronic rheumatoid arthritis with immunosuppressive drugs; With reference to 41 cases. Rev. Rhum. Mal. Osteoartic., 38:771–774, 1971.

294. Sauvezie, B., et al.: Value of the lymphoblastic transformation test (LTT) with incorporation of titrated thymidine in the supervision of immuno-suppressive treatment in rheumatology. Rev. Rhum. Mal. Osteoartic., 39:609–616, 1972.

295. Renier, J.C., Bregeon, C., Bonnette, C.: Results of immunodepressant treatment in 78 patients suffering from rheumatoid polyarthritis and having undergone treatment for more than four years. Rev. Rhum. Mal. Osteoartic., 42:399–407, 1975.

296. Krel, A., et al.: Cytopenic syndrome in patients treated with leukeran and azathioprine. Sov. Med. 9:68–72, 1979.

297. Amor, B., et al.: Follow-up study of patients and rheumatoid arthritis over a period of more than 10 years (1966–1978): Analysis of disease progression and treatment in 100 cases. Ann. Med. Interne (Paris), 132:168–173, 1981.

298. Renier, J.C., Bregeon, C., and Bonnette, C.: The evolution of patients with rheumatoid arthritis receiving immunosuppressors between 1965 and 1973. Rev. Rhum. Mal. Osteoartic., 45:453–461, 1978.

299. de Seze, S., et al.: Resultats de la therapeutique a viseé immunodepressive chez 40 malade atteint de polyarthrite rhumatoid grave. Sem. Hop. Paris, 43:3084–3091, 1967.

300. Deshayes, P., et al.: Side-effects and complications of immunosuppressive therapy in rheumatoid arthritis. Rev. Rhum. Mal. Osteoartic., 38:797–806, 1971.

301. Fosdick, W.M., Parsons, J.L., and Hill, D.F.: Long-term cyclophosphamide therapy in rheumatoid arthritis. Arthritis Rheum., 11:151–160, 1968.

302. Williams, H.J., et al.: Comparison of high and low dose cyclophosphamide therapy in rheumatoid arthritis. Arthritis Rheum., 23:521–527, 1980.

303. Fries, J.F., et al.: Cyclophosphamide therapy in systemic lupus erythematosus and polymyositis. Arthritis Rheum., 16:154–162, 1973.

304. Aymard, J.P., et al.: Acute leukemia following prolonged chlorambucil treatment of non-neoplastic disease—A study of two cases and literature review. Acta Clin. Belg., 38:228–235, 1983.

305. Townes, A.S., Sowa, J.M., and Shulman, L.E.: Controlled trial of cyclophosphamide in rheumatoid arthritis. Arthritis Rheum., 19:563–573, 1976.

306. Kahn, M.F., et al.: Chlorambucil in rheumatoid arthritis. Rev. Rhum. Mal. Osteoartic., 38:741–748, 1971.

307. Thorpe, P., Hassall, M.B., and York, J.R.: Rheumatoid arthritis treated with chlorambucil: A five-year follow-up. Med. J. Aust., 2:197–199, 1976.

308. Rudd, P., Fries, J.F., and Epstein, W.V.: Irreversible bone marrow failure with chlorambucil. J. Rheumatol., 2:421–429, 1975.

309. Mullins, G.M., and Colvin M.: Intensive cyclophosphamide (NSC-26271) therapy for solid tumors. Cancer Chemother. Rep., 59:411–419, 1975.

310. Cooperating Clinics Committee of the American Rheumatism Association: A controlled trial of cyclophosphamide in rheumatoid arthritis. N. Engl. J. Med., 283:883–889, 1970.

311. Smyth, C.J., et al.: Cyclophosphamide therapy for rheumatoid arthritis. Arch. Intern. Med., 135:789–793, 1975.

312. Bacon, A.M., and Rosenberg, S.A.: Cyclophosphamide hepatotoxicity in a patient with systemic lupus erythematosus. Ann. Intern. Med., 97:62–63, 1982.

313. O'Duffy, T.D., Robertson, D.M., and Goldstein, N.P.: Chlorambucil in the treatment of ureitis and meningoencephalitis of Behçet's disease. Am. J. Med., 76:75–84, 1984.

314. Schein, P.S., and Winokur, S.H.: Immunosuppressive and cytotoxic therapy: Long-term complications. Ann. Intern. Med., 82:84–95, 1975.

315. Marsh, F.P., et al.: Cyclophosphamide necrosis of the bladder causing calcification, contracture and reflux: Treated by colocytoplasty. Br. J. Urol., 43:324–332, 1971.

316. Johnson, W.W., and Meadows, D.C.: Urinary-bladder fibrosis and telangiectasia associated with long-term cyclophosphamide therapy. N. Engl. J. Med., 284:290–294, 1971.

317. Wall, R.L., and Clausen, K.P.: Carcinoma of the urinary bladder in patients receiving cyclophosphamide. N. Engl. J. Med., 293:271–273, 1975.

318. Pearson, R.M., and Soloway, M.S.: Does cyclophosphamide induce bladder cancer? Urology, 11:437–447, 1978.

319. Fairchild, W.V., et al.: The incidence of bladder cancer after cyclophosphamide therapy. J. Urol., 122:163–164, 1979.

320. Scheef, W., et al.: Controlled clinical studies with an antidote against urotoxicity of oxazaphorines: Preliminary results. Cancer Treat. Rep., 63:501–505, 1979.

321. Spector, J.I., Zimbler, H., and Ross, J.S.: Early-onset cyclophosphamide-induced interstitial pneumonitis. JAMA, 242:2852–2854, 1979.

322. Thorpe, P., Hassall, J.E., and York, J.R.: Cytoxic therapy in rheumatoid disease. Med. J. Aust., 2:796–798, 1971.

323. Lakin, J.D., and Cahill, R.A.: Generalized urticaria to cyclophosphamide. Type I hypersensitivity to an immunosuppressive agent. J. Allergy Clin. Immunol., 58:160–171, 1976.

324. Fairley, R.F., Barrie, J.U., and Johnson, W.: Sterility and testicular atrophy related to cyclophosphamide therapy. Lancet, 1:568–569, 1972.

325. Kumar, R., et al.: Cyclophosphamide and reproductive function. Lancet, 1:1212–1214, 1972.

326. Miller, D.G.: Alkylating agents and human spermatogenesis. JAMA, 217:1662–1665, 1971.

327. Jacobson, R.J., et al.: Leydig cell dysfunction in male patients with Hodgkins disease receiving chemotherapy. (Abstract.) Clin. Res., 26:437A, 1978.

328. Chapman, R.M., et al.: Cyclical combination chemotherapy and gonadal dysfunction. Retrospective study in males. Lancet, 1:285–289, 1979.

329. Hinkes, E., and Plotkin, D.: Reversible drug-induced sterility in a patient with acute leukemia. JAMA, 223:1490–1491, 1973.

330. Blake, D.A., et al.: Return of fertility in a patient with cyclophosphamide-induced azoospermia. Johns Hopkins Med. J., 139:20–22, 1976.

331. Tolchin, S.F., et al.: Chromosome abnormalities from cyclophosphamide therapy in rheumatoid arthritis and progressive systemic sclerosis (scleroderma). Arthritis Rheum., 17:375–382, 1974.

332. Greenberg, L.H., and Tanaka, K.R.: Congenital anomalies probably induced by cyclophosphamide. JAMA, 188:423–426, 1964.

333. Toledo, T.M., Harper, R.C., and Moses, R.H.: Fetal effects during cyclophosphamide and irradiation therapy. Ann. Intern. Med., 74:87–91, 1971.

334. Sokal, J.E., and Lessmann, E.M.: Effects of cancer chemotherapeutic agents on the human fetus. JAMA, 151:1765–1771, 1960.

335. Shotton, D., and Monie, I.W.: Possible teratogenic effect of chlorambucil on a human fetus. JAMA, 186:74–75, 1963.

336. Menkes, C.J., et al.: Acute megacaryloblastic leukemia after immunodepressive treatment of rheumatoid arthritis. Presse Med., 4:2869–2871, 1975.

337. Kahn, M.F., et al.: Acute leukemia after treatment using cytotoxic agents for rheumatologic purposes. 19 cases among 2006 patients. Nouv. Presse Med., 8:1393–1397, 1979.

338. Zittoun, R., et al.: Small intestine lymphosarcoma after treatment of rheumatoid arthritis by chlorambucil. Nouv. Presse Med., 1:2477–2479, 1972.

339. Prieur, A.M., et al.: Results of long-term risks of immunosuppressive treatment in chronic juvenile arthritis. A 40 case study. Rev. Rhum. Mal. Osteoartic., 46:85–90, 1979.

340. Lebrancha, Y., et al.: Acute monoblastic leukaemia in child receiving chlorambucil for juvenile rheumatoid arthritis. Letter. Lancet, 1:649, 1980.

341. Buriot, D., et al.: Leucemie aigue chez trois enfants atteints d'arthrite chronique juvenille traites par le chlorambucil. Arch. Fr. Pediatr., 36:592–598, 1979.

342. Dumont, J., et al.: Acute myeloid leukemia following non-Hodgkin's lymphoma. Danger of prolonged use of chlorambucil as maintenance therapy. Nouv. Rev. Fr. Hematol., 22:391–404, 1980.

343. Berk, P.D., et al.: Increased incidence of acute leukemia in

polycythemia vera associated with chlorambucil therapy. N. Engl. J. Med., *304*:441–447, 1981.

344. Aymard, J.P., et al.: Acute leukemia after prolonged chlorambucil treatment for non-malignant disease: Report of a new case and literature survey. Acta Haematol., *63*:283–285, 1980.

345. Fiere, D., et al.: Leucemies aigues myeloides apres administration de chlorambucil. Deux observations. Letter. Nouv. Presse Med., *7*:756, 1977.

346. Zittoun, R., et al.: Small intestine lymphosarcoma after treatment of rheumatoid arthritis by chlorambucil. Nouv. Presse Med., *1*:2477–2479, 1972.

347. Chaplin, H.: Lymphoma in primary chronic cold hemagglutinin disease treated with chlorambucil. Arch. Intern. Med., *142*:2119–2123, 1982.

348. Baltus, J.A., et al.: The occurrence of malignancies in patients with rheumatoid arthritis treated with cyclophosphamide: A controlled retrospective follow-up. Ann. Rheum. Dis., *42*:368–373, 1983.

349. Palmer, R.G., Drey, C.J., and Denman, A.M.: Chlorambucil-induced chromosome damage to human lymphoyctes is dose dependent and cumulative. Lancet, *1*:246–249, 1984.

350. Baker, G.L., et al.: Malignancy in cyclophosphamide-treated rheumatoid arthritis patients: A long-term followup study. (Abstract.) Arthritis Rheum., *28*(Suppl.):S37, 1985.

351. DeFronzo, R.A., et al.: Water intoxication in man after cyclophosphamide therapy: Time course and relation to drug activation. Ann. Intern. Med., *78*:861–869, 1973.

352. Herman, E.H., et al.: Comparison of the cardiovascular actions of NSC-109, 724 (ifosfamine) and cyclophosphamide. Toxicol. Appl. Pharmacol., *23*:178–190, 1972.

353. Karchmer, R.K., and Hansen, V.L.: Possible anaphylactic reaction to intravenous cyclophosphamide: Report of a case. JAMA, *237*:475, 1977.

354. Arena, P.J.: Oropharyngeal sensation associated with rapid intravenous administration of cyclophosphamide (NSC-26271). Cancer Chemother. Rep., *56*:779–780, 1972.

355. Renier, J.C., et al.: Treatment of rheumatoid polyarthritis by means of chlorambucil (in relation to 48 cases). Presse Med., *75*:2527–2530, 1967.

356. Iannuzzi, L., et al.: Does drug therapy slow radiographic deterioration in rheumatoid arthritis? N. Engl. J. Med., *309*:1023–1028, 1983.

357. Snaith, M.L., et al.: Treatment of patients with systemic lupus erythematosus including nephritis with chlorambucil. Br. Med. J., *2*:197–201, 1973.

358. Lehman, T.R., et al.: Intravenous bolus cyclophosphamide (IV-CP) therapy of lupus nephritis in children. Arthritis Rheum., *29*(Suppl.):S92, 1986.

359. Fauci, A.S., et al.: Wegener's granulomatosis: Prospective clinical and therapeutic experience with 85 patients for 21 years. Ann. Intern. Med., *98*:76–85, 1983.

360. Scott, D.G., and Bacon, P.A.: Intravenous cyclophosphamide plus methylprednisolone in treatment of systemic rheumatoid vasculitis. Am. J. Med., *76*:377–384, 1984.

361. Shelhamer, J.H., et al.: Takayasu's arteritis and its therapy. Ann. Intern. Med., *103*:121–126, 1985.

362. Skoglund, R.R., Schanberger, J.E., and Kaplan, J.M.: Cyclophosphamide therapy for severe juvenile rheumatoid arthritis. Am. J. Dis. Child., *121*:531–533, 1971.

363. El-Ghobarey, A., et al.: Dermatomyositis: Observations on the use of immunosuppressive therapy and review of the literature. Postgrad. Med. J., *54*:516–527, 1978.

364. Geltner, D., et al.: The effect of combination therapy (steroids, immunosuppressives, and plasmapheresis) on 5 mixed cryoglobulin patients with renal, neurologic, and vascular involvement. Arthritis Rheum., *24*:1121–1127, 1981.

365. Mishima, S., et al.: Behçet's disease in Japan: Ophthalmological aspects. Trans. Am. Ophthalmol. Soc., *77*:225–279, 1979.

366. Tabbara, K.F.: Chlorambucil in Behçet disease: A re-appraisal. Ophthalmology, *90*:906–908, 1983.

367. Erickson, S.B., et al.: Use of combined plasmapheresis and immunosuppression in the treatment of Goodpasture's syndrome. Mayo Clin. Proc., *54*:714–720, 1979.

368. Grupe, W.E., and Heymann, W.: Cytotoxic drugs in steroid resistant renal disease. Alkylating and antimetabolic agents in the treatment of nephrotic syndrome, lupus nephritis, chronic glomerulonephritis, and purpura nephritis in children. Am. J. Dis. Child., *112*:448–458, 1966.

369. Dau, P.C., Kaheleh, M.B., and Sagebiel, R.W.: Plasmapheresis and immunosuppressive drug therapy in scleroderma. Arthritis Rheum., *24*:1128–1136, 1981.

370. Csuka, M.E., Carrera, G.F., and McCarty, D.J.: Treatment of intractable rheumatoid arthritis with combined cyclophosphamide, azathioprine, and hydroxychloroquine. A follow-up study. JAMA, *255*:2315–2319, 1986.

371. McCarty, D.J., and Carrera, G.F.: Treatment of intractable rheumatoid arthritis with combined cyclophosphamide, azathioprine, and hydroxychloroquine. JAMA, *248*:1718–1723, 1982.

372. Butler, D., and Tiliakos, N.: Low-dose cytotoxic drug combination therapy in intractable rheumatoid arthritis. (Abstract.) Arthritis Rheum., *28*(Suppl.):S15, 1985.

373a. Tiliakos, N.A.: Single-agent versus combination cytotoxic therapy: The case for combination therapy. *In* Therapeutic Controversies in the Rheumatic Diseases. Edited by R.F. Willkens and S.L. Dahl. New York, Grune & Stratton, Inc., 1987.

373b. Biro, J.A., et al.: The combination of methotrexate (MTX) and azathioprine (AZA) for resistant rheumatoid arthritis (RA). Arthritis Rheum., *30*(Suppl.):S18, 1987.

374. Bitter, T.: Combined disease-modifying chemotherapy for intractable rheumatoid arthritis. Clin. Rheum. Dis., *10*:417–428, 1984.

375. Svartz, N.: Sulazopryin, a new sulfanilamide preparation. Acta Med. Scand., *110*:577–598, 1942.

376. Svartz, N.: The treatment of rheumatic polyarthritis with acid azo compounds. Rheumatism, *4*:56–60, 1948.

377. Sinclair, R.J.G., and Duthie, J.J.R.: Salazopyrin in the treatment of rheumatoid arthritis. Ann. Rheum. Dis., *8*:226–231, 1949.

378. Kuzell, W.C., and Gardner, G.M.: Salicylazosulfapyridine (salazopyrin or azopyrin) in rheumatoid arthritis and experimental polyarthritis. Calif. Med., *73*:476–480, 1950.

379. McConkey, B., et al.: Salazopyrin in rheumatoid arthritis. Agents Actions, *8*:438–441, 1978.

380. McConkey, B., et al.: Sulphasalazine in rheumatoid arthritis. Br. Med. J., *280*:442–444, 1980.

381. Bird, H.A., et al.: A biochemical assessment of sulphasalazine in rheumatoid arthritis. J. Rheumatol., *9*:36–45, 1982.

382. Neumann, V.C., et al.: Comparison between penicillamine and sulphasalazine in rheumatoid arthritis: Leeds-Birmingham trial. Br. Med. J., *287*:1099–1102, 1983.

383. Pullar, T., Hunter, J.A., and Cappell, H.A.: Sulphasalazine in rheumatoid arthritis: A double blind comparison of sulphasalazine with placebo and sodium aurothiomalate. Br. Med. J., *287*:1102–1104, 1983.

384. Grindulis, K.A., and McConkey, B.: Outcome of attempts to treat rheumatoid arthritis with gold, penicillamine, sulphasalazine, or dapsone. Ann. Rheum. Dis., *43*:398–401, 1984.

385. Bax, D.E., and Amos, R.S.: Sulphasalazine: A safe, effective agent for prolonged control of rheumatoid arthritis. A comparison with sodium aurothiomalate. Ann. Rheum. Dis., 44:194–198, 1985.

386. Martin, L., Sitar, D.S., Chalmers, I.M., and Hunter, T.: Sulfasalazine in severe rheumatoid arthritis: A study to assess potential correlates of efficacy and toxicity. J. Rheumatol., 12:270–273, 1985.

387. Pullar, T., Hunter, J.A., and Capell, H.A.: Effect of acetylator phenotype on efficacy and toxicity of sulphasalazine in rheumatoid arthritis. Ann. Rheum. Dis., 44:831–837, 1985.

388. Bax, D.E., Greaves, M.S., and Amos, R.S.: Sulphasalazine for rheumatoid arthritis: Relationship between dose, acetylator phenotype and response to treatment. Br. J. Rheum., 25:282–284, 1986.

389. Pinals, R.S., Kaplan, S.B., Lawson, J.G., and Hepburn, B.: Sulfasalazine in rheumatoid arthritis: A double blind, placebo-controlled trial. Arthritis Rheum., 29:1427–1434, 1986.

390. Feltelius, N., and Hallgren, R.: Sulphasalazine in ankylosing spondylitis. Ann. Rheum. Dis., 45:396–399, 1986.

391. Amor, B., Kahan, A., Dougados, M., and Delrieu, F.: Sulfasalazine and ankylosing spondylitis. Letter. Ann. Intern. Med., 101:878, 1984.

392. Dougados, M., Boumier, P., and Amor, B.: Sulphasalazine in ankylosing spondylitis: A double blind controlled study in 60 patients. Br. Med. J., 293:911–914, 1986.

393. Mielants, H., and Veys, E.M.: HLA-B27 related arthritis and bowel inflammation. I. Sulfasalazine (salazopyrin) in HLA-B27 related reactive arthritis. J. Rheumatol., 12:287–293, 1985.

394. Veys, E.M., Mielants, H., and Verbruggen, G.: Sulfasalazine (salazopyrin) in HLA-B27 related diseases. (Abstract.) Arthritis Rheum., 29(Suppl.):S56, 1986.

395. Stava, Z., and Kobikova, M.: Salazopyrin in the treatment of scleroderma. Br. J. Derm., 96:541–544, 1977.

396. Czarnecki, D.B., and Taft, E.H.: Generalized morphoea successfully treated with salazopyrine. Acta Derm. Venereol. (Stockh.), 62:81–82, 1981.

397. Dover, N.: Salazopyrin (azulfidine) treatment of scleroderma. Isr. J. Med. Sci., 7:1301–1302, 1971.

398. Ozdogan, H., et al.: Sulphasalazine in the treatment of juvenile rheumatoid arthritis: A preliminary open trial. J. Rheumatol., 13:124–125, 1986.

399. Schroder, H., Lewkonia, R.M., and Price Evans, D.A.: Metabolism of salicylazosulfapyridine in healthy subjects and in patients with ulcerative colitis. Effects of colectomy and of phenobarbital. Clin. Pharmacol. Ther., 14:802–809, 1973.

400. Das, K.M., and Dubin, R.: Clinical pharmacokinetics of sulphasalazine. Clin. Pharmacol., 1:406–425, 1976.

401. Peppercorn, M.A.: Sulfasalazine. Pharmacology, clinical use, toxicity, and related new drug development. Ann. Intern. Med., 3:377–386, 1984.

402. Azad Khan, A.K., Truelove, S.C., and Aronson, J.K.: The disposition and metabolism of sulphasalazine (salicylazosulphapyridine) in man. Br. J. Clin. Pharmacol., 13:523–528, 1982.

403. Das, K.M., Eastwood, M.A., McManus, J.P.A., and Sircus, W.: The metabolism of salicylazosulphapyridine in ulcerative colitis. Gut, 14:631–641, 1973.

404. Das, K.M., Eastwood, M.A., McManus, J.P.A. and Sircus, W.: The role of the colon in the metabolism of salicylazosulphapyridine. Scand. J. Rheum., 9:137–141, 1974.

405. Peppercorn. M.A., and Goldman, P.: The role of intestinal bacteria in the metabolism of salicylazosulfapyridine. J. Pharmacol. Exp. Ther., 181:555–562, 1972.

406. Zapp, B., Fara, J., Chowdhury, J.R., and Das, K.M.: Small bowel absorption of sulfasalazine (SASP) and its enterohepatic circulation. Clin. Res., 24:514A, 1976.

407. Pieniaszek, H.J., Jr., and Bates, T.R.: Capacity-limited gut wall metabolism of 5-aminosalicylic acid, a therapeutically active metabolite of sulfasalazine, in rats. J. Pharmacol. Sci., 68:1323–1325, 1979.

408. Schroder, H., and Price Evans, D.A.: Acetylator phenotype and adverse effects of sulphasalazine in healthy subjects. Gut, 13:278–284, 1972.

409. Das, K.M., Eastwood, M.A., McManus, J.P.A., and Sircus, W.: Adverse reactions during salicylazosulfapyridine therapy and the relation with drug metabolism and acetylator phenotype. N. Engl. J. Med., 289:491–495, 1973.

410. Das, K.M., and Eastwood, M.A.: Acetylation polymorphism of sulfapyridine in patients with ulcerative colitis and Crohn's disease. Clin. Pharmacol. Ther., 18:514–520, 1975.

411. Thayer, W.R., Charland, C., and Field, C.: Effects of sulfasalazine on selected lymphocyte subpopulations in vivo and in vitro. (Abstract.) Gastroenterology, 70(Suppl.):S033, 1976.

412. Thayer, W.R., Charland, C., and Field, C.: Effects of sulfasalazine on selected lymphocyte subpopulations in vivo and in vitro. Dig. Dis. Sci., 24:672–679, 1979.

413. Rubinstein, A., Das, K.M., Melamed, J., and Murphy, R.A.: Comparative analysis of systemic immunological parameters in ulcerative colitis and idiopathic proctitis: Effects of sulfasalazine in vivo and in vitro. Clin. Exp. Immunol., 33:217–224, 1978.

414. Laursen, M.L.: The influence of salicyl-azo-sulfapyridine on the immune response to antigenic tumour cells inoculated into the coecal lumen of C3H mice. Scand. J. Gastroenterol., 13:991–997, 1978.

415. Gibson, P.R., and Jewell, D.P.: Sulphasalazine and derivatives, natural killer activity and ulcerative colitis. Science, 69:177–184, 1985.

416. Gould, S.R.: Prostaglandins, ulcerative colitis and sulphasalazine. Letter. Lancet, 1:988, 1975.

417. Stenson, W.F., and Lobos, E.: Inhibition of platelet thromboxane synthetase by sulfasalazine. Biochem. Pharmacol., 32:2205–2209, 1983.

418. Molin, L., and Stendahl, O.: The effect of sulfasalazine and its active components on human polymorphonuclear leukocyte function in relation to ulcerative colitis. Acta Med. Scand., 206:451–457, 1979.

419. Peskar, B.M., et al.: Enhanced formation of sulfidopeptide-leukotrienes in ulcerative colitis and Crohn's disease: Inhibition by sulfasalazine and 5-aminosalicylic acid. Agents Actions, 18:381–383, 1986.

420. Franklin, J.L., and Rosenberg, I.H.: Impaired folic acid absorption in inflammatory bowel disease: Effects of salicylazosulfapyridine (azulfidine). Gastroenterology, 64:517–525, 1973.

421. Longstreth, G.F., and Green, R.: Folate status in patients receiving maintenance doses of sulfasalazine. Arch. Intern. Med., 143:902–904, 1983.

422. Swinson, C., Perry, J., Lumb, M., and Levi, A.J.: Role of sulphasalazine in the aetiology of folate deficiency in ulcerative colitis. Gut, 22:456–461. 1981.

423. Halsted, C.H., Gandhi, G., and Tamura, T.: Sulfasalazine inhibits the absorbtion of folates in ulcerative colitis. N. Engl. J. Med., 305:1513–1514, 1981.

424. Selhub, J., Dhar, J., and Rosenberg, I.H.: Inhibition of folate enzymes by sulfasalazine. J. Clin. Invest., 61:221–224, 1978.

425. Amos, R.S., et al.: Sulphasalazine for rheumatoid arthritis:

Toxicity in 774 patients monitored for one to 11 years. Br. Med. J., *293*:420–423, 1986.

426. Bateson, M.: Megaloblastic anemia associated with sulphasalazine treatment. Br. Med. J., *2*:190, 1977.

427. Kane, S., and Boots, M.A.: Megaloblastic anaemia associated with sulphasalazine treatment. Br. Med. J., *2*:1287–1288, 1977.

428. Schneider, R.E., and Beeley, L.: Megaloblastic anemia associated with sulphasalazine treatment. Br. Med. J., *2*:1638–1639, 1977.

429. West, B., Lendrum, R., Hill, M.J., and Walker, G.: Effects of sulphasalazine (Salazopyrin) on faecal flora in patients with inflammatory bowel disease. Gut, *15*:906–965, 1974.

430. Ash, G., Baker, R., Rajapakse, C., and Swinson, D.R.: Study of sulphamethoxazole in rheumatoid arthritis. Br. J. Rheum., *25*:285–287, 1986.

431. Smith, M.D., Gibson, R.A., and Brooks, P.M.: Abnormal bowel permeability in anklylosing spondylitis and rheumatoid arthritis. J. Rheumatol., *12*:299–305, 1985.

432. Mielants, H., et al.: HLA-B27 related arthritis and bowel inflammation. 2. Ileocolonoscopy and bowel histology in patients with HLA-B27 related arthritis. J. Rheumatol., *12*:294–298, 1985.

433. Azad Khan, A.K., Piris, J., and Truelove, S.C.: An experiment to determine the active therapeutic moiety of sulphasalazine. Lancet, *1*:892–895, 1977.

434. Van Hees, P.A.M., Bakker, J.H., and Van Tongeren, J.H.M.: Effect of sulphapyridine, 5-aminosalicylic acid, and placebo in patients with idiopathic proctitis: A study to determine the active therapeutic moiety of sulphasalazine. Gut, *21*:632–635, 1980.

435. Pullar, T., Hunter, J.A., and Cappell, H.A.: Which component of sulphasalazine is active in rheumatoid arthritis? Br. Med. J., *290*:1535–1538, 1985.

436. Neumann, V.C., et al.: A study to determine the active moiety of sulphasalazine in rheumatoid arthritis. J. Rheumatol., *13*:285–287, 1986.

437. Taffet, S.L., and Das, K.M.: Sulfasalazine. Adverse effects and desensitization. Dig. Dis. Sci., *28*:833–842, 1983.

438. Nielsen, O.H.: Sulfasalazine intolerance. Scand. J. Gastroenterol., *17*:1–4, 1982.

439. Block, M., Genant, H., and Kirsner, J.: Pancreatitis as an adverse reaction to salicylazosulfapyridine. N. Engl. J. Med., *282*:380–382, 1970.

440. Werlin, S., and Grand, R.: Bloody diarrhea—A new complication of sulfasalazine. J. Pediatr., *92*:450–451, 1978.

441. Schwartz, A.G., Targan, S., Saxon, A., and Weinstein, W.M.: Sulfasalazine-induced exacerbation of ulcerative colitis. N. Engl. J. Med., *306*:409–412, 1982.

442. Adler, R.D.: Sulfasalazine-induced exacerbation of ulcerative colitis. N. Engl. J. Med., *307*:315, 1982

443. Pokorney, B.H., and Nichols, T.W.: Pseudomembranous colitis. A complication of sulfasalazine therapy in a patient with Crohn's colitis. Am. J. Gastroenterol., *76*:374–376, 1981.

444. Juhl, R., et al.: Effects of sulfasalazine on digoxin bioavailability. Clin. Pharmacol. Ther., *20*:387–394, 1976.

445. Kanner, R.S. Tedesco, F.J., and Kalser, M.H.: Azulfidine-(sulfasalazine-) induced hepatic injury. J. Dig. Dis., *23*:956–958, 1978.

446. Sotolongo, R.P., Neefe, L.I., Rudzki, M., and Ishak, G.: Hypersensitivity reactions to sulfasalazine with severe hepatotoxicity. Gastroenterology, *75*:95–99, 1978.

447. Werlin, S.L., Losek, J.D.: Sulfasalazine hepatotoxicity. Am. J. Dis. Child., *135*:1070–1071, 1981.

448. Carvatti, C.M., and Hooker, T.H.: Acute massive hepatic necrosis with fatal liver failure. Am. J. Dig. Dis., *16*:803–808, 1971.

449. Rafoth, R.J.: Systemic granulomatous reaction to salicylazosulfapyridine (azulfidine) in a patient with Crohn's disease. J. Dig. Dis., *19*:465–469, 1974.

450. Pearl, R.K., et al.: Serious complications of sulfasalazine. Dis. Colon Rectum, *29*:201–202, 1986.

451. Mihas, A.A., Goldenberg, D.J., and Slaughter, R.L.: Sulfasalazine toxic reactions. Hepatitis, fever, and skin rash, with hypocomplementemia and immune complexes. JAMA, *239*:2590–2591, 1978.

452. Gulley, R.M., Mirza, A., and Kelley, C.: Hepatotoxicity of salicylazosulfapyridine: A case report and review of the literature. Am. J. Gastroenterol., *72*:561–564, 1979.

453. Callen, J.P., and Soderstrom, R.M.: Granulomatous hepatitis associated with salicylazosulfapyridine therapy. South. Med. J., *71*:1159–1160, 1978.

454. Namias, A.: Reversible sulphasalazine-induced granulomatous hepatitis. J. Clin. Gastroenterol., *3*:193–198, 1981.

455. Smith, M.D., Gibson, G.E., and Rowland, R.: Combined hepatotoxicity and neurotoxicity following sulphasalazine administration. Aust. N.Z. J. Med., *12*:76–80, 1982.

456. Chester, A.C., Diamond, L.H., and Schreiner, G.E.: Hypersensitivity to salicylazosulfapyridine. Renal and hepatic toxic reactions. Arch. Intern. Med., *138*:1138–1139, 1978.

457. Farr, M., Symmons, D.P.M., and Bacon, P.A.: Raised serum alkaline phosphatase and aspartate transaminase levels in two rheumatoid patients treated with sulphasalazine. Ann. Rheum. Dis., *44*:798–800, 1985.

458. Mitrane, M.P., Singh, A., and Seibold, J.R.: Cholestasis and fatal agranulocytosis complicating sulfasalazine therapy: Case report and review of the literature. J. Rheumatol., *13*:969–972, 1986.

459. Evans, R.S., and Ford, W.P.: Studies of the bone marrow in immunological granulocytopenia following administration of salicylazosulfapyridine. Arch. Intern. Med., *101*:244–251, 1958.

460. Roth, D.A., and Lindert, M.E.: A fatal case of azulfidine-induced agranulocytosis. Gastroenterology, *37*:787–789, 1959.

461. Ritz, N.O., and Fisher, M.J.: Agranulocytosis due to administration of salicylazosulfapyridine (azulfidine). JAMA, *172*:237–240, 1960.

462. Thirkettle, J.L., Gough, K.R., and Read, A.E.: Agranulocytosis associated with sulphasalazine (salazopyrin) therapy. Lancet, *1*:1395–1397, 1963.

463. Panitz, F.: Agranulocytosis due to administration of salicylazosulfapyridine (azulfidine). Med. Bull. U.S. Army Eur., *20*:270–271, 1963.

464. Darling, V.E.: Drug agranulocytosis: A case study. Nurs. Times, *61*:1220, 1964.

465. Cochrane, P., Atkins, P., and Ehsanullah, S.: Agranulocytosis associated with sulphasalazine therapy. Postgrad. Med. J., *49*:669–672, 1973.

466. Davies, G.E., and Palek, J.: Selective erythroid and megakaryocytic aplasia after sulfasalazine administration. Letter. Arch. Intern. Med., *140*:1122, 1980.

467. Cohen, S.M., Rosenthal, D.S., and Karp, P.J.: Ulcerative colitis and erythrocytic G6PD deficiency: Salicylazosulfapyridine-provoked hemolysis. JAMA, *205*:528–530, 1968.

468. Gabor, E.P.: Hemolytic anemia as adverse reaction to salicylazosulfapyridine. Letter. N. Engl. J. Med., *2899*:1372, 1973.

469. Pounder, R.E., Craven, E.R., Henthorn, J.S., and Bannatyne, J.M.: Red cells abnormalities associated with sulphasalazine

maintenance therapy for ulcerative colitis. Gut, 16:181–185, 1975.

470. Kaplinsky, N., and Frankel, O.: Salicylazosulphapyridine-induced Heinz-body anemia. Acta Haematol., 59:310–314, 1978.

471. Goodacre, R.L., et al.: Hemolytic anemia in patients receiving sulfasalazine. Digestion, 17:503–508, 1978.

472. Van Hess, P.A., Van Elferen, U.N., Rossum, J.M., and Tongeren, J.H.: Hemolysis during salicylazosulfapyridine therapy. Am. J. Gastroenterol., 70:501–505, 1979.

473. Dunn, A.M., and Kerr, G.D.: Pure red cell aplasia associated with sulphasalazine. Letter. Lancet, 1:1288, 1981.

474. Wheelan, K.R., Cooper, B., and Stone, M.J.: Multiple hematologic abnormalities associated with sulfasalazine. Ann. Intern. Med., 97:726–727, 1982.

475. Farr, M., Scott, D.L., and Bacon, P.A.: Sulphasalazine desenitisation in rheumatoid arthritis. Letter. Br. Med. J., 284:118, 1982.

476. Holdsworth, C.D.: Sulphasalazine desensitisation. Letter. Br. Med. J., 282:110, 1981.

477. Bax, D.E., and Amos, R.S.: Sulphasalazine in rheumatoid arthritis: Desensitizing the patient with a skin rash. Ann. Rheum. Dis., 45:139–140, 1986.

478. Strom, J.: Toxic epidermal necrolysis (Lyell's syndrome). Scand. J. Infect. Dis., 1:209–216, 1969.

479. Alarcón-Segovia, D., et al.: Lupus erythematosus cell phenomenon in patients with chronic ulcerative colitis. Gut, 6:39–47, 1965.

480. Griffiths, D., and Kane, P.: Sulphasalazine-induced lupus syndrome in ulcerative colitis. Letter. Br. Med. J., 2:1188–1189, 1977.

481. Crisp, A.J., and Hoffbrand, B.I.: Sulphasalazine-induced systemic lupus erythematosus in a patient with Sjogren's syndrome. J. R. Soc. Med., 73:60–61, 1980.

482. Reid, J., Holt, S., Housley, E., and Sneddon, D.J.C.: Raynaud's phenomenon induced by sulphasalazine. Postgrad. Med. J., 56:106–107, 1980.

483. Thomas, P., Seaton, A., and Edwards, J.: Respiratory disease due to sulphasalazine. Clin. Allergy, 4:41–47, 1974.

484. Berliner, S., et al.: Salazopyrin-induced eosinophilic pneumonia. Respiration, 39:119–120, 1980.

485. Jones, G.R., and Malone, D.N.S.: Sulphasalazine induced lung disease. Thorax, 27:713–717, 1972.

486. Davies, D., and MacFarlane, A.: Fibrosing alveolitis and treatment with sulphasalazine. Gut, 15:185–188, 1974.

487. Eade, O.E., Whorwell, P.J., Smith, C.L., and Alexander, J.R.: Pulmonary function in patients with inflammatory bowel disease. Am. J. Gastroenterol., 73:154–156, 1980.

488. Toovey, S., Hudson, E., Hendry, W.F., and Levi, A.J.: Sulphasalazine and male infertility: Reversibility and possible mechanism. Gut, 22:445–451, 1981.

489. Birnie, G.G., McLeod, T., and Watkinson, G.: Incidence of sulfasalazine-induced male infertility. Gut, 22:452–455, 1981.

490. Willoughby, C.P., and Truelove, S.C.: Ulcerative colitis and pregnancy. Gut, 21:469–474, 1980.

491. Mogadam, M., Dobbins, W.O., III, Korelitz, B.I., and Ahmed, S.W.: Pregnancy in inflammatory bowel disease: Effect of sulfasalazine and corticosteroids on fetal outcome. Gastroenterology, 80:72–76, 1981.

492. Neeman, A., et al.: Salazopyrine-induced tachycardia. Letter. Biomedicine, 33:1–2, 1980.

493. Carroll, G., et al.: A comparative study of sulphasalazine and penicillamine in the treatment of rheumatoid arthritis. (Abstract.) Aust. N.Z. J. Med., 13:212, 1983.

36

PENICILLAMINE

ISRAELI A. JAFFE

Penicillamine is a 5-carbon amino acid that is a structural analogue of cysteine, in which (CH₃) groups replace (H) at the beta-carbon position (Fig. 36–1). It is a component of penicillin, and may be prepared from it by acid hydrolysis. However, most of the penicillamine currently employed in clinical medicine is prepared synthetically. D-penicillamine (DPA) is the only isomeric form available for therapeutic use. Its chemical structure was first elucidated by Abraham and Chain,[1] and it was first demonstrated in vivo by Walshe, who identified it chromatographically in urine obtained from cirrhotic patients receiving penicillin for intercurrent infections.[2] In clinical medicine, DPA is employed as a chelating agent in treatment of Wilson's disease, where it promotes the renal excretion of the excessive tissue copper stores. It is also used in certain forms of heavy metal intoxication such as lead poisoning; however, it is not of value in the treatment of toxicity from intramuscular gold therapy in rheumatoid arthritis (RA). It is given to patients with cystinuria because it forms a soluble mixed di-

sulfide with cystine, thereby inhibiting cystine calculus formation and subsequent pyelonephritis.

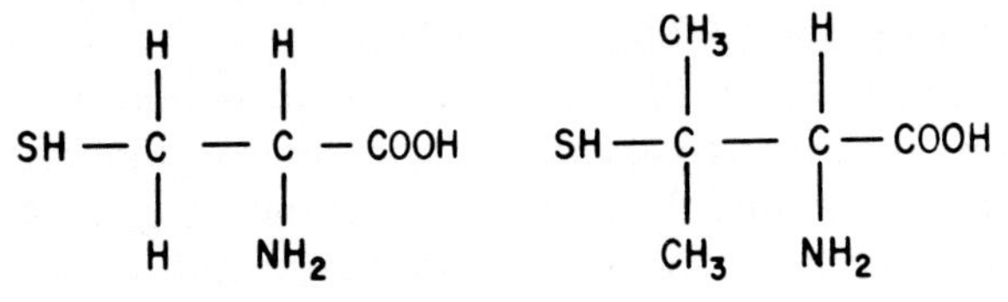

Its widest application is in the treatment of RA, where it is classified as a slow-acting (disease-modifying) agent. Anecdotal evidence supporting its use in the treatment of systemic sclerosis has appeared,[3,4] but its efficacy in this disorder has not yet been substantiated by controlled clinical trials (see Chapter 73).

METABOLISM, PHARMACOKINETICS, AND BIOCHEMICAL PHARMACOLOGY

An understanding of the metabolism and pharmacokinetics of DPA has only recently been appreciated because of the technical difficulty of measuring drug concentrations in blood and in urine. The application of high-performance liquid chromatography (HPLC)[5,6] and radioactive tracer studies in man[7] gave almost identical results in independent studies.[8–10] Orally administered DPA is rapidly absorbed, possibly by a specific amino acid carrier system.[11] It is found in the plasma within 20 minutes after ingestion,[10] and its absorption is reduced by as much as 50% if it is given postprandially.[9,12] This may be due to oxidation to the disulfide by certain dietary components, or to chelation by divalent cations in food. Oral iron, for example, reduces absorption by as much as 25%.[13]

There is a double peak in the plasma concentration of the drug with time after either oral or intravenous administration, suggesting a two-compartment model. The first plasma peak occurs 60 to 80 minutes

FIG. 36–1. Penicillamine *(right)* is an analogue of cysteine *(left)* in which hydrogen atoms are replaced by methyl groups in the β-carbon position.

593

after oral administration, and the second at 110 to 140 minutes. Plasma concentrations of 0.9 μg are achieved after 2 hours. Most of the drug measurable in the plasma is in the form of the mixed disulfide, penicillamine-cysteine, or the internal disulfide, penicillamine-penicillamine. In plasma from RA patients taking 750 mg/day, 11 μmol/l was free DPA and 23 μmol/l (68%) was disulfide. Thus, most of the DPA circulates as disulfide. Distribution studies show that radiolabeled DPA is rapidly lost from liver and kidney, but only slowly from collagen and elastin-rich tissues such as bone and skin.[14]

In the urine, only small amounts of free DPA are found, most of it existing in three biotransformed fractions, and one metabolically transformed form. The biotransformed products are the two mixed disulfides found in the plasma and homocysteine-penicillamine-disulfide.[9] The metabolically transformed metabolite is S-methyl-D-penicillamine.[15] The same urinary products, in approximately the same concentrations, are found in patients with either RA, Wilson's disease, or cystinuria, after oral administration of the drug. As indicated, radiolabeled DPA is rapidly cleared by the kidney and, within 10 hours after dosing, 80% of the final amount that will ultimately be recovered from the urine is already present.[7] The remainder is excreted slowly, with another 5% recovered after 1 to 4 days. Penicillamine-cysteine mixed disulfide has been detected in the urine 3 months after discontinuation of DPA,[16] suggesting a "depot" or tissue-bound compartment, possibly in the skin.[14] This may, in part, explain the persistence of both clinical improvement and some adverse reactions long after the drug has been stopped.

Between 16 and 30% of an orally administered dose can be recovered from the feces, as the two mixed disulfides. About half of an orally administered dose cannot be accounted for either in the urine or in feces, presumably that portion bound to plasma and tissue proteins. The measurement of plasma levels of DPA by HPLC is not generally available and is an investigative tool. In addition, the reported studies were for the most part acute, with values obtained after a single oral or intravenous dose of DPA. Similar measurements in RA patients in a steady state on long-term therapy have not been performed in a systematic, prospective fashion. Serum DPA levels have been shown to be essentially the same for good responders as well as poor or nonresponders and for patients who experienced adverse effects and those who had none.[17]

Three major *biochemical* properties of DPA occur in man.

1. *Chelation* of copper and other divalent cations is

the basis for the application of the drug in Wilson's disease and heavy metal poisoning. The elevated serum copper levels found in RA have led to a suggestion that the beneficial effects of DPA in RA are due to its copper chelating property. Most of the elevated serum copper in RA patients is ceruloplasmin copper, not free copper. It is now generally accepted that changes toward normal in ceruloplasmin levels represent a reflection of clinical improvement rather than its cause, since ceruloplasmin is an acute phase protein.

2. *Thiazolidine binding* by DPA occurs in two important areas. A thiazolidine between DPA and pyridoxal phosphate results in vitamin B_6 antagonism in man.[18] Vitamin B_6 is necessary to maintain the integrity of the immune response, and this has been considered as a possible means by which DPA might exert an immunosuppressive effect. However, attempts to reverse the effectiveness of DPA in RA by the administration of large amounts of vitamin B_6 have been without effect, and other nonsulfhydryl drugs with antivitamin B_6 properties, such as isoniazid, are ineffective in RA.[19] The second important area is the binding of DPA with the aldehyde groups of collagen, thereby inhibiting collagen cross-linking and collagen biosynthesis.[20] This property, called dermolathyrism, has led to the trial of DPA in systemic sclerosis, particularly for the sclerodermatous features (see Chapter 73). The alterations in dermal collagen by DPA with the dosages now used are of no clinical significance. However, with high doses given for prolonged periods, hemorrhagic bullae over pressure points have been encountered. As shown by a controlled trial, as well as clinical experience, DPA *does not* interfere with wound healing. It may be safely given until the time of surgery and then resumed when oral feeding is reinstituted.[21]

3. The *interchange* reaction between sulfhydryl (SH) and disulfide (S-S) groups, as exemplified by mixed disulfide formation, was the biochemical rationale for the initial use of DPA in RA. The drug was used against IgM rheumatoid factor (RF). IgM-RF is a polymer of monomeric subunits, linked by S-S bonds (see Chapter 46). In vitro, DPA and other SH compounds reduce and disrupt these S-S bonds with irreversible loss of serologic reactivity against IgG.[22] DPA was given in an attempt to produce this phenomenon in vivo in RA patients,[23] but it soon became apparent that while the RF titer usually did decrease, a direct effect of DPA on RF was not the explanation.[24] The SH-SS interchange reaction is nonetheless important in understanding the metabolism of the drug, particularly its affinity for proteins in plasma and tissues.

PENICILLAMINE IN RHEUMATOID ARTHRITIS

Although DPA was first given to RA patients to study its possible effect on IgM-RF, it was soon observed that, in addition to the titer changes, there was a favorable effect on the clinical and laboratory indices of disease activity.[19] Anecdotal studies supported these initial observations, but it was the successful completion of the United Kingdom multicenter double-blind clinical trial in 1973 that firmly established the efficacy of the drug in RA.[25] Shortly thereafter, it was registered for that indication by the Committee on Safety of Medicines in Great Britain, and in 1978 was similarly approved by the United States Food and Drug Administration. Subsequent controlled clinical trials have shown that it is at least as effective as injectable gold[26] and azathioprine.[27] A daily dose of 600 mg is statistically the equal of a daily dose of 1200 mg at the end of 1 year, with a notable decrease in adverse reactions, according to a well-executed trial.[28] DPA is not of value in ankylosing spondylitis nor in any of the HLA-B27–associated spondyloarthropathies.[29,30]

INDICATIONS AND CONTRAINDICATIONS

DPA is *indicated* for the treatment of RA, seropositive and seronegative, and has been shown to be of value in palindromic rheumatism.[31] It has been used successfully in treatment of chronic polyarthritis in children of the non-HLA-B27 type,[32] with results similar to those obtained with injectable gold.[33] DPA has been reported to be of particular value in patients with extra-articular manifestations of RA, such as vasculitis,[34] rheumatoid lung disease,[35] Felty's syndrome,[36] amyloidosis,[37] and rheumatoid nodulosis.[38] DPA is *contraindicated* if the patient is receiving gold, cytotoxic drugs, or phenylbutazone. It should be used with extreme caution in the presence of renal insufficiency, which should be regarded as a relative contraindication. DPA should not be continued if a patient becomes pregnant, although abortion is not indicated. Although there are reports of successful pregnancies in patients with Wilson's disease treated with DPA throughout gestation,[39] other reports suggest that the drug may have been responsible for fetal abnormalities.[40] Hence, patients contemplating pregnancy should not be started on DPA treatment. DPA may safely be administered to patients with a history of hypersensitivity to penicillin.[41] RA patients positive for HLA-DR3 and B8 are at greater risk for developing nephropathy, while DR2 was associated with a much reduced incidence of this toxicity.[42] RA patients positive for anti-Ro(SSA) have a greater than expected incidence of DPA side effects.[43] None of these associations is sufficiently strong to be considered a contraindication to a trial of DPA treatment.

The *positioning* of DPA in the overall therapeutic strategy in RA is similar to that for injectable gold: rheumatoid disease that is sustained, progressive, and inadequately responsive to the conventional symptomatic therapies. Gold and DPA are classified as disease-modifying, antirheumatic drugs (DMARDS) and should be considered *before* systemic corticosteroids are instituted. Whether DPA is selected before or after a trial of injectable gold is of little consequence, because the physician will generally use that agent with which he is most familiar, initially. All studies have shown that a prior failure of response, or the development of an untoward reaction to either one of these drugs, does not preclude a favorable outcome with the other.[44-47] A serious adverse reaction to gold indicates a greater likelihood for development of a major toxicity with DPA, but this is not invariable, and often a toxicity, should it occur, involves a different organ system. No time interval is required in switching from injectable gold to DPA (or the reverse), provided that there is no residual evidence of toxicity to the drug used first.

MODE OF ADMINISTRATION

As indicated earlier, all preparations of DPA currently available for clinical use are the pure (D-)isomer. The (DL) form is no longer available for pharmaceutical use. In the United States, DPA is prepared as gelatin-filled capsules of 125 mg or 250 mg, or a scored tablet of 250 mg. A 50-mg tablet is made in Great Britain.

A single daily oral dose of 250 mg is given with water in the postabsorptive state. The most effective blood level is achieved when it is given 1 to 2 hours before breakfast. When divided doses are employed, the second dose is given 2 to 3 hours after the evening meal. As indicated earlier, food markedly impairs absorption and decreases bioavailability.[9,12,17] DPA should be given after meals only if the before-meal dosage results in anorexia, nausea, or vomiting. After 8 weeks at 250 mg/day, the dose is usually doubled, for 8 weeks is the average time required for any change in dosage to be reflected clinically. Further increments are made in a similar manner, as symptoms warrant and tolerance permits. The use of 125-mg daily increments is recommended, particularly if anorexia, nausea, or pruritus is encountered during the induction phase. When the daily dose is greater than 1.0 g/day, a b.i.d. regimen should be employed.

At the end of 2 years, most patients require 750 to 1000 mg daily, and some require 750 mg twice daily. The dosage of DPA is not fixed, but must be adjusted upward or downward as the clinical picture evolves. Although the lower dosages of 500 mg/day are somewhat safer, some investigators believe that although disease activity may be reduced at these doses, disease modification as evidenced by radiographic assessment requires 1.0 g/day or more. Usually, the dosage must be increased with time, for reasons that are not understood. Although DPA is not approved for JRA in the United States, the European experience suggests that 300 to 500 mg/day is effective.[32-33] Patients receiving DPA who are on chronic hemodialysis should be given 250 mg three times a week after the completion of the hemodialysis.[48] Supplements of vitamin B_6, 50 to 100 mg/day, and trace metals, in the form of commercially available vitamin-mineral preparations, are recommended for children and adults whose nutritional status is impaired. These supplements should always be given as far apart from the DPA dosage as feasible. Clinical evidence of a vitamin B_6 deficiency produced by the drug is extremely unusual, but peripheral neuropathy has been reported, which was reversed only after vitamin B_6 administration.[49]

DRUG INTERACTIONS

Interactions between DPA and other drugs are likely because of the highly reactive nature of the molecule. Other antirheumatic drugs, analgesics, antibiotics, and vitamins should not be taken at the same time as the DPA, and ideally at least 2 hours should be allowed between DPA and any other drug. Since it is administered once or twice daily, this is easily achieved. As discussed earlier, there is a specific interaction with oral iron, which was first demonstrated by a marked decrease in DPA-induced cupruresis in the presence of oral iron.[50] Furthermore, when oral iron is taken concomitantly with DPA and is withdrawn while DPA is being continued, an excessive incidence of toxicity, particularly nephropathy, has been observed.[51] When DPA and hydroxychloroquine are given simultaneously, a decrease in both the efficacy and toxicity of the DPA occurs, suggesting the possibility of drug interaction. Although this has not been confirmed in other studies, it seems prudent not to combine these two slow-acting drugs until more data are available.[52] Large doses of ascorbic acid are thought to inactivate DPA and should be avoided.

There is no interaction between DPA and the nonsteroidal drugs or aspirin.

PATTERN OF CLINICAL RESPONSE

As with all the slow-acting drugs, up to 16 weeks may be required after the start of treatment before a clinical response is evident. All symptomatic therapies must therefore be continued as required until well into the course of DPA. In particular, corticosteroids should be maintained in constant dosage, and 1 to 2 years may be required before gradual withdrawal is attempted. When improvement begins, the favorable clinical signs are similar to those of a true natural remission or a remission induced by a successful course of gold. Patients first notice a decrease in the intensity and duration of morning stiffness. Later, as pain subsides, there is often objective evidence of a reduction in synovitis, although synovial thickening present for a long period usually remains unaltered. The quality and duration of uninterrupted sleep improve, and the easy fatigability decreases. Improvement in the laboratory parameters of disease activity, such as a decrease in the Westergren ESR, C-reactive protein, thrombocytosis, and a rise in hemoglobin, is usually seen by 6 to 9 months.[19] After 1 year, the titer of RF falls,[53] as measured by the latex fixation and sensitized sheep cell tests. With lower doses, these changes are less dramatic. Two or more years of therapy are required before there is radiologic evidence of healing of osseous lesions[54] (Fig. 36–2).

The response pattern is nonlinear, usually characterized by periods of exacerbation despite continuance of the drug. These tend to be self-limited, but often require an increase in the daily maintenance dose or conversion to a twice-daily regimen, in an attempt to regain control. Usually, these flares gradually decrease in frequency and, after several years, the improvement becomes more sustained. Rarely, a worsening of the arthritis represents a manifestation of penicillamine-induced lupus (see the section on autoimmune syndromes). This condition responds only to withdrawal of the drug and can be determined only by such a trial, for a positive test for antinuclear antibody (ANA) is not diagnostic. ANA may appear, disappear, or remain unaltered during treatment with DPA.

There is conflicting opinion regarding the optimum total duration of therapy after maximum clinical benefit has been achieved before the gradual withdrawal of the DPA. Some studies indicate that if the disease appears to be well controlled and the drug well tolerated, it should be continued indefinitely. In a pro-

FIG. 36–2.   The radiographic changes in the right hip joint of a 31-year-old woman with rheumatoid arthritis. *A*, The pretreatment roentgenogram shows considerable osteoporosis and bone destruction, with protrusio acetabuli. *B*, After 3 years of D-penicillamine treatment, which had resulted in clinical and laboratory evidence of remission, the osseous lesion has largely remineralized, with healing of the protrusio. Identical changes were noted in the left hip joint.

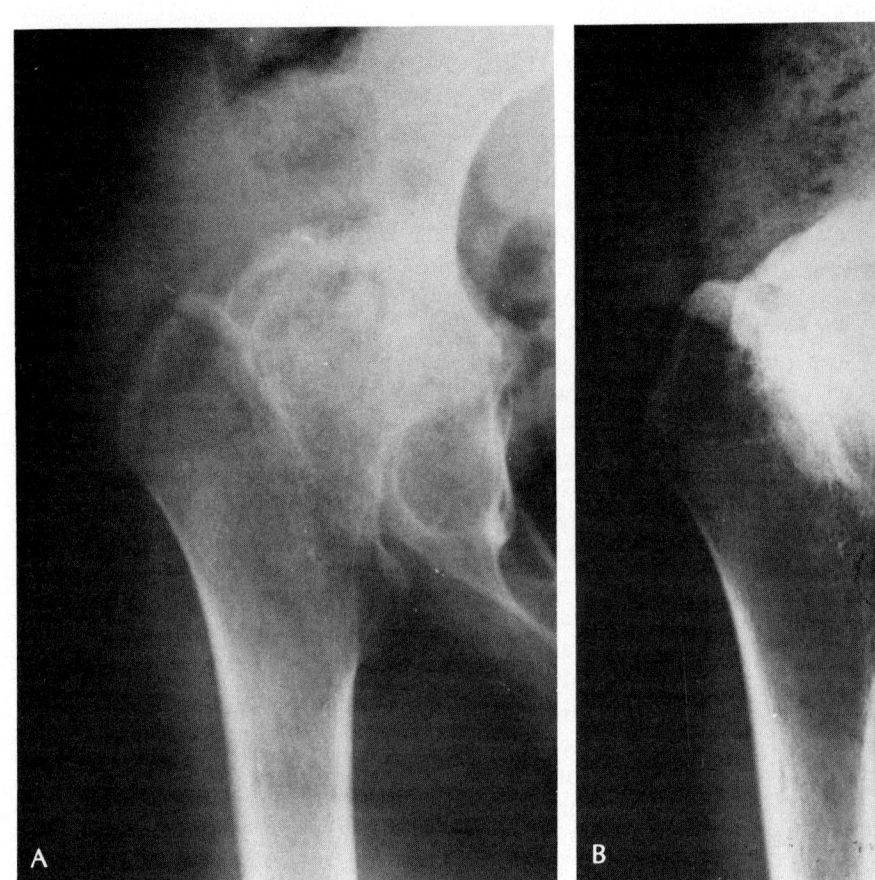

spective study, 38 RA patients judged to be in remission for more than 12 months were randomly divided into two groups: one to remain on the same dosage and the other to have the drug withdrawn by 125 mg/day at monthly intervals. Of the 19 patients continuing with the previous dosage, 17 remained in remission during a 9- to 12-month followup period. Of the 19 whose dosage was reduced, 15 experienced an exacerbation within 2 to 7 months. This represents an 80% flare rate in those in whom withdrawal was attempted.[55]

ADVERSE EFFECTS AND TOXICITY

The numerous and varied side effects that may accompany DPA therapy represent the major factor limiting its use.[56–58] Some of these are dose-related, and can often be successfully managed by brief interruptions of therapy or alterations in dosage. Others are idiosyncratic, independent of dose or duration of treatment. The latter usually preclude any attempt at reinstitution of the DPA, as the same untoward reaction will almost always recur. Because compliance and followup examinations are essential to prevent the more serious complications, prescriptions for DPA should be clearly marked nonrefillable, and the amount of drug dispensed should not exceed that required for the interval between scheduled visits. Safety monitoring requires visits to the physician at 2-week intervals for the first 6 months and monthly thereafter. A complete blood count, including a direct platelet count and a urinalysis, is performed each time, with additional laboratory tests if clinically indicated (see the section on hematologic effects).

SKIN AND MUCOUS MEMBRANES

The most frequently encountered side effects involve the skin in the form of pruritus or various rashes. Pruritus can often be controlled with a modest reduction in dosage or the addition of an antihistaminic drug such as hydroxyzine (Atarax) or cyproheptadine (Periactin). Rashes appearing early in therapy can usually be treated either by the aforementioned measures or by temporary drug withdrawal. Those rashes appearing after 1 year of therapy are more recalcitrant and often require discontinuance of DPA. Oral ulcers may appear within the first 6 months; these clear when the drug is stopped, and recur in about half the cases on rechallenge, even with very low doses. At least one attempt at retreatment is warranted if the arthritis is responding.

More serious is the development of a bullous eruption, clinically indistinguishable from pemphigus, except for the rarity of involvement of the oral mucosa. As in pemphigus, there is intraepidermal acantholysis, epidermal intercellular deposition of immunoglobulin, and circulating antibody to the intercellular region of the epidermis. Nevertheless, other histologic and immunohistologic features differ from those seen in the spontaneously occurring disease.[59] *The appearance of any bullous dermatoses during DPA treatment mandates immediate discontinuation of DPA without rechallenge.* This toxicity is usually seen during the second year of treatment but has occurred after only 2 months. Resolution generally occurs in 2 to 4 weeks after termination of drug but, in some cases, corticosteroids and immunosuppressive agents have been required.

GASTROINTESTINAL TRACT

Anorexia, nausea, and vomiting occur infrequently with the graduated dosage regimens now used. Hypogeusia or dysgeusia, a blunting, distortion, or complete loss of taste perception, is often seen. It is benign, self-limited, and not dose related, with taste normalizing within 2 to 3 months regardless of whether the DPA has been stopped. Patients should be reassured, and treatment continued. Some authors recommend the addition of copper or zinc salts to accelerate the return of taste, but their efficacy is not proved, and decreasing the bioavailability of the DPA is possible. Hepatotoxicity and cholestasis have been

reported rarely.[60,61] In both Wilson's disease and primary biliary cirrhosis, improvement in liver function has been found with DPA therapy. Diarrhea and peptic ulcer disease have not been associated with the drug.

HEMATOLOGIC EFFECTS

Marrow depression may be abrupt and may occur at any time during the course of therapy. This is the most serious toxicity and is potentially life-threatening, reinforcing the necessity for strict safety monitoring. If the white blood cell count falls below 3000/ mm^3 or the platelet counts falls below 100,000/mm^3, the drug should be stopped. Some of the pure thrombocytopenias and neutropenias are dose related, and DPA can be resumed with careful titration of the dose. This is not the case in drug-induced aplastic anemia. This condition is idiosyncratic and may occur at any time, even at the lowest doses. Differentiation can usually be made by bone marrow examination, which is characterized by marked hypocellularity in the complete aplasias. Because thrombocytopenia, agranulocytosis, and/or aplastic anemia may develop in the interval between routine laboratory tests, patients must be instructed that in the event of abnormal bleeding, menorrhagia, high fever, sore throat, or a flu-like syndrome, the drug should be temporarily discontinued, the physician contacted, and supplementary tests obtained.

The effect of penicillamine is cumulative, and patients should be told that brief interruptions of DPA do not compromise the final therapeutic result, but do provide an added measure of safety. In the dose-related depressions, the white blood cell and platelet count begin to rise in about a week, but the aplasias persist for weeks to months. There is disagreement as to whether antimicrobial drugs and antifungal agents should be administered prophylactically during this period, or whether reverse isolation alone with careful monitoring for development of infection will suffice.[62] Corticosteroids do not hasten recovery and impair host resistance to infection and hence should not be added. Blood and platelet transfusions are given as required. There may be a place for cytotoxic drugs in resistant cases of aplastic anemia.[62] Several cases of pure red cell aplasia have been caused by the drug, one of which responded to cyclophosphamide. Thrombotic thrombocytopenic purpura has been reported in an RA patient during DPA treatment.[63] Bone marrow grafts have not been successful in DPA-associated aplastic anemia.

RENAL TOXICITY

Proteinuria occurs in 15 to 20% of RA patients given DPA, owing to an immune complex mediated membranous nephropathy. The causative antigen has not been identified.[64] In the absence of nephrotic syndrome, the degree of urinary protein excretion may be titrated against the maintenance dose; often a modest reduction in dose reduces proteinuria. In general, the drug may be continued as long as the protein excretion does not exceed 2 g/24 hours. If the serum albumin falls or nephrotic syndrome appears, the drug must be stopped. Sometimes nephropathy presents as nephrotic syndrome. Proteinuria may persist for up to 1 year after the drug is discontinued, but the lesion is ultimately reversible. Rechallenge has been attempted in patients after clearing of proteinuria with variable results. Some patients can tolerate the drug without recurrence of nephropathy.

Microscopic hematuria had been considered a serious event, but incorrectly so in most instances. It is usually benign and clears despite continued DPA therapy.[65] Its cause is not known. Increasing microscopic hematuria or the appearance of gross hematuria both require that treatment be stopped, for they may portend the development of crescentic glomerulonephritis or Goodpasture's syndrome.[66] In DPA-induced Goodpasture's syndrome, staining of the glomerular basement membrane is granular not linear as in the natural disease, and antiglomerular basement membrane antibody is not detected in the serum. Some authors therefore classify this lesion as immune complex nephritis with lung hemorrhage.[67] Clinically it is indistinguishable from Goodpasture's syndrome. Plasmapheresis and intensive immunosuppressive therapy may be required to restore renal function.[66]

PULMONARY EFFECTS

The appearance of hemoptysis during DPA treatment should suggest the possibility of drug-induced Goodpasture's syndrome. Hematuria is present, and characteristic infiltrates are seen on chest roentgenogram. Another entity, fibrosing alveolitis, has been associated rarely with DPA administration. Basilar rales, a typical radiographic appearance, and rapid improvement after withdrawal of the DPA are characteristic.[68]

Bronchiolitis obliterans has been observed in some patients, but a causative role for the drug has not been established.[69] Obliterative bronchiolitis is not reversible on stopping DPA, has been described in other connective tissue diseases, and is considered to be part of the spectrum of rheumatoid lung disease.[70] Patients with RA most likely to develop extra-articular features are also most likely to be treated with DPA. Bronchiolitis obliterans has not occurred in patients with Wilson's disease given DPA, where all of its other adverse effects have appeared. Thus, obliterative bronchiolitis during treatment with DPA is considered a chance association and not an adverse reaction to the drug.

NEUROMUSCULAR SYSTEM

Myasthenia gravis (MG) may be induced by DPA in patients with Wilson's disease,[71] and RA,[72] and it is most likely to develop during the second year of treatment, similar to the time of appearance of pemphigus. Antibodies to acetylcholine receptors (AChR) are found frequently, and disappear along with clinical resolution of the MG after drug withdrawal.[73] An anticholinesterase drug is often needed, because months may elapse before the MG reverses. Corticosteroids and plasmapheresis have been needed if respiratory muscle weakness is present. Unusual muscular weakness and fatigue on repetitive acts, diplopia, and dysphagia in RA patients receiving DPA should suggest drug-induced MG. An EMG, tests for serum AChR antibody, and a Tensilon test should be performed. The DPA must be stopped because MG will recur on rechallenge. In DPA-induced MG, the AChR antibody reacts with human motor end-plate preparations, and does not have the species heterogeneity characteristic of the antibody in spontaneously developing MG.[74] A negative test result must be interpreted with caution because there is no standard end-plate preparation and many are obtained from animal muscle.

Drug-induced MG is associated with BW35, DR1, and the combination of BW35 and DR1. In spontaneous MG, B8 and DR3 predominate,[75] whereas in RA without MG, DR4 is often found. The differences in the specificity of the antibody and in the genetic associations may relate to the pathogenesis of DPA autoimmunity.

Polymyositis or dermatomyositis are well-recognized toxicities of DPA.[76] The proximal myopathy and rash are indistinguishable from the spontaneous disease. Prompt recognition is important so that the drug may be discontinued and a fatal outcome avoided.[77]

A reversible peripheral neuropathy responsive to vitamin B_6 has been alluded to previously, but this is extremely rare, and if neuropathy develops in DPA treatment of RA, other causes such as vasculitis should be entertained.

THE AUTOIMMUNE SYNDROMES

DPA induces a wide spectrum of syndromes closely simulating spontaneously occurring autoimmune diseases. Many of these have already been discussed, and they may occur in Wilson's disease and cystinuria as well as in RA. Thus, induction of autoimmunity is a property of DPA and not the abnormal immune system that might be found in RA patients.[78] In addition to causing those entities already reviewed, DPA may induce a lupus-like syndrome similar to that induced by other drugs, except that antibodies directed toward native, double-stranded DNA develop.[79] In the usual drug-induced SLE, the antibody that develops is to single-stranded (denatured) DNA (see Chapters 67 and 68). Patients develop myalgias, pleurisy, and joint pain, difficult to differentiate from an exacerbation of the underlying RA. Renal disease, however, occurs rarely.[80]

Sjögren's syndrome and chronic thyroiditis have been encountered but may have been associated with the underlying RA. The rare occurrence of breast gigantism, sometimes with galactorrhea, has been considered to be immune-mediated when secondary to DPA; however, it responds to danazol.[81] Antibodies to insulin have been observed to appear infrequently in patients receiving DPA, and they disappeared promptly on withdrawal of the drug. In one patient, symptomatic hypoglycemia developed.[82] The effectiveness of DPA in ameliorating the clinical and laboratory features of RA, while at the same time having the potential to induce autoimmunity, has raised the issue of whether these two properties might be linked, perhaps at the level of immune regulation.[83,84] Alternatively, the SH group of DPA may interact with the S-S bonds of proteins on cell surfaces (receptors) via the SH-SS interchange mechanisms, rendering them antigenic. DPA-induced MG, pemphigus, and Goodpasture's syndrome may mimic clinically the naturally occurring disease, but there are subtle differences in histology, immunohistology, and immunology.

MECHANISM OF ACTION OF DPA IN RA

The mechanism by which DPA suppresses RA is not known. In the laboratory, DPA is neither cytotoxic, anti-inflammatory, nor immunosuppressive. It does not suppress adjuvant arthritis in rats. Because it is useful only in RA, there is a connotation of disease "specificity," compared to other slow-acting agents. Marked reductions in immune complex levels in serum and synovial fluid and in both IgM and IgG RF levels are usually found with DPA (Figs. 36–3, 36–4), suggesting that the drug may be working at a fundamental level.[85] Other SH compounds with a DPA-like action in RA have been examined in the laboratory.[86] Neither chelation, antivitamin B_6 effects, induction of the collagen defect (dermolathyrism), nor mixed disulfide formation was a property of any of the other clinically useful SH drugs. Hence none of these properties of DPA seems relevant to its mode of action in RA.[86] In vitro studies of the effect of DPA on the responsiveness of lymphocytes to mitogenic

FIG. 36–3. Ultracentrifugal pattern of serum proteins before treatment *(top)* and after the patient had been taking penicillamine for 13 weeks *(bottom)*. The serum was diluted 1:1 with saline. Centrifugation was at 52,640 rpm and proceeds from left to right. Photographs were obtained at 16, 32, 48, 64, 80, and 90 minutes. The post-treatment pattern exhibits a reduction in the 22S complex, 19S macroglobulin, and in the intermediate γ-globulin complexes. (Courtesy Dr. H. Kunkel.)

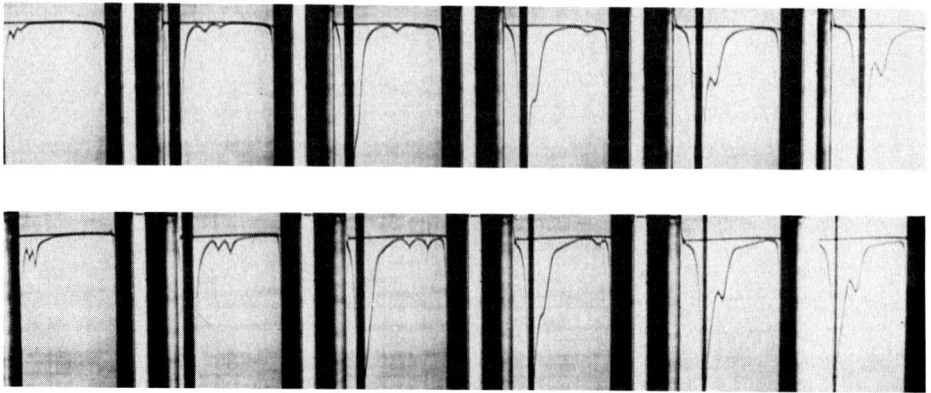

FIG. 36–4. Effect of penicillamine therapy on complexes, as measured by precipitation with purified IgM rheumatoid factor. Well 1 contains synovial fluid, and well 2 contains serum from the same patient before penicillamine therapy. Well 3 shows a decrease in the amount of complex after 6 weeks of penicillamine therapy. Wells 4 and 5 reveal the absence of demonstrable serum complexes at 3 and 6 months, respectively, after initiation of penicillamine therapy. Well C is a normal serum control. There is no post-treatment specimen of synovial fluid, because the synovial effusion had completely reabsorbed. (Courtesy Dr. R. Winchester.)

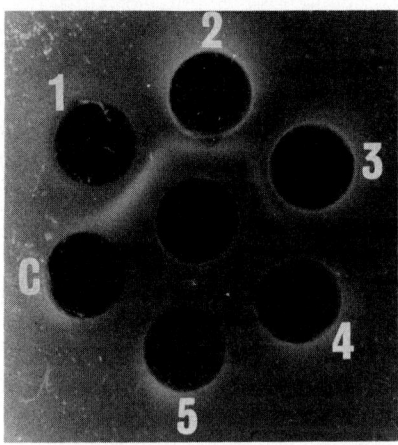

stimulation and on lymphocyte-macrophage interaction have produced results that are conflicting and difficult to interpret.[87] One in vitro study showed that DPA in the presence of copper produced a selective inhibition of human helper T-cell function; T-suppressor cells and B-lymphocytes were not affected.[88] This could explain immunosuppression but fails to account for the apparent "specificity" of DPA for RA. It is not possible to synthesize all the extensive laboratory observations into a unified hypothesis to explain mechanism. Further studies may resolve the question.

OTHER SH COMPOUNDS WITH A DPA-LIKE ACTION IN RA

Other SH compounds have been used in treatment of RA patients in an effort to find one with a more favorable therapeutic ratio.[86] In 1963, it was shown that 5-thiopyridoxine produced clinical and serologic changes similar to DPA,[89] findings that were subsequently confirmed.[90] The disulfide of this compound, pyrithioxine, is readily dissociated to the SH form and is also effective.[91] Thiopronine was comparable in efficacy to DPA in a controlled trial.[92] Another SH compound found to be effective in RA is the antihyper-

tensive drug, captopril.[93,94] Its molecular structure suggested that it might have DPA-like activity in RA. In the early studies of captopril in hypertension, when excessively high doses (by present standards) were given, a toxicity profile emerged similar to that of DPA. There was a high incidence of rash, proteinuria due to immune-complex nephritis, taste disturbances, oral ulcers, neutropenia, and pemphigus.[95] The incidence of these adverse reactions was low compared to that with DPA, and even lower with the dosages of captopril now used to treat hypertension and refractory heart failure, but the qualitative similarity of these untoward reactions led to a trial of captopril in RA.[93,94] No controlled studies have yet been performed, but the preliminary data are encouraging. In doses of 100 to 200 mg/day in normotensive RA patients, no postural hypotension was encountered, provided that diuretics and vasodilator drugs were not given simultaneously.

In all these studies with the other SH drugs, two facts emerge. First, patients with RA could respond to one of these other SH compounds, having previously failed to respond to DPA or having "escaped" from the effects of DPA.[96] Second, all these drugs had adverse effects similar to those of DPA, including the induction of autoimmunity,[97] but the same toxicity was not necessarily replicated in the same patient, nor would there necessarily be any toxicity in a particular patient to the newer drug. These findings are identical to those noted with DPA and injectable gold. Thus, an RA patient with DPA-induced proteinuria might respond well to pyrithioxine or captopril, with no proteinuria, perhaps with a rash, or possibly with no adverse effect at all. The availability of a family of these SH drugs would vastly enhance the therapeutic measures against RA.

REFERENCES

1. Abraham, E.P., et al.: Penicillamine: A characteristic degradation product of penicillin. Nature, *152*:107, 1943.
2. Walshe, J.M.: Wilson's disease: New oral therapy. Lancet, *1*:25–26, 1956.
3. Kang, B., et al.: Successful treatment of far-advanced progressive systemic sclerosis by D-penicillamine. J. Allergy Clin. Immunol., *69*:297–305, 1982.
4. Steen, V.D., Medsger, T.A., and Rodnan, G.P.: D-penicillamine therapy in progressive systemic sclerosis (scleroderma). Ann. Intern. Med., *97*:652–659, 1982.
5. Russell, A., et al.: A rapid, sensitive technique to assay penicillamine levels in blood and urine. J. Rheumatol., *6*:15–19, 1979.
6. Saetre, R., and Rabenstein, D.L.: Determination of penicillamine in blood and urine by high performance liquid chromatography. Anal. Chem., *50*:276–280, 1978.
7. Patzschke, K., et al.: Pharmakokinetische untersuchungen

nach oraler applikation von radioaktiv markiertem D-penicillamin an probanden. Z. Rheumatol., 36:96–105, 1977.

8. Kukovetz, W.R., et al.: Bioavailability and pharmacokinetics of D-penicillamine. J. Rheumatol., 10:90–94, 1983.

9. Perett, D.: The metabolism and pharmacology of D-penicillamine in man. J. Rheumatol., 8(Suppl. 7):41–50, 1981.

10. Weisner, R.H., et al.: The pharmacokinetics of D-penicillamine in man. J. Rheumatol., 8(Suppl. 7):51–55, 1981.

11. Wass, M., and Evered, D.F.: Transport of penicillamine across mucosa of the rat small intestine in vitro. Biochem. Pharmacol., 19:1287–1295, 1970.

12. Schuana, A., et al.: Influence of food on the bioavailability of penicillamine. J. Rheumatol., 10:95–97, 1983.

13. Hall, N.D., et al.: Serum SH reactivity: A simple assessment of D-penicillamine absorption. Rheumatol. Int., 1:39–41, 1981.

14. Ruocco, V., et al.: Specific incorporation of penicillamine into the epidermis of mice: An autoradiographic study. Br. J. Dermatol., 108:441–444, 1983.

15. Perett, D., Sneddon, W., and Stephens, A.D.: Studies on D-penicillamine metabolism in cystinuria and rheumatoid arthritis: Isolation of S-methyl-D-penicillamine. Biochem. Pharmacol., 25:259–264, 1976.

16. Wei, P., and Sass-Kortsak, A.: Urinary excretion and renal clearance of D-penicillamine in humans and the dog. Gastroenterology, 58:288, 1970.

17. Muijsers, A.O., et al.: D-penicillamine in patients with rheumatoid arthritis—Serum levels, pharmacokinetic aspects, and correlation with clinical course and side effects. Arthritis Rheum., 27:1362–1369, 1984.

18. Jaffe, I.A., Altman, K., and Merryman, P.: The anti-p idoxine effect of penicillamine in man. J. Clin. Invest., 43:1869–1873, 1964.

19. Jaffe, I.A.: The effect of penicillamine on the laboratory parameters in rheumatoid arthritis. Arthritis Rheum., 8:1064–1079, 1965.

20. Nimni, M.E., and Bavetta, L.A.: Collagen defect induced by penicillamine. Science, 150:905–907, 1965.

21. Ansell, B.M., Moran, H., and Arden, G.P.: Penicillamine and wound healing in rheumatoid arthritis. Proc. R. Soc. Med., 70(Suppl. 3):75–77, 1977.

22. Heimer, R., and Federico, M.: Depolymerization of the 19S antibodies and the 22S rheumatoid factor. Clin. Chim. Acta, 25:41–43, 1958.

23. Jaffe, I.A.: Comparison of the effect of plasmapheresis and penicillamine on the level of circulating rheumatoid factor. Ann. Rheum. Dis., 22:71–76, 1963.

24. Jaffe, I.A., and Merryman, P.: Effect of increased serum sulfhydryl content on titre of rheumatoid factor. Ann. Rheum. Dis., 27:14–18, 1968.

25. Multi-Centre Trial Group: Controlled trial of D(—)penicillamine in severe rheumatoid arthritis. Lancet, 1:275–280, 1973.

26. Huskisson, E.C., et al.: Trial comparing penicillamine and gold in rheumatoid arthritis. Ann. Rheum. Dis., 33:532–535, 1974.

27. Berry, H., et al.: Trial comparing azathioprine and penicillamine in rheumatoid arthritis. Ann. Rheum. Dis., 35:542–543, 1976.

28. Dixon, A. St.J., et al.: Synthetic D(—) penicillamine in rheumatoid arthritis. Double-blind controlled study of a high and low dose regimen. Ann. Rheum. Dis., 34:416–421, 1975.

29. Bird, H.A., and Dixon, A. St.J.: Failure of D-penicillamine to affect peripheral joint involvement in ankylosing spondylitis or HLA B27 associated arthropathy. Ann. Rheum. Dis., 36:289, 1977.

30. Steven, M.M., Morrison, M., and Sturrock, R.D.: Penicillamine

31. Huskisson, E.C.: Treatment of palindromic rheumatism with D-penicillamine. Br. Med. J., 11:979–980, 1976.

32. Prieur, A.M., et al.: Evaluation of D-penicillamine in juvenile chronic arthritis. A double-blind, multicenter study. Arthritis Rheum., 28:376–382, 1985.

33. Ansell, B.M., and Hall, M.A.: Penicillamine in chronic arthritis of childhood. J. Rheum., 8(Suppl. 7):112–115, 1981.

34. Jaffe, I.A.: Rheumatoid arthritis with arteritis. Report of a case treated with penicillamine. Ann. Intern. Med., 61:556–563, 1964.

35. Lorber, A.: Penicillamine therapy for rheumatoid lung disease: Effects of protein sulfhydryl groups. Nature, 210:1235–1237, 1966.

36. Lakhanpal, S. and Luthra, H.S.: D-penicillamine in Felty's syndrome. J. Rheumatol., 12:703–706, 1985.

37. Lake, B., and Andrews, G.: Rheumatoid arthritis with secondary amyloidosis and malabsorption syndrome. Effect of D-penicillamine. Am. J. Med., 44:105–115, 1968.

38. Ginsberg, M.H., et al.: Rheumatoid nodulosis. An unusual variant of rheumatoid disease. Arthritis Rheum., 18:49–58, 1975.

39. Scheinberg, I.H., and Sternlieb, I.: Pregnancy in penicillamine-treated patients with Wilson's disease. N. Engl. J. Med., 293:1300–1303, 1975.

40. Mjölnerod, O.K., et al.: Congenital connective tissue defect probably due to D-penicillamine treatment in pregnancy. Lancet, 1:673–675, 1971.

41. Bell, C.L., and Graziano, F.M.: The safety of administration of penicillamine to penicillin sensitive individuals. Arthritis Rheum., 26:801–803, 1983.

42. Stockman, A., et al.: Genetic markers in rheumatoid arthritis—Relationship to toxicity from D-penicillamine. J. Rheumatol., 13:269–273, 1986.

43. Moutsopoulos, H.M., et al.: Anti-Ro (SSA) positive rheumatoid arthritis (RA): A clinicoserological group of patients with a high incidence of d-penicillamine side effects. Ann. Rheum. Dis., 44:215–219, 1985.

44. Hala, J.T., Cassidy, J., and Hardin, J.G.: Sequential gold and penicillamine therapy in rheumatoid arthritis. Am. J. Med., 72:423–426, 1982.

45. Kean, W.F., et al.: Prior gold therapy does not influence the adverse effects of D-penicillamine in rheumatoid arthritis. Arthritis Rheum., 25:917–922, 1982.

46. Steven, M.M., et al.: Does the order of second-line treatment in rheumatoid arthritis matter? Br. Med. J., 1:79–81, 1982.

47. Webley, M., and Coomes, E.: An assessment of penicillamine therapy in rheumatoid arthritis and the influence of previous gold therapy. J. Rheumatol., 6:20–24, 1979.

48. Matthey, F., Perett, D., Greenwood, R.N., and Baker, L.R.: The use of D-penicillamine in patients with rheumatoid arthritis undergoing hemodialysis. Clin. Nephrol., 25:268–271, 1986.

49. Pool, K.D., Feit, H., and Kirkpatrick, J.: Penicillamine-induced neuropathy in rheumatoid arthritis. Ann. Intern. Med., 95:457–458, 1981.

50. Lyle, W.H., Pearcy, D.F., and Hui, M.: Inhibition of penicillamine-induced cupruresis by oral iron. Proc. R. Soc. Med., 70(Suppl. 3):48–49, 1977.

51. Harkness, J.A.L., and Blake, D.R.: Penicillamine nephropathy and iron. Lancet, 2:1368–1369, 1982.

52. Bunch, T.W., et al.: Controlled trial of hydroxychloroquine and

d-penicillamine singly and in combination in the treatment of rheumatoid arthritis. Arthritis Rheum., *27*:267–276, 1984.

53. Wernick, R., Merryman, P., Jaffe, I., and Ziff, M.: IgG and IgM rheumatoid factors in rheumatoid arthritis. Quantitative response to penicillamine therapy and relationship to disease activity. Arthritis Rheum., *26*:593–598, 1983.

54. Gibson, T., et al.: Evidence that D-penicillamine alters the course of rheumatoid arthritis. Rheumatol. Rehabil., *15*:211–215, 1976.

55. Ahern, M., Hall, N., and Maddison, P.: D-penicillamine (DPA) withdrawal in rheumatoid arthritis (RA). Ann. Rheum. Dis., *43*:213–217, 1984.

56. Stein, H.B., et al.: Adverse effects of D-penicillamine in rheumatoid arthritis. Ann. Intern. Med., *92*:24–29, 1980.

57. Stockman, A., et al.: Difficulties in the use of D-penicillamine in the treatment of rheumatoid arthritis. Aust. N.Z. J. Med., *9*:495–503, 1979.

58. Weiss, A., et al.: Toxicity of D-penicillamine in rheumatoid arthritis. Am. J. Med., *64*:114–120, 1978.

59. Troy, J.L., et al.: Penicillamine-associated pemphigus: Is it really pemphigus? J. Am. Acad. Dermatol., *4*:547–555, 1981.

60. McLeod, B.D., and Kinsella, T.D.: Cholestasis associated with D-penicillamine therapy for rheumatoid arthritis. Can. Med. Assoc. J., *120*:965–966, 1979.

61. Rosenbaum, J., Katz, W.A., and Schumacher, H.R.: Hepatotoxicity associated with use of D-penicillamine in rheumatoid arthritis. Ann. Rheum. Dis., *39*:152–154, 1980.

62. Gale, R.P., et al.: Aplastic anemia: Biology and treatment. Ann Intern. Med., *95*:477–494, 1981.

63. Trice, J.M., Pinals, R.S., and Pitman, G.I.: Thrombotic thrombocytopenic purpura during penicillamine therapy in rheumatoid arthritis. Arch. Intern. Med., *143*:1487–1488, 1983.

64. Bacon, P.A., et al.: Penicillamine nephropathy in rheumatoid arthritis. Q. J. Med., *45*:661–684, 1976.

65. Barraclough, D., Cunningham, T.J., and Muirden, K.D.: Microscopic hematuria in patients with rheumatoid arthritis on D-penicillamine. Aust. N.Z. J. Med., *11*:706–708, 1981.

66. Gavaghan, T.E., et al.: Penicillamine-induced "Goodpasture's syndrome": Successful treatment of a fulminant case. Aust. N.Z. J. Med., *11*:261–265, 1981.

67. Loughlin, G.M., et al.: Immune-complex mediated glomerulonephritis and pulmonary hemorrhage simulating Goodpasture's syndrome. J. Pediatr., *93*:181–184, 1978.

68. Eastmond, C.J.: Diffuse alveolitis as a complication of penicillamine treatment for rheumatoid arthritis. Br. Med. J., *1*:1506, 1976.

69. Editorial: Obliterative bronchiolitis. Lancet, *1*:603–604, 1982.

70. Case Records of the Massachusetts General Hospital, Case 3-1982.: N. Engl. J. Med., *306*:157–165, 1982.

71. Masters, C.L., Dawkins, R.L., and Zilco, P.J.: Penicillamine associated myasthenia gravis, anti-acetylcholine receptor and anti-striational antibodies. Am. J. Med., *63*:689–694, 1977.

72. Bucknall, R.C., Dixon, A. St.J., and Glick, E.N.: Myasthenia gravis associated with penicillamine treatment for rheumatoid arthritis. Br. Med. J., *1*:600–602, 1975.

73. Russell, A.S., and Lindstrom, J.M.: Penicillamine induced myasthenia gravis associated with antibodies to acetylcholine receptor. Neurology, *28*:847–852, 1978.

74. Garlepp, M., et al.: Heterogeneity of the acetylcholine receptor autoantigen. Muscle Nerve, *4*:282–288, 1981.

75. Garlepp, M.J., Dawkins, R.L., and Christiansen, F.: HLA antigens and acetylcholine receptor antibodies in penicillamine induced myasthenia gravis. Br. Med. J., *286*:338–340, 1983.

76. Takahashi, K., et al.: D-penicillamine-induced polymyositis in patients with rheumatoid arthritis. Arthritis Rheum., *29*:560–564, 1986.

77. Doyle, D.R., McCurley, T.L., and Sergent, J.S.: Fatal polymyositis in D-penicillamine-treated rheumatoid arthritis. Ann. Intern. Med., *98*:327–330, 1983.

78. Jaffe, I.A.: Induction of auto-immune syndromes by penicillamine therapy in rheumatoid arthritis and other diseases. Springer Semin. Immunopathol., *4*:193–207, 1981.

79. Crouzet, J., et al.: Lupus induit par la D-penicillamine au cours du traitement de la polyarthrite rheumatoid—Deux observations et Etude immunologique systematique au cours de ce traitment. Ann. Med. Interne., *125*:71–79, 1974.

80. Chalmers, A., et al.: Systemic lupus erythematosus during penicillamine therapy for rheumatoid arthritis. Ann. Intern. Med., *97*:659–663, 1982.

81. Taylor, P.J., Cumming, D.C., and Corenblum, B.: Successful treatment of D-penicillamine-induced breast gigantism with danazol. Br. Med. J., *1*:362–363, 1981.

82. Benson, E.A., Healey, L.A., and Barron, E.J.: Insulin antibodies in patients receiving penicillamine. Am. J. Med., *78*:857–860, 1985.

83. Dawkins, R.L., and Zilco, P.J.: Penicillamine: Friend and foe? Aust. N.Z. J. Med., *9*:493–494, 1979.

84. Editorial: Penicillamine—The therapeutic paradox. Lancet, *2*:1209–1210, 1981.

85. Jaffe, I.A.: Penicillamine treatment of rheumatoid arthritis: Effect on immune complexes. Ann. N.Y. Acad. Sci., *256*:330–337, 1975.

86. Jaffe, I.A.: Thiol compounds with penicillamine-like activity and possible mode of action in rheumatoid arthritis. Clin. Rheum. Dis., *6*:633–645, 1980.

87. Binderup, L., Bramm, E., and Arrigoni-Martelli, E.: D-penicillamine in vivo enhances lymphocyte DNA synthesis. Role of macrophages. Scand. J. Immunol., *11*:23–28, 1980.

88. Lipsky, P.E., and Ziff, M.: Inhibition of human helper T-cell function in vitro by D-penicillamine and $CuSO_4$. J. Clin. Invest., *65*:1069–1076, 1980.

89. Jaffe, I.A.: The effect of penicillamine and mercaptopyridoxine in rheumatoid arthritis. Abst. 243: Fifth European Congress of Rheumatic Disease. Stockholm. 1963.

90. Huskisson, E.C., et al.: 5-thiopyridoxine in rheumatoid arthritis: Clinical and experimental studies. Arthritis Rheum., *23*:106–110, 1980.

91. Camus, J.P., et al.: Etude d'une serie de 70 polyarthritis rhumatoides traitees par la pyrithioxine avec un recul de un an. Rev. Rhum., *45*:487–490, 1978.

92. Pasero, G., et al.: Controlled multicenter trial of thiopronin and D-penicillamine for rheumatoid arthritis. Arthritis Rheum., *25*:923–929, 1982.

93. Merlet, C.L., et al.: Captopril in rheumatoid arthritis. Abstract 1389: Fifteenth International Congress of Rheumatology, Paris, 1981.

94. Martin, M.F.R., et al.: Captopril: A new long-term agent for treating rheumatoid arthritis. Ann. Rheum. Dis., *42*:231, 1983.

95. Atkinson, A., and Robertson, J.: Captopril in the treatment of clinical hypertension and of cardiac failure. Lancet, *2*:836–839, 1979.

96. Camus, J.P., Koeger, A.C., Struz, P.H., and Laveant, C.: Sulfhydryl maintenance treatment in rheumatoid arthritis. A series of 120 cases followed for 10 years with a study of the possibilities of changing the drug. Rev. Rhum., *53*:31–33, 1986.

97. Jaffe, I.A.: Adverse effects profile of sulfhydryl compounds in man. Am. J. Med., *80*:471–476, 1986.

GLUCOCORTICOIDS

TIMOTHY W. BEHRENS and JAMES S. GOODWIN

Glucocorticoids are the most powerful and also the most toxic drugs available for the treatment of inflammatory disease. There is little doubt, except perhaps among the most recalcitrant skeptics, that the introduction of glucocorticoids represented a major advance in the treatment of rheumatic diseases. On the other hand, the horrible toxicities caused in the early 1950s by steroid overuse in patients with rheumatic diseases made an entire generation of rheumatologists wary of any new treatment.[1] We will trace the short history of glucocorticoids in clinical medicine, and then review the pharmacology, mechanism of action, and toxicities of these agents. The use of steroids in specific rheumatic diseases is covered in the chapters dealing with those diseases; we will focus our discussion of the clinical use of steroids to the broader issues of when to use steroids and how to stop them, and to the special considerations given to the patient treated chronically with corticosteroid who develops an intercurrent medical or surgical illness.

HISTORY OF GLUCOCORTICOIDS

Early investigations on the potential therapeutic role of adrenal cortical hormones in inflammatory diseases were stimulated by the observation by Hench in the 1920s that the constitutional symptoms of patients with rheumatoid arthritis were in many ways similar to those of patients with adrenal insufficiency. He postulated the existence of an antirheumatic compound, perhaps of adrenal origin, that was deficient

in patients with rheumatoid arthritis.[2,3] In the 1930s, Mason and his colleagues isolated cortisone (compound E) from adrenal tissue[4,5] and commenced a long endeavor to synthesize it and other adrenal cortical hormones. At about this same time, extracts of adrenal cortical tissue were shown to have some beneficial effects when injected into patients with rheumatoid arthritis.[6] Kendall reported that interest in adrenal cortical steroids in the United States was further stimulated in 1941 by a rumor that German Luftwaffe pilots were receiving injections of adrenal cortical extracts to prevent pulmonary edema from high altitude flights in unpressurized aircraft.[7]

By 1948, sufficient quantities of cortisone were synthesized to allow for clinical trials. The dramatic clinical effects of cortisone in patients with rheumatoid arthritis, and the immediate widespread acceptance of this treatment, have been chronicled by some of the participants in the process.[8,9] The enthusiasm of the medical community can be appreciated by reviewing some of the writing of that period. In the fifth edition (1953) of this textbook, Freyberg termed the use of cortisone in rheumatoid arthritis a once-in-a-lifetime "scientific bombshell."[10] Forty-eight pages of the textbook were devoted to a discussion of glucocorticoids, compared to one half a page spent on salicylates.

Hench and Kendall received the Nobel Prize for their work in 1950, 1 year after their preliminary report on the use of cortisone in rheumatic diseases.[2] By way of comparison, the discovery of the DNA double helix by Watson and Crick and the solving of the genetic

604

code by Nirenberg were recognized by the Nobel Committee after half-decade or longer delays. What was it about cortisone in rheumatoid arthritis that made it so exciting? There was a clear feeling communicated in the early papers that cortisone was more than just a new treatment, that perhaps it was a "cure." This message comes across in muted form in the title of Hench's Nobel Prize address, "The Reversibility of Certain Rheumatic and Non-Rheumatic Conditions by the Use of Cortisone or the Pituitary Adrenocorticotropic Hormone."[9] Note the use of the word "reversibility" rather than a more neutral choice, such as "treatment." The feeling that cortisone might represent a cure for rheumatoid arthritis may have stemmed from the paradigm that underlay the search by Hench and his co-workers for an anti-rheumatic factor of adrenal origin that was presumably deficient in patients with rheumatoid arthritis.[3] In that paradigm, cortisone treatment of rheumatoid arthritis represented correction of a deficiency state, much like vitamin B_{12} in pernicious anemia. The goal was to find the proper replacement dose. This optimistic view quickly faded, in part because of the rigorous fashion in which Hench and his associates screened for and recorded the toxicities of cortisone treatment.[11] Nevertheless, there was a period in the early 1950s when steroids were used in high doses for a variety of rheumatic diseases, including rheumatic fever, acute bursitis, gouty arthritis, ankylosing spondylitis, and osteoarthritis.[10,12] Even by 1953, the recommended starting and maintenance doses of cortisone in rheumatoid arthritis patients were 150 to 200 mg and 37.5 to 75 mg per day, respectively, given in divided doses.[10] This early period of the liberal use of steroids was followed by a backlash, once the serious toxicities associated with prolonged use of these drugs in these doses became apparent. Kendall characterized this period as follows: "The effective use of cortisone was retarded for a while by intemperate and unscientific extremes of exaggerated praise, bitter denunciation and emotion-laden criticism."[13]

One might reasonably ask why it is important or useful to review the history of glucocorticoid use in a modern textbook of rheumatology. We feel it is useful because some of the positive and negative attitudes of physicians today regarding steroids would appear to stem directly from the "emotion-laden" conflicts of the mid-1950s. A review of textbooks from the 1960s and 1970s reveals very few positive statements about glucocorticoids. The sixth, seventh, and eighth editions of this textbook are replete with descriptions of corticosteroid toxicity (as, indeed, this present chapter will be) and with ways of getting patients off steroids. At the same time, it was clear

that millions of patients were still receiving these drugs for rheumatic and other complaints.[14] There appeared to be a discrepancy between how rheumatologists *said* they used steroids (rarely, and with great caution) and how these drugs were actually used.[14]

Another detrimental by-product of the steroid controversy of the 1950s is that since that time there have been few clinical studies of steroid use in rheumatic diseases with results relevant to current rheumatologic practice. The controlled prospective trials in Britain of rheumatoid arthritis therapy by the Empire Rheumatism Council[15] and by the Medical Research Council[16] assigned patients to treatment with *either* aspirin *or* steroid. The results of these studies are unhelpful to the physician seeking information on the benefits and risks of *adding* low doses of steroids to patients already treated with salicylates or other nonsteroidal anti-inflammatory drugs (NSAIDs). Only one recent study addresses that question, and its small size (34 patients) and short duration (24 weeks) precluded any definite conclusions.[17] This can be compared to the hundreds of studies of NSAIDs, and of more esoteric modalities such as levamisole, plasmapheresis, or methotrexate, in the treatment of rheumatoid arthritis.

An additional factor contributing to the paucity of clinical studies of glucocorticoid therapy is that the important questions of efficacy and toxicity can be appropriately addressed only in long-term trials. Rheumatoid arthritis is a lifelong disease. A short-term study, no matter how well controlled, simply cannot address the important question of whether a given patient with active rheumatoid arthritis is likely to be better-off or worse-off in the long run if he is given steroid therapy.

Ignorance about efficacy of glucocorticoids extends even to the potentially more lethal rheumatic diseases such as systemic lupus erythematosus (SLE). Though virtually 100% of rheumatologists would agree that steroids can be lifesaving in treating complications of this disease, it is difficult to find this concept boldly and authoritatively stated in textbooks or review articles.

In summary, the catastrophies associated with overenthusiastic use of steroids in the relatively recent past would appear to have engendered a situation in which glucocorticoids are rarely mentioned in the classroom and seldom studied in the clinic.

PHARMACOLOGY AND PHYSIOLOGY

Glucocorticoids are 21-carbon steroid hormones synthesized from cholesterol. The term glucocorticoid refers to the ability of these agents to stimulate hepatic glycogen deposition and gluconeogenesis. Figure 37–1 provides the structure of the commonly used synthetic glucocorticoids. The activity of glucocorticoids depends on the presence of a hydroxyl group on carbon 11 of the steroid backbone. Two of the most commonly used glucocorticoids, cortisone and pred-

nisone, are inactive until converted in vivo to the corresponding 11-hydroxyl compounds, cortisol and prednisolone. A detailed discussion of the structure-activity relationships of glucocorticoids can be found in Haynes and Murad.[18]

The relative clinical potency of the various synthetic steroids depends upon the relative rate of absorption,

FIG. 37–1. Structure of the commonly used glucocorticoids. The arrows indicate the structural differences between cortisol and each of the other compounds.

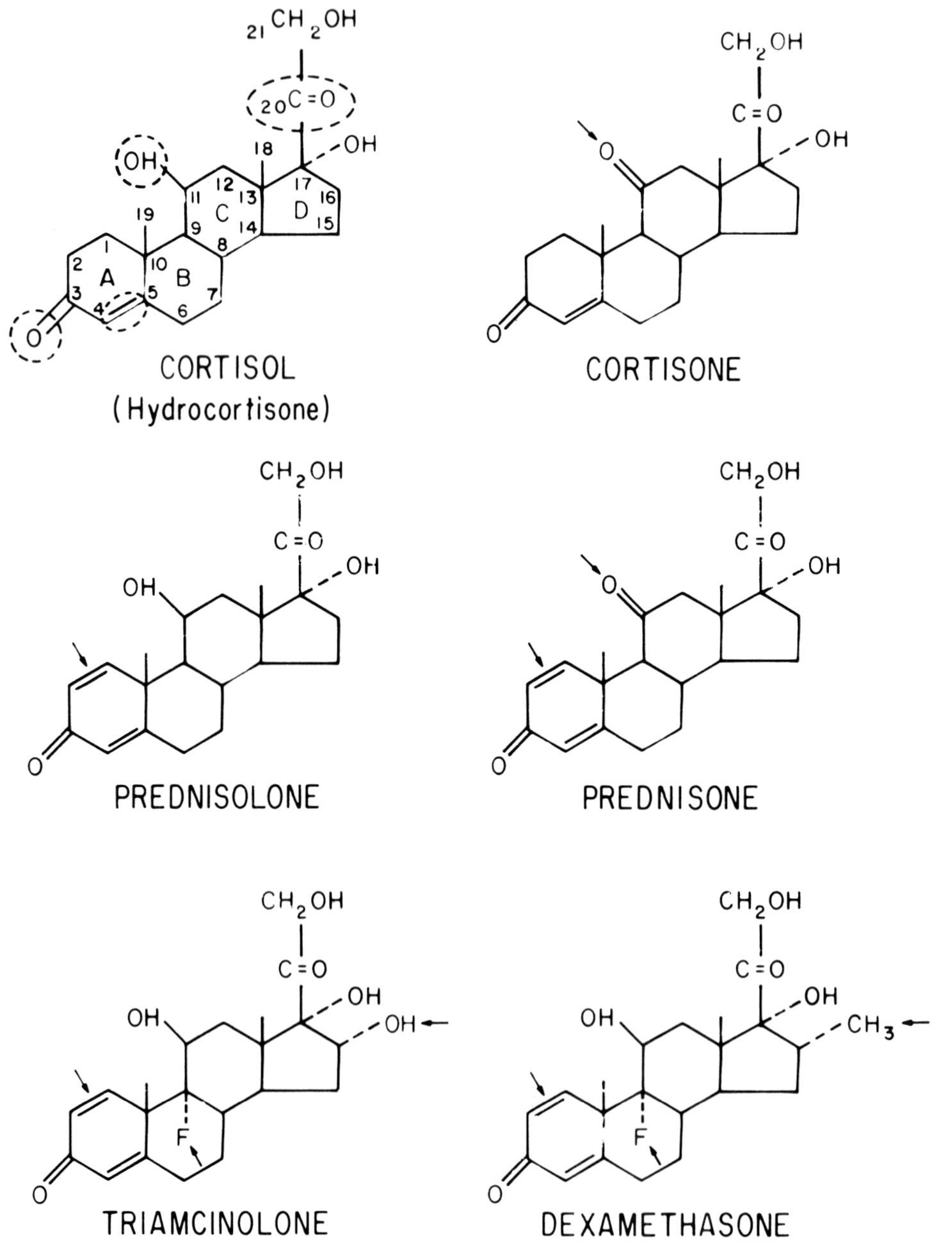

concentration at target tissues, and rate of metabolism and subsequent clearance. Consideration of these factors is essential to the rational use of glucocorticoids.

BIOAVAILABILITY

Most glucocorticoids are well absorbed after oral administration. The bioavailability of prednisolone from all forms of oral prednisone ranges from 80 to 99%,[19] and normal subjects achieve comparable plasma levels of prednisolone after receiving equivalent doses of prednisone and prednisolone.[20] Cortisol and dexamethasone are likewise well absorbed orally. Glucocorticoid uptake is not affected by most intrinsic intestinal diseases, and food intake does not influence absorption.[19]

DISTRIBUTION

Approximately 90% of endogenous circulating cortisol is bound with high affinity to the plasma protein corticosteroid-binding globulin. Another 5 to 8% is bound to albumin, which is a high-capacity, low-affinity reservoir for steroids. Only the small fraction of circulating glucocorticoids that is not protein bound is free to exert a biologic action, whereas glucocorticoids associated with proteins are inactive and protected from metabolic degradation.[21] Most synthetic steroids, with the exception of prednisolone, have a low affinity for corticosteroid-bearing globulin and are predominantly bound to albumin.[21] The volume of distribution and levels of protein binding of synthetic steroids may influence the frequency of adverse reactions with steroid therapy. Lewis et al. reported that patients with a serum albumin level less than 2.5 mg/dl who were receiving glucocorticoid therapy were twice as likely to have cushingoid side effects as a control group with normal albumin levels.[22] Individual differences in the volume of distribution of prednisolone may explain why certain patients receiving this drug are more likely to develop cushingoid side effects.[23] The increased potency of dexamethasone may in part relate to decreased plasma binding relative to other synthetic steroids.[24]

METABOLISM AND CLEARANCE

The glucocorticoids are metabolized by enzymatic modifications in the liver. Hydroxylation of the 4,5 double bond and ketone groups and subsequent conjugation with glucuronide or sulfate groups render steroids inactive and water soluble. The kidney excretes 95% of the conjugated metabolites, and the remainder are lost in the gut. The rates of metabolic degradation and clearance of steroids from the circulation are important determinants of potency. The plasma half-life is a commonly used index of the rate of clearance of glucocorticoids. However, because individuals vary considerably in both the distribution and clearance of the various glucocorticoids, the half-life often underestimates true clearance time.[19]

The decreased clearance of prednisolone and dexamethasone relative to cortisol account for much of their enhanced potency (Table 37–1). Modifications of the steroid molecule around the A ring (Fig. 37–1) decrease the rate of metabolism by the liver and delay clearance.[21] There are individual differences in the half-life of synthetic steroids, and patients with prolonged clearance of prednisolone[23] or dexamethasone[25] may be at increased risk for side effects from therapy.

Clearance rates of glucocorticoids are also affected by a variety of drugs and disease states. Phenytoin, phenobarbital, and rifampin can increase steroid clearance by inducing hepatic enzyme activity.[19] Estrogen therapy and estrogen-containing oral contraceptives impair clearance of administered steroids and may decrease the steroid requirement.[24] In liver disease, the metabolism of glucocorticoids is not significantly altered, and dosage adjustments are not necessary.[19,21] Some authors recommend the use of prednisolone rather than prednisone in chronic liver disease because of impaired hydroxylation of prednisone.[26] Dosage adjustments are generally not recommended for patients with kidney disease, although one recent study reported an increased half-life of prednisolone and an accelerated clearance of dexamethasone in renal failure.[27] In pregnancy, the clearance rate of cortisol is reduced, likely because of increased corticosteroid-binding globulin levels.[21] Glucocorticoids can lower plasma salicylate levels by enhancing renal clearance of salicylates. *Patients on fixed-dose salicylate therapy in whom glucocorticoids are withdrawn or tapered may develop rapid increases in serum salicylate levels, possibly to toxic levels.*[28]

RELATIVE POTENCY

Table 37–1 summarizes data on the half-life and relative potency of the commonly used glucocorticoid preparations.[18,24,26] It should be noted that the relative potencies are estimations based on studies measuring hypothalamic-pituitary-adrenal (HPA) axis suppression, glycogen deposition, and other parameters that

Table 37-1. Biologic Activity of Commonly Used Glucocorticoids

	Plasma Half-Life (min)	Relative Potency		Approximate Equivalent Dose (mg)
		Glucocorticoid	Mineralocorticoid	
Cortisol	80–120	1.0	1.0	20
Cortisone	80–120	0.8	0.8	25
Prednisone	200–210	3.5–4.0	0.8	5
Prednisolone	120–300	4.0	0.8	5
Triamcinolone	180–240	5.0	0	4
Dexamethasone	150–270	30–150	0	0.75

may or may not correlate with the desired clinical effect. Although the table is useful as an approximate guide, the clinician should exercise caution when calculating dose equivalents for the individual patient.[29]

CORTISOL AND THE HYPOTHALAMIC-PITUITARY-ADRENAL AXIS

Cortisol accounts for 90% of the hormonal output of the adrenal cortex. In health, secretion rates for cortisol vary from 8 to 25 mg per day in humans, with an average plasma concentration of 86 ng/ml for females and 116 ng/ml for males.[21] The production of cortisol is regulated by a neuroendocrine axis formed by the hypothalamus, the pituitary gland, and the adrenals. The hypothalamus releases a peptide, *corticotropin releasing factor* (CRF), which is a potent stimulus for the secretion of *adrenocorticotropin hormone* (ACTH) by the anterior pituitary. ACTH then stimulates the release of cortisol and other steroids from the adrenal cortex. Several mechanisms control the rate of cortisol release. Endogenous rhythms in the brain result in the pulsatile release of CRF, ACTH, and cortisol. These episodes of release are more frequent in the late evening and early morning hours and result in a circadian rhythm of plasma cortisol levels. Most endogenous cortisol is released during the last 4 hours of sleep and the first 5 hours after awakening.[21] Plasma cortisol levels may reach undetectable levels in the late afternoon. Emotions and physical factors, including hormonal and neural input, influence cortisol release and may increase plasma cortisol levels above normal. The most important control of cortisol release is feedback inhibition of CRF and ACTH release by glucocorticoids, including all the synthetic glucocorticoids. This feedback inhibition is rapid and, in the normal state, regulates cortisol levels in the physiologic range. In the patient treated with glucocorticoids, the axis may become suppressed. The degree of suppression increases progressively with continued exposure to

therapeutic doses of steroids. The axis may become unresponsive with prolonged (weeks to months) high-dose steroid therapy. Recovery of the axis after glucocorticoids are discontinued varies widely with individuals, but generally correlates with both the dosage and the duration of treatment.[30]

METABOLIC EFFECTS OF GLUCOCORTICOIDS

Like other hormones, glucocorticoids have effects on many different tissues and organ systems in the body. When glucocorticoids are present in normal levels, these various metabolic effects are presumably helpful in maintaining homeostasis. However, when steroids are present in high levels secondary to endogenous overproduction or exogenous administration, an accentuation of these same metabolic effects leads to the many toxicities associated with corticosteroid administration and Cushing's syndrome.

A summary of the metabolic effects of glucocorticoids is given in Table 37–2. In general, steroids are catabolic promoters. They block glucose uptake by tissues, enhance protein breakdown, and decrease new protein synthesis in muscle, skin, bone, connective tissue, fat, and lymphoid tissue.[24,31] DNA synthesis and cell proliferation are inhibited in fibroblasts, lymphocytes, and adipocytes.[24,31] Organisms chronically exposed to supraphysiologic levels of corticosteroids develop a type of wasting disease; they lose bone, connective tissue, and muscle, and gain water and fat. The specific metabolic effects relevant to the efficacy and toxicities of glucocorticoids in rheumatoid diseases will be discussed later.

MECHANISM OF ACTION OF CORTICOSTEROIDS

The question of the mechanism of action of corticosteroids—how they work at a molecular level—is

Table 37–2.   Metabolic Effects of Glucocorticoids

Carbohydrate Metabolism
   Impair glucose uptake and utilization by peripheral tissues
   Increase gluconeogenesis and glycogen deposition in liver

Lipid Metabolism
   Stimulate lipolysis and increase free fatty acid levels, an effect countered by increased insulin release and gluconeogenesis
   Increase fat deposition in truncal and facial areas

Protein Metabolism
   Inhibit synthesis and enhance breakdown of proteins in many tissues, leading to negative nitrogen balance
   Increase plasma free amino acid levels

Nucleic Acid Metabolism
   Stimulate RNA synthesis in liver, inhibit RNA synthesis in other tissues
   Inhibit DNA synthesis in most tissues

Fluid and Electrolyte Metabolism
   May enhance sodium retention and potassium loss, independent of mineralocorticoid action
   Increase glomerular filtration rate

Bone and Calcium Metabolism
   Decrease intestinal calcium absorption
   Decrease renal reabsorption of calcium and phosphate with resulting hypercalciuria
   Inhibit osteoblast function

exceptionally important. One of the major means of new drug development is through investigations on the mechanism of action of existing efficacious agents. For example, research on the mechanism of action of penicillin led not only to a fuller understanding of bacterial cell wall synthesis, but also to the development of other classes of powerful antibiotics. A more recent example is azidothymidine, a drug discovered in a process in which several thousand agents were screened for their ability to inhibit the replication of the acquired immune deficiency syndrome (AIDS) virus in vitro. Further work on the mechanism of action of azidothymidine revealed that it was a reverse-transcriptase inhibitor, which led to the development of whole families of reverse-transcriptase inhibitors that may prove effective in AIDS and other diseases caused by RNA viruses. One might reasonably hope that a fuller understanding of the molecular mechanisms responsible for the anti-inflammatory and other effects of corticosteroids might lead to the development of drugs with some of the actions of corticosteroids (e.g., the anti-inflammatory effect) but without the whole array of other metabolic effects and toxicities.

A major difficulty limiting early work on the mechanism of action of corticosteroids was the multitude of physiologic effects produced by these compounds. Most drugs that we understand have a single action to which we can trace the drug's efficacy and, often, much of the toxicity. Thus, a drug can inhibit an enzyme, like allopurinol; block a receptor, like propranolol or cimetidine; block ion channels, like verapamil; or mimic endogenous substrates, like morphine or diazepam. But corticosteroids have so many different therapeutic actions and toxicities that it was conceptually difficult to postulate a single mechanism of action. Corticosteroids have at least three separate therapeutic effects. First, they are clearly the most powerful anti-inflammatory agents ever discovered. Second, they are powerful antiproliferative and immunosuppressive compounds. Third, they are highly efficacious in the treatment of asthma. These three effects appear to be independent of each other. No other anti-inflammatory drug is immunosuppressive or useful in asthma, no other asthma treatment is immunosuppressive, and so on. In addition, the many powerful toxicities of corticosteroids would also appear to be independent of each other. It is difficult to relate, for example, the effect of corticosteroids in promoting negative calcium balance with their effects on the central nervous system (CNS) (see below). Drugs that have some therapeutic effects similar to corticosteroids'—for example, sodium cromolyn for asthma, or NSAIDs for inflammation—do not share the same toxicities (though they have their own).

It is easy to see how such an array of benefits and toxicities would discourage investigators from looking for *the* mechanism of action of corticosteroids. Nevertheless, progress has been made in this area. All steroid hormones (vitamin D, glucocorticoids, sex hormones, mineralocorticoids) act by binding to high-affinity receptors present in relatively low numbers (2 to 6×10^4 per cell) in the cytoplasm (Fig. 37–2). The steroid-receptor complex, in turn, has a high affinity for nuclear interphase chromosomes and thus binds to chromosomal DNA.[32] This triggers DNA transcription with the formation of messenger RNA, leading to new protein synthesis. The specific genes transcribed and proteins produced after exposure to steroid hormones varies with the different steroid hormones and also with the type of target cell. Specificity of cell response is provided for in at least two ways. First, the steroid-receptor complex binds to specific regulatory sequences that in turn lead to transcription of the particular gene containing that sequence. Presumably the receptor complex binding vitamin D attaches to regulatory sequences on different genes than the receptor complex binding glucocorticoids. Second, only a small portion of the genome is sensitive to induction by steroid hormone because it is contained in an "unraveled" portion of chromatin sensitive to digestion with DNAase. This unraveled portion will differ depending on cell type.[32]

All well-defined physiologic and pharmacologic ef-

FIG. 37–2. Model for the molecular basis of glucocorticoid action. See text for details.

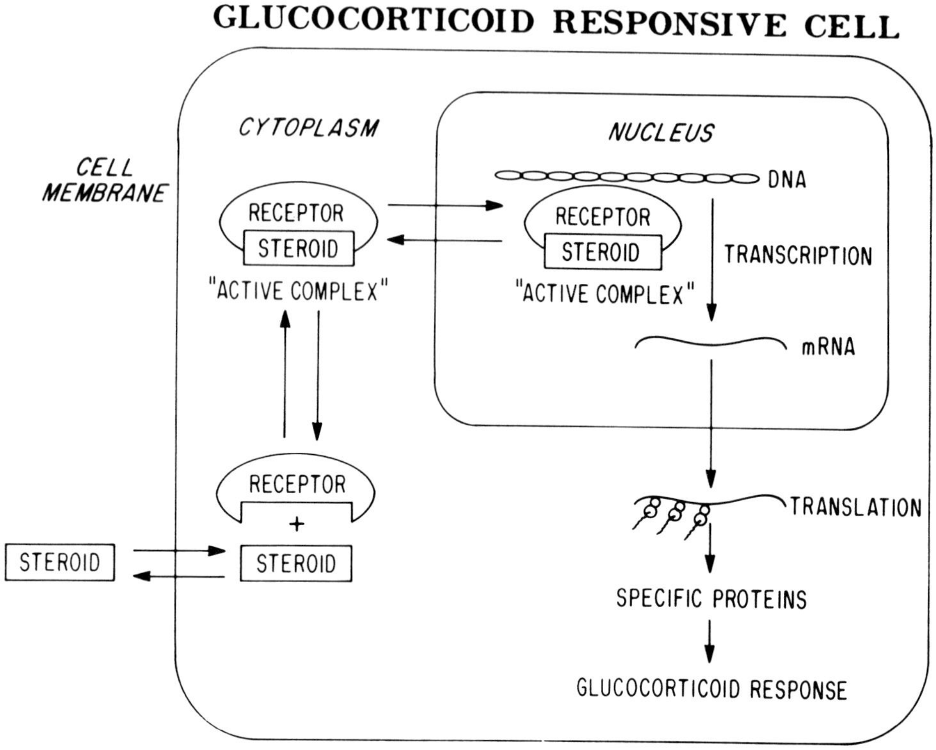

GLUCOCORTICOID RESPONSIVE CELL

fects of steroid hormones are thought to be mediated by the process outlined above. One implication of this statement is that pharmacologic or physiologic effects are separated in time from drug administration. Thus, for example, one expects to see a clinical response to intravenous hydrocortisone in acute asthma several hours or more after it is given. Another implication is that glucocorticoid action is in many ways less direct than the action of other drugs. It acts via the synthesis of other compounds. This has led to an attempt to characterize precisely which new proteins are synthesized after glucocorticoid administration. The rationale, put in an overly simplified fashion, is that if we can characterize all the proteins the synthesis of which is stimulated by glucocorticoids, and then determine the actions of those proteins, we will have delineated many new pathways that may prove useful targets for pharmacologic modulation.

One particularly rewarding path of investigation in that regard was initiated by the observation of Gryglewski et al. that prior infusion of glucocorticoids inhibited the production of prostaglandins in isolated perfused rabbit mesentery.[33] This inhibition could be overcome by the infusion of arachidonic acid. Thus, Gryglewski et al. concluded that glucocorticoids inhibited prostaglandin production by blocking the release of the precursor arachidonic acid from cellular

stores, and proposed that the anti-inflammatory properties of glucocorticoids were secondary to this effect on arachidonic acid.[33] This hypothesis was difficult for most investigators to accept, because it was already generally accepted that NSAIDs worked via inhibition of arachidonic acid metabolism,[34] and the anti-inflammatory effects of glucocorticoids were clearly different and more powerful than those of NSAIDs. The understanding of arachidonic acid metabolism at the time was essentially a straight-line pathway from membrane phospholipid to arachidonic acid to prostaglandins. Thus, if glucocorticoids and NSAIDs inhibit at different points in the same pathway, then they should have very similar actions.

This problem was clarified when Samuelsson identified the lipoxygenase metabolic pathways for arachidonic acid.[35] This more complex scheme of arachidonic acid metabolism allowed investigators to seriously consider the possibility that many of the pharmacologic and perhaps physiologic actions of glucocorticoids acted indeed through inhibition of arachidonic acid release from membrane phospholipid, because glucocorticoids would inhibit both cyclo-oxygenase and lipoxygenase products, whereas NSAIDs inhibit only cyclo-oxygenase products.

Clearly, the evidence supporting this concept has grown considerably over the past few years. Danon and Assouline showed that RNA and protein synthesis are required for steroid inhibition of prostaglandin production.[36] In 1979 and 1980, Flower and his associates,[37,38] in England, and Hirata, Axelrod, and their co-workers,[39] at the National Institutes of Health, identified a phospholipase A_2-inhibitory glycoprotein, now termed *lipocortin*, that is synthesized and released by cells on exposure to glucocorticoids. On the other hand, several investigators have failed to find an inhibition by glucocorticoids of the endogenous production of arachidonic acid metabolites in vitro[40] and in vivo.[41,42] This discrepancy exists presumably because arachidonic acid can be released from membrane phospholipid by at least two pathways, only one of which is inhibited by lipocortin. Lipocortin would appear to be a family of molecules, one of which was recently cloned and found to have potent anti-inflammatory actions.[43] Davidson et al. suggested that lipocortins are identical to calpactins, which are ubiquitous intracellular proteins that bind calcium and phospholipid.[44] If this is the case, then inhibition of arachidonic acid release by lipocortin (and by glucocorticoids) may be due to a masking of the substrate for phospholipase A_2—the membrane phospholipids—rather than inhibition of the enzyme per se.[44]

Recent reports on the physiologic and pathophysiologic roles of various lipoxygenase metabolites of arachidonic acid, particularly the leukotrienes (reviewed in Chapter 26), makes it feasible that the anti-inflammatory, and perhaps other therapeutic actions of glucocorticoids occur indeed through inhibition of arachidonic acid metabolism. Leukotriene C_4 (LTC_4) and LTD_4 were identified as the slow reactive substance of anaphylaxis (SRS-A), potentially explaining the therapeutic efficacy of glucocorticoids in asthma.[35] LTB_4 would appear to play a major role in the inflammatory response (reviewed in Chapter 26). It causes margination, chemotaxis, and aggregation of neutrophils in very small concentrations, and also stimulates pain receptors.[45,46] The potential linking of the anti-inflammatory and antiasthma properties of glucocorticoids to blockade of arachidonic acid metabolism has stimulated the pharmaceutical industry to search for specific inhibitors of the synthesis of leukotrienes and also leukotriene-receptor antagonists, with the hope that these drugs might possess a therapeutic action of glucocorticoids (for example, the anti-inflammatory or antiasthma action) but, because of their relative specificity, might not have the whole spectrum of therapeutic actions and, more importantly, the array of toxicities of glucocorticoids.

Inhibition of phospholipase A_2 by glucocorticoids also results in inhibition of platelet activating factor (PAF) production.[47] In many systems PAF would appear to have effects similar to leukotrienes. Thus, much effort is now being made in the development of PAF antagonists, with preliminary evidence that these agents may have therapeutic effects in asthma, in immediate hypersensitivity reactions, and possibly in inflammation.[47]

ANTI-INFLAMMATORY EFFECTS OF GLUCOCORTICOIDS

As mentioned earlier, the glucocorticoids are the most powerful anti-inflammatory agents available. Their administration results in a complex series of changes in the actions of cells involved in inflammatory reactions.[48] After a single dose of glucocorticoids, there is a net increase in the number of circulating neutrophils, peaking 4 to 6 hours after drug administration.[49] This increase in the number of circulating neutrophils, and increase in the half-life of neutrophils in the circulation, is accompanied by, and is presumably secondary to, a decrease in their margination, migration, and accumulation at sites of inflammation, leading to a decrease in the four cardinal signs of inflammation: heat, redness, swelling, and pain. Glucocorticoids also reduce the numbers of monocytes migrating to and accumulating in sites of inflammation, which further prevents the signs of acute inflammation and interferes with delayed-type hypersensitivity reactions.[50]

Glucocorticoids also directly suppress the action of cells involved in the inflammatory response, inhibiting phagocytosis by neutrophils and monocytes, the release of degradative enzymes such as collagenase and plasminogen activator by neutrophils and by synovial lining cells, and also the production of inflammatory lymphokines and monokines such as interleukin-1.[51-53] Other than the clear effects found in vivo and in vitro on migration and accumulation of granulocytes and monocytes, it is difficult to know which of the many other actions of glucocorticoids on inflammatory cell function actually contribute to the clinical anti-inflammatory effect. This is because most data were obtained with in vitro models using isolated cell populations. It is reasonable to assume, however, that the so-called lysosomal stabilizing effects and decreased release of inflammatory mediators and degradative enzymes probably do play a role in glucocorticoid action.[53,54]

IMMUNOSUPPRESSIVE EFFECTS OF GLUCOCORTICOIDS

The literature on effects of glucocorticoids on various immune functions is as varied as any in immunology. It is impossible to synthesize all the many observations into one coherent review, given the many apparently contradictory reports.[55]

One potential source of confusion is the marked differences in susceptibility to corticosteroids among species.[56] Steroid-sensitive species, including the mouse, rat, and rabbit, experience dramatic lymphoid depletion following steroid treatment, characterized by shrinkage of the thymus, spleen, and peripheral lymph nodes, and lysis of peripheral blood lymphocytes. In contrast, human and guinea pig lymphoid cells are resistant to the lytic effects of steroid administration.[56] This fundamental difference in steroid sensitivity should lead to cautious interpretation of the literature, especially in extrapolating data from steroid-sensitive animals to man. Another potential problem in the interpretation of early studies is that suprapharmacologic doses of steroids, clearly unobtainable in vivo, were often added to in vitro cultures.[57] We will focus here on studies investigating the effects of physiologic or pharmacologic concentrations of corticosteroids in humans.

As corticosteroids became available to investigators in the 1950s, the immunosuppressive properties of these agents were quickly recognized.[58] In general, T-lymphocytes are more sensitive to the in vivo immunosuppressive effects of corticosteroids than are B-lymphocytes. Fauci emphasized the importance of the redistribution of lymphocytes and monocytes in mediating corticosteroid action in man.[59] A single dose of corticosteroids in humans results in a 70% decline in circulating lymphocytes and a 90% decline in circulating monocytes. T-lymphocytes, especially helper T cells, are depleted from the circulation to a greater extent than B-lymphocytes in response to corticosteroids. This depletion occurs within 4 to 6 hours and reverts to normal by 24 hours.[59] A similar phenomenon occurs daily during chronic steroid administration. The lymphocytopenia appears to be because of redistribution of circulating lymphocytes to other lymphoid compartments, particularly the bone marrow, and not to cell lysis or death. The normal migration of lymphocytes from the peripheral circulation to secondary lymphoid tissues and back occurs rapidly (approximately 12 times per day) and is not random. Specific molecules present on the surface of circulating lymphocytes and the cells lining postcapillary high endothelial venules direct the lymphocyte traffic in a precise, though poorly understood, manner. Presumably, corticosteroids alter the specific recognition molecules or surface charge on the cell membranes and either enhance exit of lymphocytes from the circulation or block re-entry.

B-lymphocytes are relatively resistant to the in vivo immunosuppressive effects of corticosteroids in man. Specific antibody synthesis following inoculation with pneumococcal capsular polysaccharide, pertussis vaccine, diphtheria toxoid, and streptococcal-0-antigens are not affected by glucocorticoid therapy.[60] However, serum IgG, IgA, and IgM levels are suppressed following a brief course of daily high-dose methylprednisolone with maximal suppression at 2 to 4 weeks after treatment. In vivo steroids may augment immunoglobulin levels in certain clinical situations such as adult combined immunodeficiency by inhibiting suppressor cell function.[61]

Cell-mediated immune reactions are generally inhibited by in vivo corticosteroids. Patients on steroids are often anergic, reflecting an inability to express cutaneous delayed hypersensitivity despite previous sensitization. Bovornkitti et al. showed that 68 of 70 patients treated with 40 mg of prednisone per day converted from a positive to negative tuberculin test within 2 weeks.[62] The skin test reaction reconverted to a positive test 6 days after prednisone therapy was stopped. Steroids are believed to suppress graft rejection by inhibiting the proliferation of alloreactive T-lymphocytes and the generation of cytotoxic T-lymphocytes.[55,63] Corticosteroids suppress most in vitro T-lymphocyte proliferative responses, and they appear to interfere with early activation events.[55]

Natural killer (NK) cells and antibody-dependent cellular cytotoxicity (ADCC) effector cells are important in vivo in tumor surveillance, acute graft rejection, and lysis of virally infected cells. In vivo, Parrillo and Fauci found that 12 mg of dexamethasone suppressed NK activity at 24 and 48 hours, with normalization by 96 hours.[64]

Many of the suppressive effects of glucocorticoids would appear to be secondary to inhibition of the production and action of a variety of lymphokines and monokines. These peptides communicate between cells of the immune system, carrying messages that stimulate cells to proliferate, differentiate, or perform specific functions.

Interleukin-1 is produced by monocytes and in turn can enhance T-cell production of interleukin-2, colony stimulating factor, gamma interferon, and other lymphokines (see Chapter 42). Glucocorticoids are one of the few classes of agents capable of inhibiting the production of interleukin-1.[65] They also profoundly inhibit interleukin-2 production.[66] The observation that exogenous interleukin-2 restores proliferation of glucocorticoid-treated lymphocytes suggests that steroids do not affect the initial activation events of lymphocytes; rather, they block the passage of the cell through an early cell cycle phase.[66] Glucocorticoids also block the production of γ-interferon by T-lymphocytes, and this inhibition occurs at the level of DNA transcription.[67] By inhibiting γ-interferon production, steroids diminish Fc-receptor clearance by the reticuloendothelial system.

SIDE EFFECTS OF STEROID THERAPY

The toxicities of prolonged glucocorticoid therapy are many and are the major limiting factor in the use of these agents. One of the most puzzling aspects of glucocorticoid therapy is the wide range of susceptibility to side effects observed. Some patients on prolonged, high-dose therapy appear to tolerate glucocorticoids without adverse effects, whereas others treated with small doses for brief intervals develop devastating side effects. As noted above, part of this differential sensitivity likely relates to individual differences in plasma protein binding (with hypoalbuminemic patients at risk) and to variations in metabolism and clearance of synthetic steroids. Sensitivity to glucocorticoids in mice is closely linked to the H-2 histocompatibility region.[68,69] Differences in glucocorticoid sensitivity between different mouse strains has been associated with differences in glucocorticoid receptor content[68] and also with differences in stimulation of the phospholipase A_2-inhibitory protein lipocortin.[70] In our work involving the effects of steroids on immune function, we noted wide variations among normal individuals in the sensitivity of their lymphocytes to inhibition by steroids, and these differences in sensitivity were relatively constant over time.[71] We also found a decreased sensitivity to inhibition by steroids in lymphocytes from elderly subjects.[72] Other investigators have found decreased in vitro sensitivity of lymphocytes to hydrocortisone to be associated with poor therapeutic response to these drugs in vivo.[73,74]

The major differences between iatrogenic Cushing's syndrome and spontaneous Cushing's syndrome relate primarily to increased androgen and mineralocorticoid levels in the spontaneous syndrome.[26] A comparison is provided in Table 37–3.

As one approach to classification, we present the adverse reactions to glucocorticoids in approximate order of frequency based on a synthesis of the literature and general clinical experience (Table 37–4). Several of the adverse effects are of particular importance to rheumatologic practice and are discussed in some detail below.

OSTEOPOROSIS

(See Chapter 7 for methods of assessment of bone mineralization and Chapter 112 for discussion of prevention and treatment of steroid induced osteopenia.)

Table 37–3. Iatrogenic vs. Spontaneous Cushing's Syndrome*

Features Virtually Unique to Iatrogenic Cushing's Syndrome
  Glaucoma
  Posterior subcapsular cataract
  Avascular necrosis of bone
  Pseudotumor cerebri
  Pancreatitis
  Panniculitis

More Common in Spontaneous Cushing's Syndrome
  Hypertension
  Hirsutism/virilism
  Striae, purpura, plethora
  Altered menses
  Impotence (men)

Shared Clinical Features
  Centripetal obesity
  Psychiatric symptoms
  Poor wound healing
  Osteoporosis
  Glucose intolerance
  HPA† axis suppression

*Modified from L. Axelrod.[26]
†Hypothalmic-pituitary-adrenal.

Table 37–4. Side Effects of Glucocorticoid Therapy

Very Common and Should Be Anticipated in All Patients
  Negative calcium balance leading to osteoporosis
  Increased appetite
  Centripetal obesity
  Impaired wound healing
  Increased risk of infection
  Suppression of hypothalamic-pituitary-adrenal axis
  Growth arrest in children

Frequently Seen
  Myopathy
  Avascular necrosis
  Hypertension
  Plethora
  Thin, fragile skin/striae/purpura
  Edema secondary to sodium and water retention
  Hyperlipidemia
  Psychiatric symptoms, particularly euphoria
  Diabetes mellitus
  Posterior subcapsular cataracts

Uncommon, but Important to Recognize Early
  Glaucoma
  Benign intracranial hypertension
  "Silent" intestinal perforation
  Peptic ulcer disease (often gastric)
  Hypokalemic alkalosis
  Hyperosmolar nonketotic coma
  Gastric hemorrhage

Rare
  Pancreatitis
  Hirsutism
  Panniculitis
  Secondary amenorrhea
  Impotence
  Epidural lipomatosis
  Allergy to synthetic steroids

Osteoporosis is perhaps the most common and potentially devastating side effect of steroid therapy. Every patient treated with glucocorticoids develops negative calcium balance, and approximately 40% develop clinically significant osteoporosis.[75] Histologic studies of bone from patients undergoing prolonged treatment with various glucocorticoids have shown decreased rates of bone formation and increased rates of bone resorptive activity.[76] The decreased rate of bone formation is due to a direct effect of the hormone on osteoblasts, with studies showing impaired collagen synthesis and decreased conversion of precursors to functioning osteoblasts. Protein synthesis is greatly depressed after in vitro exposure to steroids.[31] The increased bone resorption is largely an indirect effect mediated by high levels of parathyroid hormone (PTH).[77] The stimuli for PTH release in steroid-treated patients include impaired intestinal absorption of calcium[78] and diminished tubular reabsorption of calcium in the kidney with resulting hypercalciuria.[79]

The dual effects of enhanced bone resorption and impaired bone formation may explain why steroid-induced osteopenia develops so rapidly and predictably.[80] The bone loss characteristically involves trabecular bone in the ribs, vertebrae, and distal radius, and is less severe in regions of less metabolically active cortical bone.[81] As a result, rib fractures and vertebral compression fractures of the thoracic and lumbar spine are common in steroid-treated patients. The incidence of symptomatic bone loss is most common in children and postmenopausal women.

Using single and dual photon densitometry, Dykman et al. showed that significant bone loss may accompany doses as low as 8 to 10 mg of prednisone per day and appears to correlate with length of therapy.[82] On the other hand, Sambrook et al. reported that low-dose prednisolone therapy (mean dosage 8 mg/day) over a mean of 7 years in women with rheumatoid arthritis was not associated with increased bone loss, compared to women with rheumatoid arthritis not receiving glucocorticoid.[83] In the same study, slightly higher doses of prednisolone (mean dosage 10.3 mg/day) were associated with significant bone loss in men with rheumatoid arthritis.[83] Alternate-day glucocorticoid therapy does not appear to influence the rate or degree of bone loss in patients with rheumatic disease.[75] Further discussion of steroid-induced osteoporosis and strategies for treatment and prophylaxis are presented in Chapter 112.

MYOPATHY

The myopathy associated with glucocorticoid therapy is generally insidious in onset and usually painless. The proximal muscles of the pelvic girdle are first involved, but those of the proximal upper extremity and distal limbs are also affected in more severe cases. Atrophy of the involved muscle groups is evident. Myalgias are occasionally noted and when observed in a patient receiving large dose of steroids should suggest the diagnosis.[84] An acute myopathy may (rarely) follow high dose pulse steroid therapy.[85]

Patients receiving more than 40 mg of prednisone per day are at greatest risk for developing steroid myopathy, whereas patients on alternate-day therapy appear to be relatively protected.[86] Diagnosis is most likely to present a problem when steroids are used to treat inflammatory conditions, such as systemic lupus erythematosus and polymyositis, when weakness may be due to an exacerabation of an underlying muscle disease process. Muscle biopsy and EMG are generally not helpful in differentiating among the processes.[84] Serum "muscle" enzymes (CPK, aldolase, and SGOT) are normal in steroid myopathy, and, if elevated, suggest the diagnosis of myositis.[84] Urine creatine may be elevated in steroid myopathy and should drop with reduction in steroid dose,[84] although the value of urinary creatine determinations has been questioned.[86] If a patient is suspected of having developed steroid myopathy on high-dose therapy, the dosage should be decreased to less than 30 mg of prednisone per day if possible. Alternate-day therapy should be attempted if a reduction in dose is not feasible. If a patient with muscle weakness is receiving 30 mg of prednisone per day or less *and has no other signs of glucocorticoid excess*, other causes of myopathy (endocrine, biochemical, neurologic) should be thoroughly evaluated. A physical training program, based on isokinetic exercise, may reverse steroid-induced myopathy.[87] Although this has yet to be shown for more readily available exercise modalities, physical exercise may have an important therapeutic and prophylactic role.

PEPTIC ULCER DISEASE

The true incidence of peptic ulcers as a result of glucocorticoid treatment remains controversial. Conn and Blitzer's retrospective study in 1976 of over 6000 steroid-treated patients concluded there was no significant association between steroid therapy and peptic ulcer.[88] In a similar study, Messer et al. pooled data from 71 controlled clinical trials and determined that 1.8% of steroid-treated patients developed peptic ulcers, compared to 0.8% of a control group, a significant difference.[89] These studies have been criticized; however, they offer a reasonable clinical perspective on the problem. Less than 1 in 50 patients treated with steroids should be expected to develop peptic ulcer disease, and half these patients would have developed ulcers anyway. The risk is certainly lower with steroid therapy than with treatment with aspirin or other NSAIDs.[90] It would appear that ulcer prophylaxis with antacids and/or H-2 blocking agents is not warranted if steroid therapy is the only risk factor for ulcer occurrence.[91]

PSYCHIATRIC COMPLICATIONS

Euphoria is commonly observed in patients receiving glucocorticoids. In part this may be due to the beneficial effect on the underlying disease, but there appear to be additional independent factors.[92] Depression, nervousness, insomnia, and psychotic reactions are also noted with increased frequency. The type of disorder a patient will develop is *not* predictable from the pretreatment personality, and these disorders are usually reversible with dose reduction or discontinuation. A previous history of mental disorders is not a contraindication to steroid therapy. The differentiation between steroid-induced psychosis and CNS lupus can be exceptionally difficult in a patient with a history of lupus cerebritis. Formal cognitive testing can frequently be helpful in making the distinction, as glucocorticoid-induced psychosis tends to be nonorganic.

INFECTIONS

Patients receiving more than 20 mg of prednisone per day are predisposed to developing infections.[59,93–95] Although gram-negative bacterial and fungal infections are most common, other bacterial, viral, and parasitic infections also occur with increased frequency.[93] Estimation of the true incidence of steroid-induced infections is difficult because many of the diseases for which steroids are administered (e.g., systemic lupus erythematosus) also predispose patients to infections, and many of these patients are also receiving other immunosuppressive agents concomitantly.[94]

Because glucocorticoids nonspecifically suppress the inflammatory response, detection and definitive diagnosis of infections in these patients are often delayed; a high index of clinical suspicion is therefore essential. The severity and frequency of infections appear to correlate with the dosage and length of steroid treatment. Alternate-day therapy markedly decreases the incidence of infections.[59]

Surprisingly little firm data supports the idea of prophylaxis in steroid-treated patients with a history of previous tuberculosis or a positive PPD test. An early study concluded there was no risk of tuberculosis reactivation in asthmatics receiving steroids,[96] although few patients were followed and the period of observation was short. Another study documented several episodes of tuberculous reactivation after corticosteroid therapy, but most of these patients were also receiving other immunosuppressive agents or had compromised immunity because of their underlying disease.[97] The patient with a positive PPD and either a normal chest radiogram or a single calcified nodule probably does not require prophylaxis.[98] If the chest film shows fibronodular scarring, or if the patient's immune status is otherwise significantly impaired, the risk is enhanced considerably, and prophylaxis with isoniazid is advisable.[98]

OCULAR COMPLICATIONS

Patients treated with glucocorticoids are at high risk for developing cataracts or glaucoma.[99] *Posterior subcapsular cataracts* occur frequently, and their incidence correlates with both the dosage and duration of therapy. Of patients with rheumatoid arthritis receiving 15 mg of prednisone per day for 1 year, 25% developed lenticular changes.[100] Covalent linkage of steroid molecules to crystalline proteins may be responsible for cataract formation.[101] Glucocorticoids increase intraocular pressure in up to 40% of patients.[102] Irreversible *glaucoma* and *blindness* may occur in susceptible individuals. Those at highest risk include highly myopic individuals, diabetics, and patients with primary open-angle glaucoma. Referral to an ophthalmologist for baseline measurement of intraocular pressure and for slit-lamp examination should be strongly considered in any patient when the duration of corticosteroid therapy is expected to exceed 1 month.

ATHEROSCLEROSIS

Although not traditionally recognized as a complication of steroid use, there is increasing evidence from a number of retrospective studies that atherosclerosis is more common in glucocorticoid-treated patients.[103] Steroids exacerbate many of the known coronary artery disease risk factors, including hypertension, hypercholesterolemia, hypertriglyceridemia, and glucose intolerance. Atherosclerosis of the peripheral arteries has been linked to prolonged corticosteroid use in patients with rheumatoid arthritis.[104]

PREGNANCY

In general, corticosteroid use is considered safe during pregnancy.[24] In one study of 70 pregnancies in 55 asthmatic patients treated with steroids, there were 71 live births, 1 spontaneous abortion, and a slightly increased rate of premature births.[105] There were no maternal, fetal, or neonatal deaths, and no increased incidence of toxemia, uterine hemorrhage, or congenital malformations compared to the general population. Steroids should be used cautiously, but should not be withheld if life-threatening diseases amenable to their use occurs during pregnancy.

ALTERNATE-DAY THERAPY
(See also Chapter 74)

Many of the adverse effects of steroid therapy can be decreased by administering a single dose of glucocorticoid on alternate days. This regimen decreases the incidence of infections, myopathy, obesity, excessive appetite, growth inhibition in children, cushingoid facies, glucose intolerance, suppression of the HPA axis, and other side effects.[26] For example, Fauci et al. reported that in a group of 70 patients receiving alternate-day prednisone (mean dose 55 mg) for 29 months in the treatment of a variety of collagen-vascular diseases, there were no documented infectious complications.[59] This contrasts with a 10 to 40% expected rate of infection in patients treated with daily, high-dose therapy.[93,94]

Alternate-day therapy should not be considered in the initial treatment of any disease.[26,106,107] Initial suppression of the active inflammatory and immunologic component of most diseases requires daily, divided doses of glucocorticoids.[106] Then, with the underlying disease quiescent, alternate-day therapy has been found to maintain the state of suppression. The mechanisms underlying the effectiveness of alternate-day therapy are not precisely known. In patients treated for a variety of inflammatory diseases, the lymphocytopenia and monocytopenia induced by glucocorticoids returned to normal on the day "off" prednisone, but the underlying disease remained suppressed on the "off" day.[108]

The switch to alternate-day therapy can and should be made as soon as the underlying disease is suppressed, preferably within several weeks after initiation of treatment. There are no absolute rules for the

conversion. The patient with a normal or moderately responsive HPA axis will usually tolerate an abrupt change. One suggested approach is to double the daily dose of a short-acting glucocorticoid, such as prednisone, and give it as a single morning dose on alternate days. In patients receiving long-term daily therapy who have developed a suppressed HPA axis, the change may have to be more gradual. An example of a conversion regimen is presented in Table 37–5. The pace of conversion will vary considerably with individuals. Adjunctive treatment with nonsteroidal medications on the "off" day may ease the transition; close supervision and encouragement by the physician are essential. Complaints by the patient are common on the "off" day, and the physician must determine whether these are signs due to adrenal insufficiency, loss of steroid euphoria, or recurrence of the underlying disease. If there is evidence of a flare of the underlying disease, daily therapy must be reinstituted.[106]

THERAPEUTIC USE OF GLUCOCORTICOIDS

There are no strict guidelines or dependable formulas to tell the physician when to use glucocorticoids. Like most important decisions in medicine, it is too complex to be codified. Thus, there will continue to be a large variation in glucocorticoid use among different physicians and among different academic centers in rheumatology. Nevertheless, it is possible to formulate a set of general guidelines to

Table 37–5. Protocol for Changing from a Single Daily Dose Regimen to a Single Alternate-Day Regimen*†

Day	Prednisone (mg)
1–7	60
8	60
9	40
10	70
11	30
12	80
13	20
14	90
15	10
16	95
17	5
18	95
19‡	5

*All doses taken on awakening in the morning.
†Modified from R.G. Dluhy, et al.[117]
‡The dosage on the high-dose day can be reduced at 5- to 7-day intervals.

which the majority of experienced clinicians would subscribe.

1. Give glucocorticoids for as short a time and in as low a dose as possible.
2. There are some diseases that require glucocorticoid therapy; do not try to get by with "safer" drugs. Patients with active SLE, or with giant cell arteritis, to name two examples, are not well-served by physicians who are so obsessed with glucocorticoid toxicity that the disease is allowed to progress in the face of inadequate treatment.
3. In patients requiring chronic therapy, switch to an alternate-day schedule when possible.
4. Glucocorticoids should never be the first medication used to treat rheumatoid arthritis.
5. Whenever possible, use a short- or intermediate-acting steroid and administer it in the morning to minimize suppression of the HPA axis.
6. Patients who have taken more than 10 mg prednisone, or its equivalent, daily for 3 weeks or longer should be considered to have a suppressed hypothalamic-pituitary-adrenal axis for one year following cessation of therapy and should receive supplemental glucocorticoids during surgery or severe medical illness (Table 37–6).
7. Patients must be educated about the benefits and toxicities of glucocorticoids. They must understand the trade-offs between efficacy and toxicity. Glucocorticoids make patients with rheumatoid arthritis feel good, frequently better than they have felt in a very long time. Patients ignorant of the long-term toxicities of glucocorticoids feel puzzled as to why their physician does not use this wonderful drug, just as they later feel betrayed when they encounter a serious toxicity of glucocorticoid therapy. All patients with rheumatoid arthritis who are given glucocorticoids must be prepared to stop the drug even as it is first given. As is so frequently the case in rheumatology, the physician and the patient must work together as a team, sharing common information and seeking common goals.
8. It is easier to use glucocorticoids in a patient with rheumatoid arthritis if an obvious endpoint can be identified. For example, a patient with very

active disease who is being started on parenteral gold might be given a 3-month course of low-dose glucocorticoids (e.g., 5 mg prednisone daily). Another example is a patient with long-standing, relatively well-controlled disease who has occasional flares that resolve spontaneously over several weeks. If a flare occurs during a period when the patient needs to stay very active and mobile, a short course of glucocorticoids might be considered.

9. If at all possible when using glucocorticoids to treat a serious vasculitis, try to identify an objective measurement of disease activity by which one can regulate the glucocorticoid dose. The recommended starting doses of glucocorticoids in systemic diseases such as SLE, polymyositis, or giant cell arteritis are little more than educated guesses, a distillation of combined clinical experience. These doses are quite high, and it is imperative that they be rapidly reduced to the lowest level required to control the disease activity. This is relatively easy in polymyositis or giant cell arteritis, because the laboratory tests, creatine kinase and the erythrocyte sedimentation rate (ESR), are excellent markers of disease activity.* It is frequently much more difficult in patients with SLE. The clinician must keep in mind why glucocorticoids were prescribed. For example, if they were prescribed because of glomerulonephritis with renal dysfunction, then renal function is the endpoint that should be followed. The patient may feel badly all over with diffuse myalgias when the prednisone is reduced over the course of 1 month from 50 to 25 mg per day, but the success or failure of the dose reduction should be measured by what happens in the renal function, because that was the only indication to prescribe high-dose glucocorticoids in the first place. The issue of finding an objective parameter to measure the effect of glucocorticoid therapy is the reason the management of CNS vasculitis proves so stressful to many clinicians. In that condition, the only objective endpoint is frequently catastrophic (e.g., a stroke), so the clinician is in the position of guessing whether the glucocorticoids should be raised or tapered with very little feedback. This problem underlies the continued efforts by many investigators to identify serum components such as specific autoantibodies that

Table 37–6. Glucocorticoid Replacement Regimen for Patients with Suppressed HPA Undergoing a Surgical Procedure*

Day of Operation: hydrocortisone hemisuccinate 100 mg IM every 6 hours plus maintenance dose of steroid, if any.

First to Third Postoperative Day: same as Day of Operation.

Fourth Postoperative Day: discontinue hydrocortisone, but continue maintenance dose of steroid, if any.

*Data from F.S. Plumpton, et al.[118]

*Editor's note. If the clinical status of the patient and the laboratory result are divergent, the former is always the best guide to therapy; e.g., if serum creatine kinase values or ESR remain high despite a return of normal strength or complete control of symptoms, the laboratory test should be ignored.

may prove useful as guideposts in the treatment of SLE and other vasculitic diseases.

STEROID WITHDRAWAL

The two factors that determine the rate of glucocorticoid withdrawal when indicated are the activity of the underlying disease process and the rate of recovery of the HPA axis. Patients receiving low-dose prednisone (5 mg per day or less), even when treated for up to 5 years, showed no suppression of the HPA axis.[109] With short-term, high-dose therapy, there may be suppression of basal cortisol levels and decreased responsiveness of the HPA axis and adrenals to subsequent stimulation.[110] Administration of 25 mg of prednisone twice daily for 5 days to healthy volunteers resulted in diminished cortisol responses to both insulin-induced hypoglycemia and ACTH 2 days after cessation of prednisone therapy. Within 5 days, the responses had returned to normal.[110] In patients on long-term (greater than 1 year) moderate- or high-dose glucocorticoid therapy there is profound and prolonged suppression of the HPA axis.[30] "Long-acting" steroids, such as dexamethasone, cause greater suppression than "short-acting" drugs such as cortisol, prednisone, or prednisolone.[29] The timing of the daily dose can minimize suppression of the HPA axis. Suppression is maximal if glucocorticoids are administered in the evening, because of inhibition of the early morning rise in ACTH;[111] therefore, a morning dose is preferable.*

Following 1 to 10 years of glucocorticoid therapy, suppression of the HPA axis may persist up to 1 year after complete withdrawal of drug.[26,30,112] The limiting factor in recovery is pituitary ACTH production.[21] ACTH levels generally rise above normal during recovery, stimulating adrenal growth and function. As plasma cortisol levels reach the normal range, feedback inhibition of ACTH release by hydrocortisone returns and the normal HPA axis is established.

Several difficulties may be encountered in attempting to withdraw steroid therapy. Dixon and Christy identified four types of glucocorticoid withdrawal syndromes (Table 37–7).[113] It is important to recognize the signs and symptoms of adrenal insufficiency, which include nausea and vomiting, hypotension, tachycardia, fever, and the associated metabolic abnormalities—hypoglycemia, hyperkalemia, and hyponatremia. Patients with Addisonian crisis require

*Editor's note. A small (7 mg or less prednisone) single morning dose should be *additive* to the patient's endogenous cortisol production. The same dose given in the evening would be *substitutive*.

Table 37–7.   Steroid Withdrawal Syndromes*

Type I: Symptomatic and biochemical evidence of HPA† axis suppression. Relief of symptoms with replacement doses of glucocorticoids. No recurrence of underlying disease.

Type II: Objective evidence of recurrence of underlying disease. Normal HPA axis.

Type III: Physical or psychological dependence on glucocorticoids. No recurrence of underlying disease or evidence of HPA suppression. May manifest as "pseudorheumatism."

Type IV: Biochemical evidence of HPA suppression, but no symptoms of adrenal insufficiency. No recurrence of underlying disease and no symptoms of glucocorticoid dependence.

Note: Any combination of Types I, II, and III may exist.

*Modified from R.B. Dixon and N.P. Christy.[113]
†Hypothalamic-pituitary-adrenal.

immediate treatment with intravenous corticosteroids.

Evaluating the integrity of the HPA axis is relatively easy and should be done routinely during steroid withdrawal. *Serum cortisol levels alone are of little help in evaluating function.* A normal serum cortisol does not exclude suppression, and a subnormal random serum cortisol does not prove suppression.[21] The *rapid ACTH stimulation test* is very useful in establishing secondary adrenal insufficiency. Cosyntropin (0.25 mg) is administered intravenously and plasma cortisol determinations are obtained before and 30 and 60 minutes after the injection.[114] The basal plasma cortisol level should be greater than 5 μg/dl with an ACTH-stimulated increment of at least 7 μg/dl.[21] Most normal subjects will have a peak cortisol of 20 μg/dl or greater, although patients with a high basal cortisol level may show no further increase in response to ACTH.[21] A subnormal response to the rapid ACTH stimulation test establishes the diagnosis of secondary adrenal insufficiency.

Patients may develop symptoms on steroid withdrawal that cannot be clearly related either to relapse of the underlying disease or to true adrenal insufficiency. This symptom complex, termed pseudorheumatism, is characterized by diffuse aching in the muscles, bones, and joints, anorexia, malaise, nausea, weight loss, headache, and postural hypotension.[115] Its cause is unknown, and its occurrence may require a temporary increase in steroid dosage.

Patients who have been treated with short courses of steroid therapy usually have no problems with a rapid taper. For patients who have been on long-term therapy, it is recommended that the total dosage be reduced gradually towards physiologic levels; e.g., taper the prednisone dose by 2.5 to 5.0 mg per week to a daily dose of 10 to 15 mg prednisone (or its equivalent).[116] Dosage should be consolidated as a single morning dose, and alternate-day therapy should be instituted whenever possible. When the steroid dosage has been tapered to 20 to 25 mg of cortisol or 5 mg of prednisone, the function of the HPA axis should be assessed (see above).* Serial assessment of the integrity of the HPA axis may be made at 1- to 2-month intervals. When the rapid ACTH test shows a normal response, return of normal function of the HPA axis can be assumed, and steroid therapy can be safely discontinued.

REFERENCES

1. Goodwin, J.S., and Goodwin, J.M.: Failure to recognize efficacious treatments: A history of salicylate therapy in rheumatoid arthritis. Perspect. Biol. Med., 25:78–92, 1981.
2. Hench, P.S., Kendall, E.C., Slocomb, C.H., and Polley, H.F.: The effect of a hormone of the adrenal cortex (17-hydroxy-11-dehydrocorticosterone: compound E) and of pituitary adrenocorticotropic hormone on rheumatoid arthritis: Preliminary report. Proc. Staff Meetings Mayo Clin., 24:181–197, 1949.
3. Hench, P.S., Kendall, E.C., Slocumb, C.H., and Polley, H.F.: Effects of cortisone acetate and pituitary ACTH on rheumatoid arthritis, rheumatic fever and certain other conditions. Arch. Intern. Med., 85:545–666, 1950.
4. Mason, H.L., Myers, C.S., and Kendall, E.C.: The chemistry of crystalline substances isolated from the suprarenal gland. J. Biol. Chem., 114:613–631, 1936.
5. Mason, H.L., Myers, C.S., and Kendall, E.C.: Chemical studies of the suprarenal cortex. The identification of a substance which possesses the qualitative action of cortin. J. Biol. Chem., 116:267–276, 1936.
6. Watson, E.M.: The effect of adrenal cortical extract on the serum phosphatase in chronic arthritis. Endocrinology, 27:521–522, 1940.
7. Kendall, E.C.: Some observations on the hormone of the adrenal cortex designated compound E. Proc. Staff Meetings Mayo Clin., 24:298–302, 1949.
8. Polley, H.F., and Slocumb, C.H.: Behind the scenes with cortisone and ACTH. Mayo Clin. Proc. 51:417–477, 1976.
9. Hench, P.S.: The reversibility of certain rheumatic and nonrheumatic conditions by the use of cortisone or the pituitary adrenocorticotropic hormones. Le Prix Nobel en 1950. Stockholm, P A Norstedt Soner, 1951.
10. Freyberg, R.H.: Corticotropin, cortisone and hydrocortisone. In Arthritis and Allied Conditions, 5th ed. Edited by J.L. Hollander. Philadelphia, Lea & Febiger, 1953.
11. Sprague, R.G., et al.: Observations on the physiologic effects of cortisone and ACTH in man. Arch. Intern. Med., 85:199–258, 1950.
12. Hollander, J.L.: Intra-articular injection of hydrocortisone. In Arthritis and Allied Conditions, 5th ed. Edited by J.L. Hollander. Philadelphia, Lea & Febiger, 1953.
13. Polley, H.F.: Discovery of anti-inflammatory effects of cortisone and corticotropin. In Landmark Advances in Rheumatology. Edited by D.J. McCarty. American Rheumatism Association, Atlanta, 1985, pp 10–11.
14. Wright, I., and Jacobson, W.E.: Poll on Medical Practice. Modern Medicine, Aug 75–90, 1966.
15. Empire Rheumatism Council: Multicenter controlled trial comparing cortisone acetate and acetylsalicylic acid in the long-term treatment of rheumatoid arthritis: Results of three years treatment. Ann. Rheum. Dis., 16:277–289, 1957.
16. Joint Committee of the Medical Research Council and Nuffield Foundation on Clinical Trials of Cortisone, A.C.T.H., and other Therapeutic Measures in Chronic Rheumatic Diseases: A comparison of cortisone and aspirin in the treatment of early cases of rheumatoid arthritis. Br. Med. J., 2:695–700, 1955.
17. Harris, E.D., Emkey, R.D., Nichols, J.E., and Newberg, A.: Low dose prednisone therapy in rheumatoid arthritis: A double blind study. J. Rheumatol., 10:713–721, 1983.
18. Haynes, R.C., Jr., and Murad, F.: Adrenocorticotropic hormone: Adrenocortical steroids and their synthetic analogs; inhibitors of adrenocortical steroid biosynthesis. In The Pharmacologic Basis of Therapeutics, 7th ed. Edited by A.G. Gilman, L.S. Goodman, and A. Gilman. New York, Macmillan Publishing Co., 1985.
19. Gustavson, L.E., and Benet, L.Z.: Pharmacokinetics of natural and synthetic glucocorticoids. In The Adrenal Cortex. Edited by D.C. Anderson and J.S.D. Winter. Cornwall, England, Butterworth, 1985.
20. Davis, M., et al.: Prednisone or prednisolone or the treatment of chronic active hepatitis? A comparison of plasma availability. Br. J. Clin. Pharmacol., 5:501–509, 1978.
21. Baxter, J.D., and Tyrrell, J.B.: The Adrenal Cortex. In Endocrinology and Metabolism, 2nd ed. Edited by P. Felig, J.D. Baxter, A.E. Broadus, and L.A. Frohman. New York, McGraw-Hill, Inc., 1987.
22. Lewis, G.P., et al.: Prednisone side effects and serum protein levels. Lancet, 2:778–781, 1971.
23. Kozower, M., Veatch, L., and Kaplan, M.M.: Decreased clearance of prednisone, a factor in the development of corticosteroid side effects. J. Clin. Endocrinol. Metab., 38:407–412, 1974.
24. Tyrrell, J.B., and Baxter, J.D.: Glucocorticoid Therapy. In Endocrinology and Metabolism. 2nd ed. Edited by P.Felig, J.D. Baxter, A.E. Broadus, and L.A. Frohman. New York, McGraw-Hill Inc., 1987.
25. Meikle, A.W., Clark, D.H., and Tyler, F.H.: Cushing syndrome from low doses of dexamethasone. A result of slow plasma clearance. JAMA, 235:1592–1593, 1976.
26. Axelrod, L.: Glucocorticoid therapy. Medicine, 55:39–65, 1976.
27. Kawai, S., Ichikawa, Y., and Homma, M.: Differences in metabolic properties among cortisol, prednisone, and dexamethasone in liver and renal diseases: Accelerated metabolism of dexamethasone in renal failure. J. Clin. Endocrinol. Metab., 60:848–854, 1985.
28. Klinenberg, J.R., and Miller, F.: Effect of corticosteroids on blood salicylate concentration. JAMA, 194:601–604, 1965.
29. Meikle, A.W., and Tyler, F.H.: Potency and duration of action of glucocorticoids. Effects of hydrocortisone, prednisone and dexamethasone on human pituitary-adrenal function. Am. J. Med., 63:200–207, 1977.
30. Graber, A.L., et al.: Natural history of pituitary-adrenal recovery following long-term suppression with corticosteroids. J. Clin. Endocrinol. Metab., 25:11–16, 1965.
31. Camalis, E.: Effect of glucocorticoids on type I collagen synthesis, alkaline phosphatase activity, and deoxyribonucleic acid content in cultured rat calvariae. Endocrinology, 112:931–939, 1983.

---

*Editor's note. Patients are often extremely sensitive to further reductions at this point. I have found 1-mg prednisone tablets very useful and often reduce the dose by as little as 0.5 mg per month.

32. O'Malley, B.: Steroid hormone action in eukaryotic cells. J. Clin. Invest., 74:307–312, 1984.
33. Gryglewski, R.J., et al.: Corticosteroids inhibit prostaglandin release from perfused mesenteric blood vessels in rabbits. Prostaglandins, 10:343–354, 1975.
34. Vane, J.R.: Inhibition of prostaglandin synthesis as a mechanism of action for aspirin-like drugs. Nature [New Biol.], 231:232–235, 1971.
35. Samuelsson, B.: Leukotrienes: Mediators of immediate hypersensitivity reactions and inflammation. Science, 220:568–578, 1983.
36. Danon, A., and Assouline, G.: Inhibition of prostaglandin biosynthesis by corticosteroids requires RNA and protein synthesis. Nature, 273:552–553, 1978.
37. Flower, R.J., and Blackwell, G.J.: Anti-inflammatory steroids induce biosynthesis of a phospholipase A_2 inhibitor which prevents prostaglandin generation. Nature, 278:456–458, 1978.
38. Blackwell, G.J., et al.: Macrocortin: A polypeptide causing the anti-phospholipase effect of glucocorticoids. Nature, 287:147–149, 1980.
39. Hirata, F., et al.: A phospholipase A_2 inhibitory protein in rabbit neutrophils induced by glucocorticoids. Proc. Natl. Acad. Sci. USA, 77:2533–2538, 1980.
40. Chandrabose, K.A., et al.: Action of corticosteroids in regulation of prostaglandin biosynthesis in cultured fibroblasts. Proc. Natl. Acad. Sci. USA, 75:214–217, 1978.
41. Gold, E.W., Fox, O.D., and Edgar, P.R.: The effect of long term corticosteroid administration on lipid and prostaglandin levels. J. Steroid Biochem., 9:313–316, 1978.
42. Naray-Fejes-Toth, A., Fejes-Toth, G., Fischer, C., and Frolich, J.C.: Effect of dexamethasone on in vivo prostanoid production in the rabbit. J. Clin. Invest., 74:120–123, 1984.
43. Wallner, B.P., et al.: Cloning and expression of human lipocortin, a phospholipase A_2 inhibitor with potent anti-inflammatory activity. Nature, 320:77–81, 1986.
44. Davidson, F., Dennis, E.A., Powell, M., and Glenney, J.R.: Inhibition of phospholipase A_2 by "lipocortins" and calpactins. J. Biol. Chem., 262:1698–1705, 1987.
45. Goetzl, E.J., Brindley, L.L., and Goldman, D.W.: Enhancement of human neutrophil adherence by synthetic leukotriene constituents of the slow-reacting substance of anaphylaxis. Immunology, 50:35–44, 1983.
46. Ford-Hutchinson, A.W., et al.: Leukotriene B_4: A potent chemokinetic and aggregating substance released from polymorphonuclear leukocytes. Nature, 286:264–266, 1980.
47. Braquet, P., Shen, T.Y., Touqui, L., and Vargaftig, B.B.: Perspectives in platelet-activating factor research. Pharmacol. Rev., 39:97–145, 1987.
48. Parillo, J.E., and Fauci, A.S.: Mechanism of glucocorticoid action on immune processes. Ann. Rev. Pharmacol. Toxicol., 19:179–208, 1979.
49. Dale, D.C., et al.: Comparisons of agents producing neutrophilic leukocytosis in man. J. Clin. Invest., 56:808–817, 1975.
50. Weston, W.L., et al.: Mechanism of cortisol inhibition of adoptive transfer of tuberculin sensitivity. J. Lab. Clin. Med., 82:366–374, 1973.
51. Werb, Z., et al.: Endogenous activation of latent collagenase by rheumatoid synovial cells. N. Engl. J. Med., 296:1017–1023, 1977.
52. Vane, J., and Botting, R.: Inflammation and the mechanism of action of anti-inflammatory drugs. FASEB J., 1:89–98, 1987.
53. Dinarello, C.A.: Interleukin-1. Rev. Infect. Dis., 6:51–95, 1984.
54. Weissmann, G., and Thomas, L.: Studies on lysosomes. The effect of cortisone on the release of acid hydrolases from a large granular fraction of rabbit liver induced by an excess of vitamin A. J. Clin. Invest., 42:661–669, 1963.
55. Behrens, T., and Goodwin, J.S.: Glucocorticosteroids. In The Pharmacology of Lymphocytes. Edited by J. Morley and M. Bray. New York, Springer, 1988 (in press).
56. Claman, H.N.: Corticosteroids and lymphoid cells. N. Engl. J. Med., 287:388–397, 1972.
57. Cupps, T.R., and Fauci, A.S.: Corticosteroid-mediated immunoregulation in man. Immunol. Rev., 65:133–155, 1982.
58. Billingham, R.E., Krohn, R.L., and Medawar, P.B.: Effect of cortisone on survival of skin homografts in rabbits. Br. Med. J., 4716:1157–1163, 1951.
59. Fauci, A.S., Dale, D.C., Balow, J.E.: Glucocorticosteroid therapy: Mechanisms of action and clinical considerations. Ann. Intern. Med., 84:304–315, 1976.
60. David, D.S., Grieco, M.H., and Cushman, P.: Adrenal glucocorticoids after twenty years. A review of their clinically relevant consequences. J. Chronic Dis., 22:637–711, 1970.
61. Waldmann, T.A., Blaese, R.M., Broder, S., and Krakauer, R.S.: Disorders of suppressor immunoregulatory cells in the pathogenesis of immunodeficiency and autoimmunity. Ann. Intern. Med., 88:226–238, 1978.
62. Bovornkitti, S., Kangsadal, P., and Sathirapat, P.: Reversion and reconversion rate of tuberculin skin reactions in correlation with the use of prednisone. Dis. Chest, 38:51–55, 1960.
63. Keown, P.A., and Stiller, C.R.: Control of rejection of transplanted organs. Adv. Intern. Med., 31:17–46, 1986.
64. Parrillo, J.E., and Fauci, A.S.: Comparison of the effector cells in human spontaneous cellular cytotoxicity and antibody-dependent cellular cytotoxicity: Differential sensitivity of effector cells to in vivo and in vitro corticosteroids. Scand. J. Immunol., 8:99–107,1979.
65. Synder, D.S., and Unanue, E.R.: Corticosteroids inhibit murine macrophage Ia expression and interleukin-1 production. J. Immunol., 129:1803–1805, 1982.
66. Bettens, F., et al.: Lymphokine regulation of activated (G_1) lymphocytes II. Glucocorticoid and anti-Tac-induced inhibition of human T lymphocyte proliferation. J. Immunol., 132:261–265, 1984.
67. Arya, S.K., Wong-Staal, F., and Gallo, R.C.: Dexamethasone-mediated inhibition of human T cell growth factor and gamma-interferon messenger RNA. J. Immunol., 133:273–276, 1984.
68. Gupta, C., and Goldman, A.S.: H-2 histocompatibility region: Influence on the murine glucocorticoid receptor and its response. Science, 216:994–996, 1982.
69. Gasser, D.C., Mele, L., Lees, D.D., and Goldman, A.S.: Genes in mice which affect susceptibility to cortisone-induced cleft palate are closely linked to Ir genes on chromosomes 2 and 17. Proc. Natl. Acad. Sci. USA, 78:3147–3150, 1981.
70. Gupta, C., and Goldman, A.S.: Dexamathasone-induced phospholipase A_2-inhibitory proteins influenced by the H-2 histocompatibility region. Proc. Soc. Exp. Biol. Med., 178:29–35, 1985.
71. Staszak, C., et al.: Decreased sensitivity to prostaglandin and histamine in lymphocytes from normal HLA-B12 individuals: A possible role in autoimmunity. J. Immunol., 125:181–185, 1980.
72. Goodwin, J.S.: Changes in lymphocyte sensitivity to prostaglandin E, histamine, hydrocortisone, and x-irradiation with age: Studies in a healthy elderly population. Clin. Immunol. Immunopathol., 25:243–251, 1982.

73. Bowels, L.G., et al.: Induction of steroid-resistant populations in renal dialysis patients. Transplant. Proc., *18*:281–284, 1986.

74. Langhoff, E., et al.: Recipient lymphocyte sensitivity to methyl prednisolone affects cadaver kidney graft survival. Lancet, *1*:1296–1297, 1986.

75. Gluck, O.A., et al.: Bone loss in adults receiving alternate day gluocorticoid therapy. A comparison with daily therapy. Arthritis Rheum., *24*:892–898, 1981.

76. Bressot, C., et al.: Histomorphometric profile, pathophysiology and reversibility of corticosteroid-induced osteoporosis. Metab. Bone Dis. Relat. Res., *1*:303–311, 1979.

77. Hahn, T.J., et al.: Altered mineral metabolism in glucocorticoid-induced osteopenia: Effect of 25-hydroxyvitamin D administration. J. Clin. Invest., *64*:655–665, 1979.

78. Klein, R.G., et al.: Intestinal calcium absorption in exogenous hypercortisonism. J. Clin. Invest., *60*:253–259, 1977.

79. Suzuki, Y.: Importance of increased urinary calcium excretion in the development of secondary hyperparathyroidism of patients under glucocorticoid therapy. Metabolism, *32*:151–156, 1983.

80. Baylink, D.J.: Glucocorticoid-induced osteoporosis. N. Engl. J. Med., *309*:306–308, 1983.

81. Hahn, T.J.: Corticosteroid-induced osteopenia. Arch. Intern. Med., *138*:882–885, 1978.

82. Dykman, T.R., et al.: Evaluation of factors associated with glucocorticoid-induced osteopenia in patients with rheumatic diseases. Arthritis Rheum., *28*:361–368, 1985.

83. Sambrook, P.N., et al.: Determinants of axial bone loss in rheumatoid arthritis. Arthritis Rheum., *30*:721–728, 1987.

84. Askari, A., Vignos, P.J., and Moskowitz, R.W.: Steroid myopathy in connective tissue disease. Am. J. Med., *61*:485–492, 1976.

85. Van Marle, W., and Woods, K.L.: Acute hydrocortisone myopathy. Br. J. Med., *281*:271–274, 1980.

86. Bowyer, S.L., LaMothe, M.P., and Hollister, J.R.: Steroid myopathy: Incidence and detection in a population with asthma. J. Allergy Clin. Immunol., *76*:234–242, 1985.

87. Horber, F.F., et al.: Evidence that prednisone-induced myopathy is reversed by physical training. J. Clin. Endocrinol. Metab., *61*:83–88, 1985.

88. Conn, H.O., and Blitzer, B.L.: Non-association of adrenocorticosteroid therapy and peptic ulcer. N. Engl. J. Med., *294*:473–479, 1976.

89. Messer, J., et al.: Association of adrenocorticosteroid therapy and peptic-ulcer disease. N. Engl. J. Med., *309*:21–24, 1983.

90. Goodwin, J.S.: Toxicity of nonsteroidal anti-inflammatory drugs. Arch. Intern. Med., *147*:34–35, 1987.

91. Spiro, H.M.: Is the steroid ulcer a myth? N. Engl. J. Med., *309*:45–47, 1983.

92. Ling, M.H.M., Perry, P.J., and Tsuang, M.T.: Side effects of corticosteroid therapy. Psychiatric aspects. Arch. Gen. Psychiatry, *38*:471–477, 1981.

93. Dale, D.C., and Petersdorf, R.G.: Corticosteroids and infectious diseases. Med. Clin. North Am., *57*:1277–1287, 1973.

94. Ginzler, E., et al.: Computer analysis of factors influencing frequency of infection in systemic lupus erythematosus. Arthritis Rheum., *21*:37–44, 1978.

95. Anderson, R.J., et al.: Infectious risk factors in the immunocompromised host. Am. J. Med., *54*:453–460, 1973.

96. Schatz, M., et al.: The prevalence of tuberculosis and positive tuberculin skin tests in a steroid-treated asthmatic population. Ann. Intern. Med., *84*:261–265, 1976.

97. Sahn, S.A., and Lakshiminarayan, S.: Tuberculosis after corticosteroid therapy. Br. J. Dis. Chest, *70*:195–205, 1976.

98. Iseman, M.D.: Tuberculosis prophylaxis during corticosteroid therapy-reply. JAMA, *258*:263–264, 1987.

99. Levine, S.B., and Leopold, I.H.: Advances in ocular corticosteroid therapy. *In* Steroid Therapy. Edited by D.L. Azarnoff. Philadelphia, W.B. Saunders Co., 1975.

100. Spaeth, G.L. and Von Sallmann, L.: Corticosteroids and cataracts. Int. Ophthalmol. Clin., *6*:915–920, 1966.

101. Manabe, S., Bucala, R., and Cerami, A.: Nonenzymatic addition of glucocorticoid to lens proteins in steroid-induced cataracts. J. Clin. Invest., *74*:1803–1810, 1984.

102. Dujovne. C.A., and Azarnoff, D.L.: Clinical complications of corticosteroid therapy: A selected review. *In* Steroid Therapy. Edited by D.L. Azarnoff. Philadelphia, W.B. Saunders Co., 1975.

103. Nashel, D.J.: Is atheroclerosis a complication of long-term corticosteroid treatment? Am. J. Med., *80*:925–929, 1986.

104. Kalbak, K.: Incidence of atherosclerosis in patients with rheumatoid arthritis receiving long-term corticosteroid therapy. Ann. Rheum. Dis., *31*:196–200, 1972.

105. Schatz, M., et al.: Corticosteroid therapy for the pregnant asthmatic patient. JAMA, *233*:804–807, 1975.

106. Fauci, A.S.: Alternate-day corticosteroid therapy. Am. J. Med., *64*:729–731, 1978.

107. Harter, J.G., Reddy, W.J., and Thorn, G.W.: Studies on an intermittent corticosteroid dosage regimen. N. Engl. J. Med., *269*:591–596, 1963.

108. Fauci, A.S., and Dale, D.C.: Alternate-day prednisone therapy and human lymphocyte subpopulations. J. Clin. Invest., *55*:22–34, 1975.

109. Melby, J.C.: Systemic corticosteroid therapy: Pharmacology and endocrinologic considerations. Ann. Intern. Med., *81*:505–512, 1974.

110. Streck, W.F., and Lockwood, D.H.: Pituitary adrenal recovery following short-term suppression with corticosteroids. Am. J. Med., *66*:910–914, 1979.

111. Nichols, T., Nugent, C.A., and Tyler, F.H.: Diurnal variation in suppression of adrenal function by glucocorticoids. J. Clin. Endocrinol. Metab., *25*:343–349, 1975.

112. Christy, N.P.: HPA failure and glucocorticoid therapy. Hosp. Pract., *7*:77–89, 1984.

113. Dixon, R.B., and Christy, N.P.: On the various forms of corticosteroid withdrawal syndrome. Am. J. Med., *68*:224–230, 1980.

114. May, M.E., and Carey, R.M.: Rapid adrenocorticotropic hormone test in clinical practice. Am. J. Med., *79*:679–684, 1985.

115. Amatruda, T.T., Hurst, M.M., and D'Esopo, N.D.: Certain endocrine and metabolic facets of the steroid withdrawal syndrome. J. Clin. Endocrinol. Metab., *25*:1207–1217, 1965.

116. Bynny, R.L.: Withdrawal from glucocorticoid therapy. N. Engl. J. Med., *295*:30–32, 1976.

117. Dluhy, R.G., Lauler, D.P., and Thorn, G.W.: Pharmacology and chemistry of adrenal glucocorticoids. Med. Clin. North. Am., *57*:1155–1165, 1973.

118. Plumpton, F.S., Besser, G.M., and Cole, P.V.: Corticosteroid treatment and surgery. II. The management of steroid cover. Anaesthesia, *24*:12–18, 1969.

IMMUNOREGULATION AND EXPERIMENTAL THERAPIES

38

SETH H. PINCUS

Experimental therapies offer the hope of a better future for patients with rheumatic diseases. They are also important tools for studying the underlying causes of the diseases. Many of the experimental therapies are aimed at modulating the immune system. Although it is clear that immunoregulation is not the sole mechanism of acton of antirheumatic drugs, the recent advances in our understanding of the function of the immune system and its role in the pathophysiology of rheumatic disease make this approach particularly appealing. The definition of the physiologic hormones that regulate the immune and inflammatory cells may allow for the rational development of agonist and antagonist compounds that mimic or interfere with the binding of the hormone to its cellular receptor. Current approaches to regulating the immune system are not very specific and can result in clinically significant generalized immunosuppression. It is hoped that future therapies can be directed at the disease-inciting defect(s) without altering other immune functions. In designing agents to treat diseases whose causes are only partly understood, it is important to maintain both an open mind and a high degree of skepticism. Through the use of appropriately designed clinical studies, well-defined therapeutic agents may become tools that help us to probe the cause of these diseases. With few exceptions, the agents discussed here are not currently recommended for patient use.

MECHANISMS OF ACTION OF CURRENT ANTIRHEUMATIC THERAPIES

Current therapies are the starting point for designing new forms of treatment. The potential mechanisms of action of each agent are discussed in detail in the individual chapter on that agent; however, some of the general principles are worth reviewing here. Anti-inflammatory, antiproliferative, and immunoregulatory effects are common to many of the medications used to treat rheumatic diseases. For most agents, it is not clear which effect is responsible for the improvement in disease activity. Anti-inflammatory and immunosuppressive effects are difficult to separate because inflammation is an important effector mechanism of the immune system. Our nomenclature for the medications tends to further confuse the issue. For example, nonsteroidal anti-inflammatory drugs have important effects on the immune system.[1,2] Similarly, cytotoxic drugs, such as azathioprine, cyclophosphamide, and methotrexate, are primarily antiproliferative and may also have potent anti-inflammatory effects,[3] but are frequently called immunoregulatory agents, as if that were the sole mechanism of their action.

The clinical manifestations of the rheumatic diseases are primarily the result of inflammation in a target organ. This inflammation is thought to be caused by autoimmunity. Anti-inflammatory effects can be exerted at several different levels. Agents inhibiting the accumulation or action of humoral factors and inflammatory cells at the target organ can ameliorate the disease process. Alternatively, therapies that protect the target organ from the effects of the inflammation would also be useful. These anti-inflammatory effects may be exerted without altering the immunologic signal responsible for the initiation of the inflammation.

Many drugs have immunoregulatory properties. These include all contemporary antirheumatic drugs, as well as agents given primarily for nonimmune indications, such as histamine blockers, antihypertensives, cardioactive glycosides, anticonvulsants, and polypeptide hormones. Immune actions of antirheumatic drugs include effects on the functioning of macrophages, T cells, and B cells, as well as their products. The cytotoxic drugs have strong suppressive actions on both humoral and cellular immunity, but it has never been shown convincingly that their immunoregulatory actions are the mechanism of their antirheumatic effect. Although it is appealing to think that our therapies are correcting the underlying defect in the immune system that leads to the autoimmunity, this may not necessarily be the case. As our understanding of the immunopathogenesis of the rheumatic diseases becomes clearer and as the agents we are using become better defined, this issue will be resolved.

Cellular proliferation plays an important role in rheumatic diseases. Many antirheumatic agents have antiproliferative effects. Gold compounds and D-penicillamine inhibit T-cell proliferation. Cytotoxic drugs are primarily antiproliferative agents. The generation of any immune response depends on the proliferation of antigen-specific lymphocyte clones. Inflammatory responses depend on the delivery of adequate numbers of neutrophils to the target organ. Proliferation of synovial cells is prominent in rheumatoid arthritis. Renal proliferative lesions in lupus involve at least three cell types: mesangial, epithelial, and endothelial. Therefore, antiproliferative agents can potentially affect the disease process at multiple levels. It is even possible that the primary drug effect is on the proliferative response of cells in the target organ. Highly efficacious dosing schedules of cytotoxic drugs do not correspond to the known cell cycle kinetics of hematopoietic or tumor cells. Low-dose pulse methotrexate therapy, used in both rheumatoid arthritis (RA) and psoriasis (a proliferative skin disorder), does not affect measurable cellular parameters of immunity.[4,5] Intravenous pulses of cyclophosphamide given every 3 months can suppress the development of renal disease in systemic lupus erythematosus (SLE).[6]

The proliferative cycles of synovial cells in RA or renal cells in SLE are not well studied and could be the target of these treatment schedules. The inhibition of endothelial cell proliferation has been shown to be an effect of gold compounds.[6a]

Another proposed mechanism of action for antirheumatic agents is the scavenging of toxic products by thiol-containing compounds.[7] Gold compounds and D-penicillamine can scavenge hypochlorite and inhibit its formation by myeloperoxidase. Such agents may protect the target tissues from the noxious products of inflammatory cells by this mechanism.

Most nonspecific antirheumatics in current empiric use probably act by several pathways to suppress autoimmunity, inhibit inflammation, and lessen damage to the target organ. Each drug probably has a single mechanism of action that influences each of the pathways. Agents under development for clinical testing in the near future will work through similar channels.

IMMUNOREGULATION

GENERAL CONCEPTS

The cellular basis for immune responsiveness and the regulation of antibody production and cell-mediated immunity are becoming better understood. B cells and their progeny produce antibody, the amount of which is determined by such factors as: (1) prior exposure to antigen and the generation of memory B cells; (2) the amount of help from T cells; (3) the magnitude of T-cell suppression; and (4) anti-idiotype and antibody-mediated effects, which may be indirect. If an antigen is presented in association with an immune enhancer, the response may be augmented. On the other hand, a more tolerogenic form of the antigen may specifically impair antibody production. For most antigens, antigen-presenting cells are necessary. T cells produce factors regulating the differentiation and proliferation of immune cells. An immune circuit has been constructed in which promoting and inhibiting cells and their products interact to determine the ultimate magnitude of the antibody response. A similar circuit operates in cell-mediated immunity (see Chapters 17, 19, 27, and 28).

Most of the control currently exerted over immune reactions involves control of lymphocyte proliferation and differentiation. The transition in the cell cycle from G_0 to G_1 represents activation of the cell. RNA and new protein synthesis occur, and receptors for further steps toward either proliferation or differentiation are formed at the cell membrane. The interactions of these receptors with their ligands determine whether the cell will proceed toward proliferation (S + G$_2$ + M) or differentiation (for example, immunoglobulin secretion in a B cell). Cytotoxic and cytostatic drugs interfere with events in cellular proliferation, but most of these drugs were developed as antineoplastic agents and are not specific for the receptors triggering cells to differentiate or proliferate. The antineoplastic drugs either kill cells or prevent their subsequent division. Future attempts at immunoregulation will take advantage of the receptors specific for the stages of the cell cycle.

As a result of the network of immune responses, different immunoregulatory agents theoretically could be used to interfere selectively with individual portions of the network. This possibility is tempered by the recognition that perturbation of a network at one point may produce an effect at another point. Such distant effects might operate to keep the system in balance and might negate the specific immunoregulatory interference. Thus, an "immunosuppressive" drug might actually augment the immune response if suppressor functions are inhibited to a greater extent than are helper functions.[8] Similarly, an "immune enhancer" might actually enhance suppressor circuits and impair the primary immune responses.[9–11] The recognition of the complexity of the immune system forces us to view immunoregulatory agents not only with regard to an effect on a specific pathway, but also with regard to the overall effect on an immune response and on the entire immune system. Because the immune system consists of a number of subpopulations of cells that interact with one another in a complex manner, and because both positive and negative feedback inhibition occur, interference with a given cell population may have widespread effects that might not be predicted from the properties of the administered agent. Furthermore, the timing of such interference is important. An agent given in one schedule may be an immune enhancer and may suppress tumor growth, but in another schedule the same agent may enhance suppressor cell function and encourage tumor growth.[11] Thus, drugs may enhance or suppress different immune responses, depending on (1) the cell population with which they directly interact and (2) the cells that are indirectly affected by virtue of disruption or augmentation of normal feedback control mechanisms.

In the study of immunoregulatory drugs in patients, it is often difficult to know whether observed changes should be ascribed to a direct effect of the therapeutic agent on lymphoid cells or to other effects on the underlying disease process. Peripheral blood cellular changes may reflect recirculation patterns rather than total body alterations. Another problem in evaluating the effects of immunosuppressive drugs in rheumatic diseases is determining optimal dosing schedules. Animals with autoimmune diseases respond best to immunosuppressive therapy given early and in large doses.[12] It is possible that a reevaluation of the timing (early rather than late) and method of administration (intermittent large boluses of one drug and perhaps another drug in between) may improve the effectiveness of such drugs.[13–16]

Several agents, given together, may produce varied results. With regard to immunoregulatory drugs, simultaneous treatment with two, three, or more drugs may give a greater result than would be expected by the summing of the expected results of treatment with each individual drug.[17] Such "drug synergy" has been documented in primary immune responses,[18] tolerance,[15] and treatment of autoimmune disease.[12,14,17]

Most current therapies are immunosuppressive. This fits our general understanding of the rheumatic diseases as disorders with an exaggerated immune response. However, it is possible that selective immune enhancement may be of therapeutic utility. In particular, the enhancement of suppressor circuits could be used to inhibit the disease-inciting immune response. Immunologic adjuvants have been used for many years to enhance immune responses.[19] The primary clinical use of these agents has been with vaccines to infectious agents. Many adjuvants are of bacterial origin.[20] Muramyl peptides are synthetic and naturally occurring materials that can be given orally, mimic many adjuvant effects, and interact with the central nervous system.[21] It has been shown that at least some of the effects of muramyl peptides are caused by the induction of interleukin-1 (IL-1).[22] Other interleukins and cytokines also have enhancing effects on the immune system and may offer greater target cell specificity (see below). The effects of such stimulation in human rheumatic disorders remain to be determined.

CYTOKINE REGULATION OF THE IMMUNE SYSTEM

Many of the physiologic hormones that regulate the immune system have been discovered, and their role in homeostasis and disease is being actively studied. Unfortunately, a confusing nomenclature has arisen around these proteins, which are now collectively called *cytokines*. Cytokines include interleukins, interferons, and growth factors, labels that were usually based on the first activity described for the material. Our understanding of these materials owes much to recent recombinant DNA technology.[23] The initial vague description of "factors" with certain biologic activities quickly progressed to well-defined materials whose structure, function, and pharmacologic effects are being characterized and extensively studied. The production of antibodies to these protein hormones and recognition of their cellular receptors have allowed further definition of their actions. Table 38–1 summarizes the major immunoregulatory cytokines.

The analogy between cytokine function and classic endocrinology is useful, especially because it points the way to future drug development. Cytokines may be thought of as hormones that operate between cells rather than between organs. Cytokines, like peptide hormones, are proteins that are secreted by one cell type and have an effect on another cell. The responding cell has a receptor for the cytokine. The cytokine system, like the endocrine system, is regulated by feedback inhibition and involves synergistic interactions between different hormones. But there are also differences between the actions of cytokines and classic hormones. Cytokines generally act at short distances, often between adjacent cells, and concentrations are several orders of magnitude lower than those seen with most peptide hormones. The cells that secrete cytokines are generally not organized into discrete glands that secrete hormone. Autocrine stimulation, the response of a cell to its own hormone, exists in the cytokine system but not in classic endocrinology. Other regulatory mechanisms may also differ between the systems. Although the analogy between cytokines and peptide hormones is useful in the conceptualization of these new agents, the differences must also be kept in mind.

An overview of the actions of the cytokines on the immune system is important in understanding their pharmacologic potential. T cells recognize antigen on the surface of antigen-presenting cells in association with HLA molecules. IL-1 produced by the antigen-presenting cell and acting at very short range plays an important role in this interaction, which leads to triggering of the T cell.[24] The T-cell response includes the elaboration of a number of cytokines including interleukin-2 (IL-2) and gamma-interferon (IFN-gamma). IL-2 serves to recruit additional lymphocytes to the immune response. It stimulates both T cells and B cells to proliferation, with a greater response seen in cells that are already activated and expressing a high affinity IL-2 receptor.[25–27] IFN-gamma has diverse effects on the immune response. It is a macrophage-activating factor, and it amplifies the interaction among the antigen-presenting cell, the antigen-HLA complex, and the T cell. It does this both by increasing antigen processing and by increasing the expression of HLA antigens on the surface of the antigen-presenting cell.[28,29] Other cytokines produced by activated T cells include IL-3, a multipotential stimulator of hematopoietic cells,[30] and IL-4, a B-cell differentiation and stimulation factor.[31,32] The macrophages stimulated in response to IFN-gamma secrete IL-1 and tumor necrosis factor (TNF, also called cachectin), both of which are major mediators of the acute phase and inflammatory responses.[24,33] The in-

Table 38–1. Immunoregulatory Cytokines

Name	Principal source	Biologic effects
Gamma-interferon	T cells	Macrophage activation Increased HLA expression Antiviral Antiproliferative
Interleukin-1	Macrophages	Mediator of inflammation, acute phase response, and fever T cell activation Osteoclast activation CNS, vascular, and metabolic effects
Interleukin-2	T cells	Proliferation of cells expressing IL-2 receptors, including: T cells B cells Lymphokine-activated killers
Interleukin-3	T cells	Stimulation of multiple lineages of hematopoietic precursor cells
Interleukin-4	T cells	B cell growth and differentiation
Tumor necrosis factor	Macrophages	Mediator of inflammation, acute phase response, and fever Metabolic effects, especially cachexia Lysis of tumor targets

teractions among these immunoregulatory hormones are complex and the administration of a cytokine may influence the immune system through multiple routes.

The actions of the cytokines are not restricted to the immune or the hematopoietic systems. Both IL-1 and IL-2 have effects on cells in the central nervous system.[24,34] IL-1 is even secreted by CNS cells.[35] Other organs or systems influenced by the immunoregulatory cytokines include the liver, musculoskletal system, skin, and vasculature. The pharmacologic effects of in vivo administration of these cytokines may be widespread and may limit the use of some agents, for example the capillary leak syndrome seen with IL-2.[36]

SPECIFICITY OF INTERVENTION

The immune system is regulated by a complex network of cellular and hormonal interactions. Current immunosuppressive therapies are nonspecific in their effects on the immune system and can leave patients immunologically compromised. If treatment schedules are adjusted to safe levels, the antirheumatic effects of these drugs may be diluted. The goal in developing new antirheumatic agents is to increase the specificity of the effect on the immune system and to reduce toxicity resulting from general immunosuppression. This goal may be accomplished with agents discovered through traditional discovery routes, with cytokines, with materials screened to influence cytokine effects, or with antibodies.

The use of monoclonal antibodies has resulted in major advances in our understanding of the components of the immune system[37] as well as in our knowledge of how various therapies may work. They are also agents that can be used to attack the immune system with great specificity. An example is the antibody to the CD4 antigen (this was previously designated T4; Table 38–2 reviews the nomenclature for important cellular markers). CD4 is found predominantly on helper T cells and functions in the interaction between the T cell and class II HLA antigens.[38] The proportion of T cells expressing CD4 in rheumatoid arthritis and other rheumatic diseases is increased.[39,40] Several different antirheumatic therapies either normalize this proportion or cause an absolute decrease in the number of CD4+ cells.[40–42] Similarly, administration of anti-CD4 antibody in experimental models of rheumatic diseases dramatically inhibits the development of clinical disease.[43,44] Therapies designed to target this T-cell subset may be a first step in the development of more specfic immunologic interventions. Other monoclonal antibodies may also be useful; however, this potential utility is balanced by the host response to the administered antibody.[45,46] It is likely that monoclonal antibodies will be used as tools to determine which portion of the immune system to suppress. With this knowledge, we can then devise methods of attack using other agents that are easier to administer.

THE RECEPTOR-LIGAND PARADIGM

Pharmaceutical agents can act through a variety of mechanisms; one common way drugs work is by binding to the cellular receptor for an endogenous substance. Materials bound specifically to receptors are termed ligands. Once bound to the receptor, the

Table 38–2. Lymphocyte Surface Antigens Defined by Monoclonal Antibodies

Cluster designation	Description	Other designations
CD1	Thymocyte antigen	T6
CD2	T-cell, E-rosette receptor	T11
CD3	T-cell, associated with antigen receptor	T3, Leu 4
CD4	Helper T-cell	T4, Leu 3
CD5	T-cell; B-cell subset	T1, Leu 1, Lyl
CD7	T-cell; natural killer cell	Leu 9
CD8	Suppressor T-cell	T8, Leu 2
CD16	Fc IgG receptor	Leu 11
CD20	B-cells	B1, Leu 16
CD24	IL-2 receptor	Tac, IL-2R
CDw29	Helper-inducer T-cell	4B4
CD45	Suppressor-inducer T-cell	2H4

(From Shaw, S.: Characterization of human leukocyte differentiation antigens. Immunol. Today, 8:1, 1987.)

ligand may have one of two effects: it may mimic the action of the endogenous ligand (agonist), or it may block its action (antagonist) (see Fig. 38–1). The receptor is present on the surface of the cell and is accessible to ligands in the extracellular fluid or plasma surrounding the cell. When the receptor is bound by its natural ligand, a signal is passed to the interior of the cell. In a given cell, receptors for different ligands generally use distinct signaling systems. When the signal is transmitted, a certain effect is produced in that cell. Many of the immunoregulatory cytokines induce proliferation or differentiation in their target cells.

Some of the oldest known drugs, such as digitalis and morphine, are now known to operate by receptor-ligand mechanisms. Newer drugs have been developed based on a knowledge of a receptor and its ligands, for example, beta-adrenergic and H_2-blocking agents. Current understanding of the cytokines and their cellular receptors makes it possible to devise screening assays for new pharmaceutical agents that interfere with the binding of a cytokine to its receptor or that modulate a known biologic effect of the cytokine. Such assays provide good evidence that naturally occurring inhibitors of interleukins exist.[47–49] The testing of synthetic cytokine agonists and antagonists using these assays is being actively pursued.

Antibodies can be useful probes in determining the portions of the cytokine-receptor system to target with agonist or antagonist compounds. Antibodies to different structural domains of the IFN-gamma molecule can either enhance or suppress the ability of IFN-gamma to activate macrophages.[50] Antibodies to cell surface receptors can also have either stimulatory or inhibitory effects. T cells can be activated with antibodies to the CD3/antigen-specific receptor complex.[51] Suppression of the immune response with antibody to the IL-2 receptor has been demonstrated in experimental models.[52] The IL-2 receptor is present in increased numbers on the activated T cells that circulate in the peripheral blood of patients with active rheumatic diseases.[53] Antagonism of the IL-2 receptor represents a potential mode of therapy that should be investigated. Studies of antibodies to cytokines and their receptors will indicate which systems have the greatest potential for therapeutic manipulation; then synthetic or natural analogues that interact with these systems can be developed and tested.

CLINICAL TRIALS

Experimental therapies will help us understand the underlying pathophysiology of the rheumatic diseases. Clinical trials must be designed to evaluate clinical efficacy and to determine the mechanism of action of experimental therapies. Initial discovery of agents is as likely to be the result of chance combined with good clinical observation as it is to be the result of studies based on logic and prior animal studies. The development of IFN-gamma as a potential treatment of rheumatoid arthritis began when the antiarthritic effect was first seen in cancer trials! Initial reports of efficacy must be followed up by controlled, blinded trials with well-defined endpoints. Often these agents will have been tested in neoplastic diseases before being applied to the rheumatic diseases, providing an idea of tolerable doses, but for any new agents, optimal dosing schedules need to be determined in early clinical trials. The design and interpretation of clinical trials in the rheumatic diseases have been the subject of several recent reviews[54,55] (Chapter 9) and will not be discussed here.

Immunologic monitoring represents an important adjunct to clinical trials of therapies purported to work by modulation of the immune system. The patient's immune status needs to be monitored prior to, and at several times after, the initiation of the therapy. Peripheral blood is the only body compartment readily available for serial monitoring. Although peripheral blood is not usually the site of disease activity, changes in this body compartment may reflect the systemic effects of the agent. Assays of humoral immunity are standardized, and correlations with disease status well studied (e.g., rheumatoid factor, anti-

FIG. 38–1. Receptor–ligand interactions. When a cellular receptor is bound by its endogenous ligand, a physiologic response is produced by the cell. Substances structurally related to the ligand may mimic the effect of the endogenous ligand (agonist) or block the effect of the ligand (antagonist). Understanding of the cytokines and their receptors may lead to the production of immunoregulatory molecules that are cytokine agonists or antagonists. (Reprinted by permission of the publisher from Biologically Based Immunomodulators in the Therapy of Rheumatic Diseases, edited by S. Pincus, et al., p. 11, Fig. 2, Copyright 1987 by Elsevier Science Publishing Co., Inc.)

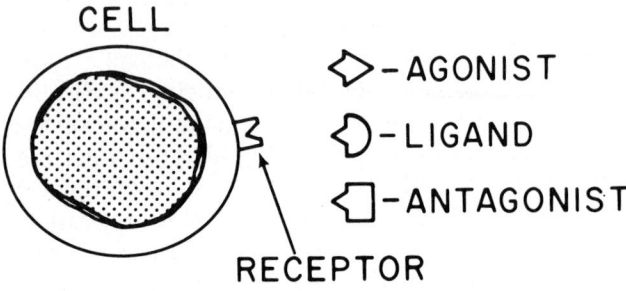

DNA antibody, complement levels). The best parameters of cellular immunity to monitor are open to debate, but the enumeration of immunocyte subsets and activation markers with monoclonal antibodies and flow cytometry[56] is rapidly becoming the most commonly used assay. With commercially available standardized antibody preparations, straightforward processing protocols, and objective (though occasionally misinterpreted) results, this technique allows comparison of results obtained in different research centers. The clinical utility of this form of analysis in individual patients remains unproven (except in extreme cases), but the changes demonstrated in populations of patients with rheumatic diseases have been repeatable in multiple different centers.[39,40,57,58] Assays of lymphocyte function are more difficult to perform, and interlaboratory variability is greater. Ultimately, for the mechanisms of action of antirheumatic therapies to be understood, functional assays will be required. The most commonly used functional assays are the proliferative responses of T cells and B cells to various mitogens and the induction of immunoglobulin secreting "plaque-forming" B cells. It remains to be established which of these different methods of assay most accurately reflects the underlying immunologic aberrations in the rheumatic diseases or can detect antirheumatic drug effects.

SPECIFIC AGENTS

The specific agents currently under development or in clinical trials as potential therapeutic agents have been divided into six groups for purposes of discussion and as a general conceptual framework. Table 38–3 lists the categories and the agents in each group. A mechanistic classification is not implied, because the mechanism of the antirheumatic or immunomodulating effect of many of these agents is not fully understood.

Most therapies described here relate to rheumatologic conditions wherein there appear to be immunoregulatory defects, primarily RA and SLE. Although osteoarthritis affects far more people than these other conditions, considerably less effort seems to be directed toward new therapies for osteoarthritis. This may reflect a lack of understanding of the underlying pathophysiology of the disease, or the feeling that osteoarthritis is primarily a degenerative process and little hope of preventing or reversing the disease exists. Of the agents discussed here, only the chondroprotective therapies relate directly to osteoarthritis.

Table 38–3. Experimental Antirheumatic Drugs and Therapies

Drugs whose primary action is upon the immune system
  Cyclosporine
  Levamisole
  Therafectin
  IMREG-1
  LS-2616
  Imuthiol
  Isoprinosine

Physical agents
  Ionizing radiation
  Therapeutic apheresis
  Splenectomy
  Radiation synovectomy

Therapies used for other indications with secondary
    immune effects
  Sex hormones
  Thalidomide
  Antihypertensives
  Neurotransmitters
  Iron-binding compounds
  Antibiotics
  Retinoids
  Tetrahydrocannabinol derivatives

Cytokines
  Interferon-gamma
  Interleukin-1
  Interleukin-2
  Tumor necrosis factor
  Thymic hormones

Antibodies
  Monoclonal antibodies
  Antilymphocyte globulin
  Placenta-eluted gammaglobulins
  Intravenous immunoglobulin

Agents whose antirheumatic effects may be nonimmune
  Dapsone
  Fish oil
  Dimethyl sulfoxide
  Chondroprotective agents

DRUGS THAT ACT ON PRIMARILY THE IMMUNE SYSTEM

Cyclosporine

Cyclosporine, originally developed as an antifungal agent, is much more useful as an immunoregulatory drug. Cyclosporine is a cyclic peptide with N-methylated amino acids that render it resistant to the low gastric pH and to intestinal proteolytic enzymes. The drug is active without further metabolism. Cyclosporine is especially effective in reducing T-cell function without important bone marrow suppression and is therefore useful in preventing allograft rejection. Used in many patients who have received renal or other organ allografts,[59,60] cyclosporine appears to have spawned an era of increased boldness in organ transplantation. The drug seems to interfere with the early stages of IL-2-dependent T-cell activation,[61-63] reducing both T-cell function and helper-T-cell-dependent B-cell function. Cyclosporine might also have a direct effect on a subset of B cells.[64] The net effect of cyclosporine therapy on antibody production in humans is *increased*, not decreased, serum IgG concentrations.[59]

Studies have been performed in animal models of autoimmune diseases. In general, such autoimmunity has been suppressed by cyclosporine.[65] MRL/lpr mice show decreased arthritis, nephritis, and lymphoproliferation in response to cyclosporine.[66] Particularly informative results have been obtained with collagen- and adjuvant-induced arthritis in rats.[67,68] Depending on the timing of cyclosporine and the collagen challenge, disease may be suppressed (cyclosporine given during the induction of the anticollagen response) or enhanced (cyclosporine administered during effector phase). Antigen-specific suppression of the arthritogenic response by cyclosporine shows that adjuvant- and collagen-induced diseases are directed against different antigenic structures. Animal studies suggest that cyclosporine may be effective in the treatment of rheumatic diseases, but these studies do not seriously address the issues of toxicity.

Cyclosporine has been used in multiple small trials in human autoimmune diseases. In all cases the patients had disease refractory to other therapies. Dosages of cyclosporine were 6 to 10 mg/kg/day, and renal abnormalities were seen in virtually all patients. Nussenblatt and co-workers have demonstrated that cyclosporine is an effective agent in suppressing various forms of uveitis,[69] but renal biopsies in 17 of these patients after 2 years of therapy showed histopathologic changes in all. These changes included interstitial fibrosis and tubular atrophy.[70] In 14 of the 17 patients, creatinine clearance declined significantly. An early report of cyclosporine use in SLE resulted in such severe toxicity that the trial was discontinued.[71] Later trials have been more favorable, with improvement in the renal biopsy seen in some patients with proliferative glomerulonephritis.[72,73] Cyclosporine is also efficacious in severe rheumatoid arthritis, but its use may be limited by renal toxicity (manifested by a decreased creatinine clearance) and hypertension.[74] In Sjögren's syndrome, cyclosporine (used at a dose of 5 mg/kg/day) was not effective, but neither was there severe toxicity.[75]

In addition to nephrotoxicity, other side effects of cyclosporine include an increased development of lymphomas, hypertrichosis, gum hypertrophy, and liver function test abnormalities. Increased susceptibility to bacterial infection does not appear to be a problem, although reactivation of Epstein-Barr virus has ben reported. Much of the toxicity of cyclosporine is dose related. Future protocols involving use of lower doses may be developed, perhaps in conjunction with other forms of chemotherapy; but at this time, renal toxicity markedly limits the use of this agent.

Levamisole

Levamisole, a three-ringed anthelmintic drug, is readily absorbed from the gastrointestinal tract and has a plasma half-life of about 4 hours in humans; peak blood levels are achieved at 2 hours.[76] In addition to its gastrointestinal absorption, levamisole is rapidly absorbed from tissue sites. It is metabolized by the liver; metabolites are excreted in the urine and to a lesser degree in the feces. Small amounts of unmetabolized levamisole may be found in urine, breast milk, tears, and respiratory secretions.

Levamisole augments nonspecific inflammation by increasing chemotaxis of polymorphonuclear leukocytes and monocytes and increasing phagocytosis.[77,78] These effects can be dramatic when these functions are impaired, but the drug has little effect on normal responses. Defective monocyte cytotoxicity seen in RA can be corrected with levamisole.[79] Although the drug may favorably alter immune effector functions in disease states, it may have no favorable effect on clinical inflammation.

In addition to levamisole's effects on effector-cell functions, it also has a more direct action on earlier stages of T-cell function, augmenting helper, amplifier, cytotoxic, and suppressor T-cell functions.[80] Patients with impaired delayed hypersensitivity show restoration of skin reactivity after levamisole therapy. Again, the drug appears to increase subnormal but not normal responses. Reported effects of levamisole on circulating lymphocyte populations appear contradictory. One study showed that levamisole increased the number of circulating T cells in patients with subnormal values, usually at the expense of non-T, non-B cells; this finding suggests maturation of pre-T cells to T cells.[81] Another study, evaluating RA patients, showed that those taking the drug for more than 3 months had a decreased number of total lymphocytes, and of CD3+ and CD4+ cells both at 6 hours and 24 hours after the drug had been injected. No such changes were seen in these parameters in patients receiving their first dose of levamisole.[82]

Levamisole has been used to treat patients with malignant diseases, aphthous stomatitis, herpes labialis, Crohn's disease, RA, and SLE.[76,83-85] Unfortunately, side effects are frequent and toxic,[85] and flulike symptoms are common. Granulocytopenia is the most dangerous untoward effect and seems especially frequent in patients with rheumatic diseases,[76,83] perhaps owing to the induction of leukoagglutinins demonstrable only after drug withdrawal. Agranulocytosis may be especially common in patients with HLA-B27.[86] It had been suggested that corticosteroids might protect against the levamisole-induced granulocytopenia, but several deaths from granulocytopenia occurred in patients receiving both drugs. Other side effects include nausea, vomiting, fatigue, drowsiness, urticarial skin rash, and drug fever. Levamisole stimulates the sympathetic and parasympathetic nervous systems, has positive chronotropic and inotropic effects on the heart, and inhibits alkaline phosphatases. Thus, despite some favorable effects in patients with RA, the side-effects probably outweigh the benefits.

Miscellaneous Agents

A number of compounds have been identified as having immune effects and are considered potential antirheumatic agents. Several have entered clinical trials. Therafectin (amiprilose HCl) is a synthetic modified hexose sugar that appears to specifically suppress the CD8 (suppressor/cytotoxic) population of T cells.[87] Several small clinical trials suggest that this agent is effective and safe in long-term RA therapy.[88,89] *IMREG-1* is a leukocyte-derived immunoregulatory substance that reverses a T-cell proliferative defect in patients with RA, although efficacy of IMREG-1 in this disease remains to be demonstrated.[90] Studies with *LS-2616*, a newly synthesized quinoline derivative, demonstrate successful treatment of autoimmunity in the MRL model of murine lupus.[91] This compound has been shown to upregulate IL-2 synthesis and enhance mixed lymphocyte reactions, but its mechanism of action in autoimmunity is not known. Imuthiol, a nickel-chelating agent, can influence the expression of T-cell surface markers both in vitro and in vivo. A small clinical study of its use in the treatment of RA suggests efficacy.[92] Isoprinosine, which may influence circulating CD8+ suppressor cells, also may be of benefit in treating RA.[92] Other agents with antirheumatic effects in animal models are now in early clinical testing. Immunoregulatory effects attributed to these agents include stimulation, restoration, and suppression; however, whether these effects on the immune system contribute to their antirheumatic actions is not known.

PHYSICAL AGENTS

Physical modalities have been used to regulate the immune response and treat rheumatic diseases. These modalities generally involve the physical removal of a portion of the immune system. Evidence also exists that these therapies may alter lymphoid recirculation or differentially induce T-cell subpopulations. Of the therapies to be discussed below, only splenectomy has a well-defined place among current treatment programs.

Ionizing Radiation

X-rays and gamma rays interact with atoms in living tissues, resulting in ejection of electrons and ionization of the affected atoms. When high-energy irradiation is used, the ejected electron may have enough energy subsequently to ionize several more atoms, resulting in the formation of reactive free radicals within cells that vigorously interact with and damage biologically important macromolecules, especially DNA. The effects on nuclear DNA frequently impair cellular reproduction. Thus, rapidly dividing cells such as those of the immune system, bone marrow, and intestinal epithelium are preferentially affected. Low doses of irradiation may selectively kill certain subpopulations of T cells and B cells. In general, precursor cells are particularly sensitive to x-rays because they have to undergo the most division.

Total lymphoid irradiation (TLI) has been effective in animal models of RA and SLE.[93,95] Experience treating humans with rheumatc diseases with TLI is growing. At least 5 different studies have been performed using TLI in intractable RA.[96] In these studies, a significant improvement resulted from TLI in doses of 2000 to 3000 rads. The largest of these studies, performed at Stanford University,[42] demonstrated a response lasting, in many cases, more than 4 years; however, serious side-effects have been reported in all studies. Prominent among these are infectious complications and an increased mortality rate following TLI (in part, this latter complication may reflect the natural history of advanced RA). Patients at high risk for morbidity following TLI include those with amyloidosis or rheumatoid lung disease and the elderly. Toxicity may be dose related, because the worst outcome was seen in the study utilizing 3000 rads.[97] One trial suggests that TLI with much lower doses of radiation (750 rads) may have as potent an antiarthritic effect as higher doses of irradiation.[98] If so, it may be possible to avoid many of the undesirable side-effects. TLI has also been used in the treatment of lupus nephritis not responsive to corticosteroids and cytotoxic drugs.[99] Therapy with 2000 rads resulted in a decrease in proteinuria, lowered titers of anti-DNA antibodies, and increased serum complement levels. Improvement persisted for more than a year. These studies indicate that TLI may have a role in the treatment of rheumatic diseases not responsive to other agents, but that with current protocols, safety is a major concern.

The immunologic effects of TLI have been well studied in humans with rheumatic diseases. Effects on the cellular immune system include the specific suppression of the CD4 (helper/inducer) population of T cells and decreased T-cell responses to alloantigens and phytohemagglutinin.[42,99] Such changes persisted for years following TLI. Effects on the humoral immune system were more varied.[100] Antibody levels in patients with RA and lupus were measured before and up to 60 weeks following TLI. Titers of antibody to diphtheria and tetanus toxoids decreased significantly following TLI, but antibody levels to pneumococcal polysaccharides were unchanged. In patients with lupus, antinuclear and anti-DNA antibody levels were decreased by TLI. In patients with RA, rheumatoid factors, antinuclear, and antigranulocyte antibodies all tended to increase. Because both lupus and RA are responsive to TLI, and yet TLI has different effects on autoantibody levels in these two diseases, these studies suggest different roles for autoantibody in the maintenance of the two disease states.

Apheresis

Therapeutic apheresis has been proposed as treatment for a variety of disorders.[101] In some, such as the treatment of hyperviscosity syndromes associated with myeloma, efficacy is clearly indicated. Autoimmune syndromes that appear responsive include myasthenia gravis and Goodpasture's syndrome. Efficacy of such therapies in the rheumatic diseases is debated. Plasma and various subpopulations of leukocytes may be removed, and often the exact component whose removal results in the improvement is unknown. In general, diseases caused by humoral factors seem most responsive to apheresis.

The effects of apheresis on RA have been mixed. Two studies, involving lymphapheresis[102] and lymphoplasmapheresis,[103] have demonstrated a beneficial effect following an intensive course of short-term therapy. A third study, involving plasma removal only, failed to show any efficacy.[104] From these results, it appears that the removal of lymphocytes, rather than a humoral factor, is responsible for the observed improvement, a similar conclusion to that regarding the mechanism of efficacy of TLI in RA. In contrast to this conclusion are the results of an ongoing uncontrolled study evaluating the effects of the specific apheretic removal of rheumatoid factor. This therapy has resulted in a decline in the titer of rheumatoid factor and an improvement in clinical status. Plasma

exchange has also been used in SLE, again with mixed results.[105,106] Given the high cost of therapeutic apheresis and the marginal clinical effect, this modality appears unlikely to play a significant role in the treatment of the rheumatic diseases.

Splenectomy

The spleen is the major site of removal of antibody-coated elements in the bloodstream and is also an important lymphoid organ. The major clinical indication for splenectomy is in patients with autoimmune leukopenias and thrombocytopenias unresponsive to less drastic forms of therapy. In particular, splenectomy has been successfully used in idiopathic thrombocytopenic purpura; however, variable results have been obtained in Felty's syndrome. Many patients with Felty's syndrome show a good short-term hematologic response, but the effect on prolonging survival and preventing infection is questionable.[107] Splenectomy is less useful in treating thrombocytopenia associated with SLE. Patients who have undergone splenectomy are particularly susceptible to overwhelming gram-positive sepsis. They should receive pneumococcal vaccine and may be candidates for prophylactic antibiotic therapy.

Radiation Synovectomy

Some believe that surgical synovectomy can provide long-term symptomatic relief in inflammatory arthritis, but its use has been limited by the expense and the long recovery time, during which joint contractures may develop. For these reasons, alternatives to this procedure have been sought. Chemical synovectomy has not obtained acceptance because of concerns regarding injury to the articular surfaces. Radiation synovectomy, consisting of the intra-articular injection of radioisotope in colloidal or particulate form, has proved to be an effective approach. But its widespread use has been inhibited by concerns regarding the leakage of radionuclide from the site of injection and accumulation in the draining lymph node. Recent attempts to circumvent this problem have resulted in the development of macroaggregate carriers coupled with very short-lived isotopes (e.g., dysprosium 165). Administration of these agents results in a long-term clinical improvement with minimal leakage of isotope from the joint space.[108] Larger clinical trials and long-term observation for delayed adverse effects will be required before this form of therapy is widely accepted.

Ultraviolet Irradiation

Ultraviolet (UV) light has many effects on the immune system, including altering lymphoid circulation, generating suppressor cells, and inhibiting antigen presentation.[108a] Short- and medium-wave UV irradiation can contribute to the induction and exacerbation of SLE. Thus, until recently the potential immunoregulatory and therapeutic role of UV light has not been explored in rheumatic diseases. However, using long wavelength UV light (320–400 nm, UV-A), investigators have shown that phototherapy of NZB/NZW mice results in improved survival, decreased anti-DNA antibody titers, and restoration of disordered immune function.[108b] Although a cautious trial of UV-A therapy in human subjects may be warranted, additional animal studies are required before patients with SLE can deliberately be exposed to UV irradiation.

THERAPIES USED FOR OTHER INDICATIONS WITH SECONDARY IMMUNE EFFECTS

Many pharmaceutical agents have immunologic effects. It is not the purpose of this section to provide a detailed list of these actions. Agents have been selected for discussion based on the demonstration or promise of antirheumatic effects.

Sex Hormones

Many of the rheumatic diseases are marked by sexual predispositions (e.g., RA and SLE in females, ankylosing spondylitis in males). Abnormalities in androgen levels have been described in lupus patients,[109] so it is only natural that some attention should be paid to the hormones that govern sexual development as potential therapeutic agents.[110] Direct administration of sex hormones can lead to distressing side effects. Synthetic analogues have been developed that avoid some of these complications and appear to have some efficacy in certain autoimmune states.

Direct effects of the hormones themselves have been studied best in animal models. Female NZB/NZW mice develop lupus nephritis more rapidly and die earlier than normal males. Castrated males die at the same age as females. Androgen treatment of females suppresses both lupus and autoantibody development.[111,112] In contrast, murine arthritis induced by type II collagen is predominantly a male disease, although there is no sexual difference in the magnitude of the antibody response to type II collagen.[113] Oophorectomy renders female mice as susceptible to collagen arthritis as are normal males.

Oral contraception can influence the clinical course of some rheumatic diseases. Administration of estro-

genic compounds may worsen SLE.[114] In contrast, there is clinical improvement in patients with RA treated with contraceptive therapy,[115] and contraceptive use may be associated with a decreased incidence of this disease.[116] These results are consistent with the animal experiments discussed above. Both lines of evidence suggest that the predominance of females afflicted by lupus is an estrogen-mediated effect although this is not the case in RA.

Danazol, a weak synthetic androgen, is of use in treating idiopathic thrombocytopenic purpura resistant to corticosteroids. It appears to decrease the number of available Fc (IgG) receptors on the surface of monocytes, which leads to a decreased clearance of antibody-coated targets.[117] Danazol does not appear to be effective in murine lupus.[118] It has some clinical efficacy in human lupus, but this is offset by a high incidence of side effects.[119]

Cyproterone acetate is a synthetic hydroxyprogesterone derivative that possesses antigonadotrophic properties. A small, open-label trial has shown that this agent is of use in lowering the number of clinical exacerbations in SLE.[120] In patients treated with cyproterone acetate, the mean plasma estradiol level decreased significantly, and side effects were few. The long-term effects on rheumatic diseases of this, and similar, agents remain to be explored.

Thalidomide

Thalidomide, a tranquilizer with an unfortunate history, has been used with some success in the rheumatic diseases. Its mechanism of action is believed to be the inhibition of circulating immune complex and neutrophil-mediated tissue damage.[121] It is used as a primary therapy in reactive lepromatous leprosy.[122] In Behçet's syndrome, mucosal ulcerations and arthritis respond well to thalidomide; uveitis is responsive in only some patients.[121,123] A flare was noted in some patients after drug withdrawal. A preliminary, open-label study in RA showed that thalidomide led to clinical improvement within several weeks.[124] In half the patients, the effect lasted long after discontinuation of the drug. Side effects of thalidomide include teratogenicity and peripheral neuropathies. The unpleasant connotations this drug has makes patient acceptance problematic.

Antihypertensives

Captopril, an angiotensin-converting enzyme inhibitor, has a molecular structure similar to D-penicillamine, having a thiol group in common. Both compounds also bind copper and have similar side effects. On this basis, an open-label trial was performed evaluating the efficacy of captopril in RA.[125] Two thirds of the patients showed improvement in both clinical and laboratory parameters. Initial improvement was seen in 6 weeks, with the maximal effect obtained by 3 months. Side effects were transient and mild. Although there was no evidence that the antirheumatic effect of captopril is due to an immunologic mechanism, it has been shown to have a suppressive effect on in-vitro lymphocyte transformation in response to mitogen.[126]

Catecholamines regulate a wide variety of cellular functions through interactions with cell surface receptors. Vasoactive amines play an important role in the delayed hypersensitivity response.[127] *Prazosin* is a specific alpha$_1$-adrenergic antagonist that suppressed the development of experimental autoimmune encephalomyelitis (EAE) in rats.[128] Brosnan and coworkers noted that this was most likely a result of drug-induced alterations in vascular permeability rather than any immune effects. Although EAE is thought to be a model of multiple sclerosis, there are implications for the rheumatic diseases as well.

Neurotransmitters

A variety of molecular structures transmit signals between different neural cells or from the neural cells to their targets. Many of these compounds play a role in the regulation of pain and the response to it. Recent evidence has demonstrated that a peptide neurotransmitter, *substance P*, may also play an important role in inflammation.[129,130] In adjuvant-induced arthritis, substance P levels in neurons innervating severely inflamed joints were higher than levels in less inflamed joints. Intra-articular injection of substance P increased the severity of arthritis. Rheumatoid synoviocytes cultured with substance P produced increased quantities of prostaglandin E$_2$ and collagenase. Substance P contributes to the severity of arthritis and may be an inflammatory mediator. *Somatostatin*, a hypothalamic-releasing factor, is a powerful inhibitor of the secretion of a number of neuropeptides.[131] Clinical trials with somatostatin analogues are being considered.

Iron-Binding Compounds

Iron and its major binding proteins, transferrin, lactoferrin, and ferritin, appear to be able to modulate immunologic functions. Cellular proliferation depends on iron, and activated T lymphocytes bear a transferrin receptor.[132] *Desferoxamine*, an iron chelator, can block T-cell proliferation in response to mitogen. This effect can be overcome by the addition of excess iron. Desferoxamine also blocks the expression of the T-cell receptor for IL-2.[133] The administration of desferoxamine can block the induction of experimental autoimmune disease.[134] Humans with severe iron deficiency have impaired immunity, but there is currently little evidence regarding the therapeutic utility of the manipulation of iron metabolism in human diseases.

Antibiotics

Many chronic rheumatic diseases may be of infectious origin (see Chaper 31); therefore antibiotics have been tried in the treatment of rheumatic diseases. Results published in peer-reviewed journals have yielded no suggestion that diseases such as RA, ankylosing spondylitis, or systemic lupus are responsive to such agents. In spite of this, *tetracycline* antibiotics have been advocated for treatment of RA at certain centers. A well-designed protocol to test the efficacy of tetracycline has been proposed. If an antirheumatic effect is demonstrated, it may not be the result of the antibacterial effect of tetracycline. It has been shown that tetracyclines are inhibitors of human synovial collagenase, both in vivo and in vitro.[135] Such activity might inhibit the tissue damage resulting from the chronic inflammatory process. Tetracyclines may also affect the immune system,[136] which could account for the putative antirheumatic effect.

Retinoids

Retinoic acid derivatives have multiple effects on cellular proliferation and differentiation. Specific stimulation of the immune system has been reported.[137] The synthesis of both collagen and collagenase is inhibited by retinoids.[138,139] These effects suggest that retinoic acid derivatives may influence rheumatic diseases. Studies on experimental systems have yielded mixed results: collagen-induced arthritis is exacerbated, while adjuvant and streptococcal cell wall-induced arthritides are suppressed.[139] A role for these agents in human disease has not been shown. The use of isotretinoin (Accutane) in treating skin disorders has been associated with skeletal hyperostosis.[140]

Tetrahydrocannabinol Derivatives

Tetrahydrocannabinol is the active ingredient of marijuana. It has been claimed that this agent has pharmacologically important effects on the immune system.[141] Marijuana is also useful in counteracting the gastrointestinal effects of cancer chemotherapy. No clinical trials have yet been performed in rheumatic diseases. Anecdotal evidence suggests a subjective improvement is noted by patients.

CYTOKINES

Large quantities of human cytokines can be produced by recombinant DNA technology. The pharmacologic utility of these agents is being probed concurrently with attempts to understand their basic physiology. Administration of cytokines to patients may help us understand the basic pathophysiology of the disease under study.

The cytokines, as well as antibodies, are macromolecular pharmaceutical agents. Because they are large biologic molecules that are easily degraded they have certain important limitations. Unless new delivery systems are developed, they must be administered parenterally. After administration, they have a limited distribution throughout the body. Macromolecules are more readily recognized by the immune system, and thus the agent may be rapidly degraded and cleared from the body, or it may induce a hypersensitivity reaction. Because of these inherent limitations, much emphasis is being placed on the development of synthetic compounds that may act as cytokine agonists or antagonists.

Interferons

The interferons were discovered because of their antiviral activity but they also have antiproliferative and immunomodulatory effects. There are three different classes of interferons: alpha, beta, and gamma. Alpha and beta interferons are structurally related, bind to the same cellular receptors, and have pronounced antiviral effects. IFN-gamma, the product of activated T cells, is noted for its immunomodulatory, rather than its antiviral, effects. IFN-gamma is primarily an upregulator of the immune system. It is a macrophage-activating factor[28] and results in an increased expression of class II histocompatibility antigens on the surface of many cells, including articular chondrocytes.[29,142] This can allow antigen presentation to T cells by cells not normally capable of this function, and may in fact precipitate an autoimmune T-cell-mediated attack.[143] Administration of IFN-gamma with immunization leads to an antigen-specific enhancement of the immune response.[144] The proliferation of synovial fibroblasts is increased by IFN-gamma.[145] Thus, there is little theoretical reason to believe that IFN-gamma would be effective in rheumatic diseases, and it may even worsen the disease process.[146]

In view of these expectations, it comes as a surprise that IFN-gamma may have a beneficial effect in RA. Initial anecdotal reports suggested improvement of arthritis in patients undergoing the treatment of malignancy with IFN-gamma. These have been followed by a series of well-designed clinical trials,[147,148] which indicate that IFN-gamma may be an effective treatment in rheumatoid arthritis. A large placebo effect (the result of frequent subcutaneous injections) complicated the analysis. Nevertheless, it appears that a subset of patients may respond to this agent. Side effects were primarily low-grade systemic symptoms related to administration of the cytokine. Antirheumatic effects of IFN-alpha and IFN-beta have not been tested. IFN-beta is effective in preventing exacerbations of multiple sclerosis, a disease sharing many characteristics with rheumatic conditions.[149]

The mechanism of action of IFN-gamma in RA is not established, but immunomodulation is an intriguing possibility. The administration of IFN-gamma resulted in an increase in the expression of HLA-DR antigens on circulating mononuclear cells, but no other pronounced change in immunoregulatory cell subsets was seen. Antiproliferative and anti-infective effects also need to be evaluated. There may be a deficiency in the production of IFN-gamma in both RA and SLE.[150,151] If this is true, the administration of IFN-gamma may function as hormone replacement therapy. Administration of interferons has been shown to reduce excessive collagen production by cultured scleroderma fibroblasts[151a] suggesting yet another potential antirheumatic effect. Further exploration of the mechanism of action of IFN-gamma and the delineation of the subset of patients who are good responders to IFN-gamma should lead to an understanding of the role of this cytokine in rheumatic disease therapy.

IL-1 and Tumor Necrosis Factor

IL-1 and tumor necrosis factor are discussed together because they have many effects in common (see Table 38–1). In particular, the role of these agents in the generation of the inflammatory response has drawn much attention. Both IL-1 and TNF are important early mediators in the generation of the inflammatory response. The development of IL-1 or TNF antagonists could represent a new class of anti-inflammatory agents. IL-1 and TNF are products of mononuclear phagocytes, although IL-1 can also be secreted by other cell types, including neural tissue[35] and polymorphonuclear leukocytes.[152] They have little structural similarity, and differences in the physiologic effects of the hormones are probably a function of the cellular distribution of the receptors for these materials.[24,33,153]

At least two distinct forms of IL-1 occur, both of which appear to bind to the same cellular receptor.[154] In the immune response, IL-1 plays an important role in T-cell activation after antigen presentation. It is also responsible for a variety of effects on other target systems.[24] Many target tissues, including endothelial, synovial, and neural cells, respond by secreting prostaglandins. Hepatocytes produce acute phase reactants in response to IL-1. Central nervous system responses include the induction of fever and increased slow wave sleep. The procoagulant activity of the vascular endothelium increases. Proliferative responses are seen in many cell types including thymocytes, synovial cells, fibroblasts, hematopoietic cells, and epithelium. Osteoclasts are stimulated by IL-1 to increase the production of collagenase. Metabolic effects include the inhibition of lipoprotein lipase and a decrease in the synthesis of albumin. Many of these activities could play an important role in the generation and persistence of an inflammatory response as seen in rheumatic diseases. In support of this concept is the finding of IL-1 in the synovial fluids of patients with RA.[155]

The multiple biologic activities of TNF have resulted in its receiving two different names: TNF and cachectin. (Both names are still used in the literature, although TNF appears to be gaining favor.) As the names imply, TNF results in the death of tumor targets and in the cachexia seen in advanced states of cancer and in certain infections.[156] Other effects include endogenous pyrogen activity, neutrophil activation, and induction of endothelial procoagulant activity.[33,153] TNF can stimulate bone resorption, through osteoclast activation and can inhibit bone formation.[157,158]

Although IL-1 and TNF are physiologic hormones, many of the responses they elicit can be toxic. Mice treated with an anti-TNF polyclonal antibody become resistant to the lethal effects of lipopolysaccharide, suggesting that death in gram-negative sepsis may be in part mediated by excess production of TNF. Pharmacologic administration of IL-1 and TNF causes anorexia, weight loss, and in high doses, shock.[153,159] In excess, the detrimental effects of these hormones may outweigh the beneficial (most likely anti-infective) effects. It thus comes as no surprise that there are naturally occurring inhibitors. IL-1 inhibitors have been found in the urine and serum of febrile patients and pregnant women and have been extracted from leukocytes.[47,46,160] The gene for one of these inhibitors has been cloned and found to be identical to the Tamm-Horsfall urinary glycoprotein, the most abundant protein of renal origin in the urine.[160] Interestingly, the immunosuppressive and IL-1 binding activities reside in the carbohydrate rather than the peptide portion of this glycoprotein. The identification and structural characterization of physiologic inhibitors suggests that pharmacologic inhibition of the activity of IL-1

and TNF is a feasible therapeutic approach. Because both IL-1 and TNF are important mediators of the inflammatory response, inhibitors of these compounds could play an important role in the future treatment of rheumatic disease.

IL-2

IL-2 has received most attention as a potential anticancer agent.[161,162] It produces proliferation of several populations of immune cells including lymphokine-activated killer cells (predominantly natural killer cells), T cells, and B cells. Other cell types, including neural cells, also can respond.[34] Techniques have been developed to avoid the fluid retention and pulmonary edema that direct administration of IL-2 can produce.[36] Among these techniques are ex vivo treatment of white blood cells with IL-2 and reinfusion of these cells into the patient, and very slow intravenous infusion. Some patients with advanced malignancy show a significant response to these therapies. The role of IL-2 therapy in rheumatic diseases is untested. A defect in the production and response to IL-2 has ben postulated in humans and experimental animals with rheumatic conditions,[163,164] although this defect has been refuted by others.[165] An IL-2 inhibitor has been found in rheumatoid synovial fluid.[49] The administration of IL-2 can overcome immune response gene defects in experimental animals.[166] Human immune response genes are one postulated mechanism for HLA-disease associations. If there is a deficiency or inhibitor of IL-2, or if there is an immune response gene defect, then it is possible that administration of IL-2 may favorably alter the course of the disease.

Human receptors for IL-2 have been well characterized.[25,26] Monoclonal antibodies have been made against them. Receptors are expressed in large numbers on activated T cells, but are also found on resting T-cells, B cells, and other responding cells. Thus, cells secreting IL-2 (activated T cells) can also respond to IL-2. Receptor expression is initially upregulated in response to IL-2 binding, increasing the sensitivity of the responding cell to this hormone. Activated T lymphocytes circulating in the peripheral blood of patients with RA express the IL-2 receptor.[53] Modulation of immune responses with monoclonal antibodies to the IL-2 receptor has been reported.[52,167,168] It may be possible to use these antibodies to treat autoimmunity as well.

Thymic Hormones

Thymosin, thymulin, and thymopoietin are factors isolated from the thymus gland that play a role in the functional development of T cells. *Thymopoietin* has been purified to homogeneity, its amino acid sequence has been deduced, and a pentapeptide (TP5) containing the biologic activity has been synthesized.[169] Administration of TP5 to thymectomized mice can reverse the development of an aging-induced immunodeficiency.[170] It can also suppress anti-red blood cell autoimmunity in mice immunized with rat red blood cells.[171] A preliminary clinical trial with TP5 in rheumatoid arthritis has been performed with promising results.[172] More definitive trials have taken place, but the results have not been published. *Thymulin* is a zinc-binding nonapeptide produced by the thymic epithelium. It has been moderately beneficial in rheumatoid arthritis.[173]

Other Cytokines

In addition to the materials discussed above, other cytokines (or inhibitors of such) have antirheumatic potential. A complete listing is not feasible. Hematopoietins including IL-3 (multipotential colony-stimulating factor) and granulocyte/monocyte colony-stimulating factors regulate the availability of inflammatory cells.[30,174] Administration of erythropoietin to RA patients reduces the disease-associated anemia and leads to an improvement in energy levels and a feeling of well-being. B-cell growth and differentiation factors may have an effect on the humoral abnormalities associated with rheumatic diseases.[31] Abnormal expression of oncogenes has been reported in rheumatic conditions,[175] and regulation of disease processes by oncogene products is possible. Growth factors[176,177] may control the proliferation of cells that accumulate in excess in the rheumatic diseases. Management of these proliferative processes may result in better control of disease activity.

ANTIBODIES

Antibody preparations can be administered for their antigen-specific effects and can also be used as replacement therapy in patients with immunoglobulin deficiencies. A third set of uses is based on the observed therapeutic efficacy of intravenous immunoglobulin (IVIG) in certain autoimmune conditions. The mechanism of action of IVIG in autoimmunity is less well understood, but may possibly relate to blockade of Fc receptor–mediated mechanisms. With few exceptions, when immune specificity is desired, monoclonal antibodies are certain to be the preparations of choice. Pooled polyclonal antibody preparations are more useful in other situations.

Monoclonal Preparations

With the introduction of monoclonal antibody technology, the specificity and reproducibility of antibody preparations has been vastly improved, leading to a resurgence of interest in antibody-based therapies. Table 38–4 lists the potential targets of monoclonal antibody therapy in the rheumatic diseases. As with the cytokines, initial studies of monoclonal antibodies have pursued applications in the treatment of cancer. As safety parameters have become established, use of these therapies in less threatening diseases has been considered.[46] Among the major concerns regarding antibody administration is the development of conditions similar to serum-sickness as a result of deposition of immune complexes containing the administered antibody. Such deposition is a particular concern in the rheumatic diseases, in which immune complex–mediated damage is one of the major pathogenic mechanisms in the disease itself. General improvements in biochemical processing have led to the production of purer preparations of antibody, with fewer antibody aggregates, than were used in the past. This has significantly decreased the host response to the administered antibody. Considerable efforts are being expended to make human monoclonal antibodies (currently most are murine), which should also limit the host response. In clinical trials with monoclonal antibodies in cancer, the major difficulty resulting from the immune response to the administered antibody has been increased clearance of the antibody and blocking of the desired therapeutic effect by anti-idiotypic antibodies.[46] Treatment with monoclonal antibody directed against CD4 at the same time antigen is administered may result in the development of long-term antigen-specific tolerance.[178] If this is also true in human systems, then the host response to administered antibody may not be a problem.

Cell surface markers on immunocytes are functional molecules, as well as labels for certain cell populations. Table 38–2 lists surface antigens that may be relevant for the rheumatic diseases. Antibodies to these structures may operate by blocking the per-

Table 38–4. Potential Targets of Monoclonal Antibody Therapy in the Rheumatic Diseases

T cell subset and activation markers
B cell subset and activation markers
Complement receptors
Fc receptors
Cytokines and cytokine receptors
Histocompatibility antigens
Idiotypic structures on autoantibodies or T cells

formance of the function, or they may serve to target the cells bearing the marker for immune-mediated destruction. This is illustrated with the antibody to CD4, which defines the helper/inducer T cell. As discussed above, this T-cell subset seems to be a particular target of immunomodulatory antirheumatic therapies.[39-42] The CD4 molecule is involved in recognition of HLA class II antigens (e.g., HLA-DR). Administration of anti-CD4 results in the suppression of disease in a number of animal models of autoimmunity.[43,44] This is associated with a profound loss in T cells bearing CD4. The same immunosuppressive effects are seen when F(ab')$_2$ fragments of the antibody are given, but cells expressing CD4 can be demonstrated in the circulation.[179] The tolerogenic potential of anti-CD4 antibody was first observed when it was noted that there was no anti-rat immune response in mice receiving rat anti-CD4 antibody.[43] This was in contrast to the sometimes lethal effects seen when antibody to a different T cell marker was used in experimental animals[45] or the oligoclonal response seen in humans to anti-CD3 antibody.[180] Appropriately timed administrations of anti-CD4 and a foreign antigen may result in specific tolerance to that antigen. Monoclonal anti-CD4 antibodies may play a future role in immunoregulation of the rheumatic diseases. To put this in perspective, however, a parallel may be drawn between the acquired immune deficiency syndrome (AIDS) and treatment with anti-CD4 antibody. Both situations eliminate the same population of cells. Use of intact antibody to eliminate permanently the CD4 population of cells may have drastic consequences, while a partial suppression may be useful. A cruel experiment of nature will be to observe those patients with rheumatic conditions who develop AIDS. The effects of AIDS may help predict the efficacy of specific immunomodulatory therapy with anti-CD4 antibodies.

Cell surface structures other than CD4 can also serve as targets of antibody-mediated immunomodulation. Monoclonal antibody to the pan T cell CD3 antigen (OKT3) has been approved by the U.S. Food and Drug Administration for use in renal transplantation. Histocompatibility antigens play an important role in cell-cell interactions. Administration of antibodies to these molecules can block the development of human responses and has been used to suppress the development of autoimmune disease in experimental animals.[181,182] Antibody to the Fc receptor on mononuclear cells has been used successfully to treat a patient with idiopathic thrombocytopenic purpura not responsive to more conventional measures.[183] Cellular activation markers can be used to target immune cells that are actively responding to an immune stim-

ulus. Human T-cell activation markers that are elevated in immune-mediated diseases include the IL-2 receptor,[53] TA-1,[184] and the very late activation (VLA) antigen.[185] Activation markers on macrophages and B cells have also been described,[186,187] but their expression on cells in rheumatic diseases has not been studied. Particular populations of cells that appear to play an important role in the development of autoimmune processes, and thus may serve as specific targets of suppression, include B cells that express the CD5 (Leu-1) antigen,[188] and helper T cells that express either the 4B4 or 2H4 antigens, markers of functional subsets of the CD4 + T cell population.[189,190] The more specific the cellular target, the less likely the chance of unwanted immunosuppressive side effects.

Antibodies to cytokines and their cellular receptors also may be used. Depending on the site of the cytokine molecule bound by the antibody, either agonistic or antagonistic effects may be seen.[50] Similarly, antibody binding to a receptor may mimic the ligand[51] or block its effect.[52] We have already discussed the effects of antibody to the IL-2 receptor. Once initial studies have (more or less empirically) defined the functional domains of the cytokines and their receptors, more sophisticated attempts to create ligand congeners with agonistic or antagonistic properties can be attempted.

Antibodies to immunoglobulin and T cell idiotypes offer the potential of highly specific immunosuppression, deleting specific clones of cells involved in the pathogenic immune response. Antibodies defining major cross-reactive idiotypes on human autoantibodies have been made.[191,192] Attempts to apply this technique in animal models of lupus have led to a transient suppression of the anti-DNA response, but eventually idiotype negative variants secreting anti-DNA antibody have arisen.[193,194] Similarly, humans with B-cell lymphomas treated with anti-idiotypic antibody develop idiotype negative tumor variants.[195] For idiotype specific therapy to be useful it will be necessary to define idiotypes that are integrally related to the combining site, so that idiotype-negative variant antibodies also lack the ability to bind to the autoantigen in question.

Recombinant DNA technology has been applied also to the production of monoclonal antibodies. The initial application has been to create chimeric antibodies, which have variable regions derived from murine hybridomas attached to human constant regions,[196] in an effort to make them less immunogenic in the host. Novel antibody constant regions with unique biologic effects may be produced as well. It will also be possible to make large quantities of antibody fragments, which can be used to induce blockade of Fc-mediated antibody effector functions.[197] Through the use of these techniques, more effective antibodies for human therapy may be produced.

Polyclonal Preparations

Three different polyclonal antibody therapies will be discussed: antilymphocyte globulin, placenta-eluted gamma globulins, and gamma globulin preparations suitable for intravenous injection (IVIG). Antilymphocyte globulin is purified from the serum of an animal immunized with human lymphocytes. The serum is rendered lymphocyte-specific by absorption on other cell types. Antibodies can also be rendered T cell-specific by similar absorptions. Antilymphocyte antibodies cause immune effects by inducing lymphopenia, resulting from direct cytotoxicity of the antibodies and from clearance of the lymphocytes by the reticuloendothelial system.[198,199] Antilymphocyte globulin has been used extensively in renal transplantation[200] and in uncontrolled trials in autoimmune disease.[198] Serum sickness is seen in a high proportion of patients receiving antilymphocyte globulins.[201] It seems likely that the use of polyclonal antilymphocyte antibodies will be replaced by more specific monoclonal antibodies directed against lymphocyte subsets.

Antibodies eluted from human placentas have been used to treat RA.[202] The preparations are purified IgG eluted under acid conditions from large pools of human placental tissues. A good clinical response, associated with a decrease in the sedimentation rate, was seen in 60% of patients treated. The most effective schedule, involving intravenous injection of antibodies seven times per month, could be maintained for years. Injection of the antibody increased lymphocyte responsiveness to mitogens and altered circulating populations of lymphocytes. A control antibody preparation made from placental blood was not effective. It is presumed that the active moiety in the placenta-eluted gamma globulin is polyspecific anti-HLA-DR antibody.[203]

IVIG preparations[204] are obtained from pooled human plasma by cold ethanol fractionation and then chromatographic separation or ultrafiltration. More than 90% of the protein in these preparations is monomer IgG, with a subclass distribution similar to that seen in human serum. The major indications for the use of IVIG are the treatment of infection in the immunocompromised host and antibody supplmentation in humoral immunodeficiency.[204,205] In these situations, the mechanism of action is straightforward: replacement of missing immunoglobulins. However, the mechanism of action of IVIG in autoimmunity is less obvious. It has been demonstrated that high-dose

IVIG (400 mg/kg daily for 5 days) is effective in the therapy of refractory idiopathic thrombocytopenic purpura,[206] and this is now an approved indication for use of the preparation. It has also been used in autoimmune neutropenia and myasthenia gravis, and in patients with autoantibodies to clotting factors.[204,207] A large clinical trial has shown that IVIG prevents the development of coronary artery disease in patients with Kawasaki disease.[208] In many pediatric centers, this has quickly become an accepted part of the therapy of Kawasaki disease. The evidence presented in support of these conclusions needs additional verification in the form of longer-term follow-up of the patients involved in this study and additional well-controlled studies. Several different mechanisms of action have been proposed for the efficacy of IVIG in autoimmunity. Blockade of Fc receptor function is the likely mechanism of IVIG function in idiopathic thrombocytopenic purpura.[209,210] Anti-idiotypic antibodies blocking the function of autoantibody have also been proposed to explain IVIG effects.[207] A decrease in circulating immune complexes has been observed following the administration of IVIG in patients with SLE, although the failure of IVIG to accomplish this in an in-vitro system raises the possibility that this is not a direct effect of IVIG.[211] Natural killer cell activity is inhibited when hypogammaglobulinemic patients receive IVIG.[212] All these different mechanisms may play a role in the efficacy of IVIG in autoimmunity. The administration of IVIG has some significant drawbacks: it is extremely expensive, and anaphylactic reactions have been reported, particularly in patients with selective IgA deficiency and anti-IgA antibodies. The decision to use this medication in patients with autoimmunity must be considered carefully.

AGENTS WHOSE ANTIRHEUMATIC EFFECTS MAY BE NONIMMUNE

4,4′ Diaminodiphenylsulfone (Dapsone)

Dapsone, a sulfone, has long been used in the treatment of leprosy. It is also effective in the treatment of bullous skin diseases, particularly those characterized by granulocyte infiltration. It is especially useful in dermatitis herpetiformis, erythema elevatum diutinum, and bullous eruptions in SLE.[213,214] Its efficacy in nondermatologic manifestations of rheumatic diseases is less well established, but it may have a role in the management of relapsing polychondritis.[215,216] In antigen-induced arthritis of mice, it has a beneficial effect, but less than that seen with azathioprine, sulfasalazine, or methotrexate.[217] In a comparative clinical trial in RA, dapsone had some efficacy, but it was less than that of chloroquine.[218] In a study to determine the reasons why patients with RA discontinued slow-acting drugs, lack of clinical effect was the most common reason for discontinuing dapsone.[219] The mechanism of action of dapsone may be to inhibit neutrophil influx to inflammatory lesions. Dapsone therapy has well-defined side effects including hemolysis, methemoglobinemia, gastrointestinal intolerance, peripheral neuropathy, and central nervous system irritability. In view of the side effects and the low degree of efficacy, dapsone is not currently recommended for the therapy of nondermatologic manifestations of rheumatic diseases.

Fish Oil (see also Chapter 65)

The dietary intake of fatty acids is reflected in the fatty acid composition of the tissues. The composition of fatty acids in marine lipids is enriched for long-chain polyunsaturated fatty acids containing double bonds at the n-3 position (omega-3 fatty acids). One of these omega-3 fatty acids, eicosapentaenoic acid, is structurally related to arachidonic acid, the precursor of prostaglandins and leukotrienes. Incorporation of eicosapentaenoic acid rather than arachidonic acid can lead to a series of prostaglandins and leukotrienes that are functionally different. One of these differences may be reflected in a decreased inflammatory response. Studies with diets high in fish oil in animal models of rheumatic diseases have been promising. The development of renal disease and mortality in lupus-prone mice can be inhibited by a diet rich in fish oil, even if not begun until after renal disease has become manifest.[220] Similarly, in murine arthritis, a diet rich in eicosapentaenoic acid can retard the development of arthritis and alter the content of fatty acids in macrophage membranes.[221] Short-term trials in patients with RA indicate that a fish oil diet may have some efficacy in decreasing symptoms and lowering leukotriene B$_4$ levels.[222] Laboratory parameters of disease activity were unchanged. The major untoward effect of diets high in fish oil is the taste of the oil supplements, eructation, and other GI complaints. Toxicity in laboratory animals has included necrotizing vasculitis,[220] and in one set of experiments a worsening of arthritis.[223] Given the well-documented effect of fish oil in preventing coronary artery disease, the benefits of fish oil supplementation may outweigh the risks. Long-term studies will be required to demonstrate definitively the utility and safety of this therapy.

Dimethyl Sulfoxide (DMSO)

DMSO is a highly polar organic solvent that is well absorbed through the skin. This chemical has received considerable attention from purveyors of "alternative cures" for rheumatoid conditions. Because of difficulties in keeping patients "blind" to this form of therapy in clinical trials, it has been difficult to define the efficacy of DMSO. Potential mechanisms of action of DMSO include anti-inflammatory effects, effects upon nerve transmission, analgesic effects, and immunomodulation.[224] Conditions that have been treated with DMSO include scleroderma, RA, and musculoskeletal pain syndromes. A controlled clinical trial in the treatment of digital ulcers in systemic sclerosis showed no efficacy and considerable toxicity associated with topical DMSO therapy.[225] Chemical grade DMSO (the form frequently sold by practitioners of this therapy) can serve as a solvent to allow the systemic absorption of contaminants in the preparation, thus adding an additional form of toxicity. Because of the high degree of toxicity and lack of efficacy, the use of DMSO in patients with rheumatic diseases should be strongly discouraged.

Chondroprotective Agents (see also Chapter 103)

RA and osteoarthritis both involve a degradation of the cartilage matrix as a prominent part of the histopathology. Agents that can prevent this degradation can ameliorate the disease process without affecting the factors that initiate the cartilage breakdown (that is, autoimmunity and inflammation). Agents that prevent loss of proteoglycans, stimulate cartilage synthesis, or inhibit the toxicity of products released from inflammatory cells might function as chondroprotective agents. Materials that purport to accomplish these goals have been developed and have undergone some degree of clinical testing.[224] Although many of these have some benefit, their effects are limited.

Glucosamine is an important precursor molecule in the synthesis of proteoglycans. The supplemental administration of glucosamine has increased proteoglycan synthesis both in vivo and in vitro.[226] Studies in osteoarthritis have shown therapeutic efficacy of glucosamine administration.[227,228] The effect was comparable to or greater than that seen with nonsteroidal anti-inflammatory agents, and two patients had histologically documented healing in cartilage lesions. The synthesis of proteoglycans can also be stimulated by the addition of proteoglycans themselves.[229] The clinical efficacy of two proteoglycan preparations has been tested: *Arteparon*, an oversulfated heparinoid, and *Rumalon*, a crude extract of calf cartilage. Both appear to be mildly effective in the treatment of osteoarthritis.[230,231]

Superoxide dismutase is a metalloenzyme that can protect mammalian tissues from the toxic effects of free oxygen radicals released by inflammatory cells.

Orgotein, the generic name given to therapeutic preparations of bovine superoxide dismutase, is most effectively administered by the intramuscular, intra-articular, or subcutaneous route. It is neither very toxic nor immunogenic, and its efficacy in osteoarthritis appears to be limited.[232] However, in RA the effect seems comparable to that obtained with gold[233] or intra-articular steroids.[234] Because superoxide dismutase appears to operate at a different level of the disease process than most second-line agents in RA, one might expect to see synergistic effects if superoxide dismutase were to be used in conjunction with immunomodulatory therapies. Clinical trials to test this possibility need to be performed.

ACKNOWLEDGMENTS

Portions of this chapter were derived from Chapter 33 in the tenth edition of this textbook, coauthored by John L. Decker and Alfred D. Steinberg.

REFERENCES

1. Goodwin, J.S., Ceuppens, J.L., and Rodriguez, M.A.: Administration of nonsteroidal antiinflammatory agents in patients with rheumatoid arthritis. JAMA, *250*:2485, 1983.
2. Ceuppens, J.L., et al.: Immunomodulatory effects of treatment with naproxen in patients with rheumatic disease. Arthritis Rheum., *29*:305, 1986.
3. Hersh, E.M., Wong, V.G., and Freireich, E.J.: Inhibition of the local inflammatory response in man by antimetabolites. Blood, *27*:38, 1966.
4. Clegg, D.O., et al.: Circulating HLA-DR bearing T cells: correlation with genetic rather than clinical variables. J. Rheumatol., *13*:870, 1986.
5. Weinblatt, M.E., et al.: Efficacy of low-dose methotrexate in rheumatoid arthritis. N. Engl. J. Med., *312*:818, 1985.
6. Austin, H.A., et al.: Therapy of lupus nephritis: controlled trial of prednisone and cytotoxic drugs. N. Engl. J. Med., *314*:614, 1986.
6a. Matsubara, T., and Ziff, M.: Inhibition of human endothelial cell proliferation by gold compounds. J. Clin. Invest., *79*:1440–1446, 1987.
7. Cuperus, R.A., Muijsers, A.O., and Wever, R.: Antiarthritic drugs containing thiol groups scavenge hypochlorite and inhibit its formation by myeloperoxidase from human leukocytes. Arthritis Rheum., *28*:1228, 1985.
8. Askenase, P.W., Hayden, B.J., and Gershon, R.K.: Augmentation of delayed-type hypersensitivity by doses of cyclophosphamide which do not affect antibody responses. J. Exp. Med., *141*:697, 1975.
9. Vladutiu, A.O.: Autoimmune thyroiditis: conversion of low-responder mice to high-responders by cyclophosphamide. Clin. Exp. Immunol., *47*:683, 1982.
10. Tripodi, D., Parks, L.C., and Brugmans, J.: Drug-induced restoration of cutaneous delayed hypersensitivity in anergic patients with cancer. N. Engl. J. Med., *289*:354, 1973.
11. Gazdar, A.F., et al.: Enhancement and suppression of murine sarcoma virus induced tumors by polyriboinosinic polyribocytidylic acid. Proc. Soc. Exp. Biol. Med., *139*:279, 1972.
12. Steinberg, A.D., et al.: Therapeutic studies in NZB/W mice. III. Relationship between renal status and efficacy of immunosuppressive drug therapy. Arthritis Rheum., *18*:9, 1975.
13. Dukor, P., and Dietrich, F.M.: Prevention of cyclophosphamide-induced tolerance to erythrocytes by pretreatment with cortisone. Proc. Soc. Exp. Biol. Med., *133*:280, 1970.
14. Gelfand, M.C., et al.: Therapeutic studies in NZB/W mice. I. Synergy of azathioprine, cyclophosphamide and methylprednisolone in combination. Arthritis Rheum., *15*:239, 1972.
15. Hyman, L.R., Kovacs, K., and Steinberg, A.D.: Drug-induced tolerance: Selective induction with immunosuppressive drugs and their synergistic interaction. Int. Arch. Allergy Appl. Immunol., *48*:248, 1975.
16. Zulman, J., et al.: Levamisole maintains cyclophosphamide-induced remission in murine lupus erythematosus. Clin. Exp. Immunol., *31*:321, 1978.
17. McCarty, D.J., and Carrera, G.F.: Treatment of intractable rheumatoid arthritis with combined cyclophosphamide, azathioprine and hydroxychloroquine. JAMA, *248*:1718, 1982.
18. Friedman, E.A., Gelfand, M.C., and Bernheimer, H.P.: Synergism in immunosuppressive drugs on tetanus antitoxin production in the mouse. Transplantation, *11*:479, 1971.
19. Freund, J., Casals, J., Hismer, E.P.: Sensitization and antibody formation after injection of tubercle bacilli and paraffin oil. Proc. Soc. Exp. Biol. Med., *37*:509, 1937.
20. Warren, H.S., Vogel, F.R., and Chedid, L.A.: Current status of immunological adjuvants. Annu. Rev. Immunol., *4*:369, 1986.
21. Kotani, S., et al.: Chemical structure and biological activity relationship of bacterial cell walls and muramyl peptides. Fed. Proc., *45*:2534, 1986.
22. Dinarello, C.A., and Krueger, J.M.: Induction of interleukin 1 by synthetic and naturally occurring muramyl peptides. Fed. Proc., *45*:2545, 1986.
23. Nagata, S., et al.: Synthesis in E. coli of a polypeptide with human leukocyte interferon activity. Nature, *284*:316, 1980.
24. Oppenheim, J.J.: There is more than one interleukin 1. Immunol. Today, *7*:45, 1986.
25. Greene, W.C., Depper, J.M., Kronke, M., and Leonard, W.J.: The human interleukin-2 receptor: Analysis of structure and function. Immunol. Rev., *92*:29, 1986.
26. Smith, K.A.: The two chain structure of high affinity IL-2 receptors. Immunol. Today, *8*:11, 1987.
27. Taniguchi, T., et al.: Molecular analysis of the interleukin-2 system. Immunol. Rev., *92*:121, 1986.
28. Svedersky, L.P., et al.: Biological and antigenic similarities of murine interferon-gamma and macrophage-activating factor. J. Exp. Med., *159*:812, 1984.
29. Steeg, P.S., Moore, R.N., Johnson, H.M., and Oppenheim, J.J.: Regulation of murine macrophage Ia antigen expression by a lymphokine with immune interferon activity. J. Exp. Med., *156*:1780, 1982.
30. Schrader, J.W.: The panspecific hemopoietin of activated T-lymphocytes (interleukin-3). Annu. Rev. Immunol., *4*:205, 1986.
31. Hamaoka, T., and Ono, S.: Regulation of B-cell differentiation: interactions of factors and corresponding receptors. Annu. Rev. Immunol., *4*:167, 1986.
32. Smith, K.A.: Draft proposals for interleukin nomenclature. Immunol. Today, *7*:321, 1986.
33. Beutler, B., and Cerami, A.: Cachectin and tumour necrosis

factor as two sides of the same biological coin. Nature, *320:*584, 1986.

34. Benveniste, E.N., and Merrill, J.E.: Stimulation of oligodendroglial proliferation and maturation by interleukin-2. Nature, *321:*610, 1986.

35. Giulian, D., Baker, T.J., Shih, L.N., and Lachman, L.B.: Interleukin 1 of the central nervous system is produced by ameboid microglia. J. Exp. Med., *164:*594, 1986.

36. Rosenstein, M., Ettinghausen, S.E., and Rosenberg, S.A.: Extravasation of intravascular fluid mediated by the systemic administration of recombinant interleukin 2. J. Immunol., *137:*1735, 1986.

37. Shaw, S.: Characterization of human leukocyte differentiation antigens. Immunol. Today, *8:*1, 1987.

38. Marrack, P., et al.: The major histocompatibility complex-restricted antigen receptor on T cells. II. Role of the L3T4 product. J. Exp. Med., *158:*1077, 1983.

39. Luyten, F., et al.: Peripheral blood T lymphocyte subpopulations determined by monoclonal antibodies in active rheumatoid arthritis. J. Rheumatol., *13:*864, 1986.

40. Karlsson-Parra, A., et al.: Peripheral blood T lymphocyte subsets in active rheumatoid arthritis—Effects of different therapies on previously untreated patients. J. Rheumatol., *13:*263, 1986.

41. Feehally, J., et al.: Modulation of cellular immune function by cyclophosphamide in children with minimal-change nephropathy. N. Engl. J. Med., *310:*415, 1984.

42. Tanay, A., Field, E.H., Hoppe, R.T., and Strober, S.: Long term followup of rheumatoid arthritis patients treated with total lymphoid irradiation. Arthritis Rheum., *30:*1, 1987.

43. Wofsy, D.O., and Seaman, W.E.: Successful treatment of autoimmunity in NZB/NZW F$_1$ mice with monoclonal antibody to L3T4. J. Exp. Med., *161:*378, 1985.

44. Ranges, G.E., Sriram, S., and Cooper, S.M.: Prevention of type II collagen-induced arthritis by in vivo treatment with anti-L3T4. J. Exp. Med., *162:*1105, 1985.

45. Wofsy, D., et al.: Treatment of murine lupus with monoclonal anti-T cell antibody. J. Immunol., *134:*852, 1985.

46. Chatenoud, L.: The immune response against therapeutic monoclonal antibodies. Immunol. Today, *7:*367, 1986.

47. Liao, Z., Grimshaw, R.S., and Rosenstreich, D.L.: Identification of a specific interleukin 1 inhibitor in the urine of febrile patients. J. Exp. Med., *159:*126, 1984.

48. Tiku, K., Tiku, M.L., Liu, S., and Skosey, J.L.: Normal human neutrophils are a source of a specific interleukin-1 inhibitor. J. Immunol., *136:*3686, 1986.

49. Miossec, P. Kashiwado, T., and Ziff, M.: Inhibitor of interleukin-2 in rheumatoid synovial fluid. Arthritis Rheum., *30:*121, 1987.

50. Schreiber, R.D., et al.: Monoclonal antibodies to murine gamma-interferon which differentially modulate macrophage activation and antiviral activity. J. Immunol., *134:*1609, 1985.

51. Chang, T.W., Kung, P.C., Gingras, S.P., and Goldstein, G.: Does OKT3 monoclonal antibody react with an antigen-recognition structure on human T cells? Proc. Natl. Acad. Sci. U.S.A., *78:*1805, 1981.

52. Kelley, V.E., et al.: Anti-interleukin 2 receptor antibody suppresses delayed-type hypersensitivity to foreign and syngeneic antigens. J. Immunol., *137:*2122, 1986.

53. Pincus, S.H., Clegg, D.O., and Ward, J.R.: Characterization of T cells bearing HLA-DR antigens in rheumatoid arthritis. Arthritis Rheum., *28:*8, 1985.

54. Bellamy, N., and Buchanan, W.W.: Interpreting clinical trials of antirheumatic drug therapy. Bull. Rheum. Dis., *36:*1, 1986.

55. Klippel, J.H., and Decker, J.L. (eds): Clinical trials in rheumatic diseases. Clin. Rheum. Dis., *9:*489, 1983.

56. Krensky, A.M., Lanier, L.L., and Engleman, E.G.: Lymphocyte subsets and surface molecules in man. Clin. Immunol. Rev., *4(1):*95, 1985.

57. Fox, R.I., et al.: Synovial fluid lymphocytes differ from peripheral blood lymphocytes in patients with rheumatoid arthritis. J. Immunol., *128:*351, 1982.

58. Goto, M., Miyamoto, T., Nishioka, K., and Okumura, K.: Selective loss of suppressor T cells in rheumatoid arthritis patients: analysis of peripheral blood lymphocytes by 2-dimensional flow cytometry. J. Rheumatol., *13:*853, 1986.

59. White, D.J.G., and Calne, R.Y.: The use of cyclosporin A immunosuppression in organ grafting. Immunol. Rev., *65:*115, 1982.

60. Merion, R.M., et al.: Cyclosporine: five years experience in cadaveric renal transplantation. N. Engl. J. Med., *310:*148, 1984.

61. Lafferty, K.L., Borel, J.F., and Hodgkin, P.: Cyclosporine-A (CsA): models for the mechanism of action. Transplant Proc., *15:*2242, 1983.

62. Kronke, M., et al.: Cyclosporin A inhibits T-cell growth factor gene expression at the level of mRNA transcription. Proc. Natl. Acad. Sci., U.S.A. *81:*5214, 1984.

63. Elliott, J.F., Lin, Y., Mizel, S.B., and Bleackley, R.C.: Induction of interleukin 2 messenger RNA inhibited by cyclosporin A. Science, *226:*1439, 1984.

64. Pisetsky, D.S.: The influence of cyclosporine on murine anti-DNA B cells. *In* Biologically Based Immunomodulators in the Therapy of Rheumatic Diseases. Edited by S.H. Pincus, D.S. Pisetsky, and L.J. Rosenwasser. New York, Elsevier, 1986, p. 153.

65. Bowles, C.A.: Clinical trials with cyclosporine in rheumatic diseases. *In* Biologically Based Immunomodulators in the Therapy of Rheumatic Diseases. Edited by S.H. Pincus, D.S. Pisetsky, and L.J. Rosenwasser. New York, Elsevier, 1986, p. 161.

66. Mountz, J.D., et al.: CS-A therapy in MRL-lpr/lpr mice: amelioration of immunopathology despite autoantibody production. J. Immunol., *138:*157, 1987.

67. Kaibara, N., Hotokebuchi, T., Takagishi, K., and Katsuki, I.: Paradoxical effects of cyclosporin A on collagen arthritis in rats. J. Exp. Med., *158:*2007, 1983.

68. Kaibara, N., et al.: Pathogenic difference between collagen arthritis and adjuvant arthritis. J. Exp. Med., *159:*1388, 1984.

69. Nussenblatt, R.B., Palestine, A.G., Chan, C.C.: Cyclosporin A therapy in the treatment of intraocular inflammatory disease resistant to systemic corticosteroids or cytotoxic agents. Am. J. Ophthalmol., *96:*275, 1983.

70. Palestine, A.G., et al.: Renal histopathologic alterations in patients treated with cyclosporine for uveitis. N. Engl. J. Med., *314:*1293, 1986.

71. Isenberg, D.A., et al.: Cyclosporine A for the treatment of systemic lupus erythematosus. Int. J. Immunopharmacol., *3:*163, 1981.

72. Miescher, P.A., and Miescher, A.: Combined cyclosporin steroid treatment of systemic lupus erythematosus. *In* Cyclosporin in Autoimmune Disease. Edited by R. Schindler. Berlin, Germany, Springer-Verlag, 1985, p. 337.

73. Feutren, G.: The effects of Cyclosporin in twelve patients with severe systemic lupus. *In* Cyclosporin in Autoimmune Diseases. Edited by R. Schindler. Berlin, Germany, Springer-Verlag, 1985, p. 366.

74. Weinblatt, M.E., et al.: Cyclosporin A treatment of refractory rheumatoid arthritis. Arthritis Rheum., 30:11, 1987.

75. Drosos, A.A., et al.: Cyclosporin A (CyA) in primary Sjogren's syndrome: A double blind study. Ann. Rheum. Dis., 45:732, 1986.

76. Symoens, J., and Rosenthal, M.: Levamisole in the modulation of the immune response: The current experimental and clinical state. J. Reticuloendothel. Soc., 21:175, 1977.

77. Hogan, N.A., and Hill, H.R.: Enhancement of neutrophil chemotaxis and alteration of levels of cellular cyclic nucleotides by levamisole. J. Infect. Dis., 138:437, 1978.

78. Mazzone, A., Baigura, R., Rossini, S., Ricevuti, G.: Immunomodulation of neutrophil chemotaxis in rheumatoid arthritis using levamisole and methisoprinol. Clin. Ther., 8:232, 1986.

79. Barada, F., O'Brien, W., and Horwitz, D.A.: Defective monocyte cytotoxicity in rheumatoid arthritis. A correlation with disease activity and reversal by levamisole. Arthritis Rheum., 25:10, 1982.

80. Sampson, D., and Lui, A.: The effect of levamisole on cell-mediated immunity and suppressor-cell function. Cancer Res., 36:952, 1976.

81. Rosenthal, M., Trabert, U., and Mueller, W.: The effect of levamisole on peripheral blood lymphocyte subpopulations in patients with rheumatoid arthritis and ankylosing spondylitis. Clin. Exp. Immunol., 25:493, 1976.

82. Veys, E.M., et al.: Influence of longterm administration of levamisole on total lymphocyte and T cell subsets in rheumatoid arthritis. J. Rheumatol., 11:398, 1984.

83. Miller, B., et al.: Double-blind placebo controlled cross-over evaluation of levamisole in rheumatoid arthritis. Arthritis Rheum., 23:172, 1980.

84. Runge, L.A., et al.: Treatment of rheumatoid arthritis with levamisole: a controlled trial. Arthritis Rheum., 20:1445, 1977.

85. Halberg, P., et al.: Double blind trial of levamisole, penicillamine, and azathioprine in rheumatoid arthritis. Dan. Med. Bull., 31:403, 1984.

86. Schmidt, K.L., and Mueller-Eckhardt, C.: Agranulocytosis, levamisole, and HLA-B27. Lancet, 2:85, 1977.

87. Weinblatt, M.E., et al.: Selective suppression of the T8-subset by therafectin in rheumatoid arthritis (RA). Arthritis Rheum., 29 (Suppl. 1):S4, 1986.

88. Ehresmann, G.R., MacLaughlin, K.E., and Horwitz, D.A.: Dose-related efficacy of therafectin (amiprilose HCl) in rheumatoid arthritis. Arthritis Rheum., 30:(Suppl)34, 1987.

89. Caldwell, J.R., et al.: Therafectin (amiprilose HCl) in rheumatoid arthritis: a six month double blind placebo controlled study, followed by a six month open extension. Arthritis Rheum., 30:(Suppl)57, 1987.

90. Kincaid, W., Tovar, Z., and Talal, N.: The immunomodulator IMREG-1 restores T cell proliferative response in rheumatoid arthritis (RA). Arthritis Rheum., 29(Suppl. 4):S28, 1986.

91. Tarkowski, A., et al.: Successful treatment of autoimmunity in MRL/1 mice with LA-2616, a new immunomodulator. Arthritis Rheum., 29:1405, 1986.

92. Renoux, G., and Renoux, M.: Immunopotentiators. In Immunology of Rheumatic Diseases. Edited by S. Gupta and N. Talal. New York, Plenum, 1986, p. 706.

93. Slavin, S.: Total lymphoid irradiation. Immunol. Today, 8:88, 1987.

94. Schurman, D.J., Hirshman, H.P., Strober, S.: Total lymphoid and local joint irradiation in the treatment of adjuvant arthritis. Arthritis Rheum., 24:38, 1981.

95. Kotzin, B.L. et al.: Treatment of NZB/NZW mice with total lymphoid irradiation: long-lasting suppression of disease without generalized immune suppression. J. Immunol., 136:3259, 1986.

96. Zvaifler, N.J.: Fractionated total lymphoid irradiation: a promising new treatment for rheumatoid arthritis? Yes, no, maybe. Arthritis Rheum., 30:109, 1987.

97. Brahn, E., et al.: Total lymphoid irradiation therapy in refractory rheumatoid arthritis: Fifteen- to forty-month followup. Arthritis Rheum., 27:481, 1984.

98. Hanly, J.G., et al.: Lymphoid irradiation in intractable rheumatoid arthritis: A double-blind, randomized study comparing 750-rad treatment with 2,000-rad treatment. Arthritis Rheum., 29:16, 1986.

99. Strober, S. et al.: Treatment of intractable lupus nephritis with total lymphoid irradiation. Ann. Intern. Med., 102:450, 1985.

100. Tanay, A., Schiffman, G., and Strober, S.: Effect of total lymphoid irradiation on levels of serum autoantibodies in systemic lupus erythematosus and in rheumatoid arthritis. Arthritis Rheum., 29:26, 1986.

101. Sjumak, K.H., and Rock, G.A.: Therapeutic plasma exchange. N. Engl. J. Med., 310:762, 1984.

102. Emery, P., Smith, G.N., and Panayi, G.S.: Lymphocytapheresis—a feasible treatment for rheumatoid arthritis. Br. J. Rheumatol., 25:40, 1986.

103. Wallace, D., et al.: A double blind controlled study of lymphoplasmapheresis versus sham apheresis in rheumatoid arthritis. N. Engl.J. Med., 306:1406, 1982.

104. Dwosh, I.L., et al.: Plasmapheresis therapy in rheumatoid arthritis: a controlled, double-blind, crossover trial. N. Engl. J. Med., 308:1124, 1983.

105. Parry, H.F., et al.: Plasma exchange in systemic lupus erythematosus. Ann. Rheum. Dis., 40:224, 1981.

106. Wei, N., et al.: Randomised trial of plasma exchange in mild systemic lupus erythematosus. Lancet, 1:17, 1983.

107. Moore, R.A., Brunner, C.M., Sandusky, W.R., and Leavell, B.S.: Felty's syndrome: long term follow-up after splenectomy. Ann. Intern. Med., 75:381, 1971.

108. Sledge, C.B., et al.: Treatment of rheumatoid synovitis of the knee with intraarticular injection of dysprosium 165-ferric hydroxide macroaggregates. Arthritis Rheum., 29:153, 1986.

108a.Daynes, R.A., and Spikes, J.D.: Experimental and Clinical Photoimmunology. Volumes I and II. Boca Raton, FL, CRC Press, 1983.

108b.McGrath, H., Bak, E., and Michalski, J.P.: Ultraviolet-A light prolongs survival and improves immune function in F1 hybrid mice. Arthritis Rheum., 30:557–561, 1987.

109. Lahita, R.G. et al.: Low plasma androgens in women with systemic lupus erythematosus. Arthritis Rheum., 30:241, 1987.

110. Ahmed, S.A., Penhale, N.J., and Talal, N.: Sex hormones, immune responses, and autoimmune diseases. Am. J. Pathol., 121:531, 1985.

111. Roubinian, J., Talal, N., Siiteri, P.K., Sadakian, J.A.: Sex hormone modulation of autoimmunity in NZB/NZW mice. Arthritis Rheum., 22:1162, 1979.

112. Steinberg, A.D., et al.: Approach to the study of the role of sex hormones in autoimmunity. Arthritis Rheum., 22:1170, 1979.

113. Holmdahl, R., Jansson, L., and Andersson, M.: Female sex hormones suppress development of collagen-induced arthritis in mice. Arthritis Rheum., 29:1501, 1986.

114. Jungers, P., et al.: Influence of oral contraceptive therapy on the activity of systemic lupus erythematosus. Arthritis Rheum., 25:618, 1982.

115. Vandenbroucke, J.P., et al.: Oral contraceptives and rheumatoid arthritis: further evidence for a preventive effect. Lancet, 2:839, 1982.

116. Allebeck, P., Ahlbom, A., Ljungstrom, K., and Allander, E.: Do oral contraceptives reduce the incidence of rheumatoid arthritis? Scand. J. Rheumatol., 13:140, 1984.

117. Schreiber, A.D., et al.: Effect of danazol in immune thrombocytopenic purpura. N. Engl. J. Med., 316:503, 1987.

118. Roubinian, J.R., et al.: Danazol's failure to suppress autoimmunity in NZB/NZW F₁ mice. Arthritis Rheum., 22:1399, 1979.

119. Agnello, V., et al.: Preliminary observation on danazol therapy of systemic lupus erythematosus: Effects on DNA antibodies, thrombocytopenia and complement. J. Rheumatol., 10:682, 1983.

120. Jungers, P., et al.: Hormonal modulation in systemic lupus erythematosus: preliminary clinical and hormonal results with cyproterone acetate. Arthritis Rheum., 28:1243, 1985.

121. Jorizzo, J.L., et al.: Thalidomide effects in Behçet's syndrome and pustular vasculitis. Arch. Intern. Med., 146:878, 1986.

122. Barnhill, R.L., and McDougall, A.C.: Thalidomide: use and possible mode of action in reactional lepromatous leprosy and in various other conditions. J. Am. Acad. Dermatol., 7:317, 1982.

123. Hamza, M.H.: Treatment of Behçet disease with thalidomide. Clin. Rheumatol., 5:365, 1986.

124. Guiterrez-Rodriguez, G.: Thalidomide: a promising new treatment for rheumatoid arthritis. Arthritis Rheum., 27:1118, 1984.

125. Martin, M.F.R., et al.: Captopril: a new treatment for rheumatoid arthritis? Lancet, 1:1325–1327, 1984.

126. Johnsen, S.A., and Aurell, M.: Immunosuppressive action of captopril blocked by prostaglandin synthetase inhibitor. Lancet, 1:1005, 1981.

127. Gershon, R.K., Askenase, P.W., and Gershon, M.D.: Requirement for vasoactive amines in delayed type hypersensitivity skin reactions. J. Exp. Med., 142:732, 1975.

128. Brosnan, C.F., et al.: Prazosin treatment during the effector stage of disease suppresses experimental autoimmune encephalomyelitis in the Lewis rat. J. Immunol., 137:3451, 1986.

129. Levine, J.D., et al.: Intraneuronal substance P contributes to the severity of experimental arthritis. Science, 226:547, 1984.

130. Lotz, M., Carson, D.A., Vaughan, J.H.: Substance P activation of rheumatoid synoviocytes: Neural pathway in the pathogenesis of arthritis. Science, 235:893, 1987.

131. Kvols, L.K., et al.: Treatment of malignant carcinoid syndrome: evaluation of a long acting somatostatin analogue. N. Engl. J. Med., 315:663, 1986.

132. Brock, J.H., and de Sousa, M.: Immunoregulation by iron-binding proteins. Immunol. Today, 7:30, 1986.

133. Carotenuto, P., Pontesilli, O., Cambier, J.C., and Hayward, A.R.: Desferoxamine blocks IL-2 receptor expression on human T lymphocytes. J. Immunol., 136:2342, 1986.

134. Bowern, N., et al.: Inhibition of autoimmune neuropathological process by treatment with an iron-chelating agent. J. Exp. Med., 160:1532, 1984.

135. Greenwald, R.A., et al.: Tetracyclines inhibit human synovial collagenase in vivo and in vitro. J. Rheumatol., 14:28, 1987.

136. Hauser, W.E., and Remington, J.S.: Effect of antibiotics on the immune response. Am. J. Med., 72:711–716, 1982.

137. Dennert, G.: Immunostimulation by retinoic acid. In Retinoids, Differentiation and Disease. Edited by J. Nugent and S. Clark. London, Pitman, 1985.

138. Oikarinen, H., et al.: Modulation of procollagen gene expression by retinoids. J. Clin. Invest., 75:1545, 1945.

139. Brinkerhoff, C.E., et al.: Effect of retinoids on rheumatoid arthritis, aproliferative and invasive non-malignant disease. In Retinoids, Differentiation and Disease. Edited by J. Nugent and S. Clark. London, Pitman, 1985.

140. Ellis, C.N., et al.: Isotretinoin therapy is associated with early skeletal radiographic changes. J. Am. Acad. Dermatol., 10:1024, 1984.

141. Klein, T.W., et al.: Effect of delta-9-tetrahydrocannabinol and 11-OH-delta-9-tetrahydrocannabinol on T and B-lymphocyte mitogen responses. J. Immunopharmacol., 7:451, 1985.

142. Jahn, B., et al.: Changes in cell surface antigen expression on human articular chondrocytes induced by gamma-interferon. Arthritis Rheum., 30:64, 1987.

143. Cowing, C., and Frohman, M.A.: Gamma interferon, class II histocompatibility antigens, and autoimmunity. In Biologically Based Immunomodulators in the Therapy of Rheumatic Diseases. Edited by S.H. Pincus, D.S. Pisetsky, and L.J. Rosenwasser. New York, Elsevier, 1986, p. 349.

144. Nakamura, M., et al.: Effect of gamma-interferon on the immune response in vivo and on gene expression in vitro. Nature, 307:381, 1984.

145. Brinckerhoff, C.E., and Guyre, P.: Increased proliferation of human synovial fibroblasts treated with recombinant immune interferon. J. Immunol., 134:3142, 1985.

146. Pincus, S.H.: Therapeutic potential of interferons: overview. In Biologically Based Immunomodulators in the Therapy of Rheumatic Diseases. Edited by S.H. Pincus, D.S. Pisetsky, and L.J. Rosenwasser. New York, Elsevier, 1986, p. 337.

147. Wolfe, F., et al.: Clinical trial with R-IFN-G in rheumatoid arthritis. In Biologically Based Immunomodulators in the Therapy of Rheumatic Diseases. Edited by S.H. Pincus, D.S. Pisetsky, and L.J. Rosenwasser. New York, Elsevier, 1986, p. 379.

148. Cannon, G.W., et al.: Double-blind trial of recombinant interferon-gamma versus placebo in rheumatoid arthritis. Arthritis Rheum., 30:S18, 1987.

149. Jacobs, L., et al.: Multicenter double-blind study of effect of intrathecally administered natural human fibroblast interferon on exacerbations of multiple sclerosis. Lancet, 2:1411, 1986.

150. Tsokos, G.C., et al.: Deficient gamma-interferon production in patients with systemic lupus erythematosus. Arthritis Rheum., 29:1210, 1986.

151. Firestein, G.S., and Zvaifler, N.J.: Interferon and rheumatoid arthritis. In Biologically Based Immunomodulators in the Therapy of Rheumatic Diseases. Edited by S.H. Pincus, D.S. Pisetsky, and L.J. Rosenwasser. New York, Elsevier, 1986, p. 369.

151a. Duncan, M.R., and Berman, B.: Persistence of a reduced-collagen-producing phenotype in cultured scleroderma fibroblasts after short term exposure to interferons. J. Clin. Invest., 79:1318, 1987.

152. Tiku, K., Tiku, M.L., and Skosey, J.L.: Interleukin 1 production by human polymorphonuclear neutrophils. J. Immunol., 136:3677, 1986.

153. Beutler, B., and Cerami, A.: Cachectin: More than a tumor necrosis factor. N. Engl. J. Med., 316:379, 1987.

154. Dower, S.K., and Urdal, D.L.: The interleukin-1 receptor. Immunol. Today, 8:46, 1987.

155. Miossec, P., Dinarello, C.A., and Ziff, M.: Interleukin-1 lymphocyte chemotactic activity in rheumatoid arthritis synovial fluid. Arthritis Rheum., 29:461, 1986.

156. Beutler, B., et al.: Identity of tumour necrosis factor and the macrophage-secreted factor cachectin. Nature, 316:552, 1985.

157. Bertolini, D.R., et al.: Stimulation of bone resorption and in-

hibition of bone formation in vitro by human tumour necrosis factors. Nature, *319*:516, 1986.

158. Thomson, B.M., Mundy, G.R., and Chambers, T.J.: Tumor necrosis factors alpha and beta induce osteoblastic cells to stimulate osteoclastic bone resorption. J. Immunol., *138*:775, 1987.

159. Asher, A., et al.: Studies on the anti-tumor efficacy of systemically administered recombinant tumor necrosis factor against several murine tumors in vivo. J. Immunol., *138*:963, 1987.

160. Pennica, D., et al.: Identification of human uromodulin as the Tamm-Horsfall urinary glycoprotein. Science, *236*:83, 1987.

161. Rosenberg, S.A., et al.: A progress report on the treatment of 157 patients with advanced cancer using lymphokine-activated killer cells and interleukin-2 or high-dose interleukin-2 alone. N. Engl. J. Med., *316*:889, 1987.

162. West, W.H., et al.: Constant-infusion recombinant interleukin-2 in adoptive immunotherapy of advanced cancer. N. Engl. J. Med., *316*:898, 1987.

163. Wofsy, D., et al.: Deficient interleukin-2 activity in MRL/Mp and C57BL/6J mice bearing the lpr gene. J. Exp. Med., *154*:1671, 1981.

164. Miyasaka, N., et al.: Interleukin-2 deficiencies in rheumatoid arthritis and systemic lupus erythematosus. Clin. Immunol. Immunopathol., *31*:109, 1984.

165. Warrington, R.J.: Interleukin-2 production and responsiveness in rheumatoid arthritis. *In* Biologically Based Immunomodulators in the Therapy of Rheumatic Diseases. Edited by S.H. Pincus, D.S. Pisetsky, and L.J. Rosenwasser. New York, Elsevier, 1986.

166. Kawamura, H., Rosenberg, S.A., and Berzofsky, J.A.: Immunization with antigen and interleukin 2 in vivo overcomes Ir gene low responsiveness. J. Exp. Med., *162*:381, 1985.

167. Diamantstein, T., and Osawa, H.: The interleukin 2 receptor, its physiology and a new approach to immunosuppressive therapy by anti-interleukin 2 receptor monoclonal antibodies. Immunol. Rev., *92*:5, 1986.

168. Kirkman, R.L., et al.: Administration of anti-interleukin 2 receptor monoclonal antibody prolongs cardiac allograft survival in mice. J. Exp. Med., *162*:358, 1985.

169. Goldstein, G., Scheid, M.P., Schlesinger, D.H., and Van Wauwe, J.: A synthetic pentapeptide with biological activity characteristic of the thymic hormone thymopoietin. Science, *204*:1309, 1979.

170. Weksler, M.E., Innes, J.B., and Goldstein, G.: Immunological studies of aging. IV. The contribution of thymic involution to the immune deficiencies of aging mice and reversal with thymopoietin. J. Exp. Med., *148*:996, 1978.

171. Lau, C.Y., Freeston, J.A., and Goldstein, G.: Effect of thymopoietin pentapeptide (TP5) on autoimmunity. J. Immunol., *125*:1634, 1980.

172. Weaver, A.L., Churchill, M.A., and Jacobs, A.J.: Treatment of refractory rheumatoid arthritis with thymopoietin pentapeptide. Arthritis Rheum., *27*:(4):s59, 1984.

173. Bach, J.F., and Dardenne, M.: Thymic hormones and rheumatoid arthritis. *In* Immunology of Rheumatic Diseases. Edited by S. Gupta and N. Talal. New York, Plenum, 1986, p. 727.

174. Cantrell, M.A., et al.: Cloning, sequence, and expression of a human granulocyte/macrophage colony stimulating factor. Proc. Natl. Acad. Sci. USA, *82*:6250, 1985.

175. Klinman, D.M., et al.: Oncogenes expression in autoimmune and normal peripheral blood mononuclear cells. J. Exp. Med., *163*:1292, 1986.

176. Stoscheck, C.M., and King, L.E.: Functional and structural characteristics of epidermal growth factor and its receptor and their relationship to transforming proteins. J. Cell. Biochem., *31*:135, 1986.

177. Shimokado, K., et al.: A significant part of macrophage-derived growth factor consists of at least two forms of platelet derived growth factor. Cell, *43*:277, 1985.

178. Benjamin, R.J., and Waldmann, H.: Induction of tolerance by monoclonal antibody therapy. Nature, *320*:449, 1986.

179. Gutstein, N.L., and Wofsy, D.: Administration of F(ab')₂ fragments of monoclonal antibody to L3T4 inhibits humoral immunity in mice without depleting L3T4 cells. J. Immunol., *137*:3414, 1986.

180. Chatenoud, L., et al.: The human immune response to the OKT3 monoclonal antibody is oligoclonal. Science, *232*:1406, 1986.

181. Wooley, P.H., et al.: Type II collagen induced arthritis in mice. 3. Suppression of arthritis using monoclonal and polyclonal anti-Ia antisera. J. Immunol., *134*:2366, 1985.

182. Adelman, N.E., Watling, D.L., and McDevitt, H.O.: Treatment of (NZB × NZW)F₁ disease with anti-I-A monoclonal antibodies. J. Exp. Med., *158*:1350, 1983.

183. Clarkson, S.B., et al.: Treatment of refractory immune thrombocytopenic purpura with an anti-Fc-gamma-receptor antibody. N. Engl. J. Med., *314*:1236, 1986.

184. Hafler, D.A., et al.: In vivo activated T lymphocytes in the peripheral blood and cerebrospinal fluid of patients with multiple sclerosis. N. Engl. J. Med., *312*:1405, 1985.

185. Hemler, M.E., Glass, D., Coblyn, J.S., and Jacobson, J.G.: Very late activation antigens on rheumatoid synovial fluid T lymphocytes. J. Clin. Invest., *78*:696, 1986.

186. Todd, R.F., and Liu, D.Y.: Mononuclear phagocyte activation-associated antigens. Fed. Proc., *45*:2829, 1986.

187. Kikutani, H., et al.: Expression and function of an early activation marker restricted to human B cells. J. Immunol., *136*:4019, 1986.

188. Casali, P., et al.: Human lymphocytes making rheumatoid factor and antibody to ssDNA belong to Leu-1⁺ B-cell subset. Science, *236*:77, 1987.

189. Morimoto, C., et al.: The isolation and characterization of the human helper inducer T cell subset. J. Immunol., *134*:3762, 1985.

190. Morimoto, C., and Schlossman, S.F.: Antilymphocyte antibodies and systemic lupus erythematosus. Arthritis Rheum., *30*:225, 1987.

191. Isenberg, D.A., et al.: The relationship of anti-DNA antibody idiotypes and anti-cardiolipin antibodies to disease activity in systemic lupus eythematosus. Medicine, *65*:46, 1986.

192. Chen, P.P., et al.: Genetic basis for the cross-reactive idiotypes on the light chains of human IgM anti-IgG autoantibodies. Proc. Nat. Acad. Sci., U.S.A. *83*:8318, 1986.

193. Hahn, B.H.: Idiotype regulation as a therapeutic approach to autoimmune diseases. *In* Biologically Based Immunomodulators in the Therapy of Rheumatic Diseases. Edited by S.H. Pincus, D.S. Pisetsky, and L.J. Rosenwasser. New York, Elsevier, 1986, p. 219.

194. Hahn, B.H., and Ebling, F.M.: Idiotype restriction in murine lupus: high frequency of three public idiotypes on serum IgG in nephritic NZB/NZW F₁ mice. J. Immunol., *138*:2110, 1987.

195. Carroll, W.L., et al.: Idiotype variant cell populations in patients with B cell lymphoma. J. Exp. Med., *164*:1566, 1986.

196. Marx, J.L.: Antibodies made to order. Science, *229*:455, 1985.

197. Hahn, G.S.: Immunoglobulin-derived drugs. Nature, *324*:283, 1986.

198. Taub, R.N., and Deutsch, V.: Antilymphocytic serum. Pharmacol. Ther., 2:89, 1977.

199. Harris, N.S., Meino, G., and Najarian, J.S.: Mode of action of antilymphocyte sera (ALS). Transplant. Proc., 3:797, 1971.

200. Sheil, A.G.R., et al.: Controlled clinical trial of antilymphocyte globulin in patients with renal allografts from cadaver donors. Lancet, 1:359, 1971.

201. Lawley, T.J., et al.: A prospective clinical and immunologic analysis of patients with serum sickness. N. Engl. J. Med., 311:1407, 1984.

202. Combe, B., et al.: Human placenta-eluted gammaglobulins in immunomodulating treatment of rheumatoid arthritis. Am. J. Med., 78:920, 1985.

203. Moynier, M., Cosso, B., Brochier, J., and Clot, J.: Identification of class II HLA alloantibodies in placenta-eluted gamma globulins used for treating rheumatoid arthritis. Arthritis Rheum., 30:375, 1987.

204. Morell, A., and Nydegger, U.E. (eds.): Clinical Use of Intravenous Immunoglobulins. London, Academic Press, 1986.

205. Pirofsky, B.: Intravenous immune globulin therapy in hypogammaglobulinemia. Am. J. Med., 76(3):53, 1984.

206. Newland, A.C., et al.: High-dose intravenous IgG in adults with autoimmune thrombocytopenia. Lancet, 1:84, 1983.

207. Sultan, Y., Maisonneuve, P., Kazatchkine, M.D., and Nydegger, U.E.: Anti-idiotypic suppression of autoantibodies to factor VIII (antihaemophilic factor) by high-dose intravenous gammaglobulin. Lancet, 2:765, 1984.

208. Newburger, J.W., et al.: The treatment of Kawasaki syndrome with intravenous gammaglobulin. N. Engl. J. Med., 315:341, 1986.

209. Kurlander, R.J., and Hall, J.: Comparison of intravenous gamma-globulin and monoclonal anti-Fc receptor antibody as inhibitors of immune clearance in vivo in mice. J. Clin. Invest., 77:2010, 1986.

210. Fehr, J., Hofmann, V., and Kappeler, U.: Transient reversal of thrombocytopenia in idiopathic thrombocytopenic purpura by high dose intravenous gamma-globulin. N. Engl. J. Med., 306:1254, 1982.

211. Lin, R.Y., and Racis, S.P.: In vivo reduction of circulating Clq binding immune complexes by intravenous gammaglobulin administration. Int. Arch. Allergy Appl. Immunol., 79:286–290, 1986.

212. Engelhard, D., Waner, J.L., Kapoor, N., and Good, R.A.: Effect of intravenous immune globulin on natural killer cell activity: possible association with autoimmune neutropenia and idiopathic thrombocytopenia. J. Pediatr., 108:77, 1986.

213. Hall, R.P., et al.: Bullous eruption of systemic lupus erythematosus. Ann. Intern. Med., 97:165, 1982.

214. Katz, S.I., et al.: Erythema elevatum diutinum: skin and systemic manifestations, immunologic studies and successful treatment with dapsone. Medicine, 56:443, 1977.

215. Martin, J., et al.: Relapsing polychondritis treated with dapsone. Arch. Dermatol., 112:1272, 1976.

216. Barranco, V.P., Minor, D.B., and Solomon, H.: Treatment of relapsing polychondritis with dapsone. Arch. Dermatol., 112:1286, 1976.

217. Hunneyball, I.M., Crossley, M.J., and Spowage, M.: Pharmacological studies of antigen-induced arthritis in BALB/c mice. II. The effects of second-line antirheumatic drugs and cytotoxic agents on the histopathological changes. Agents Actions, 18(3–4):394–400, 1986.

218. Fowler, P.D., et al.: Report on chloroquine and dapsone in the treatment of rheumatoid arthritis: A 6-month comparative study. Ann. Rheum. Dis., 43(2):200, 1984.

219. Grindulis, K.A., and McConkey, B.: Outcome of attempts to treat rheumatoid arthritis with gold, penicillamine, sulphasalazine, or dapsone. Ann. Rheum. Dis., 43:398, 1984.

220. Robinson, D.R., et al.: Dietary fish oil reduces progression of established renal disease in (NZB × NZW)F$_1$ mice and delays renal disease in BXSB and MRL/1 strains. Arthritis Rheum., 29:539, 1986.

221. Leslie, C.A., et al.: Dietary fish oil modulates macrophage fatty acids and decreases arthritis susceptibility in mice. J. Exp. Med., 162:1336, 1985.

222. Kremer, J.M., et al.: Fish oil fatty acid supplementation in active rheumatoid arthritis. Ann. Intern. Med., 106:497, 1987.

223. Prickett, J.D., Trentham, D.E., and Robinson, D.R.: Dietary fish oil augments the induction of arthritis in rats immunized with type II collagen. J. Immunol., 132:725, 1984.

224. Jimenez, R.: Innovative therapeutic agents. In Therapeutic Controversies in Rheumatic Diseases. Edited by R.F. Wilkins and S.L. Dahl. Orlando, FL, Grune & Stratton, 1987.

225. Williams, H.J., et al.: Double-blind, multicenter controlled trial comparing topical dimethyl sulfoxide and normal saline for treatment of hand ulcers in patients with systemic sclerosis. Arthritis Rheum., 28:308, 1985.

226. Vidal y Plana, R.R., Bizzarri, D., and Rovati, A.L.: Articular cartilage pharmacology. I. In vitro studies on glucosamine and non-steroidal anti-inflammatory drugs. Pharmacol. Res. Commun., 10:557, 1978.

227. Drovanti, A., Bignamini, A.A., and Rovati, A.L.: Therapeutic activity of oral glucosamine sulfate in osteoarthrosis: a placebo-controlled double-blind investigation. Clin. Ther., 3:260, 1980.

228. Vaz, A.L.: Double-blind clinical evaluation of the relative efficacy of ibuprofen and glucosamine sulphate in the management of osteoarthrosis of the knee in outpatients. Curr. Med. Res. Opin., 8:145, 1982.

229. Nevo, Z., and Dorfman, A.: Stimulation of chondromucoprotein synthesis in chondrocytes by extracellular chondromucoprotein. Proc. Nat. Acad. Sci. USA, 69:2069, 1972.

230. Siegmeth, W., and Radi, I.: Comparison of glycosaminoglycan polysulfate (Arteparon) and saline solution in arthrosis of the large joints. Z. Rheumatol., 42:223, 1983.

231. Dixon, A.S., et al.: A double-blind controlled trial of Rumalon in the treatment of painful osteoarthrosis of the hip. Ann. Rheum. Dis., 29:193, 1970.

232. Huber, W., and Menander-Huber, K.B.: Orgotein. Clin. Rheum. Dis., 6:465, 1980.

233. Menander-Huber, K.B.: Orgotein in the treatment of rheumatoid arthritis. Eur. J. Rheumatol. Inflamm., 4:201, 1981.

234. Goebel, K.M., and Storck, U.: Effect of intra-articular orgotein versus a corticosteroid on rheumatoid arthritis of the knees. Am. J. Med., 74:124, 1983.

ARTHROCENTESIS TECHNIQUE AND INTRASYNOVIAL THERAPY

39

ROBERT A. GATTER

The diagnostic value of arthrocentesis for joint fluid analysis has been amply confirmed (see Chapter 5), and the value of intrasynovial therapy has been well accepted since corticosteroid crystal injections were first described by Hollander and his colleagues in 1951.[1]

Arthrocentesis and injection therapy of joints, bursae, tendon sheaths, and soft tissues are an integral part of routine rheumatologic practice.

ARTHROCENTESIS

The examination of joint fluid is as important in the diagnosis of joint disease as the examination of urine is in the diagnosis of renal disease. Synovianalysis can be easily adapted for bedside and office use. These procedures are discussed in detail in Chapter 5.

Certain joints provide fluid frequently, while others yield fluid rarely[2] (Table 39–1).

INDICATIONS

The need for diagnostic information and the advantages of local therapy indicate the need for arthrocentesis (Table 39–2). Arthrocentesis alone can have therapeutic value by removal of offending white blood cells or crystals. However, the use of a suspension of microcrystalline corticosteroid ester for intra-articular injection provides marked therapeutic benefit. Using these long-acting suspensions, local effect is maximal with minimal systemic absorption. The duration of action is inversely proportional to the solubility of the crystal species injected. Triamcinolone hexacetonide is the least soluble compound and produces the longest local effect. However, for extra-articular soft-tissue injections, it is therefore relatively contraindicated. Prednisolone tertiary butylacetate or methylprednisolone acetate are the most versatile agents used for both joints and soft tissues. Solutions of corticosteroids, as compared with suspensions, do

Table 39–1. Estimated Success in Obtaining Fluid by Arthrocentesis

Group	Success Rate (%)	Affected Joints
A: frequent	50–90	Knee, olecranon bursa, shoulder, elbow, ankle, subtalar, first metatarsophalangeal
B: occasional	10–20	Hip, wrist, distal radioulnar, metatarsophalangeal 2–5, acromioclavicular, sternoclavicular, temporomandibular
C: rare	0–3	Carpal, tarsal, sacroiliac, spinal, proximal tibio-fibular, small joints of hands and feet

(From McCarty, D.J.: A basic guide to orthocentesis. Hosp. Med., 4:77–83, 1968.)

Table 39–2.   Indications for Arthrocentesis

Diagnostic
1. To assist in the diagnosis of arthritis
2. To provide confirmatory evidence for a clinical diagnosis
3. To serially follow the white counts, gram stains, and cultures during the treatment of septic arthritis
4. To define a source of pain as articular or extra-articular (injection of local anesthetics)
5. To provide additional diagnostic documentation in clinical studies

Therapeutic
1. Arthrocentesis alone
   a. Joint fluid evacuation of crystals to diminish inflammation in acute pseudogout
   b. Serial evacuation of white blood cells in septic arthritis to decrease destruction, i.e., drainage of pus
2. Microcrystalline corticosteroid esters may be used:
   a. To provide maximal control of sterile inflammation in key joints when systemic anti-inflammatory therapy has failed, will probably fail, or is contraindicated
   b. To provide a shortened period of morbidity in sterile inflammatory conditions that are self-limited (e.g., gout), or in post-septic arthritis when the offending organism has been eliminated
   c. To provide rapid relief of inflammatory pain
   d. To aid in physical therapy of a joint contracture

not provide local effect but rather are rapidly absorbed systemically and therefore are useless. Details are discussed under the section on Intrasynovial Therapy.

Procaine injections are not routinely used for surface anesthesia; ethyl chloride is usually sufficient, unless the patient is extremely tense or the physician is inexperienced. Procaine has two other functions. It can be injected into joints or soft-tissue structures diagnostically to determine the origin of pain, and it can be mixed with corticosteroid to dilute the steroid concentration and to increase the total volume for soft-tissue injection. Local steroid therapy is only a helpful adjunct and, except in self-limited conditions such as gouty arthritis, rarely constitutes complete treatment.

GENERAL TECHNIQUE

The joint cavity is a tissue space without a definitive limiting basement membrane. To enter the joint space, one must pierce the skin and the joint capsule, which are well supplied with nerve endings. The synovial lining with a rich capillary network is then traversed. Care must be taken not to strike the periosteum of the adjacent bone ends, again where nerve endings are present. Distended and thickened joints are more easily entered than those that are not swollen.

A careful physical examination of the affected joint and, if clinically indicated, inspection of adequate roentgenograms should precede arthrocentesis. Knowledge of the local normal anatomy and any disease-induced alterations is essential to avoid injuring vital structures such as blood vessels and nerves. The approach to most joints is via the extensor aspect, away from these structures. Ball-and-socket joints, i.e., the hip and shoulder, are exceptions. Care must be taken not to gouge the articular cartilage, which will not readily repair itself.

Sterile technique is mandatory to avoid inducing a septic joint. Standard procedures are sufficient. Iodine and alcohol are used to prepare the skin. Drapes, surgical masks, and sterile gloves are not necessary. Disposable needles and syringes are used. In my 25 years of performing arthrocenteses by this method, no infected joints have resulted.

The pain of the procedure can be decreased sufficiently by local ethyl chloride spray, except possibly in those circumstances noted earlier. Should procaine anesthesia be required, a small intradermal wheal is made through which a longer and larger gauge needle is used to reach and anesthetize the joint capsule. The needle size will depend on the joint being tapped. For the knee, a 1½-in, 21-gauge needle usually will reach the capsule. In all cases, the patient should be reminded to remain motionless during the procedure. It is good practice to have forceps present to extract the needle in the unlikely event that the needle would fracture or separate from its hub. Generally, 25-gauge needles are used for the small joints of the hands and feet, 21-gauge needles for the first metatarsals and most other joints, and a spinal needle for the hip.

CONTRAINDICATIONS AND PRECAUTIONS

The contraindications to arthrocentesis are listed in Table 39–3. Local infection of the skin or other periarticular structures constitutes a contraindication to arthrocentesis. Arthrocentesis should be withheld if bacteremia, which can be subtle, is suspected. Because it is impossible to insert a needle through the synovium without trauma to at least a few capillaries, if bacteremia were present, organisms would inoculate the joint space.

Table 39–3.   Contraindications to Arthrocentesis

Local sepsis
Bacteremia
Articular instability
Anatomical inaccessibility

Repeated injections of corticosteroid ester microcrystals into a joint may be injurious to the articular cartilage and can lead to joint destruction and instability. Injecting unstable joints therefore is likely to accelerate the process. Inaccessibility of a joint can vary with the disease process and the physician's experience. A more detailed discussion is presented under the section on Intrasynovial Therapy.

TECHNIQUE FOR SPECIFIC JOINTS

Knee. The knee is the easiest joint in the body to aspirate or inject and is one of the frequent sites of synovial effusions. Three basic approaches are presented, each for a specific circumstance.

When a small effusion is present, the knee is entered from the medial surface so that the needle enters the space between the patella and the patellar groove of the femur (Fig. 39–1). The knee is kept fully extended. The patient should not contract the quadriceps muscle because doing so will clamp the patella firmly in its groove and cause difficulty advancing the needle tip. It is rarely necessary to advance the needle to the hub; at times, ½ in. of penetration is sufficient. It is important to avoid damaging the articular cartilage with the needle. This approach can be painful if the periosteum is struck with the needle tip.

When a large amount of fluid is present, it is pref-

erable and almost painless to enter the suprapatellar bursa laterally and just superior to the patella.

The third technique is less successful, and is used only if the other approaches are not possible. The joint is entered either through the patellar tendon or just lateral to it with the knee in 90° flexion. Fluid is obtained less often with this approach; frequently the tip of the needle ends in the infrapatellar fat pad rather than in the synovial cavity.

Ankle. The ankle joint is entered with the leg-foot angle at 90°. The needle is inserted vertically at a point just medial to the extensor hallucis tendon on a line with the medial malleolus (Fig. 39–2).

Subtalar Joint. The subtalar joint is entered with the leg-foot angle kept at 90°. The needle is directed horizontally on a line with the tip of the external malleolus at a point just proximal to the sinus tarsi (Fig. 39–3).

Metatarsophalangeal Joints. Metatarsophalangeal joints are entered from the extensor surface. The space between the metatarsal head and the base of the phalanx is identified and the overlying skin marked with fingernail pressure. After the appropriate preparation and anesthetic, a 20-gauge needle is inserted into the joint. Traction on the appropriate toe facilitates entry (Fig. 39–4).

Toe Joints. The tiny toe joints require use of a 25-gauge needle. The same technique is used as for the

FIG. 39–1. Medial view at right knee (greatly simplified) showing synovial reflection. Preferred puncture site is marked by needle. (From McCarty, D.J.: A basic guide to arthrocentesis. Hosp. Med., *4*:77–83, 1968.)

FIG. 39–2. With the plane of the foot at a 90° angle to the leg, the needle is inserted vertically at a point just medial to the extensor hallucis tendon on a line with the medial malleolus. Needle marks point of insertion. (From McCarty, D.J.: A basic guide to arthrocentesis. Hosp. Med., *4*:77–83, 1968.)

LANDMARKS FOR ENTRY OF THE KNEE JOINT

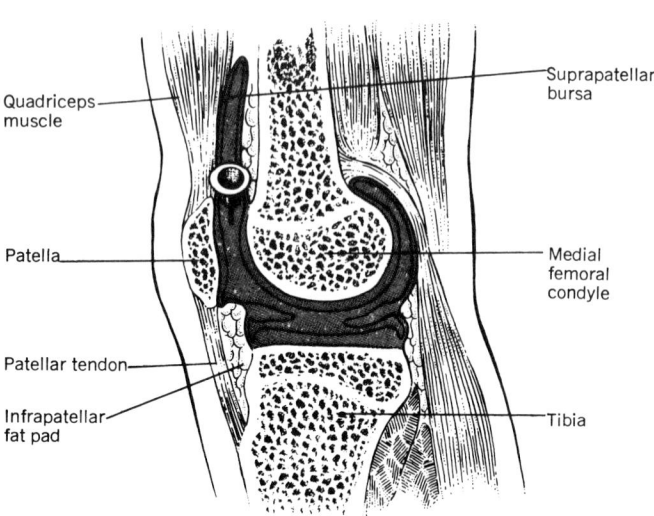

LANDMARKS FOR ENTRY OF THE ANKLE JOINT

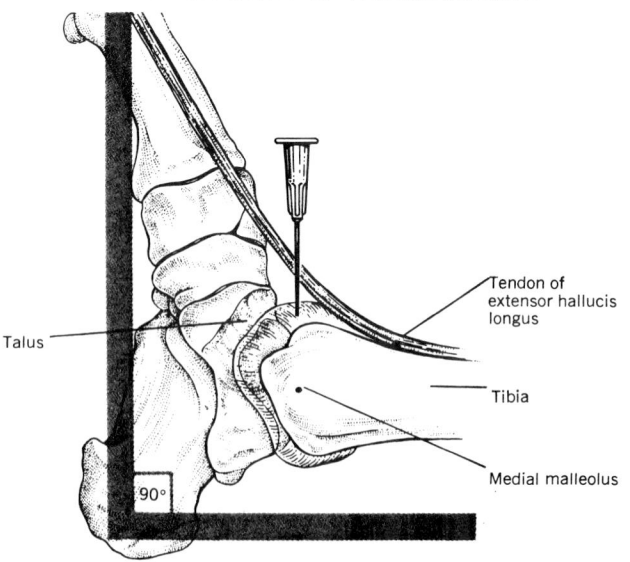

FIG. 39-3. With the leg-foot angle kept at 90°, the needle is directed horizontally on a line with the tip of the external malleolus at a point just proximal to the sinus tarsi. Needles mark point of insertion. (From McCarty, D.J.: A basic guide to arthrocentesis. Hosp. Med., *4*:77–83, 1968.)

LANDMARKS FOR ENTRY OF THE SUBTALAR JOINT

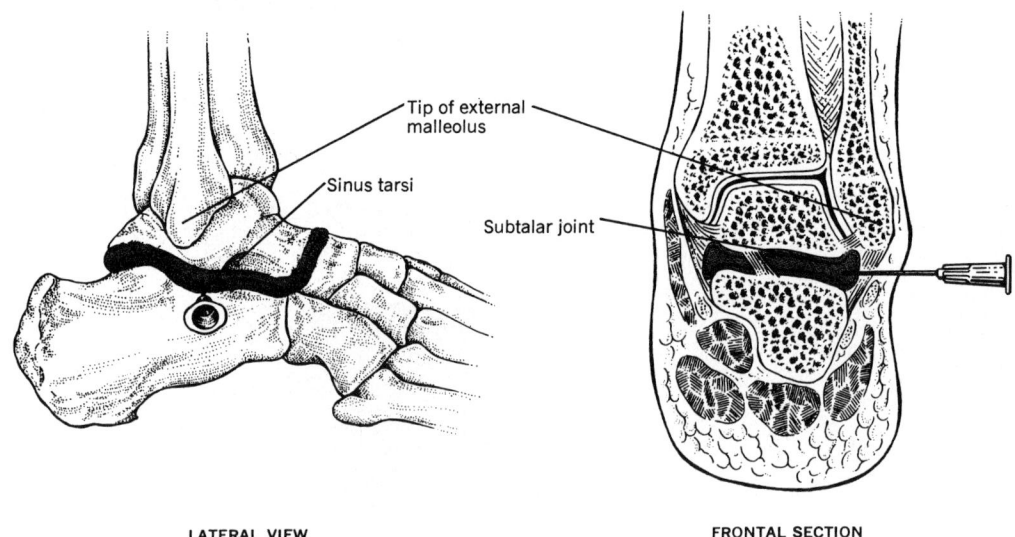

LATERAL VIEW   FRONTAL SECTION

metatarsophalangeal joints. Only rarely is injection necessary.

Hip Joint. Arthrocentesis of the hip joint is essentially a blind procedure. Close attention must be paid to the anatomic landmarks. If the hip joint architecture is severely deranged, it may be extremely difficult or even impossible to enter the joint space with a

FIG. 39-4. *A*, The space between the first metatarsal head and the base of the proximal phalanx is first identified and the overlying skin marked with fingernail pressure. *B*, After preparation of the skin and appropriate local anesthesia, a 20-gauge needle is directed into the joint space from the extensor surface just lateral to the extensor tendon. Traction on the toe facilitates entry. (From McCarty, D.J.: A basic guide to arthrocentesis. Hosp. Med., *4*:77–83, 1968.)

INJECTION OF THE FIRST METATARSOPHALANGEAL JOINT

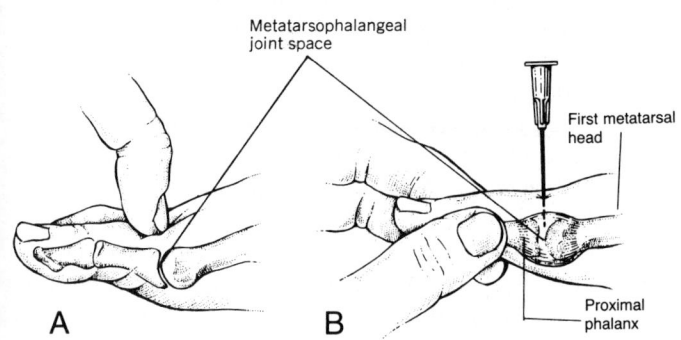

Metatarsophalangeal joint space

First metatarsal head

Proximal phalanx

A   B

needle blindly. The help of a radiologist using an image intensifier is needed in such situations. A 3½-inch spinal needle is needed to reach the joint cavity.

With the hip in external rotation, the anterior approach is used. One must identify the intersection of a vertical line from the anterior superior supine of the ilium and a horizontal line from the greater trochanter. The femoral artery is generally two fingerbreadths medial to this point and should be located before needle insertion (Fig. 39–5). The needle is directed posteromedially at the umbilicus, with the shaft of the needle making an angle of approximately 60° with the frontal plane. The tip of the needle is gently advanced until firm resistance is met (articular cartilage) and then withdrawn slightly as gentle suction is employed. Often fluid is not obtained, however, and results of corticosteroid injection are unpredictable.

Shoulder Joint. The shoulder joint is best entered from the anterior approach by directing the needle just below the tip of the coracoid process and just medial to the head of the humerus (Fig. 39–6).

Acromioclavicular Joint. The acromioclavicular joint can be easily identified by palpation along the clavicle until a defect is felt. A needle should be inserted vertically from above into the joint space (Fig. 39–6).

Sternoclavicular Joint. The sternoclavicular joint is best entered from a point directly anterior. Extreme care must be taken not to puncture the lung. The tip

FIG. 39–5. Anatomic-relationships of the hip joint in the anteroposterior direction. Needle marks the puncture site. (From McCarty, D.J.: A basic guide to arthrocentesis. Hosp. Med., *4*:77–83, 1968.)

FIG. 39–6. Synovial reflections of glenohumeral and acromioclavicular joints (anterosuperior view). (From McCarty, D.J.: A basic guide to arthrocentesis. Hosp. Med., *4*:77–83, 1968.)

LANDMARKS FOR ENTRY OF THE HIP JOINT

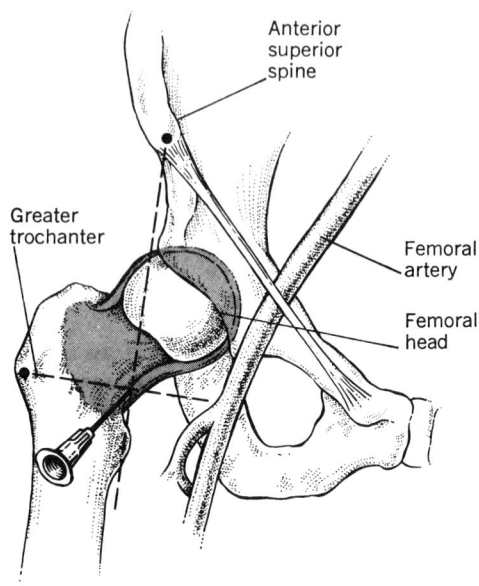

LANDMARKS FOR ENTRY OF
THE SHOULDER JOINT

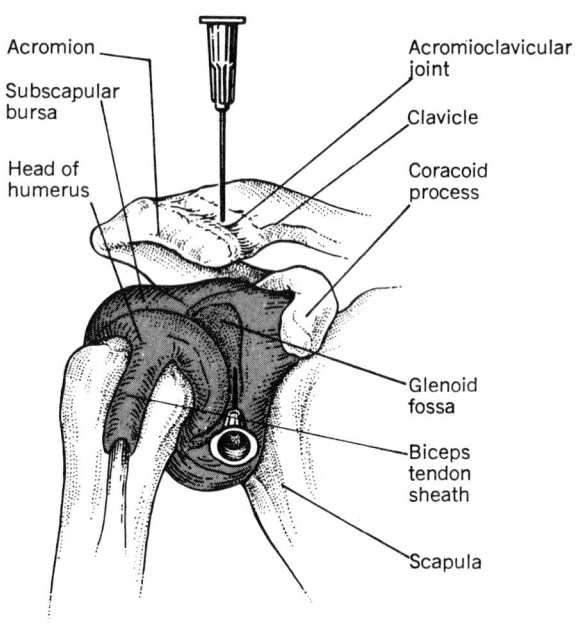

of the needle is inserted between the inferior border of the clavicle and the first rib so that the latter remains as a shield between the needle tip and the lung, avoiding pneumothorax. Suspected septic arthritis is the most common reason for arthrocentesis of this joint. Injection is rarely necessary.

Elbow Joint. With the elbow held at 90°, the needle is inserted just lateral to the olecranon and just below the lateral epicondyle of the humerus so that the shaft of the needle is parallel to the shaft of the radius (Fig. 39–7). The radiohumeral articulation can also be entered by first identifying the joint margin and then inserting the needle perpendicular to the skin (Fig. 39–8). Because these two joint spaces intercommunicate, it is usually possible to inject or aspirate both from either site.

Wrist Joint. The wrist joint proper is entered dorsally after identification of the joint line between the radial and ulnar styloid processes. The wrist is entered just distal to the radius approximately two fingerbreadths ulnar to the anatomic snuffbox (Fig. 39–9). The bursa underlying the fibrocartilaginous articular disc of the distal radioulnar joint often communicates with the distal radioulnar joint. This sac can be entered from the extensor surface at a point just distal to the ulnar bone.

Small Hand Joints. The small hand joints are best

entered from the extensor surface from either side. A distended or hypertrophic synovium almost always bulges dorsally, and it is relatively easy to slip a needle from either anteromedial or anterolateral under the extensor tendon mechanism and into the joint space (Fig. 39–10). Fluid is obtained rarely. The material to be injected will distend the joint so that one can feel and see the joint bulge on all sides. When this is accomplished, the joint space has been entered. The metacarpophalangeal joints are entered in similar fashion, or, if distention is minimal, the joint line is identified with the joint at 45–90° of flexion (Fig. 39–10). The joint is held in this position and gentle distractive force applied while the needle is being inserted.

Temporomandibular Joint. The temporomandibular joint may be entered just below the zygomatic arch at a point one fingerbreadth in front of the ear. Entry may be easier if the patient is instructed to open his mouth widely (Fig. 39–11). The temporal artery anterior to the ear should be identified prior to needle insertion. Care must be taken also to avoid the joint disc once within the joint space.

FIG. 39–7. Posterior view of flexed left elbow showing distended synovial sac. Needle marks puncture site. (From McCarty, D.J.: A basic guide to arthrocentesis. Hosp. Med., 4:77–83, 1968.)

FIG. 39–8. Lateral view of right elbow showing distended synovial sac. Needle marks puncture site. (From McCarty, D.J.: A basic guide to arthrocentesis. Hosp. Med., 4:77–83, 1968.)

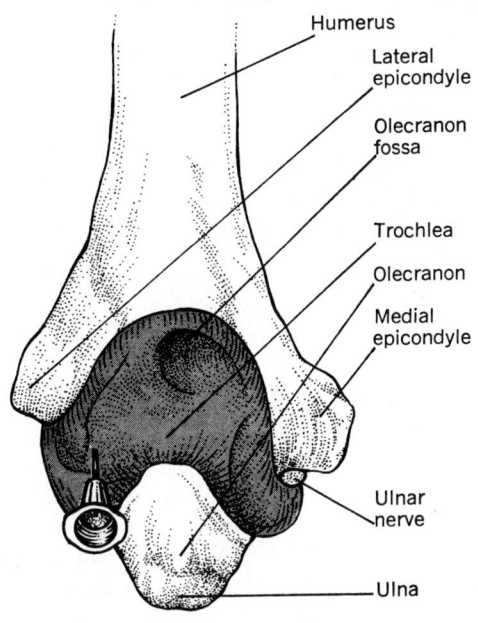

LANDMARKS FOR ENTRY OF THE ELBOW JOINT

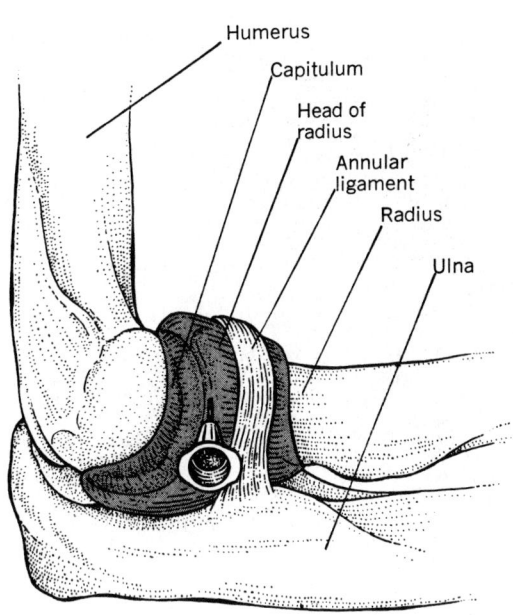

LANDMARKS FOR ENTRY OF THE RADIOHUMERAL ARTICULATION

INTRASYNOVIAL THERAPY

Historical. Over the years, a variety of materials have been injected into joints. None but corticosteroid has stood the test of time. Even intrasynovial antimicrobial therapy rarely adds to the value of their systemic administration in septic arthritis (see Chapter 114).

Therapeutic arthrocentesis alone (i.e., removal of fluid to relieve intra-articular pressure and stretching of the joint capsule and ligaments, or to remove accumulated leukocytes) may be useful for limited periods even though the joint fluid nearly always reaccumulates rapidly. Needle drainage of pus or inflammatory fluid is the chief indication for this procedure.

In 1950, noting the striking anti-inflammatory effect of cortisone used topically in the eye, Hollander injected cortisone into the inflamed knee joints of patients with RA, but the anti-inflammatory effect was minimal at best. In 1951, Hollander injected suspensions of hydrocortisone acetate crystals into affected knee joints, producing a striking reduction in tenderness, pain, swelling, and joint temperature within 24 hours. Such observations supported the notion that hydrocortisone, rather than cortisone, was the active anti-inflammatory compound. Hydroxylation of cortisone, occurring in the liver, accounted both for the benefit of cortisone given systemically and for its ineffectiveness when injected locally into joints. Injections of hydrocortisone or its derivatives are a commonly accepted form of joint and soft tissue therapy. The addition of the tertiary butyl acetate or other esters to hydrocortisone or its derivatives retarded crystal solubility and local hydrolysis, thus prolonging the anti-inflammatory effect. These suspensions must be injected into the synovial sac to be effective. Extra-articular corticosteroid crystals are resorbed slowly and are completely ineffective in treating synovitis.

Our understanding of the anti-inflammatory mechanism of local corticosteroids is still incomplete. A decreased synovial membrane permeability in osteoarthritis correlated with clinical improvement.[3]

Calcium pyrophosphate dihydrate and basic calcium phosphate crystals are rapidly cleared from joints by endocytosis followed by intracellular dissolution.[4-7] Crystalline suspensions of hydrocortisone esters almost certainly are phagocytosed by synovial lining cells from which there is slow release. It has been impossible to show this directly because these

FIG. 39–9. Posterior view of left wrist showing distended synovial sacs. Needles mark puncture sites. (From McCarty, D.J.: A basic guide to arthrocentesis. Hosp. Med., *4:*77–83, 1968.)

LANDMARKS FOR ENTRY OF
THE WRIST JOINT

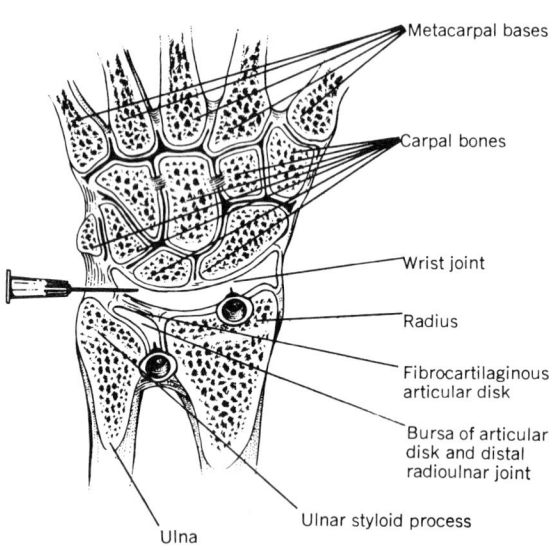

FIG. 39–10. Lateral view of finger showing distended synovial sacs. Needles mark puncture sites. (From McCarty, D.J.: A basic guide to arthrocentesis. Hosp. Med., *4:*77–83, 1968.)

LANDMARKS FOR ENTRY OF
THE SMALL HAND JOINTS

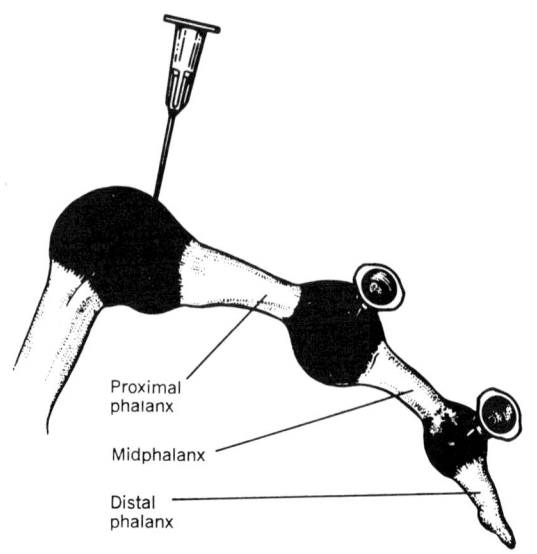

FIG. 39–11. Entry of this joint is facilitated if the patient opens his mouth wide. The needle is directed just below the zygomatic arch at a point one fingerbreadth anterior to the ear. Needle marks puncture site. (From McCarty, D.J.: A basic guide to arthrocentesis. Hosp. Med., *4:*77–83, 1968.)

LANDMARKS FOR ENTRY OF
THE TEMPOROMANDIBULAR JOINT

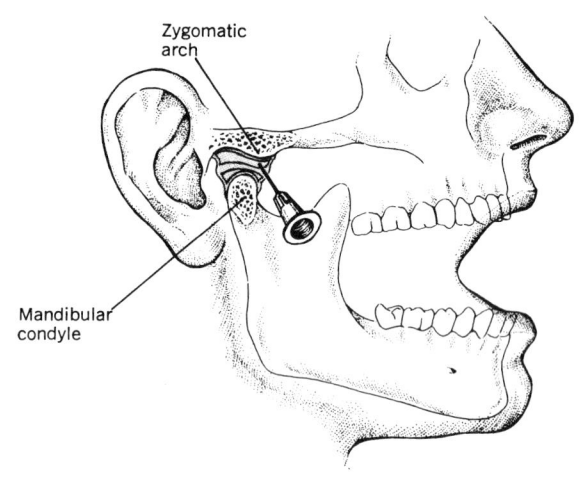

crystals cannot be labeled with a suitable gamma-emitting radionuclide. Esters of prednisolone, dexamethasone, and triamcinolone have all been prepared in microcrystalline form; each of these hydrocortisone derivatives is highly effective. Triamcinolone hexacetonide provides the most long-lasting anti-inflammatory effects of any of these intra-articular corticosteroid preparations.[8,9]

With the widespread recognition that intra-articular corticosteroids were efficacious, salicylates, phenylbutazone, indoprofen, gold compounds, orgotein, hyaluronic acid, rifamycin, and superoxide dismutase have been injected intra-articularly, but for various reasons, including local irritation and short duration of action, they are not established therapeutic agents.[10–15] "Chemical synovectomy" using various cytotoxic agents including nitrogen mustard, alone and in combination with corticosteroids to reduce the local inflammatory response, has been attempted. Triethylene thiophosphoramide (Thiotepa), osmic acid, and osmium tetroxide all have relatively short duration of beneficial effect with varying toxicity ranging from local irritation to chills, fever and liver toxicity.[16–24] These agents are no longer used.

RADIATION SYNOVECTOMY

Radiation synovectomy has been used since 1963 for treatment of persistent severe synovitis. The first radioactive agent used, *colloidal gold*, often produced suppression of pain and effusions lasting up to 1 year.[25] Newer agents have replaced radioactive gold, which emitted gamma particles as well as therapeutically useful beta irradiation. *Yttrium-90* has been favored because it emits only beta particles and has a short half-life (2 to 3 hours). Pigmented villonodular synovitis has been treated with this agent. Side effects included radionecrosis of soft tissue, needle track pigmentation, injection site tenderness, pyrexia, and lymphocyte chromosomal abnormalities.[26] Leakage from the injection site (up to 10%) of the radioactive substances was a problem noted with the older agents (e.g., radiocolloids). With the newer agents, leakage may be less than 1%. Movement of the injected joint can increase leakage. A rigid splint about the injected knee allowed yttrium-90 to be injected in outpatients with no more extra-articular spread or chromosomal damage than that found in hospitalized patients treated with bed rest for 48 hours. The results were equally good in both groups after 3 months. The increased intra-articular pressure produced by quadriceps muscle activity and knee flexion was identified as the most important factor affecting extra-articular spread of the isotope.[27]

Colloidal P32 chromic phosphate has been used in treatment of hemophilic arthropathy with encouraging results in 14 patients aged 12 to 28 years. Thirty-one "synoviortheses" were performed in these patients with chronic synovitis resistant to conventional therapy. Most patients had improved range of motion and decreased frequency and severity of bleeding episodes in the affected joint; extra-articular loss never exceeded 4% in 12 patients. Postinjection chromosomal aberrations were sought in 7 patients; none were found 2 to 5 years after treatment. Patients with high titers of factor VIII inhibitors had more recurrences of hemarthrosis and required more synoviortheses.[28]

Dysprosium 165-ferric hydroxide radioactive microaggregates have been injected into the knees of patients with seropositive RA and persistent synovitis of the knees. Seventy-three knees in 63 patients followed for 1 year revealed results that were 61% good, 23% fair, and 16% poor. A correlation with the radiographic stage of the disease was noted. The less severe the radiographic changes, the better the result. Low levels of leakage were noted. Treatment with this agent was thought to be effective, and the low leakage rates appeared to offer a definite advantage over other radioactive agents.[29]

The indications for radiation synovectomy are identical to those of surgical synovectomy (i.e., isolated refractory synovitis) despite usual comprehensive medical therapy, including modalities, rest, splinting, reduced weight bearing, and intra-articular injection of long-acting corticosteroids. Administration of radioactive substances requires special qualifications, and the use of such drugs intra-articularly mandates expert supervision.[27,30,31]

CORTICOSTEROID THERAPY

Almost always, local corticosteroid injection into a joint is *adjunctive* therapy and not a sufficient total program. A full regimen of education, systemic medication, appropriate rest, and physical therapy is the mainstay of arthritis treatment.

Corticosteroid Preparations

All hydroxycorticosteroid preparations are effective, but the various preparations are not equally potent. Tertiary butyl acetate (tebutate) esters have longer effective duration, because they are less soluble and are degraded less rapidly.[32] Triamcinolone hexacetonide has the longest biologic half-life and, therefore, the longest duration of suppression of inflammation. Fluorinated corticosteroids like triamcinolone are more likely to cause tissue atrophy. Therefore, they should be used rarely, if ever, for soft-tissue injection. With intrasynovial use, leakage along the needle track is sometimes associated with atrophy of skin and subcutaneous fat, and (rarely) with para-articular calcification.[9] Prednisolone tebutate and methylprednisolone acetate are less expensive, are effective, and are useful for soft-tissue injections. The amount of corticosteroid injected is based on the size of the joint and the potency of the chosen agent.

Contraindications. Contraindications to the use of corticosteroid therapy are listed in Table 39–3 and briefly discussed under Arthrocentesis Technique. Osteonecrotic, neurotrophic, or unstable joints generally should not be injected. Uncontrolled inflammation in more than three joints warrants a reassessment of the systemic therapeutic regimen before considering local corticosteroid therapy. If an intrasynovial corticosteroid injection was ineffective, it is likely that future injections will not be beneficial.

Although corticosteroid injection of spinal joints under fluoroscopic control, using image-intensification and the assistance of a skeletal radiologist has been performed, this form of therapy carries a definite risk of permanent nerve root or spinal cord damage.

Weight-bearing joints in patients with osteoarthritis should not be injected except on rare occasions, because benefits are transitory and frequent injections produce joint destruction.

Joint "inflammation" or pain following surgical implantation of metal or plastic components can be secondary to infection, loosening, wear fragments, fracture, or recurrence of prior synovitis. These joints are more prone to becoming infected than normal joints. Therefore, injection with corticosteroid must be approached with great caution.

Injection of nondiarthrodial joints is usually of no value because the purpose of corticosteroid is to decrease synovial inflammation, and joints without a synovial sac will not respond.

An inflamed weight-bearing joint should not be injected more frequently than every 3 to 4 months to minimize damage to the cartilage or the sustaining ligaments. A good response should suppress inflammation for 1 month or more, occasionally, for more than 1 year. A controlled trial using splinting for 3 weeks after injection of small hand joints showed that 88% of injected joints were in complete remission after 22 months.[9] Knee injections followed by 3 days of bed rest followed by 3 weeks of crutches or cane walking produced a mean benefit in 59 patients of 40.9 weeks.[9a]*

Adverse Reactions. Assuming that the indications and contraindications have been satisfied, there are very few adverse reactions as a result of local corticosteroid injections.

Infection, the most serious complication, is extremely rare. With the use of sterile technique, the incidence of infection should be negligible. Hollander reported an occurrence of only 0.005% in 400,000 injections.[33]

The most common adverse reaction to joint injection is the postinjection flare, a phenomenon related to a corticosteroid crystal-induced synovitis. Increased white blood cell count, predominantly neutrophils with many intracellular corticosteroid crystals, was found after injection of normal joints of volunteers.[34] Although at times very painful, this reaction is short-lived and can be treated effectively with oral analgesics and the local application of ice. The patient is warned at the time of injection that this reaction may occur and how to treat it. Such flares usually occur 4 to 12 hours after injection and last for 4 to 12 hours. If such a painful episode persists beyond 24 hours, the patient should be seen and evaluated; the joint should also be reaspirated and cultured to rule out infection. The incidence of postinjection flares has been estimated at 1 to 2%.

Editor's note. Treatment of rheumatoid knee joints using triamcinolone hexacetonide (40 mg) and avoidance of weight bearing for 8 weeks (crutch walking) has resulted in local remission lasting for many years in the majority of cases despite persistence of active disease in other joints. (Uncontrolled observations.)

Multiple corticosteroid injections into rabbit joints produced degenerative changes.[35-37] Such changes did not follow corticosteroid injections into monkey joints.[38] Examination of patients with osteoarthritis of the knees after weekly corticosteroid injections had been performed for many years revealed degenerative changes far in excess of those observed in a similar population from the same clinic that had not been so injected.[39] Others have made similar observations.[40,41] Avascular necrosis and Charcot's joints have been related to corticosteroid injections.[40] The mechanism underlying these observations is not clear. Initially, there may be an acute inflammatory reaction to the crystals; later, cartilage destruction may occur. This damage has been ascribed to pain relief related to overuse of the abnormal joint, the "iatrogenic Charcot joint." Prolonged suppression of protein synthesis by articular chondrocytes may follow injection of these relatively insoluble crystalline corticosteroid esters.

Repeated intraligamentous injections will weaken these structures, and calcification and rupture have been reported.[9,42,43] Penetration of the articular cartilage with the arthrocentesis needle and subsequent forceful injection will damage cartilage, as seen at surgery. Sterile technique, careful needle placement, and care not to inject against resistance will prevent such traumatic injections. *Pressure needed for injection should not exceed that generated by the extensors of the fifth digit.*

Atrophy of overlying skin can occur when corticosteroid leaks out of the joint space or is deposited extra-articularly in areas where little subcutaneous tissue exists between capsule and skin.[9] Care should be taken not to overdistend the joint space during an injection. Acute ulnar deviation of metacarpophalangeal joints caused by rapid resolution of inflamed hyperplastic synovium, which removes the support from the elongated overlying extensor tendon, has been reported.[9] Similarly, the central slip of the extensor tendon at the proximal interphalangeal joint may be ruptured, producing an acute "buttonhole" deformity.[9] The corticosteroid should flow easily from the syringe with minimal pressure on the plunger. The dose or volume of steroid injected just under or into the skin may well be a factor in the development of atrophy; dermatologists routinely use intradermal corticosteroid injections in very small doses and do not note atrophy as a common complication.

A variable fraction of injected intra-articular corticosteroid escapes from the joint into the systemic circulation in soluble form. Patients frequently note a transient improvement in other inflamed joints with decreased morning stiffness for several days following local joint injection. Elevation of blood sugar, flushing, hormonal suppression, and inhibition of ovulation also have been reported.[44-47] These systemic corticosteroid effects are proportional to the number of joints injected, the sum of the doses injected into each, and the relative solubility of the corticosteroid preparation used.

REFERENCES

1. Hollander, J.L., et al.: Hydrocortisone and cortisone injected into arthritic joints. JAMA, *147*:1629–1635, 1951.
2. McCarty, D.J.: A basic guide to arthrocentesis. Hospital Medicine,
3. Eymontt, M.J., Gordon, G.V., Schumacher, H.R., and Hansell, J.R.: The effects on synovial permeability and synovial fluid leukocyte counts in symptomatic osteoarthritis after intra-articular corticosteroid administration. J. Rheumatol., *9*:198–203, 1982.
4. McCarty, D.J., Palmer, D.W., and Halverson, P.B.: Clearance of calcium pyrophosphate dihydrate (CPPD) crystals in vivo. Studies using ¹⁶⁹Yb labelled triclinic crystals. Arthritis Rheum., *22*:718–727, 1979.
5. McCarty, D.J., Palmer, D.W., and James, C.: Clearance of calcium pyrophosphate dihydrate (CPPD) crystals in vivo II. Studies using triclinic crystals doubly labelled with ⁴⁵Ca and ⁸⁵Sr. Arthritis Rheum., *22*:1122–1131, 1979.
6. McCarty, D.J., Palmer, D.W., and Garancis, J.C.: Clearance of calcium pyrophosphate dihydrate crystals in vivo III. Effects of synovial hemosiderosis. Arthritis Rheum., *24*:706–710, 1981.
7. Palmer, D.W., and McCarty, D.J.: Clearance of ⁸⁵Sr labelled calcium phosphate crystals from rabbit joints. Arthritis Rheum., *27*:427–432, 1984.
8. Hollander, J.L.: Intrasynovial corticosteroid therapy in arthritis. Md. State Med. J., *19*:62–66, 1970.
9. McCarty, D.J.: Treatment of rheumatoid joint inflammation with triamcinolone hexacetonide. Arthritis Rheum., *15*:157–173, 1972.
9a. Neustadt, D.H.:Intra-articular therapy for rheumatoid synovitis of the knee: effects of the postinjection rest regimen. Clin. Rheumatol. In Practice, 3:65–68, 1985.
10. Caruso, I., et al.: Rheumatoid knee synovitis successfully treated with intra-articular rifamycin SV. Ann. Rheum. Dis., *41*:232–236, 1982.
11. Christophidis, N., and Huskisson, E.C.: Intra-articular drug therapy in rheumatoid arthritis. A study of indoprofen. Rheumatol. Int., *2*:129–132, 1982.
12. Goebel, K.M., and Storck, U.: Effect of intra-articular orgotein versus a corticosteroid on rheumatoid arthritis of the knees. Am. J. Med., *74*:124–128, 1983.
13. Namiki, O., Toyoshima, H., and Morasaki, N.: Therapeutic effect of intra-articular injection of high molecular weight hyaluronic acid on osteoarthritis of the knee. Int. J. Clin. Pharmacol. Ther. Toxicol., *11*:501–507, 1982.
14. Lewis, D.C., and Ziff, M.: Intra-articular administration of gold salts. Arthritis Rheum., *9*:682–692, 1966.
15. Steinbrocker, O., and Neustadt, D.H.: Aspiration and injection therapy. In Arthritis and Musculoskeletal Diseases. Edited by O. Steinbrocker and D.H. Neustadt. Hagerstown, MD, Harper & Row, 1972.
16. Scherbel, A.L., Schuchter, S.C., and Weyman, S.J.: Intra-articular administration of nitrogen mustard alone and combined with corticosteroid for rheumatoid arthritis. Cleve. Clin. Q., *24*:78–89, 1957.
17. Currey, H.L.F.: Intra-articular thiotepa in rheumatoid arthritis. Ann. Rheum. Dis., *24*:382–388, 1965.
18. Ellison, M.R., and Flatt, A.E.: Intra-articular thiotepa in rheumatoid disease. A clinical analysis of 123 injected MP and PIP joints. Arthritis Rheum., *14*:212–222, 1971.
19. Berglof, F.E.: Osmic acid in arthritis therapy. Acta Rheumatol. Scand., *5*:70–74, 1959.
20. Laine, V.: Osmic acid injected intra-articularly in rheumatoid arthritic knees. In Early Synovectomy in Rheumatoid Arthritis. Edited by W. Hijmans. Amsterdam, Excerpta Medica, 1969, p. 142–149.
21. Collan, Y., Servo, C., and Winblad, I.: An acute immune response to intra-articular injection of osmium tetroxide. Acta Rheumatol. Scand., *17*:236–242, 1971.
22. Anttinen, J., and Oka, M.: Intra-articular triamcinolone hexacetonide and osmic acid in knees. Scand. J. Rheumatol., *4*:125–128, 1975.
23. Medsger, T.A. et al. (eds.): Twenty-fifth rheumatism review. Arthritis Rheum., *26*:290–301, 1983.
24. Mancourt, D., Orloff, S., and Rao, V.H.: Synovial fluid hydroxyproline fractions before and after osmic acid treatment in rheumatoid arthritis. Scand. J. Rheumatol., *10*:43–48, 1981.
25. Topp, J.R., and Cross, E.G.: Treatment of persistent knee effusions with intra-articular radioactive gold. Preliminary report. Can. Med. Assoc. J., *102*:709–713, 1970.
26. Wiss, D.A.: Recurrent villonodular synovitis of the knee. Successful treatment with yttrium-90. Clin. Orthop., *169*:139–144, 1982.
27. Williams, P.L., et al.: Feasibility of out-patient management after intra-articular yttrium-90: A comparison of two regimens. Br. Med. J., *282*:13–14, 1981.
28. Ravard, G.V., et al.: Synoviorthesis of colloid P32 chromic phosphate in hemophiliac arthropathy. A clinical follow-up. Arch. Phys. Med. Rehabil., *66*:753–756, 1985.
29. Sledge, C.B., et al.: Treatment of rheumatoid synovitis of the knee with intra-articular injection of dysprosium 165–ferric hydroxide microaggregates. Arthritis Rheum., *29*:153–159, 1986.
30. Bridgman, J.F., Bruckner, F., and Bleehan, N.M.: Radioactive yttrium in the treatment of rheumatoid knee effusions. Ann. Rheum. Dis., *30*:180–182, 1971.
31. Lee, P.: The efficacy and safety of radiosynovectomy. J. Rheumatol., *9*:165–168, 1982.
32. Hollander, J.L.: The place of intrasynovial corticosteroid therapy. Guidelines from 27 years experience. In 1978 Symposium on Intrasynovial Therapy of Rheumatic Diseases. XVII Nordic Congress of Rheumatology. Elsinore, Lederle, 1978.
33. Hollander, J.L.: Intrasynovial therapy. In Arthritis and Allied Conditions: A Textbook of Rheumatology. 10th Ed. Edited by D.J. McCarty. Philadelphia, Lea & Febiger, 1985, p. 543.
34. McCarty, D.J., and Hogan, J.M.: Inflammatory reaction after intrasynovial injection of microcrystalline adrenocorticosteroid esters. Arthritis Rheum., *7*:359–367, 1964.
35. Behrens, F., Shepard, N., and Mitchell, N.: Metabolic recovery of articular cartilage after intra-articular injections of glucocorticoids. J. Bone Joint Surg., *58A*:1157–1160, 1976.
36. Mankin, H.J., and Conger, K.A.: Acute effects of intra-articular hydrocortisone on articular cartilage in rabbits. J. Bone Joint Surg., *48A*:1383–1388, 1966.
37. Moskowitz, R.W., et al.: Experimentally induced corticosteroid arthropathy. Arthritis Rheum., *13*:236–243, 1970.
38. Gibson, T., et al.: Effect of intra-articular corticosteroid injections on primate cartilage. Ann. Rheum. Dis., *36*:74–79, 1977.

39. Gatter, R.A.: Personal observation.
40. Chandler, G.N., and Wright, V.: Deleterious effects of intra-articular hydrocortisone. Lancet, 1:661–663, 1958.
41. Wright, V., et al.: Intra-articular therapy in osteoarthritis: Comparison of hydrocortisone acetate and t-butyl acetate. Ann. Rheum. Dis., 19:257–261, 1960.
42. Sweetnam, R.: Corticosteroid arthropathy and tendon rupture (editorial). J. Bone Joint Surg., 51B:397–398, 1969.
43. Wrenn, R.N., Goldner, J.L., and Markee, J.L.: An experimental study of the effect of cortisone on the healing process and tensile strength of tendons. J. Bone Joint Surg., 36A:588–601, 1954.
44. Koehler, B.F., Urowitz, M.B., and Killinger, D.W.: The systemic effects of intra-articular corticosteroid. J. Rheumatol., 1:117–125, 1974.
45. Gottlieb, N.L., and Riskin, W.G.: Complications of local corticosteroid injection. JAMA, 243:1547–1548, 1980.
46. Carson, T.E., et al.: Effect of intramuscular triamcinolone acetonide on the human ovulatory cycle. Cutis, 19:633–637, 1977.
47. Cunningham, G.R., Goldzieher, J.W., de la Pena, A., and Oliver, M.: The mechanism of ovulation inhibition by triamcinolone acetonide. J. Clin. Endocrinol. Metab., 46:8–14, 1978.

section **IV**

RHEUMATOID ARTHRITIS

ETIOLOGY AND PATHOGENESIS OF RHEUMATOID ARTHRITIS

40

NATHAN J. ZVAIFLER

Rheumatoid arthritis (RA), a chronic systemic and articular inflammatory disorder of unknown etiology, has a worldwide distribution and involves all racial and ethnic groups. In the United States, it is estimated to occur in 0.3 to 1.5% of the population, depending on the stringency of the criteria. Women are affected two to three times more often than men, although this female preponderance is less impressive when only those with positive serologic tests (for IgM rheumatoid factor) and erosive change on radiographs are considered. The disease can occur at any age and generally increases in incidence with advancing years. The peak incidence in women is between the fourth and sixth decades (Chapter 3).

Occasionally, many family members are affected with RA, and occurrence in monozygotic twins is greater than would be expected, but the best evidence for genetic predisposition comes from studies of the class II gene products (HLA-DR, DQ, DP) of the major histocompatibility complex. Susceptibility to a number of diseases, including RA, seems to be determined by these immune response (D region) genes (Chapter 29). In patients with seropositive RA, HLA-DR4 is the primary susceptibility haplotype in most ethnic groups.[1] Black Americans with RA are an exception. The relative risk of developing RA increases several times in DR4 individuals, but only a minority of them are afflicted. Moreover, this does not explain why all DR4 subspecificities are not equally susceptibile or why a significant number of RA patients have a haplotype other than DR4. New technologies have begun to unravel the puzzle. Both restriction endonuclease analysis of the genes coding for DR alleles and aminoacid sequencing of the polymorphic β chain of DR and DQ show families of molecules common to different haplotypes.[2,3] Likewise, certain monoclonal antibodies can identify a shared epitope present on several different classes of HLA-D, which confers a much higher relative risk for the development of RA, even in DR4-negative individuals.[2,4] Because class II molecules are involved in antigen presentation to T-lymphocyte, this type of analysis will probably lead to an identification of infectious or chemical agent(s) responsible for RA.

As a group, patients with RA have similar joint abnormalities and synovial histopathology. This similarity forms the basis for considering RA to be a single disease. Equally compelling, however, is the possibility that RA may represent a heterogeneous group of disorders. This alternative is supported by the dissimilar articular and systemic manifestations in individual patients, by variable outcomes, by the presence or absence of serum rheumatoid factors, and by the different genetic makeup of those affected. Obviously, if RA is merely one disease, identification of the cause will be easier.

ETIOLOGY

Despite many years of intensive investigation, the etiology of RA remains obscure. Endocrine, metabolic, and nutritional factors and a multitude of geographic, occupational, and psychosocial variables have all been studied. Although perhaps influencing the course of the disease, none is clearly implicated in its causation.

INFECTIOUS AGENTS

Polyarthritis occurs during many bacterial, spirochetal, and viral infections of man and animals (Chapter 31). RA resembles certain naturally occurring animal illnesses such as caprine arthritis, encephalitis caused by a lentivirus; mycoplasmal arthritis in rodents; and erysipelothrix arthritis in swine. The demonstration that Lyme disease, a multisystem disorder with a characteristic inflammatory arthritis (Chapter 119), is caused by a previously unidentified spirochete has rekindled interest in the infectious etiology of RA.

Bacteria

Evidence implicating a bacterial pathogen in RA is lacking, despite more than 50 years of intensive study. Bacteria were sought initially because of the confusion between RA and rheumatic fever. Indeed treatment of RA once included the eradication of foci of infection, particularly those containing streptococci. The streptococcal origin of rheumatic fever is unquestionable, but no evidence suggests that human RA is initiated by this microorganism. Interest then shifted to diphtheroids as etiologic agents when it appeared that these organisms were present in synovial membranes and fluids.[5] Diphtheroids, however, found as normal skin flora, were subsequently discredited as contaminants. More recently, claims have been made for the isolation of diphtheroid-like organisms, suh as Corynebacterium, now called Proprionibacterium, from rheumatoid synovium[6] and the demonstration of a polysaccharide antigen similar to that from Proprionibacterium acnes in phenol water extracts of synovial fluids and leukocytes.[7] Unfortunately, in both studies, similar organisms or antigens were found in nonrheumatoid tissues in sufficient numbers to question their etiologic significance in RA.

The fascination with mycoplasma as a cause of RA is long-standing because these organisms can induce experimental arthritis.[8] From time to time, reports have appeared of mycoplasma isolated from synovial fluid and membrane, but most studies, using a variety of sensitive detection methods, have failed to isolate these organisms. Even in experimental mycoplasma infections, however, the organisms can be isolated from the joint tissues only for a short time after the inception of the inflammatory synovitis; subsequently, they become undetectable, although the process continues as a chronic destructive arthropa-

thy.[9] This fact makes the data obtained from human RA joints difficult to interpret.

Patients with RA have large amounts of Clostridium perfringens in their feces. Most normal individuals have only small numbers of these organisms, and they are limited to the colon, whereas C. perfringens can be demonstrated in the small intestine of about two thirds of RA patients.[10] By modifying the diet of pigs, Mansson and his associates induced clostridial overgrowth and concomitantly observed the development of a rheumatoid-like arthritis in this animal.[11] Unfortunately, clostridial overgrowth can also be documented in other chronic inflammatory rheumatic diseases and in many individuals who have a larger-than-normal reservoir of enteric bacteria, but are without rheumatic complaints.[12]

Because of the failure to isolate live organisms, the emphasis has switched to the demonstration of bacterial antigens within articular tissues that are derived from the cell wall of organisms originating in the gastrointestinal tract. The idea that bacterial debris can be phagocytized by macrophages and synovial lining cells, but cannot be degraded, and thus persists as a chronic irritant is plausible and gains credibility from animal models in which the systemic administration of bacterial peptidoglycans (cell wall constituents) is followed by a chronic destructive inflammatory synovitis.[13] Attempts to detect components of bacterial cell walls in biopsies of rheumatoid synovial membranes have been unsuccessful, however, even using the unusually sensitive procedure of mass spectrometry.[14]

The inciting agents of adjuvant arthritis, a chronic destructive joint disease induced in genetically susceptible rats by injections of Freund's adjuvant, are antigens of Mycobacterium tuberculosis. One of these shows antigenic similarities to cartilage proteoglycan core protein and also causes proliferation of synovial fluid lymphocytes, sometimes to a greater amount than peripheral blood T cells and always more than controls.[15] An association of HLA-DR4, the RA-susceptibility haplotype, and the skin test response to Mycobacterium tuberculosis is also provocative,[16] but it seems unlikely that tuberculosis is responsible for RA. However, cross-reactions between common environmental infectious agents and articular antigens remains an attractive hypothesis.

Viruses

The possible viral origin of RA has been vigorously pursued. Direct viral identification, either through isolation or visualization by electron microscopy, was unrewarding.[17] As each new viral detection technique appeared, it was used to search for the putative initiating agent of RA. Sensitive methods capable of demonstrating slow viruses, noncytopathic viruses, or latent viruses, and virus rescue by co-cultivation or DNA and RNA hybridization have all been unrewarding.[18] Searching joint tissues for viral nucleic acid sequences has also proved unproductive.[19] Equally unrewarding has been the use of immunologic techniques to identify viral antigens,[20-24] virus-induced neoantigens,[25] or unique viral antibodies secreted by altered synovial B cells.[26] Despite these disappointments, the quest continues.

Given the complex biology of viruses, it is likely that almost any species could produce arthritis. On the other hand, only a limited number of mechanisms can explain a chronic inflammatory synovial disease such as RA. A few relevant pathogenetic models and the viruses that might be responsible are worth considering. In the first model, sequestration of an arthrotropic agent in articular cartilage or other joint structures could lead to arthritis, either directly or by invoking a localized immune response. The most likely pathogen in this model is rubella virus, which has a propensity for localization in cartilage when injected systemically.[27] Moreover, in humans, an inflammatory polyarthritis may follow both natural rubella infection and immunization with rubella vaccine.[28,29] Rubella virus has been recovered from peripheral blood lymphocytes and synovial tissues of several of these patients.[29-33] There are now several reports of isolates of live rubella virus from synovial effusions of adults and children with chronic inflammatory, seronegative, oligoarthritis, and polyarthritis who had no previous history of rubella infection or vaccination.[34,35] Although it appears clear that rubella virus can elicit a broad spectrum of articular responses, evidence that this virus can induce or propagate RA is still insufficient.

The recently identified human B19 strain of parvovirus causes a common exanthematous disease (erythema infectiosum, "fifth" disease) in children.[36] A few get a short-lived arthritis. Adult contacts of these children have a variety of outcomes. Most adults are unaffected, because of prior exposure, but some (10%) show serologic evidence of recent infection. Of these, about half develop an acute and sometimes protracted polyarthritis.[37] B19 parvovirus was the most frequently identified etiologic agent in patients attending an "early synovitis" clinic.[38] IgM antibodies, reflecting recent infection with the B19 strain, were found in the serum of 4 of 69 patients at or near the onset of RA.[39] A report that a different parvovirus (strain RA-1) was present in cultured synovial membrane from a patient with classic seropositive RA has yet to be confirmed.[40]

Immune complexes accompany most, if not all, viral infections in which both continuous viral replication and a continuous host response occur. Acute synovitis often results from circulating immune complexes, and occasionally they invoke a chronic arthritis. Hepatitis B infection is complicated by arthritis in 10 to 30% of cases, usually as a prodrome of recognizable liver disease.[41,42] This form of arthritis is similar to RA in that both the small joints of the hands and the larger articulations can be affected, and women have symptoms more often than men. Hepatitis B surface antigen (HBsAg) has been demonstrated by immunofluorescence in the synovium, and Dane particles can be recognized by electron microscopy, but the virus has not been propagated in tissue culture. During the prodrome, the presence of hepatitis antigen, hypocomplementemia, and cryoprecipitates containing HBsAg, anti-HB immunoglobulins, and complement components suggests that the arthritis results from intra-articular deposition of immune complexes.[43] As in other viral diseases, rheumatoid factor is often present in hepatitis B infection.[44] Sometimes, hepatitis B arthritis is complicated by persistent synovitis,[41] but only once has the subsequent development of classic RA been documented.[45] Given the relative frequency of both diseases, this association probably occurred by chance.

A third possible way in which a virus could cause a disease such as RA is viral alteration of the immune system such that potentially harmful autoantibodies, like rheumatoid factors, are produced. This hypothesis is currently popular. The prototype here is the Epstein-Barr virus (EBV), which is lymphotropic. B-lymphocytes have a membrane receptor for EBV, and this virus can both infect and trigger B-lymphocytes to proliferate indefinitely and to secrete antibodies.[46,47] No antigen is required, and EBV is considered a polyclonal B-cell activator that stimulates cells to produce their genetically programmed immunoglobulins. One consequence of EBV infection is autoantibody production; for instance, heterophile antibodies, cold agglutinins, hemolysins, antinuclear antibodies, and rheumatoid factors are often associated with acute infectious mononucleosis, a known EBV-induced disease in man.[48] Arthralgias have been noted in up to 10% of patients with infectious mononucleosis, but until recently, arthritis was considered to be a rare complication of heterophile-positive mononucleosis. In the dozen or so cases reported with EBV arthritis, radiologic findings have been limited to soft-tissue swelling. The sedimentation rate in these patients was mildly elevated, but rheumatoid factors and antinuclear antibodies were consistently absent, and all joint complaints resolved by 30 days.[49] An exception is a

19-year-old woman, followed for more than 2 years, who has a persistent symmetric polyarthritis involving the small joints of the hands, wrists, knees, and metatarsophalangeal and interphalangeal joints of the feet. This patient has remained rheumatoid-factor negative.[49]

Several other reasons for interest in the EBV are: (1) when compared with normal individuals, patients with RA have greater amounts of an unusual EBV-related antibody, that is, the rheumatoid arthritis precipitin or anti-RANA, in their serum;[50] (2) these patients may also have higher titers of antibodies to more conventional EBV-related antigens, although epidemiologic studies show that about 20% of RA patients have never been exposed to the virus, and similar increases in EBV antibody titers are found in patients with other chronic inflammatory connective tissue diseases;[51–54] and (3) RA patients appear to be defective in their ability to regulate EBV infections.[55–58]

B-lymphocytes infected in vitro with EBV transform into lymphoblastoid colonies. RA B cells develop colonies faster than normal B cells and produce more immunoglobulin and rheumatoid factor.[56,59] The rate of B-cell transformation is controlled by the interaction of a number of different mononuclear cells and their soluble products, including interferons, interleukins, and prostaglandins. A significant portion of RA patients fail to make adequate amounts of these factors and thus cannot expand a cytotoxic T-cell population necessary for the elimination of the infected B cell.[60–65] The in vivo expression of these defects may be a higher rate of spontaneous (i.e., in the absence of added EBV) transformation of RA B cells and the finding that five times more EBV is present in RA blood cells than in blood lymphocytes of normal individuals.[59,66]

Our current understanding of EBV and RA can be summarized as follows: EBV infection, serologically defined, is not necessarily present at the outset or during the course of the disease in all RA patients. EBV arthritis does exist, but it is rare and is not identical to RA. The lymphocytes of RA patients are defective in their ability to regulate an in vitro EBV infection of B cells, and this defect may explain the difference reported in the expression of antibodies to various EBV antigens in individuals with RA. The relevance of the immunoregulatory defect of RA patients for EBV is not proved, but the defect may have a role in the propagation of the disease process.

Although many facts are now available about the possible causes, epidemiology, and pathology of RA, their relationship to one another and to the disease is not clear. We shall probably not be able to understand these data until the etiologic agent responsible for the illness has been identified, but the eventual answer should explain why the disease is so common (affecting approximately 1% of all adults), ubiquitous (present in almost all populations), persistent (lasting years to decades), and intimately associated with a unique antibody (rheumatoid factor) and a particular genetic constitution (a locus related to HLA-DR4). Our future understanding should also explain the foremost question; namely, why is RA a chronic inflammatory disease of joints?

ARTICULAR INFLAMMATION

The inflammatory response is usually considered a biologic adaptation to protect the host from a hostile environment. A prerequisite is that this response occurs without significant injury to the host's own tissues. Thus, the inflammation in RA must be considered inappropriate. How this comes about is not known, but a number of factors predispose joints to injury and inflammation. Because they are moving, superficial structures, joints are subject to microtrauma almost constantly. Because the joint lining is composed, at least in part, of active phagocytic cells, it is likely that small numbers of micro-organisms are regularly extracted from the blood as it courses through the subsynovial vessels.[67] Alternatively, because the synovial lining cells are replenished by macrophage precursors in the bone marrow, organisms acquired at a distant site may be continuously transported into the joints. Equally important is the unexplained retention of immunoglobulins or antigen-antibody complexes by the macromolecules of fibrous and hyaline cartilage.[68] In most instances, articular inflammation or synovitis is self-limited. After a variable period, the joint returns to its premorbid state, but occasionally, the process persists and chronic inflammation and eventual tissue damage ensue.

A number of reasons can be proposed to account for the chronicity of articular inflammation. The first and most obvious is persistence of the initiating event or an incomplete degradation of the primary stimulus. Chronic infection with organisms such as mycobacteria or fungi are examples in humans. In some experimental forms of chronic arthritis, such as in adjuvant arthritis and the streptococcal cell wall–model, it appears that certain arthritogenic substances, such as peptidoglycans, are incriminated.[13,69] Although injected at a distant site, these substances accumulate in the joint, and because of their unique property of being biologically nondegradable, they persist as an irritative focus.

A second reason for unresolved inflammation is the

development of a cross-reacting immune response between the primary stimulus and antigens peculiar to one of the articular structures. Antibody made systemically might be retained in the joint. Examples include the shared antigens of streptococcal cell wall and human cartilage proteoglycan, or the chronic arthritis that develops in animals immunized against heterologous type II collagen.[70]

The most compelling argument, as in some other forms of chronic inflammation, is that a local immune reaction is responsible. In RA, this reaction could be an appropriate response to the putative causative agent sequestered in the articular cavity. Alternatively, it might represent autosensitization to a self-antigen rendered immunogenic within the joint. In RA, IgG is the obvious candidate. Perhaps in the course of a nonspecific synovitis, IgG is partially degraded by enzymes generated by the inflammatory process. Most individuals would not recognize the neoantigens produced, but those genetically predisposed respond with local anti-IgG production. The ensuing local antigen-antibody complex formation would beget more inflammation, resulting in further alteration of immunoglobulin and a perpetuation of the inflammatory process. The association of seropositive, but not seronegative, RA with the HLA-DR4 haplotype supports this concept. A similar model could be developed using collagen as the autoantigen.

Finally, the rheumatoid process might reflect a disturbance in the normal circulation of immunocompetent cells between intra- and extravascular compartments. Perhaps as a result of prior "activation," lymphocytes traffic into the joint in an unregulated manner or persist long after the provocative stimulus has gone. For whatever reason, the cells and products of the immune system, although probably not primarily involved in the initiation of RA, are certainly largely responsible for the perpetuation of the inflammatory response.

PATHOGENESIS

Rheumatoid synovitis, according to present concepts, is characterized by two discrete phases: (1) an exudative phase involving the microcirculation and lining cells of the synovium that allows an influx of plasma proteins and cellular elements into the joint; and (2) a chronic inflammatory phase occurring in the subsynovium and characterized by mononuclear cell infiltration. In well-established disease, both phases are present and are probably interrelated, but to simplify analysis, they are examined in sequence, first the limited information on the initiating events, then the subsequent immunologic factors that perpetuate the primary inflammatory reaction, and finally the transition of the chronic inflammatory allergic reaction in the synovium to a proliferative destructive process.

INITIATION OF SYNOVITIS

The earliest events in RA are difficult to document, but the available evidence suggests that microvascular injury and mild synovial cell proliferation are the first lesions. Synovial biopsies from patients seen during the initial weeks of an arthritis that could subsequently be classified as definite or classic RA showed only mild proliferation of synovial lining cells and perivascular lymphocytes.[71,72] Polymorphonuclear leukocytes (PMNs), when present, were seen in the superficial synovium; plasma cells were noted rarely. The small blood vessels were abnormal; they were obliterated by inflammatory cells and organized thrombi. Electron-microscopic examination disclosed gaps between vascular endothelial cells and endothelial cell injury. Evidence suggests the occurrence of phagocytosis by proliferating synoviocytes and in large mononuclear cells. Unfortunately, none of these findings are unique to RA and all are found at the inception of other acute inflammatory joint conditions. The microvascular changes, however, suggest that the etiologic factor is carried to the joint by the circulation.

INFLAMMATORY RESPONSE

In contrast to the early lesions, many excellent descriptions of the histopathologic features of established RA and the immunologic events that perpetuate the primary synovial inflammatory reaction exist[73–76] (see Chapter 41). Grossly, the synovium appears edematous and protrudes into the joint cavity as slender villous projections. Light-microscopic examination discloses a characteristic, but not pathognomonic, constellation of histologic changes. Synovial lining cells are hyperplastic and are layered to a depth of six to ten cells, in contrast to the normal thickness of one to three cell layers. Focal or segmental vascular changes are a regular feature of rheumatoid synovitis. Venous distension results from swollen endothelial cells, capillary obstruction is common, the walls of venules and arterioles are infiltrated with neutrophils, and areas of thrombosis and perivascular hemorrhage are seen. The connective tissue stroma of the normal synovial villi has few cells, but in established RA it is usually filled with mononuclear cells. PMNs, common in the early lesions, are seen only occasionally. In some places, particularly around small blood vessels, lymphocytes and dendritic-appearing cells predominate; in others, plasma cells are the major type. Transitional areas have also been identified and show an intermingling of macrophages, lymphocytes, and plasma cells.[77]

Staining of the cells in situ with fluoresceinated monoclonal antibodies shows that the majority are T-lymphocytes; many have the Ia antigen, a measure of "activation," on their surface membranes.[78,79] Controversy exists over the proportion of the T cells that display helper-inducer or suppressor-cytotoxic phenotypes. The confusion relates, in part, to the region examined, because sampling in perivascular areas shows predominantly OKT4[+] helper cells, whereas at a distance, the OKT8[+] suppressor cells may be in the majority.[80] In some biopsies, only macrophage-mononuclear cells with large amounts of Ia on their surface membrane can be seen. A simple enumeration of the cells released from enzyme-digested synovial tissues shows greater than expected T-cell populations with a modest increase in OKT8[+] cells, as compared to companion blood samples. Although plasma cells and B-lymphocytes seem under-represented,[78,80] the rheumatoid synovium makes and contains large amounts of immunoglobulin, a finding that strongly suggests the presence of large numbers of these cells.

Immunofluorescent analysis of the plasma cells located in the subsynovium shows IgG to be the predominant class of cytoplasmic immunoglobulin. The majority of the IgM is rheumatoid factor. When plasma cells in the RA synovium are treated with pepsin, many are seen to contain an IgG rheumatoid factor that combines in the cytoplasm with similar IgG molecules (self-associating IgG) (see Chapter 46). Surprisingly, pepsin-digested tissues from seronegative patients also show IgG-anti-Ig activity.[81,82]

Additional evidence that the B cells in the synovium of patients with RA can make immunoglobulins includes the demonstraton of de novo immunoglobulin production by rheumatoid synovial explants or continuous cultures of lymphocytes released from synovium.[83] In vivo measurements of IgG synthesis show that about 20% of the IgG detected in synovial fluid is made in the synovial membrane,[84] and much of it has anti-IgG activity.[85]

Excessive synovial immunoglobulin production might come about in several ways. The fault could reside in B-cell hyperactivity caused, for instance, by a polyclonal B-cell activator, such as lipopolysaccharide peptidoglycan from bacterial cell walls or EBV. An alternative explanation might be that B cells are driven

by unrestrained T helper-inducer cells. This notion is supported by two observations: first, that the synovial lining cells have abundant surface Ia-like (DR) molecules and can efficiently present antigen and serve as stimulators in the mixed leukocyte reactions;[86] and second, that in certain areas of the subsynovium, helper-inducer cells are in intimate contact with dendritic-appearing cells bearing large amounts of DR antigen.[87] Such conditions are ideal for the generation of factors that support immunoglobulin production. A lack of suppressor cells, either because of an absolute reduction in their numbers or because of compartmentalization at a distance from the helper-inducer cells, could also account for unbridled antibody production.

The cytology of a typical rheumatoid joint effusion differs from that of the synovial membrane. Total leukocyte counts range from a few thousand to tens of thousands. Mononuclear cells, although present and having surface characteristics similar to their counterparts in the synovium, are in the minority. Neutrophils usually constitute 75 to 85% of the total. All forms are represented: early, multilobed PMNs are admixed with effete white cells containing disintegrating nuclei and large cytoplasmic vacuoles. These vacuoles, when appropriately stained, can be shown to contain immunoglobulins, complement components, and antiglobulins. Similar immunoreactants are demonstrable within the cytoplasm of type A (phagocytic) synovial lining cells and in the matrix of articular cartilage.[76] Rheumatoid synovial fluids have less hemolytic complement than serum from the same patients and show evidence of activation of both the classic and alternative pathways. Complement components and biologically active fragments of the complement sequence, anaphylatoxins and chemotactic factors, have been identified in RA effusions,[88] and their presence correlates with synovial fluid immune complex levels, especially with those containing rheumatoid factors of the IgG class. Immune complexes have been isolated from rheumatoid joint effusions, and their constituent parts have been analyzed (see Chapters 27 and 46). The dominant complexes contain anti-IgGs of both the IgM (conventional rheumatoid factor) and IgG class. This second type of complex seems particularly important in the pathogenesis of local inflammation because they self-associate to form intermediate-sized complexes that activate complement.[89] Further stabilization of complexes probably occurs by interaction with conventional IgM rheumatoid factor and enhances inflammatory properties. Other relevant antibodies, many of which are directed against by-products of the inflammatory response, include antinuclear antibodies, anti-Fab$_2$, anti-C3, and antifibrinogen, and possibly, collagen–anticollagen complexes.[76]

Electron-microscopic examination of the rheumatoid synovium shows hyperplasia of the lining cells. Superficially, the synoviocytes appear to form an uninterrupted layer, but no true basement membrane separates them from the underlying connective tissue. Capillaries are particularly abundant beneath the synovial lining, and many have large fenestrations similar to those seen in the vessels of the glomerulus, choroid plexus, and endocrine tissues.[67] Thus, material traversing these capillaries has only hyaluronate and interstitial fluid hampering its diffusion throughout the entire joint cavity.

Based on the foregoing observations, it has been suggested that the as-yet-unidentified cause of RA gains access to the joint and initiates an inflammatory response. Small blood vessels are injured, and mononuclear cells accumulate in the pericapillary areas. Macrophages process the pathogenic materials and present them to lymphocytes. Local antibody production ensues. The antigens and antibodies interact in synovial tissues, fluid, and cartilage and give rise to an extravascular immune complex disease (Fig. 40–1). These complexes activate the complement cascade and generate a number of biologically active materials from the complement proteins. Some, such as C3a and C5a, increase vascular permeability and allow an influx of serum proteins and cellular blood elements into the site where the complexes reside (exudation phase). PMNs in juxtaposition to the cartilage surface or free in the joint fluid retain the complexes with cell surface receptors for IgG and C3b. Subsequent phagocytosis stimulates (1) the release of lysosomal proteinases, which have the potential to digest collagen, cartilage matrix, elastic tissues, and activate other biologically active mediators; (2) oxygen-free radicals, which directly produce cellular injury; and (3) oxidation of arachidonic acid that leads to the generation of proinflammatory byproducts of the cyclo-oxygenase and lipoxygenase pathways (see Chapters 20, 25, and 26).

CHRONIC RHEUMATOID GRANULOMATOUS RESPONSE (PANNUS)

Either simultaneously or in tandem, the proliferative and destructive stages of RA proceed (see also Chapter 42). Synovial lining cells are stimulated to replicate by mediators generated in the inflammatory response. Macrophage-derived products such as in-

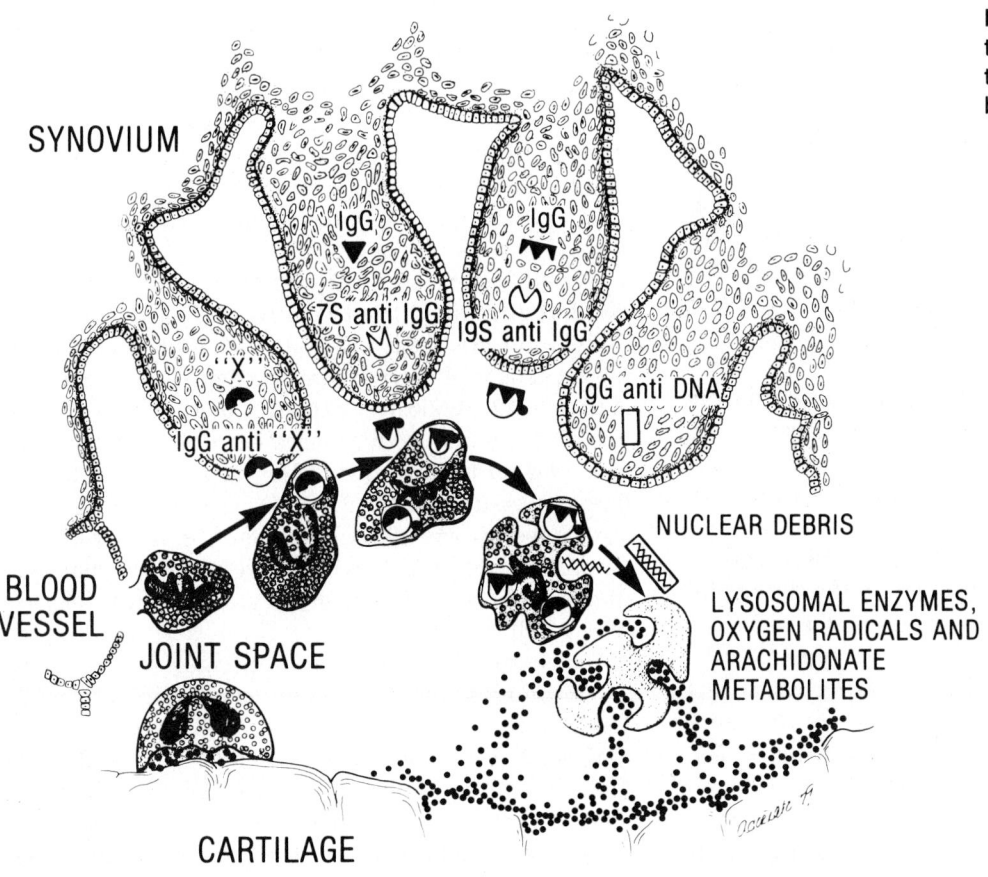

FIG. 40–1. Schematic illustration of immune complex interaction in structures involved by rheumatoid arthritis.

SYNOVIUM

IgG

IgG

7S anti IgG

I9S anti IgG

"X"

IgG anti DNA

IgG anti "X"

NUCLEAR DEBRIS

BLOOD VESSEL

LYSOSOMAL ENZYMES, OXYGEN RADICALS AND ARACHIDONATE METABOLITES

JOINT SPACE

CARTILAGE

terleukin-1 (IL-1); fibroblast-activating factor, prostaglandins, and platelet-derived growth factors participate. The neuropeptide, substance P, also stimulates synoviocytes in vitro, suggesting a link between the joint and nervous system.[90] The rheumatoid synovium contains numerous T-lymphocytes. Many of them express activation markers, like IL-2 receptor, transferrin, or 1a antigens on their surface.[78,79] Very few appear lymphoblastic.[91] Surprisingly, the usual byproducts of T-cell activation, lymphokines such as γ-interferon and IL-2, are difficult to demonstrate in the tissues or synovial fluid.[92,93] This difficulty may reflect the presence of specific IL-1 and IL-2 inhibitors[94,95] or could represent an accumulation of an unusual subset of T-helper cells. Support for the role of lymphocytes in the rheumatoid process is the observation that treatments such as thoracic duct drainage, lymphophoresis, and total lymph node irradiation may ameliorate joint inflammation and may decrease the hyperplasia of synovial lining cells.

Chronic RA is characterized by destruction of articular cartilage, ligaments, tendons, and bone. The damage results from a dual attack: from without by enzymes in the synovial fluid, and from above and below by granulation tissue.

Cartilage and other articular connective tissues are composed primarily of proteoglycans and collagen. Proteoglycans consist of repeating disaccharide subunits linked covalently to a protein core. The earliest evidence of cartilage injury is a loss of metachromatic staining due to a leaching out of the proteoglycans. Cartilage that has lost ground substance has a diminished capacity to resist deformation and may be at risk for permanent damage through mechanical disruption. Proteoglycan loss is reversible, and complete recovery is possible, but once collagen, which forms the structural skeleton, is lost, cartilage disintegration becomes irreversible.[75]

Many potentially damaging enzymes released from phagocytic synoviocytes and PMNs have been found in the fluid that continually bathes the cartilage surfaces. These enzymes include acid and neutral proteases that can split proteoglycan from its protein matrix.[96] Collagen, in its native triple-helical configuration, is resistant to degradation by these nonspecific proteases; however, collagenases derived from PMNs, macrophages, and rheumatoid synovial cells can cleave (denature) the collagen polypeptide chains specifically into two fragments, which are then rapidly degraded further by proteolytic enzymes.[75] The observation of proteoglycan depletion and collagen degradation at sites distant from the advancing margin of the proliferating synovial membrane argues for

the importance of synovial fluid enzymes in articular damage.[67,73]

The articular destruction in RA, however, begins at the periphery of the cartilage and in the "bare areas" of bone exposed to joint fluid but not covered by cartilage. It has been claimed that the earliest injury, which precedes the formation of recognizable pannus, is brought about by immature synovial cells' arising from the recesses at the margin of the joint and creeping across the surface of cartilage. Similar cells can be seen to insert themselves between the collagen fibers when the proteoglycan has been enzymatically removed. Subsequent cartilage destruction is accomplished by the release of collagenolytic enzymes.[75] These aggressive events are short-lived; occur in waves, likely in association with the exudative (inflammatory) process; and are followed by a maturation of the granulomatous response with an ingress of proliferating fibroblasts, small blood vessels, and inflammatory cells.[73]

Several different kinds of pannus have been described. The first type, which is analogous to the "activated" synovial membrane previously described, seems to destroy cartilage by enzymatic digestion. The second, "cellular" form of pannus probably operates the same way, but its similarity to granulation tissue seen at other sites of injury suggests that the cellular and fibrous infiltrate may be the result of cartilage injury, rather than the cause of it. A third type of dense fibrous, avascular, acellular pannus may act as a mantle interfering with cartilage nutrition. Although all three types of pannus can be found simultaneously in the same joint, it is not clear whether they represent a sequential phenomenon or whether each develops independently.[97]

A better understanding of the chronic synovitis of RA has developed from in vitro studies of the effects of lymphocytes, macrophages, and their products on target cells in the synovium, cartilage, and bone (see Chapter 42). Cultured explants of rheumatoid synovial fragments produce large quantities of collagenase and prostaglandins. The responsible cells are large, measuring 20 to 30 μm in diameter or greater, and have an abundant cytoplasm, a large nucleus, and dendritic processes that give them a stellate appearance. They are not monocytes, because they do not produce lysozyme, and most lack the conventional surface markers of macrophages. When placed in continuous culture, the synoviocytes initially make and secrete both collagenase and prostaglandin (PGE$_2$), but the production of these molecules decreases after trypsinization and serial passage of the cells.[98] Collagenase release is stimulated in such cultures by conditioned media from peripheral blood mononuclear cells.[99] Plant lectins, collagen, the Fc portion of IgG, and aggregated IgG can all further increase the amount of this stimulating factor.[100] Cellular fractionation studies have shown that monocytes or macrophages are responsible for the stimulating factor, which is identical to IL-1,[101] a molecule whose release from macrophages is modulated by T-cell lymphokines (see Chapter 42). A much more detailed discussion of the mechanisms of hard tissue destruction in RA is given in Chapter 42.

Another mechanism may be the destruction of cartilage brought about by the chondrocytes themselves. As noted earlier, proteoglycan loss can be observed in the absence of either pannus overgrowth or high PMN counts in synovial fluid,[67] particularly early in the disease. Histopathologic study of cartilage at this time reveals enlarged lacunae around the chondrocytes and some evidence of chondrocyte proliferation. These findings suggest that tissue degradation may result from factors released from chondrocytes. Synovium elaborates a factor called *catabolin*, which is IL-1 and stimulates chondrocytes to secrete matrix-degrading enzymes.[102] Moreover, the addition of media from cultures of normal or rheumatoid synovial explants or IL-1 to chondrocytes stimulated the release of plasminogen activator, prostaglandin E, and collagenase.[103,104]

The inciting factors in RA remain undefined, but our understanding of the cellular and molecular mechanisms leading to chronic joint inflammation and to local tissue destruction continues to increase. As seen in Figure 40–2, the central axis is the interaction between macrophage-type cells and T-lymphocytes. These cells, in concert with B cells, cause local production of antibody. Immune complexes formed locally within the joint activate complement and are phagocytized by PMNs and the macrophage-like moiety of synovial lining cells. Accompanying this ingestion, a variety of mediators are released, giving rise to the signs and symptoms of inflammation. Leukocytes adherent to cartilage can degrade proteoglycan, and perhaps collagen in their attempts to eliminate the sequestered immune complexes. Simultaneously, the macrophages and T cells communicate through soluble substances with the stellate cells in the synovial lining and stimulate the release of molecules capable of causing bone and cartilage erosion, which eventuates in characteristic rheumatoid deformities and attendant functional disability.

The same complex interaction of cells and mediators is probably involved in connective tissue turnover during repair, growth, and differentiation. As in all biologic systems, control mechanisms limit the response. Thus, antibody production and lymphokine release are modulated by suppressor cells, inhibitors, idiotype networks, and peptides derived from IgG degradation; corticosteroids and prostaglandins modify the response to mediators and the release of degradative enzymes; and inhibitors are present in plasma and articular tissues that bind and neutralize

FIG. 40–2. Schematic representation of the etiology and of the cellular and immune interactions responsible for joint inflammation and destruction in RA.

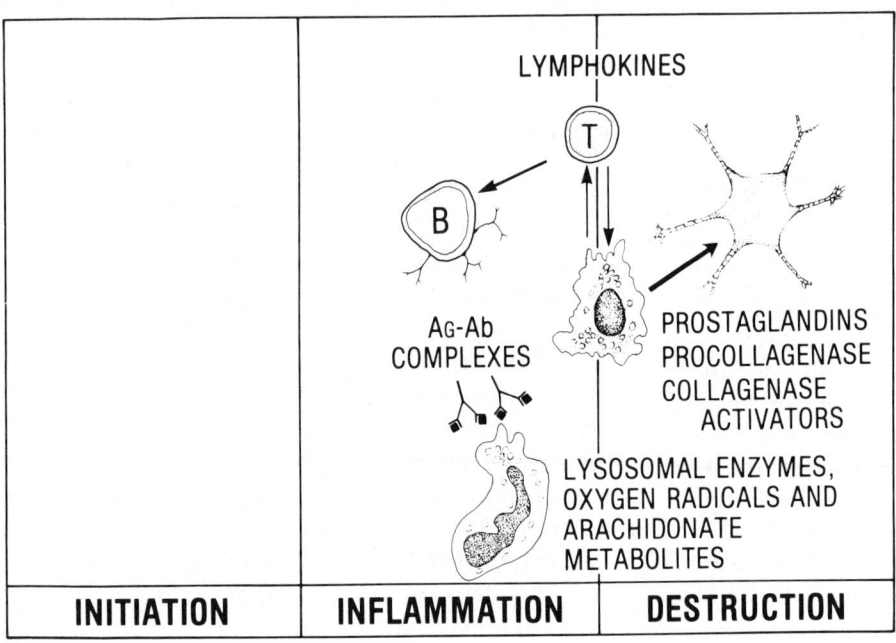

LYMPHOKINES

T

B

AG-AB COMPLEXES

PROSTAGLANDINS
PROCOLLAGENASE
COLLAGENASE
ACTIVATORS

LYSOSOMAL ENZYMES,
OXYGEN RADICALS AND
ARACHIDONATE
METABOLITES

| INITIATION | INFLAMMATION | DESTRUCTION |

metalloproteinases. Indeed, it is possible that an essential defect in RA is a failure in one or more of these normal regulatory systems.[105]

EXTRA-ARTICULAR MANIFESTATIONS

Although characteristically a joint disease, RA can affect a number of other tissues.[106] These extra-articular manifestations probably occur with considerable frequency, but are usually subclinical. The extra-articular events may, however, dominate the clinical picture. Terms such as "rheumatoid disease" and "malignant rheumatoid arthritis" have been used to describe this form of the disease (see also Chapter 44).

VASCULITIS

The spectrum of vascular lesions that accompanies RA is detailed in Chapter 44. The cause of the various vascular lesions and their relationship to one another has not been defined, but a number of observations suggest that they result from injury induced by immune complexes, especially those containing antibodies to IgG. These include (1) the generally held view that patients with high levels of serum IgM rheumatoid factor have more systemic manifestations of the disease;[107–109] (2) a correlation of depressed serum complement activity, decreased concentration of C2 and C4, and hypercatabolism of C3 with the clinical signs of vasculitis;[109–111] (3) immunofluorescent detection of deposits of IgG, IgM, and complement (C3) in the vasa nervorum of patients with rheumatoid neuropathy, and immunoglobulins and rheumatoid factor in vessel walls of vasculitis patients;[112] and an association between vasculitis and increased levels of circulating immune complexes.[113–116]

As early as 1957, Franklin and his associates identified high-molecular-weight (22S) immune complexes in the serum of RA patients. Chemical dissociation of this material revealed 7S and 19S components, the latter with anti-Ig activity.[117] Subsequently, large amounts of unusual γ-globulin complexes with sedimentation rates ranging from 9 to 17S were found in serum from patients with advanced RA.[118] These complexes, which are readily dissociated to 7S units, have been designated "intermediate complexes." Monoclonal IgM rheumatoid factors were then used to demonstrate small complexes or aggregates of IgG in the serum of approximately 50% of patients with RA.[119] This method detects aggregates that fail to precipitate with polyclonal rheumatoid factors or C1q.

A later radioimmunoassay was based on the ability of test samples to inhibit the interaction of iodinated-aggregated IgG with monoclonal rheumatoid factor and detected immune complex-like material in the serum of 12 of 51 (27%) RA patients examined. The presence of this material was associated with more severe disease, greater functional impairment, and more-advanced joint destruction. The amount of inhibiting material was inversely related to serum C4 levels but not to rheumatoid factor titers. Three fourths of the patients had extra-articular manifestations including Sjögren's syndrome, leg ulcers, Felty's syndrome, neuropathy, and pulmonary fibrosis.[120] These findings have been subsequently confirmed and extended by others, using a variety of immune complex assays including C1q binding; Raji cells, and monoclonal rheumatoid factor.[113–116,121]

Approximately 30% of an unselected group of patients with RA had significant amounts of cryoglobulins. Two thirds of the cryoprecipitable protein was polyclonal IgG and IgM, with a higher IgM/IgG ratio than found in the whole serum from which they precipitated.[122] Systemic vasculitis, present in 3 of the original 38 patients, was associated with the largest amount of cryoglobulin. Subsequently, 5 more patients with vasculitis were studied, all of whom had detectable cryoglobulins. The cryoglobulin antiglobulin (rheumatoid factor) activity was mainly by IgM. Serial studies performed on vasculitis patients treated with cyclophosphamide disclosed a close relationship between the clinical evidence of vasculitis and the presence of cryoglobulins.[122] These findings were interpreted as evidence that the widespread vascular complications of RA are mediated, at least in part, by circulating immune complexes.

Other forms of rheumatoid factor have been described in rheumatoid vasculitis.[116,123,124] Theofilopoulos and his associates detected IgG rheumatoid factor in 10 of 15 (67%) patients with rheumatoid vasculitis, but in only 3 of 33 without vasculitis.[123] Eighty percent of the patients with vasculitis, but only 18% of those without, had 7S IgM in their serum, a finding since confirmed by others.[124]

In summary, most patients with RA have circulating soluble materials with the characteristics of immune complexes. Anti-γ-globulins of the IgG and IgM classes and IgG itself are integral parts of these soluble complexes, although the clinical usefulness of their measurement is questionable.[125] Finally, whether they are responsible for vasculitis or for the other extra-articular features or are merely markers for severe disease remains a moot question.

FELTY'S SYNDROME

In 1924, Felty described a symptom complex of chronic RA associated with splenomegaly and leukopenia.[126] Subsequently, additional features have been recognized, including skin hyperpigmentation, leg ulcers, generalized lymphadenopathy, anemia, and thrombocytopenia. Commonly, such patients have high titers of rheumatoid factor and antinuclear antibodies, subcutaneous nodules, and manifestations of systemic rheumatoid disease or the sicca complex (Sjögren's syndrome).[106,127]

No single explanation for the granulocytopenia that characterizes Felty's syndrome is satisfactory. Early speculations implicated hypersplenism or splenic sequestration of neutrophils. An inability to demonstrate trapping of radiolabeled cells in the spleen and the frequent failure of splenectomy to correct the leukopenia diminished the considered importance of this organ in Felty's syndrome.[128] Consistent evidence of impaired production of granulocytes is lacking, and the bone marrow is typically hyperplastic. This finding makes the observation that serum or lymphocytes from patients with Felty's syndrome can inhibit the growth of bone marrow cells in culture less interesting.[129–130] Indeed, although neutropenia is considered the hallmark of Felty's syndrome, leukokinetic studies show that two-thirds of these patients have a normal total blood neutrophil pool. Thus, their neutropenia appears to be due to an excessive margination of neutrophils, presumably into extravascular locations.[128]

An exception may be the small group of RA patients with neutropenia, incomplete features of Felty's syndrome, and increased numbers of large granular lymphocytes (LGL) in the blood and bone marrow.[131,132] By morphology, histochemistry, and phenotyping with monoclonal antibodies, they appear to be immature T cells with nonspecific killer cell activity. In these cases, neutropenia may result from either antibody-dependent cellular cytotoxicity related to antineutrophil antibodies or to myelosuppression by the abnormal LGL.[133]

A number of observations suggest that circulating factors, particularly antibodies, play a pathogenetic role in patients with Felty's syndrome. For instance, etiocholanolone normally mobilizes granulocytes from the bone marrow. Patients with Felty's syndrome do not respond to etiocholanolone and, in one instance, infusion of plasma from a patient blocked the granulocyte-mobilizing effect of this agent.[134] Circulating IgG antibodies against neutrophils are detected in the majority of patients with Felty's syndrome.[135] Some antinuclear antibodies react only with polymorphonuclear cell nuclei. Such granulocyte-reactive antinuclear factors are said to be found in virtually all patients with Felty's syndrome, in 75% of patients with RA, and in 30% of patients with systemic lupus erythematosus. These granulocyte-reactive antibodies fix human complement, unlike the conventional organ-nonspecific antinuclear factors.[136,137]

Immune complexes containing IgG and IgM antibodies are demonstrable in the cytoplasm of circulating white blood cells and in the serum of the majority of patients with Felty's syndrome. Similar inclusions are formed when normal neutrophils are incubated with serum from patients with this condition.[138] Most such patients have significant amounts of serum cryoglobulins containing IgG, IgM, complement components, and antinuclear and anti-γ-globulin antibodies. Granulocyte-reactive antinuclear antibody was selectively concentrated in some of the cryoglobulins.[139]

Undoubtedly, multiple factors, including antibodies, immune complexes, complement activation, which influences granulocyte margination, and cellular immune reactions, either singly or in combination, are responsible for the granulocytopenia that characterizes Felty's syndrome, and it is likely that different factors or combinations of factors are operative in each patient.

REFERENCES

1. Winchester, R.G.: Genetic aspects of rheumatoid arthritis. Springer Semin. Immunopathol., 4:89–102, 1981.
2. Nepom, G.T., Hansen, J.A., and Nepom, B.S.: The molecular basis for HLA class II associations with rheumatoid arthritis. J. Clin. Immunol., 7:1–7, 1987.
3. McDaniel, D.O., et al.: Analysis of restriction fragment length polymorphisms in rheumatic diseases. Rheum. Dis. Clin. N.A., 13:353–367, 1987.
4. Gregersen, P., et al.: Molecular diversity of HLA-DR4 haplotypes. Proc. Natl. Acad. Sci. U.S.A., 83:2642–2646, 1986.
5. Stewart, S.M., Alexander, W.R.M., and Duthie, J.J.R.: Isolation of diphtheroid bacilli from synovial membrane and fluid in rheumatoid arthritis. Ann. Rheum. Dis., 28:477–487, 1969.
6. Phillips, P.E.: Infection and the pathogenesis of connective tissue diseases. In Scientific Basis of Rheumatology. Edited by G.S. Panayi. Edinburgh, Churchill-Livingstone, 1982.
7. Bartholomew, L.E., and Bartholomew, F.N.: Antigenic bacterial polysaccharide in rheumatoid synovial effusions. Arthritis Rheum., 22:969–977, 1979.
8. Cole, B.C., et al.: New models of chronic synovitis in rabbits induced by mycoplasmal: Microbiological, histopathological, immunological observations in rabbits infected with Mycoplasma arthritides and Mycoplasma pulmonis. Infect. Immunol., 16:382–396, 1977.
9. Decker, J.L., and Barden, J.A.: In Infection and Immunology in the Rheumatic Diseases. Edited by D.C. Dumonde. Oxford, Blackwell, 1976.

10. Mansson, I., and Olhagen, B.: Fecal Clostridium perfringens and rheumatoid arthritis. J. Infect. Dis., 130:444–445, 1974.

11. Mansson, I., Norberg, R., and Olhagen, B.: Arthritis in pigs induced by dietary factors microbiologic, clinical and histological studies. Clin. Exp. Immunol., 9:677–693, 1971.

12. Utsinger, P.Q., Zvaifler, N.J., and Weiner, S.B.: Etiology. In Rheumatoid Arthritis: Etiology, Diagnosis, Management. Edited by P.D. Utsinger, N.J. Zvaifler, and G. Ehrlich. Philadelphia, J.B. Lippincott, 1985.

13. Wilder, R.L.: Proinflammatory microbial products as etiologic agents of inflammatory arthritis. Rheum. Dis. Clin. N.A., 13:293–306, 1987.

14. Pritchard, D.G., Settine, R.L., and Bennett, J.C.: Sensitive mass spectrometric procedures for the detection of bacterial cell wall components in rheumatoid joints. Arthritis Rheum., 23:608–610, 1980.

15. Holoshitz, J., et al.: T lymphocytes of rheumatoid arthritis patients show augmented reactivity to a fraction of mycobacteria cross reactive with cartilage. Lancet, 2:305–309, 1986.

16. Offenhoff, T.H., et al.: Evidence for an HLA-DR4 associated immune response gene for mycobacterium tuberculosis. Lancet, 2:310–313, 1986.

17. Wilkes, P.H., et al.: Virologic studies on rheumatoid arthritis. Arthitis Rheum., 16:446–454, 1973.

18. Marmion, B.P.: Infection, autoimmunity and rheumatoid arthritis. Clin. Rheum. Dis., 4:565–586, 1978.

19. Norval, M., and Smith, C.: Search for viral nucleic acid sequences in rheumatoid cells. Ann. Rheum. Dis., 38:456–462, 1979.

20. Ghose, T., Woodbury, J.F., and Hansell, M.M.: Interaction in vitro between synovial cells and autologous lymphocytes and sera from arthritis patients. J. Clin. Pathol., 28:550–558, 1975.

21. Griffiths, M.M., Smith, C.B., and Pepper, B.J.: Susceptibility of rheumatoid and nonrheumatoid synovial cells to antibody dependent cell mediated cytotoxicity. Arthritis Rheum., 21:97–104, 1978.

22. Gruhn, W.B., and McDuffie, F.C.: Studies of serum immunoglobulin binding to synovial fibroblast cultures from patients with rheumatoid arthritis. Arthritis Rheum., 23:10–16, 1980.

23. Paget, S.A., Anderson, K., and Phillips, P.E.: Absence of complement dependent cytotoxicity of rheumatoid sera for rheumatoid synovial cell cultures. Arthritis Rheum., 21:249–254, 1978.

24. Phillips, P.E., Anderson, K., and Paget, S.A.: Lack of antibody in rheumatoid arthritis to cultured synovial cells using adherotoxicity. (Abstract.) Arthritis Rheum., 23:732, 1980.

25. Smith, C., Habermann, E., and Hamerman, D.: A technique for investigating the antigenicity of cultured rheumatoid synovial cells. J. Rheumatol., 6:147–155, 1979.

26. Paget, S.A., et al.: Studies of lymphoblastoid cell lines derived from rheumatoid arthritis synovial membrane lymphocytes: Tissue reactivity of secreted immunoglobulin. (Abstract.) Arthritis Rheum., 23:728, 1980.

27. London, W.T., et al.: Concentration of rubella virus antigen in chondrocytes of congenitally infected rabbits. Nature, 226:172–173, 1970.

28. Johnson, R.E., and Hall, A.P.: Rubella arthritis. N. Engl. J. Med., 258:743–745, 1958.

29. Ogra, P.L., and Herd, J.K.: Arthritis associated with induced rubella infection. J. Immunol., 107:810–813, 1971.

30. Chantler, J.K., Ford, D.K., and Tingle, A.J.: Persistent rubella

31. Chantler, J.K., Ford, D.K., and Tingle, A.J.: Rubella associated arthritis: Rescue of rubella virus from peripheral blood lymphocytes two years post vaccinaiton. Infect. Immunol., 32:1274–1280, 1981.

32. Hilderbrandt, H.M., and Maassab, H.F.: Rubella synovitis in a one-year-old patient. N. Engl. J. Med., 274:1428–1430, 1966.

33. Weibel, R.E., et al.: Rubella vaccination in adult females. N. Engl. J. Med., 280:682–685, 1969.

34. Grahame, R., et al.: Chronic arthritis associated with the presence of intrasynovial rubella virus. Ann. Rheum. Dis., 42:2–13, 1983.

35. Chantler, J.K., Tingle, A.S., and Petty, R.: Persistent rubella virus infection associated with chronic arthritis in children. N. Engl. J. Med., 313:1117–1123, 1986.

36. Anderson, M.J., et al.: Human parvovirus, the cause of erythema infectiosum. Lancet 1:1378–1378, 1983.

37. Woolf, A.D., et al.: An epidemiologic study of human parvovirus infection in adults. Br. J. Rheum., 25:2, 1986.

38. White, D.G., et al.: Human parvovirus arthropathy. Lancet, 1:419–421, 1985.

39. Cohen, B.J., et al.: Human parvovirus infection in early rheumatoid and inflammatory arthritis. Ann. Rheum. Dis., 45:832–838, 1986.

40. Simpson, R.W., et al.: Association of parvoviruses with rheumatoid arthritis of humans. Science, 224:1425–1428, 1984.

41. Duffy, J., Lidsky, M.D., and Sharp, J.T.: Polyarthritis, polyarteritis and hepatitis B. Medicine, 55:19–37, 1976.

42. Inman, R.D.: Rheumatic manifestations of hepatitis virus B infection. Semin. Arthritis. Rheum., 11:406–420, 1982.

43. Wands, J.R., et al.: The pathogenesis of arthritis associated with acute hepatitis B surface antigen positive hepatitis. J. Clin. Invest., 55:930–936, 1975.

44. Atwater, E.C., and Jacox, R.F.: The latex fixation test in patients with liver disease. Ann. Intern. Med., 58:419–425, 1963.

45. Morris, E.L., and Stevens, M.B.: Rheumatoid arthritis—A sequel to HBsAg hepatitis. Am. J. Med., 64:859–862, 1978.

46. Greaves, M.F., Brown, G., and Rickinson, A.B.: Epstein-Barr virus binding sites on lymphocyte subpopulations and the origin of lymphoblasts in cultured lymphoid cell lines and in blood of patients with infectious mononucleosis. Clin. Immunol. Immunopathol., 3:514–524, 1975.

47. Yefenof, E., Klein, G., and Kvarnunzk, J.: Relationship between complement activation, complement binding, and EBV absorption by human hematopoietic cell lines. Cell Immunol., 31:225–233, 1977.

48. Chervenick, P.A.: Infectious mononucleosis. Disease A Month, December 1974, pp. 955–956.

49. Utsinger, P.D., Zvaifler, N.J., and Weiner, S.B.: Etiology of rheumatoid arthritis. In Rheumatoid Arthritis. Edited by P.D. Utsinger, N.J. Zvaifler, and G.E. Ehrlich. Philadelphia, Lippincott, 1985, pp. 21–43.

50. Catalano, M.A., et al.: Antibody to the rheumatoid arthritis nuclear antigen: Its relationship to in vivo Epstein-Barr virus infection. J. Clin. Invest., 65:1238–1242, 1980.

51. Alspaugh, M.A., et al.: Elevated levels of antibodies to Epstein-Barr virus antigens in sera and synovial fluids of patients with rheumatoid arthritis. J. Clin. Invest., 67:1134–1140, 1981.

52. Ferrell, P.B., Aitcheson, C.T., and Pearson, G.R.: Antibodies to Epstein-Barr virus related antigens in the serum of patients with rheumatoid arthritis. J. Clin. Invest., 67:681–687, 1981.

53. Silverman, S.L., and Schumacher, H.R.: Antibodies to Ep-

stein-Barr viral antigens in early rheumatoid arthritis. Arthritis Rheum., *24*:1465–1468, 1981.

54. Venables, P.J.W., et al.: Titers of antibody to RANA in rheumatoid arthritis and normal sera. Arthritis Rheum., *24*:1459–1464, 1981.

55. Depper, J.M., Zvaifler, N.J., and Bluestein, H.G.: Impaired regulation of Epstein Barr virus induced outgrowth in rheumatoid arthritis is due to a T cell defect. J. Immunol., *127*:1899–1902, 1981.

56. Slaughter, L., et al.: In vitro effects of Epstein-Barr virus on peripheral mononuclear cells from patients with rheumatoid and normal controls. J. Exp. Med., *148*:1429–1434, 1978.

57. Tosato, G., Steinberg, A.D., and Blaese, R.M.: Defective EBV-specific suppressor T cell function in rheumatoid arthritis. N. Engl. J. Med., *305*:1238–1243, 1981.

58. Kahan, A., et al.: Different defects of T cell regulation of Epstein Barr virus induced B cell activation in rheumatoid arthritis. Arthritis Rheum., *28*:961–970, 1985.

59. Bardwick, P.A., et al.: Altered regulation of Epstein-Barr virus induced lymphoblast proliferation in rheumatoid arthritis lymphoid cells. Arthritis Rheum., *23*:626–632, 1980.

60. Hasler, F., Bluestein, H.G., Zvaifler, N.J., and Epstein, L.: Analysis of the defects responsible for the impaired regulation of Epstein-Barr virus-induced B cell proliferation by rheumatoid arthritis lymphocytes. I. Diminished gamma interferon production in response to autologous stimulation. J. Exp. Med., *157*:173–188, 1983.

61. Hasler, F., Bluestein, H.G., Zvaifler, N.J., and Epstein, L.: Analysis of the defects responsible for the impaired regulation of Epstein-Barr virus-induced B cell proliferation by rheumatoid arthritis lymphocytes. II. Role of monocytes and the increased sensitivity of rheumatoid arthritis lymphocytes to prostaglandin E. J. Immunol., *131*:768–772, 1983.

62. Konttinen, Y.T., Bluestein, H.G., and Zvaifler, N.J.: Regulation of the growth of Epstein Barr virus infected B cells. Growth regression of E rosetting cells from VCA positive donors is a combined effect of autologous mixed lymphocyte reaction and activation of T8+ memory cells. J. Immunol., *134*:2289–2293, 1985.

63. Lotz, M., et al.: Release of lymphokines after infection with Epstein Barr virus. II. A monocyte dependent inhibitor of interleukin-1 down regulates the production of interleukin-2 and interferon in rheumatoid arthritis. J. Immunol., *136*:3643–3648, 1986.

64. Konttinen, Y.T., Bluestein, H.G., and Zvaifler, N.J.: Regulation of the growth of Epstein Barr virus infected B cells: Temporal profile of the in vitro development of three distinct cytotoxic cells. Cell Immunol, *103*:84–95, 1986.

65. Tsoukas, C.Q., et al.: Lysis of autologous Epstein Barr virus infected B cells by cytotoxic T lymphocytes of rheumatoid arthritis patients. Clin. Immunol. Immunopathol., *24*:8–14, 1982.

66. Tosato, G., et al.: Abnormally elevated frequency of Epstein Barr virus infected B cells in the blood of patients with rheumatoid arthritis. J. Clin. Invest., *73*:1789–1795, 1984.

67. Hamerman, D., Barland, P., and Janis, R.: The structure and chemistry of the synovial membrane in health and disease. *In* The Biological Basis of Medicine. Vol 3. Edited by E.E. Bittar and N. Bittar. Philadelphia, W.B. Saunders, 1969.

68. Cooke, T.D., and Jasin, H.E.: The pathogenesis of chronic inflammation in experimental antigen-induced arthritis. I. The role of antigen on the local immune response. Arthritis Rheum., *15*:327–337, 1972.

69. Bennett, J.C.: The infectious etiology of rheumatoid arthritis: New considerations. Arthritis Rheum., *21*:531–538, 1978.

70. Trentham, D.E.: Clues provided by animal models of arthritis. Rheum. Dis. Clin. N.A., *13*:307–318, 1987.

71. Kulka, J.P., et al.: Early joint lesions of rheumatoid arthritis. Arch. Pathol., *59*:129–150, 1955.

72. Schumacher, H.R.: Synovial membrane and fluid morphologic alterations in early rheumatoid arthritis. Microvascular injury and virus-like particles. Ann. N.Y. Acad. Sci., *256*:39–64, 1975.

73. Fassbender, H.G.: Potential aggressiveness of the synovial tissue in rheumatoid arthritis. *In* Articular Synovium. Edited by P. Franchimont. Basel, S. Karger, 1982.

74. Gardner, D.L.: The Pathology of Rheumatoid Arthritis. London, Arnold, 1972.

75. Harris, E.D., Jr.: Pathogenesis of rheumatoid arthritis. *In* Textbook of Rheumatology. Edited by W.N. Kelley, E.D. Harris, S. Ruddy, and C.B. Sledge. Philadelphia, W.B. Saunders, 1985.

76. Zvaifler, N.J.: The immunopathology of joint inflammation in rheumatoid arthritis. Adv. Immunol., *16*:265–337, 1973.

77. Ishikawa, H., and Ziff, M.: Electron microscopic observations of immunoreactive cells in the rheumatoid synovial membrane. Arthritis Rheum., *19*:1–14, 1976.

78. Burmester, G.R., et al.: Ia+ T cells in synovial fluid and tissues of patients with rheumatoid arthritis. Arthritis Rheum., *24*:1370–1376, 1981.

79. Fox, R.I., et al.: Synovial fluid lymphocytes differ from peripheral blood lymphocytes in patients with rheumatoid arthritis. J. Immunol., *128*:351–354, 1982.

80. Konttinen, Y.J., et al.: Characterization of the immunocompetent cells of rheumatoid synovium from tissue sections and eluates. Arthritis Rheum., *24*:71–79, 1981.

81. Munthe, F., and Natvig, J.B.: Immunoglobulin classes, subclasses, and complexes of IgG rheumatoid factor in rheumatoid synovial cells. Clin. Exp. Immunol., *12*:55–70, 1972.

82. Natvig, J.B., and Munthe, E.: Self associating IgG rheumatoid factor represents a major response of plasma cells in rheumatoid inflammatory tissue. Ann. N.Y. Acad. Sci., *256*:88–95, 1975.

83. Smiley, J.D., Sachs, C., and Ziff, M.: In vitro synthesis of immunoglobulin by rheumatoid synovial membrane. J. Clin. Invest., *47*:624–632, 1968.

84. Sliwinski, A.J., and Zvaifler, N.J.: In vivo synthesis of IgG by rheumatoid synovium. J. Lab. Clin. Med., *76*:304–310, 1970.

85. Cecere, F., et al.: Evidence for the local production and utilization of immunoreactants in rheumatoid arthritis. Arthritis Rheum., *25*:1307–1315, 1982.

86. Klareskog, L., et al.: Immune functions of human synovial cells. Phenotypic and T cell regulatory properties of macrophage-like cells that express HLA-DR. Arthritis Rheum., *25*:488–501, 1982.

87. Janossy, G., et al.: Rheumatoid arthritis: A disease of T lymphocyte-macrophage immunoregulation. Lancet, *2*:839–842, 1981.

88. Ward, P.A., and Zvaifler, N.J.: Complement derived leukotactic factors in inflammatory synovial fluids of humans. J. Clin. Invest., *50*:606–616, 1971.

89. Winchester, R.J.: Characterization of IgG complexes in patients with rheumatoid arthritis. Ann. N.Y. Acad. Sci., *256*:73–81, 1975.

90. Lotz, M., Carson, D.A., and Vaughan, J.A.: Substance P activation of rheumatoid synoviocytes: Neural pathways and pathogenesis of arthritis. Science, *235*:893–895, 1987.

91. Kurosaka, M., and Ziff, M.: Immunoelectron microscopic study of the distribution of T cell subsets in rheumatoid synovium. J. Exp. Med., *158*:1181–1210, 1983.

92. Husby, G., and Williams, R.C., Jr.: Immunohistochemical studies of interleukin-2 and gamma interferon in rheumatoid arthritis. Arthritis Rheum., *28*:174–181, 1985.

93. Firestein, G., and Zvaifler, N.J.: Peripheral blood and synovial fluid monocyte activation in inflammatory arthritis. II. Absence of synovial fluid and synovial tissue interferon suggests that gamma interferon is not the primary MAF in arthritis. Arthritis Rheum., *30*:864–871, 1987.

94. Lotz, M., et al.: Basis for defective responses of rheumatoid arthritis synovial fluid lymphocytes to anti-CD3 (T3) antibodies. J. Clin. Invest., *78*:713–721, 1986.

95. Miossec, P., Kashiwado, T., and Ziff, M.: Inhibitors of interleukin-2 in rheumatoid synovial fluid. Arthritis Rheum., *30*:121–129, 1987.

96. Barrett A.J.: The possible role of neutrophil proteinases in damage to articular cartilage. Agents Actions *8*:11–18, 1978.

97. Kobayashi, I., and Ziff, M.: Electron microscopic studies of the cartilage pannus function in rheumatoid arthritis. Arthritis Rheum., *18*:475–483, 1975.

98. Dayer, J.M., et al.: Interactions among rheumatoid synovial cells and monocyte-macrophages: Production of collagenase stimulating factor by human monocytes exposed to concanavalin A or immunoglobulin Fc fragment. J. Immunol., *124*:1712–1720, 1980.

99. Dayer, J.M., Krane, S.M., Russell, R.G.G., and Robinson, D.R.: Production of collagenase and prostaglandins by isolated adherent rheumatoid synovial cells. Proc. Natl. Acad. Sci., U.S.A., *73*:945–949, 1976.

100. Dayer, J.M., Robinson, D.R., and Krane, S.M.: Prostaglandin production by rheumatoid synovial cells: Stimulation by a factor from human mononuclear cells. J. Exp. Med., *145*:1399–1404, 1977.

101. Dayer, J.M., et al.: Human recombinant interleukin-1 stimulates collagenase and prostaglandin E2 production by human synovial cells. J. Clin. Invest., *77*:645–648, 1986.

102. Dingle, J.T., Saklatvala, J., and Hembry, R.: A cartilage catabolic factor from synovium. Biochem. J., *184*:177–180, 1979.

103. Meats, J.E., McGuire, M.K., and Russell, R.G.: Human synovium releases a factor which stimulates chondrocyte production of PGE and plasminogen activator. Nature, *286*:891–892, 1980.

104. Ridge, S.C., Oronsky, A.L., and Kerwar, S.S.: Induction of the synthesis of latent collagenase and latent neutral protease in chondrocytes by a factor synthesized by activated macrophages. Arthritis Rheum., *23*:448–453, 1980.

105. McGuire, M.K.B., et al.: *In* Articular Synovium. Edited by P. Franchmont. S. Karger, Basel, 1982.

106. Hurd, E.R.: Extra-articular manifestations of rheumatoid arthritis. Semin. Arthritis Rheum., *8*:151–176, 1979.

107. Epstein, W.Y., and Engleman, E.P.: The relationship of the rheumatoid factor content of serum to clinical neurovascular manifestations of rheumatoid arthritis. Arthritis Rheum., *2*:250–258, 1959.

108. Gordon, D.A., Stein, J.L., and Broder, I.: The extra-articular features of rheumatoid arthritis. A systematic analysis of 127 cases. Am. J. Med., *54*:445–452, 1973.

109. Mongan, E.S., et al.: A study of the relationship of seronegative and seropositive rheumatoid arthritis to each other and to necrotizing vasculitis. Am. J. Med., *47*:23–35, 1969.

110. Franco, A.E., and Schur, P.H.: Hypocomplementemia in rheumatoid arthritis. Arthritis Rheum., *14*:231–238, 1971.

111. Weinstein, A., et al.: Metabolism of the third component of complement (C3) in patients with rheumatoid arthritis. Arthritis Rheum., *15*:49–56, 1972.

112. Conn, D.L., McDuffie, F.C., and Dyck, P.J.: Immunopathologic study of sural nerves in rheumatoid arthritis. Arthritis Rheum., *15*:135–143, 1972.

113. Gupta, R.C., et al.: Comparison of three immunoassays for immune complexes in rheumatoid arthritis. Arthritis Rheum., *22*:433–439, 1979.

114. Halla, J.T., Volanakis, J.E., and Schrohenloher, R.E.: Immune complexes in rheumatoid arthritis sera and synovial fluids. A comparison of 3 methods. Arthritis Rheum., *22*:440–448, 1979.

115. Hay, F.C., Nineham, J.L., Perumal, R., and Roitt, I.M.: Intra-articular and circulating immune complexes and antiglobulins (IgG and IgM). Ann. Rheum. Dis., *38*:1–7, 1979.

116. Scott, D.G.I., Bacon, P.A., and Tribe, C.R.: Systemic rheumatoid vasculitis. A clinical and laboratory study of 50 cases. Medicine, *60*:288–296, 1981.

117. Franklin, E.C., Holman, H.R., Muller-Eberhard, H.R., and Kunkel, H.G.: An unusual protein component of high molecular weight in the serum of patients with rheumatoid arthritis. J. Exp. Med., *105*:425–438, 1957.

118. Kunkel, H.G., Franklin, E.C., and Muller-Eberhard, H.J.:Studies on the isolation and characterization of the "rheumatoid factor." J. Clin. Invest., *38*:424–434, 1959.

119. Winchester, R.J., Agnello, V., and Kunkel, H.G.: Gamma globulin complexes in synovial fluids of patients with rheumatoid arthritis: Partial characterization and relationship to lowered complement levels. Clin. Exp. Immunol., *6*:689–706, 1970.

120. Luthra, H.S., et al.: Immune complexes in sera and synovial fluids of patients with rheumatoid arthritis. J. Clin. Invest., *56*:458–466, 1975.

121. Nydegger, U.E., et al.: Circulating complement breakdown products in patients with rheumatoid arthritis. Correlation between plasma C3d, circulating immune complexes and clinical activity. J. Clin. Invest., *59*:862–868, 1977.

122. Weisman, M.H., and Zvaifler, N.J.: Cryoglobulinemia in rheumatoid arthritis. J. Clin. Invest., *56*:725–730, 1975.

123. Theofilopoulos, A.N., Burtonboy, G., LoSpalluto, J.J., and Ziff, M.: IgG rheumatoid factor and low molecular weight IgM. Arthritis Rheum., *17*:272–284, 1974.

124. Stage, D.E., and Mannik, M.: 7S gamma M-globulin in rheumatoid arthritis. Arthritis Rheum., *14*:440–450, 1971.

125. Plotz, P.: Studies of immune complexes. Arthritis Rheum., *25*:1151–1155, 1982.

126. Felty, A.R.: Chronic arthritis in the adult, associated with splenomegaly and leucopenia. Report of 5 cases of an unusual clinical syndrome. Bull. Johns Hopkins Hosp., *35*:16–20, 1924.

127. Ruderman, M., Miller, L.M., and Pinals, R.S.: Clinical and serologic observations on 27 patients with Felty's syndrome. Arthritis Rheum., *11*:377–384, 1968.

128. Vincent, P.C., Levi, J.A., and Macqueen, A.: The mechanism of neutropenia in Felty's syndrome. Br. J. Haematol., *27*:463–475, 1974.

129. Duckham, D.J., Rhyne, R.L., Smith, F.E., and Williams, R.C.: Retardation of colony growth of an in vitro bone marrow culture using sera from patients with Felty's syndrome, SLE, RA, and other disease states. Arthritis Rheum., *18*:323–333, 1975.

130. Starkebaum, G., Singer, J.W., and Arend, W.P.: Humoral and cellular immune mechanisms of neutropenia in patients with Felty's syndrome. Clin. Exp. Immunol., *39*:307–314, 1979.

131. Wallis, W.J., et al.: Polyarthritis and neutropenia associated

with circulating large granular lymphocytes. Ann. Intern. Med., *103*:357–362, 1985.

132. Barton, J.C., et al.: Rheumatoid arthritis associated with expanded populations of granular lymphocytes. Ann. Intern. Med., *104*:314–323, 1986.

133. Newland, A., et al.: Chronic T cell lymphocytosis: A review of 21 cases. Br. J. Haematol., *58*:433, 1984.

134. Kimball, H.R., et al.: Marrow granulocyte reserves in the rheumatic diseases. Arthritis Rheum., *16*:345–352, 1973.

135. Rosenthal, F.D., Beeley, J.M., Gelsthorpe, K., and Doughty, K.: White cell antibodies and the aetiology of Felty's syndrome. Q. J. Med., *43*:187–203, 1974.

136. Faber, V., and Elling, P.: Leukocyte specific antinuclear factors in patients with Felty's syndrome, rheumatoid arthritis, systemic lupus erythematosus, and other diseases. Acta Med. Scand., *179*:257–267, 1966.

137. Wiik, A., and Munthe, E.: Complement fixing granulocyte specific antinuclear factors in neutropenic cases of rheumatoid arthritis. Immunology, *26*:1127–1134, 1974.

138. Hurd, E.R., Andreis, M., and Ziff, M.: Phagocytosis of immune complexes by polymorphonuclear leukocytes in patients with Felty's syndrome. Clin. Exp. Immunol., *28*:413–425, 1977.

139. Weisman, M.H., and Zvaifler, N.J.: Cryoimmunoglobulinemia in Felty's syndrome. Arthritis Rheum., *19*:103–110, 1975.

PATHOLOGY OF RHEUMATOID ARTHRITIS AND ALLIED DISORDERS

41

AUBREY J. HOUGH, JR., and LEON SOKOLOFF

The principal lesions of rheumatoid arthritis (RA) are found in the diarthrodial joints and, to a lesser extent, in the related tissues—tendons and their sheaths, bursae, and periarticular subcutaneous tissue. The systemic manifestations, the subject of much study during the past three decades, suggest use of the term "rheumatoid disease." Although extra-articular lesions undoubtedly occur, their incidence should not be exaggerated; they are far less frequent and severe than lesions in the joints.

Excellent descriptions of the long-standing joint changes have been published.[1] Knowledge of the morbid anatomy of RA is limited by a number of factors. The chronicity of the disease often makes tissue available for study only in its late stages. The lesions often lack histologic specificity and vary from site to site within the joints. The structures principally affected are frequently not accessible to the pathologist. For these reasons, light and immunomicroscopic study of biopsy material obtained early in the course of the illness has provided insights into the histogenesis of the lesions that have not been possible on postmortem examination.[2]

ARTICULAR LESIONS

All evidence indicates that the joint changes have their inception in the synovial tissue. Despite similarities in the character of the synovitis to that of infectious conditions and despite the prominent subchondral involvement of the bone in RA, no basis exists for believing that the synovial inflammation follows an initial seeding of the adjacent bone marrow, as it commonly does in hematogenous, infectious arthritis (Fig. 41–1).

SYNOVITIS

The microscopic appearance of the synovial tissues is variable.[3] Three pathologic elements, although integrally related and continuous, should be distinguished: (1) exudation; (2) cellular infiltration; and (3) granulation tissue development. (See also Chapter 15.)

Exudation

Congestion and the edema are most marked at the internal surface of the synovium, particularly close to margins of the articular cartilage (circulus vasculosus), and have their counterpart in effusion into the joint space. In focal areas of desquamation of synovial lining cells and of necrosis of the superficial synovial tissue, compact fibrin exudes onto the surface and, to some extent, into the swollen tissues (see Chapter 11 for evidence of synovial ischemia in RA).

Cellular Infiltration

Small numbers of polymorphonuclear leukocytes emigrate with edema fluid. Foci of necrosis and purulent exudation are seen at times in older lesions, and the concept of secondary infection need not be invoked on this score.

FIG. 41–1. Sagittal section of the knee in a patient with RA. Thickened, villous synovial tissue is seen in the suprapatellar pouch. A small Baker's cyst protrudes from the popliteal surface. A papillary pannus has completely replaced the articular cartilage of the patella and smaller segments on the femur and tibia. The dark portions of the marrow of the femur and tibia are areas of congestion and osteitis.

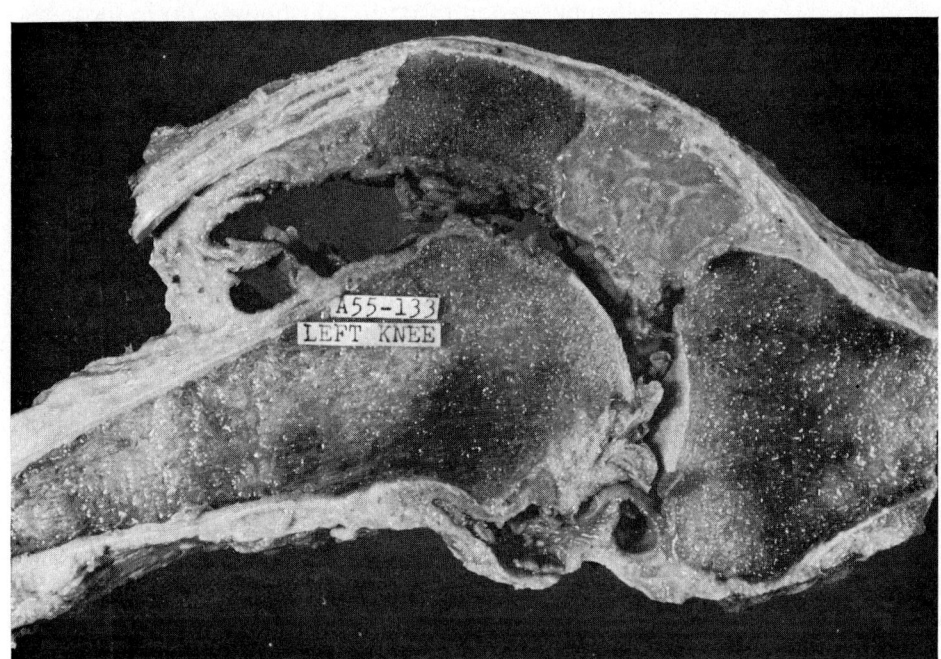

The principal infiltrating cell, particularly in early lesions, is a small lymphocyte. It is distributed in two patterns in the superficial positions of the synovium: diffusely and in small, nodular aggregates. These cells may or may not be arranged about small blood vessels. The nodular aggregates, sometimes called *Allison-Ghormley nodules,* characteristically lack the reticular framework of lymphoid nodules. In long-standing lesions, true lymphoid follicles with germinal centers are not rare (Fig. 41–2). Close cell-to-cell contacts between lymphocytes and plasma cells have been seen with electron microscopy.[4] Many of the lymphocytes in the synovial infiltrates are T cells.[5] Recently, OKT4 and OKT8 antibodies have distinguished two categories of T cells, helper-inducer and suppressor-cytotoxic, in the synovium.[6,7] The proportion of OKT8 cells is reduced in early perivenular lesions and is increased in late areas, in which macrophage-like cells are increased in numbers and lymphocyte transformation takes place. These macrophage-like cells express the DR antigen and reflect immunocompetence and mature function.[8,9] Paradoxically, the overall T-cell suppressor activity of RA synovium is decreased.[10] Natural killer (NK) activity is lower in RA synovial and synovial fluid lymphocytes than in peripheral blood, where NK cell levels are normal.[11]

In late cases, a large proportion or even a majority of the infiltrating cells are immunoglobulin-producing plasma cells.[12] When the synovium is stained with labeled aggregated immunoglobulin G (IgG), fluorescein, or ferritin tagging in electron micrographs, is found principally in the cytoplasm of the plasma cell, demonstrating a local synthesis of rheumatoid factors.[13] Areas of old hemorrhage are common, as evidenced by deposition of hemosiderin and, sometimes, by the presence of foam cells.[14]

Multinucleated giant cells are not common, but two types may be seen.[15] One is an ovoid pleomorphic cell, close to the synovial lining. It has three to eight peripheral nuclei (Fig. 41–3), as well as a basophilic cytoplasm similar to those of synovial lining cells. The other type of multinucleated cell is a foreign body phagocyte related to bone and cartilage detritus.

More-recent evidence suggests that tissue-type mast cells infiltrate the synovium in RA and that they may play a role in mediating cartilage erosion.[16,17] Sites of preferential accumulation include areas of vascular penetration and fibrosis as well as foci of cartilage erosion.[18]

FIG. 41–2. Chronic synovitis in long-standing RA. In addition to the usual diffuse infiltration of chronic inflammatory cells into the synovial tissue, a true lymphoid follicle with a germinal center is present. The larger cells, subjacent to the swollen synovial lining, are plasma cells (hematoxylin and eosin stain ×182).

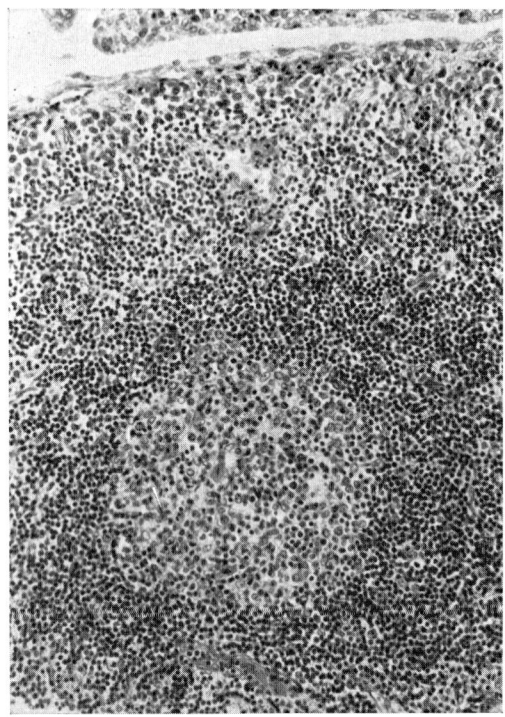

Granulation Tissue

As a result of these processes, the synovial tissue becomes grossly thickened. Proliferation of blood vessels and of synovial fibroblasts is most marked in areas of cellular infiltration and is accompanied by multiplication and enlargement of synovial lining cells. The lining cells become elongated in places and are oriented in a closely arranged palisade perpendicular to the surface. The hypertrophy has a villous character most marked near the joint cartilages. The papillary fronds may reach 2.5 cm in height and are approximately 1 to 2 mm in diameter (see Fig. 41–1). They may or may not adhere to each other. The oxygen uptake, glucose use, and lactate production of the tissue are increased as a result of both proliferation of granulation tissue and infiltration of inflammatory cells.[19] Lining cells are stained heavily by several histochemical diaphorase procedures and have a prominent endoplasmic reticulum,[20] evidence of high metabolic and secretory activity. They also contain many lysosomes and immune complex components.[15,21] Variable, sometimes extensive, ulceration of the synovial lining is a common feature of active RA. Necrotic

fronds of the villous tissue are infiltrated with fibrin or fibrin-like protein. When sloughed into the synovial cavity, they constitute rice bodies.[22] The collagen types and proportions of rice bodies are identical to those in RA synovium.[23,24] Immunohistochemical demonstration of fibrin and fibronectin in loose-textured rice bodies documents organization of exudate as a feature of their development.[25,26] Only in this sense is fibrin the defining feature of an "early" rice body and is collagen formation the defining feature of a late one. The initial source of the collagen is synovium and its granulation tissue that have undergone necrosis and ulceration.

Although these changes are typically present in RA, they lack histologic specificity. Statistical analysis has shown a correspondence between histologic features and clinical diagnosis in only 54 to 78% of chronic arthritic disorders.[3,27] Indistinguishable changes may be seen in unrelated disorders in man and in other species.[28,29]

SUBCHONDRAL BONE LESIONS

An inflammatory reaction commonly occurs in the epiphyseal bone. Its histologic character is similar to that of synovial tissue, although numbers of osteoclasts are also present. The subchondral granulation tissue is continuous with that in the synovium, through defects in the cortex of the bone near the joint. These defects are presumed originally to have been normal vascular foramina, enlarged by osteitis. Grossly, the bone marrow appears congested in these areas. The bone undergoes irregular osteolysis, which accounts for the loss of radiopacity in the para-articular tissues. In juvenile patients, the osteitis may extend into the epiphyseal plate; in such instances, bone growth is retarded, and rheumatic dwarfism results. Sizable cyst-like areas of bone destruction may be present (Fig. 41–4). Bony erosion occurs preferentially in areas not covered by articular cartilage, the so-called "bare areas." The articular cortex also is involved by the osteolysis. Side by side with the osteolysis, new bone formation occurs, and remodeling of the bone progresses under the direction of mechanical forces acting on the joint. In phalanges, "periosteitis" is frequently described as part of RA, but is not accurate, strictly speaking. The synovial recesses in the phalanges are frequently large and extend for a long distance proximally on the bone shafts. In such instances, the synovitis may evoke new bone formation in the immediately adjacent cortex. Nevertheless, periosteitis, unrelated to synovitis, is not characteristic of RA; this feature distinguishes RA from Reiter's dis-

FIG. 41–3. Synovitis in RA. Synovial lining cells are elongated and are arranged in a palisade radial to the surface. Some of the lining cells appear multinucleated, and similar giant cells are located at a slight distance from them (hematoxylin and eosin stain ×234).

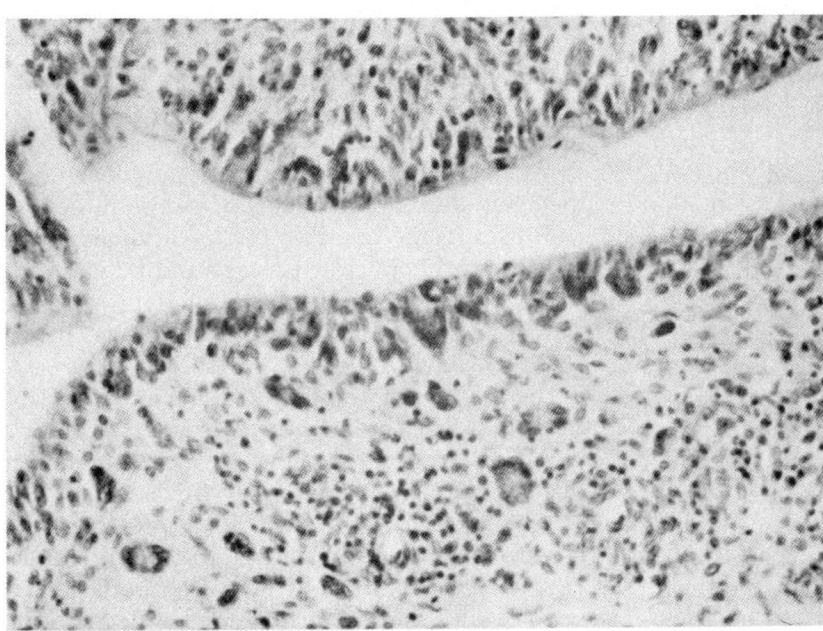

FIG. 41–4. Advanced destruction of the articular cortex of the distal femur in RA. What appear to be cystic spaces and pores in this macerated preparation are occupied in vivo by granulation tissue in the subchondral marrow and adhesions in the joint cavity.

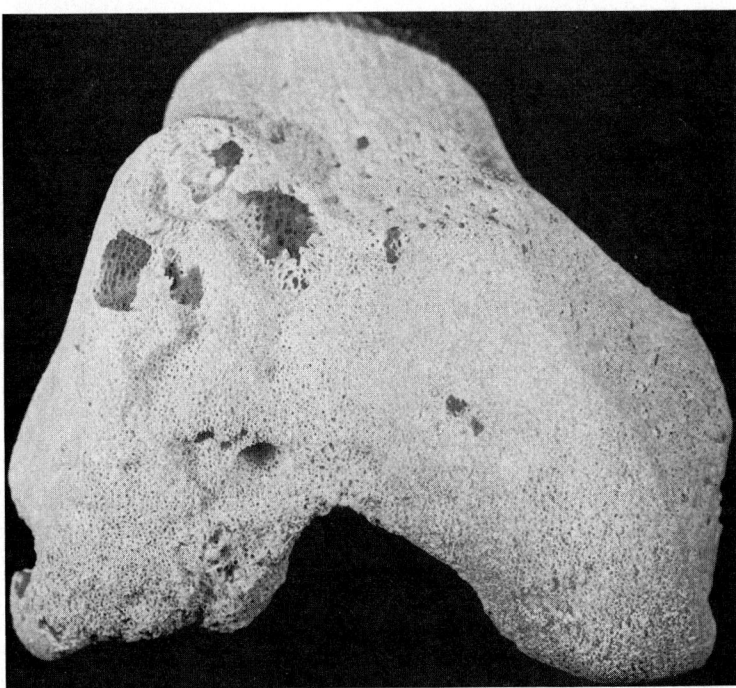

ease and from infectious arthritis. Osteoporosis often persists in burned-out, deformed specimens and may be attributed to disuse atrophy. At times, severe and widespread osteoporosis, for which no immediate explanation can be offered, is encountered.*

LESIONS OF ARTICULAR CARTILAGE

The articular cartilage is resistant to inflammatory lysis. Its surface is involved by extension of the inflammatory process from the adjacent synovium; the granulation tissue that forms a covering mantle is known as a *pannus* (see Fig. 41–1). In contemporary specimens, the pannus is usually inconspicuous, unlike that illustrated in Figure 41–1 and in classic accounts. Perhaps this change is the result of active use associated with present-day physiatric measures or better medical therapy. The destructive changes in the cartilage are most conspicuous at the junction with the synovium; in the femoral head, this means the perifoveal as well as the peripheral margin. The eroded areas have an irregular, "chewed-out" configuration, but are sharply defined. They thus differ both in quality and location from the cartilaginous lesions of osteoarthritis.

Like hypertrophic synovitis, pannus formation is not a specific feature of RA.[3,28] Concurrent with the ingrowth of the pannus and the subchondral granulation tissue, the articular cartilage disappears.[30,31] A possible mechanism for this process is provided in Chapter 42. Immediately adjacent chondrocytes are often necrotic. The fine structure of the surface is often disturbed, even when the cartilage appears normal grossly.[32] Whether granulations themselves destroy the cartilage or whether they represent a concomitant to an exudative, chondrolytic inflammation is unknown. Numerous explanations for the cartilage destruction accompanying pannus formation are supported by experimental and pathologic observations. Vascularity may allow leaching out of cartilage matrix, which normally retains its integrity by being avascular.[33] Other views are that the pannus may impede the normal, nourishing percolation of interstitial fluid through the cartilage. Several different enzymatic mechanisms have been proposed for chondrolysis. These enzymes include collagenase and neutral proteases derived from polymorphonuclear leukocytes, catheptic enzymes originating in synovial lining cells, and collagenase from the synovial granulation tis-

sue.[34–37] Cells elaborating collagenase have been characterized by a dendritic appearance in monolayer cultures of synovium.[38] Collagen fibrils have been observed in the cytoplasm of pannus cells.[39] Recently, macrophages have been shown to elaborate catabolin-like substances that stimulate chondrocytes to resorb matrix, and macrophage-like cells synthesizing prostaglandin E have been identified in RA.[40,41] Polymorphonuclear neutrophils are not readily apparent at the joint surface in conventional sections; however, they have been found in special concentrations at the pannus-cartilage interface by histochemical staining for polymorphonuclear elastase and by electron microscopy.[34,35] The presence of tissue-type mast cells in synovium and their release of histamine has been noted previously.[18]

The role of direct immune attack on articular cartilage in RA has been summarized by Cooke.[42] Using immunofluorescent staining, he found intense granular deposits of IgG and C3 in the cartilage of 85 to 92% of subjects with classic RA. Less consistent or intense amounts of IgA and IgM were present. The deposits were confined to the most superficial 0.3 mm or so of the surface. The degraded appearance of the surface was comparable to that seen in experimentally induced enzymatic digestion.

Late changes may include a dense fibrous connective tissue replacing the hyaline cartilage and penetrating the subchondral bone. This process may or may not be associated with ankylosis. Secondary osteoarthritic changes are also common in long-standing lesions.

ANKYLOSIS

The granulation tissue may form adhesions and may undergo cicatrization. The newly formed articular connective tissue has a pluripotential capacity for maturation. It may variously undergo metaplasia into synovial tissue, fibrous or hyaline cartilage, or bone; the adhesive bands may thereby cause fibrous, cartilaginous, or, rarely, bony ankylosis (Fig. 41–5).

JOINT DEFORMITIES

Several factors contribute to the deformities of RA. Most important of these is the inflammatory destruction and remodeling by the articulating surfaces under the influence of the mechanical forces of muscle pull. These changes may lead to subluxation (Fig. 41–6). Weakening of capsular and ligamentous supports by the inflammation may be of considerable

---

Editor's note. Osteoclastic activation, even at sites remote from the inflamed joints, has led to speculation that lymphokines, such as osteoclast-activating factor (OAF), are responsible (Kennedy, A.C., et al.: Clin. Sci. Mol. Med., 51:205–207, 1976.)

FIG. 41–5. Bony ankylosis of the knee in RA. A bridge of bone unites the patella of the femur and the condyles of the femur and tibial plateau to each other.

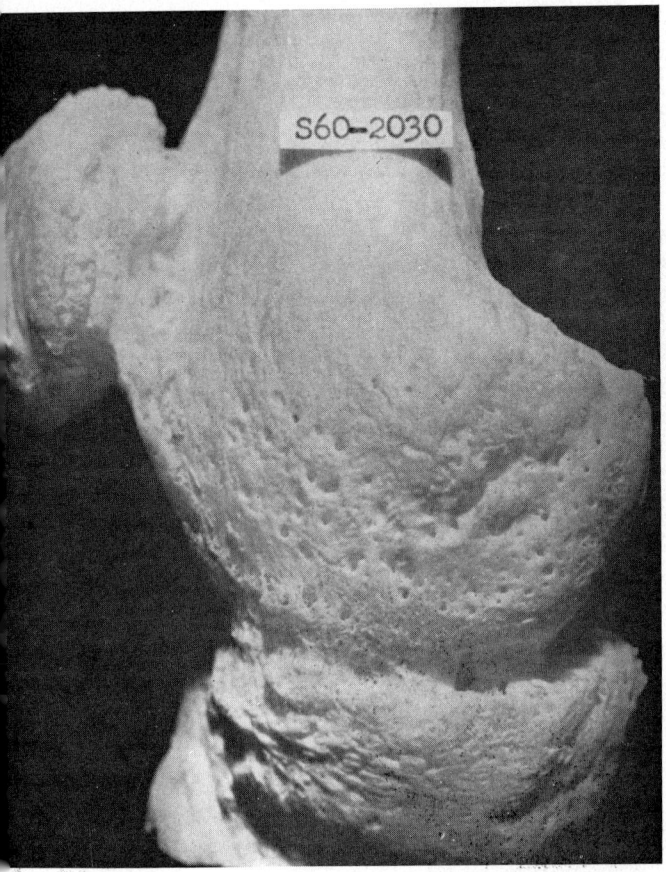

FIG. 41–6. Characteristic knuckle deformities in RA. The proximal phalanges are subluxated beneath the metacarpal heads. The tendons are displaced from their normal position over the center of the joint in association with the ulnar deviation of the fingers. No gross inflammatory change is present in the tendons, however, unlike in Figure 41–7.

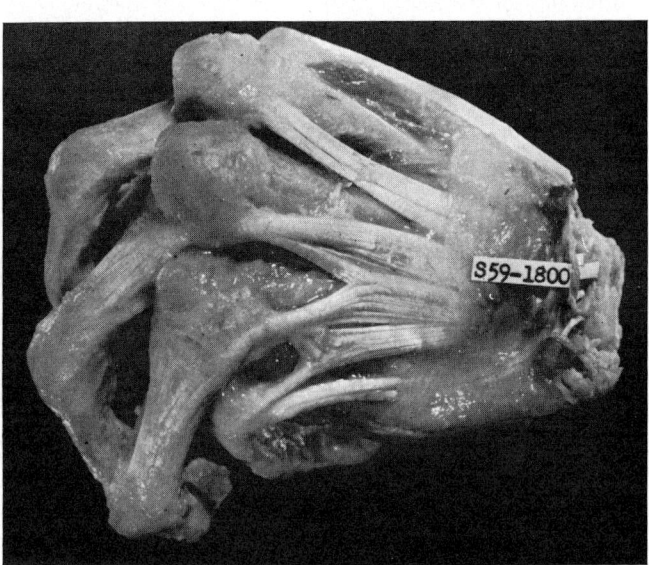

importance, particularly in small joints, where these tissues are in close proximity to the synovium. Tendon contractures and ruptures also are an important element in finger and toe deformities (Fig. 41–7). Secondary osteoarthritic changes are common in longstanding lesions, but the degree of bony proliferation is ordinarily less than that seen in primary or mechanically derived degenerative joint disease.[43]

VERTEBRAL LESIONS

In RA, the cervical spine is often affected.[44] Both the diarthrodial (apophyseal) joints and the intervertebral discs may be involved.[45] Sometimes, extensive destruction of spinal ligaments occurs as well. Ball observed the destruction of the anulus fibrosus to proceed with formation of granulation tissue from synovitis of the neurocentral (Luschka) joints in 17 of 18 unselected cases. The interspinous bursae were affected in 2 of 9 subjects studied at necropsy by By-

waters.[46] Instances of cervical spine RA with little or no peripheral joint involvement have been reported. The inflammatory changes are like those described later in this chapter with regard to the tendons and ligaments of the peripheral joints. These changes cause subluxation at times and may lead to neurologic defects or, occasionally, sudden death. Destructive lesions of lumbar vertebral bodies by rheumatoid nodules have been described on several occasions.[47] Apophyseal joint involvement in this region has also been described radiologically, but it is less frequent and less severe than in the cervical region.[45,48]

SUBCUTANEOUS NODULES

In approximately one of five patients with peripheral RA, chronic inflammatory nodules develop in para-articular subcutaneous tissue. These nodules are most common over the olecranon process of the ulna. Less frequently, they are found on the extensor aspects of the finger joints, in the achilles tendon ("pump bumps"), or in the occiput in bedridden patients. Any subcutaneous tissue subject to mechanical pressure may be involved, and individual patients show great variation in nodule development in response to pressure.

Subcutaneous nodules in RA are usually larger than

FIG. 41–7. *A* and *B,* Tendon and tendon sheath involvement in RA. *B,* White grumous exudate occupies the substance and sheaths of the anterior tibial and extensor tendons (A), and the Achilles tendon (B). The inferior extensor retinaculum (C) is irregularly infiltrated, and nodules are also present in the extensor tendons of the foot (D). The surface of the tendons is irregular and dull because of inflammatory adhesions. The changes are responsible for the cock-up deformities of the toes. A subcutaneous nodule (E) adheres to the periosteum of the fibula immediately anterior to the peroneus longus tendon.

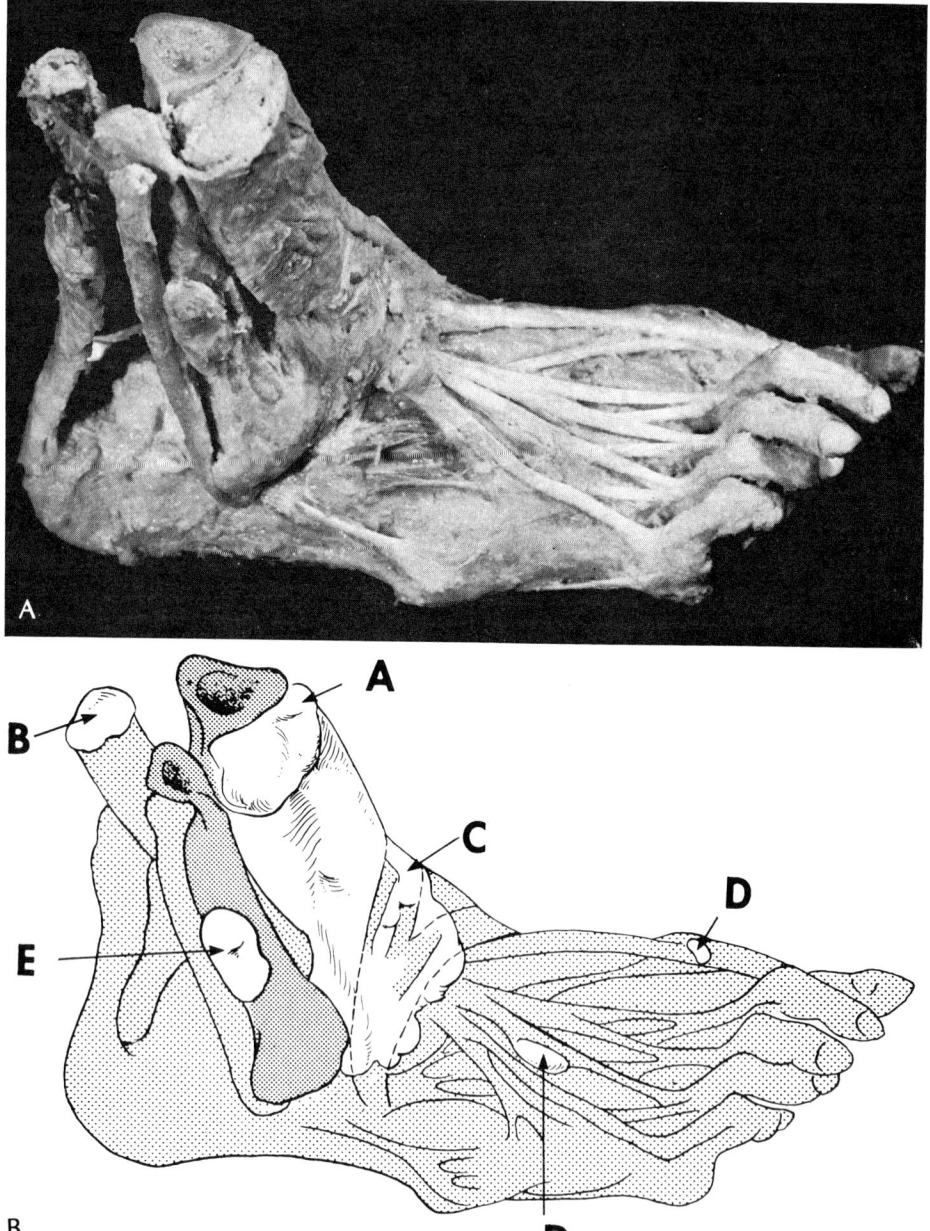

those of rheumatic fever and may reach a diameter of several centimeters. Large nodules are tough, lobulated, and multicentric. They are not encapsulated and cannot be sharply dissected from underlying articular tissue, bursae, or periosteum. Geographic areas of necrosis are recognized by their yellow color because lipochrome pigments accompany the large amounts of lipid, in the form of neutral fat, cholesterol, and phospholipids, deposited in the necrotic material.

The histologic appearance of a well-developed subcutaneous rheumatoid nodule is characteristic. It resembles many infectious or foreign body granulomas in that it has three distinct zones: (1) a central area of necrosis of subcutaneous fibrous and granulation tissue; (2) a palisade of elongated, connective tissue cells arranged radially in a corona about the necrotic zone; and (3) an enveloping granulation tissue in which chronic inflammatory cells are distributed (Fig. 41–8).

In long-standing lesions, the palisade is less apparent, and acellular fibrous tissue predominates; however, recrudescent activity may produce newer inflammatory foci adjacent to older, "mature" foci.

The necrotic centers have, to a varying extent, a "fibrinoid" appearance. This term should not be used to indicate a specific compound, a single pathogenetic significance, or identity with pathologic materials in other rheumatic or nonrheumatic disorders. It is a histologic term and simply describes the necrotic material as being oxyphilic and refractive and reacting to certain stains in the manner of fibrin rather than of collagen. The composition of the necrotic material in the rheumatoid nodule varies as the lesion progresses or "burns out." It contains collagen, lipids, nucleoproteins, acid mucopolysaccharides, serum proteins, including immunoglobulins,[49,50] and, in certain active states, material that probably is fibrin. The fibrin-like component is most prominent in active or new lesions. The lipid material may persist in an otherwise semifluid center of the nodule and may convert the nodule to a bursa-like or cystic structure. Unlike many types of persistent, lipid-rich necrotic debris, calcification of rheumatoid nodules is rare. Erosion of bone by nodules has been reported, but is also a rarity.[51]

The precise nature of the cells in the marginal palisade has not been established.[52] Although the cells to a certain degree resemble and sometimes are called epithelioid cells, as in tuberculoid granulomas, they also have fibroblastic characteristics. By electron microscopy, macrophage-like cells have been identified in the palisade zone and in the proliferating granulation tissue surrounding active nodules.[52,53] Acid phosphatase activity, indicative of a histiocytic nature, is present in these cells. Cytoplasmic fat droplets may abound in the palisaded cells and may also be present in the adjacent necrotic tissue. Whether the droplets reflect the phagocytosis of lipid, derived

FIG. 41–8. Subcutaneous nodule of RA. Although this is a long-standing lesion, the presence of nuclear fragments in the "fibrinoid" central zone is presumptive evidence of recent necrosis (hematoxylin and eosin stain × 95).

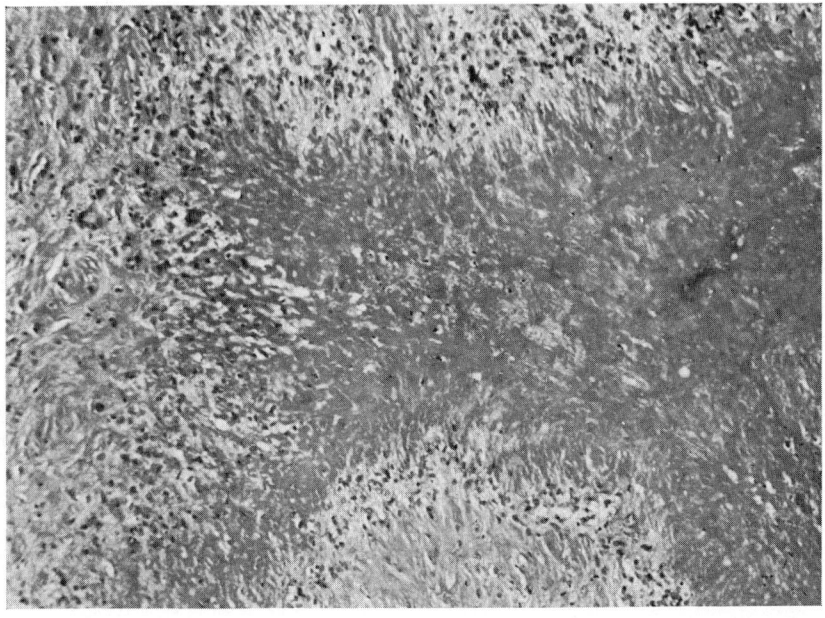

from the blood or from ground substance, or whether they are products of the cells has not been established. Multinucleated giant cells, occasionally seen in such areas, however, are usually of the Touton type and presumably are lipophages. The cells assume their radial arrangement because their axes are oriented against the fibers entering the zones of necrosis. The enveloping granulation tissue, vascular in its early stages, ultimately cicatrizes.[49] Lymphocytes and smaller numbers of plasma cells are disposed about some of the peripheral venules. In the proliferating areas of vascularity, the perivascular cells are primarily plump fibroblasts and mononuclear cells. Scattered eosinophils may be present in the earliest lesions.

The granuloma-like appearance of the subcutaneous nodule of RA is different from that usually found in the joints. A variant of RA has been described wherein synovitis is inconspicuous but many subcutaneus nodules are present.[54] Nodules can at times be confused diagnostically with tuberculous and other lesions such as necrobiosis lipoidica and granuloma annulare (Table 41–1). Granted that nodules may appear in advance of articular manifestations, para-articular lesions of this sort also occur in individuals who have no evidence of any rheumatic disease. These idiopathic subcutaneous nodules present a spectrum of appearances; they may resemble lesions of rheumatic fever, rheumatoid arthritis, and granuloma annulare.[55,56] The appearance of the early subcutaneous nodule is different from that of the older lesion, as discussed previously.

LESIONS OF TENDONS AND LIGAMENTS

The tendons and articular ligaments are involved pathologically with considerable, though undetermined, frequency. The inflammatory process is usually nonspecific; lymphocytes, mononuclear cells, and a few plasma cells infiltrate the bundles of collagen. In severe instances, focal areas of "fibrinoid" necrosis develop, and the lesion may be identical to a subcutaneous nodule. The nodular areas are at times palpable grossly (see Fig. 41–7). Ruptures may take place in such areas of necrosis.[57] Where the tendons lie in sheaths, tendinitis is accompanied by tenosynovitis. The ruptures and adhesions of the tendons to each other and to adjacent tissue are an integral part of the development of joint deformities in many instances.

Table 41–1. Differential Pathologic Diagnosis of Subcutaneous Nodules

Lesion	Depth	Common site	Histopathologic characteristics*
Rheumatoid nodule	Subcutaneous	Pressure points (e.g., olecranon)	Multicentric fibrinoid necrosis; palisading
Rheumatic fever nodule	Subcutaneous	Pressure points	Fibrinoid edema; some palisading; smaller than preceding
Granuloma annulare	Dermal	Dorsum of hands and feet	Mucoid edema; palisading
Pseudorheumatoid nodule ("deep granuloma annulare")	Subcutaneous	Anterior tibial tubercle, Achilles tendon	Similar to preceding; more nonspecific granulation tissue
Necrobiosis lipoidica	Subcutaneous	Anterior thigh, leg	Necrosis of fat and collagenous tissue; foam cell reaction and variable palisading
Erythema nodosum	Subcutaneous	Anterior leg	Chronic inflammation, often granulomatous, in veins and interlobular septa
Tophus	Subcutaneous	Olecranon, dorsum of hands	Urate crystals in amorphous matrix, with foreign body reaction
Tuberculous granuloma	Subcutaneous	Olecranon bursa	Caseous necrosis; epithelioid and Langhans cells
Epidermoid cyst	Subcutaneous	Olecranon	Keratotic material within epidermoid lining
Fibrous histiocytoma (tendon sheath xanthoma)	Subcutaneous	Flexor aspect of finger	Hemosiderin-laden mononuclear and foam cells; may co-exist with rheumatoid nodules
Xanthoma tuberosum	Subcutaneous	Dorsum of fingers, olecranon, Achilles tendon	Foam cells; cholesterol crystal granuloma

*A palisade is regarded in this context as a layer of elongated connective tissue cells oriented along the axis of collagenous fibers entering the zone of edema or necrosis.

STRIATED MUSCLE LESIONS

The skeletal muscle in severe cases of RA frequently has the histologic appearance of disuse atrophy.[58] The type 2 myofibers are affected primarily, as is usual in disuse and most other types of atrophy. An irregular diminution in the circumference of the fibers is seen, with a corresponding condensation of sarcolemmal nuclei. Immunoglobulin is localized to arteriolar walls and perimysial connective tissue in RA and in other immunologically mediated connective tissue diseases.[59,60]

In approximately two of every three patients with RA, scattered focal compact aggregates of chronic inflammatory cells, principally lymphocytes, are seen about venules in endomysium or perimysium. The lesion is lacking in diagnostic specificity, but is more common in RA and its variants than in nonrheumatic disorders. Unlike dermatomyositis, necrosis and regenerative activity are not conspicuous features.

PERIPHERAL NERVE INVOLVEMENT

Perivascular aggregates of lymphocytes and mononuclear cells, comparable to those of striated muscle, are also present in the endoneurium and perineurium of peripheral nerves in patients with RA. Myelin and axon changes are not present unless arterial disease is a complication. Entrapment of nerves by thickened inflammatory tissue is by far the most frequent cause of neuropathy in RA.[59,61] The carpal tunnel is the most common location, but other sites are also affected. The changes in the nerves result from compression rather than from intrinsic inflammation. Other than minute perivascular cellular infiltrates, lesions have not been seen in conventional sections of the sympathetic ganglia.

LESIONS OF ARTERIES

Arterial lesions of varying severity and character have been recognized in numerous studies of RA; no unanimity exists as to their significance.[62] Several anatomic factors appear reasonably certain: (1) the arteritis affects principally small segments of terminal arteries, 250 to 400 μm in external diameter; (2) the lesions are chronic and lack distinctive histologic characteristics; and (3) although these lesions may occur in many areas, the principal sites of involvement are the peripheral nerves and skeletal muscle. At one end of the spectrum of vascular lesions is the non-necrotizing, segmental arteritis of striated muscle that can be detected only when extensive serial sections have been made. This form of arteritis has been demonstrated in approximately 10% of unselected cases. At the other end of the clinical spectrum is a fulminant systemic disease that is difficult to distinguish from polyarteritis nodosa (PAN), either on clinical or on anatomic grounds. This fulminant disease is far less common than the non-necrotizing disorder.

Among the hypotheses on the nature of the arteritis is that it results from treatment of RA with corticosteroid hormones. Corticosteroid therapy of other than rheumatic disorders has, on rare occasions, also been reported to be complicated by necrotizing arteritis. Nonetheless, arteritis may be seen in patients with RA who have not received such compounds. A widespread belief that this sort of therapy has increased the incidence of vasculitis has received no support.[63]

Another view is that the arteritis is a form of PAN that reflects humoral hypersensitivity, sometimes postulated to underlie the development of RA. Several important differences between the usual vascular lesions of RA and those of PAN exist, however.[64] In RA, the lesions are usually mild, few, and affecting minute vessels. In PAN, the arteritis is widespread and involves medium-sized, rather than small, arteries. Obliteration of the lumen or ectasia and rupture are characteristic of PAN. The prognosis of PAN is often ominous, whereas the vascular lesions of RA have been known to exist for many years without causing detectable symptoms. In PAN, cutaneous gangrene of the extremities is most unusual, whereas it is frequent in RA when corticosteroid therapy has been administered. The nosologic status of PAN itself is also uncertain (see Chapter 74).

It seems likely that the vasculitis is a specific manifestation of RA that shares etiologic or pathogenetic factors with the joint disease and mediates the development of that disease. This view is based on the observation that vasculitis is an intrinsic part of the development of the granulomatous subcutaneous nodules.[49] In the early nodule, the important histologic processes are exudation of fibrin-rich edema fluid into subcutaneous fibrous tissue, formation of vascular granulation tissue,[53,62] proliferation of plump fibroblasts, and apparently also of macrophages, and necrosis of small arteries and more minute blood vessels.[52] The exudation and necrosis proceed centrifugally about the nodular buds of granulation tissue. These foci eventually coalesce to form the characteristic necrotic centers of the mature nodules. Some researchers emphasize the venular rather than terminal arterial disturbances in the genesis of these lesions. This process is histologically distinct from the superficial dermal necrosis of the legs occasionally resulting from RA. Another variant, leukocytoclastic vasculitis, is a feature of a variety of rheumatic disorders, but is infrequent in RA.[65]

Clinically manifest arteritis is frequently associated with high titers of rheumatoid factor, particularly of low-molecular-weight species,[66,67] as well as with the presence of subcutaneous nodules. The arteritis in peripheral nerves is one cause of the peripheral neuropathy that sometimes complicates RA (see Chapter 44).[68]

IMMUNOPATHOLOGY

Granular deposits of IgG, IgM, anti-IgG, C3, C4, and fibrinogen or fibrin, but not of albumin, are commonly found by immunofluorescent staining in the lining cells, matrix, and blood vessels of the synovium.[21] Their frequency is greater in seropositive than in seronegative patients and still more than in noninflammatory joint diseases. The occurrence of immunoglobulins in subcutaneous nodules has already been noted.

In overt, untreated arteritis, immunohistochemical studies have disclosed immune complex components.[69] In lesions from patients treated with corticosteroids, a proliferative endarteritis devoid of immune complex deposits has been found. Our own experience coincides with that of others that such complexes may be present at the inception of the lesion and may then be removed by leukocytes as the cellular infiltrate evolves. In other circumstances, arterioles in muscle and minute vessels in skin contain components of immune complexes,[70,71] but they are not associated with leukocytic infiltration. It is not known why such immune deposits elicit an inflammatory response in some instances and not in others.

The electron microscopic appearance of the infiltrate is consistent with an interaction among immunologic cell types involving both cellular and humoral responses.[72] A further discussion of the role of immunity in RA is found in Chapter 40.

CARDIAC LESIONS

In the past, most clinical studies found cardiac abnormalities to be uncommon; anatomic investigations, by contrast, showed frequent lesions of several sorts. The disparity has been reduced by sensitive echocardiographic techniques that yield clinical data more in accord with pathologic findings.[73–80]

RHEUMATIC HEART DISEASE

Although rheumatic heart disease was reported in many older postmortem studies in 21 to 66% of patients, most recent papers have placed the figure, exclusive of calcareous aortic stenosis, at 6 to 10%. Several reasons exist for this lack of consistency and partly account for the high frequency of rheumatic heart disease sometimes reported in studies of RA.

IDIOPATHIC PERICARDITIS

Virtually all necropsy studies have shown remote or active pericarditis in approximately 40% of cases of RA. Usually, this disorder is manifested by fibrous obliteration of the pericardial cavity. Infrequently, the lesion has a granuloma-like character resembling that of the rheumatoid nodule or synovial lesion.[78] Only the frequent association with arteritis supports the rheumatoid nature of the process. Significant clinical consequences, recognized infrequently,[81] include pericardial constriction necessitating pericardiotomy, fatal hemopericardium, and pericardial effusion with tamponade.

INTERSTITIAL MYOCARDITIS

In addition to occasional granuloma-like rheumatoid nodules in the myocardium, small infarcts secondary to coronary arteritis have been observed rarely, some surrounded by a palisade of elongated cells and some not. More often, however, focal idiopathic, nonspecific interstitial myocarditis is seen. In some instances, the leukocytic infiltrate includes many eosinophils. Whether allergic or other drug toxicity or viral infection complicating therapy, and not the rheumatoid disease, may be the etiologic basis of some of the myocarditis cannot be ascertained in the absence of appropriate differential diagnostic tests.

CORONARY ARTERITIS

Coronary arteritis, affecting scattered small vessels, is an occasional finding.[82] It has been associated with disseminated arteritis in other sites, both splanchnic and in the extremities. Myocardial infarction and aortitis may be associated with coronary involvement.[79] As in the case of peripheral arteritis, some of the variation in the frequency of coronary involvement in different laboratory studies may be influenced by selection factors. The anatomic criteria for the differential diagnosis of rheumatic heart disease are imprecise.

CALCAREOUS AORTIC STENOSIS

Whether all instances of this condition are due to rheumatic inflammation is unresolved. As in the accepted rheumatic valvular lesions, the frequency of this abnormality also was greater in several studies of patients with RA than in control subjects.

RHEUMATOID HEART DISEASE

Lesions resembling the granuloma-like subcutaneous nodules occur at times in the valve leaflets, valve rings, myocardium, or epicardium in patients with peripheral RA. Although considerable histologic variation exists, the active lesions differ from those of infectious or rheumatic carditis. Their frequency is difficult to estimate, but has been reported in various series as 2 of 19, 7 of 36, 5 of 100, and 10 of 43 necropsies. The order of frequency of involvement of the valves is as follows: (1) mitral; (2) aortic; (3) tricuspid; and (4) pulmonic. The valvular lesions differ from those of rheumatic carditis in that they are neither diffuse nor verrucous.[80] As in other viscera, the histologic appearance of cardiac rheumatoid nodules is often atypical. Clinically, some have been silent; others have produced valvular insufficiency, heart block, Adams-Stokes syndrome, and an electrocardiogram resembling that of infarction.[74]

The granuloma-like lesions may coexist with pericarditis, coronary arteritis, and interstitial myocarditis, three other frequent findings, each of which are morphologically nonspecific but lack other explanations than the rheumatoid disease. In the pathologic diagnosis of any given case, coexisting systemic lupus erythematosus (SLE) may be a possibility. The end result of burned-out lesions may be similar to those of rheumatic heart disease and may account for some reports of increased frequency of rheumatic fever in patients with RA.

AORTIC INSUFFICIENCY

In ankylosing spondylitis, an apparently specific form of aortic valve insufficiency has been recorded.[83] These lesions are grossly similar to those of syphilis in that the principal changes relate to the gross destruction of the elastic tissue of the root of the aorta and the adjacent valve rings, but they differ from syphilitic aortitis in that they are confined to the root and do not affect the ascending aorta. The commissures of the valve are separated, and the edges of the leaflets are rolled toward the ventricular cavity as a result of regurgitation. This lesion does not occur in peripheral RA, although rheumatoid valvulitis may occasionally involve the aortic valve and may render it incompetent.

MISCELLANEOUS LESIONS

Postmortem findings support the long-standing impression that hypertension and myocardial infarction occur infrequently in RA. Coronary atherosclerosis was no less frequent or severe than in control subjects, but the infarctive consequences were reduced,[84] perhaps because of the hematologic effects of aspirin therapy. Even so, atherosclerotic heart disease probably accounts for most clinical cardiac dysfunction encountered in patients with RA.[85] Secondary amyloidosis, a rare complication of RA, infrequently affects the myocardium. Aortic insufficiency has been reported as an occasional finding in spondyloarthropathy-associated psoriasis and Reiter's disease. A chronic form of rheumatic fever may lead to deformities (*Jaccoud's arthritis*) of the joints as well as of the heart valves. The existence of this condition has not been completely accepted by American rheumatologists. Takayasu's disease is not generally regarded as a rheumatic condition, but isolated instances of aortic arch syndrome have been associated with RA.[86]

PULMONARY LESIONS

Three patterns of chronic pulmonary disease have been proposed as occasional manifestations of RA: (1) Caplan's syndrome; (2) granulomatous lesions; and (3) idiopathic interstitial pneumonia or diffuse interstitial fibrosis.

CAPLAN'S SYNDROME

This term refers to unusually large, silicotic nodule formation seen in anthracite coal miners afflicted with RA. Histologically, these lesions do not resemble rheumatoid nodules. In addition to a silica, they contain much amorphous material. It has been suggested that the exuberant character of these nodules is due to an altered tissue reactivity to the silica particles; however, the condition has also been described in several other pneumoconioses.[87] Although the lesion appears frequently in Great Britain, it is not common in the United States.[88]

GRANULOMATOUS LESIONS

These lesions, resembling rheumatoid subcutaneous nodules, are infrequent findings in patients with RA. It may be difficult to distinguish them from infectious granulomas.[89] Rarely, accompanying vasculitis suggests Wegener's granulomatosis. Extension of the nodules to the visceral pleura is characteristic of pulmonary rheumatoid nodules, as opposed to variants of Wegener's granulomatosis.[90]

IDIOPATHIC INTERSTITIAL PNEUMONIA OR DIFFUSE INTERSTIAL FIBROSIS

Whether idiopathic interstitial pneumonia or diffuse interstitial fibrosis of the lungs is a fortuitous finding or a true manifestation of RA has been debated. The recorded lesions do not have anatomic characteristics distinguishing them from the pulmonary fibrosis observed in systemic scleroderma or the Hamman-Rich syndrome.[91] Although the histologic changes are nonspecific, IgM has been demonstrated in alveolar septa and capillary walls.[92] Idiopathic interstitial pneumonia or diffuse interstitial fibrosis is seen in approximately 2% of patients with RA. Abnormalities in pulmonary function are more common.[93] Biopsies also have been cited to support this entity.[94] The interpretation of these data is clouded by the effects of smoking.[95] Another possible factor is drug therapy; some drugs are known to produce interstitial pulmonary fibrosis in other circumstances. Transient interstitial infiltration of the lung has been described in occasional patients receiving gold (gold lung),[96] but long-term pulmonary effects from this agent have not been noted. Extensive pleural adhesions and fibrinous pleurisy are sometimes associated with pericardial disease in RA.

SPLEEN, LYMPHOID TISSUE, AND BONE MARROW LESIONS

Enlargement of the regional lymph nodes draining affected joints is common in RA. Although some reports to the contrary exist, generalized lymphadenopathy involving the deeper lymph chains is infrequent. Such enlargement is caused by a nonspecific hyperplasia associated with formation of prominent germinal centers. Plasma cells are usually few, but rheumatoid factor has been demonstrated in them.[97] Numerous reticulum cells may be found in the sinuses. The hypertrophy of the lymph nodes at times reaches dimensions sufficient to raise a suspicion of malignant lymphoma, and the histologic picture has all too often been confused with nodular lymphoma.[98] The pattern of immunoglobulin staining, however, is distinct from that of malignant lymphoma.[99]

Distinctive changes are not present in the spleen in RA. In the splenomegaly of Felty's syndrome, the most consistent finding is proliferation of reticuloendothelial cells in the sinusoids. The extent of this change is in proportion to the erythrophagocytosis.[100] Although hyperplasia of the white pulp has been described, the lymphoid tissue most often is atrophic. The relation of splenic immunopathology to the circulating antinuclear antibody directed against granulocytes in this syndrome is unclear.[101] Thymic hypertrophy is not characteristically present. The bone marrow may show a variety of nonspecific changes, including increased numbers of plasma cells and ineffective erythropoiesis with excessive iron.[102] In some instances, increased numbers of lymphoid nodules are present in bone marrow particle sections. Although uncommon, bone marrow aplasia, with or without subsequent acute leukemia, has developed after prolonged therapy with alkylating agents.

ENDOCRINE LESIONS

Because of the dramatic and rapid clinical response of RA to the administration of corticotropin and adrenocortical steroids, the adrenal cortex and the pituitary gland have been studied; neither shows morphologic changes different from those found in nonrheumatic diseases.

Lymphocytic thyroiditis has, in the past, been associated with some cases of RA, although some investigators have not found it to be more frequent than in a control population.[103] Some confusion may result from the development of the rheumatic disease in some patients with spontaneous hypothyroidism.[104]

OCULAR LESIONS

The episcleritis sometimes seen in RA has its inception in focal, chronic inflammatory cell infiltration and necrosis of the sclera. When these foci become larger and chronic, they may resemble the subcutaneous nodules of RA. When the scleral necrosis is sufficient to soften the wall of the eye, uveal tissue may herniate through the scleral defect, a condition known as scleromalacia perforans.[105] This condition sometimes occurs in patients with no evidence of RA.[106]

The uveitis (iridocyclitis) of juvenile RA[20] and ankylosing spondylitis does not have distinctive properties. Band keratopathy, a characteristic equatorial corneal opacity due to deposition of calcium beneath the corneal epithelium, is a sequela of the iridocyclitis, and in children it is most often, if not always, associated with the arthritic condition.[107]

Posterior subcapsular cataracts have been observed in as many as 42% of patients with RA and other rheumatic diseases during the course of corticosteroid therapy. Little is known of their pathologic anatomy. In one well-studied, early (9 months' duration) case, preservation of lens epithelium and the architecture of the lens bow distinguished the lesion from that of the usual senile cataract. Another surgically removed lens, however, had changes indistinguishable from the senile lesion.[108]

Keratoconjunctivitis sicca, associated with diminished lacrimation, is discussed more fully elsewhere (see Chapters 44 and 76).

SJÖGREN'S SYNDROME

Although its cardinal symptoms are referable to diminished secretion by the lacrimal and salivary glands, this condition is frequently associated with various rheumatic diseases and with serologic abnormalities (see Chaper 76). Classic peripheral RA is present in approximately one-third of cases, and almost all have rheumatoid factor. The classification of Sjögren's syndrome into primary, without associated connective tissue disease, and secondary, with connective tissue disease, types has been further enhanced by the discovery of serum antibodies against extractable nuclear antigens such as SS-B and RA precipitin specific for the two types.[97] Differences in histocompatibility antigens between the two types have been elucidated.[109]

Individuals with primary Sjögren's syndrome often have more widespread clinical disease, involving not only lacrimal and salivary glands, but also exocrine glands of the respiratory tract, gastrointestinal tract, skin, and pancreas. As shown by light microscopy, differences in the salivary gland involvement between primary and secondary types relate to the amount of lymphoid infiltrate and the severity of glandular effacement rather than to the character of the infiltrate.

A considerable variation is found in the salivary lesions. Four principal patterns are seen. First, the predominant finding is most often like that described in Mikulicz's disease. Two different histologic elements are distinguished.[110] The first is a peculiar metaplastic change in the epithelium of the striated ducts. The columnar cells proliferate and assume a stratified, polymorphous appearance. Their cytoplasm loses its normal oxyphilia. Because of the resemblance of the cells to the myoepithelial cells that normally lie subjacent to the duct epithelium, the ducts showing solid, heaped-up cells of this sort have been referred to as "epimyoepithelial" islands. Duct-like metaplasia of acini, with irregular ectasia and attenuation, also occurs, and the acini undergo variable degrees of atrophy. The second principal component in these lesions is infiltration of lymphocytes about the intralobular ducts. At times, germinal centers appear in the lymphoid aggregates, and acini may be obliterated by the infiltrate. Nevertheless, the lobular limits are characteristically respected by the infiltrate.

The second pattern occurs in a few instances. A localized area of lymphoid infiltration associated with duct metaplasia of the sort just noted reaches tumorlike proportions. This lesion is termed benign *lymphoepithelial lesion of Godwin*. Histologically, the differential diagnosis from malignant lymphomas of the salivary glands may be difficult. Third, the cellular infiltration may be so mild and the duct so little changed that the appearance cannot be distinguished from a control population. The fourth pattern may emerge after many years. The parenchymal lobules show extreme atrophy and replacement by adipose tissue, even though lymphocytic infiltration and duct metaplasia are no longer present.

Minor salivary and labial glands are also often infiltrated with lymphocytes and may thus be suitable for biopsy. Such studies have shown a high correlation of histologic abnormality with the presence of antibodies against certain extractable nuclear antigens.[111] Myoepithelial islands, however, are infrequently seen. Labial glands of individuals with primary Sjögren's syndrome consistently have more severe histologic changes than in patients with the secondary type of the syndrome.[112] This finding correlates with clinical observations of milder disease in those individuals with Sjögren's syndrome accompanying RA.[111] Intralobular aggregates of lymphocytes are also seen in the lacrimal glands, but they are smaller than in the salivary glands and are only rarely accompanied by epimyoepithelial islands.[113] Other glandular tissues, including the pancreas, fail to disclose a comparable pattern.

The pathologic ramifications of Sjögren's syndrome are more complicated than this account suggests. Localized tumor-like nodules of infiltrating lymphoid tissue ("pseudolymphoma") have been observed in lymph nodes and lung, more commonly in primary Sjögren's syndrome.[114] Indeed, in rare instances, unequivocal malignant lymphomas, principally diffuse histiocytic lymphomas, have developed. This complication is seen in both primary and secondary types of Sjögren's syndrome, at about 40 times the expected rate for healthy individuals.[111] Isolated instances of Waldenström's macroglobulinemia, small cell lymphosarcoma, and Hodgkin's disease have also been observed. Tissue lymphoid infiltrates in primary Sjögren's syndrome, as in RA, are primarily T-lymphocytes. The numbers of OKT4 (helper-inducer) cells are increased, whereas OKT8 (suppressor) cells are decreased.[115] Thus, the polyclonal-B-cell hyperactivity, which sometimes progresses to monoclonal pseudolymphomas or lymphoma, may reflect disordered immunoregulation.

RENAL LESIONS

Although older accounts to the contrary exist, the general experience is that glomerulitis and glomerulonephritis are infrequent in uncomplicated RA.[116,117] Membranous glomerulonephritis sometimes complicates systemic gold therapy for RA.[118] The status of analgesic nephropathy is unclear.[119] Although aspirin alone in moderation seems to cause little harm, a combination of aspirin and phenacetin is particularly likely to produce the renal papillary necrosis characteristic of this syndrome.

STILL'S DISEASE

This disorder has traditionally been considered the juvenile form of RA. It differs in several respects from the adult counterpart: (1) uncommon occurrence of circulating rheumatoid factors; (2) more frequent picture of ankylosing spondylitis; (3) greater frequency of iritis and band keratopathy; (4) lesser frequency of subcutaneous nodules; (5) frequent association with an erythematous skin eruption (see Chapter 57); and lower NK cell activity of peripheral blood lymphocytes.[12] Currently, a number of distinct subsets of Still's disease are thought to exist[120] (see Chapters 57 and 58).

ARTICULAR LESIONS

In the systemic form of the disease, with rash and high fever, variable articular manifestations occur.

The involved joints can show only a mild, nonspecific inflammation or, more rarely, a florid destructive inflammatory pannus similar to adult RA.[121] This destructive pannus, however, is more characteristic of the polyarticular form of the disease associated with rheumatoid factors and subcutaneous nodules. These patients probably have juvenile presentations of adult RA. The pauciarticular form of the disease contains a distinct subset of HLA-B27-positive male children in whom the articular inflammation and pannus are mild and are often replaced by bony ankylosis, especially in the sacroiliac and spinal joints, but frequently in the limb girdle joints as well. These patients may be victims of juvenile-onset ankylosing spondylitis; however, bony and fibrous ankylosis occurs in the polyarticular variant as well. A second subset of B27-positive girls develops spondylitis and iridocyclitis, but not sacroiliac involvement.

An additional feature of articular disease not seen in the adult RA is that the subchondral inflammatory process may arrest or distort epiphyseal bone growth and may thereby lead to so-called rheumatic dwarfism. The mandible is particularly likely to be compromised in temporomandibular arthritis because growth normally takes place in its articular condyle rather than in an epiphyseal plate. This process is the basis of the micrognathos (underslung jaw). Monarticular involvement is seen more frequently in the juvenile disorder than in the adult disease.

SUBCUTANEOUS NODULES

Subcutaneous nodules occur infrequently in all forms of Still's disease, but they are most common in the polyarticular variant.[122] The histologic appearance differs both from that of the adult rheumatoid nodule and from the nodule of rheumatic fever.[123] In material available to us, the nodules consist largely of fibrous tissue containing irregularly disposed aggregates of proliferating fibroblasts in small numbers and irregular areas of fibrinous exudation. Neither geographic areas of necrosis nor palisade formation are evident. One early lesion had proliferation of blood vessels and focal vasculitis.

OTHER LESIONS

Ocular Changes

Iridocyclitis and subsequent band-shaped keratopathy are far more frequent in Still's disease than in adult RA.[124] Macular atrophy from secondary glaucoma may result. Ocular changes occur most frequently in the pauciarticular variant of the disease.[125]

Spondylitis

The spinal changes resemble those of ankylosing spondylitis.

Cardiac Lesions

Pericardial involvement occurs in the juvenile form approximately as frequently as in adult RA, although it may be detected clinically with greater frequency.[126–128]

Skin Eruption

The erythema is transient. Histologically, only mild perivascular aggregation of mononuclear cells in the superficial dermis has been observed.[129]

ETIOLOGY AND PATHOGENESIS

The following considerations are oriented toward the pathologic findings in RA. A systematic treatment of its etiopathogenesis appears in Chapter 40.

In the past, the histologic appearance of the articular tissues suggested that rheumatoid arthritis was an infectious disease. Many types of spontaneous or induced infectious polyarthritis in species other than man have similar histologic appearances. Arthritis caused by the enteric erysipeloid organism Erysipelothrix rhusiopathiae in swine, for example, is one of the leading causes of pork condemnation in federally inspected meat plants in the United States, and it closely resembles RA histologically. Similar, but generally less chronic, synovitides occur in poultry and in pigs with species-specific types of Mycoplasma infection.[29] These minute, filtrable bacteria were formerly called pleuropneumonia-like organisms or PPLO.[29] Another type of filtrable agent causing disease in ovine species is Chlamydia. Subcutaneous nodules of the sort seen in RA have not been found in these infectious diseases, however, and serologic tests for rheumatoid factor are generally negative. The frequency of arthritis with bacteremias resulting from these organisms has prompted many microbiologic studies in RA, but most, like virologic studies, have failed to show infectious agents.[130] Recently, cross-reactive antigens common to Epstein-Barr virus-encoded proteins have been identified in RA synovium.[131] The next generation of diagnostic histopathologic procedures may well use DNA and other probes to identify such specific markers in RA synovium.

Morphologic findings in RA that might relate to hypersensitivity mechanisms include the lymphoid character of the infiltrate, the absence of demonstrable organisms, the local synthesis of rheumatoid factors,

the similarities of the "fibrinoid" necrotic material in the subcutaneous nodules and synovial surface to those of acute allergic inflammation,[132] and the resemblance of certain of the vascular lesions to those of polyarteritis nodosa and experimental serum sickness. The morphologic features of the previously described cellular infiltrate allow one to reconstruct sequence of events in accord with what is known of other chronic inflammatory processes.[133]

Both T- and B-lymphocytes enter the synovium through venules and are concentrated in compact perivascular infiltrates. Variable mobility and variable recirculation of the several cell types account for large disparities in the proportions of lymphocyte populations in synovium, synovial fluid, and peripheral blood.[8,13,134] T-lymphocytes, in particular, emigrate to adjacent portions of synovium and into synovial fluid. The migrating T cells are challenged by a currently unidentified antigen(s) in the synovium and undergo blast transformation. The uncommon T-lymphoblasts accordingly are located at a distance from the perivascular infiltrates where they synthesize and release mediators of local cellular immunity. These lymphoblasts immobilize macrophages locally and also damage adjacent fibroblasts. Plasma cells and plasmablasts are immobile and often persist in the perivascular location. The OKT8 cells are retained or proliferate in areas of increased immunologic activity. This idealized schema oversimplifies the histologic features because the cell types are distributed in a variable fashion in synovium in almost pure culture in some foci. In other places, cells are dispersed singly or in small clusters at random in the superficial or deeper portions of the synovium.

The recognition of the association between HLA-B27 and ankylosing spondylitis and DW4 and RA has led to renewed interest in genetic predisposition to rheumatic syndromes. Conceivably, microbial or other antigens lodged in the joints of genetically susceptible individuals might persist or evoke chronic inflammatory responses not shown by other animals or persons. Suitable animal models that totally recapitulate human RA are not available.[29]

Certain speculations may be offered concerning histogenesis. One of the peculiarities of the morbid anatomy of the disease is that the synovial lesions are morphologically nonspecific, whereas the subcutaneous nodules are specific. If no common histogenetic sequence of events occurred in the nodules and the joints, it would be difficult to understand how a common pathogenetic mechanism would produce both lesions. The following hypothesis is offered to account for this phenomenon: that the nodular type of reaction does at times occur in joints, particularly in the compact fibrous parts. The necrosis noted in superficial portions of the synovial tissue may be compared to the central zones in the nodules. At the base of the nodules, an ingrowth of fibroblasts and palisades of synovial lining or elongated cells also closely resembles those of subcutaneous nodules that have undergone central softening with formation of bursa-like cavities or pseudosynovial spaces. The simplest explanation for the differences between such synovial foci and the subcutaneous nodules is that the necrotic material in subcutaneous nodules is circumscribed by firm cicatrix, whereas in the synovial location, the necrotic debris is cast off into the joint space and appears as a rice body. In the joint, the inflammation thus diffuses into the articular cavity. In the synovium, the nonspecific components of the granulation tissue reaction seen about the nodules persist.

In the earliest days or weeks of their development, the subcutaneous nodules consist largely of vascular granulation tissue, in which the processes of necrosis and exudation proceed centrifugally about inflamed small arteries or islands of newly formed capillary or sinusoidal vessels.[53,62] Only later is coalescence of the areas of necrosis followed by the granuloma-like appearance that characterizes the mature nodule. Aside from this intrinsic association between the inflammatory process and the vasculitis, a principal reason for believing that blood vessels play a role in the development of the nodules is that, in these same patients, arteritis is frequent in other tissues as well. Accordingly, it may be proposed that disseminated arteritis is an integral manifestation of RA and that the development of the nodular and synovial lesions is in some manner mediated through the affected arteries to the terminal vascular bed of the target tissues. This hypothesis does not have universal acceptance,[135] but it is based on unique specimen material and provides a unitary concept of the histogenesis of the disorder.[62]

ANKYLOSING SPONDYLITIS

This disorder is an entity different from RA (see Chapter 59) as gauged by genetic, immunologic, epidemiologic, and pathologic features. In the diarthrodial joints of the spine, the sacroiliac joint, and the peripheral joints, the pathologic processes are like those of peripheral RA, except bony ankylosis is more prominent.[48,136] The initial histologic events in the intervertebral discs have not been well documented. By roentgenographic studies, osteolytic resorption of the margins of the vertebral bodies, to which the anulus fibrosus is attached, occurs early.[48,136a] Whether

an inflammatory infiltrate is present in the bone or disc tissue at this time is not known. A metaplastic ossification of the anulus fibrosus does occur, however, and penetrates from the margin of the vertebral bodies into the anulus. At times, enchondral ossification of the anulus fibrosus may occur without inflammation.[137] Although this process is commonly referred to as ossification of the spinal ligaments, the principal changes do not affect the ligaments so much as they do the anulus fibrosus (Fig. 41–9). The ankylotic bridges are located, in anteroposterior roentgenographic projections, on the lateral aspects of the vertebral bodies. The longitudinal spinal ligaments are anterolateral and posterior, but not lateral. When extensive, the bony bridges replace not only the anulus fibrosus, but also parts of the nucleus pulposus. The ossific tissue in time is remodeled to form a continuous structure. Another feature characteristic of ankylosing spondylitis, when present, is enthesopathy, that is, inflammation and eventual ossification of tendinous attachments to the pelvis and other bones at some distance from the joints.[45]

Although this picture is not observed characteristically in the vertebral involvement of RA, similar patterns may be found in patients with Still's disease, psoriatic arthritis, and Reiter's disease, but unlike in RA, subcutaneous nodules and vascular lesions are rare. Another departure from classic RA is the prevalence of histocompatibility antigen HLA-B27.[138,139] Cardiac involvement is described previously in this chapter, as well as in Chapter 59. The ocular lesions are also described previously.

PSORIATIC ARTHRITIS

The histologic changes in the joints in this condition (see also Chapter 61) are similar to those of RA, but differ in two respects: (1) the structures affected are principally the most distal rather than proximal joints (Fig. 41–10); and (2) more extensive destruction occurs in articular and adjacent bones.[140] The osteolysis is effected by a granulation tissue in which osteoclasts are present. As a result of this resorption, the bone may "telescope" within the skin of the extremity and may give rise to the so-called opera-glass hand deformity. Aside from these changes, a bulbous swelling of the periarticular soft tissue may result from proliferation of fibrous tissue in which thick-walled blood vessels are present.

The changes in the skin in psoriasis are characteristic. The papillary element of the epidermis is hypertrophied and forms coarse, club-shaped appendages, whereas the nonpapillary portion is

FIG. 41–9. Ankylosing spondylitis. Trabecular and cortical bone occupy the position of the anulus fibrosus. (Courtesy of Dr. Roger Terry.)

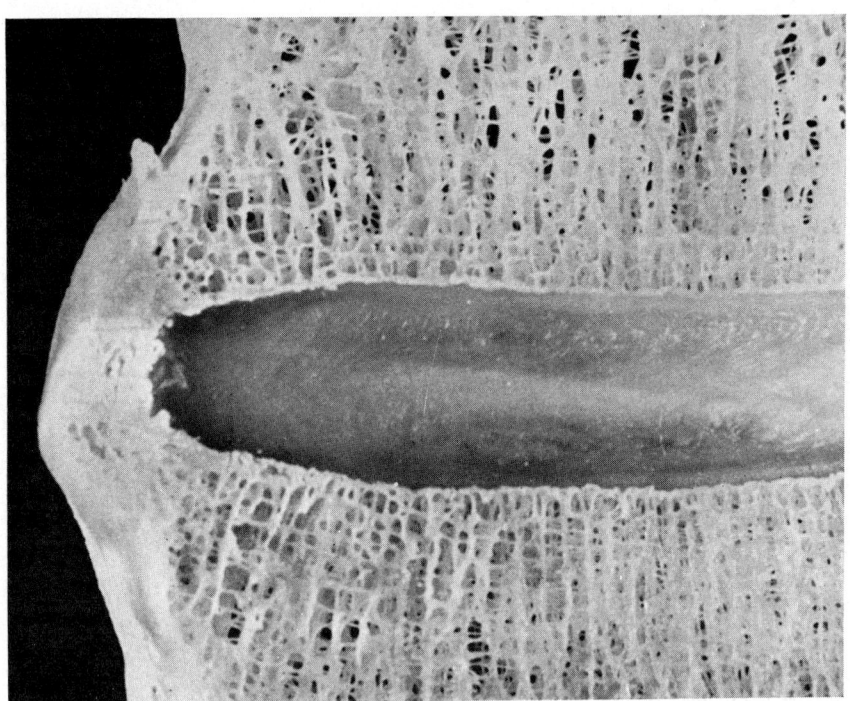

attenuated. This nonpapillary portion, however, is covered by a thick parakeratotic and keratotic scale. The superficial portions of the subjacent dermis are chronically inflamed and are infiltrated with large numbers of lymphocytes. A direct continuity between the dermal inflammation and the periarthritis or arthritis in psoriasis has not been established.

REITER'S SYNDROME

The synovitis seen in this syndrome is similar to that seen in RA, although in the early phases of the disease, it has a more purulent character.[141] The longstanding changes also are similar, but periosteal involvement, with new bone formation in attached tendons and ligaments, is much more characteristic of Reiter's disease than of RA. In this respect, the joint lesions are reminiscent of infectious arthritis. A strong association with HLA-B27 is present.[142]

The cutaneous lesions are histologically indistinguishable from those of pustular psoriasis. Such lesions are similar to those already described, except the focal purulent infiltration of the epidermis is present (see Chapter 60).

ARTHRITIS ASSOCIATED WITH WHIPPLE'S DISEASE, REGIONAL ENTERITIS, AND ULCERATIVE COLITIS

A relationship between chronic enteritic disorders and deforming arthritis exists, not only in Reiter's disease, which may be initiated by episodes of dysentery at times, but also in other entities (see also Chapter 62).[143,144] The synovium, in the arthritis accompanying ulcerative colitis and regional enteritis, shows nonspecific inflammatory changes.[2,145–147] In the arthritis accompanying Whipple's disease, the rod-like inclusions characteristic of intestinal lesions have been identified by electron microscopy in the synovium.[148,149]

ARTHRITIS ASSOCIATED WITH AGAMMAGLOBULINEMIA

Rheumatic symptoms develop in approximately 25% of patients with congenital or acquired agammaglobulinemia or hypogammaglobulinemia. Most conspicuous among these symptoms is chronic synovitis, which resembles RA in several respects. Usually, however, fewer joints are affected, and the small joints are spared more often. Histologically, the pat-

FIG. 41–10.   Psoriatic arthritis of the great toe. The extensive periarticular inflammation and destruction of bone about the distal interphalangeal joint are characteristic of this disorder. The metatarsophalangeal joint is spared (Masson's trichrome stain ×2.5).

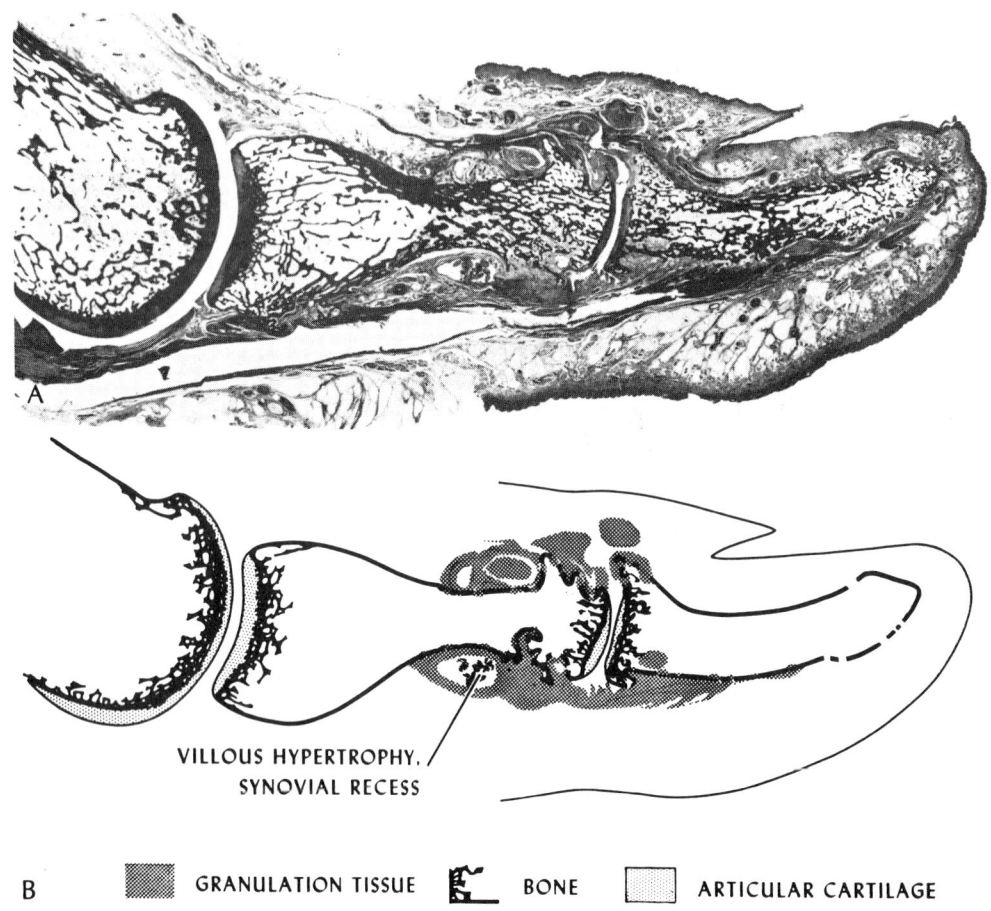

tern of synovitis is nonspecific and resembles that of RA, except plasma cells are generally absent.[150] Plasmacytes, however, have been seen in rare instances of arthritis associated with a deficiency of an isolated Ig type.[151]

Subcutaneous nodules, reported on several occasions in such patients, have a less characteristic appearance than the subcutaneous nodules of RA. Lobulated areas of proliferating fibroblasts and ill-defined palisades suggest the subcutaneous nodules seen in Still's disease. Vascular lesions of several types have also been described in rare instances.

AMYLOIDOSIS

In the past, secondary amyloidosis complicated RA, Still's disease, and ankylosing spondylitis in approximately 20% of severe cases. In the United States today, this complication is rare. This form of the dis-

order is indistinguishable from amyloidosis complicating other chronic inflammatory diseases. The principal subcomponent of amyloid in RA is the nonimmunoglobulin AA.[152] Amyloid infiltration represents the principal cause of renal dysfunction in RA, except when the joint disease co-exists with SLE[116] (see Chapter 82).

BIOPSY AS A DIAGNOSTIC AID

JOINT TISSUES

Synovial biopsy has no place in the differential diagnosis of the several conditions discussed in this chapter. It may, however, be useful in distinguishing RA from gout and from infectious arthritides.[28] Closed and open biopsy techniques are available. Punch biopsy needles have been specifically designed for this purpose. Open biopsy, carried out under local anesthesia, is often preferable because it provides more adequate samples of tissue and causes no more discomfort to the patient. This procedure is mandatory in joints that cannot easily undergo needle biopsy with the large-bone instruments. Arthroscopy is used increasingly for this purpose in large joints. In distinguishing arthritis from gout, precautions should be taken to preserve any urate crystals present by fixation of the specimen in absolute alcohol rather than in aqueous fixatives. When infection is suspected, synovial fluid and tissue should be subjected to prompt microbiologic study.

SKELETAL MUSCLE

The principal indication for muscle biopsy in this group of disorders is the demonstration of arteritis. Because of the focal nature of this lesion, it is necessary to examine adequate amounts of tissue. The surgeon must ensure that the specimen be of sufficient size; 2 × 1 × 1 cm are realistic dimensions. Disposable isometric clamps for this purpose are available commercially. Fixation should be delayed for half an hour or so after excision. Bouin's solution is a useful fixative for this tissue. In most cases, serial sections are necessary. Making 100 sections, each fifth slide stained, as routine procedure, has yielded 4 times as many positive diagnoses of arteritis as have isolated, random sections. Enzyme and immunohistochemical examinations have less diagnostic value in rheumatic diseases than do the foregoing procedures. Should these examinations be desired, the tissue should be submitted unfixed to the pathologist. Immunoglobulins usually survive at least several hours' immersion in chilled saline solution, but enzyme preparations require that the specimen be quenched immediately in low-temperature isopentane.

PERIPHERAL NERVES

Biopsy of peripheral nerves is not often indicated in RA, but when it is, the sural nerve is the site of choice.[70]

SUBCUTANEOUS NODULES

In the differential diagnosis of a tophus, fixation of the nodule in absolute alcohol may serve the same useful purpose suggested in synovial biopsy. Epidermoid cysts in the olecranon region occasionally sim-

ulate rheumatoid nodules, and diagnostic biopsy may be indicated.[153]

LYMPH NODES

The principal indications for lymph node biopsy are: (1) the differential diagnosis of specific infectious arthritides, in which case the tissue should also be cultured; and (2) the differential diagnosis of the malignant lymphomas.

AMYLOIDOSIS

Needle punch biopsies of liver, spleen, and kidney offer no difficulties to the pathologist, but have occasionally resulted in serious visceral hemorrhages. Gingival, buccal, or rectal mucosal biopsies have at times established the presence of amyloid deposits in the walls of minute blood vessels in RA, as in other types of secondary amyloidosis. In each of these procedures, the diagnosis is valid only when positive and is not excluded when negative for amyloid material. Specific immunofluorescent staining for amyloid is not yet generally useful for several reasons.[152] Reliance must still be placed on properly controlled Congo red or similar preparations.

In summary, each of the deforming arthritides discussed in this chapter has certain similarities and common pathologic features. The inflammatory reactions in the joints, although inherently indistinguishable from each other, are nonspecific. The overlapping serologic reactions in the diffuse "collagen diseases," the histologic similarities in the subcutaneous nodules, the common patterns of vertebral bridges in spondyloarthropathy, the similarity of cutaneous lesions in Reiter's disease and pustular psoriasis, and the joint disease complicating the several sorts of chronic enteritis all defy a rigid nosologic concept. Whether they are truly "variants" of RA as was once thought, or independent diseases, as most now think, or nonspecific reaction patterns, as they appear to the pathologist, awaits more specific knowledge of their etiology and pathogenesis.

REFERENCES

1. Gardner, D.L.: The Pathology of Rheumatoid Arthritis. Baltimore, Williams & Wilkins, 1972.
2. Malcolm, A.J.: Diagnostic pathology in rheumatology. Clin. Rheum. Dis., 9:27–29, 1983.
3. Cooper, N.S., et al.: Diagnostic specificity of synovial lesions. Hum. Pathol., 12:314–328, 1981.

4. Neumark, T.: Cell-to-cell contacts between lymphoreticular cells in rheumatoid synovial membrane. Acta Morphol. Acad. Sci. Hung., 25:121–135, 1977.

5. Van Boxel, J.A., and Paget, S.A.: Predominantly T-cell infiltrate in rheumatoid synovial membranes. N. Engl. J. Med., 293:517–520, 1975.

6. Duke, O., et al.: An immunohistochemical analysis of lymphatic subpopulations and their microenvironment in the synovial membrane of patients with rheumatoid arthritis using monoclonal antibodies. Clin. Exp. Immunol., 49:22–30, 1982.

7. Kurosaka, M., and Ziff, M.: Immunoelectron microscopic study of distribution of T cell subsets in rheumatoid synovium. J. Exp. Med., 158:1191–1210, 1983.

8. Iguchi, T., Kurosaka, M., and Ziff, M.: Electron microscopic study HLA-DR and monocyte/macrophage staining of cells in the rheumatoid synovial membrane. Arthritis Rheum., 29:600–613, 1986.

9. Hogg, N., Palmer, D.G., and Revell, P.A.: Mononuclear phagocytes of normal and rheumatoid synovial membrane identified by monoclonal antibodies. Immunology, 56:673–681, 1985.

10. Padula, S.J., Clark, R.B., and Korn, J.H.: Cell-mediated immunity in rheumatic disease. Hum. Pathol., 17:254–263, 1986.

11. Dobloug, J.H., et al.: Natural killer (NK) cell activity of peripheral blood, synovial fluid, and synovial tissue lymphocytes from patients with rheumatoid arthritis and juvenile rheumatoid arthritis. Ann. Rheum. Dis., 41:490–495, 1982.

12. Piatier, D., et al.: Immunofluorescence of synovial membrane: multifactorial analysis of the results. Biomedicine, 24:359–366, 1976.

13. Nowoslawski, A., and Brzosko, W.J.: Immunopathology of rheumatoid arthritis. I. The rheumatoid synovitis. Pathol. Eur., 2:198–219, 1967.

14. Ogilvie-Harris, D.J., and Fornasier, V.L.: Synovial iron deposition in osteoarthritis. J. Rheumatol., 7:30–36, 1980.

15. Grimley, P.M., and Sokoloff, L.: Synovial giant cells in rheumatoid arthritis. Am. J. Pathol., 49:931–954, 1966.

16. Crisp, A.J., et al.: Articular mastocytosis in rheumatoid arthritis. Arthritis Rheum., 27:845–851, 1984.

17. Bromley, M., and Wooley, D.E.: Histopathology of the rheumatoid lesion: identification of cell types at sites of cartilage erosion. Arthritis Rheum., 27:857–863, 1984.

18. Gruber, B., et al.: Characterization and functional studies of rheumatoid synovial mast cells. Arthritis Rheum., 29:944–955, 1986.

19. Dingle, J.T.: Lysosomal enzymes and the degradation of cartilage matrix. Etiological factors in the collagen disease. Proc. R. Soc. Med., 55:109–111, 1962.

20. Ghadially, F.N., and Roy, S.: Ultrastructure of Synovial Joints in Health and Disease. London, Butterworth, 1969.

21. Zvaifler, N.J.: The immunopathology of joint inflammation in rheumatoid arthritis. Adv. Immunol., 16:265–336, 1973.

22. Berg, E., et al.: On the nature of rheumatoid rice bodies: an immunological, histochemical and electronmicroscopic study. Arthritis Rheum., 20:1343–1349, 1977.

23. Cheung, H.S., et al.: Synovial origins of rice bodies in joint fluid. Arthritis Rheum., 23:72–76, 1980.

24. McCarty, D.J., and Cheung, H.S.: Origin and significance of rice bodies in synovial fluid. Lancet, 2:715, 1982.

25. Scott, D.L., et al.: Significance of fibronectin in rheumatoid arthritis and osteoarthrosis. Ann. Rheum. Dis., 40:142–153, 1981.

26. Popert, A.J., et al.: Frequency of occurrence, mode of development, and significance of rice bodies in rheumatoid joints. Ann. Rheum. Dis., 41:109–117, 1982.

27. Rosenberger, J.L., et al.: A statistical approach to the histopathologic diagnosis of synovitis. Hum. Pathol., 12:329–337, 1981.

28. Goldenberg, D.L., and Cohen, A.S.: Synovial membrane histopathology in the differential diagnosis of rheumatoid arthritis, gout, pseudogout, systemic lupus erythematosus, infectious arthritis and degenerative joint disease. Medicine, 57:239–252, 1978.

29. Sokoloff, L.: Animal models of rheumatoid arthritis. Int. Rev. Exp. Pathol., 26:107–145, 1984.

30. Kobayashi, I., and Ziff, M.: Electron microscopic studies of the cartilage-pannus junction in rheumatoid arthritis. Arthritis Rheum., 18:475–483, 1975.

31. Shiozawa, S., Shiozawa, K., and Fujita, T.: Morphologic observations in the early phase of the cartilage-pannus junction. Arthritis Rheum., 26:472–478, 1983.

32. Kimura, H., Tateishi, H., and Ziff, M.: Surface ultrastructure of rheumatoid articular cartilage. Arthritis Rheum., 20:1085–1098, 1977.

33. Meyers, D.B., and Brown, N.D.: Morphological and biomechanical studies of rheumatoid pannus and cartilage. J. Rheumatol., 9:502–513, 1982.

34. Menninger, H., et al.: Granulocyte elastase at the site of cartilage erosion by rheumatoid synovial tissue. Z. Rheumatol., 39:145–156, 1980.

35. Mohr, W., Westerhellwig, H., and Wessinghage, D.: Polymorphonuclear granulocytes in rheumatic tissue destruction. III. An electronmicroscopic study of PMNs at the pannus cartilage junction in rheumatoid arthritis. Ann. Rheum. Dis., 40:396–399, 1981.

36. Harris, E.D., Jr.: Role of collagenases in joint destruction. In The Joints and Synovial Fluid. Vol. I. Edited by L. Sokoloff. New York, Academic Press, 1978, pp. 243–272.

37. Wooley, D.E., Crossley, J.J., and Evanson, J.M.: Collagenase at sites of cartilage erosion in the rheumatoid joint. Arthritis Rheum., 20:1231–1239, 1977.

38. Wooley, D.E., et al.: Collagenase production by rheumatoid synovial cells: morphological and immunohistochemical studies of the dendritic cell. Ann. Rheum. Dis., 38:262–270, 1979.

39. Harris, E.D., Jr.: Intracellular collagen fibers at the pannus-cartilage junction in rheumatoid arthritis. Arthritis Rheum., 20:657–665, 1977.

40. Jasin, H.E., and Dingle, J.T.: Human mononuclear cell factors mediate cartilage matrix degradation through chondrocyte activation. J. Clin. Invest., 68:571–581, 1981.

41. Shiozawa, A., Williams, R.C., Jr., and Ziff, M.: Immunoelectron microscopic demonstration of prostaglandin E in rheumatoid synovium. Arthritis Rheum., 25:685–693, 1982.

42. Cooke, T.D.V.: The interactions and local disease manifestations of immune complexes in articular collagenous tissues. In Studies in Joint Disease. Vol. I. Edited by A. Maroudas and E.J. Holborow. London, Pittman, 1980, pp. 158–200.

43. Ilardi, C.F., and Sokoloff, L.: The pathology of osteoarthritis: ten strategic questions for pharmacologic management. Semin. Arthritis Rheum., 2(Suppl. 1):3–7, 1981.

44. Bland, J.H.: Rheumatoid arthritis of the cervical spine. J. Rheumatol., 1:319–342, 1974.

45. Ball, J.: Articular pathology of ankylosing spondylitis. Clin. Orthop., 143:30–37, 1979.

46. Bywaters, E.G.L.: Rheumatoid and other disease of the cervical interspinous bursae, and changes in the spinous processes. Ann. Rheum. Dis., 41:360–370, 1982.

47. Sims-Williams, H., Jayson, M.I.V., and Baddeley, H.: Rheumatoid involvement of the lumbar spine. Ann. Rheum. Dis., 36:524–531, 1977.

48. Bywaters, E.G.L.: The pathology of the spine. In The Joints and Synovial Fluid. Vol. II. Edited by L. Sokoloff. New York, Academic Press, 1980, pp. 427–547.

49. Fukase, M., Koizumi, F., and Wakaki, K.: Histopathologic analysis of sixteen subcutaneous nodules. Acta Pathol. Jpn., 30:871–882, 1980.

50. Nowoslawski, A., and Brzosko, W.J.: Immunopathology of rheumatoid arthritis. II. The rheumatoid nodule (the rheumatoid granuloma). Path. Europ., 2:302–321, 1967.

51. Dorfman, H.D., Norman, A., and Smith, R.J.: Bone erosion in relation to subcutaneous rheumatoid nodules. Arthritis Rheum., 13:69–73, 1970.

52. Cochrane, W., et al.: Ultramicroscopic structure of rheumatoid nodules. Ann. Rheum. Dis., 23:345–363, 1964.

53. Gieseking, R., Baumer, A., and Backmann, L.: Electronenoptische Untersuchungen an Granulomen des Rheumatismus Nodosus. Z. Rheumaforsch., 28:163–175, 1969.

54. Ginsberg, M.H., et al.: Rheumatoid nodulosis. An unusual variant of rheumatoid disease. Arthritis Rheum., 18:49–58, 1975.

55. Mesara, B.W., Brody, G.L., and Oberman, H.A.: "Pseudorheumatoid" subcutaneous nodules. Am. J. Clin. Pathol., 45:684–691, 1966.

56. Williams, J.H., et al.: Isolated subcutaneous nodules (pseudorheumatoid). J. Bone Joint Surg., 59A:73–76, 1977.

57. Ehrlich, G.E., et al.: Pathogenesis of rupture of extensor tendons at the wrist in rheumatoid arthritis. Arthritis Rheum., 2:332–346, 1959.

58. Magyar, E., et al.: Muscle changes in rheumatoid arthritis. A review of the literature with a study of 100 cases. Virchows Arch. (Pathol. Anat.), 373(A):267–278, 1977.

59. Kim, R.C., and Collins, G.H.: The neuropathology of rheumatoid disease. Hum. Pathol., 12:5–15, 1981.

60. Oxenhandler, R., Adelstein, E.H., and Hart, M.N.: Immunopathology of skeletal muscle. The value of direct immunofluorescence in the diagnosis of connective tissue disorder. Hum. Pathol., 8:321–328, 1977.

61. Nakano, K.K.: The entrapment neuropathies of rheumatoid arthritis. Orthop. Clin. North Am., 6:837–860, 1975.

62. Sokoloff, L.: The pathophysiology of peripheral blood vessels in collagen diseases. In International Academy of Pathology, Monograph No. 4, 1963, pp. 297–325.

63. Prillamin, W.W., et al.: Intestinal complications in rheumatoid arthritis and their relationship to corticosteroid therapy. J. Chronic Dis., 27:475–481, 1974.

64. Fernandez-Diez, J.: General pathology of necrotizing vasculitis. Clin. Rheum. Dis., 6:279–295, 1980.

65. Scott, D.G.I., Bacon, P.A., and Tribe, C.R.: Systemic rheumatoid vasculitis: A clinical and laboratory study of 50 cases. Medicine, 60:288–297, 1981.

66. Mongan, E.S., et al.: A study of the relation of seronegative and seropositive rheumatoid arthritis to each other and to necrotizing vasculitis. Am. J. Med., 47:23–25, 1969.

67. Theofilopoulos, A.N., et al.: IgM rheumatoid factor and low molecular weight of IgM. An association with vasculitis. Arthritis Rheum., 17:272–284, 1974.

68. Dyck, P.J., Conn, D.L., and Okazaki, H.: Necrotizing angiopathic neuropathy. Mayo Clin. Proc., 47:461–475, 1972.

69. Ghose, T., et al.: Immunopathological changes in rheumatoid arthritis and other joint diseases. J. Clin. Pathol., 28:109–117, 1975.

70. Conn, D.L., McDuffie, F.C., and Dyck, P.J.: Immunopathologic study of sural nerves in rheumatoid arthritis. Arthritis Rheum., 15:135–143, 1972.

71. Conn, D.L., Schroeter, A.L., and McDuffie, F.C.: Cutaneous vessel immune deposits in rheumatoid arthritis. Arthritis Rheum., 19:15–20, 1976.

72. Ziff, M.: Relation of cellular infiltration of rheumatoid synovial membrane to its immune response. Arthritis Rheum., 17:313–319, 1974.

73. Hernandez-Lopez, E., et al.: Echocardiographic study of the cardiac involvement in rheumatoid arthritis. Chest, 72:52–55, 1977.

74. Klein, G., and Rainer, F.: Herzmanifestationen bei rheumatischen Erkrankungen. Wien Med. Wochenschr., 4:132–135, 1977.

75. Nomeir, A.M., et al.: Cardiac involvement in rheumatoid arthritis. Ann. Intern. Med., 79:800–806, 1973.

76. Siegmeth, W., and Eberl, R.: Gelenksfernemanifestationen der chronischen Polyarthritis. Wien Klin. Wochenschr., 88:81–84, 1976.

77. Turner, R., Collins, R., and Nomeir, A.M.: Extra-articular manifestations of rheumatoid arthritis. Bull. Rheum. Dis., 29:986–990, 1979.

78. John, J.T., Hough, A.J., and Sergent, J.S.: Pericardial disease in rheumatoid arthritis. Am. J. Med., 66:385–390, 1979.

79. Reimer, K.A., Rodgers, R.F., and Oyasu, R.: Rheumatoid arthritis with rheumatoid heart disease and granulomatous aortitis. JAMA, 235:2510–2512, 1977.

80. Roberts, W.C., et al.: Cardiac valvular lesions in rheumatoid arthritis. Arch. Intern. Med., 122:141–146, 1968.

81. Kirk, J.T., and Cosh, L.: The pericarditis of rheumatoid arthritis. Q. J. Med., 38:397–423, 1969.

82. Morris, P.B., et al.: Rheumatoid arthritis and coronary arteritis. Am. J. Cardiol., 57:689–690, 1986.

83. Bulkley, B.H., and Roberts, W.C.: Ankylosing spondylitis and aortic regurgitation: description of the characteristic cardiovascular lesion from study of eight necropsy patients. Circulation, 48:1014–1027, 1973.

84. Davis, R.F., and Engleman, E.C.: Incidence of myocardial infarction in patients with rheumatoid arthritis. Arthritis Rheum., 17:527–533, 1974.

85. Bonfiglio, T., and Atwater, E.C.: Heart disease in patients with seropositive rheumatoid arthritis: a controlled autopsy study and review. Arch. Intern. Med., 124:714–719, 1969.

86. Falicov, R., and Cooney, D.F.: Takayasu's arteritis and rheumatoid arthritis: a case report. Arch. Intern. Med., 114:594–600, 1964.

87. Hunninghake, G., and Fauci, A.: Pulmonary involvement in collagen vascular diseases. Am. Rev. Respir. Dis., 199:471–503, 1979.

88. Benedek, G.: Rheumatoid pneumoconiosis: documentation of onset and pathogenetic considerations. Am. J. Med., 55:515–524, 1973.

89. Walters, M.N., and Ojeada, V.J.: Pleuropulmonary necrobiotic rheumatoid nodules. Med. J. Aust., 144:648–651, 1986.

90. Katzenstein, A.A.: The histologic spectrum and differential diagnosis of necrotizing granulomatous inflammation in the lungs. In Progress in Surgical Pathology. Vol. II. Edited by C. Fenoglio and M. Wolff. New York, Masson, 1980.

91. Katzenstein, A.A., and Askin, F.B.: Surgical pathology of non-neoplastic lung disease. In Major Problems in Pathology. Vol. 13. Edited by J.L. Bennington. Philadelphia, W.B. Saunders Co., 1982.

92. Cervantes-Perez, P., Toro-Perez, A.H., and Rodriquez-Jur-

ado, P.: Pulmonary involvement in rheumatoid arthritis. JAMA, 243:1715–1719, 1980.

93. Frank, S.T., et al.: Pulmonary dysfunction in rheumatoid disease. Chest, 63:27–34, 1973.

94. Popper, M.S., Bogdonoff, M.L., and Hughes, R.L.: Interstitial rheumatoid lung disease: a reassessment and review of the literature. Chest, 62:243–250, 1972.

95. Collins, R.L., et al.: Obstructive pulmonary disease in rheumatoid arthritis. Arthritis Rheum., 19:623–628, 1976.

96. Winterbauer, R.H., Wilske, K.R., and Wheelis, R.F.: Diffuse pulmonary injury associated with gold therapy. N. Engl. J. Med., 294:919–921, 1976.

97. McCormick, J.N.: An immunofluorescence study of rheumatoid factors. Ann. Rheum. Dis., 22:1–10, 1963.

98. Nosanchuk, J.S., and Shnitzer, B.: Follicular hyperplasia in lymph nodes from patients with rheumatoid arthritis. Cancer, 24:343–354, 1969.

99. Willkens, F.R., et al.: Immunopathological studies in lymph nodes in rheumatoid arthritis and malignant lymphomas. Ann. Rheum. Dis., 39:147–151, 1980.

100. Barnes, C.G., Turnbull, A.L., and Vernon-Roberts, B.: Felty's syndrome—A clinical and pathological survey of two patients and their response to therapy. Ann. Rheum. Dis., 30:359–374, 1971.

101. Weisman, M., and Zvaifler, N.J.: Cryoimmunoglobulinemia in Felty's syndrome. Arthritis Rheum., 19:103–110, 1976.

102. Williams, R.A., et al.: *In vitro* studies of ineffective erythropoiesis in rheumatoid arthritis. Ann. Rheum. Dis., 41:502–507, 1982.

103. Masi, A.T., et al.: Hashimoto's disease: a clinicopathological study with matched controls. Lancet, 1:123–126, 1965.

104. Dorwart, B.B., and Schumacher, H.R.: Joint effusions, chondrocalcinosis and other rheumatic manifestations in hypothyroidism. Ann. Intern. Med., 59:780–790, 1975.

105. Watson, P.G., and Hayreh, S.S.: Scleritis and episcleritis. Br. J. Ophthalmol., 60:163–191, 1976.

106. Walter, J.R., and Boldt, H.A.: Scleromalacia perforans associated with a cotton wool spot of the retina in an otherwise healthy patient. Am. J. Ophthalmol., 55:922–930, 1963.

107. Henkind, P., and Gold, D.H.: Ocular manifestations of rheumatic disorders. Rheumatology, 4:13–59, 1973.

108. Olesby, R.B., et al.: Cataracts in patients with rheumatic diseases treated with corticosteroids. Arch. Ophthalmol., 66:625–630, 1961.

109. Chused, T.M., et al.: Sjögren's syndrome associated with HLA-DW3. N. Engl. J. Med., 296:895–897, 1977.

110. Thackray, A.C., and Lucas, R.B.: Tumors of the Major Salivary Glands. Washington, D.C., Armed Forces Institute of Pathology, 1974, p. 127.

111. Moutsopoulos, H.M., et al.: Sjögren's syndrome (sicca syndrome): Current issues. Ann. Intern. Med., 92:212–226, 1980.

112. Greenspan, J.S., et al.: The histopathology of Sjögren's syndrome in labial salivary gland biopsies. Oral Surg., 37:217–229, 1974.

113. Font, R.L., Yanoff, M., and Zimmerman, L.E.: Benign lymphoepithelial lesion of the lacrimal gland and its relationship to Sjögren's syndrome. Am. J. Clin. Pathol., 48:365–376, 1967.

114. Talal, N., Sokoloff, L., and Barth, W.: Extra-salivary lymphoid abnormalities in Sjögren's syndrome (reticulum-cell sarcoma, "pseudolymphoma," macroglobulinemia). Am. J. Med., 43:50–65, 1967.

115. Fox, R.I., et al.: Use of monoclonal antibodies to analyze peripheral blood and salivary gland lymphocyte subsets in Sjögren's syndrome. Arthritis Rheum., 25:419–426, 1982.

116. Pollak, V.E., Pirani, C.L., and Kark, R.M.: The kidney in rheumatoid arthritis: studies by renal biopsy. Arthritis Rheum., 5:1–9, 1962.

117. Whaley, K., and Webb, J.: Liver and kidney disease in rheumatoid arthritis. Clin. Rheum. Dis., 3:527–547, 1977.

118. Samuels, B., et al.: Membranous glomerulonephritis in patients with rheumatoid arthritis: relationship to gold therapy. Medicine, 57:319–327, 1978.

119. Kennedy, A.: Analgesic nephropathy. J. Clin. Pathol., 28 (Suppl. 9):14, 1975.

120. Calabro, J.J., et al.: Juvenile rheumaotid arthritis: a general review and report of 100 patients observed for 15 years. Semin. Arthritis Rheum., 5:257–298, 1976.

121. Wynn-Roberts, C.R., et al.: Light and electron-microscopic findings of juvenile rheumatoid arthritis synovium: comparison with normal juvenile synovium. Semin. Arthritis Rheum., 7:287–302, 1978.

122. Simon, F.E.R., and Schaller, J.G.: Benign rheumatoid nodules. Pediatrics, 56:29–33, 1975.

123. Bywaters, E.G.L., Glynn, L.E., and Seldis, A.: Subcutaneous nodules of Still's disease. Ann. Rheum. Dis., 17:278–285, 1958.

124. Chylack, L.T., Jr.: The ocular manifestations of juvenile rheumatoid arthritis. Arthritis Rheum., 20:217–233, 1977.

125. Rosenberg, A.M., and Oen, K.G.: The relationship between ocular and articular disease activity in children with juvenile rheumatoid arthritis and associated ureitis. Arthritis Rheum., 29:787–800, 1986.

126. Brewer, E., Jr.: Juvenile rheumatoid arthritis—cardiac involvement. Arthritis Rheum., 20:231–236, 1977.

127. Leitman, P.S., and Bywaters, E.G.L.: Pericarditis in juvenile rheumatoid arthritis. Pediatrics, 32:855–860, 1963.

128. Bernstein, B., Takahashi, M., and Hanson, V.: Noninvasive techniques in the study of cardiac involvement in juvenile rheumatoid arthritis. Arthritis Rheum., 16:535–536, 1973.

129. Isdale, I.C., and Bywaters, E.G.L.: The rash of rheumatoid arthritis and Still's disease. Q. J. Med., 25:377–387, 1956.

130. Phillips, P.E.: Virologic studies in rheumatoid arthritis. Rheumatology, 6:353–360, 1975.

131. Fox, R., et al.: Rheumatoid arthritis synovial membrane contains a 62,000-molecular-weight protein that shares an antigenic epitope with the Epstein-Barr virus-encoded associated nuclear antigen. J. Clin. Invest., 77:1539–1547, 1986.

132. Poole, A.R., and Coombs, R.R.A.: Rheumatoid-like joint lesions in rabbits injected intravenously with bovine serum. Int. Arch. Allergy Appl. Immunol., 54:97–113, 1977.

133. Ishikawa, H., and Ziff, M.: Electron-microscopic observations of immunoreactive cells in the rheumatoid synovial membrane. Arthritis Rheum., 19:1–14, 1976.

134. Konttinen, Y.T., Reitamo, S., and Ranki, A.: Characterization of the immunocompetent cells of rheumatoid synovium from tissue sections and eluates. Arthritis Rheum., 24:71–79, 1981.

135. Rasker, J.J., and Kuipers, F.C.: Are rheumatoid nodules caused by vasculitis? A study of 13 early cases. Ann. Rheum. Dis., 42:384–388, 1983.

136. Pasion, E.G., and Goodfellow, J.W.: Preankylosing spondylitis. Ann. Rheum. Dis., 34:92–97, 1975.

136a. Romanus, P., and Yden, S.: Pelvo-Spondylitis Ossificans. Copenhagen, Munksgaard, 1955.

137. François, R.J.: Le rachis dans la spondyloarthrite ankylosante. Brussels, Editions Arscia, 1975.

138. Caffrey, M.F.P., and James, D.C.O.: Human lymphocyte association in ankylosing spondylitis. Nature, 242:121–123, 1973.

139. Schlosstein, L., et al.: High association of HL-A antigen W-

27 with ankylosing spondylitis. N. Engl. J. Med., *288*:704–706, 1973.

140. Moll, J.M.H., and Wright, V.: Psoriatic arthritis. Semin. Arthritis Rheum., *3*:55–78, 1973.

141. Weinberger, H.W., et al.: Reiter's syndrome, clinical and pathological observations: a long-term study of 16 cases. Medicine, *41*:35–91, 1962.

142. Morris, R., et al.: Medical intelligence. HL-A-W27—A useful discriminator in the arthropathies of inflammatory bowel disease. N. Engl. J. Med., *290*:1117–1119, 1974.

143. Haslock, I.: Enteropathic arthritis. *In* Copeman's Textbook of the Rheumatic Diseases. 5th Ed. Edited by J.T. Scott. Edinburgh, Churchill-Livingstone, 1978, pp. 567–577.

144. Macrae, I., and Wright, V.: A family study of ulcerative colitis with particular reference to ankylosing spondylitis and sacroiliitis. Ann. Rheum. Dis., *32*:16–20, 1973.

145. McEwen, C., et al.: Arthritis accompanying ulcerative colitis. Am. J. Med., *33*:923–941, 1962.

146. Soren, A.: Joint affections in regional ileitis. Arch. Intern. Med., *117*:78–83, 1966.

147. Wright, V.: A unifying concept for the spondylarthropathies. Clin. Orthop., *143*:8–14, 1979.

148. Caughey, D.E., and Bywaters, E.G.L.: The arthritis of Whipple's syndrome. Ann. Rheum. Dis., *22*:327–335, 1963.

149. Hawkins, C.F., et al.: Detection by electron microscope of rod-shaped organisms in synovial membrane from a patient with the arthritis of Whipple's disease. Ann. Rheum. Dis., *35*:502–509, 1976.

150. Rötstein, J., and Good, R.A.: Significance of the simultaneous occurrence of connective tissue disease and agammaglobulinemia. Ann. Rheum. Dis., *21*:202–206, 1962.

151. Grayzel, A.I., et al.: Chronic polyarthritis associated with hypogammaglobulinemia. A study of two patients. Arthritis Rheum., *20*:887–894, 1977.

152. Husby, G.: Amyloidosis in rheumatoid arthritis. Ann. Clin. Res., *7*:154–167, 1975.

153. Wilson, J.T., and Sokoloff, L.: Epidermoid cysts stimulating rheumatoid nodules in the olecranon region. JAMA, *214*:593–595, 1970.

MECHANISMS OF TISSUE DESTRUCTION IN RHEUMATOID ARTHRITIS

42

STEPHEN M. KRANE

In many patients with unremitting chronic rheumatoid arthritis (RA), as well as in others with non-rheumatoid chronic synovitis, disruption of the normal structure and function of the joint is a prominent feature. Indeed, much of the disability of rheumatoid disease is due to joint damage itself. Weakening of the joint capsule and ligaments, erosion of cartilage and bone, rupture of tendons, and decrease in viscosity and other alterations of the synovial fluid may be found. Under certain circumstances, during remission of the inflammatory process, the resorptive processes may diminish, and some of the connective tissue components may be renewed, although much of the damage is irreversible. Some of the pathogenetic mechanisms of joint destruction are discussed in this chapter.

The mechanical functions of the normal joint are determined by its structure. The usefulness of the joint as a bearing depends on the integrity of the opposing surfaces of the articular cartilage, the thickness and pattern of the subchondral bone, and the interaction of the cartilage with water, proteins, hyaluronic acid, and other components of the synovial fluid. The surfaces must be properly aligned, and their position must be maintained by the integrity of the joint capsule, ligaments, tendons, and muscles. The functional characteristics of each of these connective tissues are, in turn, determined by their chemical composition. Connective tissues in general are characterized by specialized component cells and by the type and abundance of extracellular material. This extracellular material may be considered in several

subclasses. The first of these subclasses comprises the fibrillar components, of which collagen and elastin are the most abundant. Then are found the components of the ground substance, of which the proteoglycans make up the greatest proportion, in addition to proteins such as glycoproteins, some of which, for example, fibronectin and laminin, are involved in adherence of cells to the extracellular matrix.[1] Bone contains a calcium-phosphate mineral phase that accounts for approximately two-thirds of its weight.[2,3] The remainder of bone matrix is predominantly type I collagen, although it also contains several noncollagenous proteins. These include two γ-carboxyglutamic acid-(GLA-)containing proteins called bone GLA protein or osteocalcin, as well as matrix GLA protein, osteonectin, and several specific proteoglycans, phosphoproteins, and sialoproteins. Another protein synthesized in the liver but present in bone in an abundance greater than expected from its concentration in plasma is α_2-HS-glycoprotein.

Little elastin is present in the joint structures; collagen is the major fibrillar component. The interstitial collagens of joint connective tissues are all basically composed of molecules aligned in the particular array characteristic of collagens in general.[2,4-7] The pattern is that of an approximately one-quarter stagger of the length of the molecule, with overlap and hole zones (see Chapter 12). The collagens of several of the joint structures differ from each other in terms of primary structure, as well as in certain post-translational modifications.[8] Types I, II, and III collagen all are composed of three polypeptide chains, arrayed in an ordered, helical configuration. This helical configuration and the formation of the collagen fibril confer certain functional properties onto these tissues, as well as a characteristic resistance to attack by proteolytic enzymes.[9,10] The further interactions of the collagen with other components of the particular connective tissue, in turn, determine the mechanical properties of these tissues and the rate at which they are degraded.

It is possible that the earliest lesion in RA is a proliferation of the lining layer of the synovium in the presence of inflammatory cells.[11,12] The collection of inflammatory cells that usually begins in the recesses of the joint at the sites of reflection of the synovium may progress over the surface of the articular cartilage (pannus) or may burrow into the subchondral bone (Figs. 42–1 and 42–2); in other areas where tendon sheaths are involved, the inflammatory mass may burrow through the surface of the tendons. If the process continues unabated, the connective tissue structures of the joint tendons will be eroded, and normal function will be interrupted. The extremes of such connective tissue destruction are seen in the rupture of extensor tendons, in the loss of entire articular cartilage down to subchondral bone, and in erosions of bone that may, on rare occasions, proceed to the resorption of entire subarticular regions. For the most part, the connective tissue destruction occurs predominantly in areas adjacent to the margin of the invading pannus. This process has been demonstrated by a variety of techniques, including electron microscopy.[13,14] The thickness of the cartilage usually remains intact in areas not immediately adjacent to the proliferating cellular granulations, but proteoglycans may be lost in areas remote from the margin of these granulations, even in early synovitis.[15]

The pannus of chronic RA (Fig. 42–3) contains a heterogeneous population of cells.[11] In the past, identification of these cells was based almost exclusively on morphologic criteria.[11,16] In addition to chronic inflammatory cells, it was thought that the pannus contained the same cell types found in the normal synovial lining, that is, phagocytic type A cells, secretory type B cells, and type C cells with features of both type A and type B cells, which was especially characteristic of RA. Both T- and B-lymphocytes and plasma cells are present to a variable extent.[17–23] T-lymphocytes predominate and are considered to be "activated." An even higher percentage (~ 90%) of these synovial T-lymphocytes have the OKT4 (CD4)

FIG. 42–1. Low-power view of typical rheumatoid arthritis of a metacarpophalangeal joint. The pannus (P) covers the surfaces of the articular cartilage (C) and in other areas has burrowed through subchondral bone (B). Bar = 400 μm.

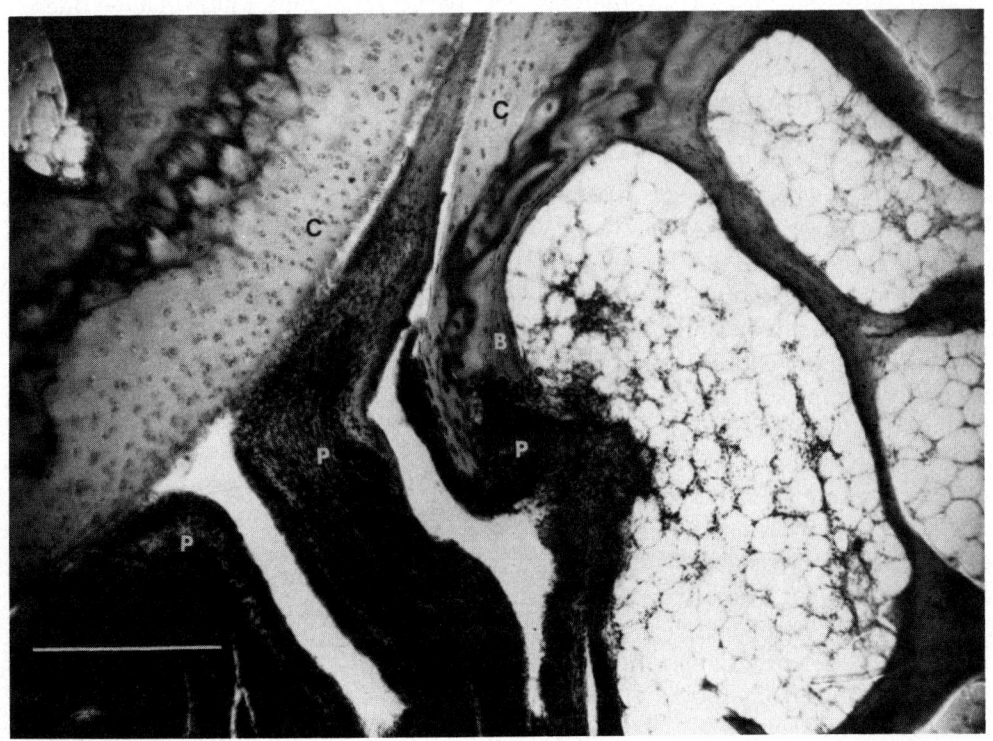

FIG. 42–2. Higher-power view of an area of rheumatoid bone erosion. Cells resembling osteoclasts (O) (artifactually pulled away from bone [B] surface) merge with other inflammatory cells. Bar = 80 μm.

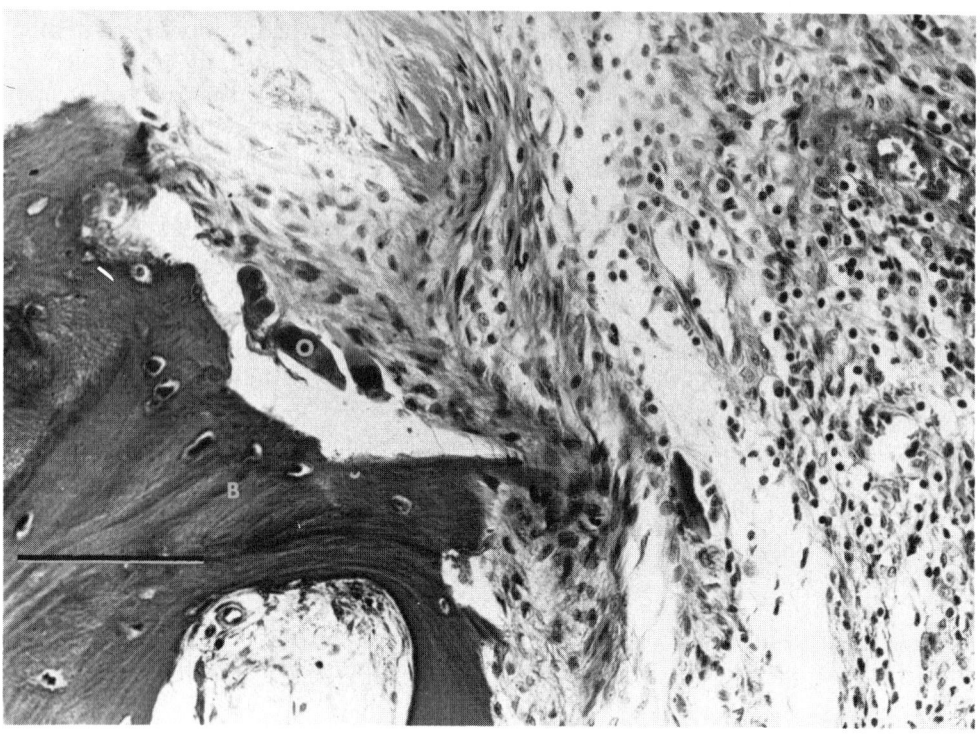

surface antigen (helper, inducer-type) than peripheral blood (~ 67%), and these are distributed differently from the OKT8+ cells.[24] Although these cells play an important function in the local inflammatory process, their specificity and function are unknown. Recently, it has been found that the T-cell populations grown from the inflammatory synovium in the presence of interleukin-2 (IL-2) are characterized by the predominance of a limited number of clones.[23] This oligoclonality probably reflects the presence of a limited number of potentially responding lymphocytes at the site of the synovial lesion. Attempts have also been made to characterize the pannus cells based on certain functions in cell culture and according to the expression of surface antigens detected by other monoclonal antibodies. The most abundant adherent cell present in primary cultures of rheumatoid synovium is a large, stellate cell frequently containing long dendritic processes.[25] These *synovial stellate cells* stain by indirect immunofluorescence using antibodies to synovial collagenase,[26] but do not have Fc receptors for immunoglobulins.[25] They are probably related to fibroblasts because they stain for type III collagen and synthesize types I and III collagens and are distinct from the strongly Ia-positive, Fc-negative, so-called *dendritic* or

accessory cells.[27,28] Some of these synovial fibroblasts express class II histocompatibility antigens (Ia) on their surface, particularly with a DR+/DQ− phenotype.[17,18] In culture, the expression of the class II antigens is lost, but that it can be reduced with interferon-γ suggests that this lymphokine functions in this role in vivo.

It has been proposed that the lining cells are divisible into three populations according to the distribution of surface antigens.[18,29] The first is an Ia-positive, Fc-positive, phagocytic cell of the monocyte-macrophage lineage. The second is a nonphagocytic, intensely Ia-positive cell that lacks Fc receptors and other monocyte-lineage antigens and is not a B- or T-lymphocyte. This is the dendritic cell particularly abundant in rheumatoid synovium. The third is usually Ia negative but always Fc negative and is probably related to fibroblasts. This third group of cells may assume a stellate shape after exposure to prostaglandin E_2 (PGE$_2$) and activation of adenylate cyclase.[30] Interferon-γ can not only induce the expression of class II antigens on these fibroblasts, but may also otherwise alter their phenotype, for example, by decreasing the expression of the genes for collagens and fibronectin through transcriptional control mechanisms.[17,31–34]

FIG. 42–3. Section of the surface of rheumatoid synovitis showing the heterogeneous population of cells. Lining cells (LC) and lymphocytes and other mononuclear cells (M) can be seen. Bar = 80 μm.

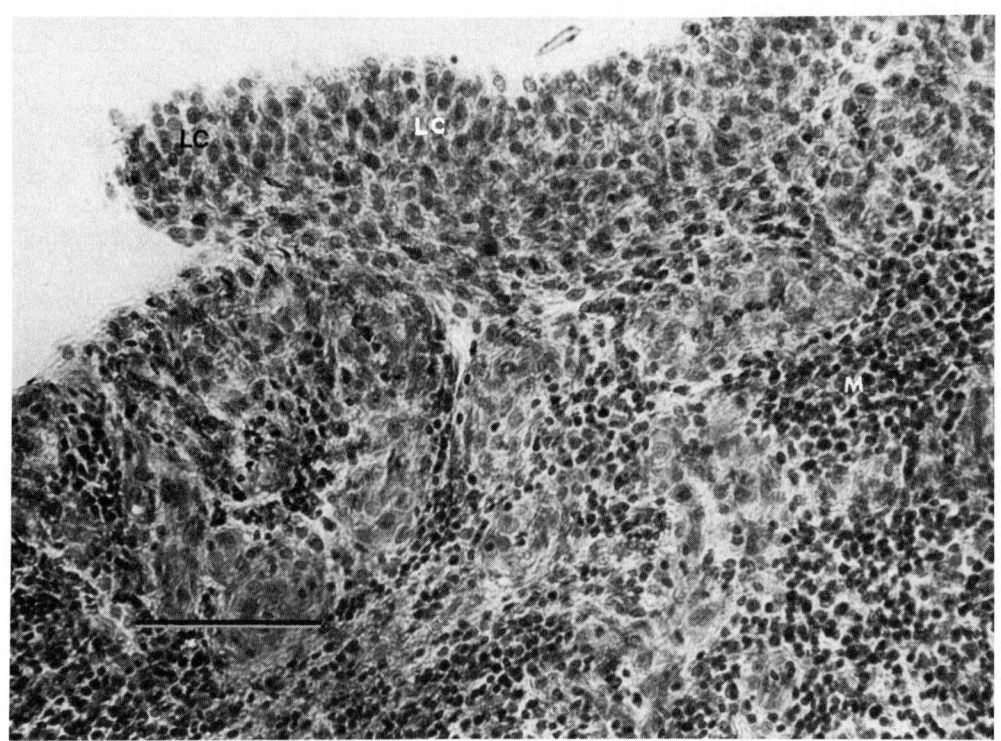

The predominant cells in rheumatoid synovial fluids are polymorphonuclear leukocytes, which are uncommon in the pannus itself,[11] although they have been found at the cartilage-pannus junction.[35] The other cells found in the pannus may also be present in synovial fluid, however. Some of the interactions among the inflammatory cells that might be important in determining the characteristics, intensity, and direction of the destructive process are considered subsequently.

COLLAGEN DEGRADATION

In its native helical form, collagen is refractory to degradation by common proteolytic enzymes such as trypsin, chymotrypsin, and pepsin.[9,10,36] Although the nonhelical region at the ends of the molecule may be attacked by these proteinases, the helical portion is less susceptible to attack. A possible exception to this generalization is type III collagen, which is cleaved at a specific site near the collagenase-cleavage site by enzymes such as neutrophil elastase.[37] Moreover, the fibril is even more resistant to proteolysis than the component molecules, presumably owing to inter-

molecular interactions that further stabilize its structure. When collagen is denatured, that is, when the helical structure is uncoiled, proteolytic enzymes can attack peptide bonds in the polypeptide chain at many different locations. No evidence suggests, however, that collagen is denatured in vivo, even in inflammatory lesions. It had been known for years that enzymes present in bacteria such as Clostridium histolyticum could attack native collagen, even the helical portion, at many different loci; however, convincing demonstration of enzymes from animal tissues that could specifically carry out such an attack was lacking until Gross and Lapiere reported their observations.[38] These workers found that certain tadpole tissues in culture produced specific enzymes that attacked helical collagen molecules in solution, as well as in fibril form, in a characteristic manner. Shortly thereafter, Evanson and co-workers demonstrated that rheumatoid synovial tissue in culture produced enzyme(s) that degraded native collagen.[39,40] This process was accomplished by implanting fragments of synovium, obtained at the time of synovectomy, directly onto reconstituted collagen gels, with resulting lysis of the gels. Furthermore, the culture media contained soluble collagenase, which could be assayed against either collagen molecules in solution or insoluble collagen fibrils.

Collagenase from rheumatoid synovial tissue culture, like that from the tadpole and other animal tissues, cleaves the collagen molecule across all three chains at a position three-quarters the distance from the amino terminal end. At 37°C, fragments cleaved from the fibril become more soluble and are then denatured. Further digestion of the solubilized fragments to smaller peptides is then accomplished, probably by neutral proteinases other than collagenase. Data obtained by many investigators, using collagenases of different sources and with types I, II, and III collagens as substrates, show that the peptide bands cleaved are between specific glycyl-isoleucyl or glycyl-leucyl residues.[9,41] Sufficient information has been accumulated to establish criteria for determining the role of collagenase in the destruction of connective tissues in inflammatory arthritis. These criteria are as follows:

Collagen degradation in RA is predominantly extracellular; this finding is consistent wih evidence in vitro that collagenase is released from cultured tissues and is present in low concentrations in tissue homogenates. Under some circumstances, phagocytosis of collagen fibrils has been observed.[14] Collagenolysis in vitro is also proportional to the collagenase activity released into the culture media, and a collagenase similar to that produced by cultured synovium is found in vivo, particularly in synovial fluids.[42,43] Some of the enzyme in rheumatoid synovial fluids is probably derived from the polymorphonuclear leukocytes.[13,42] In a minority of rheumatoid fluids, collagenase activity is present without proteolytic activation,[42] but treatment (activation) with trypsin produces activity in almost all fluids. Products similar to the specific reaction products of synovial collagenase acting on collagen in vitro have been demonstrated in vivo.[44] The pattern of inhibition of collagenase in vitro has been correlated with the pattern of collagen degradation in the rheumatoid joint; most of the collagen destruction takes place adjacent to the pannus, whereas collagen is usually preserved in regions not in contact with the pannus. Macromolecular inhibitors of collagenase are present in serum and synovial fluid and consist mainly of α_2-macroglobulin as well as lower-molecular-weight inhibitors. Finally, the putative collagen substrates degraded in the course of rheumatoid synovitis are indeed substrates for collagenase in vitro.[36,45,46]

Most collagenases, including the rheumatoid synovial enzyme, cleave the interstitial collagens (types I, II, and III), but do not degrade type IV collagen, found in basement membranes, or type V collagen, found in pericellular regions and around the interstitial collagen fibers deeper in the matrix. Types IV and V collagens are attacked, however, by several other neutral proteinases such as elastases.[47,48] The rate at which cartilage type II collagen is attacked is slower than the rate for types I and III collagens.[36,45,49] Nevertheless, both crude and purified cartilage collagens are degraded by the rheumatoid synovial collagenase. Whether proteoglycans alter the rate or extent of collagenolysis is not certain because the proteoglycan component is usually already degraded before the collagen is attacked.

Bone erosion is a characteristic accompaniment of chronic persistent RA,[11,50] but mineralized bone collagen cannot be attacked by collagenases of any source, even bacteria.[51,52] The presence of the calcium-phosphate mineral phase also protects bone collagen from thermal denaturation.[53,54] Once the calcium-phosphate phase is removed, for example, by means of chelating agents or cold dilute acid, the collagen becomes susceptible to collagenolytic cleavage. The mechanisms by which the mineral is removed in vivo are not certain. Possibilities include local decreases in pH, production of a biologic chelator such as citrate, or operation of a cellular calcium or phosphate ion pump that effectively reduces local concentration of these ions and favors dissolution of the solid phase.[54] The most likely mechanism to explain leaching of the mineral phase is production of a unique acid environment in the extracellular compartment adjacent to bone-resorbing cells. It is not certain which cells are necessary for bone resorption. For example, osteoclasts normally present on endosteal surfaces could be activated through some interactions with pannus cells, or their differentiation could be induced from the hematopoietic precursor cells.[55] Alternatively, cells derived from the inflammatory tissue itself could differentiate into osteoclasts or could be involved directly in resorbing bone, without mediation by differentiated bone cells. Currently, it is thought that osteoclasts are activated or induced to differentiate from precursors by the action of some factor released by osteoblasts or related cells. Interleukin-1 (IL-1) or tumor necrosis factor (TNF-α) or lymphotoxin (TNF-β) can induce this osteoclast activation through effects on osteoblasts.[56,57] These effects may possibly be mediated by known factors such as granulocyte-macrophage colony-stimulating factor (GM-CSF) or interleukin 3 (IL-3). Cells similar to those present in the pannus can produce these hematopoietic growth factors.[58,59] Although monocyte-macrophages can bind to mineralized bone matrix and have some capacity to resorb dead bone, it is not clear whether they have any role in resorption of living bone, and no evidence suggests that they directly form osteoclasts.

Robinson and co-workers have shown that prostaglandins, particularly PGE$_2$, are produced in large amounts by rheumatoid synovium in culture.[60–62] Such culture media have bone-resorbing activity toward mouse calvaria in vitro, accounted for by the PGE$_2$ present. The bone-resorbing activity in these studies is extractable into ether at low pH and is inhibited by indomethacin, as is the PGE$_2$ production. Bone-resorbing substances other than prostaglandins are also produced by rheumatoid synovial culture media.[54] These bone-resorbing substances are undoubtedly heterogeneous. They probably influence osteoclasts indirectly, as discussed earlier, by first acting on osteoblasts or related cells such as stromal fibroblasts.[56,57] It is reasonable to consider that the rheumatoid synovial fibroblasts would function in a similar fashion. Potential candidates for inducers of bone resorption in the rheumatoid lesion include IL-1s, TNF-α, TNF-β, the colony-stimulating factors, and transforming growth factor β (TGF-β).[63–65] So-called osteoclast-activating factor (OAF), which initially was thought to represent one protein, is best considered a term to describe one or several of the cytokines mentioned;[66–70] others may still be discovered. These resorbing factors may not only be derived from macrophages and T-lymphocytes, but also from B-lymphocytes.[71,72] For example, some B-lymphocytes secrete IL-1 and some also express TNF-β.

Collagenase, a typical neutral metalloproteinase, is secreted from cells in a latent form. The latent collagenase can be activated by limited proteolysis, as was first demonstrated by Vaes.[73] Activation in some systems can also be accomplished by organic mercurial compounds apparently incapable of cleaving peptide bonds.[74,75] In rheumatoid synovial organ cultures, the collagenase is present in an active form,[39,40] whereas in cultures of rheumatoid synovial cells, collagenase is secreted in a latent form that can be activated by trypsin.[25] The occurrence of latent collagenase in rheumatoid synovial fluids has been discussed.

Collagenase proteins are secreted from cultured rabbit synovial cells or human rheumatoid synovial cells in the form of zymogens with M$_r$ (molecular weight) of 55,000 and 60,000.[76,77] The higher-molecular-weight species is a glycosylated form of the lower-molecular-weight protein. Formation of active collagenase probably results in vivo from limited proteolysis.[78,79] The amino acid sequence of human skin and gingival fibroblast collagenase has now been deduced from the cDNA sequence, and the probable site where the zymogen is cleaved to produce active enzyme has been identified. The potential site of

cleavage would result in the removal of 81 amino acids from the amino terminal portion of the proenzyme.[80,81] The proteolytic activation of procollagenase is probably indirect and involves a specific procollagenase activator. This activator, which is also secreted in a latent form that also requires activation, may be essential for cleavage of the procollagenase zymogen.[78] The procollagenase proactivator is most likely the enzyme stromelysin (metalloproteinase 3),[82,83] which is homologous with procollagenase based on its cDNA sequence.[80,81] Collagenase and stromelysin are both induced in human fibroblasts after treatment with phorbol esters.[84–87] Another protein, originally called transin but now shown to be identical to stromelysin, is also induced in rat fibroblasts by infection with polyoma virus, Rous sarcoma virus, or transfection with the middle T oncogene or the cellular oncogene H-ras.[25,80,81,88] An invasive inflammatory lesion (rheumatoid synovitis) and some transformed cells are both characterized by major synthesis of members of this family of metalloproteinases.

Activation of the procollagenase by activator (stromelysin) first requires activation of the proactivator. Although in vitro trypsin can function in this capacity, some other proteinase system would have to operate in vivo. The plasminogen activator system, through generation of plasmin, is a likely candidate.[79,89] Other proteinases may also have this function. For example, mast cells are abundant in the rheumatoid synovium.[90–92] Some mast cells secrete tryptase, which could also act in the proactivator-procollagenase cascade.

Another important aspect of control of collagenolysis involves interactions of the active enzyme with inhibitors.[93–98] One class of these inhibitors includes a glycoprotein with an approximate molecular weight of 30,000 daltons that specifically inhibits connective tissue metalloproteinases. Some investigators have referred to this protein as tissue inhibitor of metalloproteinases (TIMP). This protein has been cloned, and its deduced amino acid sequence is identical to erythroid-potentiating activity.[99,100] The major role of erythroid-potentiating activity is probably inhibition of metalloproteinase activity rather than any specific role in augmenting the proliferation and differentiation of hematopoietic precursor cells. The inability to identify collagenolytic activity in some connective tissue cells, such as monocyte-macrophages, results from the synthesis and release of greater quantities of inhibitor than of collagenase.[101] Because proteolytic activation of procollagenases probably involves serine proteinases such as plasmin, through plasminogen activator, inhibitors of serine proteinases may also have a regulatory role. Furthermore, such enzymes could cleave the nonhelical regions of the collagen molecules and could thereby disrupt cross links. These serine proteinase inhibitors could potentially regulate the activity of enzymes such as plasminogen activator, which, by generating plasmin, could be involved in activating procollagenase by activator. An inhibitor tentatively identified in cultures of rheumatoid synovial cells is proteinase nexin. This protein interacts with serine proteinases through the active site serine and yields a complex that then binds specifically to receptors on cell surfaces and is internalized and degraded within the cell.[102] Other inhibitors that have been purified and whose cDNAs have been cloned include proteins that inhibit the activity of plasminogen activator.[89,103] All these inhibitors could play important roles in the rheumatoid synovium by regulating proteolysis.

PROTEOGLYCAN DEGRADATION

The proteoglycans are important structural constituents of connective tissue, particularly of cartilage. Enzymatic removal of the proteoglycans in vitro diminishes the capacity of cartilage to resist deformation under a mechanical load.[104,105] On the other hand, collagen is responsible for the static form of cartilage, that is, its thickness.[104] The mechanical properties of cartilage thus depend on both the collagen and the proteoglycan components. During RA, loss of proteoglycan is prominent. Even in early disease, depletion of proteoglycan may be seen in areas remote from the pannus.[15,106] Although such regions retain their form and thickness for considerable periods if the collagen network is preserved, alteration of mechanical properties is a consequence of the loss of the proteoglycans.[104]

Proteoglycan loss from articular cartilage in inflammatory joint disease probably involves cleavage of the core protein of the proteoglycan subunit. Although carbohydrases such as hyaluronidase can attack the chondroitin sulfate moiety of the proteoglycan, evidence of the presence of significant hyaluronidase activity in normal or inflamed synovial tissue is insufficient.[107] Superoxide free radical produced by polymorphonuclear leukocytes might also be involved in proteoglycan degradation, analogous to the effects of superoxide on hyaluronic acid.[108] The proteoglycan core protein is cleaved by different proteinases to yield proteoglycan subunit molecules approximately the same size as the native proteoglycan subunit molecule.[109] These fragments, however, lack the capcity to bind hyaluronic acid and diffuse out of the cartilage. Which proteinase is responsible for this effect in inflammatory joint disease?

It had been proposed that the lysosomal acid proteinase cathepsin D was the critical enzyme.[110–115] Cathepsin D at low pH can attack proteoglycan core protein. This enzyme has been found in human and other cartilage extracts and has been demonstrated extracellularly in rheumatoid synovial tissue by immunofluorescence.[113] Cathepsin D or B is unlikely to play any important role in extracellular digestion, however, because the purified enzymes have no significant activity against proteoglycan substrates at pH >6.0.[112,113] The pH in inflammatory synovial fluids is less than in noninflammatory fluids, but not <6.8.[116] Furthermore, inhibitors of cathepsin B and D have little effect on cartilage matrix depletion in model systems.[109] Enzymes such as cathepsin B1 could be important in degradation of bone collagen in the zone adjacent to the ruffled border of the osteoclast, however. The pH in this zone is low because of the function of a specialized proton pump in the osteoclast membrane.[117]

Some of the neutral proteinases described are probably responsible for degradation of proteoglycans in vivo.[109] Human granulocytes contain two different enzymes that can attack proteoglycans in solution as well as in cartilage slices. These enzymes have been characterized as an elastase and a chymotrypsin-like enzyme.[118,119] The elastase produces smaller fragments of the proteoglycan core than the chymotrypsin-like enzyme. Other proteinases active on proteoglycans at neutral pH have been described in human cartilage and fibroblasts.[109,120] The metalloproteinases can also degrade the core protein of the proteoglycans. Stromelysin (metalloproteinase 3), which has been purified from cultures of rheumatoid synovial fibroblasts, may play the most significant role in this proteolysis.[82] Polymorphonuclear leukocytes are probably responsible for at least part of the proteoglycan-degrading activity in RA. Because these enzymes are inhibited by proteins found in inflammatory synovial fluids, such as α_1-antitrypsin and α_2-macroglobulin, uncontrolled degradation of tissue constituents probably does not occur.

Although the capacity of cartilage to reconstitute itself with type II collagen is limited, cartilage has a considerable capacity to restore proteoglycan.[121] This capacity has been shown particularly in experimental carrageenin-induced arthritis in the rabbit.[122–124] Early in the lesion, proteoglycan is lost, a loss ascribable to proteolytic activity, as well as to depression of proteoglycan biosynthesis. With recovery from inflammation, proteoglycan synthesis recovers and may exceed that found in an uninvolved joint. Inhibition of proteoglycan biosynthesis might be related to soluble factors present in the inflammatory exudate, such as prostaglandins and other soluble products of lymphocytes and monocytes,[125–129] and restoration of synthesis as inflammation subsides may occur when the concentration of these factors decreases. The "overshoot" in synthetic activity might be due to a feedback control secondary to a decrease in cartilage proteoglycan concentration.

CONTROL OF TISSUE DEGRADATION

The destruction of the joint appears to be explained by the production and release of degradative enzymes. The magnitude and duration of the synovial lesion are determined by several factors, including the relative proportion and number of each cell type in the pannus, the adjacent bone marrow and synovial fluid, the activity of the responsible cells, and the interaction of these cells with the environment, mediated either by direct cell-cell contact or by release of soluble products.

Although the polymorphonuclear leukocyte contains and releases neutral proteinases capable of degrading proteoglycans, the major collagenase-producing cell is probably the synovial fibroblast. Polymorphonuclear leukocytes do contain and can release several proteinases, and it is likely that some of the proteolytic activity in inflammatory synovial fluids is derived from these cells.[13,42] These proteinases include elastase,[130] a serine proteinase, which can also cleave type III and IV collagens and gelatinase,[131] a metalloproteinase. Polymorphonuclear leukocytes are also the source of a collagenase,[124,132,133] which is a metalloproteinase distinct biochemically and immunologically from fibroblast collagenase.[134,135] As mentioned previously, however, polymorphonuclear leukocytes are scarce in the pannus. Most dermal and normal synovial fibroblasts secrete only small amounts of detectable latent collagenase activity unless they are activated with specific cytokines or exposure to reagents such as phorbol ester or cytochalasin B.[38,41,79,136] In contrast, in cultures of rheumatoid synovial fibroblasts obtained by dispersion of the synovial lining cells with proteinases, large amounts of collagenase, as well as of PGE_2, are produced spontaneously.[137] The collagenase is secreted by these cells in the form of the procollagenase zymogen previously discussed.

Cultures in which large amounts of collagenase are secreted contain many Fc-negative stellate cells.[25,26,27] These cells are positive by indirect immunofluorescence using antibodies to rheumatoid synovial collagenase.[26] Cells that retain the capacity to synthesize and to secrete collagenase persist in culture when all monocyte-macrophages are no longer detectable and when the levels of lysozyme, an enzyme marker for monocyte-macrophages, are also undetectable. Although rodent macrophages produce collagenase when stimulated, for example, with endotoxin,[138,139] macrophages derived from human peripheral blood monocytes produce low levels of this enzyme even when stimulated.[27,28] Failure to detect collagenase activity in medium conditioned by macrophages can be accounted for by excessive production of the metalloproteinase inhibitor.[101] The cells in the rheumatoid synovium that are the major source of collagenase are thus fibroblasts, possibly derived from the synovial lining B cells or similar cells in the synovial stroma. The stellate morphology can be accounted for, at least in part, by the high ambient levels of PGE_2 because this appearance can be induced by stimulating endogenous PGE_2 production or by the addition of exogenous PGE_2, with subsequent activation of adenylate cyclase.[30] Even when PGE_2 production is inhibited with indomethacin, however, and the stellate morphologic characteristics disappear, collagenase production persists. This finding indicates that the stellate shape is not essential for the expression of collagenase synthesis.

Although the term "proliferative" is frequently applied to the rheumatoid synovial lesion, it is not yet known whether the lining cells or other cells in the heterogeneous population that comprise the lesion proliferate in situ or are derived from circulating cells. Thus, attraction of a specific cell or its precursor to the lesion by chemotaxis or the enhancement of local replication of these cells would be an important control. The role of complement components and of lymphocyte factors in the inflammatory lesion is discussed in detail elsewhere (see Chapters 19 and 25), but some comment concerning control of collagenase production is in order.

We have come to understand possible cellular interactions controlling collagenase production using these synovial cell cultures.[27,28,137] Although levels of collagenase and prostaglandins are high in primary cultures, these levels decrease when the cells are maintained in culture for several weeks or after passage of the cells by trypsinization. During this period, the small cells with macrophage markers also decrease in number. It was therefore reasoned that if macrophages were added back to synovial cells in later culture, the levels of collagenase and PGE_2 could be restored. Indeed, when peripheral blood mononuclear cells or enriched populations of monocytes were co-cultivated with synovial cells, the synovial cells were stimulated to increase synthesis of collagenase, with a dose-related increase in synthesis of

PGE₂.[27,28,137,140,141] Because conditioned medium from the macrophages can produce the same effects, cell-cell contact is not essential for this stimulation. The substance(s) responsible for this stimulation was initially termed mononuclear cell factor (MCF). MCF was found to be a product predominantly of the monocyte-macrophages present in the mixed mononuclear cell population.[142] Subsequently, it was shown that MCF had structural and functional similarities to what was then called lymphocyte-activating factor (LAF).[143,144] These biologic activities can now be ascribed to IL-1, although other cytokines that must be present in the mononuclear cell-conditioned medium have some similar functional capacities. At least two IL-1 polypeptides, IL-1α and IL-1β, are products of two different genes.[145–148] In humans, IL-1β predominates, but both IL-1α and β stimulate collagenase and PGE₂ production by synovial fibroblasts.[149–151]

IL-1 polypeptides presumably act through high-affinity receptors present on target cells, although the receptors so far identified are present in low concentrations. That the effects attributed to IL-1 can be reproduced with recombinant preparations indicates that IL-1α and β are certainly two components responsible for the actions of the mononuclear cell-conditioned medium previously discussed. It is obvious from recent studies, however, that other cytokines, which have little homology to IL-1 and act through different receptors, such as TNF-α or lymphotoxin (TNF-β), also have these biologic activities.[152–154] For example, TNF-α can induce collagenase and PGE₂ production by synovial fibroblasts.[153] In our studies, however, TNF-α and β are less potent, by several orders of magnitude, than IL-1 with respect to collagenase or PGE₂ induction.[155] IL-1 and TNF-α potentiate each other and act synergistically. Although these ligands act through different receptors, a common mechanism of postreceptor signal transduction may exist.

Increases in the levels of latent collagenase in medium conditioned by synovial fibroblasts stimulated by MCF is accounted for by increased synthesis and not simply release of preformed protein.[76] Indeed, stimulation of collagenase synthesis by partially purified preparations of monocyte-conditioned medium or by recombinant IL-1 was demonstrated in experiments in which increased incorporation of [³⁵S]methionine into collagenase protein complexed with specific antibodies was found.[40] The labeled procollagenase released into culture medium under these conditions is present as a doublet, with approximate molecular masses of 57,000 and 60,000 daltons. The protein of higher molecular weight is glycosylated, as shown by retention on lectin-Sepharose columns and

its disappearance following incubation with tunicamycin.[76] Potential glycosylation sites can be predicted, based on the amino acid sequence deduced from the cDNA sequence. In addition to stimulating incorporation of [³⁵S]methionine into collagenase protein, recombinant IL-1 also increases the cellular levels of mRNA in articular chondrocytes or synovial fibroblasts, as measured by hybridization with a cDNA probe.[151,155] IL-1 probably increases transcription of the procollagenase gene, although this has not yet been demonstrated directly. It is likely that TNF-α or β also acts in this fashion.

Monocyte-conditioned medium has many profound and diverse effects on the adherent synovial target fibroblastic cells and articular chondrocytes, in addition to those described on production of collagenase and PGE₂. For example, partially purified MCF preparations stimulate replication of synovial cells,[156] as well as synthesis of types I and III collagen and fibronectin.[157] Preparations of MCF or co-cultivation with monocytes also sensitizes target cells to exogenous PGE₂ under circumstances where endogenous PGE₂ synthesis is inhibited by indomethacin.[156] Effects on cell replication are properties of the most highly purified preparations of IL-1 as well as recombinant preparations.[155] Recombinant IL-1 also reproduces the effects of MCF in augmenting PGE₂-induced increases in cellular cyclic adenosine monophosphate (cAMP) content above those resulting from incubation with indomethacin alone. These effects are not limited to IL-1 because they have also been observed using recombinant preparations of TNF-α or β. The synergism of IL-1, TNF-α, and TNF-β in augmentation of synthesis of collagenase and PGE₂ was also observed in augmentation of cellular responses to PGE₂, measured by changes in cellular content of cAMP. Phorbol ester and IL-1 have common effects on target cells in inducing procollagenase synthesis. The procollagenase is similar at the protein and DNA sequence level to two other metalloproteinases, gelatinase and stromelysin,[80,81,85] which must be involved in the degradation of the extracellular matrix components at different stages.

It was discussed previously that stromelysin can be induced in fibroblasts following infection with oncogenic viruses or transfection with oncogenes. The promoter regions of several phorbol ester-inducible genes, including those of collagenese and stromelysin, share a conserved DNA sequence motif of nine base pairs.[85] These elements are recognized by a common cellular protein, the so-called transcription factor AP-1. AP-1 may be at the receiving end of a complex pathway responsible for transmitting the effects of phorbol esters from the plasma membrane to the transcriptional apparatus. The cytokines may also act in this manner by inducing the production of factors that recognize the inducible elements in the promoter regions of the collagenase (and other metalloproteinase) genes and activating transcription of these genes. The findings that genes activated by tumor promoters, oncogenic viruses, and cellular oncogenes are also activated by cytokines produced in a chronic inflammatory lesion such as RA or infiltrates in malignant tumors may provide further clues useful in unraveling aspects of the pathogenesis of these lesions.

Monocyte-macrophages are the major source of IL-1 and TNF-α, whereas TNF-β is produced by lymphocytes. Because the release of MCF is stimulated by such diverse factors as endotoxin, aggregated immunoglobulins, the Fc portion of immunoglobulins, or self-associating IgG rheumatoid factors, effects of intermediate complexes, such as the self-associating rheumatoid factors, could provide further potential mechanisms whereby humoral influences modulate cellular immune responses in the inflammatory synovium.[158,159]

In immune-mediated reactions, most attention has been directed to the role of antigen-presenting cells in inducing proliferation of T-lymphocytes by mechanisms at least in part involving IL-1. Lymphocytes may also, in turn, be important in interactions with monocytes by modulating production of IL-1. When enriched populations of peripheral blood T-lymphocytes are co-cultured with purified monocytes in the presence of lectin, production of IL-1 is augmented, as measured by MCF biologic activity.[142,160] Because "activated" T-lymphocytes, predominantly of the CD4+ phenotype, are present in abundance in the rheumatoid synovium, it is reasonable to conclude that such "activation" of T-lymphocytes could be the initial event in RA. It is likely that several different T-lymphokines, perhaps acting in concert, could serve in the roles of inducing IL-1 production by monocytes. Candidates include GM-CSF and interferon-γ. The hormone, 1,25-dihydroxyvitamin D may also modulate IL-1 production, among other effects on cells of the immune system.[161–164] Under some circumstances, this hormone may be produced by immune cells.[165]

The possibility that interactions of monocyte-macrophages with the extracellular matrix could also regulate MCF production is suggested by studies showing that types II, III, and IX collagen increase production of MCF by peripheral blood mononuclear cells.[166,167] Components of the extracellular matrix have profound effects on cell functions such as adherence and spreading, replication, and differentiation.[1] In animal models, polyarthritis has also been induced with type II collagen in incomplete Freund's adjuvant.[168] Furthermore, patients with RA have evidence of cellular immunity to several different collagens, depending on assay system.[169] These immune effects are mediated predominantly by T-lymphocytes, whereas the effects of types II, III, and IX collagen on stimulating MCF production are observed in adherent mononuclear cells, enriched in monocytes and depleted of T-lymphocytes. Synovial fibroblast-like cells and lymphocytes are not the only targets of molecules of the IL-1 class. For example, chondrocytes also increase the production of collagenase and other proteinases capable of degrading cartilage proteoglycans when exposed to factors, released from monocytes, possibly related to IL-1.[170–178] The substance released by synovial tissue and detected by its ability to deplete cartilage of proteoglycan and termed "catabolin" has now been shown to be IL-1.[171,179] Thus, chondrocytes have a role not only in synthesis of their extracellular matrix, but also in its degradation, subject to influences of products of the cells in the inflammatory synovial fluid or the pannus.

The PGE$_2$ released by the synovial cells and macrophages can interact through specific receptors with these same cells, as well as with other cells in the environment, and can modulate their rate of replication, their morphology, and other functions. These functions include alteration in synthesis of matrix proteins, such as collagens by fibroblasts and chondrocytes, and proteinases such as plasminogen activator and collagenase, and the release of acid hydrolases.[28,30,180,181]

Connective tissue cells in the inflammatory joint lesion are also under the influence of circulating hormones and many growth factors present in serum. Receptors for parathyroid hormone are present on synovial cells, and parathyroid hormone may have a permissive role in induction of osteoclastic bone resorption near the joint.[27,162,182] As mentioned, 1,25-dihydroxy-vitamin D$_3$ may also function in inflammation through its effects on monocyte function and maturation. Substances such as platelet-derived growth factor and epidermal growth factor affect replication and function of fibroblasts and synovial cells. Castor and co-workers have described a group of factors called connective tissue activating peptides (CTAP)[183–186] (see Chapter 14). CTAP-I is derived from lymphocytes, and CTAP-III and CTAP-P2 are derived from platelets. CTAP-III has been purified, and its amino acid sequence is known. It has homologies with β-thromboglobulin. CTAP stimulate glycolysis by target cells and increase the synthesis of hyaluronic acid and proteoglycans. Of interest, particularly in view of the previous discussion, is that by analogy

CTAP-III is also similar to a major peptide expressed at high levels in embryo fibroblasts transformed with Rous sarcoma virus.[187] These peptides also potentiate prostaglandin effects on cells, as does IL-1, and may well interact with other products of mononuclear cells to affect not only the rate of cell replication and degradation of the extracellular matrix, but also repair.

The emphasis in this discussion has been on the stable prostaglandins, particularly PGE_2, because they are the most abundant products of arachidonic acid metabolism in synovial tissues. The leukotrienes, which could have several roles in synovial inflammation, such as chemotaxis, have not yet been shown to affect soft tissue matrix degradation or bone resorption.

The problem of repair is critical to the whole issue of the mechanisms of tissue destruction. The limited capacity of chondrocytes to resynthesize the appropriate (type II) collagen matrix results in an irreversible loss of cartilage thickness once the collagen has been resorbed. Even when other joint structures are destroyed and inflammation subsides, repair may be inadequate in type. For example, bone may be replaced by fibrous tissue, rather than by new bone.

The inflammatory cytokines also modulate repair. Interferon-γ, certainly one factor responsible for induction of the expression of class II antigens on inflammatory and mesenchymal cells in the rheumatoid synovium, inhibits the synthesis of collagen and fibronectin by synovial and other fibroblasts and articular chondrocytes.[17,31–34] Effects of this cytokine are probably transcriptionally controlled. Other cytokines stimulate the synthesis of various collagens by different target cells. For example, crude mononuclear cell-conditioned medium, which contains IL-1, stimulates the synthesis of types I and III collagens and fibronectin by synovial fibroblastic cells, particularly if the ambient levels of prostaglandins, which suppress collagen synthesis, are decreased by incubation with the cyclo-oxygenase inhibitor, indomethacin.[157] Furthermore, collagen synthesis in cultured synovial or articular chondrocytes is increased by IL-1, but only when the cyclo-oxygenase is blocked and ambient levels of PGE_2 are low.[188] In the absence of indomethacin, IL-1 decreases the synthesis of types I and III collagen. The levels of types I and III procollagen mRNAs in these cells parallel those of the rates of collagen synthesis. TNF-α and β probably act in a similar manner. Effects of IL-1 on type II collagen synthesis appear to be even more complex.[155] IL-1 suppresses type II collagen synthesis, as well as the levels of procollagen $\alpha 1(II)$ mRNA, but in contrast to the effects of IL-1 on types I and III collagens, the addition of indomethacin does not overcome the inhibition and even poten-

tiates it. Phorbol ester mimics the effects of IL-1 on types I and III collagen synthesis, but it is distinct from IL-1 with respect to effects on type II collagen synthesis. The effects of IL-1 and other potentially important cytokines such as TNF-α, TNF-β, and TGF-β on collagen synthesis are probably exerted at the level of transcription.

EFFECTS OF DRUGS

Although many features of the processes in degradation of joint structures have been defined, enormous gaps in our knowledge still exist. It is not yet possible to localize all effects of the drugs currently used to treat RA. The ultimate course of this disease and the natural history of a specific localized joint lesion in any individual patient are not predictable. Methods of following and interpreting biologic changes in a particular lesion, short of repeated biopsies, are inadequate. Drugs such as aspirin and the nonsteroidal anti-inflammatory compounds have multiple effects, but a major action is the inhibition of the cyclo-oxygenase reaction in prostaglandin biosynthesis.[60,61,189] This inhibition should lessen several deleterious effects attributed to prostaglandins, such as vasodilatation, edema, and pain. Because the prostaglandins can accelerate bone resorption as well, inhibition of their production would also be considered beneficial.[62] Under many conditions of cell and tissue culture, however, drugs such as indomethacin do not inhibit collagenase production,[28] but interfere with some anti-inflammatory effects of the prostaglandins.[190] Exposure of cells to cyclo-oxygenase inhibitors also has the paradoxic effect of sensitizing cells to the actions of prostaglandins.[28,156,191] If the suppression of ambient PGE_2 levels were proportional to the increase in cellular sensitivity, the overall effects of the drugs would be minimal. No data exist on the long-term effects of inhibition of prostaglandin synthesis on the progression of bone erosions or on the juxta-articular osteopenia of RA.

The glucocorticoids, on the other hand, have potent effects on many of the cellular functions and interactions previously described. Glucocorticoids, at levels approximating those achieved therapeutically, inhibit production of collagenase in synovial tissue and in synovial and chondrocyte culture,[192,193] and, in addition, block the production of cytokines such as IL-1. These steroids also suppress levels of proteinases such as plasminogen activator.[193] These effects, as well as those on collagenase, could be explained in part by specific stimulation of synthesis and release of proteins inhibitory for metalloproteinases or serine proteinases. Prostaglandin synthesis in synovial cells and tissue is also inhibited by glucocorticoids.[194–196] One mechanism proposed to explain this inhibition involved the mediation of a glucocorticoid-induced inhibitor, originally termed macrocortin or lipomodulin,[197,198] of phospholipase A_2, which is assumed to be the rate-limiting enzyme in prostaglandin synthesis. The putative inhibitor(s), now known as lipocortin, have been isolated, and their cDNAs have been cloned.[199] They represent a family of proteins induced by glucocorticoids that inhibit the phospholipase A_2 reaction, but in addition, they are substrates for the epidermal growth factor receptor and the *v-src* oncogene-kinase.[200] These substances are related to other proteins called calpactins.[201] Evidence suggests the role of these proteins in binding and depleting phospholipid substrate, rather than as phospholipase A_2 enzyme inhibitors.[202] The phospholipases are critical enzymes, but their role in inflammation is still being defined. In this regard, evidence indicates that IL-1 stimulates prostaglandin E_2 synthesis by acting on the cyclo-oxygenase,[203] rather than on phospholipase A_2. Glucocorticoids may inhibit prostaglandin E_2 synthesis at the level of cyclo-oxygenase in synovial tissue.[195]

The problem with glucocorticoids is that anabolic processes, such as synthesis of collagen and proteoglycans, are also inhibited. Furthermore, effective local concentrations of glucocorticoids may not be obtainable without systemic toxicity. Thus, that long-term use of systemic glucocorticoids decreases the rate of joint destruction has not been demonstrated convincingly, even allowing for inhibition of repair.

Less is known of the antirheumatic effects of drugs such as gold compounds or penicillamine and of the way in which they might modulate the degradative phenomena described in this chapter. Evidence suggests that these compounds function as immunosuppressive agents. Gold compounds act, at least in part, by depression of macrophage functions, whereas penicillamine inhibits several functions of T-lymphocytes.[204–207] Thus, the interaction of macrophages and T-lymphocytes, important in generating products affecting the function of other cells, would be expected to be modulated by these drugs.

REFERENCES

1. Kleinman, H.K., Klebe, R.J., and Martin, G.R.: Role of collagenous matrices in the adhesion and growth of cells. J. Cell Biol., *88*:473–485, 1981.
2. Glimcher, M.J.: Handbook of Physiology. Section 7. Vol. 8. Washington, D.C., American Physiology Society, 1976.
3. Glimcher, M.J., Bonar, L.C., and Grynpas, M.D.: Recent stud-
ies of bone mineral: is the amorphous calcium phosphate theory valid? J. Crystal Growth, *53*:100–119, 1981.
4. Bornstein, P., and Sage, H.: Structurally distinct collagen types. Annu. Rev. Biochem., *49*:957–1003, 1980.
5. Miller, E.J.: The structure of collagen. *In* Connective Tissues Diseases. Edited by B.M. Wagner, R. Fleischmajer, and N. Kaufman. Baltimore, Williams & Wilkins, 1983.
6. Piez, K.A., and Reddi, A.H. (Eds.): Extracellular Matrix Biochemistry. New York, Elsevier, 1984, pp. 1–473.
7. Prockop, D.J., Kivirikko, K.I., and Tuderman, L.: Biosynthesis of collagen and its disorders. N. Engl. J. Med., *301*:13–23, 1979.
8. Gay, S., Gay, R.E., and Miller, E.J.: The collagens of the joint. Arthritis Rheum., *23*:937–941, 1980.
9. Gross, J.: Collagen biology: structure degradation and disease. Harvey Lect., *68*:351–432, 1974.
10. Harris, E.D., Jr., and Krane, S.M.: Collagenases. N. Engl. J. Med., *291*:557–563, 605–609, 652–661, 1974.
11. Collins, D.H.: The Pathology of Articular and Spinal Disease. London, Edward Arnold, 1955.
12. Kulka, J.P., Bocking, E., and Ropes, M.W.: Early joint lesions of rheumatoid arthritis. Arch. Pathol., *59*:129–150, 1955.
13. Harris, E.D., Jr., and Dimmig, T.A.: Collagenolytic enzymes in septic arthritis: potential significance for joint destruction. Arthritis Rheum., *17*:498, 1974.
14. Harris, E.D., Jr., Glauert, A.M., and Murley, A.H.G.: Intracellular collagen fibers at the pannus-cartilage junction in rheumatoid arthritis. Arthritis Rheum., *20*:657–665, 1977.
15. Janis, R., and Hamerman, D.: Articular cartilage in early arthritis. Bull. Hosp. Joint Dis., *30*:136–152, 1969.
16. Fassbender, H.G.: Histomorphological basis of articular cartilage destruction in rheumatoid arthritis. Collagen Rel. Res., *3*:141–155, 1983.
17. Amento, E.P., Bhan, A.K., McCullagh, K.G., and Krane, S.M.: Influences of gamma interferon on synovial fibroblast-like cells. J. Clin. Invest., *76*:837–848, 1985.
18. Burmester, G.R., et al.: Differential expression of Ia antigens by rheumatoid synovial lining cells. J. Clin. Invest., *80*:595–604, 1987.
19. Decker, J.L., et al.: Rheumatoid arthritis: evolving concepts of pathogenesis and treatment. Ann. Intern. Med., *101*:810–824, 1984.
20. Goto, M., et al.: Spontaneous production of an interleukin 1-like factor by cloned rheumatoid synovial cells in long-term culture. J. Clin. Invest., *80*:786–796, 1987.
21. Kobayashi, I., and Ziff, M.: Electron microscopic studies of the cartilage pannus junction in rheumatoid arthritis. Arthritis Rheum., *18*:475–483, 1975.
22. Van Boxel, J.A., and Paget, S.A.: Predominantly T-cell infiltrate in rheumatoid synovial membranes. N. Engl. J. Med., *293*:517–520, 1975.
23. Stamenkovic, I., et al.: Clonal dominance among T lymphocyte infiltrates in arthritis. Proc. Natl. Acad. Sci. U.S.A., *85*: (in press).
24. Janossy, G., Panayi, G., and Duke, P.: Rheumatoid arthritis: a disease of T-lymphocytes/macrophage immunoregulation. Lancet, *2*:839–842, 1981.
25. Dayer, J.-M., Krane, S.M., and Russell, R.G.G.: Production of collagenase and prostaglandins by isolated adherent rheumatoid synovial cells. Proc. Natl. Acad. Sci. U.S.A., *73*:945–949, 1976.
26. Woolley, D.E., Brinckerhoff, C.E., and Mainardi, C.L.: Collagenase production by rheumatoid synovial cells: morpho-

logical and immunohistochemical studies of the dendritic cell. Ann. Rheum. Dis., *38*:262–270, 1979.

27. Krane, S.M.: Aspects of cell biology of the rheumatoid synovial lesion. Ann. Rheum. Dis., *40*:433–448, 1981.

28. Krane, S.M., Goldring, S.R., and Dayer, J.-M.: Interactions among lymphocytes, monocytes and other synovial cells in the rheumatoid synovium. Lymphokines, *7*:75–136, 1982.

29. Burmester, G.R., Dimitiriu-Bona, A., and Waters, S.J.: Identification of three major synovial lining cell populations by monoclonal antibodies directed to Ia antigen and antigens associated with monocytes/macrophages and fibroblasts. Scand. J. Immunol., *17*:69–82, 1983.

30. Baker, D.G.: Rheumatoid synovial cell morphologic changes induced by a mononuclear cell factor in culture. Arthritis Rheum., *26*:8–14, 1983.

31. Goldring, M.B., Sandell, L.J., Stephenson, M.L., and Krane, S.M.: Immune interferon suppresses levels of procollagen mRNA and type II collagen synthesis in cultured human articular and costal chondrocytes. J. Biol. Chem., *261*:9049–9056, 1986.

32. Jimenez, S.A., Freundlich, B., and Rosenbloom, J.: Selective inhibition of human diploid fibroblast collagen synthesis by interferons. J. Clin. Invest., *74*:1112–1116, 1984.

33. Rosenbloom, J., Feldman, G., Freundlich, B., and Jimenez, S.A.: Transcriptional control of human diploid fibroblast collagen synthesis by γ-interferon. Biochem. Biophys. Res. Commun., *123*:365–372, 1984.

34. Stephenson, M.L., et al.: Immune interferon inhibits collagen synthesis by rheumatoid synovial cells associated with decreased levels of the procollagen mRNAs. FEBS Lett., *180*:43–50, 1985.

35. Menninger, H., Putzier, R., and Mohr, W.: Granulocyte elastase at the site of cartilage erosion to rheumatoid synovial tissue. Z. Rheumatol., *39*:145–156, 1980.

36. Harris, E.D., and Krane, S.M.: Cartilage collagen substrate in soluble and fibillar form for rheumatoid collagenase. Trans. Assoc. Am. Phys., *86*:82–94, 1983.

37. Gadek, J.E., Fells, G.A., and Wright, D.K.: Human neutrophil elastase functions as a type III collagen "collagenase." Biochem. Biophys. Res. Commun., *95*:1815–1822, 1980.

38. Gross, J., and Lapiére, C.M.: Collagenolytic activity in amphibian tissues: a tissue culture assay. Proc. Natl. Acad. Sci. U.S.A., *48*:1014–1022, 1962.

39. Evanson, J.M., Jeffrey, J.J., and Krane, S.M.: Studies on collagenase from rheumatoid synovium in tissue culture. J. Clin. Invest., *47*:2639–2651, 1968.

40. Evanson, J.M., Jeffrey, J.J., and Krane, S.M.: Human collagenase: identification and characterization of an enzyme from rheumatoid synovium in culture. Science, *158*:499–504, 1967.

41. Gross, J., Highberger, J.H., and Johnson-Wint, B.: Mode of action and regulation of tissue collagenases. *In* Collagenase in Normal and Pathological Connective Tissues. Edited by D.E. Woolley and J.M. Evanson. Chichester, England, John Wiley & Sons, 1980.

42. Harris, E.D., Jr., BiBona, D.R., and Krane, S.M.: Collagenase in human synovial fluid. J. Clin. Invest., *48*:2104–2113, 1969.

43. Kruze, E., and Wojtecka, E.: Activation of leukocyte collagenase proenzyme by rheumatoid synovial fluid. Biochim. Biophys. Acta, *285*:436–446, 1972.

44. Nagai, Y.: Vertebrate collagenase: further characterization and the significance of its latent form in vivo. Mol. Cell. Biochem., *1*:137–142, 1973.

45. Harris, E.D., Jr., and McCroskery, P.A.: The influence of temperature and fibril stability on degradation of cartilage colla-

gen by rheumatoid synovial collagenase. N. Engl. J. Med., *290*:1–8, 1974.

46. Woolley, D.E., Glanville, R.W., and Lindberg, K.A.: Action of human skin collagenase on cartilage collagen. FEBS Lett., *34*:267–269, 1973.

47. Liotta, L.A., Abe, S., and Robey, P.G.: Preferential digestion of basement membrane collagen by an enzyme derived from a metastatic murine tumor. Proc. Natl. Acad. Sci. U.S.A., *76*:2268–2272, 1979.

48. Mainardi, C.L., Dixit, S.N., and Kang, A.H.: Degradation of type IV basement membrane, collagen by a proteinase isolated from human polymorphonuclear leukocyte. J. Biol. Chem., *255*:5435–5441, 1980.

49. Welgus, H.G., Jeffrey, J.J., and Eisen, A.Z.: The collagen substrate specificity of human skin fibroblast collagenase. J. Biol. Chem., *256*:9511–9515, 1981.

50. Mills, K.: Pathology of the knee joints in rheumatoid arthritis. J. Bone Joint Surg., *52B*:746–756, 1970.

51. Newman, W.F., Mulryan, B.J., and Martin, G.R.: A chemical view of osteoclasis based on studies with yttrium. Clin. Orthop., *17*:124–133, 1960.

52. Stern, B., Golub, L., and Goldhaber, P.: Effects of demineralization and parathyroid hormone on the availability of bone collagen to degradation by collagenase. J. Periodont. Res., *5*:116–121, 1970.

53. Bonar, L.C., and Glimcher, M.J.: Thermal denaturalization of mineralized bone collagens. J. Ultrastruct. Res., *32*:545–555, 1970.

54. Krane, S.M.: Degradation of collagen in connective tissue diseases. Rheumatoid arthritis. *In* Dynamics of Connective Tissue Macromolecules. Edited by P.M.C. Burleigh and A.R. Poole. Amsterdam, North Holland, 1975.

55. Rodan, G.A., and Martin, T.J.: Role of osteoblasts in hormonal control of bone resorption—a hypothesis. Calcif. Tissue Int., *33*:349–351, 1981.

56. Thomson, B.M., Saklatvala, J., and Chambers, T.J.: Osteoblasts mediate interleukin 1 stimulation of bone resorption by rat osteoclasts. J. Exp. Med., *164*:104–112, 1986.

57. Thomson, B.M., Mundy, G.R., and Chambers, T.J.: Tumor necrosis factors α and β induce osteoblastic cells to stimulate osteoclastic bone resorption. J. Immunol., *138*:775–779, 1987.

58. Clark, S.C., and Kamen, R.: The human hematopoietic colony-stimulating factors. Science, *236*:1229–1237, 1987.

59. Zucali, J.R., et al.: Interleukin 1 stimulates fibroblasts to produce granulocyte-macrophage colony-stimulating activity and prostaglandin E_2. J. Clin. Invest., *77*:1857–1863, 1986.

60. Robinson, D.R., Dayer, J.-M., and Krane, S.M.: Prostaglandins and their regulation in rheumatoid inflammation. Ann. N.Y. Acad. Sci., *332*:279–294, 1979.

61. Robinson, D.R., McGuire, M.B., and Levine, L.: Prostaglandins in the rheumatic diseases. Ann. N.Y. Acad. Sci., *256*:318–329, 1975.

62. Robinson, D.R., Tashjian, A.H., and Levine, L.: Prostaglandin-stimulated bone resorption by rheumatoid synovia. J. Clin. Invest., *56*:1181–1188, 1975.

63. Sporn, M.B., and Roberts, A.B.: Peptide growth factors and inflammation, tissue repair, and cancer. J. Clin. Invest., *78*:329–332, 1986.

64. Lorenzo, J.A., et al.: Colony-stimulating factors regulate the development of multinucleated osteoclasts from recently replicated cells in vitro. J. Clin. Invest., *80*:160–164, 1987.

65. Massagué, J.: The TGF-β family of growth and differentiation factors. Cell, *49*:437–438, 1987.

66. Horton, J.E., Raisz, L.G., and Simmons, H.A.: Bone resorbing

activity in supernatant fluid from cultured human peripheral blood leukocytes. Science, *177*:793–794, 1972.

67. Mundy, G.R., Luben, R.A., and Raisz, L.G.: Bone resorbing activity in supernatants from lymphoid cell lines. N. Engl. J. Med., *290*:867–871, 1974.

68. Mundy, G.R., Raisz, L.G., and Shapiro, J.L.: Big and little forms of osteoclast activating factor. J. Clin. Invest., *60*:122–128, 1977.

69. Yoneda, T., and Mundy, G.R.: Monocytes regulate osteoclast activating factor production by releasing prostaglandins. J. Exp. Med., *150*:338–342, 1979.

70. Yoneda, T., and Mundy, G.R.: Prostaglandins are necessary for osteoclast-activating factor production by activated peripheral blood leukocytes. J. Exp. Med., *149*:279–283, 1979.

71. Kahn, A.J., Stewart, C.C., and Teitelbaum, S.L.: Contact mediated bone resorption by human monocytes in vitro. Science, *199*:988–989, 1978.

72. Mundy, G.R., Altman, A.A., and Gondek, M.D.: Director resorption of bone by human monocytes. Science, *196*:1109–1111, 1977.

73. Vaes, G.: The release of collagenase as an inactive proenzyme by bone explant in culture. Biochem. J., *126*:275–289, 1972.

74. Vater, C.A., Mainardi, C.L., and Harris, E.D., Jr.: Activation in vitro of rheumatoid synovial collagenase from cell cultures. J. Clin. Invest., *62*:987–992, 1978.

75. Werb, Z., and Burleigh, M.C.: Collagenase from rabbit fibroblasts in monolayer culture. Biochem. J., *137*:373–385, 1974.

76. McCroskery, P.A., Arai, S., Amento, E.P., and Krane, S.M.: Stimulation of procollagenase synthesis in human rheumatoid synovial fibroblasts by mononuclear cell factor/interleukin 1. FEBS Lett., *191*:7–12, 1985.

77. Nagase, H., Jackson, R.C., and Brinckerhoff, C.E.: A precursor form of latent collagenase produced in a cell-free system with m-RNA from rabbit synovial cells. J. Biol. Chem., *256*:11951–11954, 1981.

78. Vater, C.A., Nagase, H., and Harris, E.D., Jr.: Purification of an endogenous activator of procollagenase from rabbit synovial fibroblast culture medium. J. Biol. Chem., *258*:9374–9382, 1983.

79. Werb, Z., Mainardi, C.L., and Vater, C.A.: Endogenous activation of latent collagenase by rheumatoid synovial cells. N. Engl. J. Med., *296*:1017–1023, 1977.

80. Goldberg, G.I., et al.: Human fibroblast collagenase. J. Biol. Chem., *261*:6600–6605, 1986.

81. Whitham, S.E., et al.: Comparison of human stromelysin and collagenase by cloning and sequence analysis. Biochem. J., *240*:913–916, 1986.

82. Okada, Y., Nagase, H., and Harris, E.D., Jr.: A metalloproteinase from human rheumatoid synovial fibroblasts that digests connective tissue matrix components. J. Biol. Chem., *261*:14,245–14,255, 1986.

83. Chin, J.R., Murphy, G., and Werb, Z.: Stromelysin, a connective tissue-degrading metalloendopeptidase secreted by stimulated rabbit synovial fibroblasts in parallel with collagenase. J. Biol. Chem., *260*:12,367–12,376, 1985.

84. Angel, P., et al.: 12-0-tetradecanoyl-phorbol-13-acetate induction of the human collagenase gene is mediated by an inducible enhancer element located in the 5'-flanking region. Mol. Cell. Biol., *7*:2256–2266, 1987.

85. Angel, P., et al.: Phorbol ester-inducible genes contain a common *cis* element recognized by a TPA-modulated *trans*-acting factor. Cell, *49*:729–739, 1987.

86. Mallick, U., et al.: 12-0-tetradecanoylphorbol-13-acetate-inducible proteins are synthesized at an increased rate in Bloom

syndrome fibroblasts. Proc. Natl. Acad. Sci. U.S.A., *79*:7887–7890, 1982.

87. Herrlich, P., et al.: The mammalian genetic stress response. Adv. Enzyme Regul., *25*:485–504, 1986.

88. Matrisian, L.M., Glaichenhaus, N., Gesnel, M.-C., and Breathnach, R.: Epidermal growth factor and oncogenes induce transcription of the same cellular mRNA in rat fibroblasts. EMBO J., *4*:1435–1440, 1985.

89. Blasi, F., Vassalli, J.-D., and Danø, K.: Urokinase-type plasminogen activator: proenzyme, receptor, and inhibitors. J. Cell Biol., *104*:801–804, 1987.

90. Bromley, M., Fisher, W.D., and Woolley, D.E.: Mast cells at sites of cartilage erosion in the rheumatoid joint. Ann. Rheum. Dis., *43*:76–79, 1984.

91. Crisp, A., Chapman, C.M., and Kirkham, S.E.: Synovial mastocytosis in adult rheumatoid arthritis. Arthritis Rheum., *26*:S52, 1982.

92. Gruber, B., et al.: Characterization and functional studies of rheumatoid synovial mast cells. Arthritis Rheum., *29*:944–955, 1986.

93. Gavrilovic, J., Hembry, R.M., Reynolds, J.J., and Murphy, G.: Tissue inhibitor of metalloproteinases (TIMP) regulates extracellular type I collagen degradation by chondrocytes and endothelial cells. J. Cell Sci., *87*:357–362, 1987.

94. Murphy, G., McGuire, M.B., and Russell, R.G.G.: Characterization of collagenase, other metallo-proteinases and an inhibitor (TIMP) produced by human synovium and cartilage in culture. Clin. Sci., *61*:711–722, 1981.

95. Murphy, G., and Sellers, A.: The extracellular regulation of collagenase activity. *In* Collagenase in Normal and Pathological Connective Tissues. Edited by D.E. Woolley and J.M. Evanson. Chichester, England, John Wiley & Sons, 1980.

96. Sellers, A., and Reynolds, J.J.: Identification and partial characterization of an inhibitor of collagenase from rabbit bone. Biochem. J., *167*:353–360, 1977.

97. Vater, C.A., Mainardi, C.L., and Harris, E.D., Jr.: Inhibitor of human collagenase from cultures of human tendon. J. Biol. Chem., *254*:3045–3053, 1979.

98. Welgus, H.G., Stricklin, G.P., and Eisen, A.Z.: A specific inhibitor of vertebrate collagenase produced by human skin fibroblasts. J. Biol. Chem., *254*:1938–1943, 1979.

99. Docherty, A.J.P., et al.: Sequence of human tissue inhibitor of metalloproteinases and its identity to erythroid-potentiating activity. Nature, *318*:66–69, 1985.

100. Gasson, J.C., et al.: Molecular characterization and expression of the gene encoding human erythroid-potentiating activity. Nature, *315*:768–771, 1985.

101. Bar-Shavit, Z., et al.: Differentiation of a human leukemia cell line and expression of collagenase inhibitor. Proc. Natl. Acad. Sci. U.S.A., *82*:5380–5384, 1985.

102. Knauer, D.J., and Cunningham, D.D.: Protease nexins: cell-secreted proteins which regulate extracellular serine proteases. Trends Biochem. Sci., *9*:231–233, 1984.

103. Ginsburg, D., et al.: cDNA cloning of human plasminogen activator-inhibitor from endothelial cells. J. Clin. Invest., *78*:1673–1680, 1986.

104. Harris, E.D., Jr., et al.: Effects of proteolytic enzymes on structural and mechanical properties of cartilage. Arthritis Rheum., *15*:497–503, 1982.

105. Kempson, G.E.: The effects of proteoglycan and collagen degradation on the mechanical properties of adult human articular cartilage. *In* Dynamics of Connective Tissue Macromolecules. Edited by P.M.C. Burleigh and A.R. Poole. Amsterdam, North Holland, 1975.

106. Lagier, R., and Taillard, W.: Softening of the cartilage and arthritis of the rheumatoid type. Acta Orthop. Scand., 40:300–316, 1969.

107. Pryce-Jones, R.H., Saklatvala, J., and Wood, G.C.: Neutral protease from the polymorphonuclear leukocytes of human rheumatoid synovial fluid. Clin. Sci. Mol. Med., 47:403–414, 1974.

108. McCord, J.M.: Free radicals and inflammation: protection of synovial fluid by superoxide dismutase. Science, 185:529–531, 1974.

109. Barrett, A.J.: Which proteinases degrade cartilage matrix? Semin. Arthritis Rheum., 11:52–56, 1981.

110. Dingle, J.T., Barrett, A.J., and Weston, P.D.: Cathepsin D: characteristics of immunoinhibition and the confirmation of a role in cartilage breakdown. Biochem. J., 123:1–13, 1971.

111. Fell, H.B., and Dingle, J.T.: Studies on the mode of action of excess of vitamin A. Biochem. J., 87:403–408, 1963.

112. Poole, A.R., Hembry, R.M., and Dingle, J.T.: Secretion and localization of cathepsin D in synovial tissues removed from rheumatoid and traumatized joints. Arthritis Rheum., 19:1295–1307, 1976.

113. Poole, A.R., Hembry, R.M., and Dingle, J.T.: Cathepsin D in cartilage: the immunohistochemical demonstration of extracellular enzyme in normal and pathological conditions. J. Cell Sci., 14:139–161, 1974.

114. Woessner, J.F.: Purification of cathepsin D from cartilage and uterus and its action on the protein-polysaccharide complex of cartilage. J. Biol. Chem., 248:1634–1642, 1974.

115. Woessner, J.F.: Cartilage cathepsin D and its action on matrix components. Fed. Proc., 32:1485–1488, 1973.

116. Falchuk, K.H., Goetzl, E.J., and Kulka, J.P.: Respiratory gases of synovial fluids. Am. J. Med., 49:223–231, 1970.

117. Baron, R., Neff, L., Louvard, D., and Courtoy, P.J.: Cell-mediated extracellular acidification and bone resorption: evidence for a low pH in resorbing lacunae and localization of a 100-kD lysosomal membrane protein at the osteoclast ruffled border. J. Cell Biol., 101:2210–2222, 1985.

118. Keiser, H., Greenwald, R.A., and Feinstein, G.: Degradation of cartilage proteoglycan by human leukocyte granule neutral proteases—a model of joint injury. J. Clin. Invest., 57:625–632, 1976.

119. Oronsky, A.L., and Perper, R.J.: Connective tissue-degrading enzymes of human leukocytes. Ann. N.Y. Acad. Sci., 265:233–253, 1975.

120. Sapolsky, A.I., Keiser, H., and Howell, D.S.: The action of cathepsin D in human articular cartilage on proteoglycans. J. Clin. Invest., 52:624–633, 1973.

121. Mankin, H.J.: The metabolism of articular cartilage in health and disease. In Dynamics of Connective Tissue Macromolecules. Edited by P.N.C. Burleigh and A.R. Poole. Amsterdam, North Holland, 1975.

122. Gillard, G.D., and Lowther, D.A.: Carrageenin-induced arthritis II. Effect of intra-articular injection of carrageenin on the synthesis of proteoglycan in articular cartilage. Arthritis Rheum., 19:918–922, 1976.

123. Lowther, D.A., and Gillard, G.C.: Carrageenin-induced arthritis. I. The effect of intra-articular carrageenin on chemical composition of articular cartilage. Arthritis Rheum., 19:769–776, 1976.

124. Lowther, D.A., Gillard, G.C., and Bacter, E.: Carrageenin-induced arthritis. III. Proteolytic enzymes present in rabbit knee joints after a single intra-articular injection of carrageenin. Arthritis Rheum., 19:1287–1294, 1976.

125. Anastassiades, T.P., and Wood, A.: Effect of soluble products from lectin-stimulated lymphocytes on the growth, adhesiveness and glycosaminoglycan synthesis of cultured synovial fibroblastic cells. J. Clin. Invest., 68:792–802, 1981.

126. Eisenbarth, G.S., Beuttel, S.C., and Lebovitz, H.E.: Inhibition of cartilage macromolecular synthesis by prostaglandin A$_1$. J. Pharmacol. Exp. Ther., 189:213–220, 1974.

127. Herman, J.H., Nutman, T.B., and Nozoe, M.: Lymphokine mediated suppression of chondrocyte glycosaminoglycan and protein synthesis. Arthritis Rheum., 24:824–834, 1981.

128. Malemud, C.J., and Sokoloff, L.: The effect of prostaglandins on cultured lapine articular chondrocytes. Prostaglandins, 13:845–860, 1977.

129. Wood, D.D., et al.: The four biochemically distinct species of human interleukin 1 all exhibit similar biologic activities. J. Immunol., 134:895–903, 1985.

130. Mainardi, C.L., Hasty, D.L., Seyer, J.M., and Kang, A.H.: Specific cleavage of human type III collagen by human polymorphonuclear leukocyte elastase. J. Biol. Chem., 255:12,006–12,010, 1980.

131. Hibbs, M.S., et al.: Biochemical and immunological characterization of the secreted forms of human neutrophil gelatinase. J. Biol. Chem., 260:2493–2500, 1985.

132. Lazarus, G.S., Daniels, J.R., and Lian, J.: Role of granulocyte collagenase in collagen degradation. Am. J. Pathol., 68:565–578, 1972.

133. Macartney, H.W., and Tschesche, H.: Latent and active human polymorphonuclear leukocyte collagenase. Eur. J. Biochem., 130:71–78, 1983.

134. Hasty, K.A., Hibbs, M.S., Kang, D.H., and Mainardi, C.L.: Heterogeneity among human collagenases demonstrated by monoclonal antibody that selectively recognizes and inhibits human neutrophil collagenase. J. Exp. Med., 159:1455–1463, 1984.

135. Hasty, K.A., Hibbs, M.S., Kang, A.H., and Mainardi, C.L.: Secreted forms of human neutrophil collagenase. J. Biol. Chem., 261:5645–5650, 1986.

136. Werb, Z., and Reynolds, J.J.: Stimulation by endocytosis of the secretion of collagenase and neutral proteinase from rabbit synovial fibroblasts. J. Exp. Med., 140:1482–1497, 1974.

137. Dayer, J.-M., and Krane, S.M.: The interaction of immunocompetent cells and chronic inflammation as exemplified by rheumatoid arthritis. Clin. Rheum. Dis., 4:517–538, 1978.

138. Wahl, L.M., Wahl, S.M., and Martin, G.R.: Collagenase production by lymphokine-activated macrophages. Science, 187:261–263, 1975.

139. Wahl, L.M., Wahl, S.M., and Mergenhagen, S.E.: Collagenase production by endotoxin activated macrophages. Proc. Natl. Acad. Sci. U.S.A., 71:3598–3601, 1974.

140. Dayer, J.-M., Robinson, D.R., and Krane, S.M.: Prostaglandin production by rheumatoid synovial cells: stimulation by a factor from human mononuclear cells. J. Exp. Med., 145:1399–1404, 1977.

141. Dayer, J.-M., Russell, R.G.G., and Krane, S.M.: Collagenase production by rheumatoid synovial cells: stimulation by a human lymphocytic factor. Science, 195:181–182, 1977.

142. Dayer, J.-M., et al.: Participation of monocytes-macrophages and lymphocytes in the production of a factor that stimulates collagenase and prostaglandin release by rheumatoid synovial cells. J. Clin. Invest., 64:1386–1392, 1979.

143. Dayer, J.-M., Krane, S.M., and Goldring, S.R.: Cellular and humoral factors modulate connective tissue disease destruction and repair in arthritic diseases. Semin. Arthritis Rheum., 11:77–81, 1981.

144. Mizel, S.B., et al.: Stimulation of rheumatoid synovial cell

collagenase and prostaglandin production by partially purified lymphocyte activating factor (interleukin I). Proc. Natl. Acad. Sci. U.S.A., 78:2474–2477, 1981.

145. Auron, P.E., et al.: Nucleotide sequence of human monocyte interleukin 1 precursor cDNA. Proc. Natl. Acad. Sci. U.S.A., 81:7907–7911, 1984.

146. Clark, B.D., et al.: Genomic sequence for human prointerleukin 1 beta: possible evolution from a reverse transcribed prointerleukin 1 alpha gene. Nucleic Acids Res., 14:7897–7914, 1986.

147. Furutani, Y., et al.: Complete nucleotide sequence of the gene for human interleukin 1 alpha. Nucleic Acids Res., 14:3167–3179, 1986.

148. Lomedico, P.T., et al.: Cloning and expression of murine interleukin-1 cDNA in Escherichia coli. Nature, 312:458–462, 1984.

149. Dayer, J.-M., et al.: Human recombinant interleukin 1 stimulates collagenase and prostaglandin E_2 production by human synovial cells. J. Clin. Invest., 77:645–648, 1986.

150. Dinarello, C.A., et al.: Multiple biological activities of human recombinant interleukin 1. J. Clin. Invest., 77:1734–1739, 1986.

151. Stephenson, M.L., et al.: Stimulation of procollagenase synthesis parallels increases in cellular procollagenase mRNA in human articular chondrocytes exposed to recombinant interleukin 1β or phorbol ester. Biochem. Biophys. Res. Commun., 144:583–590, 1987.

152. Beutler, B., and Cerami, A.: Cachectin and tumour necrosis factor as two sides of the same biological coin. Nature, 320:584–588, 1986.

153. Dayer, J.-M., Beutler, B., and Cerami, A.: Cachectin/tumor necrosis factor stimulates collagenase and prostaglandin E_2 production by human synovial cells and dermal fibroblasts. J. Exp. Med., 162:2163–2168, 1985.

154. Gray, P.W., et al.: Cloning and expression of cDNA for human lymphotoxin, a lymphokine with tumour necrosis activity. Nature, 312:721–724, 1984.

155. Krane, S.M., et al.: Modulation of matrix synthesis and degradation in joint inflammation. In The Control of Tissue Damage. Edited by A. Glauert. Amsterdam, Elsevier Science Publishers, 1988, pp. 179–195.

156. Dayer, J.-M., et al.: Effects of human mononuclear cell factor on cultured rheumatoid synovial cells. Biochim. Biophys. Acta, 586:87–105, 1979.

157. Krane, S.M., Dayer, J.-M., Simon, L.S., and Byrne, M.S.: Mononuclear cell-conditioned medium containing mononuclear cell factor (MCF), homologous with interleukin 1, stimulates collagen and fibronectin synthesis by adherent rheumatoid synovial cells: effects of prostaglandin E_2 and indomethacin. Coll. Rel. Res., 5:99–117, 1985.

158. Dayer, J.-M., et al.: Interactions among rheumatoid synovial cells and monocyte-macrophages: production of collagenase stimulating factor by human monocytes exposed to concanavalin A or immunoglobulin Fc fragments. J. Immunol., 124:1712–1720, 1980.

159. Nardella, F., et al.: Self-associating IgG rheumatoid factors stimulate monocytes to release prostaglandins and mononuclear cell factor that stimulates collagenase and prostaglandin production by synovial cells. Rheumatol. Int., 3:183–186, 1983.

160. Amento, E.P., et al.: Modulation of synovial cell products by a factor from a human cell line: lymphocyte induction of a mononuclear cell factor. Proc. Natl. Acad. Sci. U.S.A., 79:5307–5311, 1982.

161. Amento, E.P., et al.: 1α,25-dihydroxyvitamin D_3 induces mat-

uration of the human monocyte cell line U937, and, in association with a factor from human T lymphocytes, augments production of the monokine, mononuclear cell factor. J. Clin. Invest., 73:731–739, 1984.

162. Amento, E.P., et al.: Osteoclasts and arthritis. Adv. Immunopharmacol., 2:731–736, 1983.

163. Bell, N.H.: Vitamin D-endocrine system. J. Clin. Invest., 76:1–6, 1985.

164. Tsoukas, C.D., Provvedini, D.M., and Manolagas, S.C.: 1,25-dihydroxyvitamin D_3: a novel immunoregulatory hormone. Science, 224:1438–1440, 1984.

165. Fetchick, D.A., et al.: Production of 1,25-dihydroxyvitamin D_3 by human T cell lymphotrophic virus-1-transformed lymphocytes. J. Clin. Invest., 78:592–596, 1986.

166. Dayer, J.-M., Trentham, D.E., and Krane, S.M.: Collagens act as ligands to stimulate monocytes to produce mononuclear cell factor (MCF) and prostaglandins (PGE_2). Collagen Rel. Res., 2:523–540, 1982.

167. Dayer, J.-M., Richard-Blum, S., Kaufmann, M.-T., and Herbage, D.: Type IX collagen is a potent inducer of PGE_2 and interleukin 1 production by human monocyte macrophages. FEBS Lett., 198:208–212, 1986.

168. Trentham, D.E., Townes, A.S., and Kang, A.H.: Autoimmunity to type II collagen: an experimental mode of arthritis. J. Exp. Med., 146:857–863, 1977.

169. Trentham, D.E., Dynesius. R.A., and Rocklin, R.E.: Cellular sensitivity to collagen in rheumatoid arthritis. N. Engl. J. Med., 299:327–332, 1978.

170. Deshmukh-Pahdke, K., Nanda, S., and Lee, K.: Macrophage factor that induces neutral protease secretion by normal rabbit chondrocytes. Eur. J. Biochem., 104:175–180, 1980.

171. Dingle, J.T.: The role of catabolins in synovia-chondrocyte interactions. Adv. Immunopharmacol., 2:725–729, 1983.

172. Hamilton, J.A., and Slywka, J.: Stimulation of human synovial plasminogen activator production by mononuclear cell supernatants. J. Immunol., 126:851–855, 1981.

173. Hubrechts-Godin, G., Hauser, P., and Vaes, G.: Macrophage-fibroblast interactions in collagenase production and cartilage degradation. Biochem. J., 184:643–650, 1979.

174. Jasin, H.E., and Dingle, J.T.: Human mononuclear cell factors mediate cartilage matrix degradation through chondrocyte activation. J. Clin. Invest., 68:571–581, 1981.

175. Korn, J.H., Torres, D., and Downie, E.: Fibroblast prostaglandin E_2 synthesis. Persistence of an abnormal phenotype after short term exposure to mononuclear cell products. J. Clin. Invest., 71:1240–1247, 1983.

176. Meats, J.E., McGuire, M.B., and Russell, R.G.G.: Human synovium releases a factor which stimulates chondrocyte production of PGE_1 and plasminogen activator. Nature, 286:891–892, 1980.

177. Robinson, D.R., Bastian, D., and Hamer, P.J.: Mechanism of stimulation of prostaglandin synthesis by a factor from rheumatoid tissue. Proc. Natl. Acad. Sci. U.S.A., 78:5160–5164, 1981.

178. Steinberg, J., Sledge, C.B., and Noble, J.: A tissue culture model of cartilage breakdown in rheumatoid arthritis. Biochem. J., 180:403–412, 1979.

179. Saklatvala, J., et al.: Pig catabolin is a form of interleukin 1. Biochem. J., 224:461–466, 1984.

180. Clarris, B.J., and Malcolm, L.P.: Effects of prostaglandins E_1, E_2, and $F_{2\alpha}$ on N-acetyl-β-glucosaminidase activities of human synovial cells in culture. Ann. Rheum. Dis., 42:187–191, 1983.

181. Korn, J.H., Halushka, P.V., and LeRoy. E.C.: Mononuclear

cell modulation of connective tissue function. J. Clin. Invest., *65*:543–554, 1980.

182. Goldring, S.R., Dayer, J.-M., and Krane, S.M.: Rheumatoid synovial cell hormone responses modulated by cell-cell interactions. Inflammation, *8*:107–121, 1984.

183. Castor, C.W.: Synovial cell activation induced by a polypeptide mediator. Ann. N.Y. Acad. Sci., *256*:304–317, 1975.

184. Castor, C.W., Fremuth, T.D., and Roberts, D.J.: Regulation of articular cell metabolism by CTAP mediators. Semin. Arthritis Rheum., *11*:95–96, 1981.

185. Castor, C.W., Ritchie, J.C., and Scott, M.E.: Connective tissue activation-stimulation of glycosaminoglycan and DNA formation by a platelet factor. Arthritis Rheum., *20*:859–867, 1977.

186. Castor, C.W., Ritchie, J.C., and William, C.H.: Connective tissue activation. Arthritis Rheum., *22*:260–272, 1979.

187. Sugano, S., Stoeckle, M.Y., and Hanafusa, H.: Transformation by Rous sarcoma virus induces a novel gene with homology to a mitogenic platelet protein. Cell, *49*:321–328, 1987.

188. Goldring, M.B., and Krane, S.M.: Modulation by recombinant interleukin 1 of synthesis of types I and III collagens and associated procollagen mRNA levels in cultured human cells. J. Biol. Chem., *262*:16724–16729, 1987.

189. Moncada, S., and Vane, J.R.: Mode of action of aspirin-like drugs. Adv. Intern. Med., *24*:1–22, 1979.

190. Morley, J.: Anti-inflammatory effects of prostaglandins. *In* Rheumatoid Arthritis: Cellular Pathology and Pharmacology. Edited by J.L. Gordon and B.L. Hazleman. Amsterdam, North Holland, 1977.

191. Newcombe, D.S., Ciosek, C.P., Ishikawa, Y.: Human synoviocytes: activation and desensitization by prostaglandins and 1-epinephrine. Proc. Natl. Acad. Sci. U.S.A., *72*:3124–3128, 1975.

192. Dayer, J.-M., Robinson, D.R., and Krane, S.M.: Action of anti-inflammatory drugs on synovium. *In* Rheumatoid Arthritis: Cellular Pathology and Pharmacology. Edited by J.L. Gordon and B.H.L. Hazleman. Amsterdam, North Holland, 1977.

193. McGuire, M.B., Murphy, G., and Reynolds, J.J.: Production of collagenese and inhibition (TIMP) by normal rheumatoid and osteoarthritic synovium in vitro: effects of hydrocortisone and indomethacin. Clin. Sci., *61*:703–708, 1981.

194. Kantrowitz, F., Robinson, D.R., and McGuire, M.B.: Corticosteroids inhibit prostaglandin production by rheumatoid synovia. Nature, *258*:737–739, 1975.

195. Robinson, D.R., McGuire, M.B., and Bastian, D.: The effect of anti-inflammatory drugs on prostaglandin production by rheumatoid synovial tissue. Prostaglandins Med., *1*:461–477, 1979.

196. Vane, J.R., Flower, R.J., and Salmon, J.A.: Inhibitors of arachidonic acid metabolism, with especial reference to the aspirin-like drugs. *In* Prostaglandins and Cancer: First International Conference. Vol. 2. Edited by T.J. Powles, et al. New York, Alan R. Liss, 1982.

197. Blackwell, G.J., Carnuccio, R., and DiRossa, M.: Macrocortin: a polypeptide causing anti-phospholipase effects of glucocorticoids. Nature, *287*:147–149, 1980.

198. Hirata, F., Schiffman, F., and Ventasubramanian, K.: A phospholipase A₂ inhibitory protein in rabbit neutrophils induced by glucocorticoids. Proc. Natl. Acad. Sci. U.S.A., *77*:2533–2536, 1980.

199. Huang, K.-S., et al.: Two human 35 kd inhibitors of phospholipase A₂ are related to substrates of pp60^{v-src} and of the epidermal growth factor receptor/kinase. Cell, *46*:191–199, 1986.

200. Brugge, J.S.: The p35/p36 substrates of protein-tryosine kinases as inhibitors of phospholipase A₂. Cell, *46*:149–150, 1986.

201. Saris, C.J.M., et al.: The cDNA sequence fort eh protein-tyrosine kinase substrate p36 (calpactin 1 heavy chain) reveals a multidomain protein with internal repeats. Cell, *46*:201–212, 1986.

202. Davidson, F.F., Dennis, E.A., Powell, M., and Glenney, J.R., Jr.: Inhibition of phospholipase A₂ by "lipocortins" and calpactins. J. Biol. Chem., *262*:1698–1705, 1987.

203. O'Neill, L.A.J., Barrett, M.L., and Lewis, G.P.: Induction of cyclo-oxygenase by interleukin-1 in rheumatoid synovial cells. FEBS Lett., *212*:35–39, 1987.

204. Lipsky, P.E.: Immunopharmacology of remission-inducing drugs in rheumatoid arthritis. Adv. Immunopharmacol., *2*:345–350, 1983.

205. Lipsky, P.E., and Ziff, M.: Inhibition of human helper T cell function in vitro by D-penicillamine and CuSO₄. J. Clin. Invest., *65*:1069–1076, 1980.

206. Lipsky, P.E., and Ziff, M.: The effect of D-penicillamine on mitogen induced human lymphocyte proliferation synergistic inhibition by D-penicillamine and copper salts. J. Immunol., *120*:1006–1013, 1978.

207. Lipsky, P.E., and Ziff, M.: Inhibition of antigen and mitogen induced human lymphocyte proliferation by gold compounds. J. Clin. Invest., *59*:455–466, 1977.

SUGGESTED READINGS

Brinckerhoff, C.E., McMillan, R.M., Fahey, J.V., and Harris, E.D., Jr.: Collagenase production by synovial fibroblasts treated with phorbol myristate acetate. Arthritis Rheum., *22*:1109–1115, 1979.

Harris, E.D., Reynolds, J.J., and Werb, Z.: Cytochalasin B increases collagenase production by cells in vitro. Nature, *257*:243–244, 1975.

Krane, S.M.: Collagenase production by human synovial tissues. Ann. N.Y. Acad. Sci., *256*:289–303, 1975.

Krane, S.M., and Simon, L.S.: Rheumatoid arthritis: clinical features and pathogenetic mechanisms. Adv. Rheumatol., *70*:263–284, 1986.

McGuire-Goldring, M.B., et al.: In vitro activation of human chondrocytes and synoviocytes by a human interleukin-1-like factor. Arthritis Rheum., *27*:654–662, 1984.

Matrisian, L.M.: et al.: Isolation of the oncogene and epidermal growth factor-induced transin-gene: complex control in rat fibroblasts. Mol. Cell. Biol., *6*:1679–1686, 1986.

Mundy, G.R., Raisz, L.G., and Cooper, R.A.: Evidence for the secretion of an osteoclast stimulating factor in myeloma. N. Engl. J. Med., *291*:1041–1046, 1974.

Woolley, D.E., Roberts, D.R., and Evanson, J.M.: Small molecular-weight β₁ serum protein which specifically inhibits human collagenases. Nature, *261*:325–327, 1976.

43

CLINICAL PICTURE OF
RHEUMATOID ARTHRITIS

DANIEL J. McCARTY

HISTORY

The term rheumatoid arthritis (RA) was coined by Sir Alfred Baring Garrod in 1876.[1] The first convincingly clear description of the disease was that of Landre-Beauvais in 1800.[2] Garrod, Charcot, and Adams each wrote extensive clinical and anatomic descriptions of the disease; all three classified Heberden's nodes and osteoarthritis of the hip (malum coxae senilis) as variants of RA, thereby presaging the current debate on the role of inflammation in osteoarthritis. Indeed, the synovitis of osteoarthritis resembles that of RA but is confined to synovium contiguous to areas of degenerated cartilage.[3]

The term rheumatoid arthritis was officially adopted by the Empire Rheumatism Council in 1922 and by the American Rheumatism Association (ARA) only in 1941. Its use as a diagnostic label has been progressively, albeit intermittently, constricted as syndromes that superficially resemble it have been recognized as distinctive. This process is illustrated in Figure 43–1. Some investigators, including me, regard persistently seronegative polyarthritis as distinct from "true" RA. Chapter 56 is devoted to a critical evaluation of this subject.

Antiquity of Rheumatoid Arthritis. This subject is discussed fully in Chapter 2. There is no convincing evidence in paintings, in sculpture, or in skeletal remains that the disease existed in Europe or Africa before 1500 AD, in contradistinction to primary osteoarthritis, gout, spondyloarthropathy, tuberculous and septic arthritis, and ochronotic arthropathy. Skeletal evidence presented at recent ARA meetings, but still unpublished, suggests that an erosive, symmetric arthritis affecting small peripheral joints was indeed present in pre-Columbian Indians living in what is now Mexico and the United States. If this evidence passes critical scrutiny, the concept that a causative agent or agents was spread worldwide by European sailors is certainly tenable and analogous to the current worldwide epidemic caused by the acquired immune deficiency syndrome (AIDS) virus.

CLASSIFICATION

The time-honored ARA diagnostic criteria for RA[4] have been revised, as discussed in Chapter 3. The new criteria, like their predecessors, are meant to provide a disease definition that is sufficient to classify patients under clinical investigation, but they are not meant to define the disease in patients seen in everyday clinical practice. A tentative classification of RA for the purposes of this discussion is given in Table 43–1.

Rheumatoid Nodulosis. This is an uncommon variant that is usually, but not invariably, seropositive.[5-8] Such patients have little, if any, systemic reaction and often complain that they cannot grip a tennis racket or a golf club properly because of the interference by multiple nodules. Radiologists often incorrectly diagnose such cases as gout because of the punched-out bony lesions and soft-tissue nodularity. Eight of the ten reported cases were men. I have seen at least

FIG. 43–1. Syndromes once included as rheumatoid arthritis have been recognized over the years. Gouty arthritis was initially separated by Adams and Garrod from "rheumatic gout" and "rheumatoid arthritis" was coined to designate nearly all nongouty inflammatory forms of arthritis. The process of recognition of syndromes distinct from rheumatoid arthritis has occurred repeatedly for 125 years and is likely to continue. Some of these syndromes are presented here as illustrative of the process.

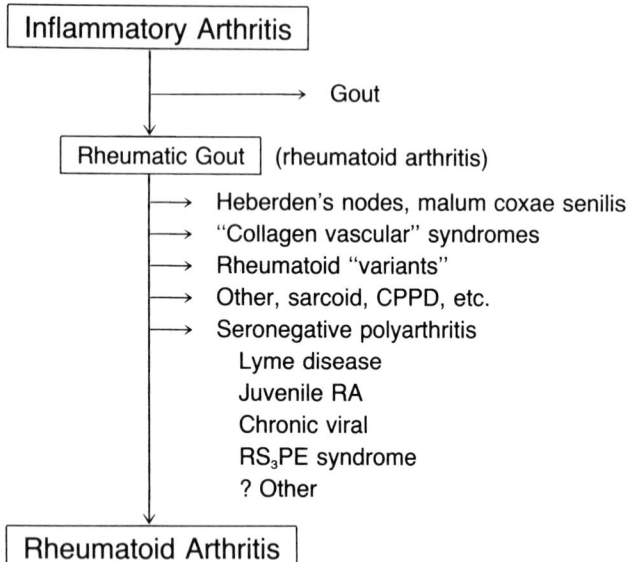

10 cases in the past 15 years. All reported cases have had acute intermittent gout-like attacks closely resembling palindromic rheumatism.[7,8] One patient actually had coexistent gout.[8] The bony lesions were shown to be due to rheumatoid nodules rather than to pannus in one reported case,[7] and I have evidence of this phenomenon in one of my patients.[9]

Palindromic Rheumatism. Palindromic rheumatism is much more common. Attacks are usually periarticular, and few joint fluids or synovial membranes have been examined.[10,11] HLA antigens were normally dis-

Table 43–1. Classification of Rheumatoid Arthritis

A. Seropositive*
  1. Erosive
    a. Bilateral, symmetric
    b. Unilateral (rare)
  2. Nonerosive (unusual)
    a. Bilateral, symmetric
    b. Unilateral

B. Seronegative
  1. Erosive
  2. Nonerosive

C. Rheumatoid nodulosis

D. Palindromic rheumatism

*For IgM rheumatoid factor.

tributed in one series of 26 cases of palindromic rheumatism.[12] Interestingly, the four patients who eventually developed RA were HLA-DR4 positive; three of these four also developed positive tests for IgM rheumatoid factor. About 20% of RA patients have a palindromic onset. The acute attacks usually but not always disappear when fixed arthritis supervenes. This condition is discussed in greater detail in Chapter 64.

Seronegative RA. Seronegative RA has various manifestations. The tests for IgM rheumatoid factor in some patients convert from negative to positive over time. Such test results change, either spontaneously or while the patients are receiving potent remission-inducing agents, from positive to negative in still other patients. Some seronegative patients clearly have the clinical features of juvenile RA, including rash and fever,[13,14] whereas others have the characteristic involvement of larger joints such as the wrist, shoulder, and knee, with lesser involvement of the small hand joints and the forefoot. Involvement is also often more asymmetric than in adult seropositive disease. The association of spondylopathic diseases with HLA-B27 has intensified interest in the residue of patients with symmetric polyarthritis associated with persistent seronegativity. With the exception of the *syndrome of remitting, seronegative, symmetric synovitis with pitting edema* (RS₃PE syndrome),[15] there is little practical reason to consider seronegative RA as a separate entity because, although the prognosis is generally better, the treatment is similar to that of seropositive disease, that is, it is empiric and often not completely effective.

Benign Rheumatoid Nodules. These need to be differentiated from rheumatoid nodulosis. Benign nodules usually occur in children or young adults and are histologically identical to the necrobiotic nodules of seropositive RA. They occur in crops, usually in the subcutaneous tissues over the shins, scalp, hands, and feet (Fig. 43–2A to D). The parents and child need reassurance that these lesions will probably disappear and that there is no increased likelihood for the development of crippling arthritis. Although this statement is probably true for the great majority of cases, there are now three recorded instances (out of about 150 reported cases) of the eventual evolution of arthritis. Joint inflammation occurred 7, 15, 50 years after the appearance of the nodules.[16,17] Only one of these three patients developed positive tests for rheumatoid factor, however.[16]

EPIDEMIOLOGY

HEREDITY

A genetic predisposition is clear. Certain histocompatibility markers, possibly related to immune-re-

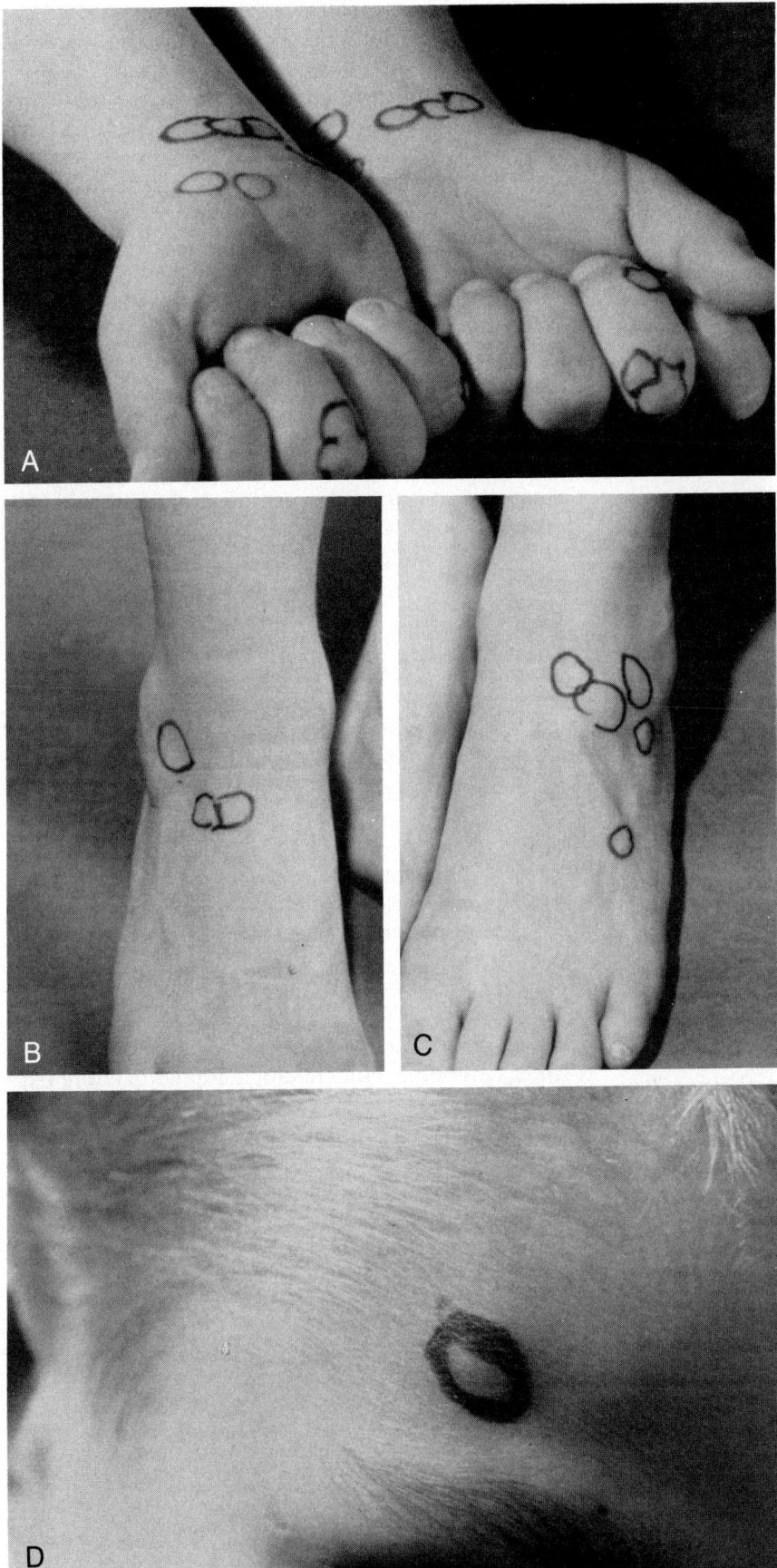

FIG. 43–2. Benign rheumatoid nodules in a child: *A*, hands; *B* and *C*, ankles; *D*, forehead. The nodules were ringed with ink for clarity.

sponse genes, appear to be linked to the expression of RA[18-20] (see Chapter 29 for fuller discussion of the immunogenetics of RA). In most populations of seropositive rheumatoid patients, the frequency of HLA-DRw4 is about twice that of the general population to which these patients belong, and the frequency of HLA-DR3 and HLA-DR7 is decreased. Jewish and Asian patients with RA show an association not with HLA-DRw4, but with HLA-DR1.[21] RA patients who were HLA-DR4 negative showed a bimodal distribution of serum IgM rheumatoid factor titers; they were either seronegative or had very high titers.[22] Furthermore, studies of identical twins, concordant or discordant for RA, clearly demonstrate a strong hereditary influence for seropositive erosive disease. A study in Finland showed that the incidence of RA was increased ninefold in monozygotic twins and threefold to fourfold in dizygotic twins,[23] compared with the thirtyfold and sixfold increases in Lawrence's study of rheumatoid arthritis in the European twin registry. Lawrence and Kellgren can account for about 80% of seropositive erosive RA through polygenic inheritance (see Chapter 3).[24]

GEOGRAPHIC DISTRIBUTION

RA presents a wide clinical spectrum of severity. Thus, patients preselected by referral or by the interests of a particular clinic do not represent a true cross section of the disease. Demographic and epidemiologic data suggest that many patients with typical disease never seek medical attention.[24] In addition, environmental, social, genetic, and economic factors may play a role in the expression of the disease. Thus, the illness may appear particularly severe in homogeneous, isolated populations such as Northwest American Indians.[25]

Information about the worldwide prevalence of RA is incomplete. Because the disease onset occurs with high frequency at about the age of 50, studies of populations in which the life expectancy is reduced, as in the era before the industrial revolution or even in the third-world countries of today, provide a false impression of lower prevalence. The prevalence of seropositive erosive RA appears to be similar all over the world, when data are corrected for the age of the population. Incidence of RA appears to be halved in women taking oral contraceptives.[26]

CLIMATE

Previous studies have reported an adverse effect of climatic changes on arthritis. Many such reports have

been based on anecdotal notations by individual patients moving from one climate to another, such as from New York to New Mexico or Arizona. Observations by Hollander and associates,[27] using a controlled climate chamber, indicated that arthritis often worsened within a few hours after a rise in humidity and fall in barometric pressure. Such patients appear to be weather sensitive. No pathogenetic mechanism has been uncovered to explain this phenomenon. In some patients, however, little relationship was noted between the climate and the activity of their disease. Later studies have yielded conflicting results. No effect of weather was noted in a 1-month study of patients with RA or with osteoarthritis who kept a daily account of pain using an analog scale.[28] A more comprehensive Dutch study of 88 RA patients over 1 year found that symptoms correlated positively with temperature and with vapor pressure and negatively with relative humidity.[29] Practically, I have never recommended a change in location as part of the treatment of RA.

CLINICAL FEATURES

RA is a systemic disease. Its onset is frequently heralded by fatigue, diffuse myalgia, fever, loss of appetite, and vague malaise. Data collected in clinics indicate that onset of the disease occurs most often between the ages of 20 and 60, with peaks at 35 and 45 years. In my own experience with 152 well-studied patients (female/male ratio, 2.6:1), the peak age of onset was perimenopausal (48 to 52 years) with a minor peak early in the third decade of life.[30] The disorder may begin at any time from the first few weeks of life to the ninth decade, however. Women are affected more frequently than men, in a ratio of 2 or 3:1, although epidemiologic studies of entire populations show a nearly equal sex ratio in patients with classic disease.[24] The ability of females in many mammalian species, including humans, to surpass males in both humoral and cellular immune response is well documented. Thus, if RA is linked to an abnormal or harmful immune response, the result may be accentuated in females.

EFFECT OF THE AGE OF ONSET ON DISEASE COURSE

A group of 55 Italian patients with onset of RA past 65 years were compared to 261 patients whose disease began at younger ages[31]; no clinical differentiating features were noted, although a subset of older patients with notably elevated erythrocyte sedimentation rates (ESR) and C-reactive protein (CRP) values was identified. In another study, the features exhibited by 78 patients with onset of RA after 60 years of age were compared with those of 134 patients with disease onset at younger ages.[32] A distinct subset of older patients with a better prognosis was clearly evident. Fully one third of the older group went into remission. And fewer elderly onset patients were seropositive (48 vs. 76%). A "polymyalgia-like" onset was four times more common in elderly patients. Only 31% of still another group of patients with onset after 60 years were seropositive for IgM rheumatoid factor.[33] The identification of an elderly subset with a favorable prognosis confirms earlier reports of a "benign" RA in the aged (reviewed in McCarty, et al.[15]).

Syndrome of Remitting Seronegative Symmetric Synovitis with Pitting Edema (RS₃PE Syndrome)

Some of these patients might have had the RS₃PE syndrome, which predominantly affects white men (male/female ratio, 4:1) living in a rural or semirural environment.[15] In this condition the onset is usually acute with symmetric involvement of the wrists, carpal joints, flexor tendon sheaths, and small hand joints, accompanied by pitting edema of the dorsum of the hand ("boxing-glove" hand). The whole hand appears puffy so that it is difficult to discern the individual swollen joints visually as can usually be done in RA (Fig. 43–3A to D). The elbows, shoulders, hips, knees, and ankles may also be involved as may the joints in the foot. Involvement of the metatarsophalangeal joints may be asymptomatic, revealed only by tenderness accompanying pressure applied to the individual joints. Pitting edema over the feet or pretibial areas may (Fig. 43–3E) or may not be present. The inflammation in all patients seen by my colleagues and me failed to respond to multiple nonsteroidal anti-inflammatory drugs used sequentially and most patients were sufficiently incapacitated to require hospitalization. Bony erosions did not occur and the disease predictably remitted completely after 3 to 36 months.

Persistent rheumatoid factor seronegativity, mild anemia, elevated ESR, and decreased serum albumin levels are the rule. There are no other distinguishing laboratory features. The edema is exquisitely sensitive to small doses (e.g., 10 mg prednisone) of corticosteroids. Hydroxychloroquine (200 to 400 mg daily) and salicylate, given in doses sufficient to produce therapeutic blood levels, are predictably effective. Remission is invariably maintained even after all drugs have been stopped, unlike in RA, in which a recrudescence

of the disease almost invariably occurs when remittive agents are withdrawn.

Limitation of motion of the affected wrists, elbows, and hands often persists indefinitely in RS₃PE patients, although the patients are generally unaware of these contractures because they are of no functional significance. Lastly, about 70% of these patients type positive for HLA-B7 versus 24% of the general population. The mean age of our 22 patients with RS₃PE syndrome is 71 years, with a range of 48 to 86 years. The onset of symptoms occurred mostly between March and November with a peak in September and October, although more data are needed on this point. Other arthritides that may be accompanied by pitting edema of the back of the hands are listed in Table 43–2.

RS₃PE syndrome has certain features that resemble those of polymyalgia rheumatica (PMR), that is, sudden onset in older white persons, nonspecific acute-phase changes in laboratory values, and great sensitivity of the inflammatory process to low doses of prednisone. PMR certainly affects joints, predominantly larger axial joints, but also the small joints of the hand. However, I have never seen this degree of appendicular synovitis, especially tenosynovitis, in any of the many patients with PMR that I have cared for over the years. The marked predominance in men, the shorter natural history, the apparent response to antimalarial agents plus aspirin, and the frequent presence of HLA-B7 all support the notion that this condition is indeed quite different from both PMR and RA.

A second group of 20 patients with an RA-like illness has been identified but not yet reported.[34] These patients were selected originally as a possible forme fruste of RS₃PE syndrome. Symmetric synovitis of the wrists and carpal joints in elderly white patients were the clinical feature that attracted our attention. The degree of synovitis was much milder than in RS₃PE syndrome and the onset of joint involvement was often gradual, over a period of a few weeks. There was no pitting edema of the hands and no patient required hospitalization. Again, men predominated. About half of these patients showed transiently positive tests for IgM rheumatoid factor. The response to hydroxychloroquine plus aspirin was uniformly excellent, but unlike in RS₃PE, some evidence of low-grade inflammation often persisted. Most patients became completely seronegative while receiving these drugs. More than half of these patients carried the haplotype B8 DR3, the classic autoimmune haplotype. This group of patients also appear to be distinct from usual seropositive RA patients.

Analysis of RA patients with antibodies to native

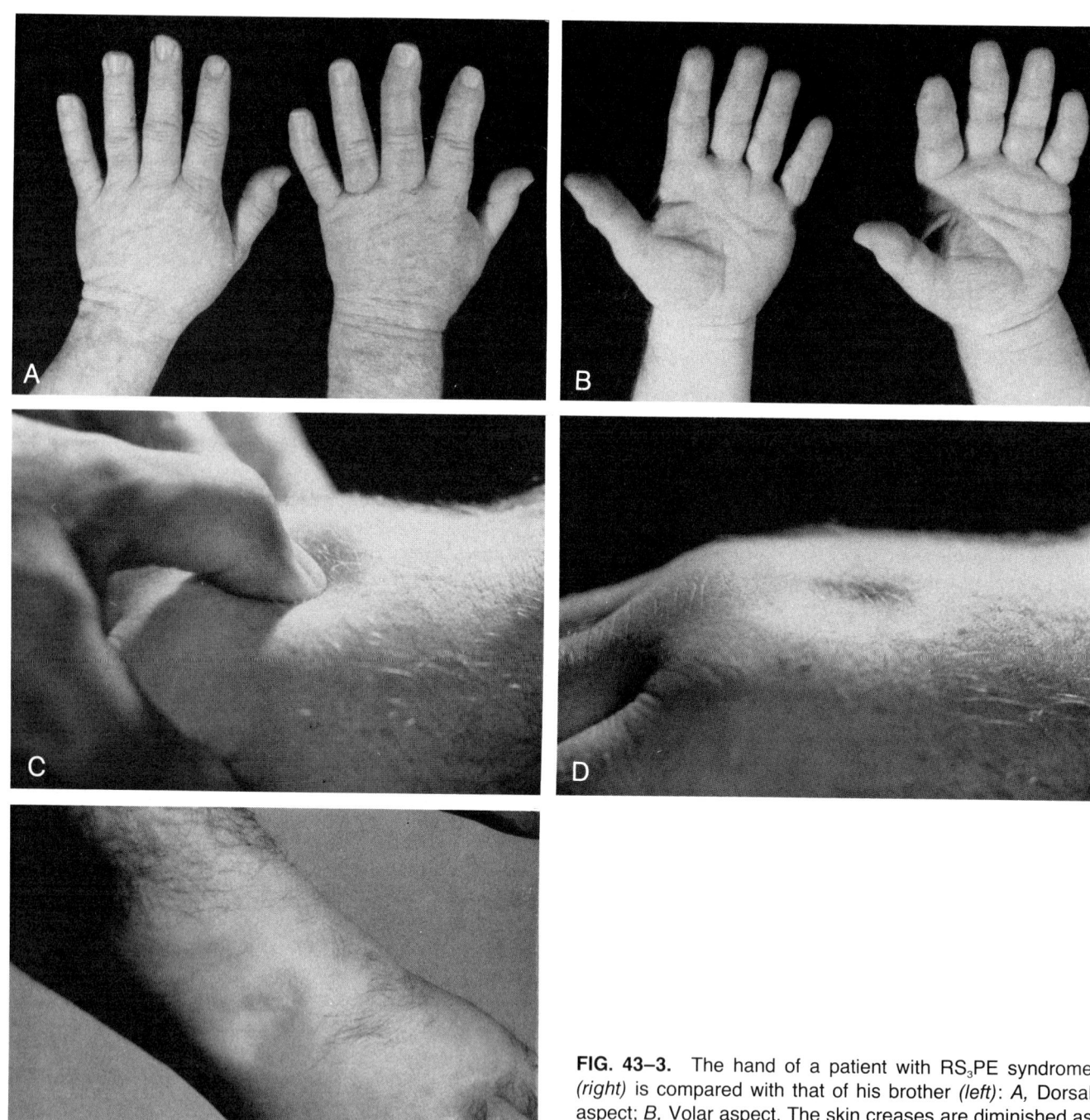

FIG. 43–3. The hand of a patient with RS$_3$PE syndrome *(right)* is compared with that of his brother *(left)*: *A,* Dorsal aspect; *B,* Volar aspect. The skin creases are diminished as a result of the generalized swelling of the hand; *C* and *D,* Pitting edema is clearly evident. *E,* Pitting edema of the feet is much less common but does occur.

Table 43–2. Conditions Associated With Pitting Edema of the Dorsa of the Hands

Condition	Differentiating Features
Shoulder hand syndrome (reflex sympathetic dystrophy)*	Stiff painful shoulders
Amyloid arthropathy*	Progressive, no response to anti-inflammatory drugs
Psoriatic arthritis	Typical skin lesions
CPPD crystal arthropathy	Radiologic chondrocalcinosis; CPPD crystals in synovial fluid
Rheumatoid arthritis†	IgM rheumatoid factor, bony erosions
Reactive arthritis (Reiter's syndrome)	Asymmetric joint involvement; gastrointestinal, genitourinary, eye, and skin symptoms and signs
Mixed connective tissue disease*	High ANA titer in speckled pattern; anti-nRNP antibodies in younger patients with Raynaud's phenomenon
Remitting seronegative symmetric synovitis	Constant feature of disease; edema sensitive to small doses of corticosteroids

*Pitting edema is often bilateral.
†Unilateral pitting edema is often associated with rupture of nearby joint.
ANA = antinuclear antibody; anti-nRNP = antinative ribonucleoprotein.

type II collagen identified them as a subset with frequent seronegativity, with more osteosclerosis, and associated with HLA-DR7 rather than with HLA-DR4.[35] The process of redefinition of "rheumatoid arthritis" as additional subsets of patients are defined and subtracted will undoubtedly continue.

PRECIPITATING EVENTS

It is often difficult to pinpoint a precipitating event in an individual patient with RA. Such events represent a variety of life stresses, including psychic, infectious, or occasionally traumatic. In most patients, the disease starts gradually and insidiously, but in some the onset is acute, occurring within 24 to 48 hours. Prodromal symptoms of fatigue, myalgias, and malaise may be present for weeks or months before the onset of joint symptoms, but in most cases, joint pain, stiffness, and swelling arise early in the disease. At times, initial joint involvement may be spotty, but a symmetric pattern of polyarthritis almost always evolves over weeks or months.[36] In one older study, a tendency for the acute pattern of onset to occur before age 40 was noted, as well as an association with fever and the presence of subcutaneous nodules.[37]

Another study of the onset of RA in 102 patients showed that in two of three patients, the disease began in the winter.[38] About 10% of patients showed an acute polyarticular onset that could be pinpointed to the day; 18% could identify the week of onset, whereas the remainder could isolate the onset only to the nearest month. The male/female ratio was about 3:4, as in population studies. Older patients fared worst during the mean 4- to 5-year followup. An insidious onset and early progression to symmetric involvement carried a poorer prognosis. More severe

disease eventually developed when the large joints were also involved initially, or when metatarsophalangeal (MTP) joints 1 and 3 were involved early. MTP joint involvement at onset also correlated with the early occurrence of erosions.[39] Still other studies, however, showed no difference in clinical progression of the disease with respect to rapidity or age of onset.[40,41]

A careful study of the effect of the removal of lymphatic tissue such as tonsils, adenoids, and the appendix on the subsequent development of RA showed no relationship,[42] in contradistinction to previous reports. Similarly, claims that RA patients were depressed, hypochondriac, or hysterical, based on standardized psychologic testing, has not been confirmed.[43] These abnormalities were thought to reflect the activity of the disease rather than underlying, premorbid psychologic traits. Another study found that psychologic depression correlated with flares in disease activity.[44] I am convinced that some patients suffer severe exacerbations of disease activity coincident with severe psychologic stress. A study of RA patient perceptions about the cause of their disease showed that 35% thought heredity was important, followed by autoimmunity (24%), behavioral problems (23%), and psychologic stress (23%).[45] Flares of disease activity were attributed to psychologic stress by 46% of patients, to weather changes in 34%, and to excessive physical activity in 34%. Because emotions have a profound influence on the endocrine system, which in turn has a modulating influence on the immune system, it is easy to conceptualize the effects of psychic stress on rheumatoid disease activity in general terms. The specific mechanisms involved remain to be clarified.

As the disease progresses, patients complain of joint pain at rest and on movement. Swelling of involved joints is prominent, and as the disorder persists, limitation of motion, accompanied by a diffuse wasting of adjacent muscles, is noted.

SYMPTOMS

Systemic complaints of weakness and fatigue and localized symptoms of pain, stiffness, weakness, and paresthesias are discussed extensively in Chapter 4, which deals with the differential diagnosis of arthritis.

Table 43–3. Symptoms and Signs of Early Rheumatoid Arthritis

	Symptoms
Joint stiffness	Found in 98% of patients; most pronounced after inactivity; its duration after arising reflects degree of synovial inflammation. Improves with physical activity.
Joint pain	Reflects severity of synovitis—may not be a prominent feature at rest.
Fatigue	Often pronounced with onset about 4.5 hours after arising; found in 80% of patients; its duration after arising varies inversely with degree of synovitis.
Weakness	Nearly universal in RA patients; often out of proportion to degree of muscular atrophy; generally proportional to degree of synovitis.
Psychological depression	Common; reflects disease activity.
	Signs
Swelling	Fusiform soft tissue enlargement of small joints and tendon sheaths in the hands, wrists, and forefeet most commonly but can affect any synovial structure in body.
Palmar erythema	Very common over palmar and thenar eminences; identical to changes found in liver disease and pregnancy; persists even in remission.
Cool moist skin	Over hands and feet; suggests excessive sympathetic tone. True Raynaud's phenomenon extremely rare.
Muscular atrophy	Occurs rapidly in severe disease.
Contracture of joints	Extension of involved joints often limited.
Nodules	Occur at sites of pressure in about 20% of patients; olecranon and over proximal ulna, over extensor surfaces of fingers, over Achilles tendon ("pump bumps") most commonly, but can occur in tendon substance, bone, sclerae, over pinna of the ear, and in visceral organs, especially the lung.
Synovial hernias	Occur through defects in capsule caused by synovitis. In hands, often mistaken for nodules.
Weight loss	May occur rarely especially with vasculitis. A sign of a poor prognosis in my experience.

The reader is referred to this discussion and to the summary in Table 43–3. Generalized fatigue is experienced by about 80% of patients with RA. It consists of a profound "bone tiredness"; in uncontrolled disease it typically occurs about 4.5 hours after arising in the morning. Pain and stiffness have a circadian rhythm and are more pronounced in the morning. Both symptoms correlate with objective measurements of decreased grip strength and increased joint swelling.[46] Rarely, visceral manifestations of the disease, such as pulmonary rheumatoid nodules, antedate joint complaints.

SIGNS

Upper Extremity (See Also Chapters 50 and 51)

Initial swelling is due to synovitis and occurs along the lines of synovial reflection, usually most pronounced over the extensor surfaces, where the articular capsule is more distensible. Involved distal interphalangeal (DIP) joints show dorsal bulging and the extensor tendon may be eroded, producing a permanently flexed DIP joint. An extensive quantitative analysis of tenderness of the small joints of the hand showed that the DIP joints were involved in about 80% of patients with RA and that tenderness in the joints varied synchronously with that in the proximal small hand joints.[47] About 20% of RA patients never showed DIP joint tenderness no matter how inflamed the other hand joints became. Systematic radiographic studies have confirmed that DIP joints are involved in RA.[48,49] Erosions were found in the DIP in 16% of patients in one study[48] and in 37% in another.[49] Erosions also occurred in 14% of hand films of control patients in the latter study. The control films had been obtained from an orthopedist's private patients and the erosions were of the type associated with inflammatory osteoarthritis.

The proximal interphalangeal (PIP) joints show a symmetric spindle-shaped swelling (Fig. 43–4). These joints may develop flexion deformities in time, particularly when flexor tenosynovitis leads to subsequent tendon contracture. The PIP joints may become hyperextended, owing to contracture of the intrinsic muscle tendons (interosseous and lumbrical). These muscles become extensors of the joint, rather than flexors. This change leads to the "intrinsicoid deflection," sometimes called the "grasshopper" deformity when associated with simultaneous DIP joint flexion.

PIP joints in flexion deformity may suffer rupture of the central slip of the extensor digitorum tendon. When this rupture occurs, little impedes the dorsal migration of the joint through the lateral slips (through the "buttonhole"). This so-called bouton-

FIG. 43–4. Second, third, and fourth fingers in a young woman with recent onset of rheumatoid arthritis. Significant fusiform swelling often occurs in the PIP joints as seen best in the finger on the extreme left.

FIG. 43–5. Extreme ulnar deviation and deformity in far-advanced rheumatoid arthritis. The base of each proximal phalange is subluxed downward.

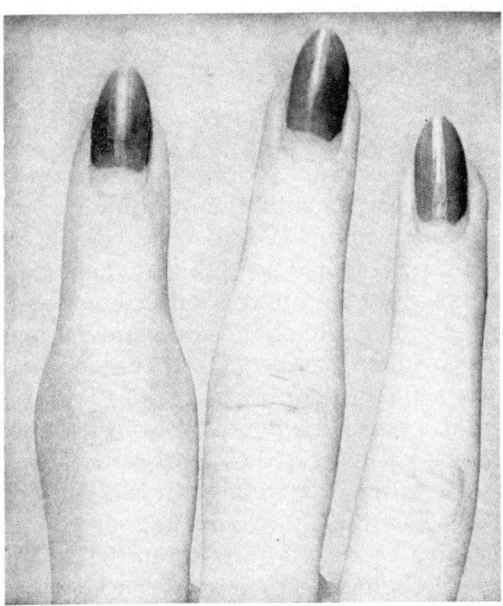

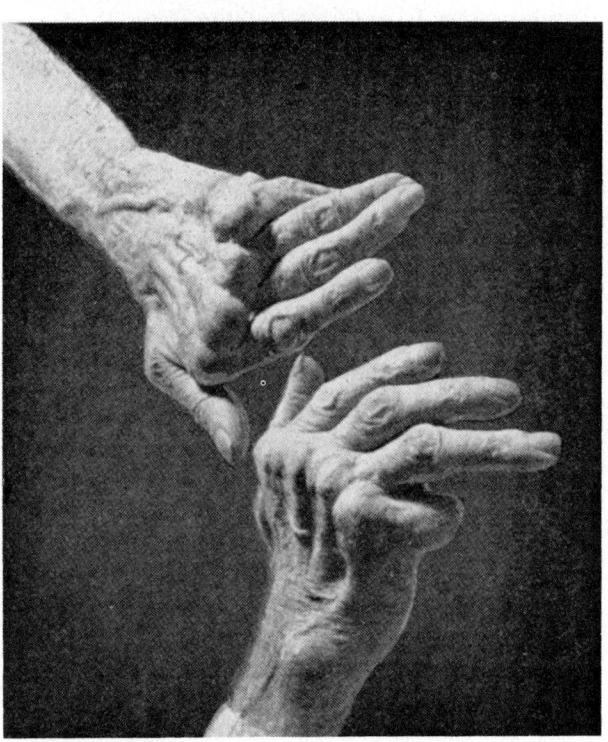

nière deformity is difficult to repair and is disabling. It is our practice to have this deformity repaired by a plastic or orthopedic hand surgeon as soon as possible. Results have been gratifying. The buttonhole deformity can occur acutely and is a distressing, although uncommon, complication of local corticosteroid injection.[50]

The metacarpophalangeal (MCP) joints swell dorsally. Their collateral ligaments become stretched, and the volar fibrocartilaginous plate to which they are attached, and on which the base of the proximal phalanx rests, drops palmward. The strong flexor muscles then pull the base of the proximal phalanx also palmward, leading to the characteristic volar subluxation (Fig. 43–5). The medial collateral ligament to the second MCP joint is often the first to be disrupted by the contiguous synovitis. The integrity of this ligament can easily be checked by flexing the second MCP joint and rocking the proximal phalanx from side to side while holding the second metacarpal firmly. Normally, the collateral ligaments are maximally tight in this position, and no side-to-side motion is possible. The tendon of the first dorsal interosseous muscle may rupture. This is associated with loss of its muscle mass, leading to formation of a hollowed-out space between the thumb and index finger (see left hand in Fig. 43–5).

With volar subluxation of the MCP joints, the ex-

tensor tendons are stretched. The pull of the forearm muscles to the ulnar side is accentuated in the presence of radial migration of the carpus. The fingers become fixed in ulnar deviation when the extensor tendons slide laterally into the groove on the ulnar side of the joint (Fig. 43–5). The entire head of the metacarpal may now be felt just beneath the skin. Volar subluxation of the first MCP joint (thumb) occurs early in the disease and is often the first evidence of deformity in the hand. Rupture of its medial collateral ligament produces the "gamekeeper's thumb" deformity, so called because it can develop in nonrheumatoid persons who frequently engage in the slaughter of birds; the thumb of the hand used to hold the birds' necks develops the deformity.

RA rarely produces bony ankylosis, except in the carpal and tarsal joints, in contradistinction to ankylosing spondylitis, psoriasis, Reiter's syndrome, and juvenile RA, all of which are associated with more bony proliferation. Osteophyte formation, even in severely destroyed rheumatoid joints with so-called secondary osteoarthritis, is almost invariably modest or absent. The only exceptions are in patients with primary osteoarthritis that antedates the onset of RA.

Flexor tenosynovitis is common in RA, and swelling

can easily be felt, and often seen, as a linear tumefaction in the palm. The soft tissues of the palm typically bulge between the swollen tendons (see Fig. 4–3). These tendons may rupture, especially if rheumatoid nodules have formed within them. Such rupture occurs generally at the level of the MCP joint at which they enter the flexor sheath.[51] Flexor tenosynovitis occurred in 55 of 100 patients with RA observed for 5 years.[52] An average of 3.1 tendons were involved per patient, with the third (the "power" flexor) most commonly inflamed, followed in order by the second, fourth, fifth, and first. In contrast, idiopathic tenosynovitis involved fewer tendons, and the first (thumb) tendon was most commonly involved.

Inflammation of the extensor digitorum tendon sheath is also common and leads to swelling over the wrist and metacarpals. This occurrence is particularly troublesome in the presence of the "caput ulnae syndrome," and tendon rupture, usually acute, is common.[53] Rupture of extensor tendons occurs at the wrist; the fifth tendon usually ruptures first, followed in order by the fourth, third, and second. Again, prompt plastic repair often gives good results (see Chapter 50). Acute ulnar deviation of the MCP joint has been described after rapid reversal of MCP joint swelling following intra-articular corticosteroid administration.[50] This disconcerting result is presumed to be due to a stretching of the extensor tendons over the swollen joint, an adaptation that proves disastrous with rapid reduction of the swelling.

The carpus is often involved, and always as a unit, because its joint spaces intercommunicate. The radiocarpal joint is also a common site of RA, as are the flexor carpi radialis, flexor carpi ulnaris, and flexor digitorum tendon sheaths at the wrist.[54] The favorite site of RA in this area is the ulnar bursa, which lies in the recess of the distal ulna and is continuous with the synovial cavity of the distal radioulnar joint. The fibrous ligament holding this joint together is weakened and destroyed by synovitis, thereby allowing the ulna to migrate dorsally so that it over-rides the radius (caput ulnae syndrome).[53] Early in the disorder, the ulna can be manually depressed by the examiner in much the same way as a piano key yields to pressure (the "piano-key sign").

The ulnar styloid and distal ulna are often covered with inflammatory rheumatoid granulation tissue that serrates the local bony cortex. That rupture of the long extensors does not occur more often as a result of this double threat to their integrity, mechanical and inflammatory, is probably a result of lessened demands on the inflamed wrist because of pain and weakness. Resnick has shown that the rheumatoid erosions of the ulnar styloid come from synovitis in the prestyloid recess of the radiocarpal joint, which attacks its tip; from the radioulnar synovitis that attacks it inferiorly; and from extensor carpi ulnaris tenosynovitis, which attacks it dorsilaterally.[55]

The wrist joint rapidly loses its full extension when inflamed. Rest splints to preserve 30° or more of extension are commonly used, with care taken to prevent fibrous ankylosis in extension. A neutral or even a slightly flexed position is least disabling in a wrist for which all hope is lost.

Treatment consists of prophylactic excision of the distal ulna together with the surrounding inflammatory tissue. This procedure, with certain caveats (see Chapter 50), should nearly always be done at the time of repair of a ruptured extensor tendon.

Both the radiohumeral and ulnohumeral joints of the elbow are often involved in RA. The elbow rapidly develops a flexion contracture. Fortunately, the shoulder is less commonly involved in RA and, like the elbow, is easily treated by local corticosteroid injection. The acromioclavicular joint is often involved and is the chief cause of complaints of pain in the shoulder area because it hurts when the patient lies on his side during sleep. The sternoclavicular and temporomandibular joints are also involved more commonly than is the shoulder. The biceps tendon sheath may be inflamed, either at the origin or at the insertion of the biceps muscle.

An exhaustive survey of conditions that might reduce hand deformities resembling those of RA has been published.[56] These include deformities caused by other joint diseases such as systemic lupus erythematosus (SLE) and chronic rheumatoid fever (Jaccoud's arthritis), as well as those produced by neurologic conditions, such as reflex sympathetic dystrophy, Parkinson's disease, Wilson's disease, and others. The general pattern of joint involvement in RA is similar to that in SLE, and the two diseases cannot be distinguished on this basis.[57]

Jaccoud's arthritis refers to hand deformities that develop as a result of chronic inflammation of the articular capsule in rheumatic fever.[58–60] Ulnar drift at the MCP joints and intrinsicoid deformities of the PIP joints develop. Aschoff bodies and focal lymphocyte collections in the capsule coexist with normal articular cartilages. The thumb may become Z-shaped. Characteristic hook-like osteophytes caused by capsular pressure remodeling have been described by Bywaters.[58] Diagnostic criteria for Jaccoud's arthropathy have been proposed.[60] Twenty cases were collected in a single French rheumatic disease center in 10 years. Changes typical of Jaccoud's arthropathy occurred in 3 of 25 cases of rheumatic fever, in 10 of 320 cases of systemic lupus erythematosus, in 2 of 56 cases of mixed connective tissue disease, in 2 of 98 cases of Sjögren's syndrome, but in only 3 of 3000 cases of rheumatoid arthritis.[59] Lupus is clearly the most common cause of most of the Jaccoud's arthropathy currently encountered by rheumatologists in Europe and North America.

Lower Extremity (See Also Chapters 53, 54, and 55)

The joints of the forefoot are commonly involved in RA. The metatarsophalangeal (MTP) joints are nearly always affected and are often the first to show erosive disease. I routinely obtain fine detail radiographs of the MTP joints as well as the hands and wrists when searching for evidence of erosive disease as a clue to early aggressive treatment.[61]

Typically, in RA, the transverse (metatarsal) arch of the foot collapses, so weight-bearing occurs on MTP heads 2, 3 and 4, rather than on 1 and 5 as in a normal foot (Fig. 43–6). The plantar fascia contracts, leading to a pes cavus deformity. The toes become cocked-up and do not fit easily into a normal shoe.

The first MTP joint undergoes a progressive valgus deformity, and a bunion develops over its medial surface. A bunionette may develop over the lateral surface of the fifth MTP joint. The hindfoot becomes

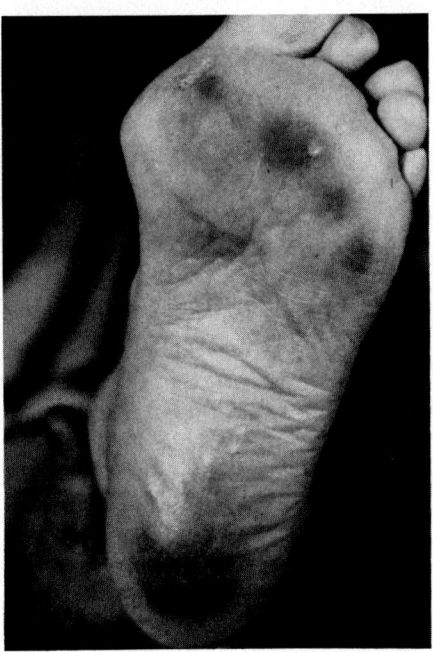

FIG. 43–6. Forefoot involvement is clearly present in this man with rheumatoid arthritis who stood on a surface lightly dusted with graphite. The weight-bearing pattern on metatarsophalangeal joints 2, 3, and 4 is abnormal. The hallux valgus, prominent bunion, high longitudinal arch, and "cocked up," overlapping toes are all typical findings in this disease.

everted. One systematic study showed that 46 of 50 hospitalized patients with RA had foot joint involvement; 42 of these showed forefoot arthritis, 68% had midfoot involvement, but only 16% showed ankle joint inflammation.[62] Another study emphasized the importance of proper shoes.[63]

The ankle and subtalar joints are sometimes troublesome but are easily injected, and once swelling subsides they can be immobilized in a walking cast for 8 weeks for maximal anti-inflammatory effect. Tenosynovitis of the tendons around the ankle is also common, especially the posterior tibial tendon as it loops under the medial malleolus, and the peroneal as it passes under the lateral malleolus. The Achilles tenosynovium may become inflamed and can become eroded at its insertion on the calcaneus. It may rupture, especially when rheumatoid nodules form within it.

The knee joints and proximal tibiofibular joints are also commonly involved in RA. Characteristically, the inflamed knee develops a flexion contracture and a progressive valgus deformity that can become so severe that the patient can hardly move one knee past the other when walking. Uniform tricompartmental narrowing (patellofemoral, medial and lateral tibiofemoral) of the joint space is visible radiologically. Ligamentous laxity, especially laxity of the medial collateral ligament and the cruciate ligaments, often develops as in other rheumatoid joints. Synovial thickening is easily felt, and effusions are the rule (Fig. 43–7). The fat pad below the patellar tendon may become enlarged[64]; this finding is especially pronounced after systemic corticosteroid treatment because the fat pad shares in the fat redistribution process that produces moon facies. An enlarged fat pad may be mistaken for an effusion. A popliteal (Adams-Baker) cyst may become prominent (see Fig. 43–12A). Quadriceps muscle atrophy occurs rapidly; a full inch of thigh muscle (circumferential measurement) may be lost in a few weeks.

Hip joint involvement in RA is fortunately uncommon. Joint space narrowing is often accompanied by central migration of the femoral head.

Axial Skeleton

Sacroiliac joints are occasionally tender in patients with seropositive erosive RA, with one side usually much more tender than the other. These patients are often HLA-B27 positive in my experience.

Involvement of the cervical spine is more common than is generally recognized.[65–68] The most frequent clinical manifestation of cervical spine involvement is painful limitation of neck motion. Radiologic evidence of cervical spine inolvement consists of intervertebral

FIG. 43–7. Rheumatoid arthritis of the knees in a middle-aged man.

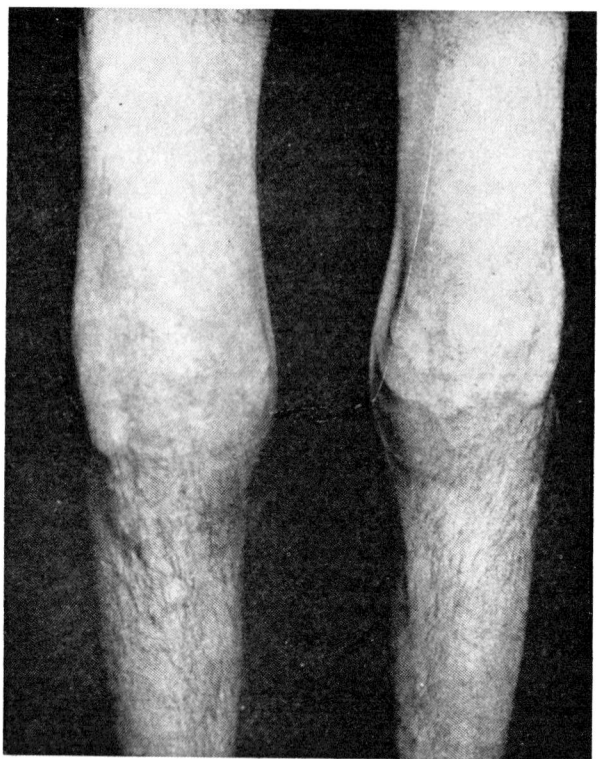

disc narrowing without much in the way of osteophytes. Narrowing and erosion of the zygapophyseal joints may occur. The ligaments of the cervical spine showed evidence of active inflammation in patients with RA who were operated on for atlantoaxial subluxation.[69] Recognition of cervical spine involvement is most important in patients with atlantoaxial joint subluxation and compression of the cervical spinal cord. This deformity is largely due to odontoid erosion from rheumatoid involvement of the bursae in front of and behind the odontoid. Such instances may represent a neurosurgical emergency,[65,67,70] and may cause signs of long-tract compression or respiratory arrest. Ligamentous distention leads to "stepladder" subluxations.[66] Subluxation of the atlantoaxial joint is usually anterior, with more than 2.5 mm between the anterior aspect of the odontoid and the posterior aspect of the atlas ring, but it can be lateral or posterior. An analysis of 194 patients with atlantoaxial subluxation or atlantoaxial imposition (upward migration of the odontoid toward or even into the foramen magnum) showed that 20 developed spinal cord compression. This serious complication, which occurred exclusively in seropositive disease, was more likely to occur (1) in men; (2) when subluxation exceeded 8 mm; (3) in the presence of atlantoaxial imposition; and (4) probably, when lateral subluxation was present. Men had a 24% chance of developing spinal cord compression, as opposed to only a 7.5% chance among the women, who constituted 83% of the patients in the series. Only 2% of those with less than 9 mm of subluxation developed neurologic symptoms. Atlantoaxial impaction tripled the chance of spinal cord compression.

Magnetic resonance imaging is an excellent noninvasive technique for detection of cervical myelopathy (see Chapter 6).[71] Treatment of cervical cord compression is obviously surgical with reduction of the deformity coupled with posterior fusion of the neural arch (see Chapter 52).[72] A series of 43 cases of cervical myelopathy associated with RA was collected over a period of 20 years in a single arthritis center in the Netherlands; 23 patients died, including all 9 cases *not* treated surgically.[70] These 9 patients all died within 1 year.

Alarm signs and symptoms suggesting the development of cervical myelopathy include (1) severe neck pain; (2) tingling or numbness in the hands and feet; (3) urinary retention or incontinence; (4) "jumping" legs (spinal automatism); and (5) "stone" or "marble" sensations in the limbs or trunk.[70] Examination of such patients reveals multiple neurologic defects.

The sternomanubrial joint and the costal cartilages are tender in some patients, usually intermittently. Painful subluxation of this joint has been reported in a number of patients.[73,74] The cricoarytenoid joints may also be involved, producing hoarseness. Rarely, respiration is compromised, and a tracheostomy becomes a lifesaving procedure.[75]

OTHER FEATURES

During the evolution of the disease, patients have little evidence of systemic reaction, except for occasional low-grade fever, slight tachycardia, anorexia, and weight loss. An occasional patient has an acute, fulminating course characterized by marked systemic reaction, elevated temperature, and warm, red, swollen joints. Such a picture can also be noted after abrupt withdrawal of corticosteroids as a rebound phenomenon. This manifestation of RA is accompanied by extensive local fibrin deposition and is rapidly reversed by a short course of systemic corticosteroids in modest (20- to 30-mg) daily doses.[76]

A striking aspect of the general clinical picture of the disease is noted in the degree and rapidity of accompanying muscular atrophy (see Figs. 43–5, 43–7). The rapidity of development of muscular atrophy is due not only to disuse, but often to an active inflammatory process in the muscles as well.

Subcutaneous nodules occur over traumatized areas such as elbows, extensor surfaces of the arms, knees, knuckles, occiput, buttocks, and medial scapular areas. About 20% of all patients with RA manifest such nodules eventually. At times, these nodules can be difficult to differentiate from gouty tophi (Fig. 43–8), and similar nodules can occur in both rheumatic fever and SLE. Histologic confirmation of typical rheumatoid nodule architecture may be diagnostically helpful. A nodule is not really a nodule until it has been histologically confirmed. The histologic differential diagnosis of subcutaneous nodules is given in Table 41–1.

Rheumatoid nodules most often develop over the forearms, distal to the olecranon process, which become traumatized as the patient uses the forearms as levers, for example, to arise from a chair (Fig. 43–9). The back of the head and ears may develop nodules owing to pressure against the mattress at night (see Fig. 43–8), the back of the heels are traumatized by shoes ("pump bumps"), the bridge of the nose by eyeglasses, and the backs of the knuckles by everyday trauma. Nodules develop in the pulps of the fingers in patients who use tools, and over the ischial tuberosities in patients who sit for prolonged periods on hard surfaces. Nodules may ulcerate or may become gangrenous as part of the picture of rheumatoid vas-

FIG. 43–8. An ulcerating rheumatoid nodule is seen on the ear of a man with severe, deforming rheumatoid arthritis.

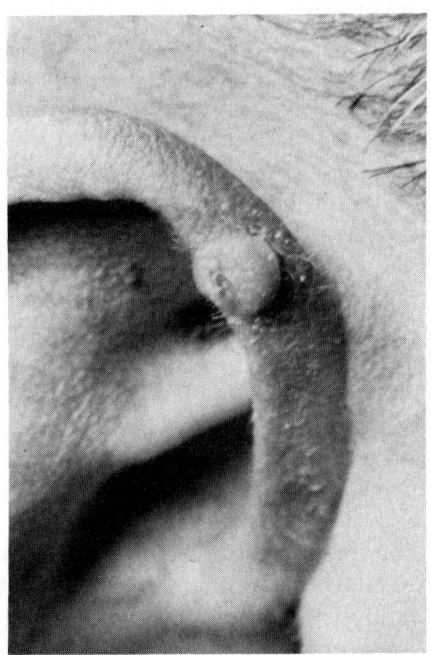

culitis. Rarely they erode bone,[77,78] but they do not calcify. They may appear as giant bone cysts.[79] These nodules may also develop in tendons or in visceral organs, such as the meninges,[80] cerebellum, cerebral cortex,[81] pleura, lung, pericardium, heart muscle, or cardiac valves. In the lung, the nodules may simulate carcinoma or, if they perforate and drain into a bronchus, an abscess. Nodules perforating the pleural space may cause pneumothorax or a bronchopleural fistula. Rarely, nodules form in the sclera from a focus of scleritis and perforate the anterior chamber, a condition called scleromalacia perforans (Fig. 43–10).

A variant of RA, rheumatoid nodulosis, has been described already (Fig. 43–11) and usually occurs in middle-aged men, some of whom are diabetic.[5-8] Few systemic features exist; radiologic changes consist of punched-out lesions in bone, but without the overhanging bony margin that occur in gout. The patient retains good grip strength and generally feels well. Most of these patients have acute attacks of palindromic rheumatism. The combination of multiple nodules and acute intermittent arthritis is often mistaken for acute and tophaceous gout.

Rheumatoid nodules are thought to form around an area of vasculitis, and Sokoloff has demonstrated arterial remnants in their center by serial sectioning. As mentioned previously, these nodules can become necrotic and may ulcerate. If this happens in a nodule near a joint that lies close to the skin, a draining fistula may develop from the synovium, so-called fistulous rheumatism. Of eight seropositive patients with this complication, seven had nodules; the fistulas were attributed to nodule necrosis in three instances, whereas four had joint sepsis and later developed fistulas, and one developed a fistula from a synovial cyst.[82]

SYNOVIAL CYSTS AND SYNOVIAL HERNIAS

The increased intra-articular pressure that occurs in rheumatoid joints tightly packed with hypertrophic, inflamed synovium or with a tense effusion is increased even further by active joint motion (see Chapter 11). As inflammatory damage occurs to cartilage and subchondral bone, especially at the "bare" areas of the synovial-bone contact, and to the articular capsule, focal areas of mechanical weakness develop. Such areas are particularly prominent in patients treated with corticosteroids. Increased intra-articular pressure may then force joint contents through the weakened spots to form cysts. Such nodular diverticula, about 5 mm in diameter, are commonly seen

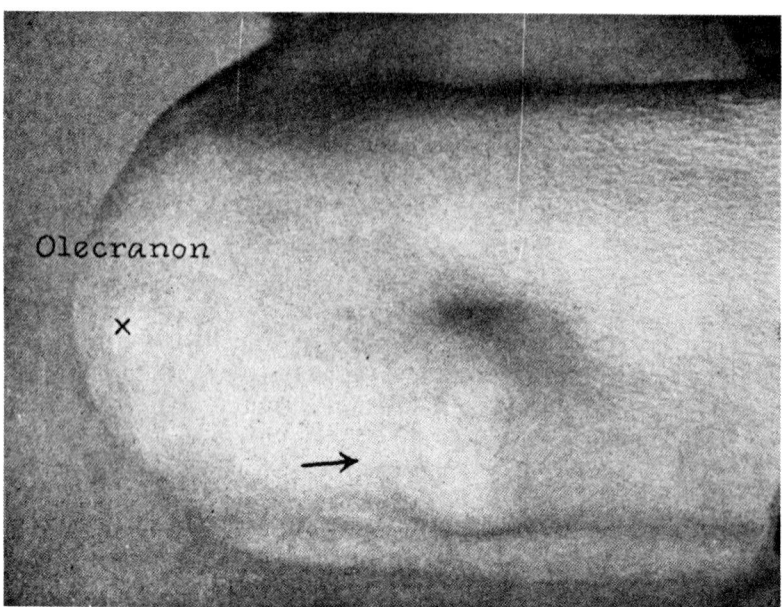

FIG. 43–9. Subcutaneous nodule on the extensor surface of the forearm distal to the elbow joint.

bulging from the dorsolateral surfaces of the PIP or MCP joints. These cysts contain diseased synovium that can be pushed back into the joint through the defect in the articular capsules, just as an inguinal hernia can be reduced through the inguinal ring. They can originate from tendons.[83] Cysts develop commonly from the knee,[84] wrist, carpal, PIP, MCP, and elbow joints[85] and rarely from ankle, shoulder, or hip joints (Fig. 43–12). In the hip, these cysts have been confused with inguinal hernias.[86] Cysts arising from the hip joint can compress the iliac vein, producing swelling of the leg.[87,88] Plantar synovial cysts also occur.[89] An apophyseal joint cyst proved to be the cause of back pain and sciatica in a patient with RA.[90] Inflamed bursae can also dissect. An olecranon bursa dissected proximally in one patient[91] and a subdeltoid

FIG. 43–10. A rheumatoid nodule is shown perforating the ocular sclera—scleromalacia perforans.

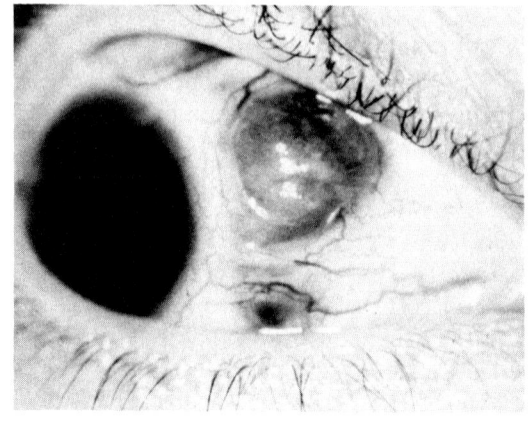

bursa extended into the clavicle and to the skin surface in another.[92] Bony erosions may lead to fractures, which in turn may rupture through the skin.[93]

The knee joint normally communicates posteriorly with the gastrocnemius-semimembranous bursa. Increased pressure in the knee forces fluid into this structure. In fully 40% of those affected, the channel between the (Adams-Baker) cyst and knee joint is long and tortuous and acts as a one-way valve, so cyst contents cannot return to the joint. Bony destruction is less apparent in knees with large cysts possibly because of decompression of the joint that these cysts afford.[94]

Acute arthritis in a previously normal joint is often accompanied by a large effusion and a nearly normal, but less compliant, fibrous articular capsule. Measurement of intra-articular pressure in the knee may reach hundreds of millimeters of mercury, even with gentle knee flexion in bed. Rupture of the joint posteriorly may result. Joint fluid leaks into the calf and simulates acute thrombophlebitis. A positive Homans' sign and calf tenderness, redness, and swelling with pitting edema may be present.[95] This has been called the *pseudothrombophlebitis syndrome.* Such leakage can occur on a long-term basis and can lead to chronc edema of the leg; with wrist or elbow joint rupture, chronic edema of the forearm or the dorsum of the hand may result.[85]

Valvular mechanisms have been implicated also in the pathogenesis of antecubital cysts and in cysts arising from other joints.[85,96] In chronic arthritis, joint rupture is unusual because the joint capsule becomes adapted by stretching. A popliteal cyst can gradually enlarge, however, dissecting distally until it nearly

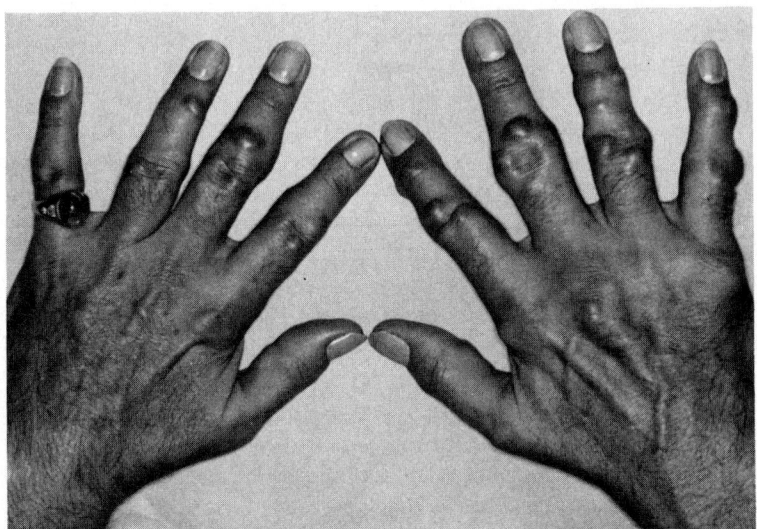

FIG. 43–11. Rheumatoid nodulosis. These multiple rheumatoid nodules and palindromic rheumatism in a diabetic man were thought at first to be gouty arthritis. A diabetologist thought the nodules were xanthomata. The patient's grip strength was nearly normal and he felt generally well.

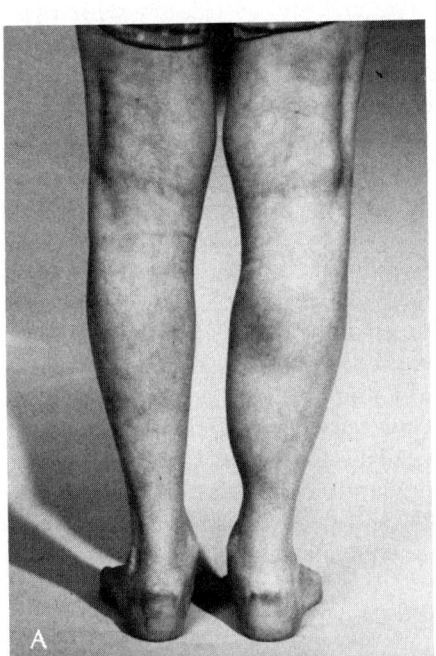

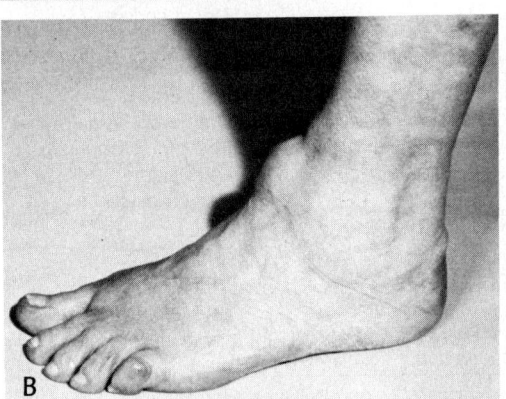

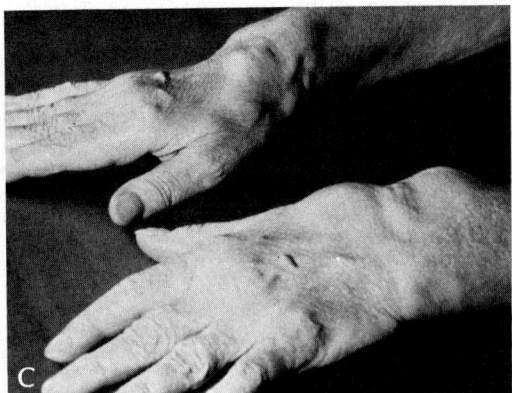

FIG. 43–12. *A,* A popliteal cyst has dissected nearly to the ankle in this woman with rheumatoid arthritis. *B,* A cyst protrudes from the ankle joint of the same patient. *C,* Cysts have developed from synovium herniated from extensor tendons at both wrists of this patient who had received corticosteroids for many years, perhaps leading to weakness of fibrous tissues.

reaches the ankle (see Fig. 43–12A). Cysts occurring near multiple joints and tendon sheaths, as in the patient shown in Figure 43–12, might suggest the term rheumatoid cystoides. Such enlargement can cause entrapment neuropathy and footdrop.[97]

Localized swelling is usually due to synovitis of joint, bursa, tendon sheath, to synovial cysts derived from these structures, or to rheumatoid nodules. Rarer causes include giant cell tumors[98] and intrasynovial fatty masses.[64] Four of five giant cell tumors in one report were derived from finger tendon sheaths.[98]

NERVE ENTRAPMENT SYNDROMES
(See Also Chapter 95)

Because RA is a proliferative disease of joint and tendon synovium, frequent entrapment of peripheral nerves by these enlarging structures might be predicted. Nerve entrapment is indeed common in RA and is important to be recognized because of its treatability, but it is not found in every case, perhaps because the ligamentous destruction caused by the disease process itself releases or prevents pressure on the nerves at risk.

Entrapment of the median nerve at the wrist (carpal tunnel syndrome) is perhaps most common, followed by entrapment of the plantar branches of the posterior tibial nerve (tarsal tunnel syndrome). Anomalous wrist muscles were thought to contribute to a carpal tunnel syndrome found in 6 of 17 patients with RA.[99] Entrapment of the ulnar nerve at the wrist or elbow, the posterior interosseous nerve just distal to the elbow,[100] the sural nerve in the leg,[97] and one or more of the common digital nerves in the foot all occur occasionally. Involvement of the posterior interosseous nerve, a branch of the radial nerve, causes extensor paralysis of all five digits, whereas pressure on the sural nerve may cause footdrop. Peroneal nerve palsy caused by posterior dislocation of the proximal tibiofibular joint has been described.[101] Such involvement must be differentiated from the neuropathy caused by rheumatoid vasculitis.

Treatment of nerve entrapment may consist of local injection of a corticosteroid suspension into the area of entrapment. If this therapy fails to provide sustained symptomatic relief and functional recovery, prompt surgical attention must be obtained. The anatomic considerations of peripheral nerves at risk from entrapment are well described and should be familiar to all those treating RA and other musculoskeletal diseases (see Chapter 95).

MISCELLANEOUS FINDINGS

In some patients, generalized lymphadenopathy is present, and splenomegaly is present in about 15%. In some persons, the palpably enlarged nodes may suggest a lymphoma. Peripheral vascular vasomotor instability is sometimes a prominent feature of the disease and is characterized by cold, clammy hands and feet with increased sweating. Very rarely, Raynaud's phenomena may accompany or may precede initial joint manifestations. Raynaud's phenomenon is much more common in scleroderma, mixed connective tissue disease, or SLE. Palmar erythema, particularly over the thenar and hypothenar areas and also associated with Laennec's cirrhosis or pregnancy, is common and is often accentuated during treatment with corticosteroids. At times, patients may show pronounced atrophy of the skin with increased pigmentation and bronzing. The cutaneous manifestations have been reviewed and include those shown in Table 43–4.[102] The arthritis associated with pyoderma gangrenosum is often seronegative.[103] Leg ulceration was twice as common in patients with RA as in those with osteoarthritis in the same clinic.[104] Tendon ruptures are common in RA, as discussed already. Ruptures in unusual sites can occur rarely.[105]

RADIOGRAPHIC CHANGES

The radiographic changes in RA have been amply described in previous editions of this book.[106] Swelling of small peripheral joints produces a periarticular radiodensity and displacement or obliteration of subcutaneous fat lines (Fig. 43–13). In larger joints, accumulation of synovial fluid can often be visualized. Joint space narrowing caused by diffuse loss of cartilage occurs later and usually affects the entire surface

Table 43–4. Cutaneous Lesions of Rheumatoid Arthritis

Nodules	Other
Typical	Lipoid nodules
Linear	Pemphigoid
	Bullous
	Cicatricial
	Dermatitis herpetiformis
Vasculitis	Granuloma annulare
Ulcers (legs, elsewhere)	Liver palms
Gangrene	Amyloidosis
Nailfold thrombi	
Purpura	
Livedo reticularis	
Urticaria	
Hemorrhagic bullae	
Pyoderma gangrenosum	

Modified from Sibbitt, W.L., and Williams, R.C.[102]

FIG. 43–13. Evolution of changes in rheumatoid arthritis. *A,* Early changes consist of mild periarticular soft tissue swelling and demineralization accompanied by minimal uniform cartilage narrowing, best seen here in the radiocarpal and third distal interphalangeal joints. *B,* Two years later, demineralization, articular destruction (arrows), and typical metacarpophalangeal and wrist deformity have occurred. Subluxation of the first metacarpophalangeal joint, an early finding, has progressed, and ulnar deviation of these joints has begun. Involvement of the distal interphalangeal joint is obvious. (From Genant, H.K.[106])

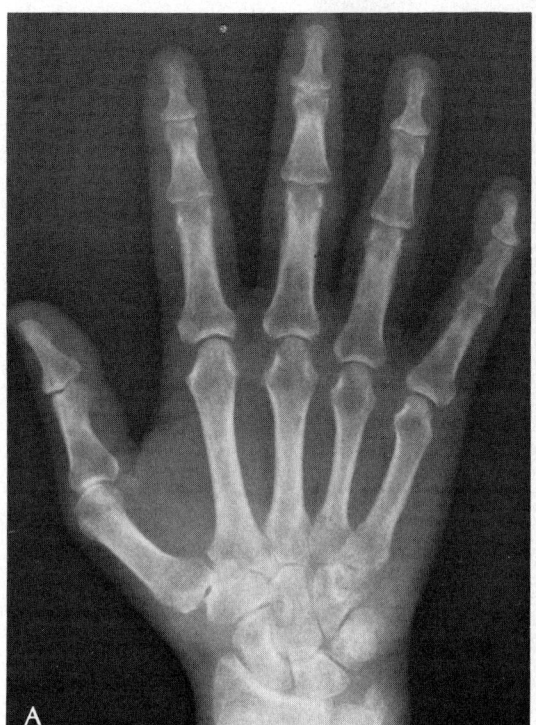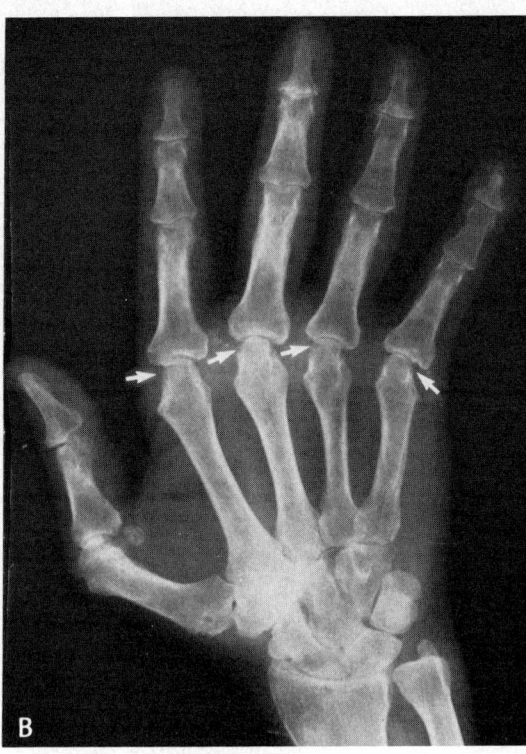

of the cartilage. Thus, in the knee joint, tricompartmental loss of joint space is the rule. Regional osteoporosis of subchondral bone also occurs, reflecting increased blood flow to the periarticular trabecular bone (Fig. 43–14A). Articular bony erosions develop at varying rates in individual patients with RA. I routinely obtain fine detail films of the hands and forefeet in early disease to detect bony erosions. They may be seen in some patients within a few months after disease onset. They are detectable within 1 year of onset in many patients, whereas in a few patients they may not ever develop, even after years of sustained joint inflammation. Their early appearance usually heralds more aggressive disease and calls for earlier use of more aggressive treatment regimens. Surface erosions occur first, producing a serrated or "dot-dash" appearance of the bony cortex (Fig. 43–15). They often occur in the "bare" areas, that is, intra-articular bone at the edges of the articular cartilage that is in direct contiguity with inflamed hypertrophic synovial tissue (pannus) (Fig. 43–16), or in extra-articular bone where

inflamed tenosynovium or bursal synovium is in direct contact with bony cortex (Fig. 43–15).

Gradually, these erosions become deeper and involve the trabecular bone, producing the "pocket" erosion (Fig. 43–14B). These are characteristic of RA but by no means specific. Severe synovitis due to many different etiologies may erode bone in a similar fashion. Bilateral symmetric pocket erosions in typical locations, however, are highly suggestive of RA, especially seropositive RA. Interestingly, erosions have been correlated with IgA but not IgG or IgM rheumatoid factor[107]; moreover, IgA rheumatoid factor predicted erosions and correlated with disease activity.[108] Serum amino-terminal type III procollagen peptide levels also correlated with disease activity and may predict erosions.[109] If either or both of these studies can be confirmed, patients at high risk for destructive disease may be identified earlier and more aggressive therapy instituted.

Occasionally the extremes of these phenomena are encountered. Thus, severe erosive disease may *not* be

FIG. 43–14.   *A,* Typical radiographic changes of moderately advanced rheumatoid arthritis with periarticular demineralization, cartilage narrowing, erosive disease showing a proximal distribution, and sparing of the distal interphalangeal joints. *B,* Magnification of the fourth proximal interphalangeal joint demonstrates fusiform soft tissue swelling and extensive erosion (arrows) of the head of the proximal phalanx. (From Genant, H.K.[106])

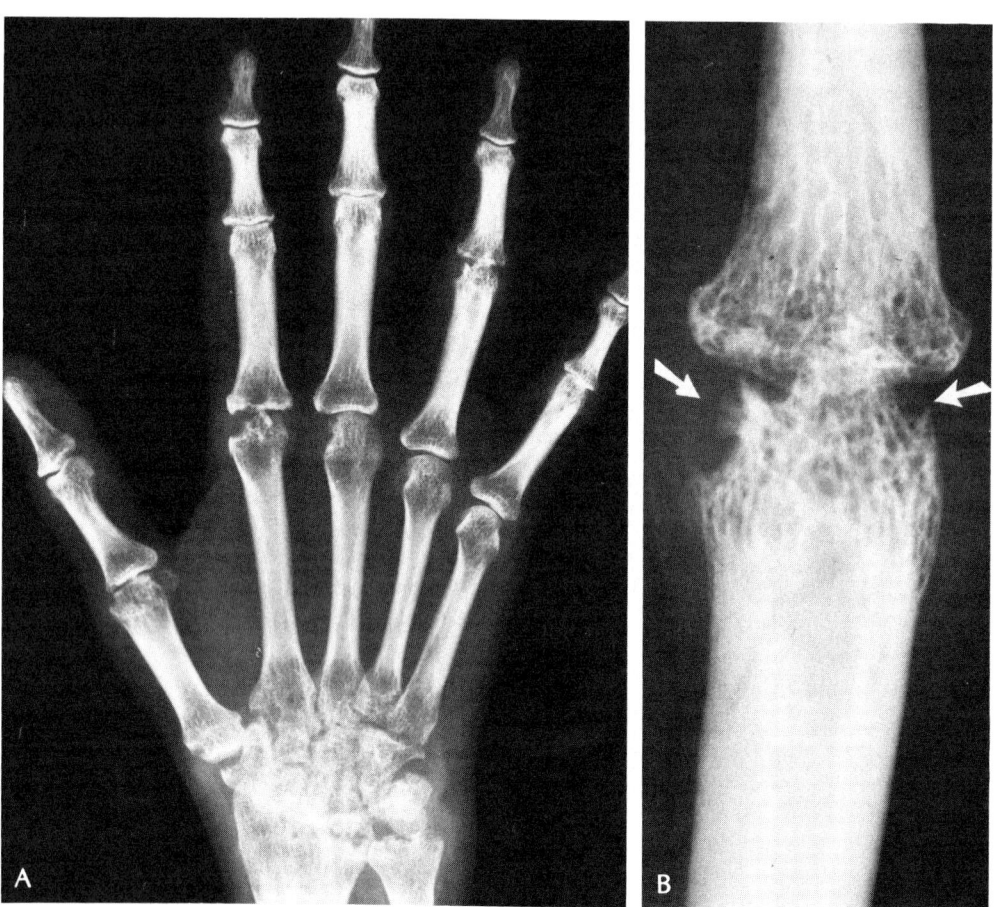

accompanied by periarticular demineralization, and vice versa. The former situation occurs in stoic individuals with strong muscles who persist in high levels of physical activity despite their disease, while severe osteopenia without erosions (but often with joint space narrowing) occurs in frail individuals with low pain thresholds who greatly reduce the use of their joints. All erosions are physically connected to the joint space, although the connection (osteum) may be difficult to appreciate radiographically. Such erosions may produce a cystic appearance sometimes called a pseudocyst or geode (Fig. 43–17). Rheumatoid nodulosis regularly produces cystic lesions, often with relatively little joint space narrowing (Fig. 43–18A and B). As discussed earlier, in several patients these have been shown to be due to the formation of rheumatoid nodules within bone itself.

In advanced disease, atrophy of soft tissues includ-

ing muscle accompanies severe bony destruction with joint subluxation (Fig. 43–19). It is easy to understand why the older term "atrophic" arthritis was an apt description for RA. As mentioned already, the atlantoaxial joint is prone to anterior subluxation, and the degree of this deformity can be ascertained by a comparison of flexion and extension views in the lateral projection (Fig. 43–20A and B). Bony destruction and subluxation occur in the cervical spine, especially in patients with such changes peripherally (Fig. 43–21 A and B).

Little has been written about healing of erosions. In most instances, the bony cortex re-forms *within the contour of a pocket erosion.* This often accompanies clinical remission, nearly always induced by a slow-acting antirheumatic drug such as gold, penicillamine, or cyclophosphamide. Occasionally, pocket erosions may become filled in with new bone. This probably

FIG. 43–15. Early changes in rheumatoid arthritis consist of soft tissue swelling adjacent to the surface erosions (arrows) at the ulnar styloid, the triquetrum, and the base of the fifth metacarpal. (From Genant, H.K.[106])

FIG. 43–17. The wrist in rheumatoid arthritis demonstrates a large subchondral cyst (geode) in the distal radius and soft-tissue swelling with erosion at the ulnar styloid. (From Genant, H.K.[106])

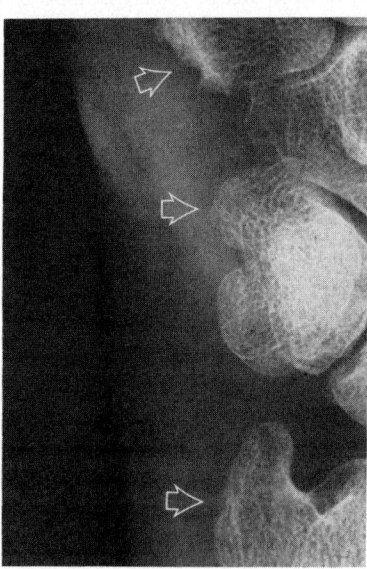

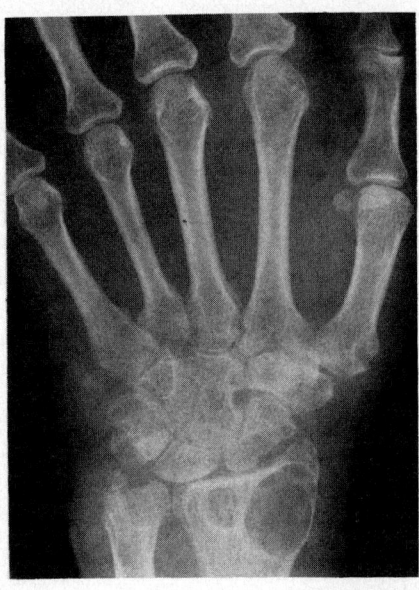

FIG. 43–16. Schematic representation of the hand demonstrating the frequent sites of early erosion in rheumatoid arthritis. (From Genant, H.K.[106])

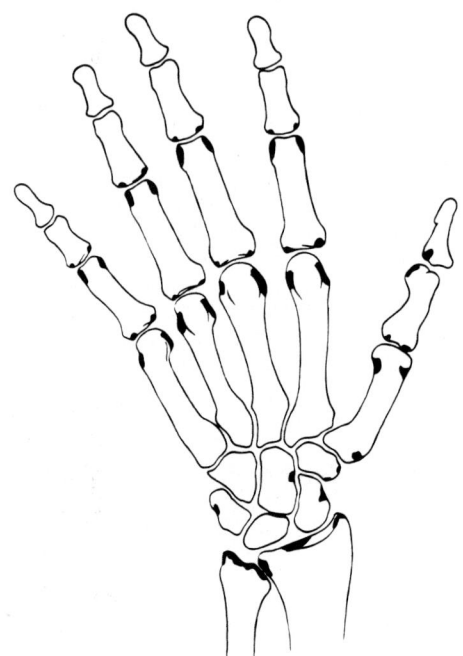

only occurs in relatively recent erosions that are filled with cellular pannus rather than with fibrous tissue scar. Bony proliferation is nearly always modest in seropositive RA; marginal osteophytes are small and effete, and periostitis is very rare, as is subchondral sclerosis. Seronegative disease is much more likely to be associated with such bony proliferative changes, and these allowed the prediction of the serologic status of 43 of 46 patients with "definite RA" from the appearance of hand radiographs alone.[110] Indeed, the only location where bony proliferation often occurs in seropositive RA accompanies healing of the ulnar styloid, which becomes mushroom-shaped.

Laboratory features of rheumatoid disease are discussed in Chapters 5 and 45. Rheumatoid factors are discussed in Chapter 46.

DISEASE COURSE AND PROGNOSIS

Inflammation of joints (fire) leads to early disability and loss of function (Fig. 43–22). Subsequent anatomic changes (ashes) gradually supervene if the inflammatory process proceeds unchecked. In the first few years of disease, the entire process is completely or nearly completely reversible, and complete restitution of function is an attainable goal. I believe that all patients with RA should be seen by a rheumatologist as early in the disease as possible, and that it is

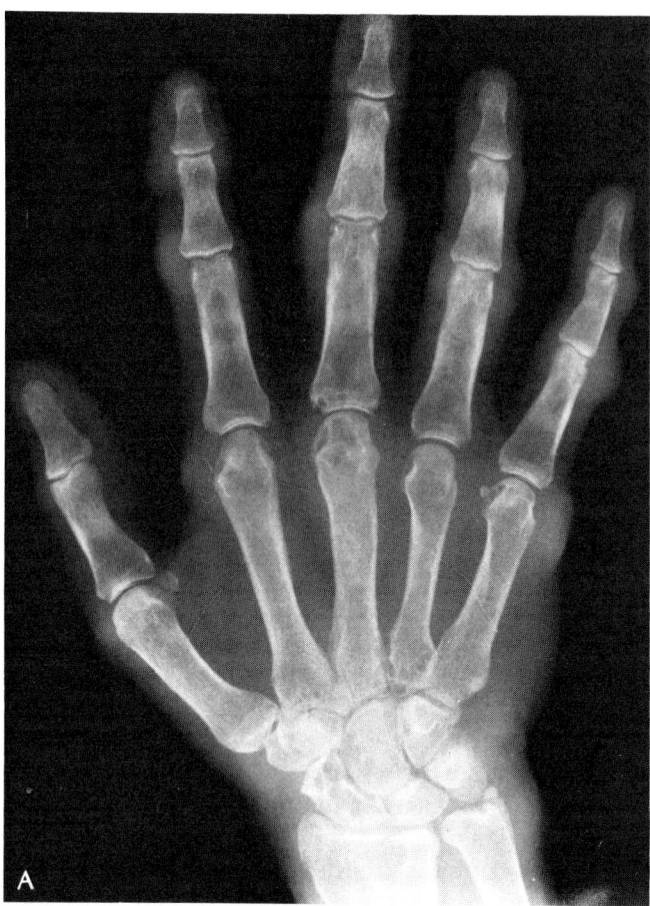

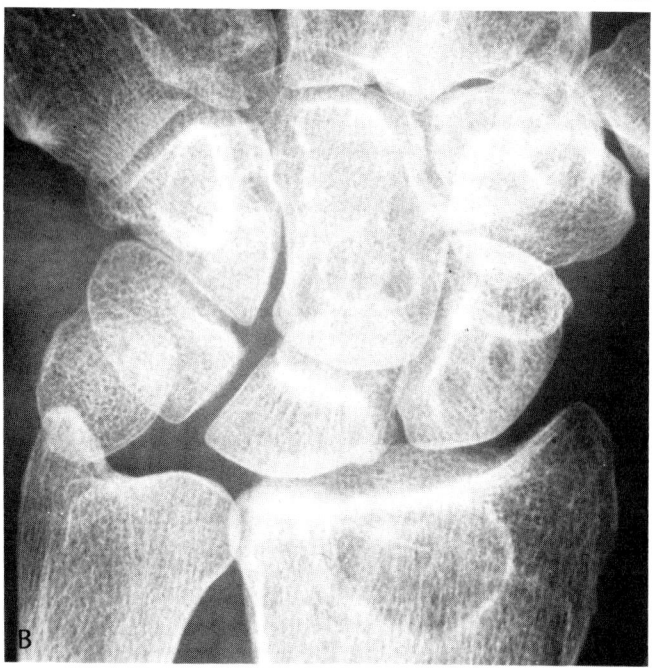

FIG. 43–18. *A,* Striking, nodular, soft tissue swelling, predominantly asymmetric and advanced, subchondral, cyst-like erosions are seen in this patient with "rheumatoid nodulosis." *B,* The left wrist of the same patient demonstrates striking geode (pseudocyst) formation with preservation of mineralization, cartilage space, and articular surfaces. (From Genant, H.K.[106])

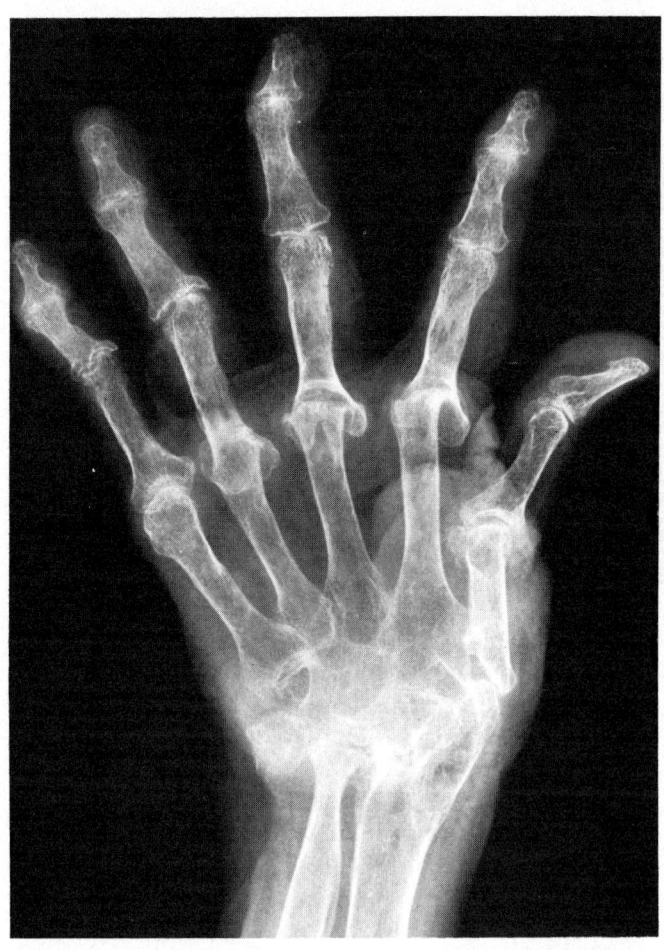

FIG. 43–19. Advanced rheumatoid arthritis showing soft tissue atrophy, severe generalized osteoporosis, resorption, and fragmentation of the metacarpophalangeal and wrist joints, accompanied by remodeling of bone. (From Genant, H.K.[106])

the rheumatologist's primary responsibility, with the help of both the patient's personal physician and the other members of the treatment team (see Chapter 48), to control the inflammatory process. The majority of patents with RA can be brought to remission or so close to remission that the development of irreversible changes proceeds very slowly.

Criteria for remission have been developed by an ARA committee.[111] These criteria have been assessed independently by a study of 458 patients with RA and were found to be 80% sensitive and 96% specific.[112] The average remission lasted 10 months, rarely lasted

more than 2 years, and was associated (86%) with the use of "remittive" drugs such as gold or penicillamine. Only 7.8% of the 1131 patient-years were spent in remission; female sex, age of onset under age 60, and the presence of erosions were associated with a lessened chance of remission. My own experience has been much more sanguine than these data suggest,[113] especially since I have been using remittive agents in combination.

But RA remains a serious threat to life-style, to livelihood, and to life itself. In one study, fully 50% of all patients with RA had to stop working within 10

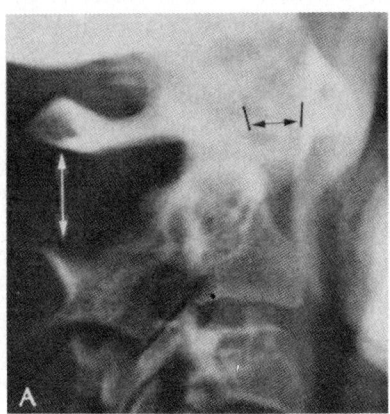
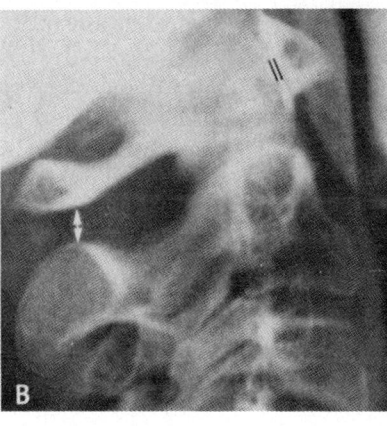

FIG. 43–20. Flexion *(A)* and extension *(B)* views of the cervical spine with C1 and C2 subluxation demonstrate increased separation between the dens (odontoid) and the anterior mass of the atlas (black arrows), as well as excessive vertical motion between the posterior arch of C1 and the spinous process of C2 (white arrows). (From Genant, H.K.[106])

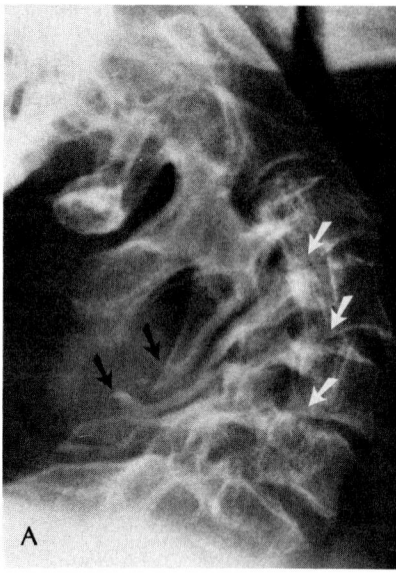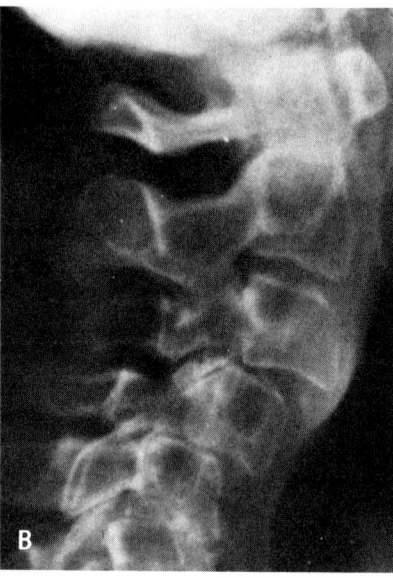

FIG. 43–21. *A,* Advanced rheumatoid arthritis (RA) of the cervical spine consisting of resorption of the dens (odontoid) and spinous processes (black arrows), ankylosis of the C2 to C3 apophyseal joints, erosions at the joints of Luschka and adjacent end plates (white arrows), moderate disc narrowing, anterior subluxation of C6 to C7, and finally, generalized demineralization. *B,* Typical "stepladder" subluxations and disc narrowing in advanced RA. (From Genant, H.K.[106])

years of diagnosis.[114] The average lifetime economic costs for each patient have been conservatively assessed at about $20,000.[115] The development of disability in a multicenter study was predicted by age (older), sex (female), and initial radiologic grade and functional class.[116] The length of time that the disease existed correlated with poor functional outcome in an older study.[117] In this study, onset of seropositive disease in childhood was associated with the worst prognosis because the time course was so prolonged.

The effect of acuteness of onset and of age on onset has been discussed already. Natural remission almost always occurred during the first year after onset. A classic study of nearly 200 patients showed that about 25% of patients followed an episodic course or remit completely, whereas the remainder had a lifelong illness, the activity of which often followed an undulating course but rarely remitted spontaneously.[37] If remission follows the use of disease-suppressing drugs, the disease will nearly always return if these are stopped.[118] Similarly, satisfactory disease control is often only temporary even if the remission-inducing agent is given continuously.[112,118] The role of psychologic stress and joint overuse have been discussed already. It is my practice to restrict physical activity until joint inflammation is controlled. No restrictions

FIG. 43–22. Diagram of disease course in R.A. Maintenance of function is the goal of therapy. See text for discussion.

FUNCTIONAL IMPAIRMENT

INFLAMMATION   STRUCTURAL (ANATOMIC) DAMAGE
(Reversible)   (Irreversible)

are prescribed for patients in remission. No flares of joint inflammation after bicycle ergometry were noted in a study of RA patients with treated RA.[119] These patients were extremely unfit and their aerobic status was greatly improved by such exercise. A stationary bicycle is an excellent exercise modality for patients without knee joint inflammation. It provides aerobic conditioning with little stress on the upper extremities or feet.

Many studies have shown that disease associated with high levels of IgM rheumatoid factor is more aggressive with regard to both joint destruction and extra-articular features such as rheumatoid nodules, vasculitis, and visceral manifestations.[117,120–122] HLA-DR4 was present in 92% of RA patients with severe joint destruction, vasculitis, or Felty's syndrome.[123] IgE rheumatoid factor was correlated with vasculitis in still another series of Japanese patients with RA.[124] IgA rheumatoid factor was found in all but one case of rheumatoid vasculitis in a group of patients studied in the Netherlands[125]; all patients with circulating IgA rheumatoid factor had active disease associated with IgM rheumatoid factor positivity. The possible prognostic significance of IgA rheumatoid factor has been mentioned already.

Seropositive progressive RA has long been thought to be associated with a reduced life expectancy, although this is masked in population studies, which include many mild cases.[126] In clinic populations, which represent a subset of more severe disease, increased mortality is clearly evident.[127–133]

In a group of 100 patients with definite or classic RA followed for up to 15 years, RA itself was implicated as the direct cause of death in 9 and as a contributor to death in 7 additional patients. Men died disproportionally, and the cause of death from RA was vasculitis, infection, and amyloidosis. Ischemic heart disease was the main cause of death in the subset of patients (11 of 27) whose death was not related directly to RA. Those who died and those who survived were younger, both at age of onset and at age of death, than the whole group.[128] Another group of 311 patients with definite or classic RA was followed for 11 years: 203 of these patients had been treated with large doses of azathioprine for a mean of 2.5 years and 52 patients had also received alkylating agents.[127] Death occurred in 46 patients; ischemic heart disease and neoplasia headed the list of causes. Again, the death rate was higher than expected (40 vs. 28) in the group aged 45 to 64 years. Death from the usual causes occurred earlier than usual. Neoplasia was not more common in patients who had received azathioprine. In this context, however, the occurrence of malignant disease in patients with RA treated with cyclophosphamide was 4 times that of a matched group of RA patients,[134] and lymphoreticular malignant disease was increased by a factor of 15. Hematologic, bladder, and skin neoplasia was increased in a case-control study of 119 RA patients treated with cyclophosphamide.[134a] This risk persists for at least 13 years after treatment.

Mortality occurred 7 years sooner than predicted in men and 3 years sooner in women in a Dutch series.[129] A retrospective study of the experience at Vanderbilt University showed that severe dysfunction in RA patients was associated with *less than a 50% 5-year survival!*[130] Mortality was associated not only with poor performance of tests of joint function but also with low socioeconomic status, with the presence of extra-articular disease, and, as expected, with rheumatoid factor positivity.[131] Another American study showed a 50% increased mortality in RA patients.[133] In contrast with European studies, men with RA died 4 years sooner than did their counterparts in the general population, while women with RA died 10 years sooner. An excellent review of studies of survival in RA has appeared.[135]

Interestingly, the only study that examined the age of death of the *parents* of patients with RA showed that they too died prematurely. These parents died 4 years earlier than expected.[136] The rate of spontaneous abortion in RA patients was increased by 50%.[137] This outcome happened even before the clinical onset of RA. This increased fetal wastage is probably related to anticardiolipin antibodies. Such antibodies were found in 33% of patients with RA, compared with 38% of patients with SLE and 12% of control subjects.[138] Interestingly, anticardiolipin antibodies in the RA patients correlated with positive antinuclear an-

tibody tests and with repeated spontaneous abortions, but not with thrombotic events (see Chapter 70).

The question of whether patients with RA are at increased risk for neoplastic disease has attracted much attention, especially since it represents a baseline against which the chronic use of immunosuppressive drug therapy must be viewed. An entire symposium has appeared on this subject.[139] Apart from a modest increase in lymphoproliferative disease, including multiple myeloma, however, no increase in neoplasms stands out. Because a generalized increase in lymphocytes and plasma cell number occurs in RA, this finding is perhaps not surprising. Data derived from the entire population of Finland is perhaps the most convincing evidence of this,[139,140] but other studies have reached similar conclusions.[141] A study of 20 cases of lymphoproliferative diseases in RA patients has appeared.[142] There is little doubt that azathioprine use is associated with increased lymphomatous disease in renal transplantation patients. Although there is no statistical evidence for this in RA, isolated case reports of non-Hodgkin's lymphoma, especially of the central nervous system, have been documented in RA patients receiving azathioprine. The use of alkylating agents in RA definitely predisposes to acute leukemia and other reticuloendothelial tumors and perhaps to an increased incidence of solid tumors as well.[134] And cyclophosphamide use carries an increased risk of bladder tumor. Anecdotally, I have been impressed that the solid tumors that do occur in patients receiving alkylating agents are extremely aggressive. This might be anticipated if normal immune surveillance mechanisms are suppressed. I know of no systematic controlled study of this apparent clinical impression, however.

Rheumatoid vasculitis is most commonly noted clinically as nailfold thrombi (Fig. 43–23) and, as mentioned already, as rheumatoid nodules. Fully expressed rheumatoid vasculitis with peripheral motor and sensory neuropathy, leg ulcers, scleritis, digital gangrene, and visceral organ involvement often leads to death (see Chapters 44 and 74). Fortunately, this syndrome, fairly common between 1950 and 1965, has once again become relatively rare as corticosteroid therapy has fallen into disfavor. Asymptomatic small vessel disease may exist in most patients with RA seen in rheumatic disease centers. Vasculitis in clinically normal skin is often found both histologically and by immunofluorescence microscopy.[143-145] These lesions have been correlated with the presence of circulating immune complexes[143] and with decreased blood flow to the fingers.[146]

In summary, published data regarding the prog-

FIG. 43–23. Nailfold thrombi in a patient with rheumatoid arthritis. These or splinter hemorrhages do not always herald severe life-threatening vasculitis, but are clearly more common in patients with systemic signs and symptoms. These thrombi represent areas of infarction due to intimal proliferation in small vessels.

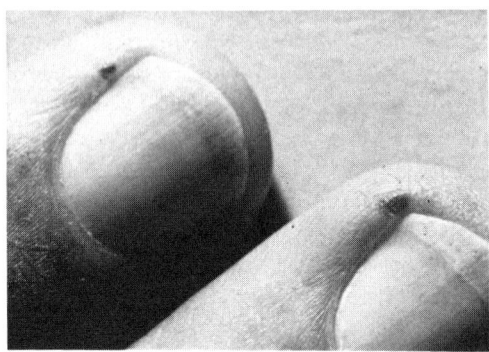

nosis in most patients with sustained seropositive active RA are depressingly pessimistic and inconsistent with my personal experience with the disease over nearly three decades. The data suggest to me that patients with severe disease should receive more aggressive therapy earlier in the course of their disease. Obviously, more specific, safer drugs are badly needed, but the monitored use of currently available slow-acting agents used singly, or if necessary, in combination, will control the inflammatory process in the great majority of patients with RA.

ASSOCIATED DISEASES

Other Arthritides. Patients with fever, leukocytosis, polyarthritis, and rash are now recognized as having adult Still's disease, an entity distinct from adult RA.[13,147,148] Some patients with RA also have features of SLE, either concurrently or sequentially.[149,150] I studied one patient with lupus and central nervous system involvement who later developed erosive seropositive RA with rheumatoid nodules. Raynaud's phenomenon, severe hypertension, and death from uremia then occurred. The classic lesions of scleroderma kidney were found at autopsy.[151]

The rarity of coexistent gout and RA still prompts isolated case reports.[152–154] The reasons for this negative association remain obscure, although one study showed that rheumatoid factor bound to urate crystals, inhibiting their interaction with neutrophils.[154]

Radiologic "chondrocalcinosis" of the knees and intrasynovial calcium pyrophosphate dihydrate (CPPD) crystals were less common in RA patients than in control subjects and when the two conditions did coincide the radiographic features of RA were atypical.[155,156] There are many problems with these studies, both in their design and interpretation.[157] I believe that the "pseudorheumatoid" form of CPPD crystal deposition was in fact diagnosed as RA, which accounts for the atypical radiographic features, that is, asymmetric disease, retained bone density, prominent osteophytosis, well-corticated bone cysts, and a paucity of progressive erosive disease.[157] I have found a 1% incidence of RA in my personal series of nearly 600 cases of CPPD crystal deposition, which is about that of the general population and about what would be expected by chance coincidence. The radiographic appearance of the affected joints in all 6 cases was quite typical of RA (see Chapter 107).

It is sometimes very difficult to distinguish RA of rapid onset from polymyalgia rheumatica, as discussed already. The diagnostic test of time usually allows differentiation. However, a few patients have persistent features of both conditions.

Septic arthritis occurs more frequently in joints already damaged by RA as well as in joints replaced by prostheses. Polyarticular septic arthritis in RA carries an extremely poor prognosis (mortality over 50%).[158]

Bone Loss. Osteopenia is frequent in RA but its mechanism remains controversial. Bone loss in early RA was found to be juxta-articular, and lumbar spine bone mass was normal by densitometry.[159] Serial study showed that generalized bone loss correlated with disease duration and loss of function.[160,161] However, serum 1,25-dihydroxyvitamin D_3 levels were twice those of control subjects even in early RA, and calcium absorption was decreased.[162] Stress fractures in RA are often associated with corticosteroid therapy.[163,164] Trabecular thinning was found in iliac crest bone biopsies from 48 patients with RA who had never received steroids.[165] It is likely that the etiology of the osteopenia of RA is multifactorial. Perhaps the effects of disease-associated metabolic factors are aggravated by disuse and corticosteroid treatment.

Liver Disease. Nodular regenerative hyperplasia of the liver may accompany systemic connective tissue diseases, including RA.[166] These patients often have overt vasculitis, which has been proposed as important in pathogenesis,[166] and the abnormal tests of liver function improve with remission induced by drugs or pregnancy. This situation may be difficult to distinguish from chronic active hepatitis with arthritis. One such patient even developed rheumatoid nodules.[167] A liver biopsy may be needed to clarify the problem.

The extra-articular manifestations of RA are discussed in Chapter 44.

REFERENCES

1. Garrod, A.B.: A Treatise on Gout and Rheumatic Gout (Rheumatoid Arthritis). 3rd. Ed. London, Longman, Green, 1876.
2. Parish, L.C.: An historical approach to the nomenclature of rheumatoid arthritis. Arthritis Rheum., 6:138–158, 1963.
3. Lindblad, S., and Hedfors, E.: Arthroscopic and immunologic characterization of knee joint synovitis in osteoarthritis. Arthritis Rheum., 30:1081–1088, 1987.
4. Ropes, M.W., et al.: 1958 revision of diagnostic criteria for rheumatoid arthritis. Bull. Rheum. Dis., 9:175–176, 1958.
5. Ginsberg, M.H., et al.: Rheumatoid nodulosis. Arthritis Rheum., 18:49–58, 1975.
6. Brower, A.C., et al.: Rheumatoid nodulosis: Another cause of juxta-articular nodules. Radiology, 125:669–670, 1977.
7. Morales-Piga, A., et al.: Rheumatoid nodulosis: Report of a case with evidence of intraosseous rheumatoid granuloma. Arthritis Rheum., 29:1278–1283, 1986.
8. Strader, K.W., and Agudelo, C.A.: Coexistence of rheumatoid nodulosis and gout. J. Rheumatol., 13:818–820, 1986.
9. McCarty, D.J.: Unpublished observations, December, 1987.
10. Schumacher, H.R.: Palindromic onset of rheumatoid arthritis. Clinical, synovial fluid and biopsy studies. Arthritis Rheum., 25:361–369, 1982.
11. Molnar, Z., Metzger, A.L., and McCarty, D.J.: Tubular structures in endothelium in palindromic rheumatism. Arthritis Rheum., 15:5523–5526, 1972.
12. Gran, J.T., Husby, G., and Thorsby, E.: HLA antigens in palindromic rheumatism, non-erosive rheumatoid arthritis and classical rheumatoid arthritis. J. Rheumatol., 11:136–140, 1984.
13. Aptekar, R.G., et al.: Adult onset of juvenile rheumatoid arthritis. Arthritis Rheum., 16:715–718, 1973.
14. McCarty, D.J.: Unpublished observations.
15. McCarty, D.J., O'Duffy, J.D., Pearson, L., and Hunter, J.B.: Remitting seronegative symmetrical synovitis with pitting edema. (RS₃PE) syndrome. JAMA, 254:2763–2767, 1985.
16. Olive, A., et al.: Evolution of benign rheumatoid nodules into rheumatoid arthritis after 50 years. Ann. Rheum. Dis., 46:624–625, 1987.
17. Rush, P.J., Bernstein, B.H., Smith, C.R., and Shore, A.: Chronic arthritis following benign rheumatoid nodules of childhood. Arthritis Rheum., 28:1175–1178, 1985.
18. Astorga, G.P., and Williams, R.C.: Altered reactivity in mixed lymphocytic culture from patients with rheumatoid arthritis. Arthritis Rheum., 12:547–554, 1969.
19. Stastny, P.: Mixed lymphocyte cultures in rheumatoid arthritis. J. Clin. Invest., 57:1148–1157, 1976.
20. Stastny, P.: Mixed lymphocyte culture typing cells from patients with rheumatoid arthritis. Tissue Antigens, 4:571–579, 1974.
21. Grennan, D.M., et al.: Family studies in rheumatoid arthritis—The importance of DR4 and of genes for autoimmune thyroid disease. J. Rheumatol., 10:584–589, 1983.
22. Walton, K., et al.: Clinical features, autoantibodies and HLA-DR antigens in rheumatoid arthritis. J. Rheumatol., 12:223–226, 1985.
23. Aho, K., Kosekenvuo, M., Tuominen, J., and Kaprio, J.: Occurrence of rheumatoid arthritis in a nationwide series of twins. J. Rheumatol., 13:899–906, 1986.
24. Population Studies in Rheumatoid Arthritis. Edited by Lawrence, J.C. and Kellren, J.H. New York Arthritis Foundation and National Institute of Arthritis and Metabolic Disease. Washington, D.C., United States Public Health Service, 1958, p. 13.
25. Beasley, R.P., Willkins, R.E., and Bennett, P.H.: High prevalence of rheumatoid arthritis in Yakima Indians. Arthritis Rheum., 16:743–748, 1973.
26. Vandenbrocke, J.P., et al.: Oral contraceptives and rheumatoid arthritis: Further evidence for a preventive effect. Lancet, 2:839–842, 1982.
27. Hollander, J.L., et al.: The controlled-climate chamber for the study of the effects of meteorological changes in human diseases. Trans. NY Acad. Sci., 24:167–172, 1961.
28. Sibley, J.T.: Weather and arthritis symptoms. J. Rheumatol., 12:707–710, 1985.
29. Patberg, W.R., Nienhuis, R.L.F., and Veringa, F.: Relation between meteorological factors and pain in rheumatoid arthritis in a marine climate. J. Rheumatol., 12:711–715, 1985.
30. McCarty, D.J.: Unpublished observations, January, 1985.
31. Ferraccioli, G.F., et al.: Clinical features, scintiscan characteristics and x-ray progression of late onset rheumatoid arthritis. Clin. Exp. Rheumatol., 2:157–161, 1984.
32. Deal, C.L., et al.: The clinical features of elderly-onset of rheumatoid arthritis. Arthritis Rheum., 28:987–994, 1985.
33. Terkeltaub, R., Decary, F., and Esdaile, J.: An immunogenetic study of older age onset rheumatoid arthritis. J. Rheumatol., 11:147–149, 1984.
34. Russell, E.B., et al.: Symmetrical synovitis of wrists (in preparation).
35. Klimiuk, P.S., et al.: Autoimmunity to native type II collagen—A distinct genetic subset of rheumatoid arthritis. J. Rheumatol., 12:865–870, 1985.
36. Bywaters, E.G.L.: Symmetrical joint involvement. Ann. Rheum. Dis., 34:376, 1975.
37. Short, C.L., Bauer, W., and Reynolds, W.E.: Rheumatoid Arthritis. Cambridge, Harvard Univerity Press, 1957.
38. Fleming, A., Crown, J.M., and Corbett, M.: Early rheumatoid disease. I. Onset. Ann. Rheum. Dis., 35:357–360, 1976.
39. Fleming, A., et al.: Early rheumatoid disease. II. Patterns of joint involvement. Ann. Rheum. Dis., 35:361–364, 1976.
40. Luukkainen, R., Isoinaki, H., and Kajander, A.: Prognostic value of the type of onset of rheumatoid arthritis. Ann. Rheum. Dis., 42:274–275, 1983.
41. Terkeltaub, R., et al.: A clinical study of older age rheumatoid arthritis with comparison to a younger onset group. J. Rheumatol., 10:418–424, 1983.
42. Linos, A.D., et al.: The effect of tonsillectomy and appendectomy on the development of rheumatoid arthritis. J. Rheumatol., 13:707–709, 1986.
43. Pincus, T., et al.: Elevated MMPI scores for hypochondriasis, depression and hysteria in patients with rheumatoid arthritis reflect disease rather than psychological status. Arthritis Rheum., 29:1456–1466, 1986.
44. Bishop, D., Green, A., Cantor, S., and Torresin, W.: Depression, anxiety and rheumatoid arthritis activity. Clin. Exp. Rheumatol., 5:147–150, 1987.
45. Affleck, G., Pfeiffer, C., Tennen, H., and Fifield, J.: Attributional processes in rheumatoid arthritis patients. Brief report. Arthritis Rheum., 30:927–931, 1987.
46. Kowanko, I.L., et al.: Domiciliary self-measurement in rheumatoid arthritis and the demonstration of circadian rhythmicity. Ann. Rheum. Dis., 41:453–454, 1982.
47. McCarty, D.J., and Gatter, R.A.: A study of distal interphalangeal joint tenderness in rheumatoid arthritis. Arthritis Rheum., 9:325–336, 1966.
48. Halla, J.T., Fallahi, S., and Hardin, J.G.: Small joint involvement: A systematic roentgenographic study in rheumatoid arthritis. Ann. Rheum. Dis., 45:327–330, 1986.

49. Jacob, J., et al.: Distal interphalangeal joint involvement in rheumatoid arthritis. Arthritis Rheum., 29:10–15, 1986.

50. McCarty, D.J.: Treatment of rheumatoid joint inflammation with triamcinolone hexacetonide. Arthritis Rheum., 15:157–173, 1972.

51. Tarrik, H.: Spontaneous rupture of tendons in rheumatoid arthritis. NZ Med. J., 79:651–653, 1976.

52. Givy, R.G., and Gottlieb, N.L.: Hand flexor tenosynovitis in rheumatoid arthritis. Arthritis Rheum., 20:1003–1008, 1977.

53. Ehrlich, G.E., et al.: Pathogenesis of rupture of extensor tendons at the wrist in rheumatoid arthritis. Arthritis Rheum., 2:332–346, 1959.

54. Ranawat, C.S., and Straub, L.R.: Volar tenosynovitis of wrist in rheumatoid arthritis. Arthritis Rheum., 13:112–117, 1970.

55. Resnick, D.: Rheumatoid arthritis of wrist: Why the ulnar styloid? Radiology, 112:29, 1974.

56. Dorwart, B.B., and Schumacher, H.R.: Hand deformities resembling rheumatoid arthritis. Semin. Arthritis Rheum., 4:53–71, 1974.

57. McCarty, D.J.: Unpublished observations.

58. Bywaters, E.G.L.: Jaccoud's syndrome: Today's view. Clin. Rheumatol. Pract., 4:148–152, 1986.

59. Kahn, M.F.: Jaccoud's syndrome in a Rheumatology unit. Clin. Rheumatol. Pract., 4:153–155, 1986.

60. Villiaumey, J., et al.: Diagnostic criteria and new etiologic events in the arthropathy of Jaccoud: A report of ten cases. Clin. Rheumatol. Pract., 4:156–175, 1986.

61. Moberg, E., Edeland, H.G., and Wikland, L.B.: Prognostic evaluation of finger joint bony lesions in rheumatoid arthritis. Scand. J. Rheumatol., 2:139–141, 1973.

62. Minaker, K., and Little, H.: Painful feet in rheumatoid arthritis. Can. Med. Assoc. J., 109:724–730, 1973.

63. Vidigal, E., et al.: The foot in chronic rheumatoid arthritis. Ann. Rheum. Dis., 34:292–297, 1975.

64. Weston, W.J.: The intra-synovial fatty masses in chronic rheumatoid arthritis. Br. J. Rheumatol., 46:213–219, 1973.

65. Isdale, I.C., and Corrigan, A.: Backward luxation of the atlas. Ann. Rheum. Dis., 29:6–9, 1970.

66. Martel, W.: Pathogenesis of cervical discovertebral destruction in rheumatoid arthritis. Arthritis Rheum., 20:1217–1225, 1977.

67. Mathews, J.A.: Atlanto-axial subluxation in rheumatoid arthritis. Ann. Rheum. Dis., 28:260–266, 1969.

68. Weissman, B.N., et al.: Prognostic features of atlanto-axial subluxation in rheumatoid arthritis. Radiology, 144:745–751, 1982.

69. Konttinen, Y.T., Bergroth, V., Santavirta, S., and Sandelin, J.: Inflammatory involvement of cervical spine ligaments in patients with rheumatoid arthritis and atlantoaxial subluxation. J. Rheumatol., 14:531–534, 1987.

70. Meijers, K.S.E., et al.: Cervical myelopathy in rheumatoid arthritis. Clin. Exp. Rheumatol., 2:239–245, 1984.

71. Breedveld, F.C., Algra, P.R., Vielvoye, J.C., and Cats, A.: Magnetic resonance imaging in the evaluation of patients with rheumatoid arthritis and subluxations of the cervical spine. Arthritis Rheum., 30:624–629, 1987.

72. Crockard, H.A., et al.: Surgical treatment of cervical cord compression in rheumatoid arthritis. Ann. Rheum. Dis., 44:809–816, 1985.

73. Holt, M.E., and Rooney, P.J.: Manubrio-sternal joint subluxation in rheumatoid arthritis. J. Rheumatol., 7:260–261, 1980.

74. Kelly, M.C., Hopkinson, N.D., and Zaphiropoulos, G.C.: Manubriosternal joint dislocation in rheumatoid arthritis: The role of thoracic kyphosis. Ann. Rheum. Dis., 45:345–348, 1986.

75. Geterud, A., et al.: Severe airway obstruction caused by laryngeal rheumatoid arthritis. J. Rheumatol., 13:948–951, 1986.

76. McCarty, D.J.: Unpublished observations.

77. Dorfman, H.D., Norman, A., and Smith, R.J.: Bone erosion in relation to subcutaneous rheumatoid nodules. Arthritis Rheum., 13:69–73, 1970.

78. Pearson, M.E., et al.: Rheumatoid nodules of the spine: Case report and review of the literature. Arthritis Rheum., 30:709–713, 1987.

79. Shapiro, J., and Laskin, R.S.: Giant bone cysts in rheumatoid arthritis. Orthop. Rev., 13:416–149, 1984.

80. Rodnan, G.P., Mathieson, G., and Chittal, S.: Clinical Pathology Conference—Rheumatoid lesions involving brain and meninges. J. Rheumatol., 11:855–861, 1984.

81. Jackson, C.G., Chess, R.L., and Ward, J.R.: A case of rheumatoid nodule formation within the central nervous system and review of the literature. J. Rheumatol., 11:237–240, 1984.

82. Shapiro, R.F., et al.: Fistulization of rheumatoid joints. Ann. Rheum. Dis., 34:489–498, 1974.

83. Martin, L.F.W., and Bensen, W.G.: An unusual synovial cyst in rheumatoid arthritis. J. Rheumatol., 14:139–141, 1987.

84. Thevenon, A., Hardouin, P., and Duquesnoy, B.: Popliteal cyst presenting as an anterior tibial mass. Arthritis Rheum., 28:477–478, 1985.

85. Gerber, N.J., Dixon, A.St.J.: Synovial cysts and juxta-articular bone cysts. Semin. Arthritis Rheum., 3:323–348, 1974.

86. Samuelson, C., Ward, J.R., Albo, D.: Rheumatoid synovial cyst of the hip. Arthritis Rheum., 14:105–108, 1971.

87. Tebib, J.G., et al.: Synovial cyst of the hip causing iliac vein and femoral nerve compression. Clin. Exp. Rheumatol., 5:92–93. 1987.

88. Atkinson, M.T.: Rheumatoid synovial cyst of the hip: An unusual cause of leg swelling. J. Rheumatol., 13:986–987, 1986.

89. Bienenstock, H.: Rheumatoid plantar synovial cysts. Ann. Rheum. Dis., 34:98–99, 1971.

90. Jacob, J.R., et al.: Reversible cause of back pain and sciatica in rheumatoid arthritis: an apophyseal joint cyst. Arthritis Rheum., 29:431–435, 1986.

91. Petrie, J.P., and Wigley, R.D.: Proximal dissection of the olecranon bursa in rheumatoid arthritis. Rheumatol. Int., 4:139–140, 1984.

92. Bassett, L.W., Gold, R.H., and Mirra, J.M.: Rheumatoid bursitis extending into the clavicle and to the skin surface. Ann. Rheum. Dis., 44:336–340, 1985.

93. Lowthian, P.J., and Calin, A.: Geode development and multiple fractures in rheumatoid arthritis. Case report. Ann. Rheum. Dis., 44:130–133, 1985.

94. Genovese, G.R., Jayson, M.I.V., and Dixon, A.St.J.: 31:179–182, 1972.

95. Schmidt, M.F., Workman, J.B., and Barth, W.F.: Dissection or rupture of a popliteal cyst. Arch. Intern. Med., 134:694–698, 1974.

96. Ehrlich, G.E., and Guttmann, G.G.: Valvular mechanism in antecubital cysts of rheumatoid arthritis. Arthritis Rheum., 16:259–264, 1973.

97. Nakano, K.K.: Entrapment neuropathy from Baker's cysts. JAMA, 239:135, 1978.

98. Reginato, A.J., Martinez, V., and Schumacher, H.R.: Giant cell tumor associated with rheumatoid arthritis. Ann. Rheum. Dis., 33:333–341, 1974.

99. Brown, F.E., Morgan, G.J., Taylor, T., and O'Connor, G.T.: Coexistence of muscle anomalies and rheumatoid arthritis in patients with carpal tunnel syndrome. Clin. Exp. Rheumatol., 2:297–302, 1984.

100. Chang, L.W., et al.: Entrapment neuropathy of the posterior interosseous nerve. Arthritis Rheum., *15*:350–352, 1972.

101. Ishikawa, H., and Hirohata, K.: Bilateral peroneal nerve palsy secondary to posterior dislocation of the proximal tibiofibular joint in rheumatoid arthritis. Rheumatol. Int., *4*:45–47, 1984.

102. Sibbitt, W.J., and Williams, R.C.: Cutaneous manifestations of rheumatoid arthritis. Int. J. Dermatol., *21*:563–572, 1982.

103. Holt, P.J.L., et al.: Pyoderma gangrenosum: Clinical laboratory findings in 15 patients with special reference to polyarthritis. Medicine, *59*:114, 1980.

104. Thurtle, O.A., and Cawley, M.D.: The frequency of ulceration in rheumatoid arthritis. A survey. J. Rheumatol., *10*:507–509, 1983.

105. Lauzon, C., Carette, S., and Mathon, G.: Multiple tendon rupture at unusual sites in rheumatoid arthritis. J. Rheumatol., *14*:369–371, 1987.

106. Genant, H.K.: Radiology of the rheumatic diseases. *In* Arthritis and Allied Conditions. 10th Ed. Edited by D.J. McCarty. Philadelphia, Lea & Febiger, 1985, pp. 88–100.

107. Arnason, J.A., et al.: Relation between bone erosions and rheumatoid factor isotypes. Ann. Rheum. Dis., *46*:380–384, 1987.

108. Withrington, R.H., Teitsson, I., Valdimarsson, H., and Seifert, M.H.: Prospective study of early rheumatoid arthritis. II. Association of rheumatoid factor isotypes with fluctuations in disease activity. Ann. Rheum. Dis., *43*:679–685, 1984.

109. Horslev-Petersen, K., Bentsen, K.D., Junker, P., and Lorenzen, I.: Serum amino-terminal type III procollagen peptide in rheumatoid arthritis: Relationship to disease activity, treatment and development of joint erosions. Arthritis Rheum., *29*:592–599, 1986.

110. Burns, T.M., and Calin, A.: The hand radiograph as a diagnostic discriminant between seropositive and seronegative "rheumatoid arthritis": A controlled study. Ann. Rheum. Dis., *42*:605–612, 1983.

111. Pinals, R.S., et al.: Preliminary criteria for clinical remission in rheumatoid arthritis. Bull. Rheum. Dis., *32*:7–10, 1982.

112. Wolfe, F., and Hawley, D.J.: Remission in rheumatoid arthritis. J. Rheumatol., *12*:245–252, 1985.

113. McCarty, D.J.: Unpublished observations, December, 1987.

114. Yelin, E., Henke, C., and Epstein, W.: The work dynamics of the person with rheumatoid arthritis. Arthritis Rheum., *30*:507–512, 1987.

115. Stone, C.E.: The lifetime economic costs of rheumatoid arthritis. J. Rheumatol., *11*:819–827, 1984.

116. Sherrer, Y.S., et al.: The development of disability in rheumatoid arthritis. Arthritis Rheum., *29*:494–500, 1986.

117. Ragan, C., and Farrington, E.: The clinical features of rheumatoid arthritis. JAMA, *181*:663–667, 1967.

118. McCarty, D.J.: Unpublished observations, December, 1987.

119. Beals, O.A., et al.: Measurement of exercise tolerance in patients with rheumatoid arthritis and osteoarthritis. J. Rheumatol., *12*:458–461, 1985.

120. Epstein, W.V., and Engelman, E.P.: The relation of the rheumatoid factor content of serum to clinical neurovascular manifestations of rheumatoid arthritis. Arthritis Rheum., *2*:250–258, 1959.

121. Mongan, E.S., Cass, R.M., and Jacox, R.F.: A study of the relation of seronegative and seropositive rheumatoid arthritis to each other and necrotizing vasculitis. Am. J. Med., *47*:23–36, 1969.

122. Duthrie, J.J.R., et al.: Course and prognosis in rheumatoid arthritis. Ann. Rheum. Dis., *16*:414–424, 1958.

123. Westedt, M.L., et al.: Immunogenetic heterogeneity of rheumatoid arthritis. Ann. Rheum. Dis., *45*:534–538, 1986.

124. Mizushima, Y., Shoji, Y., Hoshi, K., and Kiyokawa, S.: Detection and clinical significance of IgE rheumatoid factor. J. Rheumatol., *11*:22–26, 1984.

125. Westedt, M.L., et al.: IgA containing immune complexes in rheumatoid vasculitis and in active rheumatoid disease. J. Rheumatol., *12*:449–455, 1985.

126. Abruzzo, J.L.: Rheumatoid arthritis and mortality. Arthritis Rheum., *25*:1020–1023, 1982.

127. Lewis, P., et al.: Cause of death in patients with rheumatoid arthritis with particular reference to azathioprine. Ann. Rheum. Dis., *39*:457–461, 1980.

128. Rasker, J.J., and Cosh, J.A.: Cause and age of death in a prospective study of 100 patients with rheumatoid arthritis. Ann. Rheum. Dis., *40*:115–120, 1981.

129. Vandenbroucke, J.P., Hazevoet, H.M., and Cats, A.: Survival and cause of death in rheumatoid arthritis: A 25 year prospective follow-up. J. Rheumatol., *11*:158–161, 1984.

130. Pincus, T., Callahan, L.F., and Vaughn, W.K.: Questionnaire, walking time and button test measures of functional capacity as predictive markers for mortality in rheumatoid arthritis. J. Rheumatol., *14*:240–251, 1987.

131. Pincus, T., and Callahan, L.F.: Taking mortality in rheumatoid arthritis seriously—Predictive markers, socioeconomic status and co-morbidity. J. Rheumatol., *13*:841–845, 1986.

132. Cosh, J.A.: Survival and death in rheumatoid arthritis. J. Rheumatol., *11*:117–118, 1984.

133. Mitchell, D.M., et al.: Survival, prognosis and causes of death in rheumatoid arthritis. Arthritis Rheum., *29*:706–714, 1986.

134. Baltus, J.A.M., et al.: The occurrence of malignancies in patients with rheumatoid arthritis treated with cyclophosphamide. Ann. Rheum. Dis., *42*:368–373, 1983.

134a.Baker, G.L.: Malignancy following treatment of rheumatoid arthritis with cyclophosphamide. Long term case-control follow-up study. Am. J. Med., *83*:1–9, 1987.

135. Pinals, R.S.: Survival in rheumatoid arthritis. Arthritis Rheum., *30*:473–475, 1987.

136. Kaplan, D.: The age of death of the parents of patients with rheumatoid arthritis: A preliminary study. J. Rheumatol., *13*:903–906, 1986.

137. Kaplan, D.: Fetal wastage in patients with rheumatoid arthritis. J. Rheumatol., *13*:875–877, 1986.

138. Fort, J.G., Cowchock, S., Abruzzo, J.L., and Smith, J.B.: Anticardiolipin antibodies in patients with rheumatic diseases. Arthritis Rheum., *30*:752–760, 1987.

139. McDuffie, F.C. (ed): Neoplasms in rheumatoid arthritis: Update on clinical and epidemiologic data. Am. J. Med., *78*(Suppl.):1–83, 1985.

140. Laakso, M., Mutru, O., Isomaki, H., and Koota, K.: Cancer mortality in patients with rheumatoid arthritis. J. Rheumatol., *13*:522–526, 1986.

141. Prior, P., et al.: Cancer morbidity in rheumatoid arthritis. Ann. Rheum. Dis., *43*:128–131, 1984.

142. Symmons, D.P.M., et al.: Lymphoproliferative malignancy in rheumatoid arthritis: A study of 20 cases. Ann. Rheum. Dis., *43*:132–135, 1984.

143. Kozin, F., et al.: Immunoglobulin (IgG) and complement (C′) deposits in blood vessels in patients with rheumatoid arthritis. Clinical correlations. Clin. Res., *26*:503A, 1978.

144. Westedt, M.L., et al.: Rheumatoid arthritis—the clinical significance of histo- and immuno-pathological abnormalities in normal skin. J. Rheumatol., *11*:448–453, 1984.

145. McGill, P.E., Brougham, P.A., and Tulloch, J.: Immune de-

posits in the skin of patients with rheumatoid arthritis. J. Rheumatol., *11*:454–456, 1984.

146. Fischer, M., Mielke, H., Glaefke, S., and Deicher, H.: Generalized vasculopathy and finger blood flow abnormalities in rheumatoid arthritis. J. Rheumatol., *11*:33–37, 1984.

147. Fabricant, M.S., Chandor, S.B., and Friou, G.J.: Still's disease in adults. JAMA, *225*:273–276, 1973.

148. Elkon, K.B., et al.: Adult onset Still's disease: Twenty year follow-up and further study of patients with active disease. Arthritis Rheum., *25*:647–654, 1982.

149. Fischman, A.S., et al.: The co-existence of rheumatoid arthritis and systemic lupus erythematosus: A case report and review of the literature. J. Rheumatol., *8*:405–415, 1981.

150. Cohen, M.G., and Webb, J.: Concurrence of rheumatoid arthritis and systemic lupus erythematosus: Report of 11 cases. Ann. Rheum. Dis., *46*:853–858, 1987.

151. McCarty, D.J.: Unpublished observations.

152. Atbjian, M., and Fernandez-Madrid, F.: Coexistence of chronic tophaceous gout and rheumatoid arthritis. J. Rheumatol., *8*:989–992, 1981.

153. Rizzoli, A.J., Trujeque, L., and Bankhurst, A.D.: The co-existence of gout and rheumatoid arthritis: Case report and a review of the literature. J. Rheumatol., *7*:316–324, 1980.

154. Gordon, T.P., Ahern, M.J., Reid, C., and Roberts-Thomson, P.J.: Studies on the interaction of rheumatoid factor with monosodium urate crystals and case report of co-existent tophaceous gout and rheumatoid arthritis. Ann. Rheum. Dis., *44*:384–389, 1985.

155. Doherty, M., Dieppe, P., and Watt, I.: Low incidence of calcium pyrophosphate dihydrate crystal deposition in rheumatoid arthritis, with modification of radiographic features in co-existent disease. Arthritis Rheum., *27*:1002–1009, 1984.

156. Brasseur, J.P., Huaux, J.P., Devagelaer, J.P., and De-Deuxchaisnes, C.N.: Articular chondrocalcinois in seroposi-

tive rheumatoid arthritis. Comparison with a control group. J. Rheumatol., *14*:40–41, 1987.

157. McCarty, D.J.: Calcium pyrophosphate dihydrate crystal deposition in rheumatoid arthritis. (Letter to editor.) Arthritis Rheum., *28*:717–718, 1985.

158. Epstein, J.H., Zimmerman, B., and Ho, G.: Polyarticular septic arthritis. J. Rheumatol., *13*:1105–1107, 1986.

159. Sambrook, P.N., et al.: Bone turnover in early rheumatoid arthritis. 2. Longitudinal bone density studies. Ann. Rheum. Dis., *44*:580–584, 1985.

160. Sambrook, P.N., et al.: Determinants of axial bone loss in rheumatoid arthritis. Arthritis Rheum., *30*:721–728, 1987.

161. Als, O.S., Gotfredsen, A., Riis, B.J., and Christiansen, C.: Are disease duration and degree of functional impairment determinants of bone loss in rheumatoid arthritis? Ann. Rheum. Dis., *44*:406–411, 1985.

162. Sambrook, P.N., et al.: Calcium absorption in rheumatoid arthritis. Ann. Rheum. Dis., *44*:585–588, 1985.

163. Lakhanpal, S., McLeod, R.A., and Luthra, H.S.: Insufficiency-type stress fractures in rheumatoid arthritis: Report of an interesting case and review of the literature. Clin. Exp. Rheumatol., *4*:151–154, 1986.

164. Jones, G.: Another look at stress fractures in rheumatoid arthritis. J. Rheumatol., *11*:867–868, 1984.

165. Mellish, R.W.E., et al.: Iliac crest trabecular bone mass and structure in patients with non-steroidal treated rheumatoid arthritis. Ann. Rheum. Dis., *46*:830–836, 1987.

166. Reynolds, W.J., and Wanless, I.R.: Nodular regenerative hyperplasia of the liver in a patient with rheumatoid vasculitis: A morphometric study suggesting a role for hepatic arteritis in the pathogenesis. J. Rheumatol., *11*:838–845, 1984.

167. Fitz, J.G., Petri, M., and Hellmann, D.: Chronic active hepatitis presenting with rheumatoid nodules and arthritis. J. Rheumatol., *14*:595–598, 1987.

44

EXTRA-ARTICULAR
RHEUMATOID ARTHRITIS

PAUL A. BACON

Due to unforeseen circumstances the manuscript for this chapter was delayed, preventing us from placing the material in its proper sequence. Chapter 44 appears immediately after Chapter 119 on page 1967.

The Publisher and Author regret any inconvenience this situation may cause the reader.

45

LABORATORY FINDINGS IN RHEUMATOID ARTHRITIS

JOHN BAUM and MORRIS ZIFF

The laboratory findings in rheumatoid arthritis (RA) are those of a chronic inflammatory disease. No specific laboratory test exists for this condition, yet a constellation of laboratory findings can aid the experienced clinician in arriving at a diagnosis and in managing the disease. The knowledge that some laboratory tests can be abnormal in this disease can often save a patient more detailed study (Table 45–1). This chapter represents a detailed survey of the incidence and frequency of abnormal laboratory tests in RA.

HEMATOLOGIC STUDIES

ERYTHROCYTES

A recalcitrant normochromic or hypochromic normocytic anemia, usually moderate in degree, is common in RA.[1] Among Danish women with active disease, 22.7% had fewer than 10 g/dl hemoglobin; among men, 11.5% had fewer than 11 g/dl. In children, anemia is usually present,[2,3] especially in the systemic or Still's form of disease. In the series of Toumbis and co-workers, 64% of children with JRA had under 10 g/dl hemoglobin.[3]

The anemia of RA is the type seen in chronic inflammation and has been intensively studied in relation to possible contributory factors. The influence of hemolysis has been examined in detail. Early studies, using the Ashby selective agglutination technique,[4–7] indicated a reduction in the survival of erythrocytes transfused from normal donors to patients

with RA. More recent investigations have used chromium-51 to label the patient's own erythrocytes for similar studies. Although Ebaugh and co-workers[8] and Weinstein[9] found evidence of some degree of hemolysis, its magnitude could not account for the development of anemia in the presence of adequate bone marrow compensation. Three studies also using chromium-51 have confirmed these earlier reports and have disclosed only a mild hemolytic tendency of an extracorpuscular type, insufficient to explain the associated anemia.[10–12] In contrast to iron deficiency anemia, in which excretion of porphobilinogen and aminolevulinic acid is increased, porphobilinogen excretion is increased in RA.[13]

The plasma volume in patients with RA is greater than normal.[14–17] The basis for this increase is not well understood. A compensatory increase in plasma volume for a reduced corpuscular volume is probably one factor,[15,18] and another is that a larger percentage of the body weight of patients with RA is due to lean body mass than in control subjects. This phenomenon may lead to spuriously high values for the plasma volume calculated as a percentage of body weight.

Serum iron levels are sometimes decreased.[5,8,12,19–21] Results using intravenously injected tracer doses of iron for hemoglobin synthesis have been normal.[5] Although the total iron-binding capacity is usually higher than normal in simple iron deficiency anemia, it is much lower in RA.[13] Although Roberts and co-workers noted a reduced capacity to absorb iron in patients with active RA and mild anemia,[12] other studies found this function to be normal in most patients.[9]

Table 45–1. Laboratory Findings in Rheumatoid Arthritis

Test	Characteristic Results
Blood Elements	
Erythrocytes	Moderate normochromic or hypochromic, normocytic anemia; low plasma iron; moderately decreased bone marrow iron stores; normal use of plasma iron; slightly decreased survival time; inadequate release of iron from tissue stores; normal transferrin levels; decreased total iron binding capacity; increased plasma volume
Leukocytes	Normal or slightly elevated polymorphonuclear leukocytes; leukocytosis possible in severe disease; leukopenia rare (Felty's syndrome); eosinophilia with severe disease and systemic complications; thrombocytosis during active disease; normal nitroblue tetrazolium test results; reduced chemotaxis; lymphocytes—normal B, T, and null cell distribution; decreased blastogenic transformation
Acute-Phase Reactants and Immuno-globulins	
Erythrocyte Sedimentation Rate (ESR)	Increased
C-Reactive Protein (CRP)	Usually positive
Serum Amyloid Protein (SAP)	Slightly elevated
Serum Proteins	Alpha-2, fibrinogen, and gamma globulins increased; albumin decreased
Immunoglobulins	IgG increased (seropositive patients mostly); IgA and IgM increased; IgD normal or low
Cryoglobulins	Rare
Urinary Gamma Globulin	Increased IgG, IgA, and free light chains
Ceruloplasmin	Elevated
Fibronectin	Normal serum levels
Immune Factors	
LE Factor	Present in 10% of patients
Antinuclear Antibody	Present in 15%; associated with more severe disease and rheumatoid-factor positivity
Rheumatoid Factor	Usually present in adults
Biologic False Positive Serologic Test for Syphilis	Present in 5 to 10% of patients
Complement	Normal or slightly elevated levels; hypocomplementemia rare and associated with vasculitis and severe disease

Bone marrow iron stores are absent or decreased in at least one third of patients,[22,23] but no correlation has been demonstrated between the amount of iron in the bone marrow and the hemoglobin level or erythrocyte count. The refractoriness to oral iron therapy of the anemia in most patients is in accord with this observation because absorption of iron is usually normal.

An impairment of release of iron from the reticuloendothelial tissues has been proposed to explain the low plasma iron level, the most constant characteristic of the anemia of inflammation.[5] In the presence of normal use of transferrin-bound iron, such impairment would account for the low iron concentration in the plasma. This suggestion is based on the observations that (1) amounts of iron that exceed the plasma-binding capacity are deposited in the tissues and are, therefore, poorly used in patients with inflammation;[24] (2) iron injected intravenously into animals with an inflammatory reaction is diverted from normal hemoglobin formation and is deposited in storage sites;[25] and (3) the reuse of iron from senescent cells is reduced in animals with an inflammatory reaction. Insufficient release from the reticuloendothelial system would result in the low plasma iron con-

centration presumably responsible for the impaired capacity of the bone marrow to produce erythrocytes. This subject has been reviewed.[26] Intra-articular hemorrhage increases the iron content of synovial tissue in patients with RA,[27–29] and the retained iron could contribute to the low serum iron level and to the anemia of active RA. Another site of increased iron deposition in RA is striated muscle, in which mean iron levels twice those of normal muscles have been found.[30]

Although single measurements of serum ferritin levels have often failed to correlate with a number of clinical and laboratory parameters of joint activity, a longitudinal study found that serum ferritin levels rose during active synovitis and fell during remission. The highest levels were found in patients with systemic complications.[31] Thus, the clear correlation between serum ferritin and iron stores found in normal persons does not exist in patients with chronic inflammatory conditions such as RA. However, a serum ferritin level below 60 µg/L was a good indicator of iron-responsive anemia.[32]

Most patients with RA receive salicylate therapy. Occult blood in the feces has been observed in many who receive this drug.[33,34] This blood loss, although probably of minor importance, may contribute to iron deficiency, and the anemia in such patients may partially respond to iron therapy. Another factor in the anemia may be erythropoietin deficiency because serum levels in RA patients are lower than in patients with comparable degrees of iron deficiency anemia.[35]

LEUKOCYTES

Although white blood cell counts are usually in the normal range or are only slightly elevated, Short, Bauer, and Reynolds observed that about 25% of their patients had counts above 10,000/mm³.[36] Leukocytosis was noted in patients who had an acute and severe disease onset and acute exacerbations. In another study, the white blood cell was much higher in patients with severe RA.[37] Although counts in the 12,000 to 20,000 range are sometimes observed without other cause,[38] this finding suggests the presence of factors other than RA. Prednisone increases the absolute number of mature granulocytes in the circulation because of an increased inflow of cells from the bone marrow, decreased margination in the capillary blood, and a decreased emigration from the circulation.[2,3,40,41] Leukocytosis is common in juvenile RA.[39] An increased number of low buoyant density (activated) neutrophils in RA has been reported.[42] Monocytopenia, raised basophil counts, and increased numbers of neutrophils of unusually high peroxidase activity have also been described.[43]

Leukopenia is rare in RA.[36] When present, it is more likely to be observed in the chronic state of the disease. The leukopenia and splenomegaly of Felty's syndrome[44] may reflect the uptake of immune complexes by circulating polymorphonuclear cells and the subsequent removal of these cells by the spleen.[45] Neutropenia in RA has been divided into two types, one associated with splenomegaly (Felty's syndrome) and another not associated with splenomegaly but with an increased frequency of circulating immune complexes (68% versus 31%).[46] Another possible cause of the leukopenia is the uptake and destruction of polymorphonuclear leukocytes (PMNs) with attached complement-fixing antineutrophil antibodies.[47]

The differential white blood cell count is usually within normal limits, but PMNs may be increased in more acute cases.[38] Eosinophilia is not uncommon in RA. When patients in a study were selected for severity of disease or elevated rheumatoid factor titers, eosinophilia of more than 5% was found in 40% of these patients. A correlation also appeared to exist with the presence of vasculitis, pleuropericarditis,

pulmonary fibrosis, and subcutaneous nodules.[48,49] Exudative fluids in pleura or pericardium often contain eosinophils. Leukocyte elastase present in plasma as an enzyme-inhibitor complex is significantly elevated in active RA and falls in inactive disease.[50]

Correlations among thrombocytosis and disease activity, anemia, sideropenia, leukocytosis, and rheumatoid factor titer have been noted.[51] Platelets from patients with RA show lower-than-normal levels of connective tissue–activating factor.[52]

The chromosomal complement of the leukocytes of the blood in RA is normal.[53] The nitroblue tetrazolium (NBT) dye reduction test in peripheral blood leukocytes is also normal.[54] Chemotaxis of the PMNs is diminished, possibly because of prior immune complex ingestion.[55] However, recent studies of phagocytosis and migration of granulocytes of RA patients have found these functions to be normal.[56] Oxygen radical production by RA neutrophils was normal.[57] Leukotriene B$_4$ from PMNs of patients with RA was significantly higher than controls. Levels were not related to therapy with nonsteroidal anti-inflammatory drugs and had a low correlation with ESR and CRP.[58]

Lymphocytes

In recent years, many have been interested in the function of the subpopulations of lymphocytes in various diseases. For the most part, the percentages of B, T, and null cells in the blood in RA have been in the normal range.[59–62] One group found no significant difference between the percentage and the absolute number of peripheral blood T suppressor cells in RA and in control subjects.[63] In some patients, the number of OKT8$^+$ (suppressor) cells/mm³ was decreased in relation to OKT4$^+$ (helper) cells, whereas in other patients, an elevated ratio of OKT4$^+$ to OKT8$^+$ cells was due to a higher percentage of OKT4$^+$ cells and a lower percentage of OKT8$^+$ cells.[64] In another study of T-lymphocyte subpopulations in active RA, decreased Tμ (helper) cells, greatly increased T null cells, and slightly increased Fc receptor-bearing lymphocytes were found.[65] Increased levels of transferrin receptor-bearing lymphocytes and T$_4$ cells have also been observed.[66]

The function of the circulating lymphocytes has also been studied. Spontaneous lymphocyte transformation was normal in patients with RA,[67] but a decreased response to concanavalin A was observed.[68–71] In early RA of under 3 months' duration, the defect was due to a decreased generation of suppressor T cells accompanied by a decrease in the B-cell response. In a study of patients with disease activity of more than 12 months' duration, the T-cell response was normal, but the B-cell response continued to be deficient.[72] The response to phytohemagglutinin (PHA) was also depressed,[52,68,69,71,73] although in several reports the decrease was not significant.[70,74] Responsiveness of peripheral blood mononuclear cells to purified strep-tokinase-streptodornase (SK-SD) was not much depressed, nor did hyporesponsiveness predict disease activity or prognosis.[74]

Depression of the PHA response was associated with the presence of antinuclear antibodies in 16 patients, whereas 14 patients who did not have antinuclear antibodies had normal responses.[75] A decreased response to pokeweed mitogen has also been reported,[69] but two other groups did not find the decrease to be statistically significant.[68,71] Suppressor-T-cell hypofunction was found in early active RA of under 3 months' duration, but not in late RA of more than 6 months' duration or in inactive RA.[76] Overall, mitogenic transformation of RA lymphocytes appears to be decreased. Studies of RA lymphocyte responsiveness and production of IL-2 were consistent with a hyperproduction of IL-2 in RA during active disease.[77] Production of IL-2 and response to IL-2 were decreased in rheumatoid synovial fluid and circulating blood lymphocytes.[78] The reason for this is not clear.

One study of antibody-mediated lymphocyte toxicity found these antibodies to be present five times as frequently in RA as in normal controls,[79] but another study found no such difference.[80] Impaired monocyte "natural" killer activity has been reported in patients with active RA, and the impairment correlated with disease activity.[81] However, baseline natural killer (NK) cell activity and interferon-enhanced NK cell activity were the same as control levels.[82]

ACUTE-PHASE REACTANTS

These substances found in blood reflect the presence and degree of inflammation. Although nonspecifically induced, they may aid in the diagnosis of RA in patients with vague symptoms. Because their serum concentration reflects the activity of the disease, they are useful in therapeutic management. A discrepancy often exists, however, between the clinical disease severity and the magnitude of the acute-phase response. For this reason, a change in the level of an acute-phase reactant is often of greater significance in guiding therapy than the actual level itself.

ERYTHROCYTE SEDIMENTATION RATE

The erythrocyte sedimentation rate (ESR) is the single most important laboratory test of inflammatory activity. Although the increased rate of settling of erythrocytes in the blood of patients with inflammatory diseases was known for many years, it was first measured by Fahraeus in 1918. In seeking an early test for pregnancy, Fahraeus noted that the speed of sedimentation was increased not only in pregnancy, but also in many other conditions.[83,84] Measurement of the ESR was first applied to the study of acute and chronic rheumatism by Hermann in 1924.[85]

Nature of the Sedimentation Phenomenon

ESR is related to red cell rouleaux formation and increases in proportion to the size of the erythrocyte aggregates.[86] The size of the aggregates, in turn, depends on the properties of the blood plasma rather than of the cells themselves. Cellular rouleaux formation is enhanced by absorbed, large, asymmetric molecules. The plasma components that influence the ESR most are fibrinogen and α and γ globulin.

Plasma fibrinogen increases as a result of increased synthesis by the liver in the presence of inflammation elsewhere in the body. The elevation is rapid, usually detectable 48 hours after the onset of inflammation. It usually subsides within 10 days of cessation of the inflammatory process.[87]

Early observation that the plasma fibrinogen was increased when the ESR was high led to the assumption that the two were related.[88] Moreover, a linear correlation exists between the ESR and the fibrinogen level when patients with serum globulin levels over 2.5 g/dl are excluded, the coefficient of correlation being 0.90.[89] In patients in whom the serum globulin is over 2.5 g/dl, however, the correlation is only 0.60. Under circumstances in which plasma fibrinogen is low, as in liver disease, close correlation between plasma globulin concentration and the ESR has been observed.

The addition of serum fractions to defibrinated blood has confirmed that the ESR almost entirely depends on the concentration of asymmetric molecules such as fibrinogen and α-2 and γ globulins.[90] The relative effect on the ESR of these proteins, when added in equal concentration, is in the ratio 10:5:2. Detailed studies show that the closest correlation with the ESR is found when the serum concentrations of fibrinogen, α-2 macroglobulin, and IgM are summed.[91]

Another factor influencing the ESR is the sialic acid residue on the erythrocyte membrane. The sialic-acid-bearing glycoproteins contribute to the forces repelling and aggregating the red blood cells. Both red cell membrane and serum sialic acid levels are higher when the ESR is elevated, although the correlation is not quantitative.[92]

Westergren Method

The Westergren method is the most dependable of those currently used.[93] International standards have recently been developed.[94] The Westergren ESR should be performed by the classic dilution technique with citrate, or by the newer, modified technique, using ethylenediamine tetra-acetic acid (EDTA) and saline diluent. Use of undiluted whole blood has less reproducibility.[95] The upper limit of normal rises with age. A study of many normal individuals has shown the following normal limits, in millimeters/hour:[96] below age 50, 15 for men and 25 for women; above age 50, 20 for men and 30 for women. The reason for this increase with age has not been determined.[97] Higher normal levels are found in some populations.[98]

Disease Correlation

Rheumatoid Arthritis. The ESR usually is elevated and parallels the activity of the disease.[37,99] Increased values have been found in 85% of patients with RA of mild severity, and in 95% of those with moderate to severe involvement.[36] Exacerbations are usually accompanied by an increase and remissions by a decrease in the ESR. In complete remission, the values usually become normal. Nevertheless, the continuously elevated values observable in some patients with decreased joint inflammation presumably reflect the continued elevation of the serum acute phase proteins. In such circumstances, frequently repeated measurement of the ESR is unrewarding. Conversely, patients with clinically active RA may have normal sedimentation rates. This phenomenon occurred in 7.3% in one series[38] and in 5% in another.[100] In still another study, a significant correlation existed between the ESR and the plasma protein concentration and serum viscosity.[101] When a number of acute phase reactants were measured serially, the C-reactive protein and haptoglobin were more accurate than the ESR in measuring the activity of RA.[102] Treatment with disease-modifying agents significantly reduced the acute phase response in RA.[103]

Other Diseases. The ESR in primary osteoarthritis is usually normal. Nevertheless, values above 30 mm/hr were noted in 9.6% of patients by Dawson and coworkers.[38] Mild elevation of the Westergren ESR in middle-aged women with osteoarthritis is not uncommon. Thus, if the clinical findings are consistent, the diagnosis of osteoarthritis should not be excluded on the basis of a slight elevation of the ESR.

Polymyalgia rheumatica, a syndrome of pain and stiffness of the muscles of the shoulders and hip girdle appearing in the middle-aged and elderly, may be confused with RA. This disorder is characterized by high levels of the ESR. Because the symptoms usually

improve before the ESR drops, sedimentation values cannot be used as a guide to management. A rapid fall in ESR with low-dose (~10 mg daily) corticosteroid treatment is diagnostically helpful, however.

Measurement of the ESR is useful in distinguishing fibrositis from RA because sedimentation values are normal in fibrositis.[104]

Congestive Heart Failure. Congestive heart failure is believed to lower the ESR, especially in young individuals with rheumatic carditis,[105–107] as a result of a decrease in the synthesis of fibrinogen in the passively congested liver. This widely accepted tenet has been denied on the basis of an extensive analysis of the ESR in patients with rheumatic heart disease and congestive failure.[108] Numerous exceptions are also found in the data of Saghvi,[109] who noted elevation rather than depression of the ESR in patients with heart failure as a result of rheumatic activity, respiratory infection, or myocardial damage usually associated with heart failure. Nevertheless, the available evidence suggests that the effect of hepatic congestion in congestive heart failure is to retard the ESR,[105–107] although the net effect of all factors may lead to elevated values.

Unexplained Elevations. In some individuals, the ESR may be persistently elevated without obvious cause. In a group of 35 patients, 14 were eventually demonstrated to have one of the following: asymptomatic pulmonary tuberculosis, macroglobulinemia of Waldenström, hepatic cirrhosis, multiple myeloma, and systemic lupus erythematosus (SLE).[110,111] The remaining 21 patients, however, continued to have persistently elevated ESR for 3 to 20 years with an otherwise benign course. Nine of these patients also had an increased gamma globulin level. The rest had unexplained elevations of either the β lipoprotein of fibrinogen, or had paraproteins of the myeloma type on serum protein electrophoresis.

Serious illness was found on followup in 20 of 31 patients with unexplained elevation of ESR.[112] Thus, an elevated ESR as an isolated abnormality should lead to careful investigation of the patient, although it may not necessarily be associated with active disease. The ESR is elevated in the majority of patients with malignant disease.[113] In 30 of 51 elderly patients who were thought to have a known cause for a high ESR, a further possible cause was found at autopsy. Cancer was found most often,[114] and extreme ESR elevation in patients with malignant disease has been associated with skeletal metastases.[115] An elevated ESR in RA of 100 mm/hr or more, however, was associated most frequently with infection (35%), and malignant disease was found in only 15%.[116] Marked elevation of the ESR occurs in multiple myeloma because of the high concentration of paraprotein in the blood.[117]

Unexplained elevated levels have also been found in a hospitalized elderly population.[118] The ESR in elderly patients should be viewed with special precaution. In a study of almost 500 people over age 62, the ESR was found to be greater than 20 mm/hr in 20% of men and 24% of women, without apparent cause.[119] However, in the presence of an inflammatory state or monoclonal gammopathy, although the sensitivity of a rise in the ESR was only 0.55, the specificity was 0.96.[120] The ESR may be elevated in women taking oral contraceptives.[121]

C-REACTIVE PROTEIN AND OTHER TESTS

C-reactive protein (CRP) is present in practically all RA patients with clinical evidence of disease,[122] and usually parallels the ESR closely. Treatment of RA with nonsteroidal anti-inflammatory drugs produced no significant change in the ESR or the CRP after 12 weeks of therapy.[12]

Unlike rheumatic fever, salicylate and corticosteroids do not readily depress the CRP or the ESR in patients with RA. Comparison of the ESR and the CRP in 241 patients with RA showed a positive linear correlation between the measurements with a high degree of variability. The CRP was found to be a more sensitive test because gold, penicillamine, and prednisone had a greater effect on the CRP than on the ESR.[124] CRP also correlated better than ESR did with disease activity in ankylosing spondylitis (AS) and Reiter's syndrome.[125] Corticosteroids, even in small doses, suppress the CRP. Nusinow and Arnold reported that the CRP, measured nephelometrically, correlated with erosive disease in 37 patients with RA who never received corticosteroids, not even as joint injections. These researchers believe that CRP levels above 5 mg/dl (normal <0.6 mg/dl) predict erosions, and they regard the test as an indication to begin remittive therapy early in the course of the disease.[126]

Urinary excretion of sialylated low-molecular-weight saccharides increases in inflammatory disease and correlates closely with serum amyloid A protein and CRP levels in RA.[127] The serum amyloid P-component is slightly elevated in seropositive RA. In this case, this component appears to act as an acute-phase reactant.[128] The serum amyloid A protein is highly correlated with the CRP (correlation coefficient 0.85).[129]

Plasma viscosity (PV) as an index of disease activity in RA is as reliable as the ESR or the CRP.[130] The normal range for PV is independent of age and sex, and the technique is rapid and simple, with a low incidence of false positive and false negative results.[130] A new acute-phase protein, vho, has been reported in high titer in RA. Titers are higher in active and seropositive patients. Serial studies, however, did not correlate titers with disease activity.[131]

SERUM PROTEINS

Electrophoretic Studies

Increases in α-2 globulin and fibrinogen occur nonspecifically in the presence of inflammation. A rise in the γ globulin level in inflammatory disease is presumptive evidence of a response to antigenic stimulation, even though the identity of the antigen is often unknown. The electrophoretic pattern changes in RA are not specific and are often within normal limits. The albumin peak is frequently low. Serum β-2 glycoprotein 1, a protein isolated from the β globulin fraction of serum, was reduced in RA.[132] The electrophoretic pattern in SLE resembles that seen in RA, although the γ globulin elevation is usually more pronounced. Changes seen in the other connective tissue diseases are similar, but usually less marked.

The mechanism of the hypoalbuminemia in RA was studied,[133] using ^{129}I-labeled albumin for determination of pool sizes and breakdown rates in seven patients.[134] Increased albumin breakdown, a part of a general hypermetabolic state, was proportional to the activity of the RA. Other studies of albumin metabolism in RA showed that intravascular, extravascular, and total body albumin levels were lower in patients than in healthy control subjects.[135]

When a correction was made for hypoalbuminemia, 46% of studied patients with definite or classic RA had hypercalcemia.[136] One study found that total body calcium levels were reduced in 5.3% of men and in 6.8% of women with RA; it was further reduced in patients taking low doses of corticosteroids.[137] A study of serum carrier proteins and acute-phase proteins showed an 8 to 12% decrease in transferrin, an 18 to 28% increase in ceruloplasmin, a 70 to 80% increase in α-1 acid glycoprotein, and a 29% increase in α-1-antitrypsin.[138] Antichymotrypsin was elevated.[139-141]

Immunoglobulin levels determined by the radial diffusion technique in RA vary. Several studies have shown increased levels of IgM and IgA.[142,143] Little apparent correlation exists between the elevation of immunoglobulin levels and the duration of disease activity or rheumatoid factor titers. Seropositive patients have also shown increased levels of IgG.[144] In another study, IgA levels were also more likely to be increased in patients with seropositive RA.[145] In a detailed study of many patients, a significant increase in IgG was observed in 15% and an increase in IgA was noted in 20%. IgM was rarely increased; IgD levels were normal or low; and IgA was also decreased in 19%.[146]

Although serum levels of free light chains of immunoglobulin in RA were not much different from normal, higher levels, found in some seropositive patients, were related to a number of factors reflecting disease activity.[147]

Serum Cryoglobulins and Immune Complexes

In cryoglobulinemia, environmental cooling of blood before measuring the ESR may cause erroneous values because of the formation of microaggregates of cryoglobulin and fibrinogen.[148] A few patients with RA have significant amounts of mixed cryoglobulins.[149] The types found are IgM (K)/IgG, IgA (K)/IgG, and IgG/IgG. These cryoglobulins show rheumatoid factor activity. Cold insoluble globulin, a normal glycoprotein of human plasma, although found in increased amounts in SLE and secondary amyloidosis, is present in normal amounts in RA.[150]

A correlation of the concentration of immune complexes in serum with the presence of extra-articular manifestations of RA was shown in a study using C1q binding.[151] Researchers found circulating immune complexes determined by the C1q binding assay in 81% of RA patients with IgM rheumatoid factor.[152] Measurement of circulating immune complexes in RA by five different assays has shown that sensitivity, specificity, and predictive value are not sufficient to warrant their use in the management of the disease.[153] In another study, C1q binding activity was found in one third of sera and correlated with disease activity and rheumatoid factor level. Circulating immune complexes were found in 52% of sera by at least five assays.[154]

Urinary Gamma Globulin

The quantity of urinary γ globulins excreted was higher in RA than in control subjects.[155] These substances were composed of L chains, 7S γ globulin, and traces of γ A globulin. In RA the urinary excretion of IgG, IgA, and free light chains was more than three times control levels in one study.[156] The mechanism for this increased excretion is unknown.

SEROLOGIC REACTIONS AND COMPLEMENT STUDIES

NONSPECIFIC SEROLOGIC REACTIONS

Biologic false positive Wassermann reactions have been reported in 6.3% to 11.6% of patients with

RA.[157,158] Properdin assays by the zymosan technique in 24 patients with RA gave low values in 8 and showed prozone phenomena in 5.[159] Plasma fibronectin was within the normal range in RA patients (335 µg/ml).[160]

LE CELLS AND ANTINUCLEAR FACTORS

LE cells have been found in 8 to 27% of patients with RA.[157,161,162] Gamma globulins reacting with nuclear constituents (antinuclear factors) are usually demonstrated by the fluorescent antibody technique, although other methods have been used.[163] Antinuclear antibodies occur most commonly in patients with SLE, but they may be seen with varying frequency in the other connective tissue diseases, including RA. In 710 RA patients collected from the literature by Pollak,[164] 24% had positive antinuclear antibody tests. In another series, only 3% had positive LE tests, but antinuclear antibodies were found in 14%.[165] Antinuclear factors were present mainly as macroglobulin (IgM) in rheumatoid sera, but mainly as a 7S (IgG) immunoglobulin in SLE sera.[166] Antinuclear antibodies were increased in 60% of patients with RA, but in only 13% of control subjects.[167] These antinuclear antibodies were classified as follows: IgM, 41%; IgG, 40%; and IgA, 33%. Reaction with a histone nuclear antigen was found in 24%.[167] Antiperinuclear factor, an antibody reacting with cytoplasmic granules in human cheek epithelial cells, was found in 79% of patients with RA, but only in 4% of normal subjects.[168]

Studies on the significance of positive antinuclear antibody tests in patients with RA were carried out by two groups.[169,170] Both groups concluded that these patients had more severe disease. Although one study showed a higher frequency of vasculitis associated with the antinuclear antibodies,[170] this finding was not confirmed.[169] Antinuclear antibodies were more frequent in patients who were rheumatoid-factor positive. Patients with Sjögren's syndrome had a higher prevalence of antinuclear antibodies than patients with RA alone. This finding reflects a general increase of autoantibodies in Sjögren's syndrome.[171] Half of the RA patients with granulocyte-specific antinuclear factors had protein in their urine (>150 mg/ 24 hours).[172] Anti-Sm and anti-RNP antibodies, characteristic markers for SLE and mixed connective tissue disease, respectively, were not found in patients with RA.[173]

Antinuclear antibodies of the IgE class in patients with RA showed a frequency of 60% with neutropenia, but only 16% without neutropenia.[174] In another series, neutropenic patients with RA were characterized by a higher frequency of IgD granulocyte-specific antinuclear antibodies, compared to RA patients without neutropenia (67% versus 18%).[175] Antiribosomal antibodies were found in 36% of RA patients, but only in 2% of control subjects.[176] Antibody against double-stranded RNA was elevated in 33% of RA patients and was below the normal range in 11%. The lower levels were attributed to an enzyme that degraded double-stranded RNA.[177]

The occurrence in rheumatoid serum of the abnormal factors previously discussed is presumably secondary to a more fundamental process responsible for the initiation of the disease. Rheumatoid factors, antinuclear factors, and biologic false-Wassermann antibody have all been found in other conditions associated with chronic inflammation. Experimentally, prolonged hyperimmunization of rabbits with killed bacteria has resulted in the development of "rheumatoid-like" factors,[178] and even anti-DNA factors;[179] these findings suggest the relation of these antibodies to prolonged antigenic stimulation (see also Chapter 41).

BLOOD GROUPS AND HISTOCOMPATIBILITY ANTIGENS

Low isohemagglutinins have been found in RA.[180,181] No correlation was found with the antigens of the ABO, C, or E blood groups,[182,183] nor has a significant association of HLA-A or HLA-B antigens been found in RA.[184–186] The presence of HLA-B27 in RA was not associated with any specific clinical or radiographic observations.[187] Stastny, however, found a significant increase of the HLA-DRW4 antigen in patients with RA.[188] The level of HLA-DRW4 is elevated in 55% of patients with classic or definite disease, as opposed to 23% of control subjects (see Chapter 29).[189]

OTHER ANTIBODIES

Antibody titers to various autoantigens and to viruses have been examined in RA. Antibody to an RA-associated nuclear antigen (RANA) was found in 90% of patients with seropositive RA.[190] Researchers also noted an increased frequency and increased levels of other antibodies to Epstein-Barr virus.[190] In another study, however, Epstein-Barr virus and cytomegalovirus antibodies were not more frequent in patients with RA than in controls.[34] Rubella antibody titers were found in 100% of 80 patients with RA and in 86.5% of matched control subjects.[191] Sera from pa-

tients with seropositive RA showed positive precipitin reactions to streptococcal mucopeptide in 73% versus 22% in normal control sera. These reactions were due, at least in part, to precipitation enhancement by rheumatoid factor. Increases in levels of antibodies to other antigens in seropositive RA patients should be suspect unless this factor has been excluded.[192] Cathepsin D agglutinators, natural antibodies to proteolytically released IgG determinants, are normally found in low titers. Levels of these substances are elevated in seropositive RA as compared to normal controls and patients with seronegative RA.[193] Anti-β-2 microglobulin antibody was found more frequently in RA and in higher titer than in normal control subjects. The high titers were more commonly associated with pleuropulmonary lesions and nodules.[194] Factor VIII antibody, as noted clinically by reduced or absent coagulant activity, has been reported occasionally in RA.[195] Smooth muscle antibodies were found more frequently in RA than in control subjects (15.3% versus 7.6%).[196]

Antibodies to native and denatured collagen have been found in high frequency and titer in patients with RA.[197,198] Antibodies to type I were present in 13.6%, whereas antibodies to type II were found in 14.6%.[199] Antikeratin antibodies were found in 58% of patients with classic or definite RA, but not in sera from healthy people. Thus, the finding of this antibody was specific.[200] Moreover, antibody titers to the carcinoembryonic antigen (CEA) were higher in patients with seropositive RA than in a control group.[201] Negative results were found when hepatitis-associated antigen (HAA) and anti-HAA antibodies were sought.[202] A polyclonal B-cell activator has been described in rheumatoid patients, as well as in patients with other connective tissue diseases.[203]

Delayed hypersensitivity has also been investigated. One group using five antigens found decreased skin reactivity in RA patients.[34] In another investigation, 20% of patients with RA were found to be anergic. The magnitude of skin reactions and the incidence of positive reactions to multiple antigens decreased. The depression was related to age, but not to sex, duration of disease, or disease activity.[204]

SERUM COMPLEMENT

Serum complement levels in RA are usually either normal or elevated.[205–207] In contrast, the level of complement is reduced in most patients with active SLE.[205] Hypocomplementemia does occur in RA and was observed in 11 of 250 patients studied.[97] This finding is associated with severe RA and a high frequency of bacterial infection.[208] Other researchers found that serum complement activity was reduced in patients with vasculitis, and the complement levels of seropositive patients were lower than those of seronegative patients.[209] Complement is found in the dermal vessels of 60% of RA patients.[210]

An inherited deficiency of complement components is associated with connective tissue disease. When the inherited deficiency of the second component of complement (C2) was investigated, 1.4% of 134 patients who were homozygous or heterozygous for the deficiency state were found to have RA.[211] The frequency of C3 deficiency is higher in patients with RA, and especially in seropositive patients, than in the general population.[212]

Elevated levels of C3b inactivator were found in patients with seropositive RA, when compared to controls.[213] Levels of immunoconglutinin, believed to be an autoantibody to complement, are also increased in RA,[214,215] but this finding is not specific because inmunoconglutinin levels are also elevated in other rheumatic diseases.

LIVER AND GASTROINTESTINAL STUDIES

Mild-to-moderate abnormalities of liver function have been reported in RA, but these have been confined mainly to tests of liver function that reflect serum protein synthesis.[216,217] Histologic changes, found in up to 25% of biopsies, have been minimal.[217,218] These changes consist of slight-to-moderate fatty infiltration, slight evidence of fibrosis, and rarely, infiltration of portal areas with a few mononuclear cells. When liver biopsies were performed in 26 consecutive patients with RA, 1 showed cirrhosis, 1 fatty change, 1 hemosiderosis, 5 passive congestion, and 2 nonspecific changes. No correlation was found with any facet of the disease or activity, and the majority of the changes were nonspecific.[219] Alteration in liver size has been investigated by scintigraphy. In 7 of 32 patients with RA, a correlation was found between liver enlargement and the presence of rheumatoid factor, although results of the liver function tests in these patients were normal.[220] Clinical or biochemical evidence of liver disease was found only in 0.7% of 997 patients with RA.[221]

Serum alkaline phosphatase,[222] serum glutamic-oxalacetic transaminase (SGOT),[223] and serum glutamic-pyruvic transaminase (SGPT)[224] levels were normal, although 15% of patients showed an elevation of serum ornithine-carbamoyl transferase.[224] Gamma glutamyl transpeptidase (GGTP) levels, considered a sensitive indicator of liver damage, were higher in RA than in degenerative joint disease (77% versus 33%) and correlated with an improvement in disease activity after penicillamine therapy.[225] Measurements of serum bilirubin and urine urobilinogen levels were within normal limits, but urine coproporphyrin excretion was elevated.[216] Decreased bromsulphalein excretion was found in from 23 to more than 90% of patients.[226] Serum phosphatase elevation, abnormal Bromsulfalein excretion, hepatomegaly, splenomegaly, and smooth muscle antibody were observed more frequently in patients with RA than in a control group with osteoarthritis,[171] but SGPT and bilirubin levels were not different from the controls, nor was the frequency of mitochondral antibody any greater.

RA patients have a decreased amplitude of peristaltic contraction in the lower two thirds of the esophagus.[227] The lower esophageal intrasphincteric pressure is also decreased. These findings do not seem to relate to the duration or stage of the disease. Basal and maximum acid output is subnormal in RA patients.[228] Hypergastrinemia is also a feature of RA. In one study, normal mean fasting gastrin in patients with RA was three times higher than in control subjects.[229] Examination of the intestinal mucosa of patients with RA showed that histidine-methyl-esterase activity in the intestinal mucosa biopsies was increased. Other intestinal enzymes studied did not show any significant difference from normal values.[230]

Urinary excretion of glycosaminoglycans (GAG) and of hydroxyproline was higher in patients with RA than in control subjects. Patients with active disease had the highest levels.[231] Patients with RA had higher-than-normal urinary excretion levels of hydroxyproline and zinc.[232] Free GAG levels in plasma were elevated in active RA, although total GAG levels were similar to those of controls.[233] The serum levels of an intracellular enzyme of collagen biosynthesis, prolyl hydroxylase, were elevated in RA. That raised values correlated with the level of the ESR indicates that the concentration of the enzyme reflected the degree of inflammatory activity.[234] The autoantibodies to cartilage found in a few cases of RA (1.5%) were apparently related to severe erosive disease.[235]

STUDIES OF RENAL FUNCTION AND ELECTROLYTES

Urinary abnormalities are uncommon in RA. More than a faint trace of albumin was found in the urine of only 7.2% of patients in one series.[99] Urinary tract infections were not more common in RA patients than in general,[236] although patients treated with corticosteroids had an increased incidence of bacteriuria.[237] Persistent proteinuria occurred in 24 of 183 patients in another series.[238] When 20 patients were examined further, the proteinuria was explainable on the basis of unrelated renal disease in 12; in the remaining 8 patients, evidence of amyloidosis was present. Renal biopsy in 13 RA patients with persistent proteinuria disclosed normal kidneys in 3, arteriosclerosis or nephrosclerosis in 4, lupus nephritis in 2, and amyloidosis in 4.[239]

Scandinavian studies have reported a small-to-moderate decrease in the creatinine clearance in rheumatoid patients.[240–243] The average reduction was 36%.[241] Serum creatinine concentration in RA, whether measured in patients with normal or impaired renal function, was lower than in matched controls, probably because of the smaller muscle mass of RA patients.[244] Impairment of glomerular filtration was related to the stage and duration of the disease and to the presence of rheumatoid factor, but was unrelated to past history of drug intake, including phenacetin. Renal biopsies in 18 patients with classic RA but with minimal or moderate urine abnormalities showed only minimal mesangial changes in 7. Immunofluorescence studies were negative in all cases.[245] Thus, although the occurrence of occasional proteinuria and the reduction of the creatinine clearance in some patients may suggest renal abnormality in RA, histologic studies, except for those in older reports,[246] have not disclosed evidence of a specific renal abnormality other than the uncommon complication of amyloidosis.

Ammonium chloride loading experiments show normal urinary acidification in RA patients.[247] The sweat ratio of sodium to potassium increased in about half the patients in one series,[248] although information about corticosteroid therapy was not given. Increased serum copper levels have been reported,[249] but increased copper levels, associated with elevated α-2 globulin (ceruloplasmin) levels, are a nonspecific feature of inflammatory diseases. The increased levels were correlated with the ESR and with disease activity,[250] but not with the presence of rheumatoid factor or with the stage of disease.[251] The possible role of estrogen therapy has been discussed.[252] The urinary excretion of copper is higher in RA than in healthy subjects.[253] Although zinc levels in several studies were normal,[253,254] mean plasma zinc levels of 11.74 mol/L, versus 15.1 mol/L in controls, were decreased in the most recent study, particularly if the patients were treated only with nonsteroidal anti-inflammatory drugs.[255] A significant inverse relationship to the ESR was observed. In a study of serum trace-metal concentrations, the concentrations of copper, barium, cesium, tin, and molybdenum were elevated in RA.[256] Lower values of aluminum, nickel, strontium, chromium, cadmium,[256] and selenium were found.[253] Although plasma magnesium levels in RA are not much different from those in control subjects, the magnesium content of red blood cells is higher in these patients.[257]

ADRENAL FUNCTION TESTING

Adrenal cortical function has been evaluated on the basis of the excretion of 17-OH corticosteroids, 17-ketosteroids,[258] and other adrenal corticol metabolites.[259] Except for a decrease in excretion of 17-hydroxycorticosteroids in the early morning hours, the adrenal corticosteroid excretion pattern in RA is similar to that in other chronic diseases. Normal secretion rates of cortisol have been found.[1] Adrenal medullary function, as measured by the urinary excretion of epinephrine and norepinephrine, is within normal limits.[260,261]

MISCELLANEOUS LABORATORY STUDIES

URIC ACID LEVELS

Occasional studies have reported elevated levels of serum uric acid in patients with arthritides other than gout. Grayzel and co-workers,[262] who found elevated levels in 10 of 57 males with RA, ascribed this finding to the effect of low doses of salicylate. In other studies,[99,263] the levels of uric acid in RA were in the normal range.

SERUM CHOLESTEROL AND PLASMA LIPID LEVELS

In RA, as in other inflammatory arthritides, the total cholesterol level is reduced.[264] The mean reduction in rheumatoid-factor–positive patients was 53.7% in one series. The decrease was related to the severity and activity of the disease and was not affected by corticosteroid therapy. Plasma lipid levels have been reported to be within normal limits.[265,266] The difference in serum fatty acid concentration between RA patients and control subjects was not significant.[267] Oleic acid levels were elevated in patients with RA, whereas linolenic and arachidonic acid levels were decreased.[268]

Serum sulfhydryl levels have been reported to be

low in RA, especially in the presence of vasculitis.[269,270] They have been observed to predict persistent synovitis.[271] Ceruloplasmin levels have been reported to increase nonspecifically, a reflection of inflammatory activity.[253,272,273] Gerber found increased amounts of copper-binding substances in half of his rheumatoid patients.[274] The exact nature of these substances has not been determined. Patients with RA had low values of free serum histidine.[275] Adenosine triphosphatase (ATP)[276] and total serum lactic dehydrogenase[277] activities were within normal limits. Serum cholinesterase levels were variable.[278] Kininogen plasma levels and erythrocyte kininase levels were normal, but plasma kininase levels were decreased.[279] Serum plasmin activity correlated with the activity of the disease.[280] In a biopsy study of muscle ATP content, lower levels of muscle ATP were found in RA than in control subjects. No other muscle enzymes or metabolites studied were abnormal. The lowered levels of ATP were related to the duration of disease, and possibly to its severity.[281]

One study found increased capillary permeability in patients with RA. This finding was suggested as a possible cause of the occasional transient edema seen in these patients.[282]

VITAMIN LEVELS

Blood levels of vitamins are commonly decreased in patients with RA. Blood concentrations of ascorbic acid are usually low.[283] Although plasma ascorbic acid levels are low in RA, low platelet levels of ascorbic acid are found only in patients taking high doses of aspirin. The platelet ascorbic acid level is a better reflection of tissue levels, whereas serum levels are a better reflection of recent intake and are susceptible to factors that affect metabolism or excretion.[284] The levels of plasma retinol-binding protein, a specific transport protein whose plasma levels reflect the availability of vitamin A and probably of zinc, were lower in patients with RA than in matched control patients with degenerative joint disease.[285] The level of blood pantothenic acid is decreased. The amount of decrease has been correlated with the activity of the disease[286] and with an increased excretion of this vitamin.[287] Riboflavin, thiamine, and occasionally nicotinic acid levels may also be diminished;[287] but folate levels are not much different from normal.[288] In one series, a low serum folate level was found in 71% of RA patients, although the authors felt that this finding might be due to aspirin-induced alterations of folic acid binding.[289] Pyridoxin excretion has been found to be depressed.[290] Fasting serum pyridoxal levels

were below normal in 86% of RA patients, and serum folate levels were low.[291] Vitamin B_{12} levels were higher in RA patients (916 pg/ml) than in patients with degenerative joint disease (624 pg/ml) and in normal controls (440 pg/ml). The vitamin B_{12} levels increased linearly with the stage of the disease and were related more closely to the hemoglobin concentration than to the erythrocyte count.[292]

ELECTROMYOGRAPHY

Electromyographic findings in RA are not specific, but the frequency of abnormal findings is increased. Polyphasic potentials of short and long duration are often seen.[293–295] Fibrillation potentials have been reported by some authors,[293,294,296] but not by others.[297–299] Daughety and co-workers noted the presence of complicating factors such as polyneuropathy, terminal bronchopulmonary disease, and recent operation in all their patients who had fibrillation potentials.[293] Results of electrophysiologic studies of nerve conduction time in rheumatoid patients have been normal.[300]

PLEURAL FLUID STUDIES

A distinctive finding in RA is a low glucose concentration of pleural effusions. Glucose levels ranged from less than 5 mg/dl to 17 mg/dl in 10 of 11 effusions in one series;[301] values of 3, 0, and 0 mg/dl, respectively, were found in three effusions proved by pleural biopsy to be of rheumatoid origin.[302] The cause of this low glucose concentration is not known. Oral[25] or intravenous[303] administration of glucose failed to raise the glucose level in the effusions. A marked diminution of CH_{50}, C1, C1 inhibitor, and C2 was noted in the pleural fluid of rheumatoid-factor–positive RA.[304]

ELECTRODIAGNOSTIC STUDIES

On serial electrodiagnostic study, 20% of a series of patients with RA had evidence of carpal tunnel syndrome.[305]

REFERENCES

1. Pal, S.B.: The secretion rate of cortisol in patients with rheumatoid arthritis. Clin. Chim. Acta, 29:129–137, 1970.

2. Johnson, N.J., and Dodd, K.: Juvenile rheumatoid arthritis. Med. Clin. North Am., 39:459–487, 1955.

3. Toumbis, A., et al.: Clinical and serological observations in patients with juvenile rheumatoid arthritis and their relatives. J. Pediatr., 62:463–473, 1963.

4. Alexander, W.R.M., et al.: Nature of anaemia in rheumatoid arthritis. II. Survival of transfused erythrocytes in patients with rheumatoid arthritis. Ann. Rheum. Dis., 15:12–20, 1956.

5. Freireich. E.J., et al.: Radioactive iron metabolism and erythrocyte survival studies of the mechanism of the anemia associated with rheumatoid arthritis. J. Clin. Invest., 36:1043–1058, 1957.

6. Freireich, E.J., et al.: Mechanism of anaemia associated with rheumatoid arthritis. Ann. Rheum. Dis., 13:365–366, 1954.

7. McCrea, P.C.: Latent haemolysis in rheumatoid arthritis. Lancet, 1:402–405, 1957.

8. Ebaugh, F.G., et al.: The anemia of rheumatoid arthritis. Med. Clin. North Am., 39:489–498, 1955.

9. Weinstein, I.M.: A correlative study of the erythrokinetics and disturbances in iron metabolism associated with the anemia of rheumatoid arthritis. Blood, 14:950–966, 1959.

10. Lewis, S.M., and Porter, I.H.: Erythrocyte survival in rheumatoid arthritis. Ann. Rheum. Dis., 19:54–58, 1960.

11. Richmond, J., et al.: The nature of anaemia in rheumatoid arthritis. V. Red cell survival measured by radioactive chromium. Ann. Rheum. Dis., 20:133–137, 1961.

12. Roberts, F.D., et al.: Evaluation of the anemia of rheumatoid arthritis. Blood, 21:470–478, 1963.

13. Johansson, S.V., and Strandberg, P.O.: Haem biosynthesis studied in patients with rheumatoid arthritis. J. Clin. Pathol., 25:159–162, 1972.

14. Dixon, A. St.J., Ramcharan, S., and Ropes, M.W.: Rheumatoid arthritis: Dye retention studies and comparison of dye and radioactivity labelled red cell methods for measurement of blood volume. Ann. Rheum. Dis., 14:51–62, 1955.

15. Jeffrey, M.R.: Haemodilution in rheumatoid disease. Ann. Rheum. Dis., 15:151–159, 1956.

16. Kalliomaki, J.L., et al.: Extracellular fluid phase in rheumatoid arthritis. Acta Rheumatol. Scand., 4:79–85, 1958.

17. Robinson, G.L.: A study of liver function and plasma volume in chronic rheumatism by means of phenol-tetra-brom-phthalein sodium sulphonate. Ann. Rheum. Dis., 3:207–221, 1943.

18. Gibson, J.G., Harris, A.W., and Swigert, V.W.: Clinical studies of the blood volume. VIII. Macrocytic and hypochromic anemias due to chronic blood loss, hemolysis, and miscellaneous causes, and polycythemia vera. J. Clin. Invest., 18:621–632, 1939.

19. Brendstrup, P.: Serum copper, serum iron and total iron-binding capacity of serum in patients with chronic rheumatoid arthritis. Acta Med. Scand., 146:384–392, 1953.

20. Jeffrey, J.R.: Some observations on anemia in rheumatoid arthritis. Blood, 8:502–518, 1953.

21. Nilsson, F.: Anemia probelms in rheumatoid arthritis. Acta Med. Scand., 210(Suppl.):1–193, 1948.

22. McCrea, P.C.: Marrow iron examination in the diagnosis of iron deficiency in rheumatoid arthritis. Ann. Rheum. Dis., 17:89–96, 1958.

23. Richmond, J., et al.: Nature of anaemia in rheumatoid arthritis. III. Changes in the bone marrow and their relation to other features of the disease. Ann. Rheum. Dis., 15:217–226, 1956.

24. Finch, C.A., et al.: Iron metabolism utilization of intravenous radioactive iron. Blood, 4:905–927, 1949.

25. Cartwright, G.E., and Wintrobe, M.M.: Modern Trends in Blood Diseases. New York, Paul B. Hoeber, 1955.

26. Cartwright, G.E.: The anemia of chronic disorders. Semin. Hematol., 3:351–375, 1966.

27. Bennett, R.M., et al.: Synovial iron deposition in rheumatoid arthritis. Arthritis Rheum., 16:298–304, 1973.

28. Mowat, A.G., and Hothersall, T.E.: Nature of anaemia in rheumatoid arthritis: 8. Iron content of synovial tissue in patients with rheumatoid arthritis and in normal individuals. Ann. Rheum. Dis., 27:345–351, 1968.

29. Muirden, K.D.: The anaemia of rheumatoid arthritis: The significance of iron deposits in the synovial membrane. Aust. Ann. Med., 19:97–104, 1970.

30. Goldie, I.F., et al.: A comparison of the content of iron in normal and rheumatoid striated muscle. Scand. J. Rheumatol., 5:205–208, 1976.

31. Blake, D.R., and Bacon, P.A.: Serum ferritin and rheumatoid disease. Br. Med. J., 282:1273–1274, 1981.

32. Hansen, T.M., and Hansen, N.E.: Serum ferritin as indicator of iron responsive anaemia in patients with rheumatoid arthritis. Ann. Rheum. Dis., 45:596–602, 1986.

33. Dixon, A. St.J., Scott, J.T., and Harvey-Smith, E.A.: Aspirin and the anaemia of arthritis. Br. Med. J., 1:1425–1426, 1960.

34. Phillips, P.E., et al.: Virus antibody levels and delayed hypersensitivity in rheumatoid arthritis. Ann. Rheum. Dis., 35:152–154, 1976.

35. Ward, H.P., Gordon, B., and Pickett, J.C.: Serum levels of erythropoietin in rheumatoid arthritis. J. Lab. Clin. Med., 74:93–97, 1969.

36. Short, C.L., Bauer, W., and Reynolds, W.E.: Red-cell, white-cell, and differential counts. In Rheumatoid Arthritis. Edited by C.L. Short, W. Bauer, and W.E. Reynolds. Cambridge, MA, Harvard University Press, 1957, pp. 349–356.

37. Komatsubara, Y., et al.: Multi-variate analysis of serum protein in rheumatoid arthritis. Scand. J. Rheumatol., 5:97–102, 1976.

38. Dawson, M.H., Sia, R.H.P., and Boots, R.H.: The differential diagnosis of rheumatoid and osteoarthritis: The sedimentation reaction and its value. J. Lab. Clin. Med., 15:1065–1092, 1930.

39. Bishop, C.R., et al.: Leukokinetic studies. XIII. A non-steady-state kinetic evaluation of the mechanism of cortisone-induced granulocytosis. J. Clin. Invest., 47:249–260, 1968.

40. Lindjberg, I.F.: Juvenile rheumatoid arthritis. A followup of 75 cases. Arch. Dis. Child., 39:576–583, 1964.

41. Schlesinger, B.E.: The blood sedimentation rate in rheumatic fever. Practitioner, 157:38–44, 1946.

42. Hacbarth, E., and Kajdacsy-Balla, A.: Low density neutrophils in patients with systemic lupus erythematosus, rheumatoid arthritis, and acute rheumatic fever. Arthritis Rheum., 29:1334–1342, 1986.

43. Isenberg, D.A., et al.: Haematological reassessment of rheumatoid arthritis using an automated method. Br. J. Rheumatol, 25:152–157, 1986.

44. Felty, A.R.: Chronic arthritis in the adult, associated with splenomegaly and leukopenia: A report of 5 cases of an unusual clinical syndrome. Bull. Johns Hopkins Hosp., 35:16–20, 1924.

45. Hurd, E.R., and Cheatum, D.E.: Decreased spleen size and increased neutrophils in patients with Felty syndrome. Effects of gold sodium thiomalate therapy. JAMA, 235:2215–2217, 1976.

46. Bucknall, R.C., et al.: Neutropenia in rheumatoid arthritis: Studies on possible contributing factors. Ann. Rheum. Dis., 41:242–247, 1982.

47. Wilk, A., and Munthe, E.: Complement-fixing granulocyte-specific antinuclear factors in neutropenic cases of rheumatoid arthritis. Immunology, *26*:1127–1134, 1974.

48. Sylvester, R.A., and Pinals, R.S.: Eosinophilia in rheumatoid arthritis. Ann. Allergy, *28*:565–568, 1970.

49. Winchester, R.J., et al.: Observations on the eosinophilia of certain patients with rheumatoid arthritis. Arthritis Rheum., *14*:650–665, 1971.

50. Adeyemi, E.O., et al.: Circulating human leukocyte elastase in rheumatoid arthritis. Rheumatol. Int., *6*:57–60, 1986.

51. Selroos, O.: Thrombocytosis in rheumatoid arthritis. Scand. J. Rheumatol., *1*:136–140, 1972.

52. Smith, A.F., and Castor, C.W.: Connective tissue activation. XII. Platelet abnormalities in patients with rheumatoid arthritis. J. Rheumatol., *5*:177–183, 1978.

53. Bartfeld, H.: The chromosomal complement in rheumatoid arthritis. N. Engl. J. Med., *267*:551–553, 1962.

54. Wenger, M.E., and Bole, G.G.: Nitroblue tetrazolium dye reduction by peripheral leukocytes from rheumatoid arthritis and systemic lupus erythematosus patients measured by a histochemical and spectrophotometric method. J. Lab. Clin. Med., *82*:513–521, 1973.

55. Mowat, A.G., and Baum, J.: Chemotaxis of polymorphonuclear leucocytes from patients with rheumatoid arthritis. J. Clin. Invest., *50*:2541–2549, 1971.

56. King, S.L., et al.: Polymorphonuclear leukocyte function in rheumatoid arthritis. Br. J. Rheumatol., *25*:26–33, 1986.

57. Ozaki, Y., Ohashi, T., and Niwa, Y.: Oxygen radical production by neutrophils from patients with bacterial infection and rheumatoid arthritis. Inflammation, *10*:119–130, 1986.

58. Belch, J.J.F., O'Dowd, A., Ansell, B., and Storrock, R.D.: Leukotriene B4 (LTB4) production in patients with rheumatoid arthritis. Br. J. Rheumatol., *25*(Suppl. 2):43, 1986 (abstract).

59. Natvig, J.B., et al.: Different lymphocyte populations in rheumatoid arthritis and their relationship to anti-Ig activities. Ann. Clin. Res., *7*:146–153, 1975.

60. Ridley, M.G., Panayi, G.S., Nicholas, M.S., and Murphy, J.: Mechanisms of macrophage activation in rheumatoid arthritis: The role of gamma-interferon. Clin. Exp. Immunol., *63*:587–593, 1986.

61. Tannenbaum, H., and Schur, P.: The role of lymphocytes in rheumatic diseases. J. Rheumatol., *1*:392–412, 1974.

62. Van de Putte, L.B.A., et al.: Lymphocytes in rheumatoid and nonrheumatoid synovial fluids. Nonspecificity of high T cell and low B cell percentages. Ann. Rheum. Dis., *35*:451–455, 1976.

63. Mathieu, M., Mereu, M.C., and Pisano, L.: Tγ lymphocytes of peripheral blood and synovial fluid in rheumatoid arthritis. Arthritis Rheum., *24*:658–661, 1981.

64. Veys, E.M., et al.: Evaluation of T cell subsets with monoclonal antibodies in patients with rheumatoid arthritis. J. Rheumatol., *9*:25–29, 1982.

65. Meijer, C.J.L.M., et al.: T lymphocyte subpopulations in rheumatoid arthritis. J. Rheumatol., *9*:18–24, 1982.

66. Salmon, M., Bacon, P.A., Symmons, D.P.M., and Blann, A.D.: Transferrin receptor-bearing cells in the peripheral blood of patients with rheumatoid arthritis. Clin. Exp. Immunol., *62*:346–352, 1985.

67. Percy, J.S., et al.: A longitudinal study of in vitro tests for lymphocyte function in rheumatoid arthritis. Ann. Rheum. Dis., *37*:416–420, 1978.

68. Lance, E.M., and Knight, S.C.: Immunologic reactivity in rheumatoid arthritis. Response to mitogens. Arthritis Rheum., *17*:513–520, 1974.

69. Lockshin, M.D., et al.: Cell-mediated immunity in rheumatic diseases. II. Mitogen responses in RA, SLE, and other illnesses: Correlation with T- and B-lymphocyte populations. Arthritis Rheum., *18*:245–250, 1975.

70. Rawson, A.J., and Huang, T.C.: Lymphocyte populations in rheumatoid arthritis. Arthritis Rheum., *19*:720–724, 1976.

71. Silverman, H.A., et al.: Altered lymphocyte reactivity in rheumatoid arthritis. Arthritis Rheum., *19*:509–515, 1976.

72. Sakane, T., et al.: Analysis of suppressor T cell function in patients with rheumatoid arthritis. J. Immunol., *129*:1972–1977, 1982.

73. Slavin, S., and Strober, S.: In vitro T cell mediated function in patients with active rheumatoid arthritis. Ann. Rheum. Dis., *40*:60–63, 1981.

74. Runge, L.A.: In vitro lymphocyte response in early RA. J. Rheumatol., *8*:468–476, 1981.

75. Menard, H.A., Dioni, J., and Richard, C.: Antinuclear antibody: Predictive of lymphocyte response in rheumatoid arthritis. J. Rheumatol., *4*:21–26, 1977.

76. Abdou, N.I., et al.: Suppressor T cell dysfunction and anti-suppressor cell antibody in active early rheumatoid arthritis. J. Rheumatol., *8*:9–18, 1981.

77. McKenna, R.M.: Interleukin-2 production and responsiveness in active and inactive rheumatoid arthritis. J. Rheumatol., *13*:28–32, 1986.

78. Combe, B., et al.: Interleukin-2 in rheumatoid arthritis: Production of and response to interleukin-2 in rheumatoid synovial fluid, synovial tissue and peripheral blood. Clin. Exp. Immunol., *59*:520–528, 1985.

79. Steffen, C., et al.: Demonstration of lymphocytotoxins in rheumatoid arthritis in comparison with clinical course and other antibody activities. Z. Immunitaetsforsch., *145*:303–311, 1973.

80. Diaz-Jouanen, E., Bankhurst, A.D., and Williams, R.C., Jr.: Antibody-mediated lymphocytotoxicity in rheumatoid arthritis and systemic lupus erythematosus. Arthritis Rheum., *19*:133–141, 1976.

81. Barada, F.A., O'Brien, W., and Horwitz, D.A.: Defective monocyte cytotoxicity in rheumatoid arthritis. Arthritis Rheum., *25*:10–16, 1982.

82. Pedersen, B.K., Beyer, J.M., Klarlund, K., and Clemmensen, I.H.: Baseline and interferon-enhanced natural killer cell activity in rheumatoid arthritis. Acta Pathol. Microbiol. Immunol. Scand., *93*:79–84, 1985.

83. Fåhraeus, R.: The suspension stability of the blood. Physiol. Rev., *9*:241–274, 1929.

84. Fåhraeus, R.: The suspension-stability of the blood. Acta Med. Scand., *55*:1–228, 1921.

85. Hermann, H.: Die Blutkörperchensenkungsgeschwindigkeit bei arthritiden und rheumateschen Affektionen der Muskulatur. Munchen. Med. Wochenschr., *71*:1714–1716, 1924.

86. Hollinger, N.F., and Robinson, S.J.: A study of the erythrocyte sedimentation rate for well children. J. Pediatr., *42*:304–319, 1953.

87. Glynn, L.E.: Symposium on inflammation and role of fibrin in the rheumatic diseases. Bull. Rheum. Dis., *14*:323–326, 1963.

88. Gilligan, D.R., and Ernstene, A.C.: The relationship between the erythrocyte sedimentation rate and the fibrinogen content of plasma. Am. J. Med. Sci., *187*:552–556, 1934.

89. Fletcher, A.A., Dauphinee, J.A., and Ogryzlo, M.A.: Plasma fibrinogen and the sedimentation rate in rheumatoid arthritis

and their response to the administration of cortisone and adrenocorticotropic hormone. J. Clin. Invest., *31*:561–571, 1952.

90. Hardwicke, H., and Squire, J.R.: The basis of the erythrocyte sedimentation rate. Clin. Sci., *11*:333–355, 1952.

91. Scherer, R., Morarescu, A., and Ruhenstroth-Bauer, G.: Die spezifische Wirkung der Plasmaproteine bei der Blutkörperchensenkung. Eine Analyse der Korrelationskoeffizienten von Blutkorperchensen—Kungsgeschwindigkeit und den Konzentrationen von zwanzig Plasmaproteinen bei Gesunden und Kranken, insbesondere nach Herzinfarkt. Klin. Wochenschr., *53*:265–273, 1975.

92. Levinsky, H., et al.: Red blood cell membrane and serum sialic acid in relation to erythrocyte sedimentation rate. Acta Haematol., *64*:276–280, 1980.

93. Westergren, A.: Studies of the suspension stability of the blood in pulmonary tuberculosis. Acta Med. Scand., *54*:247–282, 1920.

94. International Committee for Standardization in Hematology: Recommendation for measurement of erythrocyte sedimentation rate of human blood. Am. J. Clin. Pathol., *68*:505–507, 1977.

95. Belin, D.C., Morse, E., and Weinstein, A.: Whither Westergren—the sedimentation rate reevaluated. J. Rheumatol., *8*:331–335, 1981.

96. Bottiger, L.E., and Svedberg, C.A.: Normal erythrocyte sedimentation rate and age. Br. Med. J., *2*:85–87, 1967.

97. Franco, A.E., and Schur, P.H.: Hypocomplementemia in rheumatoid arthritis. Arthritis Rheum., *14*:231–238, 1971.

98. Francis, T.I., Odusote, K., and Osuntokun, B.O.: The erythrocyte sedimentation rate in Nigerians. West Afr. Med. J., *20*:250–252, 1971.

99. Short, C.L., Dienes, L., and Bauer, W.: Rheumatoid arthritis: A comparative evaluation of the commonly employed diagnostic tests. JAMA, *108*:2087–2091, 1937.

100. Richardson, A.T.: Routine clinical pathology in rheumatoid arthritis. Proc. R. Soc. Med., *50*:466–469, 1957.

101. Crockson, R.A., and Crockson, A.P.: Relationship of the erythrocyte sedimentation rate to viscosity and plasma proteins in rheumatoid arthritis. Ann. Rheum. Dis., *33*:53–56, 1974.

102. McConkey, B., Crockson, R.A., and Crockson, A.P.: The assessment of rheumatoid arthritis: A study based on measurements of the serum acute-phase reactants. Q. J. Med., *162*:115–125, 1972.

103. Dawes, P.T.: Rheumatoid arthritis: Treatment which controls the C-reactive protein and erythrocyte sedimentation rate reduces radiological progression. Br. J. Rheumatol., *25*:44–49, 1986.

104. Decker, J.L., et al.: Primer on the rheumatic diseases. Part III. JAMA, *190*:509–530, 1964.

105. Payne, W.W., and Schlesinger, B.: A study of the sedimentation rate in juvenile rheumatism. Arch. Dis. Child., *10*:403–414, 1935.

106. Schlesinger, B.E., et al.: Observations on the clinical course and treatment of one hundred cases of Still's disease. Arch. Dis. Child., *36*:65–76, 1961.

107. Wood, P.: The erythrocyte sedimentation rate in diseases of the heart. Q. J. Med., *5*:1–19, 1936.

108. Spagnuolo, M., and Feinstein, A.R.: Congestive heart failure and rheumatic activity in young patients with rheumatic heart disease. Pediatrics, *33*:653–660, 1964.

109. Saghvi, L.M.: Sedimentation rate in heart disease. Geriatrics, *18*:382–392, 1963.

110. Liljestrand, A., and Olhagen, B.: I. Persistently high erythrocyte sedimentation rate. Acta Med. Scand., *151*:425–439, 1955.

111. Olhagen, B., and Liljestrand, A.: II. Persistently elevated erythrocyte sedimentation rate with good prognosis. Acta Med. Scand., *151*:441–449, 1955.

112. Ansell, B., and Bywaters, E.G.L.: The "unexplained" high erythrocyte sedimentation rate. Br. Med. J., *1*:372–374, 1958.

113. Mead, J., and Larson, D.L.: The erythrocyte sedimentation rate and other blood tests in terminal cancer. J. Am. Geriatr. Soc., *18*:489–490, 1970.

114. Gibson, I.I.J.M.: The value of the erythrocyte sedimentation rate in the aged. Gerontol. Clin., *14*:185–190, 1972.

115. Peyman, M.A.: The effect of malignant disease on the erythrocyte sedimentation rate. Br. J. Cancer, *16*:56–71, 1962.

116. Wyler, D.J.: Diagnostic implications of markedly elevated erythrocyte sedimentation rate: A reevaluation. South. Med. J., *70*:1428–1430, 1977.

117. Drivsholm, A.: Myelomatosis. Acta Med. Scand., *176*:509–524, 1964.

118. Boyd, R.V., and Hoffbrand, B.I.: Erythrocyte sedimentation rate in elderly hospital in-patients. Br. Med. J., *1*:901–902, 1966.

119. Milne, J.S., and Williamson, J.: The ESR in older people. Gerontol. Clin., *14*:36–42, 1972.

120. Crawford, J., Eye-Boland, M.K., and Cohen, H.J.: Clinical utility of erythrocyte sedimentation rate and plasma protein analysis in the elderly. Am. J. Med., *82*:239–246, 1987.

121. Burton, J.L.: Effect of oral contraceptives on erythrocyte sedimentation rate in healthy young women. Br. Med. J., *3*:214–215, 1967.

122. McEwen, C., and Ziff, M.: Basic sciences in relation to rheumatic diseases. Med. Clin. North Am., *39*:765–782, 1955.

123. Amos, R.S., et al.: Rheumatoid arthritis: C-reactive protein and erythrocyte sedimentation during initial treatment. Br. Med. J., *1*:1386–1387, 1978.

124. Walsh, L., Davis, P., and McConkey, B.: Relationship between erythrocyte sedimentation rate and serum C-reactive protein in rheumatoid arthritis. Ann. Rheum. Dis., *38*:362–363, 1979.

125. Nashel, D.J., et al.: C-reactive protein: A marker for disease activity in ankylosing spondylitis and Reiter's syndrome. J. Rheumatol., *13*:364–367, 1986.

126. Nussinow, S., and Arnold, W.J.: Prognostic value of C-reactive protein (CRP) levels in rheumatoid arthritis. Arthritis Rheum., *25*:524, 1982.

127. Maury, C.P.J., Teppo, A.-M., and Wegelius, O.: Relationship between urinary sialylated saccharides, serum amyloid A protein, and C-reactive protein in rheumatoid arthritis and systemic lupus erythematosus. Ann. Rheum. Dis., *41*:268–271, 1982.

128. Strachan, A.F., and Johnson, P.M.: Protein SAP (serum amyloid P-component) in Waldenström's macroglobulinaemia, multiple myeloma and rheumatic disease. J. Clin. Lab. Immunol., *8*:153–156, 1982.

129. Maury, C.P.J.: Comparative study of serum amyloid A protein and C-reactive protein in disease. Clin. Sci., *68*:233–238, 1985.

130. Pickup, M.E., et al.: Plasma viscosity—a new appraisal of its use as an index of disease activity in rheumatoid arthritis. Ann. Rheum. Dis., *40*:272–275, 1981.

131. Schwartz, M.L., et al.: The behavior of a newly described acute-phase protein in inflammatory joint disease. Inflammation, *1*:297–303, 1976.

132. Kosaka, S.: β_2-Glycoprotein I in rheumatoid arthritis. Tohoku J. Exp. Med., *122*:223–228, 1977.

133. Jeremy, R., and Wilkinson, P.: The mechanism of hypoalbuminemia in rheumatoid arthritis. Arthritis Rheum., 7:740–741, 1964.

134. Wilkinson, P., et al.: The mechanism of hypoalbuminemia in rheumatoid arthritis. Ann. Intern. Med., 63:109–114, 1965.

135. Ballantyne, F.C., Fleck, A., and Dick, W.C.: Albumin metabolism in rheumatoid arthritis. Ann. Rheum. Dis., 30:265–270, 1971.

136. Kennedy, A.C., et al.: Hypercalcaemia in rheumatoid arthritis. Ann. Rheum. Dis., 38:401–412, 1979.

137. Reid, D.M., et al.: Total body calcium in rheumatoid arthritis. Br. Med. J., 285:330–332, 1982.

138. Denko, C.W., and Gabriel, P.: Serum proteins—transferrin, ceruloplasmin, albumin, α_1-acid and glycoprotein, α_1-antitrypsin—in rheumatic disorders. J. Rheumatol., 6:664–672, 1979.

139. Brackertz, D., Hagmann, J., and Kueppers, F.: Proteinase inhibitors in rheumatoid arthritis. Ann. Rheum. Dis., 34:225–230, 1975.

140. Kosaka, S., and Tazawa, M.: Alpha-1-antichymotrypsin in rheumatoid arthritis. Tohoku J. Exp. Med., 119:369–375, 1976.

141. Swedlund, H.A., Hunder, G.G., and Gleich, G.H.: Alpha-1-antitrypsin in serum and synovial fluid in rheumatoid arthritis. Ann. Rheum. Dis., 33:162–164, 1974.

142. Barden, J., Mullinax, F., and Waller, M.: Immunoglobulin levels in rheumatoid arthritis: Comparison with rheumatoid factor titers, clinical stage and disease duration. Arthritis Rheum., 10:228–234, 1967.

143. Rhodes, K., et al.: Immunological sex differences: A study of patients with rheumatoid arthritis, their relatives and controls. Ann. Rheum. Dis., 28:104–120, 1969.

144. Veys, E.M., and Claessens, H.E.: Serum levels of IgG, IgM and IgA in rheumatoid arthritis. Ann. Rheum. Dis., 27:431–440, 1968.

145. Thompson, R.A., and Asquith, P.: Quantitation of exocrine IgA in human serum in health and disease. Clin. Exp. Immunol., 7:491–500, 1970.

146. Pruzanski, W., et al.: Serum and synovial fluid proteins in rheumatoid arthritis and degenerative joint diseases. Am. J. Med. Sci., 265:483–490, 1973.

147. Sølling, K., Sølling, J., and Rømer, F.K.: Free light chains of immunoglobulins in serum from patients with rheumatoid arthritis, sarcoidosis, chronic infectious and pulmonary cancer. Acta Med. Scand., 209:473–477, 1981.

148. Haeney, M.R.: Erroneous values for the total white cell count and ESR in patients with cryoglobulinaemia. J. Clin. Pathol., 29:894–897, 1976.

149. Mackechnie, H.L., Ogryzlo, M.A., and Pruzanski, W.: Heterogeneity of IgM/IgG cryocomplexes: Immunological-clinical correlation. J. Rheumatol., 2:225–240, 1975.

150. Fyrand, O., Munthe, E., and Solum, N.O.: Studies on cold insoluble globulin. Ann. Rheum. Dis., 37:347–350, 1978.

151. Zubler, R.H., et al.: Circulating and intra-articular immune complexes in patients with rheumatoid arthritis. Correlation of ^{125}I-C1q binding activity with clinical and biological features of the disease. J. Clin. Invest., 57:1308–1319, 1976.

152. Pope, R.M., Yoshinoya, S., and McDuffy, S.J.: Detection of immune complexes and their relationship to rheumatoid factor in a variety of autoimmune disorders. Clin. Exp. Immunol., 46:259–267, 1981.

153. McDougal, J.G., et al.: Comparison of five assays for immune complexes in the rheumatic diseases. Arthritis Rheum., 25:1156–1166, 1982.

154. Reynolds, W.J., et al.: Circulating immune complexes in rheumatoid arthritis. A prospective study using five immunoassays. J. Rheumatol., 13:700–706, 1986.

155. Gordon, D.A., Eisen, A.Z., and Vaughan, J.: Studies on urinary γ-globulins in patients with rheumatoid arthritis. Arthritis Rheum., 9:575–588, 1966.

156. Lindström, F.D.: Urinary immunoglobulins in rheumatoid arthritis and other connective tissue diseases. Ann. Clin. Res., 3:39–45, 1971.

157. Kievits, J.H., et al.: Rheumatoid arthritis and the positive L.E.-cell phenomenon. Ann. Rheum. Dis., 15:211–216, 1956.

158. Waldenström, J., and Winblad, S.: Some observations on the relationship of certain serological reactions in various diseases with hypergammaglobulinemia. Acta Rheumatol. Scand., 4:3–9, 1958.

159. Laurell, A.-B., and Grubb, R.: Complement, complement components, properdin and agglutination promoting factors in rheumatoid arthritis. Acta Pathol. Microbiol. Scand., 43:310–320, 1958.

160. Vartio, T., et al.: Fibronectin in synovial fluid and tissue in rheumatoid arthritis. Eur. J. Clin. Invest., 11:207–212, 1981.

161. Friedman, I.A., et al.: The L.E. phenomenon in rheumatoid arthritis. Ann. Intern. Med., 46:1113–1136, 1957.

162. Goldfine, L.J., et al.: Clinical significance of the LE-cell phenomenon in rheumatoid arthritis. Ann. Rheum. Dis., 24:153–160, 1965.

163. Townes, A.S., Stewart, C.R., and Osler, A.G.: Immunologic studies in systemic lupus erythematosus. *In* Mechanisms of Cell and Tissue Damage Produced by Immune Reactions. Edited by Pierre Grabar and Peter Miescher. Basel, Benno Schwabe, 1961, pp. 315–325.

164. Pollak, V.E.: Antinuclear antibodies in families of patients with systemic lupus erythematosus. N. Engl. J. Med., 271:165–171, 1964.

165. Weir, D.M., Holborow, E.J., and Johnson, G.D.: A clinical study of serum antinuclear factor. Br. Med. J., 1:933–937, 1961.

166. Baum, J., and Ziff, M.: 7S and macroglobulin antinuclear fluorescence factors in systemic lupus erythematosus and rheumatoid arthritis. Arthritis Rheum., 5:636–637, 1962.

167. Aitcheson, C.T., et al.: Characteristics of antinuclear antibodies in rheumatoid arthritis. Arthritis Rheum., 23:528–538, 1980.

168. Smit, J.W., et al.: The antiperinuclear factor: II. A light microscopical and immunofluorescence study on the antigenic substrate. Ann. Rheum. Dis., 39:381–386, 1980.

169. Condemi, J.J.: The significance of antinuclear factors in rheumatoid arthritis. Arthritis Rheum., 8:1080–1093, 1965.

170. Pitkeathly, D.A., and Taylor, G.: Antinuclear factor in rheumatoid arthritis and related diseases. Ann. Rheum. Dis., 26:1–9, 1967.

171. Webb, J., et al.: Liver disease in rheumatoid arthritis and Sjögren's syndrome: Prospective study using biochemical and serological markers of hepatic dysfunction. Ann. Rheum. Dis., 34:70–81, 1975.

172. Wiik, A., Henriksen, K., and Faber, V.: Urinary excretion of granulocyte-specific antinuclear factors in rheumatoid arthritis. Acta Pathol. Microbiol. Scand. [C], 83:273–279, 1975.

173. Hamburger, M., Nodes, S., and Barland, P.: The incidence and clinical significance of antibodies to extractable nuclear antigens. Am. J. Med. Sci., 273:21–28, 1977.

174. Permin, H., and Wiik, A.: The prevalence of IgE antinuclear antibodies in rheumatoid arthritis and systemic lupus erythematosus. Acta Pathol. Microbiol. Scand. [C], 86:245–249, 1978.

175. Wiik, A., and Permin, H.: The prevalence and possible significance of IgD granulocyte-specific antinuclear antibodies in

neutropenic and non-neutropenic cases of rheumatoid arthritis. Acta Pathol. Microbiol. Scand. [C], *86*:19–22, 1978.

176. Gordon, J., Towbin, H., and Rosenthal, M.: Antibodies directed against ribosomal protein determinants in the sera of patients with connective tissue diseases. J. Rheumatol., *9*:247–252, 1982.

177. Kalmakoff, J., et al.: Antibodies against double-stranded RNA in patients with rheumatoid arthritis, osteoarthritis and Paget's disease of bone. Aust. N.Z. J. Med., *11*:173–178, 1981.

178. Abruzzo, J.L., and Christian, C.L.: The induction of a rheumatoid factor-like substance in rabbits. J. Exp. Med., *114*:791–806, 1961.

179. Christian, C.L., DeSimone, A.R., and Abruzzo, J.L.: Anti-DNA antibodies in hyperimmunized rabbits. Arthritis Rheum., *6*:766, 1963.

180. Kornstad, L., Guldberg, D., and Kornstad, A.M.G.: Isohaemagglutinins anti-A and anti-B in rheumatoid arthritis and ankylosing spondylitis. Ann. Rheum. Dis., *29*:421–426, 1970.

181. Rawson, A.J., and Abelson, N.M.: An isohemagglutinin deficiency in relatives of rheumatoid patients. Arthritis Rheum., *7*:391–397, 1964.

182. Cohen, A.S., et al.: Correlation between rheumatic diseases and Rh blood groups. Nature, *200*:1214–1215, 1963.

183. Wood, J.W., et al.: Rheumatoid arthritis in Hiroshima and Nagasaki, Japan: Prevalence, incidence, and clinical characteristics. Arthritis Rheum., *10*:21–31, 1967.

184. Brackertz, D., et al.: Histocompatibility antigens of patients with rheumatoid arthritis. Z. Immunitaetsforsch., *146*:108–113, 1973.

185. Lies, R.B., Messner, R.P., and Troup, G.M.: Histocompatibility antigens and rheumatoid arthritis. Arthritis Rheum., *15*:524–529, 1972.

186. Seignalet, J., et al.: HL-A antigens in rheumatoid arthritis. Vox Sang., *23*:468–471, 1972.

187. Fallahi, S., Halla, J.T., and Hardin, J.G., Jr.: The influence of B27 antigen on the clinical and radiographic picture of definite or classical rheumatoid arthritis. J. Rheumatol., *9*:13–17, 1982.

188. Stastny, P.: Mixed lymphocyte cultures in rheumatoid arthritis. J. Clin. Invest., *57*:1148–1157, 1976.

189. Scherak, O., Smolen, J.S., and Mayr, W.R.: Rheumatoid arthritis and B lymphocyte alloantigen HLA-DRw4. J. Rheumatol., *7*:9–12, 1980.

190. Alspaugh, M.A., et al.: Elevated levels of antibodies to Epstein-Barr virus antigens in sera and synovial fluid of patients with rheumatoid arthritis. J. Clin. Invest., *67*:1134–1140, 1981.

191. Deinard, A.S., et al.: Rubella-antibody titres in rheumatoid arthritis. Lancet, *1*:526–528, 1974.

192. Pope, R.M., Rutstein, J.E., and Straus, D.C.: Detection of antibodies to streptococcal mucopeptide in patients with rheumatic disorders and normal controls. Int. Arch. Allergy Appl. Immunol., *67*:267–274, 1982.

193. Artmann, G., Fehr, K., and Boni, A.: Cathepsin D agglutinators in rheumatoid arthritis. Arthritis Rheum., *20*:1105–1113, 1977.

194. Falus, A., Meretey, K., and Bozsoky, S.: Prevalence of anti-beta-2-microglobulin autoantibodies in sera of rheumatoid arthritis patients with extra-articular manifestations. Ann. Rheum. Dis., *40*:409–413, 1981.

195. Green, D., Schuette, R.T., and Wallace, W.H.: Factor VIII antibodies in rheumatoid arthritis. Arch. Intern. Med., *140*:1232–1235, 1980.

196. Anderson, I., Anderson, P., and Graudel, H.: Smooth muscle antibodies in RA. Acta Pathol. Microbiol. Scand. [C], *88*:131–135, 1980.

197. Andriopoulos, N.A., et al.: Antibodies in native and denatured collagens in sera of patients with rheumatoid arthritis. Arthritis Rheum., *19*:613–617, 1976.

198. Trentham, D.E., et al.: Cellular sensitivity to collagen in rheumatoid arthritis. N. Engl. J. Med., *299*:327–332, 1978.

199. Meghlaovi, A., et al.: Mise au point d'une technique immunoenzymatique (ELISA) pour la détection des anticorps anti-collagéne de type I et II. Ann. Immunol. (Paris), *132C*:287–305, 1981.

200. Young, B.J.J., et al.: Anti-keratin antibodies in rheumatoid arthritis. Br. Med. J., *2*:97–99, 1979.

201. Unger, A., Panayi, G.S., and Lessof, M.H.: Carcinoembryonic antigen in rheumatoid arthritis. Lancet, *1*:781–783, 1974.

202. Marcolongo, R., and Debolini, A.: Incidence of hepatitis associated antigen HAA and homologous antibody in patients with rheumatoid arthritis. Vox Sang., *28*:9–18, 1975.

203. Eisenberg, G.M., et al.: Polyclonal B cell activator (PBA) in rheumatic diseases. Arthritis Rheum., *25*:S6, 1982.

204. Andrianakos, A.A., et al.: Cell-mediated immunity in rheumatoid arthritis. Ann. Rheum. Dis., *36*:13–20, 1977.

205. Ellis, H.A., and Felix-Davies, D.: Serum complement, rheumatoid factor, and other serum proteins in rheumatoid disease and systemic lupus erythematosus. Ann. Rheum. Dis., *18*:215–224, 1959.

206. Vaughan, J.H., Bayles, T.B., and Favour, C.B.: Serum complement in rheumatoid arthritis. Am. J. Med. Sci., *222*:186–192, 1951.

207. Wedgewood, R.J.P., and Janeway, C.A.: Serum complement in children with "collagen disease." Pediatrics, *11*:569–581, 1953.

208. Hunder, G.G., and McDuffie, F.C.: Hypocomplementemia in rheumatoid arthritis. Am. J. Med., *54*:461–472, 1972.

209. Mongan, E.S., et al.: A study of the relation of seronegative and seropositive rheumatoid arthritis to each other and to necrotizing vasculitis. Am. J. Med., *47*:23–35, 1969.

210. Schroeter, A.L., Conn, D.L., and Jordon, R.E.: Immunoglobulin and complement deposition in skin of rheumatoid arthritis and systemic lupus erythematosus patients. Ann. Rheum. Dis., *35*:321–326, 1976.

211. Glass, D., et al.: Inherited deficiency of the second component of complement. Rheumatic disease associations. J. Clin. Invest., *58*:853–861, 1976.

212. Brönnestam, R.: Studies of the C3 polymorphism. Relationship between C3 phenotypes and rheumatoid arthritis. Hum. Hered., *23*:206–213, 1973.

213. Whaley, K., Schur, P.H., and Ruddy, S.: C3b inactivator in the rheumatic diseases. Measurement by radial immunodiffusion and by inhibition formation of properdin pathway C3 convertase. J. Clin. Invest., *57*:1554–1563, 1976.

214. Caspary, E.A., and Ball, E.J.: Serum immunoconglutinin in multiple sclerosis, Hashimoto's diseases, and rheumatoid arthritis. Br. Med. J., *2*:1514–1515, 1962.

215. Coombs, R.R.A., Coombs A.M., and Ingram, D.G.: Formation of immunoconglutinin during disease in man. *In* The Serology of Conglutination. Edited by R.A. Coombs, A.M. Coombs and D.G. Ingram. Springfield, IL, Charles C Thomas, 1961, pp. 128–137.

216. Darby, P.W.: Liver function tests in rheumatoid arthritis. J. Clin. Pathol., *6*:331, 1953.

217. Lefkovits, A.M., and Farrow, I.J.: The liver in rheumatoid arthritis. Ann. Rheum. Dis., *14*:162–169, 1955.

218. Movitt, E.R., and Davis, A.E.: Liver biopsy in rheumatoid arthritis. Am. J. Med. Sci., *226*:516–520, 1953.

219. Dietrichson, O., et al.: Morphological changes in liver biopsies

from patients with rheumatoid arthritis. Scand. J. Rheumatol., 5:65–69, 1976.

220. Tiger, L.H., et al.: Liver enlargement demonstrated by scintigraphy in rheumatoid arthritis. J. Rheumatol., 3:15–20, 1976.

221. Whaley, K., et al.: Liver disease in Sjögren's syndrome and rheumatoid arthritis. Lancet, 1:861–863, 1970.

222. Lehman, M.A., Kream, J., and Brugua, D.: Acid and alkaline phosphatase activity in the serum and synovial fluid of patients with arthritis. J. Bone Joint Surg., 46A:1732–1738, 1964.

223. Barr, J.H., Jr., et al.: Serum glutamic oxalacetic transaminase in rheumatoid arthritis and certain rheumatoid musculoskeletal disorders. Arthritis Rheum., 1:147–150, 1958.

224. Malmquist, E., and Reichard, H.: Serum ornithine carbamoyl transferase and transaminase activity in rheumatic disease. Acta Rheumatol. Scand., 8:170–182, 1962.

225. Lowe, J.R., et al.: Gamma glutamyl transpeptidase levels in arthritis. Ann. Rheum. Dis., 37:428–431, 1978.

226. Castenfors, H., Hultman, E., and Lövgren, O.: The bromosulphthalein-test (BSP) as a measure of rheumatoid arthritis activity. Acta Rheumatol. Scand., 10:128–132, 1964.

227. Sun, D.C.H., et al.: Upper gastrointestinal disease in rheumatoid arthritis. Am. J. Dig. Dis., 19:405–410, 1974.

228. DeWitte, T.J., et al.: Hypochlorhydria and hypergastrinaemia in rheumatoid arthritis. Ann. Rheum. Dis., 38:14–17, 1979.

229. Rooney, P.J., et al.: Hypergastrinaemia in rheumatoid arthritis: Disease or iatrogenesis. Br. Med. J., 2:752–753, 1973.

230. Bergstrom, K., and Havermark, G.: Enzymes in intestinal mucosa from patients with rheumatoid diseases. Scand. J. Rheumatol., 5:29–32, 1976.

231. Mbuyi, J.-M., et al.: Relevance of urinary excretion of alcian blue-glycosaminoglycans complexes and hydroxyproline to disease activity in rheumatoid arthritis. J. Rheumatol., 9:579–583, 1982.

232. Ambanelli, U., et al.: Relation between urine zinc and hydroxyproline in rheumatoid arthritis and bone diseases. J. Rheumatol., 5:477–479, 1978.

233. Friman, C., Juvani, M., and Skrifvars, B.: Acid glycosaminoglycans in plasma. Scand. J. Rheumatol., 6:177–182, 1977.

234. Kuutti-Savolainen, E.-R., Kivirikko, K.I., and Laitinin, O.: Serum immunoreactive prolyl hydroxylase in inflammatory rheumatic diseases. Ann. Rheum. Dis., 39:217–221, 1980.

235. Ebringer, R., et al.: Autoantibodies to cartilage and type H collagen in relapsing polychondritis and other rheumatic diseases. Ann. Rheum. Dis., 40:473–479, 1981.

236. Mowat, A.G., and Camp, A.V.: Polymyalgia rheumatica. J. Bone Joint Surg., 53B:701–710, 1971.

237. Burry, H.C.: Bacteriuria in rheumatoid arthritis. Ann. Rheum. Dis., 32:208–211, 1973.

238. Fearnley, G.S., and Lackner, R.: Amyloidosis in rheumatoid arthritis, and significance of "unexplained" albuminuria. Br. Med. J., 1:1129–1132, 1955.

239. Pollak, V.E., et al.: The kidney in rheumatoid arthritis: Studies by renal biopsy. Arthritis Rheum., 5:1–9, 1962.

240. Allander, E., et al.: Renal function in rheumatoid arthritis. Acta Rheumatol. Scand., 9:116–121, 1963.

241. Sørensen, A.W.S.: Investigations of the kidney function in rheumatoid arthritis. II. Acta Rheumatol. Scand., 7:138–144, 1961.

242. Sørensen, A.W.S.: The Waaler-Rose test in patients suffering from rheumatoid arthritis in relationship to 24-hour endogenous creatinine clearance. Acta Rheumatol. Scand., 7:304–314, 1961.

243. Sørensen, A.W.S.: Investigation of the kidney function in rheumatoid arthritis. I. Acta Rheumatol. Scand., 6:115–126, 1960.

244. Nived, O., et al.: Is serum creatinine concentration a reliable index of renal function in rheumatic diseases? Br. Med. J., 286:684–685, 1983.

245. Salomon, M.I., et al.: The kidney in rheumatoid arthritis. A study based on renal biopsies. Nephron, 12:297–310, 1974.

246. Baggenstoss, A.H., and Rosenberg, E.F.: Visceral lesions associated with chronic infections (rheumatoid) arthritis. Arch. Pathol., 35:503–516, 1943.

247. Pasternack, A., et al.: Renal acidification and hypergammaglobulinaemia. A study of rheumatoid arthritis. Acta Med. Scand., 187:123–127, 1970.

248. Gronbaek, P.: The sodium/potassium ratio in thermal sweat in patients with rheumatoid arthritis. Acta Rheumatol. Scand., 6:102–110, 1960.

249. Jeffrey, M.R., and Watson, D.: Free erythrocyte porphyrin and plasma copper in rheumatoid disease. Acta Haematol., 12:169–176, 1954.

250. Youssef, A.A.R., Wood, B., and Baron, D.N.: Serum copper: a marker of disease activity in rheumatoid arthritis. J. Clin. Pathol., 36:14–17, 1983.

251. Makisara, P., et al.: Serum copper in rheumatoid arthritis and ankylosing spondylitis. Ann. Med. Exp. Biol. Fenn., 46:177–178, 1968.

252. Bajpayee, D.P.: Significance of plasma copper and caeruloplasmin concentrations in rheumatoid arthritis. Ann. Rheum. Dis., 34:162–165, 1975.

253. Aaseth, J., et al.: Trace elements in serum and urine of patients with rheumatoid arthritis. Scand. J. Rheumatol., 7:237–240, 1978.

254. Plantin, L.O., and Strandberg, P.O.: Whole-blood concentrations of copper and zinc in rheumatoid arthritis studied by activation analysis. Acta Rheumatol. Scand., 11:30–34, 1965.

255. Balogh, Z., et al.: Plasma zinc and its relationship to clinical symptoms and drug treatment in rheumatoid arthritis. Ann. Rheum. Dis., 38:329–332, 1980.

256. Niedermeier, W., and Griggs, J.H.: Trace metal composition of synovial fluid and blood serum of patients with rheumatoid arthritis. J. Chronic Dis., 23:527–536, 1971.

257. Henrotte, J.G., et al.: Modification des taux du fer sérique et du magnésium érythrocytaire au cours des rhumatismes inflammatoires chroniques. Life Sci., 9:609–612, 1970.

258. Hill, S.R., Jr., et al.: Studies on adrenal cortical activity in patients with rheumatoid arthritis: The diurnal pattern and twenty-four hour levels of urinary total 17-hydroxycorticosteroids and 17-ketosteroids. Arthritis Rheum., 2:114–126, 1959.

259. Stuart, F.S., et al.: Steroid biosynthetic and catabolic pathways in rheumatoid and non-rheumatoid chronic disease states. Clin. Res., 10:237, 1962.

260. Fruehan, A.E., and Frawley, T.F.: Adrenal medullary function in the connective tissue disorders. Arthritis Rheum., 6:698–710, 1963.

261. Smyth, C.J., and Staub, A.: Catecholamine excretion in patients with rheumatoid arthritis. Arthritis Rheum., 7:687–692, 1964.

262. Grayzel, A.I., Liddle, L., and Seegmiller, J.E.: Diagnostic significance of hyperuricemia in arthritis. N. Engl. J. Med., 265:763–768, 1961.

263. Weaver, W.F., and Smyth, C.J.: Serum urate in degenerative joint disease and rheumatoid arthritis. Arthritis Rheum., 6:372–376, 1963.

264. London, M.G., Muirden, K.D., and Hewitt, J.V.: Serum cholesterol in rheumatic diseases. Br. Med. J., 1:1380–1383, 1963.

265. Block, W.D., Buchanan, O.H., and Freyberg, R.H.: Serum lipids in patients with rheumatoid arthritis and in patients with obstructive jaundice. Arch. Intern. Med., 68:18–24, 1941.

266. Kelly, H.G., Hill, J.G., and Boyd, E.M.: The absence of effect of cortisone therapy upon plasma lipid levels in patients with rheumatoid arthritis. Can. Med. Assoc. J., 70:660–662, 1954.

267. Haataja, M., et al.: Prostaglandin precursors in rheumatoid arthritis. J. Rheumatol., 9:91–93, 1982.

268. Hagenfeldt, L., and Wennmalm, A.: Turnover of a prostaglandin precursor, arachidonic acid, in rheumatoid arthritis. Eur. J. Clin. Invest., 5:235–239, 1975.

269. Haataja, M.: Evaluation of the activity of rheumatoid arthritis. A comparative study on clinical symptoms and laboratory tests with special reference to serum sulfhydryl groups. Scand. J. Rheumatol., 7(Suppl.):1–54, 1975.

270. Lorber, A., et al.: Serum sulfhydryl determinations and significance in connective tissue diseases. Ann. Intern. Med., 61:423–434, 1964.

271. Woolf, A.D., et al.: Predictors of five-year outcome of early synovitis. Br. J. Rheumatol., 25(Suppl. 2):23–24, 1986 (abstract).

272. Rice, E.W.: Evaluation of the role of ceruloplasmin as an acute-phase reactant. Clin. Chim. Acta, 6:652–655, 1961.

273. Sullivan, J.F., and Hart, K.T.: Serum benzidine oxidase. J. Lab. Clin. Med., 55:260–267, 1960.

274. Gerber, D.A.: Increased copper ligand reactivity in the urine of patients with rheumatoid arthritis. Arthritis Rheum., 9:795–803, 1966.

275. Gerber, D.A.: Low free serum histidine concentration in rheumatoid arthritis. A measure of disease activity. J. Clin. Invest., 55:1164–1173, 1975.

276. Györki, J., and Sandell, B.-M.: Adenosine triphosphatase activity in blood in rheumatoid arthritis. Acta. Rheumatol. Scand., 7:127–130, 1961.

277. Vesell, E.S., et al.: Isozymes of lactic dehydrogenase; their alterations in arthritic synovial fluid and sera. J. Clin. Invest., 41:2012–2019, 1962.

278. Hammarsten, G., et al.: Choline esterase activity in rheumatoid arthritis. Acta Rheumatol. Scand., 5:42–48, 1959.

279. Briseid, K., Dyrud, O., and Rinvik, S.: Determination of plasma kininogen plasma kininase and erythrocyte kininase in men with rheumatoid arthritis. Acta Pharmacol., 24:179–182, 1966.

280. Anderson, R.B., and Winther, O.: Blood-fibrinolysis and activity of rheumatoid arthritis. Acta Rheumatol. Scand., 15:178–184, 1969.

281. Nordemar, R., et al.: Muscle ATP content in rheumatoid arthritis—a biopsy study. Scand. J. Clin. Lab. Invest., 34:185–191, 1974.

282. Marks, J., Birkett, D.A., and Shuster, S.: "Capillary permeability" in patients with collagen vascular disease. Br. Med. J., 1:782–784, 1972.

283. Forster, J.E., and Engleman, E.P.: The effect of adrenal corticosteroid therapy on blood ascorbic acid levels in rheumatoid arthritis. Arthritis Rheum., 4:418, 1961.

284. Sahud, M.A., and Cohen, R.J.: Effect of aspirin ingestion on ascorbic-acid levels in rheumatoid arthritis. Lancet, 1:937–938, 1971.

285. Todesco, S.: Retinol-binding protein in rheumatoid arthritis. Arthritis Rheum., 24:105–106, 1981.

286. Barton-Wright, E.C., and Elliot, W.A.: The pathogenic acid metabolism of rheumatoid arthritis. Lancet, 2:862–863, 1963.

287. Kalliomaki, J.L., Laine, V.A., and Markkanen, T.K.: Urinary excretion of thiamine, riboflavin, nicotinic acid, and pantothenic acid in patients with rheumatoid arthritis. Acta Med. Scand., 166:275–279, 1960.

288. Carr, D.T., and McGuckin, W.F.: Pleural fluid glucose. Serial observation of its concentration following oral administration of glucose to patients with rheumatoid pleural effusions and malignant effusions. Am. Rev. Respir. Dis., 97:302–305, 1968.

289. Alter, H.J., Zvaifler, N.J., and Rath, C.E.: Interrelationship of rheumatoid arthritis, folic acid, and aspirin. Blood, 38:405–416, 1971.

290. McKusick, A.B., et al.: Urinary excretion of pyridoxine and 4-pyridoxic acid in rheumatoid arthritis. Arthritis Rheum., 7:636–653, 1964.

291. Sanderson, C.R., Davis, R.E., and Bayliss, C.E.: Serum pyridoxal in patients with rheumatoid arthritis. Ann. Rheum. Dis., 35:177–180, 1976.

292. Igarai, T., et al.: Serum vitamin B_{12} levels of patients with rheumatoid arthritis. Tohoku J. Exp. Med., 125:287–301, 1978.

293. Daughety, J.S., Baum, J., and Krusen, U.: Electromyography in the connective tissue diseases: Preliminary report. Arch. Phys. Med. Rehabil., 45:224–230, 1964.

294. Graudal, H., and Hvid, N.: An electromyographic study on patients with arthritis. Acta Rheumatol. Scand., 5:34–41, 1959.

295. Steinberg, V.L., and Wynn Parry, C.B.: Electromyographic changes in rheumatoid arthritis. Br. Med. J., 1:630–632, 1961.

296. Wramner, T.: Electromyographic studies on the effect of neostigmine in rheumatoid arthritis. Acta Med. Scand., 242(Suppl.):18–23, 1950.

297. Amick, L.D.: Muscle atrophy in rheumatoid arthritis: An electrodiagnostic study. Arthritis Rheum., 3:54–63, 1960.

298. Mueller, E.E., and Mead, S.: The electromyogram in rheumatoid arthritis. Am. J. Phys. Med., 31:67–73, 1952.

299. Yates, D.A.H.: Muscular changes in rheumatoid arthritis. Ann. Rheum. Dis., 22:342–347, 1963.

300. Wells, R.M., and Johnson, E.W.: Study of conduction delay im median nerve of patients with rheumatoid arthritis. Arch. Phys. Med., 43:244–248, 1962.

301. Carr, D.T., and Mayne, J.G.: Pleurisy with effusion in rheumatoid arthritis, with reference to the low concentration of glucose in pleural fluid. Am. Rev. Respir. Dis., 85:345–350, 1962.

302. Schools, G.S., and Mikkelsen, W.M.: Rheumatoid pleuritis. Arthritis Rheum., 5:369–377, 1962.

303. Dodson, W.H., and Hollingsworth, J.W.: Pleural effusion in rheumatoid arthritis. Impaired transport of glucose. N. Engl. J. Med., 275:1337–1342, 1966.

304. Glovsky, M.M., et al.: Reduction of pleural fluid complement activity in patients with systemic lupus erythematosus and rheumatoid arthritis. Clin. Immunol. Immunopathol., 6:31–41, 1976.

305. Vemireddi, N.K., Redford, J.B., and PombeJara, C.N.: Serial nerve conduction studies in carpal tunnel syndrome secondary to rheumatoid arthritis: Preliminary study. Arch. Phys. Med. Rehabil., 60:393–396, 1979.

46

RHEUMATOID FACTORS

MART MANNIK

The term rheumatoid factor evolved from the observations of Waaler and Rose, who noted that a high proportion of serums from patients with rheumatoid arthritis (RA) agglutinated sheep erythrocytes sensitized with rabbit antibodies to erythrocytes as reviewed elsewhere.[1] Since then, the antibody nature of these factors has been proved, but the term "rheumatoid factors" (RF) has been retained. *Rheumatoid factors are now defined as antibodies specific to antigenic determinants on the Fc fragments of human or animal immunoglobulin G.* A number of antibodies to other antigenic determinants on immunoglobulins are known and are collectively referred to as the family of antiglobulins. These antiglobulins include antibodies specific to IgG digested by pepsin or by other enzymes; to idiotypes; to light chains; and to IgA, IgM, and IgE. However, these antiglobulins are not considered rheumatoid factors because they are not directed to antigenic determinants on the Fc fragments of IgG.

Rheumatoid factors commonly exist in the three major classes of immunoglobulins and possess specificities to several antigenic determinants. The general concepts of antibody structure and function (see Chapter 17) apply to rheumatoid factors and therefore are not considered in this chapter. Seropositivity of patients with RA or with other diseases is usually defined by the latex fixation test or red cell agglutination tests. These assays primarily reflect the presence of IgM rheumatoid factors (IgM-RFs). The presence of rheumatoid factors is not unique to RA, and a positive test for these antibodies should not be used as the sole criterion for the diagnosis of RA.

SPECIFICITY OF RHEUMATOID FACTORS

Like any other antibodies, rheumatoid factors have specificity to defined antigenic determinants, some of which are identified on human and animal IgG molecules. Serologic and biochemical studies on human IgG have identified some antigenic determinants for IgM-RFs and IgG-RFs. These determinants may be either genetic or nongenetic. The genetic determinants on Fc fragments are the Gm antigens of IgG or closely related antigens. The nongenetic determinants exist on certain subclasses of IgG in all persons. Thus, in a given patient, IgM-RFs may react with autologous IgG on the basis of genetic or nongenetic antigenic determinants. Finally, specificity of IgM-RFs to denatured or aggregated IgG has been considered, but the issue remains controversial.

In patients with RA, IgM-RFs exist with specificity to Gm(a) also called Gm1, and to a number of other Gm antigenic determinants. The specificities of other IgM-RFs were defined to the so-called "nonmarkers," which are antigenic determinants absent from IgG molecules with a given Gm antigen, but present in other IgG molecules of the same subclass of IgG, as well as in some of the other subclasses of IgG. For example, the antigenic determinant "non-a" is absent from Gm(a)-positive IgG1 molecules, but present on IgG1 molecules positive for GM(f), also called Gm4, as well as on IgG2 and IgG3 molecules.[2] Furthermore, some rheumatoid factors are specific to antigens common to several subclasses of IgG, regardless of genetic types. One particular antigenic determinant of this type is called the Ga antigen,[3] which constitutes a frequent antigenic determinant for IgM-RFs. This particular antigenic determinant, or one closely related to it, has now been defined in structural detail as described below. The location of some antigenic determinants on the Fc fragments of IgG subclasses is schematically depicted in Figure 46–1.

For several tested IgM-RFs and few IgG-RFs the antigenic determinants are not present on separated Cγ2 and Cγ3 domains of IgG, but require the intact Fc fragments. Furthermore, the binding of the tested IgG-RFs and some IgM-RFs to IgG was blocked by fragment D of staphylococcal protein A (SPA). Chemical modifications of histidines and tyrosines on human IgG also decreased the binding of these RFs as compared with unaltered normal IgG. The same RFs also interacted poorly with IgG3 subclass molecules similar to SPA. All these findings argue that a common antigenic determinant for RFs was the same area on IgG that interacts with SPA.[4,5] From crystallo-

graphic studies this is the cleft between the Cγ2 and Cγ3 domains and involved two amino acid sequences from Cγ2 and one amino acid sequence from Cγ3 domain.[6] This site corresponds to the subclass specificity of the Ga antigen defined serologically some time ago.[3] The complexity of antigenic determinants for RFs is not yet fully defined. Ongoing studies with monoclonal RFs from patients with essential mixed cryoglobulinemia has shown heterogeneity. Similar findings are evident in a study of polyclonal RFs from patients with RA and from patients with other disorders accompanied by the presence of RFs.[5] It remains to be established if RFs with different specificities relate to different diseases or disease outcome. The finding that SPA and other viral and bacterial proteins bind to the same area of IgG molecules as some RFs remains unexplained.[4,7–9] This finding, however, has raised the testable hypothesis that some RFs may arise as auto-anti-idiotypic antibodies secondary to an immune response to the Fc-binding viral or bacterial proteins through the internal image concept.[7,10]

Because IgM-RFs react better with aggregated IgG or with immune complexes than with monomeric IgG in agglutinating or precipitating test systems, the question of unique antigenic determinants on aggregated IgG or on immune complexes containing IgG has been raised. Monomeric IgG molecules with appropriate antigenic determinants react with IgM-RFs, but with low association constants. The best explanation for the increased reactivity of aggregated IgG or of immune complexes containing IgG is the polyvalency of the molecular aggregates with respect to IgM-RFs.

As already mentioned, the antigenic determinants for IgG-RFs have been examined only for two isolates. In both instances the IgG-RFs reacted with human and rabbit IgG, but not with fragments representing the Cγ2 and Cγ3 domains. Chemical modifications and other studies, as mentioned previously, identified the site between Cγ2 and Cγ3 domains, which also binds SPA.[7,12] The specificity of this site corresponds to the Ga antigenic determinant first identified for IgM-RFs.

The specificity of one rheumatoid factor of the immunoglobulin A class (IgA-RF) from a patient with hypergammaglobulinemic purpura is known. Because this monoclonal IgA-RF reacts with the IgG1, IgG2, and IgG4 subclasses, the antigenic determinant may well be the Ga antigen. Some rheumatoid factors that clearly react with the Fc fragments of human IgG also cross-react with DNA-histone. The immunochemical basis of this cross-reactivity remains to be determined.

FIG. 46–1. Schematic representation of antigenic determinants for RFs on the Fc fragments of human IgG subclasses. The Cγ2 and Cγ3 domains constitute the Fc fragments and the three-dimensional folding of these molecules is known. The Ga antigen for RFs on IgG1, IgG2, and IgG4 involves the same area and some of the same amino acids that bind staphylococcal protein A. This antigenic determinant consists of two amino acid sequences from the Cγ2 domain and one amino acid sequence from the Cγ3 domain, brought together into a relatively small surface area by folding of the molecule. For simplicity of representation the Ga antigen is depicted at the junction of the two domains even though the involved amino acids are not at this location in the amino acid sequence. The Gm(a)- (also called Gm1)-positive IgG1 molecules do not possess the "non-a" antigenic determinant, whereas the Gm(f)- (also called Gm4)-positive IgG1 molecules have the "non-a" antigenic determinant. Similarly, Gm(g)- (also called Gm21)-positive IgG3 molecules have the "non-b'" antigenic determinant, whereas the Gm (b')-positive IgG3 molecules lack this antigenic determinant. (Modified from Natvig, J.B., et al.[11])

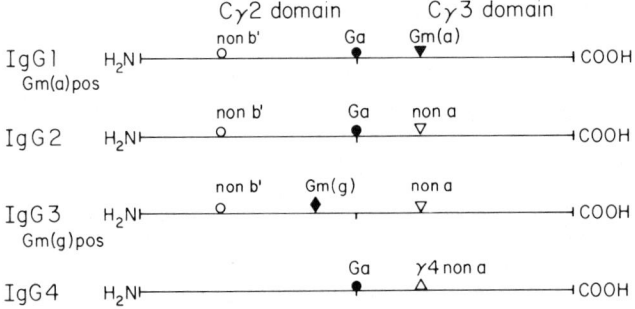

IDIOTYPES ON RHEUMATOID FACTORS

Idiotypes are antigenic determinants on the variable regions of the light and heavy chains of antibody molecules. Antibodies with a given specificity may have the same idiotypes among individuals and hence are called cross-reactive idiotypes or public idiotypes, implying common structural features on these antibody molecules. On the other hand, some idiotypes on antibodies with the same specificity vary from individual to individual and hence are called private idiotypes, implying unique structural features on each individual's antibodies with a given specificity. Specific antibodies to idiotypes can be obtained by immunizing another species with isolated antibodies yielding xenogenic anti-idiotypes. Furthermore, auto-anti-idiotypic antibodies develop during the course of a normal immune response. These auto-anti-idiotypic antibodies are thought to contribute to the regulation of the amount of antibody synthesized specific to a given antigen according to the network theory of Jerne.[13–15] Idiotypes on RFs have been extensively studied to clarify the heterogeneity of these antibody molecules, to understand the genesis of this heterogeneity, and possibly to develop alternative detection methods for RFs if public idiotypes are common.

The use of monoclonal rheumatoid factors from patients with cryoglobulinemia identified three cross-reactive idiotypes, termed Wa, Po, and Bla among these proteins.[16,17] A mouse monoclonal antibody (17.109) to a Wa group monoclonal IgM-RF was developed that reacted with kappa (κ) chains from other IgM-RFs and not with IgM proteins without RF activity.[18] Since common amino acid sequences were identified in the second and third hypervariable regions (complementarity-determining regions) of monoclonal IgM-RFs, synthetic peptides corresponding to these sequences were prepared and used to develop antibodies to these amino acid sequences. These antibodies detected apparent cross-reactive idiotypes (PSL2-CRI and PSL3-CRI), related to the Wa idiotype, on abut 80% of monoclonal RFs, and this idiotype was identified on the κ light chains of monoclonal IgM-RFs.[19] Recent studies, however, indicated that some of these antibodies to the second complementarity-determining region of κ light chains are directed to an antigen common among several monoclonal IgM-RFs and not unique to the previously identified Wa idiotype.[20] In addition, antibodies to a synthetic peptide corresponding to the third hypervariable region of the heavy chain of monoclonal IgM-RFs reacted with some monoclonal IgM-RFs, suggesting the presence of an immunodominant idiotype on mu (μ) chains.[21] These studies with monoclonal IgM-RFs suggested that a limited number of genes encoded the synthesis of monoclonal RFs. Proof has now been presented that this prediction was correct. Human B-cell hybridoma products were identified to contain the cross-reactive idiotype 17.109 present on monoclonal IgM-RFs, and this was associated with a single V_K gene or small family of closely related V_K genes.[22] Of considerable interest was that three probes specific for idiotypes on monoclonal IgM-RF were used to examine the prevalence of these idiotypes on RFs from patients with RA, Sjögren's syndrome, and apparently normal older persons with positive tests for RF. These idiotypes were found most frequently in patients with primary Sjögren's syndrome and least frequently in patients with RA.[23] These results raised the possibility that RFs in patients with RA differed from monoclonal RFs and from RFs in patients wth Sjögren's syndrome. Furthermore, using antibodies made in rabbits to individual, isolated RFs from patients with RA demonstrated the presence of cross-reactive idiotypes in a panel of serums from patients with RA.[24] These investigations, however, demonstrated that relatively small amounts of RFs accounted for this cross-reactivity. These findings suggested that patients with RA have RFs with different idiotypes and that the RFs as defined by idiotypes vary from patient to patient.

The study of idiotypes and variable region genes of human monoclonal IgM-RFs has indicated the involvement of restricted genes in the genesis of these antibodies. The same questions for polyclonal RFs in patients with RA have not yet been answered.

Interesting concepts have evolved from the study of IgM-RFs in mice. The nucleotide sequence was determined for light and heavy chains of 10 different clones of IgM-RF and translated into amino acid sequences. These RFs all bound mouse IgG1. Three families of V_K light chains were represented in these RFs but all other variable region genes were represented at random.[25] The authors argued that the κ light chains provide the amino acid sequences for specific binding to IgG1. The high homology in these κ chains was not in the complementarity-determining region but in certain framework regions of the molecule. These findings suggested to the authors that not the antigen-combining site but another surface area of IgM-RFs may be involved in the interaction with the Fc region of IgG. This is a novel concept and merits further study. In contrast, in another investigation of 20 mouse clones producing RFs with variable specificities to subclasses of mouse IgG, a restricted set of heavy chain variable region genes was identified for RF production.[26]

Thus, recent investigations of the structure of RFs,

idiotypes on RFs, and genes involved in the synthesis of these molecules have begun a new era in inquiry of RFs. Hopefully these studies on RFs in patients with RA will culminate in understanding of how the heterogeneity of RFs is generated both on the molecular and gene level.

INTERACTIONS BETWEEN RHEUMATOID FACTORS AND THEIR ANTIGENS

On a structural basis, the valence of IgM-RFs for IgG molecules should be 10 because each of the five subunits of IgM molecules possesses two binding sites (two pairs of one μ and one light chain). On analytic ultracentrifugation, however, the valence of IgM-RFs for interaction with IgG is 5, and the valence of each IgM subunit is 1. On the other hand, the Fab fragments obtained from purified IgM-RFs have antibody activity and a valence of 1.[27,28] Therefore, in each of the five subunits of these molecules, one antibody-combining site must be sterically hindered from combining with an IgG molecule. The reasons for this phenomenon are not known. The functional antigenic valence of IgG molecules for interaction with IgM-RF is 1.

The association constants for the interaction of IgM-RFs and monomeric IgG are around 10^5 L/mole.[29] Similar values exist for the interaction of IgM-RFs with specificities to known antigenic determinants on the Cγ3 domain (see Fig. 46–1), when examined with the isolated portions of IgG molecules.[30] Furthermore, the interactions of IgG myeloma proteins of several subclasses with IgM-RFs show comparable association constants for IgG1, IgG2, and IgG4, but no reaction occurs with IgG3 myeloma proteins,[31] suggesting the specificity of the used RFs is to the Ga antigen (see Fig. 46–1). The interactions of IgM-RFs with the antigenic determinants on Fc fragments of IgG are therefore weak antigen-antibody bonds.

A series of experiments has elucidated the reasons for enhanced agglutination and precipitation of IgM-RFs with aggregated IgG. First, the Fab fragments derived from IgM-RFs bind to monomeric and to heat-aggregated IgG with comparable association constants; this finding indicates that the aggregated IgG does not contain "new and better" antigen determinants. Second, the intact IgM-RFs bind to aggregated IgG about 10^6 times more effectively than the Fab fragments from IgM-RFs.[32] These findings support the concept that the enhanced agglutination and precipitation of IgM-RFs with aggregated or polymerized IgG is due to the polyvalency of the IgG and not to

the generation of new antigenic determinants on aggregated IgG molecules.

Because patients with RA may have abundant IgM-RFs reactive with autologous IgG, they may have demonstrable antigen-antibody complexes formed by these reactants.[33] These complexes sediment on analytic ultracentrifugation with 22 Svedberg units (S) and are termed 22S complexes (Figs. 46–2 and 46–3). In this interaction, each IgM-RF molecule has a valence of 5, and IgG has a valence of 1. Therefore, each IgM-RF molecule can maximally bind five IgG molecules. In the serum of patients with RA, however, the 22S complex may not contain five IgG molecules because, with the binding of five IgG molecules to one IgM-RF, the sedimentation constant would be much higher.[34] The 22S complexes usually occur in patients with high titers of IgM-RFs, but a pathogenic role for these complexes is not established.

The valence of IgG-RFs is 2 for interaction with normal IgG molecules.[35,36] On analytic ultracentrifugation, the serum of some patients with RA shows detectable quantities of the so-called *intermediate complexes* (see Fig. 46–2), sedimenting between the 7 and 19S components of normal serum, as first demonstrated by Kunkel et al.[37] These immune complexes

FIG. 46–2. Schlieren optical patterns of serum from a patient with rheumatoid arthritis on sedimentation velocity ultracentrifugation, illustrating the 22S and intermediate complexes. The serum was diluted 1:3 in top pattern at neutral pH (0.05 *M* phosphate, 0.15 *M* NaCl, pH 7.3) and 1:3 in bottom pattern at acid pH (0.05 *M* acetate, 0.15 *M* NaCl, pH 3.5). The photographs were taken 24 minutes after reaching 52,000 rpm. At neutral pH in the top pattern, 22S complexes and intermediate complexes (I.C.) are present. At acid pH in the bottom pattern, both immune complexes are dissociated, and the 19 and 6.6S peaks have increased.

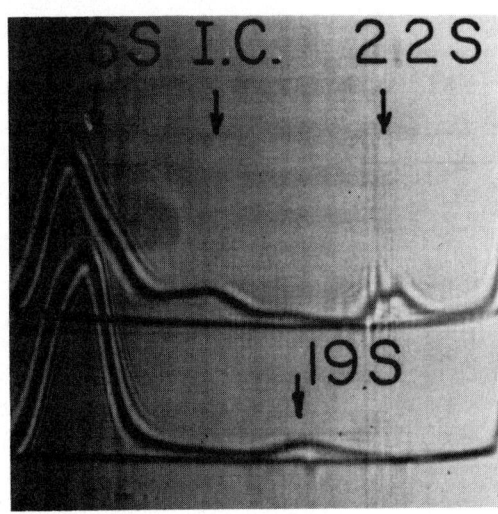

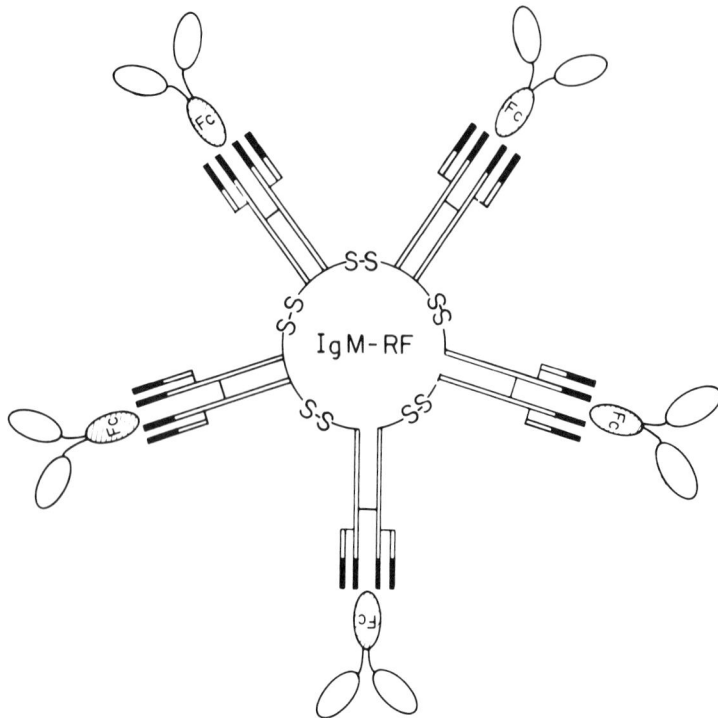

FIG. 46–3. Schematic representation of the 22S immune complex between an IgM-rheumatoid factor (IgM-RF) molecule and IgG molecules. Each IgM-RF reacts maximally with five IgG molecules, as depicted. The complexes that exist in serum most likely contain fewer than five IgG molecules. The shown position of IgG molecules does not imply an antigenic determinant at the end of the Fc fragments.

contain IgG-RFs. Comparable and larger immune complexes exist in the synovial fluids of patients with RA. The isolated IgG-RFs self-associate and form stable dimers of two IgG-RFs, provided the antibody specificity of these molecules is directed to antigenic determinants present on the same molecules.[35,36] In this dimer formation, the antibody-combining sites of each IgG-RF molecule react with the Fc fragment of the other IgG-RF molecule, thus forming two antigen-antibody bonds per dimer (Fig. 46–4). At the same time, two antibody-combining sites remain free, and antigenic determinants must be available in each dimer to allow the observed, further-concentration-dependent aggregation of the dimers, forming tetramers, octamers, and higher polymers (see Fig. 46–4) of the IgG-RFs.[35,36]

The valence of normal IgG for interaction with IgG-RF is 1, even though the valence of the Fc fragments from normal IgG or from IgG-RF is 2, as expected from the presence of two polypeptide chains. Therefore, the second antigenic determinant in intact normal IgG is not available for interaction with IgG-RF, presumably because of distortion of the molecule caused by the interaction with IgG-RF.[12] In the *self-association* of IgG-RFs, the antigenic valence of the molecules has not been examined directly, but it must be 2 because the self-association would otherwise terminate at dimer formation and would not proceed to the formation of higher polymers.

The association constant for the interaction of IgG-RFs with normal IgG, with normal Fc fragments, and with Fc fragments derived from IgG-RF, is about 10^5 L/mole.[12,36] The association constant for dimer formation of self-associating IGg-RF has not been measured directly, but by calculation it is 10^{10} L/mole.[35] This value is probably too high because energy is lost in the ring closure of dimer formation. The observed stability of the dimers is based on this high association constant and, as stated previously, unique antigenic determinants do not exist on the Fc fragments of IgG-RF. The observed association constant for further polymer formation from the IgG-RF dimers is about 10^5 L/mole.[36] The self-associating IgG-RFs thus constitute unique antibodies in that immune complexes are formed without a separate antigen molecule because these antibodies fulfill the functions both of an antibody and of an antigen.

As already discussed, the antigenic valence of normal IgG is 1 for the interaction with IgG-RFs. Therefore, the presence of large amounts of normal IgG in serum would terminate further polymer formation of self-associating IgG-RFs. In this termination, two normal IgG molecules interact with one IgG-RF dimer (see Fig. 46–4B). This reaction is consistent with the finding of intermediate complexes in serum (see Fig. 46–2). In synovial fluids of patients with RA, larger complexes exist.[38,39] Furthermore, plasma cells in synovial tissue synthesize IgG-RFs,[40,41] and in the immediate vicinity of these cells, the concentration of IgG-RFs may be even higher than in synovial fluid.

FIG. 46–4. Schematic representation of the self-association and further polymerization of IgG rheumatoid factors (IgG-RF). *A,* The formation of IgG-RF dimers is depicted. These dimers undergo concentration-dependent polymerization to tetramers, octamers, and higher polymers, owing to free antigenic determinants and free antibody-combining sites. *B,* The interaction of normal IgG molecules with the self-associated IgG-RF dimers is depicted. The dimers are stable in the presence of excess normal IgG because two antigen-antibody bonds are formed in dimerization. Because the association constants for further polymerization are comparable to the association constant for normal IgG binding to one antibody-combining site, the presence of excess normal IgG terminates the further polymerization of the dimers, particularly because normal IgG is monovalent for interaction with IgG-RFs.

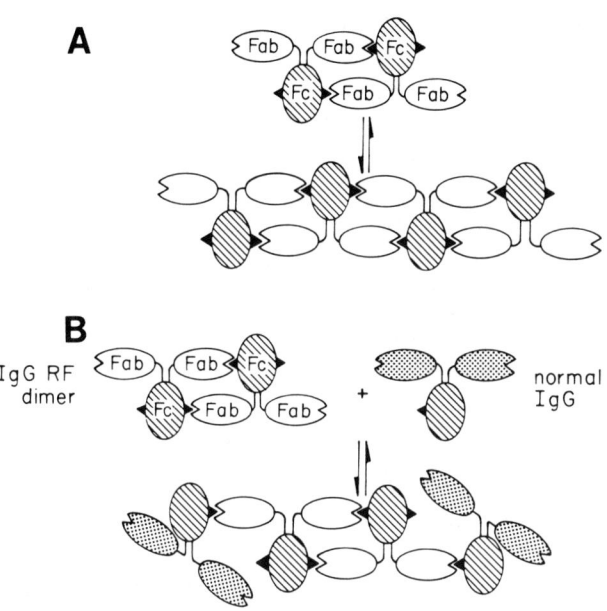

Isolated IgG-RFs precipitate from solution when concentrated at neutral pH beyond about 1.0 to 1.5 mg/ml.[35,42] Finally, the self-association of IgG-RFs occurs in the plasma cells in synovial tissues because the cytoplasm of these plasma cells binds human complement components.[40]

IgG-RFs are synthesized in the synovial tissue of patients with RA,[40,41] and no exogenous antigens can be identified in the immune complexes in synovial fluids of patients with this disease.[39,43,44] Thus, the self-associated IgG-RFs may contribute to the synovitis of RA. The MRL/1 mice that develop a synovitis similar to that of RA also have self-associating IgG-RFs in their circulation[45] (see Chapter 30).

The interactions of IgA-RFs with IgG have not been examined extensively, but detailed studies of a monoclonal IgA-RF show an association constant of 1.6×10^6 L/mole.[46]

BIOLOGIC PROPERTIES OF RHEUMATOID FACTORS

The high prevalence of rheumatoid factors in many chronic infections and in aging normal persons raises the question of the central role of these antibodies. Answers to this question have been sought by studies on activation of complement systems, generation of chemotaxis, promotion of phagocytosis, and interaction with cell receptors by rheumatoid factors.

The evaluation of biologic properties of IgM-RFs has been difficult because IgG, as antigen for these antibodies, possesses its own biologic properties, particularly when aggregated nonspecifically or when complexed with antigen to serve as a polyvalent antigen for IgM-RFs. Experiments have shown, however, that IgM-RFs activate complement. Heat-aggregated human IgG, prepared from reduced and alkylated preparations, does not fix human complement, but is an effective polyvalent antigen for IgM-RFs. When IgM-RFs are added to these aggregates, human complement is then consumed. The addition of IgM-RFs to sheep erythrocytes, sparsely sensitized with rabbit IgG antibodies, enhances complement fixation and cell lysis. Furthermore, the addition of IgM-RFs to soluble immune complexes containing IgG enhances complement fixation by these materials. Finally, red blood cells coated with aggregated human IgG, prepared from reduced and alkylated IgG or sensitized with reduced and alkylated rabbit antibodies, are lysed by the addition of IgM-RFs and human complement.[47] All these studies indicate that IgM-RFs can activate the classic complement pathway. Complement activation, in turn, explains the enhanced chemotaxis when IgM-RFs are added to aggregated IgG or to antigen-antibody complexes.

On interaction with antigen on the surface of erythrocytes, IgG-RFs activate human complement, but less efficiently than IgM-RFs in a similar system.[48] In addition, self-associating IgG-RFs in fluid phase also activate human complement, but less efficiently than other immune complexes.[49] IgG-RF-containing immune complexes from the synovial fluid of patients bind C1q and activate complement.[43] Thus, the available evidence indicates that IgG-RFs and self-associating IgG-RFs can activate complement and may thus contribute to the synovitis of RA.

The binding of IgM-RFs to immune complexes containing IgG molecules may diminish the interaction of these complexes with Fc receptors on phagocytic cells. Similarly, the binding of IgM-RFs to cells sensitized with IgG molecules may decrease the binding of these cells to phagocytes because phagocytes do not possess IgM receptors. For example, the addition of IgM-RFs to bacteria coated with an IgG class of antibodies decreases phagocytosis of these bacteria by polymorphonuclear leukocytes in the absence of complement.[50] By a comparable mechanism, IgM-RFs have blocked the killing of target cells sensitized with the IgG class of antibodies by antibody-dependent, cell-mediated cytotoxicity (ADCC). In this study, the IgM-RFs bound to the IgG molecules on target cells abrogated the reaction of IgG molecules with the Fc receptor on the killer cells.[51]

The pathophysiologic significance of some of these reactions remains uncertain. The inhibition of phagocytosis of antibody-coated bacteria by IgM-RFs may predispose patients to bacterial infections. On the other hand, the addition of IgM-RFs to antibody-coated viral particles in the presence of complement enhances the neutralization of viruses.[52]

The self-associated IgG-RFs interact with human monocytes and enhance the release of prostaglandins and a mononuclear cell factor (see Chapter 42). This factor, thought to be identical to interleukin-1, in turn acts on synovial cells in culture to increase the release of prostaglandins and collagenase.[53] Thus, these unique antibodies can contribute to the inflammatory and destructive events in synovitis. This process is likely to occur in the synovial tissue in which these antibodies are released from plasma cells and self-associate into large polymers or precipitates because of the low ambient concentration of normal IgG. In contrast, the self-association if IgG-RFs may be harmless in the plasma because the formation of high polymers is terminated by normal IgG, as explained in the preceding section. Finally, the self-associated IgG-RFs may serve as a polyvalent ligand for IgM-RFs and may thus contribute further to the inflammatory process in rheumatoid synovitis.

DETECTION OF RHEUMATOID FACTORS

Many methods have been proposed for the detection of rheumatoid factors, but few are widely employed. The purpose of this section is to consider the general principles of these methods and to discuss the nature of the rheumatoid factors detected by some of the available techniques. The details of the various methods can be found in the original articles or in works concerned with the conduct of these tests.[1,54]

The most widely used methods for detection of rheumatoid factors rely on agglutination or flocculation of IgG-coated cells or particles as the end point of the test procedure. Owing to the polyvalence of IgM-RFs, these tests emphasize the presence of IgM-RFs.

The latex test is the most common method for detection of rheumatoid factors. The bentonite flocculation test, the sensitized sheep cell test, and the sensitized human-D-cell agglutination test have been popular in certain centers. The latex test and the bentonite flocculation test use human IgG for sensitization of the test particles. For optimal results, the IgG preparations, usually Cohn fraction II, must contain some aggregated material. The coated test particles are then agglutinated or flocculated when they are linked together by IgM-RFs. The positivity of the result is expressed as a titer, following twofold serial dilution of the tested serum. As with any agglutination test, the end point can be approximated reliably only within a dilution above or below the observed end point. Therefore, these tests are not truly quantitative. Because of the use of pooled IgG, IgM-RFs of many specificities are measured. Furthermore, these tests are often not standardized from laboratory to laboratory, even though the possibilities of standardization have been debated.[55,56] Variations in the size and characteristics of latex particles cause the test results to vary. Another variable in the test system is the degree of aggregation of IgG among Cohn fraction II preparations. Low titers or false positivity results if the tested serum is not heat inactivated because C1q may cause agglutination of sensitized or unsensitized particles.

The sensitized sheep cell agglutination test for rheumatoid factors is based on the interaction of rheumatoid factors with rabbit IgG on the red blood cell. The erythrocytes are sensitized with subagglutinating doses of the rabbit antiserum to sheep erythrocytes. Heterophile antibodies must be removed from the test serum prior to testing for rheumatoid factors. This test is less sensitive than the latex and bentonite flocculation tests for rheumatoid factors but it is more specific for RA. This test detects primarily IgM-RF, for reasons already mentioned, and does not detect rheumatoid factors specific only to antigenic determinants of human IgG.

The sensitized human-D-cell agglutination test requires human red cells, preferably homozygous D cells, and carefully selected human antibodies to D cells. This test detects IgM-RFs that react with human IgG. The selection of the human serum with antibodies to D cells is critical. When antibodies to D cells are limited to a subclass of IgG (see Fig. 46–1), rheumatoid factors with limited specificity may be detected by this method.

None of the foregoing tests for rheumatoid factors are standardized among clinical laboratories. Many additional variations and modifications of these tests have been proposed. The reader interested in these tests should consult the section on rheumatoid factors in the "Rheumatism Reviews," published every 2 years in the journal *Arthritis and Rheumatism.*

In some patients with RA, the routine agglutination tests for rheumatoid factors are negative because of firm binding of autologous IgG to the IgM-RFs. When such serum is submitted to gel filtration under mildly acidic conditions (pH 4.0) to dissociate the IgM-RFs from IgG, rheumatoid factor activity is found in the IgM-containing fractions.[3] Because rheumatoid factor is not detected in unseparated serum, the term *hidden rheumatoid factor* was coined. IgM-RFs are thus detected in some seronegative adults with RA and in some seronegative children with juvenile RA.

IgM-RFs can also be detected and quantified by nephelometric methods. The real advantages are that quantitative information is obtained and the assay is quickly completed and can be automated. This approach, however, has not yet replaced the agglutination tests.

To detect and to quantify rheumatoid factors in the major classes of immunoglobulins, that is, IgG-RFs, IgM-RFs, and IgA-RFs, several solid-phase assays have been developed and tried. The basic principles of all these methods are comparable. IgG of human or animal origin is adsorbed to a test tube, is covalently linked to a solid matrix, or is solidified by chemical cross-linking. The adsorption to test tubes or microtiter plates is most frequently employed. Once the solid-phase IgG is prepared and washed, test serum is incubated with it to allow binding of all rheumatoid factors. Thereafter, the solid-phase test system is washed to remove all unbound serum proteins. The bound rheumatoid factors are then quantified by the addition of specific antiserums to IgG, IgM, or IgA, to measure the presence of IgG-RFs, IgM-RFs, or IgA-RFs, respectively. The quantitation can be accomplished by several approaches, such as by employing radiolabeled specific antibodies (radioimmunoassay) or by using enzyme-linked specific antibodies (ELISA assay). Another approach is to elute the bound rheumatoid factors, followed by quantitation of the recovered materials. This approach, however, has been fraught with problems and has been replaced by ELISA or radioimmunoassay.

Several problems are inherent in the techniques used for quantifying rheumatoid factors with solid-phase methods. The IgG bound to solid phase is prone to nonspecific adsorption of other IgG molecules and immune aggregates.[57] In addition, the washing steps used to remove the unbound serum proteins may well dissociate and discard rheumatoid factors with low association constants that were bound to the solidified IgG. As described previously, all rheumatoid factors have low association constants to monomeric IgG, and only IgM-RFs bind with strong affinity to aggregated IgG. As a consequence, only a small fraction of IgG-RFs and a higher proportion of IgM-RFs remain bound to the solid-phase IgG. This problem can be overcome in part by employing isolated IgG-RF, IgM-RF, and IgA-RF as standards, thus calculating from the bound rheumatoid factors the actual amount of rheumatoid factors present in the tested specimen. This approach assumes that all rheumatoid factors in the test serum bind to the solid-phase IgG in a manner comparable with that of the employed standard preparation. In spite of the various problems, the solid-phase assays do provide quantitative measurements.

The quantitation of rheumatoid factors by these solid-phase assays has yielded new information and should provide even more insights. A few examples from the literature are illustrative: The serum of patients with RA who were categorized as seropositive or seronegative by the routine agglutination tests contained IgM-RFs, but the concentrations in the seropositive group were higher than in the seronegative group, and both groups had significantly higher levels of IgM-RFs than the control group.[58] The level of IgG-RFs was higher than the level of IgM-RFs, expressed in mg/ml.[59] The presence of high levels of IgG-RFs was associated with active disease in patients with RA.[60] In patients with RA treated with remission-inducing drugs quantitative tests have disclosed reduction of one or more classes of RFs.[61-63] Obviously, such quantitative studies of the concentrations of rheumatoid factors during the course of the disease and during therapeutic interventions might provide additional useful insights.

These quantitative studies are also useful for the study of the production of IgM-RFs on a cellular level. For example, B cells from the blood of patients with rheumatoid factors synthesize IgM-RFs. B cells from these patients can be further stimulated with pokeweed mitogen to synthesize even more IgM-RFs per cell.[42,64]

Rheumatoid factors in low titers are found in small percentages of young adults, but the prevalence of positive tests for rheumatoid factors increases with age. A high prevalence of rheumatoid factors is also found in persons with certain infections, such as infective endocarditis, syphilis, schistosomiasis, tuberculosis, and leprosy, and transiently in persons following extensive immunizations. These observations have suggested that extensive or persistent exposure to antigens and immune-complex formation induces the synthesis of rheumatoid factors. In several lung diseases, including idiopathic fibrosis, silicosis, and asbestosis, the prevalence of rheumatoid factors is also increased. The prevalence of rheumatoid factors in various disorders was reviewed by Bartfeld in 1969.[65] IgM-RFs constitute an essential ingredient of mixed cryoglobulins, and their presence is related to the pathogenesis of the disease.[66] Furthermore, IgG-RFs are an essential component in the serum protein abnormalities of hypergammaglobulinemic purpura.[67] *Thus, a positive test for rheumatoid factors should not be used as the sole criterion for the diagnosis of RA.*

Many questions remain to be answered about the significance of rheumatoid factors in apparently normal persons and in patients with diverse disorders. Above all, we still do not know why patients with RA develop these antibodies. Hypotheses for the development of rheumatoid factors include the stimulation of synthesis by immune complexes, polyclonal B-cell activation, infection of B cells by the Epstein-Barr virus,[42] and development as auto-anti-idiotypic antibodies to the immune response to microbial Fc-binding proteins.[9,10] Evidence for the role of rheumatoid factors in maintaining the chronicity of rheumatoid arthritis, however, is mounting.

REFERENCES

1. Egeland, T., and Munthe, E.: Rheumatoid Factors. Clin. Rheum. Dis., 9:135–160, 1983.
2. Natvig, J.B., and Kunkel, H.G.: Human immunoglobulins: Classes, subclasses, genetic variants, and idiotypes. Adv. Immunol., 15:1–59, 1973.
3. Allen, J.C., and Kunkel, H.G.: Hidden rheumatoid factors with specificity for native γ globulins. Arthritis Rheum., 9:758–768, 1966.
4. Nardella, F.A., Teller, D.C., Barber, C.V., and Mannik, M.: IgG rheumatoid factors and staphylococcal protein A bind to a common molecular site on IgG. J. Exp. Med., 162:1811–1824, 1985.
5. Sasso, E.H., Barber, C.V., Nardella, F.A., and Mannik, M.: IgM rheumatoid factors (IgM RFs) bind sites at the Cγ2-Cγ3 junction (abstract). Arthritis Rheum., 30:S103, 1987.
6. Deisenhofer, J.: Crystallographic refinement and atomic model of a human Fc fragment and its complex with fragment B of protein A from Staphylococcus aureus at 2.9 and 2.8-Å resolution. Biochemistry, 20:2361–2370, 1981.
7. Schröder, A.K., et al.: Interaction between streptococcal IgG Fc receptors and human and rabbit IgC domains. Immunology, 57:305–309, 1986.
8. Johansson, P.J.H., et al.: Interaction between herpes simplex type I induced Fc receptor and human and rabbit immunoglobulin G (IgG) domains. Immunology, 58:251–255, 1986.
9. Nardella, F.A., et al.: T15 group A Streptococcal Fc receptor binds to the same location on IgC as Staphylococcal protein A and IgG rheumatoid factors. J. Immunol., 138:922–926, 1987.
10. Oppliger, I.R., Nardella, F.A., Stone, G.C., and Mannik, M.: Human rheumatoid factors bear the internal image of the Fc binding region of Staphylococcal protein A. J. Exp. Med., 166:702–710, 1987.
11. Natvig, J.B., Gaarder, P.J., and Turner, M.W.: IgG antigens of the Cγ2 and Cγ3 homology regions interacting with rheumatoid factors. Clin. Exp. Immunol., 12:177–184, 1972.
12. Nardella, F.A., Teller, D.C., and Mannik, M.: Studies on the antigenic determinants in the self-association of IgG rheumatoid factor. J. Exp. Med., 154:112–125, 1981.
13. Jerne, N.K.: Towards a network theory of the immune system. Ann. Immunol. (Paris), 125c:373, 1974.
14. Bona, C.A.: Idiotypes and lymphocytes. New York, Academic Press, 1981.
15. Kang, C-Y., and Kohler, H.: Antibodies, epibodies and homobodies: Role in autoimmunity. Concepts Immunopathol., 3:225–232, 1986.
16. Kunkel, H.G., et al.: Cross-idiotypic specificity among monoclonal IgM proteins with anti-γ-globulin activity. J. Exp. Med., 137:331–342, 1973.
17. Agnello, V., et al.: Evidence for a subset of rheumatoid factors that cross-react with DNA-histone and have a distinct cross-idiotype. J. Exp. Med., 151:1514–1527, 1980.
18. Carson, D.A., and Fong, S.: A common idiotype on human rheumatoid factor identified by a hybridoma antibody. Mol. Immunol., 20:1081–1087, 1983.
19. Chen, P.P., et al.: The majority of human monoclonal IgM rheumatoid factors express a "primary structure dependent" cross-reactive idiotype. J. Immunol, 134:3281–3285, 1985.
20. Agnello, V., et al.: Human rheumatoid factor crossidiotypes. II. Primary structure dependent crossreactive idiotype, PSL2-CRI, present on Wa monoclonal rheumatoid factors is present on Bla and other IgM K monoclonal antibodies. J. Exp. Med., 165:263–267, 1987.
21. Goldfein, R.D., Chen, P.P., Fong, S., and Carson, D.A.: Synthetic peptides corresponding to third hypervariable region of human monoclonal IgM rheumatoid factor heavy chains define an immunodominant idiotype. J. Exp. Med., 162:756–761, 1985.
22. Goldfein, R.D., et al.: Genetic analysis of human B cell hybridomas expressing a cross-reactive idiotype. J. Immunol., 138:940–944, 1987.
23. Fong, S., et al.: Expression of three cross-reactive idiotypes on rheumatoid factor autoantibodies from patients with autoimmune diseases and seropositve adults. J. Immunol., 137:122–128, 1986.
24. Nelson, J.L., Nardella, F.A., Oppliger, I.R., and Mannik, M.: Rheumatoid factors from patients with rheumatoid arthritis possess private repertoires of idiotypes. J. Immunol., 138:1391–1396, 1987.
25. Schlomchick, M.J., et al.: Variable region sequences of murine IgM anti-IgG monoclonal autoantibodies (rheumatoid factors). A structural explanation for the high frequency of IgM anti-IgG B cells. J. Exp. Med., 164:407–427, 1986.
26. Manheimer-Lory, A.J., et al.: Fine specificity, idiotype, and nature of cloned heavy-chain variable region genes of murine monoclonal rheumatoid factor antibodies. Proc. Natl. Acad. Sci. USA, 83:8293–8297, 1986.
27. Chavin, S.I., and Franklin, E.C.: Studies on antigen-binding activity of macroglobulin antibody subunits and their enzymatic fragments. J. Biol. Chem., 244:1345–1352, 1969.
28. Stone, J.M., and Metzger, H.: Binding properties of a Walden-

ström macroglobulin antibody. J. Biol. Chem., *243*:5977–5984, 1968.

29. Normansell, D.E.: Anti-γ-globulins in rheumatoid arthritis sera. I. Studies on the 22S complex. Immunochemistry, *1*:787–797, 1970.

30. Steward, M.W., Turner, M.W., and Natvig, J.B.: The binding affinities of rheumatoid factors interacting with Cγ3 homology region of human IgG. Clin. Exp. Immunol., *15*:145–152, 1973.

31. Normansell, D.E., and Young, C.W., Jr.: The IgG subclass specificity of antiIgG immunoglobulin rheumatoid factors. Immunochemistry, *12*:187–188, 1975.

32. Eisenberg, R.: The specificity and polyvalency of binding of a monoclonal rheumatoid factor. Immunochemistry, *13*:355–359, 1976.

33. Franklin, E.C., et al.: An unusual protein component of high molecular weight in the serum of certain patients with rheumatoid arthritis. J. Exp. Med., *105*:425–438, 1957.

34. Nardella, R.A., Teller, D.C., and Mannik, M.: Interaction of IgM rheumatoid factor (IgM-RF) with normal IgG (IgG) and IgG-rheumatoid factor (IgG-RF) (abstract.) Fourth Int. Congress Immunol., *13*:5–13, 1980.

35. Pope, R.M., Teller, D.C., and Mannik, M.: The molecular basis of self-association of antibodies to IgG (rheumatoid factors) in rheumatoid arthritis. Proc. Natl. Acad. Sci. U.S.A., *71*:517–521, 1974.

36. Pope, R.M., Teller, D.C., and Mannik, M.: The molecular basis of self-association of IgG-rheumatoid factors. J. Immunol., *115*:365–373, 1975.

37. Kunkel, H.G., et al.: Gamma globulin complexes in rheumatoid arthritis and certain other conditions. J. Clin. Invest., *40*:117–129, 1961.

38. Halla, J.T., Volanakis, J.E., and Schrohenloher, R.E.: Immune complexes in rheumatoid arthritis sera and synovial fluids. Arthritis Rheum., *22*:440–438, 1979.

39. Winchester, R.J., Agnello, V., and Kunkel, H.G.: Gamma globulin complexes in synovial fluids of patients with rheumatoid arthritis. Clin. Exp. Immunol., *6*:689–706, 1970.

40. Natvig, J.B., and Munthe, E.: Self-associating IgG rheumatoid factor represents a major response of plasma cells in rheumatoid inflammatory tissue. Ann. N.Y. Acad. Sci., *256*:88–95, 1975.

41. Fehr, K., et al.: Production of agglutinators and rheumatoid factors in plasma cells of rheumatoid and nonrheumatoid synovial tissues. Arthritis Rheum., *24*:510–519, 1981.

42. Carson, D.A., et al.: Physiology and pathology of rheumatoid factors. Springer Semin. Immunopathol., *4*:161–179, 1981.

43. Winchester, R.J.: Characterization of IgG complexes in patients with rheumatoid arthritis. Ann. N.Y. Acad. Sci., *256*:73–81, 1975.

44. Male, D., Roitt, I.M., and Hay, F.C.: Analysis of immune complexes in synovial effusions of patients with rheumatoid arthritis. Clin. Exp. Immunol., *39*:297–306, 1980.

45. Nardella, F.A., et al.: Self-associating IgG-rheumatoid factors in MRL/1 autoimmune mice. Arthritis Rheum., *27*:1165–1173, 1984.

46. Abraham, G.N., Clark, R.A., and Vaughan, J.H.: Characterization of an IgA rheumatoid factor: Binding properties and reactivity with the subclasses of human γG globulin. Immunochemistry, *9*:301–315, 1972.

47. Tanimoto, K., et al.: Complement fixation by rheumatoid factor. J. Clin. Invest., *55*:437–445, 1975.

48. Sabharwal, J.K., et al.: Activation of the classical pathway of complement by rheumatoid factors. Assessment by radioimmunoassay for C4. Arthritis Rheum., *25*:161–167, 1982.

49. Brown, P.B., Nardella, F.A., and Mannik, M.: Human complement activation by self-associated IgG rheumatoid factors. Arthritis Rheum., *25*:1101–1107, 1982.

50. Messner, R.P., et al.: Serum opsonin, bacteria, and polymorphonuclear leukocyte interactions in subacute bacterial endocarditis. Anti-γ-globulin factors and their interaction with specific opsonins. J. Clin. Invest., *47*:1109–1120, 1968.

51. Diaz-Jouanen, E., et al.: Serum and synovial fluid inhibitors of antibody-mediated lymphocytotoxicity in rheumatoid arthritis and systemic lupus erythematosus. Arthritis Rheum., *19*:142–149, 1976.

52. Notkins, A.L.: Infectious virus-antibody complexes: Interaction with anti-immunoglobulins, complement and rheumatoid factor. J. Exp. Med., *134*:41S–51S, 1971.

53. Nardella, F.A., et al.: Self-associating IgG rheumatoid factors stimulate monocytes to release prostaglandins and mononuclear cell factor that stimulates collagenase and prostaglandin production by synovial cells. Rheumatol. Int., *3*:183–186, 1983.

54. Linker, J.B., III, and Williams, R.C., Jr.: Tests for detection of rheumatoid factors. *In* Manual of Clinical Laboratory Immunology, 3rd Ed. Edited by N.R. Rose, H. Friedman, and J.L. Fahey. Washington, D.C., American Society for Microbiology, 1986.

55. Singer, J.M.: Standardization of the latex test for rheumatoid arthritis serology. Bull. Rheum. Dis., *24*:762–769, 1974.

56. Klein, F., Valkenburg, H.A., and Cats, A.: On standardization of the latex fixation test. Bull. Rheum. Dis., *26*:866–868, 1976.

57. Nardella, F.A., and Mannik, M.: Nonimmunospecific protein-protein interactions of IgG: Studies of the binding of IgG to IgG immunoadsorbents. J. Immunol., *120*:739–744, 1978.

58. Koopman, W.J., and Schrohenloher, R.E.: A sensitive radioimmunoassay for quantitation of IgM rheumatoid factor. Arthritis Rheum., *23*:302–308, 1980.

59. Wernick, R., et al.: Serum IgG and IgM rheumatoid factors by solid phase radioimmunoassay. Arthritis Rheum., *24*:1501–1511, 1981.

60. Allen, C., et al.: IgG antiglobulins in rheumatoid arthritis and other arthritides: Relationship with clinical features and other parameters. Ann. Rheum. Dis., *40*:127–131, 1981.

61. Wernick, R., et al.: IgG and IgM rheumatoid factors in rheumatoid arthritis: Quantitative response to penicillamine therapy and relationship to disease activity. Arthritis Rheum., *26*:593–598, 1983.

62. Rudge, S.R., Pound, J.D., Bossingham, D.H., and Powell, R.J.: Class specific rheumatoid factors in rheumatoid arthritis: Response to chrysotherapy and relationship to disease activity. J. Rheumatol., *12*:432–436, 1985.

63. Pope, R.M., Lessard, J., and Nunnery, E.: Differential effects of therapeutic regimens on specific classes of rheumatoid factor. Ann. Rheum. Dis., *45*:183–189, 1986.

64. Alarcon, G.S., Koopman, W.J., and Schrohenloher, R.E.: Differential patterns of in vitro IgM rheumatoid factor synthesis in seronegative and seropositive rheumatoid arthritis. Arthritis Rheum., *25*:150–155, 1982.

65. Bartfeld, H.: Distribution of rheumatoid factor activity in nonrheumatoid states. Ann. N.Y. Acad. Sci., *168*:30–38, 1969.

66. Meltzer, M., et al.: Cryoglobulinemia—a clinical and laboratory study. II. Cryoglobulins with rheumatoid factor activity. Am. J. Med., *40*:837–856, 1966.

67. Capra, J.D., Winchester, R.J., and Kunkel, H.G.: Hypergammaglobulinemic purpura. Studies on the unusual anti-γ-globulins characteristic of the sera of these patients. Medicine, *50*:125–138, 1971.

TREATMENT OF RHEUMATOID ARTHRITIS

47

ROBERT W. LIGHTFOOT, JR.

Specific information about the individual physical, medical, and surgical techniques for treating rheumatoid arthritis (RA) is given elsewhere in this book. This chapter describes an overall approach to the combined use of these therapies in the RA patient and provides a strategy for determining the appropriate treatment program in the individual patient.

The pyramid shown in Figure 47–1 schematically relates therapeutic regimens that may be used in the management of RA. The pyramid is interpreted as follows: (1) the lower items are often continued as higher elements are instituted and thus constitute a true "base" of the pyramid; (2) the elements toward the bottom of the pyramid are generally less toxic than those toward the top, and their usefulness has been established over many years; and (3) the elements toward the bottom are more generically applicable to the treatment of RA; they are used in virtually all patients, whereas those ranked higher are relevant only in certain patients. Although the pyramid implies a fixed relationship of these regimens to one another, treatment must be designed to meet the needs of each individual patient.

As with any standard, deviation from the ideal does occur. For example, although corticosteroids generally are not considered part of the initial conservative management of an uncomplicated case of RA, their use may be warranted under certain circumstances. Similarly, although joint reconstruction generally is considered later and in chronic, recalcitrant disease, occasional patients with relatively early inflammatory disease in many joints may nonetheless benefit from

surgical reconstruction of a single joint with more erosive involvement.

Several aspects of RA confound even the best clinician. Therapy is easy to evaluate when use of a specific drug is followed by a prompt, objectively quantifiable response. Examples are the treatment of pernicious anemia with vitamin B_{12}, the treatment of diabetic ketoacidosis with insulin, and the resolution of pneumococcal pneumonia after penicillin therapy. Unlike these disorders, RA is a chronic disease without specific therapy. Its treatment is entirely empirical. Its natural history may span decades, the results of therapy are usually not immediately apparent, and its course may fluctuate spontaneously. These factors often impair one's ability to determine the efficacy of treatment regimens. Furthermore, no universally accepted parameters permit specific measurement of disease activity. Any attempt at therapy must take the foregoing variables into account.

FIG. 47–1. The therapeutic pyramid. See text for details.

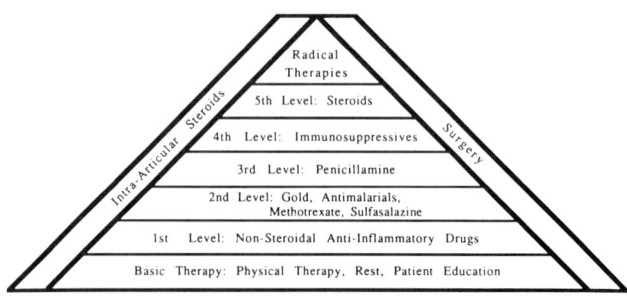

GOALS OF THERAPY

Treatment of RA is directed toward (1) alleviation of the signs and symptoms of active inflammation, both local and general; (2) prevention of tissue destruction; (3) prevention of deformity and preservation of function; and (4) reversal of phenomena threatening organ function, such as mononeuritis, myopericarditis, and lung fibrosis. Each of the elements in the therapeutic pyramid is directed toward one or more of these goals. The specific goals of a given therapy may differ among patients and with time in the same patient.

TYPES OF THERAPY

PATIENT EDUCATION

Without question, the single most important element in the management of rheumatoid disease is patient education. Most patients have only a vague notion of what RA is and how it differs from other forms of arthritis. Many believe, erroneously, that all patients with RA are destined to become crippled. They are often unaware that the symptoms of RA may partially remit and exacerbate spontaneously, sometimes from day to day. Intense anxiety and depression, common among these patients, result from fear and ignorance of what the future may hold and the inability to judge from day to day whether the disease is improving or worsening. Because these patients are unfamiliar with the concept of a chronic disease and do not know what to expect from its treatment, they often become discouraged if the initial steps taken by the physician are not immediately beneficial. The average patient is often unaware of the critical role he himself must play in disease management, especially with respect to ensuring an appropriate program of rest and physical therapy.

The patient should be told that RA is a chronic, lifelong disease for which no cure exists, but that a variety of measures, in the aggregate, can lead to significant improvement, that is, to "control" of the disease. *Relief of symptoms, preservation of joint function, and a reasonable life style* are three realistic goals. Patients must understand that the medications used in treatment generally do not provide overnight relief of symptoms, and they must be instructed to disregard the day-to-day variations and to think in terms of weeks or months in looking for evidence of improvement. If this concept is not emphasized, initial disappointment with the therapy may cause the patient

to switch physicians often or even to seek a "cure" through quackery.

In addition to familiarizing patients with the concept of chronic disease and its management, specific points must be stressed with respect to individual therapeutic regimens.

SYSTEMIC REST

The fever, weight loss, anemia, lymphadenopathy, and visceral involvement that may accompany RA attest to the systemic nature of the disease. A largely empiric body of evidence suggests that physical rest can rapidly ameliorate an acute exacerbation of rheumatoid disease. The optimal amount of rest varies from patient to patient. Some previously active patients have exaggerated fears of ultimately becoming crippled and may develop extreme anxiety if advised to quit work temporarily and take to bed. A modified rest program compatible with the patient's personality is appropriate in such an instance. Conversely, a systemically ill patient with multiple joint involvement and visceral disease may, of necessity, require nearly complete bed rest. Thus, the degree of physical rest prescribed varies from little to complete, depending on the individual circumstances. According to one study, complete bed rest is rarely indicated.[1]

In general, for patients with mild disease, a period of 2 to 4 hours in the afternoon at the time of onset of fatigue provides sufficient daily rest without interfering unduly with vocational responsibilities. The stiffness that follows periods of immobility should not dissuade patients from resting, and this phenomenon must be explained to the patient. As remission ensues, stiffness becomes less severe.

The ability to engage in periods of physical rest implies the ability to withdraw momentarily from psychosocial stress as well. The typical patient's fear about what to expect from this disease, the fear of possible loss of customary social and occupational roles in the family, and personal reaction to illness often cause a major psychologic stress reaction early in the disease. A rest program that does not permit respite from emotional stress is suboptimal.

In general, for patients with persistently active disease of recent onset or with "uncontrolled" inflammation at any point, a 2- to 3-week period of inpatient hospitalization is desirable. Physiologic studies of inflamed joints in RA (see Chapter 11) indicate that effective synovial blood flow is reduced. Because of this relative ischemia, the increased metabolic demand during joint use may cause microinfarction of synovial villi, which are the source of rice bodies found in severely involved joints.[2] Rest not only diminishes systemic stress, but probably also decreases local oxygen demand in these ischemic joints. In the study by Lee and co-workers, hospitalized patients fared much better than those managed as outpatients.[3] Hospitalization permits definitive isolation from both physical and emotional stress. It allows time for the physician and other health professionals to educate the patient fully about the nature of the illness and the programs to be used in its treatment. Hospitalization also ensures early establishment of an optimal daily medical and physical therapeutic program.

A comprehensive treatment program requires a team of diverse health-care professions including nursing, occupational and physical therapy, physiatry, orthopedic surgery, and rheumatology, as discussed in Chapters 48 through 55. The efforts of this team can be most effectively coordinated if the new patient is hospitalized. In addition, questions about whether the patient is taking proper doses of medication or receiving adequate physical therapy and rest are obviated. The majority of patients experience a gratifying improvement in symptoms during this period.[3,4] If improvement does not occur, the next level on the treatment pyramid (see Fig. 47–1) can be entered without questioning whether therapy at the preceding level has failed because of noncompliance.

PHYSICAL THERAPY

Rheumatoid synovitis is a chronic, inflammatory, destructive process that, if unchecked, proceeds to fibrosis of periarticular soft tissue with limitation of motion and contracture and to destruction of articular structures with ultimate subluxation, malalignment, and loss of function. The goals of physical therapy are to (1) maintain range of motion; (2) minimize disuse atrophy of muscle; (3) minimize deformity; (4) provide adequate systemic rest; and (5) minimize excessive articular trauma, that is, provide local rest. Although the specifics of a comprehensive physical therapy program can be obtained through consultation with an appropriate specialist (see Chapter 49), the more important elements of such a program should be initiated as soon as the diagnosis is made and should be monitored by the patient's primary physician.

The patients must be convinced that the basic program, including systemic rest, is as important a part of their treatment as any medication, and that, to succeed, the program must be followed on a daily

basis, so it becomes as habitual as brushing teeth, combing hair, or bathing.

Preservation of Range of Motion

The initial period of conservative management of RA must include a balanced program of adequate rest to decrease inflammation and appropriate therapeutic exercise to maintain range of motion, and this program should be maintained for the duration of the disease or until a complete disease remission is obtained. Patients must be educated regarding the tendency to joint contractures, and they should be instructed to move all joints gently through a full range of motion once daily. This exercise is most easily accomplished after initial morning stiffness has subsided or during or shortly after a hot bath or shower. Instruction in proper positioning of joints during rest or sleep is equally important in preventing contracture. Placing pillows under a painful knee is a major contributing factor to the development of contractures and must be actively discouraged. The patient should attempt to sleep in a position as near anatomic as possible, that is, with knees and elbows fully extended and with the neck and wrists in a near-neutral position.

Any exercise prescribed to maintain muscle strength and range of motion should minimize stress to the affected joints because such stress aggravates the inflammatory process.[4] Gentle isotonic or isometric exercises are preferable. Vigorous exercises such as jogging, bicycling, or calisthenics should be prohibited; they both worsen synovial hypoxia and increase direct joint trauma.[5] Any exercise that causes discomfort persisting for more than an hour or two should be decreased in amount. As the disease remits and physical tolerance increases, the exercise program can be escalated to include progressive resistive exercises.

Aerobic conditioning using a stationary exercise bicycle is of great value once control of synovitis in knees and hips has been achieved.[6]

Splints

Joint trauma can also be minimized by the use of splints. These appliances are especially valuable for the acutely inflamed joint, in which they relieve pain, prevent deformity, and minimize the likelihood of synovial ischemic necrosis. The study of Gault and Spyker has established objectively the benefits of joint immobilization in minimizing inflammation.[7] Splints should be removed at least once daily to permit range-of-motion exercises. Splints with which the physician should be familiar are volar wrist splints, used especially during sleep, and leg splints made of plaster or molded plastic, usually applied to the posterior aspect of the leg and foot by means of an elastic bandage to prevent knee or ankle flexion contractures.

Heat and Cold Application

The application of heat or cold to involved areas is often helpful in relieving pain and muscle spasm. Moist heat seems to be preferred by most patients and has the added advantage of relieving the "gel phenomenon," preparing the joint for subsequent range-of-motion exercises. Heat can be applied to painful areas in a variety of ways (see Chapter 49).

Cold applications are preferred if the inflammation is intense, as local hyperemia is already maximal.

Foot Support

RA is chiefly a disease of the small joints of the hands and feet (see Chapter 43). Typically, the metatarsophalangeal (MTP) joints are the worst affected in the foot, and patients often aptly describe a feeling of having stones under the forefoot when walking barefoot. The transverse arch collapses, and the forefoot spreads. The MTP joints are swollen and lie just under the skin, with weight borne chiefly by MTP joints 2, 3, and 4 instead of 1 and 5, as in a normal, healthy forefoot. The great toe develops a valgus position, and a bunion becomes prominent. The toes become "cocked-up" and do not fit easily into a shoe. The plantar fascia may contract and may lead to a pes cavus deformity. Involvement of the ankle and subtalar joints leads to eversion of the hindfoot.

Proper support must be provided for the rheumatoid foot. The physician can prescribe orthopedic (modified-last) oxfords with a heel height that is comfortable for the patient, usually 1½ to 2 inches. A medial wedge of about ⅛-inch corrects the tendency to eversion, and metatarsal bars, affixed to the leather sole of the shoe or (preferably) built into a composition sole, relieve the constant pressure on the inflamed MTP joints. If the hallux valgus is severe, the shoes can be stretched to provide a "bunion pocket." Shoes with a double toe-box provide adequate space for the patient with severe toe deformities. Overweight patients may benefit from a Thomas heel (see Chapter 89).

Axial Skeletal Support

RA often involves the cervical spine, the most mobile part of the axial skeleton. It often helps to prescribe a soft cervical collar with Velcro straps to hold the neck in midposition. This collar can be worn at night as well as during the day and acts as a splint for the neck by resting the inflamed lateral interbody joints and zygapophyseal joints.

Canes or Crutches

Canes or crutches are often helpful orthotic appliances in treating RA, despite the reluctance of many American patients to accept them. Crutches are symbolic of the cripple, just what the average RA patient fears the most. Their use must be "sold" to the patient. It is best to prescribe crutches for a short time only, to prevent weight bearing in an extremity that contains a joint recently injected with corticosteroid, especially when triamcinolone hexacetonide has been administered in an effort to produce a "medical synovectomy." In such a case, maximal therapeutic benefit can be attained by avoiding weight bearing for about 8 weeks (see Chapter 39).

The chief disadvantage of crutches is the stress they place on inflamed upper-extremity joints. This stress can be minimized by the use of platform crutches, with which weight is borne by the forearms. Aluminum crutches of the Canadian type are preferable because they have a metal band that uses the upper arm rather than the axilla as a fulcrum. Axillary crutches are dangerous because they predispose patients to brachial plexus stretching and injury.

A properly prescribed crutch should touch the floor about 3 inches in front of the foot when the patient is standing with arms straightened. A properly prescribed cane, helpful in unloading the hip joint, should touch the floor similarly and should be carried in the hand contralateral to the affected extremity.

Crutches are much more effective than canes in unloading the lower extremities. The patient must be trained to use them; three- or four-point gaits are available options and are not always easy to learn, especially for the elderly. Sometimes a walker is a better option for such patients, and this simple orthotic device may permit standing or walking for periods sufficient to allow the patient independence in self-care activities, such as cooking or getting to the bathroom.

Other Appliances

The severely handicapped patient can often be helped by simple devices such as raised toilet seats and hand rails in the bathtub and kitchen. Consultation with a physiatrist who has a special interest in arthritis can help such patients achieve or maintain independence in their usual activities of daily living (see Chapter 49). An occupational therapist can do an in-home evaluation of the need for assistive devices such as bathtub bars, special doorknobs, and raised toilet seats. These devices can be helpful to an elderly patient living alone, for whom simple modifications to the home can maintain functional independence.

MEDICAL THERAPY

All therapy with drugs, used singly or in combination to treat RA, is empirical.

Nonsteroidal Anti-inflammatory Drugs (NSAIDs)

The first line of therapy in RA is the NSAID (see Chapter 32). Salicylates, preferably as aspirin, are the cornerstone of drug treatment in RA. Their chief advantage is rapidity of therapeutic effect. A general principle of aspirin therapy is a gradual increase in the dose to produce mild toxicity, then a decrease to more tolerable doses. The most common cause of failure of aspirin therapy is reluctance of the patient to take the drug as directed. The average patient thinks of aspirin as little more than a headache remedy. To prescribe aspirin in large doses to such a patient without explaining the rationale behind its use is to invite noncompliance. The patient must be informed that salicylates in larger doses are anti-inflammatory and are not just analgesic. Patients should be advised that a regular daily dose must be taken for at least 2 weeks to maintain a blood level of between 20 and 30 mg/dl, before deciding on efficacy. Without this caution, patients often vary the dose from day to day, depending on symptoms, and thereby fail to achieve a therapeutic blood level.

The likelihood of benefit from salicylates can be maximized by hospitalization to control other variables of treatment. Aspirin is not an easy drug to use, and the average physician uses it poorly. The dose must be tailored to each patient, based on the drug kinetics discussed in Chapter 32. The primary value of obtaining serum salicylate levels in the adult is to ascertain compliance in someone with an inadequate clinical response to usually therapeutically successful doses, not to achieve a certain serum level.* In general we initiate therapy at 600 to 900 mg four times daily, increasing the dosage as needed. Toxicity may occur at any serum level. If serious toxicity occurs, salicylates are discontinued. For less serious toxicity, the dosage is decreased to the maximal tolerated. In the alert adult, symptoms of mild toxicity, such as tinnitus or decreased hearing, precede those of serious toxicity. There is no correlation of the milder, but sometimes intolerable, side effects of salicylates (e.g., tinnitus, dyspepsia) with serum salicylate levels.

Editor's note. It is my practice to measure serum salicylate levels before the first morning dose, with the goal being a level of 20 to 30 mg/dl, because I have not found symptoms of salicylism to be a reliable guide. If a patient taking an individually tailored prescribed dose of acetylsalicylic acid (ASA) experiences a flare-up of disease activity, I obtain a serum salicylate to monitor compliance and then discuss the results with the patient.[8]

Periodic serum levels are advisable in pediatric patients because young patients may not be able to articulate their symptoms of early toxicity.

The most common side effects of aspirin therapy are tinnitus in younger patients, decreased auditory activity in older individuals, and gastrointestinal distress. Tinnitus responds to lowering of the dose. Ordinary aspirin should always be taken with food. It is simplest to prescribe four doses daily with meals and a bedtime snack. The dietary habits of each patient should be known. If necessary, food must be prescribed, especially breakfast. The aspirin should be taken during the meal, between bites—not before and not after, but *during* the meal. If these measures are not successful, alternative salicylate preparations, for example, aspirin mixed with an antacid, enteric-coated aspirin,* or sodium salicylate, may be used. Patients intolerant of regular aspirin often have no gastrointestinal symptoms when taking other salicylate preparations. The newer enteric-coated preparations and zero-order release forms are well absorbed and can be substituted, if necessary, milligram for milligram, for ordinary aspirin. So effective are salicylates in the management of RA that all aforementioned agents should be tried before the physician concludes that the patient is unable to take any salicylate preparation.

A few patients experience sufficient improvement in symptoms at subtoxic doses of aspirin so that additional therapies may not be required. If, after a 2- to 4-week trial of salicylates in therapeutic doses in an optimal setting, improvement is insufficient, or if salicylates are not tolerated, another NSAID should be tried (see Chapter 32). The physician should be aware that salicylates may interfere with the absorption of some NSAIDs and vice versa. There is no documentation of an additive effect from combining aspirin with other NSAIDs, and we do not recommend this practice. In a mild case of RA, 6 or more months of NSAIDs and the basic program may be in order. In more severe cases, it may be clear after 3 weeks of NSAID administration that additional drug therapy is needed. If the disease has been present for more than 1 year, or if erosive disease is already present, it is unlikely that therapy with NSAIDs used alone will produce satisfactory suppression of joint inflammation. We routinely begin treatment of such patients with disease-remitting agents without wasting weeks of valuable time.

NSAIDs exert an analgesic effect as well. If additional analgesia is needed, acetaminophen, newer

Editor's note. I use enteric-coated preparations almost exclusively (0.975-g tablets).

non-narcotic analgesics, and propoxyphene compounds or pentazocine alone or in combination, may be added. Propoxyphene and pentazocine should be used cautiously because they may lead to drug dependency. Narcotic-containing analgesics should be used with extreme caution, if at all, in a chronic illness such as RA. Analgesic drugs should be considered as supplemental to the more important treatment regimens discussed here.

Second-Line Drugs (see Chapters 33 through 36)

If an adequate trial of aspirin or other NSAIDs provides insufficient relief, if well-established RA has been present for more than 1 year, or if erosions have already occurred, it is necessary to begin gold (Chapter 33) or antimalarial (Chapter 34) drug therapy. As mentioned previously, the precise time at which this level of the treatment pyramid (see Fig. 47–1) should be entered varies. Gold is preferred because of the more substantial documentation of its efficacy.[9–11] Retinal toxicity from antimalarial agents is minimal.[12] Chloroquine can be given safely for many years in doses not exceeding 4 mg/kg lean body weight daily. Hydroxychloroquine also can be given in doses lower than 6 mg/kg/day. Both agents have equal therapeutic and toxic effects at these doses. Light exposure accelerates ocular toxicity, and patients should be advised to wear sunglasses when in bright sunlight to minimize this effect. Patients should be advised that with gold or antimalarial treatment, improvement may not be apparent for several months. NSAIDs should be continued in full dosage throughout the period of gold or antimalarial administration.

Most patients require combined-drug treatment, not unlike the empiric drug regimens used in cancer chemotherapy. Thus, antimalarial drugs and gold are often used together in patients with uncontrolled inflammation, especially in those with erosions. Fine-detail roentgenograms enable us to identify erosions early in the disease, often only a few months after onset. Most patients with erosions have positive rheumatoid factor tests.

On the basis of several controlled trials, methotrexate has been used with increasing enthusiasm in the treatment of RA over the past 5 years.[13–15] In one multicenter controlled study of 110 patients, none experienced disease remission, major improvement occurred in 20 to 30%, and 50% had some improvement. One major advantage seems to be a relatively early onset of therapeutic effect, sometimes as early as 6 weeks.

A potential disadvantage of methotrexate is its apparent lack of remission induction. Patients well-controlled on methotrexate have flared rapidly on withdrawal of the drug.[16] Of patients in the above-mentioned multicenter study, 30% discontinued therapy because of abnormal liver function tests. Subsequent experience suggests that abnormal liver function tests often spontaneously reverse, and may not predict future hepatic fibrosis. Using the low-dose regimens discussed in Chapter 35, the short-term risk of hepatotoxicity appears negligible. The long-term risk remains undefined, but it can be minimized by avoiding the one clear additive risk—ingestion of alcohol in any amount.

Sulfasalazine, too, has been used with increasing frequency as a second-line drug in RA (Chapter 35). In blind controlled trials, it has proven effective in as little as 2 months, placing its onset of action between that of NSAIDs and the more delayed actions of gold or penicillamine.[17] About 30% of patients discontinue the drug because of side effects. Its precise position in the hierarchy of the treatment pyramid (Fig. 47–1) will continue to evolve over the next several years.

Penicillamine (see Chapter 36) may be useful in patients unresponsive to treatment with aspirin, gold, and antimalarial agents. Some clinicians even prefer penicillamine to gold, but the toxicity may be serious, even fatal. Moreover, the therapeutic effect of penicillamine may be inapparent for up to 6 months. The toxicities of gold and penicillamine, which are similar, have been linked to the HLA-DR3 antigen; if toxicity occurs in a patient who is taking both drugs, identifying the responsible agent may be impossible. It is usual to discontinue gold therapy but to continue the other drugs during the period of penicillamine treatment.

Antimalarial agents should not be given in combination with D-penicillamine because they may interfere with its adsorption. A controlled trial using both drugs found the combination inferior to either drug used alone.[18]

Immunoregulatory Drugs

Patients with active disease despite the use of the aforementioned drugs are candidates for immunoregulatory drug therapy. Considerable evidence suggests that the immunosuppressive drugs, especially cyclophosphamide and azathioprine, are effective in controlling rheumatoid disease.[19,20] Cyclophosphamide has prevented the development of joint erosions.[19] The rationale behind the use of these drugs is discussed in Chapters 35 and 38. *All use of such toxic compounds should be supervised by a rheumatologist.*

Immunosuppression by lymphophoresis, plasmapheresis, or total lymph-node irradiation is expensive and may have serious, as yet unrecognized, toxicity (Chapter 38). The duration of benefits gained is yet to be defined. Both these and combined immunosuppressive drug regimens should be considered as experimental, to be used only in cases recalcitrant to all conventional therapy, and administered as part of an approved scientific protocol.

Each of the alternate drugs already mentioned has its own set of toxic effects. In some instances, evidence of drug toxicity may be delayed for months or years. The responsible clinician must be familiar with all the toxic effects of each drug and must be prepared to monitor both short- and long-term toxicity, with proper monitoring to permit the earliest possible detection of such side effects.

Corticosteroids (see Chapter 37)

As indicated in Figure 47–1, the intra-articular injection of corticosteroids can play a major adjunctive role in controlling rheumatoid synovitis at all levels in the treatment pyramid. Details regarding the dosage, techniques for administration, frequency of injection, and contraindications are discussed in Chapter 39.

Systemic corticosteroid therapy is intentionally placed last in the treatment pyramid. Oral or intramuscular corticosteroids should be used only after a critical consideration of alternate modes of treatment and with the long-term side effects of these agents kept in mind because these drugs are much easier to start than to stop in a patient with RA. Several studies have suggested that a major subset of rheumatoid patients are prone to a dependency on corticosteroids that prevents the discontinuance of these drugs,[21,22] and the immediate improvement that often occurs may dissuade both patient and doctor from using a better-tolerated and more effective drug regimen.

Corticosteroids may be indicated in a patient who is the family breadwinner and who must continue working, or as an adjunct while waiting for clinical response to one of the remittive drugs such as gold, azathioprine, etc. Although flares severe enough to necessitate hospitalization may be rapidly controlled with a 15-mg, single daily dose of prednisone, the physician should attempt to taper this dose to no more than a 7.5 mg dose of prednisone or equivalent corticosteroid per day, and then only as a single morning dose on arising. Because the half-life of prednisone is only about 8 hours, the suppressive effect on the hypothalamic-pituitary axis is minimized, and the small dose given may be additive to the patient's endogenous corticosteroid secretion. No dose of corticosteroid is safe; even 5 mg prednisone daily can produce osteopenia (see Chapter 112). The only obvious advantage of corticosteroids is *rapidity* of action. Apart

from NSAIDs they are the only agents with this property.

No rationale exists for treatment with corticotropin (ACTH), and fluorinated corticosteroids, such as dexamethasone or triamcinolone, are to be avoided because they have long biologic half-lives and are likely to suppress the patient's endogenous corticosteroid output.

Specific indications for corticosteroid use therefore include life-threatening visceral disease, acute flares, and persistent, disabling symptoms in a breadwinner who must return to work. Additional indications and cautionary comments are detailed in Chapter 37.

TREATMENT STRATEGIES

A strategy cognizant of the five guidelines discussed in this section provides considerable assistance to the physician managing patients with RA.

TREATMENT OF SPECIFIC MANIFESTATIONS

One must determine which aspects of the disease process require treatment at a given time. RA can have protean manifestations involving many organ systems, and the preponderant manifestation may differ with time in the same patient. Figure 47–2 depicts the

FIG. 47–2. Depiction of intra- and interpatient variability of disease expression and clinical course in rheumatoid arthritis (RA). Intensity of joint inflammation and systemic involvement are represented along the lower and upper axes, respectively. Patient A had moderate synovitis and subcutaneous modules at the time shown. Patient B had little more than synovitis when first seen in 1969. After many years and several regimens, his disease manifested as severe Felty's syndrome and vasculitis, with minimal synovitis.

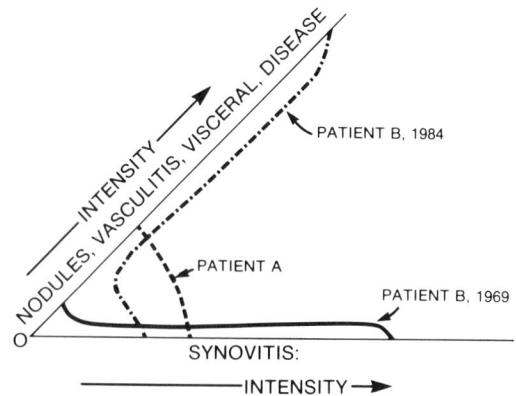

manifestations in two patients. Patient A was seen for the first time with moderate synovitis, accompanied by moderate numbers of subcutaneous nodules over the ulna and small joints of the hands. When patient B was first seen in 1969, severe incapacitating synovitis limited all activities of daily living, but more systemic features were minimal. Fifteen years later, synovitis was minimal, and the main expression of RA was severe neutropenia and digital gangrene secondary to rheumatoid vasculitis. This figure illustrates three distinct clinical presentations in two patients. It is, therefore, important to determine in advance of therapy which manifestations of RA mandate treatment. The manifestations of RA can be generally grouped as (1) signs and symptoms of joint inflammation; (2) destruction of bone and connective tissue; (3) visceral or systemic involvement; and (4) results of prior bone and soft tissue destruction.

Signs and Symptoms of Inflammation

Signs and symptoms of joint inflammation include joint pain, heat, and swelling. Systems designed to quantify these are discussed in Chapter 9.

Destruction of Bone and Connective Tissue

Although patients with sustained inflammatory symptoms usually also experience progressive joint destruction, progressive destructive disease need not always be accompanied by pain or other subjective symptoms. Rheumatoid scleritis, sometimes painless and noticed more by others than by the patient, may cause erosion through the sclera. Patients with diffuse rheumatoid nodulosis[23] who often have few or no joint complaints, may exhibit progressive, severely erosive disease in joints that have not been the seat of pain. It is of practical value therefore to consider progressive erosion and acute inflammatory signs as two possibly distinct clinical problems, one quantifiable clinically, the other often requiring serial roentgenographic measurement at annual to biennial intervals.

Manifestations of Visceral or Systemic Involvement

These manifestations include vasculitis, lung fibrosis, mononeuritis, and Felty's syndrome and are discussed at length in Chapter 44.

Results of Prior Bone and Soft-Tissue Destruction

Such destruction includes subluxations, contractures, secondary degenerative changes, and (rarely) ankylosis. These manifestations respond only to treatment with assistive devices, splints, or surgery.

Therapy should be tailored to the manifestation causing the symptoms. Gold therapy does not alleviate pain resulting from prior joint destruction, nor is surgical treatment appropriate for polyarticular inflammatory pain.

MEASUREMENT OF RESPONSE TO THERAPY

When initiating a given therapy, one must decide how the response will ultimately be measured. Methods of clinical assessment of disease activity are discussed in Chapter 9. Parameters such as joint count, ring size, grip strength, dolorimetry, articular index, duration of morning stiffness, erythrocyte sedimentation rate, walking time, and functional status questionnaires have all been used.[24] None of these is ideal, and it is customary to assess several parameters at the initiation of a new therapeutic regimen. In a multicenter study of criteria for remission in RA, duration of morning stiffness proved to be a far more reliable measure than other parameters.[24] Pain was less reliable, presumably because it partly reflects secondary degenerative disease in some patients with chronic RA. Clearly, if morning stiffness or grip weakness is absent at the initiation of a new regimen, this parameter will be a poor measure of response to treatment. In some patients with chronic RA, in whom it is difficult to separate symptoms of prior joint destruction from those of active progressive rheumatoid synovitis, serial roentgenograms may be the only reliable objective parameter. This concept is discussed further later in this chapter.

Whatever is measured, the goals of therapy are being met if there is serial improvement in values (i.e., the inflammatory response is ratcheted down until remission or disease "control" is achieved). This is possible in most cases.

TIMING OF EFFECTIVENESS OF THERAPY

One must determine in advance how long the regimen initiated generally takes before becoming effective. NSAIDs have a maximal effect within weeks. Gold, on the other hand, may not work until nearly the full 1000-mg induction regimen has been given, about 20 weeks. Obviously, one would not necessarily expect a measurable improvement after several weeks of gold therapy. Conversely, it would be unlikely to see additional improvement from adequate levels of NSAIDs after 6 to 8 weeks.

EVALUATION OF REGIMEN

Having selected parameters to be measured prior to and after initiation of therapy, one must decide, preferably in advance, what degree of change in measurements will be considered sufficient to constitute an "adequate" therapeutic response. This criterion may determine whether the regimen ultimately will be judged sufficiently successful to be continued at a maintenance level, or whether more aggressive therapy is warranted.

Criteria for a clinical remission of RA have been defined.[24] Uncontrolled RA is typically accompanied by *morning stiffness* of 4 hours' duration, *fatigue* onset within 5 hours after arising from sleep, grip strength measured with a sphygmomanometer of 100 mm Hg (women) and 120 mm Hg (men), and multiple, swollen, tender peripheral joints, all of which can be recorded rapidly on a suitable form. Serial measurements of each of these parameters and the erythrocyte sedimentation rate (ESR) should show stepwise improvement if the therapeutic regimen is effective.

COMBINATION OF THERAPIES

One must decide whether the current regimen will be continued as the next is started. This decision is more often dictated by whether their toxicities are similar, and therefore difficult to ascribe, and whether one is rapid in onset of action while the other is slow. For example, aspirin is usually continued during gold administration because the two have different rapidity of action and toxicity. Gold is not continued when penicillamine is started because their toxicities are nearly identical. Although gold and antimalarial agents are usually initiated in sequence, the first used is often continued as the other is initiated because both are slow-acting agents, and their more serious toxicities are generally distinct and are therefore easily ascribable. On the other hand, gold is usually discontinued when immunosuppressive agents are initiated because both can cause serious bone marrow depression.

Use of the foregoing guidelines minimizes the indefinite continuance of marginal therapy, a common problem in managing any chronic, complicated, multisystem disease. It also discourages the haphazard switching of drugs in an attempt to hurry a response. As an example, when aspirin or other NSAIDs alone have failed, gold therapy is started to control signs of acute inflammation and to deter joint erosion in a patient in whom salicylates are inadequate. Gold would not be given to control symptoms deemed due to irreversible secondary degenerative change or to control rheumatoid vasculitis. Parameters such as morning stiffness, grip strength, and number of swollen joints might not be expected to change drastically for as long as 20 weeks.

The patient with low-grade synovitis coexisting with severe joint destruction and deformity is a problem. It does little good to administer gold therapy in a patient with erosive disease and metacarpalphalangeal joint subluxation whose only current symptom is mild day-long pain without soft-tissue swelling, because this symptom is unlikely to reflect active inflammation, and the subluxations will not improve with gold therapy. It is often difficult to determine whether symptoms are primarily those of secondary degenerative disease, treatable only by NSAIDs or surgical intervention, or whether they reflect active synovitis, perhaps treatable with disease-modifying agents. In these patients, already functionally compromised by the abnormal joint mechanics resulting from subluxation and contracture and the discomfort of destroyed joint surfaces, even minimal worsening of joint integrity can severely threaten their ability to function independently. These patients present a formidable challenge. In many, serial roentgenograms of the involved joints at approximately yearly intervals may be the only objective parameter.

RESULTS OF THERAPY

Several studies involving many patients suggest that 50 to 70% experience significant improvement with a regimen of salicylates, rest, and physical therapy.[25–27] A similar percentage of response is found in controlled trials of gold therapy.[11,28] Thus, RA in the majority of patients can be controlled satisfactorily with well-accepted, conservative regimens. The role of more aggressive therapy, such as immunoregulatory drugs, in early or mild disease is not known. Although it has not been established scientifically that conservative management or any other therapy actually alters the course of RA, gold and cyclophosphamide, at least, have been shown to alter the rate of radiologically defined deterioration.[11,19] Although RA has not been proven to materially shorten life span, Pincus has reported a subset of RA patients, identifiable by a set of simple functional tests, whose survival potential is poorer than that of patients with Hodgkin's or with three-vessel coronary artery disease.[29] He has hypothesized that a more aggressive, less pyramidal, approach may be appropriate for such patients. The position of such an approach in the hierarchy of therapies remains to be defined.

Difficulties in diagnosing early disease, especially in initially seronegative patients, may delay the prescription of an optimal treatment regimen. The notorious spontaneous variations in disease activity make evaluation of any therapy difficult. The use of an appropriate control group is essential. Rational therapy requires that the physician use the foregoing management principles.

Use of these treatment rationales in a typical patient over time is represented in Figure 47–3. In phase I, the patient had primarily synovitis with some subcutaneous nodules, and responded gradually to NSAIDs. When the response was unacceptable, gold and, later, antimalarial agents were added, with better control of synovitis. When these agents became minimally effective, they were discontinued. Such "secondary failure" is common in RA patients. In phase III, when synovitis was minimal in this particular patient, nodulosis and vasculitis occurred. Later, synovitis recurred. Immunosuppressive agents were then added and eventually controlled the manifestations for which they were prescribed.

In conclusion, the regimens discussed in this chapter, including rest, exercise, orthotic shoes, splints, NSAIDs, and remittive agents, are all useful in managing RA. They are stratified in the treatment pyramid

(see Fig. 47–1) roughly in the order in which benefit exceeds risk. In the case of the newer regimens shown in the upper strata of the pyramid, future data may redefine the benefit-to-risk ratio, thus shifting their relative positions. Protocols using combined drug therapy may establish the effectiveness of such regimens, as in the lymphomas and leukemias. The less toxic, better-established regimens should be used before more toxic agents are employed. In the properly educated patient, the physician's attitude, more than any other factor, inspires cooperation. A *positive approach to treatment* may be the most important factor in the successful management of RA.

REFERENCES

1. Mills, J.A., et al.: Value of bed rest in patients with rheumatoid arthritis. N. Engl. J. Med., *284*:453–458, 1971.
2. Cheung, H.S., et al.: Synovial origins of rice bodies in joint fluid. Arthritis Rheum., *23*:72–76, 1980.
3. Lee, P., et al.: Benefits of hospitalization in rheumatoid arthritis. Q. J. Med., *43*:205–214, 1974.
4. Partridge, R.E.H., and Duthie, J.J.R.: Controlled trial of the effects of complete immobilization of the joints in rheumatoid arthritis. Ann. Rheum. Dis., *22*:91–99, 1963.
5. Castillo, B.A., El Sallab, R.A., and Scott, J.T.: Physical activity, cystic erosions, and osteoporosis in rheumatoid arthritis. Ann. Rheum. Dis., *29*:522–527, 1965.
6. Harcom, T.M., et al.: Therapeutic value of graded aerobic exercise training in rheumatoid arthritis. Arthritis Rheum., *28*:32–39, 1985.
7. Gault, S.J., and Spyker, J.M.: Beneficial effect of immobilization of joints in rheumatoid arthritis: A splint study using sequential analysis. Arthritis Rheum., *17*:34–44, 1969.
8. McCarty, D.J., and Csuka, M.E.: Aspirin use in chronic inflammatory arthritis. JAMA, *257*:1331, 1987.
9. Brooks, P.M., and Buchanan, W.W.: Current management of rheumatoid arthritis. *In* Recent Advances in Rheumatology. Edited by W.W. Buchanan and W.C. Dick. New York, Churchill Livingstone, 1976.
10. Tanuzzi, L., et al.: Does drug therapy slow radiographic deterioration in rheumatoid arthritis? N. Engl. J. Med., *309*:1023–1028, 1983.
11. Sigler, J.W., et al.: Gold salts in the treatment of rheumatoid arthritis. A double-blind study. Ann. Intern. Med., *80*:21–26, 1974.
12. Mackenzie, A.H.: Dose refinements in long-term therapy of rheumatoid arthritis with antimalarials. Am. J. Med., *75*:40–45, 1983.
13. Williams, H.J., et al.: Comparison of low-dose oral pulse methotrexate and placebo in the treatment of rheumatoid arthritis. A controlled clinical trial. Arthritis Rheum., *28*:721–730, 1985.
14. Andersen, P.A., et al.: Weekly pulse methotrexate in rheumatoid arthritis. Clinical and immunologic effects in a randomized, double-blind study. Ann. Intern. Med., *103*:489–496, 1985.
15. Weinblatt, M.E., et al.: Efficacy of low-dose methotrexate in rheumatoid arthritis. N. Engl. J. Med., *312*:818–822, 1985.
16. Kremer, J.M., Rynes, R.J., and Bartholomew, L.E.: Severe flare of rheumatoid arthritis after discontinuation of long-term methotrexate therapy. Am. J. Med., *82*:781–786, 1987.

FIG. 47–3. Management choices in a hypothetical patient over several years.

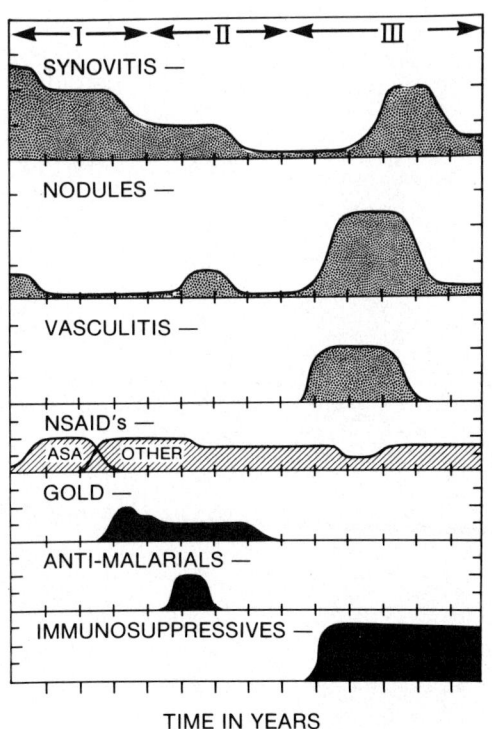

TIME IN YEARS

17. Pinals, R.S., Kaplan, S.B., Lawson, J.G., and Hepburn, B.: Sulfasalazine in rheumatoid arthritis. A double-blind, placebo-controlled trial. Arthritis Rheum., 29:1427–1434, 1986.

18. Bunch, T.W., et al.: Controlled trial of hydroxychloroquine and D-penicillamine singly and in combination in the treatment of rheumatoid arthritis. Arthritis Rheum., 27:267–276, 1984.

19. Cooperating Clinics Committee of the American Rheumatism Association: A controlled trial of cyclophosphamide in rheumatoid arthritis. N. Engl. J. Med., 283:883–889, 1970.

20. Currey, H.L.F., et al.: Comparison of azathioprine, cyclophosphamide, and gold in treatment of rheumatoid arthritis. Br. Med. J., 3:763–766, 1974.

21. Glass, D., et al.: Possible unnecessary prolongation of corticosteroid therapy in rheumatoid arthritis. Lancet, 2:334–337, 1971.

22. Moldofsky, H., and Rothman, A.I.: Personality, disease parameters and medication in rheumatoid arthritis. J. Chronic Dis., 24:363–372, 1971.

23. Ginsberg, M.H., et al.: Rheumatoid nodulosis. An unusual variant of rheumatoid disease. Arthritis Rheum., 18:49–58, 1975.

24. Pinals, R.S., Masi, A.T., and Larsen, R.A.: Preliminary criteria for clinical remission in rheumatoid arthritis. Arthritis Rheum., 24:1308–1315, 1981.

25. Duthie, J.J.R., et al.: Medical and social aspects of the treatment of rheumatoid arthritis, with special reference to factors affecting prognosis. Ann. Rheum. Dis., 14:133–149, 1955.

26. Ragan, C.: The general management of rheumatoid arthritis. JAMA, 141:174–177, 1949.

27. Short, C.L., and Bauer, W.: The course of rheumatoid arthritis in patients receiving simple medical and orthopedic measures. N. Engl. J. Med., 238:142–148, 1948.

28. Empire Rheumatism Council Research Sub-Committee Report: Gold therapy in rheumatoid arthritis. Final report of a multicentre controlled trial. Ann. Rheum. Dis., 20:315–334, 1955.

29. Pincus, T., and Callahan, L.F.: Taking mortality in rheumatoid arthritis seriously—predictive markers, socioeconomic status and comorbidity. J. Rheumatol., 13:841–845, 1986.

ROLE OF NURSING AND ALLIED HEALTH PROFESSIONS IN THE TREATMENT OF ARTHRITIS

48

JANICE SMITH PIGG

Patients with arthritis often benefit from the expertise and skills of health professionals other than physicians. Nurses, physical therapists, occupational therapists, social workers, and individuals from other disciplines can help with patient education and compliance. The growth of rheumatology has stimulated great interest in the treatment of rheumatic disease patients in such professionals.

This interest led to the development of the Arthritis Health Professions Association (AHPA), a professional section of the Arthritis Foundation. This unique multidisciplinary organization incorporates more than 14 disciplines and has nearly 2000 members. From its beginning in 1965 it was "strongly expressed that the organization not be fractionated by profession or into subgroups but that all members function and work together as in an ideal interdisciplinary clinical setting to effect a coordinated team pattern of interaction."[1] Nursing and physical therapy are the best-represented disciplines. Occupational therapy is a close third, and social work is a distant fourth (Table 48–1). Others in AHPA include health educators, psychologists, counselors, physicians, laboratory technologists, pharmacists, nutritionists and dietitians, and podiatrists.

An AHPA fellowship program was established in 1973 and a research grant program was begun in 1978. Other research support has come from the National Institutes of Health (NIH) through the Multipurpose Arthritis Centers developed as a result of the recommendations of the National Arthritis Act of 1974. All these activities have stimulated an increase in the

Table 48–1. Arthritis Health Professions Association (AHPA) Membership by Discipline

Members, by Discipline	Percentage of Total Membership (%)
Nurses	29
Physical therapists	24
Occupational therapists	20
Social workers	5
Physicians	2
Others	20

(1986–1987 Membership List of Arthritis Health Professions Association, Atlanta.)

number of general and discipline-specific publications including two discipline-specific books on rheumatology.[2,3]

With the maturing of rheumatology as a subspecialty area of nursing and some of the allied health professions, standards and competencies are being identified. The first of these was the *Outcome Standards for Rheumatology Nursing Practice* drafted by an AHPA Nursing Tasking Force and published by the American Nurses' Association in 1983.[4] A similar AHPA Occupational Therapy Task Force published a position paper on *Role and Functions of Occupational Therapy in the Management of Patients with Rheumatic Diseases* in 1986.[5] Competencies in physical therapy practice in rheumatology have also been published.[6]

The fellowship and research awards and the formulation of standards have had a definite impact on the quality of patient care. Yet, the majority of patients with arthritis are treated by nonspecialists who have not had the benefit of these advantages. A generalist in nursing or an allied health profession may have as many as 365 encounters per year with rheumatology patients.[7] Expectations of nursing and allied health rheumatology specialists and of their nonspecialized generalist colleagues should not be the same.[8] Specialists should provide service in more complex situations, serve as role models, identify standards of care, provide basic and continuing professional education in their respective areas, and conduct research.

PREPARATION

Nonphysician health professionals often have a general understanding of the rheumatic diseases but may lack the ability to apply it to a given patient.[9] Basic concepts of acute versus chronic, localized versus systemic, degenerative versus inflammatory disease may be generally understood but confusing as they inter-relate in a patient. A 1979 survey of schools of occupational and physical therapy and of nursing in the United States and Canada showed that most curricula contained minimal information about the rheumatic diseases, although training program directors believed their programs were adequate in this area.[10] A later survey of occupational and physical therapists in Arizona found that approximately half considered their academic background in arthritis poor to fair.[11]

Basic and advanced preparation of nurses and allied health professionals in the care of patients with rheumatic diseases should increase with the growing numbers of elderly persons and chronic disease patients. There has been a noticeable increasing interest in the roles of the various disciplines as evidenced by increasing numbers of symposia and research publications.

Nursing and allied health expertise in related areas such as chronic disease, pain management, medication management, patient education, counseling techniques, mobility problems, and independent living are highly applicable to the patient with arthritis.

Continuing education programs can increase in the case of rheumatology patients[12,13] by addressing the roles and functions of nurses and allied health professionals rather than placing primary emphasis on differential diagnosis and the clinical manifestations of rheumatic diseases. Written and audiovisual materials to supplement professional education efforts are available through the Arthritis Information Clearinghouse, the National Institutes of Health, which provides bibliographies on a wide variety of subjects re-

lating to rheumatic diseases, and the AHPA which has produced a slide collection and instructional guide for teachers of nurses and allied health professionals.

Attitudes and understanding of the special problems caused by arthritis influence the quality of care. A study of nurses in a rheumatology clinical rotation demonstrated the positive impact this experience had on their attitudes.[14] A tool has been developed to measure a health-care professional's attitudes toward arthritis patients.[15] A study also has been conducted showing various health professions' beliefs about people with arthritis.[16]

PRACTICE SETTINGS

Patients with arthritis are most often hospitalized in a general medical or surgical unit but specialized care can be offered in a rehabilitative, orthopedic, or rheumatic disease unit. In my experience a specialized unit best meets the rheumatic patient's unique needs by providing truly comprehensive care, including diagnosis, application of therapeutic procedures, and rehabilitation.

The general activity pattern and pace of rehabilitation in the rheumatic diseases are different from those of many other disorders. The energy and mobility limitations of many patients combined with effective learning needs, emphasis on independent function, rest and pacing requirements, and fluctuating inflammatory disease activity, require a different ratio of personnel to patients than in the general hospital population.[17]

Long-term management of an arthritis patient can take place at home where interactions with family members and assessment of the environment can be more readily appreciated. Recent restrictions on hospitalization and emphasis on early discharge have increased home care. Theoretically, patients at home have access to all the same skills and degree of expertise as found in the hospital, but in reality their care will be delivered by generalists.

Nurses and allied health professionals often provide care in a physician's office or outpatient clinic,[18] and often appear to the patient as more accessible and approachable than the physician.[19] However, routine tasks in the ambulatory setting such as scheduling appointments, handling phone calls, preparing patients for examinations, and maintaining records, may interfere with professional functions such as monitoring the patient's condition, patient education, counseling, and support.

Extended care facilities provide rehabilitation and

physical care for those patients with severe limitations. Many elderly patients in nursing homes have arthritis as only one of many infirmities.

The therapeutic needs of children with rheumatic disease are best met by a multidisciplinary team with special knowledge about normal development and growth.[20] Regional pediatric rheumatology centers are being developed.

Patients with arthritis can be seen in any health care setting; however, the current trend toward ambulatory care will require new and better networks to get patients with complicated needs and problems to those specialists that can best manage them.

PATIENT-CARE TEAM

The combined expertise of professionals with differing skills is needed to achieve optimal comprehensive management of an arthritis patient.[21] No single member of the team is capable of meeting all of the patient's needs.[22] This concept is evident in the NIH Multipurpose Arthritis Centers and in other specialized units where innovative techniques in arthritis management are being developed and evaluated. In one study a coordinated team of allied health professionals provided care that was more effective than was the episodic use of such professionals in the management of patients with mild rheumatoid arthritis (RA).[23] The problems of arthritis are diverse, and the arthritis health-care team should possess diverse skills to meet the needs of individual patients.

An interdisciplinary team working toward a common goal is more likely to produce a better therapeutic outcome than each individual member functioning separately. *The key to success lies in the coordination of efforts and in communication among the professionals and with the patient and family.* These interactions are as important as the team structure itself. No discipline can be given priority, or the interdisciplinary nature of the group is lost.

The roles of team members typically represent a distribution of responsibilities specific to a discipline by tradition and/or by a licensure restriction (e.g., the administration of medications by nurses and the use of certain modalities by physical therapists) but sharing of activities is desirable when members of more than one discipline are qualified by training or experience.[24] Although role clarification and areas of primary responsbility must be determined, in most multidisciplinary settings, the patient's physician is the designated leader of the team. The role of team coordinator may fall to any member.

Within the team, however, goals and role expectations are frequently unclear. The *Outcome Standards for Rheumatology Nursing Practice* points out that the identified patient outcomes may not be due exclusively to nursing intervention, and collaboration with members of other disciplines is often required. It is essential for those in different disciplines working together in one setting to understand each other's roles to best effect the treatment plan, but it is often impossible to define these roles generically.

A Delphi study showed that, in most cases, one discipline could be designated as primary.[25] Certain broad activities were not considered discipline specific, and team members participated according to their area of expertise modified by patient needs and the resources of the setting. All members of the team are not always available and another member can at least partially fill the gap. All patients do not need the services of all the team members.

Comprehensive treatment consists of more than a series of referrals. *Such care should be based on the patient's needs rather than on those of the "system."* The roles of the various disciplines involved in the team approach to rheumatic disease care are briefly described, based on my own experience, contributions from colleagues, and researched literature. The roles of the participants in an interdisciplinary team working for the past 18 years at a rheumatic disease center where patient care is the primary function are given in Table 48–2.

NURSE

The nurse has been called the "generalist among specialists."[26] This idea is particularly true in rheumatology, in which the nurse's role expands to fill patient's needs because of a broad expertise. Nursing responsibility for arthritis patients ranges from complete physical care for the critically ill or incapacitated patient to support and education for those with chronic illness.[27] Rheumatologic nursing has only recently emerged as a specialty.[28–31] Most nurses caring for patients with arthritis are generalists.

Hospitalization has been advocated to provide physical rest for the patient and isolation from emotional stress during times of uncontrolled exacerbation of inflammatory disease; nursing care is therefore a major reason for hospitalization.[32] The nurse should play a primary role in planning a realistic and integrated schedule for meeting the patient's pharmacotherapeutic and rehabilitation needs, in reinforcing the teaching of other disciplines, and in serving as liaison.[33]

The role of the nurse varies with the setting but

Table 48-2.   Primary Areas of Practice Accountability

PHYSICIAN AND/OR RHEUMATOLOGIST
Diagnosis
Prescription of treatment (drugs, therapy, life style)
Management (adjustment of therapeutic regimen)

PHYSIATRIST (by referral)
Consultant to medical staff
Therapeutic recommendations
Determination of impairment and disability

PSYCHIATRIST (by referral)
Consultant regarding patients' emotional problems
Recommendations of psychologic management
Diagnosis and treatment of psychiatric disorders

NURSE
Assessment of and interventions in patients' problems
Coordination based on patients' needs for consistency and continuity of care
Physical care, safety, and comfort
Emotional support
Education of patients and families (self-management of medications, life style, comfort measures)
Observations and reporting
Patients' advocate and liaison
Reinforcement of other disciplines and instructions
Medication administration and monitoring

PHYSICAL THERAPIST (per physician's order)
Evaluation of joint range of motion, muscle strength, endurance, sensation and perception, mobility, and gait
Assessment of footwear needs
Instruction in individualized exercise program, body mechanics, and transfer skills
Selection of assistive ambulation devices
Application of heat, cold, electrical, or other therapies

OCCUPATIONAL THERAPIST (per physician's order)
Evaluation of functional ability
Instruction in joint protection, energy conservation and work simplification, and individualized exercise program
Fabrication of splints
Assist patients in planning life style modification
Work evaluation

SOCIAL WORKER (by referral)
Counseling (social and emotional)
Assist patients in development of coping skills
Location and referral of patients to community resources (vocational, financial)
Identification of patients' emotional stage
Liaison to patients and families

PHARMACIST
Distribution of medications
Consultant regarding medication information
Medication instruction

DIETITIAN
Dietary assessment
Monitoring of pertinent laboratory values
Instruction to patients regarding special diet (per physician's order) and proper nutrition
Recommendation of nutritional supplements

HOME CARE COORDINATOR
Coordination with community care agencies
Provision of information on community resources
Liaison with community agencies

(Reprinted by permission from Midwest Arthritis Treatment Center, Columbia Hospital, Milwaukee.)

includes teaching, monitoring, reporting, and referral interventions. The nurse has knowledge related to human responses, the identification of patient needs, and skills in providing physical care and comfort, in observing and assessing physical signs, symptoms, and behavior, and in administering and monitoring medications.[34] Nurses have the closest and most prolonged contact with the patient and are therefore in an excellent position to teach,[35] counsel, support,[36,37] monitor for therapeutic compliance, coordinate continuity of care, communicate with the attending physicians,[38,39] and encourage patient involvement and participation in a comprehensive program.[40]

The relief of pain and provision of comfort are often considered the two main functions of the nurse.[41-43] Another major aim of the rheumatology nurse is to help the patient maintain and retain mobility.[44] Rheumatology demands aspects of both "high tech" and "high touch" nursing.

The American Nurses' Association and AHPA *Outcome Standards for Rheumatology Nursing Practice* relate problems encountered by patients and their families[45] and are in accord with the definition of nursing as "the diagnosis and treatment of human responses to actual or potential health problems."[46] The rheumatologic practice standards for which the nurse is accountable include management of pain, stiffness, fatigue, self-care, self-concept, and ineffective coping, as well as the patient's knowledge relating to mobility and self-care decisions.

The nursing care of the patient with a rheumatologic condition differs not so much by medical diagnosis but according to the individual patient's needs. For example, a patient with life-threatening visceral organ involvement requires a different type and amount of nursing intervention than does a patient with intermittently active chronic, multiple-joint involvement, a newly diagnosed patient, a patient with severe and late-stage crippling disease, a patient with a temporary, localized, problem, or a patient whose problem has a known cause and specific treatment. The medical diagnosis may be the same for each of these patients.[47]

Care also varies with the specialized role of the nurse. These functions may be specialized for certain treatments, such as surgical procedures.[48] A staff nurse has physical,[49] psychological, educational, and coordinating functions. A nurse-supervised, self-administered medication program may be instituted in the hospital.[50] A community-based public health or visiting nurse is aware of helpful community resources, can monitor the implementation of the prescribed program, can enlist family involvement, and can provide valuable feedback information concerning the home environment.[51,52] The occupational health nurse is often the first professional to see an employee with a rheumatic disease problem, and after the medical diagnosis is made, the nurse can monitor the patient's condition and compliance, provide positive reinforcement of the treatment plan and patient education, and modify the work environment.[53]

The functions of a nurse practitioner, certified by the American Nurses' Association, may include detailed physical examination, evaluation of the patient's response to the medical program and management, referral to others for special needs, coordination, and followup care.[54,55] Successful nurse-managed programs have been reported for patients receiving special drugs, such as gold, penicillamine, and methotrexate, or patients with specific conditions, such as osteoarthritis or gout.[56] Nurse "metrologists" assist in drug studies.[57,58] Patients in clinical drug trials in one study expressed a wish to remain in the nurse-run clinic because they saw the same person at each clinic visit, received more consultation time, and felt they could talk more easily to the nurse who was perceived to listen. The supportive nursing approach to chronic illness resulted in a better patient outcome.[59,60]

Nurses promote wellness by encouraging independence in activities of daily living appropriate to the patient's ability but allow an appropriate level of dependence when the patient is sickest; interdependence is the ultimate nursing goal. A sensitive, astute, and caring nurse can greatly enhance a patient's level of wellness.[61]

By the application of *nursing process* (problem solving), including *nursing diagnosis* (identification of patients' problems that lend themselves to nursing intervention), the potential role of the nurse in the care of patients with rheumatic diseases is becoming more clearly delineated.

PHYSICAL THERAPIST

Although physical therapy is an essential part of treatment of many patients with rheumatic disease, it is probably the most neglected facet in their management.[62] Physical therapy is the evaluation and treatment of disease or disability using physical modalities, therapeutic exercises, training, and education.[63] Therapists evaluate the musculoskeletal system by assessing joint range of motion, muscle strength, endurance, sensation and perception, gait, mobility, coordination development, respiratory pattern, functional ability, and the need for special footwear and mobility aids.

Physical therapists involve patients in an individ-

ualized therapeutic program directed at correcting an impairment and improving musculoskeletal or cardiovascular function. Therapeutic exercises are most often directed toward two components of function: range of joint motion and muscle strength. Range-of-motion exercises maintain the anatomic movement of a joint, while strengthening exercises improve the muscles' ability to move joints. In inflammatory joint disease, isometric exercises (contraction of muscle without changing its length) are used to minimize stress on the joint's supporting structures. Passive exercises improve mobility if a patient is unable to exercise independently. Active exercises, with and without assistance, increase strength, coordination, and function. Other exercises or activities aid endurance or posture. The physical therapist can often advise the physician in selecting the appropriate type and intensity of exercise.

The physical therapist also provides instruction in gait, body mechanics, and transfer skills. Properly selected canes, crutches, walkers, or wheelchairs often enhance mobility. Equipment must be chosen with careful consideration of all involved joints, energy conservation, convenience, and practicality. For example, painful hands or wrists may not be able to bear the load transmitted through the handle of a cane, and use of a forearm trough or platform crutches may be better. Techniques that help in transferring can increase mobility, and proper use of body mechanics can increase function and conserve limited energy. Shoe modifications often help with painful feet that limit ambulation, and shoe orthoses can prevent or correct early deformity.

The physical therapist understands the various combinations of heat, cold,[64] water,[65] and electricity that can be applied in different forms to relieve muscle spasm, to increase local circulation, or to relieve pain. Supervised movement in water is especially valuable in treatment of arthritis.[66–68]

The physical therapist plays a major role in preoperative and postoperative treatment to restore optimum function and in development of a home exercise program.[69] Society's focus on physical fitness and conditioning has stimulated physical therapists to develop recreational physical exercise recommendations and fitness center guidelines for persons with arthritis.[70]

Rheumatologic competencies have been identified as essential in seven areas:

basic knowledge (impact of rheumatic disease on the patient); *patient evaluation* (ambulation/transfer status, knowledge of disease and treatment regimen, pain status, swelling/synovitis, muscle strength, deformity/joint stability, joint range of motion, and fatigue/endurance);

design of a plan of care (plan based on history, goals, expectations, motivation, pain tolerance, deficits in muscle strength, status of joint deformities, deficits in functional activities, activity of the disease, ambulation status, ability to rest, tolerance for modalities, need for adaptive and orthotic equipment, recognize/respond to changes in physiologic status, continue, modify, or discontinue goals or treatments, design a discharge plan of care); *implementation* of a physical therapy plan of care (therapeutic exercise program, ambulation program); *patient compliance* (determining patient expectations about treatment, determining treatment based on mutual goals of patient and therapist, designing programs that have simple tasks to be done, establishing what patient knows by demonstration, providing written instructions); *patient, family, and community education* (individualize instruction in therapeutic exercise, joint protection, energy conservation, and therapeutic heat and cold; and *research activities*.[71]

Most of these competencies are not necessarily unique to rheumatic disease treatment but rather are generic to the practice of physical therapy. A study of the perceptions of physical therapists (clinical educators and arthritis health professionals) and rheumatologists showed a variance in opinions as to how essential these competencies are for entry-level therapists[71] and raised several questions: (1) Are generalist physical therapists qualified to treat complex problems of patients with rheumatic diseases? (2) Do rheumatologists know what physical therapists should be able to do? (3) What is the responsibility of physical therapists to educate rheumatologists and other physicians regarding physical therapy care of rheumatic disease patients?

OCCUPATIONAL THERAPIST

Occupational therapy personnel make a major contribution to the management of patients with rheumatic diseases. Occupational therapy for rheumatic disease patients consists of a medically prescribed evaluation and treatment directed toward improving or restoring lost functions.[72] The reference to "occupation" may be misleading unless thought of as the goal-directed use of purposeful activity.[73] The occupational therapist aids the patient in achieving optimal function by developing new adaptive skills or by improving existing performance capacity. The work of the occupational therapist falls into the categories of assessment and therapy.

Patients are appropriately referred to the occupational therapist for evaluation of performance and for help in gaining functional independence. The goals include education of the patient, physical comfort, psychosocial adjustment, and postoperative rehabilitation. To assess function, an occupational therapist evaluates motor skills, range of motion, strength, endurance, and skills of daily living, and also documents deformity.

The occupational therapist can assist the patient in gaining or in maintaining functional independence at home, at work, and at school through adaptations in activities of daily living or by the provision of assistive or adaptive equipment.[74] This goal may include physical modifications of the home, work, and school environment. In addition to vocational counseling, leisure activities and play are also analyzed. Through task analysis, occupational therapists assess the work setting and activity for incorporation of disease-management principles and exploration of alternate worksites.

Educating patients to prevent disability is part of the role of the occupational therapist.[75] This work includes instruction in energy conservation, by elimination of wasted body motion, work simplification, by means of streamlining of tasks to maximize efficiency, body mechanics, which are a component of energy conservation and joint protection concerned with posture during movement, joint protection to avoid postures or stress that cause deformities, the effect of disease on life style, and adjustment to disease or disability. The patient may also be instructed in relaxation techniques and in measures to handle emotional stress.[76,77]

The occupational therapist also addresses the psychosocial components of performance, including social interaction, self-management, decision making and problem solving, and adjustment to disability. Orthotic devices may be fabricated by the occupational therapist and may be fitted for comfort to increase function and to prevent deformity.[78–80] However, some conditions do not respond to splinting.[81] Postoperative rehabilitation, particularly of the hand and wrist, is undertaken by the occupational therapist.[82–84]

The primary goals of occupational therapy and the ways in which they are accomplished include the following: (1) the reduction of pain and inflammation through splinting or instructing the patient in positioning to rest involved joints and the protection of joints during use; (2) maintenance of motion and joint integrity by gentle passive or active range of motion, proper positioning for lying or sitting, and use of resting splints; and (3) maintenance of function by instruction in pacing, work simplification, energy conservation measures, and alternate methods of performing activities of daily living. A major role of the occupational therapist is in helping the patient to modify his life style to reach these goals.

SOCIAL WORKER

The social worker should be a part of the comprehensive management of chronic rheumatic disease by directly intervening with the patient and family and by helping other care providers to recognize the patient's emotional reactions. The social worker often acts as a liaison, aiding communication between care providers and patients and guiding the other care providers to appropriate responses.[85–87]

Through psychosocial assessment, the social worker can identify the patient's current stage of emotional response to the illness as demonstrated in denial, anger, depression, or acceptance. The patient's past and present ability to cope with stress, as well as the extent of family support, can be identified. The social worker's interventions with the patient and family include counseling on social and emotional concerns, development of coping skills, and referral to available community resources such as housing agencies, transportation resources, vocational rehabilitation programs, and financial assistance sources.

OTHER DISCIPLINES

Other disciplines may be involved in the comprehensive care of the arthritis patient. The *pharmacist* not only dispenses drugs but also may assist the physician in their selection and in considerations of dosage, optimal timing, toxicity, and interactions. Education of the staff regarding medications is yet another role of the pharmacist. The pharmacist can identify patients taking over-the-counter remedies who may need medical supervision, as well as patients who have forgotten or have neglected refills. The pharmacist can also suggest ways of reducing drug costs, and when more than one physician is prescribing, may identify potential drug interactions or prescription duplications.[88]

The *dietitian* assesses nutritional status through diet history, monitoring of pertinent laboratory values, and appropriate anthropometrics. Acutely ill patients with increased metabolic needs, increased pain, decreased appetite, and decreased ability to eat or to swallow may require nutritional supplements to ensure adequate intake. Overweight patients require individualized meal plans, education, and counseling to maximize weight loss and weight maintenance. In addition, the dietitian provides guidance through the maze of fad diets and nutritional misinformation. There is an increasing interest in the possibility of some rheumatic diseases as a manifestation of food allergy or hypersensitivity and, conversely, in the role of nutritional modification in altering immune responsiveness and thereby affecting manifestations of rheumatic diseases.[89]

Laboratory personnel contribute their efforts toward proper diagnosis and management through the performance of various qualitative and quantitative tests.[90]

Psychologists and counselors help to identify, evaluate, and manage associated emotional problems that affect the rehabilitation program. These professionals are involved in counseling and adaptation activities, including relaxation measures, and must be aware of the psychologic disorders associated with the various rheumatic diseases as well as drug-induced psychologic problems.[91,92]

The vocational rehabilitation of a person with rheumatic disease is much more complicated than that of some other physically disabled clients with more static disabilities.[93] Arthritis is often a progressive disability that may vary from day to day, and the same type of arthritis varies in severity from person to person. Arthritis can directly affect work competence and may have a significant psychologic impact. The *vocational or rehabilitation counselor* evaluates the work abilities of the patient, offers vocational counseling and guidance, and helps the individual to retrain for specific vocational skills.[94,95] The rehabilitation counselor often acts as a patient advocate in vocational settings and is skilled in locating employment opportunities.

The *podiatrist* provides routine toenail and foot care, particularly for patients with skin difficulties and deformities of the foot. In addition, the podiatrist educates patients about foot problems, including the selection of proper footwear with internal and external modifications to relieve stress areas.[96,97] Podiatrists are knowledgeable about the effects of disease and gait deviation on foot structures. The *orthotic specialist* makes and modifies prescribed appliances such as braces, splints, foot supports, and special shoes for each patient's particular needs.

Health educators and biomedical engineers are the newest professional groups in rheumatology. Although all disciplines are involved in educating the patient and his family, the health educator has the primary role and may be responsible for development and coordination of the education program. Health educators are skilled in the processes of teaching, learning, and educational psychology. Biomedical engineers have become increasingly involved in research on prostheses.

FUNCTIONS

The basic treatment goals addressed in the management of arthritis are: (1) relief of pain; (2) prevention of deformity; and (3) maintenance of function. The roles of nurses and allied health professionals stem directly from these goals. Although the physician prescribes the components of the treatment program, thereby designating participation of others, not all these functions are dependent. Each discipline also has independent, usually discipline-specific problem-solving activities. *To achieve these goals most effectively, activities should be interdependent and synergistic, so the whole is at least equal to or greater than the sum of the parts.*[98,99]

INDEPENDENT FUNCTIONS

Independent functions of nursing and allied health professionals include activities that are discipline-specific, are individualized to the patient, or require that a decision be made. A discipline-specific function is physical care. A nurse does not see a physician's order to "care for the patient." Yet nurses independently see to it that the patient has physical space of his own, a bed to sleep in, food to eat, and arrangements for hygiene and personal care. Although this function is often taken for granted, it can be of vital importance to the arthritis patient who is physically dependent on others.

As a basis not only for their independent functions, but also for individualized aspects of dependent and interdependent functions, all disciplines incorporate some sort of assessment or evaluation into their programs. The focus of the assessment or evaluation differs from one discipline to another. Whereas the physician structures history taking and physical examination to elicit data on which diagnosis or management can be based, nursing and the allied health professions are oriented toward the problems of patients, such as difficulty in walking or refusal to eat. These assessments or evaluations, in addition to health, physical, psychological, and functional status, include home environment and personal life style, as well as learning ability, financial resources, and social status. These independent assessments can be valuable because they form a more complete picture of the patient and his needs. Such combined assessments cover not only signs and symptoms and other

condition-specific information, but also the patient's ability to follow a therapeutic regimen and to adapt it to his home environment and life style.

Although specific interventions are at least partly dependent functions requiring a medical order, the way in which those interventions are performed is likely to be an independent function. As an example, pain management is a frequent problem of patients with arthritis. The physician may order an analgesic to be given when needed, but whether or not to give the medication, and when to give it, is the nurse's decision based on an assessment of the specific situation. In addition to, or in place of, the drug, the nurse may decide to apply heat or cold or to try a relaxation or distraction technique.

Education of the patient, because of its inherent individualization, is another area of independent function. The following are some examples. The nurse may teach the patient pharmacologic self-administration techniques or comfort measures based on his unique situation for a successful followup when the patient is on his own.

The occupational therapist, although often requiring a physician's order to teach, individualizes concepts and principles of work simplification, energy conservation, joint protection, and body mechanics. The occupational therapist takes into account the disease's systemic features, the general state of deconditioning, and the total needs of the patient in regard to psychosocial, recreational, and vocational demands, to determine an appropriately individualized institutional program.[100] Instruction in joint protection varies for different diseases. Increased joint activity may be helpful in some diseases, but harmful in others. Adjoining joints operate interdependently, so what may be protective to one joint may redirect the forces to another in a stressful manner. Although the physician orders instructions in joint protection, the occupational therapist determines the appropriate measures.

The physical therapist individualizes instruction in a home exercise program based on the patient's needs. Each discipline determines the best teaching opportunity, based on the patient's readiness to learn and the appropriate instructional technique.

Symptoms bring the patient into the health-care system. If the symptoms are not relieved, the patient may leave the system to seek help elsewhere. Sometimes, the symptoms cannot be totally eliminated, so the patient's understanding of and belief in the treatment become the key to satisfaction and compliance. Reaching this understanding can be time consuming and can also require special skills in relationships of nurses and allied health professionals.

Another activity of nurses and allied health professionals may be the organization of groups of patients for the purposes of education, support, or socializing.[101,102] These activities, previously thought to enhance communication, to improve compliance with medical regimens, and to promote a sense of well-being, have more recently been shown to increase patients' knowledge about their disease and to improve some patients' perception of the adequacy of their families' attitudes and behavior.[103,104] Use of accepted educational and counseling strategies to change behavior can assist patients to assume more responsibility for their own care.[105] This aspect is crucial because care providers have no control over therapeutic activities performed away from direct supervision.

As the need arises, nurses and allied health professionals are also involved with the family. Roles may have changed within the family, and the patient may no longer be the family's financial supporter or may no longer be able to care for the home. Like the patient, family members may be passing through similar stages of adjustment and may gain insight into management of their own emotional reactions by understanding those of the patient.[106] Both planned and informal opportunities enable the nurse and allied health professional to assume this independent role in assisting the family.

The areas of adaptation and coping with the problems arising from a chronic rheumatic disease are addressed by most care providers in an independent way.[107] As an example, problems relating to sexuality may involve the physical therapist if the sexual dysfunction is due to limited range of motion or to weakness; the social worker in issues of emotions, personality, body image, or interpersonal relationships; the occupational therapist in applying concepts of pacing and energy conservation to overcome fatigue; and the nurse to help the patient understand the relationship of disease or medications to sexual functioning.[108–110]

DEPENDENT FUNCTIONS

Physicians write orders that are carried out by nursing and allied health personnel. Some activities cannot be undertaken without a medical order: (1) the administration of medications by the nurse, although timing may be left to the nurse's discretion; (2) laboratory testing, although predetermined protocol may prevail; (3) splinting, although the occupational therapist or orthotist selects the splinting materials; and (4) exercise programs for a specific purpose. Physician referral establishes communication and pro-

vides a means of providing pertinent information about the patient.

INTERDEPENDENT FUNCTIONS

The role of any discipline, including medicine, is not carried out in a vacuum. A given discipline does not depend on the others, except within legal guidelines, to perform discipline-specific activities. Most functions, however, are best carried out interdependently with other care providers. Nurses and allied health professionals independently assess the patient with regard to problems, they design and implement plans to address the identified problems, and then they evaluate the results interdependently. For example, the physician notes that a patient is not responding to treatment as expected. The nurse contributes the information that the patient is not taking the medication as directed, but is taking it only as he feels the need. The social worker indicates that the patient is on a fixed income and feels that he cannot afford the medication. As a result, instructions are clarified, medication times are adapted to the patient's home schedule, and the social worker aids in seeking financial assistance. Together, the actions of the physician, the nurse and the social worker interdependently affect the outcome. The roles complement each other while approaching the patient from each discipline's unique perspective.

Confusion can exist in interdependent areas, particularly regarding the roles of physical and occupational therapists. A study of primary care physicians' perceptions of arthritis health professionals demonstrated confusion in understanding the difference between the physical and occupational therapists' roles.[111] Although many of their functions do overlap,[112–116] the roles of the physical and the occupational therapist are determined by staffing patterns, departmental philosophies, and practices, as well as by an individual therapist's skills and interests. Broadly, the physical therapist restores the function of the muscles, whereas the occupational therapist translates that function into relevant activity. *The best way to differentiate their roles in a given setting is to ask them.*

Education of the patient is an important element in management and a major independent responsibility of all health professionals who have direct contact with the patient. The interdependency of education provides consistency, reinforcement, and multiple and varied approaches to gain the patient's cooperation with the therapeutic regimen. Each discipline has areas of primary accountability, but most areas overlap disciplines (Table 48–3). An example is joint

Table 48–3.   Patient Education: Content Areas of Primary Responsibility by Discipline

NURSING
  Medications
  Pacing and rest
  Posture and positioning
  Responsibility of the patient
  Comfort measures for pain and stiffness
  Coping and adaptation
  Unproved methods of treatment
  Compliance

OCCUPATIONAL THERAPY
  Joint protection
  Energy conservation
  Use of adaptive equipment
  Relaxation
  Pacing and rest
  Exercise programs
  Posture and positioning

SOCIAL SERVICE
  Community resources
  Coping and adaptation

PHYSICAL THERAPY
  Range of motion
  Use of heat and cold therapy
  Relaxation
  Footwear
  Posture and positioning
  Exercise

MEDICINE
  Diagnosis
  Disease process
  Prognosis
  Medications

PHARMACY
  Medications
  Compliance

DIETETICS
  Nutrition
  Special diets

(Reprinted by permission from Midwest Arthritis Treatment Center, Columbia Hospital, Milwaukee.)

protection. Although the occupational therapist is most likely to teach concepts and principles, others, usually a nurse or physical therapist, provide reinforcement and instruct the patient in their applications. Therapeutic responsibilities can often be assumed by another discipline, depending on the care setting and available resources.[117]

Education of the patient involves much more than merely providing the patient with information about disease. The information must be consistent from one professional to another. This instruction should be based on the beliefs, needs, and concerns of the patient and should include educational activities aimed at assisting patients in changing their health behavior voluntarily.[118] This goal requires close communication and sharing of information among the various team members. Using needs assessment and measuring motivation, an educational program can improve cognitive knowledge and may motivate behavioral changes.

An informed patient is more likely to comply with the prescribed therapeutic regimen and usually reports more reliably the effects, good or bad, of that regimen.[119] Failure to cooperate implies that the patient has not received full benefit from the health-care provider's expertise. Failure to take the prescribed medication may exacerbate the disease. When it is assumed that the patient is taking the prescribed amount of medication without the desired results and dosage is increased, overdosage may result. Undetected failure to cooperate can lead to an incorrect evaluation of efficacy of a particular treatment regimen.[120] Regimens must be tailored to the individual characteristics of each patient and should be adjusted only when the patient is compliant. Some investigators suggest that the results of clinical trials should not be published unless they include an adequate assessment of "compliance."[121] It often takes the skills and insights of a variety of professionals to understand the reasons behind a patient's failure to comply and to then be able to help the patient.

Nurses and allied health professionals can help to identify barriers to compliance. Patients fail to adhere to therapeutic recommendations for many reasons. *Denying* patients may not believe their illness warrants extensive care. *Angry* patients may refuse to comply as a way of punishing families or the health-care provider. *Depressed* patients perceive compliance as pointless. Finances, time schedules, unrealistic family expectations, and different opinions as to an adequate therapeutic trial are other possible barriers.[122,123] The problems of noncompliance often require interdisciplinary assessment and intervention.

Discharge planning is a cooperative effort of all disciplines with emphasis on the strengths, limitations, and goals of the individual patient. When continuing care is indicated, the decision is often shared. Interdisciplinary consultation and communication demonstrate responsibility to other professionals as well as to patients.

ADMINISTRATIVE AND RESEARCH FUNCTIONS

Nurses and allied health professionals with rheumatology expertise may become chiefs of departments of therapy or head nurses. Some also hold management positions in specialized rheumatic disease programs.

Some allied health professionals and nurses are involved in independent research as principal investigators in areas such as the content and methods of programs to educate patients and families, treatment techniques, validation of measurement tools, psychosocial issues, and health status.[124-127] Others assist or coordinate research protocols under the direction of a physician.

The AHPA Fellowship Program was established in 1972 to develop research training opportunities and to grant support for professionals other than physicians engaged in the delivery of health care. The program mirrored the organization's shift in emphasis from its original purpose of providing a home for the allied health workers interested in arthritis to a more mission-oriented goal. The AHPA now emphasizes research and professional education in health-care delivery and the effective use of clinical techniques. This emphasis complements the basic biomedical research done by the members of the ARA.[124]

FACTORS INFLUENCING EFFECTIVENESS

Recommendations made by all team members must be followed to be effective. A study of recommendations made by a rheumatologist, a physical therapist, and a psychologist to the patient's primary care physician and to the patient showed that of 58 medical recommendations, 28 were acted on by the physician and 11 by the patient.[128] Only 7 of the 45 physical therapists' suggestions were acted on by the physician, but the patients followed 26. None of the counseling or psychosocial suggestions made by the team were followed by physicians, but 35 were followed by the patients. The study recommended that patients receive written copies of the suggestions and evaluations made by the allied health professionals, to encourage patient-physician dialogue regarding the suggestions.

The effectiveness of the nurse or allied health professional varies with individual, environmental, organizational, financial, and interpersonal factors. Entry-level preparation, practice experience in the discipline, as well as rheumatologic skills and expertise and individual attitudes about chronicity, deformity, and dependency all influence the care of patients with arthritis. The practice setting is another factor influencing effectiveness. When nurses, for example, care for patients other than those with arthritis, the physical care and needs of these patients may take precedence over the psychosocial and educational needs of the arthritic patient.

Support by specific departments, by hospital administrators, and by physicians is necessary for optimal function. The roles of nurses and allied health professionals in the care of patients with arthritis are often not fully understood nor are their services effectively utilized. The rheumatologist is in a position to speak to the departmental chairman or hospital administrator to request high-quality service.

The relationship between patients and nurses or allied health professionals differs from the patient-physician relationship. For various reasons, which may include physical proximity (not only the increased amount of contact time, but the intimacy of assistance provided in such tasks as bathing and toileting) and a feeling of more-equal standing, patients often confide in the nurse or allied health professional attitudes relating to compliance, financial restrictions, family relationships, and other items they did not mention to their physician. Such information is often medically relevant when conveyed to the physician.

Many of these influences on effectiveness were demonstrated in a study of primary care physicians' perceptions of nurses and allied health professionals. This study revealed a lack of understanding of roles, a concern with cost, problems in communication, lack of accessibility or availability in practice, a feeling of threat to the physician's authority, and the need for flexibility of charges.[129]

In summary, the roles and functions of nurses and allied health professionals have been defined in terms of goals, problems and interventions used to solve them, organizational structure, and the perspectives of the individual disciplines. The knowledge explosion and the demand for a "holistic" approach by patients will lead to ever-changing, flexible descriptions of the functions of nurses and allied health professionals. This change may lead to a more appropriate and effective use of their services. Rapid translation of new information into effective disease management is a challenge to the many disciplines in the health sciences.

Nurses and allied health professionals have a wide variety of unique and specialized skills and knowledge to offer in the care of the rheumatic disease patient that complement as well as supplement the offerings of the physician.

Roles of nurses and allied health professionals are best described by standards and expressed through the individual disciplines' practice. An understanding of these roles is necessary for the most effective utilization of expertise and skills of all disciplines involved in comprehensive care of the rheumatic disease patient.

REFERENCES

1. Smyth, C.J., Freyburg, R.N., and McEwen, C.: History of Rheumatology. Atlanta, Arthritis Foundation, 1985, p. 96.
2. Melvin, J.L.: Rheumatic Disease: Occupational Therapy and Rehabilitation. 2nd Ed. Philadelphia, F.A. Davis, 1982.
3. Pigg, J.S., Driscoll, P.W., and Caniff, R.: Rheumatology Nursing: A Problem Oriented Approach. New York, John Wiley and Sons, 1985.
4. Outcome Standards for Rheumatology Nursing Practice. Kansas City, American Nurses' Association, 1983.
5. Role and functions of occupational therapy in the management of patients with rheumatic diseases. Am. J. Occup. Ther., 40(12):825–829, 1986.
6. Moncur, C.: Physical therapy competencies in rheumatology. Phys. Ther., 65(9):1365–1372, 1985.
7. National Advisory Board on Research and Education. Arthritis research and education. U.S. Department of Health and Human Services, 1980.
8. Swezey, R.L.: Arthritis: Rational Therapy and Rehabilitation. Philadelphia, W.B. Saunders, 1978.
9. Bernhard, G.C.: The rehabilitation of the arthritis patient in the general hospital setting. In Rehabilitation Management of Rheumatic Conditions. 2nd Ed. Edited by G.E. Ehrlich. Baltimore, Williams & Wilkins, 1986.
10. Jette, A.M., and Becker, M.C.: Nursing, occupational therapy and physical therapy preparation in rheumatology in the United States and Canada. J. Allied Health, 9:268–275, 1980.
11. Wickersham, E.A. et al.: Arthritis: Preferred learning methods among Arizona therapists. Am. J. Occup. Ther., 36:509–514, 1982.
12. Sakalys, J., and Carter, M.: Outcomes evaluation: Continuing education in rheumatology for nurses. J. Contin. Educ. Nurs., 16(5):170–175, 1986.
13. Dickinson, G.R., Holzemer, W.L., Nichols, E.: Evaluation of an arthritis continuing education program. J. Contin. Educ. Nurs., 16:127–131, 1985.
14. Nambayan, A., McKay, J., Richards, J.M., and Brown, S.: Scale for assessing nurses' attitudes toward arthritis. Psychol. Rep., 57:138, 1985.
15. DeVallis, R.F., Cook, H.L., and Sauter, S.V.H.: Development and validation of the attitude toward arthritis patients scale (ATAPS). J. Allied Health, 15:49–57, 1986.
16. Potts, M.K., and Brandt, K.D.: Various health professions groups' beliefs about people with arthritis. J. Allied Health, 15:245–256, 1986.
17. Ogryzlo, M.A., Gordon, D.A., and Smythe, R.A.: The rheumatic disease unit (RDU) concept. Arthritis Rheum., 105:479–485, 1967.
18. Knudson, K.G., Spiegel, T.M., and Furst, D.E.: Outpatient educational program for rheumatoid arthritis patients. Patient Counsel. Health Educ., 3:77–82, 1981.
19. Bird, H.A., leGallez, P., and Hill, J.: Combined Care of the Rheumatic Patient. Berlin, Springer-Verlag, 1985.
20. Sullivan, D.B.: The pediatric rheumatology clinic. In Textbook of Pediatric Rheumatology. Edited by J.T. Cassidy. New York, John Wiley and Sons, 1982.
21. Banwell, B.F.: The role of the allied health professional in the treatment of arthritis. Symposium on Rheumatic Diseases. Primary Care, 11:219–232, 1984.
22. Ruddy, S.: The management of rheumatoid arthritis. In Textbook of Rheumatology. 2nd Ed. Edited by W.N. Kelley, et al. Philadelphia, W.B. Saunders, 1985.
23. Feinberg, J.R., and Brandt, K.D.: Allied health team management of rheumatoid arthritis patients. Am. J. Occup. Ther., 38(9):613–620, 1984.
24. Gross, M. et al.: Team care for patients with chronic rheumatic disease. J. Allied Health, 11:239–247, 1982.
25. Figley, B.A.: The roles of health professionals in management of arthritis. Clin. Rheumatol. Pract., 1:43–46, 1983.
26. Allen, K.E., Holm, V.A., and Schiefelbusch, R.L.: Early Intervention—A Team Approach. Baltimore, University Park Press, 1978.
27. Joyce, K.M., Austin, H.A., and Balow, J.E.: The patient with lupus nephritis: A nursing perspective. Heart Lung, 14:75–79, 1985.
28. White, J.F. et al.: Nursing: A specialty you can tailor to your talents. Nursing '79, 9:108–110, 1979.
29. Elliott, M.: Nursing Rheumatic Disease. New York, Churchill Livingstone, 1979.
30. Sutton, J.D.: The role of the rheumatology nurse. In Rheumatic Diseases: Rehabilitation and Management. Edited by G.K. Riggs and E.P. Gall. Woburn, MA, Butterworth Publishers, 1984.
31. Vaidyanathan, S.: Rheumatology—A challenging specialty for nurses. Nurse. J. India, 27:47, 49, 54, 1986.
32. Pigg, J.S.: Nursing care of the hospitalized patient with rheumatic disease. In Rehabilitation Management of Rheumatic Conditions. 2nd Ed. Edited by G.E. Ehrlich. Baltimore, Williams & Wilkins, 1986.
33. Sutton, J.D.: The hospitalized patient with arthritis. In Arthritis and Related Rheumatic diseases. Nurs. Clin. North Am., 19:617–627, 1984.
34. Newberger, G.B.: The role of the nurse with arthritis patients on drug therapy. In Arthritis and Related Rheumatic Diseases. Nurs. Clin. North Am., 19:593–604, 1984.
35. leGallez, P.: Patient education and self-management. Nursing (Oxford), 2:916–917, 1984.
36. Chesson, S.: Social and emotional aspects of rheumatoid arthritis. Nursing (Oxford), 2:914–915, 1984.
37. Miller, T.W., and Jay, L.L.: Multidisciplinary treatment of rheumatoid arthritis. J. Pract. Nurs., 35:57–63, 1985.
38. Beardsley, J., and Rowlands, D.: Nursing the rheumatic patient. In Essential Rheumatology for Nurses and Therapists. Edited by G.S. Panayi. London, Bailliere Tindall, 1980.
39. Horton, J.: Rheumatology nursing. Nurs. Mirror, 155:76, 1982.
40. Hawley, D., and Cathey, M.A.: Fighting fibrositis. Am. J. Nurs., 85:404–406, 1985.
41. Maycock, J.: Towards pain relief. Nurs. Mirror, 160:40–41, 1985.
42. Maycock, J.A.: Pain—A different approach. Nursing (Oxford), 2:924–925, 1984.
43. Johnson, J.A., and Repp, E.C.: Nonpharmacologic pain management in arthritis. In Arthritis and Related Rheumatic Diseases. Nurs. Clin. North Am., 19:583–591, 1984.
44. Peasnell, I.M.: Maintaining mobility and independence. Nursing (Oxford), 2:919–920, 1984.
45. Pigg, J.S., and Schroeder, P.M.: Frequently occurring problems of patients with rheumatic diseases: The ANA Outcome Standards for Rheumatology Nursing Practice. In Arthritis and Related Rheumatic Diseases. Nurs. Clin. North Am., 19:697–708, 1984.
46. Nursing—A Social Policy Statement. Kansas City, American Nurses' Association, 1980.

47. Pigg, J.S., Driscoll, P.W., and Caniff, R.: Rheumatology Nursing: A Problem Oriented Approach. New York, John Wiley and Sons, 1985.

48. Brassell, M.P.: Rehabilitation nursing and the surgical patient. In Rehabilitation Management of Rheumatic Conditions. 2nd Ed. Edited by G.E. Ehrlich. Baltimore, Williams & Wilkins, 1986.

49. Hosking, S.: Rheumatoid arthritis—Fundamental nursing care. Nursing (Oxford), 2:900–901, 1984.

50. Kallas, K.D.: Establishing a self-administered medication program. J. Nurs. Adm.,1438–1442, 1984.

51. Fligg, H., and Wright, V.: The community and hospital nurse in relation to arthritis. In Rehabilitation in the Rheumatic Diseases. Clin. Rheum. Dis., 7:321–326, 1981.

52. Dickinson, G.R.: A home care program for patients with rheumatoid arthritis. Nurs. Clin. North Am., 15:403–418, 1980.

53. Patterson, D.C.: The occupational health nurse on the arthritis team. Occup. Health Nurs., 32:350–351, 1984.

54. Brown-Skeers, V.: How the nurse practitioner manages the rheumatoid arthritis patient. Nursing '79, 9:26–34, 1979.

55. Miller, C.C.: The rheumatic disease nurse practitioner. In Rehabilitation Management of Rheumatic Conditions. 2nd Ed. Edited by G.E. Ehrlich. Baltimore, Williams & Wilkins, 1986.

56. Sutton, J.D.: The role of the rheumatology nurse. In Rheumatic Diseases: Rehabilitation and Management. Edited by G.K. Riggs and E.P. Gall. Woburn, MA, Butterworth Publishers, 1984.

57. Leatham, P.: An extended nursing role in the arthritis care team. Nurs. Times, 77:1926–1927, 1981.

58. leGallez, P.: So what's a metrologist? Nurs. Times, 77:1926–1927, 1981.

59. Hill, J.: Nursing clinics for arthritis. Nurs. Times, 81:33–34, 1985.

60. Hill, J.: Patient evaluation of a rheumatology nursing clinic. Nurs. Times, 82:42–43, 1986.

61. Bethel, T.A.: The role of the nurse in promoting high level wellness in the lupus patient. Health Values, 9:30–33, 1985.

62. Vignos, P.J.: Physiotherapy in rheumatoid arthritis. J. Rheumatol., 73:269–271, 1980.

63. Banwell, B.F.: Physical therapy in arthritis management. In Rehabilitation Management of Rheumatic Conditions. 2nd Ed. Edited by G.E. Ehrlich. Baltimore, Williams & Wilkins, 1986.

64. Banwell, B.F.: Therapeutic heat and cold. In Rheumatic Diseases: Rehabilitation and Management. Edited by G.K. Riggs and E.P. Gall. Woburn, MA, Butterworth Publishers, 1984.

65. Wickersham, B.A.: Hydrotherapy. In Rheumatic Diseases: Rehabilitation and Management. Edited by G.K. Riggs and E.P. Gall. Woburn MA, Butterworth Publishers, 1984.

66. Maloney, P.: Physiotherapy for the rheumatic patient. In Essential Rheumatology for Nurses and Therapists. Edited by G.S. Panayi. London, Bailliere Tindall, 1980.

67. Navarro, A.H.: Physical therapy in the management of rheumatoid arthritis. Clin. Rheumatol. Pract., 1:125–130, 1983.

68. Neubauer, P.: The role of the physiotherapist in a multidisciplinary arthritis program. In Rehabilitation Management of Rheumatic Conditions. Edited by G.E. Ehrlich. Baltimore, Williams & Wilkins, 1980.

69. Navarro, A.H.: The role of the physical therapist. In Rheumatic Diseases: Rehabilitation and Management. Edited by G.K. Riggs and E.P. Gall. Woburn, MA, Butterworth Publishers, 1984.

70. Banwell, B.F.: Exercise and mobility. In Arthritis and Related Rheumatic Diseases. Nurs. Clin. North Am., 19:605–616, 1984.

71. Moncur, C.: Perceptions of physical therapy competencies in rheumatology. Phys. Ther., 67:331–339, 1987.

72. Melvin, J.L.: Rheumatic Disease: Occupational Therapy and Rehabilitation. 2nd Ed. Philadelphia, F.A. Davis, 1982.

73. Sliwa, J.L.: Occupational Therapy and Management. In Rehabilitation Management of Rheumatic Conditions. 2nd Ed. Edited by G.E. Ehrlich. Baltimore, Williams & Wilkins, 1986.

74. Schweidler, H.: Assistive devices, aids to daily living. In Rheumatic Diseases: Rehabilitation and Management. Edited by G.K. Riggs and E.P. Gall. Woburn, MA, Butterworth Publishers, 1984.

75. Furst, G.P. et al.: A program for improving energy conservation behaviors in adults with rheumatoid arthritis. Am. J. Occup. Ther., 41:102–111, 1987.

76. VanDeusen, J., and Harlowe, D.: The efficacy of the ROM dance program for adults with rheumatoid arthritis. Am. J. Occup. Ther., 41:90–95, 1987.

77. Acterberg, J., McGraw, P., and Lawlis, F.: Rheumatoid arthritis: A study of relaxation and temperature biofeedback training as adjunctive therapy. Biofeedback Self Regul., 6:207–223, 1981.

78. Hanten, D.W.: The splinting controversy in RA physical disabilities. Am. J. Occup. Ther. (Special Interest Newslett.), 5:1–24, 1981.

79. Feinberg, J., and Brandt, K.D.: Use of resting splints by patients with rheumatoid arthritis. Am. J. Occup. Ther., 35:173–178, 1981.

80. Nicholas, J. et al.: Splinting in rheumatoid arthritis: Factors affecting patient compliance. Arch. Phys. Med. Rehabil., 62:92, 1982.

81. Seeger, M.W., and Furst, D.E.: Effects of splinting: the treatment of hand contractures in progressive systemic sclerosis. Am. J. Occup. Ther., 41:118–121, 1987.

82. Johnson, B.M., Flynn, M.J.G., and Beckenbaugh, R.D.: A dynamic splint for use after total wrist arthroplasty. Am. J. Occup. Ther., 35:179–184, 1981.

83. Gruen, H.: Splinting in the rheumatic diseases. In Rehabilitation Management of Rheumatic Conditions. 2nd Ed. Edited by G.E. Ehrlich. Baltimore, Williams & Wilkins, 1986.

84. Seeger, M.: Splints, braces and casts. In Rheumatic Diseases: Rehabilitation and Management. Edited by G.K. Riggs and E.P. Gall. Woburn, MA, Butterworth Publishers, 1984.

85. Ehfling, J.L.: The role of the social worker in the rehabilitation of rheumatic disease patients. In Rehabilitation Management of Rheumatic Conditions. 2nd Ed. Edited by G.E. Ehrlich. Baltimore, Williams & Wilkins, 1986.

86. Potts, M.: The role of the social worker in the management of patients with rheumatic disease. Clin. Rheumatol. Pract., 1:77–80, 1983.

87. Potts, M.G.: The role of the social worker. In Rheumatic Diseases: Rehabilitation and Management. Edited by G.K. Riggs and E.P. Gall. Woburn, MA, Butterworth Publishers, 1984.

88. Fritz, W.L.: The pharmacist's contribution to patient care. In Rheumatic Diseases: Rehabilitation and Management. Edited by G.K. Riggs and E.P. Gall. Woburn, MA, Butterworth Publishers, 1984.

89. Panush, R.S., and Webster, E.M.: Nutrition and rheumatic disease. In Rehabilitation Management of Rheumatic Conditions. 2nd Ed. Edited by G.E. Ehrlich. Baltimore, Williams & Wilkins, 1986.

90. Adams, L.E., and Hess, E.V.: Editorial: Continuing medical education in rheumatology of arthritis health professional laboratory personnel. J. Rheumatol., 7:1–4, 1980.

91. Rogal, R.A.: Psychological considerations in the management

of arthritic patients. *In* Rheumatology. Edited by R. Bluestone. Boston, Houghton Mifflin Professional Publishers, 1980.

92. Ziebel, B.: The role of the counselor. *In* Rheumatic Diseases: Rehabilitation and Management. Edited by G.K. Riggs and E.P. Gall. Woburn, MA, Butterworth Publishers, 1984.

93. Sales, A.P.: The role of the vocational counselor. *In* Rheumatic Diseases: Rehabilitation and Management. Edited by G.K. Riggs and E.P. Gall. Woburn, MA, Butterworth Publishers, 1984.

94. Spergel, P.: Vocational assessment, counseling and training. *In* Rehabilitation Management of Rheumatic Conditions. 2nd Ed. Edited by G.E. Ehrlich. Baltimore, Williams & Wilkins, 1986.

95. Cochrane, G.M.: Rheumatoid arthritis: Vocational rehabilitation. Int. Rehabil. Med., *4*:148–153, 1982.

96. Roth, R.D.: The role of the podiatrist in the rheumatology team approach. *In* Rehabilitation Management of Rheumatic Conditions. 2nd Ed. Edited by G.E. Ehrlich. Baltimore, Williams & Wilkins, 1986.

97. Snyder, M.: The role of the podiatrist, prosthetist, and orthotist. *In* Rheumatic Diseases: Rehabilitation and Management. Edited by G.K. Riggs and E.P. Gall. Woburn, MA, Butterworth Publishers, 1984.

98. Bernhard, G.C.: The rehabilitation of the arthritis patient in the general hospital setting. *In* Rehabilitation Management of Rheumatic Conditions. 2nd Ed. Edited by G.E. Ehrlich. Baltimore, Williams & Wilkins, 1986.

99. Figley, B.A.: The roles of health professionals in management of arthritis. Clin. Rheumat. Pract., *1*:43–46, 1983.

100. Shapiro-Slonaker, D.M.: Joint protection and energy conservation. *In* Rheumatic Diseases: Rehabilitation and Management. Edited by G.K. Riggs and E.P. Gall. Woburn, MA, Butterworth Publishers, 1984.

101. Kaplan, S., and Kozin, F.: A controlled study of group counseling in rheumatoid arthritis. J. Rheumatol., *8*:91–99, 1981.

102. Berg, C.E., Alt, K.J., Himmel, J.K., and Judd, B.J.: The effects of patient education on patient cognition and disease-related anxiety. Patient Educ. Couns., *7*:389–394, 1985.

103. Gross, M., and Brandt, K.D.: Educational support groups for patients with ankylosing spondylitis: A preliminary report. Patient Couns. Health Educ., *3*:6–12, 1981.

104. Potts, M.G., and Brandt, K.D.: Analysis of education support groups for patients with rheumatoid arthritis. Patient Couns. Health Educ., *4*:161–166, 1983.

105. Cave, L.: Lowering the uncertainties of arthritis with a nurse-led support group. Ortho. Nurs., *3*:39–42, 1984.

106. Gross, M.: Psychosocial aspects of osteoarthritis—Helping patients cope. Health Soc. Work, *65*:40–46, 1981.

107. Krutzen, P.: Living with and adjusting to arthritis. *In* Arthritis and Related Rheumatic diseases. Nurs. Clin. North Am., *19*:629–636, 1984.

108. Figley, B.A. et al.: Comprehensive approach to sexual health in rheumatic disease. Top. Clin. Nurs., *1*:69–74, 1980.

109. Baum, J., and Figley, B.A.: Psychological and sexual health in rheumatic diseases. *In* Textbook of Rheumatology. Vol. 1,

2nd Ed. Edited by W.N. Kelley et al. Philadelphia, W.B. Saunders, 1986.

110. Malik, C.J., and Brower, S.A.: Rheumatoid arthritis: How does it influence sexuality? Rehabil. Nurs., *9*:26–28, 1984.

111. Stephenson, V.: Occupational therapy and the nurse. Nursing (Oxford), *2*:912–913, 1984.

112. Chamberlain, M.A.: Occupational therapy. *In* Rehabilitation in the Rheumatic Diseases. Clin. Rheum. Dis., *7*:365–375, 1981.

113. Douglas, J.: Occupational therapy—Rehabilitation and resettlement. *In* Essential Rheumatology for Nurses and Therapists. Edited by G.S. Panayi. London, Bailliere Tindall, 1980.

114. Moyes, J., and Haslock, I.: Occupational therapy in rheumatic diseases. Rep. Rheum. Dis., *77*:78, 1981.

115. Yerxa, E.J.: The role of the occupational therapist. *In* Rheumatic Diseases: Rehabilitation and Management. Edited by G.K. Riggs and E.P. Gall. Woburn, MA, Butterworth Publishers, 1984.

116. Caruso, L.A., and Chan, D.E.: Evaluation and management of the patient with acute back pain. Am. J. Occup. Ther., *40*:347–351, 1986.

117. Caruso, L.A., Chan, D.E., and Chan, A.: The management of work related back pain. Am. J. Occup. Ther., *41*:112–117, 1987.

118. Lorig, K.: Arthritis patient education. *In* Rheumatic Diseases: Rehabilitation and Management. Edited by G.K. Riggs and E.P. Gall. Woburn, MA, Butterworth Publishers, 1984.

119. Fries, J.F.: General approach to the rheumatic disease patient. *In* Textbook of Rheumatology. Vol. I. 2nd Ed. Edited by W.N. Kelley et al. Philadelphia, W.B. Saunders, 1986.

120. Jette, A.M.: Improving patient cooperation with arthritis treatment regimens. Arthritis Rheum., *25*:447–453, 1982.

121. Jette, A.M.: Understanding and enhancing patient cooperation with arthritis treatments. *In* Rheumatic Diseases: Rehabilitation and Management. Edited by G.K. Riggs and E.P. Gall. Woburn, MA, Butterworth Publishers, 1984.

122. Deyo, R.A.: Compliance with therapeutic regimens in arthritis: Issues, current status, and a future agenda. Semin. Arthritis Rheum., *12*:233–244, 1982.

123. Ferguson, K., and Bole, G.G.: Family support, health belief, and therapeutic compliance in patients with rheumatoid arthritis. Patient Counsel. Health Educ., *1*:101–105, 1979.

124. Gall, E.P.: Professionalism, research and directions—The AHPA in 1983. Clin. Rheumatol. Pract., *1*:179–182, 1983.

125. Gall, E.P.: Health care research for the patient. Clin. Rheumatol. Pract., *1*:41–42, 1983.

126. Burckhardt, C.S.: The impact of arthritis on quality of life. Nurs. Res., *24*:11–16, 1985.

127. Robinson, H.S., Hildeman, J., Imrie, J., and Neubauer, P.: Evaluation of a province-wide physiotherapy monitoring service in an arthritis control program. J. Rheum., *7*:387–389, 1980.

128. Ziebel, B., Wickersham, E., and Boyer, J.A.: Team arthritis consultation. Phys. Ther., *61*:519–522, 1981.

129. Riggs, G.K.: Philosophy of rehabilitation. *In* Rheumatic Diseases: Rehabilitation and Management. Edited by G.K. Riggs and E.P. Gall. Woburn, MA, Butterworth Publishers, 1984.

49

REHABILITATION MEDICINE AND ARTHRITIS

ROBERT L. SWEZEY

Any procedure used in the management of patients is a part of the rehabilitation process. The scientific foundations of rehabilitation medicine, as well as descriptions of the rehabilitative maneuvers used in management of the rheumatic disorders, are emphasized here.

The distinctions among the terms impairment, handicap, and disability must be clear. An *impairment* is a damaged organ or extremity; a *handicap* is the disadvantaged function caused by impairment; a *disability* is the inability to function effectively as a consequence of the handicap that results from an impairment. We are challenged to minimize impairment, to lessen the burden of handicap, and to prevent disability.

The specialty of physical medicine and rehabilitation emphasizes comprehensive, multidisciplinary team care in the prevention and management of disability. Physical medicine uses various forms of physical energy such as light, heat, electricity, and exercise therapy to accomplish this end. Rehabilitation in the rheumatic diseases integrates physical medicine with surgery and medicine, occupational therapy, and new techniques for education and social, vocational, or psychologic counseling of patients. The goal of this multidisciplinary approach is to help patients to attain their maximum potential for normal living. Successful rehabilitation depends on the efforts of qualified physicians, allied health professionals specifically trained in the management of the diseases they treat, and most important, a physician coordinator responsible for all the professional services rendered.

SOCIAL AND ECONOMIC FACTORS IN REHABILITATION

Arthritis is the second leading cause of chronic disability in the United States.[1,2] Approximately two thirds of the 4 million adult Americans with rheumatoid arthritis (RA) between the ages of 35 and 50 have significant impairment; 20% of the 0.06% of children under age 15 who develop juvenile RA suffer significant crippling into adult life; approximately a million men and women over age 16 in Great Britain are disabled primarily as a consequence of rheumatic diseases; the loss of nearly one sixth of the workdays in the industrial population of England and Wales has been attributed to rheumatic complaints.[3,4] During the 1970s, approximately $426.9 million per annum were spent by the United States Veterans Administration as compensation for arthritis-related disability.[5] Also during the early 1970s, $1 billion annually was spent on disability insurance payments and aid to the permanently and totally disabled, as well $1.4 billion on "lost" homemakers' services and $4.8 billion on lost wages. Lost federal, state, and local income taxes amounted to $955 million annually.[5] In 1984 it was estimated that the lifetime cost for each patient with RA measured in 1977 dollars was $20,412.[6] The total cost of arthritis-related disability exceeds $14 billion, and several billion dollars more will be spent in the 1980s on arthritis care and rehabilitation or on quackery.

In Sweden, rheumatic conditions represent 10% of all conditions seen by primary-care physicians, comprise 15% of the country's total health expenditures, and are the cause of one third of all new disability pensions.[7] In the United States, over 30 million working days/year are lost to rheumatic diseases. The direct medical costs for a year in the population of patients with stage III RA are three times the national average, and only 58% of these expenses are covered by insurance.[8] Indirect costs due to lost income were threefold greater than direct costs, and only 42% of these losses were recoverable.[8] The psychosocial losses associated with the economic burden and the loss of job-related identity are immeasurable. The stress of unemployment is sufficient to cause physical and mental illness even in many healthy persons; unemployment should be actively avoided in those afflicted with rheumatic diseases.[9]

Economic analyses of arthritis treatment reflect the extreme difficulty of determining cost effectiveness because of the impact of many variables on estimated and actual costs.[7,8,10,11] It is equally difficult to determine the effectiveness of components of rehabilitation therapy, including exercise, rest, splinting, occupational therapy, vocational counseling, psychologic and social counseling, community support, various medical and surgical therapies, and hospitalization.[11,12] Despite the qualifications, the assumptions, and the resistance by industry to hiring people with physical handicaps, even during periods of high employment, the most critical analyses show that rehabilitation services for arthritic disorders are cost effective and that high-quality programs are likely to be accompanied not only by increased socioeconomic benefits, but also by relief of symptoms and improved psychosocial function.[8,9,12]

Many patients with severe arthritis are capable of full- or part-time work, but others need adaptive equipment, modification of work methods, and the creation of ready access to a work setting for successful employment.[13,14] Prejudice of industry, labor unions, and insurance companies toward the handicapped still often restricts opportunities for employment. Initial steps taken to eliminate restrictive underwriting provisions could increase opportunities for the handicapped worker.[5,13]

The year 1981 was designated "International Year of Disabled Persons." The International League Against Rheumatism, with its member societies in over 60 countries, was an active participant in the goals of recognition of and attention to the special needs of the disabled.[15]

Although work for compensation is an obvious goal for the handicapped, the role of homemaker is of equal importance.[16] A legitimate goal of vocational rehabilitation and Social Security is to raise the level of function of a disabled person so that even if work in the traditional "marketplace" is not possible, independence in homemaking activities can be achieved.[17]

COMPONENTS OF THE REHABILITATION PROCESS

Components of the rehabilitation process include medical and professional personnel as well as therapeutic facilities.

REHABILITATION THERAPEUTIC TEAM

The severely arthritic patient may require the diversified skills of family physicians, rheumatologists, physiatrists, and orthopedists, as well as those of the allied health care specialties (see Chapter 48).

ALLIED HEALTH PROFESSIONAL TEAM

The roles of the various health professionals are described in Chapter 48.

FACILITY CONSIDERATIONS

The most important environment is the patient's home, but the places of work and worship and the educational and recreational facilities, in addition to the physician's office, clinic, hospital or rehabilitation facility, all determine limits and provide opportunities for restoration to independence.[18,19] The patient confined to a wheelchair is confronted with many everyday impediments such as curbs, stairs, narrow doorways, insufficient space in lavatories, drinking fountains too high or too low, inaccessibility to public transportation, public telephones with coin slots out of reach, and parking spaces less than 12 feet wide or located at long distances from buildings.[18–20] The patient who is weak, who uses canes, or walks with painful joints must be concerned with the problems of uneven terrain, ice, mud, heavy doors, resistant door knobs, lack of railings, and waiting room seats that are too low, or too soft or lack arms needed to facilitate standing and to relieve joint stress while sitting.[18,19,21]

Therapeutic facilities include the gymnasium, hydrotherapy area, and the area devoted to activities of daily living (ADL). Ideally, these facilities should be adjacent, interrelated, and close to psychologic, social, and vocational counseling services.[22,23] The hospital rehabilitation area used by both inpatients and outpatients should be in the same location, for continuity of care.

A small hospital requires a therapeutic gymnasium of at least 35 m². It should include an exercise mat, an exercise table, parallel bars and corner stairs for gait training, a full-length mirror, and areas for cervical traction, paraffin application, diathermy, ultrasound, electrical stimulation, and manual therapies. A shoulder wheel, a finger "ladder," and reciprocal pulleys are desirable. A Hubbard tank, ideally a therapeutic pool, and a whirlpool are particularly useful. A hydraulic lift can facilitate transferring patients. A heavy-duty overhead wire grid accommodating a variety of pulley attachments provides flexibility when traction, reciprocal pulleys, or supporting slings are needed. More elaborate equipment, such as a standing tilt table for postural training and gravity-assisted stretching, a padded, adjustable exercise table containing cables to which graded increments of weights can be attached, or isokinetic exercise equipment facilitates a variety of stretching or strengthening exercises (often prescribed postoperatively)[5] (see the section of this chapter on strengthening exercises).

Finally, space is needed for dressing rooms, lavatories, storage, and for cleaning and sterilization facilities.[24]

The occupational therapy area should provide space for evaluation of ADL.[25] Much ADL evaluation, such as bathroom and chair transfers, feeding, toileting, and personal grooming, can be performed at the bedside or in a hospital bed in an outpatient facility. Although specific activities, such as preparation of food and performance of household tasks, can be simulated, it is preferable to provide actual household equipment and facilities to permit adequate training of patients in joint conservation and to illustrate home adaptation. A table for therapeutic exercise evaluations should be accessible to wheelchairs and should have an adjustable height capability; a drafting table works well. An area is needed to make and to test splints and adaptive equipment. Office space for the therapists and assistants and space for privacy for individual ADL evaluation, counseling, and training should be provided. Provisions for vocational assessment such as simulated factory, office, or outdoor physical labor or driving are useful extensions of occupational therapy functions, but more applicable to major rehabilitation facilities.

Socialization areas are desirable for group dining, visiting with families, education of patient and family, and for recreation.

DISABILITY AND MANAGEMENT

Disability is the inability of an individual to meet the sum or any part of his life's physical, psychologic, environmental, or socioeconomic demands. Legal definitions of disability focus on a person's inability to participate in gainful employment for a predetermined period.[26] Lawmakers recognize the difficulty in proving or disproving true disability in a court of law and instead rely on the diagnosis of a specific rheumatic disorder, presuming that the diagnosis itself will embrace a disorder of sufficient severity to justify the existence of a functional deficit.[26] This unfortunate bias toward medical diagnosis rather than functional ability in determinations of disabilities in Social Security and workers' compensation cases precludes rational disability assessments.[17,27] The Arthritis Foundation has made legal determinations easier by forming a uniform database consisting of precise definitions of disorders and their respective signs and symptoms.[28] Under any nosologic classification, however, the range of functional impairment and disability is still wide.

Outcome measures of comprehensive health status examine factors such as death, discomfort, disability, therapeutic drug toxicity, and dollar cost.[29-31] To the arthritis patient, disability is the most important issue after control of pain. Outcome measurement in any chronic disorder needs to incorporate parameters of social, physical, and mental function.[29] Older instruments to measure outcome emphasized process rather than outcome; newer ones are more sensitive to ultimate outcome.[32] No one instrument is perfect although many exist. Not all costs and benefits can be measured, functional capacity is neither absolute nor constant, and undue emphasis on measurement may distract from other critically important issues of concern to the patient.[33] The Arthritic Impact Measurement Scale (AIMS), a brief paper and pencil test, is an example of a newer instrument to measure outcome.[34] AIMS has a high level of validity and reliability.[35]

Functional assessment is important for all physicians involved in rehabilitation. A proper functional assessment plans therapeutic intervention, defines roles in caring for the patient, and designs a rehabilitation program.[36,37]

The first instrument for functional assessment of arthritis patients consists of four gradations; slight, moderate, severe, and extreme functional impairment.[38] In 1949, Steinbrocker's Committee for Therapeutic Criteria of the New York Rheumatism Association published a functional classification of arthritis patients.[39] These early crude measures of function have been used to evaluate and to justify special rehabilitation units, to help formulate function-related goals of therapy, and to highlight the crucial point that function does not always equate with the severity of disorder.[40] Refinements have created instruments that are easy to record, quantifiable, and capable of reflecting more subtle changes in function. The prototype is the ADL Scale.[41] Consideration is given to a patient's ability to bathe, feed, dress, use a toilet, and to transfer from bed to chair and from chair to toilet independently.[41] Newer ADL scales give additional emphasis to a variety of psychosexual, social, vocational, and transportation functions.[42]

One must also analyze individual components of disability.[43,44] The reason for a disability is as important to the physician as its existence. Because function and disability measures are established for many reasons,[36] one method may necessarily be better to predict outcome,[37] another to measure pain[45] or pain threshold,[32] and still another to assess patients with mild impairments such as seen in a family physician's office.[46]

It is important to quantify function as a measure of the effectiveness of therapy.[47] Improvement of function is the major goal of rehabilitation. The expense, time, and effort required to improve range of motion in any given joint should be justified by a concomitant improvement in function.[48]

A functional evaluation of a musculoskeletal condition should be brief, reproducible, quantifiable, and reasonably objective and should distinguish between upper and lower extremity dysfunctions. Although the evaluation is affected by the patient's pain and by psychologic factors, it should not directly measure them. A functional test is not a substitute for precise descriptions of mobility, strength, anatomic or radiographic features, or psychologic status, nor for attempts to quantify pain. Such a test should be designed to detect a functional deficit by the patient's failure to perform a specific task. Inability to pick up a key (a function test) may reflect a loss of sensation, a loss of index finger or thumb function in one or several joints, or muscular weakness of relevant muscles, but only the functional deficit would be noted. Further evaluation would be needed to determine the basis for the functional loss. Treatment of the basis for disability such as carpal tunnel release, splinting of the thumb, or exercise of intrinsic muscles would be reflected by improved function if the patient could then pick up the key.

Scaling of levels of function is arbitrary, and the varieties of scoring systems developed are eloquent testimony to that difficulty. Redundancies in testing may be avoided by the use of one task to measure a number of related functions. For example, picking up a key requires fingertip sensation and co-ordination of the thumb to the index fingertip. The lack of tip pinch may not prevent one from picking up a key if the patient learns to compensate by sliding the key across and off the table top into his hand. It is pertinent, then, that the evaluative measures defined in the American Rheumatism Association (ARA) Standard Data Base for Rheumatic Disease originally included only the Steinbrocker classification, grip strength, 50-foot walking time, and a description of gait as functional measures, but now include descriptors of compliance with therapeutic regimen, sexual functions, and upper and lower extremity activities, as well as self-care.[28]

Finally, what one can measure as "function" with a given instrument may not reflect a lack of the patient's functional performance in reality.[48] A patient may, while being tested, actually accomplish a given task that could not or would not normally be done as part of daily activity. For example, patients may be able to comb their hair laboriously, but may choose to arrange for others to do it on a regular basis.

Table 49–1 shows the most widely used brief functional evaluation for rheumatic disease, the Steinbrocker classification.[39] This classification does not distinguish upper- from lower-extremity problems and is insensitive to modest but useful gains in function.[23] Table 49–2 is a questionnaire detailing the patient's own assessment of function in rheumatic disease.

Recent reviews of newer instruments by which to assess function have found none to be ideal.[30,31,33,47] New measures of function, disability, and outcome are proposed at an alarming rate, far faster than the necessary followup studies of validity and reliability. All physicians should acquaint themselves with one or several measures that apply to their needs, yet may be reproduced by other physicians with minimal interobserver discrepancy. The peculiarities of "legal" methods for determining disability are also important for any physician treating arthritis patients and have been reviewed.[17,27,36]

Last, as emphasized in a recent survey of a large population of medical students of whom 69.1% had

Table 49–1. Functional Criteria of the American Rheumatism Association

1. Patient performs all usual activities without handicaps.
2. Patient performs normal activities adequately, despite occasional discomfort in one or more joints.
3. Patient is limited to few or no activities, usual occupation, or self-care.
4. Patient is largely or wholly incapacitated, is bedridden, or is confined to a wheelchair and has little or no self-care.

(From Steinbrocker, O.[39])

Table 49–2. Rheumatic Disease Self-Assessment of Function

Dear <u>(PATIENT'S NAME)</u>: In order to help us learn whether you need therapy, in addition to the medicine prescribed for you, please fill out this form.

DIAGNOSIS	PRESENT VOCATION (Housewife, carpenter, etc.)		
Please check (✔) the best answer for you			
HOW MUCH PAIN OR DIFFICULTY DO YOU HAVE WITH THE FOLLOWING ACTIVITIES:	AMOUNT OF DIFFICULTY		
	NONE	SOME	GREAT
EATING:			
Cutting meat, drinking from a cup, etc.			
DRESSING:			
Arms and upper part of body			
Legs and lower part of body			
Fastening buttons, zippers, or snaps			
GENERAL HAND ACTIVITIES:			
Using key, writing, dialing phone			
Opening jars, drawers or doors			
PERSONAL HYGIENE:			
Brushing teeth, combing hair, shaving			
Toileting			
MOBILITY:			
Getting on or off toilet			
Getting into or out of			
chair			
bed			
car			
tub			
shower			
Walking inside home			
outside home			
up or down stairs			
HOME ACTIVITIES:			
Gardening			
Cleaning			
Cooking			
Laundry			
Shopping			
OTHER ACTIVITIES?			

one to seven separate musculoskeletal abnormalities,[49] proper physical examination is important, but function is multifaceted, dynamic, and not necessarily equivalent to the sum of the physical findings.

PHYSICAL THERAPY

Physical therapists and physiatrists have an extensive array of therapeutic techniques from which to choose, including exercise therapy, electrotherapeutics, hydrotherapy, therapeutic applications of heat and cold, manipulation, traction, and ambulation-assisting devices.[50,51] Many of these therapies have their origins in antiquity and have developed their own folklore and mythology. No claim of cure or dramatic, significant improvement of a chronic rheumatic disorder by a physical therapeutic technique has ever been proved. Many current therapies have a reason-

able scientific basis, however.[52,53] The interpersonal contact between physical therapists and patient may be a significant factor in the overall outcome of the rehabilitation program.

EXERCISE THERAPY

Exercise therapy is prescribed for patients with rheumatic diseases to preserve muscle strength and joint mobility, to improve functional capability, to relieve pain and stiffness, to prevent further deformities, to improve overall physical and cardiovascular conditioning, to re-establish neuromuscular co-ordination, to mobilize stiff or contracted joints, and to prepare for functional activity and follow-through after surgery.[51,53–55] Improvement of function and pain relief are the ultimate goals.

Physicians and therapists must carefully balance

Table 49–2. Rheumatic Disease Self-Assessment of Function (Continued)

How *TIRED* are you after an average day's activity? Slightly_____ Moderately_____
Extremely_____ Not at all_____

	YES	NO

Have you ever been treated by an occupational therapist?
  If *YES*, were you last treated:
    Less than 1 year ago?_____
    More than 1 year ago?_____		

Do you perform any home exercise program?		
If *YES.* was it prescribed by a doctor or a therapist?		
Do you currently use splints		
canes or crutches		
wheelchair		
other aids		

What is your *usual* means of *TRANSPORTATION?*
  Driven by family or friend _____drive self _____
  Public transportation (taxi or bus) _____other _____

COMMENTS: _____

the roles of rest, relaxation, and exercise. Selective rest, or immobilization of affected joints and adequate general rest, can reduce the severity of inflammatory joint disease.[56-58] Fatigue, a frequent constitutional complaint in inflammatory disorders, may be used as a guide to define "sufficient rest," that is, rest sufficient to cause fatigue to disappear.[58] Immobilization of RA joints for as long as 4 weeks reduces inflammation without significant loss of mobility, although muscle strength diminishes.[58-62] Because of the mechanical stress imposed on abnormal joints by faulty posture (body alignment), a rest position in bed that prevents hip flexion contractures, or "relative" rest in the form of modification of activities that protect a painful back or joint from stress, for example, is of major importance.[63]

Proper rest and good posture require muscle relaxation. Inadequate rest or poor posture can predispose patients to muscle aches, fibromyalgia, joint contractures, and excessive fatigue.[64] Muscle relaxation is necessary before commencing stretching exercises, and techniques such as hot packs, massage, Jacuzzi whirlpools, and ultrasound are used to relax tense patients to prepare them for stretching exercises and postural training.[65,66] Brief contraction of agonist muscles to induce relaxation of antagonists (contract-relax or rhythmic stabilization) is another technique that can augment assisted stretching exercises by relaxing muscles.[23,66]

Exercise therapy is designed to achieve specific therapeutic goals over and above the psychosocial and physiologic benefits of recreational exercise activity. Exercise during an acute arthritic flare is primarily to preserve joint range of motion. During the subacute stages, restoration of active joint motion and strength are additional goals. Exercise in the patient with chronic inflammation is designed to meet specific functional goals. Therefore, the rationale for therapeutic exercise is based on functional considerations, within the limitations imposed by the disease.

Stretching Methods

Stretching exercises are used to prevent contracture or to increase range of motion in patients who already have contractures.[23] Subluxations and other deformities associated with overstretched ligaments cannot be reversed by stretching exercises. Contractures, however, may be slowly reversed at a rate of approximately 1°/day. First, the underlying factors predisposing to contractures must be corrected. For example, the patient who places a pillow under an arthritic knee for comfort risks knee, hip, and ankle flexion contractures.[67] In addition to posture instruction and such measures as prone positioning for the patient at risk of developing hip flexion contractures, seating adjustments and supportive splinting or bracing may be required as preventive postural measures. Posture correction without the addition of range-of-

Table 49–3. Functional Positions for Ankylosed Joints

Joints	Function	Position	Reference
Fingers			
Metacarpophalangeal and proximal interphalangeal	Grasping	35° flexion	68
Thumb			
Interphalangeal	Pinching	Straight	68
Metacarpophalangeal	Pinching	20° flexion	
Carpometacarpal	Apposition	50° abduction	
		20° internal rotation	
Wrist			
Unilateral	Ease in toileting	Straight	68,69
Bilateral		One straight	
		One in 5° flexion	
Elbow			
Unilateral	Feeding and grooming	70° flexion	70
Bilateral	Feeding and grooming	One in 70° flexion	
	Reaching	One in 150° extension	
Shoulder	Feeding and grooming	20° flexion	70
	Dressing	45° abduction	
		20° internal rotation	
Hip*	Smooth gait	25° flexion	68
		5° abduction	
		5° external rotation	
Knee†	Smooth gait	15° flexion	71
Ankle	10° plantar flexion for high heels	Neutral	71

*Condition of opposite hip, knees, and back, and ability to sit and walk, as well as problems of daily activity must be evaluated to determine the position.
†Full extension for stability in the knee is the goal when only limited motion can be preserved.

motion exercise or activity may result in contractures, but such correction helps to preserve the position of useful function. Table 49–3 lists the optimal position for function in joints in which contracture cannot be avoided. *It is essential to put all joints through a range of motion at least once daily to maintain mobility.* The stretching techniques chosen to maintain motion must not aggravate joint pain and inflammation.

To understand the rationale for stretching exercises, one must recognize that contractures involve the joint capsule, the synovium, and the adjacent muscles and their fasciae.[72–75] Joint capsules vary in the looseness and irregularity of the weave of the collagen fibers. In ligaments and capsules, the collagen fibers are oriented variously to permit predetermined degrees of movement, whereas in tendons, the fibers are arranged in parallel fashion. Ligamentous and capsular structures are normally "prestressed" and shorten when normal tension or stretching forces are interrupted.[76,77] Thus, a proximal interphalangeal joint undergoing hyperextension deformity (swan neck) develops a tightening of its dorsal capsular fibers.[78,79]

In the arthritic patient, contractures typically occur in an effort to avoid pain associated with active joint disease.[78,79] Contractures may also secondarily affect uninvolved joints, or they may be primarily effected by poor posture.[78] An important additional mechanism for the genesis of joint contractures is the presence of synovial effusions. A mild or moderate effusion may have little effect on the mobility of the joint in a patient whose capsular structures are lax, although stretching of the capsule may lead to instability of the joint. In a patient whose capsular structures are less yielding, however, the synovial fluid may form a mechanical block to motion. Efforts to eliminate effusions and to minimize their recurrence are important if contractures are to be avoided.

Capsular structures and muscles undergo adaptive shortening with immobilization even in the absence of an inflammatory process.[75] When inflammation occurs, connective tissue turnover and remodeling are increased, and edema and pain restrict joint movement and predispose to joint contracture.[75]

The pathogenesis of contracture formation may be multifactorial. Although most contractures have some etiologic component of trauma, pain, internal derangement, inflammation, or immobilization, additional consideration must be given to neuropathy, including neurodystrophy, psychogenic factors, and genetic predisposition.[80,81]

Several points are relevant. First, if a progressive load is applied gradually, connective tissue will slowly stretch, ultimately to the point of rupture, whereas an abrupt application of a lesser load will cause tearing without significant stretching.[55,76,77,82,83] Second, collagen is more susceptible to collagenase activity when stretched or when heated.[84-87] Third, repetitive movement aggravates the inflammatory and, ultimately, destructive process in an inflamed joint.[73,86,88,89]

Methods. Serial casting or splinting techniques induce gentle, prolonged stretching forces. These are best applied, after relieving joint effusions, in patients with moderate and long-standing contractures. When serial or wedged cases are applied, care must be taken to prevent subluxing stresses. About 5° of contracture can be overcome weekly with effective serial casting for knee contractures, and this schedule may be accelerated with traction.[73,90,91] Dynamic splinting, in which constant low-grade tension creates a corrective force, can be used in selective therapies and is particularly applicable in postoperative management. Examples of dynamic splinting are the use of spring and rubber-band tension-activated splint devices or webbed belts wound to create a low-grade dynamic tension to correct contracture deformities of a finger or elbow.[73,90-95]

Range-of-Motion Exercises. Exercise to increase joint mobility should be modified according to the degree of inflammation present and, particularly, within pain tolerance.[51] To minimize exacerbations of arthritis, exercises should be performed so that any pain incurred will subside within 2 hours; any delayed or prolonged exacerbation of pain should largely be gone by the following day. Exercises should be selected to cause the least possible stress with the fewest possible movements, done in the least stressful manner consistent with the goal of stretching. Patients usually require "warm-up" movements before an optimal stretch can be made, but once the joint has been taken through its maximal range of motion during an exercise session (anywhere from 3 to 10 repetitions of the movement), then the single exercise session is usually sufficient to maintain joint mobility for that day.[96-99] When increased joint mobility is the goal, the same precautions apply, but the exercise can be repeated more often, such as 3 to 10 exercise sessions per day.

Stretching exercises are best performed when stiffness is least. This recommendation does not preclude a "loosening up" routine on arising, but it does mean that the major exercise effort for both stretching and strengthening should be done when the patient is best able to perform. Hot applications, a warm bath or shower, and anti-inflammatory and analgesic medication can be administered to be maximally effective at the time of the exercise session. Exercises can be categorized as *passive, active-assisted, active,* and *resistive.*[50] Purely passive exercise is necessary for a paralyzed limb or when pain precludes any active motion. For most arthritic patients, active-assisted exercises are used, because the patient's participation gives some control over pain, whereas the manual or mechanical assistance encourages maximal stretching. Active stretching exercises are particularly useful to preserve range of motion, and active-resistive exercises are used to maintain or to increase muscle strength.

Passive or active-assisted range-of-motion exercises may require the assistance of another person.[68] As inflammation subsides, simple assistive devices such as a cane or "wand" can be used by the patient without requiring another person. The "good" arm can push up on one end of the wand, which is grasped above by the hand ipsilateral to a contractured shoulder, to stretch upward into forward flexion[100] (Fig. 49–1). Proper positioning of the patient ensures that movement takes place in a horizontal plane, eliminating gravity. A "powdered board" or wheels on a "skate board" to minimize friction facilitates stretching exercise in the horizontal plane. In the Codman shoulder exercises, the patient leans forward with the

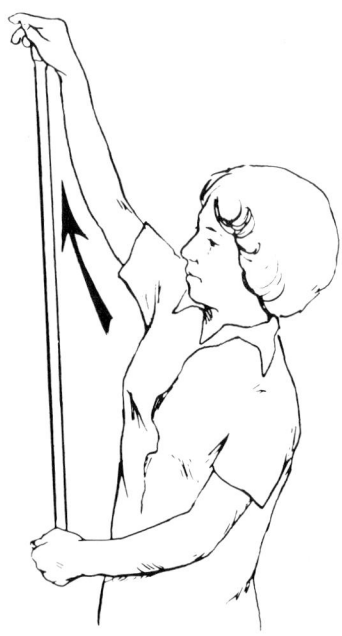

FIG. 49–1. Shoulder flexion ("wand" exercise). A stick is held with both hands approximately a shoulder's width apart. The "good" arm through the stick or wand assists the stiff shoulder in stretching. This exercise is used for subacute or chronic shoulder contractures.

FIG. 49–2. Wrist extension (dorsiflexion). The hand is placed flat on a table. The wrist is extended by leaning the body over the table.

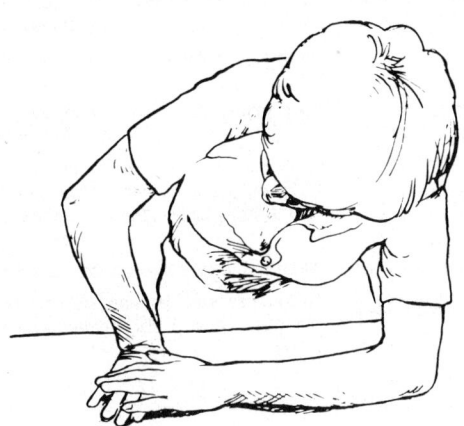

shoulder and arm hanging so that gravity actually assists the pendulum-like rotary movements of the shoulder.[71] Figure 49–2 shows assisted (body weight) dorsiflexion of the wrist, and Figure 49–3 shows gravity-assisted circumduction of the shoulder. The warmth and buoyancy of water, particularly in a pool, can be employed effectively to facilitate stretching regimens[101] (Tables 49–4 and 49–5). Active exercises are best employed in late convalescence and to maintain joint mobility.

Strengthening Exercise

Strength may be required to lift a load (isotonic or dynamic stength) or to hold or resist a load in a fixed

FIG. 49–3. Shoulder circumduction (Codman). A pendulum rotary motion is assisted by gravity and by holding a 1-kg weight. If the wrist or fingers are involved, a 1-kg wrist strap is substituted. This exercise for acute or severe restriction of shoulder motion can also be performed when the patient is lying prone, extending the arm over the side of the bed.

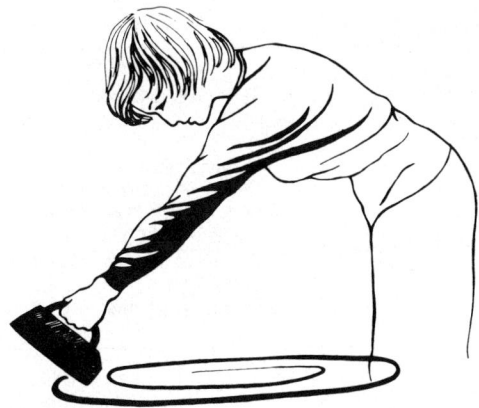

position (isometric or static strength). An isotonic stress modulated to keep the resistance throughout the range of movement constant (as the leverage changes, the load is increased or lessened to maintain a constant torque) is called an *isokinetic stress*. For example, a Nautilus machine simulates isotonic stress.

Endurance is a measure of the time that a stress can be sustained, and the duration of muscle performance may be contracted to a percentage of the level of maximum performance or to a functional assessment.[106] Static endurance is the time that a given load can be held or resisted in a fixed position (isometric contraction). Dynamic endurance is the length of time that a repetitive isotonic task can be performed and is a function of the rate of repetition, the load, and the extent to which the load is moved. Dynamic endurance is related to, but distinguishable from, power, which is the rate at which work (force × distance) is performed.

Maximal strength and endurance depend on multiple factors, including overall physical condition, muscle fiber type, motivation, pain and sensory inputs, training, learning ability, and co-ordination.[107] Although strength and endurance are interrelated, the requirements for sustaining a large weight are only minimally transferable to a low-resistance, repetitive task such as typing, and vice versa.

Muscle Fiber Morphology and Physiology. Skeletal muscle contains muscle fibers that are different anatomically, physiologically, histochemically, and biochemically.[107–110] The several classification systems of muscle fibers have proved confusing when attempts were made to correlate the classifications or to account for interspecies differences.[110] The oldest system divided muscle fibers by color into red, either slow or fast twitch, and white.[110] Peter's classification system used whole muscle and divided fibers, based on contraction time and enzyme capacity, into (1) fast-twitch glycolytic; (2) fast-twitch, oxidative, glycolytic; (3) fast-twitch, fatigue-resistant; and (4) slow-twitch, fatigue-resistant.[107,108,110] The currently accepted system, an outgrowth of a Brooke and Kaiser classification,[107–110] is as follows.

Type I Fibers. These fibers are red, slow-twitch and have the highest capacity for aerobic metabolism, with a high respiratory capacity and myoglobin content, but with a low glycogenolytic capacity and low actin-myosin adenosine triphosphatase (ATPase). These fibers can do prolonged work of moderate intensity in which ATP use matches oxidative phosphorylation.

Type IIB Fibers. These white, fast-twitch, fatigable fibers have a low respiratory capacity, a high glycogenolytic capacity, a low myoglobin content, and a

Table 49–4. Therapeutic Considerations in Exercises for Joint Diseases

	Acute/Severe		Subacute/Moderate		Chronic/Mild	
	Motion	Strength	Motion	Strength	Motion	Strength
Goal	To maintain	To defer until pain relief permits	To maintain or increase	To maintain or increase	To maintain or increase	To maintain or increase
Method	Passive or gentle	See Subacute/Moderate	Active-assisted	Isometric	Active or active-assisted	Isometric or isotonic*
Position	To preserve function, for comfort		To preserve function, for comfort	For comfort	For comfort	Antigravity acceptable if tolerated
Repetitions	1–3/session 1–2/session/day		3–10/session 1–2/session/day	6 sec/muscle 1–2/session/day	5–10/session 1/session/day to maintain or 3–5/day to increase	6 sec/muscle 1 week to maintain; 1/day to increase strength
Time	When rested, and pain and stiffness are least		When rested, and pain and stiffness are least		When rested, and pain and stiffness are least	
Preparation	Analgesics, cold, heat, hydrotherapy as needed before exercise		Analgesics, heat, cold, hydrotherapy as needed before exercise		Analgesics, heat, hydrotherapy, cold as needed; occasionally, diathermy before exercise	
Precautions	Reduce intensity of exercise if postexercise pain persists over 2 hours or if pain or swelling increases the following day		See Acute/Severe. Avoid fatigue; use prescribed working splints during activity except when exercising†		See Subacute/Moderate	

*Isotonic, low-resistance, repetitive exercises to the point of fatigue for dynamic endurance.
†Compromise between the ideal and the possible may demand selective emphasis on problem joints for maximum compliance with exercises.

Table 49–5. Range-of-Motion Exercises for Specific Joints

	Upper Extremity			
	Proximal Interphalangeal, Metacarpophalangeal	Wrist	Elbow	Shoulder
Problem	Swan neck Tight intrinsic muscles Swelling Restriction of motion	Supination loss Subluxation	Flexion of at least 70° must be preserved for useful function	Rapid loss of motion, particularly flexion, abduction, and internal rotation
Method	Manually assisted, Bunnell block	Active-assisted Use stick or door knob to assist pronation and supination; lean over hand on table top for extension*	Active, flexion-extension; best performed in horizontal plane	Gravity-assisted "Codman"† early Active-assisted pulleys, "wall walking" later Active and "wand"‡ when chronic
Comment	Forced grasp or ball-squeezing predisposes patients to joint derangement		Forceful stretching can exacerbate the disorder	Early institution of exercise prevents "frozen" shoulder
References and description	23, 68, 102–104	23, 68, 105	23, 76, 94	23, 71, 94, 104

	Lower Extremity		
	Hip	Knee	Ankle
Problem	Flexion contracture Loss of abduction Motion restricted by swelling	Maintenance of extension	Tight Achilles tendon
Method	Active Horizontal plane, side lying for extension Supine for abduction	Active Stretch on floor on mat	Active-assisted Stand with palms on wall Lean into wall to stretch heel cord of extended leg
Comment	Pool, tank or "powder board" facilitate	Pool or tub useful in acute cases	Achilles contracture requires vigorous stretching
References and description	23, 68, 94, 104	23, 68, 94, 104	23, 24, 68, 94, 104

*See Fig. 49–1
†See Fig. 49–2
‡See Fig. 49–3

high actin-myosin ATPase activity. These fibers have a capacity for short bursts of intense work, but rapidly fatigue, accumulate lactate, and require long recovery intervals.

Type IIA Fibers. These fibers are red, fast-twitch, and fatigue-resistant, with a high respiratory capacity, a high glycolytic capacity, a high myoglobin content, and a high actin-myosin ATPase activity. These fibers, intermediate between type I and type IIB, have a potential for rapid regeneration of ATP by anaerobic or aerobic metabolism.

The actual proportions of each fiber in the skeleton are fixed, and in man, approximately half are type I and half are type II.[110] Athletes often have a predominance of a single fiber type, and this factor may contribute to performance in a sport.[107] That training in man may change muscle fiber type I to type II or vice versa remains to be proved.[107]

Strength training results in (1) an increase in type II fiber area with heavy resistance training; (2) correlation of type II fiber area with maximal isometric strength; (3) no discernible metabolic changes characteristic of low-resistance endurance training; and (4) myofibrillar protein increases resulting in enlarged or hypertrophied muscle fibers.[107]

Diseases often affect one muscle fiber type more than another; thus a basis is provided for rational exercise treatment.[111] Type II fibers have a peculiar propensity to change in size, and atrophy may occur in patients receiving corticosteroid therapy, in patients with connective tissue disease with associated myopathy, and in cancer patients.[106,111] Prolonged cast immobilization does not change the proportion of muscle fiber types, but produces greater atrophy in type I fibers, unless severe joint pain has been present, as in RA.[106,107,111]

Muscle is in a constant state of simultaneous degradation and synthesis.[106] The two processes are normally balanced, but this balance may be disrupted by a number of factors.[106] With inactivity, muscle strength decreases from 1.5 to 5% per day.[26] With maximal exercise, an increase of 12% per week of muscle strength may be obtained, up to 75% of maximum, when the rate of increase declines.[112] Müller has demonstrated that, in normal human subjects, even a single contraction, for a second's duration done once a day, at half maximal strength, limits the loss of muscle strength.[112]

The effect of a muscle contraction is produced by the interaction of mechanical factors, such as fiber direction, locus of insertion, joint position, and muscle length.[113] Excessive elongation, particularly at high velocities, can produce injuries ranging from minor strain to muscle rupture.[113] Muscle rupture is more common than tendon rupture in a 2:1 ratio, and most strains and ruptures occur in muscles that cross over and interact with more than one joint, e.g. the hamstrings and rectus femoris muscles. Care must be taken with immobilization because changes in musculotendinous lengths limit range of motion. Immobilization also results in muscle atrophy[113] (see Table 49–3).

Dynamic endurance training improves the oxidative (aerobic) capacity of muscle[107] by inducing adaptive increases in mitochondrial content, respiratory capacity, in myoglobin concentration, and capillary number.[110] Another important biochemical change with endurance training is an increased ability to oxidize fat, carbohydrate, and ketones.[110]

Most functional activities such as grooming, dressing, feeding, light housekeeping, and walking are low-resistance, repetitive tasks. Fatigue occurs more rapidly in repetitious tasks requiring more than 10% of the maximal available static strength. Fatigue eventually occurs even if the task can be performed with only 5% of the maximal available static strength.[114,115] To lift and to maintain a load, such as holding a glass of water, a pot of tea, or a package of groceries, requires static strength and endurance sufficient to perform these tasks. The static endurance during grasp has been shown to be a function of the percentage of the total available grasp (static) strength used.[114,115] Repetitive, low-resistance activities, such as jogging or sawing, require additional dynamic endurance training for optimum function, if such training can be done without aggravating the joint disorder.

Methods. Two common methods for strengthening muscles are based on the concept that a stress sufficient to cause a muscle to fatigue stimulates the muscle to adapt by increasing in strength and endurance.[116,117] The DeLorme regimen uses a sequential, 10-step, graded reduction of isotonic stresses beginning with 10 repetitions of the greatest load that can be lifted. The "over-load principle" of Hellebrandt requires that the maximum isotonic load be lifted repeatedly in a paced exercise to the point of fatigue.[116,117] The muscle-fatigue stimulus can also be used advantageously in weakened patients because low-resistance activity (greater than 30% of maximum capability) also stimulates strengthening if carried to the point of fatigue.[107,112,113,117] These exercises are regularly prescribed in patients after trauma, joint operations, or when little joint inflammation exists.[116,117]

These fatiguing, strengthening methods contrast sharply with the brief, isometric contraction exercises. Daily isometric contractions at two-thirds maximum capability held for at least 1 second, and preferably for 6 seconds, are an optimal physiologic stimulus for static strengthening in healthy adults.[118] Only a slight increase in the rate of gain in strength was observed when the exercise was performed three times daily in normal subjects. In all these techniques, the stimulus must be increased proportionately to strength increase to be maximally effective. The use of a maximal contraction at each exercise session obviates this problem. Once maximal static strength is achieved, it can be maintained by one exercise session per week.[112]

Specific Considerations in Rheumatic Disease. RA patients as a group have lower than expected aerobic capacity and physical performance, and their overall muscle strength is 60% below that of age-matched control subjects.[119,120] Such patients, however, tolerate well-tailored strengthening and endurance programs, with gains in physical performance levels in as brief a time as 6 weeks.[119,121,122] Long-term exercise regimens in RA patients over many years have also been well tolerated, with resultant improvement in functional and other outcome measures.[100,123] A lessening of discomfort and a better overall emotional attitude accompany such exercise.[122,123] In healthy adults, exercise increases plasma levels of β-endorphins and β-lipotropin, and continued training augments this effect.[124] Whether this effect occurs in the less-demanding exercises of arthritic patients remains to be determined. Additionally, regular exercise training may help to relieve depression.[125]

Exercise may increase inflammation in joints, and therefore must be designed to avoid such exacerbation.[115,126] Isometric exercises are effective in increasing strength and are well tolerated by many arthritic patients.[127] In the rabbit model of acute monosodium urate arthritis, passive range-of-motion exercise exacerbated inflammation, but isometric exercise did not.[89]

Isometrics make profound cardiovascular demands, however,[128] demands great enough to compromise patients with organic heart disease. Caution should be exercised.[128] New rehabilitation techniques of "perceived exertion" allow patients with heart disease to exercise within cardiovascular restraints and still make progress.[128]

Isometric exercises should be performed with the joint positioned for comfort, to avoid pain, and to maximize the force of the muscle contraction. Pain may be reduced further by administering analgesics and by warm or cold applications before exercise. Resistance for isometric exercise can be provided by walls, floors, table tops, opposite extremities, therapists, or gymnasium equipment. A simple technique, particularly suitable for a home regimen, is the use of a minimally yielding rubber or elastic belt looped around the extremity and fixed to the opposite ex-

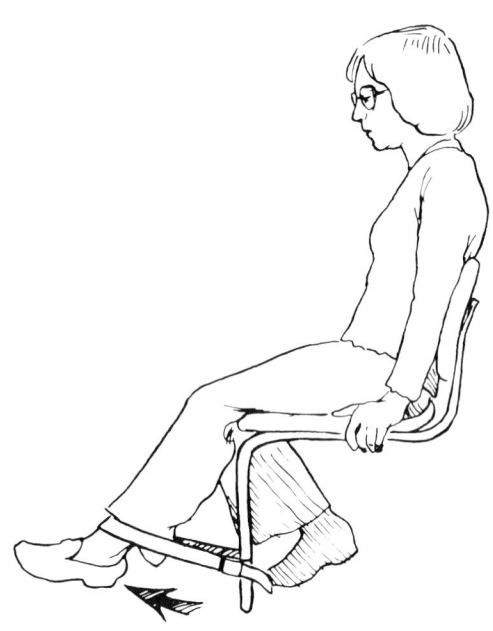

FIG. 49–4. Seated quadriceps isometric strengthening (elastic belt) exercise. An elastic belt is looped around the chair leg and the patient's ankle. The patient attempts to extend the partially flexed leg as forcibly as possible for 6 seconds (exhaling or counting to avoid increased intrathoracic pressure). The elastic belt yields minimally while providing "feedback" as it resists extension of the leg.

tremity, bed, doorknob, or chair leg (Fig. 49–4).[129] Alternatively, one can use a partially inflated beach ball, which is light, adapts comfortably to painful structures, and, like the elastic belt, moves minimally yet offers increasing resistance as force is applied and thereby reinforces the proprioceptive inputs essential for a maximum contraction[23] (Fig. 49–5). Although a maximal 6-second daily isometric exercise is an optimal strengthening stimulus, twice-daily exercise sessions are recommended when the patient's ability to contract maximally is uncertain (see Table 49–4).

Three additional muscle-strengthening methods have received increasing attention. The Nautilus continuous-resistance device was not shown to have any advantage over traditional barbells.[130] The Cybex apparatus is the prototype of devices that offer variable controlled rates of motion for isokinetic exercise. Resistance can be discontinued if pain occurs. Computerized analysis of torque makes this method advantageous compared to isometric strengthening. This has led to a growing application of variable-resistance isokinetic exercise equipment in industrial and sports rehabilitation.[131,132] Controlled studies of muscle strengthening by electrical stimulation in normal subjects have demonstrated an effect equivalent to iso-

FIG. 49–5. Biceps isometric strengthening (beach ball) exercise. A partially inflated beach ball is compressed as forcibly as possible for 6 seconds. The beach ball is lightweight, conforms to bony contours, and offers increasing resistance during compression. Counting to ensure exhalation prevents increased intrathoracic pressure.

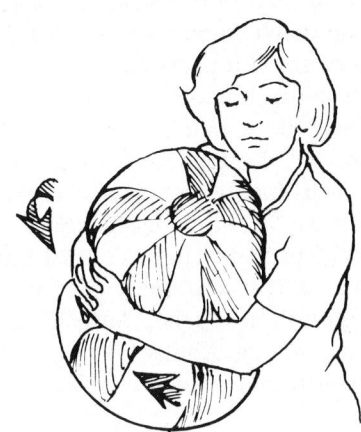

metric exercise.[133,134] The application of this method to arthritic disorders merits further study.

Specific exercise techniques are beyond the scope of this chapter, but the principles and positions used by Hines in manual muscle testing, modified for joint comfort, are readily adapted for isometric exercise, and many practical exercises for arthritic patients have been described in detail.[23]

Specfic Considerations in Muscle Disease. Physical therapy has been reported to be valuable in the management of patients with polymyositis, the prevention of contractures and stiffness, the rehabilitation of patients recovering from acute or relapsing disease, and the treatment of muscular soreness.[135] No controlled trials substantiate this finding or support the traditional belief that resistive exercises should not be done until the serum muscle enzymes are at or near normal, however. Exercise mildly elevates levels of muscle enzymes for several hours.

ELECTROTHERAPY

Electrotherapeutics have been an integral component of physical medicine and rehabilitation therapies since 1931, when the Royal Society of Medicine combined their Section of Electrotherapeutics and the Section of Balneology and Climatology to form the specialty of "Physical Medicine."[136]

The first use of electrotherapy has been attributed to the Romans, who decapitated torpedo fish and used the natural electric charge to treat various maladies including gout.[137] Erb, in 1883, wrote that "among articular affections these constitute the real field for electricity; other methods of treatment are much more often useless."[138] By the turn of the century, use of galvanic, faradic, and static currents to treat arthritis was almost as popular as treatment at spas and natural baths.[139] Notably, no proof exists that electric current may cure any rheumatic disorder, nor have controlled experiments shown that the direct application of electric current in inflammatory arthritic disorders has any effect other than that of a counterirritant.

Iontophoresis, an early addition to electrotherapy,[140] theoretically uses a direct (galvanic) current to enhance and intensify the movement of ions from drugs that may be ionized past a biologic membrane for therapeutic purposes.[140–143] Anecdotal claims of the benefits of iontophoresis in treating most forms of arthritis have appeared.[141,143,144] Scientific evaluation of iontophoresis has been attempted to determine its use in applying corticosteroid preparations to a small, anatomically defined area such as a joint or bursae.[84,145] A recent study failed to demonstrate in vivo transcutaneous migration of corticosteroids by means of iontophoresis.[146]

Electric and magnetic fields are now used by physicians and physical therapists for pain control, promotion of bone growth, stimulation of muscle groups, restoration of lost neuromuscular function, and movement retraining.[143,147–149] Further research is needed to determine what, if any, role electricity will play in the rheumatic diseases.

In 1965, Melzack and Wall proposed their gate theory of pain.[150] They suggested that intense sensory input along large-diameter nerve fibers would "close the gate" to pain sensations carried by smaller fibers. The required sensory input to the sensory mechanoreceptors could be electrical stimulation, pressure, or vibration.[150,151] The gate theory, which provided a theoretic basis for counterirritation and related pain "displacing" phenomena, has spawned a number of electrotherapeutic techniques designed to obscure pain perception by electric stimulation of cutaneous receptors, dorsal column, spinal cord, peripheral nerve, and brain.[143,149] Implantable devices, such as dorsal column and thalamic stimulators, were first used, but have largely been abandoned because of complications. The almost complication-free, easily applied, external transcutaneous electric nerve stimulators (TENS) and electroacupuncture[149,152] are now widely used as electrical stimulation for pain relief.[152] Transcutaneous nerve stimulation is done with an apparatus consisting of skin electrodes and a battery-powered, portable pulse generator.[152] Placement of electrodes is empiric, although guidelines suggest placement at trigger points or acupuncture points, which Melzack has found to be closely correlated.[153] The explanation for the analgesic action of TENS units was initially thought to be related to "gate control." Recent work suggests that endorphins may be released,[151,152,154,155] but a carefully controlled study did not show an endorphin effect.[156] Low-frequency, high-intensity TENS simulates acupuncture and generally has a slower onset and more prolonged effect on pain than does high-frequency, low-intensity TENS.[157,158] TENS has been used to treat many musculoskeletal conditions with varying success.[158,159] TENS primarily blocks C-fiber-mediated pain and, to a lesser extent, the acute pain mediated by A-δ fibers. That the periosteum, synovium, and capsule of a joint are supplied by nonmyelinated (C-fiber) sensory fibers may explain the success of TENS in reducing joint pain and in supplementing anti-inflammatory drugs during controlled trials in patients with RA, herpes zoster, and discogenic radiculopathy, and as an adjunct to the management of frozen shoulder and reflex sympathetic dystrophy.[154,160] Complications, such as interference with demand pacemakers, may occur with TENS units.

Electrical stimulation has been used to treat nonunion fractures of bone with fair success and, more germane to the arthritis patient, to treat failed arthrodesis.[82,139,161,162]

Electrical stimulation of muscle activity can retard denervation atrophy of type I fibers and, to a lesser extent, type II fibers.[163] The contraction of denervated muscle by electrical stimulation prevents the loss of oxidative enzymes and the associated atrophy,[164] although no concomitant increase in muscle strength occurs.[165] Electrical stimulation of motor nerves (faradic) to induce involuntary muscle contractions is also used as a massage technique for relief of painful muscle spasm, but no controlled trials have proved its efficacy.[39] Electrical stimulation of muscle can increase strength in normal subjects.[105,133,134]

Electroneuroprosthesis is a term describing electrical devices that stimulate the nervous system to restore lost function.[149] Such devices have been used with good results to treat footdrop, to obtain grasp in C5 fractures, to treat scoliosis, and to stimulate bowel, bladder, and diaphragmatic functions.[147,149]

Electrical stimulation has been used to facilitate muscle retraining after tendon transplants or trauma and in neurologic disorders. It is therefore a forerunner of modern biofeedback techniques.[144] Biofeedback is an outgrowth of experiments with operant conditioning done by Neal Miller showing that the effects of the autonomic nervous system are subject to training.[166] A signal, usually visual or acoustic, reflecting a physiologic "involuntary" event, is used to help the patient to gain voluntary control.[167] Electromyographic biofeedback is now used to treat upper motor neuron lesions; muscle tension headache, and neck and back pain and, particularly, to retrain muscles[168] and to induce relaxation in spastic muscles of stroke patients.[167] The mechanism may be an enhancement of awareness of small muscle contractions.[169]

Biofeedback control of skin temperature in the fingers is a new technique in the treatment of Raynaud's phenomenon.[170,171] Biofeedback training to relieve joint or back pain has been less successful, perhaps no better than a placebo.[172] Biofeedback techniques are now widely used for pain control and relief of muscle spasm in the treatment of muscle tension headache, migraine headache, "stress," and chronic neck and temporomandibular joint syndrome, although well-controlled trials are lacking.

HYDROTHERAPY

Hydrotherapy combined with heat is among the oldest rehabilitative treatments for arthritis.[65,173] Hydrotherapy provides both heat and buoyancy.[23] Arm and leg basins for single joints with or without water agitators (whirlpools) and various size tubs are used.[23] Hubbard tanks or heated swimming pools are used for patients with multiple joint problems.[65] The larger tanks permit total body immersion, heat transference, therapeutic exercise, swimming for conditioning, ambulatory training, and a popular spa technique, "Bad Ragaz."[23,51,65]

Contrast baths are used to treat small joints by producing hyperemia.[174] This cumbersome method has no known advantage over warm soaks or moist heat application

Hydrotherapy has not been subject to controlled trials.[23,51,65] It is contraindicated in patients with cardiovascular disease, because of peripheral vasodilation accompanying total immersion in water at 34°C, and in patients with infections or certain inflammatory skin diseases.[23,51,65] The larger pools are also expensive to maintain and to operate, and time in them should be used judiciously.[23,65] The feeling of freedom, relaxation, and pain relief provided by pool therapy does have important psychologic value to the arthritis patient. Arthritis clubs and YMCAs with organized exercise programs at local pools can provide recreation for arthritic patients at a much more modest cost.

THERAPEUTIC HEAT AND COLD

Superficial heating can be accomplished by conduction (direct contact with a warmed substance) or by convection (heat transferred by liquid- or gas-heated particles in motion). Deeper heating may be instituted by conversion, in which a nonthermal form of energy, such as sound waves, penetrates tissue, where the energy is converted to heat by absorption. How hot a tissue actually gets is a product of several factors, including the thermal properties of the tissues heated, the thermal conductivity, the pattern of relative heating, and neurovascular factors that locally regulate body temperature control.

Superficial heating may be done by direct contact with warmed substances such as sand, oil, wax (paraffin), mud, thermal springs, vapor bath, steam in a steam room, moist air in a moist air cabinet, hot water in a tub, hot packs, heating pad, and hydrocolator (silicate gel), or by the friction of rubbing with massage.[23,51] Regardless of source, the energy penetrates only a few millimeters through the epidermis, and thus intra-articular heating is minimal.[175] Although moist heat raises subcutaneous temperatures more than dry heat, this information does not influence any selection of a heating technique.[176]

Heat purportedly increases collagen extensibility in tendons,[177–179] decreases joint stiffness,[180–182] relieves pain,[84,175,183] elevates pain threshold,[184] relieves muscle spasm,[183,185,186] and affects intra-articular circulation in RA.[187] The effect on intra-articular circulation occurs whether the heat is superficial or is applied deep to the joint, however. Heat may also increase both inflammation and pain.[188] A controlled trial of a popular superficial heating technique, paraffin baths, in RA showed no clinical benefit.[189] The benefits of heating in the treatment of rheumatic disease patients have simply not been established.[190]

Heating of skin to temperatures greater than 109°F (43°C) causes pain, and higher temperatures may cause wheal and flare reactions. Caution must be exercised when using heat in patients with sensory neuropathies, an abnormal mental state, or cardiovascular disorders. Total immersion of women during the first trimester of pregnancy in water heated to temperatures higher than 38.9°C is contraindicated, and patients with systemic lupus erythematosus, malignant diseases, infections, and open wounds have had reported adverse reactions with heating. Table 49–6 contains a summary of precautions.[191,192]

Diathermy and Ultrasonography

Deep heat penetration of tissue sufficient to cause direct joint heating can be achieved with diathermy.[191,193,194] Diathermy, which literally means "heating through," consists of electromagnetic irradiation administered as shortwaves (11.0 M at 27.33 MHz) or as microwaves (12.2 cm at 2456 MHz).[193,194] Shortwave administration requires a direct applicator or a coil, and microwave administration uses an antenna. Ultrasonography is a deep-heating method that uses the energy of rapidly oscillating sound waves (1.0 MHz).[193,194] It provides the deepest tissue penetration, and it is the only heating technique that raises the temperature in the adult hip.[193–196] This deep penetration can be a disadvantage when ultrasonography is used over the spinal cord after laminectomy.[197] Ultrasonography is reflected from metal surfaces, rather than conducted as with diathermy, and thus is safe to use in the presence of metal implants or plates.[198–203] No information exists on the safety of ultrasonography in the presence of methyl methacrylate, used to hold joint prostheses.

Electromagnetic waves may cause burns if focused by metal or by fluid-filled spaces, such as moisture on the skin, in the eye, and in bone.[192–194,197,201] Testicular and lenticular damage from diathermy has been reported.[197,202] The use of either shortwave or microwave diathermy in patients with cardiac pacemakers is contraindicated.[203] Precautions for use of deep heat also include those for superficial heat. In addition to causing circulatory changes and increasing the threshold for pain, diathermy can alter the viscoelastic properties of collagen.[179,193,197] This heat-related effect has been the basis for advocacy of diathermy in conjunction with prolonged stretching to overcome contracture, but the relative merits of diathermy's effect on collagen over those of superficial heat to reduce pain and muscle spasm, and thus to facilitate stretching, have not been adequately studied.[183,193] Diathermy or ultrasonography has no proven advantage over superficial heating techniques for pain relief or improvement of articular disorders.[184,204,205] Indeed, evidence that heat increases collagenase activity in rheumatoid synovia raises further doubts about the use of diathermy in inflammatory joint disease.[84]

In addition to the recommendations for prescribing heat and cold therapeutic methods in Tables 49–6 and 49–7, empiric indications exist for the use of ultrasonography. Local painful areas such as fibrositic nodules, chronic ligamentous strains, neuromas, "trigger" areas in muscle, and localized tendinitis are particularly suited anatomically for focused ultrasound energy. Again, anecdotal reports of the value of treating these conditions with ultrasonography abound, but controlled studies are lacking. The special therapeutic advantage of ultrasonography attrib-

Table 49–6. Therapy Prescription Precautions

Therapeutic Method	Impaired Sensation	Circulatory Deficiency	Metal Implant or Contact	Pacemaker	Cardiac, Respiratory, or Cerebral Insufficiency	Acute Trauma or Inflammation	Infection	Tumor	Osteoporosis	Weakness or Low Endurance	Weight Bearing	Instability or Paralysis	Psychological Factors	Intellectual Factors	Economic Factors
Local superficial heat or cold*	R	R				Rʰ								R	
Ultrasonography	R	R	R			C	C	C							
Diathermy*	R	R	C	C		C	C	C							
Hydrotherapy with heat*	R	R			R		R			R		R		R	
Generalized (total body) heat*	R	R			R		R			R		R		R	
Traction	R					R	R	C	R			R			
Splint or brace	R	R					R						R	R	R
Gait training	R	R	R			R	R	R	R	R	Rʳˡ	R		R	
Exercise (passive, active, range-of-motion, strength)		R	R			R	R	R		R	R	R			
Massage or manipulation					Cᶜˢ	C	C	C	R						
Transcutaneous nerve stimulation				C										R	R

ʰ = Heat; ᶜˢ = cervical spine; ʳˡ = right or left; C = contraindication; R = relative contraindication or special consideration.
*Specific operating instructions including dosage, exposure to moisture, duration of therapy, distance of energy source, and temperature of water must be followed exactly.

utable to the specific physical effects of sound waves has not been substantiated.[197] Phonophoresis uses ultrasonography to drive molecules (medication) transdermally for local and potentially systemic purposes. Corticosteroids have been demonstrated to penetrate the dermis to a sufficient depth to be locally effective (as well as systemically absorbed).[206,207] Currently, al-though there are no controlled studies to demonstrate either safety or efficacy of corticosteroid phonophoresis, the method is being applied by therapists primarily in the treatment of painful musculotendinous disorders.[206,207]

Cold decreases electrical activity of the muscle spindle.[183,185,208] The stimulus threshold for firing is raised,

Table 49–7. Selection Factors in Techniques for Pain Relief

Severity of Pain	Technique	Localization of Pain	Comments
↑ Acute	Ice pack, cold compress, ice massage	↑ Focal*	Contraindicated in patients with cold intolerance or Raynaud's phenomenon
	Warm moist compress		Well tolerated, easy to apply
	Hydrotherapy: whirlpool, tub, tank, pool		Warmth and buoyancy assist in stretching exercises
	Dry heat: infrared bulb, heating pad	General	Inexpensive for home use, portable; danger of short circuit
	Paraffin, mud, sand		Provides palliation in PSS and rheumatoid arthritis
Chronic ↓	Diathermy: microwave, short-wave, ultrasound	Focal* ↓	Pacemaker and metal implants contraindicate use

*Transcutaneous nerve stimulation can relieve focal or regional pain

thus decreasing the afferent firing rate.[183] Cold may also reduce nerve condition velocity. Cold may be better than heat for reducing pain[184,204] and muscle spasm[183,204] and, in combination with stretching, for muscle relaxation.[183] Cold causes superficial vasoconstriction, but deep vasodilation.[209] Pain relief resulting from cold exposure may be due to counterirritant effects or to endorphin release.[183,184,209–211] Additional suggested benefits of cold include reduction of edema formation, metabolic rate, joint stiffness, muscle spasm, and joint inflammation, and enhancement of mobility.[183–185,188,209–214] Cold may be administered by immersion in cold water, application of ice or cold packs, ice massage, inflatable cold splints, or vapocoolant sprays.[183–185,188,209–211,213,215–218] Cold is contraindicated in patients with cold allergy, Raynaud's syndrome, paroxysmal nocturnal hemoglobinuria, and cryoglobulinemia and should be used cautiously in the presence of cardiovascular insufficiency.[23]

The choice of heating or cooling for symptomatic relief is empiric. Cold seems preferable in the treatment of acute inflammatory processes or injuries, whereas traditionally heat has been used to treat subacute or chronic inflammation or injury (see Table 49–7).[216,219,220]

TRACTION, MASSAGE, AND MANIPULATION

The physiotherapeutic techniques traction, massage and manipulation have been widely used in the treatment of rheumatic disease.

Traction

Traction, a basic component of orthopedic therapy, has an established place in the treatment of contractures occurring in the arthritic hip and knee.[91,93,221] Traction with modifications of Perry and Nickel's "halo" device is used in the treatment of spinal deformities, often in conjunction with surgical procedures.[222]

Traction in normal subjects can open posterior spinal articulations, disengage facet surfaces, widen intervertebral foramina, and elongate posterior muscles and ligaments.[221,223,224] Reduction of bulging discs in pathologic conditions has not been proved, however.[63,221,223] Pain is relieved by traction, especially in the treatment of cervical radiculopathy.[225–228] Detractors point out that cervical traction may incite cervical radiculopathy as well as temporomandibular joint symptoms.[229] The few controlled trials reported failed to show any influence on the rate of recovery,[225] and

results were not much better than with other treatments with the patient at bed rest.[230]

No agreement exists on the method, amount of weight, duration, or frequency of cervical traction.[223] In fact, only positioning the neck in moderate flexion is widely accepted. In healthy men, 25 pounds of traction straightens the cervical lordosis;[231] 30 pounds for 7 seconds achieves posterior vertebral separation.[224] Maximal foraminal opening occurs at 24° of cervical flexion.[232] Vertebral separation is not essential for benefit in many cases and may even do harm.[225] Because traction for no more than 20 minutes daily is the rule, it is difficult to believe that relief of nerve root pressure for so short a time is the cause of any therapeutic success, although it has been argued that facet malalignment or irritating disc fragments are occasionally reduced after distraction.[233] Traction does provide periods of supported longitudinal neck muscle stretching. The chronic state of protective muscle spasm may be overcome by traction, and this effect may explain the symptomatic relief claimed for the method. A simple method for cervical traction at home can be used for 5 minutes once or twice daily in patients with chronic cervical syndromes.[234]

The benefit of traction on the lumbar spine is equally unclear.[230,235] To separate normal lumbar vertebrae of a subject in bed, at least 25% of the body weight must be used for traction, and in lumbar disc disease, forces as high as 220 pounds for 30 minutes are frequently ineffective.[235–237] Vertebral separation has been demonstrated only with a split table designed to overcome friction of the body in bed. Variable subjective relief has been reported in patients with lumbar discogenic disease and with acute disc syndromes,[238] but treatment failures and increased root pain have been reported as well.[239] Pelvic traction, as usually applied in a hospital bed, is insufficient to cause vertebral separation, but may reinforce a regimen of bed rest in a noncompliant patient.[23] Until lumbar traction is more adequately studied, it is reasonable to use a split-table method, which requires only moderate weights in the range of 25 to 50% of body weight to relieve pain. Spinal traction is generally unsatisfactory in the presence of inflammation and is best avoided in patients with hemorrhagic states or malignant diseases.[23,221] Traction has been used in children for pain relief in both acute inflammatory joint disease and in septic arthritis of the hip. A recent wave of enthusiasm for inversion (hanging upside down) traction seems to be subsiding. Occasionally, patients with neck and back pain achieve symptomatic relief.[240] Hypertensive, ocular, and cardiovascular complications may be incurred.[240]

Massage

Massage is an ancient method for relieving musculoskeletal tension and pain and for inducing general relaxation. Therapeutic massage techniques include stroking (effleurage) for soothing effects and deep stroking for muscle relaxation; compression (pétrissage) as a means of kneading tissues to relax muscles, to stretch adhesions, and to mobilize edema; and percussion (tapotement) to create a stimulating vibration or a more vigorous percussive counterirritant effect.[221,241] A variety of exotic massage methods are currently used in nonmedical settings. Massage is useful to relieve muscle spasm and to facilitate therapeutic exercise in selected patients when less expensive and less time-consuming techniques prove ineffective.[221,223] Special techniques such as Cyriax friction massage, acupressure, and Shiatsu may yet find a place in the treatment of soft-tissue disorders.

Manipulation

Joint manipulation, with and without anesthesia, is accepted in the management of postsurgical or posttraumatic contractures, for mobilization of a "frozen" shoulder, and, to a lesser extent, for treatment of lateral epicondylitis.[208,242]

Chiropractic cervical manipulation has resulted in transient ischemia, nonfatal brain stem infarctions, and several reported cases of stroke.[243–245] The exact incidence of these complications is unknown, but with an estimated quarter of a million patients per year treated by manipulation, these findings are probably rare. No mortality has been attributed to lumbar manipulation[244] or to nonspinal manipulation. Manipulation technique uses careful positioning of the patient to achieve muscle relaxation and muscle mechanical disadvantage, so an abrupt additional manipulating stretch, "thrust," stretches tight muscles and distracts joints. This distraction is often associated with an audible "cracking" sound, thought by some to be due to reduction of facet "subluxations" or to realignment of displaced fibrocartilaginous disc material.[208,241,242,246] It is uncertain whether spinal manipulation depends on joint distraction, on muscle stretching, or on actual joint or disc realignment for pain control.

Controlled trials of manipulation in acute low-back pain showed a trend to shortened duration of pain,[238] but did not alter outcome,[247] and showed no advantage over common medical therapy[248] or other physiotherapeutic techniques.[249] Manipulation therapy is contraindicated in the presence of severe osteoporosis, bone tumor, bleeding diathesis, or sepsis.[221]

Mobilization therapies such as traction, massage, and manipulation include oscillations; alternating muscle contractions and relaxations called "muscle energy" techniques;[250,251] and joint vibrations designed to relieve muscle tension, to free minor adhesions, to increase joint and muscle motion, and to relieve pain.[23,250,251] Such "mobilizations" do not use the "thrust"; examples are Cyriax, Maitland, and Mennel methods.[221] They may play an adjunctive role in the management of articular and periarticular disorders.[221] Mobilization therapies may stimulate proprioceptive pathways and possibly more complex reflexes and may thereby diminish pain.[221] Additional effects may result from the impact of these techniques on pathologic tissues. They are generally safe if done by trained physicians or other health professionals. Various forms of mobilization are commonly and arbitrarily used by practitioners of "alternative" forms of therapy. Research is needed to define the possible role of these methods in the treatment of rheumatic diseases.

Vapocoolant Spray and Local Anesthetic Injections

Tonic focal areas of palpable, tender contracted muscle, so-called trigger areas, are commonly observed in association with painful musculoskeletal disorders.[252–255] They appear to be reflex in origin, occur in predictable locations, correlate with many acupuncture points, may themselves be a source of referred pain, and often respond promptly to local measures, such as massage, cold application, cold spray, and local anesthetic injections.[153,252–255] The use of vapocoolant sprays in the local treatment of painful musculoskeletal disorders, or as a topical anesthetic before injections, is an outgrowth of the use of cold compresses as counterirritants.[23] (Fluorimethane is nonflammable and is therefore preferred over ethyl chloride.) The use of local anesthetic trigger-area injections historically preceded that of vapocoolant sprays.[255,256] Clinically, these injections should be tried when sprays, or spray and stretch techniques, have failed. Vapocoolant sprays have the additional advantage over local injections of suitability for home use.

Tender points other than tender "trigger" points in muscles are associated with irritation at entheses and bursae. Local steroid injections into these tender points with or without a local anesthetic may prove efficacious.[257–259]

MOBILITY

A fundamental component of independent functioning for the arthritis patient is the ability to perform transfers. Modifications of bed, bath, chair, toilet, and wheelchair may be needed for the arthritic patient to transfer satisfactorily.[20,260–263] Patients unable to transfer independently depend for optimal mobility on the assistance of others. Instruction in specific techniques for the safe transfer of the patient from bed or chair to ambulatory-assist device to toilet, bath, or car must be provided to whomever is to be responsible for this activity.[260,262,263,264,265] Several excellent references provide details of transfer training.[261–263,265–267]

GAIT

Normal gait is an efficient, energy-conserving means of locomotion.[268–272] Muscle weakness, joint disease and its associated pain, swelling, instability, contracture, or deformity, leg-length discrepancy, and postural deformities may lead to awkward, inefficient gait patterns that impose excessive strains on joints and on the cardiovascular system.[269,271–274] Training in gait and in the use of properly fitted canes, crutches, walkers, and braces requires supervision by a skilled therapist. Selection of a crutch, cane, or walker that minimizes hand stress (enlarged hand grip) or wrist and elbow strain (platform crutch), or one that can be used in spite of generalized weakness (a lightweight walker), can be crucial in determining the ambulatory function of an arthritic patient.[263,275,276]

The most common ambulation-assistive device is a cane. Resistance to its use can be overcome by persuasion and demonstration of its benefits.[102] A properly fitted cane or crutch (barring modifications) when multiple joints are affected, should reach 8 inches lateral to the front of the foot when the patient is standing comfortably and holding the cane or crutch handle with the elbow flexed 15 to 30°.[23] This position permits stability on standing and an easy reach to the ground ahead during walking. The cane, grasp and arm function permitting, should be held in the hand opposite to the lower extremity joint involved by arthritis. A lightweight walking aid is particularly useful to many arthritic or elderly patients. Specific methods for gait training, including training in the use of canes and crutches, are reported.[102,277–280]

WHEELCHAIRS, DRIVING, AND PUBLIC TRANSPORTATION

When ambulation is impractical or impossible, a wheelchair must be prescribed. A variety of wheelchair options must be considered to ensure fit that provides support and function for painful or deformed joint structures.[20,264,275,281–283] Accessibility to

bathrooms, clearance under tables and desks, ease of entry and exits for transferring, durability, powered versus nonpowered models, and cost are some of the factors that require analysis when recommending purchase of a wheelchair.[20,275,281] Wheelchair manufacturers or their representatives often provide important information. However, it is advisable first to consult an experienced physical or occupational therapist. Driving an automobile is often difficult, but even a patient confined to a wheelchair may be able to drive if special provisions are made. Special instructions for the handicapped arthritic driver, automobile or van modifications, and provision of suitable parking and accessibility to home, work, and recreation make mobility independence a practical goal.[264,276,284–286]

When driving is not a practical option, public transportation is all too often inaccessible to handicapped people.[18,285,286] In some communities, special vehicles are available to meet this need.[19,285,287] Airline travel poses many problems, although many airlines have developed special policies to assist the handicapped.

Architectural barriers that often confront the handicapped or wheelchair traveler at hotels, schools, restaurants, parks, zoos, and theaters may be avoided in part by selecting places and facilities where special access for the handicapped is provided.[18,262,271,284,286]

OCCUPATIONAL THERAPY

The occupational therapist's first concern is with the patient's ability to function independently. The second concern is to provide adaptive equipment to allow function that is otherwise difficult or impossible. This goal often requires the fabrication of splints.[23,288–291] Central to the occupational therapist's evaluation of an arthritis patient is a review of the ADL (see Table 49–2).[23,289,292,293] The occupational therapist provides an arthritic patient with concepts and techniques of joint protection, energy conservation, and function-assisted methods and devices to meet needs as determined by the ADL assessment.[23,285,289,290,292,293] Several excellent reviews on assistive devices, energy-saving techniques, and protection of arthritic joints are available.[23,261–263,265,276,284,288,291,294,295]

The physician should reinforce the concepts taught by the therapist, specifically (1) joint protection, including joint "rest" with proper positioning to avoid deformity; (2) transferring skills to enable the patient to change position without stressing joints; (3) preferential use of the strongest (largest) joints for any given activity; and (4) conservation of energy by planning tasks to use involved joints to their greatest mechanical advantage.[23,289,290,292–294]

COLLARS AND CORSETS

Collars are not indicated for all neck pain, nor are corsets recommended for all back pain.[275] With the exception of the few braces that stabilize the cervical spine, collars are primarily worn for pain relief, for relief for neck muscles in spasm, and as a reminder to avoid certain movements that may exacerbate the underlying problem.[23,275] Studies on the immobilization efficiency of various cervical collars and braces have been performed on normal subjects. The lack of studies on patients with inflammatory disease of the cervical spine makes decisions regarding type of collar, duration of use, and indication for use difficult. Common practice is based on extrapolation from studies of normal subjects and from clinical experience.[23,295a,275,296] Most commonly used collars do not restrict movement at the atlantoaxial joint.[297] Scalp fixation in a halo cast[222] or Crutchfield tongs with longitudinal pull may be required.[298] Stabilization of the lower cervical spine, but not of the upper cervical spine, may be obtained with a rigid cervical collar (Philadelphia collar).[23] Although controlled studies are inadequate, soft cervical collars have been found not to affect outcome as regards episodes of acute neck pain,[225] nor have they arrested the progress of subluxation in patients with RA.[299] When a cervical collar or brace is prescribed, isometric neck exercises should also be prescribed to minimize disuse atrophy once pain is controlled and any neurologic deficit stabilized.

Corsets or spinal braces are commonly used to relieve low back discomfort and to prevent exacerbation of radiculopathy.[23] Many types of corsets and braces are available, and guidelines for individual prescriptions are described in detail elsewhere.[23] Studies of corsets show only subjective relief of pain,[300] and no available brace can effectively immobilize the lumbosacral region.[301] Pain relief with a corset may be related to an increase in abdominal pressure that relieves extensor force on the spine with an overall decrease in intradiscal pressure.[302] The indications for, and instruction in the use of braces are controversial.[303] The prolonged use of these braces has resulted in loss of spinal mobility and weakness of paraspinal muscles.

SPLINTS AND BRACES

Splints (Table 49–8) are used to relieve pain, to improve function, to prevent trauma to unstable joints, and to prevent, contain, or correct arthritic deformities.[23,61,88,103,288,290,295,309] Although deceptively simple in appearance, their proper design and appropriate application require great sophistication.

Splints can be and have been made of cloth and metal, plaster, heat-moldable plastics, and more recently, new fiberglass polymers, polyethylene, polypropylene, and air-pressure apparatus.[290,309,310] Splints should be light, durable, nonirritating, cosmetically appealing, and affordable.[9,23,88,90,103,290] The wearer should easily be able to apply, adjust, and remove the splint or brace without assistance. Splints are designed either for rest or for controlled motion of a given joint.[275] A properly designed splint should not unintentionally affect function, such as a wrist splint that prevents finger function, nor should stress be transferred to other joints (Fig. 49–6).[23,88,90,103,275,289,290,311,312] Research on splint use demonstrates better compliance if strength is enhanced more than dexterity.[291] Considerable education and encouragement are needed to convince patients to use splints during rest or relative inactivity.[291] Splint therapy of rheumatic disease patients requires frequent followup and splint adjustments.

Proved or even well-established indications for splints and braces in arthritis are few. Guidelines for postoperative splinting to maintain joint alignment and to prevent or to correct contractures, particularly in the knee and fingers, are well established.[94] Permanent reversal of joint malalignments, such as swan neck, boutonnière, or ulnar deviation, by splinting has not been demonstrated.[313] With the exceptions of contracture corrections and postoperative splinting, the indications for splints and braces should be confined to relief of pain and improvement of function (see Table 49–6).[23,61,305,309,314]

Splinting and casting can reduce joint inflammation and pain without risk of contractures if immobilization is not prolonged beyond 4 weeks.[23,61,305,314] Serial casting by a variety of techniques is an acceptable method of prevention and treatment of flexion contractures of the knee.[59,94,315] The rationale for serial or wedged casting is based on the effect of joint support on pain relief and relaxation of muscle spasm, to allow a gradual stretch of contracted connective tissue. Each cast change, which takes place every 5 to 7 days, allows for additional stretching, as well as an opportunity for range-of-motion exercise. A bi-valved cast can be removed daily for observation and exercise of the extremity. Knee contractures greater than 45° usually require traction for correction. Properly applied traction has the additional advantage of minimizing impingement and compression of a subluxed tibia on the femur.[94] When the maximum possible correction

Table 49–8. Useful Splints and Braces*

Region	Indication	Purpose	Type	Reference
Hand	Acute inflammation	Stabilize for pain relief Preserve position for function	Volar resting splint†	290,304,305
Thumb	Carpometacarpal and metacarpopha- langeal joint arthritis	Stabilize for pain relief and to permit function	Thumb post with wrist strap	90,309
	De Quervain's tenosynovitis	Relieve pain	Thumb post with wrist strap	
	Interphalangeal joint pain or instability	Improve function and relieve pain	Thumb, interphalangeal "sleeve" or "double ring"	
Wrist	Active inflammation	Improve function and relieve pain	Static "working" wrist splint‡	290
	Instability	Improve function and relieve pain	Static "working" wrist splint‡	
	Carpal tunnel syndrome	Prevent hyperflexion and nerve compression	Static "working" wrist splint‡	
Knee	Pain, instability	Relieve pain	Molded plastic hinged knee	235,290,306, 307
		Maintain position	Long leg, hinged knee with lock	
Ankle, hindfoot	Pain on weight bearing	Support foot and relieve weight- bearing stress	Cushion heel, rocker sole, below- knee weight-bearing brace	23,290
Forefoot	Pain on weight bearing	Support foot and relieve weight- bearing stress	Metatarsal pad or bar with cushion insole	307,308

*Postoperative splints not included.
†Resting splints maximally support affected joints, usually by sacrificing function.
‡Static working splints stabilize affected joints, but permit maximum function (see Fig. 49–6). Dynamic splints provide wire or elastic tension for traction or to assist weak muscles. Various dynamic splints, such as wire or rubber-band–assisted traction devices, are employed to maintain postoperative corrections. The Bunnell "knuckle bender" splints are occasionally helpful in treating an isolated finger contracture when inflammation is minimal. Splints for thumb interphalangeal stabilization, to correct swan neck, boutonnière, or ulnar deviation deformities, are available, but their efficacy is unproved.[70]

is reached, as defined by the lack of increase in motion for 2 consecutive weeks, splinting may replace serial casting to maintain range of motion.

SEXUAL, SOCIAL, AND PSYCHOLOGICAL CONSIDERATIONS IN REHABILITATION

Sexual problems are common among arthritic patients.[316] Chronic pain and inflammation; stiffness or immobility especially involving the hips, neck, hands, and knees; fatigue; malaise; and medication-related and emotional disturbances all contribute.[317–319] A recent study showed that patients preferred a physician to a psychologist or social worker for discussion of sexual concerns[320] so it is important that the physician be attuned to the sexual problems of the arthritis patient. Problems of sexual image as a consequence of perceived disfigurement, loss of sexual drive or libido due to medication or disease-related factors, physical expression of sexuality limited by pain, stiffness, and deformity, and impotence that may be due to drug effects, pain, or psychologic factors must all be addressed.[318]

The physician can advise the patient about drugs, such as the peak levels of analgesics and anti-inflammatory agents, or surgical procedures to increase mo-

bility, to relieve pain, and to improve appearance. The physician may also supervise the physical therapist's teaching of massage and hydrotherapy techniques as a prelude to sex, and the occupational therapist's use of splints for particularly painful extremities and demonstration of appropriate positions.[318,319] Alternate sexual positioning, depending on which joints are involved, and alternate forms of sexual expression may be needed.[317–319] Referral to trained sex counselors for refractory sexual dysfunction may also be indicated. Counseling regarding forms and use of contraceptive methods is often helpful.

Premarital counseling is best done with the physician and the couple together.[321] Religious, cultural, social, and disease-related histories are needed from both patient and intended spouse. Information on the specific type of arthritis, its natural course, prognosis, and how it will affect various daily activities can then be provided along with advice relative to sex.[318,321] Counseling of married couples often involves a discussion of childbirth.[318,319] Genetic counseling and concerns about the effects of the disease and medications on the bearing, nurturing, and nursing of an infant should be addressed in conjunction with the obstetrician and pediatrician.[322] The goal is an educated, confident mother and a healthy child.[322] Women afflicted with RA need help to cope with their own, often unvoiced, fears about the disease.[16] How

FIG. 49–6. Static "working" wrist splint. This heat-molded plastic splint with Velcro closures is designed to stabilize a painful or inflamed wrist in a neutral position (zero degrees of extension) while permitting free finger and thumb function. This splint is also useful for patients with carpal tunnel syndrome.

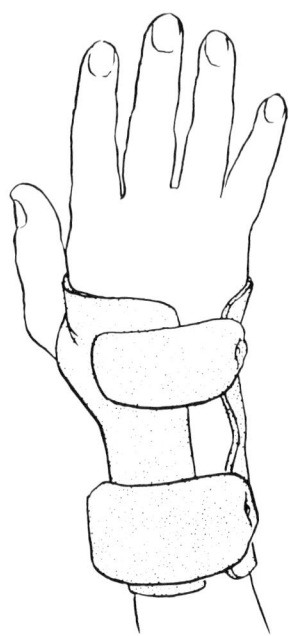

to manage a home and how to handle a spouse's anxiety? Recent studies have debunked the myth that a disability in a parent influences a child's psychologic adjustment. Psychologic development in such children is no different from that of peers with "well" parents.[323]

Attention to psychosocial factors does not alter rheumatic disease activity, but it does affect the functional results of rehabilitation.[324] A team approach helps most in social adjustment. Educational and financial background are strong "motivational" variables that influence outcome more than the team approach itself.[11,324]

Psychologic problems in patients with chronic arthritis include loss of independence and self-esteem, loss of relationships with family, friends, and lovers, loss of employment, and the stress of coping with pain and disability.[325,326] The classic sequence of adaptive psychological responses to chronic disease, that is, shock, anger, denial, resignation, and acceptance, are often altered in the arthritis patient and fluctuate with the course of the disease.[325] The approach to rehabilitation of the arthritis patient is case specific but must consider family dynamics and stress.[316,326] Technologic solutions to personal and social problems

or reluctance to accept patients as co-partners in their own rehabilitation may result in poor compliance to therapeutic regimens and poorer functional outcome.[316,324,325,327]

Newer programs to supplement an arthritis rehabilitation team's efforts to deal with all facets of the patient's life and disease include the following: (1) group counseling and educational programs;[328] (2) participation of voluntary organizations that disseminate information, aid with disability-related problems such as transportation or meal preparation, and provide group psychosocial support;[329] (3) multidisciplinary pain centers in which many psychologic, physical medicine, and drug-control approaches can be used alone or together for pain management;[184,330] and (4) recreation therapy and recreational opportunities designed for the disabled.[331]

REFERENCES

1. Colvez, A., and Blanchet, M.: Disability trends in the United States population 1966–1976: Analysis of reported causes. Am. J. Public Health, 71:464–471, 1981.
2. Kramer, J.S., Yelin, E.H., and Epstein, W.V.: Social and economic impacts of four musculoskeletal conditions. Arthritis Rheum., 26:901–907, 1983.
3. Nuki, G., Brooks, R., and Buchanan, W.W.: The economics of arthritis. Bull. Rheum. Dis., 23:726–733, 1972–1973.
4. Yelin, E., Meenan, R., Nevitt, M., and Epstein, W.: Work disability in rheumatoid arthritis: Effects of disease, social, and work factors. Ann. Intern. Med., 93:551–556, 1980.
5. Arthritis Foundation: The Arthritis 1975 Annual Report. New York, Arthritis Foundation; 1975.
6. Stone, C.: The lifetime economic costs of rheumatoid arthritis. J. Rheumatol., 11:819–827, 1984.
7. Alexander, R. McN., and Bennet-Clark, H.C.: Storage of elastic strain energy in muscle and other tissues. Nature, 265:114–117, 1977.
8. Meenan, R.F., et al.: The cost of rheumatoid arthritis: A patient oriented study of chronic disease costs. Arthritis Rheum., 21:827–833, 1978.
9. Brenner, M.H.: Health costs and benefits of economic policy. Int. J. Health Serv., 7:581–623, 1977.
10. Epstein, W.V.: Health services research in rheumatology. Bull. Rheum. Dis., 31:15–19, 1981.
11. Liang, M.H., et al.: Evaluation of comprehensive rehabilitation services for elderly homebound patients with arthritis and orthopedic disability. Arthritis Rheum., 27:258–266, 1984.
12. Johnston, M.V., and Keith, R.A.: Cost-benefits of medical rehabilitation. Arch. Phys. Med. Rehabil., 64:147–154, 1983.
13. Robinson, H.S.: Functional and social deficits—Consequences of time and disease. In Total Management of the Arthritis Patient. Edited by G.E. Ehrlich. Philadelphia, J.B. Lippincott, 1973.
14. Shelkh, K., Meade, T.W., and Mattingly, S.: Unemployment and the disabled. Rheum. Rehabil., 19:233–238, 1980.
15. Rudd, E.: International year of disabled persons, 1981. Arthritis Rheum., 24:108–109, 1981.
16. Wright, V., and Owen, S.: The effect of rheumatoid arthritis

on the social situation of housewives. Rheum. Rehabil., 15:156–160, 1976.

17. Carey, T.S., and Hadler, N.M.: The role of the primary physician in disability determination for social security insurance and workers' compensation. Ann. Intern. Med., 104:706–710, 1986.

18. Kliment, S.A.: Into the Mainstream—A Syllabus for Barrier-free Environment. Washington, D.C., Rehabilitation Services Administation. U.S. Department of Health, Education and Welfare, and American Institute of Architects, Social and Rehabilitation Services, 1975.

19. Lauri, G.: Housing and Home Services for the Disabled: Guidelines and Experiences in Independent Living. Hagerstown, MD, Harper & Row, 1977.

20. Brattstrom, M., et al.: The rheumatoid patient in need of a wheelchair. Scand. J. Rehabil. Med., 13:39–43, 1981.

21. Wild, D., Nayak, U.S.L., and Isaacs, B.: Description, classification and prevention of falls in old people at home. Rheum. Rehabil., 20:153–159, 1981.

22. Krusen, F.H., Kottke, F.J., and Ellwood, P.M.: Handbook of Physical Medicine and Rehabilitation. Philadelphia, W.B. Saunders, 1965.

23. Swezey, R.L.: Arthritis: Rational Therapy and Rehabilitation. Philadelphia, W.B. Saunders, 1978.

24. Boyle, R.W.: The Therapeutic Gymnasium. In Therapeutic Exercises. Edited by S. Licht. New Haven, CT, Waverly Press, 1965.

25. Swezey, R.L.: Arthritis rehabilitation: staff, facilities, and evaluation. In Rehabilitation of Rheumatic Conditions. Edited by G.E. Ehrlich. Baltimore, Williams & Wilkins, 1980.

26. Meenan, R.F., Liang, M.H., and Hadler, N.M.: Social security disability and the arthritis patient. Bull. Rheum. Dis., 33:1–7, 1983.

27. Gresham, G.E.: Essential considerations of the disability evaluation. J. Musculoskel. Med., 5:43–50, 1986.

28. Hess, E.V.: A uniform data base on rheumatic diseases. Arthritis Rheum., 19:645–648, 1978.

29. Fries, J.F.: Toward an understanding of patient outcome measurement. Arthritis Rheum., 26:697–704, 1983.

30. Fries, J.F., et al.: Measurement of patient outcome in arthritis. Arthritis Rheum., 23:137–145, 1980.

31. Liang, M.H., and Jette, A.M.: Measuring functional ability in chronic arthritis: A critical review. Arthritis Rheum., 24:80–86, 1981.

32. O'Driscoll, S.L., and Jayson, M.I.V.: The clinical significance of pain threshold measurements. Rheumatol. Rehabil., 21:31–35, 1982.

33. Liang, M.H., Cullen, K., and Larson, M.: In search of a more perfect mousetrap (health status or quality of life instrument). J. Rheumatol., 9:775–779, 1982.

34. Meenan, R.F.: The AIMS approach to health status measurement. Conceptual background and measurement properties. J. Rheumatol., 9:785–788, 1980.

35. Meenan, R.F., et al.: The Arthritis Impact Measurement Scales: Further investigations of health status measure. Arthritis Rheum., 25:1048–1053, 1982.

36. Harvey, R.F., and Jellinek, H.M.: Functional performance assessment: A program approach. Arch. Phys. Med. Rehabil., 62:456–461, 1981.

37. Stewart, C.P.U.: A prediction score for geriatric rehabilitation prospects. Rheumatol. Rehabil., 19:239–245, 1980.

38. Taylor, D.: A table to indicate the degree of improvement in chronic arthritis. Can. Med. Assoc. J., 36:608–610, 1937.

39. Steinbrocker, O., Traeger, C.H., and Batterman, R.C.: Therapeutic criteria in rheumatoid arthritis. JAMA, 140:659–662, 1949.

40. Conaty, J.P., and Nickel, V.L.: Functional incapacitation in rheumatoid arthritis: A rehabilitation challenge: A correlative study of function before and after hospital treatment. J. Bone Joint Surg., 53A:624–637, 1971.

41. Katz, S., et al.: Studies of illness in the aged. JAMA, 185:914–919, 1963.

42. Klein, R.M., and Bell, B.: Self-care skills: Behavioral measurements with Klein-Bell ADL Scale. Arch. Phys. Med. Rehabil., 63:335–338, 1982.

43. Kaufert, J.M.: Functional ability indices: Measurement problems in assessing their validity. Arch. Phys. Med. Rehabil., 64:260–267, 1983.

44. Williams, M.E., and Hadler, N.M.: Musculoskeletal components of decrepitude. Semin. Arthritis Rheum., 11:284–287, 1981.

45. Huskisson, E.C.: Measurement of pain. J. Rheumatol., 9:768–769, 1982.

46. Seltzer, G.B., Granger, C.V., and Wineberg, B.A.: Functional assessment: Bridge between family and rehabilitation medicine within an ambulatory practice. Arch. Phys. Med. Rehabil., 63:453–457, 1982.

47. Decker, J.L.: Conference on outcome measures in rheumatological clinical trials: Summary. J. Rheumatol., 9:802–806, 1982.

48. Huskisson, E.C.: Measurement in rehabilitation. (Editorial.) Rheum. Rehabil., 15:132, 1976.

49. Raskin, R.J., and Lawless, O.J.: Articular and soft tissue abnormalities in a "normal" population. J. Rheumatol., 9:284–288, 1982.

50. Bardwick, P.A., and Swezey, R.L.: Physical therapy in arthritis. Postgrad. Med., 72:223–234, 1982.

51. Simon, L., and Blotman, F.: Exercise therapy and hydrotherapy in the treatment of the rheumatic disease. Clin. Rheum. Dis., 7:337–347, 1981.

52. Michels, E.: Measurement in physical therapy. Phys. Ther., 63:209–215, 1983.

53. Vignos, P.J.: Physiotherapy in rheumatoid arthritis. J. Rheumatol., 7:269–271, 1980.

54. Baker, G.H.B.: Psychological management in rehabilitation. In Rehabilitation in the Rheumatic Diseases. Edited by D. Woolf. Philadelphia, W.B. Saunders, 1981.

55. Tipton, C.M., et al.: The influence of physical activity on ligaments and tendons. Med. Sci. Sports, 7:165–175, 1975.

56. Lee, P., et al.: Benefits of hospitalization in rheumatoid arthritis. Q. J. Med., 43:205–214, 1974.

57. Smith, R.D.: Effect of hemiparesis on rheumatoid arthritis. Arthritis Rheum., 22:1419–1420, 1979.

58. Smith, R.D., and Polley, H.F.: Rest therapy for rheumatoid arthritis. Mayo Clin. Proc., 53:141–145, 1978.

59. Harris, R., and Copp, E.P.: Immobilization of the knee joint in rheumatoid arthritis. Ann. Rheum. Dis., 21:353–359, 1962.

60. Mills, J.A., et al.: Value of bed rest in patients with rheumatoid arthritis. N. Engl. J. Med., 284:453–458, 1971.

61. Partridge, R.E.H., and Duthie, J.J.R.: Controlled trial of the effects of complete immobilization of the joint in rheumatoid arthritis. Ann. Rheum. Dis., 22:91–99, 1963.

62. Smith, R.D.: Bed rest at home for rheumatoid arthritis. Arthritis Rheum., 23:263–264, 1980.

63. Jayson, M.I.V.: Back pain, spondylosis and disc disorders. In Copeman's Textbook of Rheumatic Diseases. Edited by J.T. Scott. London, Livingstone, 1978.

64. Moldofsky, H., and Scarisbrick, P.: Induction of neurasthenic

musculoskeletal pain syndrome by selective sleep stage deprivation. Psychosom. Med., 38:35–44, 1976.

65. Harrison, R.A.: Hydrotherapy in rheumatic conditions. In Physiotherapy in Rheumatology. Edited by S.A. Hyde. Oxford, Blackwell Scientific Publications, 1980.

66. Kabat, H.: Proprioceptive facilitation. In Therapeutic Exercise. 2nd Ed. Edited by S. Licht. Baltimore, Waverly Press, 1965.

67. De Palma, A.F.: Diseases of The Knee. Philadelphia, J.B. Lippincott, 1954.

68. Fried, D.M.: Rest versus activity. In Arthritis and Physical Medicine. Edited by S. Licht. New Haven, CT, Waverly Press, 1969.

69. Flatt, A.E.: The Care of the Rheumatoid Hand. 3rd Ed. St. Louis, C.V. Mosby, 1974.

70. Bunnell, S.: Surgery of the Hand. 5th Ed. Revised by J.H. Bozes. Philadelphia, J.B. Lippincott, 1970.

71. Cailliet, R.: Shoulder Pain. 2nd Ed. Philadelphia. F.A. Davis, 1981.

72. Cooke, A.F., Dawson, D., and Wright, F.: Lubrication of synovial membrane. Ann. Rheum. Dis., 35:56–59, 1976.

73. Kottke, F.J., Pauley, D.L., and Ptak, R.A.: The rationale for prolonged stretching for correction of shortening of connective tissues. Arch. Phys. Med. Rehabil., 47:345–352, 1966.

74. Radin, E.L., and Paul, I.L.: Joint function. Arthritis Rheum., 13:276–279, 1970.

75. Woo, S.L., Matthews, J.V., and Akisen, W.H.: Connective tissue response to immobility. Correlative study of biomechanical and biochemical measurements of normal and immobilized rabbit knees. Arthritis Rheum., 18:257–264, 1975.

76. Tkaczuk, H.: Study of tensile properties of human lumbar longitudinal ligaments. Acta Orthop. Scand., 115:54–69, 1968.

77. Wright, D.G., and Rennels, D.G.: A study of the elastic properties of plantar fascia. J. Bone Joint Surg., 46A:482–492, 1964.

78. Swezey, R.L.: Dynamic factors in deformity of the rheumatoid arthritic hand. Bull. Rheum. Dis., 22:649–656, 1971–1972.

79. Swezey, R.L., and Fiegenberg, D.S.: Inappropriate intrinsic muscle action in the rheumatoid hand. Ann. Rheum. Dis., 30:619–625, 1971.

80. Bulgen, D.Y., Hazleman, B.L., and Voak, D.: HLA-B27 and frozen shoulder. Lancet, 1:1042–1044, 1976.

81. Risk, T.E., and Pinals, R.S.: Frozen shoulder. Arthritis Rheum., 11:440–451, 1982.

82. Allander, E., et al.: Rheumatology in perspective: The epidemiological view. Scand. J. Rheumatol., 46 (Suppl.):11–19, 1982.

83. VanBrocklin, J.D., and Ellis, D.G.: A study of the mechanical behavior of toe extensor tendons under applied stress. Arch. Phys. Med. Rehabil., 47:369–373, 1965.

84. Harris, E., Jr., and McCroskery, P.A.: The influence of temperature and fibril stability on degradation of cartilage collagen by rheumatoid synovial collagenase. N. Engl. J. Med., 290:1–6, 1974.

85. Heffman, M., and Bibby, B.G.: Effect of tension on lysis of collagen. Soc. Exp. Biol. Med. Proc., 126:561–562, 1967.

86. Nordschow, C.D.: Aspects of aging in human collagen: An exploratory thermoelastic study. Exp. Mol. Pathol., 5:350–373, 1966.

87. Rigby, B.J.: Thermal transition in the collagenous tissue of poikilothermic animals. J. Therm. Biol., 2:80–95, 1977.

88. Ehrlich, G.E.: Rest and splinting. In Total Management of the Arthritis Patient. Edited by G.E. Ehrlich. Philadelphia, J.B. Lippincott, 1973.

89. Merritt, J.L., and Hunder, G.G.: Passive range of motion, not isometric exercise, amplifies acute urate synovitis. Arch. Phys. Med. Rehabil., 64:130–131, 1983.

90. American Rheumatism Association, Arthritis Foundation and National Institute of Arthritis and Metabolic Diseases: Evaluation of splinting. Criteria for and evaluation of orthopedic measures in the management of deformities of rheumatoid arthritis. Arthritis Rheum., 7:585–600, 1964.

91. Stein, H., and Dickson, R.A.: Reversed dynamic slings for knee-flexion contractures in the hemophiliac. J. Bone Joint Surg., 57A:282–283, 1975.

92. Adamson, J.E.: Treatment of the stiff hand. Orthop. Clin. North Am., 1:467–479, 1970.

93. Karten, I., Koatz, A.O., and McEwen, C.: Treatment of contractures of the knee in rheumatoid arthritis. N.Y. Acad. Med. Bull., 44:763–773, 1968.

94. Preston, R.A.: The Surgical Management of Rheumatoid Arthritis. Philadelphia, W.B. Saunders, 1968.

95. Rhinelander, F.W., and Ropes, M.W.: Adjustable casts in the treatment of joint deformity. J. Bone Joint Surg., 27:311–316, 1945.

96. Edington, D.W., and Edgerton, V.R.: The Biology of Physical Activity. Boston, Houghton Mifflin, 1976.

97. Eysenck, H.J.: A new therapy of post-rest upswing on "warm-up" in motor learning. Percept. Motor Skills, 28:992–994, 1969.

98. Kottke, F.J.: Therapeutic exercise. In Handbook of Physical Medicine and Rehabilitation, 2nd Ed. Edited by F.H. Krusen, F.J. Kottke, and P.M. Ellwood. Philadelphia, W.B. Saunders, 1971.

99. Swezey, R.L.: Essentials of physical management and rehabilitation in arthritis. Semin. Arthritis Rheum., 3:349–368, 1971.

100. Nordemar, R., et al.: Physical training in rheumatoid arthritis: A controlled long-term study. I. Scand. J. Rheumatol., 10:17–23, 1981.

101. Zislis, J.M.: Hydrotherapy. In Handbook of Physical Medicine. Edited by F.H. Krusen, F.K. Kottke, and P.M. Ellwood. 2nd Ed, Philadelphia, W.B. Saunders, 1971.

102. Blount, W.P.: Don't throw away the cane. J. Bone Joint Surg., 38A:695–708, 1958.

103. Hyde, S.A.: Physiotherapy in Rheumatology. Oxford, Blackwell Scientific Publications, 1980.

104. Toohezu, P., and Larson, C.W.: Range of Motion Exercise: Key to Joint Mobility. Rehabilitation Publication No. 703. Minneapolis, Sister Kenney Institute, 1968.

105. Currier, D.P., and Mann, R.: Muscular strength developed by electrical stimulation in healthy individuals. Phys. Ther., 63:915–921, 1983.

106. Rothstein, J.M.: Muscle biology: Clinical considerations. Phys. Ther., 62:1823–1830, 1982.

107. Rose, S.J., and Rothstein, J.M.: Muscle mutability: Part I. General concepts and adaptation to altered patterns of use. Phys. Ther., 62:1773–1786, 1982.

108. English, A.W.M., and Wolf, S.L.: The motor unit: Anatomy and physiology. Phys. Ther., 62:10–15, 1982.

109. Herbison, G.J., Jaweed, M.M., and Ditunno, J.F.: Muscle fiber types. Arch. Phys. Med. Rehabil., 63:227–230, 1982.

110. Holloszy, J.O.: Muscle metabolism during exercise. Arch. Phys. Med. Rehabil., 63:231–234, 1982.

111. Rose, S.J., and Rothstein, J.M.: Muscle biology and physical therapy: A historical perspective. Phys. Ther., 62:1754–1756, 1982.

112. Müller, E.A.: Influence of training and of inactivity on muscle strength. Arch. Phys. Med. Rehabil., 51:449–462, 1970.

113. Soderberg, G.L.: Muscle mechanics and pathomechanics: Their clinical relevance. Phys. Ther., *63*:216–220, 1983.

114. Guniby, G., et al.: Muscle strength and endurance after training with repeated maximal isometric contractions. Scand. J. Rehabil. Med., *5*:118–123, 1973.

115. Mundale, M.O.: The relationship of intermittent isometric exercise to fatigue of hand grip. Arch. Phys. Med., *51*:532–539, 1970.

116. DeLateur, B.J., Lehmann, J.F., and Fordyce, W.E.: A test of the DeLorme axiom. Arch. Phys. Med. Rehabil., *49*:245–248, 1968.

117. Hellebrandt, F.A.: Special review; application of the overload principle to muscle training in man. Am. J. Phys. Med., *37*:278–283, 1958.

118. Edstrom, L.: Selective changes in sizes of red and white muscle fibers in upper motor lesions and parkinsonism. J. Neurol. Sci., *11*:537–550, 1970.

119. Beals, C.: A case for aerobic conditioning exercise in rheumatoid arthritis. (Abstract.) Clin. Res., *29*:780A, 1981.

120. Ekblom, B., et al.: Physical performance in patients with rheumatoid arthritis. Scand. J. Rheumatol., *3*:121–125, 1974.

121. Nordemar, R., Edstrom, L., and Ekblom, B.: Changes in muscle fiber size and physical performance in patients with rheumatoid arthritis after short term physical training. Scand. J. Rheumatol., *5*:70–76, 1976.

122. Harkom, T.M., Lampman, R.M., Banwell, B.F., and Castor, C.W.: Therapeutic value of graded aerobic exercise training in rheumatoid arthritis. Arthritis Rheum., *28*:32–39, 1985.

123. Nordemar, R.: Physical training in rheumatoid arthritis: A controlled long-term study. II. Functional capacity and general attitudes. Scand. J. Rheumatol., *10*:25–30, 1981.

124. Carr, D.B., et al.: Physical conditioning facilitates the exercise-induced secretion of beta endorphin and beta-lipoprotein in women. N. Engl. J. Med., *305*:560–566, 1981.

125. Guest, J.H., et al.: Running as a treatment for depression. Compr. Psychiatry, *20*:41–54, 1979.

126. Hollander, J.L., and Horvath, S.M.: The influence of physical therapy procedures on the intra-articular temperature of normal and arthritis subjects. Am. J. Med. Sci., *218*:543–548, 1949.

127. Machover, S., and Sapecky, A.J.: Effect of isometric exercise on the quadriceps muscle in patients with rheumatoid arthritis. Arch. Phys. Med. Rehabil., *47*:737–741, 1966.

128. Goldberg, L.I., White, D.J., and Pandolf, K.B.: Cardiovascular and perceptual responses to isometric exercise. Arch. Phys. Med. Rehabil., *63*:211–216, 1982.

129. Magness, J.L., et al.: Isometric shortening of hip muscles using a belt. Arch. Phys. Med. Rehabil., *52*:158–162, 1971.

130. Sanders, M.T.: A comparison of two methods of training on the development of muscular strength and endurance. J. Orthop. Sports Phys. Ther., *1*:210–213, 1980.

131. Scudder, G.W.: Torque curves produced at the knee during isometric and isokinetic exercise. Arch. Phys. Med. Rehabil., *61*:68–72, 1980.

132. Knapik, J.J., Mawdsley, R.H., and Ramos, M.U.: Angular specificity and test mode specificity of isometric and isokinetic strength training. J. Orthop. Sports Phys. Ther., *5*:58–65, 1983.

133. Kramer, J.F., and Mendryk, S.W.: Electrical stimulation as a strength improvement technique: A review. J. Orthop. Sports Phys. Ther., *4(2)*:91–98, 1982.

134. Laughman, R.K., Youdas, J.W., Garett, T.R., and Chao, E.Y.S.: Strength changes in the normal quadriceps femoris muscle as a result of electrical stimulation. Phys. Therapy, *63*:494–499, 1983.

135. Swash, M., and Schwartz, M.S.: Neuromuscular Diseases: A Practical Approach to Diagnosis and Management. Berlin, Springer-Verlag, 1981.

136. Nichols, P.J.R.: Rehabilitation Medicine: The Management of Physical Disabilities. 2nd Ed. Butterworth, London, 1981.

137. Senbonius Largus: De compisitione medicamentorum liber (translated by P. Kallaway.): The part played by electric fish in early history of bioelectricity and electrotherapy. Bull. Hist. Med., *20*:112–137, 1946.

138. Erb, W.: Handbook of Electro-therapeutics. New York, William Wood & Company, 1883.

139. Monell, S.H.: The Treatment of Disease by Electric Currents. 2nd Ed. New York, E.R. Pelton, 1900.

140. Kovacs, R.: Electrotherapy and Light Therapy. 2nd Ed. Philadelphia, Lea & Febiger, 1935.

141. Harris, P.R.: Iontophoresis: Clinical research in musculoskeletal inflammatory conditions. J. Orthop. Sports Phys. Ther., *4*:109–112, 1982.

142. Puttemans, F.J.M., et al.: Iontophoresis: Mechanisms of action studied by potentiometry and x-ray fluorescence. Arch. Phys. Med. Rehabil., *63*:176–179, 1982.

143. Wolf, S.L. (Ed.): Electrotherapy: Clinics in Physical Therapy. New York, Churchill Livingstone, 1981.

144. Licht, S.: History of electricity. *In* Therapeutic Electricity and Ultraviolet Radiation. Vol. 4. Edited by S. Licht. Baltimore, Waverly Press, 1969.

145. Bertolucci, L.C.: Introduction of antiinflammatory drugs by iontophoresis: Double blind study. J. Orthop. Sports. Phys. Ther., *4*:103–108, 1982.

146. Chantraine, A., Ludy, J.P., and Berger, D.: Is cortisone iontophoresis possible? Arch. Phys. Med. Rehabil., *67*:38–40, 1986.

147. Burgess, E.M.: Some applications of electrical energy for neuromuscular rehabilitation. Orthop. Digest., *4*:14–19, 1976.

148. Hong, C., et al.: Magnetic necklace: Its therapeutic effectiveness on neck and shoulder pain. Arch. Phys. Med. Rehabil., *63*:462–466, 1982.

149. Ray, C.D.: Electrical stimulation: new methods for therapy and rehabilitation. Scand. J. Rehabil. Med., *10*:65–74, 1978.

150. Melzack, R., and Wall, P.D.: Pain mechanisms: A new therapy. Science, *150*:971–979, 1965.

151. Goodman, C.E.: Pathophysiology of pain. Arch. Intern. Med., *143*:527–530, 1983.

152. Reuler, J.B., Girard, D.E., and Nardone, D.A.: The chronic pain syndrome: Misconceptions and management, Ann. Intern. Med., *93*:588–596, 1980.

153. Melzack, R., Stillwell, D.M., and Fox, E.J.: Trigger points and acupuncture points for pains: Correlations and implications. Pain, *3*:3–23, 1977.

154. Mannheimer, C., and Carlsson, C.: The analgesic effect of transcutaneous electrical nerve stimulation (TNS) in patients with rheumatoid arthritis: A comparative study of different pulse patterns. Pain. *6*:329–334, 1979.

155. Pertovaara, A., and Hamalainen, M.A.: Vibrotactile threshold elevation produced by high-frequency transcutaneous electrical nerve stimulation. Arch. Phys. Med. Rehabil., *63*:597–600, 1982.

156. O'Brien, W.J., Rutan, F.M., Sanborn, C., and Omer, G.E.: Effect of transcutaneous electrical nerve stimulation on human blood β-endorphin levels. Physical Therapy, *64*:1367–1374, 1984.

157. Lehmann, T.R., Russell, D.W., and Spratt, K.F.: The impact of patients with nonorganic physical findings on controlled trial of transcutaneous electrical nerve stimulation and electroacupuncture. Spine, *8*:625–634, 1983.

158. Fields, H.L., and Levine, J.D.: Pain—Mechanism and management. West. J. Med., *141*:347–357, 1984.

159. Melzack, R.: Prolonged relief of pain by brief, intense transcutaneous somatic stimulation. Pain, 1:357–373, 1975.

160. Kumar, V.N., and Redford, J.B.: Transcutaneous nerve stimulation in rheumatoid arthritis. Arch. Phys. Med. Rehabil., *63*:595–596, 1982.

161. Krempen, J.F., and Silver, R.A.: External electromagnetic fields in the treatment of nonunion of bones: a three-year experience in private practice. Orthop. Rev., *10*:33–39. 1981.

162. Sharrard, W.J.W., et al.: The treatment of fibrous nonunion of fractures by pulsing electromagnetic stimulation. J. Bone Joint Surg., *64B*:189–193, 1982.

163. Pachter, B.R., Eberstein, A., and Goodgold, J.: Electrical stimulation effect on denervation skeletal myofibers in rats: A light and electron microscopic study. Arch. Phys. Med. Rehabil., *63*:427–430, 1982.

164. Nemeth, P.M.: Electrical stimulation of denervated muscle prevents decreases in oxidative enzymes. Muscle Neurol., *5*:134–139, 1982.

165. Munsat, T.L., McNeal, D., and Walters, R.: Effects of nerve stimulation on human muscle. Arch. Neurol., *33*:608–617, 1976.

166. Miller, N.E., and Banuagizi, A.: Instrumental learning by curarized rats of specific visceral response, intestinal or cardiac. J. Comp. Physiol. Psychol., *65*:1–7, 1968.

167. Basmajian, J.V.: Biofeedback in rehabilitation: A review of principles and practices. Arch. Phys. Med. Rehabil., *62*:469–475, 1981.

168. Middaugh, S.J., Miller, M.C., Foster, G., and Ferdon, M.B.: Electromyographic feedback: Effect on voluntary muscle contractions in normal subjects. Arch. Phys. Med. Rehabil., *63*:254–260, 1982.

169. Middaugh, S.J., et al.: Electromyographic feedback: Effects on voluntary muscle contraction in normal subjects. Arch. Phys. Med. Rehabil., *63*:254–259, 1982.

170. Emery, H., Schaller, J.G., and Fowler, R.S., Jr.: Biofeedback in the management of primary and secondary Raynaud's phenomenon. (Abstract.) Arthritis Rheum., *19*:795, 1976.

171. Yocum, D.E., Hodes, R., Sunstrum, D.R., and Cleeland, C.S.: Use of biofeedback training in treatment of Raynaud's disease and phenomenon. J. Rheumatol., *12*:90–93, 1985.

172. Melzack, R., and Perry, C.: Self regulation of pain. Exp. Neurol., *46*:452–469, 1975.

173. Trall, R.T.: The Hydropathic Encyclopedia: A System of Hydrotherapy and Hygiene. New York, Fowlers and Wells, 1853.

174. Lehmann, J.F., and DeLateur, B.J.: Cryotherapy. In Therapeutic Heat and Cold. Edited by F. Lehmann. Baltimore, Williams & Wilkins, 1965.

175. Lehamnn, J.F., Brunner, G.D., and Stow, R.W.: Pain threshold measurements after therapeutic application of ultrasound, microwave and infrared. Arch. Phys. Med. Rehabil., *39*:560–565, 1958.

176. Abramsen, D.I., et al. Methods in training the conscious control of motor units. Arch. Phys. Med. Rehabil., *48*:12–19, 1967.

177. Gersten, J.W.: Effect of ultrasound on tendon extensibility. Am. J. Phys. Med., *34*:362–369, 1955.

178. Kennedy, A.C.: Joint temperature. Clin. Rheum. Dis., 2:177–188, 1981.

179. Waylonis, G.W., et al.: Home cervical traction: Evaluation using rat tail tendon. Arch. Phys. Med. Rehabil., *57*:122–126, 1976.

180. Bucklund, L., and Tiselius, P.: Objective measurement of joint

stiffness in rheumatoid arthritis. Acta Rheumatol. Scand., *13*:275–288, 1967.

181. Johns, R.J., and Wright, V.: Relative importance of various tissues in joint stiffness. J. Appl. Physiol., *17*:824–831, 1962.

182. Wright, V., and Johns, R.J.: Physical factors concerned with the stiffness of normal and diseased joints. Bull. Johns Hopkins Hosp., *106*:215–231, 1960.

183. Prentice, W.E.: An electromyographic analysis of the effectiveness of heat or cold and stretching for inducing relaxation in injured muscle. J. Orthop. Sports Phys. Ther., *3*:133–140, 1982.

184. Benson, T.B., and Copp, E.P.: The effects of therapeutic forms of heat and ice on the pain threshold of the normal shoulder. Rheumatol. Rehabil., *13*:101–104, 1974.

185. Don Figny, R., and Sheldon, K.: Simultaneous use of heat and cold in treatment of muscle spasm. Arch. Phys. Med. Rehabil., *43*:235–237, 1962.

186. Weidenbacker, R.A., and Smith, C.: Does heat cause relaxation? Phys. Ther. Rev., *40*:261–265, 1960.

187. Harris, R.: The effect of various forms of physical therapy on radiosodium clearance from the arthritic knee joint. Ann. Phys. Med., *7*:1–17, 1963.

188. Dorwart, B.B., Hansell, J.R., and Schumacher, H.R., Jr.: Effects of cold and heat on urate crystal-induced synovitis in the dog. Arthritis Rheum., *17*:563–571, 1974.

189. Harris, R., and Millard, J.B.: Paraffin-wax baths in the treatment of rheumatoid arthritis. Ann. Rheum. Dis., *14*:278–282, 1955.

190. Mainardi, C.L., et al.: Rheumatoid arthritis: Failure of daily heat therapy to affect its progression. Arch. Phys. Med. Rehabil., *60*:390–393, 1979.

191. Lehmann, J.F.: Diathermy. In Therapeutic Heat. Edited by S. Licht, Baltimore, Waverly Press, 1958.

192. Lehmann, J.F., and Krusen, F.H.: Biophysical effects of ultrasonic energy on carcinoma and their possible significance. Arch. Phys. Med. Rehabil., *36*:452–459, 1955.

193. Lehmann, J.F.: Diathermy. In Handbook of Physical Medicine and Rehabilitation, 2nd Ed. Edited by F.H. Krusen, F. Kottke, and P.M. Ellwood. 2nd Ed. Philadelphia. W.B. Saunders, 1971.

194. Schwan, H.P., and Piersol, G.M.: The absorption of electromagnetic energy in body tissues: Review and critical analysis: Physiological and clinical aspects. Am. J. Phys. Med., *34*:425–448, 1955.

195. Lehmann, J.F., et al.: Heating of joint structures by ultrasound. Arch. Phys. Med. Rehabil., *49*:28–30, 1968.

196. Lehmann, J.F., et al.: Comparative study of the efficiency of short-wave, microwave, and ultrasonic diathermy in heating the hip joint. Arch. Phys. Med. Rehabil., *40*:510–512, 1959.

197. Stoner, E.K.: Luminous and infrared heating. In Therapeutic Heat. Edited by S. Licht. New Haven, CT, Waverly Press, 1958.

198. Gersten. J.W.: Effect of metallic objects on temperature rises produced in tissue by ultrasound. Am. J. Phys. Med., *37*:75–82, 1958.

199. Lehmann, J.F., et al.: Ultrasonic effects as demonstrated in live pigs with surgical metal implants. Arch. Phys. Med. Rehabil., *40*:483–488, 1959.

200. Skoubo-Kristensen, E., and Sommer, J.: Ultrasound influence on internal fixation with a rigid plate in dogs. Arch. Phys. Med. Rehabil., *63*:371–373, 1982.

201. Ferris, B.G., Jr.: Environmental hazards: electromagnetic radiation. N. Engl. J. Med., *275*:1100–1105, 1966.

202. Scott, B.O.: Shortwave diathermy. In Therapeutic Heat and

Cold. 2nd Ed. Edited by S. Licht. New Haven, CT, Waverly Press, 1965.

203. Mikulic, M.A., Griffith, E.R., and Jebsen, R.H.: Clinical applications of standardized mobility tests. Arch. Phys. Med. Rehabil., 57:143–146, 1976.

204. Clark, G.R., et al.: Evaluation of physiotherapy in the treatment of osteoarthrosis of the knee. Rheumatol. Rehabil., 13:190–197, 1974.

205. Feibel, A., and Fast, A.: Deep heating of joints: A reconsideration. Arch. Phys. Med. Rehabil., 57:513–514, 1976.

206. Quillen, W.S.: Phonophoresis: A review of the literature and techniques. Athletic Training, 109–110, Summer 1980.

207. Antich, T.J.: Phonophoresis: The principles of the ultrasonic driving force and efficacy in treatment of common orthopaedic diagnoses. J. Orthop. Sports Phys. Ther., 4:99–102, 1982.

208. Mennell, J.J.: Back Pain: Diagnosis and Treatment Using Manipulative Techniques. Boston, Little, Brown, 1960.

209. Kirk, J.A., and Kersely, G.D.: Heat and cold in the physical treatment of rheumatoid arthritis of the knee. Ann. Phys. Med., 9:270–274, 1968.

210. Miglietta, O.: Electromyographic characteristics of clonus and the influence of cold. Arch. Phys. Med. Rehabil., 45:508–512, 1964.

211. Pegg, S.M.H., Litter, T.R., and Littler, E.N.: A trial of ice therapy and exercise in chronic arthritis. Physiotherapy, 55:51–56, 1969.

212. Horvath, S.M., and Hollander, J.L.: Intra-articular temperature as measures of joint reaction. J. Clin. Invest., 26:469–473, 1949.

213. Schmidt, K.L., et al.: Heat, cold and inflammation. J. Rheumatol., 38:391–404, 1979.

214. Wong, K.C.: Physiology and pharmacology of hypothermia. West. J. Med., 138:227–232, 1983.

215. DeJong, R., Hershey, W., and Wagman, I.: Nerve and conduction velocity during hypothermia in man. Anesthesiology, 27:805–810, 1966.

216. Grant, A.E.: Massage with ice (cryokinetics) in the treatment of painful conditions of the musculoskeletal system. Arch. Phys. Med. Rehabil., 45:233–238, 1964.

217. McMaster, W.G., Liddle, S., and Waugh, T.R.: Lab evaluation of various cold therapy modalities. Am. J. Sports Med., 6:291–294, 1978.

218. Travell, J.: Ethyl chloride spray for painful muscle spasm. Arch. Phys. Med. Rehabil., 33:291–298, 1952.

219. Gacker, T.: Heat and cold in orthopedics. In Therapeutic Heat and Cold. Edited by S. Licht. New Haven, CT, E. Licht, 1965.

220. Landen, R.R.: Heat or cold for relief of low back pain? Phys. Ther., 47:1126–1128, 1967.

221. Swezey, R.L.: The modern thrust of manipulation and traction therapy. Semin. Arthritis Rheum., 12:322–331, 1983.

222. Lawhon, S.M., and Crawford, A.H.: Traction in the treatment of spinal deformity. Orthopedics, 6:447–458, 1983.

223. Cailliet, R.: Neck and Arm Pain. 2nd Ed. Philadelphia, F.A. Davis, 1981.

224. Worden, R.E., and Humphey, T.L.: Effect of spinal traction on the length of the body. Arch. Phys. Rehabil., 45:318–320, 1964.

225. British Association of Physical Medicine: Pain in the neck and arm: A multicenter trial of the effects of physiotherapy. Br. Med. J., 1:253–258, 1966.

226. Caldwell, J.W., and Krusen, E.M.: Effectiveness of cervical traction in treatment of neck problems: Evaluation of various methods. Arch. Phys. Med. Rehabil., 43:214–221, 1962.

227. Puri, K., and Honet, J.C.: Cervical radiculitis: Methods and results of treatment in 82 patients. (Abstract.) Arch. Phys. Med. Rehabil., 55:585, 1974.

228. Valtown, E.J., and Kiuro, E.: Cervical traction as a therapeutic tool. Scand. J. Rehabil. Med., 2:29–36, 1970.

229. Shore, N.A.: Iatrogenic temporomandibular joint difficulty: Cervical traction may be the etiology. J. Prosthet. Dent., 41:541–542, 1979.

230. Medical Letter Staff: Traction for neck and low back disorders. Med. Lett. Drug. Ther., 17:16, 1975.

231. Judovich, B.D.: Herniated cervical disc: A new form of traction. Am. J. Surg., 84:645–656, 1952.

232. Colachis, S.C., and Strohm, B.R.: A study of tractive forces and angle of pull on vertebral interspaces in the cervical spine. Arch. Phys. Med. Rehabil., 46:820–830, 1965.

233. Farfan, A.F.: Mechanical Disorders of the Low Back. Philadelphia, Lea & Febiger, 1973.

234. Waylonis, G.W., et al.: Home cervical traction: Evaluation of alternative equipment. Arch. Phys. Med. Rehabil., 63:388–391, 1982.

235. Lehmann, J.F., and Brunner, G.D.: A device for the application of heavy lumbar traction: its mechanical effects. Arch. Phys. Med. Rehabil., 39:696–700, 1958.

236. Judovich, B.D., and Nobel, G.R.: Traction therapy, a study of resistance forces. Am. J. Surg., 93:108–114, 1957.

237. Lidsbrom, A., and Zachrisson, M.: Physical therapy on low back pain and sciatica. Scand. J. Rehabil. Med., 2:37–43, 1970.

238. Grahame, R.: Clinical trials in low back pain. Clin. Rheum. Dis., 6:143–157, 1980.

239. Chrisman, O.D., Mittnacht, A., and Snook, G.A.: A study of the results following rotary manipulation in the lumbar intervertebral disc syndrome. J. Bone Joint Surg., 46A:517–524, 1964.

240. Gianakopoulos, G., et al.: Inversion devices: their role in producing lumbar distraction. Arch. Phys. Med. Rehabil., 66:100–102, 1985.

241. Licht, S.: Massage, Manipulation and Traction. New Haven, Elizabeth Licht, 1980.

242. Maigne, R.: Orthopedic Medicine. Springfield, IL, Charles C Thomas, 1972.

243. Krueger, B.R., and Okazaki, H.: Basilar infarction following chiropractic cervical manipulation. Mayo Clin. Proc., 55:322–332, 1980.

244. Miller, R.G., and Burton, R.: Stroke following chiropractic manipulation of the spine. JAMA, 229:189–190, 1974.

245. Robertson, J.T.: Neck manipulation as a cause of stroke. Editorial. Stroke, 10:1, 1981.

246. Cyriax, J.: Textbook of Orthopedic Medicine. London, Harper & Ross, 1965.

247. Sims-Williams, H., et al.: Controlled trial of mobilization and manipulation for back pain: Hospital patients. Br. Med. J., 2:1318–1320, 1979.

248. Aoral, D.M.L., and Navell, D.J.: Manipulation in the treatment of low back pain: A multicenter study. Br. Med. J., 2:161–164, 1975.

249. Hoehler, F.K., Tobis, J.S., and Buerger, A.A.: Spinal manipulation for low back pain. JAMA, 245:1835–1838, 1981.

250. Stiles, E.G.: Safe useful manipulative techniques. Patient Care, 18:137–189, 1984.

251. Goodridge, J.P.: Muscle energy technique: Definition, explanation, methods of procedure. J. Am. Osteopath. Assoc., 81:67–72, 1981.

252. Simons, D.G.: Muscle pain syndromes—Part 2. Am. J. Phys. Med., 55:15–42, 1976.

253. Simons, D.G.: Muscle pain syndromes—Part 1. Am. J. Phys. Med., *54*:289–311, 1975.

254. Travell, J.: Myofascial trigger points: Clinical view. *In* Advances in Pain Research Therapy. Vol. I. Edited by J.J. Bonieg and D. Albe-Fessurd. New York, Raven Press, 1976.

255. Travell, J., and Simons, D.G.: Myofascial Pain and Dysfunction: The Trigger Point Manual. Baltimore, Williams & Williams, 1983.

256. Brooks, R.G., et al.: Costs of managing patients at a Canadian rheumatic disease unit. J. Rheumatol., *8*:937–948, 1981.

257. Pace, J.B., and Nagle, D.: Piriform syndrome. West. J. Med., *124*:435–439, 1976.

258. Wolfe, F., and Cathey, M.A.: The epidemiology of tender points: A prospective study of 1520 patients. J. Rheumatol., *12*:1164–1168, 1985.

259. Smythe, H.: Tender points: Evolution of concepts of the fibrositis/fibromyalgia syndrome. Am. J. Med., *81*:(3A):2–6, 1986.

260. Ferderber, M.B.: Long-term illness: Management of the chronically ill patient. Pa. Med. J., *63*:390–394, 1960.

261. Laging, B.: Furniture design for the elderly. Rehabil. Lit., *27*:130–140, 1966.

262. Lowman, E.W., and Klinger, J.L.: Aids to Independent Living: Self-Help for the Handicapped. New York, McGraw-Hill, 1969.

263. May, E.E., Waggoner, N.R., and Hotte, E.B.: Independent Living for the Handicapped and the Elderly. Boston, Houghton Mifflin, 1974.

264. Gibson, T., and Grahame, R.: Rehabilitation of the elderly arthritic patient. Clin. Rheum. Dis., *7*:485–496, 1981.

265. Haworth, R.J., and Nichols, P.J.R.: Hoists in the home: Their recommendation and use. Rheumatol. Rehabil., *19*:42–51, 1980.

266. Rehabilitative Nursing Techniques—1: Bed Positioning and Transfer Procedures for the Hemiplegic. Minneapolis, Kenny Rehabilitation Institute, 1964.

267. Travell, J.: Ladies and gentleman be seated—properly. House Beautiful, *July*:159, 1961.

268. Corcoran, P.J.: Energy expenditure during ambulation. *In* Physiological Basis in Rehabilitation Medicine. Edited by J.A. Downey and R.C. Darling. Philadelphia, W.B. Saunders, 1971.

269. Dimonte, P.C., and Light, H.: Patho-mechanics, gait deviations and treatment of the rheumatoid foot. Phys. Ther., *62*:1148–1156, 1982.

270. Frankel, V.H., and Burstein, A.H.: Orthopedic Biomechanics. Philadelphia, Lea & Febiger, 1970.

271. Inman, V.T., Ralston, H.J., and Todd, F.: Human Walking. Baltimore, Williams & Wilkins, 1980.

272. Ralston, H.J.: Energy-speed relation and optimal speed during level walking. Int. Z. Agnew Physiol., *17*:177–183, 1958.

273. Marshall, R.N., Myers, D.B., and Palmer, D.G.: Disturbance of gait due to rheumatoid disease. J. Rheumatol., *7*:617–623, 1980.

274. Saunders, J.B., Inman, V.T., and Eberhart, H.D.: The major determinants in normal and pathologic gait. J. Bone Joint Surg., *35A*:543–558, 1953.

275. Bossingham, D.H.: Wheelchairs and appliances. Clin. Rheum. Dis., *7*:395–415, 1981.

276. Klinger, J.L.: Self Help Manual for Patients with Arthritis. Arthritis Foundation, Arthritis Health Professions Section, 1980.

277. Downis, E., et al.: A comparison of efficiency of three types of crutches using oxygen consumption. Rheumatol. Rehabil., *19*:252–255, 1982.

278. Haworth, R.J., Dunscombe, S., and Nichols, P.J.R.: Mobile arm supports: An evaluation. Rheumatol. Rehabil., *17*:240–244, 1978.

279. Sankarankutty, S.M., and Rose, G.K.: A comparison of axillary, elbow and Canadian crutches. Rheumatol. Rehabil., *17*:237–239, 1978.

280. Sorenson, L., and Ulrich, P.G.: Ambulation Manual for Nurses. Minneapolis, American Rehabilitation Foundation, 1966.

281. Bossingham, D.H., and Russell, P.: The usefulness of powered wheelchairs in advanced inflammatory polyarthritis. Rheumatol. Rehabil., *19*:131–135, 1980.

282. Nichols, P.J.R., Ennis, J.A., and Norman, P.A.: Wheelchair users shoulder? Scand. J. Med. Rehabil., *11*:29–34, 1979.

283. Warren, C.G., et al.: Reducing back displacement in the powered reclining wheelchair. Arch. Phys. Med. Rehabil., *63*:447–449, 1982.

284. Buchanan, J.M., and Symons, J.: Housing and the environment for people with arthritis. Clin. Rheum. Dis., *7*:417–436, 1981.

285. Chamberlain, M.A., Buchanan, J.M., and Hanks, H.: The arthritic in the urban environment. Ann. Rheum. Dis., *38*:51–56, 1979.

286. Francis, R.A.: The development of federal accessibility law. J. Rehabil., *49*:29–33, 1983.

287. Fligg, H., and Wright, V.: The community and hospital nurse in relation to arthritis. Clin. Rheum. Dis., *7*:321–336, 1981.

288. Bennett, R.L.: Orthotic devices to prevent deformities of the hand in rheumatoid arthritis. Arthritis Rheum., *8*:1006–1018, 1965.

289. Chamberlain, M.A.: Occupational therapy. Clin. Rheum. Dis., *7*:365–376, 1981.

290. Melvin, J.L.: Rheumatic Disease: Occupational Therapy and Rehabilitation. 2nd Ed. Philadelphia, F.A. Davis, 1982.

291. Nicholas, J.H., et al.: Splinting in rheumatoid arthritis: I. Factors affecting patient compliance. Arch. Phys. Med. Rehabil., *63*:92–94, 1982.

292. Chamberlain, M.A., Thornely, G., and Wright, V.: Evaluation of bathing and toilet aids. Rheumatol. Rehabil., *17*:187–194, 1978.

293. Cordery, J.C.: Joint protection: A responsibility of the occupational therapist. Am. J. Occup. Ther., *19*:285–294, 1965.

294. Munton, J.S., et al.: An investigation into the problems of easy chairs used by the arthritic and the elderly. Rheumatol. Rehabil., *20*:164–173, 1981.

295. Tsuyuguchi, Y., Tada, K., and Kawaii, H.: Splint therapy for trigger finger in children. Arch. Phys. Med. Rehabil., *65*:75–76, 1983.

295a. Fisher, S.V., et al.: Cervical orthosis effect on cervical spine motion: Roentenographic and goniometric method of study. Arch. Phys. Med. Rehabil., *58*:109–115, 1977.

296. Hartman, J.T., Palumbo, R., and Hill, B.J.: Cineradiography of the braced normal cervical spine. A comparative study of five commonly used cervical orthoses. J. Bone Joint Surg., *59A*:332–339, 1979.

297. Althoff, B., and Goldie, I.F.: Cervical collars in rheumatoid atlanto-axial subluxations: A radiographic comparison. Ann. Rheum. Dis., *39*:485–489, 1980.

298. Hancock, D.O.: The cervical spine in rheumatoid arthritis. Clin. Rheum. Dis., *4*:443–459, 1978.

299. Smith, P.H., Sharp, J., and Kellgren, J.A.: Natural history of

rheumatoid cervical subluxations. Ann. Rheum. Dis., *31*:222–223, 1972.

300. Million, R., et al.: Evaluation of low back pain and assessment of lumbar corsets with and without back supports. Ann. Rheum. Dis., *40*:449–454, 1981.

301. Norton, P.L., and Brown, T.: The immobilizing efficiency of back braces. J. Bone. Joint. Surg., *39A*:111–139, 1957.

302. Grew, N.D.: Intra-abdominal pressure responds to loads applied to the torso in normal subjects. Spine, *5*:149–154, 1980.

303. Perry, J.: The use of external support in the treatment of low-back pain. J. Bone Joint. Surg., *43*:327–351, 1961.

304. Malick, M.H.: Manual on Static Hand Splinting. Vol. I. Pittsburgh, Harmarville Rehabilitation Center, 1972.

305. Rothstein, J.M.: Use of splints in conservative management of acutely inflamed joints in rheumatoid arthritis. Arch. Phys. Med. Rehabil., *46*:198–199, 1965.

306. Cassvan, A., Wonder, K.E., and Fultonberg, D.M.: Orthotic management of the unstable knee. Arch. Phys. Med. Rehabil., *58*:487–491, 1977.

307. Deaver, G.G.: Lower limb bracing. *In* Orthotics Etcetera. Edited by L. Licht and H. Kamenetz. New Haven, CT, Waverly Press, 1966.

308. Cracchiolo, A., III: The use of shoes to treat foot disorders. Orthoped. Rev., *8*:73–83, 1979.

309. Davis, J., and Janecki, C.J.: Rehabilitation of the rheumatoid upper limb. Orthop. Clin. North Am., *9*:559–568, 1978.

310. McKnight, P.T., and Schomburg, F.L.: Air pressure splint effects on hand symptoms of patients with rheumatoid arthritis. Arch. Phys. Med. Rehabil., *63*:560–564, 1982.

311. Gumpel, J.M., and Cannon, S.: A cross-over comparison of ready-made fabric wrist-splints in rheumatoid arthritis. Rheumatol. Rehabil., *20*:113–115, 1981.

312. Houston, M.E., and Goemans, P.H.: Leg muscle performance of athletes with and without knee support braces. Arch. Phys. Med. Rehabil., *63*:431–432, 1982.

313. Convery, F.R., Conaty, J.P., and Nickel, V.L.: Dynamic splinting of rheumatoid arthritis. Orthot. Prosthet., *21*:249–254, 1967.

314. Gault, S.J., and Spyker, J.M.: Beneficial effects of immobilization of joints in rheumatoid and related arthritis: A splint study using sequential analysis. Arthritis Rheum., *12*:34–44, 1969.

315. Rhinelander, F.W.: The effectiveness of splinting and bracing in rheumatoid arthritis. Arthritis Rheum., *2*:270–277, 1959.

316. Baum, J.: A review of the psychological aspects of rheumatic diseases. Semin. Arthritis Rheum., *11*:352–361, 1982.

317. Greengross, W.: Sex and arthritis. Rheumatol. Rehabil., *16*:(Suppl.):68–70, 1979.

318. Hamiliton, A.: Sexual problems of the disabled. *In* Rehabilitation Medicine. 2nd Ed. Edited by P.J.R. Nichols. Baltimore, Waverly Press, 1980.

319. Yoshimo, S., and Uchida, S.: Sexual problems of women with rheumatoid arthritis. Arch. Phys. Med. Rehabil., *62*:122–123, 1981.

320. Florian, V.: Sex counseling: Comparison of attitudes of disabled and nondisabled subjects. Arch. Phys. Med. Rehabil., *64*:81–84, 1983.

321. Bernardo, M.D.: Premarital counseling and the couple with disabilities: A review and recommendations. Rehabil. Lit., *42*:213–217, 1981.

322. Asrael, W.: An approach to motherhood for disabled women. Rehabil. Lit., *43*:214–218, 1982.

323. Bucks, F.M., and Hohmann, G.W.: Child adjustment as related to severity of paternal disability. Arch. Phys. Med. Rehabil., *63*:249–253, 1982.

324. Vignos, P.J., Jr., et al.: Comprehensive care and psychosocial factors in rehabilitation in chronic rheumatoid arthritis: A controlled study. J. Chronic Dis., *4*:457–467, 1972.

325. Rogers, M.P., Liang, M.H., and Partridge, A.J.: Psychological care of adults with rheumatoid arthritis. Ann. Intern. Med., *96*:344–348, 1982.

326. Vershys, H.P.: Physical rehabilitation and family dynamics. Rehabil. Lit., *41*:58–65, 1980.

327. Zola, I.K.: Social and cultural disincentives to independent living. Arch. Phys. Med. Rehabil., *63*:394–397, 1982.

328. Kaplan, S., and Kozin, F.: A controlled study of group counseling in rheumatoid arthritis. J. Rheumatol., *8*:91–99, 1981.

329. Andrews, M.C.G., and Woodford, W.F.S.: The voluntary organizations. *In* Rehabilitation in the Rheumatic Diseases. Edited by D. Woolf. Philadelphia, W.B. Saunders, 1981.

330. Swanson, D.W., et al.: Program for managing chronic pain. Mayo Clin. Proc., *51*:401–408, 1976.

331. Harsanyi, S.L.: Toward equal opportunities in recreation for the disabled. Arch. Phys. Med. Rehabil., *56*:135–137, 1975.

CORRECTION OF ARTHRITIC DEFORMITIES OF THE HAND

ADRIAN E. FLATT

Surgical procedures are an important part of the rehabilitation of the arthritic patient. The hand surgeon has a role in the team approach to the total care of the patient. Retention of function at a satisfactory level is the goal of therapy. The rate of progress and severity of disease vary, and the hand surgeon must define in each patient the type of deformity and the rate of its progression, to plan maintenance of a functional hand. Prevention of deformity is the key. The earlier the patient is seen in the disease process, the easier it is to follow the rate of functional deterioration and to intervene effectively.

Surgical treatment includes the use of various forms of dynamic splinting, hand therapy, and strategically timed operative intervention. Restoration of function in a severely debilitated hand is usually more difficult and is less successful than a preventive surgical procedure early in the disease. Appearance is only a secondary consideration. A cosmetically acceptable hand is not necessarily functional.

Arthritic hand deformity follows a spectrum of disease, with rheumatoid arthritis (RA) at one end and osteoarthritis at the other. In between are a variety of conditions such as gout, psoriatic arthritis, scleroderma, mixed connective tissue disease, and hemochromatosis. Each has its own pattern of involvement. In this chapter, I concentrate on the two main entities, RA and osteoarthritis, with only a brief discussion of the others.

RHEUMATOID DISEASE

Within the hand and wrist, the tissue primarily affected is synovium.[1] Only later are articular cartilage and subchondral bone destroyed by pannus. The intra-articular swelling of the synovium stretches and weakens the joint capsule and ligaments. This interference with joint integrity allows an imbalance of forces to occur over the joint and can eventually produce grotesque deformities.

In the upper limb, almost all operations can be performed under axillary block anesthesia. It is routine for these patients to be ambulatory the day after the operation, and now many procedures are done on outpatients. Operations on the wrist or hand are performed with a pneumatic tourniquet applied to the arm. The combination of local axillary anesthetic block and tourniquet control of bleeding produces no significant shock. Glucocorticoid therapy is not a contraindication to surgical treatment and does not produce any adverse general effects on the patients or delay local wound healing. Preoperatively, corticosteroids are reduced to the minimum maintenance dose. Once this dosage has been established, I make no effort to increase it as a precaution against the slight operative and postoperative stress in operations on the upper limb. The usual dosage is continued throughout the operative and postoperative periods. In a personal series of many hundreds of upper limb operations, I have followed this routine with excellent results.

Operative treatment can be of value to the wrist and hand, in three distinct phases of the disease. It is used (1) prophylactically, to prevent further destruction of joint surfaces when drug therapy is unable to control synovitis; (2) late in the disease, to salvage function from grossly involved tendons and joints; and (3) in the stage of adaptation (middle phase) of disease, in which it can be of value but is not as common as in the other two phases.

Operations can restore potential range of motion and can relieve pain, but it is fruitless to operate in the face of apathy, self-pity, or the general aura of despair so frequently associated with rheumatoid disease. Surgeons share a common responsibility with physicians in other disciplines to treat the disease, and the patient, as a whole. The patient must want the operation. To try to "sell" a patient an operation is a disservice, and it is my policy to try to introduce potential candidates to others who have had the proposed operation. A short, private discussion between the two patients usually answers all potential questions rapidly and allows a decision to be made without external pressures.

NONOPERATIVE TREATMENTS

The classic treatments of rest, splinting, judicious exercise, and corticosteroid injections are of value throughout the course of the disease, and their use should not be restricted to early management.[2] Inflamed, painful, swollen joints benefit from rest, but as the inflammation subsides, exercise must be introduced to prevent joint stiffness and to maintain muscle strength. Short intermittent periods of exercise are far more beneficial than prolonged vigorous workouts that can aggravate synovitis. Local intrasynovial injection of corticosteroids can diminish inflammation in joints and tendons; however, persistent use of long-acting corticosteroids in the same areas leads to local tissue reactions that can cause arthropathies and tendon ruptures. I believe that this form of treatment can become counterproductive, and I agree with others that three injections in 1 year at the same site should be the absolute maximum.[2]

Splinting is of limited value in the care of rheumatoid disease of the hands. Three major types of splints are available: passive immobilization, remedial, and assistive splints.[3] Passive immobilization splints provide rest during the acute phase of disease, remedial splints can help to overcome contractures, and assistive splints help to compensate for joint distortions and muscle weakness.

Effective splinting of the hand is an art. Much harm can be done by ill-designed or ill-fitting splints. Stiffness of the hand is inevitable if an ill-designed splint forces the fingers into a nonfunctional position, or if they are held for long periods in positions that strain the joint capsules. There is virtue in simplicity. Most ingeniously designed complex apparatus lie neglected in closets because the demands on the patient's tolerance were too great. Wide, padded Velcro straps to fasten the splints are for superior to bandages or leather, buckled straps.

WRIST

The wrist is a key joint in so many functions of the hand that its impairment influences function to a far greater degree than by merely limiting motion of the joint itself. Three joints combine to produce wrist motion: the distal radioulnar joint, the intercarpal area, and the radiocarpal joint. Rheumatoid disease frequently attacks the distal radioulnar joint, and because the joint shares a common synovial cavity with the radiocarpal joint, both are frequently involved in synovitis.

Splinting

During an acute phase of arthritis, continuous passive immobilization may be necessary. As soon as symptoms begin to subside, intermittent, properly controlled muscle-building exercises are added. Many materials are now available for making splints, none completely superior to any other. A gutter-type flexor-surface splint should be made with the wrist in a maximum of 20° of extension, with the fingers in their normal functional arches and the palm and thumb abducted at least 20°.[3] Pressure is usually more evenly distributed throughout the forearm when the splint is held in place by a bandage wrap instead of by individual straps.

Remedial splinting is infinitely more satisfactory than manipulation of contractures within the hand. The gradual pull of dynamic traction creates a gentle, persistent force to which contracted tissue yields; manipulation frequently tears tissues and causes bleeding and adhesion formation. The disorders that respond best to remedial splinting are adduction contractures of the thumb, flexion contractures of the digital joints, and stiffness of the interphalangeal joints.

Assistive and prophylactic splinting techniques are still occasionally used in the treatment of varying degrees of ulnar drift. Most patients cannot tolerate the indefinite use of these splints, and in most, hand surgeons prefer to correct the internal dynamic imbalance surgically rather than impose an external corrective framework on the hand. Dynamic splinting is of great value after such reconstructive operations, particularly when it is combined with the replacement of destroyed metacarpophalangeal joints.

Surgical Treatment

As the synovial disease progresses, it destroys the ligaments supporting the radioulnar articulation and allows dorsal dislocation of the ulna in relation to the distal end of the radius. This dislocation not only restricts pronation and supination, but also creates a hazard for the long extrinsic extensor tendons. These tendons become tightly stretched against the radial side of the distal end of the ulna. Whenever the fingers are moved, the tendons rub against any irregular surfaces of the bone, and attrition ruptures may occur.

Excision of the spurs on the distal end of the ulna removes an actual or potential hazard to the tendons. Excision of the distal ulna itself also increases the range of pronation and supination. *Care must be taken in advising this operation.* It is best performed when no signs of disease or instability of the radiocarpal joint are present. If extensive destruction of the joint has occurred, the distal end of the ulna may be a useful prop in stabilizing the wrist; its excision may so tip the balance that the wrist may be completely dislocated. The excision of bone must be conservative and should maintain the capsular attachments and the ulnar collateral ligament of the wrist joint. Silastic replacements for excision of the distal ulna are available but are used less commonly than previously. If the supporting soft-tissue structures in the area are not properly reconstituted, instability and dislocation will occur.

After the operation, therapy is directed more toward restoration of pronation and supination than to restoration of wrist motion in flexion and extension. Some discomfort can be expected at the elbow as increasing movement develops around the head of the radius, but it should not be allowed to stop treatment.

In early disease of the radiocarpal joint, the radioscaphoid-lunate ligament, or Testut's ligament, serves as a conduit for synovial invasion of the radius. Gradual dissolution of the carpal insertion of the ligament leads to the classic Terry Thomas sign* of scapholunate dissociation (Fig. 50–1).

Subsequent laxity of the intercarpal joints or the radiocarpal joint from synovial disease can often be stabilized, and pain can be diminished, by the use of a molded leather wristlet held in place by Velcro strapping. Cock-up splints made of plastic, metal, or plaster are also useful in immobilizing the wrist and in restoring some degree of function.

Tenosynovitis and Tenosynovectomy

Tenosynovitis on both palmar and dorsal surfaces of the wrist is common and, if neglected, can lead to

---

*Mr. Terry Thomas, a British comedian with upper central dental diastema. See Clin. Orthop., 129:321–322, 1977.

tendon rupture. Early synovitis may be treated by splinting of the wrist, injection of corticosteroid, and general medical management. Tenosynovectomy is the proper treatment for patients who do not respond rapidly to conservative measures. The operation is effective and has a low morbidity rate. Synovectomy of the flexor compartment effectively decompresses the median nerve and allows a surgical toilet of any spurs on the carpal bones on the floor of the canal. Rupture of the flexor pollicis longus and of the flexors of the index finger is caused by spurs arising on the palmar aspect of the scaphoid bone.[4]

Extensor tendons rupture following infiltrative and nodular disease or as a result of attrition rupture on bony spurs at Lister's tubercle or the distal ulna. Commonly, the small finger loses extensor function first, followed by the ring and then the long fingers (Fig. 50–2). The extensor pollicis longus tendon also frequently ruptures. Eventually, even wrist extensor tendons can rupture and may allow a marked flexion deformity of the wrist to develop.

Persistent dorsal synovitis or a single tendon rupture associated with synovitis should be considered an absolute indication for tenosynovectomy. During surgical exploration, any bony spurs are removed, and any intratendinous nodules are excised. Such excision may leave a ragged-looking tendon, but followup has shown that the area repairs well and tendon function is maintained. When one or two tendon ruptures have occurred, side-to-side junction or the transfer of the extensor indicis tendon is the usual treatment. Multiple ruptures need more complicated repairs, often involving the transfer of a flexor digitorum superficialis tendon through the interosseous membrane onto the dorsum of the hand. Some have criticized such tendon repairs by implying that the ability to make a fist after such an operation is restricted. If the procedure is properly done, however, the results are excellent (Fig. 50–2).

Early movement is the treatment of choice after synovectomy of flexor or extensor tendons. The patient should be encouraged to begin moving the wrist and fingers 24 hours after the operation, and a full range should be possible when the sutures are removed 12 to 14 days later.

Synovectomy of the true wrist joint is usually performed at the same time as tenosynovectomy of the extensor tendons. The operation usually increases the stability and motion of the joint and secondarily increases digital function by relieving wrist pain. Technically, it is difficult to effect complete clearance of the wrist joint synovium from the dorsal approach, and occasionally, the floor of the carpal tunnel has to be opened as well. I have not been impressed by the

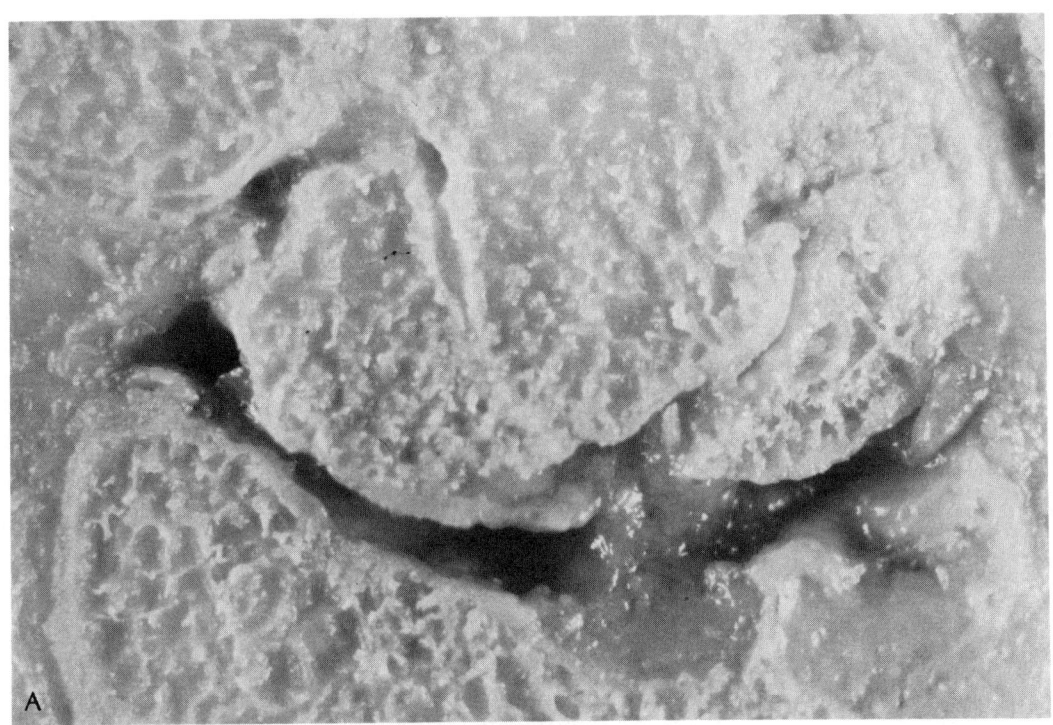

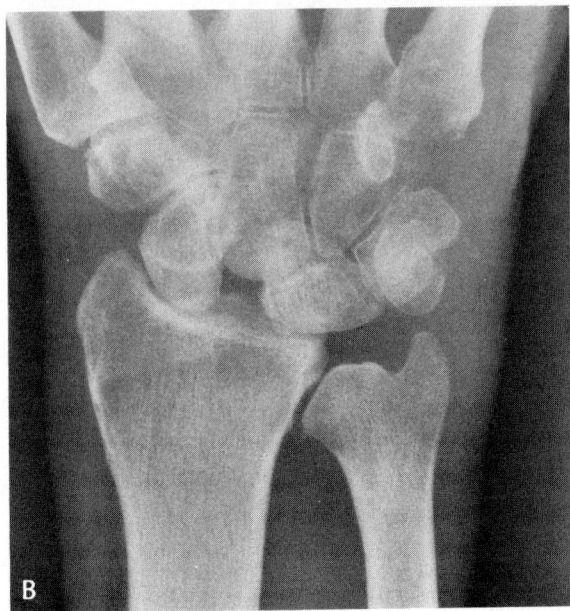

FIG. 50–1. Testut's ligament and the Terry Thomas sign. *A,* Coronal section of a rheumatoid wrist. The radius shows cavitation of its articular surface at the site of origin of Testut's ligament. The scaphoid and lunate bones are separate. *B,* The Terry Thomas sign of scapholunate dissociation. Because the lunate bone is dorsiflexed, it is superimposed on the capitate bone. (From Flatt, A.E.[3])

FIG. 50–2. Multiple tendon rupture. *A,* State of disease over the dorsum of the wrist. The proximal end of the extensor tendon to the ring finger lies on the scalpel blade, and the forceps hold the diseased synovium over the distal end of the ulna. *B,* In the repair, the extensor carpi ulnaris is used as an independent extensor for the small finger, and the intact long finger tendon is used to form a Y junction with the distal end of the ring finger tendon.

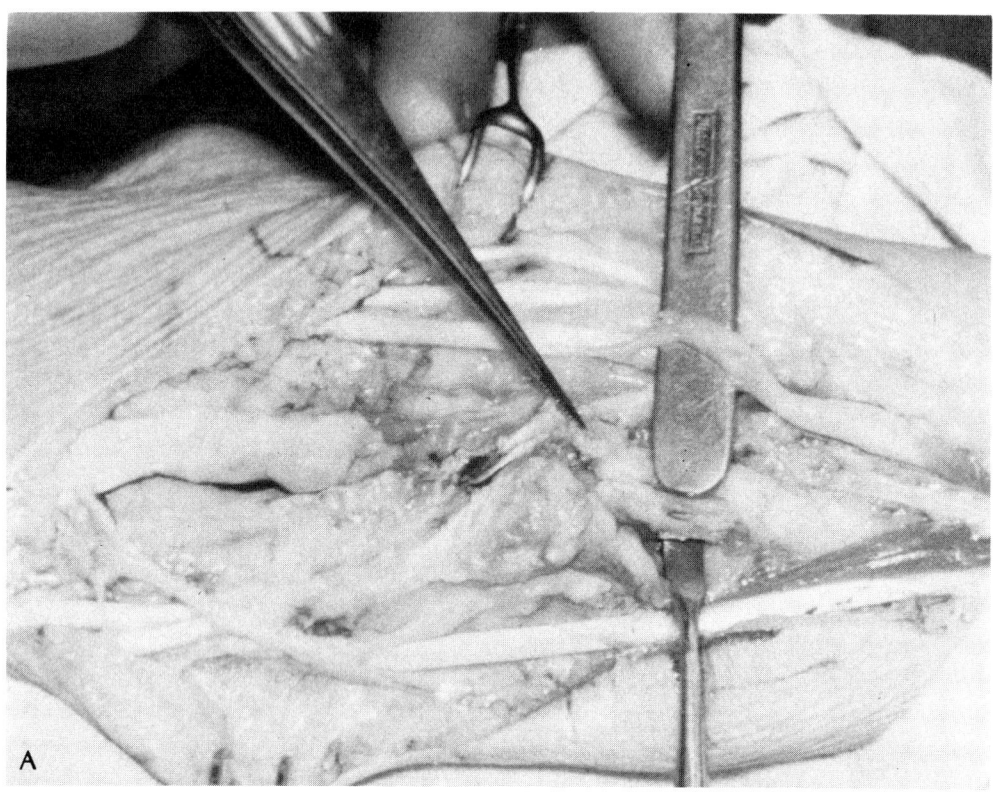

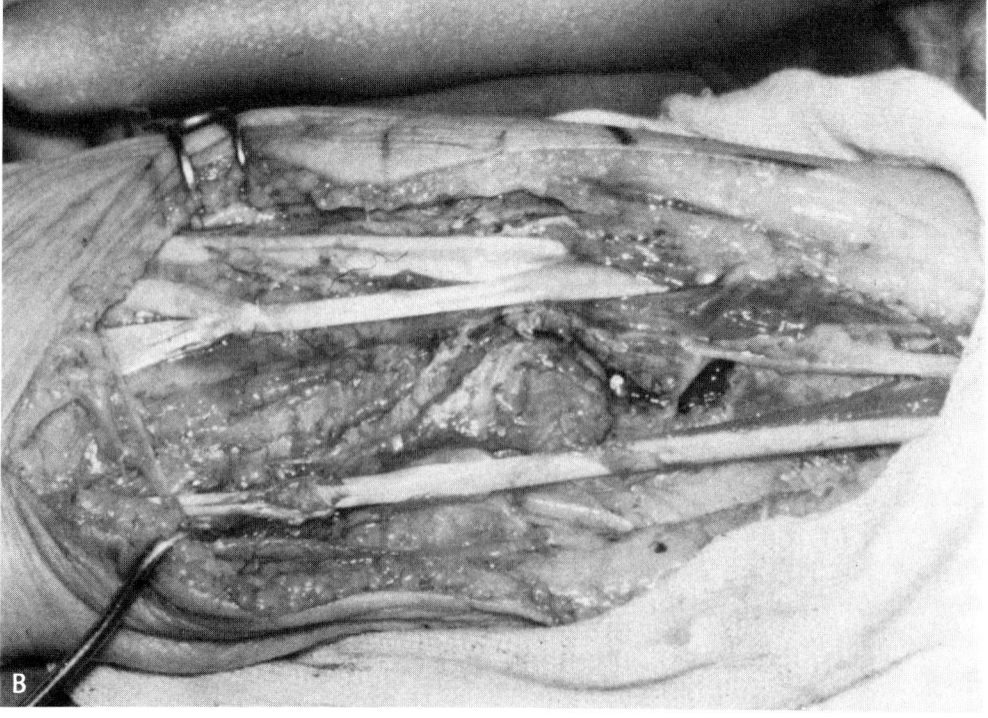

FIG. 50–2 *(Cont'd).* *C* and *D*, Two months postoperatively, a slight extensor lag exists, but the patient is able to made a good fist. (From Flatt, A.E.[3])

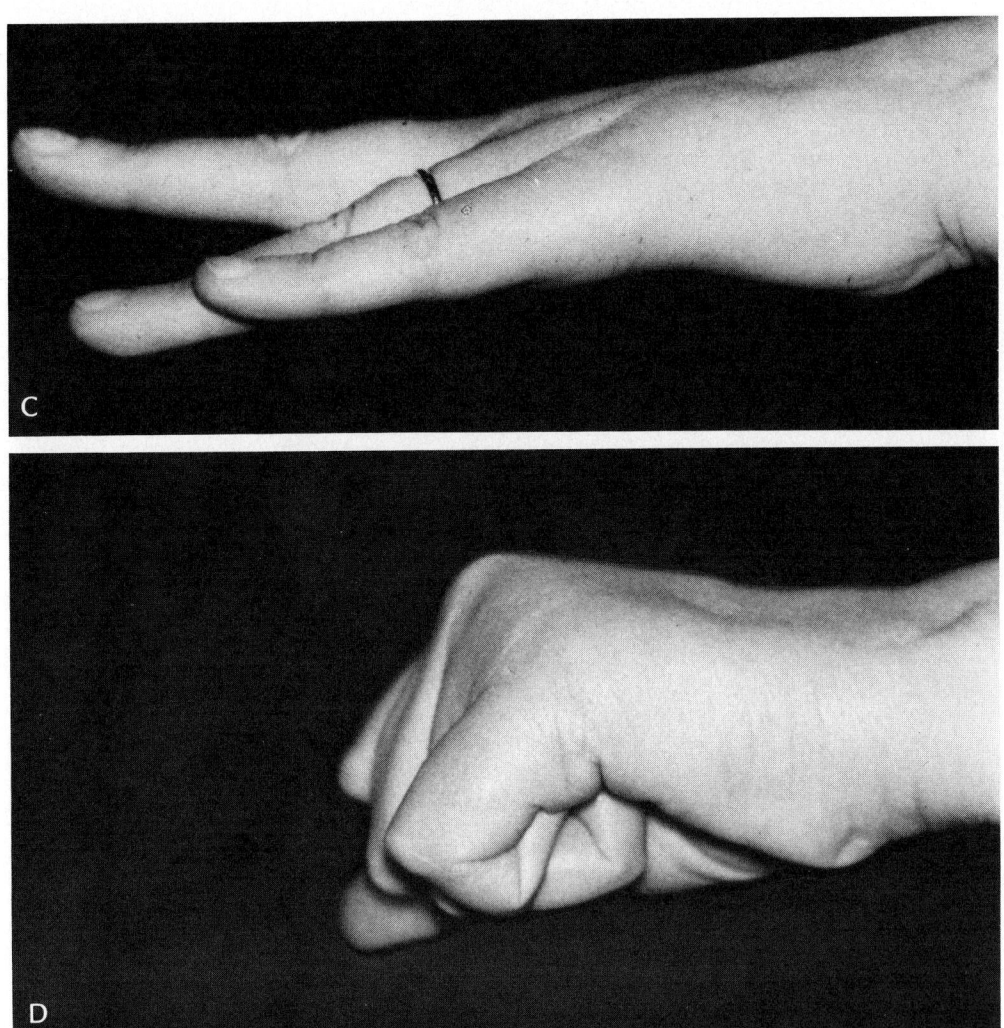

results of my attempts, or those of others, to perform intercarpal synovectomies. Theoretically, it is an admirable procedure; in practice, it is destructive and at best palliative.

Arthroplasty and Fusion

Painful or unstable wrists can be treated by arthroplasty or fusion. Retention of motion with stability is always desirable and has prompted the production of a variety of total wrist prostheses. The early results seemed encouraging, but reported problems of balancing tendon power are significant. If the device has too much mobility, the hand will assume an "end" position, usually dorsoradial or palmoulnar (Fig. 50–3). Currently, the results of total wrist replacement

are not predictable, and no device is as generally suitable as, say, the total hip. A Silastic spacer is available, but it is not a true joint substitute. No matter what device is used, most of the proximal carpal row is removed together with the end of the radius.

The reported complication rates in total wrist replacement are significant. Failure most frequently results either from an inability to balance the forces in the 22 tendons crossing the wrist or from varying forms of mechanical failure in the device used. These problems have led to restrictions in their use and greater employment of fusion of the joint.[5–7] Comparative studies[7a] of fusion and silicone implant arthroplasty show that patients with fusions have stronger wrists but decreased dexterity. Some

FIG. 50–3. *A* and *B*, Total wrist arthroplasty. Any unconstrained total wrist substitute must have its axes correctly placed to obtain a proper balance among the 22 extrinsic tendons crossing the wrist. This patient's wrist is locked into an end position. (From Flatt, A.E.[3])

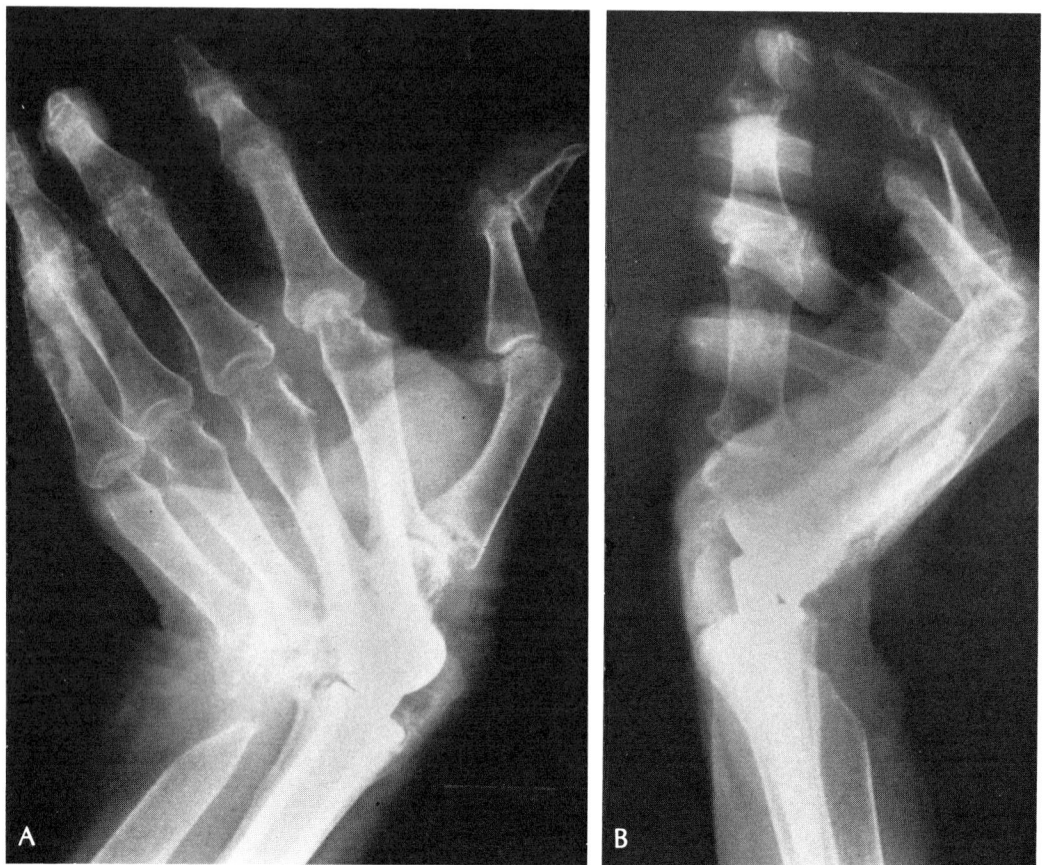

studies[7b] show complication rates up to 25% for silicone arthroplasties, but patients with arthroplasties had improved dexterity and adequate wrist strength (Fig. 50–4). In the 25% group, the chronic use of steroids, the use of ambulatory aids, and a preoperatively dislocated wrist were the main factors associated with failure.

Fusion of the wrist still has its place in the treatment of rheumatoid and degenerative disease when the patient's pain is crippling, when the wrist has stiffened in a nonfunctional position, or when the joint is completely unstable. The position of fusion is of vital importance in the planes of ulnoradial deviation and in flexion and extension. Radial inclination of metacarpal bones induces ulnar deviation of the fingers.[8] To perpetuate this zigzag deformity by fusing the wrist in radial deviation dooms any metacarpophalangeal reconstruction for ulnar drift to failure (Fig. 50–5). The third metacarpal bone must

be parallel to the long line of the radius if this deformity is to be avoided.[9]

In flexion and extension, the so-called functional position usually recommended is about 30° of extension. This position is that of the wrist in an otherwise normal limb. The limb of a patient with RA is usually far from normal, however, and the flexion deformity of the wrist occurs in part because this is the functional position for many of the most vital uses of the hand. During feeding or dressing, the wrists are almost always flexed, and perineal toilet is impossible with the wrists held in the so-called functional position.

The wrist should be fused in a neutral position and, on some occasions, in slight flexion (Fig. 50–6). The patient is usually in a below-elbow cast for about 3 months; during this time, finger movement exercises should be practiced constantly. Once the fusion is solid, exercises are done to improve pronation and

FIG. 50–4. *A,* Wrist implant resection arthroplasty. In this patient, an ulnar head replacement is judged necessary. Note the relative level of the end of the ulna, implant and the crossbar of the radial component. *B,* Wrist implant followup. These roentgenograms are taken 3 years after a wrist implant; an ulnar head replacement is not judged necessary. Fifty degrees of painless motion is possible. A trapezial implant has also been used. (From Flatt, A.E.[3])

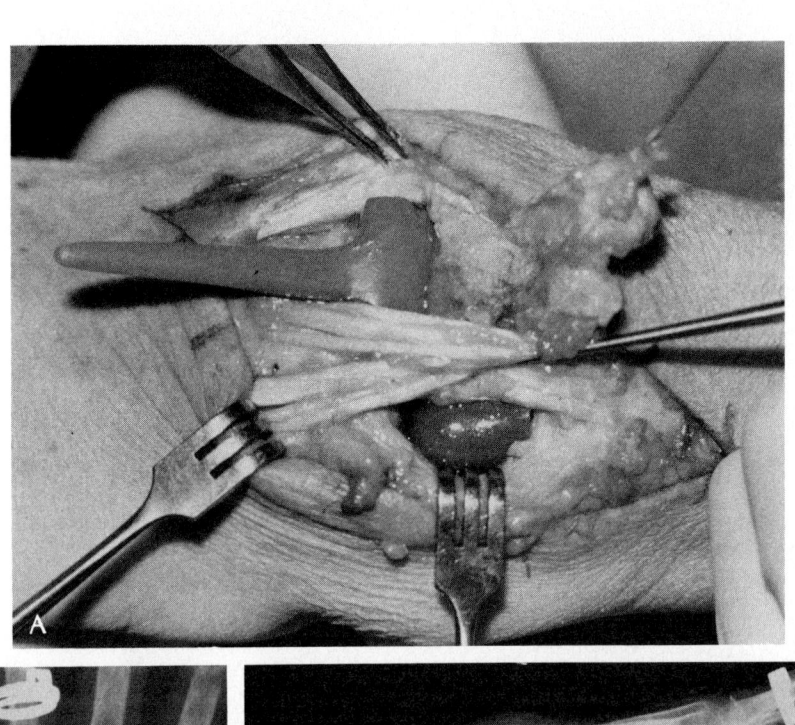

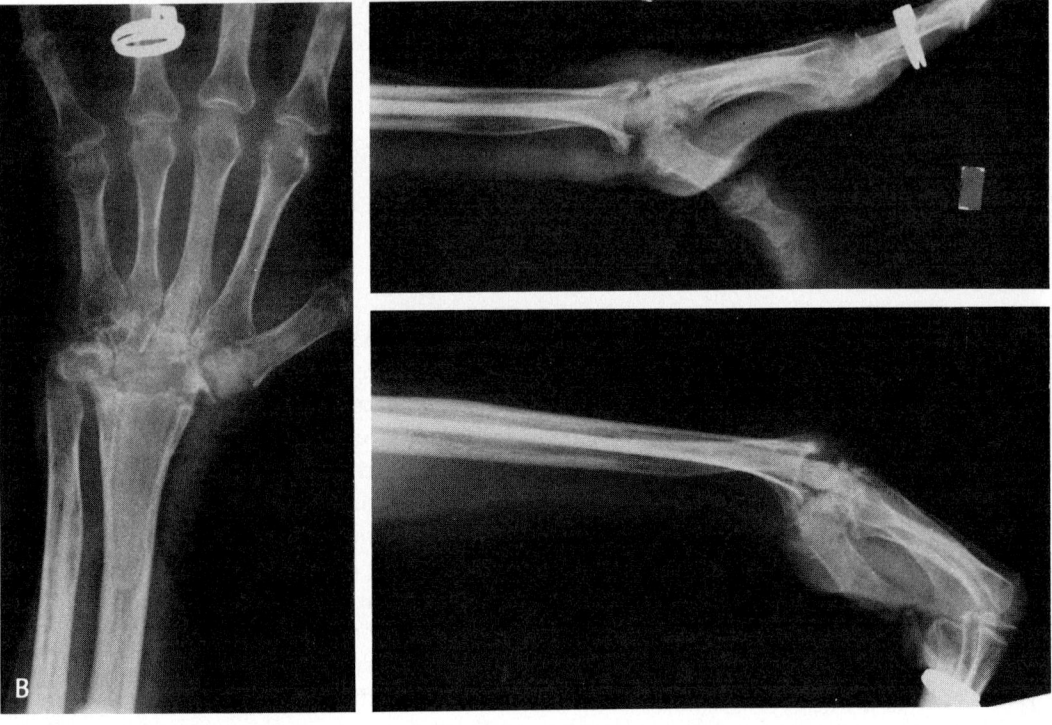

FIG. 50–5. The wrist and ulnar drift. *A*, With radial carpal collapse, the unbalanced tendon forces produce the zigzag deformity of ulnar drift. *B*, If the carpal disease is even, tendon equilibrium is not disturbed, and ulnar shift of the proximal phalangeal bases and drift of the fingers does not occur. (From Flatt, A.E.[3])

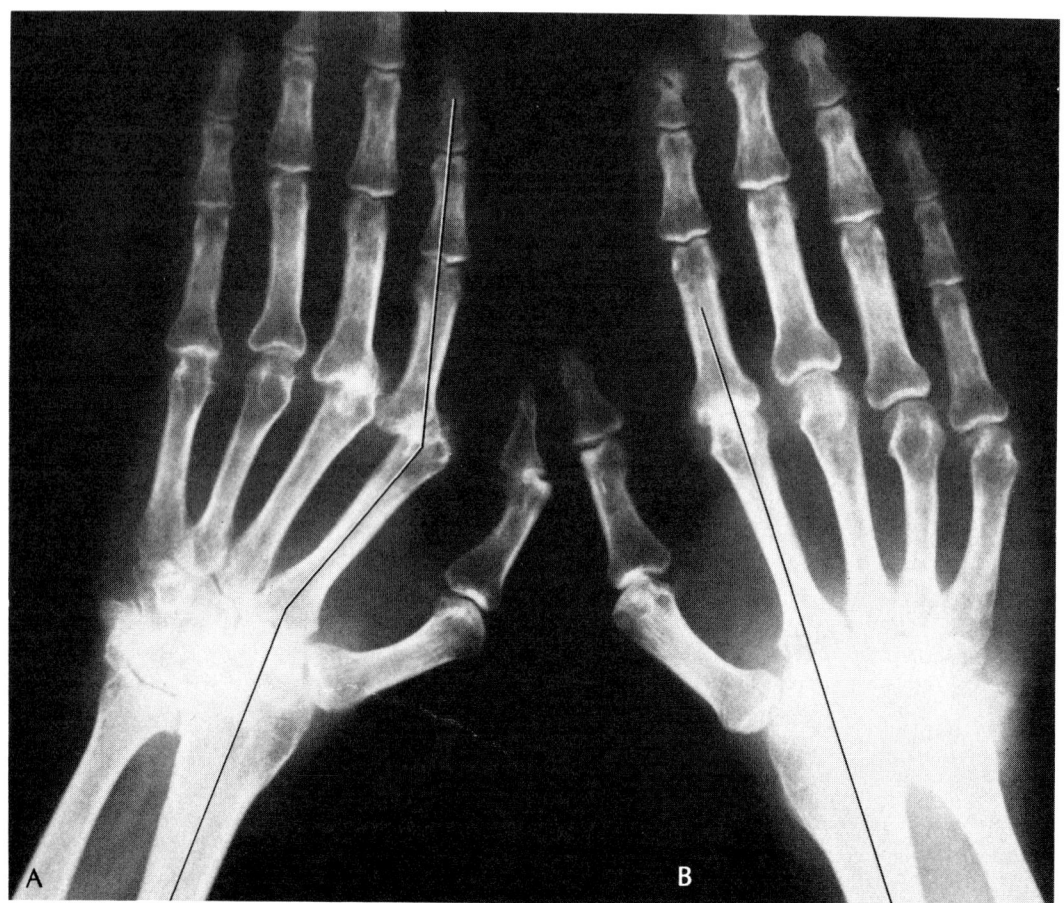

supination and the strength of grip. The fusion stabilizes the carpus on the radius and frequently adds power to the grip by allowing the extrinsic flexor and extensor tendons to act solely on the fingers, instead of wasting their power on an unstable wrist.[10]

DIGITS

Tenosynovitis within the palm and fingers causes pain, swelling, stiffness, and occasional "triggering." Surgical synovectomy yields good results, but in early disease, injection of corticosteroids into the tendon sheath can be helpful. Synovectomy within the flexor sheath is not difficult and is performed by a palmar approach (Fig. 50–7). Preservation and reconstruction of the pulleys retaining the flexor tendons against the

phalanges are vital. When doing this operation the surgeon must pull on each tendon separately to ensure that adhesions between the two flexor tendons will not restrict motion.

Localized nodular disease of the tendon may produce a "trigger" finger. Because nodules can occur on the flexor tendons from the level of the distal palmar crease to the middle of the proximal phalanx, *it is necessary to palpate the area with three fingers* (Fig. 50–8). To use the customary single finger over the entrance to the digital sheath would miss a nodule triggering in the decussation of the flexor digitorum superficialis tendon. In the thumb, the common level is the flexor crease over the metacarpophalangeal joint. Surgical treatment is frequently indicated, but a preliminary trial injection of a corticosteroid suspension intrasynovially is justified.

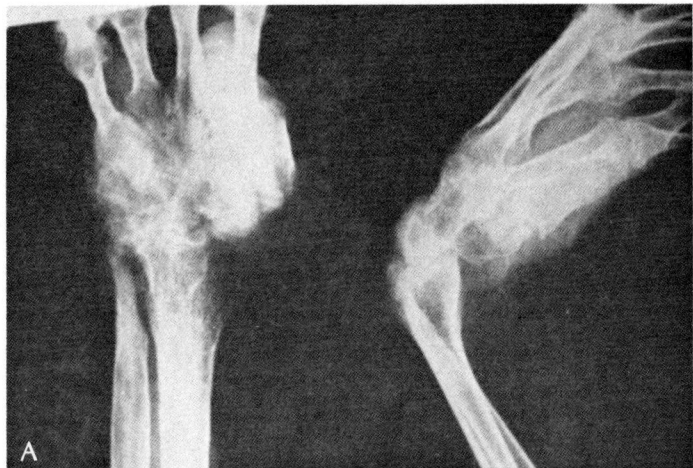

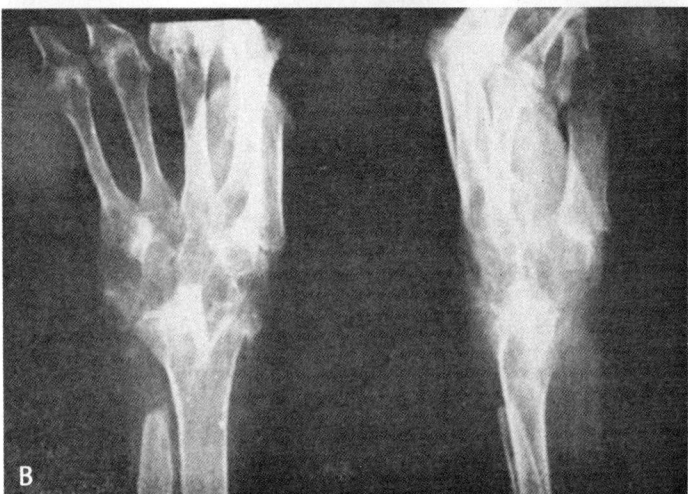

FIG. 50-6. Wrist fusion. Stabilization of the wrist is a valuable procedure, but the angle of fusion should be chosen with great care. It is not advisable to fuse the wrist in dorsiflexion because of the limitation in function imposed by such a position. *A*, Preoperative malposition in palmar flexion. *B*, Postoperative fusion in neutral position, allowing improved function of the hand. (From Flatt, A.E.[3])

The operation is usually done through a small incision with the patient under local anesthesia. The flexor tendon sheath is incised longitudinally for a sufficient length to allow free travel to the tendons. The patient can use the hand immediately after the operation.

Rheumatoid involvement of the extensor mechanism of the fingers produces two common types of deformity, both secondary to synovial disease. The normal restraints of joint motion and intrinsic muscle balance are destroyed, thereby causing deformity. In boutonnière (buttonhole) deformity, the central extensor mechanism over the proximal interphalangeal joint is eroded, and the lateral bands fall to the palmar side of the axis of the joint, with a subsequent loss of ability to extend the joint. Swan neck deformity results from the dorsal bowstringing of tight lateral bands, caused either by synovial attrition of the palmar plate or intrinsic muscle tendon contracture.

Intrinsic Muscle Disease

In the early stages of rheumatoid involvement of the intrinsic muscles, the average patient is not likely to notice any functional disturbance. Clinical detection of early disease is easy, however, using the intrinsic tightness test (Fig. 50–9). The test for this condition is conducted in two stages. In the first stage, passive flexion is applied to all three digital joints. If flexion is possible, it establishes that motion is not restricted by pathologic conditions of the extrinsic extensor tendon or the digital joints. In the second stage of the test, the intrinsic muscles are tensed by pushing the metacarpophalangeal joint into full extension and then by applying dorsal pressure to the tip of the finger, in an attempt to produce passive flexion. In the normal hand, passive flexion is still possible in this position. If rheumatoid disease is affecting the intrinsic muscles, the degree of resistance to passive

FIG. 50–7. Digital flexor tendon synovectomy. *A,* In the palm, the synovitis often bulges out as a palpable lump. *B,* The finger should be approached through a zigzag Bruner incision, which allows wide exposure. The index finger at the bottom of this illustration has been cleared of synovitis. The long finger shows the bulging synovitis prior to removal. (From Flatt, A.E.[3])

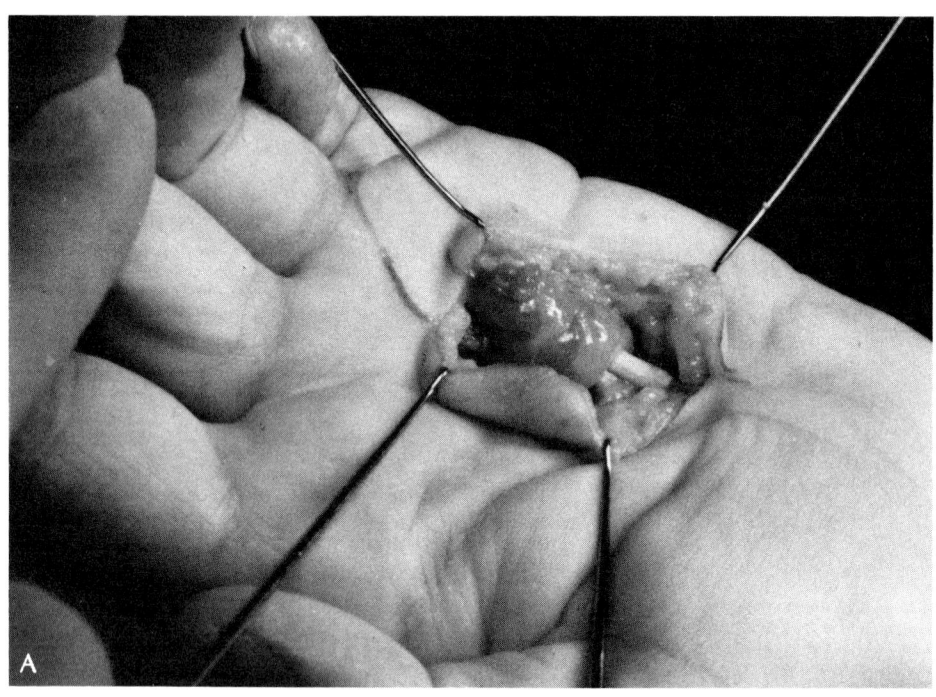

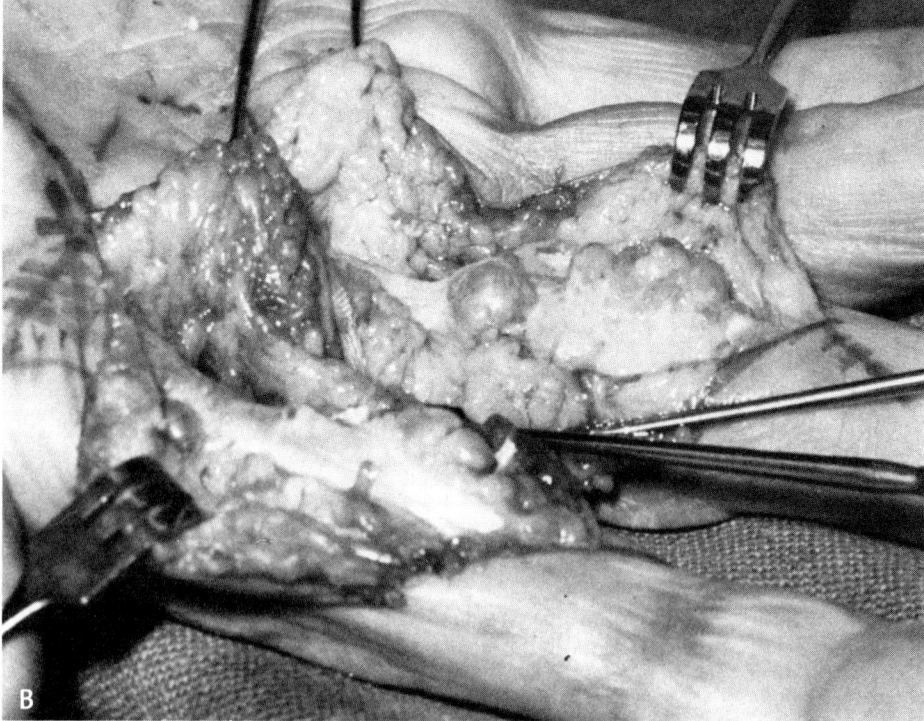

FIG. 50–8. Flexor tendon nodular disease. When a finger is "triggering," three fingers must be used to palpate a sufficient length of tendon to identify whether the nodule lies in the palm or in the area of the shaft of the proximal phalanx where the superficialis tendon decussates. (From Flatt, A.E.[3])

FIG. 50–9. Test for swan neck deformity. *A*, First stage of the test applies passive flexion to all three digital joints to exclude pathologic conditions of the extrinsic extensor tendon or the digital joints. *B*, Second stage of the test tenses the intrinsic muscles by holding the metacarpophalangeal joint in full extension and applying dorsal pressure to the tip of the finger. In patients with rheumatoid disease, the degree of resistance to passive flexion is directly proportional to the severity of the disease. (From Flatt, A.E.[3])

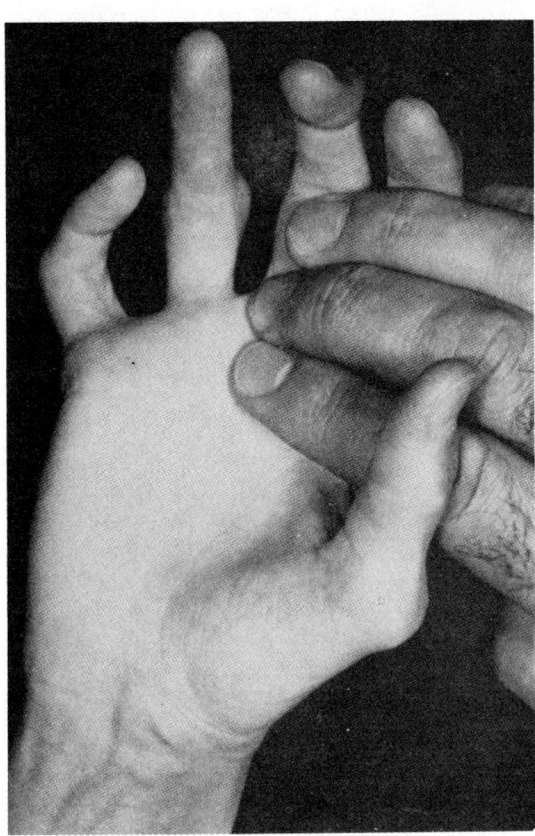

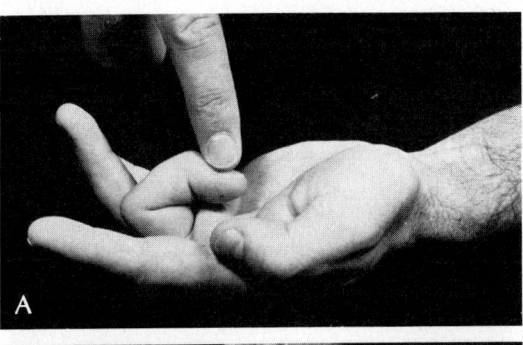

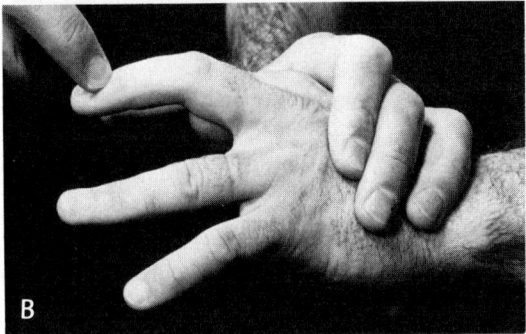

flexion is directly proportional to the severity of the disease.

This test is simple and yields valuable information and should be routine in the examination of all patients with RA. Demonstration of the differential tightness of the ulnar intrinsic muscles, as opposed to the radial intrinsic muscles, can be done by fixing the metacarpophalangeal joint in extension and passively flexing the finger with the digit first in radial deviation and then in ulnar deviation. Tightness present in radial deviation implicates the ulnar intrinsic muscles and vice versa.

The excess tension in the intrinsic muscles can be relieved by the Littler release operation. The triangular hood is excised from either side of the finger, and the pull of the intrinsic muscles on the central extensor tendon is thereby abolished. After the operation, great care must be taken to prevent the proximal interphalangeal joints from returning to their previous, hyperextended condition. Many weeks of active flexion exercises are usually needed to obtain

maximum improvement. The muscles of the thumb are subject to the same disturbance, and the metacarpophalangeal joint is held in flexion, with the interphalangeal joint in hyperextension. A similar operation at the level of its metacarpophalangeal joint improves function.

In early ulnar drift, the intrinsic muscle tightness is used to correct digital deviation by *crossed intrinsic transfer.* The tighter ulnar intrinsic muscles are released and transferred to the radial side of the next adjacent ulnar digit (Fig. 50–10). This operation of crossed intrinsic muscle transfer transforms a dynamic deforming factor into a corrective force.

Synovectomy

Synovectomy of the digital joints is a valuable operation. It is designed to relieve symptoms and to delay subsequent destruction of articular surfaces. The operation is performed most frequently at the metacarpophalangeal joints, often at the proximal interphalangeal joints, and only rarely at the distal in-

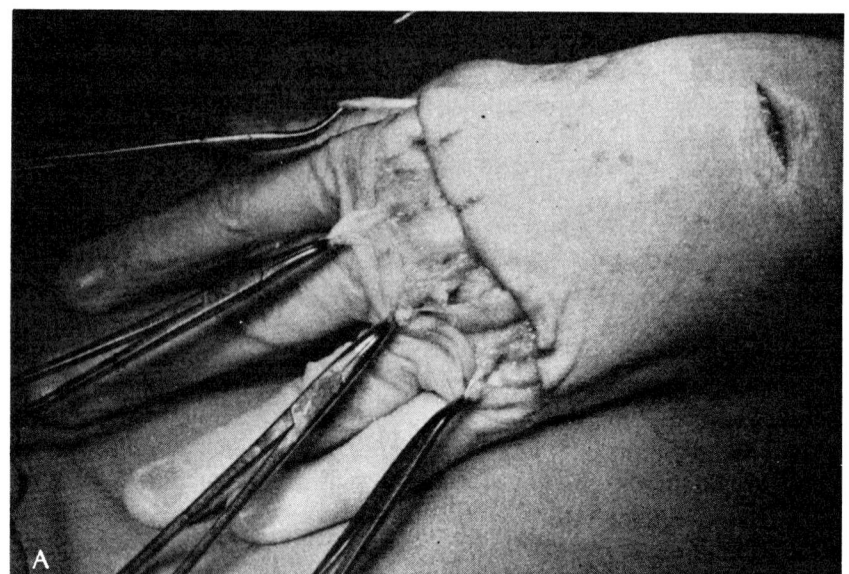

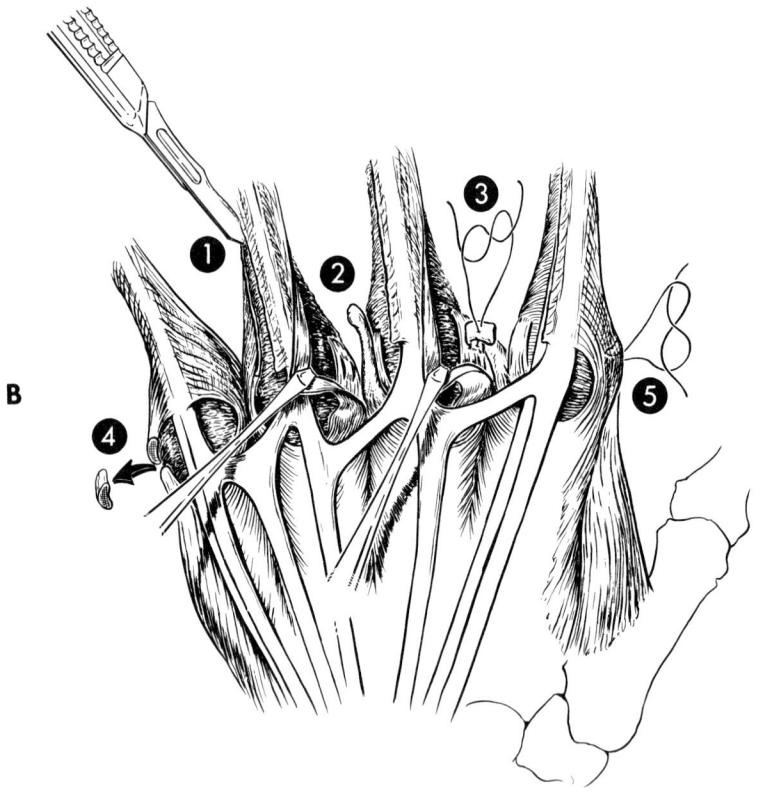

FIG. 50–10. Crossed intrinsic transfer. *A,* The detached wing of the interosseous tendon must be dissected back proximally enough to allow free excursion. Three hemostats are on the freed-up ulnar intrinsic tendons; at the top of the figure, the extensor indicis tendon is shown in a hemostat for those who wish to continue to use this transfer. *B,* Crossed intrinsic transfer. *1,* Release of the ulnar intrinsic tendon. *2,* Its mobilization to the musculotendinous junction and the slit in the radial collateral ligament of the adjacent finger through which the transfer should be passed. *3,* The sewing in of the transfer. *4,* Abductor digiti minimi release. *5,* Repositioning of the first dorsal interosseous tendon. (From Flatt, A.E.[3])

terphalangeal joints. The operation is properly indicated in the patient whose metacarpophalangeal joints continue to develop recurrent synovitis despite medical treatment and occasional corticosteroid injections. At the proximal interphalangeal joint, the need for synovectomy is more urgent because boutonnière deformity caused by the expanding synovium is difficult to treat, even in its early stages.[3]

Precise, long-term followup studies of surgical synovectomy are profoundly lacking. This gap in our knowledge is responsible for the greatest controversy in the care of the rheumatoid hand. Some workers challenge the use of the term "prophylactic" when applied to early synovectomy, and others counter that they have yet to see a sufficient number of patients early enough to test a prophylactic procedure adequately. I have no doubt that the operation gives symptomatic relief, but I believe that only in the earliest disease can one prevent irreversible joint changes. My own followup studies[11] and others in the literature[12,13] show a significant percentage of "recurrence" of rheumatoid synovitis, with higher rates in those patients suffering from more severe disease. In general, the results are more rewarding at the proximal interphalangeal joint, particularly if the operation is done early in the disease.

The operation is performed through an incision directly over the joint, and the synovium is removed when the tendons on the dorsum of the joint have been retracted laterally. The technical problem is to remove all the synovium of the joint; it is particularly important to remove completely the tongue of synovium that lies between the collateral ligaments and the neck of the proximal bone of the joint. This tongue is largely responsible for the detachment of the collateral ligament from the bone and for the destruction of the subchondral cortical bone.

Synovectomy of a digital joint is commonly combined with other procedures, but when the operation is performed by itself, the usual postoperative treatment is early active motion. Passive motion should be avoided, and the patient should be advised to exercise to the limits of discomfort. If true pain is produced, the exercise program must be reduced.

Arthroplasty

Restoration of function to digital joints destroyed by rheumatoid disease is usually provided by arthroplasty. Fusion of these joints is of value in extreme cases, but is not generally employed because it may impair necessary hand function. Arthroplasty or prosthetic replacement cannot be done unless the patient has adequate and balanced muscle control of flexion and extension of the involved joint. The extrinsic flexor muscles are frequently stronger than the extensor mechanism, and patients may need a preoperative period of strengthening exercises for the extensor muscles.

At the metacarpophalangeal joint, excisional arthroplasty is not rare because the motion and digital alignment supplied by prosthetic substitutes are superior to those provided by arthroplasty. Three generations of implants have been tried: the original metallic implants that I used in the 1950s, the silicone rubber devices introduced by Swanson[14] and Niebauer[8,15] in the 1960s, and more recently the third generation of "total" joints devised by a number of surgeons (Fig. 50–11). I no longer use the original metal implants and believe that the results achieved by the Swanson design are the standards against which other devices should be judged. I have used many of the third-generation joints and agree with Nalebuff that they are more difficult to insert, have many potential complications, and do not provide better motion or alignment than the Swanson design.[3]

The Swanson implants are not a true prosthesis, but rather are cruciform silicone rubber devices that keep the raw bone ends apart during the healing and scar encapsulation process. A properly performed operation with the correct postoperative therapy should relieve the pain, line up the digits, and provide an average of 60° of motion.

Complications such as infection, fracture of the implant, and recurrence of the ulnar drift do occur.[16] Infection is rare, and fracture probably occurs in about 5% of patients with implants. Such fractures are held together by the periarticular scarring, are usually asymptomatic, and are only detected radiographically. The ulnar drift may recur because of inadequate release of the shortened ulnar structures or inadequate repair on the radial sides. More frequently, it is caused by the uncorrected recurrence of the radial tilt of the carpometacarpal unit at the wrist joint (see Fig. 50–5).

Concern has recently been expressed regarding host tolerance and wear of silicone prosthetic implants in the wrist and digits. Reports of reactive synovitis, possibly associated with particulate silicone matter, have been reported in relation to implant substitutes for the scaphoid, lunate, trapezium, ulnar head, and wrist and finger joints.[17] The recent introduction of metal grommets around the stems may help prevent breakage in the digits and wrist. No true incidence for this problem has yet been established, and epidemiologic studies are needed to quantify the problem.

Normal motion at the proximal interphalangeal joints is over 100°, and its retention is of more func-

A

FIRST GENERATION

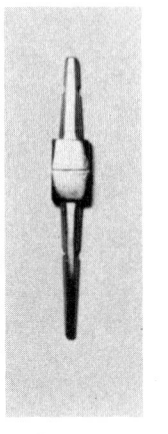

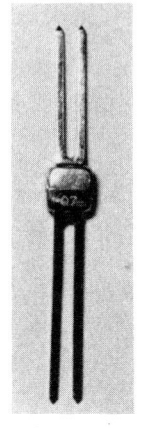

Brannon   Flatt

FIG. 50–11. The three generations of prostheses. *A,* The first generation were made of SS 316; *B,* the second of silicone rubber; and *C,* the third of a variety of metals and plastics. (From Flatt, A.E.[3])

B

SECOND GENERATION

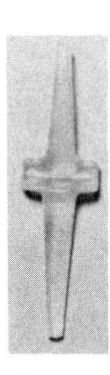

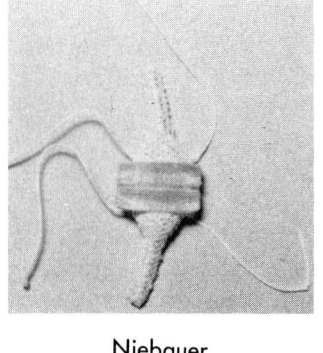

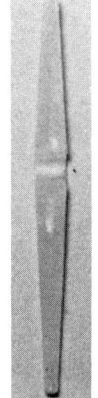

Niebauer

Swanson

Calnan

C

THIRD GENERATION

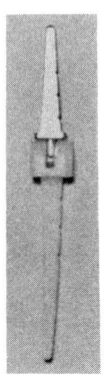

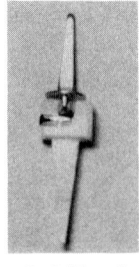

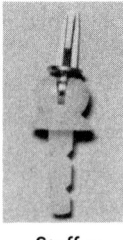

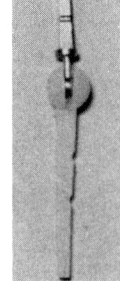

Strickland   Steffee

St. Georg-Buchholz

Schultz

tional importance in the ulnar two grasping digits than in the index and long fingers, which are used more in extension for precise activities. I am willing to fuse the index finger's proximal interphalangeal joint for stability in pinch, but I strive to maintain mobility in ring and small finger joints. Often, the choice is dictated by the state of the extensor mechanism. Long-standing synovial disease and flexion contractures impair the extensor mechanism to such a degree that extension against gravity is impossible. In such circumstances, fusion is necessary because it is useless to supply the motion provided by an implant if the balance between extensor and flexor power is absent.

At the distal interphalangeal joint, the preferred salvage operation is fusion in a neutral position or in about 5 to 10° flexion. I tend to use implants at this joint for osteoarthritis rather than in rheumatoid disease. The technical difficulties are significant, and I believe that fusion gives better and more predictable functional results.

Prosthetic replacement and other salvage procedures do not, and cannot, restore normal hand function. The greatest benefit from surgical treatment is seen in properly selected patients with early disease. Early synovectomy must still be considered a particularly valuable procedure, and its judicious use may eventually abolish the need for many current salvage procedures.

OSTEOARTHRITIS

In contrast to RA, osteoarthritis of the hand primarily involves joint cartilage and bone. Soft tissue constraints are generally normal. Involvement is usually proportional to the amount of abuse of the joints. Symptoms usually do not occur until the fifth decade and are precipitated commonly by a sprain or transmission of an unusual force through the joint. Once these symptoms occur, they are unlikely to disappear completely. The most important joint affected is the carpometacarpal joint of the thumb because the thumb carries a high proportion of the work load of the hand. In prehensile activities, the thumb is half the hand, and arthritis at its base interferes with all its functions. Conservative treatment, analgesics, and splinting are all helpful, but the symptoms are frequently so disabling that operation must be considered. Two operations are possible, fusion or arthroplasty. Neither operation is ideal; each has its advocates, and both require several months of treatment before postoperative recovery is complete.

In the younger patient (usually under age 40), fu-

sion is preferable because the small loss of mobility of the thumb is well compensated by painless stability. The operation consists of excision of the contiguous arthritic joint surfaces, impaction of the two raw bone ends, and their immobilization by a bone graft driven into both bones. Immobilization in a cast that includes the metacarpophalangeal joint of the thumb is necessary for 3 months after operation.

Arthroplasty is achieved by excision of the trapezium bone. The resulting space can be filled with local tissue such as an "anchovy" made of a strip of rolled up tendon. It can also be allowed to fill with scar, or a foreign substitute made of Silastic, metal, or high-density polyethylene can be used (see Fig. 50–4). Recent comparative studies between the "anchovy" technique and a Swanson Silastic replacement show no significant difference.[18,19] I have chosen to use the Neibauer device in which the silicone head is reinforced with Dacron and have had pleasing results over many years. No single replacement arthroplasty is superior to all others, and the best results probably are the result of superior surgical technique rather than choice of implant.

The middle and distal joints of the thumb may also become osteoarthritic, and either the metacarpophalangeal or the interphalangeal joint can be fused with little functional loss. In multiple joint disease, however, the problem is more difficult, and treatment must be individualized by the hand surgeon because multiple-joint fusions are detrimental to thumb function.

Osteoarthritis of the finger joints frequently follows trauma, usualy associated with extensive soft tissue damage (Fig. 50–12). The scarring produced by the soft tissue trauma is often of greater functional importance than the changes in the joint surfaces.

Distal joint involvement is common in osteoarthritis, and radiographs show narrowing of the joint space, subchondral sclerosis, and osteophyte formation. These osteophytes are recognized clinically as Heberden's nodes. Mucous cyst formation is commonly associated with these spurs. These cysts arise from the joint synovium beneath the dorsal skin between the joint and the eponychial fold. As the cyst increases in size, it presses on the area of the nail root and distorts the growing nail. Simple excision of the cyst is inadequate. The inciting osteophyte must also be removed (Fig. 50–13). Surgical intervention at the joint is justified in the presence of severe deformity, unrelenting pain, or instability. Cosmetic excision of Heberden's nodes is poor practice, but fusion a few degrees short of full extension is common. The condition must be distinguished from erosive osteoar-

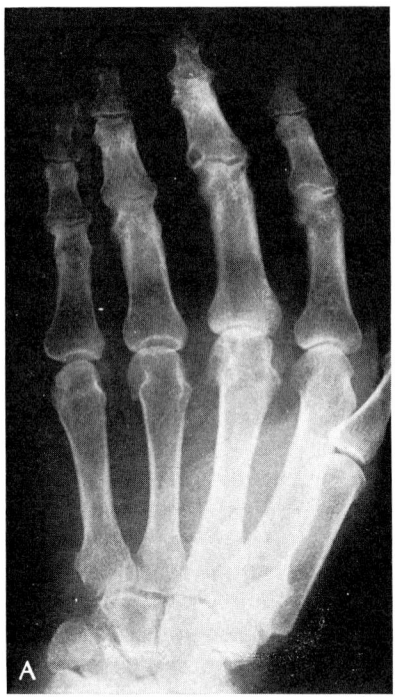
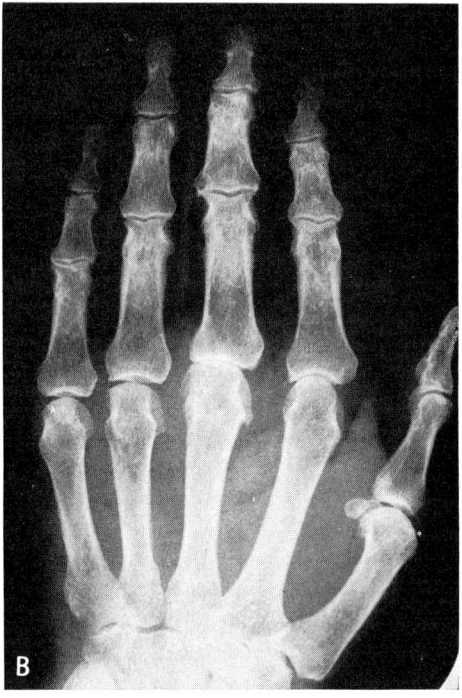

FIG. 50–12. *A* and *B*, Degenerative arthritis of fingers. This hand of a professional wrestler shows the results of repeated traumatic insults to the digital joints. (From Flatt, A.E.[3])

thritis, in which the greater degree of destruction renders the results of surgical treatment less satisfactory.

OTHER ARTHRITIC CONDITIONS

GOUTY ARTHRITIS

The synovial response to urate crystals is similar to that seen in rheumatoid disease of the small joints of the hand and wrist. The treatment for gouty arthritis is medical, and only rarely is operation indicated. I agree with Straub and co-workers in their view that indications for surgical intervention are few and are largely restricted to the excision of gouty tophi[20] (Fig. 50–14). Although increasing evidence suggests that these tophi recede with medical treatment, I believe that they should be excised if they present a mechanical block to joint motion. Draining sinuses and their causative tophi should be excised. Certainly, tophi causing nerve entrapment, as in the carpal tunnel syndrome, should be excised.

Occasionally, bony destruction or urate deposits are so massive that amputation of part or all of a finger may be required. Degenerative changes at the interphalangeal joint level may be great enough to warrant fusion in a functional position. No published reports exist of attempts at prosthetic replacement in gouty finger joints. Resorption of urate deposits, remodeling, and repair of damaged bones are often gratifying with proper medical treatment.

PSORIASIS

No definition of psoriatic arthritis is entirely satisfactory, and the true association of psoriasis and arthritis of the hand is difficult to establish. It is known that 5 to 10% of patients with rheumatoid disease have psoriasis. Moreover, radiologic changes typically seen in psoriatic arthritis precede skin lesions in 10% of patients who eventually develop psoriasis.

Clinically, excessive fibrous tissue is present around the joints, and the metacarpophalangeal joints of the hand are stiff and flexed. Severe overriding of the bones may occur, and the medullary canals of the metacarpal bones are small in diameter. The distal interphalangeal joints often stiffen in a useful position, but the proximal interphalangeal joints frequently develop boutonnière deformities. Synovial proliferation is less pronounced than in rheumatoid disease, but destruction of articular cartilage and subchondral bone does occur. Radiologically, psoriatic arthritis is characteristically asymmetric and often unilateral. It can also involve only the bones of a single digital ray. Malalignments of the digital joints are common, and subluxation occurs.

Surgical treatment of the psoriatic arthritic hand is frustrating because it is nearly impossible to provide long-term improvement of motion. Arthroplasties do not generally improve function, and fusion prevents further deformity at the expense of motion. The results of soft tissue operations and joint replacements are less satisfactory than in rheumatoid disease.

FIG. 50–13. Mucous cyst. *A,* The dorsal osteoarthritic spur frequently associated with a mucous cyst. *B,* Injection of methylene blue into the joint to fill the dorsal cyst or cysts. *C,* Dissection showing a large cyst and the presence of a small, hidden, and undiagnosed smaller cyst. (*A* and *C* Courtesy of Eugene Kilgore, II, M.D.: *B* From Flatt, A.E.[3])

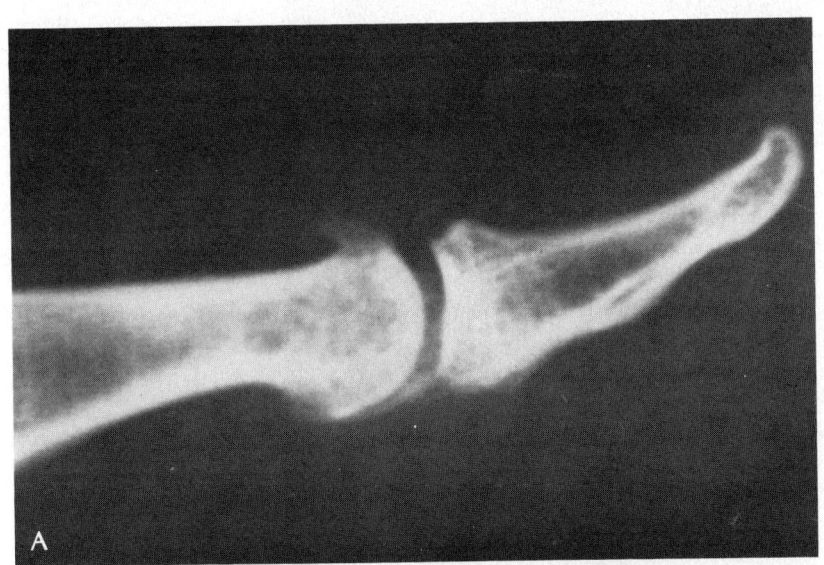

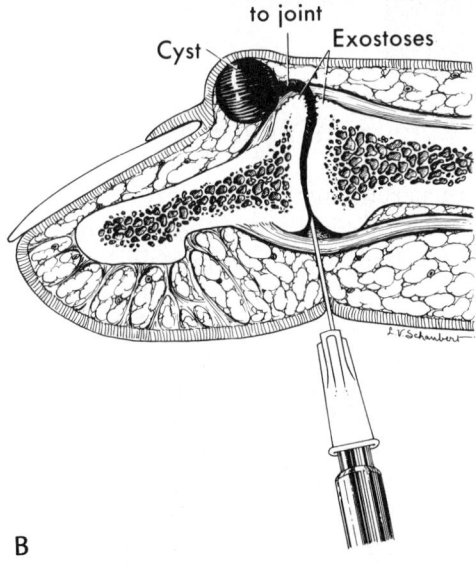

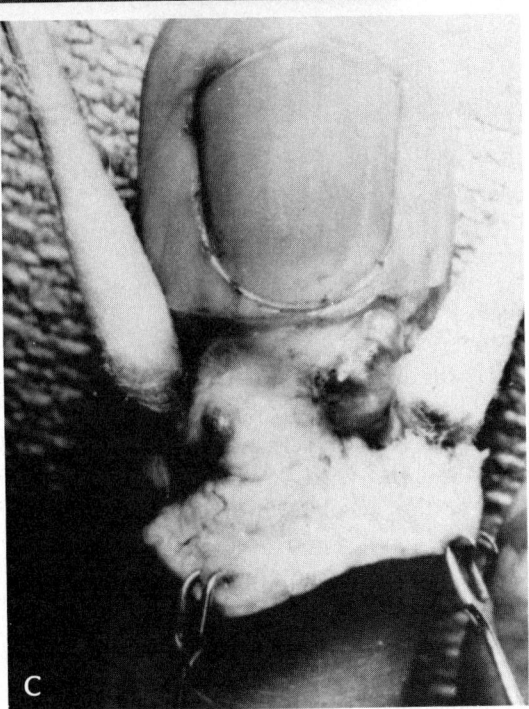

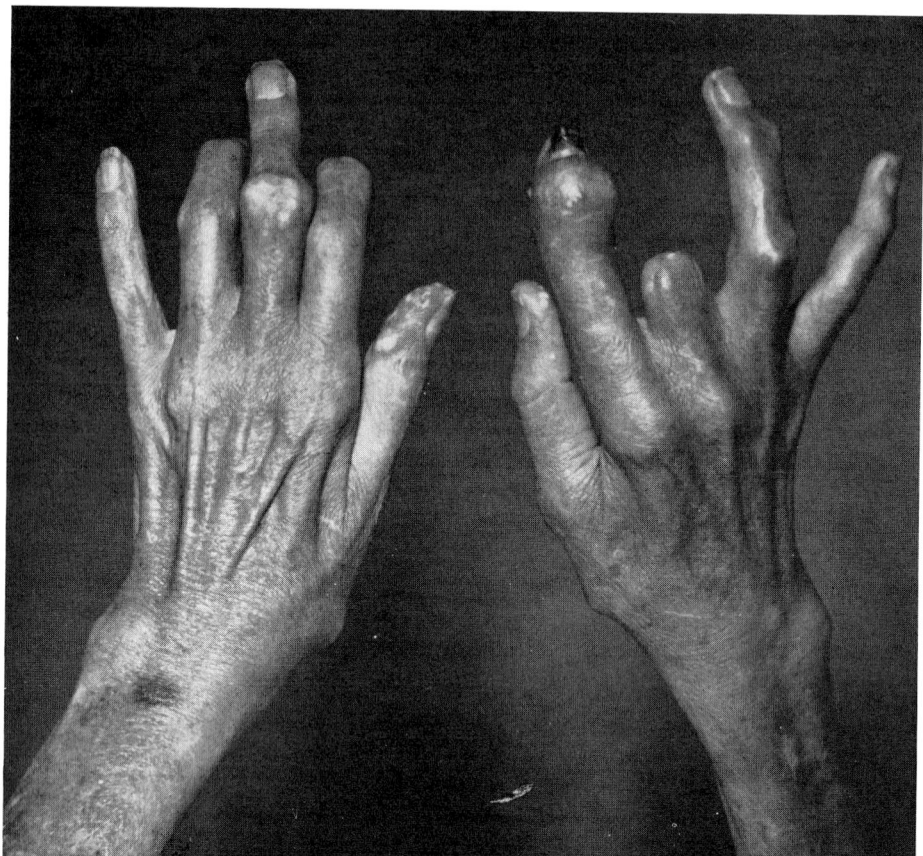

FIG. 50–14. Gout of the hand. These hands of a 53-year-old woman illustrate the classic problems encountered in the hands of both sexes. Selective amputation has already been necessary in several digits. (From Converse, J.: Reconstructive Plastic Surgery. Philadelphia, W.B. Saunders, 1977.)

SCLERODERMA

The soft tissue atrophy of the fingertips that occurs in scleroderma is usually associated with Raynaud's phenomenon. Calcification of the fingertip pulp is common in scleroderma. When calcinosis occurs, about half the cases are associated with scleroderma or some other collagen disease and with Raynaud's phenomenon. Absorption of the distal tufts of the terminal phalanges is the most common bony abnormality seen radiographically. Articular bone or cartilage destruction is seen occasionally, with absorption of bone usually involving the middle and proximal phalanges.

Surgical interventions have little to offer the victims of scleroderma. Stiffness develops in the joints of the hand, and splinting to maintain functional positions can be helpful. Assistive aids may have to be constructed for the patient. I have been able to show that digital artery sympathectomy relieves pain and aids in the healing of ulcerations.[21] I have also found that intrinsic muscle release and excision of symptomatic calcifications improve hand function.

SYSTEMIC LUPUS ERYTHEMATOSUS

Systemic lupus erythematosus (SLE) commonly involves the hand. The skin tightens, and yet deformities develop from laxity of the supporting soft tissue structures.[22] The articular cartilage is not directly involved, but it may show secondary degenerative changes following ligamentous laxity. Raynaud's phenomenon occurs in about half the patients and is the primary cause of disability, rather than the deformities caused by ligamentous laxity. Thumb carpometacarpal joint involvement is common, and replacement arthroplasty is the treatment of choice at this level. The usual treatment in recent years for metacarpophalangeal joint involvement has been Silastic arthroplasties. My results have not been as good as in rheumatoid hands because of the relentless stiffening.

Better overall results are achieved if any proximal interphalangeal joint deformities are corrected at the time of the metacarpophalangeal arthroplasties. Simple swan neck deformities are corrected by tenodesis of the superficialis tendon, and fixed deformities are treated either by arthroplasty or fusion. Boutonnière deformities can be repaired and lateral deviations can be stabilized by collateral ligament repair.

FIG. 50–15. Hemochromatosis. This surgeon's right hand has significant functional impairment because of multiple joint involvement, particularly of the metacarpophalangeal joints of the second and third digits. (From Flatt, A.E.[3])

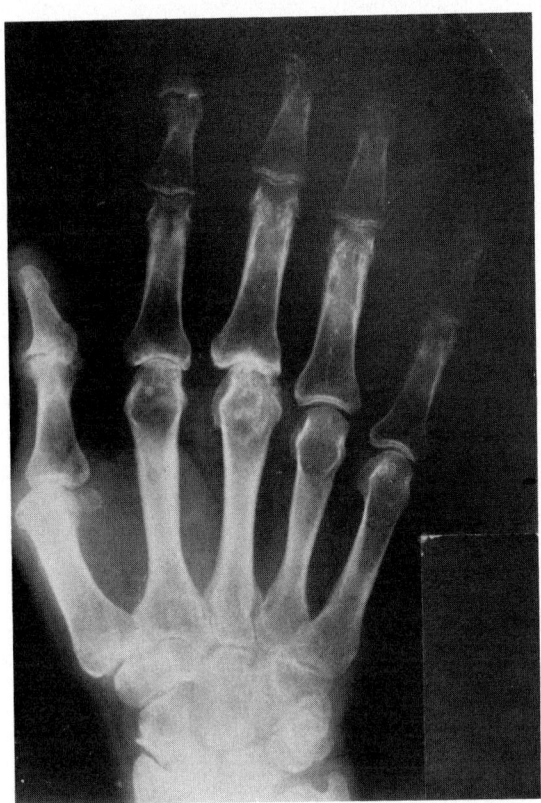

MIXED CONNECTIVE TISSUE DISEASE

The hands of these patients differ from the hands of individuals with SLE, rheumatoid disease, or scleroderma.[23] The characteristic finding is a tightness in the flexor muscles unassociated with skin or joint tightness. Occasionally, tightness of the intrinsic muscles occurs. Corticosteroid injections may be helpful, and surgical treatment may be needed to release adhesions, which occur in a high percentage of cases between the superficialis and profundus tendons. Tendon lengthening procedures are also sometimes of value.

HEMOCHROMATOSIS

A rare form of arthritis is that associated with hemochromatosis. Half these patients have arthralgia and arthritis, characteristically in their hands.[24] The proximal interphalangeal, metacarpophalangeal, and radiocarpal joints are all involved, and the triangular cartilage at the wrist may be calcified. Symptoms usually begin in the metacarpophalangeal joints, spread through the hand, and rapidly cause significant loss of function. I have seen few cases, but, to my chagrin, have been sensitized to the diagnosis by missing it in the hand of a surgical colleague (Fig. 50–15).

REFERENCES

1. Ellison, M.R., Kelly, K.H., and Flatt, A.E.: Ulnar drift of the fingers in rheumatoid disease. J. Bone Joint Surg., 53A:1061–1082, 1971.
2. Millender, L.H., and Nalebuff, E.A.: Evaluation and treatment of early hand involvement. Orthop. Clin. North Am., 6:697–708, 1975.
3. Flatt, A.E.: Care of the Arthritic Hand. St. Louis, C.V. Mosby, 1983.
4. Millender, L.H., and Nalebuff, E.A.: Preventive surgery—Tenosynovectomy and synovectomy. Orthop. Clin. North Am., 6:765–792, 1975.
5. Vahvanen V., and Tallroth, K.: Arthrodesis of the wrist by internal fixation in rheumatoid arthritis: A follow up study of 45 consecutive cases. J. Hand Surg., 9A:531–536, 1984.
6. Vicar, A.J., and Burton, R.I.: Surgical management of the rheumatoid wrist—Fusion or arthroplasty. J. Hand Surg., 11A:790–797, 1986.
7. Brase, D.W., and Millender, L.H.: Failure of silicone rubber wrist arthroplasty in rheumatoid arthritis. J. Hand Surg., 11A:175–183, 1986.
7a. Vicar, A.J., and Burton, R.I.: Surgical management of the rheumatoid wrist-fusion or arthroplasty. J. Hand Surg., 11A:790–797, 1986.
7b. Fatti, J.F., Palmer, A.K., and Mosher, J.F.: The long-term results of Swanson silicone rubber interpositional wrist arthroplasty. J. Hand Surg., 11A:166–175, 1986.
8. Niebauer, J.J.: Dacron-silicone prosthesis for the metacarpophalangeal and interphalangeal joints. In Symposium on the Hand. Vol. 3. Edited by L.H. Cramer and R.A. Chase. St. Louis. C.V. Mosby, 1971.
9. Pahle, J.A., and Raunio, P.: The influence of wrist position on finger deviation in the rheumatoid hand. A clinical and radiological study. J. Bone Joint Surg., 51B:664–676, 1969.
10. Clayton, M.L.: Surgical treatment at the wrist in rheumatoid arthritis. A review of 37 patients. J. Bone Joint Surg., 47A:741–750, 1965.
11. Ellison, M.R., Kelly, K.H., and Flatt, A.E.: The results of surgical synovectomy of the digital joints in rheumatoid disease. J. Bone Joint Surg., 53A:1041–1060, 1971.
12. Brown, P.W.: Early recurrence of rheumatoid synovium after early synovectomy in the hand and wrist. In Early Synovectomy in Rheumatoid Arthritis. Edited by W. Hjmans, W.D. Paul, and H. Herschel. Amsterdam, Excerpta Medica, 1969.
13. Vainio, K.: Synovectomies of the hand and wrist in rheumatoid arthritis. In La Main rheumatoide. Edited by R. Tugiana. Paris, Expansion Scientifique Francaise, 1969.
14. Swanson, A.B.: Flexible implant arthroplasty for arthritic finger joints. J. Bone Joint Surg., 54A:435–455, 1972.
15. Derkash, Q.S., Niebauer, J.J., and Lane, C.S.: Longterm follow-up of metacarpal phalangeal arthroplasty with silicone Dacron prosthesis. J. Hand Surg., 11A:553–558, 1986.
16. Millender, L.H., et al.: Infection after silicone arthroplasty in the hand. J. Bone Joint Surg., 57A:825–829, 1975.

17. Peimer, C.A., et al.: Reactive synovitis after silicone arthroplasty. J. Hand Surg., *11A*:624–638, 1986.
18. Pellegrini, V.D., and Burton, R.I.: Surgical management of basal joint arthritis of the thumb. I. Longterm results of silicone implant arthroplasty. J. Hand Surg., *11A*:309–324, 1986.
19. Amadio, P.C., Millender, L.H., and Smith, R.J.: Silicone spacer or tendon spacer for trapezium resection arthroplasty—Comparison of results. J. Hand Surg., *7*:237–244, 1982.
20. Straub, L.R., et al.: Surgery of gout in the upper extremity. J. Bone Joint Surg., *43A*:731–752, 1961.

21. Flatt, A.E.: Digital artery sympathectomy. J. Hand Surg., *5*:550–556, 1980.
22. Bleifield, C.J., and Inglis, A.E.: The hand in systemic lupus erythematosus. J. Bone Joint Surg., *56A*:1207–1215, 1974.
23. Lewis, R.A., et al.: The hand in mixed connective tissue disease. J. Hand Surg., *3*:217–222, 1978.
24. Jensen, P.S.: Hemochromatosis: A disease often silent but not invisible. Am. J. Roentgenol., *126*:343–351, 1976.

CORRECTION OF ARTHRITIC DEFORMITIES OF THE SHOULDER AND ELBOW

51

ALLAN E. INGLIS

Functionally, the shoulder and elbow serve to position the hand in space. Limitations of function in these two articulations therefore limit the function of the hand. The shoulder, or more broadly speaking, the pectoral girdle, serves as the basal or pivotal articulation of the upper extremity. The elbow joint allows the hand to be extended away from the body for work and, equally important, to be brought toward the body for self-care. Therefore, it is essential that these joints function smoothly and painlessly in the activities of daily life.

ANATOMIC CONSIDERATIONS

Through its design characteristics, the shoulder achieves a remarkable range of motion. Six different modalities, including combinations of motions, are achieved by the glenohumeral joint. Additional shoulder flexibility is achieved through scapulothoracic motion. A high level of stability is achieved despite this high degree of flexibility. The clavicle serves to stabilize the scapula on the thoracic wall, while at the same time permitting high levels of scapular motion. The pectoral girdle is first stabilized against the thoracic wall by the muscles passing from the spine and trunk to the scapula. Further stability is achieved from those muscles passing from the trunk to the proximal humerus. Interstabilization of the glenohumeral joint is achieved by those muscles passing from the scapula to the humerus. Disorders of these stabilizing muscles, whether simple tendinitis or a small rotator cuff tear, substantially reduce the overall coordinated movements of this joint. Further stability of the shoulder is achieved through the ligaments. The ligaments between the scapula and the clavicle, those between the coracoid process of the scapula and the humerus, as well as the glenohumeral ligaments serve to stabilize the glenohumeral joint. The ligaments act to guide the joint through a range of motion and to provide stability at the extremes of motion. The intermediate stability is achieved through the coordinated action of the surrounding muscles. Biomechanically, the joint forces across the shoulder joint at times are extremely high and equal those occurring in the joints of the lower extremity.

Four types of motion are achieved in the elbow joint: flexion, extension, pronation, and supination of the forearm. Extension of the elbow permits the hand to be used at varying distances from the trunk. Chao and associates have demonstrated that if the elbow can be extended to 35°, 90% of the activities of daily living can be accomplished.[1] Rotation of the forearm is allowed through the proximal and distal radioulnar joint. Normally, about 80° of pronation and 80° of supination are permitted by these articulations. When this range of motion is reduced, the shoulder compensates by abducting for pronation and adducting for supination. This "body English" may be embarrassing to the individual with limited pronation or supination.

Normally, there is no medial-lateral movement in the elbow. The stability of the elbow joint is achieved principally by the design of the articulating surfaces and the ligamentous support. The articulating surfaces between the semilunar notch of the ulna and the trochlea of the humerus are ridged and high-walled and are aligned perfectly. The articulation between the radius and the capitellum of the humerus allows for a small amount of laxity, enough so that the radiocapitellar joint is not constantly loaded during hand function. Force transmitted through the hand and wrist is transmitted mostly from the radius to the ulna through the interosseous membrane and thence, to the humerus, scapula and, ultimately, to the spine.[2] The important function of the radiocapitellar joint, therefore, is to provide rotation of the forearm and stability to the proximal radius.

A third articulation is also important. The proximal radioulnar joint stabilizes the proximal portions of these two bones. The annular ligament passes around the neck of the radius, securing it to the ulna. The medial-lateral stability of the elbow joint is achieved through the anterior medial ligament that passes from the humerus to the sublime tubercle of the ulna.[3] Lateral stability is largely achieved by the brachioradialis muscle, extensor muscles of the wrist and, to a lesser extent, by the lateral collateral ligament. The forces across the elbow joint are almost entirely compressional. This compression loading system occurs because many of the wrist and finger flexors and extensors originate from the humeral epicondyles. Whenever the wrist is stabilized, whether it be in grasp or release, the wrist extensors contract, thereby compressing the elbow joint. Carrying a suitcase weighing 40 lb produces a commensurate compression force across the elbow joint rather than a distraction force.

Reduced function of the shoulder and elbow occurs in a variety of situations, including pain, weakness or paralysis, instability, or stiffness. By far the most important of these is pain, and therapeutic measures must always place pain relief as the highest priority. The pain may be produced either by an inflammatory reaction, such as in RA or osteoarthritis or septic synovitis (fire), or by the anatomic destruction of the joint by these diseases (ashes). Such joint destruction produces painful instability. Stiffening of the joint, such as seen in degenerative or traumatic arthritis, may also produce pain. Whether the pain is due to an inflammatory reaction, instability, or stiffening, it is still the primary considerations in surgical therapy of the shoulder and elbow. The pain may be ameliorate by systemic medications or at times by intra-articular corticosteroid injections. For the stiff shoulder, an exercise program to increase range of motion and strength may be of benefit. The most difficult and therapeutically demanding pathologic processes are those that produce a combination of inflammation, joint destruction, and stiffness. In this situation, all three must be corrected simultaneously.

SURGICAL THERAPY

Arthritic Shoulder. Surgical therapy for the arthritic shoulder should never be instituted until conservative measures have been exhausted. These measures should always include the use of salicylates or other nonsteroidal anti-inflammatory drugs, a period of rest and, frequently, intra-articular injection of corticosteroid. The patient may be referred to a therapist for range-of-motion and strengthening exercises. These conservative measures, individually or in concert, frequently reduce symptoms to acceptable levels.

Surgical therapy for the shoulder includes synovectomy and debridement, hemiarthroplasty, arthrodesis, and total shoulder arthroplasty. Synovectomy of the shoulder is sometimes needed in rheumatoid arthritis, other primary diseases of the synovium, or secondary diseases such as hemophilia arthropathy. Open synovectomy of the shoulder is often unsuccessful and has been abandoned in most centers. The major reason open synovectomy fails is the lack of surgical accessibility to the synovium. It is extremely difficult at the time of surgery to reach the intraglenoid recess, the subscapularis pouch, and the posterior aspects of the joint. More recently, arthroscopic synovectomy has been useful through a combined anterior and posterior portal approach. Arthroscopic synovectomy can be considered when conservative measures have failed to control painful synovitis of the shoulder. If there has been any significant joint destruction, then other measures must be employed.

Debridement of the acromioclavicular joint, with acromioplasty and ligament decompression, is useful in impingement syndromes of the shoulder.[4] The glenohumeral joint is *not* opened. Surgery is directed to the area beneath the acromion process and above the supraspinous muscle. The coracoacromial ligament is incised. The acromioclavicular joint is debrided, including osteophyte removal, and a portion of the undersurface of the acromion process is removed to provide adequate space for the greater tuberosity of the humerus to move within the space between the acromion process and the remaining humerus (Fig. 51–1). Hyperplastic or exuberant tissue from the subdeltoid bursa is also removed to provide greater space between the supraspinous muscle and the acromion process. At times, it is also necessary to repair a small defect in the external rotator cuff. This operation requires prolonged convalescence during which inten-

FIG. 51–1. Osteoarthritis of the acromioclavicular joint. Note the thickening and hypertrophy of both the acromion and the end of the clavicle. Such hypertrophy irritates the subacromial bursa and injures the underlying supraspinous muscle.

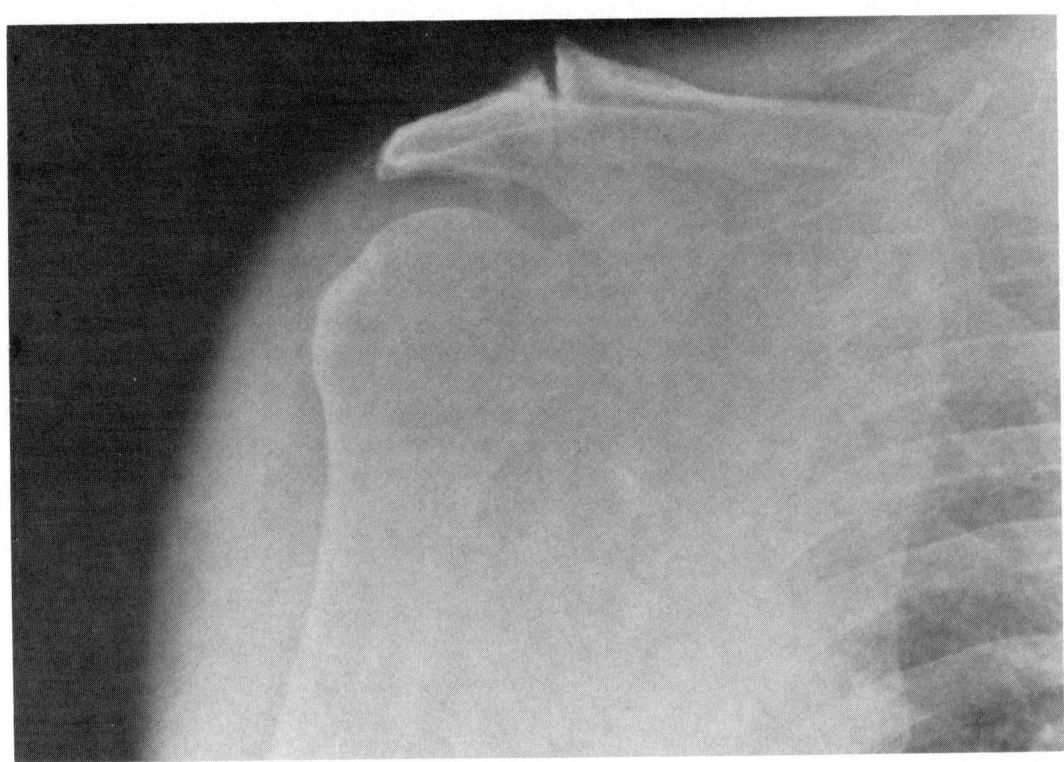

sive physical therapy is prescribed to restore functional range of motion with strength. This operation is successful in the hands of experienced surgeons. Recently, this procedure has been accomplished arthroscopically if the disease process is not too advanced. Patients can usually return to racquet sports, swimming, and other activities requiring high levels of shoulder mobility.[4]

Hemiarthroplasty of the shoulder is useful, particularly in traumatic arthritis and osteonecrosis, or when disease is confined entirely to the head of the humerus and there is an intact, functioning, rotator cuff with preservation of glenoid surface.[5] It is not necessary to cement the humeral component. Hemiarthroplasty sometimes can be used as a "salvage" procedure even when the bony glenoid process is completely destroyed. In this situation, the prosthesis articulates with the remaining glenoid labrum and remaining neck of the glenoid (Fig. 51–2). Again, intensive physical therapy is required to restore shoulder function. In a hemiarthroplasty, it is essential that a secure, functioning, external rotator cuff be established. Any tears in the cuff must be repaired at the

time of operation. When rotator cuff repair is necessary, an even more protracted period of convalescence and physical therapy is required. The results from hemiarthroplasty are salutary.[5] Full flexion, full abduction, full internal rotation, and external rotation to at least 45° are expected. Even if these results are achieved, however, return to racquet sports or other activities where the shoulder joint experiences high loading or force should not be expected.

Arthrodesis (fusion) is useful if obliteration of glenohumeral motion is desirable, as after severe recalcitrant infections where there has been complete loss of all the rotator muscles about the shoulder or gross destruction of both the humeral head and the glenoid process. This procedure is usually reserved for patients with extremely painful shoulders that do not permit use of the elbow or hand in the activities of daily living. Its major drawbacks are the long period of immobilization in a cast or splint and the occasional failure of fusion with development of a painful pseudarthrosis. Newer methods of plate and screw fixation have reduced the long period of immobilization in a plaster cast. Internal fixation with plates and screws

FIG. 51–2. *A,* Severe rheumatoid arthritis of the glenohumeral joint associated with complete destruction of the glenoid process. At surgery only a bony button of the remaining neck of the glenoid was evident; this structure was surrounded by remnants of the labrum and capsular fibrous tissue. *B,* After hemiarthroplasty, pain was completely relieved. Although the range of motion was "bench level," the shoulder joint was functional and the patient could reach her face and back.

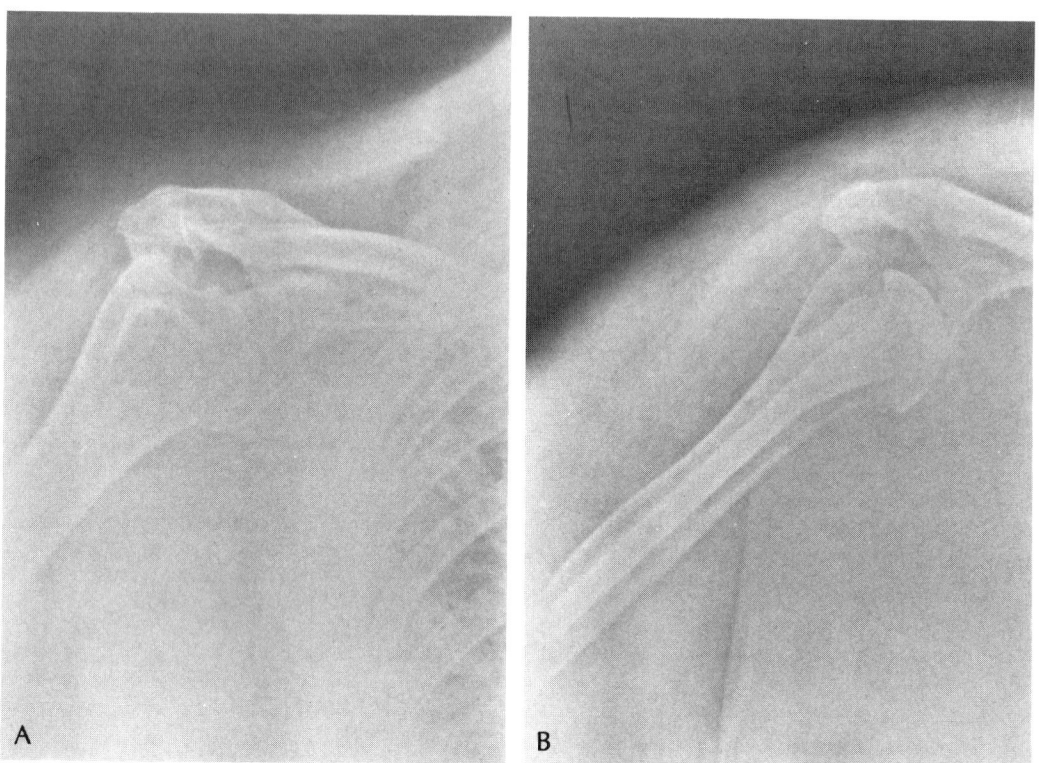

adds to the surgical procedure technical problems such as the inability to change the position of the glenohumeral joint after the application of the appliance and the increased potential for infection with such a large device. Nevertheless, these devices do show promise for a shorter, less complicated convalescence. A successful arthrodesis of the shoulder relieves pain but leaves limited motion. Such patients can move their hand to their face and ear, but probably not to the back of the head. The buttock area can be reached, but not the middle of the back. Forward flexion to 70° is expected. All activities that occur at a *bench* level should be possible.[6]

Total shoulder arthroplasty is useful when there is destruction of both the humeral head and the glenoid. In this procedure both the humeral head and the glenoid are replaced, the former with a short stemmed, metallic prosthesis and the latter with a high-molecular-weight polyethylene implant. Both components are cemented in place with polymethylmethacrylate.

There are two types of prosthetic implants: constrained and nonconstrained. A constrained prosthesis is a single unit containing glenoid and humeral components. These components are attached to one another while still allowing a high level of motion. The components of nonconstrained prostheses are not mechanically connected to one another. Stability is achieved through the newly restored capsule and the surrounding muscles. The constrained prosthesis is most useful in patients with severe irreparably damaged external rotator cuff muscles.

The constrained design produces greater stress on the cement bone bonds. The nonconstrained, total shoulder replacement achieves greater motion so that stability can be achieved and maintained through the external rotator group of muscles. The capsule of the joint must be sufficiently intact to achieve a strong repair. Stress is less at the cement bone bond. The rehabilitative program must be intensive after either type of prosthesis implant. Usually, because of pain

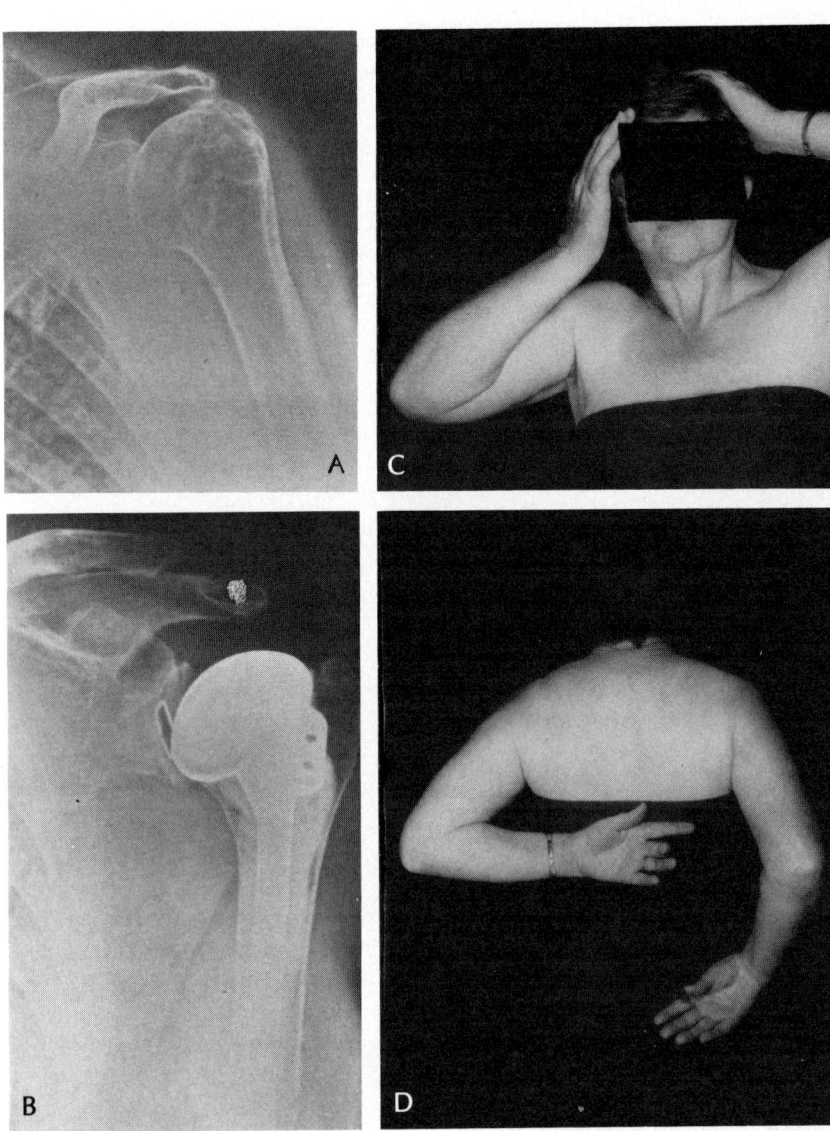

FIG. 51–3. *A,* Severe degenerative arthritis of the left shoulder with loss of cartilage from both the glenoid process and the humeral head. The patient had severe pain unrelieved by either medication or corticosteroid injections. *B,* Radiograph following total shoulder arthroplasty. Both glenoid and humeral components are secure with no evidence of loosening. *C,* Photograph obtained when the patient entered the hospital for total shoulder arthroplasty on the opposite shoulder. The left shoulder now has sufficient external rotation and abduction to permit her to reach the back of her head. *D,* Adduction and internal rotation were sufficient to enable the patient to reach the middle of her back.

relief, good patient cooperation is achieved during the rehabilitation period. Two levels of restored function can be observed. In patients with total shoulder arthroplasty, 80 to 90% restoration of function can be expected if the external rotator cuff was intact to begin with or was surgically restored (Fig. 51–3). Relief of pain with "bench level" function is expected in joints in which the external rotator cuff has been partially restored or in cases where there are other residual problems in the shoulder, such as arthritis of the acromioclavicular joint or severe muscle atrophy. Total arthroplasty is being performed with increasing frequency by surgeons experienced in reconstructive shoulder surgery.[7,8] The relief of pain and restoration of function have been gratifying to most patients.

Arthritic Elbow Joint. Conservative measures should

always be attempted first. These measures include the use of salicylates and other nonsteroidal, anti-inflammatory drugs. Intra-articular injections of corticosteroids and rest are beneficial in rheumatoid synovitis for relief of pain. Posterior splints, secured with Velcro straps, are easily prepared by occupational therapists (Fig. 51–4). Exercises, except for gentle stretching to prevent contractures, may worsen the condition because of the anatomic complexities of the elbow joint.

Surgical therapy includes: synovectomy and debridement with radial head resection, replacement arthroplasty, fascial arthroplasty, and arthrodesis.[9]

Fascial arthroplasty and arthrodesis are not used commonly for arthritic disorders of the elbow. Fascial arthroplasty is indicated when there has been a prior

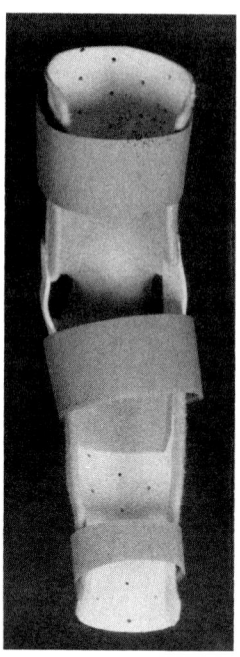

FIG. 51–4. Simple, fabricated resting splint. These splints are usually made with the elbow at 90° flexion. They are well padded with moleskin and secured with Velcro straps.

FIG. 51–5. Radiographs of a patient with uncontrolled rheumatoid synovitis of the elbow. *A,* Note preservation of joint surfaces and minimal joint margin osteophyte formation. *B,* Anterior-posterior view. The arrow points to a 1- × 1.5-cm cystic defect in the lateral epicondyle. This defect was beneath the lateral collateral ligament and was filled with rheumatoid granulation tissue. Elbow synovectomy, debridement, and evacuation of the cystic defect were performed. Postoperatively, the patient had complete relief of pain with flexion to 125° and extension to 15°.

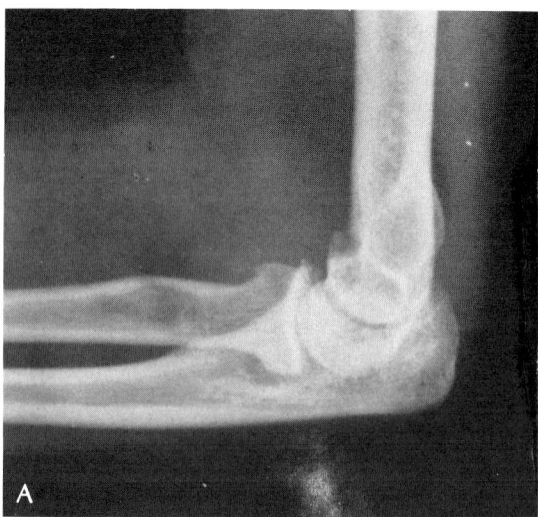
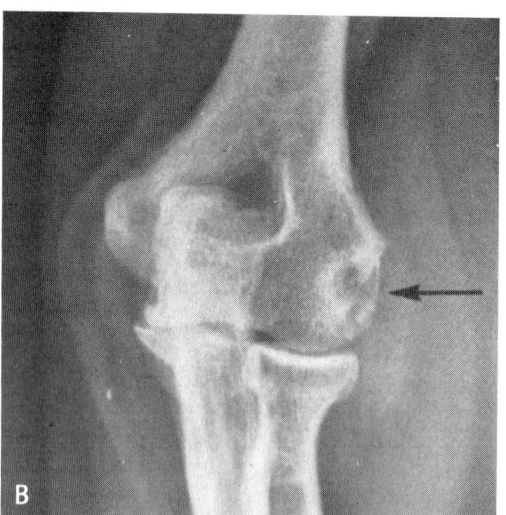

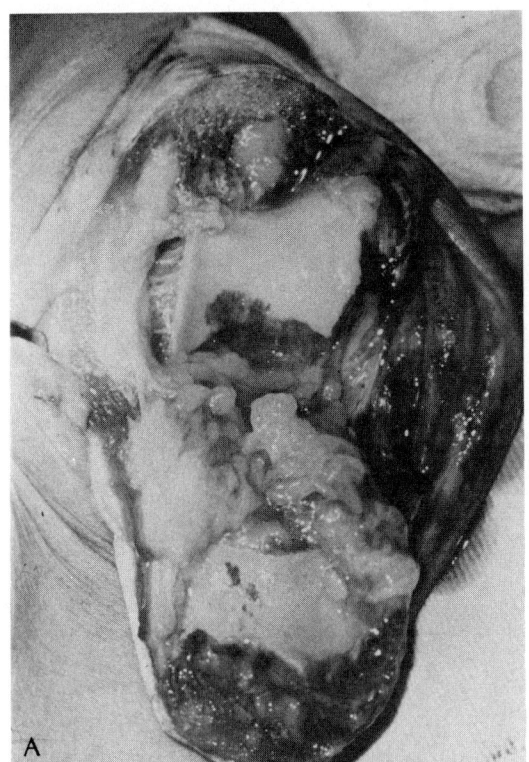

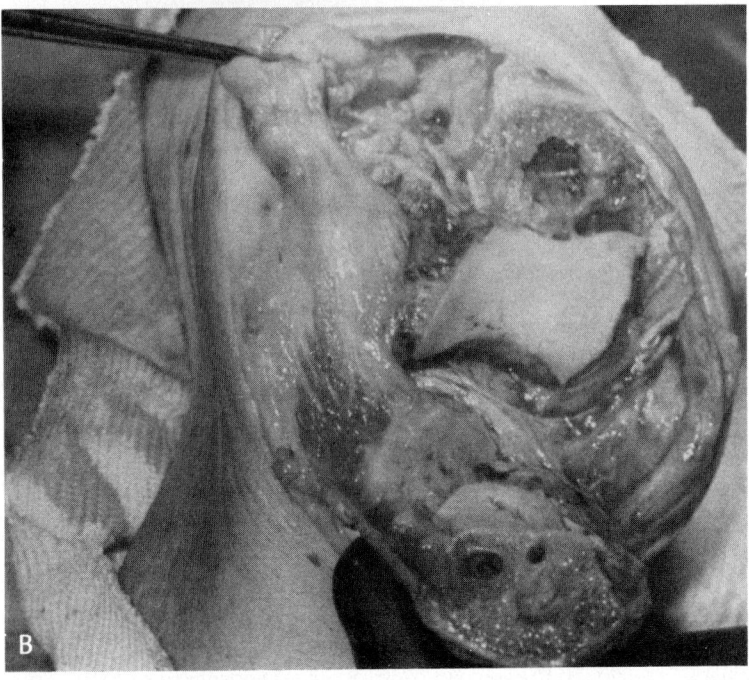

FIG. 51–6. Synovectomy and debridement of the elbow through the transolecranon approach. *A,* The osteotomized tip of the olecranon is in the foreground. Note the large rheumatoid cystic erosion in the remaining olecranon process of the ulna above. Proliferative synovitis occurs in the posterior aspect of the joint in the center of the illustration. Note the pannus formation on the surface of the trochlea of the humerus. *B,* Appearance of the joint following synovectomy and debridement. The pannus has been removed, and the joint margins debrided of all osteophytes and synovium. The radial head has been excised, following by a complete synovectomy of the anterior compartment of the joint.

infection such as tuberculosis in a stiff or painful elbow joint. A strip of fascia lata from the thigh is used to cover both the distal humerus and the ulna, thereby providing a smooth surface for motion. Although functional flexion and extension can be obtained, the medial and lateral instability that results frequently produces a weak elbow joint. Arthrodesis

is considered a salvage procedure when prior procedures have failed or if infection precludes the use of an artificial elbow joint. Arthrodesis is difficult to achieve surgically because of the long lever arm of the upper extremity. It is also difficult to determine the optimal position for the arthrodesis.

Synovectomy and joint debridement with radial

head resection are highly successful procedures in those patients with a primary disease of the synovium that has failed to respond to conservative measures.[10,11] It is particularly useful when there has been preservation of the articular surfaces of the humerus and the semilunar notch of the ulna (Fig. 51–5A,B). The synovium is excised and the joint edges are carefully debrided and restored to their normal anatomic state (Fig. 51–6A,B). The radial head is always removed to allow for normal rotation of the forearm. Ninety percent good to excellent results are expected if the appropriate indications are followed and the patient complies with the rehabilitation program. Pain and restricted motion due to degenerative arthritis can be treated by joint debridement with radial head resection with restoration of satisfactory painless function, but the results are not as predictable as in rheumatoid arthritis. Pain relief is often complete, but it may not be accompanied by a noticeable increased range of motion. To prevent disappointments in patients with degenerative arthritis of the elbow, the goals should be carefully established before the operation.

Replacement arthroplasty of the elbow is becoming more popular. The results over a 10- to 12-year period show that such arthroplasty is lasting and useful, particularly in patients with rheumatiod arthritis.[12–15] Replacement arthroplasty of the elbow may be considered in those patients who are refractory to medical management and have joint destruction. The indications for surgery in patients with traumatic arthritis and degenerative arthritis are still unclear. However, in certain centers, replacement arthroplasty is being used for painful, traumatic arthritis and in patients with severe instability of the elbow joint from fracture nonunions of the humerus and proximal ulna bones. Replacement arthroplasty is also being used with good results in patients with ankylosis of the elbow joint. Certainly, youthful patients with traumatic arthritis are not candidates for replacement arthroplasty because of their high physical demands and expectations. The situation is not unlike that seen in youthful patients with traumatic arthritis of the hip or knee.

There are two types of replacement arthroplasties available. A *nonconstrained elbow replacement* achieves stability through the design of the implant surfaces and adjacent ligaments and muscles. *Semiconstrained implants* with controlled medial and lateral movement of the prosthesis allow a reduction in the torque forces across the cement bone bond during motion, including internal and external rotation of the arm (Fig. 51–7).[16,17] Such semiconstrained implants allow full flexion and extension together with a small amount of medial-lateral laxity. Improvements in surgical

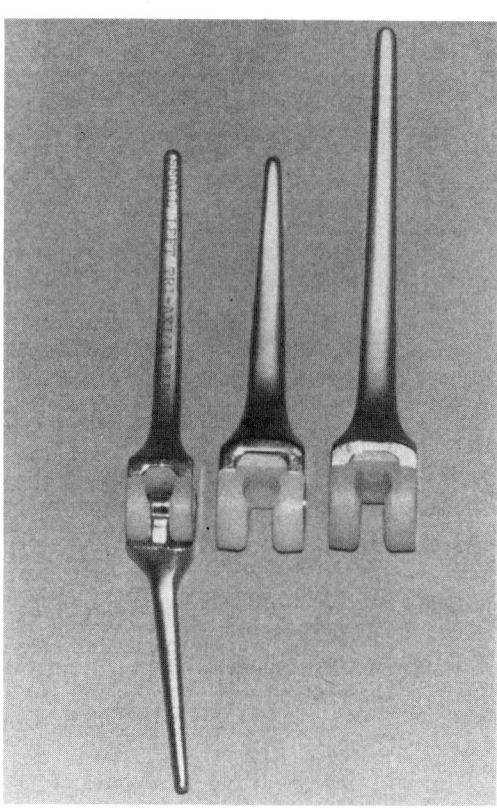

FIG. 51–7. The semiconstrained triaxial total elbow implant. The load across the implant is transmitted through the high-molecular-weight polyethylene plastic bearing. Torsional forces between the cement and the bone are reduced by the laxity in the ulnar component and the plastic bearing. This laxity reduces the potential for loosening.

technique have reduced the complication rate in both these arthroplasties to the levels expected in total hip or total knee replacement (Fig. 51–8). Rapid advancement through a therapy program can be achieved with early restoration of elbow function. Such rapid recovery is possible because of immediate intraoperative restoration of joint stability and of triceps extensor function, with retention of elbow flexion. It is expected that these patients will achieve 130° of elbow flexion and extension to 25° to 30°. Many patients achieve both full flexion and full extension.[12,14]

Complications in the shoulder and elbow are similar to those seen in implant arthroplasties of the lower extremity. The infection rate following total shoulder replacement is less than 1%, and the infection rate following total elbow arthroplasty is 3%.[18] Nonconstrained implant loosening in total shoulder arthroplasty is less than 4% after 5 years. Our experience with semiconstrained, total elbow athroplasty revealed that only 1 of 95 implants loosened during a 9-year period.[19–21] Dislocation or separation of the

FIG. 51–8. Radiograph showing total elbow arthroplasty. This joint is pain-free with flexion to 130° and extension to 5°. This patient also has an elbow replacement on the opposite side, bilateral total hip and knee replacements, and an ankle replacement. She feels that her elbows are her "most dependable joints."

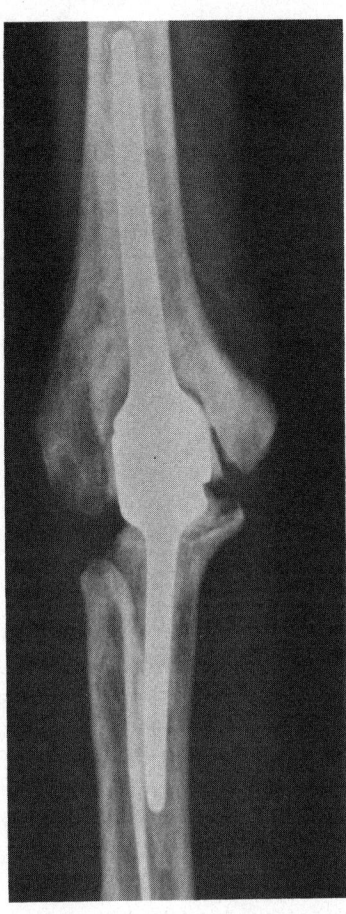

components of the implant, whether it be in the shoulder or in the elbow, occurs in about 5% of cases.

We expect a 90% return of function after total shoulder arthroplasty in patients with an intact rotator cuff, and a 90% return of function after total elbow arthroplasty. These results may be compromised by arthritic disorders in adjacent articulations such as the neck, wrist, or hand. The restoration of a painless, stable shoulder or a painless, flexible elbow is often of real value to patients in their activities of daily living.

Surgical therapy can be considered in patients whose pain and loss of function cannot be managed through rest, medications, and a controlled exercise program. The gain-versus-complications ratio is now sufficiently high that surgical therapy can be safely recommended in patients with disabling arthritis of the shoulder and elbow. The durability of these surgical procedures has been good with improvement in function and quality of life.

REFERENCES

1. Morrey, B.F., Askew, L.J., and Chao, E.Y.: A biomechanical study of normal functional elbow motion. J. Bone Joint Surg., 63A872–877, 1981.
2. Von Langer, T., and Waschmuth, W.: Prakitsche Anatomie. Berlin, Verlag von Julius Springer, 1935, p. 157.
3. Last, R.J.: Anatomy Regional and Applied. 6th Ed. Boston, Little Brown and Co., 1966, p. 111.
4. Neer, C.S.: Anterior acromioplasty for the chronic impingement syndromes of the shoulder. A preliminary report. J. Bone Joint Surg., 54A:41–50, 1972.
5. Neer, C.S.: Replacement arthroplasty for glenohumeral osteoarthritis. J. Bone Joint Surg., 56A:1–16, 1974.
6. Cofield, R.H., and Briggs, B.T.: Glenohumeral arthrodesis. Operative and long term functional results. J. Bone Joint Surg., 61A:668–677, 1979.
7. Neer, C.S., Watson, K.C., and Stanton, F.K.: Recent experiences in total shoulder replacement. J. Bone Joint Surg., 64A:319–337, 1982.
8. Warren, R.F., Ranawat, C.S., and Inglis, A.E.: Total shoulder replacement indications and results of the Neer non-constrained prosthesis. *In* Symposium on Total Joint Replacement of the Upper Extremity. Edited by A.E. Inglis. St. Louis, C.V. Mosby, 1982, pp. 56–68.
9. Koch, M., and Lipscomb, P.R.: Arthrodesis of the elbow. Clin. Orthop., 50:151, 1967.
10. Eichenblat, M., Haas, A., and Kessler, I.: Synovectomy of the elbow in rheumatoid arthritis. J. Bone Joint Surg., 64A:1074–1078, 1982.
11. Inglis, A.E., Ranawat, C.S., and Straub, L.R.: Synovectomy and debridement of the elbow in rheumatoid arthritis. J. Bone Joint Surg., 53A:652–662, 1971.
12. Coonrad, R.W.: Seven year follow-up of Coonrad total elbow replacement. *In* Symposium on Total Joint Replacement of the Upper Extremity. Edited by A.E. Inglis. St. Louis, C.V. Mosby, 1982, p. 91.
13. Ewald, F.C., et al.: Capitellocondylar total elbow arthroplasty. J. Bone Joint Surg., 62A:1259–1263, 1980.
14. Inglis, A.E.: Triaxial total elbow replacement: Indications, surgical technique and results. *In* Symposium on Total Joint Replacement of the Upper Extremity. Edited by A.E. Inglis. St. Louis, C.V. Mosby, 1982, pp. 100–111.
15. Inglis, A.E., and Pellicci, P.M.: Total elbow replacement. J. Bone Joint Surg., 62A:1252–1258, 1980.
16. Pritchard, R.W.: Long-term followup study: Semi-contrained elbow prosthesis. Orthopaedics, 4:151, 1981.
17. Schlein, A.P.: Semiconstrained total elbow arthroplasty. Clin. Orthop., 121:222, 1976.
18. Morrey, B.F., and Bryan, R.S.: Infection after total elbow arthroplasty. J. Bone Joint Surg., 65A(3):330, 1983.
19. Morrey, B.F, and Bryan, R.S.: Total Joint Replacement. *In* The Elbow and Its Disorders. Philadelphia. W.B. Saunders, 1985, p. 546.
20. Figgie, H.E., Inglis, A.E., and Mow, C.: A critical analysis of alignment factors affecting functional outcome in total elbow arthroplasty. J. Arthroplasty, 1:169–173, 1986.
21. Figgie, H.E., et al.: Critical analysis of mechanical factors correlated with bone remodelling following total elbow. J. Arthroplasty, 1:175–182, 1986.

52

CORRECTION OF ARTHRITIC DEFORMITIES OF THE SPINE

GLENN A. MEYER and JAMES E. STOLL

The commonly encountered arthritic deformities of the spine are discussed here with emphasis on those that are amenable to surgical correction. The goal is to provide medically oriented physicians with information on when and how surgical treatment may be helpful to their patients. Surgical principles are emphasized with discussions of cases in which clinical, radiologic, and electrophysiologic abnormalities indicate the need for surgical consultation.

The chapter is organized by anatomic regions starting at the C1–C2 junction and proceeding caudally. A brief description of the commonly performed operations follows.

REGIONAL DISORDERS

C1–C2 JUNCTION

Rheumatoid arthritis (RA) is second only to trauma as the most common cause of atlantoaxial instability. Mild degrees of instability, as demonstrated by lateral roentgenograms of the upper cervical spine in the flexed and extended positions, are extremely common. Movement of up to 5 mm is rarely of concern and, if necessary can be treated with a cervical collar. However, if serial films demonstrate a progressive instability, a stabilization procedure (fusion) is inevitable and should be performed before myelopathic symptoms ensue. Symptoms of particular concern are progressive lancinating pain in the C2 distribution of the occiput; Lhermitte's phenomenon (electric

shock–like sensations radiating caudally along the spine or distally in the extremities); and, rarely, evidence of intermittent vascular insufficiency in the posterior cerebral circulation caused by impingement on the vertebral arteries. Patients with instability commonly complain of a feeling of movement and/or clicking in the upper neck as they change position. This sensation may awaken the patient and may become so severe that the patient voluntarily supports his head in his hands when changing positions. Generally, any movement at the C1–C2 interspace of more than 10 mm is an absolute indication for fusion. Disabling symptoms as described or progressive instability in the 5- to 10-mm range are relative indications for fusion. Myelopathy with spastic quadriparesis is usually only incompletely reversible once established.[1]

In the rheumatoid patient, a pannus of inflammatory tissue or rheumatoid nodules may additionally compromise the intraspinal space. Magnetic resonance imaging (MRI) is rapidly replacing computed tomography (CT) imaging to visualize such lesions. The detail provided by the sagittal MRI provides precise anatomic detail necessary for surgical planning (Fig. 52–1). The same view can be provided by sagittal reconstruction of axial CT images, but this technique usually provides less anatomic detail.[2,3]

Attention to technical detail is critical in establishing a solid C1–C2 fusion. We prefer a halo vest immobilization applied a day or two before operation to ensure that the vest does not compromise the patient's respiratory status. If the rheumatic process has

856

CORRECTION OF ARTHRITIC DEFORMITIES OF THE SPINE   **857**

FIG. 52–1. This midsagittal magnetic resonance imaging of a 45-year-old patient with rheumatoid arthritis demonstrates the pathology associated with atlantoaxial instability. The fixed 10-mm displacement (between arrows) is caused by interposed inflammatory tissue. Narrowing of the spinal cord is seen where it is displaced posteriorly by the odontoid process. The tip of the odontoid protrudes upward (rostrally) into the foramen magnum.

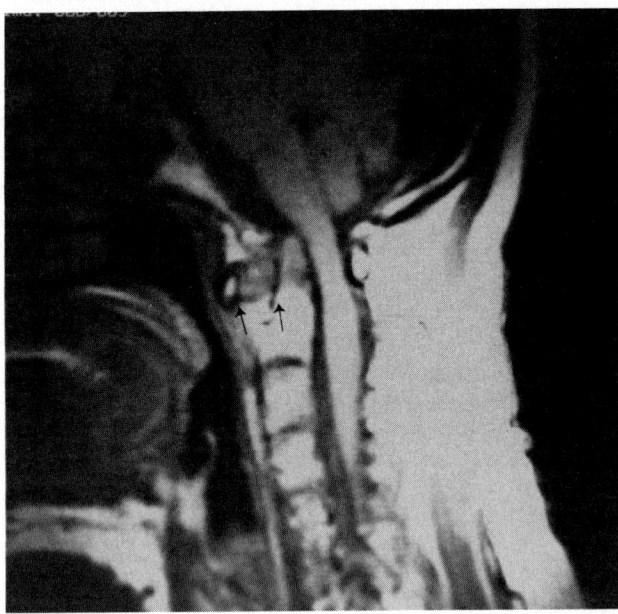

sufficiently softened or eroded the arch of C1 so that it will not hold a stabilizing wire, the occiput should be included in the fusion. Despite meticulous attention to surgical detail in performing the fusion, the rheumatoid process may involve the fusion mass and over several years destabilize a previously adequate fusion. It is important to emphasize to these patients that they should not induce pain in attempts to maintain range of motion of the cervical spine. They may require additional training in the use of mirrors in driving their automobiles or in performing other daily tasks. Generally, methylmethacrylate fusions are not recommended for RA patients.

Infrequently, bone softening may be sufficient to allow protrusion of the cervical spine, particularly of the odontoid process upward into the skull (basilar impression) with subsequent compression of the cervical medullary junction. This condition is easily demonstrated with routine radiography. Surgical decompression usually must be done via an anterior approach.[4,5]

C3–T1 SEGMENT

Similar progressive deformity, instability, and subluxation may involve any mobile segment of the cervical spine. These processes are accelerated by rheumatoid involvement and by prior laminectomy. An occasional patient may require fusion from the occiput to the thorax. Serial radiographs of the cervical spine are just as important as they are of the atlantoaxial junction. Most problems requiring surgery below C1–C2 are due to degenerative disc disease and/or osteoarthritis.

The neurologic examination of patients with extreme arthritic deformity of the upper extremity joints can be challenging. Joint replacement commonly interferes with the afferent side of the deep tendon reflex arc. Frequent serial examination of strength, reflex, and sensory functions of the upper extremity by the primary physician or rheumatologist provides the most reliable information. Often, additional useful information can be provided by the electrodiagnostic study of muscle and nerve function. If impairment of the posterior columns of the spinal cord is suspected, useful data can be obtained from somatosensory-evoked potential studies performed before and after the patient is placed in the symptom-inducing position. Serial comparison of the latencies, as well as comparisons of the data obtained on the right versus left side in both arm and leg, is most reliable. Most patients with advanced diseases who develop neurologic rheumatic dysfunction of the arms have a combination of nerve root compression at or near the intervertebral foramen and spinal cord compression.

Deformity of the spinal canal and intervertebral spaces may compromise circulation to the spinal cord with neurologic deficit of a seemingly radicular nature extending one or two segments above and/or below a mass lesion. Such intraspinal mass lesions are usually the result of a combination of osteophyte formation, disc bulging, and hypertrophy and bulging of ligamentous structures (induced by collapse of the intervertebral disc and concomitant shortening and thickening of elastic ligaments). Offending osteophytes most commonly originate from the specialized portion of the lateral area of the cervical vertebral body termed the uncovertebral joint (joint of Luschka).[6] Less frequently, osteophytes may form from the anterior aspect of the facet joint, causing further nerve root compression located posteriorly and slightly more distally along the nerve root. Both may coexist in the same patient, causing particularly severe signs of radiculopathy and segmental muscular atrophy.

Another condition that can produce myelopathy is posterior longitudinal ligament ossification.[7] Its prevalence in whites is about 0.2%, but in Japanese and certain other Orientals it is 1 to 3%. Its etiopathogenesis is obscure, although it may be associated with an equally obscure lesion, namely diffuse idiopathic skeletal hyperostosis.[8] The ossified ligament can occupy more than 50% of the spinal canal, leading to severe myelopathic signs and symptoms. The same process can occur in the anterior longitudinal ligament. Treatment consists of multilevel decompressive laminectomies and fusion.[9] The myelopathy is usually not completely reversed by decompression.

Pain alone is infrequently an indication for surgical intervention, particularly if the patient can adjust to the pain and carry on with normal activities. However, disabling sensory loss with lack of proprioceptive feedback and muscular weakness, especially with atrophy, are of great concern. Neurologic deficit of this degree is rarely completely reversible, and surgical consultation should be obtained promptly when functional deficits are first noted.

Occasionally, interspace collapse and osteophyte formation may lead to a hypomobile or completely fused vertebral segmental level. This occurrence predisposes to instability and subluxation at the next mobile segment above and/or below the relatively fixed segment. Therefore, flexion/extension lateral roentgenograms of the cervical spine should be performed in all patients for whom operative intervention is being considered.

Patients with a severe degree of osteoarthritis may have remodeling of the vertebral bodies with anterior wedging. When progressive and multisegmental, this condition may lead to reversal of the normal cervical lordosis and the swan-neck deformity. This deformity may accelerate cervical myelopathy and may be the cause for severe neck pain. Swan-neck deformity can be corrected by diskectomy of the intervertebral disc and by placement of multiple grafts to re-establish the anterior height of the vertebral canal. Figure 52–2 shows the pre- and postoperative roentgenograms of a patient successfully treated with a three-disc level technique. Generally, anterior diskectomy and fusion of more than two cervical levels is not recommended because of greater surgical morbidity rate, including nonfusion and pseudoarthrosis formation.

Fusion of the cervical spine by the anterior or pos-

FIG. 52–2. *A,* Preoperative roentgenogram of a 64-year-old woman with severe osteoporosis and degenerative osteoarthritis. She had progressive neck pain, mild myelopathy, and cervical radiculopathy. Progressive reversal of the cervical lordosis was demonstrated on serial films. *B,* The appearance following anterior diskectomy with anterior distraction of the interspace by placement of autogenous iliac bone grafts after operation at three intervertebral levels (C4–C5 through C6–C7 inclusive). The cervical lordosis was partially reestablished, and symptoms were completely relieved.

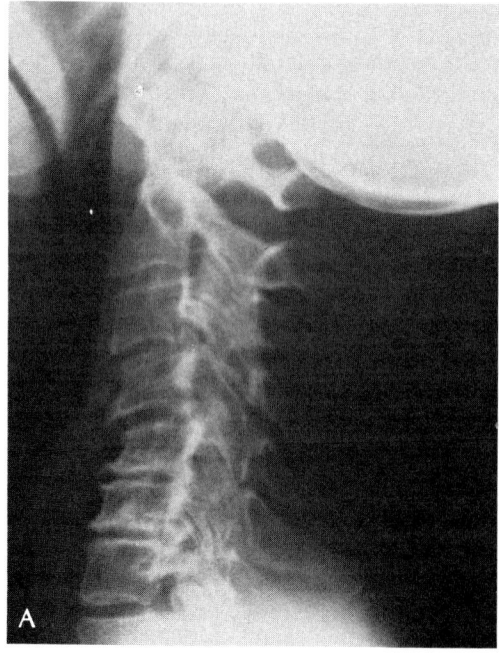
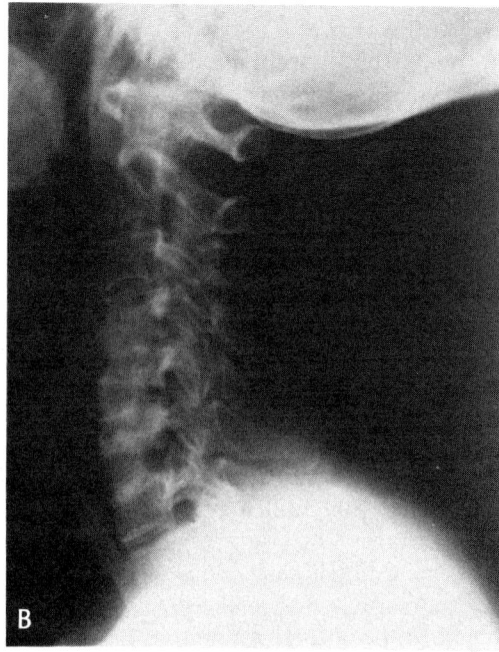

terior technique is satisfactory, depending on the clinical situation.[10] Generally, anterior diskectomy and fusion in a stenotic canal should not be performed as a primary procedure because of the risk of additional spinal cord damage and disastrous postoperative quadriplegia.

DORSAL SPINE

The marked degree of structural support of the thoracic spine by the rib cage makes arthritic deformity of the thoracic spine, which requires surgical correction, a rare condition. An increase in upper thoracic kyphosis commonly develops when osteoarthritis and osteoporosis coexist. Lesser increases in the thoracic kyphosis are occasionally seen with ankylosing spondylitis and may contribute to the fixed forward flexion of the thoracolumbar spine. Fortunately, more effective medical treatment during the active phase of this disease has made this complication infrequent. Several series[11,12] of osteotomy, usually performed at the apex of the deformity, have been reported with good results in most cases. The surgical correction of any major deformity of the thoracic spine or the thoracolumbar junction is a formidable surgical undertaking with significant risk of neurologic impairment.[11,12] In our opinion, the osteotomy should be performed via the bilateral posterolateral extracavitary approach to the spine with intraoperative monitoring by means of either somatosensory-evoked potential or intraoperative awakening of the patient to evaluate anterior spinal cord function. The relatively new technique of motor-evoked potentials, that is, evaluation of descending pathways, holds promise, but is more difficult technically. It has the advantage of monitoring the function of the anterior portion of the spinal cord, which is usually more vulnerable during the surgical correction. Correction of thoracolumbar spine angulation is a major and hazardous surgical undertaking that should be performed in larger medical centers having specialists in spine surgery.

Lesser degrees of deformity of the thoracic spine causing nerve root compression are rare. In older patients especially, neoplasia is a more common cause for localized spine pain and radiculopathy. Thoracic disc herniations with cord compression and myelopathy do occur, usually as sporadic cases not associated with arthritic conditions. The signs and symptoms of thoracic disc herniations are highly variable, and diagnosis is often delayed. Usually, the most efficient way to screen the many segments of the thoracic spine

for significant deformity causing neural compression is with MRI.

LUMBOSACRAL SPINE

During the past 15 years, arthritic deformity of the lumbar spine has been well described clinically and radiologically. Consequently, effective treatment, usually by decompression, has become commonly available. Simple uncomplicated lumbar disc ruptures are infrequent in individuals who are over 40 (Fig. 8–5).[13] The progressive collapse of disc height inevitably leads to facet joint overriding and subsequent arthritis, shortening and thickening of the elastic ligamentum flavum, and osteophyte formation from the joint margins (Fig. 8–8).[14] The clinical syndrome of neurogenic claudication of the legs secondary to lumbar spinal stenosis became commonly recognized in the early 1970s. Diagnostic radiologists then began to use pleuridirectional tomographic scanning in defining the size and shape of the lumbar spinal canal in axial cross sections.[15] In the late 1970s, use of a high-resolution CT scanning to the lumbar spine rendered tomographic equipment obsolete and made precise diagnosis routinely available. The syndrome of neurogenic claudication with position (extension) or exercise-induced radiculopathy is effectively treated by lumbar laminectomy with removal of the medial portion of the facet joints and attendant hypertrophied ligaments and osteophytes. Infrequently, a synovial cyst or ganglion will develop and compress a nerve root. Several techniques have been described to accomplish this decompression of the nerve roots of the cauda equina.[16] The lumbar spine need not be destabilized, however, by complete removal of the facet joints. Surgical undercutting, occasionally aided by the use of high-speed drills, provides neural decompression. This procedure is usually just as adequate as more radical surgery and allows continued structural support from the lateral and posterior aspects of the facet joints. On rare occasions, the facet joints may be located so far medially that they must be destabilized to allow complete decompression.

Mechanical instability may accompany and/or accelerate dural canal compression. Degenerative spondylolisthesis, most commonly at the L4–L5 level, occurs as the facet complex degenerates with sagittally oriented facet.[17] Rarely, progressive neurologic symptoms will arise at segments having previously stable idiopathic adolescent spondylolisthesis. Mechanically or surgically destabilized lumbar segments should be considered for fusion. We prefer the bilateral posterolateral technique incorporating the facet joints and transverse processes in the fusion mass.[18]

A few patients, usually middle aged, have mild disc degenerative and arthritic changes superimposed on a congenitally small spinal canal. Some of these patient have severe degeneration and bulging of all the lumbar discs, requiring extensive laminectomy, occasionally of the entire lumbar spine. However, most surgical patients are in the older age groups, and neoplasia must be considered in the differential diagnosis. Radionuclide bone scanning, in addition to a detailed history and physical examination, is routinely performed in the patient over 50.

SURGICAL PROCEDURES

LAMINECTOMY

In general, extensive laminectomies are well tolerated, provided the facet joints are surgically spared to provide stability and support.[19,20] Reversal of the cervical lordosis or swan-neck deformity has been described.[20] However, with only rare exceptions, these extensive operations are performed in cases of intramedullary tumor where denervation of paraspinous musculature coexists. Nevertheless, any individual in the younger age group, particularly children and ad-

FIG. 52–3. Postoperative roentgenograms of a 64-year-old woman with degenerative osteoarthritis. Internal fixation was used because of this patient's increased risk of nonunion. The system anchors multiple vertebrae to bilateral posterior Steffes plates using pedicle screws.

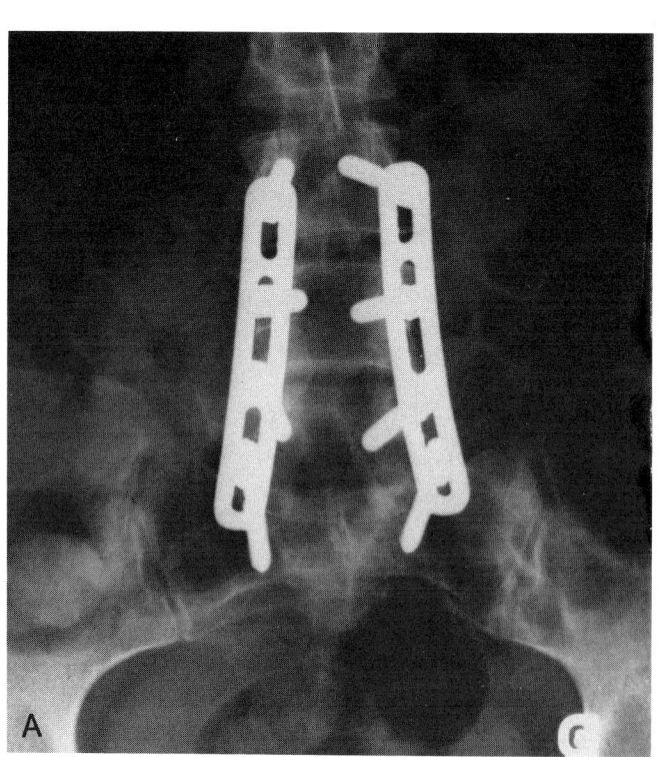
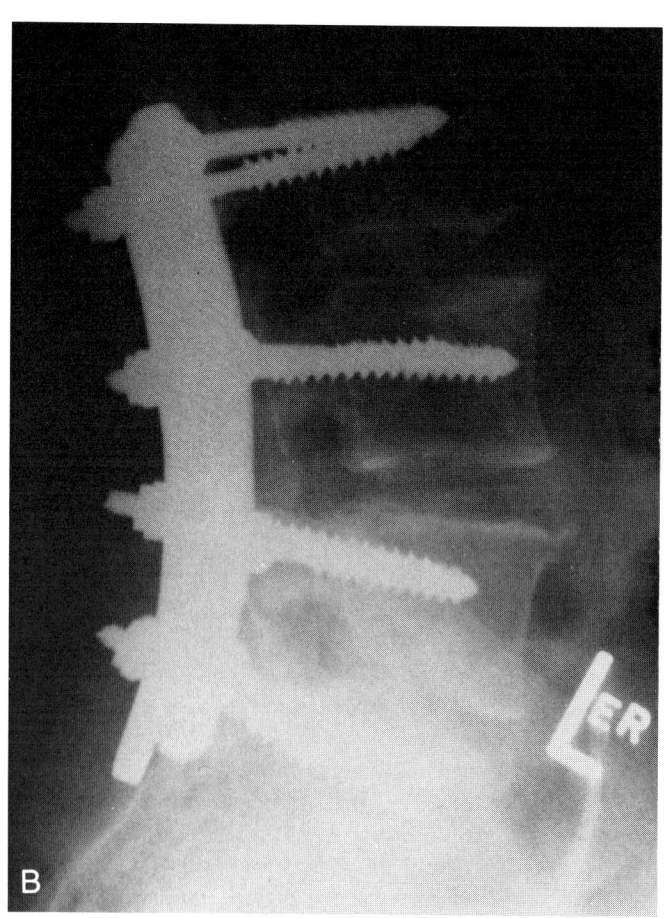

olescents, should have serial cervical spine roentgenograms taken at increasing intervals for several years to ensure that progressive deformity is not developing.

The most frequent complication of laminectomy in the older individual is disruption of the dural membrane with the risk of persistent cerebrospinal fluid fistula, pseudomeningocele, and/or infection. The dural sac becomes ectatic with age and must be clearly identified, covered with protective sponges, and gently retracted during decompressive techniques directed to the lateral portions of the spinal canal and intervertebral foramina. If the dura is torn, one should attempt to repair it with fine, nonabsorbable suture material. A few of the patients requiring cervical decompressive laminectomy for stenosis may need further decompression by opening the dural sac and sectioning the dentate ligaments. The intradural contents is protected by suturing a patch graft of fascia to the entire circumference of the dural defect.

There are several descriptions of reconstruction techniques of the laminal arch following intraspinal operative manipulations.[25] These techniques have little if any clinical applicability.

FUSION

Anterior cervical fusion using the technique described by Cloward and others is satisfactory at all levels from C2–C3 through C7–T1.[10] The use of dowel grafts in round drill holes as described by Cloward[10] is mechanically unsound, however, and a better fusion can be performed by surgical evacuation of the interspace. This procedure is aided by interspace-spreading retractors to facilitate removal of the entire cartilaginous end plate. Bone and osteophyte are removed as necessary to provide adequate neural decompression. Finally, an autogenous bone graft (cross section of the iliac crest) is placed in the interspace.

In the thoracic and upper lumbar areas, the fusion is best performed via a posterolateral exposure of the vertebral column.[21] In rare cases, a bilateral approach is required, followed by fixation instrumentation. Direct anterior approaches to the thoracic spine require chest cavity entry and, at the thoracolumbar level, incision and reconstruction of the diaphragm. Increased morbidity accompanies these extensive intracavitary approaches to the spine, and they are rarely necessary.

At lower lumbar levels, the posterolateral transverse process fusion has proved satisfactory. Single-level fusions heal with a predictably high rate in the nonsmoker.[6] Progressive levels of fusion, poor bone

stock or nutritional status, and smoking dramatically reduce the chances for a solid fusion.[22] The addition of internal fixation to these high-risk patients may improve fusion rates (Fig. 52–3). The posterior lumbar interbody fusion (PLIF) may occasionally be appropriate.[23] It does require removal of large portions of the facet joint and entails forceful dural sac and nerve root retraction. With anomalous conjoined lumbosacral nerve roots, the risk of permanent nerve root damage may make PLIF infeasible.

Fusions that rely on methylmethacrylate for their structural stability are rarely if ever indicated in nonmalignant disease. Acrylic, even when pins or wires are used, can and frequently does loosen with time. The risk of infection is also increased.[24]

REFERENCES

 1. Dirheimer, Y.: The Cranio-Vertebral Region in Chronic Inflammatory Rheumatic Diseases. New York, Springer-Verlag, 1977.
 2. Haughton, V., and Williams, A.: Computed Tomography of the Spine. St. Louis, C.V. Mosby, 1982.
 3. Lee, B.C.P., Kaza, E., and Newman, A.D.: Computed tomography of the spine and spinal cord. Radiology, 128:95–102, 1978.
 4. Menezes, A.H., Graf, J., and Hibri, N.: Abnormalities of the craniovertebral junction with cervicomedullary compression. Childs Brain, 7:15–30, 1980.
 5. VanGilder, J.C., and Menezes, A.H.: Craniovertebral junction abnormalities. Clin. Neurosurg., 30:514–530, 1982.
 6. Hall, M.C.: Luschka's Joint. Springfield, IL, Charles C Thomas, 1965.
 7. Murakami, J., et al.: Computed tomography of posterior longitudinal ligament ossification: Its appearance and diagnostic value with special reference to thoracic lesions. J. Comput. Assist. Tomogr., 6:41–50, 1982.
 8. Resnick, D.R., et al.: Association of diffuse idiopathic skeletal hyperostosis (DISH) and calcifications of the posterior longitudinal ligament. Am. J. Roentgenol., 131:1049–1053, 1978.
 9. Yonenobu, K., et al.: Choice of surgical treatment for multisegmental cervical spondylitic myelopathy. Spine, 10:710–716, 1985.
10. Cloward, R.B.: Anterior approach for removal of ruptured cervical discs. J. Neurosurg., 15:602–614, 1958.
11. Law, W.A.: Lumbar spinal osteotomy. J. Bone Joint Surg., 41B:270–278, 1959.
12. Simmons, E.J.: Kyphotic deformity of the spine in ankylosing spondylitis. Clin. Orthop., 128:65–77, 1977.
13. Meyer, G.A., Haughton, V.M., and Williams, A.M.: Diagnosis of the herniated lumbar disc with computed tomography. N. Engl. J. Med., 306:1166–1167, 1979.
14. Verbeist, H.: A radicular syndrome from developmental narrowing of the lumbar vertebral canal. J. Bone Joint Surg., 36B:230, 1954.
15. Sheldon, J.J., Russin, L.A., and Gargano, F.P.: Lumbar spinal stenosis. Radiographic diagnosis with special references to transverse axial tomography. Clin. Orthop., 115:53, 1976.
16. Ehni, G.: Significance of the small lumbar spinal canal: Cauda equina compression syndromes due to spondylosis. I. Introduction. J. Neurosurg., 31:490–494, 1969.

17. Lombardi, J.S., et al.: Treatment of degenerative spondylolisthesis. Spine, *10*:821–827, 1985.

18. Schwab, J.P., and Meyer, G.A.: Lumbar fusion. Wis. Med.J., *78*:40–42, 1979.

19. Davis, C.H., Jr.: Extradural spinal cord and nerve root compression from benign lesions of the lumbar area. *In* Neurological Surgery. Vol. 4. Edited by J.R. Youmans. Philadelphia, W.B. Saunders, 1982.

20. Rothman, R.H., and Simeone, F.A. (eds.): The Spine. Vols. 1 and 2. Philadelphia, W.B. Saunders, 1986.

21. Larson, S.J.: The lateral extrapleural and extraperitoneal approaches to the thoracic and lumbar spine. *In* Spinal Disorders: Diagnosis and Treatment. Edited by D. Ruge and L.L. Wiltse. Philadelphia, Lea & Febiger, 1977.

22. Brown, C.W.B., Orme, T.J., and Richardson, H.D.: The rate of pseudarthrosis in patients who are smokers and who are non-smokers: A comparison study. Spine, *11*:942–943, 1986.

23. Cloward, R.B.: The treatment of ruptured lumbar intervertebral discs by vertebral body fusion. J. Neurosurg., *10*:154, 1953.

24. McAfee, P.C., et al.: Failure of stabilization of the spine with methylmethacrylate. A retrospective analysis of 24 cases. J. Bone Joint Surg., *68A*:1145–1157, 1986.

25. Raimondi, A.J., Gutierrez, F.A., Di Rocco, C.: Laminotomy and total reconstruction of the posterior spinal arch for spinal canal surgery in childhood. J. Neurosurg., *45*:555–560, 1976.

53

CORRECTION OF ARTHRITIC DEFORMITIES OF THE HIP

RICHARD N. STAUFFER

Deformity of the hip joint occurs as a result of a wide variety of arthritic conditions, including degenerative, inflammatory, and infectious diseases. Degenerative disease (osteoarthritis, OA) is certainly the most common cause of hip joint disability. This category includes primary OA affecting older people, in which no predisposing causative factors can be identified, and secondary OA resulting from altered joint mechanics caused by previous trauma, osteonecrosis of the femoral head, or various other congenital or developmental conditions of the hip (e.g., congenital hip dysplasia, slipped capital femoral epiphysis, Legg-Calvé-Perthes disease). Because of the broad spectrum of these disease categories, disability from arthritis of the hip may afflict virtually all age groups, though it is most common in persons 60 years or over.

On the basis of epidemiologic studies, it is estimated that over 100,000 people undergo reconstructive surgery for hip disease in the United States each year. The surgical procedures described for correction of hip deformities can be combined and classified as joint excision, realignment (osteotomy), arthrodesis, or prosthetic arthroplasty.

Historically, reconstructions of the hip were first attempted chiefly for tuberculosis and consisted of various types of joint excision and arthrodesis. In the 1930s, there was great interest in interposition arthroplasty. Various materials (e.g., skin, fascia, Bakelite) were interposed between the acetabulum and femoral head in an attempt to produce a smooth, congruent articulation—without notable success. The development of the mold arthroplasty by Smith-Pe-

tersen (in which a Vitallium cup was interposed in the joint and provided a "mold" or scaffold for regeneration of fibrocartilage on both acetabular and femoral articular surfaces) represented a major breakthrough in reconstructive hip surgery. This procedure relieved pain, restored joint motion, and maintained stability in a *reasonably* predictable fashion, becoming the standard against which other procedures were measured for over 30 years.

Osteotomy of the proximal femur was popularized by Pauwels, and others, as a treatment for some forms of arthritic hip disorders. This technique, which redistributes the mechanical forces acting across the hip joint, has recently gained renewed interest for use in younger persons.

Prosthetic replacement of the arthritic hip joint began with the use of a Vitallium femoral head prosthesis in 1942. This procedure gained popularity during the 1950s, in spite of two commonly recognized problems: loosening of the prosthetic shaft within the intramedullary canal of the femur, and erosion of the articular surface of the acetabulum by the prosthesis. These problems were addressed by the landmark work of Charnley and others in the late 1950s. The problem of prosthetic loosening was combated by the introduction of a self-curing acrylic cement, polymethylmethacrylate, a grouting agent designed to improve fixation between prosthetic component and bone. A prosthetic acetabular component made of high-density polyethylene was added to form a "low-friction" total hip replacement, providing a dramatic breakthrough in improved function and pain relief for persons disabled by hip diseases. The rate of successful results from prosthetic hip replacement increased from about 60% to over 90%. Clinical and basic investigations in recent years have further refined the design, mechanical function, and materials of prostheses with further improvement in clinical outcome.

The reconstructive surgical procedures currently used to treat hip disease are discussed in the following sections.

OSTEOTOMY

Osteotomy is aimed primarily at relieving pain and only secondarily at improving motion. This procedure involves cutting the bone of the proximal femur and realigning the fragments to alter the distribution of forces acting across the hip, or to improve the congruency of the joint. Proximal femoral osteotomies can be grouped into two general categories, angulatory and rotational, which differ somewhat in rationale and indication.

ANGULATORY OSTEOTOMY

This procedure consists of removal of a medially or laterally based wedge of bone from the intertrochanteric region of the proximal femur, to produce either a varus or valgus angulation of the femoral neck and head (Figs. 53–1, 53–2). Careful preoperative planning is required to determine the mode (and precise degree) of angulation and to produce the maximum congruency of the arthritic femoral head within the acetabulum. After the osteotomy, the bony fragments are held with some form of internal fixation, either a fixed-angle osteotomy blade plate or a compression screw plate. Partial and progressive weight-bearing with crutches is allowed. Bony union is consistently obtained within 12 weeks.

The rationale for this procedure is that the resulting, improved congruency of the joint alters the distribution of load acting across the hip. Reducing the peak pressures that exist in the arthritic joint may allow for some biologic repair of the articular cartilage (Fig. 53–3). Purely mathematical analysis has indicated that a valgus osteotomy may decrease the magnitude and direction of the compressive load across the hip (see Fig. 53–2). An unusual case in which the primary aim of the procedure was to change the direction of the resultant hip load is shown in Figure 53–4. The pain relief from this procedure has been postulated as resulting from decompression of the increased intraosseous venous pressure noted in OA or to an interosseous neurectomy.

Angulatory osteotomy of the proximal femur was a popular form of treatment for the arthritic hip before the advent of total hip replacement. Because recent longterm followup studies have aroused grave concern regarding the durability of prosthetic hips, particularly in young people, osteotomy is again becoming more prevalent. Osteotomy has several definite advantages. There is a high incidence of pain relief.[1] Also, it is a "conservative" procedure. All bony stock is preserved, allowing subsequent surgery (including prosthetic hip replacement or arthrodesis) if necessary. No foreign material is placed in the hip joint. Postoperative disability is minimal, and formal rehabilitation is unnecessary. Its chief disadvantages are inconsistency of pain relief and pain relief of relatively

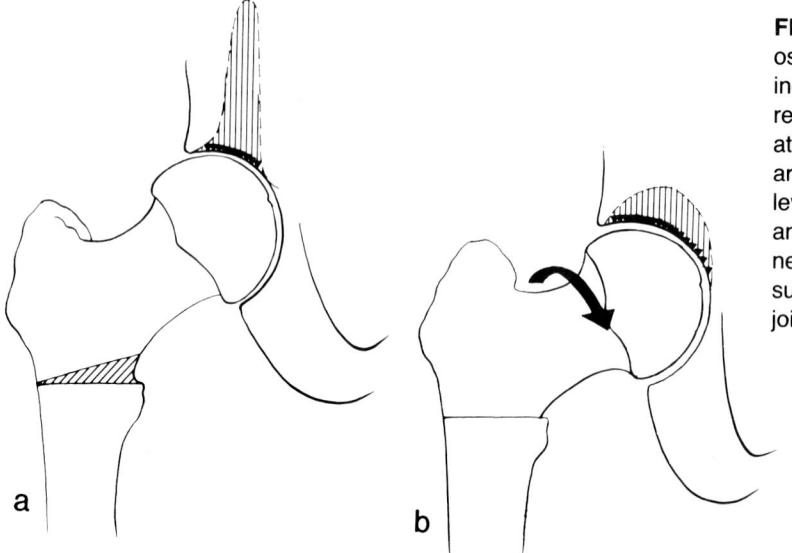

FIG. 53–1. Schematic representation of varus osteotomy of the proximal femur. *A,* Shaded area indicates the medially based wedge of bone to be removed from the intertrochanteric area. Degenerative changes in the joint have resulted in a small area of surface contact and high compressive stress levels. *B,* Medial displacement of the femoral shaft and medial (varus) rotation of the femoral head and neck have improved congruency of the articulating surfaces, increased the load-bearing area of the joint, and reduced compression stresses.

a   b

FIG. 53–2. Schematic representation of valgus osteotomy of the proximal femur. *A,* Shaded area indicates the laterally based wedge of bone to be removed from the intertrochanteric area. *B,* Lateral (valgus) rotation of the femoral head and neck. The increased congruity and enlarged surface contact area have reduced the compression stresses across the joint.

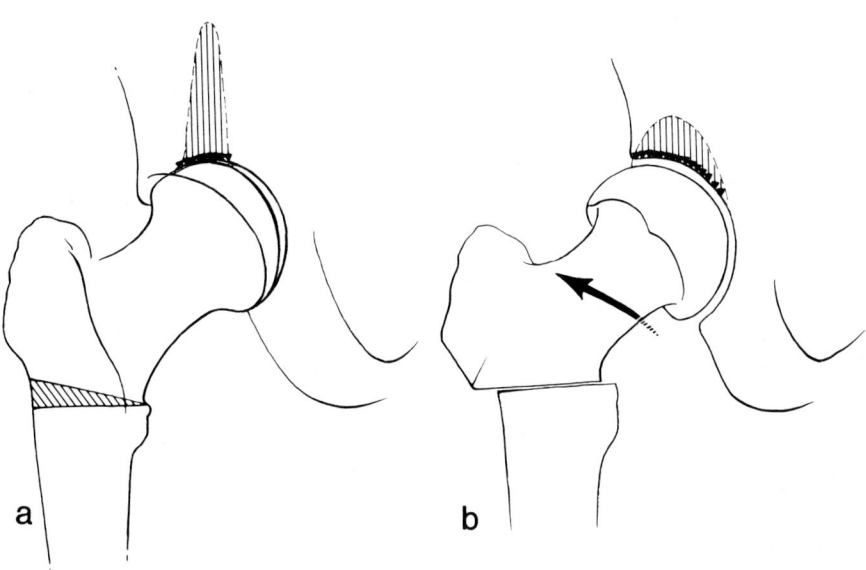

FIG. 53–3. Roentgenographic appearance of a degenerative hip joint before and after angulatory (varus) osteotomy of the proximal femur. *A,* Degenerative arthritis of the hip in a 61-year-old man. *B,* Two and one-half years after varus osteotomy. Note the definite "widening" of the joint space, and some resolution of the degenerative sclerosis and cysts. The patient had excellent relief of hip pain.

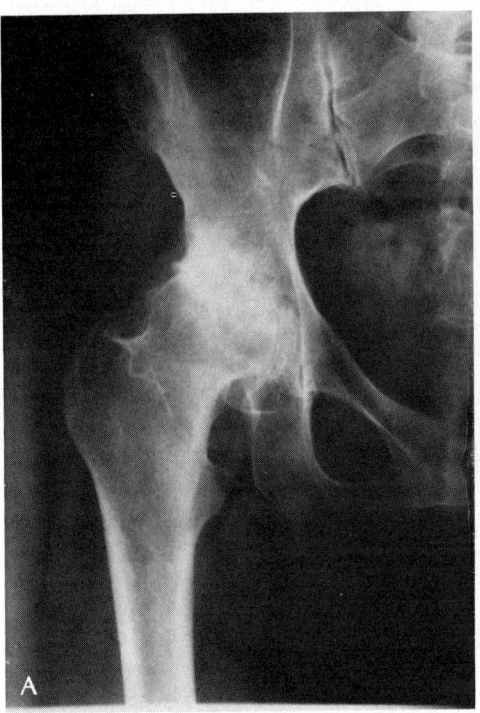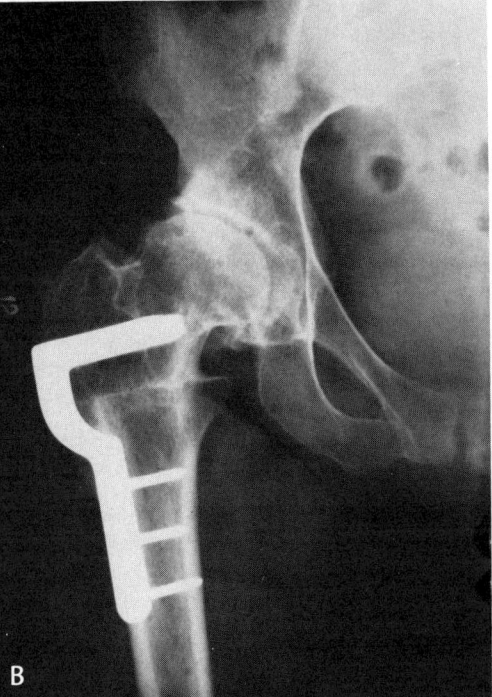

FIG. 53–4. Roentgenographic appearance of bilateral valgus osteotomies performed for protrusio acetabuli. *A*, Preoperative hip roentgenogram of a 21-year-old man with bilateral hip pain. No metabolic cause for the unusual and severe protrusion of the acetabula could be determined. The only structural abnormality was the decreased neck-shaft angle (normal is 135°). This condition is presumably the result of a developmental anomaly (coxa vara) of the hips, which resulted in an increased horizontal inclination of the resultant load acting on the hip, and gradual medial protrusion of the acetabula caused by bone remodeling. *B*, Postoperative hip roentgenograms 1 year after bilateral valgus osteotomies. The patient's hip pain was dramatically reduced. Careful long-term followup will be necessary, however, to evaluate remodeling of the acetabula and possible improvement of the protrusion.

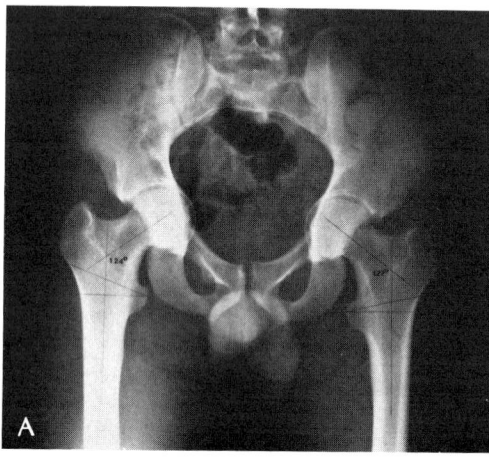

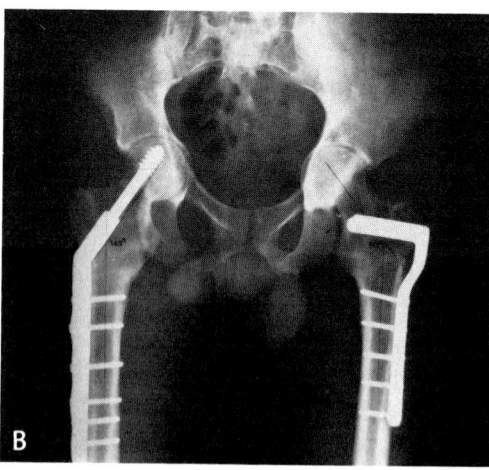

short duration (3 to 5 years) with gradual deterioration of the clinical result, until further surgery is required.

The chief indication for angulatory osteotomy of the proximal femur is OA, particularly in a younger (under 50 years) person. Success depends on the presence of adequate hip motion (at least 20° of coronal plane motion) and the probability that changing the angular relationship of the femoral head and acetabulum will result in better joint congruency.

Results are difficult to evaluate objectively because the chief aim is to relieve pain, a subjective parameter. Of 103 hips followed for more than 1 year after varus or valgus osteotomy, 83 had satisfactory pain relief, and 20 had fair or poor results.[2] In another study of 59 consecutive osteotomies, followed for an average of 2½ years, in which clinical evaluation criteria included improved range of hip motion, need for assistive gait devices, resolution of degenerative changes on roentgenograms, and pain relief, 47 (80%) were satisfactory and 12 (20%) proved unsatisfactory.[3] Pain relief closely paralleled the roentgenographic findings of increased joint space, and resolution of body sclerosis, marginal osteophytes, and subchondral cysts.

Bombelli has been largely responsible for the increased interest in angulatory osteotomy for osteoarthritis of the hip.[1] Of 170 osteotomies followed for over 10 years, 76% had good or excellent long-term pain relief and function. Improved range of hip motion was inconsistent. Several authors have noted a gradual deterioration of the pain relief obtained by this procedure. In one report, 74% of patients were pain-free at 1 year postoperatively, but only 45% at 5 years.[4] In another series, only 25% of patients still had pain relief after 10 years.[5]

Complications include problems encountered with any major hip surgical procedure, that is, cardiopulmonary disorders, thromboembolic disease, urinary retention, infection, delayed wound healing, hematoma, as well as two unique complications. Nonunion of the osteotomy site has been reported to range from 0 to 18%. An internal fixation device allowing compression of the osteotomy site greatly reduces the incidence of nonunion. The fixation device itself, however, often leads to another problem: irritation of the soft tissues and bursal formation in the trochanteric area. In one series, 17% of patients required eventual removal of the compression device because of localized lateral hip discomfort.[5] Because the angulatory osteotomy is performed in the intertrochanteric area, there is little danger of compromise of the extraosseous arterial blood supply to the femoral head, and avascular necrosis has not been reported as a complication.

ROTATIONAL OSTEOTOMY

The search continues for a satisfactory surgical treatment for avascular necrosis of the femoral head, which so frequently affects young persons. Osteonecrosis arises as a result of compromise of the intraosseous blood supply of the femoral head from various causes (see Table 86–1). Treatment by angulatory osteotomy has been disappointing.[6] Sugioka has popularized a rotational osteotomy of the femoral head and neck.[7] In this procedure, the avascular segment of the femoral head, most commonly the anterosuperior portion, is rotated anteriorly, away from the area of maximum compressive loading of the joint, preventing further collapse of the segment and allowing revascularization and repair of the necrotic bone.

The procedure is technically demanding. The osteotomy is performed through the intertrochanteric area, distal to the base of the femoral neck. Complete or circumferential division of the joint capsule is necessary. Great care is required to avoid damage to the ascending branch of the medial circumflex artery, inferiorly and posteriorly. The femoral head and neck are rotated anteriorly 50 to 70° while the necrotic portion of the head is placed anterior to the weight-bearing area of the joint. Internal fixation may be achieved by various devices, most commonly a sliding compression screw plate. Postoperatively, active range of motion exercises are started within 10 days, and nonweight-bearing ambulation with crutches is maintained for 8 to 12 weeks, followed by graduation to full weight-bearing by 6 months.

Approximately 80% relief of pain and prevention of collapse of the necrotic segment was found in one series of 100 hips followed for 2 to 7 years postoperatively.[7] The best results were obtained in those hips operated on in the early stages of the disease process. Fully 91% excellent results occurred in hips graded state I or II (see Chapter 86), before marked collapse of the femoral head or narrowing of the joint space occurred. Hips with an extensive area of necrotic involvement showed a higher failure rate; if over two thirds of the femoral heads were involved, 46% failed. Bilateral hip involvement showed a high failure rate (43%) also. The poor results with bilateral hip involvement can perhaps be explained by the difficulty in maintaining postoperative nonweight-bearing with crutches after both hips have undergone osteotomy.

The indication for rotational osteotomy of the femoral head and neck is avascular necrosis in a relatively young person. Contraindications are end stage disease with collapse of the head and degenerative changes in the acetabulum (Ficat grades III and IV),[8] more than two thirds avascular involvement of the femoral head, and bilateral hip disease.

Several reports of experience with rotational osteotomy have not supported the initial enthusiasm. Gartland and Dethoff reported successful results in about two thirds of cases at 1 to 2 years, but in 12 patients followed for over 3 years, deterioration was progressive, and only four cases were still rated as satisfactory.[9] Most of the unsatisfactory results after 3 years were in patients with corticosteroid-related avascular necrosis. Cabanela followed 17 hip cases in 16 patients for 6 to 24 months.[10] Eight hips showed a good clinical result judged by pain relief, range of motion, and ability to perform daily activities; results were fair in three hips and poor in six. Radionuclide scintigrams of the femoral heads still showed complete avascularity after the osteotomy, with no improvement with time in most cases.

Complications encountered after rotational osteotomy include those general and local problems attendant to any major hip surgical procedure. Occasional delayed unions of the osteotomy site, but no nonunion, have been reported. The procedure is technically difficult, controversial, and still in the evaluation stage. Other treatment modalities currently in clinical trial for the troublesome problem of avascular necrosis of the femoral head in young people are drilling and decompression of the avascular segment, and electrical stimulation by various techniques (see Chapter 86).

ARTHRODESIS

Arthrodesis of the hip was reportedly first performed by Albert in 1885. Over the past century, this procedure has been used primarily for hip joints destroyed by sepsis. For the past several decades, however, it has been employed more commonly to treat disability caused by post-traumatic degenerative disease in the young person. With the realization that prosthetic arthroplasty has a limited durability with unacceptable long-term results in youthful, active persons, hip arthrodesis has enjoyed increasing popularity. Although the idea of arthrodesis or "permanent stiffening" of the hip joint is often difficult for a patient to accept, it is often the best treatment alternative available, particularly in the young male laborer with disabling, unilateral post-traumatic hip disease.

Many techniques for hip arthrodesis have been described. These include various intra-articular, extra-articular, and combined methods, with and without internal fixation, and with and without adjunctive bone grafts. The reported pseudarthrosis rate for all these procedures was about 25%. The most common technique now employed is an intra-articular arthrodesis using a "cobra-head" compression plate (Fig. 53–5). This device provides rigid fixation across the joint, and pseudarthrosis rates approach zero.[11] Al-

FIG. 53–5. Anteroposterior roentgenogram of a 35-year-old man 3 years after a compression arthrodesis of the left hip for degenerative disease secondary to a slipped capital femoral epiphysis (note previous pin fixation for a similar, but less severe problem in right hip). The hip arthrodesis is solid, but the discerning observer will note an unusual serpentine stress fracture through the medial acetabular portion of the hip. The patient was treated with spica cast immobilization and an external induction-type electrical stimulator.

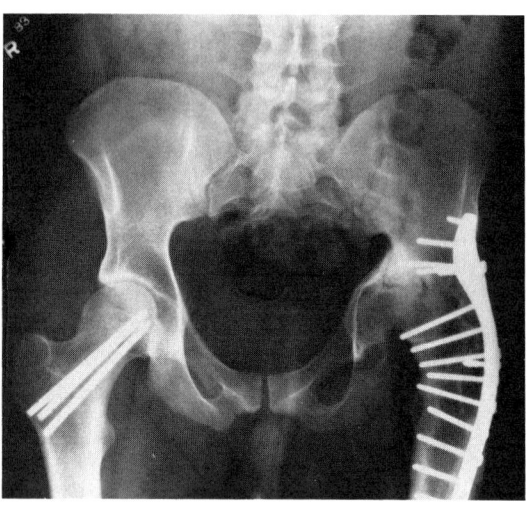

though this plate is somewhat malleable and can be conformed to the bony contours across the hip, some form of medial displacement of the femoral head is generally necessary. This can be accomplished by medial displacement innominate osteotomy, displacement of the femoral head through the medial wall of the acetabulum, or extensive reaming of the femoral head.

Although some degree of shortening of the extremity is inevitable with hip arthrodesis, it should be kept to a minimum, no more than 1 to 2 cm, if possible. The recommended position of fusion is 30° of flexion, neutral abduction-adduction, and 5 to 10° of external rotation. Postoperative immobilization in a plaster spica body cast, incorporating the trunk and the operated thigh, for 8 to 12 weeks is recommended, but may not be necessary with a cooperative patient. Partial weight-bearing with crutches is started at about 2 weeks postoperatively, with full weight-bearing allowed at 10 to 12 weeks.

The primary indications for hip arthrodesis are destruction of the joint by sepsis (pyogenic or tuberculous infection), Charcot arthropathy, or disabling unilateral degenerative disease, particularly in the youthful, active male laborer. The procedure is less desirable in the young female patient because of imposed functional difficulties associated with sexual intercourse and childbearing. Avascular necrosis of the femoral head is a relative contraindication, especially if there is extensive involvement of the head with necrotic, nonviable bone, because the disease process is frequently bilateral. D'Aubigne et al. reported a 50% pseudarthrosis rate for hip arthrodesis performed for this condition.[6] Arthrodesis of the rheumatoid hip should be avoided, because of the accompanying disease of the opposite hip and other lower extremity joints.

The long-term results reported with hip arthrodesis depend largely on achievement of ideal position of fusion and the integrity of other lower extremity joints. One report of 23 patients with unilateral hip fusion, followed for 10 to 30 years, showed that 21 were working regularly and leading active, vigorous lives.[12] Most were entirely satisfied with the long-term results of surgery, although over half experienced a discernible limp, and one third had difficulty sitting. Nearly half reported difficulties with low-back pain, and a few patients had pain in the ipsilateral knee or contralateral hip.

Gore et al. studied the gait mechanics of men with unilateral hip fusions.[13] Their gait was slower than normal, asymmetric, and arrhythmic, as might be expected. Several compensatory gait mechanisms were adopted by these patients, including increased rotation and flexion of the pelvis (i.e., increased motion of the lumbar spine), increased motion of the contralateral hip, and increased flexion of the ipsilateral knee during stance phase. Because all these compensatory gait alterations impose increased stresses on the low back and other lower extremity joints, they are likely responsible for an increased rate of degenerative change in these areas over the years.

Operative complications, in addition to those common to all major hip surgery procedures, include long-term degenerative disease of other joints and fracture of the femur; this latter complication has been reported in several series. Arthrodesis of the hip creates a long, rigid body segment from the lumbosacral joint to the knee. Because torsional or bending loads cannot be absorbed by the hip joint, fracture of the femur is therefore more likely to result from a fall or twisting injury. Most series of hip fusions have a 10 to 20% incidence of pseudarthrosis, but use of newer techniques, such as medial displacement of the femoral head, and the cobra-head plate for internal fixation, have significantly reduced this complication. No nonunions occurred in a series of 16 patients treated with these newer techniques.[11]

Conversion of a failed total hip arthroplasty to arthrodesis is possible when remaining bone stock is insufficient to permit reinsertion of prosthetic components, or when leaving a young patient with an unstable girdle stone-type hip is undesirable. This procedure is technically difficult and requires adjunctive bone grafting and a cobra-head plate for firm fixation. It also generally results in considerable shortening of the extremity.

Conversely, conversion of an arthrodesed hip to a total arthroplasty is also possible.[14] This procedure is not particularly difficult, but depends on the integrity of the abductor musculature and the absence of active sepsis. Conversion of an arthrodesed hip is most often indicated because of long-standing low-back or ipsilateral knee pain, which occurs particularly with a malpositioned hip fusion. Rehabilitation is often prolonged compared to other total hip patients. Generally, crutch walking is necessary for 6 months until the abductor muscles are strong enough to prevent a limp. Satisfactory results with an average range of hip flexion of 76° were found in 31 of 33 patients whose arthrodesed hips were converted to total hip arthroplasties.

PROSTHETIC HIP REPLACEMENT

A variety of prosthetic devices are currently used to replace arthritic hips. These devices are discussed here with those procedures that replace only the femoral side of the joint with no surgical alteration of the acetabulum (hemiarthroplasty) and those that involve replacement of both sides of the hip (total hip replacement).

HEMIARTHROPLASTY

There are two generic types of prosthetic replacement of only the femoral side of the joint. The first, the femoral head prosthesis, has been in use for over 40 years, and involves implantation of a metallic prosthesis that replaces the head and neck of the femur with fixation by a stem that fits into the medullary canal. In the past 15 years, however, the prosthesis stem has often been fixed in the medullary canal with methylmethacrylate to combat loosening (Fig. 53–6). The acetabulum is not surgically altered with this type of prosthesis, but careful sizing of the prosthesis is necessary to provide a congruent fit. A poorly fitting prosthetic femoral head may result in joint instability and "point contact" with increased localized loading and subsequent erosion of the articular cartilage of the acetabulum.[15]

The bipolar type of prosthesis, the second type, consists of a metallic femoral component, generally

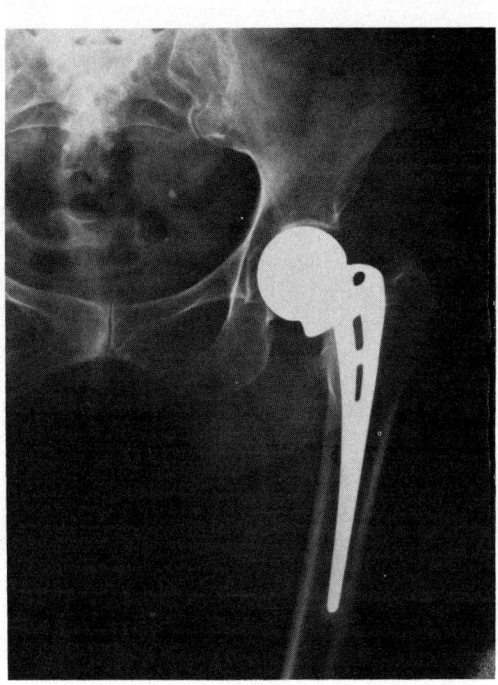

FIG. 53–6. Anteroposterior roentgenogram of a 78-year-old woman who had a femoral head prosthesis (Austin-Moore type) inserted 2 years previously for a displaced femoral neck fracture. Narrowing of the joint "space" superomedially indicates erosion of the prosthesis through the articular cartilage. The patient was experiencing progressive hip pain.

fixed into the medullary canal with methylmethacrylate, which is "snap fitted" into a high-density polyethylene socket, surrounded by a metallic shell (Fig. 53–7). The rationale behind this design is that it theoretically permits motion at both the femoral head polyethylene bearing and the interface between the metal shell and the articular cartilage of the acetabulum. Both clinical and basic laboratory studies, however, have shown that little motion actually occurs within the acetabulum because of the larger frictional properties of that interface.[16] The other theoretic advantage of this design is that later conversion into a total hip replacement is possible. Should the patient develop pain because of erosion of acetabular cartilage, the acetabular component can be replaced by one that is compatible with the femoral component and that is then cemented into the pelvis.

The indications for both types of hip hemiarthroplasty appear to be the same, namely, avascular necrosis of the femoral head, displaced (Garden type III or IV) fracture of the femoral neck, nonunion of femoral neck fractures, or certain arthritic diseases of the hip joint in which the acetabular cartilage has been relatively spared. Both procedures can be performed with minimal operating/anesthesia time because

FIG. 53–7. Appearance of the bipolar hip prosthesis. *A*, Photograph of disarticular components of bipolar hip prosthesis. *B*, Roentgenographic appearance of bipolar hip prosthesis. The femoral component is cemented in place. The acetabular component is free to rotate within the pelvis.

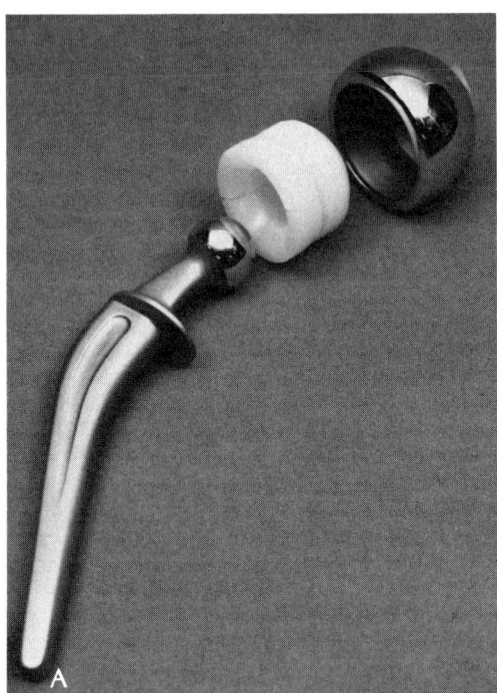
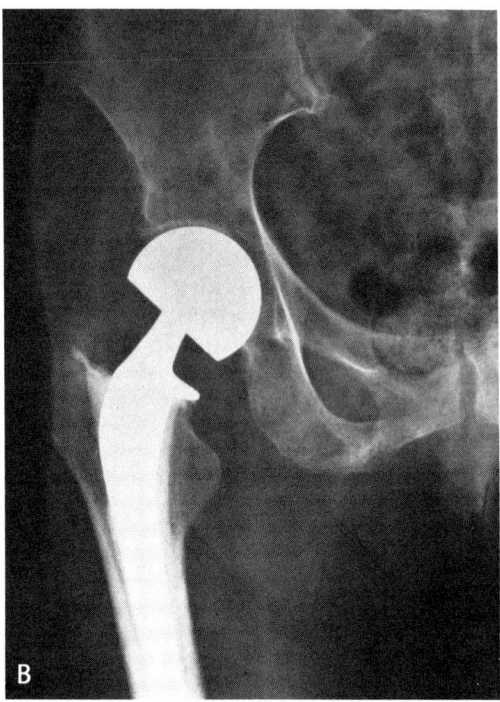

reaming, preparation, and cementing of the acetabulum, as in total hip replacement, are unnecessary. Operative time is often an important factor with hip surgery in frail, elderly patients.

Disadvantages include significant problems with residual hip pain, acetabular erosion, or protrusion, and femoral stem loosening.[17–19] The causes of these problems include the high frictional torque between the acetabular cartilage and the large, metallic head, excessive shear forces acting across the articular cartilage with joint motion, decreased damping of high-frequency vibration (loss of shock absorption) across the joint, and uneven loading patterns caused by mismatching of the radius of curvature of the acetabulum and femoral head.

The bipolar hip replacement prothesis was developed in the early 1970s in an attempt to obviate at least some of these problems. It was thought that the use of a small head size (22 mm) and a metal to polyethylene bearing surface, and the provision of compound motion between the inner and outer bearing surfaces, would decrease the frictional torque and high shear stress on the acetabular cartilage and increase the damping characteristics of the joint, and

that cementing of the femoral component would decrease the loosening problem.

Unfortunately, several other problems inherent in the design features of the bipolar device have come to light, including both outer and inner bearing separation and dislocation, and fracture of the polyethylene bearing.[20] In addition, acetabular erosion and wear, while less common with the bipolar prosthesis, have also been reported. The older designs showed a definite tendency for the acetabular component to drift into a varus position, thereby increasing the risk of dislocation or component fracture. More recent designs have largely eliminated these problems by provision of an eccentric offset between the center of the inner head and the outer component.[21] This "positive eccentricity" causes the acetabular component to assume a valgus position with vertical loading of the hip.

Yamagata et al.[22] reported a retrospective comparison of a large clinical series of patients having the two types of hip hemiarthroplasty. Femoral component loosening was slightly more frequent in the bipolar group, while acetabular erosion was more common in the femoral head replacement group. Fixation of the femoral component with bone cement led to a lower femoral component loosening and revision rate with both types of devices. By 8 years postoperatively, 23% of the femoral head replacement devices and 14% of the bipolar devices had to be revised because of hip pain. Both prosthetic devices are useful in reconstructive hip surgery, but the bipolar type appears to be indicated in younger and more active patients. The fixed head device appears to be more suitable for older persons with femoral neck fractures. Clinical results are poorer with both devices for those with osteonecrosis or osteoarthritis.

TOTAL HIP REPLACEMENT

This procedure involves prosthetic substitution for both the femoral (metallic component) and acetabular (high-density polyethylene component) joints, producing a "low-friction" arthroplasty. Although a large number of prosthetic types are currently used (that differ to some degree in design and materials), there are two basic generic types that differ in principle. The *conventional total hip replacement* (THR) employs a

FIG. 53–8. Anteroposterior roentgenogram of basic Charnley total hip replacement 5 years postoperatively. Note the slight varus position of the femoral component, the poor cement filling along the medial-distal aspects of the femoral stem, and the large intramedullary canal of the femur, which is poorly "filled" by the thin stem of the femoral component. All these factors are associated with a high rate of component loosening. The 1-mm "line" between the proximal-lateral aspect of the femoral component and the prosthesis indicates some loosening of the prosthesis in the cement. This patient, however, was completely pain free.

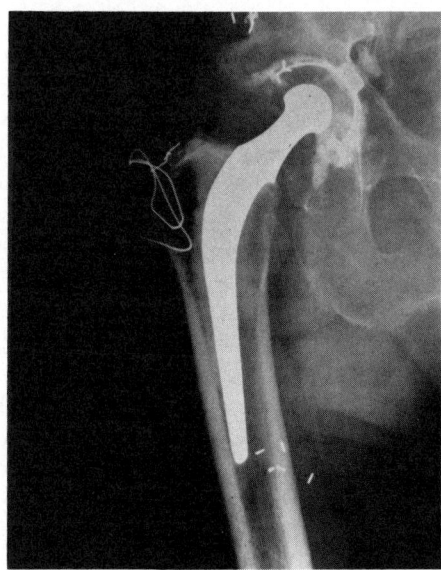

FIG. 53–9. Anteroposterior roentgenogram of a surface replacement type of THR. This patient was a 21-year-old woman with degenerative hip disease secondary to epiphyseal dysplasia. She had no signs of prosthetic loosening at 5 years after the operation.

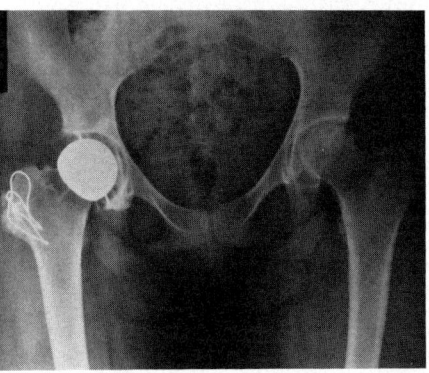

femoral component with a stem that is fixed into the medullary canal of the femur (Fig. 53–8). The *surface replacement* type employs a metal "cap," which is fixed onto the femoral head (Fig. 53–9).

The latter type was originally developed in an attempt to obviate the problem of loosening of the conventional type of femoral component stem. Its proponents believed it might be useful for the younger person with disabling disease of the hip because such patients had a high incidence of component loosening. They reasoned that if the surface type device should fail for any reason other than sepsis, adequate femoral bone stock remained to allow revision to a conventional type THR.

The surface replacement total hip enjoyed popularity for several years, starting in the late 1970s. Hip function and pain relief were excellent and equivalent to conventional THR, but several reports indicating major problems with component loosening have led to its virtual abandonment.[23-25] Failure rates of up to 34% have been reported, even over the short term (2 years), owing to loosening of the femoral component with or without avascular necrosis of the underlying femoral head, fracture of the femoral neck distal to the margin of the cup, and loosening of the acetabular component. The latter appears to be caused by the large frictional torque transmitted to the thin-walled acetabular component by the femoral component of necessarily large diameter. Revision to a conventional THR has often proved difficult because of the enormous amount of bone stock lost as a result of loosening of the large acetabular component. Failure rates have been higher in osteonecrosis, in inflammatory arthritis, and in younger patients.[26] Design and materials modifications may possibly reduce or eliminate component loosening, but for the present this technique has little to recommend it.

Conventional THR provided a major breakthrough in reconstructive hip surgery. Patients may expect greater than a 90% chance of virtually complete relief of pain and restoration of near-normal hip function. As already indicated, approximately 100,000 THRs per year are performed in the United States. The cost/benefit ratio has been found to be about 2.7 to 1 (6 to 1 under 59 years, and 2.1 to 1 from 60 to 69 years).[27] No monetary benefits are estimated in patients over the age of 70, but improvement in the *quality* of life for these elderly, retired people is undeniable and cannot be measured in monetary terms.

THR was instituted in the United States in the late 1960s, using the basic principles developed by the late Sir John Charnley (see Fig. 53–8). Since then, clinical and laboratory investigations have led to a gradual evolution in design and materials of the prosthetic devices and to improvements in surgical techniques. Currently, most THR devices include a femoral component with a stem of large cross-sectional area, a collar (to provide contact and stress transmission to the calcar femorale), a neck-shaft angle of about 130°,

FIG. 53–10. Anteroposterior roentgenogram of a total hip replacement typical of current design and surgical technique. In comparison with Figure 53–8, note the larger stem and supporting collar of the femoral component, better filling (as a result of pressurization and plugging) of the intramedullary canal with cement, and the metal-backed acetabular component. Osteotomy of the greater trochanter was not performed.

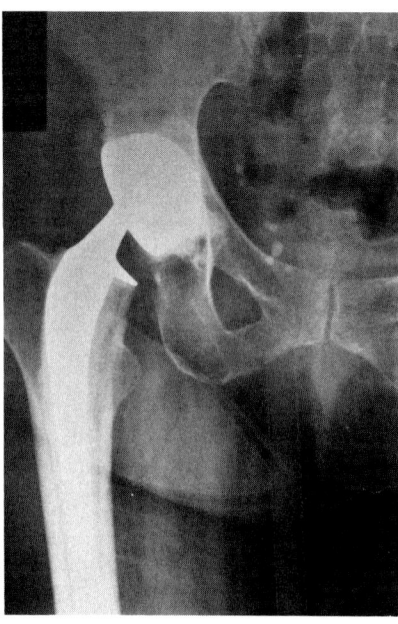

and a head diameter varying from 22 to 32 mm (Fig. 53–10). Materials most currently used include Vitallium and titanium alloys. The acetabular component is of high-density polyethylene with an outside diameter varying from 44 to 52 mm. A metal shell or "backing" of the acetabular component has been advocated. "Stiffening" of the acetabular component by addition of the metallic shell may reduce the stress transmitted to the bone and appears to decrease the incidence of component loosening.[28]

An anterolateral hip incision and exposure without removing the greater trochanter are usual. Meticulous preparation of bony surfaces, including pressurized lavage ("water-picking") to remove blood and debris, followed by thorough drying, and pressurization of cement (i.e., polymethylmethacrylate) all improve the fixation characteristics of the bone-cement interface. Pressurization is accomplished by plugging the medullary canal of the femur, thus creating a closed space, and using a cement "syringe" to deliver the cement in a low-viscosity state.

Current postoperative management consists of bed rest for 4 days, followed by gait-training and partial, progressive weight-bearing with crutches for 2 to 3 months. The average hospitalization is about 12 days. Broad-spectrum antibiotic coverage, instituted during surgery and continued for 48 hours postoperatively, has been shown to significantly reduce the infection rate. Prophylactic anticoagulation (using aspirin, sodium warfarin, or low-dose heparin), begun either before or shortly after surgery, greatly reduces the risk of thromboembolic complications.

Indications for THR include degenerative (either primary or secondary) or rheumatoid arthritis and avascular necrosis of the femoral head if there is complete collapse of the head and acetabular involvement. Contraindications include active sepsis, inadequate bony "stock" of either the pelvis or femur, and neuromuscular disease with imbalance of muscular forces acting across the hip (especially weakness of the abductor muscles, which might result in prosthetic dislocation). THR is not recommended for young, active patients with a normal life expectancy because of the high incidence of eventual prosthetic loosening.[29,30]

Complications occur in more than 30% of patients undergoing THR.[31] The more serious of these complications and their approximate incidence, as gathered from the literature, are listed in Table 53–1. In-hospital mortality is most often due to fatal pulmonary embolism, myocardial infarction, or cardiac failure. Deep infections occur as an early complication in only 0.1 to 0.3%, but many cases of deep infection, generally caused by anaerobic or other organisms of

Table 53–1. Early Complications of Total Hip Replacement

Complication	Reported Incidence (%)
Mortality	0.4
Infection	1.0
Thrombophlebitis	3.4
Pulmonary embolism	2.2
Nerve palsy	<1.0
Arterial injury	0.2
Prosthetic dislocation	3.0
Severe heterotopic bone formation	<5.0

low virulence, only become clinically obvious 1 to 3 years postoperatively. A few cases of infection occurring 5 years postoperatively have been reported. These complications are presumably caused by hematogenous "seeding" of the hip from a distant focus. Perioperative antibiotics have been shown conclusively to lower the incidence of deep infection. Modification of the operating room environment with, for example, horizontal laminar air flow, helmet-aspirator surgical attire, and ultraviolet radiation may also reduce infection rates.

The incidence of thromboembolic disease following THR depends on the sophistication of diagnostic techniques used. Clinically obvious thrombophlebitis occurs in fewer than 5% of patients, but when venograms or radioisotope techniques are employed, this complication may be detected in over 50% of patients. Pulmonary emboli occur clinically in about 2%, but when pulmonary arteriography or lung ventilation-perfusion scans are performed, they are found in 6 to 8%. Most of these patients are asymptomatic.

Dislocation of the prosthetic components is a complication that is, to a large extent, under the control of the surgeon. Posterior dislocation of the femoral head is the most common and is generally due to malpositioning (i.e., excessive retroversion) of the acetabular component. Other causes include weakness or detachment of the abductor musculature. A lower incidence of dislocation has been found with the anterolateral approach, as opposed to the posterior or lateral transtrochanteric surgical approaches.[32] Closed reduction, followed by maintenance of an abducted position of the hip in bed for 10 to 14 days with an abductor orthosis for ambulation for 8 to 12 weeks, is often successful in preventing redislocation. When revision surgery is necessary for dislocation, repeated or chronic dislocation occurs in about one third of cases.

Heterotopic bone, which may form in response to soft-tissue injury, tends to be a frequent occurrence in some persons. Heterotopic bone formation is found, to some degree, in about 30% of THR patients,

but it is severe, limiting the range of hip motion and compromising the functional result, in only 3 to 5%. It occurs more frequently in ankylosing spondylitis, in Paget's disease, and in men with the hypertrophic type of osteoarthritis. It is recommended that these high-risk patients be treated prophylactically, with low-dose irradiation[33,34] (1000 rad administered in 5 divided doses beginning 4 to 5 days postoperatively). This therapy is effective in preventing the formation of bone matrix (i.e., osteoid) in soft tissues around the hip.

Early concerns regarding wear of the polyethylene acetabular component have proved unfounded. Long-term followup studies have demonstrated wear rates of only about 0.07 mm per year. Significant wear (greater than 2 mm) detected on roentgenograms is present in fewer than .05% of cases 10 years postoperatively.[35] The apparent wear observed actually represents plastic deformation (creep or cold flow) of the polyethylene in most cases.

The primary long-term complication of THR, and a matter of great concern, is loosening of the prosthetic components within the bone. Loosening appears to be due to the inability of the polymethylmethacrylate (cement), a brittle material, to withstand the repetitive loading imposed by functional use of the joint over a long period. Although bone cement at first appeared ideal in providing rigid fixation of the prosthetic components, it now seems the obvious weak link leading to long-term failure. Ten-year followup studies show loosening of the femoral component in 30 to 50% of cases.[35–37] Factors associated with high rates of femoral loosening include heavy patients who are active, male sex, large-diameter femoral canal, varus positioning of the component, cross-sectional characteristics of the component stem (e.g., thin stem, sharp corners), and poor cement technique. Most instances of femoral component loosening occur by 5 years postoperatively, with some equilibration thereafter (i.e., few cases of femoral loosening appear between 5 and 10 years postoperatively).

Acetabular component loosening is found in 10 to 20% of patients by 10 years,[35–37] most often in younger patients (under 60 years) and in those with rheumatoid arthritis and protrusio acetabuli. This complication is associated with thin-walled polyethylene components and large-diameter prosthetic femoral heads, both of which increase the frictional torque transmitted to the bond-cement interface of the acetabulum. The rate of acetabular loosening appears to be linear with time, doubling between 5 and 10 years postoperatively. This complication may well prove to be the most common cause of THR failure 12 to 15 years after operation.

Revision of THR surgery is most often required because of component loosening. Two reports employing standard actuarial methods of statistical analysis indicate that the probability of the Charnley THR components surviving 10 years without requiring revision is 88 and 94%.[35,37]

Several recent studies have shown a remarkably lower incidence of component loosening using contemporary design, materials, and surgical techniques (as illustrated in Fig. 53–10).[38–40] Five years postoperatively, revision for component loosening is a rarity. Further developments in bone cement preparation techniques (i.e., cement centrifugation or vacuum-mixing) may decrease cement porosity and remarkably increase fatigue strength.[41] The results of these

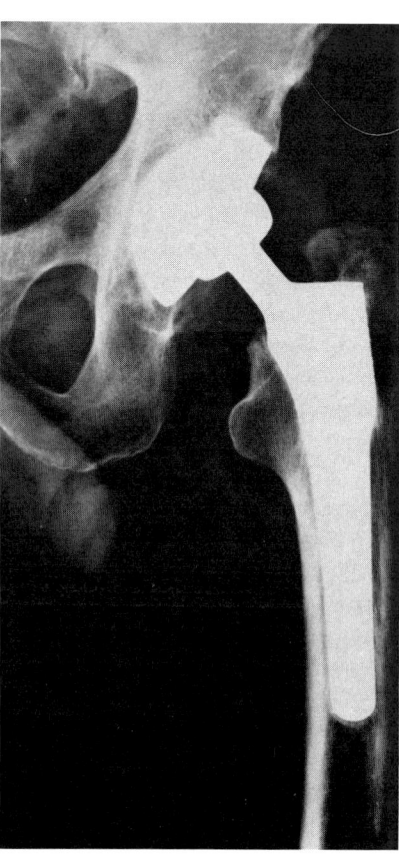

FIG. 53–11. Roentgenographic appearance of a porous-coated total hip replacement 12 months postoperatively. This 55-year-old man has gratifying pain relief and an excellent clinical result. Note the thin "shell" of cancellous bone that has formed at the distal tip of the femoral component. This common finding indicates that the prosthesis is well stabilized in the femur. Only the proximal third of this component is porous coated.

laboratory studies, however, remain controversial,[42] and clinical proof of still further reduction in component loosening has not yet been demonstrated.

Over the past 4 to 5 years considerable clinical experience has been gained using "cementless" fixation of prosthetic total hip components. These devices are coated (over all or over a portion of their surfaces) with a porous material (e.g., Vitallium beads, sintered titanium mesh, or polysulfone) (Fig. 53–11). These devices are press-fit into the bone. With a pore size of 150 to 400 μm, both laboratory and clinical studies have shown rapid bone growth into the pores within 4 to 6 weeks. It is expected that the bone–prosthesis interface should provide stable long-term fixation for the person's lifetime. Short-term clinical reports have been quite favorable. A number of unanswered questions, however, remain. What will be the effect of long-term bone remodeling on the interface? Also, because the addition of the porous coating to the prosthetic device increases the metallic surface area exposed to the body by several-hundredfold, the absorption of metallic ions is greatly increased. These ions are excreted in the urine, but also accumulate in the reticuloendothelial system. Will these absorbed ions prove toxic or even carcinogenic to persons over the long term? The use of these porous-coated total hip devices should be restricted to those persons who have been shown to have a higher incidence of failure with cemented prostheses (i.e., active persons under the age of 65) until these long-term questions are answered.

REFERENCES

1. Bombelli, R., Arsizio, B., and Santore, R.F.: Ten year results of intertrochanteric osteotomy for osteoarthritis of the hip. Presented at 50th meeting of the American Academy of Orthopaedic Surgeons, Anaheim, California, 1983.
2. Coventry, M.B.: Osteotomy of the hip for degenerative arthritis. Mayo Clin. Proc., 44:505, 1969.
3. Detenbeck, L.C., Coventry, M.B., and Kelly, P.J.: Intertrochanteric osteotomy for degenerative arthritis of the hip. Clin. Orthop., 86:73, 1972.
4. Collert, S., and Gillstrom, P.: Osteotomy in osteoarthritis of the hip. Acta Orthop. Scand., 50:555, 1979.
5. Weisel, H.: Intertrochanteric osteotomy for osteoarthritis: A long-term follow-up. J. Bone Joint Surg., 62B:37, 1980.
6. D'Aubigne, R.M., et al.: Idiopathic necrosis of the femoral head in adults. J. Bone Joint Surg., 47B:612, 1965.
7. Sugioka, Y.: Transtrochanteric rotational osteotomy of the femoral head. Hip, 8:3, 1980.
8. Ficat, R.P., and Arlet, J.: In Ischemia and Necrosis of Bone. Edited by D.S. Hungerford. Baltimore, Williams and Wilkins, 1960.
9. Gartland, J.J., and Dethoff, J.C.: Sugioka osteotomy for avascular necrosis: Results in 12 patients with over three year fol-

low-up. Presented at 96th annual meeting of American Orthopaedics Association, Hot Springs, Virginia, 1983.

10. Cabanela, M.E.: Experience with Sugioka rotational osteotomy for treatment of avascular necrosis. Unpublished data.

11. Barmada, R., Abraham, E., and Ray, R.D.: Hip fusion utilizing the cobra head plate. J. Bone Joint Surg., 58A:541, 1976.

12. Carnesale, P.G.: Arthrodesis of the hip—Long term study. J. Bone Joint Surg., 58A:735, 1976.

13. Gore, D.R., et al.: Walking patterns of men with unilateral hip fusion. J. Bone Joint Surg., 57A:759, 1975.

14. Brewster, R.C., Coventry, M.B., and Johnson, E.W., Jr.: Conversion of the arthrodesed hip to a total hip arthroplasty. J. Bone Joint Surg., 57A:27, 1975.

15. Devas, M.: Aetiology of acetabular erosion of the Thompson replacement for fractured necks of femur (abstract). J. Bone Joint Surg., 59B:128, 1977.

16. Krein, S.W., and Chao, E.Y.S.: A biomechanical analysis of bipolar proximal femoral endoprostheses. Unpublished data.

17. Beckenbaugh, R.D., Tressler, H.A., and Johnson, E.W., Jr.: Results after hemiarthroplasty of the hip using a cemented femoral prosthesis. Mayo Clin. Proc., 52:349, 1977.

18. D'Arcy, J., and Devas, M.: Treatment of fractures of the femoral neck by replacement with the Thompson prosthesis. J. Bone Joint Surg., 58B:279, 1976.

19. Whittaker, R.P., et al.: Fifteen years' experience with metallic endoprosthetic replacement of the femoral head for femoral neck fractures. J. Trauma, 12:799, 1972.

20. Drinker, H., and Murray, W.R.: The universal proximal femoral endoprosthesis: A short-term comparison with conventional hemiarthroplasty. J. Bone Joint Surg., 61A:1167, 1979.

21. Averill, R.: New concept in femoral head replacement: Mechanics of the device. Bull. Hosp. Joint Dis., 38:1, 1977.

22. Yamagata, M., et al.: Fixed head and bipolar hip endoprosthesis: retrospective clinical and roentgenographic review of 1,001 cases. J. Arthroplasty, 2, 1987.

23. Freeman, M.A.R., and Bradley, G.W.: ICLH surface replacement of the hip. An analysis of the first 10 years. J. Bone Joint Surg., 65B:405, 1983.

24. Head, W.C.: Wagner surface replacement arthroplasty of the hip: Analysis of fourteen failures in forty-one hips. J. Bone Joint Surg., 63A:420, 1981.

25. Jolley, M.N., Salvatti, E.A., and Brown, G.C.: Early results and complications of surface replacement of the hip. J. Bone Joint Surg., 64A:366, 1982.

26. Amstutz, J.C., et al.: Surface replacement of the hip with the Tharies system. J. Bone Joint Surg., 63A:1069, 1981.

27. Kelsey, J.: Total hip replacement in the United States. (NIH Consensus Conference Program, 1982). JAMA, 248:1817, 1982.

28. Harris, W.H., and White, R.E., Jr.: Socket fixation using a metal-backed acetabular component for total hip replacement. J. Bone Joint Surg., 64A:745, 1982.

29. Chandler, H.P., et al.: Total hip replacement in patients younger than thirty years old: A five-year follow-up study. J. Bone Joint Surg., 63A:1426, 1981.

30. Dorr, L.D., Takei, G.K., and Conaty, J.P.: Total hip arthroplasties in patients less than forty-five years old. J. Bone Joint Surg., 65A:474, 1983.

31. Coventry, M.B., et al.: 2012 Total hip arthroplasties: A study of postoperative course and early complications. J. Bone Joint Surg., 56A:273, 1974.

32. Woo, R.Y.G., and Morrey, B.F.: Dislocations after total hip arthroplasty. J. Bone Joint Surg., 64A:1295, 1982.

33. Coventry, M.B., and Scanlon, P.W.: The use of radiation to discourage ectopic bone. J. Bone Joint Surg., 63A:201, 1981.

34. Ayers, D.C., Evarts, C.M., and Parkinson, J.R.: The prevention of heterotopic ossification in high risk patients by low-dose radiation therapy after total hip arthroplasty. J. Bone Joint Surg., 68A:1423, 1986.

35. Stauffer, R.N.: Ten-year follow-up study of total hip replacement. J. Bone Joint Surg., 64A:983, 1982.

36. Salvatti, E.A., et al.: A ten-year follow-up study of our first one hundred consecutive Charnley total hip replacements. J. Bone Joint Surg., 63A:753, 1981.

37. Sutherland, C.J., et al.: A ten-year follow-up of 100 consecutive Mueller curved stem total hip replacement arthroplasties. J. Bone Joint Surg., 64A:970, 1982.

38. Harris, W.H., McCarthy, J.C., Jr., and O'Neill, D.A.: Femoral component loosening using contemporary techniques of femoral cement fixation. J. Bone Joint Surg., 64A:1063, 1982.

39. Roberts, D.W., Poss, R., and Kelley, K.: Radiographic comparison of cementing techniques in total hip arthroplasty. J. Arthroplasty, 1:241, 1986.

40. Russotti, G.M., Coventry, M.B., and Stauffer, R.N.: Five year results of THA using contemporary techniques. Clin. Orthop., 1988.

41. Burke, D.W., Gates, E.I., and Harris, W.H.: Centrifugation as a method of improving tensile and fatigue properties of acrylic bone cement. J. Bone Joint Surg., 66A:1265, 1984.

42. Rimnac, C.M., Wright, T.M., and McGill, D.L.: The effect of centrifugation on the fracture properties of acrylic bone cements. J. Bone Joint Surg., 68A:281, 1986.

54

CORRECTION OF ARTHRITIC DEFORMITIES OF THE KNEE

RUSSELL E. WINDSOR and JOHN N. INSALL

The knee is the largest joint in the body. It is essentially a hinge with an asymmetric arc of motion such that the tibia rotates counterclockwise (home) on the femur as the joint is extended. The joint is divided into three compartments (medial, lateral tibiofemoral, and patellofemoral) of the knee.

DEFORMITY

Most arthritic knees demonstrate some degree of instability, deformity, contracture, or a combination of these elements.

Instability initially develops because of loss of cartilage and bone, which is more or less symmetric in rheumatoid arthritis (RA) and usually asymmetric in osteoarthritis (OA). Thus, early in the course of RA a symmetric instability develops, whereas in OA knees an angular deformity soon becomes evident (Fig. 54–1). In advanced arthritis of both types, adaptive changes take place in the ligaments.

Varus Deformity. This deformity is most commonly found in OA (Fig. 54–2). The initial disorder is loss of articular cartilage from the medial compartment. The diagnosis of OA may not be made unless a weight-bearing radiograph is obtained. Unfortunately, this important examination is often omitted (Fig. 54–3A,B). As varus deformity progresses, contracture of the medial ligament produces a fixed deformity. Adaptive changes occur in the lateral ligament and capsule, which are stretched by the stresses of walking on a knee that is now in fixed varus posi-

tion. Thus, an "asymmetric instability" is now present. Extreme varus angulation may occur as a late result of Blount's disease (Fig. 54–4).

Valgus Deformity. The situation is the reverse in valgus deformity (Fig. 54–5), with contracture of the lateral capsule and iliotibial band and stretching of the medial collateral ligament. Especially in RA, there is often an associated fixed external rotation deformity of the tibia, due presumably to contracture of the iliotibial band (analogous to the similar contracture seen in poliomyelitis).

Flexion Contractures. Flexion contractures are not usually pronounced in OA; in RA the more extreme degrees are seen. In patients who have not walked for years and have spent most of their time in a wheelchair, fixed flexion deformity of 90° and more can occur. The contracture is caused by shortening of the posterior capsule with secondary contracture of the hamstring muscles.

Flexion Instability. Seen only in RA, flexion instability paradoxically is usually associated with flexion contracture. It is caused by bone loss from the posterior femoral condyles. When viewed on lateral radiographs, the lower femur looks like a drumstick or "chicken leg."

Stiff Knee. The stiff knee (extension or quadriceps contracture) usually begins by intra-articular adhesions that bind the patella to the femur. Inevitably, a secondary quadriceps shortening occurs.

In primary OA and in osteonecrosis of the medial femoral condyle, varus deformity is the most frequent (Fig. 54–6A,B), flexion contracture is mild, and the

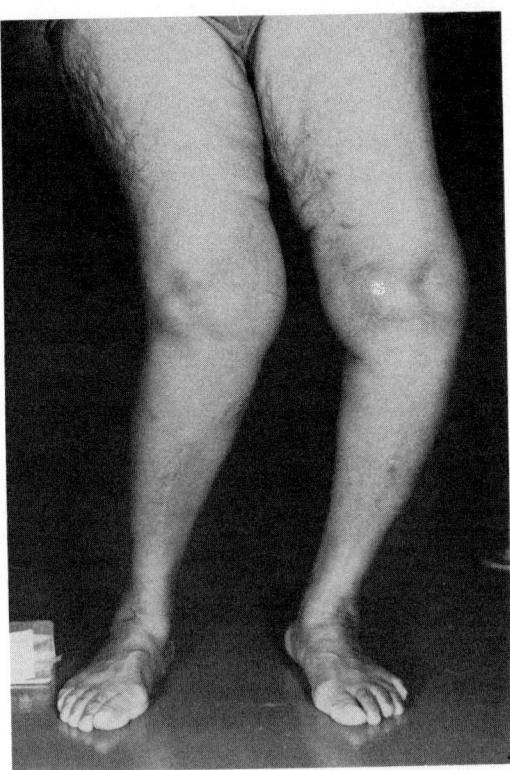

FIG. 54–1. Either varus or valgus angulation may occur in osteoarthritic knees. Both deformities have occurred in this patient, producing a "wind-swept" appearance.

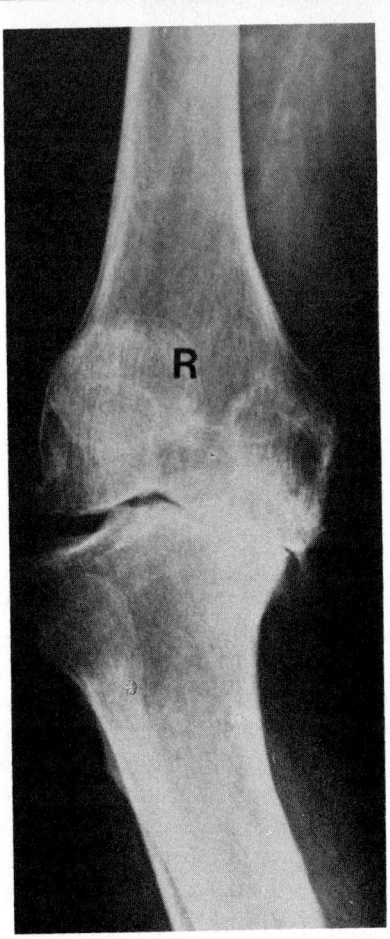

FIG. 54–2. Typical radiograph of advanced medial compartment gonarthrosis. This deformity is partially fixed by contracture of the medial soft tissues, whereas the lateral capsule is stretched.

FIG. 54–3. Weight-bearing radiographs are critical in making the diagnosis of osteoarthritis. *A,* A radiograph of a knee in the supine position. No abnormality is detectable. *B,* A radiograph of the same knee under weight-bearing conditions showing advanced narrowing of the medial compartment.

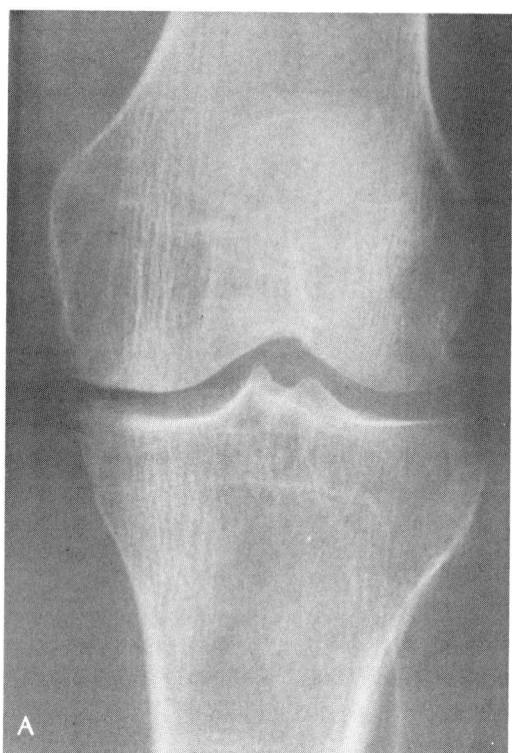 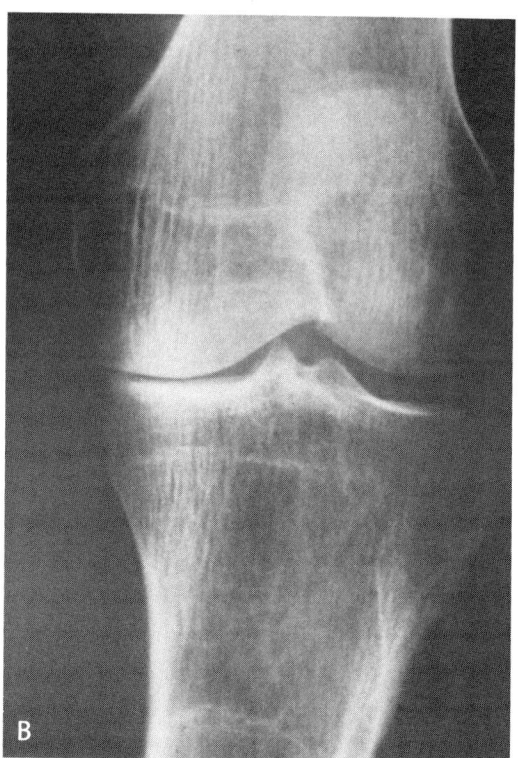

range of motion is usually well preserved. In secondary or post-traumatic arthritis, any of the deformities may be found and the knee may be stiff. In RA, lupus erythematosus, and hemophilia, flexion contracture is common, valgus deformity is frequent, and varying degrees of loss of motion can occur. External rotation deformities of the tibia are confined to this group. Loss of motion in association with deformity is seen, particularly in juvenile rheumatoid arthritis and hemophiliac arthropathy.

CONSERVATIVE TREATMENT

To some extent, the natural history of arthritic deformity can be modified.

Active exercises that maintain strength in the quadriceps and the muscles attached to the iliotibial tract minimize the development of flexion contracture and varus deformity. *Passive exercises* and *stretching* prevent the extremes of flexion contracture that are usually seen only in those patients who "give in" to their condition.

Long leg braces are needed to control angular deformity but, because of their cumbersome nature, are seldom applicable. *Elastic supports* and knee cages (short knee braces) provide only a feeling of security and will not prevent deformity.

SURGICAL CORRECTION

OSTEOTOMY

High tibial osteotomy is used to correct varus deformities secondary to OA or osteonecrosis. The operation is usually performed through the cancellous bone of the upper tibia proximal to the tibial tubercle. By removal of an appropriate sized wedge, the limb is corrected into approximately 10° of valgus.[1–5] Postoperative fixation may be accomplished by either of two methods: (1) The patient may be fitted with a cast that extends from the upper thigh to above the ankle. This method requires an accurately molded cast but otherwise is simple and virtually free of complications. The foot is exposed, and the patient can wear

FIG. 54–4. Extreme angular deformities in Blount's disease (infantile tibia vara).

FIG. 54–5. In valgus gonarthrosis, the principal bone loss occurs from the lateral femoral condyle, whereas in varus gonarthrosis, the bone loss is mostly from the tibia.

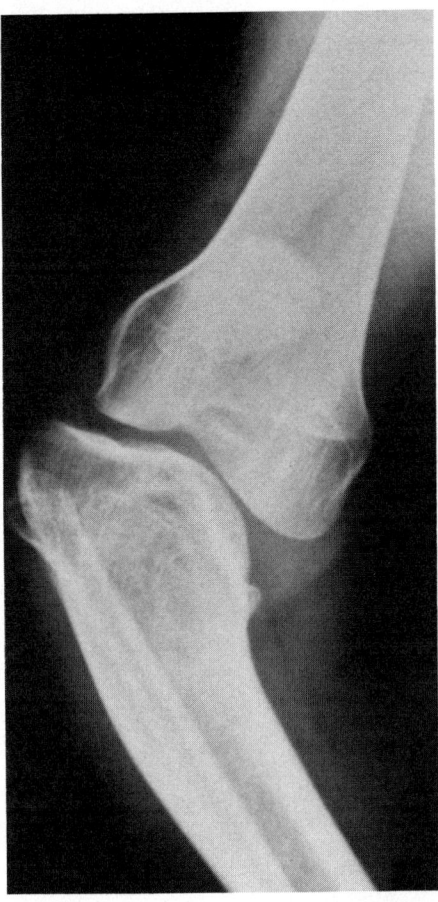

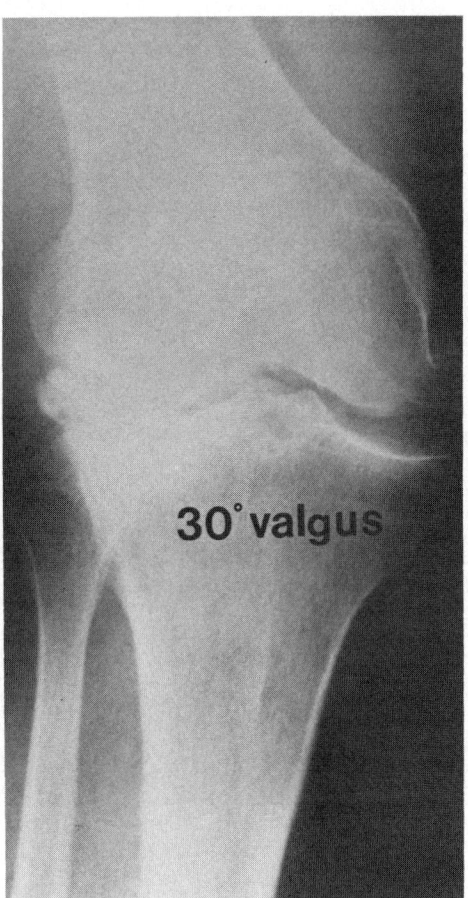

a shoe and bear weight as tolerated. Because the cast must remain in place for at least 2 months, however, troublesome stiffness in the knee may develop, and the recovery period is prolonged. (2) Internal fixation[6] by a plate and screws (Fig. 54–7) avoids the need for a cast and allows early motion. However, the operation becomes more extensive, the risk of infection is greater, and the plate interferes with an arthroplasty if this procedure is required later.

High tibial osteotomy is most suitable for knees with less than 10° of varus deformity, a well-preserved lateral compartment, and nearly normal ligamentous stability. It is mostly indicated for younger, active individuals, particularly those who wish to continue playing sports. Sedentary and overweight patients are better treated by an arthroplasty.

Supracondylar Femoral Osteotomy. For the treatment of valgus deformity in OA, supracondylar femoral osteotomy is used because the bone loss is predominantly femoral, and correction by tibial osteotomy produces an obliquity of the joint axis.[7]

Femoral osteotomies are usually fixed with a plate and screws so that early motion may begin. However, one method uses a V-shaped osteotomy without internal fixation,[8] and another author corrects valgus deformity of up to 12° with high tibial osteotomy, if there is no threat of resultant joint obliquity.[9] Crutches are required until the osteotomy is healed (approximately 2 months). The indications for femoral osteotomy are approximately the same as those for tibial osteotomy.

KNEE ARTHROPLASTY

To warrant knee joint replacement, the patient's symptoms and disability must be severe, although it is no longer true that the patient should first consent to an arthrodesis. A frank discussion with the patient concerning the consequences of failure is essential, and alternative techniques, such as tibial or femoral osteotomy, should be selected when feasible. There are four contraindications to knee replacement:

FIG. 54–6. Osteonecrosis of the medial femoral condyle (arrow). *A,* Radiograph showing well-established osteonecrosis involving most of the weight-bearing surface of the medial femoral condyle and a calcified loose fragment. Osteonecrosis differs from osteochondritis dissecans in the location of the lesion and the age group involved. *B,* Osteonecrosis often presents acutely with severe pain and swelling in the knee. In the early stages, the radiographs are negative, but the condition can be diagnosed by ^{99m}Tc diphosphonate scintigraphy.

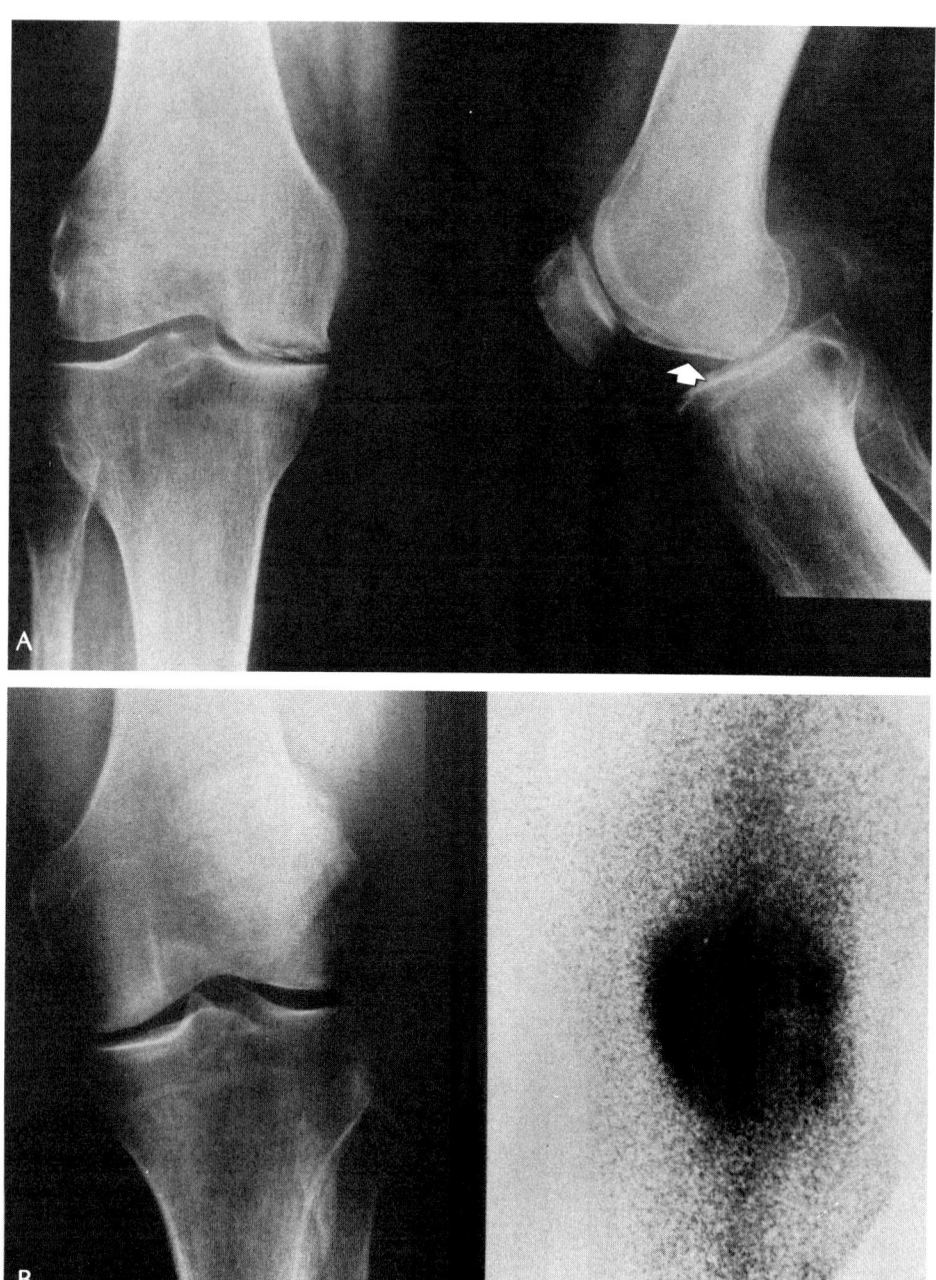

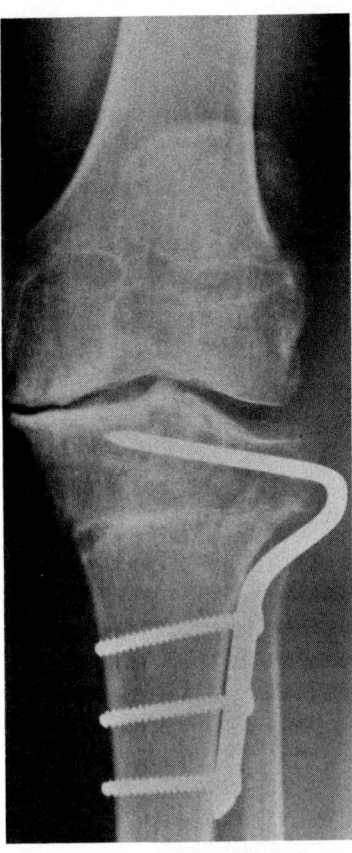

FIG. 54–7. Tibial osteotomy to correct varus angulation is a satisfactory method of surgical treatment and is the method of choice in younger, active patients. The osteotomy may be fixed with a cast or, as shown in this radiograph, by a blade plate.

1. A sound, painless arthrodesis. The prospects of a successful arthroplasty are poor.
2. Genu recurvatum associated with muscular weakness
3. Gross quadriceps weakness
4. Active sepsis

Total knee arthroplasty is indicated in the following circumstances:

1. *Rheumatoid arthritis* and *juvenile rheumatoid arthritis*, regardless of age.
2. *Osteoarthritis.* The age of the patient, occupation, level of activity, sex, and weight are all factors. In general, arthroplasty should be avoided in patients under 60 years of age, manual laborers, athletes, and those grossly overweight. Men tend to abuse the arthroplasty more than women do.
3. *Post-traumatic osteoarthritis.* Knee replacement may be rarely indicated in the younger patient following intra-articular fracture or other traumatic injuries to the joint.

4. *Failure of high tibial osteotomy.* No adverse effects due to the osteotomy have been observed with regard to fixation of the tibial component of the prosthesis.
5. *Patellofemoral arthritis.* Occasionally an elderly patient presents with severe isolated patellofemoral arthritis without significant femorotibial narrowing. Although this condition is rare, such patients fare better with total joint replacement than with any other procedure.
6. *Neuropathic joint.* Joint replacement in neuropathic states is controversial but is feasible using a surface replacement, provided the joint is thoroughly debrided (Fig. 54–8A,B).

Various prostheses used in the knee are classified in Table 54–1. Examples are shown in Figures 54–9 and 54–10. It is generally agreed that for most knees, a bicondylar surface design is most applicable. The need to preserve cruciate ligaments is debatable.[10] The place of unicompartmental replacement is controversial, and most knees suitable for unicondylar replacement are also suitable for osteotomy.

Constrained designs are needed in a small proportion of knees and particularly in revision cases. The exact percentage of knees for which this type of design is used depends on the experience of the surgeon and may range from 1 to 10%.

BICONDYLAR PROSTHESIS

Although coined as the name of a specific prosthesis, "total condylar" has been given a generic meaning to describe the whole range of prostheses that share general characteristics (see Fig. 54–10).

1. The femoral component has a grooved anterior flange, separating posteriorly into condylar runners.
2. The tibial component is made of one piece of high-density polyethylene containing two separate tibial plateaus that are biconcave and are separated by an intercondylar eminence to prevent translocation. There may be a posterior cutout for the posterior cruciate ligament, and most current designs have metallic backing or an "endo skeleton." For fixation, there is either a central stem or multiple posts.
3. The polyethylene patellar component may be (1) dome-shaped, or (2) anatomic with medial and lateral facets.

Surgical Technique

Component placement, overall alignment or "axis" and, above all, soft-tissue balance are critically important in determining the success of the arthroplasty.

FIG. 54–8. *A*, Radiograph of neuropathic joint in a patient with tabes dorsalis. Charcot joints were once thought unsuitable for joint replacement. However, provided that a complete synovectomy and debridement are performed and the joint is correctly aligned postoperatively, successful results can be obtained. *B*, Radiograph 2 years after total condylar replacement. Note that the medial defect in the tibia has been filled with a wedge-shaped custom component.

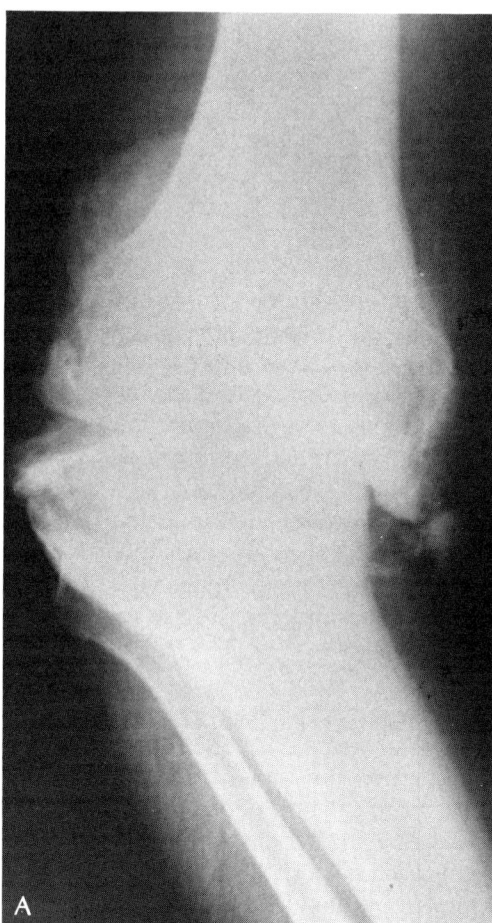

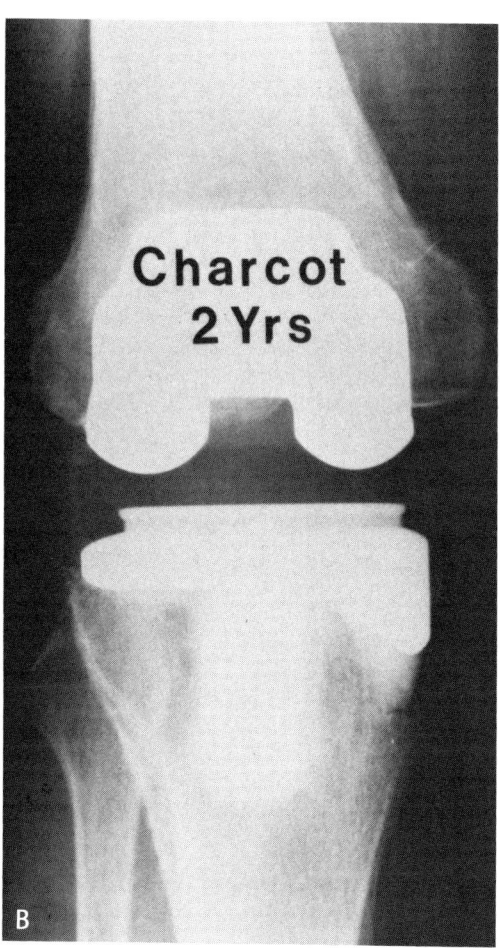

For undeformed knees, the principle is to resect the joint and reshape the bone ends so that they may be "capped" by the components to restore the original ligamentous tension. As the components themselves are almost anatomic in size and shape, subsequent function is similar to normal, although generally the range of motion is less.

In deformed and contracted knees, a surface bicondylar prosthesis may also be used if the deformity is first corrected by "soft-tissue release." This technique allows the contracted soft tissues on the concave side of deformity to be progressively released so that the limb may be stretched into correct alignment. A resurfacing prosthesis is then inserted as would be done in an undeformed knee.

Because the technique of soft-tissue release is dif-

ficult and requires experience, use of a constrained prosthesis to restore alignment and provide stability has its attractions. Although the operation is relatively simple, unfortunately, constrained prostheses are larger, invade the bone to a greater degree, and are more prone to loosening, breakage, and infection. In the event of failure, salvage is more formidable than it is for the surface replacements.

Aftercare

Intravenous antibiotics (usually oxacillin or cephalosporin) are administered preoperatively and for 48 hours postoperatively. Thromboembolism is not considered a major threat after knee arthroplasty, although fatal pulmonary emboli have been reported. Most surgeons rely on early ambulation and muscle

FIG. 54–9. Four of the early designs used for knee replacement. In a clockwise direction these designs are: a Guepar hinge, a unicondylar prosthesis, a duocondylar prosthesis, and a geometric prosthesis. A Guepar hinge was used for the most severely deformed knees and the unicondylar design for the least deformed, with the two bicondylar models occupying an intermediate position. The results obtained with these prostheses were unreliable, and there were many cases of component loosening. The operation of knee arthroplasty received a bad reputation based on the early results of designs such as these.

FIG. 54–10. The total condylar prosthesis shown in this photograph is a typical bicondylar surface replacement representative of modern prosthetic designs. The addition of a central peg to the tibial component largely eliminated the early problem of component loosening, and use of a patellar implant greatly increased the predictability of pain relief.

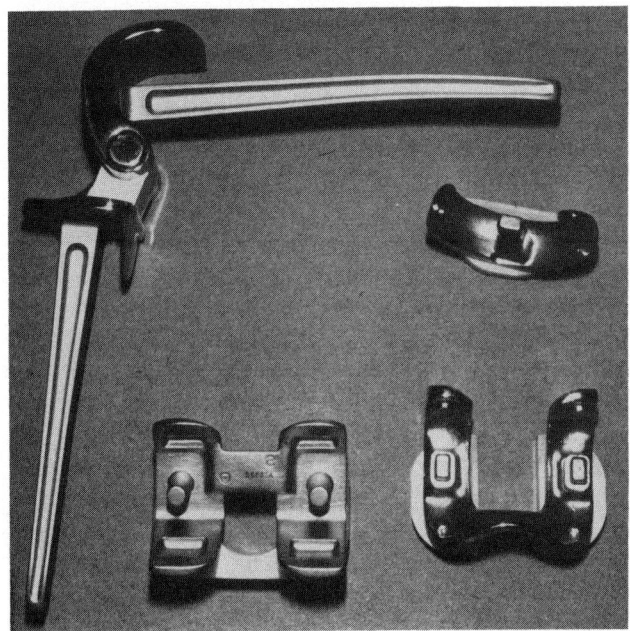

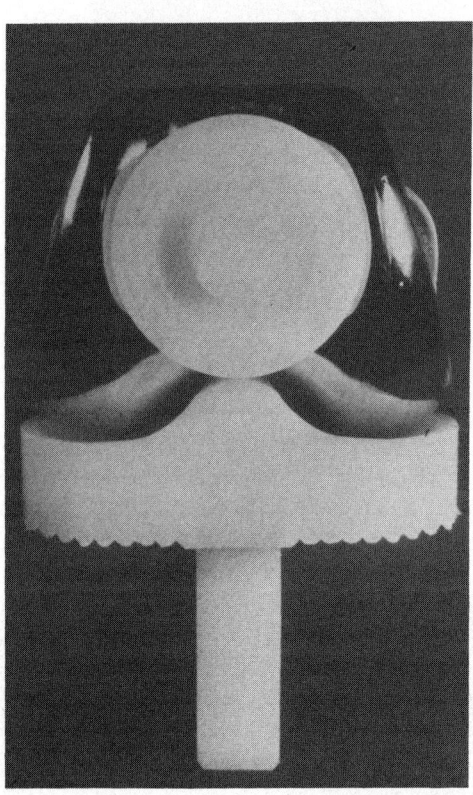

activity with perhaps the use of low doses of aspirin. Routine postoperative venography is practiced in some centers,[11] and intermittent compression stockings may also prove valuable. Patients with total knee replacement are allowed to walk on the second postoperative day using a walker or crutches with weight-bearing as tolerated. Range-of-motion exercise is usually begun in the recovery room with the assistance of a continuous passive motion machine. Manipulation under anesthesia may occasionally be necessary 2 to 3 weeks after surgery.

Complications. Urinary retention and urinary tract infections are the most frequent general complications.

The local complications include:

1. Delayed wound healing and wound drainage.
2. Vascular complications. These complications are rare, and the absence of peripheral pulses is not necessarily a contraindication to surgery.
3. Nerve palsy, usually of the peroneal nerve.[12] This condition may follow correction of severe valgus and flexion deformities. If it is recognized early, removal of the dressing and flexion of the knee may hasten recovery.
4. Stress fractures. The patella,[13] femur, and tibia are the sites of stress fractures. Usually conservative management with a cast or traction proves satisfactory, unless the components have been loosened.
5. Component breakage. This problem is rare and

Table 54–1. Classification of Knee Prostheses*

I. SURFACE REPLACEMENTS
   A. Unicondylar
   B. Bicondylar
      1. Cruciate retaining
      2. Cruciate excising
      3. Cruciate substituting

II. CONSTRAINED PROSTHESES
   A. Loose in that some rotation and varus/valgus movement are permitted
   B. Rigid, fixed axis hinges

*See also Figures 54–9 and 54–10.

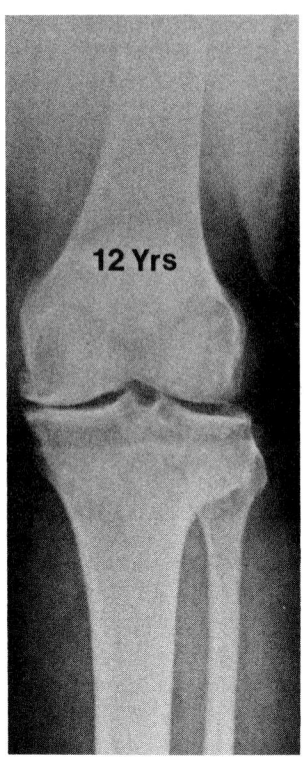

FIG. 54–11. This radiograph was taken 12 years after high tibial osteotomy in a 65-year-old woman. This knee has remained painless. Osteotomy relieves pain in most knees for about 5 years, but an increasing number of patients have recurrent pain after that time.

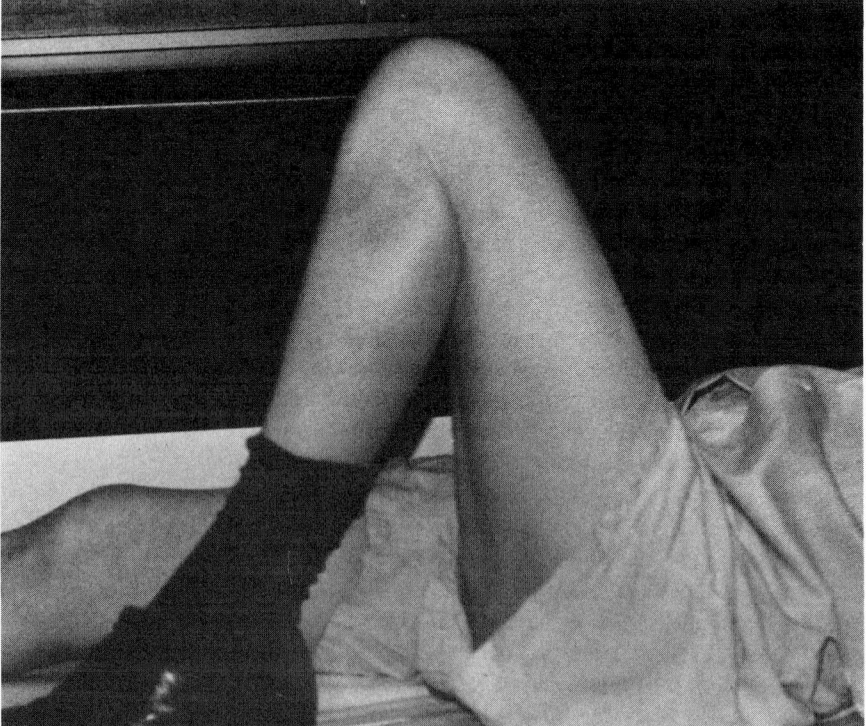

FIG. 54–12. Current designs of knee arthroplasty allow an almost normal range of motion. This photograph shows the flexion angle obtained with a posterior stabilized condylar prosthesis.

FIG. 54–13. *A, B,* Continuing followup of total condylar prostheses suggests that these models are durable. There is little evidence to suggest that late loosening or polyethylene wear will be a significant problem. These anteroposterior and lateral radiographs show the characteristic appearance of a total condylar prosthesis 12 years after implantation. There is no evidence of component loosening.

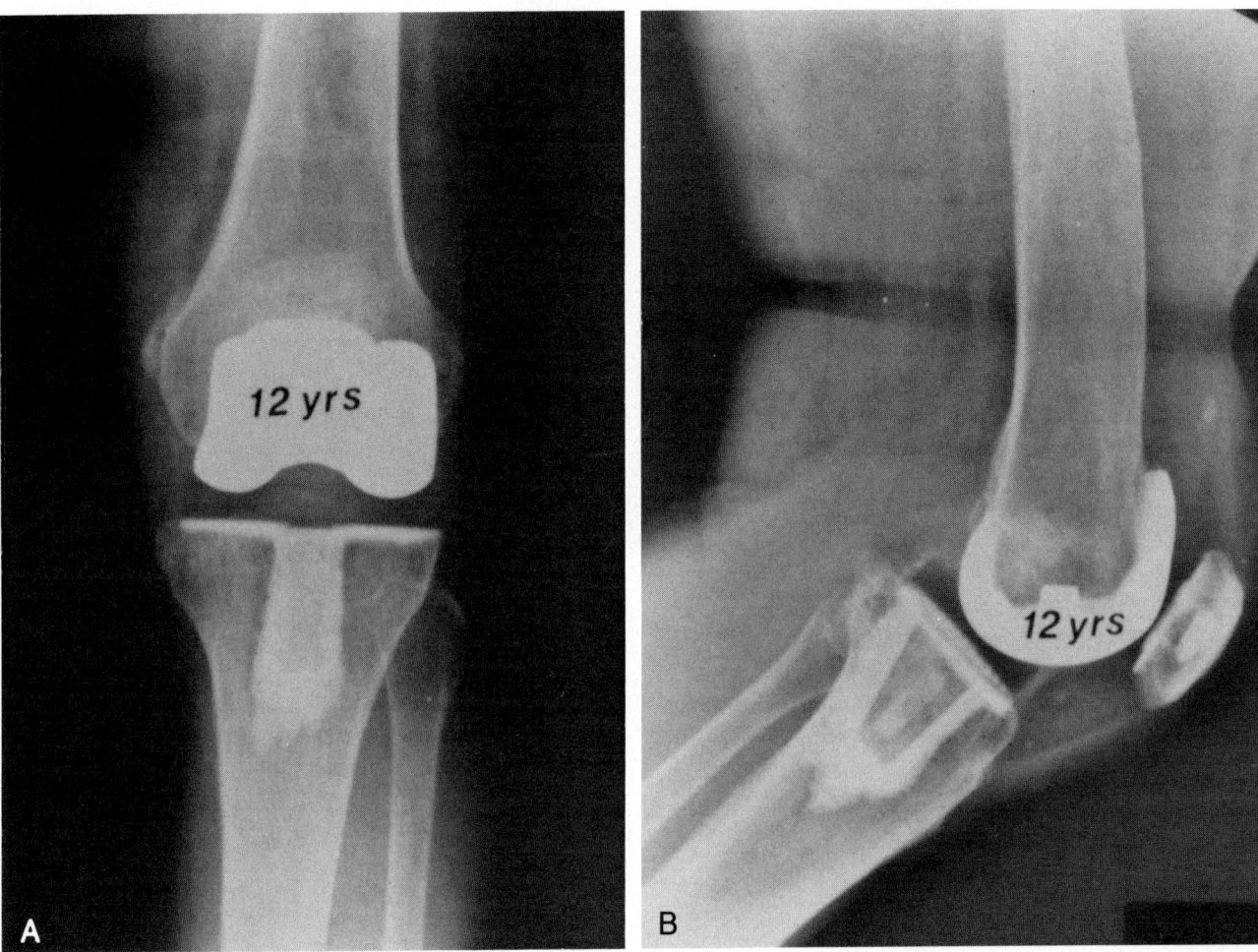

usually is restricted to hinges and linked prosthetic designs.[14]

6. Component wear. Retrieval analysis of removed total joint implants has consistently revealed polyethylene particles in the synovium. Inspection of removed components often shows imbedded cement particles with scratching, pitting, and burnishing of the articular surfaces.[15] However, clinically significant wear has not yet been demonstrated with current resurfacing designs.

7. Instability, subluxation, and dislocation. Instability after surface replacement is usually due to faulty technique, which should be recognized and corrected in the operating room.

8. Component loosening. Component loosening is now mostly a problem with constrained designs.

Most currently used surface replacements have acceptably low loosening rates, and recent modifications, such as metal backing of polyethylene components and improved cementing techniques, should further reduce the loosening rate. Malalignment of the arthroplasty due to technical error predisposes to loosening.

9. Infection. Persistent symptoms following total knee replacement in the absence of a clear mechanical explanation should suggest the possibility of infection. Infection is more common in RA and when metal-on-metal constrained hinged prostheses are selected.[16] Late infections are more common than early ones. The diagnosis is usually straightforward unless antibiotics have been given previously. Antibiotic therapy should there-

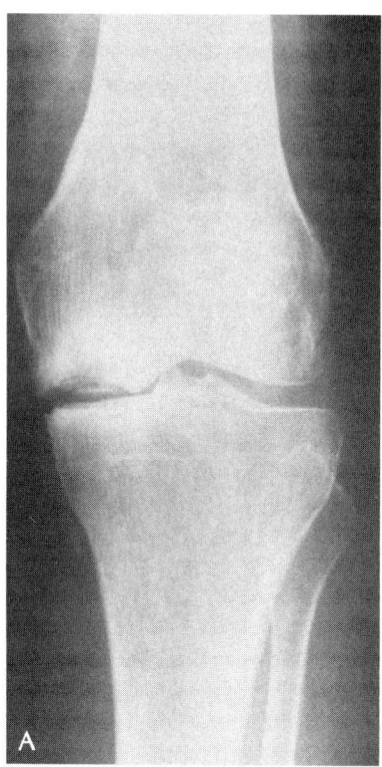 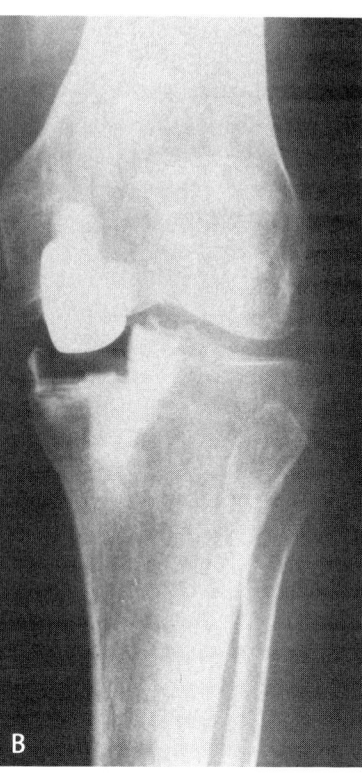

FIG. 54–14. *A, B,* Although partial or unicondylar replacement is a controversial operation, an ideal indication would be an osteonecrosis of the medial-femoral condyle in an otherwise normal knee joint as shown here.

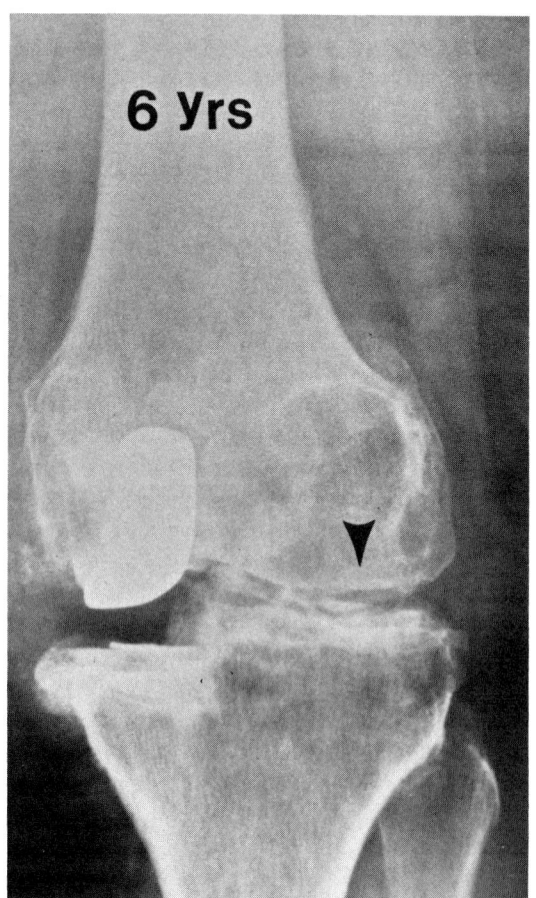

FIG. 54–15. Although unicompartmental replacement is often successful for a few years, late followup reveals an increasing incidence of progressive arthritis in other compartments of the joint (arrow). This complication is partly due to the abrasive effect of polyethylene and acrylic debris.

fore be withheld in cases of suspected infection until after diagnostic aspiration of the joint. Proven or strongly suspected late deep infection is treated by surgical removal of the prosthetic components and debridement of the involved tissues. Appropriate antibiotic therapy is then given intravenously.

After completion of approximately 6 weeks of antibiotic therapy, the following courses are open:
1. Prolonged immobilization in a supportive brace allowing a fibrous ankylosis to develop
2. Formal arthrodesis[17]
3. Reimplantation of another prosthesis. This alternative can be considered in certain cases if the wound is completely benign.[18] Usually only infections due to gram-positive organisms can be managed in this manner.

RESULTS

High Tibial Osteotomy.[4,5,19–23] Evidence is ample that high tibial osteotomy provides a successful result in 80 to 90% of properly selected cases, for 5 years (Fig. 54–11). Beyond this time, however, a significant deterioration occurs. Coventry found that 62% of the patients rated themselves as having less pain even after 10 years from the time of operation.[1] Vainionpää and co-workers found that 26 of 103 knees deteriorated after an initial good result.[24] Joseph and co-workers examined 95 knees with an average followup of 8.5 years; 83% were excellent or good at 5 years, deteriorating to 63% in these categories at the time of last followup.[3] These authors also found that patients who were under 60 at the time of osteotomy did much better than those patients over the age of 60.

Femoral Osteotomy. There is a paucity of information concerning the results. At our hospital, 12 of 15 cases were satisfactory after a followup of 1 to 10 years.

Knee Arthroplasty. Results of early attempts at knee arthroplasty were poor, and unfortunately the operation still suffers from the bad reputation earned during these early years. With the early model prostheses, there were four major problems:[25]

Component Loosening. For both surface replacements and constrained designs, the incidence of loosening, usually of the tibial component, was unacceptably high.[26,27]

Patellofemoral Pain. None of the early designs allowed for patellofemoral replacement or resurfacing.

Infection. A major complication of metallic hinged designs was infection.

Surgical Technique. The surgical procedure was extremely difficult for early surface replacements, and the instrumentation was poor. Consequently, many prostheses were poorly inserted and often malaligned. These mistakes often led to failure.[28,29]

Current resurfacing designs[30–32] can now be used for most arthroplasties, and metal hinges are obsolete. Alterations to the tibial component have reduced tibial loosening to a low level. Recent designs, such as the posterior stabilized condylar knee, permit flexion to 120° or more (Fig. 54–12). Patellofemoral resurfacing is performed routinely. Instrumentation and surgical technique have been greatly improved.[33] Consequently, the results of knee arthroplasty are now as good as those for total hip replacement, and promise to be even more durable. In a 5- to 9-year followup of the total condylar prosthesis, Insall and co-workers showed 91% excellent and good results in a series of 100 consecutive replacements.[25] Moreover, the late radiographic appearance of most of these cases remained unchanged throughout the period of followup, suggesting that component loosening will continue to be a minor problem (Fig. 54–13). In fact, only 2% showed a complete radiolucency around any of the three components compared with 25 to 50% of total hip prostheses followed for a similar time. Eighty-eight knees were subsequently followed for a minimum of 10 years, and 93.6% were functioning well by survivorship analysis.[34]

The place of unicondylar replacement is controversial (Fig. 54–14A,B). Scott and Santore studied 100 knees followed for 2 to 6 years and found satisfactory pain relief in 92.[35] However, Insall and Aglietti reported on 22 unicondylar knee replacements of similar design with a 5- to 7-year followup and found that only 36% remained satisfactory and 28% had been revised (Fig. 54–15).[36] Laskin,[37] using the somewhat different Marmor modular prosthesis,[38] found the results inferior to those for biocompartmental replacement.

The spherocentric prosthesis is probably the most frequently used constrained design. Kaufer and Matthews reviewed 82 consecutive spherocentric arthroplasties with an average followup of 4 years.[39] There was a 10% incidence of aseptic loosening and 4% infection rate. Convery and co-workers reported 8 cases of confirmed or suspected loosening in 36 spherocentric arthroplasties followed for an average of 3 years.[40] These results suggest that the spherocentric prosthesis, although an improvement over hinged designs, still loosens more frequently than do resurfacing models.[41]

REFERENCES

1. Coventry, M.B.: Upper tibial osteotomy for gonarthrosis. Orthop. Clin. North Am., *10*:191, 1979.
2. Johnson, P., Leitl, S., and Waugh, W.: The distribution of load across the knee. J. Bone Joint Surg., *62B*:346, 1980.
3. Joseph, D.M., Insall, J., and Msika, C.: High tibial osteotomy for varus gonoarthrosis. A long-term follow-up study. J. Bone Joint Surg., *66A*:1040, 1984.
4. Kettelkamp, D.B. et al.: Results of proximal tibial osteotomy. The effects of tibio-femoral angle, stance-phase flexion-extension, and medial-plateau force. J. Bone Joint Surg., *58A*:952, 1976.
5. Maquet, P.: Valgus osteotomy or osteoarthritis of the knee. Clin. Orthop., *120*:143, 1976.
6. d'Aubigne, R.M.: Joint realignment in the management of osteoarthritis. *In* Clinical Trends in Orthopaedics. Edited by L.R. Straub, and P.D. Wilson, Jr. New York, Thieme-Stratton, Inc., 1982.
7. Shoji, H., and Insall, J.: High tibial osteotomy for osteoarthritis of the knee with valgus deformity. J. Bone Joint Surg., *55A*:963,1973.
8. Aglietti, P. et al.: Correction of valgus knee deformity with a supracondylar "V" osteotomy. Clin. Orthop., *217*:214, 1987.
9. Coventry, M.B.: Proximal varus osteotomy for osteoarthritis of the lateral compartment of the knee. J. Bone Joint Surg., *69A*:32, 1987.
10. Freeman, M.A.R. et al.: Excision of the cruciate ligaments in total knee replacement. Clin. Orthop., *126*:209, 1977.
11. Stulberg, B. et al.: Deep vein thrombosis following total knee replacement: An analysis of 638 arthroplasties. J. Bone Joint Surg., *66A*:194, 1984.
12. Rose, H.A. et al.: Peroneal-nerve palsy following total knee arthroplasty. A review of the Hospital for Special Surgery experience. J. Bone Joint Surg., *64A*:347, 1982.
13. Thompson, F.M., Hood, R.W., and Insall, J.: Patellar fractures in total knee arthroplasty. Orthop. Trans., *5*:490, 1981.
14. DeBurge, A., and Guepar: Guepar hinge prosthesis: complications and results with two years' follow-up. Clin. Orthop., *120*:47, 1976.
15. Hood, R.W. et al.: Retrieval analysis of 70 total condylar knee prostheses. Orthop. Trans., *5*:319, 1981.
16. Jones, E.C. et al.: GUEPAR knee arthroplasty results and late complications of upper tibial osteotomy. Clin. Orthop., *140*:145, 1979.
17. Hagemann, W.F., Wood, G.W., and Tullos, H.S.: Arthrodesis in failed total knee replacement. J. Bone Joint Surg., *60A*:790, 1978.
18. Insall, J.N., Thompson, F.M., and Brause, B.D.: Two-stage reimplantation for the salvage of infected total knee arthroplasty. J. Bone Joint Surg., *65A*:1087, 1983.
19. Coventry, M.B.: Osteotomy about the knee for degenerative and rheumatoid arthritis. Indications, operative technique, and results. J. Bone Joint Surg., *55A*:23, 1973.
20. Coventry, M.B.: Osteotomy of the upper portion of the tibia for degenerative arthritis of the knee. A preliminary report. J. Bone Joint Surg., *47A*:984, 1965.
21. Insall, J.N., Shoji, H., and Mayer. V.: High tibial osteotomy. J. Bone Joint Surg., *65A*:1397, 1974.
22. Jackson, J.P., and Waugh, W.: Tibial osteotomy for osteoarthritis of the knee. J. Bone Joint Surg., *43B*:746, 1961.
23. Jackson, J.P., Waugh, W., and Green, J.P.: High tibial osteotomy for osteoarthritis of the knee. J. Bone Joint Surg., *51B*:88, 1969.
24. Vainionpää, S. et al.: Tibial osteotomy for osteoarthritis of the knee. A five- to ten-year follow-up study. J. Bone Joint Surg., *63A*:938, 1981.
25. Insall, J.N. et al.: The total condylar knee prosthesis in gonarthrosis: A five to nine year follow-up of the first one hundred consecutive replacements. J. Bone Joint Surg., *65A*:619–628, 1983.
26. Ducheyne, P., Kagan, A., II, and Lacey, J.A.: Failure of total knee arthroplasty due to loosening and deformation of the tibial component. J. Bone Joint Surg., *60A*:384, 1978.
27. Evanski, P.M. et al.: UCI knee replacement. Clin. Orthop., *120*:33, 1976.
28. Hood, R.W., Vanni, M., and Insall, J.N.: The correction of knee alignment in 225 consecutive total condylar knee replacements. Clin. Orthop., *160*:94, 1981.
29. Lotke, P.A., and Ecker, M.L.: Influence of positioning of prosthesis in total knee replacement. J. Bone Joint Surg., *59A*:77, 1977.
30. Ewald, F.C. et al.: Duo-patella total knee arthroplasty in rheumatoid arthritis. Orthop. Trans., *2*:202, 1978.
31. Freeman, M.A.R., and Insall, J.: Tibio-femoral replacement using two unlinked components and cruciate resection. (The ICLH and total condylar prostheses.) *In* Clinical Features and Surgical Management. Edited by M.A.R. Freeman. New York, Springer-Verlag, 1980.
32. Insall, J.N., Scott, W.N., and Ranawat, C.S.: The total condylar knee prosthesis. A report of two hundred and twenty cases. J. Bone Joint Surg., *61A*:193, 1979.
33. Insall, J.N.: Technique of total knee replacement. *In* Instructional Course Lectures. The American Academcy of Orthopaedic Surgeons. Vol. 30. St. Louis, C.V. Mosby Co., 1981.
34. Vince, K., Insall, J., and Kelly, M.: Total condylar knee arthroplasty: Twelve-year survivorship analysis. Presented at Annual Meeting of the American Academy of Orthopaedic Surgeons, San Francisco, CA, 1987.
35. Scott, R.D., and Santore, R.F.: Unicompartmental replacement for osteoarthritis of the knee. J. Bone Joint Surg., *63A*:536, 1981.
36. Insall, J.N., and Aglietti, P.: A five- to seven-year follow-up of unicondylar arthroplasty. J. Bone Joint Surg., *62A*:1329, 1980.
37. Laskin, R.S.: Unicompartmental tibiofemoral resurfacing arthroplasty. J. Bone Joint Surg., *60A*:182, 1978.
38. Marmor, L.: Results of single compartment arthroplasty with acrylic cement fixation. A minimum follow-up of two years. Clin. Orthop., *122*:181, 1977.
39. Kaufer, H., and Matthews, L.S.: Spherocentric arthroplasty of the knee. J. Bone Joint Surg., *63A*:545, 1981.
40. Convery, F.R., Minteer-Convery, M., and Malcom, L.L.: The spherocentric knee: A re-evaluation and modification. J. Bone Joint Surg., *62A*:320, 1980.
41. Insall, J.N. et al.: A comparison of four models of total knee replacement prostheses. J. Bone Joint Surg., *58A*:754, 1976.

CORRECTION OF ARTHRITIC DEFORMITIES OF THE FOOT AND ANKLE

55

MACK L. CLAYTON

Both rheumatoid arthritis (RA) and osteoarthritis (OA) are discussed in this chapter. Because the latter process tends to be more localized in a single joint and is, therefore, a less severe problem than the generalized changes found in the RA patient, more text is allotted to RA.

GENERAL CONSIDERATIONS

Seventy-five percent of patients with RA are women, and they more often have aggressive disease. The process presents in the feet in 16% and in the ankle in 4% of RA cases.[1] In the later stages of the disease, however, almost all patients have some complaints related to foot involvement. In one large series of patients, metatarsophalangeal joints were involved in 46%, tarsals in 46%, toes in 23%, ankle in 68%, knees in 78%, and metacarpophalangeal joints in 71%.

Smyth and Clayton have noted two definite clinical subtypes of chronic RA.[2] In one type, the joints tend to stiffen with gradual loss of motion and even to progress to ankylosis. These patients are generally seronegative for rheumatoid factor. Soft tissue and bursal involvement predominate in the second type. Joint destruction is slow and does not usually lead to ankylosis. The "loose" type tends to have gradual destruction of the joint with developing instability. This type predominates in seropositive patients with hand and foot involvement and is accentuated by corticosteroid treatment.

These two "subtypes" may account for the marked difference in the results obtained with reconstructive surgical procedures. In the first, ankylosis prone-type arthrodesis (fusion) is easy to obtain, but mobility may be difficult to regain after arthroplasty. In the loose type, arthrodesis is more difficult to obtain.

The statement in the older literature that "surgery should not be performed until the arthritis is 'burned out' or quiescent" has been shown to be false. Three clinical forms of RA exist with regard to progression. The first group of patients has a single inflammatory cycle lasting for a number of months and then subsiding with no further attacks of arthritis. Such patients are not considered for surgery. The second group shows periods of heightened inflammatory activity followed by partial or complete remission, and then more activity and remission, with a gradual heightening of the activity. The third group of patients has steadily progressive, active inflammation. Destructive joint changes with instability or stiffness develop at various rates in the latter two groups.

Most patients with chronic RA seen for consideration of surgical treatment have experienced such progressive deformity and disability. Inflammation continues indefinitely. Surgery can be performed at any time, provided there is no general medical contraindication. This concept is not new. In 1943 Smith-Petersen, Aufranc, and Larson recommended surgery during active disease.[3]

Surgery for arthritic feet is usually performed under general anesthesia, although regional anesthesia has been used successfully. If a patient has recently received corticosteroids, supplementary steroids must be given (see Chapter 37). The rate of wound healing is slowed, but the final result is unchanged. The tissues in such patients are often more fragile and must be handled atraumatically. I use perioperative intravenous antibiotics, usually an intravenous cephalosporin, on the day of the operation and for up to 24 hours afterward.

While the patient is in the hospital recovering from surgery, other involved joints are treated. Medical treatment using the team approach is carried out so that no time is wasted (see Chapter 47). The necessary period of rest after operation often decreases inflammation in other joints.

Upper-extremity procedures can be performed at the same time as foot surgery by using two teams of surgeons.

EVALUATION

In early RA, diagnosis may be difficult. The patient, usually female, presents with pain in the forefoot, which is usually swollen and tender. There may be mild heat, redness, and local increased sweatiness of the overlying skin. Lateral compression of the metatarsal heads increases pain. Tenderness between metatarsal heads indicates involvement of the periarticular non-weight structures, involved in RA but not in mechanical types of metatarsophalangeal disease. An exception, of course, is plantar neuroma with its characteristic findings (see Chapter 89). (Plantar neuroma also may be due to RA.) As a result of swelling of the metatarsophalangeal (MTP) joints, the toes assume a "cocked-up" position. Active and passive flexion is limited at the MTP joints. Roentgenograms may reveal only osteoporosis with soft tissue swelling (Fig. 55–1), but surface erosions of the metatarsal heads soon develop in most cases.[4]

In early disease, proper shoes and supports with a graduated exercise regimen are helpful, and some of the deformities can be prevented. Rest may be indicated in early acute exacerbations (see Chapter 47).

Despite conservative measures, some cases progress to severely painful, disabling forefoot deformities. Deformity of the knees often accentuates foot deformity. The most common deformities are hallux valgus and bunions, a spread forefoot, depressed metatarsal heads, and varying degrees of "cock-up" of the toes. The latter often becomes so pronounced that the toes no longer contact the floor when the patient stands barefoot. The proximal phalanx is dorsally subluxed on the metatarsal heads. The deformity is made even worse as the fat pad under the trans-

FIG. 55–1. Early rheumatoid arthritic changes with soft tissue swelling. Note erosion of bone at the metatarsophalangeal joints, particularly erosion of the metatarsal heads. Also note the interphalangeal joint of the great toes. Joint spaces are well preserved.

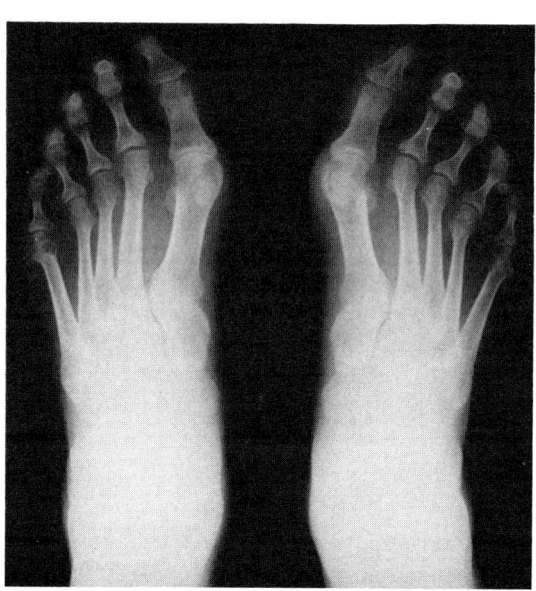

verse metatarsal arch slips anteriorly and lies under the cocked-up toes. Some toes remain slightly flexible while others are rigid with dorsal subluxation or complete dislocation of the proximal phalanges on the metatarsal heads. This condition increases the height of the forefoot and makes it difficult for the patient to wear shoes. Painful corns develop over the dorsum of the middle toe joints, and calluses develop beneath the depressed, prominent, metatarsal heads on the sole of the foot that now lies under the skin (Fig. 55–2). A painful swollen bursa often develops over the lateral aspect of the fifth MTP joint, known as a bunionette.

With walking, pain arises from abnormal pressure beneath the metatarsal heads on the sole or against the shoe on the dorsum of the toes. Attempts to support the metatarsal area often produce increased pressure on the dorsum of the toes owing to their inflexibility. There is contracture of the soft tissues, including muscles, tendons, fascia, and skin, often leading to fibrous ankylosis. *However, spontaneous bony ankylosis of the metatarsophalangeal joints is rare* (less than 1%). As synovitis continues, the intrinsic muscles are overpulled by the long extensors and flexors, and the cock-up deformity of the toes becomes similar to that often seen with paralysis of the intrinsic muscles of the foot. The flexor tendons subluxate laterally and migrate in a dorsal direction until they no longer

FIG. 55–2. Typical late severe deformities include hallux valgus *(A)*, bunions *(B)*, depressed metatarsal heads *(C)*, and cock-up (hammer) toes *(D)*.

FIG. 55–3. Late deformity with multiple metatarsophalangeal dislocations. (Note "gun barrel" sign indicating 90° dislocation of proximal phalanges over metatarsal heads.)

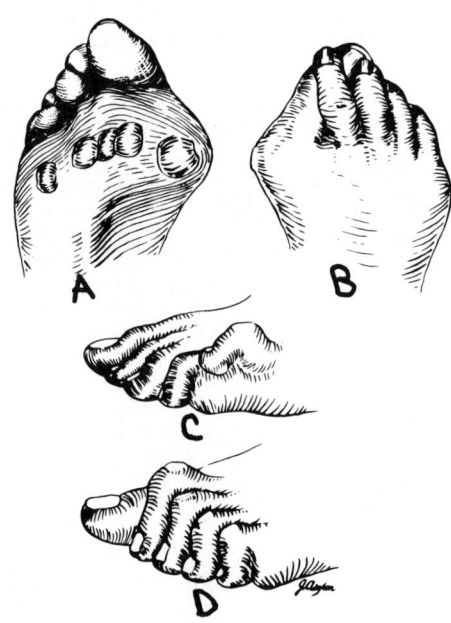

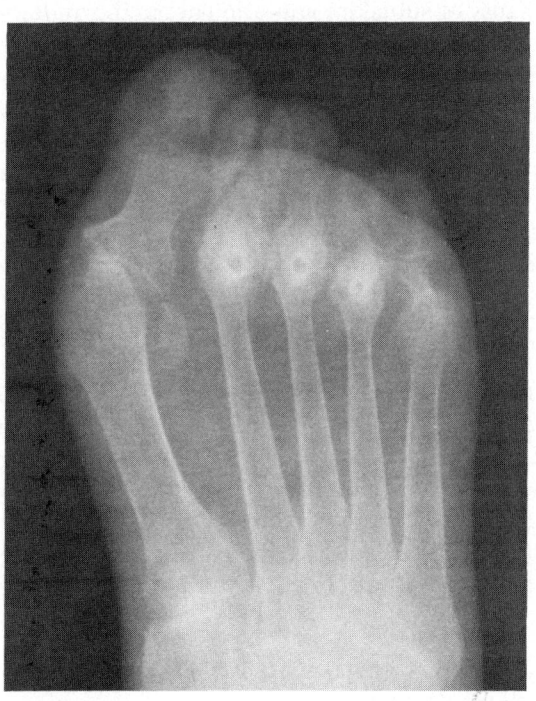

flex the proximal phalanx, again increasing the cock-up deformity. This defect does not resemble the "intrinsic plus" deformity commonly seen in rheumatoid arthritis of the hand (see Chapter 50). Many variations of pathology in the involved tissues give rise to other deformities, but most patients have the basic pattern as described.

Roentgenograms help analyze the deformities. Erosion of the metatarsal heads or bases of the proximal phalanges is nearly always greater than suspected on clinical evaluation. Joint spaces are often narrowed, and subluxation or actual dislocation of the MTP joints is often seen on anteroposterior films as the proximal phalanx overlaps the metatarsal head. When the proximal phalanx is located in marked dorsal dislocation at almost 90° to the metatarsal (Fig. 55–3), the "gun barrel" sign is seen. This sign is simply an axial view of the proximal phalanx in which the bony cortex appears as if one were peering straight down a gun barrel. Varying degrees of osteoporosis are present.

Complete spontaneous dislocation at the first metatarsophalangeal joints (Fig. 55–4) may occur as a result of rheumatoid synovial involvement of the capsule and the abductor hallucis tendon. This dislocation increases the deformity of the forefoot and increases the pressure of the bunion of the first metatarsal head. I have seen three feet with a spontaneous hallux varus. This unusual deformity was due to a rupture of the adductor hallucis tendon and

FIG. 55–4. Forefoot with dislocation of metatarsophalangeal joint of the great toe and several smaller toes. Dislocation of the first metatarsophalangeal joint without a history of trauma is pathognomonic of rheumatoid arthritis.

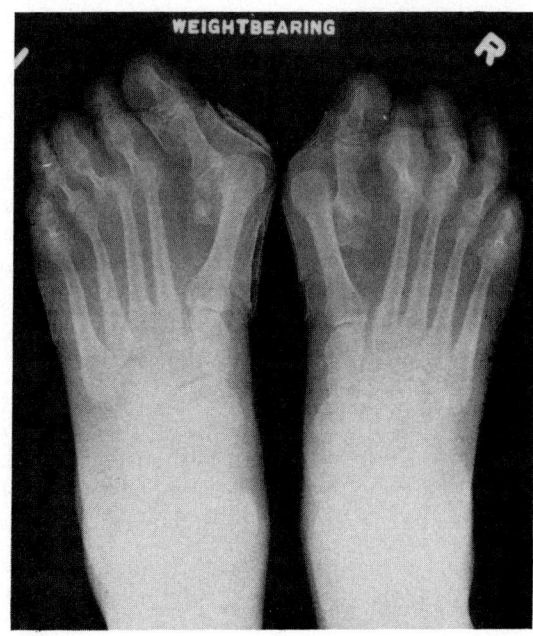

related joint capsule by synovitis. Similar tendon ruptures in the hand are well known.

The hindfoot usually shows a progressive valgus deformity (loose type) with changes first in the talonavicular or subtalar joints and later in the midtarsals. In other cases such deformity is minimal, but there is limited motion with pain in the hindfoot due to arthritic joint changes (stiff type). Cavovarus deformity is also seen most commonly in juvenile RA, but this condition is often not symptomatic until adult life. The medial longitudinal arch becomes accentuated with the development of a pes cavus deformity.

Bursitis (or tenosynovitis) may develop around the calcaneal tendon. I have seen two cases of rupture of the Achilles tendon.* Tenosynovitis also may occur near the plantar fascia insertion.

Tenosynovitis may develop in any of the tendon sheaths at the ankle level, as in the hand and wrist, and may occasionally cause tendon rupture. A ruptured posterior tibial tendon may cause rapid severe valgus of the hindfoot. Nodules often develop on the weight-bearing aspect of the os calcis and may even erode the adjacent bone.

CONSERVATIVE TREATMENT OF RHEUMATOID FOOT
(See also Chapter 89)

Proper shoes with simple ordinary orthopedic supports should be used in the early stages coupled with an exercise regimen designed to keep the toes flexible. Simple, low- to medium-heel, basic oxford shoes with closed toes and heels are recommended. Metatarsal pads, long arch pads, or heel wedges are added if needed (Fig. 55–5). Arch supports are usually made of foam rubber and covered with leather. Steel or hard plastic alone is usually too rigid for the rheumatoid foot. The supports must be custom-made for each patient and frequently require secondary alterations. Plaster impressions of the feet are often helpful to fit the arch supports precisely. Extra-depth shoes (double-toe box) are also commercially available, and special inserts of plastizoate in combination with these have been most helpful. Running shoes are useful as a pre- or postoperative walking shoe (Fig. 55–6).

Berg, using pressure-distribution footwear used successfully for insensitive neurotrophic feet, has treated many rheumatoid feet without surgery.[5] An extra-depth shoe with a plastizoate liner is useful in milder cases, but severely deformed feet required san-

*Editor's note. I have noted two cases of Achilles tendon rupture secondary to rheumatoid nodule (necrobiosis) formation within the tendon itself.

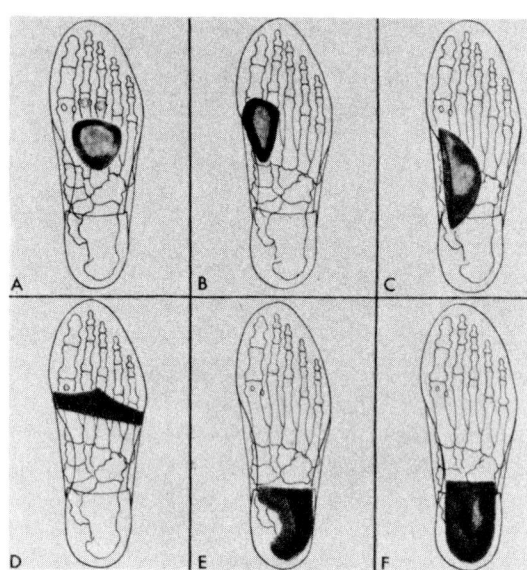

FIG. 55–5. Types of arch supports that have been helpful. The object of their use is relief of pain through mechanical realignment and pressure relief. These pads do not differ much from those used for other basic orthopedic problems, but the patient with rheumatoid arthritis requires more adjustment and "custom fitting" of the supports.

dals with special plastizoate inserts. The most severe deformities require a custom-made shoe with inserts. The principle in all cases is relief of abnormal areas of pressure, which cause the pain in long-standing deformities after the most active synovitis has passed. Success requires constant supervision of the shoe correction and close cooperation with a knowledgeable pedorthist (shoe expert). Even after proper shoeing, a number of patients may desire an operation so that

FIG. 55–6. Running shoes are useful for many patients pre- and/or postoperatively. They can be padded for pressure relief as necessary. These feet were reconstructed 6 months earlier. Fortunately, these shoes are in style, and many patients prefer them to corrective shoes.

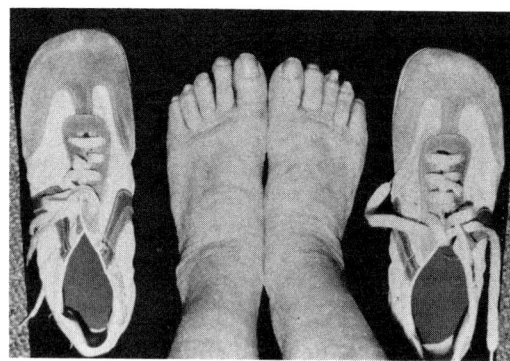

they can wear more reasonable shoes. One of the rheumatoid patient's many problems is to remain in the realm of social acceptance.

The same care must be used, however, in postoperative supports, which are necessary in practically all cases. Usually only simple metatarsal pads with or without longitudinal pads are needed. These measures are the same basic orthopedic supports used for mechanical foot deformity of any cause (see Fig. 55–5), such as marked pronation with symptoms or osteoarthritis, marked bunions, or hammer toes.

A brace may occasionally be helpful for severe valgus deformity of the hindfoot but usually provides only temporary relief. Surgical stabilization may be necessary. A simple, outside iron, short-leg brace with an inner "T" strap is prescribed when the ankle joint is not particularly painful. If the ankle is painful, a double upright brace permitting only limited ankle motion may be used. Osteoarthritis of the foot most commonly involves the MTP joints of the great toes, but it can involve any other joints.

For additional discussion of conservative treatment of the rheumatoid foot, see Chapters 47 and 89.

INDICATIONS FOR SURGERY

Surgery is indicated when there is increasing deformity of the foot or continued on weight-bearing in spite of conservative measures. In such cases, relief of the abnormal weight-bearing pressure can be obtained by surgery; the joints are extensively damaged and the feet are already "weak." The toes have lost their usual function. These patients lack the normal "takeoff" to their gait and even avoid pressure on the forefoot. Operation does not weaken the foot or impair gait further. An improved gait may decrease pain in involved knees and hips.

EVOLUTION OF SURGERY OF THE RHEUMATOID FOREFOOT

A report called "An Operation for Severe Grades of Contracted or Clawed Toes" appeared in 1912.[6] This is still an excellent paper with many valid principles. Several of the reported patients had "infectious arthritis" (now called RA). A suitable case was described as follows:

> The toes are strongly dorsiflexed at the metatarsophalangeal joints and plantar flexed at their interphalangeal ones and are retained in this position by shortening through adaptation of tendons, ligaments and

other soft structures and by bone changes due to long-continued new relationship of articular surfaces.

Operation consisted of excision of the heads and, if necessary, parts of the necks of the metatarsal bones of all the affected toes through a transverse curved plantar incision just behind the web of the toes. In the closing discussion, it was stated that:

> The operation is simply to get rid of the metatarsal heads because they make the patient's life miserable. Every step he takes hurts him so, he is afraid to get up from his chair. Mild grades of contracted toes should not be operated upon in this way.

Most of these patients had cavus feet. This finding is probably why only the metatarsal heads were resected although a considerable amount of bone was removed well back into the neck, allowing the toes to straighten and relieving the cavus deformity.

A series of patients with chronic rheumatoid arthritic feet was presented at the Boston Orthopaedic Club in 1949. Surgery had been performed with varying degrees of metatarsophalangeal joint resections through multiple dorsal incisions.

Excisional surgery has been the basic type of procedure for years, but many variations have been described. The same excisional surgery is applicable to similar painful deformities in an osteoarthritic forefoot joint.

In 1970, Raunio and Laine reviewed metatarsophalangeal joint synovectomies in 28 rheumatoid patients in many of whom the basic disease activity was judged "mild".[7] With a followup averaging 15 months, good results were found clinically and roentgenographically in up to two thirds of the cases. Overall disease activity did affect their results.

HISTORY OF HINDFOOT SURGERY IN RHEUMATOID ARTHRITIS

When the subtalar joints become inflamed, when swelling and pain occur on weight-bearing, and when planovalgus occurs, such deformity usually develops within 3 years of the onset of signs and symptoms. The most severe radiologic changes occur in the talonavicular joint, except for osteoporosis, which is most severe in the calcaneocuboid joint.

Vahvanen published a report of a controlled series of triple arthrodeses with an average follow-up of 3.7 years.[8] The symptoms of subtalar joint inflammation were usually completely resolved, and the deformity was often corrected. Slight to moderate valgus deformity (10 to 15°) commonly remained but did not cause discomfort with walking. Union usually occurred with the procedure. Nonunion occurred (9.3%) most often in the talonavicular joint. Autogenous bone grafting was recommended in the most severe cases. The use of bone graft and staples helped in the hindfoot reconstruction but did not prevent the calcaneus from slipping into a valgus position if weight-bearing was permitted sooner than 6 to 8 weeks. Triple arthrodesis did not adversely affect the stability of the ankle joint, nor did it increase progression of disease in that joint. It was recommended that the operation be performed before the hindfoot deformity became fixed. This usually occurred within 3 years of the development of progressive symptoms in the hindfoot.

The talonavicular joint is often the earliest hindfoot joint to demonstrate involvement with RA.[8a,8b] Associated peroneal muscle spasm might be the initial result, creating eversion deformity of the hindfoot. In a patient unresponsive to conservative measures but in whom the hindfoot is still flexible, *talonavicular fusion* relieves pain and corrects deformity. Progression of the deformity does not occur, and the *hindfoot is stabilized in neutral position (slight valgus) by the fusion of this single joint.*

In the hindfoot, the basic procedure is stabilization by arthrodesis. Osteoarthritic involvement of the hindfoot is treated in the same manner if supports fail to give relief.

SURGERY OF THE FOREFOOT

The marked contracture of soft tissues accompanying rheumatoid deformities demands adequate bony resection for cosmetic correction and pain relief. The MTP joints are resected with excision of enough bone to correct the deformity. In severely involved cases, I generally resect all the metatarsal heads and a portion of the necks. The proximal portion of each

FIG. 55–7. Transverse incision beginning at the dorsal aspect of the fifth metatarsophalangeal joint and extending to the medial aspect of the list metatarsal head. The shaded area of bone was excised.

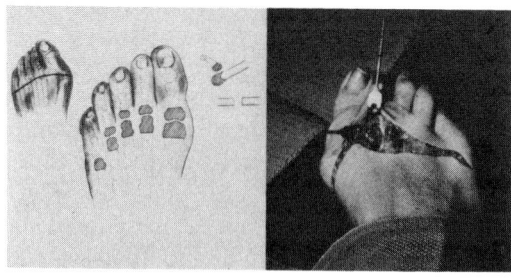

of the proximal phalanges is also removed as indicated. The toes are manipulated straight to correct the cock-up deformities, but formal fusion of the distal joints of the small toes is not performed.

All ten toes are corrected in one operation in most patients. Occasionally, in spite of the lack of underlying skin changes, such as a callus, a metatarsal head is resected because it would otherwise remain too prominent after removal of an offending adjacent head. The surgical procedure is always tailored to the individual patient. In many cases, it is preferable to operate through a transverse dorsal incision at the base of the toes (Fig. 55–7).[2] Exposure is easier than through multiple dorsal incisions. If there is a borderline circulation, however, multiple dorsal incisions are preferred. There are also indications for a plantar incision and, in general, the incision used is that with which the surgeon is most comfortable. A tourniquet, either an Esmarch bandage at the level of the ankle or a pneumatic thigh tourniquet, is used generally, but the operation can be performed without a tourniquet if nesssary.

After resection of the metatarsal heads and (usually) a portion of the proximal phalanges, the plantar aspect of each metatarsal is beveled to give a smooth weight-bearing surface. Ideally, the first and second metatarsal stumps should be approximately the same length with gradual tapering evenly across the third, fourth, and fifth. The more deformity, the more bone that is resected. The extensor tendons are usually divided except for that to the great toe, and the interphalangeal joints of the lesser toes are gently manipulated straight. The tourniquet is then released, bleeding is controlled, and drains are placed. The skin is carefully closed with fine interrupted sutures or small staples. The less trauma to these tissues, the better and more rapid the healing. Application of a large conforming dressing to hold the toes exactly in the desired position is important. In approximately 2 to 3 days, the dressings are changed and patients are permitted to take a few steps using a wooden-soled convalescent shoe. Patients are generally discharged 5 to 7 days postoperatively, and sutures are removed in the office 2 weeks later. A convalescent split shoe is fitted between 2 and 5 weeks after surgery depending on the position of the toes and/or swelling of the forefoot. Patients not needing crutches for other disability do not require crutches after forefoot surgery. A metatarsal pad, approximately $\frac{3}{16}$ inch to $\frac{1}{4}$ inch in height, is generally used postoperatively because of the altered configuration of the distal metatarsals. In some patients, a $\frac{3}{16}$ inch metatarsal bar may also be added. As a rule, no attempt is made to resect corns, calluses, or thickened bursae between

FIG. 55–8. *A, B,* Note typical deformity of forefoot. *C,* Preoperative roentgenogram. *D,*
Sole 12 days after operation.

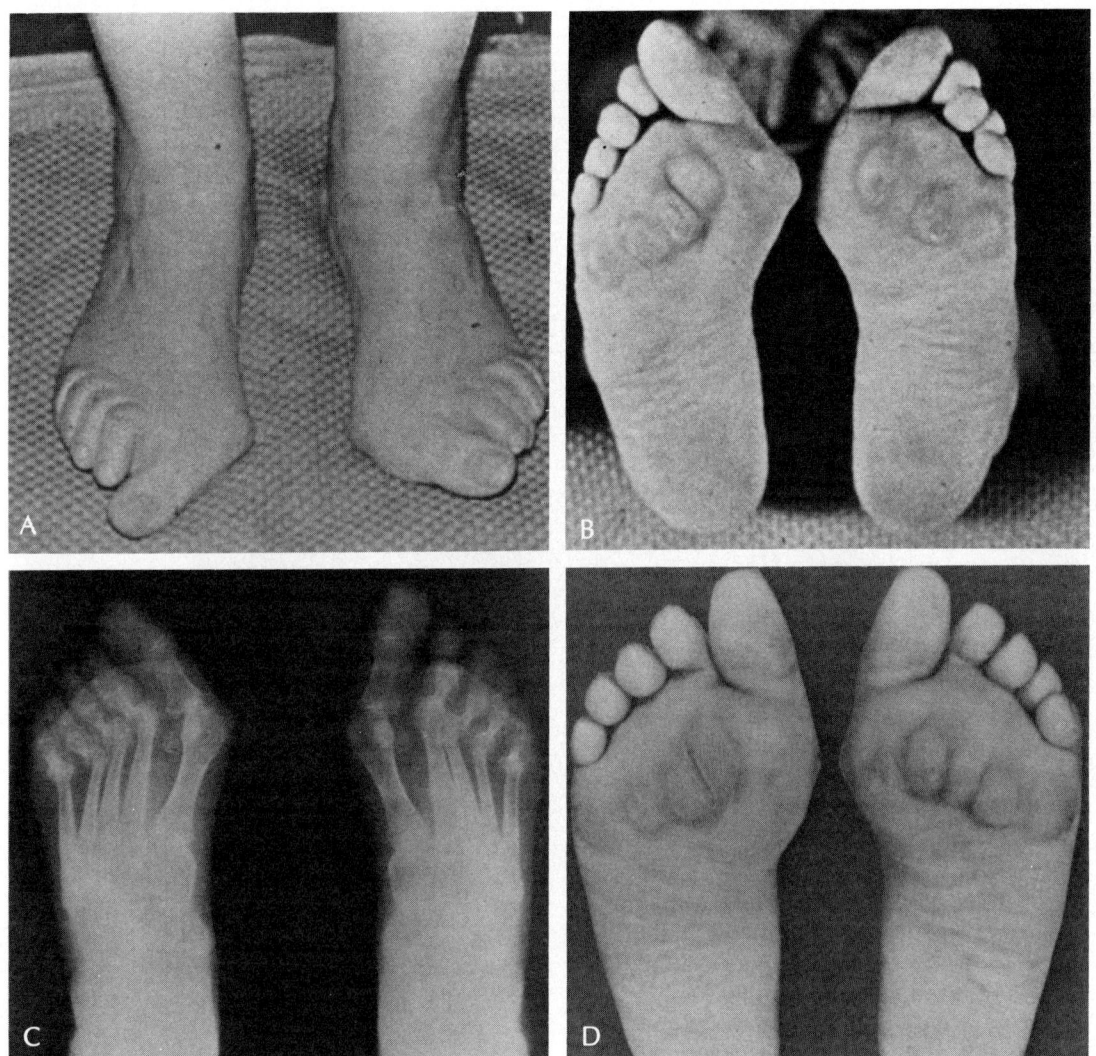

the metatarsal head at the time of surgery (Fig. 55–8*A*
to *H*) because relief of abnormal pressure allows these
to gradually disappear.

Patients should be told that 2 to 3 months are
needed for maximum recovery from bilateral forefoot
surgery, although they are usually ambulatory in 1 to
2 weeks.

The operation described previously provided good
results in 85% of patients after at least 3 years of
followup.[9–12] About 10% required additional surgery,
usually only minor procedures. These results have
been reproduced by others.[13–15] Cosmesis was not considered in reporting these results.

Other procedures used in the forefoot with less
severe deformity utilize the same basic principles of
adequate bony resection (e.g., the Keller procedure
[resection of bunion and base of proximal phalanx]
for hallux valgus and bunion [Fig. 55–9] and joint
excision for hammer toe with or without pinning [Fig.
55–10]). The basic principle of adequate bony resection holds true. However, in a rheumatoid patient, *if
more than two metatarsal heads require surgery, it is preferable to perform the entire forefoot resection so that a new
weight-bearing alignment across the entire metatarsophalangeal region is achieved.* Further decompression is obtained by resecting the base of the phalanges for
proper realignment without unnecessarily shortening
the metatarsals.

FIG. 55–8. *Continued* *E, F,* Three months after operation. *G, H,* Thirteen years after operation. Recurrent pressure problems were partially relieved by supports. Osteotomy of the second metatarsal of the right foot was performed at the time of other surgery, and symptoms were relieved.

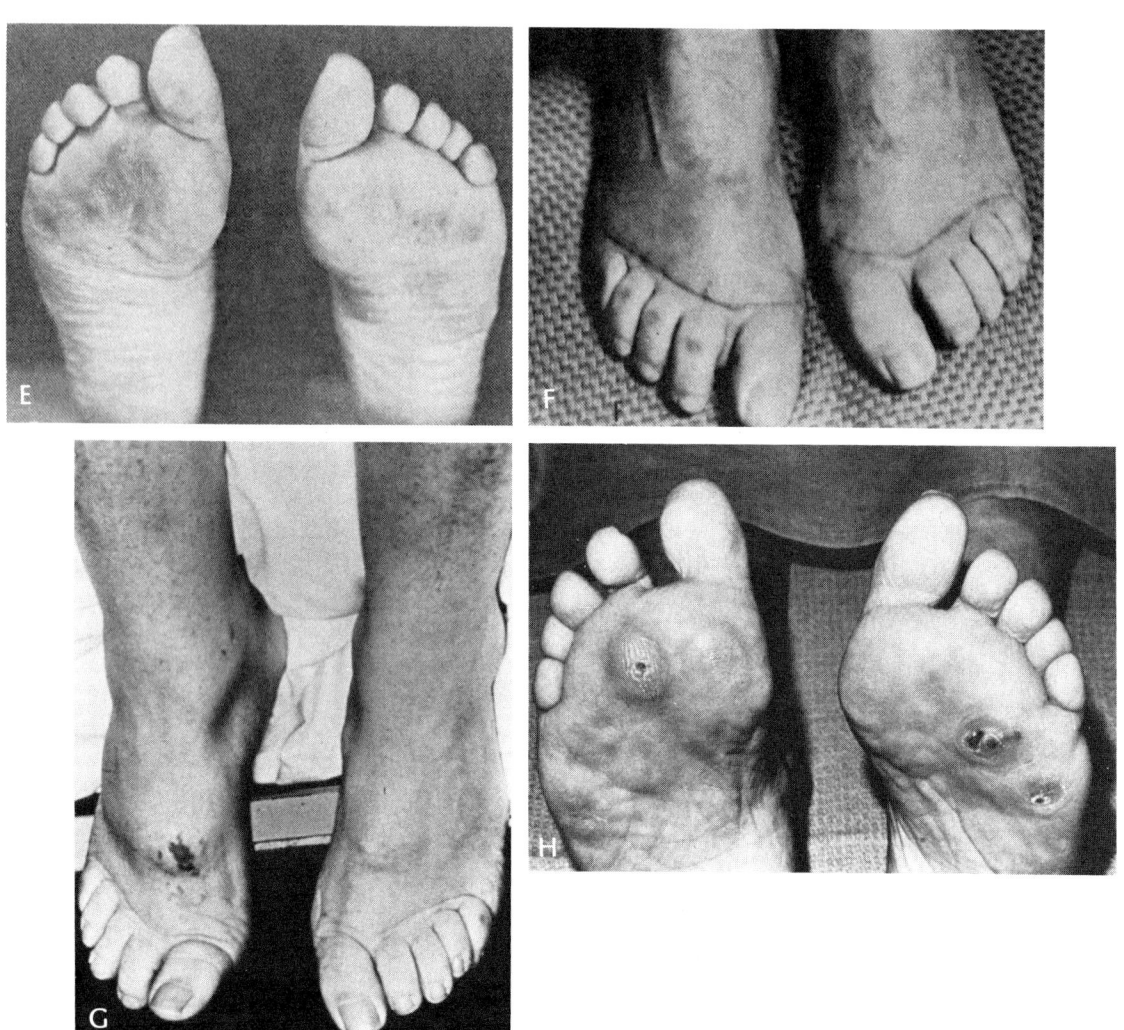

I have used a number of silicone hinge great toe implants (Swanson). Cosmetically, they are helpful and patients like them. Over 90% of my RA patients are women for whom cosmesis is important (Fig. 55–11).

The first MTP is the most common joint affected in the foot by osteoarthritis, which often produces pain and hallux rigidus as a result of loss of dorsiflexion, a motion that is necessary in the stance phase of normal gait. A resection arthroplasty (Keller procedure) is most commonly done (see Fig. 55–9); in selected cases a silicone implant may be used (Fig. 55–12). Because of a large number of cases developing silicone synovitis with the single stem prosthesis, I do not recommend its use. In a few cases in which there will not be heavy usage (e.g., running) a double stem prosthesis (Fig. 55–11) can be used for a rheumatoid great toe. Wear problems and silicone synovitis are relatively uncommon with the double hinge type prosthesis. In a very active person I do not use any artificial implant but rather use local soft tissues or banked fascia lata as necessary for interposition. After removal of the prosthesis and the reactive synovium, a resection-type arthroplasty still remains and usually gives a good functional result because of the fibrous capsule remaining around the new joint.

FIG. 55–9. Keller procedure, excision of bunion and osteophytes of the metatarsal head, and excision of proximal portion of the proximal phalanx. In addition, a hinged (silicone) implant may be used, particularly for cosmesis in women.

FIG. 55–11. Silicone hinge (Swanson) prosthesis for selected rheumatoid forefoot arthroplasty. Its use requires the same precise rebalancing of the soft tissues around the implant as it does in the hand.

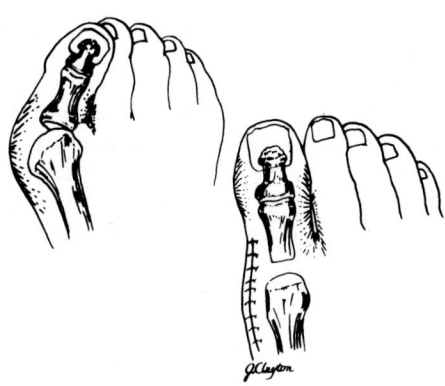

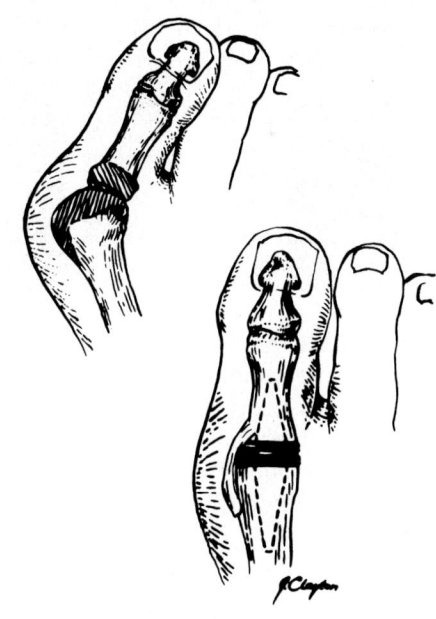

Any patient considering a joint implant or replacement should be warned that any device implanted in the body may have to be removed or revised at some future date.

Intramedullary Kirschner wires are often used to stabilize the lesser metatarsophalangeal joint resection. A plantar plate may be used to cover the weight-bearing area of the metatarsal head, providing an interposition arthroplasty (Fig. 55–13). Centralization of the flexor tendons beneath the resected end of the

FIG. 55–10. Middle joint resection for hammer toe (ankylosis of toes is neither necessary or desirable). Pin should not cross the metatarsophalangeal joint unless necessary to maintain correction. Pin is usually left in place for 3 to 4 weeks.

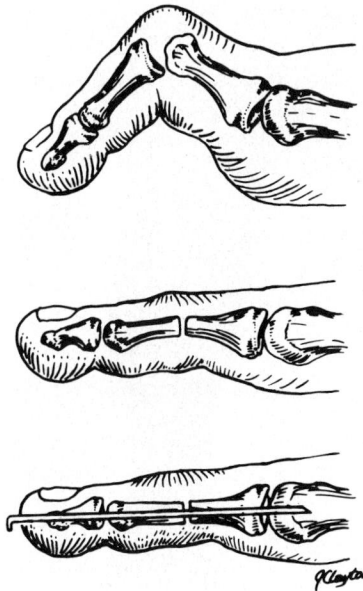

metatarsal and use of a Kirschner wire promote fibrosis in the area which prevents later subluxation. However, convalescence is slower with the use of a silicone implant or intramedullary wire fixation.

After 3 years of followup, the cosmetic results obtained from either Silastic prostheses or plantar plate arthroplasty have been good. The functional results are similar to those found after resections. (However, past experience shows that procedures that remove less bone have had more recurrences.) In general, the more cosmetic procedures are reserved for younger patients. In an older patient in whom early resumption of activities is so important, simple excisional forefoot arthroplasty without any additional fixation provides both early mobilization and pain relief (Fig. 55–14). Smyth considers this the most successful procedure in the rheumatoid lower extremity over a period of 30 years.[16]

SURGERY OF THE HINDFOOT

The valgus deformity of the hind part of the rheumatoid foot with its insidious progression often resembles a paralytic valgus deformity. Arthrodesis, the surgery of choice in the hindfoot, is indicated when pain and deformity persist despite conservative measures. Osteoarthritis of the hindfoot is usually post-

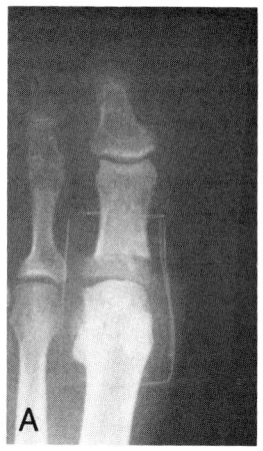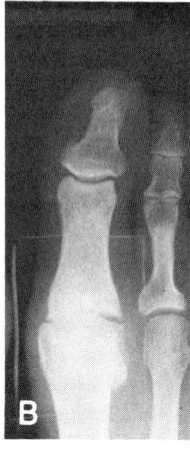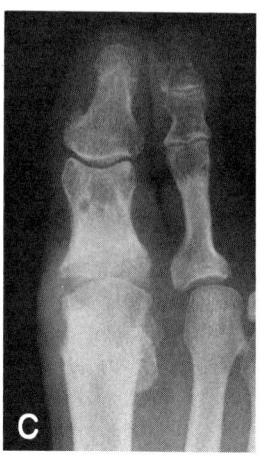

FIG. 55–12. *A,* Active, tennis-playing, 54-year-old woman with pain and limited dorsiflexion of right great toe. Note marked narrowing, sclerosis, and mild osteophytes in right first metatarsophalangeal joint. Diagnosis is osteoarthritis (hallux rigidus). *B,* Postoperative Keller procedure with silicone implant (film reversed). Patient had excellent cosmetic and functional result 7.5 years later. *C,* She then developed pain and swelling and film revealed evidence of silicone synovitis. The implant was removed, banked fascia lata was inserted, and she is again playing tennis and golf with a good cosmetic and functional result 4 months later. I no longer use single stem silicone implants.

traumatic and much rarer than RA. The indications for operation are the same.

If the deformity is not passively correctable, triple arthrodesis (subtalar, talonavicular, and calcaneocuboid) with joint excision to correct the deformity is utilized. Internal fixation is usually used and, in very unstable cases, cast immobilization is necessary without weight-bearing for 6 to 8 weeks, followed by use of a walking cast for another month. If the hindfoot is quite stable, weight can be borne sooner. It takes 4 to 6 months for complete recovery.

If the talonavicular joint is the most involved, and if the foot is in a reasonable position, fusion of this joint alone suffices to stabilize the hindfoot. Hindfoot arthrodesis gives good results in about 85% of cases, with relief of pain at the expense of motion.

Rheumatoid nodules may require excision, but recurrence is common unless recurrent pressure is prevented. Tenosynovitis appears around the foot and ankle and may require tenosynovectomy if other

FIG. 55–13. Plantar plate arthroplasty. After double resection at the metatarsophalangeal joint, the plantar plate is freed from the flexor tendon and brought up across the end of the resected metatarsal and impaled by the Kirschner wire. To provide a pad beneath the metatarsal head and to keep the important flexor tendons centralized, the extensor tendon is not sutured.

FIG. 55–14. Sixty-six year-old woman with generalized RA 3 years after bilateral forefoot reconstructions. She had no complaints referable to her feet. These feet illustrate the catch phrase, "it is a good thing the patient doesn't walk on the x-rays." Note the good overall soft-tissue contour of the feet as well as the relative length of the metatarsals.

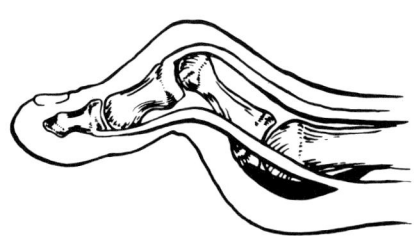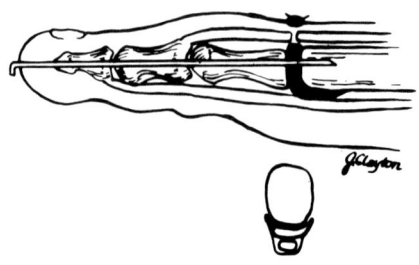

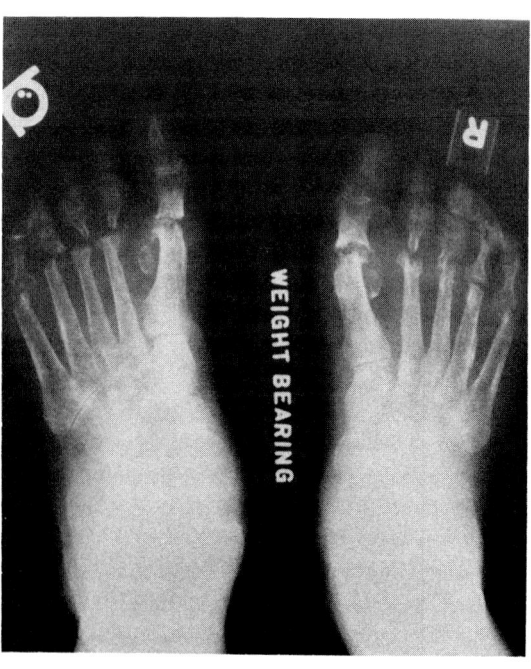

measures, such as injection of corticosteroids into the tendon sheath, fail.

CARE OF THE RHEUMATOID ANKLE

Ankle involvement of a disabling degree is unusual in RA. The patient often complains of "a painful ankle" for any pain in the hindfoot, and hindfoot deformity may increase ankle pain.

Proper shoes and supports for foot deformity are used. If no relief is obtained, a short leg double upright brace, without a joint, may be added to the shoe. Such braces may be masked by wearing boots. If relief is not obtained, surgery should be considered.

Synovectomy may help in patients with pain and marked synovial proliferation before cartilage destruction or loss of motion has occurred, but such cases are rare.

Arthrodesis of the ankle relieves pain arising from the joint, but because it often increases symptoms in the other joints of the hindfoot, it is not often indicated in RA. Rarely, if triple arthrodesis increases ankle deformity and pain, arthrodesis of the ankle is indicated.

Total ankle arthroplasty is useful in RA because of the almost uniform involvement of other joints of the hindfoot. In general, if hindfoot arthrodesis is indicated, it should be performed first and an ankle arthroplasty performed 6 weeks or more after wound healing (Fig. 55–15). Total ankle replacement is usually performed through an anterior incision using a metal-plastic articulation and methylmethacrylate (bone cement). A cast is used for a few weeks, or early motion is prescribed according to the circumstances. Protected weight bearing is usually necessary for about 3 months.

In a good result about 20 to 30° of motion are obtained. Pain relief is not as predictable as with hip or knee replacement, perhaps because of the proximity of other involved joints in the hindfoot. I have obtained only about 70% totally satisfactory results. The forces on the ankle are great (up to eight times body weight). Extreme osteoporosis is a contraindication. In the 30% unsatisfactory results there can be terrible problems. When failure results from loosening, sal-

FIG. 55–15. Total ankle arthroplasty performed 3 months after a triple arthrodesis. Note staples across subtalar and calcaneocuboid joint with fusion of these joints and the talonavicular bone. Overall alignment of the foot is good. The screw in the medial malleolus was inserted for a fracture at the time of surgery and has healed in normal alignment. The patient was immobilized for 6 weeks after the ankle surgery and has 30° of painless motion in her ankle, which is still functioning well 11 years after surgery.

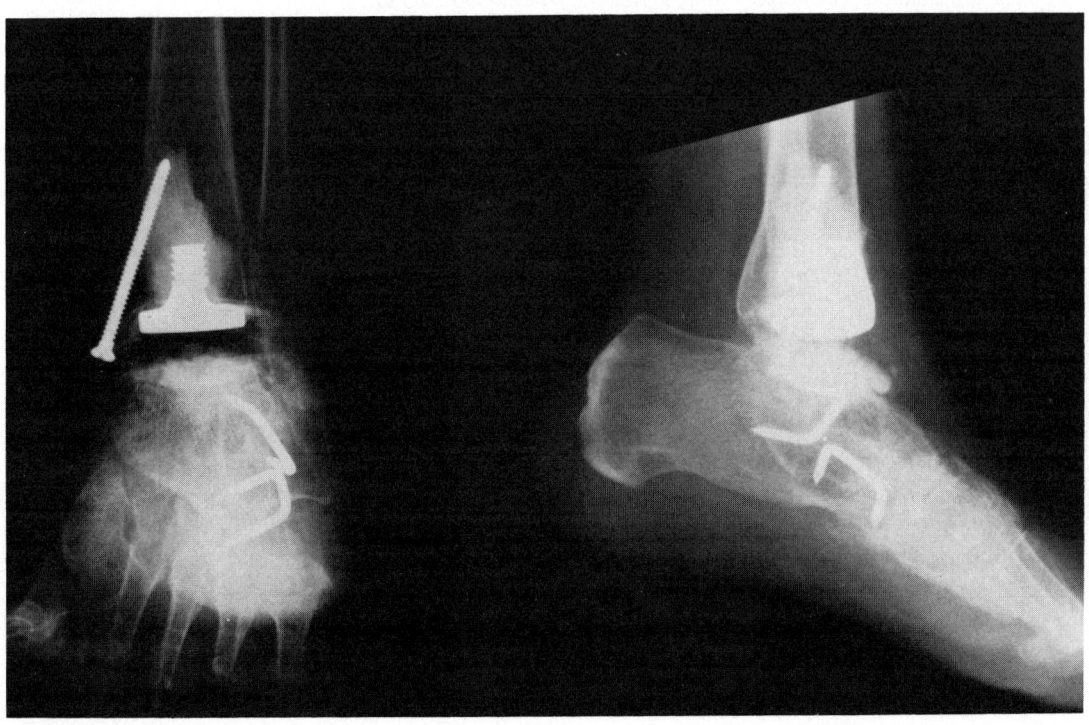

FIG. 55–16. Failed total ankle arthroplasty 7 years after procedure. Note the loosening of the tibial component and the marked bone loss and tilting into valgus of the component. The loss of bone stock makes a revision or fusion very difficult.

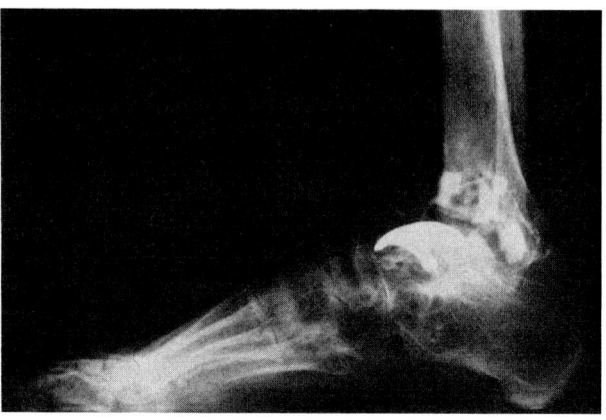

vage is extremely difficult because of bone loss around the prosthesis (Fig. 55–16). Salvage using autologous bone or bank bone with external or internal fixation and immobilization for up to 9 months have given a satisfactory fusion in two of three cases, but these are not completely free of pain. *I do not recommend total ankle replacement in RA with the use of bone cement because of the lack of a dependable salvage procedure.* It may still

be indicated in an unusual case because there have been a number of excellent results (Fig. 55–15).

Cementless total ankle replacement with press fitting and porous-coated surfaces for ingrowth now seems promising, but this is still an investigational procedure. If it should fail there would be enough bone stock remaining for salvage by fusion.

Ankle fusion is still considered the standard operation in RA until further followup data are obtained on the cementless total ankle procedure.

Fusion of the ankle and hindfoot (pantalar arthrodesis) leaves a stiff foot but relieves pain; in severe cases it is a helpful salvage procedure.

CARE OF THE OSTEOARTHRITIC ANKLE

In osteoarthritis (usually post-traumatic) in some early cases, debridement of anterior osteophytes is helpful because symptoms are often caused by impingement rather than generalized ankle osteoarthritis. In more severe cases, ankle arthrodesis is an excellent procedure that is preferable to total ankle replacement. With a normal hindfoot (triple joints), an ankle fusion in neutral position (90° angle between the foot and the tibia) still permits about 25° of plantar flexion from neutral. This result allows a normal gait

FIG. 55–17. Postoperative ankle fusion for old fracture-dislocation of ankle resulting in traumatic osteoarthritis with severe pain. Ankle fusion has been performed with a lateral approach using a living fibular graft and supplementary staple fixation. The ankle is fused in a neutral position on the lateral film. Note the normal joints in the hindfoot that allow 20 to 25° of plantar flexion and dorsiflexion and a normal gait.

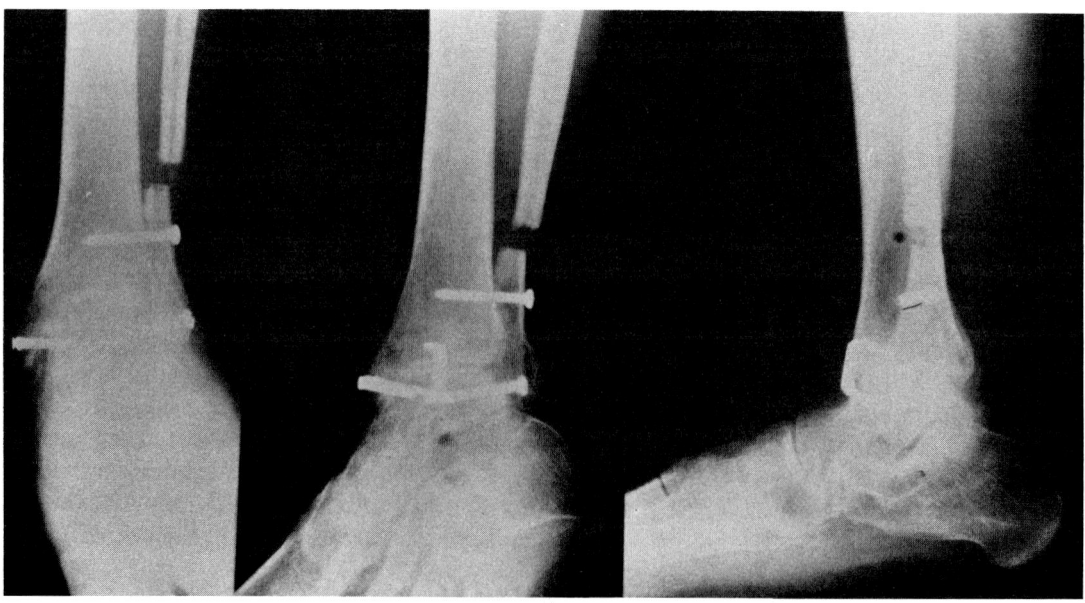

with an ordinary heel or with a one-inch dress heel for women. If the hindfoot joints are also damaged, the motion is less. Ankle arthrodesis may be performed by various approaches with or without supplementary bone grafts (Fig. 55–17). Immobilization usually lasts between 3 and 4 months with 6 to 8 weeks of non-weight-bearing. Approximately 6 months are needed for maximum recovery.

CONCLUSION

Arthritic deformities of the foot and ankle are quite common and painful. The source of the pain must be properly diagnosed.

Conservative treatment, both medical and mechanical, (shoe alterations and arch supports) should be used first. If pain is increasing and function decreasing, orthopedic consultation should be obtained regarding surgery.

With a team approach between the rheumatologist and a rheumatologically oriented orthopedic surgeon, surgery can give gratifying results.

REFERENCES

1. Short, C.L., Bauer, W., and Reynolds, W.F.: Rheumatoid Arthritis. Cambridge, Harvard University Press, 1957.
2. Clayton, M.L. Leidholdt, J.D., and Smyth, C.J.: Surgery of the forefoot in rheumatoid arthritis. Motion picture available through the American Academy of Orthopaedic Surgeons, Chicago, IL.
3. Smith-Petersen, M.N., Aufranc, O.E., and Larson, C.B.: Useful surgical procedures for rheumatoid arthritis involving joints of the upper extremity. Arch. Surg., 46:764, 1943.
4. Vainio, K.: The rheumatoid foot. A clinical study with pathological and roentgenological comment. Ann. Chir. Gynaecol. Fenn., 45:Suppl. 1, 1956.
5. Berg, E. et al.: Non-operative care of the painful rheumatoid foot. American Academy of Orthopaedic Surgeons, Exhibit. 1978.
6. Hoffman, P.: An operation for severe grades of contracted or clawed toes. Am. J. Orthop. Surg., 9:441, 1912.
7. Raunio, P., and Laine, H.: Synovectomy of the metatarsophalangeal joints in rheumatoid arthritis. Acta Rheumatol. Scand., 16:12, 1970.
8. Vahvanen, V.: Rheumatoid arthritis in the pantalar joints. Acta Orthop. Scand. Suppl. 107, Helsinki, 1967.
8a.Elabur, J.E., Thomas, W.H., Weinfeld, M.S., and Potter, T.: Talonavicular arthrodesis for rheumatoid arthritis of the hindfoot. Orthop. Clin. North Am., 7:821, 1976.
8b.Potter, T.A.: Rheumatoid arthritis of the foot. Exhibit American Medical Association Meeting. Denver, November, 1961.
9. Clayton, M.L.: Results of surgery in rheumatoid feet. Excerpta Medica Intl. Congress Series No. 165, October, 1967.
10. Clayton, M.L.: Surgery of the lower extremity in rheumatoid arthritis. J. Bone Joint Surg., 45A:1517, 1963.
11. Clayton, M.L.: Surgery of the forefoot in rheumatoid arthritis. Clin. Orthop., 16:136, 1960.
12. Clayton, M.L.: Surgery of the forefoot in rheumatoid arthritis. Arthritis Rheum., 2:84–85, 1959.
13. Funk, F.J., Jr.: Surgery of the foot in rheumatoid arthritis. Semin. Arthritis Rheum., 1:25, 1971.
14. Gschwend, N.: Surgical Treatment of Rheumatoid Arthritis. Stuttgart, New York, Georg Thieme Verlag, 1980.
15. Marmor, I.: Rheumatoid deformity of the foot. Arthritis Rheum., 6:749, 1963.
16. Smyth, C.J.: Personal communication.

section V

OTHER INFLAMMATORY ARTHRITIC SYNDROMES

56

SERONEGATIVE POLYARTHRITIS

GRACIELA S. ALARCÓN

An operational definition for the seronegative polyarthritis group of disorders is essential. *Seronegative* refers to the absence of antibodies in the serum reactive with antigenic determinants in the Fc portion of the IgG molecule, that is, rheumatoid factor(s), as determined by the latex fixation test (LFT).[1] Many disorders fulfill this definition, including the arthritides associated with some endocrinopathies (e.g., hypothyroidism); hematologic disorders (e.g., hemophilia); metabolic disorders (e.g., crystal-induced arthritis, ochronosis, hemochromatosis); connective tissue disorders (e.g., systemic lupus erythematosus, systemic sclerosis); as well as some rheumatic disorders, such as those that primarily affect the axial skeleton, the so-called spondyloarthropathies, as well as their purely peripheral forms (i.e., psoriatic arthritis without spondylitis, or the peripheral arthritis associated with inflammatory bowel disease).

Since the independent discoveries of rheumatoid factor by Waaler[2] and Rose et al.[3] in 1940 and 1948, respectively, and the widespread clinical use of the LFT,[1] it became apparent that a variable but relatively small proportion of patients with clinical rheumatoid arthritis (RA) were indeed seronegative. Despite rigorous study and classification of patients with seronegative polyarthritis, a group will remain who fulfill the American Rheumatism Association (ARA) diagnostic criteria for "definite RA"[4] (1958 ARA criteria) or RA[4a] (1987 ARA revised criteria). Disagreement exists concerning the precise proportion of seronegative polyarthritis patients who will fulfill criteria for RA after such rigorous study.[5,6] Calin[7] has argued that patients with early seronegative polyarthritis be called "undifferentiated seronegative arthritis," with the expectation that, in time, some will develop findings permitting a diagnosis other than RA, whereas others will develop "definite" (but still seronegative) RA. As a group these patients have immunologic, immunogenetic, and clinical characteristics distinguishing them from their seropositive counterparts.[8,9] As additional insight is gained into the etiology of RA and other arthritides, it may be possible to further differentiate diagnostic categories within this group of arthritides.

Unless otherwise specified, I will discuss here seronegative RA.

EPIDEMIOLOGY

The prevalence and incidence of seronegative RA as previously defined are largely unknown. Although numerous population-based studies of the prevalence and incidence of RA have been conducted, their interpretation is confounded by methodologic problems such as the inclusion of patients with other disorders (e.g., rheumatic fever or seronegative spondyloarthropathies)[10] and the definition of cases either by serologic (rheumatoid factor positivity) or radiologic status (erosive disease) with variable emphasis on the presence or absence of clinical manifestations.[11,12] These and other confounding factors have been extensively reviewed.[7,9,13,14] The prevalence and incidence of seronegative RA can only be estimated.

905

However, because patients with seronegative RA may have less severe disease (vide infra), bias *against* this group of patients probably exists in studies conducted at referral centers. Assuming prevalence figures for RA between 0.3 and 2%[15] and a frequency of seronegativity between 12 and 25%,[16,17] the estimated prevalence for seronegative RA varies between 0.03 and 0.5% for adult populations. For more accurate prevalence and incidence data, standardized criteria are clearly needed.[18] Such criteria must first be validated. Their sensitivity, specificity, and predictive positive and negative values must be established in different groups of patients.

CLINICAL MANIFESTATIONS

The recognition and study of patients with seronegative RA has obviously been possible only in the last three decades. Interpretation of published data is hampered by use of different criteria by different investigators. The serologic status of individual patients may change over time (e.g., from seronegative to seropositive in patients with early polyarthritis or vice versa in patients with long-standing RA); the characterization of a patient as "seronegative" therefore should be restricted to those consistently seronegative. In our studies we have defined seronegativity as three separate negative LFT determinations and seropositivity as two separate positive tests at a titer of $\geq$1:320.[19,20] A group of patients fulfilling neither criteria are excluded by definition. Although separate LFTs are required by our criteria, the time interval between them was not specified. Gran and Husby[18] have also included time in their definition; not less than 3 years are required before a patient is assigned to either a seropositive or a seronegative group.[18]

A consensus based on published series is that patients with seronegative RA generally have less-severe disease and a better prognosis than do seropositive patients. Seronegative RA patients have fewer extra-articular manifestations such as fever, necrotizing vasculitis, organ system involvement, and subcutaneous nodules and develop less deforming and less destructive arthritis as assessed either clinically or radiologically.[19-31] Our own studies conducted in a large number of white[19] and American black[20] patients with an average disease duration of over 10 years and in whom strict serologic status was defined corroborate this view. Pelvic roentgenograms were not obtained in all patients, however. Therefore, it could be argued that seronegative spondyloarthropathies were not conclusively excluded. None had clinical evidence of sacroiliitis or extra-articular findings associated with seronegative spondyloarthropathies; however, the B7-CREG antigens were not increased in our seronegative RA patients compared to healthy controls of the same ethnic background.[32]

Data comparing seronegative and seropositive RA are summarized in Table 56–1. Patients with seronegative RA may develop progressive and sometimes severe disease including extra-articular manifestations. Rheumatoid nodules definitely occur in a small fraction of patients with seronegative RA;[33,34] life-threatening complications such as cardiac tamponade and necrotizing vasculitis have been described.[35,36]

A small series of 10 seronegative patients with distinctive clinical features has been described recently.[37] All were white and elderly; eight tenths were men. All presented a relatively acute onset of symmetric synovitis involving the wrist, small hand joints, and flexor tendon sheaths associated with pitting edema of the dorsum of the hands ("boxing glove hand"). All patients experienced a complete remission within 3 to 36 months while taking aspirin or other nonsteroidal drugs usually coupled with hydroxychloroquine. Remissions were maintained without maintenance therapy. Most patients were positive for HLA-B7. This syndrome was designated remitting seronegative, symmetric synovitis with pitting edema (RS_3PE). Other rheumatologists have alluded to similar patients.[38,39] Whether this condition truly represents a distinct subset of seronegative polyarthritis will require longitudinal study of a larger group of patients.

IMMUNOLOGIC FEATURES

For decades immunologists and rheumatologists have been puzzled by the absence of rheumatoid factor(s) (RF) in patients otherwise fulfilling ARA criteria for the diagnosis of RA.[4,4a] Radioimmunoassays, enzyme-linked immunoassay (ELISA), and other procedures now can detect nanogram quantities of RF.[40-42] Such tests have revealed that the LFT is a relatively insensitive test. Rheumatoid factor levels in sera from normal persons, "seronegative" RA patients, and seropositive RA patients are distributed as a continuum when the more sensitive tests are used; that is, "seronegativity" is often a quantitative not a qualitative condition.

The more sensitive assays for RF have also permitted study of in vitro production of IgM and of IgM-RF by mononuclear leukocytes (MNL) from normal individuals as well as from seropositive and seronegative RA patients. MNL from approximately 40% of seropositive, but not seronegative, RA patients or

Table 56–1.   Clinical Features in Seropositive and Seronegative RA

Author, Year, Place, Ref	IgM Rheumatoid Factor Serologic Status	n	% F	DOD (Years)	EAM (%)	FC (ARA)	EA (%)	RT (%)	Comments
Dixon, 1960, England[21]	(+)	12	NA	NA	NA	Mild and severe disease observed in both sero(+) and sero(−) patients.	NA	NA	Hospital-based sample; serologic status defined at last visit
	(−)	24	NA	NA	NA		NA	NA	
Bland and Brown, 1963, United States[22]	(+)	24	46	11	58	NA	Yes	NA	Hospital-based sample; patients matched for age and sex
	(−)	23	74	9	17	NA	Yes	NA	Disease of reasonable duration
Duthie et al., 1964, England[23]	(+)	88	NA	NA	NA	Significantly better in the sero(−) patients	NA	NA	Hospital-based sample; serologic status determined at last visit
	(−)	66	NA	NA	NA		NA	NA	
Mongan and Atwater, 1968, United States[24]	(+)	216	NA	NA	43	NA	NA	NA	Hospital-based sample; patients with spondyloarthropathies included in both groups
	(−)	144	NA	NA	5	NA	NA	NA	
Mongan et al., 1969, United States[25]	(+)	107	66	NA	39	Disease was functionally and anatomically more severe in those patients with vasculitis, all of whom were sero(+)		5	Hospital-based sample
	(−)	29	66	NA	7			39	
Cats and Hazevoet, 1970, The Netherlands[26]	(+)	130	73	13	30	Significantly worse in the sero(+) patients	Yes	NA	Hospital-based sample; patients matched for age and sex
	(−)	130	73	14	5		Yes	NA	Disease of reasonable duration
Masi et al., 1976, United States[27]	(+)	20	85	0.5	20	} Similar	50	Yes	Community-based sample; patients with early polyarthritis
	(−)	30	73	0.5	3		3	Yes	Serologic status determined at entry
Esdaile et al., 1977, Canada[27]	(+)	NA	NA	NA	NA	NA	NA	NA	Hospital-based sample; study designed to determine if B27 could distinguish patients with sero(−) polyarthritis of short duration
	(−)	58	76	4	NA	NA	NA	NA	
Alarcón et al., 1982, United States[19]	(+)	80	55	12	38	2.6	65	91	Hospital-based sample; patients were consistently sero(+) or sero(−)
	(−)	30	87	13	0	2.4	41	70	Disease of reasonable duration
Alarcón et al., 1983, United States[20]	(+)	63	63	11	14	2.4	57	89	Hospital-based sample; patients were consistently sero(+) or sero(−)
	(−)	22	82	10	0	2.0	32	55	Disease of reasonable duration
Edelman and Russell, 1983, Canada[29]	(+)	30	87	6	27	NA	} Similar	77	Hospital-based sample of sequentially obtained sero(+) and sero(−) patients
	(−)	30	87	6	3	NA		57	Disease of intermediate duration
Bardin et al., 1985, France[30]	(+)	77	79	NA	42	NA	88	NA	Hospital-based sample
	(−)	46	87	12	17	NA	69	NA	Careful exclusion of other sero(−) arthritides
									Sero(−) of reasonable duration
Raspe et al., 1986, West Germany[31]	(+)	51	72	>1	NA	} Similar	33	NA	Hospital-based sample of patients with early diagnosis
	(−)	49	72	>1	NA		29	NA	

ref = reference; sero(+) = seropositive; sero(−) = seronegative; F = female; DOD = duration of disease; EAM = one or more extra-articular manifestations (subcutaneous nodules, vasculitis, Sjogren, visceral organ involvement); FC = functional capacity; ARA = American Rheumatism Association; EA = erosive arthritis; RT = remittive therapy; NA = not available.

normal persons spontaneously produce IgM-RF.[42–44] MNL from both normal individuals and seronegative RA patients, however, can synthesize IgM-RF in response to mitogens such as Epstein-Barr virus or pokeweed.[45,46] Regulatory mechanisms controlling RF production have been postulated to exist in patients with seronegative RA and normal individuals. Patients with seropositive RA are thought to have lost this regulatory function, resulting in polyclonal expansion of B-lymphocytes and enhanced production of RF.[17] Fewer B cells capable of producing RF in pa-

tients with seronegative RA is another possible explanation.[43] Anti-idiotype antibody directed against IgM-RF is another possibility explaining persistent seronegativity.[47] Perhaps different mechanisms are responsible for persistent seronegativity in different RA patients.

Whether RFs are truly pathogenic or represent an epiphenomenon is another important question. RF synthesis does occur in situ and may parallel the local inflammatory processes in patients with either seropositive RA or seronegative RA.[48] The spectrum of synovial histopathologic changes in RA ranges from a marked infiltration with mononuclear cells, predominantly lymphocytes, to one with fibroblastic and synoviocyte hyperplasia but few lymphocytes. Neither histopathologic type predicts an RA patient's serologic status.[17,49]

Local RF production occurs in both seropositive and seronegative RA patients, although it may be tightly complexed ("hidden") in the latter. Efforts to characterize hidden RFs have been undertaken by different investigators with variable degrees of success.[50,51] Hidden RFs have been uncovered after dissociation from bound IgG in some studies, while other studies have failed to detect it either in serum or in MNL supernatants from seronegative RA patients.[44]

Serum levels of immunoglobulins are generally elevated in patients with RA regardless of serologic status.[52,53] In vitro production of IgM by MNL from seropositive RA patients after mitogen stimulation is lower than that of MNL from seronegative RA patients or normal individuals, but the ratio of IgM-RF/IgM produced is greater in the seropositive patients. There appears to be preferential expansion of B-cell clones committed to IgM-RF production in seropositive RA patients.[42,44]

Patients with RA have a deficiency in IgG galactosylation, which has been postulated to trigger the production of RF by exposing antigenic determinants in the IgG molecule.[54] Although patients with seropositive RA (LFT) had more deficient IgG galactosylation than their seronegative counterparts, considerable overlap occurred between the two groups and patients with other inflammatory disorders.[55]

In summary, patients with seronegative RA appear to have a deficient number of B cells committed to RF synthesis; an intact regulatory network preventing the production of RF; or active production of anti-idiotypic antibodies that suppress RF production. Synovial histopathology and serum immunoglobulin levels cannot differentiate seropositive from seronegative RA patients. The absence of serum RF, although clearly important in disease classification and prognosis, does not exclude local production of RF in inflamed synovium from patients with seronegative RA.[48] Still other mechanisms, such as sensitization to type II collagen and production of anticollagen antibodies, may be of pathogenic significance in seronegative RA.[56]

IMMUNOGENETICS

The controversy over the immunogenetic characteristics of patients with seronegative RA most likely reflects the different inclusion and exclusion criteria used. Gran and Husby[18] have summarized most of the existing literature; nine of sixteen studies cited by these authors showed an association between HLA-DR4 and seronegative RA. From reviewing these and other studies,[19,20,30,31,57–70] the following points emerge:

1. The racial/ethnic background of the patients studied (association which may be valid for a given ethnic group, may not be for another) should be clearly stated.

2. The frequency of HLA-DR4 in patients with seronegative RA (even in those studies in which no statistically significant association was found), was generally intermediate between that of healthy controls and seropositive RA patients. Increased sample size might result in statistically significant differences. If data are pooled from studies conducted in patients and controls from the same ethnic background (e.g., whites),[19,30,57–60] the overall HLA-DR4 frequency for the Caucasian controls (n = 597) is 21.6%; for the seronegative white RA patients (n = 166), 30.7%; and for the seropositive white RA patients (n = 332), 65.9%. The differences between the frequency of HLA-DR4 between both seropositive and seronegative RA patients and controls is now statistically significant ($p < 0.02$ and < 0.05, respectively). The pooled data also permit estimation of the relative risk of HLA-DR4–positive individuals for the occurrence of seropositive RA (7.0) or seronegative RA (1.6).

3. The positive association between seronegative RA and HLA-DR4 in some studies can be partially explained by the inclusion of historically seropositive (but currently seronegative) patients, or by inclusion of patients from other ethnic groups (e.g., American blacks). The available data do not permit determination as to whether RA represents a genetically heterogeneous disorder, or a mixture of genetically distinct and relatively homogeneous subgroups.[71]

4. Other DR specificities, such as DR1, have also been associated with RA, and this association is stronger with seronegativity, especially in Jewish patients. Further, serologically determined DR4 is heterogeneous. This locus can be differentiated into at least five different specificities or subtypes (HLA-Dw4, w10, w13, w14, w15) by mixed-lymphocyte culture assays, and selected antibody typing.[72,73] These specficities associate differently with RA. For example, the lack of association of DR4 in the Jewish population appears to be related to the predominance of the Dw10 variant of DR4.[74]

DR4 has been extensively studied as a potential modulatory gene for RF expression and in vitro IgM-RF production,[75] as well as for clinical disease expression[19,20,75–79] and the occurrence of drug toxicity.[76–81]

Our own data in whites suggest that HLA-DR4–positive, seronegative RA patients (8/30) tend to have disease of similar severity to that of seropositive RA patients who were also HLA-DR4 positive.[19] HLA-DR4 has been claimed to be a possible risk factor for more severe seropositive RA,[76–79] whereas HLA-DR2 has been claimed to confer a protective effect in patients with seropositive RA who tend to have less severe disease.[76] This possible "protective" effect of HLA-DR2 has not been investigated in seronegative RA.

Whether HLA-DR3 is a marker for the occurrence of toxic reactions to gold (e.g., proteinuria, thrombocytopenia) in seronegative patients (as has been clearly shown in both whites and American black patients with seropositive RA) remains to be determined.[76,80–82] HLA-DR3 also predisposes to the occurrence of D-penicillamine–induced toxicity.[76,82] No definite association between a given genetic marker and the occurrence of either major or minor side effects to the administration of methotrexate in RA has been demonstrated.[83] Most studies have included few seronegative patients with even fewer toxic manifestations. Definite conclusions as to the importance of genetic markers and toxic reactions to drugs in patients with seronegative RA cannot be reached.

Immunogenetic studies have been conducted in the RS₃PE syndrome.[37] Eight of the ten patients studied were typed, and six possessed the CREG B7,[37] suggesting a possible link between this syndrome and the seronegative spondyloarthropathies. Again, more time and more patients are needed.

The techniques of molecular biology are being applied to the problem of the genetic basis of susceptibility to RA. DNA restriction fragment length polymorphisms analysis, permitting the detection of genetic polymorphism in chromosomes of interest in a given disease, is particularly promising. Such polymorphisms may not be detectable by more conventional serologic techniques and therefore offer a powerful tool for identifying disease-susceptibility markers in selected populations. Several DNA polymorphisms are now being studied in seropositive RA patients.[84–86] This methodology, applied to the study of patients with seronegative RA or other types of seronegative polyarthritis, may determine whether we are dealing with a single heterogeneous disease or with different but relatively homogeneous subsets.

RADIOLOGY

Despite the relative abundance of clinical data comparing seropositive with seronegative RA, the literature is relatively sparse concerning radiologic features that may help distinguish these groups of patients.[29,87] Patients with seronegative RA are often thought to have more severe involvement of the hands and feet in contrast to more involvement of large lower and upper extremity joints in seropositive disease. A systematic study of radiologic features in RA patients correlated these with serologic status.[87] Over 93% of patients with seronegative RA (n = 46) were correctly identified by their hand/wrist radiographic features. These features included (1) more significant involvement of the carpal bones, (2) relative preservation of bone alignment, (3) relatively asymmetric involvement of the hand and wrist joints, and (4) an increased frequency of subchondral bony sclerosis, periostitis, and bony ankylosis. Another study of 60 patients, however, failed to validate these findings.[29]

Characteristic hand and wrist radiographic changes in a patient with longstanding seronegative RA are shown in Figure 56–1. The radiographic features of involved large joints appear to be of little or no value in distinguishing between seropositive and seronegative RA or between these arthritides and other pannus-producing arthritis. Patients with seronegative RA, however, tend to have less destructive disease in the hips, knees, and cervical spine than do those with seropositive RA. Thus, it might be predicted that

FIG. 56–1. Posteroanterior radiograph of both hands and wrists. Advanced intercarpal cartilage loss with radioscaphoid surface erosions, left greater than right. The metacarpophalangeal and interphalangeal joints are relatively spared.

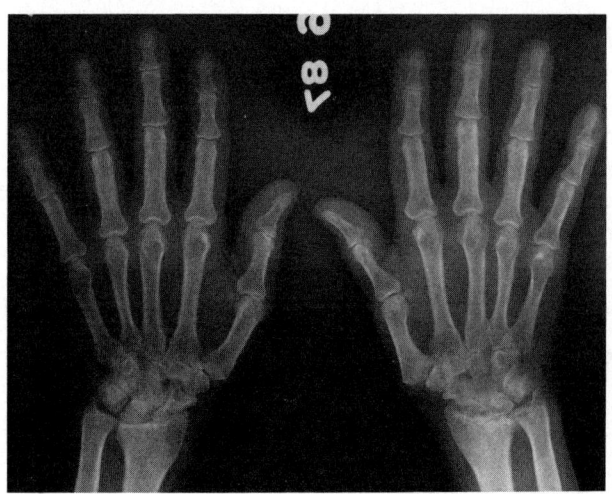

patients with seropositive RA will be disproportionately represented in surgical series dealing with total hip and knee joint arthroplasties or cervical spine fusion. In tertiary care facilities, however, where more severely affected patients predominate, this prediction may not hold. The proportion of our seronegative RA patients who have had a cervical fusion is similar to the proportion of seronegative RA patients followed by our rheumatology service.

TREATMENT

The treatment of patients with seronegative RA follows the guidelines for the treatment of patients with RA generally. Treatment should be comprehensive and aimed at maximum patient comfort with minimum functional loss. Empirical use of drugs is but one of the necessary elements to effectively treat these patients. These should be used stepwise, reserving the more potent and more toxic agents for disease unresponsive to simpler regimens. If erosions are evident early in the disease course, remission-inducing drugs should be considered. Other important therapeutic elements include patient education, physical modalities, orthotics, appropriate exercises and rest, and adequate nutrition.

Dietary manipulation (e.g., lactose-free diet) in the treatment of RA in general and seronegative RA in particular has been reported.[88,89] Alterations in dietary fatty acids (e.g., diet enriched in ω-3 fatty acids) as possible modulators of synthesis of arachidonic acid-derived inflammatory mediators have been investigated. Controlled trials have shown variable results in patients with seropositive RA.[90,91] Whether patients with seronegative RA may benefit from such dietary manipulation has not been determined.

PROGNOSIS

In general, patients who are consistently seronegative tend to have less severe disease than their seropositive counterparts but the prognosis in an individual patient must be gauged only after consideration of other known risk factors for disease severity.[92]

REFERENCES

1. Singer, J.M., and Plotz, C.M.: The latex fixation test. I. Application to the serologic diagnosis of rheumatoid arthritis. Am. J. Med., 21:888–892, 1956.

2. Waaler, E.: On the common occurrence of a factor in human serum activating the specific agglutination of sheep blood corpuscles. Acta Pathol. Microbiol. Scand., 17:172–188, 1940.
3. Rose, H.M., Ragan, C., Pearce, E., and Lipman, M.O.: Differential agglutination of normal and sensitized sheep erythrocytes by sera of patients with rheumatoid arthritis. Proc. Soc. Exp. Biol. Med., 68:1–6, 1948.
4. A Committee of the American Rheumatism Association: Revision of diagnostic criteria of rheumatoid arthritis. Arthritis Rheum., 2:16–20, 1958.
4a. Arnett, F.C. et al.: The 1987 revised ARA criteria for rheumatoid arthritis. Arthritis Rheum., 30:S17, 1987.
5. Masi, A.T., and Feigenbaum, S.L.: Seronegative rheumatoid arthritis. Fact or fiction? Arch. Intern Med., 143:2167–2172, 1983.
6. Calin, A., and Marks, S.H.: The case against seronegative rheumatoid arthritis. Am. J. Med., 70:992–994, 1981.
7. Calin, A.: The epidemiology of rheumatoid disease: Past and present. Dis. Markers, 4:1–6, 1986.
8. Alarcón, G.S.: Seronegative rheumatoid arthritis: Review of the evidence. In Current Topics in Rheumatology. A Collection from Johns Hopkins Fellows, past and present. Edited by B.H. Hahn, F.C. Arnett, T.M. Zizic, and M.C. Hochberg. New Haven, CT, Waverly Press, 1983.
9. Milazzo, S.C.: Seronegative peripheral arthritis. Clin. Rheum. Dis., 3:345–363, 1977.
10. Barter, R.W.: Familial incidence of rheumatoid arthritis and acute rheumatism in 100 rheumatoid arthritics. Ann. Rheum. Dis., 11:39–46, 1952.
11. Bremner, J.M., Alexander, W.R.M., and Duthie, J.J.R.: Familial incidence of rheumatoid arthritis. Ann. Rheum. Dis., 18:279–284, 1959.
12. Lawrence, J.S., and Ball, J.: Genetic studies on rheumatoid arthritis. Ann. Rheum. Dis., 17:160–168, 1958.
13. Hochberg, M.C.: Adult and juvenile rheumatoid arthritis: Current epidemiologic concepts. Epidemiol. Rev., 3:27–44, 1981.
14. Valkenburg, H.A.: An epidemiologist's view of rheumatoid arthritis. In Current Topics in Rheumatology. Epidemiology of the Rheumatic Diseases. Edited by R.C. Lawrence and L.E. Shulman. New York, Gower Medical Publishing Limited, 1984.
15. Alarcón, G.S.: Rheumatoid arthritis. In Rheumatology and Immunology, 2nd Ed. Edited by A.S. Cohen and J.C. Bennett. Orlando, Grune & Stratton, 1986.
16. Harris, E.D., Jr.: Rheumatoid arthritis: The clinical spectrum. In Textbook of Rheumatology. 2nd Ed. Edited by W.N. Kelley, E.D. Harris, Jr., S. Ruddy, and C.B. Sledge. Philadelphia, W.B. Saunders Company, 1985.
17. Koopman, W.J., and Schrohenloher, R.E.: Rheumatoid factor. In Rheumatoid Arthritis. Etiology, Diagnosis, Management. Edited by P.D. Utsinger, N.J. Zvaifler, and G.E. Ehrlich. Philadelphia, J.B. Lippincott, 1985.
18. Gran, J.T., and Husby, G.: Seronegative rheumatoid arthritis and HLA-DR4. Proposal for criteria. J. Rheumatol., 14:1079–1082, 1987.
19. Alarcón, G.S., Koopman, W.J., Acton, R.T., and Barger, B.O.: Seronegative rheumatoid arthritis. A distinct immunogenetic disease? Arthritis Rheum., 25:502–507, 1982.
20. Alarcón, G.S., Koopman, W.J., Acton, R.T., and Barger, B.O.: DR antigen distribution in blacks with rheumatoid arthritis. J. Rheumatol., 10:579–583, 1983.
21. Dixon, A. St. J.: "Rheumatoid Arthritis" with negative serological reaction. Ann. Rheum. Dis., 19:209–228, 1960.
22. Bland, J.H., and Brown, E.W.: Seronegative and seropositive rheumatoid arthritis. Ann. Intern Med., 60:88–94, 1963.

23. Duthie, J.J.R., et al.: Course and prognosis in rheumatoid arthritis. A further report. Ann. Rheum. Dis., 23:193–204, 1964.

24. Mongan, E.S., and Atwater, E.C.: A comparison between patients with seropositive and seronegative rheumatoid arthritis. Med. Clin. North Am., 52:533–538, 1968.

25. Mongan, E.S., Cass, R.M., Jacox, F.R., and Vaughn, J.H.: A study of the relation of seronegative and seropositive rheumatoid arthritis to each other and to necrotizing vasculitis. Am. J. Med., 47:23–35, 1969.

26. Cats, A., and Hazevoet, H.M.: Significance of positive tests for rheumatoid factor in the prognosis of rheumatoid arthritis. A follow up study. Ann. Rheum. Dis., 29:254–260, 1970.

27. Masi, A.T., et al.: Prospective study of the early course of rheumatoid arthritis in young adults: Comparison of patients with and without rheumatoid factor positivity at entry and identification of variables correlating with outcome. Semin Arthritis Rheum., 5:299–326, 1976.

28. Esdaile, J.M., et al.: HLA B27 in rheumatoid factor-negative polyarthritis. Ann. Intern. Med., 86:699–702, 1977.

29. Edelman, J., and Russell, A.S.: A comparison of patients with seropositive and seronegative rheumatoid arthritis. Rheumatol. Int., 3:47–48, 1983.

30. Bardin, T., et al.: HLA antigens and seronegative rheumatoid arthritis. Ann. Rheum. Dis., 44:50–53, 1985.

31. Raspe, H.-H., Vorbeck, A., and Robin-Winn, M.: [Does seronegative rheumatoid arthritis hold a special place? Clinical, biochemical and immunogenetic profile of early seronegative and seropositive cases of rheumatoid arthritis.] Dtsch. Med. Wochenschr., 111:1474–1478, 1986.

32. Alarcón, G.S., Barger, B.O., Acton, R.T., and Koopman, W.J.: Seronegative rheumatoid arthritis and B7-CREG: Disparate results. Arthritis Rheum., 26:1412–1413, 1983.

33. Robbins, L., Moore, T.L., and Naguwa, S.M.: IgG and IgM rheumatoid factor in active seronegative nodular rheumatoid arthritis and in children with benign rheumatoid nodules. Clin. Rheumatol., 1:104–111, 1982.

34. Kaye, B.R., Kaye, R.L., and Bobgrove, A.: Rheumatoid nodules. Review of the spectrum of associated conditions and proposal of a new classification, with a report of four seronegative cases. Am. J. Med., 76:279–292, 1984.

35. Smith, M.D., Roberts-Thomson, P.J., and Geddes, R.: Life threatening cardiac tamponade complicating a case of seronegative rheumatoid arthritis. Aust. N.Z. J. Med., 14:56–58, 1984.

36. Palacios, A., and Chavarria, P.: 24-year-old woman with seronegative arthritis and progressive neurological manifestations. Rev. Invest. Clin. (Mex), 38:65–70, 1986.

37. McCarty, D.J., O'Duffy, D., Pearson, L., and Hunter, J.B.: Remitting seronegative symmetrical synovitis with pitting edema. RS₃PE syndrome. JAMA, 254:2763–2767, 1985.

38. Zatuchni, J.: Remitting seronegative symmetrical synovitis with pitting edema. Letter to the Editor. JAMA, 255:2444, 1986.

39. Michaels, R.M., and Hochman, R.F.: Remitting seronegative symmetrical synovitis with pitting edema. Letter to the Editor. JAMA, 255:2444, 1986.

40. Vaughan, J.H., et al.: Rheumatoid factor-producing cells detected by direct hemolytic plaque assay. J. Clin. Invest., 58:933–941, 1976.

41. Koopman, W.J., and Schrohenloher, R.E.: A sensitive radioimmunoassay for quantitation of IgM rheumatoid factor. Arthritis Rheum., 23:302–308, 1980.

42. Koopman, W.J., and Schrohenloher, R.E.: Enhanced in vitro synthesis of IgM rheumatoid factor in rheumatoid arthritis. Arthritis Rheum., 23:985–992, 1980.

43. Pasquali, J.-L., et al.: Selective lymphocyte deficiency in seronegative rheumatoid arthritis. Arthritis Rheum., 24:770–773, 1981.

44. Alarcón, G.S., Koopman, W.J., and Schrohenloher, R.E.: Differential patterns of in vitro IgM rheumatoid factor synthesis in seronegative and seropositive rheumatoid arthritis. Arthritis Rheum., 25:150–155, 1982.

45. Slaughter, L., et al.: In vitro effects of Epstein-Barr virus on peripheral blood mononuclear cells from patients with rheumatoid arthritis and normal subjects. J. Exp. Med., 148:1429–1434, 1978.

46. Pasquali, J.L., et al.: Different populations of rheumatoid factor idiotypes, induced by two polyclonal B cell activators, pokeweed mitogen and Epsten-Barr virus. Clin. Immunol. Immunopathol., 21:184–189, 1981.

47. Pasquali, J.-L., Urlacher, A., and Storck, E.: Idiotypic network: Possible explanation of seronegativity in a patient with rheumatoid arthritis. Clin. Exp. Immunol., 55:281–286, 1984.

48. Munthe, E., and Natvig, J.B.: Immunoglobulin classes, subclasses and complexes of IgG rheumatoid factor in rheumatoid plasma cells. Clin. Exp. Immunol., 12:55–70, 1972.

49. Harris, E.D., Jr.: Pathogenesis of rheumatoid arthritis. In Textbook of Rheumatology. 2nd Ed. Edited by W.N. Kelley, E.D. Harris, Jr., S. Ruddy, and C.B. Sledge. Philadelphia, W.B. Saunders, 1985.

50. Bluestone, R., Goldberg, L.S., Cracchiolo, A., III: Hidden rheumatoid factors in seronegative nodular rheumatoid arthritis. Lancet, 2:878–879, 1969.

51. Waller, M., and Richard, A.J.: The frequency of 7S rheumatoid factors and 22S complexes in human sera with positive latex tests for rheumatoid factor. J. Rheumatol., 3:337–345, 1976.

52. Panush, R.S., Bianco, N.E., and Schur, P.H.: Serum and synovial fluid IgG, IgA and IgM antigammaglobulins in rheumatoid arthritis. Arthritis Rheum., 14:737–747, 1971.

53. Swierczynska, Z., et al.: [Characteristics of the humoral immune response in seronegative arthritis.] Reumatologia, 21:209–220, 1983.

54. Parekh, R.B., et al.: Association of rheumatoid arthritis and primary osteoarthritis with changes in the glycosylation pattern of total serum IgG. Nature, 316:452–457, 1985.

55. Tomana, M., Schrohenloher, R.E., Koopman, W.J., and Alarcón, G.S.: Decreased galactosylation of serum IgG from patients with rheumatoid arthritis (RA) and other chronic inflammatory diseases. Arthritis Rheum., 29:S41, 1986.

56. Townes, A.S.: Autoantibodies to Type II collagen (Editorial). Mayo Clin. Proc., 59:791–796, 1984.

57. Dobloug, J.H., et al.: HLA antigens and rheumatoid arthritis. Association between HLA-DR4 positivity and IgM rheumatoid factor production. Arthritis Rheum., 23:309–313, 1980.

58. Queirós, M.V., Sancho, M.R.H., Caetano, J.M.: HLA-DR4 antigen and IgM rheumatoid factors. J. Rheumatol., 9:370–373, 1982.

59. Terkeltaub, R., Dècary, F., Esdaile, J.: An immunogenetic study of older age onset rheumatoid arthritis. J. Rheumatol., 11:147–152, 1984.

60. Walton, K., et al.: Clinical features, autoantibodies and HLA-DR antigens in rheumatoid arthritis. J. Rheumatol., 12:223–226, 1985.

61. Panayi, G.S., Wooley, P.H., Batchelor, J.R.: HLA-DRw4 and rheumatoid arthritis. Lancet, 1:730, 1979.

62. Scherak, O., Smolen, J.S., Mayr, W.R.: Rheumatoid arthritis and B-lymphocyte alloantigen HLA-DRw4. J. Rheumatol., 7:9–12, 1980.

63. Karr, R.W., Rodey, G.E., Lee, T., Schwartz, B.D.: Association

of HLA-DRw4 with rheumatoid arthritis in black and white patients. Arthritis Rheum., 23:1241–1245, 1980.

64. Karsh, J., et al.: Histocompatibility antigen combinations in rheumatoid arthritis. Clin. Exp. Rheumatol., 1:11–15, 1983.

65. Lulli, P., et al.: HLA antigens and rheumatoid arthritis. Arthritis Rheum., 8:1053–1054, 1983.

66. Thomsen, M., et al.: HLA DRw4 and rheumatoid arthritis. Tissue Antigens, 13:56–60, 1979.

67. Gran, J.T., Husby, G., Thorsby, E.: Association between rheumatoid arthritis and the HLA antigen DR4. Ann. Rheum. Dis., 42:292–296, 1983.

68. Swiss Federal Commission for the Rheumatic Diseases, Subcommission for Research: HLA-DR antigens in rheumatoid arthritis. A Swiss collaborative study. Rheumatol. Int., 1:111–113, 1981.

69. Massardo, L., et al.: The frequency of HLA-DR4 in patients with rheumatoid arthritis. Proceedings of IX Pan American Congress of Rheumatology. Buenos Aires, Argentina. November 1986, Abstract B9.

70. Woodrow, J.C.: Analysis of the HLA association with rheumatoid arthritis. Dis. Markers, 4:7–12, 1986.

71. De Jongh, B.M., et al.: Genetic heterogeneity of rheumatoid arthritis. Dis. Markers, 4:29–33, 1986.

72. Nepom, B.S. et al.: Specific HLA-DR4–associated histocompatibility molecules characterize patients with seropositive juvenile rheumatoid arthritis. J. Clin. Invest., 74:287–291, 1984.

73. Nepom, G.T., Hansen, J.A., and Nepom, B.S.: The molecular basis for HLA class II associations in rheumatoid arthritis. J. Clin. Immunol., 7:1–7, 1987.

74. Winchester, R.J.: The HLA system and susceptibility to diseases: An interpretation. In Clinical Aspects of Autoimmunity. Edited by E. Tan. New York, Transmedica, 1986.

75. Rodriguez, M.A., et al.: Studies on the relationship between HLA-DR4 and in vitro IgM rheumatoid factor production. Clin. Immunol. Immunopathol., 27:96–109, 1983.

76. Panayi, G.S., Wooley, P., Batchelor, J.R.: Genetic basis of rheumatoid disease HLA antigens, disease manifestations and toxic reactions to drugs. Br. Med. J., 2:1326–1328, 1978.

77. Griffin, A.J., Wooley, P., Panayi, G.S., and Batchelor, J.R.: HLA DR antigens and disease expression in rheumatoid arthritis. Ann. Rheum. Dis., 43:218–221, 1984.

78. Legrand, L., et al.: HLA-DR genotype risks in seropositive rheumatoid arthritis. Am. J. Hum. Genet., 36:690–699, 1984.

79. Jaraquemada, D., et al.: HLA and rheumatoid arthritis: Susceptibility or severity? Dis. Markers, 4:43–53, 1986.

80. Bardin, T., et al.: HLA system and side-effects of gold salts and D-penicillamine treatment of rheumatoid arthritis. Ann. Rheum. Dis., 41:599–601, 1982.

81. Barger, B.O., Acton, R.T., Koopman, W.J., and Alarcón, G.S.: DR antigens and gold toxicity in white rheumatoid arthritis patients. Arthritis Rheum., 27:601–605, 1984.

82. Wooley, P.H., et al.: HLA-DR antigens and toxic reactions to sodium aurothiomalate and D-penicillamine in patients with rheumatoid arthritis. N. Engl. J. Med., 303:300–302, 1980.

83. Alarcón, G.S., et al.: Lack of association between HLA-DR2 and clinical response to methotrexate in patients with rheumatoid arthritis. Arthritis Rheum., 30:218–220, 1987.

84. McDaniel, D.O., et al.: Class II MHC restriction fragment length polymorphisms (RFLP) and HLA-DR4 in rheumatoid arthritis. Arthritis Rheum., 29:S11, 1986.

84a.Festestein, H., Awad, J., Hitman, G.A.: New HLA DNA polymorphisms associated with autoimmune diseases. Nature 322:64–67, 1986.

85. McDaniel, D.O., et al.: Increased relative risk (RR) for rheumatoid arthritis (RA) in the presence of two different restriction fragment length polymorphisms (RFLP) and the HLA-DR4 phenotype. Arthritis Rheum., 30:S36, 1987.

85a.Stephens, H.A.F., et al.: BAM H1 analysis of DR and DQβ genes in rheumatoid arthritis (RA). Arthritis Rheum., 30:S40, 1987.

86. Cutbush, S.D., et al.: New HLA DNA polymorphisms associated with rheumatoid arthritis. Dis. Markers, 4:173–183, 1986.

87. Burns, T.M., and Calin, A.: The hand radiograph as a diagnostic discriminant between seropositive and seronegative 'rheumatoid arthritis': A controlled study. Ann. Rheum. Dis., 42:605–612, 1983.

88. Stroud, R.M.: The effect of fasting followed by specific food challenge on rheumatoid arthritis. In Current Topics in Rheumatology. A Collection from Johns Hopkins Fellows, Past and Present. Edited by B.H. Hahn, F.C. Arnett, T.M. Zizic, and M.C. Hochberg. New Haven, CT, Waverly Press, 1983.

89. Ratner, D., Eshel, E., Schneeyour, A., and Teitler, A.: Does milk intolerance affect seronegative arthritis in lactase-deficiency women? Isr. J. Med. Sci., 21:532–534, 1985.

90. Kremer, J.M., et al.: Effects of manipulation of dietary fatty acids on clinical manifestations of rheumatoid arthritis. Lancet, 1:184–187, 1985.

91. Kremer, J.M., et al.: Fish-oil fatty acid supplementation in active rheumatoid arthritis. Ann. Intern. Med., 106:497–503, 1987.

92. Zvaifler, N.J.: Rheumatoid arthritis: A clinical perspective. In Current Topics in Rheumatology. Epidemiology of the Rheumatic Diseases. Edited by R.C. Lawrence and L.E. Shulman. New York, Gower Medical Publishing, 1984.

JUVENILE RHEUMATOID ARTHRITIS

57

JOHN J. CALABRO*

Juvenile rheumatoid arthritis (JRA) is a heterogeneous condition that continues to pose considerable diagnostic challenges. This situation is not surprising in a disorder as protean as JRA, with its variable modes of onset and myriad signs, symptoms, and manifestations. The historical background and classification of this major chronic rheumatic disorder of childhood are briefly reviewed.

HISTORICAL BACKGROUND, CLASSIFICATION, AND NOMENCLATURE

HISTORICAL BACKGROUND

Since childhood inflammatory arthritis was first cited in 1864 by Cornil,[1] much of the literature has been directed at clinical descriptions and efforts to classify various subgroups. As early as 1890, Diamentberger reported on the predominant involvement of large joints, the flares and remissions that characterize the course of disease, the frequent disturbances of growth, and the generally favorable prognosis.[2]

A report of 22 cases by George Frederick Still in 1897 has become the classic early description of JRA,[3] an extraordinary example of exceptional clinical observation. Moreover, Still was the first to document that joint disease could be accompanied by prominent systemic manifestations, such as high spiking fever,

lymphadenopathy, splenomegaly, hepatomegaly, pleuritis, and pericarditis. In fact, the term *Still's disease* is sometimes used to describe a systemic onset, one of the major presentations of JRA. Systemic onset may also occur in adults with RA, although less frequently. Known in the past as the *Still-Chauffard syndrome*, it has gained recent recognition as "Still's disease in the adult"[4-6] and "adult-onset JRA."[7] Systemic onset is distinctly rare in the elderly; the oldest reported case involved a 70-year-old woman.[8]

CLASSIFICATION AND NOMENCLATURE

The classification of chronic inflammatory arthritis beginning in childhood is currently undergoing widespread revision. Although JRA is the preferred term, it is commonly employed by European and British authors to describe a subgroup of children, predominantly teenage girls with a polyarticular onset, who have IgM rheumatoid factors.[9] Chronic inflammatory arthritis of childhood is also referred to as juvenile polyarthritis, juvenile chronic polyarthritis, juvenile arthritis, or juvenile chronic arthritis. The last classification, however, coined by British and European investigators, embodies several categories, including juvenile ankylosing spondylitis, psoriatic arthritis, and other childhood spondyloarthropathies, as well as the polyarthropathies associated with systemic lupus erythematosus (SLE) and other childhood connective tissue disorders.[10]

*Deceased

Table 57–1. Major Differences Between 100 Children and 100 Adults with Rheumatoid Arthritis: Consecutive Referrals to an Arthritis Clinic

	Frequency (%)	
	Children	Adults
Type of Onset		
Systemic	20	3
Pauciarticular*	32	6
Polyarticular	48	91
Characteristics		
High fever	20	3
Rheumatoid rash	40	2
Generalized lymphadenopathy	43	21
Splenomegaly	33	7
Chronic iridocyclitis	9	0
Subcutaneous nodules	8	20
Leukocytosis†	56	23
Rheumatoid factors‡	19	76

*Pauciarticular onset associated with chronic iridocyclitis and antinuclear antibodies has not been reported in adults.
†Leukocytosis is not only more frequent in children, but the level of the white cell count is also higher, usually from 15,000 to 30,000.
‡By the latex-fixation test, titer of 1:160 or greater.

As a childhood disorder with radically different kinds of onset, JRA will most certainly pose difficulties in early diagnosis. In fact, two recent surveys disclose that errors in diagnosis occur in close to half of all children referred to specialists.[11,12] In an effort to simplify the problem, a plethora of diagnostic criteria for JRA has emerged.[9,11] Those criteria designated for adult RA, even when modified,[13] are difficult to apply to children because JRA differs from adult RA in several major ways (Table 57–1).[11,14,15] As a result, separate criteria for JRA have been adopted by the American Rheumatism Association.[16] Diagnosis requires not only disease of more than 6 weeks' duration, but also exclusion of other disorders sharing similar clinical manifestations such as arthritis, fever, and rash.

PREVALENCE AND ETIOLOGY

JRA is arbitrarily confined to disease beginning before age 16. It is rare before the age of 6 months, and two onset peaks are generally observed, between ages of 1 and 3 years and between 8 and 12 years. Girls are afflicted almost twice as frequently as boys.

In an English survey, one case of JRA was noted for every 1,500 school children.[17] No comparable survey has been conducted in the United States, where there may be as many as 200,000 cases. This rough estimate is based on 5% of adults with RA, however.[18] Despite such prevalence, the cause of JRA is yet to

be clarified.[11] The roles of possible contributing factors are critically reviewed.

INFECTION, TRAUMA, AND STRESS

In the search for the origin of JRA, a variety of microorganisms have been indicted, but none has been confirmed as a cause. Suspicion of a streptococcal origin is based on elevated antistreptolysin-O (ASO) titers, found in as many as 30% of patients with JRA. These titers now appear to be nonspecific, also observed in other childhood disorders.[19] Failure to suppress these elevated titers in JRA patients with monthly intramuscular injections of benzathine penicillin appears to bear out their nonspecific nature.[19] Rubella was also suspected when rubella antibody levels were found to be higher in patients with JRA than in control subjects. The subsequent disclosure of elevations of multiple viral antibodies, including rubella, and their direct correlation with elevations of serum IgG levels suggest that these levels are also nonspecific.[20]

Upper respiratory infection, trauma, and emotional stress are often cited as factors that may trigger the disease or a recurrence.[11] These situations occur with such frequency in children that their exact roles are difficult to assess. On the other hand, emotional conflicts may result from severe restrictions imposed by the disease. Consequently, psychologic evaluations should be routine in patients, so that impending problems can be promptly identified and corrected.[21-23]

GENETIC FACTORS

Twin studies give little support of any genetic influence because of the low concordance rates reported.[24] Recently, however, a genetic basis for JRA has been disclosed.[25] When patients with JRA were compared to healthy children, certain HLA antigens were found to occur with greater frequency among the major subgroups. Systemic onset was associated with the DR5 antigen, polyarticular onset with the DR4 antigen, and pauciarticular onset with the B27, DR5, and DR8 antigens (see Chapter 9).

IMMUNOLOGIC PARAMETERS

Unlike in adults with RA, except for hidden factor,[26] IgM rheumatoid factors are observed infrequently in the sera of children with JRA.[11,15] Moreover, in contrast to previous findings, IgG rheumatoid factor levels are also normal in JRA, regardless of the type of onset.[15] On the other hand, antinuclear antibodies may be found in as many as 50% of patients with JRA.[27] Their presence may be linked to the evolution of chronic iridocyclitis.[28]

Serum immunoglobulin levels may be elevated in JRA.[29,30] When elevated levels are sustained, patients appear to have a poorer functional status and an increased incidence of hip involvement.[29] Selective IgA deficiency occurs in up to 4% of JRA patients, as compared to only 0.2% of controls.[30] IgA deficiency may thus be related to pathogenesis as a reflection of some unidentified immunologic disturbance.

TYPES OF ONSET

Early diagnosis rests on the recognition of three distinct modes of onset, *systemic, polyarticular,* and *pauciarticular,* and is based on the character, frequency, and severity of systemic and articular manifestations observed during the first 6 months of disease (Table 57–2).[31,32] Each onset type has its own differential diagnosis and each its own major hazards (Table 57–2).

Systemic onset is accompanied by prominent systemic manifestations, particularly high fever, rash, generalized lymphadenopathy, splenomegaly, and cardiopulmonary involvement. Joint manifestations are variable; occasionally, only arthralgia is present. In polyarticular onset, defined as synovitis of more than four joints, the arthritis predominates; systemic manifestations are less frequent than in systemic onset, and fever is invariably of low grade. Pauciarticular onset, with arthritis confined to a single joint (usually a knee) or to two to four joints, is the mildest form of the disease. Systemic signs are minimal or absent, with the notable exception of chronic iridocyclitis.

The major systemic manifestations of JRA are listed in Table 57–3. When viewed according to modes of onset, fever is high in patients with systemic onset and low in those with polyarticular and pauciarticular onsets. Rash, generalized lymphadenopathy, sple-

nomegaly, hepatomegaly, as well as cardiac and pleuropulmonary involvement are far more frequent in patients with systemic onset. On the other hand, subcutaneous nodules occur only in patients with a polyarticular onset, whereas chronic iridocyclitis appears primarily in those with pauciarticular disease.

SYSTEMIC ONSET

A predilection for boys is found only in this mode of onset, which occurs in about 20% of all patients with JRA.[11,32] Recognition of systemic onset is easy when the young patient has obvious arthritis in addition to characteristic systemic features (Fig. 57–1). Initially, however, when only arthralgia, fever, and an evanescent rash are present, diagnosis may be difficult. These children, frequently labeled as having fever of unknown origin, are often subjected to exhaustive diagnostic studies, trials of various antibiotics, and even exploratory laparotomy.[33]

When only arthralgia is present, the patient's appearance may provide the first diagnostic clue. Younger children usually appear toxic, listless, and irritable, with anorexia and weight loss. Even with high fever, shaking chills are rare, but seizures are unusual. Paradoxically, older children usually appear healthy, even at the time of fever spikes.

Cerebral signs, such as marked irritability, listlessness, seizures, and meningismus, may be so striking as to suggest primary central nervous system disease.[11,34] The cerebrospinal fluid is normal in these patients, but their electroencephalographic tracings, unrelated to abnormalities from aspirin therapy,[35] disclose transient, nonspecific focal and diffuse abnormalities.[34]

Joint Involvement

Such involvement varies from arthralgia alone to a florid polyarthritis (Fig. 57–1). Synovitis should always be suspected when a child appears unusually inactive or refuses to walk for the examining physician. Moreover, children attempt to protect tender joints without complaining of pain. When in bed, for

Table 57–2. American Rheumatism Association Onset Types: Differentiating Features

Onset Type	Systemic Features	Articular Findings	Major Hazard
Systemic (20%)	Frequent, including high fever	Variable, from arthralgia to florid polyarthritis	Cardiac failure from myocarditis
Polyarticular (30–40%)	Fewer, with low-grade fever	Arthritis of more than four joints	Deforming polyarthritis
Pauciarticular (40–50%)	Uncommon, except for iridocyclitis	Arthritis of one to four joints	Blindness from iridocyclitis

Table 57–3. Systemic Manifestations of 100 Patients with Juvenile Rheumatoid Arthritis According to Modes of Onset

Manifestation (No. Patients)	Systemic (20)	Polyarticular (48)	Pauciarticular (32)
Fever:			
High	20	0	0
Low-grade	0	38	16
Rheumatoid rash	18	19	3
Lymphadenopathy	17	20	6
Splenomegaly	15	11	7
Hepatomegaly	4	2	4
Pericarditis	7	3	0
Myocarditis	2	0	0
Pneumonitis or pleuritis	6	2	0
Chronic iridocyclitis	1	1	7
Subcutaneous nodules	0	8	0

instance, they sit or lie in a position of generalized flexion to ease joint discomfort (Fig. 57–1). In patients with minimal or no objective arthritis, diagnosis then depends on detection of characteristic systemic signs.

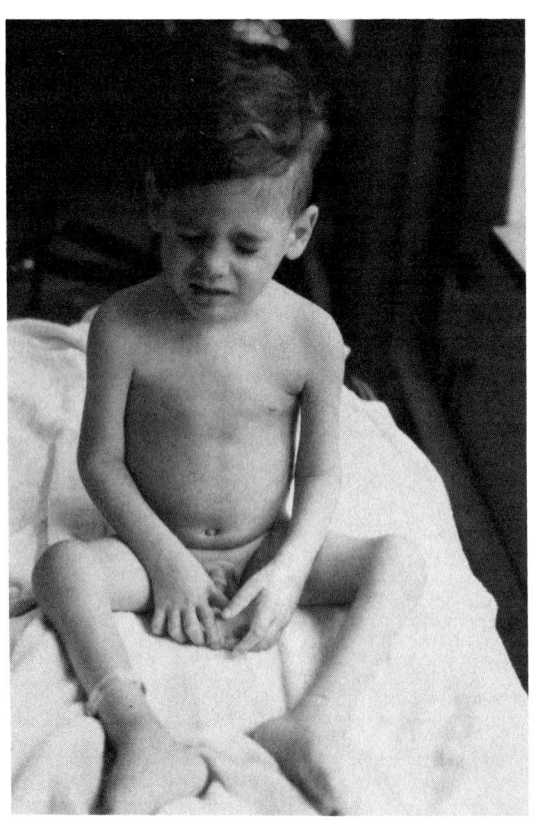

FIG. 57–1. A 4-year-old boy with systemic onset JRA with obvious polyarthritis facilitating early diagnosis. The patient assumes a position of generalized flexion to ease the discomfort of tender, swollen joints.

Systemic Signs

Of the many systemic manifestations, fever and rash are of the greatest diagnostic value. Both may be associated with generalized lymphadenopathy, splenomegaly, hepatomegaly, pericarditis, myocarditis, pneumonitis, and a striking neutrophilic leukocytosis.

High Fever. Most often, the fever pattern is quotidian (intermittent) or double quotidian.[36] One or two temperature peaks above 102°F (39°C) occur daily, whereas hyperpyrexia (fever to 105°F or 40.5°C) is observed only occasionally (Fig. 57–2). Diurnal temperatures may range as widely as 9°F (5°C), so both hyperpyrexia and subnormal temperatures occur within the same day. Consequently, in patients without detectable joint swelling, careful plotting of the fever pattern may suggest the diagnosis, especially because high fever may antedate appreciable arthritis by weeks or months, even, rarely, by years.[36] High fever usually responds to aspirin, but the daily requirement varies from 60 to 130 mg/kg body weight. When the critical dose for an individual patient is reduced, fever may promptly recur.[36]

When fever is prolonged or recurs, the pattern may be relapsing (polycyclic) or even periodic. Rarely is the febrile pattern remittent.[36] In fact, the presence of remittent fever should suggest infection, drug reaction, or other causes.

Rash. A characteristic rash[37] occurs in as many as 90% of patients with systemic onset (Fig. 57–3).[11,32] It consists of discrete or confluent macules or maculopapules found on the trunk, face, or extremities, including the soles and palms. The eruption is usually nonpruritic, but it does itch, sometimes intensely, in about 5% of patients.[11]

Occasionally constant, the rash is more often evanescent, usually appearing in conjunction with fever spikes. Individual macules migrate from day to day. The degree of erythema also varies; faint lesions may

FIG. 57–2. Typical fever pattern of systemic onset has one (quotidian) or two daily peaks (double quotidian) and wide diurnal variations. Fever is suppressed with critical daily aspirin (ASA) dosage of 110 mg/kg.

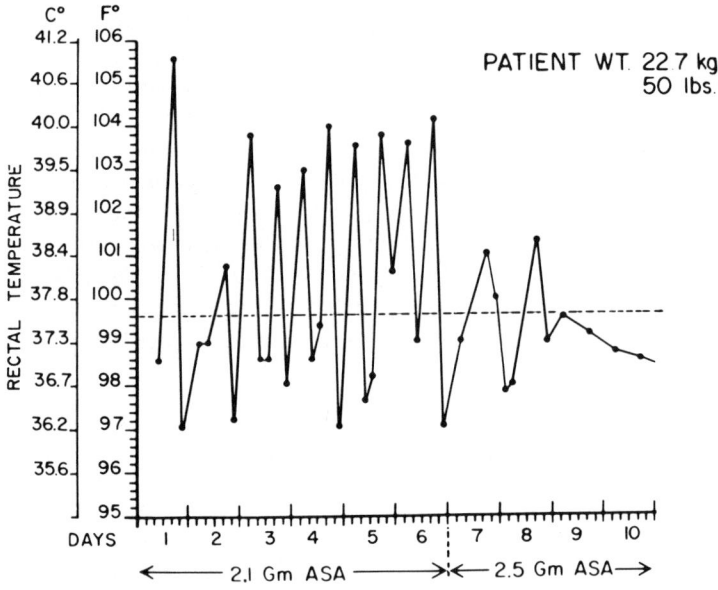

FIG. 57–3. The rheumatoid rash, present in 90% of systemic-onset patients, consists of faint macules or maculopapules occurring primarily on the trunk and extremities.

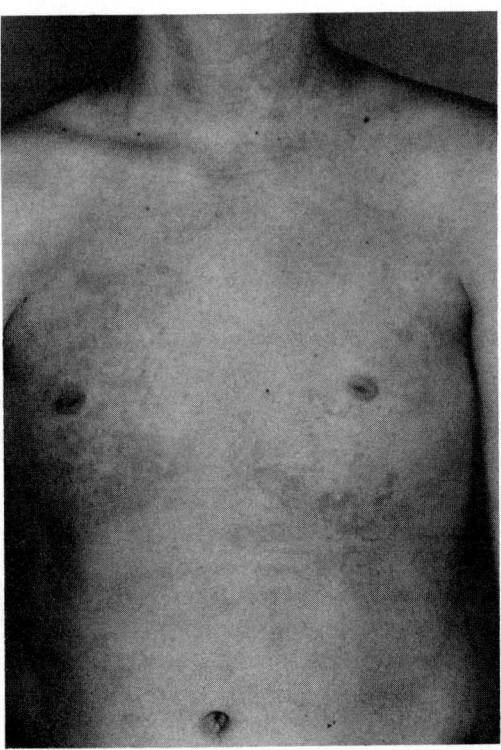

be intensified by massaging or by applying heat. The rash is most florid where the skin is rubbed or is subjected to microtrauma, such as the light pressure of underclothing. This characteristic, known as the Koebner phenomenon, may be diagnostically useful when parents report a rash that is not present when the child is examined. The typical rash may then be induced by rubbing or lightly scratching the skin at a susceptible site, an extremity or the lower abdomen.[37] Macules appear within several minutes and often persist for a day or so.

The histologic features of the rash vary;[37] however, the preponderance of perivascular mononuclear cells, rather than neutrophils, differentiates the rheumatoid rash from that of rheumatic fever.

Carditis. Although fever may be misinterpreted and the rash overlooked, cardiac involvement of an untreated child may have serious, if not fatal, consequences. Myocarditis is the most serious because it may rapidly induce cardiac enlargement and subsequent heart failure.[11,38] It should always be suspected in the presence of tachypnea, tachycardia disproportionate to the degree of fever, pericarditis, or pneumonitis.[11] Endocarditis does not seem to occur; cardiac murmurs suggesting its presence are believed to be functional.

Pericarditis, which is more frequent than myocarditis, is usually a benign manifestation that rarely produces acute cardiac tamponade,[39] but it may recur. The early detection of pericarditis is important because it may herald impending myocarditis.[11] Because precordial pain and dyspnea are rare, most attacks of pericarditis remain asymptomatic and undetected, unless the child is monitored regularly for evanescent friction rub, cardiomegaly, and electro- or echocardiographic abnormalities.[40]

Pleuropulmonary Signs. Pneumonitis or pleuritis frequently accompanies carditis, but each also occurs independently.[41] Pleuritis is often asymptomatic and is detected as an incidental finding on chest roentgenogram. Chronic pulmonary fibrosis is rare.[41]

Lymphadenopathy. Generalized lymphadenopathy is frequent and may be prominent enough, particularly in epitrochlear and axillary lymph nodes, to suggest leukemia or lymphoma. Enlarged mesenteric lymph nodes may cause abdominal pain or distention, which may suggest an acute abdominal disorder requiring surgical intervention.

Hepatosplenomegaly. Splenomegaly occurs frequently, hepatomegaly less often.[11,32] Hepatomegaly may be accompanied by abdominal pain and distention as well as abnormalities of liver function and nonspecific histologic changes.[42] In addition to direct hepatic involvement,[42] abnormalities of liver function may result from therapy with aspirin.[43,44] Progressive hepatomegaly should arouse one's suspicion of secondary amyloidosis, but this complication is rare during the initial year of disease.

Other Systemic Signs. Encephalitis and vasculitis are rare in JRA. Their presence should suggest other diagnostic possibilities, particularly polyarteritis or other forms of systemic vasculitis. Serous peritonitis is rare but constitutes another cause of abdominal pain and distention.

Differential Diagnosis

When arthritis is absent, the differential diagnosis may be difficult. Infection must always be ruled out first. Then, other causes of high fever, rash, and joint pain must be considered. Prominent among these are SLE, Kawasaki disease or another disease of the systemic vasculitides, leukemia, and inflammatory bowel disease.

Children with SLE, in contrast to adults, are more likely to have generalized lymphadenopathy, hepatosplenomegaly, and high fever,[45] features also typical of JRA. Oral mucosal lesions, renal involvement, and presence of antinative DNA antibodies support a diagnosis of SLE. Further clues include thrombocytopenia and leukopenia because these abnormalities are rare in JRA. On the other hand, the absence of antinuclear antibodies virtually excludes the diagnosis of SLE. Antinuclear antibodies may be detected in both JRA and SLE, but the titers are generally higher in SLE.[45a]

Systemic vasculitis should be suspected in the presence of purpura, hypertension, or nephritis, whereas profound anemia, purpura, or erosive changes on joint roentgenogram are clues to the possibility of malignant disease, particularly leukemia.[46–48] High spiking fever can be a prominent feature of inflammatory bowel disease, particularly regional enteritis,[49] as well as Kawasaki disease.[50] The presence of erythema nodosum and mucosal ulcers should suggest underlying inflammatory bowel disease; early features of Kawasaki disease include a strawberry tongue, red lips, conjunctivitis, erythema of the palms and soles, and an indurative edema of the hands and feet.

POLYARTICULAR ONSET

This presentation occurs in 30 to 40% of all affected children, mostly girls, and is characterized by arthritis of more than four joints that may begin either abruptly or insidiously. When abrupt, painful swelling of several joints occurs. When insidious, joint discomfort may be minimal; even early morning stiffness may be absent. Nevertheless, most patients appear ill. They are often listless, febrile, anorectic, and losing weight.

Articular Findings

Large joints such as knees, wrists, ankles, and elbows are the most frequent sites of initial involvement. Affected joints are usually swollen, tender, and

FIG. 57–4. Polyarticular onset in an 8-year-old girl with symmetric swelling of ankle, metatarsophalangeal joints, and proximal interphalangeal joints.

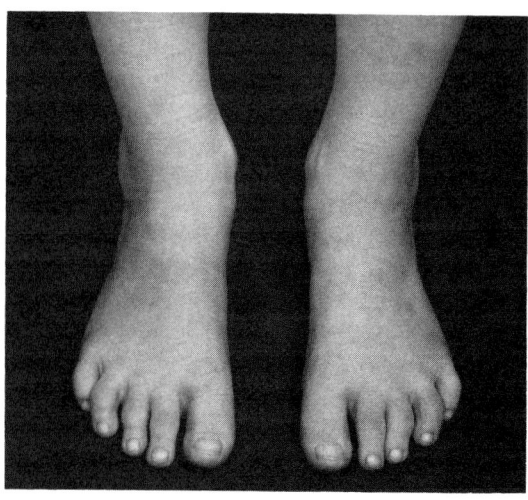

FIG. 57–5. Serial radiographs showing progressive cervical involvement. *A,* At age 12, early changes include diffuse demineralization of vertebral bodies and apophyseal fusion at C2 and C3. *B,* At age 16, one sees diffuse apophyseal fusion from C2 to C6 and underdeveloped vertebrae C2 to C6 from early closure of epiphyses.

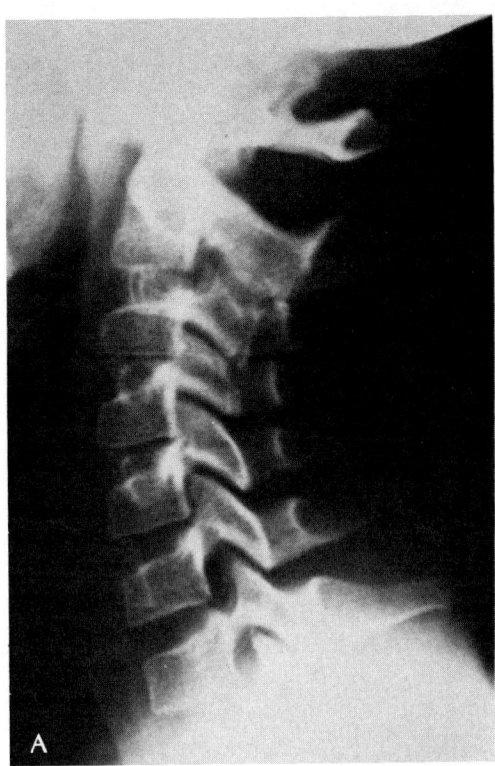
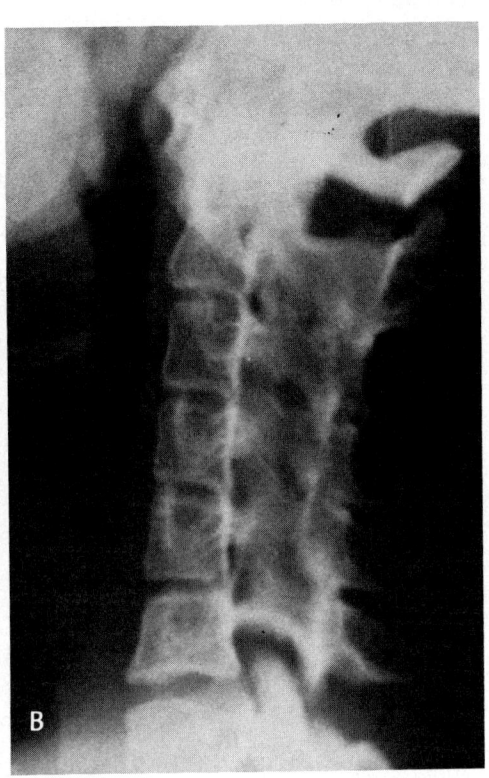

restricted in motion, and warmth and redness may or may not be present. The pattern of arthritis varies. It may be generalized, as in adult RA, with symmetric involvement of multiple joints, including the hands and feet (Fig. 57–4).[51] Polyarthritis may be confined to large joints and, when asymmetric or migratory, may be confused with other rheumatic disorders. Tenosynovitis may also occur, but it is rarely the sole presenting sign.

Hips are involved frequently; when disease is progressive, ankylosis may ensue rapidly. Affliction of the cervical spine, also frequent, causes tenderness and restriction of motion, particularly lateral flexion. Early radiographic changes include demineralization of vertebral bodies and apophyseal narrowing, primarily at C2 and C3 (Fig. 57–5). Asymptomatic sacroiliitis is an early radiographic finding that appears to correlate with hip involvement, rheumatoid factors, and the onset of disease at 10 years of age or older.[52] Axial articulations other than cervical and sacroiliac are rarely involved. Transient temporomandibular complaints are frequent, and ankylosis is a rare but difficult problem.[53]

Systemic Signs

Fever is frequent; it is low grade, with one or two daily peaks under 102°F (39°C).[36] Tachycardia may be out of proportion to the degree of fever. Systemic signs are less frequent than in JRA of systemic onset, except for subcutaneous nodules, which occur only in patients with polyarticular onset (Table 57–3).

Subcutaneous Nodules. These nodules develop in areas of excessive pressure or friction and are most frequent at the olecranon process of the elbow, the proximal ulnar aspect of the forearm, or in back of the heel (Fig. 57–6). On histologic study, the nodules of JRA resemble those of rheumatic fever more closely than they do the nodules of adults with RA.[11] Nodules impart a poor prognosis, and their presence is often associated with progressive polyarthritis and deformity.

Subcutaneous nodules also occur in SLE, rarely in other connective tissue disorders. Nodules histologically indistinguishable from those observed in adult RA may also occur in otherwise healthy children and occasionally in conjunction with granuloma annulare.[54,55] Known as *pseudorheumatoid* or *benign rheu-*

FIG. 57–6. Subcutaneous nodules occur most frequently at the olecranon process of the elbow and proximal ulnar aspect of the forearm.

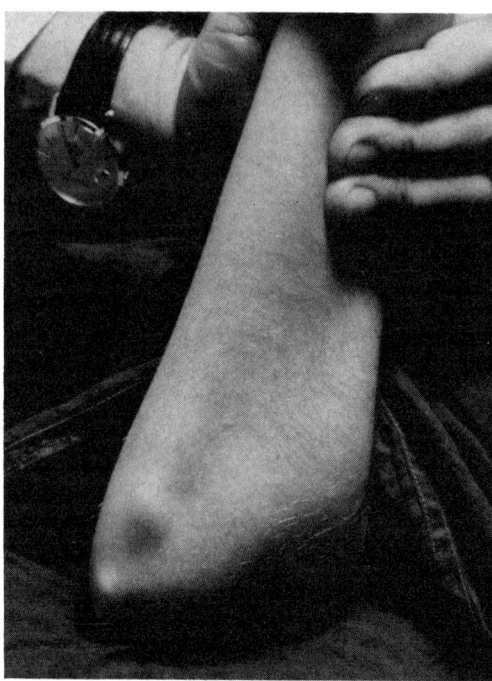

matoid nodules, they are characterized by their predilection for the pretibial areas and the scalp, by their spontaneous regression, and by their frequent recurrence, particularly following surgical removal. Consequently, surgical excision and other forms of therapy are unnecessary in this self-limited and benign syndrome (see also Chapter 43).

Polyarticular Subtypes

Two subsets of polyarticular onset must be distinguished. The first includes primarily teenage-onset patients, usually girls, who frequently have rheumatoid nodules or rheumatoid factors. As in adults with these findings, the course of arthritis is often progressive and deforming unless therapy with remission-inducing drugs, such as intramuscular gold, is instituted early.

The second subset consists of seronegative children, primarily girls, who have an atypical form of spondylitis, characterized by rheumatoid-like joint swelling of the hands and limitation of neck motion from cervical apophyseal fusion, which persists into adulthood.[56] In addition to the HLA-B27 antigen, cervical apophyseal fusion is associated with micrognathia, acute anterior uveitis, sacroiliitis, and spondylitis. Early recognition may be difficult because spondylitic features may be overshadowed by the prominence of peripheral joint involvement, including rheumatoid-like hand deformities.

Differential Diagnosis

Certain similarities make it difficult to distinguish polyarticular JRA from acute rheumatic fever.[57] Both disorders may manifest asymmetric and migratory arthritis of large joints, low-grade fever, pericarditis, abdominal pain, and elevation of ASO titers. Remittent fever, in which the daily temperature does not fall to normal levels, should suggest rheumatic fever, whereas intermittent fever characterizes JRA.[36] Several other features that help to rule out rheumatic fever are onset under age 4, cervical involvement, generalized lymphadenophathy, a poor mucin clot on synovial fluid analysis, and persistence of polyarthritis to or beyond the second month.

SLE must be considered in the differential diagnosis of polyarthritis.[45a] The salient features of this connective tissue disorder have already been cited. Serum sickness and drug reactions may also be confused with JRA because polyarthritis and fever are usually present. Presence of urticaria, remittent fever, and diminished serum complement levels favors these disorders, rather than JRA.

Viral arthritides have not been widely appreciated in the differential diagnosis of acute polyarthritis.[58] These disorders are usually self-limited. In viral hepatitis, for example, arthritis and urticaria disappear with the onset of clinical jaundice. The total serum hemolytic complement levels may be depressed in the presence of joint symptoms; hepatitis-associated antigen, immune complexes, and abnormalities of liver function may be found.[59] The arthritis that follows rubella[58] or rubella vaccination may resemble JRA. Rising or falling hemagglutination-inhibition antibody titers in sera obtained during the acute phase and in convalescence, as well as the paucity of neutrophils in synovial fluid, differentiate these disorders from JRA.

It is common for primary fibromyalgia (fibrositis) to be confused with JRA. Moreover, the frequent occurrence of fibromyalgia in the pediatric age group is not widely appreciated. Yet, in a report of 50 cases, 14 (28%) were children.[60] At onset, the youngest patient was 9 years and the oldest was 15 years. In a recent report of 36 children with fibromyalgia, more than half had been incorrectly diagnosed before referral, and most were initially believed to have JRA.[61]

Fibrositis may occur as a secondary disorder in patients with JRA. In addition to arthritis, the child has diffuse aches and pains. It would be inappropriate to alter the basic drug therapy of JRA. Instead, the primary-care physician must explain to the child and parents the basis of these additional complaints. Above all, the benign nature of the syndrome should be emphasized.

PAUCIARTICULAR ONSET

This mode of onset occurs in 40 to 50% of all cases and is manifest by arthritis of one to four joints. Girls are more frequently affected than boys. Children 5 years of age or under are often listless and irritable, have a low-grade fever, and fail to grow at a normal rate. On the other hand, constitutional symptoms are notably absent in older children.

Articular Findings

The onset of arthritis is usually insidious, with swelling and stiffness. The initial joint most often involved is the knee.[11,32] Joint pain is usually mild, but may be completely absent even in the presence of marked swelling and effusion.

Systemic Signs

Comparatively few systemic signs occur in this form of JRA (Table 57–3). Low-grade quotidian fever may be present, but cardiopulmonary involvement is notably absent. The most potentially serious manifestation is chronic iridocyclitis, which occurs in 20 to 30% of patients.[32,62–64]

Chronic Iridocyclitis. What makes this ocular manifestation so particularly treacherous is that it is so often asymptomatic, progressing quietly for weeks or months until failing vision alone compels medical attention.[65] This disorder may even occur months to years before the arthritis.

The course of iridocyclitis is usually chronic, with long periods of active ocular inflammation, remission, and subsequent recurrence. Initially, ocular pain and redness may be absent, and the process goes undetected until sight is impaired, first from synechiae or glaucoma, and later by cataract or band keratopathy (Fig. 57–7).

Pauciarticular Subtype

A subset of children with pauciarticular onset must be reclassified. It includes mostly teenage-onset boys with arthritis who are positive for the HLA-B27 antigen, but negative for both rheumatoid factors and antinuclear antibodies.[66–69] These patients usually have an asymmetric pauciarthritis of lower limb joints and are initially believed to have pauciarticular JRA. On long-term observation, however, some children eventually develop back complaints and other typical clinical and radiographic features of ankylosing spon-

FIG. 57–7. Undetected iridocyclitis may lead to band keratopathy (as shown in the upper portion of the photograph) with calcific deposits in Bowman's membrane extending horizontally as a band across the cornea.

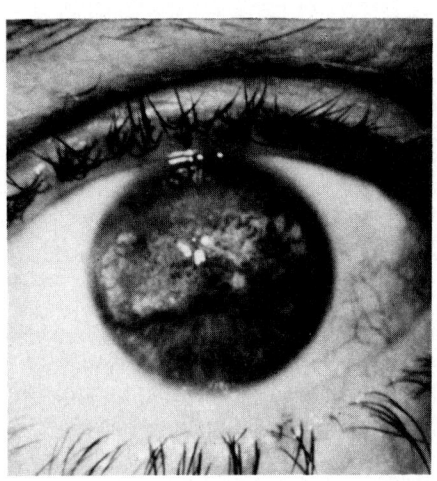

dylitis, whereas others develop Reiter's syndrome or still another of the seronegative spondyloarthropathies.[70,71]

Differential Diagnosis

When a single joint is affected, arthrocentesis and synovial fluid analysis are essential to rule out septic arthritis. This approach also aids differentiation from traumatic and tuberculous arthritis. If tuberculosis is suspected, synovial biopsy to detect the presence of caseating granulomas may be needed.[72] In JRA, histologic examination discloses nonspecific synovitis with hypertrophy, increased vascularity, and lymphocyte infiltration.

Pauciarticular arthritis may also be the initial manifestation of such diverse disorders as sarcoidosis, hemophilia, sickle cell anemia, inflammatory bowel disease, psoriasis, Reiter's syndrome, osteomyelitis, and Lyme disease.[11,73,74]

LABORATORY AND RADIOLOGIC FINDINGS

LABORATORY ABNORMALITIES

Although JRA has no consistent laboratory abnormality, each major presentation of the disease is associated with certain abnormalities that may provide additional clues for early diagnosis (Table 57–4). Elevation of the erythrocyte sedimentation rate (ESR), the presence of other acute-phase reactants, low-

Table 57–4. Laboratory Findings in Each Major Presentation

	Systemic	Polyarticular	Pauciarticular
Erythrocyte sedimentation rate	Elevated, often to striking levels	Modest elevation	Usually normal or minimally elevated
Low-grade anemia	Frequent	Frequent	Rare
Thrombocytosis	Frequent	Frequent*	Frequent†
Leukocytosis	Common, often to marked levels	Modest	Rare
Rheumatoid factor‡	Rare	10–20%	Rare
Antinuclear antibodies	Rare	10–20%	30–50%§

*The highest values of one or more million/mm³ occur with progressive polyarthritis or when secondary amyloidosis develops.
†Thrombocytosis (platelet count of 400,000/mm³ or greater) may be the only laboratory abnormality in this presentation.
‡By the latex-fixation test, titer of 1:160 or greater.
§High correlation with chronic iridocyclitis.

grade anemia, and thrombocytosis are frequently present, except in pauciarticular onset. A striking neutrophilic leukocytosis, with leukocyte values usually between 20,000 and 30,000/mm³ and occasionally higher, is usual in systemic onset.[11] Leukocytosis is modest in polyarticular onset, whereas the white blood count is often normal in pauciarticular onset. Routine urinalysis reveals little, except febrile proteinuria.

A positive latex-fixation test is seen in 10 to 20% of children. Positive tests can be correlated with late onset (ages 12 to 16), polyarticular onset, subcutaneous nodules, and a poor functional outcome.[11] Elevated antinuclear antibody titers, found in as many as 50% of patients, correlate with early onset (under age 6), pauciarticular onset, and chronic iridocyclitis.[27,28] Emergence of these antibodies may thus prove useful in identifying patients at risk for iridocyclitis.[28]

Serum protein electrophoresis may reveal low albumin levels and elevated levels of β- and γ-globulins. This test also excludes patients with the arthritis associated with agammaglobulinemia from those with JRA. The significance of serum immunoglobulin values, as well as elevated ASO titers, has already been cited. The presence of B27 on HLA typing, especially in teenage boys, may be a clue to ankylosing spondylitis.

Analysis of synovial fluid is variable and does not always correlate with the intensity of arthritis. The white blood cell count is usually between 10,000 and 20,000/mm³, but it may range from 150 to 50,000/mm³. Synovial fluid complement levels are often depressed.

ROENTGENOGRAPHIC FEATURES

Early roentgenographic abnormalities are nonspecific and include juxta-articular demineralization, radiodensities from soft-tissue swelling or effusion, and, occasionally, periosteal proliferation (Fig. 57–8). Erosions are only late findings that occur primarily in patients with progressive polyarthritis.[75]

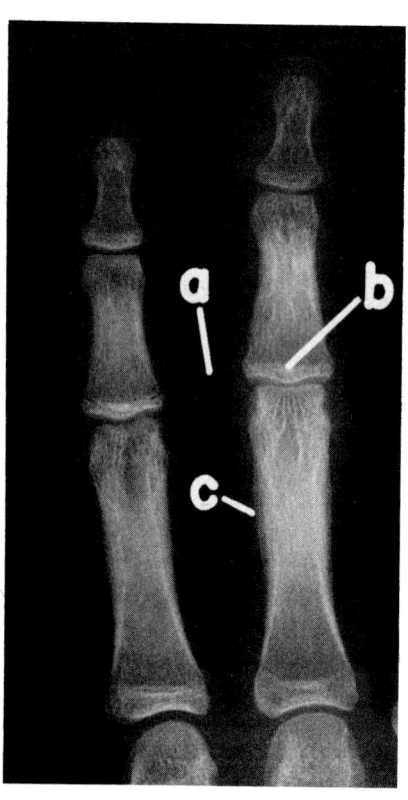

FIG. 57–8. Early roentgen features inlude soft-tissue swelling (a), early closure of epiphysis (b), and periosteal new bone along shaft of third proximal phalanx (c).

DISEASE COURSE AND PROGNOSIS

COURSE OF DISEASE

Largely determined by the mode of onset, three patterns of disease course have been observed: polycyclic systemic, polyarthritic, and pauciarthritic.[11,76]

Children with systemic onset may pursue a polycyclic systemic course, with recurrent attacks, primarily consisting of high fever and rash, but with minimal or no arthritis. Most systemic-onset patients develop polyarthritis or chronic arthritis of more than four joints; a few, however, continue to have superimposed attacks of high fever and other systemic manifestations. Patients with polyarticular onset remain polyarthritic; their course is usually characterized by flares and remissions, but occasionally by an unremitting and progressively downhill course. Of patients with pauciarticular onset, most pursue a course of pauciarthritis or chronic arthritis of one to four joints, but some develop polyarthritis. Regardless of the course, some patients may have to be reclassified when ankylosing spondylitis, psoriasis, or features of another rheumatic disorder eventually appear.

Growth Disturbances

General growth and development may be impaired in patients with JRA.[9,57,77] This impairment is related to progressively active disease as well as to the prolonged administration of corticosteroids. Once the disease becomes inactive, growth is resumed, and the child usually achieves normal proportions. If disease activity is prolonged and unremitting, however, permanent stunting of growth may occur from premature closure of epiphyses. The development of secondary sex characteristics may also be retarded.

Local abnormalities of growth include premature appearance and closure of epiphyses resulting in small hands or feet, as well as in isolated shortened metacarpals, metarsals, or phalanges. Premature epiphyseal closure may be especially striking in the mandible, in which it produces micrognathia (Fig. 57–9). Occasionally, particularly in pauciarticular JRA, overgrowth of epiphyses and metaphyses may cause one limb to be longer than the other. Such a discrepancy usually reverts to normal once disease activity is suppressed or remits.

PROGNOSIS

Of patients followed for up to 25 years, complete remission occurs in at least 50%, whereas 70% regain

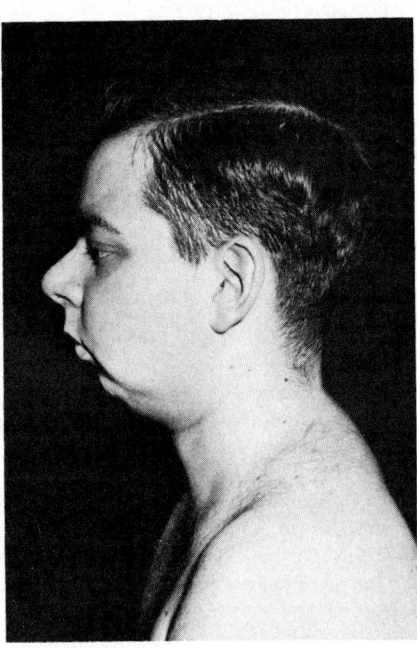

FIG. 57–9. Pronounced micrognathia in a young man with prolonged polyarthritis and progressive cervical involvement.

normal function.[9,11,70,78–81] Remission can occur at any time and does not necessarily coincide with the onset of puberty. Occasionally, however, a child in prolonged remission may as an adult have an exacerbation of the disease that results in joint destruction and severe disability for the first time.[82]

The mortality rate of JRA is 2 to 4%.[83] Most deaths occur in children with prolonged active polyarthritis and are due primarily to infection and secondary amyloidosis.[11,80,84]

REFERENCES

1. Cornil, V.: Memoire sur les coincidences pathologiques du rhumatisme articulaire chronique. C. R. Soc. Biol. (Paris), ser. 4,3:2–25, 1964.
2. Diamentberger, S.: Du rhumatisme noueux (polyarthrite déformante) chez les enfants. Paris, Lecrosnier & Babe, 1890.
3. Still, G.F.: On a form of chronic joint disease in children. Med. Chir. Trans., 80:47–59, 1897. (Reprinted in Am. J. Dis. Child., 132:195–200, 1978.)
4. Wouters, J.M.G.W., Reekers, P., and van de Putte, L.B.A.: Adult-onset Still's disease. Arthritis Rheum., 29:415–418, 1986.
5. Larson, E.G.: Adult Still's disease. Evolution of a clinical syndrome and diagnosis, treatment, and follow-up of 17 patients. Medicine, 63:82–91, 1984.
6. Cush, J.J., et al.: Adult-onset Still's disease. Arthritis Rheum., 30:186–194, 1987.
7. Aptekar, R.G., et al.: Adult onset juvenile rheumatoid arthritis. Arthritis Rheum., 16:715–718, 1973.
8. Steffe, L.A., and Cooke, C.L.: Still's disease in a 70-year-old woman. JAMA, 249:2062–2063, 1983.

9. Cassidy, J.T.: Textbook of Pediatric Rheumatology. New York, John Wiley & Sons, 1982.

10. Ansell, B.M.: Juvenile chronic polyarthritis. Series 3. Arthritis Rheum., *20(Suppl.)*:176–178, 1977.

11. Calabro, J.J., et al.: Juvenile rheumatoid arthritis. A general review and report of 100 patients observed for 15 years. Semin. Arthritis Rheum., *5*:257–298, 1976.

12. Grossman, B.J., and Mukhopadhyay, D.: Juvenile rheumatoid arthritis. *In* Current Problems in Pediatrics. Vol. 5. Edited by L. Gluck et al. Chicago, Year Book Medical Publishers, 1975, pp. 3–65.

13. Pazirandeh, M., Mackenzie, A.H., and Scherbel, A.L.: The natural course of juvenile rheumatoid arthritis. Cleve. Clin. Q., *36*:109–122, 1969.

14. Calin, A., and Calin, H.J.: Oligoarthropathy with chronic iridocyclitis—A disease only of childhood? J. Rheumatol., *9*:105–106, 1982.

15. Wernick, R., et al.: Serum IgG and IgM rheumatoid factors by solid phase radioimmunoassay. A comparison between adult and juvenile rheumatoid arthritis. Arthritis Rheum., *24*:1501–1511, 1981.

16. Brewer, E.J., Jr., et al.: Current proposed revision of JRA criteria. Arthritis Rheum., *20(Suppl.)*:195–199, 1977.

17. Bywaters, E.G.L.: Diagnostic criteria for Still's disease (juvenile RA). *In* Population Studies of the Rheumatic Diseases. Edited by P.H. Bennett and P.H.N. Wood. Amsterdam, Excerpta Medica, 1968, pp. 235–240.

18. Gewanter, H.L., Roghmann, K.J., and Baum, J.: The prevalence of juvenile arthritis. Arthritis Rheum., *26*:599–603, 1983.

19. Calabro, J.J., and Marchesano, J.M.: Medical intelligence. Current concepts. Juvenile rheumatoid arthritis. N. Engl. J. Med., *277*:696–699, 746–749, 1967.

20. Phillips, P., et al.: Virus antibody and IgG levels in juvenile rheumatoid arthritis. Arthritis Rheum., *16*:126, 1973.

21. McAnarney, E.R., et al.: Psychological problems of children with chronic juvenile arthritis. Pediatrics, *53*:523–528, 1974.

22. Rimon, R., Belmaker, R.H., and Ebstein, R.: Psychosomatic aspects of juvenile rheumatoid arthritis. Scand. J. Rheumatol., *6*:1–10, 1977.

23. Varni, J.W., and Jay, S.M.: Biobehavioral factors in juvenile rheumatoid arthritis: Implication for research and practice. Clin. Psychol. Rev., *4*:543–560, 1984.

24. Baum, J., and Fink, C.: Juvenile rheumatoid arthritis in monozygotic twins: A case report and review of the literature. Arthritis Rheum., *11*:33–36, 1968.

25. Forre, O., et al.: HLA antigens in juvenile arthritis. Genetic basis for the different subtypes. Arthritis Rheum., *26*:35–38, 1983.

26. Moore, T.L., et al.: Autoantibodies in juvenile arthritis. Semin. Arthritis Rheum., *13*:329–336, 1984.

27. Alspaugh, M.A., and Miller, J.J., III: A study of specificities of antinuclear antibodies in juvenile rheumatoid arthritis. J. Pediatr., *90*:391–395, 1977.

28. Schaller, J.G., et al.: The association of antinuclear antibodies with the chronic iridocyclitis of juvenile rheumatoid arthritis (Still's disease). Arthritis Rheum., *17*:409–416, 1974.

29. Bluestone, R., et al.: Juvenile rheumatoid arthritis: A serologic survey of 200 consecutive patients. J. Pediatr., *77*:98–102, 1970.

30. Cassidy, J.T., Petty, R.E., and Sullivan, D.B.: Abnormalities in the distribution of serum immunoglobulin concentrations in juvenile rheumatoid arthritis. J. Clin. Invest., *52*:1931–1936, 1973.

31. Calabro, J.J.: Juvenile rheumatoid arthritis. Mode of onset as key to early diagnosis and management. Postgrad. Med., *70*:120–133, 1981.

32. Schaller, J.G., and Wedgwood, R.J.: Is juvenile rheumatoid arthritis a single disease? A review. Pediatrics, *50*:940–953, 1972.

33. Calabro, J.J., Burnstein, S.L., and Staley, H.L.: Juvenile rheumatoid arthritis posing as fever of unknown origin. Arthritis Rheum., *20(Suppl.)*:178–180, 1977.

34. Jan, J.E., Hill, R.H., and Low, M.D.: Cerebral complications in juvenile rheumatoid arthritis. Can. Med. Assoc. J., *107*:623–625, 1972.

35. Brown, G.L., and Wilson, W.P.: Salicylate intoxication and the CNS with special reference to EEG findings. Dis. Nerv. Syst., *32*:135–140, 1971.

36. Calabro, J.J., and Marchesano, J.M.: Fever associated with juvenile rheumatoid arthritis. N. Engl. J. Med., *276*:11–18, 1967.

37. Calabro, J.J., and Marchesano, J.M.: Rash associated with juvenile rheumatoid arthritis. J. Pediatr., *72*:611–619, 1968.

38. Miller, J.J., III, and French, J.W.: Myocarditis in juvenile rheumatoid arthritis. Am. J. Dis. Child., *131*:205–209, 1977.

39. Majeed, H.A., and Kvasnicka, J.: Juvenile rheumatoid arthritis with cardiac tamponade. Ann. Rheum. Dis., *37*:273–276, 1978.

40. Bernstein, G., Takahashi, M., and Hanson, V.: Cardiac involvement in juvenile rheumatoid arthritis. J. Pediatr., *85*:313–317, 1974.

41. Yousefzadeh, D.K., and Fishman, P.A.: The triad of pneumonitis, pleuritis, and pericarditis in juvenile rheumatoid arthritis. Pediatr. Radiol., *8*:147–150, 1979.

42. Schaller, J.G., Beckwith, B., and Wedgwood, R.J.: Hepatic involvement in juvenile rheumatoid arthritis. J. Pediatr., *77*:203–210, 1970.

43. Athreya, B.H., Gorski, A.L., and Myers, A.R.: Aspirin-induced abnormalities of liver function. Am. J. Dis. Child., *126*:638–641, 1973.

44. Rich, R.R., and Johnson, J.S.: Salicylate hepatotoxicity in patients with juvenile rheumatoid arthritis. Arthritis Rheum., *16*:1–9, 1977.

45. Meislin, A.G., and Rothfield, N.: Systemic lupus erythematosus in childhood. Analysis of 42 cases, with comparative data on 200 adult cases followed concurrently. Pediatrics, *42*:37–49, 1968.

45a. Kornreich, H.K., Drexler, E., and Hanson, V.: Antinuclear factors in childhood rheumatic diseases. J. Pediatr., *69*:1039–1045, 1966.

46. Calabro, J.J.: Cancer and arthritis. Arthritis Rheum., *10*:553–567, 1967.

47. Calabro, J.J., and Castleman, B.: Case records of the Massachusetts General Hospital. Multiple osteolytic lesions in a 16-year-old boy with joint pains. N. Engl. J. Med., *286*:205–212, 1972.

48. Schaller, J.G.: Arthritis as a presenting manifestation of malignancy in children. J. Pediatr., *81*:793–797, 1972.

49. Schaller, J.G.: The arthritis of inflammatory bowel disease in children. Clin. Rheum. Dis., *2*:353–367, 1976.

50. Calabro, J.J.: Kawasaki disease. Clin. Rheumatol. Pract., *1*:29–35, 1983.

51. Calabro, J.J.: Rheumatoid arthritis: Diagnosis and management. Clinical Symposia. Summit, NJ: Pharmaceuticals Division, CIBA-GEIGY Corp., *38*:3–32, 1986.

52. Carter, M.E.: Sacro-iliitis in Still's disease. Ann. Rheum. Dis., *21*:105–120, 1962.

53. Ronning, O., Valiaho, M.-L., and Laaksonen, A.-L.: The involvement of the temporomandibular joint in juvenile rheumatoid arthritis. Scand. J. Rheumatol., *3*:89–96, 1974.

54. Simons, F.E.R., and Schaller, J.G.: Benign rheumatoid nodules. Pediatrics, *56*:29–33, 1975.

55. Truhan, A.P., Pachman, L.M., and Esterly, N.B.: Granuloma annulare. Arthritis Rheum., *30*:117–119, 1987.

56. Arnett, F.C., Bias, W.B., and Stevens, M.B.: Juvenile-onset chronic arthritis. Clinical and roentgenographic features of a unique HLA-B27 subset. Am. J. Med., *69*:369–376, 1980.

57. Calabro, J.J., Katz, R.M., and Maltz, B.A.: A critical reappraisal of juvenile rheumatoid arthritis. Clin. Orthop., *74*:101–119, 1971.

58. Hyer, F.H., and Gottlieb, N.L.: Rheumatic disorders associated with viral infection. Semin. Arthritis Rheum., *8*:17–31, 1978.

59. Singh, V.K., Tingle, A.J., and Schulzer, M.: Rubella-associated arthritis. II. Relationship between circulating immune complex levels and joint manifestations. Ann. Rheum. Dis., *45*:115–119, 1986.

60. Yunus, M., et al.: Primary fibromyalgia (fibrositis): Clinical study of 50 patients with matched normal controls. Semin. Arthritis Rheum., *11*:151–171, 1981.

61. Calabro, J.J.: Fibromyalgia (fibrositis) in children. Am. J. Med., *81(Suppl. 3A)*:57–59, 1986.

62. Chylack, L.T., Jr., et al.: Ocular manifestations of juvenile rheumatoid arthritis. Am. J. Ophthalmol., *79*:1026–1033, 1975.

63. Rosenberg, A.M., and Oen, K.G.: The relationship between ocular and articular disease activity in children with juvenile rheumatoid arthritis and associated uveitis. Arthritis Rheum., *29*:797–800, 1986.

64. Rosenberg, A.M.: Uveitis associated with juvenile rheumatoid arthritis. Semin. Arthritis Rheum., *16*:158–173, 1987.

65. Calabro, J.J., et al.: Chronic iridocyclitis in juvenile rheumatoid arthritis. Arthritis Rheum., *13*:406–413, 1970.

66. Bywaters, E.G.L.: Ankylosing spondylitis in childhood. Clin. Rheum. Dis., *87*:387–396, 1976.

67. Calabro, J.J., Gordon, R.D., and Miller, K.A.: Bechterew's syndrome in children: Diagnostic criteria. Scand. J. Rheumatol., *32(Suppl.)*:45–46, 1980.

68. Schaller, J.G., Bitnum, S., and Wedgwood, R.J.: Ankylosing spondylitis with childhood onset. J. Pediatr., *74*:505–516, 1969.

69. Schaller, J.: Chronic childhood arthritis and the spondylarthropathies. *In* Spondylarthropathies. Edited by A. Calin. Orlando, Grune & Stratton, 1984, pp. 187–208.

70. Calabro, J.J.: Drug therapy of juvenile rheumatoid arthritis and of the seronegative spondyloarthropathies. *In* Drug Therapy in Rheumatology. Edited by S.H. Roth. Littleton, MA, PSG Publishing Co., 1985, pp. 115–180.

71. Rosenberg, A.M., and Petty, R.E.: A syndrome of seronegative enthesopathy and arthropathy in children. Arthritis Rheum., *25*:1041–1047, 1982.

72. Konttinen, Y.T., et al.: The value of biopsy in patients with monarticular juvenile rheumatoid arthritis of recent onset. Arthritis Rheum., *29*:47–53, 1986.

73. Thomas, A.L., et al.: A case of sarcoid arthritis in a child. Arthritis Rheum., *42*:343–346, 1983.

74. Steere, A.C., et al.: The early clinical manifestations of Lyme disease. Ann. Intern. Med., *99*:76–82, 1983.

75. Williams, R.A., and Ansell, B.M.: Radiological findings in seropositive juvenile chronic arthritis (juvenile rheumatoid arthritis) with particular reference to progression. Ann. Rheum. Dis., *44*:685–693, 1985.

76. Cassidy, J.T., et al.: A study of classification criteria for a diagnosis of juvenile rheumatoid arthritis. Arthritis Rheum., *29*:274–281, 1986.

77. Ansell, B.M., and Bywaters, E.G.L.: Growth in Still's disease. Ann. Rheum. Dis., *15*:295–319, 1956.

78. Calabro, J.J., Marchesano, J.M., and Miller, K.A.: Juvenile rheumatoid arthritis. *In* Prognosis: Contemporary Outcomes of Disease. Edited by J.F. Fries and G.E. Ehrlich. Bowie, MD, Prentice-Hall, 1981, pp. 347–349.

79. Miller, J.J., et al.: The social function of young adults who had arthritis in childhood. J. Pediatr., *100*:378–382, 1982.

80. Stoeber, H.: Prognosis in juvenile chronic arthritis. Follow-up of 433 chronic rheumatic children. Eur. J. Pediatr., *135*:225–228, 1981.

81. Svantesson, H., et al.: Prognosis in juvenile rheumatoid arthritis with systemic onset. A follow-up study. Scand. J. Rheumatol., *12*:139–144, 1983.

82. Jeremy, R., et al.: Juvenile rheumatoid arthritis persisting into adulthood. Am. J. Med., *45*:419–434, 1968.

83. Baum, J., and Goutowska, G.: Death in juvenile rheumatoid arthritis. Arthritis Rheum., *20(Suppl.)*:253–255, 1977.

84. Calabro, J.J., Eyvazzadeh, C., and Weber, C.A.: Juvenile rheumatoid arthritis: Early diagnosis, management, and long-term prognosis. Advances in Therapy, *3*:97–142, 1986.

58

TREATMENT OF JUVENILE RHEUMATOID ARTHRITIS

JANE GREEN SCHALLER

Considerations in designing therapy for a child with juvenile rheumatoid arthritis (JRA) include the following: (1) recognition of the several disease subgroups of JRA; (2) identification of specific disease manifestations requiring therapy in the individual patient; (3) understanding of the long-term natural history of the disease and of its various manifestations; (4) cognizance of the overall favorable prognosis for most affected children; and (5) acknowledgment of the special burdens of chronic illness on children, adolescents, and their families.

Several subgroups can be distinguished within the "disease" now called JRA in the United States and Still's disease or juvenile chronic polyarthritis in other parts of the world.[1-12] Five possible subgroups and their characteristics are given in Table 58–1.[9-12] Whether these subgroups represent truly different diseases or only different host responses to one or more etiologic factors is not known. In any event, recognition of disease subgroups is helpful in diagnosis and in the selection of appropriate therapy in patients with JRA (see also Chapter 57).

Several distinct manifestations of JRA may require therapy. These should be identified accurately in the individual patient before planning any therapeutic program. These different disease manifestations are listed in Table 58–2 and are discussed separately in subsequent sections of this chapter.

The overall prognosis for children with JRA is better than had been previously assumed; at least 75% of affected children eventually have long remissions without significant residual damage and presumably lead normal adult lives.[1-6,8,9,11,13] Several long-term sequelae can follow JRA (Table 58–3). The risks of these sequelae vary according to disease subgroup. Children with rheumatoid-factor–positive or systemic-onset JRA are at greatest risk for chronic and destructive joint disease. Children with pauciarticular disease beginning in early childhood are at greatest risk for chronic iridocyclitis,[14-18] and those with pauciarticular disease beginning in later childhood are at some risk for subsequent ankylosing spondylitis or another spondyloarthropathy.[8,9,17,19-23] Growth retardation occurs most frequently in children with chronic systemic-onset or polyarticular disease.[24-26]

Available therapy permits control of synovitis in many children with JRA, although chronic synovitis with joint destruction, a cause of ultimate morbidity in JRA, is not always preventable. Fortunately, fewer than 20% of children with JRA have relentlessly active synovitis with resultant severe joint destruction. Synovitis can be adequately controlled in many children, especially in those with seronegative polyarthritis or with pauciarticular disease. Much of the present therapy of JRA is focused on preventing lasting deformity, and this goal can often be reached. Such residual deformities can cripple the musculoskeletal system, the eye, and the child's psychosocial outlook. Iatrogenic damage from the injudicious use of drugs and from overvigorous physical and surgical therapy must always be avoided.

Table 58–1. Subgroups of Juvenile Rheumatoid Arthritis

Type of Disease	Ratio of Girls to Boys	Age at Onset	Joints Affected	Serology	Extra-articular Manifestations	Prognosis
Systemic onset	8:10	Any age	Any joints	ANA negative; RF negative; HLA-?	High fever, rash, organomegaly, polyserositis, leukocytosis	20% severe arthritis
Polyarticular: rheumatoid factor negative	8:1	Any age	Any joints	ANA 25%; RF negative; HLA-?	Low-grade fever, mild anemia, malaise	10% severe arthritis
Polyarticular: rheumatoid factor positive	6:1	Late childhood	Any joints	ANA 75%; RF 100%; HLA-DR4	Mild fever, anemia, malaise, rheumatoid nodules	>50% severe arthritis
Pauciarticular: early childhood onset, associated with chronic iridocyclitis	7:1	Early childhood	Scattered joints, predominantly large joints; hips and sacroiliac joints spared	ANA 60%; RF negative; HLA-DRW8, -DR5, -DRW6	Few constitutional complaints; chronic iridocyclitis in 30%	Later polyarthritis in 20%, ocular damage from iridocyclitis in some
Pauciarticular: late childhood onset, associated with sacroiliitis	1:10	Late childhood	Scattered large joints; hip girdle and sacroiliac involvement common	ANA negative; RF negative, HLA-B27	Few constitutional complaints; acute iridocyclitis in 5–10%	Later spondyloarthropathy in ?% at follow-up

ANA = antinuclear antibody; RF = rheumatoid factor.

THERAPY OF ARTHRITIS AND MAINTENANCE OF MUSCULOSKELETAL FUNCTION

In planning therapy for the musculoskeletal manifestations of JRA, the physician must first assess the extent of joint involvement in the individual patient, the activity of the synovitis, the presence or absence of joint destruction, the status of muscle strength or weakness, and the amount of joint deformity and

Table 58–2. Manifestations of Juvenile Rheumatoid Arthritis Requiring Therapy

Musculoskeletal manifestations
    Active synovitis
    Joint deformity
    Muscle weakness or dysfunction
Systemic manifestations
    Fever and other manifestations of systemic-onset disease
    Constitutional manifestations of other subgroups
Iridocyclitis
Amyloidosis
Psychosocial Aspects

Table 58–3. Long-Term Sequelae of Juvenile Rheumatoid Arthritis

Persistent synovitis
    Severe, with progressive joint destruction
    Mild, with little progressive disability
Residual deformities from past disease
    Musculoskeletal dysfunction
    Ocular damage
    Growth retardation
    Amyloidosis
    Psychosocial problems
Iatrogenic damage

must determine whether observed joint deformities are due to active disease or are residua of inactive disease. In making these assessments, a careful history and physical examination, selected radiographs, and certain laboratory tests, such as the hematocrit and erythrocyte sedimentation rate, are of value.

DRUG THERAPY

To control active synovitis and the musculoskeletal manifestations of active JRA, drugs of the anti-inflammatory and antirheumatic classes are prescribed. None of these agents are curative, but synovitis can be satisfactorily suppressed with currently available drug therapy in about 80% of affected children.

Salicylates

Salicylates provide the mainstay of therapy (see also Chapter 32).[1,11,27–31] They are effective as antipyretics, analgesics, and anti-inflammatory agents. Acetylsalicylic acid (aspirin) is most commonly prescribed. Other preparations occasionally used include sodium salicylate and choline salicylate; whether these are as effective as aspirin in suppressing inflammation has not been studied adequately. Appropriate doses of aspirin are 100 mg/kg body weight/day, in four to six divided doses, for children weighing 25 kg or less. For children weighing 25 kg or more, total daily doses of 2.4 to 3.6 g/day are usually sufficient. Serious salicylate intoxication can result if doses are calculated on the basis of 100 mg/kg body weight for children weighing more than 25 kg. Serum salicylate levels between 20 and 30 mg/dl are considered adequate for therapeutic effect; such blood levels are usually achieved with the aforementioned doses. Little benefit and great potential hazard exist in giving salicylates to the point of serious toxicity. Salicylates are effective in controlling synovitis in about 75% of patients. A full therapeutic response may not occur for several months.

The major hazard of salicylate therapy is salicylism resulting from overdosage. With careful adherence to dosages and measuring blood levels if necessary, serious toxicity should not result from therapeutic use of these agents. Most children do not note or complain of tinnitus, which usually occurs with serum levels of 20 to 30 mg/dl. The first signs of salicylism are central nervous system depression or excitation or hyperventilation, which occur with serum salicylate levels over 30 mg/dl. Such signs suggest overdosage. Parents, patients, and physicians should be alert to such signs of toxicity and should react to them immediately by decreasing the dose and by checking blood levels of the drug if possible.

Other problems with salicylates include gastrointestinal irritation with gastric distress or nausea. A few patients with JRA undergoing a prolonged course of salicylate therapy have developed peptic ulcers,[32] but the relationship of these ulcers to the drug is not clear. Gastrointestinal irritation can be minimized by giving salicylates with food, by using buffered preparations, by prescribing concomitant antacids, or by administering a preparation such as choline salicylate.

Attention has been drawn to the "hepatotoxicity" of salicylates. Some children receiving salicylates in therapeutic dosages develop elevated serum transaminase levels, but not jaundice or other signs or symptoms of liver disease.[28,29,33-36] The hepatic involvement of systemic-onset JRA must be differentiated from that of other disorders.[37,38] Even with continuing use of drug, enzyme levels usually do not rise higher, and no later evidence of chronic liver disease appears. Few children develop severe acute liver disease after salicylate ingestion that precludes further salicylate usage. Although even low doses of aspirin affect platelet function and higher doses may lengthen the patient's prothrombin time,[39,40] serious bleeding problems are uncommon in aspirin-treated patients with JRA. It is wise to discontinue aspirin therapy several weeks before any surgical procedures and to substitute choline salicylate or sodium salicylate, neither of which affects hemostasis. Hypersensitivity reactions to aspirin such as hives are rare, and aspirin-related asthma and nasal polyps are unusual in JRA patients.

Small numbers of red blood cells or tubular epithelial cells may be found in the urine.[41] Although chronic renal disease has not been associated with salicylate ingestion in children, a few instances of renal papillary necrosis have been reported in children with JRA who were receiving salicylates.[42] Recent epidemiologic surveys have suggested that an association may exist between salicylate ingestion and Reye's syndrome occurring with influenza or chicken pox.[43-47]

Other Nonsteroidal Anti-inflammatory Agents

A number of other nonsteroidal anti-inflammatory agents are available for the treatment of arthritis in adults. These drugs seem to be similar to salicylates in efficacy, although some patients may respond better to one drug than to another (see also Chapter 32).

Although some of these drugs, particularly indomethacin, are widely used to treat JRA in various parts of the world, only tolmetin and liquid naproxen are currently labeled for use in children in the United States.[48-51] In patients with pauciarticular JRA beginning in late childhood who may have spondyloarthropathy, and in patients who do not respond satisfactorily to salicylates, some of these drugs might be of therapeutic benefit.

Gold Compounds

In children with progressive loss of joint function due to active synovitis after 6 months of adequate salicylate and physical therapy, gold therapy may be indicated[11,30,52,53] (see also Chapter 33). Such patients often have positive rheumatoid factors or chronic arthritis after a systemic onset. The gold preparations are the same as those used in adults. The dosage is 1 mg/kg body weight/week up to a body weight of 25 kg. For children weighing 25 to 50 kg, a dose of 25 mg/week is appropriate; for teenagers weighing more than 60 kg, doses of 25 to 50 mg/week are used. As in adults, small "test" doses of 10 or 20% of the full dose are given for 2 or 3 weeks.

Toxicity in children is similar to that in adults and is of no greater severity or frequency. Followup in children receiving gold therapy consists of weekly physical examination for evidence of rash or mucosal ulcers, a weekly white blood cell count, a hematocrit and smear for platelets, and a urinalysis for both red blood cells and protein levels. Any evidence of toxicity is cause for discontinuing the treatment with gold temporarily. When toxicity disappears, gold treatment may be resumed cautiously, perhaps at a lower dose initially. As in adults after a 6-month course of weekly doses, the patient's response to the drug is assessed. Children who respond are in full or partial remission and often have normal erythrocyte sedimentation rates. In such patients, the frequency of gold injections is reduced to once every 2 weeks, then once every 3 weeks, and then indefinitely on a once-monthly basis. It is imperative to continue surveillance for toxicity, including blood and urine tests, before each gold injection. Gold therapy probably should be abandoned in patients who do not appear to respond in 6 months. Patients with partial responses may be treated weekly for some months longer, or with doses administered at longer intervals, depending on the physician's evaluation of current status.

Oral gold has been used in the treatment of JRA,[54] and a recent study has shown its efficacy.[55]

Antimalarial Agents

As in adults, antimalarial drugs (see also Chapter 34) are a useful alternative to gold therapy in some patients. Hydroxychloroquine (Plaquenil) is the drug of choice. Doses should not exceed 200 mg/m² body surface area per day, and ophthalmologic examinations should be made every 3 months. The side effects of antimalarial agents in children are similar to those in adults, with ocular toxicity the chief hazard of prolonged administration. Antimalarial drugs are poisons with no antidote for overdosage,[56] so their inaccessibility to small children must be ensured.

Penicillamine

D-penicillamine (DPA) (see also Chapter 36) is currently being used in both adults with RA and children with JRA.[57] Some observers feel that this drug is useful to patients with severe arthritis who do not respond to nonsteroidal agents and as an alternative to gold. However, a recent controlled study of DPA, hydroxychloroquine, and placebo in children with JRA showed no significant efficacy of either drug as compared to placebo.[58,59] The toxicity of DPA is similar in children and adults. Toxic effects include rash, bone marrow suppression, nephritis, myasthenia gravis, and Goodpasture's syndrome.

Corticosteroids

Although there was once great enthusiasm for these drugs,[60,61] corticosteroids are no more curative of JRA than they are of adult RA (see also Chapter 37).[1,27,62] These agents may suppress symptoms for a time, but they do not prevent progression of joint damage in patients with severe JRA, and they may actually contribute to articular damage in some patients. Cushingoid side effects occur early after low doses of corticosteroids. Troublesome side effects other than cushingoid appearance are also common and include adrenal suppression, which may be fatal, growth suppression, osteoporosis, vertebral compression fractures, peptic ulcer disease, and cor-

ticosteroid cataracts. Few children with JRA gain much permanent benefit from corticosteroid therapy given for arthritis alone. Although the immediate relief of symptoms may be dramatic, the ultimate effect is not curative, and the long-term side effects are often horrendous. It is of little help to a patient to add chronic Cushing's syndrome and adrenal suppression to a severe destructive arthritis. In the experience of clinics managing many children with JRA, corticosteroid therapy is rarely warranted for joint disease alone and, if given, is used in the lowest possible doses, preferably on alternate days[63] and for as short a time as possible. The use of large intravenous "pulse" doses of corticosteroids in patients with JRA remains experimental.[64]

Adrenocorticotropic hormone (ACTH) has been used to advantage in some clinics[65] because it may have fewer long-term side effects than corticosteroids. Local corticosteroid injections into troublesome joints may suppress local synovitis, but no more than several injections should be made into any single joint, to avoid cartilage damage.

Immunosuppressive Drugs

Although drugs such as cyclophosphamide, azathioprine, and methotrexate have been tested and used in the therapy of adult RA,[66] no similar studies have been completed in childhood arthritis[67] (see also Chapters 35 and 38). A current controlled study is comparing methotrexate to placebo in children with severe JRA.[68] The side effects of such drugs include increased susceptibility to potentially fatal and often untreatable infections with viruses, fungi, and other agents, possible future increased risk of malignant disease, and interference with future reproductive capacity.[67,69–73] Such side effects make the use of such drugs seem rarely warranted in JRA, a disease in which most patients have a favorable prognosis. Great care must be taken in interpreting anecdotal reports of successes with these agents in JRA. Some favorable experience in England and Europe has been reported with the use of chlorambucil[74] and azathioprine in patients with JRA and amyloidosis; concomitant improvement in arthritis has been noted in such patients during therapy. No evidence suggests that any of these drugs are efficacious in the treatment of chronic iridocyclitis.

Little experience exists with experimental measures such as plasmapheresis, lymphophoresis, or total lymph node irradiation in the therapy of children with JRA.

PHYSICAL AND OCCUPATIONAL THERAPY

In general, children with JRA should be encouraged to be active and to participate in normal activities of childhood (see also Chapters 48 and 49). Activities such as tricycle riding and swimming may be valuable additions to physical therapy. Total bed rest is almost always contraindicated. Children should be trained and encouraged to function as normally as possible in a usual childhood environment.

Physical and occupational therapy are of great benefit in maintaining function and in preventing invalidism in patients with JRA.[30,52,75] Exercises to preserve joint range of motion and functional joint position, to maintain muscle strength, and to maintain normal function of the limbs and of the total child are vital. No evidence suggests that, with reasonable care, exercise damages inflamed joints. Physical and occupational therapy are invaluable, even in children with active arthritis.

All children with JRA should be instructed in range-of-motion and muscle-strengthening exercises, to be done once or twice daily at home. All joints should be put through a functional range of motion at least once daily, with particular attention to affected joints. Night splints may be useful in preserving functional joint positions, particularly in the knees and wrist. Joints should not be rigidly immobilized for long periods, because loss of joint motion may be irreversible. Exercise programs should be taught to both the patient and the parents; children older than 6 years should be largely responsible for their own exercises with minimal parental supervision. Muscle-strengthening exercises should be done when necessary for the quadriceps, hip, or shoulder girdle muscles, the gastrocnemius-soleus muscles, and the peroneal muscles. Occupational therapy can improve hand function, and it may improve overall function. Heat, in the form of a hot morning bath at home, is often valuable in alleviating morning stiffness.

Inpatient medical, physical, and occupational therapy is usually justified for children with severe musculoskeletal dysfunction who are not self-sufficient or who cannot attend school regularly. Pool therapy may be a valuable adjunct. Heat from paraffin baths may help to restore motion of small hand joints. Splinting and traction may be useful in overcoming flexion contractures.

ORTHOPEDIC THERAPY

Synovectomy plays a limited role in the early therapy of JRA.[76,77] Patients with pauciarticular disease, the most logical candidates for synovectomy, have a good prognosis for joint function without operative intervention. Synovectomy is useful occasionally in children with polyarthritis and one or few troublesome joints. Many children experience a recurrence of synovitis in operated joints, however.

Orthopedic surgery holds great promise in the late rehabilitation of children with serious disability from JRA.[78] Soft-tissue release can alleviate contractures unresponsive to nonoperative therapy.[79] Osteotomies may be useful. Total joint replacement, particularly of the hips and knees, may be of great benefit to children with serious joint damage but should be done only after adolescence and when full growth has been achieved.[78,80–84] Help is needed for younger children with serious disability, particularly from severe hip disease, because no routine surgical procedures that permit early rehabilitation are available at present.

THERAPY OF SYSTEMIC MANIFESTATIONS

SYSTEMIC-ONSET JUVENILE RHEUMATOID ARTHRITIS

The high fevers, malaise, polyserositis, organomegaly, and anemia of systemic-onset JRA can present major therapeutic problems. In the natural course of systemic-onset JRA, these manifestations usually subside spontaneously in about 6 months, regardless of treatment. Although the high fevers and malaise are debilitating, they are not generally life-threatening. Only rarely are severe pericarditis, myocarditis, or anemia potentially fatal. In treating systemic-onset JRA, it is thus imperative that the therapy be no worse than the disease. Salicylates, the drugs of choice, are effective in controlling systemic manifestations in more than half these patients. The doses used are similar to those described for treatment of arthritis: serum salicylate levels should not be higher than 40 mg/dl. Children who are seriously ill with systemic-onset JRA should be hospitalized and closely watched. If fever and other systemic symptoms remain severely incapacitating after 2 or 3 weeks of vigorous salicylate therapy, systemic corticosteroids are probably indicated. It is reasonable to begin with a high dose of corticosteroids, such as 30 to 60 mg prednisone a day, to control symptoms rapidly. A single, morning, corticosteroid dose regimen is often effective. The drug dosage can then be slowly tapered and discontinued within 6 months. Most children with severe systemic-onset disease respond rapidly to such a regimen, and corticosteroids can be withdrawn without incident. Arthritis appearing while the corticosteroid dose is being reduced should be treated with salicylates or with gold and not with more corticosteroids.

Alternate-day dosage schedules have been suggested.[63] These programs control symptoms less rapidly, but they may be effective in some patients. About half the children with systemic-onset disease experience later attacks of systemic complaints, and these should always be treated first with salicylates. Gold, antimalarial agents, and anticancer drugs are of little use in controlling systemic manifestations because all require several months for effect. The usefulness of nonsteroidal anti-inflammatory agents in controlling systemic manifestations has not been adequately explored. Because some of these drugs are effective antipyretics, some may prove effective.

EXTRA-ARTICULAR MANIFESTATIONS OF OTHER SUBGROUPS

Patients with nonsystemic-onset JRA also may have low-grade fever, malaise, mild hepatosplenomegaly, and mild anemia. These extra-articular manifestations of disease usually respond to the therapy given for the arthritis and are rarely, if ever, indications for institution of vigorous therapy with systemic corticosteroids. Anemic children with JRA should be investigated for iron deficiency and should be treated appropriately with iron if necessary.

GROWTH RETARDATION

Growth retardation is concomitant with sustained disease during the growth period.[24-26] No therapy is effective except control of the underlying disease. Growth retardation also follows therapy with corticosteroids in daily doses of more than 3 to 5 mg prednisone daily or equivalent.[62,26]

THERAPY OF IRIDOCYCLITIS

Early detection of iridocyclitis is crucial to successful therapy. At highest risk are those young-onset patients with pauciarticular disease,[14,15,17,18] particularly those with positive tests for antinuclear antibodies.[16] Patients in this high-risk group should have screening slit-lamp examinations at least every 3 months by an ophthalmologist. Iridocyclitis should be treated initially with topical corticosteroids, dilating agents, and

careful followup examinations. Should topical therapy fail, further treatment with injections of corticosteroids under the vagina bulbi or with systemic corticosteroids should be tried. Doses of systemic corticosteroids should be high enough to control ocular inflammation, as monitored by slit-lamp examinations; alternate-day dosage schedules may be effective. No evidence suggests that any of the other anti-inflammatory or antirheumatic agents, or any of the anticancer drugs, are effective in controlling chronic iridocyclitis. Surgical treatment sometimes helps to rehabilitate eyes severely damaged by chronic iridocyclitis. Band keratopathy can be chelated with topical edetate (EDTA) and may be removed surgically. Mature cataracts secondary to iridocyclitis may be extracted, but only by surgeons experienced in this procedure.

Children with older-onset pauciarticular disease with spondyloarthropathy sometimes have attacks of acute iridocyclitis.[16,17] This type of iridocyclitis is similar to that of ankylosing spondylitis in adults, as well as that of inflammatory bowel disease and Reiter's syndrome. Acute iridocyclitis is apparent early because of severe associated symptoms. Treatment with topical corticosteroids and dilating agents usually satisfactorily quiets the inflammation. Attacks are generally self-limited, and the prognosis for normal vision is excellent.

THERAPY OF AMYLOIDOSIS

Amyloidosis, a serious complication of childhood arthritis, is recognized in about 5% of patients with JRA in England, Europe, and most other parts of the world, but it is rare in the United States.[74] Reasons for this difference are not apparent. Amyloidosis is considered invariably fatal, generally from progressive renal disease. Therapy of amyloidosis with chlorambucil[74] and with azathioprine has been thought to be successful during short-term studies in several centers.

MANAGEMENT OF THE WHOLE CHILD

Appropriate management of the whole child is an important aspect of therapy.[6,67] The child and the family need to be educated about JRA and reassured that, although the disease may be chronic and unpredictable, the overall prognosis for the majority of patients is good. Children should be managed with optimism and encouragement. They should be helped to lead lives that are as full as possible, to attend regular schools, and to avoid thinking of themselves as chronic invalids. Bed rest and isolation from peers should be avoided. Children who are too ill or too disabled to be self-sufficient and to attend school should probably be hospitalized for rehabilitation. Children need constant support for the many problems of childhood and adolescence. Teenagers need appropriate counseling to help them to formulate and achieve realistic career goals.

Most children with JRA are cared for by primary physicians. For optimal care, however, the child with JRA should be seen at least periodically by a physician who understands the natural history of the disease and has had experience with needed drugs and physical therapy. Severely affected patients are best managed by such a physician directly. A team approach is optimal for care of affected children. A pediatrician or rheumatologist, a physiatrist, an orthopedist, an ophthalmologist, a physical therapist, and an occupational therapist are all needed at times. Consistent long-term followup of patients with JRA is crucial.

REFERENCES

1. Ansell, B.M.: Rheumatic disorders in childhood. *In* Postgraduate Paediatrics Series: Juvenile Chronic Arthritis. Edited by J. Apley. London, Butterworth, 1980.
2. Ansell, B.M., and Wood, P.H.N.: Prognosis in juvenile chronic polyarthritis. Clin. Rheum. Dis., 2:397–412, 1976.
3. Bywaters, E.G.L.: Categorization in medicine: A survey of Still's disease. Ann. Rheum. Dis., 26:185–193, 1967.
4. Calabro, J.J., et al.: Juvenile rheumatoid arthritis: A general review and report of 100 patients observed for 15 years. Semin. Arthritis Rheum., 5:257–298, 1976.
5. Calabro, J.J., Katz, R.M., and Maltz, B.A.: A critical reappraisal of juvenile rheumatoid arthritis. Clin. Orthop., 74:101–119, 1971.
6. Proceedings of the First American Rheumatism Association Conference on the Rheumatic Disease of Childhood. Arthritis Rheum., 20(Suppl. 2):145–636, 1977.
7. Schaller, J.G.: Juvenile rheumatoid arthritis. Pediatr. Rev., 2:163–174, 1980.
8. Schaller, J.G.: The seronegative spondyloarthropathies of childhood. Clin. Orthop., 143:76–83, 1979.
9. Schaller, J.G.: The diversity of JRA: A 1976 look at the subgroups of chronic childhood arthritis. Arthritis Rheum., 20:1519–1527, 1977.
10. Schaller, J.G., et al.: Histocompatibility antigens in childhood-onset arthritis. J. Pediatr., 88:926–930, 1976.
11. Schaller, J., and Wedgwood, R.J.: Is juvenile rheumatoid arthritis a single disease? A review. Pediatrics, 50:940–953, 1972.
12. Cassidy, J.T.: A study of classification criteria for a diagnosis of JRA. Arthritis Rheum., 29:274, 1986.
13. Ansell, B.M., and Bywaters, E.G.L.: Prognosis in Still's disease. Bull. Rheum. Dis., 9:189–192, 1959.
14. Calabro, J.J., et al.: Chronic iridocyclitis in juvenile rheumatoid arthritis. Arthritis Rheum., 13:406–413, 1970.
15. Chylack, L.T.: The ocular manifestations of juvenile rheumatoid arthritis. Arthritis Rheum., 20(Suppl. 2):217–223, 1977.
16. Schaller, J.G., et al.: The association of antinuclear antibodies with the chronic iridocyclitis of juvenile arthritis (Still's disease). Arthritis Rheum., 17:409–416, 1974.
17. Schaller, J.G., and Wedgwood, R.J.: Pauciarticular childhood arthritis: Identification of two distinct subgroups. Arthritis Rheum., 19:820–821, 1976.
18. Schaller, J.G., Kupfer, C., and Wedgwood, R.J.: Iridocyclitis in juvenile rheumatoid arthritis. Pediatrics, 44:92–100, 1969.
19. Jacobs, J.C., Berdon, W.E., and Johnson, A.D.: HLA-B27 associated spondyloarthritis and enthesopathy in childhood: Clinical, pathologic and radiographic observations in 58 patients. J. Pediatr., 100:521–528, 1982.
20. Ladd, J.R., Cassidy, J.T., and Martel, W.: Juvenile ankylosing spondylitis. Arthritis Rheum., 14:579, 1971.
21. Rosenberg, A.M., and Petty, R.E.: A syndrome of seronegative enthesopathy and arthropathy in children. Arthritis Rheum., 25:1041–1047, 1982.
22. Schaller, J.G.: Ankylosing spondylitis of childhood onset. Arthritis Rheum., 20(Suppl. 2):398–401, 1977.
23. Schaller, J.G., Bitnum, S., and Wedgwood, R.J.: Ankylosing spondylitis with childhood onset. J. Pediatr., 74:505–516, 1969.
24. Ansell, B.M., and Bywaters, E.G.L.: Growth in Still's disease. Ann. Rheum. Dis., 15:295–319, 1956.
25. Bernstein, B.H., et al.: Growth retardation in juvenile rheumatoid arthritis. Arthritis Rheum., 20(Suppl. 2):212–216, 1977.
26. Ward, D.J., Hartog, M., and Anwell, B.M.: Corticosteroid-induced dwarfism in Still's disease treated with human growth hormone. Clinical and metabolic effects including hydroxyproline excretion in two cases. Ann. Rheum. Dis., 25:416–421, 1966.
27. Ansell, B.M., Bywaters E.G.L., and Isdale, I.C.: Comparison of cortisone and aspirin in treatment of juvenile rheumatoid arthritis. Br. Med J., 1:1075–1077, 1956.
28. Doughty, R.A., Giesecki, L., and Athreya, B.: Salicylate therapy in juvenile rheumatoid arthritis: Dose, serum level, and toxicity. Am. J. Dis. Child., 134:461–463, 1980.
29. Schaller, J.G.: Chronic salicylate administration in juvenile rheumatoid arthritis: Aspirin "hepatitis" and its clinical significance. Pediatrics, 62:916–925, 1978.
30. Schaller, J.G., and Wedgwood, R.J.: Rheumatic diseases of childhood (Inflammatory diseases of connective tissue, collagen diseases). *In* Nelson Textbook of Pediatrics. 13th Ed. Edited by R.E. Behrman, V.C. Vaughan, and W.E. Nelson. Philadelphia, W.B. Saunders, 1987.
31. Stillman, J.S.: Salicylates—A review. Arthritis Rheum., 20(Suppl. 2):510–512, 1977.
32. Schaller, J.G., and Christie, D.: Peptic ulcer disease in juvenile rheumatoid arthritis. Personal communication.
33. Athreya, B.H., Gorski, A.L., and Meyers, A.R.: Aspirin-induced abnormalities of liver function. Am. J. Dis. Child., 126:638–641, 1973.
34. Miller, J.J., and Weissman, D.B.: Correlation between transaminase concentrations and serum salicylate concentrations in juvenile rheumatoid arthritis. Arthritis Rheum., 19:115–118, 1976.
35. Rich, R.R., and Johnson, J.S.: Salicylate hepatotoxicity in patients with juvenile rheumatoid arthritis. Arthritis Rheum., 16:1–9, 1973.
36. Russell, A.S., Sturge, R.A., and Smith, M.A.: Serum transaminases during salicylate therapy. Br. Med. J., 2:428–429, 1971.
37. Kornreich, K.H., Malouf, N.N., and Hanson, V.: Acute hepatic dysfunction in juvenile rheumatoid arthritis. J. Pediatr., 79:1, 27–33, 1971.
38. Schaller, J.G., Beckwith, B., and Wedgwood, R.J.: Hepatic in-

volvement in juvenile rheumatoid arthritis. J. Pediatr., 77:203–210, 1970.

39. Quick, A.J.: Salicylates and bleeding: The aspirin tolerance test. Am. J. Med. Sci., 252:265–269, 1966.

40. Sutor, A.H., Bowie, E.J.W., and Owen, C.A.: Effect of aspirin, sodium salicylates and acetaminophen on bleeding. Mayo Clin. Proc., 46:178–181, 1971.

41. Prescott, L.F., and Cantab, M.B.: Effects of acetylsalicylic acid, phenacetin, paracetamol and caffeine on renal tubular epithelium. Lancet, 2:91–95, 1965.

42. Wortmann, D.W., et al.: Renal papillary necrosis in juvenile rheumatoid arthritis. J. Pediatr., 97:37–40, 1980.

43. Starko, K.M., et al.: Reye's syndrome and salicylate use. Pediatrics, 66:859–864, 1980.

44. Fulginiti, V.A., et al.: Aspirin and Reye syndrome. Pediatrics, 69:810–812, 1982.

45. Brown, A.K., Fikrig, S., and Finberg, L.: Aspirin and Reye Syndrome. J. Pediatr., 102:157–158, 1983.

46. Rennebohn, R., et al.: Reye's syndrome in children receiving salicylate therapy for connective tissue disease. J. Pediatr., 107:877–880, 1985.

47. Hurwitz, E.S., et al.: Public health service study on Reye's syndrome and medications. N. Engl. J. Med., 313:849–857, 1985.

48. Brewer, E.J.: Nonsteroidal anti-inflammatory agents. Arthritis Rheum., 20(Suppl. 2):513–525, 1977.

49. Levinson, J.E., et al.: Comparison of tolmetin sodium and aspirin in the treatment of juvenile rheumatoid arthritis. J. Pediatr., 91:799–804, 1977.

50. Moran, H., et al.: Naproxen in juvenile chronic polyarthritis. Ann. Rheum. Dis., 38:152–154, 1979.

51. Pediatric Rheumatology Study Group: Methodology and studies of children with juvenile rheumatoid arthritis. J. Rheumatol., 9:107–155, 1982.

52. Brewer, E.J., Blattner, R.J., and Wing, H.: Treatment of rheumatoid arthritis in children. Pediatr. Clin. North Am., 10:207–224, 1963.

53. Brewer, E.J., Giannini, E.H., and Barkley, E.: Gold therapy in the management of juvenile rheumatoid arthritis. Arthritis Rheum., 23:404–411, 1980.

54. Gianni, E.H., Brewer, E.J., and Person, D.A.: Auranofin in the treatment of juvenile rheumatoid arthritis. J. Pediatr., 102:138–141, 1983.

55. Abruzzo, J.L.: Auranofin: A new drug for rheumatoid arthritis. Ann. Intern. Med., 105:274–276, 1986.

56. Cann, H.M., and Verhulst, H.L.: Fatal acute chloroquine poisoning in children. Pediatrics, 27:95–102, 1961.

57. Ansell, B.M., and Hall, M.A.: Penicillamine in juvenile chronic polyarthritis. Arthritis Rheum., 20(Suppl. 2):536, 1977.

58. Brewer, E.J., et al.: Penicillamine and hydroxychloroquine in the treatment of severe juvenile rheumatoid arthritis. N. Engl. J. Med., 314:1270–1276, 1986.

59. Cassidy, J.T.: Treatment of children with juvenile rheumatoid arthritis. Editorial. N. Engl. J. Med., 314:1312–1314, 1986.

60. Kelly, V.C.: Rheumatoid disease in childhood. Pediatr. Clin. North Am., 7:435–456, 1960.

61. Schlesinger, B.E., et al.: Observations on the clinical course and treatment of one hundred cases of Still's disease. Arch. Dis. Child., 36:65–76, 1961.

62. Schaller, J.G.: Corticosteroid therapy in childhood. Arthritis Rheum., 20(Suppl 2):537–543, 1977.

63. Ansell, B.M., and Bywater, E.G.L.: Alternate-day corticosteroid therapy in juvenile chronic polyarthritis. J. Rheumatol., 1:176–186, 1974.

64. Miller, J.J.: Prolonged use of large intravenous steroid pulses in rheumatic diseases of children. Pediatrics, 65:989–994, 1980.

65. Zutshi, D.W., Friedman, M., and Ansell, B.M.: Corticotrophin therapy in juvenile chronic polyarthritis (Still's disease) and effect on growth. Arch. Dis. Child., 46:584–593, 1971.

66. Mainland, D., et al.: A controlled trial of cyclophosphamide in rheumatoid arthritis. Cooperating Clinics Committee of the American Rheumatism Association. N. Engl. J. Med., 283:883–889, 1970.

67. Hollister, J.R.: Immunosuppressant therapy of juvenile rheumatoid arthritis. Arthritis Rheum., 20(Suppl. 2):544–547, 1977.

68. Pediatric Collaborative Study Group, "Methotrexate in Severe Juvenile Rheumatoid Arthritis." Study in progress.

69. Reimer, R.R., et al.: Acute leukemia after alkylating-agent therapy of ovarian cancer. N. Engl. J. Med., 297:177–181, 1977.

70. Sieber, S.M., and Adamson, R.H.: Toxicity of antineoplastic agents in man: Chromosomal aberrations, antifertility effects, congenital malformations, and carcinogenic potential. Adv. Cancer Res., 22:57–155, 1975.

71. Williams, H.J., et al.: Comparison of low-dose oral pulse methotrexate and placebo in the treatment of rheumatoid arthritis. A controlled clinical trial. Arthritis Rheum., 28:721–730, 1985.

72. Willkens, R.F.: Reappraisal of the use of methotrexate in rheumatic disease. Am. J. Med., 75:19–25, 1983.

73. Truckenbrodt, H., and Hafner, R.: Methotrexate therapy in juvenile rheumatoid arthritis: A retrospective study. Arthritis Rheum., 29:801–807, 1986.

74. Schnitzer, T.J., and Ansell, B.M.: Amyloidosis in juvenile chronic polyarthritis. Arthritis Rheum., 20(Suppl. 2):245–252, 1977.

75. Donovan, W.H.: Physical measures in the treatment of juvenile rheumatoid arthritis. Arthritis Rheum., 20(Suppl. 2):553–557, 1977.

76. Eyring, E.J., Longert, A., and Bass, J.C.: Synovectomy in juvenile rheumatoid arthritis. J. Bone Joint Surg., 53A:638–651, 1971.

77. Granberry, G.M.: Synovectomy in juvenile rheumatoid arthritis. Arthritis Rheum., 20(Suppl. 2):561–564, 1977.

78. Arden, G.P., and Ansell, B.M.: Surgical Management of Juvenile Chronic Polyarthritis. London, Academic Press, 1978.

79. Granberry, G.M.: Soft tissue release in children with juvenile rheumatoid arthritis. Arthritis Rheum., 20(Suppl. 2):565–566, 1977.

80. Arden, G.P., Taylor, A.R., and Ansell, B.M.: Total hip replacement using the McKee-Farrar prosthesis in rheumatoid arthritis, Still's disease, and ankylosing spondylitis. Ann. Rheum. Dis., 29:1–5, 1970.

81. Colvile, J., and Raunio, P.: Total hip replacement in juvenile rheumatoid arthritis. Analysis of fifty-nine hips. Acta Orthop. Scand., 50:197–203, 1979.

82. Singsen, B.H., et al.: Total hip replacement in children with arthritis. Arthritis Rheum., 21:401–406, 1978.

83. Sledge, C.B.: Joint replacement surgery in juvenile rheumatoid arthritis. Arthritis Rheum., 20(Suppl. 2):567–572, 1977.

84. Ruddlesdin, C., Ansell, B.M., Arden, G.P., and Swann, M.: Total hip replacement in children with juvenile chronic arthritis. J. Bone Joint Surg., 68B:218–222, 1986.

59

ANKYLOSING SPONDYLITIS

GENE V. BALL

TERMINOLOGY AND DIAGNOSIS

Ankylosing spondylitis (AS) is defined as the formation of a stiff joint by consolidation of the articulating surfaces and inflammation of the vertebral column. Despite its name, the characteristic lesion in AS is sacroiliitis. Relative to the other rheumatic diseases, diagnosis of AS is simple, yet its definition is unsettled. Some Scandinavians object to the reductionist focus on the sacroiliac joints and the spinal column, preferring the eponymic "Bechterew's syndrome," or the expansive "hereditary multifocal relapsing inflammation"[1] to emphasize the relationships among those disorders with sacroiliitis at their core, which are most often termed spondarthritides or spondyloarthropathies.[2] As an example supporting the concept of hereditary multifocal relapsing inflammation, Moller and Berg[1] have cited the relationship among acute anterior uveitis, AS, and the HLA-B27 antigen. Of their patients with acute anterior uveitis, 67% were HLA-B27 positive. Eighty-two percent were men, 50% of whom had AS. The HLA-B27–negative patients with acute anterior uveitis had no evidence of arthropathy. Moller and Berg argue that "seronegative arthropathy" incorporates only arthritic components of the syndrome, while their term encompasses the genetic factors and disease manifestations including acute anterior uveitis, cardiac conduction disturbance, aortic insufficiency, Reiter's syndrome, psoriasis, psoriatic arthropathy, enteroarthropathy, and inflammatory bowel disease.[1]

The name given to this condition has changed frequently during the 300 years since Connor's description of a skeleton with abnormalities suggestive of AS.[3] As used here, the term AS refers to idiopathic, symptomatic bilateral sacroiliitis, with or without spondylitis or uveitis, and excludes sacroiliitis that is associated with other conditions such as inflammatory bowel disease.

Connor's description[3] may portray one of the oldest known examples of a human skeleton disfigured by AS. In contrast to rheumatoid arthritis (RA), AS has been traditionally labeled an ancient disease. This view was challenged as a result of a recent examination of 560 intact skeletons and several thousand disarticulated vertebrae, of which the most ancient was of an Egyptian mummy.[4] Osteophytes were numerous, and blocks of spinal fusion were noted in 15 skeletons. Thirteen of these had features of ankylosing hyperostosis (Forrestier's disease), or diffuse idiopathic skeletal hyperostosis (DISH).[5,6] The other two were thought to most likely represent psoriatic spondylitis or Reiter's disease (the distinction between these and AS is often tenuous). A review of the relevant literature led to the conclusion that many paleopathologic specimens previously reported as AS were examples of DISH or other spondyloarthropathies.[4] Thus, AS may be a disease of "civilization".[3] The etiologic implications of relative newness, if any, are unclear.

The frequent delay of years between onset of symptoms and definitive diagnosis attests to the difficulty of establishing a diagnosis of AS and of differentiating inflammatory and noninflammatory causes of low-back pain, even though criteria for diagnosis have been promulgated, modified, and criticized.[7-9] Mild or early AS may defy detection because of the lack of sensitive and specific tests. Low-back pain of insidious onset associated with morning stiffness, improving with exercise, and persisting >3 months in a patient under 40 years old is said to denote sacroiliitis,[10] but this notion has not been tested in an open population. In an epidemiologic survey of the signs and symptoms of AS conducted in Norway, a random sample of 806 subjects was drawn from among 2908 respondents who complained of pain or stiffness of the back.[11] Out of 449 persons examined, 22 males and 5 females were found to have definite AS using New York criteria (which emphasize radiographic sacroiliitis) (Table 59–1). The symptom best differentiating AS from "non-AS" was back pain that forced the AS patient out of bed at night. Pain not relieved by

lying down was next best in sensitivity and specificity, followed by pain enduring longer than 3 months. Tenderness elicited by pressing over the sacroiliac joints was of low sensitivity and specificity. The complaint of back pain not relieved by lying but improved by exercise was highly sensitive but not very specific. Flattening of the lumbar curve, decreased Schober's index, and reduced chest expansion were not of great diagnostic significance. However, the triad of (1) reduced lateral mobility of the lumbar spine; (2) a total spinal flexion <40°; and (3) a reduced total spinal extension ≤20° increased the likelihood of AS 14-fold.[11]

In another study, 70 patients with the diagnosis of AS based on clinical symptoms and radiographic changes in the sacroiliac joints were compared to 32 patients with lumbar disc disease. Findings supporting the diagnosis of AS were low-back morning stiffness, swelling of knee joints, girdle chest pains, chest expansion <5 cm, HLA-B27 positivity, raised erythrocyte sedimentation rate, and a positive Mennell's sign (pain in the area of the sacroiliac joint on hyperextension of the thigh). Conversely, recurrent sciatic pain, limitation of all spinal movements, and a positive *Lasegue's sign* (straight leg raising) were more likely to denote lumbar disc disease.[12] Limited chest expansion is found in patients with advanced radiographic changes of sacroiliitis, and limitation of motion in the lumbar spine increases significantly in patients with increasing duration of disease. The modified New York criteria were more sensitive than the New York or Rome criteria in the diagnosis of definite AS, by a ratio of 124:115:110.[13]

The need for diagnostic criteria beyond symptomatic, radiographically verifiable, sacroiliitis has been questioned.[14] But sacroiliitis is a heterogeneous condition (Table 59–2), and in the general population, the majority of persons with this finding may be HLA-B27 negative; furthermore, the full clinical array of AS

Table 59–1.   Criteria for Diagnosing Ankylosing Spondylitis

Rome, 1961

Clinical Criteria
1. Low back pain and stiffness for more than 3 months, which is not relieved by rest
2. Pain and stiffness in the thoracic region
3. Limited motion in the lumbar spine
4. Limited chest expansion
5. History or evidence of iritis or its sequelae

Radiologic Criterion
6. Roentgenogram showing bilateral sacroiliac changes characteristic of ankylosing spondylitis (this would exclude bilateral osteoarthritis of the sacroiliac joints)

New York, 1966

Diagnosis
1. Limitation of motion of the lumbar spine in all three planes—anterior flexion, lateral flexion, and extension
2. Pain at the dorsolumbar junction or in the lumbar spine
3. Limitation of chest expansion to 1 inch (2.5 cm) or less measured at the level of the fourth intercostal space

Grading of Radiographs
   Normal 0, suspicious 1, minimal sacroiliitis 2, moderate sacroiliitis 3, ankylosis 4

Definite AS
1. Grade 3–4 bilateral sacroiliitis with at least one clinical criterion
2. Grade 3–4 unilateral or grade 2 bilateral sacroiliitis with clinical criterion 1 or with both clinical criteria 2 and 3

Probable AS
Grade 3–4 bilateral sacroiliitis with no clinical criteria

Modified New York Criteria

1. Low back pain of at least 3 months' duration improved by exercise and not relieved by rest
2. Limitation of lumbar spine in sagittal and frontal planes
3. Chest expansion decreased relative to normal values for age and sex
4. Bilateral sacroiliitis, grade 2–4
5. Unilateral sacroiliitis, grade 3–4
Definite AS if unilateral grade 3 or 4 or bilateral grade 2–4 sacroiliitis and any clinical criteria

---

Table 59–2.   Causes of Radiographic Sacroiliac Abnormalities[14a]

Osteoarthritis
Gout
Spondyloarthropathies
Hyperparathyroidism
Tuberculosis
Brucellosis
Pyogenic infections
Neoplastic metastases
Familial Mediterranean fever
Paraplegia
Relapsing polychondritis
Whipple's disease
Intestinal bypass operation
Paget's disease
Tuberous sclerosis

is uncommon in HLA-B27–negative individuals (see Chapter 29). Moreover, some relatives of HLA-B27–positive AS patients are also HLA-B27–positive and have radiographic sacroiliitis but remain asymptomatic. Studies of families of HLA-B27–positive AS probands have supported the view that clinical AS may occur in the absence of radiographic abnormalities of the spine or pelvis.[15]

The significance of these studies is uncertain, particularly because of their reliance on symptoms prejudged to be typical of AS, as evidence of chronic inflammatory back pain.[15] Radiographic changes in the lumbar spine typical of AS have been observed in six patients without radiographic sacroiliitis, although no radiographs were published.[16]

Radiographic sacroiliitis is the most objective indicator of AS, although it is arguably insufficient.[17] Changes are not always present early in the course of the disease, and oblique views of the sacroiliac joints do not significantly increase diagnostic accuracy. The interpretation of oblique views may be even more subjective than that of plain radiographs. Tomography improves the definition of the joint, but greatly increases radiation exposure. Quantitative sacroiliac scintigraphy is too nonspecific to be used for effective diagnosis. Computed tomography (CT) detects early joint abnormalities not visible on plain radiographs, but its use should be reserved for patients whose diagnoses are in doubt[18] (Fig. 59–1) (see also Chapter 8).

Laboratory testing is useful in excluding other diagnoses, as in patients whose AS begins with peripheral arthritis. An elevated erythrocyte sedimentation rate occurs in about 75% of patients with active disease.[19] Rheumatoid factors (RFs) and antinuclear antibodies (ANAs) are not found in AS, and serum complement levels are not decreased. As expected, circulating immune complexes have been detected with variable frequency. For example, positive polyethylene glycol precipitation tests were obtained in 52% of sera from patients with active disease and in 20% of those whose disease was inactive.[20]

PREVALENCE AND PATHOGENESIS

Estimates of the prevalence of AS have varied widely, depending in part on diagnostic criteria used and the importance attached to HLA-B27 positivity. Early epidemiologic studies supporting a prevalence between 0.02 and 0.22% in whites appear sound, however[21,22] (see also Chapter 29). Although 90% of patients with definite AS are HLA-B27 positive, the risk of the development of AS in individuals with this

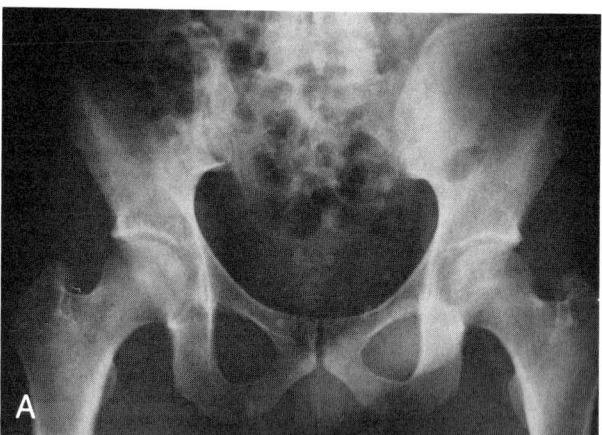
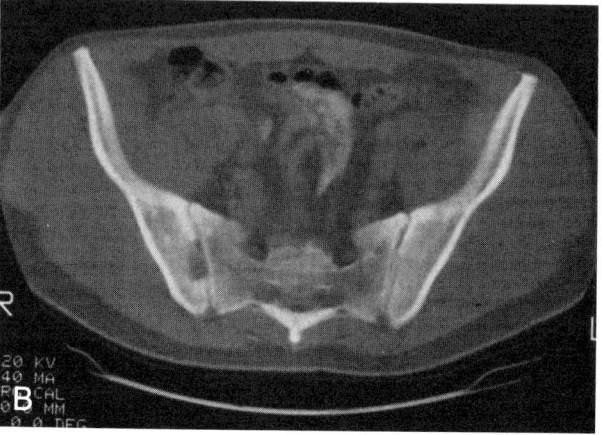

FIG. 59–1. Metastasis to the sacroiliac joint from a hypernephroma in a 32-year-old man with low back pain, limited back mobility, and tenderness over the area of the right sacroiliac joint. *A,* The iliac lesion is not seen on pelvic radiograph, *B,* but is clearly visible in the computed tomogram.

antigen is probably less than 2%. First-degree relatives of HLA-B27–positive AS patients, however, have a risk of near 20%, suggesting a major role for other factors, either genetic or environmental.[23] Genetic heterogeneity (still of unknown significance in AS) is evident in patients with the arthritis of psoriasis or inflammatory bowel disease. The patients with sacroiliitis are generally HLA-B27 positive, whereas those with peripheral arthritis without sacroiliitis are generally HLA-B27 negative, suggesting a different pathogenesis for the sacroiliitis and peripheral arthritis complicating these disorders (see also Chapters 29, 61, and 62).

The HLA-B27 antigen has stimulated research in the spondyloarthropathies. The frequent observation that HLA-B27–positive arthritis is triggered by an infection suggests an interaction between the HLA-B27 antigen and an environmental agent. A provocative experimental model has united the HLA system and enteric Klebsiella sp. in the pathogenesis of AS, beginning with reports (and denials) of increased fecal Klebsiella sp. carriage in patients with active AS.[24,25] Geczy and colleagues[26] have shown that sera raised against isolates of Klebsiella (K43) lyse the lymphocytes of HLA-B27–positive patients with AS, but not lymphocytes obtained from either HLA-B27–negative patients or HLA-B27–positive persons without AS. Culture filtrates of K43 reportedly contain a factor, apparently a plasmid, capable of specifically modifying the lymphocytes of HLA-B27–positive persons without AS to render them sensitive to anti-Klebsiella sp. antisera. Lymphocytes modified by the K43 culture filtrates become antigenically similar to lymphocytes from HLA-B27–positive and AS–positive persons. This phenomenon is restricted to certain Klebsiella strains; for example, Escherichia coli and other strains of Klebsiella do not have these properties.[27]

Cytotoxic T-lymphocytes induced by stimulating the peripheral blood mononuclear cells (PBMCs) of an HLA-B27–positive, normal individual with PBMC of an HLA identical sibling with AS, specifically lysed HLA-B27–positive and AS–positive PBMCs but not HLA-B27–positive or HLA-B27–negative and AS–negative PBMCs, or HLA-B27–negative, AS–positive PBMCs. Cytotoxic T-lymphocytes of similar specificity could also be raised by in vitro immunization of HLA-B27–positive and AS–negative cells with autologous cells modified by Klebsiella sp. culture filtrate antigens. These observations imply that cytotoxic T-lymphocytes that recognize certain bacterial antigens in association with HLA-B27 expressed by the lymphocytes of AS patients can be induced. It was postulated that such cytotoxic cells destroy target tissues bearing this antigenic complex, thereby inducing inflammation.[28] This work links HLA-B27 with the pathogenesis of AS; unfortunately, some of it has not been reproducible by others,[29] although Geczy and his colleagues[30] were able to distinguish between coded PBMC samples from normal individuals and those from AS patients.

Other indirect ways of looking at "parainfectious" etiologies of AS have been pursued. For example, the reactivity of lymphocytes from patients with AS to mitogens derived from Mycoplasma arthritidis was much greater than that of controls or of HLA-B27–positive lymphocytes from patients with Reiter's syndrome.[31] The latter observation suggests that the reactivity was not associated with the HLA-B27 per se.

The importance of the interaction of other genes with B27 in increasing susceptibility to AS is being explored. Using full length HLA-B7 cDNA probes,

different laboratories have conducted DNA restriction fragment length polymorphism (RFLP) analysis of Class I MHC genes in AS patients and controls. Cohen and colleagues found a 9.6 kb *Pvu* II fragment more often in B27+ AS+ patients than in B27− controls.[32] McDaniel and others have found a 9.2 kb *Pvu* II fragment in 73% of B27+ AS+ patients and in 27% of healthy controls. This fragment was present in 82% of AS patients with peripheral joint disease compared with 42% of those with axial disease alone. Family data show that the 9.2 kb RFLP represents a disease susceptibility marker distinct from B27. The investigators calculated a relative risk of 297 for AS in B27+ individuals with this fragment, much higher than the relative risk of 119 conferred by B27 alone.[33]

These data provide a framework toward understanding the pathogenesis of arthritis, but the reasons for the associated iritis or cardiovascular inflammation, the predilection for the sacroiliac joint and spine, and the greater prevalence in males remain obscure.

PATHOLOGIC AND RADIOGRAPHIC CHANGES

Because of the insidious early nature of AS, analyses of inchoate lesions are sparse and provide few clues to its pathogenesis. The disease process termed *enthesopathy* is thought to account for the characteristic bone lesions.[34] The enthesis is the junction of ligament and bone and the site of nongranulomatous inflammation, typically leading to local fiber disruption. Reactive bone forms a new enthesis with the eroded end of the ligament. This process occurs at the insertions of the sacrotuberous and sacrospinous ligaments, along the inferior rami of the ischia and pubis, along the superior iliac crests, the greater trochanters, and heels, producing ossified ligaments and tendons and radiographic "whiskering" (Fig. 59–2). This also occurs in the spine at the outer fibers of the annulus resulting in *syndesmophyte* formation. Ossification and ankylosis of the facet joint capsule occur at the capsular attachment of these joints and precede enchondral ossification of the residual cartilage and disc (Fig. 59–3). A similar process occurs in the sacroiliacs, where inflammation involves both the sacral and iliac cartilage in the inferior two thirds of the joint and the acartilaginous, ligamentous portion of the superior part. The cartilage on the iliac side of the joint is thinner, and bony *erosions* on that side are prominent.[35] Such erosions, filled with inflammatory tissue, create a *widened joint space* on radiographs. Bone adjacent to the inflamed areas undergoes osteoblastosis, accounting for the periarticular sclerosis that is an-

FIG. 59–2. Anteroposterior film of pelvis showing obliteration of sacroiliac joints and decrease in joint space in the hips with reactive sclerosis in the acetabulum, new bone formation, and pelvic "whiskering."

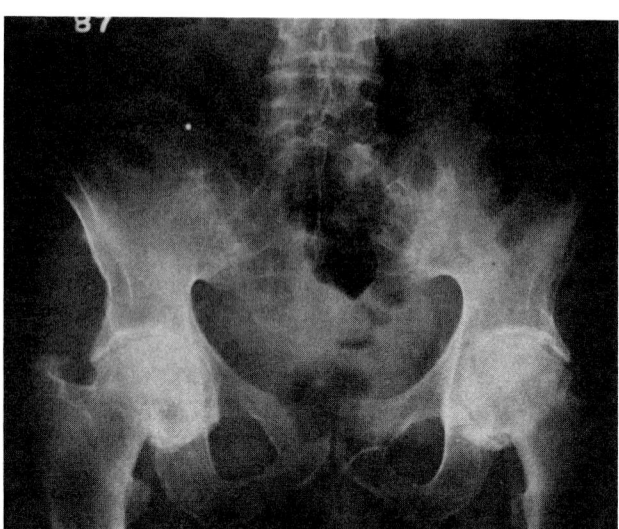

FIG. 59–3. Lateral cervical spine film showing intervertebral bony bridging, "squaring" of vertebrae and obliteration of zygapophyseal joints.

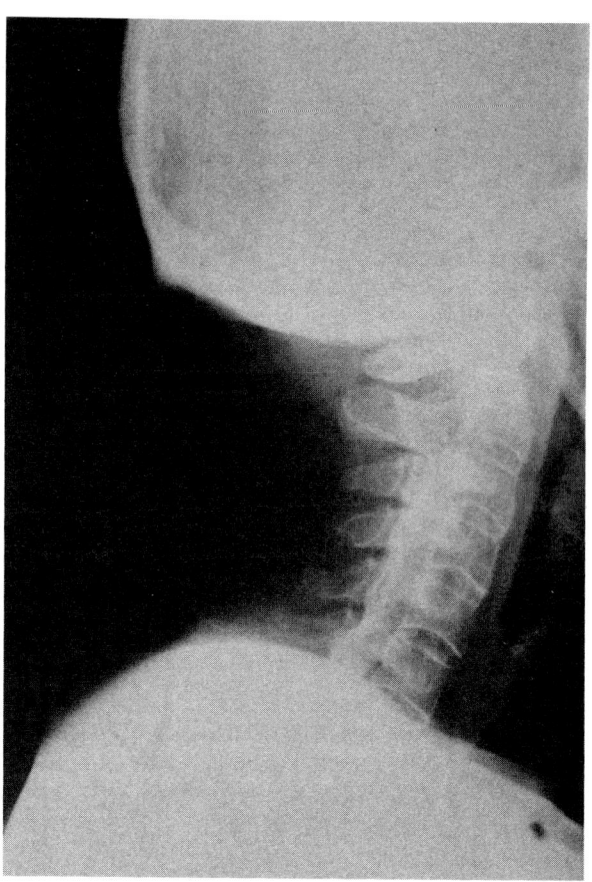

other prominent radiographic feature (Table 59–3). Replacement of inflamed cartilage by bone eventually results in *ankylosis* of the joint. It is thought that mobility inhibits the process of ankylosis, as evidenced by its rarity in the most mobile area of the cervical spine, namely, the atlantoaxial joint.[36] Synovitis occurs in peripheral joints in AS, and its pathologic features resemble those of RA and other forms of inflammatory arthritis.

SYMPTOMS

It is in the early stages of AS, when attention may be diverted from the back by complaints of aching or sharp pains in the heels, pelvis, buttocks, hips, and shoulders, and when the pain may come and go in a matter of a day or two, that an immunogenetic or other diagnostic indicator of AS is most needed. As already discussed, physical signs of disease may or may not be detectable, depending on its stage. Pain and stiffness eventually become more constant, and patients may then begin to experience early morning wakening and inability to lie in bed, and the back and spine demand more attention. The back may remain silent or at least obscured by other problems until years after the disease onset, however. In one study[37] of 100 consecutive clinic patients whose mean age was 23 years, it was estimated that 6 years had elapsed from the onset of symptoms of AS until the correct diagnosis was made. Fully 38 patients first developed

pain in areas other than the spine. In 17 it was hips; 12, knees; 4, shoulders; 2, heels; 1, hand; 1, elbow; and 1, ankle. Back symptoms occurred on the average 3 years after the onset of pain in these 38 patients.[37] Sciatic pain may be the first symptom of AS. In general the sciatica of AS is neurologically silent. The question of AS versus lumbar disc disease as a cause of sciatic pain can now be settled readily with CT myelograms or magnetic resonance imaging (MRI). (See Chapters 8 and 6.)

CHILDHOOD AS

Although clinical AS begins most often around age 20, 7% of children attending a clinic for chronic arthritis were said to have juvenile AS.[38] Certain clinical features suggest juvenile AS rather than juvenile RA; that is, late onset in childhood, male sex, relative sparing of hands and wrists, infrequent cervical spine involvement, remittent oligoarthritis, absence of RFs

Table 59–3. Radiographic Signs in Ankylosing Spondylitis[14a]

1. Pelvis
   Sacroiliac joints: Usually bilateral except early
   Blurring; adjacent bone sclerosis; widened appearance of joint space; bony irregularity; partial or complete ankylosis
   Other features: irregularity and sclerosis of symphysis pubis; whiskering and fraying of iliac crests, ischial tuberosities and trochanters
2. Thoracolumbar spine
   Erosions, sclerosis and loss of bone at anterior borders of vertebral bodies (squared off appearance)
   Bony proliferation with bridging of vertebrae beginning within outermost fibers of annulus fibrosus: syndesmophytes
   Exaggeration of syndesmophytes: bamboo spine
   Disc space narrowing, calcification of discs, and kyphosis late
   "Trolley-track" sign: Ossification of the intersupraspinous ligaments plus bilateral ankylosis of apophyseal joints, producing three vertical lines seen on frontal radiographs
3. Cervical spine
   Joint space narrowing, ankylosing multiple apophyseal joints and bony sclerosis; anterior syndesmophytes; spinous process erosions
4. Erosions metacarpal, metatarsal and humeral heads; bony ankylosis hip, wrist, and midfoot

and ANAs and HLA-B27 positivity (in about 90%). In an arthritis clinic setting, unequivocal radiographic signs of sacroiliac arthritis establish the diagnosis; however, there may be some lag in the appearance of the radiographic abnormalities vis-à-vis the clinical symptoms. Radiographs of these joints are particularly difficult to read in children, as subchondral joint margins may normally be indistinct. Blurred margins in the presence of reactive sclerosis suggest inflammatory disease.

SPINAL DISEASE

The spine, heart, aorta, and eye may be involved in AS and will be discussed in greater detail. Pain and limitation of motion in the spine have been referred to earlier. Patients with long-standing AS often lose their back pain as fusion supervenes. One important cause for new pain in the spine unrelated to trauma is the discovertebral destructive lesion, also called the *Andersson lesion* or *spondylodiscitis*.[39] Pain usually appears suddenly in an isolated spinal segment. It is sharp and intensified by exercise. Routine radiography at this time may show no evidence of these lesions. Radionuclide scans, generally featureless in longstanding AS, demonstrate an isolated level of abnormal uptake across the entire width of the vertebral column, at a level appropriate for the pain. Sterile or septic discitis, pseudarthrosis, and traumatic pseudarthrosis produce an identical picture and must be differentiated. Tomography will also reveal segmental

spinal instability at the site indicated by scintigraphy. Instability, perhaps produced by a stress fracture or isolated nonfusion of the apophyseal joints, leads to the destructive changes. Prompt, prolonged, immobilization sometimes results in healing.[40]

An ankylosed spine is vulnerable to injury from even trivial trauma. Hunter and Dubo[41] reported their experience with 20 AS patients who had 22 fractures (two patients experienced second cervical fractures).[41] Of 15 fractures in the group of 14 patients in whom diagnosis was made and management instituted immediately 9 were due to minor falls to the floor, and 2 were caused by falls down stairs. Of the 15, 14 were in the cervical region; the other involved the thoracic region. Six of the fractures caused complete cord lesions, and four produced incomplete lesions of the acute cervical central cord syndrome type. Long-term surveillance was possible in 9 of the 14 patients. Of the 8 patients with cervical fractures, 2 were treated with traction in a position of cervical flexion for 12 and 16 weeks, 1 was treated with traction for 6 weeks followed by immobilization in a cervical collar for 6 weeks, and the remaining 5 patients were treated with bed rest and a cervical collar for a mean of 12.5 weeks. Clinical and radiographic union occurred at a mean of 13 weeks, and none of the patients developed a pseudarthrosis. There was no neurologic recovery in the 3 patients with immediate, complete, spinal cord injury. The 3 patients with incomplete lesions of the acute cervical central cord syndrome type regained motor power in the lower limbs and control of bowel and bladder function. Two of the patients with complete spinal cord lesions eventually died, one from amyloidosis and the other from pulmonary embolism. The fractures of all 7 patients in whom there was a mean delay of 47 weeks from the time of fracture to diagnosis were judged to be unstable and managed variably.

Spinal fracture should be considered in any AS patient who experiences trauma. Radiographs may fail to show the fracture; tomography may be of some use, and radionuclide bone scans are particularly useful in patients with chronic pseudarthrosis. It should be kept in mind that an ankylosed spine will fracture like a long bone and is grossly unstable because of the loss of ligamentous support. Some believe that nonoperative treatment is often best, with emphasis on careful immobilization. Hunter and Dubo,[41] combining their experience with that of others, recommend laminectomy for a patient with progression of a neurologic lesion, and spinal fusion for fractures that cannot be stabilized otherwise. Regardless of management, cardiorespiratory instability and respiratory infection are major complications of spinal fractures. Spinal epidural hematomas occurred in 9 of 54 AS patients with spinal fractures, and in one AS patient who had minimal trauma and no fracture. Progressive neurologic symptoms were noted, and a myelogram showed a block at T2-3. CT and MRI were not possible because of kyphosis, which prevented entry into the gantrys of the scanners. A complete prompt evaluation is mandatory in any patient with AS and progressive neurologic symptoms.[42] Cauda equina syndrome and vertebrobasilar insufficiency have been ascribed to AS.[43,44]

THE LUNG

Pulmonary function tests on 32 patients with AS showed a reduction of total lung capacity and vital capacity to 92% and 88% of normal, respectively; normal flow values, normal functional residual capacity, and normal residual volume supported a restrictive limitation of the lung volumes, most likely due to reduced motility of the thoracic cage.[45] Compliance and diffusion capacities were normal. Speculation has centered on reduced lung volumes and a "possible" interstitial process as factors leading to the upper lobe fibrosis that is seen infrequently in AS.[45] Atypical fibrosis and cavitation occur in a few patients and simulate tuberculosis, although infection with Aspergillus sp. occurs much more commonly than with mycobacteria.[46]

HEART AND AORTA

Bulkley and Roberts[47] correlated the clinical findings with necropsy details of eight patients said to have AS (one had Reiter's syndrome). All eight were men, aged 34 to 55 years, and all had peripheral arthritis, aortic regurgitation, and congestive failure. Aortic regurgitation occurred in three before radiographic evidence of AS. The ascending aortas were mildly dilated and thickened as a result of adventitial scarring and intimal proliferation. Fibrous thickening of the aortic wall behind the unfused commissurae resulted in sagging of the cusps. Scar tissue in the root of the aorta extended below the base of the aortic valve to produce a subaortic fibrous ridge, involving the base of the anterior mitral leaflet. Extension of such scar tissue into the ventricular septum correlated with conduction disturbances. Prolonged PR intervals had been noted in four patients, and complete left bundle branch block, complete right bundle branch block, and complete heart block were each noted in one patient. Four patients died within 2 months, and

the fifth died 12 months later despite aortic valve replacement. Survival after aortic valve replacement in such patients is now improved. Differences between syphilitic heart disease and that associated with AS were noted.[47]

An association of heart block with HLA-B27 positivity has been claimed: of one group of 12 patients with spontaneous complete heart block, 8 had AS, and the remainder were HLA-B27 positive but had no clinical evidence of AS.[48] Three patients had sinus node malfunction, and six had fascicular or bundle branch block. In all 12 of these patients intermittent atrioventricular nodal block occurred. Ten were treated with a permanent pacemaker.

The subaortic "bump" of AS can be detected in vivo noninvasively using dimensional echocardiography. A prevalence of 31% was found in 25 patients with AS and 9 with Reiter's syndrome, which compares favorably to the autopsy finding of aortitis in 20 to 30% of patients *without* aortic insufficiency.[49] Long-term observation of these patients and improving technology may clarify these relationships. Aortic regurgitation has occurred in several patients less than 20 years of age.[50] AS rarely causes widespread arteritis.[51]

EYE

The uveitis of AS occurs acutely. Early episodes tend to be unilateral, but it often becomes bilateral eventually. Macular edema may reduce vision seriously during active iridocyclitis. As inflammation becomes chronic, accumulation of inflammatory debris within the vitreous may further decrease vision. Acute anterior uveitis is often associated with HLA-B27 whether or not AS is present.[52–54]

There are several reports of mesangioproliferative glomerulonephritis and IgA nephropathy in AS as well as amyloid nephropathy,[55,56] and amyloidosis is a significant cause of death.

DISEASE COURSE

The course of AS has been followed in 150 war veterans, 51 of whom were re-evaluated after a mean disease duration of 38 years. Forty-seven of the 51 were functioning well although the disease had progressed in almost one half (21) to the point of severe restriction of spinal motion. Of these 21 with severe motion restriction, 12 had early peripheral joint involvement, and 9 had iritis. Seventy-four percent of the patients with only mild loss of spinal motion after

10 years did not progress. Hips that were normal after 10 years of disease did not become affected subsequently. Thus, a predictable pattern of disease emerged within the first 10 years. Eight of 61 deaths were thought to be related to AS: two from cervical subluxation; 3 from aortic regurgitation, 2 from respiratory failure, and 1 from amyloid nephropathy. Six of these eight had peripheral joint inflammation at the onset,[57] suggesting that this feature indicates a relatively bad prognosis.

Seventy-six patients in this study were evaluated with regard to the long-term effects of radiation therapy. The survival rate in the 62 not treated with radiation was normal; but after 27 years in the men given radiotherapy, the survival rate was only 55% versus the expected 79%, a highly significant difference. Almost half died of cardiovasular causes, and three died of acute leukemia.[58] A fivefold excess of deaths from leukemia and a 62% excess of deaths from other cancers were found in patients given a single course of radiotherapy for AS in the United Kingdom.[59] In contrast, a Finnish study into the causes of death of 79 patients with AS found only one lymphoma and one chronic lymphocytic leukemia despite the radiotherapy given to almost all.[60] As expected, the single largest cause of death was cardiovascular disease (35%); the immediate cause of death in 18% was uremia secondary to amyloidosis, which contributed to the death of another 3.8% of patients.[60]

TREATMENT

Treatment consists of medications for pain relief and exercises to maintain mobility and to counteract the excessive pull of the flexor muscles. Salicylates have been found deficient in comparison with indomethacin, the nonsteroidal anti-inflammatory drug (NSAID) most used in this condition.[61] Phenylbutazone and indomethacin are about equally effective, but the latter has less serious side effects. The dose should be as low as possible. As little as 25 mg daily is sufficient in some cases, but others may require as much as 200 mg daily, a level at which side effects such as gastritis and headache appear more frequently. The 75-mg sustained-release form of indomethacin is useful taken twice daily, as the half-life of this drug is relatively short (see Chapter 32). Phenylbutazone, a long-acting NSAID, may prove useful in a patient whose disease does not respond to any of the other NSAIDs tried seriatim. If used, a monthly complete blood count is needed to detect early signs of marrow failure. This is nearly always heralded by a rash, and the patient should be instructed to stop the drug if a rash occurs. An occasional patient with severe peripheral joint arthritis may respond to a remittive agent usually reserved for RA. Controlled trials of sulphasalazine have shown its effectiveness.[62,63]

Patients often benefit from formal instruction in proper posture and exercises emphasizing mobility and ways to strengthen the spinal extensors. Proper attention to physical activities and habits may retard or prevent serious deformities. *Each patient should be committed to an exercise program under the supervision of a skilled therapist.*

Severe spinal deformities have been corrected with osteotomy of the spine,[64] although the safe induction of anesthesia can be difficult in patients with severe ankylosis.[65] Placement of a spinal or epidural needle is difficult, and in as many as 40% of patients, mouth opening is limited. Total joint replacement of the hip may be complicated by heterotopic bone formation.[66]

Of 100 patients with AS of 20 years' duration, 22% were considered disabled for daily activities. Peripheral joint involvement was a significant adverse factor. Driving was often difficult because of loss of spinal mobility, and 50% experienced a decrease of vision. Additional rearview mirrors sometimes helped with this problem.[67]

REFERENCES

1. Moller, P., and Berg, K.: Seronegative arthropathy and associated diseases—a multigenic syndrome? Br. J. Rheumatol., 22(Suppl. 2):5–11, 1983.
2. Moll, J.M.H., Haslock, I., Macrae, I.F., and Wright, V.: Associations between ankylosing spondylitis, psoriatic arthritis, Reiter's disease, intestinal arthropathies, and Behçet's syndrome. Medicine, 53:343–364, 1974.
3. Bywaters, E.G.L.: Historical perspectives in the aetiology of ankylosing spondylitis. Br. J. Rheumatol., 22(Suppl. 2):1–4, 1983.
4. Rogers, J., Watt, I., and Dieppe, P.: Palaeopathology of spinal osteophytosis, vertebral ankylosis, ankylosing spondylitis, and vertebral hyperostosis. Ann. Rheum. Dis., 44:113–120, 1985.
5. Forestier, J., and Rotes-Querol, J.: Senile ankylosing hyperostosis of the spine. Ann. Rheum. Dis., 9:321–330, 1950.
6. Resnick, D., Shaul, S.R., and Robins, J.M.: Diffuse idiopathic skeletal hyperostosis (DISH): Forestier's disease with extraspinal manifestations. Radiology, 115:513, 1975.
7. Kellgren, J.H., Jeffrey, M.R., and Ball, J. (eds.): The Epidemiology of Chronic Rheumatism. Vol. 1. Oxford, Blackwell Scientific, 1963.
8. Bennett, P.H., and Wood, P.H.N. (eds.): Population studies of the rheumatic diseases. *In* Proceedings of the 3rd International Symposium, New York, 1966. International Congress Series No. 148. New York, Excerpta Medica.
9. Moll, J.M.H., and Wright, V.: New York clinical criteria for ankylosing spondylitis. A statistical evaluation. Ann. Rheum. Dis., 32:354–363, 1973.
10. Calin, A., Porta, J., Fries, J.F., and Schurman, D.J.: Clinical

history as a screening test for ankylosing spondylitis. JAMA, 237:2613–2614, 1977.

11. Gran, J.T.: An epidemiological survey of the signs and symptoms of ankylosing spondylitis. Clin. Rheum. Dis., 4:161–169, 1985.

12. Sadowska-Wroblewska, M., et al.: Clinical symptoms and signs useful in the early diagnosis of ankylosing spondylitis. Clin. Rheum., 2:37–43, 1983.

13. The, H.S.G., Steven, M.M., van der Linden, S.M., and Cats, A.: Evaluation of diagnostic criteria for ankylosing spondylitis: A comparison of the Rome, New York and Modified New York Criteria in patients with a positive clinical history screening test for ankylosing spondylitis. Br. J. Rheumatol., 24:242–249, 1985.

14. Calin, A.: Comment on van der Linden article. Arthritis Rheum., 27:1438, 1984.

14a. Resnick, D., and Niwayama, G.: Diagnosis of Bone and Joint Disorders: With Emphasis on Articular Abnormalities. Vol. 2. Philadelphia, W.B. Saunders, 1981.

15. Khan, M.A., et al.: Spondylitic disease without radiologic evidence of sacroiliitis in relatives of HLA-B27 positive ankylosing spondylitis patients. Arthritis Rheum., 28:40–43, 1985.

16. Gran, J.T., Husby, G., and Hordvik, M.: Spinal ankylosing spondylitis: A variant form of ankylosing spondylitis or a distinct disease entity? Ann. Rheum. Dis., 44:368–371, 1985.

17. van der Linden, S., Valkenburg, H.A., and Cats, A.: Evaluation of diagnositic criteria for ankylosing spondylitis. Arthritis Rheum., 27:361–368, 1984.

18. Fam, A.G., Rubenstein, J.D., Chin-Sang, H., and Leung, F.Y.K.: Computed tomography in the diagnosis of early ankylosing spondylitis. Arthritis Rheum., 28:930–937, 1985.

19. Dixon, J.S., Bird, H.A., and Wright, V.: A comparison of serum biochemistry in ankylosing spondylitis, seronegative and seropositive rheumatoid arthritis. Ann. Rheum. Dis., 40:404–408, 1981.

20. Deicher, H., et al.: Circulating immune complexes in ankylosing spondylitis. Br. J. Rheumatol., 22(Suppl. 2):122–127, 1983.

21. Lawrence, J.S.: The prevalence of arthritis. Br. J. Clin. Pract., 17:699–705, 1963.

22. Kellgren, J.H.: Heberden Oration, 1963. The epidemiology of rheumatic diseases. Ann. Rheum. Dis., 23:109–122, 1964.

23. van der Linden, S., Valkenburg, H., and Cats, A.: The risk of developing ankylosing spondylitis in HLA-B27 positive individuals: A family and population study. Br. J. Rheum., 22(Suppl. 2):18–19, 1983.

24. Warren, R.E., and Brewerton, D.A.: Faecal carriage of Klebsiella by patients with ankylosing spondylitis and rheumatoid arthritis. Ann. Rheum. Dis., 39:37–44, 1980.

25. Ebringer, R.W., Cawdell, D.R., Cowling, P., and Ebringer, A.: Sequential studies in ankylosing spondylitis. Association of *Klebsiella pneumoniae* with active disease. Ann. Rheum. Dis., 37:146–151, 1978.

26. Seager, K., et al.: Evidence for a specific B27-associated cell surface marker on lymphocytes of patients with ankylosing spondylitis. Nature, 277:68–70, 1979.

27. Geczy, A.F., Alexander, K., and Bashir, H.V.: A Factor(s) in *Klebsiella* filtrates specifically modifies an HLA-B27-associated cell-surface component. Nature, 283:782–784, 1980.

28. Geczy, A.F., McGuigan, L.E., Sullivan, J.S., and Edmonds, J.P.: Cytotoxic T lymphocytes against disease-associated determinant(s) in ankylosing spondylitis. J. Exp. Med., 164:932–937, 1986.

29. Kinsella, T.D., Lanteigne, C., Fritzler, M.J., and Lewkonia, R.M.: Absence of impaired lymphocyte transformation to *Kleb-*

30. van Rood, J.J., et al.: Blind confirmation of Geczy factor in ankylosing spondylitis. Lancet, 2:943–944, 1985.

31. Seitz, M., Gaber, B., Nicklas, W., and Kirchner, H.: Unusual reactivity of lymphocytes from patients with ankylosing spondylitis to mitogen derived from mycoplasma arthritides. Lancet, 2:1035–1036, 1984.

32. Cohen, D., et al.: Association of class I and class II MHC restriction fragment polymorphism with HLA-related diseases. *In* Histocompatibility Testing 1984: Report of the 9th International Histocompatibility Workshop and Conference, Held in Munich, West Germany, May 6–11, 1984 and Vienna, Austria, May 13–15, 1984. Edited by E.D. Albert, M.P. Baur, and W.R. Mayr. New York, Springer-Verlag, 1984.

33. McDaniel, D.O., et al.: Association of a 9.2 kb *Pvu* II MHC Class I restriction fragment length polymorphism with ankylosing spondylitis. Arthritis Rheum., 30:894–900, 1987.

34. Ball, J.: The Heberden Oration, 1970. Enthesopathy of rheumatoid and ankylosing spondylitis. Ann. Rheum. Dis., 30:213–223, 1971.

35. Bluestone, R.: Ankylosing spondylitis. *In* Arthritis and Allied Conditions: A Textbook of Rheumatology. 10th Ed. Edited by D.S. McCarty. Philadelphia, Lea & Febiger, 1985.

36. Ball, J.: The enthesopathy of ankylosing spondylitis. Br. J. Rheumatol., 22(Suppl. 2):25–28, 1983.

37. Maltz, B.A., Sussman, P., and Calabro, J.J.: Peripheral arthritis as an initial manifestation of ankylosing spondylitis. (Abstract.) Arthritis Rheum., 12:680–681, 1969.

38. Ladd, J.R., Cassidy, J.T., and Martel, W.: Juvenile ankylosing spondylitis. Arthritis Rheum., 14:579–590, 1971.

39. Dihlmann, W., and Delling, G.: Disco-vertebral destructive lesions (so-called Andersson lesions) associated with ankylosing spondylitis. Skeletal Radiol., 3:10–16, 1983.

40. Dunn, N., Preston, B., and Jones, K.L.: Unexplained acute backache in longstanding ankylosing spondylitis. Br. Med. J., 291:1632–1634, 1985.

41. Hunter, T., and Dubo, H.I.C.: Spinal fractures complicating ankylosing spondylitis. A long-term follow up study. Arthritis Rheum., 26:751–759, 1983.

42. Murray, G.C., and Persellin, R.H.: Cervical fracture complicating ankylosing spondylitis. A report of eight cases and review of the literature. Am. J. Med., 70:1033–1041, 1981.

43. Milde, E.-J., Aarli, J., and Larsen, J.L.: Cauda equina lesions in ankylosing spondylitis. Scand. J. Rheumatol., 6:118–122, 1977.

44. Young, A., et al.: Cauda equina syndrome complicating ankylosing spondylitis: Use of electromyography and computerized tomography in diagnosis. Ann. Rheum. Dis., 40:317–322, 1981.

45. Feltelius, N., Hedenstrom, H., Hillerdal, G., and Hallgren, R.: Pulmonary involvement in ankylosing spondylitis. Ann. Rheum. Dis., 45:736–740, 1986.

46. Hillerdal, G.: Ankylosing spondylitis lung disease—An underdiagnosed entity? Eur. J. Respir. Dis., 64:437–441, 1983.

47. Bulkley, B.H., and Roberts, W.C.: Ankylosing spondylitis and aortic regurgitation. Description of the characteristic cardiovascular lesion from study of eight necropsy patients. Circulation, 48:1014–1027, 1973.

48. Bergfeldt, L., Vallin, H., and Edhag, O.: Complete heart block in HLA B27 associated disease. Electrophysiological and clinical characteristics. Br. Heart J., 51:184–188, 1984.

49. LaBresh, K.A., Lally, E.V., Sharma, S.C., and Ho, G.: Two-dimensional echocardiographic detection of preclinical aortic

root abnormalities in rheumatoid variant diseases. Am. J. Med., *78*:908–912, 1985.

50. Pelkonen, P., et al.: Rapidly progressive aortic incompetence in juvenile ankylosing spondylitis: A case report. Arthritis Rheum., *27*:698–700, 1984.

51. Ball, G.V., and Hathaway, B.: Ankylosing spondylitis with widespread arteritis. Arthritis Rheum., *9*:737–745, 1966.

52. Belmont, J.B., and Michelson, J.B.: Vitrectomy in uveitis associated with ankylosing spondylitis. Am. J. Ophthalmol., *94*:300–304, 1982.

53. Scharf, J., et al.: Anterior uveitis in ankylosing spondylitis: A histocompatibility study. Ann. Ophthalmol., *11*:1061–1062, 1979.

54. Linssen, A., et al.: Possible ankylosing spondylitis in acute anterior uveitis. Br. J. Rheumatol., *22*(Suppl. 2):137–143, 1983.

55. Mittal, V.K., Malhotra, K.K., Bhuyan, U.N., and Malaviya, A.N.: Kidney involvement in seronegative spondarthritides. Indian J. Med. Res., *78*:670–675, 1983.

56. Jennette, J., Ferguson, A.L., Moore, M.A., and Freeman, D.G.: IgA nephropathy associated with seronegative spondylarthropathies. Arthritis Rheum., *25*:144–149, 1982.

57. Carette, S., et al.: The natural disease course of ankylosing spondylitis. Arthritis Rheum., *26*:186–190, 1983.

58. Kaprove, R.E., Little, A.H., Graham, D.C., and Rosen, P.S.: Ankylosing spondylitis. Survival in men with and without radiotherapy. Arthritis Rheum., *23*:57–61, 1980.

59. Smith, P.G., and Doll, R.: Mortality among patients with ankylosing spondylitis after a single treatment course with x rays. Br. Med. J., *284*:449–460, 1982.

60. Lehtinen, K.: Cause of death in 79 patients with ankylosing spondylitis. Scand. J. Rheumatol., *9*:145–147, 1980.

61. Godfrey, R.G., Calabro, J.J., Mills, D., and Maltz, B.A.: A double blind crossover trial of aspirin, indomethacin and phenylbutazone in ankylosing spondylitis. (Abstract.) Arthritis Rheum., *15*:110, 1972.

62. Feltelius, N., and Hallgren, R.: Sulphasalazine in ankylosing spondylitis. Arthritis Rheum., *45*:396–399, 1986.

63. Dougados, M., Boumier, P., and Amor, B.: Sulphasalazine in ankylosing spondylitis: A double blind controlled study of 60 patients. Br. Med. J., *293*:911–914, 1986.

64. Camargo, F.P., Cordeiro, E.N., and Napoli, M.M.M.: Corrective osteotomy of the spine in ankylosing spondylitis. Experience with 66 cases. Clin. Orthop., *208*:157–167, 1986.

65. Sinclair, J.R., and Mason, R.A.: Ankylosing spondylitis. The case for awake intubation. Anesthesia, *39*:3–11, 1984.

66. Sundaram, N.A., and Murphy, J.C.M.: Heterotopic bone formation following total hip arthroplasty in ankylosing spondylitis. Clin. Orthop., *207*:223–226, 1986.

67. Wordsworth, B.P., and Mowat, A.G.: A review of 100 patients with ankylosing spondylitis with particular reference to socioeconomic effects. Br. J. Rheumatol., *25*:175–180, 1986.

60

REITER'S SYNDROME: REACTIVE ARTHRITIS

DENYS K. FORD

In 1818, Brodie[1] reported five case histories of arthritis associated with urethritis and conjunctivitis.[1] Almost 100 years later, Reiter[2] in Germany and Fiessinger and Leroy[3] in France described arthritis and conjunctivitis in patients having diarrhea during the Battle of the Somme in World War I. In 1942, Bauer and Engleman[4] published the first American case of Reiter's syndrome, as it has been most commonly called, and in 1945, Hollander[5] reported on 25 cases. Paronen[6] in 1948 studied the largest number of patients, from Finland, when 334 cases were observed in an epidemic of Shigella flexneri dysentery. Little has been added to the clinical description of Reiter's syndrome since the excellent reviews of Paronen[6] in 1948 and Harkness[7] in 1949. In 1963, a fortuitous "experimental" epidemic of Reiter's syndrome provided a unique opportunity to confirm the relationship between dysentery and the syndrome.[8] A U.S. Naval vessel with a complement of 1276 men celebrated the ship's anniversary with a picnic, which half the crew attended. Two cooks at the picnic concealed their own affliction with dysentery, and subsequently 606 cases of dysentery occurred among those in attendance. Nine cases of Reiter's syndrome developed in those with dysentery, but no cases occurred in those who did not attend the picnic and remained free from dysentery. Following the discovery of the relationship between Reiter's syndrome and HLA-B27 by Brewerton in 1973,[9] Calin and Fries[10] re-examined five of these nine patients and demonstrated that four had the HLA-B27 antigen,[10] so that the incidence of the

arthritis could be calculated as about 20% for HLA-B27 individuals with dysentery.

During the past 50 years, terminology has been a continuous problem in view of the "complete" or "incomplete" clinical manifestations of the triad of symptoms and also because of the alternative enteric or genitourinary origin of the syndrome. The American Rheumatism Association Diagnostic and Therapeutic Criteria Committee proposed in 1981 that Reiter's syndrome be defined as "an episode of peripheral arthritis of more than one month's duration occurring in association with urethritis or cervicitis," but the Committee did not define the enteric form of the syndrome.[11] The term *reactive arthritis* generally is becoming accepted as more precise than *Reiter's syndrome*, and the two initiating causes of the arthritis are included in the nomenclature as *sexually acquired (transmitted) reactive arthritis* and *enteric reactive arthritis*. These are often included within the broader title of *spondyloarthropathies*, and this subject has been reviewed recently.[12,13]

EPIDEMIOLOGY

SEXUALLY ACQUIRED (TRANSMITTED) REACTIVE ARTHRITIS

The precipitating event is sexually acquired nongonococcal urethritis, the usual causes of which are infection with either Chlamydia trachomatis or Ureaplasma urealyticum, each accounting for about 40%

of cases in most countries. No good evidence exists that the other rarer causes of nongonococcal urethritis such as infection by herpes simplex virus, Mycoplasma hominis, Mycoplasma gallinarum, Trichomonas vaginalis, monilia, or specific bacterial infections are related to reactive arthritis. The evidence supporting an etiologic role for chlamydia and ureaplasma in nongonococcal urethritis is derived from the isolation of the organisms from the genital tract,[14,15] the results of specific antibiotic treatment,[16] the correlation of antibiotic resistance between ureaplasma and the urethritis,[17] the detailed study of infections in conjugal partners,[18] and in the case of ureaplasma, human experimental infection.[19] The evidence supporting an etiologic role for these organisms in reactive arthritis is less certain. One or other of the organisms is usually found in the genital tract, if the isolation is attempted while the urethritis is still persisting and antibiotics have not been given. Viable organisms are not, however, found by standard culture procedures in synovial specimens. Serum antibody levels against chlamydia often show significant elevations,[20] and synovial lymphocytes show significant stimulation by chlamydial antigen.[21] Recently, convincing "proof" of causation is the finding of synovial chlamydial antigen by immunoperoxidase[22] and immunofluorescent techniques.[23] Less direct supportive data are available for a definitive ureaplasmal origin of reactive arthritis, though synovial lymphocytes respond significantly to ureaplasmal antigen in about 50% of cases of sexually acquired reactive arthritis.[21]

Nongonococcal urethritis is as common or more common than gonorrhea. Less than 1% of patients will develop reactive arthritis, and 80% of these individuals will be HLA-B27 positive; thus, the likelihood of developing reactive arthritis after contracting nongonococcal urethritis in HLA-B27–positive men is between 1:5 and 1:10. Sexually acquired reactive arthritis is almost confined to men and occurs only very rarely in women; the reasons for this are not yet defined.

ENTERIC REACTIVE ARTHRITIS

There is ample documentation that reactive arthritis follows the intestinal infections of S. flexneri,[6,8] salmonella of the different groups,[24–26] Yersinia enterocolitica of different serotypes,[27–29] and also Yersinia pseudotuberculosis[30] and Campylobacter jejuni/coli.[31–33] The cases may be of the complete or incomplete Reiter's triad; the development of urethritis or cystitis as a sequel to enteritis or colitis is not satis-

factorily explained. Women are equally susceptible to enteric reactive arthritis,[34] and it is occasionally seen in children. The data from the studies of Noer[8] and Calin and Fries[10] indicate the chance of developing reactive arthritis following shigella infection is about 1.5% for white adults and about 20% for HLA-B27 subjects. The incidence of enteric reactive arthritis in any population depends on the frequency of the intestinal infection and is increased by poor sanitation and conditions of war. Evidence exists that all the four classes of causative organisms are endemic in North America and Europe, but certain countries such as Finland seem predisposed to more widespread yersinial infection.

PATHOGENESIS

The mechanisms by which an intestinal or genitourinary infection can cause an HLA-B27–predisposed individual to develop reactive arthritis are not precisely understood.[35] The fact that some patients do not have HLA-B27 or even its cross-reactive antigens HLA-B7, HLA-B22, and HLA-B40, excludes straightforward explanations of the genetic predisposition. New findings probably must be discovered before a coherent story is acceptable.

The recent observation[36] that Reiter's syndrome is found frequently in patients having acquired immune deficiency syndrome (AIDS) raises pathogenetic questions, the answers to which will probably help in the understanding of reactive arthritis itself.

The histology of the synovial inflammation depends on the duration of the arthritis at the time of the examination. In the early stages, the synovium may resemble a low-grade pyogenic infection with hyperemia and a predominately polymorph infiltrate.[37,38] With continued arthritis, infiltration with lymphocytes and plasma cells increases so that after several months, the synovium may closely resemble that of rheumatoid arthritis (RA), which implies an immunologic contribution to pathogenesis.[37,38] The skin lesions cannot be distinguished histologically from those of psoriasis and show thickening of the horny layer, parakeratosis, and acanthosis.[37,38] Histologically, the lesions on the mucous membranes resemble those on the skin but without keratosis.

Studies over the past 8 years in my laboratory have shown that synovial lymphocytes, but not usually peripheral blood lymphocytes, are significantly, and often markedly, stimulated by antigens derived from the agents that are epidemiologically related to the reactive arthritis. In the sexually acquired Reiter's syndrome, either chlamydial antigen or ureaplasmal antigen stimulates synovial lymphocytes, as measured by the ^{3}H-thymidine uptake technique.[39] In enteric Reiter's syndrome, one or other of the enteric antigens—salmonella, shigella, Campylobacter sp., or Yersinia sp.—gives maximal stimulation, which correlates with the etiology of the preceding enteric infection.[40,41] In the recent paper of Keat et al.,[23] it was noted that chlamydial antigen was present in the synovium when standard cultures for chlamydia failed to result in the isolation of the organism. Thus, the application of similar sophisticated techniques clearly is needed for the demonstration in the synovium of antigen derived from the other organisms incriminated as likely causes of the syndrome.*

The pathogenesis of Reiter's syndrome appears to have contributed two important observations that may be applicable to the understanding of other human "aseptic" inflammatory rheumatic diseases. First, it is evident that a single clinically recognizable arthritic syndrome can be caused by at least six different infectious agents. Second, it seems that the response of synovial lymphocytes to microbial antigenic stimulation may indicate the cause of a particular patient's arthritis when this information is not available from other sources.[21]

CLINICAL MANIFESTATIONS

The typical clinical picture of arthritis and conjunctivitis developing within a month of nongonococcal urethritis or diarrhea is easy to recognize but will only occur in a minority of patients. Most commonly, the patient complains of a recent onset of arthritis, and only on direct and sometimes searching questioning are the other manifestations uncovered. The interval of 1 to 3 weeks between the antecedent infection and the onset of arthritis may prevent the patient, and even the doctor, from making the connection. The genitourinary symptoms or diarrhea may have cleared before the arthritis appears; moreover, treatment of the infection may erroneously convince the patient that no connection could exist. The initial symptoms may be mild and overlooked. Further, embarrassment may encourage the suppression of relevant history. Conjunctivitis is often transient and minimal. The mucocutaneous lesions are painless and thus often asymptomatic.†

---

*Editor's note. If these studies are confirmed and extended, the concept of "reactive" arthritis might have to be scrapped.

†Editor's note. The oral lesions can occasionally be painful in Campylobacter-reactive arthritis (personal observation).

JOINTS

Usually from one to five joints are affected, and these tend to be in the knees, ankles, or feet. The distribution is asymmetric, though both knees are often involved. Arthritis of the metatarsophalangeal joints of the feet is a common cause of pain on walking. The presence of inflammation in distal interphalangeal joints of one or two fingers is characteristic, if present. Low-back pain or sacroiliac pain from sacroiliitis is frequent and may be unilateral or bilateral. Rarely, a widespread polyarthritis resembling RA is present. The involved joints are swollen and warm in proportion to the activity of the arthritis, but the degree of acuteness is usually less than that expected for a septic arthritis, rheumatic fever, or gout.

The insertions of tendons and ligaments in the region of joints are favored locations for inflammation (enthesopathy). The classic example is plantar fasciitis giving heel tenderness and sometimes progressing to plantar spurs. The insertions of the patella and Achilles tendons may also be affected and periostitis over the rib cage with or without chondritis of the costochondral junctions is sometimes mistaken for pleurisy.

GENITOURINARY TRACT

The usual complaints from nongonococcal urethritis are dysuria and some degree of urethral discharge, which is as profuse and as purulent as that of gonorrhea only in exceptional cases. The symptoms may be mild and consequently suppressed or overlooked by the patient. The only evidence of mild urethritis may be minimal staining of underwear or a "watering can" effect on the first daily urination from the drying of exudate at the urethral meatus. The examination of the urethra before urination in the morning may be required to demonstrate the minimal urethritis. Some patients only have a cystitis, which may be evident only from the demonstration of pyuria on urinalysis.

The cause of urethritis in patients with enteric reactive arthritis is unexplained. In the study of Paronen, 80% of the 334 patients had some urogenital involvement, which most commonly was urethritis.[6]

In the sexually acquired syndrome, other genital symptoms may arise such as epididymitis and orchitis, but these are probably due to other coincidentally acquired infection. Prostatitis may regularly accompany posterior urethritis, but from the clinical and management viewpoint, it would seem that prostatitis is not important, provided the primary genital infection is appropriately treated.

In the rare case of sexually acquired Reiter's syndrome in the female, dysuria, vaginal irritation, and variable vaginal discharge may be present.

EYE

As already noted, the conjunctivitis is often so mild and transient that it may be overlooked. Occasionally, it is unilateral. The patient may have variable degrees of itchiness or burning of the eyes. The conjunctivitis usually clears in a few days.

Iritis may develop later in patients who have had one episode of Reiter's syndrome and may recur at irregular intervals, perhaps associated with the other clinical manifestations of the syndrome. Iritis can be severe and, before present treatment methods, occasionally led to blindness. In the first attack of Reiter's syndrome, iritis will not occur until some months after the onset of the illness. Keratitis has been reported[6] but is exceptional.

SKIN AND MUCOUS MEMBRANES

Circinate balanitis (Fig. 60–1) on the glans penis is virtually diagnostic of Reiter's syndrome. Small red

macules 1 to 2 mm in diameter may be the only manifestation. More commonly, shallow, painless ulcerations with serpiginous grey borders are found. These vary in size, sometimes becoming confluent and covering most or all of the glans. The lesions may be restricted to the meatal area or, alternatively, may predominate at the coronal sulcus. Apart from cosmetic appearances, the lesions are asymptomatic. Circinate balanitis occurs in 10 to 20% of patients with sexually acquired Reiter's syndrome and probably less frequently in enteric reactive arthritis.

Small, painless superficial ulcers on an erythematous base are found on the palate and dorsum of the tongue in 5 to 10% of patients with reactive arthritis (Fig. 60–2). Because patients are unaware of them, the ulcers must be specifically sought.

The skin lesions of keratodermia blenorrhagica are diagnostic if they are found on the soles of the feet (Fig. 60–3). The lesion begins as a small macule that evolves to a vesicle before the overlying epidermis becomes progressively thickened and hyperkeratinized. Usually, the lesions predominate in the region of the metatarsal heads but may also favor the heel. The lesions are painless, though keratinized crusts up to 0.5 cm thick may cause discomfort on walking. Scattered lesions of keratodermia blenorrhagica may be found on the trunk and extremities, but these are often not easily recognized. Lesions of the nails are quite common and closely resemble those of psoriasis (Fig. 60–4).

Typical keratodermia blenorrhagica on the feet persists for several weeks but eventually disappears com-

FIG. 60–1. Circinate balanitis on glans penis in a patient with sexually acquired Reiter's syndrome.

FIG. 60–2. Palatal lesion in a patient with Reiter's syndrome.

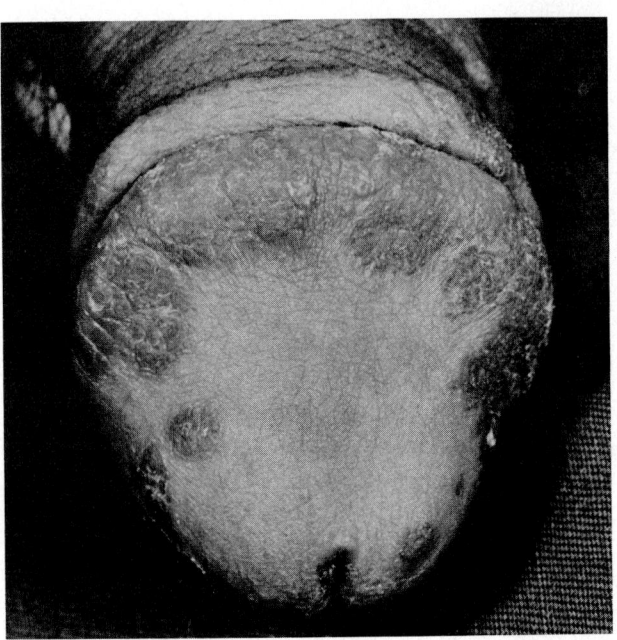

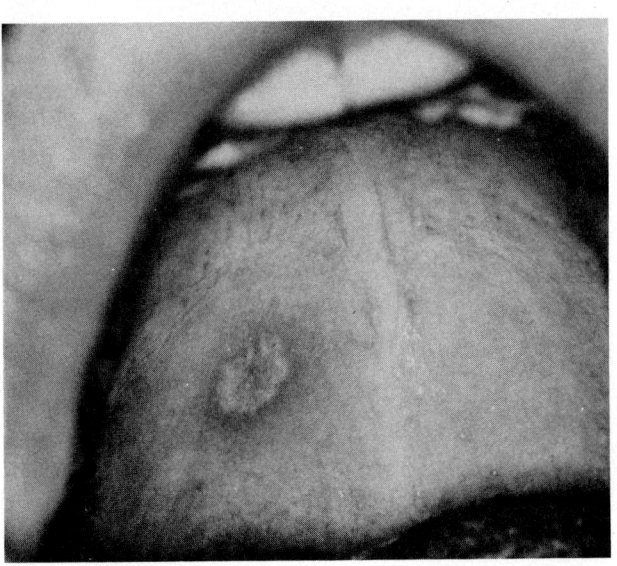

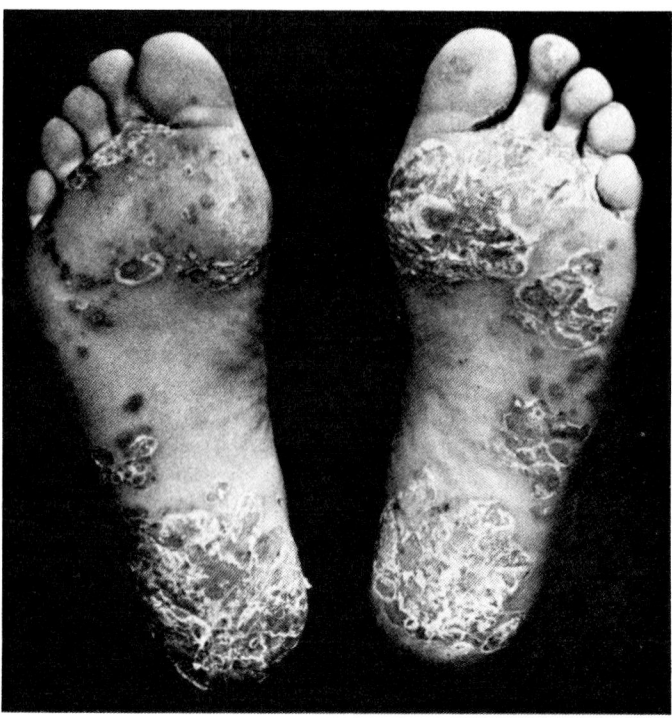

FIG. 60–3. Keratodermia blennorrhagica of feet in a patient with Reiter's syndrome.

pletely. It is seen in 5 to 10% of patients with reactive arthritis and seems to be more common in those with severe episodes.

OTHER ORGANS

Cardiac manifestations were noted many years ago;[6,7] they included myocarditis and pericarditis, but more commonly ECG abnormalities with prolongation of the PR interval, as well as ST- and T-wave changes. In 1958 a review of 519 patients with spondylitis revealed 24 with aortic incompetence, and 9 of these had had an episode of acute polyarthritis following urethritis at the onset of their disease.[42] More typical Reiter's syndrome was then noted to result in aortic incompetence.[43,44] More recently, echocardiog-

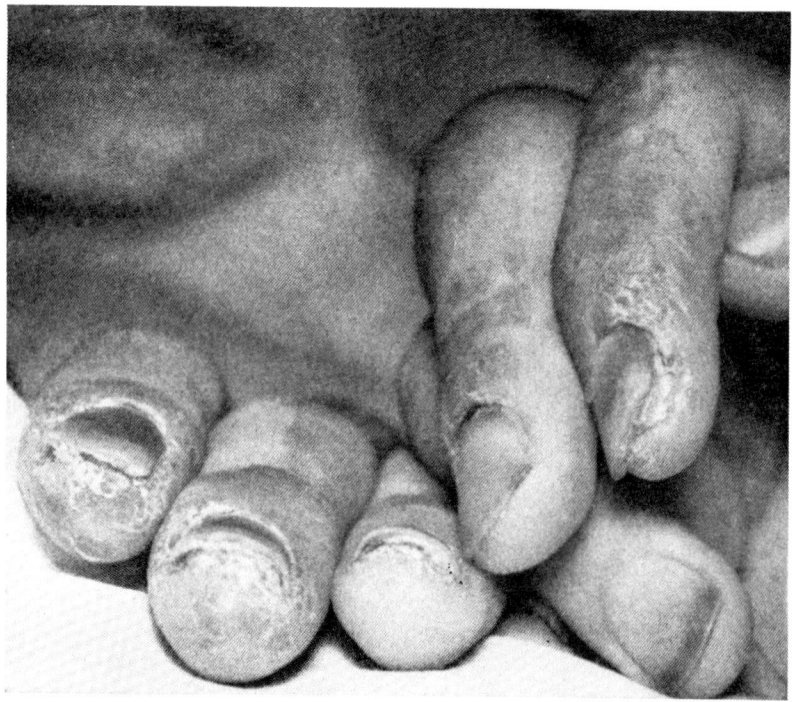

FIG. 60–4. Keratotic lesions of fingernails in a patient with Reiter's syndrome.

raphy has indicated preclinical abnormalities in the aortic root in patients with Reiter's syndrome.[45]

Neurologic abnormalities have been associated with Reiter's syndrome,[46-48] but their rarity has not permitted any precise definition.

COURSE OF ILLNESS

The clinical manifestations of Reiter's syndrome appear within a few days to about 3 weeks of the initiating nongonococcal urethritis or enteritis. Usually, the disease is at its worst in about 2 weeks, and improvement can be expected to begin within a month of onset. The speed of recovery is probably related to the degree of severity. Most patients are getting back to normal activities within 2 to 4 months after the onset of the arthritis, though some rheumatic symptoms may persist for several months afterward, particularly as painful heels, pain in the metatarsophalangeal joints, and low-back pain from persistent sacroiliitis.

Disagreement exists about the frequency of "chronic" Reiter's syndrome. Some observers believe this is a relatively common event,[49] but I think that if the causative organism of the initiating infection is eradicated and reinfection prevented, chronic Reiter's syndrome is rare.

Patients who have had one episode of Reiter's syndrome are susceptible to recurrences, which may be multiple. The importance of reinfection as their cause is the subject of debate. In my opinion, reinfection is the cause of the recurrences.

Reiter's syndrome is a precursor of spondylitis, as noted by many observers.[50-53] Varying degrees of chronic back pain and limited motion of the spine are found, mostly in patients who have had repeated or prolonged episodes. An asymmetric involvement is rather characteristic, and "skipped areas" may be present on radiography.

LABORATORY AND RADIOGRAPHIC FINDINGS

Routine laboratory tests are of little help in diagnosing or treating Reiter's syndrome. The laboratory may assist in defining the inciting genitourinary or enteric infection, and future understanding may demand that this is a requirement for optimal management. Currently, however, clinical skill unsupported by any laboratory or radiographic expenditures can provide optimal care.

The peripheral white blood cell count is usually somewhat elevated due to an increase in neutrophils. The erythrocyte sedimentation rate is variably elevated, as would be expected. The synovial fluid has a variable decrease in viscosity and elevation of cell count in proportion to the activity of the inflammation, total counts usually varying between 5000 and 30,000/μL. Neutrophils predominate, but variable numbers of lymphocytes and monocytes may be found, particularly in more persistent arthritis. The total hemolytic complement level is often elevated in both the joint fluid and the serum.* The demonstration of HLA-B27 is not clinically necessary.

Radiography is not a requirement for the clinical management of a patient with Reiter's syndrome. In the first episode, radiographs are normal, and later the expensive documentation of abnormalities is unnecessary. Areas of periostitis at tendon insertions, at the insertion of the plantar fascia (Fig. 60–5), and along phalanges were well described many years ago (Fig. 60–6),[7,51] as were the radiographic changes of sacroiliitis and syndesmophyte formation in the spine[50-53] (Fig. 60–7). Their demonstration is needed only for specific research studies.

Because both ureaplasmas and chlamydiae are sensitive to the tetracyclines, expensive "research" testing is not currently needed to demonstrate these organisms in sexually acquired reactive arthritis. As already noted, the passage of time and also prior antibiotic therapy may prevent the isolation of genital ureaplasmas or chlamydiae when the patient presents with sexually acquired reactive arthritis. Serologic investigations for both of these organisms and the study of lymphocyte responses are still research procedures. The recent demonstration of chlamydial antigen in the synovium[23] may remain a research procedure for some time, though the application of this technique and its extension to other microbial antigens may well become a standard diagnostic test, perhaps becoming a readily available, inexpensive procedure.

The bacteriologic diagnosis of enteric reactive arthritis is easy if the case appears during a documented epidemic, but is difficult in sporadic cases, as stool cultures may be negative by the time arthritis develops. The demonstration of elevated serum antibody levels against the inciting agent may be helpful if available; again the demonstration of synovial lymphocyte responses to the specific antigens is currently a research procedure.

The "Golden Rule of Rheumatology," namely that of aspirating and culturing acute monoarticular ar-

---

Editor's note. The ratio C'H$_{50}$ joint fluid/C'H$_{50}$ serum is proportional to the total protein joint fluid/serum protein. This finding is helpful diagnostically in cases of incomplete Reiter's syndrome.

FIG. 60–5. *A,* Lateral view of the calcaneus demonstrates spurs associated with proliferative erosions owing to the evident inflammation at ligamentous and fascial insertion sites of the calcaneus. These changes are most prominent in psoriatic and Reiter's arthritis. *B,* Large posterior and inferior spurs can be seen with well-corticated margins indicating chronic, inactive disease. This nonspecific finding may be seen in any of the HLA-B27–associated arthritides during later stages. *C,* Typical, well-corticated, degenerative spurs of the calcaneus, a frequent appearance in the elderly population. *D,* Linear and punctate calcifications in the Achilles tendon and plantar aponeurosis are an occasional finding in calcium pyrophosphate dihydrate crystal deposition or pseudogout. (Courtesy of H.K. Genant.)

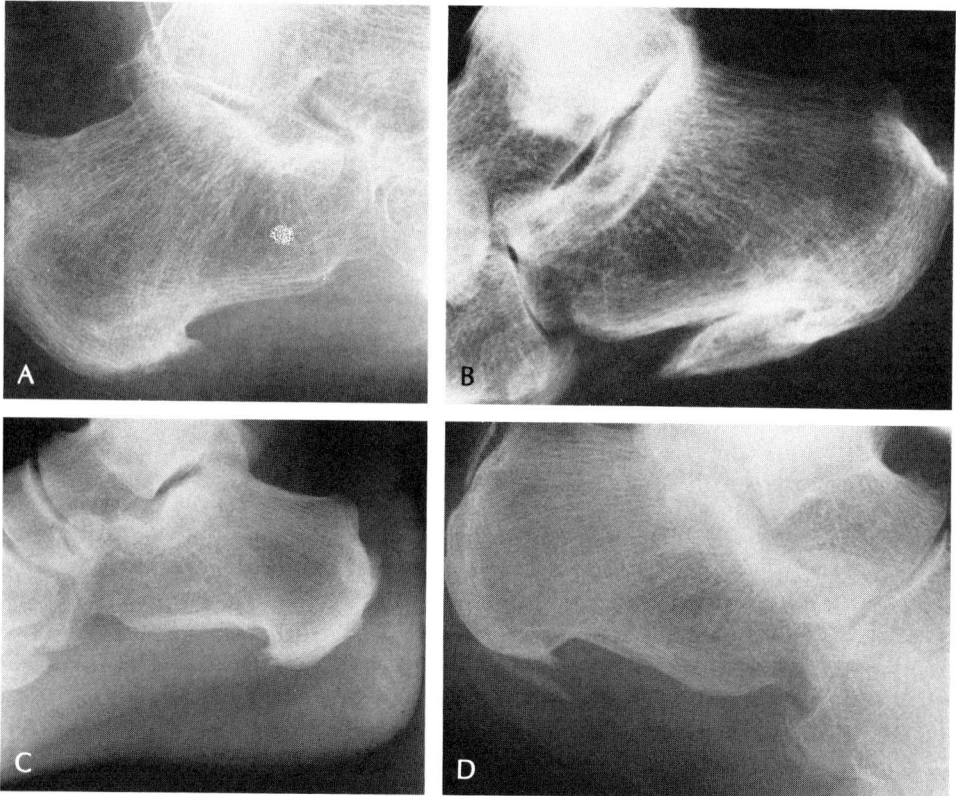

thritis, applies to some patients in whom acute septic arthritis must be excluded.

DIFFERENTIAL DIAGNOSIS

The diagnosis of Reiter's syndrome may be obvious, but patients with the incomplete syndrome may require a more open diagnosis such as arthritis associated with a recent genital (enteric) infection. A complete history is an essential ingredient for a correct diagnosis. Suspicion should be aroused by a recent asymmetric arthritis of a few joints in a man.* Some of the diagnostic features follow:

In patients with psoriatic arthritis, conjunctivitis,

Editor's note. The syndrome can occur rarely in children.

oral mucosal lesions, circinate balanitis, and diarrhea or urethritis are not found.

Circinate balanitis is painless in contrast to the lesions of genital herpes.

In gonococcal arthritis, one joint is often predominately affected, and pustular skin lesions are characteristic if present; when in doubt, aspirate and culture.

In the arthritis of ulcerative colitis and regional enteritis, chronic or recurrent diarrhea is found and erythema nodosum may be present, but the mucocutaneous lesions of Reiter's syndrome do not occur.

TREATMENT

Treatment is controversial and will remain so until the precise pathogenesis is understood. In my view,

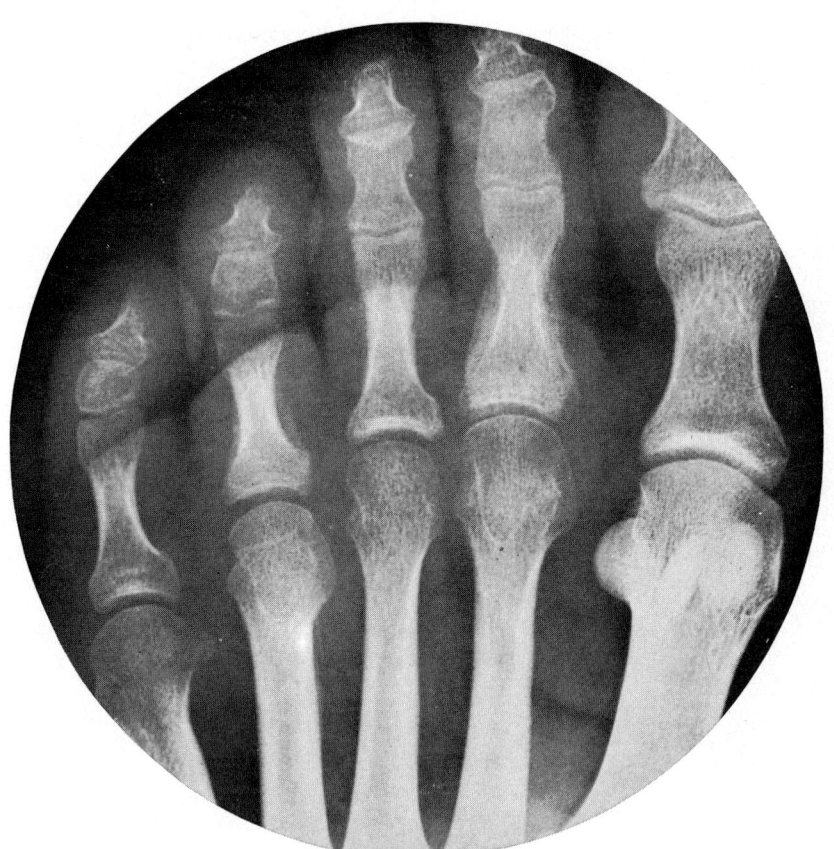

FIG. 60–6. Radiograph of the left foot of a patient with Reiter's syndrome who had complained of pain and swelling of the foot for the preceding 7 months. Periosteal new bone is visible in the shafts of the second, third, and fourth proximal phalanges and also on the medial aspect of the distal part of the shaft of the fourth metatarsal bone.

reactive arthritis is analogous to rheumatic fever, in that it is a direct consequence of an infection and the eradication of the infectious agent is essential both for satisfactory resolution and for prevention of further attacks.

The treatment of sexually acquired reactive arthritis is therefore the eradication of ureaplasmas or chlamydiae and the prevention of reinfection. Both organisms are susceptible to *tetracycline at a minimum dosage of 500 mg three times daily for 10 days.* An equivalent dosage of doxycycline is an alternative, as is an equivalent dose of erythromycin in those who cannot tolerate tetracycline. Conjugal partners must be treated with the same dosage at the same time. A condom should be employed assiduously by those who are at risk from multiple partners.

The treatment of enteric reactive arthritis has not yet been defined, because the antibiotic treatment of enteric pathogens is an evolving science. The demonstration of a negative stool culture does not prove the absence of the enteric pathogen from sites of latent infection. In consequence, I treat cases with a high-dosage course of the most appropriate antibiotic. Reinfection is unlikely to occur in cases of enteric reactive arthritis, unless the individual is living in an area of poor sanitation. *A patient with a history of enteric*

reactive arthritis is also susceptible to sexually acquired reactive arthritis.

The arthritis of an episode of Reiter's syndrome is self-limited in the absence of persistent infection or reinfection. As with rheumatic fever, antimicrobial therapy does not result in any immediate effect on the arthritis, although it may prevent a chronic disease state. The clinical manifestations of the arthritis are best treated with indomethacin in a dosage proportional to the clinical severity. If indomethacin is not tolerated, any of the other nonsteroidal anti-inflammatory drugs could be used. Physiotherapeutic measures are indicated according to standard principles.

Treatment of the conjunctivitis and mucocutaneous lesions is not required. Iritis usually requires ophthalmologic consultation and management.

Various claims have been made that some resistant chronic cases of Reiter's syndrome require management with such drugs as azathioprine, methotrexate, and cyclophosphamide. In my experience, if treatment is directed at eradicating the inciting infectious agent and preventing reinfection, the disease will remit spontaneously, and such potentially dangerous drugs will be required rarely, if ever.

FIG. 60–7. Anteroposterior view of the lumbar spine demonstrates advanced sacroiliitis with erosion and sclerosis, but with the asymmetric distribution typical of psoriatic arthritis or Reiter's syndrome. The syndesmophytes are broad, nonmarginal, and asymmetric, as is typical of these disorders.

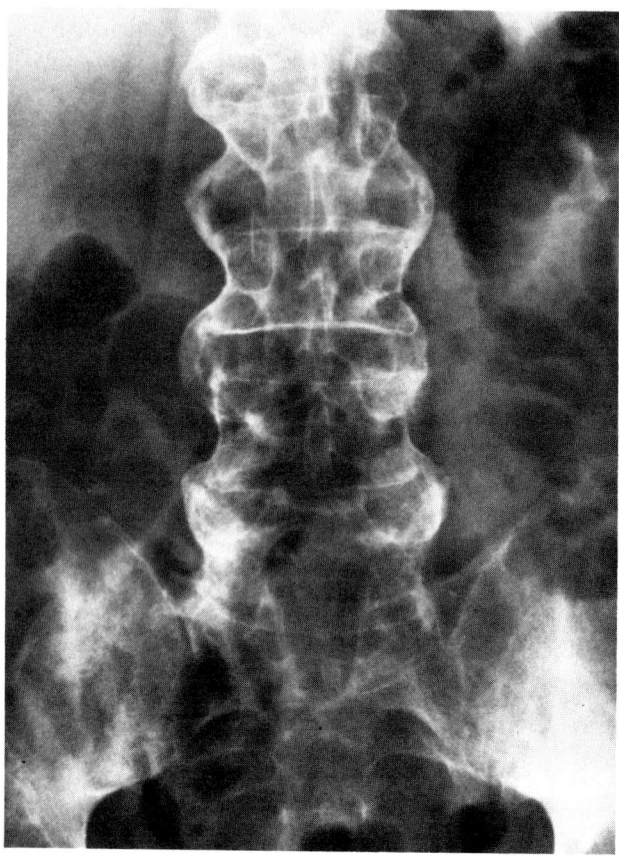

REFERENCES

1. Brodie, B.D.: Pathogenic and Surgical Observations on Diseases of the Joints. London, Longman, 1818.
2. Reiter, H.: Uber eine bisher unerkannte Spirochaeteninfektion (Spirochaetosis Arthritica). Dtsch. Med. Wochenschr., 42:1535–1536, 1916.
3. Fiessinger, N., and Leroy, E.: Contribution to the study of an epidemic of dysentery in the Somme. Bull. Mem. Soc. Med. Hop. (Paris), 40:2051–2052, 1916.
4. Bauer, W., and Engleman, E.P.: Syndrome of unknown etiology characterized by urethritis, conjunctivitis and arthritis (so-called Reiter's syndrome). Trans. Assoc. Am. Physicians, 57:307–313, 1942.
5. Hollander, J.L.: Arthritis resembling Reiter's syndrome: Observations of 25 cases. JAMA, 129:593–595, 1945.
6. Paronen, I.: Reiter's disease: A study of 344 cases observed in Finland. Acta Med. Scand., 131:(Suppl. 212):1–112, 1948.
7. Harkness, A.H.: Reiter's disease. Br. J. Vener. Dis., 25:185–201, 1949.
8. Noer, H.R.: An "experimental" epidemic of Reiter's syndrome. JAMA, 197:693–698, 1966.
9. Brewerton, D.A., et al.: Reiter's disease and HLA-27. Lancet, 2:996–998, 1973.
10. Calin, A., and Fries, J.F.: An "experimental" epidemic of Reiter's syndrome revisited: Follow-up evidence on genetic and environmental factors. Ann. Intern. Med., 84:564–566, 1976.
11. Willkens, R.F., et al.: Reiter's syndrome: Evaluation of preliminary criteria for definite disease. Arthritis Rheum., 24:844–849, 1981.
12. Ziff, M., and Cohen, S.B. (eds.): The spondyloarthropathies. Adv. Inflammation Res., 9:1–272, 1985.
13. Panayi, G.S. (ed.): Seronegative spondyloarthropathies. Clin. Rheum. Dis., 11:1–273, 1985.
14. Grayston, J.T., and Wang, S.P.: New knowledge of chlamydiae and the diseases they cause. J. Infect. Dis., 132:87–105, 1975.
15. Shepard, M.C.: Current status of Ureaplasma urealyticum in nongonococcal urethritis. ASEAN J. Clin. Sci., 1:198–209, 1980.
16. Bowie, W.R., et al.: Differential response of chlamydial and ureaplasma-associated urethritis to sulfafurazole (sulfisoxazole) and aminocyclitols. Lancet, 2:1276–1278, 1976.
17. Ford, D.K., and Smith, J.R.: Non-specific urethritis associated with a tetracycline-resistant T-mycoplasma. Br. J. Vener. Dis., 50:373–374, 1974.
18. Arya, O.P., and Pratt, B.C.: Persistent urethritis due to Ureaplasma urealyticum in conjugal or stable partnerships. Genitourin. Med., 62:329–332, 1986.
19. Taylor-Robinson, D., Csonka, G.W., and Prentice, M.J.: Human intra-urethral inoculation of ureaplasmas. Q. J. Med., 46:309–326, 1977.
20. Martin, D.H., et al.: Chlamydia trachomatis in men with Reiter's syndrome. Ann. Intern. Med., 100:207–213, 1984.
21. Ford, D.K.: Reactive arthritis: A viewpoint rather than a review. Clin. Rheum. Dis., 12:389–401, 1986.
22. Schumacher, H.R., Cherian, P.V., Sieck, M., and Clayburne, G.: Ultrastructural identification of chlamydial antigens in synovial membrane in acute Reiter's syndrome. Arthritis Rheum., 29:531, 1986.
23. Keat, A., et al.: Chlamydia trachomatis and reactive arthritis: The missing link. Lancet, 1:72–74, 1987.
24. Berglof, F.E.: Arthritis and intestinal infection. Acta Rheum. Scand., 9:144–149, 1963.
25. Vartianen, J., and Hurri, L.: Arthritis due to Salmonella typhimurium. Acta Med. Scand., 175:711–776, 1964.
26. Warren, C.P.W.: Arthritis associated with salmonella infections. Ann. Rheum. Dis., 29:483–487, 1970.
27. Ahvonen, P., Sievers, K., and Aho, K.: Arthritis associated with Yersinia enterocolitica infection. Acta Rheum. Scand., 15:232–253, 1969.
28. Laitinen, O., Tuuhea, J., and Ahvonen, P.: Polyarthritis associated with Yersinia enterocolitica infection. Ann. Rheum. Dis., 31:34–39, 1972.
29. Winblad, S.: Arthritis associated with Yersinia enterocolitica infections. J. Infect. Dis., 7:191–195, 1975.
30. Chalmers, A., et al.: Post-diarrheal arthropathy of Yersinia pseudotuberculosis. Can. Med. Assoc. J., 118:515–516, 1978.
31. Urman, J.D., Zurier, R.B., and Rothfield, N.F.: Reiter's syndrome associated with campylobacter fetus infection. Ann. Intern. Med., 86:444–445, 1977.
32. Kosunen, T.U.: Reactive arthritis after Campylobacter jejuni enteritis in patients with HLA B27. Lancet, 1:1312–1313, 1980.
33. van de Putte, L.G.A., et al.: Reactive arthritis after Campylobacter jejuni enteritis. J. Rheumatol., 7:531–535, 1980.
34. Simon, D.G., et al.: Reiter's syndrome following epidemic shigellosis. J. Rheumatol., 8:969–973, 1981.

35. Woodrow, J.C.: Genetic aspects of the spondyloarthropathies. Clin. Rheum. Dis., *11*:1–24, 1985.

36. Winchester, R., et al.: The co-occurrence of Reiter's syndrome and acquired immunodeficiency. Ann. Intern. Med., *106*:19–26, 1987.

37. Kulka, J.P.: The lesions of Reiter's syndrome. Arthritis Rheum., *5*:195–201, 1962.

38. Weinberger, H.W., et al.: Reiter's syndrome, clinical and pathologic observations. A long term study of 16 cases. Medicine, *41*:35–91, 1962.

39. Ford, D.K., da Roza, D.M., Shah, P., and Wenman, W.M.: Cell-mediated immune responses of synovial mononuclear cells in Reiter's syndrome against ureaplasmal and chlamydial antigens. J. Rheumatol., *7*:751–755, 1980.

40. Ford, D.K., da Roza, D.M., and Shah, P.: Cell-mediated immune responses of synovial mononuclear cells to sexually transmitted, enteric and mumps antigens in patients with Reiter's syndrome, rheumatoid arthritis and ankylosing spondylitis. J. Rheumatol., *8*:220–232, 1981.

41. Ford, D.K., da Roza, D.M., and Schulzer, M.: Lymphocytes from the site of disease but not blood lymphocytes indicate the cause of arthritis. Ann. Rheum. Dis., *44*:701–710, 1985.

42. Graham, D.C., and Smythe, H.A.: The carditis and aortitis of ankylosing spondylitis. Bull. Rheum. Dis., *9*:171–174, 1958.

43. Csonka, G.W., Litchfield, J.W., Oates, J.K., and Willcox, R.R.: Cardiac lesions in Reiter's syndrome. Br. Med. J., *1*:243–247, 1961.

44. Rodnan, G.P., Benedek, T.G., Shaver, J.A., and Fennell, R.M.: Reiter's syndrome and aortic insufficiency. JAMA, *189*:889–894, 1964.

45. La Bresh, K.A., Lally, E.V., Sharma, S.C., and Ho, G.: Two dimensional echocardiographic detection of pre-clinical aortic root abnormalities in rheumatoid variant disease. Am. J. Med., *78*:908–912, 1985.

46. Csonka, G.W.: Involvement of the nervous system in Reiter's syndrome. Ann. Rheum. Dis., *17*:334–336, 1958.

47. Oates, J.K., and Hancock, J.A.H.: Neurological symptoms and lesions occurring in the course of Reiter's disease. Am. J. Med. Sci., *238*:79–84, 1959.

48. Good, A.E.: Neurologic manifestations in patients with Reiter's syndrome. Arthritis Rheum., *5*:298–299, 1962.

49. Fox, R., et al.: The chronicity of symptoms and disablity in Reiter's syndrome: An analysis of 131 consecutive patients. Ann. Intern. Med., *91*:190–193, 1979.

50. Romanus, E.R.: Pelvo-spondylitis ossificans in the male and genito-urinary infection. Acta Med. Scand., *145*(Suppl. 280): 1–367, 1953.

51. Ford, D.K.: Natural history of arthritis following venereal urethritis. Ann. Rheum. Dis., *12*:177–197, 1953.

52. Marche, J.: Spondylarthrite ankylosante et syndrome de N. Fiessinger-Leroy-Reiter. France Medicale, *18*:7–30, 5–32, 1955.

53. Good, A.E.: Involvement of the back in Reiter's syndrome: Follow-up of 34 cases. Ann. Intern. Med., *57*:44–59, 1962.

61

PSORIATIC ARTHRITIS

ROBERT M. BENNETT

The association of psoriasis with inflammatory polyarthritis is generally credited to Baron Jean Louis Alibert (1768 to 1837). A connection with arthritis is mentioned in Alibert's 1818 work[1] in a brief passage, "affections arthritiques or rheumatismales," which appears under the heading *Lepre Squammeuse.*" In 1904, Menzen[2] cited several midnineteenth century case reports of a relationship between psoriasis and arthritis and described five additional cases that he had observed.

The term *psoriasis arthritique* was introduced by the French dermatologist Pierre Bazin in his book entitled *Leçon Théoriques et Cliniques sur les Affections Cutanées de Nature Arthritique et Arthreux.*[3] The first detailed description of the disease appears in the doctoral thesis of Charles Bourdillon, entitled *Psoriasis et Arthropothies*, published in 1888.[4]

The concept of *rheumatoid arthritis* (RA) as a distinct clinical entity also developed during this time as a result of Garrod's[5] and Adam's differentiation of gout from "rheumatic gout" in 1859. For about 30 years, the idea of psoriatic arthritis being a discrete entity, as opposed to the coincidental occurrence of rheumatoid arthritis and psoriasis, was not generally accepted. From the 1920s on, various authors revived the concept of psoriatic arthritis, mainly in the form of individual case reports.[6–9] Other observers were not impressed with the association, however.[10–13] It was not until the demonstration of rheumatoid factor (RF) in 1948[14] in the serum of most patients with typical RA that much nosologic progress was made. This finding divided inflammatory arthritis into seroposi-

tive and seronegative. The realization that the majority of patients with coincident psoriasis and arthritis were seronegative, coupled with the introduction of criteria for the diagnosis of RA,[15–17] was important in developing the concept of psoriatic arthritis as a disease entity.

PSORIATIC ARTHRITIS AS A DISTINCT ENTITY

In the absence of a well-defined pathogenesis, the reasons for considering a disorder as a distinct entity rest largely with a practical consideration of its natural evolution, prognosis, and response to treatment. Two questions are pertinent to considering psoriatic arthritis as a distinct entity. (1) Is there an increased prevalence of seronegative arthritis in patients with psoriasis compared to a general population? and (2) Are there any clinical features that distinguish patients with arthritis and psoriasis from those with other forms of seronegative arthritis (e.g., inflammatory bowel disease, Reiter's disease, ankylosing spondylitis).

Epidemiologic studies indicate that 20% of patients with seronegative polyarthritis but only 1.2% of patients with *seropositive* arthritis also had psoriasis.[18,19] Thus, the prevalence of psoriasis in association with seronegative arthritis is increased roughly about ten-fold. The prevalence of polyarthritis (both seronegative and seropositive) in patients with psoriasis was 6.8%;[20] this compares with a prevalence of about 1%

Table 61–1. Prevalence Data

	%	Reference
Psoriasis in general population	1.2	8
Psoriasis in seronegative polyarthritis	20.2	8
Psoriasis in seropositive polyarthritis	1.2	8
Polyarthritis in psoriasis	6.8	112
Rheumatoid arthritis in general population	1.0	111
Psoriatic arthritis in general population	0.1	214*

*In United Kingdom[90]

for RA in the general population[21] (Table 61–1). The strong association of seronegative arthritis and psoriasis has been documented in many other studies,[22–28] which is persuasive epidemiologic evidence for the concept of psoriatic arthritis. A recent study in the Netherlands, however, failed to support this association.[29–31] In a survey of two residential areas, 41 out of 3659 persons (i.e., 1.1%) had psoriasis. An inflammatory arthritis (including RA) was noted in 5% of the patients with psoriasis and in 2.2% patients without psoriasis, not a significant difference.

Family studies have provided convincing evidence of an association between psoriasis and arthritis.[32,33] Of 310 first- or second-degree relatives of 108 patients with peripheral psoriatic arthritis, 21% had psoriasis alone, 11% had a seronegative polyarthritis, 0.4% had sacroiliitis or spondylitis, and 1.8% had an erosive polyarthritis.[34] The prevalence of seronegative arthritis was significantly increased in comparison to 83 spousal controls, but that of erosive polyarthritis was similar in the two groups (1.8%). This percentage is similar to the prevalence of seropositive RA. These data suggest an 80 to 90% chance of inheritability in first-degree relatives of subjects with psoriatic arthritis.

Family studies suggest that several genetic loci might be involved in such increased susceptibility.[32,35–47] The relative risk of developing psoriasis alone or of developing psoriatic arthritis is shown in Table 61–2. A fairly strong association of psoriasis with HLA-Cw6 but the relative risk of also developing *arthritis* was not associated with this HLA genotype. Furthermore, an *absence* of HLA-Cw6 and the presence of either HLA-B39 or HLA-B7 increases the relative risk of developing psoriatic arthritis 11-fold. Psoriasis is considered to be a genetically heterogeneous disease. Various environmental "triggers" are thought to interact with different genotypes to affect clinical expression.

Most rheumatologists have accepted the concept of distinctive clinical and radiologic features of the arthritis associated with psoriasis. A recent study has challenged this assumption. The clinical features of patients with seronegative polyarthritis associated with psoriasis were compared with those of patients suffering from either seronegative or seropositive RA without psoriasis; the most prominent difference was an increased prevalence of distal interphalangeal (DIP) involvement of fingers and toes in the psoriasis group.[30] Less than 50% of the psoriatic patients with seronegative polyarthritis had involvement of these joints, which is too low a prevalence to be a sensitive marker for psoriatic arthritis. Asymmetric joint involvement and the absence of ulnar deviation of the fingers were *not* characteristic of the arthritis associated with psoriasis. However, a positive correlation between psoriatic changes in the nails and DIP joint arthritis was noted. A statistical analysis of radiographic changes showed that erosions and mutilation of the DIP and proximal interphalangeal (PIP) joints were the best criteria to distinguish patients with seronegative arthritis and psoriasis from those with seronegative arthritis without psoriasis.[29] Even when changes in the metacarpophalangeal (MCP) and metatarsophalangeal (MTP) joints were included, only 50% of patients could be classified as having psoriatic arthritis. The authors concluded that seronegative polyarthritis and psoriasis might be associated diseases in which the presence of psoriasis leads to a more severe form of arthritis. Features that are generally considered characteristic of psoriatic arthritis are given in Table 61–3.

PATHOLOGY

Psoriatic arthritis is characterized by an inflammatory synovitis macroscopically indistinguishable from

Table 61–2. Relative Risk for Developing Psoriasis and Psoriatic Arthritis Based on HLA Determinants*

Antigen Present	Antigen Absent	Relative Risk of Psoriasis Alone	Relative Risk of Psoriatic Arthritis
HLA-Cw6	—	8.10	3.2
HLA-B17	—	7.60	5.0
HLA-B27	—	0.96	3.6
—	HLA-Cw6	—	3.3
HLA-B27	HLA-Cw6	—	8.3
HLA-Bw39	HLA-Cw6	—	10.8
HLA-B7	HLA-Cw6	—	11.0

*Data taken from references 46 and 174.

Table 61-3. Clinical Characteristics Suggestive of Psoriatic Arthritis

Involvement of DIP joints in absence of primary osteoarthritis
Asymmetric joint involvement*
Absence of rheumatoid factor and subcutaneous nodules
Flexor tenosynovitis and "sausage" digits
A family history of psoriatic arthritis
Significant nail pitting (>20 pits)
Axial radiographs showing one or more of the following: (1) sacro-iliitis, (2) syndesmophytes (often "atypical"), and (3) paravertebral ossification
Peripheral radiographs showing an erosive arthritis with a relative lack of osteopenia; in particular DIP erosions with expansion of the base of the terminal phalanx and terminal phalangeal osteolysis

*See reference 30 for dissenting findings.

that of RA.[48] Synovial cell proliferation and mononuclear cell infiltration are similar in both conditions.[49-51] An excessive fibrous component was noted in the articular soft tissues of patients with psoriasis in one study,[52] a finding supported by others.[50,51] In Gardner's[53] experience the only significant histologic difference between psoriatic arthritis and RA was the predilection for a more destructive arthropathy of the feet in psoriatic patients. Psoriatic arthritis has no characteristic histopathologic features, as a similar picture is found in most other sterile inflammatory synovitis, but synovial biopsy may be useful in excluding arthritis associated with microbes, pigmented villonodular synovitis, and other tumors.

ETIOLOGY

The importance of heredity in uncomplicated psoriasis, peripheral psoriatic arthritis, and psoriatic spondylitis has already been discussed, but its pathogenetic role in leading to inflamed skin lesions and arthritis remains unclear. Note that only 70% of monozygotic twin pairs with psoriasis are concordant for the disease,[54] a similar discordance for psoriatic arthropathy in monozygotic twins, which has been observed for 40 years,[55] also is persuasive evidence that environmental factors contribute to the pathogenesis. Several morphologic, biochemical, and immunologic changes observed in uncomplicated psoriasis may also have some bearing on the pathogenesis of the associated arthritis.

The concept of a generalized abnormality of the blood capillaries in psoriasis may be relevant. Abnormal capillaries have been described in both the affected and spared areas of skin in uncomplicated psoriasis.[56] Another study found meandering capillaries with tight terminal convolutions in all patients with psoriatic arthritis but found no such changes in

patients with RA, scleroderma, morphea, systemic lupus erythematosus, or dermatomyositis.[57] Such changes appear to be a feature of psoriasis per se rather than psoriatic arthritis.[58] Plethysmographic studies have shown psoriatic patients to have an enhanced response of small vessels of the phalanges to reactive hyperemia resembling the response found in diabetes.[59] Interestingly, acro-osteolysis occurred in both diseases.[48]

Prominent endothelial cells that had a swollen appearance associated with a dilated rough endoplasmic reticulum were noted in another study.[44] Perivascular inflammatory infiltrates consisted of lymphocytes and plasma cells. In contrast with RA, synovial lining cell hyperplasia was not a prominent feature (Figs. 61-1 and 61-2). Such microvascular changes have stimulated a search for immunologic mechanisms that might mediate blood vessel damage.

Circulating immune complexes have been noted in 29 to 58% of patients with either psoriasis alone or psoriatic arthritis,[60-62] but levels were not significantly higher in the latter group. Immunofluorescence studies have shown deposits of immunoglobulins and complement components in the blood vessels of both skin and synovium in patients with psoriasis alone or with psoriatic arthritis.[63,64] IgG–anti-IgG immune complexes can be eluted from the synovial membrane of patients with psoriatic arthritis,[65] but unlike RA,

FIG. 61-1. Synovial biopsy from a patient with psoriatic arthritis (original magnification × 200) showing limited synovial cell hyperplasia, increased vascularity, and a mononuclear cell infiltration.

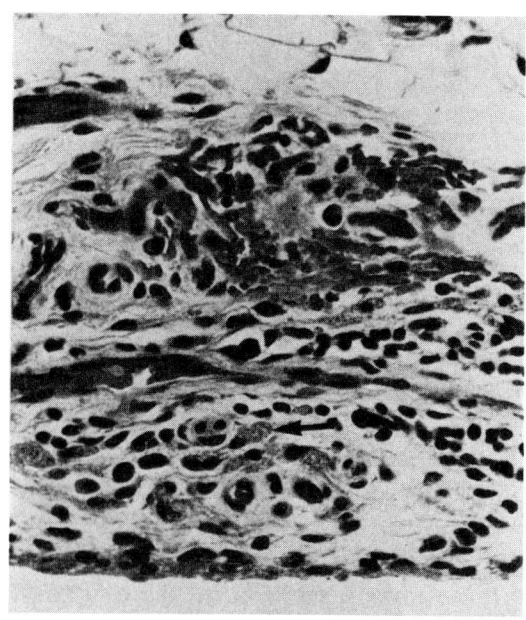

FIG. 61–2. Electronmicrograph of synovial tissue from a patient with psoriatic arthritis (original magnification ×3000) showing dilation of the rough endoplasmic reticulum and marked swelling of the endothelial cells.

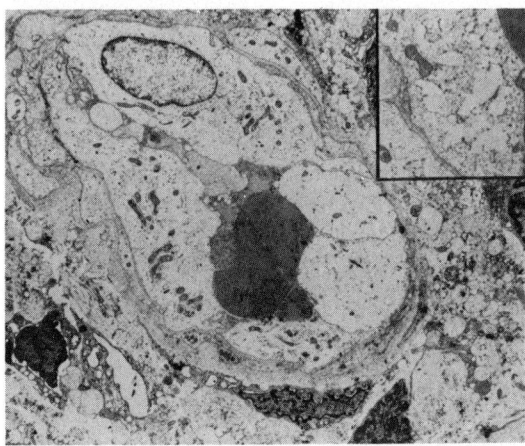

where such complexes fix complement and play an important role in joint inflammation, reduced levels of synovial fluid complement have not been observed in the effusions of psoriatic arthritis.[66] One immunofluorescent study detected RF-producing plasma cells in the synovium, albeit to a lesser degree than that usually observed in RA,[45] but another study failed to corroborate this finding.[67] The ratio of T- and B-lymphocytes in the synovial membrane of psoriatic arthritis was explored; T cells were found to be the predominant cell, with only a minority of cells staining for intra- and extracellular immunoglobulins (Fig. 61–3).[68] Studies of peripheral blood lymphocytes have not shown any impressive changes in either function[69] or subset distribution.[70]

FIG. 61–3. Immunofluorescence staining with an anti–T-cell antiserum of synovial tissue from a patient with psoriatic arthritis. The majority of mononuclear cells are seen to be T lymphocytes.

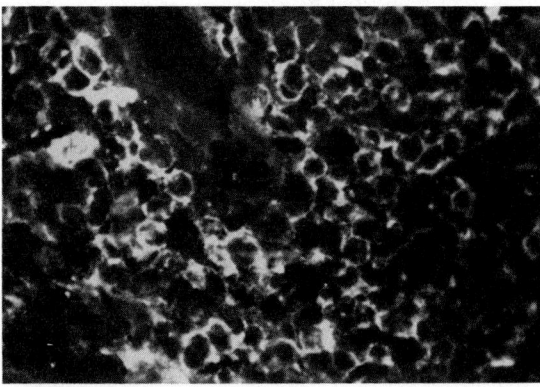

Streptococcal infections have a well-known association with flares of psoriasis, particularly guttate psoriasis in children.[71,72] Anti-DNase B antibodies (one of several exotoxins produced by group A streptococci) were found in the serum of 51% of psoriatic arthritis patients compared to 10% of controls.[73] An increased reactivity to staphylococcal α-antitoxin also has been described in patients with psoriatic arthritis.[74] The speculation that bacterial cell wall peptidoglycans cause a reactive arthritis in some psoriatic patients has stimulated such studies.

Trauma localized to a joint is well documented as "triggering" local osteolysis in psoriatic arthritis patients. In one patient, generalized acro-osteolysis developed after needle puncture of a single nail,[11] and similar associations have been reported by others.[48,75] It has been proposed that trauma may induce a "deep Koebner effect" on joint tissues.[48] A novel hypothesis that may account for flares of arthritis following trauma has been proposed by Lotz, et al.,[76] who showed that substance P, which may be released antidromically from peripheral nerve terminals, stimulates the proliferation of synoviocytes and triggers the release of PGE_2 and collagenase.

CLINICAL FEATURES

AGE OF ONSET

In the United States, the mean age of onset of uncomplicated psoriasis was found to be 28.7 years for men and 26.2 years for women.[77a] In the Faroe Islands in the northern part of Europe, which has an apparently more unfavorable climate, the age of onset was 13 years for men and 12 years for women.[77b] Psoriatic arthritis commonly first occurs between 30 and 55 years of age,[19] as does RA.[78] In one study, the age of onset of psoriatic arthritis was 44 and 46 years for men and women, respectively.[79] Childhood onset has also been noted, usually between 9 and 12 years of age.[25,80,81]

SEX RATIO

The male/female ratio in psoriatic arthritis has varied widely in different surveys. Data pooled from 10 different studies resulted in a male/female ratio of 1:1.04.[34] This contrasts to the approximately 3:1 female preponderance in seropositive RA.[15] The impression of a male predominance for psoriatic arthritis[82] is probably a reflection of more common DIP involvement in men.[83]

PATTERNS OF ONSET AND DISTRIBUTION

The classic view that the onset of arthritis occurs concurrently with the skin disease[7] has not been confirmed in subsequent studies.[19,84,85] When a simultaneous onset does occur, however, it suggests a causal relationship. An isochronous onset occurs in about 10% of patients.[86] A close temporal relationship between DIP joint involvement and psoriatic nail changes has been described.[86a] Although skin lesions usually precede the arthritis, in some 16% of patients the arthritis appears first; obviously in such cases psoriatic arthritis can be diagnosed only in retrospect. The commonly held view that psoriatic arthritis has a predilection for involvement of the DIP joints should be revised.[49,51,87] Although prominent DIP joint change is an important differentiating point vis-à-vis RA, and a strong indicator of psoriatic arthritis, it only occurs in about 16% of cases.[86] DIP joint involvement does occur in many patients with RA, although such involvement is rarely predominant. Several broad clinical surveys show a wide spectrum of presentation, ranging from mild monoarticular involvement to a rapidly destructive arthritis mutilans.[27,48,88] Five clinical patterns of psoriatic arthritis have been recognized.[89]

Group 1: Classic Psoriatic Arthritis With Predominant Involvement of Distal Interphalangeal Joints and Nail Lesions

The group 1 pattern is less common than generally appreciated; Wright gave a figure of 5% in 1959[48] and has revised this to 16.6% more recently.[90]

Group 2: Arthritis Mutilans

Arthritis mutilans is due to osteolysis of the phalanges and metacarpals. It occurs in about 5% of patients and is often associated with sacroiliitis (Fig. 61–4).

Group 3: Symmetric Polyarthritis

The presentation of symmetric polyarthritis is similar to RA and is seen in about 15% of patients (Fig. 61–5). There is a predilection for bony ankylosis of PIP and DIP joints with time, resulting in a poorly functional hand with a claw-like deformity (Fig. 61–6). Long-term followup of 131 patients with this pattern showed that 26% were seropositive for IgM RF on at least one occasion; 16% were consistently seropositive.[86a] It was thought that the majority of these patients had psoriatic arthritis and not RA.

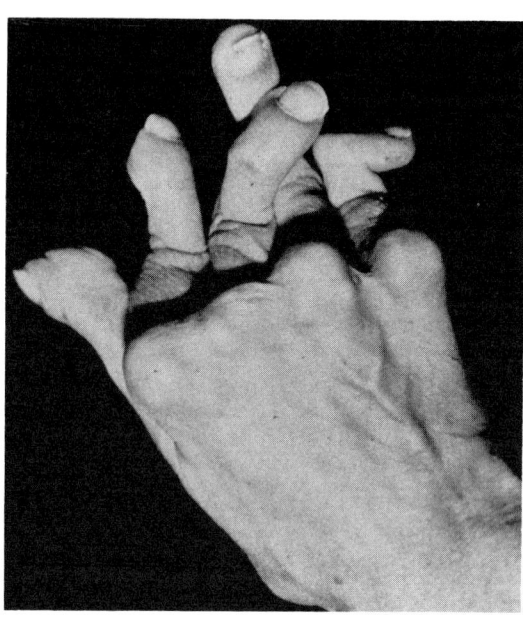

FIG. 61–4. Severe resorptive arthropathy resulting in arthritis mutilans.

Group 4: Oligoarticular Arthritis

The group 4 pattern is characteristically asymmetric, usually affecting scattered DIP, PIP, and MTP joints. Involvement of an MCP and PIP joint and a flexor tenosynovitis sometimes coincided, producing the "sausage digit" appearance (Fig. 61–7). This is the most common pattern, seen in about 70% of all cases.

Group 5: Ankylosing Spondylitis

Both sacroiliitis and/or spondylitis may be associated with psoriatic arthritis.[91,92] This is seldom the presenting complaint and usually becomes manifest after several years of peripheral joint disease.

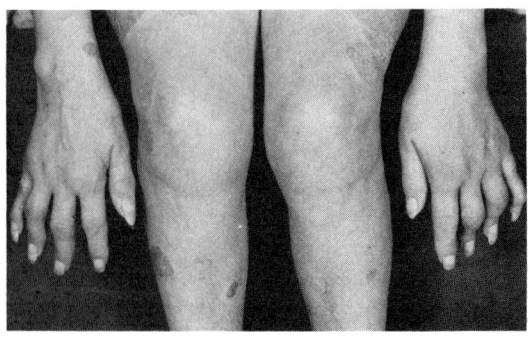

FIG. 61–5. A symmetric polyarthritis resembling rheumatoid arthritis in a patient with psoriasis.

FIG. 61–6. Longstanding psoriatic arthritis with a symmetric distribution. This patient had a "claw deformity" due to bony ankylosis of the proximal and distal interphalangeal joints.

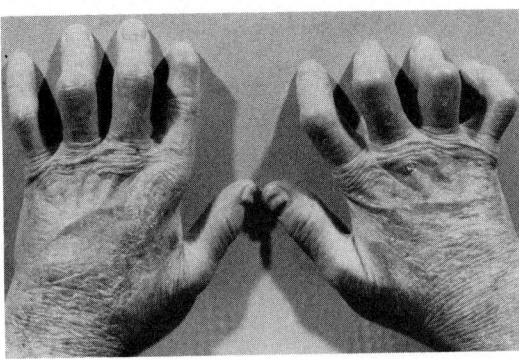

SKIN FINDINGS

No particular pattern of dermal involvement is associated with either peripheral psoriatic arthritis or spondylitis.[58] All patterns and gradations of severity of arthritis have occurred in patients with minimal skin lesions and in those with generalized exfoliative

FIG. 61–7. Psoriatic arthritis involving the metacarpophalangeal and proximal-interphalangeal joints of an index finger with an associated flexor tenosynovitis. This combination gives rise to the "sausage digit."

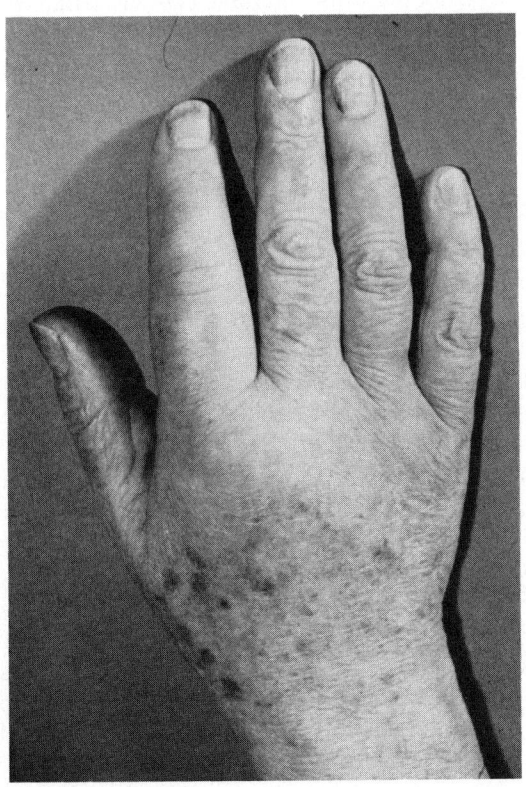

Table 61–4. Criteria for Diagnosis of Borderline Psoriasis

1. Psoriasis of the scalp must be palpable.
2. Presumed scalp psoriasis, simulating dandruff, must exhibit normal skin between plaques.
3. In the presence of eczema or seborrheic states, lesions other than classic plaques cannot be accepted as psoriasis.
4. Toenail lesions alone cannot be accepted as evidence of psoriasis.
5. In the absence of psoriasis elsewhere, only classic nail changes—i.e., pitting, onycholysis, and discoloration of the lateral nail edge—can be accepted as unequivocal psoriasis. In such cases fungal infection should be excluded by microscopy and culture.
6. Flexural lesions can only be accepted if they have the classic appearance of a psoriatic plaque. In such cases, microscopy of scrapings must be done to exclude Tinea or Candida infection.
7. Pustular lesions of the palms and soles are not acceptable unless accompanied by classic skin or nail lesions elsewhere.

psoriasis. In patients with a compatible pattern of seronegative arthritis or with a positive family history, the diagnosis may depend on finding psoriatic lesions in one of the so-called hidden areas: scalp, perineum, natal cleft, or umbilicus. In attempting to make a diagnosis of minimal psoriasis, one must avoid several pitfalls, and it is useful to bear in mind the criteria laid down by Baker[19] (Table 61–4). Psoriasis lesions typically occur on the extensor surfaces of the limbs and must be differentiated from other skin diseases associated with papulosquamous lesions.

NAIL CHANGES

It is generally accepted that there is a characteristic association between arthritis in the DIP joints and psoriatic involvement of the adjacent corresponding nails (Fig. 61–8). This takes the form of nail pitting,

FIG. 61–8. Onycholysis plus psoriasis of the nail bed in a patient who had an oligoarticular pattern of arthritis.

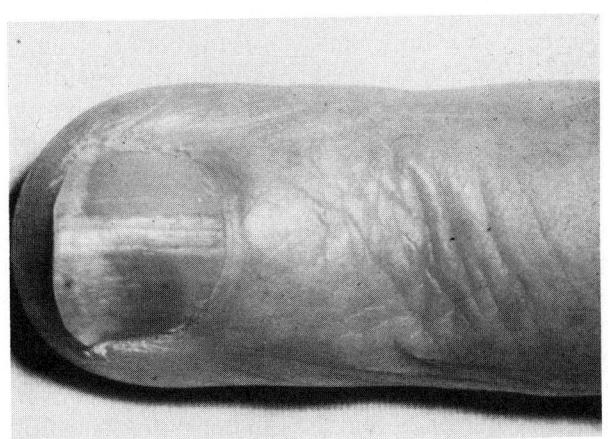

onycholysis, transverse ridges, leukonychia, crumbling, and subungual hyperkeratosis.[6,49,51,91] Wright[27] reported an incidence of nail dystrophy of 80% among patients with psoriatic arthritis compared to an incidence of 20% among patients with uncomplicated psoriasis. Baker[93] found nail involvement in 83% of patients with psoriatic arthritis, noting that the changes were not necessarily related to the pattern of distribution of joint involvement and that patients with deforming arthritis had more extensive nail changes. None of these abnormal nail findings are specific for psoriasis; conditions to be differentiated include fungal and bacterial infections, alopecia areata, lichen planus, and trauma. The most common differential diagnostic problem is fungal infection, usually caused by either Trichophyton rubrum or Trichophyton mentagrophytes. Although organisms can often be isolated from psoriatic nails, these are frequently found to be commensals,[94] possibly caused by the presence of a glycoprotein dermatophyte inhibitor in psoriatic patients.[95] Normal individuals often have some nail pitting, up to 70% according to Wright and Moll.[89] This phenomenon tends to increase with age, but the pits are less densely distributed than in psoriasis, being shallower and more irregular in outline.

ANKYLOSING SPONDYLITIS

An association between psoriasis and ankylosing spondylitis was noted much later than that with peripheral arthritis.[91,96,97] In the 1950s, the concept of *psoriatic spondylitis* as a disease sui generis gained favor.[50,51,84,98,99] This concept has been strengthened by studies showing an increased incidence of ankylosing spondylitis and sacroiliitis in patients with psoriasis.[27,90,100–102] Further credence to the concept of psoriatic spondylitis is found in some of its clinical and radiologic features in comparison to classic ankylosing spondylitis. Jajic[101] remarked on the distinct lack of back pain and stiffness as well as the poor correlation between clinical and radiologic findings. Distinctive radiologic features have been observed in some patients with psoriasis and spondylitis. The most impressive "atypical" appearance is paravertebral ossification;[103–105] other findings include vertebral fusion with disc calcification[106] and nonmarginal syndesmophytes.[96] The prevalence of these atypical features in a representative population of patients with psoriatic arthritis remain to be determined. Paraspinal ossification is certainly not unique to psoriasis, also being associated with senile ankylosing hyperostosis,[107] paraplegia,[108] fluorosis, hypoparathyroidism,[109]

familial hypophosphatemia,[110] and heredofamilial articular and vascular calcification.[111] Nonmarginal syndesmophytes have also been observed in Reiter's disease with spondylitis.[112] Spondylitis was noted in 40% of 130 patients with psoriatic arthritis;[113] only 21% had sacroiliitis, and 25% had radiologically evident syndesmophytes. Fully 60% of the latter group had radiologically normal sacroiliac joints and had no more symptoms or signs of spinal disease than those with normal spinal radiographs. Axial involvement occurred mostly in men (male/female ratio 6:1) with psoriasis onset somewhat later in life (mean age 35 years vs. 27 years for all patients).

EXTRA-ARTICULAR ASSOCIATIONS

Vasculitis and its common clinical correlates, such as subcutaneous nodules and nailfold infarcts, are not seen in psoriatic arthritis. Eye involvement has occasionally been alluded to in the past.[6,114] An incidence of eye involvement was noted in 31.2% of 112 patients with psoriatic arthritis.[115] Diagnoses included conjunctivitis, 19.6%; iritis, 7.1%; episcleritis, 1.8%; and keratoconjunctivitis sicca, 2.7%. Of the patients with iritis, 43% had sacroiliitis, and of those tested, 40% were positive for HLA-B27. Tests for antinuclear factor were negative in all the patients with iritis. Other extra-articular features that have been associated with psoriatic arthritis include myopathy,[116] Sjögren's syndrome,[117] aortic incompetence,[118–120] gastrointestinal amyloidosis,[121–123] renal amyloidosis,[124] and fever.[13]

DISEASE INTERRELATIONSHIPS

The seronegative arthritides often display certain common features, the most frequent being sacroiliitis or spondylitis, ocular inflammation, and the presence of HLA-B27. Because HLA-B27 has been strongly associated with an inherited susceptibility to both sacroiliitis[40,125] and iritis,[41] these common features may be manifestations of a shared genetic background rather than specific "complications" per se. Conditions described as associated with psoriatic arthritis include: ulcerative colitis;[102,126,127] ankylosing spondylitis;[92,98,101,102,104,128–130] Crohn's disease;[131–133] Reiter's disease;[96,98,130,134–138] and Behçet's syndrome.[139] Sometimes a striking familial clustering of these diseases is seen,[139] as shown in Figure 61–9. In this family, psoriasis, ulcerative colitis, and ankylosing spondylitis were grouped together in two generations.[139]

FIG. 61–9. Family study in which psoriasis, ulcerative colitis, and ankylosing spondylitis showed a "clustering" phenomenon. Patients DB and FB had psoriasis in addition to ankylosing spondylitis.

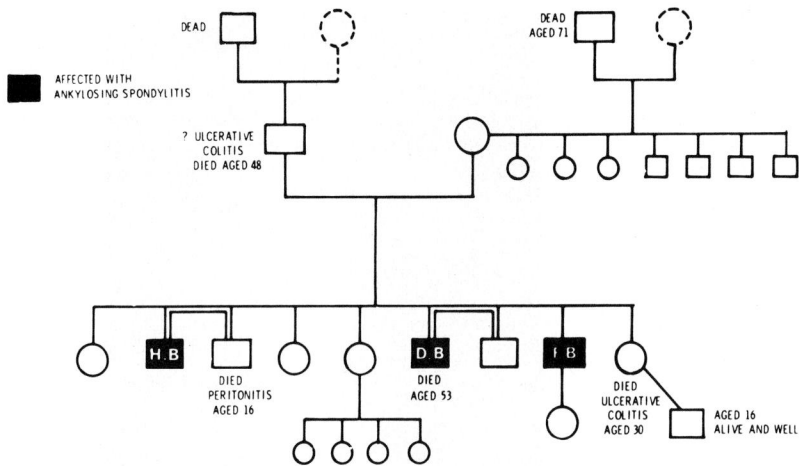

LABORATORY FINDINGS

There are no laboratory tests that aid in the diagnosis of either psoriasis or psoriatic arthritis. The most important finding is an absence of RF, including "hidden" RFs.[140] A positive RF in a typical case of psoriatic arthritis probably represents chance association.[141] Positive tests in psoriatic patients with features of RA most likely reflect the concurrent presence of these two common diseases.

Nonspecific findings include elevated acute phase reactants (e.g., fibrinogen, α-1 antitrypsin, complement components and C-reactive protein); a high erythrocyte sedimentation rate; anemia; and a transient leukocytosis.[19,60]

Hyperuricemia occurs in 10 to 20% of patients[19] and is related to the severity of the skin disease,[142–144] reflecting an increased nucleoprotein catabolism due to rapid cell turnover.[145] One study of serum uric acid in patients with psoriatic arthritis suggested that elevated uric acid may be due to concomitant therapy.[39] Elevated IgA levels occur in two thirds of patients with psoriatic arthritis and in one third with psoriasis alone.[146] Decreased IgM levels in mild psoriatic arthritis and elevated levels in more severe disease have been found.[147] Other findings have included elevated γ- and α-2-globulins,[86a] normal erythrocyte phosphoglucose isomerase activity,[148] and an absence of antinuclear antibodies.[149,150] Circulating immune complexes have been described in up to 50% of patients with both psoriasis and psoriatic arthritis,[60–62] and one recent report indicates they predominantly contain IgA.[151] Other reports indicate no specific immuno-globulin disturbance in psoriatic arthritis[152] and no correlation between disease activity and the degree of plasma protein alteration.[19] An increased adherence of granulocytes to nylon fiber columns has been noted in both psoriasis and psoriatic arthritis but the relevance of this observation is unclear.[153] Synovial fluid is usually of an inflammatory type with elevated leukocyte count, predominantly neutrophils, and a normal or elevated hemolytic complement level.[66,154] This is a useful feature in distinguishing psoriatic arthritis from RA but not from many other types of seronegative disease.

The association of psoriatic arthritis and psoriatic spondylitis with HLA antigens has already been discussed. The incidence of HLA-B27 was normal in patients with peripheral arthritis only.[10] All forms of axial involvement, however, including syndesmophytes without associated sacroiliitis, were associated with an increased incidence of HLA-B27. In the HLA-B27–negative group of patients with axial joint involvement, females preponderated (male/female, 0.06:1), the peripheral joint disease was more severe, and skin involvement tended to be greater.

RADIOGRAPHIC FINDINGS

Radiographic findings have been important in developing the concept of psoriatic arthritis as a disease entity.[27,121,155] In the majority of patients the findings are similar to those of rheumatoid arthritis but with a tendency to an asymmetric, oligoarticular distribution. However, some less common findings in both the peripheral and axial joints were considered more specific for psoriatic arthritis/spondylitis.

Findings in the peripheral joints included (1) erosion of terminal phalangeal tufts (acro-osteolysis) (Fig. 61–10); (2) "whittling" of phalanges, metacarpals, and metatarsals; (3) "cupping" of the proximal portion of the phalanges (combined with "whittling," this is the "pencil-in-cup" deformity) (Fig. 61–11); (4) bony ankylosis (Fig. 61–12); (5) destruction of isolated small joints; (Fig. 61–13); (6) predilection for DIP and PIP joints with relative sparing of MCP and MTP joints (Figs. 61–14 and 61–15); (7) osteolysis of bones (arthritis mutilans), particularly the metatarsals (Fig. 61–16); and (8) a relative lack of osteoporosis in comparison to the degree of joint involvement.

Findings in the axial skeleton include (1) paraver-

FIG. 61–11. "Whittling" of the middle phalanx and expansion of the base of the distal phalanx—the "pencil-in-cup" deformity.

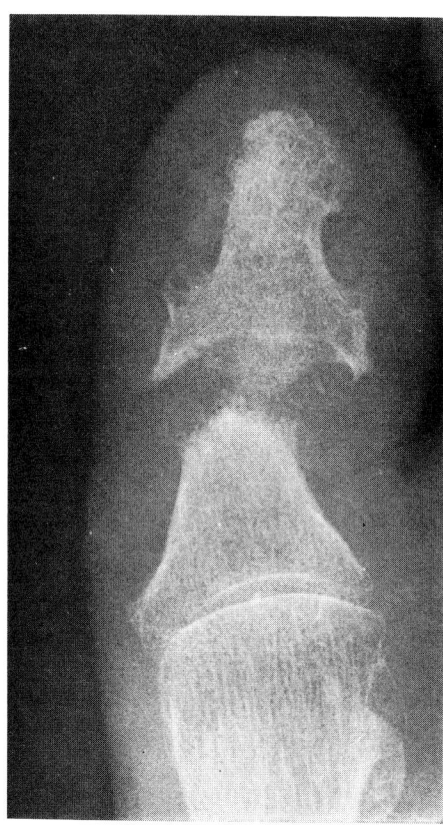

FIG. 61–10. Psoriatic arthritis with acro-osteolysis of the terminal phalanx of the great toe.

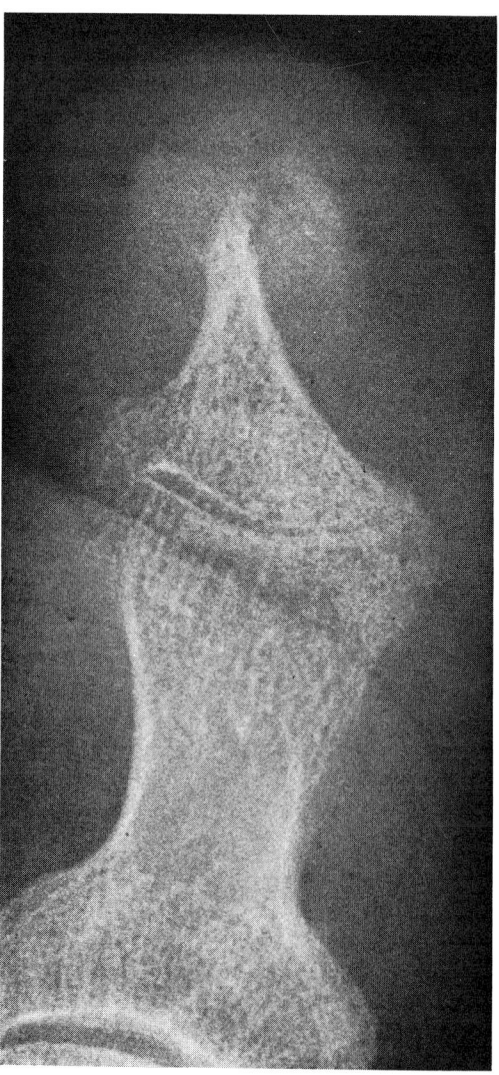

FIG. 61–12. Bony ankylosis of distal interphalangeal joints in a patient with psoriatic arthritis.

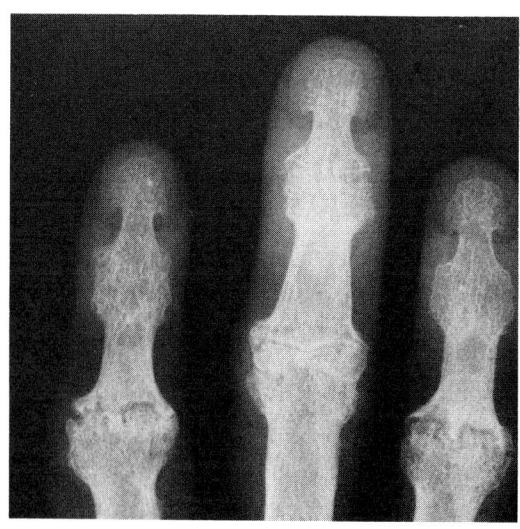

FIG. 61–13. Complete destruction of middle proximal interphalangeal joint. Also note bony ankylosis of corresponding distal interphalangeal joint.

FIG. 61–15. Osteolysis of bones of metacarphophalangeal joints with resulting subluxations.

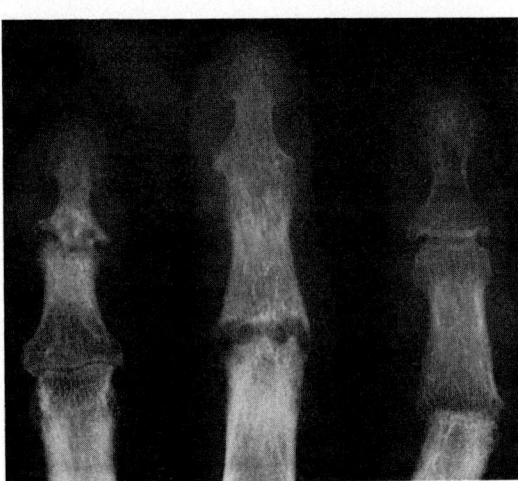

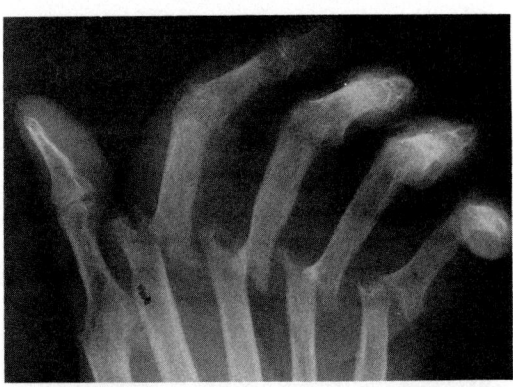

tebral ossification;[103–105] (2) atypical syndesmophytes, often present without sacroiliitis (see Fig. 61–17);[96,113] (3) asymmetric sacroiliitis;[101,113] (4) solid fusion of thoracic vertebrae;[113] (5) rarity of the typical "bamboo" spine of ankylosing spondylitis;[113] (6) a tendency for cervical spine disease to exhibit intervertebral disc space narrowing and ankylosis (Fig. 61–18), apophyseal sclerosis, and interspinous and/or anterior ligamentous calcification.[113] There is one report of spontaneous atlantoaxial fusion.[156]

FIG. 61–14. Destructive arthritis of an isolated distal interphalangeal joint with osteolysis of the proximal phalanx.

FIG. 61–16. Prominent metatarsophalangeal involvement with subluxation and cupping of the base of the proximal phalanges. The big toe distal interphalangeal joint shows characteristic marginal erosions.

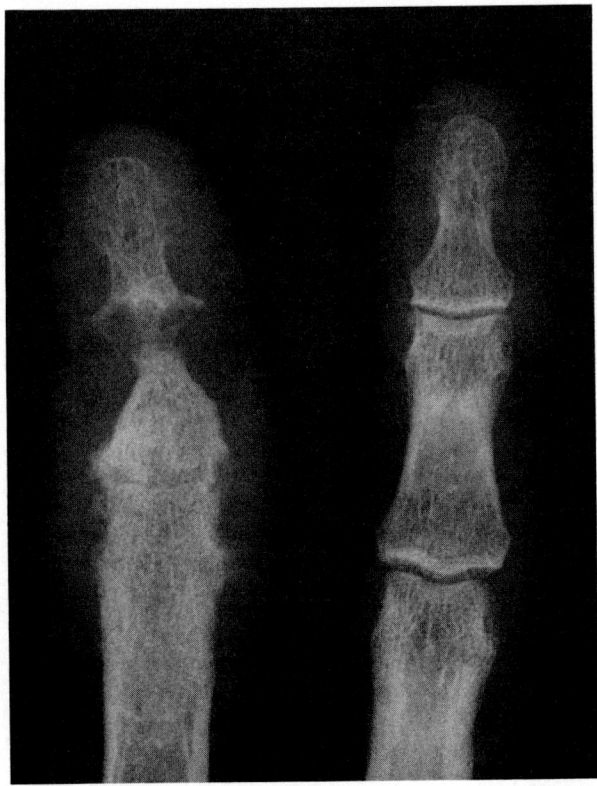

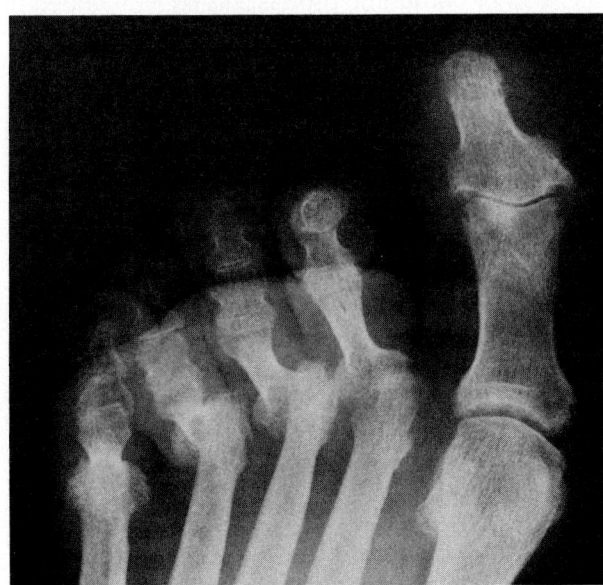

FIG. 61–17. Psoriatic arthritis with axial involvement. The patient was HLA-B27 positive and had no radiologic evidence of sacroiliitis, but atypical syndesmophytes are observed.

FIG. 61–18. Ankylosis of cervical apophyseal joints in a patient with psoriatic spondylitis in association with bilateral sacroiliitis.

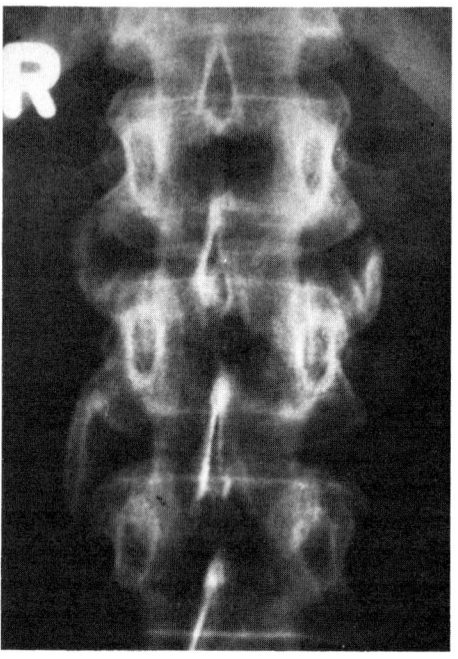

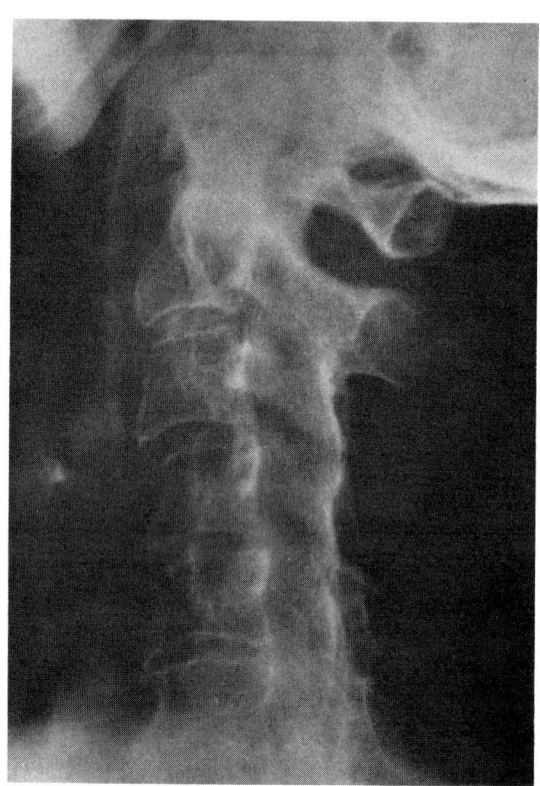

DIFFERENTIAL DIAGNOSIS

If other rheumatic diseases have been excluded, the presence of an inflammatory arthritis in association with psoriasis is usually sufficient grounds for a diagnosis of psoriatic arthritis. Problems arise when the evidence for psoriasis is lacking or equivocal; in such instances it is useful to follow the guidelines for the diagnosis of borderline psoriasis as recommended in Table 61–2. Errors may occur in relation to seborrheic dermatitis, other papulosquamous lesions, and fungal infections of the nails. Nail pitting alone lacks specificity in differentiating between psoriasis and other conditions such as exfoliative dermatitis and eczema. While isolated nail pitting is a normal occurrence, 20 fingernail pits per person suggest psoriasis, and more than 60 pits are virtually never found in the absence of psoriasis.[157] Keratodermia blenorrhagica, as seen in Reiter's syndrome, is indistinguishable both clinically and histologically from pustular psoriasis. The nail changes encountered in Reiter's syndrome are identical also and can lead to diagnostic confusion. As noted already, a mild conjunctivitis can occur in psoriasis, and this cannot be relied on to differentiate Reiter's syndrome from psoriatic arthritis. Indeed, attempts at differentiation may be artificial, because some patients presenting with a well-defined Reiter's syndrome later progress to psoriatic arthritis.[130]

Some cases of early primary osteoarthritis of the hands, especially the erosive form, may resemble psoriatic arthritis. In such instances, the presence of bony thickening of DIP and PIP joints (Heberden's and Bouchard's nodes) and the involvement of the first carpometacarpal joint helps to establish a diagnosis of osteoarthritis.

The onset of psoriatic arthritis may be very acute, and when it involves a distal joint, gout is often suspected;[49,91,158] joint aspiration for detection of urate crystals is mandatory. Both gout and pseudogout may occur in association with well-defined psoriatic arthritis.[79] Psoriatic arthritis may flare following trauma to a given joint. If such a "traumatic" arthritis fails to resolve within the usual course of a few weeks, a diagnosis of psoriatic arthritis should be made until proven otherwise. Joint aspiration showing inflammatory-type fluid may help in this situation.

JUVENILE PSORIATIC ARTHRITIS

Psoriatic arthritis has been identified as one subtype of juvenile chronic polyarthritis.[25,80,81] Unlike the adult form of the disease, there is a female/male ratio of about 3:2. The mean age of onset of both the psoriasis and the arthritis is 9 to 12 years. Arthritis antedates the skin changes in about 50% of patients. The mode of arthritis onset and its progression differ from the adult variety, in that onset often is acute, and onset is monoarticular in about one third of cases. Unlike the usual course of pauciarticular juvenile (JRA), however, most patients develop arthritis in five or more additional joints, usually in an asymmetric pattern. Another difference from adult psoriatic arthritis is hip involvement in between 30 and 40% of cases. Some children have required bilateral hip arthroplasties.[81] A "sausage" digit is the presenting feature in about 12% of patients and occurs at some stage of the disease in 23% of patients. The pattern of skin and nail involvement is similar to that seen in adults. As in the adult, extra-articular manifestations are rare in children. Iridocyclitis occurred in 8% of patients in one series,[81] causing initial confusion with pauciarticular JRA, particularly because the majority of these patients are antinuclear antibody (ANA) positive. Positive tests for ANA were found in 17% of patients.[81] These patients had an earlier onset (mean 4 years), most were girls, and tended to do poorly. In another report,[25] the arthritis was relatively benign and was generally easily controlled with nonsteroidal anti-inflammatory drugs (NSAIDs). No patient required remittive agents. In contrast, the patients described by Shore and Ansell[81] generally had severe arthritis; 35% required systemic corticosteroids at some point, and about 25% required disease-modifying agents such as gold, penicillamine, or azathioprine.

PROGNOSIS

Most patients with psoriatic arthritis have mild disease affecting only a few joints and following a rather episodic course.[84] Patients with psoriatic arthritis suffered less pain and disability than those with rheumatoid arthritis in a 10-year followup study of 227 patients;[159] only 5% of patients developed a deforming arthritis, and 97% lost less than 1 year of work. Arthritis or its treatment may have been a contributing factor in 3 of 18 fatal cases. One death was due to gastric hemorrhage, and two died with bronchopneumonia, thought to be related to immobility. Overall, the commonest cause of death was ischemic heart disease. An earlier study reported 24 deaths. Corticosteroids were implicated in 14% of these, while aminopterin was contributory in one and amyloidosis in another.[120] Death resulting from psoriasis itself is rare and is usually associated with either exfoliative dermatitis or amyloidosis. Patients with an associated spondylitis rarely develop aortic valvular incompetence or atrioventricular conduction defects.

MANAGEMENT

Psoriasis itself is a "socially difficult" disease for the afflicted, and the prospect of disability from arthritis makes it even more difficult to bear. Explaining the nature of the disease is therefore important, stressing that most cases follow a relatively benign course and that serious systemic complications, such as those of RA, are rare.

MILD DISEASE

Appropriate rest, splinting, range of motion exercises, joint protection, education, and adaptive devices, should be used in a manner similar to those employed in RA patients (see Chapter 47). Many cases of mild disease are well controlled with aspirin in anti-inflammatory doses or with one of the other NSAIDs. In patients with only a few involved joints, corticosteroids injected locally, both into joints and into tendon sheaths, are an important therapeutic modality. The least soluble preparation, triamcinolone hexacetonide (Aristospan), is the drug of choice, because systemic absorption is minimized and the local effect is prolonged. A relative contraindication to local corticosteroid therapy may be the presence of psoriatic lesions in overlying skin. One case of pyogenic arthritis of the ankle after intra-articular injection through psoriatic plaques has been reported.[89]

SEVERE OR POTENTIALLY SEVERE DISEASE

Although psoriatic arthritis is relatively mild, a small number of patients (about 5%)[86a] develop severe destructive inflammation that leads to marked disability. Most severe cases of psoriatic arthritis are referred for specialized care.

As the consensus is that the severity of the skin involvement affects the severity of the arthritis, it seems logical to maximize clearance of skin lesions. Photochemotherapy using oral 8-methoxypsoralens, followed 2 hours later by photosensitization using ultraviolet light type A (PUVA), has been successful in treating psoriasis. Such photochemotherapy suppressed the associated arthritis in one study.[160]

Antimalarials have long been considered contraindicated in the treatment of psoriatic arthritis, because they were thought to exacerbate the skin disease and even lead to life-threatening exfoliative dermatitis.[23,82,161] An uncontrolled study[162] found that 72% of patients with psoriatic arthritis improved or were stabilized while receiving hydroxychloroquine in a dose of 200 to 400 mg/day with no flare of skin lesions.

Chrysotherapy has also been linked anecdotally with an exacerbation of skin lesions[163,164] with greater toxicity than is usual in treatment of RA.[26,165] More recent studies, however, indicate that chrysotherapy is effective in suppression of psoriatic arthritis and is not accompanied by flare of the skin lesions.[159,162,166] The remission rate with chrysotherapy in psoriatic arthritis was better than that in RA (71.4% versus 59.5%), and drug toxicity was less.[166] Several uncontrolled studies have found oral gold (Ridaura) useful in the treatment of patients with moderate psoriatic arthritis.[167–169]

Systemic corticosteroids should generally be avoided, because even low doses may lead to exacerbations of the skin disease on attempted tapering, and increasing doses are then required for suppression.

Retinoids are effective in the management of psoriatic skin lesions. One recent double-blind study documented a modest improvement in psoriatic arthritis in patients treated with etretinate (Tigason) at a dose of 0.5 mg/kg/day.[170] A more optimistic, uncontrolled, study of 20 patients treated with etretinate has also appeared.[171]

Penicillamine has been used in the treatment of psoriatic arthritis,[81,162] but experience with this drug is too limited to provide reasonable guidelines on indications. Levamisole was used in six patients with psoriatic arthritis without improvement.[172]

There is now a consensus that cytotoxic drugs are of definite benefit in recalcitrant cases of psoriatic arthritis (Chapters 35 and 38). In a double-blind study of 21 patients, high-dose methotrexate (three doses of parenteral methotrexate, 1 to 3 mg/kg) was effective in suppressing both the skin and joint manifestations,[173] but there was a 30% incidence of side effects. Another study used a low-dose (5 to 15 mg/week) regimen, as shown effective in RA, and found no objective improvement as compared to placebo.[174] Perhaps higher doses of methotrexate (e.g., 20 to 25 mg/week) are required in psoriatic arthritis. Liver damage is a potential problem with methotrex-

ate,[175–178] especially in patients with psoriasis. Methotrexate is contraindicated in patients with pre-existing liver disease or who abuse alcohol. There are no specific guidelines for monitoring the development of hepatotoxicity; liver function tests do not reliably predict adverse morphologic changes as seen on biopsy.[179] It is the practice of most *dermatologists* to request a pretherapy liver biopsy with repeats at 1- or 2-year intervals, but this regimen has not been generally adopted by rheumatologists. Currently, a liver biopsy is advised at a cumulative dose of methotrexate of 1.5.[180] Other adverse reactions to methotrexate include bone marrow suppression, idiosyncratic pneumonitis, hemorrhagic enterocolitis, ulcerative stomatitis, alopecia, and dermatitis. Acute gouty arthritis may occur within 24 hours of administration of intravenous methotrexate.[181]

Intra-articular methotrexate (10 mg/5 ml of saline for a knee) had a short-term beneficial effect in psoriatic, but not RA.[182] Such therapy appears to have no advantage over the intra-articular injection of the sparingly soluble microcrystalline corticosteroid ester preparations (see Chapter 39).

Other cytotoxic agents have been used with varying success including aminopterin,[183] azathioprine,[184–186] and cyclophosphamide and triacetyl azauridine[186a] (no longer available). Good results using 6-mercaptopurine in a relatively low dose (0.36 to 2.4 mg/kg/day) have been reported in 13 patients.[187] Improvement began within 3 weeks with remission up to 10 months after treatment was stopped.[187]

Anecdotally, hydroxyurea (500 mg bid or tid) has been used successfully by Wright[83] and by myself.

Intra-articular radioactive colloids have generally proved less effective than in RA[188] or less effective than the injection of a long-acting corticosteroid preparation.[189]

Radiotherapy effectively suppresses both nail and DIP joint disease,[190] and I have used it successfully in several patients with severe DIP involvement. Its potential to cause leukemia precludes its more general use.

The indications for surgical intervention in psoriatic arthritis are similar to those for RA. Physicians sometimes are reluctant to perform surgery in patients with psoriasis because of skin colonization with pathogenic bacteria[191] and the occasional anecdotal report of an infected prosthesis.[192] Although bacterial colonies have been demonstrated to be more numerous on psoriatic plaques, the standard procedure of preoperative skin preparation is as effective at sterilizing the psoriatic plaques as the uninvolved skin.[193] Another anecdotal precautionary note is that the general tendency to fibrosis and ankylosis in psoriatic arthritis will have an adverse effect on long-term surgical results.[50,51] These fears seem ill founded, because a study of surgery in patients with psoriasis has shown that appropriate reconstructive surgery should not be withheld.[194] A review of hand surgery in psoriatic arthritis noted that the most useful procedures were MCP joint arthroplasties and fusion of fixed-flexion contractures at the PIP and DIP joints in positions of maximal function.[195]

REFERENCES

1. Alibert, J.L.: Précis Théorique et Pratique sue les Maladies de la Peau. Paris, Caille et Ravier, 1818, p. 21.
2. Menzen, J.: Über Gelenkerkrankungen bei Psoriasis. Arch. Dermatol. Syph., 70:239–240, 1904.
3. Bazin, P.: Leçons Theoriques et Cliniques sur les Affections cutanees de Nature Arthritique et Arthreux. (Monograph.) Paris, Delahaye, 1860.
4. Bourdillon, C.: Psoriasis et Arthropathies. Doctoral thesis. These de Paris, 298, 1888.
5. Garrod, A.B.: The Nature and Treatment of Gout and Rheumatic Gout. London, Walton and Maberly, 1859.
6. Hench, P.S.: Arthropathia psoriatica—Presentation of a case. Proc. Mayo Clin., 2:80–92, 1927.
7. Jeghers, H., and Robinson, L.J.: Arthropathia psoriatica: Report of case and discussion of pathogenesis, diagnosis and treatment. JAMA, 108:949–952, 1937.
8. Strom, S.: A case of arthropathia psoriatica. Acta Radiol., 1:21–34, 1921.
9. Zellner, E.: Zur Kenntnis der Arthropathia psoriatica. München Med. Wochenschr., 75:903–911, 1928.
10. Lambert, J.R., Wright, V., and Rajah, S.M.: Histocompatibility antigens in psoriatic arthritis. Ann. Rheum. Dis., 35:526–530, 1976.
11. Miller, J.L., Soltani, K., and Tourtellotte, C.D.: Psoriatic acro-osteolysis without arthritis. J. Bone Joint Surg., 53A:371–374, 1971.
12. Margolis, H.M.: Arthritis and Allied Disorders. New York, Hoeber, 1941.
13. Romanus, T.: Psoriasis from a prognostic and hereditary point of view. Acta Dermatol. Venereol. (Stockh.), 26(Suppl. 12):6, 1945.
14. Rose, H.M., et al.: Differential agglutination of normal and sensitized sheep erythrocytes by sera of patients with rheumatoid arthritis. Proc. Soc. Exp. Biol. Med., 68:1–6, 1948.
15. Ragan, C.: The clinical picture of rheumatoid arthritis. In Arthritis and Allied Conditions. Edited by J.L. Hollander and D.J. McCarty. 8th Ed. Philadelphia, Lea & Febiger, 1972.
16. Ropes, M.W., et al.: Proposed diagnostic criteria for rheumatoid arthritis. Bull. Rheum. Dis., 7:121–124, 1956.
17. Ropes, M.W., et al.: Diagnostic criteria for rheumatoid arthritis. Bull. Rheum. Dis., 9:175–176, 1959.
18. Baker, H.: Epidemiological aspects of psoriasis and arthritis. Br. J. Dermatol., 78:249–261, 1966.
19. Baker, H., Golding, N., and Thompson M.: Psoriasis and arthritis. Ann. Intern. Med., 58:909–925, 1963.
20. Leczinsky, C.G.: The incidence of arthropathy in a ten-year series of psoriasis cases. Acta Derm. Venerol. (Stockh.), 28:483–485, 1948.
21. Lawrence, J.S.: Prevalence of rheumatoid arthritis. Ann. Rheum. Dis., 20:11–17, 1961.
22. Lassus, A., Mustakillo, K.K., Laine, V., and Wager, O.: The lack of rheumatoid factor in psoriatic arthritis. Acta Rheum. Scand., 10:62–68, 1964.
23. Luzar, M.J.: Hydroxychloroquine in psoriatic arthropathy: Exacerbations of psoriatic skin lesions. J. Rheumatol., 9:462–464, 1981.
24. Mongan, E.S., and Atwater, E.C.: A comparison of patients with seropositive and seronegative rheumatoid arthritis. Med. Clin. North Am., 52:533–538, 1968.
25. Sills, E.M.: Psoriatic arthritis in childhood. Johns Hopkins Med. J., 146:49–53, 1980.
26. Sigler, J.W.: Psoriatic arthritis. In Arthritis and Allied Conditions. 8th Ed. Edited by J.L. Hollander and D.J. McCarty, Jr. Philadelphia, Lea & Febiger, 1972.
27. Wright, V.: Psoriatic arthritis: A comparative radiographic of rheumatoid arthritis associated with psoriasis. Ann. Rheum. Dis., 20:123–132, 1959.
28. Wright, V.: Proceedings of the 12th International Congress of Dermatology (Int. Congr. Series. No. 55). Amsterdam, Excerpta Medica, 1962.
29. van Romunde, L.K., et al.: Psoriasis and arthritis. III. A cross-sectional comparative study of patients with "psoriatic arthritis" and seronegative and seropositive polyarthritis: Radiological and HLA aspects. Rheumatol. Int., 4:67–73, 1984.
30. van Romunde, L.K., Cats, A., Hermans, J., and Valkenburg, H.A.: Psoriasis and arthritis. II. A cross-sectional comparative study of patients with "psoriatic arthritis" and seronegative and seropositive polyarthritis: Clinical aspects. Rheumatol. Int., 4:61–65, 1984.
31. van Romunde, L.K., et al.: Psoriasis and arthritis. I. A population study. Rheumatol. Int., 4:55–60, 1984.
32. Espinoza, L.R., Gaylord, S.W., Vasey, F.B., and Osterland, C.A.: Cell mediated immunity in psoriatic arthritis. J. Rheumatol., 7:218–224, 1980.
33. Shrank, A.B., and Blendis, L.M.: Folic acid antagonists in treatment of psoriasis. Br. Med. J., 2:156, 1965.
34. Moll, J.M.H., and Wright, V.: Psoriatic arthritis. Semin. Arthritis Rheum., 3:55–78, 1973.
35. Russell, T.J., Schultes, L.M., and Kuban, D.J.: Histocompatibility (HL-A) antigens associated with psoriasis. N. Engl. J. Med., 287:738–740, 1972.
36. White, S.H., et al.: Disturbance of HL-A antigen frequency in psoriasis. N. Engl. J. Med., 287:740–743, 1972.
37. Krulig, L., et al.: Histocompatibility (HL-A) antigens in psoriasis. Arch. Dermatol., 111:857–860, 1975.
38. Dausset, J., and Hors, J.: Some contributions of the HLA complex to the genetics of human diseases. Transplant. Rev., 22:44–74, 1975.
39. Lambert, J.R., and Wright, V.: Serum uric acid levels in psoriatic arthritis. Ann. Rheum. Dis., 36:264–267, 1977.
40. Brewerton, D.A., Coffrey, M., and Nicholls, A.: HLAB27 and the arthropathies associated with ulcerative colitis and psoriasis. Lancet, 1:956–958, 1974.
41. Brewerton, D.A., et al.: Ankylosing spondylitis and HL-A 27. Lancet, 1:904–907, 1973.
42. Medsger, T.A., et al.: HL-A antigen BW27 and psoriatic spondylitis. Arthritis Rheum., 17:322–323, 1974.
43. Metzger, A.L., et al.: HL-A BW27 in psoriatic arthropathy. Arthritis Rheum., 18:111–115, 1975.
44. Espinoza, L.R., et al.: Vascular changes in psoriatic synovium—A light and electron microscopic study. Arthritis Rheum., 25:677–684, 1982.

45. Frangione, B., Cooper, N.S., and McEwen, C.: Rheumatoid factor in rheumatoid "variants." Arthritis Rheum., *6*:772, 1963.

46. Beaulieu, A.D., et al.: Psoriatic arthritis: Risk factors for patients with psoriasis—A study based on histocompatibility antigen frequencies. J. Rheumatol., *10*:633–636, 1983.

47. Woodrow, J.C., and Ilchysyn, A.: HLA antigens in psoriasis and psoriatic arthritis. J. Med. Genet., *22*:492–495, 1985.

48. Wright, V.: Rheumatism and psoriasis—A re-evaluation. Am. J. Med., *27*:454–460, 1959.

49. Bauer, W., Bennett, G.A., and Zeller, J.W.: Pathology of joint lesions in patients with psoriasis and arthritis. Trans. Assoc. Am. Physicians, *56*:349–352, 1941.

50. Coste, F., and Solnica, J.: La polyarthrite psoriasique. Rev. Franc. Etud. Clin. Biol., *11*:578, 1966.

51. Sherman, M.: Psoriatic arthritis: Observations on the clinical, roentgenographic and radiological changes. J. Bone Joint Surg., *34A*:831–852, 1952.

52. Fassbender, H.G.: Pathology of Rheumatic Disease. New York, Springer-Verlag, 1975.

53. Gardner, D.L.: Pathology of Connective Tissue Diseases. Arnold, London, 1965.

54. Farber, E.M., Nall, M.L., and Watson, W.: Natural history of psoriasis in 61 twin pairs. Arch. Dermatol., *109*:207–211, 1974.

55. Gottlieb, M., and Calin, A.: Discordance for psoriatic arthropathy in monozyotic twins. Arthritis Rheum., *22*:805–806, 1979.

56. Ross, J.B.: The psoriatic capillary: Its nature and value in the identification of the unaffected psoriatic patient. Br. J. Dermatol., *76*:511–517, 1964.

57. Redisch, W., et al.: Capillaroscopic observations in rheumatic diseases. Ann. Rheum. Dis., *29*:244–253, 1970.

58. Zaric, D., Clemmersen, D.J., Worm, A.M., and Stahl, D.: Capillary microscopy of the nail fold in patients with psoriasis and psoriatic arthritis. Dermatologica, *164*:10–14, 1982.

59. Monacelli, M.: Koebner reaction in psoriasis. *In* Psoriasis (Proceedings of the International Symposium, Stanford University). Edited by E.M. Farber and A.J. Cox. Stanford, CA, Stanford University Press, 1971, pp. 99–104.

60. Laurent, M.R., Panayi, G.S., and Shepperd, P.: Circulating immune complexes, serum immunoglobulins, and acute phase proteins in psoriasis and psoriatic arthritis. Ann. Rheum. Dis., *40*:66–69, 1981.

61. Karsh, J., et al.: Immune complexes in psoriasis with and without arthritis. J. Rheumatol., *5*:514–519, 1978.

62. Braun-Falco, O., Manuel, C., Sherer, P.: Demonstration of immune complexes of psoriatic patients using ^{125}I–C1q deviation test. Hautarzt, *28*:658–660, 1977.

63. Ullman, S., Halberg, P., Hentzer, B., and Sylvest, J.: Deposits of complement and immunoglobulins in dermal and synovial vessels in psoriasis. Acta Derm. Venereol. (Stockh.), *58*:272–273, 1978.

64. Fyrand, O., Mellbye, O.J., Natvig, J.B.:Immuofluorescence studies for immunoglobulin and complement C3 in synovial joint membranes in psoriatic arthritis. Clin. Exp. Immunol., *29*:422–427, 1977.

65. Munthe, E.: Relationship between IgG complexes and anti IgG antibodies in rheumatoid arthritis. Acta Rheum. Scand., *16*:240–256, 1970.

66. Townes, A.S., and Sowa, J.M.: Complement in synovial fluid. Johns Hopkins Med. J., *127*:23–37, 1970.

67. Fehr, K., et al.: Production of agglutinators and rheumatoid factors in plasma cells of rheumatoid and non-rheumatoid synovial tissues. Arthritis Rheum., *24*:510–519, 1981.

68. Braathen, L.R., Fynard, O., and Mellbye, O.J.: Predominance of cells with T-markers in the lymphocytic infiltrates of synovial tissue in psoriatic arthritis. Scand. J. Rheumatol., *8*:75–80, 1979.

69. Espinoza, C.R., et al.: Association between HLA-BW38 and peripheral psoriatic arthritis. Arthritis Rheum., *21*:72–75, 1978.

70. Gladman, D.D., Keystone, E.C., Russell, M.L., and Schachter, R.K.: Impaired antigen-specific suppressor cell activity in psoriasis and psoriatic arthritis. J. Invest. Dermatol., *77*:406–409, 1981.

71. Cohentervaest, W.C., and Esseveld, H.: A study of the incidence of hemolytic streptococci in the throat of patients with psoriasis vulgaris with reference to their role in pathogenesis of this disease. Dermatologica, *140*:282–291, 1970.

72. Farber, E.M., and Nall, M.L.: Genetics in psoriasis family study. *In* Psoriasis (Proceedings of the International Symposium. Stanford University). Edited by E.M. Farber and A.J. Cox. Stanford, CA. Stanford University Press, 1971, pp. 7–11.

73. Vasey, B.F., et al.: Possible involvement of group A streptococci in the pathogenesis of psoriatic arthritis. J. Rheumatol., *9*:719–722, 1982.

74. Mustakallio, K.K., and Lassus, A.: Staphylococcal alpha-antitoxin in psoriatic arthropathy. Br. J. Dermatol., *76*:544–551, 1964.

75. Bieracki, R., Sadowska-Wroblewska, M., and Zabokrycki, J.: Acro-osteolysis in the course of ankylosing spondylitis. Rheumatologia, *6*:163–168, 1968.

76. Lotz, M., Carsen, D.A., and Vaughn, J.H.: Substance P activation of rheumatoid synoviocytes: Neural pathway in pathogenesis of arthritis. Science, *235*:893–895, 1987.

76. Coe, R.O., and Bull, F.E.: Cirrhosis associated with methotrexate treatment of psoriasis. JAMA, *206*:1515–1520, 1968.

77a.Farber, E.M., and Peterson, J.B.: Variations in the natural history of psoriasis. Calif. Med., *95*:6–11, 1961.

77b.Lomholt, G.: Psoriasis, prevalence, spontaneous course, and genetics: A census study on the prevalence of skin diseases in the Faroe Islands. Copenhagen, G.E.C., Gad, 1963.

78. Short, C.L., Bauer, W., and Reynolds, W.E.: Rheumatoid Arthritis. A definition of the disease and a clinical description based on a numerical study of 273 patients and controls. Cambridge, MA, Harvard University Press, 1957.

79. Leonard, D.G., O'Duffy, J.D., and Rogers, R.S.: Prospective analysis of psoriatic arthritis in patients hospitalized for psoriasis. Mayo Clin. Proc., *53*:511–518, 1978.

80. Lambert, J.R., Ansell, B.M., Stephenson, E., and Wright, V.: Psoriatic arthritis in childhood. Clin. Rheum. Dis., *2*:339–342, 1976.

81. Shore, A., and Ansell, B.M.: Juvenile psoriatic arthritis—An analysis of 60 cases. J. Pediatr., *100*:529–535, 1982.

82. Reed, W.B.: Psoriatic arthritis. A complete clinical study of 86 patients. Acta. Derm. Venereol. (Stockh.), *41*:396–403, 1961.

83. Wright, V.: Psoriatic arthritis. *In* Textbook of Rheumatology. Edited by W.N. Kelley, E. Harris, S. Ruddy and C. Sledge. Stoneham, MA, Butterworth, 1981.

84. Vilanova, X., and Pinol, J.: Psoriasis arthropathica. Rheumatism, *7*:197–200, 1951.

85. Wright, V.: *In* Progress in Clinical Rheumatology. London, Churchill, 1965.

86. Robillard, J.: Le Rhumatisme Psoriasique (a propos de 53 observations). Doctoral thesis, University of Lyon, France, 1968.

86a.Wright, V.: Psoriasis and arthritis. Ann. Rheum. Dis., *15*:348–353, 1956.

87. Plenk, H.D.: Psoriatic arthritis—Report of a case. Am. J. Roentgenol., *64*:635–639, 1950.

88. Chaouat, Y., et al.: Le Rheumatisme Psoriasique traitement par le Methotrexate. Rev. Rhum., *38*:453–460, 1971.

89. Wright, V., and Moll, J.M.H.: Psoriatic arthritis. *In* Seronegative Polyarthritis. Edited by V. Wright and J.M.H. Moll. Amsterdam, North Holland, 1976.

90. Moll, J.M.H., and Wright, V.: Familial occurrence of psoriatic arthritis. Ann. Rheum. Dis., *12*:181–201, 1973.

91. Dawson, M.H., and Tyson, T.L.: Psoriasis arthropathia with observations on certain features common to psoriasis and rheumatoid arthritis. Trans. Assoc. Am. Physicians, *53*:303–309, 1938.

92. Reed, W.B., and Wright, V.: Psoriatic Arthritis. *In* Modern Trends in Rheumatology. Edited by A.G.S. Hill. London, Butterworth, 1966, p 375.

93. Baker, H., Golding, D.N., and Thompson, M.: The nails in psoriatic arthritis. Br. J. Dermatol., *76*:549–554, 1964.

94. Zaias, N.: Psoriasis of the nail—a clinico-pathological study. Arch. Dermatol., *99*:567–572, 1969.

95. Van Scott, E.J., and Ekel, T.M.: Kinetics of hyperplasia in psoriasis. Arch. Dermatol., *88*:373–381, 1963.

96. Epstein, E.: Differential diagnosis of keratosis blenorrhagica and psoriatic arthropathy. Arch. Dermatol. Syph., *40*:547–549, 1939.

97. Weissenbach, R.J.: Le psoriasis arthropathique. Arch. Dermatol. Syph. (Paris), *10*:13–17, 1938.

98. Graber-Duvernay, J.: A propos de la spondylarthrite psoriasique. Rev. Rhum., *24*:288–294, 1957.

99. Wright, V.: Psoriasis and arthritis—A study on the radiographic appearances. Br. J. Radiol., *30*:113–118, 1957.

100. Bruhl, W., and Maldykowa, H.: Analiza klinicnza 50 przypadkow artropatii tuszczycowej. Pol. Tyg. Lek., *15*:525–526, 1970.

101. Jajic, I.: Radiological changes in the sacro-iliac joints and spine of patients with psoriatic arthritis and psoriasis. Ann. Rheum. Dis., *27*:1–6, 1968.

102. Moll, J.M.H.: A family study of psoriatic arthritis. Doctoral thesis, University of Oxford, 1971.

103. Bunim, J.J.: The syndrome of sarcoidosis, psoriasis and gout. Ann. Intern. Med., *57*:1018–1022, 1962.

104. Bywaters, E.G.L., and Dixon, A. St. J.: Paravertebral ossification in psoriatic arthritis. Ann. Rheum. Dis., *24*:313–331, 1965.

105. Theiss, B., et al.: Psoriasis-spondylarthritis. Z. Rheumaforsch., *28*:93–107, 1969.

106. Langeland, N., and Roass, A.: Spondylitis psoriatica. Acta Orthop. Scand., *42*:391–396, 1971.

107. Forestier, J., and Rotes-Querol, J.: Senile ankylosing hyperostosis of the spine. Ann. Rheum. Dis., *9*:321–330, 1950.

108. Abramson, D.J., and Kamberg, S.: Spondylitis, pathological ossification and calcification associated with spinal cord injury. J. Bone Joint Surg., *31A*:275–283, 1949.

109. Salvesen, H.A., and Boe, J.: Idiopathic hypoparathyroidism. Acta Endocrinol., *14*:214–226, 1953.

110. Kellgren, J.H., Stanbury, W., and Hall, L.: Proceedings of the Sixth European Congress of Rheumatology. Lisbon, Geigy, 1967.

111. Sharp, J.: Heredo-familial vascular and articular calcification. Ann. Rheum. Dis., *13*:15–27, 1954.

112. McEwen, C., et al.: Ankylosing spondylitis accompanying ulcerative colitis, regional enteritis, psoriasis and Reiter's disease. Arthritis Rheum., *14*:291–298, 1971.

113. Lambert, J.R., and Wright, V.: Psoriatic spondylitis: A clinical and radiological description of the spine in psoriatic arthritis. Q. J. Med., *46*:411–425, 1977.

114. Harkness, A.H.: Non-Gonococcal Arthritis. Edinburgh, Livingstone, 1950.

115. Lambert, J.R., and Wright, V.: Eye inflammation in psoriatic arthritis. Ann. Rheum. Dis., *35*:354–356, 1976.

116. Recordier, A.M., et al.: Les atteintes musculaires au cours du psoriasis arthropathique. Rev. Rhum., *36*:91–98, 1969.

117. Whaley, K., et al.: Sjögren's syndrome in psoriatic arthritis, ankylosing spondylitis and Reiter's syndrome. Acta Rheum. Scand., *17*:105–114, 1971.

118. Clark, W.S., Kulka, P.J., and Bauer, W.: Rheumatoid arthritis with aortic regurgitation. Am. J. Med., *22*:580–592, 1957.

119. Muna, W.F., et al.: Psoriatic arthritis and aortic regurgitation. JAMA, *244*:363–365, 1980.

120. Reed, W.B., et al.: Psoriasis and arthritis—Clinico pathological study. Arch. Dermatol., *83*:541–548, 1961.

121. Ferguson, A., and Downie, W.W.: Gastrointestinal amyloidosis in psoriatic arthritis. Ann. Rheum. Dis., *27*:245–248, 1968.

122. Willoughby, C.P., et al.: Gastrointestinal amyloidosis complicating psoriatic arthritis. Postgrad. Med. J., *57*:663–667, 1981.

123. Qureshi, M.S.A., Sardle, G.I., Kelly, H.K., and Fox, H.: Amyloidosis complicating psoriatic arthritis. Br. Med. J., *2*:302, 1977.

124. Taylor, R., Morgan, J.M., and Davie, R.M.: Renal amyloidosis secondary to psoriatic arthropathy. Br. J. Clin. Pract., *35*:410, 411, 414, 1981.

125. Calin, A., and Fries, J.F.: Striking prevalence of ankylosing spondylitis in "healthy" BW27 positive males and females. N. Engl. J. Med., *293*:835–839, 1975.

126. Jayson, M.I.V., and Boucher, I.H.D.: Ulcerative colitis with ankylosing spondylitis. Ann. Rheum. Dis., *27*:219–224, 1968.

127. Rotstein, J., Entel, I., and Zeviner, B.: Arthritis associated with ulcerative colitis. Ann. Rheum. Dis., *22*:194–197, 1963.

128. Fletcher, E., and Rose, F.C.: Psoriasis spondylitica. Lancet, *1*:695–696, 1955.

129. Lucherini, T., and Buratti, L.: Borsite reumatoide sottodeltoidea a granuli orizoidei. Rheumatismo, *17*:35–44, 1965.

130. Wright, V., and Reed, W.B.: The link between Reiter's syndrome and psoriatic arthritis. Ann. Rheum. Dis., *23*:12–20, 1964.

131. Ansell, B.M., and Wigley, R.A.D.: Arthritic manifestations in regional enteritis. Ann. Rheum. Dis., *23*:64–72, 1964.

132. Fox, T.C., and McCleod, J.M.H.: On a case of parakeratosis variegata. Br. J. Dermatol., *13*:319–346, 1901.

133. Hammer, B.P., Ashurst, P., and Naish, J.: Diseases associated with ulcerative colitis and Crohn's disease. Gut, *9*:17–21, 1968.

134. Dryll, A., et al.: Les formes de passage l'oculo-uréthro-synovite de Fiessinger-Leroy-Reiter et le rhumatisme psoriasique. Semin. Hop. Paris, *8*:499–515, 1969.

135. Dunlop, E.M., Harper, I.A., and Jones, B.R.: Sero-negative polyarthritis. The Bedsonia (Chlamydia) group of agents and Reiter's disease, a progress report. Ann. Rheum. Dis., *27*:234–239, 1968.

136. Hall, W.H., and Finegold, S.: Study of 23 cases of Reiter's syndrome. Ann. Intern. Med., *38*:533–550, 1953.

137. Maxwell, J.D., et al.: Reiter's syndrome and psoriasis. Scott. Med. J., *11*:14–18, 1966.

138. Perry, H.O., and Mayne, J.G.: Psoriasis and Reiter's syndrome. Arch. Dermatol., *92*:129–136, 1965.

139. Mason, R.M., and Barnes, G.C.: Behçet's syndrome with arthritis. Ann. Rheum. Dis., *28*:95–103, 1969.

139a. Bennett, R.M.: Familial spondylitis. Proc. Roy. Soc. Med., *64*:663–664, 1971.

140. Cracchiolo, A., Bluestone, R., and Goldberg, C.G.: Hidden

antiglobulins in rheumatic disorders. Clin. Exp. Immunol., 7:651–656, 1970.

141. Waller, M., and Toone, E.C.: Normal individuals with positive tests for rheumatoid factor. Arthritis Rheum., 15:348–359, 1968.

142. Baumann, R.R., and Jillson, D.F.: Hyperuricemia and psoriasis. J. Invest. Dermatol., 36:105–107, 1961.

143. Goldthwait, J.C., Butler, C.F., and Stillman, S.: The diagnosis of gout. Significance of an elevated serum uric acid value. N. Engl. J. Med., 259:1095–1098, 1958.

144. Tickner, A., and Mier, P.D.: Serum cholesterol, uric acid and proteins in psoriasis. Br. J. Dermatol., 72:132–144, 1960.

145. Eisen, A.Z., and Seegmiller, J.E.: Uric acid metabolism in psoriasis. J. Clin. Invest., 40:1486–1494, 1961.

146. Danielsen, L.: Immuno-electrophoretic analysis of serum proteins in psoriasis and psoriatic arthritis. Acta Rheum. Scand., 11:112–118, 1965.

147. Petres, J., and Majert, P.: Immunelektrophorese bei psoriatischer Arthropathie. Arch. Klin. Exp. Dermatol., 232:398–401, 1965.

148. Gaedicke, H., and Kaiser Ward Mathies, H.: Die Bestimmung der Phosphoglucose-Isomerase-Aktivitat in den Erythrocyten und ihre Bedeutung als diagnostisches Kriterium der Arthritis psoriatica. Klin. Wochenschr., 48:1456–1458, 1970.

149. MacSween, R.N., et al.: A clinicoimmunological study of serum and synovial fluid antinuclear factors in rheumatoid arthritis and other arthritides. Clin. Exp. Immunol., 3:17–24, 1968.

150. Sonnichsen, N.: Vergleichende immunologische Untersuchungen bei Lupus erythematodes, primar chronischer Polyarthritis and Psoriasis arthropathica. Allerg. Asthma, 15:1–8, 1969.

151. Hall, R.P., Gerber, L.H., and Lawley, T.J.: IgA-containing immune complexes in patients with psoriatic arthritis. Clin. Exp. Rheumatol., 2:221–225, 1984.

152. Zachariae, H., and Zachariae, E.: Antinuclear factors, the antihuman globulin consumption test, and Wasserman reaction in psoriatic arthritis. Acta Rheum. Scand., 15:62–66, 1969.

153. Sedgwick, J.B., Bergstresser P.R., and Hurd, E.R.: Increased granulocyte adherence in psoriasis and psoriatic arthritis. J. Invest. Dermatol., 74:81–84, 1980.

154. Kim, H.J., McCarty, D.J., Kozin, F., and Koethe, S.: Clinical significance of synovial fluid total hemolytic complement activity. J. Rheum., 7:143–152, 1980.

155. Petres, J., Klumper, A., and Majert, P.: Differentialdiagnose der psoriatischen Arthropathie auf Grund rontgen-morphologischer Befunde. Hautarzt, 21:26–29, 1970.

156. Szioba, R.B., and Benjamin, J.: Spontaneous atlantoaxial fusion in psoriatic arthritis. A case report. Spine, 10:102–103, 1985.

157. Eastmond, C.J., and Wright, V.: The nail dystrophy of psoriatic arthritis. Ann. Rheum. Dis., 38:226–228, 1979.

158. Barber, H.W.: Psoriasis. Br. Med. J., 1:219–223, 1950.

159. Roberts, M.E.T., Wright, V., Hill, A.G.S., and Mehra, A.C.: Psoriatic arthritis: A follow up study. Ann. Rheum. Dis., 35:206–208, 1976.

160. Perlman, S.G., et al.: Photochemotherapy and psoriatic arthritis. Ann. Intern. Med., 91:717–722, 1979.

161. Cornbleet, R.: Action of synthetic antimalarial drugs on psoriasis. J. Invest. Dermatol., 26:435–436, 1956.

162. Kammer, G.M., Sater, N.A., Gibson, D.J., and Schur, P.H.: Psoriatic arthritis: A clinical, immunologic and HLA study of 100 patients. Semin. Arthritis Rheum., 9:75–97, 1979.

163. Graham, W.: Comroe's Arthritis and Allied Conditions. London, Henry Kimpton, 1953.

164. Ragan, C., Tyson, T.L.: Chrysotherapy in rheumatoid arthritis. Am. J. Med., 1:252–256, 1946.

165. Rodnan, G.P., McEwen, C., and Wallace, S.L.: Primer on the rheumatic diseases. JAMA, 224(Suppl.):70–71, 1973.

166. Dorwart, B.B., Gall, E.P., Schumacher, H.R., and Krauser, R.E.: Chryotherapy in psoriatic arthritis. Efficacy and toxicity compared to rheumatoid arthritis. Arthritis Rheum., 21:513–515, 1978.

167. Dequeker, J., Verdickt, W., Gevers, G., and Vanschoubroek, K.: Long-term experience with oral gold in rheumatoid arthritis and psoriatic arthritis. Clin. Rheumatol., 3(Suppl. 1):67–74, 1984.

168. Barbieri, P., Ciompi, M.L., Bini, C., and Pasero, G.: Long term experience with oral gold in psoriatic arthritis. Clin. Rheumatol., 5:274–275, 1986.

169. Pasero, G., et al.: Psoriatic arthritis: Treatment with auranofin. Fifth SEAPAL Congress. Abstract 78P. Bangkok, 1984.

170. Hopkins, R., et al.: A double-blind controlled trial of etretinate (Tigason) and ibuprofen in psoriatc arthritis. Ann. Rheum. Dis., 44:189–193, 1985.

171. Chienagato, G., and Leoni, A.: Treatment of psoriatic arthropathy with etretinate: A two-year follow-up. Acta Derm. Venereol. (Stockh.), 66:321–324, 1986.

172. Rosenthal, M.: A critical review of the effect of levamisole in rheumatic diseases other than rheumatoid arthritis. J. Rheumatol., 5(Suppl. 4):97–100, 1978.

173. Black, R.L., et al.: Methotrexate therapy in psoriatic arthritis. JAMA, 189:743–747, 1964.

174. Willkens, R.F., et al.: Randomized, double-blind, placebo controlled trial of low-dose pulse methotrexate in psoriatic arthritis. Arthritis Rheum., 27:376–381, 1984.

175. Almeyda, J., et al.: Structural and functional abnormalities of the liver in psoriasis before and during methotrexate therapy. Br. J. Dermatol., 87:623–631, 1972.

176. Coe, R.O., and Bull, F.E.: Cirrhosis associated with methotrexate treatment of psoriasis. JAMA, 206:1515, 1968.

177. Podurgiel, B.J., et al.: Liver injury associated with methotrexate therapy for psoriasis. Mayo Clin. Proc., 48:787–792, 1973.

178. Shapiro, H.A., et al.: Liver disease in psoriatics—An effect of methotrexate therapy? Arch. Dermatol., 110:547–551, 1974.

179. Weinstein, G.D., and Frost, P.: Methotrexate for psoriasis. Arch. Dermatol., 103:33–38, 1971.

180. Robinon, J.K., Baughman, R.D., Auerback, R., and Cimis, R.J.: Methotrexate hepatotoxicity in psoriasis. Arch. Dermatol., 116:413–415, 1980.

181. Martin, J.H., Gordon, M., and Wallace, R.: Methotrexate in psoriasis. Precipitation of gout. Arch. Dermatol., 96:431–433, 1967.

182. Hall, G.H., Jones, B.J.M., Head, A.C., and Jones, V.E.: Intraarticular methotrexate. Clinical and laboratory study in rheumatoid arthritis and psoriatic arthritis. Ann. Rheum. Dis., 37:351–356, 1978.

183. Rees, R.B., et al.: Aminopterin for psoriasis. Arch. Dermatol., 90:544–552, 1964.

184. Feldges, D.H., and Barnes, C.G.: Treatment of psoriatic arthropathy with either azathioprine or methotrexate. Rheumatol. Rehab., 13:120–124, 1974.

185. Levy, J., et al.: A double blind controlled evaluation of azathioprine treatment in rheumatoid arthritis and psoriatic arthritis. Arthritis Rheum., 15:116–117, 1972.

186. duVivier, A., Munro, D.D., and Verbov, J. Treatment of psoriasis with azathioprine. Br. Med. J., *1*:49–51, 1974.

186a. Calabresi, P., and Turner, R.W.: Beneficial effects of triacetyl azauridine in psoriasis and mycosis fungoides. Ann. Intern. Med., *64*:352–371, 1966.

187. Baum, J., et al.: Treatment of psoriatic arthritis with 6-mercaptopurine. Arthritis Rheum., 16:139–147, 1973.

188. Szanto, E.: Long term follow up of ⁹⁰Yttrium-treated knee joint arthritis. Scand. J. Rheumatol., *6*:209–212, 1977.

189. Gumpel, J.M.: Synoviorthesis with erbium 169: A double blind controlled comparison of erbium 169 with corticosteroids. Ann. Rheum. Dis., *38*:341–343, 1979.

190. Popp, W.C., and Addington, E.A.: Roentgen therapy for psoriasis of nails and psoriatic arthritis. Radiology, *36*:98–100, 1941.

191. Noble, W.C., and Sarin, J.A.: Carriage of staphylococcus aureus in psoriasis. Br. Med. J., 1:417–418, 1968.

192. Kummerle, K., Wessinghage, D., and Schweikert, C.H.: Risk of alloplastic replacements in degenerative and inflammatory diseases of joints. Acta Orthop. Belg., 37:541–548, 1971.

193. Lynfield, Y.L., Ostroff, G., and Abraham, J.: Bacteria, skin sterilization and wound healing in psoriasis. N.Y. J. Med., 72:1247–1250, 1972.

194. Lambert, J.R., and Wright, V.: Surgery in patients with psoriasis and arthritis. Rheum. Rehabil., *18*:35–37, 1979.

195. Belsky, M.R., et al.: Hand involvement in psoriatic arthritis. J. Hand Surg., *7*:203–207, 1982.

62

ENTEROPATHIC ARTHRITIS

MARLENE A. ALDO-BENSON

The rheumatic syndromes associated with inflammatory bowel disease (IBD), Whipple's syndrome, intestinal bypass surgery, and pancreatitis are the subjects of this chapter.

ARTICULAR MANIFESTATIONS OF INFLAMMATORY BOWEL DISEASE

The term *IBD* encompasses both ulcerative colitis and regional enteritis. Although there are many differences in their clinical and pathologic characteristics, they both involve a chronic inflammation of the intestinal mucosa and submucosa, and the articular manifestations of both diseases are quite similar. Thus, the arthritis associated with these diseases is considered here as one entity.

Bargen[1] recognized arthritis as a complication of IBD in 1929 and differentiated it from rheumatoid arthritis (RA). *Peripheral joint arthritis* and *spondylitis* may occur separately or together. The peripheral arthritis is discussed separately from spondylitis because it differs in incidence and in its clinical course.

PERIPHERAL ARTHRITIS OF IBD

PREVALENCE

Musculoskeletal symptoms are one of the most common extra-abdominal problems occurring in IBD. From 2 to 22% of ulcerative colitis patients report ar-

thritis or arthralgias, and approximately 12% develop arthritis of peripheral joints.[2-5] The prevalence of peripheral arthritis in regional enteritis varies from 5 to 24%.[4-8] The age of onset of such arthritis is similar to the age incidence of IBD itself.[5] The mean age of appearance of arthritis in ulcerative colitis is 26 years and in regional enteritis is 31 years, but it may occur both in children and older adults.[2,3,9] The sex incidence is approximately equal;[2,4,10] the arthritis occurs most frequently in patients with more extensive and severe bowel disease.[2,5]

CLINICAL COURSE

Onset is usually acute, but it can be insidious. In over 80% of cases, arthritis coincides with the onset of the IBD or occurs within the first year.[2] Less frequently arthritis precedes clinically evident bowel disease by as much as several years.[4,7,11] The most commonly involved joints are the knees, hips, and ankles, in that order.[3,4,7] Smaller joints may also be involved, and the incidence of small-joint arthritis may be more common in regional enteritis than in ulcerative colitis.[6] The arthritis is frequently migratory, often begins as a monoarthritis, and remains oligoarticular and asymmetric in the majority of cases.[2,4,12] Those cases with acute onset often have very severe joint inflammation but mild arthritis and even arthralgias alone have been described.[12]

The course of the peripheral arthritis is usually episodic and recurrent.[5,13] In 90% of cases, the attacks are self-limiting, reaching peak severity within 2 days and resolving within 4 to 12 weeks. About 10% of cases follow a chronic course lasting more than 1 year.[5] Intervals between attacks are unpredictable and may vary from months to years.[2] In 60 to 74% of patients, exacerbation of joint symptoms correlates with a flare in their bowel disease.[5,12] This strong correlation occurs even in patients with arthritis antedating their bowel symptoms.

ASSOCIATED EXTRA-ARTICULAR FEATURES

Up to 50% of patients have some form of associated skin lesion.[2] Erythema nodosum is most common, but pyoderma gangrenosum also occurs frequently.[12,14,15] Other lesions such as erythema multiforme and exanthema occur less commonly.[16] Skin lesions accompany ulcerative colitis more frequently than regional enteritis. Iritis and, less frequently, episcleritis or uveitis can also occur.[2,12,17] Ocular problems occur more commonly in patients with spondylitis but can develop in patients with peripheral arthritis alone. Oral ulcers also occur and may be painful.[5]

LABORATORY AND RADIOLOGIC FINDINGS

There are no diagnostic laboratory tests specific for the arthritis of IBD. Normochromic normocytic anemia is often present, and the erythrocyte sedimentation rate is usually elevated;[2] a modest leukocytosis may occur. Serum hemolytic complement levels are elevated or normal but not decreased. Rheumatoid factor (RF) is absent in the serum.[2,5,12] Positive antinuclear antibody (ANA) tests may be found, but their incidence is no more frequent in the arthritis of IBD than in hospitalized sick patients without rheumatic disease.[2,5,12,18]

Synovial fluid findings are consistent with an inflammatory arthritis; leukocyte counts range from 4,000 to 40,000/μL, mostly polymorphonuclear leukocytes (PMN). Synovial fluid glucose levels are normal or slightly decreased, and bacterial cultures are negative.[6] Synovial histology is similar to that seen in RA.[12]

The peripheral arthritis is generally nonerosive and radiologic examination reveals only soft-tissue swelling and periarticular demineralization. Minimal erosions and joint space narrowing occur but are uncommon.[2]

DIFFERENTIAL DIAGNOSIS

When bowel symptoms are an obvious and major feature accompanying arthritis, other arthritis syndromes associated with bowel disease must be differentiated. Reiter's syndrome (reactive arthritis) may present as an asymmetric large-joint arthritis with or without spondylitis associated with diarrhea. However, in Reiter's syndrome, the diarrhea often remits spontaneously, stool cultures grow Campylobacter, Yersinia, Salmonella, or Shigella organisms, and attacks of arthritis seldom correspond with the severity of the bowel disease. The other characteristic features of Reiter's syndrome often develop later, making the correct diagnosis more obvious. Behçet's syndrome may be confused with arthritis accompanying IBD and associated with mouth ulcers and skin lesions. Central nervous system (CNS) lesions and the chronicity and severity of symptoms in Behçet's syndrome may help in differentiating these diseases.

When arthritis precedes IBD or when the bowel disease is mild, the correct diagnosis may be more difficult. A very acute monoarticular onset must be differentiated from septic arthritis, gout, or pseudogout by synovial fluid analysis. Ankylosing spondylitis with peripheral arthritis may be difficult to distinguish if bowel symptoms are minimal. The arthritis in those few patients with a chronic, unremitting course, may be confused with RA. In this case it may be difficult to differentiate these two diseases unless bowel symptoms develop or eventual development of RF is discovered. RA and positive tests for RF may coexist with IBD, but their incidence is no higher than in the general population.[13]

The syndrome should be considered in any patient with a seronegative sterile joint inflammation. Colonoscopy, barium enema, and small-bowel series will usually settle the issue in problem cases.

THERAPY

Because the arthritis of IBD is rarely destructive and usually resolves without loss of joint function, treatment should be symptomatic. Measures for preserving or restoring function are rarely necessary. Rest, gentle range of motion exercises, and nonsteroidal anti-inflammatory drug (NSAID) therapy usually suffice. Analgesics such as acetaminophen or propoxyphene can be used for pain relief. Systemic corticosteroids are rarely indicated for the joint disease alone, although they may be needed to control the bowel disease. Intra-articular corticosteroids are useful in relieving symptoms, especially in monoarticular disease or when large joints are involved. Gold, antimalarials, and other slow-acting agents are not particularly helpful and should be avoided.

In patients who have undergone bowel resection, the joint disease usually remits.[5] Bowel resection is rarely if ever indicated to treat the arthritis.

SPONDYLITIS ASSOCIATED WITH INFLAMMATORY BOWEL DISEASE

The association of spondylitis with IBD was first recognized about 30 years ago. Since then the characteristics of this syndrome have been more fully delineated.

PREVALENCE

The reported prevalence of spondylitis in patients with ulcerative colitis varies from 2 to 25%,[4,19–22] and in patients with regional enteritis, from 2 to 7%.[4,20,23,24] The wide variability from one series to another may be due to use of different criteria for spondylitis. About 10 to 18% of patients with IBD have only sacroiliitis, and most remain asymptomatic.[20,21] Typical symptomatic ankylosing spondylitis is less common, occurring in 4 to 6% of patients with IBD.

Reports concerning the association of genetic predisposition to the spondylitis of IBD are conflicting. Morris et al.[25] found that 75% of the patients with IBD and spondylitis were positive for the HLA-B27 haplotype. Although this is less than the prevalence of HLA-B27 in idiopathic ankylosing spondylitis (85 to 95%), it is still significantly higher than that in the general population (~10%). Another study found no significant increase in HLA-B27 in IBD patients with axial arthritis.[26] The differences in findings seem best explained by the studies of Dekker-Saeys et al.[27] All of their patients with IBD and spondylitis satisfied the New York criteria for ankylosing spondylitis, but the results showed a definite spectrum of clinical syndromes. Only those patients with features typical of classic idiopathic ankylosing spondylitis had an increased incidence of HLA-B27. Patients negative for HLA-B27 had less typical ankylosing spondylitis. The bowel symptoms predated the spondylitic symptoms in the latter group. Most patients with asymptomatic radiographic sacroiliitis were HLA-B27 negative. Thus, the spondylitis associated with IBD appears to be of two types, one of which shows no genetic predisposition. A second type is clinically and genetically identical to idiopathic ankylosing spondylitis. The prevalence of the second, classic spondylitis type,

however, is much higher in patients with IBD (3.7%) than in the general population (0.13 to 0.1%). Thus, the occurrence of classic symptomatic ankylosing spondylitis in IBD patients is not due to the coincidental occurrence of both diseases.

In most series of spondylitis associated with IBD, the male/female incidence ratio is 3:1[4,21] as contrasted to the 9:1 ratio for classic idiopathic ankylosing spondylitis.

CLINICAL COURSE

The age of onset of the spondylitis is generally similar to that of idiopathic ankylosing spondylitis.[21] Symptoms often occur before the onset of the bowel disease.[22,24] Back pain with stiffness and generalized malaise are the most common symptoms, but many patients have only mild low-back pain accompanying radiographic sacroiliitis.[20,22] Hip, knee, and shoulder arthritis may accompany spondylitis.[22] Unlike the peripheral arthritis, spondylitic symptoms do not usually parallel the activity of the bowel inflammation. Furthermore, control of the bowel disease does not measurably change the course of the spondylitis. Colectomy does not ameliorate symptoms.[2,4,21] The course of the disease is similar to that of idiopathic ankylosing spondylitis.[4] Partial or total ankylosis of the spine can occur eventually in some cases, but generally there is less physical deformity and limitation of motion in the spondylitis accompanying IBD than ankylosing spondylitis.[2]

THERAPY

Treatment is similar to that of idiopathic ankylosing spondylitis. NSAIDs and analgesics are used to relieve pain, and physical therapy is used to maintain function.

PATHOGENESIS

Although ulcerative colitis and regional enteritis have pathologic and clinical differences, they each involve abnormalities of both humoral and cellular immunity. These abnormalities may also relate to the joint and skin manifestations of the disease.

Circulating immune complexes have been found in the serum of 20 to 60% of patients with IBD as compared to controls with bacterial enteritis.[28–30] The pathogenetic significance of these complexes is unclear, however, because no immune complexes have been described in the bowel lesions or in the synovium from inflamed joints, and other features of immune complex disease such as vasculitis or glomerulonephritis are not a feature of the arthritis of IBD. Abnormalities in complement components have been described in IBD; both increased catabolism and increased synthesis of C1q, C4, C3, and properdin factor B accompany disease activity.[2,4] Again, the relationship of such changes to immunopathogenesis remains unclear.

Much experimental data suggest that IBD is an autoimmune disease.[29,30] Antibodies against epithelial cell antigens have been found in the serum and draining lymph nodes of IBD patients. From 60 to 70% of IBD patients have circulating antibodies reacting with antigens derived from the colon of germ-free rats, as compared to only 15% of controls. Such circulating antibodies react mainly with gastrointestinal epithelial cells.[31]

Abnormalities of cell-mediated immunity in IBD include circulating cytotoxic cells specific for antigens on intestinal epithelial cells[29] and antibody-mediated cellular cytotoxicity, where T cells are armed with antiepithelial cell antibodies before lysis of target cells by the complement system.[30,31] No mixed histocompatibility locus restricted cytotoxic mechanism has been definitely described as yet in IBD. Whether any of the immunologic abnormalities relate to the pathogenesis of IBD remains unclear.

ARTHRITIS ASSOCIATED WITH INTESTINAL BYPASS SURGERY

Intestinal bypass surgery for the treatment of morbid obesity was introduced in 1956. A jejunocolic shunt was performed in most of these patients but was soon abandoned because of the high incidence of life-threatening complications.[32] A jejunoileal bypass procedure was then used, but this too has multiple complications, including hepatic fibrosis and hepatic failure, cholelithiasis, calcium oxalate urinary tract stones, serum electrolyte abnormalities, increased incidence of tuberculosis, decreased absorption of fat and fat-soluble vitamins, and negative nitrogen balance.[33]

Polyarthritis has occurred in about 6 to 30% of patients after jejunoileal bypass.[33–36] The variability of incidence is probably due to the retrospective nature of most studies. A prospective study found a 28% incidence of arthritis and other connective tissue disease symptoms.[37] Arthritis occurs from 1 to 55 months following surgery. Its incidence is equal in male and females, and the peak age of onset is 30 to 35 years.

The arthritis is usually polyarticular, symmetric, and migratory in over half the cases. The knees, the metacarpophalangeal joints, and the wrist joints are most frequently involved, but any joints may become symptomatic.[36] The onset of arthritis may be either acute or insidious. In the prospective study, arthritis and other connective tissue disease symptoms were transient in 73% of the patients and chronic in only 27%.[37] Joint pain, swelling, and erythema of the overlying skin occurred with or without effusions. A few patients had only arthralgias.

Systemic features such as fatigue and morning stiffness were present, especially in the patients with skin lesions. Extra-articular symptoms, most commonly rash, occurred in approximately 80% of the patients with arthritis.[36–38] Papulopustules or erythema nodosum-like lesions developed anywhere on the body.[39–42] The papulopustules consisted of papular erythematous lesions, progressing over several days to pustular lesions, which then form crusts. Such lesions occurred in crops and sometimes disappeared completely for several months.[37] Biopsy showed a small-vessel vasculitis with immunoglobulin deposition at the dermal–epidermal junction.[40] The erythema nodosum-like skin lesions consisted of raised, tender, erythematous, indurated lesions, which occurred episodically in patients with arthritis, clinically resembling erythema nodosum. Histologically, these lesions also showed small-vessel vasculitis with features of nonsuppurative panniculitis.[36,40] Other extra-articular abnormalities included tenosynovitis, fever, malaise, pleurisy, occasionally accompanied by pleural effusion, and, less commonly, pericarditis and Raynaud's phenomenon.[36,39,43]

Synovial fluid from affected joints showed leukocyte counts ranging from 500 to 47,000/μL predominantly neutrophils.[36,39] An elevated Westergren sedimentation rate usually accompanied arthritis; RFs and complement levels were generally normal.[37,38] ANAs were rarely found, but titers were low. Cryoglobulins were found in patients with arthritis, but not in shunt patients without arthritis.[39,44] These cryoglobulins contained antibodies against bacterial antigens from Bacteroides fragilis and Escherichia coli. Another study, however, failed to confirm the presence of cryoglobulins in these patients.[36] Immune complexes have been demonstrated in the skin of shunt patients with the dermatitis syndromes, and circulating immune complexes have been found in these patients.[39,40]

A prospective study of patients undergoing bypass surgery showed circulating immune complexes in 65% of the patients who developed arthritis, as opposed to 31% of the patients who did not develop arthritis.[37] Such complexes are thought to result from stimulation of the immune system by bacteria growing in the blind loop formed by this surgical procedure. It is hardly surprising that a significant number of patients develop immune complexes after bypass surgery whether or not they develop arthritis. There are no data relating molecular size, immunoglobulin class, or other features of the immune complex to the development of arthritis. Serum IgA levels become elevated above the prebypass levels, more so in patients who develop arthritis than in those who do not.[37] Although there was one report of spondylitis with positive HLA-B27 occurring after bypass surgery, other series of patients did not show an increased incidence of this syndrome. No correlation between HLA haplotype and occurrence of arthritis has been found.[36,45]

The differential diagnosis of arthritis occurring after a bowel shunt procedure includes gout, RA, or systemic lupus erythematosus (SLE). Serum uric acid is often elevated in these patients, raising the suspicion of gout; the absence of urate crystals in the synovial fluid, however, easily refutes this diagnosis. The absence of ANAs and RF may help differentiate bypass syndrome from SLE or RA. The typical pustular or erythema nodosum-type rash in these patients can be very helpful diagnostically.

Because the arthritis is nondestructive and generally transient or episodic, treatment is symptomatic. Anti-inflammatory doses of salicylates or other NSAIDs, hot packs, physical therapy, and analgesics are helpful. Most patients respond to this regimen. Tetracycline or metromidazole may result in transient improvement of symptoms but generally are not useful in the treatment of persistent chronic arthritis.[36] If the arthritis remains chronic and becomes debilitating, prednisone, 10 to 15 mg/day, may be used. Such doses will often control both the arthritis and the dermatologic symptoms. If the arthritis remains debilitating or requires very large doses of prednisone for adequate control, reversal of the intestinal bypass procedure should be considered, because this invariably leads to remission.[45] Reversal of the bypass procedure also results in improvement of the skin lesions associated with a disappearance of immunoglobulin deposition at the dermal–epidermal junction.[40] This observation provides some indirect evidence for a pathogenetic role of immune complexes.

WHIPPLE'S DISEASE

Whipple's disease is characterized by weight loss resulting from malabsorption, fatty stools, and ar-

thritis and was first described by Whipple in 1907. Fewer than 200 cases have been reported.[46] In 1949, Black-Schaffer reported that the characteristic foamy macrophages seen in the lamina propria of the small bowel were periodic acid-Schiff (PAS) stain positive, glycoprotein-containing cells.[47] In 1960, Cohen et al, described rod-shaped particles in the intestinal mucosa, which were later recognized as bacteria.[48,49] These are probably related to disease etiology because they disappear when patients are successfully treated with antimicrobials. These typical particles are seen on an electron micrograph of intestinal mucosa in Figure 62–1.

Whipple's disease has a 9:1 male/female prevalence. Weight loss and abdominal discomfort occur in 95% of patients, but diarrhea occurs in only 70 to 78% of cases. Fever, lymphadenopathy, and darkly pigmented skin are found in about 50% of patients. Peripheral edema occurs in one third of patients and may be due to hypoalbuminemia.[50,51]

Arthritis and arthralgia are among the most common associated findings, occurring in 65 to 90% of patients. Frequently joint symptoms develop up to 10 years before the onset of abdominal or GI complaints. Thus, the true nature of the joint problems may not be obvious for many years. The associated arthritis occurs with 12:1 male/female ratio, even higher than that of Whipple's disease itself.[50,51]

FIG. 62–1. Intra- and extracellular rods in both longitudinal and cross section are evident by electron microscopy (×14,000). (Courtesy of Dr. Alan S. Cohen.)

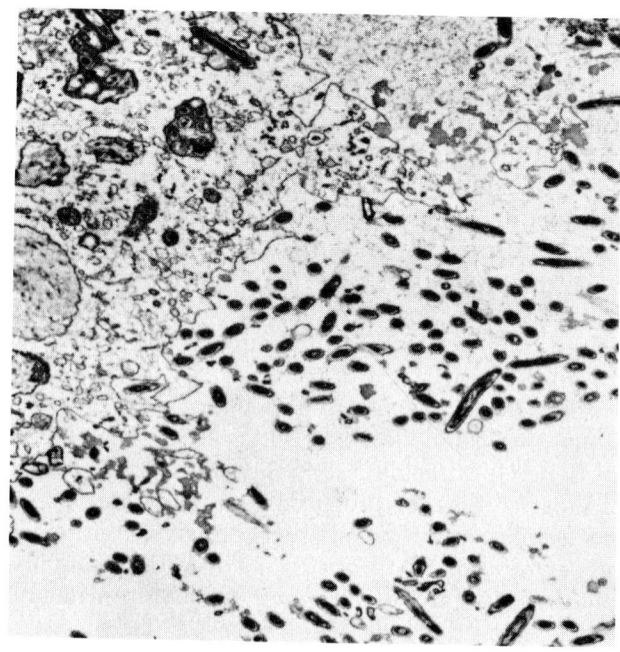

Most patients develop an overt arthritis with joint swelling, erythema, warmth, tenderness, and in some instances effusions, but 20% have arthralgia only. Arthritis is intermittent in 60% of patients with acute attacks lasting from days to weeks, but chronic arthritis lasting for several years can occur. Involvement may be either symmetric or unilateral but is usually polyarticular. The knees, ankles, and small joints of the hands are most commonly involved, but hips, wrists, and elbows may become inflamed also. Fever, lymphadenopathy, cough, dyspnea, or pleurisy occur more frequently in those Whipple's patients who develop arthritis. Pleural effusions or friction rubs have been reported in 10% of patients with this syndrome.[50,51]

The incidence of spondylitis in Whipple's disease is controversial. One retrospective series reported that 19% of arthritis patients had spondylitis, but many did not meet the diagnostic criteria for ankylosing spondylitis.[51,52] In a series from France, 11 of 36 patients with arthritis had clinical or radiologic evidence of spinal disease, but not all of these manifested classic signs and symptoms of ankylosing spondylitis.[52] Even though all of the patients with spinal involvement in Whipple's may not meet the diagnostic criteria for ankylosing spondylitis, spondylitis does occur with higher frequency than in the general population. The relationship of spondylitis to HLA haplotype has not been determined.

Laboratory findings are nonspecific and include anemia, elevated serum globulins, and hypoalbuminemia. RF tests are negative.[50] Synovial fluid is of the inflammatory type with leukocyte counts ranging from 2000 to 28,000/μL. Synovial biopsy in one case showed characteristic PAS-positive macrophages with bacilliform structures diagnostic of the disease[53] (Fig. 62–2). These cells have not been found in synovial fluid. The diagnosis of Whipple's disease is made by finding these characteristic foamy, PAS-positive macrophages containing rod-shaped bacteria in tissues from small intestine, lymph nodes, or synovium.

Both the joint and intestinal symptoms respond well to antibiotic therapy. Tetracycline given in dosages of 1 g/day over 2 to 4 weeks can result in permanent cessation of symptoms. Diarrhea may clear in 2 to 5 days, whereas arthritis may take up to 10 days to improve. Ampicillin and penicillin have also been used successfully.

ARTHRITIS ASSOCIATED WITH PANCREATIC DISEASE

Arthritis was described in patients with pancreatic disease initially in 1883. This uncommon arthritic syndrome is usually associated with subcutaneous fat necrosis and may occur in patients with acute pancreatitis or pancreatic carcinoma.[54] The arthritis may precede abdominal symptoms by many days, and in some cases no clinical pancreatic signs are found.[55] The subcutaneous fat necrosis may resemble erythema nodosum; however, the necrotic nodules may be widespread, and in some cases they become fluctuant.[56] Arthritis occurs in only 50 to 75% of patients with skin lesions. The combination of these findings in patients with pancreatitis carries a grave prognosis, with a mortality rate over 60%.[54] Patients with pancreatic carcinoma and this associated syndrome tend to have a higher incidence of the relatively rare acinar carcinoma.

Joint involvement is usually polyarticular, but occasionally a monoarticular, acute-onset arthritis may mimic gout. Ankles, knees, and small joints of the hands and wrists are most commonly involved. The arthritis tends to resolve without deformity if the acute pancreatic illness resolves. Polyserositis may accompany the arthritis and skin lesions.[54,55]

Laboratory findings are nonspecific. Eosinophilia of 5 to 20% is frequently seen in patients with pancreatic carcinoma and fat necrosis.[56] Synovial fluid analysis is quite variable and may indicate noninflammatory status or leukocytosis up to 18,000 WBC/μL with up

FIG. 62–2. PAS-positive granules in a macrophage in synovial membrane from a patient with Whipple's disease. (From Rubinow, A.G., et al. Arthritis in Whipple's disease. Isr. J. Med. Sci., *17*:445–450, 1981.)

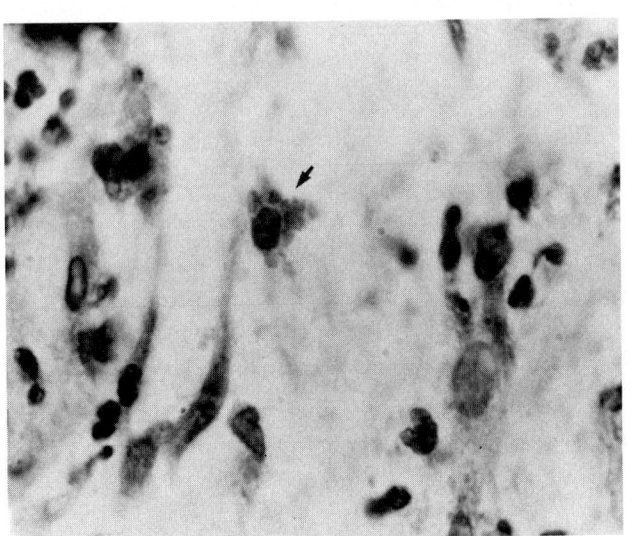

to 89% neutrophils.[57] Synovial biopsy may show acute inflammatory changes or fat necrosis.

Because of the reported fat necrosis in skin and joint, this syndrome has been thought to be due to pancreatic enzyme affecting the skin and joints.[56] Circulating immune complexes, however, have been found in about 45% of patients with acute pancreatitis; conceivably these may contribute to the arthritic syndrome associated with this disease.[58]

REFERENCES

1. Bargen, J.A.: Complications and sequelae of chronic ulcerative colitis. Ann. Intern. Med., 3:335–352, 1929.
2. Bowen, G.E., and Kirsner, J.B.: The arthritis of ulcerative colitis and regional enteritis. Med. Clin. North Am., 49:17–32, 1965.
3. Bywaters, E.G., and Ansell, B.M.: Arthritis associated with ulcerative colitis. A clinical and pathologic study. Ann. Rheum. Dis., 17:169–183, 1958.
4. Moll, J.M.: Inflammatory bowel disease. Clin. Rheum. Dis., 11:87–111, 1985.
5. Wright, V., and Watkinson, G.: The arthritis of ulcerative colitis. Br. Med. J., 2:670–675, 1965.
6. Wilske, K.R., and Decker, J.L.: The articular manifestations of intestinal disease. Bull. Rheum. Dis., 15:362–365.
7. Haslock, I., and Wright, V.: The musculoskeletal complications of Crohn's disease. Medicine, 52:217–225, 1973.
8. Ansell, B.M., and Wigley, R.A.: Arthritic manifestations in regional enteritis. Ann. Rheum. Dis., 23:64–71, 1964.
9. Ford, D.K., and Vallis, D.G.: The clinical course of arthritis associated with ulcerative colitis and regional enteritis. Arthritis Rheum., 2:526, 1959.
10. Kemper, J.W.: Arthritis accompanying ulcerative colitis and regional enteritis. Med. Rec. Ann., 54:311–316, 1961.
11. Rotstein, J., Entel, I., and Zeviner, B.: Arthritis associated with ulcerative colitis. Ann. Rheum. Dis., 22:194–197, 1963.
12. McEwen, C.: Arthritis accompanying ulcerative colitis. Clin. Orthop., 57:9–17, 1968.
13. Fernandez-Herlihy, L.: The articular manifestations of chronic ulcerative colitis. N. Engl. J. Med., 261:259–263, 1959.
14. Foster, J., and Brick, I.: Erythema nodosum in ulcerative colitis. Gastroenterology, 27:417–422, 1954.
15. Jacobs, W.H.: Erythema nodosum in inflammatory disease of the bowel. Gastroenterology, 37:286, 1959.
16. Goldgraber, M.B., and Kirsner, J.B.: Gangrenous skin lesions associated with chronic ulcerative colitis. Gastroenterology, 1:94, 1960.
17. Hammer, B., Ashurst, P., and Naish, J.: Diseases associated with ulcerative colitis and Crohn's disease. Gut, 9:17–21, 1968.
18. Taylor, K.B., and Truelove, S.C.: Immunological reactions in gastrointestinal disease. Gut, 3:277–285, 1962.
19. Palumbo, P.J., Ward, L.E., Sauer, W.G., and Scudamone, H.H.: Musculoskeletal manifestations of inflammatory bowel disease—ulcerative and granulomatous colitis and ulcerative proctitis. Proc. Mayo Clin., 48:411–416, 1973.
20. Dekker-Saeys, B.J., et al.: Prevalence of peripheral arthritis, sacro-iliitis and ankylosing spondylitis in patients suffering from inflammatory bowel disease. Ann. Rheum. Dis., 37:33–35, 1978.
21. Wright, V., and Watkinson, G.: Sacro-iliitis and ulcerative colitis. Br. Med. J., 2:675–680, 1965.
22. Zvaifler, N.J., and Martel, W.: Spondylitis and chronic ulcerative colitis. Arthritis Rheum., 3:76–87, 1960.
23. Steinberg, V.L., and Stoney, G.: Ankylosing spondylitis and chronic inflammatory lesions of the intestines. Br. Med. J., 72:1157–1159, 1957.
24. Acheson, E.D.: An association between ulcerative colitis, regional enteritis, and ankylosing spondylitis. Q. J. Med., 29:489–499, 1960.
25. Morris, R.I., Metzger, A.L., Bluestone, R., and Terasaki, P.I.: HLA-B27, a useful discriminator in the arthropathy of inflammatory bowel disease. N. Engl. J. Med., 290:1117–1119, 1974.
26. Enlow, R.W., Bias, W.B., and Arnett, F.C.: The spondylitis of inflammatory bowel disease. Evidence for a non-HLA linked axial arthropathy. Arthritis Rheum., 23:1359–1365, 1980.
27. Dekker-Saeys, B.J., et al.: Clinical characteristics and results of histocompatibility typing (HLA-B27) in 50 patients with both ankylosing spondylitis and inflammatory bowel disease. Ann. Rheum. Dis., 37:36–41, 1978.
28. Espinoza, L.R., et al.: Circulating immune complexes in the seronegative spondyloarthropathies. Clin. Immunol. Immunopathol., 22:384–393, 1982.
29. Strober, W., and James, S.: The immunologic basis of inflammatory bowel disease. J. Clin. Immunol., 6:415–432, 1986.
30. Kemler, J., and Alpert, E.: Inflammatory bowel disease associated immune complexes. Gut, 21:195–201, 1980.
31. Shorter, R.G., et al.: Effects of preliminary incubation of lymphocytes with serum on their cytotoxicity for colonic epithelial cells. Gastroenterology, 58:843–850, 1970.
32. Payne, J.H., DeWind, L.T., and Commons, R.R.: Metabolic observations in patients with jejeunocolic shunts. Am. J. Surg., 106:273–287, 1963.
33. Halverson, J.D., Wise, L., Wazna, M.F., and Ballinger, W.F.: Jejeunoileal bypass for morbid obesity. Am. J. Med., 64:461–475, 1978.
34. Bray, G.A., et al.: Intestinal bypass operation as a treatment for obesity. Ann. Intern. Med., 85:97–109, 1976.
35. Fernandez-Herlihy, L.: Arthritis after jejeunoileostomy for intractable obesity. J. Rheumatol., 4:135–138, 1977.
36. Zapanta, M., Aldo-Benson, M.A., Biegel, A., and Madura, J.: Arthritis association with jejeunoileal bypass: Clinical and immunologic evaluation. Arthritis Rheum., 22:711–717, 1979.
37. Leff, R.D., et al.: A prospective analysis of the arthritis syndrome and immune function in jejeunoileal bypass patients. J. Rheumatol., 10:612–618, 1983.
38. Ginsberg, M.D., Quismoria, F.P., DeWind, L.T., and Morgan, E.S.: Musculoskeletal symptoms after jejeunoileal shunt surgery for intractable obesity: Clinical and immunologic studies. Am. J. Med., 67:443–448, 1979.
39. Utsinger, P.D.: Systemic immune complex disease following intestinal bypass surgery: Bypass disease. J. Am. Acad. Dermatol., 2:488–495, 1980.
40. Drenick, E.J., Razzaque, A., Greenway, M.D., and Olerud, J.E.: Cutaneous lesions after intestinal bypass. Ann. Intern. Med., 93:557–559, 1980.
41. Williams, J.H., Samuelson, C.O., and Zone, J.J.: Nodular, nonsuppurative panniculitis associated with jejeunoileal bypass surgery. Arch. Dermatol., 1091–1093, 1979.
42. Goldman, J.A., et al.: Vasculitis associated with intestinal bypass surgery. Arch. Dermatol., 115:725–727, 1979.
43. Stein, H.B., et al.: The intestinal bypass arthritis-dermatitis syndrome. Arthritis Rheum., 24:684–690, 1981.
44. Wands, J.R., LaMont, J.T., Mann, E., and Isselbacher, K.J.: Arthritis associated with intestinal bypass procedure for mor-

bid obesity: Complement activation and characterization of circulating cryoproteins. N. Engl. J. Med., *294*:121–124, 1976.

45. Leff, R.D., Aldo-Benson, M.A., and Madura, J.A.: The effect of revision of the intestinal bypass on post-intestinal bypass arthritis. Arthritis Rheum., *26*:278–681, 1983.

46. Whipple, G.H.: A hitherto undescribed disease characterized anatomically by deposits of fat and fatty acids in the intestinal mesenteric lymphatic tissues. Bull. Johns Hopkins Hosp., *18*:302, 1907.

47. Black-Schaffer, B.: The tinctorial demonstration of a glycoprotein in Whipple's disease. Proc. Soc. Exp. Biol. Med., *72*:225–227, 1949.

48. Cohen, A.S., Shimmel, E.M., Holt, P.R., and Isselbacher, K.J.: Ultra-structural abnormalities in Whipple's disease. Proc. Soc. Exp. Biol. Med., *105*:411, 1960.

49. Chears, W.C., Jr., and Ashworth, C.T.: Electron microscopic study of the intestinal mucosa in Whipple's disease: Demonstration of encapsulated bacilliform bodies in the lesion. Gastroenterology, *41*:129, 1961.

50. Maizel, H.M., Ruffin, J.M., and Dobbins, W.O., III: Whipple's disease: A review of 19 patients from one hospital and a review of the literature since 1950. Medicine, *49*:175–205, 1970.

51. Kelley, J.J., III, and Weisinger, B.B.: The arthritis of Whipple's disease. Arthritis Rheum., *6*:615–632, 1963.

52. Canoso, J.J., Saini, M., and Hermos, J.A.: Whipple's disease and ankylosing spondylitis. Simultaneous occurrence in HLA-B27 positive males. J. Rheumatol., *5*:79–84, 1978.

53. Rubinow, A., et al.: Arthritis in Whipple's disease. Isr. J. Med. Sci., *17*:445–450, 1981.

54. Potts, D.E., Moss, M.F., and Iseman, M.E.: Syndrome of pancreatic disease, subcutaneous fat necrosis and polyserositis. Am. J. Med., *58*:417–423, 1975.

55. Gibson, T.J., Schumacher, H.R., Pascual, E., and Brighton, C.: Arthropathy, skin and bone lesions in pancreatic disease. J. Rheumatol., *2*:7–13, 1975.

56. Mullin, G.T., Caperton, E.M., Crespin, S.R., and Williams, R.C., Jr.: Arthritis and skin lesions resembling erythema nodosum in pancreatic disease. Ann. Intern. Med., *68*:75–87, 1968.

57. Hammond, J., and Tesar, J.: Pancreatitis associated arthritis: Sequential study of synovial fluid abnormalities. JAMA, *244*:694–696, 1980.

58. Foy, A., et al.: Immune complexes in acute pancreatitis. Aust. N.Z. J. Med., *11*:605–609, 1981.

ARTHRITIS AND LIVER DISEASE

63

JOSEPH DUFFY

Until the discovery of the hepatitis B surface antigen as a serologic marker for viral hepatitis,[1] an association between arthritic disorders and liver diseases received little attention. An excellent review by Mills and Sturrock in 1982 described the numerous clinical associations between diseases of the liver and joints.[2]

The first recognition of coexistent arthritis and liver disease dates to the mid-nineteenth century. Graves, in 1843, reported polyarthritis and rash in patients with hepatitis.[3] In 1897, Still recorded a somewhat different observation, that of improvement in patients with juvenile polyarthritis who were also afflicted with catarrhal jaundice.[4] In the 1930s Hench confirmed and extended Still's observation in adults with rheumatoid arthritis (RA) and primary fibrositis. Partial or complete relief of joint symptoms appeared before or concurrent with spontaneous jaundice of diverse causes. Remissions lasted up to 45 months, but relapse usually occurred in a matter of weeks after resolution of jaundice.[3] Attempts to reproduce this phenomenon by Hench and others were unsuccessful[5] until Thompson and Wyatt administered an empiric combination of bilirubin and bile salts by infusion, which produced the desired beneficial effects.[6] New methods of producing jaundice were constantly being sought, and in 1945 it was shown that the deliberate transmittal of viral hepatitis to rheumatoid patients was also efficacious but the benefit was short-lived.[7]

Jaundice was neither easy to induce nor reproducible by any method, however. These findings led to the search for other remittive agents. During the same era, the analogy of the spontaneous, temporary ameliorating effects of pregnancy on RA garnered attention. It was postulated that perhaps jaundice and pregnancy shared similar pathways for their beneficial effects.[8] This theory eventually led to the investigation of possible derangements in hormone metabolism and culminated in the landmark decision to administer an adrenocortical steroid preparation, compound E, to a patient with RA in 1948.[9] Additional studies showed the hypothesis of hormonal disturbances to be incorrect, and the liver has yet to reveal the secrets of its salutary effect on arthritis (see also Chapter 113).

In recent years arthritis has been described with several types of primary liver disease. This association has been observed with autoimmune and metabolic disorders as well as with viral hepatitis. Therefore, liver diseases may be associated with arthritis in some circumstances and may produce temporary remissions in others.

This chapter discusses primary liver disorders accompanied by arthritis or other connective tissue syndromes, primary articular diseases in which the liver may be affected, and liver dysfunction associated with the administration of anti-inflammatory drugs.

LIVER DISEASES

PRIMARY BILIARY CIRRHOSIS

Clinical Features

Primary biliary cirrhosis (PBC) is a rare, chronic, progressive liver disease characterized by inflammatory destruction of septal and interlobular bile ducts resulting in intrahepatic cholestasis. The disease primarily affects middle-aged women, and there appears to be an increased familial incidence. Recognition of PBC has increased worldwide because of greater physician awareness, detection of elevated serum alkaline phosphatase values through chemistry screening profiles, greater expertise in liver histopathology, and the exclusion of extrahepatic biliary obstruction through newer endoscopic techniques.

The disease may be asymptomatic or may manifest itself with pruritus, fatigue, and slowly progressive jaundice. Although the cause remains obscure, numerous documented abnormalities in humoral and cellular immune functions suggest an autoimmune pathogenesis.[10] Increased concentrations of tissue copper, especially in the liver, reflect the degree and duration of cholestasis because hepatobiliary clearance is crucial to the homeostasis of this trace metal.

The administration of D-penicillamine (DPA) for its chelating properties, however, is ineffective in reversing histologically advanced cases of PBC.[11]

In many patients, PBC is clearly a multisystem disease. In the Mayo Clinic series of 113 patients, 84% had at least one associated autoimmune disorder, and 41% had two or more such conditions in addition to PBC (Tables 63–1, 63–2).[12] The prevalence of extrahepatic involvement drops to 24% in those without liver symptoms or symptoms of less than 1 year's duration.[13] The autoimmune diseases were more common in women with PBC.[12]

Table 63–1. Autoimmune Associations in 113 Patients with Primary Biliary Cirrhosis

	Patients	(%)
Keratoconjunctivitis sicca		66
Definite	46	
Incipient	20	
Polyarthritis		19
Rheumatoid arthritis	10	
Arthritis of PBC	9	
Scleroderma and variants		18
Scleroderma	3	
CREST syndrome*	7	
Raynaud's phenomenon	8	
Thyroid disorders		19
Hashimoto's thyroiditis	7	
Hypothyroidism and/or goiter	12	
Cutaneous disorders		11
Lichen planus	7	
Discoid lupus erythematosus	2	
Pemphigus	2	
Pernicious anemia		2
Inflammatory bowel disease		1

*CREST syndrome = calcinosis, Raynaud's phenomenon, esophageal dysfunction, sclerodactyly, and telangiectasia.
(From Culp, K.S., et al.[12])

Table 63–2. Patients with Primary Biliary Cirrhosis and Two or More Autoimmune Diseases

Type of Autoimmune Disease*	No. of Patients	% of Total
KCS, thyroid disease	8	17
KCS, arthritis of PBC	6	13
KCS, CREST	5	11
KCS, RA	5	11
KCS, Raynaud's	5	11
KCS, scleroderma	3	7
KCS, Hashimoto's	2	4
KCS, CREST, Hashimoto's	2	4
RA, KCS, Hashimoto's	2	4
LP, KCS, Hashimoto's	1	2
Raynaud's, KCS, RA, Hashimoto's	1	2
LP, Hashimoto's	1	2
Raynaud's, arthritis of PBC	1	2
PA, thyroid disease	1	2
RA, KCS, thyroid disease	1	2
RA, KCS, Raynaud's	1	2
KCS, Raynaud's, arthritis of PBC	1	2
Total	46	100

*KCS = keratoconjunctivitis sicca; CREST = calcinosis, Raynaud's syndrome, esophageal dysfunction, sclerodactyly, and telangiectasia; RA = rheumatoid arthritis; LP = lichen planus; PA = pernicious anemia; Raynaud's = Raynaud's phenomenon; Hashimoto's = Hashimoto's thyroiditis.
(From Culp, K.S., et al.[12])

A unique arthropathy may be associated. Ansell and Bywaters first reported erosive bone lesions affecting large and small joints with remarkably few symptoms in three patients with PBC. Hypercholesterolemia was present, and tissue from one osseous lesion showed xanthoma cells.[14] Mills et al. described a case of PBC with fleeting episodes of inflammatory arthritis involving hands, wrists, and shoulders in the presence of hypercholesterolemia.[15] They attributed the joint inflammation to the elevated cholesterol levels, although the report showed no clear-cut demonstration of cause and effect.

In the Mayo Clinic series, 9% of patients exhibited an atypical polyarthritis termed the arthritis of PBC.[12] These patients did not meet the criteria for the diagnosis of definite or classic RA. Objective synovitis, usually symmetric, affected interphalangeal joints of the hands, wrists, ankles, and knees in various combinations. Attacks generally lasted weeks to months, resolved without deformity, and did not recur. Morning stiffness varied in duration, but was significant in fewer than half the patients.[12] Lauritsen and Diederichsen described a similar, atypical arthritis in 15 women with a positive antimitochondrial antibody test but no clinical or laboratory signs of liver disease.[16] In more than 80% of the Mayo series,[12] however, the diagnosis of the liver disorder antedated the onset of arthritis. Most patients had or developed

FIG. 63–1. Arthritis associated with primary biliary cirrhosis. Small cortical erosion in lunate. (From Marx, W.J., and O'Connell, D.J.: Arch. Intern. Med., *139*:213–216. Copyright 1979, American Medical Association.[18])

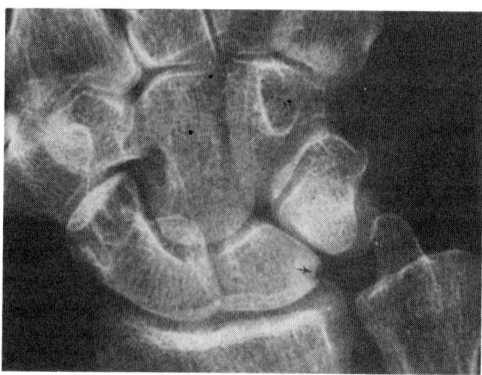

additional autoimmune disease features. Modena et al. from Italy recently confirmed these earlier observations.[17] There was no apparent relationship between the arthropathy and the histologic stage or progression of PBC.[12]

Distinctive radiographic features have been reported in some patients with PBC. In 1979 Marx and O'Connell described small, asymmetric, intracapsular, and nonarticular cortical bone erosions, mainly involving the distal small joints of the hands, accompanied by joint space narrowing in 6 of 12 PBC patients[18] (Figs. 63–1, 63–2). Subsequently, an extensive prospective radiologic survey of 42 patients with PBC confirmed the presence of articular erosions, usually in small joints, in 31% of cases. Additional

FIG. 63–2. Arthritic cortical erosion in proximal interphalangeal joint. (From Marx, W.J., and O'Connell, D.J.: Arch. Intern. Med., *139*:213–216. Copyright 1979, American Medical Association.[18])

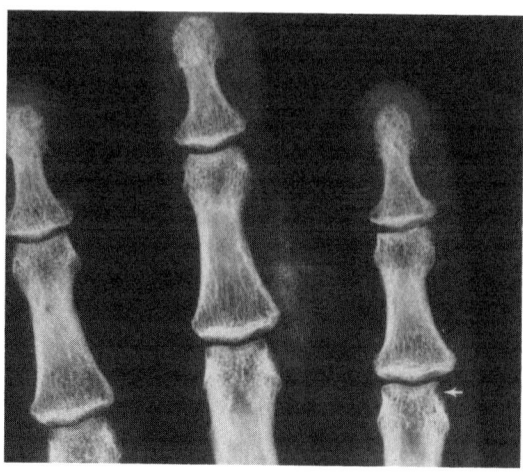

significant radiographic findings in this study included hypertrophic osteoarthropathy in 38% of the cases, osteopenia, and lytic medullary bone defects typical of cholesterol deposition.[19] One report described a surprising number of patients with avascular necrosis of femoral or humeral heads.[20] Chondrocalcinosis also has been reported in a few patients.[18]

RA coexists with PBC more often than would be expected by chance alone, with the prevalence ranging from 5 to 10% in several large series[12,15,21] and 19% in a smaller group from Sweden.[22] In the Mayo Clinic series, rheumatoid disease preceded the diagnosis of PBC in 45% of patients with the combination of RA and PBC. All patients affected by RA had additional autoimmune disease features, usually keratoconjunctivitis sicca.[12]

The sicca complex of dry eyes and dry mouth is the most common extrahepatic autoimmune disorder in patients with PBC. The prevalence varies from 66 to 100% of cases, depending on the extent of testing to make the diagnosis. Sicca symptoms usually are mild and elicited only on direct questioning. It is wise to include rose bengal staining in the ophthalmologic examinations of PBC patients because many cases of keratoconjunctivitis sicca may be discovered in a presymptomatic stage. The sicca syndrome is often associated with concurrent RA, scleroderma, and thyroid disease. It is usually preceded by the diagnosis of PBC (89%) and does not correlate with the duration or severity of liver disease.[12,23] The description of circulating Ro/anti-Ro (SSA) immune complexes and parotid deposition of anti-Ro in complexed form suggests a pathogenic potential for circulating immune complexes in the development of the sicca syndrome in patients with PBC.[24]

Since the description of scleroderma in association with PBC in 1964,[25] there have been several confirmatory reports.[12,20,26,27] The full spectrum of scleroderma has been encountered, with the prevalence varying from 3 to 31% if patients with Raynaud's phenomenon alone are excluded.[12,17,20,21] Most cases are mild and nonprogressive and constitute incomplete or complete expressions of the CREST variant.

Anticentromere antibody (ACA), an important serologic link, is present in approximately 29% of PBC patients, essentially all CREST patients, and 10% of those with diffuse scleroderma (Table 63–3). It is found rarely in other chronic liver diseases or connective tissue disorders.[28]

Although either liver disease or scleroderma may appear first, 50% of patients in one series exhibited one or more features of scleroderma before the diagnosis of PBC.[12]

A number of other autoimmune disorders have

Table 63–3. Features of CREST Syndrome in Patients with Primary Biliary Cirrhosis, with and without Anticentromere Antibody

Anticentromere	No.	C	R	E	S	T
Positive	14	5	7	3	6	6
Negative	34	0	0	1	0	0

C = calcinosis; R = Raynaud's phenomenon; E = esophageal motility abnormalities; S = sclerodactyly; T = telangiectasia. (Reprinted from Arthritis Rheum., copyright 1983. Used by permission of the American Rheumatism Association.[28])

been described in patients with PBC. Renal tubular and pulmonary diffusion defects, perhaps due to an autoimmune process, occur in 52% and 40%, respectively, of patients with PBC when appropriate tests are performed.[29] Clinical features and overt or latent thyroid function abnormalities reveal a prevalence of thyroid disease in 19 to 26% of patients. Hashimoto's thyroiditis and antithyroid antibodies are most common.[12,30] Cases of discoid and systemic lupus erythematosus (SLE) or lupus-like syndromes,[12,31,32] lichen planus, pemphigus, pernicious anemia, inflammatory bowel disease,[12] multicentric reticulohistiocytosis,[33] human adjuvant disease after silicone breast augmentation,[34] necrotizing vasculitis,[35] transverse myelitis,[36] and polymyalgia rheumatica[37] have been reported. In addition, there is a report of an extraordinary case of Churg-Strauss vasculitis with temporal arteritis, polychondritis, and PBC in a single patient.[38]

Laboratory Features

The liver disease itself may account for nonspecific hematologic changes, including anemia, variable leukocyte and platelet counts, and an elevated sedimentation rate. Serum protein abnormalities show hypoalbuminemia and hyperglobulinemia. Liver function studies are usually dominated by a marked increase in serum alkaline phosphatase levels in contrast to lesser elevations of serum transaminase values. Elevation of serum cholesterol levels has been neither significant nor consistent in patients with articular complaints or peripheral joint erosive lesions.[12,18] Numerous autoantibodies have been detected (Table 63–4), the hallmark being antimitochondrial antibody in 96% of patients.[12] Anticentromere antibody reacts with the centromeric region of metaphase chromosomes and is detected best using a human epithelial cell line (HEp2). It is present in up to 29% of patients with PBC and identifies those patients with or at risk for development of the CREST syndrome[28] (Table 63–3). Prevalence of other autoantibodies has varied from 22 to 70%.[12] Rheumatoid factor (RF), antinuclear antibody (ANA), and antibody to extractable nuclear antigens have shown no clear-cut relationship with the arthropathy of PBC.[18,39]

Serum concentrations of major immunoglobulins are elevated in almost all cases of PBC. IgM levels are increased in 95% of cases and occasionally are of monoclonal origin. Elevated IgG values are observed in about 40% of cases. In contrast, the percentage of patients with elevated IgA levels increases with histologic evidence of disease progression.[12]

Circulating immune complexes, including cryoproteins and immunoglobulin isotypes, have been described in several large series of patients with or without extrahepatic features of PBC.[17,39–41] A longitudinal study, examining levels of immune complexes over 3 years, showed a subset of PBC patients with autoimmune disease and both a greater prevalence and higher mean levels of circulating immune complexes compared with those patients without autoimmune features.[35,39] This observation supports an earlier hypothesis that defective Kupffer cell–mediated clearance of complexes may result in higher circulating levels with potential for damage to organs besides the liver.[42] No particular target organ specificity seems associated with elevated levels of immune complexes, however. Antigens in these complexes include mitochondrial[43] and hepatic canalicular and ductular[44] components. These components indicate that more than one antigen–antibody system exists that, in turn, could have some bearing on the types of clinical manifestations. Use of the C1q binding assay in patients with PBC showed complexes in 31 of 50 (62%) patients, 17 of whom had arthritis. Most cases were RF positive, but precise classification of the arthritic disorders was lacking.[45]

Evidence is abundant for activation of the complement cascade via the classic and alternative pathways.[46] Complement activation appears to be of little clinical significance, however, except for a report of reduced serum C4 levels in PBC patients with autoimmune features. C3 values in the same group of patients were normal.[38]

Past studies examining the association of tissue typing antigens with PBC have yielded conflicting re-

Table 63–4. Autoantibodies in 113 Patients with Primary Biliary Cirrhosis

	Number Tested	Positive	
		No.	%
Antimitochondrial antibodies	113	108	96
Rheumatoid factor	20	14	70
Smooth muscle antibody	29	19	66
Thyroid-specific antibodies	17	7	41
Extractable nuclear antigen	10	3	30
Antinuclear antibody	56	13	23
Antibody to native DNA	9	2	22

(From Culp, K.S., et al.[12])

sults. Recently, however, Gores et al. reported a six-fold increase in the frequency of HLA-DRw8 in patients with PBC. HLA-DQW1 was associated with the subset exhibiting Raynaud's phenomenon.[47]

CHRONIC ACTIVE HEPATITIS

Chronic active hepatitis (CAH) is a continuous inflammatory disease of the liver lasting beyond the expected period of resolution. This condition can be idiopathic or induced by several diverse agents and can progress to cirrhosis or liver failure.[48] The idiopathic disease, occurring primarily in young women with multisystem involvement, forms the basis of this discussion. Lupoid hepatitis was a popular early term because many patients had lupus erythematosus (LE) cells and clinical features of a multisystem disorder resembling SLE. Some patients with CAH may fulfill the American Rheumatism Association criteria for SLE. A recent reappraisal of CAH and SLE, however, examining clinical criteria and employing up-to-date serologic testing, concluded that, despite laboratory similarities, CAH and SLE differ substantially and are not likely to be confused.[50] Smooth muscle antibody is reported to be a reliable serologic marker because it is detectable in most patients with CAH but rarely is found in SLE or in noninflammatory liver disease.[51] ANAs are found in 70% of CAH patients without hepatitis B.[52] However, the demonstration of smooth-muscle, antimitochondrial, and antinuclear antibodies may not enhance diagnostic accuracy of CAH, because they may be undetectable in 15% of patients with severe disease.[48]

Multisystem involvement occurs in approximately 63% of patients.[29] Polyarthralgias and, less commonly, polyarthritis are observed in one fourth to one half of patients.[29,48] Large and small joints are affected. Periarticular swelling may be striking, but joint effusion is seldom encountered (Fig. 63–3). Although occasional patients exhibit erosive rheumatoid-like disease, the arthropathy is usually transient and appears to coincide with episodes of relapse of the liver disease. Synovial histology is nonspecific, with findings of hypertrophy, plasma cell infiltration, fibrosis, and vascular proliferation.[29] Fibrinoid material on the synovial surface and IgG, IgM, and C3 deposits in the surface fibrinoid have been reported.[53]

Most organ systems have been affected to a variable degree and in various combinations in chronic active hepatitis, but renal disease and neurologic disorders are seldom serious.[51]

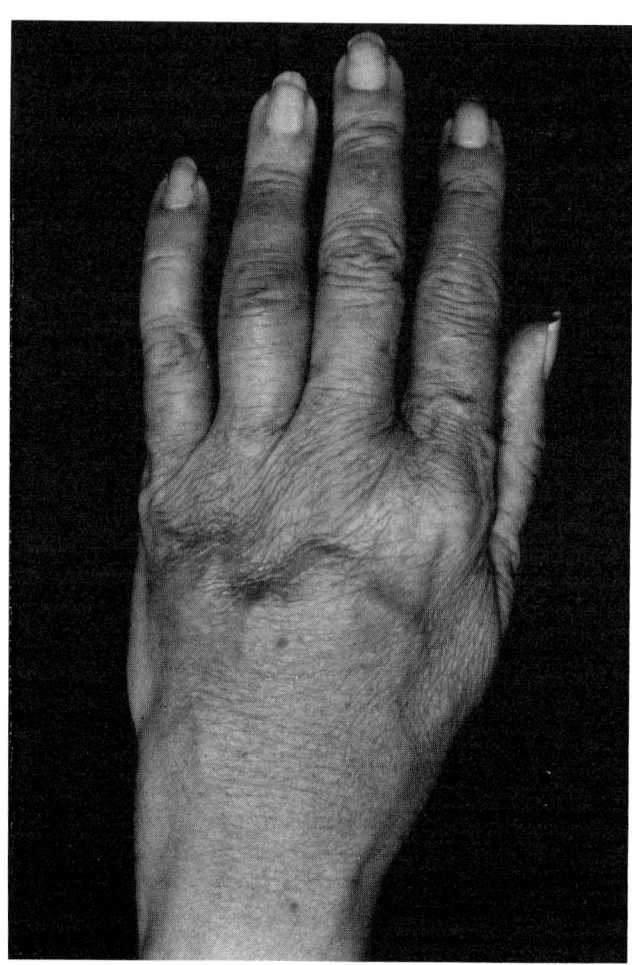

FIG. 63–3. Synovitis in the wrist and finger joints of a patient with chronic active hepatitis.

CRYPTOGENIC CIRRHOSIS

In general, multisystem disease occurs less frequently in association with cryptogenic cirrhosis (38%) than in PBC or CAH. Essentially, however, the same major organ systems are affected as with the other chronic liver diseases. Although patient numbers are small in this group, the prevalence of pulmonary diffusion defects and peripheral neuropathy is surprisingly high. Arthralgia and arthritis are encountered only rarely (3%).[29]

SCLEROSING CHOLANGITIS

Since 1975, four cases of primary sclerosing cholangitis complicated by Sjögren's syndrome and pancreatitis have been reported. Autoimmunity may be involved in this symptom complex.[54]

VIRAL HEPATITIS

Hepatitis B infection is an example of a disorder in which a single infectious agent, in combination with the host immune response, causes several immune complex syndromes. These syndromes are considered in detail in the chapter on viral arthritis (see Chapter 118).

The most common syndrome is an acute, often severe, symmetric polyarthritis involving multiple joints simultaneously or less often in a migratory or additive pattern. Involvement of large and small joints is generally the rule. Synovial fluid is often inflammatory but nondiagnostic. The arthritis is short-lived, responding rapidly to aspirin. It usually disappears coincidentally with the appearance of jaundice.

Urticarial, petechial, and/or maculopapular rashes commonly appear with the arthritis and last days to weeks. Articular pain and rash usually precede the appearance of jaundice. Many patients, however, are never jaundiced, and the illness may be indistinguishable from other connective tissue syndromes unless serial liver function tests are performed.[55]

A less common but more serious illness is necrotizing vasculitis. Patients usually are profoundly ill and exhibit involvement of more than one major organ system. Fever, joint pain, mononeuritis multiplex, renal disease, and cardiac disease are the most prominent findings initially.[55-57] In one study, joint pain occurred in 100% of vasculitis patients with hepatitis B infection in contrast to only 55% of vasculitis patients who were hepatitis B negative.[57] These patients have a prolonged illness that is fatal in some cases in spite of treatment with corticosteroids alone or in combination with immunosuppressive drugs.[55-57]

Extrahepatic manifestations of hepatitis A are recognized rarely. A recent report by Inman et al. described two patients with arthritis, vasculitis, and cryoglobulinemia complicating hepatitis A infection.[58]

HEMOCHROMATOSIS

An arthropathy can be associated with hemochromatosis in 50% of the cases[59] (see also Chapter 111). The arthropathy can be the presenting complaint. In most cases the arthropathy accompanies hemochromatosis with clinical and histologic evidence of liver involvement and elevated serum iron and transferrin levels. Characteristically it is a chronic degenerative polyarthritis. The joints that are commonly involved are the second and third metacarpophalangeal joints and the proximal interphalangeal joints of the hands, wrists, knees, and hips. This degenerative arthropathy accompanying hemochromatosis affects younger individuals with the average age 50, as compared to idiopathic primary osteoarthritis. The pattern of joint involvement is clearly different from that of "nodal" osteoarthritis. Synovium is noninflammatory, and iron is visible in articular cartilage.[60] Roentgenographic changes of the involved joints include subchondral sclerosis, cyst formation, and joint space narrowing. Chondrocalcinosis may be seen in 70% of these patients along with increases in the severity and number of joints involved with time. Chondrocalcinosis affects older patients predominantly. Attacks of acute pseudogout can occur, and calcium pyrophosphate dihydrate crystals can be demonstrated in the synovial fluid of an involved joint (see Chapters 5 and 107).

Patients have presented with a chronic arthropathy and elevated serum iron and transferrin levels before any significant liver damage can be demonstrated.[60] In addition, patients have been reported with the characteristic arthropathy and normal serum iron levels, but liver biopsies consistent with hemochromatosis.[60,61] Neither chronic arthritis nor chondrocalcinosis has been shown to regress or to demonstrate control as a result of phlebotomy treatment of the hemochromatosis, which depletes the iron stores. This treatment may be effective in those with early arthropathy and mild or subclinical liver disease.[60]

Arthropathy has been most commonly reported in association with idiopathic hemochromatosis but can also occur in secondary hemochromatosis (not necessarily the hemochromatosis secondary to alcoholic cirrhosis). There is a significant association of HLA-A3 with idiopathic hemochromatosis.[62] Whether there is a closer association with certain of the clinical features of hemochromatosis, such as the arthropathy, is doubtful.[60]

WILSON'S DISEASE

Osteoarthritis commonly accompanies Wilson's disease (see also Chapter 111) and involves the large joints and the spine.[63] Spinal osteophyte formation and squaring of the vertebral bodies can occur, simulating ankylosing spondylitis. A roentgenographic picture of osteochondritis dissecans can be present in the knee. Chondrocalcinosis has been seen but is less common than in hemochromatosis. The loss of bone density, which is the most common roentgenographic abnormality noted in Wilson's disease, is commonly demonstrated in the hands, feet, and spine. Schmorl's nodes are present, involving the midthoracic and lumbar spine. The incidence of fractures in these patients is high. Osteopenia results from loss of calcium and phosphorus in the urine as a result of a renal tubular defect. Rickets and osteomalacia can occur.

LIVER INVOLVEMENT SECONDARY TO CONNECTIVE TISSUE DISEASES

RHEUMATOID ARTHRITIS

In the past, liver involvement has not been thought to be a significant feature of RA. Hepatomegaly has been observed in about 10% of patients. However, with the routine use of serum chemistry profiles in the evaluation of rheumatoid patients, liver function abnormalities are noted frequently. From 25 to 50% of patients with RA have abnormal biochemical tests of liver function,[64] usually elevations of the liver alkaline phosphatase and the gamma glutamyl transpeptidase. These elevated serum enzymes have been correlated with the presence of associated Sjögren's syndrome and the activity of the arthritis.[65] The elevated liver alkaline phosphatase also correlates with other laboratory indicators of disease activity, such as an elevated erythrocyte sedimentation rate, diminished serum albumin, elevated serum γ-globulins, and a diminished serum iron. Patients with RA have a 1.5% prevalence of antimitochondrial antibodies. The subset of patients with antimitochondrial and smooth-muscle antibodies also has a higher prevalence of hepatomegaly, splenomegaly, and abnormal liver function tests. There have been case reports of liver rupture associated with rheumatoid vasculitis.[66] These patients have other clinical features indicating an underlying vasculitis. Study of the liver tissue in rheumatoid patients with serum enzyme abnormalities has revealed nonspecific changes of Kupffer cell hyperplasia and infiltration of the periportal regions with mononuclear cells.

Patients with RA are treated with a variety of drugs that can be potentially hepatotoxic, particularly the nonsteroidal anti-inflammatory drugs (NSAIDs). No association has been found between liver dysfunction and the use of a particular NSAID. On the contrary, patients successfully treated with anti-inflammatory agents, specifically corticosteroids, usually demonstrate improvement in liver function. Seronegative arthritis patients treated with similar NSAIDs are less likely to demonstrate liver function abnormalities than patients who are seropositive.[37]

FELTY'S SYNDROME

Felty's syndrome is associated with a characteristic liver abnormality, *nodular regenerative hyperplasia*, which may lead to gastrointestinal hemorrhage caused by portal hypertension and esophageal varices. Similar hepatic findings have been reported rarely in SLE and other connective tissue disorders.[67]

Histologic evidence of liver damage may be present in 60% of patients with Felty's syndrome.[68] An equal number of patients show liver function abnormalities, and some patients with abnormal liver histology may have normal liver function tests. The histologic abnormalities include nodular regenerative hyperplasia, portal fibrosis, lymphocytic infiltration of the sinusoids, and Kupffer cell hyperplasia. Nodular regenerative hyperplasia has been found in about 25% of patients with Felty's syndrome; it is diagnosed histologically if there are two populations of hepatocytes, large cells, and small cells, and if the nodular regions contain the large cells. Fibrous septa are not present. The diagnosis of nodular regenerative hyperplasia may not always be made by needle liver biopsy, because occasionally the nodule is not sampled and the surrounding tissue appears normal.

Portal hypertension, esophageal varices, and gastrointestinal bleeding occur most commonly in those patients with Felty's syndrome and associated nodular regenerative hyperplasia of the liver. The clinical, serologic, or extra-articular features of disease in patients with Felty's syndrome are not different in those with and those without histologic abnormalities in the liver. Patients with Felty's syndrome and significant liver changes usually do not develop the serious clinical complications of ascites and deterioration of liver function that can occur in cirrhosis. Because of the gastrointestinal bleeding, however, some patients require splenectomy and a portal shunt to control the bleeding complications.[69]

STILL'S DISEASE

Juvenile arthritis and, particularly, the acute systemic form of the disease, Still's disease, have been associated with hepatomegaly and elevation of the serum transaminases.[70] This association has not led to chronic liver disease. Likewise, similar features can occur in adult Still's disease. Patients with adult Still's disease can have hepatomegaly, splenomegaly, and elevated serum transaminase.[71] The histologic abnormalities in the liver in juvenile and adult Still's disease are similar to those seen in RA with mononuclear cell infiltration of the sinusoids and portal tracts and Kupffer cell hyperplasia.

SYSTEMIC LUPUS ERYTHEMATOSUS

Although clinically significant liver disease is uncommon in SLE, subclinical liver involvement is being recognized with greater frequency. Approximately 50% of patients with SLE have elevated serum transaminase values.[72] Liver enlargement can be detected in over 30% of patients. In some of these patients, the serum biochemical abnormality is due to the effect of drugs, particularly the NSAIDs. Patients with active lupus erythematosus can be more susceptible to the hepatotoxic effect of NSAIDs, especially aspirin. It has been estimated that in 20% of cases, the elevated serum enzymes are caused by lupus-induced liver disease.

The most common histologic finding in the liver of SLE patients is steatosis. In part, this condition can be related to the use of corticosteroids. A variety of nonspecific histologic abnormalities can be found in the liver of patients with lupus, including inflammatory cell infiltration of the portal tract, granulomatous hepatitis, CAH, and even cirrhosis.[73] As in RA, there are rare case reports of an arteritis causing liver infarction and rupture.

POLYMYALGIA RHEUMATICA AND GIANT CELL ARTERITIS

Liver function abnormalities, especially elevated serum liver alkaline phosphatase levels, occur in patients with giant cell arteritis[74] (see also Chapters 79 and 74). These abnormalities are more common in patients with severe disease as indicated by constitutional features, including fever, weight loss, anorexia, and anemia. Liver function abnormalities are detected less frequently in polymyalgia rheumatica without giant cell arteritis. The liver histologic abnormalities in patients with giant cell arteritis and liver function abnormalities include fatty changes, mild patchy liver necrosis, mononuclear cell infiltration, and granulomas.[75] The elevated enzyme levels return to normal after corticosteroid therapy.

EFFECTS OF ANTIRHEUMATIC DRUGS ON THE LIVER

SALICYLATES

Serum transaminases can be elevated as a result of treatment with aspirin in patients with RA, SLE, and

juvenile polyarthritis.[76] This elevation occurs most commonly in lupus erythematosus and juvenile polyarthritis. The serum transaminases are elevated more frequently when the salicylate level is greater than 25 mg/dl, but the transaminase elevation can occur at lower salicylate blood levels. Hepatocellular degeneration or necrosis is seen on biopsy. The abnormalities are reversible on discontinuing the salicylates. Progression to significant liver disease has not been reported.

Because salicylates have been implicated as a causal factor in Reye's syndrome, they are not recommended for children with varicella or for those suspected of having influenza.[77] A report by Rennebohm et al. of six children with Reye's syndrome receiving chronic salicylate therapy for connective tissue disorders suggests vigilance in these circumstances.[78]

NONSTEROIDAL ANTI-INFLAMMATORY DRUGS

Nonsalicylate NSAIDs in current use include several diverse compounds that rarely cause hepatic dysfunction by themselves. Toxicity can be hepatocellular or cholestatic and usually is an idiosyncratic or hypersensitivity reaction and is not dose related. Most cases occur within 2 to 12 weeks of initiation of therapy. An elevated serum transaminase level without associated clinical abnormalities is the most common finding. Biopsy features include minor mononuclear infiltrates and ultrastructural changes. Laboratory values normalize on withdrawal of the drug.

In a review by O'Brien and Bagby,[79] frank hepatitis with hepatocellular necrosis and less frequently steatosis were seen with diflunisal, indomethacin, sulindac, ibuprofen, fenoprofen, naproxen, tolmetin, and piroxicam. Cholestatic jaundice was uncommon. Rarely were the drug reactions fatal.

Hepatotoxicity with phenylbutazone has several distictive features. It occurs more frequently than with newer NSAIDs, has a mortality rate approaching 25%, and puts at greatest risk those past age 60. Hepatic injury generally appears during the first 6 weeks and about two thirds of patients exhibit additional features of hypersensitivity including fever and rash. Hepatic granulomas, mild to severe hepatocellular injury, and steatosis are the typical histologic findings.[79]

DISEASE-MODIFYING DRUGS

Gold and Penicillamine

Hepatotoxicity in RA patients taking gold and DPA is rare and usually is the subject of single case reports.

Unfortunately, many reactions to these agents are poorly authenticated, with the failure to exclude infection or other drugs administered concurrently. Nevertheless, there are bona fide reports of cholestatic jaundice caused by gold and DPA, with confirmation by inadvertent rechallenge with the offending drugs.[80,81] Gold hepatotoxicity is likely to occur early, to be self-limiting in about 3 months, and to be a hypersensitivity reaction with extrahepatic features. Data on DPA are more limited, but extrahepatic side effects reportedly occur simultaneously. Liver histology reveals cholestasis or mononuclear and eosinophilic infiltrates in portal triads. It is important to recognize this rare complication of gold and DPA treatment and to differentiate it from extrahepatic biliary tract obstruction which it may simulate.[82]

Azathioprine, Methotrexate and Cyclophosphamide

Liver function abnormalities can occur in patients treated with these drugs. Liver function abnormalities, especially elevated serum transaminase, occur in rheumatoid patients taking azathioprine. These abnormalities occur infrequently, however, and do not result in significant liver disease.[83] The liver returns to normal on discontinuation of the drug.

Serum transaminase elevations can be detected frequently in rheumatoid patients treated with methotrexate. The proliferation of papers in the past few years on methotrexate and hepatotoxicity attests to a keen interest in this topic. Elevation of aspartate aminotransferase (AST) levels as an isolated event occurs in up to 69% of patients treated using doses of methotrexate of 7.5 to 15 mg per week. Increases in AST values occur at random, are more common in the 48 hours following weekly administration, and are not predictive of liver toxicity. A prospective study by Kremer and Lee[84] failed to detect significant liver pathologic change after up to 4 years of treatment. Depressed hepatic folate levels and increased polyglutamated methotrexate stores in liver tissue are of uncertain significance but are reversible with folinic acid rescue.[85] It is not known how many of these patients will eventually develop histologically significant liver disease, but caution must be observed because of the significant liver disease that has occurred in patients with psoriasis treated with methotrexate. *In these cases, liver function tests did not predict significant histologic liver damage.* Progression to cirrhosis in the methotrexate-treated psoriatic patients was related to risk factors such as alcohol consumption and total cumulative dose. Consequently, it has been suggested that a cumulative dose of methotrexate beyond 1.5 g needs tissue surveillance.[86] The issue of whether liver biopsies should be performed routinely in rheumatoid patients receiving methotrexate is debatable.[84]

Cyclophosphamide, an alkylating agent activated by the liver, seldom causes hepatic dysfunction, with only three cases reported.[87]

Other Agents

Cyclosporine, a potent T-cell regulator, is still an investigational drug for treatment of autoimmune disorders. Limited data indicate cyclosporine hepatotoxicity is uncommon in these conditions.[88] Allopurinol hepatotoxicity is infrequent but can be severe and in some cases fatal. Hepatocellular necrosis with or without granulomas is the typical histologic finding.[89] Sulphasalazine, a drug infrequently used for RA, can cause hepatotoxicity similar to that seen in patients with ulcerative colitis treated with this agent.[90]

REFERENCES

1. Blumberg, B.S., Alter, H.J., and Visrich, S.: A "new" antigen in leukemic sera. JAMA, 191:541–546, 1965.
2. Mills, P.R., and Sturrock, R.D.: Clinical associations between arthritis and liver disease. Ann. Rheum. Dis., 41:295–307, 1982.
3. Graves, R.J.: Clinical lectures on the practice of medicine. Dublin, Fannin and Co., 1843, p. 937.
4. Still, G.F.: On a form of chronic joint disease in children. Med. Chir. Trans., 80:47–60, 1897.
5. Hench, P.S.: Effect of jaundice on chronic infectious (atrophic) arthritis and primary fibrositis. Arch. Intern. Med., 61:451–480, 1938.
6. Thompson, H.E., and Wyatt, B.L.: Experimentally induced jaundice (hyperbilirubinemia). Arch. Intern. Med., 61:481–500, 1938.
7. Gardner, F., Stewart, A., and MacCallum, F.O.: Therapeutic effect of induced jaundice in rheumatoid arthritis. Br. Med. J., 2:677–680, 1945.
8. Hench, P.S., et al.: The ameliorating effect of pregnancy on chronic atrophic (infectious arthritis) arthritis, fibrositis, and intermittent hydrarthrosis. Mayo Clin. Proc., 13:161–167, 1938.
9. Hench, P.S., et al.: The effect of a hormone of the adrenal cortex (17-hydroxy-11-dehydrocorticosterone: Compound D) and of pituitary adrenocorticotrophic hormone on rheumatoid arthritis. Mayo Clin. Proc., 24:181–197, 1949.
10. Bodenheimer, H.C., and Schaffner, F.: Primary biliary cirrhosis and the immune system. J. Gastroenterol., 72:285–296, 1979.
11. Dickson, E.R., et al.: Trial of penicillamine in advanced primary biliary cirrhosis. N. Engl. J. Med., 312:1011–1015, 1985.
12. Culp, K.S., et al.: Autoimmune associations in primary biliary cirrhosis. Mayo Clin. Proc., 57:365–370, 1982.
13. Crowe, J., et al.: Early features of primary biliary cirrhosis: An analysis of 85 patients. Am. J. Gastroenterol., 80:466–468, 1985.
14. Ansell, B.M., and Bywaters, E.G.L.: Histiocytic bone and joint disease. Ann. Rheum. Dis., 16:503–510, 1957.
15. Mills, P.R., Rooney, P.J., Watkinson, G., and MacSween, R.N.M.: Hypercholesterolemic arthropathy in primary biliary cirrhosis. Ann. Rheum. Dis., 37:179–180, 1978.
16. Lauritsen, K., and Diederichsen, H.: Arthritis in patients with

antimitochondrial antibodies. Scand. J. Rheumatol., *12*:331–335, 1983.

17. Modena, V., et al.: Primary biliary cirrhosis and rheumatic diseases: A clinical, immunological and immunogenetical study. Clin. Exp. Rheumatol., *4*:129–134, 1986.

18. Marx, W.J., and O'Connell, D.J.: Arthritis of primary biliary cirrhosis. Arch. Intern. Med., *139*:179–180, 1979.

19. Mills, P.R., et al.: A prospective survey of radiological bone and joint changes in primary biliary cirrhosis. Clin. Radiol., *32*:297–302, 1981.

20. Clarke, A.K., Gallraith, R.M., Hamilton, E.B.D., and Williams, R.: Rheumatic disorders in primary biliary cirrhosis. Ann. Rheum. Dis., *37*:42–47, 1978.

21. Sherlock, S., and Scheuer, P.J.: The presentation and diagnosis of 100 patients with primary biliary cirrhosis. N. Engl. J. Med., *289*:674–678, 1973.

22. Uddenfeldt, P., and Danielsson, A.: Evaluation of rheumatic disorders in patients with primary biliary cirrhosis. Ann. Clin. Res., *18*:148–153, 1986.

23. Alarcon-Segovia, D., Diaz-Jauonen, E., and Fishbein, E.: Features of Sjögren's syndrome in primary biliary cirrhosis. Ann. Intern. Med., *79*:31–35, 1973.

24. Penner, E., and Reichlin, M.: Primary biliary cirrhosis associated with Sjögren's syndrome: Evidence for circulating and tissue-deposited Ro/anti-Ro immune complexes. Arthritis Rheum., *25*:1250–1253, 1982.

25. Bartholomew, L.G., Cain, J.C., Winkelmann, R.K., and Baggenstoss, A.H.: Chronic diseases of the liver with systemic scleroderma. Am. J. Dig. Dis., *9*:43–55, 1964.

26. Miller, F., Lore, B., Saterakis, J., and D'Angelo, W.A.: Primary biliary cirrhosis and scleroderma. Arch. Pathol. Lab. Med., *103*:505–509, 1979.

27. Reynold, T.B., et al.: Primary biliary cirrhosis with scleroderma, Raynaud's phenomenon, and telangiectasia. Am. J. Med., *50*:302–12, 1971.

28. Makinen, D., Fritzler, M., Davis, P., and Sherlock, S.: Anticentromere antibodies in primary biliary cirrhosis. Arthritis Rheum., *26*:914–917, 1983.

29. Golding, P.L., Smith, M., and Williams, R.: Multisystem involvement in chronic liver disease. Am. J. Med., *55*:772–782, 1973.

30. Crowe, J.P., et al.: Primary biliary cirrhosis: The prevalence of hypothyroidism and its relationship to thyroid autoantibodies and sicca syndrome. Gastroenterology, *78*:1438–1441, 1980.

31. Iliffe, G.D., Naidoo, S., and Hunter, T.: Primary biliary cirrhosis associated with features of systemic lupus erythematosus. Dig. Dis. Sci., *27*:274–278, 1982.

32. Lakhanpal, S.: Unpublished observation.

33. Doherty, M., Martin, M.F., and Dieppe, P.A.: Multicentric reticulohistiocytosis associated with primary biliary cirrhosis: Successful treatment with cytotoxic agents. Arthritis Rheum., *27*:344–348, 1984.

34. Okano, Y., Nishikai, M., and Sato, A.: Scleroderma, primary biliary cirrhosis, and Sjögren's syndrome after cosmetic breast augmentation with silicone injection: A case report of possible human adjuvant disease. Ann. Rheum. Dis., *43*:520–522, 1984.

35. Terkeltaub, R., et al.: Vasculitis as a presenting manifestation of primary biliary cirrhosis: A case report. Clin. Exp. Rheumatol., *2*:67–73, 1984.

36. Rutan, G., et al.: Primary biliary cirrhosis, Sjögren's syndrome and transverse myelitis. Gastroenterology, *90*:206–210, 1986.

37. Robertson, J.C., Batstone, G.F., and Loebl, W.Y.: Polymyalgia rheumatica and primary biliary cirrhosis. Br. Med. J., *2*:1128, 1978.

38. Conn, D.C., Dickson, E.R., and Carpenter, H.A.: The association of Churg-Strauss vasculitis with temporal artery involvement, primary biliary cirrhosis, and polychondritis in a single patient. J. Rheumatol., *9*:744–748, 1982.

39. Gupta, R.C., Dickson, E.R., McDuffie, F.C., and Baggenstoss, A.H.: Immune complexes in primary biliary cirrhosis. Am. J. Med., *73*:192–198, 1982.

40. Dienstag, J.L., Savarese, A.M., Cohen, R.B., and Bhan, A.K.: Circulating immune complexes in primary biliary cirrhosis: Interactions with lymphoid cells. Clin. Exp. Immunol., *50*:7–16, 1982.

41. Wands, J.R., et al.: Circulating immune complexes and complement activation in primary biliary cirrhosis. N. Engl. J. Med., *298*:233–237.

42. Thomas, H.C., Potter, B.J., and Sherlock, G.: Is primary biliary cirrhosis an immune complex disease? Lancet, *2*:1261–1263, 1977.

43. Penner, E., et al.: Immune complexes in primary biliary cirrhosis contain mitochondrial antigens. Clin. Immunol. Immunopathology, *22*:394–399, 1982.

44. Amoroso, P., et al.: Identification of biliary antigens in circulating immune complexes in primary biliary cirrhosis. Clin. Exp. Immunol., *42*:95–98, 1980.

45. Crowe, J.P., et al.: Increased C1q binding and arthritis in primary biliary cirrhosis. Gut, *21*:418–422, 1980.

46. Jones, E.A., Frank, M.M., Jaffee, C.J., and Vierling, J.M.: Primary biliary cirrhosis and the complement system. Ann. Intern. Med., *90*:72–84, 1979.

47. Gores, C.J., et al.: Primary biliary cirrhosis: Associations with major histocompatibility complex class II antigens. Gastroenterology, *90*:1728, 1986.

48. Czaja, A.J.: Current problems in the diagnosis and management of chronic active hepatitis. Mayo Clin. Proc., *56*:311–323, 1981.

49. Mackay, I.R., Taft, L.I., and Cowling, D.C.: Lupoid hepatitis. Lancet, *2*:1323–1326, 1956.

50. Hall, S., et al.: How lupoid is lupoid hepatitis? J. Rheumatol., *13*:95–98, 1986.

51. Plotz, P.H.: Autoimmunity in hepatitis. Med. Clin. North Am., *59*:869–876, 1975.

52. Hughes, G.R., and Williams, R.: Diversity of autoantibodies in primary biliary cirrhosis and chronic active hepatitis. Clin. Exp. Immunol., *55*:553–560, 1984.

53. Bernardo, D.E., Vernon-Roberts, B., and Currey, H.L.F.: A case of active chronic hepatitis with painless erosive arthritis. Gut, *14*:800–804, 1973.

54. Montefusco, P.P., et al.: Sclerosing cholangitis, chronic pancreatitis and Sjögren's syndrome: A syndrome complex. Am. J. Surg., *147*:822–826, 1984.

55. Duffy, J., et al.: Polyarthritis, polyarteritis, and hepatitis B. Medicine, *55*:19–37, 1976.

56. Inman, R.D.: Rheumatoid manifestations of hepatitis B infections. Semin. Arthritis Rheum., *11*:406–420, 1982.

57. Sergent, J.S., Lockshin, M.D., Christian, C.L., and Gocke, D.J.: Vasculitis with hepatitis B antigenemia. Medicine, *55*:1–18, 1976.

58. Inman, R.D., et al.: Arthritis, vasculitis, cryoglobulinemia associated with relapsing hepatitis A virus infection. Ann. Intern. Med., *105*:700–703, 1986.

59. Milder, M.S., Cook, J.D., Stray, S., and Finch, C.A.: Idiopathic hemochromatosis, an interim report. Medicine, *59*:34–49, 1980.

60. Askari, A.D., et al.: Arthritis of hemochromatosis. Clinical spectrum, relation to histocompatibility antigens, and effectiveness of early phlebotomy. Am. J. Med., *75*:957–965, 1983.

61. Rosner, I.A., Askari, A.D., McLaren, G.D., and Muir, A.: Arthropathy, hypouricemia and normal serum iron studies in hereditary hemochromatosis. Am. J. Med., *70*:870–874, 1981.

62. Powell, L.W., Bassett, M.L., and Halliday, J.W.: Hemochromatosis: 1980 update. Gastroenterology, *78*:374–391, 1980.

63. Golding, D.N., and Walshe, J.M.: Arthropathy of Wilson's disease. Ann. Rheum. Dis., *36*:99–111, 1977.

64. Fernandes, L., et al.: Studies on the frequency and pathogenesis of liver involvement in rheumatoid arthritis. Ann. Rheum. Dis., *38*:501–506, 1979.

65. Webb, J., et al.: Liver disease in rheumatoid arthritis and Sjögren's syndrome. Ann. Rheum. Dis., *34*:70–81, 1981.

66. Hocking, W.G., et al.: Spontaneous hepatic rupture in rheumatoid arthritis. Arch. Intern. Med., *141*:792–794, 1981.

67. Klemp, P., Timme, A.H., and Sayers, G.M.: Systemic lupus erythematosus and nodular regenerative hyperplasia of the liver. Ann. Rheum. Dis., *45*:167–170, 1986.

68. Thorne, C., et al.: Liver disease in Felty's syndrome. Am. J. Med., *73*:35–40, 1982.

69. Blendis, L.M., et al.: Oesophageal variceal bleeding in Felty's syndrome associated with nodular regenerative hyperplasia. Ann. Rheum. Dis., *37*:183–186, 1978.

70. Schaller, J., Beckwith, B., and Wedgwood, R.J.: Hepatic involvement in juvenile rheumatoid arthritis. J. Pediatr., *77*:203–210, 1970.

71. Esdaile, J.M., et al.: Hepatic abnormalities in adult onset Still's disease. J. Rheumatol., *6*:673–679, 1979.

72. Gibson, T., and Myers, A.R.: Subclinical liver disease in systemic lupus erythematosus. J. Rheumatol., *8*:752–759, 1981.

73. Rynyon, B.A., LaBrecque, D.R., and Anuras, S.: The spectrum of liver disease in systemic lupus erythematosus. Am. J. Med., *69*:P187–194, 1980.

74. Dickson, E.R., Maldonado, J.E., Sheps, S.G., and Cain, J.A.: Systemic giant cell arteritis with polymyalgia rheumatica. JAMA, *244*:1496–1498, 1973.

75. VonKnorring, J., and Wasatjerna, C.: Liver involvement in polymyalgia rheumatica. Scand. J. Rheumatol., *5*:197–204, 1976.

76. Prescott, L.F.: Hepatotoxicity of mild analgesics. Br. J. Clin. Pharmacol., *10*:373S–79S, 1980.

77. Surgeon's General's advisory on the use of salicylates and Reye's Syndrome. Morbid. Mortal. Weekly Rep., *31*:289–290, 1982.

78. Rennebohm, R.M., Heubi, J.E., Daugherty, C.C., and Daniels, S.R.: Reye's Syndrome in children receiving salicylate therapy for connective tissue disease. J. Pediatr., *107*:877–880, 1985.

79. O'Brien, W.M., and Bagby, G.F.: Rare adverse reactions to nonsteroidal anti-inflammatory drugs. J. Rheumatol., *12*:562–567, 1985.

80. Kumar, A., et al.: D-penicillamine-induced acute hypersensitivity pneumonitis and cholestatic hepatitis in a patient with rheumatoid arthritis. Clin. Exp. Rheumatol., *3*:337–339, 1985.

81. Smith, M.D.: Hepatitis and neutropenia secondary to gold thiomalate therapy for rheumatoid arthritis. Aust. N.Z. J. Med., *16*:72–74, 1986.

82. Seibold, J.R., Lynch, C.J., and Medsger, T.A.: Cholestasis associated with D-penicillamine therapy: Case report and review of the literature. Arthritis Rheum., *24*:554–556, 1981.

83. Whisnant, J.K., and Pelkey, J.: Rheumatoid arthritis: Treatment with azathioprine (Imuran R). Clinical side effects and laboratory abnormalities. Ann. Rheum. Dis., *41*(Suppl 1):44–47, 1982.

84. Kremer, J.M., and Lee, J.K.: The safety and efficacy of the use of methotrexate in long-term therapy for rheumatoid arthritis. Arthritis Rheum., *29*:822–831, 1986.

85. Kremer, J.M., Galivan, J., Streckfuss, A., and Kamen, B.: Methotrexate metabolism analysis in blood and liver of rheumatoid arthritis patients. Association with hepatic folate deficiency and formation of polyglutamates. Arthritis Rheum., *29*:832–835, 1986.

86. Willkens, R.F., Watson, M.A., and Paxson, C.S.: Low dose pulse methotrexate therapy in rheumatoid arthritis. J. Rheumatol., *7*:501–505, 1980.

87. Goldberg, J.W., and Lidsky, M.D.: Cyclophosphamide-associated hepatotoxicity. South. Med. J., *78*:222–223, 1985.

88. Palestine, A.G., Nussenblatt, R.B., and Chan, C.-C.: Side effects of systemic cyclosporine in patients not undergoing transplantation. Am. J. Med., *77*:652–656, 1984.

89. Al-kawas, F.H., et al.: Allopurinol hepatotoxicity. Report of two cases and review of the literature. Ann. Intern. Med., *95*:588–590, 1981.

90. Farr, M., Symmons, D.P., and Bacon, P.A.: Raised alkaline phosphatase and aspartate transaminase levels in two rheumatoid patients treated with sulphasalazine. Ann. Rheum. Dis., *44*:798–800, 1985.

INTERMITTENT AND PERIODIC ARTHRITIC SYNDROMES

64

GEORGE E. EHRLICH

The intermittent entities discussed here should be regarded as syndromes rather than diseases, with the possible exception of familial Mediterranean fever, which appears to be a heritable disease. Their definitions emphasize intermittently occurring symptom complexes, and for their diagnosis, a certain number of symptoms must occur concurrently. The more that is known about a disease, the fewer symptoms are required for its diagnosis. If the cause is known, no symptoms need be present for accurate diagnosis as long as the causative agents are recoverable. Intermittent hydrarthosis is characterized by periodic monoarticular swelling with little pain. Palindromic rheumatism adds signs of local inflammation to swelling, with redness, tenderness, and heat over the joint. Familial Mediterranean fever can include joint symptoms alone accompanied by fever; however, generally other systemic features are present as well. In Behçet's syndrome and the Stevens-Johnson syndrome, joint manifestations are overshadowed by more severe involvement of other areas of the body. Sacroiliitis has been claimed as a feature of familial Mediterranean fever and Behçet's syndrome although a recent study disputes this assertion and ascribes previous reports to observer variation.[1] Allergy can play a role in eosinophilic synovitis. Other syndromes often characterized by intermittency, such as Reiter's syndrome, the arthritis of ulcerative colitis, and the arthritis of sarcoidosis, are discussed elsewhere in this volume.

INTERMITTENT HYDRARTHROSIS (PERIODIC ARTHROSIS)

The term refers to a recurrent pattern of joint effusions, usually of the knees, of long-term, even lifelong, duration. These recurrent attacks usually maintain a predictable periodicity. For the diagnosis to be tenable, evidence of neither local inflammation nor systemic signs must develop. A similar pattern can also characterize the early stages of rheumatoid arthritis or of other periodic syndromes.

Ragan attributed the first report to Perrin (in 1845).[2] A scant 200 cases have been reported since then,[3] probably because there have been few new developments. Most rheumatologists can recall a few such cases, often with the diagnosis made retrospectively. Perhaps because the condition is uncommon and benign, it has attracted little research interest.

Etiology. Nothing is known about the cause of intermittent hydrarthosis. Even feedback mechanisms fail to explain the patterned rhythmicity.[4] Although in most cases the syndrome begins early in life, it can begin at any time. Women are more susceptible than men,* and in many, the joint manifestations parallel the menses. Although familial occurrence has been claimed, other disorders might have been confused

---

*Whereas many American authors would subscribe to this statement, Bywaters considers both sexes to be equally at risk,[5] and some series actually cite a preponderance of men.

with intermittent hydrarthrosis. Because some patients have a strong allergic history, or develop giant urticaria, urticarial lesions of the joint have been suggested.[6] Unfortunately, antihistamines and other antiallergic medications have proved unsuccessful in controlling the disorder.

Symptoms. Regular periodic recurrence of effusion of joints is the rule. Usually a single knee is involved. Rarely, the disease may be bilateral, and some cases involving the elbow, hip, or ankle have been reported. Although the average interval between attacks is 1 to 2 weeks, intervals of as much as a month are not unusual, particularly when joint swelling accompanies the menses. The effusion is relatively painless, without local warmth, tenderness, or other signs of inflammation. Neither adjacent muscular spasm nor muscular atrophy occurs. However, because of the marked effusion, local mechanical difficulty in moving does occur. In some cases, the effusions cease about 20 years after onset, in others, intermittent hydrarthrosis is a lifelong condition. Generally, patients fail to consult physicians after the first few attacks because they have learned that little can or need be done about the swelling. The fluid rapidly accumulates over 12 to 24 hours; it reabsorbs more slowly, requiring a period of 2 to 4 days for restitution to the premorbid state.

Laboratory Data. Hemogram, erythrocyte sedimentation rate (ESR), and acute phase reactants all remain normal, even during the attack. Latex fixation and other rheumatoid factor tests remain negative, and antinuclear antibodies are absent. Development of abnormalities of acute phase reactants or serologic tests should cast some doubt on the validity of the diagnosis.

Joint fluid does not contain crystals. (One case in which calcium pyrophosphate dihydrate crystals were recovered from fluid aspirated from the knee has recently been reported.[7]) Cell counts vary from none to the low thousands (frequently polymorphonuclear leukocytes). The cells contain no characteristic inclusions. Serum and joint fluid complement levels are normal, although some authors claim a decrease in Cl esterase inhibitor.[3]

Typical Cases. It has become customary to illustrate this condition with case histories. One patient, aged 30, had her menarche at age 13. A year later, concurrent with the onset of a menstrual period, she experienced a swollen left knee, unaccompanied by pain or other signs of inflammation. After four days, the swelling disappeared, only to recur in 27 days, when the next menstrual period began. The pattern was thus set, with recurrent swelling of the left knee, unaccompanied by any signs of systemic disease or

local inflammation. Numerous studies were always unrewarding; therapy with salicylates, gold, and corticosteroids proved unavailing.

In another case, a 46-year-old man had for 6 years undergone regularly recurring effusions of the left knee at 14-day intervals. The effusion, unaccompanied by other signs of inflammation or pain, but interfering mechanically with the extremes of range of motion, contained normal fluid. Chrysotherapy, anti-inflammatory compounds, corticosteroids, and colchicine proved unavailing. Corticosteroids were instilled after the frequent aspirations and, ultimately, the effusion failed to subside even during the expected intercritical periods. Synovectomy ultimately was performed, the synovium displaying the features described below. Even synovectomy, however, failed to halt the recurrent effusions.

Pathology. Only few cases have come to operation, providing a dearth of material for study. Villous proliferation of the synovium has been a constant feature. Some portions of removed synovial membranes have resembled changes of early rheumatoid arthritis, with lymphocytic aggregates and large numbers of plasma cells. Ragan called these findings consistent with the first stage of rheumatoid arthritis.[2] Nevertheless, pannus has never been described.

Roentgenography. The diagnosis of intermittent hydrarthrosis demands that no abnormalities more dramatic than soft-tissue swelling be identified at the involved joint.

Prognosis. In some patients, the disorder runs a finite course whose total length is unpredictable. In others, joint swelling recurs throughout the patient's lifetime. The similarity of intermittent hydrarthrosis to an early stage of rheumatoid arthritis or related rheumatic disease makes prognostic judgment difficult even if the disorder has recurred for some time. However, the longer recurrences continue without apparent conversion to a more serious disorder, the more likely that joint damage will be avoided.

Treatment. No satisfactory treatment is available. Most of the standard treatments have been recommended at some time, including those thought to be successful in aborting acute attacks or chronic progression of other rheumatic diseases. The constant possibility of spontaneous remission and the small number of total cases invalidate most claims for successful therapy. Unfortunately, as Ragan has pointed out, sustained effusions, sometimes with evidence of inflammation, may follow enthusiastic intra-articular corticosteroid instillation.[2] Observation and optimism ultimately serve these patients best.

EOSINOPHILIC SYNOVITIS

Arthralgias and arthritis in allergy-prone individuals have long been blamed on their specific allergies, but without satisfactory proof.[8] Urticarial lesions in the joint have been hypothesized.[5] In tropical countries and other endemic areas, parasitosis has been reflected by eosinophilia in joints,[9] as in dracunculus medinensis (Guinea worm) invasion of the knee.[10] Transient eosinophilic synovitis has been described most recently[11] in connection with arthrography[12] and mild trauma[13] in individuals with strong personal and familial histories of allergy.

The clinical syndrome resembles intermittent hydrarthrosis.[13] Episodes are single or recurrent, characterized by swelling and effusion lasting 1 to 2 weeks.[14] Eosinophilic synovitis is painless or causes minimal discomfort only, and it recedes without therapeutic intervention. The patients are typically young, of either sex, with characteristic pronounced dermatographism after stroking the skin (the volar aspect of the forearm is generally used to elicit the response).[13] Limited motion of the affected joint is a result of mechanical impedence. Recurrent attacks can involve joints other than the initial target joint.

Although allergic histories are obtained, usually no dramatic allergic event precipitates an attack or is accompanied by it. IgE is elevated in blood. Eosinophilia of synovial fluid exceeds 10% and can be as high as 50%.[13] Synovial histology is normal, without increases in mast cells.

The detection of Charcot-Leyden crystals in wet preparations of synovial fluid heralds discovery of eosinophilia.[13] These crystals are hexagonal, bipyramidal, and weakly birefringent under polarized light. They may be intracellular or extracellular and should be sought in joint fluid examinations. Serving as markers, these crystals will help to increase the number of cases of eosinophilic synovitis detected and will aid in answering questions about causes of the disease and differential diagnoses that are still unresolved.

PALINDROMIC RHEUMATISM

The term *palindromic* comes from the Greek, meaning to run back or to recur. The term was chosen by Hench and Rosenberg to describe a type of rheumatism that recurs intermittently.[15,16]

Hench and Rosenberg published a detailed account of 34 cases in 1944,[16] and every investigator since then has essentially paraphrased their work. However, the definition has been made more precise, more has become known of the fate of some of the patients who have the disorder, and increased use of the diagnostic laboratory had led to speculations of etiology.

Clinical Picture. Palindromic rheumatism is characterized by intermittently recurring attacks of painful swelling of the joints. It differs from intermittent hydrarthrosis in that there are obvious signs of inflammation at the affected joint, but it resembles intermittent hydrarthrosis in that systemic manifestations are absent. Men are more likely to be affected, usually in mid or late life.[17]

Joint pain begins suddenly and resembles a gouty attack. Pain is variable, ranging from a dull ache in some patients to an intense bursting experience in others. The crescendo of pain reaches its maximum within a few hours to a few days, rarely more than 3 days. The attack commonly begins late in the afternoon. Swelling consistently accompanies pain, at least in joints where swelling is clinically detectable, and warmth and redness may be found overlying the joint. The redness is fairly characteristic, varying from a bright pink to crimson.

The diagnosis of palindromic rheumatism should not be made merely because of the recurrence of arthralgias. The cardinal signs of inflammation—pain and tenderness, redness, heat and, particularly, swelling and dysfunction—are required. Most authors have rejected the diagnosis when swelling has not been present. However, functional disability is usually mild and, in many patients, does not compromise their ability to work. Morning stiffness and gelling after rest rarely develop; when they do, they are confined to the involved joint at the time of acute involvement.[16] Generalized stiffness should direct the clinician to another diagnosis.

The pattern of joint attacks tends to be characteristic in a given patient. One or a limited number of joints is involved at a time, although symptoms may wax in new joints while waning in those affected during the previous attack. Thus, intervals between attacks may vary from none at all to months. On the whole, the established pattern continues relatively unchanged for the duration of the illness, thus satisfying both Greek definitions of palindromic: "recurrence" and "reading the same, backward and forward." Although the original description claimed a distinct predilection for finger joints,[16] the knee is probably the most frequently involved joint, followed by wrist, dorsum of the hand, metacarpophalangeal and proximal phalangeal joints of the fingers, ankle, shoulder, elbow, temporomandibular or sternoclavicular joint, hip, small joints of the foot, and cervical vertebral articulations.[18]

Para-articular attacks also occur in about one third

of the patients. These attacks consist of painful swellings of variable size at the heels, finger pads, distal phalanges, and flexor and dorsal surfaces of the forearms, thumb pads, and Achilles tendons. Although the swellings resemble angioneurotic edema, they are tender, do not pit on pressure, and do not cause itching or burning paresthesia. When present, these lesions are characteristic of palindromic rheumatism.[15,19]

Transient subcutaneous nodules are also a feature of this disorder. These nodules usually overlie the tendons in the hands and fingers, although some have been described at the proximal extensor surfaces of the forearm, the most common site for rheumatoid nodules. The main feature differentiating these nodules from rheumatoid nodules at these locations is the relatively short duration the nodules are present, in almost all cases less than a week. Isolated swelling of an olecranon bursa can also occur between attacks. Palindromic attacks occur frequently in a variant of rheumatoid arthritis called rheumatoid nodulosis.[20] Mattingly reported a strong family history of palindromic rheumatism and a high incidence of joint disease in mothers of his patients[18] (Table 64–1).

Laboratory Data. If palindromic rheumatism is to be considered as a separate entity, one should probably exclude patients with signs of systemic disease not otherwise explainable. Thus, most patients who bear this diagnosis evince no abnormalities of hemogram and, at most, show *transient* abnormalities of acute phase reactant. Erythrocyte sedimentation rates, which are normal between attacks, may be modestly elevated during attacks (rarely above 35 mm/hr, Westergren method).[18] Tests for LE cells and serum complement should be normal. No circulating immune complexes are found.[22] Uric acid likewise is normal, unless it is elevated as a result of small doses of salicylates taken for pain.

The findings in joint fluid are relatively unremarkable, with normal viscosity, mucin clot, cellular constituents, proteins,[18] and low collagenase.[23] Only few biopsy specimens have been examined, usually obtained by needle. During the acute attack, polymorphonuclear leukocyte invasion of synovial tissues characterizes the intense inflammation. The cell population changes to round cells during subsidence, and synovial tissues are normal between attacks.[19] The subcutaneous nodules and tendon nodules are nonspecific, although some investigators claim a similarity to rheumatoid nodules.[18] One synovial specimen obtained through open biopsy contained tuboreticular structures and much fibrin deposition.[24] In instances preceding rheumatoid arthritis, electrondense deposits in vessel walls suggest circulating immune complexes, which are otherwise not demonstrable.[25]

Roentgenographic Findings. Except for soft-tissue swelling at the time of the attack, no specific abnormalities result from palindromic rheumatism.

Prognosis. For the true syndrome of palindromic rheumatism, the prognosis in a given patient may be poor for recovery but good as far as potential crippling is concerned. In many patients, the attacks cease as abruptly as they began, with causes for their cessation as mysterious as those for their initiation. A followup of 140 patients with palindromic rheumatism for at least 5 years revealed that more than half (73) suffered continued attacks.[26] Eleven, or less than 10%, experienced complete remissions during the interval of observation, while more than a third (50) developed rheumatoid arthritis. Gout, systemic lupus erythematosus, and other diagnoses accounted for the remainder.

The distribution of patients reflects the hazards of this diagnosis, as an appreciable number of patients who seem to have palindromic rheumatism actually have an episodic onset of rheumatoid arthritis, for which the prognosis is obviously not as favorable. A review of 39 patients diagnosed as having palindromic rheumatism disclosed that 17 cases evolved into typical rheumatoid arthritis while 22 remained palindromic.[27] Palindromic symptoms had lasted for as long as 20 years in one patient before rheumatoid arthritis supervened, and for 2 or more years in 8 of the 17 patients. No signal differences were noted between the two populations, although those whose palindromic pattern evolved into fixed rheumatoid arthritis often were noted to have a raised ESR, a positive test for rheumatoid factor, or minor clinical or radiologic changes. The uncertainty of the diagnosis of palindromic rheumatism is thereby highlighted. Some patients develop a related rheumatic syndrome or even malignant diseases, such as multiple myeloma,[28] although it is doubtful that an episodic arthritis of such long duration can be regarded as heralding malignant tumors. In series of 59 cases

Table 64–1. Diagnostic Criteria for Palindromic Rheumatism*

Diagnostic Criteria
History of brief, sudden-onset, recurrent episodes of monoarthritis
Direct observation of one attack by a physician
More than five attacks in the last 2 years
Three or more joints involved in different attacks
Negative roentgenograms, acute phase reactants, and rheumatoid factor
Exclusion of other recurrent monoarthritides, gout, pseudogout, intermittent hydrarthrosis, and periodic arthritis

*Adapted from Pasero, G., and Barbieri, P.[21]

collected over a 5-year period, 5% stopped spontaneously, 73% persisted, and 22% converted to other diagnosable rheumatic diseases, chiefly rheumatoid arthritis.[21]

In occasional patients, palindromic rheumatism seems to be a response to an irritant or an allergen.[29] Whether such cases are perhaps examples of urticarial joint lesions remains unsettled. Ultimately, therefore, discussions of prognosis hinge on the validity of the concept of palindromic rheumatism as a separate entity. The safest course appears to be to make the diagnosis only by exclusion and after a reasonable period of observation.

Treatment. Acute attacks can end before prophylactic treatment can become effective. Claims for various drugs have been made in individual cases, but the variability of this disorder makes such claims suspect. Vacations and administration of gold compounds seem to promote the most benefit. Penicillamine, in uncontrolled trials, appears to suppress the attacks of arthritis. Various nonsteroidal anti-inflammatory drugs (NSAIDs) often seem effective prophylactically when taken daily, but again, no controlled experience is available. The attacks in a minority of patients are difficult to suppress with any anti-inflammatory drug except adrenal corticosteroids. As in most cases of acute arthritis, corticosteroids instilled into the joint may promote a more rapid return to normal, but their use is seldom justified in a disorder in which return to normal after a few days is the rule.

ARTHRITIS OF FAMILIAL MEDITERRANEAN FEVER

Familial Mediterranean fever (FMF) is a genetic disorder, apparently inherited as an autosomal recessive disorder with complete penetrance.[30] Although it occurs primarily in individuals originating in the greater Mediterranean area, chiefly Sephardic and Iraqi Jews,[31] Levantine Arabs,[32] Turks,[33] and Armenians,[34] it has been described in other groups and as isolated cases.[35,36,37,38] Many instances were undoubtedly included in series reported as periodic diseases, benign or familial paroxysmal peritonitis, or recurrent polyserositis.[34,38,39,40] The characteristic symptoms include intermittent fever and pain in the abdomen, chest, or joints. Amyloidosis (which is genetically determined) occurs in at least 40% of Sephardic Jews who have the disorder; in some, it may be the sole phenotypic expression of the disease (phenotype 2).[41] Amyloidosis develops only rarely when the disease occurs in patients other than Sephardic Jews or Turks,[33,42] and may occur early in life in predisposed groups.[43]

Clinical Picture. The disease first appears in childhood or adolescence and recurs intermittently throughout life. No true sex predilection has as yet been determined, although more men than women seem to be affected.[30] The family history may reveal siblings or other close relatives who have the disease.[30,44] Often there is a history of consanguineous marriage among the forebears.[30]

Fever probably accompanies every attack but does not give rise to shaking chills or other constitutional symptoms and usually lasts only a few hours. Temperature elevations vary from persistent and low-grade to spikes up to 103.1°F (39.5°C)[30] (Fig. 64–1).

The abdominal crises resemble acute peritonitis, lasting from 12 to 24 hours—in rare instances for 3 to 4 days.[30] Serous fluid in the abdominal cavity is the only abnormal finding on laparotomy. Occasionally, abdominal pain simulates pelvic inflammatory disease. Acute chest pain commonly involves only one hemithorax with referral to the corresponding shoulder. It is also of short duration and is usually accompanied by minimal evanescent pleural effusion[30] or pericarditis.[45,46] Many patients experience recurrent attacks of intense tenderness and redness around the ankle. This erysipelas-like erythema is probably not related to underlying joint disease.[30] Intestinal obstruction of serious proportion,[37,47] varying types of renal disease, and cyclic emotional states are sometimes considered part of the disease. Amyloidosis characteristically produces nephrotic syndrome progressing to early death in renal failure.[43,48] Periodic meningitis has been reported.[49] In some instances, Henoch-Schönlein purpura develops.[50]

The musculoskeletal attacks in FMF occur together with, or independent of, other manifestations in approximately 70% of patients. When they occur alone, the later course or the family history confirms the diagnosis. The distribution of attacks is asymmetric, with large joints more commonly involved. The affected joints, in order of decreasing frequency of involvement, are knees, ankles, hips, shoulders, feet and toes, elbows, wrists and hands, and the remaining synovial joints.[51] Isolated disease of the temporomandibular joints[52] or the sacroiliac joints[51] has been described. Arthritis is commonly monoarticular. Subsequent attacks tend to adhere to the established pattern. Attacks are intermittent, not periodic, and of varying duration. They generally last longer than other manifestations of this disease. All afflicted patients experience attacks that terminate in less than a week. Not infrequently, attacks can persist for 2 or 3 weeks, or rarely, for months.[35,51]

Localized pain is the predominant and, at times, the sole symptom. The joint and periarticular area are

THE PATTERN OF FAMILIAL MEDITERRANEAN FEVER

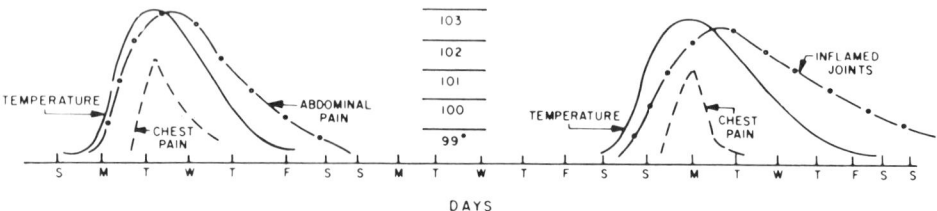

FIG. 64–1. Typical clinical pattern of attacks of familial Mediterranean fever.

usually exquisitely tender, so that the slightest touch cannot be tolerated. At the knees, ankles, elbows, and shoulders, swelling is usually present, accompanied at times by massive effusion. However, swelling is usually not as pronounced as the dramatic pain would imply. Limitation of motion and severe functional impairment result. During an attack, the muscles around the joint are in spasm. However, morning stiffness in the involved or other joints does not occur. The patients do not develop gelling of joints and muscles after rest. Although the involved joints may be somewhat warm initially, the warmth does not persist as long as the pain or functional impairment. Except for the occasional erysipelas-like erythema, redness is notable by its absence. Thus, *an intermittent asymmetric monoarthritis characterized primarily by pain, tenderness, and impaired joint function disproportionate to the amount of swelling and unaccompanied by warmth or redness should alert the physician to the possibility of arthritis of familial Mediterranean fever.*

Joint function recovers completely between attacks.[51] Disuse atrophy, which develops in prolonged attacks and may be marked, is also reversible. Demonstrable residua of attacks are extreme rarities, although occasionally destructive changes do develop.[53] However, when the hip becomes involved in a prolonged attack, functional recovery may not be as likely. In one study, 16 of 18 patients with affected hips developed moderate to marked anatomic and functional changes, with narrowing and sclerosis of the joint space and progressive limitation of motion. Destructive changes occasionally supervene, requiring surgical intervention.[44] Tendon contractures do not occur.[51]

During acute attacks, superficial vessels often dilate over the involved joints, especially at the knee, where they can be readily detected with infrared illumination.

Acute tenderness and swelling of the lower thigh or upper calf may mimic arthritis at the knee. Inflammation of bursal areas may be responsible, as has infrequently been the case at the hip.[51] Various types

of trauma may precipitate attacks. In different patients, overexertion, bruising, heat, cold, and even paracentesis of joints have been implicated. The type of trauma is specific to the patient, but many attacks are not preceded by a recognizable precipitating event.[51]

Arthrodesis occasionally has been performed when FMF was so severe as to be mistaken for tuberculous arthritis. Surgical fusion thus prevented functional recovery, which might otherwise have been inevitable.[51]

Amyloidosis is probably the basis for the frequently encountered splenomegaly. Although many patients come from the area where infectious diseases result in enlarged spleens, patients who have FMF rarely seem to develop intercurrent illnesses.[30]

Among the negative features that aid differential diagnosis are the absence of nodules, urethritis, stomatitis, balanitis, conjunctivitis, uveitis, choroiditis, and dermatitis.

Laboratory Data. Most of the laboratory findings are nonspecific (Table 64–2). ESR and fibrinogen level are elevated or at upper reaches of normal between attacks and soar precipitously with the onset of the

Table 64–2. Laboratory Features in Arthritis of Familial Mediterranean Fever

Test	Results
Blood count	Variable
Urinalysis	Variable
Latex fixation	Negative
LE preparation	Negative
Uric acid	Normal
Fibrinogen	Elevated, spiking during attack
ESR	Elevated, spiking during attack
Circulating immune complexes	Increased in about one-fourth
Cryofibrinogen	Often present
Etiocholanolone	Not elevated
Roentgenograms	Degenerative changes, retarded bone age, osteoporosis, "eggshell line," sacroiliac changes
Biopsy	Nonspecific inflammatory changes, perireticulin amyloidosis

attacks. Within days they return to previous levels.[54] Anemia may be a manifestation of chronic illness. Leukocytosis or leukopenia, the latter in the presence of splenomegaly, is an inconsistent feature. Urinary abnormalities appear only if there is amyloidosis and consist primarily of massive proteinuria. Serum albumin is often decreased. Gamma globulins may be normal or increased, but elevations of the α-2, α-2m, and β-2m globulins, haptoglobin, and lipoproteins are common. The electrophoretic pattern is similar to that seen in amyloidosis even when amyloidosis is not demonstrable.[30] Latex fixation tests for rheumatoid factor are negative, or only transiently positive in low dilutions (1:160 or less).[35,51] Other serologic tests are negative. No association with any histocompatibility (HLA) antigen has been determined.[55] Uric acid or etiocholanolone levels[56] are not elevated (but hypoaldosteronism has been unmasked after renal allotransplantation).[57] Whole serum complement and C1 esterase inhibitor may be deficient.[58] Levels of circulating immune complexes may be increased, as measured by C1q binding[59] (in one of four patients, but in half the Sephardic patients). Cryofibrinogen was present in the plasma samples in one series.[60] Evidence has been presented for C5a inhibitor deficiency in peritoneal and synovial fluids.[61] Lipoxygenase products have been identified in both serum and synovial fluid,[62] and circulating monohydroxy and dihydroxy fatty acids activate neutrophils in this disorder.[63]

Early in the attacks, the joint fluid contains many polymorphonuclear leukocytes, but these are later replaced by lymphocytes. Although viscosity is poor, the mucin clot is fairly adequate. Protein and sugar are unaltered, and cultures are negative.[35,51] Foamy cells have also been described.[30]

Roentgenography. The bone age is generally younger than the chronologic age, leading to the paradoxic finding of degenerative changes with patent epiphyses. When the FMF is prolonged, coarse trabecular metaphyseal osteoporosis forms pseudocysts. Protracted involvement of the knee leads to enlargement of the femoral condyles (Fig. 64–2). All these findings are nonspecific features of long-term immobilization during bone growth, such as occurs in poliomyelitis or hemophilia arthritis.

During the acute phases, soft-tissue enlargement can be seen. With chronicity, the joint space narrows and proliferative marginal bony changes develop. This development, which is particularly prevalent at hips and knees, is partly reversible. The changes may represent periosteal reaction to marginal destruction. True cysts are encountered only rarely. A triangular

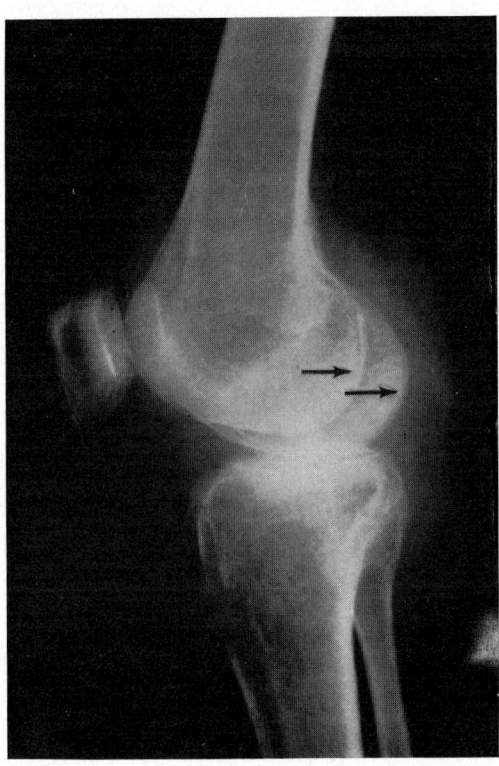

FIG. 64–2. Roentgenogram of knee. The femoral condyles are large. Soft-tissue swelling and osteoporosis are readily apparent. A double-contoured eggshell line outlines the femoral condyles. (Courtesy of Ezra Sohar, M.D., and Joseph Gafni, M.D.)

condensation of the ilium above the acetabulum characterizes chronic hip involvement[51,64] (Fig. 64–3).

In osteoporosis of the femur, the femoral condyles appear as thin eggshell lines separated from the trabecular pattern by a narrow radiolucent zone. With the arthritis of FMF, this eggshell line may be found on both sides of the radiolucent zone.[51] Although it has been described in only a few patients, it may be a specific finding. The line tends to remain even when other roentgenographic changes disappear.

Although there is no clinical evidence of ankylosing spondylitis, some sacroiliac joints are widened and others are sclerosed.[44] Rarely, patchy calcified bridges can be seen in the lower spine. Osteitis condensans ilii is frequently present. In fact, because various sacroiliac abnormalities tend to be found in a disproportionate number of patients, FMF should always be included in the differential diagnosis of radiologic abnormalities of the sacroiliac joints.[65] However, the changes may reflect more the character of the population at risk than results of the disease. The occurrence of sacroiliac changes in populations in whom

FIG. 64–3. Roentgenogram of hip (frog lateral). Marked degenerative changes include pseudocysts, periosteal proliferation and osteoporosis of the femur, and narrowing of the joint space, margin spurs, and a triangular iliac density at the acetabulum. (Courtesy of Ezra Sohar, M.D., and Joseph Gafni, M.D.)

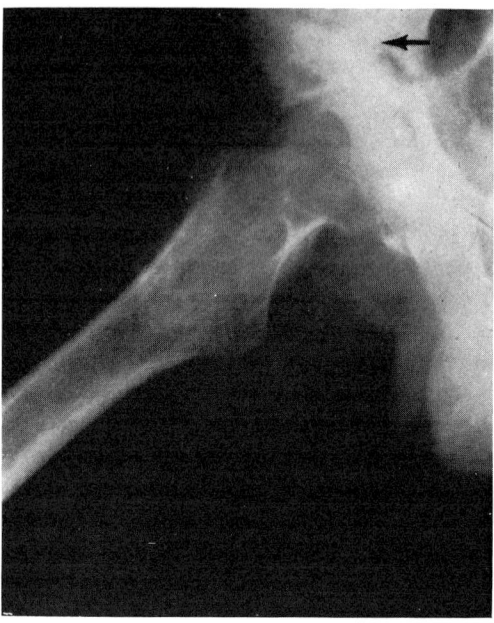

tropical diseases are prevalent[66] makes the significance of this finding questionable.

Pathologic Anatomy. The changes seen in biopsies from inflamed joints are nonspecific. Irregular aggregates of lymphocytes surround small blood vessels, but true perivascular cuffing does not occur. There is increased vascularity, and stromal fibroblasts and polymorphonuclear leukocytes are increased.[51] Lytic lesions of bone are filled with fibrous tissue. Postmortem examinations of joints that had been involved but had recovered reveal no abnormalities.[51]

The amyloidosis encountered in FMF, though primary, is distributed as if it were of the secondary variety.[67] The amyloid is deposited in the perireticular areas of blood vessels and is especially concentrated in spleen and kidney. It has occasionally been demonstrated around blood vessels in or near inflamed joints.[51] The amyloid fibrils consist of AA protein, closely related to serum amyloid A protein (SAA).[68]

Amyloidosis developed in a transplanted cadaver kidney after 4 years in an Armenian women who had intermittenty high levels of the serum precursor SAA, but renal function remained normal for at least an additional 3 years; defective degradation of amyloid precursor(s) may be important in fibril deposition as well.[69]

Treatment. Although no therapy has yet proved curative for FMF, consistent palliation has been achieved with colchicine,[70,71] perhaps because of effects on chemotaxis.[72] Long-term treatment with 0.6 mg of colchicine, two to three times daily, succeeded in reducing the number of attacks in controlled trials.[73] To avoid toxicity, intermittent colchicine therapy was attempted but was successful only in some patients.[74] It was hoped that this regimen would be more acceptable in children, but long-term treatment has now been recommended even here.[75] Steatorrhea and other more minor problems can develop.[76]

Temporary relief of joint pain has sometimes followed use of analgesic preparations. Physical therapy is recommended to avoid disuse atrophy. Corticosteroids have proved singularly ineffective, and unresponsiveness to corticosteroids has been suggested as a differential diagnostic criterion.[51] Earlier intermittent courses of colchicine and immunosuppressive drugs have not proved beneficial.[47] Fat-free diets, once recommended, have been found wanting.[77] In view of the recurrent nature of this disorder, narcotics must be assiduously avoided. Because there is usually complete functional recovery from arthritis, operative intervention is rarely indicated. However, appendectomy should perhaps be performed early because appendicitis cannot readily be distinguished from the abdominal manifestations of this disease. When renal failure complicates amyloidosis of FMF, hemodialysis has extended life for a few years,[78,79] as has renal transplantation.[80] Amyloidosis seems to be prevented by timely administration of colchicine.[81]

Prognosis. Functional recovery from individual attacks and asymptomatic remissions are the rule, except when the hip joint is involved during a protracted attack. The majority of patients in whom FMF is familial will succumb to amyloidosis at a relatively young age, but prophylactic use of colchicine prevents this complication.[48] In ethnic groups other than those commonly affected, prognosis seems more favorable.

BEHÇET'S SYNDROME

Behçet's syndrome is a multisystem disorder, generally classified as an interface between vasculitis and systemic lupus erythematosus.[82] It was originally described as a triple symptom complex consisting of recurrent oral and genital ulcerations and relapsing iritis.[83] Other systemic manifestations were soon added.[84] The original cases were described in countries bordering the Mediterranean, especially Turkey, but large series have since been collected in the rest

Table 64–3. Diagnosis of Behçet's Syndrome

MAJOR CRITERIA

1. Mouth (aphthous) ulcers
2. Iritis (with hypopyon)
3. Genital ulcers
4. Skin lesions
   pyoderma
   nodose lesions

MINOR CRITERIA

5. Arthritis
   of major joints
   arthralgias
6. Vascular disease
   migratory superficial phlebitis
   major vessel thrombosis
   aneurysms
   peripheral gangrene
   retinal and vitreous hemorrhage, papilledema
7. Central nervous system disease
   brain stem syndrome
   meningomyelitis
   confusional states
8. Gastrointestinal disease
   malabsorption
   colonic ulcers
   dilated intestinal loops
9. Epididymitis
10. Hemorrhagic pneumonitis
11. Glomerulonephritis

of Europe, the Middle East, Japan and, lately, the United States. Arthralgias and arthritis have lately been recognized as frequent and prominent manifestations.[85]

Behçet's syndrome received its eponym in 1937, after a description of three patients by the Turkish dermatologist, Professor Hulusi Behçet.[83] A previous case described in Greece by Adamantiades has caused his name to be added to the syndrome in some medical writings.[86] Individual cases were also described by Shigeta in Japan in 1924,[87] and Whitwell in England in 1934.[88] It is probable that a description of the disorder appeared in the writings of Hippocrates, who considered it an acute endemic disease and provided a fairly accurate clinical picture.[89]

The true prevalence of the disorder is difficult to estimate. Many cases go unrecognized, and others may be labeled Reiter's syndrome, Stevens-Johnson syndrome, or even periodic disease. However, Behçet's syndrome has been the subject of more medical articles than the number of cases diagnosed outside the two areas of greatest prevalence (Japan and the Middle East) would seem to warrant.

Newer discoveries have provided some rationale for the two terms, Behçet's disease and Behçet's syndrome. Behçet's disease should be reserved for those cases that clearly meet all the criteria without the presence of some concomitant disorder that might account for certain manifestations; Behçet's syndrome, probably more common in the United States, describes cases in which the classic features are present, but in which an associated disease that could be responsible is also present (e.g., ulcerative colitis or granulomatous enteritis).[90]

Etiology is unknown. Proponents of allergic or "autoimmune" causation group the disorder among the connective tissue diseases,[91] whereas some investigators see evidence for a viral etiology,[92,93] a contention that has been challenged.[94] The possibility of viral precipitation of the disease in a receptive host may reconcile the various viewpoints. Earlier, there had been some interest in blaming various environmental chemicals for Behçet's syndrome; organophosphates, organochloride pesticides, and polychlorinated biphenyls can produce a similar syndrome in swine.[95] Although chemicals and metals also have been implicated, substantive evidence remains elusive.[96]

Earlier reports linking HLA-B5 antigen with Behçet's syndrome were amplified, in that a split of this antigen, B-51, was found in 62% of patients compared with 21% of controls in Japanese studies.[97,98,99] Similar association has been proved in Turkish and British patients.[100] HLA-DR5 and MT2 are represented disproportionately among Japanese patients who have Behçet's syndrome.[98] DR7 is represented disproportionately in a British series.[94] These various antigenic markers are more common in patients who have ocular and neurologic manifestations; HLA-B12 and DR2 are frequently found in patients in whom mucocutaneous and arthritic manifestations predominate.[94] Some have hypothesized a defect in immunoregulation, thought to be under HLA control, that produces changes in cell-mediated immunity and immune complexes that are ultimately responsible for the damage in the disease. Other studies have implicated HLA-AW31 and DRW6.[101] Because MT2 is present in half the Japanese population, its increased prevalence among Behcet's patients is not necessarily of diagnostic importance. HLA-B27 has at times been implicated in arthritic manifestations of Behçet's syndrome,[102] but the possibility remains that these patients might have had a seronegative spondyloarthropathy simulating the findings of Behçet's syndrome. One major North American study failed to find an association between Behçet's syndrome and histocompatibility antigens.[103]

Clinical Picture. The combination of oral and genital ulcers and iritis is crucial to the diagnosis,[104] although some investigators have been satisfied with two of the three symptoms and at least three other accompanying systemic involvements. The major and minor

FIG. 64–4. Aphthous ulcer of the mucous membrane of the lip; note the distinct edges and the surrounding erythema. (Courtesy of the late Professor T. Shimizu.)

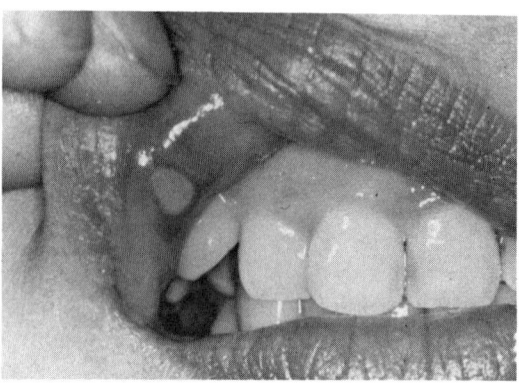

FIG. 64–6. Hypopyon iritis. Pus in the anterior chamber is a transient but important feature of Behçet's syndrome. (Courtesy of the late Professor T. Shimizu.)

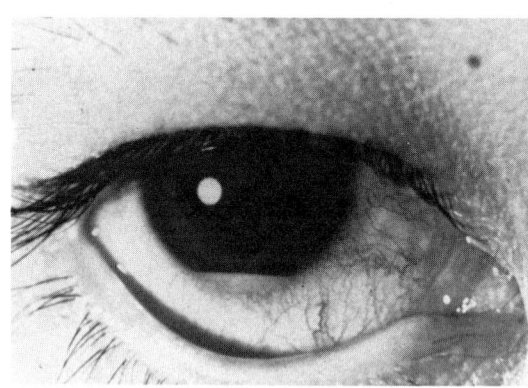

criteria are set forth in Table 64–3. These criteria do not refer to the severity of the manifestations but rather to their almost certain appearance (major) and their relatively infrequent (50% or less minor) appearance. Because Behçet's syndrome is the leading cause of acquired blindness in Japan, a research committee has been formed. The following are the major criteria developed by this committee. (1) Recurrent aphthous ulcerations of the oral mucous membranes consist of painful round or oval ulcers with sharply defined borders, located on labial, buccal, gingival, and lingual mucous membranes (Fig. 64–4). These ulcers tend to occur in crops lasting 1 to 2 weeks and recur at frequent intervals. (2) Skin lesions include erythema nodosum, superficial thrombophlebitis, fol-

FIG. 64–5. Pin prick sign. When the sterile skin is pricked by a sterile needle, a pustule with surrounding erythema develops 24 hours later in many instances of Behçet's syndrome. (Courtesy of the late Professor T. Shimizu.)

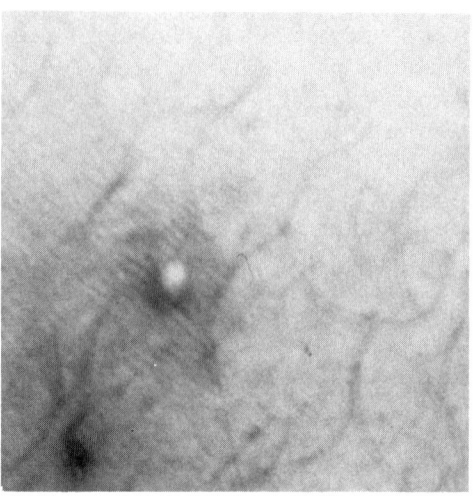

liculitis, acne-like lesions, and cutaneous hypersensitivity. Cutaneous hypersensitivity, a pathergy, is responsible for a sterile pustule with an erythematous margin that develops approximately 1 day after pricking of skin with a sterile needle. It is used as a diagnostic test, especially in Japan and Turkey (where it is positive in 90% of the patients) (Fig. 64–5). (3) Ocular symptoms include iridocyclitis, transient hypopyon iritis (Fig. 64–6), posterior uveitis, retinal detachment, chorioretinitis, and their sequels. (4) There are genital ulcers or painful punched-out lesions of the scrotum (Fig. 64–7), vulva, bladder, cervix, or glans penis (associated with balanitis).

The minor criteria include: (1) arthritis resembling rheumatoid arthritis (Fig. 64–8) or asymmetric arthritis, such as Reiter's syndrome; (2) intestinal ulcerations, especially in the right colon; (3) epididymitis; (4) obliterating thrombophlebitis or arterial occlusions and aneurysms, especially of great vessels; and (5) neuropsychiatric symptoms, including demyelinating disease. According to this committee, the complete syndrome requires that the four main symptoms appear sometime during the clinical course, whereas in the incomplete type, three of the main symptoms and four minor symptoms suffice. Interestingly, HLA-B51 is found in most patients who have the complete syndrome, and only in a slight plurality of patients with the incomplete syndrome.[96] From a diagnostic standpoint, the minor criteria assume increasing importance, as some of them are so characteristic as to point to the correct diagnosis, when the more frequent major criteria might not.

In the original series, men outnumbered women among those who developed the syndrome, but more recently, more women than men have been described.[105] The prevalence of the disorder in Japan

FIG. 64–7. Scrotal ulcer. Note resemblance to oral lesions. (Courtesy of the late Professor T. Shimizu.)

FIG. 64–8. Punched-out lesion of first metatarsal head in Behçet's syndrome. Roentgenographic changes in the joints are rare. (Courtesy of the late Professor T. Shimizu.)

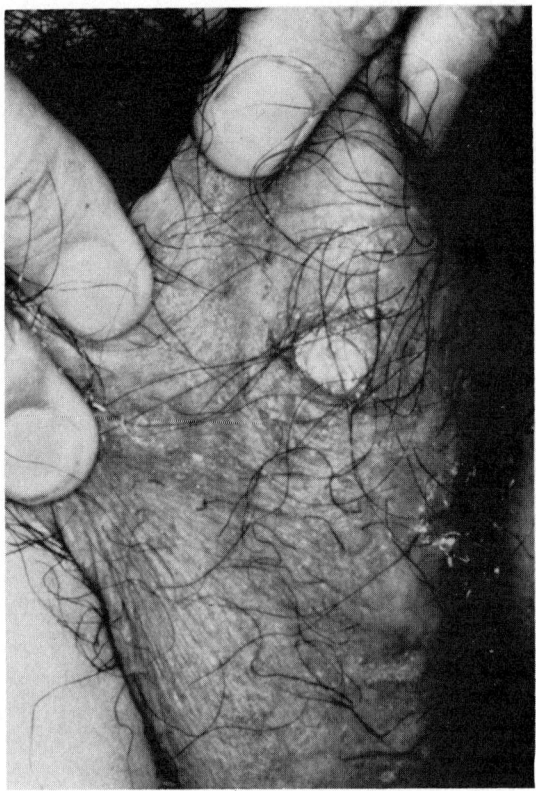

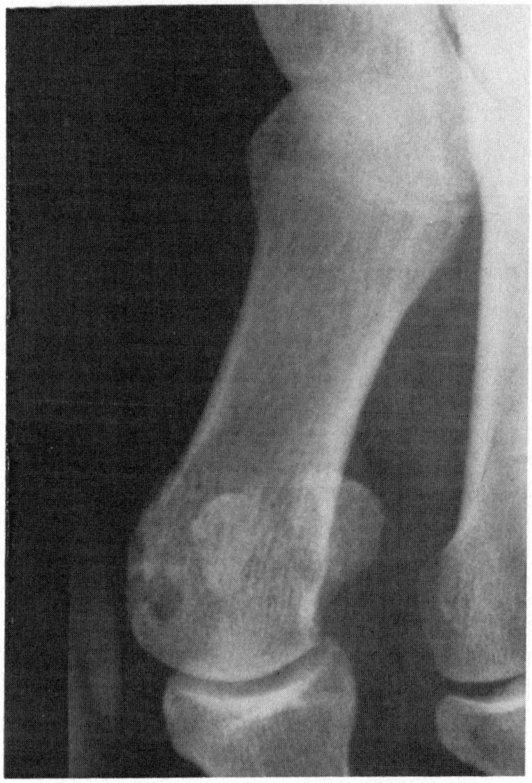

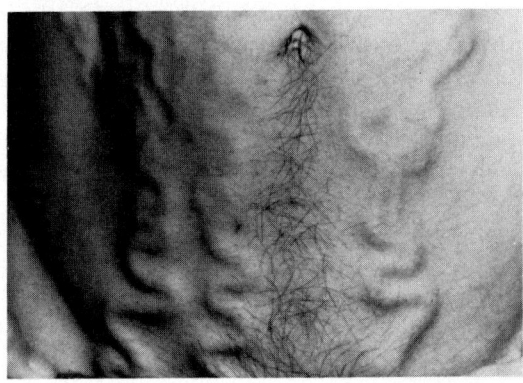

ranges from 1 in 7500 in Hokkaido to none among Japanese in Hawaii and only 6 cases in Okinawa. The distribution favors appearance in cold regions. Attacks also tend to occur during cold spells.[106]

In addition to the ulcerative lesions of the mouth, clinical descriptions include scanty fungiform papillae of the tongue, plaque-like lesions of the pharynx and larynx,[107] and considerable oral fetor.[108] In the eye, in addition to the main features noted, papilledema,[109] exudates and hemorrhages,[110] and optic atrophy[111] are encountered. Although the ulcerative lesions of the penis and scrotum tend to be painful, those of the vulva and vagina often are not, and may be missed.[95] The skin lesion can elaborate to pyoderma. Infection of surgical tracts to their full extent has been described, thought to be related to the pathergy tests.[112] Gangrene of fingertips and toes, thrombosis of superficial veins, thrombosis of the venae cavae (Fig. 64–9), aneurysms and thromboses of major arteries, small vessel vasculitis, and the consequences, including avascular necrosis of bone ends (Fig. 64–10), are dramatic manifestations of the syndrome.[90,95] In the digestive tract, nonspecific symptoms of vomiting, abdominal pain, flatulence, diarrhea, and constipa-

tion are usually noted.[113] Malabsorption and abnormal digestion are commonly seen. Erosions and ulcers are found in the large bowel, predominantly in the cecum, right colon, and occasionally in the terminal ileum. Perforation, melena, and tumor may result. Thrombosis of pulmonary arteries has been

FIG. 64–9. Caput medusae secondary to inferior vena cava occlusion in Behçet's syndrome. (Courtesy of the late Professor T. Shimizu.)

FIG. 64–10. Triangular aseptic necrosis of the femoral head secondary to occlusion of small arteries in Behcet's syndrome. (Courtesy of the late Professor T. Shimizu.)

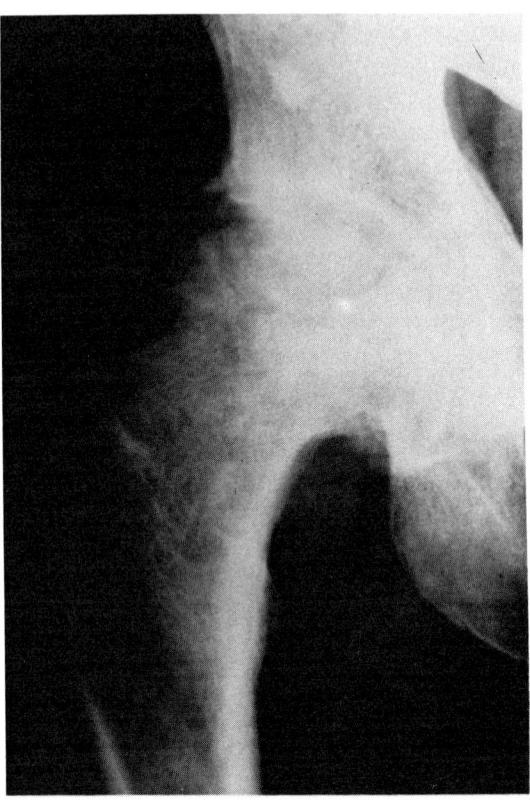

described[114] but is uncommon, as are pulmonary aneurysms[115] and hemorrhagic pneumonitis.[116] Renal involvement has been noted, especially focal glomerulonephritis,[117] but more serious forms of glomerulonephritis have also been encountered.[118,119] Many nervous system disorders, ranging from psychoneurosis through demyelinating disease, have accompanied the syndrome and are particularly likely in Japanese patients.[95] Peripheral neuropathy and myositis can also occur.[120,121]

The prognosis is influenced by the sites of involvement, the severity, and the distribution of the lesions. Recurrent morbidity is likely. In some instances, where the disease settles in, destructive consequences to specific organs will result: enucleation of an eye may be necessary, gangrene may require amputation of a peripheral part, or perforation of a viscus may require surgical removal. Deaths caused by Behçet's syndrome generally result from the central nervous system involvement, although glomerulonephritis or pulmonary involvement can also be blamed. In rare instances, amyloidosis may complicate the picture and also lead to fatality.[122]

Familial clustering has been reported frequently.[102,105,122] Although patients can belong to any racial grouping, they most likely come from inhabitants of the old silk route, extending from central Asia to Turkey and in the opposite direction to Japan via Korea. However, white and black subjects with no remote connection with these Altaic-speaking peoples develop more sporadic cases.[82]

As is true of most other intermittent and periodic syndromes, joint involvement in Behçet's syndrome tends to be monoarticular or oligoarticular, although a symmetric or asymmetric polyarthropathy may also occur. Arthralgias are always more frequent than true arthritis, but arthritis itself develops in more than half the patients.[85] This arthritis often resembles palindromic rheumatism in the context of Behçet's syndrome.[95] The knee is most commonly involved, followed by the ankle, elbow, and wrist; small joints are less commonly involved. Destruction and atrophy of bone and cartilage have been described, as has erosive arthritis,[123] but are exceedingly rare. Behçet's syndrome must be included in the differential diagnosis of sacroiliac joint disease, although sclerosis of the degree seen in ankylosing spondylitis rarely occurs. In some patients, little pain is registered, whereas in others, pain of the severity of gout is present.[124] Thus, intermittent hydrarthrosis, palindromic rheumatism, rheumatoid arthritis, gout and pseudogout, Reiter's syndrome, systemic lupus erythematosus, and enteroarthropathies figure prominently in the differential diagnosis.

Onset tends to be insidious and duration variable, with arthritis remaining from a few weeks to several years. The intervals between arthritic attacks tend to be longer than those between attacks of extra-articular manifestations. The joints are warm, tender, and slightly reddened, and morning stiffness is present. Permanent changes and disability of the joints are rare.[95]

Fever and other constitutional signs are frequently encountered. Myalgias are common. Inner ear involvement with vertigo and hearing disturbances has been added to the list of symptoms.[125]

Laboratory Findings. Acute phase reactants tend to be abnormal during an attack, including rapid sedimentation rate, strongly positive C-reactive protein, and elevation of α-2 globulins.[95] Anemia is common. Chemotactic activity of neutrophils is markedly enhanced.[126,127,128] A polyclonal gammopathy is characteristically found in this disorder. Cryoglobulins can be found in most cases,[99,129] with significant increases of C3 in the arthritic and ocular types, and of IgM and IgG in the mucocutaneous type. In sequential studies, disease remissions or exacerbations correlated with a decrease or increase in serum IgM and IgG cryoglobulins.[129] The converse was found with IgA. Serum complement level is usually high. B-lymphocytes are suppressed and T-lymphocytes are proportionately increased.[95,130] The in vitro response of T-cells to mitogens is depressed.[130] Plasmin, plasminogen activator, and fibrin degradation products are present with greater frequency in the blood of patients who have Behçet's syndrome than in any controls. Enhanced fibrinolytic activity may therefore be present.[131] Antibodies against specific organs involved, including demyelinating antibodies and antimyelin serum factors, have also been reported. Inclusion bodies can be found in various cells from patients who have Behçet's syndrome, but their significance is uncertain.[93]

Neither rheumatoid factor nor antinuclear antibodies are generally present. Rosettes of platelets surrounding neutrophils are seen in Behçet's syndrome. They appear during attacks and are absent between attacks. EDTA-anticoagulated blood, incubated at room temperature for 2 or more hours, may show this phenomenon on an ordinary differential smear.[132] In supravital preparations, the addition of heparin does not alter the phenomenon, but a later addition of calcium abolishes it.[132] This test is relatively specific but insensitive, occurring in the minority of patients. Its sensitivity can be increased by adding sera from patients to donor granulocytes and platelets, and reproducing the rosette phenomenon.[95]

Roentgenography. Significant roentgenographic changes in the joints are rare, occurring in fewer than 1% of patients. These changes resemble the lesions of reactive spondyloarthropathies. Chest radiographs often show infiltrates and rounded opacities, which may progress to excavation. The ulcers in the colon are large, discrete, and multiple, they may take ring shapes, and they often penetrate through the bowel wall. Venograms can reveal blockage of large and small vessels by thrombi, including thrombosis of renal veins and inferior and superior vena cava. Arteriograms show occlusion of major vessels, including the aorta and its branches, and aneurysms. The typical findings of aseptic necrosis of femoral heads may be seen.[95]

Differential Diagnosis. The various other oculocutaneous syndromes and the rheumatic diseases with somewhat similar manifestations have already been mentioned. There is no clear-cut way of differentiating Behçet's syndrome from other disorders it may resemble; the aphthous ulcers of the mouth, for example, are like ordinary aphthous ulcers, and only in context acquire additional significance. There may be regional differences in diagnosing Behçet's syndrome, with inclusion, in some areas, of cases that might be labeled differently in other parts of the world (especially Reiter's syndrome or systemic lupus erythematosus).

Pathology. Basic to all the ulcerative lesions of Behçet's syndrome is vasculitis, which has fueled claims for the inclusion of the disorder among the autoimmune connective tissue syndromes. Mucocutaneous lesions in rats resembling those of Behçet's syndrome in humans have been produced experimentally by injections of mycobacteria and Freund's adjuvant, which more commonly produce arthritis but can also result in dermal, genital, and ocular lesions. Organophosphate insecticides can produce similar lesions in swine. Lesions similar to those of Behçet's syndrome have been produced in man by sensitivities to English walnuts and to ginkgo-tree fruit. Skin hypersensitivity in general is found. Deep to the skin pustules, and to some of the other lesions, including nonspecific synovial involvement and arterial thromboses, are granulocyte-platelet thrombi.[90] The intestinal ulcers, even when perforating, contain minimal, if any, collections of neutrophilic leukocytes. There is superficial necrosis with signs of inflammation and prominent lymph follicles, but relatively uninvolved mucosa between lesions.[95,113] Vasculitis and platelet-granulocyte thrombi have been described in the intestines as well.[90,95]

Treatment. No uniformly effective treatment has been described. Because colchicine had proved effective in other intermittent syndromes, it was at first introduced empirically into the treatment of Behçet's syndrome, and showed much promise, although it was not capable of altering ocular or central nervous system manifestations.[133] Later, a rationale for the action of colchicine was found in its ability to reduce the enhanced granulocyte motility that is a feature of the syndrome.[131] Immunosuppressive compounds have been used; chlorambucil has fared best,[134] and is currently recommended, especially when the eye is involved.[96,135] However, as in other rheumatic diseases treated with immunosuppressants, malignant disease may eventuate.[136] Levamisole proves helpful in some cases, perhaps through its granulocyte suppressing actions.[137] Azathioprine, cyclophosphamide, and other immunosuppressive compounds seem not to be as effective. Corticosteroids provide indifferent results and, in the case of eye involvement, can actually worsen the disease.[138] Blood transfusions, at one time claimed to induce remissions, were later shown to be of no value, but not before the probable active principle, transfer factor, was adduced as likely to prove helpful. In a limited series of cases, transfer factor has brought patients through large-vessel thrombosis and other crises.[139] Fibrinolytic compounds have found some favor.[131,140] The sedative thalidomide, difficult to obtain even for experimental use since the disastrous consequences of its administration to pregnant women two decades ago, proved to be clinically effective under controlled conditions, with dramatic improvement of Behçet's syndrome, particularly of the mucosal and skin lesions.[141] Overall, however, symptomatic therapy of the various expressions of the disease is required and is moderately successful. Major surgery may be necessitated by intractable involvement of vital organs.

Prognosis. Although Behçet's syndrome does not necessarily compromise life expectancy, the advent of nervous system symptoms and signs or of ocular involvement is an ominous event. Therefore, this syndrome ought to be considered as a benign disease subject to serious or fatal complications. Behçet's disease is more likely to be progressive and destructive than Behçet's syndrome occurring in the context of other diseases.

STEVENS-JOHNSON SYNDROME

Joint and muscle involvement in Stevens-Johnson syndrome consists only of transient pains, which may be mere reflections of the severity of the disease. Because there are so many similarities or potential points of confusion between the Stevens-Johnson syndrome and Behçet's syndrome or Reiter's syndrome, however, it is discussed here.

Stevens-Johnson syndrome is included among the oculocutaneous syndromes. Most clinicians regard it as a variant of erythema multiforme exudativum with systemic manifestations and a potentially grave prognosis. Although there seem to be earlier reports, the description by Hebra is considered to be the classic depiction of the cutaneous syndrome. In 1922, Stevens and Johnson elaborated the constitutional symptoms of the syndrome that now bears their names.[142]

The onset of Stevens-Johnson syndrome is heralded by high fever and extensive stomatitis. Although this onset may superficially resemble monilial stomatitis, it rapidly develops into a series of ulcerated lesions on the oral mucous membranes, the conjunctiva, the nasal mucosa, and the genitalia and anus. Within a few days, a bullous and erythematous skin eruption develops anywhere on the body (Fig. 64–11), and erythematous plaques form on the extremities.[143] Pneumonitis is frequently present, either as a precursor or as a concomitant finding. To make the diagnosis, the eruption of erythema multiforme accompanied by bullae or vesicles and stomatitis is required. Documented fever, balanitis, vaginitis or urethritis, and conjunctivitis also occur, although they need not all be present simultaneously.

Widespread arthralgias and myalgias of relatively transient nature may be present. These symptoms are rarely accompanied by actual signs of arthritis.[144]

The syndrome is particularly prevalent in the pediatric age group, although it may occur at any age; the risk of developing the syndrome is greatly re-

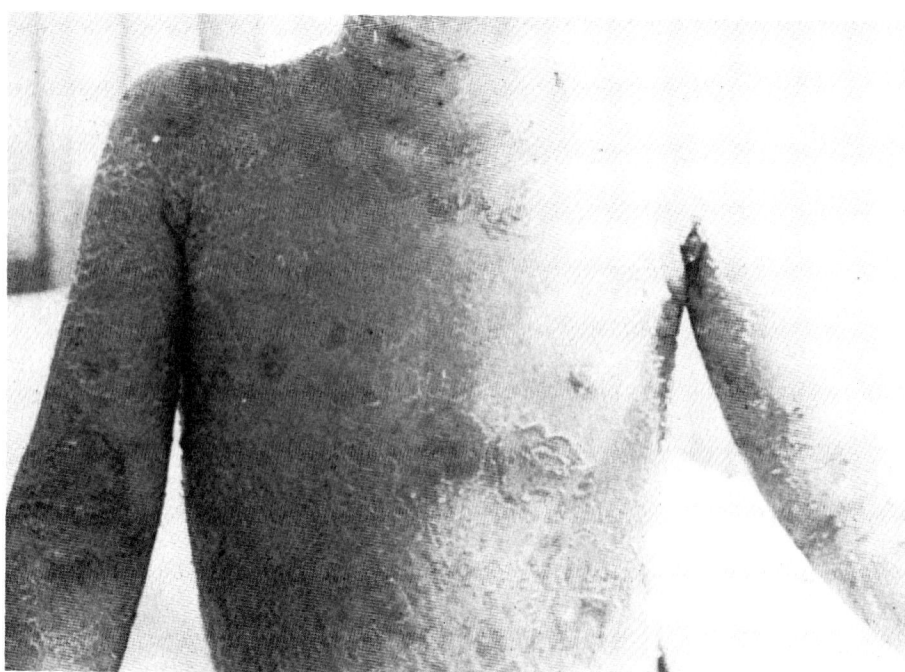

FIG. 64–11. Bullous and crusting eruption in patient with Stevens-Johnson syndrome (erythma multiforme exudativum).

duced after the age of 20. All reports emphasize a male preponderance.

The syndrome begins in one of three ways. It may appear suddenly in an individual of good health, without apparent exogenous factors. In another presentation, there may be symptoms suggestive of an upper respiratory tract[145] or urinary tract infection, for which drug therapy is initiated.[143] Whereas only about one fifth of the patients have the first pattern, half develop the syndrome after prodromata for which some treatment is afforded. In these cases, the prior illness occurs in bodily areas later to be affected by Stevens-Johnson syndrome. The third mode of presentation also follows drug treatment, but for disorders seemingly remote from the Stevens-Johnson syndrome. For example, epilepsy seems unrelated to Stevens-Johnson syndrome, but the administration of anticonvulsants can directly precede the onset of the syndrome.

Laboratory and Roentgenographic Features. No specific abnormalities of laboratry tests or roentgenographic examinations occur to support the diagnosis of Stevens-Johnson syndrome. However, in many cases, mycoplasma pneumoniae are recoverable from the pharynx,[145] sputum,[146] and exudates of the bullous lesions;[143] moreover, rises of specific hemagglutination inhibition and complement fixation antibodies are recorded during the disease, with levels of these antibodies falling during the recovery phase.[147] Leukocyte-bound immunoglobulin is also demonstrable.

Etiology. The causes of this syndrome are still the subject of controversy. Mycoplasma pneumoniae has a clear edge on other microorganisms as a provocative agent.[148,149] Other viruses, fungi, and bacteria have also been implicated. Most cases follow drug therapy, with sulfonamides clearly the major cause.[150] Warning labels have been affixed to certain long-acting sulfa drugs, naming them as potential precursors of Stevens-Johnson syndrome,[151] but careful reviews of the evidence have found it wanting. A few recorded cases have followed administration of drugs in common use for treatment of rheumatic diseases, including aspirin and phenylbutazone.[150] Laxatives and sedatives, many nonprescription, are also culpable. Measles vaccination has preceded the onset. Antibiotics, including clindamycin,[152] have been implicated. Hypoglycemic drugs, most recently chlorpropamide, have also been incriminated.[153] In many cases, no causal relationship to a preceding event can be demonstrated. Antibodies at various sites of specific provocations can be responsible and can account also for the neutropenia often seen at the same time.[154] Immune complexes then deposit in the superficial microvasculature of the skin and mucous membranes.[155]

Treatment. When a specific microorganism seems responsible for the syndrome, appropriate antibiotic therapy, usually with tetracycline, can prove beneficial.[149] In some cases, corticosteroids have been used with mixed success (it may be a matter of selection as some patients worsen while others improve). Nonspecific supportive measures should be taken.

Prognosis. Although fatalities have been recorded,[153] the outlook is not unfavorable, particularly in older patients. Infants and small children bear the greatest risk.

The *periodicity* of the syndrome results from renewed provocation by the offending factor. Recurrent episodes are likely when the syndrome is precipitated by self-administration of a nonprescription medication, which is often beyond the physician's control. Other cases recur because the patient fails to give a complete history and the offending drug is prescribed again.

Because the Stevens-Johnson syndrome occurs in conjunction with ulcerative colitis[156] and disorders of the reticuloendothelial system, including leukemias (usually in response to some therapeutic agent used for these various disorders),[143] underlying diseases should always be sought.

Provocative tests with suspected drugs should never be attempted.

OTHER INTERMITTENT SYNDROMES

Many diseases exhibiting rheumatic symptoms and signs may recur after they have seemingly run their course. Acute tropical polyarthritis, an oligoarticular disorder affecting chiefly the large joints of adults, accompanied by fever and abnormalities of the acute phase reactants, is one such disease and is described by Greenwood.[157] Although the attack is usually single and can be aborted with aspirin, recurrent attacks can develop after an indeterminate interval. Descriptions of this disease have thus far been limited to Africa, but they resemble the epidemic polyarthritis of northern Australia, which is associated with Group A arbovirus infection.

The overlapping manifestations of the syndromes discussed suggest that certain basic underlying mechanisms may be common to all. Because attention paid to esoterica often results in deeper understanding of more common problems, the periodic and intermittent syndromes may lead the way to better understanding of the mechanisms of joint inflammation and the rhythms of nature.

REFERENCES

1. Yazici, H., et al.: Observer variation in grading sacroiliac radiographs might be a cause of sacroiliitis reported in certain disease states. Ann. Rheum. Dis., 46:139–145, 1987.
2. Ragan, C.: Intermittent hydrarthrosis. In Arthritis and Allied Conditions, 7th Ed. Edited by J.L. Hollander. Philadelphia, Lea & Febiger, 1966, p. 755.
3. Reimann, H.A.: Periodic diseases in the aged. Geriatrics, 24:146–149, 1969.
4. Cronkite, E.P.: Granulopoietic models—effect on chemotherapy. N. Engl. J. Med., 282:683–684, 1970.
5. Bywaters, E.G.L., and Ansell, B.: Intermittent hydrarthrosis. In Textbook of the Rheumatic Diseases, 4th Ed. Edited by W.S.C. Copeman. London, E & S Livingstone, Ltd., 1968, p. 525.
6. Schlesinger, H.: Die intermittirenden Gelenkschwellungen. Vienna, A. Holder, Nothnagel's Specielle Pathologie und Therapie, 7:3, 1903.
7. Bukosza, M., Neumark, T., and Balint, G.P.: Calcium pyrophosphate crystals in intermittent hydroarthrosis. J. Rheumatol., 13:967–968, 1986.
8. Klofkorn, R.W., and Lehman, T.J.A.: Eosinophilic synovial effusions complicating chronic urticaria and angioedema. Arthritis Rheum., 25:708–709, 1982.
9. Bocanegra, T.S., et al.: Reactive arthritis induced by parasitic infestation. Ann. Intern. Med., 94:207–209, 1981.
10. El Garf, A.: Parasitic rheumatism: Rheumatic manifestations associated with calcified Guinea worm. J. Rheumatol., 12:976–979, 1985.
11. Al Dabbagh, A.I., and Al Irhayim, B.: Eosinophilic transient synovitis. Ann. Rheum. Dis., 42:462–465, 1983.
12. Hasselbacher, P., and Schumacher, H.R.: Synovial fluid eosinophilia following arthrography. J. Rheumatol., 5:173–176, 1978.
13. Brown, J.P., Rola-Pleszczynski, M., and Menard, H.-A.: Eosinophilic synovitis: Clinical observations on a newly recognized subset of patients with dermatographism. Arthritis Rheum., 29:1147–1151, 1986.
14. Luzar, M.J., and Friedman, B.M.: Acute synovial fluid eosinophilia. J. Rheumatol., 9:961–962, 1982.
15. Hench, P.S., and Rosenberg, E.F.: Palindromic rheumatism. Arch. Intern. Med., 73:293–321, 1944.
16. Hench, P.S., and Rosenberg, E.F.: Palindromic rheumatism: New oft-recurring disease of joints (arthritis, periarthritis, para-arthritis) apparently producing no articular residues: report of 34 cases. Proc. Mayo Clinic, 16:808–815, 1941.
17. Ansell, B.M., and Bywaters, E.G.L.: Palindromic rheumatism. Ann. Rheum. Dis., 18:331–332, 1959.
18. Mattingly, S.: Palindromic rheumatism. Ann. Rheum. Dis., 25:307–317, 1966.
19. Bywaters, E.G.L., and Ansell, B.M.: Palindromic rheumatism. In Textbook of the Rheumatic Diseases, 4th Ed. Edited by N.S.C. Copeman. London, E & S Livingstone, Ltd., 1958, p. 524.
20. Ginsberg, M.H., et al.: Rheumatoid nodulosis. Arthritis Rheum., 18:49–58, 1975.
21. Pasero, G., and Barbieri, P.: Palindromic rheumatism: You just have to think about it! Clin. Exp. Rheumatol., 4:197–199, 1986.
22. Thompson, B., et al.: Palindromic rheumatism. II. Failure to detect circulating immune complexes during acute episodes. Ann. Rheum. Dis., 38:329–331, 1979.
23. Harris, E.D., Jr., Cohen, G.L., and Krane, S.M.: Synovial collagenase: Its presence in culture from joint disease of diverse etiology. Arthritis Rheum., 12:92–102, 1969.
24. Molnar, Z., Metzger, A.L., and McCarty, D.J.: Tubular structures in endothelium in palindromic rheumatism. Arthritis Rheum., 15:553–556, 1972.
25. Schumacher, H.R.: Palindromic onset of rheumatoid arthritis. Arthritis Rheum., 25:361–369, 1982.
26. Ward, L.E., and Okihiro, M.M.: Palindromic rheumatism: Follow-up report. Arch. Inter-Am. Rheum., 2:208–222, 1959.
27. Wajed, M.A., Brown, D.L., and Currey, H.L.F.: Palindromic rheumatism. Ann. Rheum. Dis., 36:56–61, 1977.
28. Zawadzki, Z.A., and Benedek, T.G.: Rheumatoid arthritis, dysproteinemic arthropathy, and paraproteinemia. Arthritis Rheum., 12:555–568, 1969.
29. Epstein, S.: Hypersensitivity to sodium nitrate: A major causative factor in case of palindromic rheumatism. Ann. Allergy, 27:343–349, 1969.
30. Sohar, E., et al.: Familial Mediterranean fever: A survey of 470 cases and review of the literature. Am. J. Med., 43:227–253, 1967.
31. Heller, H., Sohar, E., and Sherf, L.: Familial Mediterranean fever. Arch. Intern. Med., 102:50–71, 1958.
32. Reimann, H.A.: Periodic disease. Medicine (Baltimore), 30:219–245, 1951.
33. Ozdemir, A.I., and Sokmen, C.: Familial Mediterranean fever among the Turkish people. Am. J. Gastroenterol., 51:311–316, 1969.
34. Reimann, H.A.: Periodic disease. JAMA, 136:239–244, 1948.
35. Ehrlich, G.E.: Familial Mediterranean fever. Clin. Orthop., 57:51–55, 1968.
36. Reich, C.B., and Franklin, E.C.: Familial Mediterranean fever in an Italian family. Arch. Intern. Med., 125:337–340, 1970.
37. Siegal, S.: Familial paroxysmal polyserositis. Am. J. Med., 36:893–918, 1964.
38. Siegal, S.: Benign paroxysmal peritonitis. Ann. Intern. Med., 23:1–21, 1945.
39. Priest, R.J., and Nixon, R.K.: Familial recurring polyserositis: A disease entity. Ann. Intern. Med., 51:1253–1274, 1959.
40. Rachmilewitz, M., Ehrenfeld, E.N., and Eliakim, M.: Recurrent polyserositis. JAMA, 171:2355, 1959.
41. Blum, A., et al.: Amyloidosis as the sole manifestation of familial Mediterranean fever (FMF): Further evidence of its genetic nature. Ann. Intern. Med., 57:795–799, 1962.
42. Hurwich, B.J., Schwartz, J., and Goldfarb, S.: Record survival of siblings with familial Mediterranean fever: Phenotypes 1 and 2. Arch. Intern. Med., 125:308–311, 1970.
43. Ludomirsky, A., Passwell, J., and Boichis, H.: Amyloidosis in children with familial Mediterranean fever. Arch. Dis. Child., 56:464–467, 1981.
44. Meyerhoff, J.: Familial Mediterranean fever: Report of a large family, review of the literature, and discussion of the frequency of amyloidosis. Medicine (Baltimore), 59:66–77, 1980.
45. Dabestani, A., et al.: Pericardial disease in familial Mediterranean fever: An echocardiographic study. Chest, 81:592–595, 1982.
46. Raviv, U., Rubinstein, A., and Schonfeld, A.E.: Pericarditis in familial Mediterranean fever. Am. J. Dis. Child., 116:442–444, 1959.
47. Ehrlich, G.E.: Periodic and intermittent rheumatic syndromes. Bull. Rheum. Dis., 24:746–749, 1973.
48. Heller, H., et al.: Amyloidosis in familial Mediterranean fever: An independent genetically determined character. Arch. Intern. Med., 107:539–550, 1961.

49. Vilaseca, J., et al.: Periodic meningitis and familial Mediterranean fever. Arch. Intern. Med., 142:378–379, 1982.

50. Flatau, E., et al.: Schonlein-Henoch syndrome in patients with familial Mediterranean fever. Arthritis Rheum., 25:42–47, 1982.

51. Heller, H., et al.: The arthritis of familial Mediterranean fever. Arthritis Rheum., 9:1–17, 1966.

52. Cooksey, D.E., and Girard, K.: Temporomandibular joint synovitis with effusion in familial Mediterranean fever. Oral Surg., 47:123–126, 1979.

53. Kaushansky, K., Finerman, G.A., and Schwabe, A.D.: Chronic destructive arthritis in familial Mediterranean fever: The predominance of hip involvement and its management. Clin. Orthop., 155:156–161, 1981.

54. Frensdorff, A., Sohar, E., and Heller, H.: Plasma fibrinogen in familial Mediterranean fever. Ann. Intern. Med., 55:448–455, 1961.

55. Fradkin, A., Pras, M., Zemer, D., and Gazit, E.: Familial Mediterranean fever: No association of HLA with amyloidosis or colchicine treatment response. Isr. J. Med. Sci., 21:757–758, 1985.

56. Bondy, P.K., et al.: The possible relationship of etiocholanolone to periodic fever. Yale J. Biol. Med., 30:395–405, 1958.

57. Silver, J., et al.: Unmasking of isolated hypoaldosteronism after renal allotransplantation in familial Mediterranean fever. Isr. J. Med. Sci., 18:495–498, 1982.

58. Reimann, H.A., Coppola, E.D., and Vellegos, G.R.: Serum complement defects in periodic diseases. Ann. Intern. Med., 73:737–740, 1970.

59. Levy, M., et al.: Circulating immune complexes in recurrent polyserositis (familial Mediterranean fever, periodic disease). J. Rheumatol., 7:886–890, 1980.

60. Mosesson, M.W., et al.: Evidence for circulating fibrin in familial Mediterranean fever. J. Lab. Clin. Med., 99:559–567, 1982.

61. Matzner, Y., and Brzezinski, P.: C5a inhibitor deficiency in peritoneal fluids from patients with familial Mediterranean fever. N. Engl. J. Med., 311:287–290, 1984.

62. Aisen, P., et al.: Lipoxygenase production in the serum and synovial fluid of patients with familial Mediterranean fever (FMF) (abstract). Arthritis Rheum., 27:546, 1984.

63. Aisen, P.S., et al.: Circulating hydroxy fatty acids in familial Mediterranean fever. Proc. Natl. Acad. Sci., U.S.A., 82:1232–1236, 1985.

64. Shahin, N., Sohar, E., and Delith, F.: Roentgenological findings in familial Mediterranean fever (FMF). Am. J. Roentgenol., 84:269–283, 1960.

65. Hart, F.D.: The stiff aching back: The differential diagnosis of ankylosing spondylitis. Lancet, 1:740–742, 1968.

66. Mohr, W.: Spondylitis bei Tropenerkrankungen. Verh. Dtsch. Ges. Rheumatol., 1:70–80, 1969.

67. Gafni, J., Sohar, E., and Heller, H.: The inherited amyloidoses: Their clinical and theoretical significance. Lancet, 1:71–74, 1964.

68. Knecht, A., DeBeer, F.C., and Pras, M.: Serum amyloid: A protein in familial Mediterranean fever. Ann. Intern. Med., 102:71–72, 1985.

69. Benson, M.D., Skinner, M., and Cohen, A.S.: Amyloid deposition in a renal transplant in familial Mediterranean fever. Ann. Intern. Med., 87:31–34, 1977.

70. Dinarello, C.A., et al.: Colchicine therapy for familial Mediterranean fever. N. Engl. J. Med., 291:934–937, 1974.

71. Goldstein, R.C., and Schwabe, A.D.: Prophylactic colchicine therapy in familial Mediterranean fever: A controlled double blind study. Ann. Intern. Med., 81:792–794, 1974.

72. Bar Eli, M., et al.: Leukocyte chemotaxis in recurrent polyserositis (familial Mediterranean fever). Am. J. Med. Sci., 281:15–18, 1981.

73. Wolff, S.M.: Familial Mediterranean fever: A status report. Hosp. Pract., 13:113–115, 1978.

74. Wright, D.E., et al.: Efficacy of intermittent colchicine therapy in familial Mediterranean fever. Ann. Intern. Med., 86:162–165, 1977.

75. Lehman, T.J., et al.: Long term colchicine therapy of familial Mediterranean fever. J. Pediatr., 93:876–978, 1978.

76. Ehrenfeld, M., et al.: Gastrointestinal effects of long-term colchicine therapy in patients with recurrent polyserositis (familial Mediterranean fever). Dig. Dis. Sci., 27:723–727, 1982.

77. Mellinkoff, S.M., et al.: Familial Mediterranean fever: Plasma protein abnormalities, low fat diet, and possible implications in pathogenesis. Ann. Intern. Med., 56:171–182, 1962.

78. Ari, J.B., et al.: Dialysis in renal failure caused by amyloidosis of familial Mediterranean fever. Arch. Intern. Med., 136:449–451, 1976.

79. Ilfeld, D., Weil, S., and Kuperman, O.: Correction of a suppressor cell deficiency and amelioration of familial Mediterranean fever by hemodialysis. Arthritis Rheum., 23:38–41, 1982.

80. Jacob, E.T., et al.: Renal transplantation in the amyloidosis of familial Mediterranean fever. Experience in ten cases. Arch. Intern. Med., 139:1135–1138, 1979.

81. Eliakim, M., Levy, M., and Ehrenfeld, M.: Recurrent Polyserositis. Familial Mediterranean Fever, Periodic Disease. Amsterdam, Elsevier/North-Holland, 1981, pp. 119–121.

82. Ehrlich, G.E.: Periodic and intermittent rheumatic syndromes. Bull. Rheum. Dis., 24:746–749, 1974.

83. Behçet, H.: Über rezidivierende aphthöse, durch ein virus verursachte Geschwüre am Mund, am Auge und an den Genitalien. Dermatol. Wchnschr., 105:1152, 1937.

84. Oshima, Y., et al.: Clinical studies on Behçet's syndrome. Ann. Rheum. Dis., 22:36–45, 1963.

85. Mason, R.M., and Barnes, C.G.: Behçet's syndrome with arthritis. Ann. Rheum. Dis., 28:95–103, 1969.

86. Adamantiades, B.: Sur un cas d'iritis a hypopyon recidivante. Ann. Oculist, 168:271, 1931.

87. Shigeta, T.: Recurrent iritis with hypopyon and its pathological findings. Acta Soc. Ophthalmol. Japan, 28:516, 1924.

88. Whitwell, G.P.B.: Recurrent buccal and vulvar ulcers with associated embolic phenomena in skin and eye. Br. J. Dermatol., 46:414, 1934.

89. Feigenbaum, A.: Description of Behçet's syndrome in the Hippocratic third book of endemic diseases. Br. J. Ophthalmol., 40:355–357, 1956.

90. Ehrlich, G.E.: Phagocytes and mediators of inflammation in Behçet's syndrome. *In* Behçet's Disease. Edited by G. Inaba. Tokyo, University of Tokyo Press, 1982, pp. 235–240.

91. Lehner, T.: Behçet's syndrome and autoimmunity. Br. Med. J., 1:465–467, 1967.

92. Denman, A.M., et al.: Lymphocyte abnormalities in Behçet's syndrome. Clin. Exp. Immunol., 42:175–185, 1980.

93. Dilsen, N., et al.: Virus-like particles and tuboreticular structures in kidney and eye of patients with Behçet's syndrome. *In* Behçet's Disease. Edited by G. Inaba. Tokyo, University of Tokyo Press, 1982, pp. 3–14.

94. Lehner, T.: Recent advances in cellular and humoral immunity in Behçet's syndrome. *In* Behçet's Disease. Edited by G. Inaba. Tokyo, University of Tokyo Press, 1982, pp. 357–369.

95. Shimizu, T., et al.: Behçet's disease (Behçet's syndrome). Sem. Arthritis Rheum., 8:223–260, 1979.

96. O'Duffy, J.D., Lehner, T., and Barnes, C.G.: Summary of the third international conference on Behçet's disease. J. Rheumatol., 10:154–158, 1983.

97. Ohno, S., et al.: Close association of HLA-BW51 with Behçet's disease. Arch. Ophthalmol., 100:1455–1458, 1982.

98. Ohno, S., et al.: Close association of HLA-BW51, MT2, and Behçet's disease. In Behçet's Disease. Edited by G. Inaba. Tokyo, University of Tokyo Press, 1982, pp. 73–74.

99. Scarlett, J.A., Kistner, M.L., and Yang, L.C.: Behçet's syndrome. Report of a case associated with pericardial effusion and cryoglobulinemia treated with indomethacin. Am. J. Med., 66:146–148, 1979.

100. Yazici, H., et al.: HLA antigens in Behçet's disease: A reappraisal by a comparative study of Turkish and British patients. Ann. Rheum. Dis., 39:344–348, 1980.

101. Sazazuki, T., et al.: Genetic analysis of Behçet's disease. In Behçet's Disease. Edited by G. Inaba. Tokyo, University of Tokyo Press, 1982, pp. 33–40.

102. Chamberlain, M.A.: A family study of Behçet's syndrome. Ann. Rheum. Dis., 37:459–465, 1978.

103. Moore, S.B., and O'Duffy, J.D.: Lack of association between Behçet's disease and major histocompatibility complex class II antigens in an ethnically diverse North American caucasoid patient group. J. Rheumatol., 13:771–773, 1986.

104. Shimizu, T., et al.: Behçet's disease: Guide to diagnosis of Behçet's disease. Jpn. J. Ophthalmol., 18:291, 1974.

105. Jimi, S., et al.: Epidemiological studies on Behçet's disease. In Behçet's Disease. Edited by G. Inaba. Tokyo, University of Tokyo Press, 1982, pp. 51–56.

106. Maeda, K., Agata, T., and Nakae, K.: Recent trends of Behçet's disease in Japan and some of its epidemiological features. In Behçet's Disease. Edited by G. Inaba. Tokyo, University of Tokyo Press, 1982, pp. 15–24.

107. Lehner, T.: Progress report: Oral ulceration and Behçet's syndrome. Gut, 18:491–511, 1977.

108. Chajek, T., and Fainaru, M.: Behçet disease: Report of 41 cases and a review of the literature. Medicine (Baltimore), 54:179–196, 1975.

109. Pamir, M.N., et al.: Papilledema in Behçet's syndrome. Arch. Neurol., 38:643–645, 1981.

110. Mishima, S., et al.: Behçet's disease in Japan: Ophthalmologic aspects. Trans. Am. Ophthalmol. Soc., 77:225–279, 1979.

111. Cotticelli, L., et al.: Behçet's disease: An unusual case with bilateral obliterating retinal panarteritis and ischemic optic atrophy. Ophthalmologica, 180:328–332, 1980.

112. Yazici, H., et al.: The combined use of HLA-B5 and the pathergy test as diagnostic markers of Behçet's disease in Turkey. J. Rheumatol., 7:206–210, 1980.

113. Kasahara, Y., et al.: Intestinal involvement in Behçet's disease: Review of 136 surgical cases in the Japanese literature. Dis. Colon Rectum, 24:103–106, 1981.

114. Grenier P., et al.: Pulmonary involvement in Behçet's disease. Am. J. Roentgenol., 137:565–569, 1981.

115. Durieux, P., et al.: Multiple pulmonary arterial aneurysms in Behçet's disease and Hughes-Stovin syndrome. Am. J. Med., 71:736–741, 1981.

116. Reza, M.J., and Demanes, D.J.: Behçet's disease: A case with hemoptysis, pseudotumor cerebri, and arteritis. J. Rheumatol., 5:320–326, 1978.

117. Herreman, G., et al.: Behçet's syndrome and renal involvement: A histological and immunofluorescent study of eleven renal biopsies. Am. J. Med. Sci., 284:10–17, 1982.

118. Gamble, C.N., et al.: The immune complex pathogenesis of glomerulonephritis and pulmonary vasculitis in Behçet's disease. Am. J. Med., 66:1031–1039, 1979.

119. Landwehr, D.M., Cooke, D.L., and Rodriguez, G.E.: Rapidly progressive glomerulonephritis in Behçet's syndrome. JAMA, 244:1709–1711, 1980.

120. Afifi, A.K., et al.: The myopathology of Behçet's disease—a histochemical, light- and electron-microscopic study. J. Neurol. Sci., 48:333–342, 1980.

121. Arkin, C.R., et al.: Behçet syndrome with myositis: A case report with pathological findings. Arthritis Rheum., 23:600–604, 1980.

122. Dilsen, N., et al.: Preliminary family study of Behçet's disease in Turkey. In Behçet's Disease. Edited by G. Inaba. Tokyo, University of Tokyo Press, 1982, pp. 103–111.

123. Jawad, A.S.M., and Goodwill, C.J.: Behçet's disease with erosive arthritis. Ann. Rheum. Dis., 45:961–962, 1986.

124. Giacomello, A., Surgi, M.L., and Zoppini, A.: Pseudopodagra in Behçet's syndrome. Arthritis Rheum., 24:750–751, 1981.

125. Brama, I., and Fainaru, M.: Inner ear involvement in Behçet's disease. Arch. Otolaryngol., 106:215–217, 1980.

126. Djawari, D., Hornstein, O.P., and Schotz, J.: Enhancement of granulocyte chemotaxis in Behçet's disease. Arch. Dermatol. Res., 270:81–88, 1981.

127. Fordham, J.N., et al.: Polymorphonuclear function in Behçet's syndrome. Ann. Rheum. Dis., 41:421–425, 1982.

128. Takeuchi, A., et al.: The mechanism of hyperchemotaxis in Behçet's disease. J. Rheumatol., 8:40–44, 1981.

129. Lehner, T., Losito, A., and Williams, D.G.: Cryoglobulins in Behçet's syndrome and recurrent oral ulcerations: Assay by laser nephelometry. Clin. Exp. Immunol., 38:436–444, 1979.

130. Haim, S., et al.: Leucocyte migration inhibition in Behçet's disease. Dermatologica, 159:302–306, 1979.

131. Mizushima, Y., et al.: Colchicine and anti-thrombocytic drugs in the treatment of Behçet's disease. In Behçet's Disease. Edited by G. Inaba. Tokyo, University of Tokyo Press, 1982, pp. 513–518.

132. Ehrlich, G.E., et al.: Further studies of platelet rosettes around granulocytes in Behçet's syndrome. Inflammation, 1:223–229, 1975.

133. Miyachi, Y., et al.: Colchicine in the treatment of the cutaneous manifestations of Behçet's disease. Br. J. Dermatol., 104:67–69, 1981.

134. O'Duffy, J.D.: Treatment of Behçet's disease with chlorambucil. In Behçet's Disease. Edited by G. Inaba. Tokyo, University of Tokyo Press, 1982, pp. 479–486.

135. Bonnet, M.: Immunosuppressive therapy of Behçet's syndrome: Long term follow-up evaluation. In Behçet's Disease. Edited by G. Inaba. Tokyo, University of Tokyo Press, 1982, pp. 487–498.

136. Hamza, M.: Cancer complicating Behçet's disease treated with chlorambucil. Ann. Rheum. Dis., 45:789, 1986.

137. Sampson, D.: Studies on levamisole, a potentially useful drug in the treatment of Behçet's syndrome. J. Oral. Pathol., 7:383–386, 1978.

138. Mimura, Y.: Treatment of ocular lesions in Behçet's disease. In Behçet's Disease. Edited by G. Inaba. Tokyo, University of Tokyo Press, 1982, pp. 499–512.

139. Bernhard, G.C., and Heim, L.R.: Transfer factor treatment of Behçet's syndrome (abstract). J. Rheumatol., 1:34, 1974.

140. Cunliffe, W.J., and Menon, J.S.: Treatment of Behçet's syndrome with phenformin and ethyl oestrenol. Lancet, 1:1239–1240, 1969.

141. Jorizzo, J.L., et al.: Thalidomide effects in Behçet's syndrome

and pustular vasculitis. Arch. Intern. Med., *146*:878–881, 1986.

142. Stevens, A.M., and Johnson, F.C.: A new eruptive fever associated with stomatitis and ophthalmia. Am. J. Dis. Child., *24*:526–533, 1922.

143. Bukantz, S.C.: Stevens-Johnson syndrome. DM, October 1968, pp. 1–36.

144. Coursin, D.B.: Stevens-Johnson syndrome. JAMA, *198*:113–116, 1966.

145. Fleming, P.C., et al.: Febrile mucocutaneous syndrome with respiratory involvement associated with isolation of mycoplasma pneumoniae. Can. Med. Assoc. J., *97*:1458–1459, 1967.

146. Cannell, H., Churcher, G.M., and Milton-Thompson, G.J.: Stevens-Johnson syndrome associated with mycoplasma pneumoniae infection. Br. J. Dermatol., *81*:196–199, 1969.

147. Sieber, O.F., et al.: Mycoplasma pneumoniae infection associated with Stevens-Johnson syndrome. JAMA, *200*:79–81, 1967.

148. Blattner, R.J.: Mycoplasma infection. J. Pediatr., *72*:554–555, 1968.

149. Jones, M.C.: Arthritis and arthralgia in infection with mycoplasma pneumoniae. Thorax, *25*:748–750, 1970.

150. Bianchine, J.R., et al.: Drugs as etiologic factors in the Stevens-Johnson syndrome. Am. J. Med., *44*:390–405, 1968.

151. Carroll, O.M., Bryan, P.A., and Robinson, R.J.: Stevens-Johnson syndrome associated with long acting sulfonamides. JAMA, *195*:691–693, 1966.

152. Fulghum, D.D., and Catalano, P.M.: Stevens-Johnson syndrome from clindamycin. A case report. JAMA, *223*:318–319, 1973.

153. Kanefsky, T.M., and Medoff, S.J.: Stevens-Johnson syndrome and neutropenia with chlorpropamide therapy. Arch. Intern. Med., *140*:1543, 1980.

154. Safai, B., Good, R.A., and Day, N.K.: Erythema multiforme: Report of two cases and speculation on immune mechanisms involved in the pathogenesis. Clin. Immunol. Immunopathol., *7*:379–389, 1977.

155. Kazmierowski, J.A., and Wuepper, K.D.: Erythema multiforme. Clin. Rheumat. Dis., *8*:415–426, 1982.

156. Cameron, A.J., Baron, J.H., and Priestley, B.L.: Erythema multiforme, drugs, and ulcerative colitis. Br. Med. J., *2*:1174–1178, 1966.

157. Greenwood, B.M.: Acute tropical polyarthritis. Q. J. Med., *38*:295–306, 1969.

ARTHRITIS, FOOD ALLERGY, DIETS, AND NUTRITION

65

RICHARD S. PANUSH

NUTRITION AND RHEUMATIC DISEASE

Physicians and patients alike have long been intrigued with the possibility that some foods might provoke, and others ameliorate, arthritis. If the idea is true, then arthritis might respond to appropriate nutritional therapy.[1–8] Diet therapy for rheumatic disease, however, is generally considered quackery, in pursuit of which over 90% of arthritis patients spend nearly 1 billion dollars annually.[9–11] Surprisingly, despite the skepticism of rheumatologists and the fervor of its advocates, little objective information exists about nutritional therapy for rheumatic diseases. This topic is perceived to be an important contemporary issue and has been identified by Klinenberg as among the major future clinical advances anticipated in rheumatology.[12] Most conclusions have been based on inadequate data or improper study design.[1–6]

A relationship between nutrition and rheumatic diseases could occur through two possible mechanisms that are not mutually exclusive. First, nutritional factors might alter immune and inflammatory responses and thus modify manifestations of rheumatic diseases.[1–6] Second, food-related antigens might provoke hypersensitivity responses—food allergies—leading to rheumatologic symptoms.[13] Both possibilities will be reviewed briefly.

THE INFLAMMATORY RESPONSE AND RHEUMATIC DISEASES

Eicosanoids—arachidonic acid–derived prostaglandins and leukotrienes—are important mediators of the inflammatory response.[14] Qualitative and quantitative alterations of polyunsaturated fatty acids in the diet affect endogenous cellular synthesis of eicosanoids,[15] leading to the hypothesis that modulation of dietary fatty acids can alter host responses in the rheumatic diseases. Observations in support of this notion can be summarized briefly as follows. Cold-water fish contain ω-3 (denoting the position from the methyl terminal carbon to the carbon where the first double bond occurs) polyunsaturated fatty acids, such as eicosapentaenoic dihydrate acid (EPA) (characterized by 20 carbons and 5 double bonds, 20:5) and docosahexaenoic acid (DHA, or DCHA, a 22:6, ω-3, polyunsaturated fatty acid). These are incorporated by cells and suppress leukotriene and prostaglandin synthesis from arachidonic acid, an ω-6, 20:4 polyunsaturated fatty acid, when these cells are activated. Further, EPA and DHA are metabolized to eicosanoid analogues having an extra (fifth) double bond, some of which have less biologic activities than arachidonate products.[15–19]

The effects of dietary fish oils on experimental models of rheumatic disease[20–25] are summarized in Table 65–1. Dietary EPA and DHA ingested by human subjects were incorporated by neutrophils and monocytes, blunted cellular responsiveness, and decreased elaboration of cell-derived arachidonic acid metabolites.[26]

Whether fish oils containing EPA and DHA are useful in the treatment of patients with rheumatic diseases is difficult to determine because of uncertainty regarding which components of fish oil might be most

1010

Table 65–1. Fish Oil and Experimental Rheumatic
Disease

EPA suppressed (NZB × NZW)F$_1$ murine SLE[20]
EPA suppressed B × SB murine SLE[21]
Fish oil suppressed NZW × BXSB murine SLE[22]
EPA improved renal function but increased vasculitis in MRL-1pr/1pr mice[22]
Fish oil retarded induction of secondary amyloidosis in CBA/J mice[23]
Fish oil reduced incidence and severity and delayed onset of collagen-induced arthritis in B10.R111 and B10.G mice[24]
Fish oil augmented induction of collagen-induced arthritis in Sprague-Dawley rats[25]

EPA = eicosapentaenoic acid, (NZB × NZW)F$_1$ = New Zealand
black/New Zealand white F$_1$ hybrid mice, SLE = systemic lupus
erythematosus.

effective, what dose of polyunsaturated fatty acids or fish oils should be used, what qualitative alterations of dietary fatty acids might be important, what the optimal duration of therapy should be, which diseases or patients might be responsive, or what effect other antirheumatic therapy or baseline diet might have on exogenous fatty acids.[4,6] In one controlled trial,[27] patients receiving fish oil showed a significant decrease in the number of tender joints, which number reverted toward baseline during followup; these findings are consistent with the thesis that the intake and composition of dietary fats is relevant to disease activity in patients with rheumatoid arthritis (RA).[27] A subsequent trial[28] showed improvement of arthritis symptoms as well as shortened time to fatigue and decreased number of tender joints in patients taking fish oil. A decrease in neutrophil leukotriene B$_4$ correlated with improvement in joint tenderness.[28] Another study[29] also suggested beneficial effects of fish oil on symptoms of RA.

FOOD ALLERGY AND RHEUMATIC DISEASES

Several reasons exist for considering, a priori, that food allergy might relate to rheumatic diseases. Food antigens, food antibodies, complexes of food antigens and antibodies, and lymphocytes sensitized to food antigens have all been detected in the systemic circulation of normal subjects.[30–33] Immunologically mediated symptoms closely follow food ingestion in some individuals. These symptoms are usually anaphylactic, cutaneous, respiratory, or gastrointestinal and are mediated by mechanisms of immediate-type hypersensitivity.[34–37] "Delayed" (hours to days) food reactions such as headaches, behavioral changes, gastrointestinal symptoms, or arthritis,[13] could reflect

food allergy involving mechanisms other than immunoglobulin E (IgE)-mast cell–mediated events.[35–37] Immunologic mechanisms of tissue injury are important in the pathogenesis of many of the rheumatic diseases, but the antigens triggering these mechanisms are unknown. Environmental agents, usually microbial, have received much attention,[38] but food-related antigens remain possibilities. Rheumatic diseases anecdotally associated with foods include Behçet's syndrome associated with black walnuts;[39] systemic lupus erythematosus (SLE) associated with 1-canavanine (in alfalfa)[40] and hydrazine;[41] and rheumatoid or rheumatoid-like arthritis associated with sodium nitrate,[42] dairy products,[43,44] other foods,[45–64] dust and molds,[65] petrochemicals,[65] and tartrazine.[66] Fasting had antirheumatic effects in several studies.[67–69] Lastly, gastrointestinal tract permeability is increased in some patients with RA.[3–5,7,8,69–71]

Our own initial studies of effects of food on arthritis naively used a prescription diet (no red meat, fruit, dairy products, herbs, spices, preservatives, additives, or alcohol) and found that outpatients with long-standing, progressive, active RA fared no better than when receiving a placebo diet.[7] However, some patients improved on the experimental diet and experienced recurrence of symptoms when deviating from it.

A prospective, blinded, controlled trial using our Clinical Research Center was then initiated to determine whether joint symptoms could be associated with food sensitivities in selected patients. The first patient, who had RA, had noted symptomatic exacerbations associated with dairy products and other foods. She exhibited marked consistent subjective and objective improvement during fasting, which was sustained with elemental nutrition. Four different blinded challenges with milk reproducibly exacerbated symptoms, whereas placebo and other foods were without effect. Symptoms peaked 24 to 48 hours after challenge and resolved over 1 to 3 days. Immunologic studies suggested both delayed and immediate cutaneous reactivity to milk, no elevation in antimilk IgE, marked increases of antimilk IgG and IgG4 levels, marginally increased IgG-milk circulating immune complexes, and in vitro cellular sensitivity to milk. Symptomatic exacerbation of arthritis and immunologic hypersensitivity to milk coexisted in this patient.[8]

In further, still preliminary studies we noted that 30% of our patients with RA alleged food-related ("allergic") arthritis. Fifteen patients have now completed 19 double-blind, controlled food challenge studies. Ten were negative, two were equivocal, and three clearly demonstrated subjective and objective rheumatic symptoms after double-blind, encapsulated food challenges; the three were virtually asymptomatic when on elemental nutrition or when not taking the offending foods.[72] All were seronegative with palindromic symptoms and nonerosive disease. Fasting and/or elemental nutrition also benefited several other of these patients.[72] Thus, most patients alleging food-induced rheumatic symptoms did not show these on blinded challenge, but some did. We estimate that probably not more than 5% of rheumatic disease patients have immunologic sensitivity to food(s). Such patients have been identified only by controlled challenge studies. These observations suggest a possible role for food allergy in at least some patients with rheumatic disease. In related work, we and others have noted that substituting cows' milk for water led to inflammatory synovitis in certain rabbit strains.[73]

VITAMINS, MINERALS, AND RHEUMATIC DISEASES

Ascorbic acid has interesting immunoenhancing effects, and reduced levels were found in joint fluids and blood of patients with RA,[74] but there is no convincing evidence that vitamin C has clinically evident therapeutic effects in this condition.[75–77]

Copper bracelets were used by the ancient Greeks to relieve aches and pains.[78–80] Copper salts have been used more recently, concurrent with the development of gold therapy for RA. Rheumatic disease patients treated in open trials with copper compounds showed generally favorable results but many adverse effects.[78–80] Copper in bracelets was absorbed through the dermis, and arthritis patients wearing copper bracelets experienced more subjective improvement than did wearers of identical-appearing "placebo" aluminum bracelets.[81–82] Although of theoretical interest, copper salts are unlikely to achieve an important role in rheumatic disease therapy.

Zinc was given orally to patients with RA, based on observations that serum zinc levels were low, zinc promoted wound and ulcer healing, D-penicillamine (DPA) enhanced intestinal absorption of zinc, zinc was anti-inflammatory in vitro, and zinc was necessary for the maintenance of certain cellular immune responses.[83–85] Zinc-deficient mice and cattle had impaired T-cell–mediated immune responses, and zinc deficiency was found in some children with common variable immunodeficiency; immune responses could be restored with zinc. Also, significant improvement in cellular immune responses occurred when elderly subjects were given zinc sulfate.[86,87] The initial study

of zinc in RA showed that at certain intervals the zinc-treated group fared better than did the placebo-treated patients, but improvement was small.[83] Even this modest effect was not confirmed in subsequent studies.[88,89]

L-histidine, available in health-food stores, has been used to treat patients with RA, with possible benefit in only a small subgroup of patients.[90] A decrease in serum histidine but not other amino acids was found in patients with RA compared with normal subjects, including patients' family members, and correlated with the clinical features of disease.[91–93] Histidine-cystine-copper inhibited in vitro heat-induced aggregation of human IgG.[94] A prospective randomized, placebo-controlled trial suggested possible benefit in patients older than 45 years with more active and prolonged RA.[90]

CONCLUSIONS

RA and most other forms of inflammatory joint disease remain illnesses of unknown cause for which current therapy is often inadequate. The finding that food antigens induce or perpetuate symptoms, at least in some patients, is novel, rational, and exciting. Further, the hypothesis that nutritional modification of (immunologically mediated) inflammation might ameliorate rheumatic symptoms is also of great interest but should be viewed as still experimental. Studies relating diet with arthritis appear to offer the potential of developing novel therapeutic approaches for selected patients and of new insights into disease pathogenesis.

REFERENCES

1. Panush, R.S., Kremer, J.M., and Robinson, D.R.: Dietary aspects of rheumatoid arthritis. Data Centrum, 1986 (unpublished communication).
2. Ziff, M.: Diet in the treatment of rheumatoid arthritis. Arthritis Rheum., 26:457–461, 1983.
3. Panush, R.S.: Controversial arthritis remedies. Bull. Rheum. Dis., 34:1–10, 1985.
4. Panush, R.S.: Nutritional therapy for rheumatic diseases. Ann. Intern. Med., 106:619–621, 1987.
5. Panush, R.S.: Non-traditional remedies. In Primer on the Rheumatic Diseases. 9th Ed. Edited by H.R. Schumacher. Atlanta, GA, Arthritis Foundation (in press).
6. Corman, L.C., and Panush, R.S.: Nutrition and arthritis: A perspective. Rheumatol. News, 6:3, 1985.
7. Panush, R.S., et al.: Diet therapy for rheumatoid arthritis. Arthritis Rheum., 26:462–471, 1983.
8. Panush, R.S., Stroud, R.M., and Webster, E.: Food-induced (allergic) arthritis. Inflammatory arthritis exacerbated by milk. Arthritis Rheum., 29:220–226, 1986.

9. Brown, J.H., Spitz, P.W., and Fries, J.F.: Unorthodox treatments in rheumatoid arthritis. (Abstract.) Arthritis Rheum., 23:657–658, 1980.

10. Wasner, C.K., Cassady, J., and Kronenfeld, J.: The use of unproven remedies. Arthritis Rheum., 23:759–760, 1980.

11. Arthritis, The Basic Facts. Atlanta, GA, Arthritis Foundation, 1981.

12. Klinenberg, J.R.: ARA presidential address: 1984–2034: The next half-century for American rheumatology. Arthritis Rheum., 28:1–7, 1985.

13. Panush, R.S.: Delayed reactions to foods. Food allergy and rheumatic disease. Ann. Allergy, 56:500–503, 1986.

14. Robinson, D.R.: Mediators derived from polyunsaturated fatty acids: Prostaglandins, thromboxanes, and leukotrienes. Postgrad. Adv. Rheumatol., Forum Medicus I: IX. 1–14, 1986.

15. Lee, T.H., and Arm, J.P.: Prospects for modifying the allergic response by fish oils. Clin. Allergy, 16:89–100, 1986.

16. von Shacky, C., Fischer, S., Weber, P.C.: Long-term effects of dietary marine N-3 fatty acids upon plasma and cellular lipids, platelet function, and eicosanoid formation in humans. J. Clin. Invest., 76:1626–1963, 1985.

17. Erickson, K.L.: Dietary fat modulation of immune response. Int. J. Immunopharm., 8:529–543, 1986.

18. Glomset, J.A.: Fish, fatty acids, and human health. N. Engl. J. Med., 312:1253–1254, 1985.

19. Payan, D.G., et al.: Alterations in human leukocyte function induced by ingestion of eicosapentaenoic acid. J. Clin. Immunol., 6:402–410, 1986.

20. Hurd, E.R., et al.: Prevention of glomerulonephritis and prolonged survival in New Zealand black/New Zealand white F_1 hybrid mice fed an essential fatty and deficient diet. J. Clin. Invest., 67:476–485, 1981.

21. Prickett, J.D., Robinson, D.R., and Steinberg, A.D.: Effects of dietary enrichment with eicosapentaenoic acid upon autoimmune nephritis in female NZB × NZW/F_1 mice. Arthritis Rheum., 26:133–139, 1983.

22. Robinson, D.R., et al.: Dietary fish oil reduces progression of established renal disease in (NZB × NZW) F_1 mice and delays renal disease in BXSB and MRL/1 strains. Arthritis Rheum., 29:539–546, 1986.

23. Cathcart, E.S., Leslie, C.A., Meydani, S.N., and Hayes, K.C.: A fish oil diet retards experimental amyloidosis, modulates lymphocyte function, and decreases macrophage arachidonate metabolism in mice. J. Immunol., 139:1850–1854, 1987.

24. Leslie, C.A., et al.: Dietary fish oil modulates macrophage fatty acids and decreases arthritis susceptibility in mice. J. Exp. Med., 162:1336–1344, 1985.

25. Prickett, J.D., Trentham, D.L., and Robinson, D.R.: Dietary fish oil augments the induction of arthritis in rats immunized with type II collagen. J. Immunol., 132:725–729, 1984.

26. Lee, T.H., et al.: Effect of dietary enrichment with eicosapentaenoic and docosahexaenoic acids on in vitro neutrophil and monocyte leukotriene generation and neutrophil function. N. Engl. J. Med., 312:1217–1224, 1985.

27. Kremer, J.M., et al.: Effects of manipulation of dietary fatty acids on clinical manifestations of rheumatoid arthritis. Lancet, 1:184–187, 1985.

28. Kremer, J.M., et al.: Fish-oil fatty acid supplementation in patients with active rheumatoid arthritis, a double-blind controlled crossover study. Ann. Intern. Med., 106:497–503, 1987.

29. Sperling, R.I., et al.: Effects of dietary supplementation with marine fish oil on leukocyte lipid mediator generation and function in rheumatoid arthritis. Arthritis Rheum., 30:180–187, 1987.

30. Cunningham-Rundles, C., Brandeis, W.E., Good, R.A., and Day, N.K.: Bovine antigens and the formation of circulating immune complexes in selective immunoglobulin A deficiency. J. Clin. Invest., 64:272–279, 1979.

31. Paganelli, R., Levinsky, R.J., Brostoff, J., and Wraith, D.G.: Immune complexes containing food proteins in normal and atopic subjects after oral challenges and effect of sodium cromoglycate on antigen absorption. Lancet, 1:1270–1272, 1979.

32. Cunningham-Rundles, C., Brandeis, W.E., Pudifin, D.J., and Day, N.K.: Auto-immunity in selective IgA deficiency: Relationship to anti-bovine protein antibodies, circulating immune complexes and clinical disease. Clin. Exp. Immunol., 45:299–304, 1981.

33. Paganelli, R., Levinsky, R.J., and Atherton, D.J.: Detection of specific antigen within circulating immune complexes: Validation of the assay and its application to food antigen-antibody complexes formed in healthy and food-allergic subjects. Clin. Exp. Immunol., 46:44–53, 1981.

34. Bock, S.A.: Food sensitivity: A critical review and protocol approach. Am. J. Dis. Child., 134:973–982, 1980.

35. Brostoff, J., Ed.: Food allergy. Clin. Immunol. Allergy, 2:1–260, 1982.

36. Anderson, J.A., and Sogn, D.D., Ed.: Adverse reactions to foods. Washington, D.C., U.S. Dept. H.H.S. Pub. No. 84–2442, 1984.

37. Panush, R.S., and Webster, E.M.: Food allergies and other adverse reactions to foods. Med. Clin. North Am., 69:533–546, 1985.

38. Bennett, J.C.: The infectious etiology of rheumatoid arthritis. New considerations. Arthritis Rheum., 21:531–538, 1978.

39. Marquardt, J.L., Snyderman, R., and Oppenheim, J.J.: Depression of lymphocyte transformation and exacerbation of Behçet's syndrome by ingestion of English walnuts. Cell. Immunol., 9:263–272, 1973.

40. Malinow, M.R., et al.: Systemic lupus erythematosus-like syndrome in monkeys fed alfalfa sprouts: Role of a nonprotein amino acid. Science, 216:415–417, 1982.

41. Reidenberg, M.M., et al.: Systemic lupus erythematosus-like disease due to hydrazine. Am. J. Med., 75:365–370, 1983.

42. Epstein, S.: Hypersensitivity to sodium nitrate: A major causative factor in cases of palindromic rheumatism. Ann. Allergy, 27:343–349, 1969.

43. Parke, A.L., and Hughes, G.R.V.: Rheumatoid arthritis and food: A case study. Br. Med. J., 282:2027–2029, 1981.

44. Ratner, P., Schneeyour, A., Eshel, E., and Teitler, A.: Does milk intolerance affect seronegative arthritis in lactose-deficient women? Isr. J. Med. Sci., 21:532–534, 1985.

45. Stroud, R.M.: The effect of fasting followed by specific food challenge on rheumatoid arthritis. In Current Topics in Rheumatology. Edited by B.H. Hahn, F.C. Arnett, T.M. Zizic, and M.C. Hochberg. Kalamazoo, Upjohn, 1983.

46. Otto, R., et al.: Skin-testing with cereal and pulse allergens in progressive chronic polyarthritis. Deutsche Gesundheitswesen, 28:2001–2003, 1973.

47. Rowe, A.H.: Food allergy and the arthropathies. In Food Allergy: Its Manifestations and Control. Edited by A.H. Rowe. Springfield, IL, Charles C Thomas, 1972.

48. Weatherbee, M.: Chronic arthritis. The clinical analysis of three hundred and fifty cases. Arch. Intern. Med., 50:926–944, 1932.

49. Minot, G.R.: General aspects of the treatment of chronic arthritis. N. Engl. J. Med., 208:1285–1290, 1933.

50. Bauer, W.: What should a patient with arthritis eat? JAMA, 104:1–6, 1935.

51. Hench, B.S., et al.: The problem of rheumatism and arthritis.

Review of American and English literature, 1983 (6th Rheumatism Review). Ann. Intern. Med., *13*:1838–1990, 1940.

52. Hench, B.S., et al.: Rheumatism and arthritis. Review of the American and English literature, for 1940 (8th Rheumatism Review). Ann. Intern. Med., *15*:1002–1108, 1941.

53. Rosenberg, E.F.: Diet and vitamins in rheumatoid arthritis. *In* Comroe's Arthritis and Allied Conditions. 5th ed. Edited by J.L. Hollander. Philadelphia, Lea & Febiger, 1954.

54. Turnbull, J.A.: Changes in sensitivity to allergenic foods in arthritis. Am. J. Dig. Dis., *15*:182–190, 1944.

55. Pottenger, R.T.: Constitutional factors in arthritis with special reference to incidence and role of allergic disease. Ann. Intern. Med., *12*:323–333, 1928.

56. Zeller, M.: Rheumatoid arthritis-food allergy as a factor. Ann. Allergy, *7*:200–239, 1949.

57. Kaufman, W.: Food induced allergic musculoskeletal syndromes. Ann. Allergy, *11*:179–184, 1953.

58. Zussman, B.M.: Food hypersensitivity simulating rheumatoid arthritis. South. Med. J., *59*:935–939, 1966.

59. Millman, M.: An allergic concept of the etiology of rheumatoid arthritis. Ann. Allergy, *30*:135–141, 1972.

59a. Darlington, L.G., Ramsey, N.W., and Mansfield, J.R.: Placebo-controlled, blind study of dietary manipulation therapy in rheumatoid arthritis. Lancet, *1*:276–238, 1986.

60. Lewin, P., Taub, S.J.: Allergic synovitis due to ingestion of English walnuts. JAMA, *106*:2144, 1936.

61. Berger, H.: Intermittent hydroarthrosis with an allergic basis. JAMA, *112*:2402–2405, 1939.

62. Hench, P.S., Rosenberg, E.F.: Palindromic rheumatism. Proc. Staff Meetings Mayo Clin., *16*:808–815, 1941.

63. Vaughn, W.T.: Palindromic rheumatism among allergic persons. J. Allergy, *14*:256–263, 1943.

64. Randolph, T.G.: Ecologically oriented rheumatoid arthritis. *In* Clinical Ecology. Edited by L.D. Dickey, Springfield, IL. Charles C Thomas, 1976.

65. Mandell, M., and Conte, A.: The role of allergy in arthritis, rheumatism, and associated polysymptomatic cerebro-viscero-somatic disorders: A double-blind provocation test study. (Abstract.) Ann. Allergy, *44*:51, 1980.

66. Wraith, D.G.: Allergic joint symptoms. Presented at the 4th International Food Allergy Symposium of the American College of Allergy, Vancouver, Canada, July 25–29, 1982.

67. Skoldstam, L., Larsson, L., and Lindstrom, F.D.: Effects of fasting and lactovegetarian diet on rheumatoid arthritis. Scand. J. Rheum., *8*:249–255, 1979.

68. Uden, A.M., Trang, L., Venizelos, N., and Palmblad, J.: Neutrophil functions and clinical performance after total fasting in patients with rheumatoid arthritis. Ann. Rheum. Dis., *42*:45–51, 1983.

69. Sundqvist, T., et al.: Influence of fasting on intestinal permeability and disease activity in patients with rheumatoid arthritis. Scand. J. Rheumatol., *11*:33–38, 1982.

70. Rooney, P.J., Jenkins, R.T., Goodacre, R.L., and Sivakumaran, T.: Gut permeability of small molecules in rheumatoid disease. (Abstract.) Clin. Res., *31*:160A, 1983.

71. Bjarnason, I., et al.: Intestinal permeability and inflammation in rheumatoid arthritis: Effects of non-steroidal anti-inflammatory drugs. Lancet, *11*:1171–1173, 1984.

72. Panush, R.S., et al.: Food-induced ("allergic") arthritis. Clinical and serological studies. (Abstract.) Arthritis Rheum., *29*(Suppl.):S-33, 1986.

73. Panush, R.S., et al.: Food-induced ("allergic") arthritis. A unique new model of inflammatory synovitis in rabbits. (Abstract.) Arthritis Rheum., *29*(Suppl.):S-33, 1986.

74. Panush, R.S., Delafuente, J.C., Katz, P., and Johnson, J.: Modulation of certain immunologic responses by vitamin C. III. Potentiation of in vitro and in vivo lymphocyte responses. Int. J. Vitamin Nutr. Res., *23*(Suppl.):35–47, 1982.

75. Hall, M.G., Darling, R.C., and Taylor, F.H.C.: The vitamin C requirement in rheumatoid arthritis. Ann. Intern. Med., *13*:415–423, 1939.

76. Massell, B.F., Warren, J.E., Patterson, P.R., and Lehmous, H.J.: Antirheumatic activity of ascorbic acid in large doses. Preliminary observations on seven patients with rheumatic fever. N. Engl. J. Med., *242*:614–615, 1956.

77. Abrams, E., and Sandson, J.: Effect of ascorbic acid on rheumatoid synovial fluid. Ann. Rheum. Dis., *23*:295–299, 1964.

78. Sorenson, J.R.J.: Copper complexes—A unique class of anti-arthritis drugs. Progr. Med. Chem., *15*:211–260, 1978.

79. Sorenson, J.R.J.: Development of copper complexes for potential therapeutic use. Agents Actions [Suppl.], *8*:305–325, 1981.

80. Sorenson, J.R.J., and Hangarter, W.: Treatment of rheumatoid and degenerative diseases with copper complexes. A review with emphasis on copper-salicylate. Inflammation, *2*:217–238, 1977.

81. Walker, W.R., Beveridge, S.J., and Whitehouse, M.W.: Dermal copper drugs: The copper bracelet and Cu ($\pm$I) salicylate complexes. Agents Actions [Suppl.], *8*:359–367, 1981.

82. Walker, W.R., and Keats, D.M.: An investigation of the therapeutic value of the "copper bracelet"—Dermal assimilation of copper in arthritic/rheumatoid conditions. Agents Actions, *6*:454–459, 1976.

83. Simkin, P.A.: Oral zinc sulfate in rheumatoid arthritis. Lancet, *2*:539–542, 1976.

84. Simkin, P.A.: Zinc sulfate in rheumatoid arthritis. Prog. Clin. Biol. Res., *14*:343–351, 1977.

85. Simkin, P.A.: Treatment of rheumatoid arthritis with oral zinc sulfate. Agents Actions [Suppl.], *8*:587–596, 1981.

86. Fernandez, G., et al.: Impairment of cell-mediated immunity in dietary zinc deficiency in mice. Proc. Natl. Acad. Sci. U.S.A., *76*:457–461, 1979.

87. Duchateua, J., Delepesse, G., Vrijens, R., and Collet, H.: Beneficial effects of oral zinc supplementation on the immune response of old people. Am. J. Med., *70*:1001–1004, 1981.

88. Rasker, J.J., and Kardaun, S.H.: Lack of beneficial effect of zinc sulphate in rheumatoid arthritis. Scand. J. Rheumatol., *11*:168–170, 1982.

89. Job, C., Menkes, C.J., and Delbarre, F.: Zinc sulfate in the treatment of rheumatoid arthritis. (Letter.) Arthritis Rheum., *23*:1408–1409, 1980.

90. Pinals, R.S., Harris, E.D., Burnett, J.B., and Gerber, D.A.: Treatment of rheumatoid arthritis with L-histidine: A randomized, placebo-controlled, double-blind trial. J. Rheumatol., *4*:414–419, 1977.

91. Gerber, D.A.: Decreased concentration of free histidine in serum in rheumatoid arthritis, an isolated amino acid abnormality not associated with generalized hypoaminoacidemia. J. Rheumatol., *2*:384–392, 1975.

92. Gerber, D.A.: Low free serum histidine concentration in rheumatoid arthritis. A measure of disease activity. J. Clin. Invest., *55*:1164–1173, 1975.

93. Kirkham, J., Lowe, J., Bird, A.A., and Wright, V.: Serum histidine in rheumatoid arthritis: A family study. Ann. Rheum. Dis., *40*:501–502, 1981.

94. Gerber, D.A.: Copper-catalyzed thermal aggregation of human gamma-globulin. Inhibition by histidine, gold thiomalate, and penicillamine. Arthritis Rheum., *17*:85–91, 1974.

section VI

SYSTEMIC RHEUMATIC DISEASES

INTRODUCTION TO SYSTEMIC RHEUMATIC DISEASES: NOSOLOGY AND OVERLAP SYNDROMES

66

MORRIS REICHLIN

The diffuse connective tissue diseases are a group of syndromes of unknown origin whose classification often presents formidable clinical problems. One cause of this classification problem is the large number of "overlap syndromes," which apparently exist among and between what are manifestly uncommon conditions. Dubois[1] stated that as many as 25% of all patients with diffuse rheumatic disease will have overlap features. These findings include coexistent systemic lupus erythematosus (SLE) and scleroderma; an overlap of SLE, scleroderma, and polymyositis (PM), which has been called mixed connective tissue disease (MCTD); scleroderma-PM; coexistent SLE and rheumatoid arthritis (RA); and the relationship that lymphocytic infiltration of the lacrimal and salivary glands bears to all the diffuse connective tissue diseases in what is recognized as Sjögren's syndrome.

Two current areas of investigation show promise for identifying specific biologic or biochemical markers that could be tightly linked with specific disease processes. These areas are (1) immunogenetics and (2) the identification of individual antigen–antibody reactions that exhibit disease specificity. The former subject is covered in Chapters 24 and 25, whereas the latter subject is discussed in many other chapters. Some specific aspects of this latter approach are explored here.

CLASSIFICATION OF POLYMYOSITIS

These problems are best illustrated by considering the classification of one group of these diseases, the PM syndromes. A clinical diagnosis of PM depends on the recognition of a pattern of proximal muscle weakness, on certain histopathologic findings in muscle biopsy specimens on the demonstration of characteristic findings, and on the presence in serum of elevated levels of muscle enzymes, notably creatine phosphokinase, transaminases, and aldolase (see Chapter 65). Further study of a given patient may also suggest the presence of another of the connective tissue diseases, such as RA, SLE, scleroderma, or Sjögren's (sicca) syndrome. If no features of another connective tissue disease are present, one views the patient as having PM or, if a characteristic dermatitis accompanies the muscle involvement, dermatomyositis (DM). This group of patients has long been believed to carry an increased risk for various carcinomas, although questions have been raised about the extent of this relationship.[2]

The nosology is often complicated by the variable presence in the diffuse rheumatic diseases of shared clinical features. Polyarthritis and Raynaud's phenomenon may appear in PM patients without other clinical or serologic features suggesting the presence of other connective tissue diseases. In early evaluations, one may be erroneously led to the diagnosis of either SLE or scleroderma. Opportunities for confusion abound.

Is PM one or many diseases with one or many pathogenetic mechanisms and one or many causes? PM occurring by itself is not distinguishable on clinical grounds from PM coincident with another connective tissue disease, and no solid clinical clues exist to differentiate the various forms of PM. Although nothing is known of the causes of these diseases, something is known of their pathogenesis. The pathogenesis of muscle damage has been reviewed.[3] Evidence for humoral mechanisms, either immune complex mediated or organ specific, is sparse, whereas evidence supporting a cell-mediated immune attack on muscle is strong.[3] Lymphocytes found in patients with PM are specifically cytotoxic for muscle cells and do not require serum factors for their activity. The presence and intensity of the activity of such cells correlate roughly with clinical activity. It is likely that such muscle-specific cytotoxic lymphocytes constitute the immunopathogenetic mechanism leading to muscle destruction and weakness in PM.

In the future, identification in patients with PM of the precise muscle antigens responsible for the activation of lymphocytes might shed light on the identity or nonidentity of immunopathogenetic pathways. If lymphocytes are activated by a single, unique, muscle-specific antigen, considerable importance will be given to the idea that a unitary immune mechanism exists in all PM patients. If, however, each group of lymphocytes from patients with PM, DM, or PM associated with another connective tissue disease reacts to a specific but different antigen, the alternative idea that PM is a collection of separate diseases in which the original sensitization process is characteristic for each "disease" would be more attractive. Finally, if such investigations reveal no pattern of antigenic specificity, such studies will have failed to improve our ability to classify these diseases. So far the detection of relatively specific "marker" antibodies for the various connective tissue diseases is encouraging.

SPECIFIC ANTIGEN–ANTIBODY MARKERS

Serologic reactions shown to exhibit some degree of disease specificity are listed in Table 66–1. Until recently, no antigen–antibody reaction has exhibited any specificity for the PM syndromes. Although rheumatoid factors (RFs) and antinuclear antibodies (ANAs) occur in moderate titers in about one third of such patients, these findings do not have an impact on diagnosis and are recognized as being nonspecific. At least three major antigen–antibody reactions are now recognized that show specificity for PM. The first of these involves a trypsin-sensitive nuclear antigen demonstrated initially by a modified complement fixation reaction with somewhat more specificity for DM than PM.[4] This antigen has been designated Mi, referring to the first two letters of the patient's name whose serum served as prototype for this reaction. In more recent studies using an enzyme-linked immunosorbent assay (ELISA), the specificity for DM is even more apparent.[5] The second antigen–antibody system described with specificity for patients with PM has been designated Jo_1.[6] This antibody occurs in 40% of uncomplicated PM and in <10% of DM patients, but not in sera from patients with SLE, RA, progressive systemic sclerosis (PSS), or Sjögren syndrome or in sera from normal, healthy individuals. The antigen has been identified as the enzyme histidyl tRNA synthetase.[7,8] Smaller numbers of patients with PM also make antibodies to threonyl and alanyl tRNA synthetase.[9,10] The association of antibody to Jo_1 with the DRw3 antigen suggests the involvement of specific immune response genes in its production.[11]

A third reaction involves a nucleolar antigen designated PM-Scl, because at least half the patients with antibodies to it have features of PSS as well as PM.[12] This latter system relates to a proportion of the patients originally described by Wolfe et al.,[13] whose sera contained antibody to an antigen designated PM_1. These authors reported that 60% of patients with PM had antibodies to PM_1. It is now apparent that while 60% of patients with PM have antibodies that precipitate with thymus extracts, at least three major systems (Jo_1, PM-Scl, and nRNP) and a number of minor systems account for this reactivity.[14] Studies now show that most patients without precipitins have antibodies detectable by the indirect immunofluorescence that bind to Hep-2 cells (a human epithelial tissue culture line).[14]

Such antigen–antibody reactions provide tests with diagnostic usefulness and reinforce the concept that individual antigen–antibody reactions can serve as "markers" for differentiation of the different connective tissue syndromes. Reactions that differentiate cases of PM and DM from cases of, for example, SLE and PM imply fundamental differences in the etiopathogenesis of the disease process in these two situations. Continued study of these reactions should further clarify the conceptualization of PM occurring in various clinical guises.

The disease specificity of antibodies to native DNA is the best studied antigen–antibody system. Numerous reports have shown a high correlation of antibodies to native DNA with SLE,[15] but such antibodies have been reported in the other systemic connective tissue diseases. Such reports must be interpreted with reservation because commercial "native" DNA (carbon-14–labeled KB DNA) clearly has many single-stranded regions. Ablation of these single-stranded regions with a specific enzyme (S_1 nuclease) or their removal on modified diethylaminocellulose (DEAE)

Table 66-1. Antigen–Antibody Reactions: "Markers" for Individual Connective Tissue Diseases

Antigen to Which Specific Antibody Directed	Associated Disease*
Jo$_1$	PM
Mi	DM
PM-Scl (Nucleolar)	PM–PSS overlap
Native DNA	SLE
Sm	SLE
Nuclear ribonucleoprotein (nRNP)	SLE, MCTD
Ro/SSA	SLE, Sjögren's syndrome
La/SSB/Ha	SLE, Sjögren's syndrome
Scl$_{70}$	PSS
Centromere	PSS

*DM = dermatomyositis; PM = polymyositis; SLE = systemic lupus erythematosus; MCTD = mixed connective tissue disease; PSS = progressive systemic sclerosis (systemic scleroderma).

columns leads to loss of apparent antinative DNA reactivity from non-SLE sera.[16] Thus, it is clear that the disease specificity of antibodies to native DNA rests on the use of impeccably native DNA. The crithidia lucilia assay has been of value in this regard. This immunofluorescent assay used crithidiae, which contain a giant molecule of circular double-stranded DNA in their kinetoplasts.[17]

The other antigen–antibody system exhibiting high specificity for SLE is that involving Sm, a soluble nuclear antigen, antibodies to which are detected by precipitation in agar gels.[18,19] Other antigen–antibody systems characteristically occur in SLE sera, but they are less specific, occurring to some extent in other diseases. Their disease specificity is under active investigation, and their ultimate usefulness as markers for SLE patients requires further study. These include antibodies to the soluble antigens Ro[20] and La[21] and nuclear ribonucleoprotein (nRNP).[22] Antibodies to Ro and La also occur in Sjögren's syndrome, and anti-nRNP occurs in MCTD.

Antibodies to nRNP constitute the only constant feature of patients with MCTD.[23–25] and the definition of this entity as distinct from its component diseases SLE, PM, and PSS remains controversial.[26–28] The nosologic problem can be illustrated by the following considerations. Many SLE patients lacking "overlap" features such as myositis and sclerodactyly show, as their sole precipitating serum antibody, anti-nRNP. Many such patients fulfill the American Rheumatism Association (ARA) criteria for the diagnosis of SLE. If these patients are classified as having MCTD, the clinical criteria for this diagnosis are meaningless, because overlap features are absent. Yet these patients share with the MCTD patients a low frequency of serious renal disease and a relatively favorable prognosis.[29] In my experience such "SLE" patients with anti-nRNP outnumber those showing the overlap features of MCTD by four or five to one.

A series of antigen–antibody reactions commonly

associated with Sjögren's syndrome were described by Alspaugh and Tan[30] and designated SS-A and SS-B. An antigen termed Ha that reacts with antibodies in 13% of SLE sera as well as in 68% of sera with Sjögren's syndrome has been characterized.[31,32] It is now known that the Ro antigen is identical to SSA, whereas the La antigen is identical to both SSB and Ha.[33] It is perhaps not surprising to find serologic links between the sicca syndrome and SLE in view of the demonstrable genetic link between these diseases manifested by shared Ia antigens.[34,35]

Scleroderma frequently occurs in overlap syndromes but is often difficult to recognize in the early phases of the disease. Biochemical, genetic, or serologic correlative markers would be of great nosologic value in this disease. Diverse antibodies have now been described in patients with PSS, some of which promise to show high disease specificity.[36] A precipitin reaction with a nuclear antigen of MW 70,000 Daltons present in rabbit thymus extract has been designated Scl[70] because of its relative disease specificity and its molecular weight. It occurs in sera from about 20% of patients with PSS. This antigen has been identified as the enzyme *topoisomerase 1*.[37] A second antibody that binds to the centromere of chromosomes of Hep-2 cells (anticentromere antibody) occurs in the sera of about 50% of PSS patients and seems to be more specific for the disease variant characterized by calcinosis, Raynaud's syndrome, esophageal dysfunction, sclerodactyly, and telangiectasia (CREST), which occurs in ~90% of such patients, than for diffuse scleroderma (see Chapter 73). Finally, antibodies to two nucleolar antigens, *fibrillarin*, a 34 KD protein rich in N^{G}N^G dimethyl-arginine, and *RNA polymerase 1*, show promise of being specific markers for PSS patients.[38,39] The apparent diagnostic specificity of these reactions for PSS awaits more extensive studies.

Undoubtedly, at least some of the reactions discussed here will take their place as standard tools in the diagnosis of the connective tissue diseases. Others, such as anti-nRNP, might prove less useful for diagnosis than for identifying a subset of patients with a lower frequency of serious nephritis and a better prognosis.

The ultimate resolution of the overlapping clinical features so frequently encountered in the diffuse systemic connective tissue diseases will require both better definition of pathogenetic and immunopathogenetic pathways and identification of etiologic agents.

REFERENCES

1. Dubois, E.L.: The relationship between systemic lupus erythematosus, progressive systemic sclerosis and mixed connective tissue disease. *In* Systemic Lupus Erythematosus. Edited by E.L. Dubois. Los Angeles, University Southern California Press, 1974.
2. Bohan, A., and Peter, J.R.: Polymyositis and dermatomyositis. N. Engl. J. Med., *292*:344–347, 1975.
3. Dawkins, R.L.: Experimental autoallergic myositis, polymyositis, and myasthenia gravis. Clin. Exp. Immunol., *21*:185–201, 1975.
4. Reichlin, M., and Mattioli, M.: Description of a serological reaction characteristic of polymyositis. Clin. Immunol. Immunopathol., *5*:12–20, 1976.
5. Targoff, I.N., and Reichlin, M.: The association between Mi-2 antibodies and dermatomyositis. Arthritis Rheum., *28*:796–803, 1985.
6. Nishikai, M., and Reichlin, M.: Heterogeneity of precipitating antibodies in polymyositis and dermatomyositis. Characterization of the Jo₁ antibody system. Arthritis Rheum., *23*:881–888, 1980.
7. Rosa, M.D., et al.: A mammalian tRNA histidyl-containing antigen is recognized by the polymyositis specific antibody anti-Jo-1. Nucleic Acids Res., *11*:853–870, 1983.
8. Mathews, M.B., and Bernstein, R.M.: Myositis autoantibody inhibits histidyl tRNA synthetase: A model for autoimmunity. Nature, *304*:177–179, 1983.
9. Mathews, M.B., et al.: Antithreonyl tRNA synthetase, a second myositis-related autoantibody. J. Exp. Med., *160*:420–434, 1984.
10. Bunn, C.C., Bernstein, R.M., and Mathews, M.B.: Autoantibodies against alanyl tRNA synthetase and tRNA^Ala coexist and are associated with myositis. J. Exp. Med., *163*:1281–1291, 1986.
11. Arnett, F.C., et al.: The Jo₁ antibody system. Clinical and immunogenetic associations in myositis. J. Rheumatol., *8*:925–930, 1981.
12. Reichlin, M., et al.: Antibodies to a nuclear/nucleolar antigen in patients with polymyositis overlap syndrome. J. Clin. Immunol., *4*:40–44, 1984.
13. Wolfe, J.F., Adelstein, E., and Sharp, G.C.: Antinuclear antibody with distinct specificity for polymyositis. J. Clin. Invest., *59*:176–178, 1977.
14. Reichlin, M., and Arnett, F.C.: Multiplicity of antibodies in myositis sera. Arthritis Rheum., *27*:1150–1156, 1984.
15. Reichlin, M., and Mattioli, M.: Antigens and antibodies characteristic of systemic lupus erythematosus. Bull. Rheum. Dis., *24*:756–761, 1974.
16. Locker, J.D., et al.: Characterization of DNA used to assay sera for anti-DNA antibodies. Determination of the specificities of

17. anti-DNA antibodies in SLE and non-SLE rheumatic disease states. J. Immunol., *118*:694–701, 1977.
18. Aarden, L.A., de Groot, E.G.R., and Feltkamp, T.E.W.: Immunology of DNA. III. Crithidia luciliae: A simple substrate for the detection of antibodies to dsDNA with the immunofluorescence technique. Ann. N.Y. Acad. Sci., *254*:505–514, 1975.
19. Tan, E.M., and Kunkel, H.G.: Characteristics of a soluble nuclear antigen precipitating with the sera of patients with systemic lupus erythematosus. J. Immunol., *96*:464–471, 1966.
20. Notman, D.D., Kurata, N., and Tan, E.M.: Profiles of antinuclear antibodies in systemic rheumatic diseases. Ann. Intern. Med., *83*:464–469, 1975.
21. Clark, G.C., Reichlin, M., and Tomasi, T.B.: Characterization of a soluble cytoplasmic antigen reactive with sera from patients with systemic lupus erythematosus. J. Immunol., *102*:117–122, 1969.
22. Mattioli, M., and Reichlin, M.: Heterogeneity of RNA-protein antigens reactive with sera of patients with systemic lupus erythematosus. Arthritis Rheum., *17*:421–429, 1974.
23. Mattioli, M., and Reichlin, M.: Characterization of a soluble nuclear ribonuclear protein antigen reactive with LE sera. J. Immunol., *107*:1281–1290, 1971.
24. Sharp, G.C., et al.: Association of antibodies to ribonucleoprotein and Sm antigens with mixed connective tissue diseases, systemic lupus erythematosus, and other rheumatic diseases. N. Engl. J. Med., *295*:1149–1154, 1976.
25. Sharp, G.C., et al.: Mixed connective tissue disease. An apparently distinct rheumatic disease syndrome associated with a specific antibody to an extractable nuclear antigen. Am. J. Med., *52*:148–159, 1972.
26. Sharp, G.C., et al.: Association of autoantibodies to different nuclear antigens with clinical patterns of rheumatic disease and responsiveness to therapy. J. Clin. Invest., *50*:350–359, 1971.
27. Reichlin, M.: Mixed connective disease. *In* Modern Topics in Rheumatology. Edited by G.R.V. Hughes. London, Heinemann Ltd., 1976.
28. Reichlin, M.: Problems in differentiating SLE and mixed connective tissue disease. N. Engl. J. Med., *295*:1194, 1976.
29. Maddison, P.J., Mogavero, H., and Reichlin, M.: Patterns of clinical diseases associated with antibodies to nuclear ribonucleoprotein. J. Rheumatol., *5*:407–411, 1978.
30. Reichlin, M., and Mattioli, M.: Correlation of a precipitin reaction to an RNA-protein antigen and a low prevalence of nephritis in patients with systemic lupus erythematosus. N. Engl. J. Med., *286*:908–911, 1972.
31. Alspaugh, M.A., and Tan, E.M.: Antibodies to cellular antigens in Sjögren's syndrome. J. Clin. Invest., *55*:1067–1073, 1975.
32. Akizuki, M., Powers, R., Jr., and Holman, H.R.: A soluble acidic protein of the cell nucleus which reacts with serum from patients with systemic lupus erythematosus and Sjögren's syndrome. J. Clin. Invest., *59*:264–272, 1977.
33. Kassan, S.S., et al.: Antibody to a soluble nuclear acidic antigen in Sjögren's syndrome. Am. J. Med., *63*:328–335, 1977.
34. Alspaugh, M.A., and Maddison, P.J.: Resolution of the identity of certain antigen-antibody systems in systemic lupus erythematosus and Sjögren's syndrome: An interlaboratory collaboration. Arthritis Rheum., *22*:796–798, 1979.
35. Moutsopoulos, H.M., et al.: Genetic differences between primary and secondary sicca syndrome. N. Engl. J. Med., *301*:761–763, 1979.
36. Reinertsen, J.L., et al.: B-lymphocyte alloantigens associated with systemic lupus erythematosus. N. Engl. J. Med., *229*:515–518, 1978.
37. Tan, E.M., et al.: Diversity of antinuclear antibodies in pro-

gressive systemic sclerosis: Anticentromere antibody and its relationship to CREST syndrome. Arthritis Rheum., 23:617–625, 1980.

37. Shero, J.H., et al.: High titers of autoantibodies to topoisomerase I (Sci 70) in sera from scleroderma patients. Science, 231:737–740, 1986.

38. Lischwe, M.A., et al.: Purification of a nucleolar scleroderma antigen (M^r = 34,000, pI, 8.5) rich in N^GN^G dimethylarginine. J. Biol. Chem., 260:14304–14310, 1985.

39. Reimer, G., et al.: Autoantibody to RNA polymerase I in scleroderma sera. J. Clin. Invest., 79:65–72, 1987.

SYSTEMIC LUPUS ERYTHEMATOSUS: CLINICAL ASPECTS AND TREATMENT

67

NAOMI F. ROTHFIELD

Systemic lupus erythematosus (SLE) is a disease of unknown cause that affects many organ systems and is characterized by the presence of multiple auto-antibodies that participate in immunologically mediated tissue injury.

HISTORICAL ASPECTS

During the nineteenth century, the term "lupus" described a skin disease that consisted of spreading ulcerations of the face. Acute and chronic types were distinguished in 1872 by Kaposi.[1] The concept of a systemic form of the disease was formulated by Osler in 1895 when he suggested that the basis of the disease was vasculitis.[2] He described a systemic disease with a variety of skin manifestations and recognized the involvement of joints, intestinal tract, serosal surfaces, and kidney. Osler also described the characteristic periods of exacerbation and remission. The pathologic abnormalities were later described by Libman and Sacks,[3] Gross,[4] and Baehr, Klemperer, and Schrifrin,[5] who emphasized that changes in many organs occurred even in the absence of the typical skin lesions.

In 1948, Hargraves, et al. described the lupus erythematosus (LE) cell.[6] This major advance soon led to an increased interest in the disease, to an increased frequency of diagnosis, and, eventually, to our understanding of the mechanism of the LE cell phenomenon and to the concept that antibodies were directed against nuclear antigens. Soon after the discovery of

the LE cell, corticosteroids and antimalarials were used for treatment. It became possible to prolong the life of patients and to follow the course of successfully treated patients. The discovery of antinuclear antibodies by means of the indirect fluorescence technique led to the recognition of a wide variety of antibodies and to an understanding of their clinical significance. The concept of SLE as an immune complex mediated disease evolved and the role of complement in producing tissue damage was elucidated. More recently, various B cell, T cell, and macrophage functions have been noted to be abnormal in patients with active SLE (see Chapter 69). Genetic factors have been elucidated and an abnormality of estrogen metabolism has been described (Chapters 28 and 29). No single abnormality can totally explain the disease, however. Additional environmental factors appear to be necessary for disease expression.

INCIDENCE AND PREVALENCE

SLE affects individuals of all races, but its prevalence varies in different countries (see Chapter 3). In France, the disease appears to be more common among immigrants from Portugal, Spain, North Africa, and Italy than among natives. In Hawaii, the disease is more common in Orientals or Polynesians than among whites.[7] The disease has only recently been described in black Africans[8] and appears to be more prevalent in China than in the United States.[9]

The average annual incidence in the United States

has been estimated to be 27.5 per million population for white females and 75.4 per million population for black females. The incidence of SLE among hospitalized patients was 4.6 per 100,000 per year in a Baltimore, Maryland, study,[10] and 1.8 for patients living in Rochester, Minnesota.[11] The 1.8 annual incidence rate is similar to that observed in Sweden, in New York, and in Jefferson County, Alabama, between 1955 and 1965. Incidence rates showed a steady increase beginning in early 1960, but they have stabilized since then, probably because of a greater appreciation of milder cases and improvement of diagnostic tests during the 1960s. The prevalence of SLE in a prepaid health plan for 125,000 patients indicates that SLE affects approximately 1 in 1000 women.[12] In the Rochester, Minnesota, study, which included all patients in a white population, the prevalence of definite SLE per 100,000 population on January 1, 1980, was 40.0 (53.8 for women and 19.0 for men). This figure is somewhat lower than 51 per 100,000 reported for a prepaid health group in San Francisco from 1965 to 1973.

SLE occurs in children and in the elderly, but the peak age at the onset of the first symptom is between 15 and 25 years. The mean age at diagnosis is 30 years (Fig. 67–1). In our own series of 433 patients, 90% are females. A higher percentage of males is affected among children and among the elderly SLE patients.

GENETIC FACTORS

Several cases of SLE can occur within a family (see also Chapter 29).[13] Families with members who have chronic discoid lupus and others who have SLE have been reported. Family members of some SLE patients have isolated laboratory abnormalities such as false-positive tests for syphilis, antinuclear antibodies, hypergammaglobulinemia, and deposits of immunoglobulins in their skin.[13,14] Relatives of SLE patients have an increased frequency (5%) of the disease.[15] The frequency of HLA-DR2 and DR3 in both whites and blacks is increased.[16,17,18] An association of SLE with hereditary deficiencies of several complement proteins exists, also. SLE and lupus-like syndromes have been found to be associated with genetic deficiencies of C1r, C1s, C1, INH, C4, C2, C5, and C8, with C2 being the most commonly associated deficiency. A total deficiency of C2 was found in 1 of 100 consecutive SLE patients studied by us and in one of 10,000 normal individuals studied by others.[19,20] Heterozygous (partial) deficiency of C2 is also common among patients with SLE, occurring in about 6% of patients as compared with 1% in normal individuals.[20] This genetic abnormality is associated with the presence of the histocompatibility antigens HLA-A10 and HLA-B18.

HORMONAL FACTORS

Studies have shown that both male and female SLE patients have an increased hydroxylation of estrone to 16 α-hydroxyestrone, a metabolite that is a potent estrogenic hormone.[21] The onset of SLE frequently occurs at menarche, during pregnancy, or during the postpartum period, or with the use of oral contraceptives containing estrogen.[22] Testosterone metabolism

FIG. 67–1. Sex and age at diagnosis in 356 SLE patients. (From Tan, E., and Rothfield, N.: Lupus erythematosus. *In* Immunologic Disease. 3rd Ed. Edited by M. Samter. Boston, Little, Brown and Company, 1979.)

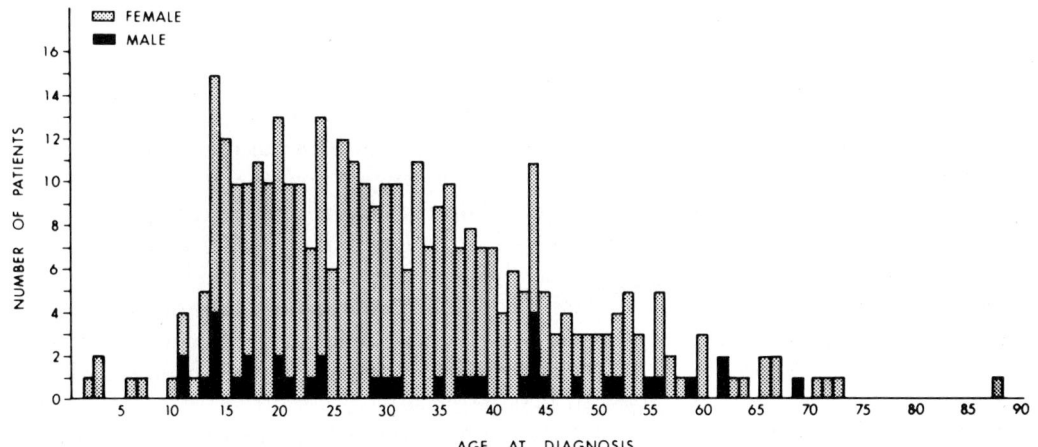

also is different in women with SLE.[23] The association of Klinefelter's syndrome with SLE has been well documented and suggests that the X chromosome may be a predisposing factor for human SLE as well as for murine lupus.[24]

ENVIRONMENTAL FACTORS

A history of sun exposure before onset of the disease is obtained in about 36% of patients. The number of new cases of SLE usually is increased during the late spring and summer months in southern New England and in New York. In other parts of the country with persistent year-round sun, the incidence of new cases may not vary in this fashion. The relative lack of sunlight in England has been postulated as an explanation for the rarity of the disease in that country. Sun exposure at the beach or swimming pools leads to rashes and to the onset of multisystem disease.

SLE patients develop exacerbations of their disease during episodes of infections. Data show that bacterial products such as lipopolysaccharides (polyclonal B-cell activators) can induce antibodies to single- and double-stranded DNA in various strains of mice.[25] Thus, during periods of infection, bacterial products might produce similar changes in individuals with the appropriate genetic background and thereby lead to the development of SLE. A variety of drugs have been implicated as capable of producing the whole or partial clinical or serologic features of SLE.

CLINICAL FEATURES AND PATHOLOGY

GENERAL FEATURES

Fatigue is present in nearly all SLE patients during periods of disease activity. It is frequently an early manifestation and can precede the appearance of objective findings such as rash or joint swelling. Corticosteroid treatment leads to a feeling of well-being and disappearance of fatigue. During subsequent periods of clinical exacerbation, fatigue usually reappears and may be the first symptom of an impending flare. The fatigue in SLE patients is similar to that felt by patients with viral hepatitis and may be the patient's major symptom.

Fever is present in about 90% of patients at the time of diagnosis. In some patients, fever is low grade, whereas in others it is spiking. It responds rapidly to corticosteroid therapy if the drug is given every 6 hours. A single daily dose of prednisone is usually not adequate to control the fever, which will return 6 to 8 hours after the daily dose has been ingested. During the course of the disease, recurrence of fever is viewed with concern because it may result from infection. *Fever in a treated SLE patient should be attributed to infection until proved otherwise.*

Weight loss has occurred in about 85% of patients at the time of diagnosis unless the nephrotic syndrome is present. Subsequent exacerbations may be preceded by a gradual or rapid loss of weight and accompanying fatigue.

DERMATOLOGIC MANIFESTATIONS

Abnormalities of the skin, hair, or mucous membranes are the second most common manifestations of SLE. Whereas arthralgia or arthritis occurs in 95% of patients, dermatologic abnormalities occur in 85%.

A rash after sun exposure (photosensitivity) is common, occurring in 33% of SLE patients. The onset of the disease frequently occurs after significant sun exposure and, in most patients, a rash will recur after sun exposure during the course of the disease.

The classic butterfly blush was present at the time of diagnosis in 52% of our patients and is nearly always located on both cheeks and across the bridge of the nose. It may be preceded by sun exposure and is initially considered by the patient to be sunburn. The blush may also occur without a history of sun exposure. The lesion heals well and leaves no scars. It may be confused with the erythematous rash of acne rosacea or seborrheic dermatitis, but the erythema of seborrheic dermatitis is particularly marked in the nasolabial folds, whereas the butterfly rash of SLE *characteristically spares the nasolabial folds.* Acne rosacea is characterized by the presence of papules and pustules, but pustules are not found in the facial rash of SLE unless secondary infection is present.

The second most common erythematous rash seen in SLE patients is a nonspecific maculopapular rash resembling a drug eruption. This rash may occur after sun exposure and may be located anywhere on the body, although it is most often found on the face and chest. Occasionally, scattered macules may also occur on the palms and fingers and less often on the soles of the feet. The rash usually heals without scarring or hyperpigmentation, but lesions occasionally persist; they become crusted and the skin may show hyperpigmentation and atrophy, although no scarring is noted. Persistent lesions with central atrophy of the skin without true scarring has been called *subacute cutaneous lupus.*

Subacute lesions differ from discoid lesions in that

they do not lead to scarring. They are erythematous at the edge and tend to be annular and widespread on the chest, back, arms, and, occasionally, legs. Subacute lesions usually begin as small erythematous, slightly scaly, papules and may evolve into either annular lesions or a papulosquamous lesion with a scaly surface, closely resembling psoriasis. Such subacute lesions are more common in patients with antibodies to Ro (SSA) who have the HLA antigens B8 and DR3.[26]

Lesions of chronic discoid lupus occurred in 19% of our patients. In about 40% of these patients, the lesions preceded the development of SLE by from 2 to 35 years. About half the lesions developed around the time of the diagnosis of SLE, and only about 10% of the patients developed discoid lesions after the diagnosis of SLE. The SLE patients with discoid lesions showed a higher incidence of Raynaud's phenomenon and photosensitive rashes than did those without discoid lesions. Discoid lesions commonly involve the scalp and may also be seen on and in the external ear. Discoid lesions begin as erythematous plaques or papules and spread outward, leaving central areas of hyperkeratosis, follicular plugging, and atrophy. The edge of an active lesion is edematous and erythematous, whereas a healed lesion may show central depigmentation with scarring and hyperpigmentation at the margin.

Alopecia occurs in about 70% of patients. The alopecia is usually diffuse, but may appear as patches of hair loss (Fig. 67–2). In about 20% of SLE patients, the diffuse alopecia is so extreme that the patients are compelled to buy wigs. The hair slowly regrows as the disease becomes inactive. It is important to reassure the patient that the loss of hair is not permanent. Alopecia usually recurs with disease exacerbation and, in some patients, may be an excellent first sign of an impending flare. Tufts of hair are easily pulled out in a patient with alopecia, and the severity

FIG. 67–2. Patchy alopecia in a man with systemic lupus erythematosus.

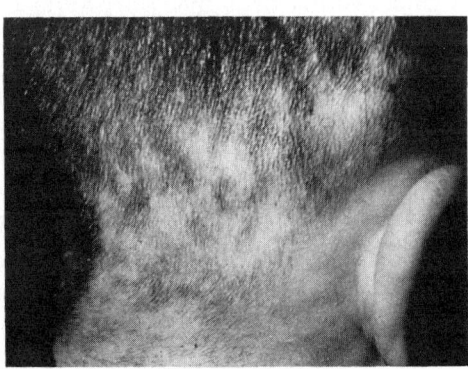

of the alopecia can be followed quantitatively by serial attempts to pull the hair out. As the new hair grows in, the patient's scalp develops a stubbled look. Patches of alopecia may occur temporarily when macular-papular lesions occur in the scalp. Lesions of discoid lupus in the scalp heal with atrophy and scarring. The permanent loss of hair follicles results in permanent areas of alopecia.

Vasculitic skin lesions are not uncommon in SLE patients and usually occur in the setting of significant disease activity in other organ systems. Vasculitic lesions with ulceration may occur on the extensor surface of the forearm. Palpable purpuric lesions may be observed especially on the lower extremity; on biopsy, these lesions reveal leukocytoclastc angiitis. Less commonly, vasculitic lesions may be noted on the backs of the hands, on the palms as blotchy and slightly purpuric lesions, near the small joints of the fingers, and on the finger pads as tender erythematous nodules. Periungual erythema is noted in about 10% of patients and palmar erythema in 20%. Splinter hemorrhages or nailfold thrombi are occasionally found. Atrophic "blanche" lesions similar to those seen in Degos' disease consist of erythematous papular or infiltrated lesions that gradually develop pearly white centers and telangiectasis at the margins.[27]

Livido reticularis is quite common in SLE patients, especially those with active disease, and is noted on the lower extremities, particularly around the knees and ankles. When the legs are dependent, the toes may take on a purplish hue. Livido reticularis is due to vasculitis of small vessels and may precede gangrene in some patients. Livido may involve not only all four extremities, but the trunk as well in some patients with active disease in other organ systems and with serologic evidence of immune complex deposition (low serum C3 and C4 and high levels of anti-DNA antibodies).

Mucosal ulcers are common (40%) in SLE patients.[28] These are most commonly found on the hard or soft palate and are asymptomatic (Fig. 67–3). Occasionally, a patient complains of pain when eating spicy foods or notes a tender area on the roof of the mouth. These palatal ulcers are present in patients with active disease and disappear within a few days of institution of corticosteroid therapy. Nasal septal ulcerations are less common. These lesions are seen on the anterior aspect of the nasal septum and will be missed if the otoscope is inserted too far into the nares. Nasal septal perforations occur in some of these patients.[29] Patients with nasal ulcerations may complain of epistaxis and nasal stuffiness caused by secretions or crusts over the ulcerated areas.

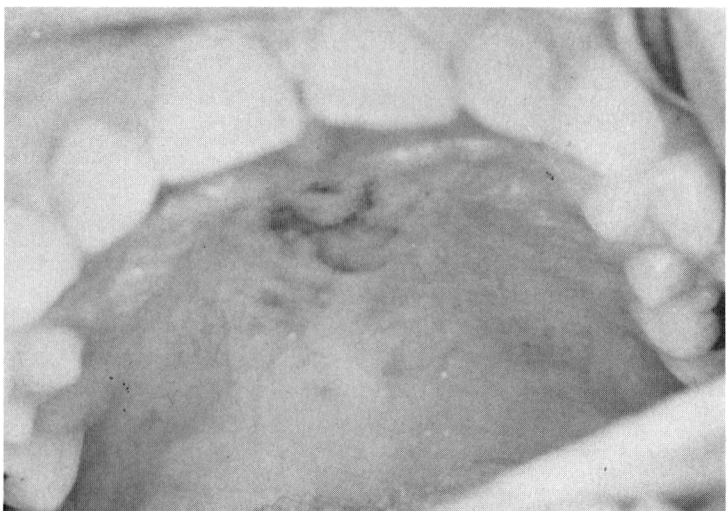

FIG. 67–3. Mucosal ulcer on hard palate.

Leg ulcers are similar to those seen in patients with rheumatoid vasculitis. They are most frequently located about the malleoli. The leg ulcers are punched-out lesions that are exquisitely tender. In a few of our patients, these leg ulcers preceded the recognition of SLE by many years.

Less common dermatologic abnormalities occur in many patients. *Bullous* lesions may be present,[30] and in patients who are thrombocytopenic, the bullae may be hemorrhagic. *Periorbital edema, urticaria,* or *erythema multiforme* may be noted. *Ecchymoses* and *petechiae* may be observed in patients with severe thromboycytopenia. Many patients complain of easy bruising prior to diagnosis of SLE and treatment with corticosteroids. *Gangrene* of the fingers or toes is uncommon and may be preceded by severe Raynaud's phenomenon or by severe livido reticularis. Occlusion of the medium-sized vessels of the legs has been noted in one such patient who eventually had a midcalf amputation because of gangrene.

Lupus profundus or *panniculitis* is occasionally noted and, in some patients, these lesions may calcify. Soft-tissue calcification occurs rarely in SLE but when present may be associated with anticentromere antibodies. The calcification appears to be present in patients with and without myositis who do not have abnormalities of calcium or phosphorous metabolism.[31] *Rheumatoid nodules* are present in about 6% of patients, usually, but not always, noted in patients with non-erosive deforming arthritis. The association of SLE with *porphyria cutanea tarda* has been reported,[32] and about 5% of our SLE patients also have psoriasis. *Dystrophic nail changes,* usually affecting only a few nails, may be found in about 10% of patients, especially those with long-standing disease. In its most extreme form, the nails are totally lost. Nail bed erythema is found in most of these patients earlier in the course of the disease. *Hypermelanosis* of skin and/or mucous membranes is observed rarely in patients treated for prolonged periods with antimalarial drugs.[33]

Histopathology of the skin lesions varies greatly. Biopsies of the typical rash of acute SLE usually show thinning of the epidermis, liquefaction degeneration of the basal layer of the epidermis with disruption of the dermal-epidermal junction, and edema of the dermis with a scattered infiltrate of lymphocytes throughout the dermis but concentrated around the upper dermal capillaries. Some biopsies reveal only a nonspecific vasculitis, however.

In some patients, the histologic picture lies between that of chronic discoid lupus and systemic lupus. Leukocytoclastic angiitis may be seen histologically in patients with palpable purpuric vasculitic lesions or with urticaria.

Immunopathologic studies of skin lesions reveal deposits of immunoglobulins and complement components at the dermal-epidermal junction in 80 to 100% of patients (Fig. 67–4).[34,35,36] This finding is not specific for lesions of SLE. Similar deposits may be found in lesions of lepromatous leprosy,[37] telangiectatic lesions from scleroderma patients, lesions of rosacea,[38] and lesions of active porphyria cutanea tarda.[39] Lesions from patients with chronic discoid lupus and without clinical or serologic evidence of SLE also have deposits of immunoglobulins and complement proteins in the dermal-epidermal junction.[40] Thus, *the diagnosis of SLE should not depend on the demonstration of deposits at the dermal-epidermal junction of skin lesions.* Because rosacea is commonly confused wth the butterfly blush of SLE, the finding of deposits in 70% of lesions of rosacea is of particular importance.[38]

Immunopathologic studies of nonlesional skin from

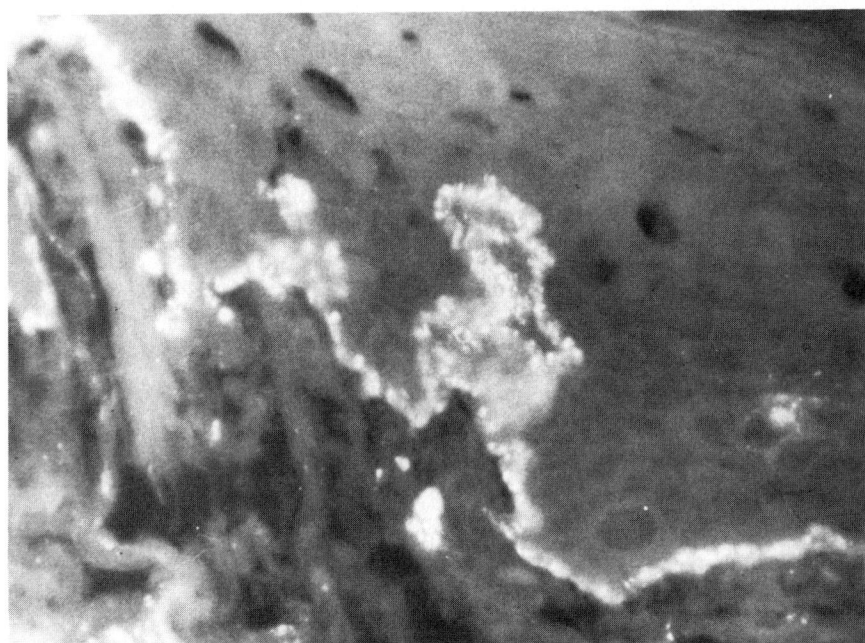

FIG. 67-4. Immunoglobulin deposits in the dermal-epidermal junction of the nonlesional skin from a patient with clinically active SLE. Anti-IgG fluorescein isothiocyanate (×500).

SLE patients also reveals the presence of immunoglobulins and complement proteins;[35,36,38] these deposits are more common in biopsies obtained during a period of clinical and serologically active disease.[35] Repeated biopsies of SLE patients have revealed that the deposits present during active disease may no longer be found later in the course when the patient has been in a sustained remission.[34] Similar deposits in normal skin have been found in patients with rheumatoid arthritis, Sjögren's syndrome, scleroderma, Raynaud's syndrome, polydermatomyositis,[41] and lepromatous leprosy.[37] We have found intermittent deposits in nonlesional skin of some patients with chronic discoid lupus and without evidence of SLE. Similarly, deposits are found in nonlesional skin from one third of patients with rosacea.[39]

Granular focal deposits have been noted in the normal skin of some relatives of SLE patients, including spouses,[14] and deposits have been found in skin of technicians handling SLE sera. The latter observation is similar to the increased lymphocytotoxic antibodies, antinuclear antibodies, and positive LE cell preparations found among workers in laboratories handling SLE sera.

MUSCULOSKELETAL MANIFESTATIONS

Involvement of the joints is the most frequent manifestation of SLE.[42] Objective evidence of pain on motion, tenderness, effusion, or periarticular soft-tissue swelling was present at the time of diagnosis of SLE in 88% of 209 patients, additional patients later developed objective evidence of joint disease so that fully 86% of all patients had arthritis at some time. Although other patients have joint pain without objective evidence of arthritis, 95% of SLE patients have either arthralgia or arthritis.

In some patients, arthralgia or arthritis precedes the onset of multisystem disease by many years. At the time of diagnosis, arthritis or arthralgia of the proximal interphalangeal joints was present in 82% of our patients; this was symmetric in all but two patients. The knees were the next most commonly involved joints (76%), followed by the wrists and metacarpophalangeal joints. Ankles, elbows and shoulders were involved less frequently (55%, 54%, and 45%, respectively). The metatarsophalangeal joints and hips were involved in 20% of patients, and the distal interphalangeal joints of the hands in 14% of patients. Involvement was symmetric in nearly all patients. Inflammation of the temporomandibular joints is rare, although several malocclusions occurred in one patient because of involvement of this joint.

Knee effusions are moderately severe in some patients, and joint aspiration usually reveals a clear (group 1) fluid. The leukocyte count is less than 3000/μL, and most of the cells are small lymphocytes. Antinuclear antibodies and LE cells may be found in the synovial fluid. Serum complement proteins and total hemolytic complement levels are usually low, reflecting similar low levels in the serum. Occasionally, opaque fluids with a higher leukocyte count and a greater percentage of neutrophils (group 2) may be found. *Inflammatory joint fluids should always be cultured, especially if the arthritis is monoarticular,* and a special culture should always be performed to rule out gonococcal arthritis. A single swollen or painful joint should be suspected as not resulting from SLE and should always be aspirated for cultures.

The histologic examination of the synovium reveals a fibrous villous synovitis. Typical pannus formation and erosions of bone and cartilage are extremely rare.[43] Arthritis disappears completely within a few days when patients are treated with corticosteroids for their systemic disease.

Although joint deformities excluded "arthritis" as one of the manifestations of SLE in the American Rheumatism Association (ARA) Preliminary Criteria for the Classification of SLE,[44] deformities certainly do occur in some SLE patients. The Revised Criteria do not exclude deformities as long as these are due to nonerosive disease[45] (Table 67–1). Typical swan-neck deformities and ulnar deviation of the fingers developed in about 10% of our SLE patients after 3 to 4 years of disease. Intermittent mild joint pains had been noted by many patients in this group, but in others no joint pain had been present since the time of diagnosis. Radiograms of the hands revealed no bony erosions or loss of joint space, although osteoporosis and joint subluxation occurred. Surgical repair of the deformities has been performed on some of these patients and normal cartilage noted in the affected joints. The joint deformities are thought to be related to chronic inflammatory involvement of the tendons of the hands and fingers and spasm of the intrinsic muscles. The presence of radiographic erosions excludes the use of "arthritis" in the Revised Criteria, however.

Morning stiffness is present in 50% of patients. Typical subcutaneous nodules occur in 10% of patients with active disease and disappear after treatment with corticosteroids. Tenosynovitis occurs in about 7% of patients. Rupture of the infrapatellar and Achilles tendons may occur, often bilaterally, and may relate to corticosteroid therapy rather than to the underlying disease.

It is extremely important to rule out two causes of joint pain that can occur in SLE patients, i.e., infectious arthritis and avascular necrosis of bone. The latter may involve the knees, elbows, shoulders, and carpal bones, as well as typically the hips. I have seen both acute and tophaceous gouty arthritis in SLE patients. Monoarticular arthritis developing in a patient with SLE should be considered to be caused by a condition other than the primary disease.

Involvement of muscles is not uncommon. Myalgia was present in 30% of patients and abnormalities of serum SGOT and SGPT were also present in 30% of patients before any treatment. The enzyme abnor-

malities probably reflect liver disease. The myalgia occurs with arthritis and, in some patients, the pain is "all over" and difficult to localize. These patients have pain in and between their joints. The muscles may be tender to palpation. Proximal muscle pain and tenderness are more common than distal. Such muscle involvement rapidly disappears, with corticosteroid doses needed to control the more significant systemic manifestations. Severe and prominent muscle involvement was noted in 8% of 228 patients studied by Tsokas, et al.[46] Biopsy usually reveals a nonspecific perivascular mononuclear infiltrate, but polymyositis with muscle necrosis can occur.[47] True polymyositis with muscle weakness, electromyographic changes typical of polymyositis, vacuolar myopathy, and necrosis have been reported in untreated SLE patients.[48] These abnormalities improved with corticosteroid therapy.

CARDIOVASCULAR MANIFESTATIONS

Clinically evident pericarditis occurs in about 25% of patients. Most often, an intermittent friction rub is heard, though massive pericardial effusions have been reported. Echocardiography revealed pericardial thickening in 29% of patients.[49] LE cells are found frequently in pericardial fluid, and a markedly acidic pH has been reported to distinguish SLE effusions from those resulting from uremia, bleeding, or unknown cause.[50] Pericardial tamponade is unusual but may be the first manifestation of SLE. Transient electrocardiographic abnormalities caused by myocardial ischemia may be seen, and tachycardia may persist for many months after the subsidence of the acute episode. Myocardial disease accompanies pericarditis. Death caused by myocardial infarction from arteritis has been reported early in the course of the disease in young patients.

Pathologically, SLE heart involvement is characterized by a pancarditis with involvement of pericardium, myocardium, endocardium, and coronary arteries.[51] Studies of hearts of patients dying from SLE have revealed a high incidence of coronary atherosclerosis in the patients treated for more than 1 year with corticosteroids.[52] Myocardial infarction late in the course of the disease in corticosteroid-treated patients represents an important cause of late death.[53] One of our patients died suddenly of a myocardial infarction while in remission in the eighth year of disease. On the other hand, studies of the hearts of young SLE patients revealed not only severe atherosclerotic coronary narrowing but also more extensive and severe lupus carditis.[54] Coronary arteritis may cause myo-

Table 67–1. The 1982 Revised Criteria for Classification of Systemic Lupus Erythematosus

Criterion*	Definition
1. Malar rash	Fixed erythema, flat or raised, over the malar eminences, tending to spare the nasolabial folds.
2. Discoid rash	Erythematous raised patches with adherent keratotic scaling and follicular plugging; atrophic scarring may occur in older lesions.
3. Photosensitivity	Skin rash as a result of unusual reaction to sunlight, by patient history or physician observation.
4. Oral ulcers	Oral or nasopharyngeal ulceration, usually painless, observed by a physician.
5. Arthritis	Nonerosive arthritis involving two or more peripheral joints, characterized by tenderness, swelling, or effusion.
6. Serositis	a) Pleuritis—convincing history of pleuritic pain or rub heard by a physician or evidence of pleural effusion. OR b) Pericarditis—documented by ECG or rub or evidence of pericardial effusion.
7. Renal disorder	a) Persistent proteinuria greater than 0.5 per day or greater than 3+ if quantitation not performed. OR b) Cellular casts—may be red cell, hemoglobulin, granular, tubular, or mixed.
8. Neurologic disorder	a) Seizures—in the absence of offending drugs or known metabolic derangements: e.g., uremia, ketoacidosis, or electrolyte imbalance. OR b) Psychosis—in the absence of offending drugs or known metabolic derangements, e.g., uremia, ketoacidosis, or electrolyte imbalance.
9. Hematologic disorder	a) Hemolytic anemia—with reticulocytosis. OR b) Leukopenia—less than 4,000/mm total on two or more occasions. OR c) Lymphopenia—less than 1,500/mm on two or more occasions. OR d) Thrombocytopenia—less than 100,000/mm in the absence of offending drugs.
10. Immunologic disorder	a) Positive LE cell preparation. OR b) Anti-DNA: antibody to native DNA in abnormal titer. OR c) Anti-SM: presence of antibody to Sm nuclear antigen: OR d) False positive serologic test for syphilis known to be positive for at least 6 months and confirmed by Treponema pallidum immobilization or fluorescent treponemal antibody absorption test.
11. Antinuclear antibody	An abnormal titer of antinuclear antibody by immunofluorescence or an equivalent assay at any time and in the absence of drugs known to be associated with "drug-induced lupus syndrome."

*The proposed classification is based on 11 criteria. For the purpose of identifying patients in clinical studies, a person shall be said to have systemic lupus erythematosus if any 4 or more of the 11 criteria are present, serially or simultaneously, during any interval of observation.

cardial infarction. Segmental myocardial perfusion abnormalities found in 39% of asymptomatic patients did not correlate with disease duration or amount of corticosteroid received but did correlate with a history of pericarditis.[55]

Aortic and mitral insufficiency caused by scarring of leaflets and thickened or ruptured chordae tendineae have been reported;[56,57] valve replacement has been used to correct these conditions.[58,59]

Verrucous endocarditis is present at autopsy in nearly all patients. The lesions are usually microscopic, but macroscopic vegetations are observed in nearly half the cases. Typical verrucous endocarditis is a pathologic diagnosis and does not correlate with the presence of cardiac murmurs. Both subacute and acute bacterial endocarditis have occurred on valves affected by lupus endocarditis.

Raynaud's phenomenon was present in 18% of our

365 patients and may precede the development of multisystem disease by many years. Cryoglobulinemia was commonly present in patients with an onset of Raynaud's phenomenon at the time of diagnosis, and such patients also often had nephritis. Unlike in systemic sclerosis, the Raynaud's phenomenon in SLE may gradually disappear after institution of corticosteroid therapy. Thrombophlebitis occurs in about 10% of patients. Large-vein thrombosis is less common. Thrombosis with occlusion of the femoral artery occurred in one of our patients, necessitating mid-thigh amputation. These episodes of thrombophlebitis occur during periods of clinical and serologic disease activity. Recurrent thrombophlebitis in the absence of active disease occurred in one of our patients who subsequently died with pancreatic carcinoma.

Thrombotic episodes clearly occur more often in patients with the lupus anticoagulant than in those without this abnormality.[60] We have found the lupus anticoagulant in our 3 patients with cerebral infarctions and in patients with venous and arterial thrombosis of other vessels. The Budd-Chiari syndrome has been described in association with the lupus anticoagulant.[61] Placental arterial thrombosis has been reported in association with the lupus anticoagulant.[62] Antiphospholipid antibodies as well as the lupus anticoagulant appear to be present in patients with venous and arterial thrombosis and in association with microscopic glomerular thrombi (see Chapter 70).

Thrombotic thrombocytopenic purpura (TTP) occurs rarely in patients with SLE. We have observed this catastrophic event in 2 of 433 patients. In one patient, TTP occurred in the fourth month of pregnancy and resulted in massive brain infarcts. In the other, TTP was recognized earlier, and the patient responded to corticosteroid therapy and plasmapheresis.

PULMONARY MANIFESTATIONS

SLE in elderly patients may present with pulmonary disease in the absence of skin and joint findings. Pleural involvement is even more common than pericardial disease. Pleural effusions occur in 40% of patients. Most are small to moderate, but massive effusions occur occasionally. LE cells may be seen in those transudates that contain the same immunoglobulin and complement proteins as the peripheral blood. Occasionally, effusions persist for months after the institution of corticosteroid therapy, leading to concern regarding cause. "Lupus pneumonitis," characterized by dyspnea, rales, and areas of plate-like atelectasis associated with elevation and fixation of the diaphragm, occurs in about 10% of patients. Infiltrates may be bilateral and associated with pleural effusions.[63] A study of the pathology of the lungs in SLE patients revealed that the most common cause of pulmonary infiltrates was infection.[64] Pneumonias caused by bacterial and fungal agents are particularly common in corticosteroid-treated SLE patients. *The diagnosis of lupus pneumonitis should be made only after a rigorous search for an infectious agent.*

Abnormalities of pulmonary function are common, even in patients without respiratory symptoms. Tests reveal a combination of pulmonary restriction, vascular obstruction, and airway obstruction.[65]

Pathologic abnormalities are extremely common in autopsied lungs and are most often nonspecific. All patients show evidence of pleural thickening, and intra-alveolar hemorrhage is not uncommon. Interstitial fibrosis was found in one third of 18 autopsied lungs by Miller, et al.[66]

"Shrinking" lung syndrome is an unusual abnormality caused by weakness of the respiratory muscles; it is seen in dyspneic patients with elevation of the diaphragm and progressive or stable loss of lung volume. This abnormality may be found in patients with otherwise inactive disease.[67]

Pulmonary hemorrhage caused by pulmonary vasculitis is a rare but life-threatening manifestation of SLE. Pulmonary hypertension rarely occurs; it is associated with Raynaud's phenomenon and may be associated with the presence of the lupus anticoagulant.[68]

RENAL DISEASE

Clinical evidence of renal disease occurs in about 50% of patients; pathologic abnormalities recognized by light microscopy are present in additional patients. Immunofluorescent studies of biopsy or autopsy material from nearly all patients reveal deposits of immunoglobulins or complement proteins. Therefore, the definition of lupus nephritis is unclear. Persistent proteinuria is the most common clinical sign of lupus nephritis.

The most characteristic pathologic abnormality is the variability of glomerular lesions and the patchy distribution of the various changes. Thus, lesions vary from one glomerulus to the other, and different structural abnormalities occur within a single glomerulus. Mesangial immune deposits are present in nearly all SLE patients. These deposits occur in all patients with clinical evidence of lupus nephritis (unless there is sclerosis of all glomeruli) and in most SLE patients without urinary abnormalities. At present, the World

Health Organization classification is used by most investigators.[69,70] This classification includes six distinctive morphologic patterns based on light, immunofluorescence, and electron microscopic findings, as briefly described below. *The type and severity of the renal disease bears no relation to the presence of other manifestations of the disease which may be either mild or severe.*

Normal. Tissue in this classification cannot be distinguished from kidney tissue of a normal healthy person.

Mesangial Lupus Nephritis. The glomeruli either appear normal or show a slight irregular increase in mesangial cells and matrix (Fig. 67–5). The diagnosis depends on the demonstration of IgG and C3 in the mesangium. Electron-dense deposits may be noted in the mesangium. Patients have normal urinary findings, transient minimal proteinuria, or minimal hematuria. Biopsy of 11 consecutive SLE patients without clinical renal abnormalities showed mesangial lupus nephritis in all.[71] A few instances of progression from the mesangial to the diffuse proliferative form have been described.[72] *It is unlikely that patients with little or no clinical evidence of renal disease at the time of diagnosis will develop progression of the condition if the disease is adequately treated and initial normalization of the serologic abnormalities is sustained over time.* The presence of IgG in the mesangium is analogous to the finding of IgG in the nonlesional skin of patients with clinically active disease. Deposits of immunoglobulins

in the dermal-epidermal junction and in the mesangium of the glomeruli occur without inflammation.

Focal Proliferative Lupus Nephritis. This condition is characterized by segmental proliferation of some glomerular tufts while others appear normal (Fig. 67–6). Mesangial proliferation may be present, but segmental proliferation is present in less than 50% of glomeruli. The glomerular abnormalities used for the index of activity score described in the section on diffuse proliferative lupus nephritis may be present but in less than 50% of glomeruli. *Thus, it is important to note the index of activity and the extent of sclerosis as well as the classification of the lesion.* For example, focal lupus nephritis with a high activity index is not uncommon, whereas diffuse proliferative lupus nephritis can have a low activity index and significant sclerosis.

In focal proliferative lupus nephritis, immunofluorescence reveals immunoglobulins and C3 in the mesangium of all glomeruli. Fine, scattered granules may be present along the capillary loops, especially in the areas of proliferation. The deposits are scattered and not evenly distributed along all capillary loops. Electron-dense deposits are noted by electron microscopy in the mesangium, and occasional deposits are also found in the subendothelial, subepithelial, and intrabasement membrane areas. Proteinuria occurs, but the nephrotic syndrome is uncommon.[73]

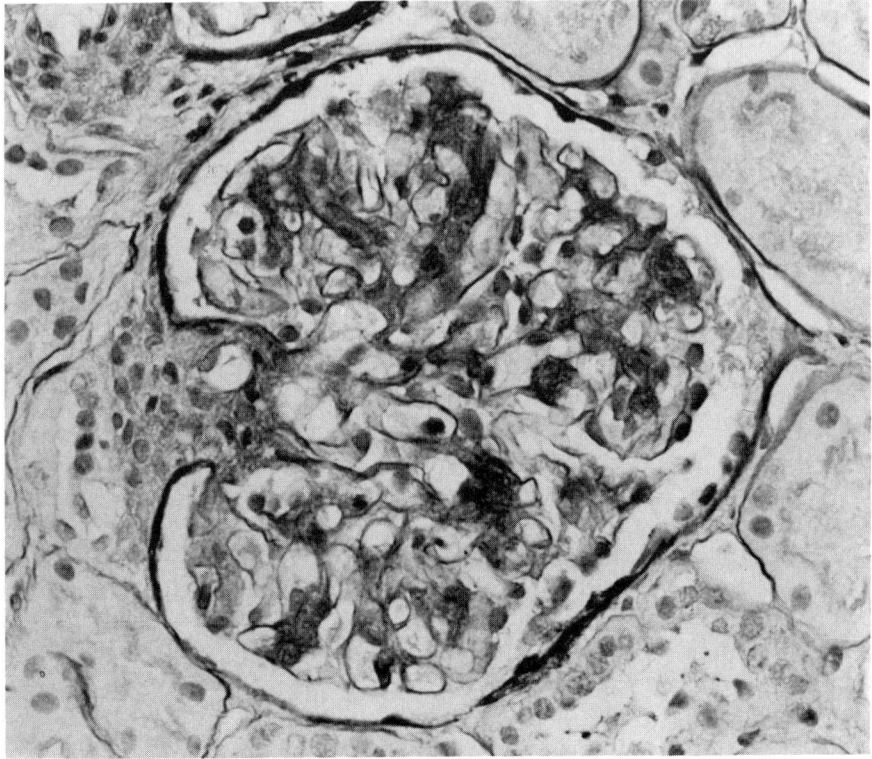

FIG. 67–5. Minimal (mesangial) lupus nephritis (hematoxylin and eosin stain ×500).

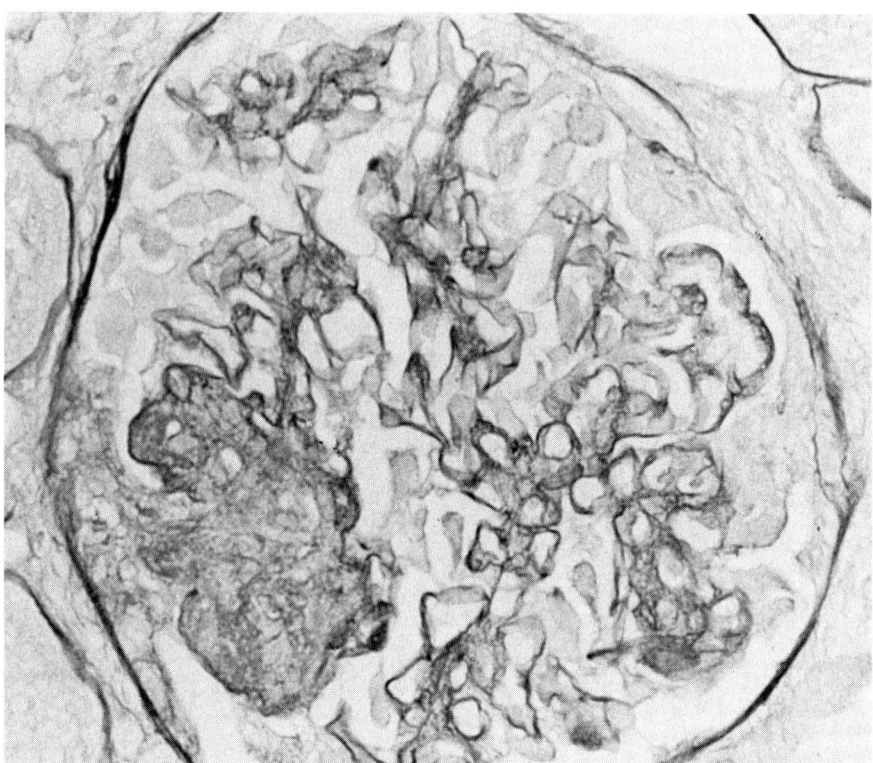

FIG. 67–6. Focal proliferative lupus nephritis (hematoxylin and eosin stain × 500).

Mild hematuria is usual, but renal insufficiency is either mild or absent.

Patients with mild (focal) lupus nephritis usually do not have mild systemic disease. They may be acutely ill with high fevers and severe extrarenal disease, including central nervous system disease. Antinative DNA antibodies and low serum complement levels may be present in those patients with active systemic disease. Treatment with corticosteroids in doses adequate to control the systemic manifestations of the disease usually leads to a clearing of the renal insufficiency, if present, and to clearing of the hematuria.[73] Proteinuria may persist for several months, but it gradually clears and the urinalysis becomes normal. Such patients do not usually develop severe renal disease later, nor do they develop renal insufficiency *if the* serologic abnormalities return to the normal range with initial therapy and *if the* patient remains in serologic and clinical remission.[73,74] If an exacerbation of the disease does occur, the same focal lesion is again found. Prompt treatment leads to remission. Death from renal disease or from other causes in the presence of renal insufficiency does not occur in these patients if no serologic or clinical disease activity occurs.

Progression from focal to diffuse lupus nephritis has been reported[72,74,75] but has occurred in only two patients in our experience. In each, corticosteroid therapy had been abruptly discontinued and a full-blown exacerbation of the clinical and serologic disease occurred at the time that severe lupus nephritis was documented. The second renal biopsy, performed during the exacerbation, revealed diffuse proliferative lupus nephritis in both of these individuals. In a review of 22 patients with focal nephritis, there was an 82% 5-year cumulative survival rate from the first sign of renal involvement[74] similar to the rate found in an earlier study.[73] Deaths occurred in patients who had normal renal function.[74] However, progression to diffuse lupus nephritis was more frequent in the patients described by Ginzler, et al.,[72] and by Zimmerman, et al.;[75] progression occurred in 9 of 31 patients (29%) in the former and 6 of 17 patients (38%) in the latter study (Table 67–2). Sclerosis may occur occasionally in patients with focal lupus nephritis, but its degree is minimal.[74] Minimal to mild sclerosis was noted in 8 of 16 patients with focal nephritis who had a stable course, and mild sclerosis was noted in the initial biopsy in half of the patients who later progressed to diffuse proliferative nephritis.[74]

Diffuse Proliferative Lupus Nephritis. In this condition there are abnormalities of more than 50% of the total area of the glomerular tufts. Although the proliferation is irregular, all glomeruli are involved, and usually most of each glomerulus is abnormal (Fig. 67–7). Sclerosis may or may not be present in the initial biopsy. The activity of the proliferative lesion

Table 67–2. Minimal Glomerular and Focal Lupus Nephritis: Clinical and Histologic Course

	Morel-Maroger et al.[69]	Ginzler et al.[39]	Zimmerman et al.[75]
No. patients	81	32	17
Stable course	77*	20†	11‡
Renal deterioration GN	4	11	5
Progression to diffuse	6 (7.4%)	9 (29%)	6 (35%)

*GN remaining focal in 16/18 cases in which biopsy was repeated (mean time of 28 mos. between first and second biopsy), having progressed to a diffuse GN in the other cases.
†GN remaining focal in the two cases in which biopsy was repeated.
‡GN remaining focal in the five cases in which biopsy was repeated.
From Morel-Maroger, L., et al.: The course of lupus nephritis: Contribution of serial renal biopsies. *In* Advances in Nephrology. Vol. 6. Edited by J. Hamburger. Copyright ©1976 by Year Book Medical Publishers, Inc., Chicago. Used by permission.

may be graded on a semiquantitative basis as originally suggested by Pirani, et al.[76] Fibrinoid necrosis, endocapillary proliferation, epithelial crescents, nuclear debris, hematoxylin bodies, wire loops, and hyaline thrombi are considered to represent active disease. Markers of active interstitial disease include interstitial cell infiltration and acute tubular epithelial lesions.[74] Necrotizing angiitis is also considered to be an active lesion. The pathologic index of activity is particularly useful if successive biopsies on the same patient are to be evaluated or if groups of patients with lupus nephritis are to be compared. Similarly, the amount of sclerosis in each biopsy can also be graded. Studies of repeated sequential biopsies in 40 patients with diffuse lupus nephritis found that the

presence of extensive sclerotic lesions indicated a poor prognosis and that high doses of prednisone given to 14 patients after the first biopsy did not prevent progression of the sclerosis in 8 of the patients, even though active lesions diminished.[74] However, patients wth active lesions had a good prognosis, responding to high doses of corticosteroids. In 19 to 25 patients with only moderate glomerular sclerosis, the initially active lesions were considerably decreased in the biopsies repeated after treatment. These conclusions are similar to those reported by Stricker, et al.[77] The 5-year survival of patients with diffuse proliferative nephritis appears to be improving. The 5-year survival was 41% of 24 patients treated before 1968,[73] and 86% of 22 patients followed thereafter. It is clear

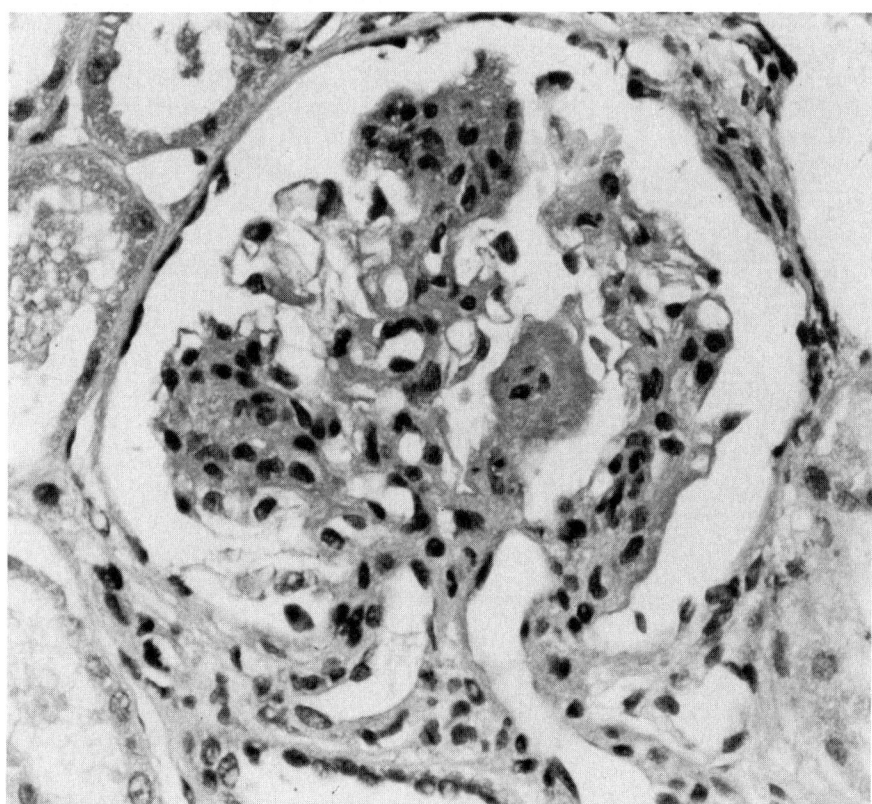

FIG. 67–7. Diffuse proliferative lupus nephritis (hematoxylin and eosin stain ×500).

that the renal biopsy provides information additional to the type of lupus nephritis. The prognosis in patients with diffuse proliferative lupus nephritis may depend greatly on the degree of activity and of sclerosis noted in the biopsy.

The immunofluorescence findings in diffuse proliferative lupus nephritis are usually striking, with granules or bumps of immunoglobulins and complement proteins, as well as mesangial deposits, noted along the peripheral capillary wall. Interstitial infiltrates and deposits of immunoglobulins and complement proteins may also be noted along the tubular basement membrane, within the walls of the peritubular capillaries, or in the interstitium.[78] Electron-dense deposits are noted in the mesangium, in the subendothelial and subepithelial areas, and within the basement membrane. The deposits are located all over the glomeruli, but are not evenly distributed.

The clinical picture is one of moderate to heavy proteinuria with nephrotic syndrome, hematuria, and mild to severe renal insufficiency. Red cell casts are not infrequent. Antibodies to native DNA and low serum C3 are usual unless the lesion is inactive, with a predominance of sclerotic glomeruli. Many patients with severe sclerosis and inactive nonsclerotic glomeruli are in clinical remission and should be treated with small doses of corticosteroids, if at all. These individuals seem to have a prolonged serologic and clinical remission and do not require treatment for the SLE, although hemodialysis has been required in some.

Membranous Lupus Nephritis. The histologic appearance of this condition is similar to that of idiopathic membranous gomerulonephritis (Fig. 67–8). Although no proliferation is noted, slight irregular increases in mesangial cells and matrix may be present. Immunofluorescence is striking in that the immunoglobulins are located in a regular fashion along all the basement membranes (Fig. 67–9). It is possible to observe on immunofluorescence the spikes of the IgG that protrude on the epithelial side of the capillary loop. Electron microscopy confirms the presence of subepithelial deposits. Patients with this form of lupus nephritis have proteinuria and may or may not have hematuria. The nephrotic syndrome is always present at onset or during the course of the disease.[75] Serologic evidence of disease activity may be absent if significant extrarenal disease activity is absent. Normal C3 levels and absence of antibodies to native DNA have been found in these patients at the time that the renal disease was noted and the biopsy performed, but we have observed some patients with hematuria, low serum C3 levels, and high titers of anti-DNA antibodies. The prognosis is variable but usually is

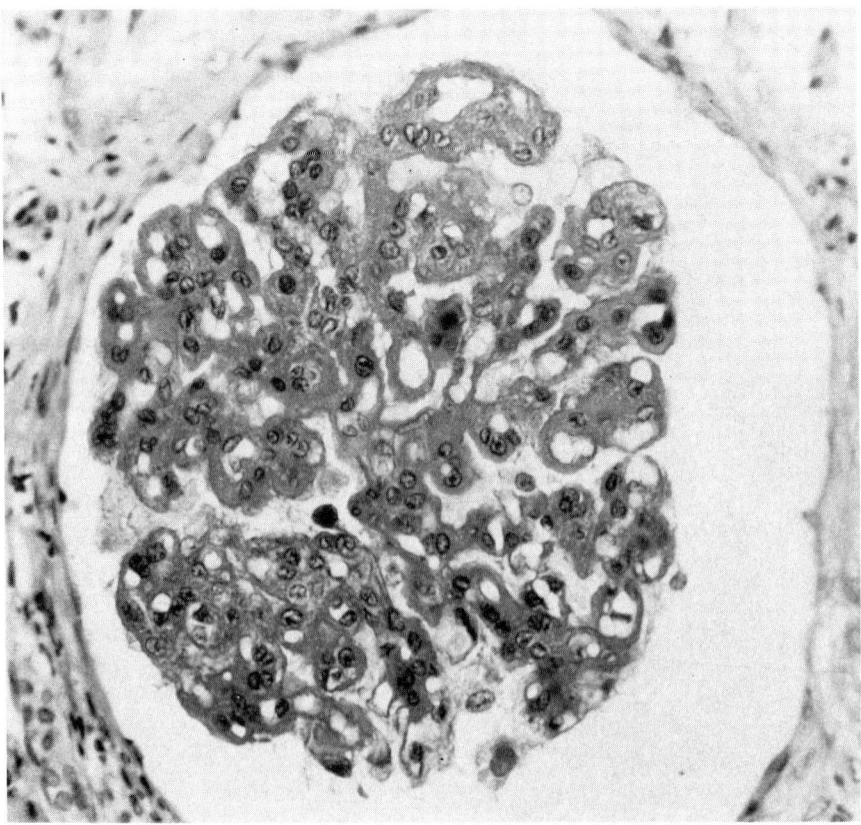

FIG. 67–8. Membranous lupus nephritis (hematoxylin and eosin stain ×500).

FIG. 67–9. Membranous lupus nephritis with granular deposits on all capillary loops. Anti-IgG fluorescein isothiocyanate (hematoxylin and eosin stain ×500).

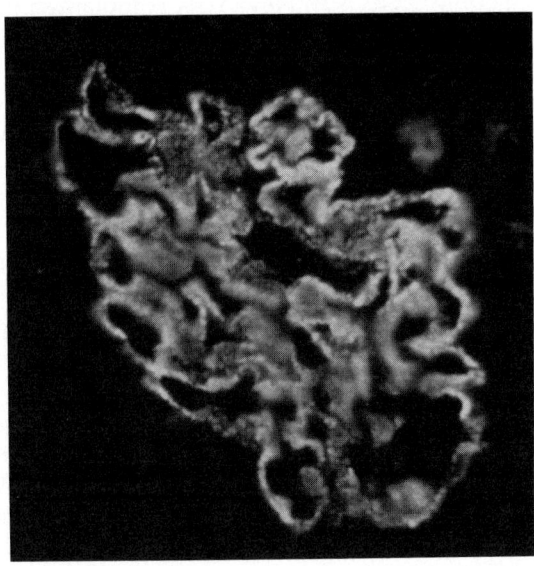

good. We have noted some patients with persistent nephrotic syndrome and slowly progressive renal insufficiency for as long as 10 years, and we have observed progression to severe renal insufficiency 14 years after the first biopsy. We observed transition to diffuse proliferative lupus nephritis in a patient who refused increased corticosteroid therapy despite clinical evidence of disease activity, persistently normal complement levels, but high levels of complement fixing anti-DNA antibody levels. The onset of severe renal disease was heralded by a severe headache and the patient was found to be extremely hypertensive with an active urinary sediment, low C3 and C4, and elevation of serum creatinine. Renal biopsy showed very active diffuse proliferative lupus nephritis. This patient, like others, has done extremely well with intravenous cyclophosphamide therapy added to daily corticosteroids.[79,80] (See also section on Treatment.)

Sclerosing Lupus Nephritis. This is seen in patients with end-stage kidneys, but as already described sclerosis may be present to a greater or lesser extent in patients with proliferative or membranous lupus nephritis.

Interstitial Nephritis. This condition has been described in approximately 50% of patients.[78] Focal or diffuse infiltrates of inflammatory cells, tubular damage, and interstitial fibrosis are observed. Immunoglobulins, complement, or both can be found in the peritubular capillaries, the interstitium, or the tubular basement membrane in a granular pattern. The interstitial abnormalities are more severe and frequent in patients with diffuse proliferative lupus nephritis, but severe interstitial nephritis with few or no glomerular abnormalities has been noted occasionally. *Renal tubular acidosis* occurs in some patients.

Prognosis. In general, most investigators agree that maleness and serum creatinine greater than 1.3 predict renal failure.[81] In our own series, most of the deaths from renal disease have occurred in our male patients. These individuals have been particularly noncompliant, refusing to take significant doses of corticosteroids, or refusing intravenous cyclophosphamide until their disease become life threatening. The data in the literature suggest that younger patients fare less well than those of middle age. The World Health Organization class of diffuse proliferative nephritis is suggestive of a poor prognosis, as is a high activity index. *The most significant factor for a poor prognosis is a high sclerosis or chronicity index.*

NERVOUS SYSTEM

Involvement of neural tissue is common in SLE.

Peripheral Neuropathy. This condition has occurred in 14% of our patients, an incidence similar to that reported by Feinglass.[82] The most common defect is sensory, but a mixed sensory-motor disturbance is seen in about 5% of patients with the typical asymmetric involvement of mononeuritis multiplex. These episodes occur most often at the time of diagnosis along with evidence of active disease in other systems. In most patients, treatment of the systemic disease with corticosteroids leads to a gradual return of function of the affected extremities. Other less common abnormalities consist of a picture suggesting the Guillain-Barré syndrome and myelopathy. Some patients with peripheral neuropathy also have evidence of cranial neuropathy.

Cranial Nerve Signs. These signs were noted in only 16 of the 140 SLE patients reported by Feinglass, et al.[82] We have noted facial weakness, ptosis, diplopia, and other evidence of cranial nerve involvement. Optic neuritis may be the first manifestation of SLE.[83] These abnormalities frequently concur with other neuropsychiatric features. One patient with optic neuritis, described by Feinglass, had transverse myelitis at the same time.[82] Peripheral neuropathy is common in patients with cranial neuropathy.

Long tract involvement occurred in 16 of 140 SLE patients described by Feinglass, et al.[82] Five of his patients had cerebrovascular accidents. Long tract signs also usually occur along with other evidence of neuropsychiatric disease.

Central Nervous System. More common and more serious than peripheral nervous system involvement, central nervous system (CNS) disease occurs as two major forms, organic psychosis and seizures. Seizures in the absence of renal insufficiency, hypertension, or infection occur in about 15% of SLE patients[82] and are usually present at the time of the original diagnosis, accompanying active systemic disease. We have not noted the onset of seizures in our patients late in the course of the disease. Grand mal seizures are most common, but we have also seen patients with chorea, Jacksonian fits, petit mal, and temporal lobe seizures. Pseudotumor cerebri may also occur with acute disease. Nearly all of these manifestations occur at the time of disease onset and, in many cases, are accompanied by other neuropsychiatric abnormalities.[82] Chorea and petit mal seizures sometimes begin at the time of diagnosis of SLE, along with other evidence of disease activity, and may persist for many years, even when no clinical evidence of disease activity elsewhere can be documented.

CNS involvement may also be manifested by organic brain disease.[84] Organic syndromes are characterized by impairment of orientation, perception, and ability to calculate. Memory deficits are common, and the patients may have difficulty remembering the name of their own physicians. In our series of patients studied at the Bellevue Medical-Psychiatric wards, 21% of the total group of 209 patients had episodes of CNS disease during the first year of diagnosis. These patients were acutely ill with multisystem disease and fever; 15% had CNS disease during the first year after diagnosis, but only 2% showed CNS findings during the fifth year through the sixth year. No episodes of CNS disease occurred in 43 patients in their eighth year or in 24 patients during their ninth year. No episodes of psychosis occurred in 25 patients during their tenth through twelfth years, although two patients had cerebrovascular accidents, one in the eleventh year and one in the twelfth year after diagnosis. Thus, CNS disease is a manifestation of severe active lupus, occurs early in the course of the disease, and coincides with evidence of disease activity in other systems.[82]

Complete recovery of the organic brain disease is usual, but some patients have residual impairment of mental processes, such as an inability to calculate as rapidly as they could before the disease episode. SLE patients with CNS disease are more likely to have evidence of vasculitis than those without such findings.[82] The 5-year survival of our 82 patients with organic brain disease at the time of diagnosis was 71% as compared to a 77% survival of the 274 patients without organic brain disease.[85] All of the patients with CNS disease were treated with high doses of corticosteroids.

Severe Headaches. At the time of diagnosis, 21 of our 209 SLE patients in New York complained of severe headaches. In five of these patients, the headache was associated with organic brain disease and in eight others it was associated with seizures. Brandt and Lessel have described 11 patients with severe throbbing headaches or with wavy or zigzag line scotomata typical of the fortification specters of migraine.[86] These phenomena either occurred for the first time after the diagnosis of SLE or occurred as an initial feature along with other manifestations of systemic disease. *Migraine headaches* or *fortification specters* have also occurred as an isolated symptom prior to the development of other clinical manifestations of SLE, but at a time when serologic abnormalities of SLE were found. Classic migraine headaches have an increased prevalence in SLE patients.[87] It is important to recognize these headaches as a manifestation of SLE because they disappear when prednisone is administered or when the dose of corticosteroid is increased, and they occur along with other manifestations of the disease during periods of exacerbation.

Cerebrovascular Accident. This occurs rarely in SLE patients. Classic strokes secondary to cerebral infarction or intracranial hemorrhage have been seen in 1 of 204 patients in my Bellevue series and in 3 of 583 patients seen in Connecticut. In all instances, patients had active SLE at the time. Polyarteritis-like lesions in cerebral vessels have been documented by angiography,[88] and embolization from Libman-Sacks vegetations on heart valves has been reported.[89] The presence of the lupus anticoagulant in patients with cerebral infarcts has been noted in our patients and reported in the literature. We have treated these patients with long-term anticoagulant therapy.

Psychologic Problems. Most SLE patients have major psychologic problems coping with their disease and with side effects of the therapy they are receiving. They become depressed and anxious. The disfigurement caused by high doses of corticosteroids is especially difficult in young women and adolescents and may lead to a major depression. Such mental abnormality is not part of the disease itself and should not be called "CNS lupus." The corticosteroid dose should not be increased in such patients. These individuals need reassurance and may require psychotherapy.

Laboratory Findings. Abnormalities of the cerebrospinal fluid (CSF) were present in 32% of episodes of neuropsychiatric illness in 37 patients studied by Feinglass.[82] Protein evaluation was noted in about half the fluids, and in a few patients, both protein and white cells were increased. Elevation of CSF pressure may be associated with papilledema. Protein elevation may be absent, modest, or even significant. Elevation of CSF IgG is relatively specific for active CNS lupus but is not very sensitive. Rarely, the cerebrospinal fluid may suggest an infectious process. Feinglass et al. have noted that death correlated with CSF abnormalities.[82] The presence of antibodies to neuronal cell membranes has been shown to correlate with the presence of neuropsychiatric lupus, but this test is not readily available.[90] Similarly, a low C4 level in the CSF is present in active CNS disease, but the test must be done immediately because the C4 protein decays rapidly even when the CSF is frozen.[91]

The electroencephalogram (EEG) is frequently abnormal during an episode of neuropsychiatric disease. Abnormal EEG may also be noted in patients without CNS abnormalities, but are more frequently abnormal in those with CNS disease. Diffuse slow-wave activity is the most common abnormality, but focal changes may also be observed. In the literature, there is conflicting data on the clinical usefulness of brain scans;[83] it is probably not wise to depend on this test to determine the presence of active CNS disease. A new technique using oxygen-15 is capable of demonstrating temporary ischemia and may be of great help in the diagnosis and management of CNS lupus.[92] At present, computed tomography (CT) is of more value than the brain scan; major areas of infarction can be visualized, especially in patients with localized findings. "Cerebral atrophy" is a term used in describing enlargement of the ventricles and cortical sulci. This enlargement may be caused by loss of water or loss of nerve cells. Cerebral atrophy is not unique to CNS lupus but is noted in a variety of conditions, including non-SLE conditions, and in patients receiving corticosteroid therapy. The significance of cerebral atrophy in an SLE patient with CNS manifestation is difficult to determine.

Pathology. Pathologic abnormalities in patients with seizures usually consist of microinfarcts.[93,94] Vasculitis is found in 35% and intracerebral hemorrhages in 22%. Focal motor seizures are associated with findings of subarachnoid hemorrhage. Pathologic changes in 12 patients with hemiparesis were similar to the changes associated with seizures, except that intracerebral hemorrhage was present in six[93] and the hemorrhage was related to the presence of brain vasculitis. Vasculitis was also present in one third of patients with subarachnoid hemorrhage and in 25% of those patients with microhemorrhages. In patients dying with lupus psychosis, researchers have found microinfarcts, vasculitis, and cerebral hemorrhages.[94]

Immunofluorescence studies have revealed deposits of immunoglobulins and C3 in the choroid plexus of SLE patients.[95]

GASTROINTESTINAL MANIFESTATIONS

The most common gastrointestinal manifestation is abdominal pain. The pain may be accompanied by nausea and less often by diarrhea. In most patients, abdominal pain occurs in association with evidence of disease activity in other systems. The cause of abdominal pain usually is not clear. Mesenteric arteritis may be noted on arteriography. Patients with mesenteric arteritis have ileal and colonic ulcers, and ileal and colonic perforations may occur.[96] We have observed three deaths from intestinal perforation in our 365 patients. Zizic, et al. described colonic perforations as the cause of four of 15 deaths occurring in 197 patients with SLE.[96] Thus, colonic perforations accounted for a significant percentage of deaths in SLE patients observed in recent years.

The pain in patients with perforations is colicky and well-localized to the lower abdomen or infraumbilical area. Abdominal pain in SLE patients without perforations is less well localized or may be localized to the epigastrium or upper quadrants. It may be either sharp or colicky. Both rebound and direct tenderness were present in our patients with perforations and in four of the five patients reported by Zizic, et al.[96] Neither rebound tenderness nor localized direct tenderness was present in SLE patients with abdominal pain without perforations. Abdominal pain is much more common in children with SLE than in adults, but perforations have not been observed. The abdominal pain in children is crampy and occurs during periods of disease activity, disappearing as other manifestations of the disease resolve.

Patients with colonic perforation usually have evidence of severe active SLE in other systems. Both our patients and those described by Zizic, et al. had highly active SLE. The only surviving patient received early surgical intervention before radiologic evidence of perforation was apparent, even though she was considered to be a poor surgical risk because of lupus nephritis with uremia.[96] Thus, early surgical intervention is strongly suggested if the diagnosis of perforation is suspected.

Some SLE patients had regional enteritis[97] with erosions and ulceration of the intestinal mucosa at the time of operation for abdominal pain.[98]

In our series, abdominal pain of acute onset with evidence of peritonitis occurred in 17 patients. The pain was due to massive ascites, ruptured ovarian cyst, perforated gastric ulcer, appendicitis, diverticulitis, and abscess of the fallopian tubes. It is wise to consider early surgical intervention in SLE patients.

PANCREATITIS

Pancreatitis occurred in seven of our 365 SLE patients when the disease was active in other systems. In one patient, pancreatitis was associated with organic brain disease as well as with other clinical and serologic evidence of active SLE. In one analysis, elevated serum amylase was found in 26 SLE patients, and pancreatitis caused by SLE was present in four patients, all of whom recovered with corticosteroid treatment.[99]

LIVER AND SPLEEN

Hepatomegaly occurs in about 30% of patients, more commonly among children than among adult-onset patients.[100] Clinically evident jaundice occurred in one of 365 patients, and hepatic insufficiency was the cause of death in one 8-year-old girl. Autopsy revealed acute fatty degeneration of the liver. Four of our 365 SLE patients had biopsy evidence of chronic active hepatitis, and all four met the ARA Preliminary Criteria for the Classification of SLE.[44] Skin manifestations, CNS lupus, and mild lupus nephritis were present in these patients. Liver enzyme elevations are noted in about 30% of patients at the time of diagnosis, when active disease is evident in many systems. In addition, aspirin may cause elevations of transaminase levels in patients with SLE. Liver biopsies from SLE patients who had either clinical liver disease or liver enzyme abnormalities revealed findings only of chronic active hepatitis, granulomatous hepatitis, cirrhosis, acute hepatitis, fatty change, or cholestasis.[101]

Slight to moderate splenomegaly is present in 20% of patients and is more common in children.[100] Splenomegaly is not usually associated with hemolytic anemia. Asplenism has been reported in SLE patients, including two of 65 patients whose functional asplenism was only detected by CT scan.[102] The onion-skin appearance of the splenic arterioles is present in 15% of patients. This change is due to concentric periarterial fibrosis, thought to be the end stage of an earlier focal arteritis.

LYMPH NODES

Lymph node enlargement occurs in about half of all SLE patients with active disease. Lymphadenop-

athy is more common in children than in adults.[100] Adenopathy is usually generalized but may be limited, and the enlarged nodes are usually nontender. One of our patients had two severe episodes of active disease, each associated with massive nontender enlargement of the occipital nodes. Microscopic changes in lymph nodes are nonspecific. They consist of follicular hyperplasia, which may be assciated with areas of necrosis, resembling giant follicular lymphoma.

OCULAR MANIFESTATIONS

Conjunctivitis or episcleritis occurred in 15% of our patients and appeared to be more common in patients with extensive cutaneous manifestations. Periorbital edema and subconjunctival hemorrhages have also been reported. Occlusion of the central retinal artery has been reported during periods of disease activity, but is a rare occurrence. Active retinal arteritis and arteriolar occlusion have been reported.[103,104] Blindness may be the first symptom of the disease.[105] Cytoid bodies, which occur in only 8% of patients, are retinal exudates appearing as hard, white lesions adjacent to retinal vessels during periods of disease activity. These exudates disappear gradually as the disease becomes inactive. Cytoid bodies may be associated with organic brain disease and seizures.

PAROTID GLAND ENLARGEMENT

Enlarged parotid glands occurred in 8% of our patients most of whom did not have xerostomia. Typical keratoconjunctivitis sicca is uncommon. Unilateral enlargement of a parotid gland may be observed during periods of disease activity in a small number of patients. One prospective study reported a high incidence of associated Sjögren's syndrome, including a positive Schirmer's test in 21%, positive parotid scan in 58%, and positive lip biopsy in 50% of patients.[106]

MENSTRUAL ABNORMALITIES AND PREGNANCY

Cessation of menses during the initial 3 to 6 months of treatment occurs frequently, but menstrual periods return as the disease goes into remission and the dose of corticosteroids is reduced. Menorrhagia occasionally occurs, possibly because of thrombocytopenia or an inhibitor of one of the clotting factors.

Stillbirths and spontaneous abortions are common in untreated patients with active disease. Normal deliveries are the rule in well-controlled patients taking low doses of corticosteroids for at least 6 months prior to conception.[107,108] Normal deliveries may be due to the suppression of maternal lupus anticoagulant.[109] However, slight exacerbations of the disease are common in the immediate prepartum and postpartum periods.[107,110] Of four deliveries during 1977, mild thrombocytopenia occurred in two patients 2 weeks prior to delivery. Hemolytic anemia occurred in one patient a few days after delivery. In each instance, prompt remissions occurred in two patients 2 weeks prior to delivery. Hemolytic anemia occurred in one patient a few days after delivery. In each instance, prompt remission occurred when corticosteroid dose was increased.

We have not observed congenital abnormalities in the children of our patients, with the exception of complete heart block. This was present in two children of one of our patients, who was one of three in the first report describing the association of congenital heart block and SLE.[111] We recently tested her banked serum and found that she had very high levels of anti-Ro. Congential heart block is clearly associated with anti-Ro antibody passively transferred to the infant from the mother. We and others have observed normal infants born to mothers with SLE and anti-Ro antibodies at the time of delivery, however.

ALLERGIC REACTIONS

SLE patients do not have a higher than normal incidence of allergic dermatitis, rhinitis, asthma, or food or drug allergies. However, instances of severe exacerbations of the disease have been observed after treatment of urinary infections with sulfasoxazole. Hives are not uncommon and are probably a manifestation of the disease rather than of allergy.

LABORATORY FINDINGS

HEMATOLOGIC ABNORMALITIES

One or more hematologic abnormalities are present in nearly all SLE patients with active disease. Most common is a mild-to-moderate normocytic, normochromic *anemia* caused by retarded erythropoiesis. Hematocrit values of less than 30% occur in about half the patients during periods of clinical disease activity. On the other hand, Coombs-positive hemolytic anemia occurred in only 10% of our 365 patients, although positive Coombs' tests occur more frequently as an isolated abnormality owing to the presence of C3 or

C4 on the erythrocyte surface without evidence of hemolysis or reticulocytosis.

Mild to moderate *leukopenia* is less common than anemia. Leukopenia of less than 4000 cells/cmm was present in 17% of our patients. Usually both lymphocyte and neutrophil numbers are decreased. Lymphopenia is usually present during periods of disease activity.[112] *Leukocytosis* is occasionally noted during episodes of active disease and may be a confusing finding if spiking fever is also present. *Leukocytosis* resulting from corticosteroid therapy also occurs in SLE patients. White blood counts of 30,000, nearly all mature neutrophils, have occasionally been observed in corticosteroid-treated, noninfected patients.

Mild *thrombocytopenia* of between 100,000 and 150,000/cmm is present in about one third of patients, but severe thrombocytopenia with purpura has occurred in only 5%. Thrombocytopenia may occur for the first time late in the course of the disease. It occurred as an isolated event in the last trimester of pregnancy in two well-controlled SLE patients taking low loses of prednisone. An antiplatelet factor on the surface of the platelets occurs in most patients even without thrombocytopenia and is found during periods of remission as well as during disease activity. Qualitative thrombocyte defects are also common.[113]

The *lupus anticoagulant* (see also Chapter 70) can be identified by the presence of a slight prolongation of the prothrombin time and more marked prolongation of the partial thromboplastin time, which is not corrected by the addition of equal volumes of normal plasma to the patient's plasma at dilutions of 1:50, 1:100, and 1:500. The lupus anticoagulant is not clinically related to increased bleeding; bleeding and clotting times are normal. Renal biopsies have been performed on individuals with the lupus anticoagulant without any bleeding.

However, there is a significant relationship between the lupus anticoagulant and thrombosis. Arterial and venous thrombosis, placental infarction, cerebral infarction, and thrombocytopenia are all more common in patients with the lupus anticoagulant. The lupus anticoagulant disappears with high-dose corticosteroid therapy, but usually recurs as the dose is lowered. If a patient has had a major thrombosis, I continue to fully anticoagulate.

Inhibitors that specifically inactivate clotting factors are more significant clinically. These are most frequently directed at factors II, VIII, IX, and XII and must be identified, because major bleeding episodes may result from renal biopsies or operative procedures. The action of these specific anticoagulants is also reversed by corticosteroid therapy. In general, bleeding problems in SLE patients occur in individuals with active disease, especially in those with vasculitis.

False positive serologic tests for syphilis were present in 25% of our patients and are frequently, but not always, associated with the lupus anticoagulant (see Chapter 70).

The ESR is elevated in nearly all SLE patients and, in most patients, falls to normal when the disease becomes inactive. However, some patients maintain a markedly elevated ESR for years in the absence of clinical or serologic evidence of active disease.

Serum C-reactive protein (CRP) levels are elevated in infections and in rheumatoid arthritis but rarely in uncomplicated SLE.[113a] CRP levels above 60 mg/L were found in 8 of 18 SLE patients with infection and in only 3 of 42 patients without infection (sensitivity = 39%; specificity = 93%). Serum acidic glycoprotein, determined as a research procedure, was 83% positive and 100% specific in differentiating active SLE from intercurrent infection.[113b]

Cryoglobulins of the mixed IgG-IgM type may be found in about 11% of patients. They are usually associated with clinical and serologic disease activity, lower serum complement levels, and clinical nephritis.

A diffuse elevation of serum gamma globulin is observed in about 80% of patients with clinically active disease. Rheumatoid factor is present in 14% of SLE patients.

Serum complement levels are usually depressed in active disease. The association of SLE-like conditions with complement component deficiencies has been discussed already.

DIFFERENTIAL DIAGNOSIS

The Preliminary Criteria for the Classification of SLE[24] have been used since 1971 and are sensitive.[44] These criteria have helped remind physicians of the major laboratory and clinical manifestations of SLE, but they were established prior to the common availability of useful serologic tests such as complement levels, antinuclear antibodies, anti-DNA, and anti-Sm antibodies. For the purpose of establishing revised criteria, a subcommittee of the ARA collected data from 20 centers on patients thought to have SLE. The Revised Criteria, published in 1982 (Table 67–1),[45] were tested against the findings in scleroderma and rheumatoid arthritis patients for specificity, and against the findings in a second group of SLE patients for sensitivity. To classify a patient as having SLE, four or more of 11 manifestations were required in the Preliminary Criteria. As noted in Table 67–1, the

Revised Criteria have the following major differences from the Preliminary Criteria: (1) The renal manifestations are grouped together, and the proteinuria item no longer requires 3.5 g per day of urinary protein; (2) alopecia has been deleted as a manifestation; (3) Raynaud's phenomenon has been deleted as a manifestation; (4) antinuclear antibodies have been added as a manifestation; (5) the LE preparation, which was a single manifestation, is included in the "immunologic" manifestation; (6) the false positive test for syphilis, which was a single manifestation, is included in the "immunologic" manifestation; and (7) anti-DNA antibodies and anti-Sm antibodies are included in the "immunologic" manifestations. Thus, the Revised Criteria group all of the relatively specific immunologic tests as one manifestation and are only marginally more sensitive and specific than are the Preliminary Criteria.[114,115]

Although not included in the Revised Criteria, serum C3 levels are of major importance in the diagnosis of an individual patient with SLE. We have shown that a low serum C3 in the presence of antibodies to native DNA is highly specific for SLE.[116] The sensitivity of the anti-DNA antibody test was 72% and the specificity 96%. The sensitivity of a low serum C3 level was 38% and the specificity 90%. Thus, in addition to studies of serum antibodies to nuclear antigens, a serum C3 level should be performed in all individuals for whom a diagnosis of SLE is considered. The most common diagnosis made in patients before definitive diagnosis of SLE is rheumatoid arthritis or "nonspecific" arthritis. Approximately one quarter of our SLE patients had this diagnosis for at least 1 year prior to the diagnosis of SLE. Young women presenting with a history of arthritis or arthralgia should be studied carefully for SLE. The onset of arthritis or arthralgia during pregnancy or the postpartum period should particularly alert the physician to the diagnosis of SLE. Diagnoses that may predate a definitive diagnosis of SLE by 2 to 10 years include rheumatic fever, chronic discoid lupus, idiopathic thrombocytopenic purpura, seizure disorder, Raynaud's phenomenon, psychosis, and hemolytic anemia.

It is important to remember that SLE can occur in elderly persons, and the diagnosis is frequently missed early in the course of their disease. Some such patients were in nursing homes because they were confused and considered senile. After SLE was finally diagnosed and the disease was treated with corticosteroids, the "senile" psychosis gradually cleared; the patients became alert and able to care for themselves once again.

Other diseases to consider in patients with multisystem disease include subacute bacterial endocarditis, infected atrioventricular shunts, gonococcal or meningococcal septicemia with arthritis and skin lesions, serum sickness, lymphoma and leukemia, thrombotic thrombocytopenic purpura, sarcoidosis, secondary syphilis, bacterial septicemia, and Acquired Immune Deficiency Disease.

MANAGEMENT

At the time of diagnosis, the severity of the disease should be determined using the history, physical examination, and laboratory workup. With rapid disease onset, the patient should be considered to have a more severe condition. The presence of both anti-DNA antibodies and low serum complement (especially C3) levels suggests more severe disease.

RENAL BIOPSY

Urinary abnormalities should lead to complete study for renal disease. Serum creatinine levels should be obtained on two occasions to determine whether renal insufficiency is present or impending. Patients with proteinuria and red cells in the urine should have a renal biopsy to determine the following: (1) the *type* of lupus nephritis, as discussed already; (2) the *activity* of the glomerular lesion; (3) the presence and extent of glomerular and/or tubular *sclerosis*; and (4) the presence and extent of tubular and interstitial disease. As described previously, the presence of sclerosis early in the course of the disease is a sign of a poor prognosis. Extensive sclerosis does not respond to any kind of aggressive therapy. The management of the various forms of lupus nephritis with corticosteroids is described in the section on renal disease. The use of other forms of therapy for lupus nephritis will be described.

Management of SLE is divided into four sections: (1) general measures that should be applied to most patients; (2) management of active disease, particularly at the onset of the illness; (3) management of the period between control of the initial episode of active disease and clinical remission; and (4) management of the patient over an extended clinical remission.

GENERAL MEASURES

Both patient and physician should become familiar with the signs and symptoms present during the time of disease onset. The early clinical recurrence of disease activity may then be recognized by the patient, who should alert the physician. For example, some patients develop an erythematous rash as the first sign of an impending serious systemic exacerbation. If the patient merely waits until the next appointment to inform the physician of the rash, the delay may result in the appearance of more serious, additional manifestations, such as hematuria or pericarditis.

The physician should be familiar with the laboratory evidence of active disease in each patient and with the response of each laboratory abnormality to corticosteroid therapy. Thus, if the ESR is initially elevated and rapidly returns to normal after therapy, future significant increase in the ESR may be viewed with concern regarding exacerbation of the disease. Similarly, initial low C3 or C4 levels, which return to the normal range as the disease becomes inactive, usually fall again either just before or when the clinical disease activity recurs.[117] Prior to treatment, the physician should know which laboratory tests were *not* abnormal during the initial episode of disease activity. Other patients have abnormal laboratory findings that do not resolve with treatment and clinical remission. For example, elevated antinative DNA antibodies have been noted over the course of 5 years in patients who are clinically well. Abnormal test results that do not respond initially to adequate treatment should probably be ignored in most patients. I have found that patients who have persistently high anti-DNA antibody levels and who are clinically well and have otherwise normal laboratory tests become acutely ill when their C3 levels fall.

All SLE patients initially need reassurance from their physician, adequate rest when the disease is active, and avoidance of sun exposure. Sunscreen creams and ointments, wide-brimmed hats, and long sleeves should be used by all SLE patients. Exercise should be encouraged at each visit after the patient has initially responded to corticosteroids with loss of fatigue, disappearance of arthritis or arthralgia, and an increase in sense of well being.

BIRTH CONTROL

Pregnancy should be avoided during the first few years of disease. Oral contraceptives should be avoided. Pregnancy has been well tolerated in our patients who have no evidence of active renal disease or sclerotic glomeruli and who are in clinical remission while taking less than 15 mg prednisone daily for at least 1 year. Exacerbations of disease during pregnancy should be managed by vigorous treatment with corticosteroids rather than by therapeutic abortion.[108]

INFECTIONS

All SLE patients should be observed carefully for infections. Patients should be instructed to inform the physician immediately if any symptoms occur or if a fever is present. Urinalysis should be performed and cultures should be performed on specimens that show bacteria. Patients should be treated prophylactically with antibiotics if scaling of the gums, teeth extraction, or major dental surgery is performed.

HYPERTENSION

Patients should be treated as aggressively as necessary to lower their blood pressure. One factor that may explain the better prognosis of severe lupus nephritis today as compared with that reported during the 1950s is the current use of antihypertensive agents to control blood pressure elevations.[73,85]

DISEASE SEVERITY

Treatment depends not only on the target organs involved but on the severity of the disease. Renal disease may be minimal or mild. Anemia may be slight or may be a severe hemolytic anemia. Mildly ill patients frequently are diagnosed at a time when arthritis and a butterfly rash are the only signs and symptoms of the disease. The laboratory evidence of severe disease is of great importance in such patients. A low serum C3 and high titers of antinative DNA antibodies are considered by many, although not all, investigators to indicate that severe clinical and/or renal disease may ensue unless the patient is treated aggressively.

Other laboratory parameters that may be present in patients whose signs and symptoms are mild include thrombocytopenia, hemolytic anemia, renal disease with more than mild proteinuria, seizures, organic brain disease, and vasculitis of the skin or other organs. If present, these parameters indicate that the disease is severe and should be treated aggressively. In our experience, pericarditis and pleuritis are also considered "severe," but others do not agree.

Initial Treatment. Patients with severe disease should be treated with corticosteroids (see Chapter 37). Most patients respond to 60 mg of prednisone given in doses of 15 mg every 6 hours. Many severely ill patients without CNS or active renal disease require a similar high dose of prednisone initially. In most patients, evidence of disease activity disappears rapidly. Large pericardial or pleural effusions, hematuria,

and, occasionally, CNS manifestations may respond more slowly and may require a higher daily dose of prednisone. In an analysis of 67 neuropsychiatric episodes, 84% had a favorable outcome, usually associated with initiation or increase in steroid dose.[82]

The use of pulse-therapy corticosteroids (intravenous infusion of large doses, usually 1 g methylprednisolone daily for 3 days) has been advocated in the management of severe SLE patients with rapidly advancing renal failure who have not responded to oral doses.[118,119] Although some investigators have described rapid fall of "nephrotic range" proteinuria, we have not found this to occur in a small number of patients so treated. Fessel described improvement in one of three patients with lupus cerebritis, in all three patients with lung disease, and in one patient with thrombocytopenia.[120]

In patients with pulmonary hemorrhage not caused by infection, pulse therapy and plasmapheresis may be the treatment of choice because these patients need as rapid a therapeutic effect as possible. It is important to continue with high-dose oral corticosteroid therapy after the 3-day pulse therapy in such an acutely ill patient. There are still no definite studies to determine whether pulse therapy provides better long-term management. The question regarding long-term side effects, such as aseptic necrosis, is not clear at present. Acute side effects have resulted from the intravenous pulse therapy, including bacteremia and sudden death, the latter presumably owing to electrolyte effects on the myocardium. In addition, hyperglycemia, hypokalemia or hyperkalemia, sodium retention, hypotension, or hypertension have been described. In some centers, intravenous pulse therapy is administered only to inpatients with continuous cardiac monitors. Infusion over at least 30 minutes is recommended.[119]

Plasmapheresis. Plasmapheresis is an experimental treatment and, in general, should be restricted to centers where controlled protocol studies are being conducted. Recorded data strongly suggest that plasmapheresis is followed by a serious rebound of both immunologic and clinical activity.[120,121] In addition, many of the reports in the literature describe a short-lived remission. Plasmapheresis together with corticosteroid therapy appears to be effective, but the response is also short-lived, as is the response to plasmapheresis and azathioprine. The most prolonged response followed plasmapheresis combined with both corticosteroids and cyclophosphamide. Patients so treated responded and had no rebound, and the improvement lasted for at least 4 months. Thus, if plasmapheresis is to be used, it should be given with corticosteroids and cyclophosphamide. Patients with pulmonary hemorrhage have responded to a combination of pulse intravenous corticosteroids, plasmapheresis, and intravenous cyclophosphamide.

Less severely ill patients respond to 20 to 40 mg of prednisone given in a regimen of 5 to 10 mg four times daily. The response is usually prompt, i.e., within 1 to 2 weeks, with disappearance of symptoms and a change in abnormal laboratory tests toward a normal range.

SLE patients with mild disease and without significantly abnormal laboratory tests may be treated with a combination of aspirin and hydroxychloroquine sulfate (Plaquenil). Aspirin is used in anti-inflammatory doses (see Chapter 32), and 200 mg of hydroxychloroquine is given twice daily (see Chapter 34). This regimen is adequate for most patients in whom arthritis and dermatologic abnormalities are the only clinical signs and symptoms and in whom laboratory tests are not "severe", e.g., in patients with subacute cutaneous lupus.

MANAGEMENT AFTER INITIAL RESPONSE

Most SLE patients respond initially to high doses of oral corticosteroids. As the clinical disease responds, resolution of laboratory abnormalities is observed. The corticosteroid dose can then be lowered. Gradual tapering with frequent monitoring of laboratory values is usually successful until the daily dose of prednisone reaches 10 to 20 mg. At this dosage, there may be evidence of serologic or clinical flare of the disease, and the prednisone dose should then be held constant temporarily or should be slightly increased.

MANAGEMENT ON LOW-DOSE PREDNISONE

In patients controlled on small doses of prednisone, repeated attempts should be made to further reduce the dose. It may be necessary to lower the dose by small increments, e.g., by 1 mg per week. In most patients, a daily dose of 10 mg or less is adequate to control the disease and to allow the patients to feel totally free of symptoms. Even in these individuals, the primary goal should be administration of no medication or of the lowest possible dose. Alternate-day therapy has been used successfully in some patients. In my experience, daily small doses (2.5 to 10 mg) lead to better prolonged control. As always, the dose

should be given early in the morning to avoid suppression of the nocturnal ACTH secretion.

ANTIMALARIALS

In patients with evidence of dermatologic manifestations, antimalarial therapy should be used. Hydroxychloroquine (Plaquenil) and chloroquine (Aralen) have been shown to significantly reduce the number of episodes of skin abnormalities.[122] Retinal toxicity occurs in SLE patients who have taken the drugs for a significant length of time in high dose.[123,124] The incidence of retinopathy is related to the total ingested dose of the antimalarial drugs. Patients should be seen by an ophthalmologist before treatment and every 6 months while receiving therapy (see Chapter 34). Hydroxychloroquine, 400 mg daily, can be used initially with eventual decrease in daily dose to 200 mg when skin lesions are no longer present. An attempt should be made to further reduce the dosage to alternate days, or three or two times per week, or to discontinue the drug. In some patients, however, relapses occur and the hydroxychloroquine must be restarted.

ASPIRIN AND NONSTEROIDAL ANTI-INFLAMMATORY DRUGS (NSAIDs) (see Chapter 32)

Anti-inflammatory doses of aspirin are of value in controlling arthritis in patients whose SLE is exacerbated by low doses of corticosteroids. Rapid dramatic control of pleural and/or pericardial effusions is sometimes achieved with indomethacin 25 mg tid. If NSAIDs are used, the physician should be aware of the reports of aseptic meningitis caused by ibuprofen, tolmetin and sulindac.[125,126]

CYCLOPHOSPHAMIDE

The use of immunosuppressive agents in the treatment of SLE is still controversial. Their use should be confined to multicenter controlled studies or to those centers with extensive experience in their use. The toxicity and long-term side effects of these drugs and their use in the management of SLE have been reviewed in Chapter 38. In my experience, cyclophosphamide is of great value in patients with medium- or small-vessel necrotizing vasculitis. Its efficacy is similar to that in patients with Wegener's vasculitis or periartertis nodosa (see also Chapters 38 and 74).

Intravenous pulse cyclophosphamide has been shown to be effective in the treatment of diffuse proliferative lupus nephritis by the National Institutes of Health group.[80] Their data suggests that intravenous cyclophosphamide reduces the tendency of the glomeruli to heal with sclerosis.[81] The need for a renal biopsy prior to using this therapy is clear, and treatment with corticosteroids is continued as necessary.

PROGNOSIS

Studies on the survival of SLE patients have shown improvement over time (Table 67–3).[47,48,85,127,128,129]

Corticosteroid-treated patients have shown 5-year survivals of 93% and 94% in two reports.[82,85] It is therefore important to consider the period of observation when patients recently treated with immunosuppressive therapy are compared with patients treated 15 to 20 years ago with corticosteroids. The improved survival rate could be due to better use of serologic parameters and antibiotics, an increased awareness of the disease on the part of both patient and physician, or a change in the natural history of the disease.

RELATED OR ASSOCIATED CONDITIONS (see also Chapter 66)

RHEUMATOID ARTHRITIS AND OTHER CONNECTIVE TISSUE DISEASES

Only a small percentage of individuals who fulfill the ARA Preliminary or Revised Criteria have definite coincident rheumatoid nodules, erosive arthritis, and rheumatoid factor.[43] Such individuals have at least 4 of the 14 manifestations of the Preliminary Criteria, excluding arthritis. Patients with classic or definitive rheumatoid arthritis occasionally develop typical multisystem SLE, including lupus nephritis. An occasional patient may have typical SLE along with one or more manifestations or another connective tissue disease. SLE patients with a typical violaceous rash of the V area of the chest and edematous violaceous upper eyelids have been observed. Necrotizing vasculitis typical of polyarteritis and plaques of scleroderma have also been observed in an occasional SLE patient, and full-blown CREST syndrome has been noted in some of our SLE patients along with anticentromere antibodies.

Myasthenia Gravis. SLE has been reported in association with myasthenia gravis either before or after thymectomy.[130]

Porphyria Cutanea Tarda. This condition has been reported in association with SLE.[32]

Chronic Discoid Lupus. This benign skin disease is not rare and is thought to be more common than SLE itself. Discoid lupus has been reported in infants and in the elderly, but most patients are between the ages of 25 and 45 at the time of onset. Although women are affected more often than men, the sex ratio is only 2:1.[131] The disease occurs in all races. Family studies have revealed more than one case in the same family, and studies of relatives of SLE patients have revealed other family members with discoid lupus.[132] Studies of antinative-DNA antibodies and complement proteins in discoid lupus patients show no increases compared to age, sex, and race-matched controls.[35] Complement proteins were normal in these studies except for increased levels of properdin found in nearly half the patients studied. It is of interest that a number of individuals with a hereditary deficiency of C2 have lesions of discoid lupus as their only clinical abnormality.

It is clear that some patients with discoid lupus develop SLE. but the percentage that does so is unknown. No serologic markers identifying patients

Table 67–3. Reported Survival in Corticosteroid-Treated SLE Patients*

Series	No. of Cases	Years of Observation	Years After Diagnosis				
			1	3	5	7	10
Johns Hopkins	99	1949–1953	78	62	..	..	..
Cleveland Clinic	299	1949–1959	89	75	69	59	54
University of Southern California	57	1950–1955	42	12	4	2	..
Sweden	54	1955–1961	82	72	70	63	51
University of Southern California	100	1956–1962	63	32	16	12	4
Group 1	209	1957–1967	89	79	70	67	63
Columbia University	150	1963–1971	98	90	77	68	59
University of Southern California	92	1963–1973	98	91	79	65	41
Group 2	156	1968–1975	99	97	93	90	84
Johns Hopkins	140	1970–1975	..	..	94	..	82

*For whom life-table analysis was employed.
From Urman, J.D., and Rothfield, N.F.[85]

who eventually develop systemic disease have been found.

Drug-Induced Lupus. This syndrome is caused by the chronic ingestion of several drugs and has been reviewed.[133] Prospective studies have revealed that procainamide-induced antinuclear antibodies develop in about 50% of individuals, about half of whom develop a lupus-like illness. Procainamide is, therefore, the most common drug inducing a lupus syndrome. Patients with this syndrome typically have joint pains and swelling, rashes, pleurisy, pericarditis, and pulmonary atelectasis. The disease clinically resembles the nondrug-induced disease in elderly individuals. In both the procainamide-induced syndrome and in SLE in elderly individuals, renal disease is uncommon, and antibodies against native DNA are usually absent. Withdrawal of procainamide gradually leads to disappearance of the clinical syndrome and eventual disappearance of the serum antinuclear antibodies.

Although drug-induced clinical disease has been described rarely after isoniazid use, the drug did induce antinuclear antibodies in 20% of individuals who received it.[134]

A prospective study on the immunologic effects of hydralazine was completed in a group of black patients. The results after 2 years revealed that antinuclear antibodies developed in 15 of the 25 patients. The antinuclear antibodies were detected in undiluted sera in 12, and a titer of 1:10 or greater occurred in three patients. Clinical symptoms of SLE developed in only one of the 25 patients.[135]

REFERENCES

1. Kaposi, M.K.: Neue Beitrage zur Kenntniss des Lupus erythematosus. Arch. Dermatol. Syph., 4:36–78, 1872.
2. Osler, W.: On the visceral manifestations of the erythema group of skin disease. Am. J. Med. Sci., 110:629–646, 1895.
3. Libman, E., and Sacks, B.: A hitherto undescribed form of valvular and mural endocarditis. Arch. Intern. Med., 33:701–737, 1924.
4. Gross, L.: The cardiac lesions in Libman-Sacks disease, with a consideration of its relationship to acute diffuse lupus erythematosus. Am. J. Pathol., 16:375–408, 1940.
5. Baehr, G., Klemperer, P., and Schrifrin, A.: A diffuse disease of the peripheral circulation usually associated with lupus erythematosus and endocarditis. Trans. Assoc. Am. Physicians, 50:139–155, 1935.
6. Hargraves, M.M., Richmond, H., and Morton, R.: Presentation of two bone marrow elements: The "tart cell" and the "LE" cell. Proc. Staff Meet. Mayo Clin., 23:25–28, 1948.
7. Serdula, M.K. and Rhoads, G.G.: Frequency of systemic lupus erythematosus in different ethnic groups in Hawaii. Arthritis Rheum., 22:328–333, 1979.
8. Taylor, H.G., and Stein, C.M.: SLE in Zimbabwe. Ann. Rheum. Dis., 45:645–648, 1986.
9. Chang, N.C.: Rheumatic diseases in China. J. Rheumatol. (special issue), November 10, 1983, 41–45.
10. Hochberg, M.C.: The incidence of SLE in Baltimore, Maryland, 1970–1977. Arthritis Rheum., 28:80–86, 1985.
11. Michet, C.J., Jr., et al.: Epidemiology of SLE and other connective tissue diseases in Rochester, Minnesota, 1950 through 1979. Mayo Clin. Proc., 60:105–113, 1985.
12. Fessell, W.J.: Systemic lupus erythematosus in the community. Arch. Intern. Med., 134:1027–1035, 1974.
13. Arnett, F.C., and Shulman, L.E.: Studies in familial systemic lupus erythematosus. Medicine, 55:313–322, 1976.
14. Lowenstein, M.B., and Rothfield, N.F.: Family study of systemic lupus erythematosus: Analysis of clinical history, skin immunofluorescence and serologic parameters. Arthritis Rheum., 20:1293–1303, 1977.
15. Block, S.R., et al.: Immunologic observations on 9 sets of twins either concordant or discordant for systemic lupus erythematosus. Arthritis Rheum., 19:545–554, 1976.
16. Gibofsky, A., et al.: Contrasting patterns of newer histocompatibility determinants in patients with rheumatoid arthritis and systemic lupus erythematosus. Arthritis Rheum., 21:134–138, 1978.
17. Reinertsen, J.H., et al.: B lymphocyte alloantigens associated with systemic lupus erythematosus. Arthritis Rheum., 21:586, 1978.
18. Kachru, R.B., et al.: A significant increase of HLA-DR3 and DR2 in SLE among blacks. J. Rheumatol., 11:471–474, 1984.
19. Glass, D., et al.: Inherited deficiency of the second component of complement. J. Clin. Invest., 58:853–861, 1976.
20. Agnello, V.: Association of systemic lupus erythematosus and systemic lupus erythematosus-like syndromes with hereditary and acquired complement deficient states. Arthritis Rheum., 21:S146, 1978.
21. Lahita, R.G., et al.: Increased 16 alpha hydroxylation of estradiol in systemic lupus erythematosus. J. Clin. Endocrinol. Metab., 53:174–178, 1981.
22. Jungers, P.J., et al.: Influence of oral contraceptive therapy on the activity of systemic lupus erythematosus. Arthritis Rheum., 25:618–623, 1982.
23. Lahita, R.G., Kunkel, H.G., and Bradlow, H.L.: Increased 17 oxidation of testosterone in SLE. Arthritis Rheum., 26:1517–1521, 1983.
24. Stern, R., Fishman, J., Brusman, H., and Kunkel, H.G.: Systemic lupus erythematosus associated with Klinefelter's syndrome. Arthritis Rheum., 20:18–22, 1977.
25. Hang, L., et al.: Induction of murine autoimmune disease by chronic polyclonal B cell activation. J. Exp. Med., 157:874–879, 1983.
26. Gilliam, J.M., and Sontheimer, R.D.: Skin manifestations of SLE. Clin. Rheum. Dis., 8:207–212, 1982.
27. Black, M.M., and Hudson, P.M.: Atrophic and blanche lesions closely resembling malignant atrophic papulosis (Degos' disease) in systemic lupus erythematosus. Br. J. Dermatol., 95:649–654, 1976.
28. Urman, J.D., et al.: Oral mucosal ulceration in systemic lupus erythematosus. Arthritis Rheum., 21:58–61, 1978.
29. Snyder, G.G., III, et al.: Nasal septal perforation in systemic lupus erythematosus. Arch. Otolaryngol., 99:456–457, 1974.
30. Rothfield, N.F., and Weissmann, G.: Bullae in systemic lupus erythematosus. Arch. Intern. Med., 107:174–180, 1961.
31. Quismorio, F.P., Dubois, E.L., and Chandor, S.B.: Soft-tissue calification in systemic lupus erythematosus. Arch. Dermatol., 111:352–356, 1975.
32. Cram, D.L., Epstein, J.H., and Tuffanelli, D.L.: Lupus ery-

thematosus and porphyria. Arch. Dermatol., *108*:779–788, 1973.

33. Tuffanelli, D.L., Abraham, R.K., and Dubois, E.L.: Pigmentation associated with antimalarial therapy: Its possible relation to ocular lesions. Arch. Dermatol., *88*:419–426, 1963.

34. Rothfield, N.F., and Marino, C.: Studies of repeat biopsies of non-lesional skin in patients with systemic lupus erythematosus. Arthritis Rheum., *25*:624–628, 1982.

35. Schrager, M.A., and Rothfield, N.F.: Pathways of complement activation in chronic discoid lupus. Arthritis Rheum., *20*:637–645, 1977.

36. Schrager, M.A., and Rothfield, N.F.: Clinical significance of serum properdin levels and properdin deposition in the dermal-epidermal junction in systemic lupus erythematosus. J. Clin. Invest., *57*:212–221, 1976.

37. Bullock, W.E., Callerame, M.L., and Panner, B.J.: Immunohistologic alternational skin and ultrastructural changes in glomerular membrane in leprosy. Am. J. Trop. Med. Hyg., *23*:78–86, 1974.

38. Baart de la Faille, H., and Baart de la Faille-Kuyper, E.H.: Immunofluorescence studies of the skin in rosacea. Dermatologica, *139*:49–54, 1969.

39. Jablonska, S., Chorzelski, T., and Maciejowska, E.: The scope and limitations of the immunofluorescence method in the diagnosis of lupus erythematosus. Br. J. Dermatol., *83*:242–247, 1970.

40. Prystowsky, S.D., and Gilliam, J.N.: Discoid lupus erythematosus as part of a larger disease spectrum. Arch. Dermatol., *11*:1448–1453, 1975.

41. Smith, D., Marino, C., and Rothfield, N.F.: The clinical utility of the "lupus band test". Arthritis Rheum., *4*:382–387, 1984.

42. Labowitz, R., and Schumacher, H.R.: Articular manifestations of systemic lupus erythematosus. Ann. Intern. Med., *74*:911–921, 1971.

43. Fischman, A.S., et al.: The coexistence of rheumatoid arthritis and systemic lupus erythematosus: A case report and review of the literature. J. Rheumatol., *8*:405–415, 1981.

44. Cohen, A.S., et al.: Preliminary criteria for the classification of systemic lupus erythematosus. Bull. Rheum. Dis., *21*:643–651, 1971.

45. Tan, E.M., et al.: Revised criteria for the classification of systemic lupus erythematosus. Arthritis Rheum., *25*:1271–1277, 1982.

46. Tsokos, G.C., Moutsopoulos, H.M., and Steinberg, A.B.: Muscle involvement in SLE. JAMA, *246*:766–768, 1981.

47. Estes, D., and Christian, C.L.: The natural history of systemic lupus erythematosus by prospective analysis. Medicine, *50*:85–96, 1971.

48. Dubois, E.L., et al.: Duration and death in systemic lupus erythematosus: An analysis of 249 cases. JAMA, *227*:1399–1402, 1974.

49. Chia, G.L., Mah, E.P.K., and Feng, P.H.: Cardiovascular abnormalities in systemic lupus erythematosus. J. Clin. Ultrasound, *9*:237–241, 1981.

50. Kindig, J.R., and Goodman, M.R.: Clinical utility of pericardial fluid pH determination. Am. J. Med., *75*:1077–1079, 1983.

51. Doherty, N.E., and Siegel, R.J.: Cardiovascular manifestations of systemic lupus erythematosus. Am. Heart J., *110*:1257–1265, 1985.

52. Bulkley, B.H., and Roberts, W.C.: The heart in systemic lupus erythematosus and the changes induced in it by corticosteroid therapy: A study of 36 necropsy patients. Am. J. Med., *58*:243–256, 1975.

53. Urowitz, M.B., et al.: The bimodal mortality pattern of systemic lupus erythematosus. Am. J. Med., *60*:221–225, 1976.

54. Haider, Y.S., Roberts, W.C.: Quantification of degrees of narrowing in 22 necropsy patients (21 women) aged 16 to 37 years. Am. J. Med., *70*:775–781, 1981.

55. Hosenpud, J.D., et al.: Myocardial perfusion abnormalities in asymptomatic patients with systemic lupus erythematosus. Am. J. Med., *77*:286–292, 1984.

56. Bernhard, G.C., Lange, R.L., and Hensley, G.T.: Aortic disease with valvular insufficiency as the principal manifestation of systemic lupus erythematosus. Ann. Intern. Med., *71*:81–87, 1969.

57. Paget, S.A., et al.: Mitral valve disease of systemic lupus erythematosus: A cause of severe congestive heart failure reversed by valve replacement. Am. J. Med., *59*:134–139, 1975.

58. Laufer, J., Frand, M., and Milo, S.: Valve replacement for severe tricuspid regurgitation caused by Libman-Sacks endocarditis. Br. Heart J., *48*:294–297, 1982.

59. Rawthshome, L., et al.: Lupus vasculitis necessitating double valve replacement. Arthritis Rheum., *24*:561–564, 1981.

60. St. Clair, W., et al.: Deep venous thrombosis and a circulating anticoagulant in systemic lupus erythematosus. Am. J. Dis. Child., *135*:230–232, 1981.

61. Averbach, M., and Levo, Y.: Budd-Chiari syndrome as the major thrombotic complication of systemic lupus erythematosus with the lupus anticoagulant. Ann. Rheum. Dis., *45*:435–437, 1986.

62. Carreras, L.O., et al.: Arterial thrombosis, intrauterine death and "lupus anticoagulant": Detection of immunoglobulin interfering with prostacyclin formation. Lancet, *1*:244–246, 1981.

63. Maathay, R.A., et al.: Pulmonary manifestations of systemic lupus erythematosus: Review of twelve cases of acute lupus pneumonitis. Medicine, *54*:397–409, 1974.

64. Haupt, H.M., Moore, G.W., and Hutchins, G.M.: The lung in systemic lupus erythematosus: Analysis of the pathologic changes in 120 patients. Am. J. Med., *71*:791–803, 1981.

65. Gibson, G.E., Edmonds, J.P., and Hughes, G.R.V.: Diaphragm function and lung involvement in systemic lupus erythematosus. Am. J. Med., *63*:926, 1977.

66. Miller, L.R., Greenberg, D., and McLarty, J.W.: Lupus lung. Chest, *88*:265–269, 1985.

67. Jacobelli, S., et al.: Inspiratory muscle dysfunction and unexplained dyspnea in systemic lupus erythematosus. Arthritis Rheum., *28*:781–788, 1985.

68. Asherson, R., et al.: Pulmonary hypertension in systemic lupus erythematosus. Br. Med. J., *287*:1024–1025, 1983.

69. Pollak, V.E., and Kant, K.S.: Systemic lupus erythematosus and the kidney chapter in systemic lupus erythematosus. Edited by R.G. Lahita. New York, Wiley Medical, 1987.

70. Baldwin, D.S.: Clinical usefulness of the morphological classification of lupus nephritis. Am. J. Kidney Dis., *2(1)*(Suppl. 1):142–149, 1982.

71. ODell, J.R., Hays, R.C.: Guggenheim, S.J., and Steigerwald, J.C.: Systemic lupus erythematosus without clinical renal abnormalities: Renal biopsy findings and clinical course. Ann. Rheum. Dis., *44*:415–419, 1985.

72. Ginzler, E.M., et al.: Progression of mesangial and focal to diffuse lupus nephritis. N. Engl. J. Med., *291*:693–969, 1974.

73. Baldwin, D.S., et al.: The clinical course of the proliferative membranous forms of lupus nephritis. Ann. Intern. Med., *73*:929–942, 1970.

74. Morel-Maroger, L., et al.: The course of lupus nephritis: Contribution of serial renal biopsies. Adv. Nephrol., *6*:79–86, 1976.

75. Zimmerman, S.W., et al.: Progression from minimal or focal

to diffuse proliferative lupus nephritis. Lab. Invest., 32:665–672, 1975.

76. Pirani, C.L., Pollak, V.E., and Schwartz, F.D.: The reproducibility of semiquantitative analyses of renal histology. Nephron, 1:230–237, 1964.

77. Striker, G.E., et al.: The course of lupus nephritis: A clinical-pathological correlation of fifty patients. In: Glomerulonephritis: Morphology, Natural History and Treatment, Vol. 2. Edited by P. Kincaid-Smith, T.H. Mathew, and L.E. Becker. New York, John Wiley & Sons, Inc., 1973, p. 1141.

78. Bretjens, J.R., et al.: Interstitial immune complex nephritis in patients with systemic lupus erythematosus. Kidney Int., 7:342–358, 1975.

79. Balow, J.E., et al.: Lupus nephritis. Ann. Int. Med., 106:79–94, 1987.

80. Austin, H.A., III, et al.: Therapy of lupus nephritis: Controlled trial of prednisone and cytotoxic drugs. N. Engl. J. Med., 314:614–619, 1986.

81. Austin, H.A., III, et al.: Prognostic factors in lupus nephritis: Contribution of renal histologic data. Am. J. Med., 75:382–391, 1983.

82. Feinglass, E.J., et al.: Neuropsychiatric manifestations of systemic lupus erythematosus: Diagnosis, clinical spectrum and relationship to other features of the disease. Medicine, 55:323–339, 1976.

83. Smith, C.A., and Pinals, R.S.: Optic neuritis in SLE. J. Rheumatol., 9:963–966, 1982.

84. Bluestein, H.G.: Neuropsychiatric disorders in systemic lupus erythematosus. In: Systemic Lupus Erythematosus. Edited by R.G. Lahita. New York, Wiley Press, 1987.

85. Urman, J.D., and Rothfield, N.F.: Corticosteroid treatment in systemic lupus erythematosus: Survival studies. JAMA, 238:2272–2276, 1977.

86. Brandt, K.D., and Lessel, S.: Migrainous phenomena in systemic lupus erythematosus. Arthritis Rheum., 21:7–16, 1978.

87. Isenberg, D.A., et al.: A study of migraine in SLE. Ann. Rheum. Dis., 41:30–32, 1982.

88. Trevor, R.P., et al.: Angiographic demonstration of major cerebral vessel occlusion in systemic lupus erythematosus. Neuroradiology, 4:202–207, 1972.

89. Fox, I.S., et al.: Cerebral Embolism in Libman-Sacks endocarditis. Neurology, 30:487–491, 1980.

90. Bluestein, H.G.: Neurocytotoxic antibodies in serum of patients with systemic lupus erythematosus. Proc. Natl. Acad. Sci. (USA), 75:3965–3969, 1976.

91. Hadler, N.M., et al.: The fourth component of complement in the cerebrospinal fluid in systemic lupus erythematosus. Arthritis Rheum., 16:507–521, 1973.

92. Bernstein, R.M., III: Cerebral lupus: A peep into Pandora's box. J. Rheumatol., 9:817–818, 1982.

93. Ellis, S.G., and Verity, M.A.: Central nervous system involvement in systemic lupus erythematosus: A review of neuropathologic findings in 57 cases, 1955–1977. Semin. Arthritis Rheum., 8:212–221, 1979.

94. Ropes, M.: Systemic Lupus Erythematosus. Cambridge, Harvard University Press, 1976.

95. Atkins, C.J., Kondan, J.J., and Quismorio, F.P.: The choroid plexus in systemic lupus erythematosus. Ann. Intern. Med., 76:65–72, 1982.

96. Zizic, T.M., Shulman, L.E., and Stevens, M.B.: Colonic perforations in systemic lupus erythematosus. Medicine, 54:411–426, 1975.

97. Shafer, R.B., and Gregory, D.H.: Systemic lupus erythematosus presenting as regional ileitis. Minn. Med., 53:789–792, 1970.

98. Tsuchiya, M., et al.: Radiographic and endoscopic features of colonic ulcers in systemic lupus erythematosus. Am. J. Gastroenterol., 64:277–283, 1977.

99. Trynolds, J.C., et al.: Acute pancreatitis in systemic lupus erythematosus. Medicine (Baltimore), 61:25–32, 1982.

100. Meislin, A.G., and Rothfield, N.F.: Systemic lupus erythematosus in childhood. Pediatrics, 42:37–49, 1968.

101. Runyon, B.A., LaBrecque, D.R., and Anuras, S.: The spectrum of liver disease in systemic lupus erythematosus. Am. J. Med., 69:187–194, 1980.

102. Dillon, A.M., Stein, H.B., and English, R.A.: Splenic atrophy in SLE. Ann. Intern. Med., 96:40–43, 1982.

103. Bishko, F.: Retinopathy in systemic lupus erythematosus: A case report and review of the literature. Arthritis Rheum., 15:57–63, 1972.

104. Coppeto, J., and Lessell, S.: Retinopathy in systemic lupus erythematosus. Arch. Ophthalamol., 95:794–797, 1977.

105. Wong, K., et al.: Visual loss as the initial symptom of systemic lupus erythematosus. Am. J. Ophthalmol., 92:238–244, 1981.

106. Matsopoulis, H.M., et al.: Correlative histologic and serologic findings of sicca syndrome in patients with systemic lupus erythematosus. Arthritis Rheum., 23:36–40, 1980.

107. Zulman, J.U., et al.: Problems associated with the management of pregnancies in patients with systemic lupus erythematosus. J. Rheumatol., 7:37–49, 1980.

108. Zurier, R.B., et al.: Systemic lupus erythematosus—management during pregnancy. Obstet. Gynecol., 51:178–189, 1978.

109. Lubbe, W.F., et al.: Fetal survival after prednisone suppression of the lupus anticoagulant. Lancet, 1:1361–1363, 1983.

110. Mund, A., Simson, L., and Rothfield, N.F.: Effect of pregnancy on course of systemic lupus erythematosus. JAMA, 183:917–920, 1963.

111. Chameides, L., et al.: Association of maternal systemic lupus erythematosus with congenital complete heart block. N. Engl. J. Med., 297:1204–1207, 1977.

112. Rivero, S.J., Diaz-Jouanen, E.: and Alarcon-Segovia, D.: Lymphopenia in systemic lupus erythematosus: Clinical, diagnostic and prognostic significance. Arthritis Rheum., 21:205, 1978.

113. Laurence, J., and Nachman, R.: Hematologic aspects of systemic lupus erythematosus. In: Systemic Lupus Erythematosus. Edited by R.G. Lahita. New York, John Wiley & Sons, Inc., 1987.

113a. Honig, S., Gorevic, P., and Weissmann, G.: C-reactive protein in systemic lupus erythematosus. Arthritis Rheum., 20:1065, 1977.

113b. Mackiewicz, S., Mackiewicz, S., Ballou, S.P., and Kushner, I.: Micro heterogeneity of c/acid glycoprotein (AGP) in detections of intercurrent infection in systemic lupus erythematosus. Proceedings of the 4th International Seminars on the Treatment of Rheumatic Diseases. (Abstract.) Israel, Nov. 2–9, 1986, p. 77.

114. Levin, R.E., et al.: A comparison of the sensitivity of the 1971 and 1982 criteria for the classification of systemic lupus erythematosus. Arthritis Rheum., 27:530–538, 1984.

115. Passas, C.P., et al.: A comparison of the specificity of the 1971 and 1982 criteria for the classification of SLE. Arthritis Rheum., 28:620–623, 1985.

116. Weinstein, A., et al.: Antibodies to native DNA and serum complement (C3) levels: Applications to the diagnosis and classification of systemic lupus erythematosus. Am. J. Med., 74:206–216, 1983.

117. Schur, P.H., and Sandson, J.: Immunologic factors and clinical activity in lupus erythematosus. N. Engl. J. Med., *278*:533–540, 1968.

118. Cathcart, E.S., et al.: Beneficial effects of methylprednisolone "pulse" therapy in diffuse proliferative lupus nephritis. Lancet, *1*:163–166, 1976.

119. Kimberly, R.P.: Pulse methylprednisolone in SLE. Clin. Rheum. Dis., *8*:261–275, 1982.

120. Fessel, W.J.: Megadose corticosteroid therapy in systemic lupus erythematosus. J. Rheumatol., *7*:846–500, 1980.

121. Jones, J.V.: Plasmapheresis in SLE. Clin. Rheum. Dis., *8*:243–260, 1982.

122. Rudnicki, R.D., Gresham, G.E., and Rothfield, N.F.: The efficacy of antimalarials in systemic lupus erythematosus. J. Rheumatol., *2*:323–330, 1975.

123. Carr, R.E., et al.: Ocular toxicity of antimalarial drugs. Am. J. Ophthalmol., *66*:737–746, 1968.

124. Henkind, P., and Rothfield, N.F.: Ocular abnormalities in patients treated with antimalarial drugs. N. Engl. J. Med., *269*:433–439, 1963.

125. Ruppert, G.B., and Barth, W.F.: Tolmetin-induced aseptic meningitis. JAMA, *245*:67–68, 1981.

126. Ballas, Z.K., Donta, S.T.: Sulindac-induced aseptic meningitis. Arch. Intern. Med., *142*:165–166, 1982.

127. Dubois, E.L.: Lupus Erythematosus, 2nd Ed. Univ. South Carolina Press, 1976.

128. Kellum, R.E., and Haserick, J.R.: Systemic lupus erythematosus: A statistical evaluation of mortality based on a consecutive series of 299 patients. Arch. Intern. Med., *113*:200–211, 1964.

129. Leonhardt, T.: Long term prognosis of systemic lupus erythematosus. Acta Med. Scand., *445*:5440, 1966.

130. Gailbraith, R.F., Summerskill, W.H.J., and Murray, J.: SLE, cirrhosis and ulcerative colitis after thymectomy for myasthenia gravis. N. Engl. J. Med., *270*:229–322, 1964.

131. Rothfield, N.F., et al.: Chronic discoid lupus erythematosus: A study of 65 patients and 65 controls. N. Engl. J. Med., *269*:1155–1161, 1963.

132. Belin, D.C., et al.: Familial discoid lupus erythematosus associated with heterozygous C2 deficiency. Arthritis Rheum., *23*:898–903, 1980.

133. Weinstein, A.: Drug-induced lupus erythematosus. *In*: Progress in Clinical Immunology, Vol. 4. Edited by R. Schwartz. New York, Grune and Stratton, 1980, pp. 1–21.

134. Rothfield, N.F., Biere, W., and Garfield, J.: The introduction of antibodies by isoniazid: A prospective study. Ann. Intern. Med., *88*:650–652, 1978.

135. Litwin, A., et al.: Prospective study of immunologic effects of hydralazine in hypertensive patients. Clin. Pharmacol. Ther., *29*:447–456, 1981.

SYSTEMIC LUPUS ERYTHEMATOSUS: IMMUNOLOGIC ASPECTS

68

ENG M. TAN

Systemic lupus erythematosus (SLE) is a disease of multiple pathogenetic mechanisms affecting many organs of the body and characterized by abnormalities of the immune system. These abnormalities are manifested primarily by the presence of many autoantibodies in the serum. The autoantibodies of greatest clinical significance are those directed against nuclear antigens (ANA). In recent years, there has been an increasing awareness of the complexity of serum ANAs in SLE and a better understanding of how these play a role in pathogenetic mechanisms. The cumulative work of several investigators has shown that some autoantibodies participate in immune complex–mediated tissue injury. Such injury may occur as immune complexes forming in the circulation or as immune complexes occurring at sites of tissue-fixed antigens (Fig. 68–1) (see Chapter 27).

ABNORMALITIES OF HUMORAL IMMUNITY

The types of autoantibodies encountered were discussed in a review by Kunkel, a pioneer in the study of immunologic aberrations in SLE (Table 68–1). Autoantibodies in SLE can be divided into two classes. The first includes those antibodies that are not tissue specific but react with antigens present in many tissues and organs. This class is exemplified in the autoantibodies to nuclear and cytoplasmic antigens. A second class of autoantibodies includes those that are tissue specific, that is, those directed against cellular ele-

ments of the hematopoietic system, such as red cells, white cells, and platelets and antibodies to tissue-specific antigens (thyroid, liver, muscle, stomach, and adrenal gland).

ANAs have received the most intensive scrutiny in SLE and can be classified in great detail (Table 68–2).

FIG. 68–1. Antibody to native DNA but no free DNA was detected in four consecutive serum samples of a patient with SLE. A relapse characterized by high fever and increased proteinuria coincided with disappearance of the antibody and the appearance of excess DNA antigen in the serum. The temporal sequence of DNA antibody followed by antigen strongly suggested immune complex formation during the period of relapse. (From Tan, E.M.[1a])

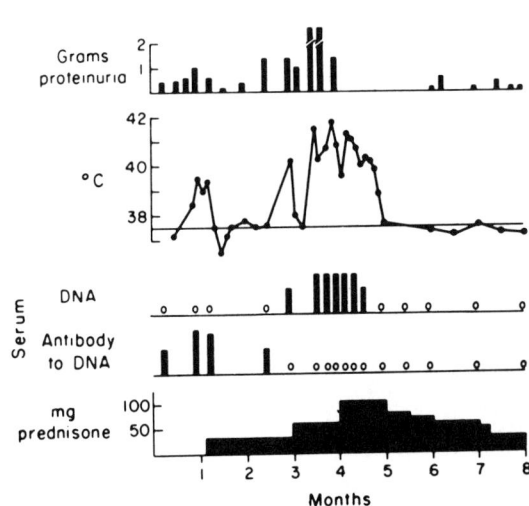

Table 68–1. Autoantibodies in SLE

Tissue Reactivity	Antibody Specificity
Nuclear antigens	DNA, nucleoprotein, histones, nonhistone (acidic) proteins
Cytoplasmic antigens	RNA, ribosomes and other RNA-protein complexes, cytoplasmic protein and liquid antigens
Clotting factors	Lupus anticoagulants
Red cell antigens	
White cell antigens	T-lymphocyte cell surface antigens, B-lymphocyte cell surface antigens
Platelet antigens	
Other tissue-specific antigens (thyroid, liver, muscle, stomach, adrenal gland)	

ANAs can be divided into four main groups: (1) those directed against double-strand DNA; (2) those directed against single-strand DNA; (3) those directed against histones, a family of basic proteins present within the nucleus; and (4) those directed against nonhistone nuclear proteins or nucleic acid–protein complexes.[2]

Antibodies to DNA were first reported in 1959.[3] Antibody to double-strand DNA reacts with an antigenic determinant present on both double-strand and single-strand DNA. This antibody is present in 50% of patients with SLE. It is generally agreed that antibody to double-strand DNA, when present in significant titer, is a diagnostic marker for SLE. It is rarely, if ever, present in other diseases. Antibody to single-strand DNA is antibody reactive with antigenic determinants that are related to the exposed purines and pyrimidines in single-strand DNA. This antibody is present in 60 to 70% of patients with SLE but may also be present in other rheumatic diseases as well as in nonrheumatic diseases. In the nonrheumatic diseases, antibody to single-strand DNA is most often seen in patients with chronic infections. Because antibody to single-strand DNA is not restricted to SLE, it is not a useful serologic marker for diagnostic purposes. However, this should not be interpreted to mean that antibody to single-strand DNA is not pathogenetically important. Indeed, it has been shown that single-strand DNA antibody can be eluted from the glomeruli of patients with SLE and that it is present in the form of immune complexes in such tissues.[4,5]

Antibodies to histones are present in approximately 70% of patients with SLE. The use of enzyme-linked immunosorbent assay (ELISA) can demonstrate that antibodies to histones are reactive with all the subclasses of histones, including H1, H2A, H2B, H3, and H4, as well as H2A/H2B and H3/H4 complexes.[6] Of great interest is the demonstration that patients with certain drug-induced lupus syndromes have antibodies to histones to the exclusion of other types of ANAs.[7]

Antibodies to nonhistone antigens have been reported with increasing frequency in SLE. Antibody to Sm antigen was the first such antibody reported.[8] Over the years, it has been confirmed repeatedly that this antibody is present almost exclusively in SLE and is a useful diagnostic marker, but it is present only in

Table 68–2. Cellular Antigens in Systemic Lupus Erythematosus

Clinical/Immunologic Designation	Structure/ Function	Molecular Characteristics	Associated RNAs	Prevalence (%)
Native DNA	Nucleic acid	Double-strand DNA	None	SLE (50%)
Denatured DNA	Nucleic acid	Single-strand DNA	None	SLE (60–70%)
Histones	Chromatin/nucleosome	H1, H2A, H2B, H3, H4	None	SLE (70%)
Sm	RNA processing	Proteins 28KD(B), 29KD(B'), 16KD(D), 13KD(E)	U1, U2, U4, U5, U6	SLE (30%)
Nuclear-RNP	RNA processing/ splicing	Proteins 68KD, 33KD(A), 22KD(C)	U1	SLE (35%)
SSA/Ro	RNA processing	Protein 60KD, 52KD	Y1–Y5 (human)	SLE (30%)
SSB/La	RNA polymerase III transcription	Phosphoproteins 46KD, 48KD	Pol III transcripts, pre-tRNA, 5S RNA, 4.5S RNA, VA-RNA, EBER RNAs	SLE (15%)
Ribosomal RNP	Protein translation	Phosphoproteins 38KD, 16KD, 15KD	None reported	SLE (10%)
PCNA/cyclin	DNA replication	Protein 36KD	None	SLE (3%)
Ku	(Nuclear protein)	Protein 86KD 66KD	None	SLE (10%)

SLE = systemic lupus erythematosus, RNP = ribonucleoprotein.

the 30 to 40% of patients with SLE. Antibody to nuclear ribonucleoprotein (RNP) was reported by Sharp, et al.[9] as a characteristic feature of patients with mixed connective tissue disease (MCTD) (see Chapter 71). It was soon apparent that this antibody was similar to an antibody described by Mattioli and Reichlin in patients with SLE.[10] Studies have elucidated the chemical nature of this antigen and have shown that it is a complex of U1-RNA and proteins.[11] Hence, the current designation for nuclear RNP is U1-RNP. Antibody to U1-RNP is present in 35 to 45% of patients with SLE and in more than 95% of patients with MCTD.

Two classes of ANAs in patients with SLE are related to ANAs seen in patients with Sjögren's syndrome. These ANAs are antibodies to SS-A/Ro and SS-B/La. Anti-SS-A/Ro is present in 30 to 40% of patients with SLE but in approximately 70% of patients with Sjögren's syndrome. Of great interest is the demonstration that anti-SS-A/Ro is related to neonatal lupus. The presence of anti-SS-A/Ro autoantibodies in maternal sera has been correlated with increased risk of skin rash and congenital complete heart block.[12] Antibody to SS-B/La is present in only 15% of patients with SLE but in 45 to 60% of patients with Sjögren's syndrome.

Antibody to ribosomal RNP is the antibody that most often accounts for cytoplasmic staining in immunofluorescence. The antigens are three proteins of 38,000, 16,000, and 15,000 MW, which are components of the large ribosomal subunit. These antibodies are present in 10% of patients.[13] The Ku antibody reacts with a doublet protein of 66,000 and 86,000 MW and is present in 10% of patients.[14] Finally, antibody to proliferating cell nuclear antigen (PCNA) is present in 3% of patients. This autoantibody, although not prevalent, reacts with a cell cycle-regulated proliferation–associated protein of 36,000 MW.[15] The antibody is useful in cell biology as a probe for identifying proliferating cells; the antigen is the auxiliary protein of DNA polymerase delta.[16]

PROFILES OF ANAs IN SLE AND OTHER SYSTEMIC RHEUMATIC DISEASES

SLE is characterized by a multitude of ANAs (see also Chapter 66). A striking feature of the profile of ANAs in SLE, which contrasts it with other systemic rheumatic diseases, is the simultaneous presence of three or four different types of ANAs in the same serum (Fig. 68–2).[17] In contrast, other systemic rheumatic diseases have two features that are different

FIG. 68–2. Distinctive profiles of ANAs occur in various autoimmune diseases. SLE is characterized by a multiplicity of ANAs occurring in different frequencies. This is in contrast to other diseases, such as MCTD, Sjögren's syndrome, and drug-induced LE, in which the ANA profile is more restricted in heterogeneity. The broken lines indicate relative absence of antibodies. (From Tan, E.M.[1a])

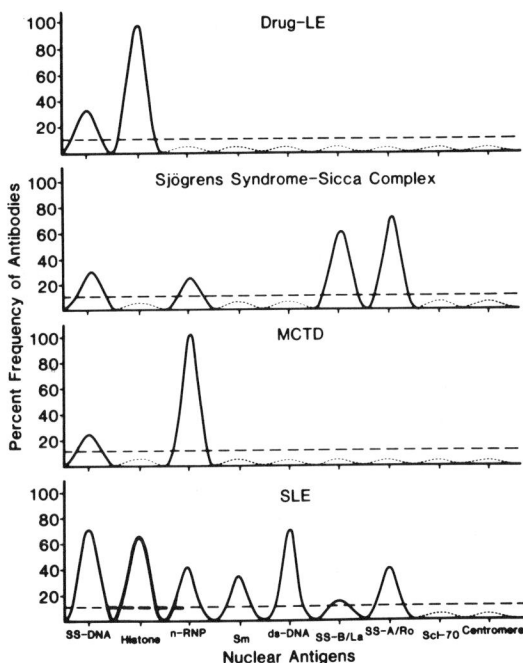

from SLE. One is the presence of antibodies of other specificities and the other is the presence of fewer types of ANAs in each individual serum. Table 68–3 describes the ANA profiles characteristic of MCTD, Sjögren's syndrome, scleroderma, and dermato- or polymyositis. It is important to compare Table 68–3 with the profile of SLE in Table 68–2. In certain syndromes, such as MCTD, antibody to U1-RNP is present in most patients, but this feature alone does not differentiate it from SLE, where it is present in 35 to 45% of patients. An equally important feature in MCTD is the absence of other ANAs, such as antibody to double-strand DNA, antibody to Sm antigen, and antibody to histones. Similarly, in Sjögren's syndrome, antibodies to SS-A/Ro and SS-B/La, characteristic of this disease, are also present in some patients with SLE. However, in Sjögren's syndrome as in MCTD, antibodies to double-strand DNA, Sm, and nuclear histones are absent.

The importance of ANAs in the clinical characterization and classification of SLE was recognized in the 1982 revised criteria for the classification of SLE.[18] In this scheme, ANA was recognized as an independent criterion, and anti-double-strand DNA and anti-Sm

Table 68–3. ANA Profiles in Certain Autoimmune Diseases

Antibodies to	Percent Frequency in				
	SLE	MCTD	Sjögren's Syndrome	Scleroderma	Dermato-polymyositis
dsDNA	50	<5*	<5	<5	<5
ssDNA	60–70	10–20	10–20	10–20	10–20
Histones	70	<5	<5	<5	<5
Sm	30–40	<5	<5	<5	<5
Ul-RNP	35–45	95–100	<5	20	<5
SS-A/Ro	30–40	<5	60–70	<5	<5
SS-B/La	15	<5	45–60	<5	<5
Scl-70	<5	<5	<5	20–30	<5
Centromere/kinetochore	<5	<5	<5	25–30	<5
Nucleolar antigen	<5	<5	5–10	50–60	5–10
PM-1	<5	<5	<5	<5	50†
Jo-1	<5	<5	<5	<5	30
Ku	<5	<5	<5	<5	55†

*<5% frequency is used to signify that the antibody is rarely observed.
†These reported frequencies are present in polymyositis-scleroderma overlap syndrome.

were included with the LE cell test and the biologically false-positive test for syphilis (anticardiolipin antibody—the "lupus anticoagulant") as four sub-items in a second immunologic criterion. (See Chapter 70 for a discussion of anticardiolipin antibodies.)

IDENTIFICATION AND CHARACTERIZATION OF NUCLEAR ANTIGENS

There has been a significant advance in the characterization of some of the nuclear antigens reactive with serum ANAs. Both Sm antigen and U1-RNP antigen are proteins, as demonstrated by the use of transfer of electrophoretically separated antigens to nitrocellulose paper and the demonstration that specific polypeptide bands react with antibodies. There are several polypeptides reactive with anti-Sm and anti-U1-RNP, and these vary from 8,000 to 70,000 Daltons in MW.[11,19] The observation that anti-Sm antibody and anti-U1-RNP antibody immunoprecipitated highly specific sets of small nuclear RNAs was interesting.[11] Anti-U1-RNP immunoprecipitated only U1-RNA, whereas anti-Sm precipitated U1 as well as four other species of small nuclear RNAs: U2, U4, U5, and U6 (Fig. 68–3). These antibodies are not reactive with the small nuclear RNAs per se, but are reactive with polypeptides complexed to these small nuclear RNAs in highly specific associations. Such studies on the molecular biology of the nuclear antigens have clarified precisely the nature of nuclear antigens and have also shown that ANAs can be used as probes to aid in identification of the structure and function of cellular constituents. Some studies have indicated that

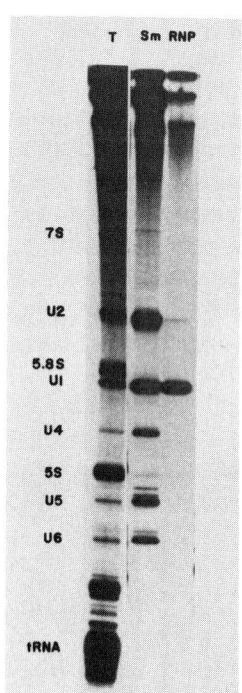

FIG. 68–3. Profiles of small nuclear RNAs immunoprecipitated by anti-Sm and antinuclear RNP sera. HeLa cells were labeled with phosphorus-32 and cell extract reacted with sera. The immunoprecipitates were solubilized and run on polyacrylamide gels to identify precipitated RNAs. Left lane represents total cellular RNA. Middle lane shows five major RNA bands precipitated by anti-Sm serum: U1, U2, U4, U5, and U6 RNAs. Right lane shows that only U1 RNA is precipitated by anti-RNP serum.

U1-RNA associated with its protein components (U1 ribonucleoprotein) is involved in processing heterogeneous nuclear RNA, the primary transcript of genomic DNA.[20]

ANTI-SS-A/RO AND NEONATAL LUPUS

The relationship between anti-SS-A/Ro and neonatal lupus was studied in three infant–mother pairs.[21] All three infants and their mothers had serum anti-SS-A/Ro antibodies. Two years later, anti-SS-A/Ro antibody had disappeared from the sera of the children but was still present in the mothers, strongly suggesting transplacental passage of antibody from mother to infant. An interesting observation was the presence of a complete heart block in one of the infants. Following this initial study, several groups of investigators confirmed these findings.[22–24] Clinical features include typical SLE skin lesions in the infants and a high association of congenital complete or partial heart block. It has been correctly pointed out that pregnant mothers with known SLE should be screened for the presence of anti-SS-A/Ro to promote awareness of the possibility of cardiac problems in the infant. However, some of the mothers with anti-SS-A/Ro antibody may not have overt clinical disease at the time of gestation or delivery.

DRUG-INDUCED LUPUS AND ANTIHISTONE ANTIBODIES

A close association exists between antihistone antibodies and drug-induced lupus, particularly those antibodies linked with ingestion of procainamide and hydralazine.[7] Owing to the increased use of sustained-release types of procainamide, the incidence of drug-induced lupus has increased.

Differentiation between drug-induced lupus and the idiopathic form of systemic lupus can be made serologically. In drug-induced lupus, ANAs are characterized by the presence of antihistone antibodies, and the absence of anti-double-strand DNA, anti-Sm, or the other SLE-related ANAs listed in Table 68–2.

Differentiation between drug-induced lupus and SLE has been notoriously difficult, although serologic analysis has helped to clarify the situation. Although both procainamide and hydralazine are characterized by antihistone antibodies, there is a difference in the subclasses of histones that are reactive in the two conditions. Table 68–4 shows that procainamide-induced antihistone antibodies are different from hydralazine-induced anti-histone antibodies. The former are more reactive with the H2A/H2B complex of histones. This involves both the immunoglobulin G (IgG) and IgM classes of antibodies. In contrast, hydralazine-induced antihistone antibodies are characterized by IgM antibodies against histone H3 and H2A. In addition, hydralazine-induced antihistone antibodies are primarily of the IgM class with few IgG antibodies. *Drug-induced ANAs are almost exclusively of the antihistone type, and there are different antihistone antibodies in procainamide- and hydralazine-induced ANAs.*

ANA-NEGATIVE LUPUS

There has been some controversy concerning ANA-negative lupus. This controversy is probably associated with two features: (1) ANA as detected with the immunofluorescence technique varies in sensitivity from one laboratory to the next; and (2) many ANA-negative lupus patients have anti-SS-A/Ro.[25] Recent studies may have clarified some of these discrepancies. The SS-A/Ro antigen, unlike Sm and U1-RNP antigens, varies remarkably in concentration from one animal species to the next.[26] SS-A/Ro antigen is present in higher concentrations in man, monkey, and dog, than in the mouse, rat, and hamster. Therefore, when tissues from species such as rat or mouse are used as substrates in indirect immunofluorescence, a serum containing anti-SS-A/Ro may not show nuclear staining. When rabbit, human, or dog tissues are used as the substrate, however, this serum is positive. Some patients with anti-SS-A/Ro antibodies have been classified into a subset of lupus called *subacute cutaneous lupus.*[27] These individuals are highly photosensitive and have prominent skin lesions, but have

Table 68–4. Types of Antihistone Antibodies Induced by Procainamide and Hydralazine

Antibody Class	Drug	Antibodies to			
		H2A	H2B	H2A/H2B	H3
IgM	Procainamide	0	0	+ +	0
	Hydralazine	+ +	+/−	+/−	+ +
IgG	Procainamide	+ +	+/−	+ + +	+/−
	Hydralazine	0	0	+/−	+/−

less involvement of other organ systems (see Chapter 67).

REFERENCES

1. Kunkel, H.G.: The immunologic approach to SLE. Arthritis Rheum., *20*:S139, 1977.

1a. Tan, E.M.: The LE cell and antinuclear antibodies. A breakthrough in diagnosis. *In* Landmark Advances in Rheumatology ARA Golden Anniversary symposium. Edited by D.J. McCarty. Arthritis Foundation, Atlanta, Ga., pp. 43–52, 1984.

2. Tan, E.M.: Autoantibodies to nuclear antigens. Their immunobiology and medicine. Adv. Immunol., *33*:167, 1982.

3. Deicher, H.R.G., Holman, H.R., and Kunkel, H.G.: The precipitin reaction between DNA and a serum factor in systemic lupus erythematosus. J. Exp. Med., *109*:97, 1959.

4. Andres, G.A., et al.: Localization of fluorescein-labeled aminonucleoside antibodies in glomeruli of patients with active systemic lupus erythematosus. J. Clin. Invest., *49*:2106, 1971.

5. Koffler, D., et al.: The occurrence of single stranded DNA in the serum of patients with systemic lupus erythematosus and other diseases. J. Clin. Invest., *52*:198, 1973.

6. Portanova, J.P., et al.: Reactivity of anti-histone antibodies induced by procainamide and hydralazine. Clin. Immunol. Immunopathol., *25*:67, 1982.

7. Fritzler, M.J., and Tan, E.M.: Antibodies to histones in drug-induced and idiopathic lupus erythematosus. J. Clin. Invest., *62*:560, 1978.

8. Tan, E.M., and Kunkel, H.G.: Characteristics of a soluble nuclear antigen precipitating with sera of patients with systemic lupus erythematosus. J. Immunol., *96*:464, 1966.

9. Sharp, G.C., et al.: Mixed connective tissue disease—An apparently distinct rheumatoid disease associated with a specific antibody to an extractable nuclear antigen (ENA). Am. J. Med., *52*:148, 1972.

10. Mattioli, M., and Reichlin, M.: Physical association of two nuclear antigens and mutual occurrence of their antibodies: The relationship of the Sm and RNA protein (Mo) systems in SLE sera. J. Immunol., *110*:1318, 1973.

11. Lerner, M.R., and Steitz, J.A.: Antibodies to small nuclear RNAs complexed with proteins are produced by patients with systemic lupus erythematosus. Proc. Natl. Acad. Sci. U.S.A., *765*:5495, 1979.

12. Tosokos, G.C., Pillemer, S.R., and Klippel, J.H.: Rheumatic disease syndromes associated with antibodies to the Ro (SS-A) ribonuclear protein. Semin. Arthritis Rheum., *16*:237, 1987.

13. Francoeur, A.M., et al.: Identification of ribosomal protein autoantigens. J. Immunol., *135*:2378, 1985.

14. Francoeur, A.M., Peebles, C.L., Gomper, P., and Tan, E.M.: Identification of Ki (Ku p70/p80) autoantigens and analysis of anti-Ki autoantibody. J. Immunol., *136*:1648, 1986.

15. Miyachi, K., Fritzler, M.J., and Tan, E.M.: Autoantibody to a nuclear antigen in proliferating cells. J. Immunol., *121*:2228, 1978.

16. Prelich, G., et al.: Functional identity of proliferating cell nuclear antigen and a DNA polymerase delta auxiliary protein. Nature, *326*:517, 1987.

17. Notman, D.D., Kurata, N., and Tan, E.M.: Profiles of antinuclear antibodies in systemic rheumatoid diseases. Ann. Intern. Med., *83*:464, 1975.

18. Tan, E.M., et al.: The 1982 revised criteria for the classification of systemic lupus erythematosus. Arthritis Rheum., *25*:1271, 1982.

19. Conner, G.E., et al.: Protein antigens of the RNA-protein complexes detected by anti-Sm and anti-RNP antibodies found in serum of patients with systemic lupus erythematosus and related disorders. J. Exp. Med., *156*:1475, 1982.

20. Yang, V.W., et al.: A small nuclear ribonucleoprotein is required for splicing of adenoviral early RNA sequences. Proc. Natl. Acad. Sci. U.S.A., *78*:1371, 1981.

21. Franco, H.L., et al.: Autoantibodies directed against sicca syndrome antigens in the neonatal lupus syndrome. J. Am. Acad. Dermatol., *4*:67–72, 1981.

22. Kephart, D.C., Hood, A.F., and Provost, T.T.: Neonatal lupus erythematosus: New serologic findings. J. Invest. Dermatol., *77*:331–333, 1981.

23. Lockshin, D.D., et al.: Neonatal lupus erythematosus with heart block: Family study of a patient with anti-SS-A and anti-SS-B antibodies. Arthritis Rheum., *26*:210–213, 1983.

24. Scott, J.S., et al.: Connective tissue disease, antibodies to ribonucleoprotein, and congenital heart block. N. Engl. J. Med., *309*:209–212, 1983.

25. Provost, T.T., et al.: Antibodies to cytoplasmic antigens in lupus erythematosus. Arthritis Rheum., *20*:1457, 1977.

26. Harmon, C.E., et al.: The importance of tissue substrates in the SS-A/Ro antigen-antibody system. Arthritis Rheum., *27*:166–173, 1984.

27. Gilliam, J.N., and Sontheimer, R.D.: Distinctive cutaneous subsets in the spectrum of lupus erythematosus. J. Am. Acad. Dermatol., *4*:471, 1981.

69

CELLULAR IMMUNITY AND IMMUNOREGULATION IN SYSTEMIC LUPUS ERYTHEMATOSUS

DAVID A. HORWITZ

The clinical manifestations of systemic lupus erythematosus (SLE) are the consequence of certain autoantibodies produced by patients with this disorder. Considerable information has accumulated during the past two decades concerning cellular mechanisms regulating antibody formation, and many abnormalities have been described in SLE. Formerly, cell-mediated immunity and T cell–mediated responses were considered synonymous. It is now recognized that in addition to T cells, non-T, non-B cells constitute a separate and important arm of cell-mediated immune reactions. The cellular components of the immune response consist of immunocompetent T-lymphocytes and B-lymphocytes, non-T non-B lymphocytes, and accessory cells. T cells and B cells each have characteristic receptors for specific antigens that provide immunologic memory, that is, recall of previous sensitization to specific antigens.[1] Non-T, non-B cells have different morphologic features. Because they lack identifiable antigen receptors they cannot be sensitized to antigens. However, they have important cytotoxic and regulatory functions.[2] Accessory (antigen-presenting) cells such as macrophages or dendritic cells are required for the initiation of a T cell-dependent response.[3] As the various cells interact in the generation of an immune response, they produce soluble regulatory factors (cytokines), including the various interleukins and interferons.

Numerous abnormalities in specific cell subsets and their cytokines have been reported in SLE. Because the patient populations studied are not uniform and laboratory methods often vary, many conflicting data have been published. Although there is considerable information regarding mechanisms leading to antibody production, less is known about suppressor cells and circuits that terminate antibody production in either healthy persons or patients with SLE. Finally, because most of the numerous immune defects described in SLE have been found in patients with active established disease, it is still not known whether a given defect is antecedent and important in pathogenesis, or whether it is a consequence of the disease itself, that is, an epiphenomenon.

The characteristic feature of SLE is the production of anti–double stranded DNA and antibodies to other self-nuclear autoantigens. The factors responsible for the breakdown in immune tolerance to self in idiopathic SLE are unknown but are thought to be central to an understanding of its pathogenesis. Formerly it was believed that B cells programmed to make autoantibodies were deleted from the lymphocyte repertoire before birth, and that their presence afterward reflected the emergence of *forbidden clones*.[4] This concept has been modified. Subjects with SLE and healthy persons have similar numbers of B cells primed to make anti-DNA antibodies,[5,6] and polyclonally activated B cells from normal subjects can produce anti-DNA autoantibodies.[7,8]

Because of the complexity of the immune response and the conflicting published information about immunologic abnormalities in SLE, it remains hazardous to construct a unifying hypothesis. However, there is a consensus that a major imbalance between the cellular and the humoral limbs of the immune response exists in SLE. B-cell hyperactivity occurs in parallel with depressed function of most T cells and non-T, non-B cells.[9] Genetic and hormonal factors contribute to this imbalance. The various immunologic abnormalities in SLE will be reviewed in this chapter, and from new information about autoreactive T cells, a multifactorial hypothesis will be developed to explain the breakdown in immune tolerance in human SLE.

SPONTANEOUS B-CELL HYPERACTIVITY

Increased activity of B cells in SLE has been demonstrated both in vivo and ex vivo. Besides the characteristic autoantibodies directed to cellular constituents as discussed in Chapter 68, antibody titers to endogenous and exogenous antigens such as blood group antigens and certain viral antigens are increased. There is spontaneous B-cell proliferation,[10] and immunoglobulin (Ig) secretion is increased in patients with either active[11-15] or inactive[16] disease. Moreover, nonaffected family members of SLE patients may have increased numbers of Ig-secreting cells.[17]

The mechanisms responsible for such spontaneous B-cell activity are not clear. This abnormality could be explained by increased numbers of B-cell precursors with aberrant maturation to Ig-secreting cells, and in fact, B-cell colony formation is increased in SLE.[18,19] However, IgM is the principal immunoglobulin class produced by B cells without T cell–dependent stimulation. In SLE, levels of IgM are normal in contrast with increased levels of IgG and IgA. Therefore the B-cell hyperactivity probably results from activation of B cells secondary to persistent T cell–dependent stimulation. Nuclear autoantibody levels are increased out of proportion to that of total IgG,[20] providing evidence for an autoantigen-induced T cell–dependent immune response.

Increased antibody production could be due to defective feedback regulation. IgG antibodies and IgG immune complexes normally shut off antibody production by an Fc receptor–dependent mechanism.[21] Although circulating immune complexes are increased in SLE, they are unable to activate suppressive mechanisms. Lymphocytes bearing Fc receptors recognized by anti-CD16 monoclonal antibodies (formerly called L cells) can suppress IgG production,[22] and this subset is decreased in patients with active SLE (see Lymphocyte Subsets below).

B-cell hyperactivity could be explained by increased production of lymphokines, which promote B-cell growth and maturation. Interleukin-1 (IL-1), interleu-

kin-2 (IL-2), interleukin-3 (IL-3), and gamma-interferon can up-regulate B-cell activity. SLE B cells may be hyper-responsive to growth factors (see Cytokine Production below). During the 1970s the prevailing view was that B-cell hyperactivity could be explained by decreased numbers or defective function of T suppressor cells.[12] It is now evident that this explanation was an oversimplification of a complex problem.

It is important to emphasize that all workers who have reported spontaneous B-cell activity in vitro have studied unseparated peripheral blood mononuclear cells or cell suspensions depleted of T cells by the sheep cell rosette method. These B cell–enriched preparations contain large numbers of non-T, non-B cells that can produce B-cell growth factors. In our laboratory, highly purified B cells prepared by both positive and negative selection lack the capacity to secrete IgG spontaneously without the addition of growth factors.[23] It is very likely that B-cell hyperactivity depends on the production of growth factors by other regulatory cells.

HYPOACTIVE B-CELL RESPONSE FOLLOWING IMMUNIZATION

The evidence of spontaneous B-cell hyperactivity notwithstanding, the antibody response of SLE patients to influenza vaccine or tetanus toxoid is not increased and may even be decreased.[24] Antibody production by cultured SLE blood mononuclear cells stimulated with pokeweed mitogen, a T cell–dependent stimulant, is decreased.[25] This defect in induced antibody production in SLE has been explained by antigenic competition. According to this concept, B cells cannot respond to an immunogen because they have already been activated in vivo.

The antigenic competition hypothesis does not adequately explain the depressed antibody response to exogenous stimulants for the following reasons: (1) The B-cell hyporesponsiveness to pokeweed mitogen can be corrected by supplementing the cultures with helper T cells or B-cell growth factors; and (2) SLE B cells can respond normally to T cell–independent stimuli such as the Epstein-Barr virus or Staphylococcus aureus bacteria. For these reasons, the impaired antibody response to T cell–dependent stimulants is best explained by decreased helper T cell function (see Helper T Cell Activity below).

LYMPHOCYTE SUBSETS

Patients with active SLE are usually both neutropenic and lymphopenic.[26,27] Peripheral blood T cells,

B cells, and non-T, non-B cells are decreased. Although non-T, non-B cells share certain surface markers with T cells, they lack identifiable antigen receptors[28,29] and can be triggered by one rather than two signals.[30] The surface markers displayed on the various peripheral blood lymphocyte subsets in SLE are shown in Table 69–1. The absolute number of T cells displaying the pan T-cell marker CD3, as well as CD4 + inducer/helper cells and CD8 + cytotoxic/suppressor cells, are decreased.[26] Although some workers have reported decreased percentages of CD8 + cells,[31,32] CD4 + cells are decreased more frequently and the *percentage* of CD8 + cells is normal or increased. This finding results in a low CD4 to CD8 ratio,[26,33] especially in lupus nephritis.[33] CD4 + cell levels are transiently decreased by corticosteroid therapy, but low levels have been found in newly diagnosed, untreated SLE patients.[26] CD4 + cells have been divided into suppressor/inducer and helper cells by several monoclonal antibodies. Suppressor/inducer cells (CD4 + 2H4 +) are significantly decreased in lupus patients with nephritis.[34] Increased numbers of SLE blood T cells display surface HLA-DR markers[35] indicating that they have been activated. Newly activated lymphocytes normally express cell surface receptors for IL-2,[36] but these receptors are usually not present on HLA-DR + SLE T cells.[35] This suggests that these cells had been activated previously and had already shed their IL-2 receptors. My colleagues and I found that the serum of patients with active SLE contained very high levels of soluble IL-2 receptors,[37] which is consistent with this idea.

Until recently, it has been difficult to separate non-T-, non-B-lymphocytes from T cells because some of the former display T-cell markers such as sheep red blood cell receptors and CD8. Non-T, non-B cells display receptors for iC3b, the type 3 complement receptor (CR3). These lymphocytes can be identified with CR3-specific anti-CD11 monoclonal antibodies[38] or with Leu 19 monoclonal antibodies (NKH-1).[38a]

The percentage of CD11 + lymphocytes is near normal in SLE, but the proportions of the two principal subsets are reversed.[38] In normal persons two thirds of CD11 + cells display high density Fc receptors for IgG. These lymphocytes were formerly called "L cells" or "Tγ cells." These Fc receptor–bearing cells can be identified by anti-CD16 monoclonal antibodies.[39] CD16 + cells are markedly decreased in patients with active SLE,[38] consistent with previous observations that Tγ cells[40] and L cells[27] are decreased in SLE. CD16 + cells are the effectors of natural killer activity and antibody-dependent cellular cytotoxicity.[41]

Although CD16 + lymphocytes bear certain T-cell markers, only rarely do these cells express CD3. There is now unequivocal evidence that CD16 + CD3− cells are *not* T cells. The genes encoding the T-cell receptor in this subset are in the germ line state,[28,29] whereas they are in the rearranged state in T cells.

In normal persons only a small percentage of CD11 + cells are T cells, but this subset is significantly increased in patients with active SLE.[38] The function of these cells is still unknown, but they could be for the human equivalent of the *autoreactive T cells* recently described in mice (see below).

Although the percentage of B cells in SLE blood lymphocytes is usually normal, their absolute number is decreased.[27] And, as already discussed, many of these cells appear to be activated. Recently, a B-cell subset has been described that displays the T-cell antigen, Leu 1, on its cell surface. This observation followed the description of an analogous B-cell subset in NZB mice. Leu 1 + B cells produce autoantibodies, mostly IgM, which include rheumatoid factor and anti–single stranded DNA.[42] This subset could reflect a separate lineage of B cells or a particular maturation state.

SOLUBLE IMMUNE MEDIATOR (CYTOKINE) PRODUCTION

Cytokines are hormone-like molecules produced by lymphocytes or monocytes that regulate lymphocyte maturation and differentiation. *Interleukin-1* (IL-1) has

Table 69–1. Lymphocyte Subsets in SLE

Population	Marker	Percentages	Absolute Numbers
Patients with active disease			
T cells (total)	CD3	Normal or decreased	Decreased
Inducer/helper	CD4	Decreased or normal	Decreased
Suppressor/inducer	CD4 2H4	Decreased	Decreased
Cytotoxic/suppressor	CD8	Increased or normal (decreased rarely)	Decreased
B cells	IgM, B1	Normal or decreased	Decreased
Non-T non-B cells	CD11 (CD3 neg)	Decreased	Decreased
Natural killer (suppressor)	CD16	Decreased	Decreased
Patients with inactive disease	—	Usually normal	Usually normal

many systemic effects besides regulating T-cell and B-cell proliferation. IL-1 is released primarily by young monocytes and its production is decreased in SLE.[43,44] The IL-1 defect may be explained by inhibitors of IL-1 production. Immune complexes bound to Fc receptors on monocytes induce prostaglandins, which inhibit IL-1 production.[45] Defective IL-1 production is largely reversed by the cyclo-oxygenase inhibitor, indomethacin.[43]

Interleukin-2 (IL-2) is the principal lymphokine responsible for T-cell and non-T, non-B cell proliferation and also influences the growth of B cells.[36,46,47] T cells, B cells, non-T, non-B cells, and even activated monocytes have receptors for IL-2.[47–49] IL-2 is produced primarily by CD4+ cells, but CD8+ subsets may also produce this lymphokine.[50,51] IL-2 production is decreased in SLE.[43,52,53] Some workers found that this defect correlated with disease activity, but others found decreased IL-2 production in patients with inactive disease as well.[43] This defect does not correlate with steroid therapy, cannot be explained by insufficient IL-1 for T-cell activation, and cannot be explained by prostaglandin inhibition, or by passive absorption of this lymphokine.[43] Two mechanisms are responsible for the IL-2 defect: (1) IL-2 production is regulated by radiosensitive CD8+ and CD16+ lymphocytes and removal of these subsets corrected the defect in patients with either active or inactive SLE[34]; and (2) IL-2 is produced predominantly by the CD4+ 2H4+ suppressor/inducer lymphocyte subset,[54] which is decreased in active SLE.[34]

The proliferative response to lymphocytes to IL-2 is also decreased in SLE.[52,55] SLE CD4+ cells and CD8+ cells have a decreased capacity to express IL-2 receptors identified with the anti-Tac monoclonal antibody. Partial depletion of monocytes did not correct the abnormality in IL-2 receptor expression, but did correct the proliferative defect in the majority of patients studied.[55]

Gamma-interferon controls the expression of MHC gene products on immune cells and inhibits lymphocyte proliferation. This lymphokine blocks the response of B cells to B-cell growth factor but augments B-cell maturation.[56] Gamma-interferon is closely related to *macrophage-activating factor.* This lymphokine has an important role in suppressor cell induction.[57] Decreased production of gamma-interferon in SLE[58] may be important in defective B-cell regulation. Paradoxically, serum levels of interferon are increased in SLE. This interferon appears to be an unusual acid-labile α-*interferon.*[59] The cellular source of this interferon is unknown.

The soluble factors that regulate B-cell function are less well characterized. Formerly, separate factors for B-cell proliferation and differentiation were described. However, interleukin-4, the principal B-cell growth factor, has both of these activities.[60] SLE lymphocytes produce increased levels of growth factors that promote B-cell proliferation and differentiation.[61–63] Moreover, the responsiveness of B cells to a high-molecular-weight B-cell growth factor is enhanced.[64] Both T cells and non-T cells can produce these factors. The identity of the mononuclear cells responsible for the production of B-cell growth factors in SLE is the subject of intense investigation.

T-CELL PROLIFERATION

The proliferative response of T cells to mitogenic lectins such as phytohemagglutinin, concanavalin A, and pokeweed mitogen is decreased in SLE.[65–72] This defect correlated with disease activity. Decreased lymphocyte proliferation was mild to severe depending on the lectin used and the patient population studied. SLE serum contains antilymphocyte antibodies and other factors that decrease proliferation,[73,74] the defect may be partially explained by residual serum factors.

The proliferative response to MHC class II antigens on both allogeneic[75–79] and autologous antigen presenting cells[80–84] is also decreased in SLE. The defect in the autologous mixed lymphocyte reaction is severe; twin studies have revealed defects in the responder T cells and in the stimulating non-T cells.[80,83] CD8+ cells develop IL-2 receptors in the presence of autologous stimulator cells, but their proliferation is decreased because of decreased IL-2 production.[84] The known functional properties of lymphocyte populations in SLE are summarized in Table 69–2.

HELPER T CELL ACTIVITY

Because B-cell hyperactivity depends on the presence of growth factors produced by T cells, it is surprising that helper T cell activity in SLE has been reported to be decreased, normal, and only rarely increased. Helper T cell activity induced by mitogenic lectins is decreased[85,86] or normal.[87,88] Helper T cell activity induced by specific antigens is decreased.[89,90] In contrast, normal or increased helper cell activity has been generated by either allogeneic or autologous mixed lymphocyte reactions.[91,92]

In mice, helper T cells producing IL-2 and γ-interferon can be distinguished from helper T cells producing the B-cell growth factor, IL-4.[93] In humans, similar T-cell subsets have not been described. Although CD4+ 2H4− lymphocytes comprise the T

Table 69–2. Lymphocyte Function in SLE

	Spontaneous	Induced
B cell		
Proliferation	Increased	Decreased
Antibody production	Increased	Decreased (in vitro)
T cell		
Proliferation	Increased	Decreased
Helper activity	Increased	Decreased
Suppression of Ig production	Decreased	Decreased
Suppression of IL-2 production	Increased	—
Cytotoxicity	—	Decreased*
Non-T non-B cell		
Natural killer antibody	Decreased	—
Antibody-dependent cellular cytotoxicity	Decreased	—

*Increased cytotoxic antibody against modified self.

helper cell subset,[31] my colleagues and I could not find quantitative differences in B-cell growth factor production between CD4+ 2H4+ and CD4+ 2H4− cells.[93a]

To the surprise of many investigators, CD8+ suppressor cells can, paradoxically, augment antibody production in SLE. CD8+ lymphocyte subsets augment rather than suppress spontaneous IgG production and anti-dinitrophenol (αDNP) production.[94] Therefore, certain CD8+ T cells in addition to helper T cells must be considered candidates for the increased production of B-cell growth factors described in SLE. Moreover, natural killer (NK) cells can produce B-cell growth factors and potentiate B-cell proliferation.[95]

SUPPRESSOR T CELL ACTIVITY

The prevailing paradigm during the 1970s was that B-cell hyperactivity in SLE was due to decreased numbers or activation of suppressor T cells. This concept has had to be revised. The decrease in lymphocytes bearing receptors for sheep erythrocytes displaying Fc receptors for IgG (so-called Tγ cells) does not signify a decrease in suppressor T cells. As stated above, the Fc receptors on these cells react with anti-CD16 monoclonal antibodies and almost all of these lymphocytes are non-T cells.

There were numerous reports of decreased suppressor cell activity in SLE generated by stimulating lymphocytes with concanavalin A[96–108] although conflicting reports also appeared.[109–110] The biologic significance of decreased concanavalin A suppressor cell activity is unclear. Whether this phenomenon truly reflects a cellular defect or reflects a decreased production of lymphokines that activate suppressor cells is unknown.

CD8+ suppressor cells have other activities besides their well-known cytotoxic properties and ability to down-regulate antibody production.[111] As stated above, the blood of SLE patients contains increased numbers of spontaneously activated CD8+ lymphocytes that suppress IL-2 production.[35] These cells also amplify polyclonal immunoglobulin and autoantibody production.[94] Thus, lymphocytes identified by the CD8 suppressor marker cell can, paradoxically, support B-cell activity. Persons with other chronic inflammatory diseases such as rheumatoid arthritis and others who are the recipients of bone marrow transplants also have impaired IL-2 production explained by CD8+ IL-2 suppressor lymphocytes.[112,112a]

By suppressing IL-2 production, these cells appear to inhibit the generation of suppressors of antibody production. This statement is based on our recent observation that when purified CD8+ cells from SLE patients are briefly exposed to IL-2 or gamma interferon, they acquire the capacity to inhibit spontaneous IgG synthesis by autologous B cells.[23] It is becoming clear, therefore, that decreased suppression of antibody production in SLE is not simply the result of insufficient numbers of suppressor cells, but may be the result of a previously unrecognized regulatory circuit.

Because both suppressors of antibody production and suppressors of IL-2 production display the same cell surface markers,[112] it is possible that all suppressor cells are derived from similar precursor cells and their ultimate effector function is determined by differentiation signals. Based on present concepts of lymphocyte activation, a model can be formulated to explain the predominance of IL-2 suppressors in SLE patients and in those with other chronic inflammatory disorders.

According to this model (Table 69–3), two differentiation signals are required for suppressor T precursor cells to become suppressors of antibody production. To suppress immunoglobulin production,

Table 69–3. Hypothesis to Explain Heterogeneity of Suppressor T-Cell Function

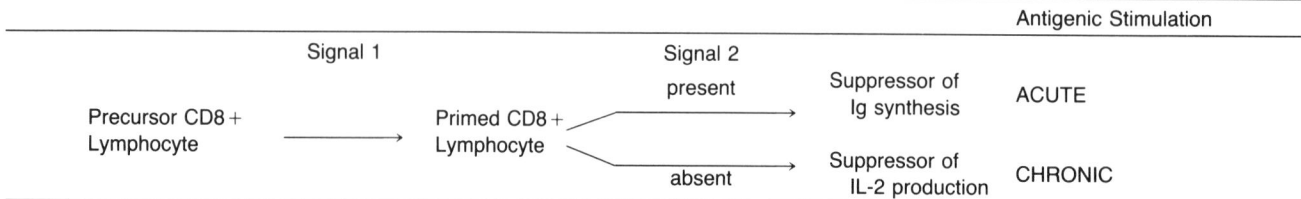

According to this model, precursor CD8+ suppressor T cells require two differentiation signals to become suppressors of antibody-producing cells. Antigen serves as signal 1, and IL-2, gamma interferon, or another soluble mediator serves as signal 2. If primed CD8+ lymphocytes do not receive signal 2, they become suppressors of IL-2–producing cells. In normal persons both signals are generated, and primed CD8+ lymphocytes usually become suppressors of antibody production. Because of chronic antigenic stimulation in SLE, signal 2 generation is defective and IL-2 suppressor cells predominate. IL-2 suppressor cells, moreover, amplify antibody production by B cells.

CD8+ precursor cells require both appropriate antigenic stimulation (signal 1) and a second signal provided by IL-2, gamma interferon, or another soluble mediator. *If the precursor suppressor cell does not receive signal 2 shortly after it is primed by signal 1, it becomes an IL-2 suppressor instead of an antibody suppressor.* The cytokines providing signal 2 are lacking in SLE, because of feedback inhibition secondary to chronic antigenic stimulation. Therefore, IL-2 suppressor cells become predominant, resulting in excessive, unregulated antibody production. If this model is correct, then the depressed production of IL-2 and γ-interferon are important factors in chronic B-cell hyperactivity.

NON-T, NON-B LYMPHOCYTE FUNCTIONS

Non-T, non-B cells are the mediators of natural killer activity and antibody-dependent cellular cytotoxicity.[41] Non-T, non-B cells also have important antigen nonspecific regulatory effects on antibody production. Natural killer (NK) cell activity is decreased in SLE, especially in patients with active disease.[113–119] In normal persons, NK-cell activity is significantly increased by interferon and IL-2, but these lymphokines are ineffective in correcting the NK-cell defect in SLE.[114,117,118] Because patients with active SLE have decreased numbers of CD16+ cells,[120] the defect in NK activity may be due to insufficient numbers of mature effector cells.

Antibody-dependent cellular cytotoxicity (ADCC) is also decreased in patients with active SLE,[121–124] also explicable by decreased numbers of effector cells. Alternatively, Fc receptors displayed on these CD16+ lymphocytes could be blocked by circulating immune complexes that would decrease ADCC.

CD16+ cells have potent antigen nonspecific suppressive activity[22] in addition to NK-cell activity.[125] The decreased numbers of these cells in patients with SLE may explain, at least in part, the failure of circulating immune complexes in this condition to down-regulate antibody production.

MONOCYTE REGULATORY ABNORMALITIES

Monocytes can either increase or decrease antibody production. Lymphocyte proliferation is increased in SLE after partial removal of monocytes. These suppressive effects have been attributed to prostaglandin production.[126] Monocytes from SLE patients can inhibit Ig production induced by pokeweed mitogen.[126,127] Nagai, et al. found decreased expression of HLA-DR antigens on the cell surface of SLE monocytes,[128] which could contribute to the reported defect in SLE helper T cell function. On the other hand, Jandl and co-workers have described adherent cell-derived factors that potentiate Ig and anti-DNA synthesis in SLE.[129]

EFFECTS OF ANTILYMPHOCYTE ANTIBODIES ON LYMPHOCYTE FUNCTION

SLE serums may contain IgG antibodies reactive with CD4+ CD8+, and non-T, non-B lymphocytes.[130–135] Although somewhat controversial, antilymphocyte antibodies react preferentially with CD4+ lymphocytes.[135] Such autocytotoxicity could be one factor responsible for the decreased percentages of CD4+ cells found in most patients with active SLE.

Antilymphocyte antibodies present in SLE serum can affect lymphocyte function. Cold-reactive IgM antilymphocyte antibodies can be found in almost all

SLE serums regardless of disease activity.[136] Warm-reactive IgG antilymphocyte antibodies are detected more often in patients with active disease. They are relatively specific for activated T cells.[137] Because of low titer and low avidity, the antigenic determinants on the cell membrane have not been well characterized. There is no evidence that they are directed against T-cell antigens and early studies suggesting that some may react with the IL-2 receptor (Tac), and Ia have not been confirmed.[138]

IgM antilymphocyte antibodies in SLE serum inhibit the lymphocyte proliferative response to soluble antigens.[138] IgG antibodies inhibit the proliferative response of small and activated T cells to mitogens,[73,137-140] and to autologous[141-145] and allogeneic stimulator[144,146,147] cells in the mixed lymphocyte reaction. IgG and IgM antilymphocyte antibodies inhibit the generation of suppressor cells.[148,149] These antibodies inhibit NK cell activity[115,150,151] and antibody-dependent cellular cytotoxicity (ADCC).[123,124] IgG antilymphocyte antibodies can sensitize cells for ADCC.[152-156] The role of antilymphocyte antibodies on immune functions in vivo is unknown, but many abnormalities of lymphocyte function reported in SLE can be reproduced by incubating normal lymphocytes with SLE serum.

SEX HORMONE AND IMMUNOGENETIC FACTORS

SLE affects females predominantly, and it is well known that sex hormones have important effects on immune regulation.[157] Estrogen receptors exist on CD8+ cytotoxic/suppressor lymphocytes.[158] Estrogens increase and androgens reduce spontaneous and immunization-induced antibodies to single-stranded DNA in mice.[159] Estradiol impairs T-cell responsiveness[160-162] and significantly decreases NK cell activity.[163] *Estrogens generally depress cell-mediated immunity in parallel with an increase in autoantibody production.*

Immune recognition and responsiveness to antigens is regulated by the major histocompatibility complex (MHC). There is an association between SLE and the class II MHC alleles HLA-D2 and HLA-D3.[164,165] There is a particularly strong association between HLA-DR2 and HLA-DR3 and the autoantibody Ro (SSA) found in SLE patients.[166-168] Class II HLA antigens regulate T-cell reactivity to tetanus toxoid,[169] mumps[170-171] and Coxsackie B4 virus.[170,171] T cells from DR3+ subjects are hyporesponsive to these antigens, and DR4+ subjects are hyper-responsive. These MHC antigens regulate the frequency of antigen-active T-lymphocytes.[171]

MHC antigens can also regulate suppressor T cell activity. Healthy subjects who are DR3+ have decreased suppressor cell function,[172] and decreased suppressor cell function has been reported in the family members of patients with the DR3-associated autoimmune chronic active hepatitis.[173] Healthy DR3+ subjects also have impaired reticuloendothelial Fc receptor function,[174] and normal DR3+ women had impaired lymphocyte proliferative responses to phytohemagglutinin.[175] All these abnormalities are found in patients with SLE.

THE RELATIONSHIP BETWEEN IMMUNOLOGIC TOLERANCE, AUTOANTIBODY FORMATION, AND CLINICAL SLE

The most consistent finding in SLE is the *imbalance between the humoral and the cellular components of the immune response.* Along with B-cell hyperactivity, there is depressed cell-mediated immunity, including impaired delayed hypersensitivity[176-178] and increased susceptibility to infections. Whether a causal relationship exists between this immunologic imbalance and the breakdown in immune tolerance leading to autoantibody formation has been a matter of speculation. There are compelling reasons for such a relationship. As discussed already, healthy subjects typing HLA-DR3+ have many of the abnormalities of immune regulation associated with SLE. Moreover, nonaffected family members of lupus patients have decreased suppressor T cell function,[179] hypergammaglobulinemia, and antinuclear antibodies.[179-182] These abnormalities in immune regulation reported in family members and in patients with inactive SLE suggest their importance in the development of B-cell hyperactivity rather than merely a consequence of the disease.

The specific mechanisms resulting in a loss of tolerance in SLE to nuclear antigens is still unknown. Recent observations in murine SLE may provide important insights. The injection of parental spleen cells into an F_1 hybrid mouse recipient can induce graft-versus-host disease in certain strain combinations.[183] Mice with chronic graft-versus-host disease develop autoantibodies and a lupus-like syndrome.[184] The immune response mounted by the recipient against parental lymphocytes is responsible for this syndrome.[185] Seamen and co-workers have made the surprising observation that T cytotoxic/suppressor (Lyt2+) cells in the recipient are required for the development of the syndrome,[186] their previous data on the crucial role of helper T cells in the pathogenesis of murine SLE notwithstanding.[187]

From studies of bone marrow transplantation in experimental animals and in humans, it has become apparent that there are autoreactive T cells that recognize self antigens and reject syngeneic bone marrow cells.[188,189] Such autoreactive killer cells might interact with resting B cells, inducing them to produce autoantibodies.

The activity of autoreactive T cells is presumably regulated by genetic, hormonal, and environmental factors. As stated above, Class II MHC genes regulate suppressor T cells and B-cell activity and these genes also regulate tolerance induction.[190] The inhibitory effects of estrogens on T and non-T, non-B suppressor (NK) cells could permit autoreactive T cells to induce autoantibodies, a finding consistent with the known association of SLE flares with the onset of menstruation.

The phenotype of the putative autoreactive T cells is unknown. They could be CD3+ CD4− CD8− cells or the CD8+ lymphocytes that augment B-cell activity in SLE. As already discussed, purified CD8+ lymphocytes from SLE patients that have IL-2 suppressor activity can also augment spontaneous IgG and anti-DNP production.[94] Because most strongly autoreactive T cells that develop in the fetal thymus are eliminated before birth, it might be predicted that their antigen receptors will be composed of γ-, δ-chains, which are found on prenatal thymic T cells before the expression of the adult type α-, β-chain T-cell receptors (see also Chapter 19).

Genetic and hormonal factors may be sufficient for the development of antinuclear antibodies, but other factors are needed to induce clinical SLE. The concordance rate of SLE in 30 identical twins was 60%,[191] but this is an overestimate of the true concordance rate. Deapen and co-workers have identified more than 200 monozygotic twins in whom one of each pair had SLE and found a concordance rate of only 27%.[192] In any case, the finding that the concordance rate is less than 100% indicates that other environmental or developmental factors are required for the expression of clinical SLE.

It is now appreciated that the diversity of antigen receptors on T cells and B cells is developmental and results from random rearrangement of the germ line genes that encode these receptors. This means that the structure of antigen receptors on lymphocytes from monozygotic twins may differ. Therefore, an immune response in one twin may differ qualitatively from the other after exposure to a common environmental antigen. This difference in antigen recognition could result in only one twin's producing an autoantibody with the appropriate characteristics (such as affinity for antigen or surface charge) capable of precipitating a clinical SLR syndrome. In conclusion, MHC genes, sex hormones, and environmental factors are all important factors in the regulation of immune tolerance and autoantibody formation, but much more information is needed to learn why susceptible persons ultimately develop clinical SLE.

REFERENCES

1. Nossal, G.J.V.: The basic components of the immune system. N. Engl. J. Med., 316:1320–1325, 1987.
2. Horwitz, D.A.: Evidence for three mononuclear populations in cellular immunity. In Scientific Basis of Rheumatology. Edited by G. Panayi. New York, Churchill Livingstone, 1982.
3. Unanue, E.R., and Allen, P.M.: The basis for the immunoregulatory role of macrophages and other accessory cells. Science, 236:551–557, 1987.
4. Burnet, F.M.: The clonal selection theory of acquired immunity. Cambridge, England, University Press, 1959.
5. Bankhurst, A.D., Torrigiani, G., and Allison, A.C.: Lymphocytes binding human thyroglobulin in healthy people and its relevance to tolerance for autoantigens. Lancet, 1:226, 1973.
6. Bankhurst, A.D., and Williams, R.C., Jr.: Identification of DNA binding lymphocytes in patients with systemic lupus erythematosus. J. Clin. Invest., 56:1378, 1975.
7. Koopman, W.J., and Schrohenloher, R.E.: In vitro synthesis of IgM rheumatoid factor by lymphocytes from healthy adults. J. Immunol., 125:934–939, 1980.
8. Dziarski, R.: Preferential induction by autoantibody secretion in polyclonal activation of peptidoglycan and lipopolysaccharide. J. Immunol., 128:1026–1030, 1982.
9. Decker, J.L., et al.: Systemic lupus erythematosus: Evolving concepts. Ann. Intern. Med., 91:587, 1979.
10. Glinski, W., et al.: Study of lymphocyte subpopulations in normal humans and patients with systemic lupus erythematosus by fractionation of peripheral blood lymphocytes on discontinuous Ficoll gradient. Clin. Exp. Immunol., 26:228, 1976.
11. Blaese, R.M., Grayson, J., and Steinberg, A.D.: Elevated immunoglobulin secreting cells in the blood of patients with active systemic lupus erythematosus: Correlation of laboratory and clinical assessment of disease activity. Am. J. Med., 69:345, 1980.
12. Fauci, A.S.: Immunoregulation in autoimmunity. J. Allergy Clin. Immunol., 66:5, 1980.
13. Ginsburg, W.W., Finkelman, F.D., and Lipsky, P.E.: Circulating and pokeweed mitogen–induced immunoglobulin-secreting cells in systemic lupus erythematosus. Clin. Exp. Immunol., 35:76, 1979.
14. Takeuchi, T., et al.: In vitro immune response of SLE lymphocytes. The mechanism involved in B-cell activation. Scand. J. Immunol., 16:369, 1982.
15. Tan, E.: Autoantibodies to nuclear antigens (ANA): Their immunobiology and medicine. Adv. Immunol., 33:167, 1967.
16. Fauci, A.S., and Moutsopoulos, H.M.: Polyclonally triggered B-cells in the peripheral blood and bone marrow of normal individuals and patients with systemic lupus erythematosus and primary Sjögren's syndrome. Arthritis Rheum., 24:577, 1986.

17. DeHoratius, R.J., and Levinson, A.I.: Increased circulating immunoglobulin secreting cells in asymptomatic family members with systemic lupus erythematosus. (Abstract.) Arthritis Rheum., 24:S92, 1981.

18. Kumagai, S., et al.: Defective regulation of B lymphocyte colony formation in patients with systemic lupus erythematosus. J. Immunol., 128:258, 1982.

19. Steinberg, A.D.: Modern concepts of systemic lupus erythematosus. Prog. Clin. Rheumatol., 1:1–31, 1984.

20. Bizar-Scheebaum, A., O'Dell, J.R., and Kotzin, B.L.: Antihistone antibody production by peripheral blood cells in SLE. Arthritis Rheum., 30:511, 1987.

21. Sinclair, N.R.: Regulation of the immune response. I. Reduction in ability of specific antibody to inhibit long-lasting IgG immunological priming after removal of the Fc fragment. J. Exp. Med., 129:1183, 1969.

22. Abo, W., Gray, J.D., Bakke, A.C., and Horwitz, D.A.: Studies on human blood lymphocytes with iC3B (type 3) complement receptors. II. Characterization of subsets which regulate pokeweed mitogen–induced lymphocyte proliferation and immunoglobulin synthesis. Clin. Exp. Immunol., 67:544–555, 1987.

23. Gray, J.D., Linker-Israeli, M., and Horwitz, D.A.: Suppression of spontaneous IgG production in systemic lupus erythematosus by autologous CD8 + lymphocytes treated with interleukin-2 and interferon γ (in press).

24. Brodman, R., Gilfillan, G., Glass, P., and Schur, P.H.: Influenzal vaccine response in systemic lupus erythematosus. Ann. Intern. Med., 88:735, 1978.

25. Bobrove, A.M., and Miller, P.: Depressed in vitro B-lymphocyte differentiation in systemic lupus erythematosus. Arthritis Rheum., 20:1326, 1977.

26. Bakke, A.C., et al.: T lymphocyte subsets in systemic lupus erythematosus. Arthritis Rheum., 26:745, 1983.

27. Horwitz, D.A., and Juul-Nielson, K.: Human blood L lymphocytes in patients with active systemic lupus erythematosus, rheumatoid arthritis, and scleroderma. Clin. Exp. Immunol., 30:370, 1977.

28. Lanier, L.L., Cwirla, S., Federspiel, N., and Phillips, J.H.: Human natural killer cells isolated from peripheral blood do not rearrange T cell antigen receptor β chains. J. Exp. Med., 163:209–214, 1986.

29. Ritz, J., et al.: Analysis of T cell receptor gene rearrangement and expression in human natural killer clones. Science, 228:1540–1543, 1985.

30. Gray, J.D., and Horwitz, D.A.: Lymphocytes expressing type 3 complement receptors proliferate in response to interleukin-2 and are the precursors of lymphokine-activated killer cells. J. Clin. Invest., 81, 1988.

31. Morimoto, C., et al.: Alteration in T cell subsets in active systemic lupus erythematosus. J. Clin. Invest., 66:1171, 1980.

32. Tsokos, G.C., and Balow, J.E.: Phenotypes of T lymphocytes in systemic lupus erythematosus: Decreased cytotoxic/suppressor subpopulation is associated with deficient cytotoxic responses rather than with concanavalin A–induced suppressor cells. Clin. Immunol. Immunopathol., 26:267, 1983.

33. Smolan, J.S., et al.: Heterogenicity of immunoregulatory T-cell subsets in systemic lupus erythematosus. Am. J. Med., 72:783, 1982.

34. Morimoto, C., et al.: A defect of immunoregulatory T cell subsets in systemic lupus erythematosus patients demonstrated with anti-2H4 antibody. J. Clin. Invest., 79:762–768, 1987.

35. Linker-Israeli, M., Bakke, A.C., Quismorio, F.P., and Hor-

36. Robb, R.J., Munck, A., and Smith, K.A.: T cell growth factor receptors: Quantitation, specificity and biological relevance. J. Exp. Med., 154:1455–1474, 1981.

37. Campen, D.H., et al.: The level of soluble interleukin 2 receptors in serum reflect activity of diseases characterized by immune system activation. (submitted for publication)

38. Gray, J.D., et al.: Studies on human blood lymphocytes with iC3b (type 3) complement receptors: Abnormalities in patients with active systemic lupus erythematosus. Clin. Exp. Immunol., 67:556, 1987.

38a. Hercerd, T., et al.: Generation of monoclonal antibodies to a human natural killer clone: characterization of two natural killer associated antigens, NKH 1a and NKH 2, expressed as subsets of large granular lymphocytes. J. Clin. Invest., 75:932, 1985.

39. Perusia, B., et al.: Human natural killer cells analyzed by B73.1, a monoclonal antibody blocking Fc receptor functions. I. Characterization of the lymphocyte subset reactive with B73.1. J. Immunol., 130:21, 1983.

40. Alarcon-Segovia, D., and Ruiz-Arguelles, A.: Decreased circulating thymus-derived cells with receptors for the Fc portion of immunoglobulin G in systemic lupus erythematosus. J. Clin. Invest., 6:1390, 1978.

41. Lanier, L.L., et al.: Subpopulations of human natural killer cells defined by expression of the Leu-7 (HNK-1) and Leu-11 (NK-15) antigens. J. Immunol., 131:1789, 1983.

42. Casali, P., et al.: Human lymphocytes making rheumatoid factor and antibody to ssDNA belong to Leu-1 + B-cell subset. Science, 236:77–81, 1987.

43. Linker-Israeli, M., et al.: Defective production of interleukin-2 in patients with systemic lupus erythematosus (SLE). J. Immunol., 130:2651, 1983.

44. Alcocer-Varela, J., Laffon, A., and Alarcon-Segovia, D.: Defective monocyte production of, and T lymphocyte response to, interleukin-1 in the peripheral blood of patients with systemic lupus erythematosus. Clin. Exp. Immunol., 54:125, 1983.

45. Arend, W.P., Joslin, F.G., and Massoni, R.J.: Effects of immune complexes on production by human monocytes of interleukin 1 or an interleukin 1 inhibitor. J. Immunol., 134:3868, 1985.

46. Smith, K.A.: T cell growth factor. Immunol. Rev., 51:337, 1980.

47. Waldmann, T.A., et al.: Expression of interleukin 2 receptors on activated human B cells. J. Exp. Med., 160:1450–1466, 1984.

48. London, L., Perussia, B., and Trinchieri, G.: Induction of proliferation in vitro of resting human natural killer cells: Expression of surface activation antigens. J. Immunol., 134:718–727, 1985.

49. Herrman, F., Cannistra, S.A., Levine, H., and Griffen, J.D.: Expression of interleukin 2 receptors and binding of interleukin by gamma-interferon induced and human monocytic cells. J. Exp. Med., 162:111–116, 1985.

50. Luger, T.A., et al.: Human lymphocytes with either OKT4 or OKT8 phenotype produce interleukin 2 in culture. J. Clin. Invest., 70:470–473, 1982.

51. Meuer, S.C., et al.: Cellular origin of interleukin 2 (IL 2) in man: Evidence for stimulus-restricted IL 2 production by T4 + and T8 + T lymphocytes. J. Immunol., 129:1076–1079, 1982.

52. Alcocer-Varela, J., and Alarcon-Segovia, D.: Decreased production and response to interleukin 2 by cultured lympho-

cytes from patients with systemic lupus erythematosus. J. Clin. Invest., *69*:1388, 1982.

53. Murakawa, Y., et al.: Characterization of T lymphocyte subpopulations responsible for deficient interleukin-2 activity in patients with systemic lupus erythematosus. J. Immunol., *134*:187, 1985.

54. Shiiba, K., Gray, J.D., and Horwitz, D.A.: Unpublished observations, Nov, 1987.

55. Kaye, H., et al.: Inhibition of high affinity IL-2 receptor expression in SLE. (Abstract.) Arthritis Rheum., *30*:S11, 1987.

56. Friedman, R.M., and Vogel, S.N.: Interferons with special emphasis on the immune system. Adv. Immunol., *34*:97, 1983.

57. Oppenheim, J.J., Ruscetti, F.W., and Faltynek, C.R.: Interleukins and interferons. *In* Basic and Clinical Immunology. 6th Ed. Edited by D.P. Stites, J.D. Stobo, and J.V. Wells. Norwalk, CT, Appleton and Lange, 1987, pp. 82–95.

58. Tsokos, G.C., et al.: Deficient gamma-interferon production in patients with systemic lupus erythematosus. Arthritis Rheum., *29*:1210, 1986.

59. Prebble, O.T., et al.: Systemic lupus erythematosus: Presence in human serum of unusual acid labile leukocyte interferon. Science, *216*:429, 1982.

60. Paul, W.E., and Ohara, J.: B cell stimulatory factor-1/interleukin 4. Annu. Rev. Immunol., *5*:429–459, 1987.

61. Alcocer-Varela, J., Martinez-Cordero, E., and Alarcon-Segovia, D.: Excessive production and response to B cell growth factor (BC6F) by cells from patients with systemic lupus erythematosus (Abstract.) Arthritis Rheum., *28*:S48, 1985.

62. Hirose, T., et al.: Abnormal production of and response to B-cell differentiation factor in patients with systemic lupus erythematosus. Scand. J. Immunol., *21*:141, 1985.

63. Martinez-Cordero, E., Alcocer-Varela, J., and Alarcon-Segovia, D.: Stimulating and differentiation factors for human B lymphocytes in systemic lupus erythematosus. Clin. Exp. Immunol., *65*:598–604, 1986.

64. Delfraissy, J.F., et al.: B cell hyperactivity in systemic lupus erythematosus: Selectively enhanced responsiveness to a high molecular weight B cell growth factor. Eur. J. Immunol., *16*:1251–1256, 1986.

65. Bell, D.A.: Cell-mediated immunity in systemic lupus erythematosus: Observations on in vitro cell-mediated immune responses in relationship to number of potentially reactive T cells, disease activity, and treatment. Clin. Immunol. Immunopathol., *9*:301, 1978.

66. Horwitz, D.A., and Garret, M.A.: Lymphocyte reactivity to mitogens in subjects with systemic lupus erythematosus, rheumatoid arthritis and scleroderma. Clin. Exp. Immunol., *27*:92, 1977.

67. Lockshin, M.E., et al.: Cell mediated immunity in rheumatic diseases. Mitogen responses in RA, SLE and other illnesses: Correlation with T and B lymphocyte populations. Arthritis Rheum., *18*:245, 1975.

68. Markenson, J.A., et al.: Suppressor monocytes in patients with systemic lupus erythematosus. Evidence of suppressor activity associated with cell free soluble product of monocytes. J. Lab. Clin. Med., *95*:40, 1980.

69. Patrucco, R., Rothfield, N.F., and Hirshhorn, K.: The response of cultured lymphocytes from patients with systemic lupus erythematosus to DNA. Arthritis Rheum., *10*:32, 1967.

70. Paty, J.G., et al.: Impaired cell mediated immunity in systemic lupus erythematosus (SLE). A controlled study of 23 untreated patients. Am. J. Med., *59*:769, 1975.

71. Rosenthal, C.J., and Franklin, E.C.: Depression of cellular-

72. Utsinger, P.D., and Yount, W.J.: Phytohemagglutinin response in systemic lupus erythematosus. Reconstitution experiments using highly purified lymphocyte subpopulations and monocytes. J. Clin. Invest., *60*:626, 1977.

73. Horwitz, D.A.: Mechanisms producing decreased mitogenic reactivity in patients with systemic lupus erythematosus and other rheumatic diseases. *In* Mitogens in Immunobiology. Edited by J.J. Oppenheim and D.L. Rosenstreich. New York, Academic Press, 1976.

74. Winfield, J.B.: Antilymphocyte antibodies: Specificity and relationship to abnormal cellular function in SLE. Edited by R. Lahitta. New York, John Wiley & Sons, 1987.

75. Dupont, B., Hansen, J.A., and Yunis, E.J.: Human mixed lymphocyte culture reaction: Genetics, specificity and biological implication. Adv. Immunol., *23*:108, 1976.

76. Suciu-Foca, N., et al.: Impaired responsiveness of lymphocytes in patients with systemic lupus erythematosus. Clin. Exp. Immunol., *18*:295, 1974.

77. Tsokos, G.C., and Balow, J.E.: Cellular immune response in systemic lupus erythematosus. J. Clin. Immunol., *1*:208, 1981.

78. Wernet, P., and Kunkel, H.G.: Antibodies to a specific surface antigen of T cells in human sera inhibiting mixed leukocyte culture reactions. J. Exp. Med., *138*:1021, 1973.

79. Kumagai, S., Steinberg, A.D., and Green, I.: Immune responses to hapten-modified self and their regulation in normal individuals and patients with systemic lupus erythematosus. J. Immunol., *127*:1643, 1981.

80. Kuntz, M.M., Innes, J.B., and Weksler, M.E.: The cellular basis of the impaired autologous mixed lymphocyte reaction in patients with systemic lupus erythematosus. J. Clin. Invest., *63*:151, 1979.

81. Sakane, T., Steinberg, A.P., and Green, I.: Failure of the autologous mixed lymphocyte reactions between T cells and non T cells in patients with systemic lupus erythematosus. Proc. Natl. Acad. Sci. USA, *75*:3464, 1978.

82. Russell, P.J., et al.: Studies of the autologous mixed lymphocyte reactions in patients with systemic lupus erythematosus. Pathology, *15*:37, 1983.

83. Sakane, T., et al.: Studies of immune functions of patients with systemic lupus erythematosus. III. Characterization of lymphocyte subpopulations responsible for defective autologous mixed lymphocyte reactions. Arthritis Rheum., *22*:770, 1979.

84. Takada, S., et al.: Abnormalities in autologous mixed lymphocyte reaction–activated immunologic processes in systemic lupus erythematosus and their possible correction by interleukin 2. Eur. J. Immunol., *15*:262–267, 1985.

85. Tan, P., Pang, G., and Wilson, J.D.: Immunoglobulin production in vitro by peripheral blood lymphocytes in systemic lupus erythematosus: Helper T cell defect and B cell hyperactivity. Clin. Exp. Immunol., *44*:548, 1981.

86. Fauci, A.S., and Moutsopoulos, H.M.: Polyclonally triggered B cells in the peripheral blood and bone marrow of normal individuals and in patients with systemic lupus erythematosus and primary Sjögren's syndrome. Arthritis Rheum., *24*:577, 1981.

87. Abe, T., et al.: Mitogenic responses to lipopolysaccharide by B lymphocytes from patients with systemic lupus erythematosus. Scand. J. Immunol., *15*:475, 1981.

88. Nies, K.M., Stevens, R.H., and Louie, J.S.: Normal T cell regulation of IgG synthesis in systemic lupus erythematosus. J. Clin. Lab. Immunol., *4*:69, 1980.

89. Delfraissy, J.F., et al.: Depressed primary in vitro antibody response in untreated systemic lupus eythematosus. J. Clin. Invest., 66:141, 1980.

90. Gottlieb, A.B., et al.: Immune function in systemic lupus erythematosus. Impairment of in vitro T-cell proliferation and in vivo antibody response to exogenous antigen. J. Clin. Invest., 63:885, 1979.

91. Chiorazzi, N., et al.: T-cell helper defect in patients with chronic lymphocyte leukemia. J. Immunol., 122:1087, 1979.

92. Volk, H.D., and Diamantstein, T.: Il-2 normalizes defective suppressor T cell function of patients with systemic lupus erythematosus in vitro. Clin. Exp. Immunol., 66:525–531, 1986.

93. Mossman, T.R., et al.: Two types of murine helper T cell clone: Definition according to profiles of lymphokine activities and secreted proteins. J. Immunol., 136:2348, 1986.

93a. Shiiba, K., and Horwitz, D.A.: Unpublished observations, June, 1987.

94. Linker-Israeli, M., Quismorio, F.Q., Jr., Gray, J.D., and Horwitz, D.A.: Modulation of the in vitro spontaneous IgG production by SLE-derived peripheral blood mononuclear cells. (Abstract.) Arthritis Rheum., 30:S125, 1987.

95. Katz, P., Mitchell, S.R., Cupps, T.R., and Whalen, G.: Enhancement of the early events in B cell activation by natural killer (NK) cells (Abstract.). Arthritis Rheum., 30:S71, 1987.

96. Alarcon-Segovia, D., and Palacios, R.: Differences in immunoregulatory T cell circuits between diphenylhydantoin-related and spontaneously occurring systemic lupus erythematosus. Arthritis Rheum., 24:1086, 1981.

97. Bresnihan, B., and Jasin, H.E.: Suppressor function of peripheral blood mononuclear cells in normal individuals and in patients with systemic lupus erythematosus. J. Clin. Invest., 59:106, 1977.

98. Coovadia, H.M., Mackay, I.R., and d'Aspice, A.J.F.: Suppressor cells assayed by three different methods in patients with chronic active hepatitis and systemic lupus erythematosus. Clin. Immunol. Immunopathol., 18:268, 1981.

99. Fauci, A.S., Steinberg, A.D., Haynes, B.F., and Whalen, G.: Immunoregulatory aberrations in systemic lupus erythematosus. J. Immunol., 121:1473, 1978.

100. Horowitz, S., et al.: Induction of suppressor T cells in systemic lupus erythematosus by thymosin and cultured thymic keithelium. Science, 197:999, 1977.

101. Ilfeld, D.N., and Krakauer, R.S.: Suppression of immunoglobulin synthesis of systemic lupus erythematosus patients by concanavalin A–activated normal human spleen cell supernatants. Clin. Immunol. Immunopathol., 17:196, 1980.

102. Miller, K.B., and Schwartz, R.S.: Autoimmunity and suppressor T lymphocytes. In Advances in Internal Medicine. Edited by G. Stollerman. Chicago, Year Book Medical Publishers, 1982, pp. 281–331.

103. Morimoto, C.: Loss of suppressor T lymphocyte function in patients with systemic lupus erythematosus. Clin. Immunol. Immunopathol., 32:125, 1978.

104. Morimoto, C., Abe, T., and Homma, M.: Altered function of suppressor T lymphocytes in patients with active systemic lupus erythematosus. Clin. Immunol. Immunopathol., 13:161, 1979.

105. Newman, B., et al.: Lack of suppressor cell activity in systemic lupus erythematosus. Clin. Immunol. Immunopathol., 13:187, 1979.

106. Ruiz-Arguelles, A., Alarcon-Segovia, D., Llorente, L., and del Gindice-Knipping, J.A.: Heterogeneity of the spontaneously expanded and mitogen-induced generation of suppressor cell

function of T cells on B cells in systemic lupus erythematosus. Arthritis Rheum., 23:1004, 1980.

107. Sagawa, A., and Abdou, N.I.: Suppressor-cell dysfunction in systemic lupus erythematosus. Cells involved and in vitro correction. J. Clin. Invest., 62:789, 1978.

108. Sakane, T., Steinberg, A.D., and Green, I.: Studies of immune functions of patients with systemic lupus erythematosus. I. Dysfunction of suppressor T-cell activity related to impaired generation of, rather than response to, suppressor cells. Arthritis Rheum., 21:657, 1978.

109. Gattringer, C., Huber, H., Michlmayr, G., and Braunsteiner, H.: Normal suppressor-cell activity in systemic lupus erythematosus. A study of 26 cases. Immunobiology, 163:48, 1982.

110. Tsokos, G.C., and Balow, J.E.: Suppressor cells in systemic lupus erythematosus. Lack of defective in vitro suppressor cell generation in patients with active disease. J. Clin. Lab. Immunol., 8:83, 1982.

111. Linker-Israeli, M., Gray, J.D., Quismorio, F.P., Jr., and Horwitz, D.A.: Characterization of lymphocytes that suppress IL-2 production in systemic lupus erythematosus. (submitted for publication)

112. Gebel, H.M., Kaizer, H., and Landay, A.L.: Characterization of circulating suppressor T lymphocytes in bone marrow transplant recipients. Transplantation, 53:258–263, 1987.

112a. Linker-Israeli, M., Ph.D., and Horowitz, D.A., M.D., Unpublished observations, June, 1986.

113. Hoffman, T.: Natural killer function in systemic lupus erythematosus. Arthritis Rheum., 23:30, 1980.

114. Katz, P., et al.: Abnormal natural killer cell activity in systemic lupus erythematosus: An intrinsic defect in the cytolytic event. J. Immunol., 129:1966, 1982.

115. Silverman, S.L., and Cathcart, E.S.: Natural killing in systemic lupus erythematosus. Inhibitory effects of serum. Clin. Immunol. Immunopathol., 17:219, 1978.

116. Tsokos, G.C., Rook, A.H., Diej, J.Y., and Balow, J.E.: Natural killer cells and interferon responses in patients with systemic lupus erythematosus. Clin. Exp. Immunol., 5:239, 1982.

117. Tsokos, G.C., et al.: Interleukin-2 restores the depressed allogeneic cell-mediated lympholysis and natural killer cell activity in patients with systemic lupus erythematosus. Clin. Immunol. Immunopathol., 34:379, 1985.

118. Sibbitt, W.L., Jr., Mathews, P.M., and Bankhurst, A.D.: Defects in effector lytic activity and response to interferon and interferon inducers. J. Clin. Invest., 10:71, 1983.

119. Oshimi, K., Sumiya, A., Gond, N., et al.: Natural killer cell activity in systemic lupus erythematosus. Lancet, 2:1023, 1979.

120. Bakke, A.C., et al.: Studies on human blood lymphocytes with iC3b (type 3) complement receptors: 1. Granular Fc-IgG receptor positive and Fc receptor negative subsets in healthy subjects and patients with systemic lupus erythematosus. J. Immunol., 136:1253–1259, 1986.

121. Diaz-Jouanen, E.E., Bankhurst, A.D., and Williams, R.C., Jr.: Antibody-mediated lymphocytotoxicity in rheumatoid arthritis and systemic lupus erythematosus. Arthritis Rheum., 19:33, 1976.

122. Feldmann, J., et al.: Antibody dependent cell-mediated cytotoxicity in selected autoimmune diseases. J. Clin. Invest., 58:173, 1976.

123. Scheinberg, M.A., and Cathcart, E.S.: Antibody-dependent direct cytotoxicity of human lymphocytes. I. Studies on peripheral blood lymphocytes and sera of patients with systemic lupus erythematosus. Clin. Exp. Immunol., 24:317, 1976.

124. Schneider, J., et al.: Reduced antibody-dependent cell-me-

diated cytotoxicity in systemic lupus erythematosus. Clin. Exp. Immunol., 20:187, 1975.

125. Lanier, L.L., et al.: Subpopulation of human natural killer cells defined by expression of Leu 11 (NK-15) antigens. J. Immunol., 131:1787, 1983.

126. Markenson, J.A., et al.: Responses of fractionated cells from patients with systemic lupus erythematosus and normals to plant mitogen: Evidence for a suppressor population of monocytes. Proc. Soc. Exp. Biol. Med., 158:5, 1978.

127. Tsokos, G.C., and Balow, M.D.: Cellular immune response in systemic lupus erythematosus. Prog. Allergy, 35:93, 1984.

128. Nagai, H., et al.: Diminished peripheral blood monocyte DR antigen expression in systemic lupus erythematosus. Clin. Exp. Rheumatol., 2:131, 1984.

129. Jandl, R.C., et al.: The effect of adherent cell-derived factors on immunoglobulin and anti-DNA synthesis in systemic lupus erythematosus. Clin. Immunol. Immunopathol., 42:344–359, 1987.

130. Morimoto, C., et al.: Studies of antilymphocyte antibody of patients with active systemic lupus erythematosus. Scand. J. Immunol., 10:213, 1979.

131. Sakane, T., Steinberg, A.D., Reeves, J.P., and Green, I.: Studies of immune functions of patients with systemic lupus erythematosus: Complement-dependent immunoglobulin-M anti-thymus derived cell antibodies to T-cell subsets. J. Clin. Invest., 64:1260, 1979.

132. Morimoto, C., et al.: Relationship between systemic lupus erythematosus T cell subsets, anti-T cell antibodies and T cell functions. J. Clin. Invest., 73:689, 1984.

133. Yamada, A., Shaw, M., and Winfield, J.B.: Surface antigen specificity of cold reactive IgM antilymphocyte antibodies in systemic lupus erythematosus. Arthritis Rheum., 28:44, 1985.

134. Yamada, A., Cohen, P., and Winfield, J.B.: Subset specificity of antilymphocyte antibodies in systemic lupus erythematosus: Preferential reactivity with cells bearing the T4 and autologous erythrocyte receptor phenotypes. Arthritis Rheum., 28:262–270, 1985.

135. Winfield, J.B., Shaw, M., Yamada, A., and Minota, S.: Reactivity with T4+ cells is associated with relative depletion of autologous T4+ cells. Arthritis Rheum., 30:162–168, 1987.

136. Winfield, J.B., et al.: Nature of cold-reactive antibodies to lymphocyte surface determinants in systemic lupus erythematosus. Arthritis Rheum., 18:1–8, 1975.

137. Litvin, D.A., Cohen, P.L., and Winfield, J.B.: Characterization of warm-reactive IgG anti-lymphocyte antibodies in systemic lupus erythematosus. Relative specificity for mitogen-activated T cells and their soluble products. J. Immunol., 13:181–186, 1983.

138. Yamada, A., and Winfield, J.B.: Inhibition of soluble antigen-induced T cell proliferation by warm-reactive antibodies to activated T cells in systemic lupus erythematosus. J. Clin. Invest., 74:1948, 1984.

139. Horwitz, D.A., and Cousar, J.B.: A relationship between cellular immunity, humoral suppression of lymphocyte function and severity of systemic lupus erythematosus. Am. J. Med., 58:829, 1975.

140. Horwitz, D.A., Garrett, M.A., and Craig, A.H.: Serum effects on mitogenic reactivity in subjects with systemic lupus erythematosus, rheumatoid arthritis and scleroderma. Clin. Exp. Immunol., 27:100, 1977.

141. Hahn, B.H., Pletcher, L.S., Muniain, M., and MacDermott, R.P.: Suppression of the normal autologous mixed lymphocyte reaction by sera from patients with systemic lupus erythematosus. Arthritis Rheum., 25:381, 1982.

142. Okudaira, K., Searles, R.P., Goodwin, J.S., and Williams, R.C., Jr.: Antibodies in the sera of patients with systemic lupus erythematosus that block the binding of monoclonal anti-Ia positive targets also inhibit the autologous mixed lymphocyte response. J. Immunol., 129:582, 1982.

143. Sakane, T., et al.: A defect in the suppressor circuits among OKT4+ cell population in patients with systemic lupus erythematosus occurs independently of a defect in the OKT8+ suppressor T cell function. J. Immunol., 131:753, 1983.

144. Stephens, H.A.F., Fitzharris, P., Knight, R.A., and Snaith, M.L.: Inhibition of proliferative and suppressor responses in the autologous mixed lymphocyte reaction by serum from patients with systemic lupus erythematosus. Ann. Rheum. Dis., 41:495, 1982.

145. Suciu-Foca, N., Buda, J.A., Thiem, T., and Reemtsa, K.: Impaired responsiveness of lymphocytes in patients with systemic lupus erythematosus. Clin. Exp. Immunol., 18:295, 1974.

146. Wernet, P., and Kunkel, H.G.: Antibodies to a specific surface antigen of T cells in human sera inhibiting mixed leukocyte culture reactions. J. Exp. Med., 138:1021, 1973.

147. Williams, R.C., Jr., Lies, R.B., and Messner, R.P.: Inhibition of mixed leukocyte culture responses by serum and gamma globulin fractions from certain patients with connective tissue disorders. Arthritis Rheum., 16:597, 1973.

148. Morimoto, C., et al.: Studies of antilymphocyte antibody of patients with active systemic lupus erythematosus. Scand. J. Immunol., 10:213, 1979.

149. Sagawa, A., and Abdou, N.I.: Suppressor-cell antibody in systemic lupus erythematosus. Possible mechanism for suppressor cell dysfunction. J. Clin Invest., 63:536, 1979.

150. Goto, M., Tanimoto, K., and Horiuchi, Y.: Natural cell mediated cytotoxicity in systemic lupus erythematosus. Suppression by antilymphocyte antibody. Arthritis Rheum., 23:1274, 1980.

151. Rook, A.H., et al.: Cytotoxic antibodies to natural killer cells in systemic lupus erythematosus. Clin. Immunol. Immunopathol., 24:179, 1982.

152. Dasgupta, M.D., et al.: Antibody-mediated cellular cytotoxicity against Raji cells ADCC (Raji): Evaluation of false positives in the detection of circulating immune complexes by Raji-cell assay. J. Clin. Immunol., 2:197, 1982.

153. Feldmann, J.-L., et al.: Antibody-dependent cell-mediated cytotoxicity in Hashimoto's thyroiditis. Clin. Exp. Immunol., 14:153, 1973.

154. Mahowald, M.L., and Dalmasso, A.P.: Lymphocyte destruction by antibody-dependent cellular cytotoxicity mediated in vitro by antibodies in serum from patients with systemic lupus erythematosus. Ann. Rheum. Dis., 41:593, 1982.

155. Wright, J., et al.: Serum-induced enhancement of peripheral blood mononuclear cell mediated cytotoxicity towards human targets in systemic lupus erythematosus. J. Clin. Lab. Immunol., 11:81, 1983.

156. Kumagai, S., Steinberg, A.D., and Green, I.: Antibodies to T cells in patients with systemic lupus erythematosus can induce antibody-dependent cell-mediated cytotoxicity against human T cells. J. Clin. Invest., 67:605, 1981.

157. Steinberg, A.D., et al.: Approach to the study of the role of sex hormones in autoimmunity. Arthritis Rheum., 22:1170–1176, 1979.

158. Cohen, J.H.M., et al.: Sex steroid receptors on peripheral T cells: Absence of androgen receptors and restriction of estrogen receptors to OKT8-positive cells. J. Immunol., 131:2767, 1983.

159. Steinberg, A.D., et al.: Studies of immune abnormalities in systemic lupus erythematosus. Am. J. Kidney Dis., 2:101–110, 1982.

160. Wyle, F.A., and Kent, J.R.: Immunosuppression by sex steroid hormones. The effect upon PHA- and PPD-stimulated lymphocyes. Clin. Exp. Immunol., 27:407–415, 1977.

161. Luster, M.I., et al.: Estrogen immunosuppression is regulated through estrogenic responses in the thymus. J. Immunol., 133:110–116, 1984.

162. Kolland, T., Strand, O., and Forsberg, J.G.: Long-term effects of neonatal estrogen treatment on mitogen responsiveness of mouse spleen lymphocytes. J. Natl. Cancer Inst., 63:413–421, 1979.

163. Seaman, W.E., et al.: Beta-Estradiol reduces natural killer cells in mice. J. Immunol., 121:2193–2198, 1978.

164. Reinersten, J.L., et al.: β-lymphocyte alloantigens associated with systemic lupus erythematosus. N. Engl. J. Med., 299:515, 1978.

165. Gibofsky, A., et al.: Disease associations of the Ia-like human alloantigens. J. Exp. Med., 148:1728, 1978.

166. Bell, D.A., and Maddison, R.J.: Serologic subsets in systemic lupus erythematosus: An examination of autoantibodies in relationship to clinical features of disease and HLA antigens. Arthritis Rheum., 23:1268, 1980.

167. Ahearn, J.M., et al.: The interrelationships of HLA-DR MB and MT phenotypes, autoantibody expression and clinical features in systemic lupus erythematosus. Arthritis Rheum., 25:1031, 1982.

168. Alvarellos, A., et al.: Relationships of HLA-DR and MT antigens to autoantibody expression in systemic lupus erythematosus (Letter.) Arthritis Rheum., 26:1533, 1983.

169. Feehally, J., et al.: Impaired IgG response to tetanus toxoid in human membranous nephropathy: Association with HLA-DR3. Clin. Exp. Immunol., 63:376–384, 1986.

170. Bruserud, O., Jervell, J., and Thorsby, E.: HLA-DR3 and -DR4 control T-lymphocyte responses to mumps and Coxsackie B4 virus: Studies on patients with type 1 (insulin-dependent) diabetes and healthy subjects. Diabetologia, 28:420–426, 1985.

171. Bruserud, O., Stenersen, M., and Thorsby, E.: T lymphocyte responses to Coxsackie B4 and mumps virus. II. Immunoregulation by HLA-DR3 and -DR4 associated restriction elements. Tissue Antigens, 26:179–192, 1985.

172. Ambindery, M., et al.: Special characteristics of immune function in normal individuals of the HLA-DR3 Type. Clin. Immunol. Immunopathol., 23:269–274, 1982.

173. Nouri-Aria, K.T., et al.: HLA A1-B8-DR3 and suppressor cell function in first-degree relatives of patients with autoimmune chronic active hepatitis. J. Hepatol., 1:235–241, 1985.

174. Lawley, T.J., et al.: Defective Fc-receptor functions associated with the HLA-B8/DRw3 haplotype: Studies in patients with dermatitis herpetiformis and normal subjects. N. Engl. J. Med., 304:185, 1981.

175. Greenberg, L.J., and Yunis, E.J.: Histocompatibility determinants, immune responsiveness and aging in man. Fed Proc., 37:1258, 1978.

176. Horwitz, D.A.: Impaired delayed hypersensitivity in systemic lupus erythematosus. Arthritis Rheum., 15:353, 1972.

177. Hahn, B.H., Babgy, M.D., and Osterland, C.K.: Abnormalities of delayed hypersensitivity in systemic lupus erythematosus. Am. J. Med., 55:25, 1973.

178. Paty, J.G., et al.: Impaired cell-mediated immunity in systemic lupus erythematosus. A controlled study of 23 untreated patients. Am. J. Med., 59:769, 1975.

179. Miller, K.B., and Schwartz, R.S.: Familial abnormalities of suppressor-cell function in systemic lupus erythematosus. N. Engl. J. Med., 3011:803, 1979.

180. Larsson, O., and Leonhardt, T.: Hereditary hypergammaglobulinaemia and systemic lupus erythematosus. I. Clinical and electrophoretic studies. Acta Med. Scand., 165:371, 1959.

181. Holman, H.R., and Deicher, H.R.: The appearance of hypergammaglobulinemia, positive serological reactions for rheumatoid arthritis and complement fixation reactions with tissue constituents in the sera of relatives of patients with systemic lupus erythematosus. Arthritis Rheum., 3:244, 1960.

182. DeHoratius, R.J., Pillarisetty, R., Messner, R.P., and Talal, N.: Anti-nucleic acid antibodies in systemic lupus erythematosus patients and their families. Incidence and correlation with lymphocytotoxic antibodies. J. Clin. Invest., 56:1149, 1975.

183. Gleichmann, E., Van Elven, E.H., and Van der Veen, J.P.W.: A systemic lupus erythematosus (SLE)-like disease in mice induced by abnormal T-B cell cooperation. Preferential formation of autoantibodies characteristic of SLE. Eur. J. Immunol., 182:129, 1982.

184. Gleichmann, E., et al.: Graft-versus-host reactions: Clues to the etiopathology of a spectrum of immunological diseases. Immunol. Today, 5:324, 1984.

185. Shearer, G.M., and Levy, R.B.: Graft-vs-host-associated immune suppression is activated by recognition of allogeneic murine Ia antigens. J. Exp. Med., 157:936, 1983.

186. Harper, S.E., Roubinian, J.R., and Seaman, W.E.: Autoimmunity during the graft-versus-host reaction requires recipient Lyt-2+ cells. Arthritis Rheum., 30:S10, 1987.

187. Wofsy, D., and Seaman, W.E.: Reversal of advanced murine lupus in NZB/NZW F$_1$ mice by treatment with monoclonal antibody to L3T4. J. Immunol., 138:3247–3253, 1987.

188. Nakano, K., Nakamura, I., and Cudkowicz, G.: Generation of F$_1$ hybrid cytotoxic T lymphocytes specific for self H-2. Nature, 289:559, 1981.

189. Rappeport, J., et al.: Acute graft-versus-host disease in recipients of bone marrow transplants from identical twin donors. Lancet, 2:717, 1979.

190. Lamb, J.R., and Feldmann, M.: Essential requirement for major histocompatibility complex recognition in T cell tolerance induction. Nature, 308:72–74, 1984.

191. Arnett, F.C.: Familial SLE, the HLA system and the genetics of lupus erythematosus. *In* Dubois' Lupus Erythematosus. 3rd Ed. Edited by D.J. Wallace and E.L. Dubois. Philadelphia, Lea & Febiger, 1987.

192. Deapen, D.M., et al.: A revised estimate of twin concordance in SLE: A survey of 138 pairs (Abstract.) Arthritis Rheum., 29:S26, 1987.

70

ANTIPHOSPHOLIPID ANTIBODIES

E. NIGEL HARRIS and GRAHAM R.V. HUGHES

Evidence shows that some patients with antibodies to phospholipids are subject to repeated episodes of venous and arterial thrombosis, repeated fetal loss, and thrombocytopenia.[1-3] Enough patients have been identified with these clinical and serologic features[4-16] to warrant cautious use of the term antiphospholipid syndrome (APS). The use of the term "antiphospholipid" seems justified because the specific serologic feature connected with this syndrome is the production of antibodies that cross-react with cardiolipin and a variety of other negatively charged phospholipids.[17-21] The term "syndrome" is used because of the constellation of clinical features, particularly thrombosis, fetal loss, and thrombocytopenia, that can occur in association with these antibodies, often in the absence of any other clinical manifestations.[1]

The APS overlaps to some extent with other connective tissue disorders, in particular systemic lupus erythematosus (SLE); many APS patients have one or more of the clinical or serologic features associated with the connective tissue disorders.[4-7] Because of this overlap, the true clinical and serologic boundaries of APS are vague and will probably remain so until these patients are studied over time. Some clinicians have already proposed that livedo reticularis,[22] migraine headaches,[22] chorea,[23,24] endocardial lesions,[25] and transverse myelopathy[1] might be features of APS.[22]

Current data show that only a minority of patients with antiphospholipid antibodies are subject to thrombosis, fetal loss, or thrombocytopenia. Approximately 30% of patients with the lupus anticoagulant appear to develop thrombosis.[12,13] Because of the high

sensitivity of anticardiolipin antibody tests, the actual percentage of patients who develop thrombosis may be small. The association of clinical complications with antiphospholipid antibodies appears to depend on specificity, isotype, level, and probably the period of time during which these antibodies are present.[2] The importance of anticardiolipin isotype and level was demonstrated in a study that showed that histories of thrombosis and fetal loss were encountered most frequently in patients with moderate to high IgG anticardiolipin antibody levels.[26]

Antiphospholipid antibodies are detected by one or more of three groups of tests. A thorough appreciation of the literature about these antibodies can only be gleaned if one understands something about these tests because most authors classify antiphospholipid antibodies according to the method used to detect them.[2] The oldest tests are the standard tests for syphilis (STS), which include the Venereal Disease Research Laboratories (VDRL) (agglutination) and Wasserman (complement fixation) tests.[27] STS levels are usually strongly positive in patients with syphilis[27] but are either weakly positive or negative in APS patients.[2,28] Patients who have a positive STS but a negative fluorescent treponema antigen-antibodies (FTA-ABS) or treponema pallidum immobilization (TPI) test are defined as having a biologic false positive test for syphilis (BFP-STS).[29]

The more useful tests for detecting antiphospholipid antibodies in APS patients are the lupus anticoagulant and the anticardiolipin antibody tests. The lupus anticoagulant test relies on the ability of some antiphospholipid antibodies to inhibit in vitro clot formation.[3,19] These antibodies probably inhibit the assembly of clotting factors on a phospholipid surface at the prothrombin activator complex stage of the clotting cascade (Fig. 70–1).[30,33] APS patients are first identified because of a prolonged partial thromboplastin time (PTT), Russell Viper Venom Time (RVVT), or prothrombin time (PT), not corrected by the addition of normal plasma.

The most sensitive test for antiphospholipid antibodies is the anticardiolipin antibody test, introduced in 1983[34] and extensively improved since that time.[35,36] This test utilizes enzyme-linked immunoabsorbent assay (ELISA)[37-42] or solid-phase radioimmunoassay techniques[17] to determine antibody binding to solid plates coated either with cardiolipin or with other negatively charged phospholipids.[21,36] It is likely that the lupus anticoagulant and anticardiolipin antibody tests detect antibodies with overlapping specificities,[2] but some investigators believe that *the results of these two tests differ frequently enough*[43,44] *to recommend that both tests be performed in patients with APS.*

OCCURRENCE

Antiphospholipid antibodies are detected in patients with a variety of autoimmune, infectious, malignant, and drug-induced disorders, as well as in some apparently healthy individuals.[2] Other than patients with APS, the single disorder in which these antibodies have been reported most frequently is SLE, in which false positive tests for syphilis are reported in 10% of cases,[45] lupus anticoagulant in 6 to 10% of cases,[46] and anticardiolipin antibodies in 15 to 40% of

cases.[2,42] The specificities of antiphospholipid antibodies probably differ in various disorders. An example of these differences was recently demonstrated in a study of antiphospholipid antibodies in patients with autoimmune disorders or with syphilis.[47] Antiphospholipid antibody specificity, isotype, and level of positivity and the period of time during which these antibodies are present may all determine clinical complications,[2] irrespective of the underlying disease in which these antibodies occur.

CLINICAL FEATURES

Thrombosis. Although some antiphospholipid antibodies can prolong in vitro clotting tests, hemorrhage is rare in patients with these antibodies, even if the patients undergo surgery.[19,48,49] When hemorrhage does occur, other causes such as thrombocytopenia[19,50] or clotting factor deficiencies, resulting from the presence of other clotting factor inhibitors,[51-54] should be excluded. The reason antiphospholipid antibodies with lupus anticoagulant activity do not cause hemorrhage is still unknown. Although these antibodies can interrupt clotting factor interactions on phospholipid micelles in vitro, they may be unable to interrupt similar interactions on platelet surfaces in vivo.[19] Others have questioned this explanation, arguing that the in vitro lupus anticoagulant reaction is observed even in the presence of plasma with high platelet counts.[12,14]

Instead of being associated with hemorrhage, antiphospholipid antibodies are paradoxically associated with thrombosis. The occurrence of venous and arterial thrombosis in a significant minority of patients

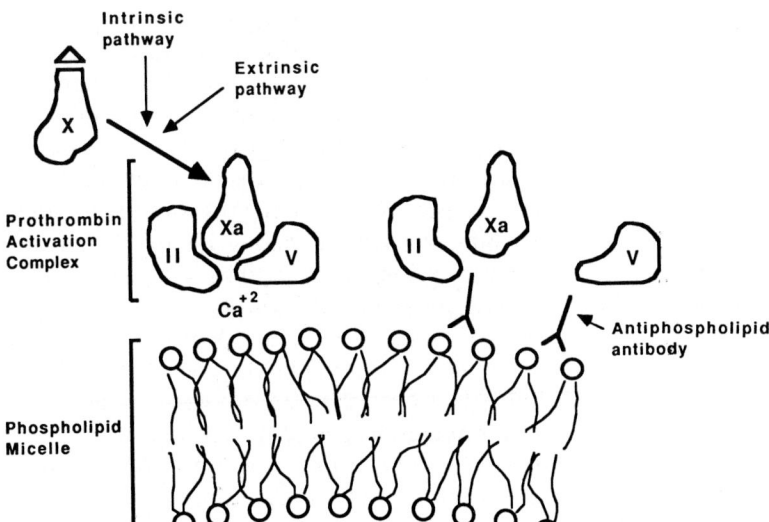

FIG. 70–1. Diagrammatic representation of *prothrombin activation complex* and proposed mechanism by which antiphospholipid antibodies can interrupt formation of the complex. The *prothrombin activation complex* (left) is believed to be formed by factor Xa (factor X is converted to Xa either by activation of the intrinsic or extrinsic coagulation pathways), prothrombin, and factor V interacting in the presence of Ca^{+2} on a phospholipid template. By binding the template, antiphospholipid antibodies may interrupt formation of the complex (right) and prolong in vitro clotting.

with lupus anticoagulant activity has been recognized by centers throughout the world.[4–17] Of the more than 800 patients reported in the literature whose plasma contained lupus anticoagulant activity, about 25 to 36% have had a history of venous or arterial thrombosis.[12,13] If patients are grouped according to anticardiolipin antibody isotype and level, the frequency of thrombosis in patients with moderate to high IgG anticardiolipin levels may exceed 50%.[26] Most figures, however, have been based on retrospective studies, and the true frequency of thrombosis in these patients must await prospective studies with properly standardized assays.[35]

Thrombosis can occur anywhere in the venous or arterial circulation and involves vessels of all sizes. In the venous circulation, thrombosis of the deep and superficial veins of the lower extremities has been reported most frequently.[4–15] Other reported venous sites of thrombosis include the axillary,[9,10,14] renal,[55] and hepatic veins[56–60] and the inferior vena cava. Some patients with lupus anticoagulant activity also have pulmonary hypertension,[61,62] perhaps caused by recurrent pulmonary emboli or intravascular thromboses.

In the arterial circulation, occlusion of the intracranial arteries has been reported most frequently, with the majority of patients presenting with stroke.[6,8–15,63–65] A few of our patients with high anticardiolipin antibody levels have dementia, perhaps caused by multiple small cerebral infarcts secondary to occlusion of intracranial vessels.[65a] Other thromboses have involved the coronary,[66,67] retinal,[68] mesenteric,[69] and peripheral arteries.[69,70]

Small vessels of the placenta may be affected, causing placental infarction[71–73] and fetal loss. Thrombosis of placental vessels and fetal loss are probably part of the generalized thrombotic diathesis present in some patients with antiphospholipid antibodies. Thrombosis of the renal glomeruli has been associated with the presence of lupus anticoagulant activity in patients with SLE, but similar histologic findings were found in tissue from SLE patients who did not have lupus anticoagulant activity in their plasma.[74]

Only a few case reports have recorded thrombosed vessels in patients with antiphospholipid antibodies. Although data are limited, because thrombosis occurred without cellular infiltration of blood vessel wall, it is unlikely that thrombotic occlusion of blood vessels in patients with antiphospholipid antibodies was due to vasculitis, which may be seen in other patients with connective tissue disorders.[69–75]

The hemostatic profile of patients with lupus anticoagulant activity has been documented in only a few series.[10,14] In these patients, no measurable parameters are apparent suggesting ongoing thrombosis or fibrinolysis. Because many of these patients have recurrent episodes of thrombosis after cessation of anticoagulant therapy, however,[7,12–15,76] it is likely that there is an ongoing thrombotic process, features of which may be undetectable using currently available analytic methods. Because of the persistent risk of thrombosis, it would seem advisable to treat affected patients with oral anticoagulants for as long as antiphospholipid antibodies are present. Since thrombosis occurs only in a minority of patients with antiphospholipid antibodies, there is no justification for prophylactic treatment of patients with these antibodies who have no history of thrombosis. We recommend that patients with moderate to high IgG anticardiolipin antibody levels and no history of thrombosis be monitored carefully because they have the greatest risk of thrombosis.

The role of steroids and immunosuppressive drugs in treatment of patients with antiphospholipid antibodies and thrombosis is uncertain. Such drugs have severe side effects when given for prolonged periods and we and others[10] have found that antiphospholipid antibodies are not always suppressed by these agents. Such treatment is probably justified only in patients with repeated episodes of thrombosis despite adequate anticoagulant therapy.

The association of antiphospholipid antibodies with thrombosis appears strong enough to justify proposals that antiphospholipid antibodies play a direct role in causation of thrombosis. Demonstration of such a role may be difficult, but a number of postulates, based on fragmentary evidence, have been advanced.[3] Thrombosis involves an interplay of clotting factors and their physiologic inhibitors, fibrinolytic proteins, platelets, and endothelial cells. One or more of these systems have been reported to be abnormal in patients with these antibodies. Immunoglobulin fractions from sera of patients with lupus anticoagulant activity inhibited prostacyclin release from the endothelium of umbilical veins and from cultured endothelial cells.[77] Inhibition of prostacyclin production was found in four of seven patients with lupus anticoagulant activity, but only two of these with prostacyclin inhibitory activity had a history of thrombosis.[10] Reduced fibrinolytic activity was recorded in 24 of 28 SLE patients, 12 of whom had the lupus anticoagulant;[78] increased factor VIII:C, von Willebrand factor and VIII:Ag activity were also noted.[14] These findings were taken as possible evidence for endothelial damage in patients with lupus anticoagulant activity.[14,78] Other proposals include inhibition of prekallikrein activity,[79] inhibition of antithrombin III activity,[80] and inhibition of protein C activation[81] and of thrombomodulin.[82] Because thrombocytopenia occurs frequently in patients with APS,[14,50,83,84] it has been postulated that these antibodies might bind phospholipids in platelet membranes, causing their activation, aggregation, and thrombosis.[2,83] Demonstrating the mechanism by which antiphospholipid antibodies cause thrombosis might prove as difficult as it has been to explain why these same antibodies cause in vitro prolongation of clotting times without causing hemorrhage in patients.

Fetal Loss. Most women with antiphospholipid antibodies and/or lupus anticoagulant activity appear to have high-risk pregnancies, with fetal loss being a frequent result.[5,8-15,26,41,72,73,85-100] Recurrent fetal loss in a woman with an "antithromboplastin" (the term once used for lupus anticoagulant activity) was first reported in 1975.[85] In 1980, reports of four women with lupus anticoagulant activity and recurrent fetal loss[86] and three women with lupus anticoagulant activity, thrombosis, and fetal loss appeared.[5] Several additional series of women with lupus anticoagulant activity and fetal loss have appeared since.[5,8-15,26,41,72,73,85-94] The introduction of solid-phase assays for detection of anticardiolipin antibodies has provided a more sensitive means of identifying women with antiphospholipid antibodies who may be prone to recurrent fetal loss.[26,41,73,94] A study of 40 women with SLE and related autoimmune disorders showed that 23 had a history of fetal loss. Anticardiolipin antibodies were present in 16 of 23 women with fetal loss but in only 3 of the 17 women with normal deliveries (p <0.01).[73] In a prospective study of 21 pregnant women with SLE, all 9 patients with midpregnancy fetal distress had elevated anticardiolipin antibody levels.[41] The anticardiolipin antibody test has a sensitive and specific indicator for fetal loss.[41] In another study of 121 patients, IgG anticardiolipin antibody level was found to be highly predictive for fetal loss.[26] An analysis of sera from women with recurrent fetal loss showed that the anticardiolipin antibody test was a more sensitive method of identifying women with antiphospholipid antibodies than were tests for the lupus anticoagulant.[94]

Although most women with plasma lupus anticoagulant activity have a poor obstetric outcome, some have normal pregnancies. In a survey of literature on women with lupus anticoagulant activity who had become pregnant, 89% of 43 women had one or more fetal losses.[90] In a series of 28 women with the lupus anticoagulant, there was a perinatal survival rate of only 14%.[90] In another series, fetal loss occurred in 73% of lupus anticoagulant–positive women.[15] In still another series, only 1 of 26 pregnancies in 7 women with the lupus anticoagulant had a successful out-

come.[10] None of 36 pregnancies in 12 women with lupus anticoagulant activity had a successful outcome without prednisone and aspirin therapy in another report.[72] However, not all investigators found that lupus anticoagulant activity is uniformly associated with a poor obstetric outcome. One report showed that only 3 of 10 pregnant women with the lupus anticoagulant had between one and three spontaneous abortions.[11] Of 50 lupus anticoagulant–positive pregnant SLE patients, 7 had histories of intrauterine fetal death, but 5 had normal pregnancies.[88] Our own experience and that of other clinicians[95] is that some patients with lupus anticoagulant activity can have uncomplicated pregnancies.

Because normal pregnancy outcome can occur in women with lupus anticoagulant activity, there appears to be no justification for prophylactic treatment with steroids during pregnancy unless the patient already has a history of fetal loss.

Fetal loss can occur at any stage of pregnancy; of 60 fetal losses in 23 women, 22 occurred in the first trimester, 31 in the second trimester, and 7 in the third trimester.[73] Of 36 episodes of fetal loss in 12 women, 24 occurred in the first trimester and 12 occurred in the second and third trimesters of pregnancy.[72] In a series of 28 women with the lupus anticoagulant, 51% of fetal losses occurred in the first trimester and 29% in the second trimester.[90] Because fetal loss can occur at any stage of pregnancy, treatment should be instituted *early* in the course of pregnancy if these women are to be treated at all.

Antiphospholipid antibodies with lupus anticoagulant activity are responsible for fetal loss, and platelets may be involved; consequently, steroids and aspirin have been used. Live births occurred in five of six women with histories of fetal loss who were treated during a subsequent pregnancy with doses of prednisone sufficient to suppress lupus anticoagulant activity (40 mg/day) and with aspirin (75 mg/day).[87] This experience has been extended to 16 treated pregnancies in 12 women, with live births in 10.[72] Another series of eight women with lupus anticoagulant activity and histories of fetal loss were similarly treated with high doses of steroids and aspirin, but three of them experienced fetal loss.[90] Of the five women with successful pregnancy outcomes, two had persistent lupus anticoagulant activity despite steroid therapy.[90] Two case reports of successful pregnancy outcomes after prednisone and azathioprine treatment have also been recorded.[97,98]

Some investigators have warned that the risks of administering steroids to pregnant women are serious and evidence of their efficacy in women with antiphospholipid antibodies is based on uncontrolled trials.[95,99] Complications of steroid therapy reported in these women include cushingoid facies,[72,90] acne,[90] impaired wound healing,[90] mycobacterial infection,[100a] and adrenal insufficiency.[90] Protocols using various combinations of steroids, aspirin, and subcutaneous heparin are currently being evaluated. If one form of therapy fails, it may be worthwhile to try another. We have managed a patient with features of APS who had a fetal loss despite treatment with prednisone and aspirin. In a subsequent pregnancy, the use of aspirin and dipyridamole alone, as well as careful supervision, resulted in a live baby at 32 weeks' gestation.[100b] Fetal loss can and does occur in women with autoimmune disorders other than APS, especially SLE.[92,101–103] Consequently, obstetricians and rheumatologists should consider other causes of fetal loss in women with autoimmune disorders. These women must be monitored carefully during pregnancy, whatever their treatment. They often benefit from close observation in a hospital during the final weeks of pregnancy.

Thrombosis of placental vessels resulting in placental infarction is the most popular explanation given for fetal loss in women with antiphospholipid antibodies;[8] however, thrombosis of placental vessels was not a uniform finding in one report, and placental infarction was not thought to be extensive enough to account for fetal loss.[41]

Because prostacyclin is a potent vasodilator, it is possible that if the lupus anticoagulant inhibits prostacyclin production by the endothelial cells of placental vessels, constriction of these vessels might occur, resulting in placental insufficiency and fetal growth retardation or death.[8]

Thrombocytopenia. Thrombocytopenia occurs frequently in patients with antiphospholipid antibodies.[5–14,26,50,83,84] First recognized as a complication in patients with lupus anticoagulant activity[5–14,50] it is now frequently noted in patients with high IgG anticardiolipin levels.[26] A survey of sera from patients presenting with idiopathic thrombocytopenic purpura found a small percentage with high anticardiolipin antibody levels.[84] This finding raises the possibility that patients with APS may present only with severe thrombocytopenia and will later develop fetal loss or thrombosis.[84]

When thrombocytopenia occurs in patients with APS, it is in the 50 to 150 × 10^6/L range and not severe enough to cause a hemorrhage. If a hemorrhage occurs in a patient with antiphospholipid antibodies, however, severe thrombocytopenia should be excluded as a cause of bleeding.[19,49,50]

The association of antiphospholipid antibodies with thrombocytopenia has prompted proposals that antiphospholipid antibodies might cause thrombosis by causing platelet activation and aggregation.[2] The platelet membrane is made up of phospholipids, which in some circumstances might be bound by antiphospholipid antibodies. Although an IgM monoclonal antiphospholipid antibody caused inhibition of factor Xa binding to phospholipid micelles in one study, it did not inhibit binding of factor Xa to platelet membranes,[18,19] leading to the statement that antiphospholipid antibodies could not attach to platelet membrane phospholipids because of steric hindrance. Others have found that partially disrupted platelets can bypass lupus anticoagulant activity[33,104,105] and that platelet membrane phospholipids can inhibit lupus anticoagulant activity.[105] We found that incubation of anticardiolipin-positive sera with freeze-thawed platelets inhibited binding to cardiolipin.[105a] Crude phospholipid extracts of platelets also inhibited cardiolipin binding activity; such inhibition was probably due to negatively charged phospholipids in the extract.

Admittedly, none of these studies proves that antiphospholipid antibodies mediate thrombosis through platelet activation, but the demonstrated binding of antibodies to platelet membranes raises the possibility that they might mediate platelet activation and even their destruction.[83,84] Such a mechanism must include a process by which the negatively charged phospholipid, located primarily on the inner leaflet of platelet membranes, flips to the outer leaflet, becoming available to the antiphospholipid antibody.[106] We could not show inhibition of cardiolipin binding activity by platelets unless the platelet membranes were first disrupted, perhaps exposing the inner-leaflet phospholipids.

OTHER POSSIBLE CLINICAL FEATURES OF APS

Sufficient data regarding patients have been published from diverse sources[5–16] to postulate the existence of the discrete clinical entity that we have labeled APS. Minimal criteria for this syndrome should be the presence of antiphospholipid antibodies, proven by the lupus anticoagulant test and/or by solid-phase anticardiolipin antibody test, together with one or more of the following clinical features: thrombosis, fetal loss, and thrombocytopenia (Table 70–1). Because neither of these serologic or clinical features is confined to these particular patients, there is certain to be debate as to the appropriateness of the term "antiphospholipid syndrome," but it seems useful to designate this group of patients to promote future clinical and

Table 70–1. Clinical and Serologic Features of Antiphospholipid Antibody Syndrome (APS)*

Clinical Features	Serologic Features
Venous thrombosis	IgG anticardiolipin antibody (>20 GPL units)
Arterial thrombosis	Positive lupus anticogulant test†
Recurrent fetal loss	IgM anticardiolipin antibody (>20 MPL units) plus positive lupus anticoagulant test
Thrombocytopenia	

*Patients with APS are defined as having at least one clinical and one serologic feature at some time in their disease course. An antiphospholipid test, performed more than eight weeks apart, should be positive on at least two occasions.

†Lupus anticoagulant activity should be confirmed by demonstrating inhibition by phospholipids or by freeze-thawed platelets (platelet neutralization procedure).[33,106,107]

laboratory studies. Several patients with APS also have other autoimmune disorders, in particular SLE, but as greater numbers of these patients are becoming identified, the proportion with clinically evident SLE is decreasing.

Given that antiphospholipid antibodies occur frequently, particularly when sensitive tests are used, and given the degree of overlap with other autoimmune diseases, the attribution of additional clinical or serologic features to APS must be done cautiously. Some clinicians who have examined patients with APS have suggested that transverse myelopathy,[1,107,108] leg ulcers,[4] splenomegaly,[10] migraine headaches,[22] pulmonary hypertension,[63] livedo reticularis,[22] chorea,[24] cardiac valvular lesions,[25] a Coombs' positive test,[26] and antimitochondrial antibodies (M5 pattern)[17,38] may all be features of this disorder. This list will undoubtedly grow. Prospective evaluation of a well-defined population of patients (Table 70–1) will enable us to determine whether these additional clinical and serologic features are truly part of the proposed syndrome.

IMMUNOLOGIC CHARACTERISTICS

Lupus Anticoagulant (LAC) and Anticardiolipin Antibodies. The possibility that lupus anticoagulant activity is attributable to antiphospholipid antibodies is based largely on deductive reasoning and was first suspected because patients with a positive LAC test often had a false positive serologic test for syphilis.[46,49,109] The VDRL, for example, uses diphosphatidylglycerol (cardiolipin) and phosphatidylcholine. In 1956, Laurell and Nilsson demonstrated that LAC activity could be partially absorbed out with the Kahn antigen, which contains cardiolipin.[110] Yin and

Gaston[111] and Lechner[112] demonstrated that it was the IgG and IgM immunoglobulin fractions of patient sera that had LAC activity. Several groups have shown that phospholipids can inhibit LAC activity in patient plasma[33,113,114] and it is known that the LAC test is most sensitive when phospholipid concentration and platelets (platelets presumably as a source of phospholipid) are low.[113,114] In 1980, Thiagarajan and co-workers isolated a monoclonal IgM antibody with lupus anticoagulant activity from a patient with Waldenström's macroglobulinemia and showed that this antibody bound negatively charged phospholipids.[18] In subsequent studies, they showed that IgG fractions from several patients with lupus anticoagulant activity cross-reacted with cardiolipin and other negatively charged phospholipids.[19,116]

The introduction of solid-phase assays to detect antiphospholipid antibodies has provided another means of examining antibodies with LAC activity. Most, but not all, patients with LAC activity have been found to have a positive anticardiolipin antibody test.[2] In a study of 20 LAC-positive patients, a statistically significant correlation was found between the degree of prolongation of the activated partial thromboplastin time and positivity of the anticardiolipin antibody test.[115,116] Antiphospholipid antibodies that were purified using cardiolipin liposomes[21,117] or phosphatidylserine-diacetyl phosphate-cholesterol liposomes[19,116] were shown to have LAC activity. Preincubation of anticardiolipin antibody-positive sera with negatively charged phospholipids (e.g., phosphatidylserine, phosphatidic acid, and phosphatidylinositol) inhibited cardiolipin binding activity.[20] Affinity-purified anticardiolipin antibody preparations and sera from patients with anticardiolipin antibodies bound ELISA plates coated with a variety of negatively charged phospholipids.[21]

Taken together, the data suggest that LAC activity is attributable to antiphospholipid antibodies that cross-react with negatively charged phospholipids. Antiphospholipid antibodies with LAC activity also have specificities in common with a subgroup of antibodies detected by the anticardiolipin antibody test.[2]

Increasing numbers of reports show discordance between the LAC and anticardiolipin antibody tests, however.[45,46] Derksen and colleagues reported a small series of pregnant women with a history of fetal loss in whom LAC activity normalized with steroid therapy without significant decrease in anticardiolipin antibody levels.[43]

One possible explanation is that antiphospholipid antibodies responsible for a positive LAC test are a subset of the antiphospholipid antibody population detected by the anticardiolipin antibody assay. In most solid-phase anticardiolipin assays, at high levels there may be a twofold to fourfold decrease in antibody levels with little measurable change in absorbance readings.[35] Therefore, significant decreases may occur in anticardiolipin antibody concentration that may escape detection in the anticardiolipin assay. Proper dilutions of high-positive sera to the sensitive range of the assay may solve this problem.[35] We recommend, however, that both tests be performed, particularly because high IgG anticardiolipin antibody levels appear to be more predictive than the LAC test for thrombosis[26] and fetal loss.[26,41,94] On the other hand, the LAC test may be a more sensitive indicator of response to steroid therapy.[43]

The reason some LAC-positive patients show a negative anticardiolipin antibody test is more difficult to explain. More than 90% of LAC-positive patients are also positive with the anticardiolipin antibody test, but there are clearly instances in which LAC-positive plasma gives a negative anticardiolipin test. Because the antiphospholipid antibody response in patients with autoimmune disorders is polyclonal,[118] it is possible that some clones of antiphospholipid antibodies are not detected in the anticardiolipin assay.[116] The LAC test is nonspecific, so it is also possible that antibodies other than antiphospholipid antibodies sometimes cause prolongation of the PTT. Nearly all patients we have seen with the APS have been identified by using the anticardiolipin antibody test. We believe that solid-phase assays for detection of antiphospholipid antibodies represent a more sensitive means of detecting these antibodies than does the LAC test.

Reagin. Although the antibodies produced in syphilis (reagin[2]) bind cardiolipin,[19–21,47,119–128] evidence shows that these antiphospholipid antibodies differ from those produced in patients with APS.[2] Unlike antiphospholipid antibodies in APS, reagin does not appear to cause LAC activity,[129,130] and there is no correlation between binding to cardiolipin-coated plates and VDRL titers.[21,37,39]

Reagin is usually detected by agglutination or complement fixation tests in which the antigen (the VDRL antigen) is a mixture of cardiolipin, phosphatidylcholine (PC), and cholesterol.[27] Although some recent reports suggest that reagin binds the PC portion of the VDRL antigen, evidence accumulated over 40 years suggests that reagin binds cardiolipin.

Demonstration of differences in binding properties between reagin and anticardiolipin antibodies has recently been made possible using an ELISA assay with VDRL-coated carbon particles as antigen.[47] Reagin bound both VDRL-coated and cardiolipin-coated plates, but binding to VDRL was always greater, a finding that was confirmed by inhibition studies.[47] Significantly less binding to plates coated with negatively charged phospholipids other than cardiolipin took place, however. Inhibition studies showed that negatively charged phospholipids caused less inhibition of reagin binding to VDRL than did cardiolipin. There was no significant binding of reagin to PC-coated plates and to phosphatidylethanolamine (PE)-coated plates. In contrast, APS sera did not bind VDRL-coated plates and, unlike reagin, APS sera bound plates coated with negatively charged phospholipids to the same extent as they did plates coated with cardiolipin.[21,36,47]

These experiments suggest that reagin binds cardiolipin best, particularly when cardiolipin is mixed with auxiliary lipids, but antiphospholipid antibodies in APS bind negatively charged phospholipids to an extent similar to cardiolipin. Mixing cardiolipin with auxiliary lipids probably alters its physical characteristics[127,131,132] in such a way that reagin binding is enhanced, whereas APS binding is decreased.[47]

The differences between reagin and APS antiphospholipid antibodies may have both clinical and immunologic significance. Cardiolipin is largely confined to mitochondrial membranes, but other negatively charged phospholipids are also present in cell membranes. Cross-reacting antiphospholipid antibodies from APS patients may be more likely to bind cell membranes and to affect cell function than reagin, which may explain why patients with APS develop complications such as thrombocytopenia and thrombosis while patients with syphilis are largely free from these complications. In addition, phospholipids used in the LAC test probably contain negatively charged phospholipids but little or no cardiolipin, which might explain why LAC activity is seen in APS but not in syphilis plasma.[129,130] These differences in specificities of reagin and APS antiphospholipid antibodies also suggest that the genes coding for the variable regions of these two groups of antibodies may differ, although both groups of antibodies bind cardiolipin. Support for this possibility comes from a study by Valesini and coworkers who showed that two monoclonal anti-idiotypic antibodies to an anticardiolipin antibody preparation cross-reacted with anticardiolipin and anti-ss DNA antibodies from patients with SLE but did not bind anticardiolipin antibodies from patients with syphilis.[133]

The Phosphodiester Group. Antiphospholipid antibodies bind a variety of negatively charged phospholipids that have only a phosphodiester group in common; thus, most investigators believe that the phosphodiester group is the epitope recognized by antiphospholipid antibodies.[18–21,122–127,134–138] Because phospholipids form micelles in aqueous solution with the glyceride portion of the molecule directed inward to the core of the micelle and with the phosphodiester groups directed outward, it is the phosphodiester group or substituted group (X) that is accessible to antibody binding (Fig. 70–2). If the epitope is the phosphodiester group, one must explain why antiphospholipid antibodies from APS patients do not bind phosphodiester groups of zwitterionic phospholipids and why they do not bind the phosphodiester-

FIG. 70–2. A phospholipid molecule as it may be oriented in aqueous solution. Phospholipid molecules align themselves so that the phosphodiester groups and substituted moiety (X) are directed toward the aqueous phase while the glyceride portion of the molecule forms the *hydrophobic core* of the micelle or membrane.

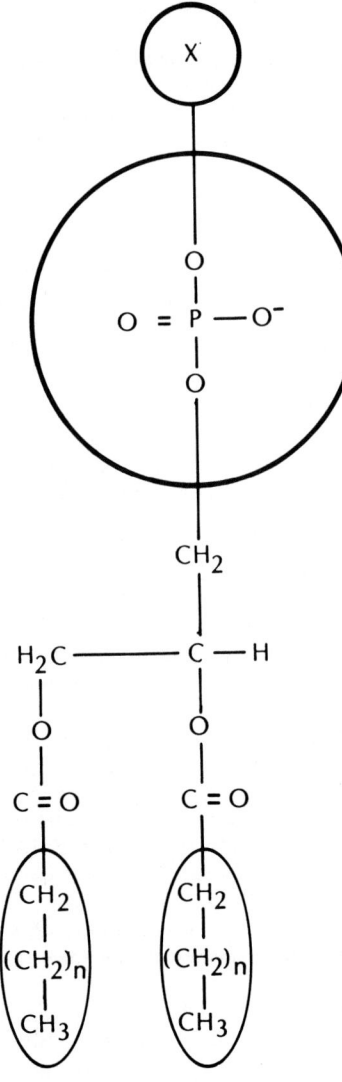

PHOSPHOLIPID

linked ribose backbone of DNA.[20,21,139] We propose that positively charged substituted groups (e.g., choline or ethanolamine) block antibody access to the phosphodiester group because of an electrostatic interaction between these two oppositely charged groups (Fig. 70–2). If the enzyme phospholipase D is used to remove the positively charged choline moiety from phosphatidylcholine so that phosphatidic acid is formed, it can be demonstrated that antiphospholipid antibodies not able to bind phosphatidylcholine will bind avidly the resulting phosphatidic acid.[47] This suggests that it is the choline moiety that blocks antibody access to the phosphodiester group of phosphatidic acid.

Although repeating negatively charged phosphodiester groups are present in the backbone of DNA, polyclonal antiphospholipid antibodies from patients with APS do not seem to bind DNA[20,21,139] and it appears that polyclonal anti-DNA antibodies from patients with SLE do not bind cardiolipin.[20,21,139,140] In contrast to these findings, some investigators have found that polyclonal antiphospholipid antibodies raised in rabbits do bind DNA,[134,139] and monoclonal anti-DNA antibodies raised in mouse-mouse hybridomas[135,136] and in human-human hybridomas[137] bind cardiolipin. Moreover, monoclonal anticardiolipin antibodies raised in mouse-mouse hybridomas bind DNA.[138] The apparent polyspecificity of these monoclonal autoantibodies and the relatively restricted specificities of polyclonal antibodies in humans with APS and syphilis seem to be the opposite of what might be expected.[141,142] Several groups of investigators are currently addressing this fascinating paradox.[142,143]

SUMMARY

Since 1980, there has been an exponential growth in publications about antiphospholipid antibodies. Although knowledge about these antibodies will increase, there will inevitably be greater confusion as claims and counter-claims are made. To minimize such confusion, we propose that patients with APS be defined as in Table 70–1. To fulfill minimal criteria for this "syndrome," patients must have both a positive antiphospholipid test and a related clinical complication. This will avoid mistreatment of patients whose sera contain antiphospholipid antibodies alone or of patients with related clinical features who may have no antiphospholipid antibodies or only slight transient increases of these antibodies, the significance of which is still uncertain. The use of one of the more recently introduced anticardiolipin antibody

ELISA tests,[35,36] calibrated with standard sera currently being distributed to laboratories that request them,[144] may enable more specific patient identification and management.

REFERENCES

1. Hughes, G.R.V.: Thrombosis, abortion, cerebral disease and the lupus anticoagulant. Br. Med. J., *287*:1088, 1983.
2. Harris, E.N., Gharavi, A.E., and Hughes, G.R.V.: Anti-phospholipid antibodies. Clin. Rheum. Dis., *11*:591, 1985.
3. Vermylen, J., Blockmans, D., Spitz, B., and Deckmyn, H.: Thrombosis and immune disorders. Clin. Haematol., *15*:393, 1986.
4. Johansson, E.A., Niemi, K.M., and Mustakallio, K.K.: A peripheral vascular syndrome overlapping with systemic lupus erythematosus. Dermatologica, *155*:257, 1977.
5. Soulier, R.P., and Boffa, M.C.: Avortements a repetition, thromboses et anticoagulant circulant antithromboplastine. Nouvelle Presse Medicale, *9*:859, 1980.
6. Mueh, J.R., Herbst, K.D., and Rapaport, S.I.: Thrombosis in patients with the lupus anticoagulant. Ann. Intern. Med., *92*:156, 1980.
7. Williams, H., Laurent, R., and Gibson, T.: The lupus coagulation inhibitor and venous thrombosis: A report of four cases. Clin. Lab. Haematol., *2*:139, 1980.
8. Carreras, L.O., and Vermylen, J.G.: "Lupus" anticoagulant and thrombosis—Possible role of inhibition of prostacyclin formation. Thromb. Haemost., *48*:28, 1982.
9. Boey, M.L., Colaco, C.B., Gharavi, A.E., et al.: Thrombosis in SLE: Striking association with the presence of circulating "Lupus anticoagulant." Br. Med. J., *287*:1021, 1983.
10. Elias, M., Eldor, A.: Thromboembolism in patients with the "lupus-like" circulating anticoagulant. Arch. Intern. Med., *144*:510, 1984.
11. Jungers, P., Liote, F., Dautzenberg, M.D., et al.: Lupus anticoagulant and thrombosis in systemic lupus erythematosus. Lancet, *i*:574, 1984.
12. Gastineau, D.A., Kazmier, F.J., Nichols, W.L., and Bowie, E.J.W.: Lupus anticoagulant: An analysis of the clinical and laboratory features of 219 cases. Am. J. Hematol., *19*:265, 1985.
13. Lechner, K., and Pabinger-Fasching, I.: Lupus anticoagulants and thrombosis. A study of 25 cases and review of the literature. Haemostasis, *15*:254, 1985.
14. Glueck, H.I., Kant, K.S., Weiss, M.A., et al.: Thrombosis in systemic lupus erythematosus: Relation to the presence of circulating anticoagulants. Arch. Intern. Med., *145*:1389, 1985.
15. Derksen, R.H., Kater, L.: Lupus anticoagulant: Revival of an old phenomenon. Clin. Exp. Rheumatol., *3*:349, 1985.
16. Gardlund, B.: The lupus inhibitor in thromboembolic diseases and intrauterine death in the absence of systemic lupus. Acta Med. Scand., *215*:293, 1984.
17. Tincani, A., Meroni, P.L., Brucato, A., et al.: Anti-phospholipid and anti-mitochondrial type M5 antibodies in systemic lupus erythematosus. J. Clin. Exp. Rheumatol., *3*:321, 1985.
18. Thiagarajan, P., Shapiro, S.S., and De Marco, L.: Monoclonal immunoglobulin M coagulation inhibitor with phospholipid specificity—Mechanism of a lupus anticoagulant. J. Clin. Invest., *66*:397, 1980.
19. Shapiro, S.S., and Thiagarajan, P.: Lupus anticoagulant. Prog. Hemost. Thromb., *6*:263, 1982.
20. Harris, E.N., Gharavi, A.E., and Loizou, S., et al.: Cross-reactivity of anti-phospholipid antibodies. J. Clin. Lab. Immunol., *16*:1, 1985.
21. Harris, E.N., et al.: Affinity purified anticardiolipin and anti-DNA antibodies. J. Clin. Lab. Immunol., *17*:155, 1985.
22. Hughes, G.R.V.: The anticardiolipin syndrome. Clin. Exp. Rheumatol., *3*:285–286, 1985.
23. Lubbe, W.F., Walker, E.B.: Chorea gravidarum with circulating lupus anticoagulant: Successful outcome of pregnancy with prednisone and aspirin therapy. Aust. N.Z. J. Med., *9*:568, 1979.
24. Asherson, R.A., et al.: Chorea in systemic lupus erythematosus and "lupus-like" disease: Association with antiphospholipid antibodies. Semin. Arthritis Rheum., *16*:253, 1987.
25. Chartash, E.K., Paget, S.A., and Lockshin, M.D.: Lupus anticoagulant associated with aortic and mitral valve disease. Arthritis Rheum. (in press).
26. Harris, E.N., et al.: Thrombosis, recurrent fetal loss, and thrombocytopenia: Predictive value of the anticardiolipin antibody test. Arch. Intern. Med., *146*:2153, 1986.
27. Catterall, R.D.: Biological false positive reactions and systemic disease. In: Ninth Symposium on Advanced Medicine. Edited by G. Walker. London, Pitman Medical, 1973, pp. 97–111.
28. Fiumara, N.S.: Biological false-positive reaction for syphilis. N. Engl. J. Med., *268*:402, 1963.
29. Moore, J.E., and Mohr, C.F.: Biologically false positive serologic tests for syphilis: Type, incidence, and cause. J. Am. Med. Assoc., *150*:467, 1952.
30. Shapiro, S.S., Thiagarajan, P., and De Marco. L.: Mechanism of action of the lupus anticoagulant. Ann. NY Acad. Sci., *370*:359, 1981.
31. Coots, M.C., Miller, M.A., and Glueck, H.I.: The lupus inhibitor: A study of its heterogeneity. Thromb. Haemost., *46*:734, 1981.
32. Exner, T.: Similar mechanism of various lupus anticoagulants. Thromb. Haemost., *53*:15, 1985.
33. Triplett, D.A., Brandt, J.T., Kaczor, D., and Shaeffer, J.: Laboratory diagnosis of lupus inhibitors: A comparison of the tissue thromboplastin inhibition procedures with a new platelet neutralization procedure. Am. J. Clin. Pathol., *79*:678, 1983.
34. Harris, E.N., et al.: Anticardioplipin antibodies: Detection by radioimmunoassay and association with thrombosis in systemic lupus erythematosus. Lancet, *ii*:1211, 1983.
35. Harris, E.N., Gharavi, A.E., Patel, S.P., and Hughes, G.R.V.: Evaluation of the anti-cardiolipin antibody test: Report of an international workshop held April 4, 1986. Clin. Exp. Immunol., *68*:215, 1987.
36. Gharavi, A.E., Harris, E.N., Asherson, R.A., and Hughes, G.R.V.: Anticardiolipin antibodies: Isotype distribution and phospholipid specificity. Ann. Rheum. Dis., *46*:1, 1987.
37. Koike, T., et al.: Anti-phospholipid antibodies and biological false positive serological tests for syphilis in patients with systemic lupus erythematosus. Clin. Exp. Immunol., *56*:193, 1984.
38. Norberg, R., et al.: Further immunological studies of sera containing anti-mitochondrial antibodies, type M5. Clin. Exp. Immunol., *58*:639, 1984.
39. Colaco, C.B., and Male, D.K.: Anti-phospholipid antibodies in syphilis and a thrombotic subset of SLE: Distinct profiles of epitope specificity. Clin. Exp. Immunol., *59*:449, 1985.
40. Meyer, O., Cyra, L., Borda-Iriarte, O., et al.: Anticorps antiphospholipids, thromboses et maladie lupique: Interet du

dosage des anticorps anticardiolipine per la methode ELISA. Revue du Rhumatisme, 52:297, 1985.

41. Lockshin, M.D., et al.: Antibody to cardiolipin as a predictor of fetal distress or death in pregnant patients with systemic lupus erythematosus. N. Engl. J. Med., 313:152, 1985.

42. Loizou, S.: et al.: Measurement of anticardiolipin antibodies by an enzyma-linked immunosorbent assay (ELISA): Standardization and quantitation of results. Clin. Exp. Immunol., 62:738, 1985.

43. Derksen, R.H.W.M., et al.: Discordant effects of prednisone on anticardiolipin antibodies and the lupus anticoagulant. Arthritis Rheum., 29:1295, 1986.

44. Lockshin, M.D.: Anticardiolipin antibody. Arthritis Rheum., 30:471, 1987.

45. Harvey, A.M., and Shulman, L.E.: Connective tissue disease and chronic biological false-positive test for syphilis. In: Lupus Erythematosus, 2nd Edition. Edited by E. Dubois. Los Angeles, University of California Press, 1974, p 196–209.

46. Feinstein, D.I., and Rapaport, S.I.: Acquired inhibitors of blood coagulation. In: Progress in Hemostasis and Thrombosis, 1st Edition. Edited by T.N. Spaet. New York, Grune and Stratton, 1972, p 75–109.

47. Harris, E.N., Gharavi, A.E., Wasley, G., and Hughes, G.R.V.: Use of an enzyme-linked immunosorbent assay and of inhibition studies to distinguish between antibodies to cardiolipin from patients with syphilis or autoimmune disorders. J. Infect. Dis., 157:23, 1988.

48. Manoharan, A., and Gottlieb, P.: Bleeding in patients with lupus anticoagulant. (Letter.) Lancet, 2:171, 1984.

49. Margolis, A., Jackson, D.P., Ratnoff, O.D.: Circulating anticoagulants: A study of 40 cases and a review of the literature. Medicine, 40:145, 1961.

50. Schleider, M.A., Nachman, R.L., Jaffe, E.A., and Coleman, H.: A clinical study of the lupus anticoagulant. Blood, 48:499, 1976.

51. Lechner, K.: Acquired inhibitors in nonhemophilic patients. Haemostasis, 3:65, 1974.

52. Loeliger, A.: Prothrombin as cofactor of the circulating anticoagulant in systemic lupus erythematosus. Thromb. et Diath. Haem., 3:237, 1959.

53. Gonyea, L., Herdman, R., Bridges, R.A.: The coagulation abnormalities in systemic lupus erythematosus. Thromb. et Diath. Haem., 20:457, 1986.

54. Rivard, G.E., Schiffman, S., Rapaport, S.I.: Cofactor of the "Lupus Anticoagulant". Thromb. et Diath. Haem., 32:554, 1974.

55. Asherson, R.A., et al.: Renal vein thrombosis in SLE: Association with the lupus anticoagulant. Clin. Exp. Rheumatol., 2:75, 1984.

56. Pomeroy, C., et al.: Budd-Chiari syndrome in a patient with the lupus anticoagulant. Gastroenterology, 86:158, 1984.

57. Hughes, G.R.V., Mackworth-Young, C.G., Harris, E.N., Gharavi, A.S.: Veno-occlusive disease in SLE: Possible association with anti-cardiolipin antibodies. (Letter.) Arthritis Rheum., 27:1017, 1984.

58. Bernstein, M.L., et al.: Thrombotic and hemorrhagic complications in children with the lupus anticoagulant. Am. J. Dis. Child., 138:1132, 1984.

59. Roudot-Thoraval, F., et al.: Budd-Chiari syndrome and the lupus anticoagulant. (Letter.) Gastroenterology, 88:605, 1985.

60. Averbach, M., and Levo, Y.: Budd-Chiari syndrome as the major thrombotic complication of systemic lupus erythematosus with the lupus anticoagulant. Ann. Rheum. Dis., 45:435, 1986.

61. Asherson, R.A., et al.: Pulmonary hypertension in systemic lupus erythematosus. Br. Med. J., 287:1024, 1983.

62. Anderson, N.E., and Ali, M.R.: The lupus anticoagulant, pulmonary thromboembolism, and fetal pulmonary hypertension. Ann. Rheum. Dis., 43:760, 1984.

63. Landi, G., Calloni, M.V., and Sabbadini, M.G.: Recurrent ischemic attacks in young adults with lupus anticoagulant. Stroke, 14:377, 1983.

64. Hart, R.G., Miller, V.T., Coull, B.M., Bril, V.: Cerebral infarction associated with lupus anticoagulant—Preliminary report. Stroke, 15:114, 1984.

65. Harris, E.N., et al.: Cerebral infarction in systemic lupus: Association with anticardiolipin antibodies. Clin. Exp. Rheumatol., 2:47, 1984.

65a. Unpublished data.

66. Asherson, R.A., MacKay, I.R., and Harris, E.N.: Myocardial infarction in young male with systemic lupus erythematosus, deep vein thrombosis, and antiphospholipid antibodies. Br. Heart J., 56:190, 1986.

67. Hamsten, A.: et al.: Antibodies to cardiolipin in young survivors of myocardial infarction: An association with recurrent cardiovascular events. Lancet, i:113, 1986.

68. Hall, S., Buettner, H., and Harvinder. L.S.: Occlusive retinal vascular disease in systemic lupus erythematosus. J. Rheumatol., 11:846, 1984.

69. Asherson, R.A., et al.: Large vessel occlusion and gangrene in systemic lupus erythematosus and "lupus-like" disease: A report of 6 cases. J. Rheumatol., 13:740, 1986.

70. Jindal, B.K., Martin, M.F., and Gayner, A.: Gangrene developing after minor surgery in a patient with undiagnosed systemic lupus erythematosus and lupus anticoagulant. Ann. Rheum. Dis., 42:347, 1983.

71. De Wolf, F., et al.: Decidual vasculopathy and extensive placental infarction in a patient with thromboembolic accidents, recurrent fetal loss and a lupus anticoagulant. Am. J. Obstet. Gynecol., 142:829, 1982.

72. Lubbe, W.F., Butler, W.S., Palmer, S.J., and Liggins, G.C.: Lupus anticoagulant in pregnancy. Br. J. Obstet. Gynaecol., 91:357, 1984.

73. Derue, G.J., Englert, H.J., Harris, E.N., and Hughes, G.R.V.: Fetal loss in systemic lupus: Association with anticardiolipin antibodies. J. Obstet. Gynaecol., 5:207, 1985.

74. Kant, K., et al.: Glomerular thrombosis in systemic lupus erythematosus: Prevalence and significance. Medicine, 60:71, 1981.

75. Asherson, R.A., et al.: Multiple venous and arterial thrombosis associated with the lupus anticoagulant and antibodies to cardiolipin in the absence of SLE. Rheumatol. Int., 5:91, 1985.

76. Asherson, R.A., et al.: Anti-cardiolipin antibody, recurrent thrombosis, and warfarin withdrawal. Ann. Rheum. Dis., 44:823, 1985.

77. Carreras, L.O., et al.: Arterial thrombosis, intrauterine death and the lupus anticoagulant: Detection of immunoglobulin interfering with prostacyclin formation. Lancet, 1:244, 1981.

78. Angeles-Cano, E., Sultan, Y., and Clauvel, J.P.: Predisposing factors to thrombosis in systemic lupus erythematosus: Possible relation to endothelial cell damage. J. Lab. Clin. Med., 94:315, 1979.

79. Sanfelippo, M.J., and Drayna, C.J.: Prekalikrein inhibition associated with the lupus anticoagulant. Am. J. Clin. Pathol., 77:275, 1982.

80. Cosgriff, T.M., and Martin, B.A.: Low functional and high antigenic anti-thrombin III level in a patient with the lupus

anticoagulant and recurrent thrombosis. Arthritis Rheum., 24:94, 1981.

81. Cariou, R., Tobelein, G., and Caen, J.: Circulating lupus-type anticoagulant, a risk factor for thrombosis by inhibition of protein C activation. C.R. Acad. Sci. (III), 303:113, 1986.

82. Comp, P.C., De Bault, L.E., Esmon, N.L., Esmon, C.T.: Human thrombomodulin is inhibited by IgG from two patients with nonspecific anticoagulants. Blood, 62 (Suppl. 1):299, 1983.

83. Harris, E.N., et al.: Thrombocytopenia in SLE and related autoimmune disorders: Association with anticardiolipin antibodies. Br. J. Haematol., 59:227, 1985.

84. Harris, E.N., et al.: Anticardiolipin antibodies in autoimmune thrombocytopenic purpura. Br. J. Haematol., 59:231, 1985.

85. Nilsson, I.M., et al.: Intrauterine death and circulating anticoagulant ("antithromboplastin"). Acta Med. Scand., 197:153, 1975.

86. Firkin, B.G., Howard, M.A., and Radford, N.: Possible relationship between lupus inhibitor and recurrent abortions in young women. Lancet, 2:366, 1980.

87. Lubbe, W.F., et al.: Fetal survival after prednisolone suppression of maternal lupus anticoagulant. Lancet, i:1361, 1983.

88. Ros, J.O., et al.: Prednisone and maternal lupus anticoagulant. (Letter.) Lancet, 2:576, 1983.

89. Prentice, R.L., et al.: Lupus anticoagulant in pregnancy. (Letter.) Lancet, 1:464, 1984.

90. Branch, W.D., et al.: Obstetric complications associated with the lupus anticoagulant. N. Engl. J. Med., 313:1322, 1985.

91. Farquharson, R.G., Pearson, J.F., and John, L.: Lupus anticoagulant and pregnancy management. (Letter.) Lancet, 2:228, 1984.

92. Clauvel, J.P., et al.: Spontaneous recurrent fetal wastage and autoimmune abnormalities: A study of fourteen cases. Clin. Immunol. Immunopathol., 39:523, 1986.

93. Cowchock, S., Smith, J.B., and Gocial, B.: Antibodies to phospholipids and nuclear antigens in patients with repeated abortions. Am. J. Obstet. Gynecol., 155:1002, 1986.

94. Lockwood, C.J., Reece E.A., Romero, R., and Hobbins, J.C.: Antiphospholipid antibody and pregnancy wastage. (Letter.) Lancet, ii:742, 1986.

95. Lockshin, M.D., and Druzin, M.L.: Antiphospholipid antibodies and pregnancy. (Letter.) N. Engl. J. Med., 313:1351, 1985.

96. Lubbe, W.F., Pattison, N., and Liggins, G.C.: Anti-phospholipid antibodies and pregnancy. N. Engl. J. Med., 313:1350, 1986.

97. Gregorini, G., Setti, G., and Remuzzi, G.: Recurrent abortion with lupus anticoagulant and pre-eclampsia: A common final pathway for two different diseases? (Case report.) Br. J. Obstet. Gynaecol., 93:94, 1986.

98. Chan, J.K.H., Harris, E.N., and Hughes, G.R.V.: Successful pregnancy following suppression of anticardiolipin antibody and lupus anticoagulant with azathioprine in systemic lupus erythematosus. J. Obstet. Gynaecol., 7:16, 1986.

99. Spitz, B., Van Assche, F.A., and Vermylen, J.: Lupus anticoagulant and pregnancy. Am. J. Obstet. Gynecol., (in press).

100. Hull, R.G., Harris, E.N., Morgan, S.H., and Hughes, G.R.V.: Anti-Ro antibodies and abortions in women with SLE. (Letter.) Lancet, 2:1138, 1983.

100a. Unpublished data.

100b. MacLachlan, N., et al. unpublished data.

101. Valesini, G., et al.: Autoimmunity and abortion. Serono Symposium No. 45, Immunological Factors in Human Reproduc-

tion. Edited by S. Shidman, F. Dondero, and M. Nicotra. London and New York, Academic Press, 1982.

102. Cowchock, S., De Horatius, R.D., Wapner, R.J., and Jackson, L.G.: Subclinical autoimmune disease and unexplained abortion. Am. J. Obstet. Gynecol., 150:367, 1985.

103. Breshihan, B., et al.: Immunological mechanism for spontaneous abortion in SLE. Lancet, 2:1205, 1977.

104. Firkin, B.G., Booth, P., Hendrix, L., and Howard, M.A.: Demonstration of a platelet by-pass mechanism in the clotting system using an acquired anticoagulant. Am. J. Hematol., 5:81, 1978.

105. Howard, M.A., and Firkin, B.G.: Investigations of the lupus-like inhibitor by-passing activity of platelets. Thromb. Haemost., 50:775, 1983.

105a. Khamashta, M. and Harris, E.N. (submitted).

106. Zwaal, R.F.A.: Membrane and lipid involvement in blood coagulation. Biochimica et Biophysica Acta, 515:163, 1978.

107. Harris, E.N., et al.: Lupoid sclerosis: A possible pathogenetic role for antiphospholipid antibodies. Ann. Rheum. Dis., 49:281, 1985.

108. Hardie, R.J., and Isenberg, D.A.: Tetraplegia as a presenting feature of systemic lupus erythematosus complicated by pulmonary hypertension. Ann. Rheum. Dis., 44:491, 1985.

109. Veltkamp, J.J., Kerkhoven, P., and Loeliger, C.A.: Circulating anticoagulant in disseminated lupus erythematosus: Proposed mode of action. Haemostasis, 2:253, 1974.

110. Laurell, A.B., and Nilsson, I.M.: Hypergammaglobulemia, circulating anticoagulant, and biological false positive Wasserman reaction: A study of two cases. J. Lab. Clin. Med., 49:694, 1957.

111. Yin, E.T., and Gaston, L.W.: Purification and kinetic studies on a circulating anticoagulant in a suspected case of lupus erythematosus. Thromb. Diathes. Haemostas., 14:88, 1965.

112. Lechner, K.: A new type of coagulation inhibitor. Thromb. Diathes. Haemorrh., 21:482, 1969.

113. Exner, T., Rickard, K.A., and Kronenberg, H.: Studies on phospholipids in the action of a lupus coagulation inhibitor. Pathology, 7:319, 1975.

114. Exner, T., Rickard, K.A., and Kronenberg, H.: A sensitive test demonstrating lupus anticoagulant and its behavioural patterns. Br. J. Haematol., 40:143, 1978.

115. Harris, E.N., et al.: Anticardiolipin antibodies and the lupus anticoagulant. Lancet, 2:1099, 1984.

116. Shapiro, S., Thiagarajan, P., and McCord, S.: Immunological specificity and mechanism of action of IgG lupus anticoagulants. Blood, 70:69, 1987.

117. Violi, F., et al.: Anticoagulant activity of anticardiolipin antibodies. Thromb. Res., 44:543–547, 1986.

118. Gharavi, A.E.: IgG subclass and light chain distribution of anti-cardiolipin and anti-DNA antibodies (submitted).

119. Pangborn, M.C.: A new serologically active phospholipid from beef heart. Proc. Soc. Exp. Biol. Med., 48:484, 1941.

120. De Bruijn, J.H.: Chemical structure and serological activity of natural and synthetic cardiolipin and related compounds. Br. J. Vener. Dis., 42:125, 1966.

121. Fowler, E., and Allen, R.H.: Studies on the production of Wasserman reagin. J. Immunol., 88:591, 1962.

122. Faure, M., and Coulon-Morelec, M.: Entre la structure clinique du cardiolipide et son activite serologique. Conservation du cardiolipide. Ann. Inst. Pasteur (Paris), 104:246, 1983.

123. Inoue, K., and Nojima, S.: Immunochemical studies of phospholipids IV: The reactions of antisera against natural cardiolipin and synthetic cardiolipin analogues-containing antigens. Chem. Phys. Lipids, 3:70, 1969.

124. Kataoka, T., and Nojima, S.: Immunochemical studies of phospholipids VI. Haptenic activity of phosphatidylinositol and the role of lecithin as an auxiliary lipid. J. Immunol., 105:502, 1970.

125. Alving, C.: Immune reactions of lipids and lipid model membranes. In: The Antigens, Vol. 4. Edited by M. Sela. New York, Academic Press, 1977.

126. Costello, P.B., and Green, F.A.: Reactivity patterns of human anticardiolipin and other antiphospholipid antibodies in syphilitic sera. Infect. Immun., 51:771, 1986.

127. Alving, C.R.: Antibodies to liposomes, phospholipids and phosphate esters. Chem. Phys. Lipids, 40:303, 1986.

128. Loizou, S., and Walport, M.J.: Antiphospholipid antibodies from patients with SLE and syphilis react homogeneously with different populations of phospholipids. (Abstract.) Br. J. Rheumatol., 25:Nov, 1986.

129. Johannson, E.A., and Lassus, A.: The occurrence of circulating anticoagulants in patients with syphilitic and biologically false positive antilipoidal antibodies. Ann. Clin. Res., 6:105, 1974.

130. Shoenfeld, Y., et al.: Circulating anticoagulant and serological tests for syphilis. Acta Derm. Venereol. (Stockh.), 60:365, 1980.

131. Takashi, T., Inoue, K., and Nojima, S.: Immune reactions of liposomes containing cardiolipin and their relation to membrane fluidity. J. Biochem., 87:679, 1980.

132. Rauch, J., et al.: Human hybridoma lupus anticoagulants distinguish between lamellar and hexagonal phase lipid systems. J. Biol. Chem., 261:9672, 1986.

133. Valesini, G., et al.: Use of monoclonal antibodies to identify shared idiotypes on anticardiolipin and anti-DNA antibodies in human sera. Clin. Exp. Immunol., 70:18, 1987.

134. Guarnieri, M., and Eisner, D.: A DNA antigen that reacts with antisera to cardiolipin. Biochem. Biophys. Res. Commun., 58:347, 1974.

135. Lafer, E.M., et al.: Polyspecific monoclonal lupus autoantibodies reactive with both polynucleotides and phospholipids. J. Exp. Med., 153:897, 1981.

136. Koike, T., et al.: Specificity of mouse hybridoma antibodies to DNA II. Phospholipid reactivity and biological false positive serological test for syphilis. Clin. Exp. Immunol., 57:345, 1984.

137. Shoenfeld, Y., et al.: Polyspecificity of monoclonal lupus autoantibodies produced by human-human hybridomas. N. Engl. J. Med., 308:414, 1983.

138. Rauch, J., Tannenbaum, H., Stoller, B.D., and Schwarz, R.S.: Monoclonal anticardiolipin antibodies bind DNA. Eur. J. Immunol., 14:529, 1984.

139. Eilat, D., Zlotnick, A.Y., and Fischell, R.: Evaluation of the cross-reaction between anti-DNA and anti-cardiolipin antibodies in SLE and experimental animals. Clin. Exp. Immunol., 65:269, 1986.

140. Edberg, J.C., and Taylor, R.P.: Quantitative aspects of lupus anti-DNA autoantibody specificity. J. Immunol., 136:4581, 1986.

141. Eilat, D.: Anti-DNA antibodies: Problems in their study and interpretation. Clin. Exp. Immunol., 65:215, 1986.

142. Emlen, W., Pisetsky, D.S., and Taylor, R.P.: Antibodies to DNA: A perspective. Arthritis Rheum., 29:1417, 1986.

143. Smeenk, R.J.T., Lucassen, W.A.M., and Swaak, T.J.G.: Is anticardiolipin activity a cross-reaction of anti-DNA or a separate entity? Arthritis Rheum., 30:607, 1987.

144. Harris, E.N., Gharavi, A.E., and Hughes, G.R.V.: Anticardiolipin antibody testing: the need for standardization. Arthritis Rheum., 30:835, 1987.

MIXED CONNECTIVE TISSUE DISEASE

71

GORDON C. SHARP and BERNHARD H. SINGSEN

Some patients have features of more than one rheumatic disease and thus do not fit into traditional classifications. Patients with a combination of clinical findings similar to those of systemic lupus erythematosus (SLE), progressive systemic sclerosis (PSS), polymyositis, and rheumatoid arthritis (RA), and with unusually high titers of a circulating antinuclear antibody with specificity for a nuclear ribonucleoprotein antigen, are considered to have *mixed connective tissue disease* (MCTD).[1]

Initial observations of MCTD suggested infrequent renal disease, a good response to corticosteroids, and a favorable prognosis.[1,2] Further study has shown, however, that renal disease occurs in 10 to 20% of patients, that some patients may require aggressive or prolonged pharmacologic intervention, and that pulmonary involvement is common. Pulmonary hypertension, associated with proliferative vascular lesions, may be a serious complication. The prognosis, therefore, is not always favorable.[3–7]

SEROLOGIC ALTERATIONS

When subjected to a sensitive passive hemagglutination test, all patients in the original study of MCTD had high titers of antibody to a nuclear antigen extractable in isotonic buffers (ENA).[1,8] Antibodies to ENA were detected in about half of a series of patients with SLE, although usually at reduced titers, and the reported incidence of ENA antibodies was also low in other rheumatic disorders.[1,8] Treatment of ENA-coated red blood cells with ribonuclease (RNase) reduced or eliminated the agglutination reaction in serum from patients with MCTD, but had little or no effect on serum from patients with SLE.[1]

Immunodiffusion studies subsequently revealed that ENA consisted of at least two distinct antigens, one sensitive to RNase and trypsin, which appeared to be a nuclear ribonucleoprotein (nRNP), and the previously described Sm antigen,[2,9–11] which is resistant to RNase and trypsin. Sera that reacted with either the nRNP antigen or the Sm antigen produced a speckled, fluorescent antinuclear antibody pattern.[1,9,12] Treatment of the tissue substrate with RNase eliminated the antinuclear antibody reaction due to anti-nRNP, however.[1,9,12]

Most investigations have shown that sera containing nRNP antibodies in high titer and no Sm antibodies are usually found in patients with MCTD, are uncommon in patients with SLE or PSS, and are rare in patients with polymyositis, RA, or other rheumatic diseases.[1,2,12–17] That some patients with high nRNP antibody titers initially appear to have another rheumatic disorder and then in several years develop additional clinical features typical of MCTD suggests a predictive value of this serologic pattern for evolving MCTD.[1,6,12,15,17,18]

The typical serologic pattern in MCTD includes high titers of speckled antinuclear antibodies, often >1:1000, high levels of antibody to RNase-sensitive ENA by hemagglutination, frequently >1,000,000, and nRNP antibody by immunodiffusion. Sm antibodies and high antinative DNA titers are infrequent in MCTD, and their appearance usually correlates with a severe flare of SLE-like features.[3,6,17,20] Rheumatoid agglutinins occur in over half the patients with MCTD, and titers are often high.[12,17] Diffuse hypergammaglobulinemia, ranging from 2 to >5 g/dl, may be present.[1,12,21] Serum complement levels are usually normal or only modestly reduced.[1,12,17,22]

Rarely, patients with clinical features of MCTD have no nRNP antibody initially.[1,3,12,23] This test may subsequently become positive, sometimes after corticosteroid therapy.[1,12,23] Such a serologic evolution may relate to the presence of circulating immune complexes, often detected by Raji cell or C1q binding assays; these immune complexes may bind available nRNP antibody, with subsequent dissociation. Once present, high titers of circulating anti-nRNP usually persist during periods of active and inactive disease, but in some patients, these antibody levels fall or become undetectable in 5 to 11 years.[6] This phenomenon is more often seen after prolonged remission, and is less frequent in active disease.

Recent studies performed in several laboratories have further elucidated the nature of the nRNP and Sm antigens. Antibodies to nRNP immunoprecipitate U1 snRNA-protein complexes, whereas anti-Sm antibodies immunoprecipitate snRNA-protein complexes containing U1, U2, U4, U5, and U6 snRNAs.[24] Immunoblotting studies have shown that anti-U1 RNP antibodies react with peptides designated 68K, A, and C, whereas anti-Sm antibodies react with the B/B' and D peptides. Several reports indicate that anti-68K peptide antibodies are associated with anti-U1 RNP antibodies in MCTD, but rarely occur in SLE.[25–27] A longitudinal study demonstrated the serologic persistence of MCTD peptide patterns over many years and their subsequent disappearance in patients who were in prolonged remission.[25]

CLINICAL FEATURES

These features include prevalence, course, and specific clinical manifestations.

PREVALENCE AND CLINICAL COURSE

MCTD occurs in patients ranging from 4 to 80 years, with a mean of 37 years; approximately 80% of patients are female.[12,15] MCTD may occur as frequently as scleroderma, more commonly than polymyositis, and less frequently than SLE. Typical clinical features of MCTD (Table 71–1) include polyarthritis, Raynaud's phenomenon, swollen hands or sclerodactyly,

pulmonary disease, muscle disease, and esophageal hypomotility.[6] Lymphadenopathy, alopecia, malar rash, serositis, and cardiac and renal disease are less frequent findings. No particular racial or ethnic distribution has been noted.

In some patients, the typical overlapping pattern is fully expressed when they are first evaluated. As physicians appreciate more fully the association of anti-U1 RNP antibody with MCTD, however, larger numbers of cases are identified at an early phase of disease. Initially, minimal symptoms such as Raynaud's phenomenon, arthralgias, myalgias, and swollen hands may be insufficient to make a definitive diagnosis. This constellation of clinical findings has been referred to as *undifferentiated connective tissue disease*.[6,28] Long-term followup study reveals that this pattern may persist for years in some patients; in others it may progress to PSS, whereas yet other patients develop additional manifestations resulting in MCTD.[3,6,15,18,22] In one prospective study, 60% of patients were initially thought to have RA, PSS, SLE, polymyositis, or undifferentiated connective tissue disease[6] (Table 71–2). At their most recent evaluation, 91% demonstrated typical overlapping features of MCTD, whereas 9% maintained their undifferentiated status.

Table 71–1. Characteristics of 34 Patients with Mixed Connective Tissue Disease

Characteristic	Number	Percentage
Raynaud's phenomenon	31	91
Polyarthritis	29	85
Swollen hands or sclerodactyly	29	85
Pulmonary disease	29	85
Inflammatory myositis	27	79
Esophageal hypomotility	25	74
Lymphadenopathy	17	50
Alopecia	13	41
Pleuritis	12	35
Malar rash	10	29
Renal disease	9	26
Cardiac disease	9	26
Anemia	8	24
Leukopenia	7	21
Diffuse scleroderma	7	21
Sjögren's syndrome	4	12
Trigeminal neuropathy	2	6
Positive antinuclear antibody	34	100
Positive ribonucleoprotein antibody	34	100
Positive rheumatoid agglutinins	20	59
Hypergammaglobulinemia	18	53
Hypocomplementemia	11	32
Positive LE cell test	6	18

(From Sullivan, W.D., et al.[6])

Table 71–2. Transitions in Mixed Connective Tissue Disease in Longitudinal Study

Disease Classification	No. Classified at Initial Medical Evaluation	No. Classified at Latest Medical Evaluation
Polymyositis	1	0
Progressive systemic sclerosis	2	0
Adult or juvenile rheumatoid arthritis	4	0
Systemic lupus erythematosus	6	0
Undifferentiated connective tissue disease	7	3
Mixed connective tissue disease	14	31

(From Sullivan, W.D., et al.[6])

DIAGNOSTIC CRITERIA AND CLASSIFICATION

At an International Symposium on MCTD and Antinuclear Antibodies (Tokyo, August, 1986), three sets of diagnostic criteria were introduced.[29–31] Major criteria included myositis, pulmonary involvement, Raynaud's phenomenon, swollen hands or sclerodactyly, and high titer anti-U1 RNP antibody. Preliminary testing has suggested high sensitivity and specificity, but more detailed testing is needed.

SPECIFIC MANIFESTATIONS

Skin

Swelling of the hands and fingers occurs in over two thirds of patients with MCTD, resulting in a tapered or "sausage" appearance[1,2,12,15,22,32] (Fig. 71–1). The skin may be taut and thick, with histologic changes of marked edema and increased dermal collagen content.[1] Scleroderma-like changes are occasionally extensive, but diffusely involved or tightly bound skin with contractures is rare.[1,12] In 40% of patients, lupus-like rashes occur, including malar eruptions; diffuse, nonscarring erythematous lesions; and chronic, scarring discoid lesions[1,12,15,22] (Fig. 71–2). Other findings include alopecia, areas of hyper- and hypopigmentation, periungual telangiectasia, "squared" telangiectasia over the hands and face, violaceous discoloration of the eyelids, and erythema over the knuckles, elbows, or knees.[1,12,15,22] Severe necrotic and ulcerative skin changes are seen only rarely.[1,12] Immunoglobulin deposits at the dermal-epidermal junction have been noted in some patients.[1,22]

FIG. 71–1. Hands of a patient with mixed connective tissue disease demonstrating the tapered or sausage appearance of fingers and erythematous discoloration over the metacarpophalangeal, proximal interphalangeal, and distal interphalangeal joints.

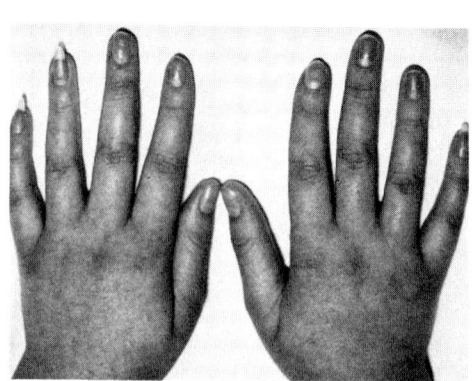

FIG. 71–2. Facial rash of MCTD; the violaceous periorbital rash is suggestive of dermatomyositis, whereas the malar rash is more commonly seen in SLE.

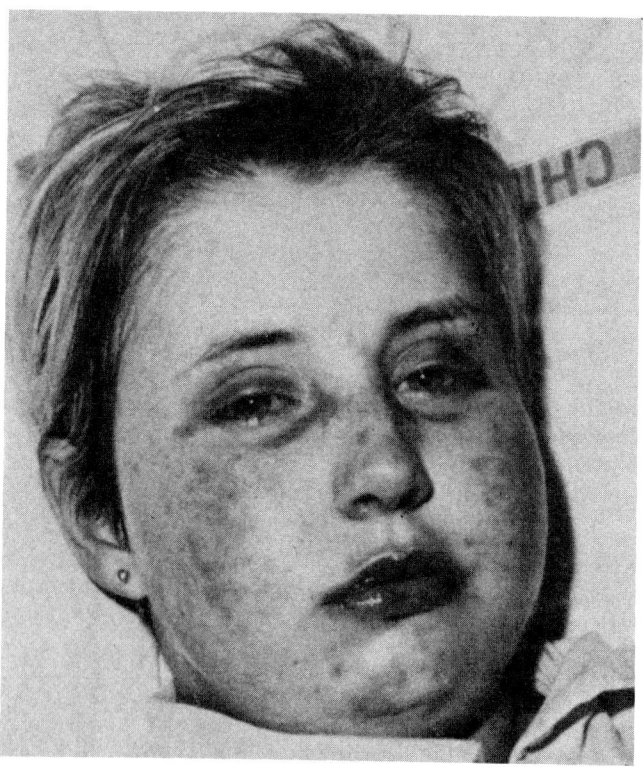

Raynaud's Phenomenon

Paroxysmal vasospasm of the fingers and, less often, the toes occurs in approximately 85% of patients with MCTD and may precede other manifestations of the disease by months to years.[1,2,12,15,22,32] Severe vasospasm and ischemic necrosis or ulceration of the fingertips, common in PSS, are rare in MCTD.[1,22,33] However, two reports showed dilated capillary changes, with avascular areas, in 50 to 90% of MCTD patients,[33,34] and a study using hand angiography revealed organic obstruction in 60% of ulnar arteries, 87% of superficial arches, and 65% of digital arteries.[33] These findings provide further evidence for vasculopathy in some patients with MCTD.

Joints

Polyarthralgias occur in most patients, and frank arthritis is seen in about three quarters of those affected.[1,12,15,35,36] Although the arthritis is often nondeforming, its features may be similar to those of RA with flexion contractures, ulnar deviation and swanneck deformities.[1,35–37] The metacarpophalangeal, proximal interphalangeal, and carpal joints are frequently affected. Subcutaneous nodules and roentgenographic evidence of erosive changes are sometimes observed.[1,18,37] Tightness of the extrinsic flexors of the hands related to volar tenosynovitis may be particularly prominent in MCTD.[38]

Muscles

Proximal muscles are commonly tender and weak, and serum levels of creatine phosphokinase and aldolase may be elevated at some point in the course of MCTD.[1,2,12,39] Electromyographic findings are typical of inflammatory myositis, and biopsies reveal muscle fiber degeneration and perivascular and interstitial infiltration of plasma cells and lymphocytes.[1,5,12,15,39] Even in patients with only mild muscular weakness, histochemical and immunofluorescent analyses reveal perifascicular atrophy, type I fiber predominance, and immunoglobulin deposition within normal-appearing vessels, within normal fibers, around or on the sarcoplasmic membrane, or within the perimysial connective tissues.[39]

Esophagus

Esophageal abnormalities are frequent in MCTD.[1,12,32,40] Systematic studies of 35 patients by cine-esophagram or manometry revealed dysfunction in 80%, but 70% of these patients had no history of esophageal problems.[40] Decreased peristaltic amplitude in the distal two thirds of the esophagus and reduced upper and lower esophageal sphincter pressures are characteristic changes. The severity of measured esophageal dysfunction appears to correlate with the duration of the disease, but not necessarily with the expression of symptoms.[15,17,40] Reflux esophagitis, sometimes leading to ulceration and stricture, may occur.

Lungs

Pulmonary dysfunction is usually clinically silent in the early phases of MCTD and may go undetected unless detailed evaluations are performed. A prospective study reported in 1976 showed that 80% of patients with MCTD had pulmonary disease, but 69% were asymptomatic.[41] Serial followup of those treated with corticosteroids revealed clinical and physiologic improvement in 12 of 14. It has since become apparent that pulmonary involvement in MCTD may lead to serious exertional dyspnea or to pulmonary hypertension, particularly in the later stages of the disease.[6] Hemoptysis and dysfunction of the diaphragm have also been reported.[42,43]

Pulmonary hypertension associated with proliferative pulmonary vascular lesions was frequent and serious in a longitudinal evaluation of 34 individuals with MCTD.[6] The most common clinical finding was dyspnea, followed by pleuritic pain and bibasilar rales. Of 11 asymptomatic patients, 8 (73%) had abnormal pulmonary function tests or chest roentgenograms. Single-breath diffusing capacity (DLCO) was abnormal in 73%, and the vital capacity was reduced in 33%. These findings have been confirmed.[44] Total lung capacity was low in 41%, and FEV_1 was abnormal in 17%; resting hypoxemia was present in 21% of patients. *Radiographic abnormalities* consisting of small, irregular opacities predominantly in the bases and middle regions occurred in 30%.[6] These findings underscore the fact that pulmonary involvement in MCTD is common and may be clinically inapparent until far advanced.

Right-heart catheterization was performed on 15 of the 34 patients in our longitudinal study.[6] Ten had elevated pulmonary vascular resistance, and ten had increased pulmonary artery pressure; wedge pressure was only abnormal in one patient. This study suggested that MCTD patients with features similar to those of PSS are more likely to develop pulmonary hypertension. Additionally, nailfold capillaroscopy in three of these patients showed severe capillary loop changes before pulmonary symptoms were present. All three patients subsequently developed pulmonary vascular disease. Thus, *nailfold changes may predict pulmonary hypertension in MCTD.*

Heart

Cardiac involvement appears to be less common than pulmonary disease in adult MCTD, but it may be frequent in children.[1,12,15] Pericarditis is the most common cardiac abnormality reported.[15,45,46] In a prospective study of 37 adults with MCTD, pericarditis or pericardial effusion occurred in 10 patients, pulmonary hypertension was present in 10 of 15, and mitral valve prolapse occurred in 9 patients. Electrocardiographic abnormalities include arrhythmias, chamber enlargement, and conduction defects.[42] The prognostic significance of these cardiac findings is unclear.

Kidneys

Longer followup suggests that renal disease is more frequent in MCTD than initially thought. When isolated case reports are excluded, recent studies give a combined incidence of renal involvement of 28%, including children.[15,47-49] Glomerular deposition of immune complexes may be observed, although the patterns differ from those of SLE.[50,51] Patients with MCTD occasionally die of progressive renal failure.[47]

In a longitudinal study of MCTD, six patients had clinical evidence of renal disease manifested by proteinuria or hematuria: one developed the nephrotic syndrome.[6] Two renal biopsies showed focal glomerulonephritis. The kidney disease responded well to corticosteroid therapy, and renal failure did not occur. At autopsy, three patients without clinical manifestations of renal disease had proliferative vascular lesions similar to those noted in other organs; the glomeruli were normal in two of these patients, and mesangial thickening and hypercellularity were noted in the third. In a recent report,[5] 7 of 15 children with MCTD had clinical or histologic evidence of renal disease, and a patient in another study had died of "scleroderma kidney."[3] Comparable levels of circulating immune complexes in MCTD and SLE are observed,[20,52] but the clinical and histologic findings suggest that vascular lesions may represent a more serious problem than immune complex nephritis in MCTD.

Nervous System

Neurologic abnormalities, noted in only 10% of patients with MCTD, are not usually major management problems.[12,15,37,53] Trigeminal neuropathy is the most frequent finding.[12,17] Other observed problems include organic mental syndromes, "vascular" headaches, aseptic meningitis, seizures, encephalopathy, multiple peripheral neuropathies, and cerebral infarction or hemorrhage, probably related to hypertension and atherosclerosis.[12,15,17,53-55]

Blood

Anemia and leukopenia are found in a third of patients with MCTD.[1,12,32] Coombs-positive hemolytic anemia and significant thrombocytopenia are rare;[1,12,56] however, in a report of 14 children with MCTD, 6 had severe thrombocytopenia.[15] Two of these patients required splenectomy because persistent, severe thrombocytopenia, which had previously responded to corticosteroids, could only be controlled by 2 mg/kg/day prednisone. One child with thrombocytopenia died of an intracranial hemorrhage. Diminished granulocyte chemotaxis also occurs in children and adults with MCTD and may be associated with the sudden onset of unexpectedly severe infections.[57]

Other Findings

Sjögren's syndrome occurs frequently in MCTD,[58] and Hashimoto's thyroiditis and persistent hoarseness are observed occasionally in both children and adults.[5,17] Fever and lymphadenopathy occur in about one third of patients.[1,12,22] Lymph nodes may be massively enlarged and may suggest a lymphoma, but biopsy reveals only lymphoid hyperplasia. Hepatomegaly and splenomegaly are possible, but serious liver function disturbances are uncommon. The intestinal tract may manifest hypomotility, pseudosacculation, dilatation, malabsorption, secretory diarrhea, sclerosis, and perforation.[59-62] In one report, three patients with MCTD had extensive gastrointestinal changes similar to those found in PSS;[63] these changes have also been observed in children.[15]

CHILDHOOD DISEASE

Since 1973, 14 reports of pediatric MCTD have been published.[15,64,65] These studies encompass 54 children, with an additional 15 patients, <16 years of age, briefly mentioned in other reports but whose clinical features and treatment responses could not be isolated from the larger groups of adults. In a large pediatric rheumatic disease service, MCTD was 10% as frequent as SLE and occurred once for every 100 children with juvenile RA (JRA). The median age of onset of MCTD in children is 10.8 years (range: 4 to 16 years); 43 girls and 11 boys have been reported.[37,66-68]

MCTD in children has several distinguishing features: (1) dermatomyositis and SLE-like rashes more common than in adults[15,50] (Fig. 71–2); (2) thrombocytopenia in about 25%; (3) a higher frequency of cardiac disease, especially pericarditis (44%), than in adults;[15,69,70] and (4) clinical and histologic evidence of renal disease, which is more common in pediatric MCTD.[15,69,71] In our experience, 6 of 19 children developed significant renal disease, including 2 who eventually required long-term hemodialysis. In all childhood cases, 18 of 37 (49%) eventually developed clinically evident renal involvement.

Deforming, painless arthritis and the presence of rheumatoid factor are common in childhood MCTD.[15,50,71] Synovitis is moderate, but complaints of discomfort are usually not marked in children; thus, responses to treatment may appear better than they actually are. Erosive disease is uncommon in children, but flexion contractures and deformity may occur.

Because Sjögren's syndrome is rare in children with rheumatic diseases, it is infrequently or incompletely sought in pediatric MCTD. At least half of carefully assessed children with MCTD have xerostomia, parotid gland enlargement, or keratoconjunctivitis sicca.[5,58] These findings suggest that salivary gland evaluation, Schirmer's test, and lip biopsy should be considered in all children with possible MCTD.

MCTD in children is frequently a sequential disease. The majority initially manifest Raynaud's phenomenon and polyarthritis. They then develop other features of MCTD, progressively but not in any particular order. Serologic findings may also change over time, commensurate with the clinical situation. Thus, the absence of antinuclear antibodies and the presence of rheumatoid factor may be associated with early polyarthropathy, whereas anti-Sm antibodies may appear along with renal disease, hypocomplementemia, and other features of SLE.[5]

Many of the features of MCTD in children are initially silent and may remain undetected unless carefully sought. The limited verbal skills, memory, and experiential understanding of children may magnify this observation. These asymptomatic features include the following: (1) minimal muscle disease with mild atrophy, moderate serum muscle enzyme elevations, and perhaps electromyographic changes, but with no significant proximal weakness; (2) esophageal dysfunction; (3) minimal alterations in bowel habits, related to early gastrointestinal tract involvement; and (4) pulmonary function test abnormalities found prior to complaints or roentgenographic changes. Children do not usually complain of dyspnea or shortness of breath. Thus, *pulmonary function testing should be part of the routine evaluation of any child in whom a diagnosis of MCTD is considered.* Overall, 23 of 38 children (61%) with MCTD have showed radiographic and pulmonary function abnormalities; 30% developed pulmonary hypertension. Pulmonary hypertension and idiopathic fibrosis must be recognized as potentially life-threatening.[15,69,72]

HISTOLOGIC AND IMMUNOPATHOLOGIC FEATURES

HISTOLOGIC MANIFESTATIONS

The first comprehensive histologic investigation of MCTD reviewed material from three autopsies and

from five additional renal biopsies.[5] The study group included 15 children with MCTD with a median age of disease onset of 10.7 years; the three who died had had the disease for 5.4 years before histologic evaluation. The age of these patients, the short duration of their disease, the absence of systemic or pulmonary hypertension, and the lack of corticosteroid treatment are relevant because, in adult patients, all would be variables that could cause, or reduce, the observed vasculopathy.

Widespread proliferative vascular lesions were the most prominent histopathologic features in the patients studied. All three children had diffuse vasculopathy; in combination, 9 organs (16%) revealed medial vessel wall thickening, and 31 of 58 organs (53%) had intimal proliferation (Fig. 71–3). These abnormalities occurred in large vessels such as the renal artery and aorta and within small arterioles. This vasculopathy has been shown angiographically in digital, radial, and ulnar arteries as well.[33]

The frequency and severity of vascular compromise in organs without overt evidence of clinical involvement was striking and included coronary vessels, myocardium, aorta, lungs, intestinal tract, and kidney (Fig. 71–4). Inflammatory infiltration of vessels was not a prominent feature.[5] Similar obstructive vascular lesions, particularly in the lungs, have now been described in MCTD in adults.[6,7,19] Thus, the presence of pulmonary hypertension in MCTD appears to be related to marked luminal vessel narrowing, rather than to interstitial fibrosis.

Other pathologic alterations in MCTD include prominent lymphocytic and plasmacytic infiltration of salivary glands, liver, and gastrointestinal tract, and a widespread inflammatory myopathy. Cardiac myopathy has been found in a few patients with MCTD,[5,45,73] but its prevalence is not yet known.

Our histopathologic understanding of MCTD is developing slowly. The absence of fibrinoid change, a predilection for large-vessel involvement, and minimal fibrosis all suggest fundamental differences from scleroderma. Evidence suggests a widespread but largely silent vasculopathy, cardiac and skeletal myopathy, membranoproliferative nephropathy, and pulmonary and gastrointestinal involvement in MCTD. Prospective histopathologic studies with serial treatment observations are necessary to determine whether current expectations of MCTD morbidity and mortality are overly optimistic.

IMMUNOLOGY

The immunologic aberrations identified in MCTD suggest that immune injury mechanisms are involved

FIG. 71–3. Photomicrograph of a section of coronary artery from a 14-year-old boy with mixed connective tissue disease, showing intimal thickening, medial proliferation, and luminal narrowing. (Hematoxylin-eosin stain; magnification ×566.)

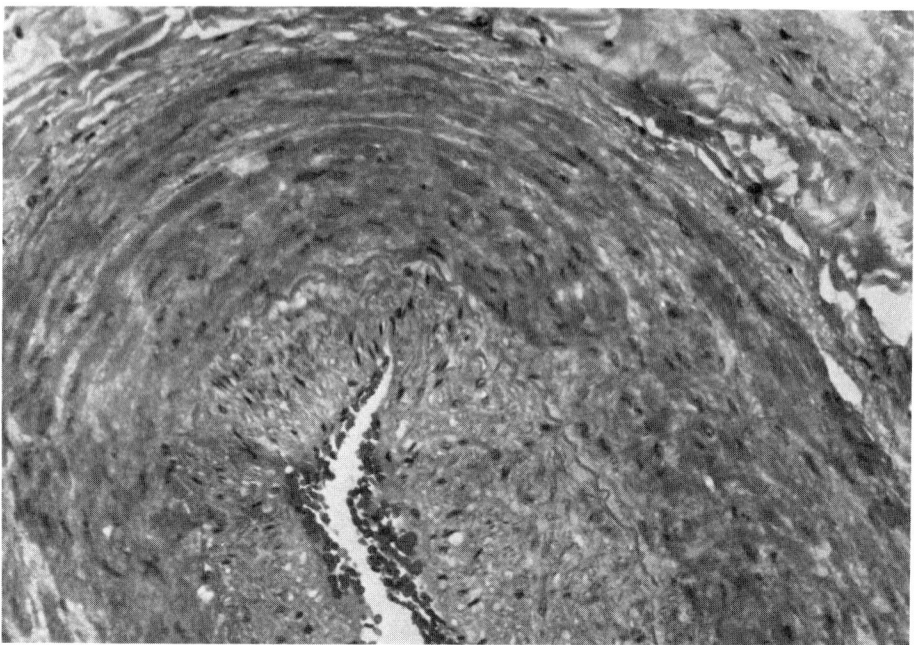

in the pathogenesis of the disease. The persistence of high titers of ribonucleoprotein antibody for many years and a marked polyclonal hypergammaglobulinemia indicate B-cell hyperactivity. Alarcon-Segovia has compared the immunoregulatory characteristics of MCTD and other connective tissue diseases.[74] MCTD patients frequently had lymphopenia and diminished total T-lymphocytes. Subpopulations of T-lymphocytes that may be diminished include T4 (helper-inducer), T8 (cytotoxic-suppressor), or both, and Tγ cells. Despite increased numbers of post-thymic precursor cells (which suggests normal serum thymic factor), concanavalin-A-induced suppression and spontaneously expanded suppression functions were both diminished. NK cell function may be normal (although less responsive to IL-2 induction), and production of IL-1, IL-2, BCGF, and BCDF was either normal or increased in MCTD. Stimulation of T-cell circuits toward increased help could result in B-cell stimulation and anti-U1 RNP antibody production. Differences in these immunoregulatory functions among MCTD and SLE, Sjögren's syndrome, PSS, and RA support the concept of MCTD as a distinct entity.[21,74]

Other observations in MCTD include reduced serum complement levels in about 25% of patients,[17] circulating immune complexes during active disease,[20,52,75] and deposition of IgG, IgM, and complement within muscle fibers, in the sarcolemmal-basement membrane region, in vascular walls, and along the glomerular basement membrane.[17,39]

Frank, et al. studied 18 patients with MCTD. Most had active disease; only 4 had defective reticuloendothelial system Fc-specific immune clearance, although 17 had circulating immune complexes detected by Raji cell and C1q binding assay.[20] The 4 patients with defective clearance had an illness that, at that time, more closely resembled typical SLE, with antibodies to Sm or DNA, higher levels of immune complexes, glomerulonephritis, and severe skin lesions. Renal disease was absent in the 14 patients with normal clearance of the reticuloendothelial system. The maintenance of normal reticuloendothelial function in classic MCTD may enable these patients to clear immune complexes and thus to avoid serious renal damage.

A solid-phase radioimmunoassay for the detection of U1 RNP immune complexes[76] showed many U1 RNP immune complexes in the pericardial fluid, but not in the serum, of an MCTD patient with acute hemorrhagic pericarditis.[77] These data suggest that locally formed U1 RNP immune complexes may have played an important role in the development of pericarditis.

TREATMENT AND PROGNOSIS

Treatment recommendations have been based largely on anecdotal information because no con-

FIG. 71–4. Small serosal artery from the ileocecal region; this child with MCTD had no signs or symptoms of gastrointestinal disturbance. There is striking intimal proliferation and luminal occlusion, but no inflammatory infiltrate. (Hematoxylin and eosin stain; magnification ×466.)

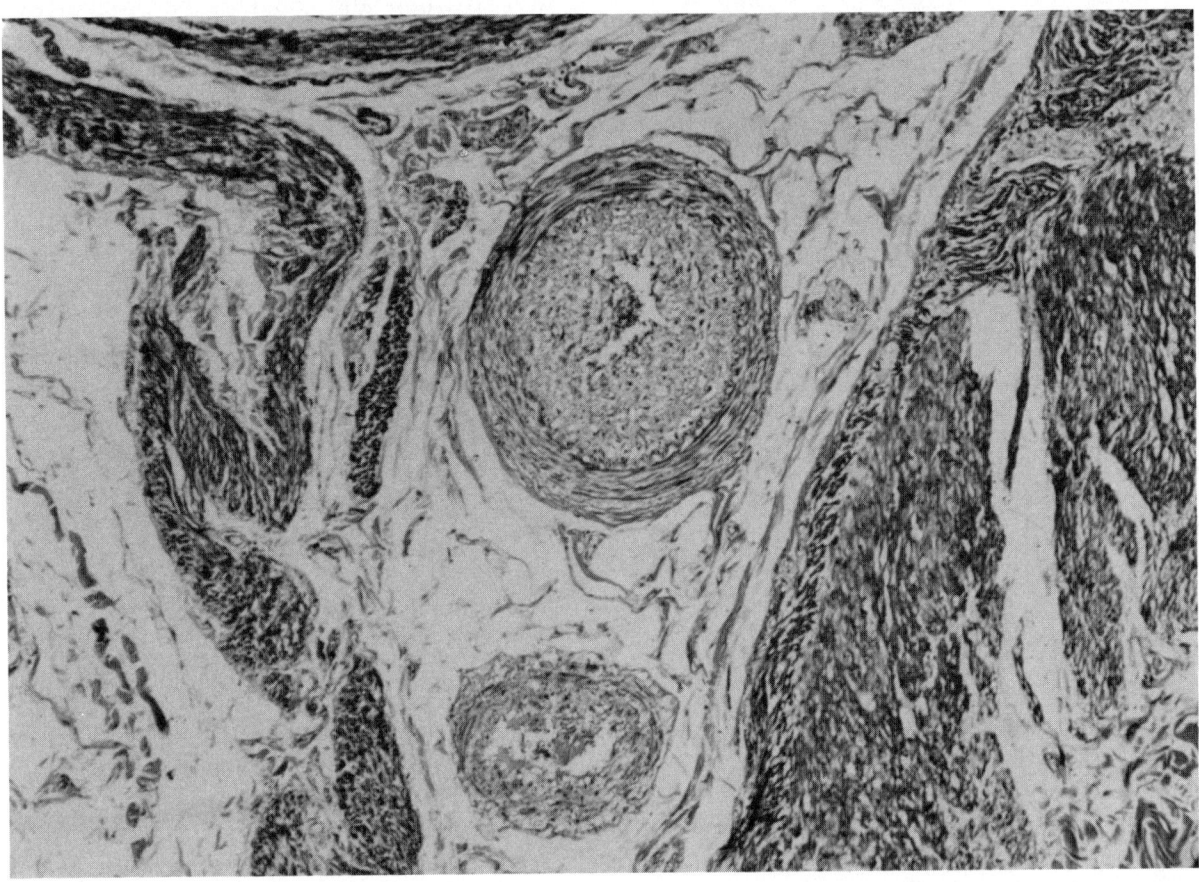

trolled, long-term evaluations exist. Because MCTD is a progressive disease, different therapies may be appropriate for the same patient over a period of several years. For example, some children and adults initially respond to intramuscular gold for RA-like or JRA-like features, then improve with corticosteroids when proximal muscle weakness develops, and finally require cytotoxic agents for renal disease.[15]

Originally, MCTD was described as responsive to corticosteroids, although a few patients who did not respond to high doses of corticosteroids improved after the addition of cyclophosphamide. Further observations do not support a uniformly optimistic outlook, however. In extended investigations, almost two thirds of patients have responded favorably to treatment.[6] Patients with scleroderma-like features are the least likely to improve. A potentially good long-term prognosis for MCTD is demonstrated by the 13 of 34 (38%) patients studied who have inactive disease, including 10 who have not required therapy for 1 to 8

years (mean 5 years). Inflammatory changes are likely to respond to corticosteroids, whereas pulmonary, sclerodermatous, and esophageal lesions are less likely to respond.

Of our patients, 36% have had less corticosteroid-responsive and more severe illness; 4 patients died. Pulmonary hypertension and widespread proliferative vasculopathy are major complications of MCTD that have emerged from several investigations. The pulmonary hypertension may or may not respond to corticosteroids or immunosuppressive agents, but without controlled studies, the most appropriate therapies remain uncertain.

Patterns of organ system involvement may be a useful guide to therapy. Arthritis may occur well before other overlapping manifestations suggest MCTD.[36] As the erosive and deforming potential of MCTD has been better recognized, so has the value of the early use of agents such as gold and penicillamine. The arthritis has responded to nonsteroidal anti-inflammatory drugs in some centers,[35] but others have not had similar success.[78] Rash, serositis, anemia, leukopenia, fever, and lymphadenopathy commonly improve within days to weeks of adding low to moderate doses of corticosteroids.[1] An inflammatory myopathy may require 1 to 2 mg/kg of prednisone, or the addition of intravenous methotrexate (1 to 2 mg/kg per week).

The therapeutic response of other organ systems is more difficult to characterize. Pericarditis and pleuritis in MCTD apparently respond well to corticosteroids.[60] Pulmonary disease in general may improve with corticosteroids,[41] interstitial and restrictive lung disease may improve,[66] or it may not.[55] In addition, pulmonary hypertension does not uniformly respond to combinations of corticosteroids and cytotoxic agents.[6,7,69,72] Renal involvement due to MCTD may lead to the use of high doses of corticosteroids, possibly in association with cytotoxic agents. Most patients show at least some response to corticosteroids, but the outcome is not uniformly predictable among the few patients treated with cytotoxic agents.

It is not clear whether gastrointestinal aspects of MCTD respond to therapy. One study showed improved esophageal motility in 8 of 14 cases as a result of corticosteroid therapy for other manifestations of the disease.[40] Several descriptions of the intestinal manifestations of MCTD exist, but indications of treatment response are lacking.[59,61,63]

Initial estimations of the prognosis of MCTD suggested a mild disease.[1] A more severe prognosis was first mentioned in the pediatric literature;[5,15] of particular concern were cardiac disease, life-threatening thrombocytopenia, and renal involvement. The proximate causes of death were infection in three, and cerebral hemorrhage in one patient. The infections, caused by encapsulated organisms (pneumococcal in two patients and meningococcal in one), were rapidly fatal, may have been associated with chemotactic abnormalities and were not related to significant corticosteroid doses.

The current prognosis for MCTD can be projected from the data in five studies with long-term, sequential assessment.[3–6,12] Nimelstein, et al. observed that six of eight deaths were not directly related to a rheumatic disorder.[4] Pulmonary hypertension, other lung disease, and heart failure were major factors in another four reported deaths;[3] a fifth death was due to squamous cell carcinoma of the lung. In another investigation, four deaths were related to MCTD; contributing factors included pulmonary hypertension and cor pulmonale in three patients, pericardial tamponade in one, perforated bowel in two, and sepsis in three. The combined mortality rate from these five

reports (194 patients) was 13%, with the mean disease duration varying from 6 to 12 years.

These observations of MCTD morbidity and mortality suggest that our early predictions must be modified. In both adults and children, the prognosis of MCTD is generally similar to that of SLE, but better than that of scleroderma. Our understanding of ideal therapy for MCTD, morbidity, and outcome all remain uncertain. Treatment protocols and longitudinal prospective assessments of this illness should all improve the care of patients with MCTD.

CONCLUSION

The International Symposium on Mixed Connective Tissue Disease and Antinuclear Antibodies determined that "on the basis of clinical, serologic, and immunologic data, mixed connective tissue disease seems to be a distinct entity."[79] Recent investigations tend to support the unique nature of this disease. Features that appear to distinguish MCTD include (1) immunoregulatory abnormalities in MCTD that differ from those found in other rheumatic diseases; (2) high titers of nuclear ribonucleoprotein antibody, usually in the absence of significant titers of other antibodies; (3) strong reactivity of nuclear ribonucleoprotein antibodies with a 68K peptide in MCTD, in contrast to infrequent 68K reactivity in SLE; (4) normal clearance by the reticuloendothelial system of immune complexes in most patients with MCTD, in contrast to SLE; (5) frequent pulmonary hypertension and a unique proliferative vasculopathy; and (6) other pathologic changes that may be restricted to MCTD, such as widespread plasmacytic and lymphocytic infiltration of tissues, an absence of fibrosis, and a distinctive hyalinization of the esophagus.

From our perspective, the status of MCTD as a distinct entity is not the most critical issue. As clinical, serologic, and pathologic characteristics of these patients have become known, and as reports of prognosis have begun to appear, certain repetitive patterns have emerged. First, the initially limited, undifferentiated connective tissue disease frequently becomes more widespread and typical of MCTD, and clinical and serologic transitions are observed during longitudinal study. Second, MCTD usually evolves gradually and, during the early phases, biopsies of tissues and functional tests often reveal abnormalities before the advent of clinical symptoms. Third, certain organs and tissues, such as the lung, the esophagus, and muscle, are at higher risk for pathologic involvement. Fourth, many manifestations of this disease initially respond to corticosteroids, but the scleroderma-like findings, which are the most resistant to treatment, may become the dominant clinical features later in the course of MCTD. Finally, although the prognosis remains favorable, a significant percentage of MCTD patients develop serious and sometimes fatal complications of pulmonary hypertension and proliferative vascular lesions.

The most significant outcome of the continuing controversy surrounding MCTD is the stimulus to further investigation. The numerous immunopathologic abnormalities of MCTD indicate that immune-injury mechanisms may play an important role. Environmental, genetic, hormonal, and immunologic factors probably determine whether patients will continue to have a prolonged, benign undifferentiated rheumatic disorder or will develop major organ-system involvement typical of MCTD, or whether the disease will become more typical of SLE or PSS. The MRL mouse model, which has some features in common with MCTD, may permit incisive investigation of some of these factors. The MRL mouse has already provided a means of producing monoclonal antibodies to U1 RNP, Sm, and other nuclear antigens.

Finally, an unexpected but remarkable consequence of the investigations stimulated by MCTD has been the demonstration that Sm, U1 RNP, and other non-histone nuclear antigens may have central roles in cell biology, such as in the processing of messenger RNA.[80,81] Thus, just as the monoclonal proteins of multiple myeloma stimulated an elucidation of immunoglobulin structure and function, the autoantibodies to antigens occurring in MCTD and other rheumatic diseases have facilitated their purification, biochemical characterization, and study of their biologic roles.

REFERENCES

1. Sharp, G.C., et al.: Mixed connective tissue disease. An apparently distinct rheumatic disease syndrome associated with a specific antibody to an extractable nuclear antigen (ENA). Am. J. Med., 52:148–159, 1972.
2. Parker, M.D.: Ribonucleoprotein antibodies: frequencies and clinical significance in systemic lupus erythematosus, scleroderma and mixed connective tissue disease. J. Lab. Clin. Med., 82:769–775, 1973.
3. Grant, K.D., Adams, L.E., and Hess, E.V.: Mixed connective tissue disease—a subset with sequential clinical and laboratory features. J. Rheumatol., 8:587–598, 1981.
4. Nimelstein, S.H., et al.: Mixed connective tissue disease: a subsequent evaluation of the original 25 patients. Medicine, 59:239–248, 1980.
5. Singsen, B.H., et al.: A histologic evaluation of mixed connective tissue disease in childhood. Am. J. Med., 68:710–717, 1980.
6. Sullivan, W.D., et al.: A prospective evaluation emphasizing pulmonary involvement in patients with mixed connective tissue disease. Medicine, 63:92–107, 1984.
7. Wiener-Kronish, J.P., et al.: Severe pulmonary involvement in mixed connective tissue disease. Am. Rev. Respir. Dis., 124:499–503, 1981.
8. Sharp, G.C., et al.: Association of autoantibodies to different nuclear antigens with clinical patterns of rheumatic disease and responsiveness to therapy. J. Clin. Invest., 50:350–359, 1971.
9. Northway, J.S., and Tan, E.M.: Differentiations of antinuclear antibodies giving speckled staining patterns in immunofluorescence. Clin. Immunol. Immunopathol., 1:140–154, 1972.
10. Reichlin, M., and Mattioli, M.: Correlation of a precipitin reaction to an RNA protein antigen and low prevalence of nephritis in patients with systemic lupus erythematosus. N. Engl. J. Med., 286:908–911, 1972.
11. Sharp, G.C., Irvin, W.S., Northway, J.D., and Tan, E.M.: Specificity of antibodies to extractable nuclear antigens (ENA) in mixed connective tissue disease (MCTD) and systemic lupus erythematosus (SLE). Arthritis Rheum., 15:125, 1972.
12. Sharp, G.C., et al.: Association of antibodies to ribonucleoprotein and Sm antigens with mixed connective tissue disease, systemic lupus erythematosus and other rheumatic diseases. N. Engl. J. Med., 295:1149–1154, 1976.
13. Notman, D.D., Kurata, N., and Tan, E.M.: Profiles of antinuclear antibodies in systemic rheumatic diseases. Ann. Intern. Med., 83:464–469, 1975.
14. Sharp, G.C.: Subsets of SLE and mixed connective tissue disease. Am. J. Kidney Dis., 2:201–205, 1982.
15. Singsen, B.H., et al.: Mixed connective tissue disease in childhood. A clinical and serologic survey. J. Pediatr., 90:893–900, 1977.
16. Tan, E.M., et al.: Diversity of antinuclear antibodies in progressive systemic sclerosis. Arthritis Rheum., 23:617–625, 1980.
17. Wolfe, J.F., et al.: Disease pattern in patients with antibodies only to nuclear ribonucleoprotein (RNP). Clin. Res., 25:488A, 1977.
18. Hench, P.K., Edgington, T.S., and Tan, E.M.: The evolving clinical spectrum of mixed connective tissue disease (MCTD). Arthritis Rheum., 18:404, 1975.
19. Esther, J.H., et al.: Pulmonary hypertension in patients with mixed connective tissue disease and antibody to nuclear ribonucleoprotein. Arthritis Rheum., 24:S105, 1981.
20. Frank, M.M., et al.: Immunoglobulin G Fc receptor-mediated clearance in autoimmune disease. Ann. Intern. Med., 98:206–218, 1983.
21. Alarcon-Segovia, D.: Mixed connective tissue disease—a decade of growing pains. (Editorial). J. Rheumatol., 8:535–540, 1981.
22. Gilliam, J.N., and Prystowsky, S.D.: Mixed connective tissue disease syndrome: The cutaneous manifestations of patients with epidermal nuclear staining and high titer antibody to RNase sensitive extractable nuclear antigen (ENA). Arch. Dermatol., 113:583–587, 1977.
23. Alarcon-Segovia, D.: Mixed connective tissue disease: Appearance of antibodies to ribonucleoprotein following corticosteroid treatment. J. Rheumatol., 6:694–699, 1979.
24. Pettersson, I., et al.: The structure of mammalian small nuclear ribonucleoproteins: identification of multiple protein components reactive with anti-(U1) ribonucleoprotein and anti-Sm autoantibodies. J. Biol. Chem., 259:5907–5914, 1984.
25. Pettersson, I., et al.: The use of immunoblotting and immunoprecipitation of (U) small nuclear ribonucleoproteins in the analysis of sera of patients with mixed connective tissue disease

and systemic lupus erythematosus. A cross-sectional, longitudinal study. Arthritis Rheum., 29:986–996, 1986.

26. Habets, W.J., et al.: Antibodies against distinct nuclear matrix proteins are characteristic for mixed connective tissue disease. Clin. Exp. Immunol., 54:265–276, 1983.

27. Habets, W.J., et al.: Quantitation of anti-RNP and anti-Sm antibodies in MCTD and SLE patients by immunoblotting. Clin. Exp. Immunol., 59:457–466, 1985.

28. LeRoy, E.C., Maricq, H.R., and Kahaleh, M.B.: Undifferentiated connective tissue syndromes. Arthritis Rheum., 23:341–343, 1980.

29. Sharp, G.C.: Diagnostic criteria for classification of MCTD. In Mixed Connective Tissue Disease and Anti-nuclear Antibodies. Edited by R. Kasukawa and G.C. Sharp. Amsterdam, Elsevier Science Publishers B.V., 1987.

30. Alarcon-Segovia, D.A., and Villarreal, M.: Classification and diagnostic criteria for mixed connective tissue disease. In Mixed Connective Tissue Disease and Anti-nuclear Antibodies. Edited by R. Kasukawa and G.C. Sharp. Amsterdam, Elsevier Science Publishers B.V., 1987.

31. Kasukawa, R., et al.: Preliminary diagnostic criteria for classification of mixed connective tissue disease. In Mixed Connective Tissue Disease and Anti-nuclear Antibodies. Edited by R. Kasukawa and G.C. Sharp. Amsterdam, Elsevier Science Publishers B.V., 1987.

32. Farber, S.J., and Bole, G.G.: Antibodies to components of extractable nuclear antigen. Arch. Intern. Med., 136:425–431, 1976.

33. Peller, J.S., Gabor, G.T., Porter, J.M., and Bennett, R.M.: Angiographic findings in mixed connective tissue disease. Arthritis Rheum., 28:768–774, 1985.

34. Maricq, H.R., et al.: Diagnostic potential of in vivo capillary microscopy in scleroderma and related disorders. Arthritis Rheum., 23:183–189, 1980.

35. Bennett, R.M., and O'Connell, D.J.: The arthritis of mixed connective tissue disease. Ann. Rheum. Dis., 37:397–403, 1978.

36. Halla, J.T., and Hardin, J.G.: Clinical features of the arthritis of mixed connective tissue disease. Arthritis Rheum., 21:497–503, 1978.

37. Bennett, R.M., and O'Connell, D.J.: Mixed connective tissue disease: a clinicopathologic study of 20 cases. Semin. Arthritis Rheum., 10:25–51, 1980.

38. Lewis, R.A., et al.: The hand in mixed connective tissue disease. J. Hand Surg., 3:217–222, 1978.

39. Oxenhandler, R., et al.: Pathology of skeletal muscle in mixed connective tissue disease. Arthritis Rheum., 20:985–988, 1977.

40. Winn, D., et al.: Esophageal function in steroid treated patients with mixed connective tissue disease (MCTD). Clin. Res., 24:545A, 1976.

41. Harmon, C., et al.: Pulmonary involvement in mixed connective tissue disease (MCTD). Arthritis Rheum., 19:801, 1976.

42. Germain, M.J., and Davidman, M.: Pulmonary hemorrhage and acute renal failure in a patient with mixed connective tissue disease. Am. J. Kidney Dis., 3:420–424, 1984.

43. Martens, J., and Demedts, M.: Diaphragm dysfunction in mixed connective tissue disease. Scand. J. Rheumatol., 11:165–167, 1982.

44. Derderian, S.S., et al.: Pulmonary involvement in mixed connective tissue disease. Chest, 88:45–48, 1985.

45. Alpert, M.A., et al.: Cardiovascular manifestations of mixed connective tissue disease in adults. Circulation, 68:1182–1193, 1983.

46. Oetgen, W.J., et al.: Cardiac abnormalities in mixed connective tissue disease. Chest, 2:185–188, 1983.

47. Bennett, R.M., and Spargo, B.H.: Immune complex nephropathy in mixed connective tissue disease. Am. J. Med., 63:534–541, 1977.

48. Bresnihan, B., et al.: Antiribonucleoprotein antibodies in connective tissue diseases: Estimation by counter-immunoelectrophoresis. Br. Med. J., 1:610–611, 1977.

49. Rao, K.V., et al.: Immune complex nephritis in mixed connective tissue disease. Ann. Intern. Med., 84:174–176, 1976.

50. Baldassare, A., et al.: Mixed connective tissue disease (MCTD) in children. Arthritis Rheum., 19:788, 1976.

51. Fuller, T.J., et al.: Immune-complex glomerulonephritis in a patient with mixed connective tissue disease. Am. J. Med., 62:761–764, 1977.

52. Halla, J.T., et al.: Circulating immune complexes in mixed connective tissue disease (MCTD). Arthritis Rheum., 21:562–563, 1978.

53. Bennett, R.M., Bong, D.M., and Spargo, B.H.: Neuropsychiatric problems in mixed connective tissue disease. Am. J. Med., 65:955–962, 1978.

54. Bernstein, R.F.: Ibuprofen-related meningitis in mixed connective tissue disease. Ann. Intern. Med., 92:206–207, 1980.

55. Cryer, P.F., and Kissane, J.M. (Eds.): Clinicopathologic Conference. Mixed connective tissue disease. Am. J. Med., 65:833–842, 1978.

56. de Rooij, D.J.R.A.M., van de Putte, L.B.A., and van Beusekom, H.J.: Severe thrombocytopenia in mixed connective tissue disease. Scand. J. Rheumatol., 11:184–186, 1982.

57. Hyslop, D.L., Singsen, B.H., and Sharp, G.C.: Leukocyte function, infection, and mortality in mixed connective tissue disease (MCTD). Arthritis Rheum., 29:S64, 1986.

58. Fraga, A., et al.: Mixed connective tissue disease in childhood. Relationship with Sjögren's syndrome. Am. J. Dis. Child., 132:263–265, 1978.

59. Cooke, C.L., and Lurie, H.I.: Case report: Fatal gastrointestinal hemorrhage in mixed connective tissue disease. Arthritis Rheum., 20:1421–1427, 1977.

60. Davis, J.D., Parker, M.D., and Turner, R.A.: Exacerbation of mixed connective tissue disease during salmonella gastroenteritis—serial immunological findings. J. Rheumatol., 5:96–98, 1978.

61. Samach, M., Brandt, L.J., and Bernstein, L.H.: Spontaneous pneumoperitoneum with pneumatosis cystoides intestinalis in a patient with mixed connective tissue disease. Am. J. Gastroenterol., 69:494–500, 1978.

62. Thiele, D.L., and Krejs, G.J.: Secretory diarrhea in mixed connective tissue disease. Am. J. Gastroenterol., 80:107–110, 1985.

63. Norman, D.A., and Fleischmann, R.M.: Gastrointestinal systemic sclerosis in serologic mixed connective tissue disease. Arthritis Rheum., 21:811–819, 1978.

64. Eberhardt, K., Svantesson, H., and Svensson, B.: Follow-up study of 6 children presenting with a MCTD-like syndrome. Scand. J. Rheumatol., 10:62–64, 1981.

65. Sanders, D.Y., Huntley, C.C., and Sharp, G.C.: Mixed connective tissue disease. J. Pediatr., 83:642–645, 1973.

66. Hepburn, B.: Multiple antinuclear antibodies in mixed connective tissue disease: report of a patient with an unusual antibody profile. J. Rheumatol., 8:635–638, 1981.

67. Peskett, S.A., et al.: Mixed connective tissue disease in children. Rheumatol. Rehabil., 17:245–248, 1978.

68. Singsen, B.H.: Mixed connective tissue disease, scleroderma and morphea in childhood. In Brenneman's Textbook of Pediatrics. Edited by R. Wedgwood. New York, Harper & Row Publishers, 1981.

69. Jones, M.B., et al.: Fatal pulmonary hypertension and resolving

immune-complex glomerulonephritis in mixed connective tissue disease. A case report and review of the literature. Am. J. Med. *65*:855–863, 1978.

70. Silver, T.M., et al.: Radiological features of mixed connective tissue disease and scleroderma-systemic lupus erythematosus overlap. Radiology, *120*:269–275, 1976.

71. Oetgen, W.J., Boice, J.A., and Lawless, O.J.: Mixed connective tissue disease in children and adolescents. Pediatrics, *67*:333–337, 1981.

72. Rosenberg, A.M., et al.: Pulmonary hypertension in a child with mixed connective tissue disease. J. Rheumatol., *6*:700–704, 1979.

73. Whitlow, P.L., Gilliam, J.N., Chubick, A. and Ziff, M.: Myocarditis in mixed connective tissue disease. Arthritis Rheum., *23*:808–815, 1980.

74. Alarcon-Segovia, D.: Immunological abnormalities in mixed connective tissue disease. *In* Mixed Connective Tissue Disease and Anti-nuclear Antibodies. Edited by R. Kasukawa and G.C. Sharp. Amsterdam, Elsevier Science Publishers B.V., 1987.

75. Fishbein, E., Alarcon-Segovia, D., and Ramos-Niembro, F.:

Free serum ribonucleoprotein (RNP) in mixed connective tissue disease (MCTD). *In* Proceedings of the Fourteenth International Congress on Rheumatology, San Francisco, 1977.

76. Negoro, N., et al.: A solid-phase radioimmunoassay for the detection of nRNP immune complexes. J. Immunol. Methods, *91*:83–89, 1986.

77. Negoro, N., et al.: Nuclear ribonucleoprotein immune complexes in pericardial fluid of a patient with mixed connective tissue disease. Arthritis Rheum., *30*:97–101, 1987.

78. Ramos-Niembro, F., Alarcon-Segovia, D., and Hernandez-Ortiz, J.: Articular manifestations of mixed connective tissue disease. Arthritis Rheum., *22*:43–51, 1979.

79. Alarcon-Segovia, D.A., and Shiokawa, Y.: Chairmen's summary. *In* Mixed Connective Tissue Disease and Anti-nuclear Antibodies. Edited by R. Kasukawa and G.C. Sharp. Amsterdam, Elsevier Science Publishers B.V., 1987.

80. Lerner, M.R., et al.: Are snRNP's involved in splicing? Nature, *283*:220–224, 1980.

81. Nyman, U., et al.: Intranuclear localization of snRNP antigens. J. Cell Biol., *102*:137–144, 1986.

72

POLYMYOSITIS/ DERMATOMYOSITIS

LAWRENCE J. KAGEN

Polymyositis and dermatomyositis are acquired, chronic, inflammatory muscle disorders of unknown cause. They occur in children and adults and are manifested by disability resulting from muscle weakness. A characteristic rash distinguishes dermatomyositis from polymyositis.

Although inflammation of muscle may develop in the course of other connective tissue disorders such as progressive systemic sclerosis, systemic lupus erythematosus, and Sjögren's syndrome, the terms polymyositis and dermatomyositis are reserved for the clinical situations in which chronic inflammatory myopathy is the dominant element in the absence of features diagnostic of other illness.

Symmetric proximal muscle weakness and histologic findings of inflammation and myofiber damage of muscle tissue, accompanied by evidence of increased amounts of certain sarcoplasmic constituents in the circulation and electrophysiologic signs of myopathy, are the chief clinical manifestations, along with characteristic changes of the skin in patients with dermatomyositis. In severe cases, impairment of deglutition and cardiorespiratory complications contribute to morbidity. Malignant neoplasms may be found in patients with myositis and may further complicate the outcome.

CLASSIFICATION

Several schemes for the classification of patients with inflammatory myopathy have been devised for the purpose of segregating patients into groups to study cause, prognosis, and response to therapy more efficiently.[1,2] Patients with polymyositis are usually grouped separately from those with dermatomyositis, malignant diseases, and other connective tissue disorders. Because of factors discussed later in this chapter, dermatomyositis of childhood also has its own category. Attempts to classify a disease without knowledge of its cause and with incomplete knowledge of its pathogenesis may be flawed and are subject to revision, however. In this light, Table 72–1 presents a grouping of patients with polymyositis, for purposes of discussion and further study.

In general, a female preponderance exists in myositis, especially in patients with features of other connective tissue disorders. This preponderance is also present in the dermatomyositis and polymyositis groups, however (Table 72–2). No female preponderance is found in childhood dermatomyositis or in adults with myositis associated with neoplasia.

Although inflammatory muscle disease may occur at any age, most cases are noted in the fifth and sixth decades of life. In a survey of 380 reported cases, 17%

Table 72–1. Classification of Inflammatory Muscle Disease

1. Polymyositis
2. Dermatomyositis
3. Dermatomyositis of childhood
4. Myositis with neoplasm
5. Myositis with other connective tissue disorders, such as progressive systemic sclerosis, systemic lupus erythematosus, Sjögren's syndrome, and rheumatoid arthritis

were age 15 or younger, 14% were from age 15 to age 30, and 60% were between the ages 30 and 60. An additional 9% of patients were over age 60.[3]

Although rare, inflammatory myopathy has been reported in infants less than a year old.[4] In this situation, recognition of myositis and its distinction from congenital myopathies are important because corticosteroid therapy is valuable in the treatment of infants with myositis.

These disorders generally occur less frequently than certain other connective tissue syndromes. The incidence of dermatomyositis and polymyositis has been estimated at 0.5 cases per 100,000 population in a racially mixed area of Tennessee over a 22-year period. Ethnic or racial factors are important, and the highest frequency is noted in black women.[5] An English survey over a 20-year period indicated an incidence of 8 cases per 100,000. The application of these figures to all populations is not precise; however, it is now estimated that one to five new cases per million people occur each year in the United States, with a frequency perhaps 4 times greater among black women.[5-7] As suggested in Table 72–2, the incidence in adults is greater than in children.

CLINICAL FEATURES

MUSCLE WEAKNESS

Muscular weakness is the dominant feature of myositis syndromes, with symmetric involvement of proximal muscles of the extremities, trunk, and neck. Difficulty with the lower extremities is often first characterized by an inability to climb stairs, to arise from a low seat or a squat, and to cross the legs. Walking may be limited, and gait may become poorly coordinated and waddling. Weakness of the upper extremities limits lifting, hanging up clothes, and combing the hair. Weakness of the anterior neck flexor muscles interferes with lifting the head from the supine position, and arising from bed becomes difficult.

Severely affected patients may have difficulty in swallowing, and liquids may be regurgitated through the nose. Along with weakness and muscle pain, soreness with tenderness may be noted, particularly in patients whose disease progresses rapidly. Although weakness may be marked, little atrophy occurs initially. With time, affected muscles may lose volume, and involvement may become more generalized and may include distal muscles. The patient's speech may be altered and may assume a nasal quality. Whereas virtually all patients have proximal muscle weakness, few progress to distal involvement or have impaired swallowing or speech. Dysphagia occurs in approximately 10 to 15% of patients.[8] Facial involvement is rare.[9]

Because weakness is the central cause of morbidity in patients with myositis, ongoing assessment of muscle strength is of prime importance in clinical evaluation. One must therefore combine careful questioning, to record changes in functional capabilities, with muscle strength testing. The most common muscle testing schemes employ a semiquantitative grading system (Table 72–3). The ability to assess muscle strength accurately is limited by several factors. First, one must be certain that the patient's effort is his best. Pain, fatigue, and malaise may interfere with full cooperation and may invalidate the results of the assessment. In addition, variables related to the observer also can be a factor. The joint position in which the test is done should be recorded because it affects muscle length and mechanical advantage and the resultant tension. For example, knee extensor muscles tested at a 60° angle of knee flexion (full extension is 0°) have greater force than at a 30° position. The differences between grades 4 and 5 of muscle strength are significant, but they are difficult to quantify precisely. The position of the examiner's hand during the procedure should also be recorded, owing to considerations of mechanical advantage and lever arm length. Finally, tests of this nature are most useful for muscle groups of the extremities. For other muscles,

Table 72–2. Distribution of Patients by Group and Sex

Group	No. of Patients	Percentage of Total (%)	Percentage of Female Patients (%)
Polymyositis	52	34	69
Dermatomyositis	45	29	58
Dermatomyositis of childhood	11	7	36
Myositis with neoplasm	13	8.5	57
Myositis with overlap features of other connective tissue disorders	32	21	90

(Based on 153 patients reviewed by Bohan, A., et al.[8])

Table 72–3. Scheme for Testing Manual Muscle Strength

Grade	
0	No evident contraction
1	Trace of contraction
2	Poor—movement with gravity eliminated
3	Fair—movement against gravity
4	Good—movement against resistance
5	Normal

(Modified from Gardner-Medwin, D., and Walton, J.N.[10])

such as of the torso, additional testing methods must be used.

To approach some of the observer-related variables, as well as to standardize and to increase reproducibility and sensitivity, several attempts have been made to introduce biomechanical methods and instruments into the clinical setting. The importance of such measurements has been stressed by Edwards and colleagues, who have reported that muscle strength correlates with metabolic studies of net losses and gains in total muscle mass and may be a better guide to progress than other laboratory measures.[11,12] Figure 72–1 demonstrates the use of biomechanical strength testing in a patient with polymyositis during initial therapy with prednisone. Torque production, an indicator of muscle strength of the quadriceps mechanism, rose after six to seven weeks of prednisone therapy and was associated with a fall in serum creatine kinase activity, as well as with gains in functional ability.

A study of polymyositis and dermatomyositis indicated a significant correlation between muscle strength and laboratory indices (serum enzymes and myoglobin) during the course of illness of some, but not all, patients.[13] Because laboratory guides are *not* correlated to disease activity in *all* patients, the need for *quantitative serial assessment of muscle strength* was emphasized.

A rapid method for evaluation of lower extremity strength has been standardized for men and women of various ages.[14] It permits "fine tuning" of therapy for myositis.

RASH

The rash of dermatomyositis appears on the face, neck, chest, and extremities (Figs. 72–2 to 72–5). It is most common over the extensor surfaces of the extremities, particularly over the dorsum of the hands and the fingers. The rash is deep red and is slightly raised in small plaques over the wrists and knuckles. A whitish scale may be seen superficially. Similar patches occur over the elbows, the knees, and the medial malleoli of the ankles. Involvement of the scalp, upper arms, and outer thighs also occurs. At the nail beds, one sees hyperemia, telangiectasia, and, with more marked involvement, destruction of the architecture of the nail bed. Dilated capillary loops at the nailfold, as well as over the knuckles and other areas of the fingers, may be seen.[15] Cutaneous vasculitis, evidenced clinically by tender nodules, periungual infarctions, and digital ulcerations, has been noted in both adult and childhood dermatomyositis. In the adult, these lesions are less common and may be associated with an underlying malignant process. In a group of 76 adults studied, 7 had lesions of this nature, and 2 of these had an underlying malignant disease (28%). Of the total number of patients with

FIG. 72–1. The use of biomechanical measurement of muscle strength during the course of polymyositis. Strength is recorded as the torque (force × lever arm) produced by the knee extensors (quadriceps femoris). This patient demonstrates an increase in strength concomitant with a fall in serum creatine kinase (CK) level after treatment with prednisone (pred). (Data from Dr. J. Otis and Mr. M. Kroll.)

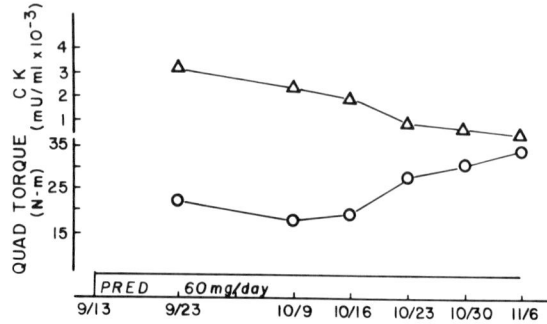

FIG. 72–2. The rash of dermatomyositis over the hand of a child. Patches of erythematous, scaly plaques over knuckles, as well as periungual changes, are evident.

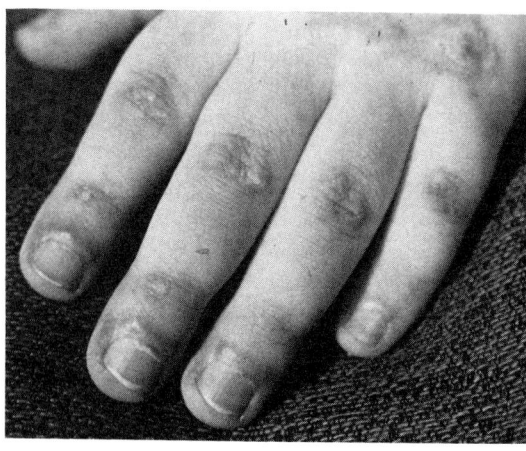

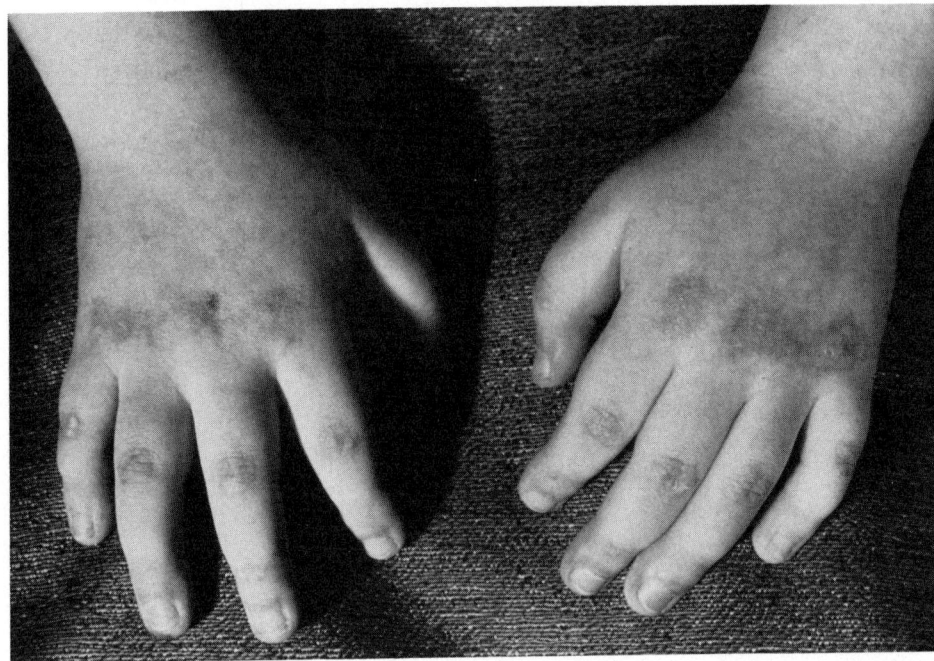

FIG. 72–3. Dermatomyositis, showing a raised, reddened rash over the dorsum of the hands.

malignant disease, 2 of 6 had these lesions.[16] A deep violet-red rash may be present on the face, particularly in the periorbital areas, which may also be edematous. Involvement is most prominent over the upper eyelids, and scaling may also occur here. Lilac suffusion or *heliotrope rash* over the upper eyelids is characteristic of dermatomyositis. A similar deep red-to-violaceous rash may appear on the forehead, neck, shoulders, and chest.

Although the heliotrope rash is characteristic, it is not absolutely diagnostic. Similar changes may occur in patients with allergic manifestations and during the course of trichinosis. A characteristic rash of this type has also been described in a patient with sarcoidosis and myopathy.[17]

Rash may appear before other signs of myopathy become manifest. As extreme examples, six patients with classic heliotrope discoloration of the periorbital area with edema and a maculopapular violaceous rash over the interphalangeal joints with periungual telangiectasia did not develop clinical evidence of muscle involvement until months to years later.[18]

Histologic evaluation of skin biopsies in dermatomyositis reveals poikiloderma, that is, epidermal atrophy with liquefaction, degeneration of the basal cell layer, and vascular dilatation. Inflammatory infiltrates, composed of perivascular accumulations of lymphocytes and histiocytes in the upper dermis, are found along with few polymorphonuclear cells and occasional infiltrates around the pilosebaceous apparatus. Hyperkeratosis, dermal edema with increased deposits of mucin, and evidence of subcu-

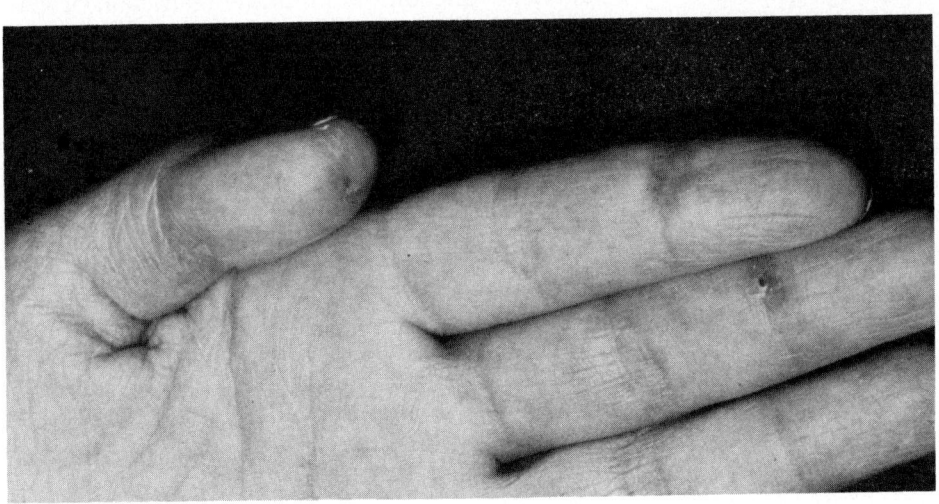

FIG. 72–4. Punched-out ulcerated skin lesions over the volar surface of the hands (at the tip of the thumb and at the terminal creases of the second and third fingers) in a patient with dermatomyositis and adenocarcinoma of the large intestine.

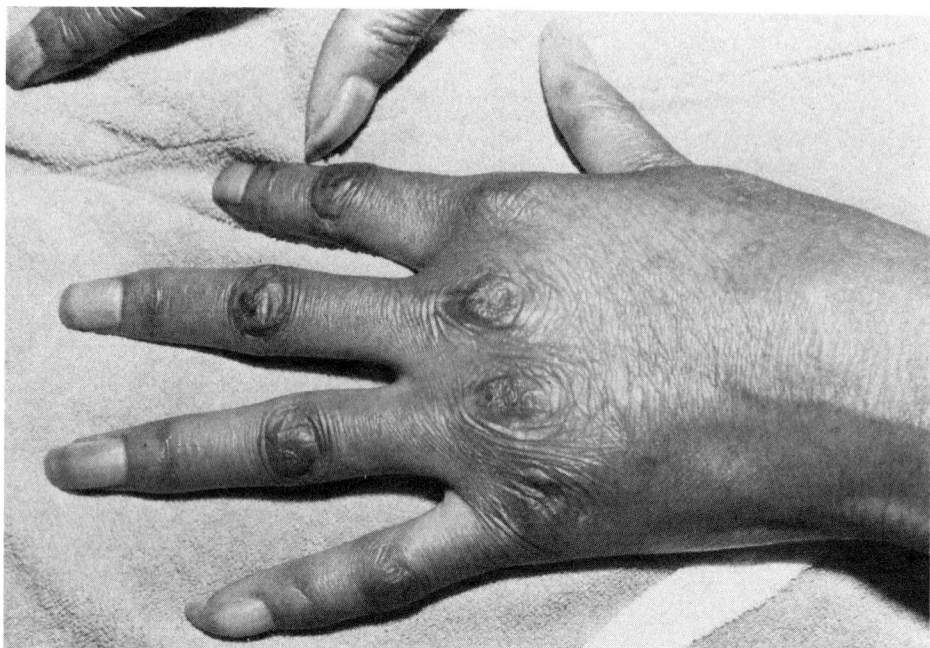

FIG. 72–5. Papular, raised rash of the knuckle above the metacarpophalangeal and proximal interphalangeal joints in a patient with chronic dermatomyositis.

taneous panniculitis may also be found.[19] Vascular endothelial changes characteristic of childhood dermatomyositis may be present in the skin (see the discussion on histology later in this chapter).

DYSPHAGIA

Difficulty in swallowing may result from several factors in patients with myositis. Decreased strength of pharyngeal contractions, disordered peristalsis, vallecular pooling, and weakness of the tongue may all interfere with normal swallowing. Patients with severe weakness of this type may also have difficulties in elevating the palate and may have nasal speech. In addition, dysfunction of the cricopharyngeus muscle with spasm and improperly timed closure may occur in some patients and may accentuate symptoms.[20] The importance of recognizing cricopharyngeal dysfunction resulting from constriction, fibrosis, or abnormal contraction lies in the possibility of surgical relief of obstruction. Appropriate investigation should be conducted in patients with dysphagia to determine to what extent cricopharyngeal dysfunction may be a complicating factor.[21]

Abnormalities of distal, as well as proximal, esophageal function and disturbances in gastric emptying have also been documented.[22,23]

Although found in only 10 to 15% of patients,[8] dysphagia is usually associated with severe disease and a poor prognosis.

PULMONARY MANIFESTATIONS

Several factors, including hypoventilation secondary to muscular weakness, infectious agents, aspiration in association with abnormalities in swallowing, and rarely, drug hypersensitivity, such as related to methotrexate,[24] may play a role in the association of pulmonary disease and myositis. In addition to these factors, interstitial pulmonary fibrosis or fibrosing alveolitis may be a significant feature of myositis syndromes.

Pulmonary fibrosis has been noted in 5 to 10% of patients, generally by roentgenography. The frequency of this disorder seems unrelated to a previous history of cigarette smoking and does not have the female preponderance seen in adults with myositis. Pulmonary function tests indicate restriction of ventilation with reduction of total lung capacity and vital capacity. Hypoxemia may be characterized by a moderate reduction in diffusing capacity. Dyspnea and cough are the major symptoms, and physical examination may reveal the presence of fine, crepitant, basilar rales. In approximately half the affected patients, pulmonary abnormalities are noted prior to the appearance of myopathy.

Alveolar septal fibrosis, interstitial mononuclear cell infiltrates containing mainly lymphocytes with smaller numbers of large mononuclear cells and plasma cells, hyperplasia of the type I alveolar epithelial cells, and increased numbers of free alveolar macrophages are seen histologically. These findings may be irregularly distributed and intermixed with areas of apparently uninvolved lung. Interstitial edema and vascular change marked by intimal and medial thickening of arteries and arterioles may also be evident. Chest roentgenograms may show diffuse, linear, interstitial thickening, with an alveolar pattern of fibrosis. Patchy consolidation and "honeycomb" changes indicate more chronic and severe involvement. These changes may be associated with right-ventricular enlargement and with prominent hilar markings. Corticosteroid therapy may be followed by relief of dyspnea and by improvements in radiographic changes and abnormalities of pulmonary function, but some patients show no improvement. Therapeutic response may be better in patients with acute illness and lung biopsies showing inflammation of the alveolar wall, whereas fibrosis in the absence of inflammation is a sign of a poorer prognosis. Rapidly progressive fatal pulmonary insufficiency may occur, despite the early introduction of corticosteroid treatment. Carefully monitored therapy with these drugs is advisable, although generally applicable, statistically validated prognostic guides are still lacking. The progression of pulmonary dysfunction resulting from fibrosing alveolitis does stop in some patients.[25-29]

Ventilatory insufficiency as a result of weakness of muscles of respiration (e.g., the diaphragm and intercostal muscles) also contributes to defects in gas exchange. Loss of respiratory muscle strength, as assessed by inspiratory and expiratory pressures at the mouth, may be associated with a tendency toward hypercapnia.[30]

As indicated above, pulmonary toxicity may occur in the course of therapy with certain agents, such as methotrexate and perhaps cyclophosphamide; such toxicity may play a role in the development of interstitial lung disease.[31] An excellent review of lung involvement in polydermatocryositis has appeared.[31]

CARDIAC MANIFESTATIONS

Cardiac abnormalities in patients with polymyositis and dermatomyositis occur frequently, but are rarely clinically symptomatic. First-, second-, and third-degree heart block, left bundle branch block, left axis deviation, and atrial and ventricular dysrhythmias have been noted. Myocarditis and congestive heart failure occur less often. At least half of patients have electrocardiographic abnormalities, with an increased frequency of mitral valve prolapse noted in one report.[32] Uncommonly, conduction abnormalities are so severe that an artificial cardiac pacemaker is required.[33] It is not certain whether the tendency to

cardiac abnormalities is greater in more severely or chronically ill patients.

Postmortem evaluations have demonstrated myocarditis, as well as myocardial fibrosis.[34,35] Myocarditis is associated with congestive heart failure. One patient with bundle branch block had inflammation and necrosis involving the conduction system. Overall, arrhythmia is estimated to occur in 6%, congestive heart failure in 3%, bundle branch block in 5%, and high-grade heart block in 2% of patients.[8] Cardiac involvement may occur in both polymyositis and dermatomyositis, but it may go unnoticed unless electrocardiographic examinations are performed. Improvement in electrocardiographic abnormality in adults rarely occurs, although this has been noted in children.[36]

CALCINOSIS

Soft-tissue calcification can be a disabling complication of inflammatory muscle disease (Figs. 72–6 to 72–8). Most commonly, it occurs during the course of chronic childhood dermatomyositis. Calcification may invest the fascia surrounding muscle groups of the proximal extremities and may lead to diffuse "woody" induration that severely limits motion. Calcified masses may also appear under the skin and may open to the surface, draining calcareous material. A review of radiographs of 40 children with dermatomyositis has suggested the occurrence of four patterns of soft-tissue calcification. Deep linear and deep calcareal deposits were most common; superficial calcareal deposits were less common. The fourth pattern, characterized by lacy, reticular, subcutaneous calcification that could be widespread, was associated with children with severe, unremitting, illness.[37] Di-

FIG. 72–6. Subcutaneous calcific masses nearing the skin surface at the elbow of a patient with dermatomyositis.

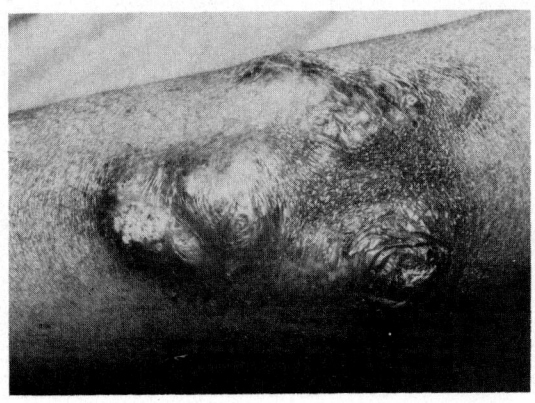

FIG. 72–7.   Subcutaneous and perimuscular calcific masses in the thigh of a child with dermatomyositis in remission.

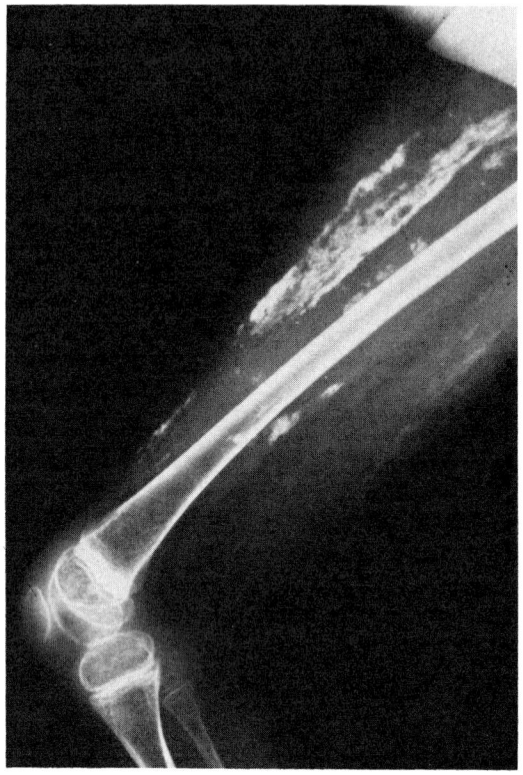

FIG. 72–8.   *A* and *B*. Subcutaneous calcification at the elbow and other areas of calcification in the upper arm of a child with dermatomyositis in remission.

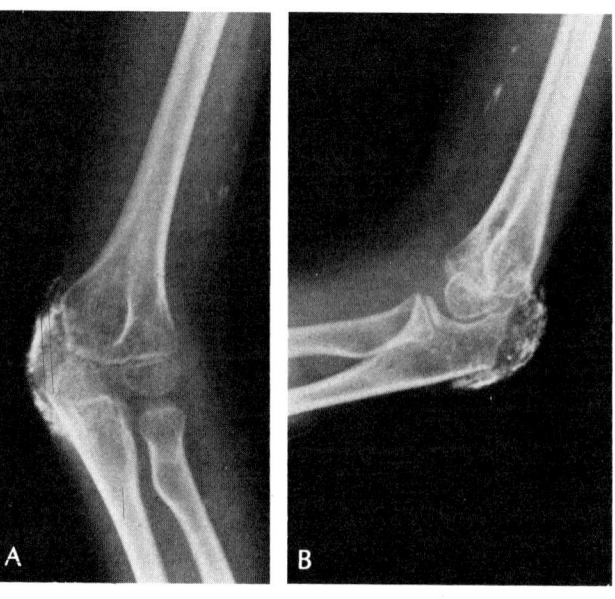

agnostic sensitivity in detecting this abnormality, prior to accumulation of masses large enough to be seen radiographically, may be increased by bone-scanning techniques with ⁹⁹ᵐtechnetium diphosphonate.[38] Treatment methods for calcinosis are generally unsatisfactory. Localized masses may be removed surgically, but extensive or more generalized involvement is a distressing problem. A number of therapies, including corticosteroids, diphosphonates, ethyl-enediaminotetra-acetate, and aluminum hydroxide gel, have been unsuccessful. Probenecid has been reported to be useful.[39] The calcific deposits are sometimes resorbed spontaneously (see Chapter 95).

RENAL INVOLVEMENT

Renal disease is rare in patients with inflammatory myopathy. Renal insufficiency in patients with severe persistent myoglobinuria has been observed.[40] This complication may occur in both polymyositis and dermatomyositis. Although rare, glomerulonephritis of the focal-mesangial type or of the progressive-crescentic type has been recorded.[41,42]

FOCAL OR NODULAR MUSCLE INVOLVEMENT

Polymyositis may begin with a single, localized, nodular swelling in muscle. This swelling may then progress over months to generalized inflammatory myopathy. This unusual variant has been described as focal or nodular myositis.[43,44] In some patients, focal myositis of the gastrocnemius muscle has simulated thrombophlebitis.[45]

CHILDHOOD DERMATOMYOSITIS

Although a female preponderance exists among adults with myositis, such is not the case in children.[46]

The signs of rash and myopathy are similar to those previously described. In addition, evidence of vascular involvement may be prominent. Abnormalities of nailfold capillaries, including dilatation, avascular areas, and tortuosity, are present in over half the affected children, especially in those with severe disease.[47] Ulcerations of the gastrointestinal tract and hemorrhage related to vascular involvement of the digestive system are serious, life-threatening complications.[48] This manifestation was described prior to the use of corticosteroid agents and represents a result of dermatomyositis rather than a complication of therapy.[2] Although vascular involvement of the gastrointestinal tract is the most prominent visceral complication of dermatomyositis, other areas may also be involved, including, rarely, the retina, in which exudates, macular edema, and visual impairment have been described.[49]

Histologic evaluation of dermatomyositis reveals distinctive abnormalities related to pathologic changes of the vessel walls, as discussed later in this chapter.

ARTHRALGIA

Joint pains without overt synovitis commonly occur during periods of active disease. Overt synovitis is sufficiently rare that its presence suggests other connective tissue syndromes.

RISK OF PREGNANCY

There are few reports of the effects of myositis on the risk of pregnancy; thus, predictive data are incomplete. The majority of these reports deal with dermatomyositis. Decreased fertility and increased fetal loss probably occur in some women with dermatomyositis. Exacerbations of disease during pregnancy have also been observed. No neonatal effects of dermatomyositis in surviving infants have been reported as yet.[50,51]

LABORATORY AND OTHER DIAGNOSTIC STUDIES

The laboratory studies most used during the course of inflammatory muscle disease involve measurement of sarcoplasmic constituents, enzymes, and myoglobin released into the circulation as a consequence of muscle damage.

ENZYMES

Measurements of serum activities of creatine kinase, lactate dehydrogenase, aldolase, and aspartate aminotransferase (glutamic-oxaloacetic transaminase) are the most common enzyme tests. Elevations occur during periods of disease activity, and values return toward normal during remission or inactive disease.

An increase in serum creatine kinase activity is the most sensitive enzyme index of active muscle disease.[52] High creatine kinase activity is found in active disease, and the level falls during remission, sometimes weeks before clinically evident improvement. The level may then rise again if the therapeutic drug dosage is reduced too quickly or if a relapse is impending. Because aldolase, transaminase, and lactate dehydrogenase may be less consistently elevated in patients with myositis, estimation of creatine kinase levels is the most reliable enzyme test.[53]

In some situations, evaluations of serum enzyme activity are of limited use. From the technical point of view, the amount of enzyme is inferred from its activity, and factors that inhibit or promote activity influence the interpretation of test results. Inhibitors of creatine kinase activity have been described in serum. Dilution of serum samples with elevated creatine kinase levels may produce artifactual increases in creatine kinase activity,[54] and certain pharmacologic agents such as barbiturates, diazepam, and morphine may alter the removal rate of creatine kinase from the circulation and may increase its activity.[55] In addition, the question whether enzyme increases are due to tissue destruction, or whether cell membranes become leaky due to disease or pharmacologic agents, is difficult to answer. For example, following exercise, elevations of creatine kinase levels may be observed in the absence of histologically demonstrable evidence of tissue necrosis. In neuromuscular disorders other than myositis, falls in creatine kinase activity may occur without clinical change,[56] so this index may not always correlate with disease activity.

Rarely, in 1 to 5% of patients with polymyositis and dermatomyositis, the serum creatine kinase level alone may be normal, and in other patients, all serum enzyme levels tested are normal throughout the course of illness.[8] One study measured serum creatine kinase levels prior to therapy and found these values to be normal in 5 of 15 patients. This finding may have been related to disease chronicity because high values were noted in all 7 patients with disease of under 3 years' duration, whereas in the 8 patients with a longer duration of illness, the creatine kinase level was normal in 5 and was only moderately elevated in 3 patients. No correlation was found between the magnitude of the enzyme elevation and the severity of the muscle weakness.[57] On the other hand, a series of seven patients without creatine kinase elevation had a poor prognosis, with five patients having had either malignancy or interstitial lung disease.[58] Taken together, therefore, the evidence suggests that serum enzyme evaluation is an important adjunct to the diagnosis and assessment of patients with myositis, but absolute correlations of strength and prognosis with the enzyme levels, particularly in patients with chronic illness, are often imprecise.

Creatine kinase exists as a dimer with three major isoenzymic forms: MM, MB, and BB. Creatine kinase-MM is the predominant form in skeletal muscle, where it represents approximately 95 to 98% of the total creatine kinase activity. The BB isoenzyme is the major component of brain and smooth muscle. The MB form is present in cardiac muscle to the extent of 20 to 30%, with the remainder as MM. The MB form may be present in skeletal muscle as well, in levels of 5% or less.[59-61] Creatine kinase-MB has been demonstrated in the circulation of patients with myositis in the absence of detectable, concomitant cardiac disease or dysfunction.[62-65] In these patients, creatine kinase-MB is probably synthesized in and released from skeletal muscle. Myofibers during embryologic development produce the B subunit and elaborate creatine kinase-MB, and skeletal muscle tissue in cell culture also produces this MB form.[66-68] These observations, combined with clinical information, suggest that regenerating myofibers within damaged skeletal muscle may be the source of the increased production of creatine kinase-MB.

MYOGLOBIN

Myoglobin, the respiratory heme protein of the muscle cell, is found in both skeletal and cardiac muscle, but not in other tissues. During the course of muscle disease or disorder, myoglobin may enter the circulation and, following renal clearance, may appear in the urine.[69] Hypermyoglobinemia is seen in most patients with dermatomyositis and polymyositis. Myoglobinuria is less frequent.[40,70] From 70 to 80% of patients with active, untreated myositis have hypermyoglobinemia, with levels falling during periods of remission. Sequential determinations of serum myoglobin levels suggest rapid reductions with response to therapy, often before the activities of serum enzymes such as creatine kinase, lactic dehydrogenase, and glutamic-oxaloacetic transaminase return to normal. It is likely that the combined use of serum myoglobin determinations with the enzymes will offer advantages for the detection and assessment of myopathic states. In a study of patients with myositis,[71] 19% had hypermyoglobinemia in the absence of elevated creatine kinase levels. Myoglobinuria, although less frequent, also occurs in patients with inflammatory muscle disease, and persistent myoglobinuria has been associated with renal failure in these patients.[40] Because levels of myoglobin may undergo

circadian variation, it is best to compare results from a standard time of day.[72]

ERYTHROCYTE SEDIMENTATION RATE

The erythrocyte sedimentation rate is often elevated in patients with active myositis in the range of 30 to 50 mm/hour as measured by the Westergren method. This value is normal, however, in many patients, and no correlation exists between the erythrocyte sedimentation rate and the grade of disability or degree of weakness.[6] During remission of the disease, this value generally approaches normal.

AUTOANTIBODIES

Patients with dermatomyositis may have circulating antibodies to certain nuclear and cellular constituents. These are discussed later, in the section on serologic factors.

ELECTROMYOGRAPHY

Patients with inflammatory muscle disease have evidence of myopathy on electromyographic examination; volitional contraction produces a pattern of activity characterized by short duration, low amplitude, and polyphasic potentials.[73] At rest, fibrillation potentials may be observed, presumably the result of involvement of terminal neural elements in the inflammatory process. Overall, 70 to 90% of patients studied have these findings; however, a few patients may have no demonstrable abnormalities. Generally, little or no correlation exists between the grade of disability at presentation and the electromyographic findings.[6,8]

Studies of patients with standard as well as single-fiber electromyography, a more specialized technique, indicate an increase in the number of muscle fibers in individual motor units, along with abnormal jitter and blocking. These findings also suggest changes in the pattern of terminal innervation of the muscle, perhaps related to involvement of intramuscular nerves by inflammation or anoxia or other factors coincident with inflammation, degeneration, and regeneration. In this connection, these changes may relate to the finding of fibrillation activity or to the occasional occurrence of fiber type grouping seen in affected tissues by histochemical techniques; these changes also suggest neural involvement.[74]

MUSCLE BIOPSY

Muscle biopsy is indicated in nearly all patients with suspected myositis before proceeding with what may be a long course of potentially hazardous therapy. Demonstration of inflammation confirms the diagnosis.

The optimal procedure for obtaining and processing muscle tissue requires coordination among clinician, surgeon, pathologist, and technologists. The site selected should be one of active involvement, but not marked by advanced atrophic or end-stage disease. In addition, sites previously traumatized by electromyography needles, intramuscular injections, or surgical procedures should be avoided. In most cases, proximal muscle tissue of the extremity is usually selected. Cases of myositis with only spinal muscle involvement have been reported. Biopsy of the erector spinae muscles may be performed. Muscle is obtained at resting length for histologic processing.

In many cases, particularly when the clinician feels histologic evaluation is all that is desired, needle muscle biopsy may be employed. Its major advantages are ease of performance and low morbidity rate. A major drawback is the small size of the sample. If needed, however, multiple samples may be obtained. Expert handling of the small bits of tissue removed is critical to ensure their proper orientation for microtome sectioning. Contraction artifacts also may be encountered in needle biopsy samples. In a series of 30 patients, the overall diagnostic yield from needle biopsy was comparable to that expected with the open-surgical procedure. Inflammation, necrosis, and degeneration were noted in most specimens studied. Two had only myofiber atrophy, and one had no abnormality. In addition, sequential needle biopsies have been employed to demonstrate response to therapy. Definite correlation in this regard may be difficult, however, because of uneven involvement of muscle tissue and because of persistent abnormalities in otherwise stable patients. In one group of patients examined by needle biopsy, failure to respond to corticosteroid therapy was associated with an increased number of myofiber internal nuclei.[75,76]

Open-surgical biopsy, the present standard, is more time-consuming and is attended with more discomfort and morbidity than needle biopsy, but it obtains larger specimens with fewer chances for artifact, and it allows biochemical or electron-microscopic studies.

HISTOLOGIC EXAMINATION

The major findings in muscle tissue of patients with inflammatory myopathy are necrosis, phagocytosis of necrotic muscle tissue, perivascular and interstitial inflammation, and myofiber regeneration (Figs. 72–9 to 72–12). Signs of regeneration include the presence of myoblasts, seen as crescentic cells with basophilic cytoplasm within the sarcolemmal sheath. Myoblasts of this type may contain one or two nuclei and either few coarse myofibrils or none. Syncytial masses of such presumed progenitor cells with basophilic cytoplasm and immature myofibrils, as well as myotubes, characterized by central nuclei, and large myofibers with peripheral basophilia may all be part of the regenerative process. Increased content of RNA and of certain enzymes such as lactate dehydrogenase and succinate dehydrogenase are noted in regenerating myofibers by histochemical techniques. The inflammatory infiltrate, the hallmark of myositis, consists of small and large lymphocytes, macrophages, and occasionally, plasma cells. Associated with the infiltrate of inflammatory cells, particularly in chronic cases, is an increase in collagen and connective tissue, which may separate bundles of myofibers as well as isolate and replace individual necrotic myofibers. Immunohistologic study has indicated that this connective tissue is rich in collagen types I to IV, and concentrations of the amino terminal propeptides of procollagen III, the precursor of type III collagen, are increased in blood serum of patients with polymyositis and dermatomyositis.[77–80]

Anastomoses between the terminal cisternae of the sarcoplasmic reticulum and the transverse tubules have been observed by electron-microscopic examination in myositis. These abnormal anastomoses may furnish pathways for the leakage of intracellular constituents such as enzymes to the extracellular space.[81]

In patients with chronic disease, inflammatory changes may be less marked, and the histologic picture may be characterized by myofiber atrophy, fibrosis, and increased deposits or accumulations of lipid.

Table 72–4 indicates the results of muscle biopsy of 103 patients, all of whom had clinical findings of polymyositis.[6] Sixty-five percent of specimens showed sufficient inflammation for the diagnosis of myositis (groups 1 and 2); however, 17% of patients had no demonstrable abnormalities. The data suggest that muscle biopsy is strong diagnostic evidence in most patients with active disease, but a negative or nonspecific biopsy does not of itself exclude the diagnosis of polymyositis.

Another review indicated an overall frequency of 5% of patients with clinically evident myositis, but normal tissue on biopsy. Interestingly, this phenomenon was more frequent in patients with associated malignancies.[82]

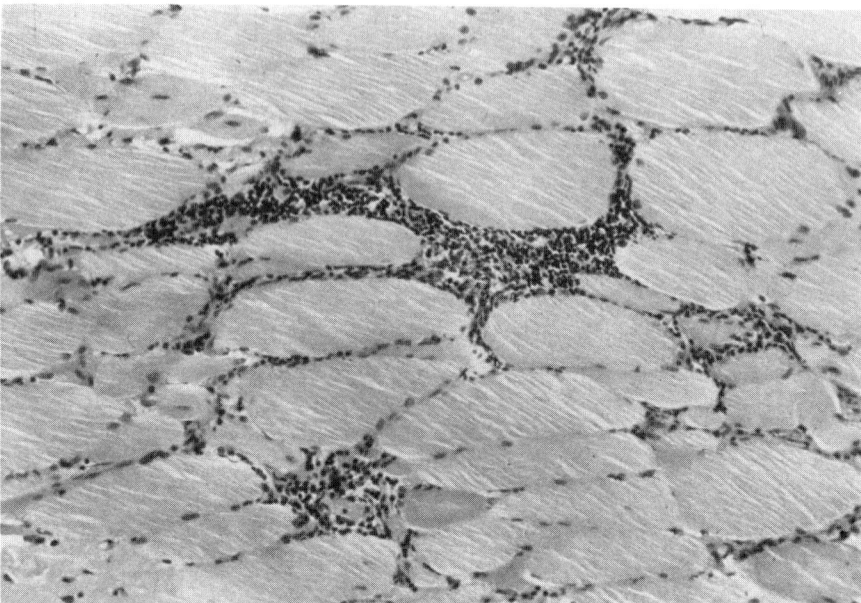

FIG. 72–9. Infiltration of inflammatory cells between fibers with necrosis and areas of loss of fibers seen on microscopic examination of a muscle biopsy specimen.

Childhood Dermatomyositis

The histologic findings of childhood dermatomyositis, characterized by zonal loss of capillaries, muscle infarction, vasculopathy, and lymphocytic infiltration of blood vessels, set this entity apart from other types of inflammatory myopathy. Vasculopathy is the striking feature. In addition to an inflammatory component, swelling, necrosis, and obliteration of vessels also occur in the absence of nearby inflammatory cells. The endothelium of small vessels may appear prominent and hyperplastic.

Electron-microscopic evaluation of endothelial cells reveals degeneration, and areas of regeneration. Affected endothelial cells appear pleomorphic and contain cytoplasmic inclusions made up of aggregates of tubular structures, both free and circumscribed by endoplasmic reticulum. The tubular structures are 250 to 280 Å in diameter, and the aggregate masses are 0.4 to 2.7 μ across. These inclusion aggregates appear to distort the endothelial cells. Gaps are present between endothelial cells. Changes in the endothelium and the loss of the normal covering of underlying collagen may be factors in the formation of thrombi in such affected vessels.

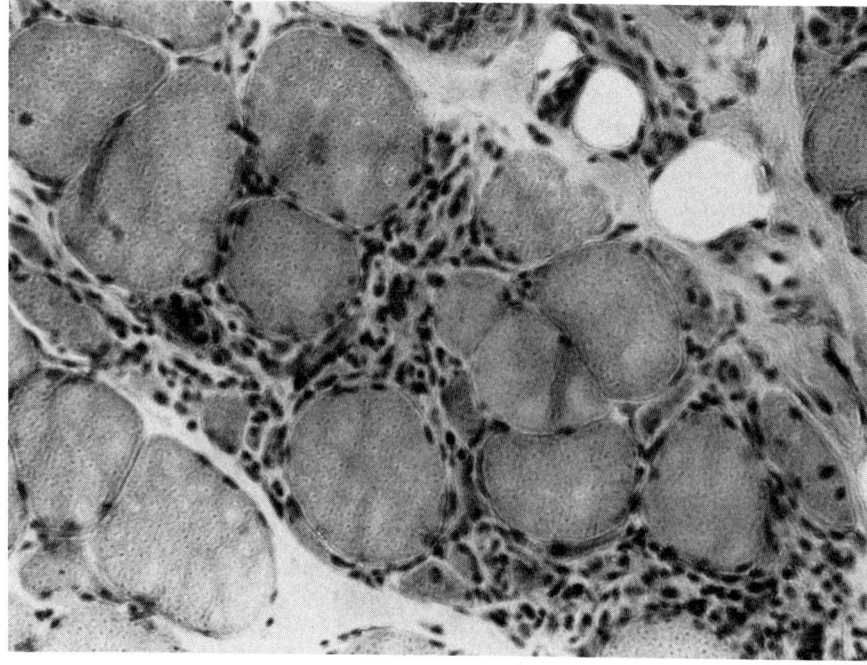

FIG. 72–10. Inflammatory cell infiltrate with areas of necrosis and an increase in connective tissue and lipid (upper right).

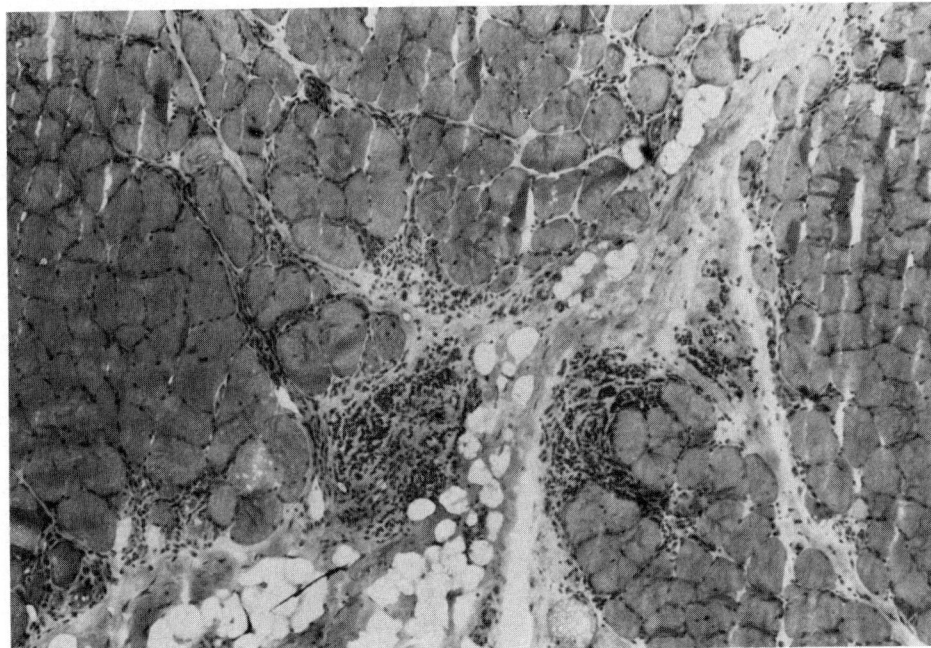

FIG. 72–11. Low-power microscopic view demonstrating zones of inflammation and an increase in connective tissue and lipid in a patient with chronic polymyositis.

Thrombosis may be seen in capillaries, small arteries, and veins in muscle tissue obtained from children with dermatomyositis. Associated with these findings of small-vessel damage and occlusion are ischemic changes in muscle. Myofiber atrophy occurs, as does infarction, particularly at the periphery of the muscle fasciculus. In addition to the changes in the blood vessels and the muscle ischemia, changes in sarcolemmal nuclei and cytoplasmic inclusions of the muscle cells are present. Signs of muscle regeneration with enlarged satellite cells are present. Immunoglobulin, fibrin, and complement components have also been identified in or near blood-vessel walls, but these constituents have not been directly related to the presence of inflammation or to the degree of vascular damage. Vasculopathy may also occur in tissue other than skeletal muscle. Endarteropathy, marked by endothelial cell abnormalities with tubuloreticular inclusions, has been found in the superficial dermis, along with dermal infiltrates of mononuclear cells.

FIG. 72–12. Perifascicular atrophy in a biopsy from a child with dermatomyositis.

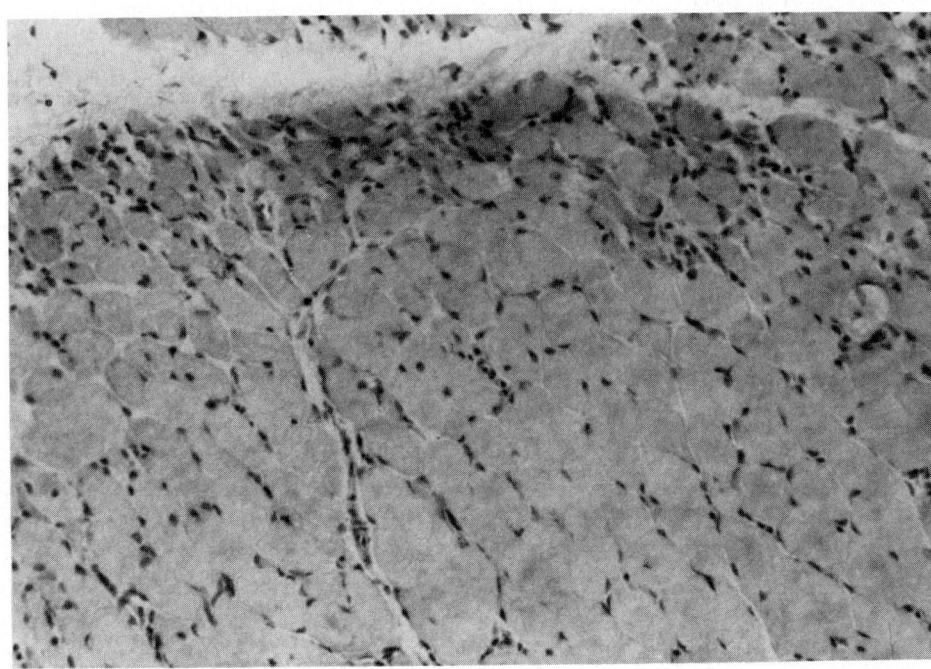

Table 72–4. Muscle Biopsy Findings in a Group of 103 Patients with Myositis

Findings	Percentage of Total (%)	
1. Fiber destruction, regeneration, perivascular and interstitial inflammation	46	65%
2. Perivascular and interstitial inflammatory infiltrate with minimal fiber destruction	19	
3. Myofiber destruction and regeneration without inflammatory cell infiltrates	8	
4. Fiber atrophy and other nonspecific changes	11	
5. Normal tissue	17	

(Data adapted from DeVere, R., and Bradley, W.G.[6])

Endarteropathy and vascular damage in the gastrointestinal tract are believed to be factors in perforation of the small intestine, a grave complication of childhood dermatomyositis.[83,84] Vascular lesions affecting the retina and skin may occur. In the skin, the dermal microvasculature may show changes of endothelial swelling and damage, as well as concentric thickening of the basement membrane. Dropout of vessels and linear deposition of collagen also may be evident. It has been suggested that children with pronounced ulcerating cutaneous vasculitis may follow a more disabling course.[85]

THEORIES OF PATHOGENESIS

The cause or causes of dermatomyositis and polymyositis are not known. Several areas, however, have served as foci for study and discussion in speculating on possible pathogenetic mechanisms. In this context, the following topics are discussed: (1) the relation of the immune system to myositis; (2) the relation of infectious disease to myositis; and (3) the association of malignant disease with myositis.

IMMUNE SYSTEM

This discussion includes aspects of humoral and cellular immunity, and genetics.

Muscle Components

Early studies demonstrated the presence of antibody with specificity for muscle tissue and its components, but such autoantibodies are not specific for patients with clinically evident myositis. Antibodies and immune reactions to myoglobin,[86] myosin,[87] and filamin and vinculin[88] have been found in higher titer in patients with inflammatory muscle disease compared to controls. Immunoglobulin and complement components have been observed deposited in muscle during the course of myositis. The presence of immunoglobulin deposits is not always correlated with the presence of inflammation in the areas in which it is found, however, nor are these deposits found only in patients with myositis.[89] Further, not all investigators have found immunoglobulins or complement components in affected muscle.[90] This topic is controversial. One study concluded that immunoglobulin associated with blood vessels, connective tissue, and necrotic fibers may be nonspecifically deposited. Using the immunoperoxidase method, the mononuclear cells of the inflammatory infiltrate were found to contain IgG and IgM in most biopsies studied.[91] Antigens of the terminal C5b-9 membrane-attack complex of the complement system were localized to the intramuscular arterioles and capillaries in muscle biopsy specimens of most patients with childhood dermatomyositis. Such vasculopathy may be of pathogenetic significance.[92]

In experimental myositis in animals, muscle-binding antibody may appear, but its presence is not correlated with the onset of illness, and no relationship exists between the titers of such antibody and the presence or severity of myositis. In this situation, muscle-binding antibody has not been demonstrated to be injurious to muscle,[93] although under other circumstances, antibody may be pathogenic.[94]

Little or no evidence exists for abnormalities in the humoral immune capabilities of most patients with inflammatory muscle disease, although the occurrence of myositis in certain patients with immunoglobulin or complement deficiency raises this issue. Hypogammaglobulinemic disorders of both the congenital and acquired types have been observed in association with dermatomyositis and polymyositis, and a patient with inflammatory myopathy associated with a deficiency of the second component of complement has been encountered.[95–97] Whether these associations suggest a relationship of myositis with a defective immune response against an unknown provoking agent is unknown at this time.

Nuclear and Cytoplasmic Antigens (see Chapters 68 and 70)

Using tissue-cultured cells as substrate for immunocytological studies, it has become evident that many patients with polymyositis have serologic reactivity. The pattern of this reactivity is nuclear in over half the tested sera, with homogeneous cytoplasmic or nucleolar staining occurring less frequently. In addition, other patterns, including centromeric and cytoplasmic filamentous, have been observed rarely.[98]

Progress toward identifying the nature of the antigens involved and the relationships of serologic reactivity to the type of disease has been great, although much remains to be done. The clearest relationships between antibody and clinical pattern are antinuclear RNP and PM-SLE overlap, anti-Jo-1 with polymyositis, and anti-Mi with dermatomyositis.[98] Several additional antibody-antigen systems have also been observed, but each specificity occurs in only a fraction of patients.

The Jo-1 antibody system is found in 20 to 30% of patients with polymyositis, but much less frequently in dermatomyositis. Antibody to Jo-1 was found in 47% of tested patients with polymyositis, but in none with dermatomyositis or myositis associated with malignancy. Fifty percent of the Jo-1-positive patients had pulmonary involvement, whereas did only 14.7% of the negative patients.[82] There may be an association between its occurrence and the presence of HLA-DR3.[99] A strong association has become apparent between the presence of this antibody and interstitial lung disease in patients with myositis. Nine of 14 patients (64%) reported from Japan had this antibody,[100] and similar findings have been reported from England and the United States. In the American series, 8 of 17 patients with polymyositis (47%), but none with dermatomyositis, had the Jo-1 antibody. An additional 2 of 13 patients with overlap syndromes also had Jo-1. Of these 10 patients, 5 had pulmonary involvement as defined by chest roentgenographs and/or diffusing capacity tests, whereas only 14.7% of the patients without the Jo-1 antibody had such involvement.[101] In the English experience, anti-Jo-1 was found in 25% of patients with myositis, but its prevalence in patients with both myositis and fibrosing alveolitis was 68% (13 of 19).[102] The Jo-1 antigen has been characterized as histidyl-tRNA synthetase.[103] Other antibodies have been detected in sera of patients with myositis against other RNA charging enzymes. Antithreonyl-tRNA synthetase was found in sera from patients with polymyositis, and one with an SLE-like syndrome.[104,105] This specificity, estimated to be present in 5% of cases, is much less common than Jo-1. Still less common is antialanyl-tRNA synthetase, estimated to occur in approximately 3% of patients with myositis.[106]

Because the antibodies of this type are present in only some patients with myositis, their pathogenic role is uncertain. Such antibodies may have been stimulated by other etiologically important molecules, and theories of molecular mimicry and viral causation have been proposed.

The Mi-antibody system has been found to consist of two components. The Mi-1 antibody cross-reacts with bovine immunoglobulin and is present in a small proportion of patients with myositis, as well as in sera from patients with other disorders.[107] The Mi-2 antibody correlates strongly with dermatomyositis, but occurs in only a minority of patients. In one study, 11 of 52 adult and pediatric patients with dermatomyositis had Mi-2 antibody demonstrated by an enzyme-linked immunosorbent assay, but it was rare or absent in other disorders or in normal individuals. The nature of the Mi antigen is not yet known.[108]

The PM-1 or PM-Scl antibody is found in about 10% of patients with myositis, approximately one half of whom also have scleroderma features, and occurs in patients with scleroderma without discernible myositis. The PM-Scl antigen is most likely a protein associated with the cell nucleus and nucleolus.[109,110]

Patients with myositis in association with other connective tissue disorders or overlap syndromes may evince a number of other antigen-antibody systems, such as anti-Ku, seen with PSS and SLE, as well as antibodies to nRNP, Ro, Scl-70, Sm, DNA, and La.

Cell-Mediated Immunity

Analysis of the inflammatory cell infiltrate in biopsy samples from patients with polymyositis suggests a role of cellular immunity in disease pathogenesis. Current data should be considered preliminary because of the relatively small numbers of patients studied and because of the lack of agreement among all investigators. Nonetheless, these data suggest differences in the composition of the cellular infiltrate among patients with different diagnoses, and among different sites in affected tissues.

Immunohistochemical studies suggest that cytotoxic T8 cells and macrophages invade, and may destroy, muscle fibers in polymyositis and inclusion body myositis, but not in dermatomyositis. In dermatomyositis, the inflammatory exudate was predominantly perivascular and perimysial, consisting chiefly of B-lymphocytes at perivascular sites and of T-lymphocytes (mostly T8) at endomysial sites. In polymyositis, the inflammatory exudate is predominantly endomysial and focal, although perimysial and perivascular infiltrates are also conspicuous. B cells again are most prominent perivascularly, whereas T cells are most abundant at the endomysium, with a particular increase of T8 cells at these sites. In both dermatomyositis and polymyositis, the relative proportions of T cells, T8 cells, and Ia bearing T cells increases from the perivascular areas to the endomysium. Conversely, the relative proportion of B cells and T4 cells decreases in this direction. It has been suggested in dermatomyositis that the high percentage of B cells and the high T4/T8 ratios reflect helper T-cell stimulation of B cells to secrete immunoglobulin, and that humoral immune mechanisms may therefore be of importance in this disorder. In polymyositis, the close apposition of lymphocytes and macrophages to membranes of myofibers and the invasion of non-necrotic muscle fibers of mononuclear cells suggest a more central role for cell-mediated immune mechanisms in pathogenesis.[111] The role of autosensitized mononuclear cells as instigators of inflammation in the myositis syndromes remains controversial, however.

Mononuclear cells from patients with either polymyositis or dermatomyositis, after incubation with autologous muscle, have been shown to release factors suppressing the ATP-dependent calcium binding of the sarcoplasmic reticulum membrane. This may play a role in the dysfunction of the sarcoplasmic reticulum of patients with myositis and, in turn, contribute to inefficiency of the contraction-relaxation mechanism.[112,113]

Genetics

The possibility of a genetic influence in dermatomyositis and polymyositis has been suggested on the basis of studies of HLA associations, but this influence is not yet understood. HLA-B8/DR3 has been noted with increased frequency in many white children with dermatomyositis,[114,115] as well as in adults with polymyositis.[116,117] Associations of disease with HLA-B14 and B-40 have also been noted.[118] A recent study of 33 patients including children and adults, however, failed to confirm any HLA associations,[119] although the possible influence of genetic factors was supported by a high incidence of putative autoimmune diseases, such as rheumatoid arthritis (RA), thyroid disease, juvenile-onset diabetes, and pernicious anemia, in first-degree relatives of patients with polymyositis. None of the relatives had polymyositis.

INFECTIOUS AGENTS

Skeletal muscle may be the site of inflammation in a number of infectious disorders caused by diverse agents including bacteria, protozoa, viruses, and parasites. None of these disorders has been linked to the development of chronic polymyositis; however, the possible role of infectious agents is considered in this section, particularly in relation to viruses and to toxoplasmosis.

Viruses

Several viruses may produce muscle damage and inflammation, usually of a transient nature. Among the best characterized of these are Coxsackie, echo- and influenza viruses. One such postviral syndrome of childhood is termed *benign acute myositis*. In this disorder, children develop severe lower extremity pain, usually in the calves, with soreness and cramps, 24 to 72 hours after an upper respiratory infection of apparent gastroenteritis. Boys are affected more frequently than girls. The average age is approximately 9 years. The prodromal illness is marked by fever, occasionally headache, and gastrointestinal or respiratory symptoms. During the period of severe myalgia, muscles may swell. Biopsy is rarely performed; however, inflammation of muscle was observed in one girl, and in another child, no abnormalities were noted. Results of virologic studies in this syndrome are consistent with recent infection, usually with influenza virus of either type A or type B. On occasion, adenovirus, and parainfluenza viruses are also implicated. Most children recover completely within a week. Creatine kinase activity of serum is elevated and returns to normal in 2 weeks.[120]

This disease has an epidemic form. In one such outbreak, 17 children developed acute myositis, chiefly involving the gastrocnemius and soleus muscles. Influenza B virus was isolated from 11 of the 17 patients. Complete recovery occurred in 4 to 5 days.[121]

Adults also have been affected with myositis following influenza virus infection. In some cases, myositis was transient; in others, severe and prolonged disease occurred with myonecrosis, myoglobinuria, and renal failure. Although documentation of viral infection is most commonly serologic, virus has been isolated from respiratory secretions, and in a 65-year-old man with inflammatory myopathy following an influenza-like syndrome, influenza B virus was recovered from affected muscle, and was seen in muscle by electron microscopy.[122]

Coxsackie virus has been seen by electron microscopy and has been isolated from muscle in children with inflammatory myopathy. Elevation of antibody titers to Coxsackie B viruses have been found in some adults and children with polymyositis and dermatomyositis.[123,124] Coxsackie B virus-specific probes prepared using molecular cloning techniques were used to detect viral RNA in skeletal-muscle biopsy samples; five of nine patients with clinical myositis tested positive, whereas no viral sequences were detected in muscle from four patients with muscular dystrophy or from six normal children.[124a]

Hepatitis B virus also has been implicated in the pathogenesis of inflammatory muscle disease. Several instances of hepatitis B infection followed by myositis have been observed, with deposition of immunoglobulin, complement, and in one case, hepatitis surface antigen in muscle.[125]

Echovirus infection also has been associated with myositis including patients with X-linked hypogammaglobulinemia. Recovery of this virus has been reported from several sites. In one patient with weakness, elevated serum enzyme levels, a myopathic electromyographic pattern, and biopsy evidence of inflamed muscle and fascia, Echovirus 11 was recovered from muscle and cerebrospinal fluid. Treatment with immunoglobulin preparations containing specific antibody was followed by dramatic clinical recovery in this patient.[126] Not all patients have responded well in this manner, however. Accurate diagnosis is important in this viral syndrome because usual treatment for polymyositis with immunosuppressive agents may be detrimental.[127]

Other viruses, including herpes and Epstein-Barr viruses, have been implicated in myopathy and myositis. Particles seen by electron microscopy, possibly related to picorna-type virus, have been noted in muscle in several patients with myositis, as well as in patients with Reye's syndrome. In such instances, viral identification has not been definite, and questions have been raised regarding other origins for these structures, such as degeneration of cellular components.

Polymyositis has also been reported in patients infected with the human immunodeficiency virus.

On the basis of available information, it is possible to conclude that viruses of several types may lodge in muscle and may lead to inflammation and myonecrosis. In some cases, as in patients with hypogammaglobulinemia, host factors may be important in viral infection and in disease severity.

Toxoplasma Gondii

This protozoan organism commonly infects individuals in the United States, and asymptomatic cysts may persist in muscle.[128,129] During the early invasion of muscle in man, it is not known whether an accompanying inflammatory response occurs; however, experimental murine infections are associated with mild focal myositis.[130] In certain cases, *Toxoplasma gondii* infection of muscle has been linked to severe myopathy. In some such patients, the diagnosis of toxoplasmosis was suggested by serologic tests, as well as by response to therapy. In others, in addition to serologic evidence, *Toxoplasma* organisms were seen in muscle biopsies. Of three patients with these organisms identified in muscle, polymyositis was the diagnosis in two, and dermatomyositis in one. Cen-

tral nervous system disease and fever are common in such patients.[131–133]

Serologic evidence of toxoplasmosis has also been obtained in studies of patients with polymyositis. In an age-, sex-, and race-matched controlled study, 60% of patients with polymyositis had positive Sabin-Feldman tests with titers higher than in control subjects. In addition, complement-fixing antibody, usually suggestive of recent infection, was present in greater frequency (35%) and at higher titers than in control subjects. Responses of this type were not found in the polymyositis patients tested for antibody against rubella, measles, parainfluenza, and Epstein-Barr viruses. Patients with serologic evidence of recent toxoplasmosis generally had polymyositis of less than 2 years' duration.[134] Declines in antibody titers over time and an improvement coincident with sulfa-pyrimethamine therapy have also been reported.[135] In addition, a high frequency of specific IgM anti-*Toxoplasma* antibody, suggestive of recent infection, is also found. In a recent study, 48% of patients with inflammatory muscle disease and positive Sabin-Feldman tests had IgM antibody.[136] Current evidence suggests high frequency of recent toxoplasmosis among certain patients with polymyositis of recent onset. It is not known, however, whether *Toxoplasma gondii* in such patients is the causative agent of polymyositis or whether dormant, persistent forms may be reactivated or reintroduced to the immune system concurrent with inflammation in muscle.

MALIGNANT DISEASE

The association of malignant disease with inflammatory myopathy may offer an important clue to the pathogenesis of myositis. The basis for this association, initially noted over 100 years ago, is still poorly understood and remains controversial. The reported frequency of malignant disease in patients with dermatomyositis varies widely; however, several series reported a rate of approximately 15 to 20% of adults. Malignant disease in children with myositis is rare, although neoplasia and coincident dermatomyositis-like syndromes have been described. One review of this aspect listed two children with leukemia, one with agammaglobulinemia followed by lymphoma, and one with pituitary adenoma.

A retrospective survey of the literature to 1976 noted 258 cases of malignant disease concurrent with myositis. Most such cases were observed in the fifth and sixth decades of life, with a mean age of 52.6 years. The most frequent tumors were cancers of the breast and lung; malignant tumors of the ovary and stomach were also common. In this group, the temporal relation of the onset of the two disorders was reported in 167 patients. In 99 of these patients, myopathy was observed first, and the malignant process was discovered later, usually within a year. In 17 patients, both diseases were noted at the same time, and in 51, the tumor appeared first, and the myopathy was recognized later, usually within a year. The frequency of malignant disease in patients with myositis was 5 to 7 times that expected in the general population. Similar results have been noted in other retrospective surveys. One study over a 20-year period noted 7 of 27 patients with both dermatomyositis and malignant disease. This frequency, 26%, was not only greater than that expected in the general population, but also was greater than that reported in patients with RA or systemic lupus erythematosus. Of this group of 7 patients, 2 had breast cancer, 2 had cancer of the colon, and 3 had cancer of an unknown primary site. In most patients, the diagnosis of malignant disease was made at the same time as the diagnosis of dermatomyositis. Adding to the general impression of the significance of this relationship are case reports of patients with multiple neoplasms in whom recurrence of dermatomyositis-like signs was observed with the recurrence of the tumor or with the appearance of a new tumor.

In another group of 35 patients with dermatomyositis seen over a 20-year period, 12 had malignant disease. Of these, 6 of 9 showed improvement in the manifestations of dermatomyositis after treatment directed toward the neoplasm, and 3 had exacerbations of dermatomyositis with progression of the neoplasm. The course of the two disorders is not always parallel, however. Although the course may not be predictable, the coexistence of these disorders generally bespeaks a grave prognosis. The types of associated malignant diseases vary, as previously indicated; most neoplasms are carcinomas originating in the lung, breast, gastrointestinal tract, nasopharynx, ovary, and uterus. Lymphomas, sarcomas, and other malignant diseases are also observed.

The reason for this concurrence is unknown. The retrospective method of enumerating published case reports may place undue emphasis on this association, and the lack of a prospective study leaves unanswered the question of the precise frequency of this association. Nonetheless, on the basis of available information, it is prudent to look for this coincidence, particularly in adults with dermatomyositis.

Because of the many kinds of malignant disorders noted, the varied times of the appearance of one disease relative to the other, and the lack of a predictable direct relationship in the short-term course of the ill-nesses, it seems unlikely that one illness is the direct cause of the other. It is possible that an alteration in host responsiveness, perhaps involving the immune apparatus, may underlie the mechanism of the expression of both illnesses.[5,82,137-141] The frequency of malignancy among adult patients with polymyositis/dermatomyositis, therefore, is in the range of 7 to 24%. If patients are excluded from analysis because the association of these disorders (e.g., malignancy and myositis) was widely separated in time, the frequency is reduced by approximately one half. It should be kept in mind, however, that if host factors predispose to this association, there may be no reason to suppose a priori that the disorders would necessarily be coincident.[5,82,137-141]

OTHER DISORDERS MARKED BY MYOSITIS

DRUG-RELATED STATES

Drugs are not usually the cause of myositis, although toxic and myopathic effects of medications are known. Myositis-like states are reported rarely in patients receiving sulfonamides, penicillin, isoniazid, and azathioprine.[142,143] One agent that may produce inflammatory myopathy, however, is D-penicillamine. Most patients with this complication have received this agent for the treatment of RA. In one reported case, a patient had two muscle biopsies; myositis was not present prior to therapy and was seen after treatment with D-penicillamine.[144-146]

OTHER CONNECTIVE TISSUE DISORDERS

Myositis may be a prominent feature of other connective tissue disorders. Progressive systemic sclerosis, in particular, may begin in a manner indistinguishable from polymyositis and may later develop its own characteristic features. In undifferentiated or mixed connective tissue disorders, inflammatory myopathy is often a prominent element. Myositis also may complicate the course of systemic lupus erythematosus and of sarcoidosis. Although patients with RA do not generally have clinical signs of inflammatory myopathy, histologic examination may reveal the presence of inflammation in skeletal muscle, particularly in severely affected patients.[147] Myalgia and muscle weakness are noted in approximately one third of patients with Sjögren's syndrome. Severe myositis with profound weakness and marked elevation of serum enzyme levels is less common.[148,149]

INCLUSION BODY MYOSITIS

This disorder is marked by chronic, progressive wasting and weakness with microscopic inclusions seen in both nuclei and cytoplasm of skeletal muscle cells. In contrast to dermatomyositis and polymyositis, this rare disorder occurs most frequently in middle-aged or elderly men. No skin rash is present. About 50 such patients have been recognized and reported. Clinical generalizations may have to be modified as more cases are documented. Although most cases have occurred in elderly men, a bimodal distribution is suggested, with younger patients being women. The disorder is usually slowly progressive and painless. Involvement of distal, as well as proximal, musculature may be marked. This feature, combined with loss of tendon reflexes and occasional asymmetric involvement at the outset, may suggest a neuropathy. Electromyographic testing, however, has revealed myopathic signs with polyphasic potentials of brief duration and neuropathic features, such as fibrillation and long-lasting, large amplitude potentials. Dysphagia has occurred, and creatine kinase elevation of a moderate degree is present in most, but not all, patients.

The distinguishing features of this disorder are seen on histologic examination of affected muscle. In addition to evidence of myonecrosis and inflammation, eosinophilic inclusions occur in the sarcoplasm, the nucleus, or both. Rimmed or lined vacuoles filled with basophilic granules are seen on cryostat sections stained with hematoxylin and eosin. These appear purplish with the Gomori trichrome stain. Paraffin sections usually do not reveal these granules, which are likely to be removed by solvents, but they do demonstrate the empty vacuoles.

By electron microscopy, the nuclear and/or cytoplasmic inclusions are seen to be masses of filamentous material, often in crystalline arrays. The diameters of the filaments range from 10 to 25 nm and are greater in the cytoplasm. The pathogenesis of the inclusions is uncertain. Recently, mumps virus antigen was demonstrated by immunohistochemical techniques in both intranuclear and cytoplasmic inclusions in eight cases. In five of these, frozen sections also showed mumps antigen-positive cytoplasmic inclusions without rimmed vacuoles.[151] These observations raise the suggestion that inclusion body myositis may be the result of chronic persistent mumps virus infection; however, serum mumps antibody ti-

ters in a few patients studied have not been found elevated.[150–155] Adenovirus type 2 was isolated from muscle tissue in one case.[155a]

Inclusion body myositis is probably under-recognized.[155b] It was documented in 17% of two large series of patients with inflammatory myopathy.[152,155c] It is important to differentiate it from polymyositis because its natural history and treatment are different.

The natural history of this disease is slow, inexorable progression. Corticosteroids, immunosuppressive drugs, or total body irradiation[155d] are ineffective in isolated inclusion body myositis. An occasional case is followed by,[155e] or associated with,[155f–155h] a diffuse connective tissue disease (e.g., SLE, Sjögren's syndrome, or immune thrombocytopenia). Some of these patients may respond to corticosteroid therapy.

TROPICAL PYOMYOSITIS

This disorder is marked by abscesses, apparently spontaneously occurring in skeletal muscle. Children and young adults chiefly in tropical areas are affected. One or more skeletal muscles such as biceps, pectoral, gluteal, or quadriceps become painful and tender. An accompanying fever is usually present. The involved area may resolve spontaneously or may swell and suppurate, yielding large numbers of microorganisms, most often *Staphylococcus aureus*. The presence of multiple abscesses suggests hematogenous spread. Occasionally, clinically involved areas may be bacteriologically sterile, and this observation has led to speculation that skeletal muscle may first be damaged by an unknown agent, and then colonized by Staphylococcus. Among candidates for such initiating agents have been tissue parasites, other bacteria and viruses, antecedent trauma, the presence of genetically variant hemoglobin, and nutritional deficiencies. The morbidity and mortality rates for tropical pyomyositis relate to the occurrence of staphylococcal septicemia and metastatic suppurative complications, suh as osteomyelitis.[156,157]

This condition is becoming recognized with increasing frequency in temperate climates: 32 cases had been recorded in the United States as of 1984,[157a] some but not all patients had traveled to the tropics before disease onset. Staphylococci predominated in these patients also, but cases resulting from Yersinia[157b] and streptococci[157c,157d] have been reported. Early recognition is important because 85% of the cases associated with the latter organism have proved fatal. Computerized tomography[157e] and gray-scale ultrasonography[157f] have been reported as useful diagnostic methods. One case occurred in association with diabetes mellitus and rheumatoid arthritis.[157g]

EOSINOPHILIC MYOSITIS AND HYPEREOSINOPHILIC SYNDROMES

Myositis with eosinophilic infiltration may be part of hypereosinophilic syndromes, along with involvement of other organs and the central nervous system. In some patients, anemia, hypergammaglobulinemia, petechiae, Raynaud's phenomenon, and pulmonary and cardiac manifestations have been observed. Cardiac complications include endocardial and myocardial fibrosis, congestive heart failure, and arrhythmias. Peripheral neuropathy may be present. Circulating eosinophilia, which may not be constant in all cases, can be marked, with relative proportions of 20 to 60% of the circulating leukocytes. Leukocytosis is common. Response to corticosteroid therapy is inconsistent or poor. One patient responded after leukapheresis.[158,159] Myositis also may occur during the course of eosinophilic fasciitis.[160–163] Eosinophilic myositis may have a relapsing course with a benign prognosis.[162,163] A single case of a new syndrome, eosinophilia associated with perimyositis and pneumonitis, has appeared.[163a]

GRANULOMATOUS MYOPATHY

This entity may be associated with other disorders such as sarcoidosis or Crohn's disease of the bowel, or it may appear without the signs of other disease. Granulomatous myopathy occurring alone is generally observed in middle-aged women who have a chronically progressive, predominantly proximal pattern of muscle weakness, occasionally complicated by dysphagia. Histologic examination reveals groups of granulomas made up of loosely packed epithelioid cells and histiocytes, often in association with lymphocytes and a surrounding rim of collagenous fibers. Reticular fibers are present in the granuloma, as well as Langerhans-type giant cells.

Myositis may occur during the course of sarcoidosis, and granulomas have been observed in muscle tissue of patients with sarcoid myopathy, as well as in patients with sarcoidosis who have no muscular symptoms.[164–166]

Myositis may also accompany *chronic enteroviral meningoencephalitis* in children with X-linked (Bruton's) agammaglobulinemia.[166a]

Metabolic muscle disorders are discussed in Chapter 110.

TREATMENT

In considering the approach to therapy, two features should be accented: the first is accuracy of diagnosis, and the second is precision of assessment of disease activity.

It is important to secure as accurate a diagnosis as possible before initiating a treatment program that may be lengthy and possibly hazardous. In this connection, the presence of an associated malignant disease or of another connective tissue disorder may affect the patient's prognosis and response to treatment.

The assessment of disease activity and of response to therapy depends on evaluating elements of the patient's medical history, physical examination, and laboratory findings. Exacerbations of disease may have manifestations similar to those present at the disease's onset. Return of rash, arthralgia, and the spread of areas of telangiectasia may be early warnings of exacerbation and increased disease activity. Renewed weakness may be difficult to evaluate, and other factors, including therapy and the possibility of altered electrolyte balance, should be considered in the ongoing assessment of the patient's muscle strength and function. Laboratory findings, particularly increases in creatine kinase, lactate dehydrogenase, and serum myoglobin levels and, to a lesser extent, erythrocyte sedimentation rate, may accompany or may precede an exacerbation of inflammatory muscle disease. These laboratory findings may be less reliable in the chronically ill patient than at the onset of disease. Active inflammation in muscle, as well as vasculitis, may be present and may continue in the absence of chemical evidence of active disease.[167] In addition, other factors such as trauma, injections, the performance of electromyographic studies, and exertion may lead to transient elevations of serum enzymes, unrelated to the progression of the disease. Patients returning to fuller schedules of activities after a period of bed rest, or those undertaking exercise programs too taxing for their clinical status, may experience muscle aching accompanied by serum enzyme elevations. All these considerations stress the need for careful analysis of changes in the patient's condition before adjusting the program of therapy.

The major approach to treatment involves the use of medications and physical measures, with a spirit of understanding and cooperation between physician and patient. The course of illness may be protracted, and periods of depression and frustration should be anticipated.

PHYSICAL THERAPY

Rest during periods of active inflammation and physical therapy to rebuild muscle strength during periods of remission are indicated. Passive range-of-motion exercises are important to prevent the development of contractures. Despite daily therapy, however, contractures may occur and may progress in severely affected patients.

PHARMACOLOGIC THERAPY

This form of treatment includes corticosteroids and immunosuppressive agents.

Corticosteroids

Corticosteroids are the mainstay of drug treatment for most patients (see Chapter 37). Although adequately controlled data are still insufficient to indicate the degree of effectiveness of agents of this class, corticosteroid therapy is generally considered beneficial and is recommended for both adults and children. One should be aware of spontaneous remissions of disease. Retrospective examinations of overall survival have not demonstrated the absolute value of corticosteroids; however, this information may be difficult to evaluate because of the lack of simultaneous comparison groups adequately matched for diagnostic classification, time of institution of therapy in relation to disease onset, variation of doses and types of treatment, and age and sex.

The usual practice is to begin oral corticosteroid therapy in the range of 40 to 80 mg/day prednisone for approximately 4 to 6 weeks or until the maximum benefit or remission of the disease is achieved. The dose may then be gradually reduced, with careful monitoring of symptoms, physical findings, and laboratory test results. For children, doses of 1 to 2 mg/ kg body weight/day are used initially. Other approaches are possible; alternate-day therapy, as well as parenteral pulse therapy, has been used.[168,169] In general, corticosteroid dosage is reduced as clinical improvement is noted.[170,171] Maintenance dosage and the need to increase therapy are decided by the patient's response and the ensuing course.

In both children and adults, one sees the usual potentially serious complications of corticosteroid therapy. Hypertension, cardiovascular decompensation, exacerbation of diabetes mellitus, gastrointestinal ulceration, sepsis, and osteoporosis, as well as changes in physical appearance and psychologic state, have been problems. Questions regarding corticosteroid-induced myopathy are sometimes difficult to analyze, although in many patients treated on a long-term basis, corticosteroid-induced weakness may cause protracted disability.

Most patients with myositis unassociated with malignant disease can be treated with corticosteroids alone; however, this treatment may not always be optimal. Two such situations are as follows: (1) life-threatening progressive illness without response to adequate corticosteroid therapy; and (2) partially responsive illness requiring doses of corticosteroids that have side effects difficult or impossible to tolerate. Under these circumstances, one should consider adding other forms of therapy, such as immunosuppressive agents.

The response of patients who received prednisone (40 mg or more daily) for at least 4 weeks was studied in a review of 81 patients. Over 60% were felt to have achieved normal or near normal muscle strength after 3 to 4 months. Morbidity among these patients included 8 with osteoporotic vertebral compression fractures, 7 with avascular necrosis of the femoral head, 7 with complicated peptic ulcer, 7 with posterior subcapsular cataracts, and 4 with diabetes mellitus.[141]

Immunosuppressive Agents (see Chapters 35 and 38)

With regard to immunosuppressive agents, two general cautions should be observed. First, adequate and complete information about the effect of these drugs in myositis is lacking. The same problems mentioned in regard to corticosteroid therapy apply here, but because these agents have been less extensively used than corticosteroids, the amount of organized, controlled data on which to base judgments is even smaller. Second, although a number of different agents are classified together by virtue of immunosuppressive activity, current evidence is insufficient to relate this factor to therapeutic effectiveness. In addition, it is not known whether any two of these agents operate in a similar manner, through similar mechanisms.

A number of agents have been used, including 6-mercaptopurine and chlorambucil, but most experience has been gained with methotrexate, azathioprine, and cyclophosphamide.

Methotrexate was first employed in the treatment of dermatomyositis many years ago;[172] since then, several reports have noted its usefulness, including its corticosteroid-sparing effects that allow reduction in corticosteroid dosage.[173] Methotrexate in conjunction with corticosteroid therapy is usually given intravenously, initially at doses of 10 to 15 mg at intervals of 5 to 7 days, then with gradually increasing doses up to 50 mg or higher. The frequency of administration is then reduced from weekly to biweekly, and finally to monthly. Stomatitis is the most common side effect. Hepatotoxicity, bone-marrow suppression (usually evident as leukopenia), gastrointestinal hemorrhage, skin effects, nephropathy, and reduction of normal host defense against infection may be other complications of therapy. Drug-induced pneumonitis has been reported in patients receiving oral therapy.[24] Methotrexate, in biweekly injections of 2 to 3 mg/kg body weight or 7 mg/kg body weight with citrovorum factor, has been used in conjunction with corticosteroid therapy in children.[174] Oral methotrexate in weekly doses of approximately 7.5 to 15 mg has been used successfully, also.

Azathioprine has been added to corticosteroid treatment. A controlled study indicated that patients treated with azathioprine and corticosteroids showed improvements in functional ability and required less prednisone for maintenance than patients treated with prednisone alone.[175] The dose was 2 mg/kg/day until the concurrent prednisone dose could be reduced to less than 15 mg/day; then the azathioprine dose was reduced as tolerated. In general, doses for active disease in most studies are in the range of 100 to 150 mg/day orally, with a decrease to 50 to 75 mg/day for maintenance therapy after remission of the disease. Doses of 50 to 125 mg/day are prescribed for children.[174] Major areas of toxicity include bone-marrow suppression, chiefly leukopenia, gastrointestinal intolerance, and increased susceptibility to infections.

Cyclophosphamide has probably been used in fewer patients than either methotrexate or azathioprine. The dose has not been completely evaluated, but a range of 100 to 200 mg/day has been used. Toxicity includes bone-marrow suppression, increased susceptibility to infection, alopecia, and hemorrhage from the urinary bladder.

Other concerns relative to the use of these agents, except methotrexate, relate to possible genetic damage and the risk of malignant disease. These associations have not been completely evaluated in patients with myositis, but they should be considered, particularly in young patients. Overall, substantial corticosteroid-sparing effects have been noted in approximately 40 to 50% of patients treated with immunosuppressive agents.[3]

Cyclosporin has been used in a few patients.

Combined Immunosuppressive Drug Therapy

Two small, uncontrolled studies have documented successful treatment of steroid-resistant dermato-myositis/polymyositis[177a,177b] using combined immunosuppressive agents.*

Plasmapheresis

Plasmapheresis is a newly developed mode of treatment in patients judged to have a poor response to corticosteroids and immunosuppressive agents. Patients undergoing plasmapheresis have continued to receive corticosteroids and immunosuppressive agents during the period of pheresis therapy, which has sometimes lasted for several months or more. Most of a group of 35 patients treated in this manner were judged to be improved. Herpes zoster developed in 7 of 35 patients subjected to plasmapheresis.[176,177]

OTHER THERAPEUTIC CONSIDERATIONS

Other areas of treatment include management of calcinosis, for which medical therapy has not been effective. Surgical removal of troublesome deposits may be helpful.

Several patients with evidence of recent *Toxoplasma gondii* infection have received therapy directed against this organism with sulfonamides, pyrimethamine, and folinic acid.

PROGNOSIS

CHILDREN

The outlook for complete remission is good in at least 50% of children, and results are best with early diagnosis and treatment. Although severe, unresponsive disease is less common, the course of such patients may be complicated by respiratory infection, cardiac failure, and gastrointestinal hemorrhage, all of which unfavorably influence prognosis. Fatalities have occurred. Approximately 30 to 40% of children have chronic active disease and need protracted therapy. Calcinosis and joint contractures are sources of disability that, along with residual weakness, limit return to normal function when remission has occurred. Physical therapy, although not always effective, should be an early part of the therapeutic program to maximize chances for mobility and to decrease the likelihood of disabling contractures. The duration of disease activity in most children is generally 2 to 4 years.[167,171,178]

---

*Editor's note. I have relied on intravenous methotrexate combined with low-dose (50 to 100 mg/day) azathioprine for many years with gratifying results.[14]

In one retrospective study, a monocyclic disease pattern was present in 25% of children, with full recovery in 2 years. The remainder had either a chronic, continuous, persistent pattern of disease or a polycyclic course with periods not requiring therapy and periods of relapses.[179] Rarely, late relapses in apparently well children may occur.[180]

ADULTS

The outlook in adult patients does not appear to be as good as in children. In general, patients with malignant disease have a poor outcome. Patients under 20 years of age have better chances for survival than those over age 55. Intercurrent infections, particularly pneumonia, severe muscle weakness, chronically active disease, and dysphagia all unfavorably influence prognosis. The overall survival rate has varied in several studied groups. One retrospective survey, which did not include patients with malignant disease, indicated a mortality rate of 39% in the first year.[181] Another smaller study disclosed a similar mortality rate after 5 years.[57] A cumulative survival rate of 53% after 7 years was observed in a group of over 100 patients,[182] whereas a lower mortality rate, 28%, was noted in another group of similar size after 6 years.[6] Taken together, the experience indicates a substantial mortality rate in adults with inflammatory muscle disease, even in groups from which patients with cancer have been excluded. In addition, most surviving patients have long-term disability and need medication. Relapses are common, and many, perhaps 20 to 30% of patients, demonstrate disease activity with deterioration of strength or elevation of serum enzyme levels and erythrocyte sedimentation rate for over 10 years. Many patients have a static clinical state with elevated serum enzyme levels for long periods.

Histologic estimate of the severity of abnormalities demonstrated by muscle biopsy is not a generally reliable indicator of outcome.

The outlook in the future may not necessarily be as gloomy as these figures suggest. In a recent large series of patients, the mortality rate was 13.7% after a mean followup period of 4.3 years; 25% of the deaths were due to malignant disease, and 20% were due to sepsis. Recognition and prompt treatment of infections as well as careful monitoring and adjustment of medications may reduce the severity of complications and may improve the overall prognosis.[8]

A retrospective review of 27 patients indicated a more favorable outcome, with 52% of patients able to discontinue steroid therapy within an average 4½ year period of followup.[183] A similar result was obtained in a Canadian series in which 42% of patients, by lifetable analysis, terminated corticosteroids within 3 years of diagnosis. Thirty-two percent of these patients died, however, and functional disability was common.[184] Mortality rates over a 10-year period studied by review of death records indicated greatest overall mortality for non-white women.[185]

Factors that have been found to affect prognosis include age, cardiopulmonary disease, and dysphagia.

Of 39 patients age 45 and older in another series, 30.8% died, compared to 2.7% of younger patients. Cardiac involvement also indicates a poor prognosis. Dysphagia occurred in the more severely ill patients, with a shortened life expectancy. The cumulative survival of all patients in this study was 73% after 8 years, which probably reflects a trend toward better outcomes in recent years.[82]

REFERENCES

1. Bohan, A., and Peter, J.B.: Polymyositis and dermatomyositis. N. Engl. J. Med., 292:344–347, 403–407, 1975.
2. Walton, J.N., and Adams, R.D.: Polymyositis. Edinburgh, E.S. Livingstone, 1958.
3. Pearson, C.M., and Bohan, A.: The spectrum of polymyositis and dermatomyositis. Med. Clin. North Am., 61:439–457, 1977.
4. Thompson, C.E.: Infantile myositis. Dev. Med. Child. Neurol., 24:307–313, 1982.
5. Medsger, T.A., Dawson, W.N., and Masi, A.T.: The epidemiology of polymyositis. Am. J. Med., 48:715–723, 1970.
6. DeVere, R., and Bradley, W.G.: Polymyositis: its presentation, morbidity and mortality. Brain, 98:637–666, 1975.
7. Pearson, C.M.: Polymyositis. Annu. Rev. Med., 17:63–82, 1966.
8. Bohan, A., et al.: A computer-assisted analysis of 153 patients with polymyositis and dermatomyositis. Medicine, 56:255–286, 1977.
9. Pearson, C.M.: Polymyositis and dermatomyositis. In Arthritis and Allied Conditions. 9th Ed. Edited by D.J. McCarty. Philadelphia, Lea & Febiger, 1979, pp. 742–761.
10. Gardner-Medwin, D., and Walton, J.N.: The clinical examination of the voluntary muscles. In Disorders of Voluntary Muscle. Edited by J.N. Walton. Edinburgh, Churchill Livingstone, 1974, pp. 517–560.
11. Edwards, R.H.T., et al.: Muscle breakdown and repair in polymyositis. A case study. Muscle Nerve, 2:223–229, 1979.
12. Young, A., and Edwards, R.H.T.: Dynamometry and muscle disease. Arch. Phys. Rehabil., 62:295–296, 1981.
13. Kroll, M., Otis, J., and Kagen, L.: Serum enzyme, myoglobin and muscle strength relationships in polymyositis and dermatomyositis. J. Rheumatol., 13:349–355, 1986.
14. Csuka, M.E., and McCarty, D.J.: A rapid method for measurement of lower extremity muscle strength. Am. J. Med., 78:77–81, 1985.
15. Maricq, H.R., and LeRoy, E.C.: Patterns of finger capillary abnormalities in connective tissue diseases by "wide-field" microscopy. Arthritis Rheum., 16:619–628, 1973.

16. Feldman, D., et al.: Cutaneous vasculitis in adult polymyositis/dermatomyositis. J. Rheumatol., *10*:85–89, 1983.
17. Itoh, J., et al.: Sarcoid myopathy with typical rash of dermatomyositis. Neurology, *30*:1118–1121, 1980.
18. Krain, L.S.: Dermatomyositis in 6 patients without initial muscle involvement. Arch. Dermatol., *111*:241–245, 1975.
19. Janis, J.F., and Winkelmann, R.K.: Histopathology of the skin in dermatomyositis. Arch. Dermatol., *97*:640–650, 1968.
20. Kagen, L.J., Hochman, R.B., and Strong, E.W.: Cricopharyngeal obstruction in inflammatory myopathy (polymyositis/dermatomyositis). Arthritis Rheum., *28*:630–636, 1985.
21. Dietz, F., et al.: Cricopharyngeal muscle dysfunction in the differential diagnosis of dysphagia in polymyositis. Arthritis Rheum., *23*:491–495, 1980.
22. De Merieux, P., Verity, M.A., Clements, R.J., and Paulus, H.E.: Esophageal abnormalities and dysphagia in polymyositis and dermatomyositis. Arthritis Rheum., *26*:961–968, 1983.
23. Horowitz, M., et al.: Abnormalities of gastric and esophageal emptying in polymyositis and dermatomyositis. Gastroenterology, *90*:434–439, 1986.
24. Arnett, F.C., et al.: Methotrexate therapy in polymyositis. Ann. Rheum. Dis., *32*:536–546, 1973.
25. Duncan, P.E., et al.: Fibrosing alveolitis in polymyositis. Am. J. Med., *57*:621–626, 1974.
26. Fergusson, R.J., et al.: Dermatomyositis and rapidly progressive fibrosing alveolitis. Thorax, *38*:71–72, 1983.
27. Frazier, A.R., and Miller, R.D.: Interstitial pneumonitis in association with polymyositis and dermatomyositis. Chest, *65*:403–407, 1974.
28. Salmeron, G., Greenberg, D., and Lidsky, M.D.: Polymyositis and diffuse interstitial lung disease. Arch. Intern. Med., *141*:1005–1010, 1981.
29. Schwarz, M.I., et al.: Interstitial lung disease in polymyositis and dermatomyositis: analysis of six cases and review of the literature. Medicine, *55*:89–104, 1976.
30. Braun, N.M.T., Arora, N.S., and Rochester, D.F.: Respiratory muscle and pulmonary function in polymyositis and other proximal myopathies. Thorax, *38*:616–623, 1983.
31. Dickey, B.F., and Myers, A.R.: Pulmonary disease in polymyositis/dermatomyositis. Semin. Arthritis Rheum., *14*:60–76, 1984.
32. Gottdiener, J.S., et al.: Cardiac manifestations in polymyositis. Am. J. Cardiol., *41*:1141–1149, 1978.
33. Henderson, A., et al.: Cardiac complications of polymyositis. J. Neurol. Sci., *47*:425–429, 1980.
34. Denbow, C.E., et al.: Cardiac involvement in polymyositis. Arthritis Rheum., *22*:1088–1092, 1979.
35. Haupt, H.M., and Hutchins, G.M.: The heart and cardiac conducting system in polymyositis-dermatomyositis. Am. J. Cardiol., *50*:998–1006, 1982.
36. Stern, R., Goodbold, J.H., Chess, Q., and Kagen, L.J.: ECG abnormalities in polymyositis. Arch. Intern. Med., *44*:2185–2189, 1984.
37. Blane, C.E., et al.: Patterns of calcification in childhood dermatomyositis. Am. J. Rad., *142*:397–400, 1984.
38. Sarmiento, A.H., et al.: Evaluation of soft-tissue calcifications in dermatomyositis with ⁹⁹ᵐTc-phosphate compounds: case report. J. Nucl. Med., *16*:467–468, 1975.
39. Dent, C.E., and Stamp, T.C.B.: Treatment of calcinosis circumscripta with probenecid. Br. Med. J., *1*:216–218, 1972.
40. Kagen, L.J.: Myoglobinemia and myoglobinuria in patients with myositis. Arthritis Rheum., *14*:457–464, 1971.
41. Dyck, R.F., et al.: Glomerulonephritis associated with polymyositis. J. Rheumatol., *6*:336–344, 1979.
42. Kamata, K., et al.: Childhood type polymyositis and rapidly progressive glomerulonephritis. Acta Pathol. Jpn., *32*:801–806, 1982.
43. Cumming, W.J.K., et al.: Localised nodular myositis: a clinical and pathological variant of polymyositis. Q. J. Med., *46*:531–546, 1977.
44. Heffner, R.R., and Barron, S.A.: Polymyositis beginning as a focal process. Arch. Neurol., *38*:439–442, 1981.
45. Kalyanaraman, K., and Kalyanaraman, U.P.: Localized myositis presenting as pseudothrombophlebitis. Arthritis Rheum., *25*:1374–1377, 1982.
46. Pachman, L.M., and Cooke, N.: Juvenile dermatomyositis: a clinical and immunological study. J. Pediatr., *96*:226–234, 1980.
47. Spencer-Green, G., Crowe, W.E., and Levinson, J.E.: Nailfold capillary abnormalities and clinical outcome in childhood dermatomyositis. Arthritis Rheum., *25*:954–958, 1982.
48. Banker, B.Q., and Victor, M.: Dermatomyositis (systemic angiopathy) of childhood. Medicine, *45*:261–289, 1966.
49. Winfield, J.: Juvenile dermatomyositis with complications. Proc. R. Soc. Med., *70*:548–551, 1977.
50. Guttierez, G., Dagnino, R., and Mintz, G.: Polymyositis/dermatomyositis and pregnancy. Arthritis Rheum., *27*:291–294, 1986.
51. King, C.R., and Chow, S.: Dermatomyositis and pregnancy. Obstet. Gynecol., *66*:589–592, 1985.
52. Pennington, R.T.: Biochemical aspects of muscle disease. *In* Disorders of Voluntary Muscle. Edited by J.N. Walton. New York, Churchill Livingstone, 1981, pp. 415–447.
53. Vignos, P.J., and Goldwin, J.: Evaluation of laboratory tests in diagnosis and management of polymyositis. Am. J. Med., *263*:291–308, 1972.
54. Farrington, C., and Chalmers, A.H.: The effect of dilution on creatine kinase activity. Clin. Chim. Acta, *73*:217–219, 1976.
55. Roberts, R., and Sobel, B.E.: Effect of selected drugs and myocardial infarction on the disappearance of creatine kinase from the circulation in conscious dogs. Cardiovasc. Res., *11*:103–112, 1977.
56. Munsat, T.L., and Bradley, W.G.: Serum creatine phosphokinase levels and prednisone treated muscle weakness. Neurology, *27*:96–97, 1977.
57. Riddoch, D., and Morgan-Hughes, J.A.: Prognosis in adult polymyositis. J. Neurol. Sci., *26*:71–80, 1975.
58. Fudman, E.J., and Schnitzer, T.J.: Dermatomyositis without creatine kinase elevation. A poor prognostic sign. Am. J. Med., *80*:329–332, 1986.
59. Dawson, D.M., and Fine, I.H.: Creatine kinase in human tissues. Arch. Neurol., *16*:175–180, 1967.
60. Jockers-Wretou, E., and Pfleiderer, G.: Quantitation of creatine kinase isoenzymes in human tissues by an immunological method. Clin. Chim. Acta, *58*:223–232, 1975.
61. Mercer, D.W.: Separation of tissue and serum creatine kinase in human tissues. Arch. Neurol., *16*:175–180, 1967.
62. Brownlow, K., and Elevitch, F.R.: Serum creatine phosphokinase iso-enzyme (CPK_2) in myositis. JAMA, *230*:1141–1144, 1974.
63. Goto, I.: Creatine phosphokinase isoenzymes in neuromuscular disorders. Arch. Neurol., *31*:116–119, 1974.
64. Larca, L.J., Coppola, J.T., and Honig, S.: Creatine kinase MB isoenzyme in dermatomyositis: a noncardiac source. Ann. Intern. Med., *94*:341–343, 1981.
65. Morton, B.D. III, and Statland, B.E.: Serum enzyme alterations in polymyositis. Am. J. Clin. Pathol., *73*:556–557, 1980.

66. Eppenberger, H.M., Richterich, R., and Aebi, H.: The ontogeny of creatine kinase isoenzymes. Dev. Biol., *10*:1–16, 1964.

67. Lough, J., and Bischoff, R.: Differentiation of creatine phosphokinase during myogenesis. Quantitative fractionation of isoenzymes. Dev. Biol., *57*:330–334, 1977.

68. Turner, D.C., Maier, V., and Eppenberger, H.M.: Creatine kinase and aldolase isoenzyme transitions in cultures of chick skeletal muscle cells. Dev. Biol., *37*:63–89, 1974.

69. Kagen, L.J.: Myoglobin: methods and diagnostic uses. CRC Crit. Rev. Clin. Lab. Sci., *9*:273–320, 1978.

70. Kagen, L.J.: Myoglobinemia in inflammatory myopathies. JAMA, *237*:1448–1452, 1977.

71. Nishikai, M., and Reichlin, M.: Radioimmunoassay of serum myoglobin in polymyositis and other conditions. Arthritis Rheum., *20*:1514–1518, 1977.

72. Bombardieri, S., et al.: Circadian variations of serum myoglobin levels in normal subjects and patients with polymyositis. Arthritis Rheum., *25*:1419–1424, 1982.

73. Daube, J.R.: The description of motor unit potentials in electromyography. Neurology, *28*:623–625, 1978.

74. Henriksson, K.-G., and Stalberg, E.: The terminal innervation pattern in polymyositis; a histochemical and SFEMG study. Muscle Nerve, *1*:3–13, 1978.

75. Edwards, R.H.T., et al.: The investigation of inflammatory myopathy. J. R. Coll. Physicians Lond., *15*:19–24, 1981.

76. Schwarz, H.A., et al.: Muscle biopsy in polymyositis and dermatomyositis. A clinicopathological study. Ann. Rheum. Dis., *39*:500–507, 1980.

77. Duance, V.C., et al.: Polymyositis—an immunofluorescence study on the distribution of collagen types. Muscle Nerve, *3*:487–490, 1980.

78. Mastaglia, F.L., and Kakulas, B.A.: A histological and histochemical study of skeletal muscle regeneration of polymyositis. J. Neurol. Sci., *10*:471–487, 1970.

79. Myllyla, R., et al.: Changes in collagen metabolism in diseased muscle. I. Biochemical studies. Arch. Neurol., *39*:752–755, 1982.

80. Peltonen, L., et al.: Changes in collagen metabolism in diseased muscle. II. Immunohistochemical studies. Arch. Neurol., *39*:756–759, 1982.

81. Chou, S.-M., Nonaka, I., and Voice, G.F.: Anastomoses of transverse tubules with terminal cisternae in polymyositis. Arch. Neurol., *37*:257–266, 1980.

82. Hochberg, M.C., Feldman, D., and Stevens, M.B.: Adult onset polymyositis/dermatomyositis: an analysis of clinical and laboratory features and survival in 76 patients with a review of the literature. Semin. Arthritis Rheum., *15*:168–178, 1986.

83. Banker, B.Q.: Dermatomyositis of childhood. J. Neuropathol. Exp. Neurol., *34*:46–75, 1975.

84. Crowe, W.E., et al.: Clinical and pathogenetic implications of histopathology in childhood polydermatomyositis. Arthritis Rheum., *25*:126–139, 1982.

85. Bowyer, S.L., et al.: Juvenile dermatomyositis: histological findings and pathogenetic hypothesis for the associated skin changes. J. Rheumatol., *13*:753–759, 1986.

86. Herrera-Esparza, R., et al.: Cell-mediated immunity to myoglobin in polymyositis. Ann. Rheum. Dis., *42*:182–186, 1983.

87. Wada, K., et al.: Radioimmunoassay for antibodies to human skeletal muscle myosin in serum from patients with polymyositis. Clin. Exp. Immunol., *52*:297–304, 1983.

88. Yamamoto, T., et al.: Anti-filamin and -vinculin antibodies in sera from patients with myasthenia gravis and polymyositis. Proc. Jpn. Acad. Ser. B., *62*:113–116, 1986.

89. Whitaker, J.N., and Engel, W.K.: Vascular deposits of immunoglobulin and complement in idiopathic inflammatory myopathy. N. Engl. J. Med., *286*:333–338, 1972.

90. Fessel, W.J., and Raas, M.C.: Autoimmunity in the pathogenesis of muscle disease. Neurology, *18*:1137–1139, 1968.

91. Fulthorpe, J.J., and Hudgson, P.I.: Immunocytochemical localization of immunoglobulins in the inflammatory lesions of polymyositis. J. Neuroimmunol., *2*:145–154, 1982.

92. Kissel, J.T., Mendell, J.R., and Rammohan, K.W.: Microvascular deposition of complement membrane attack complex in dermatomyositis. N. Engl. J. Med., *314*:329–334, 1986.

93. Dawkins, R.L., Eghtedari, A., and Holborow, E.J.: Antibodies to skeletal muscle demonstrated by immunofluorescence in experimental autoallergic myositis. Clin. Exp. Immunol., *9*:329–337, 1971.

94. Korenyi-Both, A., and Kelemen, G.: Damage of skeletal muscle in rats by immunoglobulins. Acta Neuropathol., *34*:199–206, 1976.

95. Giuliano, V.J.: Polymyositis in a patient with acquired hypogammaglobulinemia. Am. J. Med. Sci., *268*:53–56, 1974.

96. Janeway, C.A., et al.: "Collagen disease" in patients with congenital agammaglobulinemia. Trans. Assoc. Am. Physicians, *69*:93–97, 1956.

97. Leddy, J.P., et al.: Hereditary complement (C2) deficiency with dermatomyositis. Am. J. Med., *58*:83–91, 1975.

98. Reichlin, M., and Arnett, F.C.: Multiplicity of antibodies in myositis sera. Arthritis Rheum., *27*:1150–1156, 1984.

99. Arnett, F.C., et al.: The Jo-1 antibody system in myositis. Relationships to clinical features and HLA. J. Rheumatol., *8*:925–930, 1981.

100. Yoshida, S., et al.: The precipitating antibody to an acidic nuclear antigen, the Jo-1, in connective tissue diseases, a marker for a subset of polymyositis with interstitial pulmonary fibrosis. Arthritis Rheum., *26*:606–611, 1983.

101. Hochberg, M.C., et al.: Antibody to Jo-1 in polymyositis/dermatomyositis: association with interstitial pulmonary disease. J. Rheum., *11*:663–665, 1984.

102. Bernstein, R.M., et al.: Anti-Jo-1 antibody: a marker for myositis with interstitial lung disease. Brit. Med. J., *289*:151–152, 1984.

103. Mathews, M.B., and Bernstein, R.M.: Myositis autoantibody inhibits histidyl-tRNA synthetase: a model for autoimmunity. Nature, *304*:177–179, 1983.

104. Mathews, M.B., Reichlin, M., Hughes, G.R.V., and Bernstein, R.M.: Anti-threonyl—tRNA synthetase, a second myositis-related autoantibody. J. Exp. Med., *160*:420–434, 1984.

105. Okada, N., et al.: Isolation of a novel antibody, which precipitates ribonucleoprotein complex containing threonine tRNA from a patient with polymyositis. Eur. J. Biochem., *139*:425–429, 1984.

106. Bunn, C.C., Bernstein, R.M., and Mathews, M.B.: Autoantibodies against alanyl-tRNA synthetase and tRNA ala coexist and are associated with myositis. J. Exp. Med., *163*:1281–1291, 1986.

107. Targoff, I.M., Raghi, G., and Reichlin, M.: Antibodies to Mi-1 in SLE; relationship to other precipitins and reaction with bovine immunoglobulin. Clin. Exp. Immunol., *53*:76–82, 1983.

108. Targoff, I.N., and Reichlin, M.: The association between Mi-2 antibodies and dermatomyositis. Arthritis Rheum., *28*:796–803, 1985.

109. Treadwell, E.L., Alspaugh, M.A., Wolfe, J.F., and Sharp, G.C.: Clinical relevance of PM-1 antibody and physiochemical characterization of PM-1 antigen. J. Rheumatol., *11*:658–662, 1984.

110. Wolfe, J.F., Adelstein, E., and Sharp, G.C.: Antinuclear antibody with distinct specificity for polymyositis. J. Clin. Invest., 59:176–178, 1977.

111. Engel, A.H., and Arahata, K.: Mononuclear cells in myopathies. Hum. Pathol., 17:704–721, 1986.

112. Kalovidouris, A.: Mononuclear cells from patients with polymyositis inhibit calcium binding by sarcoplasmic reticulum. J. Lab. Clin. Med., 107:23–28, 1986.

113. Kalovidouris, A.E.: Dysfunction of the sarcoplasmic reticulum in polymyositis. Arthritis Rheum., 27:299–304, 1984.

114. Friedman, J.M., et al.: Immunogenetic studies of juvenile dermatomyositis. Tissue Antigens, 21:45–49, 1983.

115. Pachman, L.M., et al.: HLA-B8 in juvenile dermatomyositis. Lancet, 2:567–568, 1977.

116. Behan, W.M.H., Behan, P.O., and Dick, H.A.: HLA-B8 in polymyositis. N. Engl. J. Med., 298:1260–1261, 1978.

117. Hirsch, T.J., et al.: HLA-D related (DR) antigens in various kinds of myositis. Hum. Immunol., 3:181–186, 1981.

118. Cumming, W.J.K., et al.: HLA and serum complement in polymyositis. Lancet, 2:978–979, 1977.

119. Walker, G.L., Mastaglia, F.L., and Roberts, D.F.: A search for genetic influence in idiopathic inflammatory myopathy. Acta Neurol. Scand., 66:432–443, 1982.

120. Antony, J.H., Procopis, P.C., and Ouvrier, R.A.: Benign acute childhood myositis. Neurology, 29:1068–1071, 1979.

121. Dietzman, D.E., et al.: Acute myositis associated with influenza B infection. Pediatrics, 57:255–258, 1976.

122. Gamboa, E.T., et al.: Isolation of influenza virus in myoglobinuric polymyositis. Neurology, 29:1323–1335, 1979.

123. Christensen, M.L., et al.: Prevalence of Coxsackie B virus antibodies in patients with juvenile dermatomyositis. Arthritis Rheum., 29:1365–1370, 1986.

124. Travers, R.L., et al.: Coxsackie B neutralisation titres in polymyositis/dermatomyositis. Lancet, 1:1268, 1977.

124a. Bowles, N.E., et al.: Dermatomyositis, polymyositis and Coxsackie B virus infection. Lancet, 1:1004–1007, 1987.

125. Damjanov, I., et al.: Immune complex myositis associated with viral hepatitis. Hum. Pathol., 11:478–481, 1980.

126. Mease, P.J., Ochs, H.D., and Wedgewood, R.J.: Successful treatment of ECHO virus meningoencephalitis and myositis-fasciitis with intravenous immune globulin therapy in a patient with X-linked agammaglobulinemia. N. Engl. J. Med., 304:1278–1281, 1981.

127. Crennan, J.M., VanScoy, R.E., McKenna, C.H., and Smith, T.F.: Echovirus polymyositis in patients with hypogammaglobulinemia. Am. J. Med., 81:35–42, 1986.

128. Feldman, H.A., and Miller, L.T.: Serological study of toxoplasmosis prevalence. Am. J. Hyg., 64:320–335, 1956.

129. Remington, J.S., and Cavanaugh, E.N.: Isolation of the encysted form of Toxoplasma gondii from human skeletal muscle and brain. N. Engl. J. Med., 273:1308–1310, 1965.

130. Henry, L., and Beverley, J.K.A.: Experimental myocarditis and myositis in mice. Br. J. Exp. Pathol., 50:230–238, 1969.

131. Fonseca, R.C., et al.: Miositis toxoplasmica aguda en un adulto. Acta Med. Cost., 16:75–78, 1973.

132. Greenlee, J.E., et al.: Adult toxoplasmosis presenting as polymyositis and cerebellar ataxia. Ann. Intern. Med., 82:367–371, 1973.

133. Hendrickx, G.G.M., et al.: Dermatomyositis and toxoplasmosis. Ann. Neurol., 5:393–395, 1979.

134. Phillips, P.E., Kassan, S.S., and Kagen, L.J.: Increased toxoplasma antibodies in idiopathic inflammatory muscle disease. Arthritis Rheum., 22:209–214, 1979.

135. Kagen, L.J., Kimball, A.C., and Christian, C.L.: Serologic evidence of toxoplasmosis among patients with polymyositis. Am. J. Med., 56:186–191, 1974.

136. Magid, S.K., and Kagen, L.J.: Serological evidence for acute toxoplasmosis in polymyositis-dermatomyositis. Increased frequency of specific anti-toxoplasma IgM antibodies. Am. J. Med., 75:312–320, 1983.

137. Arundell, F.D., Wilkinson, R.D., and Haserick, J.R.: Dermatomyositis and malignant neoplasms in adults. Arch. Dermatol., 82:772–775, 1960.

138. Barnes, B.E.: Dermatomyositis and malignancy. Ann. Intern. Med., 84:68–76, 1976.

139. Callen, J.P., et al.: The relationship of dermatomyositis and polymyositis to internal malignancy. Arch. Dermatol., 116:295–298, 1980.

140. Singsen, B.H., et al.: Lymphocytic leukemia, atypical dermatomyositis and hyperlipidemia in a 4-year-old boy. J. Pediatr., 88:602–604, 1976.

141. Tymms, K.E., and Webb, J.: Dermatopolymyositis and other connective tissue diseases: a review of 105 cases. J. Rheumatol., 12:1140–1148, 1985.

142. Fayolle, J., et al.: Dermatomyosite déclenchée par l'isoniazide, avec syndrome biologique d'auto-immunisation de type lupique. Lyon Med., 233:135–138, 1975.

143. Goldenberg, D.L., and Stor, R.A.: Azathioprine hypersensitivity mimicking an acute exacerbation of dermatomyositis. J. Rheumatol., 2:346–349, 1975.

144. Fernandes, L., Swinson, D.R., and Hamilton, E.B.D.: Dermatomyositis complicating penicillamine treatment. Ann. Rheum. Dis., 36:94–95, 1977.

145. Morgan, G.L., McGuire, J.L., and Ochoa, J.: Penicillamine-induced myositis in rheumatoid arthritis. Muscle Nerve, 4:137–140, 1981.

146. Petersen, J., et al.: Penicillamine-induced polymyositis-dermatomyositis. Scand. J. Rheumatol., 7:113–117, 1978.

147. Halla, J.T., et al.: Rheumatoid myositis: clinical and histologic features and possible pathogenesis. Arthritis Rheum., 27:737–743, 1984.

148. Martinez-Lavin, M., Vaughan, J.H., and Tan, E.M.: Auto-antibodies and the spectrum of Sjögren's syndrome. Ann. Intern. Med., 91:185–190, 1979.

149. Ringel, S.P., et al.: Sjögren's syndrome and polymyositis or dermatomyositis. Arch. Neurol., 39:157–163, 1982.

150. Carpenter, S., et al.: Inclusion body myositis: a distinct variety of idiopathic inflammatory myopathy. Neurology, 28:8–17, 1978.

151. Chou, S.-M.: Inclusion body myositis: a chronic persistent mumps myositis? Hum. Pathol., 17:765–777, 1986.

152. Danon, M.J., et al.: Inclusion body myositis: a corticosteroid-resistant inflammatory myopathy. Arch. Neurol., 39:760–764, 1982.

153. Eisen, A., Berry, K., and Gibson, G.: Inclusion body myositis (IBM): myopathy or neuropathy? Neurol., 33:1109–1114, 1983.

154. Julien, J., et al.: Inclusion body myositis. J. Neurol. Sci., 55:15–24, 1982.

155. Yunis, E.J., and Samaha, F.J.: Inclusion body myositis. Lab. Invest., 25:240–248, 1971.

155a. Mikol, J., et al.: Inclusion body myositis: clinicopathological studies and isolation of an adenovirus type 2 from muscle biopsy specimen. Ann. Neurol., 11:576–581, 1982.

155b. Lazaro, R.P., et al.: Inclusion body myositis: case reports and a reappraisal of an under-recognized type of myopathy. Mt. Sinai J. Med. (NY), 53:137–144, 1986.

155c. Carpenter, S., and Karpati, G.: The major inflammatory myopathies of unknown cause. Pathol. Annu., 16:205–237, 1981.

155d.Kelly, J.J., Jr., et al.: Total body irradiation not effective in inclusion body myositis. Neurology, *36*:1264–1266, 1986.

155e.Yood, R.A., et al.: Inclusion body myositis and systemic lupus erythematosus. J. Rheumatol., *12*:568–570, 1985.

155f.Chad, D., et al.: Inclusion body myositis associated with Sjögren's syndrome. Arch. Neurol., *39*:186–188, 1982.

155g.Riggs, J.E., et al.: Inclusion body myositis and chronic immune thrombocytopenia. Arch. Neurol., *41*:93–95, 1984.

155h.Lane, R.J.M., Fulthorpe, J.J., and Hudgson, P.: Inclusion body myositis: a case with associated collagen-vascular disease responding to treatment. J. Neurosurg. Psychiatry, *48*:270–273, 1985.

156. Joseph, S.C.: Pyomyositis. Am. J. Dis. Child., *130*:775–776, 1975.

157. Taylor, J.F., Fluck, D., and Fluck, D.: Tropical myositis: ultrastructural studies. J. Clin. Pathol., *29*:1081–1084, 1976.

157a.Gibson, R.K., Rosenthal, S.J., and Lukert, B.P.: Pyomyositis: increasing recognition in temperate climates. Am. J. Med., *77*:768–772, 1984.

157b.Bremnessel, D.J., et al.: Pyomyositis caused by Yersinia enterocolitica. J. Clin. Microbiol., *20*:293–294, 1984.

157c.Moore, D.L., et al.: Per acute streptococcal pyomyositis, report of 2 cases and review of the literature. J. Pediatr. Orthop., *6*:232–235, 1986.

157d.Adams, E.M., et al.: Streptococcal myositis. Arch. Intern. Med., *145*:1020–1023, 1985.

157e.Lachiewicz, P.F., et al.: Spontaneous pyomyositis in a patient with Felty's syndrome; diagnosis using computerized tomography. South Med. J., *79*:1047–1048, 1986.

157f.Weinberg, W.G., and Dembert, M.L.: Tropical pyomyositis: delineation by gray scale ultrasound. Am. J. Trop. Med. Hyg., *33*:930–932, 1984.

157g.Caldwell, D.S., et al.: Pestoral pyomyositis: an unusual cause of chest wall pain in a patient with diabetes mellitus and rheumatoid arthritis. J. Rheumatol., *13*:434–436, 1986.

158. Ellman, L., Miller, L., and Rappaport, J.: Leukopheresis therapy of a hypereosinophilic disorder. JAMA, *230*:1004–1005, 1974.

159. Layzer, R.B., Shearn, M.A., and Satya-Murti, S.: Eosinophilic polymyositis. Ann. Neurol., *1*:65–71, 1977.

160. Bjelle, A., Henriksson, K.-G., and Hofer, P.-A.: Polymyositis in eosinophilic fasciitis. Eur. Neurol., *19*:128–137, 1980.

161. Schumacher, H.R.: A scleroderma-like syndrome with fasciitis, myositis and eosinophilia. Ann. Intern. Med., *84*:49–50, 1976.

162. Serratrice, G., et al.: Relapsing eosinophilic perimyositis. J. Rheumatol., *7*:199–205, 1980.

163. Sladek, G.D., et al.: Relapsing eosinophilic myositis. J. Rheumatol., *10*:467–470, 1983.

163a.Lakhanpal, S., Duffy, J., and Engel, A.G.: Eosinophilia associated with perimyositis and pneumonitis. Mayo Clin. Proc., *63*:37–41, 1988.

164. Hewlett, R.H., and Brownell, B.: Granulomatous myopathy: its relationship to sarcoidosis and polymyositis. J. Neurol. Neurosurg. Psychiatry, *38*:1090–1099, 1975.

165. Menard, D.B., et al.: Granulomatous myositis and myopathy associated with Crohn's colitis. N. Engl. J. Med., *295*:818–819, 1976.

166. Schimrigk, K., and Uldall, B.: The diseases of Besnier-Boeck-Schaumann and granulomatous polymyositis. Eur. Neurol., *1*:137–157, 1968.

166a.McKinney, R.E., Katz, S.L., and Wilfert, C.M.: Chronic enteroviral meningoencephalitis in agammaglobulinemic patients. Rev. Infect. Dis., *9*:334–356, 1987.

167. Miller, J.J.: Late progression in dermatomyositis in childhood. J. Pediatr., *83*:543–548, 1973.

168. Uchino, M., et al.: High single-dose alternate-day corticosteroid regimens in treatment of polymyositis. J. Neurol., *232*:175–178, 1985.

169. Yanigasawa, T., et al.: Methyl prednisolone pulse therapy in dermatomyositis. Dermatologica, *167*:47–51, 1983.

170. Dubowitz, V.: Treatment of dermatomyositis in childhood. Arch. Dis. Child., *51*:494–500, 1971.

171. Rose, A.L.: Childhood polymyositis. Am. J. Dis. Child., *127*:518–522, 1974.

172. Malaviya, A.N., Many, A., and Schwartz, R.S.: Treatment of dermatomyositis with methotrexate. Lancet, *2*:485–488, 1968.

173. Metzger, A.L., et al.: Polymyositis and dermatomyositis: combined methotrexate and corticosteroid therapy. Ann. Intern. Med., *81*:182–189, 1974.

174. Jacobs, J.C.: Methotrexate and azathioprine treatment of childhood dermatomyositis. Pediatrics, *59*:212–218, 1977.

175. Bunch, T.W.: Prednisone and azathioprine for polymyositis. Long-term follow-up. Arthritis Rheum., *24*:45–48, 1981.

176. Bennington, J.A., and Dau, P.C.: Patients with polymyositis and dermatomyositis who undergo plasmapheresis therapy. Pathologic findings. Arch. Neurol., *38*:553–560, 1981.

177. Dau, P.C.: Plasmapheresis in idiopathic inflammatory myopathy. Arch. Neurol., *38*:544–552, 1981.

177a.Tiliakos, N.A.: Low dose cytotoxic combination therapy in intractable dermatopolymyositis. Arthritis Rheum., *30*:S14, 1987.

177b.Wallace, D.J., Metzger, A.L., and White, K.K.: Combination immunosuppressive treatment of steroid-resistant dermatomyositis/polymyositis. Arthritis Rheum., *28*:590–592, 1985.

178. Hill, R.H., and Wood, W.S.: Juvenile dermatomyositis. Can. Med. Assoc. J., *103*:1152–1156, 1970.

179. Spenser, C.H., et al.: Course of treated juvenile dermatomyositis. J. Pediatr., *105*:399–408, 1984.

180. Lovell, H.B., and Lindsley, C.B.: Late recurrence of childhood dermatomyositis. J. Rheumatol., *13*:821–822, 1986.

181. Carpenter, J.R., et al.: Survival in polymyositis: corticosteroids and risk factors. J. Rheumatol., *4*:207–214, 1977.

182. Medsger, T.A., Jr., Robinson, H., and Masi, A.T.: Factors affecting survivorship in polymyositis. Arthritis Rheum., *14*:249–258, 1971.

183. Hoffman, G.S., et al.: Presentation, treatment, and prognosis of idiopathic inflammatory muscle disease in a rural hospital. Am. J. Med., *75*:433–438, 1983.

184. Baron, M., and Small, P.: Polymyositis/dermatomyositis: clinical features and outcome in 22 patients. J. Rheumatol., *12*:283–286, 1985.

185. Hochberg, M.C., Lopez-Aeuna, D., and Gittelsohn, A.M.: Mortality from polymyositis and dermatomyositis in the United States, 1968–1978. Arthritis Rheum., *26*:1465–1471, 1983.

SYSTEMIC SCLEROSIS (SCLERODERMA), LOCALIZED SCLERODERMA, EOSINOPHILIC FASCIITIS, AND CALCINOSIS

73

THOMAS A. MEDSGER, JR.

SYSTEMIC SCLEROSIS (SCLERODERMA)

Systemic sclerosis is a generalized disorder of connective tissue characterized by fibrosis and degenerative changes in the skin, synovium, muscles, and certain internal organs, notably the gastrointestinal tract, lung, heart, and kidney.[1] Although there is occasionally an early inflammatory component, the hallmark of the disease is skin thickening (scleroderma) caused by excessive accumulation of connective tissue. Proliferative vascular changes leading to Raynaud's phenomenon and other obliterative lesions of blood vessels are prominent.

CLASSIFICATION

The term "scleroderma" has traditionally been applied to the cutaneous changes of both systemic sclerosis and a heterogeneous group of conditions designated collectively as localized scleroderma. In the latter case, there is more circumscribed dermal fibrosis and absence of internal organ involvement. Only rarely is there coexistence of these entities or transition from localized to systemic disease.

Systemic sclerosis is divided into two major variants, *diffuse cutaneous* and *limited cutaneous* scleroderma, dependent primarily on the degree and extent of cutaneous involvement.[2,3] When features commonly encountered in other connective tissue dis-

eases are also present, the term "overlap syndrome" is used (Table 73–1).[4] A similar spectrum of disease is recognized in the classification systems proposed by other authors, with acrosclerosis and CREST syndrome (an acronym referring to the findings of *c*alcinosis, *R*aynaud's phenomenon, *e*sophageal hypomotility, *s*clerodactyly, and *t*elangiectasia)[5] closely analogous to limited scleroderma.

There are many distinctive demographic, clinical, laboratory, and natural history differences between

Table 73–1. Classification of Scleroderma

I. SYSTEMIC SCLEROSIS (progressive systemic sclerosis; systemic scleroderma)

With diffuse cutaneous scleroderma: symmetric widespread skin involvement, affecting the distal and proximal extremities and often the trunk and face; tendency to rapid progression of skin changes and early appearance of visceral involvement.

With limited cutaneous scleroderma: symmetric restricted skin involvement, affecting the distal extremities (often confined to the fingers) and face; prolonged delay in appearance of distinctive internal manifestations (e.g., pulmonary arterial hypertension and biliary cirrhosis); prominence of calcinosis and telangiectasia.

With "overlap": having typical features of one or more members of the connective tissue disease family.

II. LOCALIZED SCLERODERMA

Morphea: single or multiple (generalized) plaques.

Linear scleroderma: with or without melorheostosis; includes scleroderma en coup de sabre (with or without facial hemiatrophy).

III. EOSINOPHILIC FASCIITIS

1118

diffuse cutaneous systemic sclerosis, with distal and proximal extremity and truncal skin thickening, and limited cutaneous systemic sclerosis, with changes most often restricted to the fingers and distalmost portions of the extremities and the face (Table 73–2). These differences are particularly important to the patient and managing physician. Diffuse cutaneous involvement is associated with palpable tendon friction rubs, arthritis with joint contractures, serum antitopoisomerase or anti-scleroderma (Scl) 70 antibodies, and the frequent occurrence of early visceral disease (gastrointestinal tract, lung, heart, and kidney), whereas limited cutaneous disease is correlated with calcinosis, telangiectasias, serum anticentromere antibodies, and the occasional late development of pulmonary arterial hypertension and/or biliary cirrhosis.

The distinction between limited scleroderma, which is a form of systemic sclerosis, and the nonsystemic entity, localized scleroderma, should be emphasized. Additional details concerning these two illnesses are provided in subsequent sections of this chapter.

Criteria for Classification of Systemic Sclerosis. A prospective multicenter study of the American Rheumatism Association compared 264 systemic sclerosis patients with 413 persons with polymyositis-derma-

tomyositis, systemic lupus erythematosus (SLE), or isolated Raynaud's phenomenon for the purpose of developing classification criteria.[6] Sclerodermatous skin changes in any location proximal to the digits were present in 91% of systemic sclerosis cases and in fewer than 1% of the comparison patients. With the addition of any two of three minor criteria, including sclerodactyly, digital pitting scars, and bibasilar pulmonary fibrosis on chest roentgenogram, sensitivity rose to 97% and specificity was maintained at 98%.

A number of patients with limited cutaneous disease and other convincing evidence of systemic sclerosis (e.g., esophageal or small bowel abnormalities or pulmonary hypertension) do not satisfy these criteria. Modification of the criteria to more adequately include persons with limited scleroderma presents a challenge for the future. It should be remembered that these and other classification criteria are intended for description of large series of patients, and not for diagnosis of the individual patient.

EPIDEMIOLOGY

Systemic sclerosis has been described in all races and appears to be global in distribution. It occurs less

Table 73–2. Comparison of Clinical and Laboratory Features Found at Any Time During the Course of Systemic Sclerosis (University of Pittsburgh, 1972–1986)

	Diffuse Scleroderma (No. = 518)	Limited Scleroderma (No. = 506)
Demographic		
Age (<40 at onset)	30%	14%
Race (nonwhite)	10%	5%
Sex (female)	76%	84%
Duration of symptoms (years)	3.0	11.7
Organ system involvement		
Skin (total skin score)*	39.5	8.6
Telangiectases	64%	91%
Calcinosis	17%	42%
Raynaud's phenomenon	92%	98%
Arthralgias or arthritis	72%	56%
Tendon friction rubs	62%	9%
Joint contractures	89%	62%
Myositis	9%	6%
Esophageal hypomotility	73%	79%
Pulmonary fibrosis	38%	38%
Pulmonary hypertension	<1%	7%
Congestive heart failure	11%	2%
"Scleroderma renal crisis"	20%	1%
Laboratory data		
ANA positive (1:16+)	69%	63%
Anticentromere antibody positive (1:40+)	2%	46%
Anti-Scl 70 positive (any titer)	33%	15%
Cumulative survival (10 years from first diagnosis)	55%	71%

*As described in Steen, V.D., et al.[34]

frequently than systemic lupus erythematosus; two community studies detected 4.5 and 10.0 new cases per million population at risk annually.[7,8] The disease is unusual in childhood, although it does occur. Overall, women are affected approximately three times as often as men, and this sex difference is increased during the childbearing years. No significant racial differences have been found.

A number of environmental factors have been implicated as predisposing to or precipitating systemic sclerosis.[9] The disease is more common among underground coal and gold miners and others occupationally exposed to *silica dust*,[10,11] especially in those men with intense exposure.[12] Localized sclerodermatous cutaneous changes, a Raynaud-like phenomenon, and osteolysis of the distal phalanges have been described in workers exposed to unfinished plastics in the manufacture of *polyvinyl chloride*; these persons also develop an unusual form of hepatic and pulmonary fibrosis.[13,14] Use of chlorinated hydrocarbons closely related to *vinyl chloride*[15] and aromatic hydrocarbon solvents, such as *benzene* and *toluene*,[16] and exposure to the polymerization of *epoxy resins*[17] have also been associated with the development of scleroderma. *Toxic oil syndrome*, an epidemic acute illness with fever, interstitial pneumonitis and eosinophilia, followed by a chronic phase with scleroderma features and musculoskeletal involvement with joint contractures, occurred in Spain in 1981 as the result of the ingestion of adulterated cooking oil (rapeseed oil).[18,19] In Japan, systemic sclerosis has been reported to occur many years after the injection of *paraffin or silicone breast implants*.[20] Other implicated substances include the antitumor drug *bleomycin*,[21] L-5-hydroxy-tryptophan and *carbidopa*[22] and *pentazocine*.[23]

Frequently, relatives of systemic sclerosis patients are affected by other connective tissue diseases such as systemic lupus erythematosus,[24] suggesting a heritable predisposition to these disorders. The number of reports of familial scleroderma has significantly increased[25,26] and includes instances of the disease in consanguineous kindreds.[27,28] Serum antinuclear antibodies (ANA) have been found in over one fourth of blood relatives of scleroderma patients but in only 5 to 8% of controls,[29,30] suggesting that genetic factors may influence autoimmunity. In one of these studies,[29] 21 of 58 family members with ANA had one or more clinical features of connective tissue disease. Similar observations, however, in spouses of patients raise the issue of environmental contributions.[29] Immunologic studies on identical twins discordant for scleroderma showed striking abnormalities in the affected but not the normal subject, a point against a predominant genetic predisposition to disease.[31]

CLINICAL FEATURES

Initial Symptoms

Systemic sclerosis usually begins between 30 and 50 years of age, but onset in childhood and among the elderly is reported. In most cases of limited cutaneous disease, the initial complaint is Raynaud's phenomenon. In contrast, patients with diffuse scleroderma most often have skin thickening or arthritis as the first manifestation.[32] In the few remaining patients, the earliest clue is that of visceral involvement. Esophageal symptoms (dysphagia, heartburn) may long antedate the development of cutaneous changes and, in fact, the latter may be entirely absent (systemic sclerosis *sine* scleroderma).[33]

Features of Organ System Involvement

Skin. Edematous, indurative, and atrophic phases are recognized in the evolution of scleroderma. In the early or *edematous phase*, patients complain about tight, puffy fingers, especially on arising in the morning. There may be nonpitting or pitting edema of the fingers ("sausaging") and hands, which also frequently involves the forearms, legs, feet, and face. The edema lasts indefinitely (e.g., fingers in limited scleroderma) or may be replaced gradually by thickening and tightening of the skin (*indurative phase*) after several weeks or months. In limited scleroderma these changes are generally restricted to the fingers, hands, and face, whereas diffuse scleroderma first affects the distalmost extremities and then spreads at a variable rate to the forearms, upper arms, thighs, upper anterior chest, and abdomen. In diffuse scleroderma, the affected skin becomes increasingly shiny, taut, and tightly adherent to underlying subcutis, thus impairing the mobility of muscles, tendons, and joints. During this phase, the epidermis is thinned, leading to loss of skin creases, hair, sweat and oils. Facial changes may result in the development of a characteristic pinched, immobile, expressionless appearance, with thin, tightly pursed lips and reduced oral aperture (Fig. 73–1). Microstomia interferes with eating and with proper dental care. In limited disease, skin thickening is much less prominent and the most striking digital and facial finding is numerous telangiectatic lesions (Fig. 73–2). After several years, the dermis tends to soften somewhat and in many cases reverts to normal thickness, or actually becomes thinner than normal (*atrophic phase*).

The natural history of skin involvement in the two major variants of systemic sclerosis is notably different when one uses a semi-quantitative method to measure the degree and extent of cutaneous thickening in all sites combined (total skin score) (Fig.

FIG. 73–1. Face of a young woman with diffuse cutaneous systemic sclerosis. Note loss of normal skin folds and retraction of lips.

FIG. 73–2. Face of a 45-year-old woman with limited cutaneous systemic sclerosis showing multiple telangiectases.

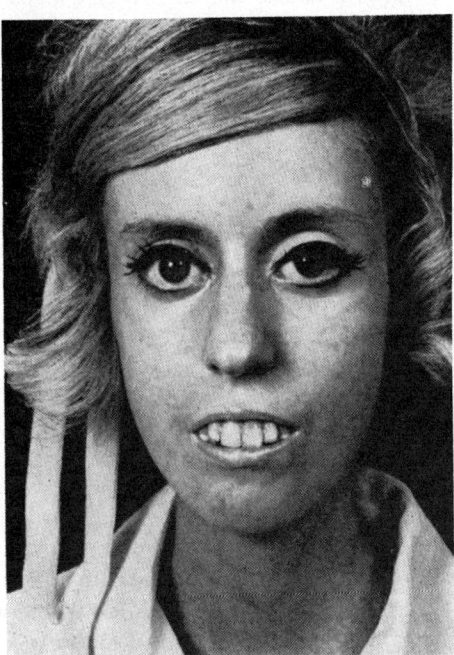

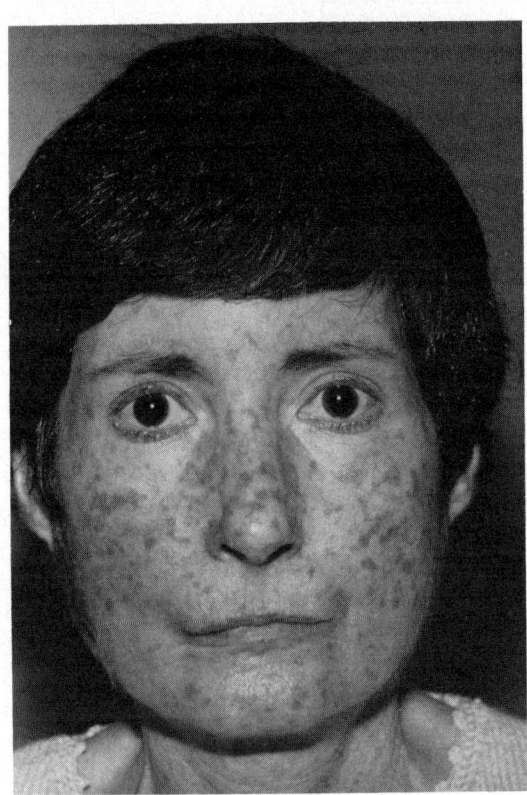

73–3).[34] In limited disease, skin thickening tends to remain minimal over many years and to have no relation to visceral sequelae. In contrast, in diffuse scleroderma, there is most often early, accelerated increase in skin thickness, which reaches a peak after 2 to 4 years and then slowly recedes. In a few instances, this regression is remarkable.[35] Rapid progression of skin thickness is associated with the development of joint contractures and several internal organ problems, including involvement of the lung, heart, and kidney.[36] Thus, although the amount of skin thickening per se does not herald a poor prognosis, the associated visceral disease is clearly life threatening.

A modified scleroderma skin scoring method has been described,[37] and a quantitative system for measuring skin elasticity has been proposed.[38] Ultrasound[39,40] and magnetic resonance imaging offer reproducible quantitative information concerning skin thickening, but are so expensive that they are not practical for office use. Other methods proposed to follow the progress of skin thickening include the measurement of urinary hydroxyproline[41] and serum levels of type III collagen aminopropeptide.[42]

Early in the disease, skin biopsy is less reliable for establishing a diagnosis than is careful physical examination. The weight and thickness of standard-diameter full-thickness skin punch biopsy cores are

significantly increased, testimony to the excessive accumulation of dermal collagen.[43] Biopsy specimens obtained during the active indurative phase disclose a striking increase of compact collagen fibers in the reticular dermis and other typical histopathologic changes, including thinning of the epidermis with loss of rete pegs, atrophy of dermal appendages, and hyalinization and fibrosis of arterioles. Variably large accumulations of mononuclear cells, chiefly T lymphocytes, are encountered in the lower dermis and upper subcutis (Fig. 73–4).[44,45] In typical cases, direct immunofluorescence is negative for immunoglobulins and complement components at the dermal-epidermal junction and in blood vessels.[46] Mast cells, which have been linked to fibrosis, are found in increased numbers and density in clinically involved skin from patients with early cutaneous disease (less than 3 years duration),[47] and may be inversely correlated with the severity of the cutaneous fibrosis.[47a] Fewer immunocompetent Langerhans cells are identified in the skin of patients with active scleroderma, along with absent dermal endothelial cell HLA-DR surface antigens.[48]

Skin thickening is frequently accompanied, and in some instances preceded, by an impressive hyper-

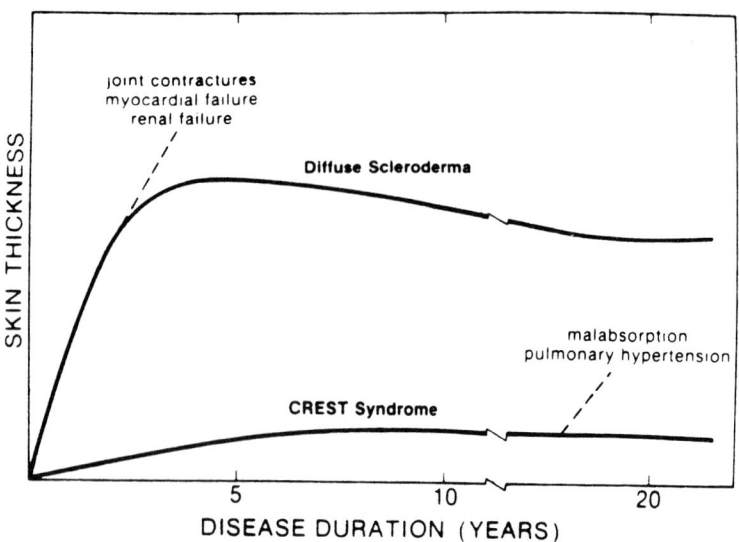

FIG. 73–3. Schematic representation of the natural history of skin thickness and timing of serious complications during the course of systemic sclerosis with diffuse cutaneous involvement and limited cutaneous involvement (CREST syndrome).

pigmentation that spares the mucous membranes. This change is most prominent in the area of hair follicles, with surrounding hypopigmentation leading to a "salt-and-pepper" appearance. Two new observations are the presence of hyperpigmentation over the course of superficial blood vessels[49] and of tendons.[49a] Increased melanin is found in the basal layer of the epidermis. Telangiectases, consisting of dilated capillary loops and venules, are frequently found on the fingers, palms, face, and lips in persons with lim-

ited scleroderma (see Fig. 73–2), and also develop late in the course of patients with diffuse scleroderma.

The skin overlying bony prominences, and especially that on the extensor surfaces of the proximal interphalangeal joints, becomes tightly stretched as a result of contractures and is extremely vulnerable to trauma. In such areas, there is cutaneous atrophy rather than thickening. Patients are often plagued by painful ulcerations at these sites and, less commonly, over the tip of the olecranon and malleoli of the ankles, which heal extremely slowly. Secondary infection may supervene. It should be noted that healing of skin in other locations is normal, including surgical incisions.

Patients with systemic sclerosis, particularly those with limited scleroderma, are liable to develop intracutaneous and subcutaneous calcification. These deposits occur chiefly in the digital pads and periarticular tissues, along the extensor surfaces of the forearms, in the olecranon bursae, and in the prepatellar area. They vary in size from tiny punctate lesions on the fingers (Fig. 73–5) to large conglomerate masses in the forearms. The latter may be complicated by ulceration of overlying skin, intermittent extrusion of calcareous material, and secondary bacterial infection. The pathogenesis of calcinosis in systemic sclerosis is unknown. Renal hydroxylation of vitamin D to the active hormone, 1,25-dihydroxyvitamin D, may be deficient.[50]

Peripheral Vascular System. Raynaud's phenomenon is defined as paroxysmal vasospasm of the fingers in response to cold exposure or emotional stress, and occurs in over 95% of patients with systemic sclerosis. Typically, the patient reports episodes of sudden pallor and/or cyanosis of the distal two thirds of the fingers, which become cold, numb, and painful. Dur-

FIG. 73–4. Photomicrograph of a skin punch biopsy obtained from the dorsum of the forearm of a 53-year-old woman with diffuse cutaneous systemic sclerosis. Skin appendages are atrophic, the dermis is significantly thickened by the deposition of dense collagenous connective tissue, and there are prominent collections of small round cells *(asterisk)* that were identified as T-lymphocytes.

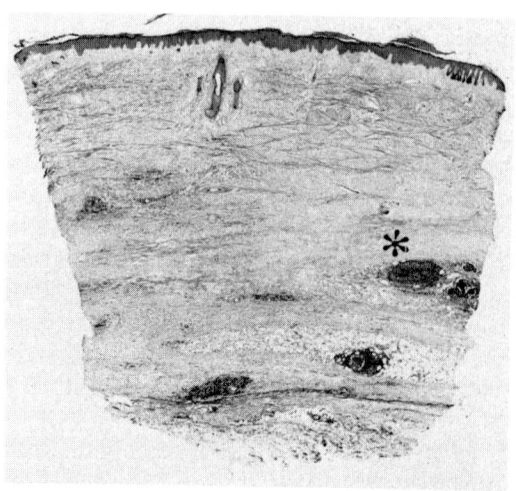

FIG. 73–5. Close-up hand roentgenogram of a 46-year-old woman with limited cutaneous systemic sclerosis. Note extensive subcutaneous calcinosis.

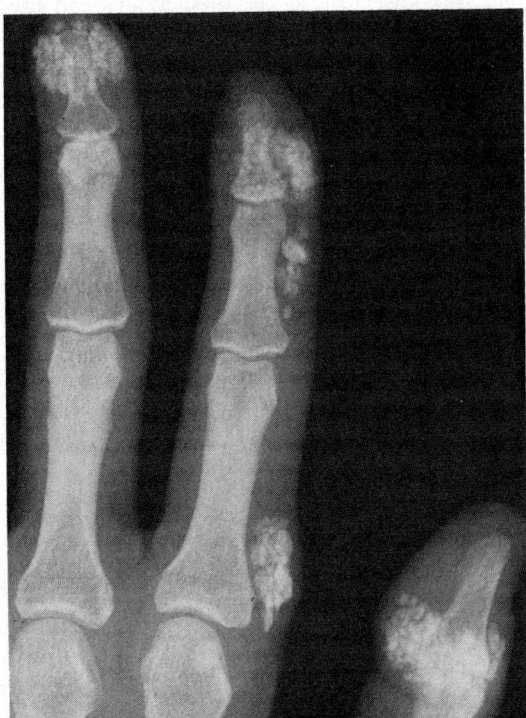

ing rewarming, reactive hyperemia is common. Small areas of ischemic necrosis or ulceration of the finger-tips leaving pitted scars are frequent, and in a few patients gangrene of the terminal portions of the pha-langes ensues. The toes also may be affected, and rarely, the tip of the nose, earlobes, or tongue. In most cases Raynaud's phenomenon begins contem-poraneously with skin changes and/or rheumatic complaints, or precedes these by a few months to a year. In patients with limited cutaneous scleroderma, Raynaud's phenomenon may antedate other evidence of systemic sclerosis by many years.[32] In contrast, when skin thickening precedes Raynaud's phenom-enon, subsequent diffuse skin thickening and an in-creased risk of renal involvement are more likely.[51]

Patients with Raynaud's phenomenon, with or without scleroderma, have a persistently reduced dig-ital pad temperature in the basal state and subnormal capillary blood flow in the fingers in both warm and cool environments.[52] Reduction in finger systolic blood pressure, unaltered by blockade of the sym-pathetic nervous system, has been observed.[53] These findings, together with delay in rewarming the fin-gers after cold exposure, suggest structural defects in the blood vessels.

In systemic sclerosis, angiographic and autopsy studies support this interpretation, disclosing nar-rowing and obstruction of the digital arteries.[54] His-tologic examination of these arteries at necropsy has revealed prominent intimal and adventitial fibrosis without evidence of inflammation. When severe, these changes lead to considerable narrowing or oc-clusion of the lumen. Recent or old thrombosis is frequently found, and one fourth of vessels examined have a distinctive type of lesion, telangiectases of the vasa vasorum (Fig. 73–6).[54] Nonatherosclerotic nar-rowing and occlusion of larger arteries is unusual;[54–56] it may be a later complication of limited cutaneous scleroderma.[55]

Concomitantly, the capillary circulation in patients with systemic sclerosis is altered by the appearance of "giant loops" and in diffuse scleroderma, a paucity of nailfold vessels on microscopy (Fig. 73–7).[57] Com-plete arrest of blood flow in these vessels has been observed following exposure to cold.[58] Capillary mi-croscopic patterns are interpreted from photo-graphs,[59] and semiquantitative grading scales have been devised for both capillary size and extent of "avascularity."[60,61] These observations may, therefore, be a useful permanent record of the state of the mi-crovasculature.[62] Nailfold biopsy has confirmed the accuracy of in vivo microscopy.[63] Such capillary changes are an early predictor of evolution to scle-roderma in persons who clinically appear to have Ray-naud's phenomenon alone,[64] and observed differ-ences in patterns may discriminate patients with other diseases, such as systemic lupus erythematosus and rheumatoid arthritis.[65] Although a relationship be-

FIG. 73–6. Photomicrograph of a digital artery obtained at autopsy from a 45-year-old woman with diffuse cutaneous systemic sclerosis who had Raynaud's phenomenon for over 20 years prior to her death. There is near occlusion of the lumen owing to subintimal proliferation and striking periad-ventitial fibrosis.

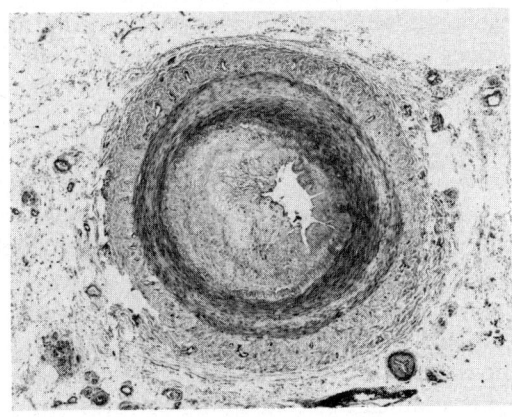

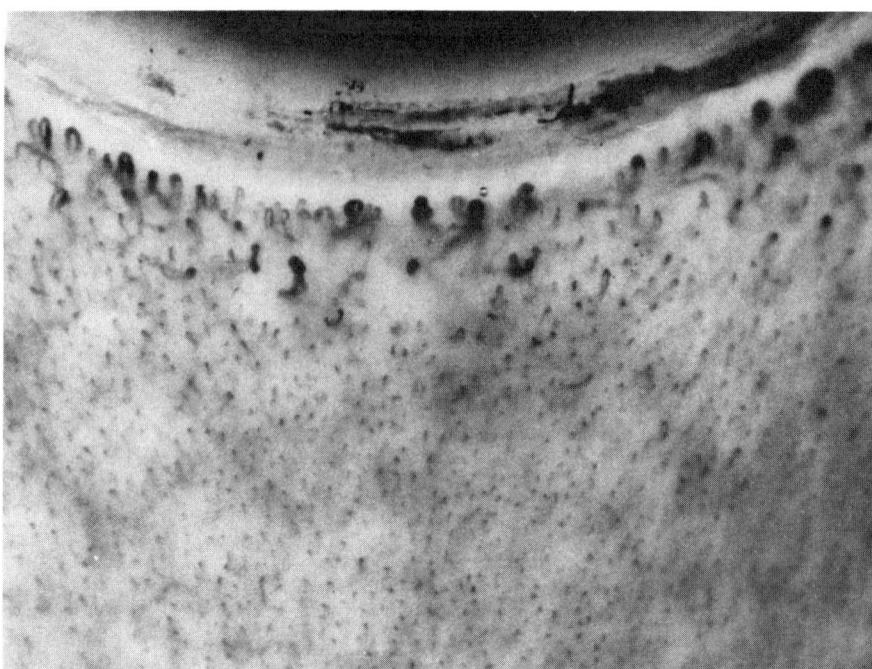

FIG. 73–7. Nailfold capillary pattern of a patient with diffuse cutaneous systemic sclerosis (× 18). Note extensive avascular area along the edge of the nailfold and grossly enlarged capillary loops. (From Maricq, H.R.[66])

tween reduced number and increased size of nailfold capillaries and visceral organ involvement in systemic sclerosis has been claimed,[66,67] not all authors agree.[68,69]

Many patients with no obvious symptoms or signs of an underlying connective tissue disease are referred to internists or rheumatologists for evaluation of Raynaud's phenomenon. In this circumstance, a small proportion of patients develop an associated disorder within the first 2 years after the onset of Raynaud's phenomenon.[70] Having passed this 2-year period, only a few patients (<5%) will develop features of scleroderma (most often limited scleroderma) or another connective tissue disease, even though twice as many have serum antinuclear antibody.[70–72a] Such signs may develop subtly even after several decades of observation.[71] Clinical clues that may antedate the late appearance of systemic sclerosis include sclerodactyly, puffy fingers, digital pitting scars, capillary microscopic abnormalities, and serum anticentromere antibodies.[71] Since it is almost always present, Raynaud's phenomenon in systemic sclerosis has little prognostic import.

Joints, Tendons, and Bones. Symmetric polyarthralgias and joint stiffness, affecting chiefly the fingers, wrists, knees, and ankles are frequent initial or early complaints in systemic sclerosis. Generalized swelling of the fingers also occurs. It may be difficult to ascertain the degree to which limitation of interphalangeal joint motion is caused by joint, periarticular, or tenosynovial disease, or by changes in the skin. Synovitis mimicking rheumatoid arthritis is uncommon, but may be the first manifestation of diffuse scleroderma. Larger peripheral joints occasionally show evidence of inflammation, with scanty synovial fluid containing fewer than 2000 leukocytes/mm³ that are predominantly mononuclear. Pathologic examination of synovium reveals variable amounts of chronic inflammatory cells, either in focal aggregates or scattered diffusely.[73] Fibrin deposition on the synovial surface is frequent. Patients with calcinosis may develop widespread calcification of the synovium and tendon sheaths.[74] The synovial fluid in the latter cases has been described as milky or chalky and containing large numbers of basic calcium phosphate crystals.[75]

Some patients are aware of creaking noises on movement of their extremities. A peculiar type of coarse, leathery crepitus (tendon friction rub) may be palpated over such areas during joint motion, particularly the elbows, wrists, fingers, knees, and ankles. These rubs, attributed to fibrinous deposits on the surfaces of tendon sheaths and overlying fascia,[76] are specific for systemic sclerosis with diffuse scleroderma and often antedate an explosive increase in skin thickening. Friction rubs occur rarely in persons with limited scleroderma or with other inflammatory rheumatic conditions. Carpal tunnel syndrome may result from flexor tenosynovitis at the wrist. Flexion contractures ("bowed fingers") are caused, at least in part, by tendinous and periarticular fibrosis and shortening.[77] These contractures, which occur commonly in the fingers, wrists, elbows, and ankles, usually become apparent within several months.

The most frequent bony radiographic abnormality

is resorption of the tufts of the terminal phalanges of the fingers (and much less often, the toes). This resorption rarely may lead to complete dissolution of the terminal phalanx. A few patients develop severe erosive changes of the fingers, radiographically more typical of osteoarthritis than of rheumatoid arthritis.[78,79] Some with joint erosions are considered to have rheumatoid arthritis as the primary rheumatic disease, but they also have scleroderma.[80] Other examples of bone resorption, which may be the result of ischemia, include "notching" of the ribs (limited to patients with diffuse scleroderma)[81] and dissolution of the condyle and ramus of the mandible.[82]

Skeletal Muscle. In most instances, weakness and atrophy of skeletal muscle found in systemic sclerosis are the result of disuse owing to joint contractures or chronic disease. However, approximately 20% of patients have a primary myopathy.[32] The minority exhibit pronounced proximal muscle weakness and electrophysiologic, biochemical, and pathologic evidence of polymyositis.[83,84] These persons have been variably classified as having systemic sclerosis with myositis or systemic sclerosis in overlap with polymyositis. In most cases, a more subtle myopathy occurs, with weakness detected only by the examining physician, mild or no serum muscle enzyme elevation, and a muscle biopsy showing focal replacement of myofibrils with collagenous connective tissue and perimysial and epimysial fibrosis without inflammatory changes. The latter condition is distinctive in that it does not occur in patients with other connective tissue diseases. Fortunately, it tends to be nonprogressive and thus does not warrant attempts at intervention.

Gastrointestinal Tract. *Oral Cavity.* Thinning of the lips (microcheilia) and atrophy of the mucous membranes are common, as is reduced oral aperture (microstomia). In the CREST syndrome, numerous lip and oral mucosal telangiectases are often noted. Atrophy of the tongue papillae, with impaired taste perception[84a] and shortening of the tongue and perioral musculature[84b] have been noted. Thickening of the peridontal membrane occurs in up to 30% of patients[84b] and loss of the lamina dura with gingivitis and subsequent loosening of the teeth is common. These events are compounded by the mechanical difficulty (hands, oral opening) of maintaining good oral hygiene, and often by the presence of Sjögren's syndrome. Temporomandibular joint involvement[82] may also be a factor in some patients.

Esophagus and Stomach. Esophageal dysfunction eventually develops in nearly 90% of patients with systemic sclerosis, thus constituting the most common internal manifestation of disease. No predilection for diffuse or limited scleroderma has been detected. In some cases, this abnormality occurs long before evidence of cutaneous disease; when it is present in the absence of skin thickening, the term systemic sclerosis *sine* scleroderma is appropriate.[33]

Solid foods tend to become "stuck" in the esophagus, requiring ingestion of fluids in order to pass. Patients often reduce their food intake and may lose appreciable amounts of weight. They may complain only about mild retrosternal burning pain, postprandial fullness, or regurgitation. Despite the frequency of peptic esophagitis, esophageal hemorrhage is surprisingly unusual.

All patients should have some assessment of esophageal function. Roentgenographic abnormalities are found in three fourths, including many who have no esophageal symptoms. *Cinefluoroscopic* examination, best performed using light barium in the recumbent position to eliminate the effects of gravity on emptying, reveals a diminution or even total absence of peristaltic activity in the distal esophagus. Gastroesophageal reflux occurs because of incompetence of the lower esophageal sphincter. With progression, the lower portion of the esophagus tends to become patulous and flaccid, but in some persons, most often those with limited scleroderma, chronic peptic esophagitis is complicated by narrowing or stricture in this location. These persons are at high risk to develop Barrett's metaplasia, a diagnosis reliably made by esophagoscopy (37% in one study of selected patients).[85] They are thus theoretically more prone to develop adenocarcinoma of the esophagus, although there is no published support for this sequence of events.[86] *Manometric* measurements, which are considerably more sensitive but limited because they are more difficult for the patient to tolerate, confirm incoordination and loss of contractile power and a reduction in the tone of the gastroesophageal sphincter.[87] *Esophageal pH-monitoring* may be useful in documenting the presence of gastroesophageal reflux.[88] *Radionuclide scintigraphy,* which is quantitative and has a high degree of patient acceptance, gives very comparable results. Reduced percentage of emptying and prolonged transit time correlate highly with abnormal distal esophageal pressure measurements.[89–92] Specificity for systemic sclerosis, however, is lacking, because abnormal radionuclide studies are reported in other connective tissue diseases[90] and normal subjects.[92]

Upper (pharyngoesophageal) dysphagia, caused by dysfunction of striated rather than smooth muscle, is frequent in polymyositis, but has also been noted in systemic sclerosis.[93] Gastric atony and dilatation may occur, but involvement of the stomach is remarkably uncommon when compared with other portions of the alimentary tract. Gastric acid secretion is unimpaired in most systemic sclerosis patients, but both hyperchlorhydria and increased basal and/or stimulated gastric acid output have been found.[94,95] In rare instances, telangiectases have been considered the source of serious bleeding from the distal esophagus, stomach, or other gastrointestinal tract sites, especially in persons with limited scleroderma.[96–98] Histologic changes are most significant in the lower two thirds of the esophagus, where there is thinning of the mucosa and increased collagen in the lamina propria and submucosa. There is a variable degree of atrophy of the muscularis, which may be almost totally replaced by fibrous tissue. The walls of small arteries and arterioles are thickened and often surrounded by periadventitial deposits of collagen. Cellular infiltrates have been noted in the submucosa. The myenteric plexuses of Auerbach, which may be conspicuously lacking in ganglion cells, usually appear to be normal. Physiologic and pharmacologic studies of esophageal blood flow have not been performed.

Small Intestine. In a small proportion of patients, the illness is dominated by intestinal complaints, consisting of severe bloating, abdominal cramps, and episodic diarrhea. A few of these persons develop malabsorption, which may result in extreme wasting. Striking hypomotility of the small intestine, documented by both radiographic and manometric methods, favors the *overgrowth of intestinal microorganisms* that consume large amounts of vitamin B_{12} and interfere with normal fat absorption as a result of their deconjugation of bile salts. There is often prolonged retention of barium in the atonic and widely dilated second and third portions of the duodenum (loop sign). In the remainder of the small intestine, one may find irregular flocculation or hypersegmentation of barium or localized areas of bowel dilatation. The mucosal pattern of the distended jejunum contains prominent transverse folds (Fig. 73–8). The valvulae conniventes remain close to one another despite pronounced dilatation of the lumen (closed accordion sign), presumably owing to excessive fibrosis of the submucosa. Similar changes are occasionally found in the ileum. Severe atony of the bowel produces a functional ileus (pseudoobstruction) with symptoms simulating mechanical obstruction. Volvulus of the greatly dilated small intestine has been observed.[99]

There are several reports of pneumatosis intestinalis in systemic sclerosis. Gas enters from the bowel lumen through small defects in the mucosa and muscularis mucosae and appears as numerous radiolucent cysts or linear streaks within the bowel wall. Rupture of these collections of air into the peritoneal space is occasionally accompanied by symptoms of partial small bowel obstruction, or those mimicking a perforated viscus. In general, however, this problem results in a benign pneumoperitoneum.

With the addition of serosal fibrosis, the pathologic changes in the intestine are similar to those described for the esophagus, that is, normal mucosa or mild villous atrophy, infiltration of the lamina propria by lymphocytes and plasma cells, fibrous thickening of the submucosa, atrophy of smooth muscle with collagenous replacement, and thickening of the walls of small arteries and arterioles. Peroral biopsy specimens of the duodenum have revealed increased amounts of collagen surrounding and infiltrating Brunner's glands. Similar periglandular fibrosis is seen involving the esophageal, minor salivary, nasal mucosal, and thyroid glands.[100–102]

Colon. Constipation, either alone or alternating with diarrhea, may signal colonic involvement. Reduced motility of this organ has been reported,[103] and in one study the frequencies of anorectal and esophageal dysmotility were similar.[104] Patchy atrophy of the muscularis leads to the development of wide-mouthed diverticula, which usually occur along the antimesenteric border of the transverse and descending colon (Fig. 73–9). They are almost entirely unique to systemic sclerosis, having been described in only a single patient with amyloidosis.[105] Ordinarily these outpouchings cause no difficulty, but rarely they may perforate or become impacted with fecal matter, producing obstruction.[106] Rectal incontinence and prolapse are rare but disabling problems.[107]

Lung. Lung involvement occurs in over 70% of patients.[108] The most prominent symptom is exertional dyspnea, which is present in nearly half. Less often there is a chronic cough, which is nonproductive unless associated with superimposed infection, and rarely one or more episodes of pleuritic chest pain. Many patients remain entirely asymptomatic, however, despite evidence of pulmonary fibrosis, possibly because their physical activity is restricted. Physical examination may reveal dry bibasilar "fibrotic" rales or pleural friction rubs, but most often examination of the lungs proves unremarkable.

In over one third of patients with both diffuse and limited cutaneous scleroderma, the chest roentgenogram discloses a reticular pattern of linear, nodular, and lineonodular densities that are most pronounced in the lower lung fields. In some persons the appearance is that of diffuse mottling or "honeycombing," indicative of cystic lesions. Large upper lobe cystic lesions have been observed, most often associated with CREST syndrome.[109]

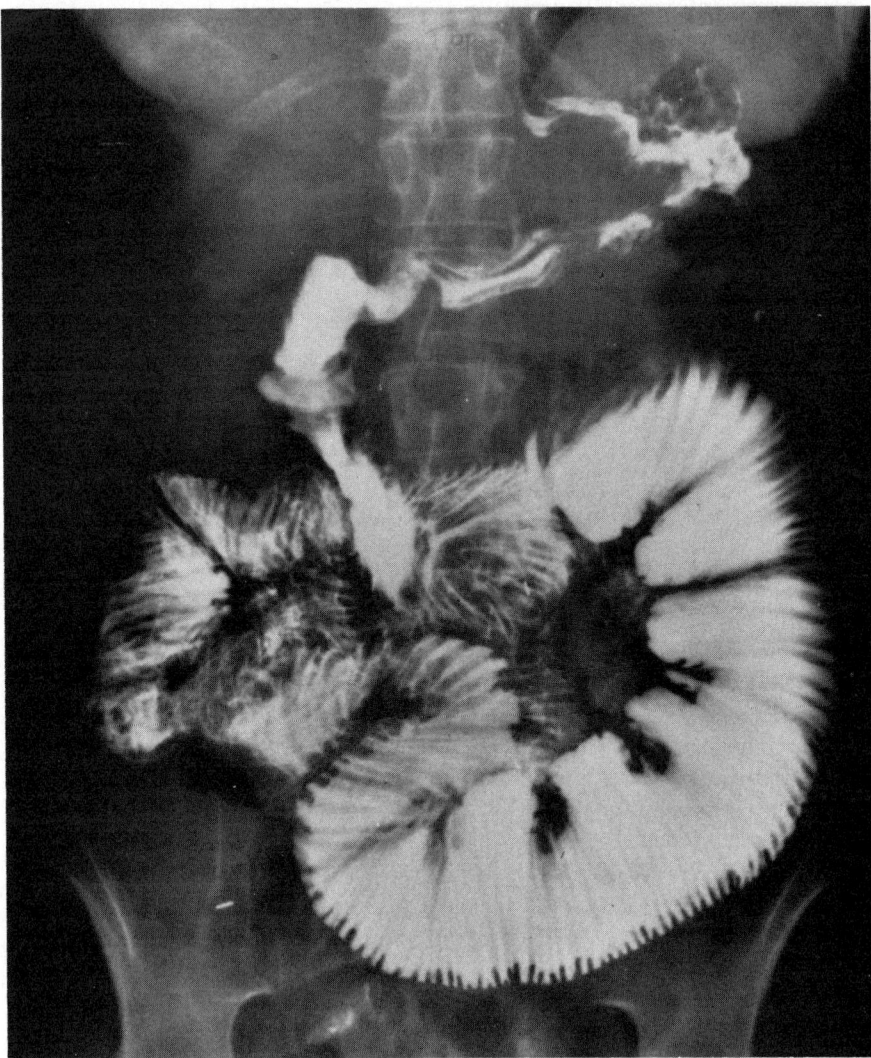

FIG. 73–8. Upper gastrointestinal tract roentgenogram in a 46-year-old woman with diffuse cutaneous systemic sclerosis. Although dilatation of the jejunum is striking, its valvulae conniventes remain closely approximated (closed accordion sign).

Pulmonary function abnormalities occur in more than two thirds of all patients, irrespective of disease variant.[81,110] A restrictive ventilatory defect, indicated by a reduction in vital capacity and decreased lung compliance, is most common. Impairment in gas exchange, evidenced by a reduced diffusing capacity for carbon monoxide, is usually present in patients with restrictive lung disease, but is also common as an isolated defect without significant alteration in ventilation or roentgenographic evidence of fibrosis. A few scleroderma patients have obstructive disease, but this finding is nearly always attributable to cigarette smoking.[111] In serial studies of pulmonary function, no excessive deterioration occurred in scleroderma patients compared with a normal population.[112–114a] An occasional patient, however, does develop progressive, fatal respiratory failure.

The predominant histologic changes, present in nearly all cases at postmortem examination, consist of diffuse alveolar, interstitial, peribronchial, and pleural fibrosis (Fig. 73–10). A moderate degree of pulmonary hypertension, with a relatively slow progression, accompanies widespread pulmonary interstitial fibrosis, which very gradually obliterates more and more of the pulmonary vascular bed. Early in the disease, an inflammatory component is present. In this stage, gallium scanning is abnormal in many patients.[115–116a] Alveolitis, with large numbers of macrophages and lymphocytes and increased proportions of neutrophils and/or eosinophils, has been documented by bronchoalveolar lavage, especially in early disease.[116–119] It is believed that mononuclear cell products are important stimulants of lung fibroblasts.

A very different clinical entity, severe pulmonary arterial hypertension with cor pulmonale, with minimal or no pulmonary interstitial fibrosis,[120] is encountered almost exclusively in patients with limited scleroderma. Less than 10% of CREST syndrome patients develop this complication after 15 to 30 years of observation.[32] In this circumstance, there is a rapid

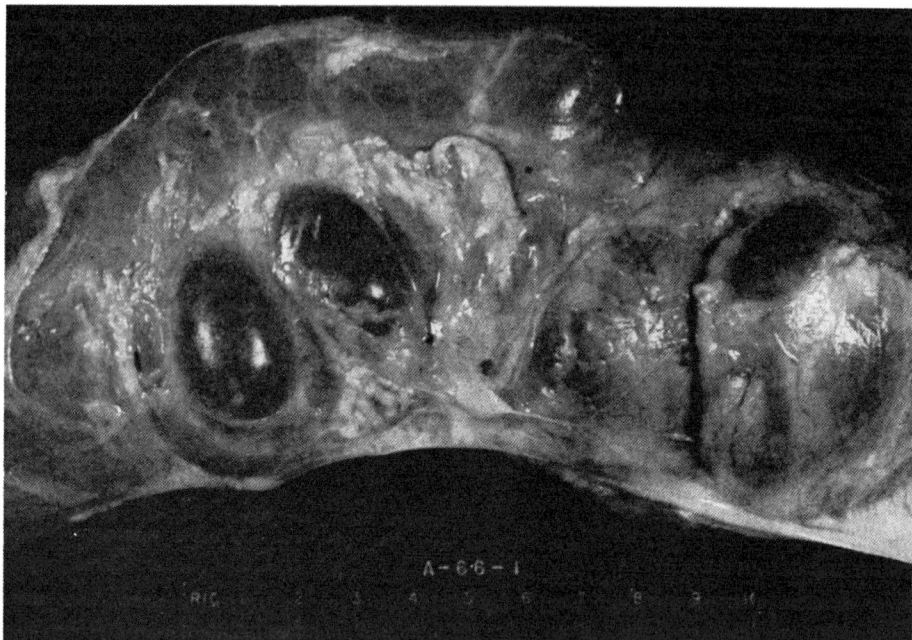

FIG. 73–9. Gross appearance of the transverse colon from a patient with limited cutaneous scleroderma and numerous large-mouthed colonic diverticula seen on barium enema.

FIG. 73–10. Photomicrograph of the lung of a 52-year-old woman with diffuse cutaneous systemic sclerosis. She died as the result of respiratory insufficiency. Note the dramatic interstitial fibrosis and dilatation of air sacs (honeycomb lung).

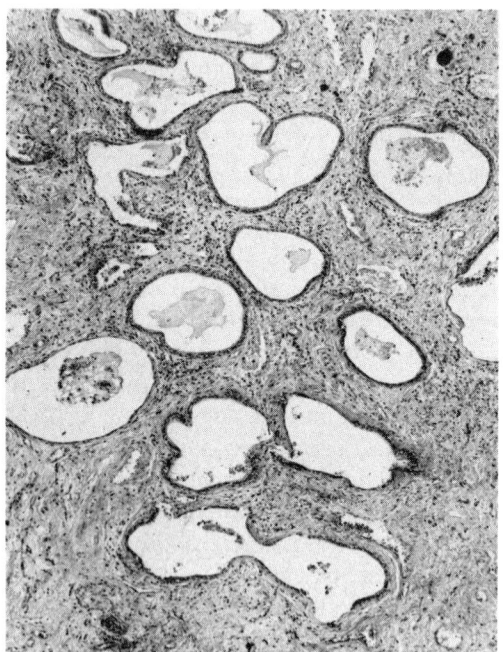

worsening of dyspnea, a markedly accentuated pulmonic component of the second heart sound, and ultimately signs of right-sided cardiac failure. The diffusing capacity is extremely low, consistent with impaired gas exchange across thickened small pulmonary blood vessels.[120–123] Diagnosis is confirmed by echocardiogram or by right-sided heart catheterization. The mean duration of survival from first clinical detection is 2 years, emphasizing the serious nature of this problem.[122] Pathologic signs include uniform narrowing and/or occlusion of small pulmonary arteries caused by subintimal proliferative changes and significant medial smooth muscle hypertrophy without evidence of vasculitis (Fig. 73–11).[122] The existence of "pulmonary Raynaud's phenomenon" is controversial.[124,125]

As expected, reduced diffusing capacity (40% of predicted or less) and an obstructive ventilatory defect were found to be associated with increased mortality.[126] Lung cancer is considered to occur with increased frequency in late stage systemic sclerosis, generally in the setting of long-standing pulmonary fibrosis with intense bronchiolar epithelial proliferation and cellular atypia, independent of smoking.[127,128]

Heart. Since the classic description of congestive heart failure caused by myocardial fibrosis,[129] cardiopulmonary and cardiovascular manifestations have been extensively reviewed.[108,130] Cardiac involvement may be classified as primary or secondary.[131,132] Primary disease consists of either pericarditis with or without effusion, left ventricular or biventricular congestive failure, or a serious supraventricular or ventricular arrhythmia. It is important to remember

FIG. 73–11. Photomicrograph of the lung of a 61-year-old woman with systemic sclerosis and limited scleroderma who died as the result of pulmonary arterial hypertension with cor pulmonale. There is significant intimal proliferation and medial hypertrophy of this small pulmonary artery and no interstitial fibrosis.

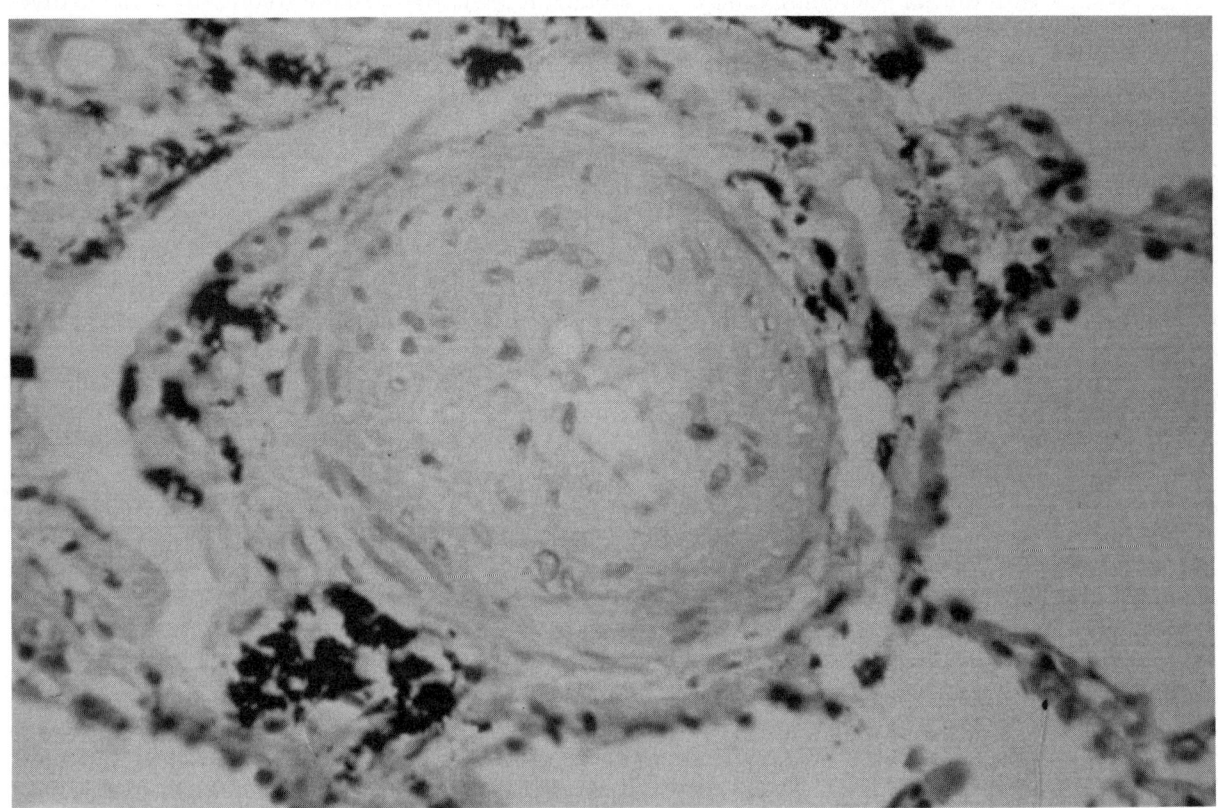

that scleroderma patients develop atherosclerosis and hypertensive heart disease with frequencies similar to their occurrence in the general population; thus attribution of cause is often a difficult decision.

Acute symptomatic pericarditis and pericardial effusion have been appreciated with increasing frequency, but cardiac tamponade is uncommon. With echocardiography, asymptomatic pericardial thickening and small effusions are readily detected.[133] Pericardial effusion may antedate renal involvement.[134] The few reported aspirates of pericardial fluid have shown exudates without evidence of immune complexes or complement activation.

Clinically apparent congestive failure owing to myocardial fibrosis occurs in fewer than 10% of patients, nearly all of whom have diffuse cutaneous scleroderma. New noninvasive radionuclide studies, however, have shown that more subtle abnormalities of ventricular function are frequent.[135–137] These changes are attributable to diffuse atrophy and fibrous

replacement of functioning myocardium. Myocarditis along with typical polymyositis has been reported in four patients.[138,139]

Although a few patients have exertional chest pain that mimics angina pectoris, coronary angiograms are most often normal. The autopsy finding of "contraction band necrosis" of the myocardium suggests that heart damage may be due to intermittent vascular spasm or "intramyocardial Raynaud's phenomenon."[133] Electrocardiographic evidence of myocardial ischemia and/or necrosis in the absence of the clinical syndrome of myocardial infarction has been noted.[140] Both resting and reversible exercise- and cold-induced myocardial perfusion defects and left ventricular dysfunction have been detected,[141–143] especially in patients with diffuse disease,[136] raising the possibility that multiple vasospastic ischemic episodes lead to myocardial fibrosis. These resting defects are reversible after administration of oral nifedipine[144] or intravenous dipyridamole.[145] The latter potent vasodilator was also used to determine coronary artery flow and resistance reserve, which were reduced in scleroderma cardiomyopathy patients compared with controls.[146,146a]

Autopsy of persons with diffuse scleroderma may also show extensive degeneration of myocardial fibers with replacement by irregular patches of fibrosis that are prominent in, but not limited to, perivascular areas (Fig. 73–12). The large extramural coronary arteries are typically normal, but focal infiltrates of round cells and considerable thickening of smaller coronary vessels may occur.[147] Myocardial infarction is unusual.

Cardiac arrhythmias including complete heart block and other electrocardiographic abnormalities are encountered, as would be expected in the case of a cardiomyopathy. Using the 24-hour continuous electrocardiogram (Holter monitor), 15 to 22% of patients had conduction defects in point prevalence studies.[148,149] One of the factors limiting exercise performance in up to one third of patients is the development of arrhythmias.[149a] Careful dissection of the conduction system of several patients with rhythm disturbances, including complete heart block, has revealed fibrous replacement of the sinus node, atrioventricular node, particularly in its proximal segment,[150,151] and bundle branches.[152] In most cases, however, no specific morphologic changes have been identified in this tissue, and arrhythmias have been attributed to disturbances of the working myocardium.

Secondary causes of heart disease are typically due to the extracardiac stresses of pulmonary and systemic arterial hypertension. The former occurs chiefly in the limited scleroderma variant, as noted previously. Severe systemic arterial hypertension associated with renal involvement frequently leads to myocardial dysfunction (see next section, Kidney). Aortic regurgitation has been reported in two cases of scleroderma,[153] but the prevalence of valvular lesions is no greater than that found in age-matched controls,[154] and thus it is difficult to exclude coincidental rheumatic heart disease.

Kidney. Renal involvement is an important aspect of systemic sclerosis and a major cause of death. Clinically evident renal disease is restricted to persons with diffuse scleroderma, especially those with rapidly progressive cutaneous involvement of less than 3 years' duration.[155] Rarely is a person with limited scleroderma affected unless the patient is misclassified during an early stage in the evolution of diffuse disease.

Twenty percent of diffuse cutaneous scleroderma patients develop a dramatic complication, termed *scleroderma renal crisis,* which is characterized by the abrupt onset of highly malignant arterial hypertension, followed immediately by the development of rapidly progressive renal insufficiency. In some populations, renal crisis is considerably less frequent, for unknown reasons.[156] The appearance of hypertension is often heralded by a variety of manifestations including severe headache, visual difficulties resulting from striking hypertensive retinopathy, seizures, or sudden left

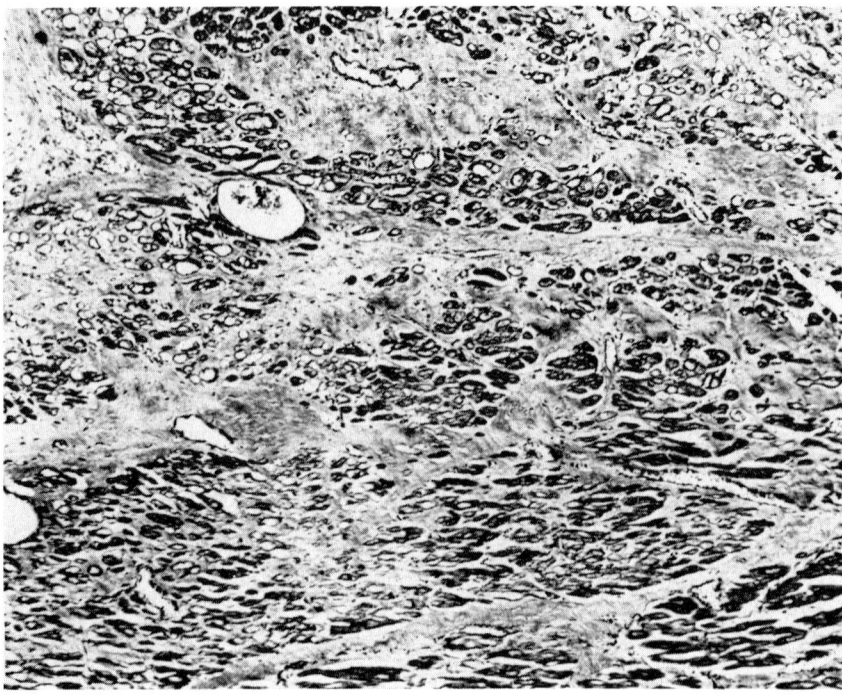

FIG. 73–12. Photomicrograph of myocardium of a 52-year-old woman with diffuse cutaneous systemic sclerosis who died of congestive heart failure. Loss of normal myocardial fibers is extensive, and interstitial fibrosis is severe.

ventricular failure. Within several days or weeks evidence of renal disease is indicated by microscopic hematuria and proteinuria, rapidly increasing azotemia, and terminally by oliguria or anuria. Proteinuria in the nephrotic range is unusual. Severe hypertension is typically associated with extremely high plasma renin levels.

On occasion the blood pressure may remain within normal limits and azotemia and severe microangiopathic hemolytic anemia are the dominant features.[157] Prior administration of adrenocorticotropic hormone (ACTH) or a corticosteroid preparation has been reported as a precipitating factor in "scleroderma kidney," but in most instances these drugs cannot be implicated. Sudden, severe volume depletion may also trigger renal crisis in the susceptible patient, who often has had clinically undetected reduced renal blood flow.

Before the last decade, survival for more than 3 to 6 months after the onset of this most dreaded complicaton was almost unknown, most patients succumbing to renal or cardiac failure or to cerebral hemorrhage despite treatment with available antihypertensive agents. However, the aggressive use of potent new drugs that block the renin-angiotensin system has dramatically improved prognosis.[158] Such therapy appears to be uniformly successful in controlling hypertension, although renal insufficiency may nevertheless progress, requiring peritoneal dialysis or hemodialysis. In some instances, it has been possible to discontinue dialysis after a number of months.[159,160] Simultaneous remarkable reduction in skin thickness has been noted in some[161,162] but not all[163] patients who have survived renal crisis.

Numerous small cortical infarcts are seen grossly in the affected kidneys with subintimal proliferative changes of the intralobular arteries. Focal microscopic alterations consist of intimal hyperplasia, with acid mucopolysaccharide deposition, and necrosis of the walls of these vessels, afferent arterioles, and glomerular tufts (Fig. 73–13). Only prominent fibrosis of the adventitia of the small vessels may distinguish this lesion from that of nonsclerodermatous malignant nephrosclerosis.[164] Identical histopathologic changes have been observed in the absence of hypertension.[165] These alterations are reminiscent of those encountered in the digital vessels, as discussed earlier.

Immunohistologic examination has revealed the regular presence of immunoglobulins (chiefly IgM), complement components (also reported in malignant hypertension not associated with systemic sclerosis), and fibrinogen in the walls of affected vessels.[166,167] Electron microscopic examination, however, has failed to reveal discrete electron-dense deposits or other features indicative of the presence of immune complexes.[166]

Renal angiography during life and postmortem injection studies have demonstrated a striking constriction of the interlobular arteries and afferent arterioles and a sharp decrease in glomerular filling (Fig. 73–14).[164] In some cases, these changes in the small vessels give rise to a "spotted" nephrogram, characterized by focal lucencies scattered throughout the kidneys, without evidence of any changes in the major arteries.[168] This disturbance in the renal circulation may be likened to Raynaud's phenomenon in the digital circulation, but is nonspecific, also occurring in the kidneys of patients with malignant hypertension of other causes.

The pathogenesis of the renal circulatory abnormalities in systemic sclerosis remains unclear. Both efferent arteriolar constriction and arteriolar hyperreactivity to stimuli such as angiotensin have been proposed. Neither supine nor standing plasma renin elevations have been found to antedate the occurrence of renal involvement.[158,169] An exaggerated increase in plasma renin levels following cold pressor testing has been reported, especially in normotensive systemic sclerosis patients with prominent vascular changes on renal biopsy.[170] Diminished[171] and normal[172] sodium excretion have both been reported. Because no consistent physiologic changes have been observed, it is likely that mechanisms other than renin-angiotensin system dysfunction are responsible for hypertension in systemic sclerosis. Some, but not all, patients with frank renal involvement show evidence of increased intravascular coagulation and increased plasma fibrinogen turnover,[173] suggesting that intraluminal events play a role in the parenchymal damage.

Symptomatic sclerodermatous involvement of the lower urinary tract is rare, although bladder wall connective tissue deposition and proliferative vascular lesions have been noted.[174]

Liver and Pancreas. Primary biliary cirrhosis occurs in some women with limited cutaneous scleroderma,[175,176] most frequently in association with Sjögren's syndrome.[177] These patients develop pruritus, jaundice, and hepatomegaly, with a pronounced elevation of serum alkaline phosphatase activity and antimitochondrial antibodies, most often directed against a 72,000-dalton M2 autoantigen.[178,179] Nodular regenerative hyperplasia of the liver has also been reported.[180] Although isolated instances of chronic pancreatitis[181] and arteritis involving this organ[182] have been described, there is no convincing clinical evidence of pancreatic exocrine or endocrine dys-

FIG. 73–13. Photomicrographs of kidneys of two women who died of malignant arterial hypertension and renal insufficiency complicating diffuse cutaneous systemic sclerosis. *A,* Intimal hyperplasia with complete luminal occlusion of an interlobular artery. Note reduplication and fraying of the internal elastic lamina (orcein stain). *B,* Fibrinoid necrosis of blood vessels in the glomerulus.

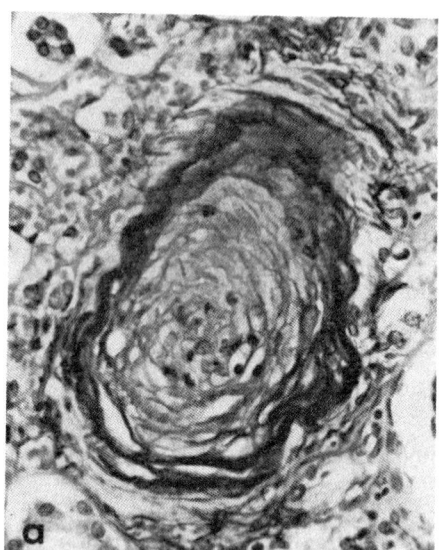
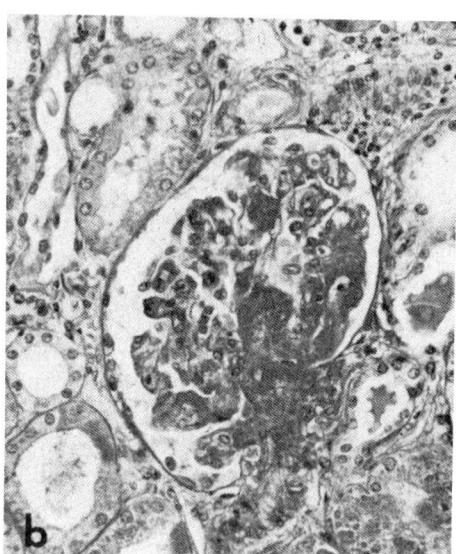

FIG. 73–14. Roentgenograms of kidneys, injected post mortem, of two patients with diffuse cutaneous systemic sclerosis. *A,* Kidney of a man who died of cardiac disease without clinical evidence of renal involvement. Filling of the interlobular and smaller cortical vessels is normal. *B,* Kidney of a man who developed "scleroderma renal crisis" with malignant hypertension and renal failure. There is irregular narrowing of the interlobular vessels and little filling of smaller vessels supplying the renal cortex.

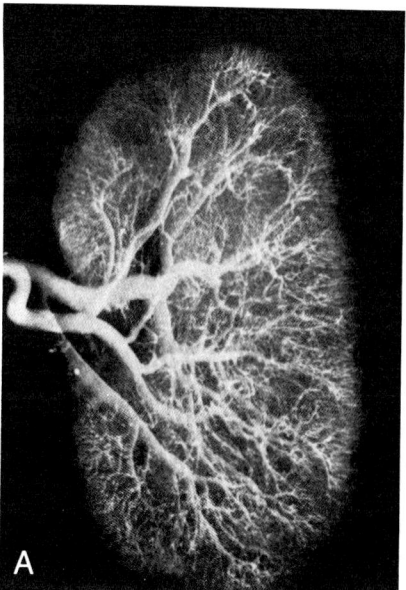
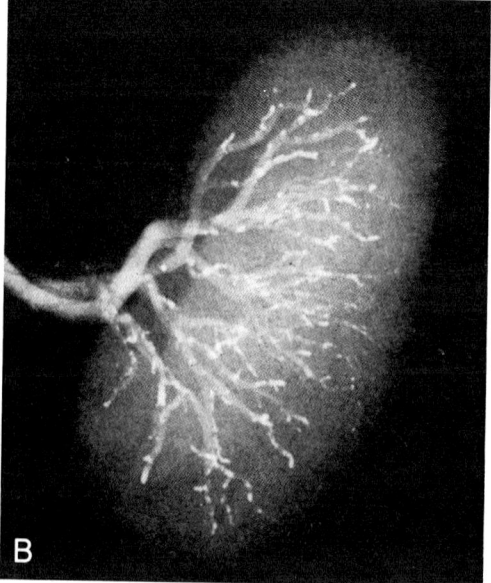

function in systemic sclerosis. The frequency of pancreatic fibrosis at autopsy has been similar in scleroderma patients[154,183] and controls.[154]

Blood. In typical systemic sclerosis, hematologic studies are normal, and abnormalities suggest either a specific complication or an associated illness.[184,185] The few patients with anemia are classified as having chronic disease, blood loss (peptic esophagitis or telangiectases), excessive destruction (microangiopathic hemolysis), or metabolic causes (intestinal malabsorption). The peripheral blood and bone marrow reflect these circumstances, and the latter is not fibrotic. Autoimmune hemolytic anemia[186] and neutropenia[187] have also been recorded. Leukopenia is often present when systemic sclerosis exists in overlap with systemic lupus erythematosus or with mixed connective tissue disease.[185] Impressive eosinophilia (500 cells/mm[3]) is unusual;[188] its presence should alert the physician to the possibility of eosinophilic fasciitis (discussed later in the chapter).

Nervous System. Primary disorders of the nervous system are seldom encountered. Most of the problems that occur are either purely coincidental or represent secondary compressive findings, for example, carpal tunnel syndrome[189] or, rarely, myelopathy[189a] or sequelae of renal or cardiopulmonary involvement. Trigeminal sensory neuropathy, an occasional finding, is associated most closely with myositis and anti-ribonucleoprotein (anti-RNP) antibodies.[190,191] Cerebral arteritis has been reported rarely.[192] Vasculitis associated with coincidental Sjögren's syndrome may rarely be detected (see below).[193] Impotence without other obvious causes has been described[194] and is most likely due to reduced penile blood flow.[195] Autonomic neuropathy has been observed in one patient and suspected in three others.[196]

Eyes and Ears. With the exception of keratoconjunctivitis sicca, most ocular disease in patients with systemic sclerosis is due to other conditions.[197] Hypertensive retinopathy found in persons with renal crisis has already been described. In addition, patchy areas of nonperfusion have been noted in the choroidal capillary bed in patients with both diffuse and limited scleroderma.[198,199] Sensorineural hearing loss was found in the majority of patients in one study and was not attributable to other factors (e.g., age, drugs, noise).[200]

Sjögren's Syndrome. Dry eyes and dry mouth are frequent complaints in systemic sclerosis. Lymphocytic infiltration of minor salivary glands on labial biopsy is present in approximately 15 to 20% of patients.[201] In many of these persons, and in some others, periglandular and intraglandular fibrosis, believed to be characteristic of scleroderma,[100] is noted.

Half the patents with systemic sclerosis and Sjögren's syndrome (SS) have serum anti-SSA and/or anti-SSB antibodies, but these autoantibodies occur almost exclusively in patients with lymphocytic infiltration rather than fibrosis.[201] As in primary Sjögren's syndrome,[202] there is an association between secondary Sjögren's syndrome and vasculitis involving the skin (palpable purpura and leg ulcers) and peripheral nervous system (sensory neuropathy and mononeuritis multiplex) in systemic sclerosis.[193]

Thyroid Gland. Hypothyroidism, often clinically unrecognized, occurs in one fourth of patients with systemic sclerosis[203] and is frequently accompanied by serum antithyroid antibodies. As in the salivary glands, fibrosis is a prominent histologic finding,[102] whereas lymphocytic infiltration typical of Hashimoto's thyroiditis is unusual. Hyperthyroidism has also been noted.[204]

DISEASE COURSE

The course of systemic sclerosis is extremely variable. Early in the illness it is difficult to judge prognosis with respect to both survival and disability. Many patients with diffuse cutaneous scleroderma experience steadily increasing sclerosis of the fingers and hands, leading to deforming flexion contractures. In others, mobility is maintained despite advancing skin changes. The most reliable early signs predicting subsequent severe diffuse skin involvement are the appearance of cutaneous thickening prior to the onset of Raynaud's phenomenon, rapid progression of scleroderma toward the more proximal parts of the extremities, palpable tendon friction rubs, and serum anti-Scl 70 antibody. Often, late in the disease, spontaneous improvement occurs, with the skin eventually returning to near-normal thickness. Such amelioration almost always begins centrally (trunk, upper arms, thighs) and proceeds distally; distal finger skin thickening seldom improves.

Most, if not all, patients eventually show evidence of visceral involvement, which can be detected by appropriate testing (e.g., pulmonary function studies, cine-esophagram, chest radiographs) before the appearance of symptoms. Internal organ dysfunction also may develop in the face of minimal or apparently stable scleroderma, and its course may be independent of the latter. Although in many instances clearcut cutaneous and/or visceral progression of disease occurs over time, the designation "progressive" is not uniformly applicable and should be abandoned.

Limited scleroderma was initially considered to represent a benign variant associated with a relatively favorable prognosis. Raynaud's phenomenon, alone or in combination with swollen, puffy fingers, is often present for a decade or more before the diagnosis of systemic sclerosis is entertained. The life span of patients with limited scleroderma is significantly longer than that of persons with diffuse scleroderma, in part because the former rarely, if ever, develop myocardial or renal involvement. Anticentromere antibody itself is often a clue to a good prognosis.[205,206] However, as noted above, limited scleroderma patients are at higher risk to acquire severe pulmonary arterial hypertension, which is independent of the presence of anticentromere antibody and almost uniformly fatal.[122]

Several large survival studies have been reported and summarized.[207] The 5-year cumulative survival rate after either first physician diagnosis or entry to study has ranged from 34 to 73%, and researchers agree that male sex, older age, and involvement of the kidneys, heart, and lungs adversely affect outcome (Fig. 73–15). To the extent that they are associated with the clinically defined subsets described

above, serum autoantibodies are also useful in predicting prognosis.[208]

Childhood Disease. Systemic sclerosis is rare in childhood.[7] Most children have diffuse cutaneous disease.[208a] Clinical findings are similar to those in adults except for an increased frequency of myocardial involvement,[208a] and possibly a reduced frequency of "renal crisis."[208a–208d] Serum antinucleolar antibodies may be more commonly found than in adults.[208e]

Pregnancy. There is controversy concerning both fertility and the frequency of spontaneous abortion.[209,210] Pregnancy appears to exert no consistent effect on the course of systemic sclerosis.[210–212] Conversely, the disease ordinarily does not interfere with pregnancy or parturition. However, instances of hypertension alone,[210] serious and fatal third-trimester or postpartum renal involvement with severe hypertension[212a,213] and nephrotic syndrome[214] have been reported but may be unrepresentative. In general, women with early diffuse disease should be advised not to become pregnant.

Cancer. The reported frequency of malignancy in

FIG. 73–15. Cumulative survival in patients with systemic sclerosis according to type of visceral involvement at first evaluation at the University of Pittsburgh from 1972 to 1986.

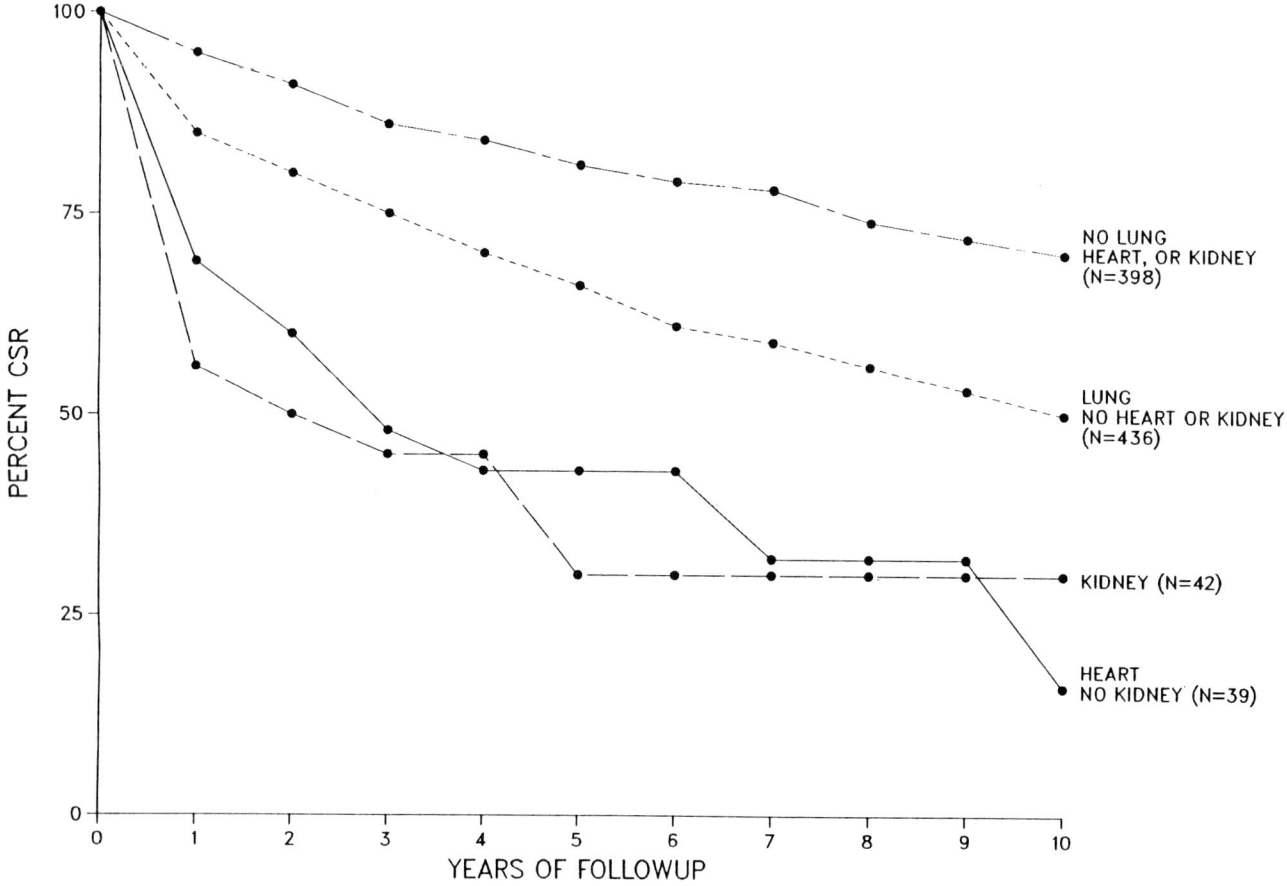

patients with systemic sclerosis in large clinical series has varied from 3 to 7%.[215–217] In the only studies in which population denominators and comparison groups have been used, several important associations have been detected. In two case series[215,218] and an epidemiologic study,[127] a subset of women developed breast cancer at or near the time of onset of scleroderma. Lung cancer is more frequent and occurs in the setting of long-standing scleroderma with pulmonary interstitial fibrosis and is independent of cigarette smoking.[127,128] Alveolar cell carcinoma, for many years believed to be a specific sequel of scleroderma[219] is only one of the lung tumors found, and does not occur more often than expected.[127,128] There are surprisingly few lymphoproliferative malignancies reported in systemic sclerosis patients.[220] However, as might be expected, the use of immunosuppressive agents may be followed by an excessive number of late lymphoproliferative neoplasms.[221]

ETIOLOGY AND PATHOGENESIS

Systemic sclerosis has been considered to be closely related to rheumatoid arthritis, systemic lupus erythematosus, polymyositis-dermatomyositis, and other connective tissue diseases because of certain epidemiologic similarities, overlapping clinical features, and involvement of blood vessels as a common target organ (see Chapter 3). The concept of immunologic and microvascular abnormalities as the common denominators in the pathogenesis of these diseases has been strengthened by evidence drawn from several different investigations. Any acceptable hypothesis concerning the pathogenesis of systemic sclerosis must account for the obvious vascular and immunologic features and link them to the overproduction of collagen and other connective tissue proteins.[222–225]

Metabolism of Connective Tissue

Both morphologic and biochemical evidence indicate that fibrosis of the skin and internal organs in systemic sclerosis is the result of overproduction of collagen. The weight and hydroxyproline content of uniform-diameter skin punch biopsy cores are significantly greater than those from normal controls, confirming the marked increase in dermal thickness so obvious on clinical and histologic examination (see Figs. 73–5, 73–17).[43] Dermal fibroblasts from patients with systemic sclerosis propagated in tissue culture synthesize increased amounts of glycosaminoglycans, chiefly hyaluronic acid, even after many generations,[226–228] and accumulate abnormally large quan-

tities of collagenase-sensitive protein (collagen).[229,230] Cells derived from the deeper portions of the dermis and subcutis are particularly active in this regard. Increased levels of mRNA for procollagen Types I and III account for this overproduction.[231] A defect in the feedback regulation of collagen synthesis by the aminopropeptide of Type I procollagen in scleroderma fibroblasts has been detected.[232] Other mechanisms, such as reduced collagen degradation, may also contribute to excessive accumulation of connective tissue components.[233] The cultured fibroblast remains an attractive model for study of the regulation of collagen synthesis.[234]

After incubation with serum from patients with early scleroderma and more extensive skin involvement, normal skin fibroblasts show increased proliferation.[235] Fibroblast growth promoting factors have been identified in scleroderma serum,[224] as has a glycosaminoglycan stimulating factor.[236] Purified platelet homogenates[237] and platelet derived growth factor,[238] but not platelet factor IV,[224] showed these activities. Cloned human fibroblasts exposed to scleroderma sera[239] and heterogeneous fibroblasts exposed to scleroderma serum for a prolonged period[240] both showed selective proliferation of high collagen–producing cells, suggesting that a specific subpopulation of cells may account for excessive collagen accumulation.

Collagen in the skin of patients with systemic sclerosis appears to be qualitatively normal. An autograft of clinically normal abdominal skin transferred to the scleroderma-involved forearm became sclerodermatous, whereas forearm skin placed in the abdominal site remained thickened.[241] In contrast, the skin changes of localized scleroderma (morphea) proved reversible after transplantation into normal areas.[242] The importance of extracutaneous factors in determining the localization and severity of cutaneous involvement in systemic sclerosis is further suggested by the following cases: (1) a finger that had been reattached following accidental amputation many years prior to the development of scleroderma remained unaffected while Raynaud's phenomenon and the resorption of terminal phalangeal bone occurred in the other digits of the same hand;[243] (2) two patients with preexisting Raynaud's phenomenon developed unilateral sclerodermatous involvement of an immobilized limb.[244]

Vascular Hypothesis

Widespread vascular disease affects the medium and small arteries and microvasculature of many organs, including the gastrointestinal tract, lungs, heart, and kidneys as well as the digital arteries. One popular concept is that systemic sclerosis is the end result of repeated insults to the vascular endothelium.[245]

The activity of a product of endothelial cells, factor VIII/von Willebrand factor antigen, was increased under basal conditions[246,247] and more so after cold exposure.[248] Decreased platelet serotonin content, indicating its release,[249] increased serotonin-induced platelet aggregation,[250] and raised levels of circulating platelet aggregates and plasma β-thromboglobulin, presumed to reflect vascular injury and repair,[246,251,251a] have been reported. The latter may separate systemic sclerosis from primary Raynaud's phenomenon.[251a] Specific endothelial cell cytotoxic activity in scleroderma serum has been described[252,253] but not confirmed.[254,255,255a] Antibody (IgG)-dependent cellular cytotoxicity to human vascular endothelial cells has been demonstrated when these cells are cocultured with non-T normal human peripheral blood mononuclear cells.[256] Activated neutrophils have been demonstrated to secrete toxic peroxides, which may contribute to vascular damage.[257]

At the level of the small artery, platelet factors are capable of stimulating proliferation and connective tissue synthesis by smooth muscle (myointimal) cells in the vessel wall. Periadventitial fibrosis may be explained by increased vascular permeability and diffusion of platelet factors. In capillaries devoid of myointimal cells, devascularization occurs and existing vessels become dilated and telangiectatic, leading to the changes observed on capillary microscopy. Interstitial fibroblasts may be stimulated to produce collagen by escape of platelet factors from such compromised capillaries. Furthermore, incubation with serum or plasma from systemic sclerosis patients results in reduced deformability and increased endothelial cell adherence of erythrocytes.[258]

Vasoconstriction could also play an important role because the aforementioned processes may be triggered by altered blood flow and resultant ischemia or intravascular coagulation. Cold exposure has been shown to cause capillary "standstill,"[259] decreased blood flow in the kidney,[164] and dysfunction of the gastrointestinal tract,[260] lung,[125] and heart.[141] Although a correlation appears to exist between the severity of skin capillary abnormalities and the extent of multisystem involvement,[57] the role of vascular disturbances in the pathogenesis of systemic sclerosis, including fibroblast activation, is unclear. For example, blood flow has been reported to be normal in the skin and subcutaneous tissue of the clinically involved forearm[261] and increased in areas of dense fibrosis from the dorsum of the hand.[262] Thus, mechanisms other than faulty nutritional blood flow must be invoked.

Immunologic Hypothesis

Association With Other Immune Disorders. A variety of "overlap" conditions have been described in which patients with systemic sclerosis also have features of rheumatoid arthritis, polymyositis-dermatomyositis, and mixed connective tissue disease. In addition, the frequencies of Sjögren's syndrome, autoimmune thyroiditis, and biliary cirrhosis are unusually high in patients with systemic sclerosis (see earlier discussion on organ system involvement).

Serum Proteins. Moderate hypergammaglobulinemia (1.4 to 2.0 g/dl) occurs in over one third of patients and is most often encountered in the setting of overlap conditions, such as mixed connective tissue disease. Typically, IgG is increased, but IgM elevation has also been observed.[263] Monoclonal gammopathy has been described in several cases of systemic sclerosis,[264,265] and a child with scleroderma, myositis, and IgA deficiency has been reported.[266] The level of serum complement is normal in all but a few patients. Mixed cryoglobulins[267] and circulating immune complexes have been either absent[268] or detected in small amounts,[269–271] but were found to be present only in association with certain autoantibodies (Scl 70, nRNP, SSA/Ro, and SSB/La).[272]

Rheumatoid Factor and LE Cell Reactions. Between one fourth and one third of patients with systemic sclerosis have positive tests for rheumatoid factor, usually in low titer. Positive lupus erythematosus (LE) cell reactions and biologic false-positive serologic reactions for syphilis have been reported, most often in overlap syndromes, but are uncommon.

Antinuclear Antibodies. With the use of multiple substrates, antinuclear antibodies have been found in the sera of over 90% of patients with systemic sclerosis.[273] The amounts are typically low, as compared with those found in SLE, but titers of 1:1000 or greater are seen occasionally. In most instances, the pattern of nuclear fluorescence is that of fine or large speckles or threads, but occasionally diffuse (homogeneous) nuclear staining occurs. Both IgG and IgM antibodies are found, but the predominant antibodies are IgG, most often of the IgG3 subclass.[274] Little if any correlation appears to exist between the presence or titer of antinuclear antibody and the clinical severity or duration of disease, although there is some disagreement in this matter. In contrast, it is widely accepted that certain specific autoantibodies have highly significant clinical associations.

Anti-topoisomerase I Antibodies. One recently identified antinuclear antibody has been found in 20% to over 50% of systemic sclerosis sera, but rarely in control specimens,[275,276] and is associated with diffuse cutaneous scleroderma and pulmonary interstitial involvement.[276–278] Originally designated anti-Scl 70,[275] it is now known that the antibody recognizes the nuclear enzyme DNA topoisomerase I.[279,280]

Anticentromere Antibodies. Antibodies morphologically appearing as fine, discrete speckles have been identified[281] as being directed against the centromeric portion of chromosomes observed in dividing cells (Fig. 73–16). Termed anticentromere antibodies, they have remarkable specificity for limited cutaneous scleroderma, where they occur in over 50% of patients, compared with fewer than 5% of patients with diffuse scleroderma.[205,278,282,283] These antibodies are found in a few persons with Raynaud's phenomenon alone, and those persons may be at increased risk to develop limited scleroderma eventually.[284] Rarely, a patient with clinical features of systemic lupus has anticentromere antibodies.[285] These predominantly IgG antibodies tend to persist in the serum for prolonged periods.[286,287] Immunoelectron microscopy has pinpointed the antigen as residing in the kinetochore region of chromosomes, but its precise identity is not yet known.[288] Three distinct antigens are recognized by nearly all anticentromere antibody positive sera,[289] but their clinical relevance is unknown.

The coexistence of anti-Scl 70 and anticentromere antibodies was reported in 2 of 121 patients,[290] but must be rare indeed since I have found no such occurrences in over 700 positive tests.

Antinucleolar Antibodies. Nucleolar immunofluorescence has been reported in 10 to 54% of scleroderma sera. These antibodies, relatively specific for systemic sclerosis, are particularly common in patients with associated Sjögren's syndrome. Several of the responsible nuclear antigens have now been identified. A few patients with anti-topoisomerase I display nucleolar staining,[291] and antibody to ribonucleic acid (RNA) polymerase I has been detected.[292] The latter autoantibody appears to identify a group of women with otherwise typical diffuse cutaneous disease.[291] Finally, anti-PM-Scl (previously termed anti-PM-1), which is also directed against a nucleolar antigen,[293] is associated with limited skin thickening and often with polymyositis.[294]

Other Antibodies. Sera of persons with systemic sclerosis contain either no antibody to native deoxyribonucleic acid (DNA), or only small quantities, and lack anti-Sm antibody. A few patients have high titers of antibody to nuclear ribonucleoprotein (anti-nRNP); these persons tend to have myositis more frequently than those without high-titer anti-nRNP.[295] Antibody directed against the nuclear antigen Ku, distinct from nRNP, has been found in a small proportion of Japanese patients, nearly all of whom had a scleroderma-polymyositis overlap syndrome.[296] Antibodies to other components of dividing cells such as metaphase chromatin[297] and centrioles[298] have also been observed in sera of systemic sclerosis patients. The latter were reported in two patients with systemic sclerosis[299,300] and in one with Raynaud's phenomenon.[299] Antilymphocyte antibodies are frequent[301,302] but their significance is unknown.

Anticardiolipin antibody has been detected in low concentration in 11 of 35 patients without vascular disease or other clinical associations.[303] Antibodies to polyuridylic acid have been noted in patients with active diffuse scleroderma.[304] Antibodies to collagen types I and IV (basement membrane), found in most

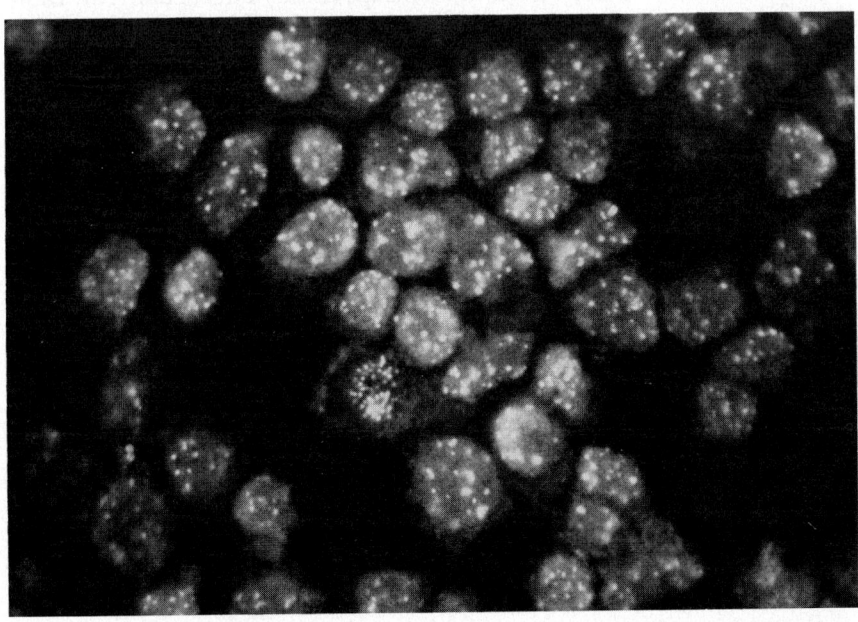

FIG. 73–16. Pattern of nuclear anticentromeric immunofluorescence on HEp-2 cells produced by serum from a patient with limited cutaneous systemic sclerosis. (From the 1981 Revised Clinical Slide Collection on the Rheumatic Diseases. Reprinted with permission of The Arthritis Foundation, Atlanta, GA)

patients in one series, were correlated with a reduction in pulmonary diffusing capacity.[305]

Lymphocyte Abnormalities. Cell-mediated immune abnormalities in systemic sclerosis have been reviewed.[306] Early in the course of disease, collections of lymphocytes and plasma cells are detected in the synovium, skin, gastrointestinal tract, lung, and other locations. The cells found in the dermis (see Fig. 73–4) are chiefly, if not wholly, T lymphocytes.[45] In the peripheral blood, the number of T cells is most often reduced, with no consistent alteration in the number of B lymphocytes. The ratio of helper T cells to suppressor T cells is elevated in one third of patients, owing to a decrease in circulating suppressor T cell lymphocytes.[45,307] The latter do not preferentially accumulate in the skin.

Lymphocytes from systemic[308] and localized[309] scleroderma patients undergo transformation in response to various human and animal skin collagen preparations. The cells of patients with diffuse scleroderma were stimulated to produce macrophage migration inhibitory factor by skin extracts of both normal and sclerodermatous skin, whereas the lymphocytes of those with limited scleroderma were not.[44]

Stimulated peripheral blood lymphocytes produce a factor that is chemotactic for human dermal fibroblasts.[310] In addition, lymphokine-rich supernatants from activated normal human and scleroderma peripheral blood mononuclear cells enhance collagen production by embryonic lung, foreskin,[311,312] and dermal[313] fibroblasts. In contrast, some supernatants of activated peripheral blood mononuclear cells actually may inhibit fibroblast proliferation and collagen production.[314] In one study, mononuclear cell supernatants from scleroderma patients caused both endothelial cell inhibition and fibroblast stimulation.[313,315] Spontaneous interleukin-1 (IL-1) release from mononuclear cells and defective T-cell response to IL-1[315a] and reduced IL-1 production has also been reported.[316] Such fibroblast-modulating factors may be implicated in the fibrosis characteristic of chronic inflammation, which occurs in many different disease states in addition to systemic sclerosis. Natural killer (NK) cells have been shown to be normal in number in the peripheral blood[317] but to have reduced activity, especially in a subset of patients with early diffuse disease[318-320] and increased visceral involvement.[320]

Soluble mediators from mononuclear cells may result in permanent alteration of a certain subpopulation of fibroblasts; these cells acquire the ability to synthesize increased quantities of collagen and glycosaminoglycans and continue to do so for many generations, even after mononuclear cell products are no longer added to the cultures.[321,322] Alterations in the clonal composition and phenotypic expression of these fibroblasts have been hypothesized.[323]

"Angiogenesis," the ability to evoke new capillary formation in an experimental circumstance, was found to be reduced by scleroderma peripheral blood mononuclear cells[324] but enhanced by a monocyte-enriched subset of these cells[325] and scleroderma sera.[326] As in rheumatoid arthritis, a subgroup of systemic sclerosis patients had defective T suppressor cell response to Epstein-Barr virus.[327]

Family Studies and Histocompatibility Antigen Testing. Although familial systemic sclerosis is unusual, reports of this circumstance have appeared with increasing frequency in recent years.[25] The disease has been described in siblings, parent and child, and second-degree relatives. Although such pairs have shown a wide variety of clinical manifestations, strikingly similar familial instances of fatal bowel involvement[328] and the coexistence of limited scleroderma and Sjögren's syndrome[329] have been encountered. Serum antinuclear antibodies have been detected in 7% of the first-degree relatives of patients with systemic sclerosis and in over 50% of those over age 60.[330] Anticentromere antibody in low titer was more common in relatives of persons with this autoantibody (3%) than in relatives of controls (none detected).[331]

Several small series of patients have been published claiming various A, B, and DR locus histocompatibility antigen associations. A strong association with null alleles at the C4a locus has recently been claimed.[332] Unfortunately, the number of patients examined in these studies has been embarrassingly small; when larger populations were examined, many HLA correlations disappeared, but meaningful clinical subsets may have been overlooked in these analyses (see Chapter 3).[333,334] Regardless of these results, a multigenic predisposition to the disease remains an attractive hypothesis.

Miscellaneous Abnormalities. An increase in random chromosomal breakage has been noted both in patients and in their siblings and children.[335] It has been suggested that this increase may constitute evidence of a familial tendency toward autoimmune disease. Scleroderma sera are toxic to B- and T-lymphocytes, monocytes, and polymorphonuclear leukocytes, suggesting the sharing of some cell surface antigens.[336] Two cases on record demonstrate an apparently fortuitous association between primary amyloidosis and systemic sclerosis.[337,338]

Experimental Models

In rats that develop homologous disease after the injection of large numbers of lymphoid cells from an unrelated strain of donor animals, a chronic dermatitis develops, characterized by an increase in dermal collagen, atrophy of the epidermis and skin appendages, and minimal or no inflammatory reaction. An analogous chronic graft-versus-host disease has been produced in mice, with mast cell degranulation accompanying, and perhaps integral to, the occurrence of fibrosis.[339] This circumstance is reminiscent of sclerodermatous skin changes in patients with chronic graft versus host reaction after bone marrow transplantation.[340] However diffuse fasciitis with eosinophilia may be a better clinical description of the type of illness that follows allogeneic bone marrow transplantation.[341]

The tight skin (TSK) mutant mouse strain has scleroderma-like cutaneous changes, with abnormal skin physical and biochemical characteristics[342] and metabolism.[343] Mast cell degranulation has been observed in this model,[344] but the vascular component appears to be lacking.[345] Cardiac and pulmonary abnormalities atypical of systemic sclerosis have also been noted.[345,346] A disease with both clinical and serologic abnormalities closely resembling systemic sclerosis has been described in white leghorn chickens; manifestations include gangrenous changes of the comb and digits and serum antinuclear antibodies.[347]

Unfortunately, no reliable experimental model of systemic sclerosis is yet available. Whether any of the above models will furnish important biochemical and immunologic insights into the pathogenesis of systemic sclerosis, or will provide a mechanism for screening of potential therapeutic agents, is unclear.

TREATMENT

The first responsibility of the physician is to discuss the nature of systemic sclerosis with the patient and family, who are often unreasonably pessimistic. When possible, classification as diffuse cutaneous or limited cutaneous scleroderma is helpful in understanding the future risk of developing visceral complications and which ones they may be. Such discussion aids in establishing a good relationship between physician and patient, which is particularly important in this chronic, demanding disease. Diagrams of the blood vessels, skin, esophagus, and other appropriate illustrations are useful in instruction.

Numerous vitamins, hormones, pharmaceuticals, and surgical procedures have been used to treat systemic sclerosis; nearly all of these therapies have been abandoned after initial enthusiasm and later critical evaluation. Improvement can hardly be expected in those manifestations that are the result of far-advanced tissue fibrosis. Too often success has been claimed solely on the basis of a diminution in subjective complaints (e.g., a reduction in frequency of Raynaud's phenomenon, which occurs with virtually any new treatment) and poorly documented "softening" of the skin.

Evaluation of the effectiveness of treatment has proved difficult for several reasons.[348] Systemic sclerosis is variable in its severity and in its rate of progression; therefore, the classification of patients into subsets is important in understanding the results of therapy. Because spontaneous improvement often occurs after several years, controlled trials are necessary. There are limitations in the availability and application of objective criteria for ascertaining improvement (or deterioration) in the condition, particularly with respect to visceral changes. Finally, the influence of psychologic factors on many of the symptoms is important.

Drugs

Figure 73–17 summarizes some current concepts of the pathogenesis of systemic sclerosis and indicates those points at which therapeutic intervention might be effective. No drug or combination of drugs has been proved to be of value in adequately controlled prospective trials or is generally accepted as being useful. Anti-inflammatory agents and corticosteroids have been disappointing. Because of their potential toxicity, I restrict the use of corticosteroids to patients with inflammatory myopathy or symptomatic serositis. On occasion, refractory arthritis and the "edematous" phase of skin involvement respond favorably to relatively small doses of corticosteroids, for example, prednisone 5 to 10 mg per day. Myositis, however, may require higher doses. There has been some concern that high-dose corticosteroid therapy may precipitate acute renal failure.[349]

In recent years, attention has been focused on D-penicillamine, a compound that interferes with the intermolecular cross linking of collagen[350] and also possesses immunosuppressive activity (see Chapter 36). Reports from England,[351] Denmark,[352,353] and the U.S.S.R.[354] have been optimistic. In a retrospective analysis of diffuse scleroderma patients with disease duration of less than 3 years, 73 patients treated with D-penicillamine for at least 6 months were compared with 45 not receiving the drug.[34] The treated group showed significantly reduced skin thickness and joint contractures after 18 to 30 months, and also better survival, primarily owing to a considerably lower frequency of subsequent renal involvement. D-penicillamine may also improve established interstitial lung disease when given for a prolonged period.[355–357] Its

FIG. 73–17. Schematic representation of immune mechanisms in the pathogenesis of skin thickening in systemic sclerosis. The proposed locations of action of immunosuppressive agents *(1)*, colchicine *(2)*, and D-penicillamine *(3)* are indicated.

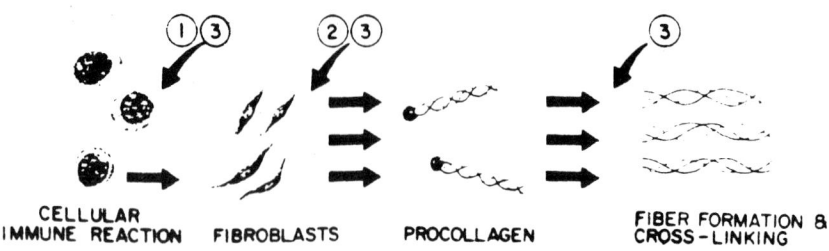

CELLULAR IMMUNE REACTION FIBROBLASTS PROCOLLAGEN FIBER FORMATION & CROSS–LINKING

use is accompanied by a disturbing plethora of potential side effects, including fever, loss of taste, nausea, anorexia, rash, leukopenia, thromobcytopenia, aplastic anemia, nephrotic syndrome, glomerulonephritis,[358] and myasthenia gravis.[359] A scleroderma-like illness was reported in a Wilson's disease patient who had taken D-penicillamine for 11 years.[360] Up to one fourth of patients may be forced to discontinue the drug.[361] Adverse reactions occur with lower frequency when the D-penicillamine is first taken in small amounts (250 mg per day) and then slowly increased over many months to 750 to 1000 mg per day. Careful monitoring of white blood cell and platelet counts and of urine protein are recommended. Despite the apparent clinical benefits, the skin fibroblasts that grow out in tissue culture retain their potential for increased collagen synthesis.[362] Chemically related compounds such as *N*-acetylcysteine[363] and *S*-adenosylmethionine[364] have also been used with limited success.

More recently, colchicine has been advocated.[365] This ancient remedy inhibits the accumulation of collagen by blocking the conversion of procollagen to collagen, probably through interference with microtubule-mediated transport,[366,367] or perhaps by stimulation of collagenase production.[368] In one long-term open trial (mean followup 39 months), improvement in skin thickening occurred in 17 of 19 patients.[365] However, another trial using similar dosage (10 mg/week), but only 1 year of treatment, resulted in no beneficial changes.[369] In some patients, progression of skin, musculoskeletal, and pulmonary involvement was documented. Several other negative studies have been published and reviewed.[348] In none of these trials was colchicine toxicity a serious limiting factor.

Considering the mounting evidence that immune processes, both humoral and cell-mediated, play an important role in the pathogenesis of systemic sclerosis, various forms of immunosuppression have been proposed. A variety of potential beneficial effects can be hypothesized, including alterations in interactions between immunocompetent cells and inhibition of fibroblast function by soluble mediators.[370] Azathioprine[371] and 5-fluorouracil[372] were considered beneficial in uncontrolled trials. Chlorambucil results have been mixed,[373,374] but a recent 3-year double-blind controlled trial was negative.[375] As in RA,[376] late-developing malignancy may be a limiting feature of the use of alkylating agents.[221] Plasmapheresis has been advocated,[377–379] but its effects are not uniformly beneficial[380] and are difficult to evaluate because of confounding immunosuppressive and corticosteroid therapy. Cyclosporine A has been used in a limited number of patients,[381] but no trials are currently ongoing owing to an unacceptably high frequency of hypertension and renal insufficiency, which could be attributable either to the drug or to scleroderma. The effects of recombinant γ-interferon, a "variant" of imunosuppression, may have therapeutic implications. This compound has been shown to inhibit the collagen production of scleroderma fibroblasts by reducing messenger ribonucleic acid (mRNA) levels.[382]

To date, there is no general agreement on the effectiveness of immunosuppressive therapy. Additional adequately controlled therapeutic trials are urgently needed.[348] I believe the use of immunosuppressive measures is justified in patients with rapidly progressive, life-threatening, or disabling disease, provided there is informed consent and close surveillance for adverse effects.

Agents designed to protect injured endothelial cells and to prevent platelet aggregation and subsequent release of platelet derived growth factors are a logical extension of the vascular hypothesis of scleroderma. Although circulating platelet aggregates and plasma β-thromboglobulin levels could be reversed by treatment with dipyridamole and aspirin,[383] a randomized, double-blind trial of these agents versus placebo for 1 to 2 years showed no significant improvement in the treatment group.[384] Lower doses of dipyridamole in this trial could conceivably account for the ineffectiveness. This approach to systemic sclerosis should not be abandoned. A controlled trial of antihypertensive therapy did not result in any clinically meaningful improvement over a 24-month period.[385]

Supporting Measures

Raynaud's Phenomenon. Thoracic sympathectomy may be followed by partial (usually transient) improvement in Raynaud's phenomenon but not by a significant or sustained influence on the course of cutaneous changes or visceral sclerosis.[386] Some patients with so-called primary Raynaud's phenomenon have developed systemic sclerosis, usually of the limited cutaneous scleroderma type, many years after sympathectomy.

Accurate measurement of digital tissue blood flow is technically difficult, results are not reproducible, and standardized cold challenge methods have not been widely used. Such methodologic problems must be addressed before progress can be made in this area. Commonsense self-management includes avoiding undue cold exposure, dressing warmly, and abstaining from tobacco. Induced vasodilatation[387] and biofeedback[388] may also be helpful. Various vasodilating drugs have been employed, including intra-arterial reserpine,[389,390] methyldopa,[391] adrenergic blocking agents, and α receptor blocking and β receptor stimulating drugs.[386] In general, these agents have proved disappointing when Raynaud's phenomenon is secondary to systemic sclerosis. Several promising new pharmacologic agents, however, have been effective in double-blind studies, including the calcium channel blocker, nifedipine[392-395]; a direct vasodilator, prazosin[396]; an oral serotonin antagonist, ketanserin[397,398]; topical nitroglycerin[399]; prostaglandin E[400-402]; and prostacyclin.[403] Whether renin-angiotensin blockade with captopril, enalapril, or minoxidil benefits vascular disease in organs other than the kidney is unknown, although captopril did not ameliorate Raynaud's phenomenon or alter digital plethysmography during cold challenge in one study.[404] When large vessels are involved, for example, radial or ulnar arteries, microvascular reconstruction should be considered.[405] Digital tip amputation may occasionally be required, although the demarcation of tissue achieved by autoamputation is preferred.[405,406]

Calcinosis. Reliable treatment to eradicate calcinosis in patients with scleroderma is not available. Surgical excision of large calcareous masses may be helpful in selected instances, depending on the degree of intracutaneous deposition.[405] Soft tissue calcinotic deposits contain increased amounts of the amino acid 4-carboxy-L-glutamic acid (Gla)[407]; long-term inhibition of Gla with low-dose anticoagulant therapy may be use-

ful.[408] Suppression of local inflammation surrounding calcinosis has been accomplished with colchicine.[409,410]

Skin. Special lotion, soaps, and bath oils should be used to relieve excessive skin dryness; taking unduly frequent baths and using household detergents may aggravate this symptom.

Digital tip ulcerations are protected by a plaster finger cast. Noninfected ulcers may respond rapidly to the use of occlusive dressings, such as Duoderm, which are also protective. If these lesions become infected (almost always with staphylococci), half-strength hydrogen peroxide soaks and gentle local debridement are employed, and oral antibiotics are sometimes recommended. Deeper infections, especially septic arthritis or osteomyelitis, must be treated vigorously, with intravenous antibiotics, excision of infected and devitalized tissue, joint fusion, and rarely, amputation.

Joints and Muscles. Articular complaints may be treated with salicylates and other nonsteroidal anti-inflammatory drugs, with careful attention to the potential for aggravation of gastroesophageal reflux symptoms. Corticosteroids are seldom necessary for musculoskeletal involvement, although polymyositis with histologic evidence of chronic inflammatory cell infiltration should be so treated. Patients with diffuse cutaneous disease often develop severe digital contractures with deformity. Dynamic splinting does not prevent the progression of this process.[411] Proximal interphalangeal joint replacement arthroplasties have been performed with improvement in hand function and appearance.[412] When extra-articular fibrosis is prominent, or septic arthritis has occurred, joint replacement will not be effective; in this circumstance, proximal interphalangeal joint fusion is preferred.[405] In considering such procedures, it must be remembered that postoperative hand functional status will depend on the amount of motion present at the metacarpophalangeal joints.

Gastrointestinal Tract. Maintenance of the oral opening requires mouth stretching exercises[412a]; the patient must also make a vigorous attempt to maintain adequate oral hygiene and make regular visits to the dentist for prophylaxis. For edentulous patients with microstomia, a flexible prosthesis has been designed to augment the exercise program.[412b] Patients who have difficulty in swallowing should learn to masticate carefully and to avoid foods likely to cause substernal dysphagia (e.g., meat, bread). Metoclopramide improves esophageal motility and is useful in some patients.[413] Cisapride stimulates both gastric and esophageal emptying.[414] Because nifedipine is capable of decreasing lower esophageal sphincter pressure and contraction amplitude in the body of the esophagus,[415,416] theoretically it could aggravate esophageal symptoms. In this respect diltiazem may be a preferable agent.[417] Reflux esophagitis can be minimized by appropriate measures, such as the upright position during and after eating, avoiding food before bedtime, raising the head of the bed on blocks to prevent nocturnal reflux, antacids 45 to 60 minutes after meals and at bedtime, histamine (H_2) receptor blockade,[418,419] and cytoprotection with carafate. The latter should be given as a slurry to avoid development of a gastric bezoar, a complication observed in some patients with reduced gastric motility. Esophageal stricture may require periodic dilatation. Successful excision of strictures and correction of gastroesophageal reflux by gastroplasty, combined with fundoplication, have been reported.[420-422]

Improvement in steatorrhea and other signs of intestinal malabsorption may follow the administration of tetracycline or other broad-spectrum antibiotics, but the underlying hypomotility is unaffected. Metoclopramide significantly increases small bowel motility,[423] but the magnitude of this change is of dubious clinical impact in patients with gross malabsorption. In advanced circumstances, one must replace calcium and fat-soluble vitamins, use medium-chain triglycerides and, often, resort to parenteral hyperalimentation.[424] In advanced malabsorption the likelihood of septicemia of catheter origin or other serious bacterial infection and premature death is high.

Lungs. Patients with pulmonary fibrosis who have infectious bronchitis or pneumonitis require prompt and vigorous antibiotic treatment. In persons with documented inflammatory alveolitis, corticosteroids (prednisone 40 to 60 mg/day for 2 to 3 months) may be efficacious short-term therapy.[425] There is mounting evidence that D-penicillamine is useful in the treatment of scleroderma interstitial lung disease.[355-357] When exercise precipitates arterial blood oxygen desaturation, and in advanced states of respiratory insufficiency, supplemental oxygen should be administered.

No effective therapy is available for the pulmonary arterial hypertension associated with limited cutaneous scleroderma. This complication typically comes to attention at a terminal stage. A variety of pharmacologic measures have been suggested, but only the serotonin antagonist, ketanserin[426] and possibly calcium channel antagonists[426a,426b] and captopril[427] hold promise. Because those who develop right-sided cardiac failure often respond poorly to digitalis and easily become intoxicated, greater reliance is placed on the use of diuretics.

Heart. Symptomatic pericarditis should be treated with nonsteroidal drugs or corticosteroids. Hemo-

dynamically significant pericardial effusion should be managed with pericardiocentesis or, if recurrent, with an open pericardial window procedure. If myocarditis can be identified clinically or by endomyocardial biopsy, glucocorticoids should be tried. The typical progressive left ventricular failure caused by myocardial fibrosis is unaffected by any therapy and is often fatal. Serious arrhythmias often complicate this situation, and respond inconsistently to antiarrhythmic drugs.

Kidney. The most important aspect of therapy of renal involvement is early detection, which is made easier by identifying and closely following the high-risk patient with rapidly progressive diffuse cutaneous scleroderma. If such a person develops any one of a number of markers of renal disease, such as hypertension, proteinuria, azotemia, microangiopathic hemolysis, or pericardial effusion, it is recommended that stimulated plasma renin levels are obtained and, if elevated, promptly treated.[428] The availability of new and more potent antihypertensive agents and of improved dialysis procedures and care has dramatically reduced mortality.[158] Captopril is the current drug of choice, but early aggressive therapy with other agents such as minoxidil, hydralazine, propranolol, or methyldopa often, but not always,[429,430] reverse this process. Failure to control azotemia may force the use of dialysis. Scleroderma patients may have inadequate vascular access and thus ineffective hemodialysis. Poor peritoneal clearance has been described,[431] but continuous ambulatory peritoneal dialysis has been successfully employed.[432]

Some patients have a slow reversal of their renal vascular damage and can be removed from dialysis after a number of months. A remarkable reduction in the degree of dermal thickening and induration has been observed in many of these patients during dialysis.[162,433] However, in one study, there was no cutaneous improvement during a 1-year followup of seven captopril-treated nondialyzed patients.[163] Many instances of successful renal transplantation have now been reported,[434] but typical scleroderma kidney histologic changes have been found in a transplanted organ[435] and in an allograft.[436]

LOCALIZED SCLERODERMA

The spectrum of localized scleroderma includes a variety of morphologic forms of skin thickening, such as morphea (patches) and linear scleroderma (bands). The clinical and histologic overlap between morphea and linear scleroderma is considerable, and patches of morphea are often found together with linear scleroderma. These conditions are most often encountered in childhood. Although the cause of localized scleroderma is obscure, in many cases the cutaneous changes appear soon after trauma and originate at the site of injury. Occurrence after mammoplasty has been reported[437] and familial occurrence has been observed.[438]

Morphea. Discrete droplike patches (guttate morphea) or plaques may begin at any age or site. The evolving lesions become sclerotic and waxy or ivory-colored and may increase to a diameter of many centimeters. The surface is smooth and hairless, and ceases to sweat. During this active phase, a surrounding erythematous or violaceous border of inflammation is often visible. After several months or years, spontaneous softening of the skin occurs with atrophy and hyperpigmentation or depigmentation; smaller patches may heal without trace. Lesions are confined entirely to the skin and subcutis, and are ordinarily of little consequence unless the face is involved or there is extensive dissemination (generalized morphea). Localized patches of morphea may be present in persons with otherwise typical systemic sclerosis,[439] but it should be emphasized that this coincidence is rare.

Early in the course the major histologic changes consist of new collagen deposition in the dermis and septa of the subcutaneous tissue and variably heavy (often intense) infiltration of lymphocytes, plasma cells, and histiocytes. This inflammatory reaction is more notable than that usually encountered in systemic sclerosis. The coexistence of morphea and lichen sclerosus et atrophicus has been reported,[440] but others feel that these two conditions are unrelated, and that confusion exists only because skin biopsies were not deep enough to show the diagnostic reticular dermis and subcutis features of morphea.[441] Inflammation and later fibrosis and atrophy of underlying subcutaneous tissue, fascia, and striated muscle may be present, suggesting an overlap with eosinophilic fasciitis,[441a] but in contrast to systemic sclerosis, muscle capillaries are normal. Treatment with D-penicillamine[442] and etretinate[443] have been reported to be of value.

Linear Scleroderma. In this form of localized scleroderma, which usually develops in childhood, a linear sclerotic band appears in the arm or leg (Fig. 73–18) and may extend the entire length of the extremity. Occasionally, multiple lesions may be present. Localized scleroderma in the frontoparietal area of the forehead and scalp ("en coup de sabre") is associated frequently with ipsilateral facial hemiatrophy,[444] and rarely with neurologic abnormalities, such as seizures attributable to hemiatrophy of the brain.[445]

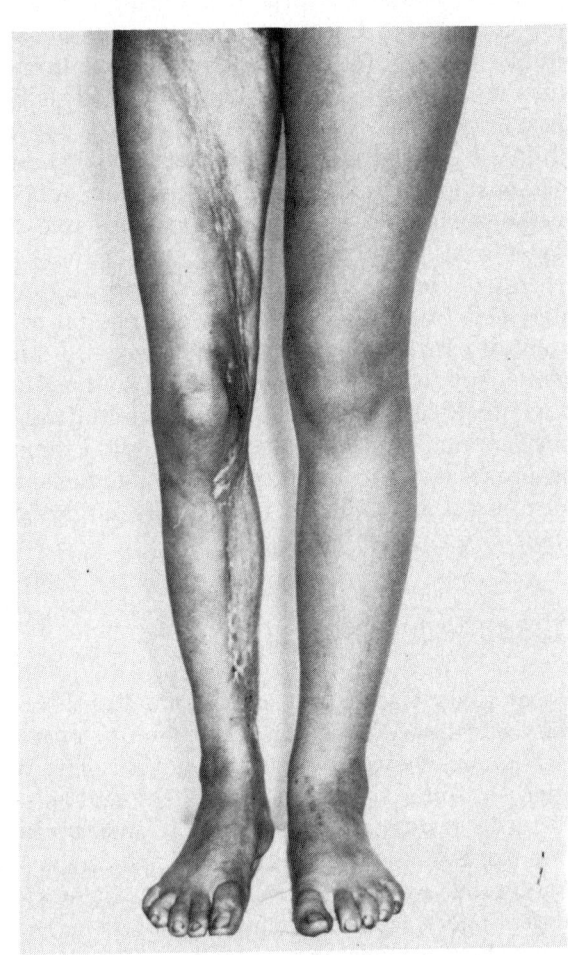

FIG. 73–18. Localized scleroderma of the linear type in the thigh and leg of a 12-year-old girl. (Courtesy of Prof. Stephanie Jablonska)

Some patients develop a nonerosive arthropathy, usually restricted to the small joints of the hands.

Inflammation and extensive fibrosis, similar to the findings in morphea, are present in the dermis, subcutis, and deep fascia and may extend into the underlying muscle, occasionally resulting in severely deforming fibrous contractures of the fingers, elbows, or knees. A noninflammatory myopathy underlying areas of linear scleroderma has been described.[446] Linear scleroderma has been reported to coexist in the same extremity with melorheostosis, a peculiar linear fibrotic hyperostosis of bone.[447]

Laboratory Features of Localized Scleroderma. The concurrence of linear scleroderma and other connective tissue diseases, especially systemic lupus erythematosus, has been reported.[448–450] Rheumatoid factor and antinuclear antibodies, including high titers of antibodies to single-stranded DNA, have been noted in the serum of patients with linear scleroderma[451–454] and morphea and its morphologic variant, generalized morphea.[454] These serologic abnormalities, and modest degrees of peripheral eosinophilia, accompany active disease and disappear during remission. Two patients with linear scleroderma and one with morphea were found to have serum anticentromere antibodies.[455] Elevated serum titers of antibody to Borrelia spirochetes have been detected in some patients with localized scleroderma,[456] raising the question of a relationship to Lyme disease. The dermal fibroblasts of persons with linear scleroderma produce excessive collagen in tissue culture.[457]

Therapy. It is important to recognize that approximately 80% of patients do not have persistent or recurrent disease activity after the first 2 years. A number of agents have been proposed for the treatment of active localized scleroderma, including D-penicillamine[442] and salazopyrin.[458] Physical therapy may prove useful in the prevention or reduction of joint contractures, but they may require surgical correction.

EOSINOPHILIC FASCIITIS

Eosinophilic fasciitis is a scleroderma-like disorder chiefly affecting adults, the rather abrupt onset of which is characterized by bilateral pain, swelling, and tenderness of the hands, forearms, feet, and legs. In contrast to systemic sclerosis, the proximal portions of the extremities (forearms, arms, legs, thighs) are considerably more affected than the distal areas (hands, fingers, feet, toes). These symptoms are soon followed by the development of induration of the skin and subcutaneous tissues of these parts with pronounced limitation of motion of the hands and feet. Flexion contractures of the fingers may result. Carpal tunnel syndrome is an early feature in many patients. The induration often remains confined to the extremities, but may spread to affect the trunk and rarely, the face. The diagnosis should be considered in a person with scleroderma-like tightening and thickening of the skin, sparing the digits, without Raynaud's phenomenon, who has peripheral eosinophilia. Although unilateral disease has been considered to be fasciitis,[459] bilaterality is almost universal and serves to distinguish this condition from linear scleroderma. Internal organ manifestations of systemic sclerosis are conspicuously absent. Some cases have been reported that suggest a close relationship to systemic sclerosis,[460] but it is my opinion that the distinction is seldom difficult. Striking peripheral eosinophilia, often 30% or more of the total peripheral white blood cell count, is present during the early

stages, but tends to decline later in the illness in parallel with serum eosinophil chemotactic activity.[461] Hypergammaglobulinemia (IgG)[462,463] and circulating immune complexes[464] have been detected in nearly half of patients and tend to parallel disease activity.

Histologic diagnosis is best confirmed using a deep, wedge, en-bloc biopsy that includes the contiguous skin, subcutis, fascia, and muscle. Both inflammation and fibrosis are found in all layers, but they are most intense in the fascia and deeper layers of the subcutaneous tissue, which are often dramatically thickened (Fig. 73–19). Large numbers of lymphocytes, plasma cells, and histiocytes are present in the affected areas, and eosinophil infiltration may be striking, particularly early in the disease.[462] Immunoglobulin and complement component C3 have been identified in the inflamed tissues.[462]

Eosinophilic fasciitis is self-limited in many patients, with spontaneous improvement and occasionally complete remission after 2 to 5 years. In my experience, however, and that of others,[465] some patients have persistent or recurrent disease, and others are left with disabling fixed joint contractures. Corticosteroids in small doses often provide prompt and substantial symptomatic relief and readily obliterate the eosinophilia. Two reports suggest that cimetidine is another potentially effective form of therapy.[466,467]

A variety of hematologic complications, including thrombocytopenia, aplastic anemia, and myelodysplastic syndromes, have developed in a small number of patients with eosinophilic fasciitis.[468–470] These con-

FIG. 73–19. Photomicrograph of an en-bloc biopsy from the leg of a 35-year-old woman with eosinophilic fasciitis. Note thickening of the dermis, subcutaneous fibrous septa, and deep fascia (asterisk). The latter is infiltrated by large collections of cells that were identified as lymphocytes, plasma cells, histiocytes, and eosinophils.

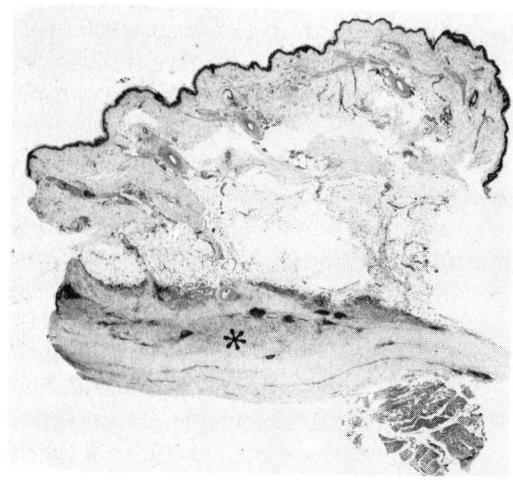

ditions, suspected to be of autoimmune cause (both humoral and cell-mediated mechanisms have been described), may occur at any time in the course of the fasciitis and do not correlate with its severity. Treatment with antithymocyte globulin has been effective in two cases of aplastic anemia associated with eosinophilic fasciitis.[471,472]

The cause of eosinophilic fasciitis is unknown. It has been preceded by unusually strenuous exertion, especially in younger men, and by allogeneic bone marrow transplantation.[341] A relationship to Borrelia burgdorferii has been suggested.[473] The blood and tissue abnormalities described previously suggest an immune pathogenesis.[462,474,475] An association with autoimmune thyroiditis has been noted.[476]

DIFFERENTIAL DIAGNOSIS OF SCLERODERMA

A number of other conditions exhibit scleroderma-like but often distinctive skin changes in the absence of typical visceral manifestations of systemic sclerosis (Table 73–3).[477,478]

Scleredema. Scleredema is characterized by symmetric, firm, painless, and edematous induration of the skin of the face, scalp, neck, trunk, and upper arms. In contrast to systemic sclerosis, the distal ex-

Table 73–3. Disorders Associated With Skin Changes That May Resemble Scleroderma (Pseudoscleroderma)

Primary cutaneous diseases
  Scleredema
  Porphyria cutanea tarda; congenital porphyria
  Scleromyxedema
  Acrodermatitis chronica
  Lichen sclerosus et atrophicus
  Lipoatrophy
*Primary systemic diseases in which cutaneous features are also
    present*
  Amyloidosis
  Juvenile onset diabetes mellitus
  Acromegaly
  Carcinoid syndrome
  Phenylketonuria
  Werner's syndrome
  Progeria
  Rothmund's syndrome
  Graft versus host disease
Chemical agents inducing scleroderma-like conditions
  Vinyl chloride
  Organic solvents, epoxy resins
  Trichloroethylene
  L-Hydroxytryptophan and carbidopa therapy
  Bleomycin
  Pentazocine
  Silicone or paraffin implantation

tremities are seldom affected. Recent streptococcal infection in childhood and diabetes mellitus[477] are the two most frequent associations of this condition, which either resolves spontaneously after 6 to 12 months or persists for many years. Other manifestations include hydrarthrosis, pleural and pericardial effusions, widespread involvement of skeletal or cardiac muscle, and macroglossia. Histochemical studies have revealed swollen collagen bundles and the accumulation of mucopolysaccharide (probably hyaluronic acid) in the dermis, subcutis, and skeletal muscle.

Porphyria Cutanea Tarda. Hypopigmented plaque-like sclerodermatous induration of the skin and pigmentary changes occur in porphyria cutanea tarda usually, but not always, in sun-exposed areas.[479,480] Particularly on the face, long-standing lesions may ulcerate and contain dystrophic calcific deposits.[481] In contrast, bullae are rare in systemic sclerosis, and uroporphyrin excretion is normal.

Scleromyxedema. Scleromyxedema (lichen myxedematosus, papular mucinosis) is an unusual disorder in which widespread lichenoid eruption of soft, pale red or yellowish papules is accompanied by diffuse thickening of the skin, especially involving the proximal extremities in a scleredema distribution. Dense deposits of acid mucopolysaccharide, without glycosaminoglycan subunits on electron microscopy,[482] are found in the upper portion of the dermis. Proximal muscle weakness, dysphagia, and vacuolar myopathy have been reported.[483] Abnormal serum immunoglobulins (M components) have been detected in several patients, suggesting a relationship of this condition to myelomatosis.[484] An unacceptably high rate of late malignancy has been associated with melphalan therapy.[484a]

Acrodermatitis Chronica Atrophicans and Lichen Sclerosus et Atrophicus. These are uncommon disorders of unknown etiology, in which cutaneous inflammation is followed by atrophy. The latter shows a high frequency of organ-specific antibodies, for example, to thyroid and gastric parietal cells. Overlap with localized scleroderma has been reported but may not be justified (see earlier discussion, Localized Scleroderma).

Amyloidosis. Infiltration of the dermis may accompany amyloidosis of either the primary (multiple myeloma associated) or secondary type.[485,486] Firm, discrete hemispheric brown or yellow papules are described, but when the deposition of amyloid is diffuse and involves the fingers, hands, and face, physical findings may mimic those of systemic sclerosis. Skin biopsies were positive for amyloid in involved skin in over one half of cases and in clinically normal skin in over one third.[486]

Juvenile Onset Diabetes Mellitus. Digital sclerosis and mild finger contractures occur in one third of patients with insulin-dependent juvenile onset diabetes mellitus.[487-489] These findings are correlated better with disease duration than with microvascular (retinal and renal) complications.[487,489]

Acromegaly. Considerable thickening of the skin and subcutaneous tissues may appear in acromegaly as a result of connective tissue hyperplasia.[43] Hypertrophy of the digital tufts is the rule, rather than the ischemic atrophy associated with systemic sclerosis.

Glycogen Storage Disease. Scleroderma-like skin induration has been observed in persons with glycogen storage disease of muscle.[490]

Carcinoid Syndrome. The occurrence of a peculiar localized scleroderma-like fibrosis in the skin of a few patients with the malignant carcinoid syndrome has suggested that 5-hydroxytryptamine (serotonin) metabolism might be deranged in systemic sclerosis.[491] There is, however, little evidence of such a disturbance, and urinary excretion of 5-hydroxyindoleacetic acid is normal in systemic sclerosis patients.[492] Persons with scleroderma (and also, in at least one case, unaffected relatives as well) have excreted excessive amounts of kynurenine and other intermediary metabolites of tryptophan. A partial deficiency in kynurenine hydroxylase may exist, but this finding appears to be nonspecific.[493] The intestinal absorption of tryptophan is normal in most patients with systemic sclerosis.[494] The finding that urinary levels of 5-hydroxyindoleacetic acid do not rise in response to increased dietary tryptophan in nearly half the cases indicates an impaired transformation of serotonin to 5-hydroxyindoleacetic acid. A disproportionately high ratio of total indoles to indoleacetic acid suggests the presence of excess tryptamine, presumably a result of impaired activity of monoamine oxidase.[492] Another abnormality in the conversion of tryptophan located at some point after the formation of hydroxyanthranilic acid has been detected in some patients with systemic sclerosis.[495] These metabolic changes remain unexplained, and may be secondary rather than primary.

Phenylketonuria. Atypical scleroderma of the trunk and extremities without visceral stigmata has been reported in children with phenylketonuria,[496,497] a disorder in which the absence of the enzyme phenylalanine hydroxylase ultimately leads to excessive urinary excretion of indolic compounds and decreased levels of plasma serotonin and urinary 5-hydroxyindoleacetic acid. Improvement follows conversion to a low phenylalanine diet. Studies of nine children with scleroderma, from 3 to 14 years of age, however, revealed normal urinary levels of both phenylalanine and D-hydroxyphenylacetic acid.[497]

Werner's Syndrome, Progeria, and Rothmund's Syndrome. The classic findings of Werner's syndrome, a rare hereditofamilial disorder, include growth retardation, premature graying of the hair and baldness, juvenile cataracts, and a high frequency of diabetes mellitus. Atrophy and hyperkeratosis of the skin with chronic ulcerations over pressure points in the feet may occur.[498,499] In progeria, a rare autosomal recessive syndrome, the corium and subcutis have been reported to be either thickened or atrophic,[500,501] and the thermal shrinkage and solubility of skin collagen resemble aged rather than normally growing connective tissue.[501] The nature of the primary defect in the development and metabolism of connective tissue in these conditions is unknown. Rothmund's syndrome is another heritable (recessive) disorder in which atrophy of the skin (poikiloderma), beginning in infancy, is associated with juvenile cataracts.

Vinyl Chloride and Epoxy Resin Associated Scleroderma. Workers who clean reactor vessels containing the polymerizing agent vinyl chloride (CH_2CHCl) may acquire a systemic illness with some features of systemic sclerosis.[502] These persons complain of soreness and tenderness of the fingertips and Raynaud's phenomenon. They develop nodular induration of skin of the dorsa of the hands and forearms, clubbing, synovial thickening of the proximal interphalangeal joints, hepatic portal fibrosis, splenomegaly, and pulmonary fibrosis. Roentgenograms reveal varying degrees of acro-osteolysis of the distal phalanges of the fingers, as well as erosive and sclerotic changes in the sacroiliac joints. Partial resorption of the mandible has been reported. Microvascular abnormalities similar to those encountered in systemic sclerosis are observed on capillary microscopy,[503] and luminal narrowing of the digital arteries has been seen on angiographic examination.[504]

The vapor of epoxy resins is believed to lead to cutaneous sclerosis and muscle weakness.[17] A biogenic amine is the suspected causative agent. Similar compounds have been implicated in other pseudosclerodermatous states, such as carcinoid syndrome[505] and L-5-hydroxytryptophan and carbidopa therapy.[22]

Bleomycin Toxicity. Administration of the tumoricidal drug bleomycin often leads to the development of nodules and/or plaques of thickened skin, the result of an increase of dense collagen deposition in the dermis.[506] More uniform induration of the skin, Raynaud's phenomenon,[507,508] and pulmonary fibrosis,[509] mimic the findings in systemic sclerosis. The dermal fibrosis tends to recede following discontinuation of bleomycin. Cultured fibroblasts from affected skin demonstrated increased collagen synthesis.[21]

Pentazocine Toxicity. Nodular cutaneous sclerosis, often associated with ulceration, has been reported to follow intramuscular injection of the non-narcotic analgesic, pentazocine.[23] "Woody," hard, and occasionally calcified skin, subcutis, and muscle have resulted. Venous and/or arteriolar thrombosis and endarteritis are described in these patients, many of whom had a personal or family history of diabetes mellitus.

Foreign Substances. In Japan, a variety of connective tissue disease syndromes have been reported to follow cosmetic surgery with injection of foreign substances (e.g., paraffin, silicone), chiefly for breast augmentation.[20] The most common clinical entity recognized in this situation is systemic sclerosis. Other examples of this association have recently been described.[510,511]

CALCINOSIS

Calcinosis, or pathologic calcification of the soft tissues, occurs in a variety of systemic and local conditions (Table 73–4). Most of these disorders are considered in detail in Chapter 108. Classification of ectopic calcification generally separates these conditions into those that result from long-continued hypercalcemia and/or hyperphosphatemia (metastatic calcification) and those following some local abnormality in the affected tissues (dystrophic calcification).

METASTATIC CALCIFICATION

Calcareous deposits, which occur commonly in hypercalcemic states, are found in the kidney (nephrocalcinosis), stomach, lung, brain, eyes (band keratopathy), skin, subcutaneous and periarticular tissues, and arterial walls. The milk-alkali syndrome and vitamin D intoxication are two such conditions that may affect rheumatic disease patients who are overzealous about the prevention of duodenal ulcer or osteoporosis.[511a] Calcification of the articular cartilage and menisci (chondrocalcinosis) and joint capsules is a well-recognized feature of hyperparathyroidism. For some persons, an attack of calcium pyrophosphate dihydrate (CPPD) crystal–induced synovitis (pseudogout) represents the first clinical manifestation of this disease. Accordingly, the possibility of primary hyperparathyroidism should be carefully considered in all patients with this arthropathy. During the immediate postoperative period, patients whose para-

Table 73–4. Diseases Associated With Calcification of the Soft Tissues in the Extremities

I. Metastatic Calcification
   Hypercalcemic conditions
     Primary hyperparathyroidism
     Hypervitaminosis D
     Milk-alkali syndrome
     Metastatic and other neoplasms of bone
     Sarcoidosis
   Hyperphosphatemic conditions
     Chronic renal failure with secondary hyperparathyroidism
     Hypoparathyroidism
     Pseudohypoparathyroidism
     Tumoral calcinosis (lipocalcinosis granulomatosis)
II. Dystrophic Calcification
   Connective tissue diseases
     Systemic sclerosis, with both diffuse and limited scleroderma
     Dermatomyositis-polymyositis
     Ehlers-Danlos syndrome
     Pseudoxanthoma elasticum
   Metabolic disorders
     Chondrocalcinosis articularis (pseudogout)
     Gout
     Diabetes mellitus
     Alkaptonuria (ochronosis)
     Porphyria cutanea tarda
     Pseudopseudohypoparathyroidism
     Werner's syndrome
     Progeria
     Myositis (or fibrodysplasia) ossificans progressiva
   Vascular diseases
     Medial sclerosis of arteries (Mönckeberg's sclerosis)
     Venous calcifications
   Parasitic infestations
   Other diseases
     Neuropathic arthropathy
     Calcific tendinitis
     Para-articular limb joint ectopic calcification associated with paralysis and other neurologic disorders

thyroid adenoma has been removed are at high risk to develop attacks of pseudogout.[512]

Soft-tissue calcification without ocular involvement and seldom affecting skin[513] is also found in normocalcemic-hyperphosphatemic hyperparathyroidism secondary to renal insufficiency, although renal calculus formation is less frequent than in the hypercalcemic states. Acute episodes of articular and periarticular inflammation, which appear to be related to the local deposition of microcrystalline calcium phosphate (and, at times, monosodium urate), have been described in patients undergoing hemodialysis for chronic renal failure.[514] The finding of subperiosteal juxta-articular bone erosions following calcinosis in the same location suggests that the calcifications may induce erosions.[515] The removal of pyrophosphate, which appears to act as a physiologic inhibitor of calcification, may be responsible for this phenomenon.[516] Treatment with phosphate binding agents has resulted in a significant reduction of serum phosphorus levels, disappearance of cutaneous calcinosis, and relief from the articular attacks,[514] although malabsorption of phosphate binders may be a problem.[517] Oxalosis secondary to end stage renal disease may be associated with chondrocalcinosis and highly inflammatory bursitis, tenosynovitis, or arthritis owing to calcium oxalate deposition.[517a]

In hypoparathyroidism, pseudohypoparathyroidism, and pseudopseudohypoparathyroidism, calcification may occur in the brain, particularly in the basal ganglia, as well as in the subcutaneous tissue. Acute calcific periarthritis in hypoparathyroidism has been reported to occur in association with a fall in serum calcium,[518] similar to the same phenomenon in surgically treated primary hyperparathyroidism[512] and gout.

Radiographically detected and biopsy proved metastatic calcification has been detected by the use of bone scan (^{99m}Tc-labeled methylene diphosphonate) in numerous areas, including the lungs, gastric wall, heart, and kidneys.[519–522] Such uptake, caused by the affinity of this tracer for the surface of hydroxyapatite crystals, has now been shown in the subcutaneous tissues and skin.[523]

Tumoral Calcinosis. Although included in the category of metastatic calcification because of frequent elevation in serum phosphorus level and occasional increase in serum calcium values, tumoral calcinosis is separable from other forms of metastatic calcification because visceral involvement is absent. This rare entity, which has also been called lipocalcinosis granulomatosis, is characterized by the rapid development of large, multilobulated calcific masses in the subcutaneous tissue and muscles surrounding the hips, shoulders, elbows, hands, and chest wall in otherwise healthy young subjects. There is no sex predilection, but there is a considerably increased prevalence among blacks and black Africans.[524] Smaller tumors occur adjacent to the spine, wrists, feet, lower ribs, sacrum, and ischium. These firm, nontender deposits may increase to a diameter of 20 cm or larger over a period of months to years. Little or no articular limitation occurs unless masses become very large or are complicated by the development of fistulous tracts caused by either infection or attempts at surgical drainage. Nerve root impingement (especially sciatica) may result. Curiously, a number of patients have angioid streaks of the retina.

Most patients with tumoral calcinosis have normal serum calcium and alkaline phosphatase values, but hyperphosphatemia[525] and elevated levels of 1,25-dihydroxyvitamin D[526] have been noted in several cases. Rapid exchange of calcium between serum and calcific masses is evident, along with an increased intestinal absorption of dietary calcium, with no defect in the turnover of skeletal calcium.[525] An intrinsic renal proximal tubular defect allowing enhanced phosphate reabsorption has been postulated. Elevated 1,25-dihydroxyvitamin D levels are present after phosphate depletion, suggesting dysregulation of its synthesis or metabolism or a yet-to-be-discovered stimulus for its production.[527] Approximately half the patients with tumoral calcinosis reported to date have had affected siblings. This observation, together with the occurrence of hyperphosphatemia, has led to the suggestion that there is a heritable disturbance in the metabolism of phosphorus.[525] Although an autosomal recessive mechanism had been postulated, the report of this condition in four generations of one family, coupled with a unique dental lesion, suggests the possibility of an autosomal dominant heredity with variable expression.[528] Affected teeth have short, bulbous roots and nearly total obliteration of pulp cavities on panoramic radiographs.

On sectioning, calcific deposits are found to be composed of multilocular cysts enclosing pockets of milky fluid or pasty microcrystalline calcareous matter. The tissue lining the walls of these cysts contains mononuclear cells rich in alkaline phosphatase and believed to be responsible for local accumulation of calcium phosphate, and it contains foreign body giant cells.[524] These mononuclear and multinuclear cells are structurally, and apparently functionally, similar to osteoblasts and osteoclasts, respectively.[525] The masses contain pure calcium carbonate and phosphate, a mixture of the two salts, or hydroxyapatite crystals.[529]

Treatment at present consists mainly of early surgical excision of the calcareous masses, which rarely recur at the same site. New deposits may appear in time around other joints. As a rule, the prognosis is good, although in some instances secondary infection of the deposits has led to multiple draining sinuses, cachexia, and amyloidosis. A low-calcium and low-phosphorus diet and large oral doses of antacids containing aluminum hydroxide have resulted in negative balances of both calcium and phosphorus with significant clinical improvement.[530] Intravenous calcitonin infusion has been reported to cause phosphaturia and a significant fall in serum phosphorus level.[531]

DYSTROPHIC CALCIFICATION

Many restrict the use of the term "calcinosis" to those patients in whom the deposition of calcium salts in the soft tissues occurs in the absence of any generalized disturbance in calcium or phosphorus metabolism.

Calcinosis Associated With Connective Tissue Disease (Fig. 73–20). In systemic sclerosis, the calcareous deposits are generally confined to the extremities and are particularly frequent on the flexor surfaces of the terminal phalanges, around joints, and near other bony eminences. Most of these patients suffer from limited scleroderma with CREST syndrome (see Fig. 73–5). In contrast, widespread encasing calcification of the skin, subcutaneous tissues, and periarticular tissues, as well as involvement of the deeper structures, occurs later in the course of polymyositis-dermatomyositis (see Chapter 72). This process includes tendons, tendon sheaths, and muscles, forming irregularly shaped plaques and nodules, and is often associated with severe joint contractures or ankylosis. This complication, more prevalent in childhood dermatomyositis (40 to 74% of cases), is associated with late, suboptimal dosage of corticosteroids and severe myopathy unresponsive to steroids.[532] The latter type of patient more frequently demonstrates a linear, reticular pattern of calcification.[533]

The standard method of detection of dystrophic calcification has been the plain roentgenogram. However, computed tomographic scanning has been reported to identify calcinosis in symptomatic but radiographically normal areas.[534] On microscopic examination, the precipitates of calcium in the skin are pleomorphic crystals, many in the shape of needles and large plates. They appear to develop in the elastic fibers of the connective tissue.[535,536] X-ray diffraction (Fig. 73–20) and electron microscopy identify these crystals as hydroxyapatite.[537]

As a rule, affected persons have normal concentrations of serum calcium, phosphorus, and alkaline phosphatase activity, but calcium balance studies have yielded conflicting data. In patients with cutaneous deposition (calcinosis cutis), increased absorption and retention of calcium have been evident, paradoxically with a more rapid disappearance rate of radiolabeled calcium injected intradermally.[538] When a woman with scleroderma and calcinosis was placed on a calcium restricted diet, the bone resorption rate increased, and urinary excretion of calcium fell normally, but the net calcium accretion rate (which included extraosseous calcium deposition) remained constant.[539] Urinary excretion of a vitamin K–dependent calcium-binding protein (γ-carboxyglutamic acid or Gla) is increased in dermatomyositis and scleroderma patients with calcinosis,[540,541] but it is premature to conclude that this substance plays a primary role in the pathogenesis of calcinosis.

The basis for the deposition of calcium salts in the dermis of patients with systemic sclerosis and dermatomyositis is unclear. A number of different forms of cutaneous, subcuticular, periarticular, and visceral calcification have been produced experimentally in

FIG. 73–20. Dystrophic calcinosis. *Left,* Roentgenogram of the hand of a woman with polymyositis showing extensive calcinosis involving both subcutaneous tissues and tendon sheaths. *Right,* X-ray diffraction patterns. The labeled spectra are derived from a hydroxyapatite control and the spectra with lower peak heights are from the patient. Correspondence of peak positions suggests the presence of hydroxyapatite (see Chapter 108 for additional information on identification of calcium phosphate crystals).

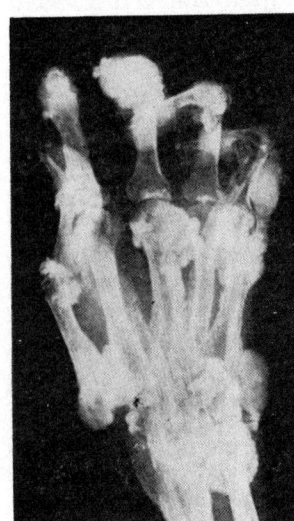

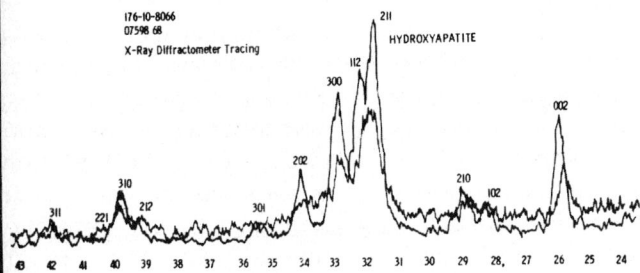

the rat by calciphylaxis, but none serve as a model of human calcinosis. It is interesting that skin of patients with systemic sclerosis contains increased numbers of mast cells.[47]

The initial precipitation of calcium salts in experimental cutaneous calcinosis in the rat occurs in areas rich in mucopolysaccharides or, in some instances, collagen fibers, which appear to act as a matrix for this calcification. Calcification of porcine cardiac valve prostheses has been shown to occur on devitalized porcine connective tissue cells and collagen fibers, and abnormal collagen cross links have been implicated in this process.[542] Because polysaccharides may "shield" reactive sites on collagen fibrils and block mineral nucleation, it is possible that the calcinosis that occurs in scleroderma may be related to the diminution of mucopolysaccharides in the affected skin during later stages of the disease.

Numerous drugs, hormones, and a host of nonspecific measures have been used unsuccessfully in the treatment of calcinosis.[543-547] Oral low-dose anticoagulant therapy has been effective occasionally in preventing and reversing subcutaneous calcinosis.[408,541] Surgical excision of large calcareous masses may be helpful in selected instances.[405,548,549] Resolution of calcinosis in juvenile dermatomyositis was accompanied by serious hypercalcemia in one case.[550] Colchicine may be effective in reducing soft tissue inflammation surrounding such deposits.[409,410]

Myositis (or Fibrodysplasia) Ossificans Progressiva. Patients with this uncommon disorder have widespread ectopic calcification and ossification in fascia, aponeuroses, and other fibrous structures related to muscle. The initial symptoms usually appear in early childhood, often preceded by local trauma (Fig. 73–21). The disease occurs in families and appears to be transmitted as an autosomal dominant trait with irregular penetrance. Associated congenital anomalies of the digits include microdactyly or total absence of the thumbs and great toes.

The initial manifestation usually consists of a localized area of swelling, redness, and warmth in the neck or paravertebral area, often associated with extreme pain. After several days the signs of inflammation subside, leaving an area of residual doughy firmness that appears fibromatous and gradually ossifies over the following weeks. Scanning with ^{99m}Tc pyrophosphate may be useful in the detection of areas of ossification prior to roentgenographic changes.[551] The replacement of the tendon and muscle by bone leads to characteristic contracture deformities. Once ossification occurs, further change is minimal. Recurring bouts of inflammation and ossification result in progressive damage to much of the striated mus-

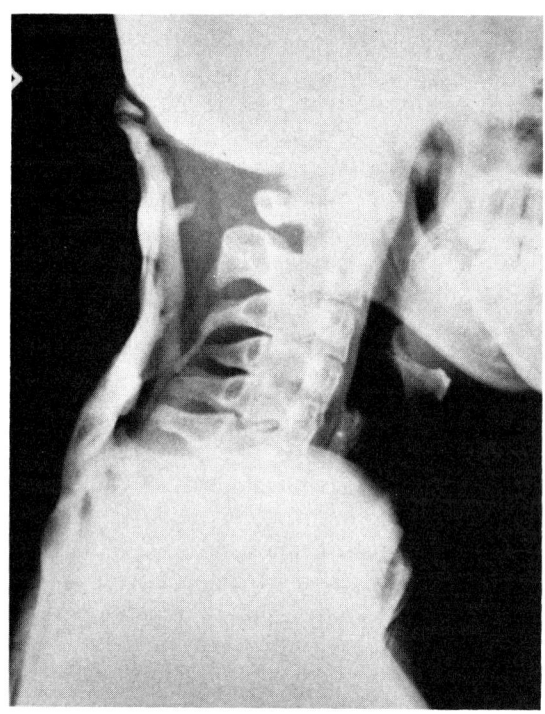

FIG. 73–21. Roentgenogram illustrating new bone formation in the cervical area of a 17-year-old woman with myositis ossificans progressiva. She first noted pain, swelling, and limitation of motion in this area after trauma 10 years previously.

culature. Involvement of the muscles of the chest wall and back may lead to restrictive pulmonary disease.[552] Death usually ensues from respiratory failure and/or pulmonary infection resulting from involvement of the muscles of the thorax or from inanition as a result of damage to the muscles of mastication.

It has been suggested that myositis ossificans progressiva may result from abnormal collagen or, alternatively, deficiency of an inhibitor material (?proteoglycan) which normally prevents the crystallization and accretion of calcium salts on collagen fibers at sites other than bone. There is no evidence of any fundamental aberration in calcium metabolism per se in this disorder. The administration of diphosphonates may suppress, at least temporarily, the development of new areas of mineralization following surgical excision of ectopic bone, but the ultimate value of these agents is as yet uncertain.[542,553] Corticosteroids may relieve the acute symptoms of inflammation and may retard progression of the disease in some patients.[554]

Other Localized Calcific Syndromes. A variety of local and regional sites of calcification have been associated with rheumatic complaints. Intra-articular[555] and periarticular[556] calcification has followed intra-articular corticosteroid injections. In addition to the common syndromes of the shoulder and hip, idiopathic calcific tendinitis and tenosynovitis has produced instances of carpal tunnel syndrome[557,558] and wrist and finger flexor tenosynovitis,[559,559a] all believed to be due to repeated minor trauma. A similar cause has been suggested for calcinosis cutis affecting the knee.[560] Synthetic retinoid therapy is associated with spinal hyperostosis, diffuse idiopathic skeletal hyperostosis (DISH), and extraspinal tendon and ligament calcification.[561] With DISH[562] and with ligamentum flavum calcification,[563] cervical myelopathy may result. Atraumatic causes of neck pain now include calcific tendinitis of the longus colli muscle[564] and retropharyngeal calcific tendinitis.[565] A genetic predisposition to calcific periarthritis of the shoulder in diabetics with HLA-B27 antigen has been suggested.[566]

REFERENCES

1. Medsger, T.A., Jr.: Systemic sclerosis (scleroderma), eosinophilic fasciitis, and calcinosis. *In* Arthritis and Allied Conditions. 10th Ed. Edited by D.J. McCarty. Philadelphia, Lea & Febiger, 1985, pp. 994–1036.
2. LeRoy, E.C., et al.: Scleroderma (systemic sclerosis): Classification, subsets, and pathogenesis. J. Rheumatol. (in press).
3. Masi, A.T.: Classification of systemic sclerosis (scleroderma). *In* Systemic Sclerosis (Scleroderma). Edited by C.M. Black and A.R. Myers. New York, Gower Medical Publishing, 1985, pp. 7–15.
4. Sharp, G.C.: Association of progressive systemic sclerosis with other connective tissue diseases ("overlap syndromes"). *In* Systemic Sclerosis (Scleroderma). Edited by C.M. Black and A.R. Myers. New York, Gower Medical Publishing, 1985, pp. 33–35.
5. Winterbauer, R.H.: Multiple telangiectasia, Raynaud's phenomenon, sclerodactyly, and subcutaneous calcinosis: A syndrome mimicking hereditary hemorrhagic telangiectasia. Bull. Johns Hopkins Hosp., 114:361–383, 1964.
6. Masi, A.T., et al.: Clinical criteria for early diagnosed systemic sclerosis: Preliminary results of the ARA Multicenter Cooperative Study. Arthritis Rheum., 21:576–577, 1987.
7. Medsger, T.A., Jr., and Masi, A.T.: Epidemiology of systemic sclerosis (scleroderma). Ann. Intern. Med., 74:714–721, 1971.
8. Michet, C.J., Jr., et al.: Epidemiology of systemic lupus erythematosus and other connective tissue diseases in Rochester, Minnesota, 1950 through 1979. Mayo Clin. Proc., 60:105–113, 1985.
9. Haustein, U.F., and Ziegler, V.: Environmentally induced systemic sclerosis-like disorders. Int. J. Dermatol., 24:147–151, 1985.
10. Erasmus, L.D.: Scleroderma in gold-miners on the Witwatersrand with particular reference to pulmonary manifestations. S. Afr. J. Lab. Clin. Med., 3:209–231, 1957.
11. Rodnan, G.P., et al.: The association of progressive systemic sclerosis (scleroderma) with coal miners' pneumoconiosis and other forms of silicosis. Ann. Intern. Med., 66:323–334, 1967.
12. Sluis-Cremer, G.K., et al.: Silica, silicosis, and progressive systemic sclerosis. Br. J. Ind. Med., 42:838–843, 1985.
13. Dinman, B.L., et al.: Occupational acroosteolysis. I. An epidemiologic study. Arch. Environ. Health, 22:61–73, 1971.
14. Veltman, G., et al.: Clinical manifestations and course of vinyl chloride disease. Ann. N.Y. Acad. Sci., 246:6–17, 1975.
15. Sparrow, G.P.: A connective tissue disorder similar to vinyl chloride disease in a patient exposed to perchlorethylene. Clin. Dermatol., 2:17–22, 1977.
16. Walder, B.K.: Do solvents cause scleroderma? Int. J. Dermatol., 22:157–158, 1983.
17. Yamakage, A., and Ishikawa, H.: Generalized morphea-like scleroderma occurring in people exposed to organic solvents. Dermatologica, 165:186–193, 1982.
18. Alonso-Ruiz, A., Zea-Mendoza, A.C., Salazar-Vallinas, J.M., and Rocamore-Ripoll, A.: Toxic oil syndrome: A syndrome with features overlapping those of various forms of scleroderma. Semin. Arthritis Rheum., 15:200–212, 1986.
19. Mateo, I.M., Izquierdo, M., Fernandez-Dapica, M.P., and Navas, J.: Toxic epidemic syndrome: Musculoskeletal manifestations. J. Rheumatol., 11:333–338, 1984.
20. Kumagai, Y., et al.: Clinical spectrum of connective tissue disease after cosmetic surgery. Observations on eighteen patients and a review of the Japanese literature. Arthritis Rheum., 27:1–12, 1984.
21. Finch, W.R., et al.: Bleomycin-induced scleroderma. J. Rheumatol., 7:651–659, 1980.
22. Sternberg, E.M., et al.: Development of a scleroderma-like illness during therapy with L-5-hydroxytryptophan and carbidopa. N. Engl. J. Med., 303:782–787, 1980.
23. Palestine, R.F., et al.: Skin manifestations of pentazocine abuse. J. Am. Acad. Dermatol., 2:47–55, 1980.
24. Flores, R.H., Stevens, M.B., and Arnett, F.C.: Familial occurrence of progressive systemic sclerosis and systemic lupus erythematosus. J. Rheumatol., 11:321–323, 1984.
25. Jablonska, S., Chorzelski, T., and Blaszczyk, M.: Familial occurrence of scleroderma. *In* Scleroderma and Pseudoscleroderma. 2nd Ed. Edited by S. Jablonska. Warsaw, Polish Medical Publishers, 1975, pp. 35–55.
26. Sheldon, W.B., et al.: Three siblings with scleroderma (systemic sclerosis) and two with Raynaud's phenomenon from a single kindred. Arthritis Rheum., 24:668–676, 1981.
27. Greger, R.E.: Familial progressive systemic sclerosis. Arch. Dermatol., 111:81–85, 1975.
28. Muralidar, K., et al.: Familial scleroderma (case report). J. Assoc. Physicians India, 26:307–309, 1978.
29. Maddison, P.J., et al.: Antinuclear antibodies in the relatives and spouses of patients with systemic sclerosis. Ann. Rheum. Dis., 45:793–799, 1986.
30. Takehara, K., Moroi, Y., and Ishibashi, Y.: Antinuclear antibodies in the relatives of patients with systemic sclerosis. Br. J. Dermatol., 112:23–33, 1985.
31. Dustoor, M.M., McInerney, M.M., Mazanec, D.J., and Cathcart, M.K.: Abnormal lymphocyte function in scleroderma: A study on identical twins. Clin. Immunol. Immunopathol., 44:20–30, 1987.
32. Medsger, T.A., Jr.: Progressive systemic sclerosis and associated disorders. *In* Principles of Rheumatic Diseases. Edited by R.S. Panush. New York, John Wiley & Sons, 1981, pp. 331–350.
33. Rodnan, G.P., and Fennell, R.H., Jr.: Progressive systemic sclerosis *sine* scleroderma. J. Am. Med. Assoc., 180:665–670, 1962.
34. Steen, V.D., Medsger, T.A., Jr., and Rodnan, G.P.: D-penicillamine therapy in progressive systemic sclerosis (scleroderma). Ann. Intern. Med., 97:652–658, 1982.

35. Black, C., Dieppe, P.K., Huskisson, T., and Hart, F.D.: Regressive systemic sclerosis. Ann. Rheum. Dis., 45:384–388, 1986.

36. Medsger, T.A., Jr.: Systemic Sclerosis. *In* Rheumatic Therapeutics. Edited by S.H. Roth, J.J. Calabro, H.E. Paulus, and R. Willkins. New York, McGraw-Hill, 1985, pp. 236–248.

37. Kahaleh, M.B., Sultany, G.L., Smith, E.A., and Huffstutter, J.E.: A modified scleroderma skin scoring method. Clin. Exp. Rheumatol., 4:367–369, 1986.

38. Bjerring, P.: Skin elasticity measured by dynamic admittance, a new technique for mechanical measurements in patients with scleroderma. Acta. Derm. Venerol., 120:83–87, 1985.

39. Akesson, A., Forsberg, L., Hederstrom, E., and Wollheim, F.: Ultrasound examination of skin thickness in patients with progressive systemic sclerosis (scleroderma). Acta Radiol. [Diagn.] (Stockh.), 27:91–94, 1986.

40. Myers, S.L., Cohen, J.S., Sheets, P.W., and Bies, J.R.: B-mode ultrasound evaluation of skin thickness in progressive systemic sclerosis. J. Rheumatol., 13:577–580, 1986.

41. Nimni, M.: A defect in the intramolecular and intermolecular cross-linking of collagen caused by penicillamine: I. Metabolic and functional abnormalities in soft tissues. J. Biol. Chem., 243:1457–1466, 1968.

42. Krieg, T., et al.: Type III collagen aminopropeptide levels in serum of patients with progressive systemic sclerosis. J. Invest. Dermatol., 87:788–791, 1986.

43. Rodnan, G.P., Lipinski, E., and Luksick, J.: Skin thickness and collagen content in progressive systemic sclerosis (scleroderma) and localized scleroderma. Arthritis Rheum., 22:130–140, 1979.

44. Kondo, H., Rabin, B.S., and Rodnan, G.P.: Cutaneous antigen-stimulating lymphokine production by lymphocytes of patients with progressive systemic sclerosis (scleroderma). J. Clin. Invest., 58:1388–1394, 1976.

45. Roumm, A.D., et al.: Lymphocytes in the skin of patients with progressive systemic sclerosis: Quantification, subtyping and clinical correlations. Arthritis Rheum., 27:645–653, 1984.

46. Connolly, S.M., and Winkelmann, R.K.: Direct immunofluorescent findings in scleroderma syndromes. Acta Derm. Venereol. (Stockh.), 61:29–36, 1981.

47. Hawkins, R.A., Claman, H.N., Clark, R.A.F., and Steigerwald, J.C.: Increased dermal mast cell populations in progressive systemic sclerosis: A link in chronic fibrosis? Ann. Intern. Med., 102:182–186, 1985.

47a. Nishioka, K., Kobayashi, Y., Katayama, I., and Takijiri, C.: Mast cell numbers in diffuse scleroderma. Arch. Dermatol., 123:205–208, 1987.

48. Andrews, B.S., et al.: Loss of epidermal Langerhans cells and endothelial cell HLA-DR antigens in the skin in progressive systemic sclerosis. J. Rheumatol., 13:341–348, 1986.

49. Jawitz, J.C., Albert, M.K., Nigra, T.P., and Bunning, R.D.: A new skin manifestation of progressive systemic sclerosis. J. Amer. Acad. Dermatol., 2:265–268, 1984.

49a. Sukenik, S., Kleiner-Baumgarten, A., and Horowitz, J.: Hyperpigmentation along tendons in progressive systemic sclerosis. (Letter.) J. Rheumatol., 13:474–475, 1986.

50. Serup, J., and Hagdrup, H.: Vitamin D metabolites in generalized scleroderma. Evidence of a normal cutaneous and intestinal supply with vitamin D. Acta Derm. Venereol. (Stockh.), 65:343–345, 1985.

51. Young, E.A., Steen, V., and Medsger, T.A., Jr.: Systemic sclerosis without Raynaud's phenomenon. (Abstract.) Arthritis Rheum., 29:S51, 1986.

52. Coffman, J.D., and Cohen, A.S.: Total and capillary fingertip blood flow in Raynaud's phenomenon. N. Engl. J. Med., 285:259–263, 1971.

53. Hendriksen, O., and Kristensen, J.K.: Reduced systolic blood pressure in fingers of patients with generalized scleroderma (acrosclerosis). Acta Derm. Venereol. (Stockh.), 61:531–534, 1981.

54. Rodnan, G.P., Myerowitz, R.L., and Justh, G.O.: Morphologic changes in the digital arteries of patients with progressive systemic sclerosis (scleroderma) and Raynaud's phenomenon. Medicine, 59:393–408, 1980.

55. Merino, J., et al.: Hemiplegia and peripheral gangrene secondary to large and medium size vessels involvement in CREST syndrome. Clin. Rheumatol., 1:295–299, 1982.

56. Furey, N.L., Schmid, F.R., Kwaan, H.C., and Friederici, H.H.R.: Arterial thrombosis in scleroderma. Br. J. Dermatol., 93:683–693, 1975.

57. Maricq, H.R., Spencer-Green, G., and LeRoy, E.C.: Skin capillary abnormalities as indicators of organ involvement in scleroderma (systemic sclerosis). Am. J. Med., 61:862–870, 1976.

58. Maricq, H.R., and LeRoy, E.C.: Capillary blood flow in scleroderma. Bibl. Anat., 11:352–358, 1973.

59. Kenik, J.G., Maricq, H.R., and Bole, G.G.: Blind evaluation of the diagnostic specificity of nailfold capillary microscopy in the connective tissue diseases. Arthritis Rheum., 24:885–891, 1981.

60. Maricq, H.R.: Widefield capillary microscopy: Technique and rating scale for abnormalities seen in scleroderma and related disorders. Arthritis Rheum., 24:1159–1165, 1981.

61. Maricq, H.R.: Comparison of quantitative and semiquantitative estimates of nailfold capillary abnormalities in scleroderma spectrum disorders. Microvasc. Res., 32:271–276, 1986.

62. Lee, P., et al.: Digital blood flow and nailfold capillary microscopy in Raynaud's phenomenon. J. Rheumatol., 13:564–569, 1986.

63. Thompson, R.P., et al.: Nailfold biopsy in scleroderma and related disorders. Arthritis Rheum., 27:97–103, 1984.

64. Harper, F.E., et al.: A prospective study of Raynaud's phenomenon and early connective tissue disease. A five-year report. Am. J. Med., 72:883–888, 1982.

65. McGill, N.W., and Gow, P.J.: Nailfold capillaroscopy: A blinded study of its discriminatory value in scleroderma, systemic lupus erythematosus, and rheumatoid arthritis. Aust. N.Z. J. Med., 16:457–460, 1986.

66. Maricq, H.R.: The microcirculation in scleroderma and allied diseases. Adv. Microcirc., 10:17–52, 1982.

67. Houtman, P.M., Kallenberg, C.G.M., Wouda, A.A., and The, T.H.: Decreased nailfold capillary density in Raynaud's phenomenon: A reflection of immunologically mediated local and systemic vascular disease? Ann. Rheum. Dis., 44:603–609, 1985.

68. Lovy, M., MacCarter, D., and Steigerwald, J.C.: Relationship between nailfold capillary abnormalities and organ involvement in systemic sclerosis. Arthritis Rheum., 28:496–501, 1985.

69. Statham, B.N., and Rowell, N.R.: Quantification of the nail fold capillary abnormalities in systemic sclerosis and Raynaud's syndrome. Acta Derm. Venereol. (Stockh), 66:139–143, 1986.

70. Sheiner, N.M., and Small, P.: Isolated Raynaud's phenomenon: A benign disorder. Ann. Allergy, 58:114–117, 1987.

71. Gerbracht, D.D., et al.: Evolution of primary Raynaud's phenomenon (Raynaud's disease) to connective tissue disease. Arthritis Rheum., 28:87–92, 1985.

72. Campbell, P.M., and LeRoy, E.C.: Raynaud phenomenon. Semin. Arthritis Rheum., *16*:92–103, 1986.

72a. Sarkozi, J., et al.: Significance of anticentromere antibody in idiopathic Raynaud's syndrome. Am. J. Med., *83*:893–899, 1987.

73. Rodnan, G.P.: The nature of joint involvement in progressive systemic sclerosis (diffuse scleroderma). Clinical study and pathological examination of synovium in twenty-nine patients. Ann. Intern. Med., *56*:422–439, 1962.

74. Devogelaer, J.P., et al.: Intra-articular calcification in progressive systemic sclerosis. Clin. Rheumatol., *5*:262–267, 1986.

75. Brandt, K.D., and Krey, P.R.: Chalky joint effusion: The result of massive synovial deposition of calcium apatite in progressive systemic sclerosis. Arthritis Rheum., *20*:792–796, 1977.

76. Schumacher, H.R., Jr.: Joint involvement in progressive systemic sclerosis (scleroderma). A light and electron microscopic study of synovial membrane and fluid. Am. J. Clin. Pathol., *60*:593–600, 1973.

77. Palmer, D.G., et al.: Bowed fingers. A helpful sign in the early diagnosis of systemic sclerosis. J. Rheumatol., *8*:266–272, 1981.

78. Baron, M., Lee, P., and Keystone, E.C.: The articular manifestations of progressive systemic sclerosis (scleroderma). Ann. Rheum. Dis., *41*:147–152, 1982.

79. Blocka, K.L.N., et al.: The arthropathy of advanced progressive systemic sclerosis: A radiographic survey. Arthritis Rheum., *24*:874–884, 1981.

80. Armstrong, R.D., and Gibson, T.: Scleroderma and erosive polyarthritis: A disease entity? Ann. Rheum. Dis., *41*:141–146, 1982.

81. Owens, G.R., et al.: Pulmonary function in progressive systemic sclerosis: Comparison of CREST syndrome variant with diffuse scleroderma. Chest, *84*:546–550, 1983.

82. Osial, T.A., Jr., et al.: Resorption of the mandibular condyles and coronoid processes in progressive systemic sclerosis (scleroderma). Arthritis Rheum., *24*:729–733, 1981.

83. Clements, P.J., et al.: Muscle disease in progressive systemic sclerosis: Diagnostic and therapeutic considerations. Arthritis Rheum., *21*:62–71, 1978.

84. Medsger T.A., Jr.: Progressive systemic sclerosis: Skeletal muscle involvement. Clin. Rheum. Dis., *5*:103–113, 1979.

84a. Foster, T.D., Fairburn, E.A.: Dental involvement in scleroderma. Br. Dent. J., *124*:353–356, 1968.

84b. Rowell, N.R., and Hopper, F.E.: The periodontal membrane in systemic sclerosis. Br. J. Dermatol., *96*:15–20, 1977.

85. Katzka, D.A., et al.: Barrett's metaplasia and adenocarcinoma of the esophagus in scleroderma. Am. J. Med., *82*:46–52, 1987.

86. Segel, M.C., Campbell, W.L., Medsger T.A., and Roumm, A.D.: Systemic sclerosis (scleroderma) and esophageal adenocarcinoma: Is increased patient screening necessary? Gastroenterology, *89*:485–488, 1985.

87. Garrett J.M., et al.: Esophageal deterioration in scleroderma. Mayo Clin. Proc., *46*:92–96, 1971.

88. Stentoft, P., Hendel, L., and Aggestrup, S.: Esophageal manometry and pH-probe monitoring in the evaluation of gastroesophageal reflux in patients with progressive systemic sclerosis. Scand. J. Gastroenterol., *22*:499–504, 1987.

89. Drane, W.E., et al.: Progressive systemic sclerosis: Radionuclide esophageal scintigraphy and manometry. Radiology, *160*:73–76, 1986.

90. Tsianos, E.B., et al.: Esophageal manometric findings in autoimmune rheumatic diseases: Is scleroderma esophagus a specific entity? Rheumatology Int., *7*:23–27, 1987.

91. Davidson, A., Russell, C., and Littlejohn, G.O.: Assessment of esophageal abnormalities in progressive systemic sclerosis using radionuclide transit. J. Rheumatol., *12*:472–477, 1985.

92. Carette, S., Lacourciere, Y., Lavoie, S., and Halle, P.: Radionuclide esophageal transit in progressive systemic sclerosis. J. Rheumatol., *12*:478–481, 1985.

93. Rajapakse. C.N.A., et al.: Pharyngo-esophageal dysphagia in systemic sclerosis. Ann. Rheum. Dis., *40*:612–614, 1981.

94. Akesson, A, Akesson, B., Gustafson, T., and Wollheim, F.: Gastrointestinal function in patients with progressive systemic sclerosis. Clin. Rheumatol., *4*:441–448, 1985.

95. Bendixen, G., et al.: Gastrointestinal involvement in systemic scleroderma. Dermatologica, *137*:26–35, 1968.

96. Allende, H.D., Ona, F.V., and Noronna, A.J.: Bleeding gastric telangiectasia: Complication of Raynaud's phenomenon, esophageal motor dysfunction, sclerodactyly and telangiectasia (REST) syndrome. Am. J. Gastroenterol., *75*:354–356, 1981.

97. Holt, J.M., and Wright, R.: Anemia due to blood loss from the telangiectases of scleroderma. Br. Med. J., *3*:537–538, 1967.

98. Rosecrans, P.C.M., et al.: Gastrointestinal telangiectasia as a cause of severe blood loss in systemic sclerosis. Endoscopy, *12*:200–204, 1980.

98a. Baron, M., Srolovitz, H.: Colonic telangiectasias in a patient with progressive systemic sclerosis. Arthritis Rheum., *29*:282–285, 1986.

99. Hendy, M.S., Torrance, H.B., and Warnes, T.W.: Small-bowel volvulus in association with progressive systemic sclerosis. Br. Med. J., *1*:1051–1052, 1979.

100. Cipoletti, J.F., et al.: Sjögren's syndrome in progressive systemic sclerosis (scleroderma). Ann. Intern. Med., *87*:535–541, 1977.

101. Elwany, S., Talaat, M., Kamel, N., and Stephanos, W.: Further observations on nasal mucosal changes in scleroderma. J. Laryngol. Otol., *98*:979–986, 1984.

102. Gordon, M.B., et al.: Thyroid disease in progressive systemic sclerosis (PSS): Increased frequency of glandular fibrosis and hypothyroidism. Ann. Intern. Med., *95*:431–435, 1981.

103. Battle, W.M., et al.: Abnormal colonic motility in progressive systemic sclerosis. Ann. Intern. Med., *94*:749–752, 1981.

104. Hamel-Roy, J., et al.: Comparative esophageal and anorectal motility in scleroderma. Gastroenterology, *88*:1–7, 1985.

105. Kemp-Harper, R.A., and Jackson, D.C.: Progressive systemic sclerosis. Br. J. Radiol., *38*:825–834, 1965.

106. Robinson, J.C., and Teitelbaum, S.L.: Stercoral ulceration and perforation of the sclerodermatous colon: Report of two cases and review of the literature. Dis. Colon Rectum, *17*:622–632, 1974.

107. D'Angelo, G., Stern, H.S., and Myers, E.: Rectal prolapse in scleroderma: Case report and review of the colonic complications of scleroderma. Can. J. Surg., *28*:62–63, 1985.

108. Owens, G.R., and Follansbee, W.P.: Cardiopulmonary manifestations of systemic sclerosis. Chest, *91*:118–127, 1987.

109. Kosaka, Y., et al.: Large cystic lesions of the upper lobes of the lungs in two patients with CREST syndrome. Arthritis Rheum., *27*:935–938, 1984.

110. Guttadauria, M., et al.: Pulmonary function in scleroderma. Arthritis Rheum., *20*:1071–1079, 1977.

111. Bjerke, R.D., et al.: Small airways in progressive systemic sclerosis (PSS). Am. J. Med., *66*:201–209, 1979.

112. Peters-Golden, M., et al.: Clinical and demographic predictors of loss of pulmonary function in systemic sclerosis. Medicine, *63*:221–231, 1984.

113. Bagg, L.R., and Hughes, D.T.D.: Serial pulmonary function

tests in progressive systemic sclerosis. Thorax, *34*:224–228, 1979.

114. Greenwald, G.I., et al.: Longitudinal changes in lung function and respiratory symptoms in progressive systemic sclerosis. Amer. J. Med., *83*:83–92, 1987.

114a.Schneider, P.D., et al.: Serial pulmonary function in systemic sclerosis. Am. J. Med., *73*:385–394, 1982.

115. Baron, M., et al.: [67]Gallium lung scans in progressive systemic sclerosis. Arthritis Rheum., *261*:969–974, 1983.

116. Edelson, J.D., et al.: Lung inflammation in scleroderma: Clinical, radiographic, physiologic and cytopathological features. J. Rheumatol., *12*:957–963, 1985.

116a.Furst, D.E., et al.: Abnormalities of pulmonary vascular dynamics and inflammation in early progressve systemic sclerosis. Arthritis Rheum., *24*:1403–1408, 1981.

117. Konig, G., et al.: Lung involvement in scleroderma. Chest, *85*:318–324, 1984.

118. Rossi, G.A., et al.: Evidence for chronic inflammation as a component of the interstitial lung disease associated with progressive systemic sclerosis. Am. Rev. Respir. Dis., *131*:612–617, 1985.

119. Silver, R.M., Metcalf, J.F., Stanley, J.H., and LeRoy, E.C.: Interstitial lung disease in scleroderma. analysis by bronchoalveolar lavage. Arthritis Rheum., *27*:1254–1261, 1984.

120. Salerni, R., et al.: Pulmonary hypertension in the CREST syndrome variant of progressive systemic sclerosis (scleroderma). Ann. Intern. Med., *86*:394–399, 1977.

121. Germain, B.F.: Cardiopulmonary function in the CREST syndrome. Arthritis Rheum., *24*(Suppl. 1):S105, 1981.

122. Stupi, A., et al.: Pulmonary hypertension (PHT) in the CREST syndrome variant of progressive systemic sclerosis (PSS). Arthritis Rheum., *29*:515–524, 1986.

123. Ungerer, R.G., et al.: Prevalence and clinical correlates of pulmonary arterial hypertension in progressive systemic sclerosis. Am. J. Med., *75*:65–74, 1983.

124. Shuck, J.W., Oetgen, W.J., and Tesar, J.T.: Pulmonary vascular response during Raynaud's phenomenon in progressive systemic sclerosis. Am. J. Med., *78*:221–227, 1985.

125. Fahey, P.J., et al.: Raynaud's phenomenon of the lung. Am. J. Med., *76*:263–269, 1984.

126. Peters-Golden, M., et al.: Carbon monoxide diffusing capacity as predictor of outcome in systemic sclerosis. Am. J. Med., *77*:1027–1034, 1984.

127. Roumm, A.D., and Medsger, T.A., Jr.: Cancer and systemic sclerosis. Arthritis Rheum., *28*:1336–1340, 1985.

128. Peters-Golden, M., et al.: Incidence of lung cancer in systemic sclerosis. J. Rheumatol., *12*:1136–1139, 1985.

129. Weiss, S., et al.: Scleroderma heart disease with a consideration of certain other visceral manifestations of scleroderma. Arch. Intern. Med., *71*:749–776, 1943.

130. Follansbee, W.: The cardiovascular manifestations of systemic sclerosis (scleroderma). Curr. Probl. Cardiol., *11*:242–298, 1986.

131. Botstein, G.R., and LeRoy, E.C.: Primary heart disease in systemic sclerosis (scleroderma): Advances in clinical and pathologic features, pathogenesis and new therapeutic approaches. Am. Heart J., *102*:913–919, 1981.

132. Bulkley, B.H.: Progressive systemic sclerosis: Cardiac involvement. Clin. Rheum. Dis., *5*:131–149, 1979.

133. Smith, J.W., et al.: Echocardiographic features of progressive systemic sclerosis (PSS). Correlation with hemodynamic and postmortem studies. Am. J. Med., *66*:28–33, 1979.

134. McWhorter, J.E., and LeRoy, E.C.: Pericardial disease in scleroderma (systemic sclerosis). Am. J. Med., *57*:566–574, 1974.

135. Duska, F., et al.: Pyrophosphate heart scan in patients with progressive systemic sclerosis. Br. Heart J., *47*:90–93, 1982.

136. Follansbee, W.P., et al.: Physiologic abnormalities of cardiac function in progressive systemic sclerosis with diffuse scleroderma. N. Engl. J. Med., *310*:142–148, 1984.

137. Gaffney, F.A., et al.: Cardiovascular function in patients with progressive systemic sclerosis (scleroderma). Clin. Cardiol., *5*:569–576, 1982.

138. West, S.G., Killian, P.J., and Lawless, D.J.: Association of myositis and myocarditis in progressive systemic sclerosis. Arthritis Rheum., *24*:662–667, 1981.

139. Carette, S., Turcotte, J., and Mathon, G.: Severe myositis and myocarditis in progressive systemic sclerosis. J. Rheumatol., *12*:997–999, 1985.

140. Todesco, S., et al.: Cardiac involvement in progressive systemic sclerosis. Acta Cardiol., *5*:311–322, 1979.

141. Long, A., Duffy, G., and Bresnihan, B.: Reversible myocardial perfusion defects during cold challenge in scleroderma. Br. J. Rheumatol., *25*:158–161, 1986.

142. Alexander, E.L., et al.: Reversible cold-induced abnormalities in myocardial perfusion and function in systemic sclerosis. Ann. Intern. Med.,*105*:661–668, 1986.

143. Ellis, W.W., et al.: Left ventricular dysfunction induced by cold exposure in patients with systemic sclerosis. Am. J. Med., *80*:385–392, 1986.

144. Kahan, A., et al.: Nifedipine and thallium-201 myocardial perfusion in progressive systemic sclerosis. N. Engl. J. Med., *314*:1397–1402, 1986.

145. Kahan, A., et al.: Pharmacodynamic effect of dipyridamole on thallium-201 myocardial perfusion in progressive systemic sclerosis with diffuse scleroderma. Ann. Rheum. Dis., *45*:718–725, 1986.

146. Nitenberg, A., et al.: Reduced coronary flow and resistance reserve in primary scleroderma myocardial disease. Am. Heart J., *112*:309–315, 1986.

146a.Kahan, A., et al.: Decreased coronary reserve in primary scleroderma myocardial disease. Arthritis Rheum., *28*:637–646, 1985.

147. James, T.N.: De subitaneis mortibus: VIII. Coronary arteries and conduction system in scleroderma heart disease. Circulation, *50*:844–956, 1974.

148. Clements, P.J., et al.: The relationship of arrhythmias and conduction disturbances to other manifestations of cardiopulmonary disease in progressive systemic sclerosis (PSS). Am. J. Med., *71*:38–46, 1981.

149. Roberts, N.K., et al.: The prevalence of conduction defects and cardiac arrhythmias in progressive systemic sclerosis. Ann. Intern. Med., *94*:38–40, 1981.

149a.Blom-Bulow, B., Jonson, B., and Bauer, K.: Factors limiting exercise performance in progressive systemic sclerosis. Semin. Arthritis Rheum., *13*:174–181, 1983.

150. Roberts, N.K.: The morphology of the atrioventricular node in scleroderma: A three-dimensional reconstruction. Eur. Heart J., *1*:361–367, 1980.

151. Roberts, N.K., and Cabeen, W.R.: Atrioventricular nodal function in progressive systemic sclerosis. Electrophysiological and morphological findings. Br. Heart J., *44*:529–533, 1980.

152. Ridolfi, R.L., Bulkley, B.H., and Hutchins, G.M.: The cardiac conduction system in progressive systemic sclerosis. Clinical and pathologic features of 35 patients. Am. J. Med., *61*:361–366, 1976.

153. Yunus, M.B., et al.: Aortic regurgitation in scleroderma. J. Rheumatol., *11*:384–386, 1984.

154. D'Angelo, W.A., et al.: Pathologic observations in systemic

sclerosis (scleroderma). Study of 58 autopsy cases and 58 matched controls. Am. J. Med., *46*:428–440, 1969.

155. Steen, V.D.: Factors predicting the development of renal involvement in progressive systemic sclerosis. Am. J. Med., *76*:779–786, 1984.

156. Sundar, A.S., et al.: Kidney in progressive systemic sclerosis. Indian J. Med. Res., *82*:534–539, 1985.

157. Salyer, W.R., Salyer, D.C., and Heptinstall, R.H.: Scleroderma and microangiopathic hemolytic anemia. Ann. Intern. Med., *78*:895–897, 1973.

158. Traub, Y.M., et al.: Hypertension and renal failure (scleroderma renal crisis) in progressive systemic sclerosis. Report of a 25-year experience with 68 cases. Medicine, *62*:335–352, 1984.

159. Lam, M., et al.: Reversal of severe renal failure in systemic sclerosis. Ann. Intern. Med., *89*:642–643, 1978.

160. Mitnick, P., and Feig, P.U.: Control of hypertension and reversal of renal failure in scleroderma. N. Engl. J. Med., *299*:871–872, 1978.

161. Markenson, J.A., and Sherman, M.L.: Renal involvement in progressive systemic sclerosis: Prolonged survival with aggressive antihypertensive management. Arthritis Rheum., *22*:1132–1134, 1979.

162. Wasner, C., Cooke, C.R., and Fries, J.F.: Successful medical treatment of scleroderma renal crisis. N. Engl. J. Med., *299*:873–875, 1978.

163. Beckett, V.L., et al.: Use of captopril as early therapy for renal scleroderma: A prospective study. Mayo Clin. Proc., *60*:763–771, 1985.

164. Cannon, P.J., et al.: The relationship of hypertension and renal failure in scleroderma (progressive systemic sclerosis) to structural and functional abnormalities of the renal cortical circulation. Medicine, *53*:1–46, 1974.

165. Moore, H.C., and Sheehan, H.L.: The kidney of scleroderma. Lancet, *1*:68–70, 1952.

166. Lapenas, D., Rodnan, G.P., and Cavallo, T.: Immunopathology of the renal vascular lesion of progressive systemic sclerosis (scleroderma). Am. J. Pathol., *91*:243–258, 1978.

167. McGiven, A.R., deBoer, W.G.R.M., and Barnett, A.J.: Renal immune deposits in scleroderma. Pathology, *3*:145–150, 1971.

168. Winograd, J., Schimmel, D.H., and Palubinskas, A.J.: The spotted nephrogram of renal scleroderma. Am. J. Roentgenol., *126*:734–738, 1976.

169. Oliver, J.A., et al.: Renal vasoactive hormones in scleroderma (progressive systemic sclerosis). Nephron, *29*:110–116, 1981.

170. Kovalchik, M.T., et al.: The kidney in progressive systemic sclerosis. A prospective study. Ann. Intern. Med., *89*:881–887, 1978.

171. D'Angelo, W.A., et al.: Functional renal involvement in normotensive patients with progressive systemic sclerosis. Impaired sodium excretion during isotonic saline infusion. Arthritis Rheum., *24*:8–11, 1981.

172. Guillevin, L., Godeau, P., and Leenhardt, A.: Renin-angiotensin system in normotensive and hypertensive patients with progressive systemic sclerosis: Hyporesponsiveness of renin during captopril test. Postgrad. Med. J., *59*(Suppl. 3):171–172, 1983.

173. Gratwick, G.M., et al.: Fibrinogen turnover in progressive systemic sclerosis. Arthritis Rheum., *21*:343–347, 1978.

174. Lally, E.V., et al.: Pathologic involvement of the urinary bladder in progressive systemic sclerosis. J. Rheumatol., *12*:778–781, 1985.

175. Reynolds, T.B., et al.: Primary biliary cirrhosis with scleroderma, Raynaud's phenomenon and telangiectasia: New syndrome. Am. J. Med., *50*:302–312, 1971.

176. Culp, K.S., et al.: Autoimmune association in primary biliary cirrhosis. Mayo Clin. Proc., *57*:365–370, 1982.

177. Clarke, A.K., Galbraith, R.M., Hamilton, E.D.B., and Williams, R.: Rheumatic disorders in primary biliary cirrhosis. Ann. Rheum. Dis., *37*:42–47, 1978.

178. Gupta, R.C., et al.: Precipitating autoantibodies to mitochondrial proteins in progressive systemic sclerosis. Clin. Exp. Immunol., *58*:68–76, 1984.

179. Alderuccio, F., Toh, B-H., Barnett, A.J., and Pedersen, J.S.: Identification and characterization of mitochondria autoantigens in progressive systemic sclerosis: Identity with the 72,000 dalton autoantigen in primary biliary cirrhosis. J. Immunol., *137*:1855–1859, 1986.

180. Russell, M.L., and Kahn, J.J.: Nodular regenerative hyperplasia of the liver associated with progressive systemic sclerosis: A case report with ultrastructural observation. J. Rheumatol., *10*:748–752, 1983.

181. Greif, J.M., and Wolff, W.I.: Idiopathic calcific pancreatitis, CREST syndrome and progressive systemic sclerosis. Am. J. Gastroenterol., *71*:177–182, 1979.

182. Abraham, A.A., and Joos, A.: Pancreatic necrosis in progressive systemic sclerosis. Ann. Rheum. Dis., *39*:396–398, 1980.

183. Cobden, I., Axon, A.T.R., and Rowell, N.R.: Pancreatic exocrine function in systemic sclerosis. Br. J. Dermatol., *105*:189–193, 1981.

184. Westerman, M.P., et al.: Anemia and scleroderma: Frequency, causes and marrow findings. Arch. Intern. Med., *122*:39–42, 1968.

185. Frayha, R.A., Shulman, L.E., and Stevens, M.B.: Hematological abnormalities in scleroderma. A study of 180 cases. Acta Haematol., *64*:25–30, 1980.

186. Sumithran, E.: Progressive systemic sclerosis and autoimmune haemolytic anemia. Postgrad. Med. J., *52*:173–176, 1976.

187. Waugh, D., and Ibels, L.: Malignant scleroderma associated with autoimmune neutropenia. Br. Med. J., *280*:1577–1578, 1980.

188. Falanga, V., and Medsger, T.A., Jr.: Frequency, levels and significance of blood eosinophilia in systemic sclerosis, localized scleroderma and eosinophilic fasciitis. J. Am. Acad. Dermatol., *17*:648–656, 1987.

189. Lee, P., Bruni, J., and Sukenik, S.: Neurological manifestations in systemic sclerosis (scleroderma). J. Rheumatol., *11*:480–483, 1984.

189a. Clement, G.B., et al.: Neuropathic arthropathy (Charcot joints) due to cervical osteolysis: A complication of progressive systemic sclerosis. J. Rheumatol., *11*:545–548, 1984.

190. Farrell, D.A., and Medsger, T.A., Jr.: Trigeminal neuropathy in progressive systemic sclerosis. Am. J. Med., *73*:57–62, 1982.

191. Teasdall, R.D., Frayha, R.A., and Shulman, L.E.: Cranial nerve involvement in systemic sclerosis (scleroderma): A report of 10 cases. Medicine, *59*:149–159, 1980.

192. Estey, E., et al.: Cerebral arteritis in scleroderma. Stroke, *10*:595–597, 1979.

193. Oddis, C.V., et al.: Vasculitis in systemic sclerosis: Association with Sjögren's syndrome and the CREST syndrome variant. J. Rheumatol., *14*:942–948, 1987.

194. Lally, E.V., and Jimenez, S.A.: Impotence in progressive systemic sclerosis. Ann. Intern. Med., *95*:150–153, 1981.

195. Nowlin, N.S., et al.: Impotence in scleroderma. Ann. Intern. Med., *104*:794–798, 1986.

196. Sonnex, C., Paice, E., and White, A.G.: Autonomic neurop-

athy in systemic sclerosis: A case report and elevation of six patients. Ann. Rheum. Dis., *45*:957–960, 1986.

197. West, R.H., and Barnett, A.J.: Ocular involvement in scleroderma. Br. J. Ophthalmol., *63*:845–847, 1979.

198. Germain, B.F., et al.: Choroidal angiopathy in the CREST syndrome. Clin. Res., *29*:164A, 1981.

199. Grennan, D.M., and Forrester, J.A.: Involvement of the eye in SLE and scleroderma. Ann. Rheum. Dis., *36*:152–156, 1977.

200. Tosti, A., Patrizi, A., and Veronesi, S.: Audiologic involvement in systemic sclerosis. Dermatologica, *168*:206, 1984.

201. Osial, T.A., Jr., et al.: Clinical and serologic study of Sjögren's syndrome in patients with progressive systemic sclerosis. Arthritis Rheum., *26*:500–508, 1983.

202. Alexander, E.L., et al.: Sjögren's syndrome: Association of anti-Ro (SS-A) antibodies with vasculitis, hematologic abnormalities, and serologic hyperreactivity. Ann. Intern. Med., *98*:155–159, 1983.

203. Kahl., L.E., et al.: Prospective evaluation of thyroid function in progressive systemic sclerosis. (Abstract.) Arthritis Rheum., *26*:S62, 1983.

204. Nicholson, D., et al.: Progressive systemic sclerosis and Graves' disease. Report of 3 cases. Arch. Intern. Med., *146*:2350–2352, 1986.

205. Powell, F.C., et al.: The anticentromere antibody: Disease specificity and clinical significance. Mayo Clin. Proc., *59*:700–706, 1984.

206. Miller, M.H., et al.: The clinical significance of the anticentromere antibody. Br. J. Rheumatol., *26*:17–21, 1987.

207. Medsger, T.A., Jr., and Masi, A.T.: Epidemiology of progressive systemic sclerosis. Clin. Rheum. Dis., *5*:15–25, 1979.

208. Giordano, M., et al.: Different antibody patterns and different prognoses in patients with scleroderma with various extent of skin sclerosis. J. Rheumatol., *13*:911–916, 1986.

208a. Suarez-Almazor, M.E., et al.: Juvenile progressive systemic sclerosis: Clinical and serologic findings. Arthritis Rheum., *28*:699–702, 1985.

208b. Singsen, B.H.: Scleroderma in childhood. Pediatr. Clin. North Am., *33*:1119–1139, 1986.

208c. Hanson, V.: Dermatomyositis, scleroderma and polyarteritis nodosa. Clin. Rheum. Dis., *2*:455–464, 1976.

208d. Cassidy, J.T., Sullivan, D.B., Dabich, L., and Petty, R.E.: Scleroderma in children. Arthritis Rheum., *20*(Suppl.):351–354, 1977.

208e. Bernstein, R.M., et al.: Autoantibodies in childhood scleroderma. Ann. Rheum. Dis., *44*:503–506, 1985.

209. Giordano, M., Valentini, G., Lupoli, S., and Giordano, A.: Pregnancy and systemic sclerosis. Arthritis Rheum., *28*:237–238, 1985.

210. Ballou, S.P., Morley, J.J., and Kushner, I.: Pregnancy and systemic sclerosis. Arthritis Rheum., *27*:295–298, 1984.

211. Mor-Yosef, S., et al.: Collagen diseases in pregnancy. Obstet. Gynecol. Surv., *39*:67–84, 1984.

212. Steen, V.D., et al.: Pregnancy in systemic sclerosis. (Abstract). Arthritis Rheum., *30*:S118, 1987.

212a. Scarpinato, L., and MacKenzie, A.H.: Pregnancy and progressive systemic sclerosis: Case report and review of the literature. Cleve. Clin. Q., *52*:207–211, 1985.

213. Sood, S.V., and Kohler, H.G.: Maternal death from systemic sclerosis. (Report of a case of renal scleroderma masquerading as pre-eclamptic toxaemia). J. Obstet. Gynecol. Br. Commw., *77*:1109–1112, 1970.

214. Palma, A., et al.: Progressive systemic sclerosis and nephrotic syndrome. Arch. Intern. Med., *141*:520–521, 1981.

215. Duncan, S.C., and Winkelmann, R.K.: Cancer and scleroderma. Arch. Dermatol., *115*:950–955, 1979.

216. Medsger, T.A., and Masi, A.T.: The epidemiology of systemic sclerosis (scleroderma) among male U.S. veterans. J. Chronic Dis., *31*:73–85, 1978.

217. Black, K.A., et al.: Cancer in connective tissue disease. Arthritis Rheum., *25*:1130–1133, 1982.

218. Lee, P., et al.: Malignancy in progressive systemic sclerosis. Association with breast carcinoma. J. Rheumatol., *10*:665–666, 1983.

219. Talbott, J.H., and Barrocas, M.: Progressive systemic sclerosis (PSS) and malignancy, pulmonary and nonpulmonary. Medicine, *58*:182–207, 1979.

220. Sugai, S., et al.: B cell malignant lymphoma in a patient with progressive systemic sclerosis and Sjögren's syndrome. Jpn. J. Med., *24*:155–163, 1985.

221. Medsger T.A., Jr.: Systemic sclerosis and malignancy—Are they related? J. Rheumatol., *12*:1041–1043, 1985.

222. Postlethwaite, A.E., and Kang, A.H.: Pathogenesis of progressive systemic sclerosis. J. Lab. Clin. Med., *103*:506–510, 1984.

223. Sternberg, E.M.: Pathogenesis of scleroderma: The interrelationship of the immune and vascular hypotheses. Surv. Immunol. Res., *4*:69–80, 1985.

224. Haustein, U.F., Herrmann, K., and Bohme, H.J.: Pathogenesis of progressive systemic sclerosis. Int. J. Dermatol., *25*:286–293, 1986.

225. Haynes, D.C., and Gershwin, M.E.: The immunopathology of progressive systemic sclerosis. Semin. Arthritis Rheum., *11*:331–351. 1982.

226. Bashey, R.E., et al.: Connective tissue synthesis by cultured scleroderma fibroblasts. II. Incorporation of 3-H glucosamine and synthesis of glycosaminoglycans. Arthritis Rheum., *20*:879–885, 1977.

227. Cabral, A., and Castor, C.W.: Connective tissue activation. XXVII. The behavior of skin fibroblasts from patients with scleroderma. Arthritis Rheum., *26*:1362–1369, 1983.

228. Bashey, R.I., Millan, A., and Jimenez, S.A.: Increased biosynthesis of glycosaminoglycans by scleroderma fibroblasts in culture. Arthritis Rheum., *27*:1040–1045, 1984.

229. Buckingham, R.B., et al.: Increased collagen accumulation in dermal fibroblast cultures from patients with progressive systemic sclerosis (scleroderma). J. Lab. Clin. Med., *92*:5–21, 1978.

230. LeRoy, E.C.: Increased collagen synthesis by scleroderma skin fibroblasts in vitro. A possible defect in the regulation or activation of the scleroderma fibroblast. J. Clin. Invest., *54*:880–889, 1974.

231. Jimenez, S.A., et al.: Co-ordinate increase in the expression of Type I and Type III collagen genes in progressive systemic sclerosis fibroblasts. Biochem. J., *237*:837–843, 1986.

232. Perlish, J.S., Timpl, R., and Fleischmajer, R.: Collagen synthesis regulation by the aminopropeptide of procollagen I in normal and scleroderma fibroblasts. Arthritis Rheum., *28*:647–651, 1985.

233. Jimenez, S.A., Yakowski, R.I., and Frontino, P.M.: Biosynthetic heterogeneity of sclerodermatous skin in organ cultures. J. Mol. Med., *2*:423–430, 1977.

234. Krieg, T., Perlish, J.S., Mauch, C., and Fleischmajer, R.: Collagen synthesis by scleroderma fibroblasts. Ann. N.Y. Acad. Sci., *460*:375–386, 1985.

235. Potter, S.R., et al.: Clinical associations of fibroblast growth promoting factor in scleroderma. J. Rheumatol., *11*:43–47, 1984.

236. Whiteside, T.L., Tsao, M., and Buckingham, R.B.: Purification of a GAG-stimulatory factor from supernatants of activated mononuclear cells. (Abstract.) Arthritis Rheum., 29:S29, 1986.

237. Falanga, V., Hebda, P.A., and Eaglstein, W.H.: Effect of platelet homogenate on *in vitro* glycosaminoglycan production by dermal fibroblasts from systemic sclerosis patients and normal controls. Br. J. Dermatol., 113:237–243, 1985.

238. Falanga, V., et al.: Transforming growth factor-beta: Selective increase in glycosaminoglycan synthesis by cultures of fibroblasts from patients with progressive systemic sclerosis. J. Invest. Dermatol., 89:100–104, 1987.

239. Botstein, G.R., Sherer, G.K., and LeRoy, E.C.: Fibroblast selection in scleroderma. An alternative model of fibrosis. Arthritis Rheum., 25:189–195, 1982.

240. Kahaleh, M.B., and LeRoy, E.C.: Effect of scleroderma serum on human fibroblast collagen production: possible selection through proliferation. J. Rheumatol., 13:99–102, 1986.

241. Fries, J.F., Hoopes, J.E., and Shulman, L.E.: Reciprocal skin grafts in systemic sclerosis (scleroderma). Arthritis Rheum., 14:571–578, 1971.

242. Haxthausen, H.: Studies in pathogenesis of morphea, vitiligo and acrodermatitis atrophicans by means of transplantation experiments. Acta Derm. Venereol., 27:352–367, 1947.

243. Scharer, L., and Smith, D.W.: Resorption of the terminal phalanges in scleroderma. Arthritis Rheum., 12:51–63, 1969.

244. Varga, J., and Jimenez, S.A.: Development of severe limited scleroderma in complicated Raynaud's phenomenon after limb immobilization: Report of two cases and study of collagen biosynthesis. Arthritis Rheum., 29:1160–1165, 1986.

245. LeRoy, E.C.: Pathogenesis of scleroderma (systemic sclerosis). J. Invest. Dermatol., 79(Suppl. 1):87S–89S, 1982.

246. Lee, P., Norman, C.S., Sukenik, S., and Alderdice, C.A.: The clinical significance of coagulation abnormalities in systemic sclerosis (scleroderma). J. Rheumatol., 12:514–517, 1985.

247. Belch, J.J.F., et al.: Vascular damage and factor-VIII-related antigen in the rheumatic diseases. Rheumatol. Int., 7:107–111, 1987.

248. Kahaleh, M.B., Osborn, I., and LeRoy, E.C.: Increased factor VIII/von Willebrand factor antigen and von Willebrand factor activity in scleroderma and in Raynaud's phenomenon. Ann. Intern. Med., 94:482–484, 1981.

249. Zeiler, J., et al.: Serotonin content of platelets in inflammatory rheumatic diseases. Correlation with clinical activity. Arthritis Rheum., 26:532–540, 1983.

250. Friedhoff, L.T., Seibold, J.R., Kim, H.C., and Simester, K.S.: Serotonin induced platelet aggregation in systemic sclerosis. Clin. Exp. Rheumatol., 2:119–123, 1984.

251. Kahaleh, M.B., Osborn, I., and LeRoy, E.C.: Elevated levels of circulating platelet aggregates and beta-thromboglobulin in scleroderma. Ann. Intern. Med., 96:610–613, 1982.

251a.Seibold, J.R., and Harris, J.N.: Plasma β-thromboglobulin in the differential diagnosis of Raynaud's phenomenon. J. Rheumatol., 12:99–103, 1985.

252. Cohen, S., Johnson, A.R., and Hurd, E.: Cytotoxicity of sera from patients with scleroderma. Effects of human endothelial cells and fibroblasts in culture. Arthritis Rheum., 26:170–178, 1983.

253. Kahaleh, M.D., and LeRoy, E.C.: Endothelial injury in scleroderma. A protease mechanism. J. Lab. Clin. Med., 101:553–560, 1983.

254. Meyer, D., et al.: Vascular endothelial cell injury in progressive systemic sclerosis and other connective tissue diseases. Clin. Exp. Rheumatol., 1:29–34, 1983.

255. Shanahan, W.R., Jr., and Korn, J.H.: Cytotoxic activity of sera from scleroderma and other connective tissue diseases: Lack of cellular and disease specificity. Arthritis Rheum., 25:1381–1395, 1982.

255a.Summers, G.D., Weiss, J.B., and Jayson, M.I.V.: Failure of sera from patients with scleroderma to exhibit cytotoxicity towards human umbilical vein endothelial cells. Rheumatol. Int., 5:9–13, 1984.

256. Penning, C.A., et al.: Antibody-dependent cellular cytotoxicity of human vascular endothelium in systemic sclerosis. Clin. Exp. Immunol., 58:548–556, 1984.

257. Maslen, C.L., et al.: Enhanced oxidative metabolism of neutrophils from patients with systemic sclerosis. Br. J. Rheumatol., 26:113–117, 1987.

258. Kovacs, I.B., et al.: Plasma or serum from patients with systemic sclerosis alters behaviour of normal erythrocytes. Ann. Rheum. Dis., 44:395–398, 1985.

259. Maricq, H.R., Downey, J.A., and LeRoy, E.C.: Standstill of nailfold capillary blood flow during cooling in scleroderma and Raynaud's syndrome. Blood Vessels, 13:338, 1976.

260. Stevens, M.B., et al.: Aperistalsis of the esophagus in patients with connective tissue disorders and Raynaud's phenomenon. N. Engl. J. Med., 270:1218–1222, 1964.

261. Coffman, J.D.: Skin blood flow in scleroderma. J. Lab. Clin. Med., 76:480–484, 1970.

262. Kristensen, J.K., and Wadskov, S.: Increased 133 xenon washout from cutaneous tissue in generalized scleroderma indicates increased blood flow. Acta Derm. Venereol., 58:313–317, 1978.

263. Barnett, A.J.: Some observations on the immunological status in scleroderma (progressive systemic sclerosis). Aust. N.Z. J. Med., 8:622–627, 1978.

264. Cazalis, P., et al.: Rheumatismes inflammatories et gammopathies monoclonales benignes: Aspects cliniques et deviner. Rev. Rhum. Mal. Osteoartic., 41:698–702, 1974.

265. Kogo, Y., et al.: A case of the progressive systemic sclerosis (PSS) with high serum concentration of M protein. Jpn. Soc. Intern. Med., 64:1167–1173, 1975.

266. Ja, S., Helm, S., and Wary, B.B.: Progressive systemic scleroderma with IgA deficiency in a child. Am. J. Dis. Child., 135:965–966, 1981.

267. Husson, J.M., et al.: Systemic sclerosis and cryoglobulinemia. Clin. Immunol. Immunopathol., 6:77–82, 1976.

268. O'Laughlin, S., Tappeiner, G., and Jordon, R.E.: Circulating immune complexes in systemic scleroderma and generalized morphea. Dermatologica, 160:25–30, 1980.

269. Seibold, J.R., et al.: Immune complexes in progressive systemic sclerosis. Arthritis Rheum., 25:1167–1173, 1982.

270. Cunningham, P.H., Andrews, B.S., and Davis, J.S.: Immune complexes in progressive systemic sclerosis and mixed connective tissue disease. J. Rheumatol., 7:301–308, 1980.

271. Chen, Z., et al.: Immune complexes and antinuclear, antinucleolar and anticentromere antibodies in scleroderma. J. Am. Acad. Dermatol., 11:461–467, 1984.

272. French, M.A.H., et al.: Serum immune complexes in systemic sclerosis: Relationship with precipitating nuclear antibodies. Ann. Rheum. Dis., 44:89–92, 1985.

273. Bernstein, R.M., Steigerwald, J.C., and Tan, E.M.: Association of antinuclear and antinucleolar antibodies in progressive systemic sclerosis. Clin. Exp. Immunol., 48:43–51, 1982.

274. Schur, P.H., Monroe, M., and Rothfield, N.: The G subclass of antinuclear and antinucleic acid antibodies. Arthritis Rheum., 15:174–182, 1972.

275. Douvas, A.S., Achten, M., and Tan, E.M.: Identification of a nuclear protein (Scl-70) as a unique target of human anti-

nuclear antibodies in scleroderma. J. Biol. Chem., 254:10514–10522, 1979.

276. Catoggio, L.J., et al.: Serological markers in progressive systemic sclerosis: Clinical correlations. Ann. Rheum. Dis., 42:23–27, 1983.

277. Jarzabek-Chorzelska, M., et al.: Scl 70 antibody—a specific marker of systemic sclerosis. Br. J. Dermatol., 115:391–401, 1986.

278. Catoggio, L.J., et al.: Autoantibodies in Argentine patients with systemic sclerosis (scleroderma). Arthritis Rheum., 28:715–717, 1985.

279. Shero, J.H., Bordwell, B., Rothfield, N.F., and Earnshaw, W.C.: High titers of autoantibodies to topoisomerase I (Scl-70) in sera from scleroderma patients. Science, 231:737–740, 1986.

280. Guldner, H.-H., et al.: Scl 70 autoantibodies from scleroderma patients recognize a 95 kDa protein identified as DNA topoisomerase I. Chromosoma, 94:132–138, 1986.

281. Burnham, T.K., and Kleinsmith, D'A.M.: The "true speckled" antinuclear antibody (ANA) pattern: Its tumultuous history. Semin. Arthritis Rheum., 13:155–159, 1983.

282. Steen, V.D., et al.: Clinical and laboratory associations of anticentromere antibody (ACA) in patients with progressive systemic sclerosis (scleroderma). Arthritis Rheum., 27:125–131, 1984.

283. Chorzelski, T.P., et al.: Anticentromere antibody: An immunological marker of a subset of systemic sclerosis. Br. J. Dermatol., 113:381–389, 1985.

284. Kallenberg, C.G.M., et al.: Antinuclear antibodies in patients with Raynaud's phenomenon. Clinical significance of anticentromere antibodies. Ann. Rheum. Dis., 41:382–387, 1982.

285. Migliaresi, S.: Infrequency of anticentromere antibody in patients without systemic sclerosis and without Raynaud's phenomenon. Arthritis Rheum., 30:358–359, 1987.

286. McCarty, G.A., et al.: Anticentromere antibody. Clinical correlations and association with favorable prognosis in patients with scleroderma variants. Arthritis Rheum., 26:1–7, 1983.

287. Tramposch, H.D., et al.: A long-term longitudinal study of anticentromere antibodies. Arthritis Rheum., 27:121–124, 1984.

288. Brenner, S., et al.: Kinetochore structure, duplication, and distribution in mammalian cells: Analysis by human autoantibodies from scleroderma patients. J. Cell. Biol., 91:95–102, 1981.

289. Earnshaw, W., Bordwell, B., Marino, C., and Rothfield, N.: Three human chromosomal autoantigens are recognized by sera from patients with anti-centromere antibodies. J. Clin. Invest., 77:426–430, 1986.

290. Ruffatti, A., et al.: Association of anti-centromere and anti-Scl 70 antibodies in scleroderma. Report of two cases. J. Clin. Lab. Immunol., 16:227–229, 1985.

291. Reimer, G., et al.: Correlates between autoantibodies to nucleolar antigens and clinical features in patients with systemic sclerosis (scleroderma). Arthritis Rheum. (in press)

292. Reimer, G., Rose, K.M., Scheer, U., and Tan, E.M.: Autoantibody to RNA polymerase I in scleroderma sera. J. Clin. Invest., 79:65–72, 1987.

293. Targoff, I.N., and Reichlin, M.: Nucleolar localization of the PM-Scl antigens. Arthritis Rheum., 28:226–230, 1985.

294. Treadwell, E.L., Alspaugh, M.A., Wolfe, J.F., and Sharp, G.C.: Clinical relevance of PM-1 antibody and physiochemical characterization of PM-1 antigen. J. Rheumatol., 11:658–662, 1984.

295. Furst, D.E., et al.: Case control study of antibodies in ENA in progressive systemic sclerosis patients. J. Rheumatol., 11:298–305, 1984.

296. Mimori, T., et al.: Characterization of a high molecular weight acidic nuclear protein recognized by autoantibodies in sera from patients with polymyositis-scleroderma overlap. J. Clin. Invest., 68:611–620, 1981.

297. Fritzler, M.J., et al.: An antigen in metaphase chromatin and the midbody of mammalian cells binds to scleroderma sera. J. Rheumatol., 14:291–294, 1987.

298. Osborn, T.G., et al.: Anticentriole antibody in a patient with progressive systemic sclerosis. Arthritis Rheum., 29:142–146, 1986.

299. Moroi, Y., et al.: Human anticentriole autoantibody in patients with scleroderma and Raynaud's phenomenon. Clin. Immunol. Immunopathol., 29:381–390, 1983.

300. Osborn, T.G., et al.: Antinuclear antibody staining only centrioles in a patient with scleroderma. N. Engl. J. Med., 307:253–254, 1982.

301. Pruzanski, W., et al.: Lymphocytotoxic and phagocytotoxic activity in progressive systemic sclerosis. J. Rheumatol., 10:55–60, 1983.

302. Labro, M.T., Perianin, A., and Kahn, M.F.: Detection of antilymphocyte antibodies in patients with scleroderma using three different techniques. Clin. Rheumatol., 3:435–442, 1984.

303. Seibold, J.R., Knight, P.J., and Peter, J.B.: Anticardiolipin antibodies in systemic sclerosis. (Letter.) Arthritis Rheum., 29:1052–1053, 1986.

304. Heinzerling, R.H., et al.: Elevated levels of antibodies to polyuridylic acid detected and quantitated in systemic scleroderma patients by solid phase radioimmunoassay. J. Invest. Dermatol., 75:224–227, 1980.

305. Mackel, A.M., et al.: Antibodies to collagen in scleroderma. Arthritis Rheum., 25:522–531, 1982.

306. Padula, S.J., Clark, R.B., and Korn, J.H.: Cell-mediated immunity in rheumatic disease. Clin. Rheum. Dis., 17:254–263, 1986.

307. Whiteside, T.L., et al.: Suppressor cell function and T lymphocyte subpopulations in peripheral blood of patients with progressive systemic sclerosis. Arthritis Rheum., 26:841–847, 1983.

308. Stuart, J.M., Postlethwaite, A.E., and Kang, A.H.: Evidence for cell-mediated immunity to collagen in progressive systemic sclerosis. J. Lab. Clin. Med., 88:601–607, 1976.

309. Fritz, J., and Sandhofer, M.: Zellulare Immunophanomene bei der Sklerodermie. Dermatologica, 154:129–137, 1977.

310. Postlethwaite, A.E., Snyderman, R., and Kang, A.H.: The chemotactic attraction of human fibroblasts to a lymphocyte-derived factor. J. Exp. Med., 144:1188–1203, 1976.

311. Cathcart, M.K., and Krakauer, R.S.: Immunologic enhancement of collagen accumulation in progressive systemic sclerosis (PSS). Clin. Immunol. Immunopathol., 21:128–133, 1981.

312. Johnson, R.L., and Ziff, M.: Lymphokine stimulation of collagen accumulation. J. Clin. Invest., 58:240–242, 1976.

313. Kahaleh, M.B., DeLustro, F., Bock, W., and LeRoy, E.C.: Human monocyte modulation of endothelial cells and fibroblast growth: Possible mechanism for fibrosis. Clin. Immunol. Immunopathol., 39:242–255, 1986.

314. Whiteside, T.L., Buckingham, R.B., Prince, R.K., and Rodnan, G.P.: Products of activated mononuclear cells modulate accumulation of collagen by normal dermal and scleroderma fibroblasts in culture. J. Lab. Clin. Med., 104:355–369, 1984.

315. Duncan, M.R., Perlish, J.S., and Fleischmajer, R.: Lymphokine-monokine inhibition of fibroblast proliferation and col-

lagen production: Role in progressive systemic sclerosis (PSS). J. Invest. Dermatol., *83*:377–384, 1984.

315a. Alcocer-Varela, J., Martinez-Cordero, E., and Alarcon-Segovia, D.: Spontaneous production of, and defective response to, interleukin-1 by peripheral blood mononuclear cells from patients with scleroderma. Clin. Exp. Immunol., *59*:666–672, 1985.

316. Sandborg, C.I., Berman, M.A., Andrews, B.S., and Friou, G.J.: Interleukin-1 production by mononuclear cells from patients with scleroderma. Clin. Exp. Immunol., *60*:294–302, 1985.

317. Miller, E.B., Hiserodt, J.C., and Medsger, T.A., Jr.: Natural killer cell numbers in systemic sclerosis. (Abstract.) Arthritis Rheum., *30*:S97, 1987.

318. Miller, E.B., Hiserodt, J.C., Steen, V.D., and Medsger, T.A., Jr.: Decreased natural killer cell (NK) function in systemic sclerosis. (Abstract.) Arthritis Rheum., *30*:S97, 1987.

319. Freundlich, B., and Jimenez, S.A.: Peripheral blood lymphocytic phenotype in patients with progressive systemic sclerosis. (Abstract.) Arthritis Rheum., *29*:S30, 1986.

320. Majewski, S.: Natural killer cell activity of peripheral blood mononuclear cells from patients with various forms of systemic sclerosis. Br. J. Dermatol., *116*:1–8, 1987.

321. Worrall, J.G., et al.: Persistence of scleroderma-like phenotype in normal dermal fibroblasts after prolonged exposure to soluble mediators from mononuclear cells. Arthritis Rheum., *29*:54–64, 1986.

322. Whiteside, T.L., et al.: Soluble mediators from mononuclear cells increase the synthesis of glycosaminoglycan by dermal fibroblast cultures derived from normal subjects and progressive systemic sclerosis patients. Arthritis Rheum., *28*:188–197, 1985.

323. Korn, J.H., Torres, D., and Downie, E.: Clonal heterogeneity in the fibroblast response to mononuclear cell derived mediators. Arthritis Rheum., *27*:174–179, 1984.

324. Kaminski, M.J., et al.: Lowered angiogenic capability of peripheral blood lymphocytes in progressive systemic sclerosis (scleroderma). J. Invest. Dermatol., *83*:238–243, 1984.

325. Marczak, M., et al.: Enhanced angiogenic capability of monocyte-enriched mononuclear cell suspensions from patients with systemic scleroderma. J. Invest. Dermatol., *86*:355–358, 1986.

326. Majewski, S., et al.: Modulatory effect of sera from scleroderma patients on lymphocyte-induced angiogenesis. Arthritis Rheum., *28*:1133–1139, 1985.

327. Kahan, A., Menkes, C.J., and Amor, B.: Defective Epstein-Barr virus specific suppressor T cell function in progressive systemic sclerosis. Ann. Rheum. Dis., *45*:553–560, 1986.

328. Strosberg, J.M., Peck, B., and Harris, E.D., Jr.: Scleroderma with intestinal involvement: Fatal in two of a kindred. J. Rheumatol., *4*:46–52, 1977.

329. Frayha, R.A., Tabbara, K.F., and Gena, R.S.: Familial CREST syndrome with sicca complex. J. Rheumatol., *4*:53–58, 1977.

330. Rothfield, N.F., and Rodnan, G.P.: Serum antinuclear antibodies in systemic sclerosis (scleroderma). Arthritis Rheum., *11*:607–611, 1968.

331. Ruffatti, A., et al.: Prevalence of anticentromere antibody in blood relatives of anticentromere positive patients. J. Rheumatol., *12*:940–943, 1985.

332. Briggs, D.C., Welsh, K., Pereira, R.S., and Black, C.M.: A strong association between null alleles at the C4A locus in the major histocompatibility complex and systemic sclerosis. Arthritis Rheum., *29*:1274–1277, 1986.

333. Birnbaum, N.S., et al.: Histocompatibility antigens in pro-

gressive systemic sclerosis (scleroderma). J. Rheumatol., *4*:425–428, 1977.

334. Whiteside, T.L., Medsger, T.A., Jr., and Rodnan, G.P.: HLA-DR antigens in progressive systemic sclerosis (scleroderma). J. Rheumatol., *10*:128–131, 1983.

335. Emerit, I.: Chromosomal abnormalities in progressive systemic sclerosis. Clin. Rheum. Dis., *5*:201–214, 1979.

336. Pruzanski, W., et al.: Lymphocytotoxic and phagocytotoxic activity in progressive systemic sclerosis. J. Rheumatol., *10*:55–60, 1983.

337. Lowe, W.C.: Scleroderma and amyloidosis. Milit. Med., *134*:1430–1433, 1969.

338. Sackner, M.A.: Scleroderma. New York, Grune & Stratton, 1966.

339. Claman, H.N., Jaffee, B.D., Huff, J.C., and Clark, R.A.F.: Chronic graft-versus-host disease as a model for scleroderma. Cell. Immunol., *94*:73–84, 1985.

340. Furst, D.E., et al.: A syndrome resembling progressive systemic sclerosis after bone marrow transplantation. A model for scleroderma? Arthritis Rheum., *22*:904–910, 1979.

341. Van Den Bergh, V., et al.: Diffuse fasciitis after bone marrow transplantation. Am. J. Med., *83*:139–143, 1987.

342. Osborn, T.G., et al.: The tight-skin mouse: Physical and biochemical properties of the skin. J. Rheumatol., *10*:793–796, 1983.

343. Jimenez, S.A., Millan, A., and Bashey, R.I.: Scleroderma-like alterations in collagen metabolism occurring in the TSK (tight skin) mouse. Arthritis Rheum., *27*:180–185, 1984.

344. Walker, M., et al.: Mast cells and their degranulation in the TSK mouse model of scleroderma. Proc. Soc. Exp. Biol. Med., *180*:323–328, 1985.

345. Russell, M.L.: The tight-skin mouse: Is it a role model for scleroderma? (Editorial.) J. Rheumatol., *10*:679–681, 1983.

346. Green, M.C., Sweet, H.O., and Bunker, L.E.: Tight-skin, a new mutation of the mouse causing excess growth of connective tissue and skeleton. Am. J. Pathol., *82*:493–507, 1976.

347. Gershwin, M.E., et al.: Characterization of a spontaneous disease of white leghorn chickens resembling progressive systemic sclerosis (scleroderma). J. Exp. Med., *153*:1640–1659, 1981.

348. Medsger, T.A., Jr.: Progressive systemic sclerosis. Clin. Rheum. Dis., *9*:655–670, 1983.

349. Helfrich, D.J., and Medsger, T.A., Jr.: Normotensive renal failure in systemic sclerosis (scleroderma). Arthritis Rheum., *31*:R41, 1988.

350. Nimni, M.: A defect in the intramolecular and intermolecular cross-linking of collagen caused by penicillamine: I. Metabolic and functional abnormalities in soft tissues. J. Biol. Chem., *243*:1457–1466, 1968.

351. Jayson, M.I.V., Lovell, C., and Black, C.M.: Penicillamine therapy in systemic sclerosis. Proc. R. Soc. Med., *70*:82–88, 1977.

352. Asboe-Hansen, G.: Treatment of generalized scleroderma: Updated results. Acta Derm. Venereol., *59*:465–467, 1979.

353. Asboe-Hansen, G.: Treatment of generalized scleroderma with inhibitors of connective tissue formation. Acta Derm. Venereol., *55*:461–465, 1975.

354. Ivanova, M.M., et al.: Treatment of systemic sclerosis with D-penicillamine. Ther. Arch., *7*:91–99, 1977.

355. Medsger, T.A., Jr.: D-Penicillamine treatment of lung involvement in patients with systemic sclerosis (scleroderma). Arthritis Rheum., *30*:832–834, 1987.

356. Steen, V.D., et al.: The effect of D-penicillamine on pulmonary

findings in systemic sclerosis. Arthritis Rheum., *28*:882–888, 1985.

357. deClerck, L.S., et al.: D-Penicillamine therapy and interstitial lung disease in scleroderma. A long-term followup study. Arthritis Rheum., *30*:643–650, 1987.

358. Ntoso, K.A., et al.: Penicillamine-induced rapidly progressive glomerulonephritis in patients with progressive systemic sclerosis: Successful treatment of two patients and a review of the literature. Am. J. Kidney Dis., *8*:159–163, 1986.

359. Tordres, C.F., et al.: Penicillamine-induced myasthenia gravis in progressive systemic sclerosis. Arthritis Rheum., *23*:900–908, 1980.

360. Miyagawa, S., et al.: Systemic sclerosis-like lesions during long-term penicillamine therapy for Wilson's disease. Br. J. Dermatol., *116*:95–100, 1987.

361. Steen, V.D., Blair, S., and Medsger, T.A., Jr.: The toxicity of D-penicillamine in systemic sclerosis. Ann. Intern. Med., *104*:699–705, 1986.

362. Shapiro, L.S., et al.: D-Penicillamine treatment of progressive systemic sclerosis (scleroderma): A comparison of clinical and in vitro effects. J. Rheumatol., *10*:316–318, 1983.

363. Furst, D.E., et al.: Measurement of clinical change in progressive systemic sclerosis: A 1 year double-blind placebo-controlled trial of N-acetylcysteine. Ann. Rheum. Dis., *38*:356–361, 1979.

364. Oriente, P., et al.: Progressive systemic sclerosis and S-adenosylmethionine. Clin. Rheum., *4*:360–361, 1985.

365. Alarcon-Segovia, D.: Progressive systemic sclerosis: Management. Part IV. Colchicine. Clin. Rheum. Dis., *5*:294–302, 1979.

366. Diegelmann, R.F., and Peterkofsky, B.: Inhibition of collagen secretion from bone and cultured fibroblasts by microtubular-disruptive drugs. Proc. Natl. Acad. Sci., U.S.A., *69*:892–896, 1972.

367. Ehrlich, H.P., and Bornstein, P.: Mictotubules in transcellular movement of procollagen. Nature (New Biol.), *238*:257–260, 1972.

368. Harris, E.D., Evanson, J.M., and Krane, S.M.: Effects of colchicine on collagenase in cultures of rheumatoid synovium. Arthritis Rheum., *14*:669–684, 1971.

369. Guttadauria, M., Diamond, H., and Kaplan, D.: Colchicine in the treatment of scleroderma. J. Rheumatol., *4*:272–275, 1977.

370. Jimenez, S.A.: Cellular immune dysfunction and the pathogenesis of scleroderma. Semin. Arthritis Rheum., *13*:104–113, 1983.

371. Jansen, G.T., et al.: Generalized scleroderma. Treatment with an immunosuppressive agent. Arch. Dermatol., *97*:690–698, 1968.

372. Casas, J.A., Subauste, C.P., and Alarcon, G.S.: A new promising treatment in systemic sclerosis (SS): 5-fluorouracil (5FU). (Abstract). Arthritis Rheum., *30*:S35, 1987.

373. Mackenzie, A.H.: Prolonged alkylating drug therapy is beneficial in systemic sclerosis. (Abstract.) Arthritis Rheum., *13*:334, 1970.

374. Steigerwald, J.C.: Chlorambucil therapy in progressive systemic sclerosis. J. Rheumatol., *1*:74, 1974.

375. Furst, D.E., et al.: Preliminary results of a double-blind parallel, randomized trial of chlorambucil vs. placebo in progressive systemic sclerosis (PSS). (Abstract.) Arthritis Rheum., *29*:S29, 1986.

376. Baker, G.L., et al.: Malignancy following treatment of rheumatoid arthritis with cyclosphophamide. Amer. J. Med., *83*:1–9, 1987.

377. Dau, P.C., Kahalen, M.D., and Sagebiel, R.W.: Plasmapheresis and immunosuppressive drug therapy in scleroderma. Arthritis Rheum., *24*:1128–1136, 1981.

378. Weiner, S.R., et al.: Preliminary report on a controlled trial of apheresis in the treatment of scleroderma. (Abstract.) Arthritis Rheum., *30*:S27, 1987.

379. Capodicasa, G., et al.: Clinical effectiveness of apheresis in the treatment of progressive systemic sclerosis. Int. J. Artif. Organs, *6*:81–86, 1983.

380. Guillevin, L., et al.: Treatment of progressive systemic sclerosis with plasma exchange. Seven cases. Int. J. Artif. Organs, *6*:315–318, 1983.

381. Zachariae, H., and Zachariae, E.: Cyclosporin A in systemic sclerosis. Br. J. Dermatol., *116*:741–742, 1987.

382. Rosenbloom, J., Feldman, G., Freunclich, B., and Jimenez, S.A.: Inhibition of excessive scleroderma fibroblast collagen production by recombinant γ-interferon. Association with a coordinate decrease in types I and III procollagen messenger RNA levels. Arthritis Rheum., *29*:851–856, 1986.

383. Kahaleh, M.D., Sherer, D.L., and LeRoy, E.C.: Endothelial injury in scleroderma. J. Exp. Med., *149*:1326–1335, 1979.

384. Beckett, V.L., et al.: Trial of platelet-inhibiting drug in scleroderma. Double-blind study with dipyridamole and aspirin. Arthritis Rheum., *27*:1137–1143, 1984.

385. Fries, J.F., et al.: A controlled trial of antihypertensive therapy in systemic sclerosis (scleroderma). Ann. Rheum. Dis., *43*:407–410, 1984.

386. Blunt, R.J., and Porter, J.M.: Raynaud's syndrome. Semin. Arthritis Rheum., *10*:282–308, 1981.

387. Jobe, J.B., et al.: Induced vasodilation as treatment for Raynaud's disease. Ann. Intern. Med., *97*:706–709, 1982.

388. Yocum, D.E., Hodes, R., Sundstrom, W.R., and Cleeland, C.S.: Use of biofeedback training in treatment of Raynaud's disease and phenomenon. J. Rheumatol., *12*:90–93, 1985.

389. McFayden, I.J., Housley, E., and MacPherson, A.I.S.: Intra-arterial reserpine administration in Raynaud's syndrome. Arch. Intern. Med., *132*:526–528, 1973.

390. Nobin, B.A., et al.: Reserpine treatment of Raynaud's disease. Ann. Surg., *187*:12–16, 1978.

391. Varadi, D.P., and Lawrence, A.M.: Suppression of Raynaud's phenomenon by methyldopa. Arch. Intern. Med., *124*:13–18, 1969.

392. Kahan, A., et al.: Nifedipine and Raynaud's phenomenon. (Letter.) Ann. Intern. Med., *94*:546, 1981.

393. Rodeheffer, R.J., et al.: Controlled double-blind trial of nifedipine in the treatment of Raynaud's phenomenon. N. Engl. J. Med., *308*:880–883, 1983.

394. Smith, C.D., and McKendry, R.J.R.: Controlled trial of nifedipine in the treatment of Raynaud's phenomenon. Lancet, *2*:1299–1301, 1982.

395. Finch, M.B., Dawson, J., and Johnston, G.D.: The peripheral vascular effects of nifedipine in Raynaud's syndrome associated with scleroderma: A double-blind crossover study. Clin. Rheumatol., *5*:493–498, 1986.

396. Surwit, R.S., Gilgor, R.S., Allen, L.M., and Duvic, M.: A double-blind study of prazosin in the treatment of Raynaud's phenomenon in scleroderma. Arch. Dermatol., *120*:329–331, 1984.

397. Seibold, J.R., and Jageneau, A.H.M.: Treatment of Raynaud's phenomenon with ketanserin, a selective antagonist of the serotonin 2 (5-HT2) receptor. Arthritis Rheum., *27*:139–146, 1984.

398. Stranden, E., Roald, D.K., and Krong, K.: Treatment of Raynaud's phenomenon with 5-HT-2 receptor antagonist ketanserin. Br. Med. J., *285*:1069–1071, 1982.

399. Franks, A.: Topical glyceryl trinitrate as adjunctive treatment in Raynaud's disease. Lancet, *1*:76, 1982.

400. Baron, M., et al.: Prostaglandin E₁ therapy for digital ulcers in scleroderma. Can. Med. Assoc. J., *126*:42–45, 1982.

401. Martin, M.F.R., and Tooke, J.E.: Effects of prostaglandin E₁ on microvascular haemodynamics in progressive systemic sclerosis. Br. Med. J., *285*:1688–1690, 1982.

402. Mizushima, Y., et al.: A multicenter double blind controlled study of lipo-PGE₁, PGE₁ incorporated in lipid microspheres, in peripheral vascular disease secondary to connective tissue disorders. J. Rheumatol., *14*:97–101, 1987.

403. Keller, J., et al.: Inhibition of platelet aggregation by a new stable prostacyclin introduced in therapy of patients with progressive scleroderma. Arch. Dermatol. Res., *277*:323–325, 1985.

404. Tosi, S., et al.: Treatment of Raynaud's phenomenon with captopril. Drugs Exp. Clin. Res., *13*:37–42, 1987.

405. Jones, N.F., Raynor, S.C., and Medsger, T.A.: Microsurgical revascularisation of the hand in scleroderma. Br. J. Plast. Surg., *40*:264–269, 1987.

406. Gahhos, F., Ariyan, S., Frazier, W.H., and Cuono, C.B.: Management of sclerodermal finger ulcers. J. Hand Surg., *9A*:320–327, 1984.

407. Lian, J.B., Skinner, M., Glimcher, M.J., and Gallop, P.M.: The presence of γ-carboxyglutamic acid in the proteins associated with ectopic calcification. Biochem. Biophys. Res. Commun., *73*:349–355, 1976.

408. Berger, R.G., et al.: Treatment of calcinosis universalis with low-dose warfarin. Am. J. Med., *83*:72–76, 1987.

409. Fuchs, D., et al.: Colchicine suppression of local inflammation due to calcinosis in dermatomyositis and progressive systemic sclerosis. Clin. Rheumatol., *5*:527–530, 1986.

410. Fuchs, D., et al.: Colchicine suppression of local inflammation due to calcinosis in dermatomyositis and progressive systemic sclerosis. Clin. Rheumatol., *5*:527–530, 1986.

411. Seeger, M.W., and Furst, D.E.: Effects of splinting in the treatment of hand contractures in progressive systemic sclerosis. Am. J. Occup. Ther., *41*:118–121, 1987.

412. Norris, R.W., and Brown, H.G.: The proximal interphalangeal joint in systemic sclerosis and its surgical management. Br. J. Plast. Surg., *38*:526–531, 1985.

412a.Naylor, W.P.: Oral management of the scleroderma patient. J. Am. Dent. Assoc., *105*:814, 1982.

412b.Naylor, W.P., and Manor, R.C.: Fabrication of a flexible prosthesis for the edentulous scleroderma patient with microstomia. J. Prosthet. Dent., *50*:536–538, 1983.

413. Ramirez-Mata, M., Ibanez, G., and Alarcon-Segovia, D.: Stimulatory effect of metaclopramide on the esophagus and lower esophageal sphincter of patients with PSS. Arthritis Rheum., *20*:30–34, 1977.

414. Horowitz, M., et al.: Effects of cisapride on gastric and esophageal emptying in progressive systemic sclerosis. Gastroenterology, *93*:311–315, 1987.

415. Hongo, M., et al.: Effects of nifedipine on esophageal motor function in humans. Correlations with plasma nifedipine concentration. Gastroenterology, *86*:8–12, 1984.

416. Kahan, A., et al.: Nifedipine and esophageal dysfunction in progressive systemic sclerosis. A controlled manometric study. Arthritis Rheum., *28*:490–495, 1985.

417. Jean, F., et al.: Effects of diltiazem versus nifedipine on lower esophageal sphincter pressure in patients with progressive systemic sclerosis. Arthritis Rheum., *29*:1054–1055, 1986.

418. Petrokubi, R.J., and Jeffries, G.H.: Cimetidine versus antacid in scleroderma with reflux esophagitis. A randomized double-blind controlled study. Gastroenterology, *77*:691–695, 1979.

419. Hendel, L., Aggestrup, S., and Stentoft, P.: Long-term ranitidine in progressive systemic sclerosis (scleroderma) with gastroesophageal reflux. Scand. J. Gastroenterol., *21*:799–805, 1986.

420. Netscher, D.T., and Richardson, J.D.: Complications requiring operative intervention in scleroderma. Surg. Gynecol. Obstet., *158*:507–512, 1984.

421. Henderson, R.D., and Pearson, F.G.: Surgical management of esophageal scleroderma. J. Thorac. Cardiovasc. Surg., *66*:686–692, 1973.

422. Orringer, M.B., et al.: Combined collis gastroplasty-fundoplication operations for scleroderma reflux esophagitis. Surgery, *90*:624–630, 1981.

423. Rees, W.D.W., et al.: Interdigestive motor activity in patients with systemic sclerosis. Gastroenterology, *83*:575–580, 1982.

424. Levien, D.H., Fiallos, F., Barone, R., and Taffet, S.: The use of cyclic home hyperalimentation for malabsorption in patients with scleroderma involving the small intestines. J. Parenter. Enter. Nutr., *9*:623–625, 1985.

425. Kallenberg, C.G.M., Jansen, H.M., Elema, J.D., and The, T.H.: Steroid-responsive interstitial pulmonary disease in systemic sclerosis. Monitoring by bronchoalveolar lavage. Chest, *86*:489–492, 1984.

426. Seibold, J.R., et al.: Acute hemodynamic effects of ketanserin in pulmonary hypertension secondary to systemic sclerosis. J. Rheumatol., *14*:519–524, 1987.

426a.Morrison, D., Goldman, S., and Alepa, F.P.: Unloading the right ventricle in the CREST syndrome variant of progressive systemic sclerosis (scleroderma). Clin. Cardiol., *7*:49–53, 1984.

426b.O'Brien, J.T., Hill, J.A., and Pepine, C.J.: Sustained benefit of verapamil in pulmonary hypertension with progressive systemic sclerosis. Am. Heart J., *109*:380–382, 1985.

427. Rouse, P.J., Lahiri, A., and Gumpel, J.M.: The CREST syndrome—Successful reduction of pulmonary hypertension by captopril. Postgrad. Med. J., *60*:672–674, 1984.

428. LeRoy, E.C.: Systemic sclerosis (scleroderma). *In* Textbook of Rheumatology. Edited by W.N. Kelley, E.D. Harris, Jr., S. Ruddy, and C.B. Sledge. Philadelphia, W.B. Saunders Co., 1985, pp. 1183–1205.

429. Brown, E.A., MacGregor, G.A., and Maini, R.N.: Failure of captopril to reverse the renal crisis of scleroderma. Ann. Rheum. Dis., *42*:52–53, 1983.

430. Waeber, B., et al.: Deterioration of renal function in hypertensive patients with scleroderma despite blood pressure normalization with captopril. Klin. Wochenschr., *62*:728–730, 1984.

431. Nolph, K.D., Stoltz, M.L., and Maher, J.L.: Altered peritoneal permeability in patients with systemic vasculitis. Ann. Intern. Med., *75*:753–755, 1971.

432. Copley, J.B., and Smith, B.J.: Continuous ambulatory peritoneal dialysis and scleroderma. Nephron, *40*:353–356, 1985.

433. Barker, D.J., and Farr, M.J.: Resolution of cutaneous manifestations of systemic sclerosis after hemodialysis. Br. Med. J., *1*:501, 1976.

434. LeRoy, E.C., and Fleischmann, R.M.: The management of renal scleroderma. Experience with dialysis, nephrectomy and transplantation. Am. J. Med., *64*:974–978, 1978.

435. Merino, G.E., et al.: Renal transplantation for progressive systemic sclerosis with renal failure. Am. J. Surg., *133*:745–749, 1977.

436. Woodhall, P.B., et al.: Apparent recurrence of progressive

systemic sclerosis in a renal allograft. J. Am. Med. Assoc., *236*:1032–1034, 1976.

437. Byron, M.A., Venning, V,A., and Mowat, A.G.: Post-mammoplasty human adjuvant disease. Br. J. Rheumatol., 23:227–229, 1984.

438. Taj, M., and Ahmad, A.: Familial localized scleroderma (morphoea). Arch. Dermatol., *113*:1132–1133, 1977.

439. Ikai, K., et al.: Morphea-like cutaneous changes in a patient with systemic scleroderma. Dermatologica, *158*:438–442, 1979.

440. Connelly, M.G., and Winkelmann, R.K.: Coexistence of lichen sclerosus, morphea, and lichen planus. J. Am. Acad. Dermatol., *12*:844–851, 1985.

441. Patterson, J.A.K., and Ackerman, B.: Lichen sclerosus et atrophicus is not related to morphea. A clinical and histologic study of 24 patients in whom both conditions were reputed to be present simultaneously. Am. J. Dermatol., *6*:323–335, 1984.

441a. Mensing, H., and Schmidt, K.-U.: Diffuse fasciitis with eosinophilia associated with morphea and lichen sclerosus et atrophicus. Acta Derm. Venereol. (Stockh.), *65*:80–83, 1985.

442. Moynahan, E.J.: Morphoea (localized cutaneous scleroderma) treated with low-dosage penicillamine (4 cases, including coup de sabre). Proc. R. Soc. Med., *66*:1083–1085, 1973.

443. Neuhofer, J., and Fritsch, P.: Treatment of localized scleroderma and lichen sclerosus with etretinate. Acta Derm. Venereol. (Stockh.), *64*:171–174, 1984.

444. Jablonska, S.: Scleroderma and Pseudoscleroderma. 2nd Ed. Warsaw, Polish Medical Publishers, 1975.

445. Rogers, B.O.: Transactions of the 3rd International Congress of Plastic Surgery (International Congress Series No. 66). Edited by T.R. Broadbent. Amsterdam, Excerpta Medica, 1963, pp. 681–689.

446. Stern, L.Z., et al.: Myopathy associated with linear scleroderma. Neurology, *25*:114–119, 1975.

447. Soffa, D.J., Sire, D.J., and Dodson, J.H.: Melorheostosis with linear sclerodermatous skin changes. Radiology, *114*:577–578, 1975.

448. Dubois, E.L., et al.: Progressive systemic sclerosis (PSS) and localized scleroderma (morphea) with positive LE cell test and unusual systemic manifestations compatible with systemic lupus erythematosus (SLE): Presentation of 14 cases including one set of identical twins, one with scleroderma and the other with SLE. Review of the literature. Medicine, *50*:199–222, 1971.

449. Mackel, S.E., et al.: Concurrent linear scleroderma and systemic lupus erythematosus: A report of two cases. J. Invest. Dermatol., *73*:368–372, 1979.

450. Tuffanelli, D.L., Marmelzat, W.L., and Dorsey, C.S.: Linear scleroderma with hemiatrophy. Report of three cases associated with collagen-vascular disease. Dermatologica, *132*:51–58, 1966.

451. Hanson, V., Drexler, E., and Kornreich, H.: Rheumatoid factor (anti-gammaglobulins) in children with focal scleroderma. Pediatrics, *53*:945–947, 1974.

452. Falanga, V., Medsger, T.A., Jr., and Reichlin, M.: High titers of antibodies to single-stranded DNA in linear scleroderma. Arch. Dermatol., *121*:345–347, 1985.

453. Takehara, K., et al.: Antinuclear antibodies in localized scleroderma. Arthritis Rheum., *26*:612–616, 1983.

454. Falanga, V., Medsger, T.A., Jr., and Reichlin, M.: Antinuclear and anti-single-stranded DNA antibodies in morphea and generalized morphea. Arch. Dermatol., *123*:350–353, 1987.

455. Ruffatti, A., et al.: Anticentromere antibody in localized scleroderma. J. Am. Acad. Dermatol., *15*:637–642, 1986.

456. Aberer, E., Neumann, R., and Stanek, G.: Is localised scleroderma a *Borrelia* infection? Lancet, *2*:278, 1985.

457. Buckingham, R.B., et al.: Collagen accumulation by dermal fibroblast cultures of patients with linear localized scleroderma. Arthritis Rheum., *19*:817, 1976.

458. Czarbecki, D.B., and Taft, E.H.: Generalized morphoea successfully treated with salazopyrine. Acta Derm. Venereol. (Stockh.), *62*:81–82, 1982.

459. Williams, H.J., Ziter, F.A., and Banta, C.A.: Childhood eosinophilic fasciitis—progression to linear scleroderma. J. Rheumatol., *13*:961–962, 1986.

460. Drosos, A.A., Papadimitriou, C.S., and Moutsopoulos, H.M.: An overlap of diffuse fasciitis with eosinophilia and scleroderma. Rheumatology, *4*:187–189, 1984.

461. Wasserman, S.I., et al.: Serum eosinophilotactic activity in eosinophilic fasciitis. Arthritis Rheum., *25*:1352–1356, 1982.

462. Barnes, L., et al.: Eosinophilic fasciitis. A pathologic study of twenty cases. Am. J. Pathol., *96*:493–507, 1979.

463. Moore, T.L., and Zuckner, J.: Eosinophilic fasciitis. Semin. Arthritis Rheum., *9*:228–235, 1980.

464. Seibold, J.R., et al.: Circulating immune complexes in eosinophilic fasciitis. Arthritis Rheum., *25*:1180–1185, 1982.

465. Shulman, L.E.: Diffuse fasciitis with eosinophilia. A new syndrome? Trans. Assoc. Am. Physicians, *88*:70–86, 1975.

466. Laso, F.J., Pastor, I., and deCastro, S.: Cimetidine and eosinophilic fasciitis. Ann. Intern. Med., *98*:1026, 1983.

467. Solomon, G., Barland, P., and Rifkin, H.: Eosinophilic fasciitis responsive to cimetidine. Ann. Intern. Med., *97*:547–549, 1982.

468. Hoffman, R., et al.: Diffuse fasciitis and aplastic anemia: A report of four cases revealing an unusual association between rheumatologic and hematologic disorders. Medicine, *61*:373–382, 1982.

469. Michet, C.J., Jr., Doyle, J.A., and Ginsburg, W.W.: Eosinophilic fasciitis. Report of 15 cases. Mayo Clin. Proc., *56*:27–34, 1981.

470. Doyle, J.A.: Eosinophilic fasciitis: Extracutaneous manifestations and associations. Cutis, *34*:259–261, 1984.

471. Balaban, E.P., et al.: Treatment of cutaneous sclerosis and aplastic anemia with antithymocyte globulin. Ann. Intern. Med., *106*:56–58, 1987.

472. Joyce, R.A., Kahl, L.E., and Rodnan, G.P.: Aplastic anemia and eosinophilic fasciitis: Demonstration of T cell inhibition of colony formation and response to antithymocyte globulin. Arthritis Rheum., *27*:S74, 1984.

473. Stanek, G., et al.: Shulman syndrome: A scleroderma subtype caused by *Borrelia burgdorferi*? Lancet, *1*:1490, 1987.

474. Cramer, S.F., et al.: Eosinophilic fasciitis: Immunopathology, ultrastructure, literature review and consideration of its pathogenesis and relation to scleroderma. Arch. Pathol. Lab. Med., *106*:85–91, 1982.

475. Kent, L.T., Cramer, S.F., and Moskowitz, R.W.: Eosinophilic fasciitis: Clinical, laboratory and microscopic considerations. Arthritis Rheum., *24*:677–683, 1981.

476. Smiley, A.M., Husain, M., and Indebaum, S.: Eosinophilic fasciitis in association with thyroid disease: A report of three cases. J. Rheumatol., *7*:871–876, 1980.

477. Fleischmajer, R., and Pollock, J.L.: Progressive systemic sclerosis: Pseudoscleroderma. Clin. Rheum. Dis., *5*:243–261, 1979.

478. Rocco, V.K., and Hurd, E.R.: Scleroderma and scleroderma-like disorders. Semin. Arthritis Rheum., *16*:22–69, 1986.

479. Kordac, V., and Semradova, H.: Treatment of porphyria cu-

tanea tarda with chloroquine. Br. J. Dermatol., *90*:95–100, 1974.

480. Ramsey, C.A., et al.: The treatment of porphyria cutanea tarda by venesection. Q. J. Med., *43*:1–24, 1974.

481. Grossman, M.E., et al.: Porphyria cutanea tarda. Clinical features and laboratory findings in 40 patients. Am. J. Med., *67*:277–286, 1977.

482. Maeda, H., Ishikaw, H., and Onta, S.: Circumscribed myxedema of lichen myxedematosus as a sign of faulty formation of the proteoglycan macromolecule. Br. J. Dermatol., *105*:239–245, 1981.

483. Verity, M.A., Troop, J., McAdam, L.P., and Pearson, C.M.: Scleromyxedema myopathy. Am. J. Clin. Pathol., *69*:446–451, 1978.

484. Lawrence, L.A., Tye, M.J., and Liss, M.: Immunochemical analysis of the basic immunoglobulin in papular mucinosis. Immunochemistry, *9*:41–49, 1972.

484a. Gabriel, S.E., and Bowles, C.A.: Scleromyxedema: A scleroderma-like disorder with systemic manifestations. (Abstract.) Arthritis Rheum., *30*:S98, 1987.

485. Jablonska, S., and Stachow, A.: Scleroderma-like lesions in multiple myeloma. Dermatologica, *144*:257–269, 1972.

486. Rubinow, A., and Cohen, A.S.: Skin inolvement in generalized amyloidosis. A study of clinically involved and uninvolved skin in 50 patients with primary and secondary amyloidosis. Ann. Intern. Med., *88*:781–785, 1978.

487. Costello, P.B., Tambar, P.M., and Green, F.A.: The prevalence and possible prognostic importance of arthropathy in childhood diabetes. J. Rheumatol., *11*:62–65, 1984.

488. Garza-Elizondo, M.A., et al.: Joint contractures and scleroderma-like skin changes in the hands of insulin-dependent juvenile diabetics. J. Rheumatol., *10*:797–800, 1983.

489. Siebold, J.R.: Digital sclerosis in children. Skin changes in insulin-dependent diabetes mellitus. Arthritis Rheum., *25*:1357–1361, 1982.

490. Jablonska, S., and Stachow, A.: Pseudoscleroderma concomitant with a muscular glycogenosis of unknown enzymatic defect. Acta Derm. Venereol., *52*:379–385, 1972.

491. Fries, J.F., Lindgren, J.A., and Bull, J.M.: Scleroderma-like lesions and the carcinoid syndrome. Arch. Intern. Med., *131*:550–553, 1973.

492. Stachow, A., Jablonska, S., and Skiendzielewska, A.: 5-Hydroxy-tryptamine and tryptamine pathways in scleroderma. Br. J. Dermatol., *97*:147–154, 1977.

493. Houpt, J.B., Ogryzlo, M.A., and Hunt, M.: Tryptophan metabolism in man (with special reference to rheumatoid arthritis and scleroderma). Semin. Arthritis Rheum., *2*:333–353, 1973.

494. Stachow, A., Jablonka, S., and Skiendzielewska, A.: Intestinal absorption of L-tryptophan in scleroderma. Acta Derm. Venereol., *56*:257–264, 1976.

495. Hankes, L.V., et al.: Metabolism of ¹⁴C-labelled L-tryptophan, L-kynurenine and hydroxy-L-kynurenine in miners with scleroderma. S. Afr. Med. J., *51*:383–390, 1977.

496. Jablonska, S., Stachow, A., and Suffczynska, A.: Skin and muscle indurations in phenylketonuria. Arch. Dermatol., *95*:443–450, 1967.

497. Kornreich, H.K., et al.: Phenylketonuria and scleroderma. J. Pediatr., *73*:571–575, 1968.

498. Epstein, C.J., et al.: Werner's syndrome. A review of its symptomatology, natural history, pathologic features, genetics and relationship to the natural aging process. Medicine, *45*:177–221, 1966.

499. Fleischmajer, R., and Nedwich, A.: Werner's syndrome. Am. J. Med., *54*:111–118, 1972.

500. Fleischmajer, R., and Nedwich, A.: Progeria (Hutchinson-Gilford). Arch. Dermatol., *107*:253–258, 1973.

501. Vilee, D.B., Nichols, G., and Talbot, N.B.: Metabolic studies in two boys with classical progeria. Pediatrics, *43*:207–216, 1969.

502. Sucio, I., et al.: Clinical manifestations in vinyl chloride poisoning. Ann. N.Y. Acad. Sci., *246*:53–69, 1975.

503. Maricq, H.R., et al.: Capillary abnormalities in polyvinyl chloride production workers. Examination by in vivo microscopy. J. Am. Med. Assoc., *236*:1368–1371, 1976.

504. Selikoff, I.J., and Hammond, E.C.: Editors and Conference Chairman: Toxicity of vinyl chloride-polyvinyl chloride. Ann. N.Y. Acad. Sci., *246*:1–337, 1975.

505. Stachow, A., Jablonska, S., and Skiendzielewska, A.: Biogenic amines derived from tryptophan in systemic and cutaneous scleroderma. Acta Derm. Venereol., *59*:1–5, 1979.

506. Cohen, I.S., et al.: Cutaneous toxicity of bleomycin therapy. Arch. Dermatol., *107*:553–555, 1973.

507. Teutsch, C., Lipton, A., and Harvey, H.A.: Raynaud's phenomenon as a side effect of chemotherapy with vinblastine and bleomyin for testicular carcinoma. Cancer Treat. Rep., *61*:925–926, 1977.

508. Vogelzang, N.J., et al.: Raynaud's phenomenon: A common toxicity after combination chemotherapy for testicular cancer. Ann. Intern. Med., *95*:288–292, 1981.

509. Yagoda, A., et al.: Bleomycin, an antitumor antibiotic. Clinical experience in 274 patients. Ann. Intern. Med., *77*:861–870, 1972.

510. Van Nunen, S.A., Gatenby, P.A., and Basten, A.: Postmammoplasty connective tissue disease. Arthritis Rheum., *25*:694–697, 1982.

511. Fock, K., Feng, P., and Tey, B.: Autoimmune disease developing after augmentation mammoplasty. Report of three cases. J. Rheumatol., *11*:98–100, 1984.

511a. Butler, R.C., Dieppe, P.A., and Keat, A.C.S.: Calcinosis of joints and periarticular tissues associated with vitamin D intoxication. Ann. Rheum. Dis., *44*:494–498, 1985.

512. Bilezikian, J.P., Auerbach, G.D., and Connor, T.B.: Pseudogout after parathyroidectomy. Lancet, *1*:445–446, 1973.

513. deGraaf, P., et al.: Metastatic skin calcifications: A rare phenomenon in dialysis patients. Dermatologica, *161*:28–32, 1980.

514. Moskowitz, R.W., et al.: Crystal-induced inflammation associated with chronic renal failure treated with periodic hemodialysis. Am. J. Med., *47*:450–460, 1969.

515. Andresen, J., and Nielsen, H.E.: Juxta-articular erosions and calcifications in patients with chronic renal failure. Acta Radiol. [Diagn.] (Stockh.), *22*:709—713, 1981.

516. Russell, R.G.G., Bisaz, S., and Fleisch, H.: Pyrophosphate and disphosphonates in calcium metabolism and their possible role in renal failure. Arch. Intern. Med., *124*:571–577, 1969.

517. Kovarik, J., et al.: Tumorous paraarticular calcifications due to undigested phosphate-binders in a patient undergoing regular hemodialysis (letter). Clin. Nephrol., *21*:141–142, 1984.

517a. Reginato, A.J., et al.: Arthropathy and cutaneous calcinosis in hemodialysis oxalosis. Arthritis Rheum., *29*:1387–1396, 1986.

518. Walton, K., and Swinson, D.R.: Acute calcific periarthritis associated with transient hypocalcaemia secondary to hypoparathyroidism. Br. J. Rheumatol., *22*:179–180, 1983.

519. Richard, A.G.: Metastatic calcifications detected through scanning with ⁹⁹ᵐTc-polyphosphate. J. Nucl. Med., *15*:1057–1060, 1974.

520. Grames, G.M., Sauser, D.D., and Jansen, C.: Radionuclide

detection of diffuse interstitial pulmonary calcification. J. Am. Med. Assoc., *230*:992–995, 1974.

521. Kim, E.E., et al.: Accumulation of Tc-99m-phosphonate complexes in metastatic lesions from colon and lung carcinomas. Eur. J. Nucl. Med., *5*:299–301, 1980.

522. Rosenthal, D.I., et al.: Uptake of bone imaging agents by diffuse pulmonary metastatic calcification. Am. J. Roentgenol., *129*:871–874, 1977.

523. Kantarjian, H.M., et al.: Uptake of ⁹⁹ᵐTc-methylene disphosphonate in calcinosis cutis. J. Amer. Acad. Dermatol., *7*:804–806, 1982.

524. McKee, P.H., Liomba, N.G., and Hutt, M.S.R.: Tumoral calcinosis: A pathological study of fifty-six cases. Br. J. Dermatol., *107*:669–674, 1982.

525. Lafferty, F.W., Raynolds, E.S., and Pearson, O.H.: Tumoral calcinosis: A metabolic disease of obscure etiology. Am. J. Med., *38*:105–118, 1965.

526. Zerwekh, J.E., et al.: Tumoral calcinosis: Evidence for concurrent defects in renal tubular phosphorus transport and in 1α,25-dihydrocholecalciferol synthesis. Calcif. Tissue Int., *32*:1–6, 1980.

527. Lufkin, E.G., Kumar, R., and Heath, H., III: Hyperphosphatemic tumoral calcinosis: Effects of phosphate depletion on vitamin D metabolism, and of acute hypocalcemia on parathyroid hormone secretion and action. J. Clin. Endocrinol. Metab., *56*:1319–1322, 1983.

528. Lyles, K.W., et al.: Genetic transmission of tumoral calcinosis: Autosomal dominant with variable clinical expressivity. J. Clin. Endocrinol. Metab., *60*:1093–1096, 1985.

529. Boskey, A.L., et al.: Chemical, microscopic, and ultrastructural characterization of the mineral deposits in tumoral calcinosis. Clin. Orthop. Rel. Res., *178*:258–269, 1983.

530. Mozarfarian, G., Lafferty, F.W., and Pearson, O.H.: Treatment of tumoral calcinosis with phosphorus deprivation. Ann. Intern. Med., *77*:741–745, 1972.

531. Salvi, A., et al.: Phosphaturic action of calcitonin in pseudotumoral calcinosis: Horm. Metab. Res., *15*:260, 1983.

532. Bowyer, S.L., Blane, C.E., Sullivan, D.B., and Cassidy, J.T.: Childhood dermatomyositis: factors predicting functional outcome and development of dystrophic calcification. J. Pediatr., *103*:882–888, 1983.

533. Blane, C.E., et al.: Patterns of calcification in childhood dermatomyositis. Am. J. Radiol., *142*:397–400, 1984.

534. Randle, H.W., Sander, H.M., and Howard, K.: Early diagnosis of calcinosis cutis in childhood dermatomyositis using computed tomography. J.A.M.A., *256*:1137–1138, 1986.

535. LeRoux, J-L., et al.: Ultrastructural and crystallographic study of calcifications from a patient with CREST syndrome. J. Rheumatol., *10*:242–246, 1983.

536. Nielsen, A.O., et al.: Dermatomyositis with universal calcinosis. A histopathological and electron microscopic study. J. Cutan. Pathol., *6*:486–491, 1979.

537. Kawakami, T., et al.: Ultrastructural study of calcinosis universalis with dermatomyositis. J. Cutan. Pathol., *13*:135–143, 1986.

538. Marks, J.: Studies with ⁴⁷Ca in patients with calcinosis cutis. Br. J. Dermatol., *82*:1–9, 1970.

539. Kales, A.N., and Phang, J.M.: Dietary calcium perturbation in patients with abnormal calcium deposition. J. Clin. Endocrinol. Metab., *31*:204–212, 1970.

540. Lian, J.B., et al.: Gamma-carboxyglutamate excretion and calcinosis in juvenile dermatomyositis. Arthritis Rheum., *25*:1094–1100, 1982.

541. Moore, S.E., Jump, A.A., and Smiley, J.D.: Effect of warfarin sodium therapy on excretion of 4-carboxy-L-glutamic acid in scleroderma, dermatomyositis, and myositis ossificans progressiva. Arthritis Rheum., *29*:344–351, 1986.

542. Sherman, F.S., et al.: Collagen crosslinks: A critical determinant of bioprosthetic heart valve calcification. Trans. Am. Soc. Artif. Intern. Organs, *30*:577–581, 1984.

543. Russell, R.G.G., and Smith, R.: Diphosphonates: Experimental and clinical aspects. J. Bone Joint Surg., *55B*:66–86, 1973.

544. Dent, C.E., and Stamp, T.C.B.: Treatment of calcinosis circumscripta wth probenecid. Br. Med. J., *1*:216–218, 1972.

545. Metzger, A.L., et al.: Failure of disodium etidronate in calcinosis due to dermatomyositis and scleroderma. N. Engl. J. Med., *291*:1294–1296, 1974.

546. Rabens, S.F., and Bethune, J.E.: Disodium etidronate therapy for dystrophic cutaneous calcification. Arch. Dermatol., *111*:357–361, 1975.

547. Russell, R.G.G., and Smith, R.: Diphosphonates: Experimental and clinical aspects. J. Bone Joint Surg., *55B*:66–86, 1973.

548. Mendelson, B.C., et al.: Surgical treatment of calcinosis cutis in the upper extremity. J. Hand Surg., *2*:318–324, 1977.

549. Ames, E.L., and Posçh, J.L.: Calcinosis of the flexor and extensor tendons in dermatomyositis—Case report. J. Hand Surg., *9A*:876–879, 1984.

550. Wilsher, M.L., Holdaway, I.M., and North, J.D.K.: Hypercalcaemia during resolution of calcinosis in juvenile dermatomyositis. Br. Med. J., *288*:1345, 1984.

551. Suzuki, Y., Bisada, K., and Takeda, M.: Demonstration of myositis ossificans by ⁹⁹ᵐTc pyrophosphate bone scanning. Radiology, *111*:663–664, 1974.

552. Buhain, W.J., Rammohan, G., and Berger, H.W.: Pulmonary function in myositis ossificans progressiva. Am. Rev. Respir. Dis., *110*:333–337, 1974.

553. Smith, R.: Myositis ossificans progressiva. A review of current problems. Semin. Arthritis Rheum., *4*:369–380, 1975.

554. Illingworth, R.S.: Myositis ossificans progressiva (Munchmeyer's disease). Brief review with report of two cases treated with corticosteroids and observed for 16 years. Arch. Dis. Child., *46*:264–268, 1971.

555. Gilsanz, V., and Bernstein, B.H.: Joint calcification following intraarticular corticosteroid therapy. Radiology, *151*:647–649, 1984.

556. Dalinka, M.K., et al.: Periarticular calcifications in association with intra-articular corticosteroid injections. Radiology, *153*:615–618, 1984.

557. Edwards, A.J., Sill, B.J., and Macfarlane, I.: Carpal tunnel syndrome due to dystrophic calcification. Aust. N.Z. J. Surg., *54*:491–492, 1984.

558. Ametewee, K.: Carpal tunnel syndrome produced by a post traumatic calcific mass. Hand, *15*:212–215, 1983.

559. Gravanis, M.B., and Gaffney, E.F.: Idiopathic calcifying tenosynovitis. Histopathologic features and possible pathogenesis. Amer. J. Surg. Pathol., *7*:357–361, 1983.

559a.Selby, C.L.: Acute calcific tendinitis of the hand: An infrequently recognized and frequently misdiagnosed form of periarthritis. Arthritis Rheum., *27*:337–340, 1984.

560. Ellis, I.O., Foster, M.C., and Womack, C.: Plumber's knee: Calcinosis cutis after repeated minor trauma in a plumber. Br. Med. J., *288*:1723, 1984.

561. DiGiovanna, J.J., Helfgott, R.K., Gerber, L.H., and Peck, G.L.: Extraspinal tendon and ligament calcification associated with long-term therapy with etretinate. New Engl. J. Med., *315*:1177–1182, 1986.

562. Sakkas, L., et al.: Cervical myelopathy with ankylosing hyperostosis of the spine. Surg. Neurol., *24*:43–46, 1985.

563. Miyasaka, K., et al.: Myelopathy due to ossification or calcification of the ligamentum flavum: Radiologic and histologic evaluations. Amer. J. Neurol. Radiol., 4:629–632, 1983.

564. Widlus, D.M.: Calcific tendonitis of the longus colli muscle: A cause of atraumatic neck pain. Ann. Emerg. Med., 14:1014–1017, 1985.

565. Benanti, J.C., Gramling, P., Bulat, P.I., and Chen, P.: Retropharyngeal calcific tendinitis: Report of five cases and review of the literature. J. Emerg. Med., 4:15–24, 1986.

566. Zervas, J., et al.: HLA antigens in diabetics with calcified shoulder periarthritis (CSP). Clin. Exp. Rheumatol., 4:351–353, 1986.

VASCULITIS

ANTHONY S. FAUCI and RANDI Y. LEAVITT

Vasculitis is a clinicopathologic process characterized by inflammation and damage to blood vessels. This process is usually associated with compromise of the vessel lumen and ischemic changes in the tissues supplied by the involved vessels.[1,2] Vasculitis may be the only manifestation of a disease. Alternatively, vasculitis may be a secondary component of another primary disease. For example, Wegener's granulomatosis and classic polyarteritis nodosa are *primary* vasculitic syndromes, whereas the vasculitides associated with underlying connective tissue diseases such as rheumatoid arthritis (RA) or systemic lupus erythematosus (SLE) are classified as *secondary* vasculitic syndromes.[1–3]

PATHOGENESIS

Most of the vasculitic syndromes are mediated, at least in part, by immunopathogenic mechanisms.[1,2] Foremost among these mechanisms is the immune complex model whereby antigen–antibody complexes either circulate and deposit in the vessel walls or are formed in situ at the area of tissue damage.[4] Although *circulating immune complexes* can be demonstrated in most of the vasculitic syndromes,[1,2] and evidence suggests deposition of complexes in various tissues, the causal role of these mechanisms in the inflammatory response of involved vessels remains unclear. In a few instances a causative antigen has been demonstrated in putative immune-complex–mediated disease. Hepatitis B antigen-associated systemic vasculitis is the

prototype of immune-complex–mediated vasculitis in which an exogenous antigen is implicated.[5] In addition to the classic immune-complex–mediated vasculitis, other types of immunopathogenic mechanisms may damage vascular tissue. One of these is cell-mediated immune reactivity, a poorly documented form of damage to vascular tissue. Nonetheless, the histopathologic features of certain types of vasculitis suggest at least a component of *cell-mediated immune injury*. Granulomatous vasculitis may indeed represent a component of classic cell-mediated immune mechanisms in certain vasculitic syndromes,[1,2] and immune complexes themselves may trigger granulomatous responses.[6] Therefore, the presence of granulomas in or near vessels may indicate immune-complex mechanisms, cell-mediated immune responses, or both. Finally, although other mechanisms, such as tissue injury mediated directly by antibodies with specificity against the vessel itself or by cytotoxic effector cells in *antibody-dependent cellular cytotoxicity*, may play a role in vascular damage, little evidence supports their contribution to the pathogenesis of any of the recognized vasculitic syndromes, with the exception of Kawasaki's disease. The production of cytotoxic antibodies directed against mediator-induced endothelial cell antigens may play a role in the vascular damage seen in this condition.[7,8]

CLASSIFICATION

The clinical spectrum of the vasculitides is characterized by heterogeneity as well as overlap among the various syndromes. Considerable confusion and difficulty have hindered the categorization of these diseases. Any categorization scheme is empiric, but we have found an approach that is helpful in prognosis and in the design of therapeutic regimens.[1,2,9] This approach emphasizes the conceptual differences between disease that is predominantly systemic, almost invariably causing irreversible organ system dysfunction and even death if untreated, and those syndromes with primarily cutaneous manifestations, rarely resulting in irreversible dysfunction of vital organs. Some syndromes may overlap these categories. A revised classification of the clinical spectrum of vasculitis is shown in Table 74–1.

The first group, systemic necrotizing vasculitis, has been the most difficult to categorize. The original *classic polyarteritis nodosa* is contained within this group.[10] Lung involvement, granulomas, eosinophilia, and a history of allergy are not characteristic of this syndrome. Another syndrome, however, called *allergic angiitis and granulomatosis or Churg-Strauss syndrome*,[11] resembles classic polyarteritis nodosa in many respects, except lung involvement is the rule, and eosinophilia, granulomas, and allergy are common. The histopathologic features of these two syndromes differ in that the vasculitic lesions of classic polyarteritis nodosa are confined to the small and medium-sized muscular arteries, whereas those of classic allergic angiitis and granulomatosis involve blood vessels of

Table 74–1. Classification of the Vasculitic Syndromes

Systemic necrotizing vasculitis
  Classic polyarteritis nodosa
  Allergic angiitis and granulomatosis of Churg-Strauss
  Polyangiitis overlap syndrome
Hypersensitivity vasculitis
  Exogenous stimuli proved or suspected
    Henoch-Schönlein purpura
    Serum sickness and serum sickness-like reactions
    Other drug-related vasculitides
    Vasculitis associated with infectious diseases
  Endogenous antigens likely involved; vasculitis associated with
    Neoplasms
    Systemic connective tissue diseases
    Other underlying diseases
    Congenital deficiencies of the complement system
Wegener's granulomatosis
Giant cell arteritis
  Temporal arteritis
  Takayasu's arteritis
Other vasculitic syndromes
  Mucocutaneous lymph node syndrome (Kawasaki's disease)
  Isolated central nervous system vasculitis
  Thromboangiitis obliterans (Buerger's disease)
  Miscellaneous vasculitides

(From Fauci, A.S.[9])

various types and sizes, including small and medium-sized muscular arteries as well as veins and venules.[1,2]

A form of systemic necrotizing vasculitis that is probably more common than classic polyarteritis nodosa or allergic angiitis and granulomatosis has been recognized. This syndrome may have features that overlap several distinct vasculitic syndromes. We call this group the *polyangiitis overlap syndrome*[1,2,9,12] (Table 74–2). This group of systemic necrotizing vasculitides has a common denominator of involvement of multiple organ systems with the overriding tendency for irreversible organ-system dysfunction. In general, the prognosis for patients with this group of disorders is poor without appropriate and aggressive therapy.

In contrast, the second broad category consists of predominantly cutaneous vasculitides and is called *hypersensitivity* vasculitides. Although these disorders may also be systemic, they most frequently remain cutaneous and do not consistently pose a threat of irreversible dysfunction of vital organs.[13–15] If the disease does remain confined to the skin and does not become systemic, aggressive therapy with high doses of corticosteroids or long-term administration of cytotoxic agents is indicated only in unusual circumstances.

The broad category of "hypersensitivity vasculitis" has been applied to a heterogeneous group of disorders thought to represent a hypersensitivity reaction to an identifiable antigenic stimulus such as a drug or an infectious agent; hence the term "hypersensitivity."[2,9] The term is often confusing because many, if not most, of the vasculitic syndromes represent hypersensitivity reactions of one form or another. As discussed later, although the proved or suspected antigenic stimuli associated with this group are heterogeneous, these disorders generally share the characteristic involvement of small vessels and a predominant, often exclusive, involvement of the vessels of the skin. Confusion has resulted from the inclusion of this group with the more serious systemic conditions. This confusion is probably related to the variable degrees of organ system involvement other than cutaneous that can occur in the hypersensitivity vasculitides. Such involvement, however, is usually much less severe than in the systemic vasculitis of classic polyarteritis nodosa or Wegener's granulomatosis. The skin is exclusively involved, or if other organ systems are involved, the cutaneous disease dominates the clinical picture.[2,9,13–15] Finally, a syndrome indistinguishable from hypersensitivity vasculitis can appear as a secondary component of another underlying disease, such as a systemic connective tissue disease or neoplasm, and may thus lead to additional confusion.

Table 74–2. Typical Clinicopathologic Features of Distinct Vasculitic Syndromes

Vasculitic Syndrome	Vessels Involved	Pathology	Distinctive Features
Polyarteritis nodosa	Small and medium-sized arteries	Necrotizing vasculitis	Angiogram showing aneurysms in renal, hepatic, and visceral vasculature
Allergic angiitis and granulomatosis (Churg-Strauss syndrome)	Small and medium-sized arteries	Granulomatous vasculitis	Allergic history, eosinophilia, pulmonary involvement
Hypersensitivity vasculitis	Arterioles, capillaries, venules, rarely small muscular arteries	Leukocytoclastic vasculitis	Skin most commonly involved, usually single type of vessel involved
Henoch-Schönlein purpura	Venules, capillaries, arterioles	Leukocytoclastic vasculitis	Usually skin, gastrointestinal, renal involvement, IgA in immune complexes
Takayasu's arteritis	Medium and large arteries	Giant cell arteritis	Predilection for aortic arch
Temporal arteritis	Medium and large arteries	Giant cell arteritis	Predilection for branches of carotid
Wegener's granulomatosis	Small arteries and veins, medium arteries	Necrotizing granulomatous vasculitis	Involves upper and lower respiratory tracts, glomerulonephritis commonly seen, varying degrees of small vessel vasculitis

(From Leavitt, R.Y., and Fauci, A.S.[12])

Most of the remainder of the vasculitic syndromes have distinctive enough clinical and pathologic features that they can readily be grouped into separate categories (Tables 74–1 and 74–2), such as Wegener's granulomatosis, temporal arteritis, or Takayasu's arteritis. Several of these distinctive syndromes are clearly systemic, but they do not appear in the polyarteritis nodosa group because they warrant separate classification.

SYSTEMIC NECROTIZING VASCULITIS (POLYARTERITIS NODOSA GROUP)

The systemic necrotizing vasculitis group includes (1) classic polyarteritis nodosa, (2) allergic angiitis and granulomatosis, and (3) the polyangiitis overlap syndrome.

CLASSIC POLYARTERITIS NODOSA

The first complete description of a vasculitic syndrome was made in 1866 by Kussmaul and Maier in an elegant clinicopathologic case report.[10] Classic periarteritis nodosa, as it was originally described[10] and further studied,[13,16] is a necrotizing vasculitis of small and medium-sized muscular arteries. The lesions are segmental, with a predilection for bifurcations of arteries with distal spread involving arterioles and, in some cases, circumferentially involving adjacent veins. This disorder is not primarily a venulitis. Histopathologically, in the acute states, polymorpho-

nuclear leukocytes infiltrate all layers of the vessel wall and perivascular areas (Fig. 74–1). Subsequently, mononuclear cell infiltration occurs as the lesions become subacute and chronic. Intimal proliferation, vessel wall degeneration with fibrinoid necrosis, thrombosis, ischemia, and infarction are seen in varying degrees. Generally, vascular lesions in various stages of development are found simultaneously. This finding may reflect the continuous deposition of immune complexes, such as one might expect in the vasculitis associated with persistent hepatitis B antigenemia.[5] Multiple organ systems are involved, and the clinicopathologic findings are consistent with the degree and location of vessel involvement and the resulting ischemic changes.[1,2]

Clinical Manifestations

The nature of the presenting problems may be nonspecific. *Vague symptoms* such as weakness, malaise, abdominal pain, extremity pain, headache, fever, and myalgias are frequent.[1,2] Less commonly, patients have signs and symptoms of neurologic and joint involvement. The nonspecific nature of the presentation and the uncommon occurrence of classic polyarteritis nodosa may contribute to the difficulty in establishing the diagnosis. The signs or symptoms and actual involvement may not correlate with those of doctumented vasculitis.

The clinical profile and manifestations in patients with classic polyarteritis nodosa are outlined in Table 74–3. These manifestations, together with the findings at autopsy summarized from several large series (Table 74–4), provide a striking witness to the scope

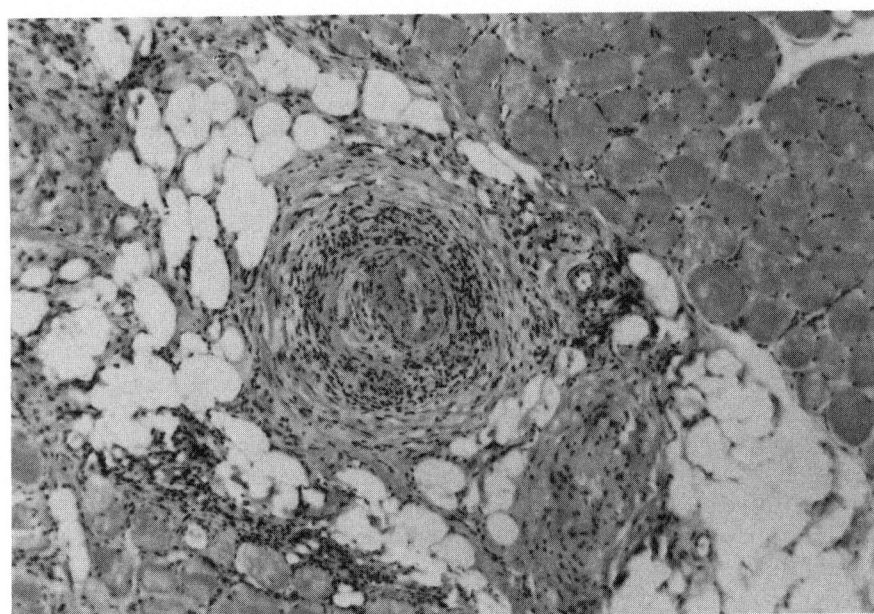

FIG. 74–1. Muscle biopsy in a 36-year-old patient with classic polyarteritis nodosa. A small muscular artery is involved, with fibrinoid necrosis and inflammatory cell infiltrate. (Hematoxylin and eosin stain; magnification ×130.)

Table 74–3. Clinical Profile and Manifestations in Patients With Classic Polyarteritis Nodosa

Clinical Parameter	Value
General considerations	
Age (mean)	45 years
Sex ratio (male to female)	2.5 to 1
	Percentage (%)
Fever	71
Weight loss	54
Organ involvement	
Kidney	70
Musculoskeletal system	64
Arthritis or arthralgia	53
Myalgias	31
Circulatory system (hypertension)	54
Peripheral nerves	51
Gastrointestinal tract	44
Abdominal pain	43
Nausea or vomiting	40
Cholecystitis	17
Bleeding	6
Bowel perforation	5
Bowel infarction	1.4
Skin	43
Rash or purpura	30
Livedo reticularis	4
Heart	36
Congestive failure	12
Myocardial infarction	6
Pericarditis	4
Central nervous system	23
Cerebral vascular accident	11
Altered mental status	10
Seizure	4

(From Cupps, T.R., and Fauci, A.S.[2])

and severity of the organ system involvement in this disease.

Variable degrees of renal involvement are seen in most patients, and this complication is a major cause of death. The renal disease may be primarily vascular with secondary ischemic changes in the glomeruli, it may be a primary glomerulitis, or it may be a combination of both. Hypertension, usually associated with elevated renin levels, may compound the severity of the renal disease or may itself be the predominant cause of renal dysfunction in the form of nephrosclerosis.[2,17,18] It was once thought that the hy-

Table 74–4. Organ Involvement at Autopsy in Classic Polyarteritis Nodosa

Organ System	Percentage (%)
Kidney	85
Heart	76
Liver	62
Gastrointestinal tract	51
Jejunum	37
Ileum	27
Mesentery	24
Colon	20
Rectosigmoid	10
Duodenum	10
Gallbladder	10
Appendix	7
Muscle	39
Pancreas	35
Testes	33
Peripheral nerves	32
Central nervous system	27
Skin	20

(From Cupps, T.R., and Fauci, A.S.[2])

pertension of polyarteritis nodosa was almost exclusively associated with the healing stages of the renal polyarteritis nodosa or glomerulonephritis,[16] but it is now clear that hypertension may occur as an independent early finding before clinically apparent functional renal disease. Hypertension may dominate the clinical picture and may be directly responsible for certain of the associated cerebrovascular, cardiovascular, or renal manifestations.

Besides hypertensive cardiovascular disease, primary involvement of the coronary arteries is common, and cardiac involvement is a major cause of death.[17,19] Areas of myocardial infarction are frequently found at autopsy in the absence of a suggestive clear-cut history.[20] Polyarteritis nodosa in children is associated with a high incidence of coronary artery involvement,[21] but most of the cases in the United States formerly reported as polyarteritis nodosa of children, with its characteristic and unusual selective involvement of the coronary arteries, were in fact the arteritis of unrecognized mucocutaneous lymph node syndrome (Kawasaki's disease).[22]

Gastrointestinal involvement is seen in over 50% of patients and usually relates to involvement of the visceral arteries.[2] Symptoms and signs include nausea, vomiting, diarrhea, ileus, abdominal pain, ulceration with bleeding, infarction, or perforation of intra-abdominal organs. Depending on the severity of involvement, manifestations range from abdominal angina or steatorrhea, associated with partial obstruction of the superior mesenteric artery or its branches, to massive bowel infarction, resulting from acute involvement of the superior mesenteric artery.[17] Bowel perforation carries a high mortality rate. Significant abdominal involvement is often masked partially or completely in patients receiving daily corticosteroids, and an ischemic segment of bowel may go undetected until actual perforation has occurred.

Liver disease varies in classic polyarteritis nodosa. When hepatitis B antigenemia accounts for the vasculitis, hepatic involvement may relate to the underlying hepatitis and ranges from subclinical diseases to chronic active hepatitis.[5] Liver disease related directly to the vasculitis may lead to massive hepatic infarction.[23]

Neurologic manifestations are common. Mononeuritis multiplex resulting from vasculitis of the vasa nervorum is the most frequent finding. In a review of the neurologic manifestations of systemic necrotizing vasculitis (Table 74–1) including polyarteritis nodosa, 80% of patients had some form of nervous system disease.[24] The peripheral nervous system was involved in 60% of this subset. Four patterns of neuropathy were seen: mononeuritis multiplex, extensive mononeuritis, cutaneous neuropathy, and polyneuropathy. The central nervous system was involved in the remaining 40%, and these patients predominantly had diffuse and focal disturbance of cerebral, cerebellar, and brain stem function.

Cutaneous Involvement. The question of the precise type of cutaneous involvement in classic polyarteritis nodosa is controversial because many cases of small-vessel "hypersensitivity vasculitis" have been included in reports of groups of patients said to have polyarteritis nodosa. Furthermore, skin involvement in the polyangiitis overlap syndrome may have features of both classic polyarteritis nodosa and hypersensitivity venulitis.[2,9,12] Skin involvement in classic polyarteritis occurs in approximately 20 to 30% of patients and is usually confined to the small muscular arteries of the subcutaneous tissues.[25] The lesions are generally manifested as painful erythematous subcutaneous nodules, which may appear in crops and may range from a few millimeters to several centimeters in size.[26] Another characteristic of skin involvement is *livedo reticularis* (Fig. 74–2). *Cutaneous polyarteritis nodosa* is characterized by a necrotizing vasculitis of small arteries of subcutaneous tissue.[27] The disease is a localized process with sparing of visceral arteries and therefore is not a true systemic vasculitic syndrome. Cutaneous polyarteritis nodosa usually runs a chronic course and has a favorable long-term prognosis. Although the histologic lesion resembles that of classic polyarteritis nodosa, this disease is clinically similar to the hypersensitivity vasculitides.

Arthralgias are common in classic polyarteritis nodosa, but frank arthritis is rare. When small and medium-sized muscular arteries in skeletal muscle are involved, the muscles are almost invariably symptomatic (see Fig. 74–1). In addition, testicular or epididymal pain is characteristic, and testicular involvement is seen in approximately 30% of autopsies in classic polyarteritis nodosa (Table 74–4). Thus, when muscular or testicular pain is present, biopsy is likely to be helpful in making the diagnosis, whereas blind biopsies of asymptomatic organs have a low diagnostic yield.

Diagnosis

No diagnostic laboratory findings are indicative of classic polyarteritis nodosa, and the many abnormalities are outlined in Table 74–5. The finding of hepatitis B antigenemia has been reported in up to 30% of patients with systemic vasculitis of the polyarteritis nodosa type,[5,28,29] but this finding in itself does not establish the diagnosis, which depends on characteristic clinical and pathologic manifestations.

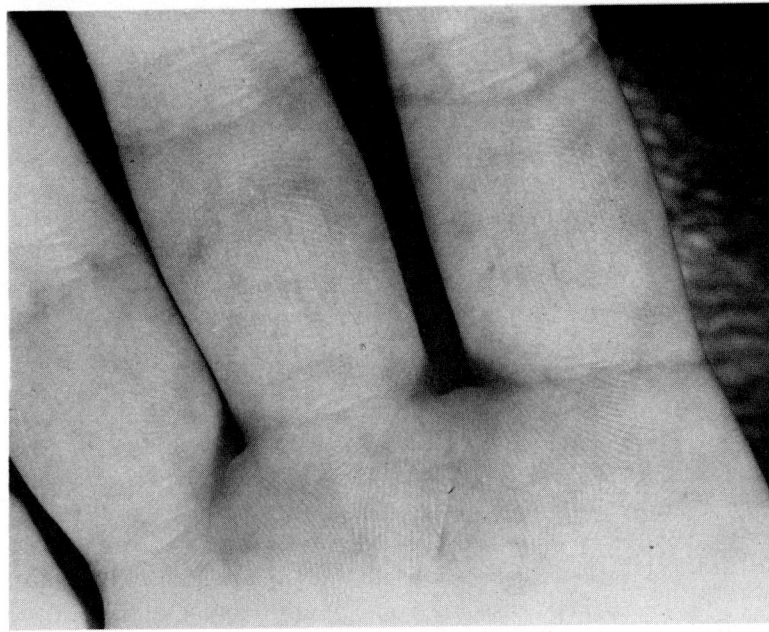

FIG. 74–2. Livedo reticularis of the volar aspect of the proximal phalanges and distal palm in a patient with systemic lupus erythematosus. The lesions are nonpalpable and may be seen in a variety of vasculitic syndromes.

The mainstay of the diagnosis of classic polyarteritis nodosa is the *histopathologic demonstration of necrotizing vasculitis of small and medium-sized arteries* in patients with *compatible clinical manifestations.* It is preferable to perform a biopsy on accessible organs such as the skin, muscle, or testis, but these structures are not invariably involved, and "blind" biopsy has only limited value.

A characteristic feature of the polyarteritis nodosa type of necrotizing vasculitis is the finding of aneurysmal dilatations up to 1 cm in size in medium-sized arteries seen by angiogram in the renal, hepatic, and visceral vasculature (Fig. 74–3). It was formerly believed that this finding was virtually pathognomonic

Table 74–5. Laboratory Abnormalities in Patients With Classic Polyarteritis Nodosa

Laboratory Abnormality	Percentage (%)
Erythrocyte sedimentation rate >10 mm/hr	94
Leukocytosis (WBC >10,000/mm³)	74
Anemia (hematocrit <35%)	66
Thrombocytosis (>400,000/mm³)	53
Renal function abnormality	70
Proteinuria	64
Hematuria	45
Casts	34
Complement abnormality	
Depressed CH_{50}	21
Depressed C3	70
Depressed C4	30
Rheumatoid factor ≥1:160	40
Immune complexes present	62.5
Cryoglobulins present	25

(From Cupps, T.R., and Fauci, A.S.[2])

of classic polyarteritis nodosa;[30–32] however, multiple aneurysms of this type are seen in overlap syndromes in which vessels of various sizes are involved,[12,33] as well as in other disorders such as SLE[34] and fibromuscular dysplasia.[35] Demonstration of involved vessels on a visceral angiogram, however, is helpful in establishing the presence of systemic vascular disease and is valuable in clinical situations in which no in-

FIG. 74–3. Renal angiogram in a patient with classic polyarteritis nodosa. Note the multiple intraparenchymal aneurysms (arrows).

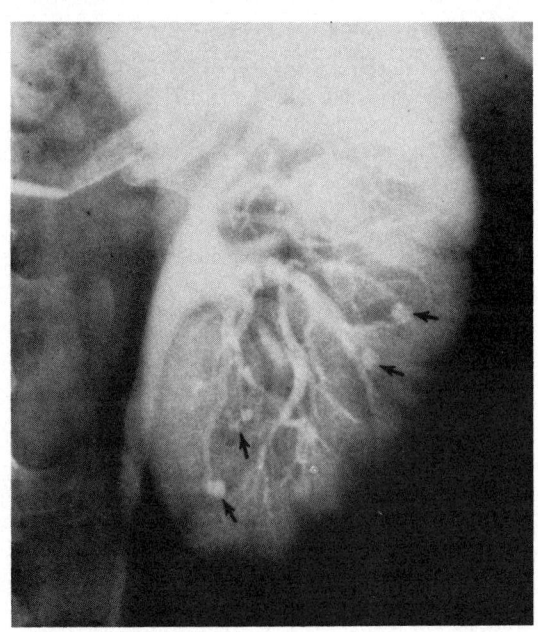

volved organ is easily accessible for biopsy. *If a patient has signs and symptoms suggestive of polyarteritis nodosa without readily accessible tissue for biopsy, the diagnosis can be made on the basis of a positive visceral angiogram.*

Prognosis

The prognosis of untreated classic polyarteritis nodosa is poor. Although some cases have resolved spontaneously, the usual course of the disease is a relentless progression with intermittent acute flares.[1,2] The grave prognosis is reflected in the 5-year survival rate of 13% reported for untreated patients.[36] With the use of corticosteroids, survival rate has improved to 48%.[36] Survival rates are lower in patients with hypertension or renal disease initially. Death usually results from renal failure or from cardiovascular or gastrointestinal involvement. Persistent and uncontrolled hypertension often contributes to the late morbidity and mortality of this disease by compounding the renal disease and by leading to late cardiovascular and cerebrovascular disorders. Treatment is considered later in this chapter.

ALLERGIC ANGIITIS AND GRANULOMATOSIS (CHURG-STRAUSS SYNDROME)

The combination of allergic angiitis and granulomatosis is a disease characterized by granulomatous vasculitis of multiple organ systems.[11,37] Although the vascular lesions may be identical to those of classic polyarteritis nodosa, this disease is unique for the following reasons: (1) frequency of involvement of *pulmonary vessels*; (2) vasculitis of blood vessels of *various types* and sizes such as small and medium-sized muscular arteries, veins, arterioles, and venules; (3) intra- and extravascular *granuloma* formation; (4) *eosinophilic tissue infiltrates*; and (5) association with severe *asthma* and *peripheral eosinophilia*. This disease can be thought of as a polyarteritis nodosa-like syndrome with strong allergic components and with pulmonary involvement as an essential element of the disease instead of a rarity.[1,37]

The clinical features of allergic angiitis and granulomatosis are listed in Table 74–6. Laboratory findings are similar to those in classic polyarteritis nodosa. An elevated erythrocyte sedimentation rate and leukocytosis are found in the majority of patients. An elevated total eosinophil count (greater than $1,000/mm^3$) is noted at some point in approximately 85% of patients. This peripheral eosinophilia is not seen in classic polyarteritis nodosa, but may be seen in the overlap syndromes described later. Elevated serum IgE levels have also been described. Unlike classic polyarteritis nodosa, no association exists with hepatitis B antigenemia.

The degree of severity of allergic angiitis and granulomatosis varies from patient to patient, and so prognosis is also variable. The overall prognosis remains poor, however, and in untreated patients, it is similar to that of classic polyarteritis nodosa. Treatment is discussed below.

Table 74–6. Clinical Profile and Manifestations in Allergic Angiitis and Granulomatosis

Clinical Parameter	Value
General considerations	
Age (mean)	44 years
Sex ratio (male to female)	1.3 to 1
Duration (mean) of pulmonary symptoms prior to systemic symptoms	2 years
Fever	Majority of patients
Organ involvement	Percentage (%)
Lungs	96
Infiltrate on chest roentgenogram	93
Wheezing	82
Skin	67
Purpura	37
Nodules	35
Peripheral nerves	63
Circulatory system (hypertension)	54
Gastrointestinal tract	42
Heart	38
Kidney	38
Lower urinary tract	10
Musculoskeletal system	10
Arthritis or arthralgia	21

(From Cupps, T.R., and Fauci, A.S.[2])

POLYANGIITIS OVERLAP SYNDROME

Many systemic necrotizing vasculitides manifest clinicopathologic characteristics that overlap classic polyarteritis nodosa and allergic angiitis and granulomatosis, as well as the hypersensitivity small vessel group of vasculitides, and it is now clear that overlap can exist among any of the well-defined vasculitic syndromes (Tables 74–2 and 74–7).[12] This subgroup of systemic necrotizing vasculitis has been referred to as the *polyangiitis overlap syndrome*.[1,2,9,12,38] This syndrome has caused the most difficulty in classification and has appeared under different designations and categories. A typical, perplexing case is that of a young person with a multisystem necrotizing vasculitis with renal involvement and mononeuritis multiplex. The patient may or may not have hypertension, and visceral and renal angiograms may or may not demonstrate multiple aneurysms. By most generally accepted criteria, this patient would be diagnosed as having classic polyarteritis nodosa.[10,13] This same patient, however, may also have significant lung involvement, a small-vessel cutaneous venulitis, or history of allergy with or without eosinophilia and granuloma, none of which occur in classic polyarteritis nodosa. Recognition of the overlap syndrome avoids confusion as to appropriate diagnosis and therapy. This subgroup is indeed a "systemic" vasculitis with the same potential for irreversible organ system dysfunction. For this reason, we categorized all three of these subgroups under the major category of *systemic necrotizing vasculitis*.

TREATMENT

Corticosteroids are still the initial treatment of choice for the systemic necrotizing vasculitides, but the addition of a cytotoxic agent, such as cyclophosphamide, to the therapeutic regimen has resulted in striking remissions in a high percentage of patients within this category.[1,29] Early reports showed an increase in survival rates from 13% in untreated patients to 48% in corticosteroid-treated patients.[36] Unlike in Wegener's granulomatosis, in which corticosteroids alone are inadequate therapy and a cytotoxic drug such as cyclophosphamide is essential for the induction of remission, treatment should be tailored to the degree, severity, and stage of the disease.[3,29] *Most patients require a combination of a cytotoxic agent and corticosteroids for maximal induction of remission*, but some treated with corticosteroids alone have a complete remission. On the other hand a few patients have such fulminant systemic vasculitis that they succumb to a devastating complication such as bowel perforation or infarction of other vital organs before any therapy has a chance to be effective. Patients with less severe forms of systemic vasculitis in whom irreversible organ system dysfunction does not appear to be imminent may be treated initially with corticosteroids alone. Initial therapy with prednisone is 1 mg/kg/day in divided doses, followed by consolidation in a few weeks to a single daily dose. Depending on the clinical response, the patient should be treated with daily prednisone for approximately 1 to 2 months, with an attempt to convert to alternate-day therapy over the next month. If conversion is accomplished without relapse, an alternate-day regimen is maintained for several months to a year. The dose is then gradually tapered until the drug is discontinued or until a maintenance dose is reached.

If patients do not improve objectively after a month of corticosteroid therapy or if they initially have fulminant disease and deteriorating organ system function, a cytotoxic regimen should be started. We have had excellent results with oral cyclophosphamide at

Table 74–7. Characteristics of the Polyangiitis Overlap Syndrome

Patient	Overlapping Syndromes
1	SNV, not classified
2	PAN and Churg-Strauss
3	PAN and Churg-Strauss
4	TA and PAN
5	PAN and Churg-Strauss
6	Takayasu's arteritis and PAN
7	SNV, not classified
8	PAN and cutaneous vasculitis
9	HSP and PAN
10	Giant cell arteritis and Churg-Strauss or Wegener's granulomatosis
11	PAN and Wegener's granulomatosis
12	PAN and cutaneous vasculitis

(Adapted from Leavitt, R.Y., and Fauci, A.S.[12])
SNV = systemic necrotizing vasculitis, PAN = polyarteritis nodosa, TA = temporal arteritis, HSP = Henoch-Schönlein purpura.

Table 74–8. Combined Cyclophosphamide-Prednisone Therapy for Severe Systemic Vasculitis

Cyclophosphamide: Initial dose of 2 mg/kg/day orally; adjust so that white blood cell count remains above 3,000 to 3,500/mm³ (neutrophil count 1,000 to 1,500/mm³); continue therapy with frequent downward adjustments of dosage, to prevent severe neutropenia; continue therapy for a year following induction of complete remission, and then taper dose by 25-mg decrements every 2 months until discontinued.

Prednisone: Initial dose of 1 mg/kg/day in 3 to 4 divided doses for 7 to 10 days; consolidate to single morning dose by 2 to 3 weeks; continue single morning daily dose until patient has had 1 month's total corticosteroid treatment; convert to alternate-day regimen for the second month; maintain alternate-day regimen for the third month, followed by gradual tapering of alternate-day dose for the next 3 to 6 months.

(From Fauci, A.S.[39])

a dose of 2 mg/kg/day. A patient who cannot tolerate oral medication or a patient with bowel vasculitis in whom intestinal absorption is questionable should receive *cyclophosphamide intravenously* at the same dose. An aggressive surgical approach to the complications of ischemic bowel with early exploratory laparotomy, appropriate removal of necrotic bowel segments, and repeated operations for observation of the retained bowel may reduce the mortality rates associated with this most serious complication of systemic vasculitis. *Prednisone should always be given together with cyclophosphamide* during the induction phase of the therapeutic protocol because it usually takes 2 to 3 weeks to achieve an immunosuppressive effect from cyclophosphamide given at these doses. The combined regimen, which we use to treat the severe corticosteroid-resistant systemic vasculitides,[39] was originally developed for the treatment of Wegener's granulomatosis,[40] and is outlined in Table 74–8. *We have induced long-term clinical remissions in most patients with systemic necrotizing vasculitis using this therapeutic protocol.*[29]

Although malignant diseases, chiefly leukemia and non-Hodgkin's lymphoma, have been noted in patients with polycythemia vera, Hodgkin's disease, or organ transplants treated with immunosuppressive drugs, only one instance of malignant lymphoma has occurred in over 200 patients treated by our group. This occurred in a patient with smoldering Wegener's granulomatosis treated for several years with cyclophosphamide. The patient developed an undifferentiated lymphoma and died.[41] In addition, there have been three cases of bladder carcinoma associated with cyclophosphamide therapy. Cyclophosphamide therapy is also rarely associated with bladder fibrosis, pulmonary fibrosis, and hypogammaglobulinemia.[38,39,41a,42] More common side effects of cyclophosphamide include bone marrow suppression, gonadal dysfunction, and hemorrhagic cystitis (see Chapter 38).[38,39,41a,42]

Other cytotoxic agents such as azathioprine, chlorambucil, and methotrexate have been used in vasculitic syndromes with variable success,[39] but cyclophosphamide is the most effective agent in the induction of long-term remission. Large, single-bolus doses of corticosteroids or cyclophosphamide, or plasmapheresis,[43,44] have been administered to certain patients with vasculitic syndromes.[39] The efficacy of these regimens is not well established, however.

HYPERSENSITIVITY VASCULITIDES

This heterogeneous group is characterized by inflammation of small vessels such as venules, capillaries, and arterioles.[13–15,25,45] The postcapillary venule is most commonly involved. Although hypersensitivity vasculitis may affect any organ system, cutaneous disease usually predominates, and life-threatening organ system dysfunction is rare.

This type of vasculitis was first described in association with a recognized antigenic stimulus such as a microbe or a drug, accounting for the term "hypersensitivity."[15] The vasculitic component of serum sickness and similar reactions falls within the category of the hypersensitivity vasculitides.[2] *The term is unfortunate because no inciting antigen can be identified or even suspected in most cases.* Moreover, virtually all the recognized vasculitic syndromes have clinical and pathologic features that suggest underlying hypersensitivity or immunologic phenomena.

Other terms used synonymously with hypersensitivity vasculitis include *allergic vasculitis*[46] and *leukocytoclastic vasculitis.* The most common histopathologic pattern is the characteristic leukocytoclastic vasculitis involving the postcapillary venules (Fig. 74–4).[14,45] Mononuclear, predominantly lymphocytic, infiltrates have been described also, however.[46] The typical macroscopic appearance of the lesion is that of *palpable purpura* caused by a combination of endothelial swelling, infiltration by leukocytes, and extravasation of erythrocytes.[1] The lesions may range in size from pinpoint to several centimeters and may take the form of *papules, nodules, vesicles, bullae, ulcers, or recurrent urticaria.*

Although vasculitic skin lesions are the major features, the syndrome may be accompanied by systemic signs and symptoms such as fever, malaise, myalgia, and anorexia, similar to the systemic vasculitides. The disease may consist of a single acute episode lasting only a few weeks, or it may be recurrent or, less commonly, chronic, lasting for months or years. Weight loss and the anemia of chronic disease may be seen in chronic hypersensitivity vasculitis. The skin lesions may be pruritic or painful, with a stinging or burning sensation. Lesions are most common in dependent areas such as the lower extremities in ambulatory patients and over the sacrum in bedridden patients, most likely as a result of hydrostatic pressure. As the lesions resolve or become chronic or recurrent, skin hyperpigmentation may result.

The hypersensitivity vasculitides comprise a number of subgroups (see Table 74–1), within which the extent of extracutaneous involvement varies. The approximate figures for extracutaneous involvement in the whole group include arthritis or arthralgias in 40%, renal involvement in 37%, gastrointestinal involvement in 15%, and peripheral neuropathy in 12% of patients.[2] Although pulmonary involvement is

FIG. 74–4. Skin biopsy in a patient with hypersensitivity vasculitis. Note the involvement of postcapillary venules with leukocytoclasis, as manifested by nuclear debris.

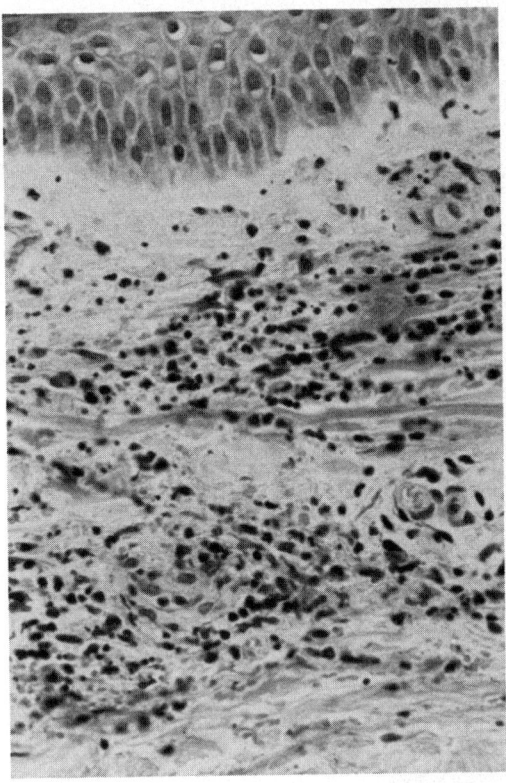

seen in up to 19% of patients with nonspecific patterns of infiltrates or effusions or both on chest roentgenograms, the significance of these findings is unclear because pulmonary vasculitis has rarely been demonstrated in these patients.[38,45] Those patients formerly diagnosed as having hypersensitivity vasculitis with significant extracutaneous involvement are now categorized within the "polyangiitis overlap" group, within the broader category of systemic vasculitis.

HENOCH-SCHÖNLEIN PURPURA

Henoch-Schönlein purpura, a distinctive subgroup of the hypersensitivity vasculitides, requires special mention not only because of its unique complex of manifestations, but also because it typifies *vasculitis that is usually confined to the skin but may have significant extracutaneous manifestations.* This disorder is characterized by the clinicopathologic complex of nonthrombocytopenic purpura, skin lesions, joint involvement, and colicky abdominal pain, sometimes associated with gastrointestinal hemorrhage and renal disease.[15,46–49] The disease usually occurs in children, but

adults of any age may be affected. The male/female ratio is 1.5:1. This disease usually remits spontaneously within a week, but may recur a number of times for some weeks to months before remission is complete. Rarely, patients have recurrent disease for years. The characteristic skin lesions are manifested as palpable purpura and represent leukocytoclastic venulitis (Fig. 74–5). Fever is seen in 75% of patients. Glomerulitis usually consists of microscopic hematuria without clinically significant functional renal impairment; rarely, renal failure occurs.[47] Hypertension is seen in 13% of patients. The organ system involvement and clinical manifestations in children with Henoch-Schönlein purpura are listed in Table 74–9.

Because of the excellent prognosis, immunosuppressive therapy is rarely indicated. Treatment usually consists of supportive, symptomatic therapy. In patients with recurrent disease, corticosteroids in daily doses of 1 mg/kg for limited periods are recommended; the dose is then tapered to an alternate-day regimen and is ultimately discontinued.[2,50] It has been difficult to evaluate the efficacy of corticosteroid therapy because of spontaneous remissions and recurrences. The few patients who develop significant renal disease may require cytotoxic therapy, according to the protocol already given for the systemic necrotizing vasculitides.

VASCULITIS ASSOCIATED WITH CONNECTIVE TISSUE DISEASES

Vasculitis may be associated with the entire spectrum of connective tissue disorders,[1,13,15,25,38,51] as discussed in other chapters devoted to the individual connective tissue diseases. Vasculitis is most common in RA, SLE and Sjögren's syndrome.[51] Although we include the vasculitis associated with other systemic connective tissue diseases under the category of hypersensitivity vasculitis, implying small-vessel disease of the skin, vasculitis in these diseases may be indistinguishable from the fulminant multisystem disorder of the systemic necrotizing vasculitis group. Cutaneous small-vessel disease is the most common associated vasculitis.[46a]

The vasculitis associated with RA usually consists of typical leukocytoclastic vasculitis of the postcapillary venules of the skin resulting in palpable purpura and cutaneous ulceration.[46a] In addition, the synovium and early rheumatoid nodules can manifest vasculitis.[52] Less commonly, patients with RA, particularly those with severely erosive and nodular disease and high-titer seropositivity for rheumatoid factor (RF),[53] develop a fulminant systemic vasculitis in-

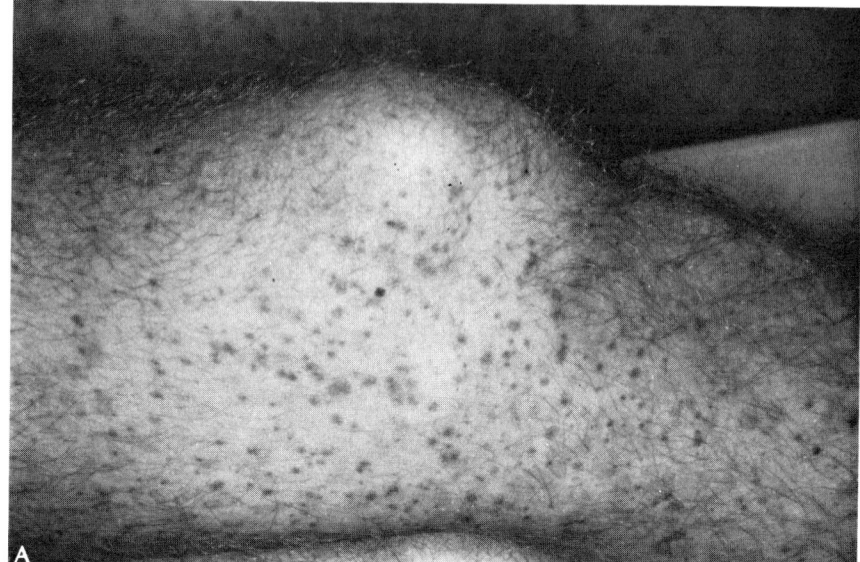

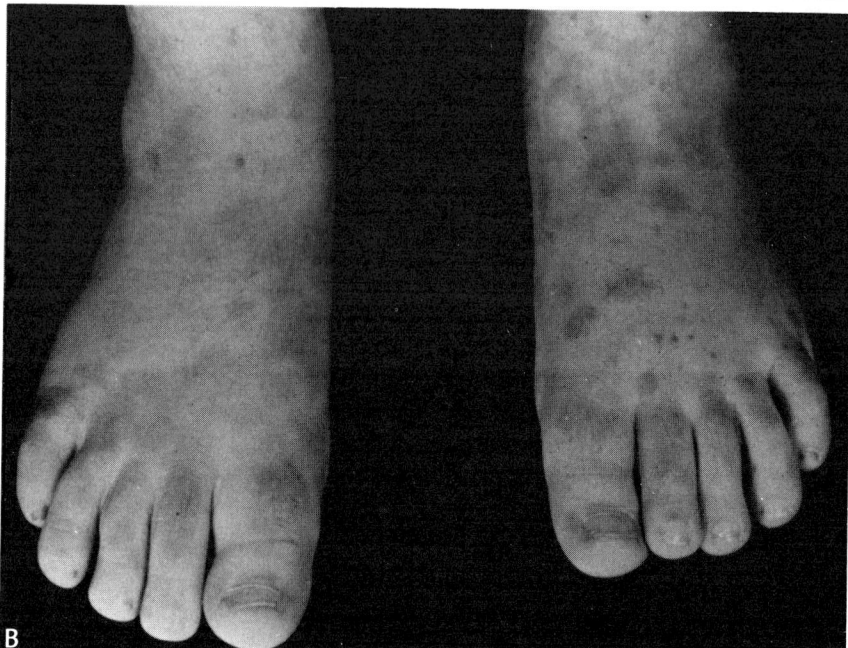

FIG. 74–5. *A*, Palpable purpura and flexion contracture of the knee in a patient with Henoch-Schönlein purpura. The flexion contracture is due to the periarthritis frequently seen with this disease. *B*, The larger, deeper, and more ecchymotic-appearing lesions seen in the dependent extremities in a patient with Henoch-Schönlein purpura. Also note the three more superficial palpable purpuric lesions over the dorsum of the distal left forefoot and the anterior aspect of the right ankle.

volving arterioles and medium-sized muscular arteries similar to that seen in the polyarteritis nodosa group of systemic necrotizing vasculitis.[54,55] Previously, it was believed that corticosteroid therapy either precipitated the development of or worsened the systemic vasculitis associated with RA;[56,57] it is now thought that systemic vasculitis merely reflects severe RA, a condition that may require corticosteroid therapy.[51]

Cutaneous vasculitis develops in approximately 20% of patients with SLE,[58] typically small-vessel vasculitis resulting in palpable purpura, although patients may develop cutaneous infarction and chronic ulceration. A serious, much less common vasculitic complication of SLE is diffuse central nervous system

vasculitis and visceral involvement similar to that seen in the polyarteritis nodosa group of systemic vasculitis.[58–60]

The mechanism is most likely immune complex deposition. The evidence for immune complex-mediated tissue damage is ample.[25,61] Treatment of most vasculitides in the diffuse connective tissue diseases is that of the primary underlying disease. If the vasculitis threatens vital organs, the treatment is as described for systemic vasculitis.

ESSENTIAL MIXED CRYOGLOBULINEMIA

Cryoglobulinemia may be present in a variety of disorders, with or without vasculitis. Indeed, cryo-

Table 74–9. Organ Involvement and Clinical Manifestations in Pediatric Patients With Henoch-Schönlein Purpura

Involvement	Percentage (%)
Skin	100
Purpura	100
Ulceration	4
Joints	71
Gastrointestinal tract	68
Pain	57
Nausea or vomiting	50
Occult blood	42
Hematemesis or melena	35
Major bleeding	5
Intussusception	3
Kidney	
Hematuria	45
Microscopic	45
Macroscopic	26
Proteinuria	35
Functional impairment	9
Localized edema	32

(From Cupps, T.R., and Fauci, A.S.[2])

globulinemia is present to a variable degree in many of the vasculitic syndromes under discussion. Several categories of cryoglobulinopathies exist, and vasculitis can be found in a number of them.[55,62] In the distinct syndrome called essential mixed cryoglobulinemia, identifiable underlying disease is not usually present.[63,64] In this syndrome, the vasculitis is generally confined to the skin, although some patients develop fulminant multisystem disease, particularly involving the kidney, with severe glomerulonephritis. Histopathologic examination of the purpuric skin lesions typically shows leukocytoclastic venulitis due to deposition of immune complexes, principally immunoglobulin M (IgM) RF directed against an IgG molecule; hence the term "mixed" cryoglobulinemia. Results of treatment are variable. When the disease remains confined to the skin, the prognosis is good. Patients with severe glomerulonephritis have a poor prognosis, however, because the disease has been reported to progress despite therapy with corticosteroids or even cytotoxic agents.[64,65] Plasmapheresis may be useful in this syndrome, but firm conclusions must await more extensive clinical trials.

VASCULITIS ASSOCIATED WITH NEOPLASMS AND OTHER PRIMARY DISORDERS

The association between small-vessel cutaneous vasculitis and certain malignant diseases is a well-recognized but rare phenomenon. Associated neo-

plasms usually are lymphoid or reticuloendothelial disorders such as Hodgkin's disease, other lymphomas, and multiple myeloma.[66-68] Although the vasculitis is usually a leukocytoclastic venulitis limited to the skin, systemic vasculitis in association with neoplasms also occurs rarely. Recent reports link hairy cell leukemia with systemic vasculitis of the polyarteritis nodosa type.[69,70] An interesting syndrome of granulomatous vasculitis of the central nervous system (CNS) is associated with lymphoproliferative disorders, usually Hodgkin's disease, in which the vasculitis is found in areas not invaded by tumor.[71] Although the cause of vasculitis associated with neoplasms is not known, it may reflect a hypersensitivity reaction to tumor or tumor-related antigen with or without the formation and deposition of immune complexes. Treatment of the vasculitis should be directed at the underlying neoplasm.

An association exists between *atrial myxoma* and systemic vasculopathy.[72] Strictly speaking, this syndrome is not a true vasculitis, because the arterial lesions result from embolization of myxomatous tissue and secondary inflammation of the arterial wall[73-75] (see Chapter 75).

Leukocytoclastic vasculitis may be a minor component of many other primary diseases.[25] Such diseases include subacute bacterial endocarditis, chronic active hepatitis, ulcerative colitis, retroperitoneal fibrosis, primary biliary cirrhosis, and Goodpasture's syndrome. As with other secondary vasculitides, therapy is directed at the underlying primary cause.

WEGENER'S GRANULOMATOSIS

Wegener's granulomatosis, a distinct clinicopathologic entity, is characterized by granulomatous vasculitis of the upper and lower respiratory tracts together with glomerulonephritis (Fig. 74–6). Variable degrees of disseminated vasculitis involving both small arteries and veins also may occur.[3,40] This disorder probably represents an aberrant hypersensitivity reaction to an unknown antigen, perhaps one that enters through the upper respiratory tract. No associations with allergic diatheses, geographic location, travel, or domestic or occupational exposure are known, however. The male/female ratio is 1.3:1, and the mean age of onset is 40.6 years.[3]

CLINICAL MANIFESTATIONS

The presenting signs and symptoms of 85 cases of Wegener's granulomatosis in a series conducted by

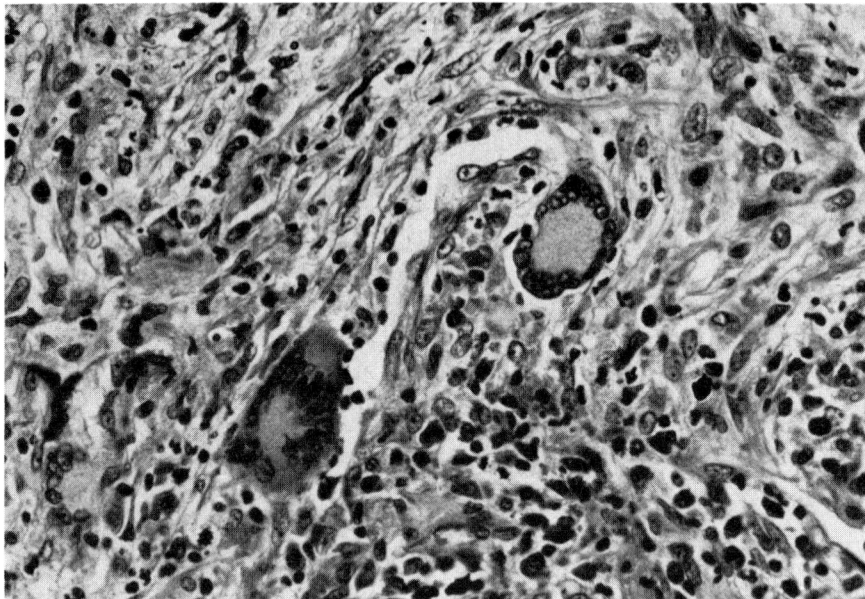

FIG. 74–6. Lung biopsy in a patient with Wegener's granulomatosis. Histopathologic study reveals granulomatous vasculitis with multinucleated giant cells infiltrating the vessel wall. (Hematoxylin and eosin stain; magnification ×200.)

Table 74–10. Presenting Signs and Symptoms in 85 Patients with Wegener's Granulomatosis

	Patients	
Sign or Symptom*	Number	Percentage (%)
Pulmonary infiltrates	60	71
Sinusitis	57	67
Arthralgia or arthritis	37	44
Fever	29	34
Otitis	21	25
Cough	29	34
Rhinitis or nasal symptoms	19	22
Hemoptysis	15	18
Ocular inflammation (conjunctivitis, uveitis, episcleritis, or scleritis)	14	16
Weight loss	14	16
Skin rash	11	13
Epistaxis	9	11
Renal failure	9	11
Chest discomfort	7	8
Anorexia or malaise	7	8
Proptosis	6	7
Shortness of breath or dyspnea	6	7
Oral ulcers	5	6
Hearing loss	5	6
Pleuritis or effusion	5	6
Headache	5	6

(From Fauci, A.S., et al.[3])

*Miscellaneous: hoarseness or stridor, saddle nose deformity, and mastoiditis, three patients each; cranial nerve dysfunction, and mastoiditis, three patients each; cranial nerve dysfunction, three patients; parotid mass or pain, two patients each; nasolacrimal duct obstruction, thyroiditis, liver function test abnormality, blindness, peripheral neuropathy, ear pinna mass, pedal edema, adenopathy, anosmia, pericarditis, asthma, diabetes insipidus, and Raynaud's phenomenon, one patient each.

my colleagues and myself are listed in Table 74–10.[3] Clinical presentations varied widely, but the typical findings related to the upper respiratory tract and included rhinorrhea, severe sinusitis, nasal mucosal ulcerations, and otitis media, usually secondary to blockage of the eustachian tube resulting from upper airway disease. Some patients had primary middle ear disease. Hearing loss was the initial complaint of several patients. A few patients had pulmonary disease without any evidence of upper airway disease. Symptoms included cough, hemoptysis, and less frequently, chest discomfort. Chest roentgenograms usually demonstrated pulmonary infiltrates. Other organ systems affected by Wegener's granulomatosis were occasionally the focus of initial complaints, often associated with the foregoing respiratory tract findings. Rarely, patients had renal failure in the absence of significant and easily detectable disease in other

Table 74–11. Organ or System Involvement in Wegener's Granulomatosis

	Patients	
Organ or System	Number	Percentage (%)
Lung	80	94
Paranasal sinuses	77	91
Kidney	72	85
Joints	57	67
Nose or nasopharynx	54	64
Ear	52	61
Eye	49	58
Skin	38	45
Nervous system	19	22
Heart	10	12

(From Fauci, A.S., et al.[3])

organ systems. Arthralgias were often present initially, as were other generalized manifestations of systemic inflammatory disease such as fatigue, malaise, anorexia, and weight loss. Fever often occurred, perhaps from the underlying inflammatory disease, although it was more commonly associated with secondary bacterial infection of the involved paranasal sinuses.

Although Wegener's granulomatosis is a generalized systemic disease with certain cardinal and characteristic features reflected in multiple organ system involvement (Table 74–11), it is essentially a true pulmonary–renal syndrome, and these two organ systems are largely responsible for the clinical course of the disease.

The characteristic and typical lung findings consist of multiple, *bilateral nodular infiltrates that usually cavitate* (Fig. 74–7). *Pleural effusions* occur in approximately 20% of patients, but hilar adenopathy is not seen, and pulmonary calcifications are rare.[40,76,77] Pulmonary function abnormalities are common and include obstruction to airflow as well as reduced lung volumes and diffusing capacity abnormalities.[78] Small areas of *atelectasis* frequently occur adjacent to parenchymal infiltrates during active pulmonary disease. Patients with documented endobronchial disease may develop atelectasis related to scarred endobronchial tissue or smoldering endobronchial disease accompanying quiescent disease in other organs.

Renal lesions range from *mild focal* and *segmental glomerulonephritis* with minimal urinary findings and little, if any, renal functional impairment to *fulminant*

FIG. 74–7. Chest roentgenogram from a patient with Wegener's granulomatosis showing multiple nodules and cavity formation.

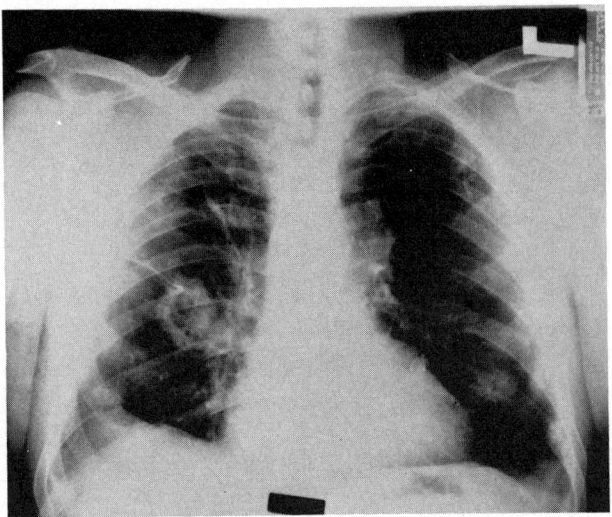

FIG. 74–8. Photomicrograph of a kidney biopsy from a patient with Wegener's granulomatosis showing extensive involvement of the glomerulus with marked increase in cellularity (hematoxylin and eosin stain; original magnification; ×400). (From Leavitt, R.Y., and Fauci, A.S.[38])

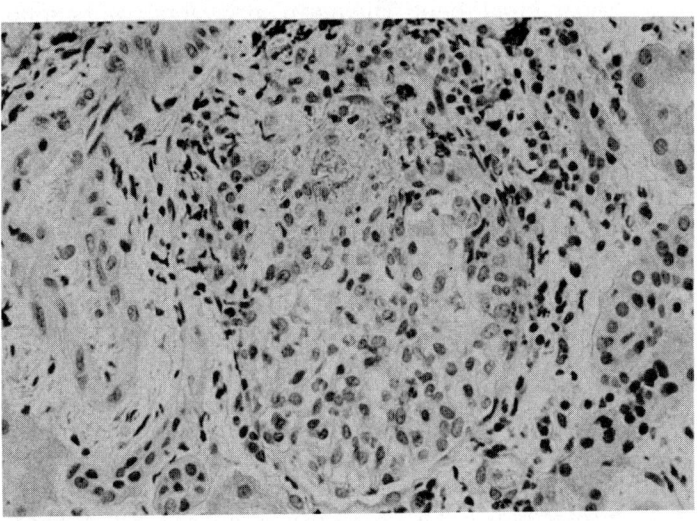

diffuse necrotizing glomerulonephritis with proliferative and crescentic changes (Fig. 74–8).[40,76,79] Granulomas and true arteritis are rarely found on renal biopsy. Once present, glomerulonephritis may rapidly progress from mild to severe and may lead to fulminant renal failure within weeks and even days of its inception. Because extrarenal manifestations usually precede functional renal disease, often by months, it is critical to establish the diagnosis early with appropriate treatment to prevent irreversible renal failure.[3]

Most patients with Wegener's granulomatosis and serious sinus or nasal disease develop *secondary infection* of these tissues, almost surely because of mucosal damage and the subsequent impairment of host defenses.[3] Staphylococcus aureus is the predominant organism cultured from the nose or sinus of infected patients. Treated patients in complete remission often have an apparent relapse because of increased sinus symptoms together with an elevation of the erythrocyte sedimentation rate. Careful evaluation shows, however, that the symptoms and the erythrocyte sedimentation rate elevation are usually related to smoldering upper airway infection, and both respond promptly to antibiotics with or without drainage procedures. *This observation is important because increasing or reinstituting immunosuppressive therapy under these circumstances is obviously contraindicated.*

TREATMENT AND PROGNOSIS

Before the use of immunosuppressive therapy, the prognosis for patients with this disease was grave. Untreated, the disease usually ran a rapidly fatal course, particularly after the recognition of functional renal impairment. The mean survival rate of patients with untreated Wegener's granulomatosis was 5 months; 82% of patients died within a year, and more than 90% died within 2 years.[80] Wegener's granulomatosis was the first vasculitic syndrome in which the use of long-term, low-dose (2 mg/kg/day) cytotoxic agents, in this case cyclophosphamide, together with alternate-day corticosteroid administration, was effective in inducing remissions in most patients.[40] We recorded complete remissions in 79 of 85 patients (93%) using this protocol.[3] The mean duration of remission for survivors was over 4 years, and some patients maintained remission without therapy for more than 10 years. This striking response of a formerly fatal non-neoplastic disease to a combination of low-dose cyclophosphamide and alternate-day corticosteroids has led to its use in other severe systemic vasculitic syndromes, as previously discussed.

LYMPHOMATOID GRANULOMATOSIS

Lymphomatoid granulomatosis is characterized by infiltration of various organs with a polymorphic cellular infiltrate consisting of atypical lymphocytoid and plasmacytoid cells together with granulomatous inflammation in an angiocentric and angiodestructive pattern.[81] Strictly speaking, lymphomatoid granulomatosis is not a vasculitis, because it is not a true inflammation of blood vessels, but it is rather an infiltration and invasion of blood vessel walls with atypical lymphoid cells in association with an intra- or extravascular granulomatous response. The disease probably represents one end of the spectrum of malignant lymphoma.[38] I include the disease here because it is often confused with certain vasculitic syndromes such as Wegener's granulomatosis.[82] The disease primarily involves the lungs, but skin, renal, and CNS disease has occurred in various patients. The characteristic inflammatory granulomas accompany lymphoproliferative disease; hence the term "lymphomatoid granulomatosis." The precise nature of this disorder remains unknown.

Patients generally have nonspecific signs and symptoms such as fever, malaise, weight loss, and fatigue. Chest roentgenograms reveal bilateral nodular infiltrates resembling metastatic cancer. The spectrum of organ system involvement in lymphomatoid granulomatosis is outlined in Table 74–12.[83]

Untreated disease is almost uniformly fatal.[81,84,85] We have treated 15 patients with lymphomatoid granulomatosis with a regimen of cyclophosphamide and alternate-day prednisone administration.[83] Approximately half the patients had a complete remission, and therapy was ultimately discontinued. Patients who did not have a remission developed the lymphoproliferative phase of the disease and ultimately died. Thus, the prognosis remains poor.

GIANT CELL ARTERITIDES

The giant cell arteritides include temporal or cranial arteritis and Takayasu's arteritis. Both are panarteritides characterized by inflammation of medium and large arteries. They are separable by the clear-cut differences in age range, the distribution of involved vessels, the associated syndromes, and the response to therapy. The characteristics of these diseases are outlined in Table 74–13.

TEMPORAL ARTERITIS

Temporal arteritis (see also Chapter 79) is well recognized by its classic clinical picture of fever, anemia, high erythrocyte sedimentation rate, and associated symptoms in a person more than 55 years old.[86,87] The diagnosis can often be made clinically and confirmed by biopsy of the temporal arteries. Because vessel involvement may be segmental and may be missed on routine biopsy, some authors have recommended local arteriography[88] and examination of multiple sections of bilateral biopsies.[88a]

Table 74–12.   Organ or System Involvement in 15 Patients with Lymphomatoid Granulomatosis

Organ or System	No. of Patients (%)
Lung	15 (100)
Skin	8 (53)
Kidney	6 (40)
Lymph nodes	6 (40)
Central nervous system	5 (33)
Bone marrow	5 (33)
Liver	4 (27)
Peripheral nervous system	3 (20)
Eyes	3 (20)
Muscle	2 (13)
Paranasal sinuses	1 (7)
Thyroid gland	1 (7)
Epididymis	1 (7)

(From Fauci, A.S., et al.[83])

Table 74–13. Characteristics of the Giant Cell Arteritides

	Temporal Arteritis	Takayasu's Arteritis
Patients	Disease of the elderly; women more than men	More prevalent in young women; more common in the Orient, but neither racially nor geographically restricted
Blood vessels	Characteristically involves branches of carotid (temporal artery), but is a systemic arteritis and may involve any medium-sized or large artery	Large and medium-sized arteries with predilection for aortic arch and its branches; may involve pulmonary artery
Histopathologic features	Panarteritis; inflammatory mononuclear cell infiltrates; frequent giant cell formation within vessel wall; fragmentation of internal elastic lamina; proliferation of tunica intima	Panarteritis; inflammatory mononuclear cell infiltrates; intimal proliferation and fibrosis; scarring and vascularization of tunica media; disruption and degeneration of elastic lamina
Clinical manifestations	Classic complex of fever, anemia, high erythrocyte sedimentation rate, muscle aches in an elderly person; possible headache; strong association with polymyalgia rheumatica syndrome	Generalized systemic symptoms; local signs and symptoms related to involved vessels; occlusive phase
Complications	Ocular (sudden blindness)	Related to distribution of involved vessels; death usually occurs from congestive heart failure or cerebrovascular accidents
Diagnosis	Temporal artery biopsy; lesions may be segmental; multiple sections, arteriography, and bilateral biopsy may aid in diagnosis	Arteriography; biopsy of involved vessel
Treatment	Corticosteroids effective	Corticosteroids not of proved efficacy; cytotoxic agents currently being tested

(From Fauci, A.S., Haynes, B.F., and Katz, P.[1])

Polymyalgia rheumatica syndrome, closely associated with temporal arteritis, is characterized by stiffness, aching, and pain in the muscles of the neck, shoulder, lower back, hips, and thighs.[86,89,90] This syndrome is discussed in Chapter 79.

A well-recognized and serious complication of temporal arteritis, particularly in untreated patients, is ocular involvement, sometimes leading to sudden blindness.[91] Although the dramatic eye manifestations may appear suddenly, most patients have complaints relating to the head or eyes for months, and so one needs to pay careful attention to symptoms and rapid use of appropriate therapy. Temporal arteritis is generally exquisitely sensitive to corticosteroid therapy.[86,89,92] Treatment should begin with 40 to 60 mg prednisone daily, followed by gradual tapering to a daily maintenance dose of 7.5 to 10 mg, with upward readjustment of dosage if symptoms recur. Therapy should be continued for at least 1 to 2 years.[86,89,92,93] Although one should not attempt to induce initial remission of temporal arteritis with alternate-day therapy, many patients can be given alternate-day therapy in preparation for discontinuing the drug after induction of remission.[93] The prognosis of this disorder is good with corticosteroid therapy, and remissions usually are maintained after withdrawal of therapy, although relapse can occur.

TAKAYASU'S ARTERITIS

Usually seen in women in the second or third decade of life, Takayasu's arteritis is characterized by inflammation and stenosis of large and intermediate-sized arteries with frequent involvement of the aortic arch and its branches.[94–100] Diagnosis is usually made angiographically. Takayasu's arteritis is often referred to as "pulseless disease" because of the frequent involvement of the subclavian artery (Fig. 74–9A). Nonetheless, it has complex manifestations ranging from generalized, often vague, symptoms characteristic of a systemic inflammatory disease to local signs and symptoms relating to the involved vessels themselves, to the characteristic manifestations of compromised blood flow to the organs perfused by the involved vessels (Fig. 74–9B). Some patients experience no apparent inflammatory symptoms and signs but have initial ischemic findings and changes related to the involved organ systems. The most common and obvious findings are absent pulses in the affected vessels. Bruits are common. The clinical course of the disease varies. Gradual deterioration is the rule, but the process may spontaneously remit, stabilize temporarily, insidiously progress, or abruptly decompensate. This variability has made it difficult to evaluate therapy. Despite reports of spontaneous remissions in untreated patients, the course is generally pro-

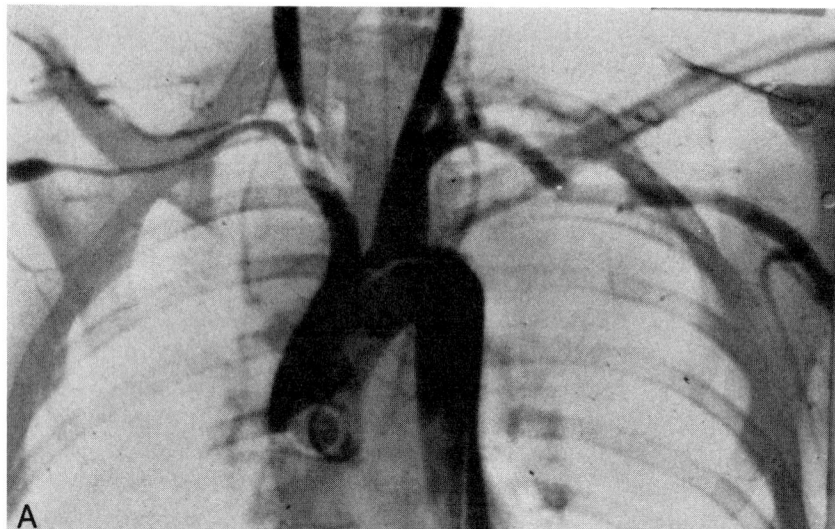

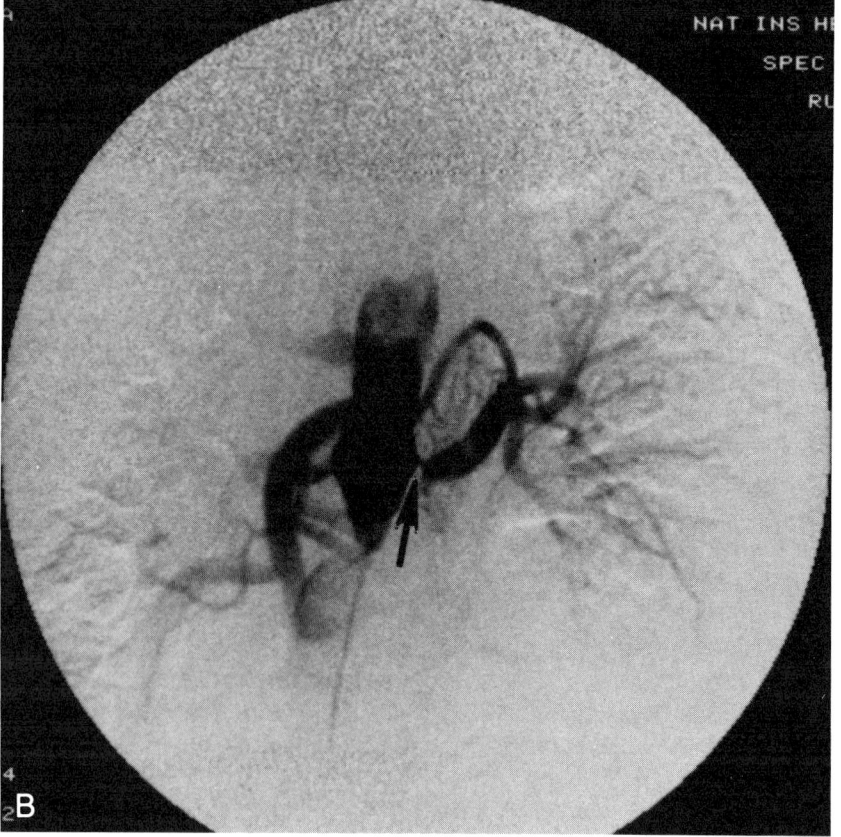

FIG. 74–9. Subtraction angiograms from two patients with Takayasu's arteritis. *A,* Angiogram demonstrates severe involvement along a large segment of the right subclavian artery, as well as involvement of the right common carotid artery. *B,* Angiogram demonstrates marked narrowing of the left renal artery (arrow) and narrowing of the infrarenal aorta.

gressive and fatal within a few years. Death usually occurs from congestive heart failure or cerebrovascular accidents.[95] Corticosteroid therapy usually results in symptomatic improvement and angiographic stabilization.[99,100] We use cyclophosphamide in patients who have persistent or progressive disease while on corticosteroid therapy.[100,101] In addition to medical treatment, we take an aggressive approach to vascular reconstructive surgery aimed at preventing ischemic damage to organs with compromised vascular flow; necessary surgery can and should be performed on patients with active arteritis.[99–101] This approach to the therapy of Takayasu's arteritis appears to improve survival and decrease ischemic complications, but longer followup is necessary.[99–101]

MUCOCUTANEOUS LYMPH NODE SYNDROME (KAWASAKI'S DISEASE)

The mucocutaneous lymph node syndrome is an acute febrile illness of infants and young children. The cause is completely unknown, and although an infectious agent has been suspected, no etiologic agent has been identified.[102] Propionibacterium acnes has been implicated as the most likely agent,[103] with house dust mites serving as its vector.[104–106] A retrovirus may play an etiologic role.[107–108] The P. acnes involvement has not been confirmed. The disease was originally described in Japan and is characterized by the following: nonsuppurative cervical adenitis; changes in the skin and mucous membranes such as edema; congested conjunctivae; erythema of the oral cavity, lips, and palms; and desquamation of the skin of the fingertips, all unresponsive to antibiotics.[109–111] The disease has recently been recognized with increasing frequency in the United States.[112] Its clinical

Table 74–14. Clinical Manifestations of Mucocutaneous Lymph Node Syndrome (Kawasaki's Disease)

Manifestations	Percentage (%)
Fever	95
Changes of the extremity	
Desquamation from finger tips	94
Erythematous palms and soles	88
Indurated edema	76
Polymorphous exanthem of body and trunk	92
Changes in lips and oral cavity	
Dry, red lips	90
Erythematous oral mucosa	90
Prominent tongue papillae	77
Congested conjunctivae	88
Swelling of cervical lymph nodes	75

(From Cupps, T.R., and Fauci, A.S.[2])

manifestations are listed in Table 74–14. The condition is usually self-limited, and most patients recover uneventfully. Approximately 1 to 2% of patients, however, develop severe and often fatal complications, resulting from vasculitic involvement of the coronary arteries. Most of the cases in the United States formerly reported as polyartertis nodosa of children, with its characteristic and unusual selective involvement of the coronary arteries, were in fact the arteritis of unrecognized Kawasaki's disease.[110] Myocarditis, endopericarditis, myocardial infarctions, and cardiomegaly are also seen. Involvement of other vessels such as the aorta and the celiac, carotid, subclavian, and pulmonary arteries occurs much less frequently. Treatment with aspirin (30 mg/kg/day) may lessen the incidence of cardiac complications. Furthermore, some evidence, as yet unconfirmed, suggests that corticosteroids are ineffective and may actually increase the incidence of cardiac complications.[113] Intravenous γ-globulin may decrease the incidence of cardiac abnormalities seen in these patients,[109] but more data are needed. At this time, intravenous immunoglobulin is not recommended in the treatment of this disorder.[109]

VASCULITIS ISOLATED TO THE CENTRAL NERVOUS SYSTEM

In addition to the granulomatous vasculitis of the CNS already discussed in association with certain lymphoproliferative malignant diseases, a syndrome of *isolated vasculitis of the CNS* exists. This uncommon entity is characterized by vasculitis restricted to the vessels of the CNS in the apparent absence of systemic vasculitis or other systemic disease.[114] Presenting manifestations include severe headaches, altered mental function, and focal neurologic defects. Systemic symptoms such as fever, myalgia, arthralgia, and arthritis, common in the systemic vasculitides, are usually not present. Diagnosis is made by the clinical presentation together with angiographic studies or biopsy of the brain parenchyma and leptomeninges, when feasible.[115] Prognosis is generally poor, but corticosteroid therapy alone or together with cyclophosphamide in corticosteroid-resistant patients used in the regimen described for systemic vasculitis may induce long-term remissions.[9,114]

BEHÇET'S DISEASE

Behçet's disease (see also Chapter 64) of unknown origin is characterized by recurrent episodes of oral ulcers, eye lesions, genital ulcers, and other cutaneous lesions.[116] The underlying pathologic lesion is a vasculitis predominantly involving venules, although vessels of any size in any organ system can be affected. No therapy for Behçet's disease is uniformly acceptable. A number of therapeutic regimens have been attempted with variable results, including topical and systemic corticosteroids, colchicine, indomethacin, transfer factor, blood transfusion, antifibrinolytic therapy, levamisole, chlorambucil, azathioprine, and sulfasalazine.[117]

THROMBOANGIITIS OBLITERANS (BUERGER'S DISEASE)

This rare inflammatory occlusive peripheral vascular disease involves the arteries and veins. The disease is seen predominantly in men, usually between the ages of 20 and 40 but it can affect women.[118–120] It primarily involves medium-sized and small arteries as well as veins in a segmental fashion. The inflammatory process is associated with a thrombus and evolves through several stages. In the acute stage, the vessel wall and thrombus are infiltrated by polymorphonuclear leukocytes. Microabscesses may be found within the thrombi.[121] A subacute stage follows, when mononuclear cells and giant cells may be seen, and ultimately a chronic stage develops, characterized by chronic inflammatory infiltrates, fibrosis, and recanalization of the vessel lumen. The entire process may be associated with migratory superficial thrombophlebitis.

Although the cause is unknown, the use of tobacco makes the disease much worse. Almost without exception, thromboangiitis obliterans occurs in heavy smokers.[118] No sufficient evidence suggests an immunologic pathogenesis.

The clinical presentation is variable and may be insidious or abrupt. Coldness of the distal extremities, color changes, dysesthesias, intense hyperemia, excruciating pain, ulceration, gangrene, and pulp atrophy are common.[118,121,122] Usually, acute attacks last 1 to 4 weeks, and the disease runs an indolent and recurrent course. Ultimately, the collateral circulation can no longer compensate for the progressive ischemia, and amputation of the involved distal extremities may be required. Various techniques such as anticoagulation, thromboendarterectomy, bypass operations, and sympathectomy have not improved the prognosis for the involved extremity.[122,123] The most effective approach to this disease seems to be meticulous local care of the involved area, together with complete abstinence from tobacco.

MISCELLANEOUS VASCULITIDES

A number of other syndromes show vasculitis as either a primary disease process or a secondary component of an underlying entity. *Erythema nodosum* is a common syndrome well recognized as a hypersensitivity manifestation of underlying disorders.[124] It is manifested as a painful, nodular, inflammatory process of the dermis and subcutaneous tissues. Vasculitis, predominantly of small venules, comprises a major component of its histopathologic picture.[125]

Other less common vasculitides that deserve mention are *erythema elevatum diutinum*,[126] *Cogan's syndrome*,[127] and *Eale's disease*.[128] Finally, some rare syndromes appear to be confined to single organs such as the vermiform appendix and the female breast.[129]

GENERAL APPROACH TO THE PATIENT

The vasculitides comprise a broad spectrum of clinicopathologic syndromes. In certain disorders, vasculitis is the predominant and most obvious manifestation in the absence of an underlying disease process. Other disorders may be characterized by a vasculitic syndrome secondary to an underlying disease. Most vasculitic syndromes are associated directly or indirectly with immunopathologic mechanisms. Using various clinical, pathologic, and

Table 74–15.   General Approach to the Patient With Vasculitis

1. Categorize the syndrome correctly (specific syndrome; primary versus secondary; localized versus systemic).
2. Determine extent of disease activity.
3. Remove offending antigen if possible.
4. If associated with underlying disease, treat underlying disease when possible.
5. Use appropriate therapeutic agents immediately in diseases in which efficacy is clearly demonstrated, such as corticosteroids in temporal arteritis and cyclophosphamide and corticosteroids in Wegener's granulomatosis.
6. Avoid immunosuppressive therapy (corticosteroids or cytotoxic agents) in diseases that: (1) do not disseminate; (2) do not usually result in irreversible organ system damage; and (3) rarely respond to such agents.
7. Institute corticosteroids immediately in patients with systemic vasculitis; add a cytotoxic agent such as cyclophosphamide if response is not prompt or if disease is known to respond only to cytotoxic agents.
8. Continually attempt to taper corticosteroids to alternate-day regimens, and discontinue when possible.
9. Have a clear-cut understanding of goals and mechanisms of the long-term use of cytotoxic agents in the treatment of non-neoplastic diseases.
10. Use other agents if clinical situation dictates (e.g., non-steroidal anti-inflammatory agents or plasmapheresis) based on results from therapeutic trials.

immunologic criteria, certain vasculitic syndromes can be clearly recognized and categorized as distinct entities, whereas others overlap different diseases within a broader category. It is important to categorize the vasculitic syndrome in a given patient, and particularly to identify disseminated systemic disease leading to irreversible organ system dysfunction if untreated or if inadequately treated. Such patients need prompt and aggressive treatment with corticosteroids and, in some cases, cytotoxic agents, such as cyclophosphamide. In contrast, patients with predominantly cutaneous disease without a high risk of systemic involvement can be treated much less aggressively. Appreciation of the scope of the vasculitic syndromes is essential for an appropriate diagnostic and therapeutic approach to individual patients (Table 74–15).

REFERENCES

1. Fauci, A.S., Haynes, B.F., and Katz, P.: The spectrum of vasculitis: Clinical, pathologic, immunologic, and therapeutic considerations. Ann. Intern. Med., 89:660–676, 1978.
2. Cupps, T.R., and Fauci, A.S.: The Vasculitides. Philadelphia, W.B. Saunders, 1981.
3. Fauci, A.S., et al.: Wegener's granulomatosis: Prospective clinical and therapeutic experience with 85 patients for 21 years. Ann. Intern. Med., 98:76–85, 1983.
4. Cochrane, C.G., and Dixon, F.J.: Antigen–antibody complex induced disease. In Textbook of Immunopathology. 2nd Ed. Vol. 1. Edited by P.A. Meischer and H.F. Müller-Eberhard. New York, Grune & Stratton, 1976.
5. Sergent, J.S., et al.: Vasculitis with hepatitis B antigenemia: Long-term observations in nine patients. Medicine (Baltimore), 67:354–359, 1976.
6. Spector, W.G., and Heesom, N.: The production of granulomata by antigen–antibody complexes. J. Pathol., 98:31–39, 1969.
7. Leung, D.Y.M., Collins, T., Lapierre, L.A., and Geha, R.S.: IgM antibodies present in the acute phase of Kawasaki syndrome lyse cultured vascular endothelial cell stimulated by gamma interferon. J. Clin. Invest., 77:1428, 1986.
8. Leung, D.Y.M., et al.: Two monokines, interleukin-1 and tumor necrosis factor, render cultured vascular endothelial cells susceptible to lysis by antibodies circulating during Kawasaki sydnrome. J. Exp. Med., 164:1958, 1986.
9. Fauci, A.S.: The vasculitis syndromes. In Harrison's Principles of Internal Medicine. 11th Ed. Edited by E. Braunwald et al. New York, McGraw-Hill, 1987.
10. Kussmaul, A., and Maier, K.: Über eine bischer nicht beschreibene eigenthümliche Arterienerkrankung (Periarteritis nodosa), die mit Morbus Brightii und rapid fortschreitender allgemeiner Muskellähmung einhergeht. Dtsch. Arch. Klin., 1:484–517, 1966.
11. Churg, J., and Strauss, L.: Allergic granulomatosis, allergic angiitis and periarteritis nodosa. Am. J. Pathol., 27:277–301, 1951.
12. Leavitt, R.Y., and Fauci, A.S.: Polyangiitis overlap syndrome: Classification and prospective clinical experience. Am. J. Med., 81:79, 1986.
13. Zeek, P.M.: Periarteritis nodosa: Critical review. Am. J. Clin. Pathol., 22:777–790, 1952.
14. Sams, W.M., et al.: Leukocytoclastic vasculitis. Arch. Dermatol., 112:219–226, 1976.
15. Alarcón-Segovia, D.: The necrotizing vasculitides. A new pathogenetic classification. Med. Clin. North Am., 61:241–260, 1977.
16. Rose, G.A., and Spencer, H.: Polyarteritis nodosa. Q.J. Med., 26:43–81, 1957.
17. Fauci, A.S.: Vasculitis. In Clinical Immunology. Edited by E.W. Parker. Philadelphia, W.B. Saunders, 1980.
18. White, R.H., and Schambelan, M.: Hypertension, hyperreninemia, and secondary hyperaldosteronism in systemic necrotizing vasculitis. Ann. Intern. Med., 92:199, 1980.
19. Holsinger, D.R., Osmundson, P.J., and Edwards, J.E.: The heart in periarteritis nodosa. Circulation, 25:610–618, 1962.
20. Sheps, S.G.: Vasculitis. In Peripheral Vascular Diseases. 4th Ed. Edited by J.F. Fairburn, J.L. Juergens, and J.A. Spittel. Philadelphia, W.B. Saunders, 1972, pp. 351–385.
21. Roberts, F.B., and Fetterman, G.H.: Polyarteritis nodosa in infancy. J. Pediatr., 63:519–529, 1963.
22. Landing, B.H., and Larson, E.J.: Are infantile periarteritis nodosa with coronary artery involvement and fatal mucocutaneous lymph node syndrome the same? Comparison of 20 patients from North America with patients from Hawaii and Japan. Pediatrics, 59:651–662, 1977.
23. Mowrey, F.H., and Lundberg, E.A.: The clinical manifestations of essential polyangiitis (periarteritis nodosa) with emphasis on the hepatic manifestations. Ann. Intern. Med., 40:1141–1155, 1967.
24. Moore, P.M., and Fauci, A.S.: Neurologic manifestations of systemic vasculitis. A retrospective and prospective study of the clinicopathologic features and responses to therapy in 25 patients. Am. J. Med., 71:517–524, 1981.
25. Gilliam, J.N., and Smiley, J.D.: Cutaneous necrotizing vasculitis and related disorders. Ann. Allergy, 37:328–339, 1976.
26. Boyle, J.A., and Buchanan, W.W.: Polyarteritis nodosa. In Clinical Rheumatology. Philadelphia, F.A. Davis, 1971.
27. Diaz-Perez, J.L., and Winkelmann, R.K.: Cutaneous periarteritis nodosa. Arch. Dermatol., 110:407–414, 1974.
28. Duffy, J., et al.: Polyarthritis, polyarteritis and hepatitis B. Medicine, 55:19–37, 1976.
29. Fauci, A.S., et al.: Cyclophosphamide therapy of severe systemic necrotizing vasculitis. N. Engl. J. Med., 301:235–238, 1979.
30. Bron, K.M., Stroot, C.A., and Shapiro, A.P.: The diagnostic value of angiographic observations in polyarteritis nodosa. Arch. Intern. Med., 116:450–453, 1965.
31. Fleming, R.J., and Stern, L.Z.: Multiple intraparenchymal renal aneurysms in polyarteritis nodosa. Radiology, 84:100–103, 1965.
32. Dornfeld, L., Lecky, L.W., and Peter, J.B.: Polyarteritis and intrarenal renal artery aneurysms. JAMA, 215:1950–1952, 1971.
33. Fauci, A.S., Doppman, J.L., and Wolff, S.M.: Cyclophosphamide-induced remissions in advanced polyarteritis nodosa. Am. J. Med., 64:890–894, 1978.
34. Longstreth, P.L., Lorobkin, M., and Palubinskas, A.J.: Renal microaneurysms in a patient with systemic lupus erythematosus. Radiology, 113:65–66, 1974.
35. Meyers, D.S., Grim, C.E., and Kertzer, W.F.: Fibromuscular dysplasia of the renal artery with medial dissection. A case simulating polyarteritis nodosa. Am. J. Med., 56:412–416, 1974.

36. Frohnert, P.P., and Sheps, S.G.: Long-term follow-up study of periarteritis nodosa. Am. J. Med., *43*:8–14, 1967.
37. Lanham, J.C., Elkon, K.B., Pusey, C.D., and Hughes, G.R.: Systemic vasculitis with asthma and eosinophilia: A clinical approach to the Churg-Strauss syndrome. Medicine (Baltimore), *63*:65–81, 1984.
38. Leavitt, R.Y., and Fauci, A.S.: Pulmonary vasculitis. Am. Rev. Respir. Dis., *134*:149–166, 1986.
39. Fauci, A.S.: Systemic vasculitis. *In* Current Therapy in Allergy and Immunology. Edited by L.M. Lichtenstein and A.S. Fauci. Philadelphia, B.C. Decker, 1983.
40. Fauci, A.S., and Wolff, S.M.: Wegener's granulomatosis: Studies in eighteen patients and a review of the literature. Medicine (Baltimore), *52*:535–561, 1973.
41. Ambrus, J.L., and Fauci, A.S.: Diffuse histiocytic lymphoma in a patient treated with cyclophosphamide for Wegener's granulomatosis. Am. J. Med., *76*:745–747, 1984.
41a. Ahmed, A.R., and Hombal, S.M.: Cyclophosphamide (Cytoxan): A review on relevant pharmacology and clinical uses. J. Am. Acad. Dermatol., *11*:1115–26, 1984.
42. Fauci, A.S.: Cytotoxic and other immunoregulatory agents. *In* Textbook on Rheumatology. Edited by W.N. Kelley, E.D. Harris, Jr., S. Ruddy, and C.B. Sledge. Philadelphia, W.B. Saunders, 1985.
43. Lockwood, C.M., et al.: Reversal of impaired splenic function in patients with nephritis or vasculitis (or both) by plasma exchange. N. Engl. J. Med., *300*:524–530, 1979.
44. Kauffmann, R.H., and Houwert, D.A.: Plasmapheresis in rapidly progressive Henoch-Schönlein glomerulonephritis and the effect on circulating IgA immune complexes. Clin. Nephrol., *16*:155–160, 1981.
45. Winkelmann, R.K., and Ditto, W.B.: Cutaneous and visceral syndromes of necrotizing or "allergic" angiitis: A study of 38 cases. Medicine (Baltimore), *43*:59–89, 1964.
46. Ackroyd, J.F.: Allergic purpura, including purpura due to foods, drugs and infections. Am. J. Med., *14*:605–632, 1953.
46a. Soter, N.A.: Clinical presentations and mechanisms of necrotizing angiitis of the skin. J. Invest. Dermatol., *67*:354–359, 1976.
46b. Lindenauer, S.M., and Tank, E.S.: Surgical aspects of Henoch-Schönlein purpura. Surgery, *59*:982–987, 1966.
47. Ansell, B.M.: Henoch-Schönlein purpura with particular reference to the prognosis of the renal lesion. Br. J. Dermatol., *82*:211–215, 1970.
48. Ballard, H.S., Eisinger, R.P., and Gallo, G.: Renal manifestations of the Henoch-Schönlein syndrome in adults. Am. J. Med., *49*:328–335, 1970.
49. Cream, J.J., Gumpel, J.M., and Peachy, R.D.G.: Schönlein-Henoch purpura in the adult. Q. J. Med., *39*:461–484, 1970.
50. Cupps, T.R., and Fauci, A.S.: Cutaneous vasculitis. *In* Current Therapy in Allergy and Immunology 1983–1984. Edited by L.M. Lichenstein and A.S. Fauci. Philadelphia, B.C. Becker, 1983.
51. Christian, C.L., and Sergent, J.S.: Vasculitis syndromes: Clinical and experimental models. Am. J. Med., *61*:385–392, 1976.
52. Glass, D., Soter, N.A., and Schur, P.H.: Rheumatoid vasculitis. Arthritis Rheum., *19*:950–952, 1976.
53. Mongan, E.S., et al.: A study of the relation of seronegative and seropositive rheumatoid arthritis to each other and to necrotizing vasculitis. Am. J. Med., *47*:23–35, 1969.
54. Sokoloff, L., and Bunim, J.J.: Vascular lesions in rheumatoid arthritis. J. Chronic Dis., *5*:668–687, 1957.
55. Brouet, J.C., et al.: The occurrence and nature of precipitating antibodies in anti-DNA sera. Clin. Immunol. Immunopathol., *2*:310–324, 1974.
56. Kemper, J.W., Baggenstoss, A.H., and Slocumb, C.H.: The relationship of therapy with cortisone to the incidence of vascular lesions in rheumatoid arthritis. Ann. Intern. Med., *46*:831–851, 1957.
57. Schmid, F.R., et al.: Arteritis in rheumatoid arteritis. Am. J. Med., *30*:56–83, 1961.
58. Estes, D., and Christain, C.L.: The natural history of systemic lupus erythematosus by prospective analysis. Medicine, *50*:85–95, 1971.
59. Klemperer, P., Pollack, A.D., and Baehr, G.: Pathology of disseminated lupus erythematosus. Arch. Pathol., *32*:569–631, 1941.
60. Mintz, G., and Fraga, A.: Arteritis in systemic lupus erythematosus. Arch. Intern. Med., *116*:55–66, 1965.
61. Conn, D.L., McDuffie, F.C., and Dyck, P.J.: Immunopathologic study of sural nerves in rheumatoid arthritis. Arthritis Rheum., *15*:135–143, 1972.
62. Grey, H.M., and Kohler, P.F.: Cryoimmunoglobulins. Semin. Hematol., *10*:87–112, 1973.
63. LoSpalluto, J., et al.: Cryoglobulinemia based on interaction between a gamma macroglobulin and 75 gamma globulin. Am. J. Med., *32*:142–147, 1962.
64. Meltzer, M., et al.: Cryoglobulinemia—A clinical and laboratory study. II. Cryoglobulins with rheumatoid factor activity. Am. J. Med., *40*:837–856, 1966.
65. Golde, D., and Epstein, W.: Mixed cryoglobulins and glomerulonephritis. Ann. Intern. Med., *69*:1221–1227, 1968.
66. McCombs, R.P.: Systemic "allergic" vasculitis. Clinical and pathological relationships. JAMA, *194*:157–164, 1965.
67. Sams, W.M., Harville, D.D., and Winkelmann, R.K.: Necrotizing vasculitis associated with lethal reticuloendothelial diseases. Br. J. Dermatol., *80*:555–567, 1968.
68. Copeman, P.W.M., and Ryan, T.J.: The problems of classification of cutaneous angiitis with reference to histopathology and pathogenesis. Br. J. Dermatol., *81*:2–14, 1970.
69. Hughes, G.R.V., et al.: Polyarteritis nodosa and hairy-cell leukemia. Lancet, *1*:678–681, 1978.
70. Goedert, J.J., et al.: Polyarteritis nodosa, hairy cell leukemia and splenosis. JAMA, *71*:323–326, 1981.
71. Rewcastle, N.B., and Tom, M.I.: Non-infectious granulomatous angiitis of the nervous system associated with Hodgkin's disease. J. Neurol. Neurosurg. Psychiatry, *25*:52–58, 1962.
72. Leonhardt, E.T.G., and Kullenberg, K.P.G.: Bilateral atrial myxomas with multiple arterial aneurysms—A syndrome mimicking polyarteritis nodosa. Am. J. Med., *62*:792–794, 1977.
73. Burton, C., and Johnston, J.: Multiple cerebral aneurysms and cardiac myxoma. N. Engl. J. Med., *282*:35–37, 1970.
74. Price, D.L., et al.: Cardiac myxoma. A clinicopathologic and angiographic study. Arch. Neurol., *23*:558–567, 1970.
75. Huston, K.A., et al.: Left atrial myxoma simulating peripheral vasculitis. Mayo Clin. Proc., *53*:752–756, 1978.
76. Wolff, S.M., et al.: Wegener's granulomatosis. Ann. Intern. Med., *81*:523–525, 1974.
77. Maquire, R., et al.: Unusual radiographic findings of Wegener's granulomatosis. AJR, *130*:133–138, 1978.
78. Rosenberg, D.M., et al.: Functional correlates of lung involvement in Wegener's granulomatosis. Am. J. Med., *69*:387–394, 1980.
79. Fauci, A.S., Balow, J.E., and Wolff, S.M.: Effect of cytotoxic therapy on the renal lesions of Wegener's granulomatosis. *In* Proceedings of the Sixth International Congress of Nephrol-

ogy. Edited by S. Giovannetti, V. Bonomini, and G. D'Amico. Basel, S. Karger, 1976.

80. Walton, E.W.: Giant-cell granuloma of the respiratory tract (Wegener's granulomatosis). Br. Med. J., 2:265–270, 1958.

81. Liebow, A.A., Carrington, C.R.B., and Friedman, P.J.: Lymphomatoid granulomatosis. Hum. Pathol., 3:457–458, 1972.

82. Fauci, A.S.: Granulomatous vasculitides: Distinct but related. Ann. Intern. Med., 87:782–783, 1977.

83. Fauci, A.S., et al.: Lymphomatoid granulomatosis: Prospective clinical and therapeutic experience over 10 years. N. Engl. J. Med., 306:68–74, 1982.

84. Israel, H.L., Patchefsky, A.S., and Saldana, M.J.: Wegener's granulomatosis, lymphomatoid granulomatosis, and benign lymphocytic angiitis and granulomatosis of lung: Recognition and treatment. Ann. Intern. Med., 87:691–699, 1977.

85. Katzenstein, A.-L.A., Carrington, C.B., and Liebow, A.A.: Lymphomatoid granulomatosis: A clinico-pathologic study of 152 cases. Cancer, 43:360–373, 1979.

86. Hamilton, C.R., Jr., Shelley, W.M., and Tumulty, P.A.: Giant cell arteritis: Including temporal arteritis and polymyalgia rheumatica. Medicine (Baltimore), 50:1–27, 1971.

87. Goodman, B.W.: Temporal arteritis. Am. J. Med., 67:839–852, 1979.

88. Hunder, G.G., et al.: Superficial temporal arteriography in patients suspected of having temporal arteritis. Arthritis Rheum., 15:561–570, 1972.

88a. Klein, R.G., et al.: Skip lesions in temporal arteritis. Mayo Clin. Proc., 51:504–510, 1976.

89. Healey, L.A., Parker, F., and Wilske, K.R.: Polymyalgia rheumatica and giant cell arteritis. Arthritis Rheum., 14:138–141, 1971.

90. Chuang, T.-Y., et al.: Polymyalgia rheumatica. A 10-year epidemiologic and clinical study. Ann. Intern. Med., 97:672–680, 1982.

91. Wagener, H.P., and Hollenhorst, R.W.: The ocular lesions of temporal arteritis. Am. J. Ophthalmol., 45:617–630, 1958.

92. Beever, D.G., Harper, J.E., and Turk, K.A.D.: Giant cell arteritis—The need for prolonged treatment. J. Chronic Dis., 26:561–570, 1973.

93. Hunder, G.G.: Temporal arteritis. In Current Therapy in Allergy and Immunology 1983–1984. Edited by L.M. Lichtenstein and A.S. Fauci. Philadelphia. B.C. Decker, 1983.

94. McKusick, V.A.: A form of vascular disease relatively frequent in the Orient. Am. Heart J., 63:57–64, 1962.

95. Nakao, K., et al.: Takayasu's arteritis. Clinical report of eighty-four cases and immunological studies of seven cases. Circulation, 35:1141–1155, 1967.

96. Vinijchaikul, L.: Primary arteritis of the aorta and its main branches (Takayasu's arteriopathy). Am. J. Med., 43:15–27, 1967.

97. Fraga, A., et al.: Takayasu's arteritis: frequency of systemic manifestations (study of 22 patients) and favorable response to maintenance steroid therapy and adenocorticosteroids (12 patients). Arthritis Rheum., 15:617–624, 1972.

98. Ishikawa, K.: Natural history and classification of occlusive thromboaortopathy (Takayasu's disease). Circulation, 57:617–624, 1978.

99. Hall, S., et al.: Takayasu arteritis: A study of 32 North American patients. Medicine (Baltimore), 64:89–99, 1985.

100. Shelhamer, J.H., et al.: Takayasu's arteritis and its therapy. Ann. Intern. Med., 103:121–126, 1985.

101. Volkman, D.J., Fauci, A.S.: Takayasu's arteritis. In Current Therapy in Allergy and Immunology. Edited by L.M. Lichtenstein and A.S. Fauci. Philadelphia, B.C. Decker, 1983.

102. Melish, M.E.: Kawasaki syndrome: A new infectious disease? J. Infect. Dis., 143:317–324, 1981.

103. Kato, H., et al.: Variant strain of *Propionibacterium acnes:* A clue to the aetiology of Kawasaki disease. Lancet, 2:1383–1388, 1983.

104. Fujimoto, T., et al.: Immune complex and mite antigen in Kawasaki disease. Lancet, 2:980–981, 1982.

105. Hamashima, Y., et al.: Mite-associated particles in Kawasaki disease. Lancet, 2:266, 1982.

106. Patriarca, P.A., et al.: Kawasaki syndrome: Association with the application of rug shampoo. Lancet, 2:575–580, 1982.

107. Burns, J.C., et al.: Polymerase activity in lymphocyte culture supernatants from patients with Kawasaki disease. Nature, 323:814–816, 1986.

108. Shulman, S.T., and Rowley, A.H.: Does Kawasaki disease have a retroviral aetiology? Lancet, 2:545–546, 1986.

109. Melish, M.E.: Intravenous immunoglobulin in Kawasaki syndrome: A progress report. Pediatr. Infect. Dis., 5:S211–S215, 1986.

109a. Kawasaki, T., et al.: Acute febrile mucocutaneous syndrome with lymphoid involvement with specific desquamation of the fingers and toes in children. Jpn. J. Allergy, 16:178–222, 1967.

110. Kawasaki, T., et al.: A new infantile acute febrile mucocutaneous lymph node syndrome (MLNS) prevailing in Japan. Pediatrics, 54:271–276, 1974.

111. Tanaka, N., Sekimoto, K., and Naoe, S.: Kawasaki disease. Relationship with infantile periarteritis nodosa. Arch. Pathol. Lab. Med., 100:81–86, 1976.

112. Bell, D.M., et al.: Kawasaki syndrome: Description of two outbreaks in the United States. N. Engl. J. Med., 304:1568–1575, 1981.

113. Kato, H., Koike, S., and Yokoyama, T.: Kawasaki disease: Effect of treatment on coronary artery involvement. Pediatrics, 63:175–179, 1979.

114. Cupps, T.R., Moore, P.M., and Fauci, A.S.: Isolated angiitis of the central nervous system. Prospective diagnostic and therapeutic considerations. Am. J. Med., 74:97–105, 1983.

115. Stein, R.L., et al.: Cerebral angiography as a guide for therapy in isolated central nervous system vasculitis. JAMA, 257:2193–2195, 1987.

116. O'Duffy, J.D., Carney, J.A., and Deodhar, S.: Behçet's disease. Report of 10 cases, 3 with new manifestations. Ann. Intern. Med., 75:561–570, 1971.

117. Allen, N., and Haynes, B.F.: Behçet's syndrome. In Current Therapy in Allergy and Immunology 1983–1984. Edited by L.M. Lichtenstein and A.S. Fauci. Philadelphia, B.C. Decker, 1983.

118. McKusick, V.A., and Harris, W.S.: The Buerger syndrome in the Orient. Bull. Johns Hopkins Hosp., 109:241–291, 1961.

119. Leavitt, R.Y., Bressler, P., and Fauci, A.S.: Buerger's disease in a young woman. Am. J. Med., 80:1003–1005, 1986.

120. Lie, J.T.: Thromboangiitis obliterans (Buerger's disease) in women. Medicine (Baltimore), 66:65–72, 1987.

121. Williams, G.: Recent views on Buerger's disease. J. Clin. Pathol., 22:573–578, 1969.

122. Hill, G.L.: A rational basis for management of patients with the Buerger syndrome. Br. J. Surg., 61:476–481, 1974.

123. Shionoya, S., et al.: Diagnosis, pathology, and treatment of Buerger's disease. Surgery, 75:195–199, 1974.

124. Blomgren, S.E.: Erythema nodosum. Semin. Arthritis Rheum., 4:1–24, 1974.

125. Winkelman, R.K., and Förstrom, L.: New observations in the histopathology of erythema nodosum. J. Invest. Dermatol., 65:441–446, 1975.

126. Katz, P., et al.: Erythema elevatum diutinum: Skin and systemic manifestations, immunologic studies, and successful treatment with dapsone. Medicine (Baltimore), *56*:443–455, 1977.

127. Cheson, B.D., Bluming, A.Z., and Alroy, J.: Cogan's syndrome: A systemic vasculitis. Am. J. Med., *60*:549–555, 1976.

128. Sheie, H.G., and Albert, D.M.: Textbook of Ophthalmology. 9th Ed. Philadelphia, W.B. Saunders, 1977.

129. Thaell, J.F., and Save, G.L.: Giant cell arteritis involving the breasts. J. Rheumatol., *10*:329–331, 1983.

75

PSEUDOVASCULITIS SYNDROMES

LEONARD H. SIGAL

Vasculitis must be considered in the differential diagnosis of any patient with a multisystem illness. Some clinical syndromes may present with features compatible with vasculitis but are ultimately related to specific underlying diseases with known pathophysiology. The embolic phenomena of subacute bacterial endocarditis[1] or other infectious diseases[2] may present in such a fashion. Atrial myxoma and multiple cholesterol embolization syndrome (MCES) are less frequently encountered mimics of systemic necrotizing vasculitis.

ATRIAL MYXOMA

Patients with cardiac myxomas typically present with and are treated for cardiac disease. They often have significant extracardiac manifestations, however, sometimes in the absence of findings referable to the heart. Uniformly fatal and usually undiagnosed antemortem until the 1950s, myxoma is now a curable entity because of early diagnosis (by echocardiography and angiography) and effective treatment (open heart surgery).

Cardiac myxoma has been reported in stillborn infants to patients 95 years old, with peak incidence in patients in the third to sixth decades, mean age of about 45 years.[3] A female predominance has been described.[4-6] Familial cardiac myxoma has been reported,[3] including a description of a family with myxoma associated with lentigines and endocrine overactivity.[7]

The incidence of primary cardiac neoplasms in unselected autopsies is between 0.0017% and 0.33%; about 80% are benign. Myxomas account for about half of these neoplasms, typically arising as solitary pedunculated tumors near the fossa ovalis. Approximately 70% are left atrial and 18% right atrial in origin.[3] Systemic manifestations of both left and right atrial myxomas are well described.[3-5] Only about 12% of myxomas arise in the ventricles. Ventricular myxomas are more often sessile and therefore less likely to cause obstruction to blood flow.[3] Extracardiac manifestations of ventricular myxomas have not been documented.

The signs and symptoms of atrial myxomas include obstructive, embolic, and systemic/constitutional manifestations. Congestive failure, systolic or diastolic murmurs (usually suggestive of atrioventricular valve dysfunction), chest pain, and dyspnea may be caused by tumoral obstruction of blood flow. Embolic disease occurs in about half of patients with left atrial myxomas,[8,9] and the brain is affected in about half of these[9,10] (Fig. 75–1). Neurologic manifestations include peripheral and cranial neuropathy, hemiparesis, seizures, syncope,[9,10] and progressive intellectual impairment.[11] Peripheral and visceral embolization also occurs.[12-15] Constitutional symptoms such as fever, weight loss, malaise, and fatigue are present in 90% of cases.[3] Isolated fever may result in evaluation of a fever of unknown origin.

In the absence of cardiac manifestations, diagnosis is often missed. Isolated fever may result in evaluation of a fever of unknown origin. Myxoma presenting

FIG. 75–1. *A*, Right internal carotid angiogram showing occlusion of the middle cerebral and pericallosal arteries; left carotid angiogram (not shown) in the same patient showed occlusion of the posterior angular branch of the left middle cerebral artery. Echocardiogram was normal, but cardiac angiography showed a filling defect in the left atrium. A left atrial myxoma was removed surgically. *B*, Right internal carotid angiogram of another patient showing a fusiform aneurysm at the bifurcation of the right middle cerebral artery. (From Roeltgen, D.P., Weimer, G.R., and Patterson, L.F.: Delayed neurologic complications of left atrial myxoma. Neurology (NY), *31*:8–13, 1981. By permission of authors and editor.)

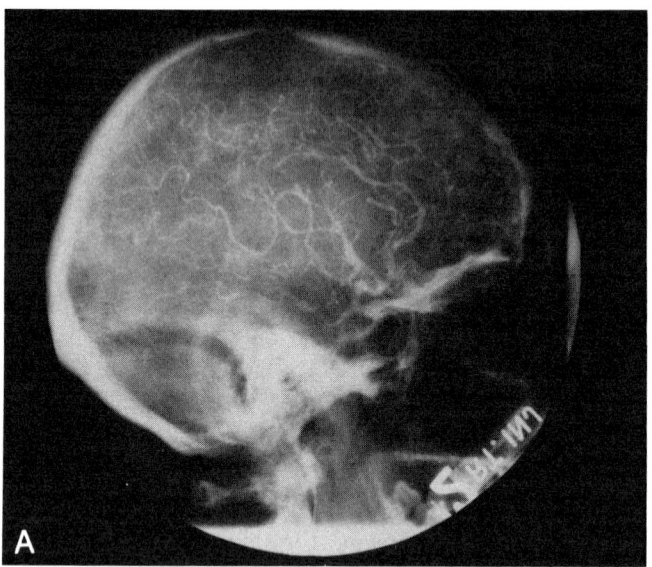 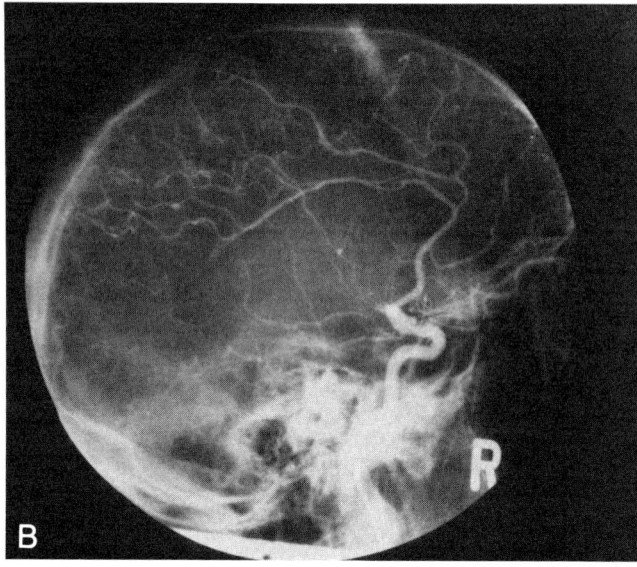

with extracardiac manifestations may mimic rheumatologic and vasculitic syndromes (Table 75–1). Patients with myxoma can experience Raynaud's phenomenon,[14–18] arthralgia or true arthritis,[12–16,18–21] petechial skin rashes,[16,22,23] and finger-pulp lesions.[12,15,16,24] The combination of embolic and constitutional findings may mimic endocarditis[12,22–29] or the Libman-Sacks lesion of systemic lupus erythematosus.[16] Tender calf muscles and elevated serum levels of muscle enzymes may suggest polymyositis or dermatomyositis.[30,31]

Systemic necrotizing vasculitis has been the clinical diagnosis in 10 reported cases of myxoma;[12–15,20,22,24,26,28,32] findings in these patients included fever, weight loss, Raynaud's phenomenon, myalgia, arthritis, central and peripheral nervous system lesions, and pleural effusions. The systemic findings may suggest polymyalgia rheumatica or giant cell arteritis,[15,28] and the importance of considering myxoma in the elderly has been stressed.[19] The isolated central nervous presentation of myxoma[9,10,33–35] may simulate isolated central nervous system vasculitis (granulomatous angiitis of the nervous system).[36]

Laboratory abnormalities (Table 75–2) are nonspecific and include elevated sedimentation rate and C-reactive protein, leukocytosis (usually granulocytic), anemia (microcytic/hypochromic or normocytic/normochromic), and abnormal urinalysis (microhematuria and proteinuria). Elevated levels of α-2 and γ-globulins are nearly universal. Polycythemia has been associated with both left and right atrial myxomas. Antibodies to double-strand DNA[24] and antibodies capable of binding to heart muscle (but not to myxoma tissue[37]) have been identified. Hypocomplementemia,[24] thrombocytopenia,[23,38] consumption coagulopathy,[32] and microangiopathic hemolytic anemia[23] have been described. Liver function abnormalities, including overt jaundice, may occur more frequently than has been appreciated.[39] Angiography of the celiac, renal, and cerebral circulation may reveal aneurysms similar to those seen in polyarteritis nodosa[10,13,15,33–35,40,41] (Fig. 75–1).

Cardiac angiography has been replaced by echocardiography as the best diagnostic tool, although the latter may be falsely negative.[34] The diagnosis also has been made by pathologic examination of muscle biopsy and embolectomy samples,[3,4,6,11,38,39] retrospectively in three instances.[14,15,35]

The immunopathogenesis of the constitutional and laboratory findings in myxoma is unclear. Tumor necrosis[42] or tissue death resulting from emboli[22] is

Table 75–1. Various Presentations of Cardiac Myxoma

Condition Mimicked	Clinical Findings	Laboratory Findings
RHEUMATOLOGIC		
Connective tissue disease*	Fever, weight loss, fatigue	Elevated ESR, CRP
	Arthralgia/arthritis	Anemia
	Myalgia	Thrombocytopenia
	Raynaud's phenomenon	Coagulopathy
	Pleuritis	Urinalysis:
	Pericarditis	proteinuria, hematuria,
	Central and peripheral nervous	hypocomplementemia
	system abnormalities	Antibodies to double-
	Petechial skin rash	stranded DNA
Polymyositis/dermatomyositis†	Tender muscles	Elevated CPK, SGOT
	Weakness	Biopsy revealing muscle
	Elevated CPK, SGOT	necrosis and vasculitis
Systemic necrotizing vasculitis‡	Fever, weight loss, fatigue	Elevated ESR, CRP
	Arthralgia/arthritis	Urinalysis:
	Myalgia	proteinuria, hematuria,
	Central and peripheral nervous	anemia, microangiopathy
	system abnormalities	Coagulopathy
	Petechial skin rash	Liver function test
	Elevated ESR, CRP	Abnormalities
		Hypocomplementemia
NONRHEUMATOLOGIC		
Subacute bacterial endocarditis§	Fever, weight loss, fatigue	Elevated ESR, CRP
	Peripheral emboli	Urinalysis:
	Petechial rash	proteinuria, hematuria,
	Arthralgia	anemia, microangiopathy
	Myalgia	Thrombocytopenia
	Heart murmur	Coagulopathy
Thrombotic thrombocytopenic purpura‖	Fever	Urinalysis:
	Peripheral emboli	proteinuria, hematuria,
	Petechial skin rash	anemia, microangiopathy
	Central and peripheral nervous	Coagulopathy
	system abnormalities	
	Urinalysis:	
	proteinuria, hematuria,	
	anemia, microangiopathy	
	Coagulopathy	

*References 12, 13, 15, 16, 18, 20, 21, 23, 25, 37.
†References 30, 31.
‡References 12–15, 20, 22, 24, 26, 28, 32.
§References 12, 22–29.
‖Reference 23.

thought to cause fever and systemic symptoms. The hyperglobulinemia has been attributed to an immune response to polysaccharide antigens released from the tumor,[8,22,23,40] and the humoral response may continue even after the tumor's surgical removal.[21] Liver dysfunction is said to be "on an immune basis."[39] Systemic autoimmune reactivity[37] and circulating immune complexes[24] have been suggested, but neither has been demonstrated. Recently, myxoma cells have been shown to produce BSF-2 (B-cell stimulatory factor-2) or BCDF (B-cell differentiation factor).[43] It seems likely that the BSF-2/BCDF molecule is identical to interferon β-2;[44] thus, myxoma cells may produce an immunologic mediator of the systemic manifestations of this tumor.

Therapy consists of surgical excision. Steroid therapy of cases mistakenly diagnosed as vasculitis has produced little or no clinical response[13–15,23] and does not substitute for surgery. Clinical and laboratory abnormalities usually resolve after tumor removal, but Raynaud's phenomenon may persist long after curative surgery.[13] Progression of cerebral aneurysmal changes may occur after tumor removal,[34] suggesting that the aneurysms result from metastatic myxoma[40] rather than from an organizing thrombus.[45] Here, primary myxoma is viewed as a neoplasm.[3] Tumor re-

Table 75–2. Laboratory Abnormalities Reported in Cardiac Myxoma

Laboratory Abnormalities
Elevated erythrocyte sedimentation rate
Elevated C-reactive protein
Elevated alpha-$_2$ and gamma globulins
Anemia: normocytic/normochromic, microcytic/hypochromic, and microangiopathic hemolytic
Polycythemia (with cyanosis and decreased arterial oxygen tension)
Thrombocytopenia
Leukocytosis (rarely eosinophilia)
Elevated liver function tests: SGOT, LDH, alkaline phosphatase, bilirubin
Elevated muscle enzymes: SGOT, CPK, aldolase
Hypocomplementemia
Antibodies to double-stranded DNA
Urinalysis: proteinuria, hematuria

currences may be associated with recrudescence of symptoms and new abnormalities of previously normalized laboratory tests.[46]

MULTIPLE CHOLESTEROL EMBOLIZATION SYNDROME (MCES)

Ulcerating plaques found in an atherosclerotic aorta may release atheromatous emboli containing cholesterol crystals.[47] Larger emboli can occlude major arteries,[48] with loss of pulse, pallor, ischemia, and, ultimately, tissue death. MCES is a result of the occlusion of smaller vessels by showers of cholesterol crystals from plaques. Therefore, MCES is typically seen in patients with severe atherosclerosis, generally men in the sixth to eighth decades,[49] but a recent report documents MCES in a 26-year-old.[50] Embolization may occur after a known event, such as abdominal trauma,[51] aortic surgery,[52] angiography,[53] or Valsalva's maneuver,[51] or during the course of anticoagulation therapy.[48,54–58] MCES may also occur spontaneously,[51,59] presenting with the multisystem manifestations and laboratory abnormalities of systemic necrotizing vasculitis,[60–66] giant cell arteritis,[67] or polymyositis.[68]

Although the lower aorta is the most common source of the crystals that cause MCES, embolization occurs throughout the body. The most obvious lesions are cutaneous (Fig. 75–2). Autopsy studies have demonstrated evidence of cholesterol crystals embolizing to the kidney, pancreas, spleen, thyroid, adrenal gland, liver, gastrointestinal tract, gallbladder, brain, spinal cord, bone marrow, and heart.[59,69–71] Such emboli may cause clinically significant damage to many of these organs (Table 75–3). Peripheral pulses are typically intact.

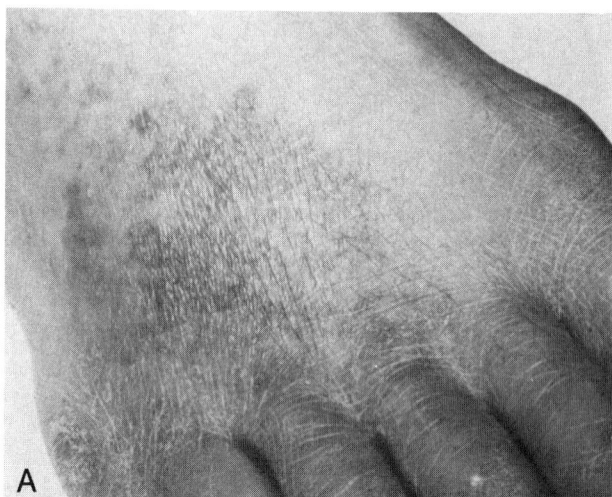

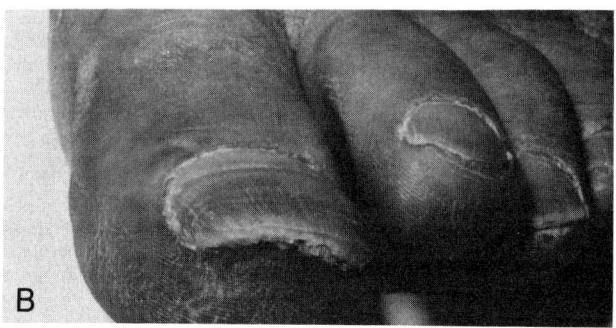

FIG. 75–2. *A,* Purpuric rash over dorsum of affected foot. *B,* Skin-discoloration at the tips of the first and second toes. (From Young, D.K., Burton, M.F., and Herman, J.F.: Multiple cholesterol emboli syndrome simulating systemic necrotizing vasculitis. J. Rheumatol., *13:*423–426, 1986. By permission of authors and editor.)

It may be difficult to distinguish the clinical manifestations of necrotizing vasculitis from those of MCES. Fever, weight loss, and fatigue are common in both. Livedo reticularis is seen in about 50% of patients with MCES,[72,73] attributed to incomplete blockage of the arteries supplying the skin,[63,74] and may be preceded by intense myalgia.[74] Petechial and purpuric lesions and localized skin necrosis are well described in both syndromes[53,65,68,73,74] (Fig. 75–2). Peripheral neuropathy has been described rarely in MCES,[65] and mononeuritis is frequent in vasculitis.[73] Retinal involvement in systemic vasculitis includes hypertensive changes, retinal artery occlusion, and vasculitis,[73] whereas in MCES, bright orange-yellow plaques, consisting of embolic cholesterol crystals, may be seen at retinal arteriolar bifurcations.[50] With the exception of true arthritis (which has been very rarely reported in MCES), all the clinical manifestations of polyarteritis frequently accompany MCES.

Table 75–3.   Manifestations of Multiple Cholesterol Embolization Syndrome

Manifestations
NEURAL*
Amaurosis fugax
Myelopathy
Stroke
Peripheral neuropathy
CARDIOVASCULAR†
Myocardial infarction (with or without preceding history of angina)
GASTROINTESTINAL‡
Abdominal pain with gastrointestinal bleeding
Pancreatitis
RENAL§
Progressive renal failure (with or without proteinuria)
Hypertension
Necrotizing glomerulonephritis
DERMAL‖
Isolated "purple toes" or "purple toes" with abdominal aortic aneurysm
Gangrene (skin, penis, and scrotum)
Petechial and purpuric lesions
Livedo reticularis
MUSCULAR¶
Tender myalgia
SYSTEMIC#
"Giant-cell arteritis"
"Systemic necrotizing vasculitis"

*References 56, 62, 64, 69, 71.
†Reference 51.
‡References 61, 70, 71.
§References 47, 49, 51, 75, 90, 91.
‖References 47, 54, 60, 68, 72, 74.
¶Reference 68.
#References 60–67.

Central nervous system deficits, including cranial nerve palsies, hemiparesis,[64] dysphasia,[60] blindness,[51,56] cerebrovascular accidents,[62,71] and declining mental function,[75] may occur in MCES. Sneddon described the association of livedo reticularis and repeated cerebrovascular accidents in young to middle-aged patients.[76] *Sneddon's syndrome* is a progressive, noninflammatory arteriopathy affecting medium-sized vessels. Intimal hyperplasia, adventitial fibrosis, irregularities of the internal elastic lamella, and thrombosis are seen in biopsies of affected vessels, not atherosclerosis.[76,77] Its pathogenesis is obscure and its treatment unsuccessful,[77] but the syndrome may mimic MCES or vasculitis.

Elevated serum glutamic oxaloacetic transaminase, creatinine phosphokinase, and aldolase in the presence of painful muscles have led to the clinical diagnosis of polymyositis; biopsy of a gastrocnemius muscle proved diagnostic of MCES.[68]

Leukocytosis,[5] eosinophilia,[47,50,54,66,78] and eosin-

ophiluria[62] have been reported in MCES. Elevated erythrocyte sedimentation rate is the rule. Hypocomplementemia and thrombocytopenia have been reported,[79] although the former has been disputed.[80] Cryoglobulins were weakly positive in the only case tested.[75] Consumption coagulopathy has also been reported.[81,82] Elevated amylase is often found, occasionally in the presence of clinical pancreatitis.[70]

Proteinuria[56,64,68,74] is common, but hematuria and red blood cell casts have not been reported. Rapidly progressive renal failure is the exception in MCES, but slow deterioration of renal function occurring approximately 2 weeks after embolization is common.[47,49] Renal failure is often severe and irreversible,[49] but it may be mild[47] and can resolve spontaneously.[47,78]

Diagnosis is usually made by muscle (quadriceps or gastrocnemius) or skin biopsy[83] (Fig. 75–3A). Routine tissue fixation dissolves the cholesterol crystals, leaving tissue "clefts" as evidence of the crystal emboli[50,51] (Fig. 75–3B). Early lesions may include eosinophils as part of the cellular infiltrate.[84] In properly fixed biopsy specimens, crystals or collections of crystals are surrounded by macrophages and foreign-body giant cells.[60,72] Biopsies of older lesions may reveal only intimal fibrosis[72] without damage to the rest of the arterial wall.[49,53,85] In experimental models of MCES using human atheroma extract,[86] the cholesterol crystals or "clefts" disappear after 1 month,[87] so that their absence in pathologic specimens probably does not rule out the diagnosis of MCES.[50] Within 1 day of embolization, a panarteritis develops.[86] Fibroblastic reaction of the intima and occasional giant cell formation effectively block the lumen within 3 days.[85] Vascular spasm may be a factor in diminished tissue perfusion,[71] although one study suggests that spasm does not contribute to decreased renal perfusion in MCES.[88]

Bone marrow[75] and prostatic[89] samples have also demonstrated tissue clefts in affected individuals. Two renal biopsies in MCES revealed necrotizing glomerulonephritis;[90,91] in one case, the linear distribution of IgG suggested the presence of antiglomerular basement membrane antibodies.[91]

MCES has occurred coincident with heparin and/or coumadin therapy of between 3 weeks' and 3 months' duration,[48,54–57,84] and 2 days after the start of streptokinase therapy.[57] Two examples of resolution of MCES after discontinuation of anticoagulants[70,92] suggests that anticoagulant-induced thrombolysis may release cholesterol crystals from atherosclerotic plaques, causing MCES.

Cholesterol, atheroma lipids, and nonlipid ather-

1194   SYSTEMIC RHEUMATIC DISEASES

FIG. 75–3. *A,* Skin biopsy from affected foot showing recent hemorrhage and a subcutaneous arteriole with medial thickening containing a cholesterol cleft (arrow) (hematoxylin and eosin stained, magnification 320 ×). *B,* Histologic section of a renal biopsy showing luminal obstruction of an interlobular artery with intimal fibroblastic proliferation surrounding cholesterol clefts (arrow) (trichrome stained, magnification 320 ×). (From Young, D.K., Burton, M.F., and Herman, J.F.: Multiple cholesterol emboli syndrome simulating systemic necrotizing vasculitis. J. Rheumatol., *13*:423–426, 1986. By permission of authors and editors.)

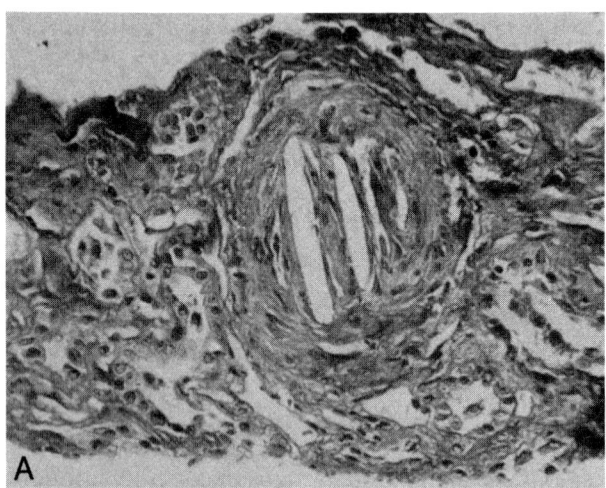

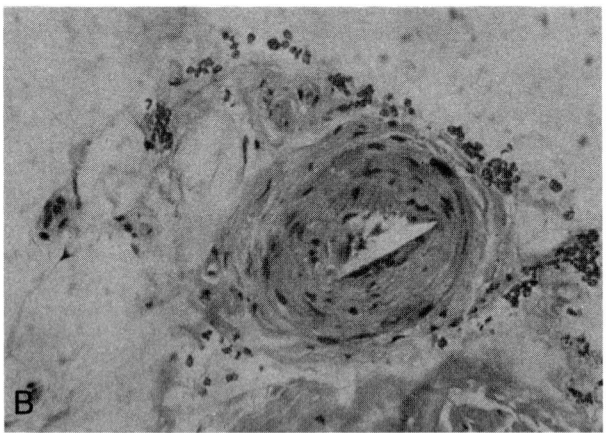

oma components have thrombogenic activity.[82,93] Atheroma contents are capable of activating complement[79] in the presence of immunoglobulin and an intact classic complement pathway.[94] Atheroma-activated complement (probably C5a) can cause aggregation of polymorphonuclear cells, perhaps contributing to local endothelial damage.[94]

Therapy should be directed at removing the atherosclerotic source of emboli.[47] Antiplatelet therapy, vasodilators, and low-molecular-weight dextran have been ineffective.[49] Discontinuation of anticoagulant therapy seems well advised, as already noted. Steroid therapy has been reported as being moderately effective[95] or of no value,[53,85] but exacerbation of MCES followed the discontinuation of steroid therapy in a case initially treated for presumed vasculitis, suggesting that steroid withdrawal may be hazardous.[60] Aggressive diagnostic workup of suspected vasculitis with MCES in mind is suggested, especially in the elderly.

REFERENCES

1. Churchill, M.A., Jr., Geraci, J.E., and Hunder, G.G.: Musculoskeletal manifestations of bacterial endocarditis. Ann. Intern. Med., *87*:754–759, 1977.
2. Manion, W.C.: Infectious angiitis. *In* The Peripheral Blood Vessels. Edited by J.L. Orbison and E.E. Smith. Baltimore, Williams and Wilkins Company, 1963, pp. 221–231.
3. Wold, L.E., and Lie, J.T.: Cardiac myxomas. A clinicopathologic profile. Am. J. Pathol., *101*:219–240, 1980.
4. Bulkley, B.H., and Hutchins, G.M.: Atrial myxomas: a fifty year review. Am. Heart J., *97*:639–643, 1979.
5. Peters, M.N., et al.: The clinical syndrome of atrial myxoma. JAMA, *230*:695–701, 1974.
6. Schechter, D.C.: Left atrial myxoma. NY State J. Med., *82*:1701–1709, 1982.
7. Carney, J.A., et al.: The complex of myxomas, spotty pigmentation, and endocrine overactivity. Medicine (Baltimore), *64*:270–283, 1985.
8. Goodwin, J.F.: Symposium on cardiac tumors. (Introduction.) The spectrum of cardiac tumors. Am. J. Cardiol., *21*:307–314, 1968.
9. Yufe, R., Karpati, G., and Carpenter, S.: Cardiac myxoma: a diagnostic challenge for the neurologist. Neurology (NY), *26*:1060–1065, 1976.
10. Steinmetz, E.F., Calanchini, P.R., and Aguiler, M.J.: Left atrial myxoma as a neurological problem: A case report and review. Stroke, *4*:451–458, 1973.
11. Frank, R.A., et al.: Atrial myxoma with intellectual decline and cerebral growths on CT scan. Ann. Neurol., *5*:396–400, 1979.
12. Buchanan, R.R.C., et al.: Left atrial myxoma mimicking vasculitis: echocardiographic diagnosis. Can. Med. Assoc. J., *120*:1540–1542, 1979.
13. Thomas, M.H.: Myxoma masquerading as polyarteritis nodosa. J. Rheumatol., *8*:133–137, 1981.
14. Leonhardt, E.T.G., and Kullenberg, K.P.-G.: Bilateral atrial myxomas with multiple atrial aneurysms—A syndrome mimicking polyarteritis nodosa. Am. J. Med., *62*:792–794, 1977.
15. Huston, K.A., Combs, J.J., Jr., Lie, J.T., and Giuliani, E.R.: Left atrial myxoma simulating peripheral vasculitis. Mayo Clin. Proc., *53*:752–756, 1978.
16. Hoffman, M.: Cardiac myxoma simulating subacute bacterial endocarditis. Minn. Med., *24*:585, 1941.
17. Potts, J.L., et al.: Varied manifestations of left atrial myxoma and the relationship pf echocardiographic patterns to tumor size. Chest, *68*:781–784, 1975.
18. Skanse, B., Berg, N.O., and Westfelt, L.: Atrial myxoma with Raynaud's phenomenon as the initial symptom. Acta Med. Scand., *164*:321–324, 1959.
19. Davidson, E.T., Mumford, D., Zaman, O., and Horowitz, R.: Left atrial myxoma in the elderly. Report of four patients over the age of 70 and review of the literature. J. Am. Geriatr. Soc., *34*:229–233, 1986.

20. Morgan, W.S., Carrington, C.B., and McFarland, W.J.: Atrial myxoma presenting without cardiac manifestations. Conn. Med., *38*:407–410, 1974.

21. Selzer, A., Sakai, F.J., and Popper, R.W.: Protein clinical manifestations of primary tumors of the heart. Am. J. Med., *52*:9–18, 1972.

22. Boss, J.H., and Bechar, M.: Myxoma of the heart. Report based on four cases. Am. J. Cardiol., *3*:823–828, 1959.

23. Vuopio, P., and Nikkila, E.A.: Hemolytic anemia and thrombocytopenia in a case of left atrial myxoma associated with mitral stenosis. Am. J. Cardiol., *17*:585–589, 1966.

24. Byrd, W.E., Matthews, O.P., and Hunt, R.E.: Left atrial myxoma presenting as a systemic vasculitis. Arthritis Rheum., *23*:240–243, 1980.

25. Gleason, I.O.: Primary myxoma of the heart. A case simulating rheumatic and bacterial endocarditis. Cancer, *8*:839–844, 1955.

26. Goodwin, J.F., Kay, J.M., and Heath, D.: Clinical pathologic conference. Am. Heart J., *70*:239–247, 1965.

27. Kendall, D., and Symonds, B.: Case reports. Epileptiform attacks due to myxoma of the right auricle. Br. Heart J., *14*:139–143, 1952.

28. Sutton, M.G. St.J., Mercier, L.-A., Giuliani, E.R., and Lie, J.T.: Atrial myxomas. A review of clinical experience in 40 patients. Mayo Clin. Proc., *55*:371–376, 1980.

29. Symbas, P., Abbott, O., Logan, W., and Hatcher, C.: Atrial myxomas: special emphasis on unusual manifestations. Chest, *59*:504–510, 1971.

30. Kaminsky, M.E., et al.: Atrial myxoma mimicking a collagen disorder. Chest, *75*:93–95, 1979.

31. McWhirter, W.R., and Tetteh-Lartey, E.V.: A case of atrial myxoma. Br. Heart J., *36*:839–840, 1974.

32. Cohen, A.I., McIntosh, H.D., and Orgain, E.S.: The mimetic nature of left atrial myxomas. Report of a case presenting as a severe systemic illness and simulating massive mitral insufficiency at cardiac catheterization. Am. J. Cardiol., *11*:802–807, 1963.

33. Maroon, J.C., and Campbell, R.L.: Atrial myxoma: a treatable cause of stroke. J. Neurol. Neurosurg. Psychiatry, *32*:129–133, 1969.

34. Roeltgen, D.P., Weimer, G.R., and Patterson, L.F.: Delayed neurologic complications of left atrial myxoma. Neurology (NY), *31*:8–13, 1981.

35. Yarnell, P.R., Spann, J.F., Jr., Dougherty, J., and Mason, D.T.: Episodic central nervous system ischemia of undetermined cause: Relation to occult left atrial myxoma. Stroke, *2*:35–39, 1971.

36. Sigal, L.H.: The isolated neurologic presentation of vasculitic and rheumatologic syndromes. A review. Medicine (Baltimore), *66*:157–180, 1987.

37. Currey, H.L.F., Matthews, J.A., and Robinson, J.: Right atrial myxoma mimicking a rheumatic disorder. Br. Med. J., *1*:547–548, 1967.

38. Willman, V.L., et al.: Unusual aspects of intracavitary tumors of the heart. Report of two cases. Dis. Chest., *47*:669–671, 1965.

39. Kluge, T.H., Ullal, S.R., and Gerbode, F.: Dysfunction of the liver in cardiac myxoma. Surg. Gynecol. Obstet., *134*:288–290, 1972.

40. Price, D.L., Harris, J.L., New, P.F.J., and Cantu, R.C.: Cardiac myxoma. A clinicopathologic and angiographic study. Arch. Neurol., *23*:558–567, 1970.

41. New, P.F.J., Price, D.L., and Carter, B.: Cerebral angiography in cardiac myxoma. Radiology, *96*:335–345, 1970.

42. Lekisch, K.: Myxoma of the left atrium: report of a case. Ann. Intern. Med., *46*:982–990, 1957.

43. Hirano, T., et al.: Human B-cell differentiation factor defined by an anti-peptide antibody and its possible role in autoantibody production. Proc. Natl. Acad. Sci. USA, *84*:228–231, 1987.

44. Sehgal, P.B., May, L.T., Tamm, I., and Vilcek, J.: Human ₂interferon and B-cell differentiation factor BSF-2 are identical. Science, *235*:731–732, 1987.

45. Salyer, W.R., Page, D.L., and Hutchins, G.M.: The development of cardiac myxomas and papillary endocardial lesions from mural thrombus. Am. Heart J., *89*:4–17, 1975.

46. Jugdutt, B.I., Rossall, R.E., and Sterns, L.P.: An unusual case of recurrent left atrial myxomas. Can. Med. Assoc. J., *112*:1099–1100, 1975.

47. Smith, M.C., Ghose, M.K., and Henry, A.R.: The clinical spectrum of renal cholesterol embolization. Am. J. Med., *71*:174–180, 1981.

48. Kempczinski, R.F.: Lower-extremity arterial emboli from ulcerating atherosclerotic plaques. JAMA, *241*:807–810, 1979.

49. Kassirer, J.: Atheroembolic renal disease. N. Engl. J. Med., *280*:812–818, 1969.

50. Kalter, D.C., Rudolph, A., and McGarran, M.: Livedo reticularis due to multiple cholesterol emboli. J. Am. Acad. Dermatol., *13*:235–242, 1985.

51. Darsee, J.: Cholesterol embolism: The great masquerader. South. Med. J., *72*:174–180, 1979.

52. Ramirez, G., O'Neill, W.M., Jr., Lambert, R., and Bloomer, H.A.: Cholesterol embolization. A complication of angiography. Arch. Intern. Med., *138*:1430–1432, 1978.

53. Kazmier, F.J., Sheps, S.G., Bernatz, P.E., and Sayre, G.P.: Livedo reticularis and digital infarct. A syndrome due to cholesterol emboli arising from atheromatous abdominal aortic aneurysms. Vasc. Diseases, *3*:12–24, 1966.

54. Drost, H., Buis, B., Haan, D., and Hillers, J.A.: Cholesterol embolism as a complication of left heart catheterization. Report of seven cases. Br. Heart J., *52*:339–342, 1984.

55. Feder, W., and Auerbach, R.: "Purple toes": an uncommon sequela of oral coumadin drug therapy. Ann. Intern. Med., *55*:911–917, 1961.

56. Moldveen-Geronimus, M., and Merriam, J.C., Jr.: Cholesterol embolization. Circulation, *35*:946–953, 1967.

57. Oster, P., Rieben, F.W., Waldherr, R., and Schettler, G.: Blood clotting and cholesterol crystal embolization. (Letter.) JAMA, *242*:2070–2071, 1979.

58. Uys, C.J., and Watson, C.E.: The effects of atheromatous embolization on small arteries and arterioles. S. Afr. Med. J., *37*:69–73, 1963.

59. Gore, I., and Collins, D.P.: Spontaneous atheromatous embolization. Review of the literature and a report of 16 additional cases. Am. J. Clin. Pathol., *33*:416–426, 1960.

60. Rosansky, S.J.: Multiple cholesterol emboli syndrome. South. Med. J., *75*:677–680, 1982.

61. Haygood, T.A., Fessel, W.J., and Strange, D.A.: Atheromatous microembolism masquerading as polymyositis. JAMA, *203*:423–425, 1968.

62. Goulet, Y., and Mackay, C.G.: Case report. Atheromatous embolism: An entity with a polymorphous symptomatology. Can. Med. Assoc. J., *88*:1067–1070, 1963.

63. Case records of the Massachusetts General Hospital. New Engl. J. Med., *315*:308–315, 1986.

64. Anderson, W.R.: Necrotizing angiitis associated with embolization of cholesterol. Case report, with emphasis on the use of the muscle biopsy as a diagnostic aid. Am. J. Clin. Pathol., *43*:65–71, 1965.

65. Retan, J.W., and Miller, R.E.: Microembolic complications of

atherosclerosis. Literature review and report of a patient. Arch. Intern. Med., *118*:534–545, 1966.

66. Young, D.K., Burton, M.F., and Herman, J.H.: Case report. Multiple cholesterol emboli syndrome simulating systemic necrotizing vasculitis. J. Rheumatol., *13*:423–426, 1986.

67. Zak, F.G., and Elias, K.: Embolization with material from atheromata. Am. J. Med. Sci., *218*:510–515, 1949.

68. Arvold, D.S.: Spontaneous atheromatous embolization. Minn. Med., *64*:141–142, 1981.

69. Maurizi, C.P., Barker, A.E., and Trueheart, R.E.: Atheromatous emboli. A postmortem study with special reference to the lower extremities. Arch. Pathol., *86*:528–534, 1968.

70. Probstein, J.G., Joshi, R.A., and Blumenthal, H.T.: Atheromatous embolization. An etiology of acute pancreatitis. Arch. Surg., *75*:566–572, 1957.

71. Winter, W.J., Jr.: Atheromatous emboli: a cause of cerebral infarction. Report of two cases. AMA Arch. Pathol., *64*:137–142, 1957.

72. Deschamps, P., Leroy, D., and Mandard, J.C.: Cutaneous crystal cholesterol emboli. Acta Derm. Venereol. (Stockh), *60*:266–269, 1980.

73. Ho, S.W.-C., Thatcher, G.N., and Matz, L.R.: Reversible renal failure due to renal cholesterol embolism. Aust. NZ J. Med., *12*:531–533, 1982.

74. Fisher, E.R., Hellstrom, H.R., and Myers, J.D.: Disseminated atheromatous emboli. Am. J. Med., *29*:176–180, 1960.

75. Leroy, D., Michel, M., and Mandard, J.: Association of disseminated intravascular coagulation and cutaneous crystal cholesterol emboli. Ann. Dermatol. Venereol., *108*:665–681, 1981.

76. Rebollo, M., et al.: Livedo reticularis and cerebrovascular lesions (Sneddon's syndrome). Brain, *106*:965–979, 1983.

77. Rumpl, E., et al.: Cerebrovascular lesions and livedo reticularis (Sneddon's syndrome)—a progressive cerebrovascular disorder? J. Neurol., *231*:324–330, 1985.

78. Cosio, F.G., Zager, R.A., and Sharma, H.M.: Atheroembolic renal disease causes hypocomplementemia. Lancet, *2*:118–121, 1985.

79. Firth, J.D., and North, J.P.: Does atheroembolic renal disease cause hypocomplementemia? (Letter.) Lancet, *2*:1133, 1985.

80. Pierce, J.R., Jr., Wren, M.V., and Cousar, J.B., Jr.: Cholesterol embolism: diagnosis antemortem by bone marrow biopsy. Ann. Intern. Med., *89*:937–938, 1978.

81. Lyford, C.L., Connor, W.E., Hoak, J.C., and Warner, E.D.: The coagulant and thrombogenic properties of human atheroma. Circulation, *36*:284–293, 1967.

82. Thurlbeck, W.M., and Castleman, B.: Atheromatous emboli to the kidneys after aortic surgery. N. Engl. J. Med., *257*:442–447, 1957.

83. Anderson, W.R., and Richards, A. MacD.: Evaluation of lower extremity muscle biopsies on the diagnosis of atheroembolism. Arch. Pathol., *86*:535–541, 1968.

84. Richards, A. MacD., et al.: Cholesterol embolism. A multiple-system disease masquerading as polyarteritis nodosa. Am. J. Cardiol., *15*:696–707, 1965.

85. Otken, L.B., Jr.: Experimental production of atheromatous embolization. AMA Arch. Pathol., *68*:685–689, 1959.

86. Flory, C.M.: Arterial occlusions produced by emboli from eroded aortic atheromatous plaques. Am. J. Pathol., *21*:549–565, 1945.

87. Cupps, T.R., and Fauci, A.S.: The vasculitides. *In* Major Problems in Internal Medicine. Edited by L.H. Smith, Jr. Philadelphia, W.B. Saunders, 1981, Vol. 21.

88. Zdon, M.J., Crawford, B., and Hermreck, A.: Renal function, microcirculation, and the role of PGI_2 following atheromatous embolization. Curr. Surg., *40*:209–211, 1983.

89. Knechtges, T.C., and Defever, B.A.: Cholesterol emboli in transurethral curettings: report of 4 cases. J. Urol., *114*:102–106, 1975.

90. Goldman, M., Thoua, Y., Dhaene, M., and Toussaint, C.: Necrotizing glomerulonephritis associated with cholesterol microemboli. Br. Med. J., *290*:205–206, 1985.

91. Hannedouche, T., et al.: Necrotizing glomerulonephritis and renal cholesterol embolization. Nephron, *42*:271–272, 1986.

92. Bruns, F.J., Segel, D.P., and Adler, S.: Case report. Control of cholesterol embolization by discontinuation of anticoagulant therapy. Am. J. Med. Sci., *275*:105–108, 1978.

93. Jeynes, B.J., and Warren, B.A.: Thrombogenicity of components of atheromatous material. An animal and in vitro model of cerebral atheroembolism. Arch. Pathol. Lab. Med., *105*:353–357, 1981.

94. Hammerschmidt, D.E., et al.: Cholesterol and atheroma lipids activate complement and stimulate granulocytes. A possible mechanism for amplification of ischemic injury in atherosclerotic states. J. Lab. Clin. Med., *98*:68–77, 1981.

95. Sayre, G.P., and Campbell, D.C.: Multiple peripheral emboli in atherosclerosis of the aorta. Arch. Intern. Med., *103*:799–806, 1959.

SJÖGREN'S SYNDROME AND CONNECTIVE TISSUE DISEASES ASSOCIATED WITH OTHER IMMUNOLOGIC DISORDERS

76

NORMAN TALAL

SJÖGREN'S SYNDROME

Sjögren's syndrome is a chronic inflammatory disease characterized by diminished lacrimal and salivary gland secretion (the sicca complex) resulting in keratoconjunctivitis sicca (KCS) and xerostomia.[1] The glandular insufficiency is secondary to lymphocytic and plasma cell infiltrations. The term *autoimmune exocrinopathy* has been introduced for Sjögren's syndrome.[2] Both a primary and a secondary form of this disease are recognized. Approximately 25% of patients with an associated rheumatoid arthritis (RA) are considered to have *secondary* Sjögren's syndrome; a small percentage may have another associated connective tissue disease. *Primary* Sjögren's syndrome is diagnosed in the absence of another connective tissue disease.

Sjögren's syndrome is particularly important among the autoimmune diseases for two reasons. First, perhaps 2 to 3 million individuals are affected in the United States, the majority undiagnosed. Second, in Sjögren's syndrome a benign autoimmune process can terminate in a malignant lymphoid disorder. Thus, it is a "crossroads" disease that offers potential insight into the mechanisms whereby immunologic dysregulation may predispose a person to a malignant transformation of B cells already involved in an autoimmune process.

HISTORICAL BACKGROUND

A number of patients with various combinations of dry mouth, dry eyes, and chronic arthritis were described by European clinicians between the years 1882 and 1925. In 1892, Mikulicz[3] reported a man with bilateral parotid and lacrimal gland enlargement associated with massive round cell infiltration. In 1925, Gougerot described three patients with salivary and mucous gland atrophy and insufficiency progressing to dryness.[3a] Two years later, Houwer emphasized the association of filamentary keratitis, the major ocular manifestation of the syndrome, with chronic arthritis.[3b] In 1933, Henrik Sjögren[4] reported detailed clinical and histologic findings in 19 women with xerostomia and keratoconjunctivitis sicca, of whom 13 had chronic arthritis. In 1953, Morgan and Castleman[5] concluded that Sjögren's syndrome and Mikulicz's disease were the same entity.

ETIOLOGIC FACTORS

Autoimmune disorders have a multifactorial origin with elements of (1) genetic control related to the activity of specific immune response genes; (2) immunologic control exerted by regulatory T-dependent lymphocytes (suppressor and helper T cells); (3) possible viral influences, although such influences are not yet clearly established; and (4) sex hormone modu-

1197

lation of immune regulation in which estrogens enhance and androgens suppress autoimmunity.[6,7]

Sjögren's syndrome is one of several autoimmune diseases associated with the histocompatibility antigens HLA-B8 and HLA-DR3. This genetic predisposition is seen in several other organ-specific autoimmune conditions such as celiac disease, dermatitis herpetiformis, myasthenia gravis, Graves' disease, chronic active hepatitis, idiopathic Addisson's disease and insulin-dependent diabetes mellitus. Recent attention has focused on the HLA-D region,[8,9] with the suggestion that gene interaction at the HLA-DQ locus is related to high-titered autoantibody responses and a more severe autoimmune disease.[10] There is also an association with HLA-DRw52 (previously known as MT2), which is a supertypic specificity encoded by an HLA-DRβ2 gene in linkage disequilibrium with HLA-DR3, -DR5, -DRw6, and -DRw8.[9] Primary Sjögren's syndrome in males is associated with HLA-DRw52 but not with HLA-B8 or HLA-DR3.[11] A familial relationship has been observed that includes an association with lymphoma.[12] Several spontaneously autoimmune mouse strains, particularly the MRL mice, have features of Sjögren's syndrome.

The presence of multiple serum autoantibodies is a characteristic feature of Sjögren's syndrome. Some of these reactions are organ-specific (e.g., against salivary duct epithelium), whereas others, such as antinuclear and rheumatoid factor (RF), are not. Two autoantibody systems, designated Ro/SSA and La/SSB, occur in the vast majority of primary Sjögren's syndrome patients and to a lesser extent in patients with systemic lupus erythematosus (SLE).[13,14] The antigens are RNA protein complexes. La/SSB binds to terminal uridine-rich regions of RNA polymerase III transcripts.

The mechanisms responsible for the glandular destruction are beginning to be understood. There are numerous HLA-DR-positive glandular epithelial cells in the Sjögren's syndrome salivary glands[14a,15] (Table 76–1). In close proximity to these HLA-Dr–positive epithelial cells are the lymphoid infiltrates in which activated T-helper cells are the most prominent population represented.[15,16] Activated T cells are also prominent in the pseudolymphoma lesions of Sjö-

gren's syndrome patients with generalized lymphoproliferation.[17] There are fewer B cells, but these too are in an activated state and produce large amounts of immunoglobulin.[18] This seems particularly important in light of the subsequent development of B-cell lymphomas in 5 to 10% of SS patients,[19] and the production of monoclonal immunoglobulins in the SS salivary glands.[18]

Natural killer cells carry the cell surface marker Leu-11b and are important for several immunoregulatory functions including natural host defense against malignancy. There is defective natural killer cell function in the blood of Sjögren's syndrome patients[20] and absent Leu-11b natural killer cells in the salivary gland lesions.[21] These results suggest that the salivary gland in Sjögren's syndrome may serve as an initial nidus for lymphoma development. This hypothesis is supported by an immunohistologic study suggesting that the myoepithelial sialadenitis of SS may contain areas of confluent lymphoid proliferation producing mostly monoclonal IgM/kappa.[22] These lesions were considered "early lymphomas," analogous to carcinoma in situ, which after a variable latent period transform into true lymphomas. β-2-Microglobulin, a component of lymphocyte membranes that may play an immunologic role, is increased in serum and saliva of patients with Sjögren's syndrome.[23]

An imbalance of helper and suppressor T cells as well as polyclonal activation of B cells are often present in autoimmunity. These abnormalities are less marked in Sjögren's syndrome than they are, for example, in SLE. The autologous mixed lymphocyte response, which may be a common denominator for both autoimmune and lymphoproliferative diseases of immunoregulation,[24] is abnormal in Sjögren's syndrome.[25]

PATHOLOGIC FEATURES

The classic lesion is a lymphocytic and plasma cell infiltrate of salivary, lacrimal, and other exocrine glands in the respiratory tract, gastrointestinal tract, and vagina. Both major (parotid, submaxillary) and minor (gingival, palatine) salivary glands are affected.[18,26,27] The term *benign lymphoepithelial lesion* has been used to describe the characteristic histologic appearance in the salivary glands.[28] These lesions may be present without xerostomia and other features of Sjögren's syndrome.[29] The earliest infiltrates may be scattered around small intralobular ducts. The histologic picture is varied and includes acinar atrophy, generally in proportion to the extent of lymphoid infiltration, occasional germinal center formation, and

Table 76–1. Immunologic Findings in the Salivary Glands in Sjögren's Syndrome

Many HLA-DR + glandular epithelial cells
Many T-helper cells expressing activation markers
Fewer activated B cells
Production of monoclonal immunoglobulins
Absence of natural killer cells

proliferative or metaplastic changes in the duct lining cells. The proliferation may progress to form the characteristic epimyoepithelial islets (Fig. 76–1), which are seen in about 40% of parotid biopsy specimens.[30] In some patients, adipose replacement may be more prominent than lymphoid infiltration. Typically, the lobular architecture is preserved; some lobules may be spared, while others are virtually destroyed.

When mucosal glands in the trachea and bronchi are involved, benign-appearing lymphoid infiltrates are again a prominent feature. More extensive lymphoid infiltrates may involve the lung, kidney, or skeletal muscle, resulting in functional abnormalities of these organs.

In some patients, the lymphoid infiltrates in salivary glands, lymph nodes, or parenchymal organs will be more pleomorphic, more primitive, or more invasive than in others, suggesting the possibility of a malignant disorder. Lymph node architecture can be destroyed, and malignant lymphoma may be diagnosed if such abnormal cells predominate. When it is not possible to distinguish a benign from a malignant process, the term *pseudolymphoma* is used.[31,32]

The immunophenotyping techniques[33] and the newly introduced immunogenotyping technique[34] now permit the diagnosis of monoclonal B-cell proliferations in tissue lymphoid infiltrates that are difficult to diagnose by conventional microscopy. Such molecular approaches may well increase diagnostic accuracy to the point where the imprecise term *pseudolymphoma* can be abandoned.

CLINICAL FEATURES[1]

More than 90% of patients are women; the mean age is 50 years. The disease occurs in all races and in

FIG. 76–1. Extensive lymphoid proliferation and formation of epimyoepithelial islets in the parotid gland of a patient with Sjögren's syndrome. (From Bloch, K.J., et al.[30])

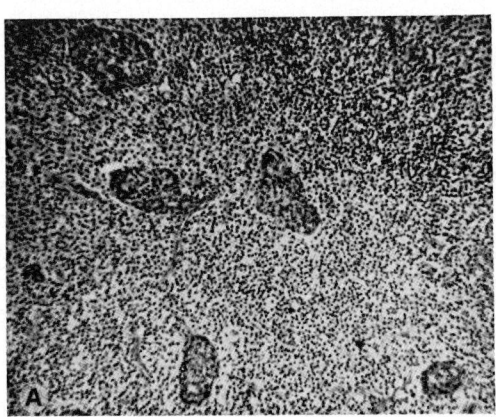

children.[35] The two most common presentations are (1) the insidious and slowly progressive development of the sicca complex in a patient with chronic RA and (2) the more rapid development of a severe oral and ocular dryness, often accompanied by episodic parotitis, in an otherwise well patient.

About 50% of patients with keratoconjunctivitis sicca have additional features of Sjögren's syndrome. The most common ocular complaint is a sensation, described as "gritty" or "sandy," of a foreign body in the eye. Other symptoms include burning, accumulation of thick, ropy strands at the inner canthus, particularly on awakening, decreased tearing, redness, photosensitivity, eye fatigue, itching, and a "filmy" sensation that interferes with vision. Patients complain of eye discomfort and difficulty in reading or in watching television. Inability to cry is *not* a common complaint. Lacrimal gland enlargement occurs infrequently. Ocular complications include corneal ulceration, vascularization, or opacification, followed rarely by perforation.

The distressing manifestations of salivary insufficiency include the following: (1) difficulty with chewing, swallowing, and phonation; (2) adherence of food to buccal surfaces; (3) abnormalities of taste or smell; (4) fissures of the tongue, buccal membranes, and lips, particularly at the corners of the mouth; (5) frequent ingestion of liquids, especially at meal times; and (6) rampant dental caries. Patients are unable to swallow a dry cracker or toast without ingesting fluids and express displeasure at the suggestion. They may carry bottles of water or other fluids with them and may awaken at night for sips of water. The dentist may notice that fillings are loosening.

Dryness may also involve the nose, the posterior pharynx, the larynx, and the tracheobronchial tree and may lead to epistaxis, hoarseness, recurrent otitis media, bronchitis, or pneumonia.

Half these patients have parotid gland enlargement (Fig. 76–2), often recurrent and symmetric and sometimes accompanied by fever, tenderness, or erythema. Superimposed infection is rare. Rapid fluctuations in gland size are not unusual. A particularly hard or nodular gland may suggest a neoplasm.

The arteritis of Sjögren's syndrome resembles classic RA in its clinical, pathologic, and roentgenographic features. Keratoconjunctivitis sicca develops in about 10 to 15% of patients with RA. Arthralgias and morning stiffness without joint deformity may occur in patients with the sicca complex. Fluctuations in the course of the arthritis are not accompanied by parallel alterations in the symptoms of the sicca complex. Splenomegaly and leukopenia suggestive of Felty's syndrome, and vasculitis with leg ulcers and pe-

FIG. 76–2. Bilateral parotid gland enlargement in a patient with severe xerostomia and Sjögren's syndrome.

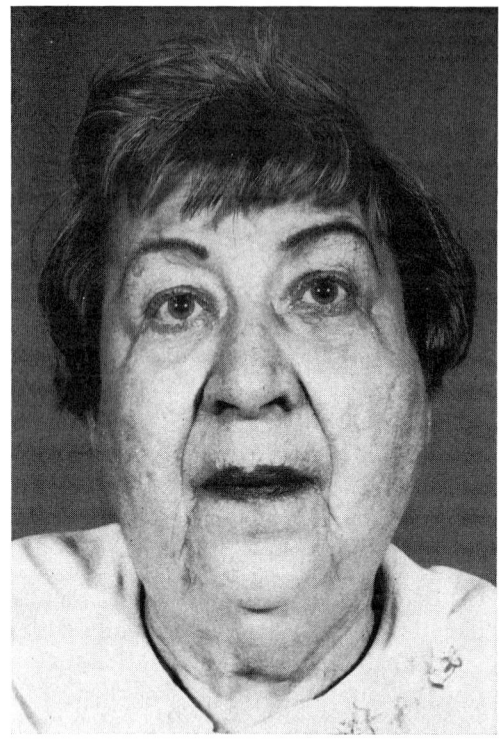

ripheral neuropathy, may appear even in the absence of RA. Raynaud's phenomenon occurs in 20% of patients.

Skin or vaginal dryness and allergic drug eruptions are frequent. Episodic lower extremity purpura, sometimes preceded by itching or other prodromal signs, may be the presenting complaint.[36] Glomerulonephritis develops rarely and should suggest either coexisting SLE or cryoglobulinemia. Cryoglobulins occur in up to a third of patients and may contain monoclonal immunoglobulin (IgM).[37] Overt or latent abnormalities of the renal tubular function, such as occurs in diabetes insipidus, renal tubular acidosis, and Fanconi syndrome, occur with greater frequency.[38–40] A variety of pulmonary disorders may be present.[41–44]

Severe proximal muscle weakness and, rarely, tenderness may be early symptoms leading to a diagnosis of polymyositis.[30] Weakness may also be associated with electrolyte imbalance, nephrocalcinosis, and the clinical findings of renal tubular acidosis. Peripheral or cranial neuropathy may cause symptoms of dysesthesia or paraesthesia. Facial pain and numbness can accompany trigeminal neuropathy[45] and may contribute to the oral discomfort caused by the dryness. Focal and diffuse central nervous system (CNS) disease may include cognitive disorders,[13,46] may

mimic multiple sclerosis,[47] and has been associated with vasculitis and CNS synthesis of immunoglobulins.

Although chronic thyroiditis of the Hashimoto type is present in 5% of patients, clinical hypothyroidism is rare. Sjögren's syndrome was found in 52% of patients with primary biliary cirrhosis and in 35% of patients with active chronic hepatitis.[48] Gastric achlorhydria, acute pancreatitis, and adult celiac disease have been reported in Sjögren's syndrome. Cervical or other lymph node enlargement may be the first indication of malignant lymphoma or pseudolymphoma (Fig. 76–3).

PHYSICAL FINDINGS

An elderly woman presenting with joint deformities, reddened eyes, and parotid gland enlargement should immediately suggest the diagnosis. In many patients, however, the findings are less obvious. The parotid glands may have any consistency, but are usually firm and nontender. Persistent bilateral parotid swelling may give rise to the so-called "chipmunk facies."

Gross inspection of the eyes may reveal nothing abnormal, a mucous thread, or conjunctival congestion. Lacrimal enlargement may not be apparent even when these glands are involved. The *Schirmer test*, in which a strip of Whatman No. 41 filter paper is folded and placed in the lower conjunctival sac, is a simple but crude measure of tear formation. Five minutes later, the moistened portion normally measures 15 mm or more. Most patients with Sjögren's syndrome moisten less than 5 mm of the test paper. More reliable diagnostic signs are obtained with rose bengal or fluorescein dye and biomicroscopic examination. Normally, no stain is visible a few minutes after dye instillation. Grossly visible or microscopic staining of the bulbar conjunctiva or cornea indicates the presence of small, superficial erosions. Biomicroscopy may also reveal increased amounts of corneal debris and attached filaments of corneal epithelium (filamentary keratitis).

The tongue and mucous membranes are characteristically dry, red, and "parchment-like." The lips may be dry and cracked. A tongue depressor adheres to oral surfaces, and the normal pool of saliva in the sublingual vestibule, visible when the tongue is elevated, is not present. A residual brownish pigmentation over the shins suggests past episodes of purpura (Fig. 76–4). Cervical or other lymph node enlargement may be the first indication of malignant

FIG. 76–3. *A,* Several hard, matted lymph nodes are present in the neck and submandibular region in this patient with Sjögren's syndrome of 20 years' duration. She has had intermittent, cervical lymphadenopathy for the last 6 years, with histologic diagnosis of pseudolymphoma made on four occasions. *B,* On biopsy, many abnormal reticulum cells with large nuclei and prominant nucleoli are found. The diagnosis is reticulum cell sarcoma. (Courtesy of Pediatric Clinics of North America.)

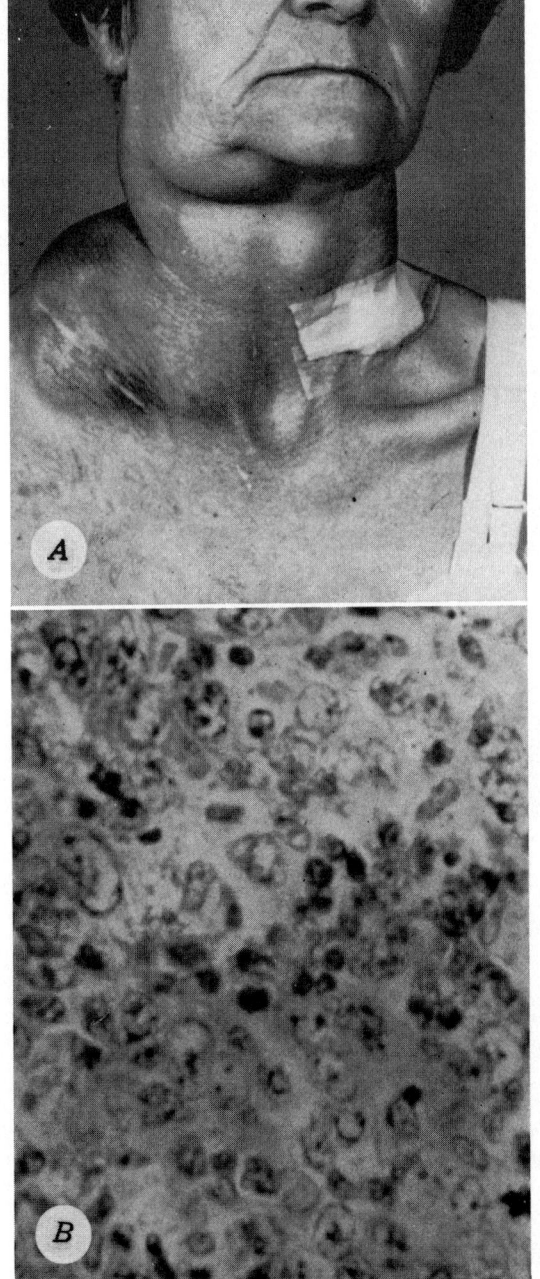

FIG. 76–4. Characteristic appearance of the legs of a patient with Sjögren's syndrome and intermittent, dependent, nonthrombocytopenic purpura.

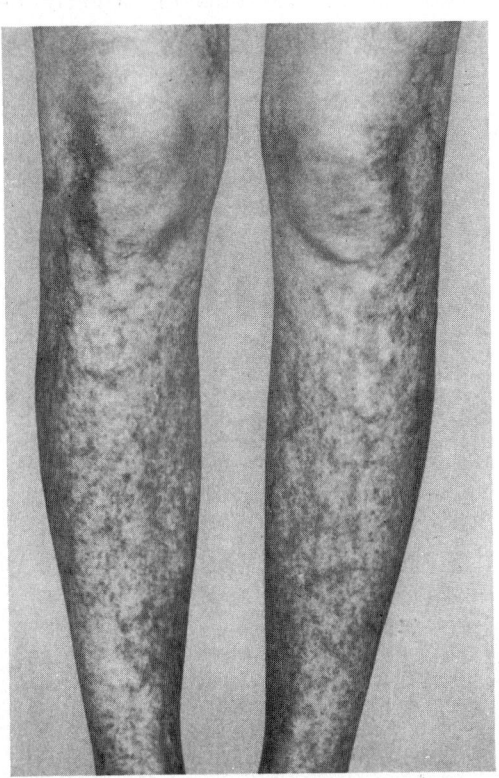

lymphoma or pseudolymphoma. Splenomegaly occurs in 25% of patients.[32]

LABORATORY FINDINGS

Parotid salivary flow rates can be measured by means of Carlson-Crittenden cups placed over the orifices of the parotid ducts and secured by suction. Flow is then stimulated by placing lemon juice on the tongue. Parotid secretion depends on age, sex, and other factors. Normal stimulated parotid flow rate should be about 0.5 to 1.0 ml/min/gland. Flow rates are reduced or unobtainable in Sjögren's syndrome.

Two techniques can be employed for visualizing the salivary glands. Secretory sialography is performed by introducing a radiopaque contrast medium through a small polyethylene catheter inserted into the orifice of the parotid duct.[49] After injection of 0.5 to 1.0 ml contrast material, the catheter is plugged, and radiographs are made (injection phase). The catheter is then removed, and emptying is encouraged by stimulation with lemon juice. Films are taken again 5 minutes later (secretory phase). A normal sialogram shows fine arborization of parotid ductules with little retention of contrast medium. In patients with Sjögren's syndrome, one sees gross distortion of the normal pattern with marked retention. The sialectasis may appear punctate, globular, or cavitary (Fig. 76–5). This procedure is performed much less frequently now than in the past.

The second method depends on the uptake, concentration, and excretion of the radionuclide ^{99m}Tc (pertechnetate) by the salivary gland. Patients are studied by sequential salivary scintigraphy in which the gland image is recorded visually on a γ-scintillation camera over 60 to 80 minutes. Both uptake and release of radionuclide are measured. Most patients show decreased function.[50] The scintigraphic findings

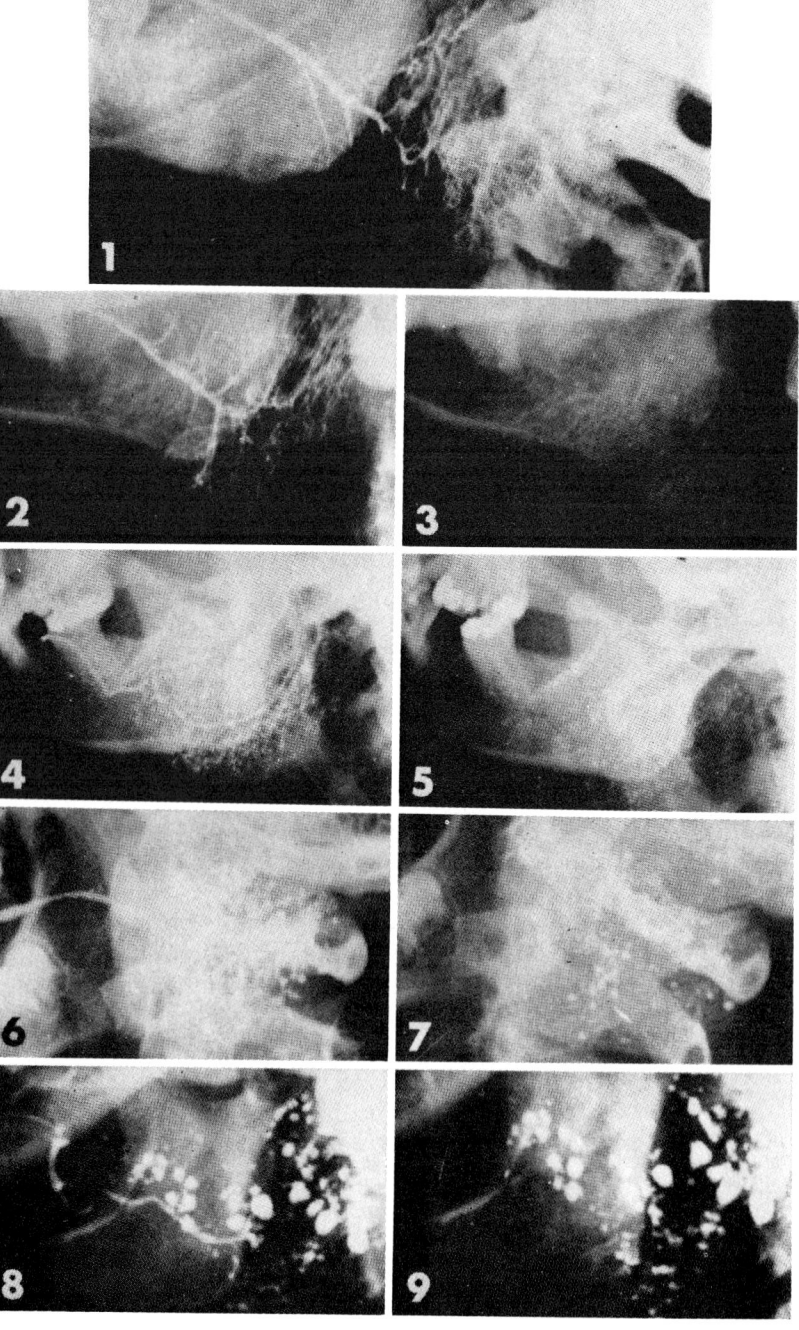

FIG. 76–5. Appearance of secretory sialography in normal individuals and in patients with Sjögren's syndrome. *1,* Injection phase, normal pattern. *2,* Injection phase, punctate sialectasis. *3,* Secretory phase, punctate sialectasis. *4,* Injection phase, punctate sialectasis with intermediate duct involvement. *5,* Secretory phase, punctate sialectasis with intermediate duct involvement. *6,* Injection phase, globular sialectasis. *7,* Secretory phase, globular sialectasis. *8,* Injection phase, cavitary and destructive sialectasis. *9,* Secretory phase, cavitary and destructive sialectasis. (From Bloch, K.J., et al.[30])

parallel the degree of xerostomia, the salivary flow rate determinations, and the results of secretory sialography (Fig. 76–6).

Involvement of minor salivary glands in the lower lip has led to the use of lower lip biopsies and histologic confirmation of the diagnosis. The procedure is performed under local anesthesia with the patient seated in a dental chair. An elliptic incision is made with a scalpel in the labial mucosa parallel to the vermillion border. Patients generally experience discomfort for 24 to 48 hours; approximately 1% complain of more persistent localized numbness. Lymphocytic infiltration can be measured by means of the focus scoring method, in which the number of foci, defined as 50 or more round cells per 4 mm^2 of sectioned tissue, is determined on the biopsy specimen. Although various authorities still disagree somewhat about precise diagnostic criteria for Sjögren's syndrome, a focus score greater than 1 is probably the best criterion for the oral component and far superior to the subjective evaluation of xerostomia.[51]

A mild normocytic, normochromic *anemia* occurs in about 25% of patients, *leukopenia* in 30%, *eosinophilia* (about 6% eosinophils) in 25%, and an elevated *erythrocyte sedimentation rate* (greater than 30 mm/hour by the Westergren method), in over 90%.

About half the patients have hyper-γ-globulinemia, which is generally a diffuse elevation of all immunoglobulin classes. The most hyperglobulinemic patients may not have RA, but rather polymyopathy, purpura, vasculitis, or renal tubular acidosis. Monoclonal IgM may be seen. Cryoglobulinemia, often of the mixed IgM–IgG type, may be present, particularly in patients with glomerulonephritis or pseudolymphoma. Hyperviscosity associated with IgG rheu-

matoid factor (RF)[51a] and intermediate complexes[52] has been reported. Some patients with lymphoma have hypo-γ-globulinemia. A mild hypoalbuminemia is common. Levels of circulating immune complexes are increased, and reticuloendothelial clearance is defective in Sjögren's syndrome.

RF is detected in over 90% of sera when pooled human F II γ-globulin is used as antigen and in 75% when rabbit γ-globulin is employed. Thus, many patients who do not have RA have RF. RF may disappear, or diminish markedly in titer when lymphoma develops.[31]

The LE cell phenomenon occurs in 20% of patients who also have RA. This phenomenon is otherwise rare, unless SLE is also present.

Antinuclear factors, giving a homogenous or speckled pattern of immunofluorescence, are seen in about 70% of patients.[30] Antibodies to native DNA are occasionally present in low titer. Thyroglobulin antibodies, detected by hemagglutination, are present in about 35% of patients.

The presence of multiple serum autoantibodies is a characteristic feature of Sjögren's syndrome as it is in SLE. Antibodies to Ro/SSA occur in the vast majority of primary Sjögren's syndrome patients (as determined by sensitive solid-phase assays) and are associated with RF, hyper-γ-globulinemia, vasculitis,[13] the neonatal lupus syndrome, and DQ heterozygosity (DQ1, DQ2). This autoantibody is often accompanied by anti-La/SSB. Both autoantibodies also occur in SLE but to a lesser extent than in Sjögren's syndrome. The relationship between Sjögren's syndrome and SLE can be confusing, not only for the sharing of these autoantibodies but also because, rarely, patients may change disease expression during the course of their

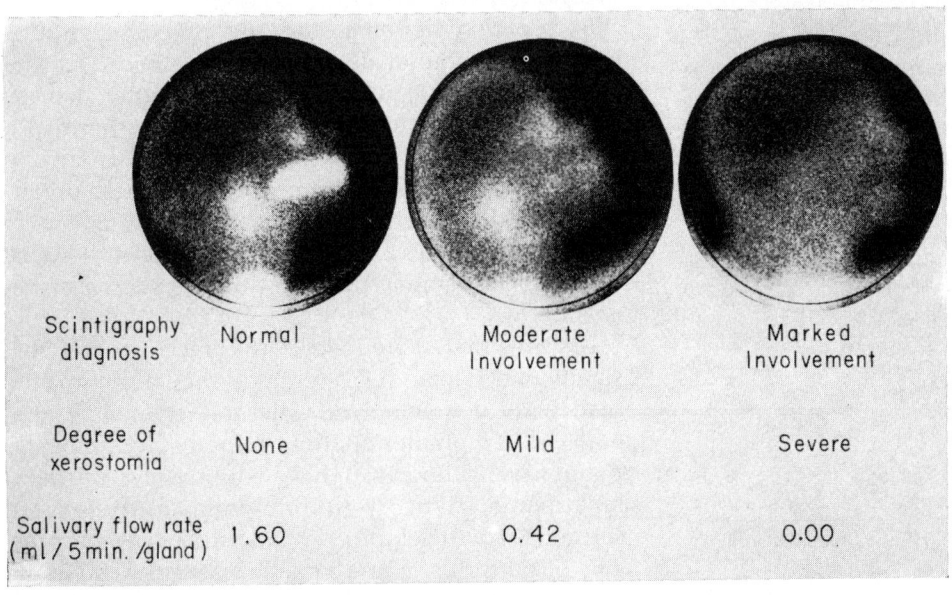

FIG. 76–6. Comparative studies of salivary function in Sjögren's syndrome illustrating the results achieved with scintigraphy employing [99mTc] (pertechnetate).

Scintigraphy diagnosis	Normal	Moderate Involvement	Marked Involvement
Degree of xerostomia	None	Mild	Severe
Salivary flow rate (ml / 5 min. /gland)	1.60	0.42	0.00

illness and therefore present a true Sjögren's syndrome–SLE overlap syndrome.[1]

The immunologic findings in the peripheral blood of patients with Sjögren's syndrome are summarized in Table 76–2. There is a marked polyclonal hyper-γ-globulinemia with the presence of RF, antinuclear antibodies (ANA), and in particular anti-Ro (SS-A) and anti-La (SS-B). Monoclonal immunoglobulins including homogenous light-chain bands are frequently found in the blood as well as in the urine by sensitive electrophoretic techniques.[53] Studies using peripheral blood lymphocytes demonstrate that many Sjögren's syndrome patients have deficient interleukin-2 (IL-2) production.[54] There is a decrease in peripheral blood T cells in about one third of patients. Abnormalities in T-cell function may be present, particularly in patients with systemic features. These patients often have alterations in T-cell subsets and decreased autologous mixed lymphocyte responses.[25] Natural killer cell activity is also diminished as a consequence of immunoregulatory abnormalities rather than intrinsic deficits.[20]

An increase in salivary β_2-microglobulin concentration correlates with the degree of lymphocytic infiltration found on labial biopsy. Serum β_2-microglobulin levels can be increased, particularly in patients with associated renal or lymphoproliferative complications.[23]

LYMPHOMA AND MACROGLOBULINEMIA

An increased incidence of non-Hodgkin's lymphoma in patients with Sjögren's syndrome was first reported over two decades ago. The chronic antigenic stimulation was suggested as a possible trigger for a malignant transformation event. There are now between 100 and 200 reported examples of this association.[19] Indeed, the risk of lymphoma development is 44 times greater in Sjögren's syndrome than in the normal population. The autoimmune disorder may precede the development of lymphoma by intervals ranging from 0.5 to 29 years. Certain extraglandular disease features (e.g., splenomegaly) as well as parotid swelling are more likely to occur in patients predisposed to lymphoma.

In most patients, significant lymphoproliferation remains confined to salivary and lacrimal tissue and has a chronic, benign course of stable or progressive xerostomia and xerophthalmia. Even after 15 years or more of benign disease, however, some patients develop an extension of lymphoproliferation to extraglandular sites such as lung, kidney, lymph nodes, skin, gastrointestinal tract, and bone marrow. Persistent or massive parotid gland enlargement may also suggest lymphoma.

When such "extraglandular" lymphoproliferation occurs, diagnosis is often difficult, and clinically and histologically the disease may simulate frankly malignant lymphoproliferative disorders such as Waldenström's macroglobulinemia or non-Hodgkin's lymphoma. Because the subsequent clinical course is frequently that of lymphoma, ending fatally, the early recognition of extraglandular lymphoproliferation in Sjögren's syndrome and the prompt institution of appropriate therapy are important.

The extraglandular lymphoid infiltrates are of two general types. They may be highly pleomorphic and include small and large lymphocytes, plasma cells, and large reticulum cells. In a lymph node the cells may distort the normal architecture and may extend beyond the capsule; the distinction between benign and malignant lesions is thereby made difficult. The term "pseudolymphoma" has been applied[32] when the lesions show tumor-like aggregates of lymphoid cells, but do not meet the usual histologic criteria for malignancy (Fig. 76–7).

In pseudolymphoma, the site of extraglandular lymphoproliferation determines the clinical presentation. Striking regional lymphadenopathy may be the predominant clinical feature. On the other hand, lymphoid infiltration may be selectively excessive in a distant organ such as kidney or lung. These organs may become functionally impaired, giving rise to renal abnormalities or pulmonary insufficiency. Renal tubular acidosis may develop through such a mechanism.

Features that should alert the clinician to the possibility of extraglandular lymphoproliferation in a patient with Sjögren's syndrome are regional or generalized lymphadenopathy, hepatosplenomegaly, pulmonary infiltrates, renal insufficiency, purpura, leukopenia, hyper-γ-globulinemia, and elevated serum β_2-microglobulin.[31,32] Vasculitis may be present, but arthritis is rare in such patients. The entity

Table 76–2. Immunologic Findings in the Peripheral Blood in Sjögren's Syndrome

Polyclonal hyper-γ-globulinemia
Autoantibodies (ANA + and RF +)
Anti-Ro (SS-A) and anti-La (SS-B)
Monoclonal immunoglobulins
Deficient IL-2 production
Impaired T-cell function
Decreased natural killer cell function

ANA + = antinuclear antibody positive, RF + = rheumatoid factor positive, IL-2 = interleukin 2.

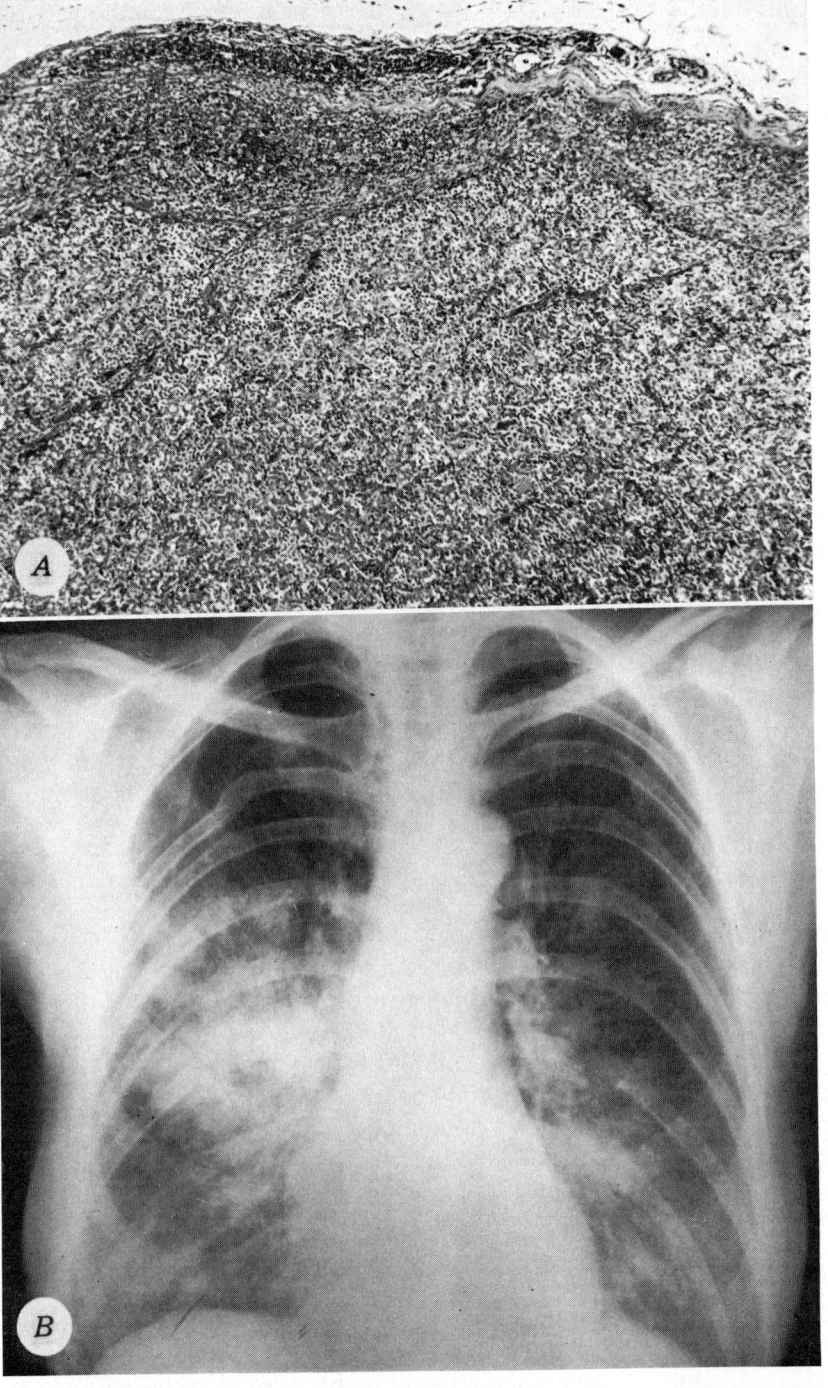

FIG. 76–7. Pseudolymphoma can distort the normal lymph node architecture with penetration of cells through (A) the capsule, or (B) it may appear as pulmonary infiltrates in chest radiogram. (From Bloch, K.J., et al.[30])

of pseudolymphoma cannot be clearly defined, but it occupies the middle portion of a spectrum ranging from benign disease to frankly malignant disease, such as Waldenström's macroglobulinemia.

The second type of extraglandular lymphoid infiltrate is histologically malignant and enables one to make the specific diagnosis of lymphoproliferative neoplasm. These lesions may also appear after several years of apparently benign disease; they may or may not be preceded by pseudolymphoma, and they are often resistant to therapy. Although the histologic diagnosis may vary, the lymphoma generally belongs to the B-cell lineage and often contains intracellular immunoglobulin.[33] Some patients may also have serum immunoglobulin spikes, which tend to be IgMκ in Western countries but non-IgM in Japan.[55]

A low IgM level may herald the presence or development of malignant lymphoproliferation and can be a sign of a poor prognosis. A fall in the serum IgM level is often accompanied by a reduction in the RF titer and may precede the onset of generalized hypo-γ-globulinemia.

DIAGNOSIS

Clinically, a "sicca-like" syndrome may be caused by a number of other disease processes including hyperlipoproteinemias IV and V, hemochromatosis, sarcoidosis, and amyloidosis.[2] The use of anticholinergic or antidepressive drugs as well as numerous other medications may cause xerostomia. Thus, it is essential to establish the presence of focal lymphoid infiltrates and autoimmunity in a patient suspected of having Sjögren's syndrome. The diagnosis of secondary Sjögren's syndrome, which should be suspected in any patient with RA, can be made when either keratoconjunctivitis sicca or a positive labial salivary gland biopsy are present. Generally, the arthritis precedes or is concurrent with the sicca complex. Other connective tissue diseases, such as scleroderma,[56] SLE,[57] or polymyositis, may substitute for RA in this definition.

Many patients have symptoms of oral or ocular dryness without an underlying connective tissue disease and appear to have primary Sjögren's syndrome. If arthritis does not develop within the first 12 months of the sicca complex, the chances are only 10% that it will appear later.

As with most diseases, obtaining the patient's medical history is the important first step in making the diagnosis. Many patients, on casual questioning, reply that their mouths feel dry. More significant is the requirement for frequent fluids during the course of the day or the admission that they awaken at night because of oral dryness. The dramatic negative response to the thought of ingesting a dry cracker is a helpful clue. Patients should be asked to describe their ocular complaints. They often use the expression "gritty" or "sandy" to characterize the discomfort of xerophthalmia.

Objective evidence of salivary or lacrimal gland insufficiency should be sought in any patient with a suggestive history. Such evidence includes a careful ophthalmologic examination with biomicroscopic examination, measurement of salivary flow, and a labial salivary gland biopsy.

The varied clinical presentation and the multisystemic nature of Sjögren's syndrome may make the diagnosis obscure. As indicated in Table 76–3, the disease may become manifest in several different ways. Unilateral or asymmetric glandular enlargement may suggest a possible tumor. Hyperglobulinemic purpura or other features of cutaneous vasculitis

Table 76–3. Clinical Presentation of Sjögren's Syndrome

1. Sicca complex—dry eyes and dry mouth
2. Rheumatoid arthritis—or other connective tissue disease
3. Salivary gland enlargement
4. Purpura—nonthrombocytopenic; hyperglobulinemic
5. Renal tubular acidosis—or other tubular disorder
6. Polymyopathy
7. Neuropathy—trigeminal
8. Chronic liver disease
9. Chronic pulmonary disease
10. Lymphoma—local or generalized
11. Immunoglobulin disorder—cryoglobulinemia; macroglobulinemia

may be prominent. The initial symptoms may be related to a renal tubular disorder such as renal gravel or calculi, or they may suggest a severe degenerative or inflammatory muscle disease. Peripheral neuropathy may be a prominent feature, and trigeminal nerve involvement can cause facial discomfort. CNS symptoms have recently been emphasized. The disease may appear initially as a chronic active hepatitis or biliary cirrhosis. Pulmonary disease may be related to dryness and infection or to lymphoid infiltration of the lung. Malignant lymphoma or an immunoglobulin disorder may first attract medical attention.

TREATMENT

Most often, Sjögren's syndrome is a relatively benign disease. Conservative management is therefore the best guide to therapy.

The sicca complex is treated with fluid replacement as often as necessary. Several readily available ophthalmic preparations, such as Tearisol, Liquifilm, and 0.5% methylcellulose, adequately replace the deficient tears. In severe situations, patients instill these drops as often as every half hour to hour. If corneal ulceration is present, patching of the eye and application of boric ointment may be necessary. Soft contact lenses are sometimes used to protect the cornea. Plastic-wrap occlusion or diving goggles may prevent tear evaporation at night. Topical corticosteroids are generally avoided unless specifically indicated because corneal thinning and subsequent perforation may occur. The use of diuretics, some antihypertensive drugs, and antidepressants may further diminish lacrimal and salivary gland function.

It is more difficult to compensate for the salivary insufficiency. Various saliva substitutes have not proved useful. Bromhexine, a mucolytic agent, has been used abroad.[58] The frequent ingestion of fluids, particularly with meals, is often the best solution.

Patients should see their dentists every 4 months and should pay scrupulous attention to proper oral hygiene. The careful use of a mouth-rinsing apparatus after eating may reduce the incidence of caries. Patients should avoid a high sucrose intake or the frequent use of sugar-containing candies to decrease oral dryness. Vigorous dental plaque control and topical application of fluoride should be routine. Oral candidiasis may be treated with nystatin tablets for a prolonged course, with separate treatment of dentures.

Proper humidification of the home environment is helpful in reducing respiratory infections and other complications of the sicca complex. Patients should be encouraged to live with their disability. They require sympathetic understanding.

The management of RA or other associated disorders is not altered by the presence of Sjögren's syndrome. No controlled studies evaluating the efficacy of corticosteroids or immunosuppressive drugs in the treatment of the sicca complex have been reported. In view of the benign nature of this problem and the potential hazards of these agents, such therapy does not seem justified.

On the other hand, corticosteroids or immunosuppressive drugs are indicated in the treatment of pseudolymphoma, particularly when the patient has renal or pulmonary involvement. Cyclophosphamide, 75 to 100 mg daily, has diminished extraglandular lymphoid infiltrates and restored salivary gland function in some patients.[59]

Malignant lymphoma should be treated with intensive chemotherapy, surgery, or radiotherapy as indicated by the location and extent of disease. These malignant and often fatal lesions require rapid and skilled intervention.

CONNECTIVE TISSUE DISEASE ASSOCIATED WITH OTHER IMMUNOLOGIC DISORDERS

HYPO-γ-GLOBULINEMIA

The functions of the immune system can be divided between those dependent on the secretion of antibody by plasma cells and those dependent on an intact thymus and specifically sensitized lymphocytes. One or both of these two functional systems, humoral and cellular immunity, respectively, may be defective in a variety of different immunodeficiency syndromes described in recent years.

A deficiency of humoral immunity results in a failure to produce specific antibody, a severe depression of serum γ-globulin concentration, and the absence of germinal center formation in lymph nodes and spleen. Five immunologically and structurally distinct classes of γ-globulin are known: IgG, IgM, IgA, IgD, and IgE. All immunoglobulin classes may be depressed simultaneously, or selective deficiencies may be present with normal or elevated levels of the remaining classes. The term "dys-γ-globulinemia" has been applied to describe the latter condition.

Hypo-γ-globulinemia may be congenital or acquired. Congenital hypo-γ-globulinemia is a sex-linked recessive disease usually heralded by recurrent pyogenic infections after the age of 6 months. Cellular immunity is generally intact, the level of IgG is usually less than 0.2 g/dl, and the other immunoglobulin classes are absent. These patients lack circulating B cells and tissue plasma cells.

Acquired hypo-γ-globulinemia, also termed the common, variable-onset form, occurs in both sexes, often becomes symptomatic between the ages of 15 and 35 years, and is frequently associated with autoimmunity,[60] as well as with pyogenic infection. Cellular immunity can be defective, and thymomas may occur. Circulating B-lymphocytes are generally normal in number, but have a diminished ability to synthesize and to secrete immunoglobulin. Suppressor T-cell function may be present.[61]

Selective IgA deficiency, the most common immunodeficiency disorder, appears to predispose persons to a variety of diseases. The incidence of IgA deficiency in the normal population varies between 1:800 and 1:600. The cause is unknown, but an arrest in B-cell maturation has been suggested. The other immunoglobulins are either normal or increased.

In addition to an enhanced susceptibility to bacterial and other infections, both congenital and acquired hypo-γ-globulinemia may be accompanied by watery diarrhea and malabsorption producing a sprue-like syndrome, a chronic polyarthritis resembling RA, or other connective tissue or lymphoproliferative disease. Frequently, the malabsorption is associated with infestation by Giardia lamblia.

CLINICAL AND DIAGNOSTIC FEATURES

The chronic polyarthritis associated with hypo-γ-globulinemia often starts in the knees and then involves the ankles, wrists, and fingers.[62-64] Pain is infrequent, but joint effusion is common. Subcutaneous nodules are rare.[65] The incidence of arthritis in patients with hypo-γ-globulinemia varies between 8 and 29%.[62,63,66]

Many characteristic features of RA, such as morning stiffness and symmetric joint swelling, are present. Radiograms show demineralization of the bones and narrowing of the joint spaces. Erosions are rare, and extensive joint destruction has not been reported. RF is absent from the serum.

Synovial biopsies may show lymphocytic infiltration, but no B-lymphocytes or plasma cells are found.[67] An excessive suppressor T-cell activity has been reported in the synovium.[68] Other patients, however, may have chronic synovitis without these features.[69] A suggestion that relatives of patients had a high incidence of RA[62] and hyper-γ-globulinemia[65] has not been substantiated.[63]

In addition to polyarthritis, other disorders that may be associated with hypo-γ-globulinemia include scleroderma,[70] SLE, dermatomyositis,[71] idiopathic thrombocytopenic purpura, Sjögren's syndrome,[72] hemolytic anemia, and pernicious anemia. Patients with the acquired form may have marked lymphadenopathy and splenomegaly, and, occasionally, autoantibodies associated with SLE or hemolytic anemia. Intestinal lymphoid nodular hyperplasia may accompany the malabsorption.[72] Lymphoreticular malignant tumors and thymomas have been reported. Three patients developed panhypo-γ-globulinemia during the course of SLE.[73,74]

Some patients have a selective IgA deficiency associated with autoimmune disease or with serologic abnormalities suggestive of autoimmunity. Recurrent sinopulmonary infections are common in these patients. Allergies, ataxia telangiectasia, gastrointestinal tract disease, and malignant tumor may be present. Immunologic abnormalities include increased serum IgA and IgM concentrations, serum 7S IgM, abnormal κ/λ ratios, and antibodies reacting with IgG, IgA, milk, bovine proteins, and human tissue antigens.[75] The clinical presentations associated with selective IgA deficiency include RA,[76,77] SLE,[78,79] Sjögren's syndrome,[79,80] dermatomyositis, pernicious anemia, chronic active hepatitis, Coombs'-positive hemolytic anemia, and thyroiditis. Cellular immunity is generally normal. Selective IgA deficiency occurs in approximately 4% of patients with SLE or juvenile RA (JRA).

Quantitative immunoglobulin determinations are essential for diagnosis. Immunoglobulin concentrations may be slightly higher in the acquired form, but are still depressed. Isohemagglutinins either are absent or are present in low titers (1:10). A failure to develop an antibody response to a specific antigenic challenge may help to establish the diagnosis if immunoglobulin levels are borderline. *Live attenuated vaccines should not be used for immunization.*

Abnormalities of cellular immunity may be seen, including absent delayed hypersensitivity skin test reactions, depressed responses to mitogenic stimulation, and decreased numbers of rosette-forming T-lymphocytes.[81]

Serum and secretory IgA may be selectively absent in IgA-deficient patients. Some subjects may have normal secretory IgA or have increased amounts of serum and secretory 7S IgM.

TREATMENT

Commercial γ-globulin is given at regular intervals, starting at doses of 0.2 ml/kg and increasing progressively. The arthritis associated with hypo-γ-globulinemia usually responds promptly to this treatment.[64,65] Anaphylactoid reactions to γ-globulin have been noted. Fresh-frozen plasma may also be used. Patients with selective IgA deficiency should not be given γ-globulin, because they may react to the foreign IgA and may develop anaphylactoid transfusion reactions.

ETIOLOGIC FACTORS

The immunologic events occurring locally in the synovium and joint space in these patients may be similar to those in typical RA, despite the hypo-γ-globulinemia and impaired ability to produce specific antibody or RF.

The pathogenesis of the autoimmune and connective tissue diseases probably depends on genetic, immunologic, and viral factors. The immunologic deficiency present in these patients predisposes them to pyogenic respiratory tract infections and to unexplained diarrhea and malabsorption, as well as to autoimmunity. Perhaps their altered immune status renders them more susceptible to disorders induced by unusual pathogens such as latent viruses. The peculiar susceptibility of patients with selective IgA deficiency supports this concept. IgA, the major secretory immunoglobulin, may play an important host defense role in the respiratory and gastrointestinal tract. Deficiency of IgA in these critical areas may permit the entry and establishment of foreign pathogens that induce antigenic alterations and contribute to the development of autoimmunity.

Knowledge of the role of suppressor cells in preventing normal B-cell maturation may help us to understand the cause of this disorder and may allow more specific immunotherapy.

HYPERGLOBULINEMIC PURPURA

Clinical Features

Hyperglobulinemic purpura affects women predominantly and is characterized by hyper-γ-globulinemia and episodes of purpura of the lower extremities. Described originally by Waldenström,[82] this disorder is not to be confused with another entity, Waldenström's macroglobulinemia. Patients often have no other associated illness, although myeloma,[83,84] arthritis, and Sjögren's syndrome may develop.[85] Prodromal symptoms such as burning or itching of the legs may precede by several hours and announce the onset of another episode of purpura. A chronic brownish pigmentation of the skin often appears as the residue of these attacks.

Laboratory Findings

The erythrocyte sedimentation rate and γ-globulin concentration are elevated. RF and antinuclear factor are frequently present in the serum.

Anti-γ-globulins of the IgG type are a feature of this disease and result in immune complexes with sedimentation properties intermediate between 7S and 19S immunoglobulins.[86] These "intermediate complexes" are formed by interactions of the IgG anti-IgG with itself and with other normal IgG molecules. The resulting pattern on serum paper electrophoresis is generally polydispersed, that is, polyclonal, but it may appear monoclonal. IgA complexes may also be involved, and the complexes may increase when the ambient temperature falls.[87]

Etiologic Factors

This disorder seems to occupy a middle ground between autoimmune and lymphoproliferative diseases. It is distinguished immunologically from RA by the frequent presence of IgG rather than IgM RF, that is, anti-IgG antibody.

The exact relation of the hyper-γ-globulinemia to the purpura is not understood. The circulating immune complexes become deposited in small blood vessels and give rise to vascular injury and extravasation of blood. The cooler skin temperature and orthostatic pressure changes may play a role in this process.

CRYOGLOBULINEMIA

Cryoglobulins are immunoglobulins with the physiochemical characteristic of precipitation in the cold followed by resolution on warming. Three types of cryoglobulins have been defined[88] as follows: (1) iso-lated monoclonal immunoglobulins produced by proliferating cells in Waldenström's macroglobulinemia or multiple myeloma; (2) mixed cryoglobulins in which a monoclonal component, usually IgM, has antibody activity against polyclonal IgC; and (3) mixed polyclonal cryoglobulins, which are usually anti-immunoglobulin immune complexes, but may also contain other molecules such as β1C or lipoprotein.

Cryoglobulins also occur in rheumatoid vasculitis,[89] cutaneous vasculitis,[90] and SLE.[64] They appear to represent circulating immune complexes and, in SLE, may contain antibodies to nucleoproteins and to lymphocyte antigens.

Clinical and Diagnostic Features

Cryoglobulins of either monoclonal or immune complex (mixed) nature may produce Raynaud's phenomenon, numbness, urticaria, vascular occlusions, tissue infarction, and digital ulcerations. Cutaneous and vasomotor symptoms are more severe in types 1 and 2 cryoglobulinemia. Types 2 and 3 are more often associated with renal and neurologic involvement, chronic vascular purpura, and Raynaud's phenomenon. Immunoproliferative disorders are associated with types 1 and 2, and autoimmunity with type 3.[88]

Mixed cryoglobulins may also be associated with a symptom complex, occurring predominantly in women, that includes arthralgias, purpura, especially involving the lower extremities, weakness, vasculitis, and diffuse glomerulonephritis.[91] RF is present and Sjögren's syndrome or thyroiditis may occur.

Forty patients with essential mixed cryoglobulins represented 32% of all cryoglobulinemic patients seen in an 18-year period.[92] Seventy percent had evidence of hepatic dysfunction, and 60% had serologic evidence of prior infection with hepatitis B virus. Many patients had severe renal disease with glomerular deposits of IgA, IgM, and complement. All cryoglobulins had RF activity. Renal involvement indicated a poor prognosis, and widespread vasculitis was found frequently during postmortem examination.

The laboratory finding that confirms the diagnosis is the cryoglobulin in the serum. From 24 to 48 hours in the cold may be required to precipitate the cryoglobulin from serum. Anywhere from 20 to 60% of the mixed cryoprecipitate is IgM. The presence of IgG is required to precipitate IgM, and IgM behaves like an antibody to IgG. Cryoprecipitation occurs in the absence of complement, although complement may be associated with the complex, and serum complement levels are generally depressed. The IgM is a fairly typical RF binding to the Fc portion of IgG. The IgM may be a monoclonal (Waldenström-type) paraprotein; mixed IgA–IgG cryoglobulinemia has also been reported.

One patient had mixed cryoglobulinemia, Sjögren's syndrome, and pulmonary lymphoid infiltrates, with an associated hypo-γ-globulinemia and increased susceptibility to bacterial infection.[93] The IgM was monoclonal and reacted specifically with IgG subclasses 1, 2, and 4 but not with subclass 3. Serum concentrations of IgG 1, 2, and 4 were 10% of normal. These three subclasses also showed reduced synthesis and shortened survival times, whereas IgG-3 had a normal synthetic rate and survival time. The hypo-γ-globulinemia was due in part to a rapid elimination of IgG through its interaction with the IgG-reactive monoclonal IgM.[93]

Hyperviscosity due to an IgM–IgG interaction has been reported in association with RA.[91]

Treatment

The treatment of mixed cryoglobulinemia has been reviewed.[66] Corticosteroids, immunosuppressive drugs, plasmapheresis, penicillamine, and splenectomy have been used with limited success.[94]

Etiologic Factors

The "mixed cryoglobulins" probably represent a special example of an immune complex phenomenon that has highly unusual physicochemical properties, both in vitro and in vivo. The cold precipitability in vitro makes it possible to identify, to isolate, and to characterize the individual components of the complex. The in vivo properties of the complex probably contribute in a major way to the findings of vascular insufficiency. The purpuric lesions may be caused by cryoprecipitation in the small skin capillaries, which reach a temperature (30°C) at which these aggregates are known to precipitate. The complexes may also induce glomerulonephritis and may be responsible for hypo-γ-globulinemia with increased susceptibility to infection.

These cryoglobulins illustrate in an impressive way the dramatic pathologic consequences of immune complex formation and deposition. They shed no light on the mechanism leading to their production, although their ready availability in serum may contribute to further investigation. If viral or tissue antigens are involved in the initial stages of their production, then the specificity of antibodies in the cryocomplex may conceivably be directed against such antigens.

MALIGNANT LYMPHOMA

Enough published reports of the association of connective tissue disease and malignant lymphoma, two rare conditions, now exist that a mere coincidental relationship may not be the best explanation. A recent report notes an increased risk of lymphoma, leukemia, and multiple myeloma in patients with RA.[95] The association of Sjögren's syndrome with lymphoproliferation was discussed earlier in this chapter.

Patients with coexisting SLE and malignant lymphoma have been reported.[96–100] Four patients had Hodgkin's disease, two had lymphosarcoma, and one each had mixed cell lymphoma, reticulum cell sarcoma, and chronic lymphocytic leukemia. All but two died of the malignant disease. Two had hypo-γ-globulinemia. One patient had hematoxylin bodies, onion-skin lesions in the spleen, and hypo-γ-globulinemia with an increase in IgM. The IgM showed cryoprecipitability, was an antinuclear factor, and contained only λ light chains.[100]

The association of RA with monoclonal gammopathies is noteworthy. In a series of 16 patients with arthritis, 6 had multiple myeloma, 8 had asymptomatic monoclonal immunoglobulin "spike" on serum protein electrophoresis, and 1 each had Waldenström's macroglobulinemia or heavy-chain disease.[101] These patients had RF, and their arthritis antedated the development of the paraprotein by as much as 26 years. Such patients should be distinguished from those with multiple myeloma or Waldenström's macroglobulinemia in whom amyloid deposition or the bony lesions themselves can mimic RA.[102,103]

The connective tissue diseases may predispose patients to the subsequent development of lymphoid or plasma cell malignant disorders, possibly as a consequence of chronic viral infection or prolonged antigenic stimulation, perhaps coupled with impaired cellular immunity and immunologic surveillance.

REFERENCES

1. Talal, N., Moutsopoulos, H.M., Kassan, S.S. (eds.): Sjögren's Syndrome: Clinical and Immunologic Aspects. New York, Springer-Verlag, 1987.
2. Strand, V., and Talal, N.: Advances in the diagnosis and concept of Sjögren's syndrome (autoimmune exocrinopathy). Bull. Rheum. Dis., 30:1046–1052, 1980.
3. Mikulicz, J.: Concerning a peculiar symmetrical disease of the lacrymal and salivary glands. Med. Classics, 2:165–186, 1937.
3a. Gougerot, H.: Insuffisance progressive et atrophie des glandes salivaires et musqueuses de la bouche, des conjonctives (et parfois des muqueuses nasale, laryngee, vulvaire) secheresse de la bouche, des conjonctives, etc. Bull. Med. (Par.), 40:360, 1926.
3b. Houwer, A.W.M.: Keratitis filamentosa and chronic arthritis. Tr. Ophthal. Soc. U.K., 47:88, 1927.
4. Sjögren, H.: Histological examinations in heratoconjunctivity sicca. Acta Ophthalmol., 11(2):1–2, 1933.

5. Morgan, W.S., and Castleman, B.: A clinicopathologic study of "Mikulicz's disease." Am. J. Pathol., 29:471–489, 1953.

6. Roubinian, J.R., Papoian, R., and Talal, N.: Androgenic hormones modulate autoantibody responses and improve survival in murine lupus. J. Clin. Invest., 59:1066–1070, 1977.

7. Ansar Ahmed, S., Penhale, W.J., and Talal, N.: Sex hormones, immune responses, and autoimmune diseases: Mechanisms of sex hormone action. Am. J. Pathol., 121:531–551, 1985.

8. Manthorpe, R., Teppa, A.M., Bendixen, G., and Wegelius, O.: Antibodies to SS-B in chronic inflammatory connective tissue diseases. Relationship with HLA-Dw2 and HLA-Dw3 antigens in primary Sjögren's syndrome. Arthritis Rheum., 25:662–667, 1982.

9. Wilson, R.W., et al.: Sjögren's syndrome. Influence of multiple HLA-D region alloantigens on clinical and serologic expression. Arthritis Rheum., 27:1245–1253, 1984.

10. Harley, J.B., et al.: Gene interaction at HLA-DQ enhances autoantibody production in primary Sjögren's syndrome. Science, 232:1145–1147, 1986.

11. Molina, R., et al.: Primary Sjögren's syndrome in men. Clinical, serologic, and immunogenetic features. Am. J. Med., 80:23–31, 1986.

12. Lichtenfeld, J.L., Kirschner, R.H., and Wiernik, P.H.: Familial Sjögren's syndrome with associated primary salivary gland lymphoma. Am. J. Med., 60:286–292, 1976.

13. Alexander, E.L., Arnett, F.C., Provost, T.T., and Stevens, M.B.: Sjögren's syndrome: Association of anti-Ro (SS-A) antibodies with vasculitis, hematologic abnormalities, and serologic hyperreactivity. Ann. Intern. Med., 98:155–159, 1983.

14. Martinez-Lavin, M., Vaughan, J.H., and Tan, E.M.: Autoantibodies and the spectrum of Sjögren's syndrome. Ann. Intern. Med., 91:185–187, 1979.

14a. Fox, R.I., et al.: Expression of histocompatibilty antigen HLA-DR by salivary gland epithelial cells in Sjögren's syndrome. Arthritis Rheum., 29:1105–1111, 1986.

15. Lindahl, G., Hedfors, E., Klareskog, L., and Forsum, U.: Epithelial HLA-DR expression and T lymphocyte subsets in salivary glands in Sjögren's syndrome. Clin. Exp. Immunol., 61:475–482, 1985.

16. Adamson, T.C., III, Fox, R.I., Frisman, D.M., and Howell, F.V.: Immunohistologic analysis of lymphoid infiltrates in primary Sjögren's syndrome using monoclonal antibodies. J. Immunol., 130:203–208, 1983.

17. Fox, R.I., et al.: Lymphocyte phenotype and function in pseudolymphoma associated with Sjögren's syndrome. J. Clin. Invest., 72:52, 1983.

18. Talal, N., Asofsky, R., and Lightbody, P.: Immunoglobulin synthesis by salivary gland lymphoid cells in Sjögren's syndrome. J. Clin. Invest., 49:49–62, 1970.

19. Talal, N.: The biological significance of lymphoproliferation in Sjögren's syndrome. In Proceedings of the XVIth International Congress of Rheumatology, ILAR'85, Sydney, Australia. The Netherlands, Elsevier Science Publishers, 1985.

20. Miyasaka, N., et al.: Natural killing activity in Sjögren's syndrome: An analysis of defective mechanisms. Arthritis Rheum., 26:954–960, 1983.

21. Fox, R.I., et al.: Salivary gland lymphocytes in primary Sjögren's syndrome lack lymphocyte subsets defined by Leu-7 and Leu-11 antigens. J. Immunol., 135:207, 1985.

22. Schmid, U., Helbron, D., and Lennert, K.: Development of malignant lymphoma in myoepithelial sialadenitis (Sjögren's syndrome). Pathol. Anat., 395:11, 1982.

23. Michalski, J.P., Daniels, T.E., Talal, N., and Grey, H.M.: Beta₂

microglobulin and lymphocytic infiltration in Sjögren's syndrome. N. Engl. J. Med., 293:1228–1237, 1975.

24. Smith, J.B., and Talal, N.: Significance of self-recognition and interleukin-2 for immunoregulation, autoimmunity and cancer. (Editorial.) Scand. J. Immunol., 16:269–278, 1982.

25. Miyasaka, N., et al.: Decreased autologous mixed lymphocyte reaction in Sjögren's syndrome. J. Clin. Invest., 66:928–933, 1980.

26. Chisholm, D.M., and Mason, D.K.: Labial salivary gland biopsy in Sjögren's syndrome. J. Clin. Pathol., 21:656–660, 1968.

27. Greenspan, J.S., et al.: The histopathology of Sjögren's syndrome in labial salivary gland biopsies. Oral. Surg., 37:217–229, 1974.

28. Godwin, J.T.: Benign lymphoepithelial lesion of the parotid gland. Cancer, 5:1089–1103, 1952.

29. Cruickshank, A.H.: Benign lymphoepithelial salivary lesion to be distinguished from adenolymphoma. J. Clin. Pathol., 18:391–400, 1965.

30. Bloch, K.J., Buchanan, W.W., Wohl, M.J., and Bunim, J.J.: Sjögren's syndrome. A clinical, pathological, and serological study of sixty-two cases. Medicine, 44:187–231, 1965.

31. Anderson, L.G., and Talal, N.: The spectrum of benign to malignant lymphoproliferation in Sjögren's syndrome. Clin. Exp. Immunol., 10:199–221, 1972.

32. Talal, N., Sokoloff, L., and Barth, W.F.: Extrasalivary lymphoid abnormalities in Sjögren's syndrome (reticulum cell sarcoma, "pseudolymphoma," macroglobulinemia). Am. J. Med., 43:50–65, 1967.

33. Zulman, J., Jaffe, R., and Talal, N.: Evidence that the malignant lymphoma of Sjögren's syndrome is a monoclonal B-cell neoplasm. N. Engl. J. Med., 299:1215–1220, 1978.

34. Cleary, M.L., et al.: Detection of lymphoma in Sjögren's syndrome by analysis of immunoglobulin gene rearrangements. In Sjögren's Syndrome: Clinical and Immunological Aspects. Edited by N. Talal, H. Mousopoulos, and S. Kassan. New York, Springer-Verlag, 1987.

35. Chudwin, D.S., et al.: Spectrum of Sjögren's syndrome in children. J. Pediatr., 98:213–217, 1981.

36. Ferreiro, J.E., Pasarin, G., Quesada, R., and Gould, E.: Benign hypergammaglobulinemic purpura of Waldenström associated with Sjögren's syndrome. Case report and review of immunologic aspects. Am. J. Med., 81:734–740, 1986.

37. Tzioufas, A.G., et al.: Cryoglobulinemia in autoimmune rheumatic diseases. Evidence of circulating monoclonal cryoglobulins in patients with primary Sjögren's syndrome. Arthritis Rheum., 29:1098–1104, 1986.

38. Morris, R.C., and Fudenberg, H.H.: Impaired renal acidification in patients with hypergammaglobulinemia. Medicine, 46:57–69, 1967.

39. Shearn, M.A., and Tu, W.H.: Latent renal tubular acidosis in Sjögren's syndrome. Ann. Rheum. Dis., 27:27–32, 1968.

40. Talal, N., Zisman, E., and Schur, P.H.: Renal tubular acidosis, glomerulonephritis and immunologic factors in Sjögren's syndrome. Arthritis Rheum., 11:774–786, 1968.

41. Constantopoulos, S.H., Papadimitriou, C.S., and Moutsopoulos, H.M.: Respiratory manifestations in primary Sjögren's syndrome. A clinical, functional, and histologic study. Chest, 88:226–229, 1985.

42. Fairfax, A.J., et al.: Pulmonary disorders associated with Sjögren's syndrome. Am. J. Med., 199:279–295, 1981.

43. Segal, I., et al.: Pulmonary function abnormalities in Sjögren's syndrome and the sicca complex. Thorax, 36:286–289, 1981.

44. Vitali, C., et al.: Lung involvement in Sjögren's syndrome: A

comparison between patients with primary and with secondary syndrome. Ann. Rheum. Dis., *44*:455–461, 1985.

45. Kaltreider, H.B., and Talal, N.: The neuropathy of Sjögren's syndrome. Ann. Intern. Med., *70*:751–762, 1969.

46. Alexander, E.L., Lijewski, J.E., Jerdan, M.S., and Alexander, G.E.: Evidence of an immunopathologic basis for central nervous system disease in primary Sjögren's syndrome. Arthritis Rheum., *29*:1223–1231, 1986.

47. Alexander, E.L.: Primary Sjögren's syndrome with central nervous system disease mimicking multiple sclerosis. Ann. Intern. Med., *104*:323–330, 1986.

48. Golding, P.L., Smith, M., and Williams, R.: Multisystem involvement in chronic liver disease. Am. J. Med., *55*:772–782, 1973.

49. Dijkstra, P.F.: Classification and differential diagnosis of sialographic characteristics in Sjögren's syndrome. Semin. Arthritis Rheum., *10*:10–17, 1980.

50. Schall, G.L., et al.: Xerostomia in Sjögren's syndrome. JAMA, *216*:2109–2116, 1971.

51. Daniels, T.E.: Labial salivary gland biopsy in Sjögren's syndrome. Arthritis Rheum., *27*:147–156, 1984.

51a. Alarcon-Segovia, D., Fishbein, E., Abruzzo, J.L., and Heimer, R.: Serum hyperviscosity in Sjögren's syndrome. Ann. Intern. Med., *80*:35–43, 1974.

52. Blaylock, W.M., Waller, M., and Normansell, D.E.: Sjögren's syndrome: Hyperviscosity and intermediate complexes. Ann. Intern. Med., *80*:27–34, 1974.

53. Moutsopoulos, H.M., et al.: Demonstration and identification of monoclonal proteins in the urine of patients with Sjögren's syndrome. Ann. Rheum. Dis., *44*:109, 1985.

54. Miyasaka, N., et al.: Interleukin 2 defect in the peripheral blood and the lung in patients with Sjögren's syndrome. Clin. Exp. Immunol., *65*:497–505, 1986.

55. Sugai, S., et al.: Non-IgM monoclonal gammopathy in patients with Sjögren's syndrome. Am. J. Med., *68*:861–866, 1980.

56. Shearn, M.: Sjögren's syndrome in association with scleroderma. Ann. Intern. Med., *51*:1352–1362, 1960.

57. Steinberg, A.D., and Talal, N.: The coexistence of Sjögren's syndrome and systemic lupus erythematosus. Ann. Intern. Med., *74*:55–61, 1971.

58. Manthorpe, R., Frost-Larsen, K., Isager, H., and Prause, J.W.: Sjögren's syndrome. A review with emphasis on immunological features. Allergy, *36*:139–153, 1981.

59. Anderson, L.G., et al.: Salivary gland immunoglobulin and rheumatoid factor synthesis in Sjögren's syndrome. Am. J. Med., *53*:456–463, 1972.

60. Ammann, A.J.: Immunodeficiency disorders and autoimmunity. In Autoimmunity: Genetic, Immunologic, Virologic, and Clinical Aspects. Edited by N. Talal. New York, Academic Press, 1977.

61. Waldmann, T.A., et al.: The role of suppressor cells in the pathogenesis of common variable hypogammaglobulinemia and the immunodeficiency associated with myeloma. Fed. Proc., *35*:2067–2072, 1976.

62. Good, R.A., and Rotstein, J.: Rheumatoid arthritis and agammaglobulinemia. Bull. Rheum. Dis., *10*:203–206, 1960.

63. Lawrence, J.S., and Bremner, J.M.: Arthritis and hypogammaglobulinaemia. Scand. J. Rheumatol., *5*:17–28, 1976.

64. Webster, A.D.B., et al.: Polyarthritis in adults with hypogammaglobulinaemia and its rapid response to immunoglobulin treatment. Br. Med. J., *1*:1314–1316, 1976.

65. Barnett, E.V., Winkelstein, A., and Weinberger, H.J.: Agam-

maglobulinemia with polyarthritis and subcutaneous nodules. Am. J. Med., *48*:40–47, 1970.

66. Lederman, H.M., and Winkelstein, J.A.: X-linked agammaglobulinemia: An analysis of 96 patients. Medicine, *64*(3):145–156, 1985.

67. Abrahamsen, T.G., et al.: Lymphocytes from synovial tissue of a boy with X-linked hypogammaglobulinemia and chronic polyarthritis. Arthritis Rheum., *22*:71–78, 1979.

68. Chattopadhyay, J., Natvig, B., and Chattopadhyay, H.: Excessive suppressor T-cell activity of the rheumatoid synovial tissue in X-linked hypogammaglobulinaemia. Scand. J. Immunol., *11*:455–459, 1980.

69. Grayzel, A.I., et al.: Chronic polyarthritis associated with hypogammaglobulinemia. Arthritis Rheum., *20*:887–894, 1977.

70. VanGelder, D.W.: Clinical significance of alterations in gamma globulin levels. South. Med. J., *50*:43–50, 1957.

71. Janeway, C.A., Gitlin, D., Craig, J.M., and Grice, D.S.: "Collagen disease" in patients with congenital agammaglobulinemia. Trans. Am. Assoc. Physicians, *69*:93–97, 1956.

72. Hermans, P.E., Diaz-Buzo, J.A., and Stobo, J.D.: Idiopathic late-onset immunoglobulin deficiency. Am. J. Med., *61*:221–237, 1976.

73. Ashman, R.F., et al.: Panhypogammaglobulinemia in systemic lupus erythematosus: In vitro demonstration of multiple cellular defects. J. Allergy Clin. Immunol., *70*:465–473, 1982.

74. Tsokos, G.C., Smith, P.L., and Balow, J.E.: Development of hypogammaglobulinemia in a patient with systemic lupus erythematosus. Am. J. Med., *81*:1081–1084, 1986.

75. Ammann, A.J., and Hong, R.: Selective IgA deficiency: Presentation of 30 cases and a review of the literature. Medicine, *50*:223–238, 1971.

76. Cassidy, J.T., Petty, R.E., and Sullivan, D.B.: Abnormalities in the distribution of serum immunoglobulin concentrations in juvenile rheumatoid arthritis. J. Clin. Invest., *52*:1931–1936, 1973.

77. Huntley, C.C., Thorpe, D.P., Lyerly, A.D., and Kelsey, W.M.: Rheumatoid arthritis with IgA deficiency. Am. J. Dis. Child., *113*:411–418, 1967.

78. Bachmann, R., Laurell, C.B., and Svenouius, E.: Studies on the serum γ1A-globulin level. Scand. J. Clin. Lab. Invest., *17*:46–50, 1965.

79. Hobbs, J.R.: Immune imbalance in dysgammaglobulinemia type IV. Lancet, *1*:110–114, 1968.

80. Claman, H.N., Merrill, D.A., Peakman, D., and Robinson, A.: Isolated severe gamma A deficiency: Immunoglobulin levels, clinical disorders, and chromosome studies. J. Lab. Clin. Med., *75*:307–315, 1970.

81. Gajl-Peczalska, K.J., Park, B.M., Biggar, W.D., and Good, R.A.: B and T lymphocytes in primary immunodeficiency disease in man. J. Clin. Invest., *52*:919–928, 1973.

82. Waldenström, J.: Clinical methods for determination of hyperproteinemia and their practical value for diagnosis. Nord. Med., *20*:2288–2295, 1943.

83. Rogers, W.R., and Welch, J.D.: Purpura hyperglobulinemia terminating in multiple myeloma. Arch. Intern. Med., *100*:478–483, 1957.

84. Savin, R.C.: Hyperglobulinemic purpura terminating in myeloma, hyperlipemia, and xanthomatosis. Arch. Dermatol., *92*:679–686, 1965.

85. Strauss, W.G.: Purpura hyperglobulinemia of Waldenström. N. Engl. J. Med., *260*:857–860, 1959.

86. Capra, J.D., Winchester, R.J., and Kunkel, H.G.: Hypergammaglobulinemic purpura. Medicine, *50*:125–138, 1971.

87. Roberts-Thomson, P.J., and Kemp, A.S.: IgA and temperature

dependent IgG complex formation in a patient with Waldenström's hypergammaglobulinaemic purpura. Clin. Exp. Immunol., 39:164–169, 1980.

88. Brouet, J.C., et al.: Biologic and clinical significance of cryoglobulins. Am. J. Med., 57:775–788, 1974.

89. Weisman, M., and Zvaifler, N.: Cryoimmunoglobulinemia in rheumatoid arthritis. J. Clin. Invest., 56:725–739, 1975.

90. Cream, J.J.: Clinical and immunological aspects of cutaneous vasculitis. Q. J. Med., 45:255–276, 1976.

91. Meltzer, M., et al.: Cryoglobulinemia—A clinical and laboratory study. Am. J. Med., 40:837–856, 1966.

92. Gorevic, P.D., et al.: Mixed cryoglobulinemia: Clinical aspects and long-term follow-up of 40 patients. Am. J. Med., 69:287–308, 1980.

93. Waldmann, T.A., Johnson, J.S., and Talal, N.: Hypogammaglobulinemia associated with accelerated catabolism of IgG secondary to its interaction with an IgG-reactive monoclonal IgM. J. Clin. Invest., 50:951–958, 1971.

94. Ristow, S.C., Griner, P.F., Abraham, G.N., and Shoulson, I.: Reversal of systemic manifestations of cryoglobulinemia. Arch. Intern. Med., 136:467–470, 1976.

95. Isomaki, H.A., Hakulinen, T., and Joutsenlahti, U.: Excess risk of lymphomas, leukemia and myeloma in patients with rheumatoid arthritis. J. Chronic Dis., 31:691–696, 1978.

96. Agudelo, C.A., et al.: Non-Hodgkin's lymphoma in systemic lupus erythematosus. J. Rheumatol., 8:69–78, 1981.

97. Cammarata, R.J., Rodman, G.P., and Jensen, W.N.: Systemic rheumatic disease and malignant lymphoma. Arch. Intern. Med., 111:330–337, 1963.

98. Canoso, J.J., and Cohen, A.S.: Malignancy in a series of 70 patients with systemic lupus erythematosus. Arthritis Rheum., 17:383–388, 1974.

99. Miller, D.G.: The association of immune disease and malignant lymphoma. Ann. Intern. Med., 66:507–521, 1967.

100. Smith, C.K., Cassidy, J.T., and Bole, G.G.: Type 1 dysgammaglobulinemia, systemic lupus erythematosus and lymphoma. Am. J. Med., 48:113–119, 1970.

101. Zawadzki, Z.A., and Benedek, T.G.: Rheumatoid arthritis, dysproteinemic arthropathy, and paraproteinemia. Arthritis Rheum., 12:555–568, 1969.

102. Calabro, J.J.: Cancer and arthritis. Arthritis Rheum., 10:553–567, 1967.

103. Goldberg, A., Brodsky, I., and McCarty, D.: Multiple myeloma with paramyloidosis presenting as rheumatoid disease. Am. J. Med., 37:653–658, 1964.

RHEUMATIC FEVER

ANGELO TARANTA

Once the most common cause of acute polyarthritis, rheumatic fever has become a rarity in the West,[1] and physicians may complete their training without having seen a single case. From recent evidence, however, the disease may be staging a comeback.[2]

HISTORY AND GEOGRAPHY

The description of rheumatic fever as a syndrome resulted from the integration of manifestations originally described independently and thought to be unrelated, that is, *acute articular rheumatism, valvular heart disease*, and *chorea* (Fig. 77–1), to which were then added *subcutaneous nodules* and *erythema marginatum*.[3] Later, a number of entities were recognized as mimics of rheumatic fever or of rheumatic heart disease and were identified separately as viral carditis, Yersinia arthritis, and mitral valve prolapse, among others.[4]

While these conceptual changes occurred, the incidence of the disease also changed. Although records from the past are poor and details are lacking, the incidence of rheumatic fever seems to have increased with industrialization and urbanization and then decreased with the consequent affluence, a process completed in the postindustrial West and still ongoing in the developing countries.[4,5]

Availability of penicillin and improvement in the standard of living (especially a decrease of crowding in the home) have been credited for the decrease of rheumatic fever in this century; yet the most striking decline may have occurred during the 1970s, when our standard of living did not improve and our use of penicillin did not increase. The strep seems to outsmart us.

PATHOLOGY AND IMMUNOPATHOLOGY

In patients dying of acute rheumatic fever, pancarditis is usually present. Tiny translucent nodules, or verrucae, form on the edge of the valves, which can no longer close properly; the valves are "regurgitant" or "incompetent." The myocardium is pale, flabby, edematous, and mildly hypertrophic; the heart chambers are dilated. Fibrin and serosanguineous fluid may be present in the pericardial cavity.

Microscopically, diffuse degeneration and swelling of muscle fibers may be apparent, along with fibrinoid degeneration of collagen. Perivascular foci of degeneration or necrosis may be surrounded by clusters of large mononuclear and giant multinuclear cells,[6] largely of monocyte or macrophage lineage.[7] These clusters, known as *Aschoff bodies*, or nodules, are considered specific for *acute* rheumatic fever, but they may persist long after any other evidence of active disease. Immunofluorescent study reveals immunoglobulins and complement in cardiac myofibers, vessel walls,[8] and pericardium.[9] Valvular lymphoid infiltrates contain a predominance of T cells.[10]

In the joints, a sterile exudate may be found that is deficient in complement components with respect to simultaneously determined serum levels;[11] there is

Acute articular rheumatism

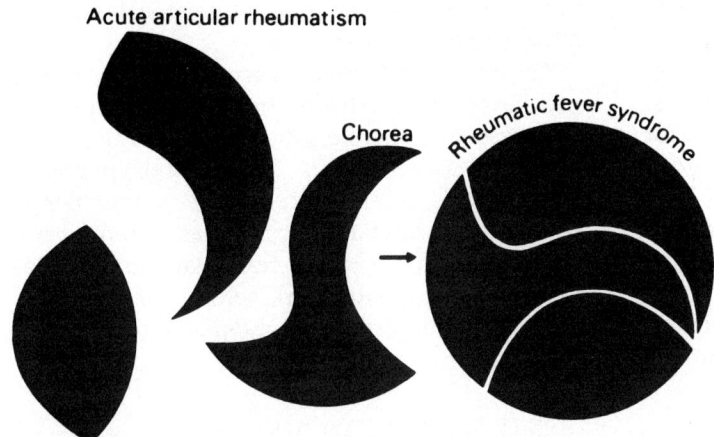

Chorea

Rheumatic fever syndrome

Heart valve deformities

FIG. 77–1. Historical development of the concept of rheumatic fever syndrome from the integration of disease manifestations previously described independently of each other. (From Taranta, A., and Markowitiz, M.[5])

no synovial hypertrophy, no bony erosion, and no cartilage loss.

Chorea affects the basal ganglia, as one would expect from the symptoms, but also, diffusely, other parts of the brain. *Subcutaneous nodules* resemble recently formed rheumatoid nodules; both consist of a central area of necrosis surrounded by parallel rows of elongated fibroblasts, as in a palisade ("palisading" fibroblasts), surrounded by loose connective tissue.[12]

INCIDENCE AND CAUSE

Like the infections that lead to it, rheumatic fever affects mostly children of 5 to 15 years of age but also is seen in young adults. In the early 1980s, its incidence in various locales in the United States was reported to be as low as 0.23 to 1.88/100,000/year among children and adolescents, but a recent report from Utah has called attention to an incidence of 18.10/100,000/year in the same age group.[2]

Sore throats accompanied by scarlatiniform rash, that is, scarlet fever, have long been known to precede some attacks of rheumatic fever. In the remainder of the patients, rheumatic fever is preceded by a sore throat without rash or by a pharyngitis without soreness of the throat, recognizable as a streptococcal infection only by antibody tests.

If streptococcal pharyngitis is treated and the organisms eradicated from the throat, rheumatic fever fails to appear;[13] if patients who have had previous attacks of rheumatic fever receive continual antistreptococcal prophylaxis, the disease does not recur.[14] In either case, the few failures to prevent rheumatic fever, whether initial attacks or recurrences, can be traced to failures to achieve the aims of prophylaxis, which are to eradicate the streptococci from the throat in the case of initial attacks, and to prevent strepto-

cocci from initiating infections in the case of recurrences.

More than 40 years ago, Kuttner and Krumwiede[15] reported that an epidemic of type 4 streptococcal pharyngitis among children convalescing from rheumatic fever failed, surprisingly, to reactivate the disease. Recently, Stollerman and co-workers have marshalled new evidence suggesting the existence of "rheumatogenic" and "nonrheumatogenic" streptococcal types;[16] and the observation that rheumatic fever seems to be coming back in some parts of the country without a concomitant increase of streptococcal infections could be explained by a shift to "rheumatogenic" streptococcal types or strains.[2]

The well-known correlation of rheumatic fever with poverty seems to be mediated mainly by crowding: the larger the number of persons per room, the higher the prevalence of rheumatic heart disease.[17] Crowding leads to multiple close contact, which facilitates streptococcal contagion and seems to favor the selection of more virulent strains. In the 1979 edition of this book, I called attention to the shrinking of family living space in this country and wondered whether it would affect rheumatic fever incidence. In the recent epidemic of rheumatic fever in Utah, the patients were not poor, but the patients' family size was double that of the average family in Utah as a whole, and the majority of patients shared bedrooms with other family members.[2]

Although all attacks of rheumatic fever follow a streptococcal infection, only a few streptococcal infections are followed by rheumatic fever, and the reason remains elusive. The severity of the infection may be a factor; although rheumatic fever follows 3% of severe infections (i.e., those accompanied by fever, exudate, swollen and tender cervical lymph nodes, persistence of positive streptococcal throat cultures, and subsequent antistreptolysin O response),[18] only

0.3 to 0.1%, or even fewer, of the less severe infections lead to rheumatic fever.[19] Still, only 3% at the most develop rheumatic fever. What accounts for the absence of rheumatic fever in the remaining 97%? Host factors may be important, as the concordance rate for rheumatic fever is seven times higher in monozygotic (18.7%) than dizygotic twin pairs (2.5%).[20] HLA type I antigens seem to have no reproducible relationship to susceptibility to rheumatic fever, but among type II antigens, HLA-DR4 may be associated with the disease among whites.[21] Moreover, certain B-cell alloantigens have been reported in the majority of rheumatic patients and in the minority of controls.[22]

PATHOGENESIS

Little is known about the chain of events that links streptococcal infections in the throat to the manifestations, distant is space and subsequent in time, of rheumatic fever. The streptococci do not migrate from the throat to the joints or to the heart, which are demonstrably sterile, but their products diffuse. Some of them are cardiotoxic in experimental animals and could be the mediators of tissue damage in rheumatic fever, but an indirect or immune pathogenesis is considered more likely.[23]

Several streptococcal antigens cross-react immunologically with human tissue antigens. As a result, the immune response to streptococci may be blunted because their antigens may be erroneously recognized as "self" by the lymphocytes, and whatever response is elicited may boomerang, in part, on the host because the host's antigens may be mistaken as foreign. The latter "mistake," which is called autoimmunity, may be the mechanism of tissue damage in rheumatic fever, especially in rheumatic carditis, as the well-studied cross-reaction of streptococcal antigens with heart antigens suggest.[23] Circulating immune complexes may also play a role.[24]

Considering the variety of manifestations of the rheumatic fever syndrome, some fleeting, others chronic, some exudative, others proliferative, it would not be surprising if more than one pathogenetic mechanism were at work.

CLINICAL FINDINGS

The natural history of rheumatic fever may be said to start with the streptococcal pharyngitis that precedes it by an interval ("latent period") of 2 to 3 weeks (mean 18.6 days). The latent period of rheumatic fever is a little longer than that of poststreptococcal glo-

merulonephritis, and is of the same length in first attacks and in recurrences.[25]

The onset of the attack is acute when the presenting manifestation is arthritis but usually gradual when the presenting manifestation is carditis alone, and the symptom is heart failure. The onset of chorea may be acute but is often preceded by subtle behavioral changes that can be interpreted as a manifestation of chorea only in retrospect. Subcutaneous nodules and erythema marginatum are seldom, if ever, the presenting manifestations of rheumatic fever.

JOINT INVOLVEMENT

In the classic, untreated case, the arthritis of rheumatic fever affects several joints in quick succession, each for a short time (Fig. 77–2). The arthritis predilects large joints and often affects the lower limbs at first and later spreads to the arms.

Joint involvement is more common, and also more severe, in young adults (nearly 100% in first attacks)[26] than in teenagers (82%) and in children (66%).[27] Rheumatic polyarthritis may be excruciatingly painful, but it is always transient. The arthritis is characteristically acute, almost like in gout, reaching its maximum intensity within a day or two in any given joint. The *pain* is usually more prominent than the objective signs of inflammation. Patients' joints are often painful, tender, and limited in motion because of pain, yet have little swelling, redness, or heat. Conversely,

FIG. 77–2. Time course of the migratory polyarthritis of rheumatic fever. Notice that even in the absence of treatment, the involvement of each joint is short-lived, but the cumulative involvement of all joints is less so. Note also that arthritis rapidly responds to aspirin.

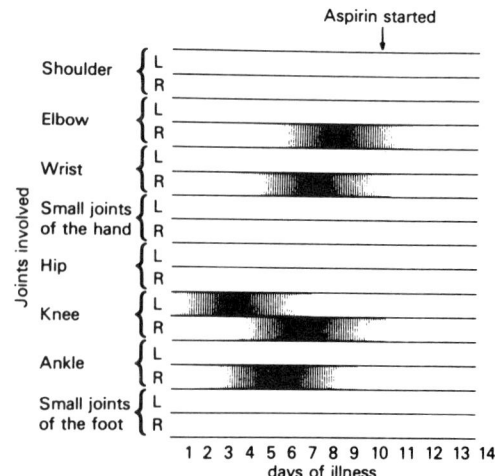

joints seldom are definitely swollen and only slightly tender.

When the disease is allowed to express itself fully, unchecked by anti-inflammatory treatment, the number of affected joints may be as high as 16, and about half of these patients develop arthritis in more than 6 joints. Each joint is maximally inflamed for only a few days, or a week at the most, when the inflammation decreases. Milder and decreasing inflammation may linger for another week or so before disappearing completely. Considering all joints, the polyarthritis may be severe for a week in two thirds of the patients, and for 2 or at the most 3 weeks in the others, and may then persist in a mild form for another week or 2.[28] Radiologic examination shows only effusion.

Under the usual circumstances of medical practice, however, many patients with joint complaints are treated empirically and prematurely with aspirin or other anti-inflammatory drugs; "migration" of the arthritis is then stopped, or the arthralgia is prevented from blooming into arthritis, depriving the clinician of useful data and the patient of a firm diagnosis. Conversely, administration of aspirin just a few days later, after the disease has declared itself, may further confirm the diagnosis of rheumatic fever by a characteristically rapid and complete therapeutic response.

Some patients may have only the subjective manifestations of joint involvement, such as arthralgia or polyarthralgia, which are very nonspecific. More often, objective evidence is present but not detected, hence the quip, "An arthralgia is an arthritis without a good physical examination."

CARDITIS

Rheumatic carditis is the most important manifestation of acute rheumatic fever, because it may lead to chronic rheumatic heart disease and even to death from heart failure during the acute attack. More commonly, however, carditis causes no symptoms, only signs, and is diagnosed by auscultation when a patient is examined because of arthritis or chorea.

Criteria for the clinical diagnosis of rheumatic carditis include organic heart murmur(s) not previously present, enlargement of the heart, congestive heart failure, and pericardial friction rubs or signs of effusion, but significant murmurs are almost always present. In some patients, Doppler echocardiography may detect a valvular lesion that cannot be picked up by auscultation.[2] Patients whose rheumatic illness consists only of asymptomatic carditis may later develop chronic rheumatic heart disease, despite the absence of a medical history of recognized rheumatic fever.

The incidence of carditis in rheumatic fever varies with age, but in a direction opposite to that of arthritis; it is present in 90 to 92% of children under the age of 3 years,[29] in 50% of children aged 3 to 6 years, in 32% of teenagers aged 14 to 17,[27] but in only 15% of adults with a first attack of rheumatic fever.[26] In addition to being less frequent, carditis is less severe in adults than in children. The mitral valve is the most common site of involvement; a high-pitched, usually loud, long, blowing apical systolic murmur indicates *mitral regurgitation*. Functional or innocent systolic murmurs may be mistaken for it, especially when their loudness is increased by fever or anemia. Unlike the murmur of mitral regurgitation, however, most functional systolic murmurs are heard best along the left sternal border, in the third to second interspace or at the lower left sternal border. The functional systolic murmurs are limited to the first two thirds of systole and usually have a midsystolic accentuation. Their pitch is generally low, and they lack the "blowing" or "steam-jet" quality of mitral regurgitation murmurs. Some functional murmurs have a "groaning" or "twanging-string" quality; they are often heard best along the lower left sternal margin or between it and the apex. Depending on its loudness, the murmur of mitral regurgitation may persist after the acute rheumatic episodes, or it may disappear.

A mid-diastolic or Carey-Coombs murmur, usually following a third heart sound, is common in patients with rheumatic fever and acute mitral regurgitation. This murmur does not indicate mitral stenosis and disappears after the edema of the leaflets subsides. Physiologic third heart sounds may be mistaken for mid-diastolic murmurs. Differentiation of the two rests mainly on the perceptible duration of the latter.

The second most common valvular lesion during acute rheumatic fever is *aortic regurgitation*. This disorder produces a high-pitched decrescendo diastolic murmur that begins immediately after the second heart sound; it may be short and faint and therefore difficult to hear.[30]

Pericarditis can be detected clinically in up to 10% of patients with acute rheumatic fever. Pericardial effusion is occasionally striking, but cardiac tamponade is rare.

Congestive failure is the most serious manifestation of rheumatic carditis. Usually, it develops in patients with severe involvement of more than one valve. It occurs in 5 to 10% of first episodes of rheumatic carditis and is more frequent during recurrences. The diagnosis is established by careful physical examination, history taking, and review of chest roentgenograms.

ELECTROCARDIOGRAPHIC FINDINGS

Prolongation of the PR interval occurs in 28 to 40% of patients with rheumatic fever, much more frequently than in other febrile illnesses,[31] and therefore is useful in diagnosis. This prolongation does not correlate with residual heart disease,[32] however, and is not useful in prognosis.

CHOREA

Sydenham's chorea, chorea minor, or "St. Vitus' dance" is a neurologic disorder consisting of involuntary movements, muscular weakness, and emotional lability. The movements are abrupt and purposeless, not rhythmic or repetitive. They disappear during sleep but may occur at rest and may interfere with voluntary activity. The movements can be suppressed by the will of the patient, for a while. They may affect all voluntary muscles, but the involvement of the hands and face is usually the most obvious. Grimaces and inappropriate smiles are common (Fig. 77–3). Handwriting usually becomes clumsy and provides a convenient way of following the patient's course. Speech is often slurred. The movements are commonly more marked on one side and occasionally are completely unilateral (hemichorea).

The muscular weakness is best revealed by asking the patient to squeeze the examiner's hands. The examiner feels that the pressure of the patient's grip increases and decreases continually and capriciously—the relapsing grip, or "milking" sign.

The emotional changes manifest themselves in outbursts of inappropriate behavior, crying, and restlessness. There are no sensory losses or pyramidal tract involvement. In doubtful cases the choreic movements can be elicited by asking patients to stretch their hands in front of them, to stretch their fingers out, to close their eyes, and to stick their tongues out, one movement added to the other. By the time patients stick out their tongues, their fingers wiggle and their eyelids flutter. When the arms are projected straight forward, one sees flexion of the wrist, hyperextension of the metacarpophalangeal (MCP) joints, straightening of the fingers, and abduction of the thumb ("spooning" or "dishing" of the hands). When patients are asked to raise their arms above their heads, they also pronate one or both hands (pronator sign).

Chorea may follow streptococcal infections after a longer latent period than that of other rheumatic manifestations. Some patients with chorea never develop other rheumatic symptoms, but other patients develop chorea weeks or months after arthritis[33] (Fig. 77–4). In either case, examination of the heart may reveal organic murmurs.

The incidence of chorea among rheumatic attacks has varied widely and seemed to be decreasing, but in the recent Utah epidemic, it was 31%.[2] Chorea is rare after puberty, and does not occur in adults, with the exception of rare cases during pregnancy ("chorea gravidarum"). Finally, it is the only manifestation with a marked sex predilection. Chorea is twice as frequent in girls as in boys; after puberty, this sex predilection increases.[34]

SUBCUTANEOUS NODULES

The subcutaneous nodules of rheumatic fever are firm and painless. The overlying skin is not inflamed and can usually be moved over the nodules. The diameter of these roundish lesions varies from a few millimeters to 1 or even 2 cm. They are located over bony surfaces or prominences or near tendons; their number varies from a single nodule to a few dozen and average three or four; when numerous, they are usually symmetric. These nodules are present for 1 or more weeks, rarely for more than a month. They are smaller and shorter lived than the nodules of rheumatoid arthritis (RA). Rheumatic subcutaneous nodules generally appear only after the first few weeks of illness, usually *only* in patients with carditis.[35] The frequency of their appearance, or rather of their detection, varies widely (from 34%[36] to 1%[27]). Rheumatic nodules are very rare in adults.

ERYTHEMA MARGINATUM

Erythema marginatum is an evanescent, nonpruritic, pink skin rash, which appears on the trunk and sometimes the proximal parts of the limbs, but not on the face. It is made up of a variable number of individual skin lesions, starting as erythematous spots that may be slightly raised. Each lesion extends centrifugally, while the skin in the center gradually returns to normal; hence the name *erythema marginatum*. The outer edge of the lesion is sharp, whereas the inner edge is soft[37] (Fig. 77–5).

The individual lesions may appear and disappear in a matter of hours, usually to return. They may change in shape and size almost as fast as smoke rings, which they resemble both in shape and in the

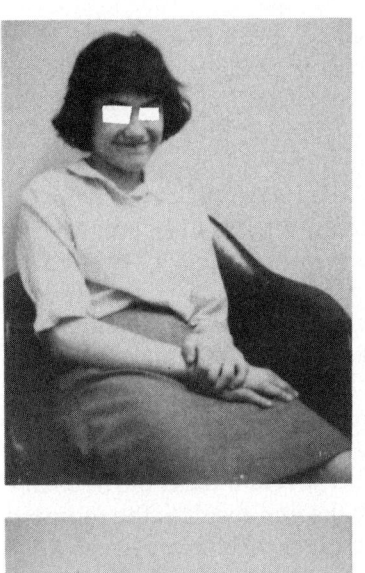
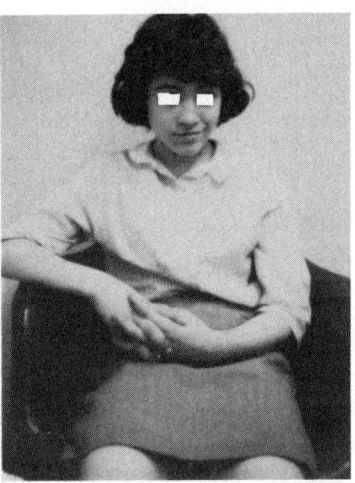

FIG. 77–3.   Grimaces and inappropriate smiles in a patient with chorea.

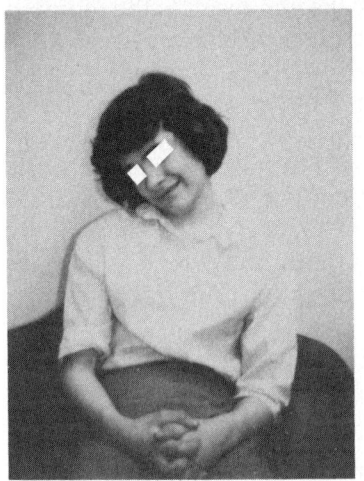
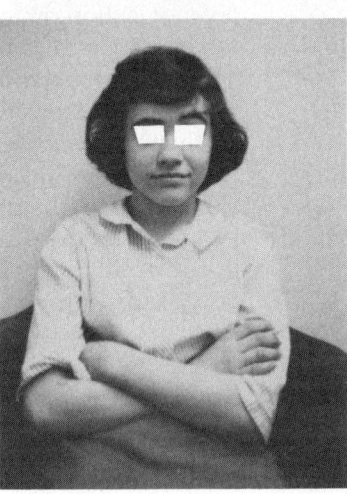

FIG. 77–4.   Chorea appearing 4 months after the onset of polyarthritis and carditis. Intercurrent streptococcal infections were ruled out by the falling titers of three streptococcal antibodies. (From Taranta, A., and Stollerman, G.H.[33])

FIG. 77–5.   Erythema marginatum.

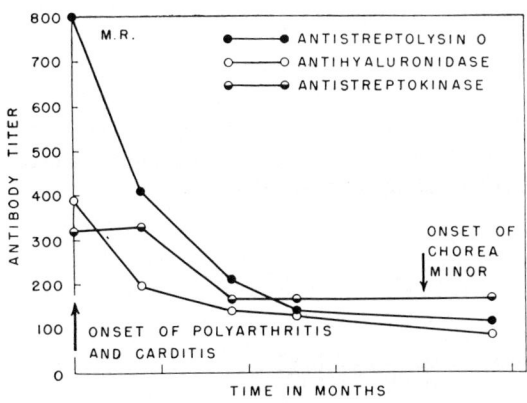

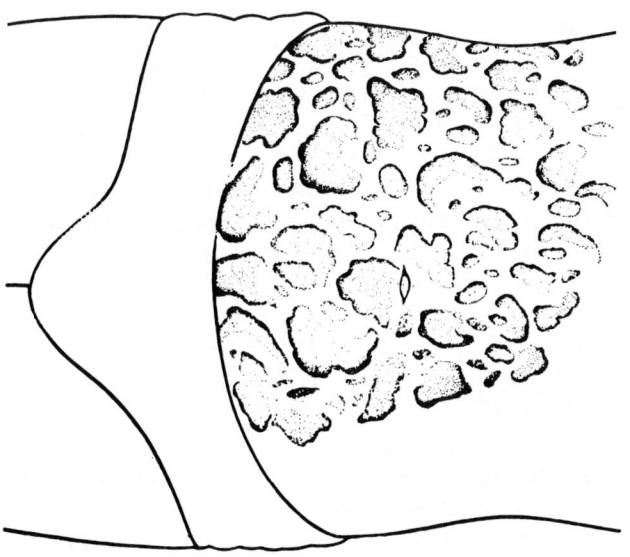

centrifugal manner in which they expand and dissolve. The lesions may coalesce while expanding and may thus acquire a circinate, gyrate, or festooned pattern. A hot bath or shower may make them more evident or may even reveal them for the first time. Erythema marginatum, like nodules, occurs *only* in patients with carditis[35] and has been reported from 13%[38] to 2%[39] of patients with rheumatic fever. Erythema marginatum is very rare in adults.

OTHER MANIFESTATIONS

Fever is regularly present in rheumatic fever with arthritis; it is often present in isolated carditis, but seldom in isolated chorea. It is a remittent type of fever (unlike the wide swings of juvenile rheumatoid arthritis) that usually does not exceed 104°F and returns to normal in 2 to 3 weeks even without treatment.[40]

Anorexia, nausea, and vomiting may occur, mostly as manifestations of congestive heart failure or salicylate intoxication. Epistaxis seems to have been frequent once, but is not common now.

DURATION OF THE ATTACK AND SEQUELAE

An episode of rheumatic fever is customarily considered to end when the patient's erythrocyte sedimentation rate returns to normal, usually several weeks after the subsidence of arthritis. By this criterion, the duration of the episode is 109 ± 57 days,[27] less than 12 weeks in 80% of cases and less than 15 weeks in 90%.[35] A few patients develop chronic rheumatic activity.[41]

Sequelae involve primarily the heart and depend on the occurrence and on the severity of carditis during the acute attack. In addition, patients who have had rheumatic fever develop it again after streptococcal infections with an attack rate much higher than in the general population (see following discussion). This propensity can also be considered a sequela.

JACCOUD'S ARTHRITIS (OR ARTHROPATHY OR SYNDROME) (see also Chapter 43)

Jaccoud's arthritis is also called, more descriptively, *chronic postrheumatic fever arthropathy*. It is a rare, indolent, slowly progressive process that deforms the fingers and sometimes the toes.[42–46] The deformity

consists of ulnar deviation of the fingers, flexion of the MCP joints, and hyperextension of the proximal interphalangeal joints, just as in RA, but without the joint pains, heat, and swelling of the latter. The ulnar deviation occurs mostly in the fourth and fifth digits and is at first correctable, but later may become fixed. The toes may be affected similarly. Although no true erosions are present, notches or "hooks," thought to be due to the mechanical effect of ulnar deviation, are sometimes seen in roentgenograms on the ulnar side of each metacarpal head ("Bywater's hooks"). Rheumatoid factor (RF) is absent; the erythrocyte sedimentation rate is normal.

In classic cases, Jaccoud's arthropathy appears after multiple, prolonged, and severe attacks of rheumatic fever. It is thought to be the end result of the repeated inflammation of the fibrous articular capsules in the small joints of the hand, perhaps depending on individual predisposition. Patients with systemic lupus erythematosus (SLE) may develop a similar arthropathy,[47,48] and some patients develop it without having either SLE or rheumatic fever.[49,50] The prognosis of Jaccoud's arthropathy is good. Patients, alarmed by the deformity, may fear that it will extend to joints in other parts of the body, but this does not happen.

RECURRENCES

The attack rates of rheumatic fever after streptococcal pharyngitis are much higher in patients who have already had a previous attack than in those who have not. The recurrence rate per infection is highest in the first year after the rheumatic attack. The rate decreases sharply in the following 2 years, and then seems to level off[51] (Fig. 77–6).

Rheumatic fever recurs only among patients who

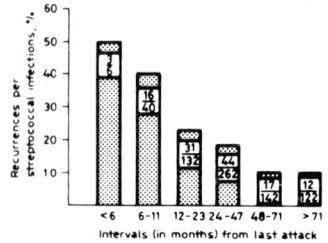

FIG. 77–6. Decrease of the rheumatic fever recurrence rate per infection with time lapsed since the latest rheumatic episode. (From Spagnuolo, M., et al.[51])

Table 77–1. Ratio of Rheumatic Fever Recurrences to Streptococcal Infections in Patients Stratified for Pre-Existing Rheumatic Heart Disease and for Rise in Antistreptolysin O (ASO)

ASO Rise in Number of Tube Dilutions	Pre-existing Heart Disease (%)	No Pre-existing Heart Disease (%)
0–1	3:24 (13)	1:79 (1)
2	10:38 (26)	3:50 (6)
3	6:16 (38)	5:34 (15)
4 +	9:16 (56)	9:26 (35)

(Data from Taranta, A., et al.[52])

develop a streptococcal antibody response, and the recurrence rate per infection increases with the magnitude of the antibody rise. At each level of antibody response, streptococcal infections are more likely to lead to recurrences of rheumatic fever in patients with pre-existing rheumatic fever attacks but without heart disease (Table 77–1).

The same clinical manifestations present in the initial episode of rheumatic fever tend to reappear in recurrences[53] (Table 77–2). Conversely, manifestations absent in the first episodes are usually absent in recurrent attacks. This is especially important in the case of the most serious manifestation, carditis.[54] Speculations on the reason(s) for this "mimetic" pattern are discussed elsewhere.[55]

In apparent contradiction to this pattern, the prevalence of heart disease increases with the number of previous episodes of rheumatic fever. Most likely, this finding is due to the increased tendency of patients with heart disease to develop recurrences,[52] rather than to the development of heart disease anew in patients originally free of it.

MORTALITY RATE

Of the many deaths ultimately caused by rheumatic fever, only a minority occur during an acute episode, and even fewer occur during the initial attack. Case-fatality rates of 0.36%,[27] 0.6%,[38] and 1.6%[35] have been reported in first episodes and rates of 2.3%[38] and 3%[27] in recurrences. None died among the 74 patients of the recent Utah epidemic.[2]

LABORATORY FINDINGS

EVIDENCE OF RECENT STREPTOCOCCAL INFECTION

Eighty percent of patients with acute rheumatic fever observed early in their course have elevated antistreptolysin O titers. The remaining 20% have elevation of one or more of the other streptococcal antibodies tested, such as antistreptokinase, anti-hyaluronidase, antideoxyribonuclease B, and antinicotinamide-adenine dinucleotidase.[56,57] All these antibody tests are based on the principle of inhibition of a specific toxic or enzymatic activity of streptococcal culture filtrate.

A simple, rapid test based on a different principle, the agglutination of sheep red blood cells coated with a mixture of streptococcal antigens, is commercially available (Streptozyme). It is more sensitive than any other single streptococcal antibody tests, simpler, and it takes only a few minutes to perform. In small series, it was positive at a dilution of 1:200 in 100% of rheumatic fever cases,[58] but there have been problems with its reproducibility.

NONSPECIFIC LABORATORY MANIFESTATIONS

Nonspecific laboratory manifestations include an elevated erythrocyte sedimentation rate, positive tests for C-reactive protein, moderate leukocytosis, and anemia. With the exception of "pure" or isolated chorea, untreated rheumatic fever is consistently accompanied by an elevated erythrocyte sedimentation rate and an elevated serum C-reactive protein.

OTHER LABORATORY ABNORMALITIES

Synovial fluid examination is useful to exclude other processes, especially septic arthritis. Synovial leukocyte counts vary (from 600 to 80,000/mm, with a mean of 16,000,[26] from 2,600 to 96,000/mm, with a

Table 77–2. Major Clinical Manifestations of Rheumatic Fever Recurrences According to Manifestations of the First Episode

Initial Manifestations (Isolated or Combined With Others)	Manifestations of Recurrences (Isolated or Combined With Others)		
	Polyarthritis No. (%)	Carditis No. (%)	Chorea No. (%)
Polyarthritis (N = 149)	110 (74)	51 (34)	18 (12)
Carditis (N = 89)	44 (49)	62 (70)	2 (2)
Chorea (N = 68)	11 (16)	10 (15)	54 (79)

(Data from Roth, I.R., Lingg, C., and Whittemore, A.[53])

mean of 29,000),[11] and polymorphonuclear leukocytes predominate (73 to 100%, with a mean of 90%,[26] 56 to 95%, with a mean of 83%).[11] The levels of C3, C4, and C1q are decreased with respect to simultaneously determined serum levels.[11] Interestingly, the viscosity of the fluid is high and gives a good mucin clot on addition of acetic acid.

Heart antibodies are demonstrable by a variety of techniques in the serum of patients with rheumatic fever but they are also found in serum of patients with uncomplicated streptococcal infections or with acute glomerulonephritis, although usually at a lower titer.[23]

Subclinical liver involvement, manifested by transient enzyme elevations, has long been known to occur in rheumatic fever patients treated with aspirin,[59] but it may also occur without therapy.[26]

DIAGNOSIS

No single manifestation is so characteristic as to be diagnostic; the greater the number of clearly recognized manifestations, the firmer the diagnosis. The most common presentation, but also the least specific, is *arthritis without carditis*. There is no diagnostic laboratory test.

Because the prognosis varies according to the manifestations of the acute attack, the diagnosis of rheumatic fever should be qualified by mention of the manifestations diagnosed, such as "rheumatic fever with polyarthritis only."

JONES CRITERIA

T.D. Jones divided the manifestations of rheumatic fever into "major" and "minor" according to their diagnostic usefulness (Table 77–3) and proposed that the presence of two major or of one major and two minor manifestations indicates a high probability of rheumatic fever. These criteria have been widely accepted and have proved useful, especially in preventing overdiagnosis.[60]

DIFFERENTIAL DIAGNOSIS

The differential diagnosis varies according to the presenting manifestations(s). It is always prudent to exclude bacteremia by blood cultures; polyarthralgia and polyarthritis, as well as heart murmurs, are frequent manifestations of infective endocarditis.[61] Disseminated gonococcal infection is a frequent cause of acute, often migratory polyarthralgia and polyarthritis in adolescents and adults. Polyarthralgia and polyarthritis occur in preicteric and anicteric viral hepatitis, which can be recognized by a high serum glutamic-oxaloacetic transaminase level, positive tests for hepatitis B surface antigen, and sometimes an accompanying urticarial rash and low serum complement.[62] RA of acute onset does not respond to aspirin as readily as does rheumatic fever; in its juvenile form, RA is often accompanied by high antistreptolysin O titers, which increase diagnostic confusion,[63] and RF tests are usually negative. The arthritis is persistent, however, and prolonged observation yields the diagnosis. Antinuclear antibody (ANA) tests, regularly positive in patients with SLE, are negative in patients with rheumatic fever, and the clinical pictures usually differ. Particularly troublesome may be the differentiation from a serum-sickness type of reaction, with fever and polyarthritis, which may occur after administration of penicillin for pharyngitis; urticaria or angioneurotic edema, if present, may help in the diagnosis.

Table 77–3. Jones Criteria (Revised) for Guidance in the Diagnosis of Rheumatic Fever

Major Manifestations	Minor Manifestations
Carditis	Clinical
Polyarthritis	Fever
Chorea	Arthralgia
Erythema marginatum	Previous rheumatic fever or rheumatic heart disease
Subcutaneous nodules	Laboratory
	Erythrocyte sedimentation rate, C-reactive protein, leukocytosis
	Prolonged P-R interval

PLUS

Supporting evidence of preceding streptococcal infection such as increased antistreptolysin O or other streptococcal antibodies; positive throat culture for group A streptococci; or recent scarlet fever.

The presence of two major criteria, or of one major and two minor criteria, indicates the probable presence of rheumatic fever if supported by evidence of a preceding streptococcal infection. The absence of the latter should make the diagnosis suspect, except when rheumatic fever is first discovered after a long latent period from the antecedent infection, as in Sydenham's chorea or low-grade carditis.

(Courtesy of the American Heart Association.)

Polyarthritis may follow a number of viral infections, especially rubella, as well as rubella vaccination.[64]

Isolated rheumatic carditis may be difficult to distinguish from viral carditis, with which it has many features in common, such as pericarditis, cardiomegaly, heart failure, and even heart murmurs.[65] In dubious cases, one should attempt viral isolation from stools and pharyngeal washings and look for an appropriate antibody response, which may help at least in a retrospective diagnosis. Left atrial myxoma may also mimic isolated rheumatic carditis.[66]

Chorea must be differentiated from tics, which are repetitive, stereotyped, localized movements, and from benign familial chorea, a rare disorder transmitted as an autosomal dominant trait and beginning in childhood.[67]

Subcutaneous nodules must sometimes be differentiated from enlarged lymph nodes, especially in rubella. Rarely, nodules clinically and histologically indistinguishable from rheumatic or rheumatoid nodules occur in an isolated fashion and are benign.[68] Erythema marginatum must sometimes be differentiated from cutis marmorata, a fixed, reticular, bluish discoloration of the skin. An evanescent rash resembling erythema marginatum has been reported in Lyme arthritis.

In Scandinavian countries, infections with Yersinia enterocolitica have been associated with acute polyarthritis, carditis, and abdominal pains, all of which may cause diagnostic confusion.[69] Febrile diarrhea, frequent in Yersinia infections, may help in the differentiation.

In doubtful cases, and maybe in all cases of acute polyarthritis in Scandinavia, the agglutination test for Yersinia should be performed.

Among blacks, another cause of diagnostic confusion is sickle cell anemia, which may mimic rheumatic fever because of heart murmurs and arthralgias but may also coexist with it.[70]

TREATMENT

GENERAL MEASURES AND BED REST

All patients with rheumatic fever should be examined daily for the first 2 weeks of the illness, primarily to watch for the development of carditis and to start treatment promptly should heart failure occur. Patients should be kept comfortable, and rest generally helps, but strict and prolonged bed rest, once the rule, appears useless.

ANALGESICS OR ANTI-INFLAMMATORY AGENTS

Patients with arthralgia alone or with mild arthritis and no carditis may be given analgesics only. This is particularly wise when the diagnosis is not definite. Patients with moderate or severe arthritis but no carditis, or with carditis but no cardiomegaly or fever, are treated with aspirin, 40 mg/lb/day for the first 2 weeks and 20 mg/lb/day for the following 4 to 6 weeks. Larger doses may be necessary to control arthritis. In patients with carditis and cardiomegaly but without congestive failure, with or without polyarthritis, treatment should be started with aspirin. In patients with marked cardiomegaly, aspirin is often insufficient to control fever, discomfort, and tachycardia, or it does so only at toxic or near-toxic doses. These patients may then be treated with corticosteroids.

Patients with carditis and heart failure, with or without polyarthritis, should receive corticosteroids, starting with a dose of prednisone, 40 to 60 mg/day, to be increased if heart failure is not controlled. In cases of extreme acuteness and severity, therapy should be started by intravenous administration of methylprednisolone, 10 to 40 mg, followed by oral prednisone. In 2 to 3 weeks, prednisone may be slowly withdrawn; one should decrease the daily dose at the rate of 5 mg every 2 to 3 days. When the dose is tapered, aspirin at standard doses may be added and continued for 3 to 4 weeks after prednisone is discontinued. This "overlap" therapy reduces the incidence of post-therapeutic clinical rebounds.

The termination of anti-inflammatory treatment may be followed in all patients with rheumatic fever by the transient reappearance, within 2 to 3 weeks, of laboratory or clinical abnormalities.[71]

Unfortunately, most well-controlled studies have failed to prove that treatment with corticosteroids decreases the incidence of residual rheumatic heart disease.[72,73] Nevertheless, such treatment is indicated in patients with severe carditis and heart failure because one may thus "tide the patient over the acute attack."[74] Patients with refractory cardiac failure may benefit from the insertion of a prosthetic valve.[2]

PREVENTION OF RECURRENCES (SECONDARY PREVENTION)

For all its simplicity, secondary prevention is the finest achievement of medicine in this disease. Its importance is out of proportion to the reduction in the number of rheumatic fever attacks because recurrences are more dangerous than first attacks.

Best results are obtained with 1.2 million U benzathine penicillin G given intramuscularly every 4 weeks. This treatment is especially useful in high-risk patients, that is, those with rheumatic heart disease, a previous rheumatic attack within the past 3 years, or multiple attacks, or in those unlikely to take daily medication. Additional risk factors are youth (childhood and adolescence), exposure to young people, and crowding in the home.

Second best is continual oral medication. Its success depends on the compliance of the patient. Sulfadiazine, at a dose of 0.5 g once daily in children weighing less than 60 pounds and 1 g in others, and oral penicillin, at a dose of 200,000 to 250,000 U twice a day, are about equally effective.

For maximum protection, continual prophylaxis may be maintained for the lifetime of the patient, particularly if rheumatic heart disease is present.[75]

PREVENTION OF INFECTIVE ENDOCARDITIS

Rheumatic heart disease predisposes patients to infective endocarditis. *It is advisable to administer appropriate antibiotics prophylactically to patients with rheumatic heart disease before they are exposed to a procedure that causes bacteremia.*[76]

PREVENTION OF INITIAL EPISODE (PRIMARY PREVENTION)

Although prevention of recurrences is both important and attainable, rheumatic fever can be eradicated only by preventing initial episodes, that is, by accurate diagnosis and appropriate treatment of streptococcal pharyngitis.[75] A relaxation of our vigilance had been suggested by the "virtual disappearance" of rheumatic fever,[1] but its return suggests otherwise.[2] Penicillin, or in the patient who is hypersensitive to it, another antibiotic, must be given *for at least 10 days* to eradicate the streptococci from the pharynx. Family members and other close contacts of the patient should have throat cultures, and if these are positive, should be treated similarly and simultaneously.

REFERENCES

1. Gordis, L.: The virtual disappearance of rheumatic fever in the United States: Lessons in the rise and fall of disease. Circulation, 72:1155–1162, 1985.
2. Veasy, L.G., et al.: Resurgence of acute rheumatic fever in the intermountain area of the United States. N. Engl. J. Med., 316:421–427, 1987.
3. Murphy, G.E.: Evolution of our knowledge of rheumatic fever: Historical survey with particular emphasis on rheumatic heart disease. Bull. Hist. Med., 14:123–147, 1943.
4. El-Sadr, W., and Taranta, A.: The spectrum and the specter of rheumatic fever in the 1980's. Clin. Immunol. Update, 1979. Edited by E.C. Franklin. Elsevier, New York, 1979, pp 183–209.
5. Taranta, A., and Markowitz, M.: Rheumatic Fever. Boston, MTP Press, 1981.
6. Murphy, G.E.: The characteristic rheumatic lesions of striated and of non-striated or smooth muscle cells of the heart. Genesis of the lesions known as Aschoff bodies and those myogenic components known as Aschoff cells or as Antischkow cells or myocytes. Medicine, 42:73–117, 1963.
7. Husby, G., et al.: Immunofluorescence studies of florid rheumatic Aschoff lesions. Arthritis Rheum., 2:207–211, 1986.
8. Kaplan, M.H., et al.: Presence of bound immunoglobulins and complement in myocardium in acute rheumatic fever. Association with cardiac failure. N. Engl. J. Med., 271:637–645, 1964.
9. Persellin, S.T., Ramirez, G., and Moatamed, F.: Immunopathology of rheumatic pericarditis. Arthritis Rheum., 25:1054–1058, 1982.
10. Raizada, V., et al.: Tissue distribution of lymphocytes in rheumatic heart valves as defined by monoclonal anti-T antibodies. Am. J. Med., 74:90–96, 1983.
11. Svartman, M., et al.: Immunoglobulins and complement components in synovial fluid of patients with acute rheumatic fever. J. Clin. Invest., 56:111–117, 1975.
12. Benedek, T.G.: Subcutaneous nodules and the differentiation of rheumatoid arthritis from rheumatic fever. Semin. Arthritis Rheum., 4:305–321, 1984.
13. Wannamaker, L.W., et al.: Prophylaxis of acute rheumatic fever by treatment of the preceding streptococcal infection with various amounts of depot penicillin. Am. J. Med., 10:673–695, 1951.
14. Taranta, A., Gordis, L.: The prevention of rheumatic fever: Opportunities, frustrations, and challenges. Cardiovasc. Clin., 4:1–10, 1972.
15. Kuttner, A.G., and Krumwiede, E.: Observations on the effect of streptococcal upper respiratory infections on rheumatic children: A three-year study. J. Clin. Invest., 20:273–287, 1941.
16. Bisno, A.L.: The concept of rheumatogenic and non-rheumatogenic group A streptococci. In Streptococcal Diseases and the Immune Response. Edited by S.E. Read and J.B. Zabriskie. New York, Academic Press, 1980, pp. 789–803.
17. Perry, B.C., and Roberts, M.A.F.: A study on the variability in the incidence of rheumatic heart disease within the city of Bristol. Br. Med. J., 22(Suppl.):154–158, 1937.
18. Rammelkamp, C.H., Jr.: Epidemiology of streptococcal infections. Harvey Lect., 15:113–142, 1955–1956.
19. Stollerman, G.H., Siegel, A.C., and Johnson, E.E.: Variable epidemiology of streptococcal disease and the changing pattern of rheumatic fever. Mod. Concepts Cardiovasc. Dis., 34:45–48, 1965.
20. Taranta, A., et al.: Rheumatic fever in monozygotic and dizygotic twins. In Proceedings of the Tenth International Congress of Rheumatology. Minerva Med., 2:96–98, 1961.
21. Ayoub, E.M., Barrett, D.J., Maclaren, N.K., and Krischer, J.P.: Association of class II human histocompatibility leukocyte antigens with rheumatic fever. J. Clin. Invest., 6:2019–2026, 1986.
22. Zabriskie, J.B., et al.: Rheumatic fever-associated B cell alloantigens as identified by monoclonal antibodies. Arthritis Rheum., 9:1047–1051, 1985.

23. Zabriskie, J.B.: Rheumatic fever: The interplay between host, genetics, and microbe. Lewis A. Conner memorial lecture. Circulation, 6:1077–1086, 1985.

24. Friedman, J., et al.: Immunological studies of post-streptococcal sequelae: Evidence for presence of streptococcal antigens in circulating immune complexes. J. Clin. Invest., 76:1027–1034, 1986.

25. Rammelkamp, C.H., Jr., and Stolzer, B.L.: The latent period before the onset of acute rheumatic fever. Yale J. Biol. Med., 34:386–398, 1961–1962.

26. Barnert, A.L., Jerry, E.E., and Persellin, R.H.: Acute rheumatic fever in adults. JAMA, 232:925–928, 1975.

27. Feinstein, A.R., and Spagnuolo, M.: The clinical patterns of acute rheumatic fever: A reappraisal. Medicine, 41:279–305, 1962.

28. Graef, I., et al.: Studies in rheumatic fever. The natural course of acute manifestations of rheumatic fever uninfluenced by "specific" therapy. Am. J. Med. Sci., 185:197–210, 1933.

29. Rosenthal, A., Czoniczer, G., and Messell, B.F.: Rheumatic fever under three years of age. A report of 10 cases. Pediatrics, 41:612–619, 1968.

30. Feinstein, A.R., and Di Masa, R.: The unheard diastolic murmur in acute rheumatic fever. N. Engl. J. Med., 260:1331–1333, 1959.

31. Mirowski, M., Rosenstein, B.J., and Markowitz, M.: A comparison of atrioventricular conduction in normal children and in patients with rheumatic fever, glomerulonephritis, and acute febrile illnesses. A quantitative study with determination of the P-R index. Pediatrics, 33:334–340, 1964.

32. Feinstein, A.R., and Spagnuolo, M.: Prognostic significance of valvular involvement in acute rheumatic fever. N. Engl. J. Med., 260:1001–1007, 1959.

33. Taranta, A., and Stollerman, G.H.: The relationship of Sydenham's chorea to infection with group A streptococci. Am. J. Med., 20:170–175, 1956.

34. Aron, A.M., Freeman, J.M., and Carter, S.: The natural history of Sydenham's chorea. Review of the literature and long-term evaluation with emphasis on cardiac sequelae. Am. J. Med., 38:83–95, 1965.

35. Massell, B.F., Fyler, D.C., and Rey, S.B.: The clinical picture of rheumatic fever: Diagnosis, immediate prognosis, course and therapeutic implications. Am. J. Cardiol., 1:436–449, 1958.

36. Bywaters, E.G.L., and Thomas, G.T.: Bed rest, salicylates, and steroid in rheumatic fever. Br. Med. J., 1:1628, 1962.

37. Perry, B.C.: Erythema marginatum (rheumaticum). Arch. Dis. Child., 12:233–238, 1937.

38. United Kingdom and United States Joint Report: The treatment of acute rheumatic fever in children: A cooperative clinical trial of ACTH, cortisone and aspirin. Circulation, 11:343–377, 1955.

39. Sanyal, S.K., et al.: The initial attack of acute rheumatic fever during childhood in North India: A prospective study of the clinical profile. Circulation, 49:7–12, 1974.

40. McMinn, F.J., and Bywaters, E.G.L.: Differences between the fever of Still's disease and that of rheumatic fever. Ann. Rheum. Dis., 18:293–297, 1959.

41. Taranta, A., Spagnuolo, M., and Feinstein, A.R.: Chronic rheumatic fever. Ann. Intern. Med., 56:367–388, 1962.

42. Bittl, J.A., and Perloff, J.K.: Chronic postrheumatic fever arthropathy of Jaccoud. Am. Heart J., 105:515–517, 1983.

43. Bywaters, E.G.L.: The relation between heart and joint disease including "rheumatoid heart disease" and chronic post-rheumatic arthritis (type Jaccoud). Br. Heart J., 12:101, 1950.

44. Girigis, F.L., Popple, A.W., Bruckner, F.E.: Jaccoud's arthropathy. A case report and necropsy study. Ann. Rheum. Dis., 37:561–565, 1978.

45. Ruderman, J.E., and Abruzzo, J.L.: Chronic postrheumatic-fever arthritis (Jaccoud's): Report of a case with subcutaneous nodules. Arthritis Rheum., 9:640–647, 1966.

46. Zvaifler, N.J.: Chronic postrheumatic-fever (Jaccoud's) arthritis. N. Engl. J. Med., 267:10–14, 1962.

47. Bywaters, E.G.L.: Jaccoud's syndrome: A sequel to the joint involvement of systemic lupus erythematosus. Clin. Rheum. Dis., 1:125–148, 1975.

48. Esdaile, J.M., et al.: Deforming arthritis in systemic lupus erythematosus. Ann. Rheum. Dis., 40:124–126, 1981.

49. Ignacak, T., et al.: Jaccoud arthritis. Arch. Intern. Med., 35:577–579, 1975.

50. Murphy, W.A., and Staple, T.W.: Jaccoud's arthropathy reviewed. AJR, 118:300–307, 1973.

51. Spagnuolo, M., Pasternak, B., and Taranta, A.: Risk of rheumatic fever recurrences after streptococcal infections. Prospective study of clinical and social factors. N. Engl. J. Med., 285:641–647, 1971.

52. Taranta, A., et al.: Rheumatic fever in children and adolescents. A long-term epidemiologic study of subsequent prophylaxis, streptococcal infections, and clinical sequelae. V. Relation of the rheumatic fever recurrence rate per streptococcal infection to pre-existing clinical features of the patients. Ann. Intern. Med., 60:58–67, 1964.

53. Roth, I.R., Lingg, C., and Whittemore, A.: Heart disease in children. A. Rheumatic Group. I. Certain aspects of the age at onset and of recurrences in 488 cases of juvenile rheumatism ushered in by major clinical manifestations. Am. Heart J., 13:36–60, 1937.

54. Feinstein, A.R., and Spagnuolo, M.: Mimetic features of rheumatic fever recurrences. N. Engl. J. Med., 262:533–540, 1960.

55. Taranta, A.: Rheumatic fever made difficult: critical review of pathogenetic theories. Pediatrician, 5:74–95, 1976.

56. Stollerman, G.H., et al.: Relationship of immune response to group A streptococci to the course of acute, chronic and recurrent rheumatic fever. Am. J. Med., 20:163–169, 1956.

57. Taranta, A., et al.: Rheumatic fever in children and adolescents. A long-term epidemiologic study of subsequent prophylaxis, streptococcal infections, and clinical sequelae. IV. Relation of the rheumatic fever recurrence rate per streptococcal infection to the titers of streptococcal antibodies. Ann. Intern. Med., 60(Suppl. 5):47–57, 1964.

58. Bisno, A.L., and Ofek, I.: Serologic diagnosis of streptococcal infection. Comparison of a rapid hemagglutination technique with conventional antibody tests. Am. J. Dis. Child., 127:676–681, 1974.

59. Manso, C., Taranta, A., and Nydick, S.: Effect of aspirin administration on serum glutamic oxaloacetic and glutamic pyruvic transaminase in children. Proc. Soc. Exp. Biol. Med., 93:84–88, 1956.

60. American Heart Association: Jones Criteria (revised) for guidance in the diagnosis of rheumatic fever. Circulation, 69:204A–208A, 1984.

61. Doyle, E.F., et al.: The risk of bacterial endocarditis during antirheumatic prophylaxis. JAMA, 201:807–812, 1967.

62. Fernandez, R., and McCarty, D.J.: The arthritis of viral hepatitis. Ann. Intern. Med., 74:207–211, 1971.

63. Roy, S.B., Sturges, G.P., and Massell, B.F.: Application of the antistreptolysin-O titer in the evaluation of joint pain and in the diagnosis of rheumatic fever. N. Engl. J. Med., 254:95–102, 1956.

64. Cooper, L.A., et al.: Transient arthritis after rubella vaccination. Am. J. Dis. Child., *118*:218–225, 1969.

65. Ward, C.: Observations of the diagnosis of isolated rheumatic carditis. Am. Heart J., *91*:545–550, 1976.

66. Lortscher, R.H., et al.: Left atrial myxoma presenting as rheumatic fever. Chest, *66*:302–303, 1974.

67. Chun, R.W.M., et al.: Benign familial chorea with onset in childhood. JAMA, *225*:1603, 1973.

68. Taranta, A.: Occurrence of rheumatic-like subcutaneous nodules without evidence of joint or heart disease. N. Engl. J. Med., *266*:13–16, 1962.

69. Laitinen, O., Leirisalo, M., and Allander, E.: Rheumatic fever and *Yersinia* arthritis; Criteria and diagnostic problems in a changing disease pattern. Scand. J. Rheumatol., *4*:145–157, 1975.

70. Mazzara, J.T., et al.: Coexistence of sickle-cell anemia and rheumatic heart disease. N.Y. State J. Med., *71*:2426–2430, 1971.

71. Feinstein, A.R., Spagnuolo, M., and Gill, F.A.: The rebound phenomenon in acute rheumatic fever 1. Incidence and significance. Yale J. Biol. Med., *33*:259–278, 1961.

72. Combined Rheumatic Fever Study Group: A comparison of short-term, intensive prednisone and acetylsalicylic acid therapy in the treatment of acute rheumatic fever. N. Engl. J. Med., *272*:63–70, 1965.

73. United Kingdom and United States Joint Report: The evolution of rheumatic heart disease in children: Five-year report of a cooperative clinical trial of ACTH, cortisone and aspirin. Circulation, 22:1503, 1960.

74. Czoniczer, G., et al.: Therapy of severe rheumatic carditis. Comparison of adrenocorticosteroids and aspirin. Circulation, *29*:813–819, 1964.

75. American Heart Association: Prevention of rheumatic fever. Circulation, *70*:1118A–1122A, 1984.

76. Shulman, S.T., et al.: Prevention of bacterial endocarditis. Circulation, *70*(6):1122A–1123A, 1984.

78

RELAPSING POLYCHONDRITIS

DAVID E. TRENTHAM

Relapsing polychondritis is an uncommon entity whose manifestations are frequently widespread and dramatic. The essential features are inflammation with progressive loss of structural integrity of some cartilaginous tissues and involvement of organs of special sense such as the eye, the middle and inner ears, and the vestibular apparatus. Aortic insufficiency can also occur.

Before 1958, the medical literature contained only 10 single case reports, but since that time the condition has become widely recognized as a distinct clinical entity.[1-6] Many of the earlier authors did not realize that similar patients had been described before, and each invented his own descriptive terms for the disease. Thus, some of the terms used for relapsing polychondritis were "systemic chondromalacia," "panchondritis," and "chronic atrophic polychondritis." "Relapsing polychondritis" best describes the undulating clinical course that this syndrome follows, although admittedly it does not take into account the frequent involvement of some noncartilaginous structures.

CLINICAL FEATURES

The earliest identifiable report of relapsing polychondritis, published in 1923 by Jaksch-Wartenhorst,[7] still provides a clear picture of the disease. His patient, a 32-year-old brewer, first became ill with arthritic swellings and pain in several finger joints and then in the wrists, left hand, right knee, and toes of the

right foot. There was also a febrile response. One-and-a-half months later, burning pain developed in both external ears, which slowly swelled and, within the next 3 months, receded and shrank, leaving a flabby deformity of both auricles. Two or three months later, without pain, the midsegment of the nose slowly collapsed, leaving a saddle-nose deformity. At that time, there was nearly complete stenosis of both auditory canals and some diminution of hearing, even when the canals were held open. Associated dizziness and tinnitus also occurred. Somewhat later, crepitation developed in both knees and in the spine.

The disease occurs equally in both sexes. It is most common in the middle decades of life, but cases have been reported in children and the elderly. Although it is often fatal, the clinical course is highly variable and may be self-limited. One study reported a 7-year average life span in 11 patients from the time of appearance of symptoms to death, but the spectrum of survival ranged widely, from 10 months to over 20 years.[3] The causes of death were usually respiratory failure due to airway stenosis (or collapse) and complicating pulmonary infection and cardiovascular failure due to intractable aortic insufficiency.[1,3] Table 78-1 summarizes many of the clinical manifestations and their incidence.

Inflammation of isolated or multiple cartilages predominates, often with an initial febrile response and involvement of one or several structures of the eye. Onset is usually acute in the first and subsequent attacks unless the latter are modified by glucocorticoid therapy. Typically, the pinnas, or cartilaginous por-

1227

Table 78–1. Incidence of Various Clinical Features in Relapsing Polychondritis*

Manifestation	No. Affected/No. Reported	Frequency (%)
Ear cartilage involvement	45/51	88
Nasal cartilage involvement	40/49	82
Fever	21/26	81
Arthropathy	40/51	78
Laryngotracheal involvement	33/47	70
Episcleritis or conjunctivitis	29/48	60
Defective hearing	21/44	48
Costochondral cartilage involvement	21/45	47
Iritis	11/41	27
Labyrinthine vertigo†	—	25
Aortic valve lesion with insufficiency‡	10/74	14

*Modified from Dolan, D.L., et al.[3]
†Rough approximation of incidence. These organ systems were not always clearly described.
‡Data from Arkin, C.R., and Masi, A.T.[1] and others.

tions of the ears, swell and become purplish-red and exquisitely tender, so that it is impossible to rest them on a pillow. The soft earlobes are always spared. The external auditory canals, especially the meatus, also swell and may close almost completely; hearing is thereby reduced. Inflammation of the inner ear producing serous otitis media and obstruction of the eustachian tube from cartilage involvement in its nasopharyngeal portion can further impair hearing.[8] A labyrinthine type of vertigo may develop. Often, the episclerae are inflamed. Joint inflammation or simple arthralgias occasionally occur during these attacks. Sometimes, the cartilaginous portion of the bridge of the nose becomes inflamed during the first or later episodes.

An attack lasts from a few days to many weeks, and may, if left untreated, progress in a subacute or smoldering fashion to involve additional cartilaginous structures and special sense organs. As the inflammatory phase subsides, the external ear may shrink, owing to the thinning of the cartilage or the loss of its structural integrity, so that the pinna droops forward from lack of support (Fig. 78–1). This condition may occur during the first episode or not until after several attacks. Similarly, the cartilaginous nasal septum may erode (Fig. 78–2), leaving a step-shaped or saddle nose, which is also characteristic for this condition.

The two most serious complications of relapsing polychondritis are: (1) an involvement of the cartilaginous structures of the respiratory tract, and (2) progressive aortic insufficiency. In the mildest forms of the disease, the respiratory tract involvement consists of hoarseness, slight cough, and minimal tenderness of the larynx and trachea. In more severe instances, there may be extensive inflammation and edema of the laryngeal and epiglottal cartilages, necessitating emergency tracheostomy. A similar process may also

involve the tracheal and bronchial rings so that diffuse narrowing of the airways may ensue. This complication may be fatal, owing to asphyxia and/or superimposed respiratory infection. Moreover, in such circumstances, tracheostomy may be inadequate to maintain adequate pulmonary ventilation. If the patient survives one or more chondrolytic attacks on the air passages, the cartilages may be left with some loss of structural support in the involved regions. The trachea and bronchi may then become diffusely or focally narrowed because of varying degrees of stenosis, or the cartilages may lose all or nearly all of their archi-

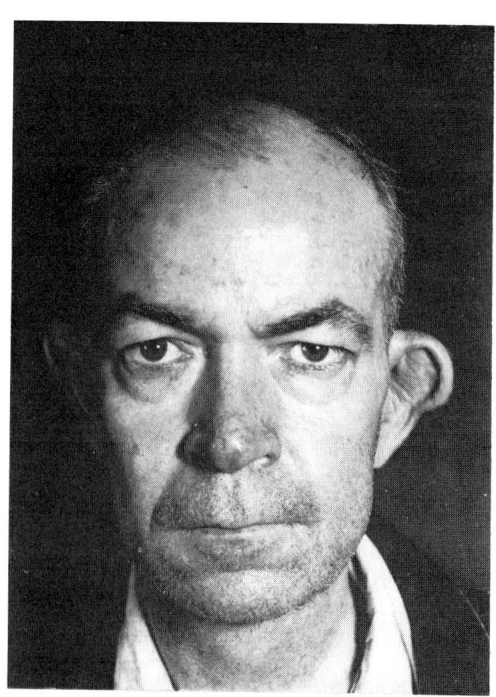

FIG. 78–1. Classic drooping of the left external ear in a man with recurrent episodes of polychondritis.

FIG. 78–2. The characteristic saddle-nose deformity had developed painlessly 3 months earlier.

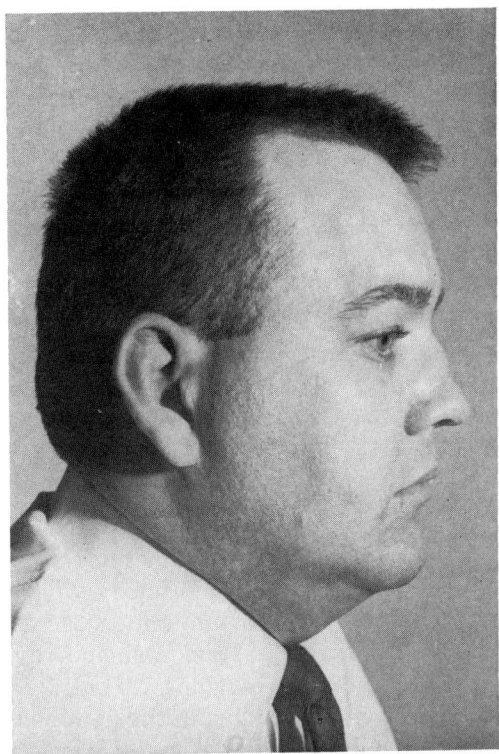

tectural support. They then appear at autopsy as floppy collapsible tubes. In such patients, intubation is useless because of the collapse throughout even the smallest bronchi.[9] As if such serious involvement of the respiratory apparatus is not enough, further embarrassment to breathing may, on occasion, be caused by tenderness and swelling of one or several costo-sternal cartilages. In rare instances, partial or complete dissolution may result, leaving a flail anterior chest plate.

Aortic insufficiency, the other life-threatening complication, has been described in approximately 10 to 15% of cases.[1,2] The aortic regurgitation is due to progressive dilatation of the aortic ring and, often, the ascending aorta, rather than to inflammation of the valve leaflets. This pattern of involvement helps to differentiate the aortic insufficiency of relapsing polychondritis from the regurgitation that occurs in ankylosing spondylitis, Reiter's syndrome, and certain other rheumatic diseases (Table 78–2). Rarely, polychondritis can be associated with dilatation of the annulus of the mitral and tricuspid valves.[2] Prosthetic valves have been inserted successfully in some patients.[1]

Eye lesions are common and include episcleritis, conjunctivitis and, less frequently, iritis. Usually, the inflammation smolders at a low level or resolves as an attack subsides. Rarely have serious sequelae resulted, but proptosis, cataracts, severe keratitis, and even blindness have occurred in isolated instances.[2]

Articular involvement is variable, usually consisting of subacute swelling and pain in one or several large joints of the extremities. The articulations of the spine, either the true apophyseal cartilages or the intervertebral discs, are rarely involved. Serious peripheral joint damage has not been a common occurrence. However, it may resemble low-grade rheumatoid arthritis (RA) or, conversely, may culminate in osteophyte formation that even limits joint mobility. In a series of 23 patients, arthritis was the presenting symptom in 35% and was a significant clinical feature during the course of relapsing polychondritis in 85% of patients.[10]

Minor hematopoietic, hepatic, and renal involvement has been described,[3] but in some cases, this may have represented another associated disease process.

The most curious clinical feature is the selectivity of the chondritic process. Not only are some cartilages and cartilaginous structures spared while others are extensively involved, but there exists in some patients a remarkable unilaterality so that only one ear or one eye may be affected, even after multiple attacks. Other disorders to be considered in the differential diagnosis of relapsing polychondritis, such as a bacterial perichondritis, trauma or frostbite, Wegener's granulomatosis, lethal midline granuloma, or Cogan's syndrome,[2] do not produce multifocal chondritic lesions. However, polychondritis may develop in patients with a variety of connective tissue diseases, including systemic lupus erythematosus, vasculitis, adult or juvenile rheumatoid arthritis, and Sjögren's syndrome.[1,2]

In a large single-institution analysis,[6] the 5- and 10-year probabilities for survival after the diagnosis of relapsing polychondritis were 74% and 55%, respectively. Infection, systemic vasculitis, and malignancy were the most frequent causes of death. Surprisingly, only 10% of the fatalities were attributable to airway involvement. Anemia at the time of diagnosis was a marker for shortened survival; a saddle-nose deformity or systemic vasculitis were additional unfavorable prognostic signs in younger patients.

LABORATORY OBSERVATIONS

As may be anticipated, aside from diagnostic biopsy findings, the laboratory features are nonspecific.[3] The most common findings are noted during the active

Table 78–2. Aortic Insufficiency

Condition	Disease Causing
Valvulitis	Rheumatic fever Rheumatoid arthritis Ankylosing spondylitis* Endocarditis Reiter's syndrome* Behçet's syndrome*
Congenital	Bicuspid aortic valve
Dilatation of valve ring	Marfan's syndrome Syphilis Relapsing polychondritis Secondary to dissecting aneurysm Idiopathic

*Also dilatation of valve ring

disease process. They consist of an increased erythrocyte sedimentation rate, some degree of leukocytosis and anemia, occasional low titer positivity for rheumatoid factor or antinuclear antibody, and modest serum protein alterations, such as a decreased albumin and increased α- and γ-globulins.

The roentgenographic finding that is of the greatest value, diagnostically, is tracheal stenosis. After mul-

FIG. 78–3. Significant stenosis of the tracheal airway as demonstrated by air tomography in a 50-year-old woman with relapsing polychondritis.

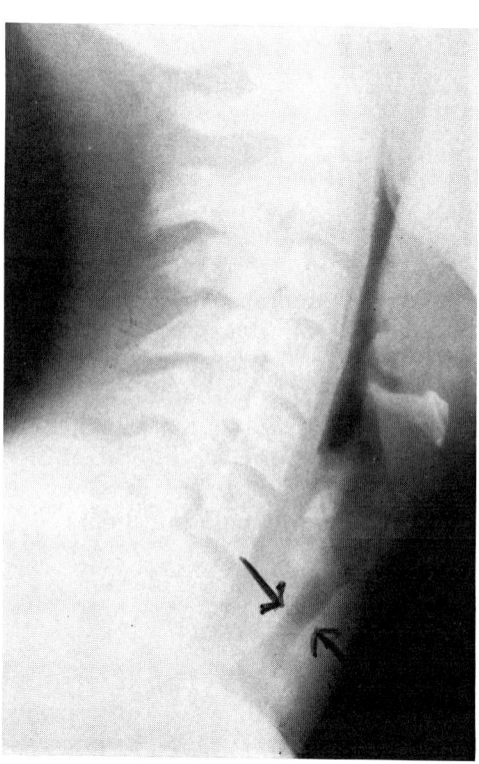

tiple inflammatory attacks, the external ears may show calcific deposits. This finding is not specific for relapsing polychondritis, however, because it may result from other inflammatory conditions such as frostbite. The joints may show moderate destructive changes, often spotty and asymmetric, but sometimes suggestive of RA. On a chest film, major airways may be narrowed. The closure may be focal or diffuse and is most clearly visualized by tracheal tomography (Fig. 78–3). In the presence of aortic insufficiency, cardiomegaly is commonly found.

PATHOLOGY

The histopathology of relapsing polychondritis is highly characteristic.[5,9,11–13] Acidophilic (pink) coloration of the cartilage matrix, in contrast to the usual basophilic (blue) hue, is seen by routine hematoxylin and eosin staining (Fig. 78–4). Focal or diffuse infiltration by predominantly mononuclear inflammatory cells, with occasional polymorphonuclear leukocytes and plasma cells in the perichondrial tissues, is associated with the dissolution of cartilage from its periphery inward (Fig. 78–5). Fibroblastic granulation tissue frequently coexists and leads to partial sequestration of the cartilage matrix (see Fig. 78–4). This vigorous reparative response may culminate in the production of new cartilage.[12] Evidence of necrotizing angiitis or thrombosis is lacking. Rarely, calcium salts are found in the cartilage. Examination of the ocular globe in one patient revealed mononuclear inflammatory cells and plasma cells scattered about the episcleral vessels.

In involved cardiac and aortic structures, the aortic valve leaflets are normal, whereas the ascending aorta, especially the aortic ring, is dilated, with a loss

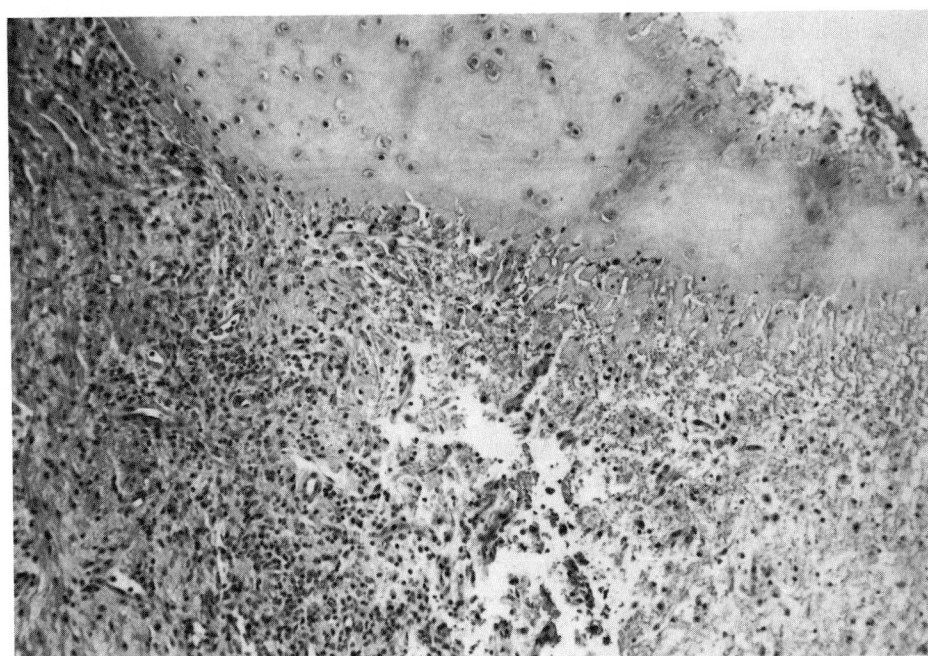

FIG. 78–4. Chondrocyte necrosis, destruction of the matrix, and loss of basophilia in the elastic cartilage of the ear, sequestration of segments of cartilage by contiguous granulation tissue, and infiltration by inflammatory cells. These histopathologic features are characteristic of the cartilage lesion in relapsing polychondritis.

of basophilia and degeneration, necrosis, and fibrosis. The primary pathologic change in the aortic ring and ascending aorta is in the media, with a loss of elastic tissue, a decrease in basophilia, and fibrosis. Associated focal acute and chronic inflammation occurs in these areas as well as in the adventitial blood vessels and in the vasa vasorum.

Histochemical studies have confirmed these findings and have revealed a loss of metachromasia in the residual cartilage matrix, with some preservation of metachromasia in the cytoplasm and in the immediate perilacunar zones around chondrocytes.[9] In the aorta,

there was a moderate loss in neutral or acidic polysaccharides by the toluidine blue, azure A (pH 2.0), or PAS-alcian blue methods. Hale's method for sulfated mucopolysaccharides showed marked depletion of these components in the abnormal aortas and aortic rings.

By electron microscopy, cartilage from patients with active relapsing polychondritis contains greatly increased numbers of "matrix granules."[14] These are small (below 10 nm in diameter) stellate granules of medium electron density and are compatible with particles of cartilage matrix composed primarily of pro-

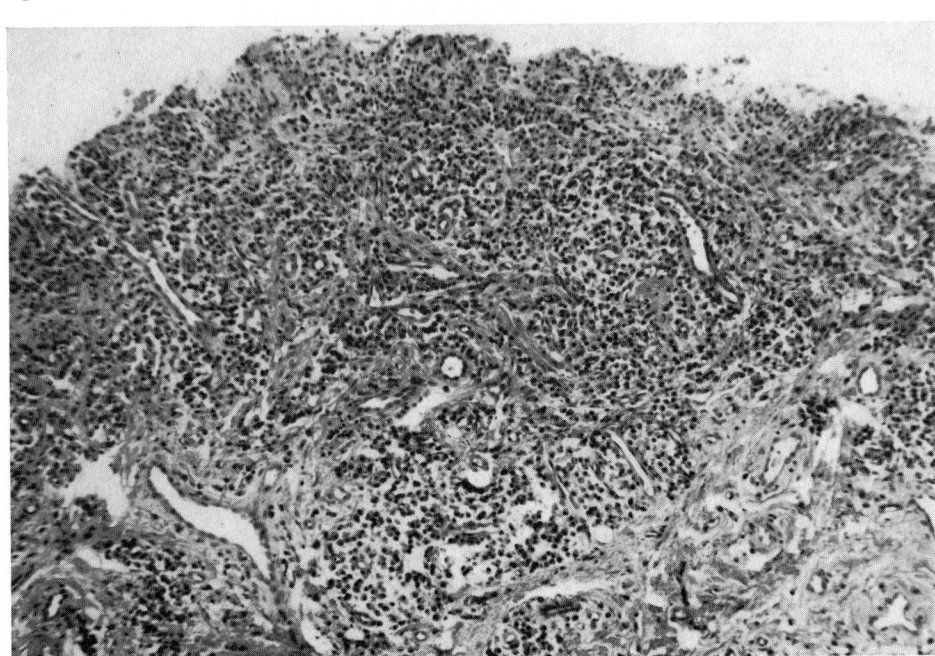

FIG. 78–5. Marked cellular infiltration composed of mononuclear inflammatory cells, plasma cells, and histiocytes in the perichondrial tissues in relapsing polychondritis. Connective tissue and blood vessel elements have proliferated, but no vasculitis is present in this exuberant granulation tissue.

teoglycan. These granules are usually not membrane limited and are seen in normal cartilage in small numbers. "Matrix vesicles," also present in these specimens, are larger than the matrix granule, measure about 1000 nm, and are located extracellularly. Ultrastructurally, the vesicles and dense granules found in the lesions are more compatible with lysosomes than typical matrix vesicles or granules, because they are usually larger and more irregular in shape, and because they often contain multiple myelin-like laminated structures. The matrix vesicles possess a significant amount of alkaline phosphatase and adenosine triphosphatase activities, but a low acid phosphatase activity, which is usually a marker for lysosomes. The origin of these cartilage matrix vesicles is uncertain. Because they are extracellular, it is likely that they are budding from cellular membranes containing cytoplasmic debris. Other investigators have recognized a few dense bodies, which they interpreted as lysosomes, in the chondrocytes of the lesion.[14] Furthermore, they observed a large number of extracellular dense bodies containing multiple vesicles. The significance of this observation is unknown.

Immunofluorescence studies of specimens from patients with relapsing polychondritis have identified granular deposits of immunoglobulin G (IgG), IgA, IgM, and C3 at the lesional junction of fibrous and cartilaginous tissue, suggesting the presence of immune complexes.[2,12,13,15]

PATHOGENESIS

The etiology of relapsing polychondritis is unknown. The loss of acid mucopolysaccharides and many of the other cartilage changes that may be secondary events could be caused by release of lysosomal enzymes, especially proteases, either from chondrocytes or from other cellular elements. Thus, it is of potential interest that intravenously administered crude papain, a proteolytic enzyme, induced a noninflammatory dissolution of the ear cartilages of rabbits within 4 hours.[16] This reaction also involved a rapid loss of cartilage metachromasia. In addition, 3 to 6 weeks after a single intravenous injection of crude papain into rabbits, focal plaque lesions due to alterations of connective tissue of the media occurred in the ascending aorta and arch. Some of these lesions progressed by metaplasia into partially developed cartilage and bone.[17] It has been postulated that these lesions resulted from the release, by papain, of large amounts of sulfated mucopolysaccharides, which are then deposited in various organs and especially in the aortic wall. A similar mechanism may be operative in

relapsing polychondritis, with an endogenous proteolytic enzyme, perhaps lysosomal, being responsible for the chondrolysis.

The identification of immunoglobulins in the lesions and the occasional coexistence of another systemic connective tissue disease are consistent with the possibility that autoimmune mechanisms cause the cartilage damage.[1,2,12,13,15,18-21] The ability of an autoimmune response to produce inflammation in both cartilage and ocular tissue could be explained by the reactivity being directed to a constituent shared by both structures. Type II collagen fulfills this requirement. Type II collagen is a brisk immunogen in rodents, and immunization with this protein can induce an inflammatory arthritis in rats or mice that resembles RA morphologically.[22] Recently, it has been observed that auricular chondritis, with immunoglobulin and complement deposits at the site of the lesion, occurred on occasion in rats with type II collagen-induced arthritis.[12,20] Because antibodies to type II collagen have been detected in the serum of patients during the acute stage of polychondritis, there is increasing, although indirect, evidence that immunologic responses to cartilage and ocular collagen participate in the pathogenesis of relapsing polychondritis.[18,19,21]

Based on these findings, a hypothetical scheme can be proposed to partially explain the pathogenesis of relapsing polychondritis. Clones of autoreactive T and/or B cells emerge, by as yet undefined mechanisms, that are sensitized to type II collagen. Autoantibodies and perhaps lymphokines induce inflammation in cartilage (and the eye), which leads to chondrocyte death and matrix dissolution. Fibroblasts and chondroblasts then attempt to repair the lesion. Occasionally, the cycle of injury and repair is repeated, accounting for the relapsing nature of the disease. Substances released into the blood during the destruction of cartilage are injurious to the structural integrity of major blood vessels and trigger the characteristic aortic lesion. Much remains to be learned about the pathogenesis of relapsing polychondritis.

THERAPY

Aside from prosthetic valve replacement for aortic insufficiency, therapy has consisted primarily of supportive measures and the use of glucocorticoids. An acute inflammatory attack on affected cartilages may be moderated or brought under complete control with prednisone, 20 to 60 mg/day.[1,2] As the attack subsides, the dosage may be reduced to a maintenance level of 10 to 15 mg daily. In some patients, the anti-inflammatory and abortive effects of prednisone diminish over months or years so that the maintenance dosage must be raised gradually in an effort to prevent further severe attacks. On occasion, it is necessary to eventually administer doses approximating 30 mg of prednisone daily in order to provide satisfactory suppression of inflammation of cartilages and episcleritis. Glucocorticoids have no obvious effect on inhibiting the development of the aortic lesions. In patients who are truly refractory to prednisone, other types of immunosuppressive drugs may be attempted.[1] Cyclosporin has been used successfully in 1 case.[21] Because the attacks are frequently self-limited and the response to prednisone is delayed, however, attempts to curtail the inflammation with glucocorticoids should not be abandoned prematurely.

REFERENCES

1. Arkin, C.R., and Masi, A.T.: Relapsing polychondritis: Review of current status and case report. Semin. Arthritis Rheum., 5:41–62, 1975.
2. Case Records of the Massachusetts General Hospital (Case 51-1982). N. Engl. J. Med., 307:1631–1639, 1982.
3. Dolan, D.L., Lemmon, G.B., and Teitelbaum, S.L.: Relapsing polychondritis: Analytical review and studies on pathogenesis. Am. J. Med., 41:285–299, 1966.
4. Hughes, R.A.C., et al.: Relapsing polychondritis: Three cases with a clinico-pathological study and literature review. Q. J. Med., 41:363–380, 1972.
5. Kaye, R.L., and Sones, D.A.: Relapsing polychondritis: Clinical and pathologic features in fourteen cases. Ann. Intern. Med., 60:653–664, 1964.
6. Michet, C.J., Jr., McKenna, C.H., Luthra, H.S., and O'Fallon, W.M.: Relapsing polychondritis: Survival and predictive role of early disease manifestations. Ann. Intern. Med., 104:74–78, 1986.
7. Jaksch-Wartenhorst, R.: Polychondropathia. Weiner Archive Innere Med., 6:93–100, 1923.
8. Moloney, J.R.: Relapsing polychondritis—Its otolaryngological manifestations. J. Laryngol. Otol., 92:9–15, 1978.
9. Verity, M.A., Larson, W.M., and Madden, S.C.: Relapsing polychondritis: Report of two necropsied cases with histochemical investigation of the cartilage lesion. Am. J. Pathol., 42:251–269, 1963.
10. O'Hanlan, M., et al.: The arthropathy of relapsing polychondritis. Arthritis Rheum., 19:191–194, 1976.
11. Kindblom, L.-G., et al.: Relapsing polychondritis: A clinical, pathologic-anatomic and histochemical study of two cases. Acta Pathol. Microbiol. Scand. (A), 85:656–664, 1977.
12. McCune, W.J., et al.: Type II collagen-induced auricular chondritis. Arthritis Rheum., 25:266–273, 1982.
13. Valenzuela, R., et al.: Relapsing polychondritis: Immunomicroscopic findings in cartilage of ear biopsy specimens. Hum. Pathol., 11:19–22, 1980.
14. Hashimoto, K., Arkin, C.R., and Kang, A.H.: Relapsing polychondritis: An ultrastructural study. Arthritis Rheum., 20:91–99, 1977.
15. Rogers, P.H., Boden, G., and Tourtellotte, C.D.: Relapsing polychondritis with insulin resistance and antibodies to cartilage. Am. J. Med., 55:243–248, 1973.
16. McCluskey, R.T., and Thomas, L.: The removal of cartilage matrix, in vivo, by papain: The identification of crystalline papain protease as the cause of the phenomenon. J. Exp. Med., 108:371–384, 1958.
17. Tsaltas, T.T.: Metaplasia of aortic connective tissue to cartilage and bone induced by the intravenous injection of papain. Nature, 196:1006–1007, 1962.
18. Foidart, J.M., et al.: Antibodies to type II collagen in relapsing polychondritis. N. Engl. J. Med., 299:1203–1207, 1978.
19. Ebringer, R., et al.: Autoantibodies to cartilage and type II collagen in relapsing polychondritis and other rheumatic diseases. Ann. Rheum. Dis., 40:473–479, 1981.
20. Cremer, M.A., et al.: Auricular chondritis in rats: An experimental model of relapsing polychondritis induced with type II collagen. J. Exp. Med., 154:535–540, 1981.
21. Svenson, K.L.G., et al.: Cyclosporin A treatment in a case of relapsing polychondritis. Scand. J. Rheumatol., 13:329–333, 1984.
22. Trentham, D.E.: Collagen arthritis as a relevant model for rheumatoid arthritis: Evidence pro and con. Arthritis Rheum., 25:911–916, 1982.

79

POLYMYALGIA RHEUMATICA AND GIANT CELL ARTERITIS

LOUIS A. HEALEY

POLYMYALGIA RHEUMATICA

Polymyalgia rheumatica is a syndrome of older patients characterized by pain and stiffness in the neck, shoulders, and pelvic girdle, persisting for at least a month, without weakness or atrophy, usually accompanied by a rapid erythrocyte sedimentation rate, and dramatically relieved by adrenocorticosteroid treatment in low doses (Table 79–1).

HISTORY

In 1957, Barber introduced the name polymyalgia rheumatica for this illness. It had previously been reported as senile arthritis, myalgic syndrome of the aged, arthritic rheumatoid disease and, dating back to 1888, senile rheumatic gout. The rapid erythrocyte sedimentation rate suggested this disease might be a specific entity, and in 1951 Porsman pointed out the similarity to the prodrome of temporal arteritis. This relation was confirmed in 1963 by Alestig and Barr

Table 79–1. Definition of Polymyalgia Rheumatica

1. Patients at least 50 years old, usually white*
2. Bilateral pain persisting for at least 1 month involving two of the following: neck, shoulder girdle, pelvic girdle
   Morning stiffness and gelling are marked
3. Erythrocyte sedimentation rate greater than 40 mm in 1 hour; often 100 mm or more
   Exclusion: Any other diagnosis except giant cell arteritis

*Editor's note. Classic cases have been reported in patients under age 50.[2]

1234

when they demonstrated giant cell arteritis on biopsy of asymptomatic temporal arteries in patients with polymyalgia rheumatica. This syndrome received little attention in the United States until 1966, but since then it has been widely recognized. The annual incidence has been estimated at 53 per 100,000 in persons over the age of 50.[1]

CLINICAL PICTURE

Polymyalgia rheumatica is rare in a patient less than 50 years old, and it has been reported twice as often in women as men. Racial predilection is striking; almost all reported patients have been white.

Patients complain of severe pain in the neck, back, shoulders, upper arms, and thighs. The onset is often abrupt. Patients may go to bed feeling well and awaken as uncomfortable as if they had chopped a cord of wood. Weakness is not prominent, but pain and gelling make rising from a chair difficult. Morning stiffness is marked. In contrast to patients with rheumatoid arthritis (RA), who describe difficulty with fine hand motions such as buttoning buttons, patients with polymyalgia rheumatica graphically describe how difficult it is to get out of bed. Some require help from a spouse, and others are forced to roll out of bed into a kneeling position and then push themselves erect. In some patients, symptoms are widespread; in others, one area, such as the pectoral or pelvic girdle, may predominate. Nonspecific symptoms may include fever, anorexia, weight loss (often marked), lassitude, apathy, and depression.

In view of the severity of the complaints, the paucity of physical findings is surprising. Patients show no rash, nodules, arteritis, muscle weakness, or atrophy. Shoulder joint tenderness may be detectable, and effusions are sometimes present in the knees. Radiographs are unrevealing. A clue to the diagnosis is found in the erythrocyte sedimentation rate, which is almost always elevated and can exceed 100 mm/h (Westergren method). Other acute-phase reactants, especially fibrinogen, are similarly increased. Rheumatoid factor and antinuclear antibodies are not present. Muscle enzyme levels in serum and electromyograms are normal, reflecting normal muscle tissue found at biopsy.

Biopsies have shown nonspecific inflammation of synovial tissue.[3] Such *synovitis* is consistent with the marked morning stiffness and gelling so characteristic of the clinical picture and explains why some of these patients have *carpal tunnel syndrome* or knee effusions.

DIFFERENTIAL DIAGNOSIS

Because the constellation of findings in polymyalgia rheumatica is not specific, the diagnosis depends on differentiation from other diseases (Table 79–2). The pain and stiffness of polymyalgia persist for at least a month in contrast to the myalgias seen with "flu syndrome" and other viral illnesses, which last several days to a week. Apathy, depression, and lack of physical findings suggest depression of the aged, but the rapid erythrocyte sedimentation rate indicates

that an additional factor is involved. The sedimentation rate also rules against a diagnosis of osteoarthritis. It may be difficult to differentiate muscle pain and stiffness from the weakness of polymyositis, but elevated muscle enzymes, abnormal electromyogram, and muscle biopsy are diagnostic of polymyositis.

Polymyalgia rheumatica may be difficult to distinguish from the onset of RA in the older patient when RF is not present. This similarity is not surprising, because both conditions are marked by synovitis. In RA, the small joints of hands and feet tend to be more involved, as opposed to the proximal distribution of polymyalgia. In some patients, only the subsequent course permits definite diagnosis. Routine biopsies of asymptomatic temporal arteries are not needed in patients with polymyalgia for the reasons discussed below.

TREATMENT

The response of polymyalgia to corticosteroids is truly dramatic. Some patients are almost entirely well the next day. The improvement is so invariable that if response is not seen within a week, the diagnosis should be doubted. The usual initial dose is 10 to 20 mg of prednisone (or equivalent) a day. After several weeks, this dose is tapered to a daily maintenance dose of 5 to 7.5 mg while the clinical response is monitored. Aspirin and other anti-inflammatory drugs are less effective.

Long-term followup has shown that polymyalgia is not always a self-limited condition, as was once thought. Seventy percent of 246 patients were still taking prednisone after 2 years.[4] With each subsequent year, more patients can stop the steroid, but a few have needed to continue it for 10 years. Despite prolonged treatment, patients were free of symptoms on 5 mg of prednisone daily and had no joint destruction. Relapse may occur years after stopping steroid, often with a normal sedimentation rate, and occasionally with symmetric synovitis of wrists and knees that resembles RA but again responds to low-dose prednisone.

ETIOLOGY

The cause of polymyalgia rheumatica is not known. No infectious agent or toxin has been found. Hypocomplementemia, increased immunoglobulins, and other serologic tests often associated with "autoimmune diseases" are lacking. The striking preponderance of the disease in whites suggests that a genetic

Table 79–2. Conditions to be Distinguished from Polymyalgia Rheumatica

1. Viral myalgia	Duration is less than a month
2. Rheumatoid arthritis	Examination detects synovitis of small joints; rheumatoid factor is often present
3. Polymyositis	Muscle enzyme levels are elevated in serum; muscle biopsy and electromyogram are abnormal
4. Multiple myeloma	Gamma globulin spike on protein electrophoresis; plasma cells in bone marrow
5. Osteoarthritis	Erythrocyte sedimentation rate is usually normal
6. Fibrositis	Normal sedimentation rate
7. Depression and psychogenic symptoms	Normal sedimentation rate
8. Occult infection	Appropriate tests needed
9. Occult cancer	Appropriate tests needed

predisposition is important, but studies of HLA antigens are inconclusive. The predilection for older patients is unexplained. Long-term followup has not shown any association of polymyalgia with other disease, either rheumatic or neoplastic. Of great interest has been the relation to giant cell arteritis.

GIANT CELL ARTERITIS

In 1932, Horton described temporal arteritis in two elderly patients who had severe headache and high sedimentation rates. As he predicted, "this was a focal localization of an unknown systemic disease." It is now recognized that giant cell arteritis may involve medium-sized and large arteries throughout the body (see also Chapter 74). The temporal artery is only the most superficial and accessible (Fig. 79–1). The aorta and most of the larger arteries may be involved, but in contrast to polyarteritis, the small arterioles are spared. Thus, pulmonary and renal manifestations are not seen in giant cell arteritis. Stroke or myocardial infarction rarely occur. The clinical manifestations can be divided into localized or systemic[5] (Table 79–3). The focal manifestations (Table 79–4) depend on the artery involved and may include the typical temporal headache (temporal); sudden unilateral blindness (ophthalmic); transient diplopia due to paralysis of an

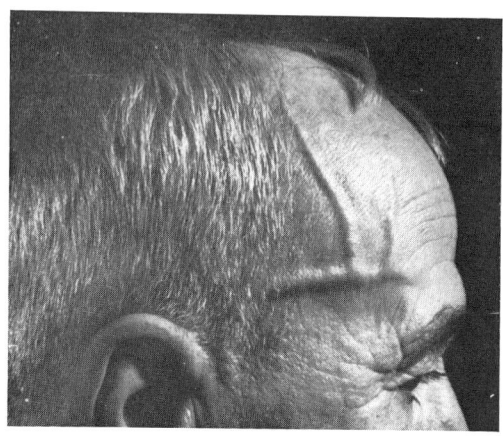

FIG. 79–1. Temporal arteritis. The swollen temporal artery is tender and painful.

extraocular muscle; pain in the jaw on chewing (facial), which is almost pathognomonic of cranial arteritis; and aortic arch syndrome, including claudication, aneurysm, and possibly rupture. The systemic manifestations may include fever, hypoproliferative anemia, weight loss, malaise, and abnormal liver function tests, particularly the *alkaline phosphatase*. At times, the systemic manifestations may predominate, posing a diagnostic problem such as fever of unknown origin, unexplained anemia, or simulation of an occult cancer. In such patients, the rapid erythrocyte sedimentation rate may provide the clue that leads to biopsy of an asymptomatic temporal artery, and establishes the diagnosis.

PATHOLOGY

Inflammation is located on either side of the internal elastic lamina, which is fragmented. Infiltrate consists of histiocytes, lymphocytes, and the giant cells for which the lesion is named. The lumen is narrowed by the thickened edematous intima and at times may be occluded (Fig. 79–2). The histologic picture is indistinguishable from Takayasu's arteritis, but the relation between the two is unknown. Electron microscopic examination reveals histiocytes and giant cells in close proximity to fragments of elastic lamina, whose ground substance is altered and appears dense and granular. Giant cell arteritis is distributed in skip fashion, interspersed with normal-appearing artery, so that often biopsy of a sizable segment of artery is necessary for diagnosis.

Table 79–3.   Manifestations of Giant Cell Arteritis

Systemic
  Fever
  Anemia
  Anorexia
  Malaise
  Weight loss (may be extreme)
  Abnormal liver function tests

Local
  Temporal headache
  Blindness
  Scalp necrosis
  Tongue gangrene
  Jaw claudication
  Neuropathic manifestations—diplopia, paresthesia, brachial paralysis
  Aortic arch syndrome—unequal pulses, claudication of arm or leg, aneurysm rupture, Raynaud's phenomenon

Table 79–4.   Symptoms Suggestive of Cranial Arteritis

  Temporal headache
  Scalp tenderness
  Amaurosis fugax
  Diplopia
  Jaw claudication
  Unexplained fever, anemia, weight loss

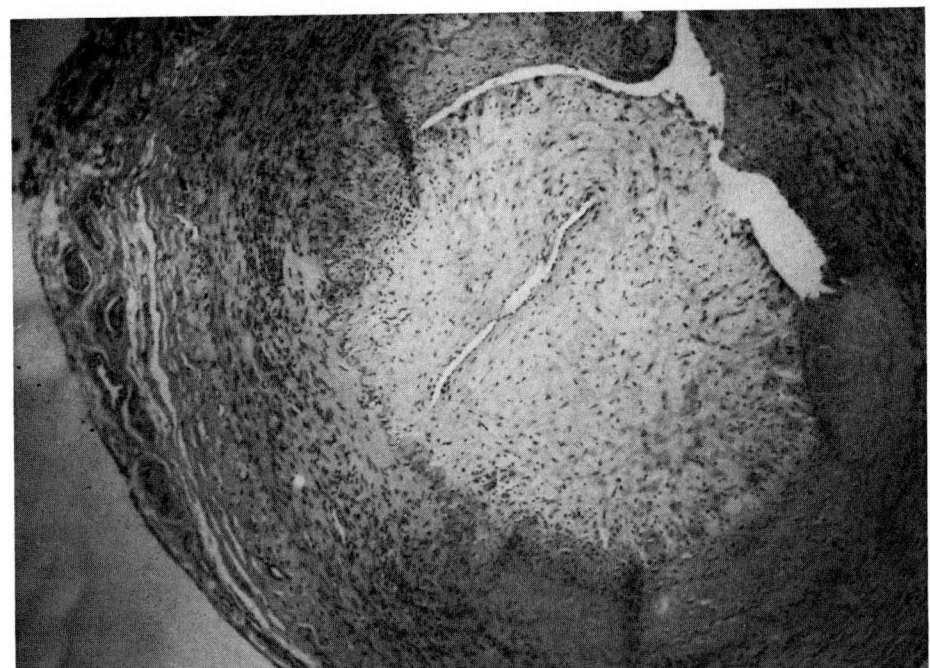

FIG. 79–2. Giant cell arteritis. Cross section of temporal artery showing inflammatory infiltrate, giant cells, fragmentation of elastic lamina, and intimal thickening; the lumen is almost occluded by thrombus. Separation at upper right is artifact.

TREATMENT

Giant cell arteritis responds to corticosteroids, but the dosage required is higher than that needed for treatment of polymyalgia rheumatica alone. Because of the risk of blindness, it is customary to treat with 60 mg of prednisone (or equivalent) a day for 1 month. Alternate-day corticosteroids are ineffective as initial therapy. There is a report of a single patient whose vision improved coincidently with the administration of 1000 mg of pulsed methyl prednisolone. At present, it is not certain that this megadose therapy, which carries significant risks for the elderly, will prove to be effective in other patients.

The use of high-dose steroid for 1 month effectively suppresses the inflammation, and no late recurrences of arteritis with vision loss have been reported in patients so treated. The dose is gradually tapered over the next 6 months. The sedimentation rate is a good indicator of inflammation initially, but in the subsequent course it does not accurately reflect the activity of the arteritis. Attempting to maintain a normal sedimentation rate will almost invariably result in steroid toxicity of osteoporosis and vertebral collapse. Unlike polymyalgia, late relapses of which do occur, giant cell arteritis has not recurred after adequate initial treatment. Most instances of what is called resistant disease are patients with an elevated sedimentation rate and nonspecific symptoms who do not require toxic doses of steroid or "steroid-sparing" drugs.

ETIOLOGY

The cause of giant cell arteritis is unknown. The histologic appearance suggests a cell-mediated immune response, but there has not been confirmatory evidence for this, whether in serologic tests, immunofluorescent staining of arterial tissue, or lymphocyte stimulation.

Relation to Polymyalgia

Although this is an important question because of the risk of blindness and other catastrophic vascular events, the exact nature of the relation of polymyalgia rheumatica to giant cell arteritis is still unclear. Both have been noted in the same patient, either concurrently or at different times, and arteritis in an asymptomatic temporal artery has been reported in some series in approximately 15% of patients with polymyalgia. However, many patients have polymyalgia rheumatica alone. They respond well to low-dose steroid therapy and never develop headache, blindness, or any other sign of giant cell arteritis. At present, if a patient with polymyalgia rheumatica shows none of the clinical manifestations of cranial arteritis described, or if a temporal artery biopsy is negative, the chance of blindness is slight. Rather than risk corticosteroid toxicity, these patients might be treated with a lower dose. They should, however, be informed of the slight, but serious, risk of blindness, alerted to symptoms that are warning signals, and instructed to increase the steroid dose and to contact their physician if these symptoms appear.

REFERENCES

1. Hunder, G.G., and Michet, C.J.: Giant cell arteritis and polymyalgia rheumatica. Clin. Rheum. Dis., *11*:471–483, 1985.
2. F. William Blaisdell: Limited utility of fibrinogen. ^{125}I leg scanning. Arch. Intern. Med., *139*:143–148, 1979.
3. Chou, C.-T., and Schumacher, H.R.: Clinical and pathologic studies of synovitis in polymyalgia rheumatica. Arthritis Rheum., *27*:1107–1118, 1984.
4. Healey, L.A.: Long-term follow-up of polymyalgia rheumatica: Evidence for synovitis. Semin. Arthritis Rheum., *13*:322–328, 1984.
5. Healey, L.A., and Wilske, K.R.: The Systemic Manifestations of Temporal Arteritis. New York, Grune & Stratton, 1978.

section VII

MISCELLANEOUS RHEUMATIC DISEASES

NONARTICULAR RHEUMATISM AND PSYCHOGENIC MUSCULOSKELETAL SYNDROMES

80

HUGH A. SMYTHE

Many patients experience deep pain that does not arise from the local joints. Disease may be clearly evident in other local structures, but often the origin of the complaints is not immediately obvious. Soreness and stiffness are described in tissues that seem normal on objective examination, except perhaps for local tenderness. In this situation, the diagnostic labels assigned, even by mature clinicians, have differed widely. The symptoms may be attributed to subtle local pathology, a referred pain syndrome, "fibrositis," or a psychogenic regional pain syndrome.

A scientific basis for the study of these patients is rapidly evolving, based on data from well-designed prospective studies of the tender sites (Table 80–1). These tender points are central to the mystery, the recognition, and the understanding of nonarticular rheumatism. Screening for nonarticular tenderness must become a routine part of the assessment of the patient in pain even if other conditions are known to be present. Many of the telltale sites are not known to the patient and not central to the areas of pain, so the evidence is only available to a skilled examiner

with a systematic approach. Problems of interpretation remain, but the most urgent challenge to rheumatologists is to transfer these skills to other physicians.

FIBROSITIS (FIBROMYALGIA) SYNDROME

Fibrositis syndrome is one of the most common conditions diagnosed in new patients seen by practicing rheumatologists.[1,2] It is most common (80 to 90%) in women and in midlife (30 to 60 years),[3–5] but it may be seen at any age, even in childhood.[6] Essential to the diagnosis of fibrositis is the discovery of localized sites of deep tenderness. This tenderness is real and measurable, but histologic studies have failed to reveal inflammation in the tissues from the tender site. Speculation as to the nature of these sites has a long history, and the early German literature has been splendidly reviewed by Simons.[7,8] In 1904 Gowers introduced the term *fibrositis* to describe hypothetical inflammatory changes in the fibrous structure of lumbar muscles.[9] Many observers described induration at the sites of tenderness, which were ". . . objective and demonstrable, although still in the minds of many they are only accessible to the finger of faith."[10,11] These sites usually represent areas of muscle spasm, fatty lumps, or variations in muscle density found equally often in control subjects. Because of the ab-

Table 80–1.   Differential Diagnosis of Nonarticular Tenderness

Normal variations in pain threshold
Local inflammation, such as bursitis, enthesopathy
Referred and "fibrositic" tenderness
Diffuse regional tenderness, as in steroid shins, or reflex dystrophy
Nerve tenderness; popliteal, femoral, carpal tunnel
Tenderness in psychogenic regional pain

1241

sence of inflammation, many authors have preferred the term *fibromyalgia*.

The fibrositis syndrome is a complex blend of features summarized in Table 80–2. The pain or aching is diffuse, generally in deep tissues in the broad regions of reference of the cervical and lumbar segments, including the shoulder and pelvic girdles, upper chest, elbow and knee regions, and hands. Headaches are common; their location can be supraorbital or temporal as well as occipital. Subjective swelling in the limbs is often described, though little is visible to the observer. A sense of numbness is common in the hands and feet. The symptoms are worse in the morning, at which time they are usually accompanied by marked stiffness and fatigue. All are aggravated by fatigue, chilling, tension, excessive use, or immobility and may be eased by heat, massage, gentle activity, or a holiday.

The patients tend to be perfectionist, demanding of themselves and others, and effective in their chosen areas of activity. Unlike classic victims of civilized tension, they dislike the effects of tranquilizers and use drugs and alcohol sparingly. Their vices are their virtues carried to excess. They hate to complain, they respectfully doubt, they forgivably fail to comply, they loyally reject. They are not abnormal, just archetypal.

It has often been suggested that these patients are depressed or suffering from "masked depression,"[12,13] and a family history of depression is reportedly common.[14] Commonly used personality inventories demonstrated differences between "fibrositics" and controls, with significant elevation in scales suggesting hysteria, hypochondriasis, and depression, using the Minnesota Multiphasic Personality Inventory (MMPI) and similar questionnaires. This finding is almost certainly artifactual,[15] due to the inclusion of questions, scored on these scales, which reflect the presence of pain and disability. The same phenomenon has been documented in patients with rheumatoid arthritis (RA)[16,17] and in those with back pain. They are concerned, frightened, frustrated, and sometimes angry. These are normal reactions, given their distress and the lack of assistance and understanding that they have previously received; they are not withdrawn or akinetic, they tolerate large doses of tricyclics poorly,

Table 80–2. Cardinal Features of Fibrositis

> A rheumatic pain syndrome
> Specific site tenderness
> High sensitivity to internal and external stimuli
> Nonrestorative sleep
> The "fibrositic" personality

and they differ in many ways from patients with depression of biochemical origin.

The patients relax poorly and are unhappy during examination. Their well-preserved musculature is in striking contrast to their account of chronic misery and disability. Active movements may be carried out slowly, with grimacing and spasmodic overactivity of antagonists as well as prime movers. Passive movements stimulate a variable plastic resistiveness, but a full range of joint motion is obtained with gentle persuasion. Grip testing reveals a weak and variable end point, approached slowly and irregularly. Tenderness not only is reported but often is demonstrated by a characteristic sudden writhing leap, called the "jump sign." Some of these features[18] suggest that the patients are dramatizing their illness and not giving their best effort.

THE TENDER POINTS

Many characteristics of the tender points argue strongly against the suggestion that the tenderness is due to psychologic factors. This is a key point, because the demonstration of tenderness becomes a semi-objective examination, in contrast to the symptoms, which are entirely subjective. The tender sites are precisely predictable in location and, being deep, are not represented in the cerebral cortex and hence are not in the body image or psychologic sense of self. They are often unknown to the patient and often not central to the area of pain. Their predictability and association with the general pain-stiffness-fatigue syndrome have been confirmed in many studies.[3,4,19,20] These sites are normally slightly tender, and their location can be verified and studied on normal subjects. Fourteen such sites have been described in detail (Fig. 80–1 and Table 80–3).[21] These sites differentiate normal from fibrositic subjects.[3] With some loss of efficiency, the list could be extended to include the origin of pectoralis minor, medial epicondyles, tip of coracoid, occiput, infraspinatus origins, rhomboids, levator scapulae, greater trochanter, the "anserine bursa" site just distal to the knee medially, the lower soleus, and the origin of the short flexor muscle to the great toe. As many as 53 sites were defined in one prospective study.[4]

It may be worth reviewing the detailed anatomy of two of these sites. The tenderness distal to the lateral epicondyle—the "tennis elbow" site—is not a round spot as pictured in Figure 80–1 but is a narrow line of tenderness, which may begin at the epicondyle and extend up to 10 cm distally, usually maximal between 2 and 5 cm along this line. It is closely related to the

FIG. 80–1. Location of 14 typical sites of deep tenderness in fibrositis. (From Smythe, H.A., and Moldofsky, H.[21])

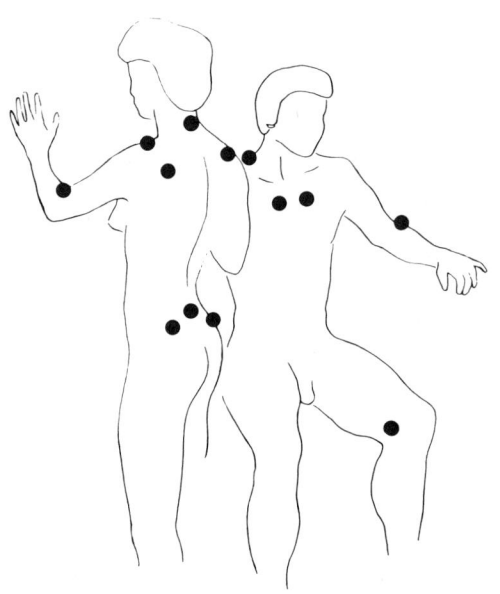

Table 80–3. Fourteen Sites of Tenderness in Fibrositis

These sites are normally somewhat tender; thus, they should be palpated with about 80% of the force used in adjacent control areas. The overlying skin is not normally tender, but may be hyperesthetic if referred pain is present.

Trapezius (R and L)
  The midpoint of the upper fold of trapezius, in a firm part of the muscle.

Second costochondral junctions (R and L)
  At or just lateral to the junction, often more marked on superior surface of rib, at the origin of pectoralis major. Overlying reactive hyperemia often develops. (Costochondral junctions may also be tender.)

Supraspinatus origins (R and L)
  Above scapular spine, near the medial border of scapula.

Lateral elbows (R and L)
  The "tennis elbow" sites, 2–5 cm distal to epicondyle, precisely located by extending and relaxing the third (long) finger. Medial epicondyle may also be tender.

Buttocks (R and L)
  In the midpart of the upper outer quadrant of buttock, in anterior portion of gluteus medius.

Knees (R and L)
  In the fat pad medial to the knee, proximal to the joint line, and overlying medial collateral ligament.

Neck
  Most marked tenderness is behind lower sternomastoid, at the anterior aspect of intertransverse ligaments at C4-C5 and C5-C6; posterior interspinous tenderness is much less.

Low Lumbar Region
  Most marked usually at L4-L5 interspinous ligament, slightly less so at L5-S1.

lateral intermuscular septum. If the examiner palpates the nontender flexor muscles with the patient's forearm supine and then slowly rotates the forearm into pronation, the patient will react sharply as the septum passes under the thumb and then relax again as the pressure moves to the extensor aspect. Clearly, the tender structure is attached to radius rather than lateral epicondyle, and lies deep, close to the attachment of the septum to bone.

The tenderness about the medial knee is even more interesting. Very commonly, the pain in the knee region is referred to the lateral or posterior aspects, which of course are not the site of the primary pathology and are not very tender; they are useful control sites. There are two sites of maximum tenderness medially, one best demonstrated by pinching the deep subcutaneous fat overlying the tendons of the medial hamstrings 3 to 6 cm proximal to the joint line and one overlying the insertion of these tendons, slightly more posterior and distal to the joint line. These two islands of tenderness usually occur together but are separated by a zone of much lesser tenderness over the joint line itself. The pinch technique shows that the tenderness is superficial to the tendons, so that the diagnosis of bursitis—anserine[22] or other—is simply wrong.

Tenderness can be detected and mapped most sensitively with the finger and scored effectively by simply counting the number of predefined points found to be tender. Better numeric definition and formal validation can be done using a dolorimeter to quantify tenderness.[23] The study of Campbell, et al.[3] (Fig. 80–2) demonstrated both the difference between normal and fibrositic individuals and also the difference between predefined fibrositic points and control sites. The dolorimeter is clearly a valuable research tool but is also useful didactically, because patients suspect that their extreme tenderness is deliberately created by the examiner. It is also useful, perhaps essential, in documenting the key findings in controversial medicolegal cases. The dolorimeter can instruct the finger; how hard should you press? Large-scale formal studies are in progress,[24] but analyses of small-scale studies (Fig. 80–3) suggest that tenderness described at less than 3 kg of force is probably abnormal and at more than 4 kg, probably normal.

Skinfold Tenderness

Skinfold tenderness over the upper scapular region may be extreme and is present in 85% of those with 12 or more tender points.[20] Testing for skinfold tenderness, or for costochondral or other deep tenderness, is often followed by a marked reactive hyperemia of the overlying skin, which speaks eloquently

FIG. 80–2. Tenderness at selected sites. Tenderness in both fibrositics and controls is shown; low values indicate increased tenderness. (After Campbell, S.M., et al.[3])

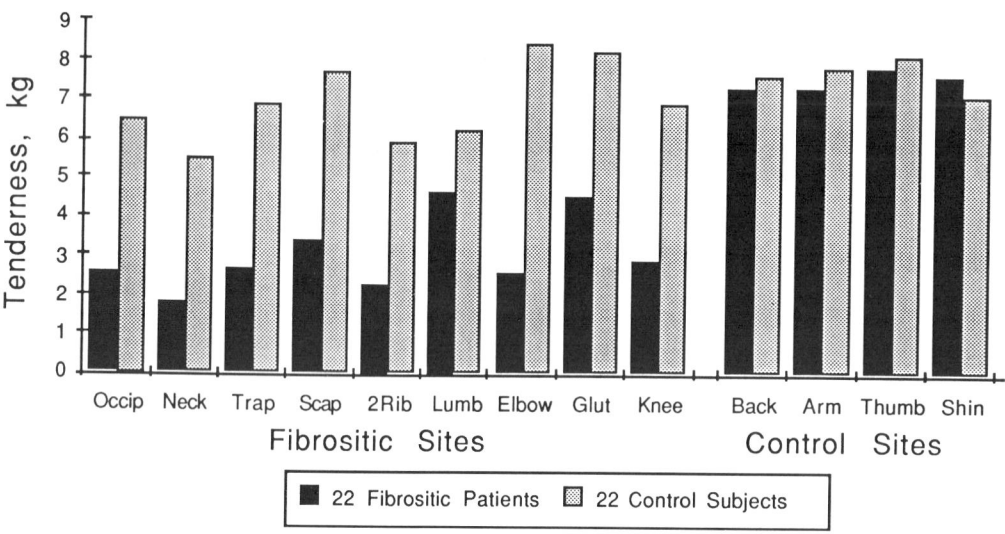

FIG. 80–3. Relative operating characteristics curve for a single dolorimeter reading. If the method had no discriminating power, the curve would have followed the 45° line of identity. Distribution of individual dolorimeter readings at eight sites by four observers, in two fibrositic individuals and two controls. Group mean tenderness in fibrositics was 2.17; controls, 6.53. Note similarity to the data of Campbell et al.[3] True positives = proportion of points in fibrositic patients with dolorimeter readings less than value shown. False positives = proportion of points in nonfibrositic patients with dolorimeter readings less than value shown.

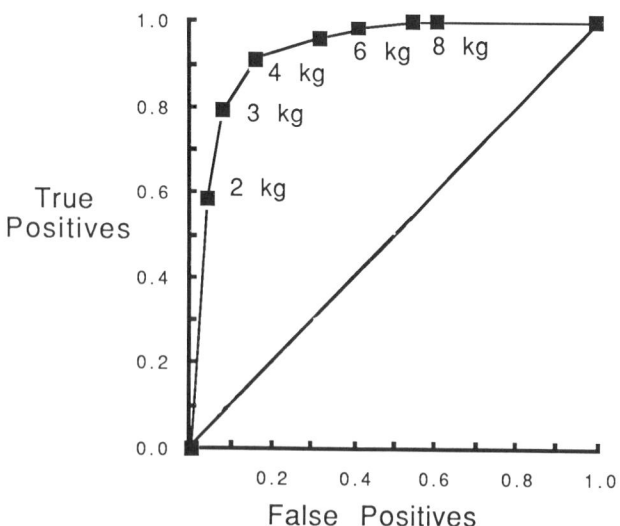

for the location and physiogenic nature of the pain. All these observations can and should be checked by similarly firm palpation of control areas, which have been shown to be normally tender in fibrositic patients[3] (see Fig. 80–2). Blood studies including cell counts, erythrocyte sedimentation rates, serum proteins, and muscle enzyme studies—a requirement by definition for the diagnosis of primary fibrositis—are usually normal.

The "Irritable Everything" Features

Not only are pain messages amplified in fibrositic patients, but these patients may also be profoundly hypersensitive to a variety of external and internal stimuli. They are sensitive to weather change, cold, drafts, cigarette smoke and other environmental irritants, and internal stimuli. They complain of dryness and a gritty sensation in their eyes in the absence of objective evidence of the sicca syndrome.[25] They may have the irritable bowel syndrome;[4] an irritable bladder with nocturia and urinary urgency and frequency; and a dry irritative cough persisting for months; they generally describe multiple symptoms.[26,27]

SLEEP DISTURBANCE

Patients who met very strict criteria for the fibrositis syndrome[28] uniformly complained of a nonrestorative sleep, with intensification of pain, stiffness, and fatigue on awakening. Key studies, still not confirmed, have provided evidence for a link between disturbed sleep and disturbed pain modulation. In the first study,[29] 10 fibrositic patients were observed, using standard electroencephalogram (EEG) techniques. All subjects showed an overnight increase in tenderness at predetermined sites, and all showed a disturbance in non–rapid-eye-movement (non-REM) sleep (see Fig. 80–3). No disturbance of REM sleep was found. These observations have since been extended in a large number of patients.

In another study, experimental reproduction of fibrositis symptoms was attempted in healthy university students.[30] After baseline studies were performed, they were deprived during 3 nights of REM sleep (seven subjects) or stage-4 slow-wave non-REM sleep (six subjects), by means of a buzzer, supplemented when necessary by hand arousal. Only those who experienced slow-wave sleep deprivation showed a significant increase in tenderness, as measured by dolorimeter scores. In addition, many of these patients suffered from anorexia, overwhelming physical tiredness, heaviness, or sluggishness to the point of experiencing difficulty with walking or standing. The symptoms disappeared during the recovery nights, and did not occur after REM sleep deprivation.[30]

Physical fitness may be an important factor. In a pilot study, three subjects who were accustomed to running 2 to 7 miles/day did not develop pain symptoms or increases in dolorimeter scores while undergoing stage-4 sleep deprivation.

The auditory stimulus used to disturb the subjects in stage-4 sleep caused an α-rhythm to appear in the EEG, superimposed on the slow-wave (δ) rhythm, much like the pattern found spontaneously in our fibrositis patients (Fig. 80–4). The spontaneous α-intrusion into the slow-wave non-REM rhythm of the fibrositis subjects was attributed to a spontaneous arousal system, analogous to the external arousal stimulus used experimentally. In Moldofsky's studies,[24,30] the frequency spectra were analyzed by computer, also illustrated in Figure 80–4. α-Intrusion into δ-sleep in high-energy bursts can be recognized by eye and was described as α–δ-sleep.[31] The author described this pattern in one patient with aching, stiffness, and fatigue relieved by amitriptyline. The effect of chlorpromazine on the fibrositis syndrome was explored in eight subjects and produced an increase in slow-wave sleep and a decrease in both subjective pain and dolorimeter scores.[32]

Apart from the experimental evidence linking fibrositic pain and tenderness to sleep disturbance, many clinical studies of the syndrome have documented the frequency of fatigue, especially in the morning.[3,4,20,25] In some, a sense of exhaustion predominates pain as the chief complaint.

The number of tender points was recorded in an unsorted group of patients presenting at an ambulatory rheumatic disease clinic (Fig. 80–5).[33] Over 30% had at least one point, 19% at least four. Most of these patients did not have the exhaustion, morning stiffness, and "irritable everything" syndrome of the classic primary fibrositis patient. At least three groups can be perceived among the patients with tender points: referred pain syndromes, "reactive" fibrositis syndrome, and chronic fibrositis syndromes (Table 80–4).

Referred Pain Syndromes

Referred pain syndromes exhibit a small number of points clustered regionally, the "localized fibrositis" of older literature. Systemic symptoms and the characteristic personality are not found. "Reactive fibrositis" is situation related, with exhaustion, stiffness, pain, and a diffuse distribution of tender points, beginning abruptly in stressful circumstances. It may be part of a normal reaction to overwhelming pressure, grief, anger, fear, or pain; it is possibly related to sleep disturbance. The prognosis is usually benign, and psychoactive drugs should be used with caution, as the victims need all their coping skills intact. Chronic fibrositic patients have an intense, perfectionist, neat but exhausting personality. They may have other diseases (secondary fibrositis) or not (primary). Inappropriate treatment is more likely and far more hazardous if they also have RA.[34]

The prevalence and clinical picture vary with the criteria employed. If one accepts the presence of 4 of 54 tender points as a key criterion,[4] nearly 20% of clinic patients are affected; if one demands 12 of 14,[28] only 3.7% are affected.[33] Information about its prevalence in the general population is not available. Very strict criteria used in older studies helped define a classic picture of the chronic fibrositic;[28] these studies required (1) widespread aching of more than 3 months' duration; (2) local tenderness at 12 of 14 specified sites; (3) skin roll tenderness over the upper scapular region; (4) disturbed sleep, with morning fatigue and stiffness; and (5) normal erythrocyte sedimentation rate, serum glutamic-oxaloacetic transaminase (SGOT), rheumatoid factor (RF) test, antinuclear antibody (ANA), muscle enzymes, and sacroiliac films. Yunus[35] has proposed criteria based on a mix of symptoms, and Campbell et al.,[3] by the use of a structured questionnaire, similarly identified a subpopulation likely to have this syndrome. These techniques successfully identified subjects with tender points, so that criteria based on symptoms and criteria based on

FIG. 80–4. *A,* Frequency spectra and raw EEG data from non-REM (stage-4) sleep in a healthy 25-year-old subject. The spectrum shows that most amplitude is concentrated at 1 cps (δ). *B,* Non-REM sleep in a 42-year-old fibrositis patient. The spectrum shows amplitude at both 1 cps (δ) and 8 to 10 cps (α). *C,* Non-REM sleep of a healthy 21-year-old subject during stage-4 sleep deprivation. The EEG shows a clear association between external arousal (auditory stimulation) and α-onset. Again, the frequency spectrum (obtained by 10-second analysis from stimulus onset) show amplitude concentrated in the δ- and α-bands. (From Moldofsky, H., et al.[29])

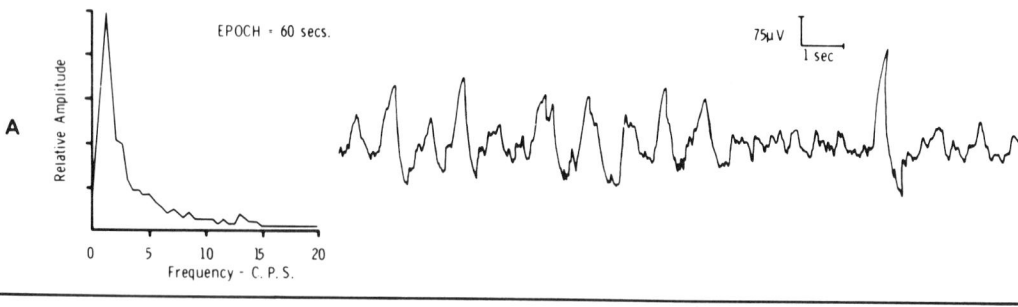

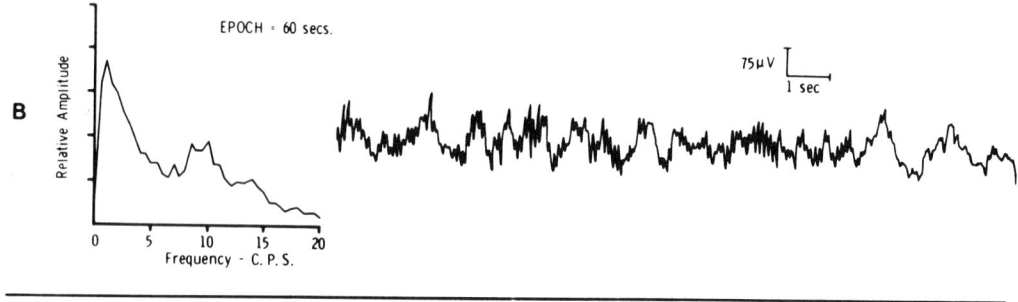

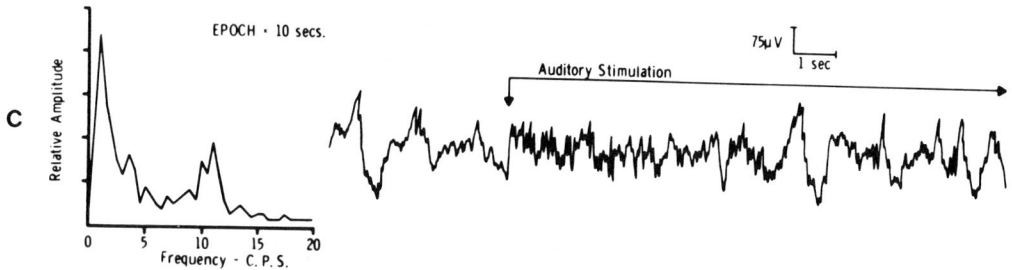

points are convergent, identifying similar populations. However, intrinsic to symptom-based criteria is a bias resulting from circular logic; there will be too many patients selected with a coincident irritable bowel syndrome if abdominal symptoms are an entry criterion. Furthermore, symptoms are subjective and might be exaggerated. Objective criteria are needed in unbiased studies, in the presence of other conditions causing pain and fatigue, and in medicolegal and other cases under dispute.

Criteria based on tender points help to differentiate fibrositic pain from pain that is malingering pretense or neurotically symbolic. The specific predictability of location of the deep tender sites, unrepresented in

the cerebral cortex, with a detailed anatomy unknown to the patient, the reactive hyperemia accompanying skinfold tenderness, and the reproduction of the syndrome in normal volunteers by slow-wave sleep deprivation, all indicate the importance of physiogenic mechanisms.

PROGNOSIS

Objective evaluation continues to indicate excellent general health, and muscle bulk and range of passive joint movement remain normal. Temporary alleviation of discomfort can be obtained with a variety of

FIG. 80–5. Prevalence of fibrositic tender points in 980 mixed rheumatic disease patients. (Data from Wolfe, F., and Cathey, M.A.[33])

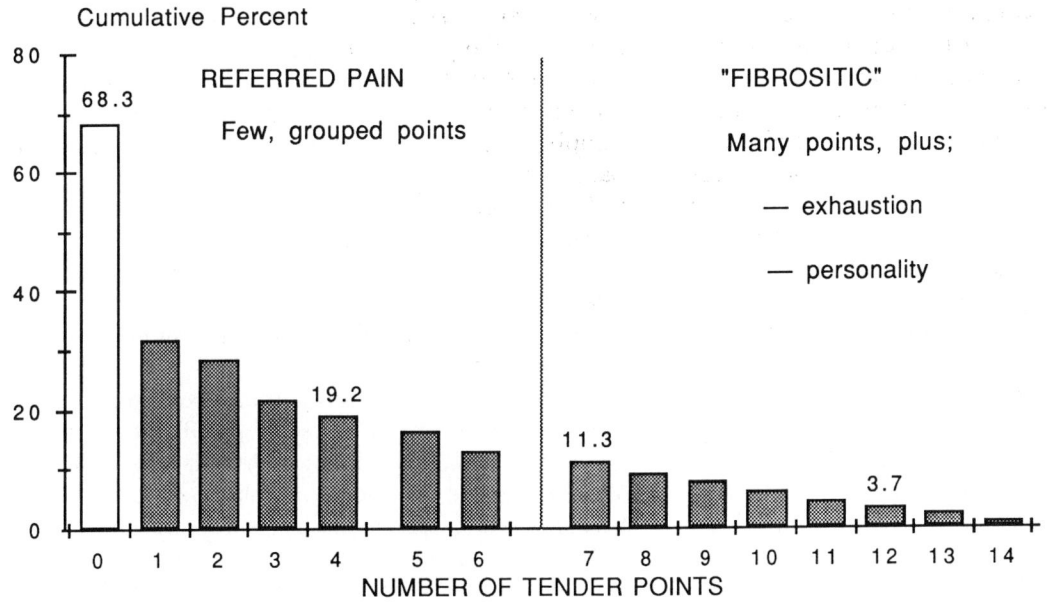

programs, but loss of all symptoms is extremely unusual.[36] In controlled trials, placebo-treated groups showed a remarkable absence of spontaneous improvement.[37–41] (These studies document the test–retest stability of tender point counts or dolorimeter scores and are valuable sources of data for validation studies and for variance estimates required for the estimation of sample sizes required in future studies.) Interruption of employment can be a disaster. Few of these patients ever return to full productive capacity if failing performance due to pain and exhaustion causes them to be fired or to resign. The meager effects of the most intensive multidisciplinary efforts at rehabilitation of these apparently fit patients is in striking contrast to the relative ease with which major functional improvement can be effected in most patients with RA, In general, the syndrome waxes and wanes for many years. Hench[42] noted 50 years ago that pregnancy or jaundice relieves the symptoms of fibrositis completely and predictably.

PATHOGENESIS

A group of patients can be identified by symptoms or solely by the presence of very tender points at sites predicted by the observer but unknown to the subject. Histologically, these sites show no changes sufficient to account for the extreme tenderness. These and other features suggest that fibrositis/fibromyalgia is a pain-amplification syndrome.

Moldofsky, et al.[43] reproduced many features of the syndrome by experimental sleep disturbance—findings that are crucial to developing a theory of pathogenesis. If these results are verified, the syndrome must be essentially a neurologic phenomenon—in these authors' terms, a "pain-modulation" disorder involving subcortical and spinal gating mechanisms. The explosion of knowledge about the down-regulation of pain mediated by endorphins has focused intense interest on the mechanisms of alterating neural message transmission and on the stimulating and inhibiting neurotransmitters. At this point, much more is known about basic mechanisms of pain relief than about pain amplification. Why are some sites and some patients particularly tender?

Table 80–4. Fibrositis (Fibromyalgia) Subtypes

Primary Fibrositis
  Chronic, sleep deprivation, typical personality (see text)
Secondary Fibrositis
  Findings as in primary but occur in association with another condition, e.g., rheumatoid arthritis
"Reactive" Fibrositis
  Situation-related, abrupt onset coincident with stressful event, disappears as stress is relieved
Referred Pain Syndrome (localized fibrositis)
  Tender points are clustered regionally, often follows trauma, especially whiplash

Deep Pain

Exact knowledge of the position in space of such structures as the hand is essential to its function, and a mental image of the hand can be summoned at any time. Thus, a body image of the superficial parts of the body exists and is based on specialized cerebrocortical representation.[44] However, no such image is formed of deeply lying structures. No cerebral cortex is assigned to keep account of deep events, and these event do not lie within the body image. Pain of deep origin must be referred, that is, misinterpreted as arising in other areas. Lewis and Kellgren[44] showed that pain localization after stimulation of deep ligaments, fascia, and muscles was grossly inaccurate, with spread of pain sensation distally to other tissues broadly sharing the same nerve supply, deep enough to share the quality of deep pain, but superficial enough to be included in the body image.

Persistent pain of any origin gives rise to protective reflex changes. These include muscle spasm, inhibition of voluntary movement, increased blood flow, and cutaneous or deep hyperalgesia. Because neural localization may be wildly inaccurate when pain is of deep origin, these reflex effects may be found in areas far removed from the original site of pathologic change.

The patient with pain due to chronic cervical strain will have marked tenderness deep in the low anterior neck but will also have referred tenderness of the unaffected intervertebral ligaments, often in the mid-trapezius, spinal muscles, and epicondyles (see Chapter 90 on the cervical spine). It is not a coincidence that these are the same sites found to be tender in the fibrositis syndrome. If reflex deep hyperalgesia is present, local anesthesia results in abolition or marked diminution of pain. The pain associated with reflex hyperalgesia may be aggravated by many factors, of which cold is the best studied.[44]

Sites of Origin of Referred Pain

Most deep pain is referred distally. Most fibrositic pain is in the areas of reference of the lower cervical and two lower lumbar levels. Acute cervical or lumbar syndromes are commonly associated with referred tenderness in the same local fibrositic points. Mechanical stresses in these two regions may therefore play a part in the production of symptoms in patients with fibrositis. These two sites are uniquely susceptible for mechanical reasons, arising from our uniquely human anatomy.

OTHER THEORIES OF ETIOLOGY

There are alternative hypotheses: a tension rheumatism, an attention rheumatism, a postviral syndrome, an immunologic disorder, or a myofascial pain syndrome caused by hypoxia, repetitive microtrauma, or other pathology.

For over a century, many investigators hypothesized that the pain arises from muscle, fat, or fascial disorder.[7,8,45,47] No histologic studies showed inflammation or necrosis, and little more than type-2 fiber atrophy was shown using standard techniques.[45] The painful muscles were usually silent electromyographically.[46] More recent studies, using electron microscopic and other newer techniques, have described subtle changes, the significance of which is not yet clear.

Trapezius muscle biopsy, studied by electron microscopy, has shown vacuolization resulting from lipid and glycogen accumulations, increases in number with variations in morphology of mitochondria, and other nonspecific changes.[46–48] Massage of tender shoulder girdle muscles was followed by release of myoglobin into the circulation.[46a] Hypoxia as a factor was supported by several studies. Oxygen tension was measured over time with an array of eight separate sensors, in subcutaneous tissue and muscle in the trapezius and nontender brachioradialis regions. The data and interpretations were complex but indicated hypoxia in *both* fat and muscle, in the tender site but not the control site.[49] Biochemical studies showed low levels of high-energy phosphate compounds, with increased low-energy phosphates, in tender trapezius muscle as compared to anterior tibial and to controls.[50]

These data are impressive, but another study illustrates the problems of study design and interpretation. Xenon-133 clearance as an index of blood flow was measured in anterior tibial muscle after 3 minutes of standardized exercise in 16 fibrositis patients and in three control groups—16 sedentary controls, 12 exercising controls, and 2 very fit controls. The results are illustrated in Figure 80–6 and indicate a clear difference between the fibrositis patients and all controls, perhaps because, as a group, the fibrositics were less fit.[51]

Apart from fitness, there may be other factors that make an individual more susceptible to pain. Biopsies from (nontender) quadriceps muscle in 13 fibrositis patients showed fine bands surrounding and joining muscle fibers, which were not seen in 7 controls. There is little information on the controls, but the patients were weaker (perhaps less fit) than the controls.[52] Reading biopsies from subjects unknown to them, Caro et al.[53] described deposits of immunoglobulin G (IgG) at the dermoepidermal junction in normal, sun-exposed skin of the distal forearm in 19 of 36 fibrositis patients and 2 of 12 controls. The pat-

FIG. 80–6. Xenon-133 clearance in anterior tibial muscle demonstrating exercising muscle blood flow after 3 minutes of standardized exercise in 16 fibrositis patients, 16 sedentary controls, 12 exercising controls, and 2 very fit controls.[7] Fitness makes a difference.

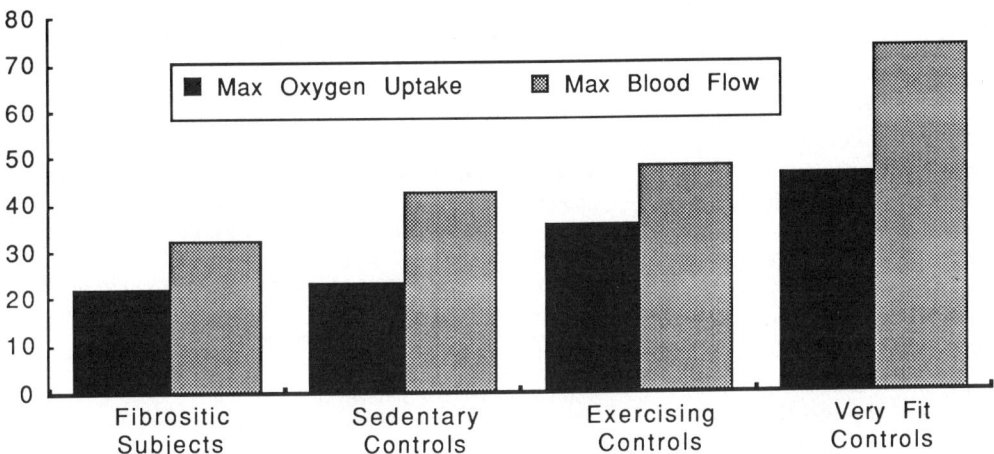

terns differed from the classic "lupus band," and albumin deposits paralleled IgG in both groups. A subset of fibrositis patients with IgG deposits showed a reticular skin pattern.

Adequate studies of the pathology of other tender points are still not available. There are no studies of nonmuscular sites, such as the fatty tissues in the medial knee region. Descriptions of the pathology at the lateral elbow still concentrate on the region between the radial neck and the lateral epicondyle and not on the more tender distal section that moves with the radius.

Trauma and Occupation

Trauma may initiate a chronic fibrositis syndrome,[20] with a frequency of 24% in one study of 95 patients. In addition, "injury" to the neck was described in 40% before the onset of symptoms and to the low back in 31%, significantly more often than in community controls (14 and 19%, respectively). This sequence is of significant medicolegal importance. In this series, the diagnosis was based on objective criteria (tender points) rather than subjective criteria. The special association with neck injury is notable because of the interaction between the cervical spine, nocturnal pain, and sleep disturbance. The chronicity of complaints after seemingly minor injury may be explained by reinjury of the affected site during sleep. Saskin, et al.[54] compared 11 fibrositis patients and 11 with "postaccident pain syndrome" and found identical diffuse pain, exhaustion point tenderness, personality scores, and sleep EEG disturbance.

Exposure

Exposure to cold, wet, drafts, and sudden changes in weather may precipitate or aggravate symptoms by mechanisms not fully understood. Kellgren[44] studied the effect of cooling on pain. He noted that when deep hyperalgesia is present, slow cooling of the affected part caused severe and prolonged pain, and the analgesia that normally accompanied cooling developed imperfectly unless the tissues were cooled to a low temperature (10°C). This phenomenon may contribute to the weather effect noted by so many patients.

Depression

Markers of depression, such as delayed sleep onset and abnormal dexamethasone suppression test, are usually absent. Low imipramine binding has been reported in depression, but elevated binding was found in fibrositis/fibromyalgia patients.[55]

Secondary Fibrositis

Discomfort similar to that of primary fibrositis is common as an accompaniment to a variety of other disorders. These range from myalgia following unaccustomed exercise or associated with viral infection,[55a] exhaustion, widespread pain, and characteristic tender points associated with a wide variety of arthropathies and other diseases.[56] An associated major sleep disturbance has been found whenever studied,[57–59] and mechanistically, it is likely that secondary fibrositis is usually the same as primary fibrositis, but associated with another disease, with each process aggravating symptoms of the other. The pain of polymyalgia rheumatica can easily be mistaken for fibrositis when the patient is first seen, but the inflammatory features, especially elevated erythrocyte sedimentation rate, permit rapid differentiation (see Chapter 79).

Treatment. A patient with fibrositis often comes to the physician feeling threatened by the illness and the associated problems and may be defensive, reacting negatively to any message interpreted as a further threat. The task of explanation may challenge the physician's skill, training, and imagination. Prescribing an analgesic regimen is relatively easy, but giving the patient an adequate account of the origins of the symptoms, in particular dealing with the relationship between pain and tension, can be extremely difficult. Patients expect physicians to use euphemisms and will examine words carefully for unfavorable underlying meanings. Thus, the suggestion that symptoms are of emotional origin or the use of the word *anxiety* may be translated by the patient into an accusation of inadequacy or willful malingering. The physician is further handicapped by the complexities of the explanation that must be given. An intelligent, curious patient may need a thorough, general discussion of referred pain and the origin of tension before his own problems are discussed. A less complex patient may need only reassurance and a positive program. The patient who is demoralized and no longer able to cope may need a brief hospitalization and a period of sympathetic protection before recovering sufficient confidence to reconstruct habits and attitudes.

A minimum initial discussion may cover (1) referred pain and deep tenderness; (2) mechanical stresses in neck and low back; (3) the sleep disturbance; and (4) attitudes and expectations (Table 80–5).

Four controlled trials have reported the effects of tricyclics in patients with the fibrositis/fibromyalgia syndrome; three documented modest improvement.[37–40] The prolonged duration of action (half-life of about 30 hours) restricts the maximum dosage usable because of daytime drowsiness or dry mouth.

Aerobic exercise may be a preferable, if difficult, long-term therapy, with documented benefit in a controlled trial.[41] Weak abdominal muscles underlying a vulnerable back should be dealt with first. Swimming in a heated pool is safest, and bicycling is effective. The patient must be encouraged to persevere, because such exercise increases symptoms at first. The exercise program should begin at modest levels and gradually be increased.

PSYCHOGENIC MUSCULOSKELETAL SYNDROMES

Four types of relationships, not mutually exclusive, between mental state and musculoskeletal symptoms

Table 80–5. Management of Fibrositis

Reassurance
    Disease is not crippling, but pain and fatigue are "real"
Explanation of Origin of Pain
    In greater or lesser detail, patients should be told:
        Referred tenderness is at constant, predictable sites
        Exaggerated reflex hyperemia indicates tissue hyperreactivity
        Condition is aggravated by cold, sleep disturbance, tension, and depression
Relief of Mechanical Stresses in Neck and Low Back
    Probably the primary source of origin or referred pain and tenderness
        Because the neck is vulnerable to stresses during sleep, support the lower neck
        Because the low back is vulnerable when locked in hyperextension, need strong abdominal muscles, flexed low back; abdominal support and an unsagging mattress may help
Medical Therapies
    Need for compliance, persistence
        Salicylates or other simple analgesics to break chronic pain cycles
        Heat, massage, liniments, or other counterirritant and relaxation therapies
        Amitriptyline, 10 to 75 mg hs or equivalent, for sleep disturbance
Attitudes and Expectations
    Recognize perfectionistic impatience
    Challenges give life meaning; accept without limitations
    Break tension with rest, diversion, exercise, or escape
    Pursue fitness (even if there is increase in symptoms)

may be seen: (1) psychosomatic production of symptoms or disease; (2) exaggeration (or denial), subconscious use of existing disease for secondary gain; (3) conversion reactions, that is, psychogenic regional pain and hysteria; and (4) malingering.

Recognizing organic disease in normally reacting individuals is relatively easy, as is recognizing that a patient is odd, but assessing organic disease in a disturbed patient can be difficult. Thus, major problems in diagnosis occur in all of the aforementioned four types.

Given accurate diagnosis, understanding the underlying processes in the last three categories is not difficult. Major controversy continues about the existence of and mechanisms involved in the psychosomatic production of structural changes in musculoskeletal syndromes.

STUDIES OF PSYCHOSOMATIC FACTORS IN RHEUMATOID ARTHRITIS

Studies of the psychosomatic aspects of RA abound,[60–69] and include numerous original and disciplined studies of the psychology of rheumatoid patients and excellent critical reviews. The various samples demonstrated a notably consistent finding of hidden anger, controlled by the patient because of insecurity in personal relations and expressed through "good" behavior, depression, and symptoms. Physiologic differences have also been identified, including a lower blood pressure but faster pulse, increased sweating, and colder extremities, with exaggeration of these differences when the subjects were stressed by angry criticism.[64] Few researchers claim that these differences are necessary for or specific for RA and intimately related to pathogenesis. The relevance of these phenomena to disease onset or exacerbations is controversial. Studies in identical twins discordant for RA suggested that stressful life events may be important,[65] but the one large, controlled study of circumstances surrounding the onset of RA showed equal frequency of such events before disease onset of 532 patients and in matched controls.[70]

There is no doubt that personality and disease course interact. Moldofsky and Chester[34] identified a subgroup of paradoxic responders among rheumatoid patients, whose moods worsened as inflammation lessened. Such patients arrived seemingly cheerful, brave, and compliant, but they developed anxiety and new complaints as therapy progressed. They therefore selected themselves for alternative therapies and were more likely to receive prolonged hospitalization, extensive investigation, and systemic steroid and surgical therapies with attendant increased morbidity and mortality. The patient's need for care held family, friends, and therapists close to them, and they had much to fear from restored health. These patients were often perfectionists, depressed, sleepless, and exhausted, and felt tenderness at the fibrositic sites as well as in their joints. The paradoxic response pattern was seen in nearly half of one group of hospitalized rheumatoid patients. Recognition of this pattern is of great therapeutic importance. The push toward advanced therapies must be recognized and controlled. The patient tends to blame the therapies for many symptoms, and the unhappy therapist is tempted to cruelly lay bare all the personal dynamics at work, shifting blame back on the patient. These patients require more time, sympathetic support, explanations, and acceptance from their therapist before they can cope with their very real symptoms of exhaustion, depression, stiffness, and RA.

PSYCHOGENIC REGIONAL PAIN SYNDROME

The symbolic use of pain and disability may be symptomatic of depression, schizophrenia, various psychoneuroses, psychopathic personality, or even organic psychoses. The term *psychogenic regional pain* has been proposed for this large clinical group,[71] reserving the term *hysteria* for the small number of patients showing all the features of classic hysteria. The diagnosis of psychopathology by no means rules out the presence of organic disease but greatly magnifies the difficulties in assessment and therapy.

The clinical presentation differs from the fibrositis syndrome. The distress tends to be concentrated in a single region that has emotional rather than segmental definition, such as the hand, back, anterior chest, or limbs. The distress is described dramatically, "The pain burns through my left breast and out my back." Spreading to adjacent areas is common, subject to manipulation by the questioner, with sharp, nonsegmental, and varying boundaries at such sites as the root of a limb or the midline. The paradoxic association of tenderness and numbness is common. Hyperalgesia to traction on skin hairs may coexist with reported numbness to pinprick.

These bizarre features allow a positive diagnosis of psychopathology to be made but unfortunately do not rule out the coexistence of organic disease. Resistance to movement may be quite stubborn, and re-examination after intravenous injection of thiopental, amobarbital, or diazepam may be helpful. Such an examination usually requires informed consent, given in the presence of a qualified anesthesiologist and other witnesses and must be carefully described in the patient's records.

ANATOMIC CHANGES

Most patients with neurotic or psychotic complaints have no clinical or radiologic abnormalities. When diffuse swelling, osteopenia, restricted movement, or changes of sclerodactyly are attributed to "disuse" of functional origin, the burden of proof is heavy on the physician responsible for the diagnosis. In many cases, reflex dystrophic reactions or even major local disease is overlooked.

OTHER SOFT-TISSUE PAIN SYNDROMES

Weak abdominal muscles underlying a vulnerable back should be dealt with first. Not all inferior heel pain is due to spondylitis. Athletes, especially runners, develop chronic pain at exactly the same site with similar late ossification of the fascial insertion, presumably in response to chronic trauma. Again, similar lesions develop in many other sites, notably the patella, greater trochanter, and elbow. Most of these patients are HLA-B27 negative and have no other stigmata of spondylitis.

The third situation in which ossification of fibrous insertions occurs is in association with ankylosing hyperostosis, otherwise known as Forestier's syndrome[72,73] or diffuse idiopathic skeletal hyperostosis (DISH).[74] Extraspinal involvement in this syndrome was also described by Forestier and involved sites including occiput, trochanters, ischia, ilia, and calcanei. In these older patients, the relationship of late ossification to earlier symptoms may be difficult to ascertain and has not yet been studied systematically (Table 80–6).

Pain at muscle–tendon junctions occurs under quite different circumstances. These lesions are not commonly associated with ankylosing spondylitis, and do not calcify or progress to ossification. The most typical example is the "tennis elbow" syndrome. Tenderness just distal to the lateral epicondyle may follow local trauma, may be associated with referred pain (usually of cervical origin) or general hyperalgesia in the fibrositis syndrome, or may occur after experimental deep sleep deprivation. Similar lesions develop in the origins of the adductor muscles of the thigh in football and hockey players or in the origin of the flexor hallucis brevis in ballet dancers. The bone–tendon and muscle–tendon lesions have in common a high tissue density, where a little swelling can cause much pain, as in a tooth socket or ear canal. If steroid injections are used in therapy, the patient should be warned that a flare of pain may occur for 1 to 2 days before relief occurs.

Table 80–6. Other Causes of Soft Tissue Pain

Bursitis
Tendonitis
Tenosynovitis

Phlebitis
Vasculitis
Panniculitis

Post-exercise myalgia
Hematoma in muscle
Myalgia in virus infections
Polymyalgia rheumatica

Referred pain syndromes
Reflex dystrophies
Nerve entrapment syndromes
Pain with central nervous system disease

Muscle–tendon junction syndromes
Bone–tendon junction syndromes
Tender shins with steroid therapy

TENDER SHINS OF STEROID THERAPY

Slocumb[75] first described myalgias occurring after administration of large doses of cortisone. Rotstein and Good[76] used the term *steroid pseudorheumatism* to describe the occurrence of striking tenderness of the muscles of the extremities in five patients on high doses of oral steroids. By dolorimetry, the tenderness is more marked in the lower than in the upper extremities. It is not confined to muscle but is diffuse in the lower leg and over bone and tendon as well as muscle. It spares the feet. It is usually associated with a shiny atrophy of skin but is usually not associated with edema, evidence of neuropathy, or tender fibrositic sites. The tenderness may lessen if the steroid can be decreased or withdrawn. Tender shins are commonly found in aged subjects of both sexes; the etiology is still obscure.

HYSTERIA

Overt conversion reactions are seen occasionally by rheumatologists, orthopedists, and others dealing

FIG. 80–7. Hysterical bent knee. The patient could straighten the knee fully while lying but not while standing. He had a bizarre gait, semi-squatting with each step.

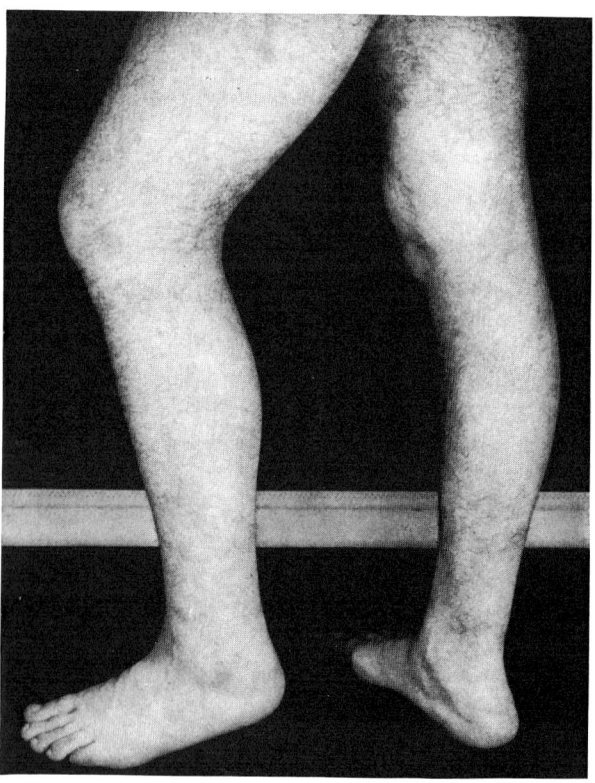

with patients with musculoskeletal complaints. These reactions can be confusing and even alarming, especially to the younger physician. The most common of these are hysterical bent back (camptocormia), hysterical bent knee (Fig. 80–7), and an inability to use one or both hands (writers' cramp). The "restless legs" syndrome is considered by some to be a depressive expression. In my experience, it often has hysterical features. The typical patient complains of boring pains in the legs or thighs at night when recumbent, relieved by walking. Placebo therapy often relieves symptoms but nearly always produces side effects such as headache and nausea.

REFERENCES

1. Bohan, A.: The private practice of rheumatology. Arthritis Rheum., 24:1304–1307, 1981.
2. Healey, L.A., et al. (ARA Committee on Rheumatology Practice): A description of rheumatology practice. Arthritis Rheum., 20:1278–1281, 1977.
3. Campbell, S.M., et al.: Clinical characteristics of fibrositis. Arthritis Rheum., 26:817–824, 1983.
4. Yunus, M., et al.: Primary fibromyalgia (fibrositis): Clinical study of 50 patients with matched normal controls. Semin. Arthritis Rheum., 11:151–171, 1981.
5. Dinerman, H., Goldenberg, D.L., and Felson, D.T.: A prospective evaluation of 118 patients with the fibromyalgia syndrome: Prevalence of Raynaud's phenomenon, sicca symptoms, ANA, low complement, and Ig deposition at the dermal-epidermal junction. J. Rheumatol., 13:368, 1986.
6. Yunus, M.B., and Masi, A.T.: Juvenile primary fibromyalgia syndrome: A clinical study of thirty-three patients and matched normal controls. Arthritis Rheum., 28:138–145, 1985.
7. Simons, D.G.: Muscle pain syndromes. Part 1. Am. J. Phys. Med., 54:289–311, 1975.
8. Simons, D.G.: Muscle pain syndromes. Part 2. Am. J. Phys. Med., 55:15–42, 1976.
9. Gowers, W.R.: A lecture on lumbago: Its lessons and analogues. Br. Med. J., 1:117–121, 1904.
10. Telling, W.H.M.: The clinical importance of fibrositis in general practice. Br. Med. J., 1:689–692, 1935.
11. Hench, P.S.: The problem of rheumatism and arthritis: Review of American and English Literature from 1935. Ann. Intern. Med., 10:880, 1936.
12. Ahles, T.A., et al.: Psychological studies in primary fibromyalgia syndrome. (Abstract.) Clin. Res., 311:801, 1983.
13. Payne, T.C., et al.: Fibrositis and psychogenic disturbance. Arthritis Rheum., 25:213–217, 1982.
14. Hudson, J.I., et al.: Fibromyalgia and major affective disorder: A controlled phenomenology and family history study. Am. J. Psychiatry, 142:441–446, 1985.
15. Smythe, H.A.: Problems with the MMPI (Editorial). J. Rheumatol., 11:939–947, 1983.
16. Bradley, L., and Wolfe, F.: MMPI scores indicate the presence of disease and not psychological abnormalities in RA. Arthritis Rheum., 29(Suppl.):S23, 1986.
17. Pincus, T., et al.: MMPI scores indicate the presence of disease and not psychological abnormalities in RA. Arthritis Rheum., 29(Suppl.):S23, 1986.
18. Leavitt, F., and Sweet, J.J.: Characteristics and frequency of malingering among patients with low back pain. Pain, 25:357–264, 1986.
19. Yunus, M.B., Masi, A.T., and Aldag, J.C.: Criteria studies of primary fibromyalgia syndrome (PFS). Arthritis Rheum., 30(Suppl.):S50, 1987.
20. Wolfe, F.: The clinical syndrome of fibrositis. Am. J. Med., 81(Suppl. 3A):7–14, 1986.
21. Smythe, H.A., and Moldofsky, H.: Two contributions to understanding of the "fibrositis" syndrome. Bull. Rheum. Dis., 28:928–931, 1977.
22. Larsson, L.-G., and Baum, J.: The syndromes of bursitis. Bull. Rheum. Dis., 36:1–8, 1986.
23. McCarty, D.J., Gatter, R.D., and Steele, A.D.: A twenty pound dolorimeter for quantification of articular tenderness. Arthritis Rheum., 11:696–697, 1968.
24. Wolfe, F.: Development of criteria for the diagnosis of fibrositis. Am. J. Med., 81(Suppl. 3A):99–104, 1986.
25. Dinerman, H., Goldenberg, D.L., and Felson, D.T.: A prospective evaluation of 118 patients with the fibromyalgia syndrome: Prevalence of Raynaud's phenomenon, sicca symptoms, ANA, low complement, and Ig deposition at the dermal-epidermal junction. J. Rheumatol, 13:368, 1986.
26. Block, S.R., Quimby, L.G., and Gratwick, G.M.: Fibromyalgia: Generalised pain intolerance and manifold symptom reporting. Arthritis Rheum., 30(Suppl.):S63, 1987.
27. Caro, X.J., Kinstead, N.A., Russell, I.J., and Wolfe, F.: Increased sensitivity to health related questions in patients with primary fibrositis syndrome. Arthritis Rheum., 30(Suppl.):S63, 1987.
28. Smythe, H.A.: Nonarticular rheumatism and the "fibrositis" syndrome. In Arthritis and Allied Conditions. 8th Ed. Edited by J.L. Hollander and D.J. McCarty. Philadelphia, Lea & Febiger, 1972.
29. Moldofsky, H., et al.: Musculoskeletal symptoms and non-REM sleep disturbance in patients with the "fibrositis" syndrome and healthy subjects. Psychosom. Med., 37:341–351, 1975.
30. Moldofsky, H., and Scarisbrick, P.: Induction of neuresthenic musculoskeletal pain syndrome by selective stage sleep deprivation. Psychosom. Med., 38:35–44, 1976.
31. Haun, P., and Hawkins, D.R.: Alpha-delta sleep. Electroencephalogr. Clin. Neurophysiol., 34:233–237, 1973.
32. Moldofsky, H., et al.: Comparison of chlorpromazine and L-tryptophan on sleep, musculoskeletal pain, and mood in "fibrositis" syndrome. Sleep Res., 5:65–71, 1976.
33. Wolfe, F., and Cathey, M.A.: Prevalence of primary and secondary fibrositis. J. Rheumatol., 10:965–968, 1983.
34. Moldofsky, H., and Chester, W.J.: Pain and mood patterns in patients with rheumatoid arthritis. Psychosom. Med., 32:309–318, 1970.
35. Yunus, M.B.: Fibromyalgia syndrome: A need for uniform classification. J. Rheumatol., 10:841–844, 1983.
36. Felson, D., Dinerman, H., and Goldenberg, D.: The natural history of fibromyalgia. Arthritis Rheum., 28(Suppl):S85, 1985.
37. Goldenberg, D.L., Felson, D.T., and Dinerman, H.: A randomized, controlled trial of amitryptiline and naproxen in the treatment of patients with fibromyalgia. Arthritis Rheum., 29:1371–1377, 1986.
38. Carette, S., McCain, G.A., Bell, D.A., and Fam, A.G.: Evaluation of amitryptiline in primary fibrositis: A double-blind, placebo-controlled study. Arthritis Rheum., 29:646–659, 1986.
39. Wysenbeek, A.J., Mor, F., Lurie, Y., and Weinberger, A.: Im-

ipramine for the treatment of fibrositis: A therapeutic trial. Ann. Rheum. Dis., 44:752–753, 1985.

40. Gatter, R.A.: Pharmacotherapeutics in fibrositis. Am. J. Med., 81(Suppl. 3A):63–66, 1986.

41. McCain, G.A.: Role of physical fitness training in the fibrositis/fibromyalgia syndrome. Am. J. Med., 81(Suppl. 3A):73–77, 1986.

42. Hench, P.S.: Effect of jaundice on chronic infectious (atrophic) arthritis and on primary fibrositis. Arch. Intern. Med., 61:451–480, 1938.

43. Moldofsky, H., et al.: Sleep-related myoclonus in rheumatic pain modulation disorder (fibrositis syndrome) and in excessive daytime somnolence. Psychosom. Med., 46:145–151, 1984.

44. Kellgren, J.H.: Deep pain sensibility. Lancet, 1:943–949, 1949.

45. Bengtsson, A., Henriksson, K.G., and Larsson, J.: Muscle biopsy in primary fibromyalgia. Scand. J. Rheumatology, 15:1–6, 1986.

46. Kraft, G.H., Johnson, E.W., and LaBan, M.M.: The fibrositis syndrome. Arch. Phys. Med., 49:155–162, 1968.

46a. Danneskiold-Samsoe, B., Christansen, E., and Andersen, R.B.: Myofascial pain and the role of myoglobin. Scand. J. Rheumatology, 15:174–178, 1986.

47. Fassbender, H.G., and Wegner, K.: Morphologie und pathogenese des weichteilrhumatismus. Z. Rheumaforsch., 32:355–374, 1973.

48. Kalyan-Raman, U.P., Kalyan-Raman, K., Yunus, M.B., and Masi, A.T.: Muscle pathology in primary fibromyalgia syndrome: A light microsopic, histochemical and ultrastructural study. J. Rheumatol., 11:808–813, 1984.

49. Lund, N., Bengtsson, A., and Throborg, P.: Muscle tissue oxygen pressure in primary fibromyalgia. Scand. J. Rheumatol., 15:165–173, 1986.

50. Bengtsson, A., Hendriksson, K.G., and Larsson, J.: Reduced high-energy phosphate levels in the painful muscles of patients with primary fibromyalgia. Arthritis Rheum., 29:817–821, 1986.

51. Bonafede, P., et al.: Exercising muscle blood flow in patients with fibrositis: A [133]Xenon clearance study. (Abstract.) Arthritis Rheum., 30:514, 1987.

52. Bartels, E.M., and Danneskjold-Samsoe, B.: Histological abnormalities in muscle from patients with certain types of fibrositis. Lancet, 1:755–777, 1986.

53. Caro, X.J., Wolfe, F., Johnston, W.H., and Smith, A.L.: A controlled and blinded study of immunoreactant deposition at the dermo-epidermal junction of patients with primary fibrositis syndrome. J. Rheumatol., 13:1086–1092, 1986.

54. Saskin, P., Moldofsky, H., and Lue, F.A.: Sleep and post-traumatic pain modulation disorder (fibrositis syndrome). Psychosom. Med., 48:319–323, 1986.

55. Russell, I.J., et al.: Imipramine receptor density on platelets of patients with fibrositis syndrome: Correlation with disease severity and response to therapy. Arthritis Rheum., 30(Suppl):S63, 1987.

55a. Buchwald, D., Goldenberg, D.L., Sullivan, J.L., and Komaroff, A.L.: The "chronic Epstein-Barr virus infection" syndrome and primary fibromyalgia. Arthritis Rheum., 30:1132–1136, 1987.

56. Hench, P.K.: Secondary fibrositis. Am. J. Med., 81(Suppl. 3A):60–62, 1986.

57. Moldofsky, H., Lue, F., and Smythe, H.: Alpha EEG sleep and morning symptoms in rheumatoid arthritis. J. Rheumatol., 10:373–379, 1983.

58. Moldofsky, H., Lue, F.A., and Saskin, P.: Sleep and morning pain in primary osteoarthritis. J. Rheumatol., 14:124–128, 1987.

59. Mahowald, K.L., Mahowald, M.W., and Ytterberg, S.R.: Sleep fragmentation in rheumatoid arthritis. (Abstract.) Arthritis Rheum., 30(Suppl.):S18, 1987.

60. Cobb, S.: Contained hostility in rheumatoid arthritis. Arthritis Rheum., 2:419–425, 1959.

61. Cobb, S., et al.: The interfamilial transmission of rheumatoid arthritis. An unusual study. J. Chronic Dis., 22:193–194, 1969.

62. Cobb, S., et al.: Some psychological and social characteristics of patients hospitalized for rheumatoid arthritis, hypertension and duodenal ulcer. J. Chronic Dis., 18:1259–1279, 1965.

63. Cobb, S., Miller, M., and Wieland, M.: On the relationship between divorce and rheumatoid arthritis. Arthritis Rheum., 2:414–418, 1959.

64. Kiviniemi, P.: Emotions and personality in rheumatoid arthritis. Scand. J. Rheumatol., 18(Suppl. 6):1–132, 1977.

65. Meyerowitz, S., Jacox, R.F., and Hess, D.W.: Monozygotic twins discordant for rheumatoid arthritis: A genetic, clinical and psychological study of 8 sets. Arthritis Rheum., 11:1–21, 1968.

66. Moos, R.H.: Personality factor associated with rheumatoid arthritis: A review. J. Chronic Dis., 17:41–55, 1964.

67. Moos, R.H., and Solomon, F.G.: Psychologic comparisons between women with rheumatoid arthritis and their non-arthritic sisters. 1. Personality test and interview data. Psychosom. Med., 27:135–149, 1965.

68. Moos, R.H., and Solomon, G.F.: Personality correlates of the rapidity of progression of rheumatoid arthritis. Ann. Rheum. Dis., 23:145–151, 1964.

69. Moos, R.H., and Solomon, G.F.: Personality correlates of rheumatoid arthritic patients; response to treatment. Arthritis Rheum., 7:331, 1964.

70. Empire Rheumatism Council: A controlled investigation into the aetiology and clinical features of rheumatoid arthritis. Br. Med. J., 1:79–805, 1950.

71. Walters, J.A.: Psychogenic regional pain alias hysterical pain. Brain, 84:1–18, 1961.

72. Forestier, J., and Lagier, R.: Vertebral ankylosing hyperostosis: Morphological basis, clinical manifestations, situation and diagnosis. In Modern Trends in Rheumatology. Vol. 2. Edited by A. Hill. London, Butterworths, 1971.

73. Forestier, J., and Rotes-Querol, J.: Senile ankylosing hyperostosis of the spine. Ann. Rheum. Dis., 9:321, 1950.

74. Resnick, D., Shall, S.R., and Robbins, J.M.: Diffuse idiopathic skeletal hyperostosis (DISH): Forestier's disease with extraspinal manifestations. Radiology, 115:513–524, 1975.

75. Slocumb, C.H.: Symposium on certain problems arising from the clinical use of cortisone. Mayo Clin. Proc., 28:655–657, 1953.

76. Rotstein, J., and Good, B.A.: Steroid pseudorheumatism. Arch. Intern. Med., 99:545–555, 1957.

NEUROPATHIC JOINT DISEASE (CHARCOT JOINTS)

81

MICHAEL H. ELLMAN

Neuropathic joint disease is a progressive degenerative arthritis with characteristic clinical and roentgenologic features. Described by J.M. Charcot in 1868[1] in patients with "l'ataxie locomotrice progressive," or tabes dorsalis, it is now most commonly seen in the mid- and forefoot of patients with diabetes mellitus (Fig. 81–1). The arthritis develops after sensory loss to a joint and continued weight bearing; for unknown reasons, however, not all patients who meet these criteria develop neuroarthropathy.

It seems fitting that the eponym *Charcot joint* be retained as synonymous with neuropathic joint disease. Jean-Martin Charcot (1825 to 1893) was a master of medicine with virtuoso contributions in neurology, psychiatry, and rheumatology.[2] He is considered a "father" of neurology, and his interest in arthritis was keen and included a thesis, written in 1853, entitled *Primary Progressive Chronic Articular Rheumatism.*[3] His progressive attitude toward medicine was revealed in a lecture at the Hospital of the Salpetriere in Paris in 1867, when he stated that the essential difference between ancient and modern medicine was that in the latter, "physicians could profit by the errors of their predecessors, which roads ought to remain closed to speculation and which, on the contrary, they may traverse without fear of losing themselves."[2]

Charcot's description of neuropathic joint disease has remained the best. He emphasized the *suddenness* of the arthritis, "most commonly without any pain whatever, or any febrile reaction." Charcot described the *swelling* of the joint and the presence of a *hydrarthrosis*. "On puncture being made, a transparent lemon-colored liquid has been frequently drawn from the joint." He also mentioned *cracking sounds* at the articular surfaces, *luxations* developing, rapid *wasting* of the muscles, the presence of *foreign bodies*, and to the etiology of this arthritis, "produced . . . by the more or less energetic movements to which the patient sometimes continues to subject the affected members. . . ." Charcot felt that the joint changes were subordinate to sclerotic changes in the spinal cord, a concept of a "trophic" injury to nerves that became known as the "French theory" of neuropathic joint disease.[1,4,5] This view was violently disputed by Volkmann and Virchow, who espoused the "German theory," that neuropathic arthritis had a mechanical origin produced by insensitive joints and repeated subclinical trauma.[4-6] Charcot also described a hyperacute variant of the disease with swelling and other signs of inflammation of such severity that joint sepsis is suspected.

Schultze and Kahler described the relationship between syringomyelia and neuropathic joint disease in 1888.[7] Dearborn,[8] in 1932, described the disease in congenital insensitivity to pain in a patient who billed himself as the "human pin cushion." Jordan,[9] in 1936, chronicled neuropathic joint disease in diabetic neuropathy. By 1964, Robillard et al.[10] reviewed 100 cases of diabetic neuropathic joint disease in the medical literature, and in 1974, Clouse and co-workers[11] reported 90 cases of neuropathic joint disease and diabetes mellitus seen at a single institution over a 13-year span. "Neuropathic-like" joint disease without neurologic deficits was described in patients receiving

FIG. 81–1. The roentgenographic appearance of neuropathic joint disease of the foot and ankle has great variety. The foot is now the most common site of neuroarthropathy. *A,* This patient with diabetes mellitus had only moderate discomfort with the dislocation of the navicular bone, which was the first indication of neuropathic joint disease. *B,* Massive soft tissue swelling surrounding the joint is common in the neuropathic ankle and is frequently seen in neuroarthropathy accompanying diabetes mellitus, tabes dorsalis, congenital insensitivity to pain, or meningomyelocele.

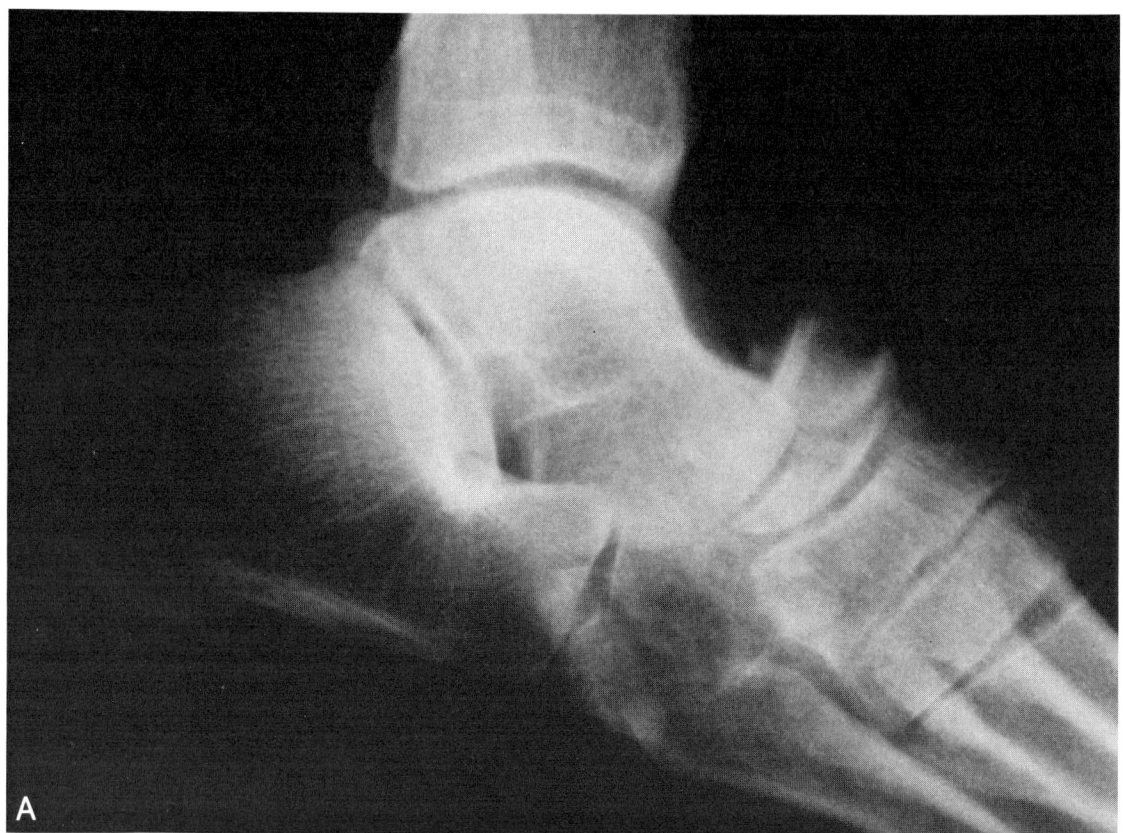

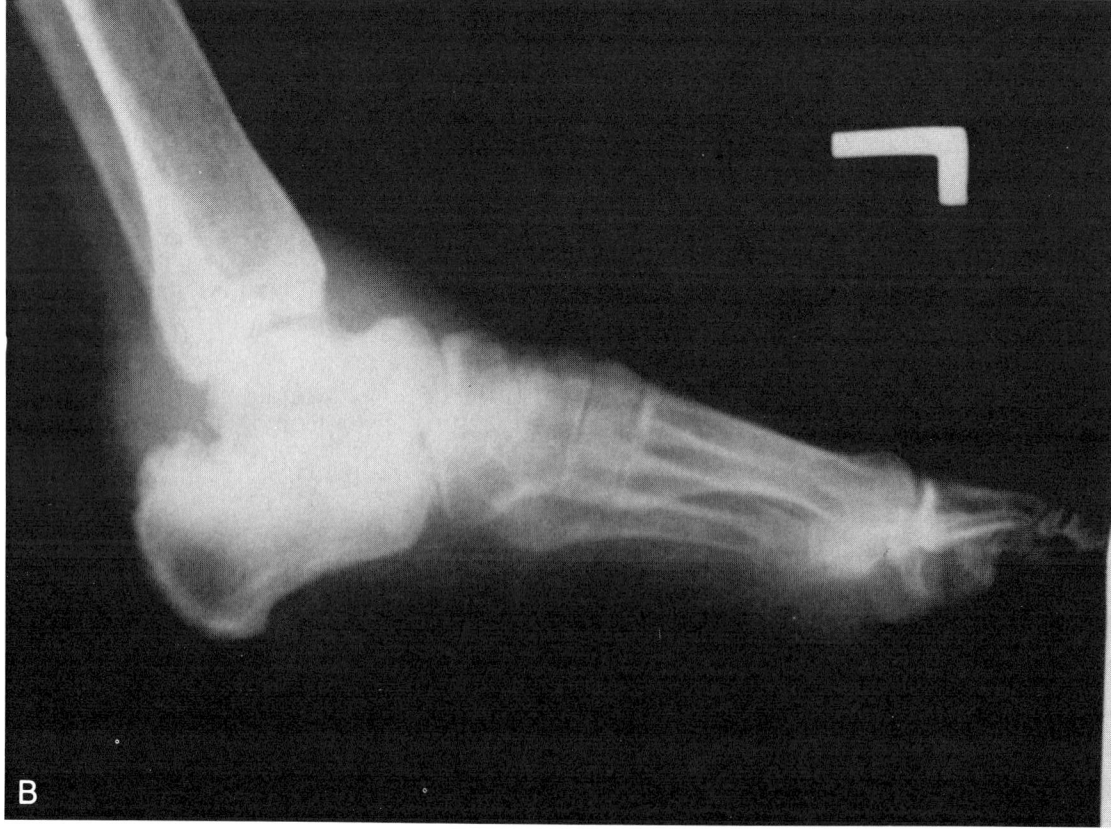

FIG. 81–1 Continued. *C,* There is striking osteolysis of the metatarsals ("sucked candy" appearance) and the phalanges in this patient with chronic diabetes mellitus. *D,* This patient with diabetes mellitus exhibits destruction, fragmentation, and displacement of the tarsometatarsal joints, which are sometimes described as "Lisfranc's fracture-dislocation" (Lisfranc actually described amputation at that site).[36,85] *E,* Another patient with diabetes mellitus with typical soft tissue swelling and fragmentation of the navicular bone. There is sharply defined osseous debris at the dorsum and posterior foot and ankle.

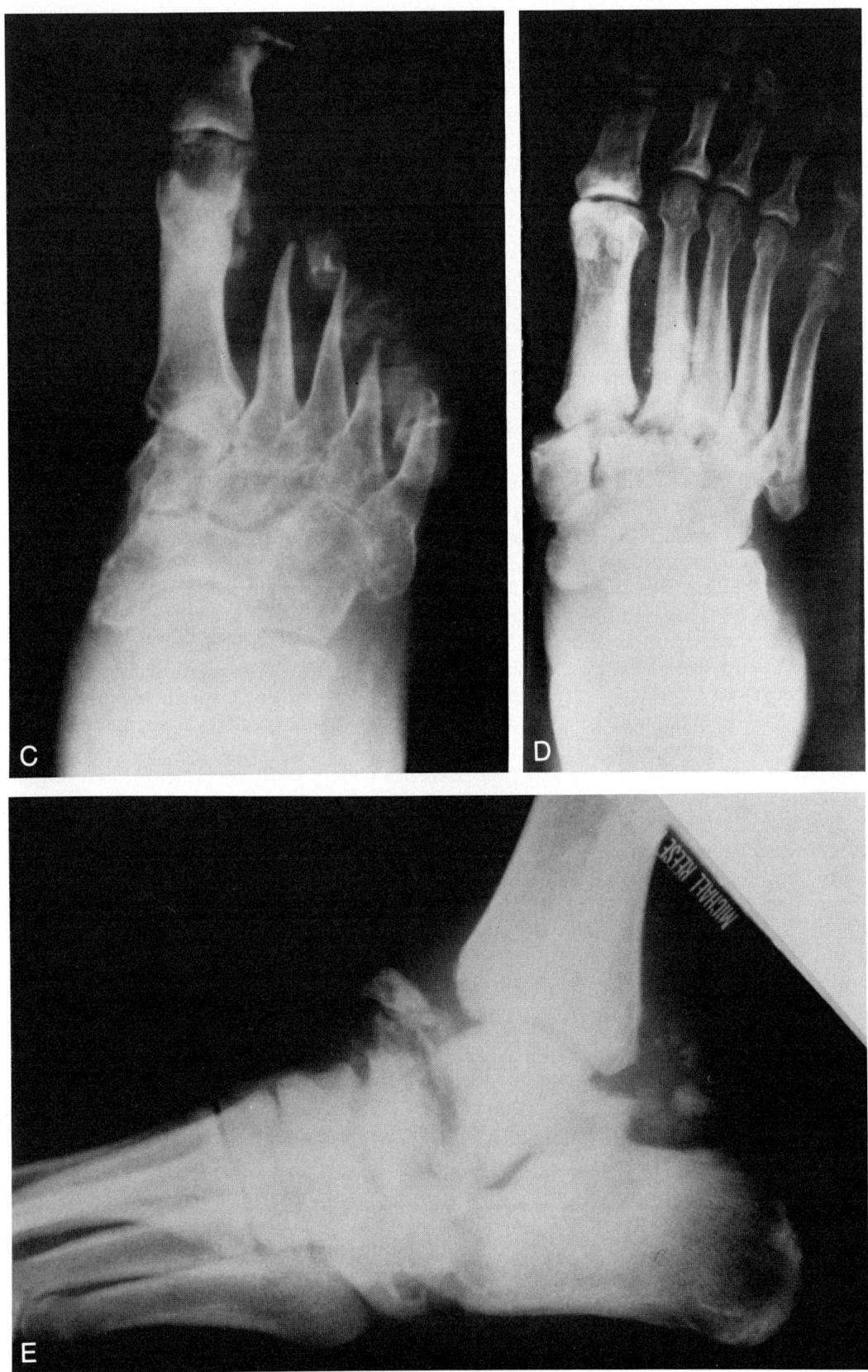

intra-articular corticosteroids[12-16] and in some individuals with calcium pyrophosphate dihydrate (CPPD) crystal deposition disease.[17-28]

Neuropathic joint disease has been described in a host of other diseases as disparate as yaws[29] and meningomyelocele.[30] It is now most frequently seen by diabetologists, podiatrists, and rheumatologists in patients with diabetes mellitus complaining of foot pain or swelling.[10,11,31-39] If the disease is diagnosed early and treatment instituted promptly, the outcome is often surprisingly successful.[10,31,33-37,39-42]

CLINICAL FEATURES

The diseases giving rise to neuropathic joint disease have changed over the last several decades, as has the clinical picture. The decline in new cases of syphilis and the success of antibiotic treatment in curing existing cases has made tabetic neuropathic joint disease uncommon. These patients typically had monoarticular involvement, usually of the knee, with the hip, ankle and lower axial skeleton less frequently involved.[5,33,43-47] A "painless" lower extremity monoarticular arthritis in a patient with a neurologic deficit was usually ascribed to neurosyphilis.[5,33,44-48] Synovitis, progressive joint instability, bony overgrowth, and fragmentation led to the characteristic "bag of bones" sensation noted when the involved joint was palpated[5,33,45,49] (Figs. 81–2 and 81–3).

Pain is often the presenting symptom, although some patients have none, even after gross joint disintegration. *Absent deep pain sensation*, tested by squeezing the achilles tendon, is the neurologic sine qua non.

Most patients with neuropathic joint disease now have diabetes mellitus with peripheral neuropathy as the underlying cause. These patients usually present to the rheumatologist with a painful and swollen mid- or forefoot or ankle with roentgenographic abnormalities demonstrating soft-tissue swelling and demineralization suggestive of early infection[11,31,32,35,39,50,51] (see Fig. 81–1).

Upper extremity neuropathic joint disease is usually caused by syringomyelia.[33,52-55] Proximal joints are most often involved, especially the shoulder (Fig. 81–4). The joints are swollen, warm, and often painful; subluxations may be seen early. In some patients, rapid dissolution of bone occurs.[56,57]

Noninflammatory (Group 1) joint fluid is frequently present when large joints are involved, although about half of the fluids obtained are grossly bloody or markedly xanthochromic.[58] Inflammatory joint fluid containing CPPD crystals has been observed in

some patients.[17,20] Such fluid without the presence of CPPD crystals should raise the possibility of sepsis. Although uncommon, infection poses diagnostic difficulties because patients may complain of only mild increases in joint pain or swelling.[59-62] Most of the reported cases of septic arthritis in large joint neuropathic disease have been caused by staphylococci, although tuberculous arthritis has been described.[59-62] Perforating ulcerations of the foot in patients with neuropathic joint disease is distressingly common and often associated with infection. This was described in 1818 as *"plantaire mal perforant."*[39,63,64]

The relative lack of pain makes a diagnosis of other complicating disorders difficult. For example, a traumatic false aneurysm developed after a hip fracture in a patient with tabes dorsalis and neuropathic joint disease. No pain was noted by the patient despite a large expanding hematoma, and the diagnosis was made only by presence of ecchymosis in the flank accompanied by a falling hemoglobin.[65]

Spontaneous fractures and dislocations are both very common in tabes dorsalis, diabetic neuropathy, congenital indifference to pain, and spinal dysraphism, and often call attention to the underlying disorder.[43,50,66-74] Untreated fractures or dislocations may hasten the development and progression of the neuroarthropathy.[69-74]

The diagnosis of neuropathic joint disease is usually considered in a patient with arthritis accompanying a neurologic disorder. Most patients experience relatively less pain than expected, allowing continued use of the joint.[5,45,75] The progression of the disease process varies widely.[4,33] Many patients have sudden and dramatic symptoms with collapse of the joint because of intra- or juxta-articular fractures.[69,72] The radiologic appearance is typical and nearly specific for the disease, although early in the course it may closely mimic the changes seen in osteoarthritis.[3,11,25] Joint disease may progress so slowly that review of serial roentgenograms correlated with the clinical features may be needed to confirm the diagnosis.[25,49] In other patients, acute fractures, dislocations, subluxations, and gross disruption of the joint confirm the diagnosis on a single roentgenogram.[25,27]

RADIOLOGIC FEATURES

The roentgenographic appearance may be the first clue to the presence of neuroarthropathy. Joint effusion, soft tissue swelling, and osteophytes difficult to distinguish from primary osteoarthritis are early changes that are not diagnostic.[25,48,49] Subluxation, para-articular debris and bony fragmentation strongly

FIG. 81–2. Neuroarthropathy of the knee joint in tabes dorsalis. *A,* This patient with tabes dorsalis was initially thought to have osteoarthritis and had been scheduled for total knee surgery, although there was minimal pain, and the large joint effusion was atypical for primary osteoarthritis. *B,* A preoperative knee roentgenogram showed sharply defined fragmentation of bone at the medial tibial joint margin and a massive joint effusion, clues to the diagnosis of neuropathic joint disease that were, unfortunately, ignored by the surgeons. *C,* Two weeks after total knee surgery, the prosthesis had subluxed, and the knee was unstable. The patient had minimal knee pain but was not able to bear weight. Total joint replacement surgery is generally contraindicated in neuropathic joints (see text).

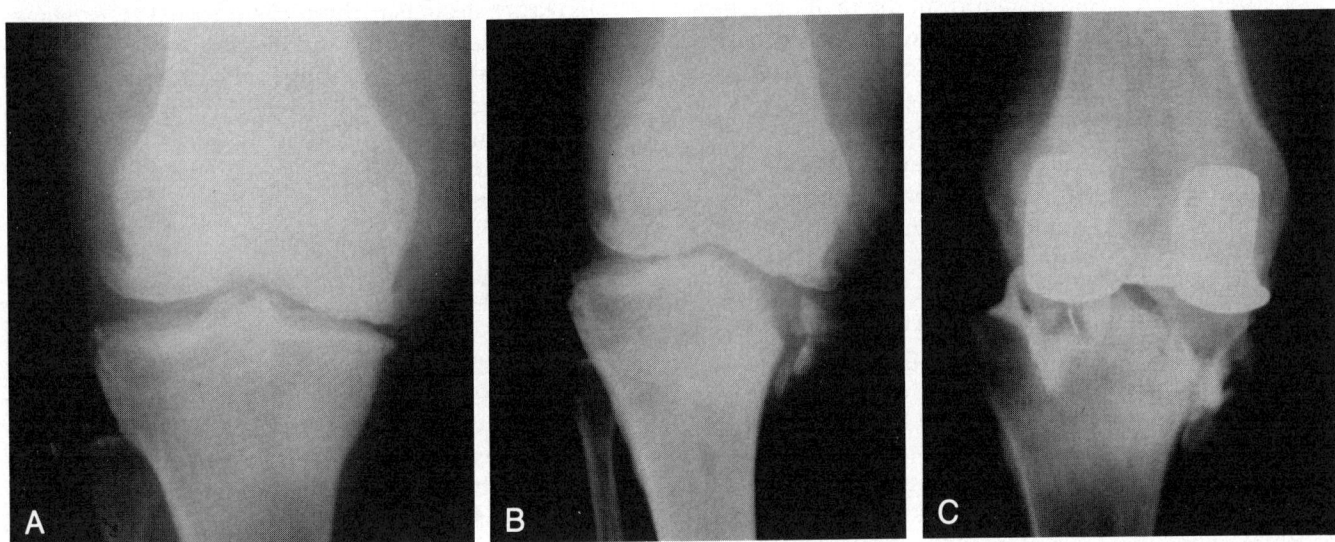

FIG. 81–3. Neuropathic joint disease of the axial skeleton may mimic osteoarthritis or ankylosing hyperostosis. Irregular narrowing of the disc spaces, a vertebral fracture, subchondral sclerosis, and bulky-headed osteophytes resembling *"les becs des parroquets"* have developed in this 78-year-old man. (From Rodnan[98].)

FIG. 81–4. Shoulder neuroarthropathy is usually due to syringomyelia. Sterile inflammatory joint fluid was observed, and this patient experienced constant pain. The osteolysis of the proximal humerus and cloudy calcification of soft tissue are typical. Some patients have painless swelling; the progression of osteolysis may be exceedingly rapid (see text).

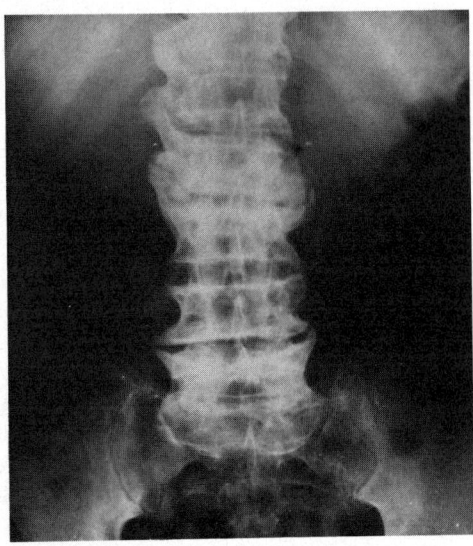

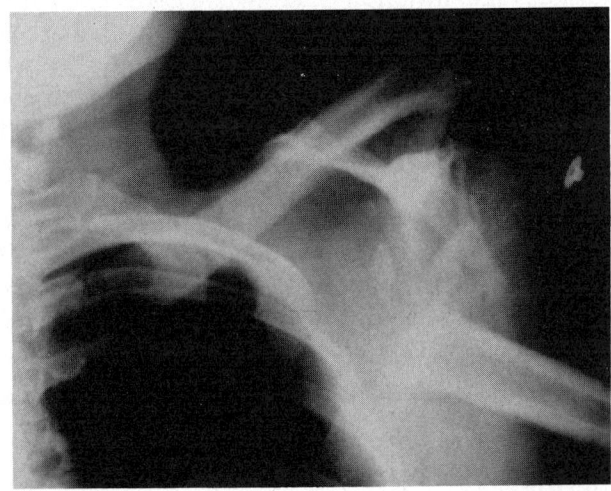

suggest the diagnosis of neuropathic joint disease.[5,25,49]

More advanced roentgenographic changes include massive soft-tissue enlargement, marked joint effusion, fractures, depression, and absorption of subchondral bone, and bony proliferation seen as osteophytes and sclerosis.[25,33,48] Fragments of bone may accumulate in tissue distant from the joint. The focal disruption of bone and cartilage with collection of debris into the synovial and para-articular tissues may produce roentgenographic clues to the diagnosis before gross fragmentation becomes evident.[25,48]

Malalignment with angular deformity and subluxation of the joint contributes to the fracturing. Pseudarthroses form at some joint surfaces as a result of fractures and deformities leading to new bone approximations.[11,25,48,49,74]

Hodgson et al., in 1948,[76] directed attention to the difficulty in separating the roentgenographic picture of neuroarthropathy from that of local infection. These authors found infection in the contiguous soft tissue in most of their patients with "neurotrophic" bone lesions and postulated that osteomyelitis contributed to the roentgenographic picture of neuropathic joint disease.[76] Resnick and Niwayama[25] emphasized that the bony margins produced by osseous fragmentation in neuropathic joint disease are well defined and sharp; "fuzzy" bony contours are atypical for neuroarthropathy and suggest infection or the presence of other inflammatory processes.

Bone scintigraphy with ^{99m}Tc-labeled diphosphonate revealed markedly abnormal uptake, even early in the disease.[77,78] Radiopharmaceutical uptake was increased within 2 minutes after injection, indicating increased local blood flow.[77] Gallium-67 accumulation may be intense and may suggest the presence of infection.[79] Of historical interest, six cases of neuropathic joint disease have been studied with angiography and three by lymphangiography.[80,81] All showed increased local vascularity by angiography, whereas lymphangiography was normal. Computed tomography (CT) has been helpful in evaluating neuroarthropathy in the axial skeleton.[82–84]

Resnick and Niwayama[25] stated, "The radiographic picture is that of a disorganized joint, characterized by simultaneously occurring bone resorption and formation. The degree of sclerosis, osteophytosis and fragmentation in this articular disorder is greater than that in any other process."

DIABETIC NEUROARTHROPATHY

The roentgenographic picture in diabetes mellitus has been divided into a *destructive* type affecting tarsal bones and an *absorptive or mutilating* type confined to the forefoot, with gradual disappearance of the epiphyseal ends with "pencil point" or "sucked candy" narrowing (see Fig. 81–1C).[10,25,32,38,39,41,51] These types are not mutually exclusive. Destructive changes at the tarsometatarsal area are sometimes referred to as a "Lisfranc fracture-dislocation"[4,85] (see Fig. 81–1D).

Forgacs[86] described three roentgenographic stages of diabetic neuropathic joint disease, with stage I (initial findings) demonstrating only osteoporosis and cortical defects leading to stage II (progression) with osteolysis and fragmentation. In stage III (healing), there is deformity, ankylosis, refilling of cortical defects, and restitution.[86]

TABES DORSALIS

The location of the joint involved may be the only differentiation between tabetic and diabetic neuropathic joint disease. Although nearly every joint has been involved in tabes dorsalis, the knee is most commonly affected, followed by the hip[5,33,47,48,66] (see Fig. 81–2). Steindler[46] found genu varum deformity in 26 of 42 tabetic Charcot knees and free joint bodies in 24. Flattening of the tibial condyles was an early sign.[44] In some cases intramuscular and ligamentous ossifications formed a sheath of bone around the knee joint.[46]

Axial neuroarthropathy is common in tabes dorsalis; 6 to 21% of tabetic neuropathic joints occur in the spine[40,43,83,87–95] (see Fig. 81–3). Syringomyelia and diabetes mellitus may also be associated with axial neuropathic joint disease, and rapid destruction of bone may occur.[84,88,92,96] The axial neuroarthropathy of tabes dorsalis occurs most often in men in the sixth and seventh decades of life. Bone atrophy and hypertrophy often co-exist, analogous to the peripheral arthropathy.[93] Local bony outgrowths have been described as *"les becs de parroquets."*[92,93] Resnick and Niwayama[25] compared the roentgenographic features of axial arthropathy in tabes dorsalis with disorders that may mimic it such as infection, degenerative disc disease and CPPD crystal deposition disease.

SYRINGOMYELIA

The neuroarthropathy in syringomyelia usually occurs in the shoulders, elbows, and cervical spine. The latter may be indistinguishable from ordinary cervical spondylosis.[25,88,97,98] Large effusions and the loss of bone, especially the proximal humerus, are characteristic[55–57,97,99] (see Fig. 81–4).

CALCIUM PYROPHOSPHATE DIHYDRATE CRYSTAL DEPOSITION DISEASE

A destructive arthropathy resembling Charcot joints has been described in CPPD crystal deposition disease per se.[17-19,21-28] Jacobelli et al. have suggested synergism between it and tabes dorsalis.[20] Typical chondrocalcinosis with subsequent joint collapse and fragmentation, especially in the knee, may suggest underlying CPPD crystal deposition[22-26] (Fig. 81–5).

PATHOPHYSIOLOGY

Charcot postulated a role for spinal cord lesions in the pathogenesis of neuropathic joint disease. Volkmann and Virchow felt that the spectacular joint destruction was primarily mechanical, caused by multiple episodes of trauma not perceived by the patient because of insensitivity of the affected joints.[4-6,100]

Eloesser[101] followed a series of cats with posterior nerve root rhizotomy on one side; the contralateral side served as a control. Charcot joints developed only on the denervated side. Cats with posterior nerve root rhizotomy followed by induction of deforming arthritis with thermocautery developed accelerated neuropathic joint disease. Bone composition and strength under a given stress load was the same on both the rhizotomy side or the control side. Neuropathic joint disease resulting from nerve resection produced in healthy cats obviously could not be as-

cribed to syphilis or other infectious causes; trauma and lack of pain and proprioception could be the only cause of neuropathic joint disease. There was no osseous atrophy produced by disturbance in the nerve roots, making Charcot's trophic theory untenable.[101]

Corbin and Hinsey[102] followed 13 cats with one hind limb completely denervated (lumbar sympathectomy and resection of L4-S3 dorsal roots) from 2 weeks to >3 years. No changes in the bones or joints were found as long as ambulation was restricted. In cats allowed to run free, hip arthritis developed. The authors concluded that activity was crucial to the development of arthritis and that nerves had no specific "trophic" function to joints.

Unilateral dorsal root ganglionectomy followed by transection of the ipsilateral anterior cruciate ligament in dogs produced remarkable gross and histologic lesions that resembled early neuroarthropathy.[103] Dogs with transection of the anterior cruciate ligament only (no ganglionectomy) had more pain, as evidenced by limping, than did those with both cruciate ligament transection and ganglionectomy. Dogs subjected only to unilateral ganglionectomy, but no joint damage, developed no evidence of degenerative joint lesions.

Finsterbush and Friedman,[104] however, found that sensory denervation of the hind limb in rabbits produced chondrocyte degeneration even in rabbits with the affected limb immobilized by a plaster cast. These cellular changes progressed over time in both rhizotomized immobilized and active rabbits. The authors postulated that the effects were mediated through altered nutrition produced by the nerve injury, not trauma, thus supporting Charcot's theory of nerve injury-mediated "trophic" changes in the joint.

Brower and Allman[105] also championed the Charcot "trophic" theory and nervous system control of bone and joint metabolism. They studied 91 roentgenograms of neuropathic joints. Approximately one half of their patients had tabes dorsalis, syringomyelia, or diabetes mellitus, but fully a third of their patients had no known underlying neurologic disease. Four of their patients were bedridden when the neuropathic joint disease developed, and the arthritis sometimes occurred with such rapidity that trauma could not be causal. They also noted striking bone resorption that also could not be adequately explained by trauma and suggested that increased bone blood flow with active bone resorption initiated by neurally controlled vascular reflex changes best explained their radiographic findings.

Evidence indicates that blood flow to Charcot joints is increased. Increased vascularity with increased venous draining and filling was shown by Kiss et al.[80] and Rabaiotti et al.[81] The latter authors commented

FIG. 81–5. This elderly patient with no neurologic disease has calcium pyrophosphate dihydrate deposition disease with rapid, painful destruction of the hips, referred to as neuropathic-like or pseudoneuropathic joint. Joint replacement is not contraindicated if the patient is otherwise well.

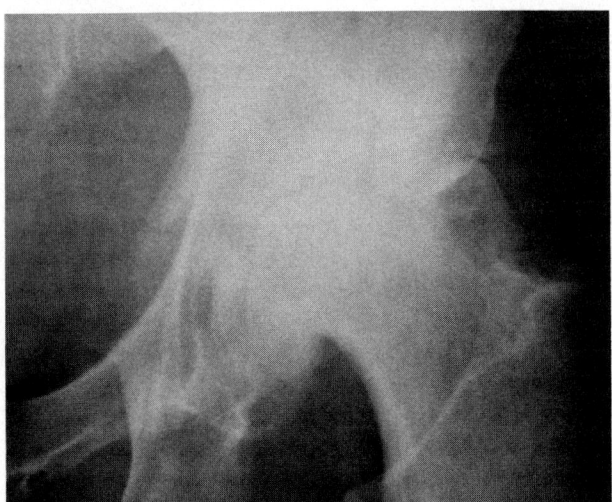

that in some respects neuropathic joint vascularity was similar to that found in certain malignancies. Bone scintigraphy in neuropathic joint disease reveals diffuse and focal increases in joint uptake both at 2 minutes and 4 hours after injection.[77,78] Scintigraphy demonstrated more extensive abnormalities than did conventional radiographs, and these sometimes preceded roentgenographic changes.[77,78] Although the increased blood flow to the neuropathic joints could be secondary to the arthritis, the disparity between the scintigrams and the roentgenograms was marked.[78] A primary autonomic nerve defect resulting in increased blood flow and increased osteoclastic activity allowing bone damage after minor trauma was postulated.[77]

The role of local anesthesia as a prerequisite for developing neuropathic joint disease remains controversial. The frequent development of neuropathic joints in patients insensitive to pain attest to the role of sensory nerves, yet many patients with neuropathic joint disease experience significant pain and near normal sensation.[5,33] The majority of these patients have neurologic disease with diminished proprioception or diminished protective reflexes.

The underlying neuropathy may be subtle. Dyck et al.[68] studied patients with neuropathic joint disease without overt neurologic signs; subclinical neuropathy and other factors such as trauma, obesity, and excessive activity were found. Sophisticated computer-assisted sensory examinations, nerve conduction velocities, and periosteal nociception testing were needed to detect the presence of the neurologic disorder in some of these patients.

The role of fractures was thoroughly studied by Johnson,[70] when he reviewed 188 cases of neuropathic joint disease, 84 of which were tabetic. Fractures were of major importance in initiating or worsening the arthritis in the majority of patients.[70] Charcot, in his original article, called attention to the frequency of spontaneous fractures in tabes dorsalis.[1] El-Khoury and Kathol[69] described unusual fractures in six diabetic patients, followed by the development of neuropathic joint disease. Even minor fractures may cause joint instability and increased susceptibility to abnormal stresses.[67,70,74] When stress fractures or sprains occur in normal persons, pain stops further injurious activities. Such warning may not happen in patients with neurologic deficits. Trauma was identified as a precipitating cause in 13 of 55 cases of neuropathic joint disease.[42] Newman[74] described spontaneous fractures of the foot and ankle in a patient with diabetic neuropathy that led to neuropathic joint disease. Neuropathic ankle joint disease developed in one patient after traumatic severance of the sciatic nerve.[106] However, in another patient, denervation of the ankle joint as treatment for unrelenting pain did not cause neuropathic joint disease.[107]

PATHOLOGY

The histologic findings in neuropathic joint disease are similar to those of osteoarthritis, with differences mainly of degree.[5,48,75,108,109] Floyd et al.[110] stated that the essential pathologic difference between the two conditions is the presence of an active pannus in neuroarthropathy. Microscopic bone and cartilage fragments in the synovium are almost universal[48,108–111] (Fig. 81–6). Horwitz[109] stressed the importance of synovial debris in the early stages of neuropathic joint disease; in three of five patients, the finding of cartilage and bone detritus "ground" into the synovium first suggested the diagnosis. Few studies have been conducted of tissues from early neuropathic joints or the underlying nerve lesions.

In contrast, many authors have provided detailed descriptions of chronic neuropathic joints.[5,45,46,48,75,105] There is degeneration and disappearance of joint cartilage followed by eburnation of the bone ends that have been denuded of cartilage. In some areas, there is proliferation of cartilage resulting in new bone formation. The coincidental occurrence of massive bony disintegration and production of exuberant quantities of new bone is striking.[5,42,46] Extra-articular bony fragments and periosteal bone production co-exist with erosions and fractures of the devitalized bone. Intra- and extra-articular osteophytes and exostosis are found on gross examination.[75]

Several authors describe a hypertrophic and atrophic form of neuropathic joint disease.[46,48,112] Extra- and intra-articular exostosis, osteocytosis, and ossification of soft tissue are predominant in the former, whereas joint displacement and bone resorption characterize the latter. King[75] postulated that the hypertrophic changes are due to the stimulation of cellular proliferation by products of bone dissolution.

The microscopic changes depend on the stage and severity of the disease and the area of tissue examined. King[75] commented on the great variety of appearances presented by the diseased bone and cartilage, and Steindler[46] described cartilage hyperplasia. Some cartilage is invaded by pannus, leading to its destruction.[46] O'Connor et al.[103] found a variety of cartilage abnormalities in dogs subjected to anterior cruciate ligament transection after dorsal root ganglionectomy. Diminution of cartilage thickness, decreased cellularity, and staining with safranin O was

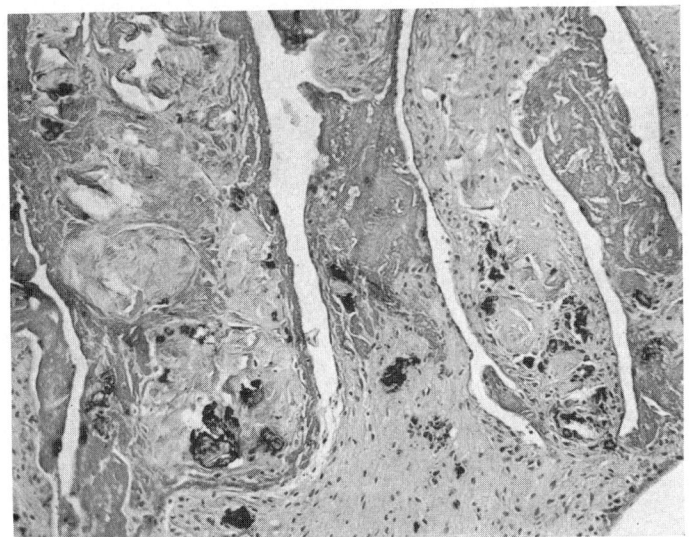

FIG. 81–6. Photomicrograph of synovium from a neuropathic hip secondary to syphilitic tabes dorsalis. Note the surface hyalinization, dense fibrosis, and scattered areas of calcification. The presence of synovial proliferation and bone and cartilage detritus is very typical of neuropathic joint disease (hematoxylin and eosin stain). (From Rodnan[98].)

common, although in other areas, hypercellularity and brood capsules were present.[103]

DIABETIC NEUROPATHIC JOINT DISEASE

It is not surprising that diabetes mellitus is the most common underlying condition in neuropathic joint disease. Perhaps 10 million Americans have diabetes mellitus, approximately 6% of the middle-aged population, and most diabetics have clinical or electromyographic evidence of neuropathy.[64,113–116] Deaths from diabetes mellitus are declining, and diabetic patients are living longer, increasing their risk of developing neuropathic joint disease.[64]

Jordan[9] reviewed the neurologic manifestations of 226 diabetic patients at the Joslin Diabetic Center in 1936. The incidence of arthropathy was estimated to be between 0.1 and 0.5%, with an approximately equal sex ratio.[64,86] The mean age at diagnosis of neuropathic joint disease is 55 years, and the mean duration of diabetes mellitus before the diagnosis of neuroarthropathy is 18 years, with a range of 8 months to 43 years.[11,39] Esses[50] described neuropathic arthritis in a 21-year-old diabetic patient. In one study of 90 diabetic patients with neuropathic joint disease, all had peripheral neuropathy.[11]

The preponderance of neuropathic joint disease occurring in diabetic rather than tabetic patients is a recent phenomenon. As late as 1964, tabes dorsalis accounted for 37 of a series of 52 cases with diabetes mellitus only accounting for four.[117]

The most common sites of neuropathic joints in diabetes are the tarsal and metatarsal joints with ankle involvement slightly less frequent.[10,11,31,32,34,35,112] The ankles were affected in 12% of 101 patients with neuropathic joint disease, while 24% had bilateral foot disease.[39] Frykberg[35] found approximately 20% bilateral foot disease in his patients. Sinha et al.[39] reported that bony deformity was most common at the tarsometatarsal joints, skin ulceration at the metatarsophalangeal joints, and soft tissue swelling at the ankle. Antecedent trauma was recalled most commonly in patients with tarsometatarsal joint disease. Neuropathic joint disease developing after fractures or dislocations in diabetic patients is common.[37,50,67,69] Diabetic neuroarthropathy uncommonly occurs in joints above the ankle, but knee, spinal, and even upper extremity joint involvement has been reported.[96,118,119] Cauda equina syndrome has complicated diabetic neuropathic joint disease.[84]

Diabetic neuropathy has been described since 1798.[64,114] Distal, bilaterally symmetric polyneuropathy, predominantly sensory, is the most common finding. The distal portions of the longest nerves are affected first, explaining the inordinate degree of foot involvement.[64,114] There is diminution of the nocifensive reflex due to loss of the small fibers responsible for pain sensation.[64,114,116] The sensory loss and recurrent everyday trauma combined with normal motor function and blood flow allow the occurrence of abnormal joint hypermobility with development of external rotation and eversion of the foot. The stress of weight bearing leads to gradual, or at times sudden, breakdown of the foot.[10,100,114]

The patient presents because of foot pain, although it is generally accepted that the pain in diabetic neuropathic joint disease is less than expected for the degree of deformity.[34,35,39,52] Swelling almost always precedes pain and may be the only manifestation of early disease.[36] Soft-tissue ankle swelling is especially typical with ankle neuropathic joint disease[11,39] (see Fig. 81–1B). Deep tendon reflexes of the ankle are diminished, with absent or diminished pain and vibration sensation and proprioception in most patients.[64,114,116] The foot is erythematous, and the pulses are usually bounding.[34,35] Increased mobility of the toes, especially in extension with crepitation on palpation, may be present.[39] Tarsometatarsal joint involvement may produce bony deformities with dorsal prominence or plantar protrusions. Downward collapse of the tarsal bones may produce convexity of the volar surface, forming a "rocker" foot or sole.[11,34,35,39] Callus formation occurs over weight-bearing areas, especially the metatarsophalangeal joints, and are frequent sites of infection. This combined surgical and medical problem of perforating ulcers in the foot with a neurologic deficit and arthritis is difficult to manage.[63]

TABES DORSALIS

The joint disorder that accompanied lesions of the central nervous system (CNS) described by Charcot was caused by tabes dorsalis; he emphasized the suddenness of the swelling and the lack of pain or fever. Swelling and hydroarthrosis would occur after a few days; and a week or 2 later "cracking sounds" developed, leaving a hypermobile joint with wearing away of the articular bones. "Besides the wearing down of the articular surfaces—you may notice the presence of foreign bodies, of bony stalactites, and in a word, of all the customary accompaniments of arthritis deformans. . . ."[1]

Late tertiary syphilis includes cardiovascular, neurologic, and gummatous lesions. The neurologic lesions may be asymptomatic (abnormal cerebral spinal fluid only) or symptomatic, including tabes dorsalis.[120] The posterior spinal column at the fasciculus gracilis is principally involved, but the fasciculus cuneatus may be affected, accounting for the loss of proprioception.[53,95] The proprioceptive loss is generally compensated by intact visual pathways.[53,95]

The VDRL or other nonspecific tests for syphilis such as the RPR (rapid reagen) test are often negative in neurosyphilis because of prior treatment or the passage of time, but the specific tests, FTA-abs and TPHA-tp, are positive in greater than 95% of patients with neurosyphilis. Testing of cerebrospinal fluid may be helpful; a positive cerebrospinal fluid VDRL usually indicates active syphilis, whereas a positive cerebrospinal fluid FTA usually indicates neurosyphilis.[120]

The best single clinical criterion for diagnosing tabetic neuropathy is the absence of deep pain sensa-

tion.[98] The Argyll Robertson pupil may be absent or the irregularity in pupil size slight.[45,46,95,110] A careful sensory examination is required. Absent knee reflexes are common.[45,46,95,100] Neuropathic joint disease may be the first sign of tabes dorsalis. The classic picture of a large, firm, painless, unstable joint is not always present, and the arthritis may remain undiagnosed for some time.[44,110,117]

Neuropathic joint disease occurs in 4 to 10% of tabetics. Key[44] considered it rare in persons less than 40 years of age. A history of syphilis is obtained in less than half the patients.[44,110] The mean interval between the onset of the syphilis and the development of the neuropathic joint is 19 years. In Key's series of 69 cases, a total of 92 joints were involved; 18 patients had two joints and 5 had three joints affected. The knee was affected in 39, the foot and ankle, 29; the hip, 15; the spine, 5; the elbow, 2; and the shoulder and wrist joint, 1 each.[44] In another series,[47] the knee was involved in 66% of the tabetic neuropathic joints and the ankle in 26%; 28% of their patients had polyarticular involvement. Women comprised one third of these cases,[47] but in most series, men outnumbered women to a greater extent.[4,45,46,66] Beetham et al.[66] also described a patient with extensive polyarticular involvement.

The onset of joint disease in neurosyphilis is not always acute, and joint swelling may continue for months or years before disintegration occurs.[44,47,66] Swelling is the prominent sign of disease onset in the knee, ankle, and foot, but in the hip, a pathologic fracture is usually the presenting finding. In the spine, deformity is frequently the first finding.[5,9,46,117]

Spinal neuroarthropathy is common.[83,87–89,91,92,94,95] As late as 1980, Wirth et al.[95] described 18 tabetic neuropathic spinal arthropathies culled from two institutions, and Campbell and Doyle[89] found eight cases within a 2-year period. The lesions are usually in the lumbar or lower dorsal vertebra with vertebral body destruction leading to posterior or lateral displacement, resulting in kyphotic and scoliotic deformity. Usually no bone tenderness occurs, but considerable discomfort may be caused by compression of nerve roots.[87,89,95] A "thud" on flexion–extension movement of the spine is said to be characteristic.[91]

The incidence of tabes dorsalis is decreasing, but the disorder has not disappeared.

SYRINGOMYELIA

Syringomyelia has been frequently associated with neuropathic joint disease,[4,52,54,56,97,99] since the original description by Schultze and Kahler in 1888.[7] Approximately 25% of syringomyelia patients have neuropathic arthritis, predominantly in the shoulders, elbows, and cervical spine, followed by the wrist, carpal, and small hand joints[25,97,99] (Fig. 81–7).

Syringomyelia (from the Greek syrinx—pipe or tube) is a chronic progressive, degenerative disorder of the spinal canal characterized clinically by weakness and atrophy of the hands and arms and segmental anesthesia of the dissociated type (loss of pain and temperature sensation but preservation of touch) especially at the neck, shoulders, and arms.[53,99] There is cavitation of the central portion of the spinal canal, usually in the cervical region.[53] The very high incidence of neuropathic joint disease in syringomyelia as compared to tabes dorsalis and diabetes mellitus is probably explained by the more profound sensory loss that occurs in syringomyelia.[4,53] Amyotrophy and

FIG. 81–7. The wrist involvement in this patient with syringomyelia resembles the tarsometatarsal changes of the foot in diabetic neuroarthropathy. The combination of bony destruction and repair is frequently seen in neuropathic joint disease.

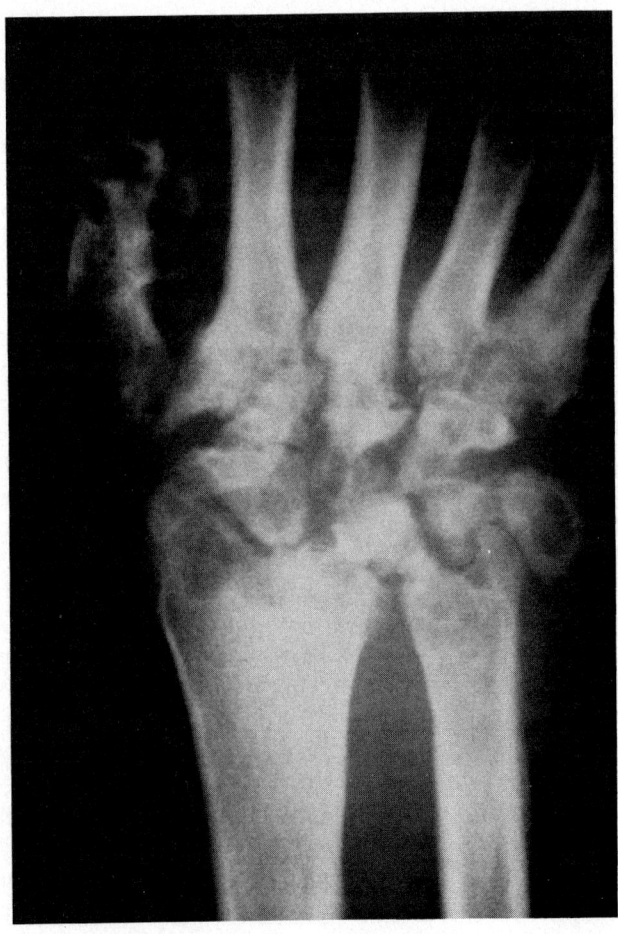

upper extremity areflexia are common in syringomyelia. Deep aching or boring pain is frequent.[53]

Neuropathic joint disease may occur early or late in the course of syringomyelia.[53,55,93,97] Painful shoulder involvement was found in two patients as the first manifestation of syringomyelia,[54] and rapid bone dissolution may occur.[56] Multiple joints may be involved, even mimicking rheumatoid arthritis (RA).[121] In one series, three patients complained of pain, while in three others, the condition was painless.[55] Swelling was so pronounced that it limited arm motion in all.[55] In two patients, no bony roentgenographic changes were found at the onset of the swelling, but gradually, extensive joint destruction and calcification in the soft tissue developed, followed by slow resorption of bone.[54] Cervical spine involvement is common in syringomyelia; early roentgenographic changes may be indistinguishable from cervical spondylosis.[25,99]

When neuropathic joint disease occurs in the upper extremity, syringomyelia should be considered the most likely cause. The loss of deep tendon reflexes in the upper extremities, analgesia, and thermal anesthesia support the diagnosis.[53] The diagnosis is confirmed by magnetic resonance imaging (MRI) of the syrinx. Unfortunately, even with early diagnosis, treatment is unsatisfactory. Decompression of the distended syrinx may temporarily alleviate the symptoms.[53]

CALCIUM PYROPHOSPHATE DIHYDRATE CRYSTAL DEPOSITION DISEASE

Jacobelli et al.[20] described the occurrence of CPPD crystal deposition and neuropathic joint disease in four patients, three with tabes dorsalis, and one with no neurologic abnormalities but with a history of syphilis and positive VDRL and FTA-abs tests. All four patients had severe arthropathy of the knees, originally considered to be only neuropathic joint disease, until careful search revealed generalized CPPD crystal deposition. The patient without neurologic deficit developed an *acute* Charcot joint with collapse of the medial tibial plateau 24 hours after his first attack of pseudogout.[17] Because only 5 to 10% of tabetic patients develop neuropathic joints and the prevalence of CPPD deposition at age 70 years is about 5%, crystal deposition and neuropathic joint disease was postulated analogous to the experimental findings of Eloesser already discussed.[20] Bennett et al.[17] suggested that the presence of CPPD crystals in joint fluid may explain some of the episodes of acute inflammation seen in some neuropathic joints.

CPPD crystal deposition and neuropathic joint disease were described in two patients without neurologic abnormalities or laboratory evidence of syphilis;[19] the destructive arthropathy was described as neuropathic-like because of the presence of pain and lack of neurologic deficit.

Menkes et al.[24] described 15 cases of neuropathic-like destructive arthropathy in 125 patients with CPPD crystal deposition collected over a 3-year period. Knees, shoulders, hips, and wrists were most commonly involved.

Resnick et al.[26] also described severe destructive arthropathy occurring frequently in his series of patients with CPPD crystal deposition. This variant has been called *pseudoneuropathic joint disease*.[21]

There is little doubt that CPPD crystal deposition alone can be associated with a destructive arthropathy,[21] but it is important to separate neuropathic-like joint disease from true neuropathic joint disease because the former patients may be candidates for prosthetic joint surgery while the latter are not.

INTRA-ARTICULAR CORTICOSTEROIDS

The possibility of iatrogenic neuropathic-like joint disease with intra-articular corticosteroids remains a concern.[12–16,122] This form of local treatment of arthritis was popularized by Hollander et al. in 1951.[123] By 1961, Hollander and associates[124] reported on more than 100,000 injections (articular and soft tissue) with careful observations on results and adverse effects. Instability of joints was noted in 0.7% of repeatedly injected weight-bearing joints. Proprioception or sensation loss was exhibited in the unstable joints, but in only four joints was "the absorption of bone extensive." Kendall[125] had even a lower incidence of untoward events in a series of 6700 injections in 2256 patients.

Chandler et al.[13] reported the rapid deterioration and development of a neuropathic-like hip joint in a patient with osteoarthritis injected at approximately monthly intervals (approximately 18 injections). Sweetnam et al.[16] described "steroid arthropathy" in four patients with rapid painless destruction of the hips; two had received intra-articular steroids and two had been treated with oral corticosteroids. Steinberg et al.[15] described neuropathic-like changes in a knee of a patient with RA treated locally with 22 corticosteroid injections over a period of 2 years. Alarcon-Segovia and Ward[12] described a similar case that developed after the patient received four to six yearly injections over a 6-year period.

Such neuropathic-like changes after local intra-articular steroid use is believed to result from the temporary suppression of pain induced by the medication, encouraging overuse of the damaged joint.[14] Hollander et al.[124] advised protection from trauma and rest of weight-bearing joints after intra-articular corticosteroid therapy.

Although reported cases of neuropathic-like joint disease with intra-articular corticosteroid use may only represent a small fraction of the actual number of cases, it still must be uncommon. It is certainly not true neuropathic joint disease, although the corticosteroids may well interfere with normal protective sensory processes.

The early reports of neuropathic-like joint disease were associated with short-lived, relatively soluble corticosteroid preparations used repeatedly in weight-bearing joints. The deleterious effects of the newer, now more commonly used, much less soluble intra-articular corticosteroids are unclear. Benefits from judicious intra-articular corticosteroids seem to greatly outweigh the risk of inducing joint instability and destruction (see also Chapter 39).

CONGENITAL INSENSITIVITY TO PAIN

Congenital insensitivity to pain, although rare, is so frequently associated with neuropathic joints that the diagnosis should be considered in children or young adults with atypical arthritis.[8,126–135] Insensitivity to pain was first described in a sideshow participant advertised as the "human pin cushion."[8] "The patient cannot recall any pain except headache—and his memory is good." The diagnostic criteria are (1) pain sensation is absent from birth, (2) the entire body is affected, and (3) all other sensory modalities should be intact or only minimally impaired, with preservation of the deep tendon reflexes.[134] Subtle varieties of the condition include *congenital insensitivity to pain with anhidrosis*[136] and *congenital sensory neuropathy* with neuropathic joint disease where all modalities of sensation are decreased.[137] Most pathologic studies of patients with congenital insensitivity to pain report an intact peripheral nervous system,[138] although neuropathologic changes have been described.[127,136]

Fractures of the metaphysis and diaphysis of long bones with epiphyseal separation and soft-tissue ulcerations occur frequently and are often unrecognized.[133] The roentgenographic appearance of injury (destruction) and repair (proliferation) of bone, occasionally complicated by infection, is similar to that seen in other causes of neuropathic joint disease.[133] The ankle is most frequently involved, with joints of the feet, elbows, spine, and hip joints less commonly involved. In a patient with bilateral leg amputation because of congenital insensitivity to pain, hand and wrist arthropathy developed after use of the upper extremities for weight bearing.[139] *Pain asymbolia*, an acquired equivalent of congenital insensitivity to pain, has not been reported in association with neuroarthropathy.

SPINAL DYSRAPHISM

The disorders of fusion of the dorsal midline structures at the primitive neural tube (especially meningomyelocele) are the most frequent cause of neuropathic joint disease in children.[30,98,133,140] Evident at birth, the neurologic findings depend on the level of the lesion.[30,53] The neuropathic joint disease most commonly affects the tarsal articulations and the ankle.[30,133,140] Lower extremity long bone fractures are common in meningomyelocele because of osteoporosis due to immobility and sensory neuropathy.[71,133,140,141] Children with myelomeningocele had less neuropathic joint disease and their fractures healed quicker than in children with congenital insensitivity to pain because children with the former walked less.[133] The joints of children with meningomyelocele often are protected by braces at an early age, which apparently decreases the incidence of neuropathic joint disease.[133]

MISCELLANEOUS

Children with thalidomide disease also may develop neuropathic joint disease.[142] Because some adults treated with thalidomide also develop severe sensory peripheral neuropathy, McCredie[142] hypothesized that the embryo developed neuropathy at the time of thalidomide exposure, which later led to the neuropathic joint disease in childhood.

Neuropathic joint disease has been reported in familial amyloid neuropathy,[143] nonfamilial amyloid neuropathy in a dialysis patient,[144] amyloidosis associated with Waldenstrom's macroglobulinemia,[145] the myelopathy of pernicious anemia,[146] spinal cord trauma,[117,147–149] familial dysautonomia,[150] multiple sclerosis,[4] paraplegia,[148] idiopathic,[151–153] arachnoiditis secondary to tuberculosis,[154] adhesive arachnoiditis,[155] and neuropathy associated with leprosy.[4] It has also been reported in acromegaly,[156] yaws,[29] juvenile RA,[157] scleroderma (with cervical osteolysis),[82] and in patients undergoing chronic hemodialysis.[158]

Neuropathic joint disease of the forefoot was described in 59 severe alcoholic patients with polyneu-

ropathy who were hospitalized at a single institution during a 3-year period.[159] Patients were excluded if diseases usually associated with neuropathic joint disease such as diabetes mellitus, amyloidosis, or syphilis were present. The patients were chronic heavy drinkers, mean age 46.7 years; painless foot ulcers, infections, chronic venous insufficiency and repeated bouts of cellulitis or lymphangitis were frequent. The association of alcohol and neuropathic joint disease had been described infrequently before this report.[4,33,63]

A variety of other neurologic disorders may be associated with neuropathic joint disease. Because the common denominator of this arthritis is sensory loss and continued weight bearing, any disease with those features may be complicated by neuropathic joint disease. Hereditary sensory neuropathy,[160–162] progressive hypertrophic polyneuritis,[163] and peroneal muscular atrophy (Charcot-Marie-Tooth disease)[164] have all been associated with neuropathic joint disease. Bruckner and Kendall[164] described seven cases of neuropathic joint disease associated with the latter. These patients had more severe muscle wasting and sensory loss than did Charcot-Marie-Tooth patients without neuropathic joint disease.[164]

MANAGEMENT

Most patients with neuropathic joint disease seen by rheumatologists will have foot involvement due to diabetic neuropathy. Either painful or painless swelling in a diabetic foot should be considered possible neuropathic joint disease. An aggressive approach to diagnosis and treatment may help the patient. Molded or contour shoes, bracing, patient education, and foot elevation bring relief to most patients when treated early.[34,35,37,41,75,100,128,165] Several authors state that control of the diabetes mellitus improves the arthropathy.[31,78]

Treatable conditions that cause neurologic disorders such as syphilis, yaws, and leprosy should always be kept in mind, but even when the underlying neurologic disease may be untreatable, prompt joint immobilization, cessation of weight bearing, accommodative foot wear, and patient education often stabilize the neuropathic joint.[37,72,100] Fractures heal with immobilization.[70] Sprains should be treated with immobilization.[36,70] Reduction of edema and treatment of infection and ulcerations are required for successful therapy of the diabetic foot.[34,35,37] Immobilization or arthrodesis of the spine often provides successful treatment in axial skeleton neuroarthropathy.[40,90,94,149] Crutch walking is usually needed for hip joint neuropathic involvement. A patellar tendon-bearing orthosis has successfully reduced weight bearing in patients with neuropathic joint disease of the ankle or foot.[32,166]

Arthrodesis of a neuropathic joint may fail because of nonunion or pin fracture,[167,168] but successful fusion is possible and is often required for treatment of the neuropathic knee.[42,126,167,169–171] Drennan et al.,[169] in 1971, described successful knee arthrodesis in eight patients. The high rate of fusion was attributed to adequate bone resection and debridement, complete synovectomy, and firm internal fixation (bleeding bone to bleeding bone). Samilson et al.[42] emphasized the need for early arthrodesis. Arthrodesis of the spine is successful in achieving stability and relieving pain in most instances.[40,90,95]

Total joint replacement is generally contraindicated in neuropathic joint disease, although pain has been relieved with hip arthroplasty even though the joints have later subluxed or loosened.[33,172,173] Charnley,[174] the innovator of total hip joint surgery, warned against total joint replacement in neuropathic joint disease. Total glenohumeral joint replacement is contraindicated.[175] The rapidity of loosening and subluxation of total joint prosthesis in neuropathic joint disease attest to the need for proprioception and deep pain sensation to stabilize even carefully reconstructed joints.

Sprenger and Foley[176] reviewed hip replacement surgery in neuropathic joint disease and described successful hip surgery in a patient with neurosyphilis. At 7-year followup, the patient was well and the hip prosthesis was stable. The authors ascribed the excellent result, contrary to the experience of other surgeons, to the lack of ataxia in their patient.

Soudry et al.[177] reported nine total knee arthroplasties in seven patients with neuropathic joint disease. Excellent results were obtained in eight and good results in one with an average followup of 3 years. The histologic and radiologic findings were diagnostic of neuropathic joint disease, but four patients with clinically apparent neurologic abnormalities had no definable neurologic disease. Posterior stabilized components, ligamentous balancing, resection of adequate bone, bone grafting if required, or the use of a custom augmented prosthesis were considered the reasons for this unusual rate of success.[177]

Lumbar sympathectomy was helpful in the diabetic foot with neuropathic joint disease in two patients with impaired circulation.[178] Amputation of the foot is occasionally required. Exostectomies, when indicated, also have been reported to be helpful.[165]

REFERENCES

1. Charcot, J.M.: Du Cerveau ou de la moelle epiniere. Arch. Physiol. Nom. Pathol., 1:161–178, 379–399, 1868.
2. Owen, A.R.G.: Hysteria, hypnosis and healing: the work of J-M. Charcot. New York, Ganett Publications, 1971.
3. Pemberton, R., and Osgood, R.B. (eds.): The Medical and Orthopaedic Management of Chronic Arthritis. New York, Macmillan, 1934.
4. Bruckner, F.E., and Howell, A.: Neuropathic joints. Semin. Arthritis Rheum., 2:47–69, 1972.
5. Delano, P.J.: The pathogenesis of Charcot's joints. AJR, 56:189–200, 1946.
6. Volkmann, R., and Virchow, R. cited by Delano, P.J.: The pathogenesis of Charcot's joints. AJR, 56:189–200, 1946.
7. Schultze, F., and Kahler, O. cited by Bruckner, F.E., and Howell, A.: Neuropathic joints. Semin. Arthritis Rheum., 2:47–69, 1972.
8. Dearborn, G.V.N.: A case of congenital general pure analgesia. J. Nerv. Med. Dis., 75:612–615, 1932.
9. Jordan, W.R.: Neuritic manifestations in diabetes mellitus. Arch. Intern. Med., 57:307–366, 1936.
10. Robillard, R., Gagnon, P.A., and Alarie, R.: Diabetic neuroarthropathy: Report of four cases. Can. Med. Assoc. J., 91:795–804, 1964.
11. Clouse, M.E., Gramm, H.F., Legg, M., and Flood, T.: Diabetic osteoarthropathy: Clinical and roentgenographic observations in 90 cases. AJR, 121:22–34, 1974.
12. Alarcon-Segovia, D., and Ward, L.E.: Charcot-like arthropathy in rheumatoid arthritis: Consequence of overuse of a joint repeatedly injected with hydrocortisone. JAMA, 193:136–138, 1965.
13. Chandler, G.N., Jones, P.T., Wright, V., and Hartfall, S.J.: Charcot's arthropathy following intra-articular hydrocortisone. Br. Med. J., 1:952–953, 1959.
14. Chandler, G.N., and Wright, V.: Deleterious effect of intra-articular hydrocortisone. Lancet, 2:661–663, 1958.
15. Steinberg, C.L., Duthie, R.B., and Piva, A.E.: Charcot-like arthropathy following intra-articular hydrocortisone. JAMA, 181:851–854, 1962.
16. Sweetnam, D.R., Mason, R.M., and Murray, R.O.: Steroid arthropathy of the hip. Br. Med. J., 1:1392–1394, 1960.
17. Bennett, R.M., Mall, J.C., and McCarty, D.J.: Pseudogout in acute neuropathic arthropathy. A clue to pathogenesis? Ann. Rheum. Dis., 33:563–567, 1974.
18. Genant, H.K.: Roentgenographic aspects of calcium pyrophosphate dihydrate crystal deposition disease (pseudogout). Arthritis Rheum., 3:307–328, 1976.
19. Helms, C.A., Chapman, G.S., and Wild, J.H.: Charcot-like joints in calcium pyrophosphate dihydrate deposition disease. Skeletal Radiol., 7:55–58, 1981.
20. Jacobelli, S., McCarty, D.J., Silcox, D.C., and Mall, J.C.: Calcium pyrophosphate dihydrate crystal deposition in neuropathic joints: Four cases of polyarticular involvement. Ann. Intern. Med., 79:340–347, 1973.
21. McCarty, D.J., Jr.: Arthritis and Allied Conditions. 10th Ed. Philadelphia, Lea & Febiger, 1985.
22. McCarty, D.J., Jr., and Haskin, M.E.: The roentgenographic aspects of pseudogout (articular chondrocalcinosis): An analysis of 20 cases. Am. J. Roentgenol. Radium Ther. Nucl. Med., 90:1248–1257, 1963.
23. Martel, W., et al.: Further observations on the arthropathy of calcium pyrophosphate crystal deposition disease. Radiology, 141:1–15, 1981.

24. Menkes, C.J., et al.: Destructive arthropathy in chondrocalcinosis articularis. Arthritis Rheum., 19:329–348, 1976.

25. Resnick, D., and Niwayama, G.: Diagnosis of bone and joint disorders with emphasis on articular abnormalities. Philadelphia, W.B. Saunders, 1981.

26. Resnick, D., et al.: Clinical, radiographic and pathologic abnormalities in calcium pyrophosphate dihydrate deposition disease (CPPD): Pseudogout. Radiology, 122:1–15, 1977.

27. Richards, A.J., and Hamilton, E.B.D.: Spinal changes in idiopathic chondrocalcinosis articularis. Rheumatol. Rehabil., 15:138–142, 1976.

28. Richardson, B.C., and Genant, H.K.: Destructive arthropathy in chondrocalcinosis: A case report. Orthopedics, 5:1482–1486, 1982.

29. Smith, F.H.: Charcot-like joints in yaws. U.S. Naval Med. Bull., 46:1832–1843, 1946.

30. Nellhaus, G.: Neurogenic arthropathies (Charcot's joints) in children. Clin. Pediatr., 14:647–653, 1975.

31. Antes, E.H.: Charcot joint in diabetes mellitus. JAMA, 156:602–603, 1954.

32. Bailey, C.C., and Root, H.F.: Neuropathic foot lesions in diabetes mellitus. N. Engl. J. Med., 236:397–401, 1947.

33. Eichenholtz, S.N.: Charcot joints. Springfield, IL, Charles C Thomas, 1966.

34. Frykberg, R.G.: Neuropathic arthropathy: The diabetic Charcot foot. Diabetes Educator, 9:17–20, 1984.

35. Frykberg, R.G., and Kozak, G.P.: Neuropathic arthropathy in the diabetic foot. Am. Fam. Physician, 5:105–113, 1978.

36. Herzwurm, P.J., and Barja, R.H.: Charcot joints of the foot. Contemp. Orthoped., 14:17–22, 1987.

37. Jackson, W.P.U., and Louw, J.H.: The diabetic foot. S. Afr. Med. J., 56:87–92, 1979.

38. Pogonowska, M.J., Collins, L.C., and Dobson, H.L.: Diabetic osteopathy. Radiology, 89:265–271, 1967.

39. Sinha, S., Munichoodappa, C.S., and Kozak, G.P.: Neuroarthropathy (Charcot joints) in diabetes mellitus. Medicine, 51:191–210, 1972.

40. Briggs, J.R., and Freehafer, A.A.: Fusion of the Charcot spine. Clin. Orthop., 53:83–93, 1967.

41. Calabro, J.J., and Garg, S.L.: Neuropathic joint disease. Am. Fam. Physician, 2:90–95, 1973.

42. Samilson, R.L., Sankaran, B., Bersani, F.A., and Smith, A.D.: Orthopedic management of neuropathic joints. Arch. Surg., 78:115–121, 1959.

43. Charcot, J.M.: Arthropathies, inxations et fractures spontanees chez une ataxique. Bull. Mem. Soc. Anat. Paris, 48:744–747, 1873.

44. Key, J.A.: Clinical observations on tabetic arthropathies (Charcot joints). Am. J. Syphilis, 16:429–447, 1932.

45. Soto-Hall, R., and Haldeman, K.O.: The diagnosis of neuropathic joint disease (Charcot joint). An analysis of 40 cases. JAMA, 114:2076–2078, 1940.

46. Steindler, A.: The tabetic arthropathies. JAMA, 96:250–256, 1931.

47. Wile, U.J., and Butler, M.G.: A critical survey of Charcot's arthropathy. Analysis of eighty-eight cases. JAMA, 94:1053–1055, 1930.

48. Potts, W.J.: The pathology of Charcot joints. Ann. Surg., 86:596–606, 1927.

49. Katz, I., Rabinowitz, J.G., and Dziadiw, R.: Early changes in Charcot's joints. AJR, 86:965–974, 1961.

50. Esses, S., Langer, F., and Gross, A.: Charcot's joints: A case report in a young patient with diabetes. Clin. Orthop., 156:183–186, 1981.

51. Kraft, E., Spyropoulos, E., and Finby, N.: Neurogenic disorders of the foot in diabetes mellitus. AJR, 124:17–24, 1975.

52. Bhaskaran, R., Suresh, K., and Iyer, G.V.: Charcot's elbow—A case report. J. Postgrad. Med., 27:194–196, 1981.

53. Rowland, L.P. (ed.): Merritt's Textbook of Neurology. Philadelphia, Lea & Febiger, 1984.

54. Sackellares, J.C., and Swift, T.R.: Shoulder enlargement as the presenting sign of syringomyelia: Report of two cases and review of the literature. JAMA, 236:2878–2879, 1976.

55. Skall-Jensen, J.: Osteoarthropathy in syringomyelia: Analysis of seven cases. Acta Radiol., 38:382–388, 1952.

56. Meyer, G.A., Stein, J., and Poppel, M.H.: Rapid osseous changes in syringomyelia. Radiology, 69:415–418, 1957.

57. Norman, A., Robbins, H., and Milgram, J.E.: The acute neuropathic arthropathy—A rapid, severely disorganizing form of arthritis. Radiology, 90:1159–1164, 1968.

58. Ropes, M.W., and Bauer, W.: Synovial fluid changes in joint disease. Cambridge, MA, Harvard University Press, 1953.

59. Bennet, K., and Hinricson, H.: A case of tuberculous infection of the knee with clinical and roentgenographic appearance of Charcot's disease. J. Bone Joint Surg., 16:463–466, 1934.

60. Goodman, M.A., and Swartz, W.: Infection in a Charcot joint: A case report. J. Bone Joint Surg., 67A:642–643, 1985.

61. Martin, J.R., Root, H.S., Kim, S.O., and Johnson, L.G.: Staphylococcus suppurative arthritis occurring in neuropathic knee joints: A report of four cases with a discussion of the mechanisms involved. Arthritis Rheum., 8:389–402, 1965.

62. Rubinow, A., Spark, E.C., and Canoso, J.J.: Septic arthritis in a Charcot joint. Clin. Orthop., 147:203–206, 1980.

63. Classen, J.N.: Neurotrophic arthropathy with ulceration. Ann. Surg., 6:891–894, 1964.

64. Marble, A., et al. (eds.): Joslin's Diabetes Mellitus. 12th Ed. Philadelphia, Lea & Febiger, 1985.

65. Boynton, E.L., et al.: False aneurysm in a Charcot hip. J. Bone Joint Surg., 68A:462–464, 1986.

66. Beetham, W.P., Jr., Kaye, R.L., and Polley, H.F.: Charcot's joints: A case of extensive polyarticular involvement, and discussion of certain clinical and pathologic features. Ann. Intern. Med., 58:1002–1012, 1963.

67. Coventry, M.B., and Rothacker, G.W., Jr.: Bilateral calcaneal fracture in a diabetic patient. J. Bone Joint Surg., 61A:462–464, 1979.

68. Dyck, P.J., et al.: Neurogenic arthropathy and recurring fractures with subclinical inherited neuropathy. Neurology, 33:357–367, 1983.

69. El-Khoury, G.Y., and Kathol, M.H.: Neuropathic fractures in patients with diabetes mellitus. Radiology, 134:313–316, 1980.

70. Johnson, J.T.H.: Neuropathic fractures and joint injuries: Pathogenesis and rationale of prevention and treatment. J. Bone Joint Surg., 49A:1–30, 1967.

71. Korhonen, B.J.: Fractures in myelodysplasia. Clin. Orthop., 79:145–155, 1971.

72. Kristiansen, B.: Ankle and foot fractures in diabetics provoking neuropathic joint changes. Acta Orthop. Scand., 51:975–979, 1980.

73. Muggia, F.M.: Neuropathic fracture: Unusual complication in a patient with advanced diabetic neuropathy. JAMA, 191:336–338, 1965.

74. Newman, J.H.: Spontaneous dislocation in diabetic neuropathy. A report of six cases. J. Bone Joint Surg., 61B:484–488, 1979.

75. King, E.J.S.: On some aspects of the pathology of hypertrophic Charcot's joints. Br. J. Surg., 18:113–124, 1930.

76. Hodgson, J.R., Pugh, D.G., and Young, H.H.: Roentgeno-

logic aspects of certain lesions of bone: Neurotrophic or infectious? Radiology, *50*:65–71, 1948.

77. Edmonds, M.E., et al.: Increased uptake of bone radiopharmaceutical in diabetic neuropathy. Q. J. Med., *224*:843–855, 1985.

78. Eymontt, M.J., Alavi, A., Dalinka, M.K., and Kyle, G.C.: Bone scintigraphy in diabetic osteoarthropathy. Radiology, *140*:475–477, 1981.

79. Glynn, T.P., Jr.: Marked gallium accumulation in neurogenic arthropathy. J. Nucl. Med., *22*:1016–1017, 1981.

80. Kiss, J., Martin, J.R., McConnell, F., and Wlodek, G.: Angiographic and lymphoangiographic examination of neuropathic knee joints. J. Can. Assoc. Radiol., *19*:19–24, 1968.

81. Rabaiotti, A., Rossi, L., Schittone, N., and Gandini, G.E.: Vascular changes in tabetic arthropathy. Ann. Radiol. Diag., *3*:115–121, 1960.

82. Clement, G.B., et al.: Neuropathic arthropathy (Charcot joints) due to cervical osteolysis: A complication of progressive systemic sclerosis. J. Rheumatol., *11*:545–548, 1984.

83. Moran, S.M., and Mohr, J.A.: Syphilis and axial arthropathy. South Med. J., *76*:1032–1035, 1983.

84. Race, M.C., Keppler, J.P., and Grant, A.E.: Diabetic Charcot spine as cauda equina syndrome: An unusual presentation. Arch. Phys. Med. Rehabil., *66*:463–465, 1985.

85. Giesecke, S.B., Dalinka, M.K., and Kyle, G.C.: Lisfranc's fracture–dislocation: A manifestation of peripheral neuropathy. AJR, *131*:139–141, 1978.

86. Forgacs, S.: Stages and roentgenological picture of diabetic osteoarthropathy. Fortschr. Rontgenstr., *126*:36–42, 1977.

87. Alergant, C.D.: Tabetic spinal arthropathy: Two cases with motor symptoms due to root compression. Br. J. Vener. Dis., *36*:261–265, 1960.

88. Brain, R., and Wilkinson, M.: Cervical arthropathy in syringomyelia, tabes dorsalis and diabetes. Brain, *81*:275–289, 1958.

89. Campbell, D.J., and Doyle, J.O.: Tabetic Charcot's spine. Report of eight cases. Br. Med. J., *1*:1018–1020, 1954.

90. Cleveland, M., and Wilson, H.J., Jr.: Charcot disease of the spine: A report of two cases treated by spine fusion. J. Bone Joint Surg., *41A*:336–340, 1959.

91. Culling, J.: Charcot's disease of the spine. Proc. R. Soc. Med., *67*:1026–1027, 1974.

92. Feldman, F., Johnson, A.M., and Walter, J.F.: Acute axial neuropathy. Radiology, *111*:1–16, 1974.

93. Holland, H.W.: Tabetic spinal arthropathy. Proc. R. Soc. Med., *46*:747–752, 1953.

94. Thomas, D.F.: Vertebral osteoarthropathy of Charcot's disease of the spine. Review of the literature and report of two cases. J. Bone Joint Surg., *34B*:248–255, 1952.

95. Wirth, C.R., Jacobs, R.L., and Rolander, S.D.: Neuropathic spinal arthropathy: A review of the Charcot spine. Spine, *5*:558–567, 1980.

96. Zucker, G., and Marder, M.J.: Charcot spine due to diabetic neuropathy. Am. J. Med., *12*:118–124, 1952.

97. Rataj, R.: Artropatic w jamistorci rdzenia. Neurol. Neurochir. Pol., *14*:439–445, 1964.

98. Rodnan, G.P.: Neuropathic joint disease (Charcot joints). *In* Arthritis and Allied Conditions. 10th Ed. Edited by D.J. McCarty. Philadelphia, Lea & Febiger, 1985.

99. Williams, B.: Orthopaedic features in the presentation of syringomyelia. J. Bone Joint Surg., *61B*:314–323, 1979.

100. Lippmann, H.I., Perotto, A., and Farrar, R.: The neuropathic foot of the diabetic. Bull. N.Y. Acad. Med., *52*:1159–1178, 1976.

101. Eloesser, L.: On the nature of neuropathic affections of the joints. Ann. Surg., *66*:201–207, 1917.

102. Corbin, K.B., and Hinsey, J.C.: Influence of the nervous system on bone and joints. Anat. Rec., *75*:307–317, 1939.

103. O'Connor, B.L., Palmoski, M.J., and Brandt, K.D.: Neurogenic acceleration of degenerative joint lesions. J. Bone Joint Surg., *67A*:562–572, 1985.

104. Finsterbush, A., and Friedman, B.: The effect of sensory denervation on rabbits' knee joints. J. Bone Joint Surg., *57A*:949–956, 1975.

105. Brower, A.C., and Allman, R.M.: Pathogenesis of the neurotrophic joint: Neurotraumatic vs neurovascular. Radiology, *139*:349–354, 1981.

106. Kernwein, G., and Lyon, W.F.: Neuropathic arthropathy of the ankle joint resulting from complete severance of the sciatic nerve. Ann. Surg., *115*:267–279, 1942.

107. Casagrande, P.A., Austin, B.P., and Indeck, W.: Denervation of the ankle joint. J. Bone Joint Surg., *33A*:723–730, 1951.

108. Collins, D.H.: The Pathology of Articular and Spinal Diseases. Baltimore, Williams & Wilkins, 1949.

109. Horwitz, T.: Bone and cartilage debris in the synovial membrane: Its significance in the early diagnosis of neuroarthropathy. J. Bone Joint Surg., *30A*:579–588, 1948.

110. Floyd, W., Lovell, W., and King, R.E.: The neuropathic joint. South. Med. J., *52*:563–569, 1959.

111. Rodnan, G.P., Yunis, E.J., and Totten, R.S.: Experience with punch biopsy of synovium in the study of joint disease. Ann. Intern. Med., *53*:319–331, 1960.

112. Raju, U.B., Fine, G., and Partamian, J.O.: Neuropathic neuroarthropathy (Charcot's joints). Arch. Pathol. Lab. Med., *106*:349–351, 1982.

113. Barrett-Connor, E.: The prevalence of diabetes mellitus in an adult community as determined by history or fasting hyperglycemia. Am. J. Epidemiol., *111*:705–712, 1980.

114. Martin, M.M.: Diabetic neuropathy: A clinical study of 150 cases. Brain, *76*:594–624, 1953.

115. Ostrander, L.D., Jr., Lamphiear, D.E., and Block, W.D.: Diabetes among men in a general population: Prevalence and associated physiological findings. Arch. Intern. Med., *136*:415–420, 1976.

116. Mulder, D.W., Lambert, E.H., Bastron, J.A., and Sprague, R.G.: The neuropathies associated with diabetes mellitus: A clinical and electromyographic study of 103 unselected diabetic patients. Neurology, *11*:275–284, 1961.

117. Storey, G.: Charcot joint. Br. J. Vener. Dis., *40*:109–117, 1964.

118. Campbell, W.L., and Feldman, F.: Bone and soft tissue abnormalities of the upper extremity in diabetes mellitus. AJR, *24*:7–16, 1975.

119. Feldman, M.J., Becker, K.L., Reefe, W.E., and Longo, A.: Multiple neuropathic joints, including wrist, in a patient with diabetes mellitus. JAMA, *209*:1690–1692, 1969.

120. Mandell, G.L., Douglas, R.G., Jr., and Bennett, J.E.: Principles and Practice of Infectious Diseases. 2nd Ed. New York, John Wiley & Sons, 1985.

121. Steinberg, V.L.: Clinical reports: Syringomyelia with multiple neuropathic joints. Ann. Phys. Med., *3*:103–104, 1956.

122. Mankin, H.J., and Congler, K.A.: The acute effects of intraarticular hydrocortisone on articular cartilage in rabbits. J. Bone Joint Surg., *48A*:1383–1388, 1966.

123. Hollander, J.L., Brown, E.M., Jr., Jessar, R.A., and Brown, C.Y.: Hydrocortisone and cortisone injected into arthritic joints. Comparative effects of and use of hydrocortisone as a local antiarthritic agent. JAMA, *147*:1629–1635, 1951.

124. Hollander, J.L., Jessar, R.A., and Brown, E.M., Jr.: Intra-syn-

ovial corticosteroid therapy: A decade of use. Bull. Rheum. Dis., *11*:239–240, 1961.

125. Kendall, P.H.: Untoward effects following local hydrocortisone injection. Ann. Physical Med., *4*:170–175, 1958.

126. Abell, J.M., Jr., and Hayes, J.T.: Charcot knee due to congenital insensitivity to pain. J. Bone Joint Surg., *46A*:1287–1291, 1964.

127. Drummond, R.P., and Rose, G.K.: A twenty-one year review of a case of congenital indifference to pain. J. Bone Joint Surg., *57B*:241–243, 1975.

128. van der Houwen, H.: A case of neuropathic arthritis caused by indifference to pain. J. Bone Joint Surg., *43B*:314–317, 1961.

129. Mooney, V., and Mankin, H.J.: A case of congenital insensitivity to pain with neuropathic arthropathy. Arthritis Rheum., *9*:820–829, 1966.

130. Murray, R.O.: Congenital indifference to pain with special reference to skeletal changes. Br. J. Radiol., *30*:2–6, 1957.

131. Petrie, J.G.: A case of progressive joint disorders caused by insensitivity to pain. J. Bone Joint Surg., *35B*:399–401, 1953.

132. Sandell, L.J.: Congenital indifference to pain. J. Fac. Radiol., *9*:50–56, 1958.

133. Schneider, R., Goldman, A.B., and Bohne, W.H.O.: Neuropathic injuries to the lower extremities in children. Radiology, *128*:713–718, 1978.

134. Silverman, F.N., and Gilden, J.J.: Congenital insensitivity to pain: A neurologic syndrome with bizarre skeletal lesions. Radiology, *72*:176–189, 1959.

135. Thrush, D.C.: Congenital insensitivity to pain: A clinical, genetic and neurophysiological study of four children from the same family. Brain, *96*:369–386, 1973.

136. Swanson, A.G., Buchan, G.C., Alvord, E.C., Jr.: Anatomic changes in congenital insensitivity to pain. Arch. Neurol., *12*:12–18, 1965.

137. Johnson, R.H., and Spalding, M.K.: Progressive sensory neuropathy in children. J. Neurol. Neurosurg. Psychiatry, *27*:125–130, 1964.

138. Feindel, W.: Note on the nerve endings in a subject with arthropathy and congenital absence of pain. J. Bone Joint Surg., *35B*:402–407, 1953.

139. Parker, R.D., and Froimson, A.I.: Neurogenic arthropathy of the hand and wrist. J. Hand Surg., *11A*:709–710, 1986.

140. Gyepes, M.T., Newbern, D.H., and Neuhauser, E.B.D.: Metaphyseal and physeal injuries in children with spina bifida and meningomyelocele. AJR, *95*:168–177, 1965.

141. Handelsman, J.E.: Spontaneous fractures in spina bifida. J. Bone Joint Surg., *54B*:381, 1972.

142. McCredie, J.: Thalidomide and congenital Charcot's joints. Lancet, *2*:1058–1061, 1973.

143. Pruzanski, W., Baron, M., and Shupak, R.: Neuroarthropathy (Charcot joints) in familial amyloid polyneuropathy. J. Rheumatol., *8*:477–481, 1981.

144. Peitzman, S.J., et al.: Charcot arthropathy secondary to amyloid neuropathy. JAMA, *235*:1345–1347, 1976.

145. Scott, R.B., et al.: Neuropathic joint disease (Charcot joints) in Waldenstrom's macroglobulinemia with amyloidosis. Am. J. Med., *54*:535–538, 1973.

146. Halonen, P.I., and Jarvinen, K.A.J.: On the occurrence of neuropathic arthropathies in pernicious anemia. Ann. Rheum. Dis., *7*:151–155, 1948.

147. Kettunen, K.O.: Neuropathic arthropathy caused by spinal cord trauma. Ann. Chir. Gynaecol., *46*:95–100, 1957.

148. Slabaugh, P.B., and Smith, T.K.: Neuropathic spine after spinal cord injury. J. Bone Joint Surg., *60A*:1005–1006, 1978.

149. Sobel, J.W., Bohlman, H.H., and Freehafer, A.A.: Charcot's arthropathy of the spine following spinal cord injury. J. Bone Joint Surg., *67A*:771–776, 1985.

150. Brunt, P.W.: Unusual cause of Charcot joints in early adolescence (Riley-Day Syndrome). Br. Med. J., *4*:277–278, 1967.

151. Blanford, A.T., Keane, S.P., McCarty, D.J., and Albers, J.W.: Idiopathic Charcot joint of the elbow. Arthritis Rheum., *21*:723–726, 1978.

152. Chillag, K.J., and Stevens, D.B.: Idiopathic neurogenic arthropathy. J. Pediatr. Orthop., *5*:597–600, 1985.

153. Meyn, M., Jr., and Yablon, I.G.: Idiopathic arthropathy of the elbow. Clin. Orthop., *97*:90–93, 1973.

154. Nissenbaum, M.: Neurotrophic arthropathy of the shoulder secondary to tuberculous arachnoiditis. A case report. Clin. Orthop., *118*:169–172, 1976.

155. Wolfgang, G.L.: Neurotrophic arthropathy of the shoulder. A complication of progressive adhesive arachnoiditis. Clin. Orthop., *87*:217–221, 1972.

156. Daughaday, W.H.: Extreme gigantism: Analysis of growth velocity and occurrence of severe peripheral neuropathy and neuropathic arthropathy (Charcot joints). N. Engl. J. Med., *23*:1267–1270, 1977.

157. Rothschild, B.M., and Hanissian, A.S.: Severe generalized (Charcot-like) joint destruction in juvenile rheumatoid arthritis. Clin. Orthop., *155*:75–80, 1981.

158. Meneghello, A., and Bertoli, M.: Neuropathic (Charcot's) joints in dialysis patients. Fortschr. Rontgenstr., *141*:180–184, 1984.

159. Thornhill, H.L., Richter, R.W., Shelton, M.L., and Johnson, C.A.: Neuropathic arthropathic (Charcot forefoot) in alcoholics. Orthop. Clin. North Am., *4*:7–20, 1973.

160. Heller, I.H., and Robb, P.: Hereditary sensory neuropathy. Neurology, *5*:15–29, 1955.

161. Murray, T.J.: Congenital sensory neuropathy. Brain, *96*:387–394, 1973.

162. Pallis, C., and Schneeweiss, J.: Hereditary sensory radicular neuropathy. Am. J. Med., *32*:110–118, 1962.

163. Russell, W.R., and Garland, H.G.: Progressive hypertrophic polyneuritis with case reports. Brain, *53*:376–384, 1930.

164. Bruckner, F.E., and Kendall, B.E.: Neuroarthropathy in Charcot-Marie-Tooth disease. Ann. Rheum. Dis., *28*:577–583, 1969.

165. Goldman, F.: Identification, treatment, and prognosis of Charcot joint in diabetes mellitus. J. Am. Podiatry Assoc., *10*:485–490, 1982.

166. Gristina, A.G., Nicastro, J.F., Clippinger, F., and Rovere, G.D.: Neuropathic foot and ankle patellar-tendon-bearing orthosis. As an adjunct to patient management. Orthop. Rev., *6*:53–59, 1977.

167. Brashear, H.R.: The value of the intramedullary nail for knee fusion particularly for the Charcot joint. Am. J. Surg., *87*:63–65, 1954.

168. Stack, J.K.: Experiences with intramedullary fixation in knee fusion. Am. J. Surg., *83*:291–299, 1952.

169. Drennan, D.B., Fahey, J.J., and Maylahn, R.J.: Important factors in achieving arthrodesis of the Charcot knee. J. Bone Joint Surg., *53A*:1180–1193, 1971.

170. Frymoyer, J.W., and Hoaglund, F.T.: The role of arthrodesis in reconstruction of the knee. Clin. Orthop., *101*:82–92, 1974.

171. Wiseman, L.W.: Neurogenic arthritis and the problems of arthrodesis of the neurogenic knee. Clin. Orthop., *8*:218–226, 1956.

172. Coventry, M.B., et al.: Geometric total knee arthroplasty. II. Patient date and complications. Clin. Orthop., *94*:177–184, 1973.

173. Ritter, M.A., and DeRosa, G.P.: Total hip arthroplasty in a Charcot joint: A case report with a six-year follow-up. Orthop. Rev., 6:51–53, 1977.

174. Charnley, J.: Present status of total hip replacement. Ann. Rheum. Dis., 30:560–564, 1971.

175. Fenlin, J.M., Jr.: Total glenohumeral joint replacement. Orthop. Clin. North Am., 6:565–583, 1975.

176. Sprenger, T.R., and Foley, C.J.: Hip replacement in a Charcot joint: A case report and historical review. Clin. Orthop., 165:191–194, 1982.

177. Soudry, M., et al.: Total knee arthroplasty in Charcot and Charcot-like joints. Clin. Orthop., 208:199–204, 1986.

178. Parsons, H., and Norton, W.S., II: The management of diabetic neuropathic joints. N. Engl. J. Med., 244:935–938, 1951.

82

AMYLOIDOSIS

ALAN S. COHEN

Although amyloid was probably described by several physicians in the 17th century,[1] Rokitansky, in 1842, observed a unique disorder causing a waxy, enlarged liver and, occasionally, similar changes in the spleen.[2] Virchow noted the more widespread recurrence of this waxy material in other organs and subsequently observed that the "lardaceous" liver and spleen stained with iodine and sulfuric acid. Because he believed that it had a certain similarity to cellulose, Virchow named the material "amyloid."[3,4] This substance was studied for many years at the autopsy table or in experimental animals, usually with amyloid induced by infection, until direct biopsy procedures and the Congo red test and stain were introduced in the 1920s.[5-7] In the subsequent 30 years, many clinical and experimental studies were done on what was then considered to be a rare "degenerative" condition. It has become apparent, however, that amyloidosis is not as rare as was thought; it is often of great clinical significance, it is associated with many diseases, and as discovered in the past several decades, it is sometimes genetically determined.[8]

Amyloidosis may be defined as the extracellular deposition of the fibrous protein amyloid in one or more sites of the body. This protein has unique ultrastructural properties, x-ray diffraction, and biochemical characteristics. The substance may be local and isolated with no clinical consequences, it may grossly involve any organ system of the body and may thus lead to severe pathophysiologic changes, or the disorder may fall between these two extremes. The natural history is poorly understood, and the clinical diagnosis may not be made until the disease is far advanced.

CLASSIFICATION

Until recently, the diagnosis of amyloidosis was rarely made during the lifetime of the patient. It is therefore not surprising that most of the older systems of classification depended on the distribution of amyloid in the various organs and on the staining properties of the deposit. Patients with heart, gastrointestinal tract, skin, nerve, and tongue involvement were considered to have "primary" amyloidosis, and those with liver, spleen, kidney, and adrenal involvement, "secondary" amyloidosis. Amyloidosis of any type can involve any organ, however, with variable severity. Furthermore, routine stains do not enable one to distinguish "types" of amyloidosis. Pirani, who has extensively reviewed the complexities of the tissue distribution of amyloid, has pointed out that we still do not know the reason that this protein is deposited repetitively in certain organs in specific syndromes.[9]

The following clinical classification is accepted by most authors: (1) *primary amyloidosis*, in which one sees no evidence of pre-existing or coexisting disease; (2) *amyloidosis associated with multiple myeloma*; (3) *secondary*, or reactive or acquired, amyloidosis, with evidence of chronic infection, such as osteomyelitis, tuberculosis, or leprosy, or chronic inflammatory disease, such as rheumatoid arthritis (RA) or ankylosing spondylitis; (4) *heredofamilial amyloidosis*, which

1273

is the amyloidosis associated with familial Mediterranean fever and a variety of neuropathic, renal, cardiovascular, and other syndromes; (5) *local amyloidosis*, in which local deposits, often resembling tumors, are seen in isolated organs without evidence of systemic involvement; and (6) *amyloidosis associated with aging*.

With the recent progress in delineating the chemical composition of various amyloid proteins, a more exact clinicoimmunochemical classification is now possible. Each of several amyloid proteins has a serum protein precursor, as follows: (1) *the light chains of immunoglobulins* in AL (primary or myeloma associated) amyloidosis, (2) *the acute-phase reactant, serum amyloid A (SAA)* in AA (secondary or acquired) amyloidosis; and (3) *prealbumin* in AF (heredofamilial) amyloidosis and others (Table 82–1). Several forms of localized amyloidosis, especially those associated with endocrine organs and with the aged heart or brain, have also been identified.

PRIMARY AMYLOIDOSIS AND THAT RELATED TO MULTIPLE MYELOMA (AL)

Although the term primary amyloidosis delineates disease in which no predisposing cause is found, it should not be misconstrued as a peculiar clinical type of amyloidosis easily distinguishable from the others. The classic distinctions between primary and secondary amyloidosis based solely on organ distribution are not completely valid. Routine staining cannot distinguish the primary from the secondary type, and under the electron microscope, all types of amyloidosis have an identical fibrillar nature. Only in the early 1970s was the biochemical composition of the amyloid

fibril in this form found to be unique and to consist of fragments of or whole immunoglobulin light chains (κ or λ) in both primary amyloidosis and that associated with multiple myeloma.[10,11] Since then it has been shown that treatment with the potassium permanganate stain, followed by Congo red staining, allows gross differentiation, because secondary amyloid deposits lose their Congo red reactivity whereas primary, myeloma, and heredofamilial deposits do not.

Certain features that alert the clinician to the diagnosis of primary amyloidosis are unexplained proteinuria, peripheral neuropathy, progressive numbness and tingling of the feet, enlarged tongue, increased heart size, unexplained electrocardiographic abnormalities, malabsorption, hepatomegaly, and orthostatic hypotension. Laboratory abnormalities are nonspecific and may or may not include proteinuria, an elevated erythrocyte sedimentation rate, and Bence Jones protein or M component in the patient's serum or urine. The patient frequently has symptoms for several years before the correct diagnosis is made. A biopsy of an involved organ is necessary to confirm the diagnosis. All patients said to have primary amyloidosis should be thoroughly investigated for evidence of other disease, to rule out unsuspected inflammatory disorders and malignant tumors.

Multiple myeloma is a malignant condition with an increased prevalence of amyloid disease. From 6 to 15% of such patients have amyloidosis, the features of which are often indistinguishable from the primary type. Whereas organ involvement in the various types of amyloidosis usually overlaps, involvement of the synovial membrane is found almost exclusively in pa-

Table 82–1. Classification of Amyloidosis

Systemic Forms	Clinical Type	Chemical Composition
AA	Secondary or acquired or reactive	AA (amyloid protein A)
AL	Primary; multiple myeloma associated	Immunoglobulin light chain or fragments
AF	Heredofamilial (dominant)	
	Familial amyloid polyneuropathy	Prealbumin(s) (variant and normal)
	Hereditary cerebral angiopathy	Cystatin C
	Heredofamilial (recessive)	
	Familial Mediterranean Fever	AA (amyloid protein A)
AH	Chronic hemodialysis associated	β_2-microglobulin
Localized Forms		
AE	Endocrine (thyroid)	Precalcitonin
	Endocrine (pancreas)	Calcitonin gene-related protein
AS	Senile (brain)	
	Alzheimer's disease	β-protein
	Senile (heart)*	Prealbumin
AD	Skin	Keratin or precursor (?)

*Possibly systemic, and more than one protein may be involved.

tients with multiple myeloma.[12] This joint disease may mimic the features of RA.

SECONDARY OR REACTIVE (AA) AMYLOIDOSIS

The frequency of amyloidosis in the general population is not known. Most available data are based on postmortem studies, which are unreliable because they are performed on a selected group of patients and special staining for amyloidosis is not routine. The prevalence of amyloid at autopsy in many general hospitals around the world is about 0.5%. In Japan, it is low (0.1%), whereas in countries such as Portugal and Israel, where hereditary amyloid syndromes are known, the prevalence is much greater. Moreover, studies in patients with chronic infectious disease who have an increased risk of developing amyloidosis, such as patients with chronic tuberculosis or leprosy, have shown a high prevalence on postmortem examination, up to 50% in some series.

Patients with chronic inflammatory conditions treated by the rheumatologist may develop amyloidosis. These rheumatic conditions include RA, ankylosing spondylitis, juvenile RA (JRA), Reiter's syndrome, the arthritis associated with psoriasis, and other miscellaneous disorders. Currently, tuberculosis, leprosy, paraplegia, and RA have the greatest incidence.[9] The development of secondary amyloidosis in a patient with one of the aforementioned diseases is often heralded by proteinuria, hepatomegaly, or splenomegaly. The interval between the onset of the rheumatic disease and the appearance of amyloid is unpredictable. Secondary amyloid deposits are composed of a protein moiety termed protein AA, which has a unique amino acid sequence and is distinct from immunoglobulin light chains.

HEREDOFAMILIAL (AF) AMYLOIDOSIS

Hereditary amyloid syndromes have been described in a number of geographic locations; each family and each type described are associated with characteristic organ involvement and clinical manifestations. Generally, the mode of transmission is autosomal dominant, with the exception of familial Mediterranean fever, a condition common in the Near East and affecting Sephardic Jews, Armenians, Turks, and Arabs, for which autosomal recessive transmission has been described. The hereditary amyloidoses represent a new field in our knowledge of amyloid disease. Classification by organ involvement is per-

haps the most useful at present. Although the biochemical nature of these disorders is rapidly being elucidated, the use of such recognizable clinical patterns in defined ethnic groups is still very helpful. Multiple kinships with hereditary amyloidosis of the peripheral nervous system are especially prevalent. Reports of such hereditary syndromes have been appearing in the literature at a rate of about one new syndrome or kinship per year. The amyloid of familial Mediterranean fever is composed of AA protein, whereas the amyloid of most other familial syndromes studied to date is composed of prealbumin.

LOCALIZED AMYLOIDOSIS

In addition to systemic deposition, amyloid may be present in small, focal amounts, sometimes resembling tumors, in any area of the body. Common locations are the lung, skin, larynx, eye, and bladder. In these patients, one rarely sees evidence of systemic disease. Blood vessel involvement is common in primary and secondary amyloidosis. If such involvement is found in a local form, one should investigate further for more widespread disease. Amyloid also occurs not uncommonly in approximation to endocrine organs.

AMYLOIDOSIS IN AGED PERSONS

For reasons not completely understood, amyloidosis occurs more frequently with aging.[13,14] In one series, virtually all consecutive autopsies in individuals over 65 years of age demonstrated small deposits of amyloid.[15] Although usually clinically inapparent, small deposits are often found in the heart, brain, pancreas, and spleen of elderly patients. Occasionally, by virtue of its specific location, such as in the conducting system of the heart, symptoms are severe. Although the pathogenesis of amyloidosis in the process of aging is not clear, the staining properties and the ultrastructure of the amyloid found in the elderly are identical to those of the other types. The major form was originally called *senile cardiac amyloid* and has subsequently been termed *senile systemic amyloid* (SSA). The amyloid protein appears to be prealbumin.[16]

HISTOPATHOLOGIC FEATURES AND STRUCTURE

GROSS APPEARANCE

Amyloid is an amorphous, eosinophilic, glassy, hyaline extracellular substance ubiquitous in distribution. It may be identified by the classic iodine and dilute sulfuric acid stain first used by Virchow. When successful, this stain imparts a blue-purple color to the amyloid, but it is inconsistent and currently only of historical interest. Small amounts of amyloid do not produce gross organ abnormalities. With larger amounts, the involved organs take on a rubbery, firm consistency. They may have a waxy, pink or gray appearance. Organ enlargement, especially of the liver, kidney, spleen, and heart, may be prominent when the deposits are large. In patients with long-standing renal involvement, however, the kidneys may become small and pale. The heart, in addition to being enlarged by the interstitial myocardial involvement, may have nodular elevations on its pericardial and endocardial surfaces, as well as lesions in the valves. Nerves are often normal, even when involved, but they may become thickened and nodular. Other gross findings are variable and depend on the presence or absence of local nodular deposits.

TINCTORIAL PROPERTIES

Microscopically, amyloid is pink when stained with hematoxylin and eosin, and shows crystal violet or methyl violet metachromasia, although it is orthochromatic when stained with toluidine blue. Collagen is stained red by the van Gieson stain, and most of the background appears yellow, but amyloid has a khaki appearance. The periodic acid Schiff (PAS) reagent gives amyloid a violaceous hue.

Congo red remains one of the most widely used stains. It is not completely specific, because it stains elastic tissue and, unless carefully decolorized, stains dense bundles of collagen. When formalin fixed, Congo-red–stained sections are viewed in the polarizing microscope, however, a unique green birefringence is present.[17] *This is the single most useful procedure for establishing the presence of amyloid.* Amyloid has also been stained with fluorochromes to produce a secondary fluorescence, and thioflavine dyes in particular are sensitive indicators of amyloid. The lack of specificity of these dyes, however, makes it mandatory to employ them primarily for screening and to follow with more specific stains. Cotton dyes, especially Sirius red, are also useful and specific. A comparative evaluation of these stains has borne out the high degree of sensitivity and specificity of the green birefringence after staining with Congo red or Sirius red.[18]

A histochemical method that is useful in differentiating AA from AL amyloid has been described by Wright,[19] who modified the Romhanyi amyloid stain.

After incubation with potassium permanganate, AA amyloid, the amyloid of the secondary disorder, loses its affinity for Congo red, whereas AL amyloid, that of primary or myeloma-related amyloidosis, does not. In addition, immunocytochemical methods, using specific anti-AA, anti-AL, and antiprealbumin antisera, allow for even more precise delineation of the type of amyloid in a tissue section.[20]

LIGHT-MICROSCOPIC APPEARANCE

By light microscopy, amyloid is almost invariably extracellular in connective tissue. The deposits may be focal in almost any area of the body, but perivascular amyloid is most often present. The amyloid may involve bone marrow, spleen, capillaries, venules, veins, arterioles, or arteries. The heart may have focal or diffuse interstitial deposits in the myocardium, endocardium, or pericardium. In the kidney, the glomerulus is primarily affected, although interstitial, peritubular, and vascular amyloid may be prominent. In early lesions, small nodular or diffuse deposits appear near the basement membrane; as the disease progresses, the glomerulus may be massively laden, with apparent occlusion of the capillary bed. Atrophic glomeruli laden with amyloid may show marked thickening in the area of Bowman's capsule. Rarely, the glomerulus is replaced almost entirely by connective tissue. Tubular dilation, casts, and interstitial amyloid deposits may be found in the medulla.

In the gastrointestinal tract, one may see perivascular deposits alone, or irregular or diffuse deposits may be found in the submucosa, in the muscularis mucosa, or in the subserosa. The amyloid may appear at any level or portion of the gastrointestinal tract, including the gallbladder and pancreas. Hepatic deposits again may be perivascular only, but more commonly, diffuse amyloid is found between the Kupffer and parenchymal cells. Primary amyloid involves the liver at least as significantly as does secondary and possibly more so.[21] In the nervous system, amyloid has been described along peripheral nerves, in autonomic ganglia, in senile plaques, and in vessels of the central nervous system (CNS). It may be found in any portion of the orbit including the vitreous humor and the cornea.

The bronchopulmonary tract may be involved focally or extensively. The unique aspect of pulmonary or pleural involvement is that although amyloid in virtually all areas of the body remains without evidence of resorption or foreign body reaction, pulmonary amyloid deposits may be accompanied by large numbers of macrophages about and within the lesions. These deposits may also contain islets of cartilage and of ossification. No area of the body is spared, and this ubiquitous distribution produces many clinical symptoms and signs.

ULTRASTRUCTURE

On direct examination under the electron microscope, amyloid consists of fine fibrils[22] (Fig. 82–1). All types of human amyloid, whether primary, secondary, or heredofamilial, no matter how classified, consist of these fine, nonbranching rigid fibrils that in tissue sections measure approximately 100 Å in diameter.[40] When distant from the cell, these fibrils are usually arranged in random array, but close to cells, they may be parallel or perpendicular to the plasmalemma with which they occasionally appear to merge. Intracellular fibrils of dimensions comparable to those outside the cell are sometimes observed. Their precise nature has not yet been established.

The amyloid fibrils are usually seen in earliest and closest relationship to the mesangial cell in the kidney,[23] although as deposits enlarge, they appear in comparable relationship to the endothelial and finally epithelial cell. In the liver, these fibrils first border the Kupffer cell, but they finally fill the space of Disse and are seen about the hepatic cell as well. In many other locations, amyloid fibrils have been found close to blood vessels, pericytes, and endothelial cells. Thus, although the cell-processing amyloid fibrils may appear to be in the reticuloendothelial or macrophage family, this complex process involves, in AA amyloid, the macrophage, the hepatocyte, and probably the reticuloendothelial system or macrophage again.

The amyloid fibrils thus visualized can be extracted from amyloid-laden tissues for more definitive ultra-

FIG. 82–1. Electron micrograph of isolated human secondary amyloid fibrils. Shadow-casted with platinum-palladium. (Magnification ×100,000.)

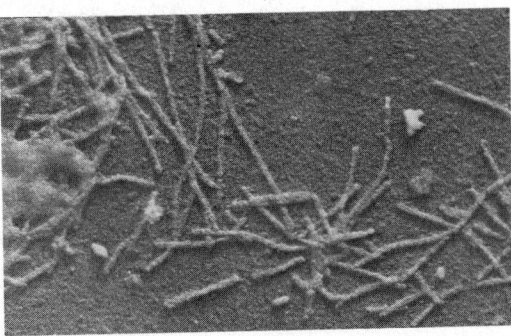

structural, chemical, and immunologic study. When isolated, these fibrils can be specially stained, either positively or negatively with phosphotungstic acid, and their delicate, thin, nonbranching fibrous character can thereby be illustrated. The individual fibril has a diameter of about 70 Å, and the fibrils aggregate laterally. Each fibril is made up of filaments, and subunit protofibrils about 30 to 35 Å in diameter have also been defined.[24] X-ray diffraction of isolated amyloid fibrils reveals a cross-β pattern, the "pleated sheet" of Pauling and Corey, indicating that the polypeptide chain runs transversely to the fiber axis of the specimen.[25,26]

A second substance, P-component (plasma component or pentagonal unit) with different ultrastructure, x-ray diffraction pattern, and chemical characteristics, has also been isolated from amyloid and is identical to a circulating α-globulin present in minute amounts. This substance is not responsible for the characteristic tinctorial properties or ultrastructure of amyloid.[27–29] Amyloid P-component (AP) is distinct on electron microscopy and consists of a pair of pentagonally structured subunits (i.e., each of the pair has five units of 22,000 daltons each, with a total molecular weight [MW] 220,000). C-reactive protein and hamster female protein have similar ultrastructural appearances, and the three belong to a family of proteins now termed *pentraxins*. The physiologic role of AP and its serum counterpart, SAP, is not known, although it has had a stable evolutionary conservation.[30]

BIOCHEMISTRY OF AMYLOID FIBRILS

Amyloid deposits are mainly composed of insoluble fibrillar material that contains a protein backbone. A more precise biochemical identification of constituent amyloid fibril proteins has been made possible with the development of appropriate isolation and purification techniques in the last two decades. Amino acid analyses have indicated that the amyloid proteins contain all of the common amino acids, with no reports of hydroxyproline, hydroxylysine, desmosine, or isodesmosine (uncommon residues present in collagen and elastin). There is a preponderance of aspartic and glutamic acid residues, which can constitute up to 20% of the total amino acid content. This tends to create a highly polyanionic environment, which is characteristic of amyloid fibrils. Identification of the major protein component of the fibril has become the basis for defining the clinical type of amyloid with certainty. Mucopolysaccharide and glycosaminoglycan residues may be present in some types of amyloid.[31-33]

AL AMYLOID

The first systemic form of amyloid to be defined biochemically was the immunoglobulin or primary type, identified in 1970,[11,34] by N-terminal sequence analysis as the variable (V_L) segment of a κ I light chain in two amyloid fibril preparations. Over the subsequent 10 years, additional sequences on this type of amyloid were performed[35-41] (Table 82–2). These sequences have shown κ I, κ II, λ IV, and λ VI and other light chains as amyloid fibril proteins. More than half of all isolated amyloid proteins have had a blocked N-terminus and have been suspected to be of a λ type with a PCA amino terminus.[42] The purified amyloid proteins vary in size from 7,500 to 23,000 daltons, and although sequence data exist for only the N-terminal region, it is assumed that the primary amyloid fibril can consist of the variable part of the light chain, the variable part and a portion of the constant region, or the whole light chain. According to the accepted classification,[43] both κ and λ types of immunoglobulins have been identified as amyloid proteins. Proteins in a λ-VI category are thought to be uniquely associated with amyloidosis, however.

In addition to the over nine amyloid preparations that have undergone partial sequence analysis and the one that has undergone total sequence analysis, data are available on at least four Bence Jones proteins isolated from patients with amyloidosis.[44-47] Two of these have sequence data from both the Bence Jones and the protein amyloid fibril and are completely identified.[44,46] This finding supports the hypothesis that an underlying immunocyte dyscrasia, manifested

by monoclonal proteins and increased bone marrow plasma cells, is of etiologic significance in this type of amyloidosis.

Because the primary proteins consist of the variable fragments of light chains, they also have idiotypic antigenic determinants. As a rule, little cross-reactivity has been noted between the amyloid proteins belonging to the different subgroups.[48,49] This lack of common antibody contributes to the diagnostic dilemma in identifying the type of amyloid in the patient with systemic disease. Tissue biopsy specimens are now analyzed for AA amyloid by radioimmunoassay or immunocytochemistry to rule out the secondary form of amyloid. If the test results are negative, the specimens can be examined for prealbumin by the same methods to exclude hereditary amyloidosis. If test results are still negative, one cannot precisely define primary amyloid short of postmortem isolation and sequence analysis of the fibrils, although the potassium permanganate stain noted earlier is of assistance.

AA AMYLOID

Another protein unrelated to any known immunoglobulin has been described in secondary amyloid deposits.[50-55] Fibrils containing AA (amyloid A) protein can be isolated from patients with secondary amyloidosis, the disorder associated with familial Mediterranean fever, and the amyloid isolated from experimental animals following casein injections. It is a unique protein with the molecular weight of about 8,500 daltons made up of 76 amino acid residues arranged in a single chain, the amino acid sequence beginning arginine-serine-phenylalanine (ARG-SER-PHE). Heterogeneity among the different species has

Table 82–2. Primary Amyloid (AL) Sequences

AL	Type	1	2	3	4	5	6	7	8	9	10	Thru	M.W.	Ref.
10	AL$_{kI}$	asp	ile	gln	met	thr	gln	ser	ala	ser	ser	(36)	7,500	10
8	AL$_{kI}$	asp	ile	gln	met	thr	gln	ser	ala	ser	ser	(35)	18,300	10
MAG	AL$_{kI}$	asp	ile	gln	met	thr	gln	ser	ala	ser	ser	(32)	11,000	67
LEP	AL$_{kI}$	asp	ile	gln	met	thr	gln	ser	ala	ser	ser	(27)	23,000	36
TEW	AL$_{kII}$	asp	ile	val	met	thr	glu	ser	pro	leu	ser	(27)	23,000	40
808	AL$_{IV}$	( )	tyr	asp	leu	thr	gln	(pro)	pro	ser	val	(21)		41
758	AL$_{IV}$	( )	tyr	asp	leu	thr	gln	pro	pro	ser	val	(27)		37
JAM	AL$_{IV}$	asp	phe	met	leu	thr	glu	pro	his	ser	val	(17)	16,000	38
AR	AL$_{IV}$	asp	phe	met	leu	thr	gln	pro	his	ser	val	(154)	16,000	39
RS	AL$_{IV}$	asp	phe	met	leu	thr	gln	pro	his	ser	val	(34)		37
LEP	BJP$_{kI}$	asp	ile	gln	met	thr	gln	ser	ala	ser	ser	(29)	23,000	44
TEW	BJP$_{kII}$	asp	ile	val	met	thr	gln	ser	pro	leu	ser	(214)	23,000	46
NIG-51	BJP$_I$	PCA	ser	val	leu	thr	gln	pro	pro	ser	ala	(214)	23,000	47
MCG	BJP$_V$	PCA	ser	ala	leu	thr	gln	pro	pro	ser	ala	(216)	23,000	45

(asp = aspartic acid; ile = isoleucine; tyr = tyrosine; phe = phenylalanine; ser = serine; gln = glutamine; val = valine; met = methionine; ala = alanine; leu = leucine; thr = threonine; glu = glutamic acid; pro = proline; his = histidine.)

Table 82–3. Amyloid A (AA) and Serum Amyloid A (SAA) Sequences

Species						1	2	3	4	5	6	7	8	9	10	Ref.
Human						arg	ser	phe	phe	ser	phe	lue	gly	glu	ala	52
Monkey						arg	ser	trp	phe	ser	phe	leu	gly	glu	ala	176
Mouse						(arg)	ser/ gly	phe	phe	ser	phe	ile	gly	glu	ala	75
Guinea pig	his	ala	lys	gly	glu	arg	ser	ile	phe	ser	phe	leu	lys	glu	ser/ ala	177
Mink						(Blocked N term-identity beginning res 17)										73
Duck	asp	asn	pro	phe	thr	arg	gly	gly	arg	phe	val	leu	asp	ala	ala	178

(his = histidine; asp = aspartic acid; ala = alanine; asn = asparagine; lys = lysine; pro = proline; gly = glycine; phe = phenylalanine; glu = glutamic acid; thr = threonine; arg = arginine; ser = serine; trp = tryptophan; ile = isoleucine; val = valine; leu = leucine.)

been described, showing that several additional residues may precede the first residue, possibly as the result of proteolysis of a larger precursor (Table 82–3).

Antisera to alkali-degraded amyloid fibrils of the AA protein have detected an antigenically related serum component, SAA.[51,56–58] The soluble protein, which appears to circulate in association with the high-density lipoprotein-3 (HDL$_3$) subclass of lipoproteins, has a total molecular weight of 160,000 to 200,000 daltons and exhibits NH$_2$-terminal homology to AA.[59,60,61] SAA is one of the most dramatic of the acute-phase reactants, that is, the production of this protein is altered tremendously (it may be increased greater than 1000-fold) in response to some inflammatory stimuli.[62,63] However, elevated amounts of SAA do not necessarily invoke amyloidosis.[64]

The current concept is that apoSAA is the putative precursor of AA protein and, in fact, studies have demonstrated the conversion of apoSAA to AA protein following COOH-terminal proteolysis in vitro and more recently in vivo.[65,66] As an acute-phase reactant, SAA is elevated in infection and inflammation.[69,70] In patients with JRA, SAA is related more to the activity and seropositivity than to the presence of amyloid. Recent data suggest that SAA is not age related.[71] SAA levels have also been suggested as potential monitors of neoplastic disease.[72]

SAA has been studied in a variety of animal species including the mink, in which endotoxin was a potent stimulus for its generation before the appearance of detectable amyloid.[73] Casein given to CBA/J mice has induced SAA as well as amyloid composed of protein AA.[74,75] A study by McAdam and Sipe showed that murine SAA has a MW of 160,000 and dissociated to a more stable 12,500 moiety on formic acid treatment.[76] These researchers found that SAA behaved as an acute-phase reactant and was elevated even in amyloid-resistant animals, either those pretreated with colchicine or a genetically resistant AJ strain, and suggested that amyloid resistance is related to the processing and catabolism of SAA. It has been suggested that SAA is a polymorphic serum protein and

may not be a simple precursor of AA.[77] It has also been suggested that SAA suppresses antibody response and may regulate such response.[78] More extensive studies of murine SAA confirmed the human studies and showed that SAA is among the apoproteins of the HDL complex.[79] Current evidence suggests that there are three isotypes of SAA and that the SAA$_2$ isotype may be the AA precursor, while SAA$_3$ may be derived from Kupffer cells and macrophages.[80–82]

OTHER AMYLOID MOIETIES

A Prealbumin

The literature on new and distinct amyloid proteins has expanded enormously. A major constituent especially in familial amyloid polyneuropathies (FAP) has been found to be prealbumin (transthyretin).[83] Amino acid sequencing has shown (in type I FAP in Portuguese, Japanese, Swedish and Greek patients) single amino acid substitutions, that is, methionine for valine at position 30 in the 127 amino acid molecule.[84–88] Type II FAP was originally described by Rukavina in a Swiss population in Indiana (carpal tunnel syndrome, vitreous opacities, and heart disease as well as neuropathy) and has a serine substitution for isoleucine at position 84.[89] A third kinship from Appalachia with late onset FAP and severe cardiac disease has a different variant prealbumin with the substitution of alanine for threonine at position 60.[90] A family of Jewish background in Poland was shown by one group to have a glycine for threonine substitution at position 49[91] and by another to have an isoleucine for phenylalanine substitution at position 33.[92] A German/American family had a tyrosine for serine at position 77, and a Danish family with severe cardiopathy, a methionine for leucine at position 110.[93] Thus, at least six variant prealbumins have been reported.

Chronic Hemodialysis-Associated Amyloid (AH)

One of the first neuropathies recognized as having an association with amyloid was the carpal tunnel syndrome. Indeed, in AL amyloid an incidence of about 20% has been reported. The carpal tunnel syndrome has also been described in certain FAP syndromes. Carpal tunnel syndrome has been increasingly associated with chronic hemodialysis (5 to 10+ years' duration) and is caused by amyloid deposits.[94] More prominent musculoskeletal lesions, including juxta-articular radiolucent bone cysts, isolated bone cysts, destructive arthropathies of large joints, and spondyloarthropathies, may also complicate long-term hemodialysis. These lesions are also caused largely by amyloid deposits.[95] Such deposits are composed of β_2-microglobulin, an 11,800-dalton molecule, whose normal level of 1 to 2 mg/L increases to 50 to 100 mg/L in patients with renal failure treated with hemodialysis.[96–98] Changes in the standard hemodialysis membranes to allow the elimination of β_2-microglobulin could potentially reduce or eliminate this complication.

Alzheimer's Disease-Related Amyloid

The lesions in the brains of patients with Alzheimer's disease consist of plaques, neurofibrillary tangles (intraneuronal), and variable blood vessel changes (congophilic angiopathy). All of these lesions stain positively with Congo red, and this reaction has been variously attributed to different proteins. These changes are also seen in the brains of individuals with Down's syndrome. A specific amyloidogenic protein variously termed β-protein[99,100] and A_4,[101,102] which has a unique amino acid sequence, has been identified in these lesions.[99–105] The genetic defect in familial Alzheimer's disease is located on chromosome 21, the location of the extra copy of Down's syndrome.

Other Amyloid Proteins

The amyloid of medullary carcinoma of the thyroid appears to be related to thyrocalcitonin,[103] while amyloid in the exocrine pancreas may be due to a peptide in the calcitonin gene-related peptide family.[104] In addition, a prealbumin-like molecule has been described in the hearts of elderly individuals with focal amyloid deposits.[105]

P-COMPONENT OF AMYLOID

In addition to the characteristic fibrils described, a minor second component, the P-component, has been noted in most amyloid deposits.[27–29] P-component (AP) has been recognized by electron microscopy as a pentagonal unit measuring about 90 Å in diameter on the outside and 40 Å on the inside. It appears to consist of five globular subunits of 25 to 30 Å, which

may aggregate laterally to form short rods. On immunoelectrophoresis, this component migrates as an α-globulin, and it possesses antigenic identity with a constituent of normal human plasma. The amino acid sequence is distinct from that of the amyloid fibrils. The N-terminal amino acid is histidine and contains large amounts of aspartic acid, glutamic acid, glycine, and leucine. Sequence to 23 residues found the protein to be unique.[29] The MW, probably that of a doublet, is about 180,000 to 220,000, and it has subunits of about 22,000 daltons. AP is associated with all types of amyloid, including that isolated from the pancreas of patients with long-standing diabetes.[106] The only exception is its absence from the amyloid plaques and neurofibrillary tangles in the brain of patients with Alzheimer's disease. It has been found in the vascular amyloid in the brain, however.[107]

Human AP has been isolated from plasma by affinity chromatography. Characterization and comparison of the isolated P-component proteins from tissue and plasma demonstrated immunologic and sequence identity[108] (Table 82–5). The AP N-terminal sequence compared from three amyloid fibril preparations, a primary κ, a primary λ, and a secondary AA, has been found to be homologous. Electron-microscopic studies have revealed that the plasma P-component has a pentagonal ultrastructure identical to that of the tissue P-component.

AP also has substantial homology in amino acid sequence, molecular appearance, and subunit composition to C-reactive protein, but differences in MW (C-reactive protein has about half the MW of SAP) and in other parameters suggest that although these substances are analogous and may have evolutionary relationships to one another, they are indeed distinct.[108–110] SAP in humans does not usually behave as an acute-phase reactant, although it does become elevated in patients with malignant disease.[111] The unique relationship between SAP and amyloid fibrils, both AA and AL, is at least partly due to a calcium-dependent binding of SAP in vitro to isolated fibrils.[112,113]

IMMUNOBIOLOGY OF AMYLOID

The origin and pathogenesis of amyloidosis are unknown. Advances in characterization of the chemical structure of amyloid may provide insight into these complex mechanisms. Ultrastructural studies of amyloid-laden tissues in an animal model have led to the concept that cytoplasmic invaginations, containing tufts of amyloid fibers, cell–amyloid interface, were the sites of amyloid formation.[117] Electron-microscopic

Table 82–4. AF Amyloid Proteins

	1	2	3	4	5	6	7	8	9	10	11	12	Ref.
Prealbumin	gly	pro	thr	gly	thr	gly	glu	ser	lys	cys	pro	leu	179
Amyloid LIN	gly	pro	thr	gly	thr	gly	glu	ser	lys	cys	pro	leu	87
Amyloid GRO													86
Amyloid SKO	gly	pro	(thr)	gly	( )	gly	glu	ser	lys	(cys)	pro	leu	91
	13	14	15	16	17	18	19	20	21	22	23	24	
Prealbumin	met	val	lys	val	leu	asp	ala	val	arg	gly	ser	pro	
LIN	met	val	lys	val	leu	asp	ala	val	arg	gly			
GRO	val	val	val	leu	asp	ala	val	arg	gly	thr	pro		
SKO	(met)	val	lys	val	leu	asp							

(gly = glycine; met = methionine; val = valine; pro = proline; thr = threonine; lys = lysine; leu = leucine; asp = aspartic acid; ala = alanine; glu = glutamic acid; ser = serine; arg = arginine; cys = cystine.)

autoradiographic studies have revealed high concentrations of fibrils adjacent to reticuloendothelial cells; this finding suggests that they may synthesize as well as degrade the fibrils. Unusual inclusions are found with the reticuloendothelial cells intimately associated with fresh amyloid deposits.[114] These inclusions are located in the areas rich in the primary lysosome type of dense bodies, and the cytoplasmic invaginations contain well-oriented fibrils. The inclusions may be transitional forms from the usual dense bodies and may constitute direct evidence of the involvement of lysosomes in amyloid fibril formation.

Excess antigenic stimulus has induced amyloid formation in animals. The basic conditions for the experimental induction have not been clearly defined, however. Marked depression of T cells with maintenance of normal B-cell function has been described, and administration of bovine thymus (thymosin) may suppress amyloid formation in mice.[118] These findings suggest that disturbances in immunoregulatory mechanisms may be important in the pathogenesis of amyloid disease.[119]

Additional studies of cellular and humoral immunity in amyloidosis have been performed.[120–122] The availability of animal models for acquired (secondary) systemic amyloidosis has advanced our understanding of this disease.[74] With these models, some important concepts regarding the pathogenesis of amyloid, such as the two-phase concept of amyloid induction,[123] transfer of amyloid,[124,125] and involvement of the reticuloendothelial system in amyloid fibril formation,[114,126] were developed.

The mechanism of acute-phase SAA elevation has also been studied. The origin of SAA as an acute-phase reactant has become a prototype for the study of the regulation of acute-phase reactant synthesis. It is believed that acute-phase proteins are produced as part of the systemic host response to localized injury, and numerous studies suggest that circulating mediators are released at the site of injury. One of the functions of these mediators is to stimulate hepatic synthesis of acute-phase reactants. Endotoxin or lipopolysaccharide stimulates the acute-phase SAA response by interacting with macrophages to produce a substance, "SAA inducer," capable of eliciting an elevated SAA concentration in mice that does not mount an SAA response to the lipopolysaccharide itself. This mediator of SAA synthesis is identical to interleukin 1 (IL-1). IL-1 is a soluble monokine elicited by inflammation and antigenic stimulation, with many target cells including T cells, hepatocytes, synovial cell fibroblasts, brain cells, and possibly B cells.[127,128]

An interesting but confusing concept, the "transfer

Table 82–5. Sequence Comparison of P-Component of Amyloid, Serum P-Component, and C-Reactive Protein

	1	2	3	4	5	6	7	8	9	10	Ref.
Human AP	his	thr	asp	leu	ser	gly	lys	val	phe	val	108
Human SAP	his	thr	asp	leu	ser	gly	lys	val	phe	val	108
Human CRP	PCA	thr	asp	met	ser	arg	lys	ala	phe	val	109
	11	12	13	14	15	16	17	18	19	20	
AP	phe	pro	arg	glu	ser	val	thr	asp	his	val	
SAP	phe	pro	arg	glu	ser	val	thr	asp	his	val	
CRP	phe	pro	lys	glu	ser	asp	thr	ser	tyr	val	

(AP = amyloid P-component; SAP = serum amyloid P-component; CRP = C-reactive protein; his = histidine; phe = phenylalanine; thr = threonine; pro = proline; asp = aspartic acid; arg = arginine; lys = lysine; leu = leucine; met = methionine; glu = glutamic acid; ser = serine; gly = glycine; val = valine; ala = alanine; tyr = tyrosine.)

of amyloid" studied by Hardt and Ranlov in the mid-1960s,[124] as well as by many others later, has recently been refined.[129] A model of accelerated amyloidosis has made it possible to relate the formation of amyloid fibrils to the normal acute-phase response. A substance called amyloid-enhancing factor, extracted from spleens of preamyloidotic mice, can alter the acute-phase response such that amyloid fibrils are deposited in spleen. This factor is localized to the extracellular portion of spleen, where amyloid is deposited. It appears that amyloid-enhancing factor, produced by repeated episodes of inflammation, plays an essential role in the formation of AA fibrils from SAA. The role of this factor in the kinetics of amyloid deposition has been defined.[125,130] Amyloidogenesis has two phases, a predeposition phase that lasts from 7 to 21 days and a deposition phase that continues as long as inflammation persists. Amyloid-enhancing factor shortens the predeposition phase to under 2 days. The spleen, although the earliest and most heavily affected tissue, is not essential for production of this factor, and in any tissue to be affected, amyloid-enhancing factor is present 1 to 2 days before the appearance of fibrils. Furthermore, the deposition phase has been subdivided into rapid deposition and plateau stages. These stages are important in defining therapy. Colchicine and dimethyl sulfoxide are most effective during the rapid deposition period, but are ineffective in the plateau stage. These studies raise an important concept of staging and prophylaxis, as well as therapy, in secondary amyloidosis. In summary then, there are two key processes involved in amyloidogenesis. First, a stimulus involves alterations in the serum concentrations of the precursor proteins (e.g., stimulus to macrophage to produce IL-1, which then induces the hepatic parenchymal cell to produce large amounts of SAA); second, a step involves processing or converting the precursor to amyloid fibrils (SAA conversion to AA).[1] Whether alterations in the local milieu (i.e., glycosaminoglycans) also occur is not yet clear.

Among many treatments purported to influence the course of amyloidosis, colchicine has played an important role in studies of the acquired systemic variety that can occur in situations of chronic and recurrent acute inflammation. Since the observation that colchicine treatment of patients with familial Mediterranean fever lessens or prevents amyloid deposition, this drug has been used to treat all types of systemic amyloidosis. Colchicine has blocked or delayed the development of AA amyloidosis in the mouse model of the disease.[131,132] The therapeutic value of dimethyl sulfoxide in amyloidosis was first reported in a mouse

model in 1976, and clinical trials have since been undertaken.[133]

Animal models for other than the AA type of amyloidosis are scarce.[48] Spontaneous amyloidosis has been reported in a few strains of mice and other species; however, in most cases, the models have been poorly defined with regard to reproducibility and the biochemical and immunologic characteristics of the amyloid. A new mouse model for spontaneous aging amyloidosis seems valuable because of the high predictable incidence of amyloidosis, the absence of apparent predisposing conditions for acquired amyloidosis, and the preliminary biochemical and immunologic findings for the uniqueness of its amyloid protein.[134]

Thus, amyloidosis the disease and amyloid the substance have been more precisely defined in modern biochemical terms. Further categorization will doubtless be possible, with clinicopathologic implications concerning pathogenesis and diagnosis. A clearer delineation of the relation of animal models of acquired amyloidosis to the other systemic and localized forms of the disease in terms of mediators and amyloid-enhancing factor will also contribute to a better understanding of the origin and pathogenesis of this complex disorder.

CLINICAL ASPECTS

DIAGNOSIS

Although the specific diagnosis of amyloidosis depends on tissue examination with appropriate stains,[22] the disease must first be suspected on clinical grounds. When a patient who has a disorder predisposing him to amyloid formation develops hepatomegaly, splenomegaly, malabsorption, cardiac disease, or, most important, proteinuria, amyloidosis should be suspected. Moreover, in heredofamilial syndromes,[8] especially those with an autosomal dominant mode of transmission and characterized by peripheral neuropathy, particularly that starting in the lower limb, nephropathy, or cardiopathy, the diagnosis of amyloidosis should be considered. Finally, primary systemic amyloidosis should be suspected in patients with a diffuse, noninflammatory, infiltrative disease involving either mesenchymal tissues such as blood vessels, heart, or gastrointestinal tract or parenchymal tissues such as kidney, liver, spleen, or adrenal gland.

For screening purposes, a subcutaneous abdominal fat-pad aspiration may be the simplest and most useful procedure[135,136] (Fig. 82–2). Complications are al-

FIG. 82–2. Light micrographs of an abdominal fat biopsy stained with Congo red and hematoxylin non-polarized (A) and polarized (B), the latter demonstrating green birefringence. (Magnification ×90.)

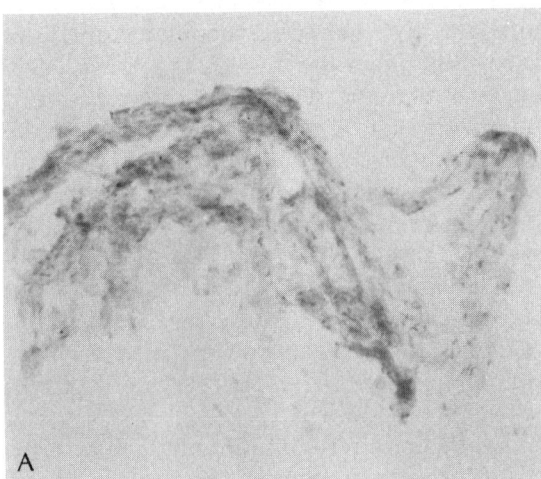
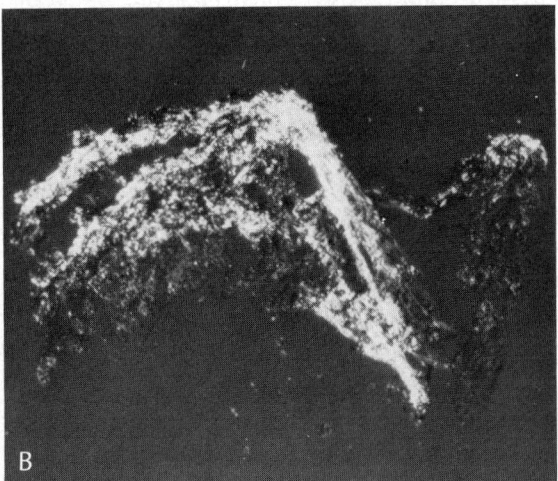

most nonexistent; no absolute contraindications exist, and with appropriate staining and interpretation, the overall sensitivity is in the range of 90%. Until this procedure is more generally used, however, it is good practice to perform a rectal biopsy for diagnosis (Fig. 82–3). If this procedure is contraindicated or if the patient refuses, gingival biopsy is recommended. Skin biopsy, of both involved and uninvolved skin, is also useful in all types of amyloidosis.[137] If results of the aforementioned procedures are negative in patients who have renal disease, hepatic disease, or other organ involvement, biopsy of the appropriate site is undertaken with the standard precautions against bleeding. All tissue obtained must be stained with Congo red and examined under a polarizing microscope for green birefringence. If a polarizing microscope is not available, a light microscope may be adapted.[17] If this is not possible, a crystal violet stain is useful. Electron-microscopic examination of tissue sections has been recommended when histochemical stains are negative. Such occasions, however, are rare, and the technique is not necessary for most routine studies.

If amyloidosis is still suspected even after negative biopsy results, a Congo red test may be performed. This test may be positive when the biopsy is negative,

FIG. 82–3. Light micrographs of a rectal biopsy stained with Congo red and hematoxylin nonpolarized (A) and polarized (B), the latter demonstrating green birefringence. (Magnification ×90.)

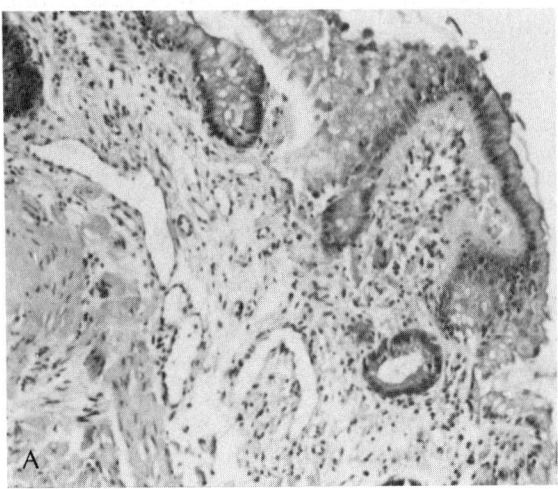
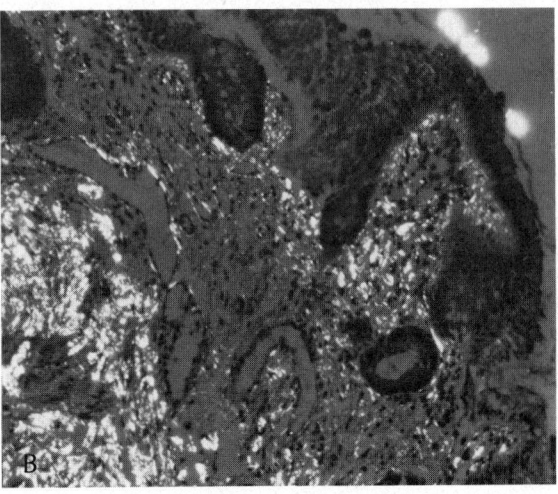

and vice versa.[138,139] The Evans blue test has been suggested as an alternative, but it does not add to results of the aforementioned test. My recommended procedures are outlined in Table 82–6, which lists the appropriate biopsy sites.

AMYLOIDOSIS AS A RHEUMATIC DISEASE

Amyloid can directly involve articular structures and may be present in the synovial membrane (Figs. 82–4, 82–5), as well as in the synovial fluid.[140] It may also occur in the articular cartilage.[141] Amyloid arthritis can mimic a number of rheumatic diseases because it can become manifest as a symmetric, small-joint arthritis associated with nodules, morning stiffness, and fatigue.[12] The diagnosis of RA can be made in error, and differentiation is imperative because of the great difference in prognosis. When diagnostic arthrocentesis is done and amorphous material is seen in the fluid, a Congo red stain should be used and the material viewed under a polarizing microscope. Individuals with nodules and no erosive disease, as well as patients whose nodules enlarge precipitously, should be looked at more critically. When excessive soft tissue boggy thickening is present, the patient may also have amyloid disease. Amyloidosis should be suspected in those patients with multiple myeloma with articular manifestations. Indeed, most, but not all, patients with amyloid arthropathy (excluding those on chronic hemodialysis) do eventually seem to have multiple myeloma.[12,142]

One might expect that amyloidosis of the joints would not be limited to multiple myeloma and would be present in patients with systemic or generalized primary amyloidosis and with generalized secondary amyloidosis. Clinical arthropathy due to amyloid in generalized secondary amyloidosis is unusual, how-ever. Few data are available from systemic analysis of joint disease for the presence of amyloid. In a report of 289 joint biopsies,[143] some suggestion of amyloid was found in 83 (28.7%). In most other autopsy series of patients with RA, either no mention is made of amyloid in joints or, in the few joints appropriately examined, none is found. Because of the widespread involvement of small blood vessels throughout the body in both primary and secondary disease, small amounts of perivascular amyloid may be found.

Amyloid has been found in association with degenerative joint disease,[144,145] as well as chondrocalcinosis.[146] Egan and associates found amyloid in 6 of 13 cartilage specimens, 4 of 18 articular capsules, and 2 of 16 synovial membranes from patients with osteoarthritis of the hip.[68] The clinical significance of such deposits is not known.

In summary, clinically significant amyloid arthritis can be characterized as follows.[12] The joints most frequently involved are shoulders, wrist, knees, and fingers.[12] The period of morning stiffness associated with the early lesions is shorter than in RA. The joints are often swollen and firm, and occasionally tender, but redness and severe tenderness have not been noted. Swelling of the shoulders may resemble shoulder pads (see Fig. 82–4). Subcutaneous nodules are present in almost 70% of cases, whereas rheumatoid factor is uncommon. Roentgenograms show soft tissue swelling. Erosions about the joints were noted only once among 20 patients studied. Generalized osteoporosis, with or without osteolytic lesions, however, is common and is seen in 80% of patients.

The synovial fluid is usually benign and appears to have the characteristics of a traumatic effusion or a low-grade inflammation. It is generally described as viscous, yellow, or xanthochromic; mucin clot is good to poor. The leukocyte count is usually low, with a median of about 1000 cells/mm³ but counts as high as 10,000 cells/mm³ have been reported. Usually, one

Table 82–6. Diagnosis of Amyloidosis

Biopsy		
Common Sites	Occasional Sites	Rare Sites
Subcutaneous abdominal fat aspirate	Small intestine	Kidney
Rectum	Muscle	Liver
Skin	Nerve	Bone marrow
Gingiva		Synovium
		Spleen

Appropriate Stain
Congo red, viewed in polarizing microscope
Others
Cotton dyes (comparable to Congo red)
Thioflavin (less specific)
Crystal violet (less sensitive)

FIG. 82–4. "Shoulder pad" sign in a 52-year-old woman with primary amyloidosis and widespread amyloid arthropathy simulating rheumatoid arthritis.

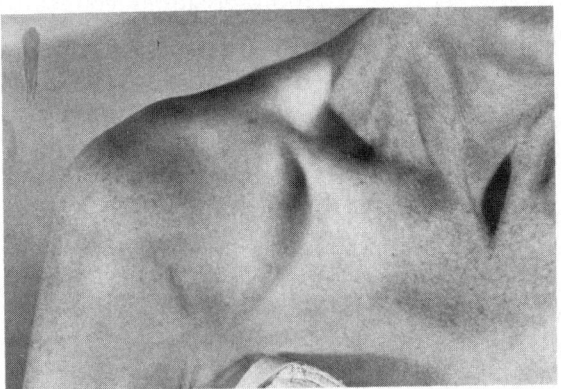

sees a predominance of mononuclear cells. Free-amyloid-containing bodies, presumably synovial villi, were found in the sediment of three fluids extensively studied, and possible free amyloid itself.[140] The synovial membrane may have lining-cell amyloid, subsynovial amyloid, or perivascular deposits. Multiple myeloma predominates. Carpal tunnel syndrome, often bilateral, is often associated with amyloid arthropathy. Congophilic deposits were found in synovial fluid from six of seven patients known to have synovial amyloidosis complicating chronic hemodialysis. Immunohistochemistry showed β_2-microglobulin in each case.[147] More extensive synovial, bone and periarticular amyloid may be present in this chronic hemodialysis amyloid syndrome.[95]

FIG. 82–5. The hands of the patient in Figure 82–4 showing flexion contractures of the fingers from synovial thickening of the metacarpophalangeal and proximal interphalangeal joints and flexor tendons.

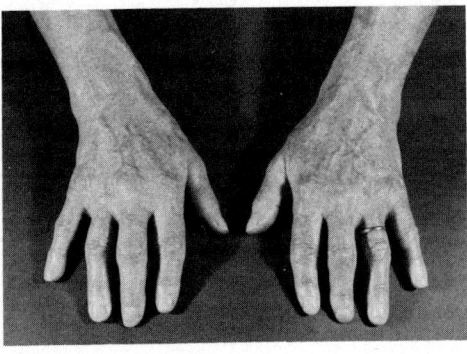

GENERAL MANIFESTATIONS

The clinical manifestations of amyloidosis vary and depend entirely on the affected structures.[3,148,149]

Renal Involvement

Renal involvement may consist of mild proteinuria or frank nephrosis, or in some cases, the urinary sediment may show only a few red blood cells.[150] The renal lesion is usually irreversible and in time leads to progressive azotemia and death. The prognosis does not appear to be related to the degree of the proteinuria. When azotemia finally develops, if it is due to the amyloid process and not to a reversible superimposed condition, the prognosis is grave. In a group of patients with secondary amyloidosis, those with some residual function remained comfortable for long periods, but once the patient's serum creatinine level was over 3 mg/dl, or the creatinine clearance was under 20 mg/ml, the prognosis was poor.[151] In another series, the mean survival after the time of biopsy was 29 months,[152] but in five cases, evidence showed regression of the disease. Hypertension is rare, except in longstanding amyloidosis. Serial films of the kidneys may or may not show a diminution in size. Renal tubular acidosis or renal vein thrombosis may occur. Localized accumulation of amyloid may be noted in the ureter, bladder, or other genitourinary tract tissue.

Hepatic Involvement

Although hepatomegaly is common, liver function abnormalities are minimal and occur late in the disease. The most useful tests of hepatic involvements with amyloid are the Bromsulphalein (BSP) extraction and the serum alkaline phosphatase level. Liver scans have variable, nonspecific results, but bone-seeking radionuclides, such as ^{99m}Tc diphosphonate, have recently shown increased liver uptake because of the high calcium content of amyloid.[153] Signs of intrahepatic cholestasis are uncommon.[154] In our series in which liver tissue from 54 patients was examined, whether the disorder was primary or secondary, all had some amyloid present, either in the parenchyma or in blood vessels.[155] The remarkable degree to which liver parenchyma can be replaced by amyloid was seen in a patient whose liver was palpable below the iliac crest and weighed 7200 g; BSP extraction during life in this patient had been 17%, with only a modest elevation of the serum alkaline phosphatase level. Splenomegaly may be massive, although usually it does not cause symptoms unless traumatic rupture occurs. Amyloidosis of the spleen is not usually associated with leukopenia and anemia.

Cardiac Involvement

Cardiac manifestations consist primarily of enlargement and congestive heart failure, either with or without murmurs and arrhythmias.[156] Although these manifestations reflect predominantly diffuse myocardial amyloid deposition, the endocardium, valves, and pericardium may be involved. Pericarditis with effusion is rare, although one must frequently distinguish between constrictive pericarditis and restrictive myocardiopathy. The clinical features and the demonstration of a left ventricular end-diastolic pressure exceeding that of the right are useful in distinguishing restrictive myocardiopathy from constrictive pericarditis, but even left heart catheterization and quantitative left ventriculography are not always enough to make the differential diagnosis.[115] Echocardiographic study has demonstrated symmetric thickening of the left ventricular wall, hypokinesia, decreased systolic thickening of the interventricular septum and left ventricular posterior wall, and the small-to-normal size of the left ventricular cavities.[157]

Hearts heavily infiltrated with amyloid may or may not exhibit an enlarged silhouette. Fluoroscopic study shows decreased mobility of the ventricular wall; angiographic studies usually show a thickened ventricular wall, decreased ventricular mobility, and the absence of rapid ventricular filling in early diastole.

The first signs of cardiac amyloid are often those of intractable heart failure. Electrocardiographic abnormalities include a low-voltage QRS complex and abnormalities in atrioventricular and intraventricular conduction, often resulting in varying degrees of heart block. Electrocardiographic abnormalities are frequent, often without previous infarct.[159] Because of their propensity to conduction defects and arrhythmias, patients with cardiac amyloidosis appear to be especially sensitive to digitalis, and this drug should be used in small doses and with caution. Binding of digoxin by isolated amyloid fibrils may play a role in such sensitivity.[158]

More recent noninvasive techniques have added to our understanding of the extent of cardiac amyloid and the associated functional abnormalities.[159] For example, ^{99m}Tc pyrophosphate or diphosphonate scintigraphy is a sensitive and specific test for amyloid in patients with congestive heart failure of obscure origin. It is not useful, however, as an indicator of early cardiac amyloid in patients without electrocardiographic or other abnormalities.[160] Although M-mode echocardiography can, by the presence of thickened ventricular walls with a small or normal left ventricle, suggest amyloid, two-dimensional echocardiography adds substantial new information. It demonstrates thickened ventricles with a normal left ventricular cavity and a unique diffuse hyperrefractile "granular" sparkling appearance.[161] Thirty-one patients with documented cardiac amyloidosis were compared to 39 control subjects with left ventricular hypertrophy to determine specific two-dimensional echocardiographic features of amyloid. In 16 patients, increased myocardial echogenicity was present when a single short-axis view was examined, and these patients had a sensitivity of 63% and a specificity of 74% for the diagnosis of amyloidosis. When complete echocardiograms were reviewed, an improved sensitivity of 87% and specificity of 81% based on increased echogenicity was seen. Increased atrial septal thickness was present in 60% of amyloid patients and in no controls. The combination of increased myocardial echogenicity and increased atrial thickness was 60% sensitive and 100% specific for the diagnosis of amyloidosis. Detailed 24-hour electrocardiographic monitoring of patients with amyloid heart disease has revealed a significant number of high-grade ventricular arrhythmias and a lesser incidence of clinically significant bradycardia.[159]

Skin Lesions

Involvement of the skin is one of the most characteristic manifestations of the so-called "primary" amyloidoses. The lesions may consist of raised, waxy, often translucent papules or plaques, usually clustered in the folds about the axillae, the anal or inguinal regions, the face and neck, or mucosal areas such as the ear or tongue. The patient may also have purpuric areas, nodules or tumefactions, alopecia, a yellowish waxy discoloration, glossitis, and xerostomia. The lesions are seldom pruritic. Involvement of the skin or mucosa may be inapparent, even on close inspection, yet may be disclosed at biopsy. Gentle rubbing of the skin with one's finger may induce bleeding (purpura). Skin involvement can also occur in secondary amyloidosis. Amyloid was demonstrated in biopsy of the skin, with or without clinical lesions, in 42% of a group of 12 patients with secondary disease and in 55% of a group of 38 patients with primary disease.[137] All of a group of 8 patients with hereditary amyloid neuropathy studied by us had positive skin biopsies.

Gastrointestinal Involvement

Gastrointestinal findings in amyloidosis are common and may result from direct infiltration at any level or from infiltration of the autonomic nervous system. Symptoms and signs include those of obstruction, ulceration, malabsorption, hemorrhage, protein loss, and diarrhea. Infiltration of the tongue may lead to macroglossia, which may become incapacitating; alternatively, the tongue, although not enlarged, may become stiffened and firm to palpation. Infiltration of the tongue is especially characteristic of primary amyloidosis or amyloidosis accompanying multiple myeloma, but it may also occur in secondary amyloidosis.

Gastrointestinal bleeding may initiate from a number of sites, notably the esophagus, stomach, or large intestine, and may be severe or even fatal. Amyloid infiltration of the esophagus or small bowel may lead to clinical and radiologic changes of obstruction. A variable pattern has been observed in esophageal motility studies.[162] Malabsorption is sometimes seen. Amyloidosis may develop in association with other entities involving the gastrointestinal tract, especially tuberculosis, granulomatous enteritis, lymphoma, and Whipple's disease. Differentiation of these conditions from diffuse amyloidosis of the small bowel may be difficult. Similarly, amyloidosis of the stomach may mimic gastric carcinoma, with obstruction, achlorhydria, and the radiologic appearance of tumor masses. Patients may also have alternating constipation and diarrhea.

Neurologic Involvement

Neurologic manifestations are common and include peripheral neuropathy, postural hypotension, inability to sweat, Adie's pupil, hoarseness, and sphincter involvement.[163] These manifestations are especially prominent in the heredofamilial amyloidoses.[8] Cranial nerves are generally spared, except for those involving the pupillary reflexes. The protein concentration of the cerebrospinal fluid may be increased. Infiltrates of the cornea or vitreous body may be present in hereditary amyloid syndromes. Amyloid may infiltrate the thyroid or other endocrine glands, but it rarely causes endocrine dysfunction. Local amyloid deposits almost invariably accompany medullary carcinoma of the thyroid. Amyloid infiltration of muscle may lead to pseudomyopathy.

Respiratory Tract Involvement

The nasal sinuses, larynx, and trachea may be involved by accumulations of amyloid that block the ducts, in the case of the sinuses, or the air passages. Amyloidosis of the lung may include diffuse involvement of the bronchi or alveolar septa. The lower respiratory tract is frequently involved in primary amyloidosis and in that associated with dysproteinemia.[164] Pulmonary symptoms attributable to amyloid are present in about 30% of patients, and in some individuals, these are the most serious disease manifestations. In secondary amyloidosis, pulmonary disease is a frequent histopathologic complication, but seldom gives rise to clinically significant symptoms. Amyloid may form a localized mass in the bronchi or alveolar tissue and may resemble a neoplasm. In such cases, local excision should be attempted; if successful, this procedure may be followed by a prolonged remission.

Hematologic Manifestations

Hematologic changes may include fibrinogenopenia, increased fibrinolysis, and selective deficiency of clotting factors, especially factor X.[165] Minor bleeding most often occurs in the absence of clotting abnormalities, however, and is due to local vessel amyloid infiltrates.[166]

PROGNOSIS

The course of amyloidosis is difficult to document because it is rarely possible to date its time of onset. Amyloidosis seldom develops in patients with RA of less than 2 years' duration. The mean duration of arthritis in one series at the time of recognition of amyloidosis was 16 years.[167]

When amyloidosis develops in patients with multiple myeloma, manifestations leading to the initial hospitalization are more apt to be related to the amyloid than to the myeloma.[148] Life expectancy is less than a year in such cases.

In amyloidosis accompanying sepsis such as osteomyelitis, at least partial remission has been reported after treatment of the primary disease. Studies of experimental amyloidosis induced in rabbits by injections of sodium caseinate show that splenic amyloid accumulation, which peaks after about 6 months of injections, is resorbed over the next 3 to 6 months, despite continuance of the caseinate injections.

Established, generalized amyloidosis in man, although usually progressive, may have a better prognosis than was once thought. Primary amyloid progresses less rapidly in women, who may also show a better response to treatment than men.[168] The chief cause of death in secondary (AA) amyloidosis is renal failure, whereas in primary amyloid, cardiac disease heads the list.[169] Sudden death may occur from arrhythmias.[70] Occasionally, gastrointestinal hemorrhage, sepsis, respiratory failure, or intractable heart failure may cause death.

TREATMENT

No specific therapy exists for any variety of amyloidosis. Rational therapy should be directed at the following: (1) decrease of chronic antigenic stimuli producing amyloid; (2) inhibition of the synthesis of the amyloid fibril; (3) inhibition of its extracellular deposition; and (4) promotion of lysis or mobilization of existing deposits.

The progression of secondary amyloidosis is apparently retarded by eradication of the predisposing disease, although many such reports are not substantiated by biopsy proof of resorption. Conclusions have often been drawn on clinical grounds or on the basis of the Congo red test, although a few patients have had biopsy-proved improvement. Despite these occasional reports, amyloidosis is generally a progressive disease. Although the average survival in most large series is 1 to 4 years, I have been treating some patients with amyloidosis for 5 to more than 10 years.

Among the most prominent of the many agents used to treat amyloidosis has been whole liver extract, but most clinicians have noted little effect on the course of the disease. Similarly, corticosteroids have little if any effect on amyloidosis. Ascorbic acid in large doses has been used, but proof of efficacy is lacking. The findings that immunoglobulin light-chain fragments are incorporated into primary amyloid and its presumed synthesis from plasma cells have led to the use of alkylating agents. These agents cause bone marrow depression, however, and acute leukemia has developed in some patients receiving melphalan.[170] Moreover, immunosuppressive agents used experimentally actually enhance amyloid deposition. Despite this, recent melphalan/prednisone regimens have suggested that this program significantly improves life expectancy in AL amyloid. In a prospective randomized study of melphalan/prednisone and of colchicine, no difference in survival was found when the groups were analyzed in aggregate. Significant differences favoring melphalan/prednisone were found when only one regimen was analyzed or when survival from the time of entry to the study to the time of death was studied.[171]

Amyloid deposition in the mouse model is inhibited by colchicine.[131,132] Colchicine prevents both acute attacks in patients with familial Mediterranean fever and deposition of the associated AA amyloid.[172] In our series of patients with AL amyloidosis, using historical controls and prospective treatment with colchicine, the mean duration of life was significantly longer in the colchicine-treated individuals (approximately doubled).[173] Because neither immunosuppressive therapy nor colchicine is a specific form of treatment, further studies of other agents are needed. At the moment, one or the other of these therapies, and possibly the combination (depending on the clinical circumstances) represent optimal therapy. Conservative, supportive measures, attention to organ in-

volvement, and avoidance of overtreatment with agents that have increased hazard in amyloidosis remain vital aspects of management.

Surgery also has a role in the management of amyloid disease.[174] This may vary from the excision of local deposits and the removal of chronic infectious lesions to kidney transplantation. Two patients with severe renal amyloidosis and azotemia had bilateral nephrectomy and renal transplantation, followed by immunotherapy.[175] One patient died of infection 5 months later, and the donor kidney showed no evidence of amyloidosis. The second patient lived 10 years after receiving a transplanted kidney. Biopsies of her kidney after 2 and 4 years showed no amyloid. Notwithstanding the hazards of operating on patients with systemic amyloidosis who may have cardiac involvement, carefully selected patients would probably benefit from kidney transplantation.

HEREDOFAMILIAL AMYLOIDOSES

No generally accepted nosology exists for the heredofamilial amyloid syndromes. Some authors emphasize the site of predominant organ involvement, such as neuropathic versus nephropathic versus cardiopathic amyloid, whereas others stress the genetic aspects. Most pedigree analyses, with one major exception, show autosomal dominant inheritance. The exception, amyloidosis of familial Mediterranean fever, is inherited as an autosomal recessive trait. The classification used here is tentative and is based largely on the major site of organ involvement, in addition to genetic data and ethnic background when available[3,8,9] (Table 82–7).

A large group of these disorders primarily involves the nervous system. Among these, a lower limb neuropathy, first described in Portugal, has a poor prognosis and is characterized by progressively severe

Table 82–7. Heredofamilial Amyloidoses

Neuropathy
    Lower limb (Portuguese; Japanese; Swedish; Other)
    Upper limb (Swiss, Indiana; German, Maryland)
Nephropathy
    Familial Mediterranean fever
    Fever and abdominal pain (Swedish; Sicilian)
    Urticaria, deafness, and renal disease
    Renal disease and hypertension
Cardiopathy
    Progressive heart failure (Danish)
    Persistent atrial standstill
Miscellaneous
    Medullary carcinoma of the thyroid
    Lattice corneal dystrophy and cranial neuropathy (Finnish)
    Cerebral hemorrhage (Icelandic) (Dutch)

neuropathy including marked autonomic nervous system involvement. This variety has also been described in Japan, in a family of Greek origin in the United States, and in Sweden. A second type of neuropathy, seen in families of Swiss origin in Indiana and of German origin in Maryland, is a milder disease often associated with a carpal tunnel syndrome and vitreous opacities. A more severe generalized neuropathy with renal amyloid has been described in Iowa in a family of English-Irish-Scottish ancestry.[8] Several of these are also noted briefly in the earlier section on the prealbumin biochemistry of the heredofamilial amyloidoses.

Several types of severe familial renal disease associated with amyloid have been described. Possibly the most remarkable is familial Mediterranean fever, a disorder subdivided into phenotype I, with irregularly occurring fever and abdominal, chest, or joint pain, preceding or accompanying renal amyloid, and phenotype II, in which amyloidosis is the first or only manifestation of the disease. This disease is most commonly seen in Sephardic Jews, Armenians, Turks, and Arabs. Other hereditary renal amyloidoses have been sporadically described, including the curious association of urticaria, deafness, and renal amyloid.

Severe familial amyloid heart disease has been described in a Danish family, and familial persistent atrial standstill has been reported in a family of Latin American origin. Miscellaneous hereditary amyloid syndromes include hereditary multiple endocrine neoplasia type 2, including medullary carcinoma of the thyroid with amyloid, and familial lattice corneal dystrophy associated with cranial neuropathy and renal disease in Finland. Finally, a syndrome of hereditary cerebral hemorrhage due to amyloid has been reported in Iceland.

REFERENCES

1. Cohen, A.S.: General introduction and a brief history of amyloidosis. *In* Amyloidosis. Edited by J. Marrink and M.H. Van Rijswijk. Dordrecht, The Netherlands, Martin Nijhoff, 1986.
2. Rokitansky, C.: Handbuch der Pathologischen Anatomie Vol. 3. Vienna, Braumuller and Seidel, 1842.
3. Cohen, A.S.: Amyloidosis. N. Engl. J. Med., *277*:522–530, 574–583, 628–638, 1967.
4. Cohen, A.S.: The constitution and genesis of amyloid. *In* International Review of Experimental Pathology, Vol. 4. Edited by G.W. Richter and M.A. Epstein. New York, Academic Press, 1965.
5. Bennhold, H.: Eine spezifische Amyloidfarbung mit Kongorot. Munchen. Med. Wochenschr., *69*:1537–1538, 1922.
6. Bennhold, H.: Ueber die Ausscheidung intravenos einverleibter Farbstoffe bei Amyloidkranken. Verh. Dtsch. Ges. Inn. Med., *34*:313, 1922.
7. Waldenstrom, H.: On the formation and disappearance of amyloid in man. Acta Chir. Scand., *63*:479–507, 1928.
8. Cohen, A.S.: Inherited systemic amyloidosis. *In* The Metabolic Basis of Inherited Disease. Edited by J.B. Standbury, J.B. Wyngaarden, and D.S. Fredrickson. New York, McGraw-Hill, 1972.
9. Pirani, C.L.: Tissue distribution of amyloid. *In* Amyloidosis. Proceedings of the Fifth Sigrid Juselius Foundation Symposium. Edited by O. Wegelius and A. Pasternack. New York, Academic Press, 1976.
10. Glenner, G.G., et al.: Amyloid fibril proteins: Proof of homology with immunoglobulin light chains by sequence analyses. Science, *172*:1150–1151, 1971.
11. Glenner, G.G., et al.: Creation of "amyloid" fibrils from Bence Jones proteins in vitro. Science, *174*:712–714, 1971.
12. Cohen, A.S., and Canoso, J.J.: Rheumatological aspects of amyloid disease. Clin. Rheum. Dis., *1*:149–161, 1975.
13. Cohen, A.S., and Kneapler, D.: Senile amyloidosis. *In* Handbook of Diseases of Aging. Edited by H.T. Blumenthal. New York, VanNostrand Reinhold, 1983.
14. Schwartz, P.: Senile cerebral, pancreatic insular and cardiac amyloidosis. Trans. N.Y. Acad. Sci., *27*:393–413, 1965.
15. Wright, J.R., et al.: Relationship of amyloid to aging. Medicine, *48*:39–60, 1969.
16. Westermark, P., Natvig, J.B., and Johansson, B.: Characterization of an amyloid fibril protein from senile cardiac amyloid. J. Exp. Med., *146*:631–636, 1977.
17. Cohen, A.S.: Diagnosis of amyloidosis. *In* Laboratory Diagnostic Methods in the Rheumatic Diseases. 2nd Ed. Edited by A.S. Cohen. Boston, Little, Brown, 1975.
18. Cooper, J.H.: An evaluation of current methods for the diagnostic histochemistry of amyloid. J. Clin. Pathol., *22*:410–413, 1969.
19. Wright, J.R., Calkins, E., and Humphrey, R.L.: Potassium permanganate reaction in amyloidosis: A histologic method to assist in differentiating forms of this disease. Lab. Invest., *36*:274–281, 1977.
20. Shirahama, T., Skinner, M., and Cohen, A.S.: Immunocytochemical identification of amyloid in formalin fixed paraffin sections. Histochemistry, *72*:161–171, 1981.
21. Chopra, S., Rubinow, A., Koff, R.S., and Cohen, A.S.: Hepatic amyloidosis. Histopathologic analysis of primary (AL) and secondary (AA) forms. Am. J. Pathol., *115*:186–193, 1984.
22. Cohen, A.S., and Calkins, E.: Electron microscopic observations on a fibrous component in amyloid of diverse origins. Nature [Lond.], *183*:1202–1203, 1959.
23. Shirahama, T., and Cohen, A.S.: Fine structure of the glomerulus in human and experimental renal amyloidosis. Am. J. Pathol., *51*:869–911, 1967.
24. Shirahama, T., and Cohen, A.S.: High resolution electron microscopic analysis of the amyloid fibril. J. Cell Biol., *33*:679–708, 1967.
25. Eanes, E.D., and Glenner, G.G.: X-ray studies on amyloid filaments. J. Histochem. Chem., *16*:673–677, 1968.
26. Bonar, L., Cohen, A.S., and Skinner, M.M.: Characterization of the amyloid fibril as a cross-B protein. Proc. Soc. Exp. Biol. Med., *131*:1373–1375, 1969.
27. Bladden, H.A., Nylen, M.U., and Glenner, G.G.: The ultrastructure of human amyloid as revealed by the negative staining technique. J. Ultrastruct. Res., *14*:449, 459, 1966.
28. Cohen, A.S.: Chemical and immunological characterization of two components of amyloid. *In* Chemistry and Molecular Biology of the Intercellular Matrix, Vol. 3. Edited by E.A. Balacz. New York, Academic Press, 1970.

29. Skinner, M., et al.: P-component (pentagonal unit) of amyloid: Isolation, characterization and sequence analysis. J. Lab. Clin. Med., 84:604–614, 1974.

30. Skinner, M., and Cohen, A.S.: Amyloid P-component. *In* Methods in Enzymology. Edited by G. DiSabato. Orlando, FL, Academic Press, In press, 1988.

31. Cohen, A.S.: Preliminary chemical analyses of partially purified amyloid fibrils. Lab. Invest., 15:66–83, 1966.

32. Newcombe, D.S., and Cohen, A.S.: Solubility characteristics of isolated amyloid fibrils. Biochim. Biophys. Acta, 104:480–486, 1965.

33. Pras, M., et al.: The characterization of soluble amyloid prepared in water. J. Clin. Invest., 47:924–933, 1968.

34. Glenner, G.G., et al.: An amyloid protein: The amino terminal variable fragment of an immunoglobulin light chain. Biochem. Biophys. Res. Commun., 41:1287–1289, 1970.

35. Cohen, A.S., et al.: Amyloid protein, precursors, mediator and enhancer. Lab. Invest., 48:1–4, 1983.

36. Lian, J.B., et al.: Fractionation of primary amyloid fibrils: Characterization and chemical interaction of the subunits. Biochim. Biophys. Acta, 491:167–176, 1977.

37. Natvig, J.B., et al.: Further structural and antigenic studies of light-chain amyloid proteins. Scand. J. Immunol., 14:89–94, 1981.

38. Skinner, M., Benson, M.D., and Cohen, A.S.: Amyloid fibril protein related to immunoglobulin lambda-chains. J. Immunol., 114:1433–1435, 1975.

39. Sletten, K., Husby, G., and Natvig, J.B.: N-terminal amino acid sequence of amyloid fibril protein AP. Prototype of a new lambda-variable subgroup, V lambda V. Scand. J. Immunol., 3:833–836, 1974.

40. Terry, W.D., et al.: Structural identity of Bence Jones and amyloid fibril proteins in a patient with plasma cell dyscrasia and amyloidosis. J. Clin. Invest., 52:1276–1281, 1973.

41. Westermark, P., et al.: Coexistence of protein AA and immunoglobulin light-chain fragments in amyloid fibrils. Scand. J. Immunol., 5:31–36, 1976.

42. Kimura, S., et al.: Chemical evidence of lambda-type amyloid fibril proteins. J. Immunol., 109:891–892, 1972.

43. Kabat, E.A., Wu, T.T., and Bilofsky, H.: Sequences of Immunoglobulin Chains: Tabulation and Analysis of Amino Acid Sequences of Precursors, V-Regions, C-region, J-Chain B₂ Microglobulins. NIH Publication 80-2008. Bethesda, MD, National Institutes of Health, 1979.

44. Block, P.J., et al.: The identity of peritoneal fluid immunoglobulin light chain and amyloid fibril in primary amyloidosis. Arthritis Rheum., 19:755–759, 1976.

45. Fett, J.W., and Deutsch, H.F.: Primary structure of the MCG lambda chain. Biochemistry, 12:4102, 1974.

46. Putnam, F.W., et al.: Amino acid sequence of a kappa Bence-Jones protein from a case of primary amyloidosis. Biochemistry, 12:3763–3780, 1973.

47. Takahashi, N., et al.: Amino acid sequence of a lambda Bence-Jones protein from a case of primary amyloidosis. Biomed. Res., 1:321–333, 1980.

48. Cohen, A.S., and Shirahama, T.: Amyloidosis, model no. 17, supplemental update. *In* Handbook: Animal Models of Human Disease. Edited by C.C. Capen, et al. Washington, D.C. Registry of Comparative Pathology, Armed Forces Institute of Pathology, 1980, fascicle 2.

49. Isersky, C., et al.: Immunochemical cross reaction of human immunoglobulin light chains. J. Immunol., 8:486–493, 1972.

50. Benditt, E.P., et al.: Guideline for nomenclature. *In* Amyloid and Amyloidosis. Edited by G.G. Glenner, P.P. Costa, and A.F. Freitas. Amsterdam, Excerpta Medica, 1980.

51. Benson, M.D., et al.: "A" protein of amyloidosis. Isolation of a cross-reacting component from serum by affinity chromatography. Arthritis Rheum., 18:315–322, 1975.

52. Levin, M., et al.: The amino acid sequence of a major non-immunoglobulin component of some amyloid fibrils. J. Clin. Invest., 51:2773–2776, 1972.

53. Ein, C., Kimura, S., and Glenner, G.G.: An amyloid fibril protein of unknown origin: Partial amino-acid sequence analysis. Biochem. Biophys. Res. Commun., 46:498–500, 1972.

54. Husby, G., et al.: Amyloid fibril protein subunit, "Protein A": Distribution in tissue and serum in different clinical types of amyloidosis including that associated with myelomatosis and Waldenstrom's macroglobulinemia. Scand. J. Immunol., 2:395–404, 1973.

55. Levin, M., Pras, M., and Franklin, E.C.: Immunologic studies of the major nonimmunoglobulin protein of amyloid. Identification and partial characterization of a related serum component. J. Exp. Med., 138:373–381, 1973.

56. Anders, R.F., et al.: Amyloid-related serum protein SAA from three animal species: Comparison with human SAA. J. Immunol., 118:229–234, 1977.

57. Linke, R.P., et al.: Isolation of low-molecular weight serum component antigenically related to an amyloid fibril protein of unknown origin. Proc. Natl. Acad. Sci. U.S.A., 72:1473, 1975.

58. Rosenthal, C.J., et al.: Isolation and partial characterization of SAA—an amyloid-related protein from human serum. J. Immunol., 116:1415–1418, 1976.

59. Benditt, E.P., and Eriksen, N.: Amyloid protein SAA is associated with high density lipoprotein from human serum. Proc. Natl. Acad. Sci. U.S.A., 74:4025–4028, 1977.

60. Eriksen, N., and Benditt, E.P.: Isolation and characterization of the amyloid-related apoprotein (SAA) from human high-density lipoprotein. Proc. Natl. Acad. Sci. U.S.A., 77:6860–6864, 1980.

61. Parmelle, D.C., et al.: Amino acid sequence of amyloid-related apoprotein (ApoSAA) from human high-density lipoprotein. Biochemistry, 21:3298–3303, 1982.

62. Rosenthal, C.J., and Franklin, E.C.: Variation with age and disease of an amyloid A protein-related serum component. J. Clin. Invest., 55:746–753, 1975.

63. Benson, M.D., et al.: Kinetics of serum amyloid protein A in casein-induced murine amyloidosis. J. Clin. Invest., 59:412–417, 1977.

64. Sipe, J.D., et al.: The role of interleukin I on acute phase serum amyloid A (SAA) and serum amyloid P (SAP) biosynthesis. Ann. N.Y. Acad. Sci., 389:137–150, 1982.

65. Lavie, G., Zucker-Franklin, D., and Franklin, E.C.: Degradation of serum amyloid A protein by surface-associated enzymes of human blood monocytes. J. Exp. Med., 148:1020–1031, 1978.

66. Husebekk, A., Skogen, B., Husby, G., and Marhaug, G.: Transformation of amyloid precursor SAA to protein AA and incorporation in amyloid fibrils in vivo. Scand. J. Immunol., 21:283–287, 1985.

67. Cohen, A.S., et al.: Ultrastructure and composition of amyloid—Variable or constant. *In* Protides of the Biological Fluids. 20th Colloquium. Edited by H. Peeters. New York, Pergamon Press, 1973.

68. Egan, M.S., et al: The association of amyloid deposits and osteoarthritis. Arthritis Rheum., 25:204–208, 1982.

69. Benson, M.D., et al.: Amyloid serum component: Relationship to aging. Fed. Proc., 33:618, 1974.
70. Rosenthal, C.J., and Franklin, E.C.: Variation with age and disease of an amyloid A protein-related serum component. J. Clin. Invest., 55:746–753, 1975.
71. Hijmans, W., and Sipe, J.D.: Levels of serum amyloid A protein (SAA) in normal persons of different age groups. Clin. Exp. Immunol., 35:96–100, 1979.
72. Rosenthal, C.J., and Sullivan, L.M.: Serum amyloid A to monitor cancer dissemination. Ann. Intern. Med., 91:383–390, 1979.
73. Husby, G., et al.: An experimental model in mink for studying the relation between amyloid fibril protein AA and the related serum protein SAA. Scand. J. Immunol., 4:811–816, 1975.
74. Benson, M.D., et al.: Kinetics of serum amyloid protein A in casein-induced murine amyloidosis. J. Clin. Invest., 59:412–417, 1977.
75. Skinner, M., et al.: Murine amyloid protein AA in casein-induced experimental amyloidosis. Lab. Invest., 36:420–427, 1977.
76. McAdam, K.P.W.J., and Sipe, J.D.: Serum precursor of murine amyloid protein: An acute phase reactant in regard to polyclonal B cell mitogens. (Abstract.) Fed. Proc., 35:1500, 1976.
77. Bausserman, L.L., Herbert, P.N., and McAdam, K.P.W.S.: Heterogeneity of human serum amyloid protein. J. Exp. Med., 152:641, 1980.
78. Benson, M.D., et al.: Suppression of in vitro antibody response by a serum factor (SAA) in experimentally induced amyloidosis. J. Exp. Med., 142:236–241, 1975.
79. Benditt, E.P., Erikson, N., and Hanson, R.H.: Amyloid protein SAA is an apoprotein of mouse plasma high density lipoprotein. Proc. Natl. Acad. Sci. U.S.A., 76:4092–4096, 1979.
80. Meek, R.L., Hoffman, J.S., and Benditt, E.P.: Amyloidogenesis. One serum amyloid A isotype is selectively removed from the circulation. J. Exp. Med., 163:499–510, 1986.
81. Meek, R.L., and Benditt, E.P.: Amyloid A gene family expression in different mouse tissues. J. Exp. Med., 164:2006–2017, 1986.
82. Sipe, J.D., et al.: Analysis of SAA gene expression in rat and mouse during acute inflammation and accelerated amyloidogenesis. In Protides Biol Fluids. Vol. 34. Edited by Peeters, H. London, Pergamon Press, 1986.
83. Costa, P.P., Figueira, A.S., and Bravo, F.R.: Amyloid fibril protein related to prealbumin in familial amyloidotic polyneuropathy. Proc. Natl. Acad. Sci. U.S.A., 75:499–503, 1978.
84. Saraiva, M.J.M., Costa, P.P., Birken, S., and Goodman, D.S.: Presence of an abnormal transthyretin (prealbumin) in Portuguese patients with familial amyloidotic polyneuropathy. Trans. Assoc. Am. Physicians, 96:261–270, 1983.
85. Tawara, S., et al.: Amyloid fibril protein in type I familial amyloidotic polyneuropathy in Japanese. J. Lab. Clin. Med., 98:811–822, 1981.
86. Benson, M.D.: Partial amino acid sequence homology between an heredofamilial amyloid protein and human plasma prealbumin. J. Clin. Invest., 67:1035–1041, 1981.
87. Skinner, M., and Cohen, A.S.: The prealbumin nature of the amyloid protein in familial amyloid polyneuropathy (FAP)—Swedish variety. Biochem. Biophys. Res. Commun., 99:1326–1332, 1981.
88. Saraiva, M.J.M., Sherman, W., and Goodman, D.S.: Presence of a plasma transthyretin (prealbumin) variant in familial amyloidotic polyneuropathy in a kindred of Greek origin. J. Lab. Clin. Med., 108:17–22, 1986.
89. Dwulet, F.E., and Benson, M.D.: Characterization of a transthyretin (prealbumin) variant associated with familial amyloidotic polyneuropathy type II (Indiana/Swiss). J. Clin. Invest., 78:880–886, 1986.
90. Wallace, M.R., Dwulet, F.E., Conneally, P.M., and Benson, M.D.: Biochemical and molecular genetic characterization of a new variant prealbumin associated with hereditary amyloidosis. J. Clin. Invest., 78:6–12, 1986.
91. Pras, M., Franklin, E.C., Prelli, F., and Frangione, B.: A variant of prealbumin from amyloid fibrils in familial polyneuropathy of Jewish origin. J. Exp. Med., 15:989–993, 1981.
92. Nakazato, M., et al.: Revised analysis of amino acid replacement in a prealbumin variant (SKO-III) associated with familial amyloidotic polyneuropathy of Jewish origin. Biochem. Biophys. Res. Commun., 123:921–928, 1984.
93. Husby, G., Ranlov, P.J., Sletten, K., and Marhaug, G.: The amyloid familial amyloidotic cardiomyopathy of Danish origin is related to pre-albumin. Clin. Exp. Immunol., 60:207–216, 1985.
94. Bardin, T., et al.: Synovial amyloidosis in patients undergoing long term hemodialysis. Arthritis Rheum., 28:1052–1058, 1985.
95. Bardin, T., et al.: Hemodialysis associated amyloidosis and beta 2 microglobulin: A clinical and immunohistochemical study. Am. J. Med., 83:419–424, 1987.
96. Gejyo, F., et al.: A new form of amyloid protein associated with chronic hemodialysis identified as β_2-microglobulin. Biochem. Biophys. Res. Commun., 129:701–706, 1985.
97. Connors, L.H., et al.: In vitro formation of amyloid fibrils from intact β_2-microglobulin. Biochem. Biophys. Res. Commun., 131:1063–1068, 1985.
98. Shirahama, T., et al.: Histochemical and immunohistochemical characterization of amyloid associated with chronic hemodialysis as β_2-microglobulin. Lab. Invest., 53:705–709, 1985.
99. Glenner, G.G., and Wong, C.W.: Alzheimer's disease: Initial report of the purification and characterization of a novel cerebrovascular amyloid protein. Biochem. Biophys. Res. Commun., 120:885–890, 1984.
100. Glenner, G.G., and Wong, C.W.: Alzheimer's disease and Down's syndrome: Sharing of a unique cerebrovascular amyloid fibril protein. Biochem. Biophys. Res. Commun., 122:1131–1135, 1984.
101. Masters, C.L., et al.: Neuronal origin of a cerebral amyloid: Neurofibrillary tangles of Alzheimer's disease contain the same protein as the amyloid of plaque cores and blood vessels. EMBO J., 4:2757–2763, 1985.
102. Masters, C.L., et al.: Amyloid plaque core protein in Alzheimer disease and Down syndrome. Proc. Natl. Acad. Sci. U.S.A., 82:4245–4249, 1985.
103. Westermark, P.: Amyloid of medullary carcinoma of the thyroid: partial characterization. Uppsala J. Med. Sci., 80:88–92, 1975.
104. Westermark, P., Wernstedt, C., Wilander, E., and Sletten, K.: A novel peptide in the calcitonin gene related peptide family as an amyloid fibril protein in the endocrine pancreas. Biochem. Biophys. Res. Commun., 140:827–831, 1986.
105. Cornwell, G.G., III, Westermark, P., Natvig, J.B., and Murdoch, J.B.: Senile cardiac amyloid: Evidence that fibrils contain a protein immunologically related to prealbumin. Immunology, 44:447–452, 1981.
106. Westermark, P., Skinner, M., and Cohen, A.S.: The P-component of amyloid of human islets of Langerhans. Scand. J. Immunol., 4:95–97, 1975.

107. Westermark, P., et al.: Immunocytochemical evidence for the lack of protein AS in some intracerebral amyloids. Lab. Invest., *46*:457–460, 1982.

108. Skinner, M., et al.: Studies on amyloid protein AP. In Amyloid and Amyloidosis. Edited by G.G. Glenner, P.P. Costa, and A.F. Freitas. Amsterdam, Excerpta Medica, 1980.

109. Oliveira, E.B., Gotschlich, E.C., and Liu, L.: Primary structure of human C-reactive protein. J. Biochem. Chem., *254*:489–502, 1979.

110. Skinner, M., et al.: Characterization of P-component (AP) isolated from amyloidotic tissue: Half-life studies human and murine AP. Ann. N.Y. Acad. Sci., *389*:190–198, 1982.

111. Skinner, M., et al.: Serum amyloid P-component levels in amyloidosis. Connective tissue diseases, infection and malignancy as compared to normal serum. J. Lab. Clin. Med., *94*:633–638, 1979.

112. Pepys, M.B., et al.: Binding of serum amyloid P-component (SAP) by amyloid fibrils. Clin. Exp. Immunol., *38*:284–293, 1979.

113. Pepys, M.B., et al.: Isolation of amyloid P component (Protein AP) from normal serum as a calcium-dependent binding protein. Lancet, *1*:1029–1032, 1977.

114. Shirahama, T., and Cohen, A.S.: Intralysosomal formation of amyloid fibrils. Am. J. Pathol., *81*:101–116, 1975.

115. Meaney, E., et al.: Cardiac amyloidosis, constrictive pericarditis and restrictive cardiomyopathy. Am. J. Cardiol., *38*:547–556, 1976.

116. Mantzouranis, E.C., et al.: Human serum amyloid P component. J. Biol. Chem., *260*:7752–7756, 1985.

117. Cohen, A.S., Shirahama, T., and Skinner, M.: Electron-microscopy of amyloid. In Electron Microscopy of Proteins. Vol. 3. Edited by J.R. Harris. London, Academic Press, 1982.

118. Scheinberg, M.A., and Cathcart, E.S.: Casein-induced experimental amyloidosis. VI. A pathogenic role for B cells in the murine model. Immunology, *31*:443–453, 1976.

119. Scheinberg, M.A., Goldstein, A., and Cathcart, E.S.: Thymosin restores T cell function and reduces the incidence of amyloid disease in casein-treated mice. J. Immunol., *116*:156–158, 1976.

120. Clerici, E., Pierpaoli, W., and Romussi, M.: Experimental amyloidosis in immunity. Pathol. Microbiol., *28*:806–815, 1965.

121. Hardt, F., and Claesson, M.H.: Quantitative studies on the T cell populations in spleens from amyloidotic mice. Immunology, *22*:677–683, 1972.

122. Scheinberg, M.A., and Cathcart, E.S.: Comprehensive study of humoral and cellular immune abnormalities in 26 patients with systemic amyloidosis. Arthritis Rheum., *19*:173–182, 1976.

123. Teilum, G.: Pathogenesis of amyloidosis: The two phase cellular theory of local secretion. Acta Pathol. Microbiol. Scand., *61*:21–45, 1964.

124. Hardt, F., and Kanlov, P.: Transfer amyloidosis. Int. Rev. Exp. Pathol., *16*:273, 1976.

125. Kisilevsky, R., Boudreau, L., and Foster, D.: Kinetics of amyloid deposition. The effects of dimethylsulfoxide and colchicine therapy. Lab. Invest., *48*:60–67, 1983.

126. Cohen, A.S., Gross, E., and Shirahama, T.: The light and electron microscopic authoradiographic demonstration of local amyloid formation in spleen explants. Am. J. Pathol., *47*:1079–1111, 1965.

127. Sipe, J.D., et al.: The role of interleukin I in acute phase serum amyloid A (AA) and serum amyloid P (SAP) biosynthesis. Ann. N.Y. Acad. Sci., *389*:137–150, 1982.

128. Sipe, J.D., et al.: Detection of a mediator derived from endo-toxin-stimulated macrophages that induces the acute phase serum amyloid A response in mice. J. Exp. Med., *150*:597–606, 1979.

129. Axelrad, M.A., and Kisilevsky, R.: Biological characterization of amyloid enhancing factor. In Amyloid and Amyloidosis. Edited by G.G. Glenner, P.P. Costa, and A.F. Freitas. Amsterdam, Excerpta Medica, 1980.

130. Kisilevsky, R., and Boudreau, L.: Kinetics of amyloid deposition. I. The effects of amyloid-enhancing factor and splenectomy. Lab. Invest., *48*:53–59, 1983.

131. Kedar, I., et al.: Colchicine inhibition of casein-induced amyloidosis in mice. Isr. J. Med. Sci., *10*:787–789, 1974.

132. Shirahama, T., and Cohen, A.S.: Blockage of amyloid induction by colchicine in an animal model. J. Exp. Med., *140*:1102–1107, 1974.

133. Osserman, E.F., Sherman, W.H., and Kyle, R.A.: Further studies of therapy of amyloidosis with dimethyl sulfoxide (DMSO). In Amyloid and Amyloidosis. Edited by G.G. Glenner, P.P., Costa, and A.F. Freitas. Amsterdam, Excerpta Medica, 1980.

134. Takeda, T., et al.: A new murine model of accelerated senescence. Mech. Ageing Dev., *17*:183–194, 1981.

135. Libbey, C.A., et al.: Diagnosis of amyloidosis and differentiation of secondary amyloid by analysis of abdominal fat tissue aspirate. Arthritis Rheum., *24*:5,125, 1981.

136. Libbey, C.A., Skinner, M., and Cohen, A.S.: The abdominal fat tissue aspirate for the diagnosis of systemic amyloidosis. Arch. Intern. Med., *143*:1549–1552, 1983.

137. Rubinow, A., and Cohen, A.S.: Skin involvement in generalized amyloidosis. A study of clinically involved and uninvolved skin in 50 patients with primary and secondary amyloidosis. Ann. Intern. Med., *88*:781–785, 1978.

138. Calkins, E., and Cohen, A.S.: The diagnosis of amyloidosis. Bull. Rheum. Dis., *10*:215–218, 1960.

139. Williams, R.C., Jr., et al.: Secondary amyloidosis in lepromatous leprosy. Possible relationships of diet and environment. Ann. Intern. Med., *62*:1000–1007, 1965.

140. Gordon, D.A., Pruzanski, W., and Ogryzlo, M.A.: Synovial fluid examination for the diagnosis of amyloidosis. Ann. Rheum. Dis., *32*:428–430, 1973.

141. Bywaters, E.G.L., and Dorling, J.: Amyloid deposits in articular cartilage. Ann. Rheum. Dis., *29*:294–306, 1970.

142. Gordon, D.A., et al.: Amyloid arthritis simulating rheumatoid disease in five patients with multiple myeloma. Am. J. Med., *55*:142–154, 1973.

143. Laine, V., Vaino, K., and Ritama, V.V.: Occurrence of amyloid in rheumatoid arthritis. Acta Rheumatol. Scand., *1*:43–46, 1955.

144. Christensen, H.E., and Sorenson, K.L.: Local amyloid formation of capsule fibrosa in arthritis coxae. Acta Pathol. Microbiol. Scand. [A], *233*:128–131, 1972.

145. Goffin, Y.A., Thoua, Y., and Potvliege, P.R.: Microdeposition of amyloid in the joints. Ann. Rheum. Dis., *40*:27–33, 1981.

146. Ryan, L.M., et al.: Amyloid arthropathy in the absence of dysproteinemia: A possible association with chondrocalcinosis. Arthritis Rheum., *21*:587–588, 1978.

147. Munoz-Gómez, J., et al.: Synovial fluid examination for the diagnosis of synovial amyloidosis in patients with chronic renal failure underlying hemodialysis. Ann. Rheum. Dis., *46*:324–326, 1987.

148. Brandt, K., Cathcart, E.S., and Cohen, A.S.: A clinical analysis of the course and prognosis of 42 patients with amyloidosis. Am. J. Med., *44*:955–969, 1968.

149. Kyle, R., and Bayrd, E.: Amyloidosis: Review of 236 cases. Medicine, 54:271–299, 1975.

150. Cohen, A.S.: Renal amyloidosis. *In* Textbook of Nephrology. Edited by S.G. Massry and R.J. Glassock. Baltimore, Williams & Wilkins, 1983.

151. Tribe, C.R.: Amyloidosis in chronic paraplegia. *In* Renal Failure in Paraplegia. London, Pitman Medical Publishing, 1969.

152. Triger, D.R., and Joekes, A.M.: Renal amyloidosis—A fourteen-year follow-up. Q. J. Med., 42:15–40, 1973.

153. Yood, R.A., et al.: Soft tissue uptake of bone seeking radionuclide in amyloidosis. J. Rheumatol., 8:760–766, 1981.

154. Rubinow, A., Koff, R.S., and Cohen, A.S.: Severe intrahepatic cholestasis in primary amyloidosis. A report of 4 cases and a review of the literature. Am. J. Med., 64:937–946, 1978.

155. Cohen, A.S., and Skinner, M.: Amyloidosis of the liver. *In* Diseases of the Liver. 6th Ed. Edited by L. Schiff and E.R. Schiff. Philadelphia, J.B. Lippincott, 1987.

156. Buja, L.M., Khoi, N.B., and Roberts, W.C.: Clinically significant cardiac amyloidosis. Am. J. Cardiol., 26:394–405, 1970.

157. Child, J.S., et al.: Echocardiographic manifestations of infiltrative cardiomyopathy. A report of seven cases due to amyloid. Chest, 70:726–731, 1979.

158. Rubinow, A., Skinner, M., and Cohen, A.S.: Digoxin sensitivity in amyloid cardiomyopathy. Circulation, 63:1285–1288, 1981.

159. Falk, R.: Cardiac involvement in amyloidosis. *In* Amyloidosis. Edited by J. Marrink and M.H. van Rijswijk. Dordrecht, The Netherlands, Martin Nijhoff, 1986.

160. Falk, R.H., et al.: Sensitivity of technetium-99m-pyrophosphate scintigraphy for the diagnosis of cardiac amyloidosis. Am. J. Cardiol., 51:826–830, 1983.

161. Siqueira-Filho, A.G., et al.: M-mode and two-dimensional echocardiographic features in cardiac amyloidosis. Circulation, 63:188–196, 1981.

162. Rubinow, A., Burakoff, R.B., Cohen, A.S., and Harris, L.D.: Esophageal manometry in systemic amyloidosis. Am. J. Med., 75:951–956, 1983.

163. Cohen, A.S., and Rubinow, A.: Amyloid neuropathy. *In* Peripheral Neuropathy. 2nd Ed., Vol. 2. Edited by P.J. Dyck, P.K. Thomas, and E.H. Lambert. Philadelphia, W.B. Saunders, 1983.

164. Celli, B.R., et al.: Patterns of pulmonary involvement in systemic amyloidosis. Chest, 74:543–547, 1978.

165. Furie, B., Greene, E., and Furie, B.C.: Syndrome of acquired factor X deficiency and systemic amyloidosis in vivo studies of the fate of factor X. N. Engl. J. Med., 297:81–85, 1977.

166. Yood, R.A., et al.: Bleeding and impaired hemostasis in 100 patients with amyloidosis. JAMA, 49:1322–1324, 1983.

167. Cohen, A.S.: Amyloidosis associated with rheumatoid arthritis. Med. Clin. North Am., 52:643–653, 1968.

168. Anderson, J.J., Mason, J.H., Skinner, M., and Cohen, A.S.: Sex differences in survival with primary amyloidosis. Arthritis Rheum., 30:S9, 1987.

169. Cohen, A.S., et al.: The life span of patients with primary (AL) amyloidosis and the effect of colchicine treatment. *In* Amyloidosis. Edited by G.G. Glenner et al. New York, Plenum Press, 1986.

170. Kyle, R.A., Pierre, R.V., and Bayrd, E.D.: Primary amyloidosis and acute leukemia associated with melphalan therapy. Blood, 44:333–337, 1974.

171. Kyle, R.A., Griepp, P.R., Garton, J.P., and Gertz, M.A.: Primary systemic amyloidosis. Comparison of melphalan/prednisone versus colchicine. Am. J. Med., 79:708–716, 1985.

172. Zemer, D., et al.: Colchicine in the prevention and treatment of the amyloidosis of familial Mediterranean fever. N. Engl. J. Med., 314:1001–1005, 1986.

173. Cohen, A.S., et al.: Survival of patients with primary (AL) amyloidosis: colchicine treated cases from 1976–1983 compared with cases seen in previous years (1961–1973). Am. J. Med., 82:1182–1190, 1987.

174. O'Doherty, D.P., Neoptolemos, J.P., and Wood, V.F.: Place of surgery in the management of amyloid disease. Br. J. Surg., 74:83–88, 1987.

175. Cohen, A.S., et al.: Renal transplantation in two cases of amyloidosis. Lancet, 2:513–516, 1971.

176. Hermodson, M.A., et al.: Amino-acid sequence of monkey amyloid protein A. Biochem., 11:2934–2938, 1972.

177. Skinner, M., Cathcart, E.S., Cohen, A.S., and Benson, M.D.: Isolation and identification by sequence analysis of experimentally induced guinea pig amyloid fibrils. J. Exp. Med., 140:871–876, 1974.

178. Gorevic, P.D., Greenwald, M., Frangione, B., and Franklin, E.C.: The amino acid sequence of duck amyloid A (AA) protein. J. Immunol., 118:1113–1118, 1977.

179. Kanda, Y., et al.: The amino acid sequence of human plasma prealbumin. J. Biol. Chem., 249:6796–6805, 1974.

83

SARCOIDOSIS

H. RALPH SCHUMACHER, JR.

Sarcoidosis is a systemic disease characterized by a noncaseating granulomatous reaction of unknown origin. Our present concept of this syndrome has evolved from the early descriptions by Hutchinson, Besnier, and Boeck,[1] as well as by Schaumann.[2] Symptoms and signs depend on the organs affected, most frequently the lymph nodes, lungs, liver, skin, and eyes. Muscle, spleen, bones, parotid glands, central nervous system, blood vessels, endocrine glands, and almost any other tissue, including the joints, may also be involved. Although generally a chronic disease, its onset can be acute, with hilar adenopathy, erythema nodosum, fever, and articular manifestations. This acute form is often termed Lofgren's syndrome.[3]

PATHOLOGIC FEATURES

The characteristic histopathologic features of epithelioid tubercles with minimal necrosis and no true caseation, in contrast to the lesions of tuberculosis, are the hallmark of sarcoidosis (Figs. 83–1, 83–2). Studies on skin (Kveim reactions) and pulmonary lesions have identified large numbers of T-lymphocytes around the epithelioid cells. At least in the lung lesions, these are enriched with T4 "helper" cells and activated cells.[5,6] Sarcoid granulomas often contain Langhans-type giant cells with three frequent types of cytoplasmic inclusions: (1) asteroid bodies, which appear to consist of criss-crossing bundles of collagen; (2) Schaumann bodies, which are round or oval, laminated calcifications containing hydroxyapatite (Fig.

83–3); and (3) irregular, poorly stained, anisotropic, glasslike fragments.[7] Such granulomas, even with the typical inclusions, are not pathognomonic for sarcoidosis. Similar granulomatous tissue reactions can be seen in histoplasmosis, coccidioidomycosis, tuberculosis, lymphoma, Hodgkin's disease, bronchogenic carcinoma, foreign body granuloma, drug reactions, beryllium poisoning, syphilis, and leprosy. Functional

FIG. 83–1. Granulomatous synovitis of the elbow in chronic sarcoid arthritis. (Hematoxylin and eosin stain, × 60.) The synovial tissue is crowded with discrete, noncaseating miliary tubercles. At the surface, the villi are hypertrophied and infiltrated with leukocytes and fibroblasts. The articular cartilage of this joint is intact, and the subchondral bone (olecranon and lateral condyle of humerus) is free of tubercles. (From Sokoloff, L., and Bunim, J.J.[4])

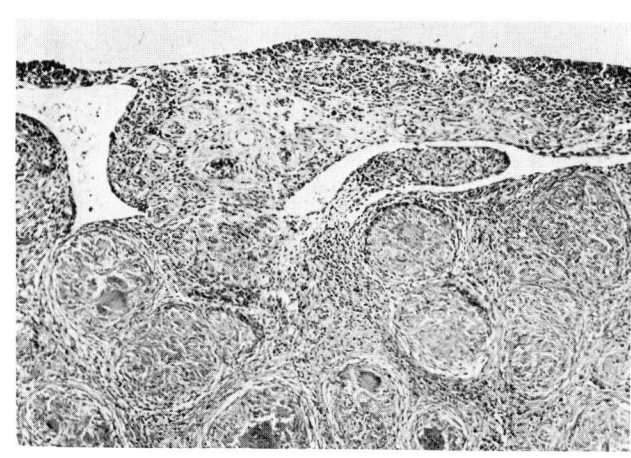

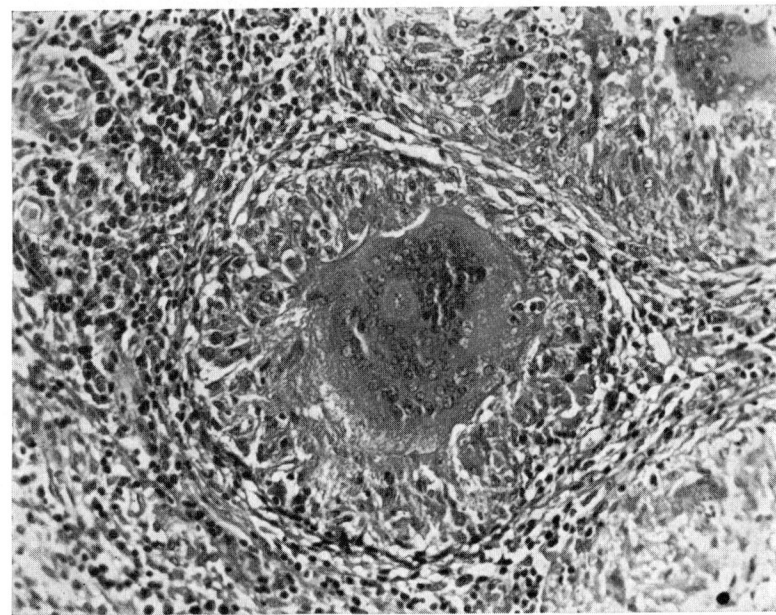

FIG. 83–2. Multinucleated giant cell in the center of a tubercle of epithelioid cells. Surrounding the tubercle is a layer of fibroblasts and a cuff of lymphocytes, plasma cells, and mononuclear cells. This figure is an area from Figure 83–1 under higher magnification. (×175.) (From Sokoloff, L., and Bunim, J.J.[4])

impairment in sarcoidosis appears to result from both the active granulomatous disease and the secondary fibrosis.

CAUSE AND PREVALENCE

Many have speculated on the possible causes of sarcoidosis. The incidence of tuberculosis in sarcoidosis is 4%, and an unusual reaction to Mycobacterium tuberculosis or to atypical mycobacteria is one suggested mechanism.[8] High titers of antibody to a number of viruses and other organisms have been reported in sarcoidosis.[14] Circulating immune complexes can be identified in up to 50% of cases, but their pathogenetic role is not clear.[14] Despite cutaneous anergy and decreased circulating T-lymphocytes, there is considerable evidence of cell-mediated immune reactivity in the pulmonary lesions.[10] Patients who have HLA antigen B8 may be more likely to express their sarcoidosis as erythema nodosum and acute arthritis.[9,11] Several series in this country show a higher incidence of sarcoidosis in black females than in the general population.[12] The disease may begin at any age, including infancy, but it is most commonly diagnosed in the third and fourth decades. Females predominate slightly over males. Sarcoidosis has a worldwide distribution, with the estimated incidence

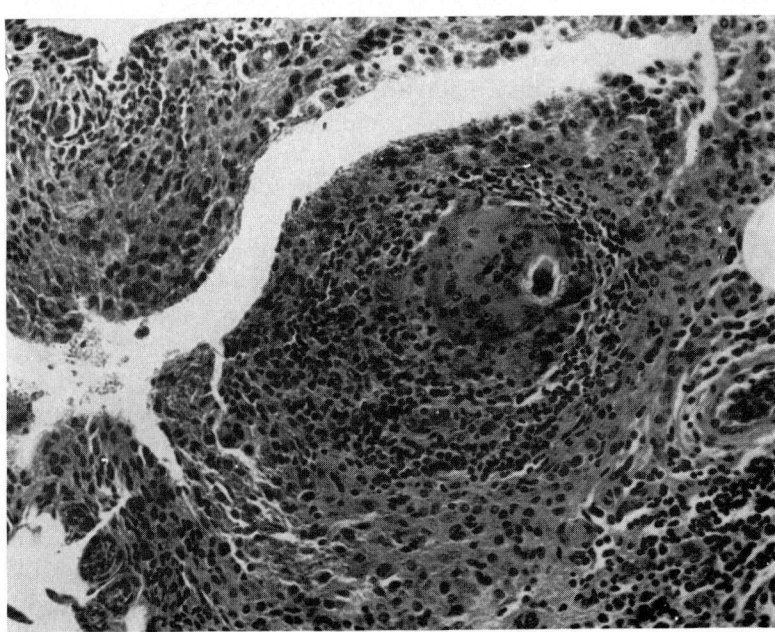

FIG. 83–3. Section of synovial tissue from the knee of a 33-year-old black woman with sarcoid polyarthritis of about 6 weeks' duration showing granulomatous synovitis and a Schaumann body. This Schaumann body appears in the cytoplasm of a giant cell as a circular clear space and consists of a colorless, crystalloid material that is doubly refractive. No bacteria or fungi are found with Brown-Brenn, Ziehl-Neelsen, or periodic acid-Schiff stains. (From Sokoloff, L., and Bunim, J.J.[4])

of the disease reaching as high as 64/100,000 in Sweden. American veterans after World War II had an incidence of 11/100,000.

GENERAL MANIFESTATIONS AND PROGNOSIS

The severity of manifestations can vary from an asymptomatic chest roentgenogram to death in approximately 4%. The most common symptoms and signs are fatigue (27%), malaise (15%), cough (30%), shortness of breath (28%), and chest pain (15%).[12] Ninety-two percent of patients have abnormal chest roentgenograms. Pulmonary parenchymal involvement is more ominous than the more frequent hilar adenopathy. Restrictive lung disease and cor pulmonale can develop. Granulomatous uveitis is the most frequent visual problem. Skin lesions occur in 30% of cases. They may be nondescript, but commonly are papular or nodular, erythematous or violaceous lesions, which show the typical granulomas on histologic examination. Erythema nodosum is common in sarcoidosis of acute onset. Liver involvement is almost always asymptomatic and is evidenced mainly by hepatomegaly. An elevated alkaline phosphatase level may suggest the presence of liver granulomas.

The acute sarcoidosis, accompanied by erythema nodosum, hilar adenopathy, and arthralgia, generally has the best prognosis. Despite the similar sarcoid tissue reaction, Truelove has urged physicians to distinguish this syndrome from sarcoidosis.[13] Certainly, most patients with this acute syndrome have a full remission within 2 years, but up to 16% may have some chronic disease.[14]

DIAGNOSIS

The diagnosis of sarcoidosis is established by the demonstration of typical noncaseating granulomas in the absence of other identifiable causes of such granulomas (Table 83–1). Impaired delayed hypersensitivity on skin testing is characteristic, but not invariable. Impaired tuberculin sensitivity after bacille Calmette Guérin vaccination may persist even after apparent recovery from sarcoidosis. Antibody production is normal. The elevated immunoglobulins are of little help in the differential diagnosis. Leukopenia, anemia, eosinophilia, hypercalcemia, and elevated erythrocyte sedimentation rates may be seen. Hypercalciuria is found in most cases. The serum level of angiotensin-converting enzyme (ACE) is typically elevated in active sarcoidosis.[15] ACE is produced by the granulomas, which also secrete 1,25 dihydrocholecalciferol, responsible for the absorptive hypercalciuria. Although increased ACE levels are seen in about 80% of patients, they are not unique to sarcoidosis and may also occur in inflammatory diseases of the liver,[16] Gaucher's disease, leprosy, silicosis, asbestosis, hyperthyroidism, and diabetes. ACE levels fall with successful therapy and may be useful in following treatment.[17] These levels can also be followed along with other findings in patients with mild disease who are not treated, to look for early clues to exacerbation.

Tissue diagnosis is most expeditiously established by biopsy of a skin lesion or an accessible superficial lymph node. With such superficial material, additional evidence of generalized disease is also needed because foreign body reactions can be difficult to distingish from sarcoidosis. Liver samples also can show granulomas, especially if the liver is palpably enlarged, but a granulomatous liver reaction is common in other liver diseases,[18] and such granulomas are not as helpful in diagnosis as lymph node lesions. Mediastinoscopy in experienced hands is a safe and reliable method of obtaining lymph node tissue for diagnosis if hilar adenopathy is present. Transbronchial lung biopsy, using the fiberoptic bronchoscope, is an attractive initial biopsy procedure yielding diagnoses in about 60% of cases in one series.[19] In typical Lofgren's syndrome with asymptomatic hilar and right paratracheal adenopathy, one can sometimes observe the patient without performing a biopsy.[20] Biopsies with serial sections often show granulomas in asymptomatic muscles.[21] Israel and Sones found muscle tissue positive in 89% of patients with erythema nodosum or arthralgia.[22]

An intradermal injection of 0.2 ml of a 10% saline suspension of sarcoid tissue (the Kveim test) has been used for diagnosis. A positive reaction consists of the development of a local sarcoid granuloma at the injection site. Positive test results can be obtained in 80% of patients with sarcoidosis, most often in those with prominent adenopathy, but standardization of

---

Table 83–1. Diagnostic Features of Sarcoidosis

1. Noncaseating granulomas on biopsy; one must exclude other causes of granulomas.
2. Hilar and right paratracheal adenopathy in 90%.
3. Skin lesions, uveitis, or involvement of almost any tissue.
4. Onset most often in third and fourth decades, but cases reported at all ages.
5. Impaired delayed hypersensitivity in 85%.
6. Frequent hyperglobulinemia.
7. Increased angiotensin-converting enzyme levels in about 80%.
8. Hypercalciuria in most; hypercalcemia in some.

preparations has been difficult, and reliable material is not generally available. Positive Kveim test results in patients with lymphadenopathy resulting from diseases other than sarcoidosis may be due to less-specific batches of antigen.[23]

[67]Gallium scintigrams can assist in evaluating activity in alveolitis,[17] and they may be abnormal even in patients with normal chest roentgenograms.[24] Bronchoalveolar lavage showing more than 35 to 45% T-lymphocytes also suggests active alveolitis. Some patients without elevated numbers of lymphocytes in lavages have also responded to corticosteroid therapy, however.[17]

SPECIFIC MUSCULOSKELETAL MANIFESTATIONS

MUSCLE

Sarcoid granulomas in muscle are often asymptomatic, but they may be accompanied by local pain and tenderness or even palpable nodules. A symmetric proximal myopathy has also been described and has been reported to occur without evident sarcoidosis in other tissues.[25,26] Involved muscles show noncaseating granulomas as well as lymphocytic infiltration, muscle necrosis, and regeneration. Calcification of muscles and other soft tissues occasionally occurs in hypercalcemic patients.

BONE

Phalangeal cysts, often considered a helpful diagnostic clue in sarcoidosis (Fig. 83–4), were described in 14% of patients in one series.[12] Although some of these cysts are due to sarcoid granulomas, others may be unrelated to the sarcoidosis. A radiologic survey of the hands of 338 patients with sarcoidosis and 342 control subjects showed cystic changes in 5% of the patients with sarcoidosis, but also in 8% of the control subjects, a group that included normal persons and patients with a variety of diseases.[27] Other bones, including the skull and vertebrae, may also develop cysts from sarcoid granulomas. Large lytic or sclerotic vertebral lesions can be seen.[28] Bone sarcoidosis is usually asymptomatic. The overlying cortex is typically intact, although cortical dissolution with scalloping or acro-osteolysis and fractures through large cysts have been described.[29] The phalangeal lesions of sarcoidosis can also be associated with osteosclerosis.[30] Cystic bone lesions only occasionally extend into the joint, in which they may cause arthritis.[4]

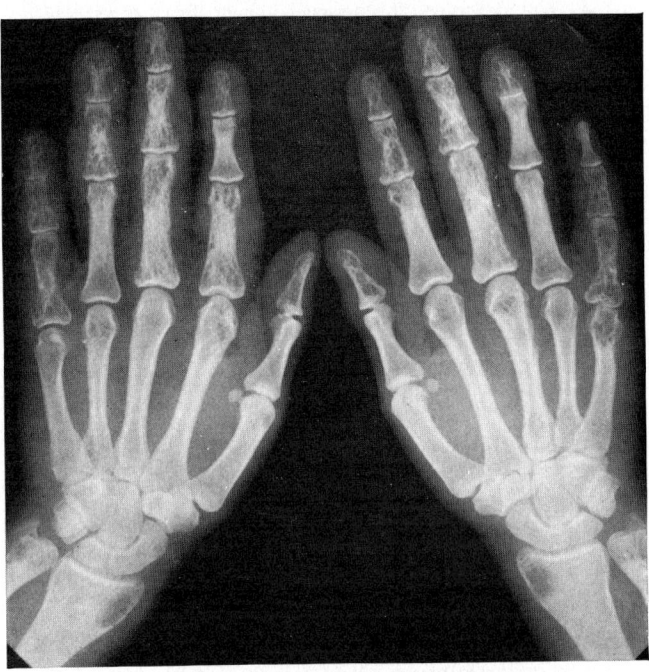

FIG. 83–4. Roentgenograms of the hands showing unusually severe bone lesions of sarcoidosis. The bone cysts have not broken through the articular cortex. The hands shown in Figure 83–5 have similar bone changes, but with extension into the distal interphalangeal joints.

Some destructive bony lesions are associated with overlying purplish red, nodular cutaneous masses, termed *lupus pernio*,[7] or with a diffuse dactylitis.[31]

JOINTS

Arthritis was first described with sarcoidosis in 1936, and since then, arthritis, periarthritis, or arthralgia has been reported in 2 to 38% of patients in various series.[12,32–34] Chronic sarcoidosis is associated with fewer joint complaints than the acute form. Table 83–2 outlines the features of sarcoid arthropathy.

In acute sarcoidosis with hilar adenopathy, fever, and erythema nodosum, up to 89% of patients have articular symptoms, and 69 and 63% had articular or periarticular swelling in the series of Lofgren[3] and James et al.,[35] respectively. Ankles and knee joints are most frequently involved in acute sarcoidosis. Most other joints are occasionally involved. Heel pad pain is common; monoarthritis is unusual.[32] The patient generally has a dramatic, tender, warm, erythematous swelling that often is clearly periarticular rather than synovial. Such changes are occasionally difficult to separate from adjacent cutaneous erythema nodosum, and the histologic appearance of the lesions

Table 83–2. Sarcoid Arthropathy

Acute Sarcoidosis (Lofgren's Syndrome)
1. Often periarticular and tender, erythematous, warm swelling.
2. Ankles and knees almost invariably involved.
3. Joint involvement possibly the initial manifestation (chest film normal).
4. Joint motion possibly normal and pain absent or minimal.
5. Synovial effusions infrequent and generally only mildly inflammatory.
6. Usually nonspecific mild synovitis on synovial biopsy.
7. Self-limited in weeks to 4 months.

Chronic Sarcoidosis
1. Arthritis possibly acute and evanescent, recurrent, or chronic.
2. Noncaseating granulomas often demonstrable in synovium.
3. Usually nondestructive, despite chronic or recurrent disease.

is identical. Joint motion is often painless; pain is much less than one would expect, considering the inflammatory signs. The frequency of a severe, localized tenderness has been emphasized.[36]

Roentgenograms show only soft-tissue swelling. Such articular findings may antedate erythema nodosum by as much as 2 weeks and suggest careful watch for the skin lesions. Both skin and joint lesions may antedate hilar adenopathy for up to several weeks. Ankle and knee involvement is often symmetric; joint involvement can be progressive. The acute inflammation often raises a suspicion of rheumatic fever, gonococcal or other infectious arthritis, and gout. Joint aspiration often yields no synovial fluid. When an effusion is aspirated, leukocyte counts can be as high as 42,500/mm³, with 90% neutrophils.[37] Most effusions are only mildly inflammatory, however, with leukocyte counts of under 1,000/mm³, predominantly lymphocytes and large mononuclear cells.

Cultures are negative, and crystals cannot be identified by compensated, polarized light. Several patients with this syndrome, including an early case described by Hutchinson, had been thought to have gout before synovial fluid crystal identification was available to confirm the presence of gouty arthritis.[38] That sarcoid arthritis may respond dramatically to colchicine further confuses the issue. Elevated uric acid levels have been noted in a small percentage of patients with sarcoidosis,[34] but recent studies suggest that hyperuricemia should not be anticipated unless it is a result of drugs or renal failure. Needle synovial biopsy specimens in acute sarcoidosis most often show only mild nonspecific synovitis and some lining-cell proliferation. Although much of the inflammation in acute sarcoidosis may be periarticular, synovial granulomas are occasionally found during open surgical biopsy.[4] Caplan et al. have described an identical periarthritis in 19 patients with hilar adenopathy,

none of whom had erythema nodosum.[39] These workers found sarcoid granulomas in the subcutaneous tissue over three of seven inflamed ankles, but no granulomas in an open joint biopsy. Angiotensin-converting enzyme levels need not be elevated in patients with acute sarcoidosis without pulmonary parenchymal involvement.[11]

The joint manifestations of acute sarcoidosis subside in 2 weeks to 4 months, although rare patients may develop chronic sarcoid arthritis. Erythema nodosum and a similar arthropathy can also be seen in lepromatous leprosy, ulcerative colitis, regional enteritis, tuberculosis, coccidioidomycosis, histoplasmosis, oral contraceptive and possibly other drug use, pregnancy, and psittacosis and other infections. Other cases are idiopathic.

In sarcoidosis of more insidious onset, joint manifestations are less common. In such cases, even with widespread systemic granulomatous disease, the arthritis may still be mild and evanescent, as in acute sarcoidosis. Arthritis can also be recurring or protracted with polysynovitis, however. Even in patients with chronic synovitis, joint destruction is infrequent, and most roentgenograms show only soft-tissue swelling. The destructive joint disease occasionally seen in sarcoidosis is illustrated in Figure 83–5. Such severe arthritis is most common in patients with multisystemic granulomatous disease. Arthritis may occur as an initial manifestation, or after years of systemic disease. Thus, such a variety of patterns can be seen that a high index of suspicion is needed to lead to biopsy and other diagnostic studies to differentiate this disorder from rheumatoid or other types of arthritis.

Reports of synovial fluid analysis are infrequent. We recently found joint-fluid leukocyte counts of 250 to 6,250/mm³ with predominantly mononuclear cells in six patients with arthritis associated with chronic sarcoidosis.[40] Sokoloff and Bunim found noncaseating granulomas in three of five surgical synovial biopsy specimens from patients with chronic arthritis.[4] In addition, the synovium showed diffuse chronic inflammation including plasma cells. None of their patients, and only 3.3% of those studied by Owen et al.,[37] had any elevation of rheumatoid factor, but others have found rheumatoid factor in as many as 38% of patients with sarcoidosis.[41] The presence of rheumatoid factor does not correlate with the presence or severity of joint disease. Tenosynovitis at the wrists and elsewhere can also be seen. Finger clubbing is an occasional complication of pulmonary sarcoidosis, but hypertrophic osteoarthropathy with joint effusions has not been reported.[42]

Arthritis in early-childhood sarcoidosis has been

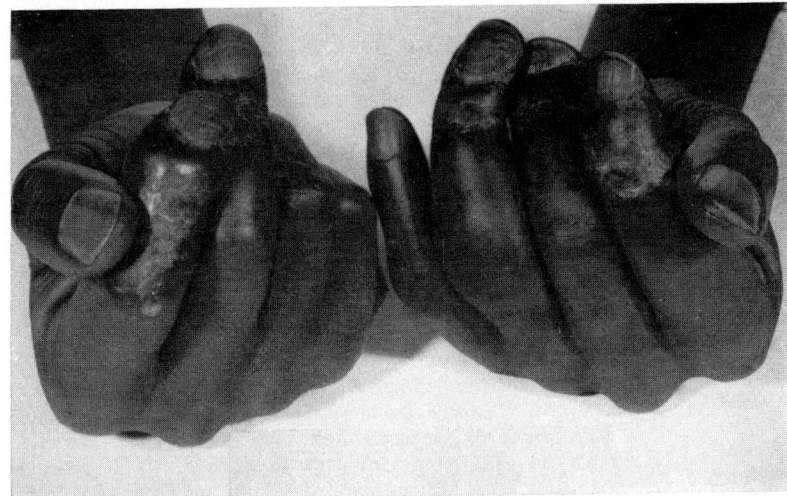

FIG. 83–5. The hands of a 33-year-old black male with sarcoidosis of 5 years' duration. Depigmented skin lesions are present on the dorsum of fingers, and the distal phalanx of the left fourth finger is displaced. Note the fusiform swelling of the proximal interphalangeal joint of the fourth and fifth fingers of left hand (asymmetric). This patient does not have psoriasis. (From Sokoloff, L., and Bunim, J.J.[4])

described, with especially large, painless, boggy synovial and tendon sheath effusions.[43] The course of the disease is indolent, and constitutional symptoms are few. Despite prolonged synovitis, no erosive radiographic changes are seen. Synovial fluid findings are not described; synovial biopsy samples show either granulomas or nonspecific inflammation. Interestingly, the sarcoidosis reported in young children is associated with uveitis, but not with hilar adenopathy.

TREATMENT

Many patients with minimal symptoms require no treatment. No curative agent exists. Adrenal corticosteroids are commonly used to try to suppress potentially serious active inflammatory reactions, such as ocular disease, pulmonary parenchymal disease, and central nervous system involvement, and are often effective. Corticosteroids can also lower persistently elevated serum calcium levels. Initial doses of 20 to 60 mg prednisone are tapered to the lowest effective maintenance dose. Alternate-day dosage seems effective for maintenance therapy. Objective long-term benefits from corticosteroids have often been difficult to demonstrate,[44] but improved vital capacity even in severe disease has been shown in one series.[45] Spontaneous remission can occur. Active articular disease almost always shows at least temporary improvement with corticosteroid therapy. When these agents are used, isoniazid coverage may be needed. Because joint disease is often self-limited, however, rest, salicylates, and other analgesics are often all that is required. Salicylates are not as dramatically effective as in rheumatic fever. Colchicine shortens attacks of acute arthritis in some patients,[36]

but it is by no means invariably effective. Chloroquine has been reported to help cutaneous sarcoidosis.[46] Uncontrolled reports of methotrexate[47] and azathioprine[48] use in sarcoidosis have suggested benefit in these patients.

REFERENCES

1. Boeck, C.: Multiple benign sarkoid of the skin. J. Cutan. Genitourin. Dis., *17*:543–550, 1899.
2. Schaumann, J.N.: Etude sur le lupus pernio et ses rapports avec les sarcoides et la tuberculose. Ann. Dermatol. Syph., *6*:357–373, 1916–1917.
3. Lofgren, S.: Primary pulmonary sarcoidosis. I. Early signs and symptoms. Acta Med. Scand., *145*:424–431, 1953.
4. Sokoloff, L., and Bunim, J.J.: Clinical and pathological studies of joint involvement in sarcoidosis. N. Engl. J. Med., *260*:842–847, 1959.
5. Hunninghake, G.W., and Crystal, R.G.: Pulmonary sarcoidosis: a disorder mediated by excess helper T-lymphocyte activity at sites of disease activity. N. Engl. J. Med., *305*:429–434, 1981.
6. Konttinen, Y.T., et al.: Inflammatory cells of sarcoid granulomas detected by monoclonal antibodies and an esterase technique. Clin. Immunol. Immunopathol., *26*:380–389, 1983.
7. Longcope, W.T., and Freiman, D.G.: A study of sarcoidosis. Medicine, *31*:1–32, 1952.
8. Vanek, J., and Schwartz, J.: Demonstration of acid-fast rods in sarcoidosis. Am. Rev. Respir. Dis., *101*:395–400, 1970.
9. James, D.G., and Williams, W.J.: Immunology of sarcoidosis. Am. J. Med., *72*:5–8, 1982.
10. Van Maarsseven, A.C.M., Mullink, H., Alons, C.L., Stam, J.: Distribution of T cell subsets in different portions of sarcoid granulomas. Hum. Pathol., *17*:493–500, 1986.
11. Fitzgerald, A.A., and Davis, P.: Arthritis, hilar adenopathy, erythema nodosum complex. J. Rheumatol., *9*:935–938, 1982.
12. Mayock, R.L., et al.: Manifestations of sarcoidosis, analysis of 145 patients, with review of 9 series selected from literature. Am. J. Med., *35*:67–89, 1963.
13. Truelove, L.H.: Articular manifestations of erythema nodosum. Ann. Rheum. Dis., *19*:174–180, 1960.

14. Neville, E., Walker, A.N., James, D.G.: Prognostic factors predicting the outcome of sarcoidosis: an analysis of 818 patients. Q. J. Med., LII:525–533, 1983.

15. Lieberman, J.: Elevation of serum angiotensin converting enzyme (ACE) level in sarcoidosis. Am. J. Med., 59:365–372, 1975.

16. Matsuki, K., and Sakata, T.: Angiotensin-converting enzyme in disease of the liver. Am. J. Med., 73:549–551, 1982.

17. Lawrence, E.C., et al.: Serial changes in markers of disease activity with corticosteroid treatment in sarcoidosis. Am. J. Med., 74:747–756, 1983.

18. Fagan, E.A., Moore-Gillon, J.C., and Turner-Warwick, M.: Multiorgan granulomas and mitochondrial antibodies. N. Engl.J. Med., 308:572–575, 1983.

19. Koontz, C.H., Joyner, L.R., and Nelson, R.A.: Transbronchial lung biopsy via the fiberoptic bronchoscope in sarcoidosis. Ann. Intern. Med., 85:64–66, 1976.

20. Winterbauer, R.H., Belic, N., and Moores, K.D.: A clinical interpretation of bilateral hilar adenopathy. Ann. Intern. Med., 78:65–71, 1973.

21. Stjernberg, N., et al.: Muscle involvement in sarcoidosis. Acta Med. Scand., 209:213–216, 1981.

22. Israel, H.L., and Sones, M.: Selection of biopsy procedures for sarcoidosis diagnosis. Arch. Intern. Med., 113:255–260, 1964.

23. James, D.G.: Editorial: Kveim revisited, reassessed. N. Engl. J. Med., 292:859–860, 1975.

24. Nosal, A., et al.: Angiotensin-1-converting enzyme and gallium scan in non-invasive evaluation of sarcoidosis. Ann. Intern. Med., 90:328–331, 1979.

25. Hinterbuchner, C.N., and Hinterbuchner, L.P.: Myopathic syndrome in muscular sarcoidosis. Brain, 87:355–366, 1964.

26. Silverstein, A., and Siltzbach, L.E.: Muscle involvement in sarcoidosis. Asymptomatic myositis, and myopathy. Arch. Neurol., 21:235–241, 1969.

27. Baltzer, G., et al.: Zur haufigkeit zystischer knochenveranderungen (Ostitis cystoides multiplex jungling) bei der Sarkoidose. Dtsch. Med. Wochenschr., 95:1926–1929, 1970.

28. Perlman, S.G., et al.: Vertebral sarcoidosis with paravertebral ossification. Arthritis Rheum., 21:271–277, 1978.

29. Sartoris, D.J., Resnick, D., Resnick, C., Yaghmai, I.: Musculoskeletal manifestations of sarcoidosis. Semin. Roentgenol., 20:376–386, 1985.

30. McBrine, C.S., and Fisher, M.S.: Acrosclerosis in sarcoidosis. Radiology, 115:279–281, 1975.

31. Liebowitz, M.R., et al.: Sarcoid dactylitis in black South African patients. Semin. Arthritis Rheum., 14:232–237, 1985.

32. Gumpel, J.M., Johns, C.J., and Shulman, L.E.: The joint disease of sarcoidosis. Ann. Rheum. Dis., 26:194–205, 1967.

33. Siltzbach, L.E., and Duberstein, J.L.: Arthritis in sarcoidosis. Clin. Orthop., 57:31–50, 1968.

34. Spilberg, I., Siltzbach, L.E., and McEwen, C.: The arthritis of sarcoidosis. Arthritis Rheum., 12:126–137, 1969.

35. James, D.G., Thomson, A.D., and Wilcox, A.: Erythema nodosum as a manifestation of sarcoidosis. Lancet, 2:218–221, 1956.

36. Kaplan, H.: Sarcoid arthritis with a response to colchicine. N. Engl. J. Med., 268:778–781, 1960.

37. Owen, D.S., et al.: Musculoskeletal sarcoidosis and rheumatoid factor. Med. Coll. VA Q., 8:217–220, 1972.

38. Kaplan, H., and Klatskin, G.: Sarcoidosis, psoriasis, and gout: syndrome or coincidence? Yale J. Biol. Med., 32:335–352, 1960.

39. Caplan, H.I., Katz, W.A., and Rubenstein, M.: Periarticular inflammation, bilateral hilar adenopathy and a sarcoid reaction. Arthritis Rheum., 13:101–111, 1970.

40. Palmer, D.G., and Schumacher, H.R.: Synovitis with non-specific histologic changes in synovium in chronic sarcoidosis. Ann. Rheum. Dis., 43:778–782, 1984.

41. Oreskes, I., and Siltzbach, L.E.: Changes in rheumatoid factor activity during the course of sarcoidosis. Am. J. Med., 44:60–67, 1968.

42. West, S.G., Gilbreath, R.E., and Lawless, O.J.: Painful clubbing and sarcoidosis. JAMA, 246:1338–1339, 1981.

43. North, A.F., et al.: Sarcoid arthritis in children. Am. J. Med., 48:449–455, 1970.

44. Young, R.J., et al.: Pulmonary sarcoidosis: a prospective evaluation of glucocorticoid therapy. Ann. Intern. Med., 73:207–212, 1970.

45. Emirgil, C., Sobol, B.J., and Williams, M.H.: Long-term study of pulmonary sarcoidosis. The effect of steroid therapy as evaluated by pulmonary function studies. J. Chronic Dis., 22:69 86, 1969.

46. Morse, S.I., et al.: The treatment of sarcoidosis with chloroquine. Am. J. Med., 30:779–784, 1961.

47. Lacher, M.J.: Spontaneous remission or response to methotrexate in sarcoidosis. Ann. Intern. Med., 69:1247–1248, 1968.

48. Krebs, P., Abel, H., and Schonberger, W.: Behandling der boeckschan sarkoidose mit immunosuppressiven substanzen. Erfahrungen mit Azatioprin (Imurel). Munchen. Med. Wochenschr., 111:2307–2311, 1969.

ARTHRITIS ASSOCIATED WITH HEMATOLOGIC DISORDERS, STORAGE DISEASES, DISORDERS OF LIPID METABOLISM, AND DYSPROTEINEMIAS

84

MICHAEL H. WEISMAN

The importance of recognizing articular manifestations originating from underlying systemic illness cannot be overemphasized. If a complaint or sign is a presenting manifestation, a delay in diagnosis can be avoided. Conversely, some osteoarticular complications may become the dominant clinical manifestation of a systemic illness, hemophilia for example. Rheumatic signs and symptoms have been recognized and characterized in a diverse collection of hematologic conditions, storage diseases, disorders of lipoprotein metabolism, and of immunoglobulin production.[1-7] Current clinical and relevant pathophysiologic aspects of these conditions are summarized here as a basis for rational diagnostic and therapeutic decisions.

LEUKEMIAS

The earliest manifestations of leukemia often include rheumatic signs and symptoms.[8-11] Children with leukemia are often misdiagnosed as having acute rheumatic fever, juvenile rheumatoid arthritis (JRA), or Still's disease.[8,12,13] The clinical picture may be confused further by the presence of a nondiagnostic or preleukemic (cytopenic) peripheral smear or the absence of radiographic evidence of the skeletal changes of leukemia despite severe bone pain. Most patients with leukemia show a combination of arthritis and periarthritis in a polyarticular distribution with knee and ankle joint predominance. In very young children a diffuse dactylitis resembling sickle cell disease may occur;[14] in others the findings may be monoarticular or oligoarticular.[9,10,11,15,16] Synovial fluid analysis is almost always nondiagnostic, with leukocyte cell counts ranging from noninflammatory (50 cells/mm³) to very inflammatory (45,000 cells/mm³).[17]

Unfortunately, delay in diagnosis is all too often the hallmark of leukemic arthropathy. In children, bone pain out of proportion to objective evidence of arthritis, lymph node enlargement, and hematologic abnormalities have been stressed as distinguishing diagnostic features.[15] Bone pain is most likely a consequence of leukemic involvement of the periarticular periosteum; however, leukemic infiltration into synovium or juxta-articular bone, as well as hemorrhage, may play a role.[10,11,18] Other, still unknown, mechanisms must be involved because several carefully done histopathologic studies in patients with arthritis associated with leukemia have shown no synovial, periosteal, or periarticular bony leukemic infiltration.[17,19]

Articular involvement also occurs in the chronic leukemias;[10] it is seldom dramatic and may appear late in the disease course, heralding disease exacerbation or transformation to a blast crisis. Patients with acute as well as chronic leukemias have a higher than expected frequency of positive tests for antinuclear antibodies and rheumatoid factor;[10,15,20-22] the signifi-

1301

cance of this finding is unknown. Chronic lymphocytic leukemia of T-cell origin has produced a picture of nonerosive polyarthritis resembling seronegative rheumatoid arthritis with skin nodules; T-cell infiltration of skin, synovial tissues, and bone marrow has been demonstrated.[23] Polymyositis has been reported in association with leukemias.[24]

Bone scintigraphy may show increased juxta-articular uptake as an important clue to the diagnosis of leukemic arthropathy.[25] Conventional roentgenograms reveal a multiplicity of abnormalities in acute leukemia[11,26-29] including osteopenia, lytic lesions, cortical and periosteal defects, distortion of trabecular patterns, pathologic fractures, osteosclerosis, and periosteal new bone. Children may display juxta-epiphyseal radiolucent bands in actively growing metaphyseal cortices at the ends of long bones. However, this particular abnormality is nonspecific and associated with other disturbances of osteogenesis.[29] Similar radiographic abnormalities occur in the chronic leukemias with the proximal portions of the femora and humeri, the pelvic bones, and the vertebrae most often affected.[30] Osteolytic and sclerotic changes in these areas may represent foci of a blastic crisis.[25]

Hairy cell leukemia (HCL), felt to be B cell in origin and presenting in middle-aged men with associated splenomegaly and cytopenias, may be accompanied by vasculitis and/or arthritis.[6] Systemic vasculitis follows usually within 2 years of the onset of HCL.[31] Most cases resemble polyarteritis nodosa (PAN), but a few display cutaneous small vessel vasculitis alone; mononuclear cells in the vessel walls are the predominant histologic feature.[32] A substantial number of patients with HCL have been reported to manifest arthritis or arthralgia. Oligoarthritis, dermal vasculitis, or erythema nodosum was found in 10 of 37 HCL patients in one series, suggesting an autoimmune mechanism for these rheumatic findings.[33] The actual pathogenetic link between HCL and vasculitis has not been explained, and studies to date have failed to reveal signs of immune-complex mechanisms.[34] Hairy cell infiltration of vessel walls has been demonstrated in a few cases.[32] Further confounding our understanding is the absence of a parallel clinical relationship between activity of HCL and the nonleukemic manifestations such as vasculitis or other "autoimmune" features.[33] Finally, destructive bone involvement, a direct manifestation of HCL, has been reported in 11 cases and may be favorably affected by radiation therapy.[35]

Two rare hematologic conditions may be associated with osteoarticular signs and symptoms. *Sinus histiocytosis with massive lymphadenopathy* (SHML) is a be-nign childhood entity presenting with cervical adenopathy, leukocytosis, and hypergammaglobulinemia; osseous abnormalities resembling leukemia or metastatic neuroblastoma have produced large joint arthropathy.[36] A patient with agnogenic myeloid metaplasia developed a chronic inflammatory elbow effusion; myeloid elements were noted in the deeper portions of the synovium with a nonspecific synovitis in the more superficial elements. The arthritis was attributed to *extramedullary hematopoiesis*.[37]

Treatment of articular signs and symptoms in general should be aimed at management of the underlying malignancy, but joint symptoms in some patients with acute leukemia have been temporarily suppressed by salicylates or other anti-inflammatory agents. Such good therapeutic responses have further confused the diagnosis.[11] The disappearance of bone and joint pain is often one of the first indications of a positive response to antileukemic therapy.

MALIGNANT LYMPHOMAS

Skeletal involvement is commonly seen in the malignant lymphomas.[27,28,30,38,39] Bone defects, which can be seen roentgenographically in as many as 15% of patients with *Hodgkin's disease*, have been found at postmortem examination in up to 50% of such patients.[18,40,41] Sites of involvement include the spine, pelvis, ribs, femur, skull, and shoulder. Symptoms referable to these lesions include deep pain, which is unremitting and worse at night, as well as pain caused by pathologic fracture, particularly when the disease occurs within vertebrae. Diagnostic difficulty, however, may exist when articular signs or symptoms occur in the absence of overt, radiographically evident bone lysis or lymph node enlargement directly suggesting a lymphoma. In one patient with reticulum cell sarcoma and articular involvement, the diagnosis was established by the demonstration of malignant cells in the synovial fluid at a time when these cells were absent from the peripheral blood and initial bone marrow specimen.[42] Such direct involvement of the actual joint tissues is unusual.[43] One patient with malignant lymphoma of a poorly differentiated, diffuse type initially had sternoclavicular joint arthritis. The joint was surrounded by grayish neoplastic tissue; marginal erosions and lysis of the adjacent clavicle and manubrium sterni were present.[44]

Six cases of *non-Hodgkin's lymphoma* primarily in joint tissues (capsule and/or synovium) have been reported.[45] Patients may present with either polyarticular disease resembling rheumatoid arthritis or with monoarthritis. Lymphadenopathy and splenomegaly may not be apparent, and conventional radiographs typically do not reveal malignant bone destruction in the vicinity of the involved joint. A synovial and/or bone biopsy was required for the diagnosis.[45]

Primary non-Hodgkin's lymphoma of bone or *reticulum cell sarcoma of bone* without involvement of regional lymph nodes or distant viscera is a morphologically diverse condition affecting primarily young men. Involvement is usually localized to the ends of long bones.[46–48] One patient, a middle-aged woman, presented clinically with monoarthritis. Radiographs revealed a fine periosteal reaction along the distal femoral metaphysis. The synovial fluid was bloody and of the non-inflammatory type. Bone and synovial biopsy revealed a malignant large cell infiltrate within the medullary canal and hyperplastic synovial villi; this lymphoma arose in bone and expanded to involve the contiguous synovium, but did not extend into the joint space.[49] Conventional synovial fluid analyses as well as cytologic examinations appear nondiagnostic in these cases of early tumor involvement, reflecting the periarticular nature of the process. Computerized tomography and/or bone scintigraphy may suggest a periarticular focus. Tissue examination, of either synovium or bone, is critical to establishing a diagnosis.

Angioimmunoblastic lymphadenopathy with dysproteinuria (AILD) is a lymphoproliferative disease with unique histopathologic features and a fatal prognosis.[50,51] A 70-year-old man with sicca syndrome displayed extranodal histologic features of AILD on lip and kidney biopsies. It was concluded that a Sjögren's-syndrome-like condition may occur secondary to widespread manifestations of AILD.[52] In another case the generalized manifestations of a nodular, poorly differentiated, lymphocytic lymphoma (or follicular small cleaved cell lymphoma) produced prominent polymyalgia rheumatica symptoms and an extensive perivascular lymphomatous infiltrate of the temporal arteries, without frank vasculitis.[53] This patient displayed prominent features of temporal or giant cell arteritis at the time the lymphoma was disseminating.

MULTIPLE MYELOMA AND AMYLOID ARTHROPATHY (see also Chapter 82)

In most cases pain in the back or proximal extremities, often the earliest symptom of multiple myeloma, is attributable to disease of the bone, and roentgenograms often reveal osteoporosis and osteolytic defects.[18,27,28,39,54,55] Persons with multiple myeloma may develop amyloid arthropathy. Pain and swelling of the joints, most commonly the shoulders, wrists,

knees, and fingers, is the hallmark of the disease. One may note prominent enlargement of the shoulders (shoulder-pad sign) and a rubbery, hard consistency of the periarticular connective tissue resulting from deposition of amyloid protein.[56–58] Amyloid deposits can be identified by histochemical and electron-microscopic techniques in articular cartilage, in perichondrocytic lacunae, in synovium (Fig. 84–1), and in synovial fluid debris including fragments of synovial villi (see Chapter 5).[59,60]

The presence of morning stiffness, fatigue, polyarticular involvement, periosteal nodular deposits of amyloid, and occasional bony erosion and destruction may closely simulate the clinical features of rheumatoid arthritis (RA).[54,58,60–65] However, the duration of morning stiffness is shorter and fatigue is more prominent than in RA, and the synovial fluid findings are completely inconsistent with RA. In amyloid arthropathy the synovial fluid is viscous and contains comparatively few leukocytes (200 to 4500/mm^3), predominantly mononuclear cells.[59–61,63–66] Synovial fluid

FIG. 84–1. Photomicrograph of synovium obtained from the right shoulder of a 56-year-old woman with multiple myeloma who had developed pain in this shoulder and inability to use her arm 10 days earlier, following a fall. The humerus was dislocated. At the time of open reduction of this dislocation, large deposits of amyloid were found in the glenoid fossa. Note the mass of amyloid covered by a thin rim of synovium. The material in this nodule stained metachromatically with crystal violet.

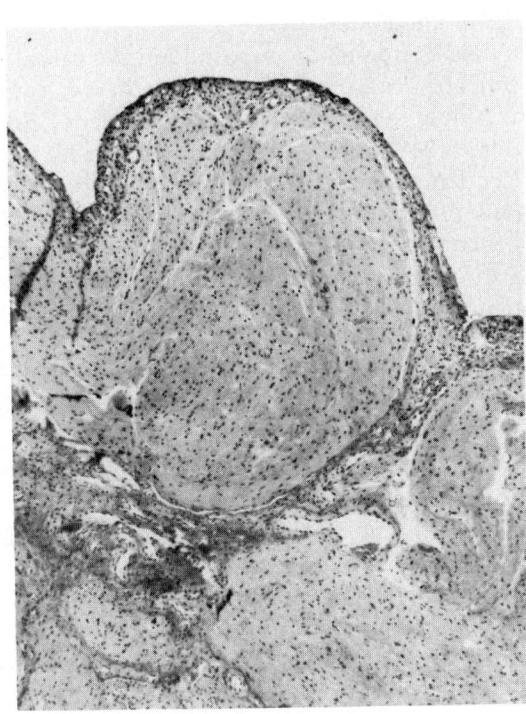

pellets, stained with Congo red and viewed under polarized light, demonstrate intracellular and extracellular amyloid. Although the radiographic findings of amyloid arthropathy may be superficially reminiscent of RA, extensive soft tissue nodular masses, well-defined cystic lesions with or without surrounding sclerosis, and preservation of joint space are more characteristic of amyloid joint disease.[55] Many of these lesions resemble gouty arthritis. Lucencies, cysts, and osteolytic defects are usually present but do not directly abut the articular surface. An exceptional case has been reported with multiple myeloma and the usual physical findings of amyloid joint disease but whose radiographs revealed typical rheumatoid-like articular erosions of the carpus and ulnar styloid, as well as joint space narrowing of the metacarpophalangeal and proximal interphalangeal joints; synovial biopsy revealed amyloid deposits without any evidence of synovial inflammation.[67]

Amyloidosis occurs in association with all forms of myeloma, including the IgD and pure Bence Jones varieties,[57,58,64] but it is found most frequently in patients with pure light-chain disease or with IgA myelomas.[62,64,68] Typical amyloid arthropathy is found most frequently in association with multiple myeloma, but it has also been reported with primary amyloidosis.[63,69] In contrast, it is rare and indeed may not occur in those with generalized secondary amyloidosis.[62] The incidence of typical amyloid arthropathy in multiple myeloma is estimated to be about 5%.[60] Amyloid deposits may be seen in small quantities from synovial biopsy specimens in some patients with secondary amyloidosis.[70]

Amyloid is frequently deposited in the carpal tunnel and may compress the median nerve, causing carpal tunnel syndrome.[54,63,65,71,72] Prevalence figures range from 20% of all cases of amyloid itself[61] to 45% of all patients with amyloid arthropathy reported in a review of the literature from 1931 to 1975.[62] Thus, the concurrence of multiple myeloma, symmetric polyarthropathy, and carpal tunnel syndrome suggests amyloidosis.

A discussion of amyloidogenic proteins, the chemical structure of the fibrils, and information about the molecular biology of the amyloidoses is covered in Chapter 8 and in several recent reviews.[73,74]

Skeletal involvement in multiple myeloma may be limited to diffuse osteoporosis, but one may also see circumscribed lytic areas, expansile lesions, or ill-defined diffuse areas of bone destruction ("moth-eaten" bone).[75] Scintigraphic examination of bone may be helpful by demonstrating osseous lesions not detected by conventional radiography.[76] In patients with amyloidosis, osteoporosis with or without lytic le-

sions is common.[62] When light-chain myeloma is accompanied by amyloidosis, the patient has fewer lytic lesions of bone, but the prognosis is worse than when amyloid is absent.[68] Patients with Waldenström's macroglobulinemia may also exhibit bony changes including osteoporosis, isolated or multiple osteolytic defects resembling those seen in multiple myeloma, and multilocular cyst-like lesions found in the supraacetabular portions of the iliac bones.[77] A single example of typical amyloid arthropathy has been described in a patient with Waldenström's macroglobulinemia,[78] as has another case of Waldenström's disorder with neuropathic joint disease secondary to amyloid neuropathy.[79]

POEMS syndrome is an acronym suggested for the combination in a single patient of plasma cell dyscrasia with *p*olyneuropathy, *o*rganomegaly, *e*ndocrinopathy, *M* protein, and *s*kin changes.[80] Other findings include hyperhidrosis, skin thickening, hyperpigmentation, gynecomastia or amenorrhea, and hirsutism. In addition to the radiographic presence of sclerotic plasmacytomas in the spine and pelvis, bony proliferation is apparent at sites of tendon and ligament attachment to bone, often with associated irregular bony excrescences involving the posterior elements of the spine.[81,82] The significance of paraproteinemia in the pathogenesis of this disorder, including the endocrine manifestations, is unknown.

An acquired form of amyloidosis is now recognized as a frequent accompaniment of long-term hemodialysis.[83] Amyloid in this syndrome has thus far been demonstrated primarily in articular and periarticular structures with generally negative results obtained from abdominal fat aspirations.[84,85] A recent report of 15 patients, however, with an average period of 10.8 years of dialysis revealed positive fat aspirates in 3 of 12 and several had amyloid deposited in colon mucus and rectal biopsy specimens. These findings suggest that, with time, patients may develop systemic amyloidosis.[86]

Arthralgias, knee swelling, painful stiff shoulders, and carpal tunnel syndrome are prominent and frequent features.[83,86,87] Studies of synovial fluid are not extensive; available data suggest that the fluid is generally noninflammatory or grossly bloody.[83,86,88,89] Synovial fragments staining with Congo red dye are common and helpful diagnostically.[88] The overall frequency of dialysis-related amyloid appears to relate directly to the length of time on dialysis. Many of the pathologic features are similar to those observed in the amyloid arthropathy of myeloma, including erosions and radiolucent cysts in the hand and wrist, a destructive arthropathy needing surgery, or femoral neck cysts leading to pathologic fractures.[90,91] Subchondral bone cysts and/or erosions may be present for years, followed by relatively rapid narrowing of cartilage and collapse of subchondral bone.[83]

Hemodialysis-related amyloid is composed of β_2-microglobulin.[92,93] In renal failure the serum level of this protein increases in conjunction with the serum creatinine, and its gradual accumulation in the tissues is the major factor felt to be responsible for the syndrome.[83] Use of the standard cuprophane dialysis membrane appears to have been important for the accumulations of amyloid seen in patients dialysed for the past 10 or 15 years.[94] Hemofiltration with more highly permeable membranes are able to reduce serum levels of this molecule and its attendant amyloidosis.[94,95] The factors responsible for the largely articular and osseous accumulation, and the molecular mechanisms responsible for its deposition remain to be elucidated.

Synovial amyloid obtained at the time of knee arthroscopy has been shown to contain β_2-microglobulin,[89] confirming other studies[92,96,97] isolating amyloid from tissues obtained from carpal tunnel decompression or from bone. The clinical spectrum of osteoarticular manifestations has broadened to include a destructive spondyloarthropathy.[98,99,100] Of 80 patients undergoing long-term hemodialysis 9% had developed an erosive spondyloarthropathy with intervertebral disc space narrowing and major erosions at the vertebral end plates.[101,102] The prevalence of lesions attributable to renal osteodystrophy was almost identical to the prevalence of amyloid-related osteoarthropathy.[101] The increasing prevalence of this problem as well as its potential nonskeletal effects has caused great concern in terms of the prognosis of patients undergoing dialysis therapy.

SICKLE CELL DISEASE AND OTHER HEMOGLOBINOPATHIES

Sickle cell crisis is frequently associated with severe periarticular pain and objective signs of arthritis manifested by warmth, swelling, and tenderness.[5,103] Joint involvement is almost always monoarticular or pauciarticular, and the knees and elbows are most commonly involved. Synovial fluid is not usually inflammatory and is often clear with a normal viscosity and a leukocyte count of fewer than 1000 cells/mm[3], containing a low percentage of polymorphonuclear leukocytes.[103] Sickled erythrocytes can be seen in these effusions. A few reports note sterile inflammatory effusions with high cell counts and no crystals.[104–107] Crystal-induced synovitis has been documented in a

few reports[108–111]; the mechanism for secondary gout in sickle cell disease is discussed in Chapter 104.

Synovial biopsies obtained at the time of acute joint disease show little cellular infiltrate, prominent congestion of small blood vessels, and, in a few cases, definite microvascular thrombosis.[103] Microvascular obstruction probably leads to infarction of synovium and adjacent bone and may account for joint effusions and inflammation. The painful crisis very likely results from ischemia of bone marrow in an intermediate zone of blood supply between the main nutrient artery and the perforating synovial vessels. Maximal intensity of bone pain in juxta-articular areas supports this hypothesis.[112]

Bone marrow scans using ^{99m}Tc sulfur colloid and other isotopes reveal diminished uptake in the bone marrow adjacent to painful joints; such a finding suggests infarction.[113–115] Scintigraphic defects occur in the absence of roentgenographic evidence of marrow or bone infarction and may precede these findings by many months. A normal scan in a symptomatic area may suggest another process, such as infection. On occasion, however, joint inflammation is followed by a rapid destruction of the articular cartilage. The presence of prominent lymphocytic and plasma cell infiltrates in these patients suggests a possible immune mediated mechanism. Cryoprecipitable immune complexes have been implicated in sickle cell nephropathy,[116] and an abnormality of the alternate pathway of complement activation has been demonstrated in the serum of patients with sickle cell disease.[117] However, no direct evidence for the participation of immune mechanisms in sickle cell arthropathy has yet been uncovered.

The skeletal lesions characteristic of this hemoglobinopathy may be separated into those related to hyperplasia of bone marrow and those resulting from local thrombosis and infarction.[39,104,118–123] Bone marrow proliferation is associated with widening of medullary cavities, thinning of cortices, coarsening and irregularity of trabecular markings, and cupping of vertebral bodies. Lesions believed to result from sickle cell thrombosis and infarction include cortical bone infarcts with periostitis and periosteal elevation, bone marrow lysis, sclerosis and fibrosis, and most notably, avascular necrosis of the femoral and humeral heads. Less commonly, one sees infarction in the distal portion of the femur, the radius, patella, and the vertebrae.[39,104,118,124,125]

Subchondral and intraosseous hemorrhages contribute to the destruction of articular cartilage in the hip.[126] Avascular necrosis of the femoral head has been reported in patients with S-S (sickle cell) disease and sickle cell trait, as well as in those with hemoglobin S-C disease, sickle cell–thalassemia, and hemoglobin S-F disease.[124,127–132] Avascular necrosis occurs in 20 to 68% of patients with S-C disease, but in only 4 to 12% of those with S-S disease.[124] In one study, the incidence of avascular necrosis was not increased in patients with sickle cell trait, when compared with age-matched control subjects with A-A hemoglobin.[133] Total hip replacement has been successful in some patients with these hemoglobinopathies.[127,134]

Although it has generally been assumed that infarction of the femoral head is caused by sickle cell thrombosis of the fine epiphyseal vessels, occlusion may be the result of fat emboli. Systemic fat embolization, apparently originating in the necrotic bone marrow, has been reported in hemoglobin S-C disease, as well as in sickle cell (S-S) anemia (see Chapter 98).[135,136]

Although the pathogenesis of sickle cell arthropathy is thought to be ischemic in origin, it remains unclear if the associated noninflammatory synovial effusions represent "sympathetic effusions," that is, a secondary response to bone damage, or occur as a result of synovial ischemia. The incidence and pattern of articular disease was studied prospectively for 2½ years in 37 consecutive patients attending a sickle cell clinic in Jamaica.[112] Gout and ischemic bone necrosis were excluded. Twelve patients developed arthritis during a painful crisis; 13 patients had miscellaneous causes of arthritis, and 12 others displayed noninflammatory ankle effusions associated with the spontaneous development or deterioration of leg ulcers. Painful crises were associated with arthritis 20% of the time. The leg ulcers were felt to be vaso-occlusive in origin and the chronic ankle joint effusions resolved with improvement of the leg ulcers. It was hypothesized that synovial ischemia occurs in parallel with the ischemic leg ulcers, supporting the concept of primary synovial involvement.[112] If small synovial vessels participate in this process as has been demonstrated during crises,[103] the resultant ischemia could conceivably cause permeability changes in synovial capillary endothelium and subsequent leakage of plasma proteins.

Young children with sickle cell disease may have transient swelling and tenderness of their hands and feet as a result of periostitis of the metacarpal, metatarsal, and proximal phalangeal bones, a condition known as *sickle cell dactylitis*.[39,104,105,118,137,138] Dactylitis may occur even before the diagnosis of sickle cell disease is established. In addition to periosteal elevation and subperiosteal new bone formation, roentgenograms reveal radiolucent areas intermingled with areas of increased density, giving a moth-eaten appearance. These changes have been interpreted as

representing infarction.[104] In most cases, the integrity of the affected bones is restored to normal in several months without residual deformity or alteration in growth. The rarity of this "hand-and-foot" syndrome after the fourth year of life is explained by the recession of red marrow from the cooler distal bones and its replacement by fibrous tissue.[104]

Another striking skeletal complication of sickle cell disease is salmonella osteomyelitis, which may be multifocal.[104,125,139] The first radiographic signs of this infection, which usually starts in the medullary cavity of the long tubular bones, is periosteal proliferation. Bony destruction extending throughout the shaft then follows.[118] Septic arthritis, although less common than osteomyelitis, has been reported to be due to a number of organisms, including salmonellae,[104] staphylococci, Escherichia coli, Fusobacterium varium,[140] and Serratia liquefaciens.[141] Staphylococci and Serratia organisms have also been responsible for osteomyelitis in these patients.[104] After successful treatment with antibiotics, the bones usually heal with minimal deformity. The serum of many patients with sickle cell anemia is deficient in opsonins for salmonellae and pneumococci and their leukocytes are therefore limited in their ability to phagocytose these microorganisms.[142] This impairment has been attributed to a defective alternative complement pathway.[117,143] Local vascular insufficiency associated with sickling may also adversely affect the host response to infection and the efficacy of antibiotic treatment.[144]

Although the pattern and prognosis of septic arthritis in sickle cell disease varies in different parts of the world, a large Nigerian experience emphasizes several important points.[145] In 50 septic joints in 31 patients the following observations were made: the hip was the most common site; polyarticular involvement occurred in 39% of cases; and contiguous osteomyelitis was present in 84%. Severe complications occurred in 76% of cases, mostly relating to a delay in diagnosis and to the high frequency of hip joint infection. In contrast to most American studies, septic arthritis was not uncommon. This complication represented 12% of a total of 266 skeletal events seen in 207 consecutive patients over 5 years. In contrast, a recent American series of 600 children followed for 10 years reported only three cases of septic arthritis. All three patients had contiguous osteomyelitis of adjacent bone and two of these involved the hip or shoulder.[115] The hip or shoulder is a rare site for sickle cell arthropathy accompanying hemolytic crises.

A specific osteoarthropathy has been described in patients with β-thalassemia major, as well as in those with thalassemia minor.[146,147] Twenty-five of 50 patients between the ages of 5 and 33 years with β-thalassemia major had evidence of periarticular disease marked by pain and swelling of the ankles and pain on compression of the malleoli, calcaneus, and forefoot.[146] Synovial fluid obtained from the ankle joint in two of these patients was of the noninflammatory type. Hyperplasia of the synovial lining cells and a heavy deposition of hemosiderin were found. Radiographic changes included osteopenia, widened medullary spaces, thin cortices with coarse trabeculations, and evidence of microfractures. The presence of microfractures was confirmed histologically; increased osteoblastic and resorptive (osteoclastic) surfaces, with iron deposits at the calcification front and cement lines, were noted. The arthropathy in these persons appears to be related to the underlying bone disease, although the role of iron overload in the pathogenesis remains to be fully evaluated. A similar form of pauciarticular, nonerosive, seronegative arthropathy was observed in persons with thalassemia minor.[143] Bilateral avascular necrosis of the femoral heads has been reported in a patient with this condition.[148]

The recurrent episodes of arthritis in thalassemia minor have been described as gout-like, lasting less than 10 days, and self-limited but recurrent.[149] The erythrocyte sedimentation rate (ESR) is always normal and the synovial fluid from four cases showed 1500 to 8000 leukocytes/mm³, mostly mononuclear cells, and no crystals. Synovial biopsy revealed nonspecific, mildly inflammatory synovitis with local infiltration by lymphocytes and plasma cells and lining cells one to three layers thick. The authors speculated that the synovial inflammation followed primary compromise of the microvasculature. No evidence of bone disease was uncovered in contrast to thalassemia major, in which arthropathy is related to juxta-articular bone disease.

STORAGE DISEASES

The lysosomal storage diseases are uncommon inborn errors of metabolism resulting from the deficiency or absence of specific lysosomal hydrolytic enzymes. Since the lysosome functions to break down aging macromolecules, the enzyme deficiencies result in accumulation and storage of large amounts of substrate in multiple organ systems and connective tissue, including the skeleton. The target tissues are related to the sites of normal degradation of the specific macromolecule. Most cases represent inherited autosomal recessive traits, with the notable exception of Fabry's disease, an X-linked disorder with manifestations in females. The lysosomal storage diseases include most of the lipid storage disorders, the mu-

copolysaccharidoses, the mucolipidoses, glycoprotein storage diseases, and others. In-depth discussions of the specific disorders, their diagnosis, heterogenic expressions, management, and prevention have been published.[150,151] Skeletal features of the most common gangliosidoses and certain other storage diseases are discussed here.

GAUCHER'S DISEASE

Gaucher's disease, described by P.C.E. Gaucher in 1882, is a heritable lysosomal sphingolipid storage disease characterized by the accumulation of the glycolipid glucocerebroside, or glucosylceramide, in reticuloendothelial cells in the bone marrow, spleen, liver, lymph nodes, and other internal organs.[152,153] Glucocerebroside, a complex glycolipid membrane constituent, accumulates because of a deficiency of the enzymes β-glucocerebrosidase and β-glucosidase, which catalyze the hydrolytic cleavage of glucocerebroside into ceramide and glucose.[152,153] Three clinical forms of Gaucher's disease are recognized. Type 1, by far the most common, is the chronic, nonneuronopathic, "adult" form of the disease; type 2 is the infantile or acute neuronopathic form, with an average survival rate of less than a year; and type 3 is the juvenile or subacute neuronopathic form. All are transmitted as autosomal recessive disorders. In the adult form, type 1, the patient is deficient in lysosomal glucocerebrosidase, whereas in type 2, both this enzyme and a soluble β-glucosidase are lacking.[152] The adult form is 30 times more frequent among Ashkenazi Jews; this form may be diagnosed at any age but it is one of the lysosomal storage diseases most likely to present in the practice of internal medicine.[151]

Osteoarticular complaints are an important feature in both type 1 and type 3 Gaucher's disease. Symptoms result from infiltration of the bone marrow by lipid-laden histiocytes (Gaucher's cells) and are often the earliest manifestation of Gaucher's disease.[4,153-155] The most common rheumatic complaint is acute, severe pain in the extremities, particularly in the hip, knee, and shoulder. Such painful bone crises are more common in children, but they occur in both juvenile and adult forms of the disease. When accompanied by signs of inflammation and fever, such episodes may mimic pyogenic osteomyelitis and have been called "pseudo-osteomyelitis."[155,156] In many ways, these crises resemble those of sickle cell anemia. The exact cause of these exacerbations is unknown, but vasospasm or vascular occlusion of end arteries within bone may result from deposition of Gaucher's cells and may increase the intramedullary pressure.

This process may, in turn, lead to ischemia, necrosis, and local hemorrhage. Symptoms last from days to weeks, but they eventually resolve spontaneously.

The patient may also have pathologic fractures of long bones, as well as compression deformity of vertebrae causing low back pain.[157] In rare cases, the patient has migratory polyarthritis, the nature of which is poorly understood. Joint disease is usually monoarticular or pauciarticular and involves the large joints, in which it appears to be related to changes in adjacent bone.[39,155] Small joint involvement, including the proximal interphalangeal joints, is most uncommon.[158] A number of reports cite severe degenerative hip disease as a result of avascular necrosis and collapse of the head of the femur (Fig. 84–2).[39,155,159] Total hip arthroplasty has been successful in such patients, but it is associated with increased intraoperative blood loss; the likelihood of loosening of the prosthesis may also be greater, perhaps because infiltration of the medullary cavity by Gaucher's cells prevents adequate cement fixation.[160] Recurrent avascular necrosis of the capital femoral epiphysis has been observed.[154]

Changes in the femoral neck may lead to pathologic fracture or to coxa vara deformity. On occasion, in-

FIG. 84–2. Roentgenogram of the left hip joint of a 22-year-old man with Gaucher's disease illustrating avascular necrosis of the head of the femur. This roentgenogram was obtained 2 years after the onset of pain in the hip.

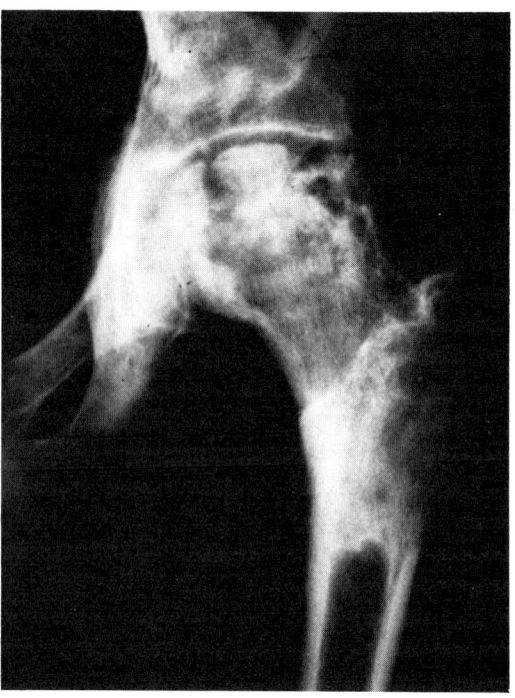

vasion of the head of the humerus gives rise to degenerative arthropathy of the shoulder.[155,161]

Splenectomy, performed on some persons with thrombocytopenia, with hypersplenism, or with mechanical problems resulting from an enlarged spleen, may be followed by accelerated skeletal manifestations,[162] although this latter point is controversial. Following splenectomy, cerebroside storage may occur at an increased rate in liver and bone and may lead more rapidly to osteoarthritis, aseptic necrosis, and pathologic fractures.[163] Many patients with longstanding disease have elevated serum immunoglobulin levels, often monoclonal.[164] Some patients with Gaucher's disease appear to progress from monoclonal dysproteinemia to overt multiple myeloma.[165,166]

One of the most consistent roentgenographic features of Gaucher's disease is widening of the distal portion of the femur. This process usually occurs just superior to the femoral condyles and creates the well-known "Erlenmeyer flask" appearance.[155] Similar flaring is less common in the tibia and humerus, together with changes in the other long bones, pelvis, skull, vertebrae, and mandible.[39,155] Characteristically, areas of rarefaction are mingled with patchy sclerosis and cortical thickening, resulting from new bone formation. The diagnosis of Gaucher's disease can be established by demonstrating large, kerasin-filled Gaucher's cells in the bone marrow, as well as by analyzing peripheral blood leukocytes for residual β-glucocerebrosidase and β-gluosidase activities.[167,168] Administration of purified glucocerebrosidase to patients with Gaucher's disease produces a significant reduction of glucocerebroside in the liver and a reduction to normal levels of this substance in the erythrocytes.[152,153,169,170] Enzyme replacement therapy is under active investigation and holds the greatest future promise for these patients.

FABRY'S DISEASE

Fabry's disease, or glycolipid lipidosis, was first described by J. Fabry in 1898. This hereditary, X-linked disorder of glycosphingolipid metabolism is characterized by the progressive accumulation of birefringent deposits of a trihexosylceramide in endothelial, perithelial, and smooth muscle cells of blood vessels, in ganglion and perineural cells of the autonomic nervous system, in epithelial cells of the cornea, and in kidney, bone marrow, and many other tissues.[171,172] This pathologic storage is due to a defect in the activity or absence of the lysosomal enzyme L-galactosidase A (ceramide trihexosidase), required for the normal catabolism of trihexosylceramide, which is derived from kidney and the membranes of senescent erythrocytes. Death usually occurs in the fifth or sixth decade as a result of renal failure or from the cardiac and cerebral complications of arterial hypertension or vascular disease. Heterozygous women may exhibit the disease in an attenuated form.

The disorder is characterized by a typical rash, known as *angiokeratoma corporis diffusum universale,* consisting of widespread telangiectasia or angiokeratoma. These pinpoint lesions, which occupy the dermal papillae, are venules with multiple layers of basement membrane in the vascular walls and may represent the ectopic placement of small collecting veins. They are thought to arise by alteration of the existing microvasculature rather than as a result of newly proliferating microvessels (neovascularization).[173] Vasospasm similar to that seen in Raynaud's disease, induced by changes in temperature and associated with paresthesias and burning in the extremities, are seen in many patients and are caused by deposits in the cells of the autonomic nervous system.[171,174] A study of forearm hemodynamics in eight patients with Fabry's disease revealed increased vascular resistance, decreased venous capacitance, and decreased forearm blood flow.[174]

The patient may also have painful swelling of the fingers, elbows, and knees.[172] A characteristic deformity consisting of limitation in extension of the distal interphalangeal joints of the fingers has been described.[171,175,176] Avascular necrosis of the head of the femur[177] or talus[178] and multiple, small, infarct-like opacities in the femoral head may occur.[179] Involvement of the metacarpal and metatarsal bones and of the temporomandibular joint has been reported,[180] as well as osteoporosis of the dorsal vertebrae.[181] The diagnosis of Fabry's disease is established by demonstration of the characteristic birefringent lipid material in skin and also by enzymatic assay. Efforts have been made to determine whether an allograft, in the form of a kidney transplant, might provide a sufficient amount of L-galactosidase A to correct the metabolic defect. This question, as well as that of the value of other forms of enzyme replacement therapy, remains controversial.[182-185]

FARBER'S DISEASE

Farber's disease, or disseminated lipogranulomatosis, was first described in 1952 by S. Farber. This rare, progressive sphingolipidosis of early childhood is characterized by painful and swollen joints, periarticular and subcutaneous nodules, dysphonia, pul-

monary infiltrations, and retardation of mental and motor development.[186-191] The patient has an accumulation of ceramide, a glycolipid, in the cytoplasm of neurons and certain other cells attributable to a heritable deficiency in the lysosomal enzyme acid ceramidase, which catalyzes the conversion of ceramide to sphingosine and fatty acids.[188,190] Ceramide may accumulate in lysosomes of cultured diploid fibroblasts from persons with Farber's disease who are deficient in acid ceramidase.[192]

Articular disease, usually appearing between 2 weeks and 4 months of age, has been the dominant initial manifestation in the handful of patients recognized to date. Typically, pain and swelling of the interphalangeal and metacarpophalangeal joints, the ankles, wrists, knees, and elbows occur. Nodular masses develop on tendon sheaths and in para-articular tissues, as well as at points of pressure such as the occiput and the lumbosacral region. Nodules have also been found in the conjunctiva, the external ear, and the external nares. These patients often develop flexion contractures of the fingers and other joints. Ankylosis may follow. Swelling and granuloma formation in the epiglottis and larynx are responsible for a disturbance in swallowing and episodes of lung infection. Few children survive past the age of 2 years, and the usual cause of death is pulmonary disease. The data on familial occurrence of Farber's disease are compatible with autosomal recessive inheritance.[190]

Fibroblasts, histiocytes, and macrophages with foamy cytoplasm-containing material having the staining properties of glycolipid are found in granulomatous deposits in the larynx, pleura, myocardium, pericardium, synovium, bones, liver, spleen, lymph nodes, cerebral cortex, and lung. Abnormal lipid is also present in the cytoplasm or neurons of the central nervous system. Roentgenographic changes consist of generalized bony demineralization, juxta-articular erosions of long bones, and irregular disruption of trabeculae in the metacarpal bones and phalanges.[187]

LIPOCHROME HISTIOCYTOSIS

This rare, familial disorder is marked by pulmonary infiltrates, splenomegaly, hypergammaglobulinemia, increased susceptibility to infection, and lipochrome pigment granulation of the histiocytes. In the first report of this syndrome, one of three affected sisters had rheumatoid arthritis with typical nodules, and a second had transient episodes of joint inflammation; the serum of all three contained rheumatoid factor in high titer.[193] The peripheral blood leukocytes of these patients have impaired respiration and hexose monophosphate shunt activity after phagocytosis and are deficient in their capacity to kill staphylococci.[194]

MULTICENTRIC RETICULOHISTIOCYTOSIS

Multicentric reticulohistiocytosis (MR) or lipodermatoarthritis, is a rare disorder seen in adults and characterized by a profusion of histiocytic nodules in the skin (Fig. 84–3A) and mucous membranes and by severe, often mutilating polyarthritis.[195–208]

To date just over 80 cases have been reported.[205,208,209] The disease affects women three times as often as men, and has a worldwide distribution. There is no evidence that the disorder is heritable.[195,205] Isolated lesions can occur, so-called solitary reticulohistiocytoma.[205]

Although the disorder has been thought to represent a lipid storage disease,[210] definitive evidence has not been presented. It is most likely that the histiocytes and giant cells contain a variety of nonspecifically accumulated lipid; it is not known with certainty whether this event is primary or secondary. Most lipid studies in MR reveal a varied and inconsistent pattern, suggesting a secondary accumulation. This latter phenomenon is generally referred to as a storage histiocytosis, defined by an accumulation of a normal or abnormal substance secondary to an alteration or disturbance in its metabolism by the mononuclear-phagocytic system.[211]

The disease appears to be inflammatory in nature, and the lesions in skin and synovium resemble experimentally produced granulomas, containing activated histiocytes that fuse to form cells of increasing size. These larger cells, or megalocytes, may eventually coalesce to form giant cells and may have granules that contain a variety of lipids, including triglycerides, cholesterol esters, and phospholipids.[201,203,212–214]

The role of lymphocyte/histiocyte interaction in the pathogenesis of MR is suggested by recent histochemical, immunochemical, and ultrastructural investigations. Staining techniques indicate that abundant lymphocytes are present in early nodules with reduction in their numbers as the nodule matures. The MR cell appears to be an activated macrophage.[207]

Severe bone and joint destruction is the hallmark of MR. This may occur without cartilage loss or with less cartilage loss than occurs in rheumatoid arthritis. Bony sites other than joints are destroyed, in addition to the typical areas of damage in the distal interphangeal joints and the posterior facet joints of the lumbosacral spine. The severe bone and joint destruction is probably due to erosion of cartilage and bone by collagenase, elastase, and other degradative enzymes released by the proliferating, activated histio-

FIG. 84–3. Photomicrograph of *A*, a skin nodule, and *B*, synovium (knee) from a 54-year-old woman with multicentric reticulohistiocytosis. Numerous histiocytes and multinucleated giant cells contain large amounts of periodic-acid-Schiff-positive material. (× 185)

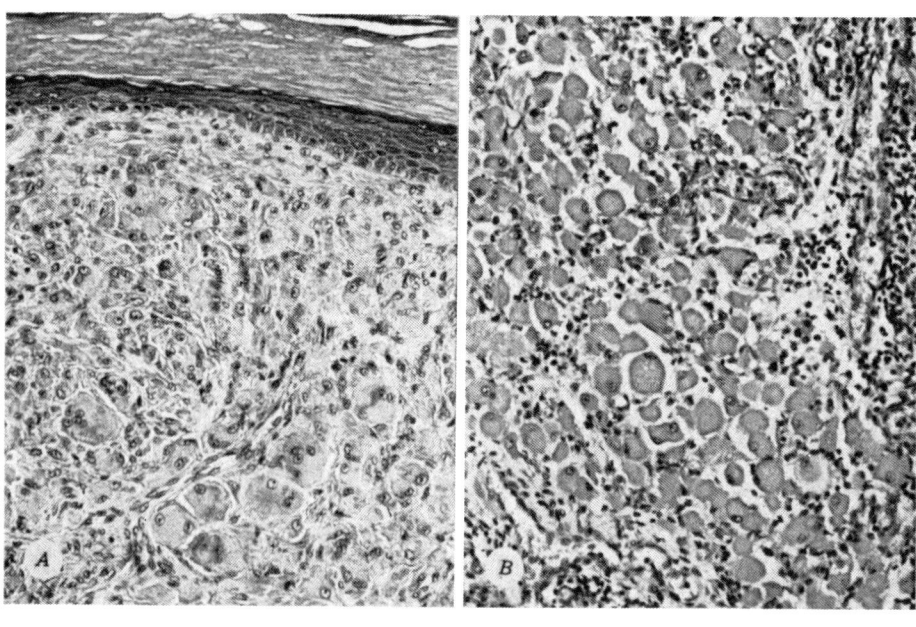

cytes, although direct evidence for such enzymatically mediated damage is still lacking.

The major difference between rheumatoid arthritis and MR is seen in the synovium. In MR microscopic examination shows dense infiltrations of the dermis and synovium by a granulomatous proliferation of histiocytes and multinucleated giant cells containing large amounts of periodic-acid-Schiff-positive material (Fig. 84–3B). Similar cells have been observed in the bone marrow, lymph nodes, bone and periosteum, muscle, larynx, and endocardium.[204] There is no characteristic composition of the synovial fluid in MR; a wide range of cell counts are noted with protein content usually above 4 g/dl. In the few synovial fluid samples examined the cell count has varied from 700 to 93,000 cells/mm[3,186,197,198,205,210,215] with predominance of either mononuclear[210] or polymorphonuclear cells.[198] Foamy giant cells have been found in the synovial fluid as well as in the synovium.[210,213] The presence of these large cells, known as megalocytes, may be a helpful early diagnostic clue.[213] Pericardial or pleural effusions may occur.[215] Electron microscopic study of these unusual macrophages reveals the presence of inclusions resembling the Golgi apparatus and seemingly developing from smooth endoplasmic reticulum.[210]

In approximately two thirds of patients, the first sign of the disease is polyarthritis, followed months to years later (average 3 years) by a nodular skin eruption. In the remaining patients, nodules appear first or are noted at the same time as the joint symptoms. The polyarthritis is usually symmetric, often simulates rheumatoid arthritis, and may involve all of the peripheral joints, including the distal interphalangeal (DIP) joints of the fingers, as well as the spinal and temporomandibular joints. Joint stiffness may be a prominent early complaint. The joints are swollen, tender, and may be inflamed. Large joint effusions may be present.[197] The most frequent joints affected are (in decreasing order): the interphalangeal joints, shoulders, knees, wrists, hips, feet, ankles, elbows, and spine. Marked DIP joint destruction is one of the distinguishing features of this disease.[205] In one half of cases severely deforming arthritis mutilans appears. It has been suggested that the degree of destruction is inversely related to age of onset.[205]

Although the disease may enter a spontaneous remission, chronic active disease is the rule. Many patients suffer severe destructive changes, particularly of the fingers (main en lorgnette) and less often of the hip and toe joints. The tendon sheaths on the flexor and extensor surfaces of the wrists may be involved,[197] and Dupuytren's contracture or carpal tunnel syndrome has been described.[198]

The skin lesions consist of firm, reddish brown or yellow papulonodules, most commonly on the face and hands, ears, forearms, and elbows, scalp, neck, and chest.[195] Small tumefactions resembling coral beads are seen around the nailfold (Fig. 84–4).[195] These lesions may remain discrete, or they may coalesce into diffuse plaques. They may be pruritic.[215] The nodules usually wax and wane and may disappear without a trace. Xanthelasma is noted in a third of these patients. About half the patients develop mucosal papules on the lips, tongue, buccal membrane, nasal septum, and gingiva, as well as on the pharynx and larynx. Fever, weakness, and weight loss may occur during the disease course. Mild anemia, monoclonal gammopathy, or erythrocyte sedimentation rate elevation may occur.[215] Endocardial tissue (at post mortem) and pleural biopsy specimens as well as perirenal fat have shown involvement.[205]

Roentgenograms reveal rapidly progressive, symmetric joint destruction with loss of cartilage and absorption of subchondral bone, disproportionately severe when compared with the mildness of the symptoms.[216] Characteristic features of the arthropathy of multicentric reticulohistiocytosis include

1. Well-circumscribed erosions spreading inward from the joint margins
2. Widened joint spaces
3. Predominance of changes in the interphalangeal, metacarpophalangeal, and metatarsophalangeal joints
4. Early and severe atlantoaxial joint involvement with erosion of the odontoid process leading to subluxation[217]
5. Erosion of the distal ends of the clavicles
6. Absent or minimal periosteal reaction
7. Absent or disproportionately mild osteopenia when compared with the severity of erosive changes
8. Prominent, uncalcified soft tissue nodules[216]

These findings are in direct contrast to typical radiographic features of osteoarthritis (where erosions begin centrally), rheumatoid arthritis (prominent cartilage loss and periarticular osteopenia occur early), and the seronegative spondyloarthropathies (periostitis with ill-defined margins).[218]

Patients with multicentric reticulohistiocytosis (MR) have an increased incidence of coexistent malignant disease. Perhaps as many as 25% develop a neoplasm.[213,215] Twenty-eight cases of associated neoplasm were reported in 82 subjects with MR; the papulonodular skin involvement was the initial manifestation (alone or concurrent with the arthritis) in 90% of the reviewed cases and a firm diagnosis of MR

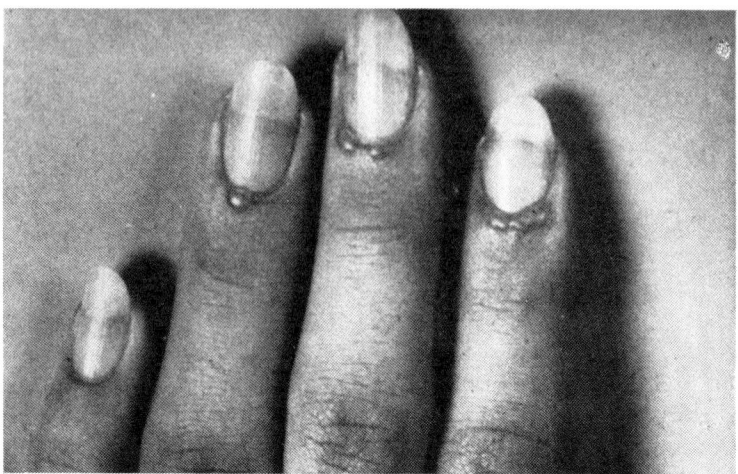

FIG. 84–4. The fingers of a 16-year-old girl who had polyarthritis for 8 months and reddish brown "coral beads" around the nailfold for 5 months. Typical infiltrates of multicentric reticulohistiocytosis were found in biopsy specimens of both skin and synovium. (From Barrow and Holubar.[195])

was made before the neoplasm was discovered in 73% of the subjects.[208] A wide spectrum of tumors appear to be associated with MR. In some situations MR has served as a marker for tumor recurrence, and therapy directed at the tumor caused regression of MR.[208] The frequency of tumor association should sharply heighten the index of suspicion for neoplasm, especially during the first year after the diagnosis of MR.

As mentioned already, MR may become spontaneously quiescent. Although the mucocutaneous nodules may shrink or even disappear completely, the patient is often left with serious joint disability and, at times, a disfigured, leonine facies.[195] Treatment with anti-inflammatory corticosteroids may cause temporary regression of the cutaneous lesions, but these agents have little effect on the arthritis.[203] A few reports cite dramatic clinical response to cytotoxic drug therapy. Both nodule formation and joint disease abated in one patient after treatment with cyclophosphamide.[200] The skin lesions were successfully treated with topical nitrogen mustard in another patient, who later responded to cyclophosphamide by an improvement in both joint and skin disease.[219] Treatment with nitrogen mustard and chlorambucil in still other patients has been reported to be effective.[220] Two cases of coexisting multicentric reticulohistiocytosis and primary biliary cirrhosis, successfully treated with cyclophosphamide, have been reported.[221] In the first case, chlorambucil was substituted when the patient developed hematuria, and improvement continued. A patient with multicentric reticulohistiocytosis with salivary gland involvement and pericarditis with effusion responded to a regimen of prednisone, cyclophosphamide, and vincristine administered simultaneously.[222] In still other cases azathioprine was used, but controlled neither the arthritis nor the size and number of cutaneous nodules.[210,215] The presence of hypothyroidism, bi-

opsy proved Sjögren's syndrome, and anti-Ro (SS-A) in a patient with MR has led to speculation about the association of MR and autoimmune diseases.[223]

In one report, four family members developed a reticulohistiocytosis-like disorder during childhood or adolescence.[224] The disease was characterized by a histiocytic papulonodular eruption on the face and hands, symmetric destructive polyarthritis, chiefly of the hands and wrists, and ocular involvement with cataract, uveitis, and glaucoma. The histologic changes in these patients differed from those of multicentric reticulohistiocytosis in a number of respects, however, including the absence of typical multinucleated giant cells and histiocytes with a "ground-glass" appearance of the cytoplasm.

HYPERLIPOPROTEINEMIAS

Articular and tendinous manifestations are important features of certain heritable disorders of lipid transport or lipoprotein metabolism.[4,225–227] The hyperlipoproteinemias are a result of a defect in either the synthesis or the degradation of lipoprotein particles.[227] These often dramatic articular signs and symptoms may be the first indication of the lipid disease and should alert the physician to an underlying disorder that may respond to dietary modification or drug therapy.

Patients with *type II hyperlipoproteinemia* exhibit tendinous, tuberous, and periosteal xanthomas as well as xanthelasma, corneal ulcers, and early, rapidly progressive atherosclerosis. Tendinous xanthomas are located in Achilles and patellar tendons and in the extensor tendons of the hands and feet.[225,228,229] Tendon xanthomas have also been found in the plantar aponeurosis, in the fascia, and in periosteum overlying the lower tibia and the peroneal tendons. Xanthomas are situated within the tendon fibers and not on the tendon sheath, and they cannot be separated from the tendon on movement. They contain large, lipid-lined histiocytes within the collagenous connective tissue. Tendon xanthomas are composed of cholesterol and phospholipid.[228,230] Tuberous xanthomas are soft, subcutaneous masses occurring over extensor surfaces, especially of the elbows, knees, and hands, as well as on the buttocks. Persons homozygous for type II hyperlipoproteinemia develop extensive xanthomas in childhood, whereas those who are heterozygous develop tendinous xanthomas after age 30 and lack tuberous xanthomas.

Tendinous and tuberous xanthomas also occur in type III and type IV hyperlipoproteinemia.[226,227] A distinctive clinical feature of the type III disorder is lipid deposition, or plane xanthomas, in the palms of the hands.[226] Types I, IV, and V hyperlipoproteinemia are characterized by eruptive xanthomas over the knees, buttocks, shoulders, and back.[227,231]

Several studies have described individual rheumatic syndromes associated with type II hyperlipoproteinemia.[232-236] Recurrent episodes of migratory polyarthritis have been reported in about 50% of patients homozygous for type II hyperlipoproteinemia.[233] Arthritis occurs chiefly in large peripheral joints, and inflammation varies from mild to severe. Severely inflamed joints are swollen, warm, and red, and joint involvement is symmetric. Episodes of arthritis are self-limited, resembling acute attacks of gout, lasting several days to 2 weeks. In some patients, the illness resembles rheumatic fever because of the evanescent arthritis, the presence of (atherosclerotic) aortic valvular disease, an elevated erythrocyte sedimentation rate, and a false-positive increased titer of antistreptolysin O caused by hyperlipoproteinemia. The valvular disease and the elevated erythrocyte sedimentation rate may occur in persons without arthritis and are presumably a direct result of the elevated lipoproteins.

In patients heterozygous for type II hyperlipoproteinemia, recurrent Achilles tendinitis is a common problem. This finding has been reported in adults, adolescents, and children.[229,232,234,235] In addition to Achilles tendinitis, monoarticular arthritis involving the knee or great toe is seen,[229] and in some heterozygous type II patients, migratory "polyarthritis" involving up to six joints has been reported.[234] Affected joints include the knee, the proximal interphalangeal joints, the ankle, the wrist, the elbow, the shoulder, and the hip. Some evidence suggests that the polyarthritis actually represents an inflammatory periarthritis or peritendinitis.[234] Synovial fluid from these

joints contains no crystals, and the cell counts are low (less than 200 neutrophils/mm³).

A recent review of heterozygotes with familial hypercholesterolemia reveals a 40% prevalence of symptoms in 73 cases; the observed manifestations included four types: Achilles pain (18%), Achilles tendinitis (11%), oligoarticular arthritis (7%), and polyarticular or rheumatic fever–like arthritis (4%).[236] Symptoms appear quite diverse, recurrent, even incapacitating, yet they are short-lived and no progression to joint damage is noted, unlike that observed in some homozygous patients. Attacks are "gout-like" with symptom-free intervals. Tendon xanthomas were present in many of these patients but they may be absent before the onset of symptoms.[236] Since symptoms may occur long before appearance of xanthomata or coronary artery insufficiency, the recognition of the significance of these unique joint complaints may lead to an early diagnosis of familial hypercholesterolemia and primary prevention of its consequences. A patient with high concentrations of low-density lipoprotein (LDL) cholesterol (type IIa) and gout-like attacks of periarthritis was treated with a low-cholesterol diet and colestipol with resolution of the joint abnormality and lowering of cholesterol.[237]

An arthropathy resembling that seen in type II hyperlipoproteinemia occurs in patients with *type IV hyperlipoproteinemia*.[238,239] These persons have predominantly an asymmetric oligoarthritis involving both small and large joints, including the proximal interphalangeal and metacarpophalangeal joints in the hands, wrists, shoulders, knees, ankles, tarsus, and metatarsophalangeal joints. In some cases, the inflammatory disease is mild and persistent, and in others it is episodic and recurrent.

Morning stiffness and para-articular hyperesthesia have been described in these patients.[239] Synovial fluid is noninflammatory and is free of crystals. Radiographs in a number of these patients show prominent para-articular bone cysts (Fig. 84–5). One such cyst was grossly yellow and mucinous and on microscopic examination showed only fibrous tissue and fat cells (Fig. 84–6). There were no granulomata, no cholesterol deposits and no lipid-laden histiocytes. Synovial biopsy in one case revealed moderate hyperplasia of the synovial villi, prominent stromal vessels, and a moderate mononuclear infiltrate. Four patients experienced decreased severity of articular symptoms after reduction or normalization of serum lipid levels.[238]

Skeletal lesions associated with other hyperlipoproteinemias have been reported also. A person with probable *type V hyperlipoproteinemia* had cystic lesions in both proximal femurs. Curettage yielded yellowish

FIG. 84–5. *A,B,* Roentgenograms showing prominent para-articular bone cysts in the fingers of two patients with arthritis associated with type IV hyperlipoproteinemia. Both patients had polyarticular inflammatory disease.

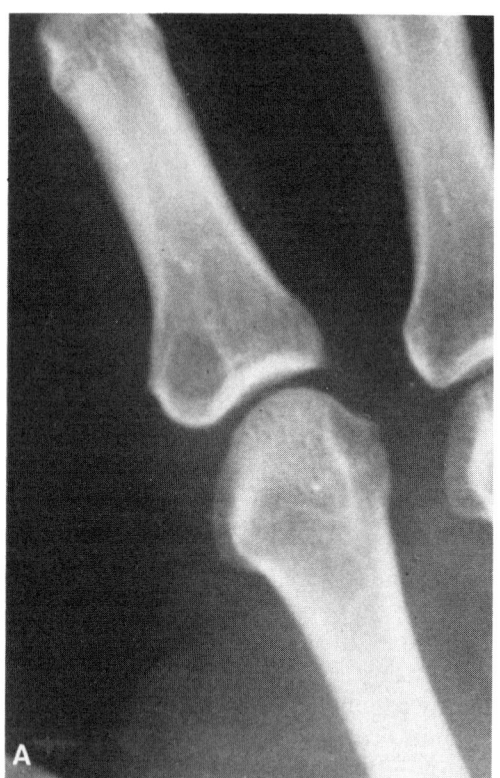
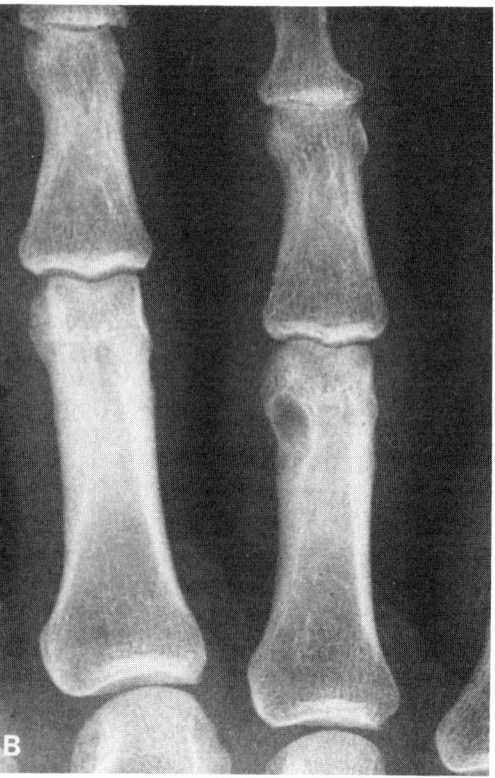

fragments that on microscopic examination showed foamy histiocytes and a granulomatous reaction around cholesterol clefts.[240] Secondary hyperlipoproteinemia can occur in association with the nephrotic syndrome, pancreatitis, alcoholism, hypothyroidism, and diabetes mellitus, and may be associated with musculoskeletal complaints. Joint changes secondary to infiltration of foam cells in subchondral bone in secondary hyperlipoproteinemia resemble those developing in patients with biliary cirrhosis.[241]

Cerebrotendinous xanthomatosis (CTX) is a rare autosomal recessive disorder characterized by progressive cerebellar ataxia, dementia, spinal cord paresis, subnormal intelligence, tendon xanthomas, and cataracts.[242,243] Cholestanol, or dihydrocholesterol, accumulates in the nervous tissue, tendons, and other tissues throughout the body. The underlying defect involves a deficiency of a hepatic enzyme involved in bile acid synthesis; treatment with chenodeoxycholic acid inhibits the abnormal bile acid synthesis, reduces plasma cholestanol concentrations, and offers the promise of preventing progression of the disease.[242] Tendon xanthomas may appear as early as the second

decade, but usually they are first noted in the third or fourth decade. The Achilles tendons are the most common sites, but xanthomas may also occur in the triceps tendons, at the tibial tuberosities, and in the extensor tendons of the hands. Tuberous xanthomas and xanthelasma may also occur.

Tendon xanthomas constitute a feature of *sitosterolemia with xanthomatosis,* another rare, newly recognized familial lipid storage disease marked by the accumulation of plant sterols in the blood and tissues.[242,244,245] These persons have an increased intestinal aborption of dietary sitosterol coupled with decreased removal, but the underlying metabolic defect has not yet been defined. The patient's serum cholesterol level may be normal or moderately elevated.[245] Inheritance is autosomal recessive. Tendon xanthomas indistinguishable histologically from those found in hyperlipoproteinemia appear during childhood, initially in the extensor tendons of the hands and later in the patellar, plantar, and Achilles tendons. Sitosterolemia should be considered in the differential diagnosis of a patient who presents with xanthomas in childhood and who does not have familial hypercholesterolemia or the CTX syndrome. Since some of

FIG. 84–6. A patient with arthritis associated with type IV hyperlipoproteinemia and prominent knee symptoms had a large cyst in the proximal tibia *(A)*. Tissue removed from the cyst at biopsy *(B)* was yellow and mucinous and on microscopic examination showed fibrous tissue and many fat cells (× 400).

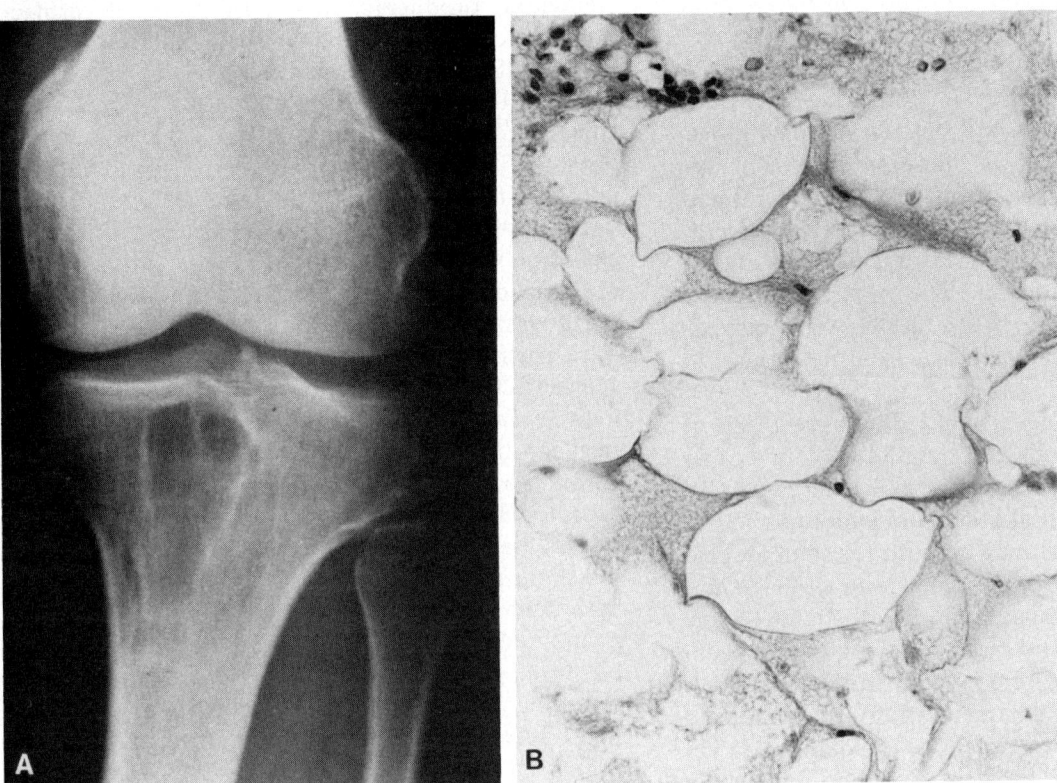

these persons may have an elevated cholesterol level, measurement of plasma sterols are necessary to establish this diagnosis.[242]

BLEEDING DISORDERS

Hemophilia is the collective designation for a group of hereditary hemorrhagic diseases in which there is a qualitative or quantitative deficiency of plasma procoagulant proteins.[246–248] Hemophilia A is an X-linked recessive disorder secondary to decreased levels of properly functioning factor VIII (also known as antihemophilic factor, or AHF). This disorder accounts for 80% of true hemophilias; hemophilia B is also X-linked and is not clinically distinguishable from hemophilia A.[249] For hemophilia B the deficiency resides in factor IX (also known as plasma thromboplastin component, PTC, or Christmas factor). Von Willebrand's disease and factor XI (plasma thromboplastin antecedent [PTA]) deficiency account for a very small number of cases. Patients are subject to abnormal bleeding, the frequency and intensity varying with

the level of the deficient factor. In addition to skin bruising, patients experience recurrent bleeding into the gastrointestinal and genitourinary tracts and hemorrhage into the musculoskeletal system.[1,3,250] Hemarthrosis is the bleeding manifestation most commonly requiring treatment;[251] it has been described in all of the hereditable coagulation disorders (except factor V deficiency) and as a complication of anticoagulant drugs.[252–255] Recurrent hemarthroses are painful, acute episodes that may lead ultimately to a self-sustaining synovitis and result in a deforming joint disease with permanent disability.[1,250,251,256–258]

PATHOGENESIS AND ANATOMIC FINDINGS

Hemophilic hemarthrosis usually but not always follows trauma. The injury is often trivial and is apparent neither to the young patient nor to his parents. The results of joint hemorrhage have been well studied in naturally hemophilic dogs, which develop an arthropathy comparable with that encountered in man.[259] The initial lesion consists of synovial or subsynovial hemorrhage. Rupture of blood into the joint cavity provokes an inflammatory reaction characterized by effusion, villous hypertrophy, hyperplasia of the lining cells, and infiltration by lymphocytes and plasma cells. This reaction gradually subsides several days to weeks after the cessation of hemorrhage. Hemoglobin is released once lysis of erythrocytes into the joint cavity and synovial tissues has occurred. Hemosiderin remains in the synovium for an indefinite period, appearing as finely particulate matter within the phagocytic lining cells.[260] Additional coarser aggregates of this iron-containing pigment, lying free or within macrophages, are found in deeper portions of the synovium. The presence of large amounts of hemosiderin in this location distinguishes this variety of synovial siderosis from that found in hemochromatosis.

Repeated hemorrhage is marked by hyperplasia of the synovial lining cells and by gradually increasing synovial fibrosis and hemosiderosis, leading to rigidity of the subsynovial tissue and joint capsule. Although these changes may account for some degree of limitation in motion, the damage to cartilage and bone, eventually, is most harmful to the joint.[256,261,262] Marginal erosion of the cartilage owing to encroachment of the hyperplastic synovium and more central, irregular, "map-like" degeneration attributable to subchondral hemorrhage occur.[263] The demonstration of plasmin, or fibrinolysin, in joint fluid during the course of acute hemarthrosis and the finding of numerous siderosomes suggest that the loss of cartilage may in part result from enzymatic degradation. Siderosomes are membrane-bound bodies with aggregates of iron-containing particles believed to be lysosomal organelles in which hemoglobin or its derivatives are digested.

One sees a marked increase in cathepsin-D and acid phosphatase activity in synovial tissue and a lesser increase in acid phosphatase activity in the joint fluid of patients with chronic hemophilic arthropathy.[3,250] These enzymes are inactive at neutral pH and probably contribute little to extracellular connective tissue degradation. Nevertheless, such findings indicate that the synovial tissue is "activated" and may release other degradative enzymes or may form pannus and directly invade and destroy contiguous cartilage and bone. Supporting this concept are studies of synovium isolated from a young hemophilic boy with proliferative synovitis revealing secretion of latent collagenase in amounts equal to those secreted by rheumatoid synovium.[264] In addition, isolated hemophilic synovium and synovial cells secrete a proteinase, active at neutral pH, that can degrade the protein core of the glycosaminoglycan component of cartilage.

In tissue culture hemophilic synovium generates prostaglandin E at high rates, similar to rheumatoid synovium, producing brisk breakdown of cartilage proteoglycans.[265] Immunopathologic mechanisms for perpetuation of the chronic synovitis in hemophilia have not been demonstrated; joint tissue from seven subjects showed no immune deposits.[266] Activated hemophilia synovium, therefore, appears to have the potential for considerable connective tissue destruction and a marked degradative effect on cartilage. In experimental hemarthrosis in rabbits, the synthesis of both ribonucleic acid and protein by articular cartilage was initially unimpaired despite repeated daily intra-articular injection of autologous blood.[267] When such injections were continued for several weeks or months, however, definite alterations occurred in the cartilage matrix, consisting at first of altered metachromasia, followed by superficial and deep erosions, accompanied by a reduction in proteoglycan concentration and a depression in the synthetic activity of the chondrocyte.[262] The deposition of iron pigment in both synovium and cartilage plays a significant role in the pathogenesis of the degeneration of articular cartilage.[3,268] Degradation of ground substance surrounding chondrocytes containing iron suggests that local release of degradative enzymes may be prompted by the retained pigment.[269] Proteoglycan loss alters the resilience and compressibility of normal cartilage and may accelerate its destruction.

Articular cartilage damage caused by repeated joint hemorrhage is accompanied by the development of cavities or "cysts" in the subchondral bone. These lesions can become large and have been thought to be the result of intraosseous bleeding (Fig. 84–7). In a study of hemophilic dogs, these cysts communicated with the synovial cavity at a point of cartilage and subchondral bone erosion, at the margin of the articular cartilage, or at the site of ligamentous attachments.[259] These and similar observations in human hemophilic joint disease suggest that the development of these cysts is related more to secondary degenerative changes in articular cartilage and subchondral bone than to intraosseous bleeding.[260,270]

The final answer on the cause of the hemophiliac subchondral cyst is far from complete. Pathoanatomic evidence suggests that an expanding cyst is produced primarily through biomechanical forces. The initial event may be a subchondral hematoma beneath the load-bearing surface; centrifugal expansion of its developing fibrous wall destroys bone and cartilage with the end result producing a large osteochondral defect displaying discrete vertical margins and a depressed

FIG. 84–7. Sagittal section of the knee joint of a 49-year-old man with advanced hemophilic arthropathy. The femoral condyle appears flattened and the patella has virtually disappeared. The head of the tibia has undergone massive cystic resorption. The articular cartilage has disappeared from most of the joint surfaces, which have undergone partial fibrous ankylosis on the popliteal aspect on the right and have been replaced by fibrous tissue. The cyst in the tibia is lined by loose-textured fibrous tissue. The synovial and capsular tissues are thickened and infiltrated with many hemosiderin-laden mononuclear cells. (From Sokoloff.[300])

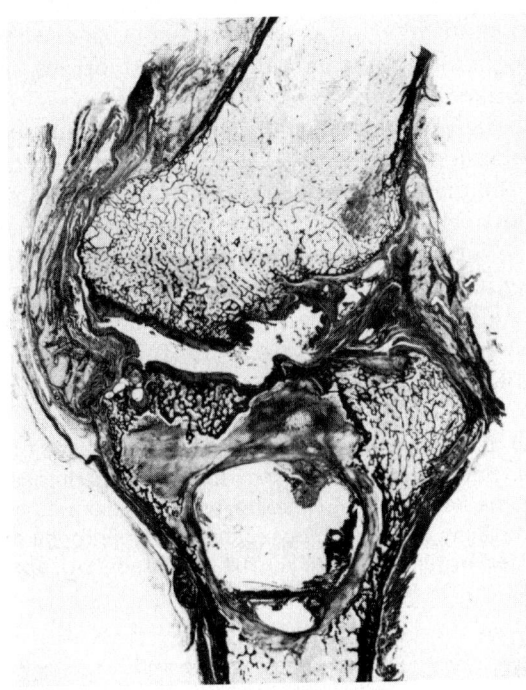

sclerotic bony base. The process proceeds from within to without or toward the joint surface. Characteristic knee intercondylar widening noted radiologically is felt to be the evolution of these cysts in the load-bearing portion of the patellofemoral articulation.[271]

A striking but less specific finding in young patients is accelerated maturation and hypertrophy of the epiphyses adjacent to affected joints. Chronic hyperemia of the epiphyseal cartilage, induced by repeated hemarthrosis, may be responsible for this change.

In addition to hemarthrosis, bleeding into muscle and bone may occur. The terms "hemophilic pseudotumor" and "hemophilic cyst" have been applied to the destructive lesions that follow massive muscle, subperiosteal, or intraosseous hemorrhages. Such hematomas, if not optimally treated, subsequently organize, become vascular, and are locally destructive to soft tissue and bone. In the adult, these hematomas occur most often in the pelvis, thigh, or leg,[272–278,279,280]

whereas in children they occur distal to the elbow or knee and are less destructive.

Soft tissue bleeding may be dangerous because of neurovascular compression, severe destruction and contracture of muscle, including Volkmann's contracture,[275,280–282] cyst rupture, sinus formation, or chronic infection.[275] One of the most dramatic examples of hemophilic bleeding involves the iliopsoas muscle.[283,284] Hemorrhage into the closed fascial compartment that contains the iliopsoas muscle and the femoral nerve is marked by the development of sudden, severe pain in the groin and thigh, followed by the appearance of a tender mass, a hematoma, in the iliac fossa and the groin, flexion contracture of the hip, and signs of femoral nerve palsy. Bleeding into the gastrocnemius or soleus muscle, or both may lead to a talipes equinus deformity. Repeated bleeding in and around the joints and associated muscle atrophy inevitably lead to instability of the weight-bearing articulations.

CLINICAL FEATURES

Hemarthrosis occurs in approximately 80 to 90% of patients with hemophilia,[1,251,256,258,285,286] and constitutes the most common major hemorrhagic event in the disease. Bleeding into the joints is particularly frequent when the patient's level of antihemophilic globulin is less than 1 to 2% of normal.[285,287,288] Most patients first experience articular symptoms between the ages of 1 and 5 years, and they usually have repeated hemarthroses during the remainder of the first decade of life; thereafter, these episodes ordinarily become less and less frequent.[281,286] Patients with levels of antihemophilic globulin greater than 5% of normal generally experience fewer episodes of hemarthrosis, and these occur only after more severe trauma.

A clinical and radiologic survey of 139 hemophiliac patients provides some unique observations on the prevalence of arthropathy because of the inclusion of many with mild to moderate disease (factor levels 6 to 60%); in contrast to earlier observations, a significant (one third) prevalence of definite arthritis was seen in this mild to moderate group although it was less severe, mostly affecting one or two joints.[251] This study pointed out that even subjects with factor levels up to 20% may experience arthropathy; those with factor levels of less than 5% are at risk for severe polyarthritis. In addition, some persons without a history of bleeding demonstrated severe articular changes radiographically. The presence of this anomaly suggests that subclinical bleeding may occur and if it does, the hemorrhage may remain confined to the synovium.

Joint hemorrhage occurs most commonly in a knee, ankle, or elbow and less frequently in the shoulders, hips, wrists, fingers, and toes.[251,286,289] Generally, only a single joint is involved in each episode, but two joints may be affected simultaneously. The patient often has repeated hemorrhaging at the same site.[286]

The affected joint is swollen, warm, and often exquisitely painful and tender. Associated muscle spasm leads to flexion of the extremity. In instances of milder bleeding, the normal configuration and full motion of the joint may be restored within a matter of days, and the patient may experience little more than transient stiffness on reambulation. In the case of protracted bleeding, and particularly when repeated injury of the joint leads to renewed hemorrhage, symptoms may persist for many weeks to months. Thermograms and radionuclide scanning have been used to assess the effects of acute hemarthrosis,[290] and it has been suggested that ^{99m}Tc scintigraphy may be useful to follow patients sequentially.[291] Ultrasonographic studies have proved useful in demonstrating deeper bleeding, such as retroperitoneal hemorrhage.[292]

After repeated severe hemarthrosis, the joint gradually fails to return to full normal form and function, and loss of muscle power and mass is progressive. Examination discloses thickening of the periarticular soft tissues, crepitation, atrophic muscle accentuating the bony enlargement of the joint, and various deformities, the most common of which are flexion contractures of the elbow and knee. Flexion contracture of the knee is frequently accompanied by posterior subluxation of the tibia. Occasionally, joints develop fibrous or (rarely) bony ankylosis.[256,281]

Bleeding into the hip joint during childhood may lead to dislocation,[281] as well as to flattening and destruction of the capital epiphysis and deformity of the femoral neck, with resultant shortening of the extremity. Synovial hyperemia may be accompanied by epiphyseal hyperemia and epiphyseal overgrowth. In growing children, this process causes axial deviations including cubitus valgus, coxa valga, genu valgum, and pes valgus, and any one of these structural abnormalities may be asymmetric.

Bleeding episodes necessitate long periods of bed rest, which, in turn, delay neuromotor maturation.[293] Approximately one half of all patients with hemophilia have some permanent changes in their peripheral articulations, and only the rare person with severe hemophilia (less than 2% of the normal level of antihemophilic globulin) escapes some residual deformity.[251,288] In many cases, only a few joints are involved in this chronic arthropathy, usually knees and

elbows, and many other joints remain normal despite repeated bleeding episodes. Although hemarthroses were noted to be equally common in both factor VIII and IX deficiencies in a large referral hemophiliac clinic, arthritis was more frequently present in those with factor VIII deficiency. Hemarthroses and arthritis were exceptional in von Willebrand's disease.[251]

In addition to muscle atrophy as a result of joint inflammation and disuse, hemophiliacs have demonstrated other features of a neuromyopathy. Electromyographic assessments reveal reduced numbers of functioning motor units and a "myopathic" motor unit potential; serum creatine phosphokinase levels are frequently increased, and muscle biopsies show type 2 fiber atrophy.[294]

Although the presence of hemophilia is suspected readily in a person with a recognized bleeding tendency, the diagnosis may be much less obvious in the occasional child or adult in whom hemarthrosis is the initial symptom of the disease or in whom minor hemorrhagic episodes have been overlooked. It is especially important to recognize this condition, because unsuspecting surgical intervention has disastrous consequences.[263]

FIG. 84–8. *A* and *B*, Roentgenograms of the knee of a 9-year-old boy with hemophilia and repeated hemarthroses involving the left knee *(B)*. Note the loss of articular cartilage, the irregularity of bony surfaces, and the hypertrophy of the epiphyses of femur and tibia. The right knee *(A)* appears normal.

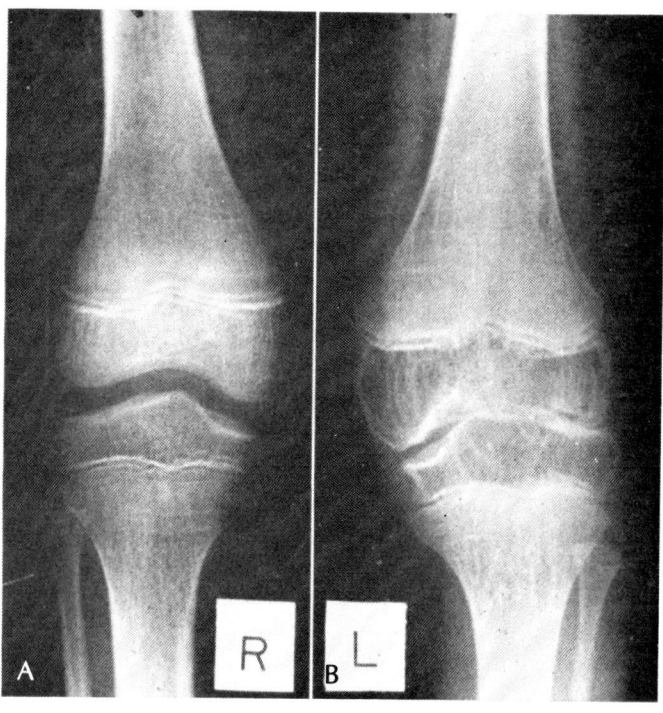

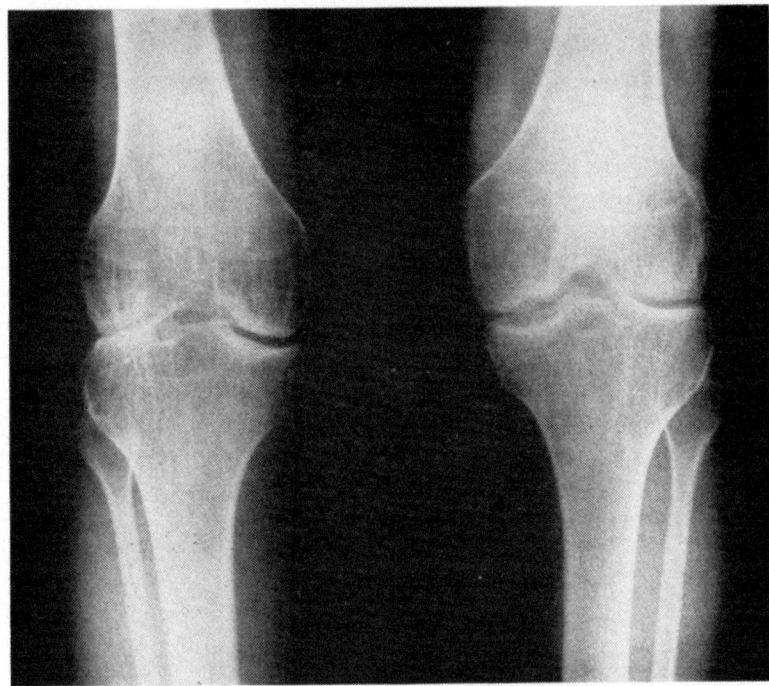

FIG. 84–9. Roentgenograms of the knees of the patient in Figure 84–8 at the age of 17 years. During the 8 years since the roentgenograms in Figure 84–8 were obtained, the patient had many more episodes of joint hemorrhage involving both knees. Note the irregular narrowing of the joint space and early osteophyte formation.

ROENTGENOGRAPHIC FINDINGS

In acute intra-articular hemorrhage, one sees distention of the joint capsule and increased density of the soft tissues. An accompanying subperiosteal hemorrhage, which is followed by thickening or, in some cases, by atrophy of the underlying cortex may be evident. Subchondral hemorrhage may lead to defects in epiphyseal ossification centers.

Chronic hemophilic joint disease is characterized by irregular narrowing or obliteration of the joint space and later by marginal spurring and sclerosis of bone, which often contains one or more areas of cystic translucency[39,256,276,295,296] (Figs. 84–8 through 84–15). These cystic areas may be quite large. The periarticular soft tissues may be thickened and increased in density, and they occasionally contain fine opacities. These opacities were traditionally attributed to the

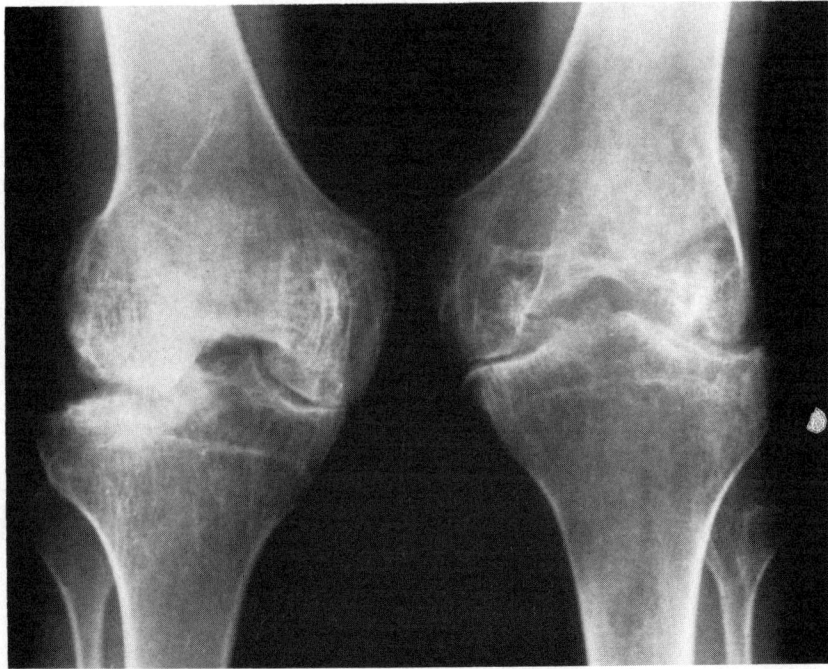

FIG. 84–10. Roentgenogram of the knees of a 23-year-old man with hemophilia illustrating severe secondary degenerative joint disease.

FIG. 84–11. Roentgenogram of the right hip of the patient in Figure 84–10 illustrating severe degenerative joint disease and protrusio acetabuli.

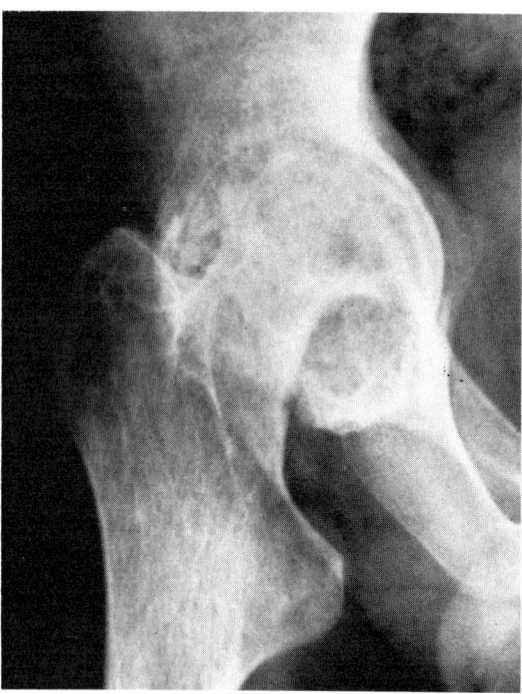

FIG. 84–12. Roentgenogram of the ankle of a 26-year-old man with hemophilia. Note the loss of cartilage and subchondral sclerosis in both ankle and subtalar joints.

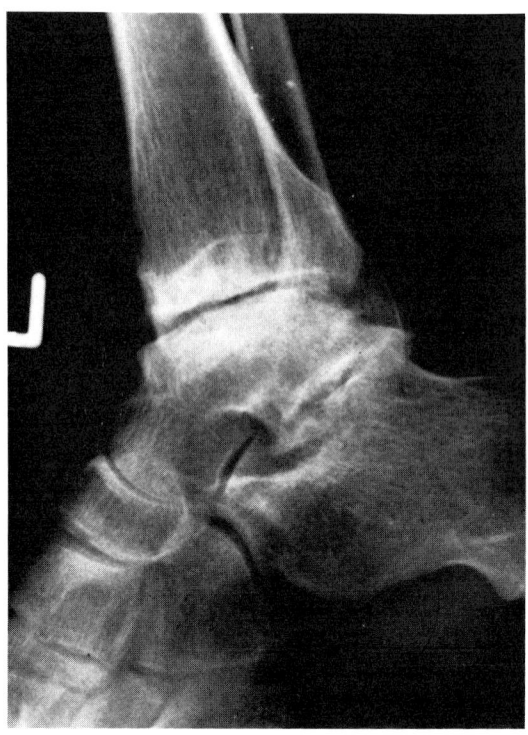

deposition of hemosiderin in the synovium, a view that has been disputed. Certain roentgenographic features are characteristic but not pathognomonic of chronic hemophilic arthropathy. These findings include enlargement of the head of the radius in patients with elbow involvement;[256,288] flattening of the inferior portion of the patella, or "squared-off" patella, in advanced disease of the knee;[39,295] widening of the intercondylar notch of the femur; and flattening of the talus. Aseptic necrosis of the femoral head,[39] as well as of the talus,[256] may also be seen. In rare cases, chondrocalcinosis has been described in hemophiliacs,[297] and in one person, an episode of acute pseudogout, masquerading as hemarthrosis, was proved by arthrocentesis and demonstration of calcium pyrophosphate dihydrate (CPPD) crystals.[298]

MANAGEMENT

Has modern treatment of hemophilia (e.g., demand therapy, home treatment programs) reduced the long-term morbidity of the associated arthropathy? A study using historical controls suggests a reduction in prevalence as well as severity of arthropathy.[251] A review of demand therapy in classic (factor VIII) disease pa-

FIG. 84–13. Roentgenogram of the elbow of a 27-year-old man with hemophilia illustrating large subchondral erosion in the ulna.

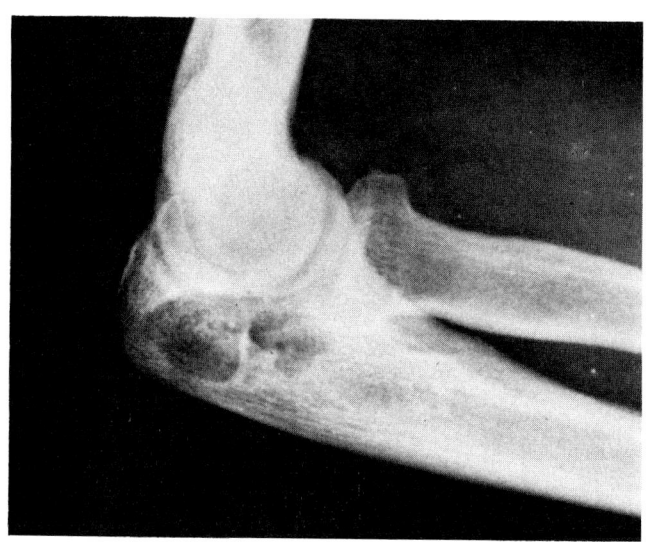

FIG. 84–14. Roentgenogram of the shoulder of a 24-year-old man with hemophilia illustrating the loss of articular cartilage and large defects in the subchondral bone of both the humerus and the glenoid fossa.

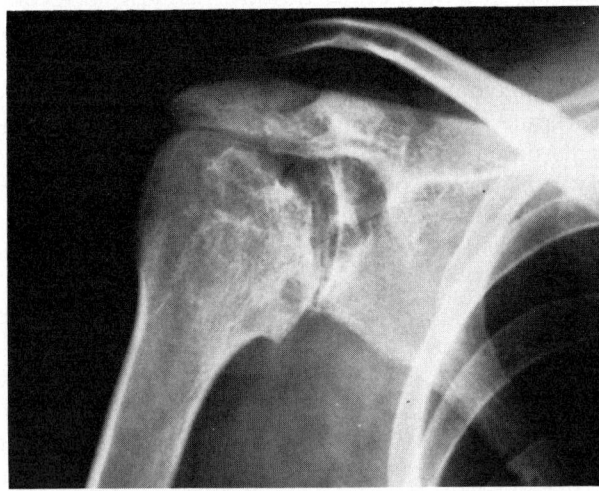

tients indicates that those with normal range of motion and those with marked or severe limitation can maintain their range of motion for over 6 years. Nevertheless some people with mild disease at the outset showed progression in spite of demand therapy.[299] The proof for an optimistic viewpoint is not yet at hand. Clearly the unchecked use of factor VIII

replacement from human sources is not without risk and there is a need to identify subsets of patients who have additional requirements or expected benefits from more aggressive therapy.

Approximately a dozen cases of septic arthritis complicating hemophilia have been reported,[300–308] as has a review[309] comparing pyogenic arthritis with spontaneous hemarthrosis in hemophiliac subjects. Although this complication is relatively uncommon, it carries serious morbidity. Key clinical features suggesting sepsis include monoarticular involvement, most often the knee; association with an underlying arthropathy; presence of Staphylococcus aureus; invariable fever, leukocytosis (white blood cell count >10,000 mm³); and presence of factors predisposing to sepsis (intravenous drug use, hemodialysis, prior aspirations, or surgical procedures).[309] Based on a comparison with the findings in spontaneous hemarthrosis it has been recommended that a patient with fever of 1° C (1.8° F) and acute symptoms of joint inflammation should have an aspiration to rule out infection.[309] Arthrocentesis in uncomplicated hemarthrosis does not modify the clinical course and may increase the risk for additional bleeding; the choice to perform the procedure should be based on the need to rapidly diagnose joint sepsis in the proper clinical setting, that is, when there is a high probability that the patient has a septic joint. The diagnosis of pyogenic arthritis should be entertained when joint

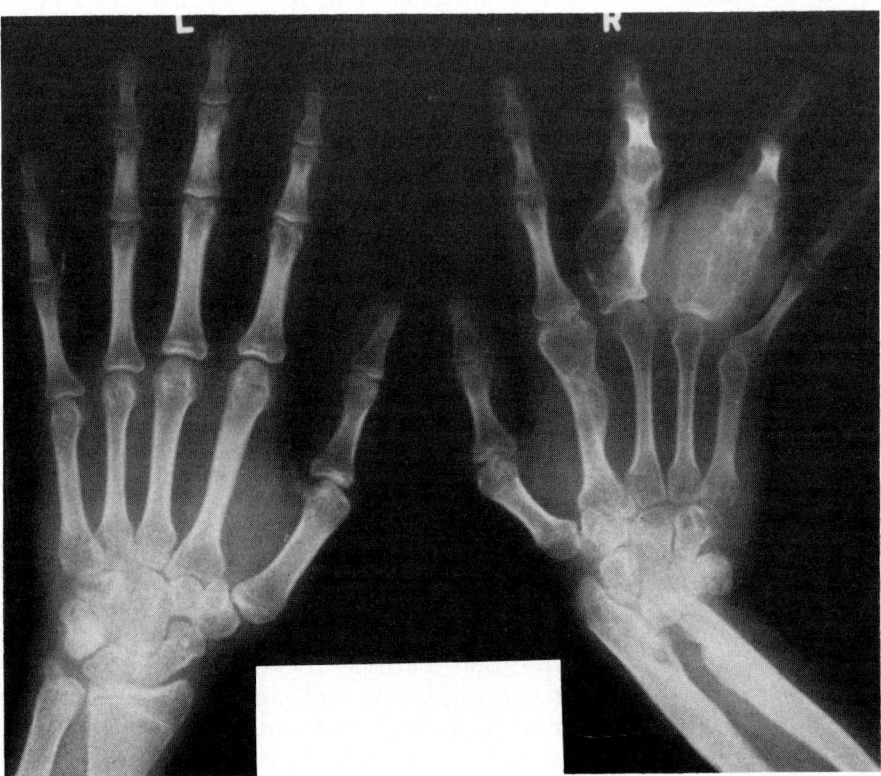

FIG. 84–15. Roentgenogram of the right hand of a 16-year-old boy with hemophilia illustrating the destruction of bone of the proximal phalanges of the fourth and fifth fingers resulting from hemophilic pseudotumor (normal left hand for comparison).

symptoms appear prolonged despite standard replacement therapy. Although hemophiliac patients are thought not to be predisposed to joint infection, it being a rare problem considering their degree of joint damage, frequent trauma, and bleeding,[306] the number of episodes of pyogenic arthritis in hemophilia equaled the number of episodes of joint sepsis in rheumatoid arthritis in an admission survey from a Denver hospital.[309]

Hemarthroses and chronic arthropathy are reported in factor XIII deficiency[310] and von Willebrand's disease (VWD).[311] Bleeding does not appear to be rare in factor XIII deficiency, which is characterized by a qualitatively unstable clot. Articular hemorrhage in factor XIII deficiency occurs usually 12 to 36 hours after trauma; destructive joint sequelae, however, are uncommon.[310] Although earlier reports indicated that hemarthrosis occurred in only 5 to 10% of severe VWD patients, 4 out of 35 subjects in a more recent study were affected, 3 of 4 were girls, none had violent trauma, and bleeding into the ankle predominated.[311] Recurrent hemarthrosis in the shoulder of a 56-year-old man taking warfarin produced a destructive arthropathy in the absence of a pre-existing joint abnormality.[255]

CHRONIC HEMOPHILIC JOINT DISEASE

The knee is most often affected by the development of a chronic flexion contracture. This defect may be corrected by physical therapy and stable weight-bearing may be achieved by means of traction, wedging casts, quadriceps setting exercises, and later, active resistive exercises.[256,289,295,312–314] The use of a long leg-extension brace and crutches may be required for many months or years to prevent recurrence of the contracture.[250,256,277]

The use of surgical procedures for the correction of chronic joint deformities was limited because of the risk of uncontrollable postoperative hemorrhage until potent concentrates of antihemophilic factors became available. The prospect of orthopedic rehabilitation is excellent.[277] Many procedures are now successful, including arthroplasty of the hip,[315] supracondylar wedge osteotomy or correction of valgus deformity of the knee,[250,289,312] wedge osteotomy of the tibia,[312] lengthening of the Achilles and other tendons of the feet for correction of equinus contracture,[250,278,281,286,312,316] compression arthrodesis of the knee, hip, and ankle,[278,316] and total knee and total hip replacement.[1,250,317–320] Heroic operations, such as drainage or radical excision of hematoma and pseudotumor and the amputation of an extremity in cases

of uncontrollable, life-threatening bleeding, or infection are now also possible.[275,277,278,321–325] An analysis of 76 individual operative procedures revealed three that were particularly successful: (1) supracondylar correction of knock knee; (2) intertrochanteric correction of coxa valga; and (3) evacuation of iliacus hematoma in patients with femoral nerve paralysis.[293]

Synovectomy should be viewed as a hemostatic procedure. It should probably be limited to those patients under the age of 20 with radiographically less advanced arthropathy, and when conservative therapies are not successful.[326] The procedure has proved successful in control of repeated or intractable hemorrhage.[3,250,327–329]

Synoviorthesis with osmic acid is less effective than synovectomy in preventing recurrent hemarthrosis, but because of its simplicity, it has been recommended for use in younger patients.[330] Intra-articular radioactive gold (^{198}Au) also decreases the bleeding frequency and halts the progression of the disease if used early when the arthropathy is still reversible.[331]

In a study of 50 joints treated with radioactive gold (^{198}Au) or rhenium (^{186}Re),[30] 60% displayed no further bleeding and 88% were improved overall. The authors felt that the procedure reduces AHF requirements, has low cost and can be repeated. The danger of extra-articular spread with chromosomal damage was thought to be minimal.[332]

Hemophilic pseudotumor has been treated successfully surgically, as well as with x-irradiation.[250,333,334] A number of uncontrollable, destructive pseudotumors have been excised successfully.[323,324,333] In the management of fractures in the hemophilic patient, rigid immobilization has been essential. In addition to the maintenance of hemostasis during healing, internal stabilization may be required.[335]

The acquired immune deficiency syndrome (AIDS) has now been reported in a number of patients with hemophilia, all of whom have been exposed to factor VIII or factor IX concentrates as well as other blood components. AIDS in hemophiliacs appears to be reaching epidemic proportions, and all evidence suggests that it is imperative to attempt to limit further occurrence of the syndrome in this apparently high-risk group. Most of the patients with hemophilia who have AIDS have died of opportunistic infections within a short time. Hemophiliacs are more difficult to manage than the usual patients with AIDS because diagnostic and therapeutic procedures may be complicated by their bleeding diathesis.[336]

Purification methods (heat, lyophilization, pasteurization, organic solvent and detergent) and donor screening have greatly reduced the risk of virus transmission in commercial factor preparations. A formulation of factor VIII purified by affinity chromatography has been approved for marketing by the United States Food and Drug Administration (FDA).[337] Nevertheless, until plasma-free factor VIII manufactured by recombinant DNA techniques becomes available, the risk of viral transmission is still present and should be considered when making clinical decisions.

Management of Chronic Hemophilic Joint Disease

A detailed discussion of factor replacement therapy and the specific treatment of spontaneous hemarthroses is available in general excellent recent reviews.[249,338–340] Certain principles, however, are well established and deserve reiteration. *Acute hemarthrosis should be recognized early and treated with intensive infusion therapy.* It is essential that both the patient and parents be instructed in this process to minimize joint damage and loss of schooling. Chronic joint disease should be managed with aggressive factor VIII or factor IX replacement as well as orthopedic and physical therapy measures for muscle building and increased joint stability, intervals of non-weight-bearing, and correction of flexion contractures.[249] However, the cornerstone to therapy in hemophilia is to immediately and adequately correct the hemostatic defect once bleeding is suspected.[341] The majority of severe and moderately severe hemophiliacs can achieve that goal through a comprehensive multidisciplinary program of intensive self-education and a supervised self-therapy program at home.[342]

The use of factor replacement therapy is governed by the overriding general principle to achieve hemostasis quickly and with sufficient duration to allow wound healing. The amount required depends on the location, severity, duration, and nature of the bleeding episodes, as well as the long-term goals of the individual patient. The optimum or ideal dosage of factor VIII or IX varies.[340] A recent recommendation for factor replacement therapy suggests that infusions be given every 24 hours to achieve a minimal hemostatic level of 30% for mild hemorrhages (early hemarthrosis) and 50% for a major bleeding episode (advanced hemarthrosis) to be maintained for one to several days until resolution of the lesion; management includes repeated laboratory measurements of factor VIII levels.[249]

Oral corticosteroid administration may facilitate the resolution of hemarthrosis. A 5-day course of prednisone, in doses of up to 80 mg/day, has reduced the amount of specific replacement factor necessary for the treatment of acute hemarthrosis and has increased the number of favorable responses to single infusions of factor VIII.[343]

Nonsteroidal anti-inflammatory drugs have been used with caution in hemophiliac patients. No change in platelet function, bleeding time, or coagulation measures occurred with benoxaprofen, or salsalate; a prospective study demonstrated that ibuprofen did not affect the frequency of bleeding episodes or replacement concentrate used while significantly reducing pain compared to placebo.[344] D-Penicillamine reduced chronic inflammation in a rabbit model of hemarthrosis-induced arthritis and reduced the number of joint bleeding episodes in three of four hemophiliacs with chronic synovitis.[345]

REFERENCES

1. Duthie, R.B., and Rizza, C.R.: Rheumatological manifestations of the haemophilias. Clin. Rheum. Dis., 1:53–93, 1975.
2. Easton, J.A.: Musculo-skeletal aspects of haematological disorders. Clin. Rheum. Dis., 2:459–491, 1976.
3. Hilgartner, M.W.: Hemophilic arthropathy. Adv. Pediatr., 21:139–165, 1974.
4. Rooney, P.J., Ballantyne, D., and Buchanan, W.W.: Disorders of the locomotor system associated with abnormalities of lipid metabolism and the lipoidoses. Clin. Rheum. Dis., 1:163–193, 1975.
5. Schumacher, H.R.: Rheumatological manifestations of sickle cell disease and other hereditary haemoglobinopathies. Clin. Rheum. Dis., 1:37–52, 1975.
6. Isenberg, D.A., and Shoenfeld, Y.: The rheumatologic complications of hematologic disorders. Semin. Arthritis Rheum., 12:348–358, 1983.
7. Caldwell, D.S., and McCallum, R.M.: Rheumatologic manifestations of cancer. Med. Clin. North Am., 70:385–417, 1986.
8. Bichel, J.: Arthralgic leukemia in children. Acta Haematol., 1:153–164, 1948.
9. Fink, C.W., Windmiller, J., and Sartain, P.: Arthritis as the presenting feature of childhood leukemia. Arthritis Rheum., 15:347–349, 1972.
10. Spilberg, I., and Meyer, G.J.: The arthritis of leukemia. Arthritis Rheum., 15:630–635, 1972.
11. Thomas, L.B., et al.: The skeletal lesions of acute leukemia. Cancer, 14:608–621, 1961.
12. Aisner, M., and Hoxie, T.B.: Bone and joint pain in leukemia, simulating acute rheumatic fever and subacute bacterial endocarditis. N. Engl. J. Med., 238:733–737, 1948.
13. Hallidie-Smith, K.A., and Bywaters, E.G.L.: The differential diagnosis of rheumatic fever. Arch. Dis. Child., 33:350–357, 1958.
14. Case Records of the Massachusetts General Hospital. N. Engl. J. Med., 314:973–981, 1986.
15. Schaller, J.: Arthritis as a presenting manifestation of malignancy in children. J. Pediatr., 81:793–797, 1972.
16. Silverstein, M.N., and Kelly, P.J.: Leukemia with osteoarticular symptoms and signs. Ann. Intern. Med., 59:637–645, 1963.
17. Weinberger, A., Schumacher, H.R., and Schimmer, B.M.: Arthritis in acute leukemia: Clinical and histopathological observations. Arch. Intern. Med., 141:1183–1187, 1981.
18. Jaffe, H.L.: Tumors and Tumorous Conditions of the Bones and Joints. Philadelphia, Lea & Febiger, 1958.

19. Luzar, M.J., and Sharma, H.M.: Leukemia and arthritis: Including reports on light, immunofluorescent and electron microscopy of the synovium. J. Rheumatol., *10*:132–135, 1983.

20. Seligmann, M., Cannat, A., and Hamad, M.: Studies on antinuclear antibodies. Ann. N.Y. Acad. Sci., *124*:816–832, 1965.

21. Lane, J.J., Jr., and Decker, J.L.: Latex particle slide tests in rheumatoid arthritis. J. Am. Med. Assoc., *173*:982–985, 1960.

22. Sherry, M.G.: The incidence of positive RA tests in Hodgkin's disease and leukemia. Am. J. Clin. Pathol., *50*:398–400, 1968.

23. Soebergen, E.M., et al.: T cell leukemia presenting as chronic polyarthritis. Arthritis Rheum., *25*:87–91, 1982.

24. Evans, F.J., and Hilton, J.H.B.: Polymyositis associated with acute monocytic leukemia: Case report and review of the literature. Can. Med. Assoc. J., *91*:1272–1275, 1964.

25. Valimaki, M., Vuopio, P., and Luewendahl, K.: Bone lesions in chronic myelogenous leukemia. Acta Med. Scand., *210*:403–408, 1981.

26. Pear, B.L.: Skeletal manifestations of the lymphomas and leukemias. Semin. Roentgenol., *9*:229–240, 1974.

27. Greenfield, G.B.: Radiology of Bone Diseases. 4th Ed. Philadelphia, J.B. Lippincott, 1986.

28. Hudson, T.L.: Radiologic-Pathologic Correlation of Musculoskeletal Lesions. Baltimore, Williams & Wilkins, 1987.

29. Resnick, D., and Haghighi, P.: Myeloproliferative disorders. *In* Diagnosis of Bone and Joint Disorders. 2nd Ed. Edited by D. Resnick and G. Niwayama. Philadelphia, W.B. Saunders Co., 1988, pp. 2459–2496.

30. Kellerhouse, L.E., and Limarzi, L.R.: Bone manifestations of hematologic disorders. Med. Clin. North Am., *49*:203–228, 1965.

31. Elkton, R.B., Hughes, G.R.V., and Catovsky, D.: Hairy cell leukemia with polyarteritis nodosa. Lancet, *2*:280–282, 1979.

32. Gabriel, S.E., et al.: Vasculitis in hairy cell leukemia: Review of literature and consideration of possible pathogenetic mechanisms. J. Rheumatol., *13*:1167–1172, 1986.

33. Westbrook, C.A., and Golde, D.W.: Autoimmune disease in hairy cell leukemia: Clinical syndromes and treatment. Br. J. Haematol., *61*:349–356, 1985.

34. Weinstein, A.: Systemic vasculitis and hairy cell leukemia. J. Rheumatol., *9*:349–350, 1982.

35. Demames, D.J., Lane, N., and Beckstead, J.H.: Bone involvement in hairy-cell leukemia. Cancer, *49*:1697–1701, 1982.

36. Puczynski, M.S., Demos, T.C., and Suarez, C.R.: Sinus histiocytosis with massive lymphoadenopathy: Skeletal involvement. Pediatr. Radiol., *15*:259–261, 1985.

37. Heinicke, M.H., Zarrabi, M.H., and Gorevic, P.D.: Arthritis due to synovial involvement by extramedullary haematopoiesis in myelofibrosis with myeloid metaplasia. Ann. Rheum. Dis., *42*:196–200, 1983.

38. Fucilla, I.S., and Hamann, A.: Hodgkin's disease in bone. Radiology, *77*:53–60, 1961.

39. Moseley, J.E.: Bone Changes in Hematologic Disorders. New York, Grune & Stratton, 1963.

40. Rosenberg, S.A., et al.: Lymphosarcoma: A review of 1269 cases. Medicine, *40*:31–84, 1961.

41. Newcomer, L.N., et al.: Bone involvement in Hodgkin's disease. Cancer, *49*:338–342, 1982.

42. Emkey, R.D., et al.: A case of lymphoproliferative disease presenting as juvenile rheumatoid arthritis: Diagnosis by synovial fluid examination. Am. J. Med., *54*:825–828, 1977.

43. Martin, V.M., et al.: Lymphosarcomatous arthropathy. Ann. Rheum. Dis., *32*:162–166, 1973.

44. Adamsky, A., Varetzky, A., and Klajman, A.: Malignant lymphoma presenting as sternoclavicular joint arthritis. Arthritis Rheum., *23*:1330–1331, 1981.

45. Dorfman, H.D., Siegel, H.L., Perry, M.C., and Oxenhandler, R.: Non-Hodgkin's lymphoma of the synovium simulating rheumatoid symptoms. Arthritis Rheum., *30*:155–161, 1987.

46. Dosovetz, D.E., et al.: Primary lymphoma of bone. Cancer, *51*:44–46, 1983.

47. Dosovetz, D.E., et al.: Primary lymphoma of bone. Cancer, *50*:1009–1014, 1982.

48. Reimer, R.R., et al.: Lymphoma presenting in bone: Results of histopathology, staging, and therapy. Ann. Intern. Med., *87*:50–55, 1977.

49. Rice, D.M., et al.: Primary lymphoma of bone presenting as monoarthritis. J. Rheumatol., *11*:851–854, 1984.

50. Frizzera, G., Moran, E.M., and Rappaport, H.: Angio-immunoblastic lymphoadenopathy: Diagnostic and clinical course. Am. J. Med., *59*:803–818, 1975.

51. Pangalis, G.A.,et al.: Angio-immunoblastic lymphoadenopathy: Long-term follow-up study. Cancer, *52*:318–321, 1983.

52. Bignon, Y.J., et al.: Angioimmunoblastic lymphoadenopathy with dysproteinaemia (AILD) and sicca syndrome. Ann. Rheum. Dis., *45*:519–522, 1986.

53. Webster, E., Corman, L.C., and Braylan, R.C.: Syndrome of temporal arteritis with perivascular infiltration by malignant cells in a patient with follicular small cleaved cell lymphoma. J. Rheumatol., *13*:1163–1166, 1986.

54. Hamilton, E.B.D., and Bywaters, E.G.L.: Joint symptoms in myelomatosis and similar conditions. Ann. Rheum. Dis., *20*:353–362, 1961.

55. Resnick, D.: Plasma cell dyscrasias and dysgammaglobulinemias. In Diagnosis of Bone and Joint Disorders. 2nd Ed. Edited by D. Resnick. Philadelphia, W.B. Saunders Co., 1988, pp. 2358–2403.

56. Katz, G.A., et al.: The shoulder-pad sign—A diagnostic feature of amyloid arthropathy. N. Engl. J. Med., *288*:354–355, 1973.

57. Kavanaugh, J.H.: Multiple myeloma, amyloid arthropathy, and pathological fracture of the femur: A case report. J. Bone Joint Surg., *60A*:135–137, 1978.

58. Nashel, D.J., Widerlite, L.W., and Pekin, T.J., Jr.: IgD myeloma with amyloid arthropathy. Am. J. Med., *55*:426–430, 1973.

59. Gordon, D.A., Pruzanski, W., and Ogryzlo, M.A.: Synovial fluid examination for the diagnosis of amyloidosis. Ann. Rheum. Dis., *32*:428–430, 1973.

60. Hickling, P., Wilkens, M., and Newman, G.R.: A study of arthropathy in multiple myeloma. Q.J. Med., *200*:417–433, 1981.

61. Hall, S., and Luthra, H.S.: Rheumatologic manifestations of amyloid disease. Minn. Med., *66*:631–632, 1983.

62. Cohen, A.S., and Canoso, J.J.: Rheumatological aspects of amyloid disease. Clin. Rheum. Dis., *1*:149–161, 1975.

63. Goldberg, A., Brodsky, I., and McCarty, D.: Multiple myeloma with paraamyloidosis presenting as rheumatoid disease. Am. J. Med., *37*:653–658, 1964.

64. Gordon, D.A., et al.: Amyloid arthritis simulating rheumatoid disease in five patients with multiple myeloma. Am. J. Med., *55*:142–154, 1973.

65. Wiernik, P.H.: Amyloid joint disease. Medicine, *51*:465–479, 1972.

66. Bernhard, G.C., and Hensley, G.T.: Amyloid arthropathy. Arthritis Rheum., *12*:444–453, 1959.

67. Leonard, P.A., Clegg, D.O., and Lee, R.G.: Erosive arthritis

in a patient with amyloid arthropathy. Clin. Rheumatol., 4:212–217, 1985.

68. Stone, M.J., and Frenkel, E.P.: The clinical spectrum of light chain myeloma: A study of 35 patients with special reference to the occurrence of amyloidosis. Am. J. Med., 58:601–619, 1975.

69. Grossman, R.E., and Hensley, G.T.: Bone lesions in primary amyloidosis. A.J.R., 101:872–875, 1967.

70. Laine, V., Vaino, K., and Ritama, V.V.: Occurrence of amyloid in rheumatoid arthritis. Acta Rheumatol. Scand., 1:43–46, 1955.

71. Bastina, F.O.: Amyloidosis and the carpal tunnel syndrome. Am. J. Clin. Pathol., 61:711–717, 1974.

72. Grossman, L.A., et al.: Carpal tunnel syndrome—Initial manifestation of systemic disease. J. Am. Med. Assoc., 176:259–261, 1961.

73. Husby, G., and Sletten, K.: Chemical and clinical classification of amyloidosis, 1985. Scand. J. Immunol., 23:253–265, 1986.

74. Glenner, G., et al. (eds): Amyloidosis. New York, Plenum Press, 1986.

75. Gompels, B.M., Votaw, M.L., and Martel, W.: Correlation of radiological manifestations of multiple myeloma with immunoglobulin abnormalities and prognosis. Radiology, 104:509–514, 1972.

76. Neufeld, A.H., Morton, H.S., and Halpenny, G.W.: Myelomatosis with xanthomatosis multiforme. Can. Med. Assoc. J., 91:374–380, 1964.

77. Vermess, M., et al.: Osseous manifestations of Waldenstrom's macroglobulinemia. Radiology, 102:497–504, 1972.

78. Goldberg, L.S., et al.: Amyloid arthritis associated with Waldenstrom's macroglobulinemia. N. Engl. J. Med., 281:256–257, 1969.

79. Scott, R.B., et al.: Neuropathic joint disease (Charcot joints) in Waldenstrom's macroglobulinemia with amyloidosis. Am. J. Med., 54:535–538, 1973.

80. Bardwick, P.A., et al.: Plasma cell dyscrasia with polyneuropathy, organomegaly, endocrinopathy, M protein and skin changes: The POEMS syndrome. Medicine, 59:311–322, 1980.

81. Resnick, D., et al.: Plasma-cell dyscrasia with polyneuropathy, organomegaly, endocrinopathy, M-protein, and skin changes: The POEMS syndrome. Radiology, 140:17, 1981.

82. Resnick, D., Haghighi, P., and Guerra, J., Jr.: Bone sclerosis and proliferation in a man with multisystem disease. Invest. Radiol., 19:1, 1984.

83. Bardin, T.: Dialysis related amyloidosis. J. Rheumatol., 14:647–649, 1987.

84. Varga, J., Felson, D., Skinner, M., et al.: Absence of amyloid in fat aspirates of long-term dialysis patients. (Abstract.) Arthritis Rheum., 29:S514, 1986.

85. Noel, L.H., et al.: Tissue distribution of dialysis amyloidosis. Clin. Nephrol., 27:175–178, 1987.

86. Munoz-Gomez, J., Gomez-Perez, R., Llopart-Buisan, E., and Sole-Arques, M.: Clinical picture of the amyloid arthropathy in patients with chronic renal failure maintained on haemodialysis using cellulose membranes. Ann. Rheum. Dis., 46:573–579, 1987.

87. Brown, E.A., Arnold, I.R., and Gower, P.E.: Dialysis arthropathy: Complication of long term haemodialysis. Br. Med. J., 292:163–166, 1986.

88. Munoz-Gomez, J., Gomez-Perez, R., Sole-Arques, M., and Llopart-Buisan, E.: Synovial fluid examination for the diagnosis of synovial amyloidosis in patients with chronic renal failure undergoing haemodialysis. Ann. Rheum. Dis., 46:324–326, 1987.

89. Bruckner, F.E., et al.: Synovial amyloid in chronic haemodialysis contains B2 microglobulin. Ann. Rheum. Dis., 46:634–637, 1987.

90. Huaux, J.P., et al.: Erosive azotemic osteoarthropathy: Possible role of amyloidosis. Arthritis Rheum., 28:1075–1076, 1985.

91. Bardin, T., et al.: Synovial amyloidosis in patients undergoing long term hemodialysis. Arthritis Rheum., 28:1052–1058, 1985.

92. Gejyo, F., et al.: A new form of amyloid protein associated with hemodialysis was identified as β_2 microglobulin. Biochem. Biophys. Res. Commun., 129:701–706, 1985.

93. Gorevic, P.D., et al.: Polymerization of intact beta-2 microglobulin in tissue causes amyloidosis in patients on chronic hemodialysis. Proc. Natl. Acad. Sci. USA, 83:7908–7912, 1986.

94. Vandebroucke, J.M., et al.: Possible role of dialysis membrane characteristics in amyloid osteoarthropathy. Lancet, 1:1210–1211, 1986.

95. Chanard, J., et al.: β-2 microglobulin associated amyloidosis in chronic haemodialysis patients. Lancet, 1:1212, 1986.

96. Casey, T.T., Stone, W.J., and Di Raimondo, C.R.: Tumoral amyloidosis of bone of β2 microglobulin origin in association with long term hemodialysis. Hum. Pathol., 17:731–738, 1986.

97. Gorevic, P.D., et al.: Beta-2 microglobulin is an amyloidogenic protein in man. J. Clin. Invest., 76:2425–2429, 1985.

98. Kuntz, D., et al.: Destructive spondylarthropathy in hemodialyzed patients. Arthritis Rheum., 27:369–375, 1984.

99. Sebert, J.L., et al.: Destructive spondylarthropathy in hemodialyzed patients: Possible role of amyloidosis. Arthritis Rheum., 29:301–303, 1986.

100. Munoz-Gomez, J., and Estrada Laza, P.: Destructive spondylarthropathy in hemodialyzed patients. Arthritis Rheum., 29:1171–1172, 1986.

101. Hardouin, P., et al.: Current aspects of osteoarticular pathology in patients undergoing hemodialysis: Study of 80 patients. Part 1. Clinical and radiological analysis. J. Rheumatol., 14:780–783, 1987.

102. Hardouin, P., et al.: Current aspects of osteoarticular pathology in patients undergoing hemodialysis: Study of 80 patients. Part 2. Laboratory and pathologic analysis. Discussion of the pathogenic mechanism. J. Rheumatol., 14:784–787, 1987.

103. Schumacher, H.R., Andrews, R., and McLaughlin, G.: Arthropathy in sickle-cell disease. Ann. Intern. Med., 78:203–211, 1973.

104. Diggs, L.W.: Bone and joint lesions in sickle-cell disease. Clin. Orthop., 52:119–143, 1967.

105. Espinoza, L.R., Spilberg, I., and Osterland, C.K.: Joint manifestations of sickle cell disease. Medicine, 53:295–305, 1974.

106. Goldberg, M.A.: Sickle cell arthropathy: Analysis of synovial fluid in sickle cell anemia with joint effusion. South. Med. J., 66:956–958, 1973.

107. Hanissian, A.S., and Silverman, A.: Arthritis and sickle cell anemia. South. Med. J., 67:28–32, 1974.

108. Reynolds, M.D.: Gout and hyperuricemia associated with sickle-cell anemia. Semin. Arthritis Rheum., 12:404–413, 1983.

109. Ball, G.V., and Sorensen, L.B.: The pathogenesis of hyperuricemia and gout in sickle cell anemia. Arthritis Rheum., 13:846–848, 1970.

110. Leff, R.D., Aldo-Benson, M.A., and Fife, R.S.: Tophaceous gout in patient with sickle cell-thalassemia: Case report and a review of the literature. Arthritis Rheum., 26:928–929, 1983.

111. Rothschild, B.M., et al.: Sickle cell disease associated with uric acid deposition disease. Ann. Rheum. Dis., 39:392–395, 1980.

112. de Ceulaer, K., et al.: Non-gouty arthritis in sickle cell disease: Report of 37 consecutive cases. Ann. Rheum. Dis., 43:599–603, 1984.

113. Alavi, A., et al.: Bone marrow scan evaluation of arthropathy in sickle cell disorders. Arch. Intern. Med., 136:436–440, 1976.

114. Hammel, C.F., et al.: Bone marrow and bone mineral scintigraphic studies in sickle cell disease. Br. J. Haematol., 25:593–598, 1973.

115. Rao, S.P., Miller, S., and Solomon, N.: Acute bone and joint manifestations of sickle cell disease in children. N.Y. State J. Med., 86:254–260, 1986.

116. Strauss, J., et al.: Cryoprecipitable immune complex nephropathy and sickle cell disease. Ann. Intern. Med., 81:114–115, 1974.

117. Johnston, R.B., Jr., Newman, S.L., and Struth, A.G.: An abnormality of the alternate pathway of complement activation in sickle cell disease. N. Engl. J. Med., 288:803–808, 1973.

118. Carroll, D.S.: Roentgen manifestations of sickle cell disease. South. Med. J., 50:1486–1490, 1975.

119. Goldring, J.S.R., MacIver, J.E., and Went, L.N.: The bone changes in sickle cell anaemia and its genetic variants. J. Bone Joint Surg., 41B:711–718, 1959.

120. Hewett, B.W., and Nice, C.M., Jr.: Radiographic manifestations of sickle cell anemia. Radiol. Clin. North Am., 2:249–259, 1964.

121. Reynolds, J.: A re-evaluation of the "fish vertebra" sign in sickle cell hemoglobinopathy. A.J.R., 97:693–707, 1966.

122. Reynolds, J.: The Roentgenological Features of Sickle Cell Disease, and Related Hemoglobinopathies. Springfield, IL, Charles C Thomas, 1965.

123. Reynolds, J.: An evaluation of some roentgenographic signs in sickle cell anemia and its variants. South. Med. J., 55:1123–1128, 1962.

124. Chung, S.M., and Ralston, E.L.: Necrosis of the femoral head associated with sickle-cell anemia and its genetic variants: A review of the literature and study of thirteen cases. J. Bone Joint Surg., 51A:33–58, 1969.

125. Serjeant, G.R.: The clinical features in adults with sickle cell anaemia in Jamaica. West Indian Med. J., 19:1–8, 1970.

126. Sherman, M.: Pathogenesis of disintegration of the hip in sickle cell anemia. South. Med. J., 52:632–637, 1959.

127. Golding, J.S.: Conditions of the hip associated with hemoglobinopathies. Clin. Orthop., 90:22–28, 1973.

128. Hurwitz, D., and Rhot, H.: Sickle cell-thalassemia presenting as arthritis of the hip. Arthritis Rheum., 13:422–425, 1970.

129. Nachamie, B.J., and Dorfman, H.D.: Ischemic necrosis of bone in sickle cell trait. Mt. Sinai. J. Med. (N.Y.), 41:527–536, 1974.

130. Rothermel, J.E., and Raney, R.B.: The changing prognosis in hemophilic arthropathy. South. Med. J., 62:1340–1342, 1969.

131. Smith, E.W., and Conley, C.L.: Clinical features of the genetic variants of sickle cell disease. Bull. Johns Hopkins Hosp., 104:17–43, 1959.

132. Smith, E.W., and Krevans, J.R.: Clinical manifestations of hemoglobin C disorders. Bull. Johns Hopkins Hosp., 104:17–43, 1959.

133. Dorwart, B.B., et al.: Absence of increased frequency of bone and joint disease with hemoglobin AS and AC. Ann. Intern. Med., 86:66–67, 1977.

134. Gunderson, C., D'Ambrosia, R.D., and Shoij, H.: Total hip replacement in patients with sickle-cell disease. J. Bone Joint Surg., 59A:760–762, 1977.

135. Ober, W.B., et al.: Hemoglobin S-C disease with fat embolism. Am. J. Med., 27:647–658, 1959.

136. Shelley, W.M., and Curtis, E.M.: Bone marrow and fat embolism in sickle cell anemia and sickle cell-hemoglobin C disease. Bull. Johns Hopkins Hosp., 103:8–26, 1958.

137. Watson, R.J., et al.: The hand-foot syndrome in sickle-cell disease in young children. Pediatrics, 31:975–982, 1963.

138. Worrall, V.T., and Butera, V.: Sickle-cell dactylitis. J. Bone Joint Surg., 58A:1161–1163, 1976.

139. Hughes, J.G., and Carroll, D.S.: Salmonella osteomyelitis complicating sickle cell disease. Pediatrics, 19:184–191, 1957.

140. Moxley, G.F., Owne, D.S., and Irby, R.: Septic arthritis due to Fusobacterium varium in patient with sickle-cell anemia. J. Rheumatol., 10:161–162, 1983.

141. Harden, W.B., et al.: Septic arthritis due to Serratia liquefaciens. Arthritis Rheum., 23:946–947, 1980.

142. Hand, W.L., and King, N.L.: Serum opsonization of Salmonella in sickle cell anemia. Am. J. Med., 64:388–395, 1978.

143. Wilson, W.A., Hughes, G.R., and Lachmann, P.J.: Deficiency of factor B of the complement system in sickle cell anaemia. Br. Med. J., 1:367–369, 1976.

144. Palmer, D.W.: Septic arthritis in sickle-cell thalassemia: Pathophysiology of impaired response to infection. Arthritis Rheum., 18:339–345, 1975.

145. Ebong, W.W.: Septic arthritis in patients with sickle-cell disease. Br. J. Rheumatol., 26:99–102, 1987.

146. Gratwick, G.M., et al.: Thalassemic osteoarthropathy. Ann. Intern. Med., 88:494–501, 1978.

147. Schlumph, U., et al.: Arthritis in thalassemia minor. Schweiz. Med. Wochenschr., 107:1156–1162, 1977.

148. Abou Rizk, N.A., Nasr, F.W., and Frayha, R.A.: Aseptic necrosis in thalassemia minor. Arthritis Rheum., 20:1147–1148, 1977.

149. Gerster, J.C., Dardel, R., and Guggi, S.: Recurrent episodes of arthritis in thalassemia minor. J. Rheumatol., 11:352–354, 1984.

150. Stanbury, J.B., et al. (eds.): The Metabolic Basis of Inherited Disease. 5th Ed. New York, McGraw-Hill, 1983.

151. Beaudet, A.L.: Lysosomal storage diseases. In Harrison's Principles of Internal Medicine. 11th Ed. Edited by E. Braunwald, et al. New York, McGraw-Hill, 1987, pp. 1661–1671.

152. Peters, S.P., Lee, R.E., and Glew, R.H.: Gaucher's disease: A review. Medicine, 56:425–442, 1977.

153. Brady, R.O., and Barranger, J.A.: Glucosylceramide lipidosis: Gaucher's disease. In The Metabolic Basis of Inherited Disease. 5th Ed. Edited by J.B. Stanbury, et al. New York, McGraw-Hill, 1983, pp. 842–856.

154. Amstutz, H.C., and Carey, E.J.: Skeletal manifestations and treatment of Gaucher's disease: Review of twenty cases. J. Bone Joint Surg., 48A:670–701, 1966.

155. Silverstein, M.N., and Kelly, P.J.: Osteoarticular manifestations of Gaucher's disease. Am. J. Med. Sci., 253:569–577, 1967.

156. Schubiner, H., Lefourdeau, M., and Murray, D.L.: Pyogenic osteomyelitis versus pseudo-osteomyelitis in Gaucher's disease. Clin. Pediatr., 20:667–669, 1981.

157. Seinsheimer, F., 3d, and Mankin, H.J.: Acute bilateral symmetrical pathologic fractures of the lateral tibial plateaus in a patient with Gaucher's disease. Arthritis Rheum., 20:1500–1555, 1977.

158. Wrizman, Z., Tennenbaum, A., and Yatziv, S.: Interphalangeal joint involvement in Gaucher's disease, Type I, resembling juvenile rheumatoid arthritis. Arthritis Rheum., 25:706–707, 1982.

159. Groen, J., and Garrer, A.H.: Adult Gaucher's disease with special reference to the variations in its clinical course and the

value of sternal puncture as an aid to its diagnosis. Blood, 3:1221–1237, 1948.

160. Lan, M.M., et al.: Hip arthroplasties in Gaucher's disease. J. Bone Joint Surg., 63A:591–601, 1981.

161. Adler, E., and Maybaum, S.: Rare features in a case of Gaucher's disease. Ann. Rheum. Dis., 13:229–232, 1954.

162. Rose, J.S., et al.: Accelerated skeletal deterioration after splenectomy in Gaucher type I disease. A.J.R., 139:1202–1204, 1982.

163. Shiloni, E., et al.: The role of splenectomy in Gaucher's disease. Arch. Surg., 118:929–932, 1983.

164. Pratt, P.W., Estren, S., and Kochwa, S.: Immunoglobulin abnormalities in Gaucher's disease: Report of 16 cases. Blood, 31:633–640, 1968.

165. Garfinkle, B., et al.: Coexistence of Gaucher's disease and multiple myeloma. Arch. Intern. Med., 142:2229–2230, 1982.

166. Pinkhas, J., Djeldetti, M., and Yaron, M.: Coincidence of multiple myeloma with Gaucher's disease. Isr. J. Med. Sci., 1:537–540, 1965.

167. Kudoh, T., and Wenger, D.A.: Diagnosis of metachromatic leukodystrophy, Krabbe disease, and Farber's disease after uptake of fatty acid labeled cerebroside sulfate into cultured skin fibroblasts. J. Clin. Invest., 70:89–97, 1982.

168. Pouard, A.C., et al.: Enzymological diagnosis of a group of lysosomal storage diseases. Med. J. Aust., 2:549–553, 1980.

169. Beichetz, P.E., et al.: Treatment of Gaucher's disease with liposome-entrapped glucocerebroside-beta-glucosidase. Lancet, 1:116–117, 1977.

170. Brady, R.O., et al.: Replacement therapy for inherited enzyme deficiency: Use of purified glucocerebrosidase in Gaucher's disease. N. Engl. J. Med., 291:989–993, 1974.

171. Wise, D., Wallace, H.J., and Jellinek, E.H.: Angiokeratoma corporis diffusum. Q. J. Med., 31:177–206, 1961.

172. Desnick, R.J., and Sweeley, C.C.: Fabry's disease: β-Galactosidase A deficiency. In The Metabolic Basis of Inherited Disease. 5th Ed. Edited by J.B. Stanbury, et al. New York, McGraw-Hill, 1983, pp. 906–944.

173. Braverman, I.M., and Ken, Y.A.: Ultrastructure and three dimensional reconstruction of several macular and papular telangiectases. J. Invest. Dermatol., 81:489–497, 1983.

174. Seino, I., et al.: Peripheral hemodynamics in patients with Fabry's disease. Am. Heart J., 105:783–787, 1983.

175. Garcin, R., et al.: Neurologic aspects of Fabry's angiokeratosis: Apropos of 2 cases. Presse Med., 75:435–440, 1967.

176. Johnston, A.W., Weller, S.D., and Warland, B.J.: Angiokeratoma corporis diffusum: Some clinical aspects. Arch. Dis. Child., 43:73–79, 1968.

177. Pittelkow, R.B., Kierland, R.R., and Montgomery, H.: Angiokeratoma corporis diffusum. Arch. Dermatol., 72:556–561, 1955.

178. Fone, D.J., and King, W.E.: Angiokeratoma corporis diffusum (Fabry's syndrome). Aust. Ann. Med., 13:339–348, 1964.

179. Lacroux, R.: Angiokeratome diffusum (angiokeratoma corporis diffusum) de Fabry. Bull. Soc. Fr. Dermatol. Syphilol., 67:474–478, 1960.

180. Spaeth, G.L., and Frost, P.: Fabry's disease: Its ocular manifestations. Arch. Ophthalmol., 74:760–769, 1965.

181. Bethune, J.E., Landrigan, P.L., and Chipman, C.D.: Angiokeratoma corporis diffusum universale (Fabry's disease) in two brothers. N. Engl. J. Med., 264:1280–1285, 1961.

182. Ahlmen, J., et al.: Clinical and diagnostic considerations in Fabry's disease. Acta Med. Scand., 211:309–312, 1982.

183. Brady, R.O., et al.: Replacement therapy for inherited enzyme

184. Clarke, J.T.R., et al.: Enzyme replacement therapy by renal allotransplantation in Fabry's disease. N. Engl. J. Med., 287:1215–1218, 1972.

185. Philippart, M., Franklin, S.S., and Gordon, A.: Reversal of an inborn sphingolipidosis (Fabry's disease) by kidney transplantation. Ann. Intern. Med., 77:195–200, 1972.

186. Abul-Haz, S.A., et al.: Farber's disease: Report of a case with observations on its histogenesis and notes on the nature of the stored material. J. Pediatr., 61:213–221, 1962.

187. Berman, S.M., et al.: Farber's disease: A disorder of mucopolysaccharide metabolism with articular, respiratory, and neurologic manifestations. Arthritis Rheum., 9:620–630, 1966.

188. Dulaney, J.T., Moser, H.W., and Sidbury, J.: The biochemical defect in Farber's disease. In Current Trends in Sphingolipidoses and Allied Disorders. Edited by B.W. Volk and L. Schneck. New York, Plenum Press, 1976, pp. 403–411.

189. Farber, S., Cohen, J., and Uzman, L.: Lipogranulomatosis: A new lipo-glyco-protein "storage" disease. J. Mt. Sinai Hosp., 24:816–837, 1957.

190. Moser, H.W., and Chen, W.W.: Ceramidase deficiency. In The Metabolic Basis of Inherited Disease. 5th Ed. Edited by J.B. Stanbury, et al. New York, McGraw-Hill, 1983, pp. 820–830.

191. Moser, H.W., et al.: Farber's lipogranulomatosis: Report of a case and demonstration of an excess of free ceramide and ganglioside. Am. J. Med., 47:869–890, 1969.

192. Chen, W.W., and Deeker, G.L.: Abnormalities of lysosomes in human diploid fibroblasts from patients with Farber's disease. Biochim. Biophys. Acta, 718:185–192, 1982.

193. Ford, D.K., et al.: Familial lipochromic pigmentation of histiocytes with hyperglobulinemia, pulmonary infiltration, splenomegaly, arthritis and susceptibility to infection. Am. J. Med., 33:478–489, 1962.

194. Rodey, G.E., et al.: Defective bactericidal activity of peripheral blood leukocytes in lipochrome histiocytosis. Am. J. Med., 49:322–327, 1970.

195. Barrow, M.V., and Holubar, K.: Multicentric reticulohistiocytosis: A review of 33 patients. Medicine, 48:287–305, 1969.

196. Bortz, A.L., and Vincent, M.: Lipoid dermato-arthritis and arthritis mutilans. Am. J. Med., 30:951–960, 1961.

197. Ehrlich, G.E., et al.: Multicentric reticulohistiocytosis (lipoid dermatoarthritis): A multisystem disorder. Am. J. Med., 52:830–840, 1972.

198. Flam, M., et al.: Multicentric reticulohistiocytosis: Report of a case with atypical features and electron microscopic study of skin lesions. Am. J. Med., 52:841–848, 1972.

199. Goltz, R.W., and Laymon, C.W.: Multicentric reticulohistiocytosis of the skin and synovia. Arch. Dermatol. Syphilol., 69:717–731, 1954.

200. Hanauer, L.B.: Reticulohistiocytosis: Remission after cyclophosphamide therapy. Arthritis Rheum., 15:636–640, 1972.

201. Lyell, A., and Carr, A.J.: Lipoid dermatoarthritis (reticulohistiocytosis). Br. J. Dermatol., 71:12–21, 1959.

202. Melton, J.W., 3d, and Irby, R.: Multicentric reticulohistiocytosis. Arthritis Rheum., 15:221—226, 1972.

203. Orkin, M., et al.: A study of multicentric reticulohistiocytosis. Arch. Dermatol., 89:640–654, 1964.

204. Warin, R.P., et al.: Reticulohistiocytosis (lipoid dermatoarthritis). Br. Med. J., 1:1387–1391, 1957.

205. Lesher, J.L., Jr., and Allen, B.S.: Multicentric reticulohistiocytosis. J. Am. Acad. Dermatol., 11(No. 4, Pt. 2):713–723, 1984.

206. Hansen, E., Nilsen, R., and Milde, E.J.: Multicentric reticu-

lohistiocytosis: A case report. Acta Derm. Venereol. (Stockh.), *63*:175–176, 1983.

207. Heathcote, J.G., Guenther, L.G., and Wallace, A.C.: Multicentric reticulohistiocytosis: A report of a case and a review of the pathology. Pathology, *17*:601–608, 1985.

208. Nunnink, J.C., Krusinski, P.A., and Yates, J.W.: Multicentric reticulohistiocytosis and cancer: A case report and review of the literature. Med. Pediatr. Oncol., *13*:273–279, 1985.

209. Belaich, S.: Multicentric reticulohistiocytosis. J. Ital. Dermatol., *115*:77, 1980.

210. Krey, P.R., Comerford, F.R., and Cohen, A.S.: Multicentric reticulohistiocytosis: Fine structural analysis of the synovium and synovial fluid cells. Arthritis Rheum., *17*:615–633, 1974.

211. Nezelof, C., and Barbey, S.: Histiocytosis: Nasology and pathology. Pediatr. Pathol., *3*:1–41, 1985.

212. Barrow, M.V., et al.: Identification of tissue lipids in lipoid dermatoarthritis (multicentric reticulohistiocytosis). Am. J. Clin. Pathol., *47*:312–325, 1967.

213. Freemont, A.J., Jones, C.I.P., and Denton, J.: The synovium and synovial fluid in multicentric reticulohistiocytosis—A light microsopic, electron microscopic and cytochemical analysis of one case. J. Clin. Pathol., *36*:860–866, 1983.

214. Tani, M., et al.: Multicentric reticulohistiocytosis: Electromicroscopic and ultracytochemical studies. Arch. Dermatol., *117*:495–499, 1981.

215. Hall, S., et al.: Multicentric reticulohistiocytosis. Arthritis Rheum., *27*:S79, 1984.

216. Gold, R.H., et al.: Multicentric reticulohistiocytosis (lipoid dermato-arthritis). An erosive polyarthritis with distinctive clinical, roentgenographic and pathologic features. A.J.R., *124*:610–624, 1975.

217. Martel, W., Abell, M.R., and Duff, I.F.: Cervical spine involvement in lipoid dermato-arthritis. Radiology, *77*:613–617, 1961.

218. Scutellari, P.N., Orzincolo, C., and Trotta, F.: Case report 375: Multicentric reticulohistiocytosis. Skeletal Radiol., *15*:394–397, 1986.

219. Brandt, F., et al.: Topical nitrogen mustard therapy in multicentric reticulohistiocytosis. J. Am. Acad. Dermatol., *6*:260–262, 1982.

220. Davies, N.E.: Multicentric reticulohistiocytosis: Report of a case with histochemical studies. Arch. Dermatol., *97*:543–547, 1968.

221. Doherty, M., Martin, M.F.R., and Dieppe, P.A.: Multicentric reticulohistiocytosis associated with primary biliary cirrhosis: Successful treatment with cytotoxic agents. Arthritis Rheum., *27*:344–348, 1984.

222. Furey, N.D., et al.: Multicentric reticulohistiocytosis with salivary gland involvement and pericardial effusion. J. Am. Acad. Dermatol., *8*:679–685, 1983.

223. Carey, R.N., et al.: Multicentric reticulohistiocytosis and Sjögren's syndrome. J. Rheumatol., *12*:1193–1195, 1985.

224. Zayid, I., and Farraj, S.: Familial histiocytic dermatoarthritis: A new syndrome. Am. J. Med., *54*:793–800, 1973.

225. Goldstein, J.L., and Brown, M.S.: Familial hypercholesterolemia. *In* The Metabolic Basis of Inherited Disease. 5th Ed. Edited by J.B. Stanbury, et al. New York, McGraw-Hill, 1983, pp. 672–712.

226. Brown, M.S., Goldstein, J.L., and Fredrickson, D.S.: Familial Type 3 hyperlipoproteinemias. *In* The Metabolic Basis of Inherited Disease. 5th Ed. Edited by J.B. Stanbury, et al. New York, McGraw-Hill, 1983, pp. 655–671.

227. Brown, M.S., and Goldstein, J.L.: The hyperlipoproteinemias and other disorders of lipid metabolism. *In* Harrison's Prin-

ciples of Internal Medicine. 11th Ed. Edited by E. Braunwald, et al. New York, McGraw-Hill, 1987, pp. 1650–1661.

228. Fahey, J.J., et al.: Xanthoma of the Achilles tendon. J. Bone Joint Surg., *55A*:1197–1211, 1973.

229. Shapiro, J.R., et al.: Achilles tendinitis and tenosynovitis: A diagnostic manifestation of familial type II hyperlipoproteinemia in children. Am. J. Dis. Child., *128*:486–490, 1974.

230. Harlan, W.R., Jr., et al.: Familial hypercholesterolemia: A genetic and metabolic study. Medicine, *45*:77–110, 1966.

231. Nikkila, E.A.: Familial lipoprotein lipase deficiency and related disorders of chylomicron metabolism. *In* The Metabolic Basis of Inherited Disease. 5th Ed. Edited by J.B. Stanbury, et al. New York, McGraw-Hill, 1983, pp. 622–642.

232. Glueck, C.J., Levy, R.I., and Fredrickson, D.S.: Acute tendinitis and arthritis: A presenting symptom of familial type II hyperlipoproteinemia. J. Am. Med. Assoc., *206*:2895–2897, 1968.

233. Khachadurian, A.K.: Migratory polyarthritis in familial hypercholesterolemia (type II hyperlipoproteinemia). Arthritis Rheum., *11*:385–393, 1968.

234. Rooney, P.J., et al.: Transient polyarthritis associated with familial hyperbetalipoproteinemia. Q. J. Med., *187*:249–259, 1978.

235. Walker, R.E.: Hyperlipoproteinemia and symptoms of the lower extremity. J. Am. Podiatry Assoc., *69*:370–375, 1979.

236. Mathon, G., et al.: Articular manifestations of familial hypercholesterolaemia. Ann. Rheum. Dis., *44*:599–602, 1985.

237. Carroll, G.J., and Bayliss, C.E.: Treatment of the arthropathy of familial hypercholesterolaemia. Ann. Rheum. Dis., *42*:206–209, 1983.

238. Buckingham, R.B., Bole, G.G., and Bassett, D.R.: Polyarthritis associated with type IV hyperlipoproteinemia. Arch. Intern. Med., *135*:286–290, 1975.

239. Goldman, J.A., et al.: Musculoskeletal disorders associated with type-IV hyperlipoproteinaemia. Lancet, *2*:449–452, 1972.

240. Siegelmann, S.S., et al.: Hyperlipoproteinemia with skeletal lesions. Clin. Orthop., *87*:228–232, 1972.

241. Ansell, B.M., and Bywaters, E.G.L.: Histiocytic bone and joint disease. Ann. Rheum. Dis., *16*:503–510, 1957.

242. Salen, G., Shefer, S., and Bergener, V.M.: Familial diseases with storage of sterols other than cholesterol (cerebrotendinous xanthomatosis and sitosterolemia with xanthomatosis). *In* The Metabolic Basis of Inherited Disease. 5th Ed. Edited by J.B. Stanbury, et al. New York, McGraw-Hill, 1983, pp. 713–730.

243. Truswell, A.S., and Pfister, P.J.: Cerebrotendinous xanthomatosis. Br. Med. J., *1*:353–354, 1972.

244. Battacharyya, A.K., and Connor, W.E.: Beta-sitosterolemia and xanthomatosis: A newly described lipid storage disease in two sisters. J. Clin. Invest., *53*:1033–1043, 1974.

245. Shulman, R.S., et al.: Beta-sitosterolemia and xanthomatosis. N. Engl. J. Med., *294*:482–483, 1976.

246. Biggs, R. (ed.): The Treatment of Haemophilia A and B and von Willebrand's Disease. Oxford, Blackwell Scientific Publications, 1978.

247. Biggs, R., and Rizza, C.R. (eds.): Human Blood Coagulation, Haemostasis, and Thrombosis. 3rd Ed. Oxford, Blackwell Scientific Publications, 1984.

248. Colman, R.W., Hirsh, J., Marder, V.J., and Salzman, E.W. (eds.): Hemostasis and Thrombosis: Basic Principles and Clinical Practice. 2nd Ed. Philadelphia, J.B. Lippincott, 1987.

249. Levine, P.H.: Clinical manifestations and therapy of hemophilia A and B. *In* Hemostasis and Thrombosis: Basic Principles and Clinical Practice. 2nd Ed. Edited by R.W. Colman,

J. Hirsh, V.J. Marder, and E.W. Salzman. Philadelphia, J.B. Lippincott, 1987, pp. 97–111.

250. Arnold, W.D., and Hilgartner, H.W.: Hemophilic arthropathy: Current concepts of pathogenesis and management. J. Bone Joint Surg., 59A:287–305, 1977.

251. Steven, M.M., et al.: Haemophilic arthritis. Q. J. Med., 58:181–197, 1986.

252. Katz, A.L., and Alepa, F.P.: Hemarthrosis secondary to heparin therapy. (Letter.) Arthritis Rheum., 19:996, 1976.

253. McLaughlin, G.E., McCarty, D.J., Jr., and Segal, B.L.: Hemarthrosis complicating anticoagulant therapy: Report of three cases. J. Am. Med. Assoc., 196:1020–1021, 1966.

254. Wild, J.H., and Zvaifler, N.J.: Hemarthrosis associated with sodium warfarin therapy. Arthritis Rheum., 19:98–102, 1976.

255. Andes, W.A., and Edmunds, J.O.: Hemarthroses and warfarin: Joint destruction with anticoagulations. Thromb. Haemost. 28:187–189, 1983.

256. DePalma, A.F.: Hemophilic arthropathy. Clin. Orthop., 52:145–165, 1967.

257. Kisker, C.T., Perlman, A.W., and Benton, C.: Arthritis in hemophilia. Semin. Arthritis Rheum., 1:220–225, 1971.

258. Rodnan, G., et al.: Hemophilic arthritis. Bull. Rheum. Dis., 8:137–138, 1957.

259. Swanton, M.C., and Mepocki, G.P.: Pathology of joints in canine hemophilia A. In Handbook of Hemophilia. Edited by K.M. Brinkous and H.C. Hemker. Amsterdam, Excerpta Medica, 1975, pp. 313–332.

260. Rodnan, G., et al.: Postmortem examination of an elderly severe hemophiliac, with observations on the pathologic findings in hemophilic joint disease. Arthritis Rheum., 2:152–161, 1959.

261. Convery, F.R., et al.: Experimental hemarthrosis in the knee of the mature canine. Arthritis Rheum., 19:59–67, 1976.

262. Mankin, H.J.: The reaction of articular cartilage to injury and osteoarthritis. N. Engl. J. Med., 291:1285–1292, 1974.

263. Key, J.A.: Hemophilic arthritis (bleeder's joints). Ann. Surg., 95:198–225, 1932.

264. Mainardi, C.L., et al.: Proliferative synovitis in hemophilia: Biochemical and morphologic observations. Arthritis Rheum., 21:137–144, 1978.

265. McLardy Smith, P.D., Ashton, I.K., and Duthie, R.B.: A tissue culture model of cartilage breakdown in haemophilic arthropathy. Scand. J. Haematol. (Suppl.), 40:215–220, 1984.

266. Andes, W.A., Walker, P.D., Edmunds, J.O., and Wulff, K.M.: Hemophilic arthropathy—An immunologic study of the synovium. Scand. J. Haematol. (Suppl.), 40:221–224, 1984.

267. Wolf, C.R., and Mankin, H.J.: The effect of experimental hemarthrosis on articular cartilage of rabbit knee joints. J. Bone Joint Surg., 47A:1203–1210, 1965.

268. Sokoloff, L.: Biochemical and physiological aspects of degenerative joint diseases with special reference to hemophilic arthropathy. Ann. N.Y. Acad. Sci., 240:285–290, 1975.

269. Hough, A.J., Banfield, W.G., and Sokoloff, L.: Cartilage in hemophilic arthropathy. Arch. Pathol. Lab. Med., 100:91–96, 1976.

270. Landells, J.W.: The bone cysts of osteoarthritis. J. Bone Joint Surg., 35B:643–649, 1953.

271. Speer, O.P.: Early pathogenesis of hemophilic arthropathy: Evolution of the subchondral cyst. Clin. Orthop., 185:250–265, 1984.

272. Abell, J.M., Jr., and Bailey, R.W.: Hemophilic pseudotumor: Two cases occurring in siblings. Arch. Surg., 81:559–581, 1960.

273. Fraenkel, G.J., Taylor, K.B., and Richards, W.C.D.: Haemophilic blood cysts. Br. J. Surg., 46:383–392, 1959.

274. Ghormley, R.K., and Clegg, R.S.: Bone and joint changes in hemophilia: With report of cases of so-called hemophilic pseudotumor. J. Bone Joint Surg., 30A:589–600, 1948.

275. Steel, W.M., Duthie, R.B., and O'Connor, B.T.: Haemophilic cysts: Report of five cases. J. Bone Joint Surg., 51B:614–626, 1969.

276. Stoker, D.J., and Murray, R.U.: Skeletal changes in hemophilia and other bleeding disorders. Semin. Roentgenol., 9:185–193, 1974.

277. Tarnay, T.J.: Surgery in the Hemophiliac. Springfield, IL, Charles C Thomas, 1968.

278. Trueta, J.: Orthopaedic management of patients with haemophilia and christmas disease. In Treatment of Haemophilia and Other Coagulation Disorders. Edited by R. Biggs and R.G. Macfarlane. Oxford, Blackwell Scientific Publications, 1966, pp. 279–323.

279. Biggs, R., and Rizza, C.R.: The control of haemostasis in haemophilic patients. In The Treatment of Haemophilia A and B and von Willebrand's Disease. Oxford, Blackwell Scientific Publications, 1978, pp. 127–152.

280. Duthie, R.B., et al.: The Management of Musculoskeletal Problems in the Hemophilias. Oxford, Blackwell Scientific Publications, 1972.

281. Eyring, E.J., Bjornson, D.R., and Close, J.R.: Management of hemophilia in children. Clin. Orthop., 40:95–112, 1965.

282. Thomas, H.B.: Some orthopaedic findings in ninety-eight cases of hemophilia. J. Bone Joint Surg., 18:140–147, 1936.

283. Brower, T.D., and Wilde, A.H.: Femoral neuropathy in hemophilia. J. Bone Joint Surg., 48A:487–492, 1966.

284. Goodfellow, J., Fearn, C.B., and Matthews, J.M.: Iliacus haematoma: A common complication of haemophilia. J. Bone Joint Surg., 49B:748–756, 1967.

285. Ramgren, O.: Haemophilia in Sweden. IV. Symptomatology, with special reference to differences between haemophilia A and B. Acta Med. Scand., 171:237–242, 1962.

286. Stuart, J., et al.: Haemorrhagic episodes in haemophilia: A 5-year prospective study. Br. Med. J., 2:1624–1626, 1966.

287. Landbeck, G., and Kurme, A.: Hemophilic arthropathy of the knee joint: Treatment of hemorrhages of the knee joint and their consequences. Monatsschr. Kinderheilkd., 118:29–41, 1970.

288. Webb, J.B., and Dixon, A. St. J.: Haemophilia and haemophilic arthropathy: an historical review and a clinical study of 42 cases. Ann. Rheum. Dis., 19:143–157, 1960.

289. Ahlberg, A., Nilsson, I.M., and Bauer, G.C.H.: Use of antihemophilic factor (plasma fraction I-O) during correction of knee-joint deformities in hemophilia A. J. Bone Joint Surg., 47A:323–332, 1965.

290. Forbes, C.D., et al.: A comparison of thermography, radioisotope scanning and clinical assessment of the knee joints in haemophilia. Clin. Radiol., 26:41–45, 1975.

291. Steven, M.M., et al.: Radio-isotopic joint scans in haemophilic arthritis. Br. J. Rheumatol., 24:263–268, 1985.

292. McVerry, B.A., et al.: Ultrasonography in the management of haemophilia. Lancet, 1:872–874, 1977.

293. Hofmann, P., Menge, M., and Brachman, H.H.: Reconstructive surgery in the lower limb in hemophiliacs. Isr. J. Med. Sci., 13:988–994, 1977.

294. Defaria, C.R., Demelo-Souza, S.E., and Pinheiro, E.D.: Haemophilic neuromyopathy. J. Neurol. Neurosurg. Psychiatry, 42:600–605, 1979.

295. Jordan, H.H.: Hemophilic Arthropathies. Springfield, IL, Charles C Thomas, 1958.

296. Resnick, D.: Bleeding disorders. In Diagnosis of Bone and

Joint Disorders. 2nd Ed. Edited by D. Resnick and G. Niwayania. Philadelphia, W.B. Saunders, 1988, pp. 2497–2522.

297. Jensen, P.S., and Putnam, C.E.: Chondrocalcinosis and haemophilia. Clin. Radiol., 28:401–405, 1977.

298. Leonello, P.P., Cleland, L.G., and Norman, J.E.: Acute pseudogout and chondrocalcinosis in a man with mild hemophilia. J. Rheumatol., 8:841–844, 1981.

299. Brettler, D.B., et al.: A long-term study of hemophilic arthropathy of the knee joint on a program of Factor VIII replacement given at time of each hemarthrosis. Am. J. Hematol., 18:13–18, 1985.

300. Reference deleted.

301. Houghton, G.R.: Septic arthritis of the hip in a hemophiliac. Clin. Orthop., 129:223–224, 1977.

302. Moseley, P., et al.: Hemophilia, maintenance hemodialysis, and septic arthritis. Arch. Intern. Med., 141:138–139, 1981.

303. Rosner, S.M., and Bhogal, R.S.: Infectious arthritis in a hemophiliac. J. Rheumatol., 8:519–521, 1981.

304. Wilkins, R.M., and Wiedel, J.D.: Septic arthritis of the knee in a hemophiliac. A case report. J. Bone Joint Surg., 65:267–268, 1983.

305. Goldsmith, J.C., Silberstein, P.T., Fromm, R.E., Jr., and Walker, D.Y.: Hemophilic arthropathy complicated by polyarticular septic arthritis. A case report. Acta Haematol. (Basel), 71:121–123, 1984.

306. Cobb, W.B.: Septic polyarthritis in a hemophiliac. J. Rheumatol., 11:87–89, 1984.

307. Scott, J.P., Maurer, H.S., and Dias, L.: Septic arthritis in two teenaged hemophiliacs. J. Pediatr., 107:748–751, 1985.

308. Hofmann, A., Wyatt, R., and Bybee, B.: Septic arthritis of the knee in a 12-year-old hemophiliac. J. Pediatr. Orthop., 4:498–499, 1984.

309. Ellison, R.T., 3rd, and Reller, L.B.: Differentiating pyogenic arthritis from spontaneous hemarthrosis in patients with hemophilia. West J. Med., 144:42–45, 1986.

310. Thakker, S., McGehee, W., and Quismorio, F.P., Jr.: Arthropathy associated with factor XIII deficiency. Arthritis Rheum., 29:808–811, 1986.

311. Sankarankutty, M., and Evans, D.I.: Chronic arthropathy in von Willebrand's disease. Clin. Lab. Haematol., 5:149–156, 1983.

312. Ahlberg, A.: Treatment and prophylaxis of arthropathy in severe hemophilia. Clin. Orthop., 53:135–146, 1967.

313. Crock, H.V., and Boni, V.: The management of orthopaedic problems in haemophiliacs: A review of 21 cases. Br. J. Surg., 48:8–15, 1960.

314. Dietrich, S.L.: Rehabilitation and nonsurgical management of musculoskeletal problems in the hemophilic patient. Ann. N.Y. Acad. Sci., 240:328–337, 1975.

315. Bellingham, A., et al.: Hip arthroplasty in a haemophiliac and subsequent prophylactic therapy with cryoprecipitate. Br. Med. J., 4:531–532, 1967.

316. Mazza, J.J., et al.: Antihemophilic factor VIII in hemophilia: Use of concentrates to permit major surgery. J. Am. Med. Assoc., 211:1818–1823, 1970.

317. D'Ambrosia, R.D., et al.: Total hip replacement for patients with hemophilia and hemorrhagic diathesis. Surg. Gynecol. Obstet., 139:381–384, 1974.

318. McCollough, N.C., et al.: Synovectomy or total replacement of the knee in hemophilia. J. Bone Joint Surg., 61A:69–75, 1979.

319. Marmor, L.: Total knee replacement in hemophilia. Clin. Orthop., 125:192–195, 1977.

320. Small, M., et al.: Total knee arthroplasty in hemophilic arthritis. J. Bone Joint Surg., 65:163–165, 1983.

321. Hall, M.R.P., Handley, D.A., and Webster, C.U.: The surgical treatment of haemophilic blood cysts. J. Bone Joint Surg., 44B:781–789, 1962.

322. Lewis, J.H., Cottington, M., and Brower, T.D.: The use of plasma fraction 1 to maintain hemostasis following amputation for hemorrhagic cysts of the thigh in a severe hemophiliac. J. Bone Joint Surg., 47A:333–339, 1965.

323. Post, M., and Telfer, M.C.: Surgery in hemophilic patients. J. Bone Joint Surg., 57A:1136–1145, 1975.

324. Rosenthal, R.L., Graham, J.J., and Selirio, E.: Excision of pseudotumor with repair by bone graft or pathological fracture of femur in hemophilia. J. Bone Joint Surg., 55A:827–832, 1973.

325. Stas, W.E., Jr., et al.: Lower extremity amputation in hemophilia: Case report and review of surgical principles. J. Bone Joint Surg., 54A:1514–1522, 1972.

326. Matsuda, Y., and Duthie, R.B.: Surgical synovectomy for haemophilic arthropathy of the knee joint: Long-term follow-up. Scand. J. Haematol (Suppl.), 40:237–247, 1984.

327. Dyszy-Laube, B., et al.: Synovectomy in the treatment of hemophilic arthropathy. J. Pediatr. Surg., 9:123–125, 1974.

328. London, J.T., et al.: Synovectomy and total joint arthroplasty for recurrent hemarthroses in the arthropathic joint in hemophilia. Arthritis Rheum., 20:543–545, 1977.

329. Mannucci, P.M., et al.: Role of synovectomy in hemophilic arthropathy. Isr. J. Med. Sci., 13:983–987, 1977.

330. Gamba, G., Grignani, G., and Ascari, E.: Synoviorthesis versus synovectomy in the treatment of recurrent haemophilic haemarthrosis: Long term evaluation. Thromb. Haemost., 45:127–129, 1981.

331. Ahlberg, A., and Pettersson, H.: Synoviorthesis with radioactive gold in hemophiliacs. Acta Orthop. Scand., 50:513–517, 1979.

332. Fernandez-Palazzi, F., de Bosch, N.B., and de Vargas, A.F.: Radioactive synovectomy in haemophilic haemarthrosis: Follow-up of fifty cases. Scand. J. Haematol. (Suppl.), 40:291–300, 1984.

333. Ahlberg, A.: On the natural history of hemophilic pseudotumor. J. Bone Joint Surg., 57A:1133–1136, 1975.

334. Hilgartner, M.W., and Arnold, W.D.: Hemophilic pseudotumor treated with replacement therapy and radiation: Report of a case. J. Bone Joint Surg., 57A:1145–1146, 1975.

335. Fell, E., Bentley, G., and Rizza, C.R.: Fracture management in patients with haemophilia. J. Bone Joint Surg., 56B:643–649, 1974.

336. Evatt, B.L., et al.: The acquired immunodeficiency syndrome in patients with hemophilia. Ann. Intern. Med., 100:499–504, 1984.

337. The Medical Letter, vol. 29, Jan. 1, 1988, pp. 1–4.

338. Biggs, R., and Rizza, C.R.: The control of haemostasis in hemophiliac patients. In The Treatment of Haemophilia A and B and von Willebrand's Disease. Edited by R. Biggs. Oxford, Blackwell Scientific Publications, 1978, pp. 127–152.

339. Dietrich, S.L., Luck, J.V., and Martinson, A.M.: Musculoskeletal problems. In Hemophilia in the Child and Adult. Edited by M.W. Hilgartner. New York, Masson Publishing, 1982, pp. 85–98.

340. Rizza, C.R., and Matthews, J.M.: The management of patients with coagulation factor deficiencies. In Human Blood Coagulation, Hemostasis, and Thrombosis. 3rd Ed. Edited by R. Biggs and C.R. Rizza. Oxford, Blackwell Scientific Publications, 1984, pp. 273–318.

341. Levine, P.H.: Efficacy of self therapy in hemophilia: A study

of 72 patients with hemophilia A and B. N. Engl. J. Med., *291*:1381–1384, 1974.

342. Levine, P.H.: The Home Therapy Program at the New England Area Hemophilia Center. Scand. J. Haematol., *31*:37–51, 1977.

343. Kisker, C.T., et al.: Double-blind studies on the use of steroids in the treatment of acute hemarthrosis in patients with hemophilia. N. Engl. J. Med., *282*:639–642, 1970.

344. Steven, M.M., et al.: Non-steroidal anti-inflammatory drugs in haemophilic arthritis. A clinical and laboratory study. Haemostasis, *15*:204–209, 1985.

345. Corrigan, J.J., Jr., et al.: Treatment of hemophilic arthritis with D-penicillamine: A preliminary report. Am. J. Hematol., *19*:255–264, 1985.

HERITABLE AND DEVELOPMENTAL DISORDERS OF CONNECTIVE TISSUE AND BONE

85

REED E. PYERITZ

Theoretically, any disorder can be described or studied by two fundamental approaches: etiology and pathogenesis. Either can be useful, depending on the need. Understanding causes leads to reliable classification, diagnosis, and prevention; understanding mechanisms leads to effective prognosis and treatment. Unfortunately, the two approaches are often thought to be similar or even interchangeable—misconceptions that confuse nosology, management, and clinical investigation. Knowledge of etiology, no matter how refined, may shed no light on how the clinical manifestations (the phenotype) develop. For example, the "cause" of sickle cell disease is known at the highest level of resolution possible, the specific nucleotide mutation, whereas the mechanisms by which the diverse clinical features appear remain largely obscure. Conversely, the pathogenesis of acute gout is far better understood than is the etiology in most cases.

Consideration of the role of genetic factors in the disorders of a given system perforce focuses on etiology. The traditional approach has been to divide all disorders into mendelian, chromosomal, and multifactorial categories. This scheme retains some didactic utility, provided one recognizes that no disorder is purely genetic or environmental in cause, and that all involve some interaction of genes and environment to produce the abnormal phenotype.

In *mendelian disorders,* a single mutant gene is of overriding importance, although its effect may be modulated by other genetic and environmental factors. These conditions occur in families in simple in-heritance patterns, that is, autosomal dominant, autosomal recessive, or X-linked. Nearly all these disorders are individually rare (prevalences of $1/10^4$ to $1/10^6$ in the general population), but because so many are now known (close to 4000 in one tabulation[1]), in the aggregate they represent a substantial category of disease. The heritable disorders of connective tissue are all examples.

Chromosomal disorders are those in which an abnormal phenotype is associated with a chromosome aberration visible with the light microscope. For example, Down's syndrome is caused by the presence of three copies of chromosome 21 (trisomy 21), or by the patient's having two normal chromosomes 21, and an additional copy of a short segment of the long arm of chromosome 21, usually attached to one of the other chromosomes. The number of syndromes associated with chromosome aberrations continues to grow as improved cytogenetic techniques enhance resolution,[2] resulting in blurring of the distinctions between mendelian and cytogenetic disorders. For example, susceptibility to retinoblastoma and the Wilms tumor–aniridia syndrome are inherited as autosomal dominant traits, but in some cases such susceptibility is due to deletions of chromosomes 13 and 11, respectively.[3] In one instructive family, the Greig cephalopolysyndactyly syndrome occurred only in relatives having an apparently balanced translocation between chromosomes 3 and 7.[4] Disruption of the gene responsible for this rare condition by the breakage and reunion of chromosome segments, without the visible loss of chromosomal material, is the most likely causal explanation.

The term *multifactorial* has a specific and a general meaning. Disorders such as pyloric stenosis, clubfoot, and idiopathic scoliosis, which conform to empiric predictions of recurrence, concordance in monozygotic twins, and prevalence between sexes, are classified as multifactorial in the narrow sense.[5] On the other hand, any condition in which genes are a necessary, but insufficient, part of the cause and that is distributed in families in ways that do not fulfill any mendelian pattern can be described as multifactorial in the broad sense. Disorders in this latter category tend to be relatively common and include much of what is diagnosed as rheumatoid arthritis, osteoarthritis, and the "acquired" disorders of connective tissue (e.g., lupus and scleroderma).

Several excellent texts provide comprehensive coverage of genetic principles fundamental to an understanding of these concepts and those that will emerge from review of individual disorders.[6,7]

HERITABLE DISORDERS OF CONNECTIVE TISSUE AND BONE

This category of human disease was defined in 1955 by McKusick,[8] and in its first incarnation included only osteogenesis imperfecta, Marfan syndrome, Ehlers-Danlos syndrome, pseudoxanthoma elasticum, and gargoylism. Over more than three decades, 140 distinct, mendelian disorders of connective tissue have been described and are now subject to periodic review by international committees, charged with consensus development of diagnostic criteria and nosologic boundaries (Table 85–1).[9,10] Although their classification remains rooted in phenotypic distinctions, study of the causes of these disorders at the biochemical and nucleic acid level is providing greatly increased understanding of their genesis.

The complexity of connective tissue is emphasized in Chapters 12–16 and in recent reviews.[11,12] Discovery of specific biochemical defects has only begun to be instructive about the pathogenesis of the heritable disorders of connective tissue and how the macromolecular components interact.[13–18] These disorders are as much inborn errors of metabolism as are the familial defects in amino acid and carbohydrate metabolism first investigated by Garrod at the turn of the century, and with careful study, each of these disorders can serve as a window to normal structure and function of connective tissue. The disorders chosen for description in this chapter are relatively common and important in clinical rheumatology, highly instructive as to general principles, or both.

MARFAN SYNDROME

Patients with the Marfan syndrome tend to have major abnormalities in the skeletal, ocular, cardiovascular, and pulmonary systems.[19,20] The diagnosis is based solely on the clinical features and the autosomal dominant inheritance pattern.[19] Although a variety of biochemical abnormalities have been described, none has proven to be the long-sought basic defect. Attention has been focused on elastic fibers because they are highly disorganized and even fragmented in the aortic media and dermis,[21–22] but if the defect were in elastin, the pathogenesis of increased length of long bones and dislocated lenses would be difficult to explain. A recently discovered, 350,000-dalton glycoprotein, fibrillin, is a constituent of both elastic fibers and the microfibrils that are so ubiquitous throughout connective tissue.[23] Preliminary studies of Marfan patients and their relatives suggest that defects in synthesis of fibrillin account for some cases.[24] However, given the wide interfamilial variation in the phenotype of the Marfan syndrome and the precedent with other hereditary disorders, genetic heterogeneity is anticipated.[25]

Skeletal Features. Patients with the Marfan syndrome are excessively tall, or at least taller than unaffected relatives (Fig. 85–1). Body proportions are irregular (dolichostenomelia), with an abnormally low ratio of the upper segment to the lower segment (US/LS). In practice, two measurements are made with the patient standing: height and lower segment (top of the pubic symphisis to floor). In normal adult white persons, the mean ratio is about 0.92; in adult black persons, it is about 0.87. The excessive length of the lower extremities is primarily responsible for the abnormally low US/LS in the Marfan syndrome. The US/LS varies with age, race, sex, and degree of vertebral column deformity in all persons, so that an isolated determination in a suspected patient must be interpreted with caution. The arms also show excessive length, with the span of adult patients usually exceeding their height by more than 3%. The metacarpal index, based on the ratio of length to width of metacarpals, is said to be useful but requires a radiograph of the hands.

The ribs undergo excessive longitudinal growth as well. Depression of the sternum (pectus excavatum), protrusion (pectus carinatum; see Fig. 85–1), or an asymmetric combination thereof often results.

The vertebral column is frequently deformed. Most

Table 85–1. General Classification of the Heritable Disorders of Connective Tissue and Bone

Categories	Basic Defect(s)
Marfan syndrome	A component of microfibrils (? fibrillin)
Stickler syndrome	Type II collagen
Ehlers-Danlos syndromes	Types I and III collagen in some disorders
Familial articular hypermobility syndromes	?
Osteogenesis imperfecta	Various defects in type I collagen
Skeletal dysplasia with predominant joint laxity	?
Cutis laxa	?
Pseudoxanthoma elasticum	Calcification of elastic fibers
Osteochondrodysplasias	Most ?
Epidermolysis bullosa	Increased collagenase in one form
Disorders secondary to metabolic defects	
Alcaptonuria	Homogentisic acid oxidase deficiency
Homocystinuria	Cystathionine β-synthase deficiency
Disorders of copper transport	
Occipital horn syndrome	Decreased serum copper and ceruloplasmin
Menkes syndrome	Excess copper bound to metallothionein
Heteroglycanoses	
Mucopolysaccharidoses	Deficiencies of lysosomal hydrolases
Phosphotransferase deficiencies	Inability to modify lysosomal hydrolases
Fucosidosis	Deficiency of α-fucosidase
Mannosidosis	Deficiency of α-mannosidase
Aspartylglucosaminuria	Deficiency of aspartamido-N-Ac-glucosamine-amidohydrolase
GM₁ gangliosidosis	Deficiency of β-galactosidase
Sialidoses	Deficiency of various neuraminidases
Sialuria	Intralysosomal neuraminic acid retention
Galactosialidosis	Deficiency of β-galactosidase and neuraminidase
Mucosulfatidosis	
Miscellaneous disorders	
Buschke-Ollendorff syndrome	?
Familial cutaneous collagenoma	?
Wrinkly skin syndrome	?

often, the normal thoracic kyphos is lost, resulting in a "straight back" or an outright thoracic lordosis. Scoliosis may involve multiple segments and may progress rapidly, particularly during the adolescent growth spurt.

Loose-jointedness is often striking in patients with the Marfan syndrome. Flat feet (pes planus), hyperextensibility at the knees (genu recurvatum), elbows, and fingers, congenital dislocation of the hip, and recurrent dislocation of the patellae are manifestations of the loose-jointedness. A relatively narrow palm of the hand, long thumb, and longitudinal laxity of the hand are the bases for the *Steinberg thumb sign* (Fig. 85–2): the thumb apposed across the palm extends well beyond the ulnar margin of the hand. Another simple, but nonspecific, test is the *wrist sign*: the first and fifth digits, when wrapped around the contralateral wrist, overlap appreciably in the Marfan syndrome (Fig. 85–3).

Joint laxity is so variable, even among relatives affected by the Marfan syndrome, that for a time distinct disorders were suspected. About 10% of patients have some restriction of extension at one or more joints, usually of congenital onset; while a separate congenital contractural arachnodactyly syndrome undoubtedly exists,[26] all patients with this signal feature should be evaluated as if they had the Marfan syndrome so that serious problems in other systems are not overlooked.[27] Similarly, the "marfanoid hypermobility syndrome"[28] is not worth distinguishing as a separate entity.

Other Features. Most patients with the Marfan syndrome have myopia, and about half have subluxation of the lenses (ectopia lentis). The ascending aorta bears the main stress of ventricular ejection, leading to progressive dilatation beginning in the sinuses of Valsalva. Resultant aortic regurgitation, dissection, or both are the main causes of death.[29] Before the development of reliable surgical procedures and their early application,[30,31] life expectancy was reduced, on

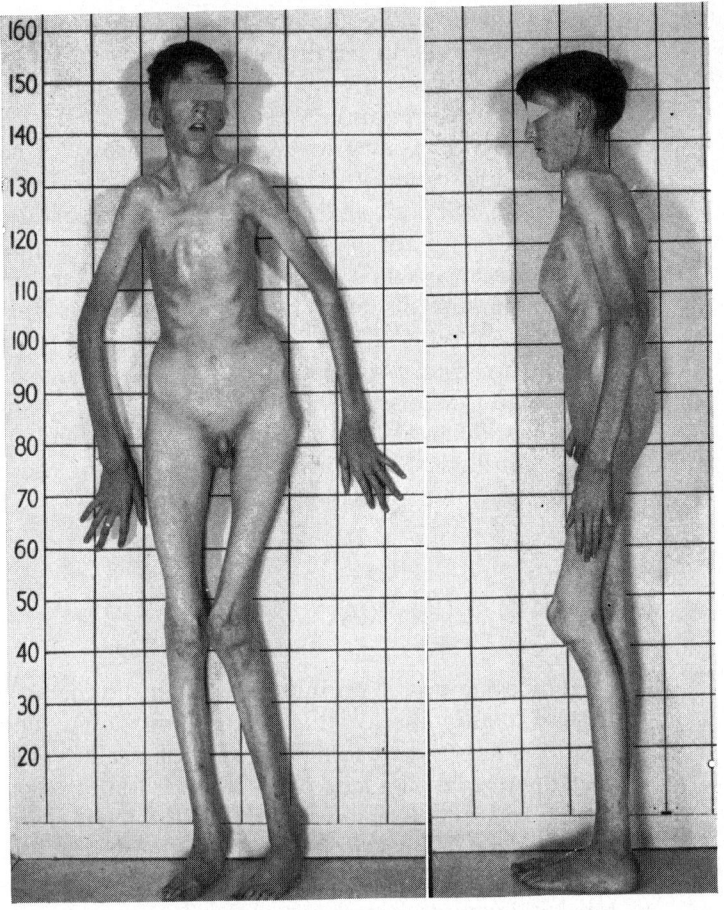

FIG. 85–1. Marfan syndrome in a 14-year-old boy. Note arachnodactyly, relatively long limbs (dolichostenomelia), pectus carinatum, sparse subcutaneous fat, unilateral genu valgum, and pes planus. Ectopia lentis and scoliosis were also present. This patient died of aortic rupture at 15 years of age.

average, by one third in patients with the Marfan syndrome. Mitral valve prolapse occurs in 80% of patients and leads to severe mitral regurgitation in about 10%. Hernias are frequent, cystic changes in the lungs lead to pneumothorax,[32] and striae distensae over the pectoral and deltoid areas and thighs are often first noticed in adolescence. Dural ectasia is usually an incidental finding on computed tomography (CT) or magnetic resonance imaging (MRI) of the vertebral column; occasional patients have problems with spinal fluid dynamics or spinal anesthesia as a consequence.

Management of the Skeletal Manifestations. Most Marfan patients can lead long and productive lives, especially now that the success of cardiovascular surgery in repairing the aorta has improved.[30,32] Thus, all patients deserve aggressive and prophylactic management of all organ systems at risk. For the skeletal

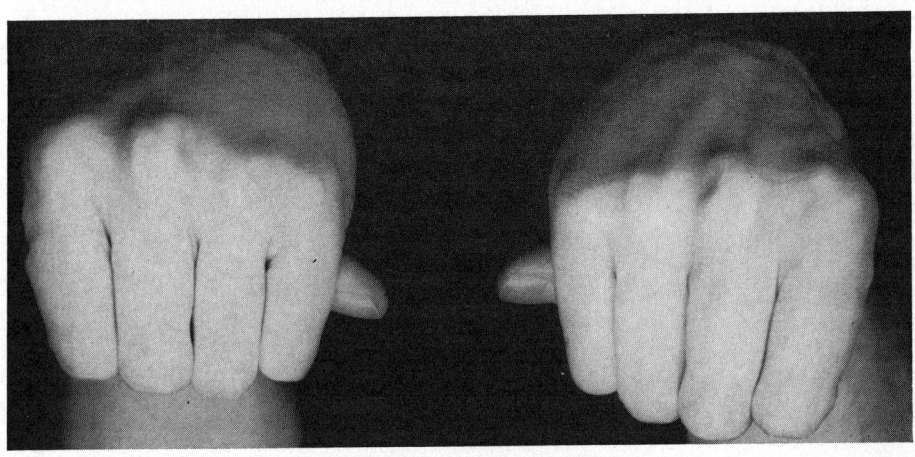

FIG. 85–2. The Steinberg thumb sign in a patient with Marfan syndrome. A positive test, such as this, consists of the distal phalanx of the thumb protruding beyond the ulnar border of the clenched fist and reflects both longitudinal laxity of the hand and a long thumb.

FIG. 85–3. The wrist sign in a patient with Marfan syndrome. In a positive test, the first phalanges of the thumb and fifth digit substantially overlap when wrapped around the opposite wrist.

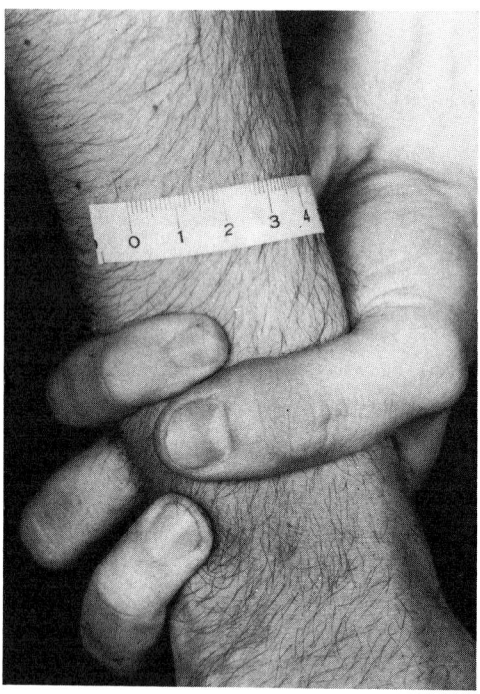

system, management must begin in childhood, because most problems are progressive during the years of growth.

Initial management of vertebral column deformity is by bracing. If abnormal curves can be stabilized, persistent bracing may be necessary until the skeleton matures. The presence of thoracic lordosis, rather common in the Marfan syndrome, unfortunately limits the effectiveness of most braces. Whenever scoliotic curves exceed 40 to 45°, surgical stabilization and fusion are required.

Tall stature per se is usually not a problem in males. Girls, on the other hand, often suffer much psychosocial turmoil as a result of their height. Analysis of growth shows that the average height for girls parallels the ninety-fifth percentile of the normal female growth curve; the average adult height is thus close to 6 feet.[33] Early induction of puberty by administration of ethinyl estradiol (0.05 mg/10 kg in a single oral dose daily) and medroxyprogesterone (2.5 mg/10 kg on days 25 to 28) results in accelerated skeletal maturation. If therapy is begun well before the age of physiologic menarche (I begin around 8 years of age) then adult height is clearly lessened.[33] Furthermore, by accelerating the "adolescent" growth spurt, there

is less time for scoliosis to progress, and deformity is mitigated. Once the epiphyses are nearly fused or once the girl attains the age of physiologic menarche, hormonal therapy can be discontinued.

Deformity of the anterior chest also tends to worsen during adolescence as a result of rapid rib growth. Repair of either pectus excavatum or pectus carinatum for cosmetic indications should thus be delayed until midadolescence, when the defect is not likely to recur.

Uncommonly disability can result from hyperextensibility at other joints. Dislocation of the patellae and the first metacarpal-phalangeal joints, severe pes planus, and metatarsus valgus are the most frequent problems. Physical therapy, muscular strengthening, and well-fitted shoes are useful. Surgery for these problems should be avoided if possible.

HOMOCYSTINURIA

Homocystinuria is an inborn error in the metabolism of methionine in which activity of the enzyme cystathionine β-synthase is deficient. Clinical features are superficially similar to those of the Marfan syndrome and include ectopia lentis, dolichostenomelia, arachnodactyly, and chest and spinal deformity (Fig. 85–4).[34] Generalized osteoporosis, "tight" joints, arterial and venous thrombosis, malar flush, psychiatric disturbance, and mental retardation are features of homocystinuria usually not found in the Marfan syndrome.[35,36] Aortic aneurysm and mitral prolapse are not features of homocystinuria. Homocystinuria is an autosomal recessive disorder, unlike the Marfan syndrome, which is a dominant trait. The hand in homocystinuria has none of the longitudinal laxity present in the Marfan syndrome, and the appendicular joints tend to have reduced mobility. Back pain resulting from osteoporosis occurs in some patients.

The pathogenesis of the three cardinal groups of manifestations—mental retardation, connective tissue disorder (ectopia lentis, osteoporosis, reduced joint mobility), and thrombosis—is not understood. Perhaps the reduced sulfhydryl groups of homocysteine or other substances that accumulate proximal to the block interfere with collagen cross linking, thus accounting for the connective tissue manifestations. Such a mechanism occurs in the thiolism caused by prolonged administration of penicillamine, a compound structurally similar to homocysteine. An alternative, but not necessarily exclusive, hypothesis focuses on the deficiency of cysteine that results from the inability to join homocysteine with serine. Cysteine is one of the three amino acids that forms glu-

FIG. 85–4. Homocystinuria in a 12-year-old girl. Note the excessive height, long, narrow feet, and mild anterior chest deformity. The teeth were crowded, ectopia lentis was present, and the joints showed moderate restriction of motion. Despite several episodes of pulmonary embolism and thrombophlebitis, she was active at 40 years of age.

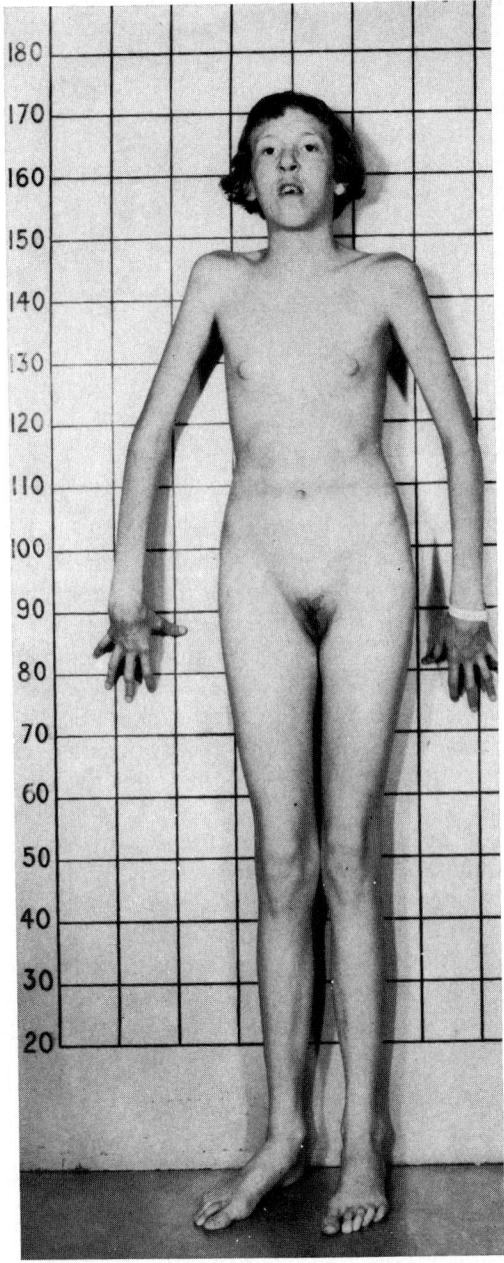

tathione, the deficiency of which predisposes to damage from free radicals.

Over half the patients with homocystinuria respond to large doses of vitamin B₆ (pyridoxine) with clearing of homocystine from the urine, lowering of plasma methionine and cysteine, raising of cystine to normal,

and reducing the likelihood of developing clinical manifestations.[37] Pre-existent mental retardation and ectopia lentis are not improved by pyridoxine treatment in patients who show biochemical correction, emphasizing the need for early diagnosis and therapy. Because most states include testing for elevated blood methionine as part of the newborn screening program, early treatment is possible. Newborns, however, with B₆-responsive cystathionine β-synthase deficiency may have sufficient pyridoxine from maternal sources to prevent hypermethioninemia during the first week of life, and thereby escape detection.[37] With supplementary folic acid (1 mg daily), as little as 20 mg of pyridoxine daily may be effective, although usually a dosage of 100 to 300 mg is required. In vitamin B₆-nonresponders, a low methionine diet is the mainstay of management,[38] although pyridoxine and folate should be included because of a tendency for unsupplemented patients to develop deficiency of these cofactors. In addition, sulfinpyrazone, dipyridamole, or aspirin, singly or in combination, may be useful in preventing thrombotic episodes in all homocystinurics, even though platelet survival is normal in most patients.[35,39]

WEILL-MARCHESANI SYNDROME

The Weill-Marchesani syndrome is another systemic disorder with ectopia lentis as a conspicuous feature (Fig. 85–5). The skeletal features are the antithesis of those in the Marfan syndrome: the patients are short, with particularly short hands and feet, and have stiff joints, especially in the hands. The hands sometimes show atrophy of the abductor pollicis brevis muscle consistent with carpal tunnel compression.[34] The Weill-Marchesani syndrome is autosomal recessive, but heterozygotes are shorter of stature than average.[40]

THE EHLERS-DANLOS SYNDROMES

The Ehlers-Danlos syndromes (EDS) are a group of disorders of considerable diversity of phenotypes, largely caused by extensive genetic heterogeneity. The cardinal and unifying features relate to the joints and skin; hyperextensibility of skin, easy bruisability, dystrophic scarring, increased joint mobility, and abnormal tissue fragility. Internal manifestations, which include rupture of great vessels, hiatal hernia, diverticulum of the gastrointestinal and genitourinary tracts, spontaneous rupture of the bowel, and spon-

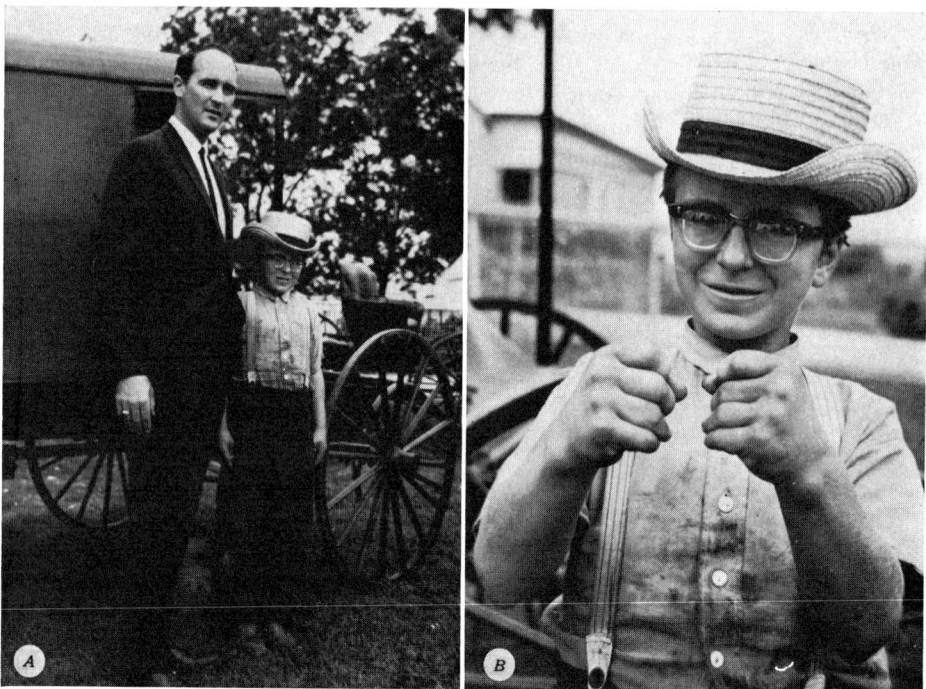

FIG. 85–5. Weill-Marchesani syndrome in a 15-year-old Amish boy. *A*, Shown with normal adult male. Ectopia lentis was present, and attacks of acute glaucoma had occurred. *B*, The fingers were short with knobby joints and restricted flexion. Flattening of the thenar eminence was consistent with carpal tunnel compression.

taneous pneumothorax, tend to occur only in specific types of EDS.

The classification of EDS has been set at nine general types on the basis of phenotypic and inheritance characteristics (Table 85–2).[9] Biochemical studies have demonstrated considerable heterogeneity within individual types.[13,14,41,42] This extensive phenotypic and biochemical characterization nonetheless fails the clinician as often as it helps; nearly half of all patients who have at least one "cardinal" manifestation defy categorization.[43]

EDS I (Gravis Form) and EDS II (Mitis Form). Generalized hyperextensibility of joints (Fig. 85–6), together with stretchability of skin, leads to characterization of the affected persons as "India rubber men." Other features are bruising and fragility of the skin, with gaping wounds caused by minor trauma and

with poor retention of sutures.[34,44] Congenital dislocation of the hips in the newborn, habitual dislocation of selected joints in later life, joint effusions, clubfoot deformity of the feet, and spondylolisthesis are all consequences of the loose-jointedness. Hemarthroses and "hemarthritic disability" have been described and are analogous to bruising of the skin. Scoliosis is sometimes severe. Severe leg cramps occurring at rest and of unclear cause are troublesome to some patients.

Both of these types are inherited as autosomal dominant traits and tend to breed true within a family. They differ from one another only in severity; hence, the differentiation is somewhat subjective (Fig. 85–7). The biochemical defects have not been characterized in either type, although abnormalities of the collagens most common in skin (types I and III) have long been suspected.

Table 85–2.   Ehlers-Danlos Syndromes

Type	Inheritance	Skeletal Features	Other Features	Basic Defect
I	AD	Marked joint hypermobility	Skin hyperextensibility and fragility	?
II	AD	Less severe than type I		?
III	AD	Marked joint hypermobility	None	?
IV	AD, AR	Hypermobile digits	Arterial and bowel rupture	Deficient type III collagen
V	X-L	Similar to type II		?
VI	AR	Marked joint hypermobility	Rupture of globe	Lysyl hydroxylase
VII	AD, AR	Marked joint hypermobility and dislocations; short stature	Minimal skin change	Defect in procollagen cleavage
VIII	AD	Variable joint hypermobility	Periodontitis	?
X	AD	Mild joint hypermobility	Mild skin changes; MVP	Defect in fibronectin

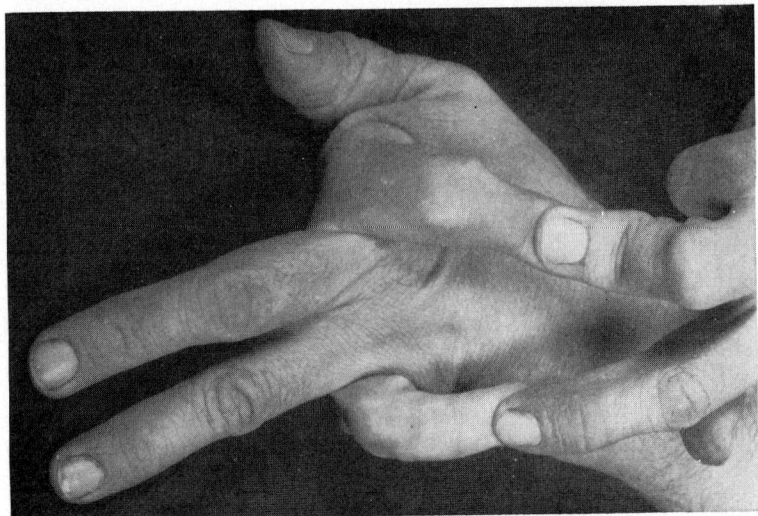

FIG. 85–6. Joint hypermobility in the Ehlers-Danlos syndrome, type I.

Management of both EDS I and EDS II stresses prevention of trauma and great care in treating wounds. Some patients, particularly young boys, wear shin guards to protect their lower legs from the repeated minor injuries that lead to frequent hemorrhage, unsightly scars, and absence from school. Patients should be dissuaded from demonstrating their joint laxity as entertainment for their friends. Because the ligaments and joint capsules are lax, joint stability can be improved only by developing the mus-

cles. Care must be employed, however, in weight lifting and other forms of exercise because of fragility of tendons.

EDS III (Benign Hypermobility Form). This condition has moderate dermal hyperextensibility and minimal fragility. The joint hyperextensibility ranges from extreme to bordering on normal.[44] All too often, patients with mild joint laxity without joint instability or skin manifestations are labeled as EDS III, particularly if relatives show a similar manifestation. In some cases,

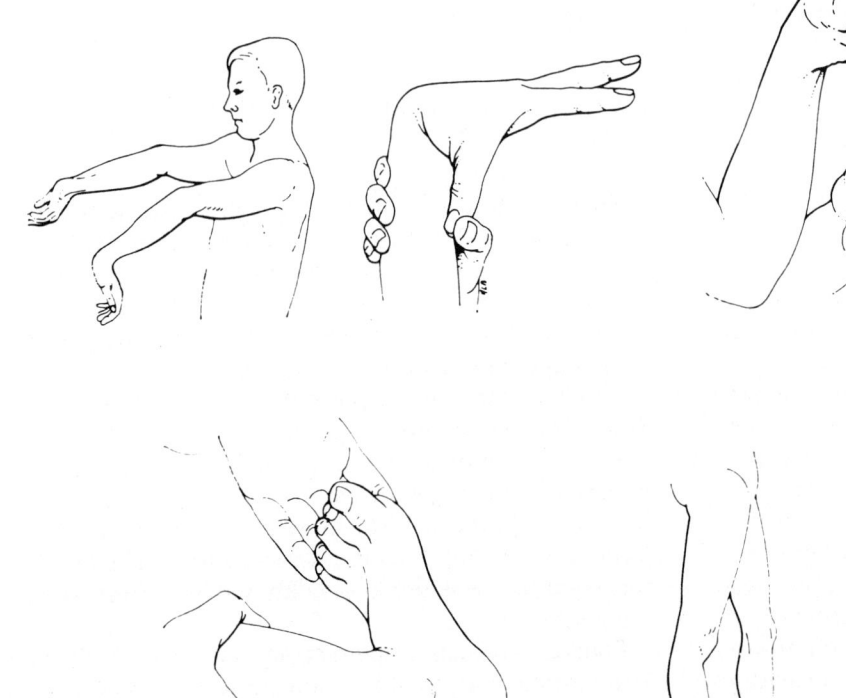

FIG. 85–7. A method for evaluating joint mobility.[57] Excessive joint laxity is judged to exist when at least three of the following five conditions are present: (1) elbows and (2) knees extend beyond 180°; (3) thumb touches the forearm on flexing the wrist; (4) fingers are parallel to the forearm on extending the wrist and metacarpal joints; and (5) foot dorsiflexes to 45° or more.

such labeling causes more harm than good, unless one makes it clear that little if any disability is likely to result.

EDS IV (Arterial Form). This condition is by far the most serious type of EDS because of a propensity for spontaneous rupture of arteries and bowel.[34,44,45] This type is particularly heterogeneous genetically, the unifying theme being abnormal production of type III collagen.[46,47] Skin involvement is variable, with thin, nearly translucent skin present in some, and mildly hyperextensible skin the only feature in others. Joint laxity is also variable, but is generally limited to the digits. Inheritance is usually autosomal dominant.

EDS V. The phenotype of this rare, X-linked form resembles EDS II most closely.[48,49] Although a deficiency of lysyl oxidase was claimed in one pedigree, this deficiency has not been confirmed or found in any other family.

EDS VI (Ocular-Scoliotic Form). Fragility of the ocular globe and a propensity to severe scoliosis, in addition to the skin and joint involvement seen in EDS I, are the hallmarks of this autosomal recessive form of EDS.[34] This is the first of the heritable disorders of connective tissue to have its basic defect elucidated, by Krane and colleagues in 1972.[50] Collagen in this condition contains little hydroxylysine because of deficiency of the enzyme that hydroxylates selected lysyl residues in the nascent collagen chains. Because hydroxylysine is normally involved, along with lysine, in cross linking of collagen, the clinical feature of EDS VI is readily explained. Vitamin C is a necessary cofactor of lysyl hydroxylase and, in high doses, may be beneficial in some cases of EDS VI[51] (comparable to the benefit of vitamin B6 in some cases of homocystinuria).

EDS VII (Arthrochalasis Multiplex Congenita). Profound loose-jointedness with congenital dislocations dominates the clinical picture. The patients are moderately short of stature and the skin is variably, but usually mildly, involved.[34,52] An inability to convert type I procollagen to mature collagen, by cleavage of the N-propeptide, has been found in all patients who have been studied.[13,15,53,54] The genetic heterogeneity of EDS VII is instructive. Deficiency of procollagen N-peptidase, the enzyme that cleaves the propeptide from the amino-terminal end of type I procollagen, was said in one report to be deficient in fibroblasts from several patients.[53] But at least one of these, and all other patients, have had normal N-peptidase activity but an amino acid sequence alteration around the site of the procollagen molecule where cleavage occurs. Two general types of mutations have been seen thus far. At the cleavage site, an amino acid in either the α1(I) or the α2(I) procollagen chain is mu-

tated, disrupting the α-helix conformation requisite for peptidase activity. Alternatively, a deletion (or theoretically an insertion) of amino acids anywhere in either of the procollagen chains proximal to the N-peptidase cleavage site causes misregister of the three chains and disruption of the α-helix. Deficiency of peptidase activity would likely be an autosomal recessive trait. In distinction, the mutations causing amino acid alterations have all affected only one allele for either α1(I) or α2(I) procollagen. Because neither parent was affected in any of the cases examined biochemically so far, the mutation occurred in a parental gonad. The patients, however, should they choose to reproduce, will have a 50% chance of having an affected offspring, and their condition will thus satisfy criteria for an autosomal dominant trait.

EDS VIII (Periodontitis Form). This rare condition is characterized by severe periodontal disease, with early loss of both primary and permanent teeth. Presence of EDS I–like manifestations has varied in the few reported kindreds.[34] The basic defect is unknown, and inheritance is autosomal dominant.

EDS IX. This disorder has been reclassified as a disorder of copper transport (see Table 85–1).

EDS X (Fibronectin Deficiency). One pedigree was reported with a phenotype inherited as an autosomal recessive, characterized by features of EDS II, and associated with abnormal platelet aggregation.[55] The platelet defect was corrected by exogenous plasma fibronectin.

FAMILIAL ARTICULAR HYPERMOBILITY SYNDROMES

This is a newly created category of disorders that includes generalized articular hypermobility with or without subluxation.[9] Specifically excluded are the skeletal dysplasias with joint hypermobility (e.g., the Larsen syndrome) and the EDS syndromes (which all have some degree of skin involvement).

Familial Articular Hypermobility, Uncomplicated Type. This is a relatively common, autosomal dominant condition of unknown biochemical defect. Joint hypermobility is generalized, but rarely causes dislocation or disability.[56] The incidence of congenital dislocation of the hip may be increased in families with this condition,[57] which is also known as familial simple joint laxity.

Familial Articular Hypermobility, Dislocating Type. The cardinal feature of this autosomal dominant condition is instability of multiple appendicular joints; recurrent dislocation is the usual clinical finding. Joint hyperextensibility is variable but usually mild, and skin involvement is uncommon.[58] This condition, which has been called both familial joint instability syndrome and Ehlers-Danlos type XI, may cause considerable disability. Clinical variability within a family is the rule, emphasizing the need for a comprehensive family history, including examination of close relatives if possible (Fig. 85–8).

This is an extremely difficult condition to manage successfully. For most patients, diagnosis is established only after multiple orthopedic surgical attempts (usually disappointing) to prevent recurrent dislocation of shoulders, knees, or elbows. As in EDS I and II, physical therapy of affected joints to increase periarticular muscle strength should be attempted first.

SKELETAL DYSPLASIAS WITH PREDOMINANT JOINT LAXITY

Many of the osteochondrodysplasias have variable degrees of joint laxity or instability as part of the overall phenotype. Several disorders, however, have such prominent joint hypermobility as to be the cardinal sign, and have been grouped in one category.

Larsen Syndrome. The Larsen syndrome is characterized by multiple congenital dislocations and characteristic facies: prominent forehead, depressed nasal bridge, and widely spaced eyes.[59] Dislocation occurs at the knees (characteristically anterior displacement of the tibia on the femur), hips, and elbows. The metacarpals are short, with cylindrical fingers lacking the usual tapering. Cleft palate, hydrocephalus, abnormalities of spinal segmentation, and moderate-to-severe short stature have occurred in some. Several instances of multiple affected sib-

lings with normal parents are known, suggesting autosomal recessive inheritance, but parent-child involvement also occurs, consistent with dominant inheritance. Thus, two clinically indistinguishable forms of the Larsen syndrome may exist.[60]

Radiographic features that are helpful in diagnosis, in addition to congenital segmentation anomalies of the spine and congenital hip dislocation, are multiple ossification centers in the calcaneus and carpus.[61]

Desbuquois Syndrome. Desbuquois and colleagues described patients with short stature, joint laxity, prominent eyes, broad terminal phalanges, and supernumerary digits. The most characteristic radiographic features are extracarpal ossification centers and prominence of the lesser trochanter of the femur.[62] This rare condition can be inherited as an autosomal recessive trait, but may be genetically heterogeneous, so that sporadic cases should not be counseled that they have no risk of having an affected offspring.

OSTEOGENESIS IMPERFECTA SYNDROMES

Several phenotypically distinct osteogenesis imperfecta (OI) syndromes, and even more classification schemes, exist.[63–65] The disorders share osseous, ocular, dental, aural, and cardiovascular involvement. The classification enjoying current application is based on clinical and inheritance pattern criteria (Table 85–3).[9,65,66] At the current rapid pace of defining basic biochemical defects in collagen, a nosology grounded in objective data is a reasonable expectation.[13–15]

FIG. 85–8. Pedigree of a family with familial articular hypermobility, dislocating type. The autosomal dominant transmission and variability of the phenotype are both well illustrated. Pedigree symbols: ◐ = joint hypermobility; ● = hip dislocation; ◑ = patella dislocation; ▨ = possibly affected; ◌̇ = examined by authors; ⊘ = deceased. From Horton, W.A., et al.[58] Reprinted with permission.

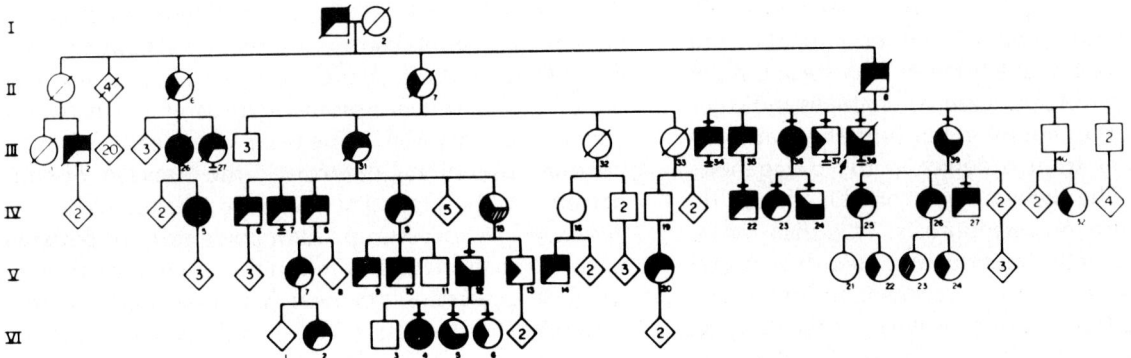

Table 85–3. Osteogenesis Imperfecta Syndromes

Type	Inheritance	Skeletal Features	Other Features
IA	AD	Variable bone fragility and short stature, wormian bones	Blue sclerae, opalescent teeth, hearing loss
IB	AD	Variable bone fragility and short stature, wormian bones	Blue sclerae, normal teeth, hearing loss
II	Most sporadic, due to heterozygosity for a new mutation in type I collagen	In utero fractures, little calvarial calcium	Blue sclerae, pulmonary hypertension, neonatal death usual
III	Most sporadic; some AR	Moderately severe fragility, variable deformity, scoliosis, joint laxity	Variable sclerae, some with opalescent teeth
IVA	AD	Variable bone fragility and short stature, wormian bones	Normal sclerae, opalescent teeth, hearing loss
IVB	AD	Variable bone fragility and short stature, wormian bones	Normal sclerae and teeth, hearing loss

Type 1 OI is the most common form and is associated with wide intrafamilial variability.[34,67,68] One patient might be extremely short of stature, with frequent fractures and much disability, whereas an affected relative leads an unencumbered, vigorous life. Type II encompasses the classic "OI congenita" variants, most of which are lethal in infancy, if not in utero.[34,69,70] Molecular characterization of type II is progressing rapidly, at both the collagen and the DNA level. Most cases arise as the result of a new mutation (the phenotype thus being transmissible as a dominant, if the patient could live and reproduce) while a few have affected siblings and normal but sometimes consanguineous parents, consistent with autosomal recessive inheritance. Type III OI comprises miscellaneous phenotypes that cannot be classified better.[71] Most cases include severe skeletal deformity and short stature as distinguishing features. Most occur sporadically. Type IV OI is similar to type I, only rarer and not associated with blue sclerae.[72,73]

Skeletal Features. "Brittle bones" are a familiar and dramatic feature of all the OI variants. Sometimes fractures occur in utero, particularly in type II, and permit radiographic antenatal diagnosis. In such cases, the limbs are likely to be short and bent at birth. Multiple rib fractures give a characteristic "beaded" appearance on radiographs.[69] Other patients with types I or IV have few fractures or may escape them entirely, although blue sclerae or deafness indicates the presence of the mutant gene. Brittleness and deformability result from a defect in the collagenous matrix of bone. The skeletal aspect of OI is, therefore, a hereditary form of osteoporosis. "Codfish vertebrae" (scalloping of the superior and inferior vertebral bodies by pressure from the expansile intervertebral disc) or flat vertebrae are observed, particularly in older patients in whom senile or postmenopausal

changes exaggerate the change, or young patients immobilized after fracture or orthopedic surgery. Usually the frequency of fractures decreases at puberty for patients with types I, III, and IV. Because of failure of union of fractures, pseudarthrosis (especially of humerus or femur) occurs in some. Hypertrophic callus occurs frequently in patients with OI and is often difficult to distinguish from osteosarcoma. Debate continues as to whether the risk of true osteosarcoma is increased in any form of OI; regardless, the risk is not great, but worthy of consideration whenever skeletal pain occurs in the absence of fracture, particularly in an older patient. Loose-jointedness is sometimes striking in type I OI; dislocation of joints can result from deformity secondary to repeated fracture, ligamentous laxity, or rupture of tendons (especially the Achilles and patellar).

Ocular Features. Blue sclerae are present in types I, II, and III OI and represent a valuable clue to the diagnosis. The cornea, like the sclera, is abnormally thin. The ocular features are usually not of great functional importance.

Aural Features. Hearing loss becomes detectable in many patients by the second or third decade of life. It was long assumed that deafness in OI was the result of precocious otosclerosis; alternatively, otosclerosis is such a common disorder that many OI patients are likely to develop it. A variety of aural abnormalities occurs in OI, and symptomatic hearing loss is nearly always multifactorial.[74] The tympanic membrane may be thin, the pinna deformed, the ossicles disconnected, or the stapedial footplate thickened or degenerated. A surprisingly high percentage of patients have a sensorineural component, owing in part to cochlear deformity, cochlear hair loss, and tectorial membrane distortion.[74] Thus, each patient must be evaluated in considerable detail to determine whether hearing impairment is present and whether it is conductive, sensorineural, or mixed.

Dental Features. The characteristic dental manifestation of OI is opalescent teeth caused by a defect in dentin morphogenesis.[75] This finding is easily ascertained by direct observation of the blue or brown opalescent deciduous or permanent teeth or by the typical radiographic changes. This dental abnormality can be useful diagnostically because opalescent teeth, of all of the pleiotropic OI manifestations, breeds true in families.[65] It thus forms the basis for subdividing types I and IV into disorders with and without opalescent teeth. Affected teeth wear poorly; enamel loss is secondary to fracture of the underlying dentin.

Other Features. Unusual bruising occurs in some patients, probably owing to a defect in the connective tissue in the walls of small blood vessels or in the supporting connective tissues. No consistent defect of the coagulation mechanism has been demonstrated.

Mitral valve prolapse occurs in about 15% of patients with OI type I, several times more frequently than in the general population, and occasionally may progress to mitral regurgitation. Aortic dilatation and regurgitation also occur but are infrequent.[76–78]

The differential diagnosis of osteogenesis imperfecta includes idiopathic juvenile osteoporosis,[79] juvenile osteoporosis with ocular pseudoglioma and mental retardation,[80] Cheney syndrome (osteoporosis, multiple wormian bones, acro-osteolysis),[81] pycnodysostosis (dwarfism, brittle bones, absent ramus of mandible, persistent cranial fontanelles, acro-osteolysis),[82] and hypophosphatasia.[83] When children with unrecognized OI are taken to the emergency room on account of a new fracture, and radiographs show multiple healed fractures, the possibility of child abuse may be raised and the parents unjustly accused. Conversely, we encountered a patient who was clearly abused and battered, but whose parents tried repeatedly and nearly successfully to have their child diagnosed as having a variant of OI.

STICKLER SYNDROME

The cardinal features of this relatively common (at least 1 per 10,000 in the population) autosomal dominant condition are severe, progressive myopia, vitreal degeneration, retinal detachment, progressive sensorineural hearing loss, cleft palate, mandibular hypoplasia, hypermobility and hypomobility of joints, epiphyseal dysplasia, and variable disability resulting from joint pain, dislocation, or degeneration.[84,85] In one large clinic for craniofacial anomalies,

6.6% of all patients with cleft palate but without cleft lip had Stickler syndrome.[86] This condition, also called progressive arthro-ophthalmopathy, is clearly underdiagnosed, in part because patients often do not have the full syndrome and in part because the physician fails to obtain a detailed family history that might suggest a hereditary condition. Some nosologic confusion persists as well. The ocular features, first described in 1938, have been called the Wagner syndrome by ophthalmologists.[87] Some patients with typical ocular and aural features have severe midfacial hypoplasia (not just flat malae), a thick calvarium, and abnormal frontal sinuses, findings termed the Marshall syndrome[88]; while nosologic splitting is supported by some,[89] most ascribe the phenotypic differences to the variable expression of a single mutation.[90,91] Recently the Weissenbacher-Zweymüller syndrome has been recognized as a severe, neonatal form of the Stickler syndrome.[91,92] The Stickler syndrome should be strongly considered in any infant with "swollen" wrists, knees, or ankles, the Robin sequence (hypognathia, cleft palate, and glossoptosis), or flared ("dumbbell"-shaped) femoral metaphyses; in any adult with precocious degenerative arthritis of the hip, especially if relatives are similarly affected; and in any person with spontaneous retinal detachment.

The Stickler syndrome has been linked to the α1(II) procollagen locus.[93] This is the first human disease shown to be due to a heritable defect in the principal collagenous component of cartilage.

CUTIS LAXA

The cardinal feature of these conditions is dermatologic: the skin is lax and loose, with none of the hyperelasticity seen in the Ehlers-Danlos variants. Beyond childhood, the prominent skinfolds and excessive wrinkling give a prematurely aged appearance. Both congenital (usually autosomal recessive) and late-onset (autosomal dominant) forms occur, and the basic defects, which presumably affect elastic fibers, are unclear.[34] The skeletal system is largely unaffected, but the condition is of importance to rheumatologists on account of the *phenocopy* that the disease may inadvertently cause in the offspring of their patients. A phenocopy is a disorder of nongenetic cause that mimics a hereditary disorder. Some fetuses exposed to D-penicillamine, as a result of maternal treatment of acquired connective tissue disorders, Wilson's disease, or cystinuria, develop a congenital syndrome indistinguishable from the severe, autosomal recessive form of cutis laxa.[94] Neither the susceptible period of pregnancy nor the threshold dosage has been established.

PSEUDOXANTHOMA ELASTICUM

The characteristic features occur in the skin, retina, and arteries.[34] In areas of flexural stress, yellowish papules develop over time, giving the skin the appearance of that of a plucked chicken. As Bruch's membrane fragments, angioid streaks develop in the retina; hemorrhages lead to progressive visual loss. An arteriolarsclerosis, similar histopathologically to that of Mönckeberg, develops and leads to loss of peripheral pulses, myocardial infarction, and gastrointestinal hemorrhage. The skeleton is not involved in any obvious way. Both autosomal recessive (the most common) and autosomal dominant forms occur.[95,96] The basic defect is unclear, but the pathognomonic dermatopathologic finding is calcification of elastic fibers. Restriction of nutritional calcium intake in early life may retard progression of the disease.[97]

CONSTITUTIONAL DISEASES OF BONE

In addition to the disorders of connective tissue already discussed, a wide array of hereditary conditions affect the skeleton. According to a standard nomenclature,[10] they are classified broadly as osteochondrodysplasias, dysostoses, idiopathic osteolyses, and primary metabolic abnormalities. The most common or instructive examples will be presented here.

OSTEOCHONDRODYSPLASIAS

These disorders affect cartilage or bone growth and development. This category is divided into defects primarily of tubular bones, defects primarily of the spine, or defects of both the appendicular and axial skeleton. In some conditions, such as multiple epiphyseal dysplasia (MED), only the skeleton is involved. In others, such as spondyloepiphyseal dysplasia (SED) congenita, other organs are affected as well; the Stickler syndrome can be classified among this group. Achondroplasia merits special attention because it is the most common of the skeletal dysplasias.

Multiple Epiphyseal Dysplasia (MED). This group of disorders is defined by disordered growth of the epiphyses of one or more pairs of joints that leads to a strong predisposition to early degenerative arthritis.

Because of diversity in clinical phenotype and inheritance pattern among affected families, MED is undoubtedly heterogeneous, but subgroups cannot be reliably differentiated. The most common form is autosomal dominant and comes to attention when a child is evaluated for short stature, abnormalities of gait, or hip pain. Occasionally the diagnosis is not made until the third or fourth decade, when degenerative arthritis of the hips, or occasionally other joints occurs.

The most characteristic radiographic features occur in epiphyses of the limbs, with mild to no involvement of the spine and a normal skull. Joints are symmetrically involved. Appearance of ossification is delayed, and the centers then become irregular or even fragmented.[61] Cone-shaped epiphyses of the metacarpals and phalanges may lead to brachydactyly and deformity of the interphalangeal joints, but surprisingly little pain or disability. The hips are nearly always affected, with abnormal ossification of the capital femoral epiphyses leading to a flattened femoral head (Fig. 85–9). The acetabulum is often affected, and protrusio acetabuli is often seen.

The differential diagnosis is usually Legg-Perthes disease, which is distinguished by being asymmetric, involving the metaphysis, sparing the acetabulum, and usually improving spontaneously. Other considerations include the spondyloepiphyseal dysplasias (especially in males, the tarda form), in which the spine is more severely affected than the limbs, and untreated hypothyroidism.

Spondyloepiphyseal Dysplasia (SED) Congenita. As the name implies, short stature and gross skeletal deformity is obvious at birth.[98] Platyspondyly contributes more to reduced height than does dysplasia of the limbs, which tends to be more severe proximally. Associated clinical features are cleft palate, pectus carinatum, kyphoscoliosis, vitreoretinal degeneration, myopia, and retinal detachment. The cervical spinal cord is vulnerable to subluxation of C1 on C2. In some respects, SED congenita is a more severe phenotype of the Stickler syndrome. The two disorders may have the same biochemical basis. As noted above, type II collagen has been implicated by linkage analysis as being defective in the Stickler syndrome,[93] and cyanogen bromide peptides of type II collagen from patients with SED congenita have shown overmodification consistent with a problem in forming the triple helix.[99] Many cases of SED congenita are sporadic, with little likelihood that the affected women will reproduce because of the significant restriction in abdominal size. Pedigrees with autosomal dominant transmission, however, suggest that most mutations that cause this disorder are heterozygous.

FIG. 85–9. Multiple epiphyseal dysplasia (MED) in father and son. Both were short of stature, the father being 153.7 cm (61.5 inches) tall. *A,* Hips in the father at 44 years of age showing advanced degenerative changes. *B,* Hips in the son at 10 years of age showing small femoral capital epiphyses and irregularities of the acetabula. *C,* Hands of the father showing brachydactyly, a short carpus, and degenerative joint disease. *D,* Hands of the son at 10 years of age showing dysplastic epiphyses and delayed development of the carpal bones. *E,* Sloping of the distal tibia is a clue to the diagnosis of MED in the adult.

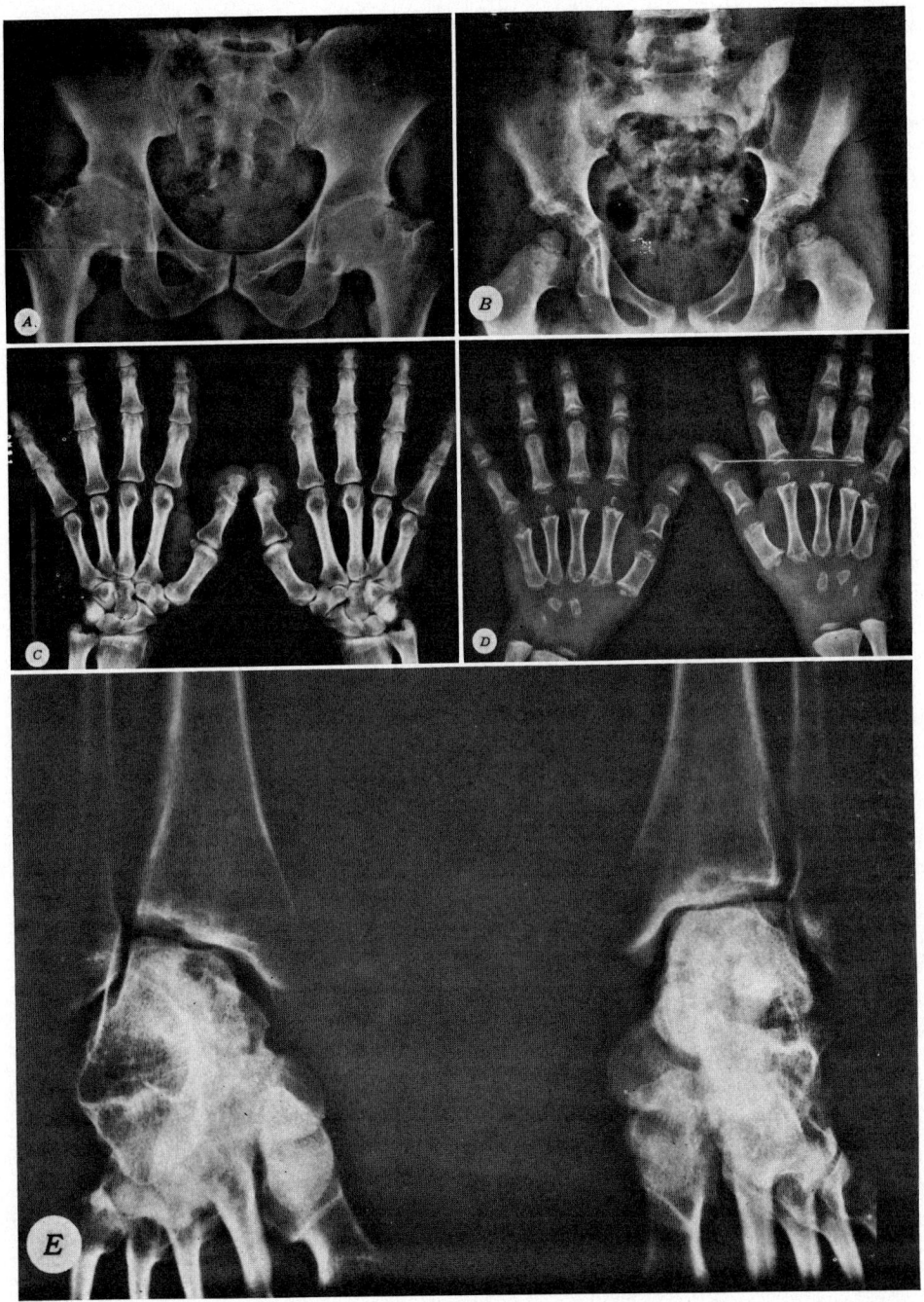

FIG. 85–9. (Cont'd)   *F*, Family pedigree, in which cases 1 and 2 are the father and son illustrated here, demonstrates typical autosomal dominant inheritance of MED.

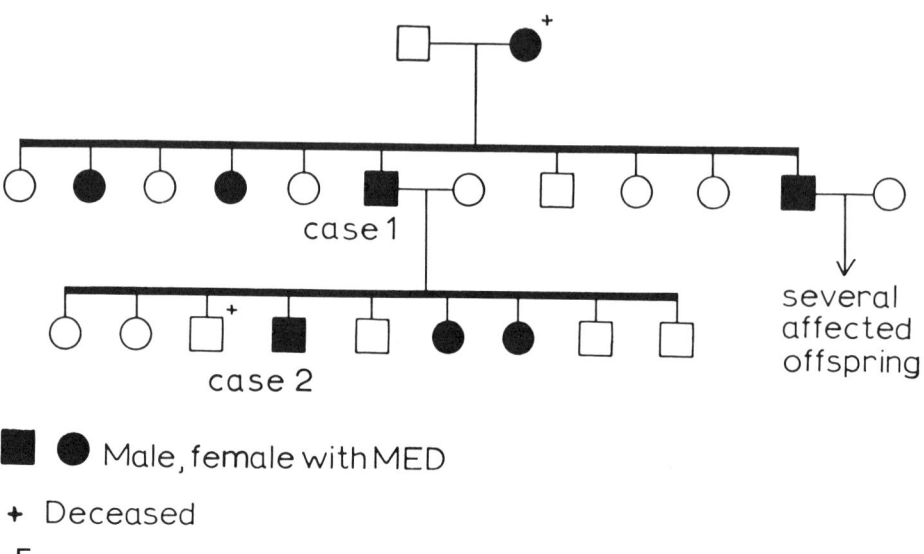

■ ● Male, female with MED

✛ Deceased

F

The radiographic features include a normal skull; platyspondyly; delayed ossification of a dysplastic odontoid; severe disorganization and delay in limb ossification centers, more severe proximally and especially so at the femoral capital epiphyses; irregular, horizontal acetabula; mild involvement of the carpus; and minimal involvement of the digits.[61] Whether two clinical subgroups can be distinguished based on the severity of coxa vara is unconfirmed.[100]

Premature degenerative arthritis can be crippling; early, aggressive realignment of the legs may have a role, but long-term followup is still in progress.

Spondyloepiphyseal Dysplasia Tarda. Although several types of late-onset SED may occur, the vast majority of patients are male and occur in pedigrees consistent with X-linked recessive inheritance.[101] The condition is often not diagnosed until degenerative arthritis develops in the shoulders and hips in late childhood or early adulthood. The radiographic findings in the femoral capital epiphyses and proximal humeral epiphyses are difficult to distinguish from MED. The spine, however, is not only more severely affected, but characteristic (Fig. 85–10).

Achondroplasia. This most common of the osteochondrodysplasias may occur as frequently as 1 per 50,000 births, and is the classic form of "short-limbed" dwarfism. In the medical literature before 1950, one has to view a diagnosis of "achondroplasia" with a healthy degree of skepticism because many conditions that affected the limbs more than the spine were so diagnosed. Achondroplasia is evident at birth,[61,103]

is heritable as an autosomal dominant trait (but most cases arise through sporadic mutation in a parental gamete), and affects other organ systems only secondarily. Midfacial hypoplasia produces a characteristic facies. General habitus and appearance are typified by rhizomelic (proximal) shortening of the limbs, flexion contractures of the elbows, bowed legs, hyperlordosis of the lumbosacral spine, and excessive body weight. Constriction on the craniocervical junction, particularly from a small foramen magnum,[104] can produce quadriparesis, sleep apnea, and sudden death in infants.[105] The entire vertebral canal is constricted, and many patients develop neurologic problems from impingement of the cord, roots, or cauda equina at ages ranging from early adolescence to late adulthood.[106,107] The entire range of neurologic complications is only partly understood.[108] Joint laxity of the shoulders and the knees can precipitate recurrent subluxation and predispose to degenerative arthritis.

The basic defect, which is not yet understood, affects enchondral bone and produces diagnostic radiographic features. The skull base is short and the face small compared to the cranium; megalencephaly is part of the syndrome[103] but may be accentuated by hydrocephalus.[108] The posterior border of the vertebrae is scalloped and the pedicles are short. In the lumbar spine, the interpedicular distance narrows caudally. In infants, a thoracolumbar gibbus is common, and if it persists, anterior vertebral wedging results. The pelvis has square ilia with horizontal ace-

FIG. 85–10. X-linked spondyloepiphyseal dysplasia tarda. *A,* Partially updated pedigree of family reported by Jacobsen.[102] *B* to *D,* Radiographic changes in the spine are progressive; the heaping up of the posterior portion of the superior vertebral plate *(B)* is particularly distinctive. At first glance, the late changes *(D)* suggest those of alkaptonuria.

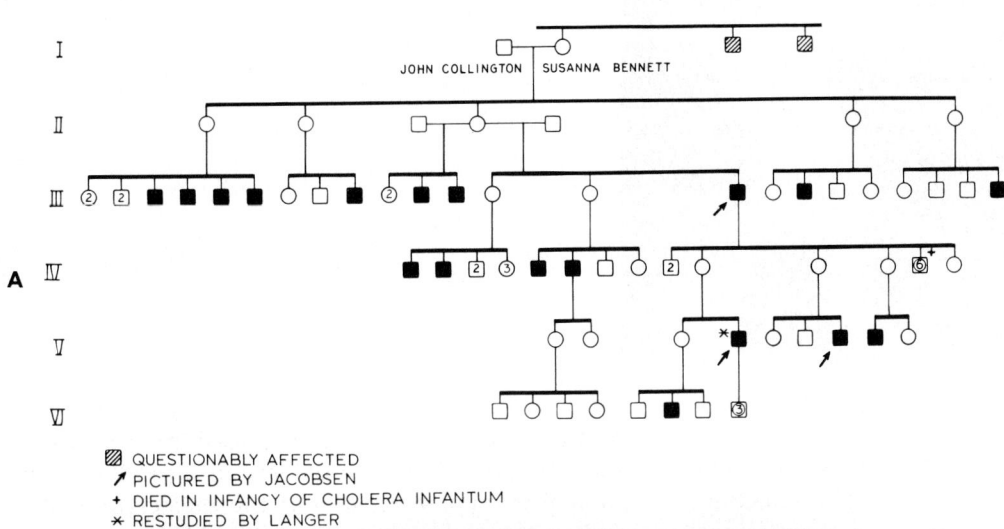

QUESTIONABLY AFFECTED
PICTURED BY JACOBSEN
+ DIED IN INFANCY OF CHOLERA INFANTUM
* RESTUDIED BY LANGER

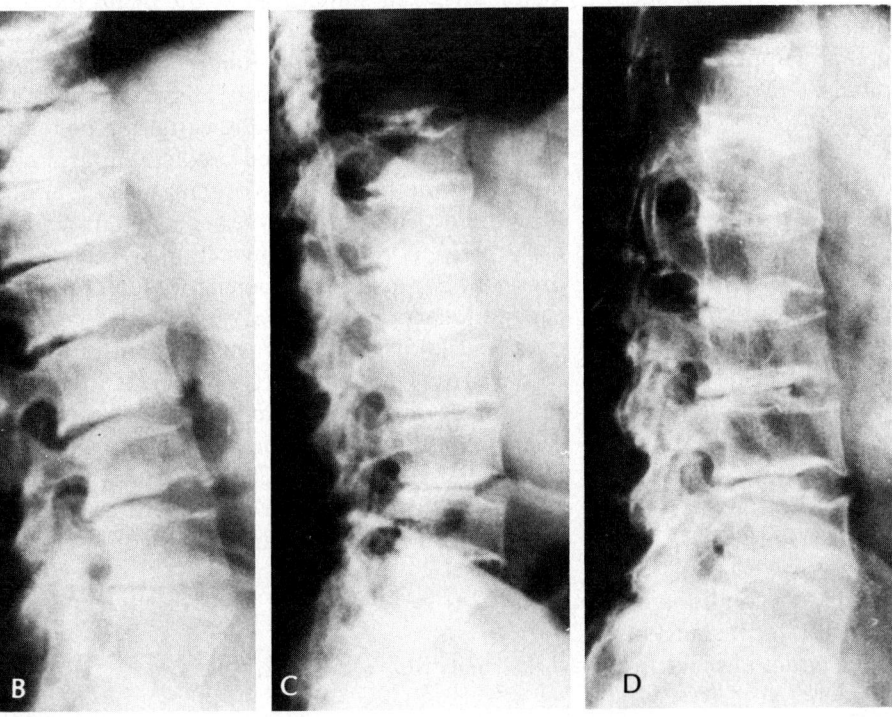

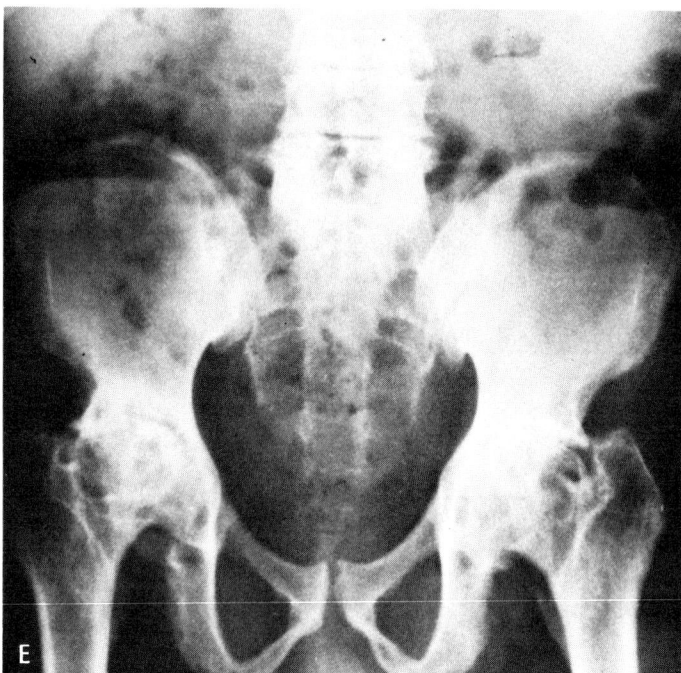

FIG. 85–10. (Cont'd) *E,* Late changes in the hips. Note the deep acetabula. (Radiographs courtesy of Dr. Leonard O. Langer, Jr., Minneapolis.)

tabular roofs and small sciatic notches. The metaphyses of the limbs are widened.[61]

Many patients benefit greatly from occupational and physical therapy, back braces, weight reduction, and various surgical procedures. Suboccipital craniectomy can be lifesaving in infancy. Straightening bowed legs can improve both gait and appearance.[109] Extended laminectomy for spinal stenosis, if performed early in the evolution of neurologic complications, can restore function.[110]

DYSOSTOSES

This group of disorders involves malformations of individual bones, either singly or in combination. Some involve primarily the cranium and face (e.g., mandibulofacial dysostosis[111]), others the spine (e.g., Klippel-Feil deformities), and others the extremities (e.g., brachydactyly, symphalangism, polydactyly, and syndactyly[112]).

Symphalangism

Harvey Cushing applied this term to a condition of hereditary ankylosis of the proximal interphalangeal joints.[113] Fusion of carpal and tarsal bones also occurs in this autosomal dominant disorder.

Camptodactyly

Limited extension of the digits is a feature of over 25 syndromes, incuding the Marfan syndrome, but occasionally is an isolated abnormality inherited as an autosomal dominant trait.[114] Permanent flexion contractures are present at the proximal interphalangeal joints without limitation of flexion, typically accompanied by hyperextension at the metacarpophalangeal joints, and sometimes at the distal interphalangeal joints. Camptodactyly may be limited to the fifth finger, or other fingers. Rarely the thumb may be involved as well, with severity decreasing in the radial direction. A contracture band can often be felt on the volar surface of the affected proximal interphalangeal joint, and the transverse skin crease is invariably absent there. Camptodactyly is present from birth or early childhood and shows little tendency to progression. Because of compensatory hyperextension at the metacarpophalangeal joints, the contracture causes little disability. As was pointed out by Archibald Garrod, camptodactyly, when it involves multiple fingers, is often accompanied by "knuckle pads," thickened skin on the dorsal aspect of the proximal interphalangeal joints.[114] Camptodactyly is sometimes confused with Dupuytren's contracture, which is late in onset and has its primary site of contracture in the palm.

IDIOPATHIC OSTEOLYSES

In the several rare heritable conditions that belong to this category,[115,116] progressive dissolution of bone occurs, with predictable debilitating and disfiguring consequences. In no case is either the cause or the pathogenesis understood.

PRIMARY METABOLIC ABNORMALITIES

In each of the disorders in this category, an inborn error disrupts metabolism of a constituent of cartilage or bone. In many cases, the constituent is also present in the connective tissue of other organs, and associated features of each syndrome may be either primary or secondary to skeletal involvement.

Mucopolysaccharidoses

The conditions in this subgroup of the heteroglycanoses are the result of inborn errors of mucopolysaccharide metabolism. Although phenotypically diverse, the individual disorders share mucopolysac-

chariduria and deposition of mucopolysaccharides in various tissues. Numerous distinct types of mucopolysaccharidoses (MPS) can be distinguished on the basis of combined phenotypic (i.e., clinical), genetic, and biochemical analysis.[117] Table 85–4 summarizes the distinctive features of each. Additional biochemical and clinical variants undoubtedly remain to be described. All these disorders are recessive, one being X-linked and the others autosomal.

Glycosaminoglycans (acid mucopolysaccharides) are the major constituents of the relatively amorphous part of the extracellular matrix that has been in the past referred to as "ground substance." The size, composition, and structure of proteoglycans vary

Table 85–4. The Genetic Mucopolysaccharidoses

Number	Eponym	Clinical Manifestations	Genetics	Urinary MPS	Enzyme-Deficient
MPS I H (25280)*	Hurler	Clouding of cornea, grave manifestations, death usually before age 10	Homozygous for MPS IH gene	Dermatan sulfate, heparan sulfate	α-L-iduronidase
MPS I S	Scheie	Stiff joints, cloudy cornea, aortic valve disease, normal intelligence and (?) lifespan	Homozygous for MPS IS gene	Dermatan sulfate, heparan sulfate	α-L-iduronidase
MPS I H/S	Hurler-Scheie	Intermediate phenotype	Genetic compound of MPS IH and MPS IS genes	Dermatan sulfate, heparan sulfate	α-L-iduronidase
MPS II-XR severe (30990)	Hunter, severe	No corneal clouding, milder course than in MPS IH, death before 15 years	Hemizygous for X-linked gene	Dermatan sulfate, heparan sulfate	Iduronate sulfatase
MPS II-XR, mild	Hunter, mild	Survival to 30s to 60s, fair intelligence	Hemizygous for X-linked allele	Dermatan sulfate, heparan sulfate	Iduronate sulfatase
MPS III A (25290)	Sanfilippo A	Indistinguishable phenotype: Mild somatic, severe central nervous system effects	Homozygous for Sanfilippo A gene	Heparan sulfate	Heparan N-sulfatase (sulfamidase)
MPS III B (25292)	Sanfilippo B		Homozygous for Sanfilippo B gene	Heparan sulfate	N-acetyl-α-D-glucosaminidase
MPS III C (25293)	Sanfilippo C		Homozygous for Sanfilippo C gene	Heparan sulfate	Acetyl-CoA: α-glucosaminide N-acetyltransferase
MPS III D (25294)	Sanfilippo D		Homozygous for Sanfilippo D gene	Heparan sulfate	N-acetylglucosamine-6-sulfate sulfatase
MPS IV A (25300)	Morquio A	Severe, distinctive bone changes, cloudy cornea, aortic regurgitation, thin enamel	Homozygous for Morquio A genes	Keratan sulfate	Galactosamine-6-sulfate sulfatase
MPS IV B (25301)	Morquio B (O'Brien-Arbisser)	Mild bone changes, cloudy cornea, hypoplastic odontoid, normal enamel	Homozygous for Morquio B gene	Keratan sulfate	β-galactosidase
MPS V	No longer used				
MPS VI, severe (25320)	Maroteaux-Lamy, classic severe	Severe osseous and corneal change; valvular heart disease, striking WBC inclusions; normal intellect; survival to 20s	Homozygous for Maroteaux-Lamy (M-L) gene	Dermatan sulfate	Arylsulfatase B (N-acetylgalactosamine 4-sulfatase)
MPS VI, intermediate	Maroteaux-Lamy, intermediate	Moderately severe changes	Homozygous for allele at M-L locus or genetic compound	Dermatan sulfate	Arylsulfatase B (N-acetylgalactosamine 4-sulfatase)
MPS VI, mild	Maroteaux-Lamy, mild	Mild osseous and corneal change, normal intellect; aortic stenosis	Homozygous for allele at M-L locus	Dermatan sulfate	Arylsulfatase B (N-acetylgalactosamine 4-sulfatase)
MPS VII (25323)	Sly	Hepatosplenomegaly dysostosis multiplex, mental retardation, WBC inclusions	Homozygous for mutant gene at β-glucuronidase locus	Dermatan sulfate, heparan sulfate	β-glucuronidase
MPS VIII (25323)	DiFerrante	Short stature, mild dysostosis multiplex, ring-shaped metachromasia of lymphocytes	Homozygous for MPS VIII gene	Keratan sulfate, heparan sulfate	Glucosamine-6-sulfate sulfatase

*Entry number in McKusick, V.A.[1]

widely in the human body (Chapter 13), but the hyaluronate backbone, core protein side chains, and link proteins that bind the glycosaminoglycan moieties are common to all. Proteoglycans, regardless of structural nuances and tissue distribution, share catabolic pathways; in particular, glycosaminoglycan degradation is largely catalyzed by lysosomal hydrolases. Thus, a deficiency of one enzyme will affect the metabolism of a variety of glycosaminoglycans in a variety of tissues and is largely responsible for the pleiotropism of the MPS disorders, that is, the diversity of phenotypic features associated with a single mutant gene. All the MPS disorders are characterized by abnormal urinary excretion of glycosaminoglycans—"mucopolysacchariduria" of dermatan sulfate, heparan sulfate, and keratan sulfate—which is useful in screening and specific diagnosis.

Mucopolysacchariduria can be identified by one of several standard screening tests, at least one of which is part of the standard battery performed when a "metabolic screen" is ordered. Fractionation and characterization of the urinary mucopolysaccharides are useful in separating the several types of MPS. For example, MPS III (Sanfilippo syndrome—the heparan sulfate excretors) and MPS IV (Morquio syndrome—the keratan sulfate excretors) in young subjects may be distinguished from the other types, especially MPS IH (Hurler syndrome—dermatan sulfate excretors), mainly by chemical analysis.

Studies with radioactive sulfate indicate accumulation of label in cultured fibroblasts and delayed washout, compatible with the conclusion that these disorders are due to a degradative defect. The specific lysosomal enzyme deficient in each is now known (see Table 85–4). Like other lysosomal disorders, MPS have six distinctive characteristics:

1. Intracellular storage of material occurs.
2. The storage material is heterogeneous because the degradative enzymes are not strictly specific, for example, in MPS IH, ganglioside is deposited in brain and predominantly mucopolysaccharide in the liver, and two glycosaminoglycans are excreted in the urine.
3. Deposition is vacuolar, that is, membrane-bound, when viewed with the electron microscope.
4. Many tissues are affected.
5. The disorder is clinically progressive.
6. Replacement therapy is at least theoretically possible, through replacing the missing enzyme by the process of endocytosis.

The possibility of replacement therapy in MPS is more than theoretic. Normal cells or the medium in which they have grown, when mixed with MPS fibroblasts, correct the metabolic defect.[118] This finding indicates the production of a diffusible correction factor by normal cells, which is found also in normal urine. The correction factor is the enzyme specially deficient in the given disorder. Several trials of enzyme replacement therapy, by plasma exchange and fibroblast transplantation, have been attended by limited success, however, particularly in reversing established neurologic defects.[119]

Bone marrow transplantation has been used in patients with MPS disorders that do and do not affect the brain.[120,121] In either case, some improvement in somatic features (such as corneal clouding and joint stiffness) may occur, but mental retardation or other severe neurologic problems have been resistant to the presence of enzyme in the bloodstream. Also at this time, the complications of bone marrow transplantation, particularly graft versus host disease, preclude early intervention with this method when prevention of somatic features, rather than their reversal, might be possible.

The differential features of MPS are summarized in Table 85–4, and the clinical features of MPS IH, MPS IS, and MPS II are illustrated in Figures 85–11, 85–12, and 85–13, respectively. The nosologic validity of this classification is supported by the findings of coculti-

FIG. 85–11. Mucopolysaccharidosis IH (Hurler syndrome) in a 2-year-old girl. Note the coarse facial features, prominent abdomen from hepatosplenomegaly, claw hands, and short stature. The joints generally had moderate restriction of motion. The patient died of congestive heart failure at 12 years of age.

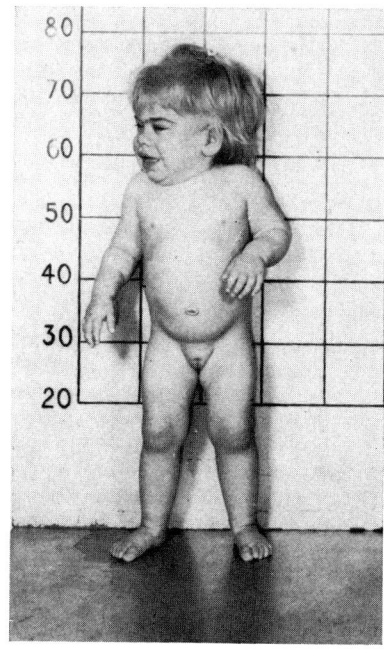

FIG. 85–12. Mucopolysaccharidosis IS (Scheie syndrome) in a 54-year-old attorney. *A*, Clouding of the cornea was densest peripherally. *B*, The hands were clawed; atrophy of the lateral aspect of the thenar eminences indicated carpal tunnel compression.

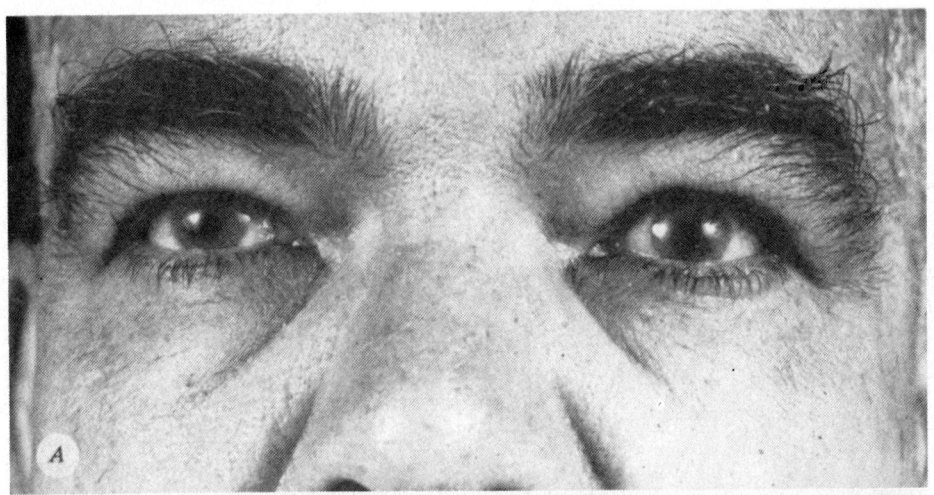

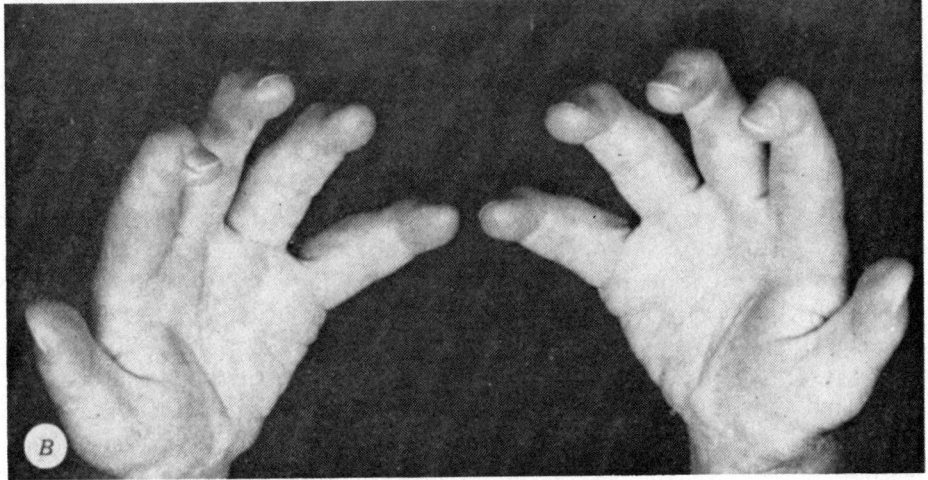

vation of fibroblasts. Mutual correction of their metabolic defects occurs when fibroblasts from MPS I and MPS II, MPS I and MPS III, and other combinations are mixed. Failure of cross-correction between cultured fibroblasts of two patients indicates that they have the same enzyme deficiency, and that the mutations underlying them at a minimum are allelic, if not identical.[117]

MPS V does not exist in the present classification. It was previously the numeric designation for the Scheie syndrome, a disorder distinct clinically from the other MPS (Fig. 85–12). In vitro studies, however, showed no cross-correction between Hurler and Scheie fibroblasts, and the same enzyme, α-L-iduronidase, was subsequently found deficient in the two disorders.[122] Our interpretation is that the Hurler and Scheie syndromes are due to homozygosity for two

different mutations at the gene locus determining the structure of α-L-iduronidase. Thus, both are designated MPS I. The Hurler syndrome, MPS IH, is analogous to hemoglobin SS disease, a severe disorder, and the Scheie syndrome, MPS IS, to hemoglobin CC disease, a mild disorder. If the notion that MPS IH and MPS IS are due to allelic genes is correct, then a Hurler-Scheie genetic compound comparable to SC disease should exist. Indeed, patients with phenotypic features intermediate to MPS IH and MPS IS have been identified and are designated MPS IH/S. Some are likely true genetic compounds, whereas others are likely homozygotes (because of parental consanguinity) for other mutant alleles at the α-L-iduronidase locus.[123] Allelic forms of MPS II and MPS VI presumably account for the severe and mild forms of those disorders.

FIG. 85–13. Mucopolysaccharidosis II, mild (the Hunter syndrome, mild variant) in brothers, 7 and 6 years of age. Note the short stature, coarse facies, prominent abdomen, and clawed hands. Intellect was normal.

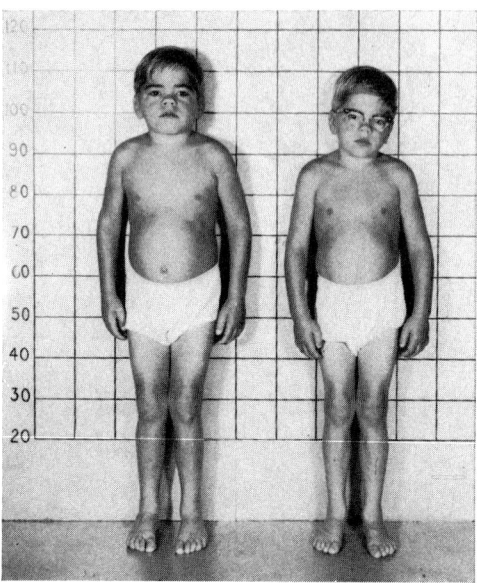

Skeletal Features. Relative short stature is the rule in all patients with the MPS disorders, and can be profound in MPS IH. MPS II, MPS IV (the Morquio syndrome being the prototype "short trunk" form of dwarfism), and MPS VI. Radiographically, the skeletal dysplasia is similar in character in all but MPS IV, differing among the others largely in severity. The term dysostosis multiplex has been applied, but is not specific for MPS, similar changes occurring in a variety of storage disorders. The chief radiographic features are a thick calvaria, an enlarged J-shaped sella turcica, a short and wide mandible, biconvex vertebral bodies, hypoplasia of the odontoid, broad ribs, short and thick clavicles, coxa valga, metacarpals with widened diaphyses and pointed proximal ends, and short phalanges.[61]

For the disorders compatible with survival to adulthood without severe retardation (MPS IS, MPS II mild, MPS IV, MPS VI), progressive arthropathy and transverse myelopathy secondary to C1-C2 subluxation account for considerable disability. Cervical fusion should be considered whenever upper motor neuron signs appear. Joint replacement, particularly of the hips, has been beneficial in MPS IS.[124]

Stiff joints are a more or less striking feature of all forms except MPS IV. Like other somatic features, such as coarse facies, reduced joint mobility is less striking in MPS III. In the Scheie syndrome, stiff hands, together with clouding of the cornea, lead to

the main disability. In that condition, as in the others, carpal tunnel syndrome contributes to the disability. Early decompression can be beneficial.

Regardless of the presence or severity of mental retardation or of the average life span, the major causes of death have as their pathogenesis the accumulation of glycosaminoglycan in soft tissues. The myocardium, cardiac valves, and coronary arteries are prime sites, and death from cardiac failure secondary to restrictive cardiopathy, severe valvular disease, or myocardial infarction is common (but often unrecognized) in MPS IH and MPS IIA.[29] Infiltration of the oropharynx and middle airways progresses to cause major clinical problems in most patients who survive cardiac disease.[125,126] When attempting any procedure that requires sedation or anesthesia in a patient with an MPS disorder, maximal precautions to protect the airway must be employed. If possible, procedures should be performed under local anesthetic. Intubation of the airway should be attempted only after careful assessment of the anatomy, and with full respect for the possibility of atlantoaxial instability.

Phosphotransferase Deficiencies

Mucolipidosis II (ML II) is also called I-cell disease (because of conspicuous inclusions in cultured cells). Mucolipidosis III (ML III) is also called pseudo-Hurler polydystrophy. Neither shows mucopolysacchariduria despite lysosomal storage of mucopolysaccharide and a demonstrable defect in degradation of mucopolysaccharides. Both are inherited as autosomal recessive conditions and some forms are likely allelic. The basic biochemical defect rests with an enzyme. UDP-N-acetylglucosamine:lysosomal enzyme, N-acetylglucosaminylphosphotransferase, responsible for posttranslational modification of lysosomal enzymes.[127] This defect results in multiple enzyme deficiencies and accumulation in tissues of both mucopolysaccharides and mucolipids.

ML II is a severe Hurler-like disorder. ML III is a distinctive disorder with stiff joints, cloudy cornea, carpal tunnel syndrome, short stature, coarse facies, and sometimes mild mental retardation, compatible with survival to adulthood[128] (Fig. 85–14).

Mannosidosis

Deficiency of α-mannosidase, one of the many acid hydrolases found in lysosomes, causes phenotypic abnormalities of widely varying severity. Males and females are affected with equal frequency, and parents of patients have reduced levels of α-mannosidase, both features of autosomal recessive inheritance. Although the clinical conditions were initially thought to be limited to a severe and a mild form

FIG. 85–14. Mucolipidosis III (pseudo-Hurler polydystrophy) in a 6-year-old girl. *A*, Note the short stature and coarse facies. The corneas were clouded, motion of all joints was restricted, a murmur of aortic regurgitation was present, and intellect was mildly deficient. *B* and *C*, The hands were clawed, and atrophy of the thenar eminences indicated carpal tunnel compression, for which operation was performed at 13 years of age, with some benefit.

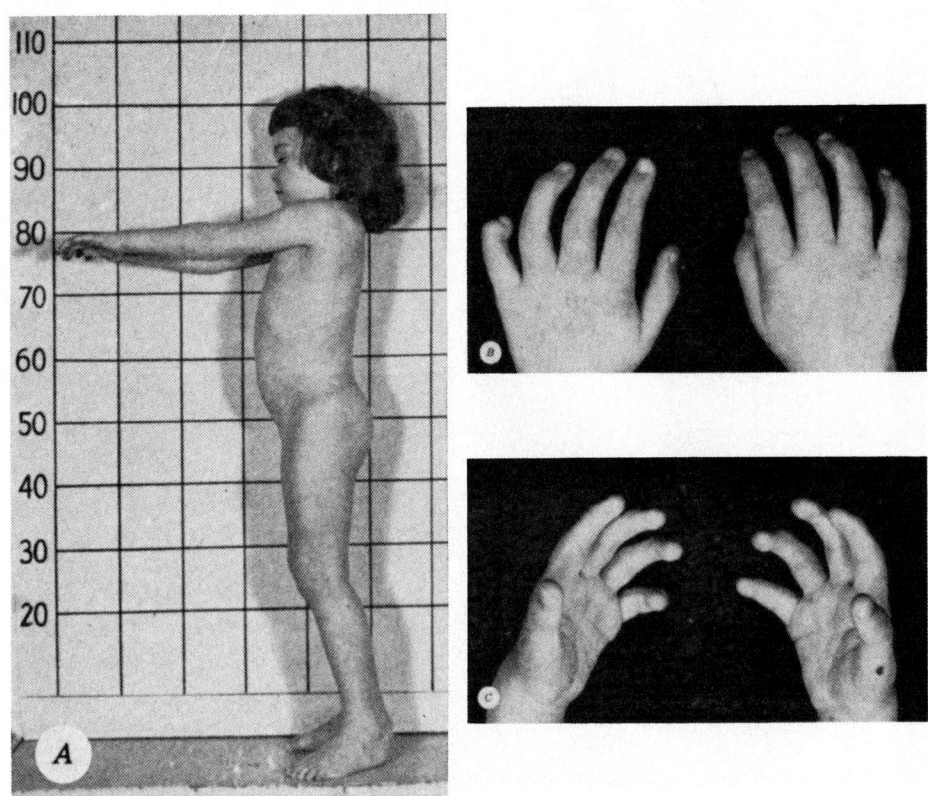

(labeled types I and II), enough variation has been described to suggest a spectrum of phenotypes, presumably caused by an allelic series of mutations.[129,130]

The most severe phenotype resembles the Hurler syndrome (MPS IH) in terms of coarse facial features, short stature, mental and motor retardation, hepatomegaly, and skeletal changes of dysostosis multiplex. Patients with severe mannosidosis have typical spoke-like posterior cataracts and lymphocytes with clear cytoplasmic vacuoles, however. Death in infancy from recurrent respiratory infections is common.[131] At the other end of the phenotypic continuum, patients may not be diagnosed until adulthood, have mild coarsening of facies, clear corneas, IQs in the borderline normal range, and joint hypermobility; they come to medical attention because of degenerative arthritis of the hips or cardiac problems similar to those described in the mucopolysaccharidoses.[130,132]

The diagnosis is suggested by screening urine for oligosaccharides and confirmed by documenting de-

creased activity of α-mannosidase in cultured fibroblasts.

OTHER DISORDERS THAT SIMULATE ARTHRITIDES

Hypophosphatemic Bone Disease. At least three distinct hereditary disorders have short stature, bowed legs, and reduced serum phosphate as cardinal features. The autosomal dominant and recessive forms are uncommon; the former responds to (hydroxycholecalciferol) 1,25-$(OH)_2D_3$ supplementation and the latter to oral phosphate.

Rickets has largely been eliminated as a medical concern because of supplementation of the diet with vitamin D and exposure to sunlight. As a result, the cases that are seen are highly likely to have a genetic basis. Fuller Albright and colleagues[133] described the first instance of a patient with rickets who responded

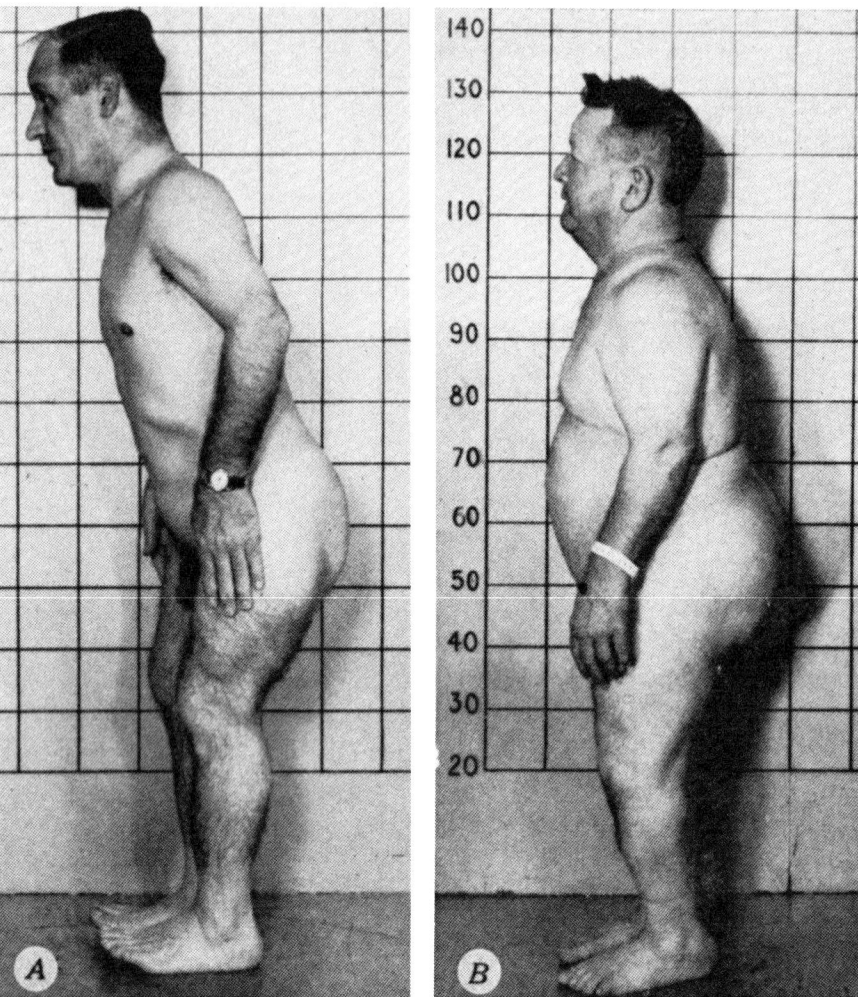

FIG. 85–15. Ankylosing arthropathy in two men with vitamin D–resistant rickets. *A*, 41-year-old man. *B*, 61-year-old man. The younger man is the more severely affected, but both have almost complete ankylosis of the spine and similar changes in some peripheral joints. Note the short stature.

only to supraphysiologic doses of vitamin D. This condition, now termed *familial hypophosphatemic rickets* or vitamin D–resistant rickets, is inherited as an X-linked dominant trait. Males and females both have reduced renal tubular reabsorption of phosphate that results in hypophosphatemia; however, serum calcium remains normal and patients do not develop muscle weakness or tetany. The skeletal features, which are more severe in males (Fig. 85–15), are those of rickets and osteomalacia. In infancy and childhood, the epiphyses are broad and the metaphyses cupped; the epiphyses fuse early, the limbs bow, and the endplates of the vertebrae become sclerotic; in adults, generalized bony sclerosis, scoliosis, protrusio acetabuli, and spinal stenosis from calcification of the ligamentum flavum are features.[61] Therapy with both oral phosphate and vitamin D can prevent skeletal changes.

Fibrodysplasia Ossificans Progressiva. This disorder, formerly called myositis ossificans progressiva and commonly abbreviated FOP, is uncommon and its biochemical defect is unknown. Characterized by

progressive ossification of ligaments, tendons, and aponeuroses, FOP begins an inexorable, progressive course in the first year or so of life, usually with a seemingly inflammatory process and nodule formation on the back of the thorax, neck, or scalp. Local heat, as well as leukocytosis and elevated sedimentation rate, is observed at this stage. Acute rheumatic fever is sometimes diagnosed. A valuable clue to the correct diagnosis is a short great toe with or without a short thumb; this is the leading cause of congenital hallux valgus.[134]

Most cases of this autosomal dominant disorder are the consequence of new mutation. Life expectancy is considerably reduced, with progressive restriction in lung capacity contributing to respiratory insufficiency and terminal pneumonia.[135]

Arthrogryposis Multiplex Congenita (AMC). The syndrome of congenital rigidity of multiple joints is of complex etiology, pathogenesis, and phenotype.[136,137] In many instances, the disorder is a deformation of joints resulting from immobilization of the developing fetus, so that the proper stimulus for joint develop-

FIG. 85–15. (Cont'd) *C,* Lateral radiograph of the lower spine in the older patient. *D,* Left femur of the younger patient. Pseudofractures were situated symmetrically in the subtrochanteric area of both femurs. *E,* Pelvis of the 41-year-old patient.

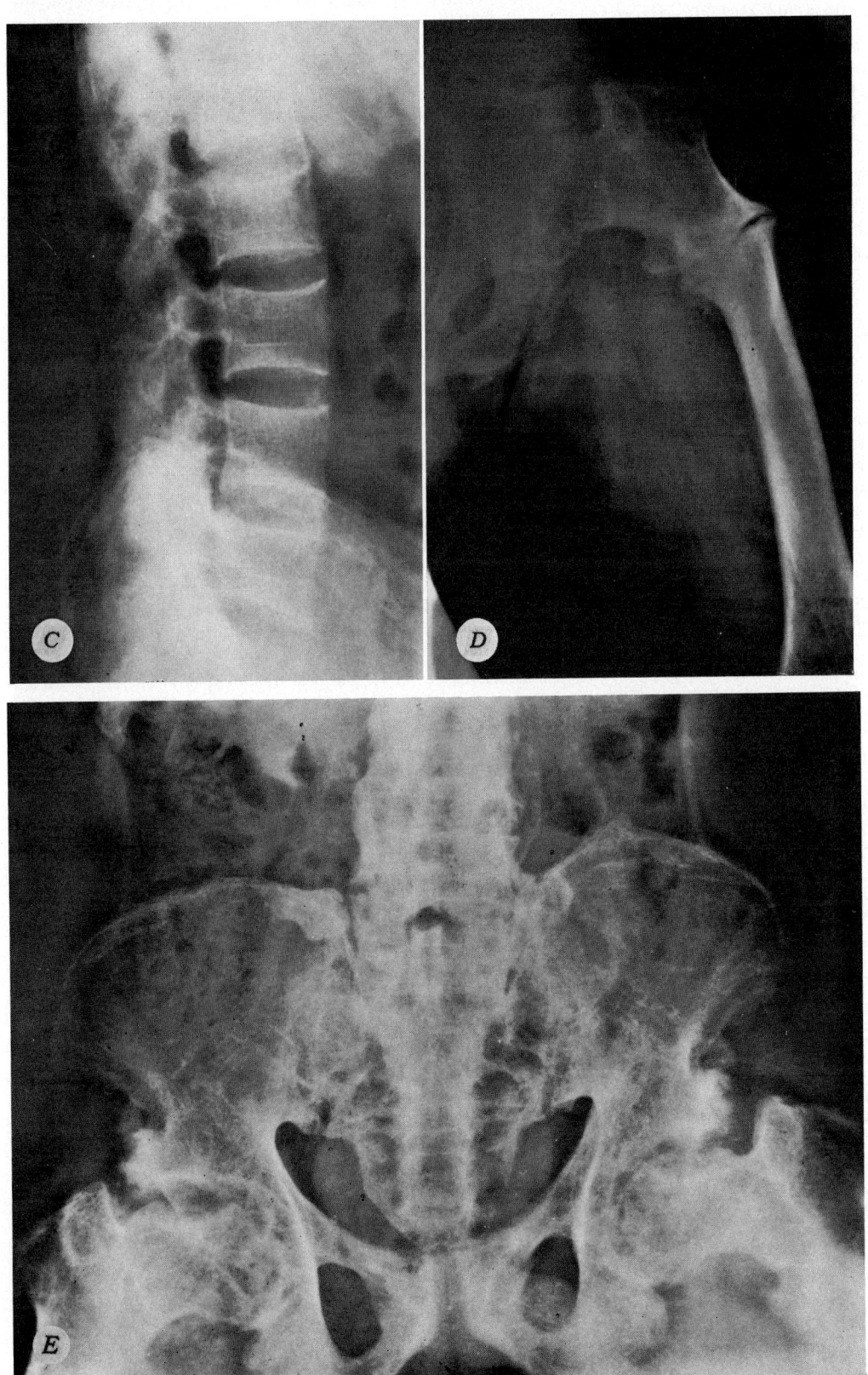

ment is lacking.[136,138] The cause of the immobilization may be a prenatal disorder of the brain, spinal cord, peripheral nerves, vasculature, or muscle. The affected baby is born with the arms and legs fixed in postures dictated by the position of the embryo and fetus in development. In addition to joint rigidity, dislocation of the hips and micrognathia are frequent findings. The Drachman theory of fetal immobilization as the "cause" of AMC was developed from studies of the effects of neuromuscular blocking agents on chick embryos. His theory is supported by observation of AMC in an infant born of a mother who received tubocurarine in early pregnancy for treatment of tetanus.[136]

REFERENCES

1. McKusick, V.A.: Mendelian Inheritance in Man. Catalogs of Autosomal Dominant, Autosomal Recessive and X-linked Phenotypes, 7th Ed. Baltimore, Johns Hopkins Press, 1986.
2. De Grouchy, J., and Turleau, C.: Clinical Atlas of Human Chromosomes. 2nd Ed. New York, John Wiley, 1984.
3. Cavenee, W.K., et al.: Prediction of familial predisposition to retinoblastoma. N. Engl. J. Med., 314:1201–1207, 1986.
4. Tommerup, N., and Nielsen, F.: A familial reciprocal translocation t(3;7)(p21.1;p13) associated with the Grieg polysyndactyly-craniofacial anomalies syndrome. Am. J. Med. Genet., 16:313–321, 1983.
5. Holmes, L.B.: Inborn errors of morphogenesis: A review of localized hereditary malformations. N. Engl. J. Med., 291:763–773, 1974.
6. Emery, A., and Rimoin, D.L.: Principles and Practice of Medical Genetics. London, Churchill Livingstone, 1983.
7. Vogel, F., and Motulsky, A.G.: Human Genetics, 2nd Ed. New York, Springer-Verlag, 1986.
8. McKusick, V.A.: The cardiovascular aspects of Marfan's syndrome: A heritable disorder of connective tissue. Circulation, 11:321–342, 1955.
9. Beighton, P., et al.: Classification of the heritable disorders of connective tissue. Am. J. Med. Genet., 29, 1988 (in press).
10. Rimoin, D.L.: International nomenclature of constitutional diseases of bone with bibliography. Birth Defects, 15(10):30, 1979.
11. Furthmayr, H. (ed.): Immunology of the Extracellular Matrix. Boca Raton, CRC Press, 1982.
12. Fleishmajer, R., Olsen, B.R., and Kuch, K. (eds.): Biology, Chemistry, and Pathology of Collagen. New York, New York Academy of Sciences, 1985.
13. Prockop, D.J., and Kivirikko, K.L.: Heritable diseases of collagen. N. Engl. J. Med., 311:376–386, 1984.
14. Prockop, D.J.: Mutations in collagen genes. Consequences for rare and common diseases. J. Clin. Invest., 75:783–787, 1985.
15. Pyeritz, R.E.: Heritable defects in connective tissue. Hosp. Pract., 22:153–168, 1987.
16. Holbrook. K.A., and Byers, P.H.: Structural abnormalities in the dermal collagen and elastic matrix from the skin of patients with inherited tissue disorders. J. Invest. Dermatol., 79:7s, 1982.
17. Uitto, J., et al.: Elastin in diseases. J. Invest. Dermatol., 79:160s–168s, 1982.
18. Sandberg, L.B., Soskel, N.T., and Leslie, J.G.: Elastin structure, biosynthesis, and relation to disease states. N. Engl. J. Med., 304:566–579, 1981.
19. Pyeritz, R.E., and McKusick, V.A.: The Marfan syndrome: Diagnosis and management. N. Engl. J. Med., 300:772–777, 1979.
20. Pyeritz, R.E.: The diagnosis and management of the Marfan syndrome. Am. Fam. Physician, 34:83–94, 1987.
21. Perejda, A.J., et al.: Marfan's syndrome: Structural, biochemical, and mechanical studies of the aortic media. J. Lab. Clin. Med., 106:376–383, 1985.
22. Halme, T., et al.: The borohydride-reducible compounds of human aortic elastin. Biochem. J., 232:169–175, 1985.
23. Sakai, L.Y., Keene, D.R., and Engvall, E.: Fibrillin, a new 350-kD glycoprotein, is a component of extracellular microfibrils. J. Cell Biol., 103:2499–2509, 1986.
24. Hollister, D.W., Sakai, I.Y., and Pyeritz, R.E.: Marfan syndrome: Abnormality of the microfibrillar array. Clin. Res., 35:211A, 1987.
25. Pyeritz, R.E., and McKusick, V.A.: Basic defects in the Marfan syndrome (editorial). N. Engl. J. Med., 305:1011–1012, 1981.
26. Beals, R.K., and Hecht, F.: Congenital contractural arachnodactyly: A heritable disorder of connective tissue. J. Bone Joint Surg., 53A:987–993, 1971.
27. Gruber, M.A., et al.: Marfan syndrome with contractural arachnodactyly and severe mitral regurgitation in a premature infant. J. Pediatr., 93:80–82, 1978.
28. Walker, B.A., Beighton, P.H., and Murdoch, J.L.: The marfanoid hypermobility syndrome. Ann. Intern. Med., 71:349–352, 1969.
29. Pyeritz, R.E.: Cardiovascular manifestations of heritable disorders of connective tissue. Prog. Med. Genet., 5:191–302, 1983.
30. Gott, V.I., et al.: Surgical treatment of aneurysm of the ascending aorta in the Marfan syndrome: Results of composite repair in 50 patients. N. Engl. J. Med., 314:1070–1074, 1986.
31. Crawford, E.S.: Marfan's syndrome: Broad spectral surgical treatment of cardiovascular manifestations. Ann. Surg., 198:487–505, 1983.
32. Hall, J., Pyeritz, R.E., Dudgeon, D.L., and Haller, J.A., Jr.: Pneumothorax in the Marfan syndrome: Prevalence and therapy. Ann. Thorac. Surg., 37:500–504, 1984.
33. Pyeritz, R.E., Murphy, E.A., Lin, S.J., and Rosell, E.M.: Growth and anthropometrics in the Marfan syndrome. In Endocrine Genetics and Genetics of Growth. Edited by C.J. Papadatos and C.S. Bartsocas. New York, A.R. Liss, 1985, pp. 355–366.
34. McKusick, V.A.: Heritable Disorders of Connective Tissue, 9th Ed. St. Louis, C.V. Mosby Co., 1972.
35. Mudd, S.H., and Levy, H.L.: Disorders of trans-sulfuration. In The Metabolic Basis of Inherited Disease. Edited by J.B. Stanbury, et al. New York, McGraw-Hill Book Co., 1983, pp. 522–559.
36. Abbott, M.H., Folstein, S.E., Abbey, H., and Pyeritz, R.E.: Psychiatric manifestations of homocystinuria due to cystathionine beta-synthase deficiency. Am. J. Med. Genet., 26:959–969, 1987.
37. Mudd, S.H., et al.: The natural history of homocystinuria due to cystathionine beta-synthase deficiency. Am. J. Hum. Genet., 36:1–31, 1985.
38. Valle, D., et al.: Homocystinuria due to cystathionine beta-synthase deficiency: Clinical manifestations and therapy. Johns Hopkins Med. J., 146:110–117, 1980.
39. Hill-Zobel, R.L., et al.: Kinetics and biodistribution of [111]In-

labeled platelets in homocystinuria. N. Engl. J. Med., *307*:781–786, 1982.

40. Kloepfer, H.W., and Rosenthal, J.W.: Possible genetic carriers in the spherophakia-brachymorphia syndrome. Am. J. Hum. Genet., *7*:398–425, 1955.

41. Cupo, L.N., et al.: Ehlers-Danlos syndrome with abnormal collagen fibrils, sinus of Valsalva aneurysms, myocardial infarction, panacinar emphysema, and cerebral heterotopias. Am. J. Med., *71*:1051–1058, 1981.

42. Pinnell, S.R.: Molecular defects in the Ehlers-Danlos syndome. J. Invest. Dermatol., *798*:90s–92s, 1982.

43. Hollister, D.W.: Heritable disorders of connective tissue: Ehlers-Danlos syndrome. Pediatr. Clin. North Am., *25*:575–591, 1978.

44. Beighton, P.: The Ehlers-Danlos Syndrome. London, William Heinemann Medical Books Ltd., 1970.

45. Pyeritz, R.E., Stolle, C.A., Parfrey, N.A., and Myers, J.C.: Ehlers-Danlos syndrome IV due to a novel defect in type III procollagen. Am. J. Med. Genet., *19*:607–622, 1984.

46. Byers, P.H., et al.: Clinical and ultrastructural heterogeneity of type IV Ehlers-Danlos syndrome. Hum. Genet., *47*:141–150, 1979.

47. Stolle, C.A., Pyeritz, R.E., Myers, J.C., and Prockop, D.J.: Synthesis of an altered type III procollagen in a patient with type IV Ehlers-Danlos syndrome. A structural change in the alpha 1(III) chain which makes the protein more susceptible to proteinases. J. Biol. Chem., *260*:1937–1944, 1985.

48. Beighton, P.: X-linked recessive inheritance in the Ehlers-Danlos syndrome. Br. Med. J., *2*:9–11, 1968.

49. Beighton, P., and Curtis, D.: X-linked Ehlers-Danlos syndrome type V: The next generation. Clin. Genet., *27*:472–478, 1985.

50. Krane, S.M., Pinnell, S.R., and Erbe, R.W.: Lyso-protocollagen hydroxylase deficiency in fibroblasts from siblings with hydroxylysine deficient collagen. Proc. Natl. Acad. Sci. U.S.A., *69*:2899–2903, 1972.

51. Elsas, L.J., II, Miller, R.L., and Pinnell, S.R.: Inherited human collagen lysyl hydroxylase deficiency: Ascorbic acid response. J. Pediatr., *92*:378–384, 1978.

52. Hass, J., and Hass, R.: Arthrochalasis multiplex congenita: Congenital flaccidity of the joints. J. Bone Joint Surg., *40A*:663–674, 1958.

53. Lichtenstein, J.R., et al.: Defect in conversion of procollagen to collagen in a form of Ehlers-Danlos syndrome. Science, *182*:298, 1973.

54. Steinmann, B., et al.: Evidence for a structural mutation of procollagen type I in a patient with the Ehlers-Danlos syndrome type VII. J. Biol. Chem., *155*:8887–8893, 1980.

55. Arneson, M.A., et al.: A new form of Ehlers-Danlos syndrome: Fibronectin corrects defective platelet function. JAMA, *244*:144–147, 1980.

56. Kirk, J.A., Ansell, B.M., and Bywaters, F.G.L.: The hypermobility syndrome: Musculoskeletal complaints associated with generalized joint hypermobility. Ann. Rheum. Dis., *26*:419–425, 1967.

57. Wynne-Davies, R.: Acetabular dysplasia and familial joint laxity: Two etiologic factors in congenital dislocation of the hip. J. Bone Joint Surg., *52B*:704–716, 1970.

58. Horton, W.A., et al.: Familial joint instability syndrome. Am. J. Med. Genet., *6*:221–228, 1980.

59. Latta, R.J., et al.: Larsen's syndrome: A skeletal dysplasia with multiple joint dislocations and unusual facies. J. Pediatr., *78*:291, 1971.

60. Trigueros, A.P., Vazquez, J.L.V., and De Miguel, G.F.D.: Lar-

sen's syndrome: Report of three cases in one family, mother and two offspring. Acta Orthop. Scand., *49*:582–588, 1978.

61. Wynne-Davies, R., Hall, C.M., and Apley, A.G.: Atlas of Skeletal Dysplasias. Edinburgh, Churchill Livingstone, 1985.

62. Sconyers. S.M., et al.: A distinct chondrodysplasia resembling Kniest dysplasia: Clinical, roentgenographic, histologic, and ultrastructural findings. J. Pediatr., *103*:898–904, 1983.

63. Smith, R., Francis, M.J.O., and Houghton, G.R.: The Brittle Bone Syndrome. London, Butterworth, 1983.

64. Sillence, D.O.: Osteogenesis imperfecta: An expanding panorama of variants. Clin. Orthop., *159*:11–25, 1981.

65. Levin, L.S., Salinas, C.F., and Jorgenson, R.J.: Classification of osteogenesis imperfecta by dental characteristics. Lancet, *1*:332–333, 1978.

66. Sillence, D.O., Senn, A., and Danks, D.M.: Genetic heterogeneity in osteogenesis imperfecta. J. Med. Genet., *16*:101–116, 1979.

67. Paterson, C.R., McAllion, S., and Miller, R.: Heterogeneity of osteogenesis imperfecta type I. J. Med. Genet., *20*:203–205, 1983.

68. Rowe, D.W., Shapiro, J.R., Poirier, M., and Schlesinger, S.: Diminished type I collagen synthesis and reduced alpha 1(I) collagen messenger RNA in cultured fibroblasts from patients with dominantly inherited (type I) osteogenesis imperfecta. J. Clin. Invest., *76*:604–611, 1985.

69. Sillence, D.O., et al.: Osteogenesis imperfecta type II. Delineation of the phenotype with reference to genetic heterogeneity. Am. J. Med. Genet., *17*:407–423, 1984.

70. Cohn, D.H., et al.: Lethal osteogenesis imperfecta resulting from a single nucleotide change in one human pro alpha 1(I) collagen allele. Proc. Natl. Acad. Sci. U.S.A., *83*:6045–6057, 1986.

71. Sillence, D.O., et al.: Osteogenesis imperfecta type III. Delineation of the phenotype with reference to genetic heterogeneity. Am. J. Med. Genet., *23*:821–832, 1986.

72. Paterson, C.R., McAllion, S., and Miller, R.: Osteogenesis imperfecta with dominant inheritance and normal sclerae. J. Bone Joint Surg., *65B*:35–39, 1983.

73. Tsipouras, P., et al.: Molecular heterogeneity in the mild autosomal dominant forms of osteogenesis imperfecta. Am. J. Hum. Genet., *36*:1172–1179, 1984.

74. Bergstrom, L.V.: Fragile bones and fragile ears. Clin. Orthop., *159*:58–63, 1981.

75. Levin, L.S.: The dentition in the osteogenesis imperfecta syndromes. Clin. Orthop., *159*:64, 1981.

76. Pyeritz, R.E., and Levin, L.S.: Aortic root dilatation and valvular dysfunction in osteogenesis imperfecta. Circulation, *64*:IV-311, 1981.

77. White, N.J., Winearls, C.G., and Smith, R.: Cardiovascular abnormalities in osteogenesis imperfecta. Am. Heart J., *106*:1416–1420, 1983.

78. Hortop, J., et al.: Cardiovascular involvement in osteogenesis imperfecta. Circulation, *73*:54–61, 1986.

79. Dent, C.E., and Friedman, M.: Idiopathic juvenile osteoporosis. Q. J. Med., *34*:177–210, 1965.

80. Neuhauser, G., Kaveggia, E.G., and Opitz, J.M.: Autosomal recessive syndrome of pseudogliomatous blindness, osteoporosis, and mild mental retardation. Clin. Genet., *9*:324–332, 1976.

81. Weleber, R.G., and Beals, R.K.: The Hadju-Cheney syndrome. J. Pediatr., *88*:243–249, 1976.

82. Meredith, S.C., Simon, M.A., Laros, G.S., and Jackson, M.A.: Pycnodysostosis: A clinical pathological, and ultramicroscopic study of a case. J. Bone Joint Surg., *60A*:1122–1128, 1978.

83. Rasmussen, H.: Hypophosphatasia. *In* The Metabolic Basis of Inherited Disease. Edited by J.B. Stanbury, et al. New York, McGraw-Hill Book Co., 1983, pp. 1497–1507.

84. Herrmann, J., et al.: The Stickler syndrome (hereditary arthro-ophthalmopathy). Birth Defects, *11*:76–103, 1975.

85. Liberfarb, R.M., Hirose, T., and Holmes, L.B.: The Wagner-Stickler syndrome: A study of 22 families. J. Pediatr., *99*:394–399, 1981.

86. Shprintzen, R.J., Siegel-Sadewitz, V.L., Amato, J., and Goldberg, R.B.: Anomalies associated with cleft lip, cleft palate, or both. Am. J. Med. Genet., *20*:585–595, 1985.

87. Wagner, H.: Ein bischer unbekanntes Erbleiden des Auges (Degeneratio hyaloideo-retinalis hereditaria) beobachtet im Kanton Zurich. Klin. Monatsbl. Augenheilkd., *100*:840–857, 1938.

88. Marshall, D.: Ectodermal dysplasia: Report of kindred with ocular abnormalities and hearing defect. Am. J. Ophthalmol., *45*:143–156, 1958.

89. Ayme, S., and Preus, M.: The Marshall and Stickler syndromes: Objective rejection of lumping. J. Med. Genet., *21*:34–38, 1984.

90. Baraitser, M.: Marshall/Stickler syndrome. J. Med. Genet., *19*:139–140, 1982.

91. Winter, R.M., et al.: The Weissenbacher-Zweymüller, Stickler, and Marshall syndromes: Further evidence for their identity. Am. J. Med. Genet., *16*:189–199, 1983.

92. Kelley, T.E., Wells, H.H., and Tuck, K.B.: The Weissenbacher-Zweymüller syndrome: Possible neonatal expression of the Stickler syndrome. Am. J. Med. Genet., *11*:113–119, 1982.

93. Francomano, C.A., et al.: The Stickler syndrome: Evidence for close linkage to the structural gene for type II collagen. Genomics, *1*, 1987 (in press).

94. Solomon, I., Abrams, G., Dinner, M., and Berman, L.: Neonatal abnormalities associated with D-penicillamine treatment during pregnancy. N. Engl. J. Med., *296*:54–55, 1977.

95. Pope, F.M.: Two types of autosomal recessive pseudoxanthoma elasticum. Arch. Dermatol., *110*:209–212, 1974.

96. Pope, F.M.: Autosomal dominant pseudoxanthoma elasticum. J. Med. Genet., *11*:152–157, 1974.

97. Renie, W.A., Pyeritz, R.E., Combs, J., and Fine, S.L.: Pseudoxanthoma elasticum: High calcium intake in early life correlates with severity. Am. J. Med. Genet., *19*:235–244, 1984.

98. Horton, W.A., et al.: Growth curves for height for diastrophic dysplasia, spondyloepiphyseal dysplasia congenita, and pseudoachondroplasia. Am. J. Dis. Child., *136*:316–319, 1982.

99. Murray, L.W., and Rimoin, D.L.: Type II collagen abnormalities in the spondyloepi- and sponyloepimetaphyseal dysplasias. Am. J. Hum. Genet., *37*:A13, 1985.

100. Wynne-Davies, R., and Hall, C.: Two clinical variants of spondyloepiphyseal dysplasia congenita. J. Bone Joint Surg., *64B*:435–441, 1982.

101. Bannerman, R.M., Ingall, G.B., and Mohn, J.F.: X-linked spondyloepiphyseal dysplasia tarda: Clinical and linkage data. J. Med. Genet., *8*:291–301, 1971.

102. Jacobsen, A.W.: Herediary osteochondro-dystrophia deformans. JAMA, *113*:121–124, 1939.

103. Horton, W.A., et al.: Standard growth curves for achondroplasia. J. Pediatr., *93*:435–438, 1978.

104. Hecht, J.T., et al.: Computerized tomography of the foramen magnum: Achondroplastic values compared to normal standards. Am. J. Med. Genet., *20*:355–360, 1985.

105. Reid, C.S., et al.: Cervicomedullary compression in young patients with achondroplasia: Value of comprehensive neu-rologic and respiratory evaluation. J. Pediatr., *110*:522–530, 1987.

106. Lutter, I.D., and Langer, I.O.: Neurological symptoms in achondroplastic dwarfs—surgical treatment. J. Bone Joint Surg., *59A*:87–92, 1977.

107. Pyeritz, R.E., Sack, G.H., Jr., and Udvarhelyi, G.B.: Thoracolumbosacral laminectomy in achondroplasia: Long-term results in 22 patients. Am. J. Med. Genet., *28*:433–444, 1987.

108. Hurko, O., Pyeritz, R.E., and Uematsu, S.: Neurologic considerations in achondroplasia. *In* Proceedings of the First International Conference on Human Achondroplasia. Edited by E. Ascani, B. Nicoletti, V.A. McKusick, and S.E. Kopits. New York, Plenum, 1987 (in press).

109. Kopits, S.E.: Correction of bowleg deformity in achondroplasia. Johns Hopkins Med. J., *146*:206–209, 1980.

110. Streeten, E.A., et al.: Extended laminectomy for spinal stenosis in achondroplasia. *In* Proceedings of the First International Conference on Human Achondroplasia. Edited by E. Ascani, B. Nicoletti, V.A. McKusick, and S.E. Kopits. New York, Plenum, 1987 (in press).

111. Rovin, S., et al.: Mandibulofacial dysostosis, a familial study of five generations. J. Pediatr., *65*:215–221, 1964.

112. Temtamy, S., McKusick, V.A.: The Genetics of Hand Malformations. New York, AR Liss, 1978.

113. Strasburger, A.K., et al.: Symphalangism: Genetics and clinical aspects. Bull. Johns Hopkins Hosp., *117*:108–127, 1965.

114. Welch, J.P., and Temtamy, S.A.: Hereditary contractures of the fingers (camptodactyly). J. Med. Genet., *3*:104–113, 1966.

115. Renie, W.A., and Pyeritz, R.E.: Idiopathic multicentric osteolysis in a 78-year-old woman. Johns Hopkins Med. J., *148*:165–171, 1981.

116. Carnevale, A., Canun, S., Mendoza, L., and del Castillo, V.: Idiopathic multicentric osteolysis with facial anomalies and nephropathy. Am. J. Med. Genet., *26*:877–886, 1987.

117. McKusick, V.A., and Neufeld, E.F.: The mucopolysaccharide storage diseases. *In* The Metabolic Basis of Inherited Disease. Edited by J.B. Stanbury, et al. New York, McGraw-Hill Book Co., 1983, pp. 751–777.

118. Fratantoni, J.C., Hall, C.W., and Neufeld, E.F.: Hurler and Hunter syndromes. Mutual correction of the defect in cultured fibroblasts. Science, *162*:570–572, 1968.

119. Brown, F.R., III, et al.: Administration of iduronate sulfatase by plasma exchange to patients with the Hunter syndrome: A clinical study. Am. J. Med. Genet., *13*:309–318, 1982.

120. Hobbs, J.R., et al.: Reversal of clinical features of Hurler's disease and biochemical improvement after treatment by bone-marrow transplantation. Lancet, *2*:709–712, 1981.

121. Krivit, W., et al.: Bone-marrow transplantation in the Maroteaux-Lamy syndrome (mucopolysaccharidosis type VI): Biochemical and clinical status 24 months after transplantation. N. Engl. J. Med., *311*:1606–1611, 1984.

122. Wiesmann, U., and Neufeld, E.F.: Scheie and Hurler syndromes: Apparent identity of the biochemical defect. Science, *169*:72–74, 1970.

123. Mueller, C.T., Shows, T.B., and Optiz, J.M.: Apparent allelism of the Hurler, Scheie, and Hurler/Scheie syndromes. Am. J. Med. Genet., *18*:547–556, 1984.

124. Pyeritz, R.E., and McKusick, V.A.: Genetic heterogeneity and allelic variation in the mucopolysaccharidoses. Johns Hopkins Med. J., *146*:71–72, 1980.

125. Young, I.D., and Harper, P.S.: Long-term complications in Hunter's syndrome. Clin. Genet., *16*:125–132, 1979.

126. Semenza, G.L., and Pyeritz, R.E.: Respiratory complications

of the mucopolysaccharide storage disorders. Medicine, 1988 (in press).

127. Neufeld, E.F., and McKusick, V.A.: Disorders of lysosomal enzyme synthesis and localization: I-cell disease and pseudo-Hurler polydystrophy. *In* The Metabolic Basis of Inherited Disease. Edited by J.B. Stanbury, et al. New York. McGraw-Hill Book Co., 1983, pp. 778–787.

128. Kelly, T.E., et al.: Mucolipidosis III (pseudo-Hurler polydystrophy): Clinical and laboratory studies in a series of 12 patients. Johns Hopkins Med. J., *137*:156–175, 1975.

129. Yunis, J.J., et al.: Clinical manifestations of mannosidosis—a longitudinal study. Am. J. Med., *61*:841–848, 1976.

130. Montgomery, T.R., Thomas, G.H., and Valle, D.L.: Mannosidosis in an adult. Johns Hopkins Med. J., *151*:113–117, 1982.

131. Desnick, R.J., et al.: Mannosidosis: Clinical, morphologic, immunologic, and biochemical studies. Pediatr. Res., *10*:985–996, 1976.

132. Vidgoff, J., Lovrien, E.W., Beals, R.K., and Buist, N.R.M.: Mannosidosis in three brothers—a review of the literature. Medicine, *56*:335–348, 1977.

133. Albright, F., Butler, A.M., and Bloomberg, E.: Rickets resistant to vitamin D therapy. Am. J. Dis. Child., *54*:529–, 1937.

134. Schroeber, H.W., Jr., amd Zasloff, M.: The hand and foot malformations in fibrodysplasia ossificans progressiva. Johns Hopkins Med. J., *147*:73–78, 1980.

135. Conner, J.M., and Evans, D.A.P.: Fibrodysplasia ossificans progressiva: The clinical features and natural history of 34 patients. J. Bone Joint Surg., *64B*:76–83, 1982.

136. Drachman, D.B.: The syndrome of arthrogryposis multiplex congenita. Birth Defects, *7*:90–97, 1971.

137. Hall, J.G., Reed, S.D., and Greene, G.: The distal arthrogryposes: Delineation of new entities—review and nosologic discussion. Am. J. Med. Genet., *11*:185–239, 1982.

138. Smith, D.W.: Recognizable Patterns of Human Deformation. Philadelphia, W.B. Saunders Co., 1981.

86

HYPERTROPHIC OSTEOARTHROPATHY

ROY D. ALTMAN

Few clinical abnormalities are as old as clubbing, yet little more is known of its etiopathogenesis today than when it was recorded circa 400 BC by Hippocrates.[1,2] The association of clubbing to bone and joint changes was noted by von Bamberger in 1899 and Marie in 1890.[2,3] *Hypertrophic osteoarthropathy* (HPO) is a syndrome that includes clubbing of fingers and toes, periostitis of long bones, and arthritis. HPO has also been called familial idiopathic hypertrophic osteoarthropathy, Marie-Bamberger syndrome, osteoarthropathic hypertrophiante pneumique, and secondary hypertrophic osteoarthropathy.

HPO is classified as *primary* or *secondary.* The primary form is hereditary and most often appears during childhood. The secondary form is often associated with neoplasms or infectious diseases and can appear at any age. Although the original scope of associated disease was intrathoracic, hypertrophic osteoarthropathy is now recognized as possibly being associated with numerous extrathoracic diseases. Insidious development of symptoms and signs with mild rheumatic complaints over a period of months or years generally characterizes hypertrophic osteoarthropathy associated with suppurative disease, especially of the lungs. In contrast, a rapidly progressing syndrome with prominent joint pain and stiffness is commonly associated with malignant diseases.

CLINICAL FEATURES

CLUBBING

Clubbing is unsightly but rarely produces symptoms. Hence, the physician generally observes the deformity before the patient. When it does produce symptoms, there may be occasional clumsiness, stiffness, and burning or warmth of fingertips. HPO almost always includes clubbing, whereas periostitis and synovitis may not.[4-6] Whether isolated clubbing is a separate condition or a *forme fruste* of hypertrophic osteoarthropathy is unclear.[4,7] Increased blood flow through the digits is a universal feature of clubbing, whether or not periostitis or synovitis is present. The presence of isolated clubbing does not distinguish primary from secondary disease.

Initially, there is softening of the nail bed, causing a fluctuant and rocking sensation to palpation of the proximal nail. This is accompanied by periungual erythema with periungual telangiectasias, local warmth, and sweating. Increased convexity of the nail in sagittal and cross-sectional planes is noted, with loss of the normal 15° angle between the proximal portion of the nail and dorsal surface of the phalanx (Fig. 86–1). Later, excessive distal phalangeal resorption of fingers and toes may lead to acrolysis.[8]

Excessive sweating or warmth of the fingertips, eponychia, paronychia, breaking or loosening of the nail, hangnails, and accelerated nail or cuticle growth are frequent. In advanced stages, the fingers may assume a drumstick appearance and the distal interphalangeal joints show hyperextensibility (Fig. 86–1). Similar changes occur in the toes. A spade-like enlargement of the hands and feet may occur. Clubbing most often evolves over months or years. Clubbing without periostitis is more often idiopathic.

A useful clinical calibration method is to measure

1360

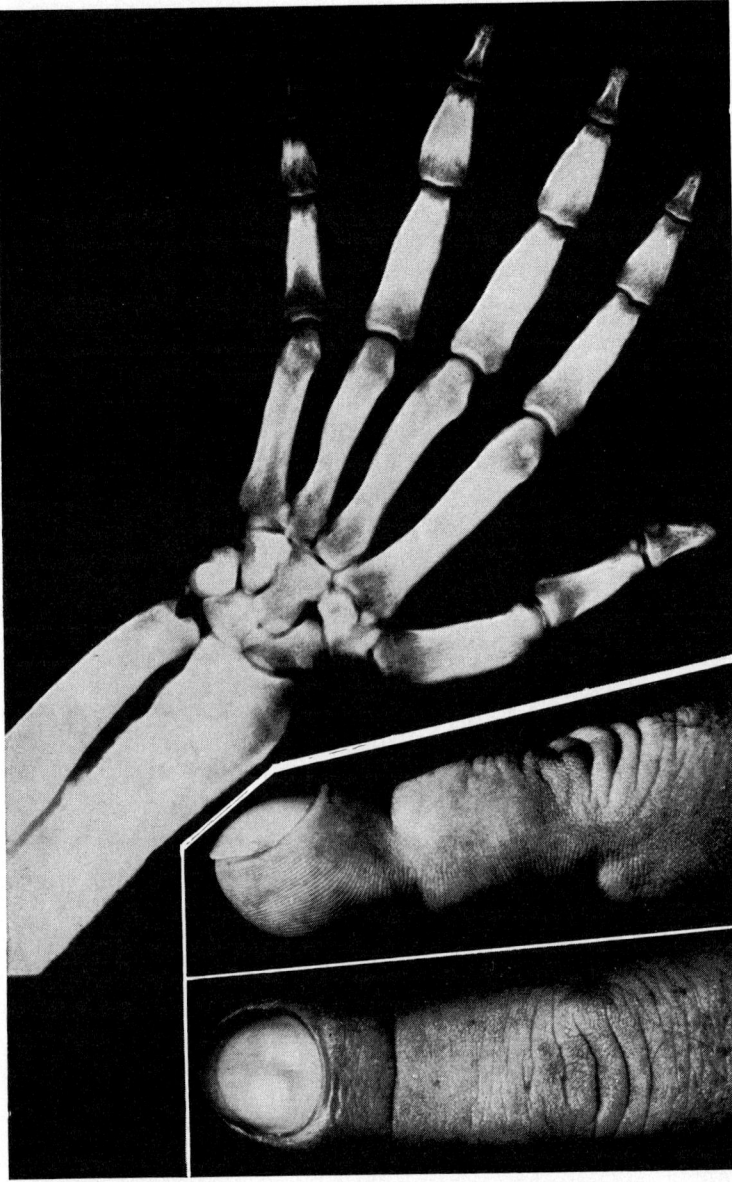

FIG. 86–1. Hippocratic finger and roentgenogram of hand showing the characteristic features of hypertrophic osteoarthropathy. (From Campbell, et al.)

the diameter of the finger at the base of the nail at the index finger and to divide the measurement by the diameter of the distal interphalangeal joint. If the ratio is greater than 1, it is abnormal and signifies clubbing. The normal ratio is independent of race, age, or sex.[9,10] A shadowgram technique has been proposed for measurement of the hyponychial angle.[11] Another method was proposed by Schamroth, who suggested placing the dorsal surfaces of the contralateral fingers together (the ring finger is preferred).[12] A gap normally appears between the fingers at the nail bed; with clubbing, as the nail bed expands, the gap disappears.

Isolated cases of unilateral clubbing have been reported.[4] Unilateral clubbing also has been associated with aneurysms of the aorta and with the subclavian or innominate artery, as well as with axillary tumors, subluxations of the shoulder, apical lung cancer, brachial arteriovenous aneurysm, and hemiplegia.[13,14] Unidigital clubbing is reported following injury to the median nerve, in sarcoidosis, and in tophaceous gout. "Paddle fingers" occasionally develop in bass viol players. Unidigital clubbing is most often related to trauma.[4] Clubbing of the toes but not the fingers has accompanied infected abdominal aortic aneurysm.

PERIOSTITIS

Periostitis may be asymptomatic or may produce mild aching pain to deep-seated, severe aching or burning pain and tenderness over the long bones.

Aggravation of bone pain on limb dependency is a unique feature of this disease and suggests that local vascular stasis may play a role in production of pain. Conversely, the discomfort is often relieved by limb elevation. The extent of periostitis depends on its duration and is not a factor of primary or secondary disease. It is not uncommon to observe a patient reversed in a hospital bed with feet elevated at the head of the bed.[15] The patient may complain of heat and swelling over the feet and legs. The distal extremities often appear broadened with a palpable, firm, mildly pitting edema. There is often tenderness to pressure over the bone and warmth of the skin over the distal shin (tibia), feet, radius, and ulna.

ARTHRITIS

The arthritis may be an oligosynovitis or a polysynovitis. Joint symptoms range from arthralgias to severe joint pain. Joint pain usually involves knees, metacarpophalangeal joints, wrists, elbows, and ankles symmetrically.[16] Concomitant with these symptoms is variable heat, erythema, restricted joint motion, and swelling. Ingestion of alcohol may worsen joint pain and swelling.[17] Hypopigmentation of the skin and induration of the subcutaneous tissue around the affected joint may suggest scleroderma.[18] Effusions may be huge, even grotesque, particularly in HPO accompanying cyanotic congenital heart disease.

ADDITIONAL FINDINGS

The syndrome may be associated with signs of autonomic dysfunction such as flushing, blanching, and profuse sweating, most severe in hands and feet. Coarsening of the facial features and thickened furrowed skin of the face (leonine facies) and scalp may develop. Occasionally, patients will develop gynecomastia, often associated with elevation of urinary estrogen excretion.[19,20]

CLINICAL SUBSETS

PRIMARY HPO

Primary HPO is also referred to as pachydermoperiostosis or Touraine-Solente-Golé syndrome. Symptoms usually begin in teenage years, affecting boys more often than girls.[21] The disease occurs within families, and appears to be transmitted by an autosomal dominant gene with variable expression.

Symptoms are usually limited to 1 or 2 decades.[17,22–25] An insidious onset of clubbing occurs, with spade-like enlargement of hands and feet. Symptoms include reduced dexterity and awkwardness of the hands. Vague joint and bone pain can occur,[24] both of which may be exacerbated by alcohol.[17]

Examination reveals marked clubbing with cylindric thickening of forearms and legs of both bony and soft-tissue origin.[22,24] Recurrent, mildly symptomatic joint effusions may occur.[25] Acrolysis may involve the distal phalanges of hands and feet.[8,26] Excessive sweating, particularly of the hands and feet, often occurs. The facial skin thickens and furrows, causing deep nasolabial folds and a corrugated scalp, which creates the classic leonine appearance. The skin of the face and scalp is often greasy. (The leonine face, greasy skin, and sweating are uncommon in secondary hypertrophic osteoarthropathy, however.) Gynecomastia, female hair distribution, striae, acne vulgaris, and cranial suture defects occur rarely.[6]

SECONDARY HPO

By definition, this syndrome appears secondary to another condition, particularly pulmonary neoplasms or suppurative conditions of the lungs, mediastinum, and pleura.

HPO accompanies 5 to 10% of intrathoracic neoplasms,[27–29] most frequently bronchogenic carcinoma[30–31] and pleural tumors.[32] Secondary HPO can also accompany lung abscess, bronchiectasis, chronic bronchitis, or empyema, but with modern therapy of chronic infections, HPO is now more often associated with chronic pneumonitis, pneumoconiosis, pulmonary tuberculosis, mediastinal Hodgkin's disease, sarcoidosis, or cystic fibrosis.[33–35] Many other neoplasms have been reported with secondary HPO, often in association with intrathoracic metastases,[36–44] but metastatic lesions, per se, are an uncommon cause of the syndrome.

Congenital malformations of the heart that cause cyanosis may be accompanied by HPO. Other cardiac diseases that may be associated with HPO include patent ductus arteriosus[46] and cardiac rhabdomyosarcoma.[47] HPO with cyanotic congenital heart disease is related directly to the degree of right-to-left-sided blood shunting.[48] Clubbing, a sign of bacterial endocarditis, may indicate embolization.

Various gastrointestinal diseases can lead to HPO, including ulcerative colitis, regional enteritis, amebic colitis, subphrenic abscess, cirrhosis, idiopathic steatorrhea, sprue, neoplasms of the small intestine, multiple colonic polyposis, and carcinoma of the colon, esophagus, or liver.[49] The syndrome may accompany relatively rare diseases, e.g., primary cholangiolitic cirrhosis,[50,51] secondary hepatic amyloidosis (perhaps related to infection), or biliary atresia.[4,52] HPO confined to the lower extremities has been reported in association with an infected abdominal aneurysm.[53]

Clubbing has been associated with diverse miscellaneous disorders such as post-thyroidectomy for Graves' disease, hyperthyroidism, pregnancy, purgative abuse, connective tissue diseases, and hyperparathyroidism.[4,27,54–57]

THYROID ACROPACHY

Thyroid acropachy is generally considered a secondary form of HPO.[58,59] This uncommon condition is characterized by clubbing of the fingers and asymptomatic periosteal proliferation of the bones of the hands and feet. It is associated with either treated or active hyperthyroidism (Graves' disease), with accompanying exophthalmos and localized nonpitting soft-tissue swelling of the extremities or pretibial myxedema. Serum long-acting thyroid stimulator (LATS) has been identified in these cases.[60]

LABORATORY AND ROENTGENOGRAPHIC FINDINGS

No specific laboratory tests exist for HPO, although the erythrocyte sedimentation rate is often elevated. Synovial fluids are group I (noninflammatory), and are clear with good mucin clot and high viscosity. Leukocyte counts are usually below 2000/mm³, and fewer than 50% are neutrophils.[30,61,62] Serum and synovial fluid C3 and C4 levels are normal in secondary HPO.[62]

Radiography is important in the diagnosis of HPO. Subperiosteal symmetric new bone layering characteristically appears in the distal diaphyseal regions of the long bones, especially of the legs and forearms, and less commonly of the phalanges (Fig. 86–2). Rarely, active clinical disease occurs in the *absence* of any radiologic changes.[63] The characteristic radiopaque subperiosteal new bone can be reduplicated in multiple layers, producing an "onion skin" appearance.

The diagnosis can also be suggested by the characteristic abnormal pattern seen on skeletal imaging using ⁹⁹ᵐTc diphosphonate.[64,65] A pericortical linear accumulation of radiotracer along the long bones (Fig. 86–3) and proximal phalanges is noted along with increased periarticular uptake, disclosing synovitis. Involvement of the skull, scapulae, clavicles, and patellae is frequently noted. Asymmetric or irregular distribution is seen in fewer than 20% of patients. HPO can be easily differentiated from metastatic disease by bone scanning because of the diffuse pattern of radionuclide distribution in the former. After tumor removal, resolution of the abnormal tracer pattern may occur.[39]

PATHOLOGY

Histopathologic changes are similar in the hereditary and secondary forms of HPO. In clubbed phalanges, there is edema of the distal digital soft parts, thickening of the blood-vessel walls, cellular infiltration, fibroblastic proliferation, and growth of new collagenous tissue. These changes account for the uniform enlargement of the terminal segments. Nail bed and finger pulp mast cell counts were lower in clubbed fingers compared to control fingers.[66]

The pathologic changes of periostitis develop predominantly at the distal end of metacarpals, metatarsals, and the long bones of the forearms and legs.[67] In severe disease, ribs, clavicles, scapulae, pelvis, and malar bones may be involved. The earliest histologic alterations are round-cell infiltration and edema of the periosteum, synovial membrane, articular capsule, and neighboring subcutaneous tissues. These changes are associated with elevation of the periosteum, deposition of subperiosteal osteoid matrix, and subsequent mineralization. As such foci enlarge, the distal long bones eventually become ensheathed with a cuff of new bone (Fig. 86–4). Concurrent with thickening, there is accelerated resorption of endosteal and haversian bone. The resultant structure is weakened, and pathologic fractures may occur occasionally. With advancing disease, the pathologic alterations spread proximally along the bony shafts.

Synovial membranes adjoining the involved bones are often edematous, hypervascularized, and infiltrated with lymphocytes, plasma cells, and a few neutrophils. Advancing proliferative fibrous tissue at joint margins is sometimes associated with cartilage degeneration. Electron microscopic studies of the synovial membranes have shown alterations of the microcirculation, with dilatations of capillaries and venules, endothelial cell gaps, and multilamination of small-vessel basement membranes.[61] Subendothelial electron-dense deposits have been described in the synovial membranes of five patients with secondary

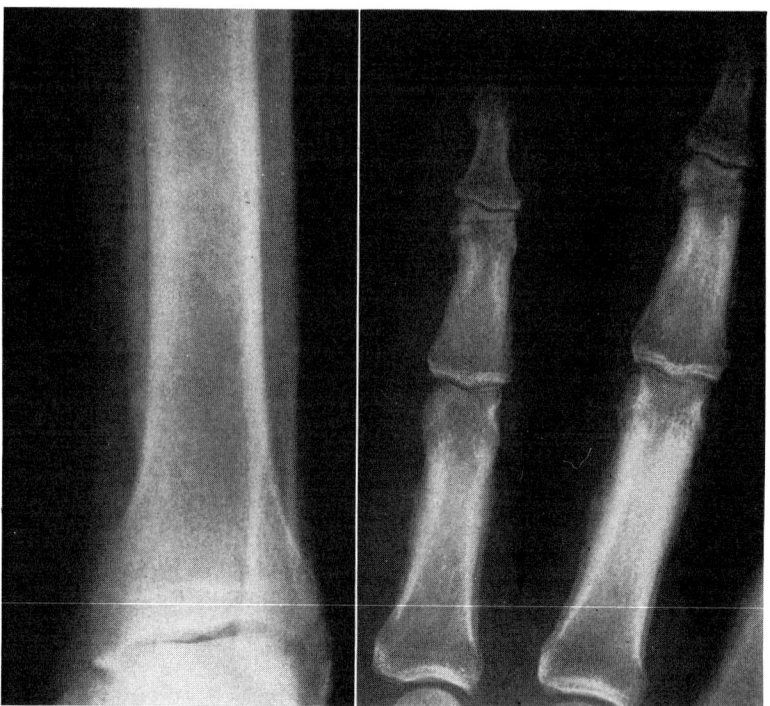

FIG. 86–2. Hypertrophic osteoarthropathy. Radiodense bands along a margin of the shaft indicate new osseous formation beneath the elevated periosteum. Appearance of these typical lesions is similar in phalanges *(right)* to that of long bones *(left)*. (Courtesy of the late Dr. J.J. Bunim.)

HPO,[61] but their significance is still unclear. Negative immunofluorescent staining for γ globulins and complement was reported in three HPO synovia.[62]

ETIOLOGY AND PATHOGENESIS

The nature of the genetic factors operative in the idiopathic form of HPO is unknown, although angiographic studies have demonstrated hypervascularization of the finger pads.[68] In secondary HPO, it has been postulated that the vascular proliferation and osteogenesis is produced by (1) obscure autonomic reflexes stimulated at the site of underlying disease; (2) a high level arteriolar pulse pressure, possibly also involving autonomic reflexes; (3) toxins liberated by primary malignant lesions; and (4) osteoblast-stimulating agents released at the site of malignant pulmonary lesions or by the pluripotential cells of pleural membranes.

Another theory hypothesizes the development of pulmonary arteriovenous shunts such that a substance (hormone or toxin) normally inactivated in the lungs enters the systemic circulation to produce the characteristic changes. One suspected vasoactive substance is reduced ferritin.

Factors conditioning the susceptibility of an individual with intrathoracic disease to develop HPO are unknown, but there is evidence for the participation of a local circulatory disorder.[4,69] A locally-acting circulating vasodilator has been identified in some patients.[70] Increased vascularity of clubbed fingers in

secondary HPO has been well documented by measurement of skin temperature, infrared photography, nail bed capillarioscopy, and postmortem arteriography.[71,72] In his classic studies, using digital plethysmography, Mendlowitz found elevated digital pulse pressure and blood flow in patients with the condition and a return to normal pressures following removal of pulmonary lesions.[4,73] Growth hormone production by bronchogenic carcinomas provides a possible explanation for the joint marginal bony overgrowth observed in some patients.[74–76] Elevated urinary estrogens were found in three patients with pulmonary lesions.[77] Decarboxylation of a polypeptide differing from immunoreactive growth hormone but related to somatotropin has been suggested as the mediator of HPO.[78] Abnormal vascular responses to intravenous infusion of epinephrine disappeared after excision of lung tumor.[19] Striking resolution of symptoms and signs followed simple denervation of the hilum or pulmonary vagotomy on the same side as the lesion.[27,28,79] Thoracotomy alone was ineffective.

Circulating tumor antigen-antibody complexes have been described in patients with a variety of tumors, including lung carcinomas. The electron microscopic findings seem equivocal, but raise the possibility that the synovitis seen in HPO associated with bronchogenic carcinoma might be immune complex mediated.

DIFFERENTIAL DIAGNOSIS

The presence of clubbing accompanying HPO simplifies diagnosis, and a primary disease must be

FIG. 86–3. Bone scintiphoto utilizing ^{99m}Tc labeled methylene diphosphonate demonstrating periosteal localization of the nuclide to the anterior tibiae and radius *(arrows).*

FIG. 86–4. Cross section through a metatarsal of a patient with hypertrophic osteoarthropathy. The periosteum shows thickening with an irregular cuff of new bone deposited over the cortex. (From Bartter, F.C., and Bauer, W. In Cecil and Loeb. Textbook of Medicine. Edited by Cecil and Loeb. Philadelphia, WB Saunders Co.)

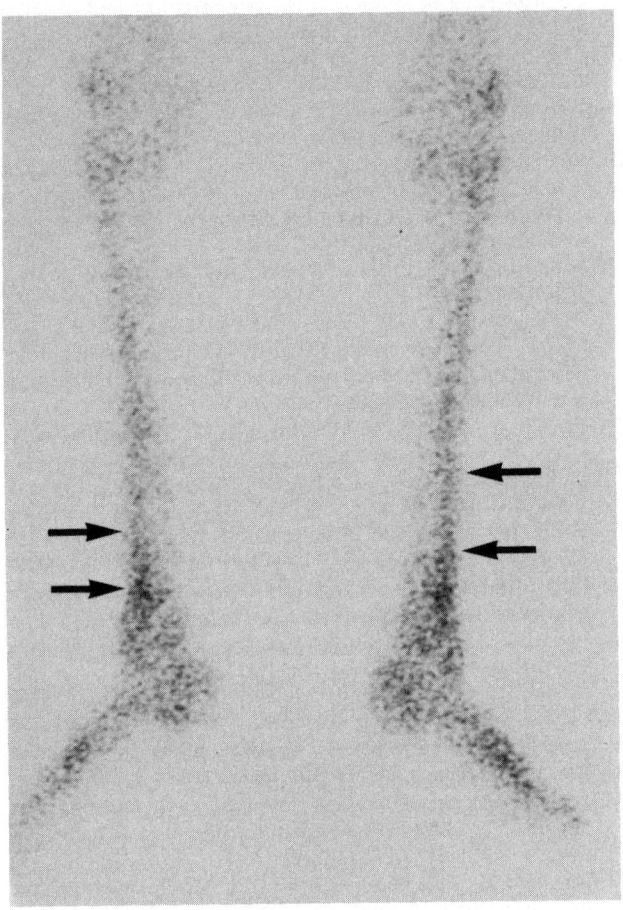

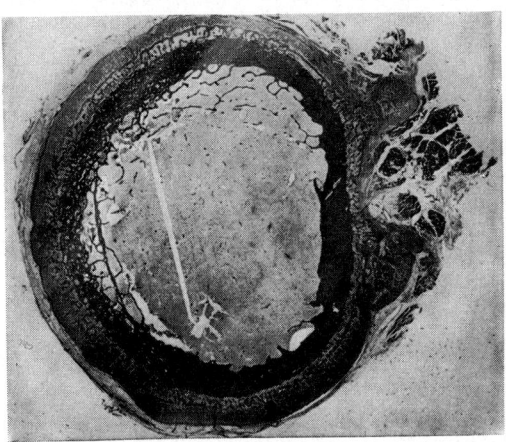

mary and secondary HPO is not difficult because the hereditary or idiopathic syndromes begin after puberty, follow a self-limited course of 1 to 2 decades, and often occur in other members of the family.[22]

sought. If acute polyarthritis precedes clubbing, however, a search for an asymptomatic pulmonary neoplasm might be neglected and the problem mislabeled as rheumatoid arthritis.[80,81] In most instances, roentgenograms will reveal elevation of the periosteum and evidence of new bone growth.[82] Periosteal elevation of HPO must be differentiated from that resulting from local tumors, lymphangitis, syphilis fractures, and the hemorrhages of trauma or scurvy. Swelling and tenderness of the lower legs may falsely suggest thrombophlebitis, and bony pains may be misinterpreted as peripheral neuritis. The spoon-shaped nails of hypochromic anemia should be readily distinguishable. HPO may have features suggestive of scleroderma.[18]

An associated disease should be excluded before a patient is assigned to the ill-defined hereditary or idiopathic groups. This point is emphasized because of the danger of overlooking infection, a resectable tumor, or another treatable condition. Separation of pri-

TREATMENT

Clubbing is usually asymptomatic, requiring no treatment. Disabling symptoms related to periostitis and synovitis in secondary HPO usually respond dramatically to removal of the primary pulmonary lesion or to intrathoracic vagotomy.[27,83,84]

Anti-inflammatory agents have been beneficial in reducing the discomfort. Aspirin in modest doses is frequently effective,[44] as are the propionic acid derivatives, but indomethacin is most often effective.[15] Chemical vagotomy by atropine[13,85] or propantheline also has provided relief of symptoms.[86] Analgesics are often appropriate. Adrenocortical steroid therapy may be useful in some patients.[83] Radiotherapy to the primary tumor site[87] or to metastatic lesions,[88] as well as chemotherapy,[89] has relieved joint symptoms. Symptoms usually resolve after successful therapy of bacterial endocarditis.[90] Complete disappearance of HPO has followed appropriate therapy for empyema, lung abscess, bronchiectasis, or pneumonia.[90]

Treatment of the idiopathic form of the syndrome must necessarily be symptomatic.

REFERENCES

1. Hippocrates (c. 400 BC): The Genuine Works of Hippocrates. Vol. I. Translated by F. Adams. Syndenham Society, 1849, p. 249.
2. Marie, P.: De l'osteoarthropathie hypertrophiante pneumique. Rev. Med., 10:1–36, 1890.
3. von Bamberger, E.: Uber Knochen veranderungen bei chronishen Lungenund. Herzkran Kenheiten Klin. Med., 18:193, 1890–1891.
4. Mendlowitz, M.: Clubbing and hypertrophic osteoarthropathy. Medicine, 21:269–306, 1942.
5. Fischer, D.S., Singer, D.H., and Feldman, S.M.: Clubbing, a review, with emphasis on hereditary acropachy. Medicine, 43:459, 1965.
6. Reginato, A.R., Schinpachasse, Y., and Guerrero, R.: Familial idiopathic hypertrophic osteoarthropathy and cranial suture defects in children. Skeletal Radiol., 8:105–109, 1982.
7. Seaton, D.R.: Familial clubbing of fingers and toes. Br. Med. J., 1:614, 1938.
8. Hedayati, H., Barmada, R., and Skosey, J.L.: Acrolysis in pachydermoperiostosis. Arch. Intern. Med., 140:1087–1088, 1980.
9. Sly, R.M., et al.: Objective assessment for digital clubbing in Caucasian, Negro and Oriental subjects. Chest, 64:687–689, 1973.
10. Waring, W.W., et al.: Quantitation of digital clubbing in children. Measurements of casts of the index finger. Am. Rev. Respir. Dis., 104:166–174, 1971.
11. Sinniah, D., and Omar, A.: Quantitation of digital clubbing by shadowgram technique. Arch. Dis. Child., 54:145–146, 1979.
12. Schamroth, L.: Personal experience. S. Afr. Med. J., 50:297–300, 1976.
13. Day, W.H., and Hagelsten, J.O.: Blocking of the vagus nerve relieving osteoarthropathy in lung diseases. Dan. Med. Bull., 11:131–133, 1964.
14. Denham, M.J., Hodkinson, H.M., and Wright, B.M.: Unilateral clubbing in hemiplegia. Gerontol. Clin., 17:7–12, 1975.
15. Personal observation.
16. Shulman, L.E., Hypertrophic ostearthropathy. Bull. Rheum. Dis., 7:135–136, 1957.
17. Mueller, M., and Trevarthen, D.: Pachydermoperiostosis: Arthropathy aggravated by episode alcohol abuse. J. Rheumatol., 8:862–864, 1981.
18. Gray, R.G., and Gottlieb, N.L.: Pseudoscleroderma in hypertrophic osteoarthropathy. JAMA, 246:2062–2063, 1981.
19. Ginsburg, J.: Observations on the peripheral circulation in hypertrophic pulmonary osteoarthropathy. Q. J. Med., 27:335–352, 1958.
20. Jao, J.Y., Barlow, J.J., and Krant, M.J.: Pulmonary hypertrophic osteoarthropathy, spider angiomata and estrogen hyperexcretion. Ann. Intern. Med., 70:581–584, 1969.
21. Rimoin, D.L.: Pachydermoperiostosis (idiopathic clubbing and periostosis): Genetic and physiologic considerations. N. Engl. J. Med., 272:923–931, 1965.
22. Touraine, A., Solente, A., and Golé, L.: Un syndrome osteodermopathique. La pachydermie plicaturee avec pachyperiostose des extremites. Presse Med., 43:1820–1824, 1935.
23. Vogl, A., Blumenfeld, S., and Gutner, L.B.: Diagnostic significance of pulmonary hypertrophic osteoarthropathy. Am. J. Med., 18:51–65, 1955.
24. Vogl, A., and Goldfischer, S.: Pachydermoperiostosis. Primary or idiopathic hypertrophic osteoarthropathy. Am. J. Med., 33:166–187, 1962.
25. Lauter, S.A., Vasey, F.B., Huttner, I., and Osterland, C.K.: Pachydermoperiostosis: studies on the synovium. J. Rheumatol., 5:85–95, 1978.
26. Fam, A.G., Chin-Sang, H., and Ramsay, C.A.: Pachydermoperiostosis: scintographic, plethysmographic, and capillarscopic observations. Ann. Rheum. Dis., 42:98–102, 1983.
27. Christian, C.L., Chairman Editorial Committee. 19th Rheumatism Review. Arthritis Rheum., 13:615, 1970.
28. Lansbury, J.: Connective tissue manifestations of neoplastic disease. Geriatrics, 9:319–324, 1954.
29. Wierman, W.H., Clagett, O.T., and McDonald, J.R.: Articular manifestations in pulmonary diseases: an analysis of their occurrence in 1,024 cases in which pulmonary resection was performed. JAMA, 155:1459–1463, 1954.
30. Calabro, J.J.: Cancer and arthritis. Arthritis Rheum., 10:553–567, 1967.
31. Freeman, M.H., and Tonkin, A.K.: Manifestations of hypertrophic pulmonary osteoarthropathy in patients with carcinoma of the lung. Demonstration by 99mTc-pyrophosphate bone scans. Radiology, 120:363–365, 1976.
32. Briselli, M., Mark, J., and Dickersin, G.R.: Solitary fibrous tumors of the pleura: eight new cases and review of 360 cases in the literature. Cancer, 47:2678–2689, 1981.
33. Athreya, B.H., Gorske, A.T., and Myers, A.R.: Aspirin-induced abnormalities of liver functions. Am. J. Dis. Child., 129:638–641, 1973.
34. Matthay, M.A., et al.: Hypertrophic osteoarthropathy in adults with cystic fibrosis. Thorax, 31:572–575, 1976.
35. West, S.G., Gilbreath, R.E., and Lawless, O.J.: Painful clubbing and sarcoidosis. JAMA, 246:1338–1339, 1981.
36. Martin, C.L.: Complications produced by malignant tumors of the nasopharynx. Am. J. Roentgenol., 41:377–390, 1939.
37. Temple, H.L., and Jaspin, G.: Hypertrophic osteoarthropathy. Am. J. Roentgenol., 60:232–245, 1948.
38. Trivedi, S.A.: Neurilemmoma of the diaphragm causing severe hypertrophic pulmonary osteoarthropathy. Br. J. Tuberc. Dis. Chest., 52:214–217, 1958.
39. Ali, A., et al.: Distribution of hypertrophic pulmonary osteoarthropathy. Am. J. Roentgenol., 134:771–780, 1980.
40. Lofters, W.S., and Walker, T.M.: Hodgkin's disease and hypertrophic pulmonary osteoarthropathy. West Indian Med. J., 227–230, 1978.
41. McNeil, M.M., Sage, R.E., and Dale, B.M.: Hypertrophic osteoarthropathy complicating primary bone lymphoma association with invasive Phycomyosis and Aspergillus infections. Aust. NZ J. Med., 11:71–75, 1981.
42. Solimbu, C., Marchetta, P., Firooznnia, H., and Rafu, M.: Hypertrophic osteoarthropathy in metastatic renal cell carcinoma. J. Urol., 22:669–672, 1983.
43. Arlson, K.S., and Naidoo, A.: Hypertrophic osteoarthropathy. Mayo Clin. Proc., 59:208–209, 1979.
44. Lokich, J.J.: Pulmonary osteoarthropathy; association with mesenchymal tumor metastases to the lungs. JAMA, 238:37–39, 1977.
45. McLaughlin, G.E., McCarty, D.J., Jr., and Downing, D.F.: Hypertrophic osteoarthropathy associated with cyanotic congenital heart disease. Ann. Intern. Med., 67:579–587, 1967.
46. Williams, B., Ling, J., Leight, L., and McGaff, C.J.: Patent ductus arteriosus and osteoarthropathy. Arch. Intern. Med., 111:346–350, 1963.
47. Pascuzzi, C.A., Parkin, T.W., Bruwer, A.J., and Edwards, J.E.: Hypertrophic osteoarthropathy associated with primary rhabdomyosarcoma of the heart. Mayo Clin. Proc., 32:30–41, 1957.

48. Martinez-Lavin, M., et al.: Hypertrophic osteoarthropathy in cyanotic congenital heart disease. Arthritis Rheum., 25:1186–1192, 1982.

49. Peirce, T.H., and Weir, D.G.: Hypertrophic osteoarthropathy associated with a non-metatasising carcinoma of the oesophagus. J. Ir. Med. Assoc., 66:160–162, 1973.

50. Buchan, D.J., and Mitchell, D.M.: Hypertrophic osteoarthropathy in portal cirrhosis. Ann. Intern. Med., 66:130–135, 1967.

51. Kieff, E.D., and McCarty, D.J.: Hypertrophic osteoarthropathy with arthritis and synovial calcification in a patient with alcoholic cirrhosis. Arthritis Rheum., 12:261–268, 1969.

52. Epstein, O., Dick, R., and Sherlock, S.: Prospective study of periostitis and finger clubbing in primary biliary cirrhosis and other forms of chronic liver disease. Gut, 22:203–206, 1981.

53. Sorin, S.B., Askari, A., and Rhodes, R.S.: Hypertrophic osteoarthropathy of the lower extremities as a manifestation of arterial graft sepsis. Arthritis Rheum., 23:768–770, 1980.

54. Souders, C.R., and Manuell, J.L.: Skeletal deformities in hyperparathyroidism. N. Engl. J. Med., 250:594–597, 1954.

55. Lovell, R.R.H., and Scott, G.B.D.: Hypertrophic osteoarthropathy in polyarteritis. Ann. Rheum. Dis., 15:46–50, 1956.

56. Borden, E.C., and Holling, H.E.: Hypertrophic osteoarthropathy and pregnancy. Ann. Intern. Med., 71:577–580, 1969.

57. Prabhu, R., Berger, H.W., Subietas, A., and Lee, M.: Lymphomatoid granulomatosis, report of a patient with severe anemia and clubbing. Chest, 78:883–885, 1980.

58. Diamond, M.T.: The syndrome of exophthalmos, hypertrophic osteoarthropathy and localized myxedema: a review of the literature and report of a case. Ann. Intern. Med., 50:206–213, 1959.

59. Kinsella, R.A., Jr., and Back, D.K.: Thyroid acropachy. Med. Clin. North Am., 52:393–398, 1968.

60. Lynch, P.J., Maize, J.C., and Sisson, J.C.: Pretibial myxedema and nonthyrotoxic thyroid disease. Arch. Dermatol., 107:107–111, 1973.

61. Schumacher, H.R.: Articular manifestations of HPO in bronchogenic carcinoma. A clinical and pathologic study. Arthritis Rheum., 19:629–636, 1976.

62. Vidal, A.F., et al.: Structural and immunologic changes of synovium of hypertrophic osteoarthropathy (HPO). Arthritis Rheum., 20:139, 1977.

63. Horn, C.R.: Hypertrophic pulmonary osteoarthropathy without radiographic evidence of new bone formation. Thorax, 35:479, 1980.

64. Donnelly, B., and Johnson, P.M.: Detection of hypertrophic pulmonary osteoarthropathy of skeletal imaging with ^{99m}Tc-labeled diphosphonate. Radiology, 114:389–391, 1975.

65. Rosenthal, L., and Kirsh, J.: Observations on radionuclide imaging in hypertrophic pulmonary osteoarthropathy. Radiology, 120:359–362, 1976.

66. Marshal, R.: Observations of the pathology of clubbed fingers with special reference to mast cells. Am. Rev. Respir. Dis., 113:395–397, 1976.

67. Gall, E.A., Bennett, G.A., and Bauer, W.: Generalized hypertrophic osteoarthropathy. Am. J. Pathol., 27:349–381, 1951.

68. Jajic, I., et al.: Primary hypertrophic osteoarthropathy (HPO) and changes in the joints. Scand. J. Rheumatol., 9:89–96, 1980.

69. Mendlowitz, M., and Leslie, A.: Experimental simulation in dogs of cyanosis and hypertrophic osteoarthropathy which are associated with congenital heart disease. Am. Heart J., 24:141–152, 1942.

70. Shneerson, J.M.: Digital clubbing and hypertrophic osteoarthropathy: the underlying mechanisms. Br. J. Dis. Chest, 75:113–131, 1981.

71. Harter, J.S.: Joint manifestations (discussion). J. Thorac. Surg., 9:505, 1939–1940.

72. Rominger, E.: Ein fall von morbus caeroleus mit demonstration der hautkapillaren am lebenden nach weibund elektro kardiographischen untersuchungen. Dtsch. Med. Wochenschr., 46:168, 1920.

73. Mendlowitz, M.: Measurement of blood flow and blood pressure in clubbed fingers. J. Clin. Invest., 20:113–117, 1941.

74. Cameron, D.P., et al.: On the presence of immunoreactive growth hormone in a bronchogenic carcinoma. Aust. Ann. Med., 18:143–146, 1969.

75. Dupont, B.: Plasma growth hormone and hypertrophic osteoarthropathy in carcinoma of the bronchus. Acta Med. Scand., 188:25–30, 1970.

76. Martinez-Lavin, M.: Digital clubbing and hypertrophic osteoarthropathy: a unifying hypothesis. J. Rheumatol., 14:6–8, 1987.

77. Ginsburg, J., and Brown, J.B.: Increased oestrogen excretion in hypertrophic pulmonary osteoarthropathy. Lancet, 2:1274–1276, 1961.

78. Audebert, A.A., et al.: Osteoarthropathie hypertrophiante pneumique associee a une quadruple secretion hormonale paraneoplastique. Sem. Hop. Paris, 458:529–530, 1982.

79. Semple, T., and McCluskie, R.A.: Generalized hypertrophic osteoarthropathy in association with bronchial carcinoma. Br. Med. J., 1:754–759, 1955.

80. Holmes, H.H., Bauman, E., and Ragan, C.: Symptomatic arthritis due to hypertrophic pulmonary osteoarthropathy in pulmonary neoplastic disease. Report of seven cases. Ann. Rheum. Dis., 9:169–173, 1950.

81. Polley, H.F., et al.: Articular reactions with localized fibrous mesothelioma of the pleura. Ann. Rheum. Dis., 11:314, 1952.

82. Greenfield, G.B., Schorsch, H.A., and Ahkoln, A.: The various roentgen appearances of pulmonary hypertrophic osteoarthropathy. Am. J. Roentgenol. Rad. Ther. Nucl. Surg., 101:927–931, 1967.

83. Holling, H.E., and Brodey, R.S.: Pulmonary hypertrophic osteoarthropathy. JAMA, 178:977–982, 1961.

84. LeRoux, B.T.: Bronchial carcinoma with hypertrophic pulmonary osteoarthropathy. S. Afr. Med. J., 42:1074–1075, 1968.

85. Lopez-Enriquez, E., Morales, A.R., and Robert, F.: Effect of atropine sulfate in pulmonary hypertrophic osteoarthropathy. Arthritis Rheum., 23:822–824, 1980.

86. Schwartz, H.A.: Pro-Banthine for hypertrophic osteoarthropathy. Arthritis Rheum., 23:1588, 1981.

87. Steinfeld, A.D., and Munzenrider, J.E.: The response of hypertrophic pulmonary osteoarthropathy to radiotherapy. Radiology, 113:709–711, 1974.

88. Rao, G.M., et al.: Improvement in hypertrophic pulmonary osteoarthropathy after radiotherapy to metastases. Am. J. Radiol., 133:944–946, 1979.

89. Evans, W.K.: Reversal of hypertrophic osteoarthropathy after chemotherapy for bronchogenic carcinoma. J. Rheumatol., 7:93–97, 1980.

90. Shapiro, C.M., and Mackinnon, J.: The resolution of hypertrophic pulmonary osteoarthropathy following treatment of subacute bacterial endocarditis. Postgrad. Med. J., 56:513–515, 1980.

REGIONAL DISORDERS OF JOINTS AND RELATED STRUCTURES

TRAUMATIC ARTHRITIS AND ALLIED CONDITIONS

87

ROBERT S. PINALS

In its broadest sense, the term "traumatic arthritis" circumscribes a diverse collection of pathologic and clinical states that develop after single or repetitive episodes of trauma (Table 87–1). Although these conditions may be encountered frequently by the rheumatologist, interest in the area has been casual, and studies of basic mechanisms of disease have been few as compared with those in the other rheumatic diseases. Because surgeons are more likely to deal with the sequelae of trauma, it is not surprising that the most significant contributions are to be found in the orthopedic literature. The credulous assignment of etiologic roles to trauma in early writings stands in sharp contrast to modern attitudes on the subject. Rheumatoid arthritis, tuberculous arthritis, gout, and other rheumatic diseases were formerly attributed to trauma, which might alter the structural integrity of joints, predisposing them to inflammation.[1] As other pathogenetic mechanisms have been revealed, it has become less necessary to invoke "unrecognized trauma," which was previously such a convenient explanation for poorly understood disorders. Even in osteoarthritis, once the bellwether of traumatic disorders, considered by some to be synonymous with traumatic arthritis, increasing emphasis is being placed on altered cartilage metabolism, leaving an even smaller role for "multiple microtraumata."

ACUTE TRAUMATIC SYNOVITIS

Following a direct blow or forced inappropriate motion to a joint, swelling and pain may develop. Be-cause the knee is most commonly affected, the following discussion will be directed at that joint, but one might follow a similar approach for a traumatic synovitis in the elbow, shoulder, or ankle. On examination, an effusion is usually evident, which should be aspirated to determine whether hemarthrosis is present and to aid in further examination of the joint. Hemarthrosis is usually present if fluid appears within 2 hours after the injury.[2] In about half the cases, swelling occurs within 15 minutes.[3] On the other hand, nonbloody effusions generally appear 12 to 24 hours after injury.[3] With hemarthrosis there is usually more pain, and at times a low-grade fever. Fractures, internal derangements, or major ligamentous tears must be ruled out by examination and radiographs, which should include stress, skyline, and intercondylar views. In one series of patients with traumatic hemarthrosis, 66 had fractures or ligamentous rupture, and 20 did not.[2] Detachment or laceration of cartilage and capsular tears may not be discovered in this manner. It has been suggested, on the basis of calcification that developed later in the median parapatellar area, that lateral subluxation of the patella, tearing the medial retinaculum, may be the source of joint hemorrhage in some cases.[2] Partial or complete anterior cruciate ligament tears, often undetected on physical examination, were confirmed by arthroscopy in 72% of a group of patients with traumatic hemarthrosis.[4] The presence of fat globules floating on the surface of bloody fluid usually indicates a fracture. At times, sufficient fat may be present to be detectable on a lateral knee radiograph as a

1371

Table 87–1. Classification of Traumatic Arthritis and Allied Conditions

I. Articular trauma, single episode.
   A. Traumatic synovitis, without disturbance of articular cartilage or disruption of major supporting structures. This type includes acute synovitis, with or without hemarthrosis, and most sprains. Healing is expected within several weeks, without permanent tissue damage.
   B. Disruptive trauma, with infraction of the articular cartilage or complete rupture of major supporting structures. This type includes intra-articular fractures, meniscal tears, and severe sprains.
   C. Post-traumatic osteoarthritis. This type includes cases of disruptive trauma in which major residual damage is present. Patients may have deformity, limited motion, or instability of joints.
II. Repetitive articular trauma. This type includes a variety of conditions related to occupation or sports and results in localized chronic arthritis.
III. Induction or aggravation of another specific rheumatic disease by acute or repetitive trauma.
IV. Conditions in which trauma may be one of several etiologic factors, or in which a relationship has been suggested but not established: osteochondritis dissecans, osteitis pubis, Tietze's syndrome, and hypermobility syndrome.
V. Disorders of extra-articular structures, such as tendons, bursae, and muscles, in which trauma commonly plays an etiologic role.
VI. Nonmechanical types of trauma, such as arthropathy following frostbite, radiation, and decompression.

radiolucent layer in the suprapatellar pouch[5] (Fig. 87–1). A similar appearance has been described in the anterior compartment of the elbow.[6] Hemorrhagic fluid usually does not clot; coagulation may indicate more profound tissue damage and a poorer prognosis. Rarely, a chylous effusion may occur, either with or without an intra-articular fracture or hemarthrosis.[7,8]

In the absence of gross bleeding, examination of the fluid reveals a variable number of red blood cells and 50 to 2000 white blood cells, of which only a few are neutrophils. The protein content, mostly albumin, is two or three times that of normal fluid. Viscosity is slightly reduced, but the mucin clot is good.[9] Synovial biopsy reveals some vasodilatation, edema, and an occasional small focus of synovial cell proliferation with mild lymphocytic infiltration. An electron-microscopic study has shown evidence of increased pro-

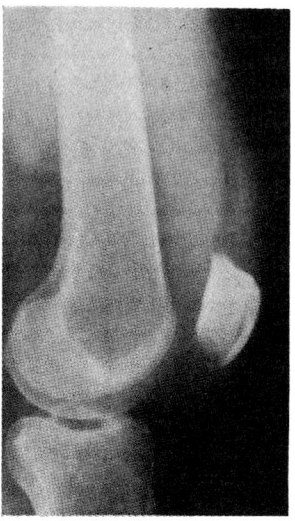

FIG. 87–1. Traumatic hemarthrosis. Liquid fat and a fat-blood level are visible in the joint. (From Berk, R.N.[5])

tein synthesis by synovial cells, perhaps accounting for a portion of the excessive protein content in post-traumatic effusions.[10]

Rarely, a high leukocyte count in traumatic synovial effusions is accompanied by intra- and extracellular lipid globules, suggesting that lipid droplet phagocytosis might have provoked an inflammatory reaction.[11] This hypothesis was supported by studies of dog knees subjected to blunt trauma, which resulted in clear effusions containing fat globules. Intra-articular injection of autologous fat was shown to induce phagocytosis and mild inflammation[12] (see Chapter 109).

Treatment may include such measures as cold packs initially and heat later; compression dressings or posterior splints; graded quadriceps exercises; repeated aspiration if significant volumes of fluid reaccumulate; and a period of bed rest or partial weight-bearing, depending upon the severity of the injury. Early arthroscopic surgery is being advocated with increasing frequency, particularly in athletes with cruciate ligament or meniscal disruption.[13] Prognosis is excellent in the absence of improper treatment, such as cylinder cast immobilization, which may result in muscle atrophy and loss of motion, or premature weight-bearing, which may lead to an extended duration of synovitis. A study of experimental hemarthrosis in rabbits has shown that there is no deleterious effect on articular cartilage, even from repeated hemarthroses, although the synovium may show a mild inflammatory process and iron accumulation.[14]

SPRAINS

A sprain may be defined as a stretching or tearing of a supporting ligament of a joint by forced movement beyond its normal range. In its simplest form, there is minimal disruption of fibers, swelling, pain, and dysfunction. Severe sprains may cause total rupture of ligaments, marked swelling and hemorrhage, and joint instability, which may be permanent if untreated. Sprains occur most frequently in the ankle, but are also common in the knee, low back, and neck.

Ankle Sprains. Most ankle sprains result from unintentional weight-bearing on the inverted, plantar-flexed foot. There is partial or total disruption of one or more of the three main lateral supporting structures, which unite the fibula above with the calcaneus and talus below (Fig. 87–2). Rupture of the anterior talofibular ligament is most common; this structure prevents anterior displacement of the talus out of the ankle joint mortise. With additional force, the calcaneofibular ligament, which prevents excessive inversion, may also rupture. The third ligament, the posterior talofibular ligament, is seldom torn with the usual type of injury. If it also tears, a completely unstable ankle results. Stretching of the medial supporting structures usually results in fracture and avulsion of the medial malleolus rather than a sprain.

The patient presents with severe pain and swelling on the outer aspect of the foot and ankle. Much of the early swelling is due to hemorrhage, resulting in ecchymosis several hours later. A history of something snapping, giving away, or slipping out of place may suggest a complete ligament rupture. The nature of the treatment is largely dependent upon assessment of the integrity of these ligaments. This is most easily accomplished soon after the injury, before swelling and pain make forced motion difficult. Local anesthesia may be required for proper examination.

FIG. 87–2. A severe ankle sprain, occurring in equinus and inversion, may result in rupture of the anterior talofibular ligament (arrow). (From Pipkin, G.: Clin. Orthop., 3:8, 1954.)

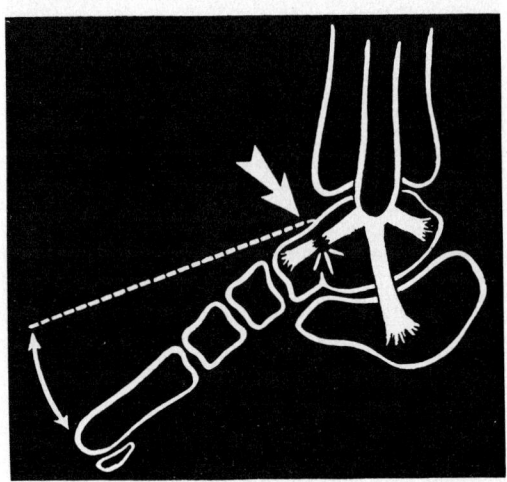

Some orthopedists insist upon stress roentgenograms after all severe sprains.

Early treatment of simple sprains may include elevation, ice packs, and compression dressing to prevent swelling; injection of local anesthetics to permit early motion; and adhesive strapping. Full weight-bearing is permitted on the following day. A lift on the outer border of the heel will maintain eversion and prevent strain on the injured ligament. Strapping, or later an elastic support, is continued until healing is complete.[15]

Severe sprains may demand additional treatment, such as walking plaster for 4 to 6 weeks when the anterior talofibular ligament is ruptured, and early or late surgical repair for marked instability.[15] A followup study of patients with long-standing lateral ligament instability demonstrated a high incidence of degenerative changes in the articular cartilage of the medial joint surface.[16]

Other Sprains. Knee sprains are considered in Chapter 88, and low back sprains in Chapter 92. Shoulder "sprain" is actually a subluxation of the acromioclavicular joint, commonly seen in body contact sports. Wrist "sprain" is usually a fractured navicular bone, often missed on initial roentgenograms. Traumatic torticollis may be called a neck sprain. Following a sudden twist or wrenching of the neck, pain and muscle spasm may result in involuntary assumption of a "wry neck" position. Spontaneous remission occurs after 1 to 2 weeks. Measures such as a cervical collar, traction, and heat may be helpful. The actual structures involved in neck sprain have not been well defined.

PELLEGRINI-STIEDA SYNDROME; PERIARTICULAR OSSIFICATION

A linear calcific density may develop in the area of the medial collateral ligament after acute knee trauma. A hematoma may be the initial event. Calcification is noted on roentgenograms obtained as early as 3 or 4 weeks after the injury.[17] Few biopsies have been obtained in the early stages; those performed later show bone rather than a calcific deposit. The initial injury may be minor or may produce a fracture, torn meniscus, or ligamentous rupture. Initial signs and symptoms, as well as subsequent disability, are related more to this associated trauma than to the Pellegrini-Stieda lesion itself.[18] Persistent tenderness and some swelling are often found on the medial aspect of the knee, however. Local corticosteroid injections have been advocated for these patients.

ECTOPIC BONE FORMATION AFTER SPINAL CORD INJURY

Paraplegic and quadriplegic patients may develop ossification in soft tissues adjacent to joints that are located below the level of the neurologic lesion. The hips and knees are most commonly involved. This complication occurs in 16 to 53% of patients with spinal cord injury[19] and occasionally in other neurologic conditions.[20] Although some of the milder cases may not be detected by physical examination, many patients have swelling, warmth, and erythema in the affected area, suggesting alternative diagnoses, such as cellulitis and thrombophlebitis. These signs may appear as early as 3 weeks after the injury, when radiographic findings are minimal or absent.[21] At this stage, serum alkaline phosphatase may be elevated, and soft tissue uptake of radionuclide may be increased on a bone scan.[20] Over a period of weeks or months, a firm mass of trabeculated bone may be detected on physical examination and demonstrated radiologically. This finding is often accompanied by loss of joint motion and occasionally by complete ankylosis. Serious functional impairment may result; for instance, the patient may be unable to sit because hip flexion is lost. The osseous deposit may be excised when it reaches maturity, but it recurs in most patients.

The pathogenesis of this condition is unknown, but it has been suggested that these immobile patients develop areas of ischemic tissue necrosis at pressure points near joints, leading to an inflammatory reaction and subsequent bony metaplasia.[22] The areas of ectopic bone formation correlated with decubitus ulcerations of the overlying skin in one report.[23] Vigorous passive exercise, advocated to prevent loss of joint motion, does not appear to increase the ossification process.[22] Patients with spinal cord injury may also develop hydrarthrosis or hemarthrosis of the knee, presumed to be of traumatic origin.[24] The effusion, which may precede the ossification, has a normal cell count but a discordantly high protein concentration.[25]

DISRUPTIVE ARTICULAR TRAUMA: POST-TRAUMATIC OSTEOARTHRITIS

Permanent joint damage may be the end result of various types of trauma, including fractures through the articular surface, dislocations, internal derangements, major ligamentous ruptures, and wounds, often with sepsis and foreign body implantation (Fig. 87–3). There may be permanent or progressive struc-tural alterations, e.g., deterioration of articular cartilage, limitation of joint motion, instability, or angular deviation. Detailed consideration of these injuries and their treatment is beyond the scope of this book. Pathologically and radiographically, the condition has most of the characteristics of osteoarthritis. However, a specific traumatic episode should not be definitely accepted as etiologically related to osteoarthritis unless there is evidence establishing the following points: (1) the joint was normal prior to injury; (2) records document either an effusion or structural damage shortly after the injury; and (3) similar disease has not occurred in nontraumatized joints. Other points favoring a traumatic origin are the occurrence of significant isolated osteoarthritis in a joint not usually involved by the idiopathic variety (such as ankle, wrist, elbow, or metacarpophalangeal joint) and radiologic demonstration of foreign bodies and healed fractures near the joint in question.

REPETITIVE ARTICULAR TRAUMA

Osteoarthritis may develop in joints that are repeatedly traumatized as a result of certain occupations

FIG. 87–3. Arthritis due to foreign body. A piece of steel lodged in this index finger of the patient 4 years earlier. Swelling of the finger began about 2 years later and has continued to date. Roentgenograph shows marked deformity of the proximal interphalangeal joint of the right index finger. This consists of marked hypertrophic changes with possible ankylosis of the joint. There are two small opaque foreign bodies in relation to the palmar and radial aspects of the joint.

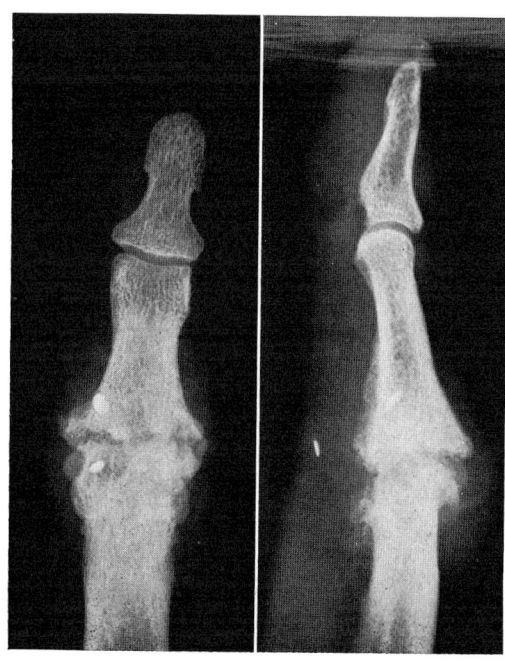

and sports. Radiographic abnormalities, such as joint space narrowing, subcortical cysts, and marginal osteophytes, are common in some groups studied, but many of the affected individuals are asymptomatic. These changes occur in the hands and wrists of boxers and stone workers using pneumatic hammers, in the ankles of soccer players, in the first metatarsophalangeal joints of ballet dancers, and in the elbows of foundry workers.

ROLE OF TRAUMA IN OTHER TYPES OF ARTHRITIS

Trauma plays an important role in the development of neuropathic joint disease (see Chapter 81). Attacks of gouty arthritis and pseudogout often develop in recently injured joints. Rheumatoid arthritis occasionally begins in a joint that has been injured or subjected to a surgical procedure. In a followup study of patients who had sustained a serious fracture, the incidence of rheumatoid arthritis was found to be greater than in control subjects.[26] A history of recent or old trauma to the affected joint is sometimes obtained from patients with septic or tuberculous arthritis. The evidence in these situations is anecdotal and difficult to evaluate, however. Data have not been gathered in an organized fashion, and the mechanisms involved are not well understood. In many instances, the trauma has been minimal, perhaps representing an unrelated antecedent to the joint disease.[27]

Williams and Scott have reported three patients in whom trauma to a finger joint was followed by chronic polyarthritis with most prominent involvement of the injured joint.[28] In the absence of appropriate studies, however, the putative etiologic or precipitating role of trauma in rheumatoid arthritis remains speculative.

Pre-existing arthritis may certainly be aggravated by trauma, but the dimensions of this statement are an unknown quantity, and each case must be considered on its own merits.[29] Only minor force would be required to cause rupture of a frayed wrist extensor tendon or collateral ligament in a patient with rheumatoid arthritis. Other acute episodes, such as abrupt increase in joint swelling or rupture of the posterior knee joint capsule, are commonly associated with unusual resistive exercise. Sanguineous joint fluid is sometimes aspirated from a knee or shoulder in patients with rheumatoid arthritis who report sudden increase in pain and swelling following relatively minor trauma. It is presumed that pinching or compressing the hypertrophied synovium may result in

bleeding. In such cases, the synovial fluid hematocrit is fairly low, usually less than 10%.

BENIGN HYPERMOBILITY SYNDROME

Generalized joint hypermobility due to ligamentous laxity occurs in about 5% of the population. The condition is regarded by some as a familial disorder that predisposes the affected individual to articular injuries, leading to chronic or recurrent arthralgia. The term "hypermobility syndrome" was introduced by Kirk et al. to describe healthy subjects with joint laxity in the absence of major features of the Marfan or Ehlers-Danlos syndromes, and arthralgia for which no other explanation could be found.[30] The syndrome has a marked female preponderance. Symptoms first appear in children or young adults.[31] Hypermobile individuals are often able to hyperextend the knee and elbow beyond 10°, to achieve sufficient lumbar flexion to place both palms on the floor without bending the knees, and to passively oppose the thumb to the flexor aspect of the forearm. Lacking the stability afforded by normal ligaments, hypermobile subjects are said to be more vulnerable to the adverse effects of injury and overuse, including sprains, traumatic synovitis, recurrent dislocations, tendinitis, and premature degenerative arthritis.[32] An associated systemic connective tissue abnormality is possible. A group of patients with mitral valve prolapse in one study had a higher frequency of joint hypermobility than controls.[33] A marfanoid habitus,[34] thin skin, and uterine prolapse[35] may also be associated with hypermobility. In a recent study of skin biopsies from selected patients with hypermobility, most of whom also had mitral valve prolapse, an increased content of type III collagen was demonstrated.[36]

The relationship between benign hypermobility and joint symptoms or systemic features is supported by several studies,[31,37,38] but is not universally accepted. In one study of healthy blood donors, no differences were found between hypermobile individuals and controls in the frequency of arthralgias, dislocations, mitral valve prolapse, or thin skin.[39]

ACUTE BONE ATROPHY (SUDECK'S ATROPHY; REFLEX DYSTROPHY)

After trauma to an extremity, a few patients develop severe pain, edema, vasomotor abnormalities, and atrophy of bone, muscle, and skin. Many labels have been applied to this syndrome, depending upon the feature of particular interest to the describer: *Su-*

deck's atrophy, Leriche's post-traumatic osteoporosis, Weir Mitchell's causalgia, peripheral trophoneurosis, reflex dystrophy, and *chronic traumatic edema.* The term "causalgia" should probably be reserved for cases in which there has been injury to a major nerve trunk, but the resulting intense burning pain is not confined to the distribution of the nerve and may not differ from that which occurs in reflex dystrophy without nerve injury.[40,41] Most patients are adults, but the condition can occasionally occur in children, resulting in growth arrest in the involved limb.[42] Another variant, the "shoulder-hand syndrome," is usually not related to trauma and is described in detail in Chapter 97.

The antecedent injury may be a fracture, but it is often fairly trivial, such as a sprain or laceration, and it may occur with about equal frequency in an upper or lower extremity.[43] Pain, of a quality and degree inappropriate for the injury, may begin immediately or not until several weeks after the trauma.[41,43] Disinclination to move the extremity is also an early feature that is inextricably linked to the pain. The limb is painful on motion and may have striking cutaneous hyperalgesia and cold sensitivity. A hyperemic stage may be noted in some cases, but a cold, moist, cyanotic, edematous hand or foot is more typical after 2 or 3 months. Roentgenograms, usually normal during the first month, later show patchy osteopenia, often periarticular in distribution initially, but diffuse later. With continued immobility, muscle and skin atrophy occur and joint motion is lost.

Pathogenesis and management are discussed in Chapter 97. It should be emphasized that early identification of patients and restoration of active motion are the keys to successful treatment. Early treatment with simple, conservative measures, including graded active exercises, heat, and elevation, may produce good results. Long-standing disease, with advanced atrophy of skin, muscle, and bone, may be largely irreversible. To obviate this irreversibility, more aggressive therapies have been proposed, but none has been studied in controlled trials. These measures include oral corticosteroids, sympathetic nerve blocks, and regional intravenous injection of corticosteroids, analgesics, or sympatholytic agents.[41,43]

Another syndrome characterized by pain and osteopenia has been described in several reports since 1959[44-47] as *migratory osteolysis, regional migratory osteoporosis,* and *transient osteoporosis of the hip.* The condition was first described during pregnancy,[44] but subsequently has been noticed most often in middle-aged men, who develop a painful swelling in one region of a lower extremity, rarely with preceding trauma.[47] Either the hip, knee, or foot may be involved. Pain is often severe, especially on motion and weight-bearing. Although radiographs may be normal during the first 2 or 3 weeks of symptoms, severe osteoporosis in the painful region is readily apparent thereafter. This condition is unlikely to be related to disuse because uptake of a bone-seeking radioisotope is increased in the affected area during the first week, prior to immobilization of the extremity.[48] This disorder is self-limited, with resolution of signs and symptoms in several months and eventual return of bone density to normal. Subsequent attacks may occur in other areas but not in previously involved joints. Nothing is known of the pathogenesis of this syndrome, but its resemblance to Sudeck's atrophy has been noted[46,47] and a strong association with type IV hyperlipoproteinemia has been demonstrated.[49]

OSTEOCHONDRITIS DISSECANS

This local disorder of subchondral bone is most commonly found in the knees of adolescents and young adults. A devitalized fragment of bone, with its articular cartilage still present, demarcates from its original site, usually on the lateral portion of the medial femoral condyle. Partial or complete detachment may occur eventually, with resulting signs and symptoms of a "loose body" in the joint; less frequently, the fragment may lodge in the intercondylar notch and may remain clinically silent.

Antecedent trauma, though common, seems to be only one of several etiologic factors. Anomalous ossification centers, locally deficient blood supply, and genetic factors[50] are particularly important in the younger age group, whereas trauma plays a greater role in adults. In histologic studies, no evidence of ischemic necrosis was found, however.[51,52] The trauma involved may be "endogenous," such as repeated contact between an unusually prominent tibial spine or aberrantly situated cruciate ligament and the femoral condyle.

The clinical picture in patients with knee involvement consists of mild discomfort rather than pain. This discomfort is aggravated by exercise, but there may also be some aching at rest. With separation of the fragment, the patient may complain of instability or "giving-way." Often an unusual stance, due to external rotation of the tibia, may be noted.[53] This stance diminishes contact between the tibial spine and the usual site of osteochondritis on the medial condyle, near the intercondylar notch. A sign that correlates with this may be demonstrated by forcing the tibia into internal rotation while slowly extending the knee from 90° of flexion. At about 30°, the patient complains of pain, which is relieved immediately by external rotation of the tibia.

Roentgenograms may be normal for as long as 6 months after the injury; the typical picture is that of a bony sequestrum lodged in a sharply defined cavity (Fig. 87–4). The lesion has a similar appearance when it occurs in other locations, such as the elbow (capitellum), ankle (talus), hip, and metatarsal head.[54,55] Occasionally, multiple sites are involved particularly in individuals from predisposed families.[50]

Treatment is conservative if the fragment remains in place. Loose fragments may be treated surgically, with either removal or fixation.[55] The immediate prognosis is good, but some patients may develop osteoarthritis later in life.

Epiphyseal Osteochondritis. Necrosis of an entire epiphysis is a common localized disorder in childhood. Vascular insufficiency is thought to be the most significant etiologic factor; trauma is often mentioned, but seldom established as a primary cause. Experimental evidence suggests that compression fractures may lead to disorderly epiphyseal ossification characteristic of osteochondritis.[56] In the hip (*Legg-Calvé-Perthes disease*), osteochondritis occurs in younger children (2 to 10 years of age), usually presenting with a limp rather than with pain. In the knee (*Osgood-Schlatter disease*), older children (9 to 15 years of age) develop pain and swelling in the tibial tubercle; this condition may result from a traction injury.[56] Osteochondritis of the vertebrae (*Scheuermann's disease*) presents with kyphosis and is described in Chapter 92.

FIG. 87–4. Osteochondritis dissecans. Arrow indicates osseous fragment.

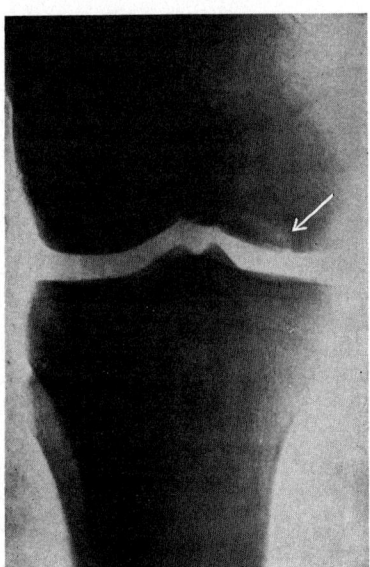

Generalized osteochondritis involving small joints in the hands and wrists, as well as the joints already mentioned, is a rare but definite entity. This condition must be differentiated from the polyarthritides.[57]

TIETZE'S SYNDROME; COSTOCHONDRITIS

Tietze's syndrome is a benign condition in which painful enlargement develops in the upper costal cartilages. The syndrome occurs with the same frequency in both sexes and on both sides of the chest. Involvement of only a single costal cartilage is found in 80% of patients, the second and third being most affected. Onset of pain is either acute or insidious, usually without prior injury, with the exception of trauma, which may have occurred during vigorous coughing in a minority of cases. Pain is sometimes severe, is aggravated by motion of the rib cage, and may radiate to the shoulder and arm. Palpation of a firm tender fusiform swelling of the costal cartilage confirms the diagnosis. Biopsy usually shows normal cartilage, occasionally some edema of the perichondrium, and, rarely, nonspecific chronic inflammation in the surrounding tissues. The duration is variable, from a week to several years. Some patients have multiple episodes, but spontaneous remission is the rule. The swelling has been attributed to cartilaginous hypertrophy by some and to abnormal angulation by others, but nothing is known of the pathogenesis. Treatment may include analgesics, heat, local infiltration with corticosteroid, intercostal nerve block, and reassurance that symptoms are not due to heart disease.

Other disorders may produce pain, tenderness, or evidence of inflammation in the costochondral joints, but not a hard swelling as in Tietze's syndrome. They include rheumatoid arthritis, fibrositis, gout, pyogenic infection, and the anterior chest wall syndrome that may follow myocardial infarction.

The most common cause of chest wall pain in individuals who do not have a generalized rheumatic disease is an ill-defined condition usually called *costochondritis*.[58] The pain may be severe, radiating widely, but is often worse on the left side. In some cases it is aggravated by coughing, deep respiration, and motion of the thorax. Anxiety and hyperventilation are common accompaniments. Some episodes are brief and self-limited, but others are chronic, recurrent, and disabling. Tenderness over the costal cartilages, simulating or accentuating the spontaneous pain, is the main physical finding. The xiphoid may be tender in patients with generalized costochondritis, but there is also a syndrome of *isolated xiphoidalgia,* which may result in epigastric pain suggestive of various intra-abdominal disorders. Reproduction of the pain by pressing over the xiphoid is the essential diagnostic maneuver. Little is known of the etiology and pathology of these conditions. In most cases there is no evidence for a traumatic cause, but emotional factors are frequently involved. Care must be taken to rule out coronary artery disease, which may occasionally be associated with chest wall hyperalgesia.

Sudden episodes of sharp pain at the costal margin may be caused by the *rib-tip syndrome.*[59,60] This condition is due to hypermobility of the anterior end of a costal cartilage, usually that of the tenth rib, as a result of past trauma. The patients, usually middle-aged of either sex, complain of upper abdominal pain, precipitated by movement and by certain postures. A snapping sensation and point tenderness at the rib tip, relieved by a local anesthetic injection, will confirm the diagnosis.

OSTEITIS PUBIS

Surgical trauma in the retropubic area may occasionally provoke an inflammatory process in the pubic symphysis and adjacent bone.[61] Osteitis pubis may occur after prostate or bladder surgery and, more rarely, following herniorrhaphy or childbirth. Several weeks postoperatively, the patient develops pain over the symphysis radiating down the inner aspects of the thighs, often aggravated by coughing and straining. Physical findings include an antalgic gait, point tenderness over the symphysis, spasm in the abdominal and hip adductor muscle groups, and a low-grade fever. Radiographs may be normal initially, but rarefaction and osteolysis develop around the symphysis within 2 to 4 weeks. A sterile chronic inflammatory process is usually noted on biopsy,[61] but a true osteomyelitis may be discovered in a minority of patients, generally those with more marked bone destruction and fever.[62] Tuberculosis and metastatic disease must also be considered in the differential diagnosis. Similar radiographic findings may be observed in ankylosing spondylitis and occasionally in chondrocalcinosis or in other types of polyarthritis, but pain is minimal or absent. Although spontaneous remission may be expected in osteitis pubis, disabling symptoms may persist for many months. The gamut of anti-inflammatory drugs has been used with varying success. Other measures, such as immobilization, wearing a tight pelvic belt, surgical debridement, and radiotherapy, have been advocated. The pathogen-

esis is uncertain, but there is general agreement that one or more factors, in addition to trauma, may contribute.

Traumatic osteitis pubis in athletes, particularly soccer players, may be a result of an avulsion stress fracture at the origin of the gracilis muscle near the symphysis.[63]

SYNOVIAL CYSTS OF THE POPLITEAL SPACE: "BAKER'S CYSTS"

Six primary bursae are associated with muscles and tendons on the posteromedial aspect of the knee. Communications between two bursae and between a bursa and the knee joint are common. Popliteal cysts may arise in three ways: (1) accumulation of fluid in a noncommunicating bursa; (2) distention of a bursa by fluid originating as a result of a lesion in the knee joint; and (3) posterior herniation of the joint capsule in response to increased intra-articular pressure. The communication between joint and cyst is generally narrow and the anatomy such that a flap-valve mechanism may be operative, allowing free passage of fluid from knee to cyst, but not in the opposite direction.[64]

Popliteal cysts may be seen at all ages. Those in children are usually unassociated with joint disease and are often bilateral. Most disappear spontaneously.[65] In about half of all cases, some abnormality is evident in the knee joint. In one study of 198 patients, 40 had osteoarthritis, 27 had rheumatoid arthritis, 11 had cartilage tears or osteochondromatosis, and 11 had a variety of other conditions.[66] Only 10 patients had a history of trauma. In most patients with knee joint disease, a connection between the cyst and joint could be demonstrated. The cyst itself usually causes only mild discomfort; other symptoms may be related to the associated joint lesions. A fluctuant swelling is present in the popliteal area, occasionally extending well into the calf and presenting superficially at the medial border of the gastrocnemius. The differential diagnosis includes aneurysms, benign neoplasms, varicosities, and thrombophlebitis. Arthrograms may be helpful if the cyst communicates with the knee joint.[67] The histopathologic characteristics of the cysts are varied and do not particularly correspond to the presumed origin, bursal or hernial.[66] Most have a thin fibrous wall, lined by a single layer of flat cells. Others have structural characteristics of a synovial membrane, particularly those occurring in patients with rheumatoid arthritis. A few have a thickened, inflamed wall coated with fibrin, but no villus formation.

Definitive treatment is essentially surgical. In some

cases, correction of knee joint pathology (such as synovectomy in a patient with rheumatoid arthritis) may result in spontaneous disappearance. Aspiration of the cyst and corticosteroid injections are often palliative.

Synovial cysts in rheumatoid arthritis are seen in many other joints.[68] Occasionally, a communicating cyst of traumatic or nonspecific origin may be seen elsewhere. For instance, a cyst connecting with the hip joint may present anteriorly as a mass in the groin or posteriorly with sciatic pain.

GANGLION

A ganglion is a cystic swelling that may be found near, and often attached to, a tendon sheath or joint capsule, and is believed to be derived from these structures. A slender connection may be demonstrated histologically[69] and radiographically.[70] The thick mucoid material within the ganglion contains hyaluronic acid, although no true synovial membrane lines the cavity.[71] The most common location is on the dorsum of the wrist (Fig. 87–5), but ganglia are also frequently noted on the volar aspect of the wrist, the fingers, and the dorsum of the foot. Ganglia of the flexor tendon sheaths, at the base of the fingers, are common in typists.[72] They have been reported near many other joints and also attached to the tibial periosteum.[73] In most instances, there has been no definite relationship to trauma. Small ganglia are more likely to be painful than larger ones, probably because they are in the process of expanding. Most patients have few symptoms other than unsightly swelling and slight discomfort on motion.

Ganglia may disappear spontaneously. Treatment is not necessarily required, but is often demanded by the patient for cosmetic reasons. Successful treatment in about 80% of cases has been reported after multiple punctures of the cyst wall with a large bore needle, aspiration of the contents, and injection of a corticosteroid preparation.[74] If the ganglion recurs after this procedure, surgical excision may be performed.[75]

TENOSYNOVITIS; STENOSING TENOVAGINITIS

Tenosynovitis is an inflammation of the cellular lining membrane of the fibrous tube (vagina) through which a tendon moves. It may be produced by various diseases (e.g., rheumatoid arthritis, gout, gonococcal arthritis), but even more commonly by trauma. Such trauma may occur from a direct blow, from abnormal pressure upon a tendon (such as from the stiff counter of a new shoe on the Achilles tendon) or, most often, from a short period of unusual activity involving a certain muscle-tendon unit. In one industrial study of 88 cases, the wrist and thumb extensors were involved in 71% and the dorsiflexors at the ankle in 18%. Most were related to a new type of repetitive work or to resumption of work after vacation.[76] The condition is identified by tenderness, swelling, and palpable crepitus over the tendon as it is moved (peritendinitis crepitans). Remission usually occurs if the affected part is rested for a few days.

Stenosing tenovaginitis is primarily a disorder of the fibrous wall of the tendon sheath, particularly at locations where the tendon passes through a fibrous ring or pulley. Generally, an osseous groove comprises part of the ring, which is completed by a thickening of the tendon sheath. Such arrangements are found over bony prominences, such as the radial styloid and the flexor surfaces of the metacarpal and metatarsal heads. With prolonged mechanical stress from either tendon motion under an excessive load

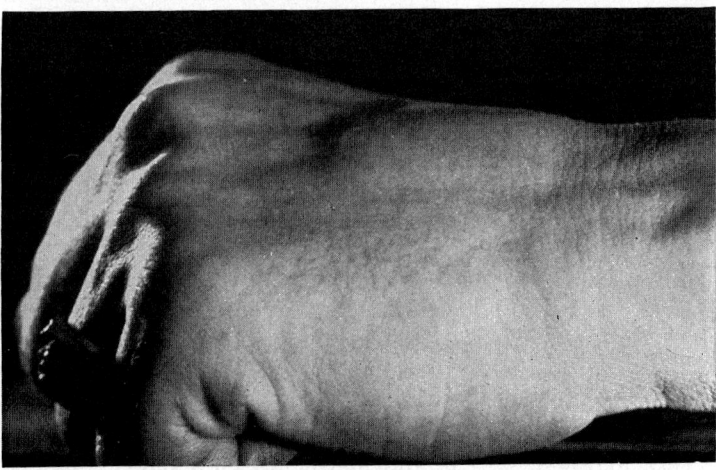

FIG. 87–5. Ganglion arising from extensor tendon sheaths. An oval and flattened cystic mass is on the dorsum of hand.

or external pressure, such as from the handles of pruning shears, abnormal proliferation of fibrous tissue in the ring constricts the lumen of the tendon sheath. Secondary changes may then occur in the tendon, usually with enlargement distal to the constriction. There may be a snapping sensation with movement of the enlarged segment of tendon through the narrowed ring ("trigger finger" and "snapping thumb"). Further progression may produce locking in flexion; the tendon may be pulled through the constriction by its own flexor muscle but not by its weaker extensor antagonist. When extension is forced, the bulbous portion suddenly pops back through the constriction, and the digit "unlocks." Tenosynovitis due to mechanical stress may also contribute to pain and loss of motion.

Stenosing tenovaginitis of the abductor pollicis longus and extensor pollicis brevis at the radial styloid is known as *de Quervain's disease*.[77] It is a common disorder among women who perform repetitive man-

FIG. 87–6. *Top,* Wrist and thumb in neutral position, tendons relaxed. *Center,* Radial deviation of wrist and thumb relaxed, minor tearing stress applied to retinaculum. *Bottom,* Radial deviation of wrist while gripping, strong tearing stress applied to retinaculum. (From Muckart, R.D.[77])

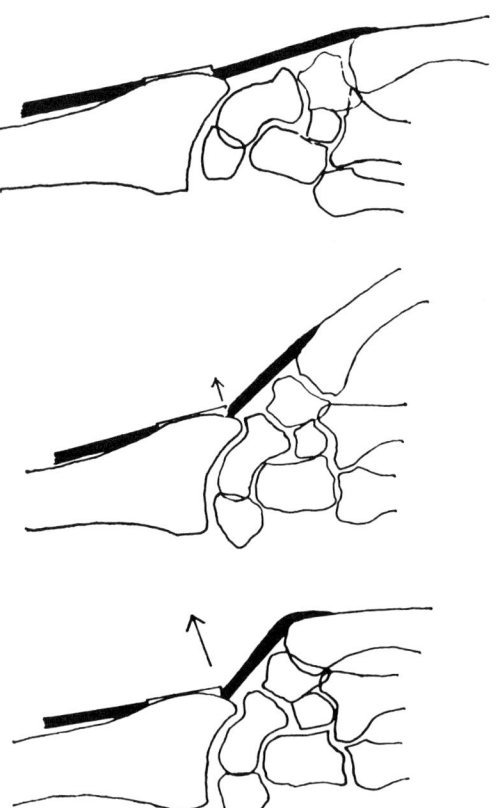

ual tasks involving grasping with the thumb accompanied by movement of the hand in a radial direction (Fig. 87–6). Occurrence during pregnancy, followed by spontaneous resolution, has also been reported.[78] Symptoms include pain in the area of the radial styloid and weakness of grip. Examination reveals tenderness and thickening over the involved tendons and limited excursion of the thumb; locking and snapping seldom occur. The classic test is the demonstration of *Finkelstein's sign.* The thumb is placed in the palm of the hand and grasped by the fingers; ulnar deviation of the wrist elicits a sharp pain if inflammation of the tendon sheath is present.

The most common locations for stenosing tenovaginitis are the thumb flexor and extensor tendons and the finger flexors, but occasionally other sites are involved. These sites include the flexor carpi radialis tendon, resulting in pain at the base of the thenar eminence,[79] the common peroneal sheath, causing pain on the lateral aspect of the ankle,[80] and the tibialis posterior tendon,[80] presenting with pain below and behind the medial malleolus after prolonged standing and walking.

Treatment of Stenosing Tenovaginitis. Conservative measures such as (1) cessation of the repetitive activity thought to have provoked the condition, (2) immobilization with splints, and (3) local corticosteroid injections often result in improvement, but recurrences are common. Tenosynovitis may subside, but the area of fibrous constriction is unlikely to be greatly altered by this approach, particularly when the duration of symptoms exceeds 4 months.[81] It is sometimes necessary to resort to surgical excision of this portion of the sheath. In all the locations, the operation is simple and results in permanent remission, even allowing resumption of full activity in most cases.

Carpal and Tarsal Tunnel Syndromes. Tenosynovitis in the flexor compartment of the wrist, where the tendons are enclosed in a bony canal, roofed by a rigid transverse carpal ligament, may result in compression and degeneration of the medial nerve that shares this space. Trauma is only one of many causes of this syndrome; others include rheumatoid arthritis, amyloidosis, myxedema, benign tumors, pregnancy, acromegaly, polymyalgia rheumatica, and diabetes.[82,83] In one report, about half of the patients had been engaged in prolonged activity involving forceful flexion of the fingers with the wrist held in flexion or moving through an arc of flexor motion.[83] In another larger series, only 16% of patients had a history of possible related trauma, including fractures and sprains, as well as excessive use.[82]

An entrapment neuropathy of the posterior tibial nerve behind and below the medial malleolus may be caused by tenosynovitis of the tendons that accompany the nerve through an osseofibrous tunnel.[84] These and other nerve entrapment syndromes are described in Chapter 95.

OTHER FORMS OF TENDINITIS AND BURSITIS

Painful conditions attributed to strain or injury of tendons and their attachments to bone are often loosely described by the term tendinitis. The supraspinatus and bicipital tendons of the shoulder, which are commonly affected, are discussed in Chapter 97. Frequently, tendinitis is related to a particular occupation or sport. For instance, a baseball pitcher, at the end of his delivery, stretches the attachment of the long head of the triceps to the inferior glenoid rim. This movement results in pain in the posterior axillary fold. It is presumed that inflammatory changes occur in the tendon attachment; treatment includes rest, local corticosteroid injections, and ultrasound. Baseball pitchers and golfers may also develop a similar condition at the *medial* epicondyle of the elbow. Jumper's knee refers to tendinitis of the patellar tendon, usually at its attachment to the lower pole of the patella.[85]

Injections of corticosteroid ester crystals into the tendon substance should be avoided, especially in athletes, because subsequent severe loading may result in a tear and severe disability.

TENNIS ELBOW (EPICONDYLITIS)

This is a common condition, most often found in middle-aged men, in which pain derives from the origin of the wrist and finger extensors at the lateral epicondyle. Although first described in tennis players, most cases are not related to that sport, but may be provoked by any exercise or occupation that involves repeated and forcible wrist extension or pronation-supination. The right elbow is involved more often than the left; the condition is seldom bilateral. Pain is usually gradual in onset, but is sometimes related to a specific traumatic incident. It often radiates to the forearm and dorsum of the hand. Physical examination reveals point tenderness at or near the lateral epicondyle, with little or no swelling. Elbow joint motion is unrestricted and painless, but resisted wrist extension results in accentuation of pain. Many possibilities have been expressed for the pathogenesis,[86] including tendon rupture, radiohumeral synovitis, periostitis, neuritis, aseptic necrosis,

and displacement of the orbicular ligament. A detailed pathologic study, including a control group of individuals with apparently normal elbows, revealed no evidence of a bursa in the area of the common extensor insertion, but rather a subtendinous space containing loose areolar connective tissue. In patients with tennis elbow, this space showed granulation tissue, increased vascularity, and edema. Periostitis and tendon tears were not noted.[86]

Management should be directed toward modifying the provocative activity. Many treatments have been proposed, including massage, ultrasonography, anti-inflammatory drugs, braces, and several surgical procedures. The most common approach, local corticosteroid injection, is usually successful. In a recent study, 10% of patients continued to have symptoms after initial therapy with ultrasonography or corticosteroid injection.[87] The rate of response was greater with local injection, but recurrences were more common.

BURSITIS

Bursae are closed sacs, lined with a cellular membrane resembling synovium. They serve to facilitate motion of tendons and muscles over bony prominences. There are over 80 bursae on each side of the body.[88] Many are nameless, and additional ones may form at almost any point subjected to frequent irritation. Excessive frictional forces or, at times, direct trauma may result in an inflammatory process in the bursal wall, with excessive vascularity, exudation of increased amounts of viscous bursal fluid, and fibrin-coating of the lining membrane. Only small numbers of inflammatory cells are found in bursal fluid in traumatic bursitis, but there may be a greater leukocyte response in bursitis secondary to other rheumatic diseases, such as rheumatoid arthritis or gout. Septic bursitis is usually caused by organisms introduced through punctures, wounds, or cellulitis in the overlying skin. Traumatic bursitis may be complicated by infection or hemorrhage. "Beat knee" and "beat shoulder" in miners are examples of this condition. Continuous abrasion of the skin with stone dust results in cellulitis, and repeated scraping of the bursa against rough stone surfaces leads to hemorrhage. With modification of occupations and habits, many of the classic forms of bursitis are encountered less frequently, e.g., "housemaid's knee," "weaver's bottom," and "policeman's heel." Sports-related bursitis (e.g., "wrestler's knee," a prepatellar bursitis found in 10% of college wrestlers) is receiving greater emphasis.[89]

Subdeltoid bursitis, which is described in detail in Chapter 97, is a very common bursitis. The following other types are also frequently seen.

Trochanteric Bursitis. Trochanteric bursitis is an inflammation of one or more of the bursae about the gluteal insertion on the femoral trochanter. This condition is most common in females and usually has insidious onset, preceded by apparent trauma in only about a fourth of the cases.[90,91] Aching pain on the lateral aspect of the hip and thigh is aggravated by lying on the affected side. The patient experiences tenderness posterior to the trochanter and pain with external rotation of the hip and with active abduction against resistance, but not with flexion and extension.

Olecranon Bursitis. An inflammation with effusion at the point of the elbow occurs frequently with rheumatoid arthritis and gout as well as after trauma. Pain is usually minimal, except when pressure is exerted on the swollen bursa. Elbow motion is unimpaired and usually painless. The swelling often subsides if additional trauma is prevented with a sponge ring. Fluid from the bursa is often serosanguineous with a low leukocyte concentration. Septic bursitis here is common.

Achilles Bursitis. In this condition, an inflammation of the bursa occurs just above the attachment of the Achilles tendon to the os calcis. Achilles bursitis is often related to trauma from tight shoes ("pump bumps") and perhaps to an unusual configuration of the posterior calcaneus (see Chapter 89).

Calcaneal Bursitis. An inflammation of a bursa occurs at the point of attachment of the plantar fascia to the os calcis (see Chapter 89).

Bunion. A painful bursitis occurs over the medial surface of the first metatarsophalangeal joint, usually with a hallux valgus (see Chapter 89).

Ischial Bursitis. An inflammation of the bursa separating the gluteus maximus from the underlying ischial tuberosity is usually produced by prolonged sitting on hard surfaces ("weaver's bottom").

Prepatellar Bursitis. This type of bursitis is a swelling between the skin and lower patella or patellar tendon, resulting from frequent kneeling (Fig. 87-7). Pain is usually slight unless there is direct pressure on the swollen area.

Anserine Bursitis. This inflammation of the sartorius bursa on the medial aspect of the tibia is said to occur in women whose legs are disproportionately large. The characteristic complaint is pain with stair climbing. In a recently reported series of bursitis in various locations, anserine bursitis was found to be the most common.[91] Inflammation in another, nameless bursa located at the anterior edge of the medial collateral

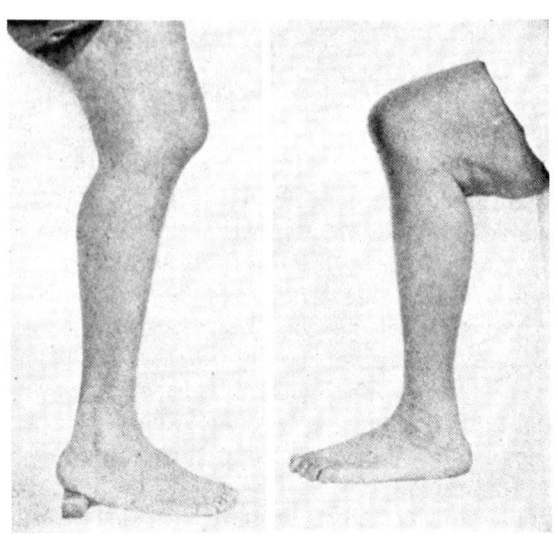

FIG. 87-7.   Bilateral prepatellar bursitis (housemaid's knee) in a scrubwoman. (From Lewin: Orthopedic Surgery for Nurses. Philadelphia, W.B. Saunders Co.)

ligament also gives pain on the inner aspect of the knee, but with point tenderness in a different area.

Iliopectineal Bursitis. With this inflammation of a bursa between the iliopsoas and inguinal ligament, the patient complains of groin pain radiating to the knee. He often adopts a shortened stride to prevent hyperextension of the hip while walking. Examination reveals tenderness just below the inguinal ligament, lateral to the femoral pulse, and pain on hyperextension of the hip.

Treatment. In general, therapy includes protection from irritation and trauma, either by modifying the patient's activities or by using appropriate padding. Anti-inflammatory drugs, heat, and ultrasound are also commonly employed. Local corticosteroid injections are usually successful, but there are occasional local complications such as infection and skin atrophy, particularly with olecranon bursitis.[92] Surgical excision is reserved for refractory cases.

CALCIFIC TENDINITIS AND PERIARTHRITIS

Some cases of tendinitis and bursitis are associated with calcific deposits, most commonly with subdeltoid bursitis and trochanteric bursitis, but occasionally with tendinitis, bursitis, or periarthritis around the wrist, knee, or elbow. In these instances, the attacks are less likely to be preceded by recognized trauma. The attacks tend to be abrupt in onset, with intense local inflammatory signs resembling an attack of gout.

These episodes, which may be examples of crystal-induced inflammation, are described further in Chapters 97 and 108.

INJURIES TO MUSCLES AND TENDONS

The following clinical features are suggestive of rupture of muscles and tendons:

1. The patient has a history of sudden sharp pain or a snapping sensation that occurs during vigorous muscular effort.

2. The patient is unable to perform certain definite movements following this pain or snapping sensation.

3. The diagnosis is more certain if a defect is apparent in the belly of the muscle or in the tendon, with subsequent ecchymosis.

4. Roentgenogram of soft tissues often reveals a defect in the shadow cast by the muscle; in some cases, a small chip of bone is seen attached to a tendon that has been torn from its insertion.

5. Electrical stimulation of the muscle causes it to contract and produce pain at the site of a tear in either the muscle or tendon.

6. Local anesthetic injection eliminates pain and permits testing of muscular function in those patients in whom the diagnosis is difficult.

The supraspinatus muscle or tendon is the most likely to be torn in the upper extremity. The calf muscles and the quadriceps are the most vulnerable in the lower extremity.

Because of their great tensile strength, rupture seldom occurs in the tendons, but rather at the muscle-tendon junction or at the bony insertion.[88] Attrition of the musculotendinous cuff, secondary to local trauma by pulley systems and bony prominences, may lead to necrobiotic changes that predispose to rupture. Trauma is the immediate and direct cause of rupture; sudden application of a stretching force on a strongly contracting muscle results in tearing of muscle fibers, followed by hemorrhage, edema, and localized spasm ("charley horse"). In some cases, the primary mechanism is extreme passive stretching of a tendon attachment, such as the avulsion of the adductor insertion in the groin in a water skier falling with widely abducted hips. Muscle fatigue results in incomplete relaxation and predisposes to stretch injuries. Therefore, these injuries are more likely to occur in poorly conditioned athletes.

Tendon rupture, common in rheumatoid arthritis, is caused by the lytic effect of tenosynovial inflammation and, in addition, mechanical abrasion of tendons due to disruption of the contiguous bone. In-jection of corticosteroids for tendinitis has also been said to predispose to tendon rupture, especially in the Achilles tendon.[93]

Tears in the supraspinatus tendon occur in older individuals. It is presumed that attrition and trauma both contribute to the rupture (see Chapter 97).

Rupture of the long head of the biceps may be the final result of chronic frictional attrition of the tendon within the bicipital groove (see Chapter 97). The rupture may be accompanied by transient pain over the anterior aspect of the shoulder. The belly of the muscle assumes a spherical shape and lies closer to the elbow than normal. Surgical repair is often possible, but not mandatory since disability is generally mild.

The greater or lesser rhomboid muscles may be strained by a sudden uncoordinated movement of the shoulder. This injury occurs frequently in industrial practice. These muscles arise from the ligamentum nuchae and the spinous process of the seventh cervical of the fifth dorsal vertebrae, and they insert into the vertebral border of the scapula. Contraction of these muscles draws this border of the scapula upward.

Following injury to the rhomboid muscles, there is a localized tenderness between the mid-dorsal spine and the scapula. Pain occurs at this point if the shoulder is passively flexed forward or if it is extended against resistance. Treatment consists of partial immobilization of the scapula by drawing it backward and upward with adhesive. Physical therapy (heat and light massage) should be started when the signs of injury have disappeared.

Other muscles arising from the spinous processes and inserting on the scapula or humerus include the levator scapulae, latissimus dorsi, and trapezius muscles. Strains of these muscles give a clinical picture somewhat similar to that for injury to the rhomboids.

Rupture of the pectoralis major muscle is usually caused by an abrupt traction injury, with sudden sharp pain in the shoulder and a snapping sensation.[94] A tender mass is felt in the muscle, and there is ecchymosis of the overlying skin. Evacuation of the hematoma and surgical repair are the treatments of choice.

Rupture of the rectus abdominus muscle may at times be mistaken for intraperitoneal disease (such as appendicitis). Rupture of this muscle may occur following a severe bout of coughing or sneezing, during pregnancy or labor, or following influenza or typhoid fever (with degeneration of the muscle fibers). A large hematoma may form as a result of tears of branches of the epigastric vessels. The hematoma may require evacuation surgically.

Rupture of the quadriceps muscle or tendon is relatively common. This injury occurs at the point of attachment of the tendon to the patella or at the musculotendinous junction; occasionally, a tear may occur through the purely tendinous or muscular portions. The usual cause of this condition is a violent contraction of the muscle, such as falling on a flexed knee. The injury occurs in both young and aged individuals. The patient is unable to actively extend the knee, and a hiatus is seen in the tendon or muscle. Partial tears of the muscle may leave only a depression in the muscle substance without permanent disability. The depressions usually heal readily following splinting of the leg in full extension for 3 or 4 weeks, followed by gradual mobilization. Complete tears of the quadriceps muscle or tendon should be repaired surgically.

When the patellar tendon is ruptured, the patella lies higher than usual, a gap is noted, active knee extension is lost, and joint effusion is usually present. A roentgenogram will confirm the diagnosis.

Partial rupture of one of the calf muscles, termed "tennis leg," usually involves a belly of the gastrocnemius muscle. Symptoms include a snap with sudden burning pain in the calf during a strong muscular contraction. The pain may extend to the popliteal space; it is aggravated by passive dorsiflexion of the ankle and may be confused with thrombophlebitis.[95] Treatment includes adhesive strapping to immobilize the ankle in plantar flexion for several weeks, followed by heat, massage, and exercises.

Spontaneous rupture of the posterior tibial tendon results in pain, tenderness, and swelling behind and below the medial malleolus, with loss of stability of the foot.[96] This injury is usually preceded by chronic symptoms suggestive of tenosynovitis and is often associated with planovalgus feet. Treatment is either surgical repair, in cases diagnosed early, or an arch support.

Injury to the Achilles tendon may occur in runners or in middle-aged men unaccustomed to exertion who indulge in weekend athletics involving jumping (such as basketball and volleyball). There may be rupture at the musculotendinous junction or avulsion at the attachment to the calcaneus. Examination reveals a depression over the tendon and inability to flex the ankle against resistance. In partial rupture, the pain may be mild. Swelling and ecchymosis may conceal the depression usually noted with complete tears. Partial rupture may be treated conservatively with immobilization of the foot in plantar flexion; complete tears usually require surgical intervention.[97]

The anterior tibial compartment syndrome is an ischemic necrosis of muscle caused by swelling after unaccustomed exercise. The muscles in this compartment are confined by a tight fascial sheath, resulting in a compromised blood supply when swelling occurs. Examination shows a marked weakness of the involved muscle and local swelling and erythema. Sensation in the first two toes is often lost because of compression of the deep peroneal nerve. Immediate fasciotomy must be performed to prevent irreversible destruction of the muscle. Less frequently, similar problems may arise from high pressure in other muscle compartments of the lower leg.[98]

FIBROTIC INDURATION AND CONTRACTURE OWING TO REPEATED INTRAMUSCULAR INJECTIONS

Certain drugs may cause local destruction of muscle tissue at injection sites, leading to fibrosis and contracture. Self-administration of pentazocine (Talwin) by patients with chronic pain has resulted in the most striking examples of this condition.[99] The characteristic features are woody induration of the quadriceps, deltoids, and other muscles; needle marks and ulcerations in the overlying skin; and marked muscle shortening.

RUNNING INJURIES

The extraordinary popularity of running has engendered special interest in associated injuries and increased awareness of biomechanical aspects, including running techniques, conditioning, and equipment. These activities are often centered in special runners' clinics, in which the therapeutic goals may differ from those of conventional medicine. Emphasis is placed on continued participation and enhanced performance, in addition to the traditional aims of symptomatic relief and prevention of permanent tissue damage. The spectrum of running injuries encompasses virtually all the categories of musculoskeletal trauma (Table 87–2). About one third of running injuries involve the knee; heel pain is next in frequency. Certain pre-existing conditions may predispose the runner to injury. For instance, a high-arched foot (pes cavus) does not pronate sufficiently to absorb shock during running, leading to Achilles tendinitis or plantar fasciitis. Running on a hyperpronated or flat foot may result in lateral ankle pain. Incongruity, faulty tracking, or laxity in the patellofemoral joint may predispose to patellar pain or chondromalacia. Recrudescent symptoms from virtually any previous articular derangement may develop when the individual begins to run regularly. Ill-fitting or poorly constructed footwear, hard or irregular running surfaces, poor running posture or technique, and inadequate warmup or tendon stretching also

Table 87–2. Common Disorders in Runners

Disorder	Sites of Involvement
Stress fracture	Tibia, fibula, metatarsus, femur
Compartmental syndromes	
Sprains	
Bursitis	Retrocalcaneus, anserine, ischium, trochanter
Fasciitis	Plantar area, iliotibial band
Tendinitis	Achilles, anterior and posterior tibial, peroneal, quadriceps, patella
Tendon and muscle rupture	Achilles, hamstrings
Intra-articular disorders	Chondromalacia, meniscal tears, plica, "overuse" synovitis, osteoarthritis
Cervical and lumbar disc degeneration	

increase the likelihood of injury. Detailed discussion of these matters is available elsewhere.[100,101]

Stress fractures, also called fatigue fractures, are partial, cortical fractures related to prolonged, repetitive mechanical loading. A complete fracture may eventually result if the activity is continued. Currently, running is probably the most common cause. The presenting symptom is pain, which is generally aggravated by weight-bearing and relieved by rest. In some areas, such as the tibia and fibula, tenderness, warmth, and swelling may occur over the fracture. The diagnosis is usually made radiographically, but typical findings of a linear cortical radiolucency or a localized area of periosteal new bone formation may not be present during the first week or two of symptoms. Therefore, negative radiographs should be repeated if a stress fracture is strongly suspected. A radionuclide scintigram shows increased uptake at the stress fracture site at this early stage,[102] but this expensive procedure is seldom justified in typical cases. The treatment of stress fractures depends upon their location and severity. If the fibula is involved, continuation of running at a reduced level may be possible. At the other extreme, femoral fractures occasionally require surgical intervention.

Knee problems represent about a third of running injuries. They most frequently involve tracking abnormalities of the patella, often in relation to underlying anatomic and biomechanical factors (see Chapter 88). Internal derangements are seldom caused by running, but patients with pre-existing, asymptomatic lesions are likely to develop pain and swelling under the stress of running. *"Overuse" synovitis* in the apparent absence of intra-articular pathology is noted occasionally with rapid increases in mileage. This condition should be managed with temporary cessation until the effusion resolves, with gradual resumption of the running program later. Lateral knee pain may result from the *iliotibial band friction syndrome.*[103] A thick strip of fascia lata, which inserts into the lateral tibial condyle, may impinge on the femoral condyle

during repeated flexion and extension of the knee, particularly in individuals with tibia vara and hyperpronated feet.

Heel pain, the second most frequent complaint among runners, results from various conditions that can usually be distinguished by physical examination and radiographs. These conditions include plantar fasciitis, calcaneal bursitis, Achilles tendinitis and/or rupture and calcaneal stress fractures. Treatment includes instruction in running technique to avoid excessive heel strike, heel pads and orthotic devices, stretching exercises, temporary cessation or reduction in running, and anti-inflammatory drugs.

Degenerative arthritis and disc disease may produce pain and limited activity among older runners, but there is little evidence that running causes osteoarthritis in previously normal hips and knees. Substitution of an alternative exercise program with less impact loading, such as swimming or walking, may be recommended in such cases.

REPETITION STRAIN INJURY

Vague regional symptoms that are difficult to ascribe to a specific musculoskeletal injury may be encountered in patients whose occupations require fixed positions and repetitive movements, such as musicians,[104,105] assembly line workers, or accounting machine operators.[106] The complaints include muscular fatigue, stiffness and aching, weakness, paresthesia, and incoordination. Mental stress, various environmental factors, and adverse working conditions may influence the symptoms. Multiple pathogenetic factors may be involved, including muscle fatigue, tenosynovitis, nerve entrapments, compartment syndromes, synovitis, and ligamentous strain. Treatment usually depends on careful analysis and modification of performing techniques and may include rest, anti-inflammatory drugs, and local injections.

FIG. 87–8.   Radiation necrosis of acetabulum with protrusio acetabuli resulting from pathologic fractures.

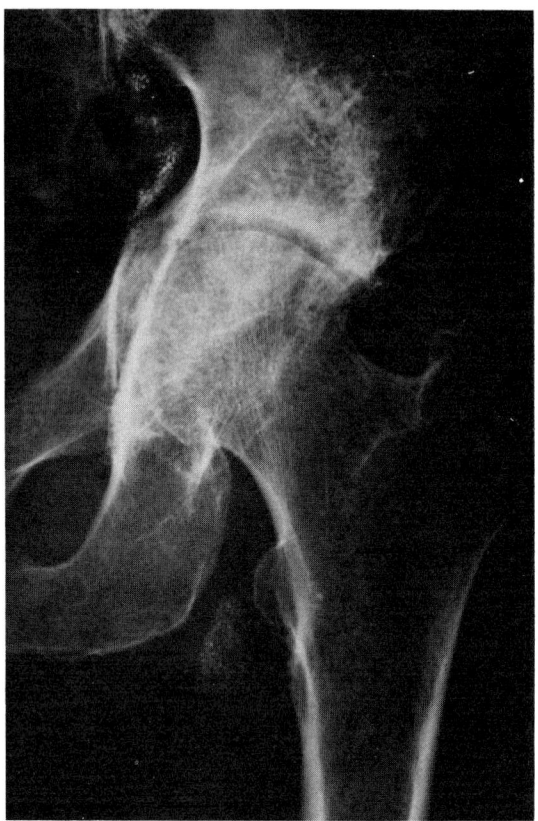

RADIATION ARTHROPATHY FOLLOWING NONMECHANICAL TRAUMA

Because articular cartilage is relatively radioresistant, the effects of radiation on joints are usually secondary to destruction of osteoblasts.[107,108] Vascular damage (endarteritis) may also contribute to osteonecrosis. Since the field of radiotherapy is more likely to include the axial skeleton than the extremities, radiation arthropathy is usually seen in the hips, shoulder, spine, and sacroiliac and temporomandibular joints. Radiation changes are dose-related; the threshold is 3000 rads, with cell death occurring at 5000 rads. Their occurrence depends not only on dosage, but on age, various technical factors, and superimposed trauma or infection. The time of onset of clinical manifestations is generally greater than 1 year, and is often several years after irradiation. Adults may present with aseptic necrosis, fracture, or protrusio acetabuli[109] (Fig. 87–8). Children may develop slipped capital femoral epiphysis,[110] and scoliosis or kyphosis[111] resulting from injury to the epiphyseal plates, leading subsequently to wedge deformities of the vertebral bodies.

Changes resembling degenerative arthritis are occasionally found only in joints that had been included in the field of radiation many years previously.[112] Radiographic findings include narrowing of the joint space, marginal new bone formation, and periarticular osteoporosis. Occasionally, chondrocalcinosis and ankylosis may occur. A few examples of "rheumatoid-like" arthritis with soft tissue swelling have been noted. The spine may be involved, showing narrowing and calcification of intervertebral discs.

Irradiation of the rib cage may result in osteochondritis, with pain and swelling in the costal cartilages. These symptoms may suggest cancer or Tietze's syndrome, but, in contrast to these conditions, erythema exists in the tender area.[113] High-dose ultrasound[114] and diathermy have been reported to cause exacerbations of synovitis in rheumatoid arthritis (see Chapter 49).

FROSTBITE ARTHROPATHY

Frostbite injury to the distal extremities may occasionally involve the joints, in addition to overlying soft tissues. Skeletal changes are not apparent until several months after frostbite, and include demineralization, juxta-articular cysts, and joint space narrowing. The late development of osteophytes results in a clinical picture closely resembling that of osteoarthritis, with Heberden's and Bouchard's nodes.[18] In children, destruction of the phalangeal epiphyses may lead to premature closure and digital growth impairment.[115] These changes may be the result of direct chondrocyte injury during cold exposure.

REFERENCES

1. Thomas, H.O.: Diseases of the Hip, Knee and Ankle Joints. 3rd Ed. London, H.K. Lewis, 1878.
2. Wilkinson, A.: Traumatic haemarthrosis of the knee. Lancet, 2:13–15, 1965.
3. Davie, B.: The significance and treatment of haemarthrosis of the knee following trauma. Med. J. Aust., 1:1355–1359, 1969.
4. Noyes, F.R., et al.: Arthroscopy in adult traumatic hemarthrosis of the knee; incidence of anterior cruciate tears and other injuries. J. Bone Joint Surg., G2A:687–695, 1980.
5. Berk, R.N.: Liquid fat in the knee joint after trauma. N. Engl. J. Med., 277:1411–1412, 1967.
6. Yousefzadeh, D.K., and Jackson, J.H., Jr.: Lipohemarthrosis of the elbow joint. Radiology, 128:643–645, 1978.
7. Reginato, A.J., Feldman, E., and Rabinowitz, J.L.: Traumatic chylous knee effusion. Ann. Rheum. Dis., 44:793–797, 1985.
8. White, R.E., Wise, C.M., and Agudelo, C.A.: Post-traumatic chylous joint effusion. Arthritis Rheum., 28:1303–1306, 1985.

9. Ropes, M.W., and Bauer, W.: Synovial Fluid Changes in Joint Disease. Cambridge, Harvard University Press, 1953.

10. Roy, S., Ghadially, F.N., and Crane, W.A.J.: Synovial membrane in traumatic effusion. Ultrastructure and autoradiography with tritiated leucine. Ann. Rheum. Dis., 25:259–271, 1966.

11. Graham, J., and Goldman, J.A.: Fat droplets and synovial fluid leukocytosis in traumatic arthritis. Arthritis Rheum., 21:76–80, 1978.

12. Weinberger, A., and Schumacher, H.R.: Experimental joint trauma: Synovial response to blunt trauma and inflammatory reaction to intra-articular injection of fat. J. Rheumatol., 8:380–389, 1981.

13. Zarins, B., and Nemeth, V.A.: Acute knee injuries in athletes. Orthop. Clin. North Am., 16:285–302, 1985.

14. Wolf, C.R., and Mankin, H.J.: Effect of experimental hemarthrosis on articular cartilage of rabbit knee joints. J. Bone Joint Surg., 47A:1203–1210, 1965.

15. Cass, J.R., and Morrey, B.F.: Ankle instability: current concepts, diagnosis and treatment. Mayo Clin. Proc., 59:165–170, 1984.

16. Harrington, K.D.: Degenerative arthritis of the ankle secondary to longstanding lateral ligament instability. J. Bone Joint Surg., 61A:354–361, 1979.

17. Nachlas, I.W.: The Pellegrini-Stieda para-articular calcification. Clin. Orthop., 3:121–127, 1954.

18. Glick, R., and Parhami, N.: Frostbite arthritis. J. Rheumatol., 6:456–460, 1979.

19. Venier, L.H., and DiTunno, J.F.: Heterotopic ossification in the paraplegic patient. Arch. Phys. Med. Rehabil., 52:475–479, 1971.

20. Furman, R., Nicholas, J.J., and Jivoff, L.: Elevation of the serum alkaline phosphatase coincident with ectopic bone formation in paraplegic patients. J. Bone Joint Surg., 52A:1131–1137, 1970.

21. Nicholas, J.J.: Ectopic bone formation in patients with spinal cord injury. Arch. Phys. Med. Rehabil., 54:354–359, 1973.

22. Stover, S.L., Hataway, C.J., and Zeiger, H.E.: Heterotopic ossification in spinal cord injured patients. Arch. Phys. Med. Rehabil., 56:199–204, 1975.

23. Hassard, G.H.: Heterotopic bone formation about the hip and unilateral decubitus ulcers in spinal cord injury. Arch. Phys. Med. Rehabil., 56:355–358, 1975.

24. Varghese, G., and Chung, T.: Benign hydrarthrosis of the knee in patients with spinal cord injury. Arch. Phys. Med. Rehabil., 57:468–469, 1976.

25. Yue, C.C., Regier, A., and Kushner, I.: Heterotopic ossification presenting as arthritis. J. Rheumatol., 12:769–772, 1985.

26. Julkunen, H., Rasanen, J.A., and Kataja, J.: Severe trauma as an etiologic factor in rheumatoid arthritis. Scand. J. Rheumatol., 3:97–102, 1974.

27. Gelfand, L., and Merliss, R.: Trauma and rheumatism. Ann. Intern. Med., 50:999–1009, 1959.

28. Williams, K.A., and Scott, J.T.: Influence of trauma on the development of chronic inflammatory polyarthritis. Ann. Rheum. Dis., 26:532–537, 1967.

29. Durman, D.C.: Arthritis and injury. J. Mich. Med. Soc., 51:301–303, 1955.

30. Kirk, J.A., Ansell, B.M., and Bywaters, E.G.L.: The hypermobility syndrome. Ann. Rheum. Dis., 26:419–425, 1967.

31. Biro, F., Gewanter, H.L., and Baum, J.: The hypermobility syndrome. Pediatrics, 72:701–706, 1983.

32. Beighton, P.H., Grahame, R., and Bird, H.: Hypermobility of Joints. New York, Springer-Verlag, 1983.

33. Pitcher, D., and Grahame, R.: Mitral valve prolapse and joint hypermobility: Evidence for a systemic connective tissue abnormality? Ann. Rheum. Dis., 41:352–354, 1982.

34. Grahame, R., et al.: A clinical and echocardiographic study of patients with the hypermobility syndrome. Ann. Rheum. Dis., 40:541–546, 1981.

35. Al-Rawi, Z.S., and Al-Rawi, Z.T.: Joint hypermobility in women with genital prolapse. Lancet, 1:1439–1441, 1982.

36. Handler, C.E., et al.: Mitral valve prolapse, aortic compliance, and skin collagen in joint hypermobility syndrome. Br. Heart J., 54:501–508, 1985.

37. Al-Rawi, Z.S., Al-Aszawi, A.J., and Al-Chalabi, T.: Joint mobility among university students in Iraq. Br. J. Rheumatol., 24:326–331, 1985.

38. Gedalia, A., et al.: Hypermobility of the joints in juvenile episodic arthritis/arthralgia. J. Pediatr., 107:873–876, 1985.

39. Jessee, E.F., Owen, D.S., and Sagar, K.B.: The benign hypermobility joint syndrome. Arthritis Rheum., 23:1053–1056, 1980.

40. Schott, G.D.: Mechanisms of causalgia and related clinical conditions. Brain, 109:717–738, 1986.

41. Schutzer, S.F., and Gossling, H.R.: The treatment of reflex sympathetic dystrophy syndrome. J. Bone Joint Surg., 66A:625–629, 1984.

42. Rush, P.J., et al.: Severe reflex neurovascular dystrophy in childhood. Arthritis Rheum., 28:952–956, 1985.

43. Poplawski, Z.J., Wiley, A.M., and Murray, J.F.: Post-traumatic dystrophy of the extremities: a clinical review and trial of treatment. J. Bone Joint Surg., 65A:642–655, 1983.

44. Curtiss, P.H., Jr., and Kincaid, W.E.: Transient demineralization of the hip in pregnancy: A report of three cases. J. Bone Joint Surg., 41A:1327–1333, 1959.

45. Hunder, G.G., and Kelly, P.J.: Roentgenologic transient osteoporosis of the hip. A clinical syndrome? Ann. Intern. Med., 68:539–552, 1968.

46. Lequesne, M.: Transient osteoporosis of the hip. A nontraumatic variety of Sudek's atrophy. Ann. Rheum. Dis., 27:463–471, 1968.

47. Swezey, R.L.: Transient osteoporosis of the hip, foot and knee. Arthritis Rheum., 13:858–868, 1970.

48. O'Mara, R.E., and Pinals, R.S.: Bone scanning in regional migratory osteoporosis. Radiology, 97:579–581, 1970.

49. Guenee, B., et al.: Type IV hyperlipoproteinemia in patients with algodystrophy. Clin. Exp. Rheumatol., 3:49–52, 1985.

50. Phillips, H.O., and Grubb, S.A.: Familial multiple osteochondritis dissecans. J. Bone Joint Surg., 67A:155–156, 1985.

51. Chiroff, R.T., and Cooke, C.P.: Osteochondritis dissecans: A histologic and microradiographic analysis of surgically excised lesions. J. Trauma, 15:689–696, 1975.

52. Milgram, J.W.: Radiological and pathological manifestations of osteochondritis dissecans of the distal femur. Radiology, 126:305–311, 1978.

53. Wilson, J.N.: A diagnostic sign in osteochondritis dissecans of the knee. J. Bone Joint Surg., 49A:477–480, 1967.

54. Lindholm, T.S., Osterman, K., and Vankka, E.: Osteochondritis dissecans of the elbow, ankle and hip. Clin. Orthop., 148:245–253, 1980.

55. Pappas, A.M.: Osteochondrosis dissecans. Clin. Orthop., 158:59–69, 1981.

56. Douglas, G., and Rang, M.: The role of trauma in the pathogenesis of the osteochondroses. Clin. Orthop., 158:28–32, 1981.

57. Duthie, R.B., and Houghton, G.R.: Constitutional aspects of the osteochondroses. Clin Orthop., 15B:19–27, 1981.

58. Peyton, F.W.: Unexpected frequency of idiopathic costochondral pain. Obstet. Gynecol., *62*:605–608, 1983.

59. McBeath, A.A., and Keene, J.S.: The rib-tip syndrome. J. Bone Joint Surg., *57A*:795–797, 1975.

60. Wright, J.T.: Slipping-rib syndrome. Lancet, *2*:632–634, 1980.

61. Coventry, M.B., and Mitchell, W.C.: Osteitis pubis: Observations based on a study of 45 patients. JAMA, *178*:898–905, 1961.

62. Rosenthal, R.E., et al.: Osteomyelitis of the symphysis pubis: A separate disease from osteitis pubis. J. Bone Joint Surg., *64A*:123–128, 1982.

63. Wiley, J.J.: Traumatic osteitis pubis: the gracilis syndrome. Amer. J. Sports Med., *11*:360–363, 1983.

64. Rauschning, W.: Anatomy and function of the communication between knee joint and popliteal bursae. Ann. Rheum. Dis., *39*:354–358, 1980.

65. Dinham, J.M.: Popliteal cysts in children, the case against surgery. J. Bone Joint Surg., *57B*:69–71, 1975.

66. Burleson, R.J., Bickel, W.H., and Dahlin, D.C.: Popliteal cyst: A clinicopathological survey. J. Bone Joint Surg., *38A*:1265–1274, 1956.

67. Harvey, J.P., Jr., and Corcos, J.: Large cysts in lower leg originating in the knee occurring in patients with rheumatoid arthritis. Arthritis Rheum., *3*:218–228, 1960.

68. Palmer, D.G.: Synovial cysts in rheumatoid disease. Ann. Intern. Med., *70*:61–68, 1969.

69. Tophoj, K., and Henriques, U.: Ganglion of the wrist—a structure developed from the joint. Acta Orthop. Scand., *42*:244–250, 1971.

70. Andren, L., and Eiken, O.: Arthrographic studies of wrist ganglions. J. Bone Joint Surg., *53A*:299–302, 1971.

71. Ghadially, F.N., and Mehta, P.N.: Multifunctional mesenchymal cells resembling smooth muscle cells in ganglia of the wrist. Ann. Rheum. Dis., *30*:31–42, 1971.

72. Matthews, P.: Ganglia of the flexor tendon sheaths in the hand. J. Bone Joint Surg., *55B*:612–617, 1973.

73. Byers, P.D., and Wadsworth, T.G.: Periosteal ganglion. J. Bone Joint Surg., *52B*:290–295, 1970.

74. Lapidus, P.W., and Guidotti, F.P.: Report on the treatment of 102 ganglions. Bull. Hosp. Joint Dis., *28*:50–57, 1967.

75. Angelides, A.C., and Wallace, P.F.: The dorsal ganglion of the wrist: its pathogenesis, gross and microscopic anatomy, and surgical treatment. J. Hand Surg., *1*:228–235, 1976.

76. Wilson, R.N., and Wilson, S.: Tenosynovitis in industry. Practitioner, *178*:612–615, 1957.

77. Muckart, R.D.: Stenosing tendovaginitis of abductor pollicis longus and extensor pollicis brevis at the radial styloid (de Quervain's disease). Clin. Orthop., *33*:201–207, 1964.

78. Schumacher, H.R., Jr., Dorwart, B.B., and Korzeniowski, O.M.: Occurrence of DeQuervain's tendinitis during pregnancy. Arch. Int. Med., *145*:2083–2084, 1985.

79. Weeks, P.M.: A cause of wrist pain: Non-specific tenosynovitis involving the flexor carpi radialis. Plast. Reconstr. Surg., *62*:263–266, 1978.

80. Norris, S.H., and Mankin, H.J.: Chronic tenosynovitis of the posterior tibial tendon with new bone formation. J. Bone Joint Surg., *60B*:523–526, 1978.

81. Rhoades, C.E., Gelberman, R.H., and Manjarris, J.F.: Stenosing tenosynovitis of the fingers and thumb. Clin. Orthop., *190*:236–238, 1984.

82. Phalen, G.S.: The carpal tunnel syndrome. J. Bone Joint Surg., *48A*:211–228, 1966.

83. Tanzer, R.C.: The carpal tunnel syndrome: A clinical and anatomical study. J. Bone Joint Surg., *41A*:626–634, 1959.

84. Lam, S.J.S.: Tarsal tunnel syndrome. J. Bone Joint Surg., *49B*:87–92, 1967.

85. Martens, M., et al.: Patellar tendinitis: Pathology and results of treatment. Acta Orthop. Scand., *53*:445–450, 1982.

86. Goldie, I.: Epicondylitis lateralis humeri (epicondylalgia or tennis elbow). A pathogenetical study. Acta Chir. Scand. (Suppl.), *339*:1+, 1964.

87. Binder, A., et al.: Is therapeutic ultrasound effective in treating soft tissue lesions? Br. Med. J., *290*:512–514, 1985.

88. Bywaters, E.G.L.: Lesions of bursae, tendons and tendon sheaths. Clin. Rheum. Dis., *5*:883–925, 1979.

89. Mysnyk, M.C., et al.: Prepatellar bursitis in wrestlers. Am. J. Sports Med., *14*:46–54, 1986.

90. Rasmussen, K.-J.E., and Fanø, N.: Trochanteric bursitis: treatment by corticosteroid injection. Scand. J. Rheumatol., *14*:417–420, 1985.

91. Larsson, L.-G., and Baum, J.: The syndromes of bursitis. Bull. Rheum. Dis., *36*:1–8, 1986.

92. Weinstein, P.S., Canoso, J.J., and Wohlgethan, J.R.: Long-term follow-up of corticosteroid injection for traumatic olecranon bursitis. Ann. Rheum. Dis., *43*:44–46, 1984.

93. Sweetnam, R.: Corticosteroid arthropathy and tendon rupture. J. Bone Joint Surg., *51B*:397–398, 1969.

94. Park, J.Y., and Espiniella, J.L.: Rupture of pectoralis major muscle. J. Bone Joint Surg., *52A*:577–581, 1970.

95. McClure, J.G.: Gastrocnemius musculotendinous rupture: a condition confused with thrombophlebitis. South. Med. J., *77*:1143–1145, 1984.

96. Johnson, K.A.: Tibialis posterior tendon rupture. Clin. Orthop., *177*:145–147, 1983.

97. Wills, L.A., et al.: Achilles tendon rupture: a review of the literature comparing surgical versus nonsurgical treatment. Clin. Orthop., *207*:156–163, 1986.

98. Matsen, F.A., Winquist, R.A., and Klugmire, R.B.: Diagnosis and management of compartmental syndromes. J. Bone Joint Surg., *62A*:286–291, 1980.

99. Oh, S.J., Rollins, J.I., and Lewis, I.: Pentazocine-induced fibrous myopathy. JAMA, *231*:271–273, 1975.

100. D'Ambrosia, R., and Drez, D., Jr.: Prevention and Treatment of Running Injuries. Thorofare, New Jersey, Charles B. Slack, Inc., 1982.

101. James, S.L., Bates, B.T., and Ostering, L.R.: Injuries to runners. Am. J. Sports Med., *6*:40–50, 1978.

102. Norfray, J.F., et al.: Early confirmation of stress fractures of joggers. JAMA, *243*:1647–1649, 1980.

103. Renne, J.W.: The iliotibial band friction syndrome. J. Bone Joint Surg., *57A*:1110–1111, 1975.

104. Fry, H.J.H.: Overuse syndrome in musicians: prevention and management. Lancet, *2*:728–731, 1986.

105. Hochberg, F.H., et al.: Hand difficulties among musicians. JAMA, *249*:1869–1872, 1983.

106. McDermott, F.T.: Repetition strain injury: a review of current understanding. Med. J. Aust., *144*:196–200, 1986.

107. Dalinka, M.K., and Bonavita, J.A.: Radiation changes. In Diagnosis of Bone and Joint Disorders. Edited by D. Resnick, and G. Niwayama. Philadelphia, W.B. Saunders Co., 1981, pp. 2341–2362.

108. Howland, W.J., et al.: Postirradiation atrophic changes of bone and related complications. Radiology, *117*:677–685, 1975.

109. Hasselbacher, P., and Schumacher, H.R.: Bilateral protrusio acetabuli following pelvic irradiation. J. Rheumatol., *4*:189–196, 1977.

110. Libshitz, H.I., and Edeiker, B.S.: Radiotherapy changes of the pediatric hip. Am. J. Roentgenol., *137*:585–588, 1981.

111. Mayfield, J.K.: Postradiation spinal deformity. Orthop. Clin. North Am., *10*:829–844, 1979.

112. Kolar, J., Vrabec, R., and Chyba, J.: Arthropathies after irradiation. J. Bone Joint Surg., *49A*:1157–1166, 1967.

113. Lau, B.P.: Postirradiation costal osteochondritis simulating metastatic cancer. Radiology, *89*:1090–1092, 1967.

114. Tiliakos, N.A., and Wilson, C.H., Jr.: Ultrasound-induced arthritis (abstract). Arthritis Rheum., *26*:549, 1983.

115. Carrera, G.F., Kozin, G., and McCarty, D.J.: Arthritis after frostbite injury in children. Arthritis Rheum., *22*:1082–1087, 1979.

88

MECHANICAL DISORDERS OF THE KNEE

ROGER P. JOHNSON

A mechanical disorder of the knee is defined as any condition that interferes with normal joint motion or mobility. Strictly speaking, an internal derangement of the knee is a mechanical disorder due to an intra-articular pathologic process. An external derangement, a term not commonly used but certainly appropriate, implies a disorder external to the joint proper that creates abnormalities in motion and function. Examples include cruciate and collateral ligamentous tears, quadriceps or hamstring insufficiency or contractures, masses outside the joint cavity such as popliteal cysts and tumors, and extensor tendon malalignment. Many of these external disorders can cause sudden or long-term loss of motion of the knee, and they may mimic or may even cause internal derangements, such as ligamentous instability leading to meniscal tears.

INTERNAL DERANGEMENTS OF THE KNEE

William Hey, of Leeds, England, coined the term "internal derangement of the knee" in the late 1700s.[1] He noted that "trifling accidents" could unexpectedly lock the knee and lead to an inability to "freely bend or extend the limb in walking." If the knee remained locked for months or even years, Hey indicated that it could become a "serious misfortune" leading to a "considerable degree of lameness," a condition he suffered with himself for almost 50 years. He reasoned that "some slight derangement of the semilu-

nar cartilages may probably be sufficient to bring on the complaint," and if caught in the joint, would prevent the "os femoris from moving truly in the hollow formed by the semilunar cartilages and articular depression of the tibia."

Hey also stated that a loose body or fragment of meniscus locked in the joint could cause "an unequal tension of the lateral (collateral) or cross (cruciate) ligaments of the knee." He advised manipulation "without surgical assistance." In a case presentation of a young lady who suffered from a locked knee, Hey noted that three days after manipulation, "she danced at a private ball without inconvenience."

From this statement, we conclude that Hey clearly understood the essential features of internal derangement of the knee, as follows: (1) incarceration or entrapment of bony or soft tissue fragments between the condyles and the tibial plateau causing the knee to lock; (2) circumscription by the tibia of an abnormal arc about the femur, causing painful stretching of the ligaments of the knee and capsule; (3) sudden loss of motion, usually of full extension; (4) sudden loss of function of the knee, often associated with a minor injury; (5) possible restoration of the knee to normal function by manipulation; and (6) significant long-term disability if the condition remains uncorrected. To these features we add: (7) recurrent locking; (8) the reflex "pseudoparalysis" of the hamstring and quadriceps muscles at the time of locking, causing the knee to buckle during weight bearing; (9) subjective complaints of "something moving around in the knee," the "knee skipping over one track'' and ''jumping out of the groove;'' and finally (10) the history of a remote, more severe injury, such as a ''sprain'' of the knee or patellar dislocation, that left the patient disabled for at least a few weeks, followed by a return to normal or near-normal activities.

A fragment of bone or soft tissue that suddenly becomes interposed between the articular surfaces is the classic cause of internal derangement. This misplaced fragment can be radiolucent or radiopaque. The most frequent cause of locking is entrapment of the radiolucent meniscus. Osteochondritis dissecans and patellar disorders are the most common conditions that generate radiopaque osteocartilaginous loose bodies. Other causes of fragment generation with incarceration and internal derangement are discussed briefly in this chapter. Current methods used to define accurately the precise cause of mechanical disorders of the knee are also discussed in this chapter.

MENISCAL TEARS AND INSTABILITY

The best-known internal derangement of the knee is the torn meniscus.[2-6] Partial rings of fibrocartilage fill the marginal triangular space between the convex condyles and the flat posterior sloping tibial plateaus. As load-dispersing structures and stabilizers of the knee, the menisci are subject to considerable compression.[7] The medial meniscus is typically narrower and less mobile and is torn three to six times more commonly than the lateral meniscus.

Subtle instability, often secondary to old anterior cruciate ligament insufficiency,[8-15] previously diagnosed as a ''sprained knee,'' allows the condyle to deviate from its normal plane of motion and to encroach on the margin of the meniscus. Because its peripheral attachments are stretched, the meniscus migrates closer to the center of the knee and renders it more susceptible to trapping and peripheral tears, the so-called ''hypermobile meniscus.''

Such stretching tugs on the joint capsule and peripheral attachments with minute bleeding, irritation, and synovitis causing joint-line tenderness, an important sign in patients with trapping, tearing, or shredding of a meniscus. Condylar or tibial plateau degeneration or other causes of knee irritation with synovitis may also produce joint-line tenderness, a sign that becomes less reliable when these chronic conditions antedate the meniscal tear.

The many types of tears are classified as longitudinal, vertical, transverse, ''parrot-beak,'' horizontal or cleavage, or pedunculated[5] (Figs. 88–1 to 88–4). Under direct vision through an arthroscope, rotation of the knee can produce wrinkles in a meniscus. If the condyle should impinge on a wrinkled meniscus, a transverse or parrot-beak tear can occur. External rotation of the tibia brings the medial tibial plateau anteriorly and the posterior horn of the medial meniscus under the condyle (see Fig. 88–4). This characteristic explains the posterior medial horn tears of the medial meniscus commonly associated with anteromedial instability.

Longitudinal vertical tears can involve the knifelike edge of the meniscus or a major portion of its body (see Fig. 88–3). When torn and separated, the inner margin displaces into the intercondylar notch, a condition referred to as a ''bucket-handle tear'' (see

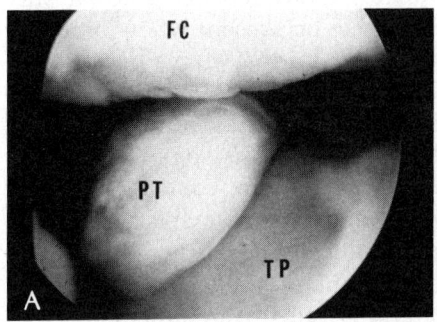
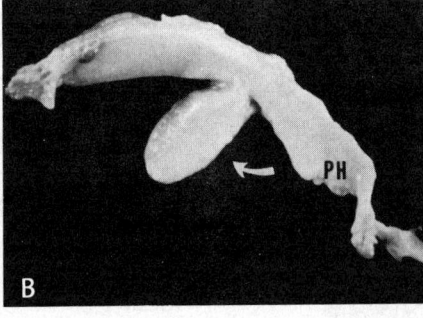

FIG. 88–1. *A,* This arthroscopic view demonstrates pedunculated tear (PT) of the medial meniscus incarcerated between the femoral condyle (FC) and the tibial plateau (TP). The patient is a 27-year-old athletically active man who had to give up all sports because of sudden locking and giving way of his knee. Note the damage to the cartilage covering the femoral condyle, as evidenced by the irregularity of the surface, which is normally perfectly smooth. *B,* This surgical specimen demonstrates the pedunculated tear shown in *A.* This pedunculated part (arrow) arose from a longitudinal tear of the posterior horn (PH), which became detached and protruded into the joint cavity, to become intermittently caught between the femoral condyle and the tibial plateau.

FIG. 88–2. This specimen is from a 27-year-old man who had three painful incidents of locking of his left knee in one year. Three longitudinal tears (arrows) of the lateral meniscus were found at operation.

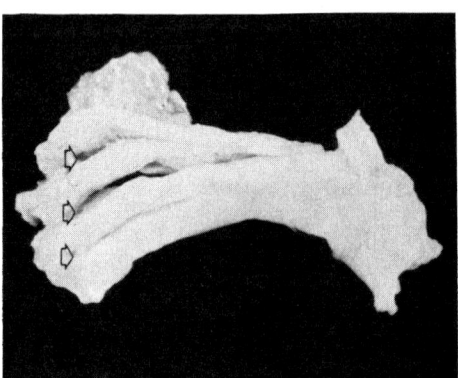

FIG. 88–4. Anteromedial instability is the most common form of instability of the knee. It has components of valgus and anterior motion of the medial tibial plateau, which is a manifestation of external rotation of the tibia on the femur (arrow). For this reason, tears of the medial meniscus typically start posteromedially and extend anteriorly into bucket-handle tears with forceful extension of the knee when the meniscus is trapped.

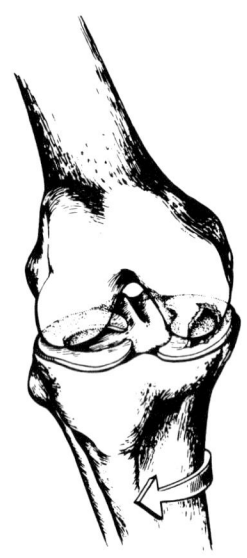

Fig. 88–4). This tear locks the knee in flexion. The patient may notice that the knee is becoming progressively straighter. Such a finding indicates anterior extension of the tear.

"Locking" is classically defined as sudden loss of extension. A torn meniscus may also block flexion, but the end point may be more difficult to define because the knee is less restrained in flexion.

Loss of extension should be assessed by comparing the affected and normal knees. With the patient supine, the legs are lifted by the heels to equal levels. The patella is higher on the side with a loss of extension. Any passive attempt to straighten the knee is resisted. The mechanical block forces the tibia to circumscribe an abnormal arc, to stretch the ligaments and joint capsule, and to cause pain. Effusion and protective muscle spasm can also suddenly prevent full extension. Usually, one notes a soft, spongy feel-

FIG. 88–3. This arthroscopic view of a longitudinal tear of a medial meniscus demonstrates the smoothness of the femoral condyle (FC), the vascular margin of the meniscus (VM), and the longitudinal tear of the meniscus (arrow).

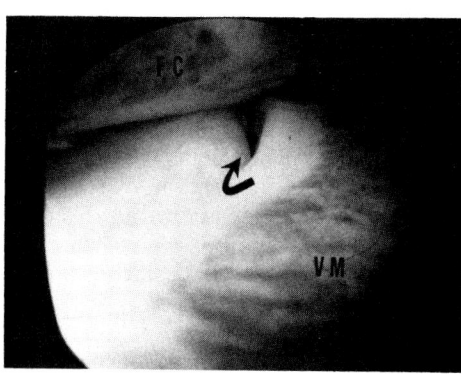

ing at extension, which I call "soft locking." When the extension stop is abrupt, definite, and repeatable, I call this "hard locking."

The relationship between a torn meniscus and knee instability becomes clear when we recognize that the primary purpose of the ligaments of any joint is to direct the motion of one articular surface in a prescribed plane or planes about another articular surface.[16] Instability is said to be present when joint motion occurs outside this normal domain. As Hey noted,[1] the condyles normally ride "in the hollow formed by the semilunar cartilages and articular depression of the tibia." When instability is present, and it is often subtle, the femoral condyle rides out of the meniscal hollow and over the meniscus. Should weight bearing occur and the meniscus not slide out from under the condyle, it will be torn. A torn fragment free on one end is called a pedunculated tear (see Fig. 88–1). Such fragments can be easily trapped in the joint without any abnormal motion of the condyle or the body of the meniscus. If the joint is then forced into extension, it will be pried apart, stretching the ligaments and further aggravating instability and damaging the articular surfaces.

The complex interplay between instability, torn menisci, athletic activities, muscle control, and repeated trauma ultimately leads to a degenerative knee.[17] It is difficult to evaluate studies of meniscectomy and instability because it is often unclear whether the original injury, the repeated locking, the instability, the high athletic demands of the patient, the powerful muscular contractions, the repeated microtrauma, or the altered mechanics[18] (most likely a combination of these factors) caused the disabled knee.

Terminology describing instability of the knee is as for dislocations, that is, according to the motion or abnormal position of the distal articulation or bone (Table 88–1).[19–22] *Anterior instability* indicates anterior displacement of the tibia on the femur and generally means at least anterior cruciate insufficiency. *Posterior instability* means posterior displacement of the tibia on the femoral condyles and usually indicates at least posterior cruciate ligament insufficiency. *Medial instability* means that the medial compartment opens with valgus stress, and *lateral instability*, opening laterally with varus stress. A comparison of mobility of affected and opposite knees is important because considerable "normal" variation occurs.

Basically, two types of rotational instability exist, internal and external. *Anteromedial*[23] and *posterolateral*[20,24] instability are forms of external rotational instability. When the tibia rotates externally,[25] the medial tibial plateau moves anteriorly and the lateral moves posteriorly to an excessive degree. Excessive *posteromedial* and *anterolateral* mobility can be thought

Table 88–1. Tests of Knee Instability

Anterior Instability
    Anterior drawer test[19,20,30]
    Ritchey-Lachman test[14,27,29]

Posterior Instability
    Posterior drawer test[19,20,28]

Medial Instability
    Abduction stress test (20–30° flexion)[19,20]

Lateral Instability
    Adduction stress test (20–30° flexion)[19,20]

Internal Rotary Instability
    Pivot shift[26]
    Losee test[30a]
    ALRI test[30b]
    Jerk test[19,20]
    Crossover test[8]
    Flexion-rotation drawer test[32,72]
    Posterior medial displacement of medial
       tibial plateau with valgus stress

External Rotary Instability
    Posterolateral drawer test[30c,30d]
    External rotational recurvatum test[30c,30d]
    Reversed pivot shift[30c]
    Anterior drawer with foot externally
       rotated[30e]

of as internal rotational instability. In the anterolateral disorder, a "pivot shift"[17,26] or sudden anterior subluxation of the tibial plateau occurs as the knee is extended. Another sign of anterior cruciate ligament insufficiency is the anterior "drawer sign" wih the knee at 90°.[21] *The Ritchey-Lachman* test,[14,27–29] which consists of anterior subluxation of the tibia with the knee at 0 to 20°, is a more sensitive sign of anterior cruciate ligament damage, especially if no anterior drawer sign is present at 90° of flexion.

Obviously, many combinations, degrees, and variations in anatomic involvement can accompany instability.[8,21] Although most students of the knee acknowledge that instability is "bad," it is difficult to say whether the injury, the "scrubbing" action of the articular surfaces, the indentation of the articular surface by the loose fragment, the loss of muscular control, or the ligamentous laxity is the ultimate cause of articular cartilage degeneration, the final common denominator of most arthritides.[18]

The relationship between instability and torn menisci is inherent in understanding the concept of the knee with a deficient anterior cruciate ligament.[9,15,30] An acute injury, usually of the internal or external rotational type, bowstrings the anterior cruciate ligament across the medial or lateral femoral condyles and attenuates or ruptures this ligament. The injury, often diagnosed as a "sprained knee," is the most common cause of hemarthrosis in the active adolescent or young adult.[31,32] In 2 or 3 weeks, the hemarthrosis subsides, and many patients return to normal activities within a month or two. Often, no clinical instability or evidence of knee dysfunction is present at that time. Usually, a few years later, the burden of stabilization, formerly borne by the anterior cruciate ligament, is absorbed by the remaining ligamentous structures, which gradually stretch, especially if the patient participates in competitive athletics without adequate muscular control.[28,33,34] Trivial injuries or simple twisting produce fleeting sensations of giving way, "skipping over one track," or sudden loss of control. These clinical manifestations suggest instability and trapping, but not necessarily cutting or tearing of the meniscus.

When the meniscus is ultimately torn, repair[3,15] or meniscectomy[6] is considered. Meniscectomy, which removes the "spacer effect" of the meniscus, can aggravate or potentiate the instability[15,35] and may hasten degeneration of the femoral condyle and, secondarily, the tibial plateau. With this series of events in mind, Allman has dubbed anterior cruciate ligament rupture as "the beginning of the end" of the knee.[14]

OSTEOCHONDRITIS DISSECANS

Osteochondritis dissecans is a prototype for conditions producing osteocartilaginous loose bodies. It was named by Konig in 1887,[36] but had been described by Sir James Paget in 1870 as "quiet necrosis" as compared with the more dramatic suppurative necrosis of bacterial infection. Although the term denotes inflammation of bone and cartilage, little inflammation is present. The term as used here means an island in the femoral condyle consisting of subchondral bone with its articular cartilage. This island, usually 1 to 2 cm in diameter often "dissects" from the main condylar mass and can be thought of as a small fracture that develops chronic nonunion. Eighty-five percent of such lesions are found in the knee, but they have been reported in many sites,[37,38] including the femoral head, the dome of the talus, and the capitulum humeri.

Osteochondritis dissecans is a condition of unknown origin in which 85% of the lesions appear on the medial or central portion of the medial femoral condyle and 15% occur laterally.[37] These lesions are possibly shear fractures, but their occasional "mirror-image," bilateral occurrence suggests other anatomic or developmental disorders. Prominent tibial spines have been associated with the condition and have been implicated as sites of impingement with rotation of the tibia against the condyles.[39] Fairbank failed to find any evidence to dispute the hypothesis that the separation is caused by "trauma and trauma alone."[40]

This lesion is most common in adolescents and young adults, less common in patients in their thirties and forties, and rare in the elderly, in whom degeneration overshadows the primary cause. In the skeletally immature, the lesions heal without surgical intervention if the affected area is immobilized for a long enough time.[41] In children, I prefer multiple drilling of these lesions transversely through the femoral condyle distal to the epiphyseal plate with immobilization. This process seems to hasten the healing time if the articular surface is intact, as it usually is. In adults, excision gives favorable results,[42-44] although some prefer to pin the fragment in place.[45-47]

Osteochondritis dissecans is three times more common in males than in females. Shed or free fragments of bone loose in the knee joint are common in adults and rare in children. Smillie called it a "mysterious condition . . . never seen in the recent state."[46] True spontaneous healing was not observed in his five pediatric patients.

The small bony island is probably alive at the time of separation or fracture. The edges of the bony fragment become necrotic, but the overlying articular cartilage remains alive.[48] Studies on the blood supply of the condyles indicate a rich, anastomotic arterial network that makes localized infarction an unlikely cause.[40] The lesion has been reported in families as an autosomal dominant condition.[48-51] Osteochondritis dissecans of the patella, at least in some cases, appears to be due to a tangential or shear fracture secondary to subluxation. Osteochondritis dissecans of the femoral condyles, patellar fractures, and lateral femoral condylar fractures secondary to patellar dislocation are the three most common generators of "loose bodies," also called arthrophytes, "joint mice," corpora mobile, or arthroliths, in the knee (Fig. 88–5).

Long-term followup studies have revealed that many patients with osteochondritis dissecans develop degenerative arthritis. Thirty-eight of 48 patients seen at an average of 33 years after diagnosis had arthritis.[42] At least 20 years of observation are often required before arthritis is manifest. The process is accelerated in athletes.[37]

FIG. 88–5. The three small arrows point to longitudinal grooves or excoriations in the medial femoral condyle in this 21-year-old dock worker. These lesions were the result of repeated trapping with impingement of a single loose body. The large arrow points to early osteophyte formation along the medial border of the femoral condyle.

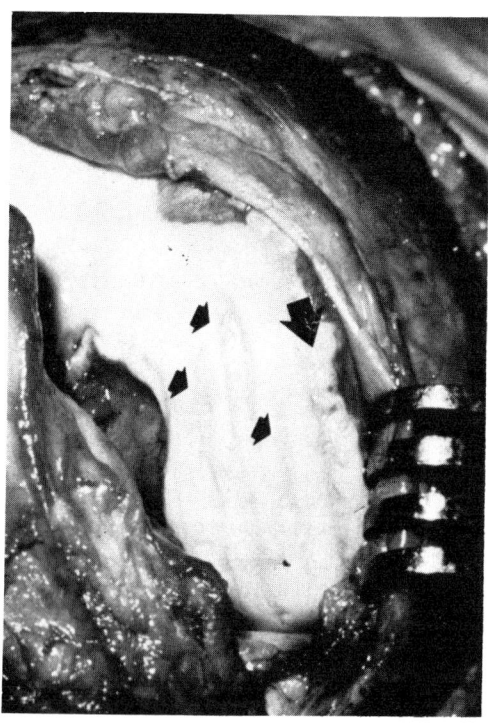

LATERAL FACET SYNDROME OF THE PATELLA

Lateral facet syndrome is a compressive arthropathy of the lateral patellofemoral joint. Pain is the most common symptom. Activities requiring quadriceps activity in knee flexion such as athletics, ascending or descending stairs, running, jumping, squatting, and progressive resistive exercises cause patellar pain. A notable feature of the condition is that the pain is often delayed until after activity has ceased. It is most commonly seen in teenage female athletes and often erroneously diagnosed as "chondromalacia patellae."

Physical findings include (1) lateral patellofemoral joint line tenderness, (2) tenderness over the insertion of the vastus lateralis obliquus tendon, and (3) apprehension and resistance to passive medial and lateral patellar displacement with the knee in 30° of flexion. Crepitation is frequently present and indicates chondromalacia patellae secondary to mechanical imbalance. Roentgenograms, bone scans, and arthroscopy are of little diagnostic use except to document other pathology in the knee.

Conservative treatment consists of nonsteroidal anti-inflammatory drugs, activity modification, improvement of quadriceps excursion through deep knee flexion, quadriceps medialis strengthening, and occasional patellar bracing. Effective surgical treatment consists of complete resection of a ribbon of tissue adjacent to the lateral patellar margin, which comprises the distal vastus lateralis obliquus tendon, the lateral retinaculum, and the anterior terminal portion of the iliotibial band.[52,53]

The vastus lateralis obliquus tendon is the primary lateral restraint in 50% of all knees with lateral facet syndrome. The iliotibial band is the primary lateral restraint in 16% of the knees, and the lateral retinaculum is the primary lateral restraint in 5% of the knees. All three structures contribute significantly or equally to lateral restraint in 29% of the knees.[53]

The lateral restraint of the vastus lateralis has dynamic and static components. With knee flexion, its pull becomes increasingly perpendicular to the lateral patellar facet. Its static tension is typically due to surgically evident hypertrophy or contracture. The same is true of the iliotibial band. Dynamically, its anterior terminal fibers migrate posteriorly with knee flexion and pull the patella laterally. Contracture of these fibers causes static lateral tethering.

Cadaveric dissection and testing demonstrated that the dynamic component of the vastus lateralis obliquus provides 6% of total quadriceps force.[53] Lateral resection diminishes extensor force by 6 to 10%. I have used this procedure in athletes who returned to athletics postoperatively. They have reported little or no decrease in performance.

The exact cause of pain remains unclear.[54] Pain could result from an increase of patellar or femoral intraosseous pressure in response to increased articular pressure between the lateral patellar facet and the lateral femoral condyle.[53,55,56] Other theories include subchondral bone microfractures, marginal synovitis above the patella, excessive tension in the lateral structures, patellar or quadriceps tendonitis, and even chondromalacia patellae. The last is the most common condition confused with the lateral facet syndrome.

SYNOVIAL PLICA SYNDROME

A plica is a synovial fold, pleat, or band that is usually soft, mobile, thin, pliable, asymptomatic, and more prominent in flexion.[56a,56b,56c] Occasionally, embryonic remnants of intrasynovial septa persist into adult life and become thickened, fibrotic, and often hemorrhagic cords causing snapping, clicking, or "catching" along the medial or lateral side of the patella.

The medial suprapatellar plica and the less-common lateral suprapatellar plica are the most prominent. These structures can also cause localized tenderness or a click as they snap over the anterior femoral condyles, usually at repeatable positions when the knee is extended or flexed.

Double-contrast arthrography can identify these folds[57,58] (Fig. 88–6), although arthroscopic visualization with documentation of synovitis, hemorrhage, and thickening and actual catching over the condyle is more conclusive evidence that the plica is the cause of the symptoms. Initially, nonoperative management consisting of rest, heat, and anti-inflammatory drugs may control the patient's symptoms. If this regimen fails, partial resection of the cord arthroscopically or through arthrotomy cures the condition.

RECURRENT LATERAL DISLOCATION OF THE PATELLA

Sudden "giving way" of the knee mimicking locking can occur with subluxation of the patella. True locking can result from an osteochondral fracture of the patella (Fig. 88–7) or of the lateral femoral condyle (Fig. 88–8) from a recent or remote dislocation of the patella.[59] I agree with Macnab that most patellar subluxations and dislocations begin at or near full extension.[60] When the patella is subluxed laterally at full extension and sudden uncontrolled flexion occurs,

FIG. 88–6.   Double-contrast arthrographic study documents a suprapatellar plica (arrow).

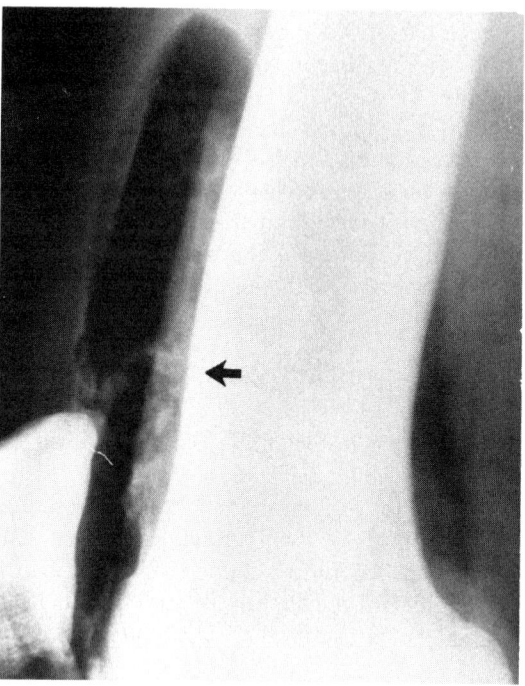

the patella is drawn along the lateral femoral condyle. With progressive flexion, the vastus medialis muscle and the medial retinaculum can become progressively taut, so as the patella is forcibly returned to the sulcus, fracture of the medial facet of the patella or lateral condylar margin can occur. If the patella does not snap back but continues to ride the lateral margin of the

FIG. 88–7.   The large radiopaque loose body (arrows) can be seen in both the anteroposterior *(A)* and lateral *(B)* projections in the suprapatellar pouch. Note the sclerotic margin on the undersurface of the patella in the lateral view, the site of origin of the loose body.

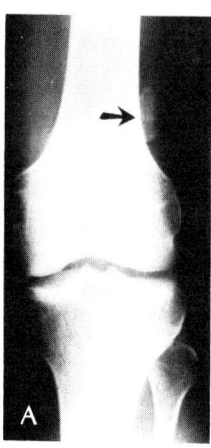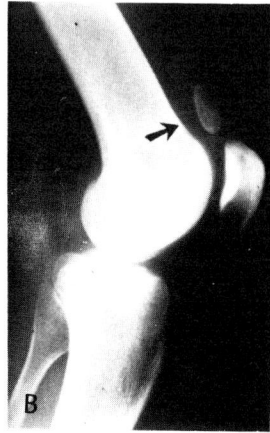

FIG. 88–8.   The single arrow points to a loose body in the intercondylar notch from a "corner fracture" of the lateral femoral condyle (double arrows).

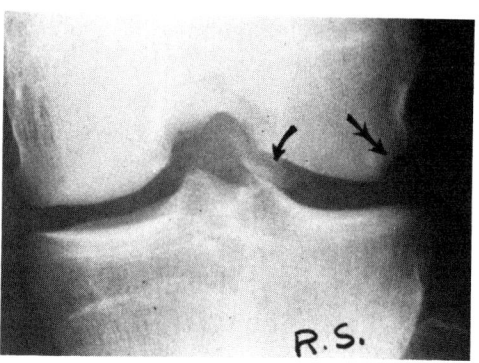

condyle to full flexion, the medialis muscle and retinaculum will be torn or severely stretched. When this process occurs and the scar does not retract to repair it, medialis muscle insufficiency ensues. With the medial restraints gone and further contracture laterally, patellar tilt becomes evident.[61,62]

Many factors have been implicated in the cause of malalignment of the extensor mechanism of the knee.[59,63,64] These can be divided into *intrinsic* factors, those directly located to the patellofemoral articulation, and *extrinsic* factors.

The intrinsic factors, usually more evident in severe forms of patellofemoral instability, include the following: (1) hypoplasia of the patella;[65] (2) high-riding patella, also called patella alta;[28] (3) enlarged lateral patellar facet; (4) flat articular surface of the patella; (5) flat lateral femoral condyle;[28] and (6) shallow intercondylar groove.[28]

Extrinsic factors that may contribute to instability of the patella include the following: (1) insufficiency of the vastus medialis muscle, from disuse, prior rupture, or an anomalous high position of insertion on the patella;[28] (2) over-pull or contracture of the vastus lateralis muscle;[52,53] (3) contracture of the iliotibial band;[28] (4) contracture of the lateral retinaculum; (5) tethering through the patellofemoral and patellotibial ligaments;[28] (6) lateral fat pad scarring from repeated arthroscopy; (7) an excessive "Q" angle (line of quadriceps force) creating a "bowstring" effect on the patella accentuated by external rotation of the tibia near full extension; (8) a laterally positioned tibial tubercle; (9) a valgus deformity of the knee; and (10) generalized hyperlaxity. Turner's syndrome, nail-patella or Fong's disease, and Down's syndrome[66] are three genetic conditions of which patellar dislocation is a clinical manifestation.

Surgical treatment progresses from lateral release

to medial reefing or plication and, finally, to tibial tubercle transplantation medially if severe malalignment is present. Occasionally, patellar and intercondylar groove reshaping are necessary if the groove is shallow, flat, or convex and the patella is flat.

CHONDROMALACIA PATELLAE

Chondromalacia patellae is a morbid softening, fissuring, degenerative process of the articular surface of the knee cap owing to many causes[63] (Fig. 88–9). It can result from overuse during athletic activity,[67] from disuse following prolonged traction or cast immobilization,[68,69] from direct injury such as a blow to the patella from a car dashboard, or from an old patellar fracture with imperfect reduction. The disorder is accompanied by quadriceps muscle contractures with loss of flexion, frequently with malalignment of the quadriceps muscles and a laterally riding or chronically dislocating patella.[59,63] This common form of internal derangement of the knee is present in the majority of patients over the age of 30 who have a history of one of the aforementioned conditions. Athletic adolescent girls seem especially prone to chondromalacia.

Symptoms consist of bone pain on ascending or descending stairs. Localized aching also occurs after periods of immobility with the knee in the flexed position, such as while watching television or working at a desk. The symptoms of crepitation and grinding usually correspond directly to the degree of surface cartilaginous disruption. I grade this into three degrees: (I) fine fibrillation with yellowing (xanthochromia) and softening; (II) surface degeneration with a "crabmeat" appearance; and (III) exposure of the subchondral bone.

Crepitation, a sound resembling that of dry leaves underfoot, and grating, a palpatory sensation of roughness, are best demonstrated by active extension of the knee against resistance. These signs can be enhanced by direct manual compression of the patella against the femoral groove, with active resistive extension of the knee. Tenderness is often elicited along the inferior patella on the medial and lateral margins of the patellar ligament. I think that this sign is caused by a mild synovitis from the chips of chondromalacic fragments.

If chondromalacia is secondary to quadriceps muscle malalignment, the frightening "apprehension test" will be positive; this test produces a feeling of uneasiness with passive medial or lateral displacement of the patella. It is unusual to see an effusion of the knee due to chondromalacia patellae, unless the fibrillated surface has rapidly degenerated and has shed many fragments into the joint cavity over a short time, a phenomenon called "snowstorm knee." Therefore, an effusion in a patient with chondromalacia patellae is an ominous sign. These patients often obtain dramatic relief when the fragments and their products of digestion are arthroscopically irrigated from the joint.

The pathologic changes in chondromalacia may be precursors to osteoarthritis and may consist of a localized softening, discoloration, and loss of normal off-white sheen.[70] Surface signs of progressive degeneration include fine fibrillation, fissuring, fragmentation, and finally, exposure of subchondral bone. The exact relationship between chondromalacia, primarily seen in the central and inferior part of the patella, and patellar osteoarthritis, which is primarily lateral facet degeneration, remains unclear. Few of my patients with severe chondromalacia have developed severe lateral facet arthritis without concomitant medial or lateral compartment degeneration. The roentgenographic findings of a degenerative patellofemoral joint include loss of mainly lateral facet cartilage space and roughening on the superficial surface, the so-called hair-on-end appearance of the patella seen best in the "sunrise view."[62] The lateral projection shows superior and inferior pole osteophytes adjacent to the articular surface. If the compartments of the knee have moderate-to-severe degeneration in comparable degrees, the medial compartment will be the most symptomatic, the lateral compartment will be less symptomatic, and the patellofemoral compartment will be symptomatic in 20 to 30% of patients.

FIG. 88–9. This operative view of the undersurface of the patella shows typical chondromalacia with fissuring (arrow) of the medial facet (MF). The surface of the lateral facet (LF) appears unaffected.

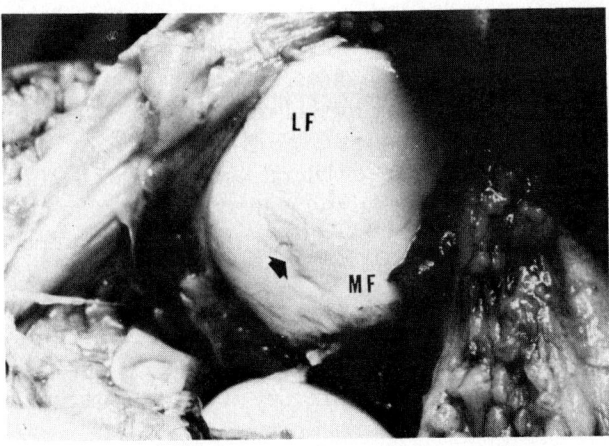

The treatment of chondromalacia patellae is difficult because of the multiple causes and the general irreversibility of this degenerative process. The inherent constant loading of the patellar articular surface with three to six times body weight during athletic activity further frustrates recovery.

Repair of identifiable mechanical defects such as malalignment of the extensor mechanism, lateral capsular release, and tibial tubercle elevation (Maquet technique) can be helpful.[70a,70b] Chondroplasty or debridement of the patellar articular surface is a nonphysiologic operation. Other than narrowing the articular surface by patellar decompression and preventing debris from falling into the joint cavity, this procedure offers little long-term relief. Patellectomy results in a 30 to 40% loss of quadriceps muscle power and is the last resort.[71]

DIAGNOSTIC METHODS

An adequate medical history, physical examination,[72] and roentgenographic evaluation of the knees consisting of at least anteroposterior and lateral views should be obtained. One may also consider patellar axial, sunrise, or sunset views for further evaluation of malalignment of the patella,[28,61,62] oblique views for occult lesions or fractures, and tunnel views to see the posterior portion of the femoral condyles more clearly, when looking for osteochondritis dissecans. Arthrography has been especially useful in demonstrating posterior horn tears of the medial meniscus and has been used to document anterior cruciate ligament tears.[72a]

Ultrasonography has been used to delineate Baker's cysts.[73] Computed tomographic (CT) scanning is helpful in showing the size and anatomic configuration of masses about the knee,[74,75] as well as in evaluating the configuration and anatomic features of the patellofemoral joint.[76] Recently, triple-phase bone scintigraphy has been especially useful in determining the presence of active bony lesions of the condyles, tibial plateaus, and patella, as well as synovial hyperemia.[77] This technique has also been helpful in determining industrial and legal cases in which claims of serious dysfunction do not seem to correspond to the physical examination and the physician does not feel arthroscopy is indicated.

Aspiration of the knee to look for free fat in a patient with acute hemarthrosis may aid in discovering an occult fracture not radiographically visible, *but of all diagnostic procedures, arthroscopy has added more to our understanding of the knee than any other technique.*[28,78–83] Its great diagnostic usefulness lies in the direct vision of the articular surfaces of the knee, the synovium, the anterior cruciate ligament, and the menisci. Various selections in angle of viewing with scopes of 0, 30, 70, and 110° are available. Many portals including suprapatellar, medial, lateral, and transpatellar tendon, and posterior have been described. The use of fiberoptics with more intense illumination has led to the ability to document intra-articular disorders in color. Miniature television cameras have expanded the capabilities of arthroscopy as an educational and operative tool.

Intra-articular arthroscopic surgery, without formal arthrotomy,[84,85] permits lateral plica release, patellar shaving, irrigational debridement, removal of loose bodies, debridement of the lesions of osteochondritis, synovectomy, plical resection,[56c,86,87] meniscectomy,[84] and closed fixation of small intra-articular fractures.

The complications of arthroscopy are few. With sterile, continuous irrigation, small portals, minimal tissue retraction, and limited dissection, infections are rare. Leakage of irrigation fluid from the synovial cavity into the soft tissues about the knee and transient swelling and discomfort are occasionally encountered. Intra-articular seeding of extra-articular tumor arthroscopically has been reported.[80]

I can say without reservation that the arthroscope has taught us more about the knee than any other development in diagnosis. Nevertheless, it is not what is seen but what is understood that counts.

MECHANICAL DISORDERS AND OSTEOARTHRITIS

Many osteoarthritic knees began with a minor insult leading to degeneration of one of its three compartments, that is, the medial, patellofemoral, or lateral. The injured compartment sheds debris and spreads the "seeds" of arthritis ("wear particles") to the other compartments; the result is triple-compartment disease. Most commonly, the first affected knee compartment in women is the patellofemoral joint, and in men, it is the medial compartment.[88]

The lateral compartment can be injured by instability, meniscal tear, or lateral tibial plateau fracture, but degeneration beginning in this compartment is much less common than in the other two compartments. It is known as the "silent compartment" both because degeneration rarely begins there and because it is often asymptomatic even in the presence of a significant pathologic process.

The following case history illustrates a typical course of a degenerative knee:

CASE HISTORY

A 16-year-old boy sprained his right knee while playing football; he was clipped from the "blind side." The knee became massively swollen a few hours after injury, it was wrapped in an elastic bandage, and crutches were obtained from a friend. Three weeks later, the patient's knee felt much improved, and he resumed playing football without seeking medical attention.

Interpretation

The twisting injury resulted in a tear of the anterior cruciate ligament, the most common cause of hemarthrosis in young athletes.[31,32] Because the knee was swollen, no tear could have been present in the capsule. With acute anterior cruciate ligament rupture, signs of knee instability are often absent, and the patient thereby had the impression that nothing was seriously wrong.

Case History Continued

Four years later, while playing basketball in college, the same patient turned to throw the ball. His knee suddenly gave way and he fell to the floor. He tried to extend the knee, but could not. The trainer applied traction, and the knee suddenly became free, but the patient was unable to return to the game because of pain. Two weeks later, the same thing occurred again when the patient simply turned to talk to a friend. This time, he could straighten his knee to a greater degree. Once again, traction and slight twisting of the leg suddenly "released it." For the first time, the patient saw a physician, who made the diagnosis of a torn medial meniscus and surgically removed it. The patient returned to sports with no further problems.

Interpretation

The insufficiency of the torn anterior cruciate ligament led to increased loading and attenuation of the other ligamentous structures, stabilizing the knee. The combined ligamentous insufficiency caused an instability manifested by a subtle anterior motion of the medial tibial plateau in relation to the femoral condyle, with the knee in flexion and the leg and foot in external rotation. This aberrant motion brought the posterior horn of the medial meniscus forward underneath the femoral condyle during most turning or "cutting" activities, eventually trapping the meniscus and finally causing a longitudinal tear (see Fig. 88–4). Repeated incidents of trapping and progressive tearing, allowing greater extension with each episode, gave the false impression that the knee was improving with each locking event.

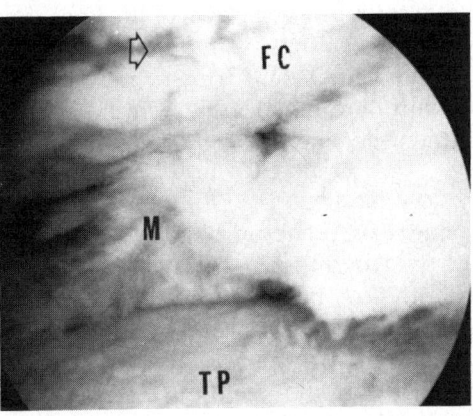

FIG. 88–10. This arthroscopic view demonstrates end-stage degeneration of the femoral condyle (FC), the meniscus (M), and the tibial plateau (TP). The arrow points to an ulceration of the articular cartilage extending to subchondral bone.

Case History Continued

At age 46, the patient was still active in athletics, refereeing basketball and coaching soccer. He noticed that his right knee was beginning to bow, and the inner medial side of the knee ached after standing on it all day. The patient also noted intermittent swelling, heat, and deep bone pain with weather changes. He had tried some of the new "antiarthritic medications," which took the edge off the discomfort but did not seem to halt the progression of the disorder. His physician recommended "taking a wedge out of the tibia," to shift some of the weight to the lateral compartment and to correct the bowing.

Interpretation

Medial femoral condylar degeneration is common after meniscectomy.[28,89] Progressive degeneration with wearing of the medial condylar cartilage places

Table 88–2. Conditions That Mimic or Produce Symptoms of Internal Derangement of the Knee

Avascular necrosis of the femoral condyles[89,90]
Chondromalacia patellae[63]
Cystic degeneration of the lateral meniscus[91]
Discoid lateral meniscus[92,93,94]
Heterotopic calcification[95]
Lipoma arborescens[96]
Localized pigmented villonodular synovitis[97]
Osteochondromatosis[98]
Pigmented villonodular synovitis[99]
Posterior cruciate ligament rupture[100]
Segond fracture[101]
Synovial cyst[102]
Synovial hemangioma[103]
Tibiofibular instability[104]
Tumors about the knee[105]

more stress on the medial compartment of the knee and causes further varus. This process initiates the vicious cycle of medial compartment overload-further degeneration-greater compartment overload, and it ultimately leads to a "loss of medial joint space" on standing anteroposterior views of the knee. Proximal valgus tibial osteotomy shifts the weight from the medial to the lateral compartment and is often effective in controlling most of the symptoms of medial compartment degeneration.

Case History Continued

The patient was relieved of pain by the osteotomy until age 65, when he retired as a school teacher. He continued to golf, but had to ride a cart because he was unable to walk 18 holes, owing to severe right knee discomfort. The patient had almost continual swelling, heat, grinding, and discomfort during minimal activity (Fig. 88–10). Soon thereafter, he underwent total knee replacement.

In summary, I have reviewed internal and external derangements of the knee, using the torn meniscus and its relationship to instability as the prototype for soft tissue entrapment and osteochondritis and patellar dislocation as prototypic conditions that generate osteochondral loose bodies. Other conditions can mimic internal derangements (Table 88–2). Finally, I have reviewed current diagnostic methods and have presented a typical case history of degenerative osteoarthritis of the knee.

REFERENCES

1. Rang, M. (Ed.): Anthology of Orthopaedics. Internal Derangement of the Knee: William Hey. London and Edinburgh, E. and S. Livingstone Ltd., 1966.
2. Daniel, D., Daniels, E., and Aronson, D.: The diagnosis of meniscus pathology. Clin. Orthop., 163:218–224, 1982.
3. Hamberg, P., Gillquist, J., and Lysholm, J.: Suture of new and old peripheral meniscus tears. J. Bone Joint Surg., 65A:193–197, 1983.
4. Jones, R.E., Smith, E.C., and Resich, J.S.: Effects of medial meniscectomy in patients older than forty years. J. Bone Joint Surg., 60A:783–786, 1978.
5. Noble, J., and Erat, K.: In defense of the meniscus. J. Bone Joint Surg., 62B:7–11, 1980.
6. Sonne-Holm, S., Fledelius, I., Ahn, N.: Results after meniscectomy in 147 athletes. Acta Orthop. Scand., 51:303–309, 1980.
7. Walker, P.S., and Erkman, M.J.: The role of the menisci in force transmission across the knee. Clin. Orthop., 109:184–192, 1975.
8. Arnold, J.A., et al.: Natural history of anterior cruciate tears. Am. J. Sports Med., 7:305–313, 1979.
9. Feagin, J.A.: The syndrome of the torn anterior cruciate ligament. In Symposium on disorders of the knee joint. Orthop. Clin. North Am., 10:81–90, 1979.
10. Fetto, J.F., and Marshall, J.L.: The natural history and diagnosis of anterior cruciate ligament insufficiency. Clin. Orthop., 147:29–38, 1980.
11. Grove, T.P., et al.: Non-operative treatment of the torn anterior cruciate ligament. J. Bone Joint Surg., 65A:184–192, 1983.
12. Noyes, F.R., et al.: The symptomatic anterior cruciate-deficient knee. Part II. The results of rehabilitation activity modification and counseling on functional disability. J. Bone Joint Surg., 65A:163–174, 1983.
13. Noyes, F.R., et al.: The symptomatic anterior cruciate-deficient knee. Part I. The long term functional disability in athletically active individuals. J. Bone Joint Surg., 65A:154–162, 1983.
14. Torg, J.S., Conrad, W., and Kalen, V.: Clinical diagnosis of anterior cruciate ligament instability in the athlete. Am. J. Sports Med., 4:84–93, 1976.
15. DeHaven, K.E.: Meniscus repair in the athlete. Clin. Orthop., 198:31–35, 1985.
16. Warren, R.F., and Levy, I.M.: Meniscal lesions associated with anterior cruciate ligament injury. Clin. Orthop., 172:32–37, 1983.
17. Symposium on the anterior cruciate ligament. Part I. Orthop. Clin. North Am., 16:29–39, 127–134, 1985.
18. Frankel, V.H., Burstein, A.H., and Brooks, D.B.: Biomechanics of internal derangement of the knee—Pathomechanics as determined by analysis of the instant centers of motion. J. Bone Joint Surg., 53A:945–962, 1971.
19. Hughston, J.C., et al.: Classification of knee ligament instabilities. Part I. The medial compartment and cruciate ligaments. J. Bone Joint Surg., 58A:159–172, 1976.
20. Hughston, J.C., et al.: Classification of knee ligament instabilities. Part II: The lateral compartment. J. Bone Surg., 58A:173–179, 1976.
21. Marshall, J.L., and Baugher W.H.: Stability examination of the knee: A simple anatomic approach. Clin. Orthop., 146:78–83, 1980.
22. Marshall, J.L., Getto, J.F., and Botero, P.M.: General orthopaedics: Knee ligament injuries: A standardized evaluation method. Clin. Orthop., 123:115–129, 1977.
23. Parker, H.G.: Chronic anteromedial instability of the knee. Clin. Orthop., 142:123–130, 1979.
24. Hughston, J.C., and Jacobson, K.E.: Chronic posterolateral rotatory instability of the knee. J. Bone Joint Surg., 67A:351–359, 1985.
25. Nicholas, J.A.: The five-one reconstruction for anteromedial instability of the knee: Indications, technique, and the results in fifty-two patients. J. Bone Joint Surg., 55A:899–922, 1973.
26. Galway, H.R., and MacIntosh, D.L.: The lateral pivot shift: A symptom and sign of anterior cruciate ligament insufficiency. Clin. Orthop., 147:45–50, 1980.
27. Ritchey, S.J.: Ligamentous disruption of the knee. U.S. Armed Forces Med. J., 11:167–176, 1960.
28. Symposium on the Knee. Clin. Sports Med., 4:231–265, 275–278, 295–324, 1985.
29. Frank, C.: Accurate interpretation of the Lachman test. Clin. Orthop., 213:163–166, 1986.
30. Indelicato, P.A., and Bittar, E.S.: A perspective of lesions associated with ACL insufficiency of the knee. A review of 100 cases. Clin. Orthop., 198:77–80, 1985.
30a. Losee, R.E., Johnson, T.R., and Southwick, W.O.: Anterior subluxation of the lateral tibial plateau. J. Bone Joint Surg., 60A:1015–1030, 1978.

30b.Slocum, D.B., et al.: Clinical test for anterolateral rotary instability of the knee. Clin. Orthop., *118*:63–69, 1976.

30c.Baker, C.L., Norwood, L.A., and Hughston, J.C.: Acute posterolateral rotatory instability of the knee. J. Bone Joint Surg., *65A*:614–618, 1983.

30d.Hughston, J.C., and Norwood, L.A.: The posterolateral drawer test and external rotational recurvatum test for posterolateral rotatory instability of the knee. Clin. Orthop., *147*:82–87, 1980.

30e.Jakob, R.P., Hassler, H., and Staeubli, H.U.: Observations on rotatory instability of the lateral compartment of the knee. Acta Orthop. Scand. [Suppl. 191], *52*:1–32, 1981.

31. DeHaven, K.E.: Diagnosis of acute knee injuries with hemarthrosis. Am. J. Sports Med., *8*:9–14, 1980.

32. Noyes, F.R., et al.: Arthroscopy in acute traumatic hemarthrosis of the knee. J. Bone Joint Surg., *62A*:687–695, 1980.

33. Witvoet, J., and Christel, P.: Treatment of chronic anterior knee instabilities with combined intra- and extra-articular transfer augmented with carbon-PLA fibers. Clin. Orthop., *196*:143–153, 1985.

34. Lipscomb, A.B., and Anderson, A.F.: Tears of the anterior cruciate ligament in adolescents. J. Bone Joint Surg., *68A*:19–28, 1986.

35. Hughston, J.C., and Barrett, G.R.: Acute anteromedial rotatory instability. J. Bone Joint Surg., *65A*:145–153, 1983.

36. Nagura, S.: The so-called osteochondritis dissecans of Konig. Clin. Orthop., *18*:100–122, 1960.

37. Aichroth, P.: Osteochondritis dissecans of the knee: A clinical survey. J. Bone Joint Surg., *53A*:440–447, 1971.

38. Ribbing, S.: The hereditary multiple epiphyseal disturbance and its consequences for the aetiogenesis of local malacias—Particularly the osteochondrosis dissecans. Acta Orthop. Scand., *24*:286–299, 1955.

39. Giorgi, B.: Morphologic variations of the intercondylar eminence of the knee. Clin. Orthop., *8*:209–217, 1956.

40. Fairbank, H.A.T.: Osteochondritis dissecans. Br. J. Surg., *21*:67–82, 1933.

41. Green, W.T., and Banks, H.H.: Osteochondritis dissecans in children. J. Bone Joint Surg., *35A*:26–47, 1953.

42. Linden, B.: Osteochondritis dissecans of the femoral condyles. J. Bone Joint Surg., *59A*:769–776, 1977.

43. Linden, B., and Nilsson, B.E.: Strontium-85 uptake in knee joints with osteochondritis dissecans: Acta Orthop. Scand., *47*:668–671, 1976.

44. O'Donoghue, D.H.: Chondral and osteochondral fractures. J. Trauma, *6*:469–481, 1966.

45. Johnson, E.W., and McLeod, T.L.: Osteochondral fragments of the distal end of the femur fixed with bone pegs. J. Bone Joint Surg., *59A*:677–679, 1977.

46. Smillie, I.S.: Treatment of osteochondritis dissecans. J. Bone Joint Surg., *39B*:248–260, 1957.

47. Hughston, J.C., Hergenroeder, P.T., and Courtenay, B.G.: Osteochondritis dissecans of the femoral condyles. J. Bone Joint Surg., *66A*:1340–1348, 1984.

48. Ahuja, S.C., and Bullough, P.G.: Osteonecrosis of the knee: A clinico-pathological study in twenty-eight patients. J. Bone Joint Surg., *60A*:191–197, 1978.

49. Stougaard, J.: Familial occurrence of osteochondritis dissecans. J. Bone Joint Surg., *46B*:542–543, 1964.

50. Stougaard, J.: The hereditary factor in osteochondritis dissecans. J. Bone Joint Surg., *43B*:256–258, 1961.

51. Wagoner, G., and Cohn, B.N.E.: Osteochondritis disssecans: A resume of the theories of etiology and the consideration of heredity as an etiologic factor. Arch. Surg., *23*:1–25, 1931.

52. Johnson, R.P.: Lateral resection for moderate patellofemoral instability. Orthop. Trans., *7*:196, 1983.

53. Johnson, R.P.: The lateral facet syndrome of the patella. Lateral restraint analysis and use of lateral resection. Clin. Orthop., *233*:61–71, 1988.

54. Ficat, R.P., and Hungerford, D.S. (Eds.): Disorders of the Patellofemoral Joint: The Excessive Lateral Pressure Syndrome. Baltimore, Williams & Wilkins, 1977.

55. Hejgaard, N., and Arnoldi, C.C.: Osteotomy of the patella in the patellofemoral pain syndrome. The significance of increased intraosseous pressure during sustained knee flexion. Int. Orthop., *8*:189–194, 1984.

56. Waisbrod, H., and Treiman, N.: Intraosseous venography in patellofemoral disorders—A preliminary report. J. Bone Joint Surg., *62B*:454–456, 1980.

56a.Pitkin, G.: Knee injuries: The role of the suprapatellar plica and surapatellar bursa in simulating internal derangement. Clin. Orthop., *74*:161–174, 1971.

56b.Pitkin, G.: Lesions of the suprapatellar plica. J. Bone Joint Surg., *32A*:363–369, 1950.

56c.Hardaker, W.T., Whipple, T.L., and Bassett F.H., III: Diagnosis and treatment of the plica syndrome of the knee. J. Bone Joint Surg., *62A*:221–225, 1980.

57. SanDretto, M.A., et al.: Suprapatellar plica synovialis: A common arthrographic finding. J. Can. Assoc. Radiol., *33*:163–166, 1982.

58. SanDretto, M.A., and Carrera, G.F.: The double fat fluid level: Lipohemarthrosis of the knee associated with suprapatellar plica synovialis. Skeletal Radiol., *10*:30–33, 1983.

59. Larson, R.L.: Subluxation-dislocation of the patella. In The Injured Adolescent Knee. Edited by J.C. Kennedy. Baltimore, Williams & Wilkins, 1979.

60. Macnab, I.: Recurrent dislocation of the patella. J. Bone Joint Surg., *34A*:957–967, 1952.

61. Laurin, C.A., et al.: The abnormal lateral patellofemoral angle: A diagnostic roentgenographic sign of recurrent patellar subluxation. J. Bone Joint Surg., *60A*:55–60, 1978.

62. Merchant, A.C., et al.: Roentgenographic analysis of patellofemoral congruence. J. Bone Joint Surg., *56A*:1391–1396, 1974.

63. Insall, J.: Current concepts review: Patellar pain. J. Bone Joint Surg., *64A*:147–152, 1982.

64. Kettelkamp, D.B.: Current concepts review: Management of patellar malalignment. J. Bone Joint Surg., *63A*:1344–1348, 1981.

65. Scott, J.E., and Taor, W.S.: The "small patella" syndrome. J. Bone Joint Surg., *61B*:172–175, 1979.

66. Smith, D.W.: Recognizable Patterns of Human Malformation. Vol. 7. Major Problems in Clinical Pediatrics. Philadelphia, W.B. Saunders, 1970.

67. Gruber, M.A.: The conservative treatment of chondromalacia patellae. In Symposium on disorders of the knee joint. Orthop. Clin. North Am., *10*:105–115, 1979.

68. Paukkonen, K., Jurvelin, J., and Helminen, H.J.: Effects of immobilization on the articular cartilage in young rabbits. Clin. Orthop., *206*:270–280, 1986.

69. Jurvelin, J., Koviranta, I., Tammi, M., and Helminen, H.J.: Softening of canine cartilage after immobilization of the knee joint. Clin. Orthop., *207*:246–252, 1986.

70. Mankin, H.J.: Biochemical changes in articular cartilage in osteoarthritis. In Symposium on Osteoarthritis. St. Louis, C.V. Mosby, 1976.

70a.Ferguson, A.B., Jr., et al.: Relief of patellofemoral contact stress by anterior displacement of the tibial tubercle. J. Bone Joint Surg., *61A*:159–172, 1979.

70b. Maquet, P.G.J.: Biomechanics of the Knee: With Application to the Pathogenesis and the Surgical Treatment of Osteoarthritis. Berlin, Springer-Verlag, 1976.

71. Wendt, P.P., and Johnson, R.P.: A study of quadriceps excursion, torque, and the effect of patellectomy on cadaver knees. J. Bone Joint Surg., *67A*:726–732, 1985.

72. Paulos, L., Noyes, F.R., and Malek, M.: A practical guide to the initial evaluation and treatment of knee ligament injuries. J. Trauma, *20*:498–506, 1980.

72a. Freiberger, R.H., and Kaye, J.J.: Arthrography. New York, Appleton-Century-Crofts, 1979.

73. Beals, R.K., et al.: Ultrasound as a diagnostic aid in the evaluation of popliteal swelling. Clin. Orthop., *149*:220–223, 1980.

74. Paul, D.F., Morrey, B.F., and Helms, C.A.: Computerized tomography in orthopedic surgery. (Section II. General orthopaedics.) Clin. Orthop., *139*:142–149, 1979.

75. Pavlov, H., et al.: Computer-assisted tomography of the knee. Invest. Radiol., *13*:57–62, 1978.

76. Delgado-Martins, H.: A study of the position of the patella using computerized tomography. J. Bone Joint Surg., *61B*:443–444, 1979.

77. Mauer, A.H., et al.: Utility of three-phase skeletal scintigraphy in suspected osteomyelitis: Concise communication. J. Nucl. Med., *22*:941–949, 1981.

78. Casscells, S.W.: The place of arthroscopy in the diagnosis and treatment of internal derangement of the knee: An analysis of 1000 cases. Clin. Orthop., *151*:135–142, 1980.

79. Curran, W.P., and Woodward, E.P.: Arthroscopy: Its role in diagnosis and treatment of athletic knee injuries. Am. J. Sports Med., *8*:415–418, 1980.

80. Joyce, M.J., and Mankin, H.J.: Caveat arthroscopos: Extra-articular lesions of bone simulating intra-articular pathology of the knee. J. Bone Joint Surg., *65A*:289–292, 1983.

81. McGinty, J.B., and Freedman, P.A.: Arthroscopy of the knee. Clin. Orthop., *121*:173–180, 1976.

82. Minkoff, J.: The philosophy and application of arthroscopy in non-meniscal problems of the knee. *In* Symposium on disorders of the knee joint. Orthop. Clin. North Am., *10*:37–50, 1979.

83. Patel, D., Fahmy, N., and Sakayan, A.: Isokinetic and functional evaluation of the knee following arthroscopic surgery. Clin. Orthop., *167*:84–91, 1982.

84. O'Connor, R.L.: Arthroscopy. Philadelphia, J.B. Lippincott, 1977.

85. Watanabe, M.: Arthroscopy: The present state. Orth. Clin. North Am., *10*:505–522, 1979.

86. Reference deleted.

87. Munzinger, U., et al.: Internal derangement of the knee joint due to pathologic synovial folds: The mediopatellar plica syndrome. Clin. Orthop., *155*:59–64, 1981.

88. Klunder, K.B., Rud, B., and Hansen, J.: Osteoarthritis of the hip and knee joint in retired football players. Acta Orthop. Scand., *51*:925–927, 1980.

89. Ahlback, S., Bauer, G.C.H., and Bohne, W.H.: Spontaneous osteonecrosis of the knee. Arthritis Rheum., *11*:705–733, 1968.

90. Rozing, P.M., Insall, J., and Bohne, W.H.: Spontaneous osteonecrosis of the knee. J. Bone Joint Surg., *62A*:2–7, 1980.

91. Barrie, H.J.: The pathogenesis and significance of meniscal cysts. J. Bone Joint Surg., *61B*:184–189, 1979.

92. Hall, F.M.: Arthrography of the discoid lateral meniscus. AJR, *128*:993–1002, 1977.

93. Resnick, D., and Niwayama, G.: Discoid meniscus. *In* Diagnosis of Bone and Joint Disorders. Vol. I. Arthrography, Tenography, and Bursography. Philadelphia, W.B. Saunders, 1981.

94. Dickhaut, S.C., and DeLee, J.C.: The discoid lateral-meniscus syndrome. J. Bone Joint Surg., *64A*:1068, 1982.

95. Tibone, J., et al.: Heterotopic ossification around the hip in spinal cord-injured patients. J. Bone Joint Surg., *60A*:769–775, 1978.

96. Hermann, G., and Hockberg, F.: Lipoma arborescens: Arthrogrpahic findings. Orthopedics, *3*:19–21, 1980.

97. Granowitz, S.P., and Mankin, H.J.: Localized pigmented villonodular synovitis of the knee: Report of five cases. J. Bone Joint Surg., *49A*:122–218, 1967.

98. Milgram, J.W.: Synovial osteochondromatosis: A histopathological study of thirty cases. J. Bone Joint Surg., *59A*:792–801, 1977.

99. Rosenthal, D.I., Coleman, P.K., and Schiller, A.L.: Pigmented villonodular synovitis: Correlation of angiographic and histologic findings. Am. Roentgen Ray Soc., *135*:581–585, 1980.

100. Clancy, W.G., et al.: Treatment of knee joint instability secondary to rupture of the posterior cruciate ligament. J. Bone Joint Surg., *65A*:310–322, 1983.

101. Segond, P.: Pathologie externe. Recherches cliniques et experimentales sur les epanchements sanguins du genou par entorse test. Le Progres Medical, *7*:319–321, 1879.

102. Kilcoyne, R.F., Imray, T.J., and Stewart, E.T.: Ruptured Baker's cyst simulating acute thrombophlebitis. JAMA, *240*:1517–1518, 1978.

103. Moon, N.F.: Synovial hemangioma of the knee joint. Clin. Orthop., *90*:183–190, 1973.

104. Ogden, J.A.: Subluxation and dislocation of the proximal tibiofibular joint. J. Bone Joint Surg., *56A*:145–154, 1974.

105. Johnston, A.D., and Parisien, M.V.: Soft tissue tumors about the knee. Symposium on disorders of the knee joint. Orthop. Clin. North Am., *10*:263–284, 1979.

89

PAINFUL FEET

JOHN S. GOULD

Painful foot disorders have been classified according to relative anatomic areas, for example, metatarsalgia, arch strain, heel pain, with empiric efforts made to treat these nonspecific entities. The modern orthopedist evaluates the foot for biomechanical, vascular, neurogenic (local and referred), infectious, neoplastic, traumatic, developmental, and acquired disorders. Each area of the anatomy may be the source of the disorder, or a reflection of an underlying problem involving the skin, bursae, tendons, nerves, fasciae, blood vessels, joints, and bone.

Evaluation begins with the history and physical examination, includes the use of foot mirrors and footprint papers in the office, and may require noninvasive vascular analysis, nerve conduction studies and electromyography, plain radiographs, computed tomography (CT), magnetic resonance imaging (MRI), sophisticated gait analysis (force plate) examination, and routine or specialized laboratory tests. Management of the problems, of course, include medical and surgical solutions, but also may involve simple or sophisticated pedorthic prescriptions, pedicare (nail, corn, and callus trimming), and physical therapy. The pedorthist (trained and certified in the fabrication of orthotic devices for the foot and the modification and custom design of shoes), the skilled foot-care nurse, and the physical therapist have collaborated with the orthopedist, rheumatologist, dermatologist, and peripheral vascular specialists to provide a multidisciplinary approach to optimal foot care.

PAINFUL TOES

Painful toes or areas of the toes may result from trauma or from an underlying acquired or congenital deformity, which becomes painful after contact with certain types of footwear.

ATHLETIC INJURIES

Various athletic activities may also be associated with toe injuries. Acute or chronic trauma to toenails often occurs in skiers, who may bruise the nail to the great or long second toe in a new, hard boot. The subungual hematoma is obvious and requires treatment with a longer or better-fitting boot, and occasional drainage of the hematoma when exquisitely painful. More subtle, repetitive trauma occurs in tennis players, whose nails simply become white after a low-grade injury, and eventually slough (tennis toe). A similar injury occurs in ballet dancers.[1]

CORNS

Persons with fixed flexion contractures of the distal interphalangeal joint from an acquired hammer or mallet toe or from a congenital mallet toe can develop an apical corn on the tip of the toe. Shoes with a higher or increased depth of the toe box and lower heels will help, but loafers and fashionable shoes with the usual

1403

tapered toe cause pain. Resection of the distal middle phalanx condyles, with or without formal fusion, resolves the problem.

Corns develop typically on the dorsum of the joints, which are acutely angled dorsally, as over a claw toe when contact is made with a hard shoe (Fig. 89–1). The underlying problem may be congenital clawing, or an acquired phenomenon associated with crowding of the second toe by the great toe in a bunion deformity, congenital overlapping of the fifth toe, and dislocation or subluxation of the metatarsophalangeal (MTP) joints from synovitis. The dorsum of the joint contacts the shoe, producing callus formation. As the callus grows, it causes pain on contact. Pedicare by trimming or "paring" or by abrading the corn with a pumice stone is helpful; moleskin cutouts (corn pads), higher toe boxes in shoes, stretching the contacting area of shoe leather (use of the shoemakers' wand), and dynamic correction of a flexible deformity with a toe crest (Fig. 89–2) are all conservative approaches to the problem.[2] Surgical correction of bunions, overlapping toes, and claw toes may be needed. Joint resection, fusions, and dynamic corrections with tendon transfers may be indicated.

Soft corns (Fig. 89–3) develop between toes when contacting condyles of the adjacent toes cause extremely painful callus formation. Toe separators help, but simple condylectomies relieve the problem, which originated during toe crowding from certain footwear.[3]

FIG. 89–1. Claw toes with corns over proximal interphalangeal joints.

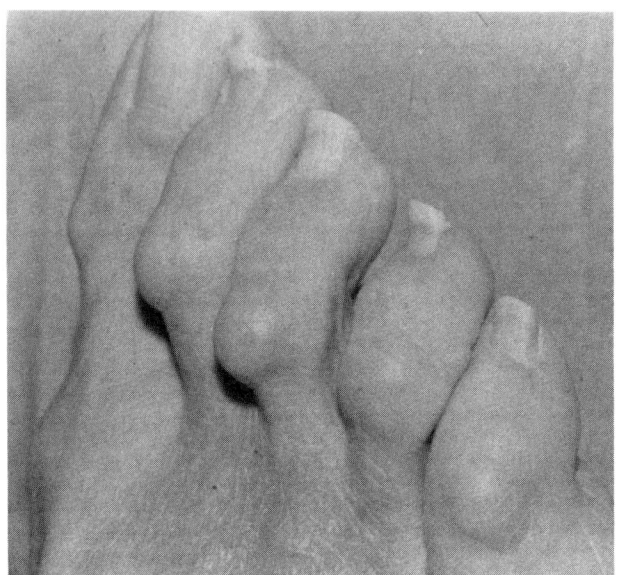

FIG. 89–2. Use of a toe crest to correct a claw toe.

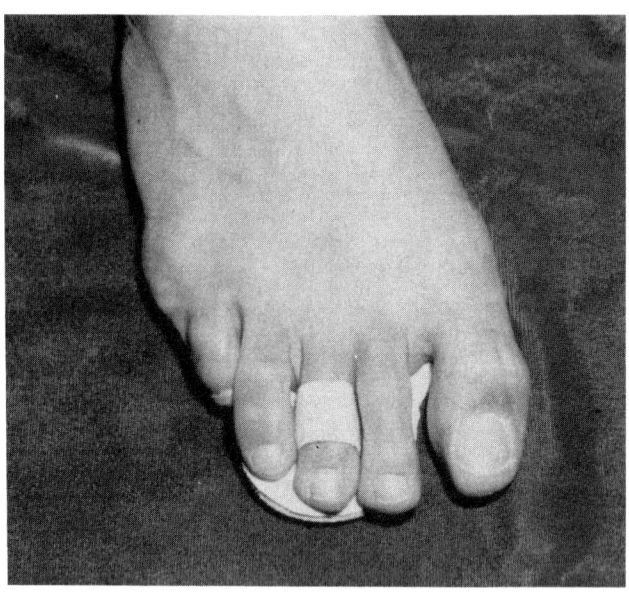

FIG. 89–3. *A,* Soft corn between toes secondary to contacting adjacent condyles. *B,* Artist's depiction of soft corn pathodynamics.

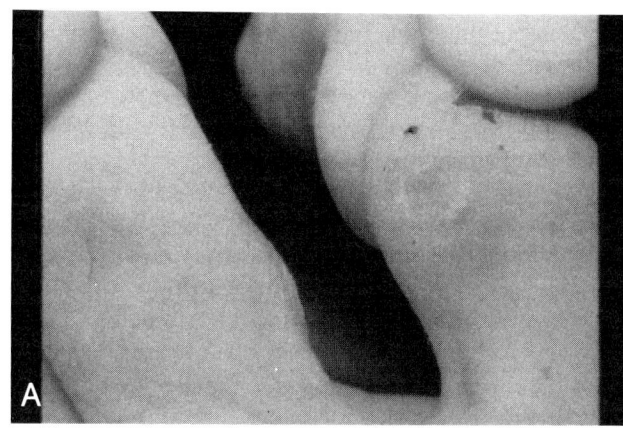

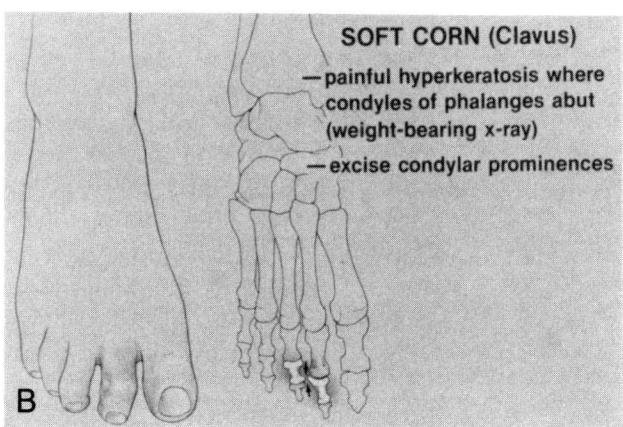

SOFT CORN (Clavus)

—painful hyperkeratosis where condyles of phalanges abut (weight-bearing x-ray)

—excise condylar prominences

INGROWN TOENAILS

Ingrown toenails may occur from inappropriate short trimming or may follow trauma with secondary infections. In mild cases, the nail grooves are gently packed with cotton to allow the nail to grow out normally. More refractory problems may require *partial matrixectomies* performed mechanically, chemically (phenol), or most recently with lasers; or *wedge resections* of nail and matrix.[4] Recalcitrant cases are treated by *total matrixectomy*, with and without skin grafting, or by *excision of nail and distal phalanx tuft* (terminal Syme's procedure).

SYNOVITIS

"Jamming" and hyperextension injuries, particularly to the great toe joint, may occur on artificial athletic field surfaces (turf toe). Such traumatic synovitis is effectively treated with splinting, rest, and nonsteroidal anti-inflammatory drugs (NSAIDs). Osteochondral fractures may be found in refractory cases and require surgical intervention.

MORTON'S NEUROMA

Toe pain emanating from the web space, particularly from compression of an interdigital nerve, occurs frequently in athletes or middle-aged patients. So-called Morton's neuroma,[5] pain from perineural fibrosis, results from compression of an interdigital nerve under the intermetatarsal ligament. The patient presents with shooting pain into the toes, or paresthesias or numbness in the involved toes and localized pain with compression of the metatarsal heads. Tenderness is specifically localized between the involved metatarsal heads, typically between the third and fourth, less frequently between the second and third. More-specific findings include palpation of a mass, divergence of the toes, and a clicking sensation when the adjacent toes are flexed and extended. In acute cases, a metatarsal pad (Fig. 89–4) behind the involved heads may help. An association with a pronated foot may require longitudinal arch support as well. More resistant cases are treated with local corticosteroid injections; the most refractory cases require neurectomy (Fig. 89–5).[6] Simple division of the intermetatarsal ligament alone has had some recent interest.[7]

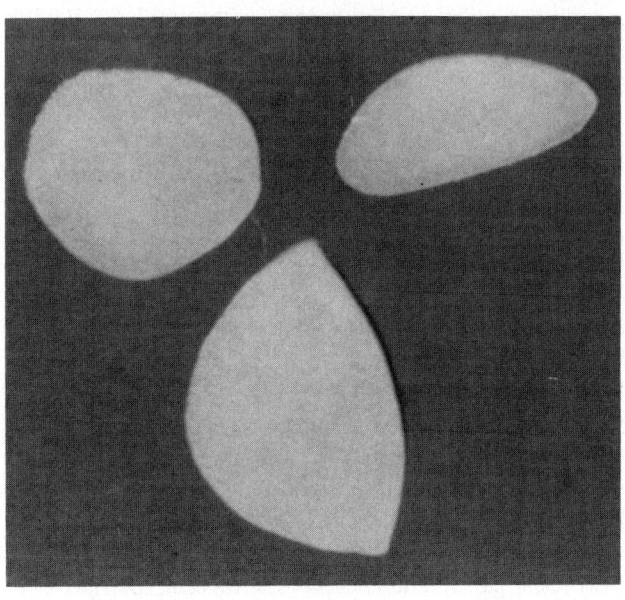

FIG. 89–4. A variety of metatarsal felt pads may be shaped and cemented to the insole of the shoe behind painful lesions.

METATARSALGIA

Metatarsal pain, frequently plantar, may be isolated to a specific joint or generalized across the ball of the foot.[8] As already discussed, Morton's neuroma may present as pain in the metatarsal area. Other localized problems are delineated below.

FIG. 89–5. *A*, Artist's rendition of the thickened interdigital nerve (Morton's neuroma). *B*, The resected interdigital nerve. Note the marked enlargement of the nerve.

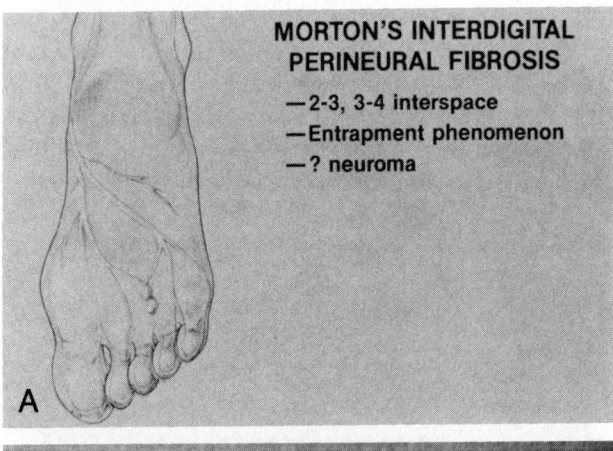

MORTON'S INTERDIGITAL PERINEURAL FIBROSIS

—2-3, 3-4 interspace
—Entrapment phenomenon
—? neuroma

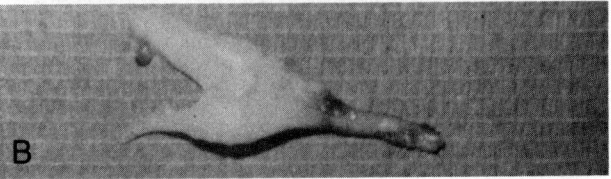

BUNIONS

Hallux valgus, usually associated with *metatarsus primus varus*, or "splay" between the first and second metatarsals, is not in itself painful. However, patients seek medical help for the correction of appearance and for the relief of pain caused by footwear. Although some MTP joints become secondarily arthritic, the pain usually occurs over the medial prominence of the first metatarsal head, under the second metatarsal head, or over the proximal interphalangeal joint of the second toe that has become clawed through contact with footwear. Unshod populations also develop bunion deformities but rarely request medical help, apparently because of lack of pain.[9] The medial first MTP pain may be secondary to an inflamed bursa (Fig. 89–6) or to pressure on the medial branch of the superficial peroneal nerve, which is stretched over the bunion and compressed. The painful corn over the second proximal interphalangeal joint has already been described. The callosity (intractable plantar keratosis) under the second metatarsal head is secondary to altered weight-bearing (Fig. 89–7). As the first metatarsal moves into varus at its joint with the first cuneiform, its head also moves dorsally, resulting in a transfer of weight to the second metatarsal head. This

FIG. 89–6. Bunion (hallux valgus) deformity with medial bursa.

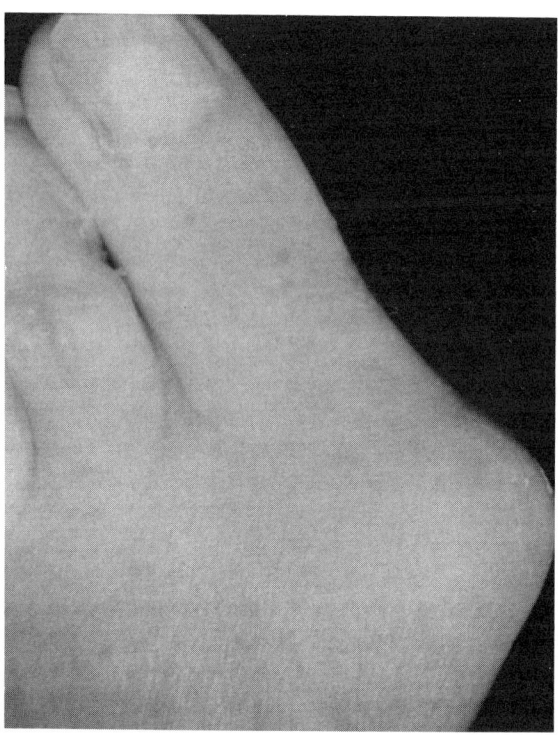

FIG. 89–7. Intractable plantar keratosis (IPK) under second metatarsal head (transfer lesion).

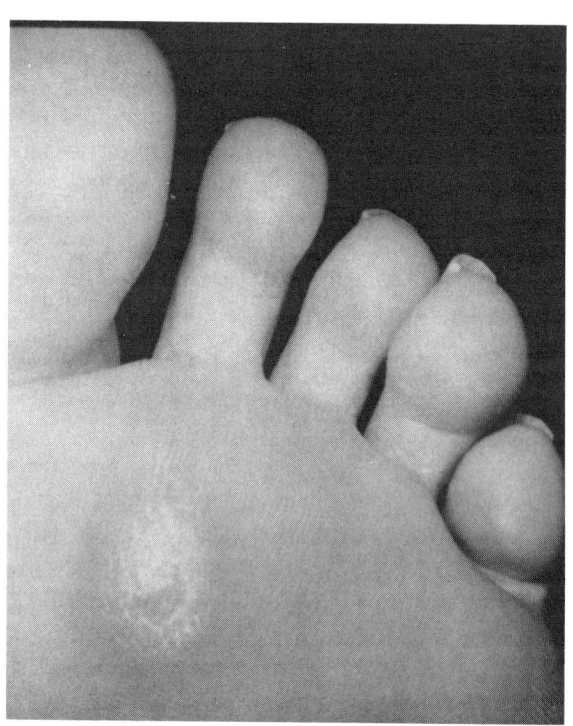

is known as a "transfer lesion," and it is further accentuated as the second MTP joint hyperextends. Biomechanically, with the toe now positioned dorsally, further downward force is exerted on the metatarsal head.

Bunion pain can be managed using a shoe with a wider toebox and increased depth (made on a bunion last), and with a "total contact" insert proximal to the painful second metatarsal head, around it, and particularly under the first metatarsal head ("Morton's extension") (Fig. 89–8). Paring an associated callus is also helpful.

Surgical treatment of more severe cases is by osteotomy, which moves the first metatarsal back to the neutral position, decreases the angle between the first and second metatarsals to less than 8° (normal), and depresses the first metatarsal head slightly plantarward. I perform a concentric-shaped osteotomy at the first metatarsal base.[9] Distally, the medial prominence of the first metatarsal is excised (ostectomy), the soft tissue is released laterally, and the capsule is imbricated medially with realignment of the sesamoids. The toe is thus realigned, and the bunion corrected. The deformity of the second toe is also corrected,

FIG. 89–8. Total contact insert with relief around IPK.

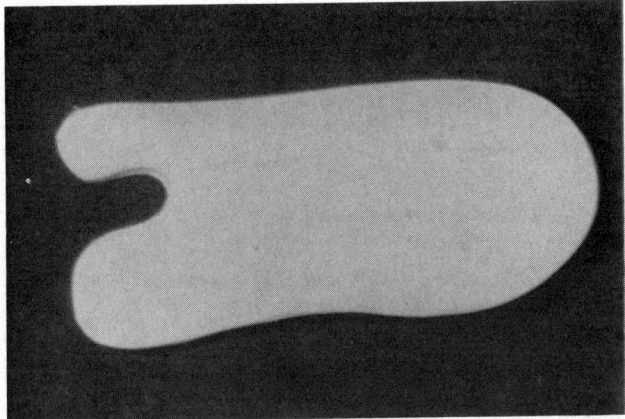

often with a capsulectomy and tenotomy at the MTP joint. I resect the proximal phalanx distal condyles in a fixed deformity at the proximal interphalangeal joint, with a flexor to extensor tendon transfer. A transfer alone may be sufficient to correct a flexible deformity.

BUNIONETTE

A *bunionette* (tailor's bunion) is the reverse of the first MTP joint bunion, involving the fifth MTP joint. A bursa forms over the lateral prominence of the fifth metatarsal head. Again, a wider toebox and a moleskin cutout may help. Surgical correction can usually be accomplished by simple resection of the fifth metatarsal prominence. If splay between the fourth and fifth metatarsals is significant, an osteotomy (usually an oblique diaphyseal type) is done to narrow the foot, along with the ostectomy.

HALLUX RIGIDUS

Other painful afflictions around the hallux (great toe) include hallux rigidus, a degenerative arthritis of the first MTP joint, typically occurring in relatively young men, characterized by localized dorsal spurring on the first metatarsal head (Fig. 89–9), but not generalized MTP joint arthritis. Dorsiflexion of the first MTP joint is limited, as is motion in the first cuneiform–first metatarsal joint, thought to be the primary source of the problem.

Traumatic arthritis or osteoarthritis of the first MTP joint also results in pain and loss of motion, but here the process is generalized. Primary osteoarthritis is

FIG. 89–9. *A,* Clinical appearance of hallux rigidus. *B,* Radiograph of hallux rigidus. Note dorsal spurring at first MTP joint.

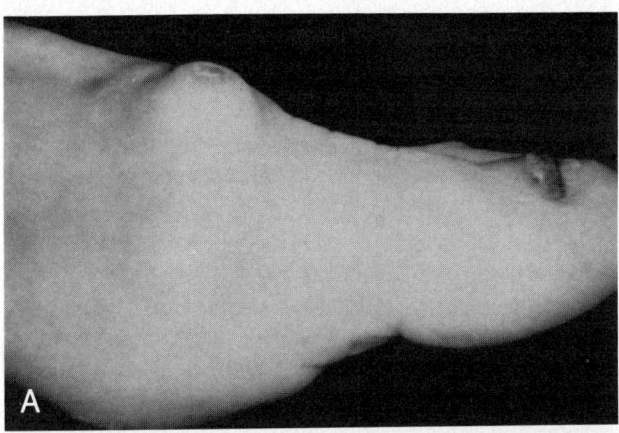

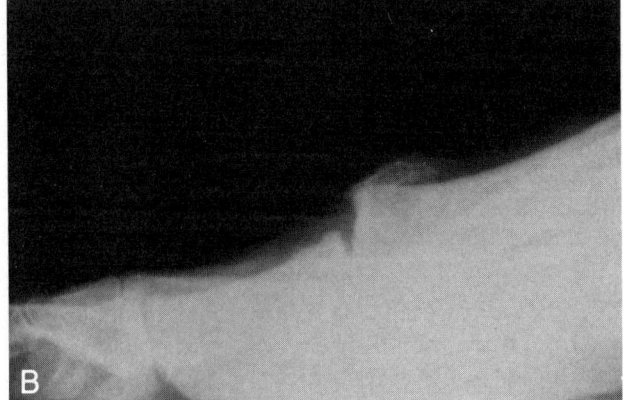

common in this joint, but more frequently afflicts the first cuneiform–first metatarsal joint.

Conservative treatment includes NSAIDs and the use of stiff-soled shoes. An extended steel shank between the outsole and midsole or insole may be needed from the heel to the distal end of the sole. This eliminates the normal sole break and a rocker sole must be added to the shoe. This dramatically relieves the pain in most cases. If it does not, resection of the dorsal half of the first metatarsal head will allow increased motion and is the procedure of choice. More extensive arthritis is treated by hemiresection of the joint (Keller arthroplasty), prosthetic replacement, or arthrodesis.[10] The latter procedure is generally favored by most foot surgeons today, because pain, including transfer lesion pain, is relieved, and weight can again be borne on the first ray.

SESAMOIDITIS

Pain under the great toe sesamoids may arise from prominence of the tibial sesamoid (Fig. 89–10), from

FIG. 89–10. Callus (IPK) under tibial sesamoid.

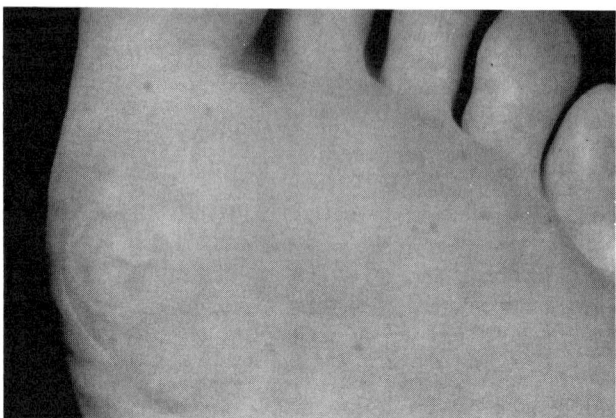

FIG. 89–11. Plantar aspect of the rheumatoid foot.

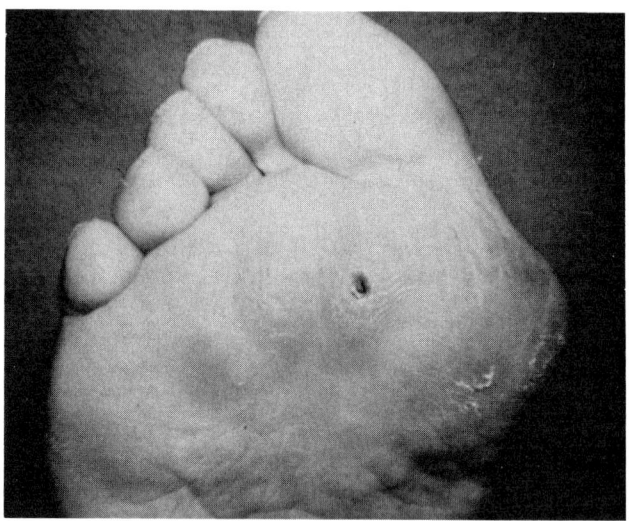

chondromalacia, or from osteoarthritis between the sesamoid and its articulation with the plantar condyles of the metatarsal head. With a localized prominence under a single sesamoid, paring of the associated callus and a total contact insert under the painful area will help. Shaving the plantar surface of the prominent sesamoid is often sufficient, but a total sesamoidectomy is usually necessary when advanced chondromalacia or osteoarthritis has developed and nonoperative means have failed. This is not done frequently today because imbalance of alignment of the toe from disruption of one tendon of the flexor brevis may occur. One sesamoid can usually be safely removed, unless bunionectomy is required also. Here the balance is more delicate and sesamoidectomy should be avoided.

SYNOVITIS OF THE MTP JOINTS

Inflammation of the MTP joints can be significantly relieved by the use of an extended steel shank and rocker sole. In rheumatoid arthritis, the problem may be extensive with upward subluxation of the proximal phalanx, forward shift of the plantar fat pad under the toes, and significant loss of articular cartilage (Fig. 89–11). Clawing of the toes may occur, with development of calluses, corns, and adventitial bursae. In such cases the patient requires an extra-depth shoe, usually made with a pliable leather upper such as deerskin. Polyethylene foam (Plastazote) may be bonded to the leather and heat-molded to the patient's foot. A total contact insert is made with polyethylene foam of various grades (e.g., Plastazote, Pelite) (Fig. 89–12), built up behind the heads and relieved under them. In areas of breakdown or impending ulcer, the relieved area may be filled with a

viscoelastic polymer, which is particularly effective in preventing tissue breakdown. An extended steel shank and rocker sole completes the prescription.[11] Surgical treatment (see Chapter 55) usually consists of resection of the metatarsal heads and, often, the proximal condyles of the proximal phalanges. The first MTP joint is resected, fused, or replaced with a prosthesis. I prefer the latter two approaches.[12]

METATARSAL PAIN ASSOCIATED WITH CAVUS DEFORMITY

Cavus deformity is discussed later in the section on the midfoot, but may be associated with pain in the metatarsal heads. In such cases, the flexible orthotic includes a total contact insert to diffuse the pressure both proximal to and over the metatarsal heads.

FIG. 89–12. The total contact insert made with various grades of polyethylene foam (Plastazote).

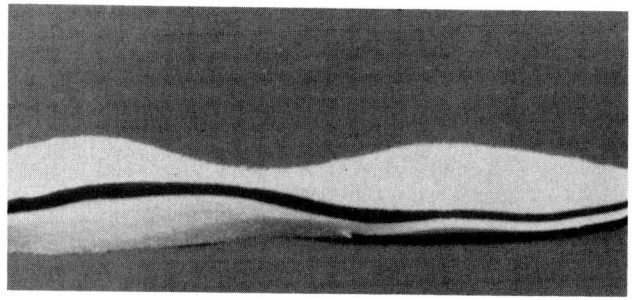

FIG. 89–13. The micropore rubber insert.

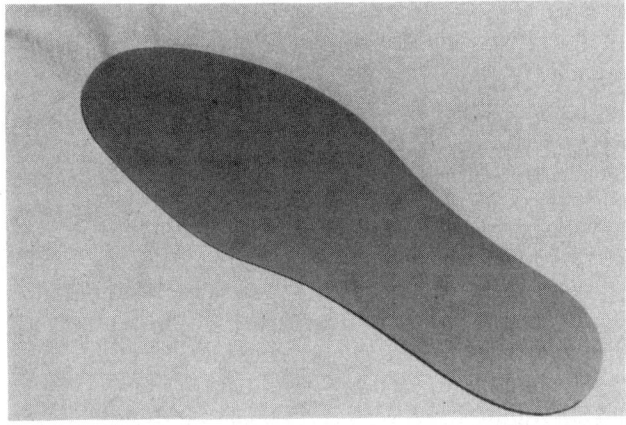

NONSPECIFIC PAIN IN THE METATARSALS

Patients with biomechanically normal feet may develop pain in the metatarsal area under certain circumstances, such as changes in walking surfaces (e.g., steel- or concrete-reinforced floors), hard running surfaces, use of shoes with poorly cushioned soles, and excessive wearing of high-heeled shoes. Recommendations include lower heels; an ankle strap, which will decrease forward shifting of the foot when in high heels; more cushioned soles (e.g., crepe rubber, or Vibram); mild rocker soles, which shift weight-bearing behind the metatarsal heads; and thin micropore rubber (Spenco) inserts (Fig. 89–13). Thicker inserts are not tolerated in ordinary depth shoes. Ready-made metatarsal pads sometimes help, and, traditionally, a metatarsal bar (Jones bar) (Fig. 89–14) is inserted on the sole to place weight-bearing behind the heads. The bar is less well tolerated than

FIG. 89–14. The metatarsal (Jones) bar.

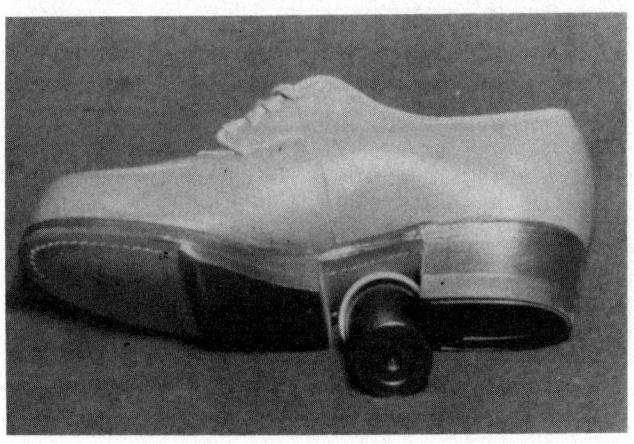

the mild rocker, and felt pads in normal shoes may become quite uncomfortable.

MIDFOOT AND LONGITUDINAL ARCH PAIN

FLAT FEET

Flexible flat feet (pes planus) are not necessarily painful, nor are congenitally relatively stiff flat feet, seen in various barefoot populations such as African blacks and American Indians. However, hard surfaces, noncushioning shoes, weight gain, and other unknown factors may lead to complaints of pain in a pronated foot. The flat-footed marcher or runner does not necessarily develop pain more commonly than his companions with normal arches. The normal biomechanics of gait begins with heel strike, and then a supple phase where the foot pronates as a shock absorber with weight-bearing along its lateral border and then on all the metatarsal heads evenly. As the weight moves forward, the foot supinates, becomes more rigid, and toe-off is completed. If, in the foot-flat position, the longitudinal arch is flat or very low, but reforms as the patient goes up on his toes the foot is functioning relatively normally.

If the arch does ache, an orthotic such as a Plastazote-lined device, reinforced (or "posted") in the arch with cork can be used. This device is comfortable, well tolerated, and can be worn in most shoes, including running shoes. If the medial leather of the shoe is too flexible, the orthotic will be less effective. Steel (Whitman plates) or hard plastic orthotics are more durable but often not well tolerated. I do not prescribe them. The hyperpronated foot[13] with excessive medial motion of the talar head at the talonavicular joint may also be a source of arch pain and is usually successfully treated with a semirigid, well-molded orthotic device.

THE COLLAPSED FOOT

Spontaneous unilateral collapse of the foot is a painful condition usually caused by rupture of the posterior tibial tendon.[14] From behind, the observer sees "too many toes" laterally. The patient cannot stand on tiptoes when standing on the involved foot. The condition usually begins with posterior tibial tendonitis. The sheath may be swollen and tender, but no fixed deformity has occurred. The patient cannot toe-up without pain. NSAIDs and a longitudinal arch orthotic device are often curative. If they are not, surgical decompression of the tendon sheath and subsequent use of the orthotic are sufficient. If rupture has occurred direct repair is rarely possible, and a tendon transfer using the flexor digitorum or the flexor hallucis longus is performed. An orthotic device is used postoperatively. In a chronic case subtalar arthritis has occurred, and a subtalar arthrodesis is the appropriate surgical maneuver.

THE SPASTIC FLAT FOOT

A spastic flat foot is a rigid painful deformity. It is said to be due to inflammation of the subtalar joint, caused by a local or generalized condition. A tarsal coalition (usually calcaneonavicular or talocalcaneal) may become symptomatic and is often refractory to drugs and immobilization. Resection of the bar with soft tissue interposition is routinely performed for calcaneonavicular coalition, and is now attempted frequently for a talocalcaneal bar, because this can be well delineated by CT and three-dimensional imaging.[15] A subtalar arthrodesis is an effective salvage procedure.

THE CAVUS FOOT

The cavus or rigid high-arched foot is a significant problem for runners and distance walkers.[16] Normal talonavicular motion is impaired and the foot will not normally pronate after heel strike. This results in poor shock absorption and pain in the arch and over the dorsal midfoot. Better cushioned soles (crepe rubber) are useful, with a semirigid or flexible orthotic to cushion the foot. These help with normal rates of gait, but a symptomatic distance runner frequently has to find another source of exercise. Surgical procedures to lower the arch and relieve the accompanying varus heel have included release of the plantar fascia and osteotomies of the os calcis and metatarsals. Although the foot will fit into a shoe better postoperatively, it is still rigid and unfit as a shock absorber.

STRESS FRACTURES

A metatarsal stress fracture must be suspected when a history of localized pain and tenderness follows an overuse situation such as running an increased distance and hiking. If plain films are normal, bone scintigraphy confirms the diagnosis. Periosteal reaction and eventual callus will be seen on later radiographs. A stiff-soled shoe, avoidance of the stress-provoking situation, and (possibly) casting are appropriate treatment.

HEEL PAIN

PLANTAR FASCIITIS

The plantar fascia is a static functional structure, described as a windlass mechanism. During toe-off it helps the arch to reform and the foot to become more rigid. Stress on this structure at its narrow proximal origin on the os calcis with repetitive microtrauma results in an inflammatory condition known as *plantar fasciitis*. Bone may form at this site (spur) secondary to the inflammatory response. On examination, there is point tenderness at the origin of the fascia, and hyperextension of the toes at the MTP joints increases the discomfort. Heel cutouts and heel cups along with local steroid injections constitute the most common treatment. I feel that these approaches are often either insufficient or, in the case of steroids, ill-advised. A heel cup encloses the plantar heel fat pad, providing a cushion around the inflamed area. A cutout may result in "window" edema, so it is usually filled with a viscoelastic polymer. The longitudinal arch is supported to relieve the tension on the plantar fascia. Hence, a combination of a posted longitudinal arch (cork and polyethylene foam liner), an attached heel cup, and filled cutout are effective treatment (Fig. 89–15). I avoid steroid injections, because they cause atrophy of fat, which in the heel can result in a new, far more pernicious, lesion.* NSAIDs are often helpful. If the problem is refractory to a conservative ap-

FIG. 89–15. Combination of heel cup, longitudinal arch support, and cutout filled with viscoelastic polymer.

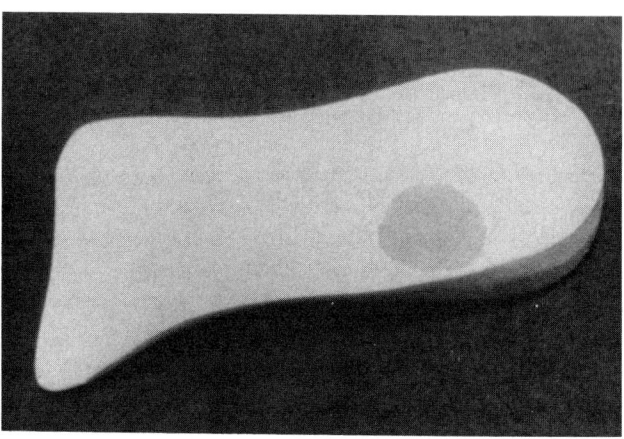

Editor's note. I agree strongly with the author's view.

proach the origin of the plantar fascia is released through a short longitudinal arch incision.

TARSAL TUNNEL SYNDROME
(See Also Chapter 95)

Compression of the posterior tibial nerve, and its branches, the median and lateral plantar, results in heel and plantar foot pain. The laciniate ligament behind the medial malleolus, the superior fibrous edge of the abductor hallucis, and varicosities[17] have each been implicated as the source of the compression. Compression of the calcaneal branch by local fascia and a motor branch of the abductor digiti minimi off the lateral plantar nerve,[18] under the origin of the plantar fascia, have also been implicated as causes of pain. Pain and paresthesias in the course of the nerves help with the diagnosis, as does localized tenderness and, specifically, a localized paresthesia with percussion (Tinel's sign). A nerve conduction study, particularly the sensory component, will confirm the diagnosis. A semirigid longitudinal arch orthotic with relief over the nerve medially will relieve acute conditions. Surgical decompression is done, but a determination of the site of the compression preoperatively, with a localizing Tinel's sign, carries a better prognosis for relief.

OTHER SOURCES OF HEEL PAIN

Other causes of heel pain include stress fractures of the os calcis, detected by plain radiographs, tomograms, or bone scintigraphy;[19] osteoid osteoma, characterized by night pain and relieved specifically with aspirin; and heel pad attrition and heel bruising (stone bruise). A fracture responds to immobilization, osteoid osteoma to excision, and heel pad attrition or bruising to polyethylene foam inserts and solid action cushion heels (SACH).

Painful bursae may occur behind the heel deep to the Achilles tendon. These lesions respond to cushioning, NSAIDs, occasional injections with steroids, and at times, surgical excision. Avascular necrosis of the tarsal navicular (Köhler's disease), the second metatarsal (Freiberg's infraction), and the apophysis of the os calcis are well-known sources of pain. Ordinary films demonstrating dense areas of bone are not conclusive for diagnosis. MRI scans can determine avascularity (see Chapter 6).

BURNING PAIN IN THE FOOT

The complaint of burning pain in the foot provides a diagnostic and therapeutic challenge. Dermatologic causes include a mixed fungal and bacterial infection (athlete's foot) or neurodermatitis.

A vasogenic cause may be large-, or more typically, a small-vessel disease. If noninvasive vascular studies reveal satisfactory pulse pressures and pulse volume recordings in the toes, and if the skin of the foot has a purplish discoloration, empiric treatment may be initiated. This includes physical modalities such as contrast baths (alternating cold water and hot whirlpool), swimming pool walking, and medications to improve local perfusion. Controlled studies to determine the efficacy of these modalities are lacking despite promising anecdotal accounts.

Neurogenic causes may be local or referred. Local compressions and "neuromas" may be primary, traumatic, or iatrogenic.[20] Interdigital (Morton's) neuroma, pressure over the medial branch of the superficial peroneal or the saphenous nerve associated with a bunion, and tarsal tunnel syndrome have been described already. The superficial peroneal nerve is also vulnerable over the dorsum of the foot as it crosses potentially arthritic joints, such as the talonavicular, naviculocuneiform, or cuneiform–first metatarsal. Pressure from the joint below and the shoe above can account for the entrapment. The sural nerve may be compressed and entrapped with and after os calcis fractures, and all nerves are subject to damage from surgical procedures. Referred pain from lumbosacral spinal root compression can result in a burning pain in the appropriate dermatome. Although referred pain areas classically lack localized tenderness, the affected dermatomes may develop local hyperpathia.

Mechanical sources of pain are ruled out because nerve pain is typically not relieved by non-weight-bearing, and indeed, is often accentuated at night.

CONCLUSION

This review is brief but covers most causes of foot pain. All components of the anatomy, alone and in various combinations, may be involved, Medical, surgical, pedorthotic, and physical modalities may all be needed to provide relief. Definitive treatment may occasionally be surgical, as with an osteoid osteoma, but in general, nonoperative approaches are most appropriate initially. It is important, however, to carry out these approaches properly. If a patient fails to respond, the accuracy of the diagnosis must be reassessed and it must be determined that orthotic appliances or shoes have been properly prescribed and fabricated. Lastly, the physician must determine whether the patient has been compliant in following the prescribed program.

REFERENCES

1. Sammarco, G.J., and Miller, E.H.: Forefoot conditions in dancers. Foot Ankle, 3:85–98, 1983.
2. Smith, R.W.: Calluses: Nonsurgical treatment. *In* The Foot Book. Edited by J.S. Gould. Baltimore, Williams & Wilkins, 1988.
3. Shereff, M.J.: Acquired disorders of the toes. *In* The Foot Book. Edited by J.S. Gould. Baltimore, Williams & Wilkins, 1988.
4. Dixon, G.L.: Treatment of ingrown toenail. Foot Ankle, 3:254–260, 1983.
5. Morton, T.G.: A peculiar and painful affection of the fourth metatarsophalangeal articulation. Am. J. Med. Sci., 71:37–45, 1876.
6. Mann, R.A., and Reynolds, J.C.: Interdigital neuroma—a critical clinical analysis. Foot Ankle, 3:238–243, 1983.
7. Gauthier, G.: Thomas Morton's disease: A nerve entrapment syndrome. Clin. Orthop., 142:90–92, 1979.
8. Scranton, P.E.: Metatarsalgia: A clinical review of diagnosis and management. Foot Ankle, 1:229–234, 1981.
9. Mann, R.A., and Coughlin, M.J.: Hallux valgus and complications of hallux valgus. *In* Surgery of the Foot. Edited by R.A. Mann. St. Louis, The C.V. Mosby Co., 1986.
10. Gould, N.: Hallux rigidus: Cheilectomy or implant? Foot Ankle, 1:315–320, 1981.
11. Gould, J.S.: Conservative management of the hypersensitive foot in rheumatoid arthritis. Foot Ankle, 2:224–229, 1982.
12. Cracchiolo, A.: Rheumatoid arthritis of the foot and ankle. *In* The Foot Book. Edited by J.S. Gould. Baltimore, Williams & Wilkins, 1988.
13. Gould, N.: Graphing the adult foot and ankle. Foot Ankle, 2:213–219, 1982.
14. Mann, R.A.: Tendon injuries. *In* Surgery of the Foot. Edited by R.A. Mann. St. Louis, The C.V. Mosby Co., 1986.
15. Herzenberg, J.E., Goldner, J.L., Martinez, S., and Silverman, P.M.: Computerized tomography of talocalcaneal tarsal coalition: A clinical and anatomic study. Foot Ankle, 6:273–288, 1986.
16. Lutter, L.D.: Cavus foot in runners. Foot Ankle, 1:225–228, 1981.
17. Gould, N., and Alvarez, R.: Bilateral tarsal tunnel syndrome caused by varicosities. Foot Ankle, 3:290–292, 1983.
18. Baxter, D.E., and Thigpen, C.M.: Heel pain—operative results. Foot Ankle, 5:16–25, 1985.
19. Graham, C.E.: Painful heel syndrome: Rationale of diagnosis and treatment. Foot Ankle, 3:261–267, 1983.
20. Kenzora, J.E.: Symptomatic incisional neuromas on the dorsum of the foot. Foot Ankle, 5:2–15, 1985.

90

CERVICAL SPINE SYNDROMES

HUGH A. SMYTHE

Though a great variety of diseases can affect the cervical spine, by far the most common are degenerative and probably predominantly mechanical.

Because pain of deep origin is referred elsewhere, the cervical origin of confusing symptoms is often missed. Clinical study and treatment of neck problems is unsatisfactory though not really difficult. With appropriate assessment techniques, diagnosis is easy; and with understanding of the pathogenetic factors, rational therapy readily follows.

ETIOLOGY AND MECHANICAL FACTORS

A variety of epidemiologic studies[1-4] have shown an intense concentration of clinical and radiographic findings in the lower cervical spine, predominantly C5-C7, with some extension to the segments immediately above and below; rarely is there involvement in the upper cervical spine (Fig. 90–1). This frequency is analogous to the frequency of involvement of the two lowest lumbar segments and the relative rarity of major problems above L4. The segments between T1 and L3, and above C4, share the same inheritance, the same movement for work and play activities, the same biochemical environment, and the same aging process, but they rarely present with major neurologic or chronic pain syndromes of a mechanical nature. Most physicians have seen evidence of C6 or C7 root involvement, but loss of the pectoral reflex (C2-4) is extremely rare.

Kellgren and Moore extended this observation in their classic paper on generalized osteoarthritis and Heberden's nodes. The degenerative changes were not generalized, but concentrated at just eight sites: the proximal and distal interphalangeal joints of the hands, the base of the thumb, the lower neck, the lower back, the hip, the knee, and the base of the great toe. The striking relative sparing of joints such as the wrist or ankle does not occur in the presence

FIG. 90–1. Hult[9] studied 277 males doing heavy work, ages 35 to 49; all radiographic changes were counted. The data from Hayashi et al.[6] are for anterior osteophytosis in 100 subjects over age 60, male to female ratio was 46:54.

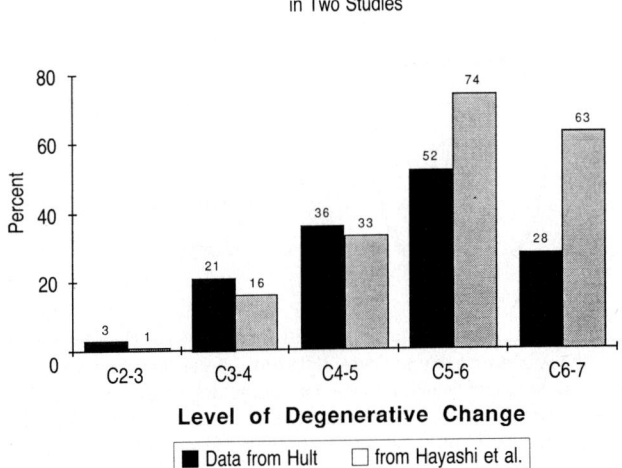

Distribution of X-ray Changes in the Neck in Two Studies

1413

of chondrocalcinosis or other conditions in which there may be an inherited and diffusely acting defect of cartilage metabolism.

This pattern of degenerative involvement is uniquely human, and each of the sites affected has a unique structure and function in humans Homo habilis et erectus.[4]

What is different about human structure and function that stresses the lower cervical spine? Humans not only have unique hands, they have unique shoulders, held up and far to the side. They can not only climb, they can also throw, and with great efficiency. They can swing their arms through a complete 360° circle; no dog or horse can make this motion.

The anatomic basis for these abilities is the clavicles and the shape of the rib cage (Fig. 90–2). Four-footed animals do not have clavicles. Their scapulae are connected to the often crested sternum by muscles and are free to glide forward and back during a long running stride. In evolution, clavicles begin to appear in monkeys, presumably in adaptation to the needs of climbing. In gorillas and chimpanzees the clavicles are strong, but still relatively short compared with humans, and are located above a barrel-shaped chest.*

FIG. 90–2. Humans have a long clavicle and broad chest to hold the shoulder laterally. Quadrupeds are adapted for running, and scapular movement is unconstrained.

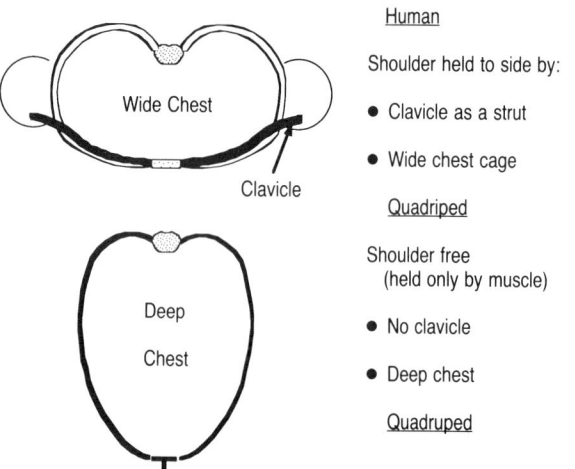

Comparative Anatomy of Upper Thorax

Wide Chest

Clavicle

Deep Chest

Human

Shoulder held to side by:

- Clavicle as a strut
- Wide chest cage

Quadriped

Shoulder free
(held only by muscle)

- No clavicle
- Deep chest

Quadruped

*I have been unable to find a full study of the comparative anatomy of the clavicle, and these comments are based on personal observations in museums, especially Le Musée de Paleontologie in the Jardin des Plantes, Paris. None of the hundreds of skeletons there showed degenerative changes concentrated in the neck or low back (perhaps because of selection criteria).

Humans have long clavicles (the Latin word *clavicula* means key) and their ribs have become broad transversely. These changes do not make humans breathe better than a dog or horse, but they do position human shoulders to give much more freedom of hand and upper limb function.

What humans cannot do is lie on their side during the night. A dog can stretch out on a flat surface, comfortable on a rug in front of a fire, with uniform support to all parts of its spine, because of its narrow chest, thickly muscled neck, and narrow skull. Humans cannot do this without subjecting the lower neck to major shearing and compressive stresses at the junction of the supported thoracic and unsupported cervical spine. The thoracic spine is generally supported by the ribs, but T1 is thrust upward even more strongly, because stresses are transmitted from the shoulder, through the long scapula to the sternum, to T1 by our strong, short first rib. Because of bony shoulders (and hips), many young persons sleep belly down with the neck in forced rotation. Humans breathe better this way, but at the cost of neck stresses. As the neck stiffens, the belly-down posture becomes no longer possible, and over 80% of people at midlife sleep on their sides, enduring the problems discussed. Eventually, as the neck gets stiffer, many can be comfortable only lying on the back, despite possible adverse effects on the airway. This is a major reason why old men snore and young men do not.

SYMPTOMS

These mechanical forces can give rise to any of three problems, each with different clinical manifestations. *Pain* or its equivalents may appear early (or not at all), and is usually reversible when the pathogenetic forces are neutralized. *Degenerative changes* appear late and result in stiffness and radiologic change, are generally poorly responsive to therapy and poorly correlated with pain. *Neurologic complications* are of several kinds, which are discussed in more detail later in the chapter.

PAIN

Although the degenerative and neurologic changes are easily shown to be concentrated at C5-7, it is much less obvious to the patient and therapist that the pain also comes from these levels. These patients *never* complain of pain in these vertebral structures. They cannot, because there is no representation of these deep structures in the cerebral cortex, and therefore in the body image. The pain must be referred, that is, misinterpreted as arising in other structures that generally share the same nerve supply, and that are at least vaguely represented in the conscious brain. The pain is most commonly felt posteriorly and laterally. Massage of these painful areas gives comfort, but the key inference may be missed. These areas, although painful, are not particularly tender; they are not the source of the symptom. The tenderness is highly characteristic and located at the site of the pathology, in the low anterior neck, but this site is usually asymptomatic.

The patterns of referred symptoms from the cervical spine are complex and variable, even in the same patient. The arm and hand develop from the cervical segments, and any of the structures of the arm or controlling the arm can be the target for referred symptoms. Interscapular pain is common, because the muscles that control the position of the scapula are functionally and neurologically part of the arm. Anterior chest pain and tenderness are common, because the pectoralis major and minor muscles control the shoulder and share its nerve supply. Patients complaining of breast (anterior chest) heaviness and discomfort will often be found to have significant tenderness deep to the breast, in the origin of the pectoralis minor muscle, and not in the breast itself. The breast, derived from skin, has thoracic innervation, as do the ribs and pleura. Only the muscles have cervical innervation, and the finding of referred tenderness at characteristic sites within the muscles argues strongly for a cervical origin of the symptoms, and against disease of the breast, ribs, pleura, or viscera.

Dizziness, more an unsteadiness or "swimming" feeling than a rotational vertigo, is another common symptom,[7] less well known and understood. *The neck muscles function as extraocular muscles and are closely integrated with all the apparatus of balance.* Imagine the complex interactions that take place when a golfer or baseball batter swings, keeping the eyes fixed on the ball while aggressively pivoting the trunk.

Often the referred discomfort is not felt as pain, but as a stiffness, a swelling, or, even more confusingly, a numbness or tingling. These complaints are often nocturnal, and nerve compression syndromes are often suspected. The numbness is not a true loss of sensation. While feeling the symptom, the patient can still appreciate the tactile difference between cloth and paper, neurologically a very demanding task. These and other symptoms are grouped as *pain equivalents* and discussed further in Chapter 80.

INCIDENCE AND PREVALENCE OF SYMPTOMS

Large-scale studies in Sweden[1] in the 1950s, in Britain in the 1960s,[8] and in the United States in the 1970s and 1980s[9,10] give similar and complementary information. About 10% of adult populations have neck pain at any given time. This prevalence matches that of low-back pain, but is less likely to result in loss of time from work. At least one attack of stiff neck was reported in 25% of men in their twenties and nearly 60% of men in their fifties in Hult's study[1] of 1200 male workers. Even higher incidences had been reported in his earlier study of men doing very heavy work,[5] but in this study light work was not protective. Arm pain was reported by 262 persons, 36% of them with neck pain, and 13% of them reporting no neck pain. Of those with arm pain, 33% reported pain or numbness in the fingers, 25% had "frozen" (stiff) shoulders, 11% had headache, and 11% had anterior chest pain. Neurologic signs were recorded in less than 1% of those with neck pain, 7% of those with a history of arm pain, but in 23% of those with arm pain at the time of examination. Preceding trauma was described by 10%. More "usually the patient awakens with a stiff neck and blames the attack on an uncomfortable sleeping position; . . . the symptoms sometimes disappear in a few hours, although they usually persist for two or three days and occasionally for a week or so." Loss of time was reported in only 3% performing light work, and 15% of those doing heavy work.

Lawrence surveyed 1803 males and 1572 females.[8] The incidence of remembered attacks was similar to that in the Swedish study. He also linked neck, shoulder, and arm pain, which was present in 9% of male and 12% of female subjects at the time of the survey. Only 8% reported time loss, and neurologic complications were uncommon. Hadler[9,10] has reviewed the HANES data, arising from a structured survey of health problems, effects, and care utilization based on a carefully designed random subsample of the U.S. population. The study included 6913 subjects, a 70% completion rate for 9881 persons selected as a national probability sample. Again, about 10% of American adults were experiencing neck pain, often associated with arm pain, and 30% recalled such an episode in the past year. Severe disability was uncommon, and relatively few sought medical advice. About 70% noted symptomatic improvement within 1 month.

These data are remarkably consistent but do not focus on the 30% who do not improve quickly, and who make up an important proportion of patients with chronic musculoskeletal complaints. They are often unhappy with the medical help they receive, and either demand more and more referrals and investigation, or seek help from alternative caregivers.

SIGNS

The classic objective signs of a cervical spine disorder are restricted movement, obviously associated with muscle guarding; tenderness at the interspinous spaces posteriorly; and reproduction of pain by vertical compression. None of these signs are very sensitive or reliable (although formal studies are lacking). Neck pain in young or hypermobile subjects is commonly associated with a range of movement well within normal limits, and posterior tenderness is neither striking nor reliably present. (Normal range, correlated with age, sex, race, and general skeletal mobility, has not been defined.) The patient complaining of pain, but with a normal range, and little obvious tenderness posteriorly, is in danger of being dismissed as a chronic complainer, or referred for behavior modification.

In our studies,[4,14,16] the best of the classic measures was *restriction of lateral flexion.** Because of the odontoid peg, no lateral flexion occurs between the occiput and C2, so that this range is more sensitive than others to lower cervical disease. It is an excellent screening test but does not discriminate between the effects of pain, diffuse idiopathic skeletal hyperostosis (DISH), other degenerative change, or spondylitis, because all of these affect the same levels. Observer variation is a problem, as it is with all other available measures. We have used a Latin square design to analyze sources of variance with this and other proposed diagnostic measures; typical results are shown in Figure 90–3.

TENDERNESS IN THE LOW ANTERIOR NECK

We have advocated a search for typical sites of tenderness, not only in the generalized fibrositis/fibromyalgia syndrome, but also in patients with a more localized distribution of symptoms, such as those that might be related to cervical spine problems. In the simplest situation, the patient complains of neck pain or stiffness but locates these symptoms laterally and

---

**Editor's note.* In my experience, lateral flexion and rotation are often restricted, but predominantly, pain or severely limited motion upon *flexion* or *extension* is not compatible with degenerative lesions. Infections and tumors must be strongly considered in this situation.

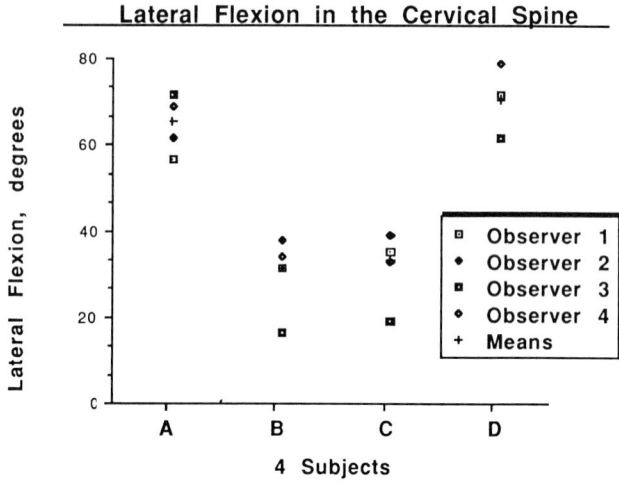

FIG. 90–3. Variation among 4 patients and 4 observers in a 4*4 study. The standard deviation among observers within patients was 15°.

posteriorly. Massage (i.e., deep palpation) of these sites, progressing from gentle to firm, is appreciated as giving comfort. As the patient relaxes, lateral gliding movements with gentle manual traction can move each set of posterior facet joints in turn and show that these structures are also not tender. The patient denies pain in the low anterior neck and is astonished when the examiner's palpating thumb reveals significiant tenderness in the low anterior neck, most specifically in the anterior aspects of the intertransverse spaces between C5 and C7, located centrally, close to the vertebral body. The anterior tubercles and lateral aspects of the transverse processes are much less tender. This region is often somewhat tender in normal subjects, although quantitatively less so than in patients with symptoms. Perhaps the best control group is the small number of spondylitic patients with complete fusion of the cervical spine, who lose this normal tenderness. The target site lies behind the lower sternomastoid muscle, just above the clavicle. It is important to relax this muscle, which means that the patient must be supine and the examiner's touch reassuring.

The thumb is a better tool for finding and evaluating this tenderness than is the dolorimeter,[11] giving better interobserver agreement (Fig. 90–4), but the latter gives numeric values, which serve to allay suspicion that the examiner is deliberately creating the discomfort by excessive pressure. The methods correlate, but with important, still unexplained variance (Fig. 90–5). Interobserver and intraobserver variations have been found by others in the course of methodologic and therapeutic studies, although detailed reports with

FIG. 90–4. Interobserver variation on assessing tenderness by scored palpation. This was part of a study of possible outcome measures, so that the two readings were separated by a number of other assessments.

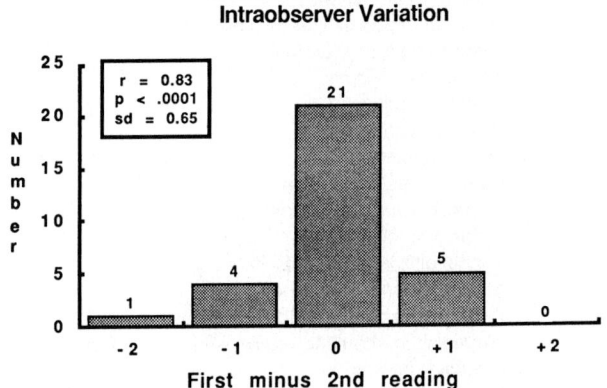

Tenderness, Scored 0 – 4
Intraobserver Variation

$r = 0.83$
$p < .0001$
$sd = 0.65$

this information are few.[12] Campbell is one of the few researchers to systematically study anterior neck tenderness. In a dolorimeter study comparing tenderness (tolerance), he found a threshold of 1.8 ± 1.3 kg in fibrositic patients, and 5.5 ± 2.7 kg in control subjects, yet in his discussion he stated that "the intertransverse ligament in the neck was fairly tender in both groups."[13]

FIG. 90–5. Scoring of low anterior cervical tenderness by scored palpation using thumb pressure, and by dolorimetry. There is good agreement at the extremes, but problems at borderline values.

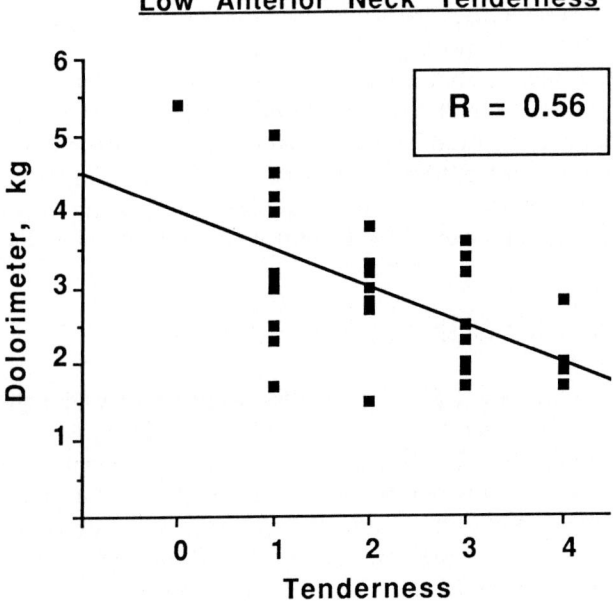

Low Anterior Neck Tenderness

$R = 0.56$

REFERRED TENDERNESS

Besides direct local cervical tenderness, there is very often referred tenderness, at precisely the same sites found to be tender in "fibrositic" patients, but in a clumped, asymmetric distribution.[14] To identify a diffuse pain amplification syndrome it is sufficient and useful to consistently check a relatively small number of highly reliable points. The presence of multiple tender points is an important issue, and in referred pain syndromes it is helpful to know additional, commonly involved points. A multiplicity of points makes less credible the alternative diagnoses of imaginary local diseases, such as costochondritis, bicipital groove tendinitis, or lateral epicondylitis. And because the points are localized, prospectively predictable in location, and largely unknown to the patient, they rule out exaggeration operating at the psychologic level. The most important additional points in cervical syndromes involve the slips of origin and insertion of the pectoralis major and minor muscles (Fig. 90–6). The tenderness of the medial and inferior aspect of the coracoid process is of special importance. It can be confused with shoulder syn-

FIG. 90–6. Clumped distribution of tender points in a patient with pain of cervical origin.

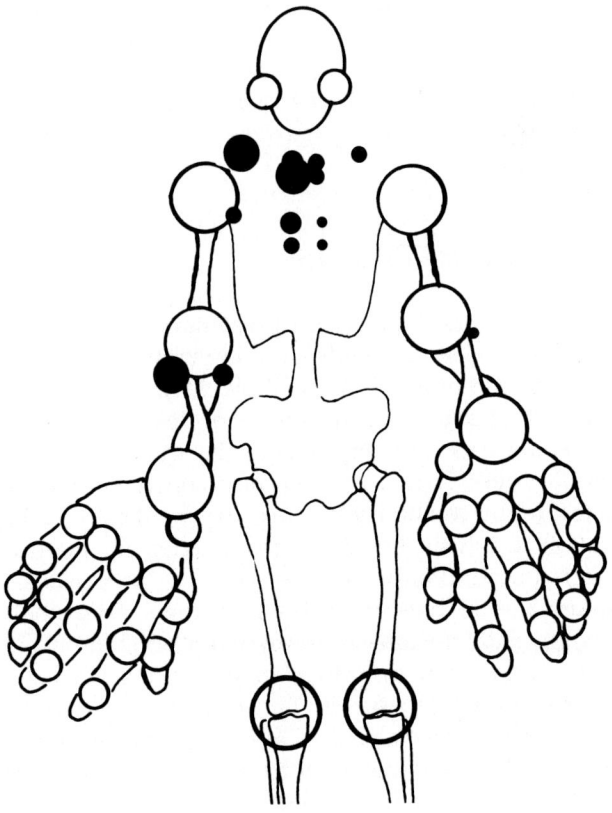

ovitis or with bicipital tendinitis, but palpation after lateral rotation of the humerus shows that the tenderness remains with the coracoid, and does *not* involve the synovium or the bicipital groove.

REFLEX DYSTROPHIES
(See also Chapter 97)

The association of shoulder stiffness with cervical problems was noted by Hult[1] and many others. The importance of cervical factors, however, in the pathogenesis of shoulder or shoulder-hand syndromes can easily be overlooked because of the dominance of the more peripheral symptoms, and the symptomatic silence in the lower neck. Unless the low anterior neck is examined specifically, neither patient nor therapist will be aware of the notable tenderness there. I have never seen a case of shoulder-hand syndrome that did not have significant neck tenderness, and therapy directed toward the neck problem (in addition to other measures) may be essential for success.

In addition to shoulder stiffness, some patients develop diffuse cervical stiffness, a "frozen neck." Cervical fusion at one level has only a small effect on overall cervical movement. Loss of range at multiple cervical levels cannot be attributed to the effects of a one- or two-level mechanical lesion and is analogous to the diffuse reaction of the shoulder girdle muscles in a "frozen shoulder." Steroid therapy may be indicated and successful when such general pain and stiffness is severe and persistent despite other therapies.

CLINICAL PATTERNS

A wide variety of clinical presentations can result from cervical strain syndromes; in many, the cervical origin is not at all obvious (Table 90–1). Apart from our lack of subjective awareness of deep neck structures, the lack of symptoms in the site targeted by pathogenetic forces, and the firm conviction by the interpreting cerebral cortex that the problem is in the region to which the discomfort is referred, there is often a separation in time between the precipitating injury and the time of greatest symptoms. This is best seen in acute flexion-extension (whiplash) injuries, in which immediate symptoms may be minor but build after days or even weeks. Part of this delay may be due to the development of reflex changes, and part may be due to aggravation by nocturnal forces, and the effects of a superadded nonrestorative sleep syn-

Table 90–1.   Cervical Syndromes: Clinical Presentations

Neck syndromes
  Acute wry neck
  Chronic neck pain
  Whiplash syndrome
Shoulder girdle syndromes
  Shoulder pain, stiffness
  Localized fibrositis/fibromyalgia
  Pseudoangina syndrome
  Interscapular pain
  Costochondritis
  Tietze's syndrome
Arm syndromes
  Carpal tunnel syndrome
  Thoracic outlet syndromes
  Bicipital tendinitis
  Tennis elbow syndrome
  Shoulder-hand syndrome
  Writer's and other occupational cramps
  "Arthritis" in shoulder, elbow, wrist, and hand
Cranial syndromes
  Morning headaches
  Temporomandibular joint (TMJ) syndrome
  Benign postural vertigo
Neurologic syndromes
  Acute radiculopathy
  Chronic radiculopathy
  Chronic cervical myelopathy

drome, each changing the nervous system's processing pain inputs and responses.

DIAGNOSIS OF NECK PROBLEMS IN THE PRESENCE OF OTHER DISEASES

Patients with other diseases, for example, rheumatoid arthritis or cancer, often complain of severe neck pain. If the pain is due to the associated disease, aggressive therapies may be indicated. If the pain is due to the more common mechanical lesions, then steroids, radiation, or chemotherapy are inappropriate. The restricted tenderness in the low anterior neck seems highly characteristic of pain of mechanical origin, and patients with disease of other etiologies show tenderness elsewhere. Newer imaging techniques can be extremely helpful when doubt persists.

NEUROLOGIC COMPLICATIONS

Acute Radicular Syndromes. Acute radicular syndromes generally involve the C5, C6 or C7 roots; less commonly, T1. They are not supposed to occur, because the uncovertebral joints (joints of Luschka) block posterolateral disc herniations, but they occur nevertheless, and often in youth and midlife. Loss of the biceps and triceps reflex is of concern, but as with low-back syndromes, the problem usually subsides without the need for surgical intervention. It is much more difficult to document the recovery process in cervical than in low-back syndromes, because signs equivalent to the straight leg raising test are much less reliable. Obvious weakness of the appropriate muscle usually occurs, and numeric measures of strength to document clinical progress are the most valuable outcome measurement. We urge the use of the modified blood pressure cuff for this application.[15]

Chronic Radicular Syndromes and Cervical Myelopathy. These syndromes usually result from degenerative changes, generally in the levels showing maximum radiologic change. There may be no pain, and the cervical origin of lower limb spasticity may not be obvious, however. With age and degenerative change, the C5-C6 level, previously most mobile of all, becomes less mobile, and abnormal mobility may develop in the level above. Listhesis on forward flexion can produce important narrowing of the spinal canal between the upper corner of C5 and the posterior elements of C4.[6] Apart from bony change, fibrous proliferation can occur extensively, resulting in root sleeve fibrosis and in hypertrophy of the annulus and dura. This is often associated with other features of DISH, along with maleness, obesity, and type 2 diabetes. Evidence for generally acting growth stimuli in the form of hyperinsulinemia[16] or elevated retinoic acid levels[17,18] have been reported in these syndromes, in which these substances act on fibrous tissue as well as bone.

TREATMENT OF PAIN OF MECHANICAL ORIGIN

Heat, massage, traction, and counterirritant therapies (e.g., transcutaneous electrical nerve stimulation [TENS], acupuncture, liniments) all give real if temporary relief, which may be adequate if the illness runs its usual benign course.

Traction may often aggravate symptoms but can be helpful if great attention is paid to the details of this therapy. The patient must be completely relaxed, or else muscle contraction nullifies the therapeutic effect. Traction force in excess of 5 kg commonly causes discomfort to the jaw or site of pull of the harness, and reactive muscle spasm. Because the weight of the head averages about 7 kg, the patient must be supine; vertical traction too often makes things worse. The harness must fit comfortably, and pull from the occiput rather than from the chin. The angle of pull is important, and must primarily be comfortable. This is most often achieved if the neck is in midposition,

with the vertebral end plates parallel. Because the upper thoracic spine is relatively stiff, the angle of the upper surface of T1 determines the inclination of the neck; more flexion in those with a rounded thoracic spine, and a flatter line of pull in those with a straight thorax. Sedation is helpful, and it is useful to begin with brief and gentle sessions, progressing only when the patient feels more comfortable in traction than out of traction.

Manipulation can be modestly to dramatically beneficial, especially in young, hypermobile patients with symptoms of acute onset and obvious, asymmetric restriction of range of movement. Because of the uncommon but real danger of precipitating or aggravating neurologic complications, the techniques should not involve sudden, forceful twists or thrusts. Gentle but persistent mobilization during manual traction imposes no compressive forces, and can result in major relief and increased range of motion in a few moments. The techniques require skill and practice; the account of Mennell is recommended.[3]

None of these measures are directed at the cause.

FIG. 90–7. Arrow shows stresses in the unsupported neck during sleep (upper drawing), and the corrective effect of adequate lower neck support (lower drawing). Note that the lower shoulder tends to rise toward the chin, displacing upward the support given by usual pillows. This occurs because of rotation of the clavicle at the sternoclavicular joint.

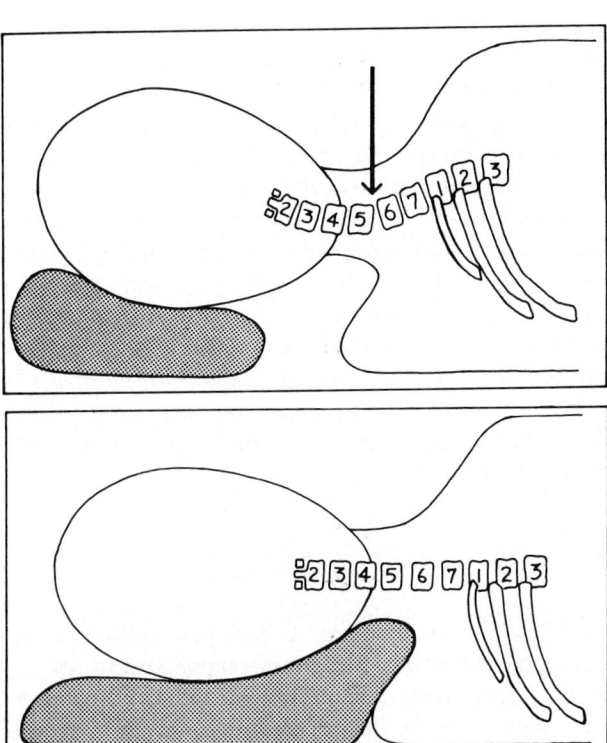

If it is accepted that stresses in the unsupported lower neck are central to the primary cause, and to persistence or recurrence of symptoms in structurally normal necks, then it follows that provision of reliable support to the lower neck during sleep is central to therapy. With an *extremely* painful neck, soft rolls may be most comfortable and reliable. The support must be given to the *lower* neck (Fig. 90–7.) The shoulder tends to rise during sleep, and the upper roll keeps the lower one in place. This therapy is effective—for a time. The rolls are hot, sweaty, choking, and unattractive, so this treatment, although effective, is often abandoned. Neck support pillows provide a more comfortable long-term alternative, but again must support the *lower* neck. Because patients are unaware of the low neck origin of the pain, they often have to be taught the need to target the support to the vulnerable area, just above the collar bone.

THERAPEUTIC STUDIES AND OUTCOME MEASURES

Most studies have not shown one therapy to be convincingly superior to others or to placebo. One study found neck support superior to traction.[19] All of the published studies had major design flaws. This is a difficult area of clinical research, and none of the previous studies have addressed design issues adequately. The most difficult tasks are to choose an appropriate outcome measure and to predetermine an adequate sample size. Because the pain is referred and the location varies, the visual analogue scale performs inconsistently. The use of multiple outcome measure increases the probability of finding at least one spuriously "statistically significant" result and requires a predetermined strategy for pooling information, or for making corrections for multiple comparisons after the study. Finally, one must consider type 2 error: the risk of rejecting a useful treatment because a significant difference was not shown. This risk is high when the spontaneous remission rate is high, so that quite large sample sizes may be required. The data in Figures 90–2 and 90–3 may assist future researchers.

COURSE AND PROGNOSIS

Although most episodes of neck pain settle in a few weeks, some persist for years, representing an important proportion of patients with chronic pain. At this stage there is debate about the relative contributions of continuing mechanical factors (nobody has prescribed neck support), related and interacting nonrestorative sleep patterns, learned pain behavior, or depression and neuroticism as determinants of the chronic disability. Adversarial relationships with insuring agencies or physicians are not helpful, and the therapist should avoid implying that the problem is the patient's fault. Appropriate therapy often gives valuable help, and the therapist's role is to develop and explain an effective strategy. It is then the patient's responsibility to follow the advice given, and develop the expectation of a return to full function.

INVOLVEMENT OF THE NECK BY OTHER DISEASE PROCESSES

Although neck problems of mechanical origin are overwhelmingly dominant in clinical practice, other rheumatic and nonrheumatic conditions obviously can involve the cervical spine. This account cannot review these in detail, and the reader is referred to the chapters on rheumatoid arthritis, ankylosing spondylitis, juvenile arthritis, psoriatic arthritis, and diffuse idiopathic skeletal hyperostosis (DISH) for fuller accounts. The value of computed tomography and magnetic resonance imaging, new noninvasive imaging techniques, in assessing patients with complex problems involving the cervical spine are discussed in Chapters 8 and 6 respectively.

REFERENCES

 1. Hult, L.: Cervical, dorsal and lumbar spinal syndromes. Acta Orthop. Scand. (Suppl.), *17*:1–102, 1954.
 2. Kellgren, J.H., and Moore, R.: Generalized osteoarthritis and Heberden's nodes. Br. Med. J., *1*:181–187, 1952.
 3. Mennell, J.M.: Back Pain: Diagnosis and Treatment Using Manipulative Methods. Boston, Little, Brown, & Co., 1960.
 4. Smythe, H.A.: The mechanical pathogenesis of generalized osteoarthritis. J. Rheumatol., *10*(Suppl. 9):11–12, 1983.
 5. Hult, L.: The Munkfors Investigation. Acta Orthop. Scand. (Suppl.), *16*:1–76, 1954.
 6. Hayashi, H., et al.: Etiologic factors in myelopathy: A radiographic evaluation of the aging changes in the cervical spine. Clin. Orthop., *214*:200–209, 1987.
 7. Toglia, J.V.: Acute flexion-extension injury of the neck. Electronystagmographic study of 309 cases. Neurology, *26*:808–814, 1976.
 8. Lawrence, J.S.: Disc degeneration: Its frequency and relation to symptoms. Ann. Rheum. Dis., *28*:121–138, 1969.
 9. Hadler, N.M.: Illness in the workplace: The challenge of musculoskeletal symptoms. J. Hand Surg., *10A*:451–456, 1985.
10. Hadler, N.M.: Osteoarthritis as a public health problem. Clin. Rheum. Dis., *11*:175–185, 1985.
11. McCarty, D.J., Jr., Gatter, R.A., and Steele, A.D.: A twenty-pound dolorimeter for quantification of articular tenderness. Arthritis Rheum., *11*:696–698, 1968.

12. Zylbergol, R.S., and Piper, M.C.: Cervical spine disorders: A comparison of three types of traction. Spine, *10*:867–871, 1985.
13. Campbell, S.M.: Is the tender point concept valid? Am. J. Med., *81*(Suppl. 3A):33–37, 1986.
14. Smythe, H.A.: Referred pain and tender points. Am. J. Med., *81*(Suppl. 3A):90–92, 1986.
15. Helewa, H., Goldsmith, C.H., and Smythe, H.A.: Patient, observer, and instrument variation in the measurement of strength of shoulder abductor muscles in patients with rheumatoid arthritis using a modified sphygmomanometer. J. Rheumatol., *13*:1044–1049, 1986.
16. Smythe, H.A.: Osteoarthritis, insulin, and bone density. J. Rheumatol., *14*(S-14):91–93, 1987.
17. Arlet, J., et al.: Vitamin A et hyperostose vertébral ankylosante. Rev. Rhum., *50*:63–65, 1983.
18. Abitéboul, M., et al.: Hyperostose vertébral et troubles du métabolism du retinol. Rev. Rhum., *52*:141–143, 1985.
19. Steinberg, V.L., and Mason, R.M.: Cervical spondylosis: Pilot therapeutic trial. Ann. Phys. Med., *5*:37–47, 1959.

PAINFUL TEMPOROMANDIBULAR JOINT

91

DORAN E. RYAN

The tempororomandibular joint (TMJ), like other central joints, is paired and cannot function alone. This rotating, sliding joint must function in total harmony with its counterpart on the opposite side of the horseshoe-shaped mandible. The articulating surfaces of the bone are not covered by hyaline cartilage as are most other joints of the body, but rather by an avascular fibrous connective tissue that may contain chondrocytes and hence is designated fibrocartilage.[1] The fifth cranial nerve, which supplies the muscles that move the joint, also provides sensory protection and innervates the overlying skin.

ANATOMIC FEATURES

This joint is complex, with an articulating fibrous connective tissue disc interposed between the temporal and the mandibular bones, separating the articular space into superior and inferior compartments. The articulating surface of the mandible is the antero-superior surface of the condylar head. This surface measures approximately 16 to 20 mm mediolaterally and 8 to 10 mm anteroposteriorly. The disc is ovoid with distinct anterior, central, and posterior zones and is firmly attached to the medial and lateral poles of the condylar head. Its average measurements are 27.5 mm mediolaterally and 9 mm anteroposteriorly. The posterior band is its thickest part (3 mm). The central zone is only 1 mm thick, and the anterior band is about 2 mm thick. Chondrocytes can be found in

the disc with aging, and cartilage will form when the disc is displaced and abnormal forces exerted.[1]

The fibrous capsule is frail, although its lateral surface is strengthened into a distinct temporomandibular ligament. The joint capsule is attached to the border of the temporal articulating surface and to the neck of the mandible. It is directly fused to the medial anterior and lateral circumference of the articulating disc. Posteriorly, however, the disc and the capsule become integrated into the posterior attachment, or "bilaminar zone." This area is generously innervated and vascularized, with large sinusoids that fill and empty during joint function. The zone is termed "bilaminar" because it splits, with one attachment on the posterior condyle neck and the other on the anterior wall of the auditory canal.

The only muscle directly attached to the TMJ is the lateral (external) pterygoid. It has two points of origin, the superior portion from the infratemporal crest and the undersurface of the greater wing of the sphenoid bone. Its bundles converge to attach to the capsular ligament and directly into the articular disc. The inferior portion of the muscle is larger and arises from the lateral surface of the pterygoid process, from the pyramidal process of the palatine bone, and from the maxillary tuberosity. Its bundles converge to insert on the condylar head and neck. As the head rotates and then translates, the interior belly of the muscle contracts, helping to pull the condyle forward and inferiorly along the posterior slope of the eminentia articularis. The superior belly of the muscle remains flaccid on opening and the disc moves in concert with the head of the condyle by mechanical action. On closing, the superior belly of this muscle contracts to maintain the disc in proper relation to the head of the condyle.

SIGNS AND SYMPTOMS

Examination of the patient with TMJ symptoms begins when the patient enters the room. Note should be made of the posture, stride, and general carriage.

When did symptoms first appear and under what circumstances? Was the onset acute or insidious? Was there a specific incident, or did the patient simply wake up one morning with symptoms? How do the symptoms relate to time of day and physical activity? What can be accomplished to increase or decrease the severity of symptoms? Where are the symptoms located? Has treatment of any kind been instituted? If so, has the treatment helped?

The examiner should put the patient at ease and should watch mandibular function as the conversation proceeds, noting particularly thrusting, limited function, or deviation of the mandible. Once normal or abnormal function of the mandible has been established, specific voluntary movements are requested. The interincisal distance is measured at the midline with the patient's mouth open. A range of approximately 38 to 42 mm is normal, although this distance varies with sex and general physical build. Lateral excursions are requested, and measurements are made as the jaw moves into right lateral, left lateral, and protrusive positions. Normal lateral excursions are 5 to 10 mm, and normal protrusion is 4 to 6 mm. Function of the mandible is then ascertained while the joints are palpated. A smooth rotation followed by translation of the condylar head without pops, clicks, or crepitus is normal. At the same time, the examiner questions the patient about pain and local tenderness determined by digital pressure over the joint or through the external auditory canal.

A stethoscope is used to auscultate the joints during function; one should listen for the character of the noise, if noise is present. A pop or click signifies malposition of the disc, whereas grating or crepitus usually indicates bone-on-bone contact. The muscles of mastication are then palpated, beginning with the temporalis muscle and proceeding to the masseter, digastric, and medial and lateral pterygoid muscles. Accessory muscles of mastication such as the suprahyoid and infrahyoid, digastric, and sternocleidomastoid muscles are also palpated. Muscle spasm in the sternocleidomastoid or the hyoid muscles or in the muscles of mastication may occur in patients with limited mandibular function. Spasm in some or all of the vertebral muscles may cause the patient to have difficulty in moving the head.

Examination of the dentition follows, with special attention to the skeletal relationship of the arches, as well as the tooth-bone relationship. This determination is important because persons with a class II (retrognathia) skeletal and dental malocclusion frequently have TMJ symptoms. Internal joint derangements are rare in patients with class I (normal) and class III (prognathic) skeletal relationships. Finally, the patient is asked to point to the area of pain. The pointing finger frequently distinguishes between muscular disorders and internal joint derangements.

DIAGNOSTIC MODALITIES

RADIOGRAPHIC EXAMINATION

Roentgenograms of the painful TMJ give a wealth of information and are particularly useful in patients with possible internal joint derangements. Screening films are important, but definitive diagnosis should not be attempted using these alone. The most common views are the panoramic and the transcranial or transpharyngeal views in both opened and closed positions. These views reveal the general shape and condition of the bony condylar head, but they do not show its position relative to the glenoid fossa. It is possible to obtain these data with corrected tomograms. If the clinical exmaination and screening radiographic examination suggest internal joint derangement, further specific radiographic studies are indicated.

ARTHROGRAPHY

Arthrography is the standard diagnostic tool for internal TMJ derangement.[2-4] An iodized dye is injected into the inferior joint spaces or into both the inferior and superior spaces. If both joint spaces are injected, the disc will be outlined between the two pools of dye (Fig. 91–1). With a single inferior joint space injection, the disc is outlined by dye between the inferior compartment and the eminentia articularis (Fig. 91–2). As multiple sequential films are exposed with the patient opening and closing the mouth, the dye shifts from anterior to posterior as the condyle first rotates and then translates. In a person with an anterior displacement of the disc, the dye concentrates anterior to the condylar head. As the disc is captured by forward movement of the condyle, the

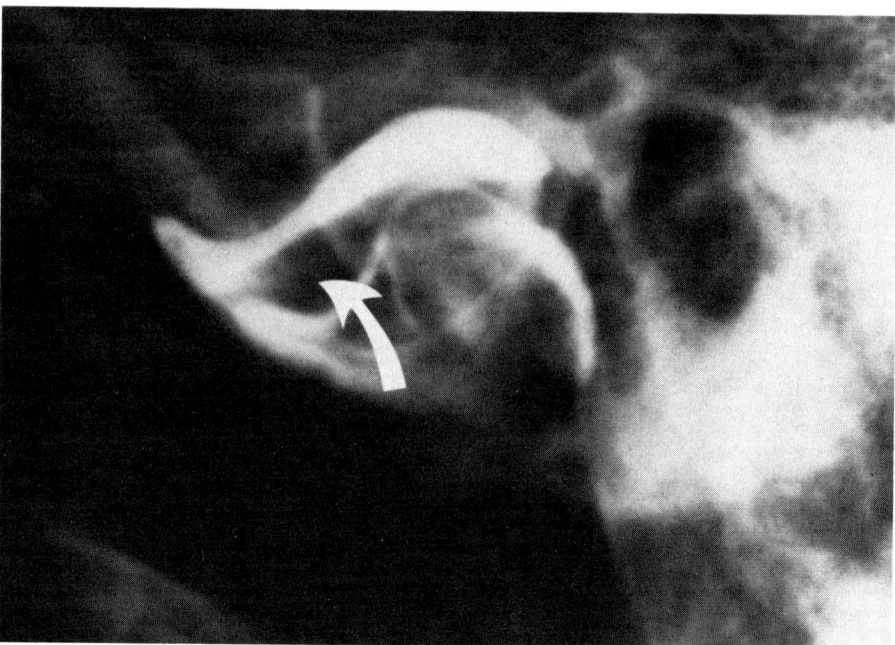

FIG. 91–1. Disc *(arrow)* outlined by dye in both the superior and inferior joint compartments.

dye flows rapidly posterior to the condylar head. At maximal joint opening, little dye is evident in the anterior portion of the inferior joint space. In the anterior closed lock, the disc is not recaptured, and a pool of dye remains in the anterior compartment of the inferior joint space, with the disc bunched superior to the dye concentrations and inferior to the eminentia articularis (Fig. 91–3).

Arthrographic views of the TMJ are now recorded dynamically on videotape and are far easier to interpret because the action of the condylar head in relation to the disc and dye is viewed in its entirety. One can watch the immediate and rapid shift of dye from

anterior to posterior as the disc is captured, or the concentrated anterior pools of dye with forced displacement of the disc anterior to the articular eminence. In a static arthrogram, in which the disc is recaptured at midfunction, the series of pictures may well show abnormal position of the disc on two or three views, followed by normal position of the disc on the remaining views.

SCINTIGRAPHY

Single photon emission computed tomography (SPECT) is an excellent noninvasive technique for de-

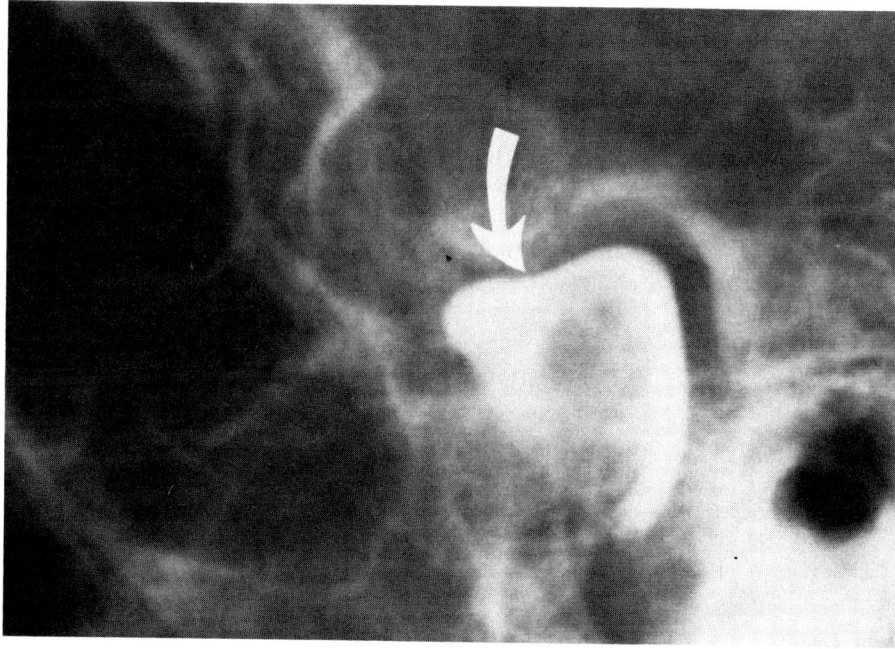

FIG. 91–2. Disc *(arrow)* outlined by dye between the inferior joint compartment and the articular eminence.

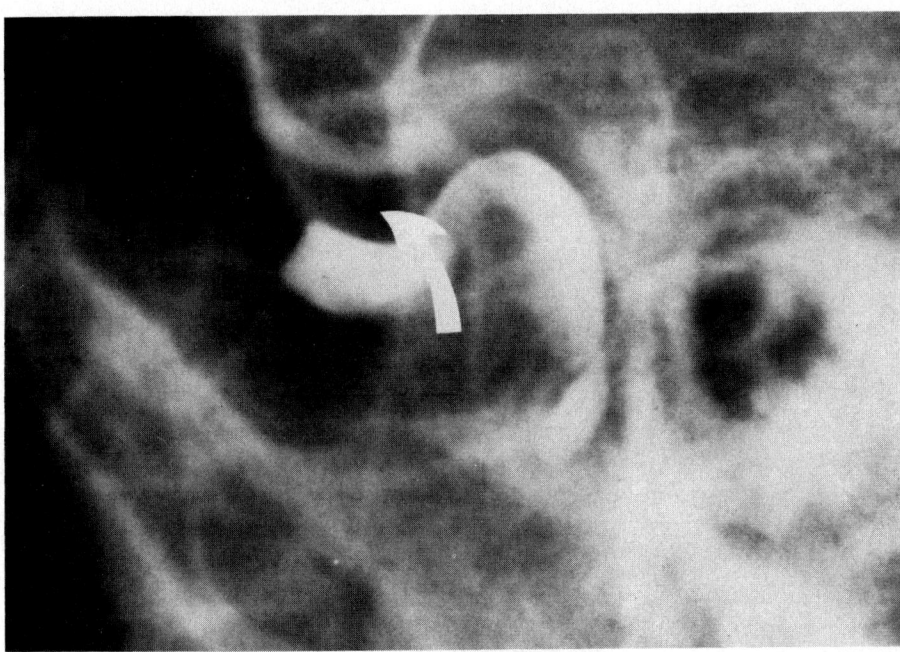

FIG. 91–3. Disc bunching ahead of the condyle as the condyle head attempts to move anteriorly *(arrow)*.

termining the presence or absence of TMJ disorders.[5] When internal joint derangement is present, condylar remodeling takes place and bone scintiscans using ^{99m}Tc MDP are positive before either conventional radiographs or x-ray tomograms demonstrate joint space narrowing, bony sclerosis, or disc degeneration.[6] Radionuclide angiography is performed with 10 sequential 3-second anterior-view images of the head, followed by a 50,000-count image 3 hours later. Anterior, right-lateral, and left-lateral planar bone scintigrams (500,000 count) of the head are obtained using

a large-field-of-view gamma camera equipped with a high-resolution collimator. A right lateral view demonstrates increased bone uptake over the right TMJ (Fig. 91–4). Tomographic studies in the coronal and transaxial planes can confirm the marked increase in radionuclide activity over the right TMJ (Figs. 91–5, 91–6). Quantitative analysis of the bone uptake over both joints and intervening bony structures also shows the sharp peak of increased activity over the right TMJ (Fig. 91–6), caused by subchondral bone

FIG. 91–4. Increased radionuclide activity *(arrow)* over the right TMJ joint.

FIG. 91–5. Coronal slice through the head of the TMJ joint showing a marked increase in activity on the right side *(arrow)*.

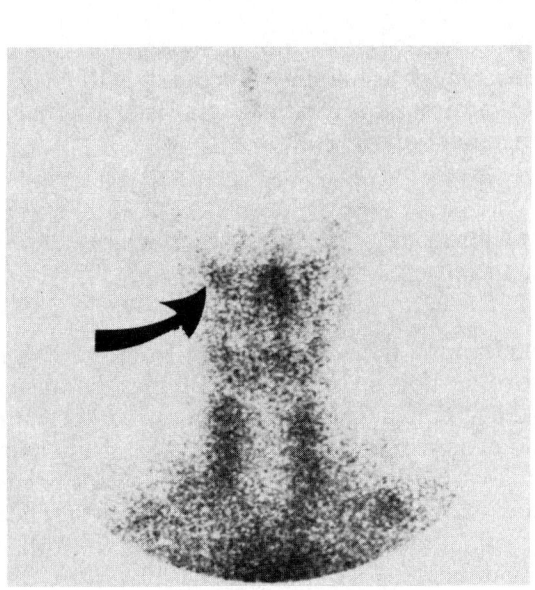

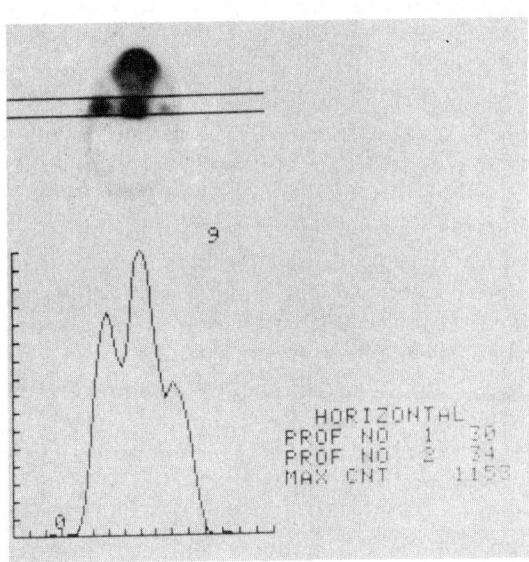

FIG. 91–6. Transaxial slice in a single photon emission computed tomogram confirms increased radioactivity in the right TMJ (upper part of the figure). Quantitative analysis shows a sharp peak of activity in the right TMJ (lower part of the figure).

FIG. 91–7. Magnetic resonance image of the left TMJ in closed position. Condyle (C), articular eminence (AE), external auditory canal (EAC), bilaminar zone (BZ), posterior band of disc (PB), intermediate zone (IZ), anterior band of disc (AB), lateral pterygoid muscle (PT). (Courtesy Bruce Kneeland, MD, Medical College of Wisconsin, Milwaukee)

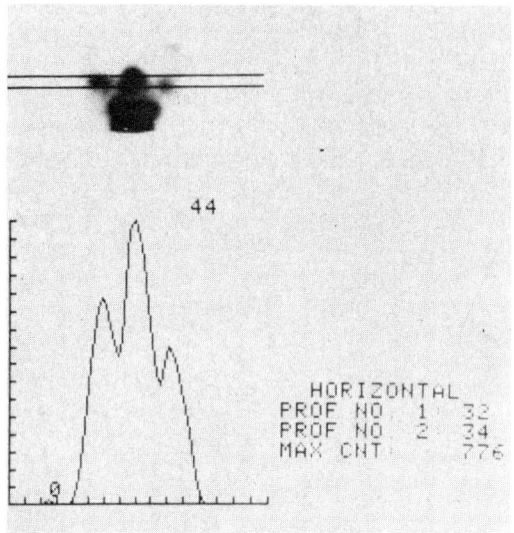

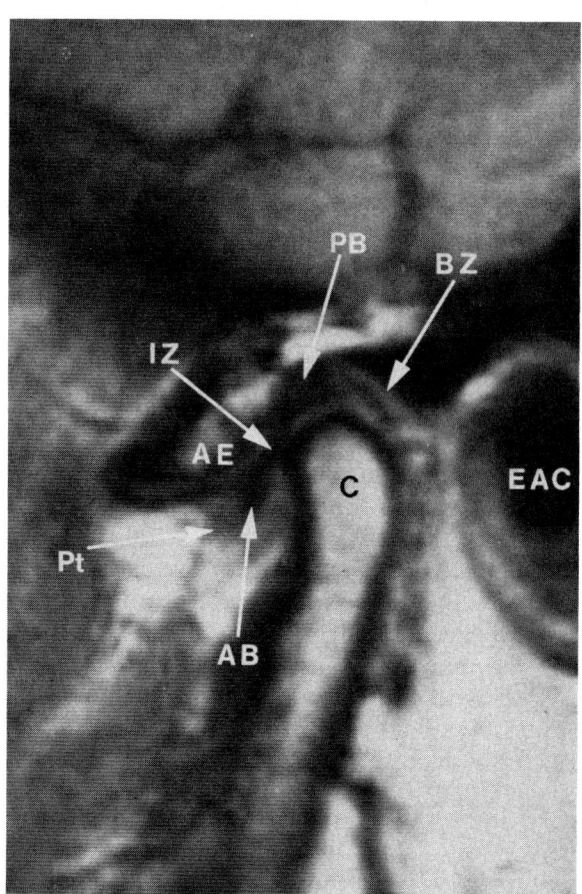

changes from anterior displacement of the disc noted on clinical examination.

MAGNETIC RESONANCE IMAGING

The usefulness of high-resolution magnetic resonance imaging (MRI) obtained with surface coil for imaging of the disc and of replacement implants of the TMJ has been well documented in the recent literature and unpublished data.[7,8]

In a normal TMJ, the condyle and eminence are easily visualized because of the high-intensity signal from the marrow spaces and the low-intensity signals from the cortical bone (Fig. 91–7). The posterior attachment, or bilaminar zone, is a mixed vascular and connective tissue structure with medium intensity and can therefore be distinguished from the low-intensity avascular disc (Fig. 91–7). In the anterior displaced disc of internal joint derangement, the disc will be located anterior to the condyle and below the articular eminence with the posterior attachment stretched over the condyle (Fig. 91–8).

MRI is a noninvasive, painless imaging technique that does not use ionized radiation. Unfortunately MRI provides static images, which in its present state of development cannot reproducibly demonstrate perforations of the soft tissues of the TMJ. The long scanning time (8 to 12 minutes per image) makes MRI

a more expensive procedure than other imaging techniques, but as technology advances, MRI may well replace arthrograms for the diagnosis of internal joint derangement of the TMJ.

DIFFERENTIAL DIAGNOSIS AND TREATMENT

Determining the source of pain from the TMJ and its surrounding structures is complex because the maxillofacial region has the highest sensory innervation density in the body, and the cranial nerves do not follow the orderly segmentation typically found in other joints of the body. Because of this complicated innervation, the diagnosis of diseases of the TMJ joint can be difficult.

FIG. 91–8. Magnetic resonance image of the left TMJ in closed position showing an anteriorly displaced disc *(arrows)*. (Courtesy Bruce Kneeland, MD, Medical College of Wisconsin, Milwaukee)

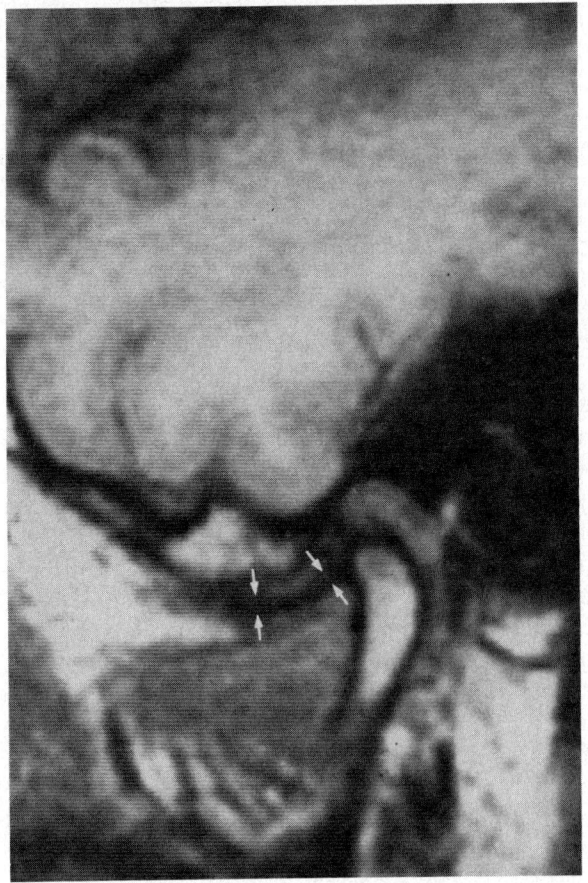

REFERRED OTALGIA AND ODONTALGIA

The symptom of earache is common with lesions of the TMJ. The auricle, external auditory canal, and tympanum are supplied by sensory fibers from the fifth, seventh, ninth, and tenth cranial nerves, in addition to the second and third cervical nerves. Earache caused by pain referred from other sites is more common than that resulting from disorders of the ear itself. Because the sensory innervation varies widely and overlaps, it is often difficult for the patient to localize the pain to a particular area of the ear. For these reasons, diagnosis of lesions of both the external and the inner ear is made mainly by clinical evaluation. If the patient's pain is localized within the meatus of the auditory canal and if pain is produced by palpation or passive movement of the auricle, a lesion of the external ear or auditory canal should be suspected. Diseases of the middle ear usually produce symptoms of hearing impairment, low-pitched tin-

nitus, and pain that varies from mild discomfort or pressure sensation, as seen with an early, acute serous or purulent otitis media, to a deep, boring pain, as seen late in these diseases. If the earache is modified in any way by movement of the lower jaw, and if the auricle, external auditory canal, and tympanic membrane appear normal on examination, the diagnosis of TMJ disease should be considered.

Pain of dental origin is commonly referred to the TMJ through the fifth cranial nerve, primarily the auriculotemporal branch. It is often difficult for the patient to determine whether the offending tooth is in the mandible or the maxilla, and the pain may be felt diffusely throughout the teeth, jaw, face, and head. Because of the variability and the diffuse nature of the pain it is wise to consider all diffuse pain in the head and neck, including the oral cavity, to be of dental origin until proved otherwise. In most cases, clinical evaluation reveals a large carious lesion or a fractured tooth to be the source of pain. Palpation of the affected tooth with a tongue blade elicits pain and is thereby a dependable means of diagnosis. The surrounding soft tissues may also show signs of inflammation.

Radiographic Findings. In dental disease, radiographs are helpful and often diagnostic. The panoramic radiograph and the periapical radiograph taken in a dental office are most frequently used.

Laboratory Findings. Except in the case of acute infection, when the white blood cell count is elevated, the laboratory examination does not contribute to the diagnosis.

MYOFASCIAL PAIN DYSFUNCTION SYNDROME

As many as 85% of all patients seen with "TMJ syndrome" really have myofascial pain dysfunction of the muscles of mastication. The TMJ is implicated because pain occurs when it is mobilized. The female-to-male sex ratio is 8:1, with an age range from puberty to 40 years, although it can occur at any age. The cardinal signs and symptoms of this syndrome include pain on movement of the jaw, limited ability to open the jaw, deviation of the open jaw toward the affected side, and clicking or popping heard in the TMJ during motion. Two negative findings are important: (1) No tenderness on palpation of the TMJ, and (2) normal bony radiographic findings.[9] Classically, the patient describes the pain by placing the whole hand over the affected side of the face. The description of pain varies from a sensation of pressure to severe and lancinating, occurring both spontaneously and in response to movement of the involved muscles. Pain occurs when chewing and when clenching the teeth. The pain is often more severe in the morning, on awakening, secondary to nocturnal bruxism. A period of emotional stress often precedes the onset of symptoms.

Clinical Findings. No pain is present in the TMJ during movement or on palpation of the condylar head. The "clicking" sometimes felt during early movement of the joint is related to spasm of the superior belly of the lateral pterygoid muscle. If clicking is detected during extreme excursion, a diagnosis of internal joint derangement should be considered. At least one of the muscles of mastication is tender to palpation on the painful side, and when the patient bites, pain is experienced in the same muscles. If a tongue blade is placed between the incisors and the patient is asked to bite, the pain should decrease. If the tongue blade is placed on the posterior teeth, and the patient is asked to bite, the pain will probably increase.

Treatment. Initial treatment consists of muscle relaxants, anti-inflammatory drugs, moist heat, and a soft diet. If the symptoms persist for more than 2 weeks, the patient should be referred to a dentist for construction of an acrylic splint to help to disocclude the teeth. Because bruxism or clenching of the teeth is a primary cause of this syndrome, the splint may interrupt the cycle of jaw clenching and muscle spasm. Psychologic counseling may be indicated because emotional stress often initiates the problem. If these measures are not successful, physical therapy, biofeedback, hypnosis, and formal psychotherapy may be tried.

INTERNAL TEMPOROMANDIBULAR JOINT DERANGEMENT

By definition, this disorder is an abnormal relationship of the disc with the condyle when the teeth are in maximal occlusion.[10] The abnormal position of the disc is usually anteromedial because of the direction of contraction of the superior belly of the lateral pterygoid muscles toward the pterygoid plates. Internal derangements are subdivided into the following categories: (1) anteromedial displacement of the disc with reduction; (2) anteromedial displacement of the disc without reduction (close lock); and (3) perforation of the disc or the posterior attachment of the disc. These derangements are also classified by the amount of movement of the mandible necessary to reposition or "capture" the disc, as evidenced by the clicking sound. Thus, *early, midphase,* or *late reductions* are

classified by measurement of the interincisal opening. If the reduction takes place during the first 15 mm of interincisal opening, it is considered an early reduction; if it takes place during 15 to 30 mm of interincisal opening, it is a midphase reduction; and if it happens after 30 mm, it is classified as a late reduction. If the patient can open the mouth only to 27 to 30 mm with deviation toward the affected side and no clicking is heard or palpated, a "close lock" must be considered. With close lock, the disc is wedged in front of the condyle and prevents foward motion of the mandible. The pathophysiologic features of the abnormality are compared with its unpredictable clinical progression (Table 91–1).[10-12] The disorder may progress in a period of several months to years, or it may not follow the full sequence of clinical events.

Clinical Findings. The ratio of women to men affected with the disorder is 8:1, and the condition is most commonly seen in the second or third decade, but it can occur at any age. The cardinal signs and symptoms of internal joint derangement include pain on palpation of the condylar head, and popping, clicking, or crepitus in the TMJ. One also sees limited range of motion, as in close lock, deviation toward the affected side before the pop takes place, and finally, return to midline at maximal opening. Other, more variable symptoms include temporal or frontal headaches, retro-orbital pain, otalgia, tinnitus, dizziness, and varying degrees of myofascial pain dysfunction syndrome. A history of asymptomatic clicking is important, especially when the patient has limited and noiseless joint opening.

Radiographic Findings. Routine radiographic examination is not diagnostic. Arthrography is invaluable in the diagnosis of internal joint derangement and is the definitive test of choice. More recently, MRI has also become a useful diagnostic tool.[7,8]

Treatment. Treatment depends on the severity of the condition. The patient with painless joint clicking is informed of the possible progression of the disease, but no treatment is indicated. If a patient has early clicking and pain, nonsurgical techniques are used,

Table 91–1.   Internal Temporomandibular Joint Derangement

Clinical Progression of Disease	Pathophysiology
Clicking	Stretching of lateral attachment
	Stretching and loss of elasticity of posterior attachment
Clicking with intermittent locking	Thickening of posterior ridge of disc
Close lock	Metaplasia of disc tissue to cartilage or permanent deformation of disc
Crepitus	Perforation of posterior attachment

including splint therapy to recapture the disc followed by alteration of the occlusion to hold the position.[4,13,14] With late reduction or with nonreduction (close lock) of the disc or in patients unsuccessfully treated by nonsurgical means, a surgical procedure is indicated. If the disc is of normal shape and texture and is easily pulled posteriorly and laterally into a normal relationship with the condyle head, a diskoplasty is performed. The posterior and lateral attachments are shortened, and the disc is reattached to the condyle.[3,13] If the disc has undergone metaplasia or is scarred in an anteromedial position, a diskectomy is indicated, with implantation of a soft silicone implant. Because a fibrous capsule is formed around the implant in approximately 3 months, the implant can be removed either prophylactically or if it has become torn or perforated. The fibrous capsule then functions as a "disc-like" structure to separate the condyle from the temporal bone.[15] At present, fractured implants can be imaged *only* with MRI (Fig. 91–9). Patients tolerate these surgical procedures well; diskoplasty is successful in 80 to 90%; the success rate of the diskectomy with implantation is about 70 to 90%.

Arthroscopic examination and surgery is now being used in the treatment of internal joint derangement.[16] Indications for arthroscopy of the TMJ include acute hemarthrosis, acute locking unresponsive to manipulation, and chronic scarring of the disc to the temporal bone. An arthroscope between 1.5 and 2.3 mm is introduced into the superior joint space, and changes such as synovial hypertrophy, hyperemia of the posterior attachment, perforation of the disc, and adhesions of the disc to the temporal bone can be identified. Surgically, adhesions can be lysed, the disc mobilized by sweeping the superior compartment, and mobile foreign bodies removed with copious irrigation. Corticosteroid esters, either triamcinolone or betamethasone, can be injected to decrease the inflammatory process and its accompanying pain.

DEGENERATIVE JOINT DISEASE

Unlike other diarthrodial joints, the articular surface of the TMJ is covered with fibrocartilage rather than with hyaline cartilage. The progression of degenerative disease in the TMJ is also different from that in other joints. Initially, erosion is seen in the subchondral bone, followed by thinning and destruction of the fibrocartilage, with some attempts at repair. Degenerative joint disease is traditionally divided into primary and secondary types.[17] Primary disease is idiopathic, whereas secondary disease is related to trauma or, most important, to chronic internal joint

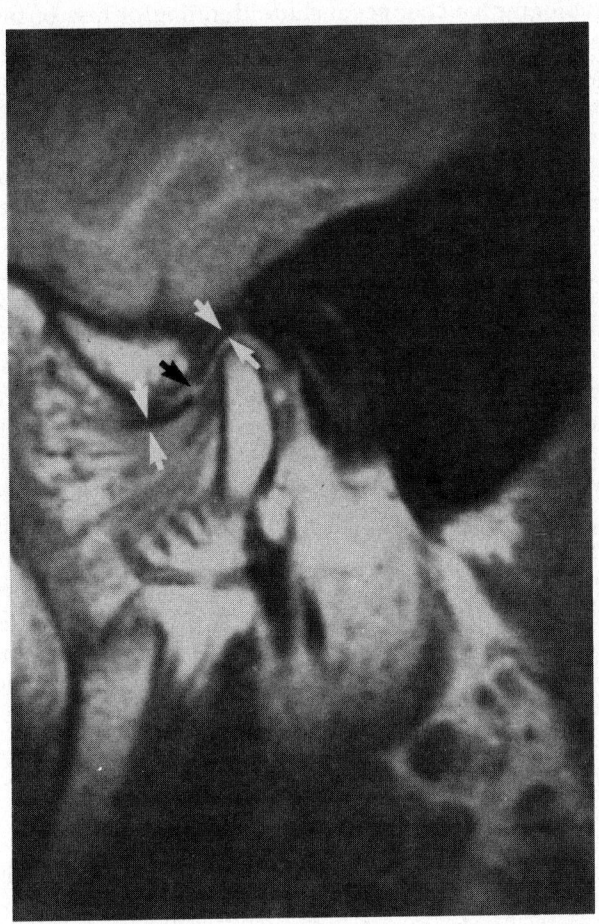

FIG. 91–9. Magnetic resonance image showing a silicone implant *(white arrows)* with discontinuity *(black arrow)*, representing a fracture. (From Kneeland, J.B. et al.[8] Reprinted with permission of the Journal of Computer Assisted Tomography)

derangement. In patients with primary disease, with an intact articular disc, the clinical course of pain and dysfunction is short and is usually followed by repair, with diminution or resolution of symptoms. In secondary disease, the disc is either destroyed or damaged beyond repair, symptoms become chronic, and natural repair is only partial.

Clinical Findings. The onset of this disorder is usually insidious. The initial symptom is stiffness of the involved joint. Pain on joint motion becomes worse by progressive activity during the day. Patients are least symptomatic on arising in the morning. Coarse crepitus is often felt in the affected joint late in the disease process, especially in secondary degenerative joint disease.[18]

Radiographic Findings. A screening radiograph is first obtained. Tomograms can be used to delineate the extent of the bony changes if a surgical procedure is contemplated. Arthrograms are of great value in determining whether the disc is displaced or torn, a finding that determines therapy. Bone scanning with tomography is also of diagnostic value and can be used to evaluate the effectiveness of treatment. Early radiographic changes include thinning or loss of the cortical bone in the area of articulation. As the disease progresses, one sees a roughened and irregular bony surface, which can lead to loss of normal condylar anatomic features. Flattening of the superior and anterior aspects with anterior lipping of the condyle are evidence of natural repair, and cortical margins develop when repair is complete.

Treatment. Primary degenerative joint disease is usually a self-limiting process, often treated symptomatically and nonsurgically. If the disc remains intact, normal healing by fibrocartilaginous proliferation will take place on the condylar surface, and the disease generally runs its course in approximately 2 years. In secondary disease, in which the disc is destroyed or torn and displaced, the condition progresses, and surgical treatment is indicated. This treatment consists of diskectomy, smoothing of the articular surfaces, and placement of an implant between the condylar head and glenoid fossa. Corticosteroid injections have been used to create a "chemical smoothing" of the articular surfaces of the condyle with moderate success.[19]

RHEUMATOID ARTHRITIS

Involvement of the TMJ in rheumatoid arthritis (RA) varies from 1 to 60%. Affected women outnumber affected men 3 to 1. The disease usually affects both TM joints. Only the condylar head is affected, and the glenoid fossa is seldom involved. Initial bony destruction occurs in the neck of the condyle inferior to the fibrocartilaginous cover of the head. It then involves the cartilaginous surface and the subchondral spaces of the bone.[20] The disc is usually destroyed in the process.

Clinical Findings. Signs and symptoms of RA in the TMJ are similar to those in other affected joints. Pain and stiffness on arising in the morning are prominent features. These symptoms decrease with moderate activity, and stiffness recurs with inactivity. Pain becomes more severe during strenuous activity. On palpation there is tenderness over the joint, and limitation of motion becomes progressive as the disease develops. Later in the disease process, crepitus may be found.

Radiographic Findings. A screening radiograph is used for initial evaluation. Erosions of the neck and head, marginal proliferations of bone, flattening of the superior and anterior surfaces of the condylar head, and eventually, gross deformities are evident. Although not as diagnostic, limitation of joint excursions and narrowing of the joint space are also seen. More detailed evaluation can be accomplished by the use of tomography or corrected tomography. Tomographic bone scanning is diagnostic for RA, and arthrograms can be valuable in determining the status of the disc.

Laboratory Findings. Rheumatoid factor test is positive in 70 to 80% of patients, and other findings are identical to those described in Chapter 43.

Treatment. The usual treatment is conservative, as described in Chapter 47. With successful management of the systemic disease, symptoms in the TMJ usually subside. Rest is prescribed for the joints during the acute phase of the illness, along with mild exercises to maintain function. Occasionally, an acrylic splint is useful to remove the mandible from tooth function or replace missing teeth, thereby decreasing trauma to the joint. Ankylosis is rare. If it does occur, the procedure of choice consists of creating a joint space, lining the joint space with silicone implant, and instituting motion soon after the operation. Occasionally, a total joint replacement is necessary to maintain a functioning mandible.

GOUTY ARTHRITIS

Gout of the TMJ is rare but painful. As in other joints of the body, urate crystals precipitate in the synovial tissues and fluid. Left untreated, degenerative joint disease develops.[21,22]

Clinical and Laboratory Findings. Sudden onset of symptoms, frequently at night and for no apparent reason, is characteristic. A warm sensation over the joint is common, and the patient notes limitation of mandibular movement because of the acute pain and swelling. The patient may also experience headache, fever, and general malaise.

Radiographic Findings. In the acute phase of the disorder, no radiographic changes are seen. If the disease becomes chronic, radiographic changes resemble those of degenerative joint disease.

Treatment. Aspiration of the joint gives temporary symptomatic relief; medical management of the acute attack is uniformly successful (see Chapter 93).

OTHER DISEASES

The temporomandibular joints can be affected by any disease that involves the joints. Short- or long-term symptoms in this joint may be due to the deposition of calcium pyrophosphate dihydrate crystals, as discussed in Chapter 107. Crystal masses may occur in areas of chondroid metaplasia in the synovium as an isolated finding, resembling osteochondromatosis. Acute temporomandibular gout or pseudogout was thought to be precipitated by bruxism in one patient.[23]

Two other categories that cause extreme joint symptoms, only mentioned here, are trauma and either benign or malignant tumors. Trauma can cause pain and can limit movement in the TMJ, but diagnosis is straightforward, by history, examination, and standard facial radiographs. Tumors are rare. Pain usually occurs late in the course of the disease. Limited function and grossly abnormal radiographic changes often precede pain. Biopsy is needed for diagnosis, and treatment is determined by the nature of the lesion.

In summary, pain in the TMJ is often misdiagnosed and frequently attributed to a psychologic cause. With the introduction of arthrography, scintigraphy, and MRI, as well as a better understanding of the anatomy and physiology of this joint, most patients can now be helped.

REFERENCES

1. Dolwick, M.F., Aufdemorte, T.B., and Cornelius, J.D.: Histopathlogic findings in TMJ internal derangements. J. Dent. Res., 63:267 (Abstract 865), 1985.
2. Bronstein, S.L., Tomasetti, B.J., and Ryan, D.E.: Internal derangement of the temporomandibular joint: Correlation of arthrographic and surgical findings. J. Oral Surg., 39:572–584, 1982.
3. Dolwick, M.F.: Surgical management in internal derangements of the temporomandibular joint. *In* Internal Derangement of the Temporomandibular Joint. Edited by C.A. Helms, R.W. Katzberg, and M.F. Dolwick. San Francisco, Radiology Research and Education Foundation, 1983.
4. Dolwick, M.F., et al.: Arthrotomographic evaluation of the temporomandibular joint. J. Oral Surg., 37:793–799, 1979.
5. Krasnow, A.Z., et al.: Comparison of high resolution MRI and SPECT bone scintigraphy for noninvasive imaging of the temporomandibular joint. J. Nucl. Med., 28:1268–1274, 1987.
6. Collier, D., et al.: Detection of internal derangement of the temporomandibular joint by single photon emission computed tomography. Radiology, 149:557–561, 1983.
7. Katzberg, R.W., et al.: Normal and abnormal temporomandibular joint: MR imaging with a surface coil. Radiology, 158:183–189, 1986.
8. Kneeland, J.B., et al.: Magnetic resonance imaging of temporomandiular disc prosthesis: A case report. J. Comput. Assist. Tomogr., 11:199–200, 1987.
9. Laskin, D.M.: Etiology of pain dysfunction syndrome. J. Am. Dent. Assoc., 79:147–153, 1969.
10. Dolwick, M.F., and Sanders, B.: TMJ internal derangement and arthrosis surgical atlas. 1st Ed. St. Louis, The C.V. Mosby Co., 1985, pp. 27–50.
11. Farrar, W.B.: Diagnosis and treatment of anterior dislocation of the articular disc. N. Y. J. Dent., 41:348–351, 1971.
12. Scapino, R.P.: Histopathology associated with malposition of the human temporomandibular joint disc. Oral Surg., 55:382–397, 1983.
13. McCarty, W.L., Jr., and Farrar, W.B.: Surgery for internal derangement of the temporomandibular joint. J. Prosthet. Dent., 42:191–196, 1979.
14. McNeill, C., et al.: Craniomandibular (TMJ) disorders—the state of the art. J. Prosthet. Dent., 44:434, 1980.
15. Eriksson, L., and Westesson, P.L.: Deterioration of temporary silastic implants in the temporomandibular joint: A clinical and arthroscopic follow-up study. Oral Surg., 62:2–6, 1986.
16. Sanders, B.: Arthroscopic surgery of the temporomandibular joint: Treatment of internal derangement with persistent closed-lock. Oral Surg., 62:361–372, 1986.
17. Toller, P.A.: Osteoarthrosis of the mandibular condyle. Br. Dent. J., 134:223–231, 1973.
18. Kreutziger, K.L., and Mahan, P.E.: Temporomandibular degenerative joint disease. I. Anatomy, pathophysiology and clinical description. Oral Surg., 40:165–182, 1975.
19. Poswillo, D.: Experimental investigation of the effects of interarticular hydrocortisone and high condylectomy on the mandibular condyle. Oral Surg., 30:161, 1970.
20. Ogus, H.: Rheumatoid arthritis of the temporomandibular joint. Br. J. Oral Surg., 12:275–284, 1975.
21. Kleinman, H.Z., and Ewbank, R.L.: Gout of the temporomandibular joint: Report of three cases. Oral Surg., 27:281–282, 1969.
22. Rodnan, G.P.: Gout and other crystalline forms of arthritis. Postgrad. Med., 58:6, 1978.
23. Good, A.E., and Upton, L.G.: Acute temporomandibular arthritis in a patient with bruxism and calcium pyrophosphate deposition disease. Arthritis Rheum., 25:353–355, 1982.

92

THE PAINFUL BACK

DAVID B. LEVINE

The syndrome of low-back pain, with or without radiation, is one of the most common disorders affecting humans. Although great advances have been made in understanding the complexities of the pathogenesis of this syndrome, medical knowledge is still not advanced sufficiently to clarify the origin of low-back pain.

Anatomic focus is on the lower lumbar spine (L3–L5), the lumbosacral junction, the sacrum, the sacroiliac joints, and finally, the sacral-coccygeal region. Although symptoms in these regions often stem from local disease, etiologic factors may be present elsewhere.

Physicians should plan an orderly approach to the patient with low-back syndrome. They should first attempt to determine whether the cause is primarily musculoskeletal, neurologic, or visceral. A differential diagnosis should then be established by medical history, physical examination, routine radiographs, and laboratory analysis. Precise diagnosis may be reached by repeated examinations and special tests. Only then can logical management be formulated.

PREVALENCE

The worldwide prevalence of low-back pain is becoming known. It has been estimated that 80% of the population will experience low-back pain at some time.

The painful low back is a major cause of loss of time from work. Workdays lost are reported to be 1400 per thousand workers in the United States and 2600 per thousand workers in Great Britain.

The prevalence of low-back pain is directly influenced by various social and psychologic factors. Consequently, psychologic evaluation has become a necessary part of the clinical examination.

DIFFERENTIAL DIAGNOSIS

The list of possible diagnoses of the low-back syndrome seems endless, yet the physician must make every effort to arrive at a specific presumptive diagnosis. Although such terms as "lumbago" and "sciatica" were common labels in the past, they should be avoided because of their ambiguity. The diagnosis of "strain" alone is meaningless unless applied to a certain anatomic part.

The differential diagnosis may be reached by a logical and reasonable approach, based on appropriate anatomic and potential etiologic factors. The following outline provides a basis for differential diagnosis:

ANATOMIC FACTORS
Vertebra (hard)
  Body
  Neural arch
  Spinous process
  Lamina
  Facet
  Pedicle
  Transverse process

Vertebra (soft)
Supraspinous ligament
Infraspinous ligament
Ligamentum flavum
Posterior longitudinal ligament
Anterior longitudinal ligament
Intervertebral disc
Minor ligaments
Vertebra (articulation)
Anterior (disc)
Posterior (facets)
Lateral (sacroiliac joints)
Vertebra (orifices)
Neural canal
Intervertebral foramina
Vertebra (alignment)
Paravertebra (muscular)
Anterior
Posterior
Lateral
ETIOLOGIC FACTORS
Traumatic
Acute
Chronic
Congenital
Degenerative
Inflammatory
Infectious
Noninfectious
Neoplastic
Developmental
Metabolic
Toxic
Psychoneurotic
Nerves
Primary (local)
Primary (general)
Coverings
Vessels
Arterial
Venous
Visceral organs

ANATOMIC CONSIDERATIONS

VERTEBRAL COLUMN

Each vertebra is composed of an anterior portion, the body, and a posterior portion, the neural arch (Fig. 92–1). From the neural arch, several processes are important: the transverse processes, one on each side; the superior and inferior articular processes (facets), one above and one below on each side; and one

FIG. 92–1. Anatomy of the lumbar vertebrae and their articulations. *A,* Superior view of a stripped lumbar vertebra. *B,* Lateral view of two articulated lumbar vertebrae. *C,* Superior view of a horizontal section of a lumbar disc. *D,* Lateral view of a sagittal section of two articulated lumbar vertebrae. B = Body of the vertebra; SC = spinal column; IVF = intervertebral foramen; IF = inferior articular facet; SF = superior articular facet; P = pedicle; TP = transverse process; SP = spinous process; L = lamina; AF = anulus fibrosus; NP = nucleus pulposus; CP = cartilage plate; ALL = anterior longitudinal ligament; PLL = posterior longitudinal ligament; LF = ligamentum flavum; IL = interspinous ligament.

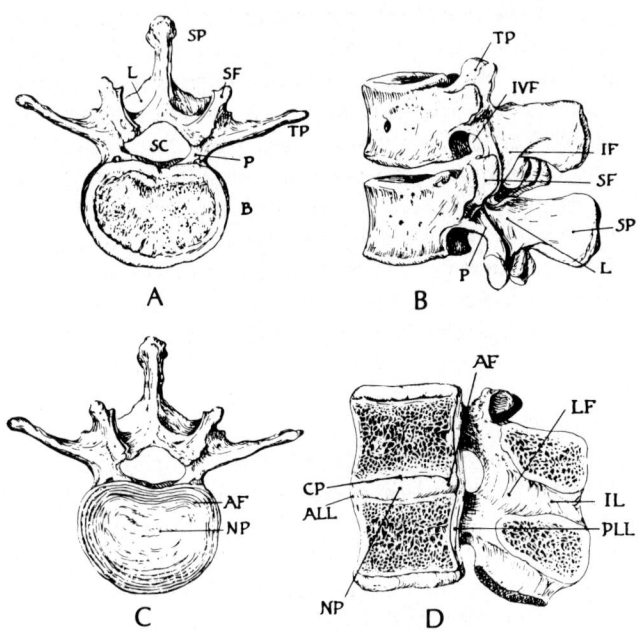

spinous process. The portion of the neural arch connected to the body and anterior to the articular processes is called the root or pedicle; that posterior to it is called the lamina; that part between the superior and inferior articular facets has come to be known as the pars interarticularis, or isthmus.

The vertebrae are articulated together by a system of joints, three for each level. The disc lies between two adjacent vertebral bodies and is composed of a tough fibrocartilaginous outer ring, the anulus fibrosus, with a central viscous core, the nucleus pulposus. It is bounded superiorly and inferiorly by hyaline cartilaginous plates that blend with the anulus fibrosus. The transitions from cartilaginous plate to anulus and from anulus to nucleus are gradual. The fibers of the anulus fibrosus are arranged concentrically and in multiple layers. In the lumbar discs, the layers are thicker anteriorly and laterally than posteriorly, and the nucleus pulposus is closer to the posterior aspect of the disc. Posteriorly, one for each side, are true diarthrodial joints, which lie between the inferior facets of one vertebra above and the superior facets of the next below.

The ligamentous support of the spine is provided by the massive anterior longitudinal ligament and the narrow posterior longitudinal ligament. In a study of 35 autopsy specimens at the level of the L5 vertebral body, the average width of the anterior longitudinal ligament was 2 cm and the average thickness 1.9 mm, whereas the average width of the posterior longitudinal ligament was 0.7 cm and the average thickness 1.3 mm. These ligaments are situated around the margins of the vertebral bodies and lend strong support to the discs, except posteriorly on either side of the midline, where their fibers are much attenuated or nonexistent. In contrast to the anterior ligaments, which can be easily separated from the underlying anulus fibrosus, the posterior longitudinal ligament is strongly attached to the anulus fibers. Additional support is provided by the ligamentum flavum, an elastic structure that bridges the interlaminal spaces and reinforces the facet joint capsules, and the interspinous, intertransverse, and iliolumbar ligaments.

Embryology

The anlage of the spine forms in a right and left column on each side of the primitive notochord, just anterior to the neural tube. At a later stage of development, the two halves fuse anteriorly and posteriorly around the developing spinal cord. A failure of this process accounts for the frequent incidence of fusion defects, various degrees of spina bifida when development fails posteriorly, and various degrees of platyspondylisis and butterfly vertebrae when anteriorly. Anterior fusion defects are much rarer than posterior defects.

At the same time, the vertebrae are formed, also from a fusion of two embryonic parts in another plane, that is, the inferior portion of one sclerotome with the subjacent superior part of another. Disturbances of this stage of development produce incomplete and asymmetric segmentation and hemivertebrae.

As the lateral halves of the vertebral body fuse in the midline, the notochord is forced superiorly and inferiorly, where its remnants concentrate to aid in the formation of the nucleus pulposus. This process, when imperfect, leads to defects in the cartilaginous plates. The anulus fibrosus, which encloses the nucleus pulposus, originates in the mesenchyme left as the cephalad and caudad portions of the sclerotome separate to form the vertebral bodies.

SACRUM AND PELVIS

The anatomic details of the sacrum do not warrant special description. The articulation between it and the fifth lumbar vertebra follows the pattern previously described. The sacrum articulates with the pelvis by means of the two sacroiliac joints, which are partly fibrous and partly diarthrodial. The surfaces of the fibrous portion of these joints are irregular and fit closely together. The female pelvis has less bony apposition than the male, and the ligaments are stronger. The cartilaginous surface of the sacrum is thicker and hyaline, that of the ilium thinner and fibrous. In both sexes, some motion can and does take place, but with the exception of the late stages of pregnancy, the range is small and physiologically insignificant. The motion is in a rotary plane and is resisted in one direction by the wedge shape of the sacrum and in the other by the sacrotuberous and sacrospinous ligaments. Increased compensatory motion can occur at the sacroiliac joints in patients who have had surgical fusions of the lumbar spine. Because the joint is supported by some of the densest ligaments of the body, it is doubtful that sacroiliac strain or "slipping" can occur except in cases of extensive injury, pregnancy, or disease. That portion of the joint lined, although imperfectly, by synovium is subject to all the diseases of diarthrodial joints, however, and is a common site of involvement for arthritic disease, whether infectious, rheumatoid, or degenerative.

COCCYX

This part of the vertebral column is composed of four segments, the first one of which is often free from the others. Motion can and does take place between the sacrum and the coccyx. This joint has little ligamentous support and it is vulnerable to injury, but its anatomic situation protects it.

NEURAL STRUCTURES

The neural arch of each vertebra encloses the spinal cord, together with its supporting structures. Originally, the distal end of the spinal cord extends to the caudal end of the dural sac at about the level of the third sacral segment, but it retracts superiorly as the spine grows in length to reach a final adult position at the level of the first lumbar vertebra. The nerve roots of the lumbosacral plexus are drawn up with the spinal cord and lie within the dura, to form the cauda equina. A slender filament, the filum terminale, loosely anchors the distal end of the spinal cord to the coccyx. Cephalad, the spinal cord is held by its origin from the brain. It is also fixed by the succession of spinal nerves, which pass out through the intervertebral foramina. It is supported everywhere by its dural and arachnoidal membranes. Over this immobile neural tube, the spinal segments must move smoothly to perform their physiologic functions.

Each nerve root leaves the spinal canal inferior to its corresponding vertebral arch, except in the cervical spine, where it leaves superiorly. That is, the first cervical nerve root passes out superior to the first cervical vertebral arch, whereas the fifth lumbar nerve root leaves the canal inferior to the fifth lumbar vertebral arch. The difference is made up by the presence of eight cervical nerves, as opposed to seven cervical vertebrae, the eighth cervical nerve passing out of the intervertebral foramen between C7 and T1.

A nerve root is in an intimate relationship with several parts of the vertebra and discs as it passes from the dural sac to outside the neural canal. In the lower lumbar spine, each nerve root, together with a sheath of dura, becomes separated from the remainder of the cauda equina at the level of the superior disc, courses laterally as it passes distally across its corresponding vertebral body, and reaches the intervertebral foramen at a point opposite its disc of the same numerical designation. For instance, the fifth lumbar nerve leaves the cauda equina just superior to the level of the fourth lumbar disc (the disc between L4 and L5) and passes diagonally laterally, posterior to the fifth lumbar body to reach the intervertebral foramen between L5 and the sacrum. In the foramen, it is held against the medial and inferior surfaces of the pedicle (in this case, of L5) lying in a groove called the sulcus nervi spinalis. Anteriorly lies the body (of L5), inferiorly the bulging fifth lumbar disc, and posteriorly, shielded by the ligamentum flavum, the inferior facet (of L5). Although the nerve root moves freely in the intervertebral foramen, pathologic or traumatic disturbances of any of these structures (pedicle, body, or facet) can obstruct its passage and may cause pressure. More recently, transforaminal ligaments, reducing available space for passage of the nerve root through the lumbar intervertebral foramina, have been described. The extradural courses of the lower lumbar nerve roots are related to two discs: the one superior to and the one inferior to their corresponding vertebrae.

VASCULAR SUPPLY

Arnoldi reported that interosseous hypertension may be a cause of lumbar spine pain.[1] The blood sup-

ply of the lumbar spine is derived from four lumbar arteries, arising in pairs from the abdominal aorta and traversing close to the anterior and lateral portions of the vertebral bodies.[2] The middle sacral artery, a small vessel, arises from the back of the aorta superior to the bifurcation and occasionally produces a fifth pair of segmental vessels. Each lumbar artery divides into three main branches: anterior, intermediate, and posterior.

The anterior branches supply the abdominal wall. The intermediate branches divide and supply mainly the neural structures, including the nerve roots and the cauda equina. The posterior branches come in contact with the laminae and enter the sacrospinalis muscles. The division of the segmental arteries occurs at the "distribution point" at the level of the intervertebral foramina. This anatomic landmark is important when anterior spinal surgical procedures are contemplated.

The veins draining the vertebral column form intricate plexuses, which may be divided into external and internal, according to their position inside or outside the vertebral canal. Lumbar veins accompany the lumbar arteries and drain into the venae cavae and the left common iliac vein. Through ascending lumbar veins, drainage continues into the lumbar azygous or hemiazygous system. Because the vertebral plexuses have few valves and communicate with veins in the body wall and pelvis, they are a potential pathway by which metastasis from other areas may involve the vertebral column. Variations in pressure on arteries, veins, and capillaries may interfere with nerve condition.

BIOMECHANICAL CONSIDERATIONS

In utero, the spine is formed in one long curve, with its convexity directed posteriorly. After birth and with the gradual assumption of vertical posture, this curve is altered. Because of the immobility of the thoracic segment and because of its attached ribs, the kyphosis (curve with convexity posteriorly) persists in this area. As strength develops to allow the infant to raise his head and then to sit and finally to stand, however, lordoses (curves with their convexities directed anteriorly) develop first in the cervical segment and then in the lumbar segment. By this means, balance is achieved, and the weight of the trunk is carried directly over its base. As long as the curves anteriorly and posteriorly balance each other, the erect position can be maintained with surprisingly little muscular effort. The lordotic curves are entirely functional and can be reversed by bending forward, in contrast to the kyphotic thoracic curve, which is structural.

Two essential forces are responsible for the development of these curves. One is the anterior tilt of the pelvis produced by the downward pull of the iliopsoas muscles and the hip capsules, and the other is the extending force of the massive erector spinae muscle. Once the spine is balanced in the erect position, however, the muscular forces in various directions become purely stabilizing. Thus, if the normal erect posture is not disturbed, it is possible to stand with little or no muscular effort, and the ligaments act mainly as check-reins to prevent excessive motion.

Lordosis of the lumbar spine varies among different races, age groups, and sexes. Standardized values of lumbar lordosis in the normal population for these different groups are not available. An average value for the lumbosacral angle is about 135° (Fig. 92–2).[3] Of course, the angle depends on the load on the spine and the position at the time of measurement, whether recumbent, sitting, or standing.

Because of the relative fixation of the pelvis, the lumbosacral junction is subject to a high level of stress. Axial compression can cause flexion, lateral bend, and rotation. Similarly, deformation such as lateral bend may cause rotation, flexion, and axial compression. Most important, depending on the lumbosacral angle, such forces promote shear. The

amount of shear is related to the stiffness of the area. The load on the third lumbar disc is four times greater in an upright than in a recumbent patient. This load becomes six times greater when the patient is standing and is partially bent forward. More recently, lumbar disc pressure and myoelectric activity of spinal muscles have been recorded in subjects in different sitting positions.[4] In the lumbar spine, motion is largely flexion and extension. On bending forward, lumbar lordosis is reversed, and on extension, it is increased. Lateral inclination and rotation occur mainly at the thoracolumbar junction.

Generally speaking, muscles that lie anterior to the small posterior articulations, especially the abdominal muscles, act as flexors, and those posterior act as extensors. The actions of the muscle groups on one side result in lateral inclination. Rotation is produced by more complex muscle combinations. Because many of the spinal motions are performed in the erect position, however, the force of gravity cannot be discounted, and once the motion is started, the opposing muscles are called into play to prevent loss of balance. For instance, on bending to the right, the muscles on the left side of the spine must act to prevent falling to the right. This description of function represents a great oversimplification of spinal kinesiology, but it serves as a basis for understanding the principles discussed elsewhere in this chapter.

FIG. 92–2. The angle between L5 and the sacrum is commonly known as the lumbosacral angle, obtained by measuring the intersection of two lines drawn through the midbodies of L5 and the sacrum and perpendicular to their endplates. The intersection of vertical lines parallel to the anterior border of L5 and the sacrum is known as the promontory angle.

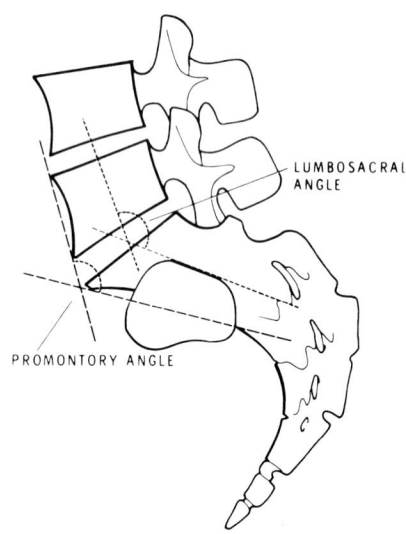

PHYSIOLOGIC CONSIDERATIONS

Another basic consideration is the source and character of the pain itself. Pain from deep skeletal structures and pain from direct nerve pressure must be differentiated. Almost everyone is familiar with direct nerve pressure as the "funny" or "crazy bone" sensation when the ulnar nerve is suddenly bumped. Faradic stimulation of a peripheral mixed nerve causes the same sensation. The onset of pain is rapid; it follows the distribution of the sensory portion of the ulnar nerve and is associated with numbness and tingling when severe. Stimulation of a single spinal nerve root produces a sensation that is the same in character, but is confined to the peripheral representation or dermatome of that nerve root. The pain is sharp, lancinating, and accompanied by paresthesia and numbness. It may also be accompanied by muscle cramps. This is the condition known as neuralgia.

If the pressure is severe and prolonged, the nerve will be deadened, and the property of conduction will be lost even though the fibers are still in continuity. The larger nerve fibers, which mediate touch and motor stimuli, lose their function first, followed by the progressively smaller nerve fibers. Pain fibers, although both large and small, are in general smaller than those for touch and motor conduction, and their function may be unimpaired if pressure is relieved soon enough.

The foregoing properties hold only for sudden forceful pressure on a nerve. In the case of gradual or intermittent pressure, the stimulus may not be sufficient at any time to excite the nerve tissue, and its presence may remain undetected until paresis develops. Such is frequently the case in gradually developing gibbus consequent to tuberculosis.

The pain produced by stimuli within deep skeletal structures, such as a ligament, fascia, muscle, and periosteum, is different. Here the pain is vaguely localized, aching in character, radiating over great distances, slow in onset, and long in duration. When severe, it is often accompanied by sweating, nausea, and vomiting. The patterns of radiation are consistent for one point of stimulation, but the extent of radiation depends on the intensity of stimulation. According to results of experiments, the pattern of radiation is consistent from one individual to another. Although these "sclerotomes" appear to have a segmental representation, they do not follow the patterns of corresponding dermatomes. The sclerotome and dermatome coincide more nearly in the midportion of the trunk than they do in the extremities.

The pain thresholds of different somatic structures are variable. The periosteum is most sensitive, followed by ligaments and fibrous joint capsules, tendons, fasciae, and muscles. Ligaments and capsules are particularly sensitive at points close to their osseous attachments. Bone is usually insensitive, although its endosteal surface apparently contains some pain-perceptive nerves.

The difference between this "deep" pain and the "superficial" pain that can be elicited from touching the skin is important. This difference can be readily demonstrated by pinching a small piece of skin (superficial pain) and by squeezing a web space between the fingers (deep pain). This simple experiment is not completely accurate because touching the skin helps to localize the deep pain elicited. Experimental evidence suggests that the more superficially situated deep structures allow accurate localization of a pain source. Thus, stimulation of periosteum overlying the subcutaneous surface of the tibia can be identified accurately by the subject. Pain from deeply situated periosteum, however, as in the spine, is poorly localized and is diffuse, with radiation to areas distant from the source.

Various kinds of pain may be mediated by changes in the intervertebral disc itself and may result from a decrease in pH or leakage of connective tissue breakdown products. Naylor et al. have reported that lysosomal enzymes present in the nucleus pulposus of the prolapsed intervertebral disc degrade protein polysaccharides,[5] and they postulated a possible autoimmune basis for these biochemical changes. Others have suggested a cellular immune response in patients who have sequestrated discs.[6] The relationship of pain originating from pathologic intervertebral discs with local biochemical changes needs further investigation.

MEDICAL HISTORY AND PHYSICAL EXAMINATION

A general appraisal should include sex, age, race, economic and social background, family and past medical history, and a general review. The patient's type of work and daily habits are important.

ANALYSIS OF THE PATIENT'S PAIN

An analysis of the pain should proceed along two lines: one concerned with the chronologic aspect, such as onset, development, and reaction to previous treatment; the other with the character of this pain. Chronologically, one should ascertain when and where the pain began. Was its onset associated with injury or illness? If the patient was injured, was it on the job or did it involve liability? Has the pain remained the same, worsened, or lessened? Is it intermittent, or has the patient had periods of amelioration or exacerbation? Has the site of pain changed, or has it extended to involve hitherto painless areas? Have any aggravating incidents occurred since its onset? Has the patient had any kind of treatment, self-administrered or otherwise, and with what effect?

The character of the pain may be analyzed in various ways, as follows:

1. *Severity,* an individually variable factor that should be interpreted with caution. Useful indices include inability to work, confinement to bed, and sleeplessness.
2. *Quality,* which is variable and depends much on previous experience. Therefore, its usefulness is questionable. One should differentiate somatic from nerve root pain insofar as possible.
3. *Localization,* a most important criterion, although it is often difficult for the patient to locate the pain accurately. A point of origin is usually recognized. Distal radiation is often present. The extent of radiation in many instances may be used as a

rough index of the severity of the lesion. The type of radiation should be distinguished again, whether it is a nerve root type or the vaguely localized, deep, aching pain so characteristic of irritation of skeletal structures.

4. *Duration*, whether steady or intermittent. If steady, is it at all times the same, or does it have periods of exacerbation? If intermittent, at what times does pain seem to occur? Is it a night or early morning pain suggesting a joint source? Is it a pain associated with work or with activity, suggesting strain, or does it occur only during certain movements?

5. *Reduplication*, either by the patient or by some technique of examination.

6. *Aggravation*. Is the pain aggravated by coughing or sneezing or by bending or lifting, and if so, is it reproduced in full or only in part?

7. *Alleviation*. Is the pain relieved by rest or by any particular types of medication? Is it relieved by manipulation, by gentle activity, or by vigorous exercise?

GENERAL PHYSICAL APPRAISAL

In general, it is sufficient to note whether the person is stocky and heavy-set with heavy musculature, strong ligaments, and tight joints, or whether he is sthenic, tall, and lithe, with a relaxed joint structure, ligaments, and muscles. Are the legs well aligned? Are the feet pronated? Are the knees bowed, straight, or in some valgus position? Are abnormal or suggestive skin pigmentations visible? A café-au-lait mark may signify an underlying neurofibromatosis.

If, in taking the patient's medical history, any points of suspicion have come up relative to systemic diseases, these should be investigated before proceeding with the specific examination of the back.

STANCE AND POSTURE

The posterior aspect of the back is first viewed. It should be noted whether the iliac crests are level, whether the spine is straight or curved, and whether the patient lists to one side or the other. Humans have a strong reflex to keep the head centered over the feet and the eyes level. Thus, in the normal individual, a deviation of the spinal column from the vertical is compensated by an opposite deviation elsewhere whenever possible (Fig. 92–3). From the point of view of the spine, full compensation signifies that the first thoracic vertebra is centered over the sacrum, no mat-

FIG. 92–3. Compensated and uncompensated deviations of posture. *A*, A plumb line dropped from the first thoracic spinal process indicates a right list. *B*, A compensated right thoracolumbar scoliosis. *C*, An uncompensated right thoracic, left lumbar scoliosis with right list. List or decompensation causes prominence of the hip opposite to the direction of the list.

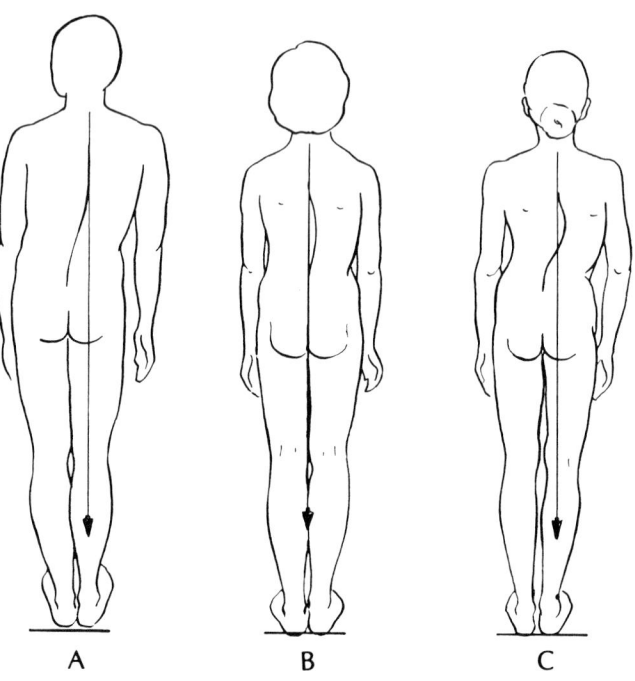

ter what the spine does in between. If the spine is uncompensated, that is, if the first thoracic vertebra is not centered over the sacrum, the patient is spoken of as having a *list*. A convenient measurement of list is to drop a perpendicular line from the first thoracic vertebra and to measure how far to the right or left of the gluteal cleft it falls. If a list is present, a lateral curvature of the spine (scoliosis) must also be present. Scoliosis may be classified as structural or nonstructural. In the former, intrinsic structural changes of the vertebral column and thoracic rib cage are present and may be detected by asking the patient to bend forward and by viewing the trunk from posteriorly. Asymmetry is then noted, with the high side on the convex side of the curve. In nonstructural scoliosis, no intrinsic anatomic changes occur, and no asymmetry is found on forward bending. Nonstructural scoliosis commonly occurs secondary to pain and may be termed "sciatic scoliosis."

Scoliosis is designated right or left, depending on the direction of its convexity; right scoliosis indicates a curve convex to the right. The curve pattern of the scoliosis is designated by the apex of the curve. A thoracic curve has its apex at the thoracic level; a thoracolumbar curve has its apex at the junction of the thoracic and lumbar spine; and a lumbar curve has its apex at the lumbar level. Usually, the pelvis is level in nonstructural and structural scoliosis. If not, some other causes for the pelvic obliquity should be sought, such as a gross decompensation of the curves or a short leg or a hip contracture.

The patient is then viewed from the side, and the posture is noted. It is normal to stand with a slight degree of lumbar lordosis and thoracic kyphosis. Increase or decrease of these curves should be noted. Muscle spasm in acute low-back pain often causes flattening of the lumbar lordosis. In the sagittal plane, as well as in the transverse plane, man usually maintains balance, that is, has the head centered over the feet. The curves in between generally balance one another. Thus, if the thoracic kyphosis is increased, the lumbar lordosis is usually increased. Sometimes, such a state of affairs does not exist, and to balance an increased thoracic kyphosis, the patient stands with a posterior *overcarriage,* that is, leaning backward. Overcarriage is to the sagittal plane what list is to the transverse plane.

The degree of forward inclination of the pelvis should be noted. Is the abdomen pendulous and is the chest well-developed, or does the patient stand with a narrow anteroposterior thoracic diameter? Persons of the thin body type often have a narrow chest, and those of the heavy body type often have the opposite.

An analysis of stance is completed by a brief survey from anteriorly. Again, list may be noted, and the anterior superior iliac spines should be palpated to check whether the pelvis is level. Slight degrees of curvature of the spine are difficult to detect, especially in heavy-set persons. Certain signs may lead one to suspect the presence of a structural scoliosis, that is, a prominent hip, a flank crease on one side or the other, prominence of one side of the chest or of the opposite shoulder blade, or a high shoulder.

SPINAL MOTIONS

The spine is now analyzed in motion (Figs. 92–4, 92–5). One again views the patient from posteriorly. He is asked to bend forward. The lordotic curve of the lumbar spine should first flatten and should then reverse slightly as the degree of forward bending increases. If it does not do so, motion will be limited, even though the patient is able to touch the floor. The patient should be watched to see whether he bends straight forward or whether he lists to one side as he bends forward. Listing may suggest restriction of

straight leg raising on the opposite side. If scoliosis has been detected in the erect position, the flexed position should be checked to determine whether it is structural. The associated rotation of the vertebrae produces a prominence of the thorax and overlying scapula on the side of convexity. In lumbar scoliosis, the rotation is not so readily evident, but it can be detected by prominence of the paravertebral muscles on the side of the convexity and a depression of those on the opposite side. In patients with a slight degree of scoliosis, forward flexion is the best position for detection because it accentuates the deformity. When the patient is bent forward, it is also wise to view his back from the side. Usually, one sees a smooth curve with its convexity posteriorly extending from the base of the skull to the sacrum. If the curve is broken and becomes more sharply angular at any point, it should be recorded. Such is often the case in structural round back, that is, "epiphysitis" of the spine.

The degree of backward bending is then determined. This bending is accompanied by an increase in the lordotic curve. If the degree of lordosis does not increase, the motion is limited. On returning to the upright position, the patient is asked to bend to one side and then to the other. The normal spine has an equivalent degree of bending to both sides with a smooth curve starting at the sacrum. Limitation of motion can be detected in one of two ways. The maximal degree of motion may not be as much to one side as to the other, or the curve on bending to one side may be broken and may begin at a higher level than it does to the other side.

In examination of the lower back, the motions of flexion, extension, and lateral bending are the most important. It is often wise, however, to check the whole spine, and the patient should be asked to demonstrate the degree of rotation by placing his fingers behind his neck. This motion occurs chiefly in the thoracic region. The degree of cervical lordosis and cervical motions should also be noted. The findings are rechecked in the sitting position, where normally the lordosis flattens and scoliosis, if functional, disappears.

MEASUREMENTS

The patient is next asked to lie supine on the examining table. A patient in acute pain can be made more comfortable if a pillow is placed under the knees. Measurements of the thigh and calf at equivalent points superior and inferior to the patellae should be made and recorded. Atrophy may be due to disuse or to neuromuscular disease. The patient is

THE DORSAL AND LUMBAR SPINE (FLEXION)

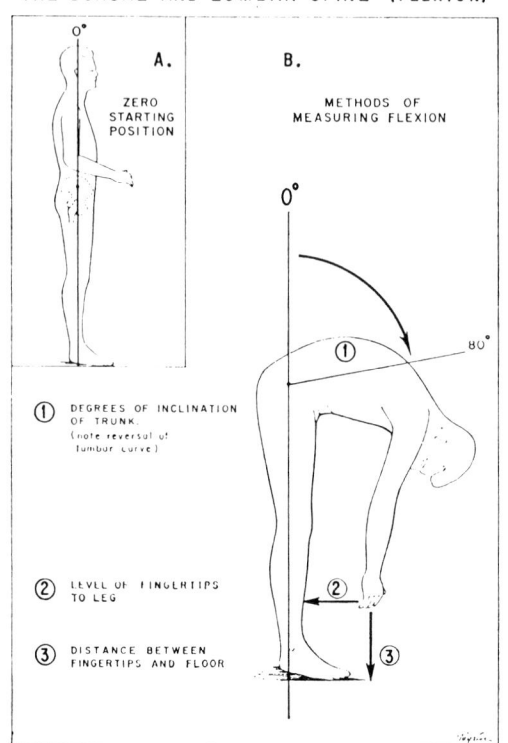

A.

ZERO
STARTING
POSITION

B.

METHODS OF
MEASURING FLEXION

0°

80°

① DEGREES OF INCLINATION
OF TRUNK.
(note reversal of
lumbar curve)

② LEVEL OF FINGERTIPS
TO LEG

③ DISTANCE BETWEEN
FINGERTIPS AND FLOOR

THE DORSAL AND LUMBAR SPINE
LATERAL BENDING

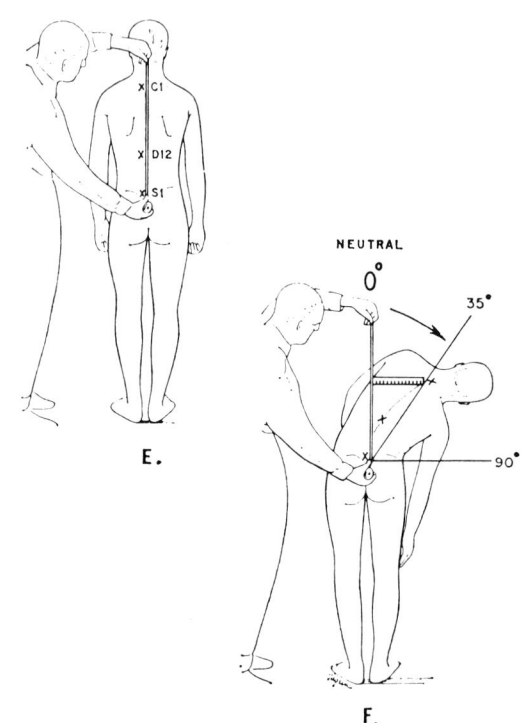

E.

NEUTRAL

0°

35°

90°

F.

(Continuation)
METHODS OF
MEASURING
SPINAL
FLEXION

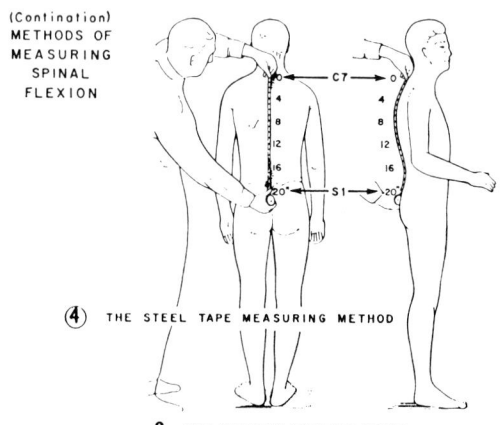

④ THE STEEL TAPE MEASURING METHOD

C. THE PATIENT STANDING ERECT

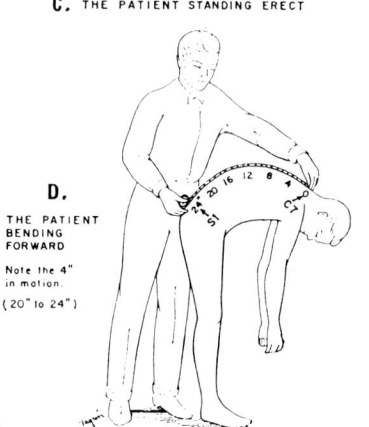

D.

THE PATIENT
BENDING
FORWARD

Note the 4"
in motion.
(20" to 24")

THE DORSAL AND LUMBAR SPINE (EXTENSION)

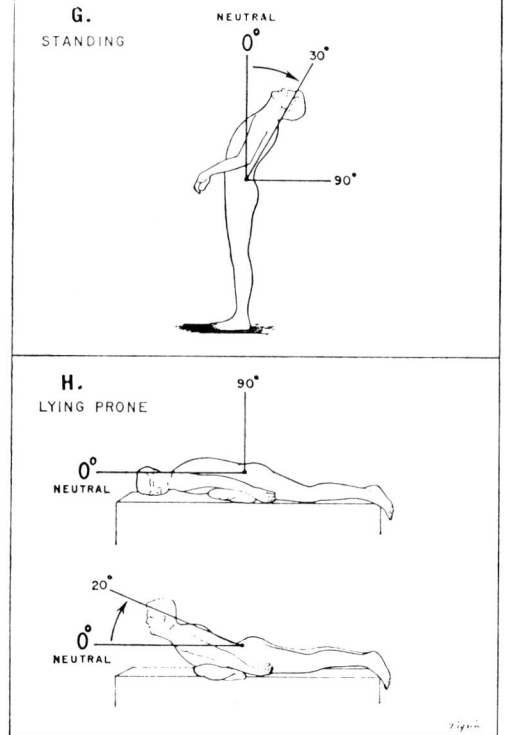

G.
STANDING

NEUTRAL

0°

30°

90°

H.
LYING PRONE

90°

0°
NEUTRAL

20°

0°
NEUTRAL

FIG. 92–4. (Legend on Facing Page)

FIG. 92–4. Measurement of spinal motion. *A,* Zero starting position, the correct standing position. *B,* Flexion. Four clinical methods of estimating the range of spinal flexion are used: (1) by measuring the degrees of forward inclination of the trunk in relation to the longitudinal axis of the body; the examiner should "fix" the pelvis with his hands; the loss (or not) of lordosis should also be noted; (2) by indicating the level the fingertips reach along the patient's leg; for instance, fingertips to the patella or fingertips to the midtibia; (3) by measuring the distance in inches or centimeters between the fingertips and the floor; and (4) by the steel or plastic tape measure method. *C,* The steel tape measure method (4), perhaps the most accurate clinical method of measuring true motion of the spine in flexion. The flexible steel or plastic tape adjusts accurately to the thoracic and lumbar contours of the spine. *D,* As the patient bends forward, the reversal of the lumbar curve and the spread of the spinous processes can be indicated by lengthening the tape measure. The normal healthy adult has an average increase of 4 inches in forward flexion. If the patient bends forward with his back straight (as in ankylosing spondylitis), the tape measure will not record motion. One is able to record motion of the thoracic spine itself by taping from the spinous process of C7 to T12. Similarly, motion of the lumbar spine can be measured from the spinous process of T12 to S1. Usually, if the increase in the total spine in flexion is 4 inches, the examiner will find that 1 inch occurs in the dorsal spine and 3 inches occur in the lumbar spine. *E* and *F,* Lateral bending. The vertical steel tape, if held firmly and straight, may also aid in measuring the motion of lateral bending. This can be estimated by: (1) the degrees of lateral inclination of the trunk; (2) noting the position of spinous process of C7 with relation to the pelvis; (3) using the level of lumbar spine as a reflection of the base of lateral motion; this level may be lumbosacral or higher and may vary from right to left in the same patient; and (4) using the knee joint as a fixed point; one should record the distance of the fingertips from the knee joint on lateral bending. *G,* Extension standing. The range of extension is recorded by degrees. *H,* Extension lying prone. The range of motion in this position is measured by degrees, in relation to the position of the spinous process of C7. *I,* Rotation. To estimate the degrees of rotation of the spine, the pelvis must be held firmly by the examiner's hands, and the patient is instructed to rotate to the right or left. This motion is recorded in degrees, or in percentages of motion, as compared to persons of similar age and physical build.

I. THE SPINE — ROTATION

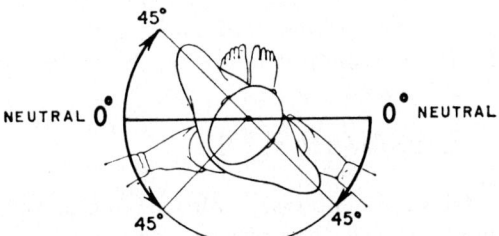

next carefully positioned so that the pelvis is level and the hips are placed in a neutral degree of abduction and adduction. The leg lengths are then recorded, using the bony landmarks of the anterior superior iliac spine and medial malleolus. In the presence of a fixed deformity of one hip, the measurement loses some significance. For measurements to be accurate, the lower extremities must have equivalent relationships with the pelvis.

HIP MOTIONS

The hip movements are now analyzed (Fig. 92–6). Flexion contracture is noted by maximally flexing the opposite hip to flatten the lumbar lordosis and by measuring the degree of the angle between the horizontal surface of the table and the maximally extended extremity. The movements of each hip in abduction, adduction, and internal and external rotation should be measured. The arcs of rotation are usually most easily obtained by rotating the foot and leg inward (external rotation) and outward (internal rotation) with the hips flexed to 90°.

PASSIVE SPINAL MOVEMENTS

Movements of the lumbar spine are now performed passively by grasping the patient's legs with the knees bent and by flexing the spine maximally. With the patient's hips flexed to 90°, the pelvis is then inclined laterally and is rotated on the spine. Note is made if these motions produce pain.

PALPATION AND TENDERNESS

The patient is next asked to lie prone with a pillow under his abdomen (Fig. 92–7). The thickness of the pillow should be sufficient to flatten the lumbar lordosis. The lower spine and the structures of the back are carefully palpated. Tightness or spasm of paravertebral muscles is noted. At all times, the patient must be fully relaxed. Just as in examination of the abdomen, the anatomic structures under the examining finger must constantly be kept in mind. The spine of each lumbar vertebra is pressed, and the interspaces between are palpated. It is sometimes advantageous to examine the flexed patient lying on his side, to palpate more easily the bony spinous processes and the interspinous ligaments. Adjacent spinous processes can be grasped from the side by the examiner and can be rotated in opposite directions to

FIG. 92–5. Forward bending. *A,* Normally on forward bending, one sees an even contour of the spine when viewed laterally. *B,* An accentuation of the thoracic kyphosis indicates a thoracic round back, especially when the apex of the curve is sharp and angular. *C,* A persistence of the angular lordotic curve in the position of forward bending indicates that the lumbar spine has lost its flexibility. The flexion is all taking place at the hip joints. *D,* When viewed posteriorly, minor degrees of structural scoliosis can readily be detected in the position of forward bending. The convex rotation of the thoracic vertebrae is easily recognized because it is accentuated by the rib deformity or hump. Similar rotation of the lumbar segment is more difficult to detect.

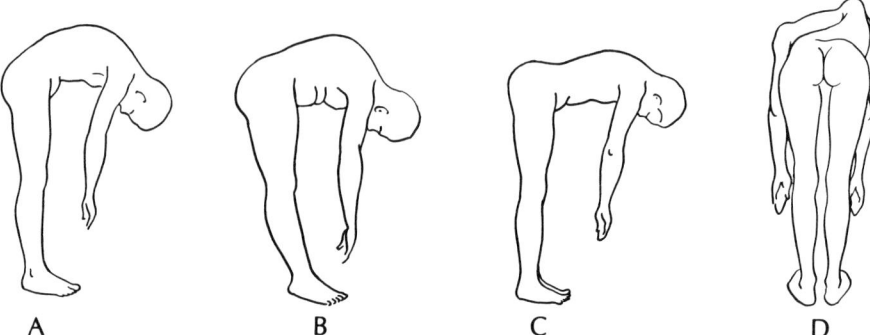

FIG. 92–6. Lumbar lordosis and hip flexion contracture. An inability to fully extend one or both hips may produce an increase in the lumbar lordosis in the standing or lying positions. The angle of the deformity can be determined by flattening the lordosis, by maximum flexion of the opposite hip. *A,* Normal, *B,* Flexion deformity of the hip masked by an increase in the lumbar lordosis. *C,* Flexion of the opposite hip flattening the lumbar spine to the table and indicating the true situation.

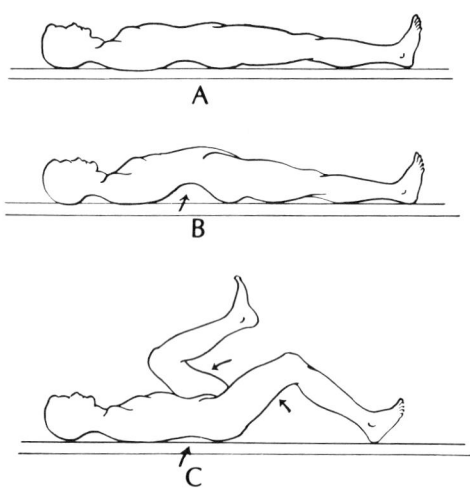

determine the source of pain. Useful landmarks are the iliac crests, where a horizontal line bisects the fourth lumbar process, and the posterior superior iliac spines, which lie opposite the second sacral spine. The sacrosciatic notch is palpated when tenderness may indicate irritation of one or more roots of the sciatic nerve. The patient's thighs and calves must also be palpated when pain extends into the legs. The region of the trochanters should also be examined.

PERCUSSION TENDERNESS

Pressure or percussion over the interlaminal spaces may, in patients with disc herniation, produce sharp, lancinating pain radiating to the lower extremities. Because lumbar lordosis is increased in the position of extension, the vertebral spinous processes are brought closer together, and it is difficult to distinguish the separate processes. For this reason, it is most important to have the patient's back flattened or the lumbar lordosis reversed. If this effect cannot be achieved in the prone position with a pillow under the abdomen, the patient may be asked to bend over the examining table (Fig. 92–8). He can usually do this despite the presence of pain, if the knees are flexed and the weight is borne on the abdomen.

RECTAL EXAMINATION

A rectal examination is usually advisable, especially in patients with coccygeal pain. The coccyx may be

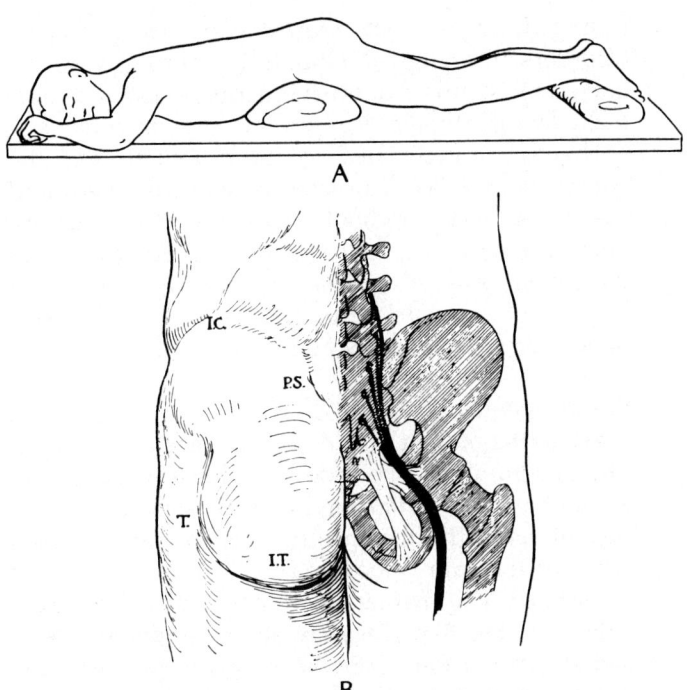

FIG. 92–7. Palpation of the back. *A,* Proper positioning is necessary for adequate examination. When the lumbar spine is flat, the bony elements are more easily distinguished from one another. The interspinous and interlaminal spaces are opened. *B,* Useful landmarks include the iliac crest (I.C.), the posterior superior iliac spine (P.S.), the greater trochanters (T), and the ischial tuberosities (I.T.). The position of the sacrosciatic notch and the course of the sciatic nerve should be kept in mind. The lumbar roots are shielded from palpation in their extraspinal course.

FIG. 92–8. Percussion test. With the patient positioned as shown, the interlaminal spaces are opened as much as possible. In the case of irritation of a nerve root, sharp percussion or deep pressure may reproduce the sciatic distribution of pain, especially in the presence of disc herniation because the nerve root is forced posteriorly in the spinal cord. This position is also useful for palpation of the back, particularly for examination of the sacroiliac joints.

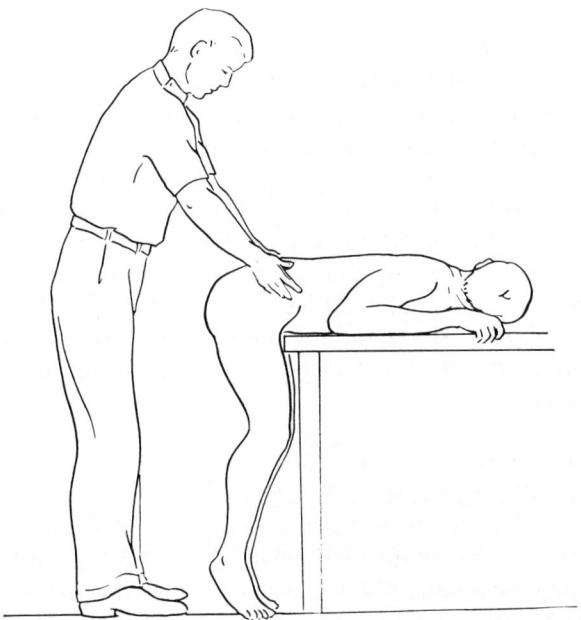

grasped between the finger in the rectum and the thumb outside, and it can be moved about. One should note the angle of inclination of the coccyx, its freedom of movement, and the presence of pain on movement. The levator ani and coccygeus muscles and the sacrotuberous and sacrospinalis ligaments are palpated on either side of the sacrum, and tenderness is noted. In thin persons, the region of the sacrosciatic notch can often be reached, and bimanual palpation of this region is possible. The rectal examination is completed with palpation of the pelvic viscera. Tenderness in the sacroiliac joint may be elicited by pressure exerted over it. This joint lies between the posterior inferior spine and superior border of the sciatic notch. Bimanual vaginal examination with cytologic smear should be performed when indicated.

NEUROLOGIC EXAMINATION

It is important to analyze the knee and ankle jerks. The best position for eliciting knee jerks is having the patient sitting with the legs hanging free; that for ankle jerks is having the patient kneeling on a chair with a pillow under the legs and the feet projecting outward from the edge of the seat. If necessary, the reflexes can be reinforced if the patient contracts the muscles of the upper extremities with the fingers locked together. In reflexes tested carefully in this fashion, small discrepancies are of much greater significance than when testing is done casually. Gluteus maximus, medial hamstring, and posterior tibial reflex responses should also be determined, but they are more difficult to elicit and, therefore, are most significant when absent on one side and present on the other. Babinski's sign is also tested.

Sensory examination is performed with the point of a pin and light stroke of the finger or cotton. Significant zones of sensory disturbance may be found in this manner, and if so, the examination can be repeated in more detail, including heat and cold sensation.

Atrophy of the buttocks is determined by inspection and palpation. Although atrophy of thigh and calf muscles may be seen, circumferential measurements are helpful to document the degree of atrophy and to follow the response to therapeutic exercises. The ability to walk on tiptoe and on the heel, the ability to do a deep knee bend, and the ability to stand on one leg alone should be tested. The manner of walking should be observed, and the cause of limp, if one is present, should be determined. More accurate analysis of motor function is done by testing the strength of muscle action in various planes, but such an evaluation may be omitted for practical purposes unless some previous point of the patient's medical history or physical examination leads one to suspect nerve root compression. The power of dorsiflexion of the great toe, of the lateral four toes, and of the entire foot should be analyzed and should be compared on the two sides. Similarly, the forces of inversion, eversion, and plantar flexion of the foot and of the toes can be tested. Powers of hip flexion when sitting and of knee extension when supine are easily determined. When the patient is in pain or when movement is accompanied by pain, weakness of function should be given less significance. Moreover, the inability of some patients, especially older ones, to coordinate may interfere with muscle examinations of this kind.

SPECIAL TESTS

Straight Leg Raising Test of Lasegue

This test is one of the most useful maneuvers in analysis of low-back disorders (Fig. 92–9). First, it stretches the roots of the lumbosacral plexus by putting tension on the sciatic nerve, a tension that increases as the leg is raised higher. Second, it flattens the lumbar spine by putting tension on the extensor muscles of the hip and hamstrings as they pass from the pelvis to the femur and tibia. Thus, a nerve root lesion is not prerequisite for painful or restricted leg raising. On the other hand, restriction of straight leg raising is usually much more marked in lesions af-

fecting the nerve roots than it is in purely skeletal disorders. The angle of straight leg raising, which is limited by tightness of the hamstring muscles, is normally less in sthenic than it is in asthenic persons.

The test is performed by the examiner, and the patient must relax. The knee is held extended, and the leg is raised gradually from the table until the point of pain is reached. This point is recorded, and the patient is asked to describe the extent and radiation of the pain. In nerve root lesions, the typical pattern of radiation may be reproduced.

Sitting Knee Extension Test

While the patient is sitting, one knee is extended. The patient should be observed to see whether and at what angle of extension he leans backward. If the patient finds the test painful, he should be asked whether the pain is localized to his back or whether it radiates. The maneuver is repeated on the other side, and the two sides are then compared. Occasionally, extension of one knee aggravates "sciatica" in the opposite leg. This test is similar to straight leg raising, but with one major difference; that is, in the sitting position, the lumbar lordosis is usually largely obliterated.

Popliteal Compression Test

Radiating pain produced either by sitting knee extension or by straight leg raising can often be aggravated by pressure over the course of the tibial nerve through the popliteal space. This finding also suggests nerve root compression.

Jugular Compression Test (Naffziger Test)

This test should be performed whenever one suspects involvement of the spinal cord or nerve roots. A blood pressure cuff around the neck is inflated to 40 mm Hg and is held in place for a minute. The cerebrospinal fluid pressure is increased. The patient is asked to indicate when and if the pain is reproduced and if it is reproduced accurately. When the exact pattern of the patient's leg pain is reproduced, the test is practically pathognomonic of an intraspinal lesion. A negative test result, however, is not as significant.

Iliac Compression Test

Of all the tests described as pathognomonic of sacroiliac disease, the test of iliac compression is the most sensitive. It is performed most easily with the patient lying on his side. The examiner applies firm pressure against the uppermost iliac crest. When the test is positive, pain will be produced in the region of the involved sacroiliac joint. Other signs of sacroiliac dis-

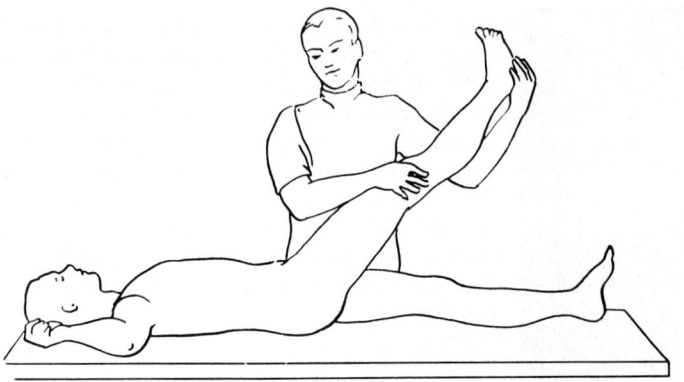

FIG. 92–9. Straight leg raising. The leg being tested should be relaxed and should rest in the examiner's hand. The knee is fully extended and is kept from flexing by gentle pressure against the patella.

ease are pain in the region of the sacroiliac joint on passive abduction of one or both hips while flexed, tenderness along the superior bony margin of the sacroiliac notch, lower quadrant abdominal tenderness, and tenderness in the region of the sacroiliac joint on rectal examination. (See also Chapter 4 for the technique of determining tenderness in this joint.)

Passive Extension Test

This test is performed with the patient lying on his back at the foot of the examining table. The extremities are supported by the examiner with the hips and knees flexed. First, the uninvolved lower extremity is lowered. No pain is produced. The involved leg is then gradually lowered, to extend the spine, and pain develops. The unaffected extremity is then flexed maximally, thus flattening the lumbar spine, and the pain is relieved. If this test produces pain with radiation similar to that which the patient experiences spontaneously, it is suggestive of nerve root compression. Other lesions of the back, however, may be associated with pain on hyperextension.

The back examination is now finished. It requires considerable exertion by the patient and may not be possible to complete. After a day or two of rest and sedation, a more satisfactory analysis can often be made, however.

DIAGNOSTIC MODALITIES

RADIOGRAPHIC EXAMINATION

A routine examination of the back is not complete unless roentgenograms have been made. To the trained observer, anteroposterior and lateral views of the entire lumbar spine and sacrum often suffice. First, anteroposterior and lateral views are made of the lumbar spine, with the x-ray tube centered at the upper lumbar region and inclined slightly distally (10°) (Fig. 92–10). A true or 45° anteroposterior view

of the lumbosacral region is then obtained (Fig. 92–11). For this view, the direction of the x-ray tube is adjusted to the inclination of the sacrum. The actual angle of the tube is usually nearer 30° than 45°. The x-ray tube itself is centered opposite the third or fourth lumbar vertebra. Details of the vertebral bodies, the sacrum, and the sacroiliac and intervertebral joints should be adequate to detect significant abnormalities, including defects of the neural arch and facets.

Special roentgenographic views are used to obtain better detail of spinal parts or to detect the presence of specific pathologic processes. Oblique views show the intervertebral foramina and lesions of the neural arch and facets exceptionally well, but the technique is difficult (Fig. 92–12). A posteroanterior film made with the patient standing, bending first to the right and then to the left, is often helpful in diagnosing the level of a disc lesion. If the restriction of lateral movement is diffuse throughout the lumbar spine, such views are of no help, but if the restriction of lateral bending is confined to one disc space and to one side only, it suggests a pathologic condition at this level. Lateral roentgenograms of the lumbosacral spine in full flexion and extension are occasionally useful to demonstrate an anteroposterior instability in the early stages of disc degeneration, but they are mainly indicated for postoperative study of spinal lesions.

Myelography

Radiologic visualization of neural structures of the spinal canal is obtained by myelographic examination. Myelograms are used to determine compression of the spinal cord or nerve roots by tumor, intervertebral disc herniation, osteophyte formation, or other bony ridges. Complete blocks or narrowing of the neurocanal by spinal stenosis may also be seen. The accepted technique in the past was to introduce an oil-contrast medium into the subarachnoid space (iophendylate [Pantopaque] myelography) (Fig. 92–13). The oil-contrast medium has a minimal immediate

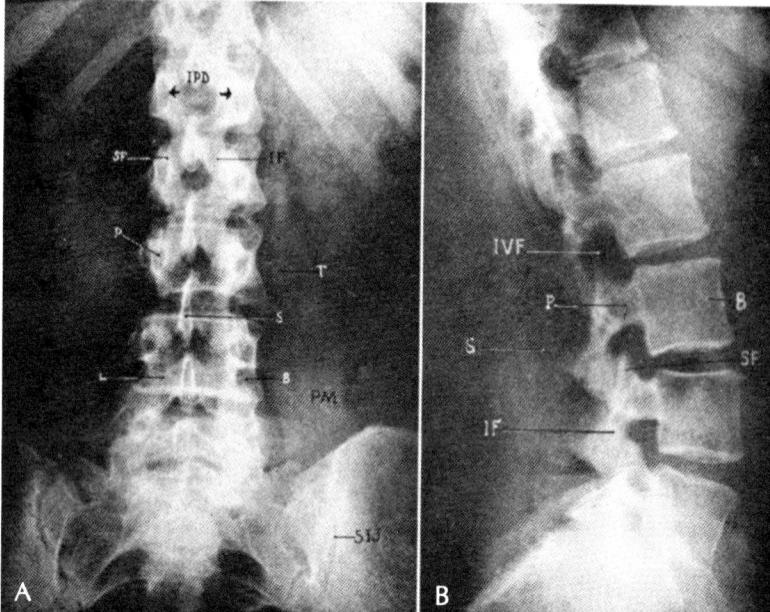

FIG. 92–10. Roentgenograms of the normal spine. *A,* Anteroposterior and *B,* lateral films of the lumbar spine. Note the detail of most of the lumbar spine, but the obscurity of the lumbosacral region. B = Body; D = disc space; I = isthmus, or pars interarticularis; IF = inferior facet; IVF = intervertebral foramen; L = lamina; P = pedicle; PM = psoas margin; S = spinous process; SF = superior facet; SIJ = sacroiliac joint; T = transverse process; and IPD = interpedicular diameter.

neurotoxic effect, but if allowed to remain in the spinal canal for extended periods, it may cause arachnoiditis. Consequently, at the end of the procedure the contrast material is generally removed. The dye is usually introduced by injection into the lower lumbar spine and may be used to visualize the neurocanal from the lumbar to the cervical spine. Few side effects occur other than transient headaches. The technique is safe when performed by experienced physicians. Usually, myelograms are indicated only when surgical treatment is considered.

Because oil has a high density, the nerve root sheaths may be incompletely filled. Water-soluble contrast agents have a lower viscosity and allow better filling of the nerve root sheaths. Such agents do not have to be removed because they are rapidly absorbed from the subarachnoid space. Presently a water-soluble medium, metrizamide, is used (Fig. 92–14).

Metrizamide Myelography

Of the many water-soluble agents used as contrast media in myelography today, metrizamide (Amipaque) is still the most popular (Fig. 92–14). Metrizamide was developed by the Norwegian company Nyegaard on the theory that a nonionic compound would result in lower osmolarity and would produce

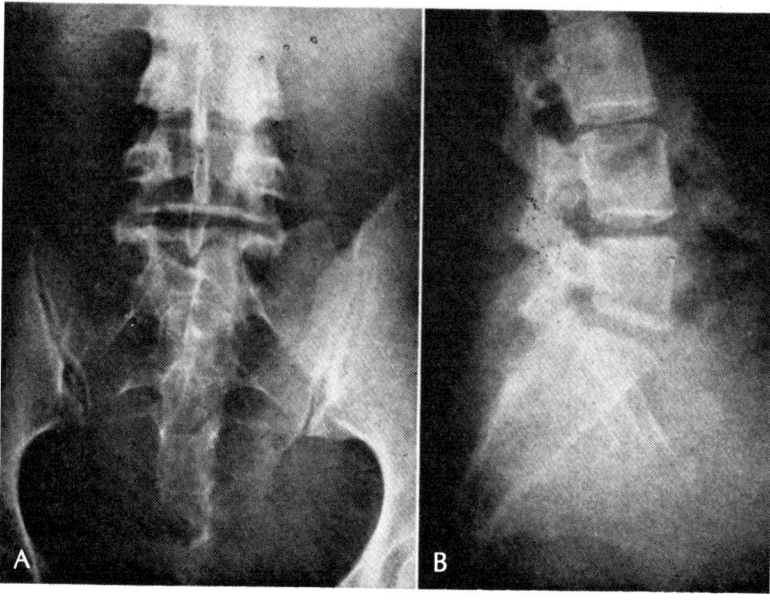

FIG. 92–11. Forty-five degree anteroposterior *(A)* and lateral *(B)* roentgenograms of the lumbosacral level and the sacrum. Note the detail of the fifth lumbar vertebra, sacrum, lumbosacral disc space, and sacroiliac joints.

FIG. 92–12. Oblique roentgenogram of the lumbar spine. Note the detail of the facets and the pars interarticularis. SF = Superior facet; T = transverse process; P = pedicle; I = isthmus, or pars interarticularis; and IF = inferior facet.

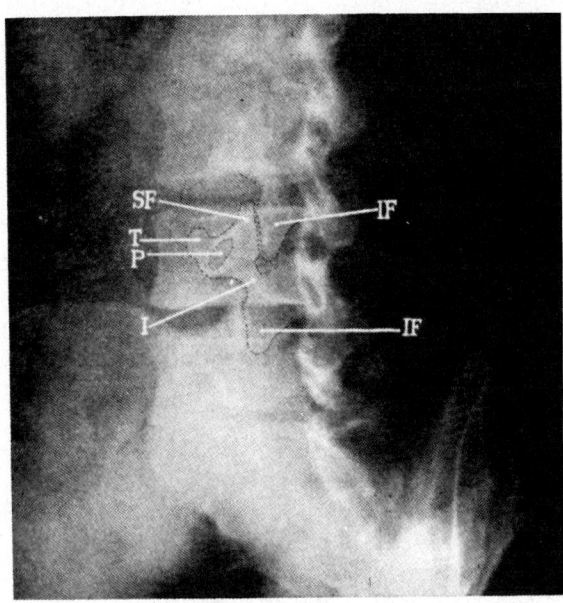

fewer adverse effects. Nonetheless, the two major possible complications are grand mal seizures and arachnoiditis.[7]

A nonionic water-soluble opaque medium (iohexol) has been introduced for clinical use.[8] This contrast agent, used extensively in European countries, may eventually replace metrizamide because of its safety and diagnostic advantages.

We prepare patients for metrizamide myelography by hydration the night before and after the procedure. Phenothiazine derivatives, which interact with this contrast medium by lowering the convulsion threshold, should be withheld for at least 48 hours prior to the myelogram. Other drugs with similar effects are monoamine oxidase inhibitors, tricyclic antidepressants, analeptic agents, and central nervous system stimulants. Patients are positioned with their head elevated at least 30° following the procedure. If the patient has to be supine, the neck is maintained flexed to prevent the agent from traveling above the cervical spine. An aqueous technique may be used for lumbar myelograms as well as for thoracic and cervical myelograms. The agent provides less contrast ability in the superior spine, but it is satisfactory.

The use of computed tomography (CT) with aqueous myelograms has been rewarding in establishing more definitive diagnoses of tumors, spinal stenosis, and congenital anomalies.

Discography

Visualization of the internal structures of a disc by the injection of radiopaque absorbable compounds may be helpful in the diagnosis of disc degeneration. Lumbar discography is still controversial, but is used by many physicians. The examination is performed under local anesthesia with premedication. The contrast medium is a mixture of 50% diatrizoate (Hypaque) and 1% procaine. The normal disc accepts as much as 2 ml fluid, depending on its size. If the disc is ruptured, the contrast material escapes. The technique and interpretation vary according to experience.

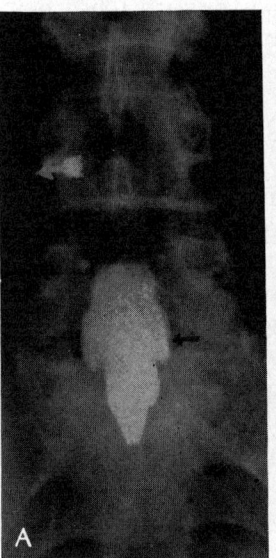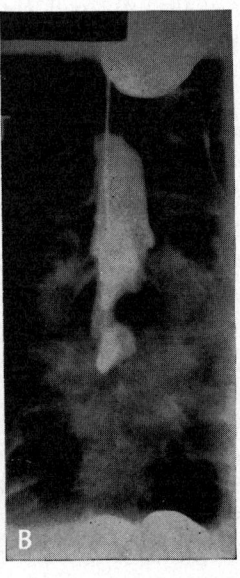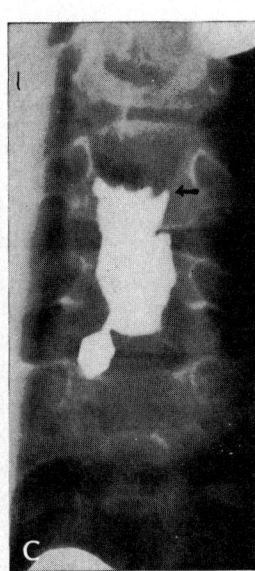

FIG. 92–13. Myelogram. *A,* Normal filling of the lower end of the dural sac. The axillary pouches (nerve root sheaths) are well visualized at the lumbosacral level *(black arrow).* To complete the examination, each intervertebral level must be similarly visualized until the interior end of the spinal cord is reached. *B,* A filling defect on the left side at the level of the fifth lumbar disc. A disc herniation is likely, although a cyst or a tumor is possible. *C,* Complete block of the spinal canal *(arrow)* through which the contrast material cannot pass. Such a block indicates a tumor of the cauda equina. It is rarely seen in disc herniation.

FIG. 92–14. Metrizamide myelogram. A filling defect is noted at the L4-L5 interspace. The arrow points to blunting of the L5 nerve root sleeve from a protruding disc.

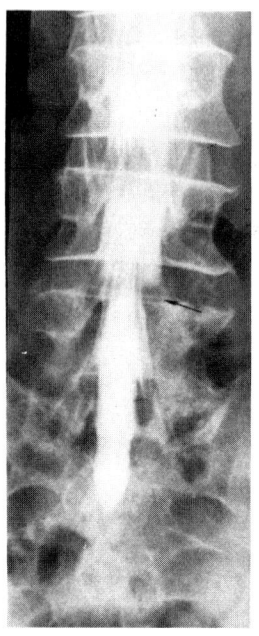

FIG. 92–15. [99m]Technetium diphosphonate scan of the vertebral column. The dark area in the upper spine illustrates an area of increased radioactive uptake confirming an osteoid osteoma of the thoracic spine. Note the spinal curvature (scoliosis) characteristically associated with this lesion.

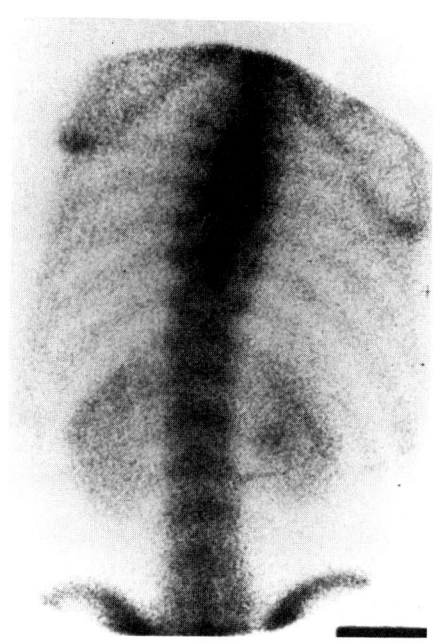

Radioactive Scanning

Radionuclides have been used extensively in the diagnosis of bone diseases associated with increased calcium turnover. Scanning agents such as [85]Sr and ^{18}F have been used.[9] The diagnosis of osteoid osteoma has been facilitated by scintimetric examination.[10] At present, the scanning agent of choice is [99m]technetium-Sn-polyphosphate (or diphosphonate) (Fig. 92–15).

MAGNETIC RESONANCE IMAGING (MRI)

Magnetic resonance imaging (MRI) has recently been used in the evaluation of the spine for normal anatomy and pathological disorders.[11] MRI is a noninvasive technique with many potentials for evaluating spinal conditions. Its complete role at this time is not well-defined because of lack of sufficient experience. Of the 16 posterior disc ruptures found by CT scan in one study, 12 were also recognized by MRI.[12]

The role of MRI as an adjunct to or replacement of invasive methods of evaluation of spinal disorders will become better defined with time.

ELECTROMYOGRAPHY

Electromyography is the study of spontaneous involuntary electric waves generated in a motor unit and recorded by a coaxial electrode attached to an oscilloscope. In a typical nerve root compression syndrome, muscles innervated by the involved roots show fibrillation potentials. The technique is a useful adjunct in the diagnosis of nerve root compression and in localizing its level. It may be particularly helpful in patients with questionable neurologic findings.

SOMATOSENSORY EVOKED POTENTIALS

The technique of stimulating peripheral nerves in the extremities and recording electrical potentials in the scalp was first described by Dawson.[13] In the past 10 years, this technique has been used by Nash and his colleagues for monitoring spinal cord function during spinal operations on patients with scoliosis.[14,15] Modifications of this technique using surface electrodes on the spine provide spinal evoked potentials that may be helpful as a noninvasive test for evaluating spinal cord and cauda equina lesions. We have used this technique at the Hospital for Special Surgery in a small group of patients with congenital spinal deformities as a screening test in evaluating spinal cord or peripheral nerve lesions. Once greater familiarity with this technique is gained, it should help physicians to localize low back pain with nerve root involvement.

CONDITIONS PREDISPOSING PATIENTS TO SPRAIN SYNDROMES

FAULTY POSTURE

Poor posture is prevalent and can be classified into two groups. The first type is *functional*, in which the position of faulty posture is correctable. It is common in children and is progressively less frequent in older age groups. The second is a *structural* group, in which the deformity is fixed. The cervical lordosis is increased; the thoracic spine is rounded, and its motion is limited. An exaggerated lordotic lumbar curve may become fixed owing to shortening of the sacrospinalis muscles. If so, the interspinous ligaments become contracted so that the tips of the spinous processes and facets "kiss." Conversely, the abdominal muscles overstretch and relax, a process that may be accelerated by pregnancies and obesity. The pelvis tilts more anteriorly than normal, and the hip flexor muscles shorten. The lumbosacral angle increases. When the patient is asked to bend forward, he cannot obliterate his lumbar curve as he normally would. Often, one sees secondary degenerative changes on x-ray examination.

In the purely functional state, faulty posture is rarely painful; at most, it may cause fatigue and backache. When the position becomes fixed, however, the symptoms are more likely to be bothersome.

SPONDYLOLISTHESIS

Generally, this term means a slipped vertebra, but clinically it is associated only with anterior displacement of one vertebra on the next inferior vertebra (Figs. 92–16, 92–17). The classification of spondylolisthesis that is now generally accepted is dysplastic, degenerative, traumatic, and pathologic.[16]

Dysplastic Type
A congenital dysplasia of the upper sacrum or neural arch of L5 allows the upper lumbar vertebra to slip forward.

Isthmic defects are present in the portions of the vertebral arch lying between the superior and inferior articular processes (pars defects). The defect may be unilateral or bilateral. Three types of defects have been recognized: (1) lytic, with fatigue fracture of the pars interarticularis; (2) with an elongated but intact pars; and (3) involving acute fracture of the pars interarticularis.

When bilateral defects are present, the anterior vertebral body may slip forward while the posterior arch remains behind; the result is a true spondylolisthesis. If the pars defect occurs without forward slip, the condition is termed *spondylolysis*.

The cause of the basic neural arch defect is still the subject of some controversy. Willis found spondylolysis in 4% of adult skeletal specimens, but not in fetal skeletons.[17] We have encountered it in identical twins and in several members of the same family. These findings indicate a predisposing factor, such as vulnerability of the pars interarticularis, which is congenital and may be genetically determined, whereas the final condition is produced by wear and tear or trauma.[18]

Spondylolisthesis is usually qualified by the amount of forward displacement, first degree for one-quarter anteroposterior-vertebral-diameter displacement and fourth degree for full-diameter displacement. Although it is uncommon to see the condition progress in adults, it is not unusual in children. The fibrous tissue bridging the defects, the structure of the disc, and the intervertebral ligaments must give and stretch, so the vertical body, pedicles, and superior facets can slip away from the detached portion of the neural arch, which includes the laminae, spinous process, and inferior facets. Pseudarthroses may develop in the sites of defective ossification if the degree of slipping is minimal because movements of the spine cause false motion between the two vertebral segments.

Several syndromes are caused by spondylolisthesis. First, the condition may be silent or the symptoms associated with it may be inconsequential. Second, back pain may arise from the pseudarthrosis or from the wear and tear of the disc joint, which has slipped. In this connection, herniation of such a disc has been described, but we have not encountered it. Third, unilateral or bilateral sciatica may be caused by root impingement resulting from hypertrophy of the fibrous tissue in one or both defects, or by traction on the roots secondary to forward displacement, especially when the defects are situated low in the superior articular processes. Fourth, the displacement may be so severe that a lesion of the whole cauda equina is produced, in part from traction and in part from compression. The most severe syndrome is usually seen in adolescents.

Although the astute clinician can often make the

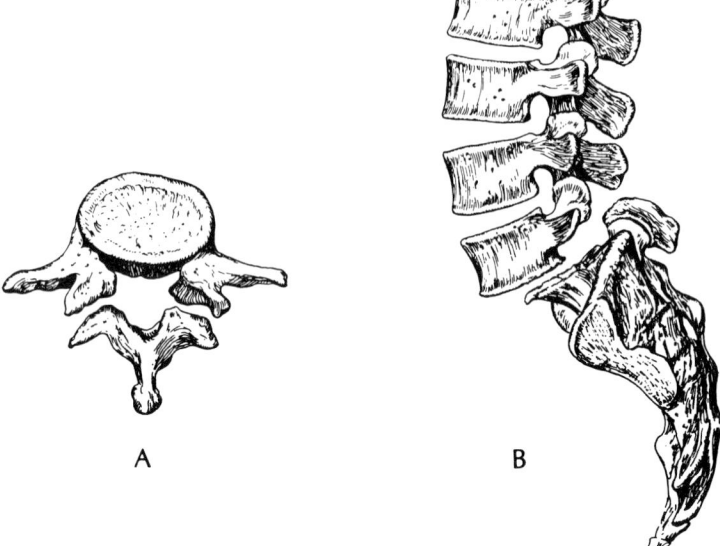

FIG. 92–16. Spondylolisthesis. *A,* Vertebra showing failure of ossification of the interarticular portions of the neural arch. Without forward slip of the involved vertebra, this disorder is called spondylolysis. (From Willis.[17]) *B,* The deformity (spondylolisthesis), which may occur as the result of the foregoing disorder. The defect is in the arch of L5. The posterior portion of the arch including the inferior facets remains with the sacrum while the rest of the fifth lumbar vertebra slips forward, carrying with it the entire spine. All degrees of slipping are seen.

FIG. 92–17. Identical twins with spondylolisthesis of L5 to S1. *A,* Lateral roentgenogram of the lumbosacral area of K.R., who had progressive back pain requiring spinal fusion. *B,* Lateral roentgenogram of twin, D.R., who had no back symptoms.

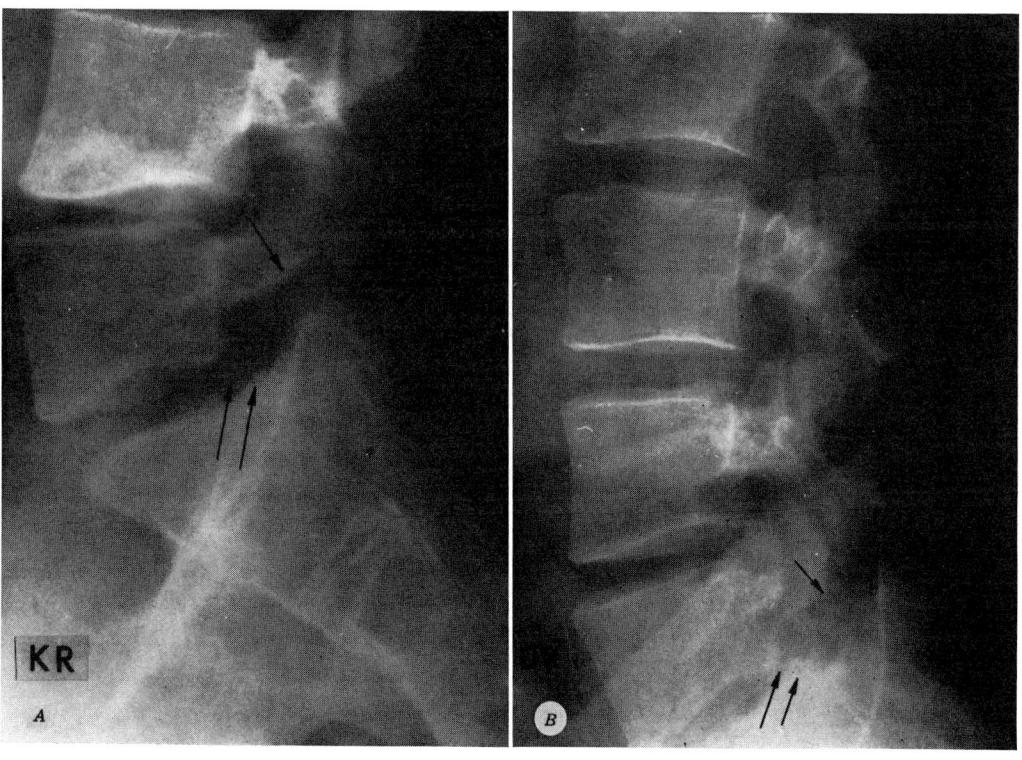

diagnosis from a visible or palpable prominence of the spine of the affected vertebra, noticed most readily when the patient is bent forward, final diagnosis depends on radiographic demonstration of the neural arch defects. When slipping is sufficient, these defects may be visible in a routine lateral film if the x-ray tube is well centered (Fig. 92–17). In the presence of minimal slipping, however, oblique views are necessary (see Fig. 92–12). Occasionally, although a defect is present, slippage may not be evident on the routine lateral recumbent film of the lumbosacral junction, but if the films are taken with the patient standing, slippage becomes apparent.

Treatment varies with the syndrome. Postural measures sometimes suffice for patients with minimal symptoms, especially if no nerve involvement has occurred. Spinal fusion, however, is indicated when the symptoms of sprain are severe or persistent or begin before maturity. When the nerve roots or the cauda equina are involved, decompression is the most important part of the operation and is indicated at the time of, or before, spinal fusion. Occasionally, simple removal of the loose neural arch and hypertrophic tissue in the defects (foraminotomy) affords relief, but in our experience the outcome is too uncertain to recommend this procedure routinely.

Degenerative Type

The most common acquired form is one in which osteoarthritic changes of the facets combined with disc degeneration result in forward displacement. This condition is diagnosed radiographically, especially by oblique views (Fig. 92–18). Treatment is much the same as for dysplastic spondylolisthesis. Complicating compression of nerve roots or cauda equina should be looked for and should be given precedence in the therapeutic plan.

Traumatic Type

This type is secondary to an acute injury with a fracture of some portion of the posterior arch. Treated early with immobilization, these injuries often heal.

Pathologic Type

Because of local or generalized bone disease, the posterior arches may become incompetent and may allow spondylolisthesis.

TRAUMA

Each spinal injury weakens the spine and predisposes the patient to further injury, regardless of type and extent of damage. This phenomenon is especially true when protection of the injured part is not adequate. Ligaments and muscles heal only by scar formation, and the anulus fibrosus is almost powerless to heal tears of its substance. These circumstances, unfortunately, are beyond the control of the physician, but the patient should be warned to protect his back following injury.

DISC DEGENERATION

The pathologic aspects of this condition are also discussed later in this chapter. Besides predisposing a patient to herniation, disc degeneration also weakens the structure of the intervertebral joint and increases the risk of sprain syndromes. When the degeneration is localized, little stability is lost, and the normal width of the disc space may be preserved. A patient with such a condition may have few or no symptoms, and some patients therefore do well after simple removal of herniated disc material.

When the degeneration is more massive, however, narrowing of disc space follows. If this condition occurs slowly over the course of years, the patient may have little pain or few other symptoms. Stability and vertebral alignment are preserved by marginal spur formation and by adaptive changes in the facets and intervertebral ligaments. Occasionally, such patients have a history of several acute episodes of back pain

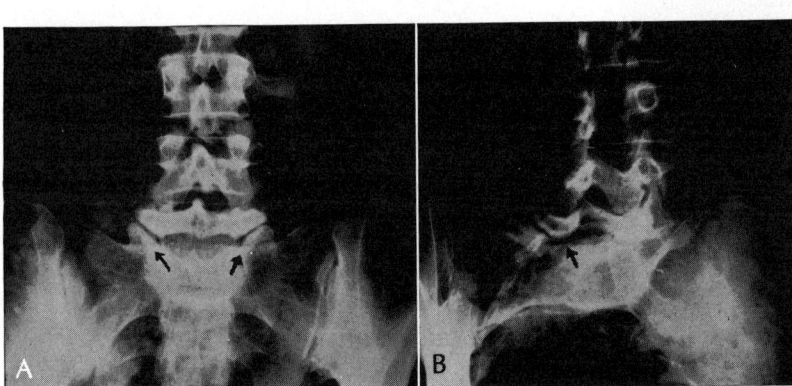

FIG. 92–18. Abnormal facets. Anteroposterior *(A)* and oblique *(B)* films in a patient with low back pain. Note the abnormal plane of the facets between the fifth lumbar vertebra and the sacrum. Less bony stability is present, and actual spondylolisthesis may occur. The instability may sometimes be detected roentgenographically only during flexion or extension of the spine.

many years prior to examination, but frequently they are unaware of any previous back trouble.

Massive disc degeneration occurring rapidly is likely to be continuously painful, whether or not herniation and root compression are associated. Instability of such joints leads to either backward shift of the superior vertebra on the inferior as the facets telescope on each other (Fig. 92–19) or forward displacement as the structure of the articular facets gives way, that is, degenerative spondylolisthesis.

During the course of collapse of the disc space, not only the disc itself but also the intervertebral joint is *unstable* and is therefore prone to give symptoms of sprain. When the intervertebral space becomes narrowed and arthritic, however, it again becomes stable, and back pain may subside, although later symptoms may develop from projection of marginal osteophytes against the nerve roots, either posteriorly in the neural canal or laterally in the narrowed intervertebral foramina.

PHYLOGENETIC SHORTENING OF THE SPINE

The structure of the lowest lumbar vertebra and of the first sacral segment is variable. Either may take on some or all of the characteristics of the other. When this happens the vertebrae are spoken of as *transitional*. Certainly, complete fusion or sacralization of the fifth lumbar vertebra does not predispose a patient to strain. It is also difficult to see how complete lumbarization of the first sacral segment could cause strain.

When the changeover is complete, however, the situation is different. One finds a unilaterally enlarged transverse process articulating with the sacrum and asymmetric facets (Fig. 92–20); that is, the facets are in different planes on the two sides. These changes reduce intervertebral mobility and therefore may predispose a patient to sprain. They are not incompatible, on the other hand, with normal existence, and if trouble occurs, the superiorly placed joint is often involved. Pain from a transitional vertebra itself probably arises from sclerosing osteitis of the pseudarthrosis between the enlarged transverse process and the sacrum.

SPINA BIFIDA OCCULTA

This condition is a failure of fusion between the right and left halves of the neural arch and may occur at any level of the vertebral column. The most common site for spina bifida occulta is S1, where the incidence has recently been reported to be 9% in women and 13% in men.[19] The condition is in no way a predisposing factor to low-back pain. When spina bifida occulta occurs at L5, further evaluation should be made to rule out a spondylolisthesis or spondylolysis.

CLINICAL PICTURE OF SPRAIN SYNDROMES

Low-back sprain may be acute, subacute, or chronic. The acute syndrome usually follows an injury or a trivial strain, is of short duration, and is self-

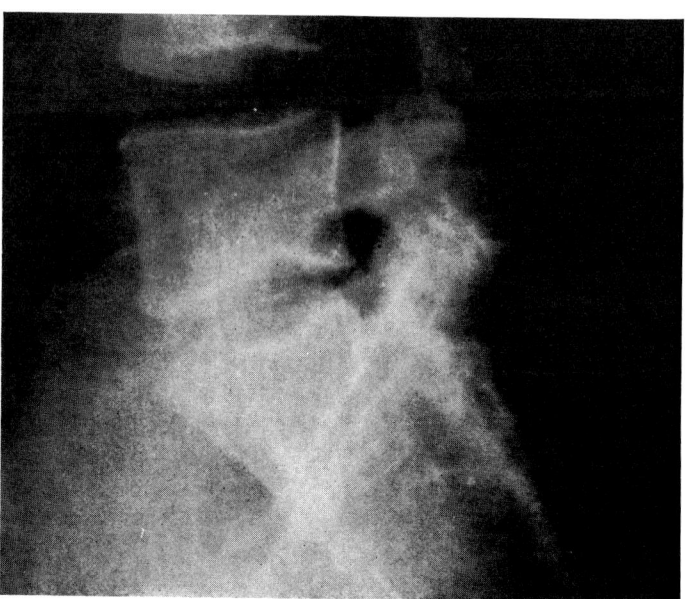

FIG. 92–19. Retrodisplacement. Lateral roentgenogram showing slight narrowing of the fifth lumbar disc and retrodisplacement of the fifth lumbar vertebra on the sacrum. This condition, often called reverse spondylolisthesis, is generally painful.

FIG. 92–20. Articulating transverse process. *A,* An incompletely sacralized fifth lumbar vertebra is shown with an articulating transverse process on the right. The intervertebral disc is usually congenitally narrow in these patients. *B,* An articulating transverse process on the left side of the fifth lumbar vertebra. The articulation is usually fibrous. This common congenital anomaly is not necessarily associated with pain.

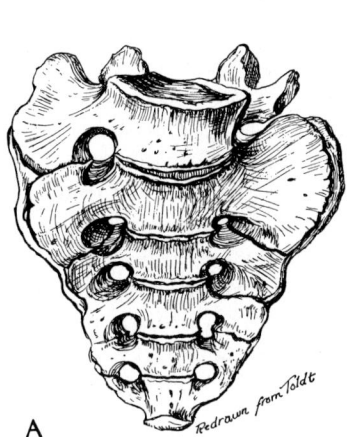

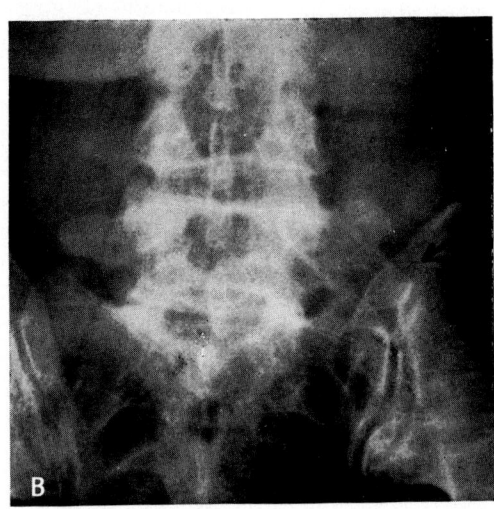

limited enough to respond well to treatment of any type. The chronic form, on the other hand, is usually of long duration, often occurs without an initiating trauma, and is refractory to treatment. Recurrences of the acute form are common.

ACUTE SPRAIN

The pain is usually severe and diffuse over the lower back and is associated with paravertebral muscle spasm. The patient adopts a protective attitude of moderate flexion and perhaps some list. Any motion is painful and aggravates the spasm.

Examination obviously cannot be complete but is carried as far as possible. Roentgenograms should be made if the patient can cooperate well enough. If not, they can be safely deferred until later.

The patient should be put to bed, preferably a bed with a thin sponge-rubber or hair mattress reinforced by an underlying board (Fig. 92–21). If such a board is not available, shifting the mattress to the floor often substitutes. A pillow behind the knees may assist in relaxation. "Muscle relaxants" and salicylates are usually helpful, but narcotics are sometimes necessary. No particular drug combination is effective in all patients. Heat in the form of hot moist packs applied to the back relieves muscle spasm. Light massage is often helpful, but deep massage should be avoided. Sometimes, procaine infiltration of the tight muscles is effective, but injection of a locally acting cortico-

steroid into the disc has questionable value. Traction has been used for acute low-back symptoms for many years, to keep a restless patient still. If applied directly to the pelvis, such forces no doubt may be transmitted to the spine and may have a stretching effect. Countertraction may be provided by positioning the patient with the foot of the bed elevated or by applying countertraction on the head. In the routine management of scoliosis, the effects of head and pelvic traction have been documented by x-ray films of the spine showing the stretching effect. Constant pelvic traction may be used with weights up to 35 to 40 lb (15.7 to 18 kg), whereas intermittent pelvic traction to 65 to 70 lb (29 to 31.5 kg) has been of value in treating patients with acute back symptoms. If traction is necessary, I believe that it should be instituted while the patient is hospitalized. It is difficult to instruct a patient initially in the correct use of traction unless he is in the hospital.

As the pain subsides, a complete examination can be done. As soon as straight leg raising is free through an arc of 45° or more, the patient may be allowed up. His back must be protected until symptoms have subsided completely. If the sprain has been severe, a brace or lumbosacral corset may be advisable. Before normal activities are resumed, the patient should be checked to see whether he has regained full motion. Exercises should be instituted not only to restore motion and strength, but also to stretch contracted muscles and ligaments. Exercises must be started gradually and gauged to pain tolerance.

FIG. 92–21. Postural principles. Patients should be instructed in some simple principles to avoid unnecessary back strain. *A*, The bed should be hard, to avoid sagging of the buttocks with increase in the lumbar lordosis. *B*, A hard, straight-back chair is desirable. Arm rests are not contraindicated. *C*, Lifting should be avoided whenever possible. When it is unavoidable, the legs should do most of the work; the elbows can be buttressed by the thighs.

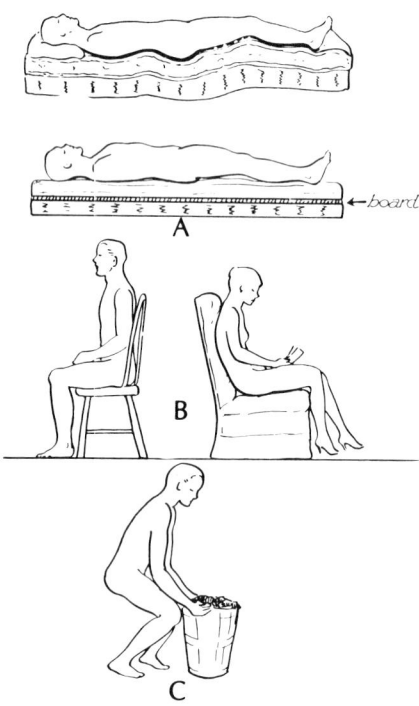

Many acute episodes are not so severe as the one described. In less-severe cases, ambulatory treatment may be sufficient. Immobilization with a brace of adhesive strapping, procaine injection, and heat and massage are all useful measures. Again, one should watch for developing contractures, which should be corrected with exercises.

CHRONIC SPRAIN

This syndrome, probably the most common of low-back conditions, has variable clinical manifestations. In its milder form, it is characterized by a mild low backache aggravated by bending and lifting and improved by rest. In other cases, the pain may be more severe and may cause true discomfort. Rarely is it severe for more than short periods, and it subsides to a nagging, diffuse low backache with radiation into one or both thighs. It is aggravated by activity and is improved by rest.

The physical signs of this syndrome are also vari-

able. In patients with mild cases, motion may not be limited, but the extremes of motion are usually painful. The patient notes tenderness at some point over the lower spine. As the severity of the syndrome increases, one notes additional signs such as partial restriction of straight leg raising, loss of motion, abnormal postural attitudes, and muscle spasm, particularly in response to movement.

In patients with severe cases, a period of bed rest may be indicated; therapeutic measures are as described for acute low-back pain. In milder cases, the patient should be instructed in proper postural principles. Proper sleeping and sitting positions should be demonstrated, and he should be taught to avoid bending and lifting or to bend and lift in such a way as to minimize the pressure on his back. He is instructed in postural exercises, which have as their principles the reduction of lumbar lordosis and the strengthening of the trunk. Stretching of shortened hamstring and sacrospinal muscles may be advisable but should be done cautiously.

Frequently, external support is helpful, and many different types of braces have been designed to achieve the desired goals of abdominal compression and restricted spinal movement (Fig. 92–22). These braces should reach from the pubic level to the lower costal margins and should support the abdomen, particularly the lower abdomen. The central back uprights, if present, should be contoured to fit comfortably when the patient is seated erect. Pressure into the lumbosacral hollow is not necessary and in fact should be avoided.

When conservative therapy fails, lumbosacral fusion should be considered. In this operation, two or more vertebrae are induced to grow together, to put the intervening joint at rest. Many techniques have been devised. Although newer methods have shortened the period of morbidity, the incidence of pseudarthroses is still bothersome; and rarely, following a successful fusion, the intervertebral joint superior to the operation site may become painful as a result of the additional stress placed on it. Because the operation is elective, the decision should be left up to the patient, once the advantages and disadvantages have been explained.

NERVE ROOT COMPRESSION SYNDROMES

DEGENERATIVE DISC DISEASE AND HERNIATED DISC

Since Mixter and Barr first clearly described the syndrome of nerve root compression resulting from her-

FIG. 92–22. *A, B, C,* Lumbosacral corset. Steel stays are incorporated into the back of the support, which must extend from the iliac crests to just over the costal margins.

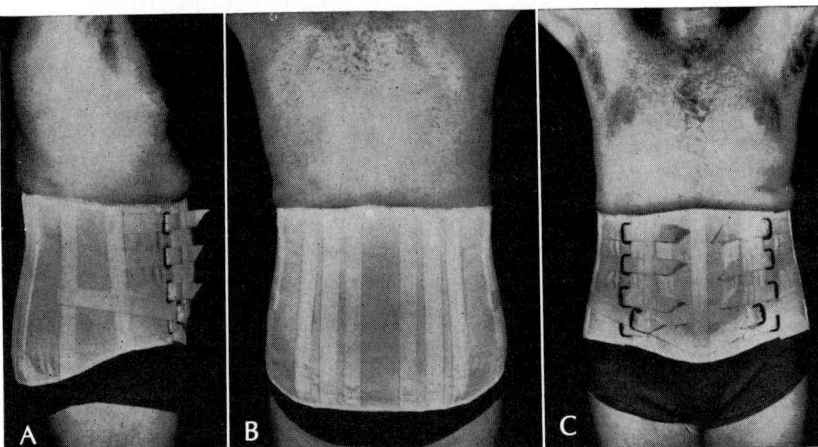

niated disc in 1934, it has become clear that lesions of the disc are responsible for much of idiopathic low-back pain (Fig. 92–23).

Pathogenesis

Although a single trauma, if severe enough, can rupture a hitherto normal anulus fibrosus and can allow prolapse of disc substance with disastrous effect on the cauda equina, this occurrence is rare. More commonly, the trauma of strain acts only as a triggering mechanism. Underlying asymptomatic biomechanical and biochemical changes usually first weaken the disc structure. The course of these changes has been traced anatomically, and alteration and weakening of the discs are part of the aging process. Because the discs have no innervation and no blood supply, such degeneration can take place silently and with little appreciable repair. When the anulus has weakened enough, the interior disc sub-

stance, that is, the nucleus pulposus and the degenerating annular fibers, prolapse in the direction of greatest weakness. Because of these forces and certain anatomic factors already described, the directions of greatest weakness for the lumbar discs are to the right and left of the posterior midline. Lumbar disc herniations, therefore, follow these two directions. They are favored by radially oriented annular tears or fissures, which develop either as a result of normal wear and tear or as the result of one or more excessive strains.

Herniations that approach the surface distend the superficial fibers and longitudinal ligaments, where pain-perceptive nerve endings are situated. This deep pain is poorly localized and can radiate into the buttocks and perhaps even into the lower extremities. The source of the pain is further obscured by the frequent development of spasm of the lumbar and hamstring muscles, and this spasm in itself is painful.

FIG. 92–23. *A* and *B,* Roentgenograms showing an advanced stage of degenerative disc disease.

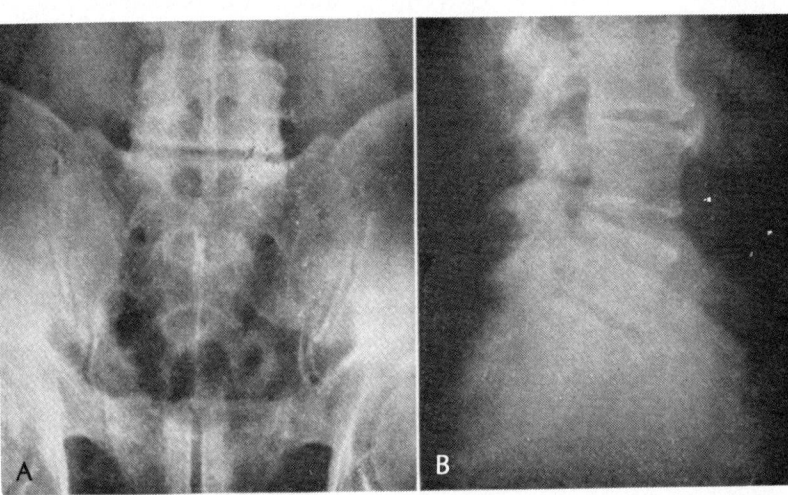

If herniation proceeds, the lumbar nerve roots or the cauda equina may next become involved; the smaller the diameter of the neural canal and the larger the herniation, the more likely this disorder is to occur and to affect nerve root functions. If the herniation does not rupture through the longitudinal ligament, it is called *protrusion,* and if it does, *extrusion.* In either case, the nerve root or roots are displaced and compressed. Disc fragments may herniate from the disc space and may lie superior or inferior to it and still not extrude.

Because of all these variables, the manifestations of disc herniation differ from one patient to the next. Most commonly, nerve root compression is localized, and the neurologic deficit is minor. In rare instances, however, the prolapse may be massive and may involve several nerve roots or the entire cauda equina. As the site of herniation comes closer to the midline, the more likely is multiple nerve root involvement; as the site shifts laterally, the more likely is involvement confined to one nerve root.

Clinical Picture

Although any of the lumbar discs can herniate, one or both of the most inferior (L4-L5 and L5-S1) are usually responsible for symptoms. The level L3-L4 is involved occasionally; other lumbar levels, rarely.

Minimal nerve root compression may have no localizing physical or roentgenographic manifestations, and conclusive diagnosis depends on CT or myelographic findings. In many instances, however, symptoms and signs may subside with bed rest, and these studies can be deferred. I recommend myelograms only when the syndrome is atypical or operative intervention is contemplated. In any event, CT study is preferred, for it is safe and noninvasive.

Classic cases of root compression caused by herniated disc are difficult to overlook. Patients are otherwise healthy and are often vigorous men or women in middle age. Patients often have a previous history of backache or of one or more acute lumbosacral sprains from which recovery has been complete. Usually, the onset of the present pain follows a back injury, but not necessarily a severe injury; in fact, it is sometimes so minor that it is difficult for the patient to recall it. Frequently, a snap is felt before the back pain begins. Once started, the pain increases in intensity and, after an interval, radiates distally into one or the other lower extremity. As radiation begins, the back pain may subside, but the radiating pain typically increases and is associated with numbness and paresthesia. The patient cannot stand straight, and the involved leg is too sensitive to bear weight. Examination shows a patient in great pain, with par-

avertebral muscle spasm, who stands with a flattened lumbar lordosis and a list to the side opposite the pain and who walks only with difficulty. All spinal movements are limited, particularly bending to the side of the pain. Straight leg raising is restricted on the involved side, and often this leg cannot be straightened. The patient prefers the sitting or flexed position to any other. In addition, the patient has pronounced paravertebral tenderness with reproduction of sciatica on percussion or deep palpation.

Neurologic signs are variable for the reasons already described, but certain combinations suggest specific nerve root involvements. Loss or suppression of ankle jerk, sensory deficit in the lateral border and sole of the foot and toes, and weakness and atrophy of the calf suggest S1 nerve root compression. Unchanged reflexes, sensory deficit in the lateral leg and mediodorsal aspect of the foot, and weakness of the toe extensors suggest L5 nerve root compression. Loss or suppression of the knee jerk, sensory deficit along the shin, and weakness of knee extension suggest L4 nerve root compression. Most commonly, S1 nerve root compression is the result of herniation of the L5 to S1 disc, L5 root compression of the L4 to L5 disc, and L4 root compression of the L3 to L4 disc. When neurologic findings are profound, however, it is wise to suspect multiple nerve root involvement. CT and (perhaps) myelography are obtained to confirm the level of involvement when an operation is contemplated.

Treatment

Thanks to improvement of diagnostic technique, diagnosis can be definitely established in most patients. Operative intervention is elective unless the patient has an important nerve deficit or is in intractable pain. Even in the presence of definite signs of nerve root compression, the majority of patients respond to conservative treatment. A trial of 2 to 3 weeks of bed rest in the hospital is indicated for most patients with acute symptoms before operation is recommended. When the syndrome is subacute, bed rest may be less valuable, but a sustained course of outpatient treatment is indicated before operation is considered.

When pain is relieved by conservative treatment, the relief is probably due to subsidence of root edema and to limited repair of the superficial layers of the anulus fibrosus and the posterior longitudinal ligament. It is doubtful that the herniated disc material is ever fully absorbed, but it may shrink or become pocketed in the neural canal, no longer compressing nerve tissue. This phenomenon is more likely when the lumbar neural canal is proportionately larger than the cauda equina. Along with subsidence of pain, the neurologic picture often improves, but some neurologic changes of little functional significance may persist.

Chymopapain and Chemonucleolysis. Intradiscal injection of chymopapain in a chemonucleolysis technique was reported by Lyman Smith in 1964 to treat herniated lumbar intervertebral discs.[20] Chymopapain, derived from papaya latex, is a proteolytic enzyme that catalyzes rapid hydrolysis of the noncollagen ground substance of the nucleus pulposus.[21] Based on this pharmacologic effect, chemonucleolytic treatment of low-back pain with nerve root irritation was used in clinical trials in this country and in Canada until 1975, when the efficacy and safety of the method came into question. The technique was discontinued in this country, but it was still used by Canadian orthopedic and neurologic surgeons. In 1980, a double-blind, randomized trial was conducted to compare the efficacy of chymopapain injection with placebo injection in patients with a herniated lumbar disc.[22] The United States Food and Drug Administration (FDA) approved the use of this enzyme for intradiscal injections in this country in January 1983. The American Academy of Orthopaedic Surgeons and the American Association of Neurological Surgeons then began a cooperative educational program to instruct their members in the clinical use of chymopapain injections.

Patients considered suitable for intradiscal injection are as follows: (1) those with clear-cut lumbar radiculopathy who have had an appropriate trial of conservative treatment for 2 to 4 weeks and who have not responded well; and (2) those with an abnormal myelogram confirming disc protrusion. Patients with a large, extruded fragment are not likely to benefit.

Certain contraindications are as follows: (1) major weakness in a muscle group; (2) sphincter disturbance; (3) extensive spondylosis or spinal stenosis; (4) pregnancy; and (5) allergy to papaya or to any meat tenderizer.

Less clear-cut contraindications include patients who (1) have had previous operations at the current symptomatic level; and (2) have workmen's compensation claims, are in litigation related to their back disorder, or have a psychiatric disturbance.

The major adverse effect of this treatment is anaphylaxis. In a worldwide series of 40,000 cases, the incidence of this complication was 1%, with 2 deaths reported.[23] The incidence of anaphylaxis in women was approximately 2.5%, whereas in men it was approximately 0.18%. Women had a greater risk of reaction if their erythrocyte sedimentation rate was above 20 or if treatment occurred during the menstrual period.

While chemonucleolysis is generally viewed with great suspicion by most neurosurgeons and orthopedists,[24] some still believe that chemonucleolysis plays a significant role in the treatment of herniated lumbar discs, with changing criteria for patient selection and with significant change in technique.[25] A newly employed monoclonal antibody test for immunoglobulin is now being used to screen for possible allergic reactions. The ultimate role, if any, of this controversial method of treatment is still unclear.

Operative Treatment. When operative treatment is advised, the question is whether to be content with nerve root decompression only or whether to proceed with spinal fusion. Should the degenerative disc process be controlled by fusing the involved joint at the same time that loosened disc tissue is removed? On this point opinion still differs, and arguments on both sides are convincing. In cases of rupture of the intervertebral discs in adolescence, in acute ruptures for the first time, and in intervertebral disc ruptures with a previous history of symptoms but with little radiologic change, when operation becomes necessary I prefer to decompress the involved disc space without fusion. If a repeat operation is necessary or if the patient has advanced changes of degenerative arthritis, however, spinal fusion may be considered. In questionable cases, I prefer not to perform spinal fusion because the decompression operation is less extensive, convalescence is usually easier, and if a fusion fails to heal properly and a pseudarthrosis develops, the situation may be worse than if no fusion had been done. I review these various aspects of the problem with the patient and, if he is still uncertain, I request his permission to make the final decision at the time of operation.

Complications. If the indications for operative intervention are conservative, and if the type of operation is precisely fitted to the circumstances, the results will be satisfying. Complications are rare, but one deserves particular mention. Spondylitis or discitis sometimes develops in the operated disc space. It is manifested by recurrence of back pain, which begins 3 or 4 weeks after operation, and elevation of the patient's erythrocyte sedimentation rate. Other manifestations of inflammation such as fever and leukocytosis are absent, and infection, the primary concern, cannot be demonstrated. In time, roentgenograms show sclerosis of the adjacent vertebral margins and localized areas of bone absorption. The cause of this complication has not been definitely established, but the condition is usually self-limited and subsides with bed rest.

Recurrences of nerve root compression from fresh herniation of degenerated disc tissue can occur, but are infrequent. Because the mobility of the nerve root and the dura is reduced by postoperative scarring, such herniations do not have to be large to irritate the nerve tissue. In such cases, treatment by bed rest is well worth a trial. If it fails, however, reoperation for decompression is indicated, and a spinal fusion should be carefully reconsidered. It is probably wise to advise a fusion operation, especially if the degenerative disease is still localized to one disc level.

SPINAL STENOSIS

This important syndrome is discussed in Chapter 93.

OTHER CONDITIONS PRODUCING LOW BACK PAIN

INFECTIONS

Backache may occur as part of the toxemia of a generalized infection. In these cases, diagnosis usually is not a problem. Except for muscle soreness, few if any localizing signs exist. More important is the back pain that accompanies meningeal irritation. Usually, one may detect a generalized spasm of the erector spinae muscle by Kernig's maneuver or by limitation of straight leg raising. When severe, as in infectious meningitis, this spasm produces opisthotonos.

Infections may cause backache by direct involvement of spinal structures. Nontubercular infections are now more prevalent and are seen most commonly in the aged. The infection usually begins in the disc space and spreads to involve the bone secondarily. Roentgenographic changes may be slow to develop. At first, the shadow of an abscess may appear, followed by gradual destruction of the contiguous vertebral margins, with final obliteration of the disc space.

The infecting organism may be obtained from culture of blood or from aspiration biopsy of the disc space itself. Sometimes, the spine may be involved by an infection elsewhere, such as the urinary tract; culture from the suspected source may reveal the organism. Treatment by bed rest, spinal bracing, and suitable chemotherapy is best. Operation is rarely necessary because the involved vertebrae often undergo spontaneous fusion.

Perhaps of greater interest in the differential diagnosis are the granulomatous infections. By far the most important of these is tuberculosis, although brucellosis and fungal, particularly coccidioidomycosis, infections also occur (see Chapter 117).

Pott's Disease (Tuberculosis)

Symptoms vary because of the marked individual patterns of resistance. Back pain may be present for several months before other characteristic changes of the disease occur. Systemic signs, particularly otherwise *unexplained weight loss*, should make one suspicious. Night pain, night cries, fever, and previous pulmonary tuberculosis all help one to make the diagnosis. Paraplegia is a common complication. *Elevation of the erythrocyte sedimentation rate* is the most helpful laboratory clue. A tuberculin test should always be done. Even though a positive test result is not conclusive evidence, a negative result excludes this diagnosis.

Roentgenographic changes are usually present, although early in the disease they may be difficult to find (Fig. 92–24). Tomograms may be helpful, as are bone scans. Narrowing of the disc space with destruction of neighboring vertebrae and *soft-tissue abscess* are the most typical changes. Diagnosis can be made from culture of aspirated pus.

This disease often involves the sacroiliac joints. Here again, roentgenographic evidence of bone destruction is the most important diagnostic finding.

Herpes Zoster

Infection of the dorsal lumbar root ganglions by the herpes zoster virus may cause severe sciatica. Early diagnosis is difficult, but the absence of trauma and the presence of fever should make one suspicious. As soon as the vesicular eruption appears, the diagnosis becomes evident.

FRACTURES AND DISLOCATIONS

Characteristic wedge fractures of the vertebral bodies caused by injuries of flexion are not difficult to recognize or to treat. Fractures of the posterior elements, such as the pedicles, laminae, and articular processes, may be complicated by severe spinal cord or nerve root damage, however, especially when such fractures are accompanied by subluxation or dislocation. Immediate exploration and fixation of the region of injury are indicated, and these patients require around-the-clock care to avoid pressure sores, urinary tract infection, and increased neurologic damage, all of which can take place quickly with improper management. Later, rehabilitation is also necessary.

Fractures of the spinous processes are rare in the

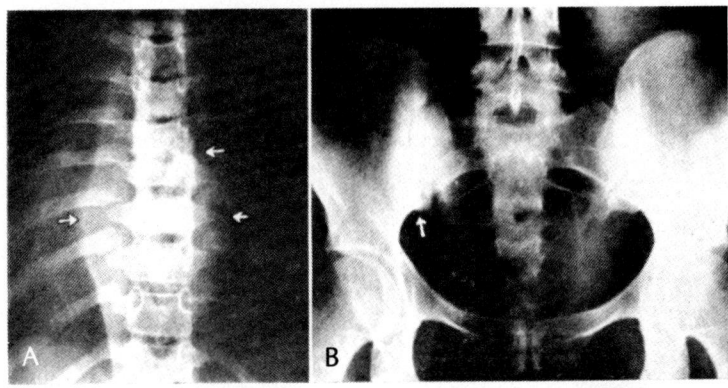

FIG. 92–24. Tuberculosis. *A,* Tuberculous spondylitis; note the abscess *(arrow).* Destruction of the sixth dorsal intervertebral disc space has occurred. This case is too high to cause pain in the lower back. When involvement is in the lumbar spine, the abscesses frequently follow the plane of the psoas muscle, and roentgenograms show distention of the muscle border. *B,* Sacroiliac tuberculosis; note the sclerosis and irregularity *(arrow)* of the right sacroiliac joint.

lumbar spine. Separations of the posterior elements, with or without fractures of the vertebral body or neural arch, have occurred in persons involved in automobile accidents when wearing the lap-type seat belt. Fractures of one or more transverse processes are common, however. These injuries are usually caused by simultaneous local contusion and strain and generally respond well to supportive treatment such as rest, sedation, and strapping. Sometimes, injection of the injured area with procaine provides remarkable relief.

Fractures of the sacrum usually result from direct trauma. Localized tenderness and superficial hematomas help one to make the diagnosis. These fractures are difficult to demonstrate roentgenographically. Fractures of the pelvic ring are sometimes associated with dislocation of the sacroiliac joints; proper roentgenographic evaluation is not difficult.

Pathologic Fractures

Because of the great forces brought to bear on the spine, it is not surprising that destruction or weakening of the vertebral trabecular structure is followed by vertebral fracture. It is surprising, however, that much bone substance may be lost without roentgenographic evidence. The pain of the fracture is frequently the first indication of the pathologic process. Lack of adequate trauma should cause one to suspect this diagnosis. The following lesions are most likely to lead to collapse of a vertebra: (1) *metastatic malignant disease,* such as breast, kidney, thyroid, or lung cancer in the adult or neuroblastoma in children; occasionally the primary source cannot be found; (2) *primary neoplasms, such as multiple myeloma; (3) metabolic dyscrasias,* particularly senile, postmenopausal, or "steroid-induced" osteoporosis; rarely, osteomalacia or hyperparathyroidism; (4) *tuberculosis;* and (5) *other conditions,* such as Gaucher's disease and eosinophilic granuloma.

Differential diagnosis of these conditions depends on a complete medical history and physical examination and full use of laboratory and radiographic techniques. As previously discussed, radioactive bone scanning is effective in distinguishing various lesions of the spine. Differentiation can now be made between recent and old compression fractures, one can now detect occult metastasis to the spine, and activity of an infectious spondylitis may be evaluated.[26] Biopsy of the lesion itself should be performed whenever possible. If the lesion is accessible without hazard to adjacent viscera, blood vessels, or nerves, needle biopsy is a practical method of obtaining material for section. If not, open biopsy is necessary unless clinical, laboratory, and radiographic findings are conclusive.

RHEUMATIC DISEASES

Ankylosing Spondylitis

This common cause of low-back pain in young men involves the sacroiliac joints early in the disease. It can be diagnosed by diminished chest expansion and reuced spinal mobility. A useful sign is the contraction of the ipsilateral spinal musculature when bending to the side (Forestier's bowstring sign). Normally, the contralateral musculature tightens (see also Chapter 59).

Osteitis Condensans Ilii

This term is applied to the roentgenographic demonstration of sclerotic changes on the iliac sides of the sacroiliac joints. It is particularly common post partum and may be related to the strain that delivery places on these joints. When such changes occur, however, a more exact diagnosis should be sought because these lesions are also seen in osteoarthritis, in early ankylosing spondylitis, and in the presence of a nearby osteoid osteoma. Osteitis condensans ilii is not associated with the HLA-B27 antigen.[27] The clinical picture is not characteristic, and the condition

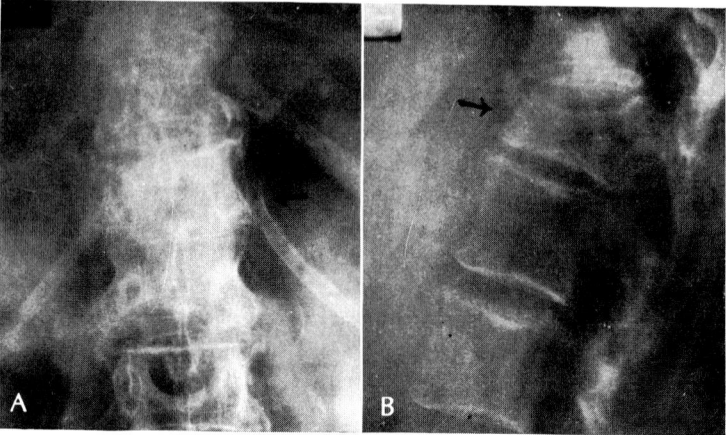

FIG. 92–25. *A* and *B*, An osteolytic metastasis with a pathologic compression fracture of D12 *(arrow)*. These lesions may be difficult to recognize before collapse occurs. The source of the metastasis was carcinoma of the breast, surgically treated 20 years previously.

is said to respond to conservative therapy identical to that used for low-back sprain.

Occasionally, late in pregnancy, women develop low-back pain as the result of relaxation of the sacroiliac joints. The pubic symphysis is also involved and is tender. Symptoms can be troublesome, and the pain may be severe enough to force the patient to bed. Although it may be aggravated during delivery, such pain usually subsides afterward, and the joints resume their former stability. Rarely, pain and instability persist, requiring sacroiliac fusion.

METABOLIC BONE DISEASE

Metabolic disorders of bone are discussed in Chapter 112.

NEOPLASTIC DISEASE

Certain tumors show a predilection for the spine.

Intraspinal Lesions

Physicians experienced in spinal surgery have, at one time or another, encountered an intraspinal tumor causing backache and sciatica. A report from the Mayo Clinic has shown the incidence of various lesions. Neurofibroma and ependymoma each occurred three times in over 1000 cases. Carcinoma metastatic to the spinal cord and its supporting structures occurs, as do primary tumors. These conditions develop frequently in the *absence* of neurologic signs. Myelographic or CT examination is needed for diagnosis.

Lesions of the Vertebral Column

Of the malignant tumors, by far the most common are *multiple myeloma* and *metastatic carcinoma*. They often have a similar roentgenographic appearance

and both can cause extensive bone destruction. Myeloma spares the neural arch, which does not contain red bone marrow. Both diseases are often widespread. Differentiation depends on the demonstration of a primary source such as prostate, breast, kidney, thyroid, and lung, most frequently, in the case of metastatic disease and of abnormal gamma globulins in the case of multiple myeloma. Plasma and urine protein electrophoresis and bone marrow aspiration are valuable in the early diagnosis of multiple myeloma. One often sees an associated anemia. Rarely, both metastatic carcinoma and multiple myeloma cause spinal cord and nerve root compression (Fig. 92–25). *Chordoma*, a rare malignant tumor largely confined to the sacrococcygeal and cranial portions of the axial skeleton, arises from remnants of the primitive notochord and is locally invasive. It is resistant to both surgical treatment and radiotherapy.

Benign tumors of the spine are less common. Giant cell tumor, bone cysts, osteochondromas, and chondromas may occur, but *hemangiomas, aneurysmal bone cysts,* and *osteoid osteomas* are seen more frequently. It is probably wrong to classify all hemangiomas as benign because some lead to extensive bone destruction. Many of these tumors respond favorably to irradiation. The typical roentgenogram is easily recognized and has vertical striations in the vertical body, which is often partially crushed and broadened in all dimensions but the vertical. Aneurysmal bone cysts involve the posterior vertebral elements and form large paraspinal masses with scattered calcific deposits. Although biopsy is required for definitive diagnosis, these cysts are best treated by irradiation.

Osteoid osteoma is a painful tumor in which a small focus of osteogenetic activity develops and leads to extensive surrounding sclerosis of bone.[28] This tumor usually arises in the posterior vertebral elements and is therefore difficult to demonstrate roentgenographically. Tomograms are helpful to demonstrate the typical lesion, a zone of dense bone surrounding a small, radiolucent nidus. The pain, which may be severe and often occurs at night, is so dramatically relieved by aspirin or other nonsteroidal anti-inflammatory drugs that this response is a helpful diagnostic aid.

EPIPHYSITIS

Also known as Scheuermann's disease, epiphysitis is a painful back condition of adolescence, the cause of which is obscure. It is more common in boys than in girls and involves the thoracic spine much more frequently than the lumbar. Although structural round back, increased anteroposterior diameter of the chest, and tight hamstrings form part of the syndrome, this triad frequently occurs without pain. I have seen it most often without pain, and the usual presenting complaint is poor posture. The so-called typical roentgenographic findings of several mildly wedged vertebrae, narrowed disc spaces, and irregular vertebral margins are also not exclusively limited to patients in pain. These radiographic lesions are caused by faults in the cartilaginous end plates and permit herniation of the disc material into the spongiosa.

Treatment for patients whose primary problem is deformity differs from therapy for those who are in pain. A firm mattress, a bed board, and postural exercises are recommended when the deformity is mild. When thoracic kyphosis is significant and the patient has not completed growth, the use of a Milwaukee brace gives gratifying results. Frequently, after wearing this brace full-time for only 6 months and part time for 6 months more, one sees a noticeable improvement of the round back. In patients in pain but with little deformity, more simplified bracing or the use of a plaster jacket for a few months may be all that is necessary.

The intent of postural treatment is not to correct deformity, but to prevent its progression. Whether this end can actually be achieved is open to question because the condition is often self-limiting. The goal of treatment is to reduce the thoracic or thoracolumbar kyphosis and not merely to increase the lumbosacral lordosis. When an exercise program is considered, therefore, the usual lumbar flattening exercises are recommended, but in addition, a special one is added to extend the thoracic spine. The patient is asked to flatten his lumbar spine by flexing his hips over the end of a hard table and to hold this position while he raises his head and shoulders.

If a plaster jacket or brace is used, the same principles apply: the lumbar lordosis must first be flat-tened and then the thoracic kyphosis extended. Immobilization of this kind is more likely to be helpful to patients with subacute pain. For those whose pain is severe, spinal fusion should not be delayed because it is the best way of relieving the pain and the most effective means of controlling progression of deformity. Operative reduction of kyphosis is difficult, but it may take place with further spinal growth, once a strong fusion is obtained.

SCOLIOSIS

I have found that 40% of patients with adolescent idiopathic scoliosis are in pain.[29] The problem of pain in the older patient with scoliosis is often challenging. Pain may exist at the level of the apex of the curve secondary to osteoarthritis, which occurs in the growing child. In lumbar curves, low-back pain with leg radiation simulates disc symptoms. The usual operative management of excision of the disc fails. Such patients should be treated by external support with lumbosacral corsets. If no relief is obtained, a course of traction, supplemented by a more rigid brace, is often helpful. In patients not responding to conservative treatment, reduction of the curve and spinal fusion relieve the pain.

Although idiopathic scoliosis does not usually progress after full maturation of the spine, I have seen several patients in whom lumbar curves worsened during middle age. Such symptomatic curves may best be treated initially by correction and fusion because they continue to progress throughout life. Patients with untreated, progressive, painful scoliosis past 65 years old are the most difficult to manage.

COCCYGODYNIA

Pain in the coccygeal area is often difficult to diagnose and to treat. It may be of three separate types:
1. *Primary coccygeal abnormality.* As the result of direct trauma or childbirth, the coccyx may be fractured or the sacrococcygeal joint may be severely strained.
2. *Primary low back disorder.* Coccygodynia commonly develops as a secondary phenomenon in a patient with low-back pain. The mechanism is not understood, and the pain is most likely to be referred.
3. *Visceral lesion.* It is common for patients with rectal or genitourinary disease to develop coccygeal pain. This pain is of a referred type and is sometimes associated with "spasm" of the muscles of the pelvic floor.

It is only by careful evaluation that these three entities may be separated. The back must always be examined because trauma to the coccyx cannot usually occur without simultaneously involving the low back. Rectal examination should include palpation of pelvic structures as well as of the coccyx and its adjacent structures, that is, the coccygeus and levator ani muscles and the sacrospinous and sacrotuberous ligaments.

Proctologic, gynecologic, and urologic evaluations may be indicated. When examination points to primary disease in the sacrococcygeal articulation, coccygectomy may be effective if conservative therapy fails. Every effort should be made to avoid irritation of the painful area. Soft chairs are usually worse than hard, and the patient should sit with good posture. A rubber ring may be necessary. Sometimes, a strapping or "sacroiliac belt" helps by pulling fatty tissues over the nonpadded coccygeal region.

CAMPTOCORMIA

Hysterical back pain characterized by extreme flexion of the spine and by pain in the lumbar area has been termed *camptocormia*. The diagnosis is made by normal findings on orthopedic and neurologic examinations and a deformity that disappears in recumbency or by suggestion.

Although this condition is not common, psychologic overlay in the patient with back pain is almost always present. Such anxiety frequently confuses the clinical picture and is often transferred to the treating physician, making diagnosis and successful treatment difficult (see also Chapter 80).

When evaluating the patient with low-back pain, the physician must be aware of the possibility of secondary gain, as with liability cases, compensation cases, avoidance of military draft, and malingering.

STENOSIS OF THE AORTIC BIFURCATION AND ILIAC ARTERIES

When pain is centered in the buttocks, groin, and thighs and is brought on by walking but relieved quickly by rest, one should consider the possibility of intermittent claudication caused by stenosis of the iliac arteries. Palpation of the femoral arteries should provide a quick diagnosis. The condition is common enough so that *palpation of the arterial trunks should be included as part of the routine back examination.*

HIP JOINT DISEASE

Occasionally, it is difficult to distinguish the pain of hip disease from that of the spine because both may radiate along the same pathways. Intra-articular disease often causes pain radiating down the inner aspects of the thighs to the knees, whereas the pain of trochanteric bursitis may follow the more usual "sciatic" distribution. For this reason, it is important to analyze hip joint movements in all patients with sciatica and especially those in whom the findings in the lower back are equivocal.

REFERRED PAIN FROM VISCERAL STRUCTURES

A lesion in one of the pelvic organs or the retroperitoneal structures can cause pain referred to the back. In women, the most usual condition is a retroverted uterus, but disease of the ovaries and fallopian tubes may also be the cause. The pain is usually worse during menses. In men, referred low-back pain is usually the result of a prostatic lesion. Stones within the urinary tract are easily diagnosed in the presence of typical ureteral colic, but at other times, they may be a more obscure cause of back pain. In the presence of associated anorexia and weight loss, a retroperitoneal neoplasm must be considered. In most such patients, the back findings are insufficient to explain the symptoms, but in elderly patients, associated lower back lesions may complicate the picture and may test the diagnostic acumen of the attending physician.

HERNIATED FAT SYNDROME

As pointed out by Copeman many years ago, fibrofatty nodules may develop by herniation through the dense fascia of the lower back. These nodules may become tender, especially in patients lying in bed for prolonged periods. Symptomatic relief may be obtained by infiltration with corticosteroid ester crystal suspensions diluted 1:10 in 1% procaine.

REFERENCES

1. Arnoldi, C.C.: Intraosseous hypertension: A possible cause of low back pain? Clin. Orthop., *115*:30, 1976.
2. Crock, H.V., and Hoshizawa, H.: The blood supply of the lumbar vertebral column. Clin. Orthop., *115*:6, 1976.
3. Schmorl, G., and Junghanns, H.: The Human Spine in Health and Disease. New York, Grune & Stratton, 1971.

4. Anderson, B.J., et al.: The sitting posture: An electromyographic and discometric study. Orthop. Clin. North Am., 6:105, 1975.

5. Naylor, A., et al.: Enzymic and immunological activity in the intervertebral disk. Orthop. Clin. North Am., 6:51, 1975.

6. Gertzbein, S., et al.: Autoimmunity in degenerative disc disease of the lumbar spine. Orthop. Clin. North Am., 6:67, 1975.

7. Baker, R.A., et al.: Sequelae of metrizamide myelography in 200 examinations. A.J.R., 130:499, 1978.

8. Kendall, B., Schneidau, A., Stevens, J., and Harrison, M.: Clinical trial of iohexol for lumbar myelography. Br. J. Radiol., 56:539, 1983.

9. Asnis, S., Blau, L., and Bohne, W.: A comparison of ^{18}F and ^{85}Sr scintimetric patterns by computerized data analysis and display. Radiology, 106:607, 1973.

10. Bohne, W.H., Levine, D.B., and Lyden, J.P.: ^{18}F scintimetric diagnosis of osteoid osteoma of the carpal scaphoid bone. Clin. Orthop., 107:156, 1975.

11. Modic, M.T., Masaryk, T., and Paushter, D.: Magnetic resonance imaging of the spine. Radiol. Clin. North Am., 24:229, 1986.

12. Chafetz, N.I., et al.: Recognition of lumbar disk herniation with NMR. A.J.R., 141:1153, 1983.

13. Dawson, G.D.: Cerebral responses to electrical stimulation of peripheral nerve in man. J. Neurol. Neurosurg. Psychiatry, 10:137, 1947.

14. Nash, C.L., Brodsky, J.S., and Croft, T.J.: A model for electrical monitoring of spinal cord function in scoliosis patients undergoing correction. In Proceedings of the Scoliosis Research Society. J. Bone Joint Surg., 54A:197, 1982.

15. Nash, C.L., Schatzinger, L., and Lorig, R.: Intraoperative monitoring of spinal cord function during scoliosis spine surgery. J. Bone Joint Surg., 56A:1765, 1974.

16. Wiltse, L.L., Newman, P.H., and MacNab, I.: Classification of spondylolisis and spondylolisthesis. Clin. Orthop., 117:23, 1976.

17. Willis, T.A.: The separate neural arch. J. Bone Joint Surg., 13:709, 1931.

18. Wiltse, L.L.: American Academy of Orthopaedic Surgeons Symposium on Spine. St. Louis, The C.V. Mosby Co., 1969.

19. Cowell, M.J., and Cowell, H.R.: The incidence of spina bifida occulta in idiopathic scoliosis. Clin. Orthop., 118:16, 1976.

20. Smith, L.: Enzyme dissolution of the nucleus pulposus in humans. JAMA, 187:137, 1964.

21. Stern, I.J.: Biochemistry of chymopapain. Clin. Orthop., 67:42, 1969.

22. Javid, M.J., et al.: Safety and efficacy of chymopapain (chymodiatin) in herniated nuclear pulposus with sciatica. JAMA, 249:2489, 1983.

23. Nordby, E.J., Long, D.M., and Dawson, E.G.: Postgraduate Syllabus on Intradiscal Therapy. Chicago, American Academy of Orthopaedic Surgeons and American Association of Neurological Surgeons, 1983.

24. Merz, B.: The honeymoon is over: Spinal surgeons begin to divorce themselves from chemonucleolysis. JAMA, 256:317, 1986.

25. Goldstein, T.B.: Chemonucleolysis: Still controversial, but worthwhile for selected patients. J. Musculoskel. Med., 3:21, 1986.

26. DeFiore, J.C., Linderg, L., and Ranawat, N.S.: ^{85}Strontium scintimetry of the spine. J. Bone Joint Surg., 52A:21, 1970.

27. Singal, D.P., et al.: HLA antigens in osteitis condensans ilii and ankylosing spondylitis. J. Rheumatol., 4:105, 1977.

28. Freiberger, R.H.: Osteoid osteoma of the spine. Radiology, 75:232, 1960.

29. Nastasi, A.J., Levine, D.B., and Veliskakis, K.P.: Pain patterns associated with adolescent idiopathic scoliosis. J. Bone Joint Surg., 54A:199, 1972.

Spinal stenosis is a syndrome resulting from pressure on the spinal cord or cauda equina by a narrowed spinal canal.[1-6] Typically such compression occurs in the cervical and lumbar spine in persons over age 50. In each case the end result is a disorder of gait. The two clinical syndromes of spinal stenosis are *cervical myelopathy caused by cervical spondylosis*[5,6] and *caudal compression with neurogenic claudication caused by lumbar stenosis.*[1,2-4,7] Each of these syndromes is a manifestation of regional osteoarthritis. Whether these patients have more extensive nonspinal osteoarthritis than age-matched controls is not known.

HISTORY

An early description of lumbar spinal stenosis appeared in 1893 by the London surgeon Sir William Arbuthnot Lane.[8] His patient, a 35-year-old servant, complained of "weakness of her back and insecurity of her legs" and had reduced sensation in her feet. Lane noted an unusual convexity of the lumbar spine. At laminectomy he observed that the spine of L5 was "buried" as a consequence of spondylolisthesis. Since he noted that the neural arch was intact he assumed that the listhesis was degenerative. The idea that spondylolisthesis, with or without a defect in the neural arch, might cause sciatica was later developed by Junghanns,[9] MacNab,[10] and Stewart.[11]

"Congenital stricture of the spinal canal" was the term used by M.A. Sarpyener, a Turkish orthopedic surgeon, who in 1945 described 12 children with severe and varied neurologic sequelae to a congenital narrowing of the spinal canal.[12] In 1954 Verbiest, a Dutch surgeon, described patients having "signs of disturbance of the cauda equina, i.e., bilateral radicular pains, and disturbances of sensation and impairment of motor power in the legs" upon standing and walking, with relief of symptoms upon recumbence.[1] Verbiest used myelography to demonstrate extradural compression. Van Gelderen had antedated (1948) Verbiest's description and had proposed that a hypertrophied ligamentum flavum was responsible.[13] In contrast, Verbiest championed the contribution of congenital narrowing of the lumbar vertebral canal even though the mean age in his seven patients was 51 years.[1] The debate over the relative contributions of congenital narrowing versus hypertrophic changes persists. The history of lumbar stenosis has been reviewed by Kirkaldy-Willis.[3]

Verbiest's descriptions of lumbar stenosis coincided with reports from English neurologists of spondylotic cervical myelopathy.[6,14-16] Just as lumbar disc protrusion entered the medical consciousness ahead of lumbar stenosis, so had Stookey described cervical disc protrusion[17] many years before cervical myelopathy caused by advanced cervical spondylosis was proposed by Brain and colleagues.[6]

CERVICAL SPONDYLOSIS WITH MYELOPATHY

ETIOLOGY AND PATHOLOGY

After decades of attrition caused by trauma and central dehydration, one or more cervical discs degenerates. At the adjacent posterior margins of the vertebral bodies, posterior protrusions of exostotic bone and degenerated anulus fibrosus and disc cause "spondylotic bars" compressing the cord anteriorly.[5,15,18] Thickening of the ligamentum flavum encroaches on the cord from behind.[5] The lateral corticospinal tracts are demyelinated at and below the level of compression, whereas the ascending dorsal sensory columns are demyelinated above this level.[5] Frequently there are deep indentations of the cord by several spondylotic bars (Fig. 93–1). Because the bars can extend into the intervertebral foramina, the cervical nerve roots often become compressed. This compression results in fibrosis of the dural sleeves of the nerve roots. The theory that the myelopathy is due to ischemia has no foundation.[18]

Nurick discussed the various contributions to such a squashed cervical cord.[15,16] As with lumbar stenosis, controversy exists regarding the relative importance of a congenitally narrow canal versus the end results of degenerative disc disease, that is, osteophytes, sub-

luxations, thickened yellow ligament, and impaired blood supply through the anterior spinal artery.[15,19] Hindering a resolution of this conflict are the imprecision of radiographic measurements and the considerable overlap between the anteroposterior (AP) spinal diameters of patients with cord compression and those of controls. Thus the mean minimum AP diameter of myelopathic cervical spines, as determined radiologically by Nurick, was 14.6 mm, whereas that of controls was 16.2 mm.[15] The average AP diameter of the cervical cord itself in the normal adult is abut 10 mm.

INCIDENCE

The peak age at onset of symptoms is in the range of 40 to 60 years.[14,16] Males predominate in a ratio of 60:40, and to an even greater extent beyond age 60. Although cervical disc degeneration is present in 50% of persons at age 45 and in over 90% after age 60, only a few patients with spondylosis develop cervical myelopathy.[14,19] Among a group of 51 patients with cervical spondylosis followed for over 6 years, none developed symptoms or signs of cord compression.[14] Those who did develop cord symptoms and signs seldom recalled previous discrete episodes of cervical radiculopathy.

FIG. 93–1. *A,* Posterior aspect of bodies of cervical vertebrae showing transverse bosses and bars. *B,* Same patient as in *A,* showing indentations of anterior cervical cord and nerve roots corresponding to the bosses and bars. (From Wilkinson, M.: Pathology: Cervical myelopathy. *In* Cervical Spondylosis. Edited by M. Wilkinson. Philadelphia, W.B. Saunders Co., 1971, pp. 49–51. Reproduced with permission.)

SYMPTOMS AND SIGNS

The clinical manifestations of spondylotic cervical myelopathy are presented in Table 93–1. Typically the patient has a spastic gait, hyper-reflexia in the lower limbs, and Babinski signs. There may be upper and/or lower motor neuron signs in the upper extremities depending on the site of compression.[5,14,19] Neck pain may be absent, but restricted neck motion is usual. Cervical radicular pains are often present. Disturbances of sensation can include dysesthesias and clumsiness in the hands, while impaired vibration and joint-position sense can occur in the lower extremities. Weakness and wasting of the small muscles of the hands are common. The site of the lesion can sometimes be deduced from the pattern of upper motor neuron change. Thus, absence of biceps deep tendon reflexes combined with hyperactive triceps tendon reflexes can signify cord compression at C6. Fasciculations can be seen in upper extremity muscles, especially in the small muscles of the hands. Urinary incontinence is uncommon. While there is usually no history of discrete neck trauma, sometimes

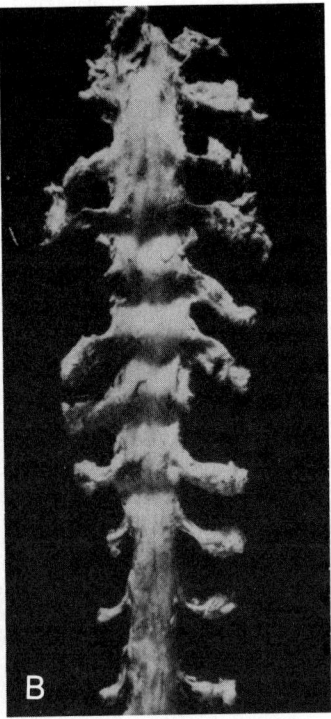

A B

Table 93–1. Symptoms and Signs of Myelopathy Caused by Spondylotic Cervical Myelopathy in 32 Patients*

Type	Percent
Motor	
Hyper-reflexia	87
Babinski sign	54
Spastic gait	54
Sphincter disturbance	49
Arm weakness	31
Paraparesis	21
Quadriparesis	10
Brown-Sequard	10
Hand atrophy	13
Fasciculation	13
Sensory	
Vague sensory level	41
Proprioceptive loss	39
Cervical dermatome sensory loss	33
Pain	
Radicular, arm	41
Cervical pain	26

*From Lundsford, L.D., Bissonette, D.J., and Zarub, D.S.: Anterior surgery for cervical disc disease. Part 2: Treatment of cervical spondylotic myelopathy in 32 cases. J. Neurosurg., 53:12–19, 1980.

sudden worsening of neurologic signs may follow a mild neck injury.[14]

DIAGNOSIS

Roentgenograms of the cervical spine show narrowed disc spaces and osteophytes, especially at C5-6 and C6-7 (Fig. 93–2A). Oblique views show encroachment of intervertebral foramina by spurs of Luschka joints. The myelogram suggests distortion of the cord with interruptions in the column of radiocontrast material, often with complete subarachnoid block. Computed tomography (CT) with myelography reveals cross-sectional anatomy (Fig. 93–2C). Although the diagnosis may be suspected by CT or magnetic resonance imaging (MRI), myelographic features remain most helpful. MRI is a useful noninvasive test that can *rule out* nonspondylotic causes of cord compression. The corkscrew shape of the cervical cord that is compressed at several levels is seen well in T2-weighted images (Fig. 93–2B) and gives an approximate sense of the amount of impingement into the subarachnoid space and consequently on the cord itself. Scoliosis can lead to a false MRI impression of a narrowed cervical cord; otherwise, MRI is almost as useful as myelography. Cerebrospinal fluid (CSF) from below the block may show protein content above 50 mg/dl.[19]

Myelography can usually distinguish cervical cord tumors, cervical disc herniation, and arteriovenous malformations from spondylotic myelopathy. However, multiple sclerosis, amyotrophic lateral sclerosis, and neurosyphilis, as well as subacute combined degeneration of the cord with vitamin B_{12} deficiency, must also be considered in the differential diagnosis.

NATURAL HISTORY

Most authors describe an indolent course with little progression of disability from the time of diagno-

FIG. 93–2. *A,* Cervical spondylosis, showing disc degeneration at C5-6 and C6-7, and mild subluxation of C3 and C4. *B,* MRI T2-weighted image with CSF (appearing white) showing beaded stenosis worst at C3-4 and C6-7 *(arrows). C,* CT-metrizamide myelogram showing a spondylotic bar *(arrow)* protruding posteriorly that resulted in squashed canal contents at C4-5.

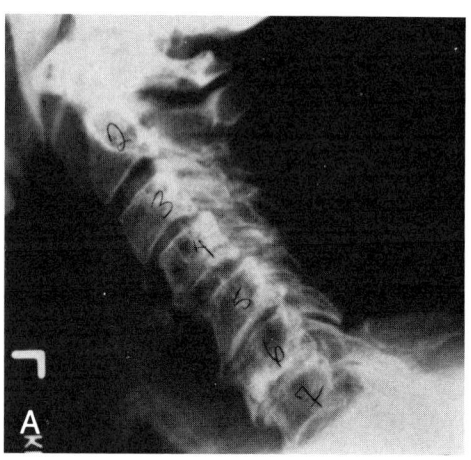
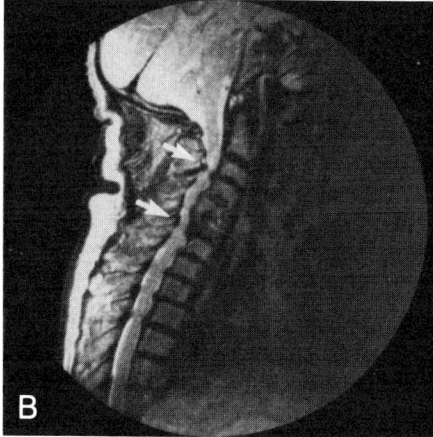
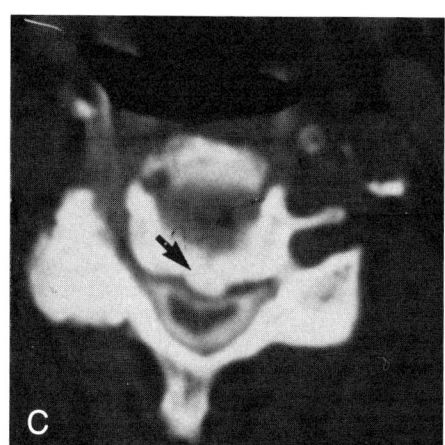

sis.[14,15] Lees and Turner followed 44 of 51 well-documented, and mostly unoperated on, patients for 5 or more years.[14] An injury often preceded the onset of symptoms, and the indolent course was punctuated at long intervals by one or more episodes of neurogenic exacerbation. Disability in these 44 patients, although rated "severe" in over half, did not change appreciably during observation.[14] Nevertheless, Nurick, while extolling the virtues of nonoperative measures, found that about 20% of their patients worsened.[16]

TREATMENT

Because the neurologic status might not change much after surgical laminectomy and because the conservative measures of physiotherapy and the use of a cervical collar are of unproven benefit, controversy exists over the value of an operation in spondylotic myelopathy.[5,14,20] A laminectomy, which is usually multilevel, decompresses the cord and results in improvement in 56 to 61% of patients.[5,16] Multilevel foraminotomies to decompress nerve roots are usually done also. Anterior fusion has not been shown to relieve symptoms.[20a] Surgical results do not appear to be influenced by the age of the patient, but patients left with "stable" cervical spines appeared to fare better than those left with an increased range of movement.[20] The upper extremity sensory symptoms may improve less than the gait disturbance. Appropriate guidelines for extensive laminectomy are not yet defined. When patients are told of the uncertain results of surgical treatment, some decline. At present the best surgical candidates are those with demonstrated recent progression in gait disturbance.

LUMBAR STENOSIS

DEFINITION

The definition of lumbar stenosis invokes a description of symptoms and myelographic findings, because there are no widely acceptable criteria based on the AP diameter of the spinal canal.[3,4,21] This diameter may range from 10 to 15 mm in symptomatic patients.[21] It is generally agreed that there is "an incongruity between the capacity and the contents of the lumbar spinal canal [that] may give rise to compression of the roots of the cauda equina".[7] The clinical syndrome consists of symptoms of compression of the roots of the cauda equina.[1,3,22,23] These symptoms are *intermittent claudication* brought on by walking and

pain or *paresthesias* in the legs evoked by standing and accentuated by exercise, but relieved by sitting or lying down.[1,10,22,24-26] The diagnosis is confirmed by demonstrating a blockage to the flow of myelographic contrast material and by the surgical finding of compression of the caudal sac.

PATHOPHYSIOLOGY (Table 93–2)

The laminae and facets are dense and thickened, creating difficulty in performing spinal puncture.[27] The pathology is diagrammatically shown in Figure 93–3, in which a normal-sized spinal canal is compared with a congenitally narrow one and with the more-commonly encountered canal that is compromised by hypertrophic changes. *Synovial cysts* from the hypertrophic apophyseal joints may be encountered. Degeneration of discs, although not the immediate cause of radiculopathies, along with apophyseal joint disease contributes to the syndrome.[22,27] The liagmentum flavum, which should not exceed 4 mm in thickness, may be up to 7 or 8 mm thick.[3,22] The apophyseal joint hypertrophy is the key to narrowing of the lateral recesses and contributes to the *spondylolisthesis* that occurs in at least one third of patients.[26] Lumbar stenosis has been described in achondroplasia,[28] in Paget's disease of the bone, in diffuse intervertebral skeletal hyperostosis,[29] and after surgical lumbar fusion.[25] In one study calcium pyrophosphate crystals were encountered in four patients, but all had previously undergone surgery.[30] Because the dura is not normally opened at laminectomy, the nerve roots are seldom seen. In one patient who died after laminectomy there was segmental demyelination from compressions of the roots of the cauda equina at regular intervals in accordance with the myelographic findings.[26] This finding and the abnormal electromyographic findings at rest suggest that mechanical pressure rather than ischemia causes the symptoms.[26] Proof of ischemia as a cause of symptoms is lacking.[23,31]

Table 93–2.   Causes of Lumbar Stenosis

Degenerative
   Lumbar spondylosis with or without spondylolisthesis

Iatrogenic (previous fusion)

Paget's disease of the bone

Congenital
   Narrow lumbar canal
   Achondroplasia

FIG. 93–3. Types of lumbar spinal canal. *A,* Normal. *B,* Congenital narrowing. Stippled line shows normal dimensions. *C,* Hypertrophy of ligamentum flavum, apophyseal joints, and vertebral body *(arrows).* This is the most common pathology in lumbar stenosis.

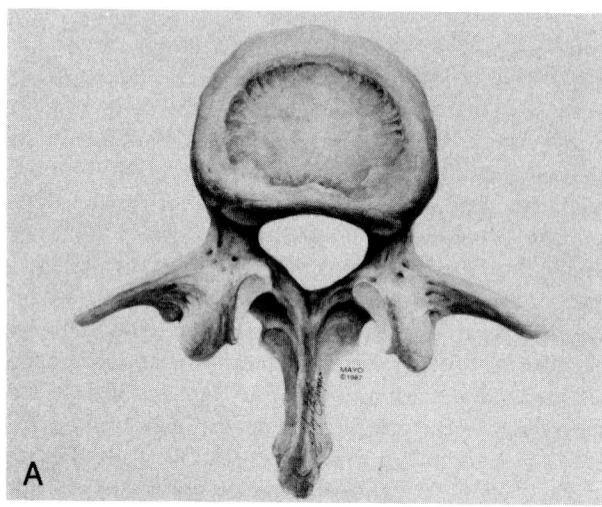

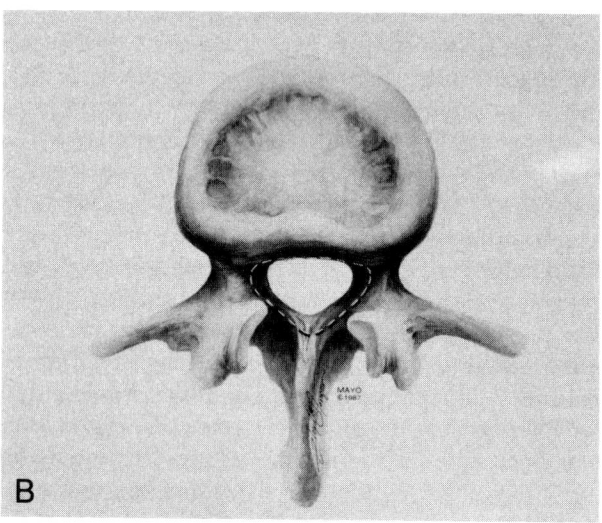

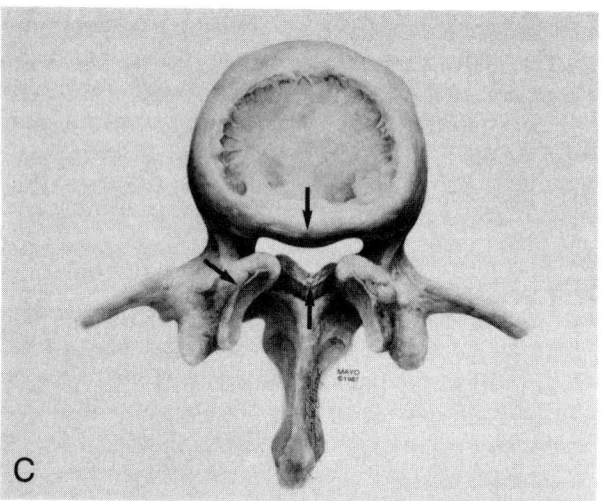

SYMPTOMS AND SIGNS

The cardinal symptom is *neurogenic claudication.*[1,3,23,26] This "pseudoclaudication" is usually bilateral and consists of discomfort or weakness in the buttocks, thighs, legs, and calves brought on by standing or walking and relieved by sitting or lying down.[3,22,23,25,26] The symptoms and signs are listed in Table 93–3. Patients describe "numbness" or "tingling" and "weakness" in the legs,[23,26] which symptoms are relieved by adopting a flexed position.[26] To alleviate symptoms patients will lean against a wall or, more typically, lean forward on a shopping cart or a church pew (Fig. 93–4). In advanced cases not only is the pain provoked by standing and walking a brief distance, but it may come on even when patients are lying supine. Lying on one side, curled in a fetal position, relieves the pain.

Neurogenic claudication differs from vascular claudication. In vascular claudication leg pain is provoked by walking and is relieved by standing, whereas in neurogenic claudication the symptoms are provoked by standing as well as by walking, and paresthesias often accompany the pain.[23] Typically, symptoms come on after walking 100 to 200 yd (90 to 180 m) and usually are felt in the entire lower extemities.[26] Sometimes the symptoms are confined to either above or below the knee; in the case of one-sided lateral recess stenosis, they may be unilateral. Patients often describe their symptoms with a sweeping downward motion of the hands, indicating buttock to heel sciatica. Seldom do patients experience acute radicular symptoms with aggravation by a Valsalva maneuver. If they do, they are probably experiencing discogenic sciatica. Hip stiffness is absent, but spinal stenosis has been confused with hip disease.[24]

Most patients experience lumbar pain that is mechanical and mild.[22,25,26] In our series, only 19% previously had well-defined discogenic sciatica.[26] Patients often complain of leg weakness[3] and may actually fall down. In contrast to other causes of cauda equina compression, sphincter disturbances are rare.

CLINICAL SIGNS

On examination few physical signs are present.[26,31] Pedal pulses are normal unless atherosclerosis coexists with lumbar stenosis as it does in about 9% of patients.[26] Deep tendon reflexes were reduced at the ankle in 29 of 68 (43%) and at the knee in 12 of 68 (18%) patients.[26] Mild, often unilateral, weakness in the lower limbs is found in about one third of patients and usually in the distribution of L5 and S1 roots.

Table 93–3. Symptoms and Signs of Lumbar Stenosis

	Neurogenic Claudication	Vascular Claudication
Distribution	Buttock, thigh or calf (often, the entire leg)	Buttock (aortoiliac) or calf (femoropopliteal)
Symptoms	Cramping pain, numbness, loss of power	Cramping, pain
Inciting factors	Exercise in the erect position, prolonged standing	Exercise in any posture
Relieving factors	Bending forward, sitting or lying down	Standing or sitting
Pulses	Usually normal	Diminished or absent
Electromyogram	Abnormal	Normal

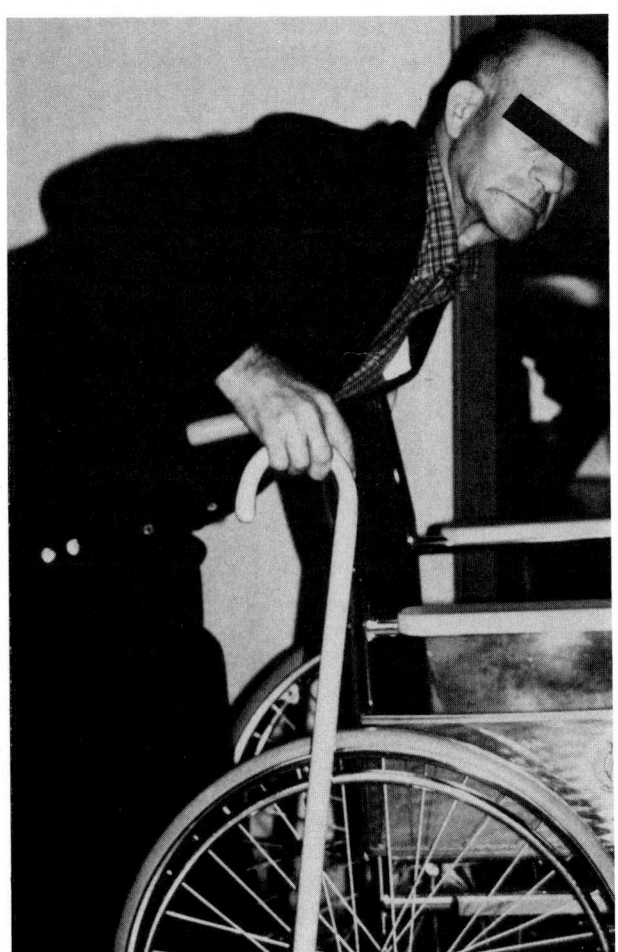

FIG. 93–4. Typical posture of severe lumbar stenosis (simian stance).

This weakness is best evoked by attempts to walk on the heels and toes, respectively. Straight leg raising should not evoke back pain in the Lasègue test.[23,26] Range of motion of the lumbar spine, which is difficult to estimate in any age group, may be reduced or normal.[3,26] The best test is to provoke the symptoms by having the patient stand up or walk for a few minutes and noticing if he adopts a flexed position. Typically, standing up for several minutes will cause the patient to bend forward and lean on the nearest support. Continuous walking for several minutes should induce leg distress (see Fig. 93–4). Occasionally, rechecking the deep tendon reflexes after the symptoms develop will show a reduction as compared with sitting.[23] The frequency of coexisting severe osteoarthritis in the limb joints has not been studied in patients with lumbar stenosis.

The differential diagnosis of lumbar stenosis is (1) vascular claudication caused by atherosclerosis, (2) osteoarthritis of the hips,[24] knees, or both, (3) lumbar disc disease with radiculopathy, and (4) chronic neurologic disease, that is, intraspinal tumor or arteriovenous malformation, multiple sclerosis, and peripheral neuropathy.

LABORATORY FINDINGS

Electromyography (EMG) can be diagnostically helpful showing evidence of chronic neurogenic changes in the distribution of several lumbosacral nerve roots, often bilaterally.[26] The muscles supplied by the L5 and S1 nerve roots are most commonly affected. In our series, 34 of 37 patients (92%) undergoing EMG showed neurogenic abnormalities compatible with nerve root compression. However, all of our patients had complete blocks on myelography and thus had advanced disease.[26] Although testing of somatosensory evoked potentials (SEP) has been proposed as a more sensitive test than EMG, in a study proposing this test only 1 of 11 patients tested by EMG had a positive EMG, while all 11 had abnormal SEPs.[32] At the Mayo Clinic, EMG is done in only half of spinal stenosis patients presenting for surgery,[26] and SEP is omitted.

If the CSF is examined below the level of myelographic block, the CSF protein will be elevated, whereas it is usually normal if measured above a block.[23]

RADIOLOGY

Plain radiographs of the lumbar spine show dense bony structures and one or more degenerative discs.[26] The oblique views show narrowing and sclerosis of apophyseal joints. Chondrocalcinosis is occasionally seen.[30] Over one third of patients have spondylolisthesis, typically L4 on L5.[1,26] This results from partial subluxation of the apophyseal joints. The myelogram is usually done at L2 and typically is technically difficult.[25] *Myelography is the most important diagnostic test and is essential when laminectomy is being considered.* The distal flow of contrast material is blocked either completely or subtotally in the usual position of myelography, that of spinal extension (Fig. 93–5A).[1,27] Flexion of the spine, however, will usually allow the iodinated contrast material to flow (Fig. 93–5B).[22,23,26] About 30% of spinal stenosis patients have multilevel block.[26,27] An hourglass deformity signifies the dual contribution from the apophyseal joints and ligamentum flavum behind and from the degenerated disc in front of the cauda equina (Fig. 93–5A).[3]

Water-soluble agents such as metrizamide are now preferred over iophendylate (Pantopaque), which is not readily absorbed and therefore must be removed after the procedure lest it cause arachnoiditis.[33,34] Because important stenotic or neoplastic lesions at higher levels, typically in the cervical canal, can coexist with lumbar stenosis, *complete myelography is advised.*[25,26]

Myelography does not allow good visualization of the neural foramina of the spinal canal and lateral recesses, especially at the levels below a block.[35] For this reason, CT, with its ability to show a cross section of bone and soft tissues, has gained favor.[4,36–39] CT allows accurate three-dimensional examination of the spine with multiplanar reconstruction techniques. Although CT is widely used, is noninvasive, can show inadequate previous operations, and distinguishes scar from block, its contribution to the diagnosis is controversial.[36,37] Many CT study reports have had serious flaws in design.[36] The problems with relying on CT alone for a diagnosis of lumbar stenosis include

FIG. 93–5. *A,* The myelographic block at L4-5 is due to compression of the dural sac by the liagmentum flavum behind and bulging anulus in front *(arrows).* Diagnosis was grade I spondylolisthesis of L4 on L5. *B,* Block is largely overcome by mild flexion.

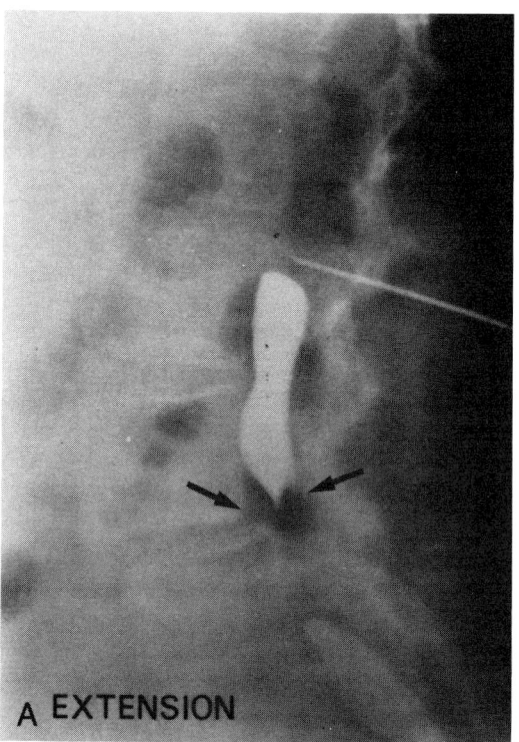

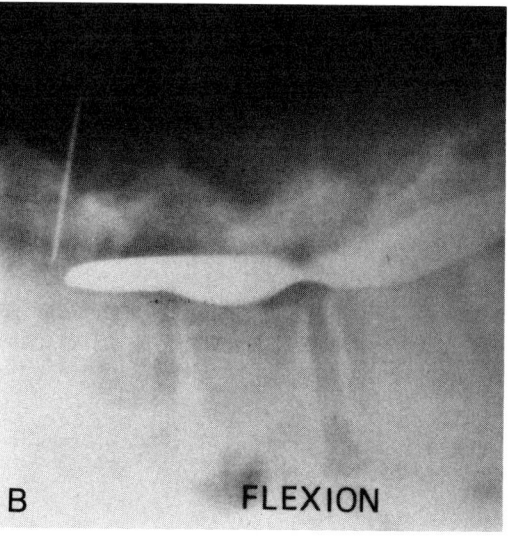

lack of clear guidelines for defining stenosis,[38] false positive interpretations,[37] and the fact that CT may not visualize the spinal canal above L3.[26] *Of our 68 patients, 6 (9%) had stenosis only at L1, L2, or both,*[26] *that is, sites that are not routinely examined on CT of the lumbosacral spine.* In one prospective study of surgically operated patients in which an attempt was made to compare diagnostic techniques, metrizamide myelography proved superior to CT.[36] At present, CT is combined with myelography to enhance diagnosis.[35] CT allows inspection of the lateral recesses and neural foramina, areas that are poorly seen with myelography.[35] Although MRI has also been proposed as a diagnostic test,[40] its expense and unproven diagnostic validity[41] in the lumbar canal have hindered its usefulness in lumbar stenosis.

TREATMENT

There is little evidence that conservative treatment with bracing, exercises, and analgesics is effective. Patients find that using a short cane or walker and wearing padded shoes help. Only those patients with severely restricted activities and otherwise in good health are offered surgery. Myelography is done only as a prelude to planned surgery. *Patients are told to expect little or no improvement in back pain.*

Surgery is extensive.[7] Most patients require multilevel bilateral laminectomy.[26] The average operation is a three-level procedure, while the range in levels operated is from one to five.[26] Foraminotomies for lateral recess stenosis may be needed, in which case, owing to the width of the laminectomy, the medial part of the hypertrophied facet joint is trimmed, that is, a hemifacetectomy is performed. A few patients also need to have large discs or disc fragments removed.[26]

Adding to the difficulty of surgery is the thickness and density of the bones and ligaments.[3,7,22,25] The surgeon notices absence of dural fat and dural pulsations as well as a ligamentum flavum that is up to 8 mm thick.[3,22,25] Indications for fusion are not clearly defined. When spondylolisthesis of L4 on L5 is so advanced that it has slipped forward by a half or more of its AP diameters, that is, grade-2 slip or more, then laminectomy is combined with lateral interbody fusion.[42]

RESULTS

In a mean followup of 4 years, two thirds of the 68 patients operated on at the Mayo Clinic in a 30-month period reported excellent to good relief of their lower limb symptoms while about one third reported little or no improvement.[26] Causes of the disappointing results in the minority appear to be restenosis,[43] inadequate unroofing of the spinal canal, or an increase in mechanical back pain from instability[44,45] especially if a spondylolisthetic slip was worsened.[3,45] Nevertheless, at present there is more enthusiasm for surgical treatment of lumbar stenosis than there is for operation for cervical myelopathy.

REFERENCES

1. Verbiest, H.: A radicular syndrome from developmental narrowing of the lumbar vertebral canal. J. Bone Joint Surg., *36B*:230–237, 1954.
2. Jones, R.A.C., Thomson, J.L.G.: The narrow lumbar canal. J. Bone Joint Surg., *50B*:595–605, 1960.
3. Kirkaldy-Willis, W.J., et al.: Lumbar spinal stenosis. Clin. Orthop., *99*:30–50, 1974.
4. Uden, A., et al.: Myelography in the elderly and the diagnosis of spinal stenosis. Spine, *10*:171–174, 1985.
5. Wilkinson, M.: Pathology: cervical myelopathy. *In* Cervical Spondylosis. Its Early Diagnosis and Treatment. Edited by M. Wilkinson. Philadelphia, W.B. Saunders, 1971, pp. 49–55.
6. Brain, W.R., Knight, G.C., and Bull, J.W.D.: Discussion on rupture of the intervertebral disc in the cervical region. Proc. R. Soc. Med., *41*:509–516, 1948.
7. Epstein, J.A., Epstein, B.S., and Lavine, L.: Nerve root compression associated with narrowing of the lumbar spinal canal. J. Neurol. Neurosurg. Psychiatry, *25*:165–176, 1962.
8. Lane, W.A.: Case of spondylolisthesis associated with progressive paraplegia; laminectomy. Lancet, *1*:991, 1893.
9. Junghanns, H.: Spondylolisthesen ohne spalt im 3 weischengelenkstuck (Pseudospondylolisthesen). Arch. Orthop. Trauma Surg., *29*:118–127, 1930.
10. MacNab, I.: Spondylolisthesis with an intact neural arch: The so-called pseudo-spondylolisthesis. J. Bone Joint Surg., *32B*:325–333, 1950.
11. Stewart, T.D.: Spondylolisthesis without separate neural arch (pseudospondylolisthesis of Junghanns). J. Bone Joint Surg., *17*:640–648, 1935.
12. Sarpyener, M.A.: Congenital stricture of the spinal canal. J. Bone Joint Surg., *27*:70–79, 1945.
13. Van Gelderen, C.: Ein Orthotisches (Lurdotisches) Kaudasyndrom. Acta Psychiatr. Neurol., *23*:57–68, 1948.
14. Lees, F., and Turner, J.W.A.: Natural history and prognosis of cervical spondylosis. Br. Med. J., *2*:1607–1610, 1963.
15. Nurick, S.: The pathogenesis of the spinal cord disorder associated with cervical spondylosis. Brain, *95*:87–100, 1972.
16. Nurick, S.: The natural history and the results of surgical treatment of the spinal cord disorder associated with cervical spondylosis. Brain, *95*:101–108, 1972.
17. Stookey, B.: Compression of the spinal cord due to ventral extradural cervical chondromas. Arch. Neurol. Psychiatry, *20*:275–291, 1928.
18. Dunsker, S.B.: Cervical spondylotic myelopathy: Pathogenesis and pathophysiology. *In* Seminars in Neurological Surgery. Cervical Spondylosis. Edited by Stewart Dunsker. New York, Raven Press, 1980, pp. 119–134.
19. Rowland, L.P.: Cervical spondylosis. *In* Merritt's Textbook of Neurology. 7th Ed. Edited by L.P. Rowland. Philadelphia, Lea & Febiger, 1984, pp. 310–312.
20. Adams, C.B.T., and Logue, V.: Studies in cervical spondylotic myelopathy, Parts I, II and III. Brain, *94*:557–594, 1971.
20a. Lunsford, L.D., Bissonette, D.J., and Zarub, D.S.: Anterior surgery for cervical disc disease. Part 2: Treatment of cervical

spondylotic myelopathy in 32 cases. J. Neurosurg., 53:12–19, 1980.

21. Naylor, A.: Factors in the development of the spinal stenosis syndrome. J. Bone Joint Surg., 61B:306–309, 1979.

22. Yamada, H., et al.: Intermittent cauda equina compression due to narrow spinal canal. J. Neurosurg., 37:83–88, 1972.

23. Blau, J.N., and Logue, V.: Intermittent claudication of the cauda equina. Lancet, 1:1081–1086, 1961.

24. Bohl, W.R., and Steffee, A.D.: Lumbar spinal stenosis: A cause of continued pain and disability in patients after total hip arthroplasty. Spine, 4:168–173, 1979.

25. Pennal, G.F., and Schatzker, J.: Stenosis of the lumbar spinal canal. Clin. Neurosurg., 18:86–105, 1971.

26. Hall, S., et al.: Lumbar spinal stenosis: Clinical features, diagnostic procedures and results of surgical treatment in 68 patients. Ann. Intern. Med., 103:271–275, 1985.

27. Ehni, G.: Significance of the small lumbar canal: Cauda equina compression syndromes due to spondylosis. Part 1. J. Neurosurg., 31:490–494, 1969.

28. Pyeritz, R.E., Sack, G.H., and Udvarhelyi, G.B.: Cervical and lumbar laminectomy for spinal stenosis in achondroplasia. Johns Hopkins Med. J., 146:203–209, 1980.

29. Karpman, R.R., et al.: Lumbar spinal stenosis in a patient with diffuse idiopathic skeletal hypertrophy syndrome. Spine, 7:598–603, 1982.

30. Ellman, M.H., et al.: Calcium pyrophosphate dihydrate deposition in lumbar disc fibrocartilage. J. Rheumatol., 8:955–958, 1981.

31. Ciric, I., and Mikhael, M.A.: Lumbar spinal lateral recess stenosis. Neurol. Clin., 3:417–423, 1985.

32. Keim, H.A., et al.: Somatosensory evoked potentials as an aid in the diagnosis and intraoperative management of spinal stenosis. Spine, 10:338–355, 1985.

33. Herkowitz, H.N., et al.: Metrizamide myelography and epidural venography. Spine, 7:55–64, 1982.

34. McIvor, G.W.D., and Kirkaldy-Willis, W.H.: Pathologic and myelographic changes in the major types of lumbar spinal stenosis. Clin. Orthop., 115:72–76, 1976.

35. McAfee, P.C., et al.: Computed tomography in degenerative spinal stenosis. Clin. Orthop., 161:221–234, 1981.

36. Bell, G.R., et al.: A study of computer-assisted tomography: Comparison of metrizamide myelography and computed tomography in the diagnosis of herniated lumbar disc and spinal stenosis. Spine, 9:552–556, 1984.

37. Wiesel, S.W., et al.: A study of positive CAT scans in an asymptomatic group of patients. Spine, 9:549–551, 1984.

38. Hammerschlag, S.B., Wolpert, S.M., and Carter, B.L.: Computed tomography of the spinal canal. Radiology, 121:361–367, 1976.

39. Sheldon, J.J., Russin, L.A., and Gargano, F.P.: Lumbar spinal stenosis. Radiographic diagnosis with special reference to transverse axial tomography. Clin. Orthop., 115:53–67, 1976.

40. Modic, M.T., et al.: Lumbar herniated disc disease and canal stenosis: Prospective evaluation by surface coil MR, CT and myelography. Am. J. Neuroradiol., 7:709–717, 1986.

41. Han, J.S., et al.: NMR imaging of the spine. A.J.R., 141:1137–1145, 1983.

42. Onofrio, B.: Personal communication, May, 1987.

43. Levy, W.J., Dohn, D.F., and Duchesneau, P.M.: Recurrence of lumbar canal stenosis. A decade after decompressive laminectomy. Surg. Neurol., 17:96–98, 1982.

44. Shenkin, H.A., and Hack, C.J.: Spondylolisthesis after multiple bilateral laminectomies and facetectomies for lumbar spondylosis. J. Neurosurg., 50:45–47, 1979.

45. Johnsson, K.E., Willner, S., and Johnsson, K.: Postoperative instability after decompression for lumbar stenosis. Spine, 11:107–110, 1987.

FIBROSING SYNDROMES: DIABETIC STIFF HAND SYNDROME, DUPUYTREN'S CONTRACTURE, AND PLANTAR FASCIITIS

94

WILMER L. SIBBITT, JR.

The expansion of fibroblasts and related cells into areas of tissue damage is a normal consequence of the healing process. Indeed, new connective tissue with its network of collagen fibrils, fibroblasts, and vascular elements is essential to the integrity of the organism after injury.

Certain diseases, however, are characterized by *fibrosis*, defined as the invasion and replacement of normal tissue by increased quantities of soft connective tissue or, alternatively, replacement of normal connective tissue by altered connective tissue. Fibrosis is a pathologic process that may distort the architecture of affected normal tissue and thus, can interfere with normal function.[1] A disorder characterized by an overaccumulation of fibrous tissue is termed a *fibrosing or sclerosing disease*. A partial list of diseases characterized clinically by fibrosis is shown in Table 94–1.

PATHOGENESIS OF FIBROSIS

Tissue injury, chronic inflammation, vascular ablation, alterations in collagen type, and chemical modifications of existing collagen can all induce what is clinically recognized as fibrosis. All of these mechanisms can be considered variations of the normal healing process.[2]

THE HEALING PROCESS

The normal healing process is classically divided into four phases:[2] (1) tissue injury, (2) secondary inflammation; (3) tissue proliferation; and (4) tissue remodeling (Table 94–2). Type I and type III collagens exposed by tissue injury react with platelet fibronectin, resulting in platelet adhesion and aggregation.[3] Platelets release vasoactive amines, adenine nucleotides, arachidonic acid metabolites, and cytokines, all of which enhance fibroblast proliferation and promote leukocyte chemotaxis.[4-6] Platelets also activate the coagulation system and, subsequently, the complement and kinin cascades[7] (see Chapter 24).

The preceding events are followed by chemotactic factor-induced invasion by blood neutrophils and eosinophils and, later, by monocytes.[2] The monocytes differentiate into tissue macrophages in the site.[8] Of these inflammatory cells, only the monocyte and macrophages are thought to be essential to the reparative process[9] (see Chapter 18).

CONNECTIVE TISSUE INVASION

Fibroblasts, myofibroblasts, and capillary endothelial cells derived from local tissue appear in the area of injury 24 to 48 hours after the migration of white cell elements.[2,10] This cellular proliferation is controlled largely by resident macrophages and monocytes, both of which secrete a variety of factors that

1473

Table 94–1. Fibrosing Diseases

Skin and Musculoskeletal System
Progressive systemic sclerosis
Morphea
Graft–host reaction
Diabetic stiff-hand syndrome
Dupuytren's contracture
Plantar fasciitis
Keloids

Lungs
Pulmonary fibrosis
Chronic pleural reaction

Cardiovascular
Constrictive pericarditis
Vascular plaques
Intimal proliferation

Gastrointestinal
Chronic active hepatitis
Primary biliary cirrhosis
Sclerosing cholangitis
Esophageal stricture
Collagenous colitis

Genitourinary
Nephritis
Nephrosclerosis
Interstitial cystitis
Peyronie's disease

Other
Pseudotumor
Retroperitoneal fibrosis
Reidel's struma
Cancer
Sjögren's syndrome

enhance fibroblast proliferation and vascular ingrowth.[11–17] The fibroblasts then secrete collagen, fibronectin, reticulin, and proteoglycans, creating a stabilizing matrix in the area of the injury.[18]

Once fibroblast proliferation and collagen synthesis have stabilized the area, remodeling of the extracellular matrix occurs.[19] This involves resorption of collagen fibers and secretion of new collagen along lines of stress to provide the greatest strength to the healed wound. When resident fibroblasts migrate through tissues, they leave extracellular strand-like arrays; these structures may help the fibroblast anchor itself in tissue and sense the direction of external stresses.[20,21]

CONTRACTION OF CONNECTIVE TISSUE

Important in the last phase of tissue remodeling is contraction of the new connective tissue.[20,22] This is mediated by epithelial cells in the early wound and later by fibroblasts and myofibroblasts in the mature granulation tissue.[23] Myofibroblasts differentiate from fibroblasts and contain large amounts of the contractile protein actin.[24] These cells migrate through tissue, produce anchoring strands composed of fibronectin, allow the formation of collagen fibrils, and then contract to bring the margins of the injury as close to complete apposition as possible.[25] The degree of tension on adjoining normal tissues is dependent on the amount of contraction by the myofibroblasts. The contractures and distorted microscopic and macroscopic anatomy of fibrosing diseases are largely due to the contraction of the myofibroblasts in the affected area.[26]

ABNORMALITIES OF COLLAGEN

The most obvious abnormality associated with fibrosis is an increase in the total amount of collagen. This usually occurs from increased local production of collagen but can also occur from a relative resistance of resident collagen to collagenase.[27] Increased local production of collagen occurs in the presence of most chronic inflammatory diseases, in areas of massive tissue necrosis, and in the presence of chronic vas-

Table 94–2. The Normal Healing Process

Phase of Wound Healing	Microscopic Characteristics	Days after Injury
1 Tissue injury	Exposure of hidden proteins	0
	Release of mediators	0
	Release of chemoattractants	0–2
	Platelet activation	
	Coagulation	
2 Secondary inflammation	Neutrophils and eosinophils	1–4
	Monocytes	2–6
3 Tissue proliferation	Fibroblast migration	3–7
	Vascular ingrowth	6–10
	Collagen secretion	2–21
4 Tissue remodeling	Modification by proteases	3–21
	Collagen cross linking	7–72

cular insufficiency.[28] Macroscopic and microscopic vascular ablation has been increasingly recognized as a major mechanism for the induction of fibrosis.[28] Hypoxia in areas of injury may stimulate the production of collagen by fibroblasts.[29] Vascular ablation may also be a critical mechanism of fibrosis in progressive systemic sclerosis[30] and Dupuytren's contracture[28] and may be independent of fibrosis mediated by infiltrative mononuclear cells, as occurs in inflammatory diseases.[31]

The molecular type of collagen may also change, inducing profound changes in the physical properties of the tissue (Chapter 12). Alterations in the type of collagen are common in many fibrosing diseases and are characterized by changes in the ratio of type I to type III collagen.[32] An example is pulmonary fibrosis, in which the total amount of collagen is not increased, but the amount of type I collagen is increased relative to that of type III.[33,34] In Dupuytren's contracture, both total collagen and type III collagen are increased.[32] Similarly, post-translational chemical changes such as glycosylation may increase the hydrophilic characteristics of the collagen and change its physical properties.[35] These molecular changes may influence both the amount of collagen and its tensile properties.[36]

The number of diseases associated with fibrosis is quite large (Table 94–1). A discussion of all diseases characterized by fibrosis is beyond the scope of this chapter; only those fibrosing conditions affecting regional areas of the musculoskeletal system are discussed in detail here. Progressive systemic sclerosis and scleroderma variants are discussed in great detail in Chapter 73 and are mentioned here only in relationship to other diseases.

DUPUYTREN'S CONTRACTURE

PATHOLOGY AND BIOCHEMISTRY

Dupuytren's contracture is a clinical condition characterized by nodular thickening of the palmar fascia and flexor contracture of the digits (Fig. 94–1). It was first described in the seventeenth century and later was given a full and accurate description by the French surgeon Baron Guillaume Dupuytren.[37] Because anatomy of the hand is distorted by the diseased fascia, treatment of this disorder is complex and hazardous.[38]

Dupuytren's contracture is an active fibrotic process characterized by fibroblast proliferation and accelerated production of collagen in and around the palmar fascia. The fibrotic tissue coalesces into *palmar nodules, cords,* and *bands,* all of which are composed of con-

FIG. 94–1. This is an early stage of Dupuytren's contracture characterized by a puckering of the skin and the presence of a nodular thickening of the palmar fascia. The contracture of the fourth metacarpophalangeal joint is in an incipient stage but should progress with time. Similar lesions may be present in the plantar fascia (plantar fibromatosis).

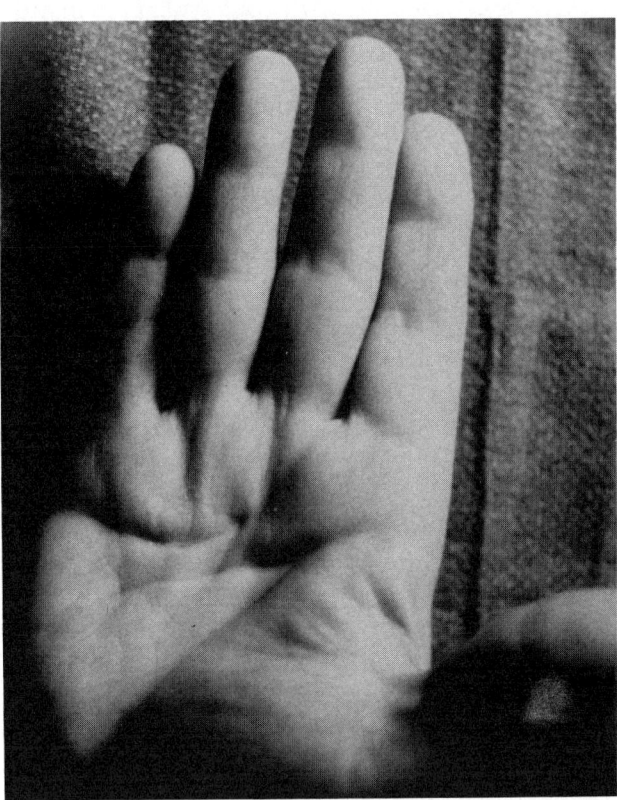

tractile connective tissue.[39] Commonly, the nodules are confined to the palmar aponeurosis, the bands may extend into the digital fascia, and the cords are discrete connective tissue structures extending into the digits.[40] All of these abnormal connective tissue growths can contract, resulting in the development of fixed deformities and contractures. Such traction applied to the palmar aponeurosis, flexor tendons, neurovascular bundles, skin, and periarticular structures results in pain, deformity, and loss of function.[39]

The *early* or *proliferative* stage begins with the clinical appearance of a palmar nodule but no contracture. Microscopically, this stage demonstrates endothelial cell swelling, proliferation of the layers of basal laminae, vessel occlusion, and fibroblast hypertrophy.[28] These findings suggest that vascular occlusion may be the initiating factor in Dupuytren's contracture, as may also occur in scleroderma.[30]

The *active phase* follows, characterized by further growth of nodules and thickened cords in the fascia.[41] In this stage, traction of the skin and flexor tendons is noted first, followed by frank contracture.[42] Pathologically, thickening of the palmar fascia is noted without an obvious antecedent inflammatory event.[41] The nodules contain dense connective tissue and are essentially avascular.[28] *Myofibroblasts* are present in huge numbers in the involved tissue.[43] These cells contain large amounts of the contractile protein actin and may be responsible for the marked contracture of adjacent tissue.[25]

The active phase is characterized by increased amounts of collagen and alterations in the type of resident collagen. The ratio of type I to type III is markedly altered with an enormous increase in type III collagen relative to normal surrounding tissues.[32] Importantly, the collagen from a Dupuytren's contracture binds water more avidly, contributing to connective tissue swelling and further impingement of surrounding structures.[32,41] This sign is shown clearly on magnetic resonance imaging (MRI) (Fig. 94–2). As can be seen, Dupuytren's contracture is the result of a large mass of abnormal connective tissue obscuring the palmar fascia and distorting the flexor tendons of the fourth digit, resulting in an angular deformity. The proton intensity is increased, confirming the accentuated hydration of the involved connective tissue.

The advanced or residual stage of Dupuytren's disease is characterized by chronic contractures with thick cords and nodules consisting mainly of type I collagen.[41] Disuse atrophy of muscles of the hand and forearm is often present. This stage can be quite disabling, and surgery is usually indicated.

ETIOLOGY

Heredity and genetics have important roles in the predisposition to Dupuytren's contracture (Table 94–3). Northern Europeans, especially Celts, have a prevalence of 25% in populations greater than 60 years old,[44–46] while the disease is completely unknown in pure African or Asian peoples.[47] The incidence is increased in younger men, but the prevalence in women older than 75 approaches that of men the same age.[44,45] Chromosomal abnormalities and mosaicism have been described, further emphasizing the importance of genetic considerations.[48,49]

The relationship of Dupuytren's contracture and predisposing diseases appears to be real (Table 94–3). The association with diabetes mellitus is quite strong, and Dupuytren's contracture can occur in as many as 42% of all diabetic patients, although it is unknown whether metabolic derangements or genetic patterns create this association.[50] Injury to the palmar struc-

FIG. 94–2. A magnetic resonance image of the hand shown in Fig. 94–1 demonstrates the invading mass of connective tissue extending along the palmar fascia into the adjoining structures in Dupuytren's contracture. The contractile mass of tissue (arrows) has enmeshed itself around the flexor digitorum profundus and superficialis tendons and exerts traction, resulting in a angular deformity of the tendon and a clinical contracture. The proton intensity (as manifested by increased brightness) is greater than surrounding connective tissue, indicating markedly increased hydration. (Courtesy Dr. Randy R. Sibbitt.)

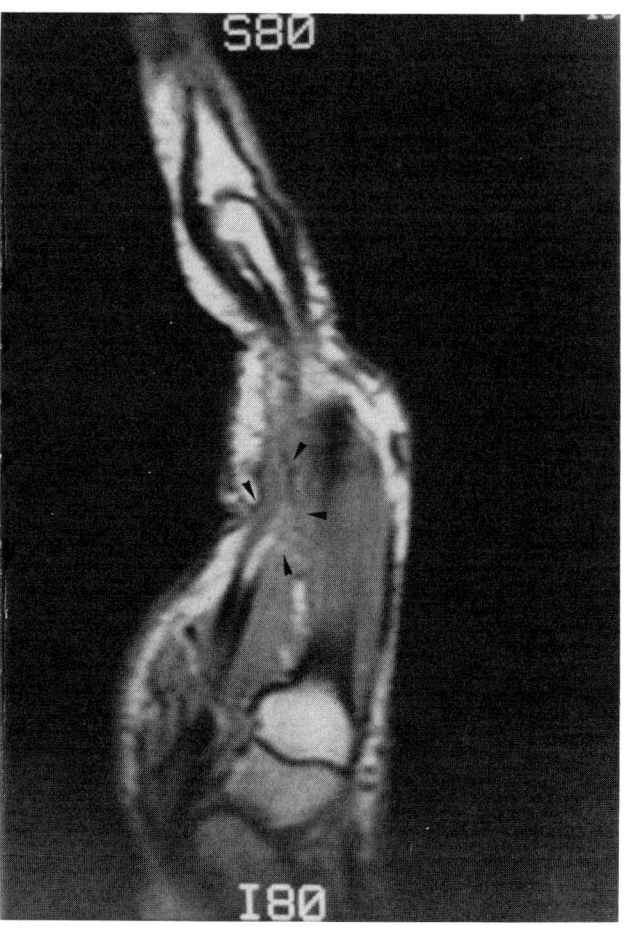

tures, epilepsy, hepatic disease, carpal tunnel syndrome, trigger finger, alcoholism, and rheumatoid arthritis have all been associated with Dupuytren's disease.[41,51] *Dupuytren's diathesis* consists of Dupuytren's contracture, nodules in the plantar fascia (Ledderhose disease), Peyronie's disease, and pads in the popliteal fossa, shoulder, knuckles, and other areas.[52,53] Affected individuals usually have more severe disease and tend to have postsurgical recurrences.

Table 94–3.   Associations With Dupuytren's Contracture

Intrinsic Associations	Extrinsic Associations
Male gender	Injury to palmar aspect of hand
Northern European descent	Pulmonary tuberculosis
Increasing age	Alcoholism
Family history	
Chromosomal abnormalities	
Disease Associations	
Diabetes mellitus	
Chronic liver disease	
Epilepsy	
Plantar fasciitis	
Peyronie's disease	
Knuckle pads	
Carpal tunnel syndrome	
Trigger finger	
Rheumatoid arthritis	

CLINICAL FINDINGS

Patients typically note some decreased mobility in the affected fingers and may complain of pain in the palm or digits.[54] Commonly, both hands are affected, and similar lesions can occur in the feet.[55] In the hands, involvement is most common in the ring finger but can also occur in the fifth, third, and second digits, in order of frequency. Clinically, a nodular thickening is present in the palmar fascia. However, unlike the nodules associated with tenosynovitis, the nodule of Dupuytren's is less discrete, does not move in the exact track of the tendon, and typically dimples the overlying skin (see Fig. 94–1).

The restriction of the flexor tendons is not altered by flexing the wrist (as in congenital or spastic contractures) or by flexing the metacarpophalangeal joints (as in contracture of the intrinsic muscles). If any question remains concerning the identity of the process, MRI study will clearly delineate the presence of the typical fibrotic mass (see Fig. 94–2).

THERAPY

For patients with pain in the nodule, reassurance, local heat, or an intralesional corticosteroid injection may alleviate the symptoms and may improve function.[54,55] Certainly, stretching exercises are indicated in all patients but may not be effective as the disease progresses. Eventually, the contracture may become disabling, and surgery may be necessary to remove the mass of hypertrophied connective tissue from the entrapped flexor tendons of the affected digits. If a contracture greater than 10° is present in the proximal interphalangeal joint, some authors recommend early surgical release to prevent permanent deformity.[41]

Surgery in the treatment of Dupuytren's contracture must be cautious, because the fibrotic tissue often surrounds the neurovascular bundles as well as the fascia and tendons. Not surprisingly, surgery is not uniformly successful. Approaches include nodule excision, fasciotomy, regional fasciotomy, and radical fasciotomy.[38,41,54–58] Of these procedures, radical fasciotomy is the most extensive and involves the removal of the diseased fascia and as much of the surrounding tissue as possible, including the overlying dermis. Skin grafts are usually necessary to close these large wounds.

Complications associated with the surgical treatment of Dupuytren's contracture approach 20% and include flexion contractures, hematoma, skin necrosis, infection, and reflex sympathetic dystrophy.[41] Even after removal of the affected palmar fascia, isolated digital cords may contract and require further therapy.[40]

THE SYNDROME OF LIMITED JOINT MOBILITY

DEFINITION

The *syndrome of limited joint mobility* (SLJM) in patients with diabetes mellitus has been recognized in one form or another for more than a century.[58–61] This disorder is characterized by limitation of motion of the joints of the hands and wrists in a patient with diabetes without the presence of an underlying inflammatory joint disease.[62] SLJM has also been termed *cheiroarthropathy, stiff hand syndrome, diabetic contractures,* and *diabetic sclerodactyly.*[59,63] Although there has been some effort to differentiate these diabetes-associated conditions on the basis of skin, joint, or tendon involvement,[63] it has become increasingly clear that diabetes affects both the skin and periarticular structures and results in a condition that superficially resembles progressive systemic sclerosis.[64]

SLJM is clearly associated with diabetes mellitus, although the range of motion of the small joints in the hands may vary considerably in different populations and may be related to aging.[65,66] SLJM is most common in patients with type I diabetes but has also been reported in type II patients.[67,68] It is not rare and can affect as many as 40% of all insulin-dependent diabetics.[59,68] Most patients are completely asymptomatic in the early phases of this disease, although considerable disability may occur later.

CLINICAL FINDINGS

SLJM is often accompanied by *diabetic sclerodactyly*, a thickening of the skin with loss of elasticity that clinically resembles scleroderma. Thickening begins distally but can affect the wrists, elbows, and neck. A prominent feature of SLJM is the presence of contractures involving the small joints of the hands including the proximal and distal interphalangeal joints and the metacarpophalangeal joints (positive "prayer sign") (Fig. 94–3). Some authors have described a palpable thickening of the joint capsule in addition to the obvious contractures.[63] Diabetic conditions that must be differentiated from SLJM include carpal tunnel syndrome, reflex sympathetic dystrophy, diabetic neuropathy, Dupuytren's contracture, and flexor tenosynovitis with trigger finger (Table 94–4).[63]

In the early stages of SLJM, the patients are often asymptomatic, although accompanying aching, neuropathy, or vascular phenomena can occur. SLJM often occurs in those patients predisposed to the development of retinopathy, nephropathy, and neuropathy, and this group of patients should be carefully examined for a limitation of joint movement.[67] When the contractures are severe, the condition can be completely disabling. Examination typically demonstrates contractures in the proximal interphalangeal, metacarpophalangeal, and wrist joints. Other than the presence of an elevated blood glucose, laboratory evaluation is not of use. Antinuclear antibodies and rheumatoid factor are negative.[62] Careful examination may disclose restrictive pulmonary disease consistent with a more generalized disorder of connective tissue.[69]

PATHOLOGY

The cause of SLJM is unknown but appears to be related to the hyperglycemia that occurs even in

FIG. 94–3. This diabetic patient is suffering from syndrome of limited joint mobility with contractures of the metacarpophalangeal, proximal interphalangeal, and distal interphalangeal joints, resulting in a prominent positive "prayer sign." The skin is also thickened and has lost many of its fine wrinkles, simulating true sclerodactyly.

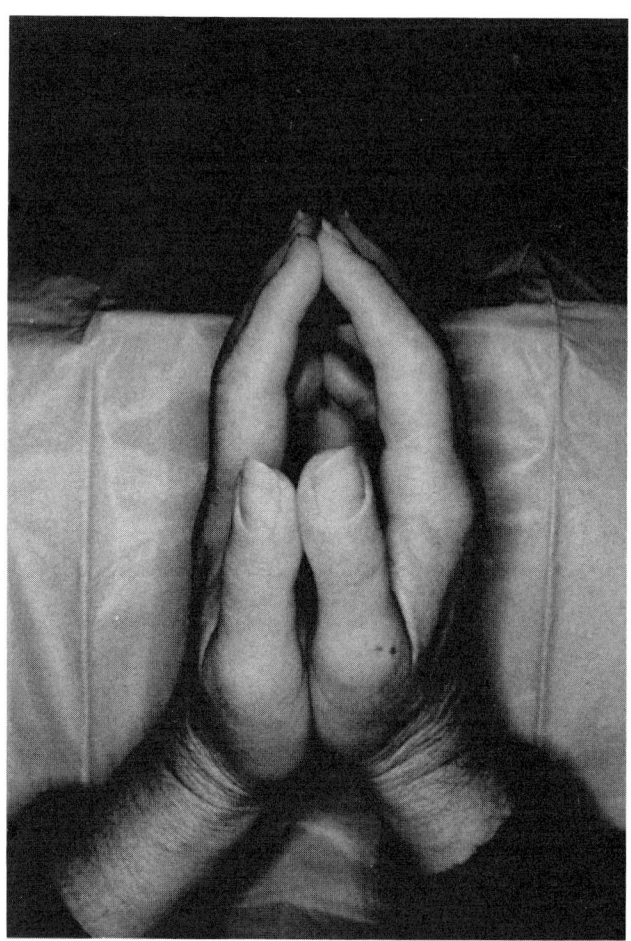

tightly controlled diabetics.[70–76] Biopsies from these patients have demonstrated increased amounts of collagen in the dermis.[71] This collagen appears to have increased cross linking and glycosylation, both of which may change its physical properties with greater resistance to degradation and subsequent accumulation.[36,72,73] Hyperglycemia may also induce increased collagen production by fibroblasts.[71]

Eaton[76] has suggested that SLJM is related to increased hydration of connective tissue and has proposed a mechanism by which glucose is converted into sorbitol, which accumulates intracellularly, resulting in connective tissue swelling. If connective tissue collagen is also altered chemically by nonenzymatic glycosylation, such changes in hydration may be even more impressive.[32,74] MRI has confirmed that

Table 94–4. Classic Hand Syndromes of Diabetes Mellitus

Condition	Typical Joints Involved	Comments
Dupuytren's contracture	3rd, 4th, 5th MCP, PIP	Palpably thickened palmar fascia, flexion contracture of involved digits
Flexor tenosynovitis	1st, 3rd, and 4th MCP, PIP	Trigger finger; thickened tendon sheath; pain
Carpal tunnel syndrome	MCP and PIP	Often associated with true diabetic neuropathy, prominent pain, slowed conduction velocity
Reflex sympathetic dystrophy	Contracture and edema involving entire hand	More often bilateral in diabetes (42%) than other conditions (5%); positive bone scan
Diabetic sclerodactyly	Distal fingers, but may extend to entire hand	Thickened, waxy skin
Syndrome of limited joint mobility	MCP and PIP, and wrist contractures	Decreased range of motion of small joints; often associated with diabetic sclerodactyly
Diabetic neuropathy	Variable contractures	Dysesthesias, pain, muscle atrophy, abnormal nerve conduction

MCP = Metacarpal phalangeal joint; PIP = proximal interphalangeal joint.

the skin is truly thickened in some patients with SLJM and that the connective tissue of the dermis contains greater proton intensity, implying the presence of increased hydration (Fig. 94–4). Increased cross linking of collagen and increased hydration may both be important in the development of SLJM.[70]

TREATMENT OF SLJM

Treatment of SLJM is controversial. Strict control of blood glucose is indicated, and insulin pump therapy may be ameliorative, although this modality has failed in some series.[62] Range-of-motion exercises are essential to maintain function but do not reverse established contractures.[62] Perhaps the most hopeful approach to SLJM is the use of aldose reductase inhibitor agents. Eaton, et al. treated three patients with the experimental agent sorbinil, which greatly improved hand function and reduced contracture.[61,62]

Because increased cross linking of collagen may also be important in the expansion of connective tissue in diabetes mellitus, agents that inhibit cross linking may be of some use. Such agents, including penicillamine, aminoguanidine, and β-amino propionitrile, remain experimental and are not indicated for the treatment of SLJM.*

---

*Editor's note. I have noted marked relief of symptoms with an objective decrease in swelling and increased grip strength after injections of corticosteroids into the volar tendon sheaths in several patients with SLJM.

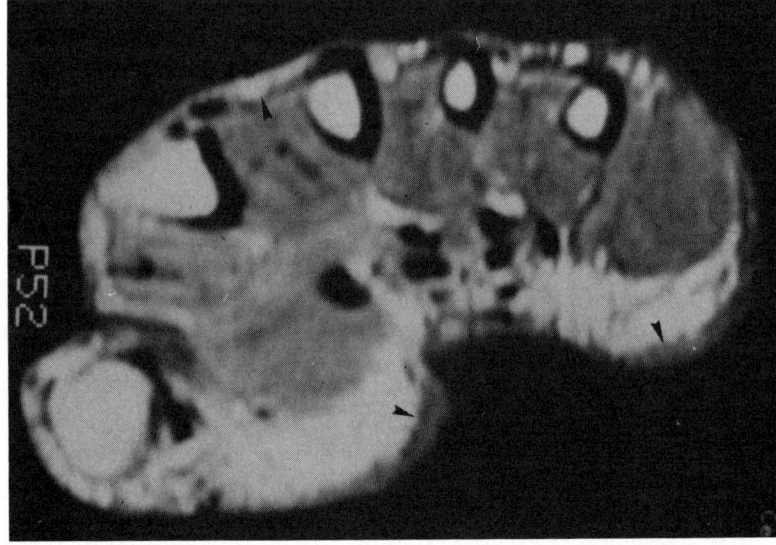

FIG. 94–4. A magnetic resonance image of the hands of the diabetic patient with syndrome of limited joint mobility shown in Fig. 94–3 shows thickened dermal connective tissue resembling that found in progressive systemic sclerosis (arrows). The increased proton density (brightness) indicates increased hydration of the resident connective tissue. (Courtesy Dr. Randy R. Sibbitt.)

PLANTAR FASCIITIS

DEFINITION

Painful heel is a common musculoskeletal complaint. *Plantar fasciitis* refers specifically to a clinical syndrome characterized by pain and morning stiffness involving the heel and plantar surface of the foot with maximum tenderness to palpation localized at the insertion of the plantar fascia on the calcaneal tuberosity. Radiologic studies will often show small calcifications anterior to the calcaneal tuberosity or the presence of an exuberant anterior calcaneal ostosis (spur) (Fig. 94–5).

ETIOLOGY

Plantar fasciitis is one of the most common disorders affecting the foot and is responsible for over 15%

FIG. 94–5. This patient, a long-distance runner, continued to run despite severe calcaneal pain secondary to plantar fasciitis. A large calcaneal hyperostosis extends anteriorly, following the plantar fascia. The patient responded to 8 months of abstinence from long-distance running and eventually was able to resume running at reduced distances with the use of antipronator running shoes. (Courtesy Dr. Randy R. Sibbitt.)

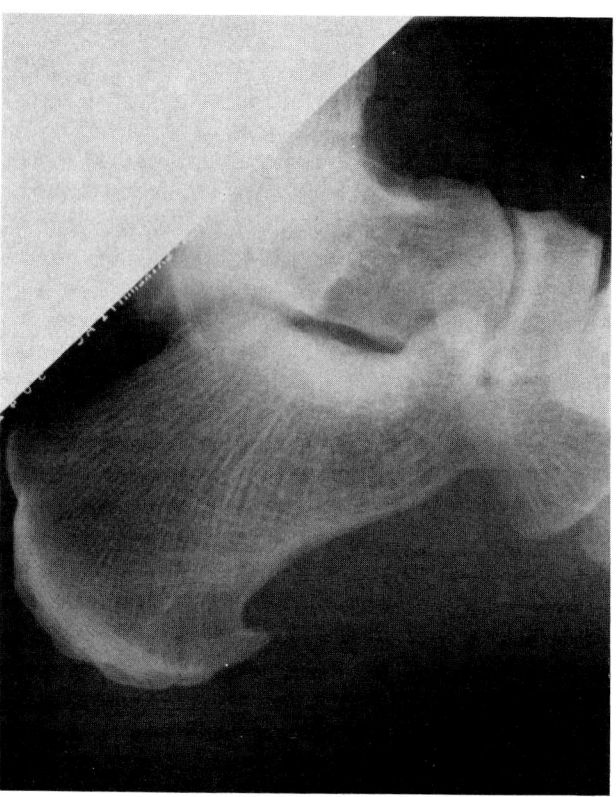

of all foot complaints.[77–79] It may be associated with other inflammatory diseases (Table 94–5), including Reiter's syndrome, ankylosing spondylitis, RA, Dupuytren's contracture, lupus, and gout.[80–82] Plantar fasciitis and other inflammatory heel disorders are often found in the seronegative spondylarthropathies.[83] Indeed, inflammation may be a major inciting factor in the induction of plantar fasciitis.[84,85]

The most common causes of plantar fasciitis are related to abnormal stresses applied to the foot, particularly conditions resulting in unusual torsion of or tension on the plantar fascia.[82,84,86] Such forces are magnified in the foot with an inherent tendency to pronate (evert). This is called the *"flexible flat foot"* and is associated with excessive motion at the talonavicular and naviculocuneiform joints.[87]

Excessive motion at these joints pronates the foot and stretches the plantar fascia, resulting in increased tension across the fascia after heel strike and before toe-off. This chronic traction on the plantar fascia results in microscopic avulsion of a portion of the fascia or an actual fascial tear. Continued injury to the plantar fascia results in chronic inflammation and replacement with connective tissue elements.[78,88]

PATHOLOGY

Surgical specimens obtained from plantar fascial releases show a wide variety of changes including collagen degeneration, angiofibroblastic hyperplasia, chondroid metaplasia, and calcification of degenerated matrix.[88] Periosteal inflammation is almost ubiquitous and may result in the growth of an anterior heel spur, which follows the course of the fascia.[78] The presence of an anterior heel spur is not necessary for the diagnosis of plantar fasciitis but often confirms it and implies that the process has already become chronic (see Fig. 94–5). The spur usually remains after the inflammation and symptoms have abated, indicating that it was not the original cause of pain.

DIAGNOSIS OF PLANTAR FASCIITIS

Inflammatory conditions, particularly the seronegative spondylarthropathies, should be excluded by physical examination, appropriate radiologic studies, and laboratory tests. Other causes of heel pain, noted in Tables 94–5 and 94–6, should also be excluded. The patient should be questioned about overuse, particularly long-distance running. The structure and motion of the foot, ankle, knee, and hip should be carefully examined for a tendency to pronate the foot.

Table 94–5.   Conditions Associated with Plantar Fasciitis

Inflammatory Conditions	Overuse	Other
Frequently	Long-distance running	Diabetes mellitus
Reiter's syndrome	Prolonged walking or standing	Gout
Ankylosing spondylitis	Aerobic dance	Obesity
Psoriatic arthritis		Calcaneal spurs
Intestinal arthropathies		Dupuytren's contracture
Behçet's disease		Achilles tendonitis
Less commonly		
Rheumatoid arthritis		
Systemic lupus erythematosus		
Structural abnormalities		
Pes valgus		
Increased pronation		
Flexible "flat foot"		

Neurologic dysfunction as a cause of heel pain should be considered, and tarsal tunnel syndrome in particular should be excluded.[89]

THERAPY

The treatment of plantar fasciitis should first be directed at reducing torsion and injury to the plantar fascia and its bony insertion. Long-distance running and other activities contributing to overuse should be suspended until the symptoms have completely resolved, which typically requires months of inactivity. The compulsive athlete should be told that rest is the best treatment. Another endurance exercise such as bicycling or swimming can be substituted until the heel symptoms have resolved. Continued overuse of

Table 94–6.   Intrinsic Causes of Heel Pain

Disorder	Complaints	Diagnostic Sign
Plantar fasciitis	Plantar foot, anterior heel	Tenderness over calcaneal tuberosity and anterior osteophyte
Achilles tendon		
Tenosynovitis	Tendon, posterior heel	Diffuse pain and swelling along tendon
Tendonitis	Tendon, posterior heel	Diffuse pain along tendon and calcaneal insertion
Subtendinous bursitis	Tendon, posterior heel	Pain, swelling of superior posterior calcaneus
Subcutaneous bursitis	Tendon, posterior heel	Pain, swelling of inferior posterior calcaneus
Rupture	Weakness, pain often not present	Pain and absence of tendon in area of rupture
Calcaneal		
Apophysitis	Posterior heel	Tenderness insertion of Achilles tendon on roentgenogram
Calcaneal stress fracture	Heel	Stress fracture, on roentgenogram
Flexor hallucis		
Longus tendonitis or tenosynovitis	Anterosuperior heel and posteromedial malleolus into plantar foot	Pain and swelling posterior to medial malleolus into plantar foot
Tibialis posterior		
Tendonitis or tenosynovitis	Same as above	Same as above
Calcaneal periostitis	Tenderness in heel or erosion	Radiologic diagnosis, inflammatory arthritis
Osteomyelitis	Heel pain	Radiologic diagnosis
Calcaneal spur	Heel pain	Nonanterior calcaneal ostosis, pain directly over ostosis
Tarsal tunnel syndrome	Heel and midfoot	Neurologic abnormalities of heel and plantar foot

a predisposed foot will result in chronic, intractable pain and the development of a calcaneal hyperostosis.

Nonsteroidal anti-inflammatory drugs (NSAIDs) are often effective in diminishing the pain and stiffness of plantar fasciitis but are not curative. If a month trial of rest and NSAIDs has not markedly improved the patient's symptoms, injection of the plantar fascia with nonfluorinated corticosteroid esters may temporarily improve symptoms.[88] Injection of the plantar fascia should be attempted through a lateral or medial approach, not through the plantar surface of the foot. The plantar approach is very painful and, if the corticosteroid flows back along the needle track, may induce atrophy and fragility of the plantar skin, a condition that may predispose to injury, infection, and atrophy of the fatty heel pad, leaving the calcaneus under the skin.

If these measures are ineffective, orthotic devices can be constructed to reduce the tension in the plantar fascia by preventing eversion. These devices, the simplest of which is the varus wedge, can consist of a plastic heel cup and medial arch support or may be customized from plaster foot moldings and adjusted to the appropriate degree of correction.[84,88] Prolonged therapy with these devices is required before permanent improvement is noted.[90]

Finally, for cases resistant to conservative therapy, surgical intervention can be considered. Both fasciectomy and fasciotomy (fascial release) have been successful,[84,88] although these procedures might increase the instability in the foot. The symptomatic effectiveness of surgical therapy may be related to hypesthesia of the heel secondary to obliteration of the lateral plantar nerve. In spite of the protracted course of plantar fasciitis, most cases eventually resolve spontaneously. Hence, surgical intervention should be employed only in intractable cases.

REFERENCES

1. Sporn, M.B., and Harris, E.D.: Proliferative diseases. Am. J. Med., 70:1232–1236, 1981.
2. Schilling, J.A.: Wound healing. Surg. Clin. North Am., 56:859–874, 1976.
3. Gordon, J.L.: Mechanisms regulating platelet adhesion. In Cell Adhesion and Mobility (Third Symposium of the British Society for Biology). Edited by A.S.G. Curtis and J.D. Pitts. Cambridge, England: Cambridge University Press, 1980.
4. Turner, S.R., Tainer, J.A., and Lynn, W.S.: Biogenesis of chemotactic molecules by the arachidonate lipoxygenase system of platelets. Nature, 257:680–681, 1975.
5. Ward, P.A.: Complement-derived leukotactic factors in biological fluids. J. Exp. Med., 134:109–113, 1971.
6. Melmon, K.L., and Cline, M.J.: Interaction of plasma kinins with granulocytes. Nature, 213:90–92, 1976.
7. Born, G.U.: Platelets in hemostasis and thrombosis. In Cellular Response Mechanisms and Their Biological Significance. Edited by A. Rotman et al. New York, Wiley Interscience, 1980.
8. Galiman, T.: On some aspects of collagen formation in localized injury and in diffuse fibrotic reactions to injury. In Treatise on Collagens. Vol. 2B. Edited by B.S. Gould. London: Academic Press, 1968.
9. Leibovich, S.J., and Ross, R.: The role of the macrophage in wound repair: Study with hydrocortisone and antimacrophage serum. Am. J. Pathol., 78:71–100, 1975.
10. Leibovich, S.J., and Ross, R.: A macrophage dependent factor stimulates the proliferation of fibroblasts in vitro. Am. J. Pathol., 84:501–514, 1976.
11. Jimenez, S.A., McArthur, W., and Rosenbloom, J.: Inhibition of collagen synthesis by mononuclear cell supernates. J. Exp. Med., 156:1421–1431, 1979.
12. O'Hare, R.P., et al.: Isolation of collagen stimulating factors from healing wounds. J. Clin. Pathol., 36:707–711, 1983.
13. Johnson, R.L., and Ziff, M.: Lymphokine stimulation of collagen accumulation. J. Clin. Invest., 58:240–252, 1976.
14. Wahl, S.M., Wahl, L.M., and McCarthy, J.B.: Lymphocyte-mediated activation of fibroblast proliferation and collagen production. J. Immunol., 121:942–946, 1978.
15. Hibbs, M.S., et al.: Alterations in collagen production in mixed mononuclear leukocyte-fibroblast cultures. J. Exp. Med., 157:47–59, 1983.
16. Hunt, T.K., et al.: Studies on inflammation and wound healing: angiogenesis and collagen synthesis stimulated in vivo by resident and activated wound macrophages. Surgery, 96:48–54, 1984.
17. Kahaleh, M.B., DeLustro, F., Bock, W., and LeRoy, E.C.: Human monocyte modulation of endothelial cells and fibroblast growth: Possible mechanism for fibrosis. Clin. Immunol. Immunopathol., 39:242–255, 1986.
18. Forrest, L.: Current concepts in soft connective tissue wound healing. Br. J. Surg., 70:133–140, 1983.
19. Grillo, H.C., and Gross, J.: Collagenolytic activity during mammalian wound repair. Dev. Biol., 15:300–317, 1967.
20. Baur, P.S., et al.: Wound contractions, scar contractures, and myofibroblasts: A classical case study. J. Trauma, 18:8–22, 1978.
21. Hedman, K., Vaheri, A., and Wartiovaara, J.: External fibronectin of cultured human fibroblasts in predominately a matrix protein. J. Cell Biol., 76:748–760, 1978.
22. Carrico, T.J., Mehrhof, A.I., Jr., and Cohen, I.K.: Biology of wound healing. Surg. Clin. North Am., 64:721–732, 1984.
23. Baur, P.S., Jr., Parks, D.H., and Hudson, J.D.: Epithelial mediated wound contraction in experimental wounds—The purse-string effect. J. Trauma, 24:713–720, 1984.
24. Vande Berg, J.S., and Rudolph, R.: Cultured myofibroblasts: A useful model to study wound contraction and pathological contracture. Ann. Plastic Surg., 14:111–120, 1985.
25. Squier, C.A., Leranth, C.S., Ghoneim, S., and C.R. Kremenak: Electron microscopic immunochemical localization of actin in fibroblasts in healing skin and palate wounds of beagle dog. Histochem., 78:513–522, 1983.
26. Tomasek, J.J., Schultz, R.J., Episalla, C.W., and Newman, S.A.: The cytoskeleton and extracellular matrix of the Dupuytren's disease "myofibroblast": An immunofluorescence study of a nonmuscle cell type. J. Hand Surg., 11A:365–371, 1986.
27. Vater, C.A., Harris, E.D., Jr., and Siegal, R.C.: Native cross-links in collagen fibrils induce resistance to human synovial collagenase. Biochem. J., 181:639–645, 1979.
28. Kischer, C.W., and Speer, D.P.: Microvascular changes in Dupuytren's contracture. J. Hand Surg., 9A:58–62, 1984.

29. Kischer, C.W.: Fine structure of granulation tissues from deep injury. J. Invest. Dermatol., 72:147–152, 1979.

30. LeRoy, E.C.: Pathogenesis of scleroderma (systemic sclerosis). J. Invest. Dermatol., 79(Suppl. 1):875–895, 1982.

31. Kischer, C.W., and Shetlar, M.R.: Microvasculature in hypertrophic scars and the effects of pressure. J. Trauma, 19:757–764, 1976.

32. Bazin, S., et al.: Biochemistry and histology of the connective tissue of Dupuytren's disease lesions. Eur. J. Clin. Invest., 10:9–16, 1980.

33. Seyer, J.M., Hutcheson, E.T., and Kang, A.H.: Collagen polymorphism in idiopathic chronic pulmonary fibrosis. J. Clin. Invest., 57:1498–1507, 1976.

34. Kirk, J.M.E., et al.: Biochemical evidence for an increased and progressive deposition of collagen in lungs of patients with pulmonary fibrosis. Clin. Science, 70:39–45, 1986.

35. Kohn, R.R., Cermani, A., and Monnier, V.M.: Collagen aging in vitro by nonenzymatic glycosylation and browning. Diabetes, 33:57–59, 1984.

36. Golub, L.M., Greenwald, R.A., Zebrowski, E.J., and Ramamurthy, N.S.: The effect of experimental diabetes on the molecular characteristics of soluble rat-tail tendon collagen. Biochim. Biophys. Acta, 534:73–81, 1978.

37. Lindskog, G.E.: Guillaume Dupuytren: 1777 to 1835. Surg. Gynecol. Obstet., 145:746–754, 1977.

38. Watson, H.K., Light, T.R., and Johnson, T.R.: Checkrein resection for flexion contracture of the middle joint. J. Hand Surg., 4:67–77, 1979.

39. Stack, H.G.: The palmar fascia, and the development of deformities and displacement in Dupuytren's contracture. Ann. R. Coll. Surgeons Engl., 48:238–251, 1971.

40. Strickland, J.W., and Bassett, R.L.: The isolated digital cord in Dupuytren's contracture: Anatomy and clinical significance. J. Hand Surg., 10A:118–124, 1985.

41. Legge, J.W.H.: Dupuytren disease. Surg. Ann., 45:355–368, 1985.

42. Chiu, H.F., and McFarlane, R.M.: Pathogenesis of Dupuytren's contracture: A correlative clinical-pathological study. J. Hand Surg., 3:1–10, 1978.

43. Iwasaki, H., Mueller, H., Stutte, H.J., and Breenscheidt, U.: Palmar fibromatosis (Dupuytren's contracture): Ultrastructural and enzyme histochemical studies in 43 cases. Virchows Arch. [A], 405:41–53, 1984.

44. Hueston, J.T.: The incidence of Dupuytren's contracture. Med. J. Aust., 47:999–1006, 1960.

45. Hueston, J.T.: Further studies on the incidence of Dupuytren's contracture. Med. J. Aust., 49:586–588, 1962.

46. Ling, R.S.M.: The genetic factor in Dupuytren's disease. J. Bone Joint Surg., 45B:709–718, 1963.

47. Rosenfeld, N., Mavor, E., and Wise, L.: Dupuytren's contracture in a black female child. Hand, 15:82–84, 1983.

48. Sergovick, F.R., Botz, J.S., and MaFarlane, R.M.: Nonrandom cytogenetic abnormalities in Dupuytren's disease (Letter). N. Engl. J. Med., 308:162–163, 1983.

49. Madden, J.S.: Chromosome abnormalities in Dupuytren's disease (Letter). Lancet, 1:207, 1976.

50. Noble, J., Heathcote, J.G., and Cohen, H.: Diabetes mellitus in the aetiology of Dupuytren's disease. J. Bone Joint Surg., 66:322–325, 1984.

51. Bradlow, A., and Mowat, A.G.: Dupuytren's contracture and alcohol. Ann. Rheum. Dis., 45:304–307, 1986.

52. Mikkelsen, O.A.: Knuckle pads in Dupuytren's disease. Hand, 9:301–305, 1977.

53. Wheeler, E.S.: Case report of popliteal fasciitis. Plast. Reconstr. Surg., 68:781–783, 1981.

54. Hueston, J.T.: Operative plastic and reconstructive surgery. In Dupuytren's Disease in the Hand. Edited by J.N. Barron and M.N. Saad. New York, Churchill Livingstone, 1980.

55. Pentland, A.P., and Anderson, T.F.: Plantar fibromatosis responds to intralesional steroids. J. Am. Acad. Dermatol., 12:212–214, 1985.

56. Curtis, R.M.: Capsulectomy of the interphalangeal joints of the fingers. J. Bone Joint Surg., 36A:1219–1232, 1954.

57. McCash, C.R.: The open palm technique in Dupuytren's contracture. Br. J. Plast. Surg., 17:271–280, 1964.

58. Hill, N.A.: Dupuytren's contracture. J. Bone Joint Surg., 67A:1439–1443, 1985.

59. Leden, I., Schersten, B., and Svensson, B.: Rheumatic hand syndromes: An early or late manifestation of diabetes mellitus. Pract. Cardiol., 9:209–227, 1983.

60. Cambell, R.R., Hawkins, S.J., Maddison, P.J., and Reckless, J.P.D.: Limited joint mobility in diabetes mellitus. Ann. Rheum. Dis., 44:93–97, 1985.

61. Eaton, R.P.: Aldose reductase inhibition and the diabetic syndrome of limited joint mobility: Implications for altered collagen hydration. Metabolism, 35:119–121, 1986.

62. Eaton, R.P., Sibbitt, W.L., Jr., and Harsh, A.: The effect of an aldose reductase inhibiting agent on limited joint mobility in diabetes mellitus. JAMA, 253:1437–1471, 1985.

63. Rosenbloom, A.L.: Joint contractures preceding insulin-dependent diabetes mellitus. (Letter.) Arthritis Rheum., 26:931, 1983.

64. Eversmeyer, W.H.: Digital sclerosis in adult insulin-dependent diabetes. (Letter). Arthritis Rheum., 26:932, 1982.

65. Larkin, J.G., and Frier, B.M.: Limited joint mobility and Dupuytren's contracture in diabetic, hypertensive, and normal populations. Br. Med. J., 292:1494, 1986.

66. Wright, V.: The rheology of joints. Br. J. Rheum., 25:243–252, 1986.

67. Lawson, P.M., Maneschi, F., and Kohner, E.M.: The relationship of hand abnormalities to diabetes and diabetic retinopathy. Diabetes Care, 6:140–143, 1983.

68. Slama, G., et al.: Quantification of early subclinical limited joint mobility in diabetes mellitus. Diabetes Care, 8:329–332, 1985.

69. Schuyler, M.R., Niewoehner, D.E., Inkley, S.R., and Kohn, P.: Abnormal lung elasticity in juvenile diabetes mellitus. Am. Rev. Resp. Dis., 113:37–41, 1976.

70. Brownlee, M., Vlassara, H., and Cerami, A.: Nonenzymatic glycosylation and the pathogenesis of diabetic complications. Ann. Intern. Med., 101:527–537, 1984.

71. Buckingham, B.A., et al.: Scleroderma-like changes in insulin-dependent diabetes mellitus: Clinical and biochemical studies. Diabetes Care, 7:163–169, 1984.

72. Hamlin, C.R., Kohn, R.P., and Luschin, J.H.: Apparent accelerated aging of human collagen in diabetes mellitus. Diabetes, 24:902–904, 1975.

73. Schnider, S.L., and Kohn, R.R.: Effects of age and diabetes mellitus on the solubility and nonenzymatic glucosylation of human skin collagen. J. Clin. Invest., 67:1630–1635, 1981.

74. Means, G.E., and Chang, M.K.: Nonenzymatic glycosylation of proteins: Structure and function changes. Diabetes, 31(Suppl.):1–4, 1982.

75. Rowe, D.W., Starman, B.J., Fujimoto, W.Y., and Williams, R.H.: Abnormalities in proliferation and protein synthesis in skin fibroblast cultures from patients with diabetes mellitus. Diabetes, 26:284–290, 1977.

76. Eaton, R.P.: The collagen hydration hypothesis: A new para-

digm for the secondary complications of diabetes mellitus. J. Chronic Dis., 39:763–766, 1986.

77. DuVries, H.L.: Heel spur (calcaneal spur). Arch. Surg., 74:536–542, 1957.

78. Furey, J.G.: Plantar fasciitis. The painful heel syndrome. J. Bone Joint Surg., 57A:672–673, 1975.

79. Gerster, J.C., et al.: The painful heel. Ann. Rheum. Dis., 36:343–348, 1977.

80. Calabro, J.J.: A critical evaluation of diagnostic features of the feet in rheumatoid arthritis. Arthritis Rheum., 5:19–29, 1962.

81. Calabro, J.J.: Chiropody and arthritis. Bull. Rheum. Dis., 23:692, 1972.

82. Cozen, L.: Bursitis of the heel. Am. J. Orthop., 3:372–374, 1961.

83. Gerster, J.C.: Plantar fasciitis and Achilles tendinitis among 150 cases of seronegative spondarthritis. Rheum. Rehab., 19:218–222, 1980.

84. Lester, D.K., and Buchanan, J.R.: Surgical treatment of plantar fasciitis. Clin. Orthop., 186:202–204, 1984.

85. Sewell, J.R., et al.: Quantitative scintigraphy in diagnosis and management of plantar fasciitis (calcaneal periostitis): Concise communication. J. Nucl. Med., 21:633–636, 1980.

86. Taunton, J.E., Clement, D.B., and McNicol, K.: Plantar fasciitis in runners. Can. J. Appl. Sport Sci., 7:41–44, 1982.

87. Scranton, P.E., Pedegana, L.R., and Whitesel, J.P.: Gait analysis: Alterations in support phase forces using supportive devices. Am. J. Sports Med., 10:6–10, 1982.

88. Snider, M.P., Clancy, W.G., and McBeath, A.A.: Plantar fascia release for chronic plantar fasciitis in runners. Am. J. Sports Med., 11:215–219, 1983.

89. Lam, J.S.: The tarsal tunnel syndrome. J. Bone Joint Surg., 49B:87–92, 1967.

90. Campbell, J.W., and Inman, V.T.: Treatment of plantar fasciitis and calcaneal spurs with the UC-BL shoe insert. Clin. Orthop., 103:57–62, 1974.

91. Przylucki, H., and Jones, C.L.: Entrapment neuropathy of the muscle branch of lateral and plantar nerve. J. Am. Podiatry Assoc., 7:119–124, 1981.

NERVE ENTRAPMENT SYNDROMES

95

NORTIN M. HADLER

The major peripheral nerves of healthy individuals, with the few exceptions discussed later here, withstand compromise in spite of their length and soft-tissue shielding. Blunt trauma, fractures, and lacerations are the usual culprits and are the purview of trauma surgeons. Rheumatologists, however, often care for the systemically ill in whom the soft-tissue shielding of the peripheral nerves and the nerves themselves are often involved by synovitis and vasculitis, respectively. The challenge is to discern the symptoms and signs of peripheral neuropathy in a more general inflammatory setting.

THE CLINICAL PRESENTATION

This chapter considers entrapment neuropathies of the major peripheral nerves as they course through the upper and lower extremities. The chapter focuses on those lesions likely to present to the rheumatologist; rare and exceptional sites of compression neuropathy require a more encyclopedic treatment.[1] The differential diagnosis of peripheral compression neuropathies includes more proximal neurologic disease. Cervical and lumbar radiculopathies are discussed in Chapters 90, 92, and 93, thoracic outlet syndrome and diseases of the brachial plexus in Chapter 97, and complementary essays are readily available.[2,3] Rather than re-emphasize the hallmarks of these confounding diagnoses, the distinctive features of peripheral entrapment neuropathies are emphasized here. Several of these features are common to all peripheral

entrapment neuropathies and are discussed in the following paragraphs.

1. Dysesthesias are characteristic; they are often localized to the sensory distribution of the involved nerve.

2. The discomfort is variously described as burning, tingling, "pins and needles," or even "itchy" skin. Sometimes an aching pain is noted in the muscles, even the proximal muscles, innervated by the involved nerve.

3. The discomfort is not prominently use related. Tenderness in the distribution of the dysesthesias is not a feature; on the contrary, dysesthesias occurring at night and at rest plague these patients. The response is to attempt to rub or move the distal extremity, leading to further dismay if the patient has coincident inflammatory arthritis.

4. *Tinel's sign* is elicited by tapping the nerve at the site of entrapment. Focal tenderness is usually present but nonspecific, particularly in the setting of synovitis. The more specific response is to elicit pain and dysesthesias radiating into the sensory distribution of the nerve distal to the point of damage. The sensitivity of a Tinel's sign approaches 90% for some forms of entrapment such as carpal tunnel syndrome and is nearly as sensitive for most others. The sign is important both in the clinical diagnosis of entrapment neuropathy and in the localization of the compression.

5. The dysesthesias and associated symptoms reflect the greater vulnerability of the sensory fibers in the peripheral nerve to compressive damage. The

1485

process, however, rarely progresses to severe hypesthesia such that traditional testing with a pin is clearly abnormal. More-subtle tests of tactile compromise such as sensory thresholds are useful when performed by experienced investigators, but a normal sensory examination does not militate against the diagnosis of an entrapment neuropathy.

6. With severe and prolonged compression, the motor function of the nerve is compromised as well. In instances of insidiously progressive compression, motor compromise may be present with insignificant dysesthesias. In the upper extremity, motor compromise is manifest as clumsiness and decreased hand function. In the lower extremity, a gait disorder may eventuate. Atrophy and weakness becomes evident in muscles innervated by the compressed nerve.

7. Discerning entrapment neuropathies in the setting of rheumatoid or other inflammatory arthritis is obviously particularly difficult. With many idiopathic entrapments, particularly those occurring after subtle trauma, the involvement is often unilateral. Idiopathic carpal tunnel syndrome is an important exception. Symmetry of proliferative synovitis, however, can lead to symmetric entrapment neuropathies. Discerning the historical features of entrapment neuropathy among the more familiar inflammatory complaints is crucial. Inspecting the distal musculature is important, seeking asymmetry in the typical pattern of periarticular muscle atrophy, both between and within hands and feet, that might provide a clue to a peripheral neuropathy.

8. Although the patient may perceive that the involved distal extremity is "swollen," objective swelling or vasomotor phenomena are unusual in entrapment neuropathies, and their presence should lead to a restructuring of the differential diagnosis.

9. Entrapment neuropathies should be treated conservatively, unless symptoms become recalcitrant or weakness or atrophy supervenes. Atrophy is often obscured in the setting of inflammatory synovitis. Before considering surgical decompression, the physician should attempt to confirm the clinical diagnosis of entrapment and localize the compression by electroneurography.[4] The sensitivity of these techniques varies depending on the lesion; for some, such as carpal tunnel syndrome, it can approach 90%.

ENTRAPMENT NEUROPATHIES OF THE UPPER EXTREMITY

The three major nerves of the upper extremity are protected from external compression short of that consequent to a humeral fracture or similar trauma.

At the elbow, all three are at risk. Their course is more superficial at the elbow, even subcutaneous; they traverse synovial reflections that can proliferate in rheumatoid arthritis (RA); and they are sandwiched at points between long bones and muscles. At the wrist, they again are at risk for all of the preceding reasons except that the sandwich is between bony prominences and tendons. Each nerve is considered separately in the following sections.

MEDIAN NERVE

The median nerve approaches the antecubital fossa lying medial to the brachial artery and separates from the artery at the artery's bifurcation. The nerve passes beween the two heads of the pronator teres (the ulnar artery is deep to this muscle) and courses through the forearm lying between the flexores digitorum superficialis and profundus. It then passes through the carpal tunnel just beneath the transverse carpal ligament deep to the tendon of the palmaris longus. The median nerve supplies all the superficial and deep muscles of the volar forearm except the flexor carpi ulnaris. It also supplies nearly all the muscles of the thenar eminence: the abductor pollicis brevis, the opponens pollicis, and the superficial head of the flexor pollicis brevis. The sensory distribution is illustrated in Figure 95–1A.

Entrapment neuropathy of the median nerve is the most common of entrapment neuropathies. In fact, it is the most common peripheral neuropathy. Regardless of the clinical setting, the most common site of compression is within the carpal tunnel. Thus, the carpal tunnel syndrome is the prototype entrapment neuropathy most likely to exhibit all of the preceding clinical features. Motor compromise involves the thenar eminence, with weakness and atrophy best detected by inspecting the contour of the abductor pollicis brevis (Fig. 95–2). There is less uniformity of opinion regarding the sensitivity of provocative tests and the sensory examination. Some clinicians,[5] including me, find the Tinel's and Phalen's signs (symptoms reproduced on flexion at the wrist) useful, whereas most clinicians find sensory examinations very insensitive and provocative tests with a blood pressure cuff useless.[6]

Extension splints are often useful, especially to relieve symptoms that occur at night when the wrist assumes the flexed position, increasing the pressure in the carpal tunnel.

Idiopathic carpal tunnel syndrome is often bilateral. In cases severe enough to warrant carpal tunnel release, the pressure to which the nerve is subjected is

FIG. 95–1. Distribution of the cutaneous nerves to the extremities. *A,* Sensory innervation of the palm and dorsum of the hand. *B,* Sensory innervation of the anterior aspect of the leg. *C,* Cutaneous innervation of the sole.

FIG. 95–2. The lateral contour of the thenar eminence is the abductor pollicis brevis. Abduction against resistance allows one to assess the power of this muscle and inspect its bulk as a bulge (arrow). Since the innervation of this muscle is exclusively the median nerve, weakness and atrophy is a specific sign of median neuropathy.

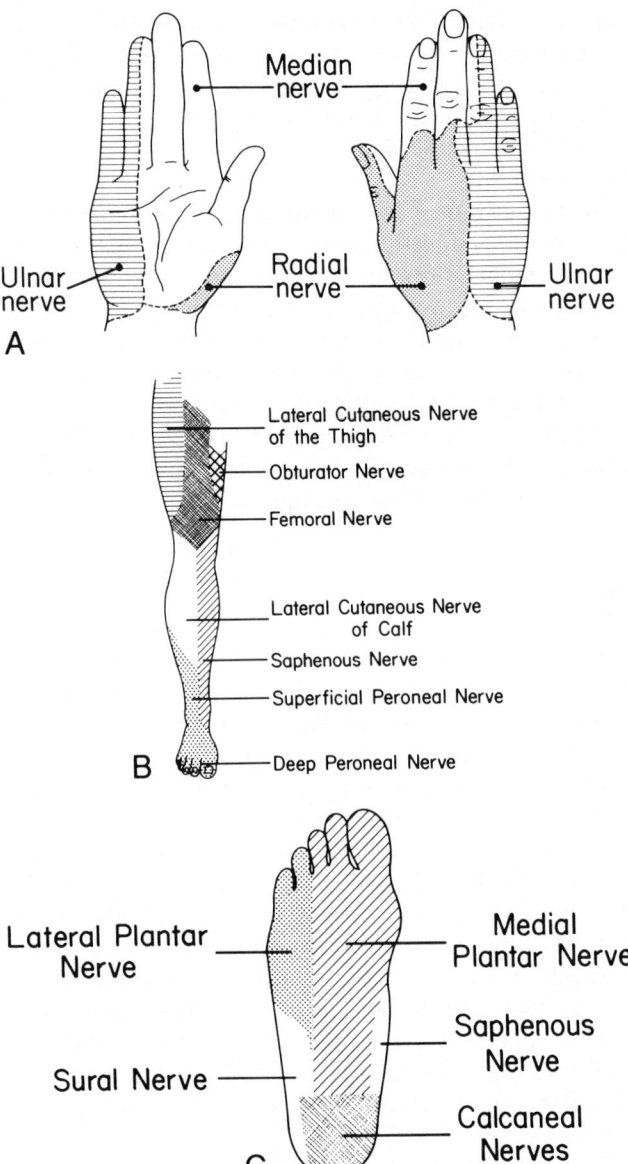

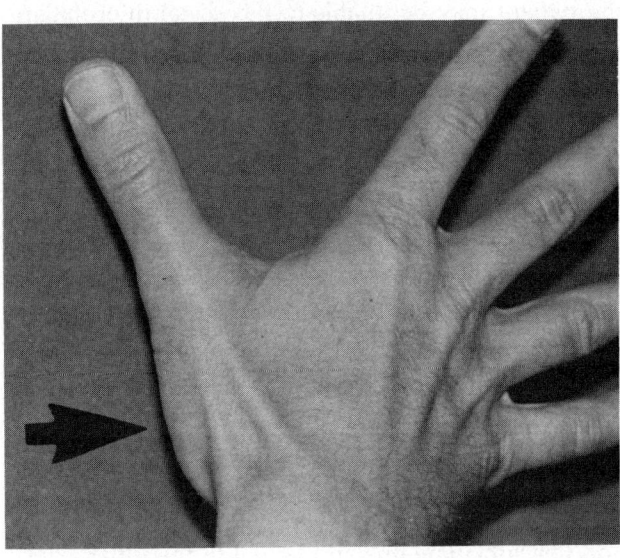

increased.[7] The treatment of idiopathic carpal tunnel syndrome has been studied systematically.[8] In those patients with persistent symptoms despite extension splinting, injection of corticosteroid esters into the carpal tunnel provides complete relief in the majority, although up to 78% will relapse within 18 months. Thenar atrophy is a consensus indication for surgical intervention; recalcitrant symptoms, particularly atypical symptoms, call for perspicacity, good judgment, and unequivocal electroneurographic confir-

mation of the diagnosis.* It is important to emphasize that valid idiopathic carpal tunnel syndrome is not prevalent, is not use related, and does not cluster.[3]

Carpal tunnel syndrome can complicate RA, even early in the course and with bilateral involvement.[9] Here, too, steroid injection can prove palliative with two provisos: first, thenar muscle atrophy secondary to median nerve compression can be obscured by that caused by articular inflammation, mandating close observation and ready recourse to surgical consultation. Second, injection therapy by the usual volar route carries greater risk of nerve infiltration and damage because of anatomic distortion secondary to articular destruction. Injecting the proximal radiocarpal joint by the dorsal approach carries no such risk and may produce the same end result.

The differential diagnosis of carpal tunnel syndrome is broad and lengthy,[1–3] but aside from pregnancy, most associated entities are exceedingly rare.[10] Nonetheless, consideration and, on occasion, appropriate laboratory tests are germane because interventions vary considerably. Myxedema, tuberculous wrist, and gout are examples of medically treatable entities. Amyloid and multiple myeloma may not respond even to carpal tunnel release.

The median nerve is only rarely subjected to

Editor's note. I have found serial evaluation of hand grip strength (sphygmomanometer) useful in following these patients.

compression at sites other than the carpal tunnel. Compression between the heads of the pronator teres is suspected by a localizing Tinel's sign, confirmed by electrodiagnosis, and can be treated by constraining forceful pronation.[11] Such a proximal median neuropathy may compromise the long flexors to the digits; the patient may be unable to flex distal interphalangeal joints as confirmed in the clinical test of opposing the tips of the first and second digits to the thumb to form a circle.

ULNAR NERVE

The ulnar nerve parts from the brachial artery in the middle of the arm. It courses dorsally, piercing the medial intermuscular septum, and it lies in the condylar groove behind the medial epicondyle at the elbow. The nerve then courses in a volar direction, and 2 cm into the forearm, it enters the "cubital tunnel," the floor of which is the medial ligament of the elbow joint; the roof is the aponeurosis of the flexor carpi ulnaris muscle. It courses beneath this muscle and lies subcutaneous and lateral to the ulnar artery in the distal half of the forearm. The ulnar nerve enters the wrist superficial to the flexor retinaculum (here called the pisohamate ligament) between the pisiform and the hook of the hamate and deep to the superficial volar carpal ligament in a conduit called *Guyon's canal*. The ulnar nerve supplies the flexor carpi ulnaris and, with the median, the profundus in the forearm. In the palm it supplies the muscles of the hypothenar eminence, all the interossei, the third and fourth lumbricals, the adductor pollicis, and part of the flexor pollicis brevis. Its cutaneous distribution is shown in Figure 95–1.

The ulnar nerve is at risk of compression at the condylar groove, in the cubital tunnel, and in Guyon's canal. Furthermore, all three sites are potential targets of proliferative synovitis in RA. The presentation can have all the features of compression neuropathy, but it is notoriously variable. Insidiously progressive atrophy can occur with little discomfort and even little sensory loss, the so-called "tardy ulnar palsy." Discerning early motor compromise is difficult and particularly challenging in the setting of RA. Weakness in apposition of the fourth and fifth digits and *Froment's sign* (Fig. 95–3) can be helpful along with inspection of the hypothenar eminence for atrophy. Localization of the site of the compressive lesion can be challenging, particularly because the sensitivity of electrodiagnostic testing for ulnar neuropathy does not equal that for median neuropathies.

Ulnar neuropathies must be distinguished from lesions that involve the lower trunk of the brachial plexus. In these cases, the symptoms often extend proximal to the elbow. Pancoast tumors must be sought; a Horner syndrome may offer a clue. "Thoracic outlet syndrome" is an often abused and often tenuous concept.[2] In an undisputed *axonopathic* form of neurogenic thoracic outlet syndrome, there is weakness and atrophy of median and ulnar innervated muscles of the hand and forearm with sensory disturbance in the ulnar, but *not* the median, distribution.[3]

In the setting of RA, treatment of ulnar neuropathies includes injections of corticosteroids into the elbow or wrist joints to decrease the synovitis. Such maneuvers are of unproven benefit, however, in idiopathic ulnar neuropathies. In the absence of joint deformities, conservative management focuses on preventing trauma to the nerve at the elbow with padding and by restricting flexion. The decision to attempt "decompression" or nerve transposition will tax the judgment of any surgeon.

RADIAL NERVE

The radial nerve leaves the axilla, passes posterior to the humerus, through the lateral intermuscular septum just distal to the deltoid insertion to lie superficially in the lateral arm. The nerve then passes between the brachialis and brachioradialis to the front of the lateral epicondyle near where it divides into two branches. The deep branch, the posterior interosseous nerve, passes into the supinator muscle through the arcade of Frohse and courses within the muscle in the supinator canal, from which it emerges to supply the extensor muscles of the digits and some of the wrist. The superficial radial nerve passes over the supinator and pronator teres muscles and descends along the lateral border of the forearm to provide the sensory distribution of the radial nerve (see Fig. 95–1).

The radial nerve is at risk of compression on the humerus as it courses through the radial groove. Generally, compression is the result of prolonged improper positioning during anesthesia or sleeping on the arm, often when inebriated or sedated ("Saturday night palsy") and results in wristdrop; sensory involvement is variable.

The posterior interosseous nerve is at risk of entrapment at the elbow by the proliferative synovitis of RA. Entrapment is manifest by weakness in the finger extensors more than in the wrist extensors and needs to be distinguished from compromise in the integrity of extensor tendons by dorsal synovitis at

FIG. 95–3. Froment's sign is the inability to maintain extension of the interphalangeal joint of the thumb during forceful pinching. It is a subtle sign of intrinsic muscle compromise in ulnar palsy.

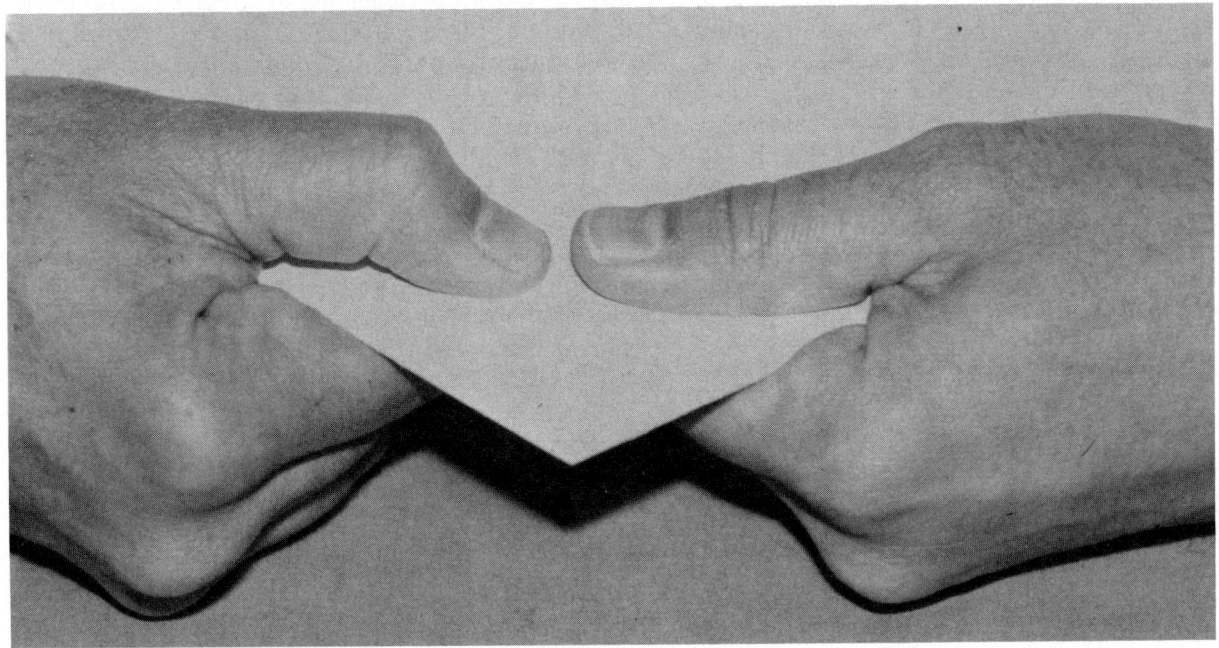

the wrist. Neither lesion produces a sensory deficit. It has been argued,[12] though not convincingly,[2] that entrapment of the posterior interosseus nerve in the arcade of Frohse or in the supinator canal is common and mimics lateral epicondylitis ("tennis elbow"). Such a clinical hypothesis would suggest surgical remediation, but electrodiagnosis should be a prerequisite.

The superficial radial nerve is subject to external trauma, often resulting in distressing dysesthesias. Rarely, rupture of a rheumatoid elbow effusion can similarly compromise the nerve.[13]

ENTRAPMENT NEUROPATHIES OF THE LOWER EXTREMITY

Compression or entrapment of the peripheral nerves in the absence of external force occurs less frequently in the lower extremity than in the upper. Lower extremity entrapment neuropathy is seldom recognized in RA. Nonetheless, there are a few examples that are themselves important and enter into a differential diagnosis relevant to rheumatologic practice.

FEMORAL NERVE

The femoral nerve exits the pelvis beneath the medial aspect of the inguinal ligament to supply the quadriceps and the skin of the anterior thigh (see Fig. 95–1B). It terminates at the saphenous nerve, which courses through the subsartorial canal before emerging through the fascia above the knee to supply the cutaneous innervation of the medial leg (see Fig. 95–1). Aside from trauma and hematomas, femoral or saphenous entrapment is exceedingly rare. Saphenous entrapment is seen occasionally as a consequence of scarring from surgery on the venous system.

LATERAL CUTANEOUS NERVE OF THE THIGH

The lateral cutaneous nerve of the thigh exits the pelvis either through or beneath the lateral inguinal ligament. The nerve is purely sensory (see Fig. 95–1). Compression causes burning paresthesias and hyperpathia along the lateral aspect of the thigh, the syndrome of *meralgia paresthetica* or *Bernhardt's disease* ("meralgia" derives from the Greek for pain in the thigh). The symptoms are worsened by standing and walking or by prolonged adduction or extension of the leg. The pathogenesis is thought to be entrapment of the nerve either at the inguinal ligament or when it pierces the fascia to reach the skin.*[14] The differential diagnosis includes an L3 radiculopathy or a femoral neuropathy though both of these cause more anterior symptoms and rarely hyperesthesia. Rarely, retroperitoneal compression of the lumbar plexus by lymphoma or other neoplasms can provoke meralgia paresthetica. The diagnosis is based on the clinical features because there is no reliable electrodiagnostic test. Treatment is conservative because spontaneous regression of symptoms is the rule. Attempts should be made to eliminate compression by tight garments; weight loss is often advised.

SCIATIC NERVE

The sciatic nerve exits the pelvis through the sciatic notch and lies between the greater trochanter and the ischial tuberosity deep to the gluteus maximus muscle. It courses deep to the hamstrings and supplies the posterior thigh muscles. Aside from overt trauma, the nerve is well cushioned throughout its course once it exits the pelvis, and compression is exceedingly rare. The sciatic nerve is at some risk at the pyriform fossa, particularly with prolonged sitting on a hard surface or in a wheelchair. In the upper popliteal fossa, the sciatic nerve divides into the common peroneal nerve and the tibial nerve.

Common Peroneal Nerve

The common peroneal nerve courses obliquely around the lateral aspect of the proximal fibula to pass through the superficial head of the peroneus longus muscle in the "fibular tunnel." On emerging, it divides into the superficial (musculocutaneous) and deep (anterior tibial) peroneal nerves. The former courses beside and supplies the peroneal muscles and supplies cutaneous innervation to the lateral and distal portion of the leg and dorsum of the foot (see Fig. 95–1B). The deep peroneal nerve runs in the anterior compartment of the leg between the tibialis anterior and extensor hallucis longus muscles and tendons. It passes beneath the extensor retinaculum at the ankle and supplies most of the ankle and toes and the skin between the first and second toes.

The common peroneal nerve is peculiarly susceptible to compression in its superficial course around the fibula. Plaster casts and leg braces are frequent culprits, although prolonged pressure, prolonged

---

*Editor's note. This syndrome occurs most often in pregnancy and in obese individuals, especially if constricting garments are worn. The classic victim is the fat Army sergeant with a tight gun belt.

squatting, and even habitual leg crossing have been implicated when no other explanation is patent. The syndrome includes footdrop and sensory compromise. The deep peroneal nerve can be compressed in the very rare anterior tibial syndrome. After trauma, or even excessive exercise, this compartment can become inflamed to the point of which timely surgical decompression is mandatory (i.e., a surgical emergency).

Tibial Nerve

The tibial nerve branches in the popliteal fossa to give off the sural nerve, which descends in the midline of the calf and passes the lateral malleolus to supply the skin over the lateral ankle and foot (see Fig. 95–1C). The tibial nerve continues through the popliteal fossa and deep to the gastrocnemius to emerge at the medial aspect of the Achilles tendon. It then passes deep to the flexor retinaculum at the medial malleolus to enter the sole. This retinaculum forms the roof of the tarsal tunnel, which also contains the tendons of the tibialis posterior, flexor digitorum longus, and flexor hallucis longus muscles, as well as the posterior tibial artery and veins. The tibial nerve branches from the tarsal tunnel into two plantar nerves and calcaneal sensory branches. The tibial nerve supplies the flexors of the ankle and toes and provides cutaneous innervation (see Fig. 95–1C).

The tibial nerve is at risk of entrapment beneath the flexor retinaculum, the tarsal tunnel syndrome. Although this syndrome is often described after trauma, rheumatoid synovitis is also a frequent setting. Paresthesias and, to a lesser extent, pain are the presenting complaints with the features previously listed. Occasionally, specific muscular atrophy can be discerned, though this is usually obscured by rheumatoid foot deformities. The distribution of paresthesias and a Tinel's sign suggest the diagnosis, which can be confirmed electrodiagnostically. The plantar and digital nerves are also subject to compression neuropathy, but specific diagnosis and differentiation from the tarsal tunnel syndrome is difficult if not elusive. Initial treatment is conservative with systemic and local anti-inflammatory agents and orthotic devices.

Surgical decompression is reserved for the rare patient with recalcitrant symptoms or compromised muscle strength. The procedure is tricky, because the tarsal tunnel is cone-shaped. The tunnel's narrow inlet is formed by a thickening of the deep fascia of the leg, which forms the flexor retinaculum; the tunnel's exit is an oval (double-lumened) structure, through which the medial and lateral plantar nerves pass.[15] Decompression of the entire tunnel, including excision of the septum forming the double-lumened exit seems important. The calcaneal branch of the medial tibial nerve may or may not be compressed, depending on whether it divides proximal to the flexor retinaculum. It should be identified in every case at surgery. Patients with "failed" or recurrent tarsal tunnel syndrome have usually had inadequate surgery, that is, incomplete release of the tunnel. Such patients often have severe intraneural fibrosis, requiring adjunctive intraneural neurolysis at reexploration.[15]

REFERENCES

1. Stewart, J.D., and Aguayo, A.J.: Compression and entrapment neuropathies. *In* Peripheral Neuropathy. Edited by P.J. Dyck, P.K. Thomas, E.H. Lambert, and R. Bunge. Philadelphia, W.B. Saunders, 1984.
2. Hadler, N.M.: Medical Management of the Regional Musculoskeletal Diseases. Orlando, FL, Grune & Stratton, 1984.
3. Hadler, N.M. (ed.): Clinical Concepts in Regional Musculoskeletal Illness. Orlando, FL, Grune & Stratton, 1987.
4. Kimura, J.: Electrodiagnosis in Diseases of Nerve and Muscle: Principles and Practice. Philadelphia, F.A. Davis, 1983.
5. Pfeffer, G.B., and Gelberman, R.H.: The carpal tunnel syndrome. *In* Clinical Concepts in Regional Musculoskeletal Illness. Orlando, FL, Grune & Stratton, 1987.
6. Golding, D.N., Rose, D.M., and Selvarajah, K.: Clinical tests for carpal tunnel syndrome: An evaluation. Br. J. Rheum., 25:388–390, 1986.
7. Gelberman, R.H., et al.: The carpal tunnel syndrome: A study of carpal canal pressures. J. Bone Joint Surg., *63A*:380–383, 1981.
8. Gelberman, R.H., Aronson, D., and Weisman, M.H.: Carpal tunnel syndrome: Results of a prospective trial of steroid injection and splinting. J. Bone Joint Surg., *62A*:1181–1184, 1980.
9. Chamberlain, M.A., and Corbett, M.: Carpal tunnel syndrome in early rheumatoid arthritis. Ann. Rheum. Dis., 29:149–152, 1970.
10. Phillips, R.S.: Carpal tunnel syndrome as a manifestation of systemic disease. Ann. Rheum. Dis., 26:59–62, 1967.
11. Morris, H.H., and Peters, B.H.: Pronator syndrome: Clinical and electrophysiological features in seven cases. J. Neurol. Neurosurg. Psychiatr., 39:461–464, 1976.
12. Roles, N.C., and Mauldsley, R.H.: Radial tunnel syndrome. J. Bone Joint Surg., *54B*:499, 1972.
13. Fernandes, L., Goodwill, C.J., and Srivatsa, S.R.: Synovial rupture of rheumatoid elbow causing radial nerve compression. Br. Med. J., 2:17, 1979.
14. Jefferson, D., and Eames, R.A.: Subclinical entrapment of the lateral femoral cutaneous nerve: An autopsy study. Muscle Nerve, 2:145–151, 1979.
15. Mackinnan, S.E., and Dellon, A.L.: Homologies between the tarsal and carpal tunnels: Implications for treatment of the tarsal tunnel syndrome. Contemp Orthop., 14:75, 1987.

TUMORS OF JOINTS AND RELATED STRUCTURES

ALAN S. COHEN and JUAN J. CANOSO

Neoplasms and other tumorous conditions of the articular structures are uncommon in rheumatologic practice. Nevertheless, it is important to give these disorders prominent consideration in patients with monoarticular and focal tenosynovial disease, lest proper diagnosis and treatment be delayed. The diagnosis of these lesions has been facilitated by techniques such as arthroscopy,[1] arteriography,[2] computed tomography (CT),[3] and magnetic resonance imaging (MRI).[4–6]

BENIGN TUMORAL CONDITIONS

Benign tumoral conditions comprise a heterogeneous group of disorders of joints, bursae, and tendon sheaths. They include pigmented villonodular synovitis, which is a chronic inflammatory lesion of unknown origin, synovial chondromatosis and other cartilaginous metaplasias of the subsynovial tissue, vascular malformations, fat growths, and fibromas.

PIGMENTED VILLONODULAR SYNOVITIS

The term pigmented villonodular synovitis denotes a group of interrelated, benign, tumorous disorders that involve the lining of joints, bursae, and tendon sheaths.[7–14] These lesions consist of villous or nodular growths, which are covered by a thin layer of synovial lining cells. The connective tissue stroma contains a heterogeneous and variably dense collection of cells,

collagen bundles, and blood vessels. The cellular infiltrate consists of polyhedral, histiocytic-like cells, lipid-laden cells appearing as foam cells on routine histologic preparations, hemosiderin-laden macrophages, and multinucleated giant cells (Fig. 96–1). Early lesions are highly vascular, whereas old lesions are less vascular, exhibit more fibrosis and hyalinization, and may contain cholesterol crystals.[7,15] The color of the lesion, ranging from yellow to tan to dark brown, depends on the proportion of lipid and hemosiderin. Bone invasion results from direct penetration through vascular foramina, extension through the chondro-osseous junction at the articular margin, and pressure erosion.[16–18]

Electron-microscopic studies in both villous and nodular forms usually revealed a predominance of cells resembling fibroblasts (type-B cells) and a lesser number of cells resembling both macrophages (type-A cells) and intermediate cells, consistent with a derivation from normal synovium.[19–24] The iron tends to be deposited within lysosomal bodies (siderosomes) in deep type-B cells.[25] So far, pigmented villonodular synovitis has only been detected in humans. Reported cases in horses bear little resemblance to the human disease.[26,27]

Clinical Findings

Involvement of the affected joint, tendon sheath, or bursa may be either diffuse or localized. The condition is typically monotopic and lacks systemic symptoms or findings. The patient's erythrocyte sedimentation rate is usually normal.[23,28,29] Rarely are two

FIG. 96–1.   Circumscribed nodular synovitis; photomicrographs of a nodular lesion. *A*, Large deposits of hemosiderin pigment in richly cellular connective tissue stroma. *B*, Multinucleated giant cells amid dense infiltrate of small round cells and large cells with pale, spindle-shaped nuclei (× 175).

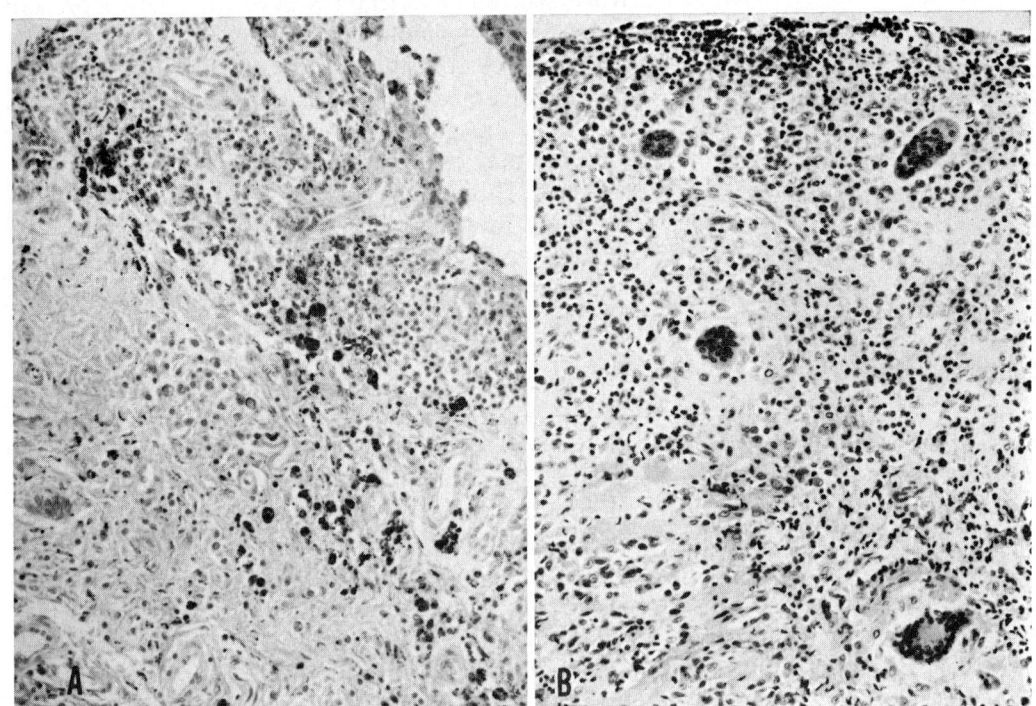

or more joints affected.[30–36] Several cases have been observed in association with rheumatoid arthritis (RA)[19,37–39] or psoriatic arthritis.[24] It is unclear whether this connection represents a true association or whether it is the result of a detection bias.

It is useful to classify pigmented villonodular synovitis according to its location, articular, tenosynovial, or bursal, and to the lesional type, either diffuse or nodular.

Articular, Diffuse.   This condition occurs chiefly in young adults and is equally frequent in both sexes.[29,38] The joint usually affected is the knee; much less commonly involved are the hip, ankle, elbow, carpus, hand, and tarsus.[7,9,10,40] Rare locations include the temporomandibular joint[41–43] and the vertebral facet joint.[44–46] The principal symptoms are pain and swelling, which may be mild and intermittent for a long period, and gradual swelling of the joint due to effusion and synovial proliferation. Focal masses are usually palpable in or about the joint. A popliteal cyst often develops.[23] The joint fluid is usually sanguineous or dark brown, not viscous, and does not usually clot.[23,38,47] One report noted an average white blood cell count of 3110/mm³, with an average of 26% polymorphonuclear cells. The red blood cell count

varied from 43,000 to 1,780,000/mm³. Mucin clot tests varied from fair to good.[47] The glucose content was normal.[38,47]

Roentgenographic examination, in addition to showing increased amounts of joint fluid, may reveal lobulation and thickening of the synovial tissues. Narrowing of the joint space and periarticular demineralization occur late in the disorder.[48] There is a peculiar lack of hypertrophic spurs.[18]

In the hip, elbow, and shoulder, and on occasion the wrist, finger, and temporomandibular joint, one may see considerable narrowing of the joint space, bony erosions, and uni- and multiloculated cysts in the subchondral bone.[29,40,41,48–50] Erosions and cysts usually involve both sides of the joint, and their peripheral location around and just proximal to the articulating surfaces parallels the distribution of the perforating blood vessels (Fig. 96–2).[16,51,52] Arthrograms, preferably with air contrast, demonstrate enlargement and distortion of the suprapatellar pouch with numerous recesses and filling defects.[48] Similar features have been shown by sonography.[53] The high iron content of the lesion can be determined by CT scanning, although the specificity of this finding is still unknown.[54] The diagnostic procedure of choice

FIG. 96–2. Cartilage narrowing and cystic erosive changes in the acetabulum and femoral head and neck from pigmented villonodular synovitis.

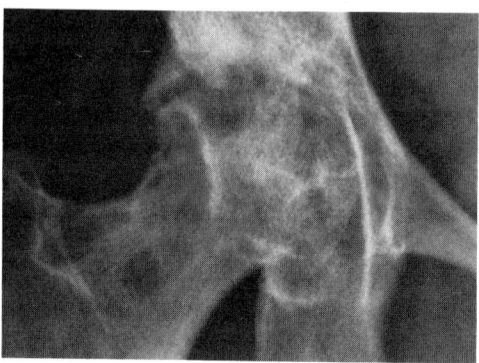

is arthroscopy.[1] The synovium is stained brown and appears shaggy and proliferative. Representative biopsies can be obtained for pathologic and bacteriologic studies, including mycobacterial and fungal cultures.

Articular, Circumscribed (Nodular). Localized involvement of the synovium occurs less frequently than the diffuse form of the disease, with a ratio of 1:4.[29,38] Here again, the knee is most commonly affected, and the patient is usually an adult with symptoms for many months or years before the diagnosis is established. The symptoms are often episodic and consist of pain, swelling, locking, and "giving way" of the joint.[38] Acute symptoms may follow torsion and infarction.[55] Small to moderate effusions and occasional limited range of motion are found. The synovial fluid is less likely to be sanguineous. Radiograms of the joint usually show no abnormalities.[29,38,56] Arthrographic examination may demonstrate an intra-articular bulge.[57,58] The true nature of the process is not suspected until one or more sessile or stalked yellow-brown nodular growths are found at arthroscopy or at operation.

Tenosynovial, Circumscribed (Nodular). This type constitutes by far the most common form of this disorder,[10,13,14,38] and it is 10 times more common than circumscribed nodular synovitis.[38] It is the second most common soft-tissue tumor of the hand, outnumbered only by ganglia.[59] The majority of patients are young or middle-aged adults. Women are affected more often than men, and the incidence is higher in the dominant hand. Most frequently involved is a finger, more often the index or middle, on the volar (60%) or dorsal or lateral aspect of which a firm, slow-growing, painless nodular mass develops. Less often, this lesion is found near a metacarpophalangeal joint, wrist, ankle, or toe. Larger lesions may cause exten-

sive pressure erosion of adjacent bone.[48] The origin of lesions arising in sites devoid of tendon sheaths, such as the lateral or dorsal aspect of fingers, is controversial. Some authors believe that they represent outgrowths of silent joint lesions.[60]

Tenosynovial, Diffuse. Occasionally, one sees diffuse involvement of the tendon sheaths of the hand and foot, in which the lesions may grow to a large size and may erode neighboring bone.[7]

Bursal. This uncommon lesion, usually diffuse, may be found in a deep bursa such as the iliopsoas, the gastrocnemius-semimenbranosus, the suprapatellar, and the anserine.[7,10,61,62] No instances have been described involving the subcutaneous bursae.

Pathogenesis

Whether this condition represents a true neoplasm of synovial tissue or some form of obscure chronic inflammation is still not clear. The frequent erosion of adjacent bone by these lesions, their recurrence after synovectomy, and the presence of clefts and spaces surrounded by synovial lining cells have been thought to support the theory of neoplasm. In fact, many lesions have been considered neoplastic at operation, leading to amputation.[9,51] Strict histologic criteria of malignant lesions are lacking, however, and no case has been known to metastasize. Malignant transformation is exceptional.[10,63]

Fragments of the lesion grown in culture have shown a metabolic rate far in excess of rheumatoid synovium and a significant rise in the activity of glycolytic and lysosomal enzymes.[64] Such tissue, like hemophilic synovitis, may produce large amounts of collagenase or other proteolytic enzymes,[65] and PGE_2,[25] and such findings may explain the destructive nature of many of these lesions.

Similarities between pigmented villonodular synovitis and the findings in hemophilia and intra-articular hemangioma have led many to consider that the lesion might result from recurrent hemarthrosis.[66,67] In support of this view, changes resembling those of the human disease have been produced experimentally in dogs and in rhesus monkeys by repeated intra-articular injection of blood and colloidal iron.[68,69] Moreover, multiple lesions in children have been associated with cutaneous or synovial hemangiomas; this finding suggests a pathogenetic role of recurrent hemarthrosis.[30,33,34]

No evidence of vascular malformation exists in most instances of pigmented villonodular synovitis, however, and foam cells do not occur in hemosideric synovitis induced experimentally[69] or in hemophilic joints.[66] It has been suggested that recurrent lipohemarthrosis would explain the deposition of both hemosiderin and lipids.[70] This view is supported by the finding that, in over 50% of patients, acute or repetitive local trauma seemingly precedes the appearance of the lesion.[38]

A microbial cause of the lesion has been sought but not found. Cultures are routinely negative. Tubular structures resembling myxovirus nucleoprotein were found in only one of many cases studied by electron microscopy.[71] A primary proliferation of synovial cells has also been proposed.[23] Although the exact nature of pigmented villonodular synovitis is unknown at present, the condition appears to be an inflammatory granuloma, rather than a true neoplasm. The possibility remains that the lesion, defined on clinical, radiologic, and histopathologic grounds, may result from more than one causative mechanism.[23]

Treatment

Although pigmented villonodular synovitis appears to be a benign lesion usually confined to a single joint or soft-tissue structure, the results of surgical treatment are often disappointing. Resection of nodular synovitis of tendon sheath has a recurrence rate of approximately 20%, presumably owing to incomplete removal of the lesion.[8] In localized nodular synovitis of the knee, results have been better.[8,28,29,56] Major difficulties are encountered in the treatment of the diffuse form of pigmented villonodular synovitis in the knee. Extensive synovectomy has been followed by a 30 to 40% recurrence rate.[8,29] In the event of recurrence, radiotherapy has been instituted, but the response to this therapeutic technique is also uncertain.[8,72] Arthroscopic surgical procedures[1] and intra-articular administration of radiocolloids[73,74] hold promise in the treatment of recurrent disease. In the hip, the destructive lesions of pigmented villonodular synovitis can be eradicated by total hip arthroplasty,[29,49] but the youth of the patients raises questions about the long-term results of the prosthesis. Followup studies have shown that chronic pain and limitation of motion are frequent sequelae of the disease.[28,29]

SYNOVIAL CHONDROMATOSIS

Synovial chondromatosis arises from focal metaplasia of subsynovial tissue producing nodules of normal-appearing cartilage, or rarely in bursa, tendon sheath, joint capsule, or para-articular connective tissue.[7,10,11,75,76] These nodules become pedunculated and often detach from the synovium and grow as viable loose bodies within the joint cavity.[77] These cartilage nodules may calcify or even ossify, leading to the term *osteochondromatosis*. The origin of the disorder is unknown. The lesion is benign and rarely undergoes malignant change.[10]

Synovial chondromatosis occurs most often as a monoarticular disturbance in young or middle-aged adults and is more common in men than in women. Pediatric cases are rare.[78,79]

The joint most frequently involved is the knee, followed by the hip, the elbow, and the shoulder.[10,75,80,81] Osteochondromatosis of the temporomandibular joint has been reported.[82–85] In the uncommon case of multiple joint involvement, both knees are usually affected.

Clinical Findings

Patients may have pain, swelling, and limitation of joint motion, or they may be asymptomatic, with the lesion discovered by accident. Examination of the joint often reveals the presence of loose bodies and increased amounts of synovial fluid, which is viscous and normal in all other characteristics.[47]

The diagnosis, usually established by roentgenographic examination, discloses multiple stippled calcifications within the confines of the joint capsule in approximately 90% of patients (Fig. 96–3).[10,48] Extrinsic erosions can be noted, particularly in the femoral neck and proximal humerus.[17,86] The joint otherwise appears normal.

The differential diagnosis of synovial chondromatosis includes several other conditions associated with loose joint bodies, such as severe osteoarthritis with intra-articular osteophytic fragments, osteochondritis dissecans, neuropathic arthropathy, and the "Milwaukee" shoulder.[48,87] Synovial calcification mimicking osteochondromatosis can also occur in calcium pyrophosphate dihydrate crystal deposition disease.[88]

Pathogenesis

Gross examination of the affected joint reveals variably large and compact clusters of flat or pedunculated cartilaginous nodules protruding from the thickened synovial membrane, as well as loose bodies within the joint cavity. Microscopic study indicates that the cartilage found in synovial chondromatosis develops as a result of metaplastic transformation of the subsynovial connective tissue (Fig. 96–4). An imperceptible transition between subsynovial fibrocytes and fully developed chondrocytes has been shown by electron microscopy.[89] Predictably, the collagen of the nodules is type II.[90]

Detailed analysis of operative and histologic findings in loose bodies and synovial membrane has permitted a reconstruction of the natural history of the disease.[77] At first, cartilage metaplasia occurs in the

FIG. 96–3. *A,* Primary synovial osteochondromatosis with multiple loose bodies extruded into a Baker's cyst. *B,* Advanced degenerative joint disease with effusion and secondary osteochondromatosis.

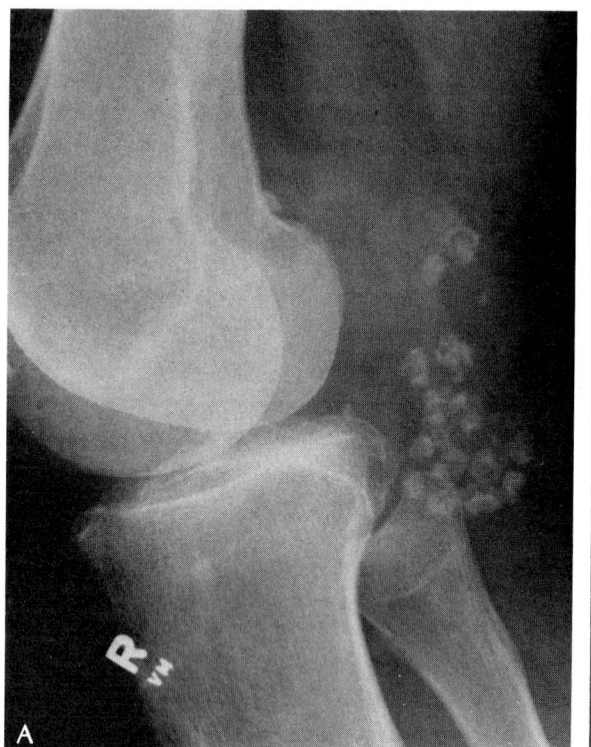

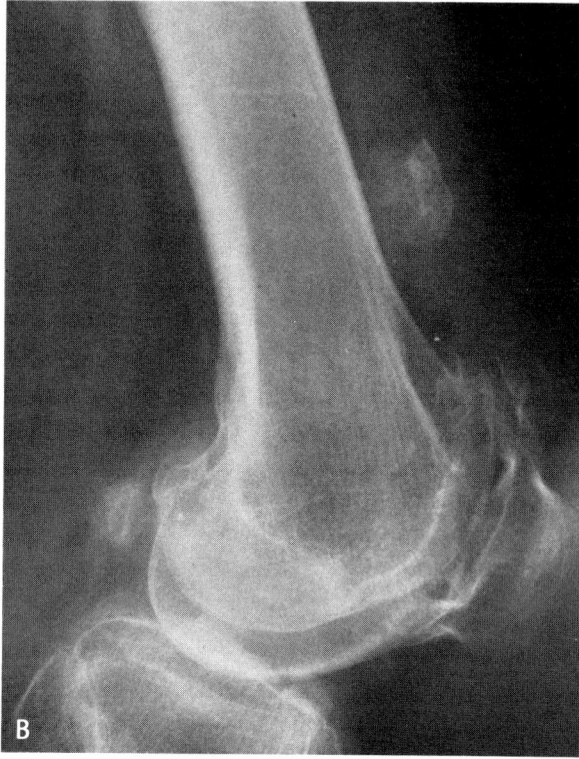

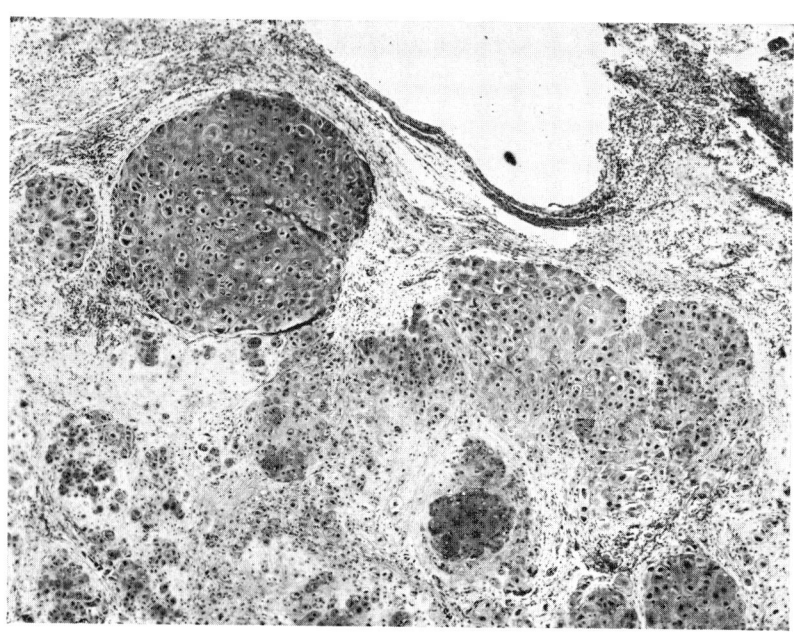

FIG. 96–4. Synovial chondromatosis; photomicrograph of synovium showing several small islands of cellular cartilage lying just beneath the surface of the membrane (×25).

subsynovial tissue in a multifocal fashion. In a later stage, some of the growing nodules become pedunculated and are finally released as loose joint bodies, whereas others remain buried in the membrane. Finally, the synovial membrane resumes its normal morphologic features, probably by resorption of residual foci of cartilaginous metaplasia, while the loose bodies undergo further remodeling. Calcification and ossification of the nodules can occur either before or after their release into the joint cavity.[77,91] Although this view is based on pathologic findings rather than a longitudinal study of individual cases, it has gained wide acceptance. Spontaneous regression of calcified bodies has been reported in one patient.[79]

Treatment

When the condition is suspected, arthroscopy or arthrotomy should be undertaken to remove the loose bodies, to determine the condition of the synovial membrane, and to assess the integrity of the articular cartilage. Synovectomy is indicated in extensive synovial disease.[75] Minor synovial metaplasia can be treated arthroscopically,[1] provided the articular cartilage is still normal.

INTRACAPSULAR, EXTRASYNOVIAL CHONDROMA

Intracapsular, extrasynovial chondroma is an unusual lesion that occurs most frequently in the knee. The patient has discomfort and a firm mass distal to the patella and deep to the patellar tendon.[92] Lateral radiographs reveal a calcified lesion within the infrapatellar fat pad.[48] Treatment is surgical excision.

HEMANGIOMA

The tissue usually affected by hemangioma is the synovial membrane of the knee.[7,10,11,93–96] When the joint capsule is diseased, the adjacent soft tissues and bone may become involved. Hemangiomas occur most often in adolescents or in young adults, many of whom have had symptoms since childhood; this feature suggests that the lesion may represent a congenital vascular malformation.[67] The affected joint is periodically painful and swollen and often contains blood or bloody fluid. Intra-articular hemangioma should be suspected in a patient with recurrent episodes of hemarthrosis of the knee in the absence of a clear explanation. Hemangiomas may be seen in the skin overlying the affected joint.

An arteriovenous shunt in a patient with a heman-gioma may be associated with increased leg length. In some cases, a tender, doughy joint mass decreases in size on elevation of the limb. The roentgenographic examination may show a tumor containing phlebolithic densities of differential diagnostic value. Patients with a hemangioma of long standing can exhibit enlarged epiphyses, joint-space narrowing, and enlargement of the intercondylar notch resembling hemophilic arthropathy.[97] When hemangioma is suspected, arteriography, phlebography,[2,97,98] or radionuclide angiography, and blood pool imaging[99] may help to localize the lesion and to rule out arteriovenous shunt.

A hemangioma within the joint can be localized in the form of a dark, grape-like mass, or it can be diffuse. Circumscribed lesions commonly originate from the infrapatellar fat pad. It may be difficult to differentiate diffuse hemangiomatous involvement of the synovium from pigmented villonodular synovitis.[30,33,34] In circumscribed lesions, the histologic pattern is usually that of a capillary or cavernous hemangioma, whereas in the diffuse variety, the vascular channels appear to be venous. Surgical excision, which is usually simple and effective in patients with a circumscribed hemangioma, is often unsatisfactory in patients with diffuse involvement of the synovial membrane and regional soft tissues, and the likelihood of recurrence is high.

Hemangiomas may also occur in tendon sheaths and may grow to involve both the tendon itself and the surrounding structures.[10] One usually notes a soft, compressive swelling, which changes when the limb is elevated or when a tourniquet is placed proximal to the mass. The roentgenographic examination frequently reveals many calcified phleboliths. The hand, forearm, and ankle are the sites favored by this lesion, which is treated by surgical excision.

FAT TUMOR

Intra-articular lipomas are rare. Almost all examples have been found in the knee joint in relation to the subsynovial fat on either side of the patellar ligament or the anterior surface of the femur.[7,10,100] Lipomas are also found in the tendon sheaths of the hand, wrist, feet, and ankles.[101] Extensor tendons appear to be affected more often than flexor tendons, and involvement may be bilateral.

The term lipoma arborescens represents a villous or polypoid synovial proliferation in response to chronic mechanical irritation of the synovium. This disorder can also occur in seemingly normal joints.[7,102]

Arthrographic examination reveals sharply marginated filling defects.[103]

The term Hoffa's disease designates the traumatic inflammation of the infrapatellar fat pad.[104] Patients are in pain, and the usual finding is swelling in the infrapatellar region, deep to the patellar tendon. The differential diagnosis includes pretendinous bursitis, deep infrapatellar bursitis, and intracapsular chondroma. Hoffa's disease is now classified in the broader category of plica syndromes, as defined arthroscopically (see Chapter 88).[1]

FIBROMA

Intra-articular fibroma is definitely rare.[105] Fibroma of tendon sheath is frequently seen.[106–108] The lesion consists of a firm, lobulated tumor attached to tendon or tendon sheath. The majority (98%) of lesions occur in the hand and wrist. The nodules are composed of fibroblasts and dense collagen and are frequently divided by narrow clefts. The lesion is benign, but recurrences are frequent following local excision.

MALIGNANT NEOPLASMS OF JOINTS

These neoplasms may be either primary or secondary. Primary tumors are uncommon and are represented almost solely by synovial sarcoma. Other malignant tumors with an origin in the fascial tissues of the extremities, and probably related to synovial sarcoma, are the clear cell sarcoma of tendons and aponeuroses and the epithelioid sarcoma. Secondary involvement of joints occurs as a complication of the contiguous spread of malignant bone tumors, metastases of carcinoma, leukemia, or lymphoma. Rheumatologic manifestations of hematologic malignant diseases are discussed in Chapter 84.

SYNOVIAL SARCOMA

Clinical Findings

Synovial sarcoma is a malignant and histologically complex neoplasm of connective tissue that is generally found near a large joint. The tumor seldom originates within the joint itself (Table 96–1). This lesion has been described by many different names, including malignant synovioma, synovial fibrosarcoma, sarcoendothelioma, and mesothelioma, and has been observed in certain domestic animals, such as the dog and cow.

Synovial sarcoma occurs most often in adolescents or in young adults, but it has been observed at all ages from birth to 80 years. A preponderance is seen in men. The lower limb (thigh, leg, foot, and knee) is more commonly the site of primary involvement than the upper limb (arm, forearm, and hand).[11,109–114] Other primary sites have included the buttocks, trunk (back), chest or abdominal wall, retroperitoneum,[115] orbit,[116] mouth and face,[117] neck,[118] and esophagus.[119] The characteristic history is that of a slowly growing mass that, in the case of a deeply situated lesion, may reach a considerable size before detection. When located on the hand or foot, the tumor may resemble a ganglion or a distended tendon sheath. Pain is not marked, except in unusual lesions or when the tumor interferes with the normal movement of the joint.

The typical roentgenographic appearance of malignant synovioma is that of a para-articular soft-tissue mass of homogeneous water density,[48] possibly lobulated, with a sharp, discrete border. Less often, the mass is irregular in outline and is not clearly separable from the surrounding tissues. In 30% of patients, the tumor contains clusters of small foci of calcification. Secondary invasion of contiguous bone produces osteolytic defects in 10 to 20% of patients. A nearby periosteal reaction may occur. Increased uptake of bone-seeking radionuclides has been shown in a partially calcified lesion,[120] but this finding is probably nonspecific. Arteriographic examination has shown increased vascularity, particularly in rapidly growing tumors.[2,121,122] Angiography, CT scanning, and MRI are useful in the initial evaluation of patients with synovial as well as other types of soft-tissue sarcoma, before biopsy.[2,4] Angiography gives better information when tumors occur distally, where little fat is present. CT scanning and MRI provide more precise information in the assessment of size, location, axial extent, and relationships of more centrally placed primary or locally recurrent lesions, as well as in the detection of metastases.

Although the rate of growth and the rapidity of metastatic spread vary, the disease characteristically follows a malignant course.[123] As is true of other connective tissue sarcomas, the synovial sarcoma spreads by direct extension along tissue planes, by invasion of regional lymph nodes (possibly a later phenomenon), and by way of the vascular system. The rate of local recurrence, particularly after simple excision, is high.[124] The most common site of visceral metastasis is the lung,[112,125] in which the lesions appear as multiple large densities or as a diffuse infiltrate. The pleura, diaphragm, pericardium, and skin are also frequently involved. Osteolytic lesions are more common than sclerotic changes in skeletal metastases.

Table 96–1.   Characteristics of Malignant Synovial Tumors[11,132–135,143,147]

	Synovial Sarcoma	Epithelioid Sarcoma	Clear Cell Sarcoma of Tendons and Aponeuroses (Malignant Melanoma)
Age			
Median	26.5	26	27
Greatest prevalence	15–35	15–35	20–40
Sex, male/female	1.2:1	2:1	1:1
Clinical features	Deep mass related to joints; most frequent in lower extremities	Slow-growing nodule in finger, hand, forearm, knee, lower leg Rare in other locations Central necrosis common; ulceration	Deep-seated nodule adherent to tendon or aponeurosis Most frequent in foot and ankle
Radiologic calcification	30%	Occasional	Not seen
Histology	Biphasic (epithelial cells, spindle-cell stroma); monophasic; undifferentiated*	Large ovoid to plump spindle cells arranged in a nodular pattern	Nests or fascicles of fusiform or rounded cells with clear cytoplasm
Immunohistochemistry	Keratin	Keratin	S-100 protein
Electron microscopy	Basal lamina, maculae adherens, desmosomes	Maculae adherens, desmosomes, watertight junctions	Melanosomes or premelanosomes
Histologic grade†	2 or 3; 1	2 or 3	2 or 3
Metastases	Lung, lymph nodes, bone marrow	Lymph nodes, lung, skin	Lung, lymph nodes, bones
Recurrence rate	28–49%	76%	50%
5-year survival	25–63%	NA	NA

*In all types, a biphasic cellular pattern is required in at least one portion of the neoplasm.
†Grade is determined by a combined assessment of cellularity, cellular anaplasia or pleomorphism, mitotic activity, expansive or infiltrative growth, and necrosis.
NA = not available; S-100 protein = a neuroectodermal marker.

Histopathologic Findings

Synovial sarcomas most commonly originate in peri- and para-articular tissues including the joint capsule, tendon sheaths, intermuscular septa, and fascia separating muscles and ligaments.[110,112,126]

Rarely does this neoplasm lie within a joint cavity, and joint involvement is usually secondary.[10,48,110] Unequivocal origin in a synovial structure is rare.[127]

The gross appearance of a synovial sarcoma depends on its place of origin, the duration and rapidity of its growth, and its cellular composition. The color of the tumor, which may be 1 to 20 cm or more in diameter, varies from a pale gray-yellow to a deep red, usually the result of hemorrhage. The tumor may feel uniformly firm when spindle cell elements predominate, or it may be soft and contain cystic spaces filled with mucoid secretions when epithelial-like cells predominate. Compression of the surrounding tissue may give rise to the mistaken belief that the tumor is encapsulated.

Synovial sarcomas are pleomorphic tumors. Some are characterized by a biphasic cellular pattern that includes epithelial-like cells arranged in nests, tubules and acini, and a stroma of spindle cells and abundant reticulin fibers with the appearance of a fibrosarcoma (Fig. 96–5). Other tumors are monophasic, most commonly of the spindle-cell type and less commonly of the epithelial-like type, in which the cells are arranged in sheaths and cords in a tenuous reticular stroma.[112,116,126]

Finally, an undifferentiated type is also recognized.[11] Regardless of the type, the diagnosis of synovial sarcoma requires the presence of a biphasic cellular pattern in at least one portion of the tumor. Mast cells are common in the spindle cell areas. There is prominent vascularity, and vascular invasion is often apparent.

The most distinctive histologic feature of synovial sarcoma is the presence of clefts and cystic spaces, lined by cuboidal or columnar cells and containing a mucin-rich secretion that stains intensely with periodic acid-Schiff, mucicarmine, colloidal iron, and alcian blue and is resistant to hyaluronidase.[11,128] Calcification of the spindle cell areas is common.

FIG. 96–5.   Biphasic synovial sarcoma. Note the irregular spaces lined with columnar cells, in addition to the spindle-cell stroma ($\times$100).

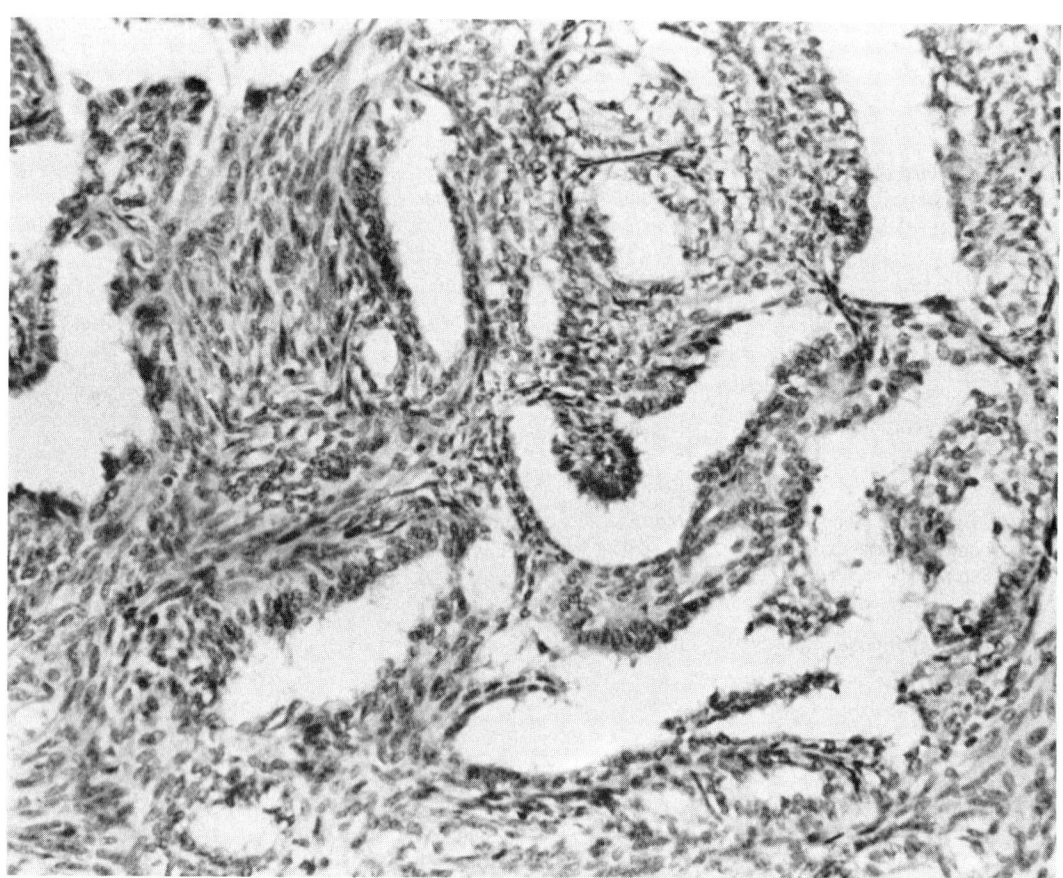

The ultrastructural characteristics of these tumors are intriguing.[70,129–133] For instance, the epithelial-like cells, which under light microscopy resemble the synovial lining cells, are connected by desmosomes and maculae adherens, which are not present in normal synovial tissue. Most observations have revealed the presence of a basal lamina at the epithelial-stromal junction, a structure also absent from normal synovial tissue. To complicate the issue, anti-intermediate filament antibodies demonstrate keratin in the epithelial-like cells,[132–135] consistent with epithelial derivation or differentiation.

The random location of synovial sarcoma in relation to joints, the lack of effect of hyaluronidase on the tinctorial characteristics of the mucinous material, and the presence of structures that do not occur in normal synovial tissue raise questions regarding the histogenesis of these tumors, although some nonmalignant inflammatory lesions of synovial tissue also share some of these characteristics, probably from cellular crowding. A proposal to abandon the name *synovial sarcoma* has been made.[136]

Diagnosis and Treatment

The principles of therapy in synovial sarcoma are based on current concepts of growth and spread of soft-tissue sarcomas. These tumors are poorly circumscribed, and even if invested by a pseudo-capsule, their enucleation inevitably leaves behind microscopic tumor. In addition, their rapid extension along soft-tissue planes explains the local recurrence rates of 18% after en bloc soft part resection and of 4% after amputation.[124] The possibility of synovial sarcoma should be suspected in patients with any tumor in the soft parts of the hand or foot or in the vicinity of the knee, elbow, and shoulder joints, especially. Once considered, the diagnosis should be confirmed by histologic examination. Plain roentgenograms of the region should be followed by angiographic examination, CT scanning, or MRI. Only then should biopsy be performed.[113,123] Although surgical and needle biopsies both have advocates, a surgical biopsy has the advantage of a larger sample, which can be used for prognostic studies, such as the mitotic index.

If the results of biopsy are positive, a wide resection

is undertaken, depending on the extent and location of the tumor. In superficial lesions of the hands and feet and in lesions emerging from extra-articular connective tissues and tendons, a wide local excision with a margin of at least 6 cm of normal tissue has been recommended. The entire muscle group in which the tumor grows should be resected. Deeper tumors of hands and feet and tumors developing in the vicinity of joints usually require amputation of the limb. Radical dissection of regional lymph nodes is optional, except when nodal metastases are obvious or in proximal lesions, as part of the en bloc resection.[124] Interest in preserving a functional limb has stimulated the use of adjuvant perfusion chemotherapy as well as radical radiotherapy in association with local excision in various types of soft-tissue sarcoma,[137,138] and short-term results are encouraging. Postoperative chemotherapy may also hold promise.

Prognosis

Features of the tumor or the host that may affect prognosis have been investigated. The most important determinant of prognosis appears to be the size of the tumor at the time of initial therapy. The 5-year survival rate for patients with tumors under 5 cm in diameter is much better than for patients with larger tumors. Other favorable features include (1) the extremes of age; (2) occurrence in an "exposed" area such as the foot, ankle, forearm, wrist, and neck; (3) female sex; (4) biphasic histologic pattern;[112,116] and (5) calcification within the tumor.[139] Recent experience has indicated overall 5- and 10-year actuarial survival rates of 58% and 48%, respectively, in patients treated with en bloc, wide, soft part resection and amputation. The possible beneficial effects of newer techniques for the control of the primary tumor, such as isolation-perfusion chemotherapy and radical radiotherapy in association with surgical excision, as well as prevention of recurrence and metastasis by postoperative chemotherapy, remain to be determined.

CLEAR CELL SARCOMA OF TENDONS AND APONEUROSES (MALIGNANT MELANOMA OF SOFT PARTS)

A peculiar neoplasm arising from tendons or aponeuroses is termed *clear cell sarcoma* (Table 96–1).[140–144] A more accurate designation based on current knowledge is malignant melanoma of soft parts.[142] This painless mass is usually present for long periods. Many such tumors arise from the lower limb in the region of the foot (Achilles tendon, ankle, and plantar fascia) and the knee (patellar tendon and aponeuroses about

the knee). The tumor is peculiarly composed of compact nests and fascicles of round or fusiform, pale-staining cells with vesicular nuclei and prominent nucleoli.

Melanin and S-100 protein (a neuroectodermal marker) are present in the majority of these tumors.[141–144] Clear cell sarcoma has been postulated to derive from potentially melanogenic cells that migrated from the neural crest into the vicinity of tendons and fasciae during embryonal life.[143]

Surgical excision is only temporarily beneficial. Local recurrences and metastases are common, and the prognosis is generally poor.

EPITHELIOID SARCOMA

The epithelioid is a distinctive sarcoma that occurs predominantly in young adults (Table 96–1). Common sites include the hand, wrist, forearm, and lower leg, where the lesion arises from tendon and fascial structures. Necrosis of the tumor nodule with skin ulceration often leads to the erroneous diagnosis of a chronic inflammatory process, granuloma, or squamous cell carcinoma. Microscopically, the tumor includes large, acidophilic polygonal cells and spindle cells arranged in irregular nodules, where central necrosis frequently occurs.[145] Electron-microscopic, enzyme histochemical, and immunohistochemical findings resemble those of synovial sarcoma.[146–148]

SYNOVIAL ANGIOSARCOMA

Angiosarcomas usually involve skin, soft tissues, the heart, or the liver. Primary synovial angiosarcoma is truly exceptional.[149]

INVOLVEMENT OF JOINTS BY PRIMARY BONE TUMORS

Metaphyseal bone tumors, chiefly osteosarcoma, fibrosarcoma, and chondrosarcoma, often invade joints.[150] Articular (hyaline) cartilage is thought to act as a barrier to local tumor extension by means of tissue factors that inhibit tumor angiogenesis.[151] Tumor penetration eventually occurs, however, whether peripherally beneath the joint capsule, at the bone attachment of intracapsular ligaments such as the cruciate ligaments of the knee, or across cartilage itself.[150] Bland synovial effusions may indicate early invasion of the joint.[152]

CARCINOMATOUS SYNOVITIS

That metastases to synovium are clinically rare is surprising given the high frequency of disseminated carcinomas and the rich vascular supply of synovial tissue.[52] Knees are most commonly affected.[153,154] Other evidence of disseminated tumor is usually present, but, rarely, joint metastases are the first indications of malignant disease or of tumor dissemination.[153,155] Radiographic studies of such joints demonstrate lytic lesions of the patella, femur, or tibia, but patients with early cases may lack abnormal findings.[155,156]

Bone scanning may reveal increased local radionuclide uptake.[157,158] Multiple focal lesions of increased activity throughout the skeleton provide further evidence of metastatic disease. Synovial fluid is hemorrhagic, with 100 to 8000 WBCs/mm[3], predominantly mononuclear cells. The fluid of one patient exhibited eosinophilia.[156] Tumor cells are found in synovial fluid in 80% of patients;[153,155,157,158] arthrotomy or closed synovial biopsy reveals carcinomatous involvement of the synovium. Arthroscopy is valuable in the diagnosis of synovial metastases when the results of other tests are inconclusive.

METASTASES TO BONES OF THE HANDS AND FEET

Bone metastasis of the hands and feet is an unusual form of "arthritis" that occurs in patients with disseminated carcinoma. Metastases occur in small bones, particularly the distal phalanges and the tarsal bones. The clinical syndromes resemble paronychia or gout. Lytic lesions, sometimes with pathologic fractures, are usually present.[159–162]

METASTASES TO SHOULDERS

Bone metastases in renal cell carcinoma exhibit a curious predilection for the clavicle, acromion, and proximal humeral head.[163] Painful lytic lesions in these areas should direct attention to the kidney. An instance of nasopharyngeal carcinoma metastatic to both acromioclavicular joints is on record.[164]

LYMPHOMA

Musculoskeletal manifestations of lymphoma, both Hodgkin's[165] and non-Hodgkin's,[166,167] include pain caused by bone metastasis or primary involvement of bone, hypertrophic osteoarthropathy in patients with intrathoracic lesions, and very rarely arthritis caused by lymphomatous synovial infiltration. The latter is usually monoarticular, but polyarticular cases have been confused with RA.

NONMETASTATIC SYNDROMES

The nonmetastatic syndromes comprise a variety of conditions.[168]

HYPERTROPHIC OSTEOARTHROPATHY

The well-known association of intrathoracic tumors and hypertrophic osteoarthropathy is discussed separately (see Chapter 86). It can be considered the prototype of tumor-associated arthritis; its onset often leads to the discovery of an unsuspected intrathoracic malignant process.[169–172]

PANCREATIC CANCER WITH ARTHROPATHY AND FAT NECROSIS

Panniculitis resembling erythema nodosum accompanied by synovitis and serositis is a well-known accompaniment of pancreatic carcinoma, particularly of the acinar-cell type, as well as of pancreatitis. Its pathogenesis includes fat necrosis in subcutaneous tissue, bone marrow, and subsynovial fat, as a result of high levels of circulating pancreatic lipase.[173–176]

CANCER ARTHRITIS

Several observers have described a syndrome resembling RA with typical or atypical features,[177–179] having its onset a few months before the discovery of a tumor. The atypical form is characterized by explosive onset, asymmetry of joint involvement, sparing of wrists and small joints of the hand, absence of subcutaneous nodules, and seronegativity. All patients in one series were in their fifth decade or older. Removal or successful treatment of the tumor was associated with remission of the arthritis in approximately half these patients. Remission was more frequent in the atypical than in the typical RA-like arthritis. The validity of these associations has not been definitely established by epidemiologic methods.

Supporting evidence of a causal association between carcinoma and rheumatic disease has been provided by individual observations, in which removal of carcinoma has been followed by complete clinical and serologic remission of the syndrome.

The tumors inolved included lung carcinoma,[180,181] esophageal carcinoma,[182,183] gastric carcinoma,[184] colonic carcinoma,[185] breast carcinoma,[186] and ovarian dysgerminoma.[187,188]

HYPERURICEMIA AND GOUT

The degree of hyperuricemia in patients with carcinoma correlates with extensiveness of the disease, involvement of the liver, and presence of hypercalcemia. Gout occurred in only 5 of 70 patients studied. In 2 of these patients, the gout preceded the tumor.[189] The frequency of hyperuricemia and gout in a cancer patient population remains to be elucidated. Interestingly, hypouricemia has also been described in association with disseminated carcinoma.[190]

CARCINOID ARTHROPATHY

This peculiar form of arthropathy characterized by arthralgias, juxta-articular demineralization, erosions, and subchondral cysts was observed in four of five consecutive patients with the carcinoid syndrome.[191,192]

LYMPHOMATOID GRANULOMATOSIS

Arthralgia may be associated with this peculiar lymphoproliferative disorder, which is characterized by angiodestructive lymphoreticular proliferative granulomata. A case presenting with polyarthritis has been recorded.[193]

MULTICENTRIC RETICULOHISTIOCYTOSIS

An association may well be present between multicentric reticulohistiocytosis and cancer; 28% of the 82 cases in one review had an associated neoplasm.[194]

PALMAR FASCIITIS AND POLYARTHRITIS ASSOCIATED WITH CARCINOMA

Medsger et al.[195] have described a unique syndrome including palmar fasciitis and polyarthritis in six patients with ovarian carcinoma predominantly of the endometrioid type. Other tumors also produce this syndrome.[196] The palmar changes ranged from dif-

Table 96–2. Rheumatologic Syndromes Associated with Nonhematologic Malignant Diseases

By Direct Extension or Metastatic
Primary bone tumors
Carcinomatous (metastatic) synovitis
Metastases to small bones
Nonmetastatic (Paraneoplastic)
Articular
Hypertrophic osteoarthropathy
Subcutaneous nodules, arthritis, and serositis (fat necrosis) in pancreatic cancer (as in pancreatitis)
Cancer arthritis
Hyperuricema and gout; hypouricemia
Carcinoid arthropathy
Multicentric reticulohistiocytosis
Palmar fasciitis and polyarthritis associated with carcinoma
Coincidental arthritis of any type
Muscular
Polymyositis (dermatomyositis)
Eaton-Lambert syndrome
Carcinoid myopathy
Type II muscle fiber atrophy
Coincidental myopathy of any type
Cutaneous
Carcinoid "scleroderma"
As Complications of Therapy
Aseptic necrosis of bone
Septic arthritis
Corticosteroid myopathy
Chemotherapy-induced fibrotic syndromes

fuse, globular swelling with warmth and erythema to typical Dupuytren's contracture. The shoulders and the metacarpophalangeal and proximal interphalangeal joints were most frequently involved and exhibited painful limitations of motion and flexor contractures. Morning stiffness was prominent. Although two of these patients had the carpal tunnel syndrome, none had Raynaud's phenomenon, dermal or pulmonary fibrosis, or evidences of myositis. In five patients, the articular symptoms preceded the diagnosis of malignant disease by several months to 2 years. In the remaining patient, the articular symptoms preceded tumor recurrence. In all patients, the ovarian tumor was extensive and gave evidence of intra- and extraperitoneal spread. The median survival time after diagnosis of the tumor was six months. The pathogenesis of this syndrome, which resembled reflex sympathetic dystrophy, remains unexplained.

OTHER RHEUMATOLOGIC SYNDROMES

Polymyositis (dermatomyositis) and other muscle syndromes associated with tumors are discussed in Chapter 72. Other nonmetastatic rheumatologic or neuromuscular syndromes associated with malignant disease are listed in Table 96–2.

COMPLICATIONS OF CANCER TREATMENT

Tumor involvement of joints is occasionally suggested when a patient is receiving corticosteroid or immunosuppressive therapy, which alone can be associated with secondary joint manifestations. These manifestations include *aseptic necrosis of bone* (see Chapters 37 and 98), *septic arthritis* (see Chapters 114 and 115), and *steroid myopathy* (see Chapter 37). In addition, chemotherapy with bleomycin can give rise to a *fibrotic syndrome* resembling systemic sclerosis (see Chapter 73).

REFERENCES

1. Cassells, S.W.: Arthroscopy, Diagnostic and Surgical Practice. Philadelphia, Lea & Febiger, 1984.
2. Yaghmai, I.: Angiography of Bone and Soft Tissue Lesions. Berlin, Springer-Verlag, 1979.
3. Soye, I.: Computed tomography in the preoperative evaluation of masses arising in or near the joints of the extremities. Radiology, *143*:727–732, 1982.
4. Petasnick, J.P., et al.: Soft-tissue masses of the locomotor system: Comparison of MR imaging with CT. Skeletal Radiol., *160*:125, 1986.
5. Sundaram, M., et al.: Magnetic resonance imaging of lesions of synovial origin. Skeletal Radiol., *15*:110, 1986.
6. Hartzman, S., et al.: MR imaging of the knee. II. Chronic disorders. Radiology, *162*:553, 1987.
7. Jaffe, H.L.: Tumors and Tumorous Conditions of the Bones and Joints. Philadelphia, Lea & Febiger, 1958.
8. Granowitz, S.P., D'Antonio, J., and Mankin, H.L.: The pathogenesis and long-term end results of pigmented villonodular synovitis. Clin. Orthop., *114*:335–351, 1976.
9. Nilsonne, U., and Moberger, G.: Pigmented villonodular synovitis of joints. Acta Orthop. Scand., *40*:448–460, 1969.
10. Schajowicz, F.: Tumors and Tumorlike Lesions of Bone and Joints. New York, Springer-Verlag, 1981.
11. Enzinger, F.M., and Weiss, S.W.: Soft Tissue Tumors. St. Louis, Mosby, 1983.
12. Rao, A.S., and Vigorita, V.J.: Pigmented villondular synovitis (giant-cell tumor of the tendon sheath and synovial membrane). A review of eighty-one cases. J. Bone Joint Surg., *66A*:76–94, 1984.
13. Ushijima, M., Hashimoto, H., Tsuneyoshi, M., and Enjoji, M.: Pigmented villonodular synovitis. A clinicopathologic study of 52 cases. Acta Pathol. Jpn., *36*:317–326, 1986.
14. Mizuno, K., Ishikura, H., and Aizawa, M.: Giant cell tumor of tendon sheath. An immunohistochemical study of 28 cases. Acta Pathol. Jpn., *36*:1487, 1986.
15. Rosenthal, D.I., Coleman, P.K., and Schiller, A.L.: Pigmented villonodular synovitis: Correlation of angiographic and histologic findings. A.J.R., *135*:581–585, 1980.
16. Scott, P.M.: Bone lesions in pigmented villonodular synovitis. J. Bone Joint Surg., *50-B*:306–311, 1968.
17. Goldberg, R.P., Weissman, B.N., Naimark, A., Braunstein, E.: Femoral neck erosions: Sign of hip joint synovial disease. AJR, *141*:107, 1983.
18. Dorwart, R.H., Genant, H.K., Johnston, W.H., and Morris, J.M.: Pigmented villonodular synovitis of synovial joints: Clinical, pathologic, and radiologic features. AJR, *143*:877, 1984.
19. Reginato, A., Martinez, V., Schumacher, H.R., and Torres, J.: Giant cell tumor associated with rheumatoid arthritis. Ann. Rheum. Dis., *33*:333–341, 1974.
20. Alguacil-Garcia, A., Unni, K.K., and Goellner, J.R.: Giant cell tumor of tendon sheath and pigmented villonodular synovitis. An ultrastructural study. Am. J. Clin. Pathol., *69*:6–17, 1978.
21. Gaucher, A., et al.: Pigmented villonodular synovitis of the hip: Ultrastructure and scanning electron microscopy (Fr). Rev. Rhum. Mal. Osteoartic., *43*:357–362, 1976.
22. Ghadially, F.N., Lalonde, J.M., and Dick, C.E.: Ultrastructure of pigmented villonodular synovitis. J. Pathol., *127*:19–26, 1979.
23. Schumacher, H.R., Lotke, P., Athreya, B., and Rothfuss, S.: Pigmented villonodular synovitis: Light and electron microscopic studies. Semin. Arthritis Rheum., *12*:32–43, 1982.
24. Archer-Harvey, J.M., Henderson, D.W., and Papadimitriou, J.M.: Pigmented villonodular synovitis associated with psoriatic polyarthropathy: An electron microscopic and immunocytochemical study. J. Pathol., *144*:57–68, 1984.
25. Morris, C.J., Blake, R.D., Wainwright, A.C., and Steven, M.M.: Relationship between iron deposits and tissue damage in the synovium: An ultrastructural study. Ann. Rheum. Dis., *45*:21, 1986.
26. Nickels, F.A., Grant, B.D., and Lincoln, S.D.: Villonodular synovitis of the equine metacarpophalangeal joint. J. Am. Vet. Med. Assoc., *168*:1043–1046, 1976.
27. Barclay, W.P., White, K.K., and Williams, A.: Equine villonodular synovitis: A case survey. Cornell Vet., *70*:72–76, 1980.
28. Donde, R., and Funding, J.: Pigmented villonodular synovitis: A follow-up study. Scand. J. Rheumatol., *9*:172–174, 1980.
29. Johansson, J.E., et al.: Pigmented villonodular synovitis of joints. Clin. Orthop., *163*:159–166, 1982.
30. Bobechko, W.P., and Kostuik, J.P.: Childhood villonodular synovitis. Can. J. Surg., *11*:480–486, 1968.
31. Brown-Crosby, E., Inglis, A., and Bullough, P.G.: Multiple joint involvement with pigmented villonodular synovitis. Radiology, *122*:671–672, 1977.
32. Gehweiler, J.A., and Wilson, J.W.: Diffuse biarticular pigmented villonodular synovitis. Radiology, *93*:845–851, 1969.
33. Leszczynski, J., et al.: Pigmented villonodular synovitis in multiple joints: Occurrence in a child with cavernous haemangioma of lip and pulmonary stenosis. Ann. Rheum. Dis., *34*:269–272, 1975.
34. Lindenbaum, B.L., and Hunt, T.: An unusual presentation of pigmented villonodular synovitis. Clin. Orthop., *122*:263–267, 1977.
35. Wagner, M.L., et al.: Polyarticular pigmented villonodular synovitis. AJR, *136*:821–823, 1981.
36. Wendt, R.G., et al.: Polyarticular pigmented villonodular synovitis in children: Evidence for a genetic contribution. J. Rheumatol., *13*:921–926, 1986.
37. Torisu, T., and Watanabe, H.: Pigmented villonodular synovitis occurred in a rheumatoid patient. Clin. Orthop., *91*:134–140, 1973.
38. Myers, B.W., Masi, A.T., and Feigenbaum, S.L.: Pigmented villonodular synovitis and tenosynovitis: A clinical epidemiology study of 166 cases and literature review. Medicine, *59*:233–238, 1980.
39. Vigorita, V.J.: Pigmented villonodular synovitis-like lesions in association with rare cases of rheumatoid arthritis, osteone-

crosis, and advanced degenerative joint disease. Report of five cases. Clin. Orthop., *183*:115, 1984.

40. Danzig, L.A., Gershuni, D.H., and Resnick, D.: Diagnosis and treatment of diffuse pigmented villonodular synovitis of the hip. Clin. Orthop., *168*:42–47, 1982.

41. Lapayowker, M.S., Miller, W.T., Levy, W.M., and Harwick, R.D.: Pigmented villonodular synovitis of the temporomandibular joint. Radiology, *108*:313–316, 1973.

42. Rickert, R.R., and Shapiro, M.J.: Pigmented villonodular synovitis of the temporomandibular joint. Otolaryngol. Head Neck Surg., *90*:668, 1982.

43. Curtin, H.D., Williams, R., Gailla, L., and Meyers, E.N.: Pigmented villonodular synovitis of the temporomandibular joint. Comput. Radiol., *7*:257, 1983.

44. Campbell, A.J., and Wells, I.P.: Pigmented villonodular synovitis of a lumbar vertebral facet joint. J. Bone Joint Surg., *64A*:145–146, 1982.

45. Pulitzer, D.R., and Reed, R.J.: Localized pigmented villonodular synovitis of the vertebral column. Arch. Pathol. Lab. Med., *108*:228–230, 1984.

46. Weidner, N., et al.: Giant cell tumors of synovium (pigmented villonodular synovitis) involving the vertebral column. Cancer, *57*:2030–2036, 1986.

47. Ropes, M.W., and Bauer, W.: Synovial Fluid Changes in Joint Disease. Cambridge, Harvard University Press, 1953.

48. Wilner, D.: Radiology of Bone Tumors and Allied Disorders. Philadelphia, W.B. Saunders, 1982.

49. Aglietti, P., DiMuria, G.V., Salvati, E.A., and Stringa, G.: Pigmented villonodular synovitis of the hip joint. Ital. J. Orthop. Traumatol., *9*:487, 1983.

50. Moroni, A., Innao, V., and Picci, P.: Pigmented villonodular synovitis of the hip. Study of 9 cases. Ital. J. Orthop. Traumatol., *9*:331, 1983.

51. Jergesen, H.E., Mankin, H.J., and Schiller, A.L.: Diffuse pigmented villonodular synovitis of the knee mimicking primary bone neoplasm. A report of two cases. J. Bone Joint Surg., *60A*:825–829, 1978.

52. Liew, M., and Dick, W.C.: The anatomy and physiology of blood flow in a diarthrodial joint. Clin. Rheum. Dis., *7*:131–138, 1981.

53. Kaufman, R.A., Towbin, R.B., Babcock, D.S., and Crawford, A.H.: Arthrosonography in the diagnosis of pigmented villonodular synovitis. AJR, *139*:396–398, 1982.

54. Rosenthal, D.I., Aronow, S., and Murray, W.T.: Iron content of pigmented villonodular synovitis detected by computer tomography. Radiology, *133*:409–411, 1979.

55. Howie, C.R., Smith, G.D., Christie, J., and Gregg, P.J.: Torsion of localised pigmented villonodular synovitis of the knee. J. Bone Joint Surg., *67B*:564–566, 1985.

56. Granowitz, S.P., and Mankin, H.J.: Localized pigmented villonodular synovitis of the knee. Report of five cases. J. Bone Joint Surg., *49A*:122–128, 1967.

57. Goergen, T.G., Resnick, D., and Niwayama, G.: Localized nodular synovitis of the knee: A report of two cases with abnormal arthrograms. AJR, *126*:647–650, 1976.

58. Lowenstein, M.B., Smith, J.R.V., and Cole, S.: Infrapatellar pigmented villonodular synovitis: Arthrographic detection. AJR, *135*:279–282, 1980.

59. Bogumill, G.P., Sullivan, D.J., and Baker, G.I.: Tumors of the hand. Clin. Orthop., *108*:214–222, 1975.

60. Crawford, G.P., and Offerman, R.J.: Pigmented villonodular synovitis in the hand. Hand, *12*:282–287, 1980.

61. El-Khoury, G.Y. Corbett, A.J., and Summers, T.B.: Case report 303: A complete plica synovalis suprapatellaris, with dif-

fuse pigmented villonodular synovitis limited to an isolated, non-communicating suprapatellar bursa. Skeletal Radiol., *13*:164, 1985.

62. Present, D.A., Bertoni, E., and Enneking, W.F.: Case report 348: Pigmented villonodular synovitis arising from bursa of the pes anserinus muscle, with secondary involvement of the tibia. Skeletal Radiol., *15*:236, 1986.

63. Ushijima, M., et al.: Malignant giant cell tumor of tendon sheath. Report of a case. Acta Pathol. Jpn., *35*:699, 1985.

64. Henderson, B., et al.: Metabolic alterations in human synovial lining cells in pigmented villonodular synovitis. Ann. Rheum. Dis., *38*:463–466, 1979.

65. Mainardi, C.L., et al.: Proliferative synovitis in hemophilia: Biochemical and morphological observations. Arthritis Rheum., *21*:137–144, 1978.

66. Duthie, R.B., and Rizza, C.R.: Rheumatological manifestations of the hemophilias. Clin. Rheum. Dis., *1*:53–93, 1975.

67. Hawley, W.L., and Ansell, B.M.: Synovial hemangioma presenting as monoarticular arthritis of the knee. Arch. Dis. Child., *56*:558–560, 1981.

68. Roy, S., and Ghadially, F.N.: Synovial membrane in experimentally produced chronic hemarthrosis. Ann. Rheum. Dis., *28*:402–414, 1969.

69. Singh, R., Grewal, D.S., and Chakravarti, R.N.: Experimental production of pigmented villonodular synovitis in the knee and ankle joints of Rhesus monkeys. J. Pathol., *98*:137–142, 1969.

70. Ghadially, F.N.: Diagnostic Electron Microscopy of Tumors. London, Butterworths, 1980.

71. Molnar, Z., Stern, W.H., and Stoltzner, G.H.: Cytoplasmic tubular structures in pigmented villonodular synovitis. Arthritis Rheum., *14*:784–787, 1971.

72. Friedman, M., and Schwartz, E.E.: Irradiation therapy of pigmented villonodular synovitis. Bull. Hosp. Joint Dis., *18*:19–32, 1957.

73. Robert D'Eshoughes, J., Delcambre, B., and Delbart, P.: Pigmented villonodular synovitis and radioisotopic synoviorthesis. (Fr.) Lille Med., *20*:438–446, 1975.

74. Wiss, D.A.: Recurrent villonodular synovitis of the knee. Successful treatment with Yttrium-90. Clin. Orthop., *169*:139–144, 1982.

75. Murphy, F.P., Dahlin, D.C., and Sullivan, C.R.: Articular synovial chondromatosis. J. Bone Joint Surg., *44A*:77–86, 1962.

76. Sim, F.H., Dahlin, D.C., and Ivins, J.C.: Extra-articular synovial chondromatosis. J. Bone Joint Surg., *59A*:492–495, 1977.

77. Milgram, J.W.: Synovial osteochondromatosis. A histopathological study of thirty cases. J. Bone Joint Surg., *59A*:792–801, 1977.

78. Carey, R.P.L.: Synovial chondromatosis of the knee in childhood. A report of two cases. J. Bone Joint Surg., *65B*:444–447, 1983.

79. Pelker, R.R., Drennan, J.C., and Ozonoff, M.B.: Juvenile synovial chondromatosis of the hip. J. Bone Joint Surg., *65A*:552–554, 1983.

80. DeBenedetti, M.J., and Schwinn, C.P.: Tenosynovial chondromatosis of the hand. J. Bone Joint Surg., *61A*:898–903, 1979.

81. Paul, G.R., and Leach, R.E.: Synovial chondromatosis of the shoulder. Clin. Orthop., *68*:130–135, 1970.

82. Rosen, P., et al.: Synovial chondromatosis affecting the temporomandibular joint. Arthritis Rheum., *20*:736–740, 1977.

83. Blankestijn, J., Panders, A.K., Vermey, A., and Scherpbier, A.J.J.A.: Synovial chondromatosis of the temporomandibular

joint. Report of three cases and review of the literature. Cancer, 55:479–485, 1985.

84. Thompson, K., Schwartz, H.C., and Miles, J.W.: Synovial chondromatosis of the temporomandibular joint presenting as a parotid mass: Possibility of confusion with benign mixed tumor. Oral Surg. Oral Med. Oral Pathol., 64:377, 1986.

85. Manco, L.G., and De Luke, D.M.: CT diagnosis of synovial chondromatosis of the temporomandibular joint. AJR, 148:574, 1987.

86. Norman, A., and Steiner, G.C.: Bone erosion in synovial chondromatosis. Radiology, 161:749–752, 1986.

87. McCarty, D.J., et al.: "Milwaukee shoulder"—Association of microspheroids containing hydroxyapatite crystals, active collagenase, and neutral protease with rotator cuff defects. I. Clinical aspects. Arthritis Rheum., 24:464–473, 1981.

88. Ellman, M.H., Krieger, M.I., and Brown, N.: Pseudogout mimicking synovial chondromatosis. J. Bone Joint Surg., 57A:863–865, 1975.

89. McCarthy, E.F., and Dorfman, H.D.: Primary synovial chondromatosis. an ultrastructural study. Clin. Orthop., 168:178–186, 1982.

90. Ryan, L.M., Cheung, H.S., Schwab, J.P., and Johnson, R.P.: Predominance of Type II collagen in synovial chondromatosis. Clin. Orthop., 168:173–177, 1982.

91. Milgram, J.W.: The development of loose bodies in human joints. Clin. Orthop., 124:292–303, 1977.

92. Smillie, I.S.: Diseases of the Knee Joint. 2nd Ed. Edinburgh, Churchill Livingstone, 1980.

93. Lewis, R.C., Coventry, M.B., and Soule, E.H.: Hemangioma of the synovial membrane. J. Bone Joint Surg., 41A:264–270, 1959.

94. Halborg, A., Hansen, H., and Sneppen, H.O.: Haemangioma of the knee joint. Acta Orthop. Scand., 39:209–216, 1968.

95. Moon, N.F.: Synovial hemangioma of the knee joint. Clin. Orthop., 90:183, 1973.

96. Rosales Wynne-Roberts, C., Anderson, C., Turano, A.M., and Baron, M.: Synovial haemangioma of the knee: Light and electron microscopic findings. J. Pathol., 123:247–254, 1977.

97. Resnick, D., and Oliphant, M.: Hemophilia-like arthropathy of the knee associated with cutaneous and synovial hemangiomas. Radiology, 114:323–326, 1975.

98. Forrest, J., and Staple, T.W.: Synovial hemangioma of the knee. Demonstration by arthrography and arteriography. AJR, 112:512–516, 1971.

99. Sty, J., Simons, G., and Becker, D.: Radionuclide angiography and blood pool imaging: Synovial hemangioma. Clin. Nucl. Med., 5:517, 1980.

100. Pudlowski, R.M., Gilula, L.A., and Kyriakos, M.: Intraarticular lipoma with osseous metaplasia: Radiologic–pathologic correlation. AJR, 132:471–473, 1979.

101. Rodriguez, J.M., and Phalen, G.S.: Lipomas in the hand and wrist. Diagnosis and treatment. Cleveland Clin. Q., 37:201–205, 1970.

102. Weitzman, G.: Lipoma arborescens of the knee: Report of a case. J. Bone Joint Surg., 47A:1030–1033, 1965.

103. Burgan, D.W.: Lipoma arborescens of the knee. Another cause of filling defects on a knee arthrogram. Radiology, 101:583–584, 1971.

104. Hoffa, A.: The influence of the adipose tissue with regard to the pathology of the knee joint. JAMA, 43:795–796, 1904.

105. Ogata, K., and Ushijima, M.: Tenosynovial fibroma arising from the posterior cruciate ligament. Clin. Orthop., 215:153, 1987.

106. Chung, E.B., and Enzinger, F.M.: Fibroma of tendon sheath. Cancer, 44:1945, 1979.

107. Cooper, P.H.: Fibroma of tendon sheath. J. Am. Acad. Dermatol., 11:625, 1984.

108. Sarma, D.P., Weilbaecher, T.G., and Rodriguez, F.H., Jr.: Fibroma of tendon sheath. J. Surg. Oncol., 32:230, 1986.

109. Buck, P., Mickelson, M.R., and Bonfiglio, M.: Synovial sarcoma: A review of 33 cases. Clin. Orthop., 156:211–215, 1981.

110. Cadman, N.L., Soule, E.H., and Kelly, P.: Synovial sarcoma. An analysis of 134 tumors. Cancer, 18:613–627, 1965.

111. Crocker, D.W., and Stout, A.P.: Synovial sarcoma in children. Cancer, 12:1123–1133, 1959.

112. Hajdu, S.I., Shiu, M.H., and Fortner, J.G.: Tendosynovial sarcoma. A clinicopathological study of 136 cases. Cancer, 39:1201–1217, 1977.

113. Enneking, W.F.: Musculoskeletal Tumor Surgery. New York. Churchill Livingstone, 1983.

114. Dreyfuss, U.V., Boome, R.S., and Kranold, D.H.: Synovial sarcoma of the hand. A literature review. J. Hand Surg. (Br.), 11:471, 1986.

115. Shmookler, B.M.: Retroperitoneal synovial sarcoma. Am. J. Clin. Pathol., 77:686–691, 1982.

116. Wright, P.H., Sim, F.H., Soule, E.H., and Taylor, W.F.: Synovial sarcoma. J. Bone Joint Surg., 64A:112–122, 1982.

117. Shmookler, B.M., Enzinger, F.M., and Brannon, R.B.: Orofacial synovial sarcoma. A clinicopathologic study of 11 new cases and review of the literature. Cancer, 50:269–276, 1982.

118. Roth, J.A., Enzinger, F.M., and Tannenbaum, M.: Synovial sarcoma of the neck: A followup study of 24 cases. Cancer, 35:1243–1253, 1975.

119. Bloch, M.J., Iozzo, R.V., Edmunds, L.H., Jr., and Brooks, J.J.: Polypoid synovial sarcoma of the esophagus. Gastroenterology, 92:229, 1987.

120. Horne, T., Mogle, P., Finterbush, A., and Gordin, M.: Increased uptake of 99mTc-MDP in calcified synovial sarcoma. Eur. J. Nucl. Med., 8:75–76, 1983.

121. Lindell, M.M., Jr., et al.: Diagnostic technique for the evaluation of soft tissue sarcoma. Semin. Oncol., 8:160–171, 1981.

122. Lois, J.F.: Angiography of histopathologic variants of synovial sarcoma. Acta Radiol. [Diagn.] (Stockh.), 27:449, 1986.

123. Russell, W.O., et al.: Staging system for soft tissue sarcoma. Semin. Oncol., 8:156–159, 1981.

124. Shiu, M.H., McCormack, P.M., Hajdu, S.I., and Fortner, J.G.: Surgical treatment of tendosynovial sarcoma. Cancer, 43:889–897, 1979.

125. Ryan, J.R., Baker, L.H., and Benjamin, R.S.: The natural history of metastatic synovial sarcoma. Clin. Orthop., 164:257–260, 1982.

126. Tsuneyoshi, M., Yokohama, K., and Enjoji, M.: Synovial sarcoma. A clinicopathologic and ultrastructural study of 42 cases. Acta Pathol. Jpn., 33:23–36, 1983.

127. Dardick, I., et al.: Synovial sarcoma arising in an anatomical bursa. Virchows Arch. [A], 397:93–101, 1982.

128. Nakamura, T., et al.: Histochemical characterization of mucosubstances in synovial sarcoma. Am. J. Surg. Pathol., 8:429, 1984.

129. Gabbiani, G., et al.: Synovial sarcoma: Electron microscopic study of a typical case. Cancer, 28:1031–1039, 1971.

130. Dische, F.E., Darby, A.J., and Howard, E.R.: Malignant synovioma: Electron microscopical findings in three patients and review of the literature. J. Pathol., 124:149–166, 1978.

131. Mickelson, M.R., et al.: Synovial sarcoma. An electron microscopic study of monophasic and biphasic forms. Cancer, 45:2109–2118, 1980.

132. Abenoza, P., Manivel, J.C., Swanson, P.E., and Wick, M.R.: Synovial sarcoma: Ultrastructural study and immunohistochemical analysis by a combined peroxidase-anti-peroxidase/avidin-biotin-peroxidase complex procedure. Hum. Pathol., *17*:1107, 1986.

133. Fisher, C.: Synovial sarcoma: Ultrastructural and immunohistochemical features of epithelial differentiation in monophasic and biphasic tumors. Hum. Pathol., *17*:996–1008, 1986.

134. Miettinen, M., Lehto, V.-P., Badley, R.A., and Virtanen, I.: Expression of intermediate filaments in soft-tissue sarcomas. Int. J. Cancer, *30*:541–546, 1982.

135. Corson, J.M., Weiss, L.M., Banks-Schlegel, S.P., and Pinkus, G.S.: Keratin proteins and carcinoembryonic antigen in synovial sarcomas: An immunohistochemical study of 24 cases. Hum. Pathol., *15*:615–621, 1984.

136. Miettinen, M., Virtanen, I.: Synovial sarcoma—A misnomer. Am. J. Pathol., *117*:18, 1984.

137. Carson, J.H., et al.: The place of radiotherapy in the treatment of synovial sarcoma. Int. J. Radiat. Oncol. Biol. Phys., *7*:49–53, 1981.

138. Eilber, F.R., et al.: Is amputation necessary for sarcomas? A seven-year experience with limb salvage. Ann. Surg., *192*:431–438, 1980.

139. Varela-Duran, J., and Enzinger, F.M.: Calcifying synovial sarcoma. Cancer, *50*:345–352, 1982.

140. Enzinger, F.M.: Clear-cell sarcoma of tendons and aponeuroses. An analysis of 21 cases. Cancer, *18*:1163–1174, 1965.

141. Tsuneyoshi, M., Enjoji, M., and Kubo, T.: Clear cell sarcoma of tendons and aponeuroses. Cancer, *42*:243–252, 1978.

142. Chung, E.B., and Enzinger, F.M.: Malignant melanoma of soft parts. A reassessment of clear cell sarcoma. Am. J. Surg. Pathol., *7*:405, 1983.

143. Kindblom, L.G., Lodding, P., and Angervall, L.: Clear-cell sarcoma of tendons and aponeuroses. An immunohistochemical and electron microscopic analysis indicating neural crest origin. Virchows Arch. [A], *401*:109, 1983.

144. Mukai, M., et al.: Histogenesis of clear cell sarcoma of tendons and aponeuroses. Am. J. Pathol., *114*:264, 1984.

145. Enzinger, F.M.: Epithelioid sarcoma. A sarcoma simulating a granuloma or a carcinoma. Cancer, *26*:1029–1041, 1970.

146. Lombardi, L., and Rilke, F.: Ultrastructural similarities and differences of synovial sarcoma, epithelioid sarcoma, and clear cell sarcoma of the tendons and aponeuroses. Ultrastruct. Pathol., *6*:209, 1984.

147. Chase, D.R., Weiss, S.W., Enzinger, F.M., and Langloss, J.M.: Keratin in epithelioid sarcoma. An immunohistochemical study. Am. J. Surg. Pathol., *8*:435, 1984.

148. Mukai, M., et al.: Cellular differentiation of epithelioid sarcoma. An electron-microscopic, enzyme-histochemical, and immunohistochemical study. Am. J. Pathol., *119*:44, 1985.

149. Case 43-1983. N. Engl. J. Med., *309*:1042–1049, 1983.

150. Simon, M.A., and Hecht, J.D.: Invasion of joints by primary bone sarcomas in adults. Cancer, *50*:1649–1655, 1982.

151. Folkman, J., and Klagsburn, M.: Angiogenic factors. Science, *235*:442, 1987.

152. Lagier, R.: Synovial reaction caused by adjacent malignant tumors: Anatomopathological study of three cases. J. Rheumatol., *4*:65–72, 1977.

153. Fam, A.G., Kolin, A., and Lewis, A.J.: Metastatic carcinomatous arthritis and carcinoma of the lung: A report of two cases diagnosed by synovial fluid cytology. J. Rheumatol., *7*:98–104, 1980.

154. Murray, G.C., and Persellin, R.H.: Metastatic carcinoma presenting as monoarticular arthritis: A case report and review of the literature. Arthritis Rheum., *23*:95–100, 1980.

155. Weinblatt, M.E., and Karp, G.I.: Monoarticular arthritis: Early manifestations of a rhabdomyosarcoma. J. Rheumatol., *8*:685–688, 1981.

156. Goldenberg, D.L., Kelley, W., and Gibbons, R.B.: Metastatic adenocarcinoma of synovium presenting as acute arthritis: Diagnosis by closed synovial biopsy. Arthritis Rheum., *18*:107–110, 1975.

157. Khan, F.A., Garterhouse, W., and Khan, A.: Metastatic bronchogenic carcinoma: An unusual cause of localized arthritis. Chest, *67*:738–739, 1975.

158. Speerstra, F., et al.: Arthritis caused by metastatic melanoma. Arthritis Rheum., *25*:223–226, 1982.

159. Colson, G.M., and Willcox, A.: Phalangeal metastases in bronchogenic carcinoma. Lancet, *1*:100–102, 1948.

160. Vaezy, A., and Budson, D.C.: Phalangeal metastases from bronchogenic carcinoma. JAMA, *239*:226–227, 1978.

161. Amadio, P.C., and Lombardi, R.M.: Metastatic tumors of the hand. J. Hand Surg., *12A*:311, 1987.

162. Zindrick, M.R.: Metastatic tumors of the foot. Clin. Orthop., *170*:219–225, 1982.

163. Ritch, P.S., Hansen, R.M., and Collier, D.: Metastatic renal cell carcinoma presenting as shoulder arthritis. Cancer, *51*:968, 1983.

164. Rozboril, M.B., Good, A.E., Zarbo, R.J., and Schultz, D.A.: Sternoclavicular joint arthritis: An unusual presentation of metastatic carcinoma. J. Rheumatol., *10*:499, 1983.

165. Barton, A., and Hickling, P.: Synovial involvement in Hodgkin's disease. Br. J. Rheumatol., *25*:391, 1986.

166. Rice, D.M., et al.: Primary lymphoma of bone presenting as monoarthritis. J. Rheumatol., *11*:851–854, 1984.

167. Dorfman, H.D., Siegel, H.L., Perry, M.C., and Oxenhandler, R.: Non-Hodgkin's lymphoma of the synovium simulating rheumatoid arthritis. Arthritis Rheum., *30*:155–161, 1987.

168. Caldwell, D.S., and McCallum, R.M.: Rheumatologic manifestations of cancer. Med. Clin. North Am., *70*:385, 1986.

169. Schumacher, H.R., Jr.: Articular manifestations of hypertrophic pulmonary osteoarthropathy in bronchogenic carcinoma. Arthritis Rheum., *19*:629–636, 1976.

170. Shneerson, J.M.: Digital clubbing and hypertrophic osteoarthropathy: The underlying mechanisms. Br. J. Dis. Chest, *75*:113–131, 1981.

171. Segal, A.M., and MacKenzie, A.H.: Hypertrophic osteoarthropathy: A 10-year retrospective analysis. Semin. Arthritis Rheum., *12*:220–232, 1982.

172. Martinez-Lavin, M.: Digital clubbing and hypertrophic osteoarthropathy: An unifying hypothesis. J. Rheumatol., *14*:6, 1987.

173. Good, A.E., et al.: Acinar pancreatic tumor with metastatic fat necrosis. Dig. Dis. Sci., *21*:978–987, 1976.

174. Mullin, G.T., et al.: Arthritis and skin lesions resembling erythema nodosum in pancreatic disease. Ann. Intern. Med., *68*:75–87, 1968.

175. Simkin, P.A., et al.: Free fatty acids in the pancreatic arthritic syndrome. Arthritis Rheum., *26*:127–132, 1983.

176. Wilson, H.A., et al.: Pancreatitis with arthropathy and subcutaneous fat necrosis. Arthritis Rheum., *26*:121–126, 1983.

177. Mackenzie, A.H., and Sherbel, A.L.: Connective tissue syndromes associated with carcinoma. Geriatrics, *18*:745–753, 1963.

178. Sheon, R.P., et al.: Malignancy in rheumatic disease: Interrelationships. J. Am. Geriatr. Soc., *25*:20–27, 1977.

179. Strandberg, B.: Rheumatoid arthritis and cancer arthritis. Scand. J. Rheumatol. [Suppl.] 5:1–14, 1974.

180. Litwin, S.D., Allen, J.C., and Kunkel, H.G.: Disappearance of the clinical and serological manifestations of rheumatoid arthritis following a thoracotomy for a lung tumor. Arthritis Rheum., 9:865, 1966.

181. Bradley, J.D., and Pinals, R.S.: Carcinoma polyarthritis: Role of immune complexes in pathogenesis. J. Rheumatol., 10:826, 1983.

182. Cayla, J., Rondier, J., Leger, J.M., and Giraudon, C.: Esophageal carcinoma revealed by acute polyarthritis. (Fr.) Rev. Rhum. Mal. Osteoartic., 48:595, 1981.

183. Burki, F., and Treves, R.: Polyarthritis and esophageal carcinoma. (Fr.) Rev. Rhum. Mal. Osteoartic., 53:547, 1986.

184. Chaun, H., Robinson, C.E., Sutherland, W.H., and Dunn, W.L.: Polyarthritis associated with gastric carcinoma. Can. Med. Assoc. J., 131:909, 1984.

185. Simon, R.D., and Ford, L.E.: Rheumatoid-like arthritis associated with colonic carcinoma. Arch. Intern. Med., 140:698–700, 1980.

186. Chan, M.K., Hendrickson, C.S., and Taylor, K.E.: Polyarthritis associated with breast carcinoma. West. J. Med., 137:132, 1982.

187. Kahn, M.F., et al.: Systemic lupus erythematosus and ovarian dysgerminoma: Remission of the systemic lupus erythematosus after extirpation of the tumor. Clin. Exp. Immunol., 1:355–359, 1966.

188. Bennett, R.M., Ginsberg, M.H., and Thomsen, S.: Carcinomatous polyarthritis: The presenting symptom of an ovarian tumor and association with a platelet activating factor. Arthritis Rheum., 19:953–958, 1976.

189. Ultman, J.E.: Hyperuricemia in disseminated neoplastic disease other than lymphomas and leukemias. Cancer, 15:122–129, 1962.

190. Ramsdell, C.M., and Kelley, W.N.: The clinical significance of hypouricemia. Ann. Intern. Med., 78:239–242, 1973.

191. Plonk, J.W., and Feldman, J.M.: Carcinoid arthropathy. Arch. Intern. Med., 134:651–654, 1974.

192. Crisp, A.J.: Carcinoid arthropathy. Br. J. Radiol., 56:782, 1983.

193. Bergin, C., et al.: Lymphomatoid granulomatosis presenting as polyarthritis. J. Rheumatol., 11:537, 1984.

194. Nunnink, J.C., Krusinski, P.A., and Yates, J.W.: Multicentric reticulohistiocytosis and cancer: A case report and review of the literature. Med. Pediatr. Oncol., 13:273, 1985.

195. Medsger, T.A., Jr., Dixon, J.A., and Garwood, V.F.: Palmar fasciitis and polyarthritis associated with ovarian carcinoma. Ann. Intern. Med., 96:424–431, 1982.

196. Pfinsgraff, J., et al.: Palmar fasciitis and arthritis with malignant neoplasms: A paraneoplastic syndrome. Semin. Arthritis Rheum., 16:118, 1986.

PAINFUL SHOULDER AND THE REFLEX SYMPATHETIC DYSTROPHY SYNDROME

97

FRANKLIN KOZIN

Evolutionary development of the prehensile upper extremity and upright posture in man was accompanied by structural changes in the shoulder girdle and its musculature. Unlike the weight-bearing lower extremity, which remained firmly fixed to the axial skeleton, the upper extremity became loosely joined to the trunk at the small sternoclavicular joint. The result was a tremendous increase in mobility providing a wide range of efficient hand function. This freedom of motion was achieved only by sacrificing stability.

EVOLUTIONARY CHANGES

The origins of the upper limb and shoulder girdle can be traced to the lateral fin folds of early fish.[1,2,3] The first true pectoral girdle is found in later fish, however, in which it is attached to the skull and buttresses the bilateral pectoral fins and their cartilaginous radials (limb forerunners). As these structures were adapted for weight bearing and terrestrial locomotion in amphibians and reptiles, the shoulder girdle separated from the skull and migrated to a more caudal position to provide increased support. Failure of scapular separation and descent in human ontogeny is reflected in congenital anomalies such as Sprengel's deformity.

Acquisition of prehensile function in mammals and upright posture in primates evoked new changes in the shoulder. The greatest change occurred in the structure and position of the scapula. The scapular

spine appeared, creating the infraspinous and supraspinous segments, and gradually the infraspinous segment elongated. The distal end of the scapular spine, the acromion, enlarged in size and mass to accommodate a growing deltoid muscle. With these changes, the scapula migrated from its lateral position on the chest wall to a posterior position and, at the same time, rotated, maintaining the anterior and lateral planes of arm movement. A new bone, the clavicle, developed and assumed its present position in the shoulder girdle, where it functions primarily as a buttress to prevent medial and forward displacement of the scapula and arm. The humerus elongated and twisted along its shaft, bringing the hand into a more functional position relative to the arm and trunk.

Parallel modifications evolved in the shoulder musculature. The scapulohumeral muscles, including the supraspinatus, infraspinatus, teres major and minor, subscapularis, and deltoid, which subserve arm rotation and elevation, underwent the most pronounced changes. The deltoid muscle doubled in relative mass and its insertion on the humerus migrated distally. These factors increased its leverage and established the deltoid muscle as a prime abductor and extendor of the arm. The lower fibers of the deltoid gave rise to a new muscle not found in lower animals, the teres minor. It and the other short rotator muscles formed the musculotendinous (rotator) cuff of the shoulder, so important in stabilizing the joint. Less-pronounced changes occurred in the axioscapular (trapezius, rhomboids, levator scapulae) and axiohumeral (pectoralis major and minor, latissimus

1509

dorsi) muscles, which help to suspend the arm and to fix the scapula during movement.

FUNCTIONAL ANATOMY

Normal shoulder motion is the result of complex, integrated movement in four separate joints: the glenohumeral, acromioclavicular, sternoclavicular, and scapulothoracic joints. This last structure, although not a true joint anatomically, is concerned with scapular motion around the thoracic wall. The three diarthrodial joints allow movement of the shoulder girdle as a whole and a wide range of glenohumeral motion. Although these joints are considered individually, all four joints normally move simultaneously and synchronously to produce smooth, uninterrupted shoulder motion or "scapulothoracic rhythm."

The sternoclavicular joint unites the shoulder girdle to the trunk and is formed by the first rib, the clavicle, and the manubrium sterni. A fibrocartilaginous disc is interposed between the bones to provide stability and to ensure a smooth articulation. A thick, fibrous capsule and several surrounding ligaments strengthen this important joint. The acromioclavicular joint also has an intra-articular fibrocartilaginous disc, but unlike that of the sternoclavicular joint, it is inconstant and often rudimentary and may predispose the joint to degenerative arthritis.[1] Adjacent to this joint is the coracoacromial arch (Fig. 97–1), which consists of the acromium and coracoacromial ligaments and protects the humeral head and rotator cuff superiorly. The sternoclavicular and acromioclavicular joints allow the clavicle to rotate along its long axis and permit elevation or depression (as in shrugging the shoulders) and extension or flexion (as in forward or backward thrusting of the shoulders) of the entire shoulder girdle (Fig. 97–2).[1-4] These movements are essential to full elevation of the arm in abduction or extension.

The glenohumeral joint is formed by the articulation of the humerus and scapula at the shallow glenoid fossa, which is deepened by an encircling rim of fibrocartilage, the labrum glenoidale or glenoid lip. The articular capsule is loose and redundant inferiorly (Fig. 97–3); its surface area is twice that of the humeral head.[1,5] Anteriorly, it is usually thickened into two or three glenohumeral ligaments that support the humerus at its least stable point.[6] The coracohumeral ligament and the long bicipital tendon, which passes through the capsule and functions as an accessory ligament,[2] further support the joint. Despite this organization, most of the dynamic stability of the joint is derived from the surrounding short rotator muscles of the humerus, the supraspinatus superiorly, the infraspinatus and teres minor posteriorly, and the subscapularis anteriorly. The relative position of these muscles may change with glenohumeral motion,[7] although no stabilizing structures are present inferiorly. The short rotator muscle tendons insert radially on the proximal humerus (Fig. 97–4); they are joined by loose connective tissue to form a layer, the rotator cuff, that is closely applied to the underlying capsule. Overlying the rotator cuff, and separated from it by the subacromial bursa, is a second layer of muscle composed of the deltoid and teres major (Fig. 97–3).

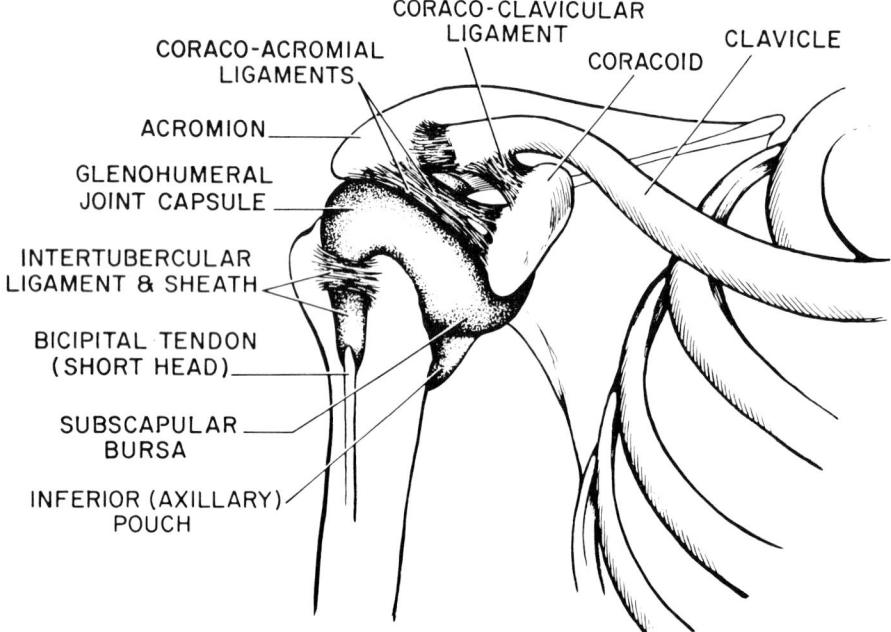

CORACO-ACROMIAL LIGAMENTS
CORACO-CLAVICULAR LIGAMENT
CORACOID
CLAVICLE
ACROMION
GLENOHUMERAL JOINT CAPSULE
INTERTUBERCULAR LIGAMENT & SHEATH
BICIPITAL TENDON (SHORT HEAD)
SUBSCAPULAR BURSA
INFERIOR (AXILLARY) POUCH

FIG. 97–1. The glenohumeral joint capsule and surrounding structures.

FIG. 97–2. *A* and *B*, Movements of the sternoclavicular and acromioclavicular joints.

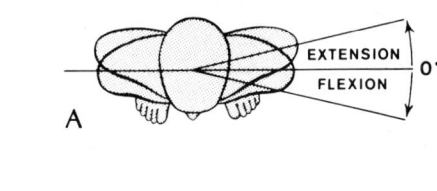

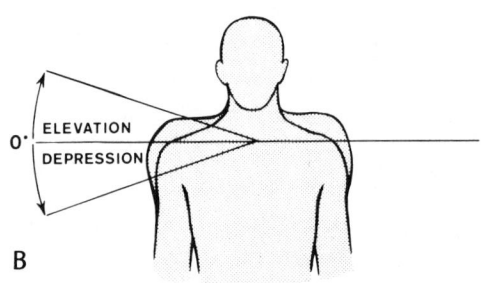

Thus, the joint capsule is supported and protected by two musculotendinous layers: the inner rotator cuff and the outer deltoid and teres minor.

Normal movement in the glenohumeral joint is accompanied by scapulothoracic motion. During the initial 30 to 60° of humeral elevation, that is, abduction or extension, scapular motion is variable and apparently unique to each individual.[3] Thereafter, depending on the precise plane in which it is studied, the ratio of glenohumeral to scapulothoracic movement is constant and ranges from 1.25 to 2.00; in other words, for every degree of glenohumeral motion there is 0.5 to 0.8° of scapulothoracic motion.[3,8] It is possible to fix or to immobilize the scapula and still elevate the arm 90° actively or 120° passively, when further movement is blocked by the acromion. This movement results in a significant loss of power, however, and is not physiologically important.[3,9]

The chief muscles producing glenohumeral joint motion are the deltoid, pectoralis major and minor, teres major, latissimus dorsi, and those in the rotator cuff.[10] Abduction is accomplished by the rotator cuff muscles acting with the deltoid and, occasionally, the long head of the biceps. The down-and-in action of the rotator muscles and the up-and-down action of the deltoid muscle produce a "force couple," in which the off-setting vertical forces stabilize the humeral head within the glenoid while the lateral forces cause abduction.[3,6,9] During abduction, maximum forces on the glenohumeral joint are attained at 90° of elevation.[11] The chief adductors are the pectoralis major and latissimus dorsi, with assistance from the deltoid. Internal and external rotation are produced by the short rotator (cuff) muscles and the latissimus dorsi and deltoid muscles, respectively. Flexion is due primarily to the action of the pectoralis major and deltoid muscles, although both heads of the biceps muscle also are active, and extension is produced by the deltoid, pectoralis major, and latissimus dorsi muscles.

Many of our daily activities require the arm to be used in forward flexion and elevation, especially in the scapular plane.[12] These movements are produced by the concerted function of the supraspinatus, infraspinatus, and deltoid muscles. When these muscles are paralyzed by loss of suprascapular and axillary nerve function, the shoulder is essentially immobile.[13] The supraspinatus and deltoid contribute equally to the force of these movements.[12]

PHYSICAL EXAMINATION OF THE PATIENT

A detailed medical history and physical examination are essential in all patients with shoulder com-

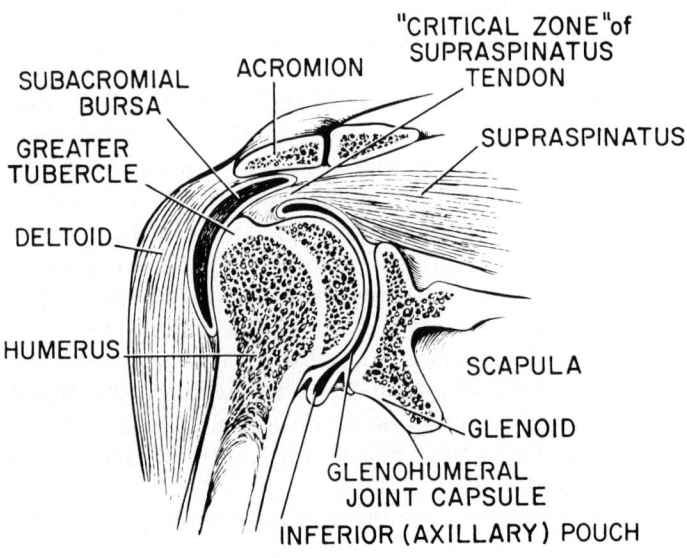

FIG. 97–3. Coronal section of the shoulder, illustrating the relationships of the glenohumeral joint, the joint capsule, the subacromial bursa, and the rotator cuff (supraspinatus tendon).

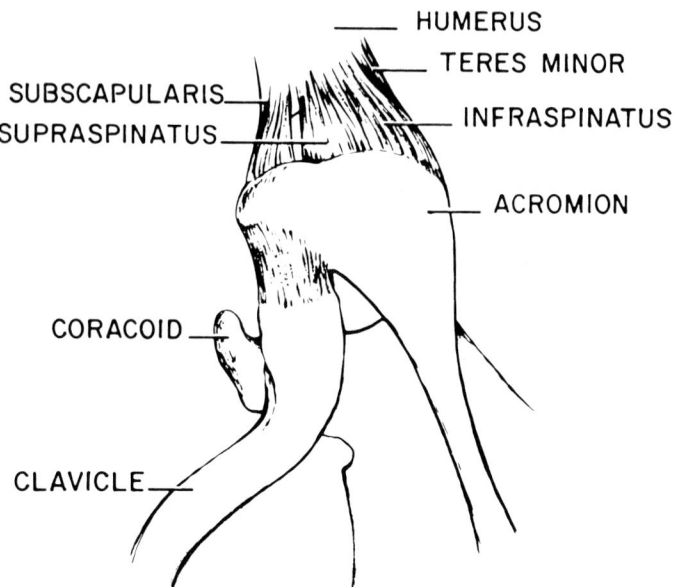

SUBSCAPULARIS

SUPRASPINATUS

CORACOID

CLAVICLE

HUMERUS

TERES MINOR

INFRASPINATUS

ACROMION

FIG. 97–4. The musculotendinous (rotator) cuff viewed from above.

plaints to determine whether these symptoms arise from local injury, from systemic disease, or from pain referred from another location.[1,14,15] Particular attention should be given to a patient's occupation or avocation; the presence of chronic illness, particularly diabetes mellitus (see below); and general mental attitude. Impairment of shoulder motion can lead to significant disability,[16] especially in the elderly.

The shoulder is examined with the patient standing or sitting and undressed to the waist, to permit a thorough inspection and comparison of both sides. Joint swelling, abnormality of bony structure, such as inequality or malposition, or muscle fasciculation or atrophy may be apparent. Atrophy of the infraspinatus or supraspinatus muscles, detected as diminished fullness of the respective scapular fossae, usually indicates chronically painful shoulders or acute, severe rupture of the rotator cuff. Arthritis involving the synovial joints of the shoulder may produce soft tissue or bony swelling or effusions; in the glenohumeral joint, an effusion may be detected by swelling along the bicipital tendon as it traverses the bicipital groove. Fullness or fluctuance beneath the deltoid muscle suggests subacromial (subdeltoid) bursitis. The patient's posture should be noted.

Shoulder motion is evaluated next. The normal shoulder is capable of a wide range of movement including abduction and adduction (raising or lowering the arm in the coronal plane), flexion and extension (backward or forward movement of the arm in the sagittal plane), internal and external rotation, circumduction, and other remarkable combinations of these motions (Fig. 97–5). Movements of the shoulder girdle as a unit include elevation and depression, as in shrugging, or extension and flexion, as in protrusion (Fig. 97–2). Active range of motion may be determined quickly and accurately by asking the patient to perform the following movements, keeping in mind that minor variations of the "normal range" exist, depending on the age and sex of the patient: (1) raise both arms to the side until the hands touch overhead, return them to the side, and cross them in front (abduction and adduction); (2) extend both arms forward until the hands touch overhead and extend them behind the back (flexion and extension); (3) place both hands behind the neck (external rotation) and behind the back, as high as possible (internal rotation) (Fig. 97–6); and (4) shrug and protrude the shoulders (sternoclavicular and acromioclavicular joints). Careful observation during these movements is essential because patients with shoulder pain often learn to achieve full abduction or extension by hunching the shoulder to reverse the normal scapulohumeral rhythm.

Assessment of passive shoulder motion may provide additional diagnostic clues when active movements are limited. As with active motion, particular attention is given to abduction and rotation because these movements are frequently the best indicators of early glenohumeral disease. Passive abduction is measured by fixing the scapula with one hand while the other supports the arm at the partially flexed elbow and abducts it; normally, 90 to 120° of abduction is possible. To measure passive rotation, the arm is abducted with the elbow flexed to 90° and is slowly rotated (Fig. 97–5B); a 180° arc can usually be achieved.

Patients who complain of pain during arm eleva-

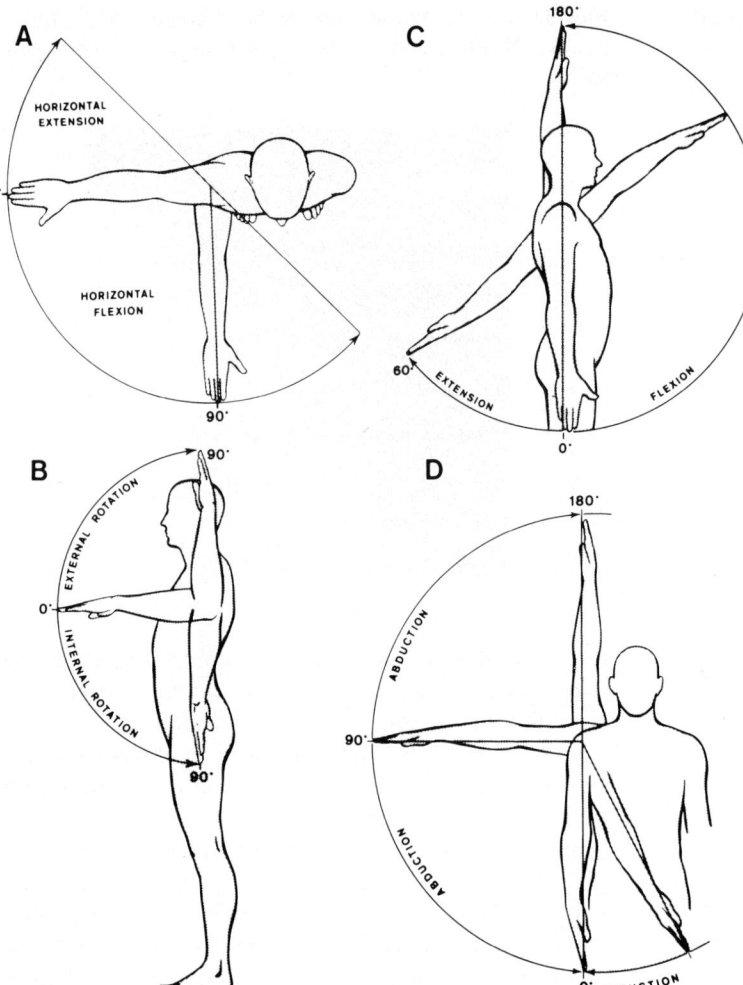

FIG. 97–5. Movements of the shoulder. *A*, "Horizontal" flexion and extension. *B*, Internal and external rotation. *C*, "Vertical" flexion and extension. *D*, Abduction and adduction.

tion, usually from 60 to 120° of abduction or extension (a "painful arc"), should be assessed with several specific maneuvers. The *impingement sign* is elicited by immobilizing the scapula while forcibly elevating the arm. Subjects with the impingement syndrome experience pain when the greater tuberosity impinges against the coracoacromial arch;[17] on occasion, concomitant popping or "clunking" can be palpated or heard. Injection of 3 to 10 ml 1% xylocaine beneath the acromium may produce relief during this maneuver, thereby conferring some specificity to this test.[17] The *supraspinatus test* is performed by placing the arm in 90° of abduction and internal rotation and by angling the arm 30° forward to isolate the supraspinatus muscle. Muscle strength is tested against resistance to indicate weakness or pain in the supraspinatus. A *subluxability test* also may be useful, especially in elderly individuals with poorly localized pain. Patients are asked to lie supine with the shoulder over the edge of the examination table; the shoulder is then tested for ease of subluxation.[18] During this test, the glenoid lip should be palpated to disclose tenderness, which may be the only physical finding in tears of this structure.

Assessment of resisted movements in the arm may help isolate the painful structure(s). Thus, pain on resisted abduction suggests supraspinatus tendinitis; pain on resisted external rotation, infraspinatus tendinitis; pain on resisted internal rotation, subscapularis tendinitis. This approach may be helpful in diagnosis of difficult shoulder problems, especially when pain is not reproduced by simple active range of motion.

Finally, the shoulder must be palpated to determine the exact site of tenderness and to identify areas of increased heat, swelling, fluctuation, muscle spasm or atrophy, or, on occasion, frank tears within the rotator cuff. Although shoulder pain may be deep and widely radiating, the patient often suggests the diagnosis by identifying a specifically painful point.

RADIOLOGIC EXAMINATION

Certain studies that should be considered in many patients with shoulder pain are discussed in this section.

FIG. 97–6. Internal and external rotation of the shoulder (active).

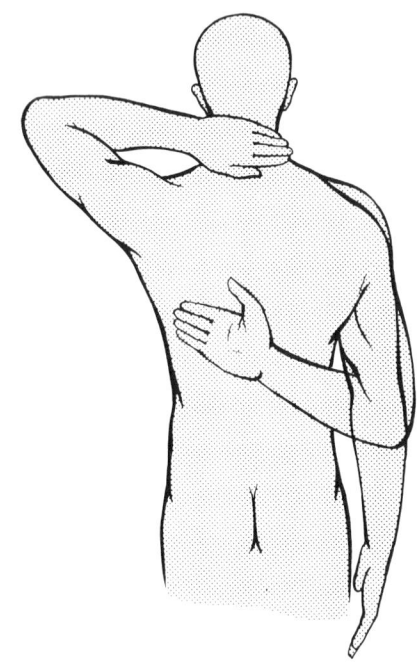

FIG. 97–7. Plain radiograph of the shoulder, illustrating humeral cysts and sclerosis, particularly about the greater tuberosity.

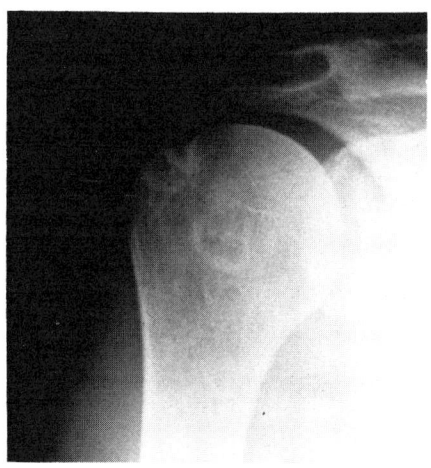

PLAIN RADIOGRAPHY

Proper positioning is essential in visualizing specific structures such as the glenohumeral, sternoclavicular, and acromioclavicular joints, the scapula and clavicle, the humeral head or greater tuberosity, and the bicipital groove. Arthritic changes, fractures and dislocation, and soft-tissue calcification may be identified and localized more readily when the appropriate projection is used. Although of little direct benefit in the diagnosis of soft-tissue lesions such as tendinitis, bursitis, or rotator cuff tears, plain radiography may show degenerative changes in the tuberosities or the humeral head and avulsion fractures at tendon insertions, which frequently accompany these conditions (Fig. 97–7). Soft-tissue xeroradiography may be of considerable value in the recognition of soft-tissue lesions and localized areas of tendon calcification.[19,20]

ARTHROGRAPHY

Contrast studies of the glenohumeral joint are helpful in diagnosing adhesive capsulitis, bicipital tenosynovitis or tendon rupture, rotator cuff tears, and shoulder dislocations.[21-24] The normal arthrogram demonstrates the bicipital sheath, the redundant inferior joint capsule, and the subscapular bursa (Fig. 97–8A). The cartilage of the glenoid lip appears as a negative shadow. Because no communication normally exists between the joint cavity and the subacromial bursa, the bursa is not visible.

Complete rotator cuff tears (full-thickness tears) are seen readily as extravasation of contrast material into the subacromial bursa or, occasionally, soft tissues (Fig. 97–8B). Incomplete tears (partial-thickness tears) are more difficult to recognize, although they may be suggested by irregularities or small clefts in the rotator cuff. Bicipital tendon tenosynovitis or rupture may produce irregularity in the bicipital sheath or leakage of the contrast material into the soft tissues of the upper arm. Shoulder dislocations and subluxations that tear the capsule away from the glenoid lip may be demonstrated by excessive capsule laxity (ballooning) or by leakage of dye.

The arthrogram in adhesive capsulitis is characteristic. Joint volume is reduced, and the normal anterior and inferior pouches are obliterated. As a result, *the volume of contrast material that can be injected is reduced from the usual 15 to 35 ml to only 5 to 10 ml.*

Double-contrast arthrography, in which a small amount of radiopaque contrast material and a larger amount of air are instilled into the glenohumeral joint, improves the resolution of the rotator cuff structures and the articular cartilage,[22] and it may cause less joint irritation than other methods.[25] Although it appears to be extremely sensitive,[26] this technique is more difficult to perform and to interpret than the conventional method.[27] When this technique is combined with tomography (arthrotomography), it is possible to visualize abnormalities of the glenoid lip effectively and to diagnose avulsion or tears of the cartilaginous rim.[28,29]

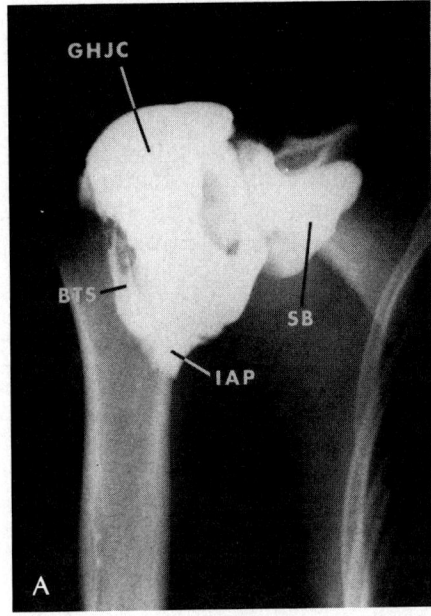
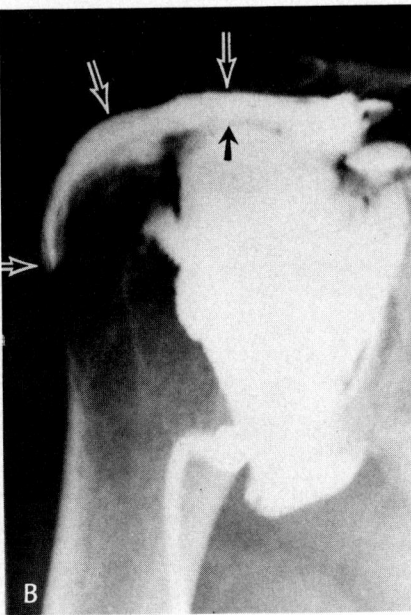

FIG. 97–8. *A,* Arthrogram of the normal shoulder, showing the glenohumeral joint capsule (GHJC), the subscapular bursa (SB), the inferior axillary pouch (IAP), and the bicipital tendon sheath (BTS). *B,* Arthrogram of the shoulder in a patient with a complete rotator cuff rupture, demonstrating contrast in the subacromial bursa (arrows).

Subacromial bursography is used with increasing frequency, particularly for diagnosis of adhesive subacromial bursitis, in which the bursal volume is reduced from 4 to 6 ml to 1 to 2 ml,[30] and in the shoulder impingement syndrome discussed later in this chapter.[24,30]

SCINTIGRAPHY

Inflamed joints can be readily detected by scintigraphy,[31,32] and it may be useful in mildly or even noninflammatory articular disease.[31,33] Studies in adhesive capsulitis[34] and polymyalgia rheumatica[33] show abnormal shoulder uptake, but such findings must be interpreted cautiously because increased local radioactivity is common in patients without symptoms or radiographic abnormalities relating to the shoulder,[35,36] or in patients with injury of the rotator cuff.[37]

ULTRASONOGRAPHY

Ultrasonography appears to be a sensitive and specific means of evaluating the rotator cuff, demonstrating excellent correlation with arthrography and surgical findings.[38–40] It can be effective for visualizing changes in the bicipital tendon.[40]

COMPUTED TOMOGRAPHY (CT)

CT is useful for evaluating the unstable shoulder. This technique may be preferable to arthrography or arthrotomography.[41,42] CT may be useful for assessing rotator cuff integrity.[43]

MAGNETIC RESONANCE IMAGING (MRI)

Although MRI has not been critically evaluated for shoulder imaging, early reports indicate that it provides superb anatomic detail of the shoulder and rotator cuff.[44–46] Improved techniques will be necessary before MRI can be used for general assessment of the shoulder.[47]

PAINFUL SHOULDER

Shoulder pain is among the most common complaints in medical practice. Such pain may be caused by local problems within the shoulder region or by remote disorders, especially heart, lung, and cervical spinal disease, or systemic conditions. A variety of classifications have been devised to aid in differential diagnosis; it seems most useful to divide shoulder pain into two broad etiologic categories: intrinsic (local) and extrinsic (remote and systemic) disorders (Table 97–1). Intrinsic conditions, which account for most shoulder complaints, are emphasized here. Extrinsic disorders may account for up to 20% of shoulder pain.[48]

IMPINGEMENT SYNDROME

The coracoacromial arch (Fig. 97–1) protects the humeral head and the rotator cuff from direct trauma.

Table 97–1.   Differential Diagnosis of the Painful Shoulder

Intrinsic Disorders
　Impingement Syndrome
　Specific Lesions of the Rotator Cuff
　　Degenerative tendinitis
　　Calcific tendinitis
　　Subacromial bursitis
　　Rotator cuff rupture
　Lesions of the Bicipital Tendon
　Adhesive Capsulitis ("Frozen Shoulder")
　Fibrositis and Fibromyalgia
　Arthritis
　　Degenerative
　　"Milwaukee shoulder"
　　Neurotrophic
　Traumatic and Athletic Injuries
　　Subluxation or dislocation
　Neurologic
　　Peripheral neuropathy
　　Brachial plexus injury
　Postural Effects
　Infection
　Neoplasia, Benign and Malignant

Extrinsic Disorders
　Inflammatory Conditions
　　Rheumatoid arthritis
　　Spondyloarthritides
　　Myopathies
　　Polymyalgia rheumatica
　Avascular Necrosis
　Metabolic and Endocrine
　　Gout and pseudogout
　　Diabetes mellitus
　　Hyperparathyroidism
　　Other
　Neurologic
　　Cervical nerve root compression (C4, C5, C6)
　　Lesions of the spinal cord
　　"Viscerosomatic" and referred pain
　　Peripheral neuropathy
　Neurovascular
　　Thoracic outlet syndrome
　　Axillary arterial and venous thrombosis
　Reflex Sympathetic Dystrophy Syndrome(s)

The arch is rigid and may limit full arm elevation. The impingement syndrome occurs when the supraspinatus tendon and the subacromial bursa are caught between the humerus and the overlying coracoacromial arch.[17,49] Repeated impingement may result in attrition of rotator cuff tendons or frank rotator cuff tears. A number of sports appear to increase the incidence of impingement.[50]

Subjects with the impingement syndrome often complain of a painful arc in the range of 60 to 120° of arm elevation. The impingement sign, described previously in this chapter, is a specific test for diagnosis.[17] Radiographs often show bony spurs on the undersurface of the acromion,[46] although the frequency of this finding varies considerably.[51,52] Subacromial bur-

sography demonstrates reduced volume and abnormal configuration of the bursa.[53]

Neer proposes three stages of impingement.[49] *Stage 1* typically is seen in subjects younger than 25 years who are active athletically or frequently use their arm overhead. The subacromial bursa demonstrates edema and hemorrhage. *Stage 2* affects individuals ages 25 to 40 and presumably results from repeated or subacute impingement. Thickening and fibrosis are present in the bursa and rotator cuff. In *Stage 3*, subjects are older, usually over 40 years, and have chronic impingement. Degenerative changes or frank tears in the rotator cuff may be present. Calcific deposits are often observed in the rotator cuff tendons or bursa.[52]

Conservative therapy is sufficient to control symptoms and limit progression in earlier or milder cases.[17,52] Surgical intervention with acromioplasty or bursectomy may be necessary in later or more severe cases.[49,54,55] Significant reduction in pain was found in athletic individuals who required surgery; however, only 40% of subjects were able to return to their preinjury level of function.[56]

DEGENERATIVE TENDINITIS ("SUPRASPINATUS SYNDROME")

Origin and Pathogenesis

Degenerative changes in the rotator cuff tendons appear to represent the normal aging process.[15] Twenty-five percent of unselected subjects have attritional changes in the rotator cuff by their fifth decade, and the incidence increases progressively thereafter.[15] The supraspinatus tendon is affected most frequently, especially in the so-called critical zone of Codman, a site approximately 1 to 2 cm medial to the tendon's insertion at the greater tuberosity. Several factors may combine to explain the increased susceptibility of this region:[57,58] (1) it is a relatively avascular zone where the osseous and tendinous blood supplies anastomose; (2) the few blood vessels in this area are compressed when the arm is hanging down normally;[57] and (3) repeated impingement of this area may occur between the acromion and the humeral head during abduction. In contrast, the vascular supply of the other flat tendons of the rotator cuff is greater, nonanastomotic, and unimpeded by arm motion.[57] These observations also may explain the high frequency of degenerative tendinitis in subjects with repeated occupational stresses to the shoulder, such as carpenters, painters,[15] and welders,[59] or with a compromised neurologic or vascular supply, such as alcoholics and diabetics.[15,60,61] Experimentally, it is difficult to tear a normal tendon, but it is easy to tear an ischemic tendon.

Clinical Features

The patient with degenerative tendinitis is most likely to be a man in his fifth decade or older, to work as a laborer, and to localize his complaints to the dominant side. The condition is generally asymptomatic until provoked by minor trauma or exertion; however, careful questioning often elicits a history of recurrent shoulder problems.

The patient complains of a dull ache in the shoulder that is not easily localized. It may be more severe at night and may interfere with sleep. On examination, active shoulder movements are restricted, especially abduction. A painful arc from 70 to 100° of abduction is characteristic, probably reflecting supraspinatus involvement because at this range supraspinatus activity is maximal and the greatest force is applied across the glenohumeral joint.[3,8,10,11] Many patients learn to avoid this painful arc by reversing the scapulohumeral rhythm, that is, by hunching their shoulder to position the scapula before initiating glenohumeral motion. Often, passive movements are normal because force across the joint is minimal when the arm is supported. Weakness is uncommon unless the pain is chronic, the pain is of more than 3 weeks' duration, or an associated rotator cuff tear is present. In patients with severe pain, it may be necessary to inject an anesthetic agent into the rotator cuff before attempting to assess strength.[62] Palpation is helpful in identifying the source of pain. Tenderness over the bicipital groove suggests bicipital tendinitis. Subscapularis tendinitis may be detected by tenderness at its insertion on the lesser tuberosity. Similarly, tenderness localized to the superior or inferolateral aspects of the greater tuberosity suggests supraspinatus tendinitis or injuries of the infraspinatus or teres minor tendons, respectively. Location of the area of maximal tenderness is important in guiding therapy.[63]

Radiologic Examination

A radiograph of a shoulder with an early tendon lesion generally is normal. In patients with chronic disease, degenerative changes such as bony fragments, pseudocysts, sclerosis, and osteophytes may develop in the greater tuberosity and the humeral head (Fig. 97–7).[1,15] Unless the disorder has progressed to a frank rotator cuff tear, the arthrogram is usually normal, although small irregularities on the undersurface of the tendon may be noted.

The treatment of this disorder is discussed later in this chapter, under "Bursitis."

CALCIFIC TENDINITIS

Origin and Pathogenesis

Many have assumed that tendon calcification occurs as a consequence of degenerative tendinitis.[1,15,64] Yet considerable evidence from studies in experimental animals,[65,66] as well as from observations of patients with uremia,[67] hypervitaminosis D,[68] and multiple sites of "calcific periarthritis,"[69,70] suggests that calcium deposits in tendon may occur in the apparent absence of local degeneration.

Most studies of the pathogenesis of this condition have focused on local factors that predispose tendons to calcification. Although the precise mechanism still remains uncertain, a number of hypotheses have evolved.[71-76] Altered tendon physiologic features, possibly produced by changes in blood flow, minor trauma, or mild inflammation, may promote a direct interaction between tendon matrix and calcium ion.[71,72] Phospholipids and various proteins have been implicated in the process of calcification in bone,[77-80] and they may subserve this function in tendon as well. The resultant calcium complex then may react with phosphorus, to produce a series of intermediate salts until hydroxyapatite is formed.[74] This crystalline substance has been identified in shoulder tendons,[1,81] just as in other forms of calcific periarthritis.[69] Four histologic phases have been described in "primary" calcific tendinitis that occurs typically in the aforementioned critical zone.[82,83] These phases are: (1) "precalcific," in which metaplastic fibrocartilage is observed within the tendon; (2) "calcific," in which deposits of calcium are found within a fibrocartilaginous nodule in a close relationship with matrix vesicles, without reactive changes; (3) "resorptive," in which reactive changes consist of phagocytic cells and increased vascularity; and (4) "repair," which is characterized by the appearance of abundant mesenchymal cells within the tendon. The natural history of primary calcific deposits is spontaneous resorption. The majority of patients in a recent study had no reactive or reparative changes associated with tendon calcification.[83] "Secondary" calcification occurs at the torn edges of the rotator cuff or in a degenerated tendon insertion into the greater trochanter, that is, an enthesopathy distal to the critical zone. Such calcific deposits do not resorb spontaneously and elicit little repair reaction.

Once deposited, the calcified material exists in two states, or possibly phases, that seem to correlate with the clinical stage of the condition. In the chronic stage, the deposits are usually hard and dry (inspissated), with a gritty consistency; in the acute stage, the material is creamy white and paste-like (hydrated).[15,83]

Clinical Features

The prevalence of calcific tendinitis is high, occurring in 2.7 to 8.0% of the general population.[84] The highest incidence appears to be in the fifth decade, and the association with various chronic diseases, particularly diabetes mellitus, is strong.[15,60] Unlike degenerative tendinitis, this condition is seen in both sexes equally and often affects subjects in sedentary occupations.[1,15,84] Like degenerative tendinitis, the supraspinatus tendon is most commonly involved (approximately 50% of cases), followed by the infraspinatus, teres minor, and subscapularis tendons and the subacromial bursa. Multiple sites of calcification and bilateral involvement are also common.[1,70,84]

Three clinical states are recognized and resemble those of the other crystal-induced arthritides (see Chapters 91, 94, 95).[1,15,85] The first, asymptomatic stage is found incidentally on radiographs usually obtained for other reasons.[84] Little or no inflammatory reaction is present, possibly because the calcium deposit is small and located in the avascular critical zone.[1] Radiologically, the borders of the deposit are smooth. The calcium may be resorbed spontaneously, often correlating with symptoms of pain and inflammation. The borders of the calcific deposit appear scalloped. Other symptoms develop later. These stages might be likened to acute or "tophaceous" gout, both clinically and pathologically, because a granulomatous reaction with chronic inflammation and giant cells is present as part of the resorptive process.[15,82] Chronic symptoms and physical signs are indistinguishable from those of degenerative tendinitis, previously described, and the course of the disorder is characterized by exacerbations and remissions. The acute stage resembles the acute gouty or pseudogouty attack: pain is sudden and severe, often following minimal trauma or effort. This diffuse pain may radiate into the subdeltoid (bursa) area; a few patients develop features of a reflex sympathetic dystrophy in the ipsilateral hand.[1,15] Because the rotator cuff muscles are in spasm, the arm is held rigidly in a neutral or an adducted position. Even the slightest movement evokes a painful outcry. Complete examination of the patient is virtually impossible, although gentle palpation may reveal a point of maximal tenderness. As in acute gout and pseudogout, colchicine therapy often has dramatic results. The relation of calcific tendinitis to a more advanced form of crystal-induced shoulder disease, Milwaukee shoulder, is uncertain.

Standard radiographs show the typical ovoid calcific deposit (Fig. 97–9A), although special views may be needed to identify the exact site of calcification.[86] Rupture into the subacromial bursa is noted in about 5% of cases (Fig. 97–9B).[84] When rupture occurs, the calcium salt is usually rapidly resorbed. Such rupture may leave a hole in the rotator cuff, designated as a tear.

The treatment of this disorder is discussed in the following section, "Bursitis."

BURSITIS

Origin and Pathogenesis

A number of bursae or thin-walled, usually closed sacs lined with synovial tissue strategically placed to minimize friction between moving parts are found in the shoulder region. The largest and most constant is the subacromial bursa, located between the rotator cuff inferiorly and the deltoid and teres major muscles superiorly (Fig. 97–3). Its lateral extension beneath the deltoid muscle is termed the subdeltoid bursa. Other bursae include the subscapular and supracoracoid and those found in relation to the insertion of various muscles, such as the trapezius, pectoralis major, teres major, and latissimus dorsi muscles. Except for the systemic arthritides, which may affect the bursae primarily, bursitis of the shoulder area is usually secondary to traumatic, degenerative, or calcific disease in the rotator cuff. The subacromial bursa is most commonly involved because of its large size and its anatomic position.

Clinical Features

Symptoms of subacromial bursitis or "deal-runner's shoulder" are similar to those of the primary disease. Pain and tenderness may extend distally to the superior third of the arm because of the subdeltoid extension of the bursa. Active and passive abduction are usually reduced, but active motion is disproportionately limited, probably because of the added force of the contracting abductor muscles on the bursa.

Depending on the primary disease, plain radiographs may demonstrate bony changes,[87,88] calcific deposits,[84] or actual enlargement of the bursa. An arthrogram may show a communication with the glenohumeral joint capsule when bursitis is caused by complete rupture of the rotator cuff.[23,62,89] Bursography may be useful in demonstrating the impingement syndrome, adhesive bursitis, or rotator cuff tears.[30]

Treatment

Treatment of degenerative or calcific tendinitis and subacromial bursitis is directed at pain relief, maintenance of maximal shoulder function, prevention of complications such as adhesive capsulitis or the reflex sympathetic dystrophy syndrome, early rehabilitation, and education of the patient in methods of

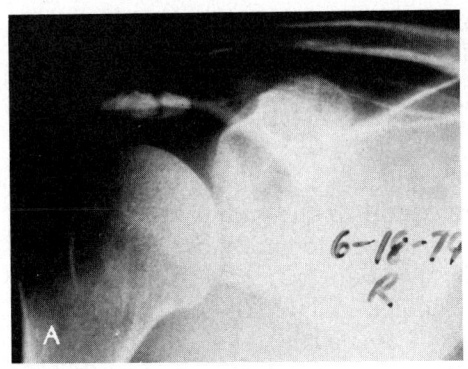 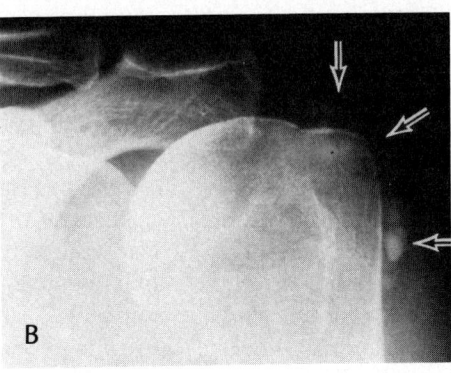

FIG. 97–9. Plain radiographs of the shoulder in a patient with calcification in the supraspinatus tendon, *A*, and in the subacromial bursa, *B*. Note the calcium extending into the subdeltoid area in *B* (arrows).

avoiding recurrent attacks.[1,15] The vast number of therapeutic programs that have been advocated attest to their lack of specificity and to the unavailability of a uniformly successful program.

A standard conservative program should be instituted first (Table 97–2). Rest of the acutely painful shoulder is essential. Immobilization of the arm in partial adduction with a sling may help. Salicylates or other nonsteroidal anti-inflammatory drugs (NSAIDs) in adequate doses are useful for their analgesic and anti-inflammatory properties,[90] although convincing evidence of their beneficial effect is lacking.[91,92] Concomitant administration of simple analgesics, such as acetaminophen or propoxyphene, or narcotic analgesics may be required. Muscle relaxants are of doubtful value. Any of a variety of local physical modalities that provide heat or cold to the affected area may assist in reducing pain. These modalities include moist hot-packs, such as hydrocollator packs, ultrasonography,[93,94] other such methods,[95] or simple ice packs.[93] These techniques may raise the local pain threshold,[93] promote local blood flow, enhance tissue

repair,[96,97] reduce muscle spasm, or simply exert a placebo effect.[98,99] Controlled studies suggest that some of these approaches have no effect.[100] Treatment with local radiotherapy, dimethyl sulfoxide (DMSO),[101] or acupuncture,[98] although recommended by some, does not appear to be any more effective than treatment with the other measures discussed and is not recommended.

Early mobilization of the painful extremity is important in minimizing disability and the risk of adhesive capsulitis or reflex dystrophy. Passive movements immediately after local heat or cold applications or 1 to 2 hours after analgesic drug administration may be instituted. These movements may be extended gradually, and active exercises may be started as symptoms subside. Often, the simple pendulum exercise of Codman, which uses the effect of gravity, is a good starting point. The trunk is flexed at the hips and lumbar spine, and the arm allowed to hang in approximately 90° of flexion; as the patient swings the body, the arm moves back and forth like a pendulum. This exercise is done first in the sagittal

Table 97–2. Conservative Treatment Program for Painful Shoulder*

1. Limited use of extremity during acute painful period
   Complete rest for hyperacute symptoms
   Arm in adduction sling; hand and forearm elevated
2. Anti-inflammatory and analgesic agents (and muscle relaxants)
   Salicylates and other NSAIDs
   Acetaminophen and propoxyphene derivatives
   Narcotic analgesics for severe pain only
   Muscle relaxants not recommended
3. Physical Therapy
   Heat or cold (cold for acute conditions; heat for subacute or chronic symptoms)
      Home: heating pad, hot packs, ice packs
      Physician's office or hospital: ultrasound, diathermy, hydrocollator packs
   Exercises
      Initially, as acute pain subsides: passive range of motion
      Later, when pain is mild to moderate: pendulum swinging (Codman), when possible; active exercises with
         resistance or assistance
4. Treatment of associated or underlying condition
5. Psychologic support in the form of reassurance and encouragement
6. Education for self-help and avoidance of provocative activities

*Objectives: Relief of pain and muscle spasm, maintenance and restoration of motion, and prevention of secondary changes.

plane (flexion-extension) and later in the coronal plane (abduction-adduction). Eventually, full, active range-of-motion exercises can be encouraged, with or without assistance or resistance.[102]

Failure of these basic measures to control symptoms and to restore movement requires a more aggressive approach. The usual first step is the local instillation of corticosteroids. One should mix 25 to 100 mg hydrocortisone acetate or equivalent amounts of the newer preparations with 5 to 10 ml 1% procaine and inject into the point(s) of maximal tenderness. Local corticosteroids are not without potentially serious side effects, however.[97,103–105] In addition to the possible complication of systemic adsorption and the risk of infection,[106] intratendinous or peritendinous corticosteroids may interfere with healing,[107] may reduce the tensile strength of unaffected tendon, and ultimately may cause tendon rupture.[108] A transient, 24- to 48-hour increase in symptoms may follow local injection.[109] Little critical evidence suggests that corticosteroid injections are more or even equally effective as the basic conservative measures.[110] Empirically, however, when conservative treatment fails to produce satisfactory results, corticosteroid injections may be useful. Systemic administration of corticosteroids or adrenocorticotrophic hormone (ACTH) has also been advocated, but it should be reserved for the most difficult therapeutic problems, in view of serious potential side effects. Operative intervention for degenerative tendinitis is rarely necessary.

In most cases, considerable improvement occurs within 2 to 6 weeks of therapy. Persistence of pain beyond this time should suggest a serious rotator cuff tear, and a thorough re-evaluation, including arthrographic study, is indicated. After improvement, the physician should make every effort to identify the source(s) of shoulder trauma, such as employment or avocational abuse, and to suggest appropriate modifications in these activities to prevent recurrence.

Calcific tendinitis or bursitis presents a special problem. Acute symptoms probably represent a form of crystal-induced synovitis, so local corticosteroids early in the disease appear justified,[81] especially if conservative therapy, including NSAIDs, proves ineffective within the initial 24 to 72 hours of symptoms. Spontaneous resolution occurs in at least 30 to 40% of such patients, however. In those with chronic symptoms or recurrent attacks, removal of the calcific deposit may be indicated, achieved by needling the affected area, with or without concomitant instillation of corticosteroids and local anesthetics.[1,111] On occasion, surgical removal of the deposit is useful in providing relief,[83] but this procedure should be delayed

as long as possible because recovery with resorption of the deposits is the rule in most patients.[1,84]

RUPTURE OF THE ROTATOR CUFF

Origin and Pathogenesis

Because of its critical role in stabilizing the glenohumeral joint, the musculotendinous (rotator) cuff may be torn by a variety of forces applied to the joint.[1,15,112] In younger individuals, as considerable force is necessary, tears usually follow direct trauma, unexpected falls on an outstretched arm, or the extreme stress of modern athletics. Much less force is required in older individuals, possibly as a result of pre-existent degenerative tendinitis and decreased vascularity that weakens the tendon structure. In such patients, tears are usually idiopathic or follow minor falls or the lifting of a weight with the arm fully extended or abducted.

Lesions of the rotator cuff are divided into complete or partial tears. Complete tears involve the full thickness of the cuff and the overlying subacromial bursa. As in degenerative tendinitis, the supraspinatus tendon is affected most commonly. Partial tears produce incomplete rents in the cuff, usually on the undersurface of the tendon near its insertion, and communication with the subacromial bursa does not occur.

Both conditions are more common than generally believed; partial tears are found in as many as 30% of cadavers.[1,15] The condition frequently goes unrecognized because the clinical and radiographic features of other forms of rotator cuff disease are so similar.

Clinical Features

The classic history of a fall or direct shoulder trauma in a patient complaining of shoulder pain and limitation of motion generally suggests the diagnosis of rotator cuff tear. Often, however, a specific event is not apparent, even after careful questioning. Persistence of symptoms in the shoulder of a patient who was previously diagnosed as having tendinitis, bursitis, or "strain" for more than 6 to 8 weeks should suggest a rotator cuff tear, especially in an older patient.

Acute full-thickness rupture produces immediate pain and muscle spasm. Weakness of the arm may be marked within hours to days of the injury, and both pain and weakness may persist for many months. On examination, motion is limited by pain and muscle spasm; in mild cases, pain may be present during active abduction in an arc between 70 and 100°. Local infiltration of an anesthetic agent abolishes pain, but not weakness. Although this finding is not entirely specific, it is suggestive of a rotator cuff tear. Frequently, the *drop arm sign* is positive: the arm is passively abducted to 90°, but it falls to the side when no longer supported by the examiner.[15,113] The patient cannot usually hold the arm in abduction at 90°, or the arm collapses to the side with just a little push downward by the physician. Occasionally, the actual tear can be palpated directly by an experienced examiner.

Diagnosis of the small complete tear or partial tear is more difficult. Persons engaged in overhead work, such as paperhangers and painters, or in lifting with extended arms, such as nurses and waitresses, appear to be predisposed to those lesions, just as they are to degenerative tendinitis. Although shoulder pain or discomfort is often present, it may be minimal. Frequently, the only complaint or physical finding is weakness in elevation of the arm, an important clue to diagnosis.

The symptoms and signs of rotator cuff rupture are similar to those of older "degenerative diseases" of the rotator cuff, but persistent pain and, especially, weakness in arm elevation, often with early (2 to 4 weeks) muscle atrophy, suggest this diagnosis. Full-thickness tears can be present for years without any symptoms, especially in the elderly person who demands little from his body.

Radiologic Examination

The plain radiograph in rotator cuff ruptures in younger individuals is usually normal. That it is abnormal in as many as 60% of older individuals may reflect pre-existent degenerative tendinitis.[87,88] Changes consist of erosion, sclerosis, pseudocysts, and osteophytes about the greater tuberosity at the site of insertion of the supraspinatus tendon. These changes are indistinguishable from those of degenerative tendinitis (Fig. 97–7). Narrowing of the space between the humeral head and the acromion is a useful radiologic sign of superior subluxation of the humerus. This condition may be so extreme as to produce a "pseudoarticulation."

Complete ruptures of the rotator cuff may be confirmed by arthrography.[21,62,89] Leakage of contrast material into surrounding soft tissues or into the subacromial bursa is diagnostic of this condition (Fig. 97–8B). In partial ruptures, however, the arthrogram is normal, although, rarely, small irregularities or clefts are seen.[112] Partial rotator cuff tears or degenerative changes in the cuff are best visualized by double-contrast arthrography[22] or bursography.[30]

Treatment

Early surgical repair of the acute, complete rupture, before granulation tissue forms and the edges of the torn capsule retract or calcify, appears to provide the best long-term result.[1,15,88,113–115] Treatment of patients with chronically torn rotator cuffs remains an unresolved problem.[54,115] Conservative therapy, as outlined in Table 97–2, may be effective, especially when supplemented with local corticosteroid injection.[116] Sixty percent of patients so treated show significant improvement,[115] although this figure may depend on which factors are assessed.[110] Newer surgical approaches have produced satisfactory results with reduction in pain and improvement in function in the majority of patients.[54,117–120] Although the greater size of the tear,[103,121,122] longer duration of symptoms,[117] or greater severity of symptoms[120] has been reported to adversely affect outcome, agreement on these issues is lacking.[118] Only one third of professional athletes who require surgical repair of a torn rotator cuff return to professional competition.[119] It should be emphasized that complete pain relief or return to full function are uncommon after surgery.[120–122]

BICIPITAL SYNDROMES

Origin and Pathogenesis

The long head (tendon) of the biceps brachii extends from its origin on the supraglenoid tubercle and posterior rim of the glenoid lip, through the articular capsule and intertubercular (bicipital) groove, and inserts on the posterior portion of the radial tuberosity. Within the joint capsule, the tendon functions as an accessory ligament and prevents upward and outward displacement of the humeral head. The tendon remains ensheathed in synovial tissue as it leaves the articular capsule until it traverses the bicipital groove (Fig. 97–1). The biceps supinates the forearm and assists in abduction and flexion of the arm.

The following four conditions are included in the category of bicipital syndromes: (1) tendinitis and tenosynovitis, (2) elongation of the tendon, (3) rupture, and (4) dislocation and subluxation.[15] Bicipital tendinitis or tenosynovitis is usually produced by constant friction within the intertubercular groove that causes attrition and inflammation of the tendon and its sheath. When these attritional changes are severe, the tensile strength of the tendon is lost, and elongation occurs. This condition may progress to frank rupture following even minimal effort. Dislocation or subluxation of the bicipital tendon is usually related to a congenitally shallow intertubercular groove or to traumatic disruption of the intertubercular ligaments that hold the tendon in the groove (Fig. 97–1).

Clinical Features

Bicipital tendinitis produces pain in the anterior shoulder that may radiate along the biceps into the forearm. Limitation of abduction or internal rotation may be present. Occasionally, a history of repetitive arm movements can be elicited, but it is not generally possible to identify a specific cause. On examination, a number of signs are useful in differential diagnosis. Manual side-to-side displacement of the bicipital tendon ("twanging") or simple palpation of the tendon in the bicipital groove during arm rotation may be associated with marked tenderness, indicating bicipital tendinitis. Pain along the course of the tendon produced by resisted supination of the forearm (Yergason's supination sign) or by resisted flexion at the elbow also suggests bicipital tendinitis. When elongation has occurred, pain may be minimal, but bicipital weakness is prominent. Absence of a palpable tendon and loss of normal bicipital contraction during resisted supination confirm this diagnosis. This syndrome can be differentiated from frank rupture, which causes persistent swelling of the biceps in the upper arm; in acute rupture, extravasation of blood is noted in the upper arm. Dislocation and subluxation are recognized by palpation of the tendon as it snaps or slides in and out of the bicipital groove.

Radiologic Examination

Radiographic studies of the shoulder in this condition are usually normal. Special views of the bicipital groove may show irregularity or osteophytes of the tuberosities in tendinitis or a shallow groove in a case of subluxation of the tendon. Arthrograms are rarely abnormal, but they may demonstrate irregularity or blockage of contrast medium within the tendon sheath. Ultrasonography may be useful in assessing this condition,[40,123] although data are incomplete.

Treatment

The initial program consists of the measures outlined in Table 97–2. In resistant cases, local instillation of corticosteroids into the tendon sheath is indicated and often produces a good result. Operative intervention is rarely necessary, but in persistent cases it may prove beneficial.[124] When a lax, elongated tendon does not respond to conservative therapy, resection of the intra-articular portion of the tendon with fixation of the distal end may restore useful function.

Pain from a dislocating or subluxing tendon may also respond to a conservative program and exercises. Surgical treatment may be necessary, however, to fix the tendon within the groove or to the proximal humerus. In acute bicipital rupture in younger patients, early surgical repair is indicated. If several weeks have passed or if the patient is elderly, a conservative approach may be better.

ADHESIVE CAPSULITIS

This disorder is also known as frozen shoulder, scapulohumeral periarthritis, periarthritis of Duplay, periarthritis of the shoulder, and check-rein shoulder.

Origin and Pathogenesis

Adhesive capsulitis is a clinical entity apparently unique to the shoulder. It is characterized by pain and stiffness in the absence of any recognized intrinsic abnormality, although it may complicate any of the conditions previously discussed. In addition to following local soft-tissue injuries, adhesive capsulitis may result from such problems as other trauma, coronary artery disease, chronic lung disease, pulmonary tuberculosis, diabetes mellitus, and cervical spinal syndromes.[34,125,126a,126b] The common denominator appears to be prolonged immobility of the arm.[1,127] A third factor, the "periarthritic personality," has been suggested as a necessary component for the development of the full syndrome, but psychologic testing of a large group of patients has failed to confirm this hypothesis.[34] A possible immunologic basis for adhesive capsulitis and an association of this syndrome with HLA-B27 has not been confirmed.[128–131]

The pathologic findings have been described by several investigators.[1,23] The joint capsule is thickened and is loosely adherent to the underlying humeral head; the normal capsular folds are obliterated. Microscopic changes include proliferation of synovial lining cells, fibrosis, and a mild, chronic inflammatory cell infiltrate. Such findings are inconstant, and at least 20% of cases have a normal histologic appearance.[23] As in other immobilized joints,[132] biochemical studies of the joint capsule have shown diminished glycosaminoglycan and water content.[132,133]

Clinical Features

Adhesive capsulitis is more common in women than in men, occurs in the fifth decade or later, and bears no relation to occupation.[1,15,34] The associated clinical conditions have already been enumerated. Both shoulders may be affected simultaneously or successively in some patients.[1,134]

The patient characteristically complains of the insidious onset of a diffusely painful and stiff shoulder. A specific precipitating event is rarely identified. The patient is unable to sleep because of pain and, perhaps as a result, is often anxious and irritable; hence the "periarthritic personality." Objective findings include diffuse tenderness about the glenohumeral joint and restricted active and passive motion in all planes. Injection of anesthetic agent locally may reduce pain but fails to improve mobility.

Three phases of the disease have been described.[1,134] The first, characterized primarily by pain and by gradually increasing stiffness, usually last 2 to 9 months. In the second phase, pain is less severe, and the patient often describes a vague discomfort in the shoulder, but stiffness is marked ("frozen shoulder"). This phase persists from 4 to 12 months. The final phase, lasting an additional 5 to 26 months, is one of gradual recovery of function ("thawing") and resolution of pain. *The natural progression of a frozen shoulder is a thaw.* The majority of patients are often fully improved within 12 to 18 months of the onset of this disorder,[15,127,134] although symptoms may persist for many more months.[15,134]

Radiologic Examination

Except for localized osteopenia in the shoulder after 1 to 2 months of disuse, the plain radiograph in adhesive capsulitis is generally normal.[23,135] An arthrogram may be useful in differentiating this disorder from other painful conditions, however.[21,24] The joint capsule typically appears contracted, with absence of the normal inferior reflection (axillary pouch), bicipital tendon sheath, and subscapular bursa.[15,21,24,89] The injectable volume of contrast material may be reduced by 60 to 90%. One report demonstrated some volume loss in 67% of cases, but marked volume loss ($\geq$50%) was found in only 43%.[136] Intra-articular adhesions were not observed. It has been suggested that scintigraphy of the shoulder may be helpful in the diagnosis of adhesive capsulitis and related conditions and in predicting response to local corticosteroid injection.[31,126] Confirmatory studies and further characterization of scintigrams in normal shoulders,[36,112] as well as in injured shoulders,[37] are needed before this approach can be recommended, however. Over 90% of patients with adhesive capsulitis were reported to have abnormal scintigrams, but a number of them were found to have rotator cuff tears, indicating a mixed population.[137]

Treatment

The best treatment of adhesive capsulitis is prevention. Early mobilization of the shoulder(s) in any painful condition or chronic illness is essential, although this approach may not be effective in patients with hemiparesis.[30,138] Once the disorder is established, little critical evidence suggests that any therapeutic approach shortens the natural course of the disease. A conservative program should be instituted as early as possible (Table 97–2); however, if symptoms persist or worsen, a variety of therapeutic techniques have been advocated. These include local corticosteroid injections,[104,127,139,140] stellate ganglion blockade,[140] systemic corticosteroids or ACTH, antidepressant medications,[141] and exercises combined with transcutaneous nerve stimulation.[142]

In the patient with a resistant case or in those who have had symptoms for several months, I have achieved good to excellent responses with injection into the joint of a mixture containing 2.5 to 3.0 ml 1% procaine, 20 to 40 mg of prednisolone tertiary butyl acetate microcrystalline suspension, and 20 ml sterile saline solution, using maximum pressure on the injecting syringe, followed immediately by exercises.[143] A similar procedure, termed infiltration brisement, has been used successfully by others,[85] and simple pressure distension during arthrography appears to yield similar gratifying results.[144,145] Unfortunately, none of these regimens have been studied under controlled conditions. Manipulation of the shoulder under general anesthesia has been used in refractory cases with varied success,[146] but this form of therapy remains controversial because of the risk of considerable soft-tissue damage, shoulder dislocation, or even humeral fracture.[85]

FIBROSITIS (FIBROMYALGIA)

Fibrositis, a poorly defined entity of unknown cause, appears to be most common in women between the ages of 35 and 50 years who are anxious and often fatigued. An aching pain, usually aggravated by stress or cold, damp weather, is reported in soft tissues between the shoulder and neck. Frequently, painful trigger points or actual small nodules can be found on careful palpation. Treatment by injection of local anesthetic agents with or without corticosteroids may be helpful, especially when accompanied by considerable reassurance and support. This condition is more fully discussed in Chapter 80.

ARTHRITIS

Although arthritis is an uncommon cause of isolated shoulder pain,[97] each of the shoulder girdle joints and bursae can be affected by the various arthritides described in this book. By far the most frequent is degenerative arthritis, which is found in the shoulders of approximately 30% of elderly subjects.[15] This disorder is almost always asymptomatic and is an incidental radiographic abnormality,[147,148] but unless it is considered in the differential diagnosis of shoulder pain, especially in patients of advanced age, error in diagnosis and treatment may occur.

Acromioclavicular Joint

The acromioclavicular joint is particularly prone to degenerative arthritis because of its rudimentary intra-articular disc,[1] which apparently has a protective function, and because of the repeated stresses to which this joint is exposed during overhead arm movements. The patient usually complains of shoulder pain, but often cannot localize it specifically; sleeping on the affected side may increase the pain. That elevation of the arm above shoulder level produces pain is an important clue to diagnosis because rotator cuff lesions cause pain at or below this level.

Inspection of the shoulder may reveal a distorted contour with prominence of the affected joint. Direct palpation over this area elicits tenderness. Active shrugging of the shoulder, passive adduction and flexion of the arm across the chest, and forcing of the humerus by passively raising the arm against a fixed clavicle isolate the movement of this joint and aid in diagnosis when pain or crepitus is found. Confirmation of the diagnosis by plain radiography is helpful, but degenerative changes, although frequently present, are often asymptomatic.

Treatment consists of the standard conservative approach (Table 97–2) and restriction of the patient's movements to a painless, and usually functional, arc. Occasionally, intra-articular corticosteroid injections are of benefit. In difficult cases, arthroplasty may be necessary; this procedure generally provides a satisfactory result. Osteolysis of the distal clavicle may resemble acute arthritis of the acromioclavicular joint. This condition may follow traumatic shoulder injuries[149] or repeated minor traumas such as occur in weight lifters or those who work with arms extended.[150]

Sternoclavicular Joint

Arthritis in this small but important joint is rare. Post-traumatic arthritis, degenerative arthritis, and rheumatoid arthritis (RA) are the most common forms, although this joint is also affected in ankylosing spondylitis and related diseases. Two unusual forms of arthritis, *pustulotic arthro-osteitis,* reported in Japanese patients, and *sternoclavicular hyperostosis,* appear to involve the sternoclavicular joint particularly frequently. These entities are probably identical, differing only in the frequency of associated pustular lesions of the palms and soles.[151–153]

Patients often complain of pain, tenderness, and swelling of the sternoclavicular joint, although a careful history and examination may disclose an inflammatory polyarthritis. Maximal pain in the sternoclavicular joint is present during the midrange of arm elevation or on protrusion of the shoulders. Pustular lesions are found on the palms and soles in many patients.

Laboratory studies are normal or nonspecific and synovial tissue is moderately inflamed in this condition.[154] The plain radiograph is often difficult to interpret because of overlying shadows. Scintigraphy may help localize the site of inflammation, and polytomography or computed tomography (CT) may be necessary to identify erosive changes. Changes resembling diffuse idiopathic skeletal hyperostosis (DISH) or ankylosing spondylitis may be present elsewhere.[153]

Conservative treatment with NSAIDs or intra-articular corticosteroids is usually sufficient for symptomatic relief. Concomitant use of antibacterial agents may be of benefit.[154]

A number of other disorders may affect the sternoclavicular joint, as noted above.[155] Erosive changes occur in polymyalgia rheumatica (see Chapter 79) with variable frequency.[156,157] These also respond to conservative measures or treatment of the underlying condition. Surgical intervention is required occasionally, especially in post-traumatic arthritis.[158]

Glenohumeral Joint

Degenerative arthritis of the glenohumeral joint, which is uncommon, generally involves the glenoid rather than the humeral side of the joint.[1,159] This feature may be due to its nonweight-bearing nature, although considerable force is exerted across the joint.[1] On occasion, ischemic (avascular) necrosis or neurotropic arthropathy, usually secondary to syringomyelia, causes identical symptoms. Pain is rarely severe, and the patient is more likely to be concerned by the cosmetic appearance of the joint, such as after fracture and malunion, or by the restricted motion. Functional limitation can usually be overcome by increased movement in accessory joints and by avoidance of painful motion. Examination discloses a crepitant joint with diminished mobility, but minimal pain. Radiography may reveal an old fracture site or characteristic changes of osteoarthritis. Severe degenerative arthropathy is often associated with calcium pyrophosphate or basic calcium phosphate crystal deposits in synovial tissues or in shoulder joint cartilage; the shoulder is not involved in primary generalized osteoarthritis.

Again, treatment is conservative and symptomatic for the most part. Arthrodesis or arthroplasty may be indicated in certain instances, but the results, except pain relief, are less than ideal.

Milwaukee shoulder is a form of advanced degenerative arthritis involving the glenohumeral joint,[160] as well as other large joints.[161] Patients are usually elderly women who complain of weakness and loss of motion in the dominant shoulder, but who are in little pain. Massive rotator cuff tears are present. Microcrystalline basic calcium phosphates are found in synovial fluids and have been implicated in the pathogenesis of this syndrome (see Chapter 108). This arthropathy resembles *dislocation, or cuff-tear, arthropathy* in some respects,[162,163] and both conditions seem related to shoulder joint instability. This condition may be associated with stress fractures of the acromion.[164]

OTHER "INTRINSIC" CAUSES OF SHOULDER PAIN

Athletic and Other Traumatic Injuries

A detailed discussion of traumatic injuries to the shoulder, whether produced by blunt or by penetrating forces, is beyond the scope of this chapter. Although such injuries are diagnosed with relative ease from the patient's medical history, cautious examination is essential to avoid overlooking associated soft-tissue, bony, or neurovascular complications.

In addition to many of the conditions discussed previously, trauma may result in capsular ruptures with or without associated hemarthrosis, subluxation or dislocation, fractures, tendon avulsion (especially in adolescents), nerve injuries, and a variety of sprains and contusions. Obviously, knowledge of the type and mechanism of injury provides important clues to diagnosis; several of the more common injuries are considered briefly. Chronic repetitive trauma may lead to advanced degenerative changes in the glenohumeral joint.[165]

Falls. During unexpected falls, the arm is usually extended to cushion the impact, thereby transmitting the force upward to the shoulder and either anteriorly, as in backward falls, or posteriorly, as in forward falls. As a result, the rotator cuff or the joint capsule itself can be torn, or if sufficient force is applied, subluxation (dislocation), neurovascular injury, or actual fracture may be present.

Dislocation of the glenohumeral joint is common, especially in athletic young men. Anterior dislocation occurs in 95% of these cases because the humeral head is usually thrust forward against the weak anteroinferior portion of the joint capsule. Posterior dislocations, although rare, are more likely to be overlooked.

Acute dislocation is readily diagnosed. The patient provides a history of recent injury followed by sudden, severe pain in the shoulder. He supports the injured arm at the forearm with the elbow angled outward. The deltoid muscle is often tense on palpation. A depression is observed on palpation just inferior to the acromion. Neurovascular injuries may accompany shoulder dislocation in up to 25% of cases;[166] careful examination of the neurologic and vascular systems is essential whenever dislocation is suspected. Characteristic radiographic changes are present, although special views may be required.

Treatment consists of closed reduction within the first hours after dislocation. Thereafter, increasing restriction in shoulder motion may necessitate surgical repair.

Recurrent or habitual dislocations may follow the acute dislocation, especially in subjects under 20 years of age. Each subsequent dislocation may require less and less force, so even routine tasks, such as combing the hair, may cause it. A number of reasons for recurrent dislocation have been proposed, including an incompetent glenoid labrum, poor capsular ligament development, an enlarged humeral head, or a shallow glenoid fossa. A number of surgical approaches have been advocated for this problem.[1]

Direct Impact. The shoulder girdle is a prime target for falling objects, in part because of the protective flexion reflex of the neck and head. Depending on the point of impact, fractures, severe contusions, or nerve root or neurovascular injuries may occur.

Throwing. The overhead throw in baseball or football is a complex, coordinated series of movements. The shoulder girdle acts first as a base and then as a fulcrum to support and propel the object. The throw has four phases: (1) the preparation, in which the arm is extended, abducted, and externally rotated; (2) the phase of forward flexion and release; (3) the follow-through; and (4) the braking phase. Shoulder pain may result from repeated impingement, as well as from injury during the braking phase, because the joint capsule and rotator cuff are maximally stretched to prevent humeral dislocation. Tears may result, and when they occur repeatedly or are not allowed to heal, a periosteal reaction and, later, osteophytes develop.

The underhand throw, as in softball, bowling, or curling, is not as forceful, and injuries to the shoulder are far less common. Because this motion brings the anterior capsular mechanism and the bicipital apparatus into play, injuries to these structures may result. They are rarely serious, and rest is sufficient for complete healing in most cases.

Golfing. Usually considered a "safe" sport, golfing may result in injuries to the shoulder girdle. The most common injuries, resulting from recurrent stress at or superior to the horizontal plane, are those of the acromioclavicular joint. Symptoms and findings relating to this joint have previously been discussed; rest and other conservative measures are usually adequate.

Contact Sports. The causes of injury in the various

contact sports such as football, hockey, basketball, and soccer are apparent. In addition to those injuries already discussed, fracture and dislocation, subluxation, and soft-tissue tears are common.

Congenital and Developmental Anomalies

Many bony, muscular, and articular anomalies of the shoulder region have been recognized.[1,167,168] Although they rarely cause serious pain, they may produce functional or cosmetic problems requiring medical intervention.

The most common congenital anomaly of the shoulder, *Sprengel's deformity*, or congenital elevation of the scapula, is often associated with other skeletal and soft-tissue abnormalities. It is caused by a failure of the scapula to descend normally during ontogeny. Surgical treatment is arduous and is often less than satisfactory, and it is warranted only if the deformity produces serious functional disability or psychologic problems.[167]

Another congenital anomaly that occasionally produces shoulder pain is the Klippel-Feil syndrome, or congenital brevicollis, in which failure of segmentation or fusion of two or more cervical vertebrae may be associated with a cervical rib, other bony abnormalities, or an anomalous nerve and blood supply to the head, neck, and upper extremities.

Posture

Poor posture, a frequent cause of shoulder and neck pain, often goes unrecognized. It may result from working in a slumped position, from spinal malformation such as kyphosis or spondyloarthritis, from psychologic difficulties, from chronic illness with reduced muscle tone, or from a combination of these and other factors. Whatever the cause, abnormal posture places undue stress on the suspensory or mooring muscles of the upper extremity, especially the trapezius, rhomboid, and latissimus dorsi muscles. It may be difficult to identify this cause of shoulder pain because symptoms often develop hours after the patient has left work, and only a careful medical history reveals the source. Chronic aberrant posture is readily apparent. The patient complains of pain in the shoulder girdle, although this pain may radiate widely.

Correction of work or living habits, postural instruction, and physiotherapy usually produce improvement, but braces or supports are occasionally required.

NEUROLOGIC CAUSES OF SHOULDER PAIN

Brachial Plexus Injuries

Trauma is the most common cause of isolated brachial plexus lesions.[1,169,170] These injuries may result from penetrating wounds such as stab or gunshot wounds; blunt trauma, as from falling objects; external pressure, such as from backpacks; or stretch injuries, either obstetric or from machines. Surgery and radiotherapy also may produce brachial plexus injuries.[171] The clinical picture varies, depending on the specific site and branch affected; however, loss of motor function, rather than pain, is usually the predominant complaint. Involvement of cervical roots 5 and 6 is common and produces weakness in the deltoid, biceps, and rotator cuff muscles, so abduction and rotation of the arm are altered. When pain does occur in brachial plexus injuries, it often has a burning or causalgic quality, which represents an adverse prognostic sign.

Peripheral Neuropathy

Localized peripheral nerve lesions are usually traumatic in origin, but other factors may contribute to or produce them directly, such as vasculitis, metabolic derangements, heavy-metal toxicity, and vitamin deficiencies.[1] As with brachial plexus injury, peripheral neuropathies generally result in loss or decrease in motor function, but rarely in pain. The *suprascapular nerve* may be *entrapped* during scapular fractures or by compression of the nerve as it traverses the notch of the scapula.[1,172,173] Lesions of the axillary nerve are most often produced by blunt or penetrating trauma,[174] as well as by traumatic shoulder dislocation. Injuries of the suprascapular nerve, which supplies the infraspinatus and supraspinatus muscles, or of the axillary nerve, which supplies the deltoid muscle, weaken abduction but do not eliminate it.

Neuralgic Amyotrophy (Brachial Plexitis, Parsonage-Turner Syndrome)

This rare disorder has received scant attention in the literature in the United States.[14,175] It appears to be an actual peripheral neuropathy with "causalgic" features in patients recovering from a variety of serious illnesses. Characteristically, the patient has sudden pain in and about the shoulder, followed in several days to weeks by muscle weakness or paralysis, again usually in the shoulder region. Spontaneous recovery generally occurs, and no specific treatment exists.

EXTRINSIC CAUSES OF SHOULDER PAIN

Few causes of shoulder pain are truly extrinsic, except referred pain. A variety of systemic inflammatory or metabolic diseases are considered under this category because shoulder pain or disability is a single manifestation of the broader disease process. Such diseases in fact produce intrinsic shoulder lesions.

Arthritis

Virtually all forms of generalized arthritis can, and often do, affect the shoulder girdle joints and the bursae. RA and osteoarthritis are most common. These and the other arthritides are discussed elsewhere and need not be considered here. Over 90% of unselected patients with RA have had shoulder pain and 30 to 40% have erosive disease in the glenohumeral, acromioclavicular, and sternoclavicular joints.[147,176,177] Similarly, radiographic evidence of osteoarthritis in these joints is common, especially in patients with osteoarthritis in other joints.[147]

Avascular Necrosis

Avascular (ischemic, aseptic) necrosis of the humeral head is rarely an isolated finding in the shoulder. It usually occurs in patients with other diseases, as discussed in Chapter 98.

Polymyalgia Rheumatica

Polymyalgia rheumatica, a chronic systemic disease of unknown origin, primarily affects individuals in their sixth decade or older and is discussed in Chapter 79. Pain and stiffness occur in both the shoulder and the pelvic girdles, but symptoms may be present in only one girdle. Erosive changes may be present in the sternoclavicular joints.[156,157]

Muscular Diseases

Polymyositis, the muscular dystrophies, and various other myopathies frequently affect the upper limb girdle muscles. Pain is rarely a major symptom, but weakness and disability may cause the patient to seek medical attention.

Metabolic Diseases

Diabetes Mellitus. The prevalence of certain disorders of the shoulder, such as degenerative and calcific tendinobursitis,[60,61,146,178] degenerative arthritis,[60] and adhesive capsulitis,[125,126] is increased in patients with diabetes mellitus. Limitation of shoulder mobility has been found in 50% of unselected diabetic patients.[179] Adhesive capsulitis was diagnosed in 19% of these patients (versus 5% of normal control subjects). Adhesive capsulitis often is associated with *cheirarthropathy* in diabetic subjects. The latter condition is characterized by waxy skin, skin and connective tissue induration, and finger flexion contractures.[180] The recent observation of improved joint mobility following aldose reductase administration[181] supports the hypothesis that reversible metabolic changes in periar-

ticular connective tissues account for the joint changes observed in diabetes mellitus (see Chapter 94).

Gout and Pseudogout. Crystal-induced synovitis may occur in any of the shoulder girdle joints. Gouty arthritis is rare,[182] whereas pseudogout is seen in 25 to 50% of affected subjects, at least by the radiographic findings of calcium pyrophosphate deposition (see Chapter 107).[183]

Hyperparathyroidism. Patients with hyperparathyroidism may develop a number of musculoskeletal complaints. In addition to a distinct hyperparathyroid arthropathy, these patients may have pseudogout, resorption of the distal clavicle, or formation of cystic brown tumors in the clavicle, humerus, or other long bones. With the greater use of biochemical screening studies and the earlier recognition of this disease, articular complications are far less common than formerly.

Other Disorders. Shoulder arthropathy may be found in patients with other metabolic diseases including hemachromatosis, alkaptonuria, ochronosis, Wilson's disease, and amyloidosis.

Neurologic Diseases

Perception of pain at a site remote from the area of irritation is considered referred pain. Attention was focused on this cause of pain by the classic experiments of Kellgren and Lewis, who injected hypertonic saline solution into interspinous ligaments or specific muscle groups and mapped out the location and extent of resulting pain. These researchers found that pain frequently radiated distally, but always within the same sensory root segment. The various causes of neurologic pain discussed under the category of "extrinsic" are all examples of referred pain.

Cervical Nerve Root Compression. Compression of a cervical nerve root is commonly a result of degenerative arthritis or spondylopathy. Other causes include spinal infection, especially tuberculosis, primary or secondary neoplasms, spondyloarthritis, fractures, subluxations, or congenital anomalies.

Because the fifth and sixth cervical vertebrae are usually affected, complaints of shoulder and neck stiffness and aching are common. Pain may be increased by moving the neck and by coughing and sneezing, which stretch the affected nerve root. Objective evidence of motor or sensory nerve involvement, of changes in tendon reflexes, and of muscle wasting provides clues to diagnosis.

Radiographic evidence of degenerative arthritis is common in subjects beyond the age of 50 years and must be interpreted cautiously unless definite neuroforaminal encroachment is present. In patients with a herniated disc, the plain radiograph may be entirely normal, and diagnosis depends on myelographic or CT study.

These and other features of the cervical syndrome, which represents the most common extrinsic cause of shoulder pain, are discussed fully in Chapter 90.

Spinal Cord Lesions. Other lesions of the cervical spine and of the spinal cord itself may cause pain to be referred to the shoulder. These lesions include traumatic injuries; infections such as tuberculosis, herpes zoster, and poliomyelitis; syringomyelia; tumors; and various vascular anomalies. Patients with herpes zoster also may lack shoulder abduction when the C5-C6 nerve roots are affected.

Viscerogenic (Viscerosomatic) Pain. Pain is referred to the shoulder from deeper somatic or visceral structures by intrasegmental transmission. Most common are lesions along the course of the phrenic nerve, originating from C4 primarily, with fibers from C3 and C5, or from the diaphragm, which it supplies. The diaphragm can be irritated by many conditions involving the mediastinum, the pericardium, the inferior pulmonary segments, the liver, and especially the biliary tract. Other visceral diseases that refer pain to the shoulder are myocardial ischemia, pulmonary infarction or neoplasm, perforated intra-abdominal or pelvic viscera, peptic esophagitis or esophageal spasm, and dissecting aortic aneurysm (Fig. 97–10). Referred pain to the shoulder may be the sole symptom of serious distant disease.

THORACIC OUTLET SYNDROME(S)

The region through which the neurovascular supply of the upper extremity exits the neck and thorax to enter the axilla constitutes the thoracic outlet.[184,185] It actually represents a series of narrow, fixed passages, each of which affords opportunity for compression of the neurovascular bundle. Symptoms and signs vary, depending on the nature and position of the obstruction. The manifestations include a cervical rib, anomalies of the first rib, interscalene muscle compression, and other rarer entities collectively termed the thoracic outlet syndrome.

ANATOMY AND PATHOPHYSIOLOGY

The anatomic relationships of the thoracic outlet are complex, but are considered briefly.[1,184] The clavicle conveniently divides the region into three segments, supraclavicular, retroclavicular, and infraclavicular. Each is associated with certain structural or functional abnormalities that may compress the neurovascular bundles.

In the supraclavicular segment, in the posterior triangle of the neck, the subclavian artery and the brachial plexus lie between the anterior and posterior scalenic muscle masses. The subclavian vein is situated in front of the anterior scalene muscle here and therefore is separated from the artery and the plexus; it joins them at the level of the clavicle. Two major sources of neurovascular compression are seen in this segment. Interscalenic compression, also known as *scalenus anterior syndrome* or Naffziger's syndrome, is caused by minor variations in the size, contour, or sites of insertion of the scalene muscles, with resultant narrowing of the already small interscalenic triangle. The presence of a cervical rib, found in approximately .6% of the population,[184] may also compromise the neurovascular supply in this segment by angulating the bundle or by narrowing the interscalene triangle (Fig. 97–11).

In the retroclavicular space, the neurovascular bundle, now joined by the subclavian vein, passes between the clavicle anteriorly and the first or thoracic rib posteriorly (Fig. 97–11). Compression in this segment is produced by a variety of conditions that narrow this space, such as clavicular fracture or its complications of malunion or exuberant callus formation, congenital anomalies of the clavicle or first rib, external pressure from heavy weights or packs, and poor

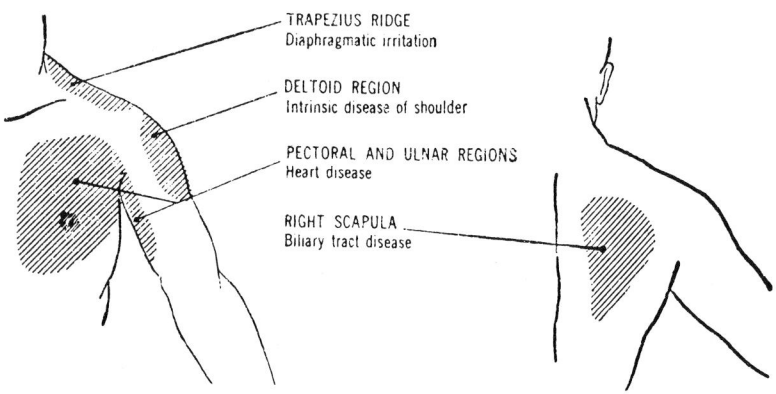

TRAPEZIUS RIDGE
Diaphragmatic irritation

DELTOID REGION
Intrinsic disease of shoulder

PECTORAL AND ULNAR REGIONS
Heart disease

RIGHT SCAPULA
Biliary tract disease

FIG. 97–10. Sites of reference about the shoulder in viscerogenic pain. (From Morgan. Courtesy of Modern Medicine.)

FIG. 97–11. Thoracic outlet syndrome produced by a cervical rib; poststenotic dilatation of the subclavian artery is present.

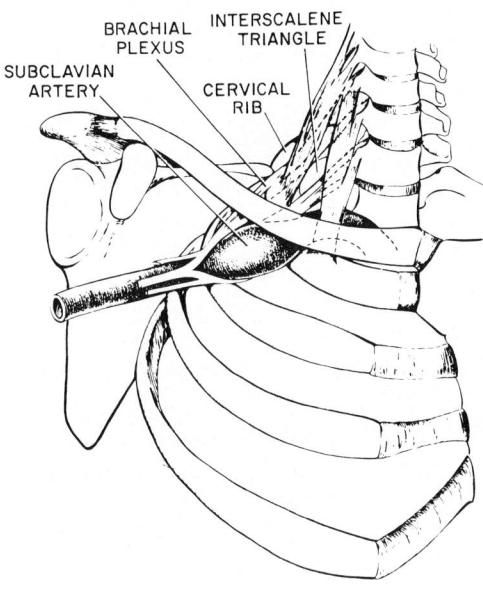

posture. These conditions are termed the *costoclavicular disorders.*

The infraclavicular segment of the neurovascular bundle is situated behind (beneath) the pectoralis minor tendon and the clavipectoral fascia and in front of the subscapularis, from which it is separated by abundant areolar tissue. The considerable variation in the structural relationships of this region that occurs with normal arm motion may result in neurovascular compression, the so-called clavipectoral disorders. The most common is the hyperabduction syndrome, in which the neurovascular bundle is pulled around the pectoralis minor tendon during abduction, to create a pulley-like effect (Fig. 97–12). This hyperabducted position was well known to soldiers in the past as a method of controlling upper extremity bleeding. It is usually seen in patients who sleep with arms hyperabducted, that is, folded under the head, or who are engaged in occupations requiring this position for prolonged periods, such as automobile mechanics and painters.

Clinical Features

Symptoms of the thoracic outlet syndrome may be variable and intermittent, depending on the role of fixed anatomic abnormalities, shoulder movement, or combinations of these factors.[184–186] Pain in the shoulder or arm is characteristic of the syndrome, although it is present in only 70% of patients.[186] When neural in origin, the pain is segmental in distribution, usually in the ulnar segment because its roots, C8 and T1, are lowermost and more readily compressed, and is often described as a dull aching or burning sensation. This pain is almost always associated with paresthesias and numbness. Objective findings include diminished sensation, muscle weakness, or atrophy. When the pain is vascular in origin, it is vague and poorly localized and is described as a fullness or numbness. One may see associated objective findings of edema, color and temperature change, Raynaud's phenomenon, and dilatation of the superficial veins of the arm, shoulder, and neck.

A careful medical history may reveal typical patterns of aggravation and relief of symptoms. For example, symptoms present on awakening may be produced by placing the hands beneath the head or pillow during sleep. Occupation may be a factor when symptoms develop during the day or early evening in those who work overhead, such as automobile mechanics and painters. Symptoms that occur on weekends or vacations may be traced to sporting habits, as with backpackers who compress their costoclavicular space with heavy shoulder weights. Certain large-breasted women also may experience compressive symptoms as a consequence of brassiere-strap pressure.[187] Although poor upper back and neck posture have long been recognized to contribute to compression of the neurovascular bundle, a particular group of subjects with long necks and low-set shoulders that appears to be at increased risk has recently been described.[188]

The presenting complaint may represent a complication of neurovascular compression. A cool, cyanotic, or pallid extremity, with or without Raynaud's phenomenon, ulceration, or frank gangrene, may occur consequent to arterial obstruction or thrombosis. Postobstructive arterial dilatation may be recognized as a supraclavicular mass. Venous obstruction produces edema, an increased girth in the affected arm, dilation and tortuosity of superficial veins, or venous thrombosis (Paget-Schroetter syndrome).

Diagnosis and Differential Diagnosis

Diagnosis depends on a thorough medical history and physical examination to reveal the typical clinical features of neurovascular compression.[184,185] Several special tests may be helpful in confirming the diagnosis and in localizing the site of obstruction. The *Adson maneuver,* which narrows the interscalene triangle, is performed with the patient holding his breath in full inspiration and then fully extending his neck and rotating it toward the side examined. The *costoclavicular maneuver* diminishes the costoclavicular space and is effected by bracing the shoulders pos-

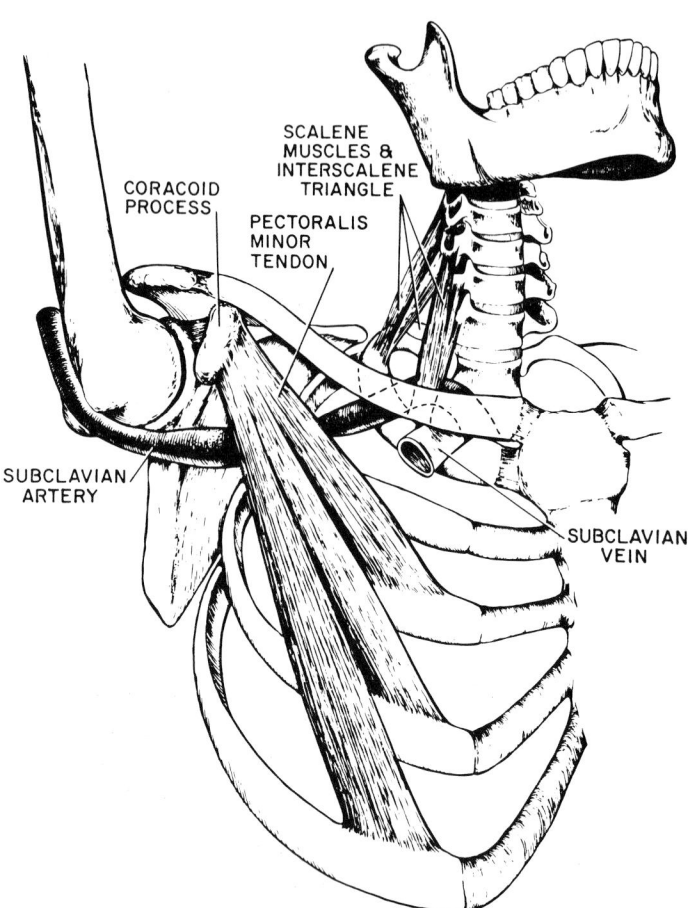

FIG. 97–12. Thoracic outlet syndrome produced by hyperabduction maneuver; note compression beneath the pectoralis minor tendon.

teriorly and inferiorly, the exaggerated military posture. The *hyperabduction maneuver* for hyperabduction syndrome is performed by abducting the arms 180° in external rotation. A positive test result reproduces the patient's symptoms and obliterates or dampens the radial artery pulse. Because the radial pulse is often reduced in normal subjects during these maneuvers,[185,186,189] this sign alone is insufficient for diagnosis.

Other studies may be useful in diagnosis and differential diagnosis. The plain radiograph of the chest, cervical spine, and entire shoulder area may disclose specific bony abnormalities, such as cervical rib or clavicular fracture, that explain the patient's symptoms. Doppler studies, venography, arteriography, and plethysmography may be useful as well, especially when performed during the foregoing postural maneuvers.[186,189,190] Determination of nerve conduction velocities across the thoracic outlet, elbow, and wrist may also help in diagnosis and differential diagnosis, but must be interpreted cautiously.[191] Somatosensory-evoked potentials across the thoracic outlet (Erb's point) may reveal poorly formed waves, supporting the diagnosis.[192]

Depending on whether neurologic or vascular signs predominate, a number of conditions may enter into the differential diagnosis. Some of these are listed in Table 97–3. When the thoracic outlet syndrome is suspected, it is essential that the diagnosis be established promptly, so appropriate therapy can be initiated.

Treatment

Unless the disorder is complicated by serious obstructive vascular disease or neurologic findings, initial therapy of the thoracic outlet should be conservative. Reassurance, education, and postural retraining to reduce thoracic outlet compression are of prime importance and are sufficient in most patients.[185,186,193] Usually, these measures are combined with physiotherapy to reduce muscle spasm and to strengthen the suspensory muscles, such as the rhomboid, levator scapulae, and trapezius muscles. In patients with severe or refractory disease, operative intervention is indicated. Careful preoperative assessment is imperative, however, because more than one site of obstruction may be present.

REFLEX SYMPATHETIC DYSTROPHY SYNDROME

The unusual complex of symptoms constituting this syndrome was first isolated by S. Weir Mitchell and

Table 97–3. Differential Diagnosis of Thoracic Outlet Syndrome

Primarily Neurologic Symptoms
 Cervical spine syndromes
 Spinal cord tumors
 Syringomyelia
 Entrapment neuropathy
  Ulnar nerve (elbow)
  Medial nerve (carpal tunnel)
 Peripheral neuropathy
 Brachial plexus neuropathy
 Herpes zoster and postherpetic neuralgia
Primarily Vascular Symptoms
 Arterial
  Granulomatous arteritis, Takayasu's disease
  Atherosclerosis
  Embolic disease
  Arterial aneurysms
  Raynaud's phenomenon or disease
 Venous
  Thrombophlebitis
  Obstruction, benign or malignant
Neurovascular Symptoms
 Reflex sympathetic dystrophy syndrome

his colleagues Moorehouse and Keen during the American Civil War,[194] although several cases with similar features had been reported earlier. Later, Mitchell introduced the term "causalgia," derived from the Greek words for "heat" and "pain," to describe the peculiar burning pain so characteristic of this disorder.[195–197] Unfortunately, the confusing array of terms and designations for the syndrome that appeared in the years following Mitchell's classic studies created considerable uncertainty as to its very nature and existence (Table 97–4).

The exact prevalence of the reflex sympathetic dystrophy syndrome is unknown. Data from several studies suggest that it is frequent in patients with coronary artery disease (5 to 20%),[198,199] in patients with hemiplegia (12 to 21%),[200,201] in patients with

Table 97–4. Synonyms for the Reflex Sympathetic Dystrophy Syndrome

Causalgia, major or minor
Acute atrophy of bone
Sudeck's atrophy
Sudeck's osteodystrophy
Peripheral acute thromphoneurosis
Traumatic angiospasm
Traumatic vasospasm
Post-traumatic osteoporosis
Postinfarctional sclerodactyly
Shoulder-hand syndrome
Shoulder-hand-finger syndrome
Reflex dystrophy
Reflex neurovascular dystrophy
Reflex sympathetic dystrophy
Algodystrophy
Algoneurodystrophy

Colles' fracture (.2 to 11%),[202–204] and in patients with peripheral nerve injury (3%) or other forms of traumatic injury (.5%).[205] Although emphasis on early mobilization following fractures, myocardial infarction, and stroke has reduced the frequency of this complication, it has not been eliminated.[200,203,206]

ORIGIN

A number of diseases, precipitating events, or drugs have been associated with this syndrome (Table 97–5). They are thought to provoke the syndrome through reflex neurologic mechanisms, although their exact role in its pathogenesis remains obscure. It is difficult, if not impossible, to determine the relative frequency of these factors in initiating the syndrome because of selection factors in reported series. In surgical practice, trauma is clearly the most common precipitant, especially fractures or peripheral nerve injuries. In medical practice, although trauma, often minor, still ranks as the leading provocative event, myocardial ischemia, cervical spinal or spinal cord disorders, and a variety of cerebral lesions are also common. These findings are shown in Table 97–6, in which several studies are compared. Two points are worthy of note. First, in over 25% of patients, a definitive precipitating event could not be identified. Second, cervical discogenic disease is so common in this age group that its significance remains uncertain; before considering this as an "associated disease," definite evidence of nerve root impingement should be present.

Table 97–5. Conditions Associated with the Reflex Sympathetic Dystrophy Syndrome

Trauma, major or minor
Fractures, especially Colles' fracture
Primary central nervous system disorders
Cerebrovascular disease with hemiplegia
Hemiplegia of other causes
Convulsive disorders (?)
Spinal cord lesions
Cervical spine disease, such as arthritis or discogenic
 disorders
Peripheral neuropathy
Herpes zoster with postherpetic neuralgia
Ischemic heart disease
Painful lesions of the rotator cuff
Pulmonary tuberculosis
Antituberculous drug administration
Barbiturate and other anticonvulsive drug administration
Hysterical personality (?)

Table 97–6. Estimated Frequency of Associated Conditions in the Reflex Sympathetic Dystrophy Syndrome

Study	No. of Patients	Age	Bilateral Involvement (%)	Fracture	Peripheral Nerve Injury	Other Trauma	Myocardial Ischemia	Central Nervous System Disease	Spinal Injury or Discogenic Disease	Idiopathic or Miscellaneous Conditions
Acquaviva et al.[207]*	585	51	10	216	23	179	3	16	0	148
Evans[208]	57	—	—	12	1	26	0	1	2	15
Johnson and Pannozzo[209]	76	59†	18	6	0	15	10	18	13	14
Kozin et al.[210]	11	56	18	0	0	1	1	2	3	4
Kozin et al.[197]	32‡	—	—	4	3§	10§	0	6	2	7
Pak et al.[206]	140	54	—	28	0	40	12	3	3	43
Patman et al.[211]	113	44†	—	41	0	57	0	0	0	15
Rosen and Graham[212]	73	63	30	1	0	5	27	9	14	17
Steinbrocker and Argyros[139]	146	>50	25	0	0	15	30	11	29	61
Subbarao and Stillwell[213]	125	54‖	10	31	24	25	4	6	0	35
Thompson[214]	17	>50	47	0	0	1	2	7	1	6
Totals										
Number:	1375	—	—	339	51	374	89	79	67	376
Percentage:	—	—	23	25	4	27	6	6	5	27

*Patients diagnosed as "algodystrophy"; number with "definite" diagnosis uncertain.
†Estimated average age.
‡Definite and probable diagnosis.
§Two patients had peripheral nerve injury associated with fractures.
‖Median age.

CLINICAL FEATURES

Both sexes are affected equally in this syndrome, except when the provocative cause is sex-related, such as myocardial ischemia in men. No predilection exists for the dominant side. In medical practice, the syndrome is far more common in patients over the age of 50 years (Table 97–6), probably because of the

Table 97–7. Classification and Clinical Criteria for the Reflex Sympathetic Dystrophy Syndrome

Definite
1. Pain and tenderness in an extremity
2. Symptoms or signs of vasomotor instability
   Raynaud's phenomenon
   Cool, pallid skin (vasoconstriction)
   Warm, erythematous skin (vasodilatation)
   Hyperhidrosis
3. Swelling of the extremity
   Pitting or nonpitting edema
4. Dystrophic skin changes
   Atrophy
   Scaling
   Hypertrichosis or hair loss
   Nail changes
   Thickened palmar fascia

Probable
1. Pain and tenderness
2. Signs or symptoms of vasomotor instability
3. Swelling of the extremity

Possible
1. Symptoms or signs of vasomotor instability
2. Swelling of the extremity

foregoing disease associations. Children and younger individuals are not spared,[215–220] although the syndrome has been described in large series of children only recently.[215,220]

The fully developed syndrome is usually characterized by pain and swelling in the distal extremity, trophic skin changes, and signs and symptoms of vasomotor instability (Table 97–7). The pain is often severe and burning, or causalgic, and it generally involves the entire hand or foot. Other sites are less commonly affected; the syndrome may be segmental in distribution, involving one or two rays of the hand or foot (radial form),[221,222] knee,[223–225] or hip,[226,227] or a portion of bone (zonal form), such as part of the femoral head.[221] Patients may wrap an extremity in wet dressings to protect it and to reduce the pain. Objective examination may disclose an exquisitely tender hand or foot, which the patient withdraws at the slightest touch. Tenderness is generalized, but is most severe in the periarticular tissues.[228] Tenderness may be further characterized by *allodynia*, pain due to "non-noxious stimuli" (light touch), or *hyperpathia*, pain persisting or increasing after mild or light pressure.[229,230] Several investigators have suggested that the presence of severe, burning pain, allodynia, and hyperpathia may be sufficient for diagnosis.[231,232] Pitting or nonpitting edema is usually present and is localized to the painful and tender region; again, this feature appears to be more pronounced in the periarticular areas.[228,230] When the reflex sympathetic dystrophy syndrome occurs in the upper extremity, the patient may have associated pain and limitation of motion in the ipsilateral shoulder (*shoulder-hand syndrome*) (Fig. 97–13).

Vasomotor or sudomotor disturbances vary from patient to patient or within the same patient at different times. Occasionally, frank Raynaud's phenomenon occurs, but vasodilation or vasoconstriction is more common. Locally, increased sweating, hyperhidrosis, may be noted or reported by the patient and is an important diagnostic sign. Dystrophic changes in the skin gradually develop (Table 97–7). Ultimately, atrophy of the skin and of the subcutaneous tissue produces a shiny, thinned appearance. Contractures of the fingers and palmar fascia, Dupuytren's contracture, may eventually occur, leaving a claw-like, deformed hand.

The clinical course of this syndrome has been divided into three overlapping stages.[233,234] The first,

FIG. 97–13. *A*, A patient with shoulder-hand syndrome who has limited shoulder motion and diffuse swelling of the hand. *B*, Note the flexion contractures of the hands and the presence of pitting edema.

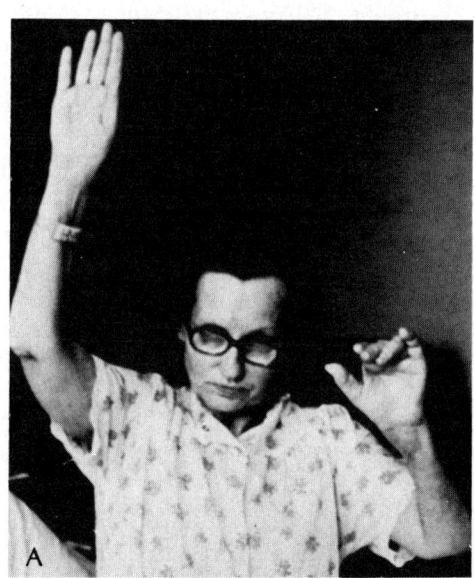

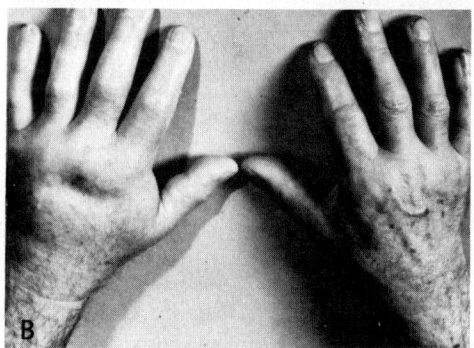

"acute" stage lasts 3 to 6 months and is characterized primarily by pain, tenderness, swelling, and vasomotor disturbances. In the second, "dystrophic" stage, these features resolve completely or partially, and trophic changes develop in the skin. This phase persists an additional 3 to 6 months. A third, "atrophic" stage then gradually evolves, in which skin and subcutaneous tissue atrophy and contractures predominate. Once this stage occurs, substantial reversal is uncommon, and the patient is left with a shiny, cool, contracted, and usually painless extremity.

Although staging of this syndrome is useful, it is often difficult to distinguish specific stages in an individual patient. More often, fluctuation between the first two stages occurs for weeks or months, until the atrophic and contractural changes gradually supervene. Therapy during the "active" period (stages 1 and 2) is essential; therapy during the last stage is rarely of benefit.

Incomplete (partial, limited, abortive, circumscribed) forms of this syndrome exist.[235] These types may include such diverse conditions as transient painful osteoporosis or osteolysis,[223,226,236] juvenile osteoporosis,[237,238] major or minor causalgia, segmental causalgia as in postherpetic syndromes, adhesive capsulitis or frozen shoulder, and idiopathic carpal tunnel syndrome or Dupuytren's contracture, especially when associated with a painful shoulder. Until the pathogenic mechanisms are understood and until more specific diagnostic tests are developed, the relation of these conditions to the reflex sympathetic dystrophy syndrome must remain uncertain. The incomplete category also includes patients who do not manifest all four clinical features evident in the classic syndrome (Table 97–6).[210] My colleagues and I have proposed criteria that allow such patients to be distinguished clinically and to be compared with others having overlapping symptoms or signs (Table 97–7).[210]

Bilateral involvement is generally thought to be present in 18 to 50% of patients (Table 97–6). Careful analysis of a small group of patients with the fully developed syndrome, however, has disclosed bilateral changes in all instances by clinical and radiologic methods.[210,239] This finding supports the concept that the syndrome is, in fact, "reflex" and is mediated by central neurologic mechanisms.

Laboratory studies, such as blood count and erythrocyte sedimentation rate, and other special studies are usually normal or show changes consistent with other associated conditions. The prevalence of hyperlipoproteinemia may be increased.[240,241] Unless the patient has had a specific nerve injury, electromyography and nerve condition velocity studies are normal.[211,242] Thermography,[242–245] as well as skin potential measurements,[246] have been advocated as diagnostic tests for this disorder. Diagnosis depends on the clinical and radiologic features (see below). Differential diagnosis includes local injury or inflammation, infection, or early RA and scleroderma. Either reflex sympathetic dystrophy syndrome or a condition that resembles it, termed palmar fasciitis and arthritis, may develop as a paraneoplastic syndrome.[247–249]

RADIOLOGIC FEATURES

These features include those evident on plain roentgenograms, as well as those requiring newer radiographic techniques.[197,218,221,228,239,250–253]

Plain Radiography

The characteristic radiographic appearance of the reflex sympathetic dystrophy syndrome is a patchy or mottled osteopenia (Fig. 97–14), a finding recognized since the early descriptions of Sudeck[254,255] and Kienbock.[256] This appearance is not found in all cases,[210,212,228] however, nor is it pathognomonic of the syndrome because it may be present in simple disuse osteopenia, such as from hemiparesis or immobilization, or in other conditions.[250] Its patchy character is caused by irregular resorption of cancellous or trabecular bone.[250,253] In addition, fine-detail radiographic techniques have disclosed resorption of subperiosteal, intracortical, endosteal, and subchondral and marginal bone.[243] Subchondral bone resorption produces a form of "erosive" articular disease manifested either as cortical breaks, surface erosions, as may be seen in early RA, or a peculiar fragmenta-

FIG. 97–14. Fine-detail radiographs of a patient with the reflex sympathetic dystrophy syndrome illustrating progressive osteopenia at three months (right) and eight months (left) after the onset of symptoms.

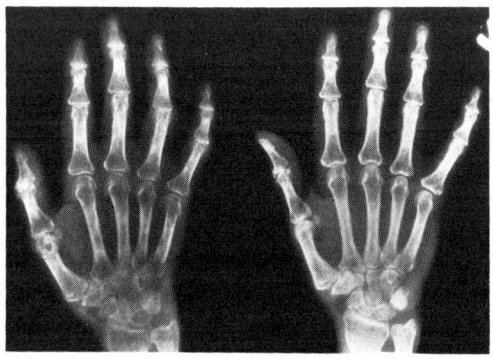

tion of marginal bone, "crumbling" erosion (Fig. 97–14).[228,253] Late in the course of the illness, diffuse osteopenia occurs and gives the radiograph a ground-glass appearance.

In adults, once these changes are established, they appear to be irreversible, although this feature may depend on the duration of the disease.[252] In children, the potential for healing appears to be greater.[218]

Quantitative Bone Mineral Analysis

In this syndrome, one sees an average loss of one third of the entire bone mineral content or cortical thickness in the affected extremity.[253] Treatment halts progression of the osteopenia, but it does not reverse it.

Scintigraphic Studies

The use of technetium-99m (^{99m}Tc) as the pertechnetate, which depends on the local blood pool, demonstrates increased periarticular uptake in the affected extremity (Fig. 97–15).[210,228,229,257–260] Frequently, uptake in the contralateral extremity is also increased, suggesting subclinical bilateral involvement.[202,229] Technetium-99m–labeled diphosphonate or polyphosphate uptake, which depends on local blood flow immediately after injection and on adsorption to bone later on, is also increased in the metaphysial regions of the bones on the affected, and to a lesser extent, on the contralateral side. In several reported cases, diminished radionuclide uptake was found in the affected extremity.[210,261] Scintigraphy may also be valuable in detecting incipient or subclinical reflex dystrophy.[262]

Rapid-sequence imaging immediately after radionuclide injection often demonstrates enhanced uptake in the affected extremity in patients with this syndrome,[210,239] and these findings indicate increased local blood flow.[253,263]

A number of studies have confirmed the value of scintigraphy in the diagnosis,[210,239,257,258,264] and possibly in the therapy,[210] of this syndrome. Studies are abnormal in 68 to 87% of subjects,[210,264] as well as in virtually all patients with transient osteoporosis syndromes, which often are clinically indistinguishable from the reflex sympathetic dystrophy syndrome.[226] Nuclide uptake was reported to be normal in certain patients responsive to corticosteroid therapy.[210]

PATHOLOGY AND PATHOPHYSIOLOGY

The skin and subcutaneous tissues are usually normal or exhibit minor, nonspecific changes. Dupuytren's contracture is frequently present. Affected bone

FIG. 97–15.   A three-phase bone scintigram in a patient with reflex sympathetic dystrophy syndrome affecting the left hand is illustrated. *A,* The characteristic changes are shown in the flow study in which there is more rapid accumulation of radionuclide in the left hand, and *B,* in the 2.5-hour delayed bone scan in which increased radionuclide is present in the periarticular tissues.

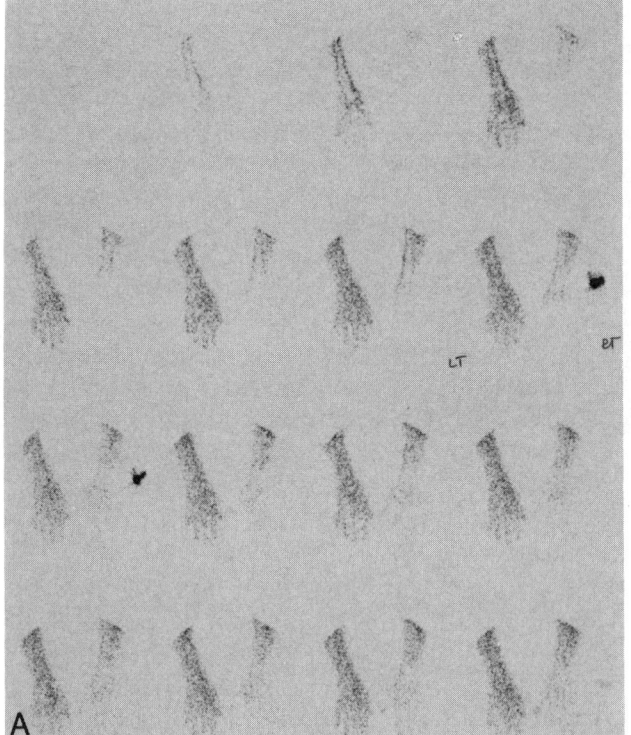

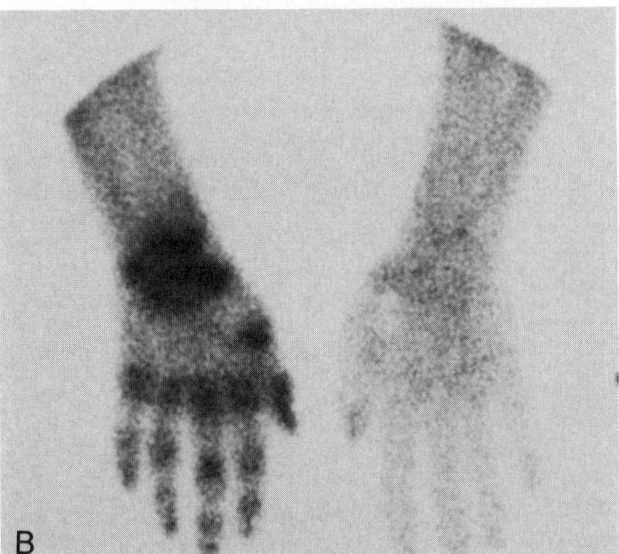

is hyperemic, and prominent osteoclastic activity is seen in the areas of patchy osteoporosis.[233,254,255,265] Fibrosis of the surface of affected cartilage may be observed.[265] Synovial tissue is abnormal and generally resembles that of the shoulder in adhesive capsulitis.[197] The histologic changes consist of proliferation of synovial lining cells and small blood vessels, synovial edema, and subsynovial fibrosis (Fig. 97–16). Little or no inflammatory cell infiltrate is present.

Any explanation of the pathophysiologic features of the reflex sympathetic dystrophy syndrome must account for its peculiar clinical features, such as nonsegmental pain, trophic skin changes, and vasomotor instability, its radiographic findings of patchy osteopenia, and its evidence of increased local blood flow.[233,243,266,267] Although a number of theories have been proposed, most suggest a disturbance of autonomic nervous system regulation to explain these diverse findings. Little true evidence of autonomic nerve dysfunction exists, however.

Moberg attributes the reflex sympathetic dystrophy syndrome primarily to a mechanical disturbance of venous and lymphatic flow.[268] He suggests that shoulder and hand movements are essential for fluid removal from the extremity, and any interference in this mechanism produces edema, further limitation of motion, disuse osteopenia, and, eventually, contracture formation. A second factor, sympathetic nervous system stimulation, occasionally contributes to the pain and limitation of motion when the syndrome is initiated by a traumatic, usually painful, injury. Although intriguing, especially with regard to the shoulder-hand syndrome, this hypothesis fails to account for the syndrome after painless, nonimmobilizing events, such as drug ingestion,[269,270] after myocardial ischemia with pain in the opposite arm,[212] or in isolated regions, for example, the hand or the patella.[223]

Theories supporting the primary involvement of the sympathetic nervous system are more popular and have been reviewed recently.[223,224] These may be divided into either the peripheral or the central hypothesis, depending on the site of injury. The central hypothesis was favored by De Takats and Steinbrocker and their co-workers,[234,235,265,271] who championed the theory of Livingston,[272] who originally proposed that a painful peripheral stimulus produced excessive, repetitive excitation of the internuncial neuron pool in the spinal cord. Spread of these impulses to adjacent areas in the spinal cord then activates efferent autonomic and motor nerves and results in increased blood flow, vasomotor changes, and other "dystrophic" changes in bone and soft tissues. These factors, in turn, produce further sensory input and establish a vicious cycle between central and pe-

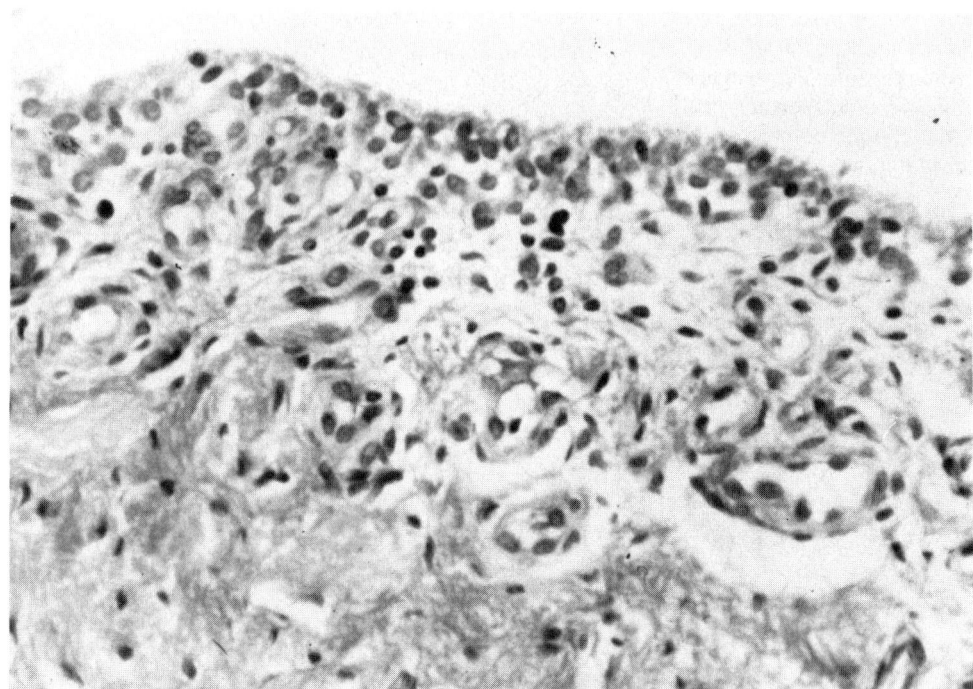

FIG. 97–16. Photomicrograph of synovium of a metacarpophalangeal joint from a patient with the reflex sympathetic dystrophy syndrome, illustrating synoviocyte and vascular proliferation.

ripheral mechanisms of pain and response. Livingston's theory may explain the reflex sympathetic dystrophy syndrome in any location and may be extended to precipitants other than pain because changes in the central regulatory mechanism may be caused by drugs, stroke, or other provocative stimuli.

Noordenhos and others have offered an intriguing variant of this mechanism.[273] Two types of nerve fibers are suggested to exist: small fibers that carry the painful impulse and large fibers that inhibit its transmission. Normally, a delicate balance exists under central control, but a shift in this balance may result in excessive pain, either real or imagined, and may establish the vicious cycle already described. The beneficial effects of selective large-fiber stimulation in certain patients with causalgia support this proposal.[274,275]

More recently, the gate-control theory of pain, which combines many features of the aforementioned mechanisms, has achieved prominence.[276,277] In this model, a dynamic balance that exists between large, inhibitory and small, effector neurons is influenced by cognitive and perceptual processes in the central nervous system. Because the sympathetic nervous system impulses also feed into the same receptor center(s), stimulation of efferent sympathetic fibers may produce the reflex sympathetic dystrophy syndrome, by ascending "painful" sources such as trauma; by descending cognitive or perceptual mechanisms such as stroke, drugs, or trauma; or by direct irritation of the receptor center(s) such as by stroke, drugs, or cervical spine or spinal cord lesions.

Roberts extended this view by proposing that nociceptive inputs may excite wide-dynamic-range neurons in the spinal cord, causing these neurons to become sensitized to subsequent afferent input.[231] Afferent stimuli may be initiated by sympathetic nerves to produce a painful state or to maintain a painful state following injury. Alternatively, increased sympathetic activity may lower the threshold of nociceptor or mechanoreceptor function.

TREATMENT

Because the natural history of this syndrome is so variable and unpredictable, results of the usual therapeutic approaches are difficult to interpret. Therapy appears to have little relation to the initiating or provocative event, the severity of trauma, or the stage of disease. It is generally thought that the earlier the institution of therapy, the better the result.[206,212] Rosen and Graham examined this problem carefully and found that only 20% of patients symptomatic for 6 months or longer had a good or excellent response to treatment, as compared with 43% of those with symptoms of shorter duration.[212] The overall response rate was poor, however; over 50% of their patients had significant pain or disability 2 to 6 years later. Other authors suggest that most patients recover in 6 to 24 months.[278,279]

Clearly, avoidance of the syndrome is the best treatment. Early mobilization following trauma[280] or myocardial infarction[199] may be helpful in this regard, although even this concept is controversial.[138,281] Once the disease process is established, a number of therapeutic approaches have been advocated, including exercises, various physical therapeutic techniques, sympathetic blockade, local or systemic corticosteroids, vasodilator drugs, α- or β-adrenergic drugs, and continuous elevation of the involved extremity. None are specific; all are most effective when used early. Unfortunately, even today, prolonged delays in recognition of the syndrome and in institution of therapy are common.[211]

The basic treatment program should consist of analgesic medications, local heat or cold packs, and exercises of the affected and contralateral extremities to improve motion. A favorable result may be expected in a majority of patients with these conservative measures if treatment is started early in the course of the disease,[206,209] especially in children.[215,220] More aggressive therapy is indicated if a satisfactory result is not obtained within 1 to 4 weeks. The most effective therapeutic measures are sympathetic blockade and administration of systemic corticosteroids.

Sympathetic blockade represents a rational attempt to block the vicious cycle of pain at an accessible site in the efferent pain pathway. Results of this approach are variable, although the patient may have partial or transient relief of pain.[208,211,282] Satisfactory control of symptoms, defined as a 50% relief of pain or a significant reduction in disability, can be expected in only 14 to 25% of patients,[142,172,199,208,211,283] although several authors report response rates as high as 50 to 100%.[204,282,284] My own experience with stellate ganglion blockade has been discouraging,[210] and Patman et al. found that all 41 causalgic patients treated with sympathetic blockade later required surgical sympathectomy.[211] Frequently, a series of daily or alternate-day sympathetic blocks are required;[282] this approach should be abandoned if 3 to 5 successive blocks fail to provide lasting symptomatic relief. Patients who benefit from sympathetic blockade appear to be excellent candidates for surgical sympathectomy. Results of this procedure appear to be rewarding, both in reduction of pain and in restoration of motion.[208,211,285]

Other methods for interrupting sympathetic tone appear to be effective as well, including regional intravenous reserpine,[286–288] or guanethidine, which is not approved by the United States Food and Drug Administration,[83,289–291] or oral phenoxybenzamine.[292] β-adrenergic blocking agents have been beneficial in some,[293,294] but not all,[286] patients.

Systemic corticosteroids are effective in controlling the reflex sympathetic dystrophy syndrome,[197,200,210,212,295–297] although the use of these agents is not without controversy.[298] Studies of high-dose corticosteroid treatment, using sensitive, quantifiable methods of assessment, showed improvement in a majority of patients with a reflex dystrophy.[197,210,296] These findings have been confirmed.[266] Although not all patients had a complete recovery, most experienced marked, lasting pain relief and restoration of function. Furthermore, progression of osteopenia appeared to be reduced in adults,[197] as well as reversed in a child.[218] Patients with positive scintigraphic evidence of the disease appeared to respond best to corticosteroids.[210]

Initial therapy should consist of 60 to 80 mg prednisone or an equivalent preparation daily *in 4 divided doses*. In 1 to 2 weeks, one can rapidly reduce the dose, with the aim of discontinuing corticosteroids entirely after 3 to 4 weeks of treatment. One often sees a mild, "poststeroid" exacerbation, which usually resolves within 10 days.[197,210] Occasionally, patients require retreatment, in which case a longer period of high-dose therapy, lasting 2 to 4 weeks, and a more gradual tapering program, lasting 4 to 8 weeks, are indicated. Rarely, a maintenance dose of prednisone, 5 to 10 mg on alternate days or 5 mg daily, is required to control symptoms permanently. Lower doses have been used successfully.[266] Intravenous injection of corticosteroids into the affected extremity may be an effective approach.[299]

Unlike the interruption of sympathetic pathways, no currently known theoretic mechanisms explain the efficacy of corticosteroids in the reflex sympathetic dystrophy syndrome. It is possible that these agents interfere with the action of peripheral mediators, which perhaps are prostaglandin-like substances, or they may modulate the transmission of neural impulses in the gate-control system or the internuncial pool.

Other agents, including griseofulvin and calcitonin, have been used effectively in patients with algodystrophy;[261] it is not clear whether all patients with this diagnosis fulfill the rigorous criteria of the reflex sympathetic dystrophy syndrome.

Recent studies employing transcutaneous nerve stimulation in patients with causalgia following nerve injuries have been encouraging,[300,301] although this technique has failed on occasion.[286] Again, the best responses were obtained in patients symptomatic for brief periods prior to treatment.

REFERENCES

1. DePalma, A.F.: Surgery of the Shoulder. 3rd ed. Philadelphia, J.B. Lippincott, 1983.

2. Boileau Grant, J.C., and Basmajian, J.V.: Grant's Method of Anatomy. 7th ed. Baltimore, Williams & Wilkins, 1965.

3. Inman, V.T., Saunders, J.B., and Abbott, L.C.: Observations on the function of the shoulder joint. J. Bone Joint Surg., 26:1–30, 1944.

4. Conway, A.M.: Movements in the sternoclavicular and acromioclavicular joints. Phys. Ther. Rev., 41:421–432, 1975.

5. Rothman, R.H., Marvel, J.P., and Heppenstall, R.B.: Anatomic considerations in the glenohumeral joint. Orthop. Clin. North Am., 6:341–352, 1975.

6. Saha, A.K.: Dynamic stability of the glenohumeral joint. Acta Orthop. Scand., 42:491–505, 1971.

7. Turkel, S.J., et al.: Stabilizing mechanisms preventing anterior dislocation of the gleno-humeral joint. J. Bone Joint Surg., 63A:1208, 1981.

8. Poppen, N.K., and Walker, P.S.: Forces at the glenohumeral joint in abduction. Clin. Orthop., 135:165–170, 1978.

9. Lucas, D.B.: Biomechanics of the shoulder joint. Arch. Surg., 107:425–432, 1973.

10. Basmajian, J.V.: Muscles Alive: Their Functions Revealed by Electromyography. Baltimore, Williams & Wilkins, 1962, pp. 161–178.

11. Poppen, N.K., and Walker, P.S.: Normal and abnormal motion of the shoulder. J. Bone Joint Surg., 58A:195–201, 1976.

12. Howell, S.M., Imobersteg, A.M., Seger, D.H., and Marone, P.J.: Clarification of the role of the supraspinatus muscle in shoulder function. J. Bone Joint Surg., 68A:398–404, 1986.

13. Colachis, S.C., Jr., and Strohm, B.R.: Effect of suprascapular and axillary nerve blocks on muscle force in upper extremity. Arch. Phys. Med. Rehabil., 52:22–29, 1971.

14. Booth, R.E., and Marvel, J.P.: Differential diagnosis of shoulder pain. Orthop. Clin. North Am., 6:353–379, 1975.

15. Moseley, H.F.: Shoulder Lesions. 3rd ed. Edinburgh, Churchill Livingstone, 1969.

16. Badley, E.M., Wagstaff, S., and Wood, P.H.N.: Measures of functional ability (disability) in arthritis in relation to impairment of range of joint movement. Ann. Rheum. Dis., 43:563–569, 1984.

17. Neer, C.S.: Anterior acromoplasty for the chronic impingement syndrome in the shoulder. J. Bone Joint Surg., 54A:41–50, 1972.

18. Jobe, F.W., and Jobe, C.M.: Painful athletic injuries of the shoulder. Clin. Orthop., 173:117–124, 1983.

19. Gerster, J.C., et al.: Tendon calcification in chondrocalcinosis. Arthritis Rheum., 20:717–722, 1977.

20. Reichmann, S., et al.: Soft tissue xeroradiography of the shoulder joint. Acta Radiol. (Diagn.), 21:572–576, 1975.

21. Freiberger, R.H., and Kaye, J.J.: Arthrography. New York, Appleton-Century-Crofts, 1979.

22. Goldman, A.B., and Ghelman, B.: The double-contrast shoulder arthrogram. Radiology, 127:655–663, 1978.

23. Neviaser, J.S.: Adhesive capsulitis of the shoulder: A study of the pathological findings in periarthritis of the shoulder. J. Bone Joint Surg., 27:211–222, 1945.

24. Reeves, B.: Arthrographic changes in frozen and post-traumatic stiff shoulders. Proc. R. Soc. Med., 59:827–830, 1966.

25. Hall, F.M., et al.: Morbidity from shoulder arthrography: Etiology, incidence, and prevention. Am. J. Roentgenol., 136:59–62, 1981.

26. Mink, J.H., Harris, E., and Rappaport, M.: Rotator cuff tears: Evaluation using double-contrast shoulder arthrography. Radiology, 157:621–623, 1985.

27. Resnick, D.: Shoulder arthrography. Radiol. Clin. North Am., 19:243–253, 1981.

28. Braunstein, E.M., and O'Connor, G.: Double-contrast arthrotomography of the shoulder. J. Bone Joint Surg., 64A:192–195, 1982.

29. McGlynn, F.J., El-Khoury, G., and Albright, J.P.: Arthrotomography of the glenoid labrum in shoulder instability. J. Bone Joint Surg., 64A:506–518, 1982.

30. Lie, S., and Mast, W.A.: Subacromial bursography. Radiology, 144:626–630, 1982.

31. Bekerman, C., et al.: Radionuclide imaging of the bones and joints of the hand: A definition of normal and a comparison of sensitivity using ^{99m}Tc-pertechnetate and ^{99m}Tc-diphosphonate. Radiology, 118:653–659, 1976.

32. Maxfield, W.S., Weiss, T.E., and Shirler, S.E.: Synovial membrane scanning in arthritic disease. Semin. Nucl. Med., 2:50–70, 1972.

33. O'Duffy, J.D., Wahner, H.W., and Hunder, G.G.: Joint imaging in polymyalgia rheumatica. Mayo Clin. Proc., 51:519–531, 1976.

34. Wright, V., and Haq, A.M.M.M.: Periarthritis of the shoulder. I. Aetiological considerations with particular reference to personality factors. Ann. Rheum. Dis., 35:213–219, 1976.

35. Genoe, G.A., and Moeller, J.A.: Normal shoulder variations in the technetium 99m polyphosphate bone scan. South. Med. J., 67:659–662, 1974.

36. Sebes, J.I., Vasinrapee, P., and Friedman, B.I.: The relationship between radiographic findings and asymmetrical radioactivity in the shoulder. Radiology, 120:139–142, 1976.

37. Stodell, M.A., et al.: Radio-isotope scanning in the painful shoulder. Rheumatol. Rehabil., 19:163–166, 1980.

38. Middleton, W.D., et al.: Sonographic detection of rotator cuff tears. Am. J. Roentgenol., 144:349–353, 1985.

39. Mack, L.A., et al.: US evaluation of the rotator cuff. Radiology, 157:205–209, 1985.

40. Middleton, W.D., et al.: Ultrasonographic evaluation of the rotator cuff and biceps tendon. J. Bone Joint Surg., 68A:440–450, 1986.

41. Deutsch, A.L., et al.: Computed and conventional arthrotomography of the glenohumeral joint: Normal anatomy and clinical experience. Radiology, 153:603–609, 1984.

42. Rafii, M., et al.: Athlete shoulder injuries. CT arthrographic findings. Radiology, 162:559–564, 1987.

43. Beltran, J., et al.: Rotator cuff lesions of the shoulder: Evaluation by direct sagittal CT orthography. Radiology, 160:161–165, 1986.

44. Kieft, G.J., et al.: Normal shoulder: MR imaging. Radiology, 159:741–745, 1986.

45. Seeger, L.L., et al.: MR imaging of the normal shoulder: Anatomic correlation. Am. J. Roentgenol., 148:83–91, 1987.

46. Middleton, W.D., et al.: High resolution MR imaging of the normal rotator cuff. Am. J. Roentgenol., 148:559–564, 1987.

47. Kneeland, J.B., et al.: Rotator cuff tears: Preliminary application of high resolution MR imaging with counter rotating current loop-gap resonators. Radiology, 160:695–699, 1986.

48. Anderson, B.C., and Kaye, S.: Shoulder pain: Differential diagnosis. West. J. Med., 138:268–269, 1983.

49. Neer, C.S.: Impingement lesions. Clin. Orthop., 173:70–77, 1983.

50. Penny, J.N., and Welch, R.P.: Shoulder impingement syndromes in athletes and their surgical management. Am. J. Sports Med., 9:11–15, 1981.

51. Cone, R.O., Resnick, D., and Danzig, L.: Shoulder impingement syndrome: Radiographic evaluation. Radiology, 150:29–33, 1984.

52. Hardy, D.C., Vogler, J.B., III, and White, R.H.: The shoulder

impingement syndrome: Prevalence of radiographic findings and correlation with response to therapy. Am. J. Roentgenol., *147*:557–561, 1986.

53. Strizak, A.M., et al.: Subacromial bursography. J. Bone Joint Surg., *64A*:196–201, 1982.

54. Ha'eri, G.B., and Wiley, A.M.: Advancement of the supraspinatus muscle in the repair of ruptures of the rotator cuff. J. Bone Joint Surg., *63A*:232–238, 1981.

55. Post, M., and Cohen, J.: Impingement syndrome. A review of late stage II and early stage III lesions. Clin. Orthop., *207*:126–132, 1986.

56. Tibone, J.E., et al.: Shoulder impingement syndrome in athletes treated by an anterior acromioplasty. Clin. Orthop., *198*:134–140, 1985.

57. Rathburn, J.B., and Macnab, I.: The microvascular pattern of the rotator cuff. J. Bone Joint Surg., *52B*:540–553, 1970.

58. Rothman, R.H., and Parke, W.W.: The vascular anatomy of the rotator cuff. Clin. Orthop., *41*:176–186, 1965.

59. Herberts, P., et al.: Shoulder pain in industry: An epidemiological study on welders. Acta Orthop. Scand., *52*:299–306, 1981.

60. Campbell, H.L., and Feldman, F.: Bone and soft tissue abnormalities of the upper extremity in diabetes mellitus. Am. J. Roentgenol., *124*:7–16, 1975.

61. Trapp, R.G., Soler, N.G., and Spencer-Green, G.: Musculoskeletal abnormalities of the upper extremities and neck in insulin dependent diabetics: symptomatology and physical findings. (Abstract.) Arthritis Rheum., *26*:547, 1983.

62. Kerwein, G.A., Roseberg, B., and Sneed, W.R.: Aids in differential diagnosis of the painful shoulder syndrome. Clin. Orthop., *20*:11–20, 1961.

63. Kessel, L., and Wastson, M.: The painful arc syndrome: clinical classification as a guide to management. J. Bone Joint Surg., *59B*:166–172, 1977.

64. Pedersen, H.E., and Key, J.A.: Pathology of calcareous tendinitis and subdeltoid bursitis. Arch. Surg., *62*:50–63, 1951.

65. McClure, J., and Gardner, D.L.: The production of calcification in connective tissue and skeletal muscle using various chemical compounds. Calcif. Tissue Res., *22*:129–135, 1976.

66. Selye, H., Goldie, I., and Strebel, R.: Calciphylaxis in relation to calcification in periarticular tissues. Clin. Orthop., *28*:151–158, 1963.

67. Parfitt, A.M., et al.: Disordered calcium and phosphorus metabolism during maintenance hemodialysis. Am. J. Med., *51*:319–330, 1971.

68. Christensen, W.K., Liebman, C., and Sosman, M.C.: Skeletal and periarticular manifestations of hypervitaminosis D. Am. J. Roentgenol., *65*:27–41, 1951.

69. McCarty, D.J., and Gatter, R.A.: Recurrent acute inflammation associated with focal apatite crystal deposition. Arthritis Rheum., *9*:804–819, 1964.

70. Pinals, R.S., and Short, C.L.: Calcific periarthritis involving multiple sites. Arthritis Rheum., *9*:566–574, 1966.

71. Luben, R.A., and Wadkins, C.L.: Studies of the relationship of proton production and calcification of tendon matrix in vitro. Biochemistry, *10*:2183, 1971.

72. Luben, R.A., Sherman, J.K., and Wadkins, C.L.: Studies of the mechanism of biological calcification. IV. Ultrastructural analysis of calcifying tendon matrix. Calcif. Tissue Res., *11*:39–55, 1973.

73. Urist, M.R., Moss, M.J., and Adams, J.M.: Calcification of tendon: A triphasic local mechanism. Arch. Pathol., *77*:594–608, 1964.

74. Fisher, L.W., and Termine, J.D.: Noncollagenous proteins influencing the local mechanisms of calcification. Clin. Orthop., *200*:362–385, 1985.

75. Addadi, L., and Weiner, S.: Interactions between acidic proteins and crystals: Stereochemical requirements in biomineralization. Proc. Natl. Acad. Sci. USA, *82*:4110–4114, 1985.

76. Poole, A.R., Rosenberg, L.C.: Chondrocalcin and the calcification of cartilage. Clin. Orthop., *208*:114–118, 1986.

77. de Bernard, B.: Glycoproteins in the local mechanism of calcification. Clin. Orthop., *162*:233–244, 1982.

78. Neuman, W.F., et al.: Blood:bone disequilibrium. VI. Studies of the solubility characteristics of brushite:apatite mixtures and their stabilization by noncollagenous proteins of bone. Calcif. Tissue Int., *34*:149–157, 1982.

79. Termine, J.D., Eanes, E.D., and Conn, K.M.: Phosphoprotein modulation of apatite crystallization. Calcif. Tissue Int., *31*:247–251, 1980.

80. Yaari, A.M., Shapiro, I.M., and Brown, C.E.: Evidence that phosphatidylserine and inorganic phosphate may mediate calcium transport during calcification. Biochem. Biophys. Res. Comm., *105*:778–784, 1982.

81. Quigley, T.B.: The nonoperative treatment of symptomatic calcareous deposits in the shoulder. Surg. Clin. North Am., *6*:1495–1503, 1963.

82. Lippmann, R.K.: Observations concerning the calcific cuff deposit. Clin. Orthop., *20*:49–60, 1961.

83. McKendry, R.J.R., et al.: Calcifying tendinitis of the shoulder: Prognostic value of clinical, histologic, and radiologic features in 57 surgically treated cases. J. Rheumatol., *9*:75–80, 1982.

84. Bosworth, B.M.: Calcium deposits in the shoulder and subacromial bursitis: a survey of 12,122 shoulders. JAMA, *116*:2477–2482, 1941.

85. Simon, W.H.: Soft tissue disorders of the shoulder. Orthop. Clin. North Am., *6*:521–539, 1975.

86. ViGario, G.D., and Keats, T.E.: Localization of calcific deposits in the shoulder. Am. J. Roentgenol., *108*:806–811, 1970.

87. Kotzen, L.M.: Roentgen diagnosis of rotator cuff tear: Report of 48 surgically proven cases. Am. J. Roentgenol., *112*:507–511, 1971.

88. Wolfgang, G.L.: Surgical repair of tears of the rotator cuff or the shoulder. J. Bone Joint Surg., *56A*:14–26, 1974.

89. Killoran, J.R., Marcone, R.C., and Freiberger, R.H.: Shoulder arthrography. Am. J. Roentgenol., *103*:658–668, 1968.

90. Soave, G., et al.: Indoproten versus indomethacin in acute painful shoulder and other soft-tissue rheumatic complaints. J. Int. Med. Res., *10*:99–103, 1982.

91. Bulgen, D.Y., et al.: Frozen shoulder: Prospective clinical study with an evaluation of three treatment regimens. Ann. Rheum. Dis., *43*:353–360, 1984.

92. Ward, M.C., Kirwan, J.R., Norris, P., and Murray, N.: Paracetamol and diclofenac in the painful shoulder syndrome. (Letter.) Br. J. Rheumatol., *25*:412, 1986.

93. Benson, T.B., and Copp, E.P.: The effects of therapeutic forms of heat and ice on the pain threshold of the normal shoulder. Rheumatol. Rehabil., *13*:101–104, 1974.

94. Berry, H., et al.: Clinical study comparing acupuncture, physiotherapy, injection and oral-anti-inflammatory therapy in shoulder-cuff lesions. Curr. Med. Res. Opin., *7*:121–126, 1980.

95. Binder, A., Parr, B., and Fitton-Jackson, S.: Pulsed electromagnetic field therapy of persistent rotator cuff tendinitis. A double-blind controlled assessment. Lancet *1*:695–698, 1984.

96. Harvey, W., et al.: The stimulation of protein synthesis in human fibroblasts by therapeutic ultrasound. Rheumatol. Rehabil., *14*:237, 1975.

97. Richardson, A.T.: The painful shoulder. Proc. R. Soc. Med., 68:731–736, 1975.

98. Moore, M.E., and Berk, S.N.: Acupuncture for chronic shoulder pain: An experimental study with attention to the role of placebo and hypnotic susceptibility. Ann. Intern. Med., 84:381–384, 1976.

99. Hashish, I., Harvey, W., and Harris, W.: Anti-inflammatory effects of ultrasound therapy: Evidence for a major placebo effect. Br. J. Rheumatol., 25:77–81, 1986.

100. Downing, D., and Weinstein, A.: Ultrasound therapy of subacromial bursitis: A double blind trial. (Abstract.) Arthritis Rheum., 26:S87, 1983.

101. Symposium: DMSO in musculoskeletal conditions. Ann. N.Y. Acad. Sci., 141:493, 1967.

102. McMillan, J.A.: Therapeutic exercise for shoulder disabilities. J. Am. Phys. Ther. Assoc., 46:1052–1060, 1966.

103. Fitzgerald, R.H.: Intrasynovial injection of steroids: Uses and abuses. Mayo Clin. Proc., 51:655–659, 1976.

104. Roy, S., and Oldham, R.: Management of painful shoulder. Lancet, 1:1322–1324, 1976.

105. Steinbrocker, O., and Neustadt, D.H.: Aspiration and Injection Therapy in Arthritis and Musculo-Skeletal Disorders. Hagerstown, MD, Harper & Row, 1972.

106. Koehler, B.E., Urowitz, M.B., and Killinger, D.W.: The systemic effects of intra-articular corticosteroid. J. Rheumatol., 1:117–125, 1974.

107. Asboe-Hansen, G.: Influence of corticosteroids on connective tissue. Dermatologica, 152:127–132, 1976.

108. Sweetham, R.: Corticosteroid arthropathy and tendon rupture. J. Bone Joint Surg., 51B:397–398, 1969.

109. McCarty, D.J., and Hogan, J.: Inflammatory reaction after intrasynovial injection of microcrystalline adrenocorticosteroid esters. Arthritis Rheum., 7:359–367, 1964.

110. Darlington, L.G., and Coombs, E.N.: The effects of local steroid injection for supraspinatus tears. Rheumatol. Rehabil., 16:172–179, 1977.

111. Comfort, T.H., and Arafiles, R.P.: Barbotage of the shoulder with image-intensified fluoroscopic control of needle placement for calcific tendinitis. Clin. Orthop., 135:171–178, 1978.

112. Nixon, J.E., and DiStefano, V.: Ruptures of the rotator cuff. Orthop. Clin. North Am., 6:423–447, 1975.

113. Neviaser, J.S.: Ruptures of the rotator cuff of the shoulder. Arch. Surg., 102:483–485, 1971.

114. Bakalim, G., and Pasila, M.: Rotator cuff tears. Acta Orthop. Scand., 46:751–757, 1975.

115. Samilson, R.L., and Brider, W.F.: Symptomatic full thickness tears of the rotator cuff: An analysis of 292 shoulders in 276 patients. Orthop. Clin. North Am., 6:449–466, 1975.

116. Weiss, J.J.: Intra-articular steroids in the treatment of rotator cuff tear: reappraisal by arthrography. Arch. Phys. Med. Rehabil., 62:555–557, 1981.

117. Post, M., Silver, R., and Singh, M.: Rotator cuff tear: Diagnosis and treatment. Clin. Orthop., 173:78–91, 1983.

118. Hawkins, R.J., Misamore, G.W., and Hobeika, P.E.: Surgery for full-thickness rotator-cuff tears. J. Bone Joint Surg., 67A:1349–1355, 1985.

119. Tibone, J.E., et at.: Surgical treatment of tears of the rotator cuff in athletes. J. Bone Joint Surg., 68A:887–891, 1986.

120. Ellman, H., Hanker, G., and Bayer, M.: Repair of the rotator cuff. End-result of factors influencing reconstruction. J. Bone Joint Surg., 68A:1136–1144, 1986.

121. Gore, D.R., Murray, M.P., Sepic, S.B., and Gardner, G.M.: Function after surgical repair of full-thickness rotator cuff tears. Long-term follow-up of fifty-one patients. Orthop. Trans., 9:466–467, 1985.

122. Cofield, R.H., and Lanzer, W.L.: Rotator cuff repair, results related to surgical pathology. Orthop. Trans., 9:466, 1985.

123. Middleton, W.D., et al.: US of the biceps tendon apparatus. Radiology, 157:211–215, 1985.

124. Neviaser, T.J., et al.: The four-in-one arthroplasty for the painful arc syndrome. Clin. Orthop., 163:107–112, 1983.

125. Bridgeman, J.F.: Periarthritis of the shoulder and diabetes mellitus. Ann. Rheum. Dis., 31:69, 1972.

126a. Withrington, R.H., Girgis, F.L., and Seifert, M.H.: A comparative study of the aetiological factors in shoulder pain. Br. J. Rheumatol., 24:24–26, 1985.

126b. Wright, M.G., Richards, A.J., and Clarke, M.B.: ^{99m}Tc-pertechnetate scanning in capsulitis. Lancet, 2:1265–1266, 1975.

127. Lee, P.N., et al.: Periarthritis of the shoulder, trial of treatments investigated by multivariate analysis. Ann. Rheum. Dis., 33:116–119, 1974.

128. Bulgen, D.Y., et al.: Immunological studies in frozen shoulder. Ann. Rheum. Dis., 37:135–138, 1978.

129. Bulgen, D.Y., Hazelman, B.L., and Voak, D.: HLA-B27 and frozen shoulder. Lancet, 1:1042–1044, 1976.

130. Noy, S., et al.: HLA-B27 and frozen shoulder. Tissue Antigens, 17:251, 1981.

131. Seignalet, J., et al.: Lack of association between HLA-B27 and frozen shoulder. Tissue Antigens, 18:364, 1981.

132. Akeson, W.H., et al.: The connective tissue response to immobility: Biochemical changes in periarticular connective tissue of the immobilized rabbit knee. Clin. Orthop., 93:356–362, 1973.

133. Lundberg, B.J.: Glycosaminoglycans of the normal and frozen shoulder-joint capsule. Clin. Orthop., 69:279–284, 1970.

134. Reeves, B.: The natural history of the frozen shoulder syndrome. Scand. J. Rheumatol., 4:193–196, 1975.

135. Wright, V., and Haq, A.M.M.M.: Periarthritis of the shoulder. II. Radiological features. Ann. Rheum. Dis., 35:220–226, 1976.

136. Ha'eri, G.B., and Maitland, A.: Arthroscopic findings in the frozen shoulder. J. Rheumatol., 8:149–152, 1981.

137. Binder, A.I., et al.: Frozen shoulder: An arthrographic and radionuclear scan assessment. Ann. Rheum. Dis., 43:365–369, 1984.

138. Brockelhurst, J.C., et al.: How much physical therapy for patients with stroke? Br. Med. J., 1:1307–1310, 1978.

139. Steinbrocker, O., and Argyros, T.G.: Frozen shoulder: Treatment by local injections of depot corticosteroids. Arch. Phys. Med. Rehabil., 55:209–213, 1974.

140. Williams, N.E., et al.: Treatent of capsulitis of the shoulder. Rheumatol. Rehabil., 14:236, 1975.

141. Tyler, M.A.: Treatment of the painful shoulder syndrome with amitriptyline and lithium carbonate. Can. Med. Assoc. J., 111:137–140, 1974.

142. Rizk, T.E., et al.: Adhesive capsulitis (frozen shoulder): A new approach to its management. Arch. Phys. Med. Rehabil., 64:29–33, 1983.

143. Kozin, F.: Painful shoulder and the reflex sympathetic dystrophy syndrome. In Arthritis and Allied Conditions, 9th ed. Edited by D.J. McCarty. Philadelphia, Lea & Febiger, 1979, pp. 1322–1355.

144. Older, M.W.H., McIntyre, J.L., and Lloyd, G.J.: Distension arthrography of the shoulder joint. Can. J. Surg., 19:203–207, 1976.

145. Gilula, L.A., Schoenecker, P.C., and Murphy. W.A.: Shoulder arthrography as a treatment modality. Am. J. Roentgenol., 131:1047–1048, 1978.

146. Thomas, D., Williams, R.A., and Smith, D.S.: The frozen shoulder: A review of manipulative treatment. Rheumatol. Rehabil., 19:173–179, 1980.

147. McNair, M.M., et al.: A clinical and radiological study of rheumatoid arthritis with a note on the findings in osteoarthrosis. I. The shoulder joint. Clin. Radiol., 20:269–277, 1969.

148. Zanca, P.: Shoulder pain: Involvement of the acromioclavicular joint. Am. J. Roentgenol., 112:493–506, 1971.

149. Quinn, S.F., and Glass, T.A.: Post-traumatic osteolysis of the clavicle. South. Med. J., 76:307–308, 1983.

150. Kaplan, P.A., Resnick, D.: Stress-induced osteolysis of the clavicle. Radiology, 158:139–140, 1986.

151. Sonozaki, H., et al.: Clinical features of 53 cases with pustulotic arthro-osteitis. Ann. Rheum. Dis., 40:541–553, 1981.

152. Nilsson, B.E., and Uden, A.: Skeletal lesions in palmar-plantar pustulosis. Acta Orthop. Scand., 55:366–370, 1984.

153. Sartoris, D.J., et al.: Sternocostoclavicular hyperostosis: A review and report of 11 cases. Radiology, 158:125–128, 1986.

154. Chigira, M., et al.: Sternoclavicular hyperostosis. A report of nineteen cases, with special reference to etiology and treatment. J. Bone Joint Surg., 68A:103–112, 1986.

155. Kofold, H., Thomsen, P., and Lindenberg, S.: Serous synovitis of the sternoclavicular joint. Differential diagnostic aspects. Scand. J. Rheumatol., 14:61–64, 1985.

156. Paice, E.W., Wright, F.W., and Hill, A.G.S.: Sternoclavicular erosions in polymyalgia rheumatica. Ann. Rheum. Dis., 42:379–383, 1983.

157. Healey, L.A.: Long-term follow-up of polymyalgia rheumatica: Evidence for synovitis. Semin. Arthritis Rheum., 13:322–336, 1984.

158. Pierce, R.: Internal derangement of the sternoclavicular joint. Clin. Orthop., 141:247–250, 1979.

159. Meachim, G.: Effect of age on the thickness of adult articular cartilage at the shoulder joint. Ann. Rheum. Dis., 30:43–46, 1971.

160. McCarty, D.J., et al.: "Milwaukee shoulder"—Association of microspheroids containing hydroxyapatite crystals, active collagenase, and neutral protease with rotator cuff defects. I. Clinical aspects. Arthritis Rheum., 24:464–473, 1981.

161. Halverson, P.B., McCarty, D.J., Cheung, H.S., and Ryan, L.M.: Milwaukee shoulder syndrome: Eleven additional cases with involvement of the knee in seven (basic calcium phosphate crystal deposition disease). Semin. Arthritis Rheum., 14:36–44, 1984.

162. Samilson, R.L., and Preito, V.: Dislocation arthropathy of the shoulder. J. Bone Joint Surg., 65A:456–460, 1983.

163. Neer, C.S., II, Craig, E.V., and Fukuda, H.: Cuff-tear arthropathy. J. Bone Joint Surg., 65A:1232–1244, 1983.

164. Dennis, D.A., Ferlic, D.C., and Clayton, M.L.: Acromial stress fractures associated with cuff-tear arthropathy. J. Bone Joint Surg., 68A:937–940, 1986.

165. Hellmann, D.B., Helms, C.A., and Genant, H.K.: Chronic repetitive trauma: A cause of atypical degenerative joint disease. Skeletal Radiol., 10:236–242, 1983.

166. Pasila, M., et al.: Recovery from primary shoulder dislocation and its complications. Acta Orthop. Scand., 51:257–262, 1980.

167. Chung, S.M.K., and Nissenbaum, M.M.: Congenital and developmental defects of the shoulder. Orthop. Clin. North Am., 6:381–392, 1975.

168. Tachdjian, M.O.: Pediatric Orthopedics. Philadelphia, W.B. Saunders, 1972.

169. Leffert, R.D.: Brachial plexus injuries. N. Engl. J. Med., 291:1059–1067, 1974.

170. Meyer, R.D.: Treatment of adult and obstetrical brachial plexus injuries. Orthopedics, 9:899–903, 1986.

171. Clodius, L., Uhlschmid, G., and Hess, K.: Irradiation plexitis of the brachial plexus. Clin. Plast. Surg., 11:161–165, 1984.

172. Garcia, G., and McQueen, D.: Bilateral suprascapular-nerve entrapment syndrome. J. Bone Joint Surg., 63A:491–492, 1981.

173. Ganzhorn, R.W., et al.: Suprascapular nerve entrapment. J. Bone Joint Surg., 63A:492–494, 1981.

174. Berry, H., and Bril, V.: Axillary nerve palsy following blunt trauma to the shoulder region: A cervical and electrophysiological review. J. Neurol. Neurosurg. Psychiatry, 45:1027–1032, 1982.

175. Gathier, J.C., and Bruyn, G.W.: Neuralgic amyotrophy. In Handbook of Clinical Neurology. Vol. 8. Diseases of Nerves. Part II. Edited by P.J. Vinkin and G.W. Bruyn. New York, American Elsevier, 1970, pp. 77–85.

176. Petersson, C.J.: Painful shoulders in patients with rheumatoid arthritis: Prevalent clinical and radiological features. Scand. J. Rheumatol., 15:275–279, 1986.

177. Kalliomaki, J.L., Viitanen, S.-M., and Virtama, P.: Radiological findings of sternoclavicular joints in rheumatoid arthritis. Acta Rheumatol. Scand., 14:223–240, 1968.

178. Kaklamanis, P., et al.: Calcification of the shoulders and diabetes mellitus. N. Engl. J. Med., 293:1266–1267, 1975.

179. Pal, B., Anderson, J., Dick, W.C., and Griffiths, I.D.: Limitation of joint mobility and shoulder capsulitis in insulin- and non-insulin-dependent diabetes mellitus. Br. J. Rheumatol., 25:147–151, 1986.

180. Fisher, L., Kurtz, A., and Shipley, M.: Association between cheiroarthropathy and frozen shoulder in patients with insulin-dependent diabetes mellitus. Br. J. Rheumatol., 25:141–146, 1986.

181. Eaton, R.P.: Aldose reductase inhibition and the diabetic syndrome of limited joint mobility: Implications for altered collagen hydration. Metabolism, 35(Suppl 1):119–121, 1986.

182. Hadler, N.M., et al.: Acute polyarticular gout. Am. J. Med., 56:715–719, 1974.

183. Okazaki, I., et al.: Pseudogout: clinical observations and chemical analysis of deposits. Arthritis Rheum., 19:293–306, 1976.

184. Rosati, L.M., and Lord, J.W.: Neurovascular Compression Syndromes of the Shoulder Girdle. New York, Grune and Stratton, 1961.

185. Tyson, R.R., and Kaplan, G.F.: Modern concepts of diagnosis and treatment of the thoracic outlet syndrome. Orthop. Clin. North Am., 6:507–519, 1975.

186. Dunant, J.H.: The diagnosis of thoracic outlet syndrome. In Pain in the Shoulder and Arm. Edited by J.M. Greep, et al. The Hague, Martinus Nijhoff, 1979.

187. De Sliva, M.: The costoclavicular syndrome: A "new cause." Ann. Rheum. Dis., 45:916–920, 1986.

188. Swift, T.R., and Nichols, F.T.: The droopy shoulder syndrome. Neurology, 34:212–215, 1984.

189. Gergoudis, R., and Barnes, R.W.: Thoracic outlet arterial compression: Prevalence in normal persons. Angiology, 31:538–541, 1980.

190. Stallworth, J.M., Quinn, G.J., and Aiken, A.F.: Is rib resection necessary for relief of thoracic outlet syndrome? Ann. Surg., 185:581–589, 1979.

191. Wilborn, A.J., and Lederman, R.J.: Evidence for a conduction delay in thoracic outlet syndrome is challenged. N. Engl. J. Med., 310:1052, 1984.

192. Yiannikas, C., and Walsh, J.C.: Somatosensory evoked re-

sponses in the diagnosis of thoracic outlet syndrome. J. Neurol. Neurosurg. Psychiatry, 46:234, 1983.

193. Stallworth, J.M., and Horne, J.B.: Diagnosis and management of thoracic outlet syndrome. Arch. Surg., 119:1149–1151, 1984.

194. Mitchell, S.W.: Injuries of Nerves and Their Consequences. Philadelphia, J.B. Lippincott, 1872.

195. Richards, R.L.: The term 'causalgia.' Med. Hist., 11:97–99, 1967.

196. Mitchell, S.W., Moorehouse, G.R., and Keen, W.W.: Gunshot Wounds and Other Injuries of Nerves. Philadelphia, J.B. Lippincott, 1864.

197. Kozin, F., et al.: The reflex sympathetic dystrophy syndrome. I. Clinical and histologic studies: Evidence for bilaterality, response to corticosteroids, and articular involvement. Am. J. Med., 60:321–331, 1976.

198. Johnson, A.C.: Disabling changes in the hands resembling sclerodactylia following myocardial infarction. Ann. Intern. Med., 19:443–456, 1943.

199. Russek, H.I.: Shoulder-hand syndrome following myocardial infarction. Med. Clin. North Am., 42:1555–1556, 1958.

200. Davis, S.W., et al.: Shoulder-hand syndrome in a hemiplegic population: 5-year retrospective study. Arch. Phys. Med. Rehabil., 58:353–356, 1977.

201. Eto, F., et al.: Shoulder-hand syndrome as a complication of hemiplegia. Jpn. J. Geriatr., 12:245–251, 1977.

202. Bacorn, R.W., and Kurtzke, J.F.: Colles' fracture: A study of two thousand cases from the New York State Workman's Compensation fund. J. Bone Joint Surg., 35A:643–658, 1953.

203. Cooney, W.P., Dobyns, J.H., and Linscheid, R.L.: Complications of Colles' fracture. J. Bone Joint Surg., 62A:613–619, 1980.

204. Dunningham, T.H.: The treatment of Sudeck's atrophy in the upper limb by sympathetic blockade. Injury, 12:139–144, 1981.

205. Plewes, L.W.: Sudeck's atrophy in the hands. J. Bone Joint Surg., 38B:195–203, 1956.

206. Pak, T.J., et al.: Reflex sympathetic dystrophy—A review of 140 cases. Minn. Med., 53:507–511, 1970.

207. Acquaviva, P., et al.: Reflex dystrophies: Background and etiological factors. Rev. Rhum. Mal. Osteoartic., 49:761–766, 1982.

208. Evans, J.A.: Reflex sympathetic dystrophy: Report on 57 cases. Ann. Intern. Med., 26:417–426, 1947.

209. Johnson, E.W., and Pannozzo, A.N.: Management of shoulder-hand syndrome. JAMA, 195:152–154, 1966.

210. Kozin, F., et al.: The reflex sympathetic dystrophy syndrome (RSDS) III. Scintigraphic studies, further evidence for the therapeutic efficacy of systemic corticosteroids, and proposed diagnostic criteria. Am. J. Med., 70:23–30, 1981.

211. Patman, R.D., Thompson, J.E., and Perrson, A.V.: Management of post-traumatic pain syndromes: Report of 113 cases. Ann. Surg., 177:780–786, 1973.

212. Rosen, P.S., and Graham, W.: The shoulder-hand syndrome: Historical review with observations on seventy-three patients. Can. Med. Assoc. J., 77:86–91, 1957.

213. Subbarao, J., and Stillwell, G.K.: Reflex sympathetic dystrophy syndrome of the upper extremity: Analysis of total outcome of management of 125 cases. Arch. Phys. Med. Rehabil., 62:549–554, 1981.

214. Thompson, M.: Shoulder-hand syndrome. Proc. R. Soc. Med., 54:679–682, 1961.

215. Bernstein, B.H., et al.: Reflex neurovascular dystrophy in childhood. J. Pediatr., 93:211–215, 1978.

216. Carron, H., and McCue, F.: Reflex sympathetic dystrophy in a ten year old. South. Med. J., 65:631–632, 1972.

217. Fermaglich, D.R.: Reflex sympathetic dystrophy in children. Pediatrics, 60:881–883, 1977.

218. Kozin, F., Houghton, V., and Ryan, L.N.: The reflex sympathetic dystrophy in a child. Pediatrics, 90:417–419, 1977.

219. Matles, A.I.: Reflex sympathetic dystrophy in a child: A case report. Bull. Hosp. Joint. Dis., 32:193–197, 1971.

220. Ruggeri, S.B., et al.: Reflex sympathetic dystrophy in children. Clin. Orthop., 103:225–230, 1982.

221. Lequesne, M., et al.: Partial transient osteoporosis. Skeletal Radiol., 2:1–30, 1977.

222. Helms, C.A., O'Brien, E.T., and Katzberg, R.W.: Segmental reflex sympathetic dystrophy syndrome. Radiology, 35:67–68, 1980.

223. Corbett, M., Colston, J.R., and Tucker, A.K.: Pain in the knees associated with osteoporosis of the patella. Am. Rheum. Dis., 36:188–191, 1977.

224. Kim, H.J., et al.: Reflex-sympathetic dystrophy of the knee following meniscectomy: Report of three cases. Arthritis Rheum., 22:177–181, 1979.

225. Tietjen, R.: Reflex sympathetic dystrophy of the knee. Clin. Orthop., 209:234–243, 1986.

226. Gaucher, A., et al.: The diagnostic value of ^{99m}Tc-diphosphonate bone imaging in transient osteoporosis of the hip. J. Rheumatol., 6:774, 1979.

227. Langloh, N.D., et al.: Transient painful osteoporosis of the lower extremities. J. Bone Joint Surg., 55A:1188–1227, 1973.

228. Kozin, F., et al.: The reflex sympathetic dystrophy syndrome. II. Roentgenographic and scintigraphic evidence of bilaterality and periarticular accentuation. Am. J. Med., 60:332–338, 1976.

229. International Association on the Study of Pain. Subcommittee on Taxonomy Pain Terms: A list with definitions and notes on usage. Pain, 6:249–252, 1979.

230. Tahmoush, A.J.: Causalgia: Redefinition as a clinical pain syndrome. Pain, 10:187–197, 1981.

231. Roberts, W.J.: A hypothesis on the physiological basis for causalgia and related pains. Pain, 2400:297–311, 1986.

232. Kozin, F.: The reflex sympathetic dystrophy syndrome. Bull. Rheum. Dis., 36:1–8, 1986.

233. Miller, D.S., and de Takats, G.: Post-traumatic dystrophy of the extremities. Surg. Gynecol. Obstet., 125:558–582, 1941.

234. Steinbrocker, O., and Argyros, T.G.: The shoulder-hand syndrome: Present status as a diagnostic and therapeutic entity. Med. Clin. North Am., 42:1533–1553, 1958.

235. Steinbrocker, O., Spitzer, N., and Friedman, H.H.: The shoulder-hand syndrome in reflex dystrophy of the upper extremity. Ann. Intern. Med., 29:22–52, 1947.

236. Naides, S.J., Resnick, D., and Zvaifler, N.J.: Idiopathic regional osteoporosis: A clinical spectrum. J. Rheumatol., 12:763–768, 1985.

237. Dent, C.E., and Friedman, M.: Idiopathic juvenile osteoporosis. Q. J. Med., 34:177–210, 1965.

238. Jowsey, J., and Johnson, K.A.: Juvenile osteoporosis: Bone findings in seven patients. J. Pediatr., 81:511–517, 1972.

239. Kozin, F., et al.: Bone scintigraphy in the reflex sympathetic dystrophy syndrome. Radiology, 138:437–443, 1981.

240. Amor, B., et al.: Algodystrophies et hyperlipemies. Rev. Rhum. Mal. Osteoartic., 47:353–358, 1980.

241. Pinals, R.S., and Jabbs, J.M.: Type IV hyperlipoproteinemia and transient osteoporosis. Lancet, 2:929, 1972.

242. Uematsu, S., et al.: Thermography and electromyography in the differential diagnosis of chronic pain syndromes and reflex sympathetic dystrophy. Electromyogr. Clin. Neurophysiol., 21:165–182, 1981.

243. Sylvest, J., et al.: Reflex dystrophy: Resting blood flow and

muscle temperature as diagnostic criteria. Scand. J. Rehabil. Med., 9:25–29, 1977.

244. Ecker, M.A.: Contact thermography in diagnosis of reflex sympathetic dystrophy. In Thermography. Edited by A. Fischer. Philadelphia, W.B. Saunders, 1984.

245. Hendler, N., Uematsu, S., and Long, D.: Thermographic validation of physical complaints in "psychogenic pain" patients. Psychosomatics, 23:283–287, 1982.

246. Cronin, K.D., and Kirsner, R.L.G.: Diagnosis of reflex sympathetic dysfunction: Use of skin potential response. Anaesthesia, 37:847–852, 1982.

247. Pfinsgraff, J., et al.: Palmar fasciitis and arthritis with malignant neoplasms: A paraneoplastic syndrome. Semin. Arthritis Rheum., 16:118–125, 1986.

248. Medsger, T.A., Dixon, J.A., and Garwood, V.F.: Palmar fasciitis and polyarthritis associated with ovarian carcinoma. Ann. Intern. Med., 96:424–431, 1982.

249. Michaels, R.M., and Sorber, J.A.: Reflex sympathetic dystrophy as a probable paraneoplastic syndrome: Case report and literature review. Arthritis Rheum., 27:1183–1185, 1984.

250. Allman, R.M., and Brower, A.C.: Circulatory patterns of deossification. Radiol. Clin. North Am., 19:553–569, 1981.

251. Herrmann, L.G., Reincke, H.G., and Caldwell, J.A.: Posttraumatic painful osteoporosis: A clinical and roentgenological entity. Am. J. Roentgenol., 47:353–361, 1942.

252. Jones, G.: Radiological appearances of disuse osteoporosis. Clin. Radiol., 20:345–353, 1969.

253. Genant, H.K., et al.: The reflex sympathetic dystrophy syndrome: A comprehensive analysis using fine-detail radiography, photon absorptiometry and bone and joint scintigraphy. Radiology, 117:21, 1975.

254. Sudeck, P.: Uber die akute (reflektorishe) Knockenatrophie nach Entzundungen und Verletzungen an den Extrematation and ihre Klinischen Ersheinungen. Fortschr. Gebd. Roentgen., 5:277–293, 1901–1902.

255. Sudeck, P.: Uber die akute entzundlicke Knockenatrophie. Arch. Klin. Chir., 62:147–156, 1900.

256. Kienbach, R.: Über akute knochenatrophie bie Enuyndungprocessen an den Extrematatun (Falschlich sagenannage inactivitats atrophie die Knochen) und ihre Diagnose nach dem Roentgen-Bild. Wien Med. Wochenschr., 5:1345–1360, 1901.

257. Holder, L.E., and MacKinnon, S.E.: Reflex sympathetic dystrophy in the hands: Clinical and scintigraphic criteria. Radiology, 152:517–522, 1984.

258. MacKinnon, S.E., and Holder, L.E.: The use of three-phase radionuclide bone scanning in the diagnosis of reflex sympathetic dystrophy. J. Hand Surg., 9A:556–563, 1984.

259. Charkes, N.D.: Skeletal blood flow: Implications for bone-scan interpretation. J. Nucl. Med., 21:91–98, 1980.

260. McKinstry, P., et al.: Relationship of 99m Tc-MDP uptake to regional osseous circulation in skeletally immature and mature dogs. Skeletal Radiol., 8:115–121, 1982.

261. Doury, P., Dirheimer, Y., and Pattin, S.: Algodystrophy. New York, Springer-Verlag, 1981.

262. Carlson, D.H., Simon, H., and Wegner, W.: Bone scanning and diagnosis of reflex sympathetic dystrophy secondary to herniated lumbar discs. Neurology, 27:791–793, 1977.

263. Deutsch, S.D., Gandsman, E.J., and Spraragen, S.C.: Quantitative regional blood-flow analysis and its clinical application during routine bone-scanning. J. Bone Joint Surg., 63A:295–305, 1981.

264. Simon, H., and Carlson, D.H.: The use of bone scanning in the diagnosis of reflex sympathetic dystrophy. Clin. Nucl. Med., 5:116–121, 1980.

265. Arlet, J., et al.: Histopathology of bone and cartilage lesions in reflex sympathetic dystrophy of the knee: Report of 16 cases. (French.) Rev. Rhum. Mal. Osteoartic., 48:315–321, 1981.

266. Christensen, K., Jensen, E.M., and Noer, I.: The reflex dystrophy syndrome: Response to treatment with systemic corticosteroids. Acta Chir. Scand., 148:653–655, 1982.

267. Stolte, B.H., Stolte, J.B., and Leyten, J.F.: De pathofysiologie van het shoulder-handsyndroom. Med. Tijdschr. Geneeskd., 114:1208–1209, 1980.

268. Moberg, E.: The shoulder-hand-finger syndrome. Surg. Clin. North Am., 40:367–373, 1960.

269. Good, A.E., Green, R.A., and Zorafonetis, C.J.D.: Rheumatic symptoms during tuberculosis therapy: A manifestation of isoniazid toxicity. Ann. Intern. Med., 63:800–807, 1965.

270. van der Korst, J.K., Colenbrauder, H., and Cats, A.: Phenobarbital and the shoulder-hand syndrome. Ann. Rheum. Dis., 25:553–555, 1966.

271. DeTakats, G.: Reflex sympathetic dystrophy of the extremities. Arch. Surg., 34:939–956, 1937.

272. Livingston, W.K.: Pain Mechanisms. New York, Macmillan, 1943.

273. Noordenhos, W.: Pain. Amsterdam, Elsevier, 1959.

274. Meyer, G.A., and Fields, H.L.: Causalgia treated by selective large fibre stimulation of peripheral nerve. Brain, 95:163–168, 1972.

275. Richlin, D.M., et al.: Reflex sympathetic dystrophy: Successful treatment by transcutaneous nerve stimulation. J. Pediatr., 93:84–86, 1978.

276. Melzack, R.: The Puzzle of Pain. New York, Basic Books, 1973.

277. Melzack, R., and Wall, P.D.: Pain mechanisms: A new theory. Science, 150:971–979, 1965.

278. Doury, P., et al.: Algodystrophy with hypofixation of technetium 99m pyrophosphate on bone scintigraphy. (French.) Sem. Hop. Paris, 57:1325–1327, 1981.

279. van der Korst, J.B.: Shoulder-pain as a rheumatologic problem. In Pain in the Shoulder and Arm. Edited by I.M. Green, et al. The Hague, Martinus Nijhoff, 1979.

280. Frykman, G.: Fracture of the distal radius including sequelae—Shoulder-hand-finger syndrome, disturbance in the distal radioulnar joint, and impairment of nerve function. Acta Orthop. Scand., 108 (Suppl.):1–153, 1967.

281. Lind, K.: A synthesis of studies on stroke rehabilitation. J. Chronic Dis., 35:133–149, 1982.

282. Steinbrocker, O., Neustadt, D., and Lapin, L.: Sympathetic block compared with corticotropin and cortisone therapy. JAMA, 153:788–791, 1953.

283. Drucker, W.R., et al.: Pathogenesis of post-traumatic sympathetic dystrophy. Am. J. Surg., 97:454–465, 1979.

284. Wang, J.K., Johnson, K.A., and Ilstrup, D.M.: Sympathetic blocks for reflex sympathetic dystrophy. Pain, 23:13–17, 1985.

285. Buker, R.H., et al.: Causalgia and transthoracic sympathectomy. Am. J. Surg., 124:724–727, 1972.

286. Benzon, H.T., Chomka, C.M., and Brunner, E.A.: Treatment of reflex sympathetic dystrophy with regional intravenous reserpine. Anesth. Analg., 59:500–502, 1980.

287. Chuinard, R.G., et al.: Intravenous reserpine for treatment of reflex sympathetic dystrophy. South. Med. J., 74:1481–1484, 1981.

288. Chuinard, R.G., et al.: Intravenous reserpine for treatment of reflex sympathetic dystrophy. South. Med. J., 74:1481–1484, 1981.

289. Hannington-Kiff, J.G.: Relief of Sudeck's atrophy by regional intravenous guanethidine. Lancet, 1:1132–1134, 1977.

290. Hannington-Kiff, J.G.: Relief of causalgia in limbs by regional intravenous guanethidine. Br. Med. J., 2:367–368, 1979.

291. Bonelli, S., Conocente, F., et al.: Regional intravenous guanethidine vs. stellate ganglion block in reflex sympathetic dystrophies: A randomized trial. Pain, 16:297–307, 1983.

292. Ghostine, S.Y., et al.: Phenoxybenzamine in the treatment of causalgia. A report of 40 cases. J. Neurosurg., 60:1263–1268, 1984.

293. Simson, G.: Propanolol for causalgia and Sudeck's atrophy. JAMA, 227:327, 1974.

294. Visitsunthorn, U., and Prete, P.: Reflex sympathetic dystrophy of the lower extremity. West. J. Med., 135:62–66, 1981.

295. Glick, E.N., and Helal, B.: Post-traumatic neurodystrophy: treatment by corticosteroids. Hand, 8:45–48, 1976.

296. Mowat, A.G.: Treatment of the shoulder-hand syndrome with corticosteroids. Ann. Rheum. Dis., 33:120–123, 1974.

297. Russek, H.I., et al.: Cortisone treatment of shoulder-hand syndrome following acute myocardial infarction. Arch. Intern. Med., 91:487–492, 1953.

298. Glick, E.N.: Reflex dystrophy (algoneurodystrophy): results of treatment by corticosteroids. Rheumatol. Rehabil., 12:84–88, 1973.

299. Poplawski, E.J., Wiley, A.M., and Murray, J.F.: Post-traumatic dystrophy of the extremities. J. Bone Joint Surg., 65A:642–649, 1983.

300. Prough, D.S., et al.: Efficacy of oral nifedipine in the treatment of reflex sympathetic dystrophy. Anesthesiology, 62:796–799, 1985.

301. Wall, P.D., and Sweet, W.H.: Temporary abolition of pain in man. Science, 155:108–109, 1967.

98

OSTEONECROSIS

JOHN P. JONES, JR.

The terms osteonecrosis, avascular (aseptic) necrosis, and osseous ischemia indicate death of the cellular constituents of both bone and bone marrow. The etiology is multifactorial.

PATHOPHYSIOLOGIC FEATURES

TRAUMATIC (MACROVASCULAR) DAMAGE

Traumatic osteonecrosis usually involves bones covered extensively by cartilage, with few vascular foramina and limited collateral circulation. For example, 8% of posterior hip dislocations without fractures develop femoral necrosis.[1] The incidence increases to 13 to 18% with associated fractures of the acetabulum or the femoral head.[2] Dislocations usually rupture the ligamentum teres.[3]

Rarely does necrosis of the femoral head complicate extracapsular intertrochanteric hip fractures, noted in only 11 of 3839 (0.29%) reported cases.[4] Intracapsular femoral neck fractures, however, interrupt most blood flow through the subsynovial retinacular vessels, including the important lateral epiphyseal arteries to the femoral head. Because blood to the superolateral two thirds of the femoral head comes almost entirely from these lateral epiphyseal arteries, this area is particularly susceptible to osteonecrosis. The only other blood available to the femoral head flows through the ligamentum teres (medial epiphyseal artery),[5] which anastomosed with the lateral epiphyseal vessels in only 5 of 17 (29.4%) reported cases.[6]

NONTRAUMATIC (MICROVASCULAR) DAMAGE

Cytotoxicity

Chemotherapy is known to cause osteonecrosis. Corticosteroids, however, are unable to directly kill osteoblasts or osteocytes in tissue culture; this inability suggests an indirect mechanism for the production of corticoid-induced osteonecrosis. However, radiation necrosis is linked to both cellular cytotoxicity and to endarteritis because preferential bone absorption increases with secondary irradiation during orthovoltage therapy. Osteonecrosis may occur in patients with leukemia or lymphoma after irradiation or after radiotherapy for carcinoma of the prostate. Osteonecrosis can also result from thermal injuries, including burns, electrical injuries, or frostbite.

Various miscellaneous conditions are also associated with osteonecrosis, including Gaucher's disease[7] and Leriche's syndrome.[8]

Fat Embolism

Osteonecrosis associated with fat embolism of bone[9] was first demonstrated clinically in 1965[10,11] and first confirmed experimentally in 1966.[12,13] In one epidemiologic study, for example, 89% of 269 patients with nontraumatic osteonecrosis had disorders known to be complicated by disturbed fat metabolism or fat embolism.[14]

FIG. 98–1. Schematic representation of three mechanisms potentially capable of producing intraosseous fat embolism and triggering a process leading to focal intravascular coagulation and osteonecrosis. (From Jones, J.P.: Fat embolism and osteonecrosis. Orthop Clin. N. Am., *16*:601, 1985.)

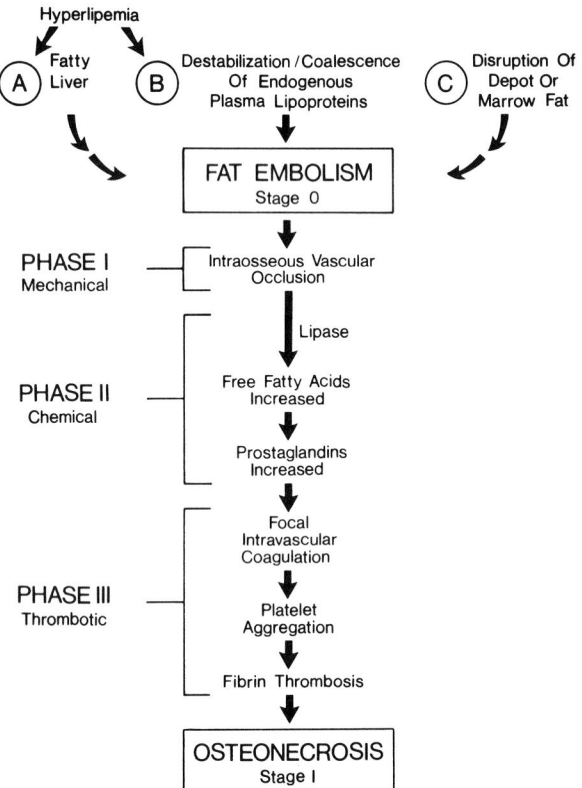

MECHANISMS OF LIPID METABOLISM RESULTING IN FAT EMBOLISM AND OSTEONECROSIS

Table 98–1. Conditions Associated with Osteonecrosis Related to Fat Embolism

Condition	Suspected Mechanism*		
Alcoholism	A		
Carbon tetrachloride poisoning	A		
Diabetes mellitus	A	B	
Dysbaric phenomena		B	C
Hemoglobinopathies			C
Hypercortisonism (or Cushing's syndrome)	A		
Hyperlipemia (type II or IV)	A	B	
Obesity	A	B	
Oral contraceptives (estrogen)	A	B	
Pancreatitis		B	C
Pregnancy	A	B	
Unrelated fractures			C

*A = fatty liver; B = coalescence of plasma lipoproteins; C = disruption of fatty bone marrow.

Corticosteroids caused hyperlipemia, especially increased very-low-density, pre-β lipoproteins, after 4 to 7 days; fatty liver and significant systemic fat embolism to the subchondral arterioles and capillaries of femoral heads, similar to the findings in humans occurred after 2 to 3 weeks; significant bone marrow necrosis[22] took place as early as 3 weeks; increased intrafemoral head pressure,[24] with decreased blood flow,[25] occurred after 6 to 8 weeks.

There was fat embolism to the subchondral capillary beds of both the humeral and femoral heads.[18] Steroid therapy caused an increased number of nonfunctioning, probably dead, osteocytes; 84% took up H3 cytidine in the control group and 50% did so in the treated group.[15] In another study, the large number of empty lacunae, which became evident during the second and third weeks, was noted, along with an accumulation of necrotic debris within the marrow spaces, which persisted throughout the 18 weeks of the study.[17]

Wang and associates demonstrated a progressive decrease in blood flow in the rabbit femoral head, which was reduced 24% at 8 weeks and 32% after 10 weeks of steroid treatment.[25] They previously had shown enlargement of marrow fat cells and volume, and an increase in intrafemoral head pressure in the hips of steroid-treated rabbits, already impaired 3 weeks earlier by intraosseous fat embolism.[23,24]

Fat emboli may arise from a fatty liver (*Mechanism A*), destabilization and coalescence of plasma lipoproteins (*Mechanism B*), and/or disruption of fatty bone marrow or other adipose tissue depots (*Mechanism C*) (Fig. 98–1). Fat embolism occurs in several clinical disorders that are also associated with osteonecrosis (Table 98–1). Alcoholism and hypercortisonism are the two most common diseases associated with nontraumatic osteonecrosis, however; together, they account for about two thirds of the cases.

Experimental Confirmation

Experiments have been conducted in corticosteroid-treated rabbits from nine laboratories[15–23] with follow-ups from 21 to 365 days. All instances involved hyperlipemia, fatty liver, pulmonary fat embolism, systemic fat embolism, and fat embolism of the femoral heads. Focal osteocyte death in the femoral heads occurred in six of the eight series studied (Table 98–2).

POPULATION AT RISK

DYSBARISM-RELATED OSTEONECROSIS

Those individuals exposed to changes in atmospheric pressure in the course of their occupations,

Table 98–2. Corticoid-Induced Fat Embolism and Osteocyte Death: Summary of Experimental Studies in Rabbits

Investigator(s) (Year)	Days of Followup	Hyperlipemia	Fatty Liver	Fat Embolism Femoral Head	Osteocytic Death
Fisher et al. (1972)	150	Yes	Yes	Yes	Yes
Jaffe et al. (1972)	63	—	—	Yes	No
Cruess et al. (1975)	56	Yes	Yes	Yes	Yes
Wang et al. (1977)	140	Yes	Yes	Yes	—
Kenzora (1978)	365	—	Yes	Yes	No
Gold et al. (1978)	126	Yes	—	Yes	Yes
Paolaggi et al. (1984)	21	Yes	Yes	Yes	Yes
Surat (1984)	90	Yes	Yes	Yes	Yes
Kawai et al. (1985)	56	Yes	Yes	Yes	Yes

principally compressed-air workers, divers, and, to a lesser extent, aviators, are at risk.

Compressed-Air Workers (Tunnel or Caisson)

"Caisson disease" was first described in 1911.[26] Virtually all caisson and tunnel workers in the United States were once decompressed according to modifications of the New York code of 1922, which required workers to split shifts. Unfortunately, inadequate surface time permitted considerable nitrogen gas to remain dissolved in the workers' tissues at the start of their second shift, with a resultant high incidence of decompression sickness and osteonecrosis.

The Washington State Decompression Tables were used first in 1964 during the Seattle tunnel construction and later in the San Francisco Bay Area Rapid Transit (BART) project. These tables became the United States Occupational Safety and Health Administration (OSHA) standard in 1971 and have minimized the development of osteonecrosis at pressures up to 34 psig (pounds per square inch gauge pressure), but the incidence of the disorder at pressures over 36 psig is still unacceptable. Roentgenograms and bone scintigrams of 23 men working at pressures of up to 43 psig (using the OSHA schedules) revealed 9 (39%) with osteonecrosis.[27] The risk of decompression sickness is minimal if working pressures are maintained below 11 psig, but pressures greater than 17 psig increase the incidence of this illness and the risk of osteonecrosis.[28]

Femoral lesions are distributed differently in compressed-air workers than in commercial divers. Only 38% of 977 lesions in 383 compressed-air workers appeared in the lower femoral shaft, as compared to 54% of 114 lesions in 60 commercial divers; in the compressed-air workers, 12% of the lesions developed in the femoral head, as compared to only 0.9% in the divers. Of the lesions in both compressed-air workers and commercial divers, 24% involved the humeral head, however.[29] Therefore, the skeletal distribution of lesions in dysbaric osteonecrosis, in contrast to other causes of osteonecrosis, involves the humeral head much more frequently than the femoral head.

Divers

In 1941, Grutzmacher first described osteonecrosis in a diver.[30] Today, advances in diving research and operations permit safe and effective underwater work in depths to 1600 feet. Four groups of divers are considered: (1) skin divers, in whom osteonecrosis is nonexistent, and sport scuba divers, in whom it is virtually nonexistent; (2) United States, British, French, Japanese, and Canadian navy divers, who have a 1 to 3% incidence of osteonecrosis, using standard tables; (3) commercial divers, who have a 4.2% overall and a 1.2% juxta-articular incidence; and (4) Hawaiian and Japanese diving fishermen, who have a 50 to 65% incidence of osteonecrosis. Dysbaric osteonecrosis is not a risk at depths of less than 30 m. Divers with the most experience, and "saturation" divers, rather than "bounce" divers, are more prone to develop bone lesions.

The British Decompression Sickness Panel studied 4980 commercial divers. At least one definite bone lesion was found in each of 207 divers (4.2%), but only 62 divers (1.2%) had juxta-articular lesions.[29] In contrast, 13 of 20 Hawaiian diving fishermen, who neither followed conventional diving procedures nor used standard oxygen decompression schedules, had 43 osteonecrotic lesions, with 44% of these in juxta-articular regions.[31] Osteonecrosis was found in 268 of 450 (59.5%) Japanese diving fishermen.[32]

OSTEONECROSIS ASSOCIATED WITH OTHER CONDITIONS

Hypercortisonism

Corticosteroid treatment[33] has been complicated by osteonecrosis. One patient developed osteonecrosis after only 700 mg prednisolone in 7 days.[34] Another patient received only 16 mg prednisolone daily for 30 days.[35] The at-risk threshold for the adult is generally considered to be about 2000 mg of prednisone or its equivalent.

Osteonecrosis was found in 26 of 520 (5%) patients with systemic lupus erythematosus;[36] an even higher incidence (40%) occurs in childhood. No relationship exists between osteonecrosis and the severity of systemic lupus erythematosus. Another series of 365 lupus patients showed osteonecrosis in 17 (4.7%). More prednisone was consumed during the initial 6 months of therapy by patients who developed osteonecrosis (6.4 g) than by those who did not (3.0 g).[37] Vasculitis has not been found in resected femoral heads from patients with systemic lupus erythematosus, or similar diseases and is no longer considered an etiologic mechanism. The capitellum, carpal scaphoid and capitate, metacarpal and metatarsal heads, distal femoral condyles, patella, talus, and tibial plateau, as well as the femoral and humeral heads, have been involved by osteonecrosis in systemic lupus erythematosus.

Osteonecrosis complicating renal transplantation was reported in 1964.[38] Osteonecrosis occurred in 299 of 2285 (13%) patients from 18 renal-transplant centers.[39] Kidney-transplant recipients frequently also have osteoporosis, osteomalacia, and secondary hyperparathyroidism, but heart-transplant recipients with osteonecrosis do not have these coexistent diseases; these findings further implicate corticosteroids.

As with treatment for systemic lupus erythematosus, a correlation existed between the total steroid dose during the first few weeks after transplantation and the incidence of osteonecrosis. Osteonecrosis developed in 16 of 50 (32%) patients receiving higher doses (2960 mg prednisone in 3 weeks), as compared with only 2 of 101 (2%) patients receiving lower doses (1180 mg prednisone in 3 weeks). Immunosuppression with cyclosporin A has required less prednisone and reduced the incidence of osteonecrosis.

Alcoholism

The first report of osteonecrosis in an alcoholic patient appeared in 1928. The alcohol-induced fatty liver is conceivably the most common source of continuous, low-grade, and relatively asymptomatic showers of systemic fat emboli.[41] In 26 alcoholic patients with osteonecrosis of the femoral head, 38 hips showed elevated intraosseous pressures in the early stages.[42] Of 38 alcoholics with osteonecrosis, 24 (63%) had type II or type IV hyperlipemia and biopsy-proven fatty livers.

Hyperlipemia

Hyperlipidemia was linked with osteonecrosis in 1960,[43,44] with hypertriglyceridemia in 18 of 22 patients. Type IV, or rarely, type II or type V, is present. Type IV hyperlipemia is characterized by increased pre-β-lipoprotein, elevated triglyceride, and normal or slightly elevated cholesterol levels. Patients with osteonecrosis often had increased pre-β-lipoproteins and other type II and type IV abnormalities.[45,46] Eight family members had type IV hyperlipidemia and osteonecrosis of the femoral heads. Seven were affected bilaterally.[47]

Hyperlipidemia is frequently accompanied by hypothyroidism, diabetes, obesity, or hyperuricemia. Hyperuricemia is a frequent finding in both osteonecrosis and hyperlipemia. Obesity, which increases the risk of osteonecrosis and contributes to hyperlipemia, was reported in 20% of 150 patients with osteonecrosis. Fat embolism in diabetes was first described in 1880.[48]

The most dramatic elevations of serum triglycerides occur in types I and V; osteonecrosis is most common in type IV. Management of the type IV disorder includes diet management, treatment of diabetes or hypothyroidism, restriction of alcohol, avoidance of corticoids and oral contraceptives, and a therapeutic trial of clofibrate. Used experimentally, clofibrate tempered the rise of serum cholesterol and the degree of fatty liver, but did not significantly reduce fatty emboli in subchondral arteries.[49,50]

Pregnancy

Osteonecrosis of the femoral head can develop in an otherwise uncomplicated pregnancy;[51] this disorder has been found by biopsy in six instances.[52] Acute fatty liver, first noted in 1934, often occurs in the third trimester of pregnancy.[53] A number of recorded deaths associated with fatty livers are now known to be associated with increased plasma cortisol and aggravated by high-dose tetracycline administration.[54] Plasma lipid levels also increase after the third month of gestation. Femoral head osteonecrosis has been linked to the use of oral contraceptives.[14]

Pancreatitis

Bone marrow fat involvement was found in a fatal case of acute pancreatitis in 1872.[55] Pancreatitis may be associated with subcutaneous fat necrosis, polyarthritis, and bone lesions.[56] Macroscopic evidence of fat necrosis in bone was found in 10.4% of 67 necropsied cases of acute pancreatitis.[57]

Hemoglobinopathies

Femoral head abnormalities in patients with sickle cell disease were first recognized in 1937.[58] Bone necrosis resulting from combined sickle cell–thalassemia disease was reported in 1953,[59] and it was reported later in patients with sickle cell anemia.[60] Osteonecrosis was also associated with sickle cell trait. The incidence of femoral head involvement in sickle cell anemia varied from 0% in 120 cases studied in West Africa to 12% in 51 cases studied in the United States,[61] whereas hip involvement in hemoglobin SC disease varied from 20 to 68%.[62] The prevalence of SS hemoglobin in the American black population is approximately three times greater than that of other sickle cell variants, but the incidence of osteonecrosis is higher in hemoglobin SC disease, in which, paradoxically, hemolytic crises are fewer and milder, but fat embolism is more common.[63]

Halogenated Hydrocarbon Poisoning

Osteonecrosis has been reported with carbon tetrachloride poisoning and liver disease, unrelated to either alcohol or corticosteroid use. A second case has also been studied by Jacobs.[14] Alcoholics are especially sensitive to carbon tetrachloride because of the synergism of alcohol and carbon tetrachloride in producing fatty liver. The blood of another patient with carbon tetrachloride poisoning contained 60% fat. The liver weighed 2600 g, and the central and mid-zones of the lobules were filled with fat globules; fat emboli were present in hepatic veins and pulmonary arteries.[64]

PATHOGENESIS OF NONTRAUMATIC OSTEONECROSIS

I have divided the pathophysiology of osteonecrosis into five stages: 0, I, II, III, and IV. Thermal injuries, chemotherapy, and radiation cause osteonecrosis by direct cytotoxicity (stage 0) and by obliterative endarteritis. Necrosis is also caused by occlusive vascular disease with thrombosis.[8] In addition, it is now considered, particularly in hypercortisonism, that intraosseous fat embolism (stage 0)[9] may trigger a three-phase process leading to focal intravascular coagulation, which may result in focal osteonecrosis (stage I) (Fig. 98–1).

Stage I lesions show dead bone marrow and dead bone trabeculae *without repair*, either pathologically or radiographically. The repair process starts in stage II with recanalization of thrombosed vessels and revascularization (resorption, followed by reossification), but without subchondral collapse or articular incongruity. Late segmental collapse initiates stage III, which is usually followed by stage IV and secondary degenerative arthritis.

STAGE 0

Phase 1: Mechanical (Intraosseous Vascular Occlusion). The dynamics of intraosseous fat embolism were originally studied experimentally using Lipiodol.[12] In 1965 I found prelabeled intravascular fat that had extended circumferentially through canaliculi to become deposited within individual osteocytic lacunae. More recently, Kawai and associates demonstrated a progressive accumulaiton of lipid in osteocytes that subsequently became necrotic.[19] In another experimental animal preparation, intra-arterial injection of neutral fat produced pulmonary hypertension, decreased pulmonary wedge pressure, and increased pulmonary resistance. The arterial oxygen tension fell and was accompanied by metabolic acidosis.[65] Pulmonary hypertension opens up right-to-left shunts.[66] In another study, the injection of depot fat into rabbits produced hypoxemia and pulmonary edema. A biphasic response was suggested: an early mechanical effect and a later, presumably chemical, effect.[67] Similar events are likely to occur after intraosseous vascular occlusion.

Phase 2: Chemical (Inflammatory). Neutral marrow fat itself produces little or no thrombotic reaction in the isolated venous segment, but neutral embolic fat is indirectly thrombogenic, through its ability to generate free fatty acids. Because the complete breakdown of intraosseous fat emboli may be a slow process, experimentally requiring up to 5 weeks,[12] there is a delay, or latent period, between the mechanical and chemical phases.

Oleic acid is the main fatty acid component of neutral trioleum (glyceryl trioleate), which is the most abundant marrow fat.[68] Oleic acid causes a marked stripping of capillary endothelium, passive congestion, and edema formation. Oleic acid also produces local thrombosis when injected into an isolated vein segment. Marked platelet aggregation and fibrin deposition occur in the vicinity of the fat.[69,70] If oleic acid is injected into the pulmonary circulation of dogs, thrombocytopenia occurs secondary to intravascular coagulation, with deposition of labeled fibrinogen and platelets.[71]

Free fatty acids liberated as a result of lipase activity most likely cause a toxic, inflammatory response in the marrow. Increased levels of circulating free fatty acids may lead directly to increased production of prostaglandins,[72] powerful mediators of inflammation, which may cause intramedullary edema and increased intraosseous pressure. Twofold to threefold elevations in both unbound free fatty acids and plasma prostaglandins began 1 to 2 weeks after initiation of corticoids in rabbits.[17] Elevated serum total lipids and free fatty acids, as well as intraosseous fat emboli and increased prostaglandins, were found in the necrotic femoral heads of steroid-treated rabbits. The PGE_2-like activity was increased 8-fold and 16-fold, after 30 and 90 days of prednisolone administration, respectively.[21]

It is not known whether the hydrolysis of triolein leads to a local accumulation of free fatty acids in the femoral or humeral head, whether free-unemulsified triolein remains unbound, or whether the free fatty acids produced bind to albumin at the site of production.[65,69,70] Fat macroglobules (emboli) in the blood and elevated free fatty acids afford valuable diagnostic clues of fat embolism.[73,74]

The precise mechanism by which fat produces thrombosis is unknown. The thrombogenic potential of fat is probably counterbalanced by an antithrombotic system, which also relies, at least in part, on precursors of free fatty acids.[75] Both venous stasis and arterial ischemia result in the local formation and release of the antithrombotic prostaglandin (prostacyclin, PGI_2), which inhibits platelet aggregation. This mechanism can be exhausted by prolonged or repetitive insults, however, so that, ultimately, there is no protection against thromboxane (TXA_2), which initiates local platelet aggregation.[76]

Phase 3: Thrombotic (Focal Intravascular Coagulation). A relatively common subclinical form of fat embolism is associated with intravascular coagulation, and vice versa.[77] Focal intravascular coagulation may be defined as active blood coagulation within the circulation, with secondary activation of fibrinolysis. Stagnant blood flow in the femoral head may lead to focal intravascular coagulation (as initially recognized by elevated plasma fibrinopeptide A).

Thrombosis of large vessels distal to an arterial embolus has been demonstrated. Widespread clotting of capillaries and terminal arterioles after mechanically induced ischemia (stage 0, phase 1) may result in venous thrombosis and retrograde thrombosis of major extraosseous arteries because of vascular stasis and edema causing vascular compression (intraosseous hypertension).[78,79] The result may be hypoxia of the underperfused femoral heads.

Platelet aggregation and fibrin thrombi are associated with fat emboli.[80,81] Intravascular coagulation may be precipitated by endothelial damage and fat embolism.[82] Elevated plasma lipids may accelerate blood clotting and increase platelet adhesiveness and aggregation.[81] Toyoshima demonstrated fat embolism and associated intraosseous thromboses in the femoral head of a patient treated with corticoids.[83]

Treatment

There is no known way to prevent corticosteroid-induced osteonecrosis. Although still investigational, clofibrate (Atromid-S) could possibly prevent steroid-induced osteonecrosis by its antilipidemic action (stage 0, phase 1).[49,50] Aprotinin (Trasylol) may possibly prevent steroid-induced osteonecrosis by inhibiting tissue kallikrein activity, and inhibiting platelet aggregation, while preventing contact activation of focal intravascular coagulation (stage 0, phase 3).[21]

DIAGNOSIS AND MANAGEMENT OF OSTEONECROSIS

Early diagnosis has been a serious obstacle to treating potentially reversible lesions. This discussion focuses on management of lesions affecting the juxta-articular or epiphyseal regions because metadiaphyseal lesions, such as calcified intramedullary fat necrosis or bone infarction, are neither symptomatic nor disabling.

STAGE I LESION

The patient is asymptomatic, with no physical or radiographic findings. Histologically, localized stage I lesions show dead bone trabeculae and dead bone marrow, without any evidence of repair. The generalized stage I lesion occurs with physiologic death of the skeleton and appears in nonfossilized archeologic specimens.

All osseous tissues do not die at the same rate after fat embolism.[13] Hematopoietic marrow cells die first, because they are most sensitive to acute anoxia. Death of hematopoietic cellular elements, especially capillary endothelial cells and, later, marrow lipocytes, is the most reliable evidence of osteonecrosis.[84] More than 200 core biopsy specimens of early lesions indicated interstitial edema and necrosis of fatty and hematopoietic marrow and rupture of lipocytes, pro-

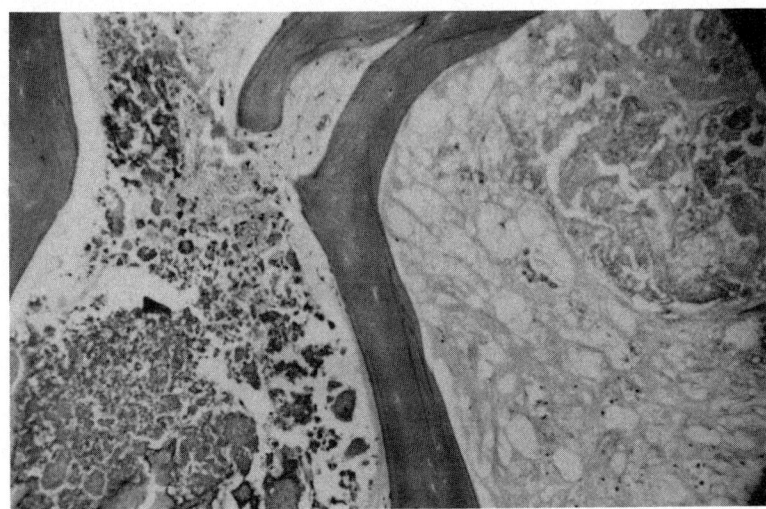

FIG. 98–2. Photomicrograph of femoral head specimen showing stage I lesion with liquefaction necrosis of marrow fat *(right)* separated from amorphous granular marrow debris *(left)* by a trabeculum with ischemic-appearing osteocytes.

ducing large, fatty cysts and liquefaction necrosis (Figs. 98–2 and 98–3), amorphous debris, sinusoidal distension, and arteriolar thrombosis.[52] Marrow changes occurred before alterations in the trabeculae. Osteocytes were the last cells to show histologic and cytologic changes. In experimental animals, bone ischemia lasting longer than 6 hours produced cellular death,[85,86] although osteocytes may retain radioactive amino acids and glucose for up to 48 hours.[86] Thus, the presence or absence of osteocyte nuclei (empty lacunae) is variable, because of wide variations in autolytic rates after functional death.

Laboratory Tests

Certain selected tests may be useful for persons suspected of having an associated condition discussed previously.

FIG. 98–3. Graph demonstrating prolonged reduction in marrow adipose cells beginning 5 days after intraosseous Lipiodol fat embolism of the proximal rabbit femur.

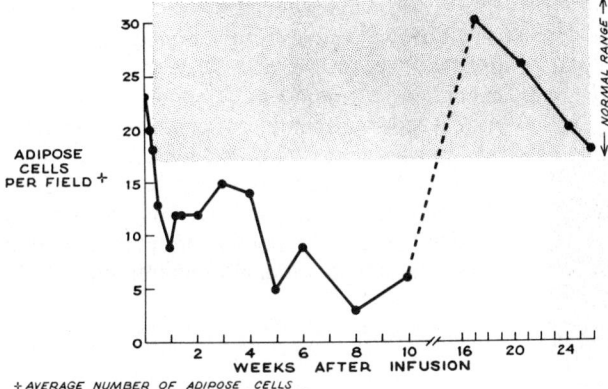

+ AVERAGE NUMBER OF ADIPOSE CELLS
COUNTED IN TEN CONSECUTIVE 45X FIELDS
OF METAPHYSEAL MARROW (PROXIMAL RIGHT FEMUR)

Imaging

The early diagnosis of osteonecrosis can be established in stage I (and subsequently confirmed by biopsy) with a combination of *decreased* signal intensity on magnetic resonance imaging, *decreased* radionuclide uptake on ^{99m}Tc-methylene diphosphonate scintigrams,[87–91] and the demonstration of an *interruption* of the medial femoral circumflex artery or its lateral epiphyseal tributaries on superselective angiography.[92–94] Computed tomography (CT), even with multiplanar reconstructions, will not show any abnormalities in stage I.

Because osteonecrotic damage is selective, *radiographs* should concentrate on the shoulder, hip, and knee joints with two rotational views of each shoulder, and an anteroposterior and lateral projection of each hip and knee. Conventional radiography is not satisfactory for early diagnosis of osteonecrosis because death of bone and marrow, *without repair*, produces no radiologic abnormality. Tomograms are similarly unhelpful.

Magnetic Resonance Imaging (MRI) (See Chapter 6). MRI is the most sensitive, specific, low-risk, noninvasive test for the early (stage I) localization of osteonecrosis. In one study, biopsies were available in 55 of 90 patients with suspected osteonecrosis. MRI was 96% accurate when compared with biopsy findings. Isotope studies and CT scans correlated with biopsy findings in 71% and 54%, respectively.[95] In another study, MRI suggested osteonecrosis in 26 hips. Of 13 MRI-positive hips with normal radiographs, only 4 had abnormal technetium diphosphonate scintigrams.[96] Other investigators compared the results of MRI in 20 patients with bone scintigraphy in 12 patients and conventional radiographs in 14 patients. In five cases, MRI was abnormal, but the bone scintigraphy was normal.[97]

In MRI images acquired with a T1-weighted, spin-echo pulse sequence, the normal bone marrow is characterized by a signal of high intensity, resulting from the high content of hydrogen-rich marrow fat.[98] Normally, there is high signal intensity (white) on coronal images of the humeral[99] and femoral heads. Fat cells may remain viable for 2 to 5 days (Fig. 98–3). In stage I the necrotic zone will retain high signal intensity (isointense with viable marrow fat) if the nonviable fat cells and fatty cysts have not yet saponified. However, the necrotic zone will have homogeneous low signal intensity on T1-weighting if liquefaction necrosis and saponification have resulted in degradation of the pre-existing fat into amorphous granular debris (Fig. 98–2). Heterogeneous hypointensity (Fig. 98–4A) most likely occurs when only a portion of the nonviable fat undergoes saponification.

Coronal images provide information that is most easily correlated with radiographs and is the best for displaying the subcortical cancellous bone in the superior femoral head. Direct coronal, axial, and sagittal imaging using T1 and T2 weighting is the most accurate method of osteonecrosis staging because there is equal resolution in all planes. High-resolution studies also can reveal focal, minimal bone infarctions. Axial or coronal multiecho images may show subtle abnormalities not evident with the partial saturation technique.

Few false negative results exist with MRI. If there is preservation of normal signal in the superolateral portion of the femoral head, the diagnosis of osteonecrosis becomes quite unlikely. No patients with a normal MRI image have developed osteonecrosis in 300 hips, with up to a 30-month followup.[100]

Recently by MRI I classified 15 hips with precollapse osteonecrosis. Thirteen femoral heads already had evidence of repair with bands of decreased intensity (stage II). However, two femoral heads had no obvious reparative response (stage I) at that time. These two patients had fatty livers *(mechanism A)* with arterial fat embolism, which most likely triggered focal intravascular coagulation, as evidenced by increased plasma fibrinopeptide A (Fig. 98–5) and interruption (probable retrograde thrombus propagation from intraosseous to extraosseous) of the lateral epiphyseal arteries (partial femoral head lesion) (Fig. 98–4B), or continued retrograde thrombosis to involve the medial femoral circumflex artery (complete femoral head lesion) (Figs. 98–6 and 98–7).

Scintigraphy. Scintigraphy using bone-seeking isotopes is more sensitive than radiography but not as sensitive as MRI. Technetium ^{99m}-methylene diphosphonate adsorbs to the surface of newly forming bone crystals. Interpretation of scintigrams is generally based on asymmetric radioisotope uptake, so diagnosis becomes more difficult in patients with bilateral involvement; the less affected side is often overlooked.[91] Experimental osteonecrosis has been detected consistently within 12 weeks.[101] Abnormal scintigrams usually precede the earliest radiographic changes by 3 to 4 months.

Although theoretically a cold spot resulting from *decreased* radioactive uptake should be seen in the affected bone, cold spots are rare.

Intraosseous Pressure and Venography

Because of their invasive nature and lack of specificity compared to MRI, these procedures may become obsolete. Elevation of intraosseous pressure and impaired venous drainage[24,102,103] have been documented in early osteonecrosis.

Superselective Angiography

If the MRI image is abnormal, superselective angiographic studies may reveal an abrupt interruption

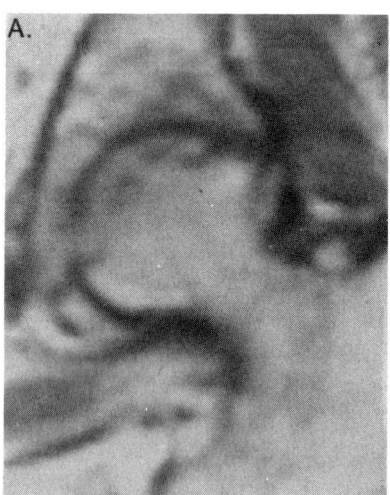
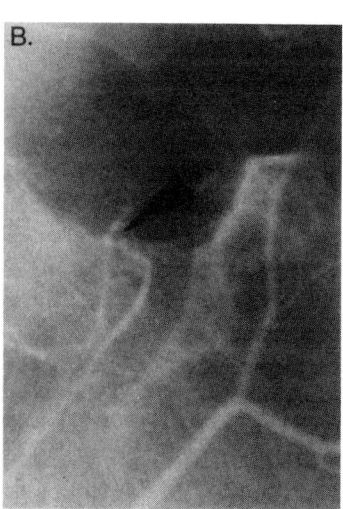

FIG. 98–4. Patient treated with corticosteroids for asthma had obesity, diabetes, hyperlipemia, fatty liver, arterial fat embolism, elevated serum lipase, and evidence of intravascular coagulation with elevation of plasma fibrinopeptide A to 9.0 nM (normally less than 2.0 nM) and increased fibrinogen split products. Although conventional radiographs and tomograms of her asymptomatic left hip were normal, (A) MRI indicated a stage I lesion with a subchondral region of multifocal, heterogeneous hypointensity; (B) angiography revealed an extraosseous interruption of one or more lateral epiphyseal arteries (arrow).

FIG. 98–5. This patient had obesity, diabetes, fatty liver, arterial fat embolism, and increased free fatty acids. Probable focal intravascular coagulation occurred with a transient decrease in platelets and fibrinogen and a sharp elevation in the plasma fibrinopeptide A (435 nM) as depicted on this graph. (From Jones, J.P.: Fat embolism and osteonecrosis. Orthop. Clin. N. Amer., *16*:601, 1985.)

FIG. 98–6. MR image of left hip from same patient shown in Fig. 98–5, showing a stage I lesion with homogeneous decreased signal intensity diffusely involving nearly the entire left femoral head, but terminating abruptly at the neck, with loss of the normal, bright, homogeneous, high-intensity signal. (From Jones, J.P.: Fat embolism and osteonecrosis. Orthop. Clin. N. Am., *16*:609, 1985.)

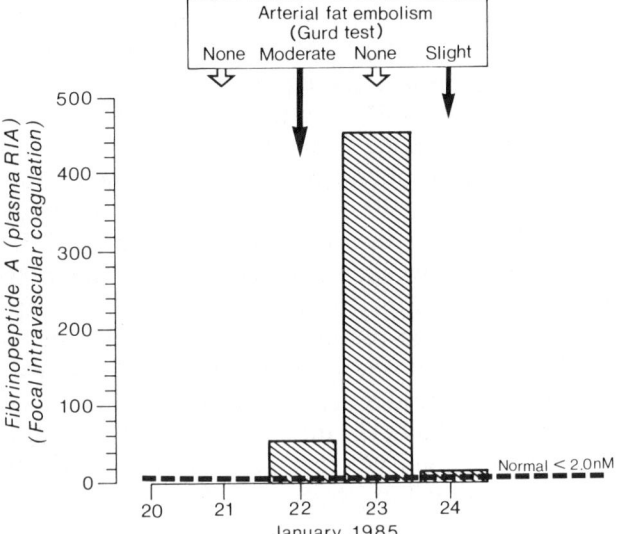

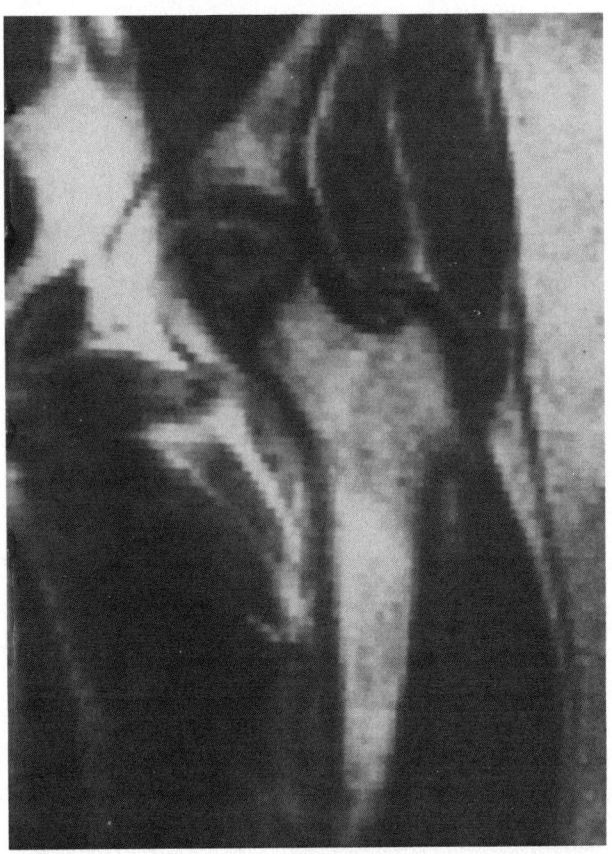

of the medial femoral circumflex artery (Fig. 98–7),[92,93] absence of its lateral epiphyseal (superior retinacular) branches (Fig. 98–4),[94] or absence of anastomoses between the circumflex vessels and branches of the obturator artery, presumably the result of intraosseous, retrograde thrombus propagation extending from the femoral head to involve the extraosseous vessels.

Biopsy

A biopsy should be obtained to confirm a diagnosis of osteonecrosis if the MRI image is abnormal. A trephine is introduced into the subchondral bone of the femoral or humeral head under radiologic control, and the tissue is examined both microscopically and microroentgenographically.[104]

STAGE II LESION

The patient is usually asymptomatic and still has no physical findings. The bony lesion shows repair without collapse.

Pathologic Features

There is a lag period before the repair response is activated. Presumably, collateral circulation is stimulated and fibrinolysis occurs. Angiogenesis may be

signaled by platelet-derived growth factor, and osteoclast migration (chemotaxis) may be stimulated by necrotic collagen degradation products. Because the osteonecrotic segment is avascular, repair can begin only along its outer perimeter, at the junction of the ischemic zone surrounding the dead area and the viable area with intact circulation (the *hyperemic* zone). Primitive, undifferentiated mesenchymal cells and capillary buds, containing endothelial cells, proliferate and differentiate to fibroblasts, which begin synthesizing collagen. Subsequently, these mesenchymal cells differentiate to osteoblasts. This process is retarded in corticoid-treated transplant patients. The dead trabeculae are partially or completely resorbed by osteoclasts and are replaced or covered with new appositional bone, resulting in thickened, reinforced trabeculae.

Reossification usually occurs distal to the revascu-

FIG. 98–7. Superselective angiogram of hip shown in Figs. 98–5 and 98–6 showing complete interruption *(arrow head)* and nonvisualization of the medial femoral circumflex artery and its lateral epiphyseal branches to the femoral head. There is no evidence of any collateral vessels, despite a normal-appearing lateral femoral circumflex artery. The entire femoral head had photopenia on radionuclide imaging. (From Jones, J.P.: Fat embolism and osteonecrosis. Orthop. Clin. N. Amer., *16*:623, 1985.)

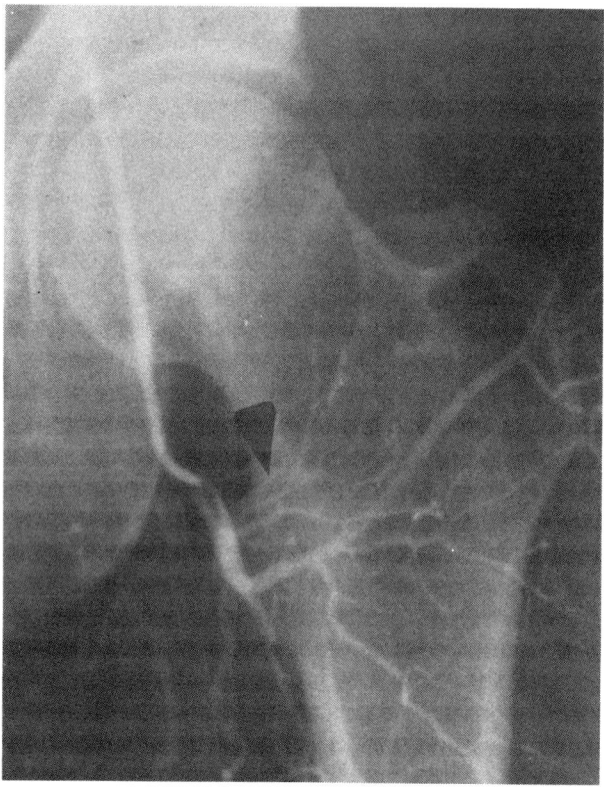

larization and resorption front. The revascularization front includes osteoclasts, fibroblasts, and capillaries. Narrowed, attenuated, and serrated trabeculae are resorbed (Fig. 98–8).

Radiographic Features

Radiographic changes produced by infarcted bone and marrow vary according to location.[105] Areas of focal demineralization beneath an intact articular surface first appear on conventional radiographic examination as less dense areas, the result of subchondral bone resorption (radiolucency) and surrounding appositional new bone formation (radiosclerosis). Metaphyseal lesions often appear as irregular lucencies or linear or mottled densities. Shaft or diaphyseal lesions often show serpentine calcification. No evidence of secondary subchondral fracture exists; the radiolucent "crescent" sign is not yet seen.

Magnetic Resonance Imaging. In general, stage II lesions, which repair without collapse, show either rings (focal smaller lesions) (Fig. 98–9) or bands (larger lesions) (Fig. 98–10A–D) of low signal intensity, representing the combined revascularization/ reossification front surrounding the necrotic zone.

Once an enlarging revascularization (repair) front begins penetrating into the necrotic zone (Fig. 98–8), there is a further delay before a discrete band is obvious on MRI. In stage II, a repair (revascularization) front appears as a single band or ring of decreased signal intensity on T1-weighting. This band is composed of viable tissue without fat cells and includes two parts, a resorption front, which is usually proximal, and a formation front, which is usually more distal. These two parts may be visualized with T2-weighting, the so-called double-line sign. The high-intensity proximal part of this sign most likely represents granulation tissue with inflammatory edema and hyperemia (the resorption front), and the low-intensity distal band represents thickened trabeculae. By performing both T1- and T2-weighted imaging, it can be determined whether an area of avascularity exists surrounded by hypervascularity or reactive change.[100]

Joint effusions can be diagnosed by hyperintensity from the synovium using very heavily T2-weighted images.[106] If there are no areas of low intensity in the femoral head on T1-weighting, but hyperintensity is noted on T2-weighting, it is likely that the patient has *synovitis* without avascularity. *Regional osteoporosis* will also give a false positive MRI with a diffusely diminished signal. Other false positive cases can occur with *metastatic disease, leukemia, myeloma,* or various *storage or metabolic diseases. Bone islands* or *subchondral degenerative cysts* have focal decreased intensity and may also give false positive results.

Scintigraphy. Stage II lesions usually show increased radionuclide uptake (Fig. 98–11). In one study, 12 of 27 (45%) patients with biopsy-proven stage I–II osteonecrosis had false negative radionuclide scintigrams; most of these patients had bilaterial disease.[107] In the transition from a stage I "cold" lesion to a stage II "hot" lesion is an intermediate stage II "cold/hot" lesion in which the revascularization front surrounds the necrotic zone. This cold/hot lesion must be defined because it is prone to collapse into stage III; it is best visualized by single photon emission computed tomography (SPECT) scintigrams.

Single Photon Emission Computed Tomography. In this method of imaging, the radionuclide is administered as in ordinary scintigraphy. A tomographic image is then obtained using a rotating camera, and computer reconstruction, as in CT scanning is per-

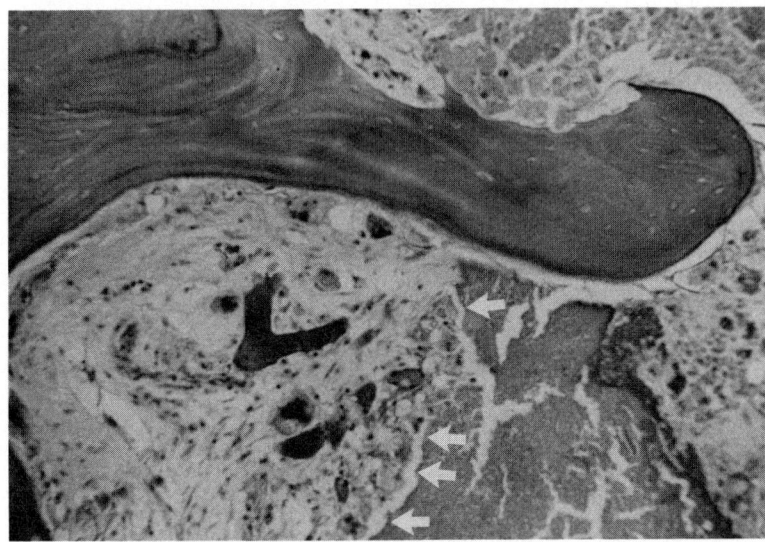

FIG. 98–8. Photomicrograph of femoral head specimen with stage II lesion demonstrating the present ischemic margin of the infarction *(arrows)*; the revascularization front is removing necrotic marrow debris, and there is osteoclastic resorption of a necrotic trabeculum.

formed, The advantage of SPECT over planar imaging is that "cold" spots are not obscured by overlying or contiguous "hot" areas. In stage II lesions, osteonecrosis is diagnosed by SPECT when an area of no uptake or an area of diminished uptake is surrounded by an area of increased uptake. One study compared MRI to SPECT results in 29 hips and found MRI to be more sensitive (96%/54%), more specific (100%/77%), and more accurate (98%/63%) than SPECT.[108]

Computed Tomography with Multiplanar Reconstruc-

FIG. 98–9. MR image in coronal plane showing two well-demarcated, focal stage II lesions in the right femoral head, appearing as revascularization/reossification *rings* of low signal intensity, surrounding central areas of increased intensity.

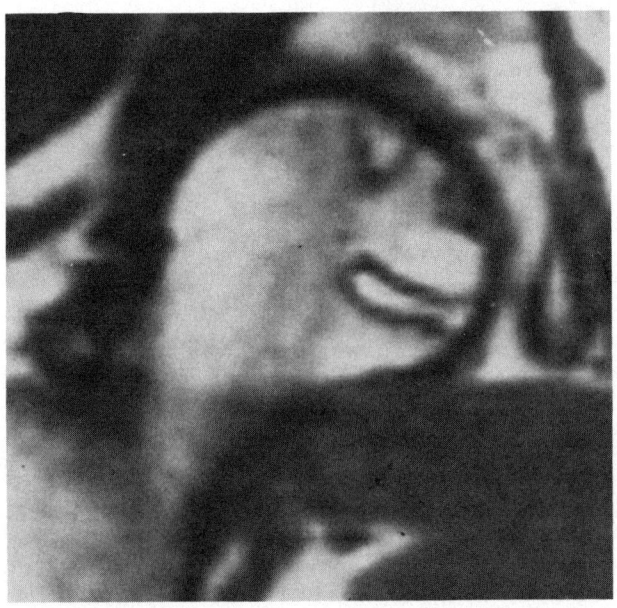

tions (CT/MPR). This method of imaging the hip is also effective in the diagnosis of stage II osteonecrosis, because it is sensitive to small changes of contour and differences in radiographic density. It has a marked advantage over conventional radiographs by assessing either gross (Fig. 98–12) or subtle trabecular coarsening ("asterisk sign").[109] With conventional transaxial CT, it is difficult to evaluate the superior pole of the femoral head and the superior joint space because of a partial volume effect. This problem can be alleviated by systematic reformatting into multiple coronal and sagittal images.[110] Unsuspected osteonecrosis of the contralateral hip was found by CT/MPR in 16% (9/55 patients), most of whom had stage II lesions.[111]

Estimation of the extent of involvement can also be refined by the use of grid-area mapping, planimetry, and concentric circles to detect subtle alterations in sphericity. Forty-five hips in 26 patents were studied with CT/MPR and compared with plain film radiographs. CT/MPR studies upgraded the disease staging in 14 of 45 hips (30%). The increased bone density on CT/MPR usually corresponds in both pattern and location to regions of decreased signal intensity on MR image sections.[98]

Superselective Angiography. Bone scintigrams and superselective angiography of the medial circumflex femoral artery, when performed in hips with stage II–III lesions, indicate hypervascularity of the femoral head by probable reconstituted (recanalized) lateral epiphyseal vessels about a subchondral zone of devascularization.[92,94] Ultimately, there may also be some collateral circulation of the lateral epiphyseal vessels derived from the uninvolved lateral femoral circumflex arterial tributaries, the inferior gluteal vessels, and the obturator artery and its medial epiphy-

FIG. 98–10. Femoral head specimen removed at surgery from a 31-year-old woman with progressive hip pain following steroid treatment and chemotherapy for Hodgkin's disease. *A*, 5 mm-thick, coronal MRI image section (TR = 1150 msec, TE = 40 msec). *B*, Line drawing outlining areas of varying MRI signal intensity that had been correlated with histological evaluation. Area I (high signal): nonviable trabeculae and marrow fat; area II (low signal) combination of dead bone, thickened living trabeculae with dead cores, and intertrabecular fibrous tissue; areas III and V (high signal): viable trabeculae and marrow fat with scattered hematopoietic marrow; area IV (intermediate signal): living bone with thickened longitudinal trabeculae. *C*, Radiograph of corresponding 5 mm-thick slice of gross specimen. *D*, Histologic section prepared from gross specimen slice. (From H.E. Jergesen, P. Lang, and H.K. Genant.)

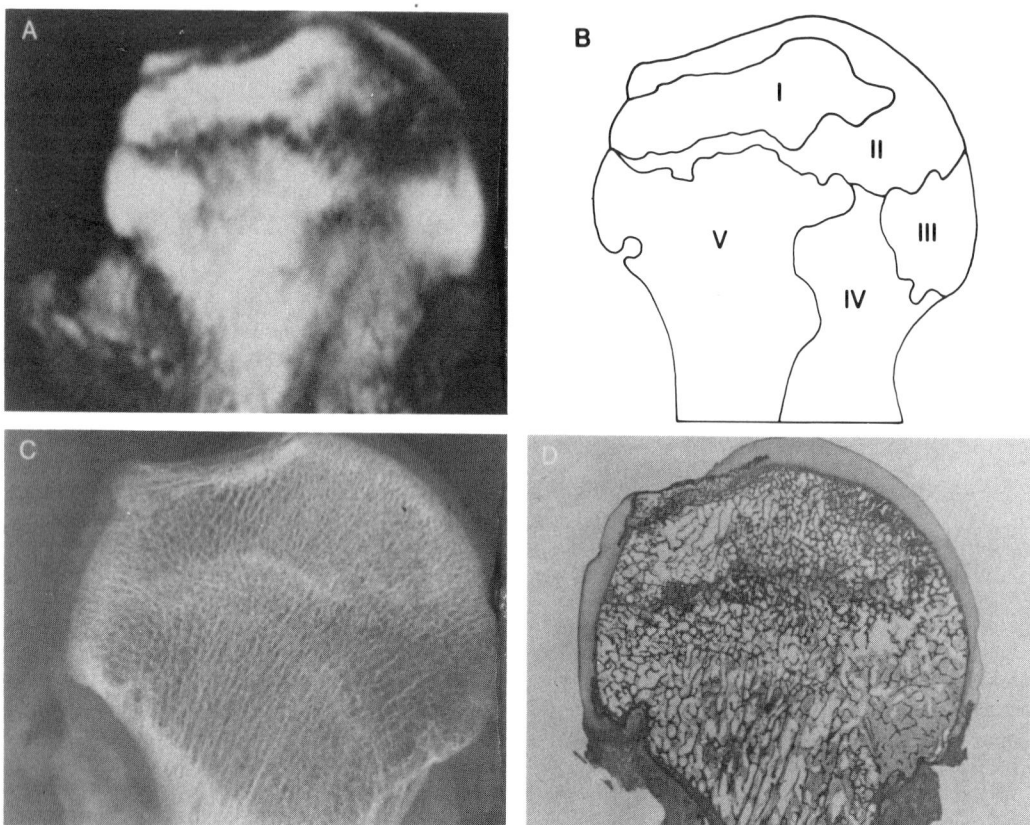

seal branches traversing the ligamentum teres. These are known to anastomose with lateral epiphyseal (superior retinacular) vessels to a limited extent.

Noninvasive Treatment

Focal lesions (IIA) measuring 10 to 15 mm in diameter may spontaneously heal. In order to prevent larger lesions (IIB) from collapsing during repair, it is recommended that an external pin fixator (iliofemoral) be used to distract the hip joint while the patient is nonweight-bearing.

Electrical stimulation: A relationship exists among mechanical forces, bioelectricity, and enhanced osteogenesis. A study of osteogenesis stimulation to heal early necrotic lesions of the femoral head is under way, using either capacitive coupling or pulsing electromagnetic fields.[112]

Invasive Treatment

Core decompression in Ficat stage I disease is followed by a 76% survival rate of the femoral head after 5 to 10 years; in stage II disease, there was a 64% survival.[113] Others have found that 60 to 79% of the core decompressions performed in the pre-collapse stages failed to prevent progressive collapse, however.[114,115] Because of *deleterious effects on the distribution of stress to the femoral head, core biopsy decompression without cortical grafting is discouraged.*[116] Revascularization of segmental necrotic lesions of the femoral head from the cancellous region is possible, within certain limits, if the patient has no evidence of sec-

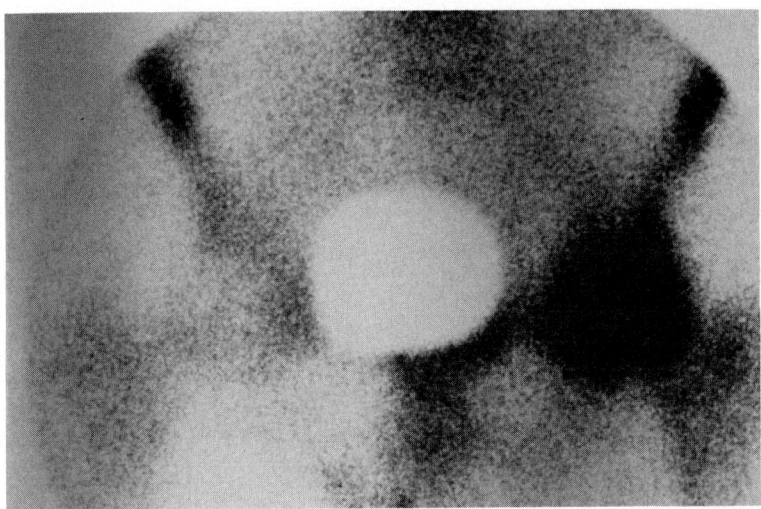

FIG. 98–11. Conventional ^{99m}Tc methylene-diphosphonate bone scintigram of the pelvis showing asymmetrically increased uptake in a necrotic left femoral head ("hot" lesion) and possible "cold/hot" lesion in right femoral head.

ondary subchondral fracture. To augment intrinsic revascularization, the necrotic area in the femoral head is excavated. Some surgeons transfer iliac bone on circumflex vascular pedicles, or free vascularized fibular grafts,[117] others fill the excavated cavity with iliac bone grafts,[117] and others introduce square autogenous bone pegs from the tibial cortex through round holes created in the femoral neck and head (Phemister-type graft);[118] 70% of stage II hip lesions so treated responded satisfactorily in two separate studies.[119]

STAGE III LESIONS

The patient usually remains asymptomatic until the articular surface undergoes late segmental collapse, when a stage II lesion becomes a stage III lesion. The patient reports symptoms of acute joint pain, and

occasionally spasm, usually aggravated by weight bearing and relieved by rest. Joint tenderness and slight limitation of motion are often present. Before MRI was available, over 90% of lesions were first diagnosed in stage III.

Pathologic Features

Late segmental collapse is essentially a result of the repair process. If repair were prevented entirely, the necrotic femoral head, covered with viable cartilage, would not collapse because dead bone (stage I) is essentially as strong as living bone. In stage III lesions, however, the radiolucent revascularization front has resorbed subchondral bone and uncalcified articular cartilage. Intracapital *fractures* begin in a focal area of osteoclastic resorption at the chondro-osseous junction. *Stress risers* are created by focal resorption of the subchondral plate.

Impulse loading, especially if applied while the hip

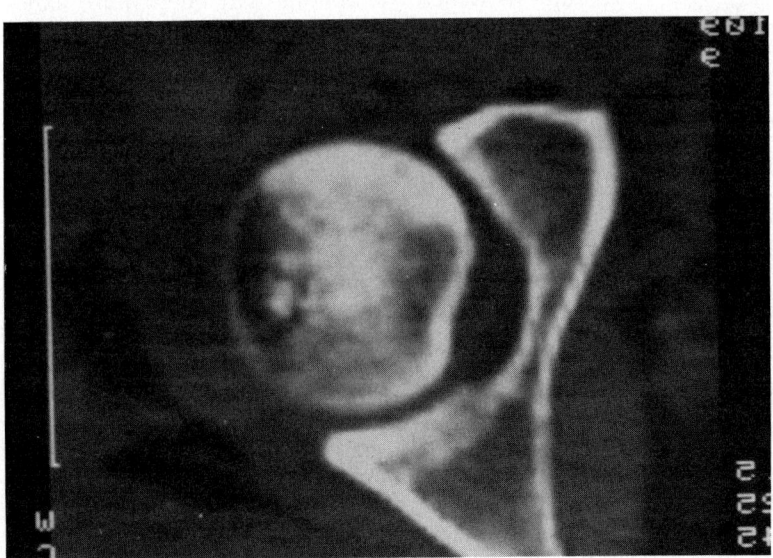

FIG. 98–12. CT of femoral head revealing a typical anterior-quadrant lesion (stage II) with diffuse sclerosis in a V-shaped configuration.

is in abduction,[120] leads to shear-induced microfractures of the pre-existing necrotic trabeculae, beginning at the stress risers, which propagate into the femoral head as a subchondral "saucer." In post-traumatic osteonecrosis, these intracapital fractures usually propagate deeper into the femoral head.[121] Finally, there is buckling and collapsing of the anterosuperior portion of the femoral head or the central portion of the humeral head.

Fibrocartilaginous metaplasia often occurs beneath the subchondral fracture, (Fig. 98–13) blocking further revascularization. This metaplasia probably develops as a result of micromotion or terminal hypoxia at the revascularizaiton front. Articular hyaline cartilage overlying severely osteonecrotic femoral heads, even with gross deformity of the underlying bone structure, shows surprisingly few histologic, bio-

FIG. 98–13. Photomicrograph of stage III lesion in a corticoid-treated cardiac transplant recipient revealing fibrocartilaginous metaplasia *(top)* immediately beneath the secondary subchondral fracture and the ischemic margin of the revascularization front *(bottom)* separated by a fibrous tissue barrier (A-B).

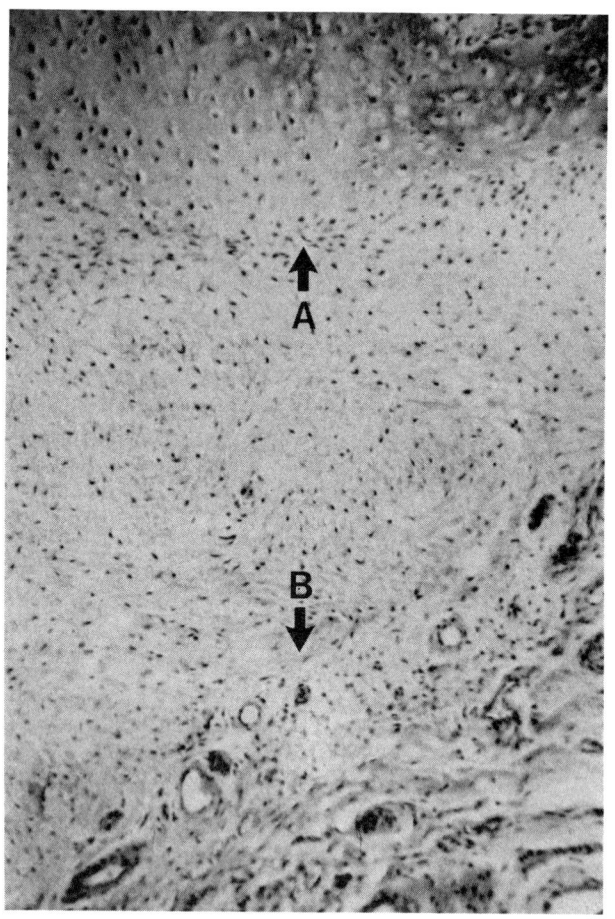

chemical, or metabolic changes because joint cartilage in mature adults derives most of its nutrition from synovial fluid.[122,123]

Radiographic Features

Radiographic examination, particularly external rotation views of the shoulder and lateral views of the hip, indicate architectural failure and structural collapse. A unipolar or bipolar subchondral fracture is often apparent (Fig. 98–14). A positive, radiolucent, crescent (meniscus) sign indicates a stage III lesion.[124] Once a break has occurred in the smooth, spherical articular cartilage and in subchondral bone; the necrotic lesion is *irreversible*, inevitably progressing to further collapse, with articular incongruity and secondary degenerative changes. *Focal* lesions (Fig. 98–14) are *spontaneously* reversible if their maximal diameter is less than 15 mm, however.

Treatment

The humeral or femoral head is not salvable at this point. The humeral head can be replaced by a metal prosthesis held in the humeral shaft by a stem (hemiarthroplasty) if the glenoid is normal.[125] Some patients with stage III lesions have been treated successfully by replacement of the collapsed segment with fresh osteochondral allographs.[27]

Using a varus or valgus trochanteric osteotomy, the necrotic area is moved so that maximal stress may fall on the uninvolved surface of the femoral head. If the lesion involves less than 25% of the femoral head and is confined entirely to the anterosuperior quadrant, a transtrochanteric rotational osteotomy may be successful. Although excellent results were obtained in 98 of 128 (77%) hips in one study, progressive collapse in the newly created weight-bearing area occurred in 25 hips in which the lesions had been more extensive.[127,128] Hemiarthroplasty is indicated for patients with extensive involvement of the femoral head when the acetabulum appears normal.

STAGE IV LESIONS

These patients have continuous joint pain, limpness, stiffness, and weakness. Physical findings include tenderness, deformity, crepitation, contracture, and limited motion.

Pathologic Features

As subchondral collapse continues, joint destruction occurs with advanced changes typical of osteoarthritis, including a narrowed, incongruous joint space, diffuse hypertrophy with extensive marginal

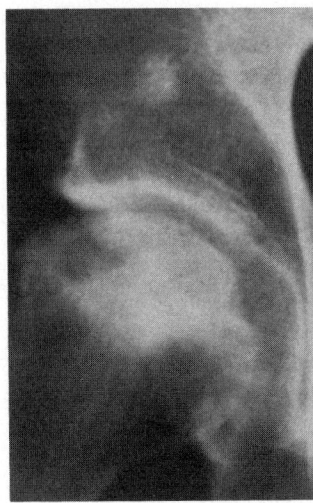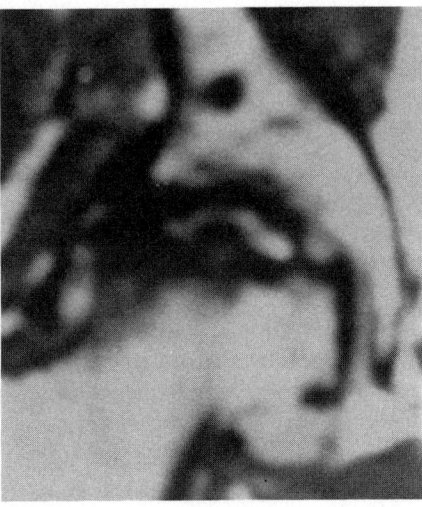

FIG. 98–14. Anteroposterior roentgenogram of the right hip revealing a probable focal sclerotic infarct in the supra-acetabular region and a stage III lesion in the femoral head with late segmental collapse *(left);* MR imaging indicates focal decreased signal intensity in the supra-acetabular infarct; collapse occurred laterally through the resorption front, in the band of decreased signal intensity in the femoral head *(right).*

osteophytic proliferation, and degenerative cyst formation of either side of the joint. Malignant fibrous histiocytoma and osteogenic sarcomas have been associated (rarely) with bone infarcts.

Treatment

Total joint replacement is the recommended treatment for stage IV lesions.

REFERENCES

 1. Upadhyay, S.S., Moultoj, A., and Srikrishnamurthy, K.: An analysis of late effects of traumatic posterior dislocation of the hip without fractures. J. Bone Joint Surg., *65B*:150–152, 1983.
 2. Roeder, L.F., Jr., and DeLee, J.C.: Femoral head fractures associated with posterior hip dislocations. Clin. Orthop., *147*:121–130, 1980.
 3. Kelly, R.P., and Yarbrough, S.H., III: Posterior fracture dislocation of the femoral head with retained medial head fragment. J. Trauma, *11*:97–108, 1971.
 4. Mann, R.J.: Avascular necrosis of the femoral head following intertrochanteric fractures. Clin. Orthop., *92*:108–115, 1973.
 5. Sevitt, S.: Avascular necrosis and revascularization of the femoral head after intracapsular fracture: a combined arteriographic and histologicaly study. J. Bone Joint Surg., *46B*:270–296, 1964.
 6. Sevitt, S., and Thompson, R.G.: The distribution and anastomoses of arteries supplying the head and neck of the femur. J. Bone Joint Surg., *47B*:560–573, 1965.
 7. Hermann, G., et al.: Gaucher's disease type 1: assessment of bone involvement by CT and scintigraphy. A.J.R., *147*:943–948, 1986.
 8. Hughes, E.C., Schmacher, H.R., and Sbarbaro, J.L.: Bilateral avascular necrosis of the hip following Leriche syndrome. J. Bone Joint Surg., *53A*:380–382, 1974.
 9. Jones, J.P., Jr.: Fat embolism and osteonecrosis. Orthop. Clin. North Am., *16*:595–633, 1985.
10. Jones, J.P., Jr., et al.: Fat embolization as a possible mechanism producing avascular necrosis. Arthritis Rheum., *8*:449, 1965.
11. Jones, J.P., Jr., Engleman, E.P., and Najarian, J.S.: Systemic fat embolism after renal homotransplantation and treatment with corticosteroids. N. Engl. J. Med., *273*:1453–1458, 1965.
12. Jones, J.P., Jr., and Sakovich, L.: Fat embolism of bone. A roentgenographic and histological investigation, with use of intra-arterial Lipiodol, in rabbits. J. Bone Joint Surg., *48A*:149–164, 1966.
13. Jones, J.P., Jr., Sakovich, L., and Anderson, C.E.: Experimentally produced osteonecrosis as a result of fat embolism. *In* Dysbarism-Related Osteonecrosis. Edited by E.L. Beckman, D.H. Elliot, and E.M. Smith. Washington, D.C., U.S. Department of Health Education and Welfare, 1974, pp. 117–131.
14. Jacobs, B.: Epidemiology of traumatic and nontraumatic osteonecrosis. Clin. Orthop., *130*:51–67, 1978.
15. Cruess, R.L., Ross D., and Crawshaw, E.: The etiology of steroid-induced avascular necrosis of bone. A laboratory and clinical study. Clin. Orthop., *113*:178–183, 1975.
16. Fisher, D.E., et al.: Corticosteroid-induced aseptic necrosis. II. Experimental study. Clin. Orthop., *84*:200–206, 1972.
17. Gold, E.W., et al.: Corticosteroid-induced avascular necrosis: an experimental study in rabbits. Clin. Orthop., *135*:272–280, 1978.
18. Jaffe, W.L., et al.: The effect of cortisone on femoral and humeral heads in rabbits. An experimental study. Clin. Orthop., *82*:221–228, 1972.
19. Kawai, K., Tamki, A., and Hirohata, K.: Steroid-induced accumulation of lipid in the osteocytes of the rabbit femoral head. A histochemical and electron microscopic study. J. Bone Joint Surg., *67A*:755–763, 1985.
20. Kenzora, J.E.: The effect of high dose corticosteroids on kidney, liver and bone tissues of rabbits. Unpublished data, 1978.
21. Surat, A.: Isolation of prostaglandin E2-like material from osteonecrosis induced by steroids and its prevention by kallikrein-inhibitor, aprotinin. Prostaglandins Leukotrienes Med., **13**:159–167, 1984.
22. Paolaggi, J.B., et al.: Early alterations of bone and marrow after high doses of steroids: results in two animal species. *In* Bone Circulation. Edited by J. Arlet, R.P. Ficat, and D.S. Hungerford. Baltimore, Williams & Wilkins, 1984, pp. 42–47.
23. Wang, G.-J., et al.: Fat-cell changes as a mechanism of avascular necrosis of the femoral head in cortisone-treated rabbits. J. Bone Joint Surg., *59A*:729–735, 1977.
24. Wang, G.-J., et al.: Cortisone-induced intrafemoral head pressure change and its response to a drilling decompression method. Clin. Orthop., *159*:274–278, 1981.

25. Wang, G.-J., et al.: Femoral head blood flow in long-term steroid treatment (study of rabbit model). In Bone Circulation. Edited by J. Arlet, R.P. Ficat, and D.S. Hungerford. Baltimore, Williams and Wilkins, 1984, pp. 35–37.

26. Bornstein, A., and Plate, E.: Chronic joint changes due to compressed air sickness. Fortschr. Gebiete Roentgenstr., 18:197–206, 1911.

27. Kindwall, E.P., Nellen, J.R., and Spiegelhoff, D.R.: Aseptic necrosis in compressed air tunnel workers using current OSHA decompression schedules. J. Occup. Med., 24:741–745, 1982.

28. Jones, J.P., Jr., and Behnke, A.R., Jr.: Prevention of dysbaric osteonecrosis in compressed-air workers. Clin. Orthop., 130:118–128, 1978.

29. Decompression Sickness Panel, Medical Research Council: Aseptic bone necrosis in commercial divers. Lancet, 8243:384–388, 1981.

30. Grutzmacher, K.T.: Changes of the shoulder as a result of compressed air sickness. Roentgenpraxis, 13:216–218, 1941.

31. Wade, C.E., et al.: Incidence of dysbaric osteonecrosis in Hawaii's diving fishermen. Undersea Biomed. Res., 5:137–147, 1978.

32. Kawashima, M., et al.: Pathological review of osteonecrosis in divers. Clin. Orthop., 130:107–117, 1978.

33. Pietrograndi, V., and Mastromario, R.: Osteopathia de proluregato trattemento cortisonico. Ital. J. Orthop. Traumatol., 25:791–810, 1957.

34. Anderton, J.M., and Helm, R.: Multiple joint osteonecrosis following short-term steroid therapy: case report. J. Bone Joint Surg., 64A:139–141, 1982.

35. Fisher, D.E., and Bickel, W.H.: Corticosteroid-induced avascular necrosis: a clinical study of seventy-seven patients. J. Bone Joint Surg., 53A:859–873, 1971.

36. Dubois, E.L.: Lupus Erythematosus. 2nd Ed. Los Angeles, University of Southern California Press, 1974, pp. 332–342.

37. Abeles, M., Urman, J.D., and Rothfield, N.F.: Aseptic necrosis of bone in systemic lupus erythematosus: relationship to corticosteroid therapy. Arch. Intern. Med., 138:750–754, 1978.

38. Starzl, T.E., et al.: Renal homotransplantation. Late function and complications. Ann. Intern. Med., 61:470–497, 1964.

39. Ibels, L.S., Alfrey, A.C., and Huffer, W.E.: Aseptic necrosis of bone following renal transplantation: experience in 194 transplant recipients and review of the literature. Medicine, 57:25–45, 1978.

40. Harrington, K.D., et al.: Avascular necrosis of bone after renal transplantation. J. Bone Joint Surg., 53A:203–215, 1971.

41. Jones, J.P., Jr.: Alcoholism hypercortisonism, fat embolism and osseous avascular necrosis. In Idiopathic Ischemic Necrosis of the Femoral Head in Adults. Edited by W.M. Zinn. Stuttgart, Georg Thieme, 1971, pp. 112–132.

42. Hungerford, D.S., and Zizic, T.M.: Alcoholism associated ischemic necrosis of the femoral head: early diagnosis and treatment. Clin. Orthop., 130:144–153, 1978.

43. Lequesne, M., Cloarec, M., and DeSeze, S.: Le terrain bioloqique de la necrose primitive de la tete femorale: hyperuricemie, hyperlipidemie. Dixieme Congres de la ligue internationale contre la rhumatism, Rome, 1961. Turin, Minerva Medica, 1961.

44. DeSeze, S., Welfling, J., and Lequesne, M.: L'osteonecrose primitive de la tete femorale chez l'adulte: etude de 30 cas. Rev. Rhum. Mal. Osteoartic., 27:117–127, 1960.

45. Blotman, F., et al.: Epreuve d'hyperlipemie, provoquee en crus, et osteonecrose. Rev. Rhum. Mal. Osteoartic., 43:419–424, 1976.

46. Mielants, H., et al.: Avascular necrosis and its relation to lipid and purine metabolism. J. Rheumatol., 2:430–436, 1975.

47. Palmer, A.K., et al.: Osteonecrosis of the femoral head in a family with hyperlipoproteinemia. Clin. Orthop., 155:166–171, 1981.

48. Starr, L.: Lipemia and fat embolism in diabetes mellitus. Med. Rec., 17:477–481, 1880.

49. Wang, G.-J., et al.: Steroid-induced femoral head pressure changes and their response to lipid-clearing agents. Clin. Orthop., 174:298–302, 1983.

50. Wang, G.-J.: Improvement of femoral head blood flow in steroid-treated rabbits using lipid-clearing agent. In The Hip. St. Louis, Mosby Publications, 1987, pp. 87–93.

51. Kay, N.R.M., Park, W.M., and Bark, M.B.: The relationship between pregnancy and femoral head necrosis. Br. J. Radiol., 45:828–831, 1972.

52. Ficat, R.P., and Arlet, J.: Ischemia and Bone Necrosis. Baltimore, Williams & Wilkins, 1980.

53. Peters, R.L., Edmondson, H.A., and Kunelis, C.T.: Acute fatty metamorphosis of the liver in pregnancy. JAMA, 180:767, 1962.

54. Kahil, M.E., et al.: Acute fatty liver of pregnancy; report of two cases. Arch. Intern. Med., 113:113–119, 1964.

55. Ponfick, E.: Ueber die sympathischen Erkrankungen des Knochenmarkes bei inneren Krankheiten. Virchows Arch. (Pathol. Anat.), 56:534, 1872.

56. Gerle, R.D., et al.: Osseous changes in chronic pancreatitis. Radiology, 85:330–337, 1965.

57. Boswell, S.H., and Baylin, G.J.: Metastatic fat necrosis in lytic bone lesions in a patient with painless acute pancreatitis. Radiology, 106:85–86, 1973.

58. Diggs, L.W., Pulliam, H.N., and King, J.C.: Bone changes in sickle cell anemia. South. Med. J., 30:249–259, 1937.

59. Reich, R.S., and Rosenberg, N.J.: Avascular necrosis of bone in Caucasians with chronic hemolytic anaemia due to combined sickling and thalassemia traits. J. Bone Joint Surg., 35A:894–904, 1953.

60. Golding, J.S.R., MacIver, J.E., and Went, L.N.: The bone changes in sickle cell anemia, and its genetic variants. J. Bone Joint Surg., 41B:711–718, 1959.

61. Tanaka, K.R., Clifford, G.O., and Axelrod, A.R.: Sickle cell anemia with aseptic necrosis of the femoral head. Blood, 11:998–1010, 1956.

62. Barton, C.J., and Cockshott, W.P.: Bone changes in hemoglobin SC disease. Am. J. Roentgen., 88:523–532, 1962.

63. Chung, S.M.K., and Ralston, E.L.: Necrosis of the femoral head associated with sickle cell anemia and its genetic variants: a review of literature and study of 13 cases. J. Bone Joint Surg., 51A:33–58, 1969.

64. MacMahon, H.E., and Weiss, S.: Carbon tetrachloride poisoning with macroscopic fat in the pulmonary artery. Am. J. Pathol., 5:623–630, 1929.

65. Sikorski, J., et al.: The pathophysiological changes of experimental fat embolism. Early pre-hypoxaemic changes. Br. J. Surg., 64:6–10, 1977.

66. Kellos, T.: Impaired arterial oxygenation associated with the use of bone cement in the femoral shaft. Anesthesiology, 42:210–216, 1975.

67. Collins, J.A., and Caldwell, M.C.: Relationship of depot fat embolism to pulmonary structure and function of rabbits. Am. J. Surg., 119:581–584, 1970.

68. Peltier, L.F., et al.: Fat embolism: II. The chemical composition of fat obtained from human long bones and subcutaneous tissue. Surgery, 40:661–664, 1956.

69. Sikorski, J.M.: Venous thrombosis produced by the local injection of fat. J. Bone Joint Surg., *65B*:340–345, 1983.

70. Sikorski, J.M., and Bradfield, J.W.: Fat and thromboembolism after total hip replacement. Acta Orthop. Scand., *54*:403–407, 1983.

71. King, E.G., et al.: Consumption coagulopathy in the canine oleic acid model of fat embolism. Surgery, *69*:533–541, 1971.

72. Collier, H.O.J., McDonald-Gibson, W.J., and Saeed, S.A.: Stimulation of prostaglandin biosynthesis by capsaicin, ethanol and tyramine. Lancet, *1*:702, 1975.

73. Gurd, A.R.: Fat embolism: an aid to diagnosis. J. Bone Joint Surg., *52B*:732–737, 1970.

74. Treiman, N., Waisbrod, V., and Waisbrod, H.: Lipoprotein electrophoresis in fat embolism: a preliminary report. Injury, *13*:108–110, 1981.

75. Kernoff, P.E., et al.: Antithrombotic potential of dihomo-gammalinolenic acid in man. Br. Med. J., *2*:1441–1444, 1977.

76. Serneri, G.C., et al.: Release of prostacyclin into the blood stream and its exhaustion in humans after local blood flow changes (ischemia and stasis). Thromb. Res., *17*:197–208, 1980.

77. Halleraker, B.: Fat embolism in intravascular coagulation. Acta Pathol. Microbiol. Immunol. Scand., *78A*:432–436, 1970.

78. Hartsock, L.A., Seaber, A.V., and Urbaniak, J.R.: Intravascular thrombosis in skeletal muscle microcirculation after ischemia. Trans. 33rd Ann. Meeting Ortho. Res. Soc., *12*:259, 1987.

79. Saldeen, T.: The importance of intra-vascular coagulation and inhibition of the fibrinolytic system in experimental fat embolism. J. Trauma, *10*:287–298, 1970.

80. Bradford, D.S., Foster, R.R., and Nossel, H.L.: Coagulation alterations, hypoxemia, and fat embolism in fracture patients. J. Trauma, *10*:307–321, 1970.

81. Philp, R.B.: A review of blood changes associated with compression-decompression: relationship to decompression sickness. Undersea Biomed. Res., *1*:117–150, 1974.

82. Lasch, H.G.: Therapeutic aspect of disseminated intravascular coagulation. Thrombosis Diathesis Haemorrh., *36(Suppl.)*:281–293, 1969.

83. Toyoshima, H.: Steroid-induced avascular necrosis of the femoral head. A histological investigation with use of bone fat staining technique. Bone Metab. (Japanese), *11*:291–294, 1978.

84. Kenzora, J.E., et al.: Experimental osteonecrosis of the femoral head in adult rabbits. Clin. Orthop., *130*:8–46, 1978.

85. Roesingh, G.E., and James, J.: Early phases of avascular necrosis of the femoral head in rabbits. J. Bone Joint Surg., *51B*:165–176, 1969.

86. Kenzora, J.E., et al.: Tissue biology following experimental infarction of the femoral heads. Part I. Bone studies, J. Bone Joint Surg., *51A*:1021, 1969.

87. Alavi, A., McCloskey, J.R., and Steinberg, M.E.: Early detection of avascular necrosis of the femoral head by [99m]technetium diphosphonate bone scan: a preliminary report. Clin. Orthop., *127*:137–141, 1977.

88. Bauer G.C.H., Weber, D.A., and Cedar, L.: Dynamics of technetium-99m methylene diphosphonate imaging of the femoral head after hip fracture. Clin. Orthop., *152*:85–92, 1980.

89. Goergen, T.G., et al.: "Cold" bone lesion: a newly recognized phenomenon of bone imaging. J. Nucl. Med., *15*:1120–1124, 1974.

90. MacLeod, M.A., et al.: Functional imaging in the early diagnosis of dysbaric osteonecrosis. Br. J. Radiol., *55*:497–500, 1982.

91. Nishioka, J.: The diagnosic value of bone scintiscanning in aseptic osteonecrosis of femur — comparative study between bone scintigram and histological findings. J. Jpn. Orthop. Assoc., *53*:429–440, 1979.

92. Atsumi, T.: Hemodynamic study of the idiopathic necrosis of femoral head using superselective angiography. J. Jpn. Orthop. Assoc., *57*:353–372, 1983.

93. Camargo, F.P., Godoy, R.M., Jr., and Tovo, R.: Angiography in Perthes' disease. Clin. Orthop., *191*:216–220, 1984.

94. Atsumi, T., et al.: A study of the vascular changes of Perthes' disease. Trans. 33rd Ann. Meeting. Ortho. Res. Soc., *12*:254, 1987.

95. Mitchell, M.D., et al.: Avascular necrosis of the hip: comparison of MR, CT, and scintigraphy. Amer. J. Roentgen., *147*:67–71, 1986.

96. Bassett, L.W., et al.: Magnetic resonance imaging in the early diagnosis of ischemic necrosis of the femoral head: preliminary results. Clin. Orthop., *214*:237–248, 1987.

97. Totty, W.G., et al.: Magnetic resonance imaging of the normal and ischemic femoral head. Amer. J. Roentgen., *143*:1273–1280, 1984.

98. Jergesen, H.E., Heller, M., and Genant, H.K.: Magnetic resonance imaging in osteonecrosis of the femoral head. Orthop. Clin. North Am., *16*:705–716, 1985.

99. Huber, D.J., et al.: MR imaging of the normal shoulder. Radiology, *158*:405–408, 1986.

100. Easton, E.J., Jr., and Powers, J.A.: Musculoskeletal magnetic resonance imaging. Slack Inc., Thorofare, NJ, 1986, pp. 21–46.

101. Gregg, P.J., and Walder, D.N.: Scintigraphy versus radiography in the early diagnosis of experimental bone necrosis, with special reference to caisson disease of bone. J. Bone Joint Surg., *62B*:214–221, 1980.

102. Johnson, L.C.: Histogenesis of avascular necrosis. *In* Proceedings of the Conference of Aseptic Necrosis of the Femoral Head. U.S. Public Health Service. St. Louis, Missouri, 1964, pp. 55–79.

103. Zizic, T.M., et al.: The early diagnosis of ischemic necrosis of bone. Arthritis Rheum., *29*:1177, 1986.

104. Arlet, J., and Ficat, P.: Biopsy drilling as a means of early diagnosis. *In* Idiopathic Ischemic Necrosis of the Femoral Head in Adults. Edited by W.M. Zinn. Stuttgart, Thieme, 1971, pp. 152–157.

105. Heard, J.L., and Schneider, C.S.: Radiographic findings in commercial divers. Clin. Orthop., *130*:129–138, 1978.

106. Mitchell, D.G., Rao, The., Dalinka, M., et al.: MRI of joint fluid in the normal and ischemic hip. Amer. J. Roentgen., *146*:1215, 1986.

107. Bieber, E., Hungerford, D.S., and Lennox, D.W.: Factors in diagnosis of avascular necrosis of the femoral head. Adv. Orthop. Surg., *10*:93, 1985.

108. Miller, I.L.: The use of magnetic resonance imaging and single photon emission computed tomography in evaluation of osteonecrosis of the femoral head. Exhibit, 54th Ann. Meet., AAOS, San Francisco, January 24, 1987.

109. Dihlmann, W.: CT analysis of the upper end of the femur: the asterisk sign and ischemic necrosis of the femoral head. Skeletal Radiol., *8*:251, 1982.

110. Fishman, E.K., et al.: Multiplanar (MPR) imaging of the hip. Radio-Graphics, *6*:7, 1986.

111. Magid, D., et al.: Computed tomography with multiplanar reconstructions in the assessment in staging of avascular necrosis of the femoral head. Radiology, *157*:751, 1985.

112. Basset, C.A.L., Schink, M.M., and Mitchell, S.N.: Treatment of osteonecrosis of the hip with specific, pulsed electromagnetic fields (PEMFs): a preliminary clinical report. *In* Bone

Circulation. Edited by J. Arlet, R.P. Ficat, and D.S. Hungerford. Baltimore/London, Williams & Wilkins, 1984, pp. 343–354.

113. Hungerford, D.S.: Symposium: osteonecrosis of the femoral head. Contemp. Orthop., *14*:119–124, 1987.

114. Camp, J.F., and Colwell, C.W., Jr.: Core decompression of the femoral head for osteonecrosis. J. Bone Joint Surg., *68A(9)*:1313–1319, 1986.

115. Steinberg, M.E., et al.: Electrical stimulation in the treatment of osteonecrosis of the femoral head: a 1-year followup. Orthop. Clin. North Am., *16*:747–756, 1985.

116. Penix, A.R., et al.: Femoral head stress following cortical bone grafting for aseptic necrosis: a finite element study. Clin. Orthop., *173*:159–165, 1983.

117. Wagner, H.: Treatment of idiopathic necrosis of the femoral head. *In* Idiopathic Ischemic Necrosis of the Femoral Head in Adults. Edited by W.M. Zinn. Stuttgart, Georg Thieme, 1971, pp. 202–204.

118. Bonfiglio, M., and Bardenstein, M.B.: Treatment by bone-grafting of aseptic necrosis of the femoral head and non-union of the femoral neck (Phemister technique). J. Bone Joint Surg., *40A*:1329–1346, 1958.

119. Wang, G.-J., and Thompson, R.C.: Treatment of aseptic necrosis of the femoral head with Phemister-type bone grafts. South. Med. J., *69*:305–308, 1976.

120. Brown, T.D., and Ferguson, A.B., Jr.: The development of a computational stress analysis of the femoral head: mapping tensile, compressive, and shear stress for the varus and valgus positions. J. Bone Joint Surg., *60A*:619–629, 1978.

121. Kenzora, J.E., and Glimcher, M.J.: Osteonecrosis. *In* Textbook of Rheumatology. Edited by Kelley, et al. Philadelphia, W.B. Saunders Co., 1981, pp. 1755–1779.

122. Glimcher, M.J., and Kenzora, J.E.: The biology of osteonecrosis of the human femoral head and its clinical implications: I. Tissue biology. Clin. Orthop., *138*:284–309, 1979.

123. Mankin, H.J., Thrasher, A.Z., and Hall, D.: Biochemical and metabolic characteristics of articular cartilage from osteonecrotic human femoral heads. J. Bone Joint Surg., *59A*:724–728, 1977.

124. Waldenstrom, H.: The first stages of coxa plana. J. Bone Joint Surg., *20*:559–566, 1938.

125. Cruess, R.L.: Experience with steroid-induced avascular necrosis of the shoulder and etiologic considerations regarding osteonecrosis of the hip. Clin. Orthop., *130*:86–93, 1978.

126. Meyers, M.H.: Allografts with the muscle pedicle technique. Clin. Orthop., *130*:202–209, 1978.

127. Kotz, R.: Avascular necrosis of the femoral head: a review of the indications and results of Sugioka transtrochanteric rotational osteotomy. Int. Orthop., *5*:53–58, 1981.

128. Sugioka, Y., Katsuki, I., and Hotokebuchi, T.: Transtrochanteric rotational osteotomy of the femoral head for the treatment of osteonecrosis: follow-up statistics. Clin. Orthop., *169*:115–126, 1982.

99

UVEITIS

JAMES T. ROSENBAUM

Many diseases associated with joint inflammation also have the potential to cause *uveitis,* inflammation within the eye. An understanding of uveitis can aid greatly in the differential diagnosis of rheumatologic disease.

The richly vascular uvea develops during embryogenesis as the middle layer of the eye (Fig. 99–1). Anteriorly, it includes the iris and the ciliary body and continues posteriorly as the choroid. Inflammation may affect all or part of the uveal tract and its adjacent structures. Thus, the terms *iritis, iridocyclitis* (inflammation of the iris and ciliary body), *choroiditis, retinochoroiditis,* and *panuveitis* (inflammation throughout the uveal tract) describe subsets of uveitis.

FIG. 99–1. Schematic diagram of the eye. The uveal tract (shown in black) includes the iris, ciliary body, and choroid.

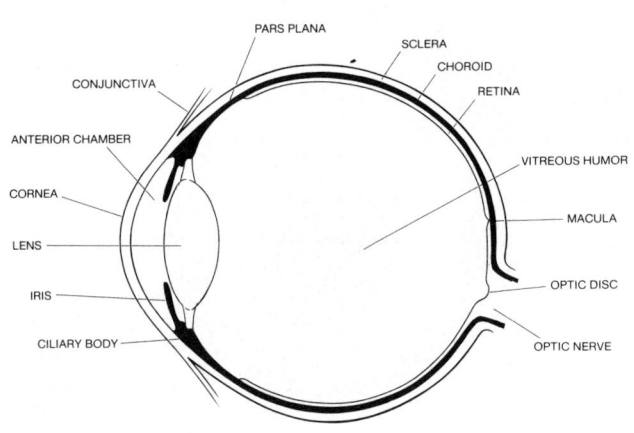

Some of the more common diseases associated with uveitis are listed in Table 99–1. The listed diseases have been assigned to one of four classes: (1) infectious diseases, (2) syndromes restricted primarily to the eye, (3) entities with a suspected immune-mediated pathogenesis, and (4) "masquerade" syndromes that mimic inflammation. This classification is somewhat arbitrary, and the classes do not have absolute boundaries. For example, some of the syndromes limited to the eye such as sympathetic ophthalmia may be immune mediated, and some of the immune-mediated diseases may ultimately be shown to have an infectious cause. This list is also not meant to be all-inclusive. For example, many common viral infections are associated with a mild iritis; also one of the most common diagnoses is omitted, so-called idiopathic (nonclassifiable) disease. Just as a particular pattern of joint involvement may suggest a specific rheumatologic diagnosis, the characteristics of the eye inflammation may indicate a most likely diagnostic entity.

THE CHARACTERIZATION OF UVEITIS

The subsets of uveitis can be distinguished by such features as location (anterior vs. posterior or both); chronicity; tendency to recur; laterality; occurrence of complications including cataract, glaucoma, band keratopathy (Fig. 99–2) (the deposition of calcium in cornea), or synechiae (Fig. 99–3) (fibrous adhesions such as occur between the iris and lens); and the appear-

Table 99–1.   Diagnostic Categorization of Uveitis

Infectious Causes
  Viral
    Herpes simplex
    Herpes zoster
    Cytomegalovirus
  Bacterial or spirochetal
    Tuberculosis
    Leprosy
    Proprionobacterium
    Syphilis
    Whipple's disease
  Parasitic (protozoan or helminthic)
    Toxoplasmosis
    Toxocariasis
    Cysticercosis
  Fungal
    Histoplasmosis
    Coccidioidomycosis
    Candidiasis

Suspected Immune Mediated
  Ankylosing spondylitis
  Behçet's syndrome
  Crohn's disease
  Drug or hypersensitivity reaction
  Juvenile rheumatoid arthritis
  Kawasaki disease
  Psoriatic arthritis
  Reiter's syndrome
  Relapsing polychondritis
  Sarcoidosis
  Sjögren's syndrome
  Systemic lupus erythematosus
  Ulcerative colitis
  Vasculitis
  Vitiligo
  Vogt Koyanagi Harada syndrome

Syndromes Confined Primarily to the Eye
  Acute multifocal placoid pigmentary epitheliopathy
  Birdshot choroidopathy
  Fuch's heterochromic cyclitis
  Glaucomatocyclitic crisis
  Lens-induced uveitis
  Serpiginous choroiditis
  Sympathetic ophthalmia
  Trauma

Masquerade Syndromes
  Leukemia
  Lymphoma
  Melanoma
  Retinitis pigmentosa
  Retinoblastoma

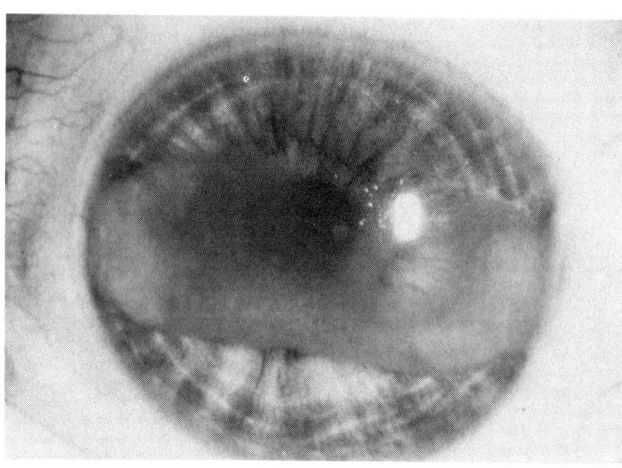

FIG. 99–2.   Band keratopathy results from the deposition of calcium in the cornea. Although any chronic anterior uveal inflammation can result in band keratopathy, this complication is most characteristic of the chronic iritis associated with juvenile arthritis.

trate and increased vascular permeability. The white cells are seen directly through the microscope. Permeability can be quantitated as "flare." Normal aqueous humor contains only minimal amounts of protein. As vascular permeability increases, the protein in the aqueous humor increases; the beam of light from the slit lamp becomes smokey as it passes through this proteinaceous fluid. This smokiness or "flare" is akin to the effect of fog on a car headlight; particles in fog or protein in aqueous humor diffract the light beam and make it visible.

Although an internist lacks the technology used by

FIG. 99–3.   Posterior synechiae forming between the iris and anterior lens capsule have given this pupil a cloverleaf appearance.

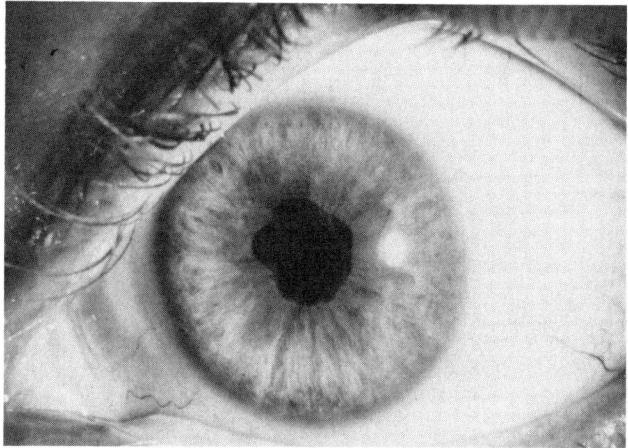

ance of keratic precipitates (Fig. 99–4) (concretions of cells on the endothelial surface of the cornea). An ophthalmologist uses instruments including the slit-lamp biomicroscope, the indirect ophthalmoscope, the gonioscope, and the fluorescein angiogram to help characterize the uveitis. If the iris is involved, the slit lamp allows visualization of the two universal hallmarks of inflammation, namely a leukocytic infil-

FIG. 99–4. Concretions of cells on the corneal endothelium are called keratic precipitates. The distribution and size of these deposits can aid in the differential diagnosis of iritis.

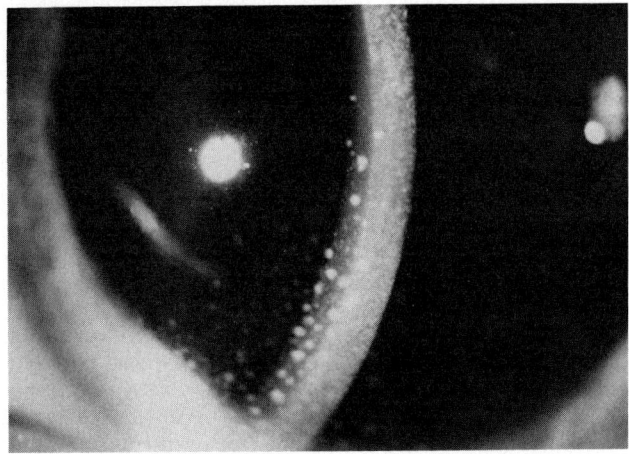

an ophthalmologist during an eye examination, the history and physical examination can characterize uveitis to a significant degree. Acute anterior uveitis or iritis, for example, provokes redness and pain, whereas chronic anterior uveitis causes much less redness or pain. Posterior uveitis generally causes neither. Symptoms of posterior uveitis will depend on the location of the inflammation. Inflammation in the peripheral choroid and adjacent retina may be asymptomatic, whereas inflammation near the macula or optic nerve distorts vision or reduces acuity. Posterior uveal inflammation associated with leukocytes in the vitreous humor will generally result in large or numerous "floaters" when these traverse the visual axis.

UVEITIS AND SYSTEMIC DISEASE

Approximately 35% of all patients with uveitis have an identifiable systemic disease, but a far higher percentage have laboratory abnormalities such as an elevated erythrocyte sedimentation rate or an alteration in lymphocyte subsets.[1] Many diseases that cause joint inflammation have a propensity to affect the uveal tract as well. Some of the characteristics of uveitis associated with rheumatologic disease are shown in Table 99–2. By far the most common disease associated with uveitis is spondyloarthritis.

The incidence rate of anterior uveitis is approximately four times that of posterior uveitis.[2] Acute anterior uveitis has a 50 to 75% likelihood of association with the antigen HLA-B27.[3,4] Greater than 90% of the episodes of HLA-B27 associated uveitis are unilateral.[5] Frequently, however, episodes are recurrent,

and alternate between the right eye and the left. Episodes of iritis associated with HLA-B27 are generally self-limited, resolving completely within 2 to 4 months. Choroidal inflammation is *not* linked to HLA-B27. Rarely, a marked vitreous cellular infiltrate occurs in association with HLA-B27. About 30 to 90% of patients with iritis associated with HLA-B27 also have spondyloarthritis.[5–7] In my experience, the figure approaches 90% because many of these patients have previously undiagnosed axial or peripheral inflammatory joint disease. Spondyloarthritis should be sought in any patient with acute, primarily anterior, unilateral uveitis associated with redness and pain.

Patients with HLA-B27–associated iritis differ in many respects from those who are HLA-B27 negative. The eye inflammation in the former group is generally of shorter duration, has a greater likelihood of recurrence in the other eye, is more likely to develop complications such as synechiae, and is far more likely to be associated with joint inflammation.[5,8] Because knowledge of HLA-B27 status has diagnostic, prognostic, and therapeutic implications, many authorities recommend routine HLA-B27 typing for patients with acute, anterior, unilateral uveitis.[8] HLA-B27 typing, however, is inappropriate for a patient with chronic or bilateral uveitis; chorioretinitis; or little associated redness or pain. Neither Reiter's syndrome nor ankylosing spondylitis is typically associated with uveitis that is bilateral, chronic, or posterior.

An appreciation of the subsets of uveitis can be helpful in the differential diagnosis of rheumatic disease. For example, oral mucosal ulcers, arthritis, diarrhea, and uveitis are features of Behçet's syndrome as well as Reiter's syndrome. The iritis of Reiter's syndrome, however, should rarely be confused with the uveal involvement seen with Behçet's syndrome because the latter is frequently bilateral, chronic, posterior as well as anterior, and associated with retinal vasculitis.

Several juvenile rheumatoid arthritis (JRA) subsets are associated with iritis. In the HLA-B27 positive subsets such as juvenile ankylosing spondylitis[9] or polyarticular peripheral joint disease associated with C_2–C_3 apophyseal joint fusion,[10] the iritis is acute, self-limited, and frequently recurrent. In contrast, the antinuclear antibody (ANA)-positive, pauciarticular, early onset, generally female subset of JRA is associated with a chronic, bilateral iridocyclitis,[11,12] which is often insidious and painless. The iritis frequently develops after the joint disease. Although the joint disease may be self-limited, the chronic iritis can become the most salient feature of the syndrome, frequently complicated by glaucoma, cataract, and band keratopathy.

Table 99–2. Rheumatologic Diseases Associated With Uveitis

Disease	Usual Characteristics of Uveitis	Likelihood of Uveitis During Disease Course	Reference
Ankylosing spondylitis	Acute, anterior, unilateral, recurrent	29%	16
Reiter's syndrome	Acute, anterior, unilateral, recurrent	20%	15
Juvenile rheumatoid arthritis (HLA-B27+ subset, axial or peripheral joint disease)	Acute, anterior, unilateral, recurrent	25%	9, 10
Psoriatic arthritis	Acute, anterior, unilateral	8%	26
Ulcerative colitis	Acute, anterior, unilateral	2%	27
Crohn's disease	Acute, anterior, unilateral*	2%	27
Kawasaki disease	Acute, anterior, bilateral	78%	14
Familial granulomatous juvenile arthritis	Acute, anterior, bilateral, recurrent	Common	28
Juvenile rheumatoid arthritis (pauciarticular, ANA positive, early onset subset)	Chronic, anterior, bilateral	53%	11
Sjögren's syndrome	Chronic anterior and posterior, bilateral	Rare	21
Sarcoid	Acute or chronic, anterior and/or posterior, unilateral or bilateral	32%	17
Behçet's syndrome	Acute or chronic, anterior and posterior, bilateral	66%	13
Relapsing polychondritis	Anterior, recurrent, often with associated scleritis or episcleritis	9%	29
Vasculitis†		Rare	30
Systemic lupus erythematosus‡		Rare	18

ANA = antinuclear antibody.
*Uveitis associated with this disease may sometimes be posterior or bilateral.
†Uveitis has been described in association with many forms of vasculitis including Wegener's granulomatosis, polyarteritis nodosa, temporal arteritis, and leukocytoclastic vasculitis. In all of these examples, uveitis is rare and too infrequent to characterize the typical presentation.
‡Systemic lupus causes uveitis too infrequently to characterize a typical presentation. Other ocular manifestations such as xerophthalmia and cotton wool spots are far more common.

Some diseases involve both the uveal tract and the joint in 50 to 80% of all cases. Examples include the pauciarticular, ANA-positive subset of JRA,[11] Behçet's syndrome,[13] and Kawasaki disease.[14] About 20% of patients with Reiter's syndrome,[15] ankylosing spondylitis,[16] or the HLA-B27–positive subset of JRA[9] develop uveitis. A few diseases commonly cause uveitis and occasionally cause arthritis, for example, sarcoid.[17] Finally, a long list of arthritic conditions may rarely involve the uvea along with the other systemic manifestations. Systemic lupus erythematosus[18] and several types of vasculitis, such as Wegener's granulomatosis[19] and leukocytoclastic vasculitis,[20] fall within this category.

Most forms of vasculitis can also involve the retinal vessels. *Retinal vasculitis* can be a manifestation of uveitis as in sarcoid or Behçet's syndrome. Retinal vasculitis can also occur without evidence for inflammation either in the eye or systemically. Rheumatoid arthritis is not usually associated with uveal tract involvement, although it can be associated with scleritis, which if severe can affect the entire thickness of the sclera, resulting in secondary uveitis.

EVALUATION OF THE UVEITIS PATIENT: THE INTERNIST'S ROLE

A thorough history and physical examination are an essential first step. Behçet's syndrome, spondyloarthritis, or ulcerative colitis should be readily apparent. Other diseases such as sarcoidosis could be overlooked by history but might be suggested by physical findings such as a typical skin lesion. In many instances, the onus for diagnosis rests squarely with the ophthalmologist, for whom history and examination of the eye should be sufficient to arrive at diagnoses such as histoplasmosis, toxoplasmosis, or sympathetic ophthalmia. If no diagnosis is evident, a chest roentgenogram to look for hilar and mediastinal lymph nodes and a serologic test for syphilis are obtained. In approximately 20% of patients with sarcoid, an eye abnormality will be the initial manifestation of the disease.[17] Sarcoid can involve the uveal tract in many different ways and is second only to spondyloarthritis as a systemic disease associated with uveitis.

Syphilis is now rare, but it can involve any portion of the uveal tract usually in the late secondary stage. Nearly a third of patients with luetic uveitis therefore may have a negative VDRL, so the fluorescent treponemal antibody test (FTA) should be used. All uveitis patients with a positive FTA test should be treated with antimicrobial agents. Those who truly have syphilis can be distinguished by a good therapeutic response and a fall in their VDRL titer if this is positive.

An association has been suggested between Sjögren's syndrome and chronic, bilateral, anterior, and posterior uveitis.[21] Such patients have dry eyes by Schirmer testing, focal lymphocytic infiltration of minor salivary glands, an elevated erythrocyte sedimentation rate, and often a positive ANA titer with a speckled pattern. These patients are almost all female, usually have associated xerostomia, and frequently have associated systemic findings such as arthralgias, fatigue, depression, or neuropathy. Unlike most patients with Sjögren's syndrome, these patients generally lack rheumatoid factor or autoantibodies to Ro or La. Therefore, a Schirmer's test and rose bengal staining of the conjunctiva may prove useful as initial screening tests in the differential diagnosis of a subset of patients with uveitis.

Even in experienced hands, as many as one third of all patients with uveitis seen at a referral clinic may have idiopathic disease; that is, no findings allow any diagnosis such as those given in Table 99–1.[22]

ETIOLOGY

In most patients with uveitis, the precise etiopathogenesis is uncertain. In laboratory animals, uveal inflammation can be induced by a variety of methods, including the Arthus reaction, a cell-mediated immune response, an "autoimmune" response against a self-antigen such as lens protein or retinal S antigen, and local or systemic injection of bacterial products including endotoxin or peptidoglycan.[22] Rats developing adjuvant arthritis also frequently develop uveitis.

The reason for the frequent coexistence of eye and joint inflammation remains obscure. Type II collagen is present in both eye and joint, and hyaluronic acid is commmon to both vitreous humor and synovial fluid. A cross-reactive immune mechanism is one possible explanation for the concomitant inflammation in these two locations.

TREATMENT

The treatment of uveitis depends on the diagnosis, the location of the inflammation, and its complications. Antibiotics with adjunctive corticosteroids are often indicated for toxoplasmosis associated with chorioretinitis. Antiviral therapy is becoming the mode for acute retinal necrosis, a fulminant panuveitis associated with herpes simplex or herpes zoster.[23] Iritis is usually treated by topical corticosteroids and a mydriatic to reduce the likelihood of synechiae and relieve pain by decreasing spasm in the ciliary muscle. For control of inflammation posterior to the lens, corticosteroids must be given either systemically or by periocular injection. Inflammation refractory to steroids may respond to systemic immunosuppressive therapy such as chlorambucil or methotrexate.[24] Cyclosporine appears effective in controlling uveal inflammation,[25] but its role is presently limited by nephrotoxicity (see Chapter 38). It must be given continuously to control uveitis, that is, it does not induce remission.

REFERENCES

1. Deschenes, J., et al.: Uveitis: Lymphocyte subpopulation studies. Trans. Ophthalmol. Soc. U.K., 105:246–251, 1986.
2. Darrell, R.W., Wagener, H.P., and Kurland, C.T.: Epidemiology of uveitis. Incidence and prevalence in a small urban community. Arch. Ophthalmol., 68:502–514, 1962.
3. Brewerton, D.A., et al.: Acute anterior uveitis and HLA B27. Lancet, 2:994–996, 1973.
4. Ehlers, N., Kissmeyer-Nielsen, F., Kjerbye, K.E., and Lamm, L.U.: HLA27 in acute and chronic uveitis. (Letter.) Lancet, 1:99, 1974.
5. Feltkamp, T.E.W.: HLA B27, Acute anterior uveitis, and ankylosing spondylitis. Adv. Inflamm. Res., 9:211–216, 1985.
6. Beckingsale, A.B., Davies, J., Gibson, J.M., and Rosenthal, A.R.: Acute anterior uveitis, ankylosing spondylitis, back pain and HLA B27. Br. J. Ophthalmol., 68:741–745, 1984.
7. Vinje, O., Dale, K., and Moller, P.: Radiographic changes, HLA B27 and back pain in patients with psoriasis or acute anterior uveitis. Scand. J. Rheumatol., 12:219–224, 1983.
8. Rothova, A., et al.: Clinical features of acute anterior uveitis. Am. J. Ophthalmol., 103:137–145, 1987.
9. Ansell, B.M.: Chronic arthritis in childhood. Ann. Rheum. Dis., 37:107–120, 1978.
10. Arnett, F.C., Bias, W.B., and Stevens, M.B.: Juvenile-onset

chronic arthritis. Clinical and roentgenographic features of a unique HLA B27 subset. Am. J. Med., 69:369–376, 1980.

11. Glass, D., et al.: Early-onset pauciarticular juvenile rheumatoid arthritis associated with human leukocyte antigen-DRw5, iritis, and antinuclear antibody. J. Clin. Invest., 66:426–429, 1980.

12. Kanski, J.J.: Anterior uveitis in juvenile rheumatoid arthritis. Arch. Ophthalmol., 95:1794–1797, 1977.

13. Colvard, D.M., Robertson, D.M., O'Duffy, J.D.: The ocular manifestations of Behçet's disease. Arch. Ophthalmol., 95:1813–1817, 1977.

14. Ohno, S., et al.: Ocular manifestations of Kawasaki's disease (mucocutaneous lymph node syndrome). Am. J. Ophthalmol., 93:713–717, 1982.

15. Oates, J.K., and Young, A.C.: Sacro-iliitis in Reiter's disease. Br. Med. J., 1:1013–1015, 1959.

16. Lenoch, F., Kralik, V., and Bartos, J.: "Rheumatic" iritis and iridocyclitis. Ann. Rheum. Dis., 18:45–48, 1959.

17. Obenauf, C.D., Shaw, H.E., Sydnor, C.F., and Klintworth, G.K.: Sarcoidosis and its ophthalmic manifestations. Am. J. Ophthalmol., 86:648–655, 1978.

18. Gold, D.H., Morris, D.A., and Henkind, P.: Ocular findings in systemic lupus erythematosus. Br. J. Ophthalmol., 56:800–804, 1972.

19. Haynes, B.F., Fishman, M.L., Fauci, A.S., and Wolff, S.M.: The ocular manifestations of Wegener's granulomatosis. Fifteen years experience and review of the literature. Am. J. Med., 63:131–141, 1977.

20. Ryan, L.M., Kozin, F., and Eiferman, R.: Immune complex uveitis: A case. Ann. Intern. Med., 88:62–63, 1978.

21. Rosenbaum, J.T., and Bennett, R.M.: Chronic anterior and pos-terior uveitis is associated with primary Sjögren's syndrome. Am. J. Ophthalmol., 104:346–352, 1987.

22. Henderly, D.E., Genstler, A.J., Smith, R.E., and Rao, N.A.: Changing patterns of uveitis. Am. J. Ophthalmol., 103:131–136, 1987.

23. Rosenbaum, J.T., and Cousins, S.: Uveitis and arthritis: Experimental models and clinical correlates. Semin. Arthritis Rheum., 11:383–389, 1982.

23. Freeman, W.R., et al.: Demonstration of herpes group virus in acute retinal necrosis syndrome. Am. J. Ophthalmol., 102:701–709, 1986.

24. Andrasch, R.H., Pirofsky, B., and Burns, R.P.: Immunosuppressive therapy for severe chronic uveitis. Arch. Ophthalmol., 96:247–251, 1978.

25. Nussenblatt, R.B., et al.: Treatment of intraocular inflammatory disease with cyclosporine. Lancet, 2:235–238, 1983.

26. Lambert, J.R., and Wright, V.: Eye inflammation in psoriatic arthritis. Ann. Rheum. Dis., 35:354–356, 1976.

27. Korelitz, B.I., and Coles, R.S.: Uveitis (iritis) associated with ulcerative and granulomatous colitis. Gastroenterology, 52:78–82, 1967.

28. Jabs, D.A., Houk, J.L., Bias, W.B., and Arnett, F.C.: Familial granulomatous synovitis, uveitis, and cranial neuropathies. Am. J. Med., 78:801–804, 1985.

29. Isaak, B.L., Liesegang, T.J., and Michet, C.J.: Ocular and systemic findings in relapsing polychondritis. Ophthalmology, 93:681–689, 1986.

30. Gold, D.M.: Ocular manifestations of connective tissue (collagen) diseases. In Clinical Ophthalmology. Vol. 5. Edited by T.D. Duane. Hagerstown, MD, Harper & Row, 1980.

section IX

OSTEOARTHRITIS

PATHOLOGY OF OSTEOARTHRITIS

100

AUBREY J. HOUGH, JR. and LEON SOKOLOFF

Despite the almost ubiquitous occurrence of osteoarthritis in the adult population, many elements of its pathogenesis are not understood. Although the term *osteoarthritis* is a misnomer because it implies an inherently inflammatory process, it has been in common use in the English-speaking world for many years and will probably continue to be because it has greater appeal than the more accurate term, *degenerative joint disease*. The term *arthrosis* or *osteoarthrosis* frequently is employed in Europe. There is no consensus on its definition. Osteoarthritis is not a single entity but a pattern of reaction of joints to injury. The etiology involves the interaction of diverse mechanical and biologic factors and is the basis for several schemes of classification and subsets. Our preferred definition is that osteoarthritis is an inherently non-inflammatory disorder of movable joints characterized by deterioration and abrasion of articular cartilage, as well as by formation of new bone at the joint surfaces. Two different views of the relationship between the bone changes and the joint changes have been argued over the years.

OSTEOARTHRITIS AS A REMODELING PROCESS

Remodeling is the alteration of the internal and external architecture of the skeleton, dictated by Wolff's law, in response to variation in mechanical loading. It involves removal of bony tissue at certain points and simultaneous formation of new bone elsewhere.

The concept has been expanded to include changes in shape of joints with age and osteoarthritis.[1] These mechanisms in bone have been the subject of much thought. Only recently has the question even been formulated in the case of the remodeling of cartilage. Changes in the shape of joints from loading have been shown by Thompson and Bassett,[2] who produced abnormal pressures on the articular surfaces of the knees in rabbits by excising one of the femoral condyles. In the joint compartment with the reduced pressure, the calcified layer of the tibial cartilage was resorbed by invading blood vessels. On the side subjected to increased pressure, the articular cartilage proper showed loss of metachromasia and necrobiosis of its chondrocytes.

The usual accounts of the pathologic features of osteoarthritis state that the lesions begin with fibrillation of articular cartilage. Fibrillation is the earliest gross change seen on the surface of the opened joint (Fig. 100–1). It is not necessarily the first change, however, if the adjacent bony structure is also examined. The sequences in the remodeling of osteoarthritis can be reconstructed only hypothetically. The recognition of the complexity of the pathologic sequences is important because several pharmacologic strategies for treating osteoarthritis are based on the assumption that loss of cartilage is at its heart.[3]

Three general hypotheses of the relationships between cartilaginous and bony changes have been proposed at various times, but all seem overly simple. First, osteoarthritis is a *degeneration of articular cartilage that progressively leads to denudation of the joint surface.*

1571

FIG. 100–1. Osteoarthritis of the knee. Large areas of erosion of articular cartilage are present on the patellar facet and on the condyles of the femur. These erosions occupy principally the central portions of the joint surfaces and spare the marginal regions. The cartilage at the eroded edges is fibrillated. The irregular elevations at the periphery of the surfaces are osteophytic.

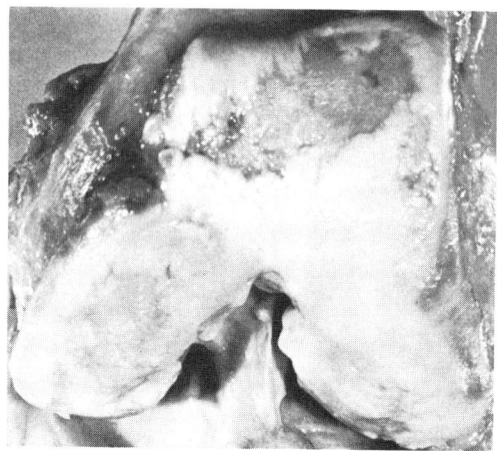

If this statement were valid, little or no remodeling of bone would occur. Only rarely is extensive eburnation seen in surgically resected femoral heads that retain their sphericity.[4] Concentric osteoarthritis has been attributed to inflammatory lysis, as distinct from mechanical overloading of the cartilage.[5,6] The degree of deformity in surgically resected femoral heads is generally greater in osteoarthritis than in rheumatoid arthritis (RA).[3] Lagier has made analogous observations on the sparing of the contour of the hip joint in ochronotic arthropathy, in which the destruction of the cartilage is related to inherent metabolic deterioration of the cartilage rather than to mechanical remodeling.[7]

The second hypothesis states that osteoarthritis begins as *fibrillation of articular cartilage that leads to secondary remodeling of the bony components of the joint.* This view is held most commonly (see Fig. 100–3*A*). A principal difficulty with the concept is that it is difficult to isolate any individual finding as a unique morphologic event that precedes others in the complicated changes seen in histologic section. It does not take into account, for example, the remodeling of the osteochondral junction as an early age-related change in the cartilage.[8,9] The changes ordinarily coexist.

The third hypothesis is that osteoarthritis is the *consequence of changes in the stiffness of subchondral bone.* Radin et al. proposed that microfractures of subchondral bone precede cartilage damage.[10] This idea is predicated on the observations that bone, rather than

cartilage, absorbs most of the energy of impact stress on the extremities. Repair of the fractures leads to a net local increase in stiffness of the bone that, in turn, causes the overlying cartilage to absorb excess energy. The process, it is argued, leads to the degeneration of the cartilage. This hypothesis has a distinct mechanical logic as well as some experimental support, but it suffers from the same limitations as the preceding hypothesis.

The degenerative and remodeling changes are so intimately associated that it seems unrealistic to attempt to identify a unique initial event in the osteoarthritic process. The structural disintegration of the osteoarticular junction and abrasion lead to the loss of substance of the articular surface. These processes are also responsible for the proliferative phenomena, including the formation of new cartilage at the surface of the osteoarthritic joint (Fig. 100–2). The generation of new cartilage in defects in the joint surface that penetrate into the subjacent bone marrow has been documented experimentally.[11,12]

In advanced osteoarthritis, overt microfractures and osteoclastic resorption of the subchondral plate are seen together with osteoblastic foci and sclerotic new bone. Irregularity of the accretion lines indicates that the sclerotic process occurs in bursts, at least some of which arise through repair of microfractures. Islands of cartilaginous proliferation interdigitate with new bone formation in the subchondral marrow.[13] These changes represent abortive attempts at repair of infractions of the joint surfaces.

It would be an error to conclude that osteophytes represent late changes in the evolution of the lesions. In osteoarthritis produced experimentally in canine knee joints by incising the anterior cruciate ligament, remodeling of the bone occurs by the end of the first week, no later than changes in the composition of the cartilage.[14] Osteoarthritis in this sense is not so much an inherent biologic inability of the joint surface to repair itself as it is a failure of the repair to be successful.

ARTICULAR CARTILAGE

EARLY CHANGES

The earliest changes observed microscopically in the cartilage have been described differently by various investigators.

Focal Chondromucoid Softening

In their historic study of the knee joint, Bennett and co-workers concluded that the initial abnormality is

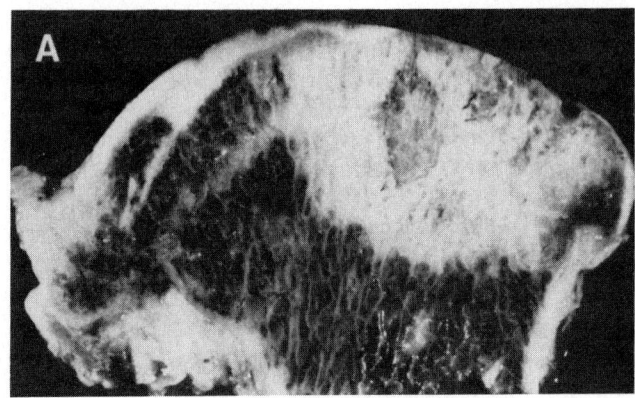

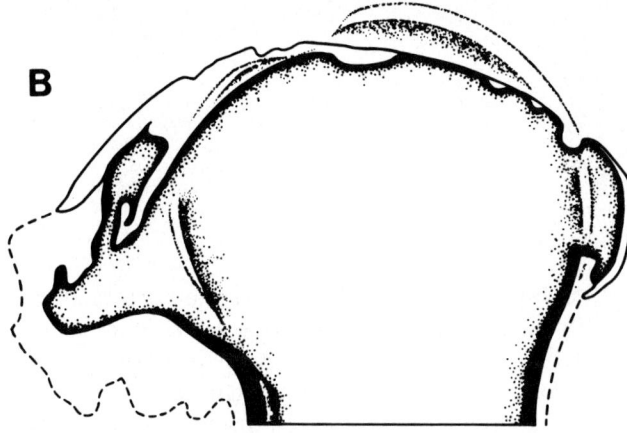

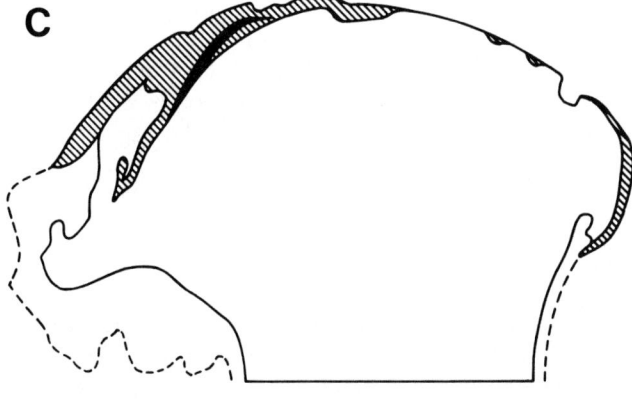

■ ORIGINAL   ▨ NEWLY FORMED

FIG. 100–2. Advanced osteoarthritis of the head of the femur. *A,* The contour has been deformed both by abrasion of the bearing surface and by formation of marginal osteophytes. The large inferomedial spur at the left has grown not only to the side but also into the original joint cartilage. Subchondral pseudocysts approach the eroded surface through slender crevices. The pallor of the eburnated zone reflects the condensation of bony trabeculae and compact fibrous tissue, in contrast to the darker, vascular hematopoietic marrow. *B,* Schematic representation of the remodeling. The outline of the gross specimen is superimposed on a best-fit contour of a normal femoral head of corresponding size. Bone appears black; cartilage, white outlined by a solid line. The broken line demarcates retinacular synovium. The loss of substance affects both articular cartilage and the immediately subjacent bone. *C,* Newly formed cartilage as deduced from the difference in the corresponding outlines in *B.* Only a minute residue of the original cartilage (black) persists at the base of the inferomedial osteophyte. The bulk of the cartilage must have therefore formed in the retinaculum or the subchondral bone marrow.

a focal swelling of cartilage matrix associated with increased affinity for hematoxylin.[15] This mucoid transformation takes place close to the surface of the cartilage. Cellular changes are also present in relation to this alteration: Chondrocytes adjacent and superficial to the softened matrix are more numerous than normal.

Focal Loss of Metachromasia

Loss of metachromatic material, presumably chondroitin sulfate, from all but the deepest portion of the radial zone of the articular cartilage, has been proposed as the morphologic counterpart of chondromalacia followed by osteoarthritis. The diminution of metachromasia corresponds to a loss, rather than an increase, of affinity for hematoxylin, as proposed in the preceding view.

Proliferation of Chondrocytes

Small clusters of chondrocytes are common at the margin of minute fissures in the surface of the cartilage. These chondrocytes have proliferated in response to the dehiscence of the tissue (Fig. 100–3).

Diminution of Chondrocytes

The unit number of chondrocytes is lower in adult than in young joint cartilage, but the cell count alters little in aging articular cartilage once adulthood is reached, unless osteoarthritis is present.[16] Electron-microscopic evidence of chondrocyte loss has been found in all layers of aging human and other mam-

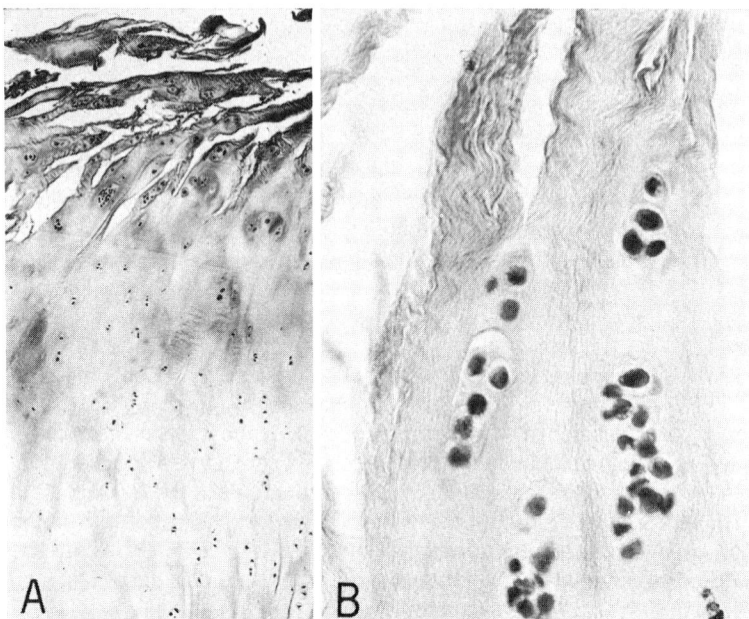

FIG. 100–3. Fibrillation of articular cartilage. *A,* The most superficial dehiscences are oriented parallel to the surface and then arch downward in a more vertical direction. This pattern corresponds to the fibrous planes of the cartilage. (Hematoxylin and eosin stain, × 40.) *B,* Higher magnification (× 240) of the fibrillated edge. The collagen fibrils at the surface have been "unmasked" from the hyaline matrix and appear frayed. Clusters of chondrocytes have proliferated to form so-called brood capsules.

malian articular cartilage. This evidence takes the form of microscars in which relics of disintegrated cells are associated with fragmentation, disarrangement, and great variation in the girth of adjacent collagen fibrils.[17] Lipid droplets are often present in these foci.

Fatty Degeneration

Fine fat deposits in the interterritorial matrix have been described as an early degenerative change in cartilage; these deposits may become larger and may form coarse droplets at the "capsule" of the chondrocytes. The content of triglyceride and complex lipids increases with age in the cells and the matrix of cartilage even before fibrillation. The increase of arachidonic acid, the precursor of prostaglandins, is confined to the tangential layer.

Alteration of Collagen Fibrils

In aging articular cartilage, the general architecture and appearance of the collagen fibrils are preserved, although looser packing and occasional fragmentation are sometimes seen in the superficial layers. The aforementioned microscars increase in number as osteoarthritis evolves. Some of the fragmented fibrils in these areas have a large diameter. A progressive radial reorientation of the collagen has been noted, both by electron-microscopic study and by x-ray diffraction methods. Although *amianthoid* (asbestos-like) degeneration of the matrix has been described as a late feature of the disorder,[18] this process is typical of costal and other extra-articular cartilage rather than of joint cartilage.[19]

Surface Irregularities

Age-dependent irregularities in the surface of articular cartilage have been proposed to evolve into fibrillation.[20] Although several types of evidence support this concept, data are inconclusive because the various analytic procedures themselves may involve technical artifacts.[21]

Weichselbaum's Lacunar Resorption

Focal dissolution of matrix by chondroclastic cells in the cartilage lacunae was once regarded as a feature of osteoarthritis (Fig. 100–4). This change is more characteristic of RA, however.

GROSS CHANGES

Localized areas of softening of the cartilage are associated with a fine, velvety disruption of the surface. In these areas, one sees a dehiscence of the cartilage along the axis of the matrix collagen. When the disruption is confined to the tangential layer of the surface, the process is referred to as *flaking;* when the process extends to the deeper radial layer, it is described as *fibrillation* (see Fig. 100–3). Because these minute discontinuities in the surface are readily stained grossly by India ink,[22] they lend themselves to quantitative study. Abrasion of the fibrillated cartilage takes place with progressive denudation of the underlying bony cortex (see Fig. 100–1). The sites of predilection for destruction of the joint surface are those subject to greatest load bearing or shearing stress. Earliest fibrillation, however, is often present

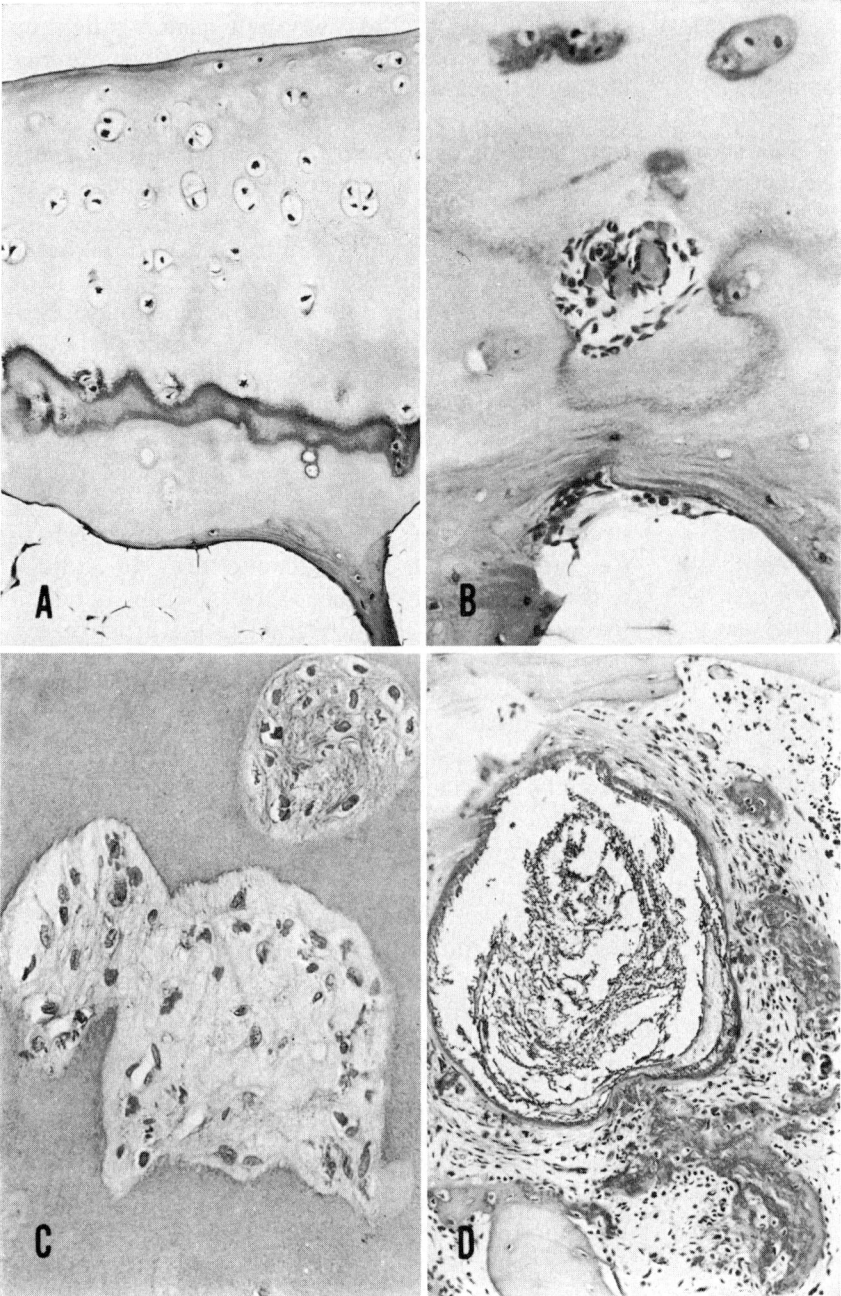

FIG. 100—4. Miscellaneous remodeling and degenerative changes; all sections are stained with hematoxylin and eosin. *A,* Reduplication of calcification "tidemark" (×95). *B,* Vascularization of base of articular cartilage; the dark-stained material in the capsules of the chondrocytes is calcific (×183). *C,* Weichselbaum's lacunar resorption; small, geographic areas of hyaline cartilage are replaced by loose-textured, cellular fibrous tissue (×210). *D,* Early subchondral "cystic" degeneration; a small true cyst, filled with mucoid material, has a fibrous border. New bone formation is seen in the adjacent marrow (×90).

in regions with presumably low compressive stress, such as the infrafoveal portion of the femoral head. In the patella, the central facets are the sites most prone to erosion.[23] Although not a weight-bearing joint, the patella is subjected to enormous loads by leverage when the knee is flexed, such as while climbing stairs or in the squatting position.

LATE HISTOLOGIC CHANGES

In fibrillated regions, continuity of the surface of the articular cartilage is disrupted. The height of the fronds is in the range of 20 to 150 μm.[24] Ground-substance metachromasia is reduced, and the matrix has a fibrillary, disheveled appearance. Birefringence of the collagen is increased. Clusters of chondrocytes, long known as brood capsules, are located close to the margins of the clefts (see Fig. 100–3B). The proliferative and proteoglycan-producing activities of these cells have been amply documented by autoradiography. Little or no collagen is seen within the clones, and it must be presumed that chondrolytic enzymes, including collagenases, have been generated to make room for the new cells (see Chapter 101).

Some investigators regard these cellular clusters as doomed to fail and die.[25] Only small segments of necrobiosis are seen, however, and these segments are not necessarily confined to the cell clusters. Focal proliferation of chondrocytes is also seen in deeper areas of disrupted cartilage in severe lesions. The matrix in such lesions has a pale, myxoid appearance.

Mitrovic and others have described *activation* of articular chondrocytes in osteoarthritis; that is, a generalized increase of biosynthetic activity in the same joint even at a distance from overt damage to the tissue.[26] This judgment is based on advanced lesions in which the bulk of the cartilage studied is of a new, immature type. The morphologic character of early lesions indicates that activation is a focal rather than a generalized phenomenon. Reparative cartilage has a mixed hyaline and fibrocartilaginous character. Fibrillary collagen typically is more conspicuous than normal. In osteophytes, much of the covering is fibrocartilaginous, and overt fibrous tissue covers segments of the latter. Variable degrees of secondary degenerative change and fibrillation are superimposed in reparative cartilage. The histochemical features of the matrix, accordingly, are heterogeneous.[27,28]

Reduplication of the tidemark is exaggerated in the vicinity of the fibrillated cartilage and, more remotely, at the margin of the joint. Calcium-containing crystals are deposited in the territorial matrix of the adjacent chondrocytes as forward remodeling occurs. These crystals appear as basophilic granules in demineralized sections (see Fig. 100–4B) and within or around matrix vesicles in electron micrographs.[8,29]

BONE

New bone formation occurs in two separate locations in relation to the joint surface: in exophytic growths at the margins of the articular cartilage and in the immediately subjacent bone marrow (see Fig. 100–2). Marginal osteophytes have two patterns of growth. One is a protuberance into the joint space; the other develops within capsular and ligamentous attachments to the joint margins. In each circumstance, the direction of the osteophyte is governed by the lines of mechanical force exerted on the area of growth and generally corresponds to the contour of the joint surface from which the osteophyte protrudes. The osteophyte consists in large part of bone that merges imperceptibly with the other cortical and cancellous tissue of the subchondral bone. The osteophyte is capped by a layer of hyaline and fibrocartilage, continuous with the adjacent synovial lining. In advanced lesions, the landmarks are

obliterated because the osteophyte itself is caught up in the degenerative process. Not only does the proliferative tissue occupy the fovea of the ligamentum teres, but also it extends along the femoral neck to form buttress osteophytes.[30] In most resected specimens, little or no demonstrably native articular cartilage is present.

The proliferation of bone in the subchondral tissue is most marked in areas denuded of their cartilaginous covering.[31–34] In these regions, the articulating surface consists of bone that has been rubbed smooth. The glistening appearance of this polished sclerotic surface suggests ivory, hence the name *eburnation*. Nubbins of newly proliferated cartilage usually protrude through minute gaps in the eburnated bone.[13] Most of the osteocytes in the eburnated surface undergo necrobiosis, as indicated by empty lacunae. Perhaps this process results from frictional heat. In addition to this alteration, two other variants of new bone formation are also seen in relation to the articular cartilage.

"Cystic" areas of rarefaction of bone are commonly seen immediately beneath the eburnated surfaces in the hip joint (see Fig. 100–2), but they are much less frequent in other joints. Both femoral and acetabular components are affected. Most often, the lesions are present on the superolateral weight-bearing surface, but in severe instances, they involve other regions of the hip as well.[35] In a few cases, these lesions appear roentgenographically before narrowing of the joint space, which is evidence of cartilage destruction. The lesions only infrequently contain pockets of mucoid fluid and thus are not truly cystic (see Fig. 100–4D). The trabeculae in the affected areas disappear, and the bone marrow undergoes fibromyxoid degeneration. Fragments of dead bone, cartilage, and amorphous debris are often interspersed within them. In time, the entire area is encircled by a rim of reactive new bone and compact fibrous tissue (see Fig. 100–2). Minute gaps in the overlying articular cortex, resulting from microfractures, are commonly seen at the apex of the pseudocysts (Fig. 100–5). These findings are consistent with an intrusion of pressure, if not of synovial fluid, from the joint cavity through a defect in the articular cortex into the subchondral bone marrow. Intra-articular pressures exceeding 1000 mm Hg have been calculated to occur in hip joints with effusions. The increased pressure is dissipated radially into the adjacent bone marrow, compresses the medullary blood vessels, and thereby leads to the retrogressive changes. This mechanism is not contradicted by observations that the intraosseous pressure is not elevated in osteoarthritic femoral heads at the time of arthroplasty.[36] In these specimens, bulk pressures,

FIG. 100–5. Relationship between a pseudocyst and a microfracture of the subchondral plate. This fortuitous slab section is from a recently fractured femoral head of a 77-year-old woman. Although moderate fibrillation is present elsewhere in the cartilage surface, the sole pseudocyst is located immediately beneath the minute discontinuity in the otherwise intact cartilage and osteochondral junction. A, Gross appearance (approximately ×4). B, Roentgenogram, showing the gap in the subchondral plate and the sclerotic wall of the "cyst."

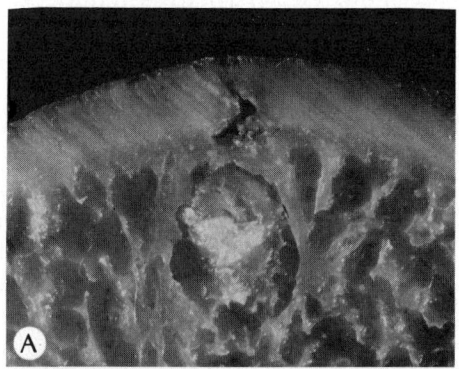

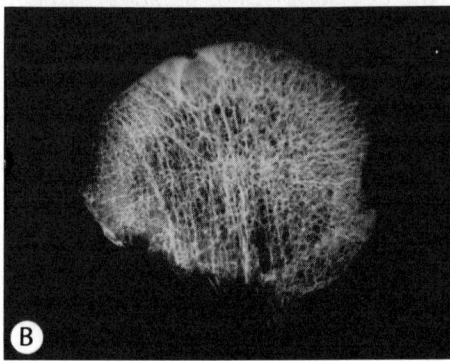

rather than localized gradients, are measured. Furthermore, internal remodeling compensates for the presumptive pressure gradients. The "punched-out" lesions observed roentgenographically in gout and the bone "cysts" in hemophilic arthropathy correspond pathologically to the pseudocysts in osteoarthritis, except the specific exudates of the former arthropathies also lie within the degenerated bone marrow space.

The other type of new bone formation in this location is a focal ossific metaplasia of the base of the articular cartilage. This metaplasia is part of the remodeling of the joint contour through which bone is added to a portion of the articular cortex, whereas other areas in the joint surface undergo focal resorption. The junction between the articular cartilage and the subchondral plate of bone is occupied by a zone of calcified cartilage. During the years of skeletal

growth, the epiphysis and the articular cartilage participate in the enlargement of the bone. During this period, the epiphysis is expanded by endochondral ossification of the calcified cartilage. The interface between calcified and noncalcified hyaline articular cartilage is demarcated in usual histologic preparations by the *tidemark*, which is a thin, wavy hematoxyphil line (see Fig. 100–4A). In joints of older persons, a number of such discontinuous parallel lines are commonly found in this region. The presence of these lines is clear evidence of progression of calcification of the basal portion of the articular cartilage.[8,37] The possibility that basilar calcification may lead to a thinning of articular cartilage (senile atrophy) has received no support.[9]

Much of the deformity in symptomatic osteoarthritis results from collapse of the joint surface. Localized areas of necrosis are seen frequently in this location, and occlusion of minute intramedullary arteries has been demonstrated by angiography. Small secondary infarcts of eburnated bone are seen in approximately 6% of surgically resected femoral heads.[13,38,39] Nevertheless, Streda's suggestion that all osteoarthritis of the hip is secondary to osteonecrosis exceeds the evidence.[40] The new bone formation of the remodeling process is accompanied by increased vascularity and is the basis for scintigraphic studies using bone-seeking radionuclides in this disorder.[41]

CHONDROCALCINOSIS

There are divergent views on the relationship of osteoarthritis with chondrocalcinosis. Calcium pyrophosphate dihydrate (CPPD) deposition has been variously considered (1) to have no relationship to osteoarthritis;[42] (2) to favor development of osteoarthritis[43] or its inflammatory manifestations;[44] (3) to result from osteoarthritis or other derangement of cartilage in the aged;[45] or (4) to be another but separate manifestation of articular aging. The significance of basic calcium phosphate (apatite-like) versus CPPD crystals in synovial fluid has also been debated. One suggestion[46] is that the former finding is a feature of osteoarthritis; the latter, of aging per se.

Our experience[47] indicates that meniscal chondrocalcinosis is present in roughly half of knees treated surgically for osteoarthritis after age 68. In fact, the risk for meniscal calcinosis in surgically removed knees was sixfold that of an age- and sex-adjusted postmortem population.[47] By contrast, CPPD crystals are rarely found in femoral heads removed for osteoarthritis. Chondrocalcinosis also is relatively infrequent in fractured hips below the age of 85. The view of Pritzker et al.[42] that basic calcium phosphate crystals (apatite) in osteoarthritic synovial fluid arise predominantly from abrasion of the eburnated surface or the remodeling basal cartilage, whereas CPPD crystals are part of the meniscocalcinosis, is attractive from the pathologist's perspective. Why the meniscus is the predominant site of involvement in osteoarthritis of the knee, while the articular cartilages are largely spared, remains a matter of conjecture. Ordinarily, the deposition of CPPD in the osteoarthritic knee engenders no inflammatory reaction. Several observers have noted that joint mice are more frequent in osteoarthritic specimens affected by chondrocalcinosis than in those that are not.

CHANGES IN SOFT TISSUE

During recent years, the inflammatory aspects of osteoarthritis have aroused discussion.[48–51] Although osteoarthritis is inherently not inflammatory by definition, villous hypertrophy and fibrosis are the rule in clinically symptomatic cases (Fig. 100–6). Moderate, focal, chronic synovitis is seen in about one fifth of surgically resected specimens.[39] This synovitis is characterized by hyperplasia and enlargement of lining cells and by mild infiltration of lymphocytes and mononuclear cells. Polyclonal B cells compose part of the infiltrate, and extracellular deposits of C3 have also been described.[52–54] Fibronectin is deposited in exudative foci.[55] Hemosiderin,[56] foreign-body reaction to joint detritus, and even xanthoma-cell aggregation about foci of fat necrosis may be seen. Occasionally, the inflammation is severe enough to raise the question of RA. Some observers suggest that, in one or more subsets of osteoarthritis, anti-inflammatory medication may be helpful. The inflammatory reaction probably is a secondary phenomenon. It is seen equally in other deforming joint diseases in which no primary phlogistic origin is likely, such as acromegalic arthropathy.[57] Autosensitization to joint detritus is an attractive possibility and receives some experimental support from studies in rabbits.[58] Lymphokines are occasionally found in the synovial fluid and constitute supportive evidence for such a mechanism.

Cooke has emphasized the presence of immune complex components in the surface of the cartilage in primary, but not in secondary, osteoarthritis.[59] Doyle relates the inflammation to calcific crystals.[49] Minute quantities of hydroxyapatite and CPPD occur both in the synovium and in the synovial fluid (see Chapters 5, 107, and 108). Such crystals may arise as part of the basilar remodeling of the cartilage that accompanies the osteoarthritis. Synovitis must be respon-

sible for the effusion as well as some of the accompanying pain. Minute tears in capsular tissue appear as slender, fibrovascular seams disrupting the principal axis of the collagen bundles. Secondary osteochondromatosis occurs only infrequently. The ligamentum teres commonly disintegrates. In the knee joint, cruciate ligaments and menisci also become frayed. Although substantial clinical evidence suggests that meniscectomy leads to osteoarthritis, no correlation has been found in autopsy material between tears or other lesions of the semilunar cartilages and osteoarthritis.[60] Fibrillation and fibrosis of the synovial surface and even mild cartilaginous metaplasia of patellar tendon occur at times in such cases. Analysis of hand and bilateral knee radiographs of 150 subjects who had undergone unilateral meniscectomy 19 or more years earlier showed a striking correlation between degeneration in the finger joints and in both operated and opposite knees.[61] Degeneration was more severe on the operated side and was independent of age and sex. This study suggests that the predisposition to primary osteoarthritis influences the development of secondary degeneration and makes a clear distinction between these two subsets of the disease more difficult.

Amyloid deposits have been reported in the joint capsule in osteoarthritis, but they also occur in nonosteoarthritic joint capsules, in articular cartilage, and in intra-articular discs of older individuals.[62–66] It may not be entirely gratuitous to question whether green birefringence following alkaline Congo red staining, the usual histochemical method for demonstrating amyloid, is a reliable measure for this material in cartilage.

A progressive increase in the amount of fibrous tissue separating the synovial capillaries from the joint space has been described as an age-related finding, but it is unlikely that this condition interferes with the nourishment of the cartilage. Hyaline sclerosis of minute vessels is a common, although focal, finding in joints even of young individuals that is not directly related to osteoarthritis. Periarticular muscle undergoes atrophy; type 2 myofibers are affected primarily.[67]

COMPARATIVE PATHOLOGIC FEATURES

Osteoarthritis occurs widely in the vertebrate kingdom, regardless of the position of the species in the taxonomic scale.[68] Osteophytic lesions, sometimes leading to ankylosis, were common in certain giant dinosaurs 100 million years ago. The disorder has

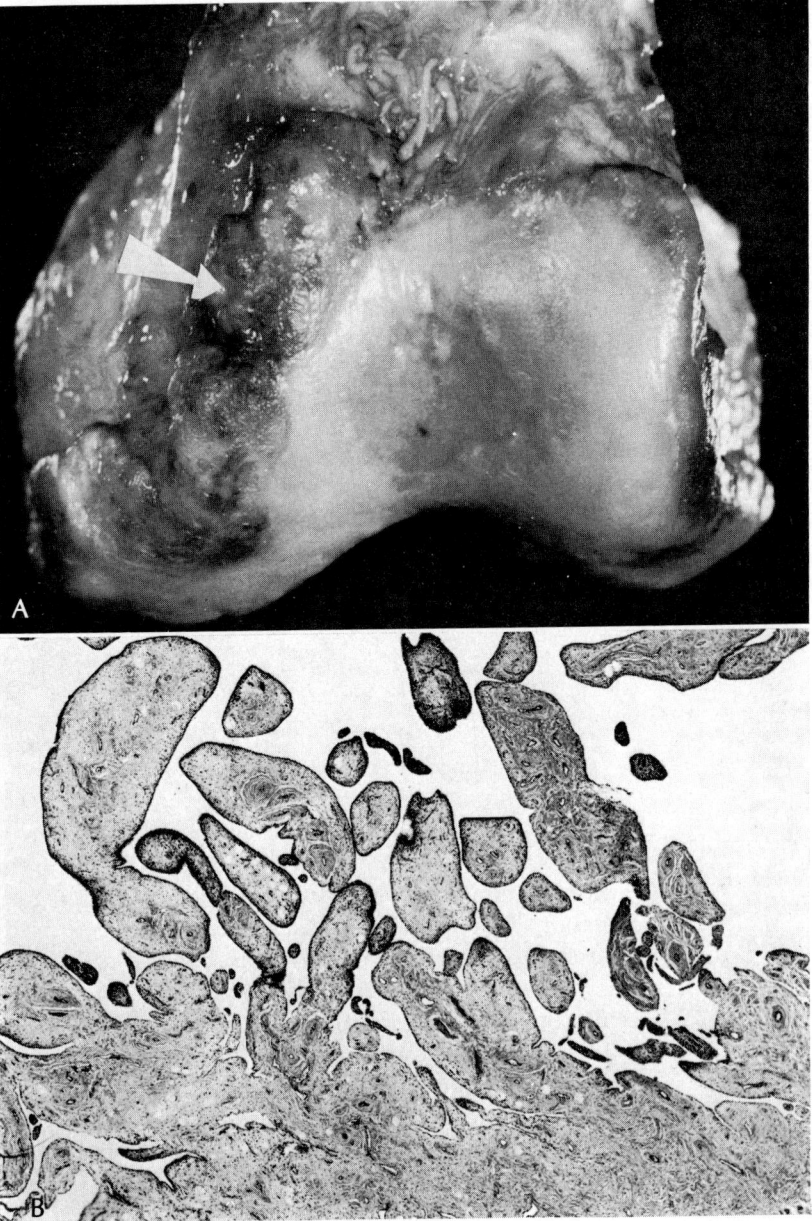

A

B

FIG. 100–6. Synovial hypertrophy in severe osteoarthritis. The patient is a 63-year-old man whose left knee had been enlarged for 23 years following an automobile accident. *A*, A massive osteophyte (arrow) is seen at the medial border of the articular surface. The adjacent synovial tissue has undergone prominent papillary thickening. *B*, Histologically, the villous processes are made up of compact fibrous tissue not infiltrated by inflammatory cells. (Hematoxylin and eosin stain, ×16.)

been observed in large and small mammals, in animals that swim (cetaceans) rather than bear their weight on their extremities, and also, to a mild degree, in birds. It is of considerable economic importance in livestock commerce, the horse-racing industry, and veterinary practice.

In small laboratory animals, it has been possible to study a number of pathogenetic concepts of osteoarthritis. The importance of genetic factors has been established in mice.[68,69] The inheritance appears to be polygenic and the overall behavior, recessive. No evidence suggests major sex linkage. Male mice consistently develop more severe osteoarthritis than do females. Obesity is not an important factor.[70] In lab-

oratory rodents, the knee and elbow joints are most commonly severely affected, and the hips rarely. That heritable biochemical defects are major factors in the development of osteoarthritis is indicated by the frequency of osteoarthritic lesions in blotchy (BLO) mice, in which a mutant gene leads to inadequate cross-linking of collagen.[71] In another strain of mouse, STR/ORT, widely studied for its predisposition to osteoarthritis, Walton attributes osteoarthritis of the knee to spontaneous subluxation of the patella.[72] By containing the subluxation surgically, this investigator prevented the development of the osteoarthritis, and implies that the susceptibility to osteoarthritis in these animals is due to abnormal mechanical loading rather than to some metabolic peculiarity of the cartilage. These data are impressive but difficult to reconcile with our observations that lesions in STR/1N mice are not confined to the knee but are more generalized. The broader principle is that *genetic factors that influence the development of osteoarthritis may operate at many levels, local and generalized, mechanical and metabolic.*

The genetic aspect of the disorder is also manifested by the variable susceptibility of different species to its development. Rats, for example, are generally resistant, whereas another rodent, *Mastomys natalensis,* develops severe generalized osteoarthritis by the time it is 2 years old. Genetic contributions also are found in certain breeds of cattle and swine. The fundamental pathogenetic problem is whether these genetic factors are local and articular, related to the configuration and mechanical forces exerted on the joint, as in the dysplastic hips of German shepherd dogs, or whether they are more generalized metabolic properties of the articular tissues.

DEGENERATIVE DISEASE OF THE SPINAL COLUMN

Degenerative changes in the spine affect two discrete intervertebral articular systems: the diarthrodial or apophyseal joints and the synchondroses or intervertebral discs. The term *spinal osteoarthritis* describes the changes in the apophyseal joints, whereas the term *spinal osteophytosis* or *spondylosis deformans* applies to degenerative disc disease. This distinction should not lead to a fundamental dichotomy between the pathologic processes in these two sets of joints. It is common, in the cervical region, to find both lesions, albeit on neighboring rather than the same vertebrae. The pathologic findings in the two sets of joints are similar. The nucleus pulposus becomes fissured and deformed. Fibrillary disintegration of the hyaline cartilage plates, through which the disc is attached to the vertebral bodies, cannot be distinguished histologically from the changes in diarthrodial osteoarthritis. Eburnation of the subchondral bony plate develops in like manner. Marginal osteophytes arise under the mechanical stimulus of horizontal pulsion of the anulus fibrosus and its periosteal attachments attending collapse and spreading out of the nucleus pulposus. Traction forces of spinal muscles on the tendinous insertions in this region also have been implicated in this disorder. These mechanisms are not qualitatively different from those in the more movable joints.

Although the marginal osteophytes develop most often on the anterolateral aspects of the vertebral bod-

ies, posterior osteophytic protrusions also occur and may affect the spinal cord and its roots. In the cervical region, antecedent spondylosis constitutes a principal neurosurgical hazard of injuries among older patients.[73] Osteophytes in the Luschka (uncovertebral, neurocentral) joints have been shown by anatomic and angiographic means to compromise the neighboring vertebral arteries (see Chapter 90). The narrowing of the vascular lumen is most marked during rotation of the head and provides the basis for the posterior cervical sympathetic or *Barre-Lieou* syndrome.

Osteoarthritis does not characteristically lead to ankylosis; however, in at least three forms of segmental disease of the senescent spine, bony bridges unite the vertebral bodies. The proclivity for ankylosis may be related to the inherent limited mobility of the intervertebral disc.

HYPEROSTOTIC SPONDYLOSIS

The best-known entity goes by several names: *hyperostotic spondylosis, senile ankylosing hyperostosis of Forestier and Rotés-Querol, spondylorrheostosis.* Hyperostotic spondylosis nominally is distinguished from ordinary spondylosis by the absence of disc degeneration.[74] The distal thoracic spine is the site of predilection. The ankylotic bridges are located on the anterolateral portions of the vertebral bodies and extend into the anterior longitudinal ligaments. The appearance has often led to confusion with ankylosing spondylitis, also known as Marie-Strümpell disease. In some instances, at least, the vertebral lesion is accompanied by excessive osteophyte formation in peripheral joints. From this feature comes still another term for this condition, *diffuse idiopathic skeletal hyperostosis* (DISH).[75,76] Currently, no consensus exists on the bounds of the DISH syndrome.

ANKYLOSIS

Ankylosis may accompany severe spondylosis in man and other species (Fig. 100–7). The disc space is narrowed. Destructive changes are present in the cortex of the anterior portion of the vertebral bodies. Dense new bone formation is seen in the anterior longitudinal ligament. The appearance suggests that the ligament is first avulsed from the osteophyte and then is repaired.

FIG. 100–7. Hyperostotic ankylosing spondylosis in thoracic vertebrae of a 72-year-old man. Unlike the Marie-Strümpell lesion, marked degenerative changes occur in the intervertebral disc. The space between the vertebral bodies is narrowed, and the articular lamella is irregular as a result of both focal resorption and protrusion of new bone into the disc. The cortex on the anterolateral surface of the vertebra (right) has blended with the bony bridge.

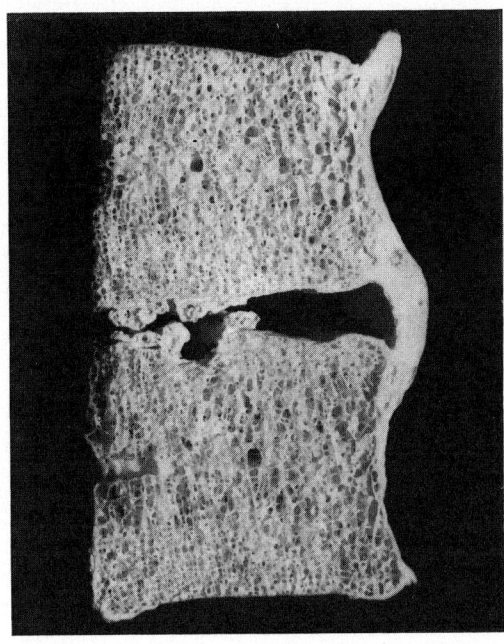

OTHER SEGMENTAL DISEASE

Several patterns of dorsal protrusion and bridging of cervical vertebrae (posterior spondylotic osteophytes) may cause life-threatening cervical myelopathy. The relation of *physiologic vertebral ligamentous ossification* to the preceding disorder and to hyperostotic spondylosis is uncertain. It occurs in 7% of Japanese[77] and 0.3% of U.S. adults.[78] These lesions are asymptomatic in individuals with large spinal canals, but they require surgical decompression when spinal canals are small.

Baastrup's syndrome, an osteoarthritis-like change in the distal portions of "kissing" dorsal spinous processes,[79] is usually associated with severe spondylosis and is primarily of roentgenographic interest.

Degeneration of intervertebral discs occurs normally with aging and apparently is exaggerated in instances of herniation. It is characterized microscopically by a depletion of metachromatic ground substance from the matrix and partial fibrous transformation of the nucleus pulposus. In electron micrographs of herniated nucleus pulposus, the collagen fibers are disorderly and attenuated, the cross-striations are often indistinct, and the periods are shortened. Although swelling of the nucleus pulposus has sometimes been considered to cause acute herniation, evidence suggests that the water content and the swelling pressure of the disc are reduced, rather than increased, in the disorder.[80] The herniation ultimately depends on the development of tears in the anulus fibrosus. The direction of displacement of the nucleus pulposus in quadrupeds differs from that in man. In dogs, for example, displacement often occurs dorsally and, particularly in chondrodysplastic breeds, leads to spinal cord paralysis. In man, the upright posture leads more characteristically to displacement toward the vertebral bodies. The common development of nodules of cartilaginous and fibrous tissue beneath the subchondral plate of the vertebral bodies, the *Schmorl nodes*, is usually attributed to the displacement of nucleus pulposus into the vertebral body.[81] These islands are often surrounded by a shell of bone and, except for their greater content of cartilage, are reminiscent of the subchondral "cysts" in osteoarthritic peripheral joints. Schmorl's nodes are not a particular feature of vertebral osteoporosis.

SPECIAL FORMS OF OSTEOARTHRITIS

HEBERDEN'S NODES

Despite the great frequency of these nodes, little systemic information is available on the morbid anatomic features of these common marginal osteophytes at the base of the distal finger phalanges. In advanced cases, the lesions cannot be distinguished from osteoarthritis in other locations (Fig. 100–8). Some specimens have, however, a different appearance and are of considerable theoretic interest. In these, the articular cartilage, rather than displaying degenerative fibrillation and erosion, is actually hypertrophic. Ossific transformation of the insertion of the tendons into joint capsule and periosteum accounts for the exophytosis. Whether these two forms correspond, as has been suggested,[82] to two clinically different types of Heberden node, the traumatic acquired and the genetically governed, cannot be determined without further clinicopathologic information. In other instances, mucoid transformation of the periarticular fibroadipose tissue is associated with proliferation of myxoid fibroblasts and cyst formation. Hyaluronic acid has been found in the cyst fluid. This finding is not a unique anatomic feature of Heberden nodes. Indistinguishable changes may be present in other osteoarthritic joints in other species. The process has certain morphologic similarities to ganglion formation

FIG. 100–8.   Heberden's node. The articular cartilage has completely disappeared from the surfaces of the distal interphalangeal joint. Bony osteophytes, directed toward the base of the finger, are present on the dorsal and palmar aspects of both articulating surfaces. Advanced osteoarthritic changes also are present in the proximal interphalangeal joint and form a so-called Bouchard node. (Hematoxylin and eosin stain, ×20.)

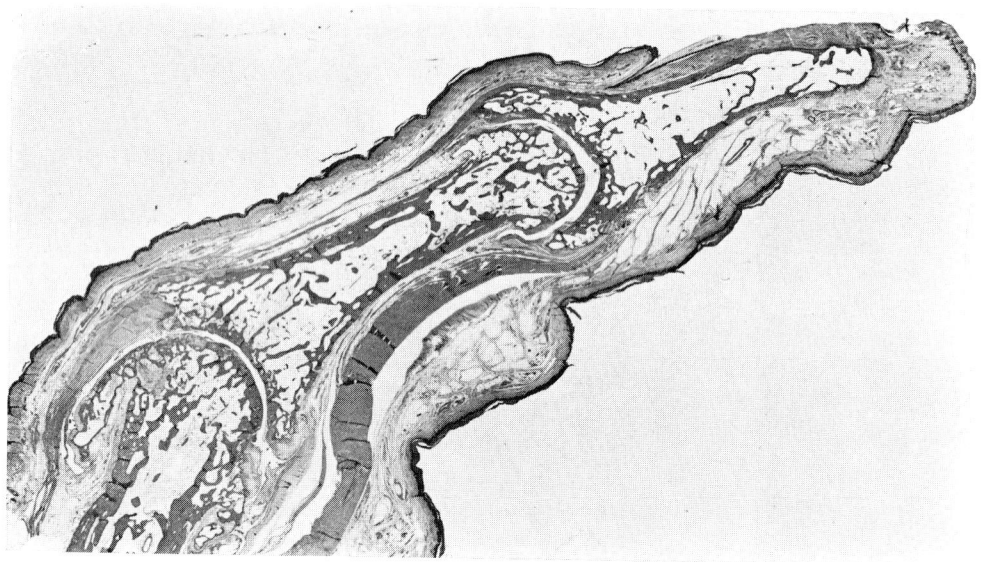

or to cystic degeneration of the semilunar cartilages and the subchondral pseudo-cysts of osteoarthritis. Unilateral sparing from Heberden node formation following hemiplegia has been reported on numerous occasions,[83] and this observation suggests the possibility of neurovascular contributions to the development of the lesion without excluding a biomechanical explanation.

The association of the para-articular mucoid cysts ("synovial cysts") of the distal interphalangeal joints with osteophytes has been emphasized because the cysts are likely to recur following excision unless the osteophytes are also removed.[84]

The term *erosive osteoarthritis* has been applied to a disorder resembling osteoarthritis in its predilection for the distal and proximal interphalangeal joints, but in which a distinct inflammatory component exists.[85] A nonspecific, chronic, lymphocytic and mononuclear cell infiltrate is present in the synovium. The nosologic status of the disorder is uncertain. One possibility is that this entity represents osteoarthritis with a prominent, detritic synovitis. In a few cases, the lesion is disseminated to other joints and may evolve into RA.[86]* We may therefore be dealing with two separate conditions. Bony ankylosis occurs in rare instances in association with Heberden's nodes.[87]

*Editor's note. Such patients are generally seronegative and radiologically different from seropositive RA in that osteophyte formation is prominent.

PRIMARY GENERALIZED OSTEOARTHRITIS

The concept of a pattern of primary osteoarthritis affecting multiple joints was first formulated by Kellgren and colleagues.[88] These workers found that Heberden node formation was a conspicuous feature of this disorder, as was involvement of the first carpometacarpal and knee joints; the hip was less often affected. Inflammatory manifestations were common, and the onset often occurred at menopause. Radiologic examination of the joints suggested that the primary events were not erosion of the articular cartilage, but proliferation of adjacent bone. Only limited anatomic material was available to document the nature of the pathologic process.

The status of primary osteoarthritis remains controversial. The pattern is encountered far more often in rheumatologic than in orthopedic practice. The association of Heberden's nodes with osteoarthritis of the hips has been affirmed by some,[39,61,89,90] but denied by others.[91] Discrimination of subsets of osteoarthritis may resolve some of these contradictions. Heberden's nodes, particularly those associated with inflammatory manifestations, more often coexist with concentric or nondeforming than with deforming osteoarthritis of the hip. This form of hip disease has been referred to by some as postinflammatory,[5,6] whereas others consider it to be part of primary generalized osteoarthritis.[89,92]

MALUM COXAE SENILIS

A variety of structural abnormalities of the hip joint in childhood, such as congenital dysplasia, Legg-Perthes disease, slipped capital epiphysis, and congenital coxa vara, lead to premature osteoarthritic degeneration. In other patients, however, no precursors are clinically overt. Roentgenographic analysis of the contour of the hip joint has suggested to some investigators that low-grade dysplasia is the basis for most of these cases.[93] The validity of this retrospective view may be questionable because subluxation has been documented roentgenographically as a late manifestation of the joint deformity.

OSTEOARTHRITIS ASSOCIATED WITH HERITABLE ARTICULAR DISEASES

Precocious osteoarthritis develops with great frequency in *multiple epiphyseal dysplasias*. In these rare diseases, epiphyseal growth and maturation of variable portions of the axial and appendicular skeleton are defective. In some instances, the anatomic changes are indistinguishable from those of banal osteoarthritis; in others, eburnation is absent and the articular surface is covered by a shaggy reparative cartilage.[94] Allison and Blumberg have reported the development of osteoarthritis in patients with a rare form of heritable osteochondrosis of the digits.[95] The *nail-patella syndrome (hereditary osteo-onychodysplasia, Turner-Kieser syndrome, iliac horn syndrome)* is also frequently complicated by osteoarthritis. The hereditary component of *congenital dysplasia of the hip* has been argued several ways. In dogs, evidence seems to support significant genetic contribution to the disorder because certain breeds, such as German shepherds, commonly develop it, whereas others, such as American greyhounds, do not. Shepherd dogs are also prone to dysplasia and secondary osteoarthritis of the elbows.

CHONDROMALACIA PATELLAE

This term is used loosely to describe a clinically distinctive, post-traumatic softening of the articular cartilage of the patella in young persons (see Chapter 88). It is usually difficult to distinguish the anatomic lesions from those of early osteoarthritis. Subtle differences have been described by some authors. The changes are not confined to the cartilage, but also involve subchondral bone.[96,97] Softening, swelling, and an increased water content of the cartilage have been reported in early chondromalacia. These changes presumably result from localized dehiscence of the collagen in the cartilage.

CHARCOT JOINTS

The morphology of neuropathic arthropathies varies with the duration and underlying sensory defect.[98] Extensive detritic synovitis is characteristic and may be accompanied by secondary osteochondromatosis. Advanced lesions resemble severe osteoarthritis in which the destructive and hypertrophic elements are exaggerated by trauma. The often postulated primary role of neurovascular reflexes on the para-articular circulation has received some support from experimental studies.[99] In the diabetic foot, currently the most frequent form of Charcot joint, landmarks of tarsal bones are often obliterated.[100] The pattern thus differs from the characteristically nonankylosed lesions in other joints and may reflect inflammatory complications in the diabetic foot (see Chapter 81). Experimental findings[101] suggest the possibility that subclinical sensory defects may underlie some cases of idiopathic osteoarthritis.

ASSOCIATED OSTEONECROSIS

A considerable literature describes osteoarthritis as a late sequela of bone infarction (see also Chapter 98). The epiphyseal ends of the bones are involved primarily in osteonecrosis. Articular cartilage, deriving nutrition from synovial fluid, does not become infarcted, whereas the subchondral bone does. Nevertheless, weakening of the bony support of the joint over the course of a year or so leads to mechanical fracture and collapse of the joint surface. Proliferative remodeling results in variable osteophyte formation. In late stages of this disorder, the articular cartilage is sloughed off, and the apposed articulating member remodels. In some patients, overt osteoarthritis ensues, but eburnation is ordinarily inconspicuous. Evidence suggests that when osteonecrosis is associated with osteoarthritis of the hip, the arthritis is the primary and the necrosis is the secondary event.[13,38,39] Thus, ischemic necrosis of bone must be an infrequent cause of osteoarthritis.

"Gonarthrosis," supervening on a special form of osteonecrosis of the medial femoral condyle, is a frequent finding in elderly persons.[102] Clinical onset is sudden, and the initial event may be segmental fracture with depression of the articular cortex. Norman and Baker have associated this disorder with a torn medial meniscus.[103] Osteoarthritis has been described as a late consequence, but the available data are not persuasive. When segmental infarction occurs in osteoarthritic knee specimens,[104] it probably is a secondary phenomenon, as in the hip.

Osteonecrosis is a common occupational disease in sandhogs, pearl divers, and submariners. Dysbaric release of dissolved gases from the adipose tissue in the bone marrow is responsible for the death of bone tissue. Despite this association, a history of "bends" (caisson disease) often cannot be elicited. Several cases of authentic osteoarthritis have been reported, but in most published accounts, eburnation has not been documented.

GOUT

The articular lesions of gout are related to the deposition of monosodium urate monohydrate crystals in or about the joint tissues (see Chapters 104 and 106). The form that these lesions take varies with the amount, location, and duration of the deposits. Aside from massive disorganization of the articular structures by tophaceous deposits, the most common lesion is osteoarthritis. Urate crystals are deposited not only on and in the surface of the articular cartilage, but also in the subchondral cysts, where they constitute the so-called "punched-out" lesions. In the areas of crystal deposition in the cartilage, chondrocytes are characteristically necrotic, and the matrix is exceptionally oxyphilic.

OCHRONOTIC ARTHROPATHY

The articular and spinal lesions associated with alkaptonuria are similar to those of osteoarthritis (see Chapter 111). External remodeling is less prominent than in ordinary osteoarthritis.[7] The hyaline articular cartilage and the nucleus pulposus become discolored by the ochronotic pigment, and their material properties are grossly altered. These structures become remarkably brittle despite a normal water content. Necrosis of chondrocytes is more conspicuous than in osteoarthritis. Splitting off of fragments of the brittle cartilage is much more evident in ochronotic than in nonochronotic osteoarthritis, and these fragments may be found in joint fluid (see Chapter 5). With these exceptions, the processes are similar. Although "cal-

cification" of the nucleus pulposus is frequently described in ochronosis, probably ossific replacement of degenerated, pigmented tissue, is seen, rather than calcium deposition in the disc. Furthermore, the radiologically recognized, so-called "loose bodies" in the peripheral joints actually represent a reactive polypoid secondary osteochondromatous response of the synovial tissue to the articular detritus. Both calcium pyrophosphate and basic calcium phosphate (apatite) crystals have been identified in ochronotic cartilage.

ENDEMIC OSTEOARTHRITIS

Special types of noninflammatory deforming joint disease occur frequently in several parts of the world. These disorders share several features with generalized osteoarthritis, but they are distinguished from the latter by, among other things, stunted growth. Despite extensive research, their cause is obscure. These diseases are discussed in the following paragraphs.

Kashin-Beck Disease

Kashin-Beck disease, also known as *endemic osteoarthrosis deformans*, affects approximately 2 million persons in northern China and adjacent regions of Siberia. The changes appear during childhood and develop with varying severity in different individuals. Initially, the articular cartilage shares with the growth plate a zonal necrosis of chondrocytes.[105] For many years, the predominant Soviet view was that the condition results from poisoning by a fungal toxin. Contemporary Chinese investigators are more inclined to an explanation based on a dietary deficiency of selenium. Neither hypothesis is supported by experimental evidence.

Mseleni Disease

Mseleni disease is a crippling arthropathy that is endemic in northern Zululand. The hip is particularly susceptible. In surgically resected femoral heads, the lesions differed from those of ordinary osteoarthritis in that the joint surface was covered by a heterogeneous regenerated and degenerated cartilage. Eburnation was conspicuously absent.[106] Some investigators believe that Mseleni disease actually is heterogeneous, and that one subset is secondary to a hereditary spondyloepiphyseal dysplasia.[107]

HEMOPHILIC ARTHROPATHY

The joint disease that complicates the hemophilias may also be regarded as a variation of osteoarthritis.

Erosion of articular cartilage occurs early and is accompanied by eburnation and marginal osteophyte formation. The subchondral pseudo-cysts are filled with hemorrhagic material, but otherwise are analogous to those of osteoarthritis. Although hemosiderin deposition in synovial tissue reaches great proportions, only minute quantities are found in articular chondrocytes.[108,109] How the iron enters the chondrocytes is unknown because excessive iron is not detectable in the matrix. The pathogenesis of the cartilage destruction is not understood, although it obviously is related to the articular hemorrhages (see also Chapter 84).

Two general hypotheses are entertained currently: (1) elaboration of chondrolytic enzymes by hemosiderin-laden synovial cells[110] and (2) damage to the cartilage by toxic products of hemoglobin degradation. For example, free radicals, generated from ionic hemoglobin-derived iron, may damage the cartilage. The iron may also chelate with proteoglycans and may thereby alter the elastic properties of the matrix.[108,109] In advanced lesions, destruction of the joint passes beyond osteoarthritic limits; disintegration and fibrous ankylosis are then seen.

CHEMICAL CHANGES

The biochemistry of osteoarthritis has made rapid strides in recent years and is reviewed in Chapter 101. Several comments from the perspective of the pathologist are necessary to avoid making erroneous conclusions from the chemical findings. These comments principally concern problems of sampling and a discrimination between changes associated with osteoarthritis and those simply related to chronologic age in the cartilage.

Living tissue is required for studies involving incorporation of metabolic tracers or in vitro culture. Surgically resected femoral heads are most often used. Major discrepancies in published data have arisen from the sampling of reparative rather than degenerated native cartilage. How else does one account for the disparity in the biochemical data of Santer et al.,[111] based on cartilage obtained at routine necropsy, with data from numerous reports (reviewed in the following chapter) based on cartilage taken from surgically resected specimens? A warning concerning the use of fractured femoral heads as a source of control cartilage is also in order because this tissue undergoes secondary changes following the injury.[112]

Changes should be studied in articular rather than in other types of cartilage because important biologic differences exist among various types of cartilage. For example, the vascularity, amianthoid degeneration,[19] and pigmentation that occur in adult costal cartilage are not characteristic of old articular cartilage.[4] Although the costal cartilage of human adults has approximately 20% less water by weight than that of children, the difference in patellar cartilage is only about 2% less. Corresponding differences are found in the histochemical, elastic, and chemical properties of the two tissues.

Even within a single joint, areas that are fibrillated or are otherwise disintegrated differ from those that are not. It is therefore necessary to denote as aging changes only those found in the intact portions of such cartilage.

REPAIR OF ARTICULAR CARTILAGE AND POTENTIAL REVERSIBILITY

The persistent erosion of articular cartilage in osteoarthritis has long aroused interest in the limited ability of this tissue to grow. By all aspects studied, the metabolic activity of hyaline cartilage is low. In general, experimentally induced gaps in articular cartilage show little tendency to be filled in with new cartilage, as long as they do not penetrate into the subchondral vascular bone marrow. These observations provide the basis for the common view that the inability of cartilage to repair itself is responsible for the irreversible development of osteoarthritis.

A number of reasons for re-examining the validity of this concept exist. The cornerstone of the wear-and-tear theory of osteoarthritis is a putative inability of articular chondrocytes to undergo mitotic division. Nevertheless, these cells, isolated from mature individuals, divide, grow, and synthesize phenotypic glycosaminoglycans and collagen under proper conditions of culture in vitro.[113] The clue to this process is the release of the chondrocytes from their imprisoning matrix by enzymic means. The matrix thus serves ordinarily to switch off the cell-replicative mechanism. The clones of chondrocytes illustrated in Figure 100–3 are analogous to the in vitro cell division previously described. Autoradiographic studies demonstrate that the proliferating cells in osteoarthritis not only incorporate thymidine as a precursor of DNA synthesis,[114,115] but also show an increased rather than a diminished uptake of sulfate.[116] The rate of repair of articular cartilage by this mechanism is low, but it may not be negligible over time.

A more obtrusive mechanism of repair exists, that is, formation of new cartilage from pluripotential granulation tissue in subchondral bone marrow. The experimental data,[11,117] as well as the morphologic features of osteoarthritis already described, illustrate this mechanism. Surgical experience offers two sorts of limited evidence relevant to this potential for restoring the joint surface. First, following arthroplasties in which devitalized tissue is removed, a new articular surface forms beneath the prosthesis. The metallic device presumably protects the reparative granulation tissue from mechanical abrasion. Most such reparative tissue is bony and fibrous,[118] but foci of hyaline and fibrocartilaginous metaplasia also are seen.[4] Second, wedge osteotomies and other procedures designed to relieve mechanical stresses on osteoarthritic hips have frequently widened the radiologic joint space. Although much of the radiologic change may be an artifact caused by the repositioning of the weight-bearing surface, in a few, well-documented anatomic instances, fibrocartilaginous recovering of the joint surface has been noted.

EXPERIMENTAL INDUCTION

Numerous efforts have been made to establish possible mechanisms in the pathogenesis of osteoarthritis through induction of osteoarthritis by diverse local manipulations,[119] as discussed in the following paragraphs.

SURGICAL DISCONTINUITY IN THE ARTICULAR SURFACE

Although the literature on the subject is not wholly consistent, minute defects in the articular cartilage generally do not result in osteoarthritis. On the other hand, larger defects, which deform the joint contour, may.

PHYSICAL OR CHEMICAL INJURY TO ARTICULAR CARTILAGE

Heat, freezing,[120] and traumatic insults to the cartilage may also cause osteoarthritis. Necrosis of chondrocytes and associated degenerative changes have also been induced by the topical application of caustic agents. Synovitis, induced by intra-articular instillation of acids or other irritants or infectious materials, may also be accompanied by certain osteoarthritic changes, but these same agents may act on the cartilage as well as on the synovium.

SUBLUXATIONS AND LUXATIONS

Protracted displacements of the patella and of the hip have resulted in early remodeling and in later degenerative changes in the articular tissues.

INSTABILITY

Surgical disruption of the cruciate ligaments or partial excision of the menisci result in the rapid development of lesions that are frequently used as experimental models of osteoarthritis.

PROLONGED COMPRESSION

When the articular cartilages remain compressed for even a few days, death of chondrocytes may be followed by the development of osteoarthritis. Under these circumstances, the compression is presumed to hinder the normal percolation of interstitial fluid on which the nutrition of the chondrocytes depends.

RESTRICTION OF JOINT MOTION

Altered mobility is often associated with changes in the loading of joints. Failure to distinguish between the two phenomena accounts for some of the contradictions in the literature. Older studies indicated that experimental restriction of motion leads to degenerative changes with varying similarities to osteoarthritis, but Palmoski et al. found that motion in the absence of weight bearing does not maintain normal articular cartilage.[121] Immobilization itself leads to reversible depletion of aggregatable proteoglycan. In humans immobilized for prolonged periods by paralysis or by other means, contracture and fibrous ankylosis occur, rather than osteoarthritis.[122]

IMPULSIVE LOADING

Minor degenerative changes have been produced in rabbit joints by repetitive-impact forces. These findings support the contention that the destruction of cartilage in osteoarthritis results from compressive insults to subchondral bone, rather than from shearing of the surface cartilage.

FOREIGN BODY ABRASION

Degenerative changes in the superficial layer of articular cartilage have resulted from the intra-articular instillation of carborundum. These particles, like cartilage detritus, also evoke a foreign-body reaction in the synovium and joint capsule. Exostoses develop in the vicinity of the attachments of the joint capsule to the articular surface.

INJECTION OF CHONDROLYTIC ENZYMES

Intra-articular injection of papain into rabbits causes degenerative changes in articular cartilage associated with low-grade synovitis, and then eburnation of the surface.

It thus appears that a variety of procedures that impair the viability of articular chondrocytes and the integrity of the collagenous framework can lead to osteoarthritic changes. The procedures placing abnormal mechanical stresses on the cartilage also evoke structural remodeling of the joint contours.

PATHOGENESIS

With this background, we can attempt to formulate some concepts on the nature of osteoarthritis.

PRIMARY VERSUS SECONDARY OSTEOARTHRITIS

Osteoarthritis often supervenes on a pre-existing structural abnormality of joints. Such instances are classified as secondary, in contradistinction to primary osteoarthritis, in which no traumatic origin or predisposition can be assigned. In primary osteoarthritis, intrinsic aging or other alteration of the articular tissue is presumed to underlie development of the disease. The previously noted paucity of external remodeling in ochronotic or postinflammatory arthropathies is consistent with the idea that cartilage damage is responsible for concentric osteoarthritis, whereas biomechanical overloading is responsible for the common varieties in which one sees much joint deformity. The localization of the areas of greatest joint-space narrowing in the hip, such as the superolateral or medial area, and the configuration of osteophytes have been proposed as guides to a particular etiologic abnormality in roentgenograms,[123] as well as in excised specimens.[124] In surgically resected femoral heads, however, the changes are usually so far advanced and so diverse that it is difficult to sustain these interpretations.[39] Stulberg et al. are confident that they can identify a structural basis for at least

85% of cases of osteoarthritis of the hip.[93] They speculate that the bulk of osteoarthritis in other joints is also of a secondary type. Other workers report a much lower percentage and recognize primary osteoarthritis as a valid and frequent entity.[6,39,59,89] The recent study of Doherty et al., previously cited, complicates the traditional classification of osteoarthritis as either "primary" or "secondary."[61]

DOES OSTEOARTHRITIS BEGIN PRIMARILY IN THE BONE OR IN CARTILAGE?

If the view that the earliest events in osteoarthritis take place in articular cartilage is correct, then the bony remodeling results from the loss of energy-absorbing function of the cartilage. Transmission of mechanical forces to more labile para-articular tissues transduces the abortive attempts at repair. A different view emphasizes primary alteration in the bone. One formulation is that growth does not completely cease at the articular ends of bones in the adult; furthermore, remodeling takes place, under the aegis of functional demand, independently of degeneration of the cartilage.[8] Accordingly, only when the rate of remodeling exceeds that of orderly cartilage repair would osteoarthritis develop. Evidence supporting the view that bony changes underlie the deterioration of the cartilage includes the following: (1) articular cartilage is so much thinner than the length of bone that it has little measurable impact-absorbing function; (2) in experimental and clinical lesions, microfractures and sclerosis of subchondral trabeculae precede measurable changes in the cartilage; and (3) the cartilage is mechanically more susceptible to disintegration by impact-loading than by shearing stresses.[10]

Ordinarily, the degree of osteophyte formation corresponds to that of cartilage damage, but such is not always the case. Osteophytes themselves are not reliable indicators of the prognosis of osteoarthritis in the hip or knee.[125] Nevertheless, even in early osteoarthritis of the hip with joint-space narrowing, marginal osteophytosis is present.[126] This finding corresponds with the experimental data of Gilbertson described earlier.[14]

In the absence of more-definitive methods for resolving these divergent concepts, it seems useful to attempt to reconcile them: Both are likely true and are intimately related to each other. This formulation denies neither the possible role of metabolic factors in deterioration of the cartilage nor the significance of mechanical factors in inducing or treating osteoarthritis. The relative importance of the cartilage degeneration to bone remodeling may, of course, vary in different joints and in the different types of osteoarthritis.

SYSTEMIC CONTRIBUTIONS

Systemic factors include age, metabolic and genetic influences, and obesity.

Age

An outstanding feature of osteoarthritis is its relation to age. As an etiologic factor, senescence can have two different meanings. It may simply represent a series of cumulative insults to the articular tissue or, more biologically, it may suggest time-dependent molecular alterations that take place independent of acquired lesions. In the case of the articular cartilage, for example, a long-protracted, low-grade thermal degradation of the collagen or interaction of the collagen with cross-linking metabolites might represent such a biologic aging of cartilage. Dehydration does not occur as a progressive phenomenon of aging in articular cartilage. Chemical alterations presumably would change the biomechanical properties of the cartilage on which its functional integrity depends.

One way in which to assess the contribution of aging is to compare the severity of the clinically obtrusive lesions with the changes found in a general, aging population.[127] A quantitative time curve of the severity of osteoarthritis in routine necropsies is not readily obtained. The available data are limited, but they indicate that the deterioration of the joint surfaces progresses linearly with age.[4] The slope is greater in the patellofemoral than in the hip joint. The changes in surgically resected specimens fall far outside the scatter in the natural history of the aging hip. This finding suggests that some local or systemic factors aside from aging itself are of major etiologic importance, at least in the hip.[128]

Metabolic Factors

Other differences in the occurrence of osteoarthritis have aroused speculation about systemic-modifying factors. Ochronotic arthropathy is a striking prototype of a metabolic factor. We can easily conceive of metabolic patterns of osteoarthritis that remain unknown because the metabolites are colorless. Endocrine factors have been invoked. The arthropathy complicating acromegaly is an extreme example of damage to articular cartilage by somatotropin, through somatomedin-induced stimulation.[57] In one report, fasting levels of growth hormone were higher in patients with primary osteoarthritis than in control subjects.[129]

Little convincing evidence suggests that thyroidal dysfunction plays a role in human degenerative joint disease. In addition to favoring neurogenic arthropathy, diabetes mellitus has been found to predispose patients to the development of osteoarthritis.[130] Although gonadal hormones contribute to osteoarthritis in mice, menopausal changes probably do not affect the development of osteoarthritic lesions. Osteoarthritis of the hip, however, is twice as frequent in women as in men.

Osteoporosis

Although both osteoporosis and osteoarthritis are diseases of the aging skeleton, they do not frequently coexist in the same individual. Osteoporosis may actually protect against articular degeneration.

Genetic Factors

Genetic factors that contribute to osteoarthritis in other species may have systemic, metabolic, or, as in the case of the dysplasias, simply local effects on the joint disease. In humans, one investigation has yielded evidence of a genetic influence on the development of Heberden's nodes. The data were interpreted as indicating involvement of a single gene; its behavior in females appeared to be dominant, whereas it was recessive in males.[82] This type of inheritance is different from that described previously in mice. In another study in humans, degenerative joint disease of other peripheral and spinal joints also gave evidence of genetic influence, but of a recessive, polygenic type.[88] Several remarkable familial occurrences of chondromalacia patellae have also suggested heritable factors.

Obesity

Obesity has generally been accepted as a definite contributory factor because it seems self-evident that excessive weight imposes a mechanical burden on the joints undergoing abrasion. Several studies indicate that the situation is not so simple. In mice, obesity itself does not have an important, harmful effect on osteoarthritis.[70,131] Obesity does not contribute to the formation of Heberden's nodes[82] or, apparently, to osteoarthritis of the hip.[132,133] Some reports affirm a degree of correlation between overweight and osteoarthritis of the knee,[134] whereas others deny this association.[135] In certain epidemiologic studies, osteoarthritis and spondylosis were more common in obese persons than in those of normal weight.[136] In these studies, the affected joints were not necessarily those that bear weight, and the contribution of overloading was unclear. Perhaps the impact of obesity was greater on the symptomatic than the anatomic expressions of osteoarthritis.[132]

Ligamentous Laxity

In addition to congenital dysplasia of the hip, a variety of postural abnormalities of joints associated with laxness of the ligamentous structures also predispose patients to osteoarthritis. These abnormalities include recurrent luxations of the patella and shoulder, genu recurvatum or back-knee, and genu valgum or knock-knee. Laxness has been described as a feature of several systemic disorders, including Ehlers-Danlos and Marfan's syndromes. Howorth observed that general relaxation of the ligaments is common in children growing up in New York City, but not in youngsters in many less-privileged parts of the world.[137] Whether this finding reflects different genetic substrates or is an untoward acquired consequence of urban life remains to be determined.

"UNMASKING" OF COLLAGEN

One feature common to osteoarthritic alteration of joint cartilage, degeneration of intervertebral discs, and senescent change in costal cartilage is a diminution of chondroitin sulfate content relative to the collagen in the matrix. This chemical change has its histologic counterpart in the depletion of metachromatic ground substance and in a more conspicuous fibrillary appearance under polarized light. One would anticipate that this change would alter the material properties of the cartilage with respect to wear and tear: the matrix sol ordinarily dissipates applied stresses hydrostatically. In the absence of such protection, flexural and torsional forces might lead the unmasked collagen fibrils to rupture. Several processes probably are involved. Enzymatic mechanisms for selective removal of proteoglycan are reviewed in Chapter 101. Escape of interfibrillar components must be facilitated by disruption of the collagen. It has also been suggested that excessive percolation of fluid associated with vascularization of the base of the cartilage may enhance the leaching process. Another contributor may be synthesis of collagen types not usually found in cartilage. Minute amounts of abnormal (type I) collagen have been found by immunohistochemical means in the immediate vicinity of some chondrocytes in osteoarthritic cartilage.[117]

MECHANICAL FACTORS

Medicolegal agencies deal constantly with occupational injuries as mechanical factors in osteoarthri-

tis. In many publications on this subject opinions differ widely. The type of loading (for example, sustained rather than impulsive) does not itself account for the disparities of the findings. Osteoarthritis of the elbow has been observed in foundry workers who use long tongs to lift hot metals and so exert great leverage on this joint. Some investigators affirm[138] and others deny[139] that vibratory pressure causes osteoarthritis in the hands and arms of pneumatic drill workers. The occurrence of osteoarthritis in runners has not been found to be greater than in control populations.[140,141] This sort of information is vitiated by sampling problems: it excludes a priori persons who are unfit for running. Retired soccer players had more radiologically visible osteoarthritis of the hips than an age- and weight-matched control group.[142] Single injuries probably do not cause osteoarthritis unless they are severe enough to disorganize the joint surface or its major stabilizing components (see Fig. 100-6).

It is not known whether articular cartilage turns over normally through desquamation of its surface layer. Electron-microscopic studies have not disclosed a progressive death of cells proceeding toward the tangential layer. Evidence for mechanical abrasion of the cartilage in osteoarthritis is provided by the anatomic findings in the joint surface and by the demonstration of shards of cartilage in the synovial fluid. Information on the mechanics of such changes is sparse.

The articular cartilage of animal joints that is oscillated in vitro in the absence of synovial fluid undergoes rapid frictional destruction. Instillation of testicular hyaluronidase also leads to in vitro scoring of the joint surface. Although the results of this second group of experiments suggested that depolymerization of synovial mucin accounted for the friction, it is possible that the hyaluronidase may also have acted on the cartilage. Recently developed concepts of lubrication make untenable the widely accepted views of the importance of the viscosity of synovial fluid in maintaining the low friction.[143,144]

The volume, hyaluronate content, and relative viscosity of synovial fluid are usually normal in osteoarthritis and may even be greater than normal. Several studies have shown diminished polymerization of synovial mucin in osteoarthritis, as measured by the intrinsic and dynamic viscosities, as well as a reduction of the hyaluronate content.[131] The contradictory data arise in part because truly normal synovial fluids are not readily obtained for comparison. Synovial fluid obtained at necropsy differs from that aspirated clinically because the clinical specimen is often complicated by synovitis.

The principal contribution of synovial fluid to joint lubrication, other than the simple supply of water and salts to the cartilage, is the provision of a specific lubricating glycoprotein,[145] which adheres to the cartilage surface and makes it slippery. Using a synthetic bearing test system, no deficiency in the boundary-lubricating ability of synovial fluid has been found in osteoarthritis.[146]

The stresses on diarthrodial joints have never been measured directly. Rough estimates have been made in artificial models,[147] as well as through analyses of the forces between the feet and the ground, in concert with the rate and magnitude of excursion of the center of gravity of the body during walking.[148] The computation of moments from roentgenograms provides a clinical approximation of the distribution and magnitude of compressive loading of the hip and knee and underlies the design for osteotomy in the surgical treatment of osteoarthritis. Direct measurement of the stress in intervertebral discs has been made in vivo and in vitro.[80] The nucleus pulposus, through its hydrostatic properties, distributes the loads uniformly on the surrounding tissues. This purpose is effectively preserved even in the presence of moderate degenerative changes in the disc; only in severe disease is the hydrostatic function of the disc decreased.

The elastic properties and the strength of the articular cartilage are important factors governing its resistance to wear. The elasticity is determined largely by the water-binding capacity of the matrix. Neither the water content nor the elasticity, measured either as stiffness or recovery from a standard deformation, is altered in aging, as long as fibrillation is absent.[131]

The stiffness of the underlying bone has also been considered in relation to the development of osteoarthritis. Although osteoporosis and osteoarthritis affect the same age groups, no association exists between these two common senescent processes. Indeed, osteoporosis seems to militate against development of the joint disease.[129] Considerable veterinary evidence suggests that metabolic states in which mineralized bone is insufficient may adversely affect the articular cartilage.[68] The arthropathy that complicates hyperparathyroidism may, in part, reflect a lack of mechanical support from the subchondral, articular lamella.[131] This interpretation is complicated by the additional joint lesions: infractions of the surface and calcification of the cartilage. The obverse bone disease, osteopetrosis, also favors premature osteoarthritic degeneration.[149] The excessive stiffness of the bone may interfere with the normal nutritive movement of fluid in the cartilage during joint function.

In Paget's disease, the pathologic process sometimes extends into the base of the articular cartilage and wrinkles its surface. Mixed patterns of Paget's disease and osteoarthritis are frequently present in the hip.[150,151] Protrusio acetabuli develops in approximately 25% of such patients.

PATHOLOGIC BASIS OF CLINICAL COMPLAINTS

A general correlation exists between the clinical features and the anatomic manifestations of peripheral osteoarthritis.[132,152] Patients' complaints fall into two groups: pain and loss of motion. The sources of pain include synovitis, localized circulatory disturbances associated with subchondral microfractures, capsular tears, and impingement of the deformed bony structures on adjacent soft tissues. Loss of mobility must be attributed to the abnormal configuration of the joints, to muscle atrophy, and to capsular fibrosis. Anterolateral osteophytes in lumbosacral spondylosis are quite asymptomatic. Spurs located close to the neural foramina do, however, account for radicular pain.

CONCLUDING REMARKS

In recent years, our understanding of the pathogenesis of osteoarthritis, as of other fields of rheumatic disease, has progressed. This progress has largely taken the form of inquiry into an area of disease formerly regarded as incomprehensible to the pathologist and hopeless for the patient. Apparently divergent biomechanical and biochemical concepts of the nature of the lesions seem to reaffirm an interdependence between the wear-and-tear process and the metabolic state of the articular tissues.[131] The pathologic findings should not be interpreted as proof that degenerative joint disease is an inevitable concomitant of aging or that the lesions have no biologic potential for reversibility. By the same token, clinical trials of medications for osteoarthritis, based on the biologic features of articular cartilage, are premature and are conceivably hazardous.[3]

REFERENCES

1. Bullough, P.G.: The geometry of diarthrodial joints, its physiological maintenance and the possible significance of age-related changes in geometry to load distribution and the development of osteoarthritis. Clin. Orthop., *156*:61–66, 1981.
2. Thompson, R.C., Jr., and Bassett, C.A.L.: Histological observations on experimentally induced degeneration of articular cartilage. J. Bone Joint Surg., *52A*:435–443, 1970.

3. Ilardi, C.F., and Sokoloff, L.: The pathology of osteoarthritis: Ten strategic questions for pharmacologic management. Semin. Arthritis Rheum., 11(Suppl. 1):3–7, 1981.

4. Sokoloff, L.: Aging and degenerative diseases affecting cartilage. In Cartilage. Vol. 3. Edited by B.K. Hall. New York, Academic Press, 1987.

5. Fabry, G., and Mulier, J.C.: Biochemical analyses in osteoarthritis of the hip: A correlative study between glycosaminoglycan loss, enzyme activity and radiologic signs. Clin. Orthop., 153:253–264, 1980.

6. Solomon, L.: Patterns of osteoarthritis of the hip. J. Bone Joint Surg., 58B:176–183, 1976.

7. Lagier, R.: The concept of osteoarthrotic remodeling as illustrated by ochronotic arthropathy of the hip: An anatomico-radiological approach. Virchows Arch. [A], 385:293–298, 1980.

8. Bullough, P.G., and Jagannath, A.: The morphology of the calcification front in articular cartilage. J. Bone Joint Surg., 65B:72–78, 1983.

9. Lane, L.B., and Bullough, P.G.: Age-related changes in the thickness of the calcified zone and the number of tidemarks in adult human articular cartilage. J. Bone Joint Surg., 62B:372–375, 1980.

10. Radin, E.L., et al.: Response of joints to impact loading. III. Relationship between trabecular microfractures and cartilage degeneration. J. Biomech., 6:51–57, 1973.

11. Cheung, H.S., et al.: In vitro synthesis of tissue specific type II collagen by healing cartilage. 1. Short term repair of cartilage in mature rabbits. Arthritis Rheum., 23:211–219, 1980.

12. Furukawa, T., et al.: Biochemical studies on repair cartilage resurfacing experimental defects in the rabbit knee. J. Bone Joint Surg., 62A:79–89, 1980.

13. Milgram, J.W.: Morphologic alterations in the subchondral bone in advanced degenerative arthritis. Clin. Orthop., 173:293–312, 1983.

14. Gilbertson, E.M.M.: Development of periarticular osteophytes in experimentally induced osteoarthritis in the dog. Ann. Rheum. Dis., 34:12–25, 1975.

15. Bennett, G.A., Waine, H., and Bauer, W.: Changes in the Knee Joint at Various Ages. New York, Commonwealth Fund, 1942.

16. Vignon, E., Arlot, M., and Vignon, G.: Etude de la densité cellulaire du cartilage de la tète femoral en fonction de l'age. Rev. Rhum. Mal. Osteoartic., 43:403–405, 1976.

17. Weiss, C.: Ultrastructural characteristics of osteoarthritis. Fed. Proc., 32:1459–1466, 1973.

18. Ghadially, F.N., Lalonde, J.M., and Yong, N.K.: Ultrastructure of amianthoid fibers in osteoarthrotic cartilage. Virchows Arch. (Cell Pathol.), 31:81–86, 1979.

19. Hough, A.J., Mottram, F.C., and Sokoloff, L.: The collagenous nature of amianthoid degeneration of human costal cartilage. Am. J. Pathol., 73:201–216, 1973.

20. Longmore, R.B., and Gardner, D.L.: The surface structure of aging human articular cartilage: A study by reflected light interference microscopy (RLIM). J. Anat., 126:353–365, 1978.

21. Ghadially, F.N.: Fine structure of joints. In The Joints and Synovial Fluid. Vol. 1. Edited by L. Sokoloff. New York, Academic Press, 1978.

22. Meachim, G.: Light microscopy of Indian ink preparations of fibrillated cartilage. Ann. Rheum. Dis., 31:457–464, 1972.

23. Meachim, G.: Age-related degeneration of patellar articular cartilage. J. Anat., 134:365–371, 1982.

24. Minns, R.J., Steven, F.S., and Hardinge, K.: Osteoarthrotic articular cartilage lesions of the femoral head observed in the scanning electron microscopy. J. Pathol., 122:63–70, 1977.

25. Dustmann, H.O., Puhl, W., and Krempien, B.: Phänomen der Cluster im Arthroseknorpel. Arch. Orthop. Unfallchir., 79:321–333, 1974.

26. Mitrovic, D., et al.: Metabolism of human femoral head cartilage in osteoarthrosis and subcapital fracture. Ann. Rheum. Dis., 40:18–26, 1981.

27. Christensen, S.B., and Reimann, I.: Differential histochemical staining of glycosaminoglycans in the matrix of osteoarthritic cartilage. Acta Pathol. Microbiol. Scand., 88:61–68, 1980.

28. Getzy, L., et al.: Factors influencing metachromatic staining in paraffin-embedded sections of rabbit and human articular cartilage: A comparison of the safranin O and toluidine blue techniques. J. Histotechnol., 5:111–116, 1982.

29. Ali, S.Y.: Matrix vesicles and apatite nodules in arthritic cartilage. In Perspectives in Inflammation. Edited by D.A. Willoughby, J.P. Giroud, and G.P. Velo. Baltimore, University Park Press, 1978.

30. Jeffery, A.K.: Osteophytes and the osteoarthritis femoral head. J. Bone Joint Surg., 57B:314–324, 1975.

31. Christensen, P., et al.: The subchondral bone of the proximal tibial epiphysis in osteoarthritis of the knee. Acta Orthop. Scand., 53:889–896, 1982.

32. Havdrup, T., Hulth, A., and Telhag, H.: The subchondral bone in osteoarthritis and rheumatoid arthritis of the knee: A histological and microradiographical study. Acta Orthop. Scand., 47:345–350, 1976.

33. Reimann, I., and Christensen, S.B.: A histochemical study of alkaline and acid phosphatase activity in subchondral bone from osteoarthrotic human hips. Clin. Orthop., 140:85–91, 1979.

34. Reimann, I., Mankin, H.J., and Trahan, C.: Quantitative histological analysis of articular cartilage and subchondral bone from osteoarthritic and normal human hips. Acta Orthop. Scand., 48:64–73, 1977.

35. Resnick, D., Niwayama, G., and Coutts, R.D.: Subchondral cysts (geodes) in arthritic disorders: Pathologic and radiographic appearance of the hip joint. AJR, 128:799–806, 1977.

36. Termansen, N.B., et al.: Primary osteoarthritis of the hip: Interrelationship between intraosseous pressure, x-ray changes, clinical severity and bone density. Acta Orthop. Scand., 52:215–222, 1981.

37. Green, W.T., Jr., et al.: Microradiographic study of the calcified layer of articular cartilage. Arch. Pathol., 90:151–158, 1970.

38. Hardt, C.F., and Sokoloff, L.: Secondary osteonecrosis in osteoarthritis of the femoral head: A pathological study. Hum. Pathol., 15:79–83, 1984.

39. Meachim, G., et al.: An investigation of radiological, clinical and pathological correlations in osteoarthrosis of the hip. Clin. Radiol., 31:565–574, 1980.

40. Streda, A.: Participation of osteonecrosis in the development of severe coxarthrosis. Acta Univ. Carol. (Med. Monogr.), 46:103–153, 1971.

41. Christensen, S.B., and Arnoldi, C.C.: Distribution of 99mTc-phosphate compounds in osteoarthritic femoral heads. J. Bone Joint Surg., 62A:90–96, 1980.

42. Pritzker, K.P., Cheng, P.T., and Renlund, R.C.: Calcium pyrophosphate crystal deposition in hyaline cartilage: Ultrastructural analysis and implications for pathogenesis. J. Rheumatol., in press.

43. Menkes, C.J., Decraemer, W., Poste, M., and Forest, M.: Chondrocalcinosis and rapid destruction of the hip. J. Rheumatol., 12:130–133, 1985.

44. Gordon, G.V., Villanueva, C., Schumacher, H.R., and Gohel, V.: Autopsy study correlating degree of osteoarthritis, syn-

ovitis and evidence of articular calcification. J. Rheumatol., 11:681–686, 1984.

45. Dieppe, P.A., and Watt, I.: Crystal deposition in osteoarthritis: An opportunistic event? Clin. Rheum. Dis., 11:367–392, 1985.

46. Halvorsen, P.B., and McCarty, D.J.: Patterns of radiographic abnormalities associated with basic calcium phosphate and calcium pyrophosphate dihydrate deposition in the knee. Ann. Rheum. Dis., 45:603–605, 1986.

47. Sokoloff, L., and Varma, A.A.: Chondrocalcinosis in surgically resected joints. Arthritis Rheum., in press.

48. Arnoldi, C.C., Reimann, I., and Bretlau, P.:The synovial membrane in human coxarthrosis. Light and electron microscope studies. Clin. Orthop., 148:213–220, 1979.

49. Doyle, D.V.: Tissue calcification and inflammation in osteoarthritis. J. Pathol., 136:199–216, 1982.

50. Goldenberg, D.L., Egan, M.S., and Cohen, A.S.: Inflammatory synovitis in degenerative joint disease. J. Rheumatol., 9:204–209, 1982.

51. Soren, A.: Osteoarthritis—An arthritis? Z. Rheumatol., 41:1–6, 1982.

52. Fritz, P., et al.: Beitrage zum enzymhistochemischen Nachweis von Immunoglobulinen in Gelenkkapsel bei chronischer Polyarthritis und entzündlich aktivierter Arthrose. Z. Rheumatol., 39:331–342, 1980.

53. Ghose, T., et al.: Immunopathological changes in rheumatoid arthritis and other joint diseases. J. Clin. Pathol., 28:109–117, 1975.

54. Pringle, J.A., Byers, P.D., and Brown, M.E.A.: Immunofluorescence in osteoarthritis and rheumatoid arthritis. Nature, 274:84, 1978.

55. Scott, D.L., et al.: Significance of fibronectin in rheumatoid arthritis and osteoarthrosis. Ann. Rheum. Dis., 40:142–153, 1981.

56. Ogilvie-Harris, D.J., and Forasier, V.L.: Synovial iron deposition in osteoarthritis and rheumatoid arthritis. J. Rheumatol., 7:30–49, 1980.

57. Johanson, N.A., et al.: Acromegalic arthropathy of the hip. Clin. Orthop., 173:130–139, 1982.

58. Champion, B.R., Sell, S., and Poole, A.R.: Immunity to homologous collagens and cartilage proteoglycans in rabbits. Immunology, 48:605–616, 1983.

59. Cooke, T.D.V.: The interactions and local disease manifestations of immune complexes in articular collagenous tissues. Stud. Joint Dis., 1:158–200, 1980.

60. Fahmy, N.R., Williams, E.A., and Noble, J.: Meniscal pathology and osteoarthritis of the knee. J. Bone Joint Surg., 65B:24–28, 1983.

61. Doherty, M., Watt, I., and Dieppe, P.A.: Influence of primary generalized osteoarthritis on development of secondary osteoarthritis. Lancet, 2:8–11, 1983.

62. Egan, M.S., et al.: The association of amyloid deposits and osteoarthritis. Arthritis Rheum., 25:204–208, 1983.

63. Goffin, Y.A., Thoua, Y., and Potvliege, P.R.: Microdeposition of amyloid in the joints. Ann. Rheum. Dis., 40:27–33, 1981.

64. Ladefoged, C.: Amyloid in osteoarthritis hip joints: A pathoanatomical and histological investigation of femoral head cartilage. Acta Orthop. Scand., 53:581–586, 1982.

65. Ladefoged, C., Christensen, H.E., and Sorensen, K.H.: Amyloid in osteoarthritis hip joints: Deposition in cartilage and capsule. Acta Orthop. Scand., 53:587–590, 1982.

66. Uchino, F., et al.: Amyloid-like substance in cartilage of the sternoclavicular joints. In Amyloid and Amyloidosis. Edited by G. Glenner, P. Pinho e Costa, and A. Falcao de Freitas. Amsterdam, Excerpta Medica, 1980.

67. Sirca, A., and Sucec-Michieli, M.: Selective type II fibre muscular atrophy in patients with osteoarthritis of the hip. J. Neurol. Sci., 44:149–159, 1980.

68. Sokoloff, L.: Comparative pathology of arthritis. Adv. Vet. Sci., 6:193–250, 1960.

69. Wigley, R.D., et al.: Degenerative arthritis in mice: Study of age and sex frequency in various strains with a genetic study of NZB/B1, NZY/B1, and hybrid mice. Ann. Rheum. Dis., 36:249–253, 1977.

70. Walton, M.: Obesity as an aetiological factor in the development of osteoarthrosis. Gerontology, 25:165–172, 1979.

71. Silberberg, R.: Epiphyseal growth and osteoarthrosis in *blotchy* mice. Exp. Cell Biol., 45:1–8, 1977.

72. Walton, M.: Patella displacement and osteoarthrosis of the knee joint in mice. J. Pathol., 127:165–172, 1979.

73. Wilkinson, M.: Pathology. In Cervical Spondylosis. Its Early Diagnosis and Treatment. Edited by M. Wilkinson. Philadelphia, W.B. Saunders, 1971.

74. Utsinger, P.D., Resnick, D., and Shapiro, R.: Diffuse skeletal abnormalities in Forestier disease. Arch. Intern. Med., 136:763–768, 1976.

75. Resnick, D., et al.: Diffuse idiopathic hyperostosis (DISH) (ankylosing hyperostosis of Forestier and Rotes-Querol). Semin. Arthritis Rheum., 7:153–187, 1978.

76. Vernon-Roberts, B., Pirie, C.J., and Trenwith, V.: Pathology of the dorsal spine in ankylosing hyperostosis. Ann. Rheum. Dis., 33:281–288, 1974.

77. Ono, K., et al.: Ossified posterior longitudinal ligament: A clinicopathological study. Spine, 2:128–138, 1977.

78. Firooznia, H., et al.: Calcification and ossification of posterior longitudinal ligament of spine. N.Y. State J. Med., 82:1193–1198, 1982.

79. Bywaters, E.G.L.: The pathology of the spine. In The Joints and Synovial Fluid. Vol. 2. Edited by L. Sokoloff. New York, Academic Press, 1980.

80. Andersson, G.B.J.: Measurements of loads on the lumbar spine. In American Academy of Orthopaedic Surgeons Symposium on Low Back Pain. Edited by A.A. White, III, and S.L. Gordon. St. Louis, C.V. Mosby, 1982.

81. Hilton, R.C., Ball, J., and Benn, R.T.: Vertebral endplate lesions (Schmorl's nodes) in the dorsolumbar spine. Ann. Rheum. Dis., 35:127–132, 1976.

82. Stecher, R.M.: Heberden's nodes: A clinical description of osteoarthritis of the finger joints. Ann. Rheum. Dis., 14:1–10, 1955.

83. Goldberg, R.P., Zulman, J.I., and Genant, H.K.: Unilateral primary osteoarthritis of the hand in monoplegia. Radiology, 135:65–66, 1980.

84. Eaton, R.C., Dobranski, A.I., and Littler, J.W.: Marginal osteophyte excision in treatment of mucous cysts. J. Bone Joint Surg., 55A:570–574, 1973.

85. Utsinger, P.D., et al.: Roentgenologic, immunologic, and therapeutic study of erosive (inflammatory) osteoarthritis. Arch. Intern. Med., 138:693–697, 1978.

86. Ehrlich, G.E.: Pathogenesis and treatment of osteoarthritis. Compr. Ther., 5:36–40, 1978.

87. Smukler, N.M., Edeiken, J., and Giuliano, V.J.: Ankylosis in osteoarthritis of the finger joints. Radiology, 100:525–530, 1971.

88. Kellgren, J.H., Lawrence, J.S., and Bier, F.: Genetic factors in generalized osteoarthritis. Ann. Rheum. Dis., 22:237–255, 1963.

89. Marks, J.S., Stewart, I.M., and Hardinge, K.: Primary osteoarthrosis of the hip and Heberden's nodes. Ann. Rheum. Dis., 38:107–111, 1979.

90. Stewart, I.M., Marks, J.S., and Hardinge, K.: Generalized osteoarthrosis and hip disease. *In* Epidemiology of Osteoarthritis. Edited by J. Peyron. Paris, Geigy, 1981.

91. Yazici, H., et al.: Primary osteoarthrosis of the knee or hip. JAMA, 231:1256–1260, 1975.

92. Cooke, T.D.V.: The polyarticular features of osteoarthritis requiring hip and knee surgery. J. Rheumatol., 10:288–290, 1983.

93. Stulberg, S.D., et al.: Unrecognized childhood hip disease: A major cause of osteoarthritis of the hip. *In* The Hip. St. Louis, C.V. Mosby, 1975.

94. Stanescu, V., Stanescu, R., and Maroteaux, P.: Articular degeneration as a sequela of osteochondrodysplasia. Clin. Rheum. Dis., 11:239–270, 1985.

95. Allison, A.C., and Blumberg, B.S.: Familial osteoarthropathy of the fingers. J. Bone Joint Surg., 40B:538–545, 1958.

96. Abernethy, P.J., et al.: Is chondromalacia patellae a separate clinical entity? J. Bone Joint Surg., 60B:205–210, 1978.

97. Goodfellow, J., Hungerford, D.S., and Wood, C.: Patello-femoral joint mechanics and pathology. 2. Chondromalacia patellae. J. Bone Joint Surg., 58B:291–299, 1976.

98. Brower, A.C., and Allman, R.M.: The neuropathic joint: A neurovascular bone disorder. Radiol. Clin. North Am., 19:571–580, 1981.

99. Finsterbush, A., and Friedman, B.: The effect of sensory denervation on rabbits' knee joints: A light and electron microscopic study. J. Bone Joint Surg., 57A:949–956, 1975.

100. Raju, U.B., Fine, G., and Partemian, J.O.: Diabetic neuroarthropathy (Charcot's joint). Arch. Pathol. Lab. Med., 106:349–351, 1982.

101. Connor, B.L., Palmoski, M.J., and Brandt, K.D.: Neurogenic acceleration of degenerative joint lesions. J. Bone Joint Surg., 67A:562–572, 1985.

102. Bauer, G.C.H.: Osteonecrosis of the knee. Clin. Orthop., 130:210–217, 1978.

103. Norman, A., and Baker, N.D.: Spontaneous osteonecrosis of the knee and medial meniscal tears. Radiology, 129:653–656, 1978.

104. Ahuja, S.A., and Bullough, P.G.: Osteonecrosis of the knee: A clinicopathological study in twenty-eight patients. J. Bone Joint Surg., 60A:191–197, 1978.

105. Sokoloff, L.: Endemic forms of osteoarthritis. Clin. Rheum. Dis., 11:187–202, 1985.

106. Sokoloff, L., Fincham, J.E., and du Toit, G.T.: Pathological features of the femoral head in Mseleni disease. Hum. Pathol., 16:117–120, 1985.

107. Solomon, L.: Distinct types of hip disorder in Mseleni joint disease. S. Afr. Med. J., 69:15–17, 1986.

108. Hough, A.J., Banfield, W.G., and Sokoloff, L.: Cartilage in hemophilic arthropathy: Ultrastructural and microanalytical studies. Arch. Pathol. Lab. Med., 100:91–96, 1976.

109. Rippey, J.J., et al.: Articular cartilage degradation and the pathology of hemophilic arthropathy. S. Afr. Med. J., 53:345–351, 1978.

110. Mainardi, C.L., et al.: Proliferative synovitis in hemophilia: Biochemical and morphological observations. Arthritis Rheum., 21:137–144, 1978.

111. Santer, V., White, R.J., and Roughley, P.J.: Proteoglycans from normal and degenerate cartilage of adult human tibial plateau. Arthritis Rheum., 24:691–700, 1981.

112. Hirotani, H., and Ito, T.: The fate of the articular cartilage in intracapsular fractures of the femoral neck. Arch. Orthop. Unfallchir., 86:195–199, 1976.

113. Sokoloff, L.: *In vitro* culture of joints and articular tissues. *In* The Joints and Synovial Fluid. Vol. 2. Edited by L. Sokoloff. New York, Academic Press, 1980.

114. Havdrup, I., and Telhag, H.: Mitosis of chondrocytes in normal adult cartilage. Clin. Orthop., 153:248–252, 1980.

115. Hirotani, H., and Ito, T.: Chondrocyte mitosis in the articular cartilage of femoral heads with various diseases. Acta Orthop. Scand., 46:979–986, 1975.

116. Meachim, G., and Collins, D.H.: Cell counts of normal and osteoarthritic articular cartilage in relation to the uptake of sulphate ($^{35}SO_4$) *in vitro*. Ann. Rheum. Dis., 21:45–50, 1962.

117. Gay, S., et al.: Immunohistologic study on collagen in cartilage-bone metamorphosis and degenerative osteoarthrosis. Klin. Wochenschr., 54:969–976, 1976.

118. Milgram, J.W., and Rana, N.A.: The pathology of the failed cup arthroplasty. Clin. Orthop., 158:159–179, 1981.

119. Adams, M.E., and Billingham, M.E.: Animal models of degenerative joint disease. Curr. Top. Pathol., 71:265–297, 1982.

120. Simon, W.H., Lane, J.M., and Beller, P.: Pathogenesis of degenerative joint disease produced by *in vivo* freezing of rabbit articular cartilage. Clin. Orthop., 155:259–268, 1981.

121. Palmoski, M.J., Colyer, R.A., and Brandt, K.D.: Joint motion in the absence of normal loading does not maintain normal articular cartilage. Arthritis Rheum., 23:325–334, 1980.

122. Enneking, W.F., and Horowitz, M.: The intra-articular effects of immobilization on the human knee. J. Bone Joint Surg., 54A:973–985, 1972.

123. Gofton, J.P.: Studies in osteoarthritis of the hip. Part I. Classification. Can. Med. Assoc. J., 104:679–683, 1971.

124. Resnick, D.: Patterns of migration of the femoral head in osteoarthritis of the hip: Roentgenographic-pathologic correlation and comparison with rheumatoid arthritis. AJR, 124:62–74, 1975.

125. Hernborg, J.S., and Nilsson, B.E.: The relationship between osteophytes in the knee joint, osteoarthritis and aging. Acta Orthop. Scand., 44:69–74, 1973.

126. Wroblewski, B.M., and Charnley, J.: Radiographic morphology of the osteoarthritic hip. J. Bone Joint Surg., 64B:568–569, 1982.

127. Casscels, S.W.: Gross pathological changes in the knee joint of the aged individual: A study of 300 cases. Clin. Orthop., 132:225–232, 1978.

128. Byers, P.D., Contempomi, C.A., and Farkas, T.A.: Post-mortem study of the hip joint. III. Correlations between observations. Ann. Rheum. Dis., 35:122–126, 1976.

129. Dequeker, J.: The relationship between osteoporosis and osteoarthritis. Clin. Rheum. Dis., 11:271–296, 1985.

130. Waine, H., et al.: Association of osteoarthritis and diabetes mellitus. Tufts Fol. Med., 7:13–19, 1961.

131. Sokoloff, L.: The Biology of Degenerative Joint Disease. Chicago, University of Chicago Press, 1969.

132. Jerring, K.: Osteoarthritis of the hip: Epidemiology and clinical role. Acta Orthop. Scand., 51:523–530, 1980.

133. Saville, P.D.: Age and weight in osteoarthritis of the hip. Arthritis Rheum., 11:635–644, 1968.

134. Hartz, A.J., et al.: The association of obesity with joint pain and osteoarthritis in the HANES data. J. Chronic Dis., 39:311–320, 1986.

135. Goldin, R.H., et al.: Clinical and radiological survey of the incidence of osteoarthrosis among obese patients. Ann. Rheum. Dis., 35:349–353, 1976.

136. Lawrence, J.S.: Rheumatism in Populations. London, William Heinemann, 1977.
137. Howorth, M.B.: General relaxation of the ligaments with special reference to the knee and shoulder. Clin. Orthop., *30*:133–143, 1963.
138. Bovenzi, M., Petronio, L., and Di Marino, F.: Epidemiological survey of shipyard workers exposed to hand-arm vibration. Int. Arch. Occup. Environ. Health, *46*:251–266, 1980.
139. Burke, M.D., Fear, E.C., and Wright, V.: Bone and joint changes in pneumatic drillers. Ann. Rheum. Dis., *36*:276–279, 1977.
140. Lane, N.E., et al.: Long distance running, bone density and osteoarthritis. JAMA, *255*:1147–1151, 1986.
141. Panush, R.S., et al.: Is running associated with degenerative joint disease? JAMA, *255*:1152–1154, 1986.
142. Klünder, K.B., Rud, B., and Hansen, J.: Ostoarthritis of the hip and knee in retired football players. Acta Orthop. Scand., *51*:925–927, 1980.
143. Davis, W.H., Jr., Lee, S.L., and Sokoloff, L.: A proposed model boundary lubrication by synovial fluid: Structuring of boundary water. J. Biomech. Eng., *101*:185–192, 1979.
144. McCutchen, C.W.: Lubrication of joints. *In* The Joints and Synovial Fluid. Vol. 1. Edited by L. Sokoloff. New York, Academic Press, 1978.
145. Swann, D.A.: Macromolecules of synovial fluid. *In* The Joints and Synovial Fluid. Vol. 1. Edited by L. Sokoloff. New York, Academic Press, 1978.
146. Davis, W.H., Jr., Lee, S.L., and Sokoloff, L.: Boundary lubricating ability of synovial fluid in degenerative joint disease. Arthritis Rheum., *21*:754–760, 1978.
147. Rushfeldt, R.D., Mann, R.W., and Harris, W.H.: Improved techniques for measuring *in vitro* the geometry and pressure distribution in the human acetabulum. II. Instrumental endoprosthesis measurement of articular surface pressure distribution. J. Biomech., *14*:315–323, 1981.
148. Paul, J.P.: Joint kinetics. *In* The Joints and Synovial Fluid. Vol. 2. Edited by L. Sokoloff. New York, Academic Press, 1980.
149. Milgram, J.W., and Jasty, M.: Osteopetrosis: A morphological study of twenty-one cases. J. Bone Joint Surg., *64A*:912–929, 1982.
150. Altman, R.D., and Collins, B.: Musculoskeletal manifestations of Paget's disease of bone. Arthritis Rheum., *23*:1121–1127, 1980.
151. Roper, B.A.: Paget's disease involving the hip joints. Clin. Orthop., *80*:33–38, 1971.
152. Gresham, G.E., and Rathery, U.K.: Osteoarthritis in knees of aged persons. Relationship between roentgenographic and clinical manifestations. JAMA, *233*:168–170, 1975.

ETIOPATHOGENESIS OF OSTEOARTHRITIS

101

DAVID S. HOWELL

Our understanding of the etiopathogenic pathways in primary and, to a lesser extent, in secondary osteoarthritis has advanced over the last two decades. Recent concepts derived from expanding information on the cell biology and metabolism of chondrocytes and of the biochemical structure of cartilage are emphasized here, but some biomechanical aspects also are considered. I presuppose familiarity with the terminology and concepts presented in the section of this volume on the scientific basis for the study of arthritis. Many of the hypotheses relating to the pathogenesis of osteoarthritis stem from combined morphologic, biomechanical, and epidemiologic observations, as reviewed in Chapters 3, 10, and 100, respectively.

Problems multiply when one studies a given osteoarthritic lesion from living tissues. Careful morphologic data are needed on the site and stage of the lesion, its depth in the cartilage, and the presence or absence of inflammation. Biochemical etiologic pathways have been considered in relation to failure of the biomaterial properties of cartilage matrix or as a failure in the biomechanical aspects of joint development. Such errors may occur during pre- or postnatal growth, maturation, or aging. We need to know more about the biology of the chondrocyte (see Chapter 16). Metabolic control by local and systemic hormones, feedback control from matrix products regulating molecular synthesis, and types and numbers of membrane receptors are subjects still in their infancy.

EARLY BIOCHEMICAL EVENTS AND THE "FINAL COMMON PATHWAY"

We currently have more information on the pathogenesis of osteoarthritis than on etiologic factors. Both morphologic and biochemical data indicate a similar pattern by which cartilage expresses a degenerative response in both human disease and in animal models. Working hypotheses linking these observations have been described in various reviews.[1-14] Multiple etiologic factors are thought to result in chondrocyte injury, leading to a disturbance in its synthetic and degradative processes (Fig. 101–1). The net result is accelerated matrix breakdown by chondrocytic and perhaps synovial enzymes, followed by altered repair. Products of this tissue response stimulate chondrocytic proliferation and accelerated matrix synthesis at the local site. Breakdown products from cartilage are phagocytized by the surrounding synovial tissue, inducing a remodeling phenomenon involving new cartilage and bone production.

Various theories concerning the so-called final common pathway have been advanced as follows: (1) Injurious stimuli might lead to faulty cartilage matrix metabolism and inadequate repair as the major defective mechanism. (2) Trauma or other factors, such as hormones, may directly initiate the hypertrophic remodeling at marginal synovial membrane and ligament attachment sites, with accelerated cartilage breakdown as a secondary event. (3) Direct traumatic injury of the collagen network could lead to unrav-

1595

FIG. 101–1. Etiopathogenic factors in osteoarthritis.

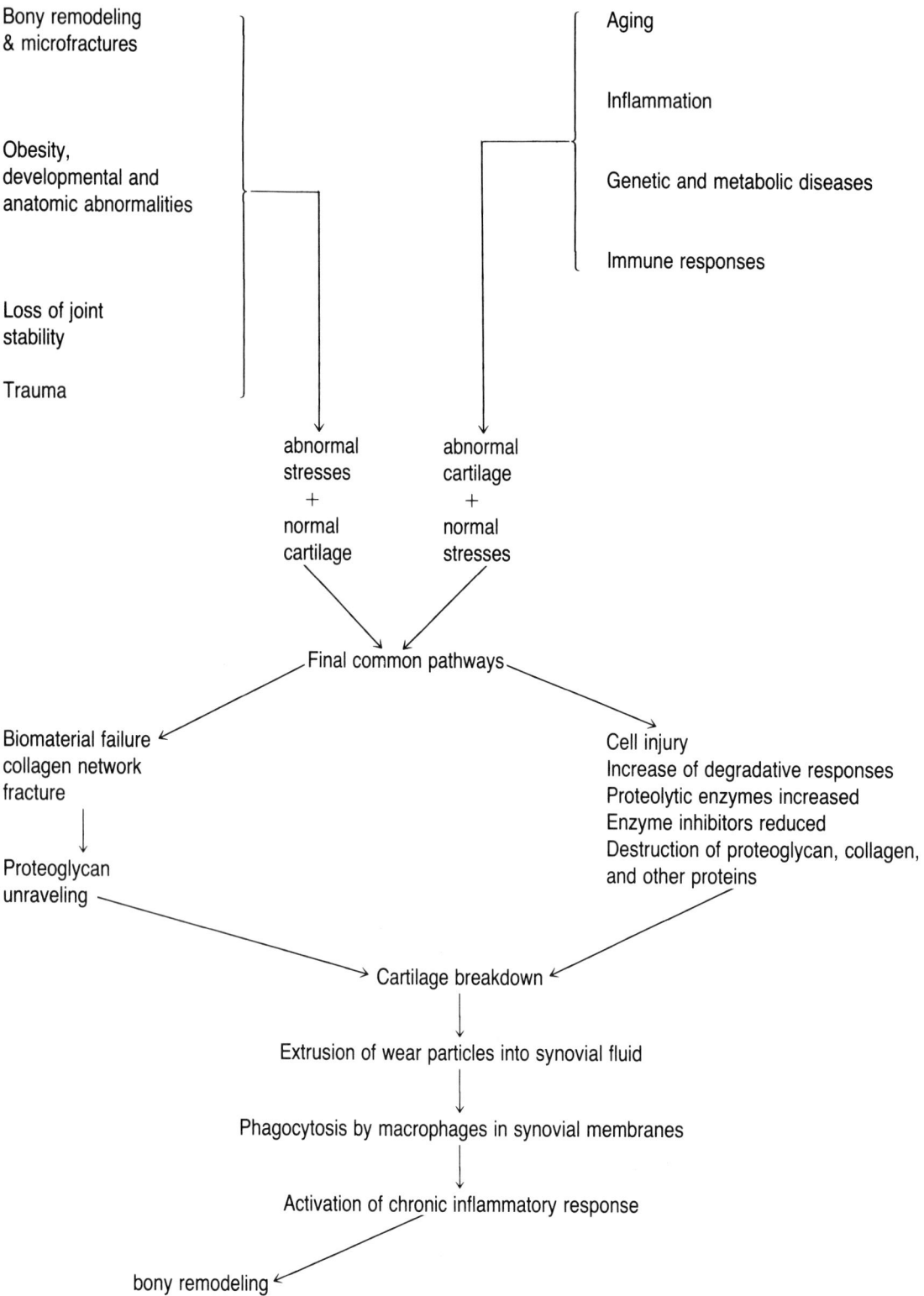

eling of proteoglycans and secondary tissue breakdown.

In *secondary osteoarthritis* from a variety of causes, cartilage breakdown may be the result of accumulation of abnormal biochemical products in the cartilage matrix, such as homogentisic acid in ochronosis, blood products in hemophilia, or urate crystals in gout.

Chondromalacia, the development of "soft spots" in unloaded or nonweight-bearing margins of articular cartilage, probably results from lack of normal physical stimulus to the regionally affected chondrocytes, as well as reduced local nutrition. The biochemical changes and histologic appearance are similar to those of early, aggressive lesions. *Chondromalacia patellae* develops most often on the medial patellar facet, an unloaded surface. Such lesions usually appear in young adults and can heal spontaneously, remain as localized spots, or progress to patellofemoral osteoarthritis, depending on the applicable biomechanical factors, such as the degree of lateral pull of the quadriceps tendon, the shallowness of the intertrochlear fossa, or inadvertent injury during unusual load carriage by the medial facet. Factors that permit advancement or restriction of such lesions probably involve a balance of injury and repair responses and are both biomechanical and biochemical.

BIOCHEMICAL STRUCTURE OF ARTICULAR CARTILAGE AND OSTEOARTHRITIC CHANGES

Throughout a lifetime, cartilage maintains an unusual relative isolation from exposure to endogenous and exogenous agents normally carried to extracellular tissues by the circulation. This isolation stems largely from an absence of capillaries and an abundance of proteoglycans, huge molecules with strong negative charges. The diffusion of macromolecules into the cartilage is thereby limited. On a dry-weight basis, cartilage contains about 35% proteoglycan and electrolytes, 60% collagen, and 5% noncollagenous, nonproteoglycan protein.[8] Its water content varies from 65 to 80% of its wet weight. The striking progress in elucidation of heterogeneities of cartilage proteoglycan and collagen structure in cartilage and metabolism was reviewed recently.[7,15-21]

Verification of proteoglycan molecular structure predicted by biochemical analysis was obtained directly by electron microscopy. These molecules looked like a cluster of Christmas trees. The "trunk" of each "tree" constituted a hyaluronate molecule, with branches of core protein of the proteoglycan subunits; linear glycosaminoglycans, as well as O-linked and mannose-containing oligosaccharides, were attached at intervals along the protein core. The proteoglycan subunits were attached to the hyaluronate molecule, stabilized by "link" glycoprotein (see Chapter 13). The proteoglycan subunits contain a core protein of about 250,000 daltons, to which the linear glycosaminoglycan molecules, weighing 11,000 to 36,000 daltons, are attached. In adult articular cartilages, about 90% of these glycosaminoglycan molecules are a mixture of chondroitin-6 sulfate and keratan sulfate, and the rest is mostly chondroitin-4 sulfate. The existence of such aggregates in vivo has been established by their associative extraction from cartilage and by their presence in samples of extracellular fluid obtained from cartilage by micropuncture. In such samples, ultramicrobiochemical analysis has demonstrated the existence of these aggregates.[22]

The importance of the aggregates to the function of normal articular cartilage has been shown in studies in which compressive and tensile moduli of the aggregates were much higher than those of monomers.[23] In fact, the biomechanical properties of cartilage appeared to depend partly on the presence of these aggregates. The shape of cartilage, even when the cartilage lacks proteoglycans, such as occurs following protease degradation, is still maintained by the collagen network, but all elastic properties are lost.[24] Proteoglycans confer elastic properties because of their large size and their high level of sulfation. The resultant high density of negative charges causes these molecules to repel each other and keeps the branches of glycosaminoglycans extended, thereby encompassing water and contained solutes. Such properties make the proteoglycans excellent "stuffing material" for the interstices in the collagen fiber network of cartilage. Although large linear macromolecules such as the monomers themselves can slowly diffuse through cartilage, plasma proteins, except for traces of albumin, are excluded under normal conditions.[8]

Normal nutrition of cartilage requires delivery of nutrients almost completely through the synovial fluid,[25] with passage of low-molecular-weight compounds such as glucose and amino acids directly to the cartilage cells[8] (see Chapters 10 and 11). Cyclic loading of joints probably increases the flow of nutrients to the cartilages; conversely, the supply of nutrients is reduced during immobilization.

The following changes have been observed in the biochemical composition of cartilage in osteoarthritis; with some exceptions, the total proteoglycan content was reduced in rough proportion to the histologic severity of the lesion sampled. The ratio of keratan sulfate and chondroitin-6 sulfate to chondroitin-4 sulfate was decreased. Controversial or variable changes included a shortened length of the proteoglycan subunit core protein, either in the chondroitin sulfate or the hyaluronate (HA) binding region, a shortened glycosaminoglycan chain length, decreased hyaluronic acid polymer size and content, variable capacity to form aggregates by proteoglycan subunits, and increased concentrations of nonproteoglycan, noncollagen proteins. Whether the size of the macromolecules and their component subunits was reduced by enzymatic degradation or by errors of synthesis is unclear. Reviews of these studies have appeared.[9,18,26–34]

Aging changes in articular cartilage are often *opposite* to those seen in osteoarthritis. For example, with aging, cartilage water content is reduced[8] and the concentration of hyaluronic acid is increased.[34] The importance of quality and quantity of link protein, of proteoglycan subunits, and of hyaluronate contributes to size-distribution profiles of proteoglycan aggregates[30–33] and probably to biomechanical properties in normal and osteoarthritic cartilages.[23] Sensitive monoclonal antibody techniques have extended greatly the capacity to study proteoglycan structure and metabolism.[35]

Heterogeneity of proteoglycan molecular populations has been found in human articular cartilage with respect to core protein epitopes[36] and two populations of dermatan sulfate-containing proteoglycans.[37] Such heterogeneities might significantly influence cartilage rheologic properties as a function of aging. Use of sensitive methods for quantitating biomechanical properties from the kinetic biomaterial standpoint has extended old and still largely valid views regarding biomechanical behavior of normal and osteoarthritic cartilage.[38–42] These results have been explained in terms of a biphasic flow theory.[38]

Whether osteoarthritic cartilage is characterized by low, normal, or increased metabolism of key matrix constituents remains controversial. The rates of glycosaminoglycan and DNA synthesis, measured by the uptake of small precursor molecules, were positively correlated with the severity of the osteoarthritic process in one study. This correlation abruptly failed when the most severe osteoarthritic changes were noted histologically. These findings were reviewed and corroborated in a subsequent study from the same laboratory,[43] and partial confirmation was obtained from other laboratories.[44,45] Other investigators, however, found no such increased metabolism or found lower turnover rates of macromolecules in osteoarthritic cartilage.[29]

Suggestions that cartilage collagen might be in-creasingly cross linked with aging have not been supported by studies quantitating reducible cross links,[16] or the nonreducible (hydroxypyridinium) cross links. Type II collagen is predominant in osteoarthritic cartilage.[17] Tiny amounts of type I, VI, and IX collagen were seen around cartilage cells, and small amounts of newly discovered minor collagen types, that is 1α, 2α, 3α (type XI), have been found in cartilage.[15] Fibronectin has also been found to accumulate in human and canine osteoarthritic cartilages.[46]

Reviews of cartilage repair and potential pharmacologic chondral protection have appeared.[47–49] Natural repair of osteoarthritic ulcerations seems to be almost impossible. For example, the arcade of collagen fibers visualized by polarizing light microscopy, or to some extent by scanning electron microscopy, is not duplicated in the healing lesions. This failure to re-create the correct "basket weave" of tissue collagen probably accounts for the inadequate biomechanical properties of repair cartilage.[49] After experimentally damaging knee cartilage in rabbits, researchers noted that repair cartilage lacked the mechanical strength of the original tissue, despite elaborate measures to promote healing. Clinical and laboratory experience with the fibrocartilage layers formed after a tenotomy and osteotomy procedure, however, indicates that a functional weight-bearing surface can develop under defined conditions, despite the aforementioned limitations.[49] Thus, hope remains that even the weaker tissue arising from a limited repair response may suffice as a resurfaced weight-bearing joint. Proper pharmaceutical or physical stimulation might encourage such regenerated cartilage to function satisfactorily.[47,48]

A prototype of this approach to treatment is seen in patients with acromegaly, in whom a thickened layer of apparently normal articular cartilage results from overproduction of growth hormone.[50] Although this disease is often attended by arthritis resulting from mechanical stresses due to overthickened joint cartilage, control of cartilage thickness seems a prerequisite to adequate cartilage replacement. Growth hormone itself was reportedly inactive in direct stimulation of articular cartilage cell proliferation or increased matrix synthesis.[51] Growth hormone treatment seems feckless, but insulin-like growth factor 1 (IGF1), stimulated in part by growth hormone, is a potential candidate for such experimentation because it is partly responsible for the effects of growth hormone on cartilage.[52] Still other important growth-stimulating factors active on cartilage are under study.[53–55]

Our understanding of the role of growth factors is changing as a result of new information gained largely from studying the effect of these factors on chondrocytes in cell culture.[13] The response of these cells seems to depend on the matrix adhesion of the cells. Chondrocyte adherence to matrix collagens may partly depend on such factors as anchorin CII, chondronectin, heparan sulfate proteoglycan, and colligin.[7] A role for fibronectin as an adhesive agent in cartilage is not supported. Repair responses are conditioned first by matrix hindrance of diffusion of growth factors to reach chondrocytes. Theoretically, hindrance to permeability of growth factors, such as connective tissue-activating peptides, platelet-derived growth factor, pituitary-fibroblast growth factor, and IGF1, is reduced as the matrix becomes degraded in osteoarthritis. Depending on local conditions, these factors then may amplify repair responses (see Chapter 14).

Insulin appears to be essential for adequate synthetic responses. IGF1 (somatomedin C) appears to amplify such responses and reacts with its own receptors, as well as with insulin receptors, on chondrocytes. Pituitary-fibroblast growth factor appears to stimulate chondrocyte proliferation but not matrix production.[9,14] Certain cytokines appear to enhance, and other cytokines to inhibit, cartilage repair responses.[56]

Chondroitin sulfate injected into canine knee joints has stimulated the production of peripheral cartilage and of bony spurs.[9] Obviously, potential therapeutic use of such factors must result in healing of the osteoarthritic erosions without promoting unwantd marginal bony and cartilaginous overgrowth.

CARTILAGE-DEGRADATIVE MECHANISMS

No consistent findings have been recorded regarding breakdown products of collagen in osteoarthritic tissues. In cultures of osteoarthritic human cartilages, however, a small but significant elevation of collagenase activity has been found to correlate positively with histologic severity of the lesions.[57] Incubates of human osteoarthritic cartilage elaborated hydroxyproline-containing products into the culture medium, and these products could be used to assess the activity of endogenous collagenolytic enzymes.[58] In these experiments also, collagenase activity was positively correlated with the histologic severity of the lesions.[58] Collagenase activity was higher in the erosion sites than in the margins or in sites distant from the erosions.

In the Pond-Nuki dog model of osteoarthritis, the same methods showed elevated collagenolytic enzyme activity in the erosive lesions.[59] The enzyme collagenase was postulated to be the cause of these changes on the basis of the response to inhibitors.[59] Whether the collagenolytic enzymes produce the erosions themselves, whether they enlarge the lacunae to accommodate proliferating chondrocytes or both remains unknown.

Proteoglycans are believed to be degraded early in the genesis of osteoarthritis. Although lysosomes of cultured chondrocytes contain exo-B-n-D-hexosaminidase and exo-B-d-glucuronidases capable of degrading oligosaccharides, no enzyme capable of cleaving the chains of chondroitin sulfate and releasing sulfated oligosaccharides has been found in adult cartilage. Hyaluronidase has been isolated from adult articular cartilage, but it was not active at physiologic pH.[60] This enzyme failed to break down chondroitins, which seem to be cleaved mainly in the liver.[61]

Evidence for increased neutral metalloprotease and serine proteinase activity, but not thiol proteinase, was found in human osteoarthritic and Pond-Nuki experimental osteoarthritic cartilages compared to controls.[62]

Lysosomal enzymes, cathepsin D, B, and F, are believed to be involved in terminal degradation of matrix proteins.[63,64] These enzymes are probably also active on the outside or margin of chondrocyte plasma membranes, where a surprisingly acid pH has been demonstrated.[65] Over the last decade, a neutral metalloproteinase in human articular cartilage has been partially purified and characterized with great difficulty because of its small amounts.[66] Subsequently, with new methods for extraction and purification, this enzyme activity has been greatly enhanced and distributes as two neutral proteinases active at neutral pH.[67] An acidic metalloproteinase, previously documented,[66] has been partially purified and characterized.[68] It has a wide pH range of activity from the acid into the neutral range and is probably the enzyme that is increased after interleukin 1 (IL1) stimulation of chondrocytes. These enzymes (and possibly serine proteases) are elaborated by cultured chondrocytes into the media[69,70] and act on proteoglycan matrix distant from the chondrocytes, and therefore could clip the hyaluronate binding region of unaggregated monomers[71] and probably degrade the outer end (c-terminal) of protein cores in proteoglycan aggregates. Roughley et al.[72] found evidence in aging human cartilage of nonaggregatable hyaluronate because of the presence of HA binding region stubs of core protein attached to hyaluronate. These degraded products increased with aging.

Little controversy has arisen over the source of these enzymes because no pannus invades osteoarthritic cartilage, and no lymphocytic or other cellular infiltrates occur within the cartilage to provide a possible alternative source for these proteases found in early disease. Although these enzymes are considered to play some role in early cartilage matrix destruction, the picture becomes more complicated once an osteoarthritic erosion develops and thereby permits an influx of synovial fluid. Despite its content of potent enzyme inhibitors, such as α-2-macroglobulin, synovial fluid could deliver enzymes deleterious to the matrix originating from leukocytes or from synovial lining cells. Synovial lining cells can elaborate serine and metalloneutral proteases, cathepsin D, and collagenase, probably very similar to those of cartilage.[73]

Protease tissue degradation must be closely regulated. Evidence indicates that collagenase is secreted as a proenzyme and then activated by another factor of about the same molecular weight.[73,74] Treatment with a mercurial organic compound aminophenylmercuric acetate (APMA), or trypsin can reduce the molecular weight of the enzyme from studies of synovial cell culture, but its activation requires the presence of this new factor. Thus, the reduction of molecular weight (MW) by about 11,000 daltons occurs with APMA, but procollagenase activator is still required. The activated enzyme is then vulnerable to irreversible binding to the endogenous tissue inhibitor of metalloproteases (TIMPs).[75,76] TIMP was purified originally in Reynold's laboratory from human cartilage and has since been synthesized by recombinant DNA technology.[77] Quantification of TIMP in osteoarthritic cartilage revealed levels thought to be inappropriately low.[75] Inhibitors of other proteases, particularly serine protease,[78,79] as well as an antitumor invasion factor,[80] have been characterized in cartilage. Once cartilage matrix is degraded by one or more proteases or, possibly under certain circumstances, by free radicals,[81,82] its permeability to large molecules, hitherto effectively excluded, is lost, and exogenous enzymes can possibly penetrate and amplify the matrix degradation.

The cationic protein lysozyme is abundant in cartilage. Regardless of whether its origin is endogenous or exogenous, a growing body of evidence suggests that lysozyme can regulate the size of proteoglycan aggregates.[63] The presence of aggregates appears to reduce the vulnerability of proteoglycans to enzymatic attack. Once a minute amount of neutral protease attacks a proteoglycan monomer, it may clip selectively the HA-binding region. Such degraded fragments can rapidly diffuse from an incubated piece of cartilage, leaving behind the normal proteoglycans capable of aggregation.[9,83] This important finding may explain why so few breakdown products of proteo-glycans have been found in osteoarthritic cartilage; as soon as degradation occurs, the products are either further degraded by the chondrocytes, or they rapidly diffuse into the synovial fluid. Such proteoglycan degradation products have been identified in synovial fluid of osteoarthritis patients.[84] A hallmark sugar of cartilage proteoglycan degradation, keratan sulfate, has been found significantly elevated in the sera of patients with osteoarthritis. The potential usefulness of these methods is apparent.[85]

WATER CONTENT AND THE COLLAGEN NETWORK

The actual role of proteases in cartilage breakdown in osteoarthritis remains controversial because remodeling phenomena cannot be separated from genuine primary tissue breakdown. It is still possible that most cartilage destruction proceeds mechanically.[3,8] Increased water content, one of the earliest changes in osteoarthritis, is apparently caused by disruption of collagen network and exposure of water-binding proteoglycans.[8,86] The collagen network in articular cartilage is a "sealed type," that is, the proteoglycan aggregates are confined in a concentrated, semidehydrated state.[8,86] After rupture of this network by enzymes, physical forces, or both, the proteoglycans expand and imbibe water. The collagen fibers can take up some water as well.[87] As a result, not only do proteoglycans become more exposed to enzymatic attack, but their cushioning effect is lost, and the cell and matrix are injured further.

ROLE OF INFLAMMATORY PRODUCTS

As osteoarthritis progresses, wear particles gain access to synovial fluid and are phagocytized by synovial membrane macrophage-like cells. The responses of these cells to wear particles have been examined in tissue culture with respect to the release of inflammatory mediators. Such studies may relate to clinical work showing a frequent inflammatory component in osteoarthritis. Nearly 75% of a series of osteoarthritic joints showed some evidence of inflammatory response,[2,6] a finding that might explain the remarkable symptomatic improvement of most patients with osteoarthritis after treatment with nonsteroidal anti-inflammatory drugs (NSAIDs). Vascular and synovial cell hyperplasia and spotty, low-grade infiltration with mononuclear cells have been commonly observed in osteoarthritic synovium. Studies on leukocytes from patients with osteoarthritis have shown cytokines either stimulating or suppressing chondrocytic synthesis of proteoglycans.[88]

Thus, increasing evidence for the potential role of cytokines in amplifying cartilage destruction has been reported wth special reference to IL1 (α and β) and historically closely related factors, catabolin and mononuclear cell factor. These molecules stimulate chondrocytes to produce degradative enzymes in organ culture, with inhibition of repair and elaboration of degradation products.[5,88–94] In osteoarthritis, wear particles stimulate synovial cells to produce collagenase and probably lead to cytokine production. These results have led to increasing research on the influence of cell–cell communication in joint tissues–with characterization of regulators "upstream," to the mechanisms of elaboration and activation of proteases.[5] Characterization of chondrocyte receptors for IL1, second-messenger systems, and final target enzyme responses, and/or inhibition of synthetic responses, have been sought in various explant and cell culture systems.[5,88] Circulating antibodies and cellular immunologic responses have been documented in some patients with osteoarthritis.[1]

Immunogenicity of cartilage matrix constituents[1] and "switching on" of inflammatory responses[95,96] is probably a secondary event in amplifying osteoarthritic synovial inflammation and cartilage breakdown. Cooke et al.[1] found C3, immunoglobulin G (IgG), and IgA deposits within the surfaces of osteoarthritic cartilage.[1] Clinical characterization of such patients, in comparison to those lacking these deposits, has not led to any well-defined syndrome. Most of these studies were conducted on patients with osteoarthritis involving hips or knees that required surgery.

Crystals can play an important role in causing secondary inflammation in secondary osteoarthritis involving calcium pyrophosphate dihydrate crystal deposition disease or basic calcium phosphate arthropathy. (For a discussion of the role of crystals in synovial inflammation, see Chapters 106 to 109.) Certainly, crystals destabilize plasma membranes of synovial fibroblasts, engender synthesis or release of PGE$_2$ collagenase and neutral protease,[97] and can effect such processes without a classic inflammatory response.[98,99] An example is the "Milwaukee shoulder syndrome" reviewed in Chapter 108.[98]

ENDOCRINE FACTORS

Animal models of osteoarthritis have been studied extensively for effects of hormones, but direct application of findings to the human disease is difficult.

Adrenocorticosteroids in dosages comparable to those injected into human joints had no effect on osteoarthritic erosions in the Moskowitz rabbit model, but these agents seemed to prevent spur formation.[100] When delivered in larger doses, corticosteroids can cause severe cartilage damage by interfering with matrix repair.[101] An estrogen antagonist, tamoxifen, has blocked osteoarthritic erosions in this animal model, but whether through reduced degradation or improved synthetic repair is still unclear.[102] Most NSAIDs, including the currently marketed proprionic acid derivatives, fenamates, salicylates, and some acetic acid derivatives, appear to reduce synthetic rates of proteoglycans in incubates of articular cartilage from normal dogs and from Pond-Nuki dogs with osteoarthritis.[103] The possibility of unfavorable effects on cartilage repair of these agents remains to be demonstrated by human in vivo studies, but these results certainly deserve further consideration (see Chapter 103).

Hyaluronic acid, previously considered the main lubricant in joints, is a poor lubricant of cartilage-to-cartilage bearings, and hydrolysis of synovial hyaluronic acid with hyaluronidase does not lessen synovial fluid lubrication.[104] A glycoprotein called *lubricin* probably contributes the most to lubrication of joints by its adsorption on cartilage surfaces.[105] In contrast, in periarticular soft tissues in which resistance to joint motion predominates, hyaluronic acid still seems to be an effective lubricant (see Chapters 10 and 100). Whether abnormalities exist in joint lubrication in osteoarthritis is unknown.

REFERENCES

1. Cooke, T.D.V.: Which comes first: Inflammation or osteoarthritis? Relationship of immune deposits in articular cartilaginous tissues to synovitis in osteoarthritis. *In* Clinical Pathological Osteoarthritis Workshop. Edited by T.D.V. Cooke, I. Dwosh, and J. Cossairt. J. Rheumatol., *10*(Suppl. 9):55–56, 1983.
2. Dieppe, P.: Osteoarthritis: Are we asking the wrong questions? Br. J. Rheumatol., 23:161–163, 1984.
3. Freeman, M.A.R.: Adult Articular Cartilage. 2nd Ed. Tunbridge Wells, England, Pitman Medical, 1979.
4. Gardner, D.L.: The nature and cause of osteoarthritis. Br. Med. J., *286*:418–424, 1983.
5. Hamerman, D., Klagsbrun, M.: Osteoarthritis: Emerging evidence for cell interactions in the breakdown and remodelling of cartilage. Am. J. Med., *78*:495–499, 1985.
6. Howell, D.S., and Talbott, J.H. (eds.): Osteoarthritis Symposium. Semin. Arthritis Rheum., *11*(Suppl. 1):1–147, 1981.
7. Kuettner, K.E., Schleyerbach, R., and Hascall, V.C.: Articular Cartilage Biochemistry. New York, Raven Press, 1986.
8. Maroudas, A., and Holborow, E.J.: Studies in Joint Disease. Vols. 1 and 2. Tunbridge Wells, England, Pitman Medical, 1980.

9. Moskowitz, R.W., Howell, D.S., Goldberg, V.M., and Mankin, H.J., Jr.: Osteoarthritis: Diagnosis and Management. Philadelphia, W.B. Saunders Company, 1984.

10. Muir, H.: Current and future trends in articular cartilage research and osteoarthritis. *In* Articular Cartilage Biochemistry. Edited by K.E. Kuettner, R. Schleyerbach, and V.C. Hascall. New York, Raven Press, 1985.

11. Peyron, J.G.: Osteoarthritis: Current Clinical and Fundamental Problems. Paris, Ciba-Geigy, 1985.

12. Radin, E.L., et al.: Mechanical factors influencing articular cartilage damage. *In* Osteoarthritis: Current Clinical and Fundamental Problems. Edited by J. G. Peyron. Paris, Ciba-Geigy, 1985.

13. Sokoloff, L.: Aging and degenerative diseases affecting cartilage. *In* Cartilage. Vol. 3. Edited by B. Hall. New York, Academic Press, 1984.

14. Verbruggen, G., and Veys, E.M.: Degenerative Joints. Vol. 2. International Congress Series. Edited by G. Verbruggen and E.M. Veys. Amsterdam, Excerpta Medica, 1985.

15. Apone, S., Wu, J.J., and Eyre, D.R.: Collagen heterogeneity in articular cartilage: Identification of five genetically distinct molecular species. Trans. Orthop. Res. Soc., *12*:109, 1987.

16. Eyre, D.R., et al.: Studies on the molecular diversity and cross-linking of cartilage collagen. *In* Osteoarthritis: Current Clinical and Fundamental Aspects. Edited by J.G. Peyron. Paris, Ciba-Geigy, 1985.

17. Gay, S., Gay, R., and Miller, E.J.: The collagen of the joint. Arthritis Rheum., *23*:937–941, 1980.

18. Hascall, V.C.: *In* Biology of Carbohydrates. Vol. 1. Edited by V. Ginsburg. New York, John Wiley & Sons, 1981.

19. Mankin, H.J., and Brandt, K.: Biochemistry and metabolism of cartilage in osteoarthritis. *In* Osteoarthritis: Diagnosis and Management. Edited by R. Moskowitz, D.S. Howell, V.M. Goldberg, and H.J. Mankin. Philadelphia, W.B. Saunders, 1984.

20. Nimni, M.E.: Collagen: Structure, function, and metabolism in normal and fibrotic tissues. Semin. Arthritis Rheum., *13*:1–86, 1983.

21. Sandell, L., Upholt, W.B., and Kuettner, K.E.: Structure of the type II (cartilage) collagen gene: Implications for regulation of collagen gene expression. Trans. Orthop. Res. Soc., *9*:209, 1984.

22. Pita, J.C., Muller, F.J., Morales, S., and Alarcon, E.J.: Ultracentrifugal characterization of proteoglycans from rat growth cartilage. J. Biol. Chem., *254*:10313–10320, 1979.

23. Mak, A.F., et al.: Assessment of proteoglycan–proteoglycan interactions from solution biorheological behaviors. Trans. Orthop. Res. Soc., *7*:169, 1982.

24. Harris, E.D., Jr., et al.: Effects of proteolytic enzymes on structural and mechanical properties of cartilage. Arthritis Rheum., *15*:497–503, 1972.

25. McKibbin, B.: The nutrition of articular cartilage and its relationship to development. *In* Normal and Osteoarthrotic Articular Cartilage. Edited by S.Y. Ali, M.W. Elves, and D.H. Leaback. London, Institute of Orthopaedics, 1974.

26. Muir, H.: Heberden oration: Molecular approach to the understanding of osteoarthrosis. Ann. Rheum. Dis., *36*:199–208, 1977.

27. Byers, P.D., et al.: Histological and biochemical studies on cartilage from osteoarthritic femoral heads with special reference to surface characteristics. Connec. Tiss. Res., *5*:41–49, 1977.

28. McDevitt, C.A., and Muir, H.: Biochemical changes in the cartilage of the knee in experimental and natural osteoarthritis in the dog. J. Bone Joint Surg., *58B*:94–101, 1976.

29. Bayliss, M.T., and Venn, M.: Chemistry of human articular cartilage. *In* Studies in Joint Disease. Vol. 1. Edited by A. Maroudas and E.J. Holborow. Tunbridge Wells, England, Pitman Medical, 1980.

30. Buckwalter, J.A., et al.: The effect of link protein concentration on proteoglycan aggregation. Trans. Orthop. Res. Soc., *11*:98, 1986.

31. Manicourt, D.H., Pita, J.C., Pezon, C.F., and Howell, D.S.: Characterization of the proteoglycans recovered under nondissociative conditions from normal articular cartilage of rabbits and dogs. J. Biol. Chem., *261*:5426–5433, 1986.

32. Manicourt, D.H., et al.: Studies of cartilage proteoglycans in an osteoarthritic rabbit model. *In* Osteoarthritis: Current Clinical and Fundamental Problems. Edited by J.G. Peyron. Paris, Ciba-Geigy, 1984.

33. Pita, J.C., Manicourt, D.H., and Howell, D.S.: Heterogeneity of normal and osteoarthritic articular cartilage as determined by proteoglycan aggregation. Trans. Orthop. Res. Soc., *11*:100, 1986.

34. Bayliss, M.T., Holmes, M.W.A., and Muir, H.: Hyaluronic acid: Age-related changes in human articular cartilage. Trans. Orthop. Res. Soc., *12*:110, 1987.

35. Caterson, B., Hampton, A., Hascall, V.C., and Stevens, J.: The production and characterization of monoclonal antibodies to the hyaluronic acid binding region of cartilage proteoglycan. Trans. Orthop. Res. Soc., *9*:189, 1984.

36. Glant, T.T., Mikecz, K., Roughley, P.J., and Poole, A.R.: Differences in protein-related epitopes of proteoglycans from human articular cartilage of different ages. Trans. Orthop. Res. Soc., *12*:63, 1987.

37. Rosenberg, L., et al.: Separation of dermatan sulfate proteoglycans from mature articular cartilages by hydrophobic chromatography. Trans. Orthop. Res. Soc., *12*:59, 1987.

38. Akizuki, S., et al.: Knee joint cartilage: I. Influence of ionic conditions, weight bearing, and fibrillation on the tensile modulus. J. Orthop. Res., *4*:379–392, 1986.

39. Armstrong, C.G., and Mow, V.C.: Variations in the intrinsic mechanical properties of human articular cartilage with age, degeneration and water content. J. Bone Joint Surg., *64A*:88–94, 1982.

40. Mow, V.C., Mak, A.F., and Lai, W.M.: Viscoelastic properties of proteoglycan subunits and aggregates in varying solution concentrations. J. Biomech., *17*:325–338, 1984.

41. Kempson, G.E., et al.: Correlations between stiffness and the chemical constituents of cartilage of the human femoral head. Biochim. Biophys. Acta, *215*:70–77, 1970.

42. Altman, R.D., et al.: Biomechanical and biochemical properties of dog cartilage in experimentally-induced osteoarthritis. Ann. Rheum. Dis., *43*:83–90, 1984.

43. Mankin, H.J., Johnson, M.E., and Lippiello, L.: Biochemical and metabolic abnormalities in articular cartilage from osteoarthritic human hips. II. Distribution and metabolism of amino sugar containing macromolecules. J. Bone Joint Surg., *63A*:131–134, 1981.

44. Thompson, R.C., Jr., and Oegema, T.R., Jr.: Metabolic activity of articular cartilage in osteoarthritis: An in vitro study. J. Bone Joint Surg., *61A*:407–416, 1979.

45. Vignon, E., et al.: Hypertrophic repair of cartilage in osteoarthritis. Ann. Rheum. Dis., *42*:82–88, 1983.

46. Wurster, N.B., et al.: Presence of fibronectin in articular cartilage in two animal models of osteoarthritis. J. Rheumatol., *13*:175–182, 1986.

47. Burkhardt, D., and Ghosh, P.: Laboratory evaluation of glycosaminoglycan polysulfate ester for chondroprotective activity: A review. Curr. Therap. Res., *40*:1034–1053, 1986.

48. Salter, R.B., et al.: The biological effect of continuous passive motion on the healing of full-thickness defects in articular cartilage: An experimental investigation in the rabbit. J. Bone Joint Surg., *62A*:1232–1250, 1980.

49. Radin, E.L., and Burr, D.B.: Hypothesis: Joints can heal. Semin. Arthritis Rheum., *13*:293–302, 1984.

50. Detenbeck, L.C., et al.: Peripheral joint manifestations of acromegaly. Clin. Orthop., *91*:119–127, 1973.

51. Mankin, H.J., et al.: Dissociation between the effect of bovine growth hormone in articular cartilage and in bone of the adult dog. J. Bone Joint Surg., *60A*:1071–1075, 1978.

52. Zeulak, K.M., and Green, H.: The generation of insulin-like growth factor-1-sensitive cells by growth hormone action. Science, *233*:551–553, 1986.

53. Davidson, J.M., et al.: Accelerated wound repair, cell proliferation, and collagen accumulation are produced by a cartilage-derived growth factor. J. Cell Biol., *100*:1219–1227, 1985.

54. Castor, C.W., et al.: Regulation of synovial cell metabolism by growth factors. *In* Rheumatology-85. Edited by P.M. Brooks and J.R. York. Amsterdam, Elsevier Science Publishers, 1985.

55. Sporn, M.B., Roberts, A.B., Wakefield, L.M., and Assoian, R.K.: Transforming growth factor-B: Biological function and chemical structure. Science, *233*:532–534, 1986.

56. Herman, J.H.: Lymphokines: Potential role in the immunopathogenesis of osteoarthritis. Semin. Arthritis Rheum., *11*(Suppl. 1):104–107, 1981.

57. Ehrlich, M.G., et al.: Correlation between articular cartilage collagenase activity and osteoarthritis. Arthritis Rheum., *21*:761–766, 1981.

58. Pelletier, J.-P., et al.: Collagenase and collagenolytic activity in human osteoarthritic cartilage. Arthritis Rheum., *26*:63–68, 1983.

59. Pelletier, J.-P., et al.: Collagenolytic activity and collagen matrix breakdown of the articular cartilage in the Pond-Nuki dog model of osteoarthritis. Arthritis Rheum., *26*:866–874, 1983.

60. Stack, M.T., and Brandt, K.D.: Identification and characterization of articular cartilage hyaluronidase (HAase). (Abstract 70.) Arthritis Rheum., *25*(Suppl.):S100, 1982.

61. Wood, K.M., Wusterman, F.S., and Curtis, C.G.: The degradation of intravenously injected chondroitin-4 sulfate in the rat. Biochem. J., *134*:1009–1013, 1973.

62. Pelletier, J.-P. (Chairman): Symposium on osteoarthritis—proteases: Their involvement in osteoarthritis. J. Rheum., *14*(Suppl.):1–133, 1987.

63. Woessner, J.F., Jr., and Howell, D.S.: Hydrolytic enzymes in cartilage. *In* Studies in Joint Disease. Vol. 2. Edited by A. Maroudas and E.J. Holborow. Tunbridge Wells, England, Pitman Medical, 1983.

64. Poole, A.R., Hembry, R.M., and Dingle, J.T.: Cathepsin D in cartilage: The immunohistochemical demonstration of extracellular enzyme in normal and pathological conditions. J. Cell Sci., *14*:139–161, 1974.

65. Dingle, J.T., and Knight, G.: The role of the chondrocyte microenvironment in the degradation of cartilage matrix. *In* Degenerative Joints. Vol. 2. Edited by G. Verbruggen and E.M. Veys. Amsterdam, Elsevier Science Publishers, 1985.

66. Sapolsky, A.I., et al.: Metalloproteases of human articular cartilage that digest cartilage proteoglycan at neutral and acid pH. J. Clin. Invest., *58*:1030–1041, 1976.

67. Woessner, J.F., Jr., and Selzer, M.G.: Two latent metallopro

68. Azzo, W., and Woessner, J.F., Jr.: Purification and characterization of an acid metalloproteinase from human articular cartilage. J. Biol. Chem., *261*:5434–5441, 1986.

69. Sapolsky, A.I., et al.: Neutral proteinases from articular chondrocytes in culture: 2. Metal-dependent latent neutral proteoglycanase and inhibitory activity. Biochim. Biophys. Acta, *658*:138–147, 1981.

70. Malemud, C.J., et al.: Neutral proteinases from articular chondrocytes in culture. 1. A latent collagenase that degrades human cartilage type II collagen. Biochim. Biophys. Acta, *657*:517–529, 1981.

71. Sapolsky, A.I., and Howell, D.S.: Further characterization of a neutral metalloprotease isolated from human articular cartilage. Arthritis Rheum., *25*:981–988, 1982.

72. Roughley, P.J., Poole, A.R., Campbell, I.K., and Mort, J.S.: The proteolytic generation of hyaluronic acid-binding regions derived from the proteoglycans of human articular cartilage as a consequence of aging. Trans. Orthop. Res. Soc., *11*:209, 1986.

73. Harris, E.D., Jr., Welgus, H.G., and Krane, S.M.: Regulation of the mammalian collagenases. Coll. Rel. Res., *4*:493–512, 1984.

74. Vater, C.A., Nagase, H., and Harris, E.D., Jr.: Purification of an endogenous activator of procollagenase from rabbit synovial fibroblast culture medium. J. Biol. Chem., *258*:9374–9382, 1983.

75. Dean, D.D., et al.: Levels of metalloproteases and tissue inhibitor of metalloproteases in human osteoarthritic cartilage. J. Rheumatol., *14*:(Suppl.):43–44, 1987.

76. Morales, T.I., Kuettner, K.E., Howell, D.S., and Woessner, J.F., Jr.: Characterization of the metalloproteinase inhibitor produced by bovine articular chondrocytes in culture. Biochim. Biophys. Acta, *760*:221–229, 1983.

77. Doherty, A.J.P., et al.: Sequence of human tissue inhibitor of metalloproteinases and its identity to erythroid-potentiality factor activity. Nature, *318*:66–68, 1985.

78. Killackey, J.J., Roughley, P.J., and Mort, J.S.: Proteinase inhibitors of human articular cartilage. Coll. Rel. Res., *3*:419–430, 1983.

79. Ghosh, P., Andrews, J., Osborne, R., and Lesjak, M.: Variations with aging and degeneration of serine and cysteine proteinase inhibitors of human articular cartilage. Agents Actions, *18*(Suppl.):69, 1986.

80. Kuettner, K.E., Pauli, B.U., and Soble, L.: Morphological studies on the resistance of cartilage to invasion by osteosarcoma cells in vitro and in vivo. Cancer Res., *38*:277–287, 1978.

81. Greenwald, R.: Effects of oxygen-derived free radicals in connective tissue degradation: III. Studies on hyaluronic acid depolymerization in inflamed synovial fluids. Semin. Arthritis Rheum., *11*(Suppl. 1):97, 1981.

82. Bates, E.J., Lowther, D.A., and Handley, C.J.: Oxygen free radicals mediate an inhibition of proteoglycan synthesis in cultured articular cartilage. Ann. Rheum. Dis., *43*:442–446, 1984.

83. Carney, S.L., Billingham, M.E.J., Muir, H., and Sandy, D.: Demonstration of increased proteoglycan turnover in cartilage explants from dogs with experimental osteoarthritis. J. Orthop. Res., *2*:201–206, 1984.

84. Witter, J.P., Roughley, P.J., Caterson, B., and Poole, A.R.: The isolation and characterization of proteoglycan fragments derived from articular cartilage in human arthritic synovial fluid. Trans. Orthop. Res. Soc., *9*:313, 1984.

teases of human articular cartilage that digest proteoglycan. J. Biol. Chem., *259*:3633–3638, 1984.

85. Thonar, E.J.-M., et al.: Quantification of keratan sulfate in blood as a marker of cartilage catabolism. Arthritis Rheum., *28*:1367–1376, 1985.

86. Maroudas, A.: Balance between swelling and pressure in collagen tension in normal and degenerate cartilage. Nature, *260*:808–809, 1976.

87. Mankin, H.J., and Thrasher, A.Z: Water content and binding in normal and osteoarthritic human cartilage. J. Bone Joint Surg., *57A*:76–80, 1975.

88. Hess, E.V., and Herman, J.H.: Cartilage metabolism and antiinflammatory drugs. Am. J. Med., *81*:36–43, 1986.

89. Dayer, J.-M., Robinson, D.R., and Krane, S.M.: Prostaglandin production by rheumatoid synovial cells: Stimulation by factor from human mononuclear cells. J. Exp. Med., *145*:1399–1404, 1977.

90. Phadke, K.D., and Lawrence, M.N.: Synthesis of collagenase and neutral protease by articular chondrocytes: Stimulation by a macrophage-derived factor. Biochem. Biophys. Res. Commun., *85*:490–496, 1978.

91. Dingle, J.T.: The role of catabolin in arthritic damage. Semin. Arthritis Rheum., *11*:82–83, 1981.

92. Jasin, H.E., and Dingle, J.T.: Human mononuclear cell factors mediate cartilage matrix degradation through chondrocyte activation. J. Clin. Invest., *68*:571–581, 1981.

93. Gowan, M., et al.: Stimulation by human interleukin-1 of cartilage breakdown and production of collagenase and proteoglycanase by human chondrocytes but not by human osteoblasts in vitro. Biochem. Biophys. Acta, *797*:186–193, 1984.

94. Radcliffe, A.R., Tyler, J.A., and Hardingham, T.E.: Articular cartilage cultured with interleukin-1: Increased release of link protein, hyaluronate binding region and other proteoglycan fragments. Biochem. J., *238*:571–580, 1986.

95. Utsinger, P.D., and Fife, F.L.: Immunologic evidence for inflammation in osteoarthritis: High percentage of IA & T lymphocytes in the synovial fluid and synovium of patients with erosive osteoarthritis. Arthritis Rheum., *25*(Suppl.):S44, 1982.

96. Golds, E.E., and Poole, A.R.: Connective tissue antigens stimulate collagenase production in arthritic disease. Cell Immunol., *86*:190–205, 1984.

97. McCarty, D.J., and Cheung, H.S.: Prostaglandin (PG)E$_2$ generation by cultured canine synovial fibroblast exposed to microcrystals containing calcium. Ann. Rheum. Dis., *44*:316–320, 1985.

98. McCarty, D.J., et al.: Milwaukee shoulder: Association of microspheroids containing hydroxyapatite crystals, active collagenase and neutral protease with rotator cuff defects. Arthritis Rheum., *24*:464–491, 1981.

99. Dieppe, P., and Calvert, P.: Crystals and Joint Disease. New York, Chapman and Hall, 1983.

100. Moskowitz, R.M., et al.: Specific drug therapy of experimental osteoarthritis. Semin. Arthritis Rheum., *11*(Suppl. 1):127–129, 1981.

101. Gray, R.G., and Gottlieb, N.L.: Intra-articular corticosteroids: An update assessment. Clin. Orthop., *177*:235–263, 1983.

102. Fife, R.S., and Brandt, K.D.: Experimental modes of therapy in osteoarthritis. *In* Osteoarthritis: Diagnosis and Management. Edited by R.W. Moskowitz, D.S. Howell, V.C. Goldberg, and H.J. Mankin. Philadelphia, W.B. Saunders, 1984.

103. Brandt, K.D., and Palmoski, M.: Effects of nonsteroidal antiinflammatory drugs on proteoglycan metabolism in articular cartilage. Semin. Arthritis Rheum., *11*:(Suppl. 1):133–134, 1981.

104. Swann, D.A.: Macromolecules of synovial fluid. *In* The Joints and Synovial Fluid. Vol. 1. Edited by L. Sokoloff. New York, Academic Press, 1978.

105. Swann, D.A.: The lubricating activity of synovial fluid glycoproteins. Arthritis Rheum., *24*:22–30, 1981.

CLINICAL AND LABORATORY FINDINGS IN OSTEOARTHRITIS

102

ROLAND W. MOSKOWITZ

Osteoarthritis (OA) is a slowly evolving articular disease characterized by the gradual development of joint pain, stiffness, and limitation of motion. The terms *degenerative joint disease* or *osteoarthrosis* may be more precise because degeneration of cartilage is the most prominent pathologic change. Both experimental[1] and clinical[2] studies have shown mild to moderate synovitis, however. Some favor a particular form of nomenclature, but at present, the terms osteoarthritis, osteoarthrosis, and degenerative joint disease are used interchangeably. Although this disease is often benign, severe degenerative changes may cause serious disability. Newer concepts of pathogenesis suggest that osteoarthritis is not an inevitable consequence of aging itself, and raise the possibility of rational preventive and therapeutic methods in the future.

CLASSIFICATION

Classification of OA is difficult because of its varying forms of presentation. Increasing support exists for the concept that OA may represent a number of disease subsets leading to similar clinical and pathologic alterations, rather than being one specific disorder. The disease is classified as *primary* or idiopathic when it occurs in the absence of any known underlying predisposing factor. In contrast, *secondary* OA is that form of the disease following an identifiable underlying local or systemic pathogenetic factor. The distinctions on which this simple classification is based may be artificial, however. Studies on OA of the hip, for example, show that many cases of "primary" OA are actually secondary to anatomic abnormalities that result in articular incongruity and premature cartilage degeneration, such as congenital hip dysplasia and slipped capital femoral epiphysis of childhood.[3]

Classification criteria for various forms of OA are currently undergoing review by the American Rheumatism Association (ARA). Initial efforts have been directed at defining criteria for idiopathic OA of the knee[4] and determining their sensitivity and specificity based on clinical, clinical and laboratory, or clinical and radiographic parameters. Using clinical findings alone, the presence of knee pain with at least three of six variables, including age >50 years, joint stiffness <30 minutes, crepitus, bony tenderness, bony enlargement, and no palpable warmth provided 95% sensitivity and 69% specificity. Criteria were 92% sensitive and 75% specific when clinical and laboratory parameters were used. These parameters included knee pain and at least five of nine variables including those listed above as well as erythrocyte sedimentation rate <40 mm/hour, latex fixation test <1:40 titer, and minimal or absent inflammatory changes on synovial fluid analysis. The presence of osteophytes and knee pain, and at least one of three variables including age >50 years, joint stiffness <30 minutes, and crepitus provided 91% sensitivity and 86% specificity (Table 102–1). These classification criteria should not be used as diagnostic criteria; they have value in standardization of reporting series of cases, perform-

Table 102–1. Criteria for Classification of Idiopathic Osteoarthritis of the Knee

Clinical*	Clinical and Laboratory	Clinical and Radiographic
Knee pain plus at least 3 of 6: age >50 years stiffness <30 minutes crepitus bony tenderness bony enlargement no palpable warmth	Knee pain plus at least 5 of 9: age >50 years stiffness <30 minutes crepitus bony tenderness bony enlargement no palpable warmth ESR <40 mm/hr† RF <1:40 SF OA	Knee pain plus at least 1 of 3: age >50 years stiffness <30 minutes crepitus plus osteophytes
95% sensitive 69% specific	92% sensitive 75% specific	91% sensitive 86% specific

*Alternative for the clinical category would be 4 of 6, which is 84% sensitive and 89% specific.
†ESR = erythrocyte sedimentation rate (Westergren); RF = rheumatoid factor; SF OA = synovial fluid signs of OA (clear, viscous, or white blood cell count <2,000/mm³).
Modified with permission from Altman, R., et al. Development of criteria for the classification and reporting of osteoarthritis. Classification of osteoarthritis of the knee. Arthritis Rheum., 29:1047, 1986.

ing investigational studies, and improving consistency in communication.

The subcommittee of the ARA elected to design separate sets of criteria for use under different circumstances. For example, criteria not involving radiographs can be used in screening in an office practice. Clinical trials in which radiographs are routinely obtained and other parameters are frequently present allow use of criteria based on clinical examination, laboratory tests, and radiographs. Criteria based on clinical examination alone are useful for population surveys and other epidemiologic studies.

As usual, increased sensitivity was achieved at the sacrifice of specificity. For this reason, algorithms that allow the use of surrogate variables when the primary variables are not available were developed by recursive partitioning for each of the classification groups. The algorithms give high sensitivity and specificity, and cross-validated sensitivity and specificity rates for the classification tree were considerably higher than those obtained by traditional methods of analysis. The complexity of the algorithms, on the other hand, requires an understanding of, familiarization with, and training in the sophisticated methods used.

Various forms of the disease, such as primary generalized OA, erosive inflammatory OA, diffuse idiopathic skeletal hyperostosis (DISH), and chondromalacia patellae, have different clinical, pathologic, and radiologic findings and are generally considered distinct syndromes. Alternatively, because of fundamental ignorance in pathogenesis, these syndromes may merely reflect various clinical extremes of the disease. A working classification of OA based on known anatomic and etiologic mechanisms is presented in Table 102–2.

Table 102–2. Classification of Osteoarthritis

Primary (Idiopathic)
    Peripheral joints
    Spine
        Apophyseal joints
        Intervertebral joints
    Subsets
        Generalized osteoarthritis
        Erosive inflammatory osteoarthritis
        Diffuse idiopathic skeletal hyperostosis
        Chondromalacia patellae
Secondary
    Trauma
        Acute
        Chronic (occupational, sports)
    Underlying joint disorders
        Local (fracture, infection)
        Diffuse (rheumatoid arthritis)
    Systemic metabolic or endocrine disorders
        Ochronosis (alkaptonuria)
        Wilson's disease
        Hemochromatosis
        Kashin-Beck disease
        Acromegaly
        Hyperparathyroidism
    Crystal deposition disease
        Calcium pyrophosphate dihydrate (pseudogout)
        Basic calcium phosphate (hydroxyapatite-octacalcium phosphate-tricalcium phosphate)
        Monosodium urate monohydrate (gout)
    Neuropathic disorders (Charcot joints)
        Tabes dorsalis
        Diabetes mellitus
    Intra-articular corticosteroid overuse
    Miscellaneous
        Bone dysplasia (multiple epiphyseal dysplasia; achondroplasia)
        Frostbite

PRIMARY OSTEOARTHRITIS

Interpretation of data regarding the natural history of primary OA is complicated by the different case-finding techniques, whether clinical, radiologic, or pathologic, used in many of the reported studies. Moreover, studies focused on different joints cannot be compared, even when similar case-finding methods are used. Variations due to interobserver error may be significant, despite the use of essentially identical protocols. Nevertheless, sufficient data permit a reasonable approximation of the natural course of the disease.

EPIDEMIOLOGIC FEATURES

A comparison of epidemiologic surveys undertaken to characterize the prevalence and clinical characteristics of OA requires close attention to variations in analytic techniques and populations studied[5] (see Chapter 3). Such variations may have a major impact on the data obtained. Studies derived from autopsy analyses, for example, define earlier disease manifestation than clinical studies based on symptoms that develop later. In clinical surveys, disease definitions must be clear, and the use of prospective or retrospective techniques must be taken into account. Data obtained from roentgenographic studies depend on the number and location of joints studied.[6] Surveys of hospitalized patients, in contrast to those in the general population, are narrow in scope, but they may be useful in identifying certain disease subsets.

Prevalence

Autopsy studies show that degenerative joint changes begin in the second decade.[7] By age 40, 90% of all persons have such changes in their weight-bearing joints, even though clinical symptoms are generally absent. Roentgenographic manifestations of the disease are common in the third decade, and involvement increases progressively with age. In a survey of roentgenograms of the hands and feet, 40.5 million (37 of each 100) adult United States citizens living outside institutions had some evidence of OA.[8] The prevalence rate increased from 4 per 100 among persons 18 to 24 years of age to 85 per 100 at age 75 to 79 years, and 23% had moderate or severe disease. Under age 45, nearly all cases were mild. A roentgenographic survey of a larger number of joints showed OA in approximately 52% of an adult English population.[9] When minimal disease was excluded, the prevalence of OA was about 20%. In persons age

55 to 64 years, 85% of these studied had some degree of OA in one or more joints.

Signs and symptoms suggestive of OA of the knee were evaluated in 682 elderly people.[10] The frequency of signs and symptoms and their degree of severity remained constant in the seventh, eighth, and ninth decades, suggesting that OA of the knee was indeed common in the elderly but not inevitably progressive. In contrast to these observations, however, OA of the knee in 1581 subjects over age 63 (Framingham heart study cohort) increased progressively with age.[11] This difference might be related to the diagnostic use of roentgenographic, in addition to clinical, findings.

In all studies, the relation of OA to aging is striking. When individuals with severe grades of OA only are considered, the increase with age is exponential.[9] Several possible explanations have been advanced. Release of cartilage matrix molecules from their normally isolated locale relative to the vascular system may lead to a progressively enhanced autoimmune response. Alternatively, mild, early degeneration may be augmented by superimposed mechanical instability.

Sex, Race, and Heredity

Men and women were equally affected by OA in one study when all ages were considered.[8] Under age 45, prevalence was greater among men, whereas prevalence was greater in women than in men after age 55. Moderate and severe grades of OA were seen to a greater extent in women than in men. In radiographic studies in Great Britain on population samples from the age of 15 years,[12] the number of joints involved and severity were similar in men and women to age 54; thereafter, the disease was more severe and more generalized in women. The pattern of joint involvement was also similar in men and women under age 55, but in older persons, distal interphalangeal, proximal interphalangeal, and first carpometacarpal joints were more frequently affected in women, and hips were more commonly affected in men. The sex difference in patterns of joint involvement suggests that, although the same basic etiologic mechanisms may be involved in osteoarthritis in both sexes, the pattern in men may be affected by trauma, occupational stress, and mechanical factors. Clinical symptoms appear to be more common in women.

Differences in the prevalence of OA in black and white races have been noted, particularly when patterns of joint involvement are analyzed.[13,14] The differences can often be attributed to variations in occupation and life-style. Differences in certain predisposing genetic factors, such as congenital subluxation of the hip, may also play a role.

Southern Chinese,[15] South African blacks,[16] and

East Indians[17] have a lower incidence of OA of the hip than European or American whites. In the Chinese, the hip joint may be protected by the extreme range of motion required for frequent squatting. A decreased frequency of predisposing factors such as rheumatoid arthritis (RA), congenital dysplasia of the hip, and slipped capital femoral epiphysis, all believed to be uncommon in the Chinese, may also explain some of the differences.[15] In contrast, Japanese have a high incidence of secondary OA of the hip, related to antecedent congenital hip disease, especially dislocation or acetabular dysplasia.[18] Painful arthropathy of the hips described in the black population around Mseleni in southern Africa appears to be the result of two distinct abnormalities: protrusio acetabuli, affecting mainly women and increasing in frequency with age; and hip dysplasia, which does not increase in frequency with age.[19] Degenerative joint disease was *more* prevalent in American Indians than in the general population.[8]

Genetic factors in generalized OA have been evaluated in a series of studies in England.[12,20,21] Patients with generalized OA comprise two clinical groups, differentiated by involvement of the distal interphalangeal joints of the hands (Heberden's nodes). Patients with generalized disease and involvement of these joints were said to have "nodal" osteoarthritis. Involvement of proximal interphalangeal, first carpometacarpal, spinal apophyseal, hip, knee, first tarsometatarsal, and first metatarsophalangeal joints was frequent. *Nodal generalized OA* was more common in women and had an inheritance pattern similar to that described by Stecher and colleagues for Heberden's nodes alone.[22] This pattern is consistent with a single autosomal gene, dominant in females and recessive in males. Generalized OA in the absence of Heberden's nodes, "non-nodal OA," showed polygenic inheritance. Statistically significant associations with seronegative inflammatory polyarthritis,[12] hyperuricemia,[21] and hypertension[20] have been observed.

Climate

Geographic studies in Northern Europe and America suggest that OA is less frequent farther north.[13] The prevalence of OA may be lower in Alaskan Eskimos[23] and less prevalent in Finland than in the Netherlands.[24] Studies comparing populations in Jamaica and Great Britain, however, revealed an equal frequency in the two climates.[13] Factors such as race, culture, and environment complicate comparisons of climatic effects on disease prevalence. Symptoms may be less severe in a warmer climate, related perhaps to higher temperatures, greater amounts of sunshine, and lighter-weight clothes.

Obesity, Body Somatotype, and Bone Density

The role of *obesity* in the etiology of OA remains controversial. Some experimental[25] and clinical[26,27] studies suggest that obesity itself is not a factor in the induction or aggravation of degenerative joint disease; other studies have demonstrated an increased frequency of OA in the obese, particularly in weight-bearing joints.[28–30] A study based on data from the National Health and Nutrition Examination Survey (HANES) found that obesity was associated with OA of the knee, especially in women.[31] The suggested principal reason for the association was the obvious additional mechanical stress. Another study using HANES data found a strong association between knee OA and significant *past* or present obesity.[32]

Obese persons have an increased incidence of OA in nonweight-bearing joints, such as the sternoclavicular and distal interphalangeal joints.[29] It has been suggested that obesity in OA patients may be secondary to the relative inactivity brought on by joint pain and limitation of motion.[26]

In addition to the possible biomechanical effects of obesity in the origin of OA, a *metabolic* role for fat in disease pathogenesis has been suggested.[33] Studies in strains of mice that develop OA showed that diets enriched with lard, a saturated fat, increased the frequency and severity of the degenerative lesions. When unsaturated fat was fed to achieve the same body weight, however, no adverse effect was noted. Perhaps obesity in humans is related to OA not only through its biomechanical effects, but also as a result of still obscure metabolic changes in cartilage.

OA has been associated with specific somatotypes; its prevalence is greater in stout individuals than in thin ones.[34] Patients with OA of the hip or femoral neck fractures were compared; 94% of the former were endomorphic mesomorphs, whereas the majority of patients with fractures were ectomorphic.[35]

Bone density is associated with OA. In studies of the femoral head, a diminished bone mass was associated with femoral neck fracture; increased bone mass, on the other hand, showed a positive correlation with osteoarthritis.[36–38] Quantitative bone density by photon absorption study of the proximal phalanx of both hands was greater than normal in a group of 25 patients with degenerative arthritis of the hip or knee associated with calcium pyrophosphate dihydrate (CPPD) crystal deposition *and* in a group of 22 patients with similar degenerative changes not associated with crystal deposition.[39] Reduction in bone mass increases the shock-absorbing capacity of subchondral bone and protects articular cartilage against stress. Conversely, stiffer, denser subchondral bone increases the mechanical forces acting through cartilage, with a resultant predisposition to degenerative change, according to the hypothesis formulated by Radin.[39a]

Increased ligamentous laxity correlates positively with joint degeneration. Patients with joint hypermobility had an increased prevalence of generalized OA compared to age- and sex-matched control subjects.[40] Conversely, when patients with OA were evaluated, the prevalence of generalized joint hypermobility was higher than in matched control subjects. Synovial effusions and chondrocalcinosis were common in patients with hypermobility syndrome.

Occupation and Sports

Stress related to occupation or sports activities has been implicated in the induction of OA. In one study, OA of the hips, knees, and shoulders was more common in miners than in porters or clerks.[41] Dock workers showed a higher prevalence of OA of the fingers, elbows, and knees than age-matched civil servants.[42] The joints in the right hand are more commonly involved than those in the left hand. Repetitive manual work performed by women in a weaving factory confirmed that the right hand was more severely involved; this study also noted that the pattern of hand and finger lesions could be directly related to the type of work done by each group, and the joints used most repetitively were also the most involved by disease.[43] Prolonged or repeated, heavy overuse of joints has been related to an increased frequency of OA in bus drivers[21] and foundry workers.[44]

Some studies, however, have failed to show a consistent relationship between OA and the trauma related to overuse. Pneumatic-hammer drillers had no increased risk of elbow disease. The prevalence of OA in shipyard laborers, all of whom had been working for decades in heavy industry, was compared to that in white-collar workers and in a random population sample.[45] All groups were males of the same age. OA of the hip occurred in about 3% of both the laborers and their white-collar controls.

Involvement of millions of individuals in aerobic exercise of various sorts, especially running, has intensified interest in the possible relationships of joint overuse to OA. An older study showed no increase in OA of the hip in Finnish running champions as compared to age- and sex-matched controls.[46] A later study comparing knee roentgenograms of long-distance runners age 50 to 72 years to those of community controls revealed a statistically significant increase in knee sclerosis in women but not in men and no differences in joint-space narrowing, crepitus,

joint stability, or symptomatic OA.[97] A study of men who ran many miles per week over many years showed no evidence of premature OA in the lower extremities.[48] Unfortunately, these studies represent *retrospective* investigations of the prevalence of OA in self-selected individuals with a demonstrated ability to maintain active running. Selection bias cannot be excluded in any of these studies; that is, individuals with a predisposition to OA (because of obesity, habitus, or metabolic or structural connective tissue abnormalities) may not have chosen this particular form of exercise. In addition, individuals who developed OA early may have discontinued running. Further longitudinal studies of a prospective nature should provide more definitive information regarding the relationship, if any, of increased susceptibility to OA and running or other exercise programs.

A number of studies have suggested that osteoarthritis is common in soccer players.[49,50] Many of these studies, however, used osteophytes alone as an indication of OA. In summary, *there is no evidence suggesting that exercise is deleterious to normal joints when the criterion used is the loss of roentgenographic joint space.*[46]

SYMPTOMS AND SIGNS

The symptoms of OA are localized to the affected joints (Table 102–3). Involvement of a number of joints may suggest a systemic form of arthritis. Frequently, little or no correlation exists between the joint symptoms and the extent or degree of pathologic or radiologic change. Only about 30% of persons with roentgenographic evidence of OA complained of pain at the relevant sites.[51] Except for lumbar apophyseal joints, persons with radiographic OA were predisposed to develop related symptoms.[9] Similarly, a positive correlation between clinical symptoms and roentgenographic evidence of OA of the knee was noted.[52] Some of the apparent disparity between symptoms and radiologic abnormalities may relate to the roentgenologic definition of OA. For example, the use of osteophytes alone as a diagnostic feature has been questioned. Long-term radiographic studies of the hip and knee suggest that the presence of osteophytes does not imply later development of other structural changes of OA, such as joint-space narrowing, subchondral bone cysts, and eburnation.[53] Correlation of symptoms with these more definitive structural abnormalities might well provide evidence of a positive interrelationship.

The cardinal symptom of OA is pain, which at first occurs after joint use and is relieved by rest. The pain

Table 102–3. Clinical Profiles of Osteoarthritis

Factor	Characteristics and Occurrence
Age	Usually advanced; symptoms uncommon before age 40, unless due to secondary cause
Joint involvement	Commonly, distal interphalangeal, proximal interphalangeal, first carpometacarpal, hip, knee, first metatarsophalangeal joints and lower lumbar and cervical vertebrae Rarely, metacarpophalangeal, wrist, elbow, or shoulder joints, except after trauma
Joint effusion	Little or none
Onset	Usually insidious
Systemic manifestations	Rare
True bony ankylosis	Uncommon
Symptoms	Pain on motion (early); pain at rest (later); pain aggravated by prolonged activity, relieved by rest; localized stiffness of short duration ("gelling") relieved by exercise; possibly painful muscle spasm; limitation of motion; "flares" associated with crystal-induced synovitis
Signs	Localized tenderness; crepitus and crackling on motion; mild joint enlargement with firm consistency from proliferation of bone and cartilage; synovitis (less common), gross deformity (later)

is usually aching in character and is poorly localized. As the disease progresses, pain may occur with minimal motion or even at rest. In advanced cases, pain may awaken the patient from sleep because of the loss of protective muscular joint splinting, which during the waking hours limits painful motion. Because cartilage has no nerve supply and is insensitive to pain, the pain in OA must arise from noncartilaginous intraarticular and periarticular structures. The pain is usually multifactorial and may result from elevation of the periosteum accompanying marginal body proliferation, pressure on exposed subchondral bone, venous engorgement with intramedullary hypertension, trabecular microfractures, involvement of intraarticular ligaments, capsular distension, and pinching or abrasion of synovial villi. Additional contributory factors may be synovitis and capsulitis. Although prostaglandins released from synovial tissues and chondrocytes may theoretically contribute to pain response, a parallel between the inflammatory response and joint fluid prostaglandin concentrations has not been described.[54] Periarticular tissues, such as tendons and fascia, are supplied with sensory nerves and are an important source of pain. Muscle spasms around the joint or pressure on contiguous nerves may be more painful than the pain of articular origin. Frequently, as with other types of joint disease, the pain is intensified just before weather changes.

OA is sometimes associated with acute or subacute inflammation. This response is most common in erosive (inflammatory) osteoarthritis of the hands, but it may occur in other peripheral joints. When seen in peripheral joints other than the hands, such inflammatory "acute flares" have been attributed to various degrees of trauma or to crystal-induced synovitis in response to calcium pyrophosphate or other crystals.[55]

Stiffness on awakening in the morning and after periods of inactivity during the day is a common complaint. Such stiffness is of short duration, rarely lasting for more than 15 minutes. *Articular gelling*, a transient stiffness lasting only for several flexion-extension cycles, is extremely common, especially in the lower extremity joints of elderly patients. This occurs often in the absence of other symptoms of OA and follows prolonged inactivity. The initial few steps of a grandparent going to the television set to change the channel is a familiar example. The physiologic basis for gelling is poorly understood. Gelling needs to be distinguished from the more prolonged stiffness associated with inflammation (see Chapter 4). Limitation of motion develops as the disease progresses, owing to joint-surface incongruity, muscle spasm and contracture, capsular contracture, and mechanical block from osteophytes or loose bodies. In weight-bearing joints, abrupt *giving way* may occur. Objectively, joints may show *localized tenderness*, especially if synovitis is present. *Pain on passive motion* may be a prominent finding even without local tenderness. *Crepitus*, a crackling or grating sound as the joint is moved, may result from cartilage loss and joint-surface irregularity. Enlargement of the joint may be caused by secondary synovitis, an increase in synovial fluid, or marginal proliferative changes in cartilage or bone (osteophytes). Osteophytes can be readily palpated along the margins of the affected joint. Late stages of the disease are associated with gross deformity and subluxation due to cartilage loss, collapse of subchondral bone, formation of bone cysts, and gross bony overgrowth. Although these symptoms and signs are common to OA in general, the clinical picture and course depend on the particular joint involvement.

SPECIFIC JOINT INVOLVEMENT

Heberden's Nodes

One of the most common manifestations of primary OA, *Heberden's nodes*[56] (Figs. 102–1, 102–2), represent cartilaginous and bony enlargement of the dorsolateral and dorsomedial aspects of the distal interphalangeal joints of the fingers, often associated with flexion and lateral deviation of the distal phalanx. Similar nodes may be seen in the proximal interphalangeal joints, where they are called *Bouchard's nodes* (Fig. 101–3). Heberden's nodes may be single, but they usually are multiple. They begin most often after age 45 years, but can begin in the 3rd decade of life. Women are affected much more frequently than men, at a ratio of approximately 10 to 1.[57] Heredity plays a large part in the origin of these lesions, particularly in the female side of the family, in mothers, daughters, and sisters.[58] Heberden's nodes were twice as common in mothers and three times as common in sisters of affected women than in the general population.[22] Stecher postulated a single autosomal gene, sex-influenced, dominant in females and recessive in males, with complete penetrance by age 70, because all who have this gene develop the lesions. Although idiopathic Heberden's nodes undoubtedly have a genetic origin, the exact mode of transmission remains open to question because several genetic patterns fit the available data.

Clinically, Heberden's nodes may develop gradually with little or no pain and may progress essentially unnoticed for months or years. In other cases, they appear rapidly with redness, swelling, tenderness, and aching, particularly after use. Afflicted individ-

uals may complain of paresthesias and loss of dexterity. A number of joints may be involved almost simultaneously, or one or two joints may be involved for a long time before others develop similar changes. The swollen joints may feel either soft and fluctuant or hard. Small, gelatinous cysts may appear, generally on the dorsal aspects of the joint or just proximal to it. These cysts, which are often attached to tendon sheaths and resemble ganglia, may recede spontaneously or may persist indefinitely. At times, they precede the appearance of Heberden's nodes themselves. The cysts' cause is uncertain. Studies have demonstrated communication of the cysts with the distal interphalangeal joint space.[59] This communication may later be pinched off, but at some stage in development the cysts are in direct communication with the joint space. As stated, the *proximal interphalangeal joints* of the fingers may also be involved, usually after several distal joints are affected. Horizontal deviation of the distal and proximal interphalangeal joints may lead to a snake-like configuration of the fingers. Metacarpophalangeal joint involvement is rare; when it does occur, it involves the joints of the second and third fingers.

Carpometacarpal and Trapezioscaphoid Joints. Degenerative changes involving the first carpometacarpal joint are often present. Pain and localized tenderness may suggest a stenosing tenosynovitis. The patient often has a tender prominence at the base of the first metacarpal bone, and the joint in this area may have a squared appearance (shelf sign) (Fig. 102–4). Motion is often limited and painful. Radiographic examination may reveal subluxation of the base of the first metacarpal bone in addition to joint-space narrowing and osteophyte formation.

Osteoarthritic changes in the *trapezioscaphoid joint* of the wrist are common.[60] Such changes may occur in association with OA of the first carpometacarpal and distal interphalangeal joints, or they may be an isolated finding. Symptoms and signs include pain in the wrist and thumb base, radial and volar swelling, and tenderness over the scaphoid bone.

Metatarsophalangeal Joints. One of the most common sites of primary OA is the first metatarsophalangeal joint of the foot; OA at the other metatarsophalangeal joints occurs to a lesser degree. The onset is usually insidious, with gradual progression of swelling and pain. Symptoms may be aggravated by wearing tight shoes. A sudden increase in swelling and pain may accompany inflammation of the bursa at the medial aspect of the joint (bunion). The irregular contour of the involved joint can be felt. Foot symptoms may also result from OA of the subtalar and other tarsal joints. Pain of subtalar origin is ag-

FIG. 102–1. Typical Heberden's nodes, the cardinal sign of primary OA. Note their characteristic position at the distal interphalangeal joints. The proximal interphalangeal joints may be involved later.

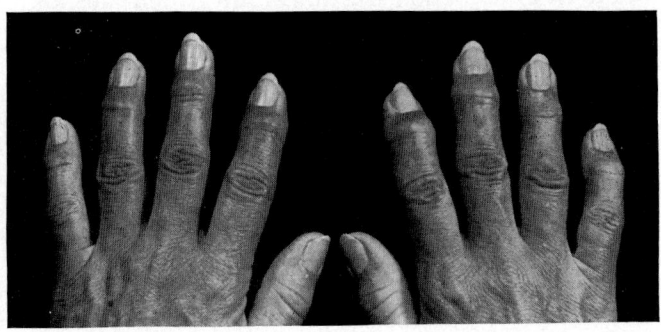

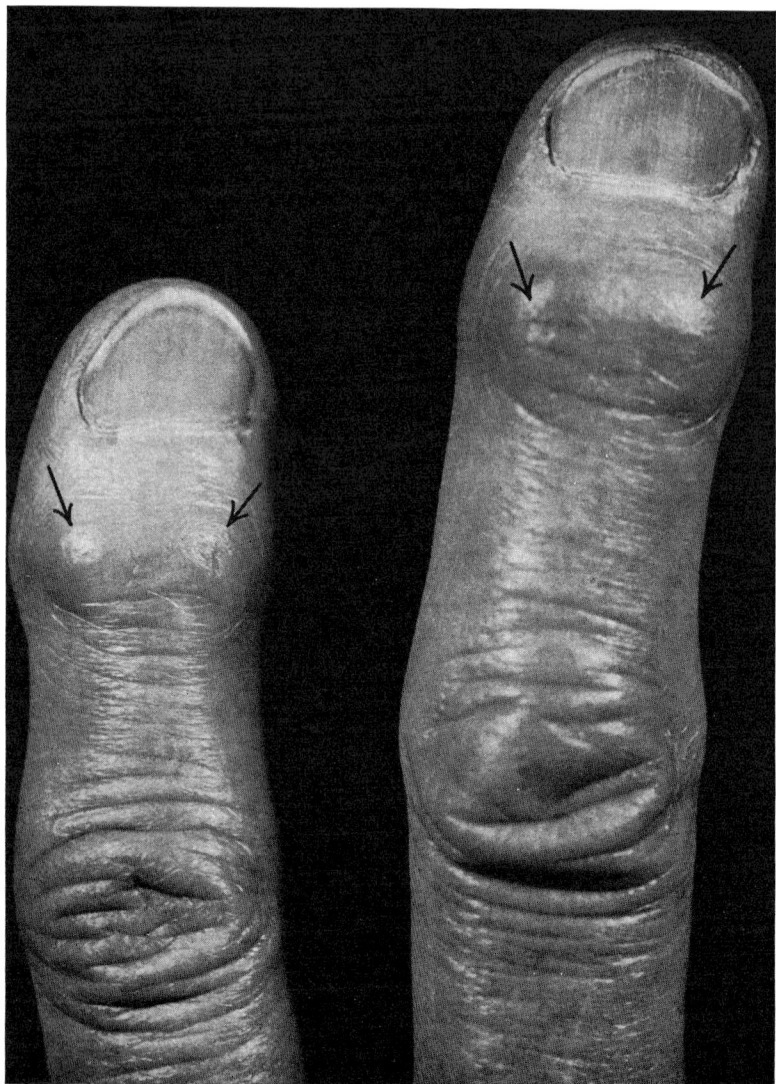

FIG. 102-2. Close-up view of Heberden's nodes (arrows) affecting the index and middle fingers.

gravated by inversion and eversion of the foot, and symptoms may make walking difficult.

Acromioclavicular Joint. OA of the acromioclavicular joint is common and frequently overlooked as a cause of shoulder pain and disability. Symptoms are usually poorly localized to the joint, and shoulder motion is nearly normal, although painful. Tenderness localized to the joint is the key finding. Roentgenographic changes of degeneration are often minimal. OA of the *manubriosternal joint* is rare, but it may result in chest pain and tenderness.

Temporomandibular Joints. OA produces symptoms of crepitus, stiffness, and pain in chewing (see Chapter 91). Similar symptoms may be caused by disturbances in temporomandibular joint dynamics (temporomandibular dysfunction syndrome), rather than by structural degenerative change. The patient may complain of joint noise and pain, masticatory muscle tenderness, limited motion, and deviation of the jaw to the affected side. The distinction between

OA and other causes of jaw pain are discussed in detail in Chapter 91.

Knee. The knee joint is frequently affected by primary OA, with involvement of one or more of its three compartments (medial femorotibial, lateral femorotibial, and patellofemoral) (Fig. 102–5). Symptoms consist of pain on motion, relieved by rest; stiffness, particularly after sitting or rising in the morning; and crepitus on motion. Little objective change might be found on examination. At times, the patient has localized tenderness over various aspects of the joint and pain on passive motion. Marginal osteophytes may be seen and felt. These are often more prominent on physical examination than they are on roentgenography. Mild synovitis and joint effusion may be present. Crepitus can often be detected when the examiner's hand is held over the patella as the knee is flexed. Pain may be elicited by the examiner, by holding the patella tight against the femur with the quadriceps relaxed and then requesting that the patient

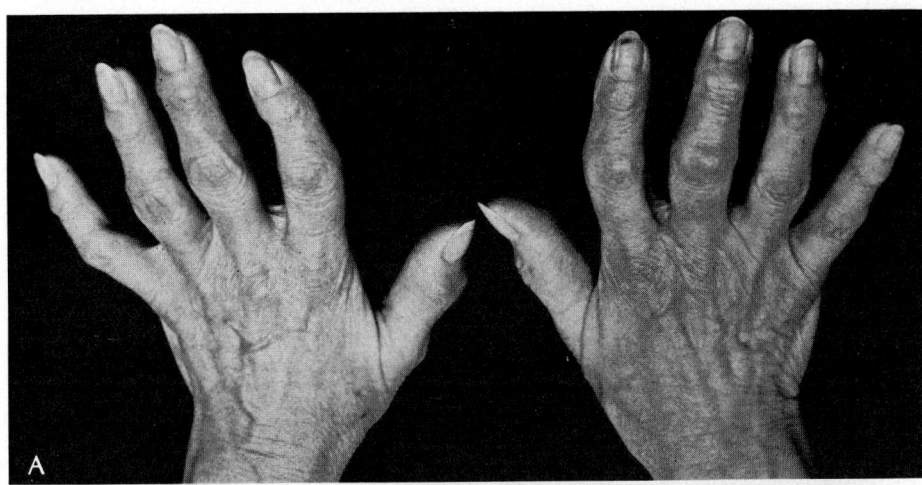

FIG. 102–3. *A*, Primary OA of the hands with marked proximal interphalangeal joint involvement (Bouchard's nodes), as well as distal interphalangeal joint involvement (Heberden's nodes). *B*, Roentgenographic appearance of the same hands.

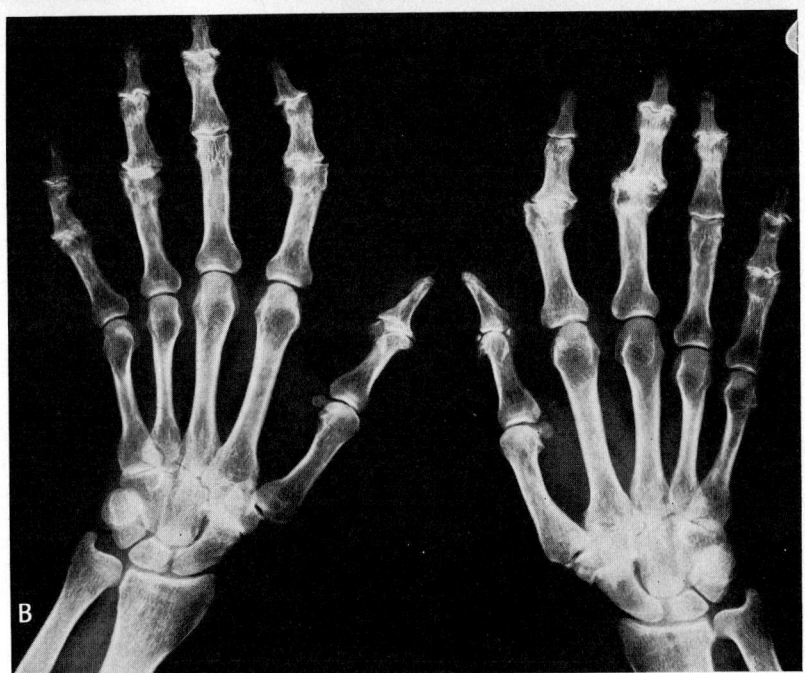

FIG. 102–4. Severe osteoarthritis of the first carpometacarpal joint leads to a prominent squaring (shelf sign) at the base of the thumb (arrow). Heberden's nodes are also seen.

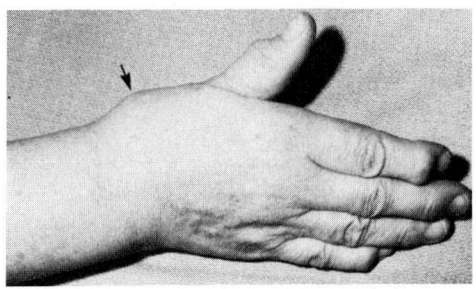

contract this muscle. Limitation of joint motion, usually extension, on both active or passive motion may be noted. Muscle atrophy about the knee may occur rapidly, especially with disuse. Disproportionate degenerative changes localized to the medial or lateral compartment of the knee may lead to secondary genu varus or, much less commonly, to genu valgus with joint instability and subluxation. Instability is further aggravated by laxity of the collateral ligaments. Isolated patellofemoral compartment or tricompartmental involvement should alert the clinician to underlying calcium pyrophosphate dihydrate (CPPD) crystal deposition. Joint fluid basic calcium phosphate (BCP) crystals were associated with lateral tibiofemoral disease in patients with concomitant (Milwaukee) shoulder joint disease.[60a] Ike et al. found erosions of the articular cartilage of the lateral compartment

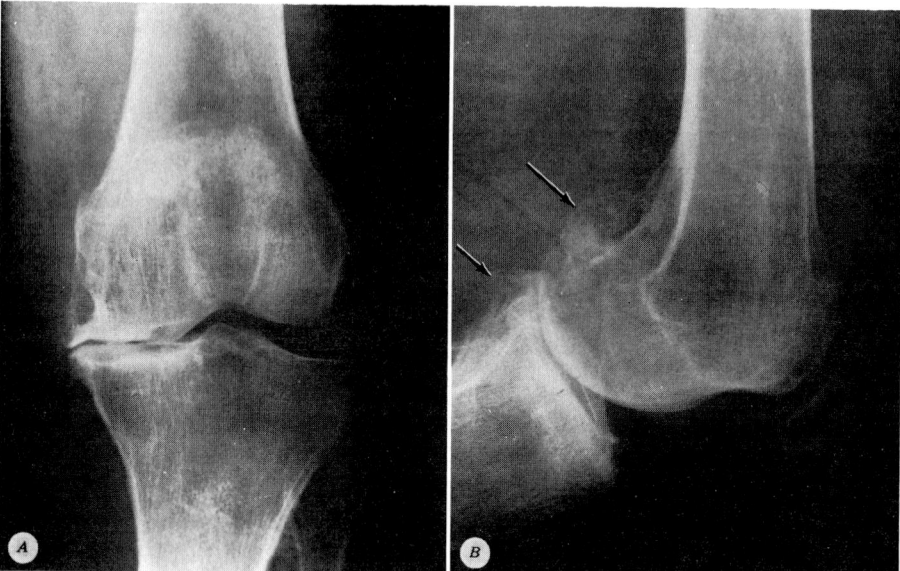

FIG. 102–5. *A*, OA of the knee; medial joint-space narrowing is prominent and is associated with subchondral bony sclerosis (eburnation) and osteophyte formation. *B*, Lateral view of the same knee; large osteophytes can be seen at the posterior aspects of the femur and tibia (arrows).

arthroscopically in all patients with lateral tibiofemoral joint-space narrowing by roentgenographic examination, and all had CPPD deposits.[60b] They also found medial meniscal degeneration and cartilage erosions in all patients with medial tibiofemoral compartment narrowing.

Hip. OA of the hip, also known as malum coxae senilis or morbus coxae senilis, may be disabling (Fig. 102–6). Symptoms usually first appear in older individuals. This condition occurs more frequently in men than in women and may be unilateral or bilateral. In a study of the natural history of hip OA, Evarts noted that over 8 years, 10% of patients with unilateral hip degeneration developed bilateral disease.[61]

Data on the frequency of right and left hip involvement in unilateral disease are conflicting. One study

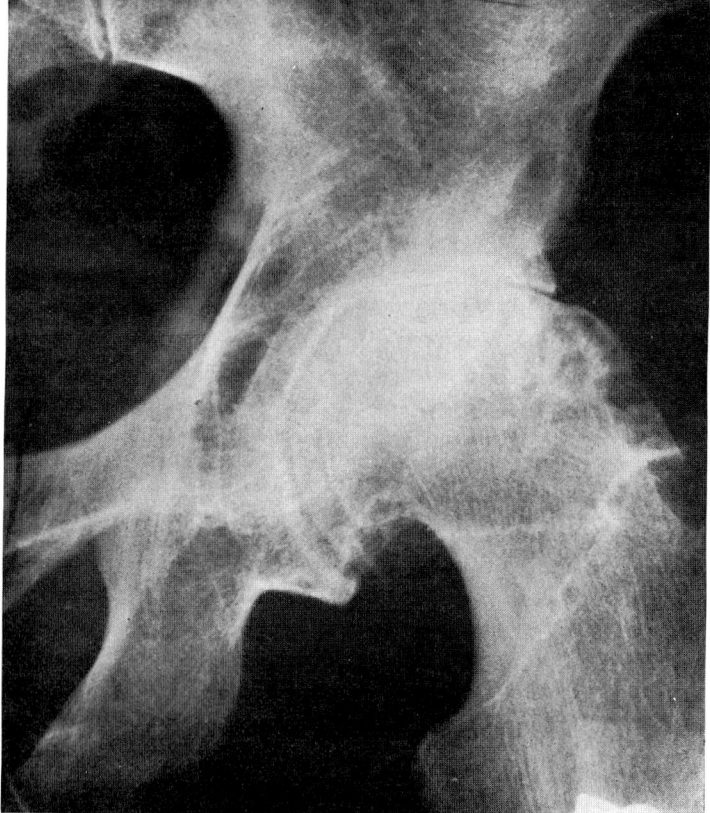

FIG. 102–6. OA of the hip. Note the almost complete loss of articular cartilage, flattening of the femoral head, and small cystic areas in the head and neck of the femur. Subchondral bone is sclerotic.

of 54 patients with idiopathic OA of the hip noted that the two sides were affected with equal frequency when disease was unilateral.[62] Another study of 175 patients found that 13% of men and 29% of women had unilateral disease.[63] The latter patients had a significant predilection for a particular side; 20 right and 10 left hips were involved, a 2:1 ratio. In those with the onset of symptoms after age 60, the ratio of right to left hip involvement was even more marked, 7:1.

The main symptom of OA of the hip is insidious pain followed by a characteristic limp *(antalgic gait)*. Pain in the "hip" may often not originate there, and pain actually arising in the hip joint may be referred to other areas. True hip pain is usually felt on its outer aspect, the groin, or along the inner aspect of the thigh. It may be referred to the buttocks or sciatic region and is often referred down the obturator nerve to the knee. Occasionally, most of the pain is in the knee, and its true origin is overlooked. The degree of pain varies widely and does not always correlate with the extent of cartilaginous and osseous changes. *Trochanteric bursitis,* caused by inflammation of the bursa over the greater trochanter, produces pain and tenderness at the lateral aspect of the hip; symptoms and physical findings may simulate those seen in patients with OA of the hip. Pain is exaggerated by weight bearing, and a mild limp is common, however, *hip motion is normal, in contrast to the invariable limitation of motion seen in OA of the hip joint.* Localized tenderness over the bursa is characteristic. Rapid relief of symptoms following bursal injection with local corticosteroids and procaine is diagnostically helpful.

Stiffness is common and increases after inactivity. Examination reveals varying degrees of limited motion. The leg is often held in external rotation with the hip flexed and adducted. *Severe backache* may result from the compensatory lordosis accompanying flexion contracture. Functional shortening of the extremity may occur. The gait is frequently awkward with shuffling or waddling. Sitting is difficult, as is rising from this position, owing to limitation of motion.

Spine. (See Chapters 90, 92, and 93.) OA of the spinal joints is common (Fig. 102–7). It often results from degenerative changes in the intervertebral fibrocartilaginous discs, from damage to vertebral bodies, or from degeneration in the posterior apophyseal articulations themselves. Disc narrowing may cause subluxation of the posterior apophyseal joints (see Chapter 90). Lipping or spur formation (osteophytosis) on the vertebral bodies is a prominent finding (Fig. 102–8). Anterior spurs are most prevalent. Although usually asymptomatic, large anterior osteophytes in the cervical spine may give rise to symptoms of dysphagia.[64] Respiratory symptoms such as hoarse-

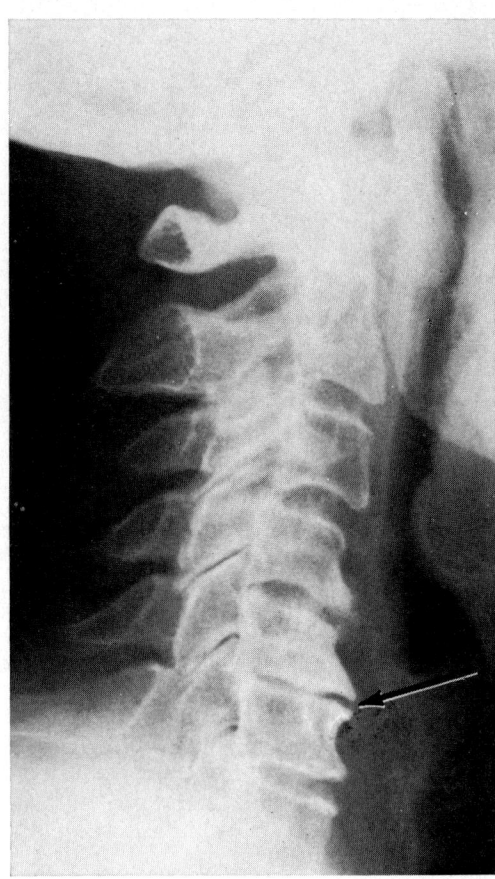

FIG. 102–7. Osteoarthritic changes in the lower cervical spine. Spur formation is prominent. Note the marked narrowing of the intervertebral disc between C5 and C6 vertebrae (arrow) and subluxation at C3-C4.

ness, coughing, and aspiration may be noted. Joint-space narrowing, bony sclerosis, and spur formation are often seen in apophyseal joints. Some authors make a distinction between degenerative changes involving the discs and vertebral bodies, for which they use the term *spondylosis,* and degenerative changes of the apophyseal joints, which are classified as true OA, because radiologic abnormalities more closely resemble those seen in other diarthrodial joints.

Degenerative changes of all types are most frequent in the areas of the lordotic and kyphotic apices, C5, T8, and L3 to L4, and correlate in general with the areas of maximal spine motion. In some older individuals, however, osteophytes may extend along the entire length of the spine, with prominent involvement of the thoracic region (Fig. 102–9). These osteophytes may be striking, and coalescence with fusion may occur (Fig. 102–10). Forestier et al. have suggested the name *ankylosing hyperostosis* for these severe cases, which may be associated with moderate-

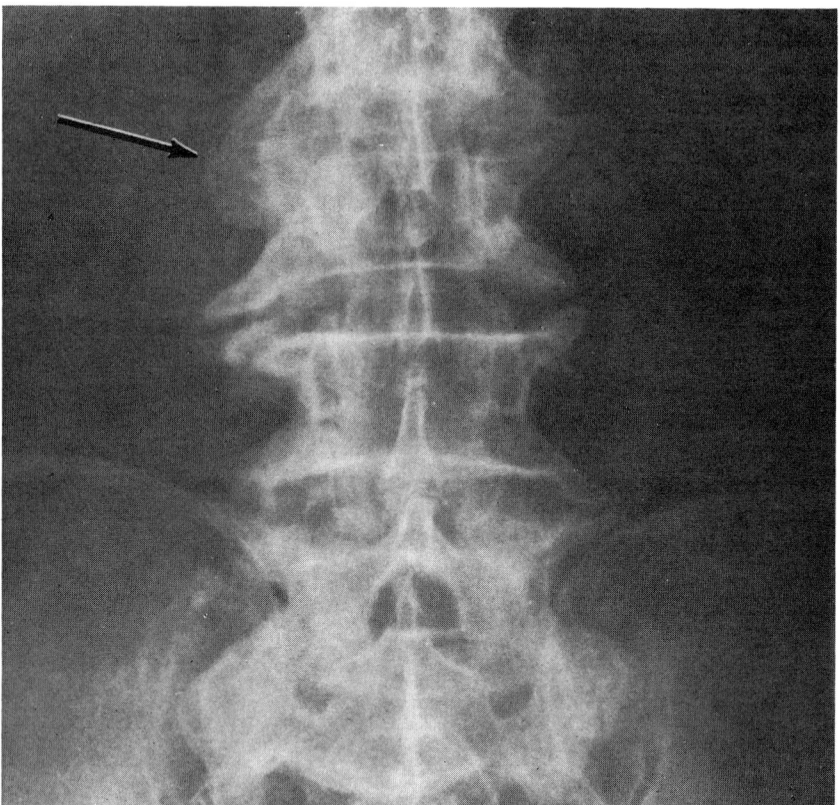

FIG. 102–8. OA of the lumbar spine. Note the marked osteophyte formation with bridging of spurs between L2 and L3 on the right (arrow).

to-severe spinal limitation.[65] The frequent extraspinal manifestations of "Forestier's disease" have led to the term *diffuse idiopathic skeletal hyperostosis*,[66,67] discussed later in this chapter.

Symptoms of spinal OA include localized pain and stiffness and radicular pain. Localized pain has been assumed to originate in paraspinal ligaments, joint capsules, and periosteum. Such changes may explain spontaneous fluctuations of symptoms in the presence of persistent or progressive cartilage degeneration and spur formation. Spasm of paraspinal muscles is common and may be a major cause of pain. Radicular pain may be due to compression of nerve roots, or it may represent pain referred along dermatomes related to the primary local lesion.

Nerve root compression causing neuropathy is common. This disorder may result from impingement on the nerve root by spurs that compromise the foraminal space (Fig. 102–11), by lateral prolapse of a degenerated disc, or by foraminal narrowing from apophyseal joint subluxation. Pressure on nerve roots may cause radicular pain, paresthesias, and reflex and motor changes in the distribution of the involved root. Neurologic complications of this type occur most frequently in the neck because of its small spinal canal and intervertebral foramina, but they can occur in other areas of the spine. Nerve root compression in

the dorsal spine may result in radicular pain radiating around the chest wall in a girdle distribution. This must be differentiated from symptoms caused by other disorders. Involvement of nerve roots in the lumbosacral area is associated with low back pain and neurologic signs and symptoms, which frequently allow localization of specific nerve root compression. Involvement of the L3 or L4 nerve roots is associated with a diminished or absent patellar reflex; an absent ankle jerk indicates involvement of the S1 nerve root. Sensory loss over the anteromedial aspect of the leg is consistent with L4 nerve root compression. A lesion at L5 causes sensory changes at the anterolateral aspect of the leg and the medial aspect of the foot and weakness of dorsiflexion of the foot and great toe. S1 nerve root compression results in sensory changes at the posterolateral aspect of the calf and the lateral foot. Gastrocnemius muscle weakness may be evident.

Further neurologic symptoms may be associated with cervical OA if large posterior spurs or protruded discs compress the spinal cord. In these cases, upper-motor-neuron and other long-tract signs may be observed. Compression of the anterior spinal artery may produce a central cord syndrome. The blood supply to the brain may be compromised if large spurs compress the vertebral arteries. The spectrum of clinical

FIG. 102–9. OA of the thoracic spine. Note the pronounced exostoses at the anterior vertebral margins and the narrowed intervertebral disc spaces.

FIG. 102–10. Florid hyperostosis of the spine in a patient with Forestier's disease (diffuse idiopathic skeletal hyperostosis). A flowing mantle of ossification from ligamentous calcification and coalescence of osteophytes is seen at the anterior aspect of the spine. (Courtesy of Dr. Donald Resnick.)

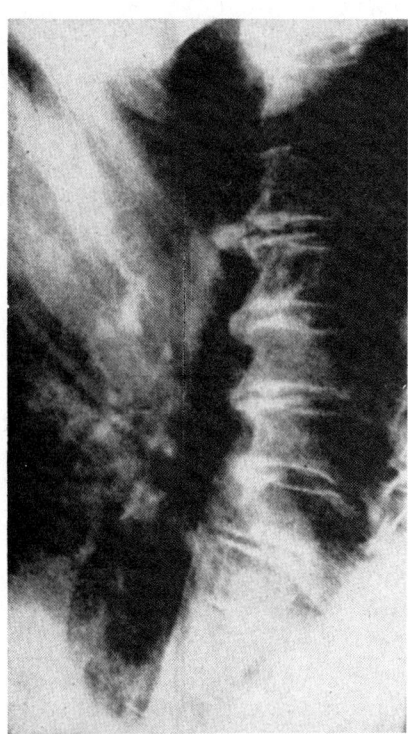

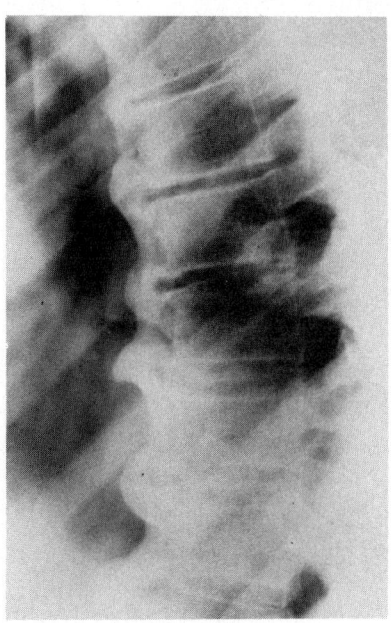

signs and symptoms is similar to that in basilar artery insufficiency. Exacerbations are often associated with postural neck changes from compression of vertebral arteries by osteophytes. Angiographic studies of carotid and vertebral arteries are diagnostically helpful.

OA of the atlantoaxial joint has been described in 31 patients.[68] Radiologic signs consisted of joint-space narrowing, marginal cortical thickening, and osteophyte formation. Involvement of the lateral atlantoaxial joint, the articulation of the atlas with the odontoid, or mixed involvement was found. Patients complained of occipital pain, stiffness of the shoulder, and paresthesias of the fingers. Conservative treatment provided satisfactory relief of symptoms, except in one patient who required a transoral atlantoaxial fusion.

Spinal cord lesions as a result of OA of the dorsal spine are rare. Spinal cord compression is not seen in patients with lumbosacral lesions because the spinal cord ends at the level of L1, but *cauda equina syndrome* with sphincter dysfunction may develop.

Spinal stenosis (Chapter 93) may produce symptoms in the lower back and the lower extremities. Pain may be constant or intermittent. It is often worsened by exercise, simulating intermittent claudication. Hy-

perextension of the spine often exacerbates symptoms; relief is noted with flexion. The patient may stand with knees, hips, and lumbar spine flexed (simian stance). Sensory changes may be present, and motor power in the legs may be diminished. Stenosis is usually caused by combined anatomic abnormalities because congenital narrowing alone is generally asymptomatic.[69] Commonly associated causes include degenerative spurs, disc herniation, ligamentous hypertrophy, and spondylolisthesis. Trauma, postoperative fibrosis, Paget's disease, and fluorosis are less commonly associated.

Radiological evidence of degenerative disease in the spine may be extensive but may still bear little relation to the patient's symptoms. On the other hand, severe symptoms may develop with minor spur formation if the spur is located in a critical area. Roentgenographic changes of marginal lipping, sclerosis of the articular margins, and narrowing have been found in sacroiliac joints with increasing age, but it is unlikely that such changes lead to symptoms.

LABORATORY FINDINGS

No specific diagnostic laboratory abnormalities exist in primary OA (Table 102–4). The erythrocyte sed-

FIG. 102–11. OA of cervical spine, oblique radiologic view. The foraminal space between C3 and C4 (arrow) is compromised by marked posterior spur formation.

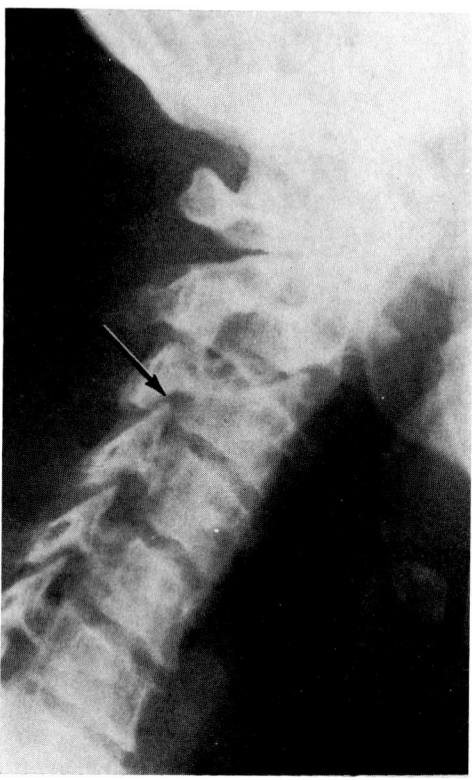

imentation rate, routine blood counts, urinalyses, and blood chemical determinations are normal in patients with primary disease but are important in excluding other forms of arthritis considered in the differential diagnosis, and they may identify systemic metabolic disorders associated with secondary OA. For example, patients with associated CPPD crystal deposition disease may have evidence of underlying primary hyperparathyroidism with elevation of serum calcium and an increase in serum parathyroid hormone level. Patients with Paget's disease exhibit elevated serum alkaline phosphatase levels and increased urinary hydroxyproline excretion. In patients with joint disease associated with ochronosis, the presence of homogentisic acid metabolites in the urine darkens the urine on standing or causes a false positive Benedict's test result for glycosuria.

Synovial fluid in primary OA is "noninflammatory" with no abnormalities other than a slight increase in white cells. Viscosity is good, and the mucin clot formed after addition of glacial acetic acid is normal. Synovial fluid fibrils, morphologically indistinguishable from sloughed collagen fibers, are often seen. The collagen fibers seen in synovial fluid in osteoar-

thritis appear to be type II, derived from articular hyaline cartilage.[70] CPPD or basic calcium phosphate crystals may be present. Cholesterol crystals have been identified by light microscopy in synovial fluids of patients with recurrent OA knee effusions.[71,72] Although evidence of altered cellular and humoral immune mechanisms has been described,[73,74] its significance remains to be determined. Immune complexes have been detected in hyaline articular cartilage of OA joints, but not in synovial fluid.[75]

Histologic examination of the synovium in primary OA reveals nonspecific changes of chronic mild inflammation, particularly in more advanced disease.

SCINTIGRAPHY

Bone and joint scintigraphy using technetium 99m (^{99m}Tc) as the pertechnetate has been of limited diagnostic value,[76] but studies using 4-hour ^{99m}Tc coupled with bone-seeking diphosphonates correlated with radiographic abnormalities in OA of hand joints.[77,78] Abnormalities predicted the development of radiographic signs, and joints abnormal on scintigraphy showed the greatest progression in followup studies. Some joints were abnormal on either roentgenogram or scan alone, and others showed a marked disparity in the degree of abnormality on radiographic evaluation compared with isotopic evaluation. These discrepancies suggested that scintigraphy offered a different way of assessing OA changes, perhaps useful in evaluating response to therapeutic strategies. Expanded studies may further define its role in the evaluation of OA.

Intraosseous phlebography reveals impaired drainage from the juxta-articular bone marrow.[79,80] Venous stasis and engorgement are generally associated with intramedullary hypertension. Thermography, a method of constructing photographic images of surface temperatures, may be normal or, in the presence of mild synovitis, may show a pattern of heat emission. Arthrography may be useful in differential diagnosis. The role of these techniques in the routine diagnosis of OA remains limited and poorly defined. They usually add little to observations evident on routine physical examination.

ROENTGENOGRAPHIC APPEARANCE

The roentgenographic appearance may be normal if the pathologic changes leading to clinical symptoms are sufficiently mild. Many gradations of abnormality may be noted as the disease progresses (Table 102–4).

Table 102–4. Laboratory and Radiologic Findings in Primary Osteoarthritis

Laboratory Tests	Results
Erythrocyte sedimentation rate	Usually normal
Routine blood counts	Normal
Rheumatoid factor	Negative
Antinuclear antibody	Negative
Serum calcium, phosphorus, alkaline phosphatase, serum protein electrophoresis	Normal
Synovial fluid analysis	Good viscosity with normal mucin clot; modest increase in leukocyte number
	Presence of fibrils and debris (wear particles)

Radiologic Findings	Causes
Narrowing of joint space	Articular cartilage ulceration
Subchondral bony sclerosis (eburnation)	New bone formation
Marginal osteophyte formation	Proliferation of cartilage and bone
Bone cysts and bony collapse	Subchondral microfractures
Gross deformity with subluxation and loose bodies	Ligamentous laxity as a result of mechanical forces

Joint-space narrowing occurs as a result of degeneration and disappearance of articular cartilage. *Subchondral bony sclerosis* (eburnation) is noted as increased bone density. *Marginal osteophyte formation* takes place as a result of proliferation of cartilage and bone. *Cysts,* varying in size from several millimeters to several centimeters, are seen as translucent areas in periarticular bone. Gross *deformity* and *subluxation* and *loose bodies* may occur in advanced cases.

Although osteophytes are usually regarded as a manifestation of OA, the use of this feature alone in diagnosis has been questioned, as noted earlier in this chapter. Osteophytes correlate with aging and are not necessarily an early sign of OA.[53,81] Some authors suggest that the diagnosis of OA of the peripheral joints should be based on radiologic findings of structural abnormalities in cartilage (decreased joint space) or in subchondral bone (cysts and eburnation) or in both.

The origin of the subchondral "detritus" cysts has been explained as follows: (1) a failure in the bone remodeling process, in which local osteoclastic activity outstrips that of osteoblasts; or (2) the result of pressure transmitted from the joint surface to subarticular bone through cracks in the subchondral plate (trabecular microfractures). The cysts may contain fluid, nonspecific detritus, or a primitive mesenchymal tissue that undergoes fibrosis. *These cysts may be prominent even in joints with adequately preserved joint space when seen radiographically.*

Ankylosis in osteoarthritis is uncommon. It is seen occasionally in OA of the hands, especially in its erosive inflammatory form.

Osteophytes are usually located on the anterior and anterolateral borders of the vertebral bodies and are best visualized on lateral roentgenograms. The amount of bony overgrowth varies. Spurs arising from the posterior margins of the vertebral bodies or

from the margins of the articular facets are less common but are of greater clinical importance, owing to their proximity to neural structures. Narrowing of intervertebral joint spaces results from disc degeneration; this is most frequent and usually most marked in the lower cervical and lower lumbar regions. Sclerosis of adjacent bone is common, and one sometimes sees wedging of the anterior borders of the vertebral bodies. Apophyseal joints may show joint-space narrowing, sclerosis, and associated spur formation. Osteoporosis is not a component of OA.

Many of the previously mentioned radiologic abnormalities may be visualized on routine posteroanterior and lateral views. Oblique views of the cervical and lumbar spine should be performed routinely, if degenerative changes involving intervertebral foramina and apophyseal joints are to be accurately delineated. Myelography may be of help when symptoms are severe and a surgical procedure is contemplated. Computed tomography (CT) scanning is particularly useful diagnostically in patients with OA of the spine, especially when spinal stenosis or lumbar facet disease is suspected (see Chapter 8). Diagnostic evaluation of disc herniation is enhanced, especially when the procedure is combined with myelography. Magnetic resonance imaging (MRI) promises to provide significant advances in noninvasive diagnostic imaging of both the spinal and peripheral articulations (Chapter 6).

Roentgenographic study of Heberden's and Bouchard's nodes reveals joint-space narrowing, bony sclerosis, and cyst formation. Spur formation, best seen radiologically on routine posteroanterior views, is prominent and appears to develop at the attachments of the flexor and extensor tendons to the distal phalanx. In some patients, however, spurs may be directed anteroposteriorly rather than mediolaterally, and lateral views with the fingers spread may be necessary to demonstrate changes. Although the nodes may feel hard, only minimal spur formation may be visible radiographically, and the enlargement may consist of soft tissue and cartilage. OA of metacarpophalangeal joints is uncommon, but *hook-like osteophytes* were noted on the radial side of the head of the metacarpal bones in 7 of 100 patients with nodal OA.[82] These changes, seen primarily in patients over 65 years of age, may result from tension on capsular ligaments caused by contraction of interosseous muscles at the radial side of the metacarpal head.

Anteroposterior views of the pelvis should be obtained routinely when OA of the hip is suspected. This view is especially informative in that the hips, sacroiliac joints, symphysis pubis, and pelvic bones are visualized. Special views of the hips, including lateral views and tomograms, may be of value when pathologic changes are suspected but not seen by routine techniques. Advanced disease may demonstrate striking abnormalities such as *protrusio acetabuli* (arthrokatadysis), a condition in which the floor of the acetabulum is displaced medially by the head of the femur, so that the femoral head may bulge into the pelvis ("Otto's pelvis").

Although OA changes of the knee are usually readily seen on routine anteroposterior and lateral views, special views are often helpful. *Tunnel views* taken with the knee in flexion expose the intercondylar notch and enable one to identify loose bodies, intraarticular spurs, and changes in the tibial spines. Tunnel views may best reveal loss of the joint space.[83] Its effectiveness in delineating cartilage loss may relate to the visualization of a more posterior portion of the femoral condyles, where cartilage loss may be significant. *"Skyline"* (Hughston) views taken from above allow more detailed study of the patellofemoral compartment. Films obtained when the patient is *bearing weight* allow optimal demonstration of genu varus or genu valgus and medial or lateral compartment narrowing. Roentgenograms of the contralateral joint are helpful in evaluating observed changes.

VARIANT FORMS

The clinical, radiologic, and pathologic findings in certain patients with primary OA are sufficiently different from those usually seen to warrant consideration of these cases as distinct symptom complexes.[66,67,84–88] One such group, characterized by diffuse polyarticular involvement, has been termed *primary generalized osteoarthritis.*[84] A second group demonstrating similar features has been given the name *ankylosing hyperostosis or diffuse idiopathic skeletal hyperostosis.*[66,67,88] A third group, characterized by inflammatory synovitis of interphalangeal joints of the hands in association with juxta-articular bone erosions, has been termed *erosive inflammatory osteoarthritis.*[85–87] Finally, a fourth group of patients may exhibit evidence of *chondromalacia patellae* with variable degrees of progression to full forms of osteoarthritic change.[89,90]

Primary Generalized Osteoarthritis

This pattern of "nodal" OA occurs predominantly in middle-aged women.[84] Distal and proximal interphalangeal joints and first carpometacarpal joints are sites of predilection and are often affected in succession. Other peripheral joints including knees, hips, and metatarsophalangeal joints are frequently involved, as are joints of the spine. An acute inflammatory phase commonly precedes chronic articular symptoms. The erythrocyte sedimentation rate is normal or slightly elevated; serum rheumatoid factor is absent. Although the overall pattern of radiologic changes is similar to that usually seen in localized OA certain differences are notable. Articular facets, neural arches, and spinous processes of the vertebral column are often enlarged leading to the radiologic designation of "kissing spines." Knee films show marked joint-space narrowing with "molten wax" osteophytes as opposed to ordinary, sharply pointed osteophytes. Patients with advanced cases show radiologic changes in excess of the clinical findings. Joint function is often only mildly affected despite severe anatomic changes.

The concept of primary generalized OA as a distinct subset is still controversial. This form may simply reflect more severe disease differentiated only by polyarticular involvement.

In some patients with generalized OA, chondrocalcinosis has been noted.[55,91,92] Studies have demonstrated the presence of diffuse deposits of CPPD crystals.[93,94] A familial form of chondrocalcinosis associated with "apatite" crystal deposition has been described in patients exhibiting symptoms indistinguishable from those seen in generalized OA alone.[95]*

Erosive Inflammatory Osteoarthritis

Erosive inflammatory OA[85,87] is another variant of "nodal" disease and involves primarily the distal and proximal interphalangeal joints. The metacarpophalangeal joints may also be involved. The disease is

Editor's note. Synovial fluid BCP crystals (apatite-type) correlated well with the severity of radiographic joint degeneration, and synovial fluid CPPD crystals correlated with patient age but not with degeneration.[95a]

usually hereditary. Painful inflammatory episodes eventually lead to joint deformity and sometimes to ankylosis. Postmenopausal women are most frequently affected. Acute flares may occur for years, but eventually, the affected joints often become asymptomatic. Gelatinous cysts, variably painful and tender, may develop over the involved joints. Inflammation and swelling may be sufficiently severe to suggest a diagnosis of RA. Roentgenographic examination reveals loss of joint cartilage, spur formation, and subchondral bony sclerosis. Bony erosions are prominent. Bony ankylosis, commonly seen, may be the result of synovial inflammation and pannus formation, healing of denuded cartilage surfaces, or coalescence of adjacent osteophytes. Studies of synovium may reveal an intense proliferative synovitis, often indistinguishable from that of RA. The erythrocyte sedimentation rate is usually normal or only slightly elevated. In one study of this disorder,[86] later changes more characteristic of RA were noted in 15% of cases.

Rheumatoid factor and antinuclear antibodies are absent. The presence of abnormal immune mechanisms has been suggested, however, by the demonstration of immune complexes in involved synovium.[96] Synovial fluid and synovial specimens from patients with erosive osteoarthritis have increased numbers of Ia$^+$ T-lymphocytes, similar to those seen in specimens from patients with RA.[97] These findings are not present in patients with OA of other types. Evidence of sicca syndrome in patients with erosive OA suggests the presence of some immunologic abnormality.[98,99] Such individuals may well represent a subset of erosive inflammatory OA with an autoimmune background.

Diffuse Idiopathic Skeletal Hyperostosis (DISH); Ankylosing Hyperostosis

This syndrome is characterized by an unusual type of florid hyperostosis of the spine, with large spurs or marginal bony proliferations in the form of anterior osseous ridges.[66,67,88] Fusion of these ridges often has a flowing appearance (Fig. 102–10). Ossification occurs in the connective tissue surrounding the spine, such as the anterior longitudinal ligament and peripheral disc margins. A predilection exists for involvement of the dorsal spine, although all levels of the spine may be affected. Lesions are most marked at the anterior and right lateral aspects of the vertebral column. The observation of left-sided vertebral bridging in patients with situs inversus suggests that the descending thoracic aorta plays a role in the location of vertebral calcification.[100] Although most common in older patients, the disease has been noted in younger persons. Despite extensive anatomic abnor-

malities, pain is often minimal or absent, and spinal motion is only moderately limited. Physiologic vertebral ligamentous calcification is probably a variant of this same process.[101]

Subsequent studies have further defined the clinical and pathologic features of this syndrome[66,67] and have demonstrated extraspinal manifestations.[66] Resnick and co-workers defined specific criteria for vertebral involvement, to allow differentiation of this disorder from degenerative disc disease or ankylosing spondylitis.[102] The criteria include flowing ossification along the anterolateral aspect of at least four contiguous vertebral bodies; preservation of disc height; absence of vacuum phenomena or vertebral body marginal sclerosis; and absence of apophyseal joint ankylosis or sacroiliac joint erosions, sclerosis, or fusion. Frequently, radiolucency is apparent between the abnormal calcification and the underlying vertebral body. Extraspinal manifestations include irregular new bone formation or "whiskering," large bony spurs, seen particularly on the olecranon process and the calcaneus (Fig. 102–12), and severe ligamentous calcification, seen mainly in the sacrotuberous, iliolumbar (Fig. 102–13), and patellar ligaments. Periarticular osteophytes were conspicuous.

Spinal stiffness is a prominent clinical complaint despite surprising maintenance of spinal motion with minimal pain. Dysphagia related to severe cervical osteophytosis has been reported. Peripheral joint symptoms include pain in involved elbows, ilium, shoulders, hips, knees, and ankles. Heel pain related to a calcaneal spur is common. The diffuse radiographic findings involving both spinal and extraspinal structures have led to the suggestion that this disorder represents an "ossifying diathesis," rather than merely a localized disorder of the spine.

FIG. 102–12. DISH. The calcaneus demonstrates large, irregular spurs at its posterior and plantar aspects (straight arrows). Associated irregularity at the area of the cuboid and fifth metatarsal bones is seen (curved arrow). (Courtesy of Dr. Donald Resnick.)

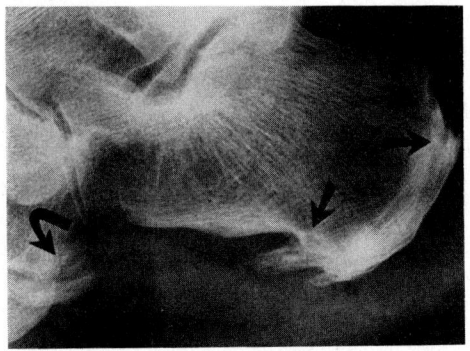

FIG. 102–13. Radiogram of the pelvis in a patient with DISH reveals iliolumbar (straight arrow) and sacrotuberous (curved arrow) ligament ossification and para-articular sacroiliac osteophyte formation (open arrows). (From Resnick, D., et al.[79]).

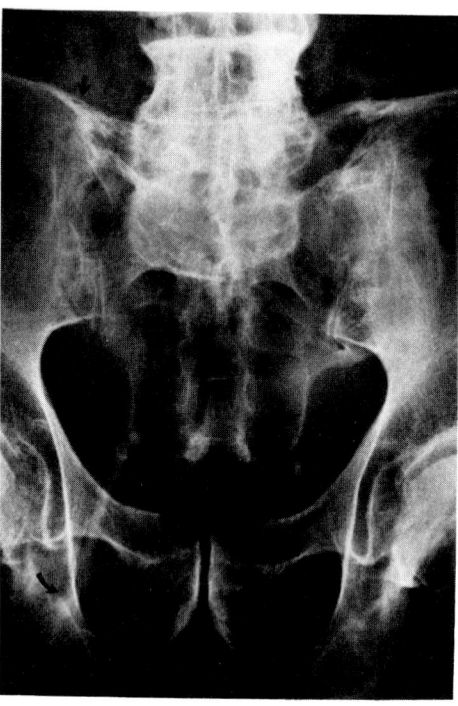

Hyperglycemia is the commonest laboratory abnormality noted in patients with this syndrome, with an incidence of abnormal glucose tolerance tests about twice that seen in an age-, sex-, and weight-matched populations. In a recent study, diabetes mellitus was present in 40% of these patients.[103] Growth hormone and somatomedin (insulin-like growth factor) levels are normal in DISH, but insulin levels have been shown to be elevated.[104,105]

The etiopathogenesis of DISH is unknown. In one report, 16 of 47 patients with this syndrome were HLA-B27 positive.[106] In other studies, however, a statistically significant increase in HLA-B27 has not been confirmed. Studies of Pima Indians have shown this syndrome to be present in 50% of all individuals, with a 20% frequency of HLA-B27.[107] No significant association was seen, however, with B-locus antigens when Pima Indians with the syndrome were compared to age-matched control subjects. Patients with DISH have increased levels of serum vitamin A.[108] Of special interest in this regard is the observation that patients receiving high doses of synthetic vitamin A derivatives, retinoids, develop an ossification disorder resembling DISH.[109,110] Radiographic features may simulate vertebral and extravertebral manifestations

of DISH syndrome, or may be limited to extraspinal tendon and ligament calcification with minimal or absent vertebral involvement. In a limited report, 5 patients with DISH syndrome were noted to have elevated plasma and urine fluoride levels.[111] Abnormal levels of fluoride were, however, not noted in other studies.[67,112]

A syndrome characterized by *ossification of the posterior longitudinal ligament* has been described, occurring mainly in Japanese.[113] It has been estimated that over 4000 patients in Japan are afflicted with this disorder. Roentgenographic study of the spine reveals lumpy or linear bony masses across one or more disc spaces, sometimes extending from the superior cervical spine to the thoracic region. Ankylosing hyperostosis of the type seen in DISH may be associated. Clinical manifestations may be severe because of spinal cord compression.

Chondromalacia Patellae
(see also Chapters 87 and 88)

This disorder is characterized by degenerative changes of the cartilage of the patella and is included in those conditions associated with OA changes in the knee. Although in the past it was identified as a specific entity, chondromalacia patellae is now thought to result from many conditions affecting the knee that lead to cartilage degeneration.[89,90] The malacic changes are considered to be simply the final common pathway through which articular cartilage of the patella degenerates. The specific conditions effecting these changes, such as primary meniscal disease, knee laxity, or abnormal patellar positions such as patella alta, may lead to a similar end-stage complex of symptoms. The syndrome is often associated with repeated trauma, as occurs in recurrent lateral subluxation of the patella. Radiologic changes may be limited or absent. Pain is present about the patella and is aggravated by activity such as ascending or, particularly, descending stairs. Paradoxically, vague knee pain may occur after periods of inactivity in the flexed position, such as watching a movie. The disease is typically seen in young adults, especially women, and may be a precursor to the development of patellofemoral compartment OA.

Although the findings described in the foregoing discussion support the existence of various forms of OA, the validity of classifying these as distinct symptom complexes or entities remains open to question. OA may affect one or a number of joints in any given patient, so generalized involvement may merely reflect one end of the spectrum of clinical severity. Inflammation may occur in early OA, whether localized or generalized, and its use as a differentiating characteristic is not definitive. In some patients, it is difficult to rule out the coexistence of seronegative RA and OA.[86] Ankylosing hyperostosis has many characteristics that distinguish it from the more common forms of OA. The pathologic changes may be indistinguishable, however, especially in early disease.

PROGNOSIS

The outlook for patients with primary OA is variable, depending on the extent and site of the disease. Involvement of the distal interphalangeal joints, for example, may be associated with a moderate amount of pain, but usually causes little limitation of function unless fine finger motion is required occupationally, such as in typing or in playing musical instruments. Involvement of weight-bearing joints, on the other hand, may lead to marked disability. Similarly, OA of the cervical spine may not only give rise to distressing symptoms, but may also lead to severe objective neurologic deficits and disability.

Studies of disease progression in specific joints suggest that not all cases of OA inevitably deteriorate.[27,114] In a study of 6321 patients who had undergone roentgenographic examination of the colon, 4.7% had OA of the hip.[115] Only half of these patients with roentgenographic evidence of hip OA actually needed treatment and 20% were entirely free of symptoms.

Occasional patients may develop a rapidly progressive, destructive OA of the hip.[116–118] Severe changes are seen both in the acetabulum and in the femoral head. Degenerative pseudocysts and lack of osteophyte formation are characteristic findings. Synovitis noted at operation is of a low grade. Such rapid deterioration of hip joints may be associated with use of nonsteroidal anti-inflammatory drugs (NSAIDs).[119–121] Such an association, if real, might be related to increased joint use permitted by the analgesic action of these drugs, to a direct effect of these drugs on cartilage with inhibition of proteoglycan synthesis, or both.[122] Similar rapid destructive changes have been described unrelated to the use of analgesic agents,[29] and the overall clinical experience with these agents over many years in the treatment of various forms of arthritis is reassuring.

Some studies of the natural course of OA of the knee suggest a worse prognosis than in disease of the hip.[81] Most patients worsened during the 10- to 18-year period of followup, with increased pain, deformity, and instability and decreased function. Most patients were unable to use public transportation because of pain on walking. Marked radiologic deterioration was noted, usually limited to the compart-

ment first affected. Varus deformity and early development of pain were unfavorable prognostic factors. Other data suggest that OA of the knee affects only a limited portion of the population and is not inevitably progressive.[12]

Treatment may retard the progression of the disease and is of further value in protecting the contralateral joints exposed to increased stress. Patients should be reassured that the general outlook is favorable and disability is uncommon, in contrast to the threat of crippling seen in patients with RA. Patients should be told that involvement of certain joints may be associated with localized pain, stiffness, and limitation of motion. OA is certainly not always benign.

DIFFERENTIAL DIAGNOSIS

The differentiation of primary OA from other disorders of the musculoskeletal system depends on a correlation of clinical, laboratory, and roentgenographic findings. OA may be confused with other forms of arthritic disease because pain, stiffness, and limitation of motion are common features in all these disorders. Differential diagnosis is further complicated by the high radiologic prevalence of OA in the general population that often bears no relation to the musculoskeletal complaints of a given patient.

In most patients, the diagnosis is simple. In others, however, atypical disease presentation and behavior may require extensive differential diagnostic considerations. Examples of such presentations include OA occurring in an atypical site such as the shoulder, association with a significant inflammatory element, coexistence with other entities such as CPPD crystal deposition, precocious occurrence in young individuals, and OA of the spine with neurologic findings that simulate other underlying neurologic disorders.

RA can usually be differentiated on the basis of its more inflammatory nature and the characteristic pattern of joint involvement. If RA begins as monarticular disease of the knee or hip, however, differentiation from OA may be difficult without prolonged followup study. An increase in the erythrocyte sedimentation rate, a positive test for rheumatoid factor, and synovial fluid analysis are helpful (see Chapter 5). RA may be particularly difficult to differentiate from erosive OA. The pattern of joint involvement is of diagnostic value because the latter is limited mainly to the distal and proximal interphalangeal joints of the hands; RA usually affects the metacarpophalangeal and the wrist and carpal joints and peripheral joints elsewhere. *Joints afflicted with active seropositive RA rarely develop osteophytes.* Some patients with Heberden's nodes or erosive OA may later develop RA, in which case osteophytes *precede* rheumatoid involvement, and a careful clinical history is necessary to identify the presence of a "mixed" arthritis. Mixed disease may also be present when RA leads to secondary degenerative change, but bony overgrowth occurs only in "burned out" disease, and even then, osteophyte formation is abortive. Proximal or distal interphalangeal joint involvement in juvenile RA or psoriatic arthritis is frequently accompanied by nodal formation in these joints.

Rheumatic syndromes characterized by involvement of the distal interphalangeal joints of the hands, such as psoriatic arthritis, Reiter's syndrome, and the arthritis of chronic ulcerative colitis, may be confused with OA of the nodal type. The associated clinical findings of the underlying disease in these patients usually suffice to clarify the diagnosis. Pseudogout syndrome, or chondrocalcinosis articularis, may simulate OA when low-grade arthralgias result from the presence of CPPD crystals in synovial fluid. The pattern of arthritis is clearly different in these patients; the metacarpophalangeal joints, wrists, elbows, shoulders, knees, hips, and ankles are often affected (see Chapter 107). Symptoms related to early manifestations of localized joint disorders such as osteonecrosis, pigmented villonodular synovitis, and chronic infectious arthritis may be mistakenly attributed to degenerative changes seen as coincidental radiographic findings. Neurologic symptoms secondary to spinal OA must be differentiated from those that result from other neurologic disorders. The symptoms of OA of the cervical spine may simulate those of multiple sclerosis, syringomyelia, amyotrophic lateral sclerosis, progressive spinal atrophy, and spinal cord tumors.

SECONDARY OSTEOARTHRITIS

The term "secondary OA" describes those cases that follow a recognizable underlying local or systemic factor, some of which are noted in Table 102–2. A diagnosis of secondary OA should be considered particularly when the disease develops at an early age.

ACUTE TRAUMA

Joint degeneration may follow acute injury. The history includes the injurious event followed by redness, soft tissue swelling, and pain over the involved joint. In several months, the inflammatory changes subside and are replaced by a hard, painless enlargement. The

deformity is localized to the injured joint. The anatomic changes are similar to those seen in primary OA. Injury of this nature involving the distal interphalangeal joints of the hands may lead to traumatic Heberden's nodes.[57] Acute trauma to any of the interphalangeal joints of the hands may lead to the common "baseball finger" (Fig. 102–14).

CHRONIC TRAUMA

An increased prevalence of OA is associated with chronic trauma related to certain occupations. Although exposure of a joint to subtle chronic trauma, or microtrauma, has been suggested as an etiologic factor in the development of primary OA, the relationship between trauma and joint changes, as described previously, seems more clear cut and supports the classification of such lesions as secondary.

OTHER JOINT DISORDERS

Such disorders may be either local or diffuse. Secondary localized OA may follow local joint disorders of other causes, such as fractures, aseptic necrosis, or acute or chronic infection. Early age OA in the knee may be the result of torn menisci, patellar dislocation, strain resulting from obesity, or poor mechanics as a result of genu varus, or tibial torsion. Localized OA of the hip may follow childhood disorders such as congenital dysplasia of the hip, slipped capital epiphysis, and Legg-Calvé-Perthes disease. OA of the midfoot or hindfoot may result in patients with congenital calcaneonavicular and talocalcaneal coalition.

Diffuse secondary degenerative changes may supervene in patients with RA, in patients with bleeding dyscrasias in whom repeated hemarthroses may occur, or in dwarfs with achondroplasia.

SYSTEMIC METABOLIC OR ENDOCRINE DISORDERS

OA changes may follow several metabolic or endocrine disorders (see also Chapters 111 and 113).

Alkaptonuria (Ochronosis)
This inherited metabolic disease, associated with an absence of homogentisic acid oxidase and characterized by excretion of homogentisic acid in the urine and by a binding of its metabolic products to connective tissue components, is associated with gen-

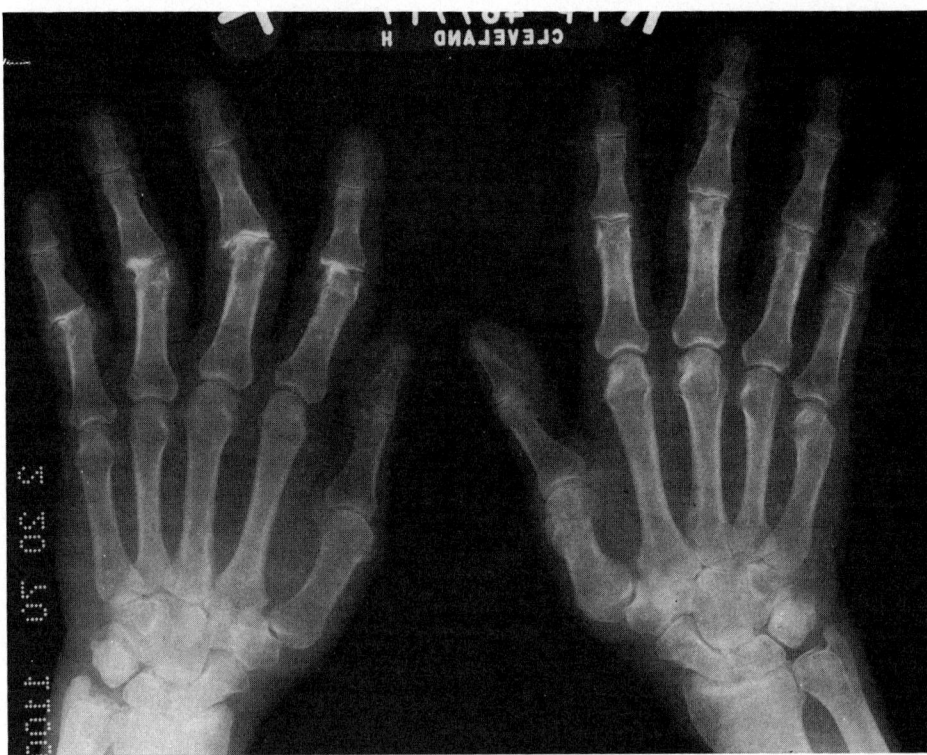

FIG. 102–14. Secondary OA of the second, third, fourth, and fifth proximal interphalangeal joints of the left hand ("baseball fingers") in a patient with recurrent episodes of acute trauma while a semiprofessional baseball player.

eralized osteoarthritis.[123] Tissue deposition of brown-black pigment, or ochronosis, is seen primarily in cartilage, skin, and sclera. Degenerative disease of the spine occurs frequently; calcification of numerous intervertebral discs is a characteristic finding. Arthritis of peripheral joints such as hips, knees, and shoulders is less common and develops later.

Wilson's Disease

Hepatolenticular degeneration, or Wilson's disease, is an inherited disorder characterized by excessive retention of copper, with degenerative changes in the brain and hepatic cirrhosis. Premature OA has been described as one component of associated articular manifestations of this disorder.[124]

Hemochromatosis

This chronic disease is associated with excessive deposition of iron and fibrosis in a variety of tissues. Although it can result from long-term overingestion of iron and from multiple transfusions, the disease is most often idiopathic. OA changes occur in 20 to 50% of patients.[125,126] Hands, knees, and hips are most commonly involved, although virtually any joint, including those in the feet, can be affected. Involvement of the second and third metacarpophalangeal joints of the hands is particularly characteristic. Synovial tissue shows a striking deposition of iron, most prominently in the synovial lining cells. Roentgenograms reveal joint-space narrowing and irregularity, subchondral sclerosis, cystic erosions, bony proliferation, and at times, subluxation. Chondrocalcinosis with deposits of calcium pyrophosphate dihydrate is seen in up to 60% of patients.

Kashin-Beck Disease

This disorder, characterized by disturbances in growth and maturation in children, is endemic in eastern Siberia, northern China, and northern Korea.[127] Abnormalities in enchondral bone growth lead to dystrophic changes in epiphyseal and metaphyseal areas. Severe secondary OA involves the peripheral joints and the spine. Various causes have been suggested, including a relation to a fungus ingested with cereal grains, iron excess, or selenium deficiency.[127a]

Acromegaly

Hypersecretion of growth hormone by the anterior pituitary gland in adults leads to a slowly progressive overgrowth of soft tissue, bone, and cartilage. Peripheral and spinal OA is common. Peripheral joint symptoms occur in about 60% of patients.[128] Most commonly involved are the knees, hips, shoulders, and elbows. Carpal tunnel syndrome is frequently seen. Backache is common, but back motion is often normal or increased because of the thickened intervertebral discs and the laxity of acromegalic ligaments. Early, increased cartilage thickness gives wide joint spaces on roentgenograms. Later, joint-space narrowing, osteophyte formation, and subchondral sclerosis occur.

Hyperparathyroidism

Increased levels of parathyroid hormone, whether primary or secondary, can produce many rheumatic problems. It has been postulated that degenerative changes result from damage to cartilage related either to CPPD crystal deposition or to subchondral bony erosion from the resorptive effects of parathyroid hormone. Roentgenograms classically show subperiosteal bone resorption, cystic or sclerotic changes in bones, and chondrocalcinosis.

CRYSTAL DEPOSITION DISEASE

Generalized OA has been reported in patients with idiopathic articular chondrocalcinosis.[129] Large joints of the lower limbs and intervertebral joints of the lumbar spine are especially involved. Although a destructive arthropathy has been described in patients with articular chondrocalcinosis,[130] these changes appear to be much more common when generalized OA and chondrocalcinosis coexist.[131] Weight-bearing joints are frequently affected, but involvement of nonweight-bearing joints such as the elbow, shoulder, wrist, and metacarpophalangeal joints also occurs.

Several mechanisms have been postulated to relate the increased association of CPPD crystal deposition to OA.[132,133] In certain patients, obvious crystal deposition antedates significant OA; alterations in calcium matrix in these patients may predispose them to degenerative changes. In other patients, OA is present for a prolonged period and crystal deposition disease occurs later in the disorder. Whether changes in cartilage matrix as a result of OA may favor the deposition of these crystals is still unclear.

An association between BCP (apatite-type) crystal deposition and OA has been described.[134-136] The disease in patients with identifiable BCP crystals in synovial fluid is similar to other forms of OA, except the presence of crystals correlates with more severe roentgenographic change. Whether apatite crystals are a result of or a cause of OA is unknown. Severe degenerative changes of the shoulder in association with basic calcium phosphate crystal deposition have been described by Halverson and McCarty and colleagues and termed Milwaukee shoulder.[135,136] Similar changes have been seen in other joints, such as the knee.[134,137]

NEUROPATHIC DISORDERS

Severe OA occurs in association with neuropathic disorders, as first described by Charcot.[138] The loss of proprioceptive or pain sensation, or both, relaxes the normal protective mechanisms of the joint and leads to articular instability and an exaggerated response to normal daily stresses. Although first described in patients with tabes dorsalis, similar lesions may be seen in other diseases associated with neuropathy including diabetes mellitus, syringomyelia, meningomyelocele, and peripheral nerve section (see Chapter 81).

OVERUSE OF INTRA-ARTICULAR CORTICOSTEROID THERAPY

The development of localized OA has been ascribed to the repeated use of intra-articular injections of adrenal corticosteroids.[139] In these patients, pain relief may allow overuse of already damaged joints and may thereby promote degenerative change. Studies have demonstrated a direct, deleterious effect of corticosteroids on cartilage, suggesting a second mechanism for the development of those degenerative changes.[140]

MISCELLANEOUS ASSOCIATIONS

OA, often polyarticular, is associated with a number of *bone dysplasias*. These disorders are uncommon and include multiple epiphyseal dysplasia, spondyloepiphyseal dysplasia, and osteo-onychodystrophy, or nail-patella syndrome. Mechanisms for OA are related to the severe distortion of articulating bone. The primary defects leading to bone dysplasia and the possible contributions of the primary metabolic defect are as yet unknown.

Severe cold injury with *frostbite* may lead to premature OA when cold exposure occurs prior to epiphyseal closure.[148] Joint pain may begin months to years later.

Symptoms and signs, laboratory findings, and roentgenographic abnormalities of secondary OA are generally similar to those seen in the primary form of the disease. Additional findings related to associated underlying disease states are also present. The management of secondary OA is similar to that of the primary form of the disease.

REFERENCES

1. Moskowitz, R.W., Goldberg, V.M., and Berman, L.: Synovitis as a manifestation of degenerative joint disease: An experimental study. Arthritis Rheum., 19:813, 1976.
2. Goldenberg, D.L., Egan, M.S., and Cohen, A.S.: Inflammatory synovitis in degenerative joint disease. J. Rheumatol., 9:204–209, 1982.

3. Murray, R.O.: The aetiology of primary osteoarthritis of the hip. Br. J. Radiol., *38*:810–824, 1965.

4. Altman, R., et al.: Development of criteria for the classification and reporting of osteoarthritis. Classification of osteoarthritis of the knee. Arthritis Rheum., *29*:1039–1049, 1986.

5. Peyron, J.G.: Epidemiologic and etiologic approach of osteoarthritis. Semin. Arthritis Rheum., *8*:288–306, 1979.

6. Bland, J.H., et al.: A study of inter- and intra-observer error in reading plain roentgenograms of the hands: 'To err is human.' Am. J. Roentgenol., *105*:853–859, 1969.

7. Lowman, E.W.: Osteoarthritis. JAMA, *157*:487–488, 1955.

8. Roberts, J., and Burch, T.A.: Prevalence of osteoarthritis in adults by age, sex, race, and geographic area, United States—1960–1962. [National Center for Health Statistics: vital and health statistics: data from the national health survey.] United States Public Health Service Publication No. 1000, Series 11, No. 15, 1966. Washington, D.C.: United States Government Printing Office.

9. Lawrence, J.S., Bremner, J.M., and Bier, F.: Osteoarthrosis. Prevalence in the population and relationship between symptoms and x-ray changes. Ann. Rheum. Dis., *25*:1–24, 1966.

10. Forman, M., Malamet, R., and Kaplan, D.: A survey of osteoarthritis of the knee in the elderly. J. Rheumatol., *10*:283–287, 1983.

11. Felson, D., et al.: Knee osteoarthritis (OA) in the elderly: The Framingham study. Arthritis Rheum., *29*:S26, 1986.

12. Kellgren, J.H., Lawrence, J.S., and Bier, F.: Genetic factors in generalized osteo-arthrosis. Ann. Rheum. Dis., *22*:237–255, 1963.

13. Bremner, J.M., Lawrence, J.S., and Miall, W.E.: Degenerative joint disease in a Jamaican rural population. Ann. Rheum. Dis., *27*:326–332, 1968.

14. Solomon, L., Beighton, P., and Lawrence, J.S.: Rheumatic disorders in the South African Negro. Part II. Osteoarthrosis. S. Afr. Med. J., *49*:1737–1740, 1975.

15. Hoaglund, F.T., Yau, A.C.M.C., and Wong, W.L.: Osteoarthritis of the hip and other joints in Southern Chinese in Hong Kong. J. Bone Joint Surg., *55A*:645–657, 1973.

16. Solomon, L., Beighton, P., and Lawrence, J.S.: Rheumatic disorders in the South African Negro, Part II. Osteo-arthrosis. S. Afr. Med. J., *49*:1737–1740, 1975.

17. Mukhopadhaya, B., and Barooah, B.: Osteoarthritis of hip in Indians: An anatomical and clinical study. Indian J. Orthop., *1*:55–62, 1967.

18. Hoaglund, F.T., Shiba, R., Newberg, A.H., and Leung, K.Y.K.: Diseases of the hip. A comparative study of Japanese oriental and American white patients. J. Bone Joint Surg., *67*:1376–1383, 1985.

19. Solomon, L., et al.: Distinct types of hip disorder in Mseleni joint disease. S. Afr. Med. J., *69*:15–17, 1986.

20. Lawrence, J.S.: Hypertension in relation to musculoskeletal disorders. Ann. Rheum. Dis., *34*:451–456, 1975.

21. Lawrence, J.S.: Generalized osteoarthrosis in a population sample. Am. J. Epidemiol., *90*:381–389, 1969.

22. Stecher, R.M., Hersh, A.H., and Hauser, H.: Heberden's nodes: Family history and radiographic appearance of large family. Am. J. Hum. Genet., *5*:46–60, 1953.

23. Blumberg, B.S., et al.: A study of the prevalence of arthritis in Alaskan Eskimos. Arthritis Rheum., *4*:325–341, 1961.

24. Lawrence, J.S., DeGraff, R., and Laine, V.A.I.: Degenerative joint disease in random samples and occupational groups. *In* The Epidemiology of Chronic Rheumatism, Vol. 1. Edited by J.H. Kellgren, M.R. Jeffrey and J. Ball. Oxford, Blackwell, 1963.

25. Sokoloff, L., et al.: Experimental obesity and osteoarthritis. Am. J. Physiol., *198*:765–770, 1960.

26. Goldin, R.H., et al.: Clinical and radiological survey of the incidence of osteoarthrosis among obese patients. Ann. Rheum. Dis., *35*:349–353, 1976.

27. Seifert, M.H., Whiteside, C.G., and Savage, O.: A 5-year follow-up of fifty cases of idiopathic osteoarthritis of the hip. Ann. Rheum. Dis., *28*:325–326, 1969.

28. Kellgren, J.H.: Osteoarthrosis in patients and population. Br. Med. J., *2*:1–6, 1961.

29. Kellgren, J.H., and Lawrence, J.S.: Osteo-arthrosis and disk degeneration in an urban population. Ann. Rheum. Dis., *17*:388–397, 1958.

30. Leach, R.E., Baumgard, S., and Broom, J.: Obesity: Its relationship to osteoarthritis of the knee. Clin. Orthop., *93*:271–273, 1973.

31. Hartz, A.J., et al.: The association of obesity with joint pain and osteoarthritis in the HANES data. J. Chron. Dis., *39*:311–319, 1986.

32. Anderson, J., and Felson, D.: Factors associated with knee osteoarthritis (OA) in a national survey. Arthritis Rheum., *29*:S16, 1986.

33. Silberberg, M., and Silberberg, R.: Osteoarthritis in mice fed diets enriched with animal or vegetable fat. Arch. Pathol, *70*:385–390, 1960.

34. Acheson, R.M., Collart, A.N.: New Haven survey of joint diseases XIII. Relationship between some systemic characteristics and osteoarthrosis in a general population. Ann. Rheum. Dis., *34*:379–387, 1975.

35. Solomon, L., Schnitzler, C.M., and Browett, J.P.: Osteoarthritis of the hip: The patient behind the disease. Ann. Rheum. Dis., *41*:118–125, 1982.

36. Foss, M.V.L., and Byers, P.D.: Bone density, osteoarthrosis of the hip and fracture of the upper end of the femur. Ann. Rheum. Dis., *31*:259–264, 1972.

37. Roh, Y.S., Dequeker, J., and Mulier, J.C.: Bone mass in osteoarthrosis, measured in vivo by photon absorption. J. Bone Joint Surg., *56*:587–591, 1974.

38. Weintroub, S., et al.: Osteoarthritis of the hip and fractures of the proximal end of the femur. Acta Orthop. Scand., *53*:261–264, 1982.

39. McCarty, D.J., et al.: Diseases associated with calcium pyrophosphate dihydrate crystal deposition—A controlled study. Am. J. Med., *56*:704–714, 1974.

39a. Radin, E.L., et al.: Effects of mechanical loading on the tissues of the rabbit knee. J. Orthop. Res., *2*:221–234, 1984.

40. Bird, H.A., Tribe, C.R., and Bacon, P.A.: Joint hypermobility leading to osteoarthrosis and chondrocalcinosis. Ann. Rheum. Dis., *37*:203–211, 1978.

41. Schlomka, G., Schroter, G., and Ocherwal A.: Uber der bedeutung der beruflischer Belastung fur die entsehung der degenerativen Gelenkleiden. Z. Gesamte. Inn. Med., *10*:993–999, 1955.

42. Partridge, R.E.H., and Duthie, J.J.R.: Rheumatism in dockers and civil servants: A comparison of heavy manual and sedentary workers. Ann. Rheum. Dis., *27*:559–568, 1968.

43. Hadler, N.M., et al.: Hand structure and function in an industrial setting. Influence of three patterns of stereotyped repetitive usage. Arthritis Rheum., *21*:210–220, 1978.

44. Mintz, G., and Fraga, A.: Severe osteoarthritis of the elbow in foundry workers. Arch. Environ. Health, *27*:78–80, 1973.

45. Lindberg, H., and Danielson, L.G.: The relation between labor and coxarthrosis. Clin. Orthop., *191*:159–161, 1984.

46. Puranen, J., et al.: Running and primary osteoarthrosis of the hip. Br. Med. J., 2:424–425, 1975.
47. Lane, N.E, et al.: Long-distance running, bone density, and osteoarthritis. JAMA, 255:1147–1151, 1986.
48. Panush, R.S., et al.: Is running associated with degenerative joint disease? JAMA, 255:1152–1154, 1986.
49. Brodelius, A.: Osteoarthrosis of the talar joints in footballers and ballet dancers. Acta Orthop. Scand., 30:309–314, 1961.
50. Solonen, K.A.: The joints of the lower extremities of football players. Ann. Chir. Gynaecol. Fenn., 55:176, 1966.
51. Cobb, S., Merchant, W.R., and Rubin, T.: The relation of symptoms to osteoarthritis. J. Chronic Dis., 5:197–204, 1957.
52. Gresham, G.E., and Rathey, U.K.: Osteoarthritis in knees of aged persons: Relationship between roentgenographic and clinical manifestations. JAMA, 233:168–170, 1975.
53. Hernborg, J., and Nilsson, B.E.: The relationship between osteophytes in the knee joint, osteoarthritis and aging. Acta Orthop. Scand., 44:69–74, 1973.
54. Tokunaga, M., et al.: Change of prostaglandin E level in joint fluids after treatment with flurbioprofen in patients with rheumatoid arthritis and osteoarthritis. Ann. Rheum. Dis., 40:462–465, 1981.
55. Schumacher, H.R., et al.: Osteoarthritis, crystal deposition, and inflammation. Semin. Arthritis Rheum., 11(Suppl.):116–119, 1981.
56. Heberden, W.: Commentaries on the History and Cure of Diseases, 2nd ed. London, T. Payne, 1803.
57. Stecher, R.M., and Hauser, H.: Heberden's nodes: Roentgenological and clinical appearance of degenerative joint disease of fingers. Am. J. Roentgenol., 59:326–327, 1948.
58. Stecher, R.M.: Heberden's nodes: Heredity in hypertrophic arthritis of finger joints. Am. J. Med. Sci., 201:801–809, 1941.
59. Eaton, R.G., Dobranski, A.I., and Littler, J.W.: Marginal osteophyte excision in treatment of mucous cysts. J. Bone Joint Surg., 55A:570–574, 1973.
60. Patterson, A.C.: Osteoarthritis of the trapezioscaphoid joint. Arthritis Rheum., 18:375–379, 1975.
60a. Halverson, P.B., Cheung, H.S., and McCarty, D.J.: Milwaukee shoulder syndrome (MSS): Description of predisposing factors. Arthritis Rheum., 30:S131, 1987.
60b. Ike, R.W., Arnold, W.J., and Simon, C.: Correlations between radiographic (XR) changes, meniscal chondrocalcinosis and other intra-articular (IA) abnormalities (ABN) in patients (PT) with osteoarthritis of the knee (OAK) undergoing arthroscopy (AR). Arthritis Rheum., 30:S131, 1987.
61. Evarts, C.M.: Challenge of the aging hip. Geriatrics, 24:112–119, 1969.
62. Meachim, G., et al.: An investigation of radiological, clinical and pathological correlations in osteoarthrosis of the hip. Clin. Radiol., 31:565–574, 1980.
63. Macys, J.R., Bullough, P.G., and Wilson, P.D., Jr.: Coxarthrosis: A study of the natural history based on a correlation of clinical, radiographic, and pathologic findings. Semin. Arthritis Rheum., 10:66–80, 1980.
64. Prince, D.S., et al.: Osteophyte-induced dysphagia: Occurrence in ankylosing hyperostosis. JAMA, 234:77–78, 1975.
65. Forestier, J., Jacqueline, F., and Rotes-Querol, J.: Ankylosing Spondylitis: Clinical Considerations, Roentgenology, Pathologic Anatomy, Treatment. Springfield, Charles C Thomas, 1956.
66. Resnick, D., Shaul, S.R., and Robins, J.M.: Diffuse idiopathic skeletal hyperostosis (DISH): Forestier's disease with extraspinal manifestations. Radiology, 115:513–524, 1975.
67. Utsinger, P.D., Resnick, D., and Shapiro, R.: Diffuse skeletal abnormalities in Forestier disease. Arch. Intern. Med., 136:763–768, 1976.
68. Harata, S., Tohno, S., and Kawagishi, T.: Osteoarthritis of the atlanto-axial joint. Int. Orthop., 5:277–282, 1981.
69. Arnoldi, C.C., Brodsky, A.E., and Cauchoix, J.: Lumbar spinal stenosis and nerve root entrapment syndromes—Definition and classification. Clin. Orthop., 115:4–5, 1976.
70. Cheung, H.S., et al.: Identification of collagen subtypes in synovial fluid sediments from arthritic patients. Am. J. Med., 68:73–79, 1980.
71. Fam, A.G., et al.: Cholesterol crystals in osteoarthritic joint effusions. J. Rheumatol., 8:273–280, 1981.
72. Stastny, P., et al.: Lymphokines in the rheumatoid joint. Arthritis Rheum., 18:237–243, 1975.
73. Moskowitz, R.W., and Kresina, T.F.: Immunofluorescent analysis of experimental osteoarthritic cartilage and synovium: Evidence for selective deposition of immunoglobulin and complement in cartilaginous tissues. J. Rheumatol., 13:391–396, 1986.
74. Kresina, T.F., Malemud, C.J., and Moskowitz, R.W.: Analysis of osteoarthritic cartilage using monoclonal antibodies reactive with rabbit proteoglycan. Arthritis Rheum., 29:863–871, 1986.
75. Cooke, T.D.V., et al.: Identification of immunoglobulins and complement in rheumatoid articular collagenous tissues. Arthritis Rheum., 18:541–551, 1975.
76. Tanaka, S., Ito, T., Hamamoto, K., and Torizuka, K.: Clearance of technetium pertechnetate from the hip joint with arthrosis deformans. Am. J. Roentgenol. Radium Ther. Nucl. Med., 118:870–875, 1973.
77. Hutton, C.W., et al.: ^{99m}Tc HMDP bone scanning in generalised nodal osteoarthritis. I. Comparison of the standard radiograph and four hour bone scan image of the hand. Ann. Rheum. Dis., 45:617–621, 1986.
78. Hutton, C.W., et al.: ^{99m}Tc HMDP bone scanning in generalised nodal osteoarthritis. II. The four hour bone scan image predicts radiographic change. Ann. Rheum. Dis., 45:622–626, 1986.
79. Arnoldi, C.C., et al.: Intraosseous phlebography, intraosseous pressure measurements and ^{99m}Tc-polyphosphate scintigraphy in patients with various painful conditions in the hip and knee. Acta Orthop. Scand., 51:19–28, 1980.
80. Arnoldi, C.C., Linderholm, H., and Müssbichler, H.: Venous engorgement and intraosseous hypertension in osteoarthritis of the hip. J. Bone Joint Surg., 54B:409–421, 1972.
81. Hernborg, J.S., and Nilsson, B.E.: The natural course of untreated osteoarthritis of the knee. Clin. Orthop., 123:130–137, 1977.
82. Swezey, R.L., Peter, J.B., and Evans, P.L.: Osteoarthritis of the metacarpophalangeal joint: Hook-like osteophytes. Arthritis Rheum., 12:405–410, 1969.
83. Resnick, D., and Vint, V.: The "tunnel" view in assessment of cartilage loss in osteoarthritis of the knee. Radiology, 137:547–548, 1980.
84. Kellgren, J.H., and Moore, R.: Generalized osteoarthritis and Heberden's nodes. Br. Med. J., 1:181–187, 1952.
85. Crain, D.C.: Interphalangeal osteoarthritis. JAMA, 175:1049–1053, 1961.
86. Ehrlich, G.E.: Inflammatory osteoarthritis. II. The superimposition of RA. J. Chronic Dis., 25:635–643, 1972.
87. Ehrlich, G.E.: Inflammatory osteoarthritis. I. The clinical syndrome. J. Chronic Dis., 25:317–328, 1972.
88. Forestier, J., and Lagier, R.: Ankylosing hyperostosis of the spine. Clin. Orthop., 74:65–83, 1971.

89. DeHaven, K.E., Dolan, W.A., and Mayer, P.J.: Chondromalacia patellae in athletes. Am. J. Sports Med., 7:1–5, 1979.

90. Goodfellow, J.W., Hungerford, D.S., and Woods, C.: Patellofemoral mechanics and pathology. II. Chondromalacia patellae. J. Bone Joint Surg., 58B:291–299, 1976.

91. Dieppe, P.A., et al.: Mixed crystal deposition disease in osteoarthritis. Br. Med. J., 1:150–152, 1978.

92. Doyle, E.V., Huskisson, E.C., and Willoughby, D.A.: A histological study of inflammation in osteoarthritis: The role of calcium phosphate crystal deposition. Ann. Rheum. Dis., 38:192, 1979.

93. Alexander, G.M., et al.: Pyrophosphate arthropathy: A study of metabolic associations and laboratory data. Ann. Rheum. Dis., 41:377–381, 1982.

94. Dieppe, P.A., et al.: Pyrophosphate arthropathy: A clinical and radiological study of 105 cases. Ann. Rheum. Dis., 41:371–376, 1982.

95. Marcos, J.C., et al.: Idiopathic familial chondrocalcinosis due to apatite crystal deposition. Am. J. Med., 71:557–564, 1981.

95a. Halverson, P.B., and McCarty, D.J.: Patterns of radiographic abnormalities associated with basic calcium phosphate and calcium pyrophosphate dihydrate crystal deposition in the knee. Ann. Rheum. Dis., 45:603–605, 1986.

96. Ohno, O., and Cooke, T.D.: Electron microscopic morphology of immunoglobulin aggregates and their interaction in rheumatoid articular collagenous tissues. Arthritis Rheum., 21:516–517, 1978.

97. Utzinger, P.D., and Fite, F.L.: Immunologic evidence for inflammation (I) in osteoarthritis (OA): High percentage of Ia$^+$ T lymphocytes (L) in the synovial fluid (SL) and synovium (S) of patients with erosive osteoarthritis (EOA). Arthritis Rheum., 25:S44, 1982.

98. Singleton, P.T., Cervantes, A.G., and McKoy, J.: Sicca complex and erosive osteoarthritis: Immunologic implications of a new osteoarthritis subset. Arthritis Rheum., 25:S33, 1982.

99. Shuckett, R., Russell, M.L., and Gladman, D.D.: Atypical erosive osteoarthritis and Sjögren's syndrome. Ann. Rheum. Dis., 45:281–288, 1986.

100. Bahrt, K.M., Nashal, D.J., and Haber, G.: Diffuse idiopathic skeletal hyperostosis in a patient with situs inversus. Arthritis Rheum., 26:811–812, 1983.

101. Smith, C.F., Pugh, D.G., and Polley, H.F.: Physiologic vertebral ligamentous calcification: Aging process. Am. J. Roentgenol., 74:1049–1058, 1955.

102. Resnick, D., et al.: Diffuse idiopathic skeletal hyperostosis (DISH) [ankylosing hyperostosis of Forestier and Rotes-Querol]. Semin. Arthritis Rheum., 7:153–187, 1978.

103. Robbes-Ruy, E., Rojo-Mejia, A., Harrison-Garcin Calderon, J., and Discoya-Arbanil, J.: Diffuse idiopathic skeletal hyperostosis: Clinical and radiologic manifestations in 50 patients. Arthritis Rheum., 25:S101, 1982.

104. Littlejohn, G.O., and Smythe, H.A.: Marked hyperinsulinemia after glucose challenge in patients with diffuse idiopathic skeletal hyperostosis. J. Rheumatol., 8:965–968, 1981.

105. Littlejohn, G.O.: Insulin and new bone formation in diffuse idiopathic skeletal hyperostosis. Clin. Rheum., 4:294–300, 1985.

106. Shapiro, R., Utsinger, P.D., and Wiesner, K.B.: The association of HLA-B27 with Forestier's disease (vertebral ankylosing hyperostosis). J. Rheumatol., 3:4–8, 1976.

107. Spagnole, A., Bennett, P., and Terasaki, P.: Vertebral ankylosing hyperostosis (Forestier's disease) and HLA antigens in Pima Indians. Arthritis Rheum., 21:467–472, 1978.

108. Abiteboul, M., et al.: Hyperostose vertébral ankylosante et métabolisme de la vitamine A. Rev. Rhum., 9:8–9, 1981.

109. Pittsley, R.A., and Yoder, F.W.: Retinoid hyperostosis. N. Engl. J. Med., 308:1012–1025, 1983.

110. Di Giovanna, J.J., Helfgott, R.K., Gerber, H.L., and Peck, G.L.: Extraspinal tendon and ligament calcification associated with long-term therapy with etretinate. N. Engl. J. Med., 315:1177–1182, 1986.

111. Mills, D.M., et al.: Association of diffuse idiopathic skeletal hyperostosis and fluorosis (Abstract.) Arthritis Rheum., 26(Suppl.):S11, 1983.

112. Utsinger, P.D.: A clinical and laboratory analysis of 200 patients with DISH. Clin. Exp. Rheumatol. (in press).

113. Ono, K., et al.: Ossified posterior longitudinal ligament, a clinicopathologic study. Spine, 2:126–138, 1977.

114. Nilsson, B.E., Danielsson, L.G., and Hernborg, S.A.J.: Clinical feature and natural course of coxarthrosis and gonarthrosis. Scand. J. Rheumatol., 43(Suppl.):13–21, 1982.

115. Jorring, K.: Osteoarthritis of the hip. Epidemiology and clinical role. Acta Orthop. Scand., 51:523–530, 1980.

116. Edelman, J., and Owen, E.T.: Acute progressive osteoarthropathy of large joints: Report of three cases. J. Rheumatol., 8:482–485, 1981.

117. Keats, T.E., Johnstone, W.H., O'Brien, W.M.: Large joint destruction in erosive osteoarthritis. Skeletal Radiol., 6:267–269, 1981.

118. Bouvier, M., Bonvoisin, B., Colson, F., and David, P.H.: Les coxarthroses destructrices rapides. Etude radioclinique de neuf cas. Ann. Radiol., 28:549–553, 1985.

119. Moskowitz, R.W.: Use of nonsteroidal antiinflammatory drugs in rheumatology: A review. Semin. Arthritis Rheum., 15:1–10, 1986.

120. Ronningen, H., and Langeland, N.: Indomethacin treatment in osteoarthritis of the hip joint. Acta Orthop. Scand., 50:169–174, 1979.

121. Newman, N.M., and Ling, R.S.M.: Acetabular bone destruction related to non-steroidal anti-inflammatory drugs. Lancet, 2:11–13, 1985.

122. Palmoski, M.J., and Brandt, K.D.: Effect of some nonsteroidal anti-inflammatory drugs on proteoglycan metabolism and organization in canine articular cartilage. Arthritis Rheum., 23:1010–1020, 1980.

123. O'Brien, W.M., La Du, B.N., and Bunim, J.J.: Biochemical, pathologic and clinical aspects of alcaptonuria, ochronosis and ochronotic arthropathy: Review of world literature (1584–1962). Am. J. Med., 34:813–838, 1963.

124. Golding, D.N., Walshe, J.M.: Arthropathy of Wilson's disease: Study of clinical and radiological features in 32 patients. Ann. Rheum. Dis., 36:99–111, 1977.

125. Hamilton, E., et al.: Idiopathic hemochromatosis. Q. J. Med., 145:171–182, 1968.

126. Schumacher, H.R.: Articular cartilage in the degenerative arthropathy of hemochromatosis. Arthritis Rheum., 25:1460–1468, 1982.

127. Nesterov, A.I.: The clinical course of Kashin-Beck disease. Arthritis Rheum., 7:29–40, 1964.

127a. Wei, X.W., Wright, G.C., and Sokoloff, L.: The effect of sodium selenite on chondrocytes in monolayer culture. Arthritis Rheum., 29:660–664, 1986.

128. Bluestone, R., et al.: Acromegalic arthropathy. Ann. Rheum. Dis., 30:243–258, 1971.

129. Atkins, C.J., et al.: Chondrocalcinosis and arthropathy: Studies in haemochromatosis and in idiopathic chondrocalcinosis. Q. J. Med., 39:71–82, 1970.

130. Richards, A.J., and Hamilton, E.B.D.: Destructive arthropathy in chondrocalcinosis articularis. Ann. Rheum. Dis., 33:196–203, 1974.
131. Gerster, J.C., Vischer, T.L., and Fallet, G.H.: Destructive arthropathy in generalized osteoarthritis with articular chondrocalcinosis. J. Rheumatol., 2:265–269, 1975.
132. Hernborg, J., Linden, B., and Nilsson, B.O.E.: Chondrocalcinosis: A secondary finding in osteoarthritis of the knee. Geriatrics, 32:123–126, 1977.
133. Wilkins, E., Dieppe, P., Maddison, P., and Evison, G.: Osteoarthritis and articular chondrocalcinosis in the elderly. Ann. Rheum. Dis., 42:280–284, 1983.
134. Halverson, P.B., and McCarty, D.: Patterns of radiographic abnormalities associated with basic calcium phosphate and calcium pyrophosphate dihydrate crystal deposition in the knee. Ann. Rheum. Dis., 45:603–695, 1986.
135. McCarty, D.J., et al.: "Milwaukee shoulder"—Association of microspheroids containing hydroxyapatite crystals, active collagenase, and neutral proteases with rotator cuff defects. I. Clinical aspects. Arthritis Rheum., 24:464–473, 1981.
136. Halverson, P.G., et al.: "Milwaukee shoulder"—Association of microspheroids containing hydroxyapatite crystals, active collagenase, and neutral protease with rotator cuff defects. II. Synovial fluid studies. Arthritis Rheum., 24:474–483, 1981.
137. Halverson, P.B., et al.: Milwaukee shoulder syndrome: Eleven additional cases with involvement of the knee in seven (basic calcium phosphate crystal deposition disease). Semin. Arthritis Rheum., 14:36–44, 1984.
138. Charcot, J.M.: Sur quelques arthropathies qui paraissent dépendre d'une lésion du cerveau ou de la moelle épinière: arthrites dans l'hémiplégie de cause cérébrale. Arch. Physiol. Norm. Pathol., 2:379–400, 1868.
139. Gottlieb, N.L., and Risken, W.G.: Complications of local corticosteroid injections. JAMA, 243:1547–1548, 1980.
140. Moskowitz, R.W., et al.: Experimentally induced corticosteroid arthropathy. Arthritis Rheum., 13:236–243, 1970.
141. Glick, R., and Parhami, N.: Frostbite arthritis. J. Rheumatol., 6:456–460, 1979.

TREATMENT OF OSTEOARTHRITIS

103

KENNETH D. BRANDT

FITTING THE TREATMENT TO THE PATIENT

Management of the patient with osteoarthritis begins appropriately with an assessment of the goal of that individual's treatment program. Is it to relieve pain? To increase mobility? To prevent progression of disease in the involved joint? To reduce disability? Each of these aims is not equally relevant to all patients with osteoarthritis.

Obviously, success in attaining any of these objectives requires accurate analysis of the pathogenetic factors underlying the patient's problem. Patients with osteoarthritis are all different, and optimal management cannot be based on a "cookbook" approach to treatment. Is the patient's pain due to synovitis, periarticular muscle spasm, mechanical instability of the joint, or end-stage disease, with bone rubbing against bone? Or, is it perhaps due to bursitis, rather than to intra-articular disease? The type of treatment will be influenced by the answer.

Is loss of joint motion due to soft-tissue contracture or a restrictive osteophyte? Does sufficient cartilage remain on the osteoarthritic joint so that measures aimed at preventing further damage can be recommended? Or is the joint so badly destroyed that such measures will accomplish nothing? The approach to treatment cannot be the same in both cases.

Because disability is defined in terms of the handicapped person's ability to relate to his environment,[1] it is important to determine whether treatment will reduce the patient's handicap and thus enable him to deal more effectively with obstacles presented by his workplace or home. Additionally, perhaps the environment can be altered to lessen the consequences of the handicap.

Both patient and physician should understand what can and cannot be accomplished. The physician needs to know what the patient expects from treatment, and the patient needs to know if his expectations are realistic. Chances of successful management[2,3] and patient satisfaction[4] are greatest when the views of patient and physician about the importance of various facets of a treatment program are congruous.

For the individual with advanced disease and chronic pain and disability, especially in the hip or knee, an aggressive, multidisciplinary, comprehensive program of management is warranted.[5,6] On the other hand, for many patients with mild osteoarthritis, all that is required is reassurance that the disease is not likely to become generalized or crippling, instruction in principles of joint protection, and prescription of a mild analgesic. Such reassurance is important; patients with mild osteoarthritis involving only one or two joints often are greatly (and unnecessarily) concerned that they have a disease that will become more widespread and increasingly painful and limiting. They anticipate a life of pain, confinement, and dependency. Indeed, a recent survey of senior citizens in Indianapolis showed that some believe that osteoarthritis may be fatal.[7]

The preceding conservative management of the pa-

1631

tient with mild disease can be fully justified in view of the following considerations:

First, the drugs currently prescribed for treatment of osteoarthritis are analgesic and/or anti-inflammatory. Although they may provide effective symptomatic relief, they will not arrest or reverse the pathologic changes of the disease in articular cartilage or bone. Indeed, some may contribute to these changes.

Second, joint pain in individuals with osteoarthritis is often episodic and not necessarily crippling.[8] The natural history of osteoarthritis is not one of inevitable progression of pain or disability. Thus, although radiographic evidence of osteoarthritis of the knee was present in about 10% of those surveyed at age 50 and rose steadily thereafter so that it was present in about 50% at age 80, at all ages only about half of those with radiologic changes reported episodic knee pain.[8] However, few in any age group reported crippling knee pain, and the proportion of those with crippling pain showed no tendency to increase between ages 60 and 80.

Similarly, a recent study of nearly 700 elderly people surveyed for signs and symptoms suggestive of osteoarthritis of the knee indicated that neither the prevalence of these features nor their severity increased with age, but remained constant between the seventh and ninth decades.[9] A lack of progressive degeneration of the knee has been noted recently also in an autopsy study.[10] Patients with osteoarthritis of the hip may show no radiologic progression over years; in some cases joint space narrowing may even lessen.[11,12] Even in the face of radiologic progression, pain may diminish, although this is often accompanied by loss of mobility, associated with the development of buttressing osteophytes or fibrosis of the capsule. Similarly, a longitudinal radiologic analysis emphasizes the slow rate of progression of osteoarthritis of the hand, especially in proximal interphalangeal joints.[13]

DRUG THERAPY

ANALGESICS

Although articular cartilage lacks pain receptors, pain in osteoarthritis may arise from the fibrous capsule, the subchondral bone (due to microfractures or to venous congestion resulting from the remodeling of subchondral trabeculae),[14] periarticular muscle, or ligaments. Ligamentous sprains are common, especially in the unstable joint, and local pain receptors may become hypersensitive.[15]

In patients with osteoarthritis who have mild or intermittent pain without clinical evidence of inflammation (e.g., joint warmth, synovial effusion) an analgesic, taken as needed, and instruction in general measures of joint protection (see following discussion) may be all that are required for satisfactory symptomatic relief.

Acetylsalicylic acid (aspirin), in a dose of 650 mg every 4 to 6 hours, as needed, is an effective analgesic for many patients with osteoarthritis. At this dose, the drug has little or no anti-inflammatory effect.

Aspirin should always be taken with food. Even when taken with meals, however, as a buffered preparation, or with antacids, aspirin can produce dyspepsia. Enteric-coated aspirin, Zorprin (aspirin encapsulated in a special matrix to control its rate of release), or one of the nonacetylated salicylate preparations (e.g., Disalcid, Trilisate, Arthropan) cause less gastric distress than standard aspirin. Although enteric-coated aspirin has been criticized for years for lack of efficacy, the shellac coatings used formerly are no longer employed, and newer preparations dissolve more reliably and can provide excellent bioavailability of acetylsalicylic acid.[16]

Some individuals with osteoarthritis, because of dyspepsia or ototoxicity, are unable to tolerate salicylate in any form. For these patients, acetaminophen, 650 mg every 4 to 6 hours, as needed, or propoxyphene hydrochloride, 32 to 65 mg every 4 to 6 hours, as needed, provides comparable analgesia. Taken in excess, acetaminophen may cause toxic hepatitis. It is thus relatively contraindicated in patients with pre-existing liver disease.[17–19] Propoxyphene can cause drowsiness, lightheadedness, or gastrointestinal upset. *With chronic propoxyphene therapy, drug dependence can develop.* Codeine or other narcotics are rarely required in osteoarthritis. If used, they should be prescribed for only a brief period.

Recently, additional analgesics have been marketed that have been reported to be useful in osteoarthritis—naproxen sodium (Anaprox) and several preparations of ibuprofen that are available over-the-counter (e.g., Advil, Medipren, Nuprin). They may provide more effective analgesia than aspirin, with a somewhat longer duration of action. These are all nonsteroidal anti-inflammatory drugs (NSAIDs), which inhibit the cyclo-oxygenase pathway of arachidonate metabolism. In the patient who is also taking salicylate or another cyclo-oxygenase inhibitor, their analgesic effect can be less obvious than when they are given alone. Furthermore, because undesirable side effects, such as gastric irritation or renal insufficiency (see following discussion), can be additive, naproxen sodium or over-the-counter preparations of ibuprofen should not be taken concurrently with aspirin or other cyclo-oxygenase inhibitors.[20]

ANTI-INFLAMMATORY DRUGS

Synovial inflammation, although usually much less intense than that seen, for example, in rheumatoid arthritis (RA), occurs in osteoarthritis and may contribute significantly to the patient's pain. Hence, some patients with osteoarthritis exhibit greater preference for anti-inflammatory drugs than for comparably analgesic agents that lack anti-inflammatory properties.[21] Thus, if the patient's pain is not alleviated by an analgesic, or if signs of joint inflammation (e.g., warmth, effusion) are present, an anti-inflammatory dose of a cyclo-oxygenase inhibitor is indicated.

In the elderly, ototoxicity may develop with a relatively low salicylate dose, precluding maintenance therapy with anti-inflammatory levels of *any* salicylate preparation in some patients. Furthermore, the older patient may develop gastrointestinal upset from salicylate more readily than the younger individual.

Several NSAIDs currently available in the United States (fenoprofen, ibuprofen, indomethacin, meclofenamic acid, naproxen, piroxicam, sodium tolmetin, sulindac) are effective in osteoarthritis. The average daily dose for treatment of osteoarthritis is often only one half, or less, of that required for treatment of RA. Because these agents are generally well tolerated and tend to produce dyspepsia less frequently than aspirin, a strong case may be made that they should be the first choice when anti-inflammatory therapy is elected for the patient with osteoarthritis. They are, however, considerably more expensive than aspirin.

Because gastrointestinal and neurologic side effects are more frequent with indomethacin than with the other agents mentioned here, it should be considered separately. Indomethacin may produce dyspepsia and peptic ulcer, headache, depression, and a variety of other symptoms of central nervous system (CNS) dysfunction, including muzziness (altered sensory perception).

Despite these limitations of higher doses of indomethacin, a low dose (e.g., 25 to 50 mg) is usually well tolerated and, if taken at bedtime, may be particularly helpful for patients with nocturnal pain. A newly available sustained-release formulation of indomethacin appears to produce fewer side effects than the standard preparation and provides a much longer therapeutic effect.

Salicylate and all other cyclo-oxygenase inhibitors are relatively contraindicated in the patient with peptic ulcer disease. All of these agents affect platelet aggregation to some extent, although the inhibition of platelet function by NSAIDs other than aspirin is reversible and may be less profound clinically than the irreversible inhibition of platelet cyclo-oxygenase caused by aspirin. In the patient who is at particular risk of bleeding, nonacetylated salicylate preparations, which have no effect on platelets, may be preferable to the preceding agents.

Certain risk factors (e.g., cardiac decompensation, cirrhosis and ascites, administration of diuretics, clinically apparent renal disease)[22] are clearly associated with the development of reversible renal insufficiency in patients taking NSAIDs. Even in the osteoarthritic patient who exhibits none of these risk factors, age alone—presumably because of the presence of subclinical glomerulosclerosis[23]—can cause renal blood flow to depend on local prostaglandin production and hence to be vulnerable to the effects of cyclo-oxygenase inhibitors.[22] In such cases, serum creatinine and urea nitrogen concentrations can rise rapidly after initiation of treatment. The serum potassium concentration can also rise, occasionally to alarming levels, reflecting inhibition of the renin-angiotensin-aldosterone mechanism.[24,25] Body weight may increase because of fluid retention, which may precipitate congestive heart failure.

Phenylbutazone (which is *not* a cyclo-oxygenase inhibitor) is a potent anti-inflammatory agent and may be very effective in providing symptomatic relief in acute flare-ups of osteoarthritis. When it is given for only brief periods, its ulcerogenic potential is usually not a concern. However, it may cause fluid retention, potentiate the action of coumadin derivatives, and enhance the activity of oral hypoglycemic agents. Thus, it may cause problems, particularly in the elderly patient with osteoarthritis, who often provides a fertile milieu for drug interactions.

Notably, the agranulocytosis and aplastic anemia associated with phenylbutazone, although uncommon, may be idiosyncratic and thus unrelated to the dose or duration of treatment. The risk of serious side effects with this agent, and the availability of the alternative compounds mentioned previously (which, although somewhat less potent are clearly less toxic), markedly limit the role of phenylbutazone in treatment of osteoarthritis. Its use in acute attacks of osteoarthritis should be considered only after other therapeutic measures have been tried and found to be inadequate.

It is worth considering that all of the cyclo-oxygenase inhibitors described previously were designed principally for use as anti-inflammatory compounds for patients with RA, without consideration of the pathophysiology of osteoarthritis. Recently, attempts have been made to develop drugs for treatment of osteoarthritis that take into account our current understanding of the mechanisms of cartilage damage in this disease.[26] Thus, compounds that stimulate chondrocyte metabolism or inhibit enzymes capable of degrading articular cartilage matrix have become available, for example, glycosaminoglycan sulfate peptide (Rumalon) and glycosamine sulfate polypeptide (Arteparon). Some of these have achieved a certain amount of popularity, particularly in Europe. In experimentally induced osteoarthritis, Arteparon diminished the severity of the morphologic changes in the articular cartilage, even when instituted following their initiation.[27] In a long-term study of a large number of patients treated in Czechoslovakia with glycosaminoglycan sulfate peptide, it was concluded that such therapy retarded radiographically observed disease progression and resulted in less frequent orthopedic intervention.[28] The study, however, was neither blinded nor adequately controlled. Unfortunately, no "chondroprotective" drug has yet been shown in a well-designed controlled study to alter the natural history of osteoarthritis in man. This area of research can be expected to receive much more attention over the next few years.

Can anti-inflammatory drugs aggravate osteoarthritis? A retrospective radiographic analysis of osteoarthritis of the hip suggested that indomethacin administration may be associated with greater joint destruction than that seen in controls.[29] It is conceivable that the symptomatic relief produced by indomethacin (and, perhaps, also by other analgesic or anti-inflammatory drugs) leads to greater usage of the affected joint, inciting further damage. In addition, agents that inhibit prostaglandin synthetase (cyclooxygenase) can interfere with the repair of microfractures in subchondral bone.[30] This could account for the radiologic evidence of increased subchondral cyst formation and joint destruction observed in patients treated with indomethacin.[29] However, in a carefully studied series of 17 patients with hip roentgenograms typical of analgesic arthropathy, no evidence implicated NSAIDs in the development of the disease.[31]

In vitro studies employing organ cultures of normal canine articular cartilage have shown that salicylates[32] and several other NSAIDs that inhibit prostaglandin synthetase[33] can suppress proteoglycan biosynthesis. Not all prostaglandin synthetase inhibitors exhibited this effect, however; diclofenac, indomethacin, piroxicam, and sulindac sulfide did not significantly reduce proteoglycan metabolism under identical experimental conditions.

Notably, the suppressive effect of salicylate in the preceding in vitro studies was much greater in osteoarthritic cartilage—where basal levels of proteoglycan synthesis are increased three- to fivefold—than in normal cartilage.[34] Furthermore, it did not reflect a general toxic effect on the chondrocyte, because net protein synthesis was unaffected by salicylate concentrations that markedly suppressed proteoglycan synthesis. Presumably, this effect of salicylate is due to inhibition of enzymes involved in the early stages of chondroitin sulfate synthesis (e.g., UDP glucose dehydrogenase, which is required for conversion of UDP-glucose to UDP-glucuronic acid).[35]

Recent evidence indicates that salicylate can inhibit proteoglycan metabolism in articular cartilage in vivo as well as in vitro.[36,37] Thus, feeding aspirin in reasonable doses to dogs developing osteoarthritis[36] or to dogs in whom articular cartilage atrophy was being induced by immobilization of the ipsilateral limb[37] aggravated the degeneration of articular cartilage. Salicylate had no apparent in vivo effect on normal articular cartilage.

The effect of salicylate on degenerating cartilage in vivo is related to the proteoglycan concentration of the matrix and the resultant decrease in the fixed negative charge density of the glycosaminoglycans, which permits greater diffusion of the weakly anionic NSAIDs into the cartilage.[38,39] There is no evidence that the osteoarthritic chondrocyte is inherently more susceptible to the effects of these drugs on proteoglycan metabolism.[40]

Furthermore, the effects of these agents on proteoglycan metabolism can be unrelated to their actions on prostaglandin biosynthesis.[41] Notably, the in vitro data suggest that differences among various NSAIDs regarding their effects on joint cartilage may be related to differences in the synovial fluid concentration of the various agents. This, in turn, is related to the dose administered, which is based on the clinical potency of the drug.

While these experimental data are interesting, it is important to note that they have been derived only from studies in animals. While they suggest the possibility that chronic administration of salicylates and, perhaps, other NSAIDs may be injurious to articular cartilage in arthritic joints, the effects of these drugs on the pathophysiology of human osteoarthritic joints cannot confidently be deduced from these animal data. A 2-year clinical trial comparing naproxen with acetaminophen has been undertaken in an attempt to examine this issue. Whether the drop-out rate will be sufficiently low to permit meaningful conclusions from this trial remains to be seen.

ADRENAL CORTICOSTEROIDS

There is no place for systemic corticosteroids or adrenal corticotrophic hormones in the management of osteoarthritis. The side effects associated with prolonged use of these agents outweigh any potential benefits.

Intra-articular injection of adrenal corticosteroids, however, may be helpful. Hollander, in a review of nearly 1000 patients with osteoarthritis of the knee who were treated over a 9-year period with repeated intra-articular steroid injections, as needed, found that nearly 60% became sufficiently free of pain so as to require no further injections, and about 20% achieved sufficient temporary benefit so that they continued to receive intra-articular injections, while the remainder did not benefit from the treatment or had been lost to follow-up.[42] These data must be judged against the results of other studies, which have shown similar benefits following a single injection of procaine,[43] saline,[43] or the suspending vehicle.[44] Furthermore, pain relief following intra-articular steroid injection is usually temporary. For example, by 4 weeks following injection, the response of patients receiving an intra-articular steroid injection may be indistinguishable from that of controls.[45]

Although some evidence suggests that intra-articular corticosteroid injections lessen the severity of the pathologic changes of osteoarthritis in experimental animals,[46,47] no such evidence exists in man. On the other hand, amelioration of pain may lead to overuse of the damaged joint, aggravating the breakdown of cartilage. Furthermore, corticosteroids can cause direct cartilage injury. Thus, repeated injections of corticosteroid into the joints of normal rabbits depressed biosynthesis of collagen and proteoglycans[48] and caused cartilage degeneration.[49] Although little histologic change occurred in non-weight-bearing joints, fibrillation and cystic degeneration were prominent in weight-bearing cartilage. For the preceding reasons, intra-articular steroids should generally be used at intervals not more frequent than 4 to 6 months for a given joint. In addition, on the basis of the preceding evidence it appears prudent *to caution the patient to minimize joint loading for some time after an intra-articular steroid injection.* Notably, injection of corticosteroids into ligaments and painful pericapsular sites often produces excellent symptomatic relief in patients with osteoarthritis and is not associated with the potential hazards of intra-articular injection.*

REDUCTION OF JOINT LOADING

Analysis of the vocational and avocational demands imposed on the arthritic joint is an integral part of the

Editor's note. I have not found intra-articular corticosteroid injections very useful in treating osteoarthritis, especially in weight-bearing joints.

patient's evaluation, and joint usage must be taken into account in designing the treatment program. Indeed, the pattern of usage may have influenced the development of osteoarthritis. Activities that lead to excessive loading of the involved joint should be avoided where possible. Rest periods, for 30 to 60 minutes in the morning and afternoon, may help reduce pain in lower extremity joints or lumbar spine. Activities requiring loading of the diseased joint should be fractionated, rather than performed in a sustained fashion. Several shorter periods of standing or walking are preferable to a single prolonged period for the patient with osteoarthritis of the weight-bearing joints in the lower extremity.

The patient might consider recommendations for modification of his activities in the workplace to be impractical. One of the goals of treatment should be to assist him to maximize his potential for employment. This requires, as an initial step, assessment of his functional capacity. Occupational and physical therapists may provide valuable input regarding the amount and type of work the patient can perform and the feasible type of employment.

In many instances, the solution to employment problems may be simple, for example, having the patient use principles of joint protection or modify the pace of his work. In some cases, it may be helpful for the physician or another health care professional to contact the patient's employer to discuss desirable modifications of the workplace. Some patients may benefit by referral to a state department of vocational rehabilitation for job counseling, retraining, aid in establishing an independent business, and/or assistance in seeking further formal education. It is incumbent on the physician to inform the vocational rehabilitation counselor about the patient's limitations, diagnosis, and other relevant factors.

In some cases, poor body mechanics may be etiologic in the development of osteoarthritis; in others, they are an aggravating factor. Poor posture should be corrected. Supports are useful for the excessively lordotic lumbar spine or for the pendulous abdomen or breasts. Pronated feet and varus and valgus deformities of the knee, all of which create excessive loading on the tibiofemoral joint, can be corrected with orthotics or by osteotomy. A cane (which should be held in the contralateral hand) is helpful if hip or knee involvement is unilateral. If involvement is bilateral, a pair of crutches or a walker is preferable.

Obesity contributes to the excessive loading of articular cartilage. It may aggravate symptoms and possibly accelerate cartilage breakdown in the lumbar spine and joints of the lower extremity.

In the Framingham study, obesity was associated

with osteoarthritis of the knee, even when the obesity antedated radiologic evaluation by more than 20 years.[50] The United States Health and Nutrition Examination Survey (HANES) found an association between obesity and osteoarthritis of the hands and knees, but not of the hips or ankles.[51]

Whether weight reduction by the obese patient with osteoarthritis will lead to a reduction in joint pain or retard joint breakdown has not been examined in a controlled fashion. Nonetheless, it is reasonable to recommend that the obese osteoarthritic patient adhere to a weight reduction diet. Such patients often find weight loss difficult to achieve, however, because of the degree of inactivity imposed by their disease. Participation in a mutual support group (e.g., Weight Watchers, TOPS) may be helpful.

PHYSICAL THERAPY

The recommendation to the patient to reduce usage of an osteoarthritic joint to minimize wear-and-tear may not be accepted readily because of the patient's concern that the joint will become stiffer unless it is used. Some of this concern arises because the patient with osteoarthritis, especially in a lower extremity joint, may experience a sensation of gelling in the involved joint following periods of inactivity (e.g., an automobile trip or airplane ride). Putting the involved joint through its range of motion intermittently during such periods of inactivity will minimize gelling. Informing the patient that prescribed exercises are important and are an integral component of his treatment program will reassure some individuals who balk at a recommendation to curtail activities that stress the diseased joints.

Physical therapy is an indispensable component of the treatment plan for most patients with osteoarthritis. It involves, principally, the use of heat or cold and an exercise program tailored to the individual.

Usually, it is helpful to precede each exercise session with application of moderate heat for 15 to 20 minutes to relieve joint pain and diminish stiffness. Liniment should be removed from the skin before application of heat, and the patient should be instructed to avoid lying on the heat source, because this may impede skin blood flow, leading to a burn. A variety of modalities are available, such as electric pads, paraffin baths, hydrocolator packs, ultrasonography, diathermy, and infrared bakers. Practicality and cost should be considered. Often, in selecting the heat modality, the view that "the simpler the better" is best. Many patients find moist heat more effective than dry heat; a warm bath or shower may prove to

be the most convenient form of providing heat to the involved joint. For deep-seated joints (e.g., hips, spine), ultrasonography or diathermy can be especially helpful, although they often provide no greater benefit than cheaper, simpler methods. Occasionally, the patient's pain may be aggravated by use of heat, and ice packs will provide more effective analgesia.

The exercise program is designed to preserve or improve range of motion and strengthen periarticular muscles. Periarticular muscle atrophy is common in osteoarthritis, probably because of decreased activity.[52] Isometric exercises, which minimize joint stress, are preferable to isotonic exercises.

For the patient with lower extremity involvement who requires an ambulatory aid (e.g., cane, crutches, walker), consultation with a physical therapist is desirable. The therapist may assist with education of the patient concerning the mechanical advantage to be derived from the device, oversee a trial usage to permit the patient to experience the pain relief that it will afford, and help ensure that the patient is using the assistive device correctly. The physical therapist can also assist the physician in educating the patient about principles of joint protection.

ORTHOPEDIC SURGERY

For patients with advanced disease who have intractable pain or significantly impaired function, orthopedic surgery may be extremely helpful. For example, tibial or femoral osteotomy in the patient with genu varum or valgum and osteoarthritis of the knee may be of great value, especially when the disease is only moderately advanced (see Chapter 54). Osteotomy may produce excellent pain relief by altering stresses of loading and creating a more normal alignment of the opposing cartilage surfaces. Debridement of the joint, with removal of free cartilage fragments (joint mice), may prevent locking, eliminate pain, and reduce the wear of joint surfaces. Resection of large osteophytes may also improve the range of motion but may accelerate the breakdown of articular cartilage.

In advanced disease, arthroplasty or arthrodesis may be required. Both generally can be expected to provide relief of pain; often, arthroplasty will also improve the range of motion. Arthrodesis is generally not indicated in weight-bearing joints, such as the hip or knee. However, in patients whose future activities will necessitate heavy usage of the diseased joint, arthroplasty is associated with a high failure rate, so that arthrodesis may be preferable even though it eliminates joint motion permanently.

TREATMENT OF OSTEOARTHRITIS IN SPECIFIC JOINTS

THE HAND

The patient with osteoarthritis in the first carpometacarpal joint may be afforded considerable symptomatic relief by an occasional intra-articular injection of corticosteroids. A simple hand splint, which immobilizes the first carpometacarpal and the metacarpophalangeal joint of the thumb, will often reduce pain during activity.[53] In more severe cases, with pain unresponsive to the above measures, arthroplasty or arthrodesis may be indicated. Arthroplasty will permit retention of motion but will result in subnormal grip strength. Arthrodesis will provide excellent grip strength but will eliminate motion.

In many patients, Heberden's nodes develop insidiously and asymptomatically and are of no consequence. In some individuals, however, they develop rapidly and are associated with localized swelling, erythema, acute pain, and marked tenderness. Such patients often require reassurance that they do not have a crippling form of arthritis or a disease that is likely to become more generalized. They are grateful for reassurance that their nodes will eventually become painless and present minimal disability. For relief of pain from Heberden's nodes, heat (hot soaks, paraffin baths, contrast baths, electric pads, etc.) is usually helpful. Analgesics or NSAIDs may be useful. Occasionally, local injection of a corticosteroid preparation into or around the joint may be of benefit, especially when the node is acutely inflamed. Trauma to the hands, which may exacerbate the pain and aggravate the deformity, should be avoided.

Instruction of the patient in measures to reduce stress on the involved joints is important. Often, the occupational therapist can provide a useful analysis of the patient's activities of daily living and recommend measures to minimize joint trauma during such activities. Nylon-spandex stretch gloves, used at night, may relieve pain and stiffness in patients with osteoarthritis of the interphalangeal joints.[54]

THE FOOT

Osteoarthritis of the metatarsophalangeal joint of the great toe is a common problem. It produces pain, limits mobility, and causes bony enlargement, because of proliferation of osteophytes at the joint margins. In patients with only mild or moderate discomfort, metatarsal pads, or metatarsal bars may be helpful. Use of metal to stiffen the sole of the shoe to minimize dorsiflexion of the joint with walking may also be useful.* Inflammation of the bursa medial to the first metatarsophalangeal joint may be treated effectively by a local steroid injection. If these measures are ineffective, surgery may be required.

Osteoarthritis of the subtalar joint is often resistant to the preceding general measures. When pain is aggravated by weight-bearing, a cane or crutches may be helpful. Triple arthrodesis may be indicated in patients with severe disease of the subtalar joint.

THE KNEE

A program of analgesic or anti-inflammatory medication, heat, and prescribed exercises, periods of rest, and adherence to principles of joint protection will often provide effective relief of pain and stiffness in the patient with osteoarthritis of the knee. If the patient is obese, as is often the case, weight reduction is indicated. Other measures to decrease joint loading should also be recommended. For example, jogging and participation in racket sports should be discouraged. Swimming or cycling are excellent alternatives. The patient should be advised to avoid stairs whenever possible and, in general, to sit rather than stand. Use of a high stool will be helpful if the patient is required to work at a counter. Chairs with high seats should be used rather than low sofas. The patient should avoid kneeling or squatting. He should be instructed *not to sleep with pillows placed behind the knees,* because this may lead to flexion contractures. Isometric quadriceps exercises should be prescribed. Knee cages (hinged braces that lace up the front) or elastic supports may increase stability.

Often, the patient with knee osteoarthritis may complain of knee pain caused by anserine bursitis. In this case, injection of a depot corticosteroid preparation into the area of the bursa will often eliminate the discomfort. In flare-ups of the joint disease, with increased pain, warmth, tenderness, effusion, elimination of weight-bearing by bed rest or temporary use of an assistive device (e.g., a cane) is indicated. Aspiration of a knee effusion, if present, and an intra-articular injection of corticosteroid may also be beneficial.

In advanced cases, surgery may be warranted. Total knee arthroplasty has not, in general, enjoyed a success rate as high as that of total hip arthroplasty. Nonetheless, in many patients it can afford excellent pain relief, increase mobility, and enhance function.

Editor's note. Use of well-padded jogging shoes is often very helpful in this situation.

THE HIP

Measures to reduce loading of the involved joint should be considered an integral component of the treatment program. A cane, crutch, or walker should be recommended if the patent has pain with ambulation. The obese patient should be encouraged to reduce. Principles of joint protection should be outlined. Those described here for patients with osteoarthritis of the knee are equally applicable to the patient with hip osteoarthritis. Rest periods, heat, analgesics, NSAIDs, and isometric exercises to strengthen the supporting muscles in the lower extremity, as well as exercises to maintain normal range of hip motion, are indicated. Flexion contractures may be prevented, and mild ones corrected, by having the patient lie prone for 30 minutes two or three times daily. Elevated toilet seats will be helpful for the patient who has difficulty with a low commode. If muscle spasm is severe, traction may be required. Because capsular fibrosis is a significant cause of loss of motion in patients with hip osteoarthritis, exercises to strengthen adduction, extension, and external rotation are indicated. Intra-articular injections of corticosteroid may be helpful during flare-ups.

For the patient with severe disease who is a candidate for surgery, total hip arthroplasty is generally the procedure of choice. In most instances, it will provide pain relief and will restore hip motion. Intertrochanteric osteotomy may also be very effective.[55,56] However, later, conversion to total hip replacement may not be technically feasible, limiting the role of this procedure.

THE SPINE

Pain from osteoarthritis of the cervical spine may also respond to local heat and analgesics and/or NSAIDs (see also Chapter 90). If acute muscle spasm or evidence of nerve root irritation is present, a cervical collar may be helpful. Severe muscle spasm or nerve root compression may require traction. To decrease stress on the cervical spine, the patient should avoid postures in which the neck is maintained in a fixed position for prolonged periods, as with shampooing, sitting near the screen in a movie theater, or watching television while lying on a sofa. For patients with neurologic complications that do not respond to the above measures, surgery may be indicated.

Pain from osteoarthritis of the lumbar spine also will generally respond to heat, rest, and analgesics and/or NSAIDs. Adherence to joint protection principles is particularly important. In general, patients should avoid leaning over a desk or work surface for prolonged periods. When driving a car they may find it helpful to move the seat forward sufficiently so that the knees are flexed and lumbar lordosis diminished. A lumbosacral corset with abdominal support, and weight reduction if the patient is obese, are advisable. A firm mattress or a board placed beneath the mattress is often helpful.* Local heat, massage, or muscle relaxants can be employed to relieve spasm. An exercise program to strengthen the anterior abdominal muscles and correct faulty posture should be instituted after acute symptoms subside. Surgery, such as laminectomy, discectomy, or fusion, may be indicated when symptoms are severe or neurologic deficits occur.

MANAGEMENT OF PSYCHOSOCIAL PROBLEMS

EMOTIONAL ISSUES

Osteoarthritis, by imposing loss of mobility, function, and independence, often causes major changes in life-style. To the extent that the patient's identity depends on his body-image, major impairment of physical function can result also in a loss of self-esteem. Notably, patients with osteoarthritis have been found to be less satisfied with their present life than patients undergoing renal dialysis.[57] The emotional reactions to these losses of mobility and independence experienced by people with osteoarthritis are similar to those of people with other chronic illness,[58] and include denial, depression, and anger.

Denial serves as a buffer against threatening information, such as the initial diagnosis of arthritis. It is marked by the patient's tendency to minimize the severity of the symptoms, the chronicity of the disease, and/or the importance of following medical recommendations. It may lead the patient to "shop around" for an alternative diagnosis or to search for a miracle cure through quackery.

The denying patient should be approached supportively. Questions about disease management and prognosis should be answered truthfully but with only minimal detail. Because the denying patient may have a limited ability to absorb information about his treatment, the physician should be prepared to repeat his instructions during subsequent appointments.

As the patient with osteoarthritis recognizes the full impact of his situation and the extent of his limita-

Editor's note. A waterbed can provide dramatic symptomatic relief in these patients.

tions, depression may develop. Mild, temporary depression should be considered normal. Low self-esteem is a factor in depression, and the patient may believe he has nothing of value to contribute to others. In addition, isolation and withdrawal are characteristic at this stage. Regression may also occur and is evidenced by dependent behavior.

Because the depressed patient may be unable to relate to the hope of future improvement, immediate positive feedback is more appropriate than discussion of the long-term goals of treatment. To counteract the patient's low self-esteem, the physician might encourage him to emphasize valuable traits that are not affected by the disease, for example, "You may no longer be able to climb the steps in the football stadium, but your terrific tenor voice can still enhance the church choir." Isolation from others should be discouraged. If depression is severe or interferes with function, antidepressant drugs are indicated.

The realization that a "quick cure" does not exist may lead to anger, which may be projected toward physically healthy people. Other patients may blame God or fate, saying, "Why me?" If anger is not expressed openly, it may be manifested indirectly through passive-aggressive, manipulative behavior.

Before a meaningful discussion of treatment can begin, it may be necessary to allow the patient to ventilate feelings of anger. Focusing on the patient's feelings is often preferable to reacting to the content of a hostile comment. When confronted with a patient who is angry about his slow improvement, for example, a response such as "What you are really telling me is that you are very concerned about your future" may be more helpful than a lecture concerning the nature of the patient's medications. Passive-aggressive patients, who manifest their anger by refusing to comply with treatment plans, failing to keep appointments, and so on, should be confronted, and the feelings behind their behavior should be discussed.

SEXUALITY

Sexuality is a normal lifetime phenomenon. Disease and disability do not preclude sexual needs.[59] Because patients are often reluctant to express sexual concerns, it may be incumbent on the physician to initiate a discussion of sexual functioning. This can be accomplished as a component of the physical examination, as the physician ascertains the impact of the disease on other aspects of function. For example, during the hip examination the physician may include such questions as "Can you raise and lower yourself from a toilet seat? Can you climb a flight of stairs? Can you engage comfortably in sexual intercourse?"

Because of mechanical problems, sexuality may be particularly problematic for patients with osteoarthritis of the hips, knees, or spine. In a survey of 121 patients with osteoarthritis of the hip, 67% expressed sexual difficulties, the most frequent of which were joint pain (40%) and stiffness (75%).[60] For the patient with reduced mobility or joint pain, a side-by-side position for intercourse may be most comfortable. Approaches to the assessment and management of sexual problems in the elderly have been recently reviewed.[61] In addition, the Arthritis Foundation's patient education pamphlet, "Living and Loving with Arthritis," describes a variety of sexual problems and provides suggestions for their solution.[62]

FINANCIAL ASPECTS

Financial concerns may lead patients with osteoarthritis to refuse certain treatment recommendations. If the patient is unable to work and ineligible for retirement benefits, disability benefits may be obtained through the Social Security Administration. Patients with osteoarthritis may be eligible for Social Security Disability or Supplemental Security Income (SSI) Disability benefits if their disabling condition is expected to last for at least 12 months and if they are unable to engage in any substantial gainful employment. Laboratory and radiographic findings, functional ability, age, and educational and vocational background all may be considered in determining the patient's eligibility. The Social Security Administration provides a booklet for physicians that describes in detail the medical criteria used to assess the extent of disability.[63] To reduce the likelihood that patients who are legitimately disabled by osteoarthritis will be denied disability benefits, the physician must provide the Society Security Administration specific information about the claimant's ability to perform work-related tasks and must document the patient's objective clinical findings.[64]

Patients who have received Social Security Disability benefits for 2 years, or who are age 65 or over, may receive Medicare benefits. With the exception of the deductible and certain copayments, Medicare hospital insurance (Part A) pays the "allowable" charges (based on the average cost of the services provided in the locale) for inpatient hospital care, including physical and occupational therapy, laboratory tests and roentgenograms, posthospitalization skilled home health care. Medicare medical insurance (Part B) pays the allowable charges for physician services and outpatient treatment, including diagnostic tests and procedures, roentgenograms, drugs that cannot be self-administered, durable medical equipment, physical and occupational therapy, and skilled home health care. Medicare will *not* pay, however, for drugs that can be self-administered, patient education, or orthopedic shoes, unless they are a component of a leg brace.

Patients who are "medically indigent," that is, whose income beyond a certain subsistence allowance is less than their medical expenses, may qualify for Medicaid (MedCal in California). This is administered by county departments of human services or departments of welfare or public assistance. Although the services paid for by Medicaid vary from state to state, this program generally pays for a large proportion of a wide variety of medical expenses, for example, hospital and outpatient care, prescribed medication, home care, nursing home care, and transportation to health care providers. A recent review emphasizes the special problems of older adults with arthritis, and the governmental and private resources available to elderly arthritis patients, and details the physical, financial, and social barriers to appropriate treatment that exist for this growing segment of the population.[65]

REFERENCES

1. World Health Organization: Technical Report No. 419. Geneva, World Health Organization, 1969.
2. Starfield, B., et al.: Patient-doctor agreement about problems: Influence on outcome for care. JAMA, 242:344–346, 1979.
3. Starfield, B., et al.: The influence of patient–practitioner agreement on outcome of care. Am. J. Pub. Health, 71:127–131, 1981.
4. Larsen, D.E.: Physician role performance and patient satisfaction. Soc. Sci. Med., 10:29–32, 1976.
5. Pigg, J.S.: Presentation at the Forum on Arthritis Research and Education in Nursing and Allied Health, National Arthritis Advisory Board, Washington, D.C., 1980.
6. Gross, M., et al.: Team care for patients with chronic rheumatic disease. J. Allied Health, 11:239–247, 1982.
7. Potts, M., Yngve, D.N., Weinberger, M., and Brandt, K.D.: Educational needs of ambulatory arthritics attending senior citizens centers. Clin. Rheum. Pract., 1:255–259, 1983.
8. Kellgren, J.H., and Lawrence, J.S.: Osteoarthrosis and disc degeneration in an urban population. Ann. Rheum. Dis., 17:388–397, 1958.
9. Forman, M.D., Malamet, R., and Kaplan, D.: A survey of osteoarthritis of the knee in the elderly. J. Rheum., 10:282–287, 1983.
10. Casscells, S.W.: Gross pathological changes in the knee joint of the aged individual. Clin. Orthop., 132:225–232, 1978.
11. Danielsson, L.: Incidence and prognosis of coxarthrosis. Acta Orthop Scand. [Suppl.], 66:9–87, 1964.
12. Seifert, M.H., Whiteside, C.G., and Savage, O.: A 5 year follow-up of fifty cases of idiopathic osteoarthritis of the hip. Ann. Rheum. Dis., 28:325–326, 1969.
13. Plato, C.C., and Norris, A.H.: Osteoarthritis of the hand: Longitudinal studies. Am. J. Epidemiol., 110:740–746, 1979.
14. Lempberg, R.K., and Arnoldi, C.C.: The significance of intraosseous pressure in normal and diseased states with special reference to intraosseous engorgement pain syndrome. Clin. Orthop., 136:143–156, 1978.
15. Kellgren, J.H.: Some painful joint conditions and their relation to osteoarthritis. Clin. Sci., 4:193–201, 1939.
16. Orozlo-Alcala, J.J., and Baum, J.: Regular and enteric coated aspirin: A reevaluation. Arthritis Rheum., 22:1034–1037, 1979.
17. Ameer, B., and Greenblatt, D.J.: Acetaminophen. Ann. Intern. Med., 87:202–209, 1977.
18. Barker, J.D., deCarle, D.J., and Anuras, S.: Chronic excessive acetaminophen use and liver damage. Ann. Intern. Med., 87:299–301, 1977.
19. Johnson, G.K., and Tolman, K.G.: Chronic liver disease and acetaminophen. Ann. Intern. Med., 87:302–304, 1977.
20. Brandt, K.: Warning: Over-the-counter ibuprofen as an analgesic in patients with arthritis. Indiana Med., 78:37, 1985.
21. Doyle, D.V., Dieppe, P.A., Scott, J., and Huskisson, E.C.: An articular index for the assessment of osteoarthritis. Ann. Rheum. Dis., 40:75–78, 1981.
22. Blackshear, J.L., Davidman, M., and Stillman, T.: Identification of risk for renal insufficiency from nonsteroidal anti-inflammatory drugs. Arch. Intern. Med., 143:1130–1134, 1983.
23. Kaplan, C., et al.: Age-related incidence of sclerotic glomeruli in human kidneys. Am. J. Pathol., 80:227–234, 1975.
24. Tan, S.A.Y., et al.: Indomethacin-induced prostaglandin inhibition with hyperkalemia. Ann. Intern. Med., 90:783–785, 1979.
25. Galler, M., Folkert, V.W., and Schlondorff, D.: Reversible acute renal insufficiency and hyperkalemia following indomethacin therapy. JAMA, 246:154–155, 1981.
26. Fife, R., and Brandt, K.: Experimental modes of therapy in osteoarthritis. In Osteoarthritis Diagnosis and Management. Edited by R.W. Moskowitz, D.S. Howell, V.M. Goldberg, and H.J. Mankin. Philadelphia, W.B. Saunders, 1984, pp. 549–559.
27. Howell, D.S., Carreno, M.R., Pelletier, J.-P., and Muniz, O.E.: Articular cartilage breakdown in a lapine model of osteoarthritis. Clin. Orthop., 213:69–76, 1986.
28. Rejholec, V.: Long-term studies of antiosteoarthritic drugs: an assessment. Semin. Arthritis Rheum., 17(2)(Suppl. 11):35–53, 1987.
29. Ronninger, H., and Langeland, N.: Indomethacin treatment in osteoarthritis of the hip joint. Does the treatment inferfere with the natural course of the disease? Acta Orthop. Scand., 50:169–174, 1979.
30. Doherty, M., et al.: Reappraisal of analgesic hip. Ann. Rheum. Dis., 45:272–276, 1986.
31. Sudmann, E., Dregelia, E., Bessesen, A., and Morland, J.: Inhibition of fracture healing by indomethacin in rats. Eur. J. Clin. Invest., 9:333–339, 1979.
32. Palmoski, M., and Brandt, K.: Effects of salicylate on proteoglycan metabolism in normal canine articular cartilage *in vitro*. Arthritis Rheum., 22:746–754, 1979.
33. Palmoski,M., and Brandt, K.: Effects of some nonsteroidal anti-inflammatory drugs on articular cartilage proteoglycan metabolism and organization. Arthritis Rheum., 23:1010–1020, 1980.
34. Palmoski, M., Colyer, R.A., and Brandt, K.: Marked suppression by salicylate of the augmented proteoglycan synthesis (? matrix repair) in osteoarthritic cartilage. Arthritis Rheum., 23:83–90, 1980.
35. Palmoski, M., and Brandt, K.: Partial reversal by beta-D-xyloside of salicylate-induced inhibition of glycosaminoglycan syn-

thesis in articular cartilage. Arthritis Rheum., 25:1084–1093, 1982.

36. Palmoski, M., and Brandt, K.: In vivo effect of aspirin on canine osteoarthritic cartilage. Arthritis Rheum., 26:994–1001, 1983.

37. Palmoski, M., and Brandt, K.: Aspirin aggravates the degeneration of canine joint cartilage caused by immobilization. Arthritis Rheum., 25:1333–1342, 1982.

38. Palmoski, M., and Brandt, K.: Relationship between matrix proteoglycan content and the effects of salicylate and indomethacin on articular cartilage. Arthritis Rheum., 26:528–531, 1983.

39. Palmoski, M.J., and Brandt, K.D.: Proteoglycan depletion, rather than fibrillation, determines the effects of salicylate and indomethacin on osteoarthritic cartilage. Arthritis Rheum., 28:548–553, 1985.

40. Slowman, S.D., and Brandt, K.D.: Salicylate effects on glycosaminoglycan synthesis by chondrocytes from normal and osteoarthritic dogs. Arthritis Rheum., 30(Suppl.):S19, 1987.

41. Palmoski, M., and Brandt, K.: Effects of salicylate and indomethacin on glycosaminoglycan and prostaglandin E_2 synthesis in intact canine knee cartilage ex vivo. Arthritis Rheum., 27:398–403, 1984.

41a. Williams, J., and Ward, J.: Personal communication.

42. Hollander, J.L.: Treatment of osteoarthritis of the knees. Arthritis Rheum., 3:564–566, 1960.

43. Traut, E.F.: Procaine and procaine amide hydrochloride in skeletal pain. JAMA, 150:785–789, 1952.

44. Wright, V., Chandler, G.N., Morrison, R.A.H., and Hartfall, S.J.: Intra-articular therapy in osteoarthritis. Comparison of hydrocortisone acetate and hydrocortisone tertiary butylacetate. Ann. Rheum. Dis., 19:257–261, 1960.

45. Friedman, D.M., and Moore, M.A.: The efficacy of intraarticular corticosteroid for osteoarthritis of the knee. Arthritis Rheum., 21:556, 1978.

46. Moskowitz, R.W., Goldberg, V.M., Schwab, W., and Berman, L.: Effects of intraarticular corticosteroids and exercise in experimental models of inflammatory and degenerative arthritis. Arthritis Rheum., 18:417, 1975.

47. Butler, M., et al.: A new model of osteoarthrosis in rabbits. III. Evaluation of antiarthrosic effects of selected drugs administered intraarticularly. Arthritis Rheum., 26:1132–1139, 1983.

48. Behrens, F., Shepard, H., and Mitchell, N.: Alteration of rabbit articular cartilage by intra-articular injections of glucocorticoids. J. Bone Joint Surg., 58A:1157–1160, 1976.

49. Moskowitz, R.W., et al.: Experimentally induced corticosteroid arthropathy. Arthritis Rheum., 13:236–243, 1970.

50. Felson, D.T., et al.: Obesity and symptomatic knee osteoarthritis: Results from the Framingham study. Arthritis Rheum., 30(Suppl.):S130, 1987.

51. Acheson, R.M.: Epidemiology and the arthritides. Arthritis Rheum., 41:325–334, 1982.

52. Sirca, A., and Susec-Michieli, M.: Selective type II fibre muscular atrophy in patients with osteoarthritis of the hip. J. Neurol. Sci., 44:149–159, 1980.

53. Melvin, J.L.: Splinting for arthritis of the hand. In Rheumatic Disease, Occupational Therapy and Rehabilitation. 2nd Ed., Philadelphia. F.A. Davis, 1982.

54. Ehrlich, G., and DiPierro, A.M.: Stretch gloves: Nocturnal use to ameliorate morning stiffness in arthritic hands. Arch. Phys. Med. Rehab., 52:479–480, 1971.

55. Mogensen, B.A., Zoega, H., and Marinko, P.: Late results of intertrochanteric osteotomy for advanced osteoarthritis of the hip. Acta Orthop. Scand., 51:85–90, 1980.

56. Langlais, F., Roure, J.L., and Maquet, P.: Valgus osteotomy in severe osteoarthritis of the hip. J. Bone Joint Surg., 61B:424–431, 1979.

57. Laborde, J.M., and Powers, M.J.: Satisfaction with life for patients undergoing hemodialysis and patients suffering from osteoarthritis. Res. Nursing Health, 3:19–24, 1980.

58. Gross, M.: Psychosocial aspects of osteoarthritis: Helping patients cope. Health Soc. Work, 6:40–46, 1981.

59. Ehrlich, G.E.: Sexual problems of the arthritic patient. In Total Management of the Arthritic Patient. Edited by G.E. Ehrlich. Philadelphia, J.B. Lippincott, 1973.

60. Currey, H.L.F.: Osteoarthrosis of the hip joint and sexual activity. Ann. Rheum. Dis., 29:488–493, 1970.

61. Brandt, K.D., and Potts, M.K.: Arthritis in the elderly: Assessment and management of sexual problems. Med. Aspects Hum. Sex., 21(Suppl.):S767, 1987.

62. Living and Loving: Information about Sex. Arthritis Foundation, Atlanta, GA, 1982.

63. Disability Evaluation Under Social Security: A Handbook for Physicians. U.S. Department of Health and Human Services, Social Security Administration, Publication No. (SSA) 79-10089, August, 1979, pp. 1–62.

64. Meenan, R.F., Liang, M.H., and Hadler, N.M.: Social Security disability and the arthritis patient. Bull. Rheum. Dis., 33:1–6, 1983.

65. Brandt, K.D., Potts, M.K., Barton, R., and Sokolek, C.: Arthritis in the elderly: Problems in procurement of care. Geriatrics (in press).

section X

METABOLIC BONE AND JOINT DISEASES

CLINICAL GOUT AND THE PATHOGENESIS OF HYPERURICEMIA

104

DENNIS J. LEVINSON

Gout is defined as the presence of tissue deposits of crystalline monosodium urate monohydrate (MSU) resulting from antecedent and often longstanding hyperuricemia. The clinical spectrum includes *asymptomatic hyperuricemia; acute gouty arthritis*, in which MSU crystals are found in synovial fluid; *tophaceous gout*, in which aggregated deposits of MSU crystals may produce destruction of hard tissues about joints; and *uric acid urolithiasis*. Athough renal disease is common in gouty individuals, current evidence suggests that nephropathy in gout is usually secondary to associated conditions such as hypertension, vascular disease, or infection, rather than to MSU crystals. Hyperuricemia, the biochemical hallmark and the prerequisite of gout, arises chiefly through two mechanisms: increased uric acid production and diminished uric acid clearance by the kidney. Both hyperuricemia and gout are classified as *primary* when they occur in the absence of a predisposing disorder, and *secondary* when they occur as a consequence of another disorder.

HISTORY OF GOUT

The earliest evidence of tophaceous deposits was found in the great toe of an Egyptian mummy, although Hippocrates, in the fifth century B.C., recognized the distinctive clinical features of gouty arthritis, which he inscribed in the oldest recorded medical text.[1] Celsus, in the first century A.D., and Galen in the second century, who was also the first to describe

gouty tophi, both recognized that gouty arthritis often afflicts the rich and powerful, who are in a position to be bibulous, gluttonous, and successfully lecherous. Aretaeus, also a Roman physician, recognized that the tendency to gout might be inherited, calling this the "gouty diathesis." The word *gout* can be traced to the tenth century Latin *guta* (a drop), which has its origin in the belief that the disease was caused by a poisonous *noxa* falling drop-by-drop into the joint. Anton van Leeuwenhoek, the Dutch upholsterer and inventor of the optical microscope, in 1679 described needle-shaped crystals obtained from a gouty tophus.[2] A century later, Scheele, a Swedish chemist and apothecary, identified urolithic (uric) acid from a urinary calculus.[3] In 1797, the same substance was found in a gouty tophus by the British chemist Wollaston, a nephew of Heberden, who reportedly removed the tophus from his own ear.[4] Fifty years later, the British physician Alfred Baring Garrod demonstrated by the murexide test and his simple "thread test" an increased amount of uric acid in the blood of gouty subjects.[5] In 1907, Emil Fisher established uric acid to be a purine compound.[6] Garrod also recognized asymptomatic hyperuricemia, the cause-and-effect relationship of urate deposition and gouty inflammation, the implication of impaired renal function in gout, the relation of hyperuricemia to gout, and treatment changes in urate levels preceding gouty attacks. The MSU crystals were first specifically identified in 1961 by McCarty and Hollander.[7] Over the past quarter of a century a unified concept of gout

1645

centering on the pathologic role of urate deposits has been established by a number of investigators.[8-10]

Colchicine, an alkaloid obtained from the corm of the autumn crocus, has a long and interesting history. Guttman and Yu[11] and Talbot et al.[12] provided evidence of the clinical effectiveness of the caronomide derivative, probenecid, in lowering serum urate values and diminishing the size of tophi. In 1963, Rundles and his colleagues[13] showed the effectiveness of allopurinol in the treatment of gouty patients.

DEFINITION OF HYPERURICEMIA

Hyperuricemia has been defined physiochemically and also on the basis of epidemiologic studies. Based on the solubility product of sodium urate at 37° C (Fig. 104–1) and allowing an additional 0.4 mg/dl for urate bound to plasma proteins, the solubility of sodium urate in plasma is about 6.8 mg/dl.[14] Above this value, the potential for precipitation of urate crystals exists. The solubility of sodium urate in plasma at 30° C is only 4 mg/dl, which may explain why crystals form preferentially in cooler acral regions of the body.

The epidemiologic definition of hyperuricemia is based on the mean ± 2 SD with a given analytic method applied to a randomly chosen sample population. With the colorimetric or specific uricase enzymatic spectrophotometric methods, the upper limits of normal are about 7 mg/dl in men, and 6 mg/dl in premenopausal women.[15,16] Automated colorimetric methods give values about 0.4 to 1.0 mg/dl higher

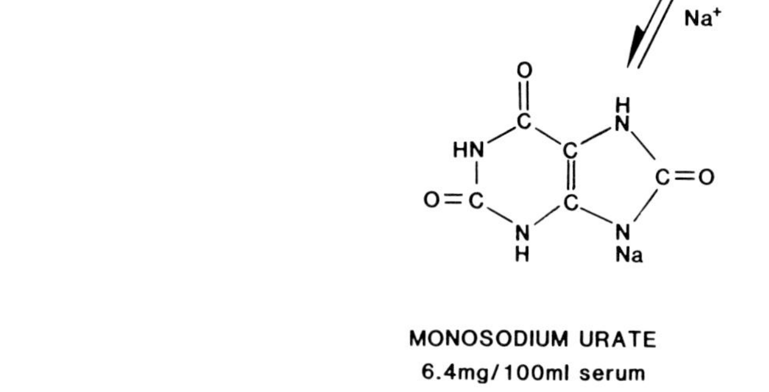

than specific enzymatic methods.[17] This difference reflects the measurement of chromogens other than uric acid. Colorimetric methods historically have been easier to adapt to automation and mass testing and in a normal population are highly correlated with results obtained with specific enzymatic methods. In uremic subjects, or in urine, however, the colorimetric methods often give higher values because of the inclusion of variable quantities of nonurate chromogens.* The physiochemical definition is preferable because the distribution of plasma urate values from population studies is not symmetric about the mean but is skewed so that the majority of values outside of the 2 SD range are high. Serum urate values in children are lower but rise with puberty in boys.[18,19] Serum urate values in postmenopausal women approach or equal those of men. Alteration in urate renal clearance accounts for some of the changes seen in serum urate values at both puberty and menopause.[20,21]

ASYMPTOMATIC HYPERURICEMIA

Asymptomatic hyperuricemia, a laboratory finding but not a disease, represents a raised serum urate level in a patient without arthritis, tophi, or uric acid urolithiasis. Asymptomatic hyperuricemia may last a lifetime without recognizable consequence, or gout may develop in patients who have had hyperuricemia only after many decades. In men at risk for primary gout, hyperuricemia begins at puberty, whereas in women it is usually delayed until menopause.

Few epidemiologic studies have assessed the risks of asymptomatic hyperuricemia. In a cohort of 2046 initially healthy men followed for 15 years with serial measurements of urate levels, the annual incidence rate of gout was 4.9% for a serum urate of 9 mg/dl or more.[22] The rate fell to 0.5% for values between 7.0 and 8.9 mg/dl, and 0.1% for values below 7.0 mg/dl. Throughout this prospective study there was no evidence of renal deterioration attributable to hyperuricemia. This observation was supported by a study of 3693 subjects enrolled in a hypertension detection and followup program.[23] Therapy with thiazide-type diuretics tended to increase both serum urate and creatinine values. However, lowering urate values with drug therapy did not influence creatinine values. Also, the incidence of gouty attacks in subjects at risk was only 2.7% over a 5-year period. Fessel has concluded that azotemia is of no clinical importance until serum urate levels reach 13 mg/dl in men and 10 mg/

FIG. 104–1. Solubility of uric acid species.

URIC ACID
Solubility 6.5mg/100ml H₂O

URATE ION
120mg/100ml H₂O

Na⁺

MONOSODIUM URATE
6.4mg/100ml serum

Editor's note. Most hospital laboratories now use automated specific uricase methods for both serum and urinary uric acid measurement. Colorimetric methods are of historic interest only.

dl in women.[23a] The rarity of urolithiasis in asymptomatic hyperuricemic individuals was also noted; the annualized incidence rate was 0.4% compared to 0.9% in gouty patients. In the Framingham study, gout developed in only 12% of patients with urate levels between 7 and 7.9 mg/dl.[24] Values greater than 9 mg/dl had a sixfold greater predictive value but represented only 20% of the gouty population. In a population study of individuals 79 years old, 17% were hyperuricemic, whereas only 1% had gouty arthritis.[25]

The limited data available do not justify therapy for most patients with asymptomatic hyperuricemia. Despite its apparent benignity, however, asymptomatic hyperuricemia does predispose individuals to both articular gout and nephrolithiasis. After the hyperuricemic patient experiences one of these complications, medical management of hyperuricemia might be indicated. (See Chapter 105.)

CLINICAL DESCRIPTION OF GOUT

Acute gouty arthritis, intercritical gout, and chronic tophaceous gout represent the three stages in the progression of urate crystal deposition disease. Attacks of exquisitely painful arthritis, at first usually monoarticular and with few constitutional symptoms, typify the basic pattern of clinical gout.

ACUTE GOUTY ARTHRITIS

The patient goes to bed and sleeps quietly till about two in the morning when he is awakened by a pain which usually seizes the great toe, but sometimes the heel, ankle, or instep. The pain resembles that of a dislocated bone . . . and is immediately preceded by a chillness and slight fever in proportion to the pain which is mild at first but grows gradually more violent every hour; sometimes resembling a laceration of ligaments, sometimes the gnawing of a dog, and sometimes a weight and constriction of the parts affected, which becomes so exquisitely painful as not to endure the weight of the clothes nor the shaking of the room from a person walking briskly therein.[26]

The acute gouty attack, as vividly described by Sydenham,[26] lasts from a few days to several weeks in untreated patients and recurs at progressively shorter intervals, producing chronic inflammation, which may progress to a crippling arthritis. Superimposed acute exacerbations then occur with decreasing frequency and severity. Various studies cite the peak age of onset of gouty arthritis to be between the fourth and sixth decades.[27–29] Onset before age 30 should

raise suspicion of a specific enzyme defect or, occasionally, intrinsic renal disease. In classic gout, there is a marked male predominance with a peak age of onset at 50 years.

While fully 90% of gouty patients experience acute attacks in the great toe at some time during the course of their disease, the first metatarsophalangeal joint is involved in about 50% of first attacks and constitutes classic podagra (pain in the foot). Although only 3% of initial attacks were polyarticular in 143 men, in 40 women 26% were polyarticular.[27] In another series of 76 patients (29% women), 14.5% of first attacks involved multiple joints.[30] In another series of 92 women with gout, 70% of attacks were polyarticular, and 35% of the patients gave no history of preceding monoarthritis.[30a] Other common initial sites include the instep, ankle, heel, knee, wrist, fingers, and elbows, although rarely involved sites include the shoulders, sternoclavicular joints, hips, spine, and sacroiliac joints. The manubriosternal joint may also be affected.[31] Conceptually, acute gout is predominantly a disease of the lower extremities; the more distal the site of involvement, the more typical is the attack. This localizing may relate to the marked temperature dependency of sodium urate solubility. Unusual sites of urate deposition are almost always preceded by typical attacks in the usual distal joints.

Trivial episodes of pain ("the petite attack") lasting only hours and sometimes going back over several years may precede the first dramatic gouty attack. The initial attack of gout occurs with explosive suddenness, typically awakening the patient or noted when the foot is placed on the floor on arising. The skin over the affected joint soon becomes reddened and warm; extreme tenderness of the affected joint and periarticular tissues are noted (Fig. 104–2). The slightest pressure produces exquisite pain. Fever, leukocytosis, and elevation of the erythrocyte sedimentation rate often occur.

The course of untreated acute gout is variable. Mild attacks can subside in several hours or can persist for only a day or two and not reach the intensity described by Sydenham. Severe attacks can last many days to several weeks.

The skin over the joint may desquamate as the episode subsides. On recovery, the patient re-enters an asymptomatic phase termed the *intercritical period*. Even though the attack may have been incapacitating with excruciating pain and swelling, resolution is usually complete and the patient is once again well. The complete freedom from symptoms during the intercritical period is an important diagnostic feature, as noted by Aretaeus 17 centuries ago. He recorded that

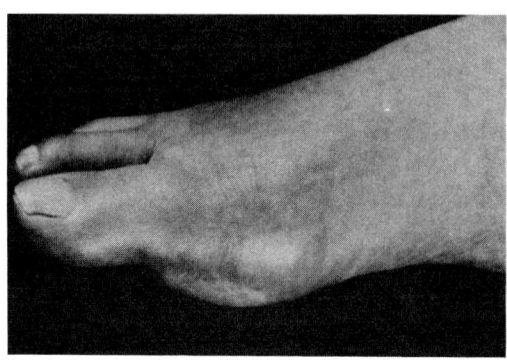
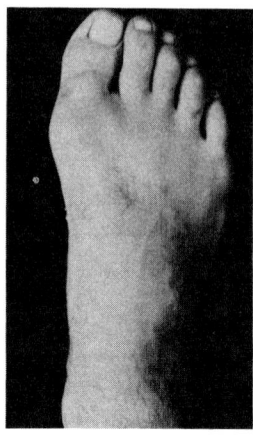

FIG. 104–2. Acute gouty arthritis of the first metatarsophalangeal joint. (From Dieppe, P.A., et al. (Eds): Gout. *In* Slide Atlas of Rheumatology. London, Gower Medical Publishing Ltd., 1985.)

an athlete had won an Olympic Marathon between gouty attacks.

PROVOCATIVE OR POSSIBLE ETIOLOGIC FACTORS

Provocative factors of acute gouty arthritis include trauma, exercise, alcohol ingestion, certain drugs, other medical illnesses, and surgery. Although these factors may be important in the incidence and sites of predilection of gouty attacks, their relationship to the disease is less clear. For example, the first metatarsophalangeal joint is a primary weight-bearing area and subject to considerable microtrauma; yet, the severity of the gouty attacks are out of proportion to the severity of injury, an important point of differentiation from traumatic arthritis or fracture. Alcohol ingestion predisposes to both hyperuricemia and gout. In predisposed individuals, gouty attacks may be precipitated by various drugs such as the use of thiazide diuretics in the treatment of hypertension, in vitamin B$_{12}$ administration in patients with pernicious anemia,[32] or following specific treatment of hyperuricemia with urate-lowering medications. Both starvation and hyperalimentation in patients with a gouty diathesis can cause hyper- or hypouricemia resulting in gouty attacks.[33] Thus, *in predisposed individuals, changes in serum urate concentration in either direction can result in acute arthritis.**

In patients with a history of gout, acute attacks are common in the postoperative period or in association with the stress of an acute medical illness. In 22 gouty patients undergoing surgical procedures without colchicine prophylaxis, gouty attacks occurred in 86%,

**Editor's note.* A rapid *fall* in serum urate level seems to best correlate with the onset of acute gouty arthritis. Aldermanic gout, following a binge of eating and excessive alcohol consumption, correlated best not with the initial rise in serum urate but with its subsequent rapid return to baseline levels.[33a]

usually between the third and fifth postoperative day.[34] By comparison, post-surgical attacks of pseudogout are more common on the first or second postoperative day.[35]

INTERCRITICAL GOUT AND RECURRENT EPISODES

A clear description of the initial attack and the completely asymptomatic (intercritical) interval between this and subsequent attacks are valuable diagnostic clues. Although some patients never experience a second attack, most do so within 6 months to 2 years. In Gutman's series, 62% had recurrences within the first year and 78% within 2 years, whereas, only 7% had no recurrences for 10 years or more.[36]

As the disease progresses in the untreated patient, acute attacks occur with increasing frequency and often become polyarticular, more severe, longer lasting, and associated with fever. Affected joints usually recover completely, but erosive bony changes may develop. One third of a series of patients with late polyarticular attacks reported that their initial attack was also polyarticular.[37,38] Various joints may flare in sequence in a migratory pattern, or as in pseudogout, a number of neighboring joints may be involved simultaneously in a *cluster attack*.[39] Frequently, extra-articular sites such as bursae and tendons are also involved.

Eventually, the patient may enter a phase of chronic polyarticular gout without pain-free intercritical periods. Gout at this stage may be confused with rheumatoid arthritis (RA). Unlike RA, in which inflammation in affected joints is synchronous, inflamed gouty joints are out of phase, flaring in one joint coinciding with subsidence in another. On occasion, the disease can progress from initial podagra to a chronic deforming arthritis without remissions and with synovial thickening and the early development of tophi.

Tophi may be mistaken for rheumatoid nodules, especially in patients treated with systemic corticosteroids. Conversely, subcutaneous nodules in patients with "rheumatoid nodulosis" are easily confused with tophi.[40] One third of patients with tophaceous gout had positive tests for rheumatoid factor (RF).[41] The titers are generally lower than in RA. Low-titer RF in gouty patients has been correlated with the presence of liver disease.[42] In a study of 160 patients with RA, hyperuricemia was found in 7.5% and correlated inversely with disease activity.[43]

CHRONIC TOPHACEOUS GOUT

The deposition of solid urate crystals (tophi) in extra-articular and articular structures leading to a destructive arthropathy, often with secondary degenerative changes, characterizes chronic tophaceous gout (Fig. 104–3). In the untreated patient, the interval from an initial gouty attack to the beginning of chronic arthritis or visible tophi is highly variable, ranging from 3 to 42 years with an average of 11.6 years.[44] A retrospective analysis of 1165 patients in the pretreatment era found that 70% were free of demonstrable tophi within 5 years of the first gouty attack; about 50% were nontophaceous at 10 years; but by 20 years, the proportion of nontophaceous cases had declined to 28%.[45] The percentage of patients with severe tophaceous gout reached appreciable proportions (24%) some 20 years after the first attack. In a population of 4110 gouty Japanese subjects followed over 19 years, 9.2% had tophaceous deposits.[46]

Tophaceous gout is often associated with an early age of onset, a long duration of active but untreated disease, frequent attacks, higher serum urate values, and a predilection for upper extremity and polyarticular episodes.[47] Bony tophi occur before subcutaneous tophi.[47] If the latter are found, the clinician may predict the radiologic findings. Exceptions to these general rules, of course, are encountered.

Of 60 consecutive gouty patients presenting to a rheumatology unit, 15% were elderly women (mean age 82 years), all of whom were receiving diuretic drugs, and most had tophi in osteoarthritic fingers (Fig. 104–4).[48] Acute inflammation was less common than in men (mean age, 52 years), whereas renal disease was more frequent. The combination of diuretic-induced hyperuricemia, age, and nodal osteoarthritis appears to predispose these women to tophaceous gout arising in nodal tissue. The disease has been referred to as *impostumous gout.*[49]*

In Gutman's series, the rate of urate deposition in joint tissue correlated with both the duration and degree of hyperuricemia.[45] In nontophaceous patients, the mean serum urate concentration was 9.2 mg/dl. Values of 10 to 11 mg/dl were found in subjects with minimal to moderate deposits, and levels >11 mg/dl were noted in patients with extensive tophaceous deposits.

Occasionally, tophi are present at the time of the initial gouty attack. This presentation is unusual in primary gout but has been observed in 0.5% of subjects with gout secondary to myeloproliferative disease,[50] in gout complicating glycogen storage disease,[51] or the Lesch-Nyhan syndrome.[52] Tophi rarely develop in gout secondary to primary renal disease.

The helix of the ear is a classic location for tophaceous deposits, where they form small white excrescences (Fig. 104–5). Other sites include the olecranon

*Editor's note. Simkin has also recorded the predilection of gouty tophi for Heberden's nodes. This phenomenon also occurs in men.

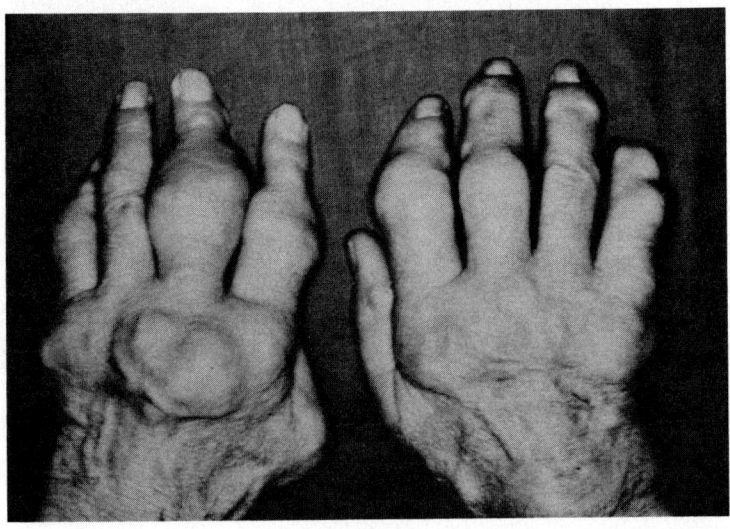

FIG. 104–3. Chronic tophaceous gout with grotesque tumescences of hands. (From Dieppe, P.A., et al. (Eds): Gout. *In* Slide Atlas of Rheumatology. London, Gower Medical Publishing Ltd., 1985.)

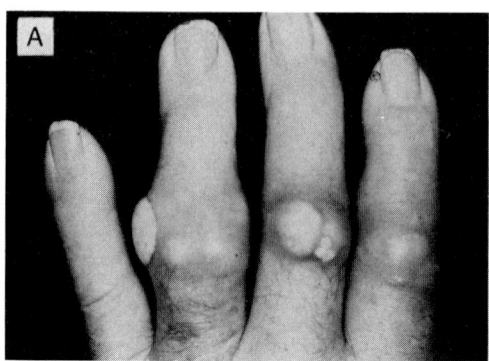

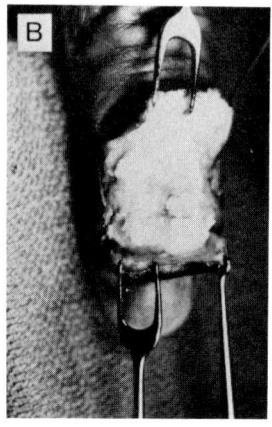

FIG. 104–4. *A,* Impostumous gout involving osteoarthritic joints of an elderly woman on diuretic therapy for hypertension. *B,* Note the extensive urate deposits in periarticular tissue from a similar patient. (Courtesy Dr. Michael Jablon, Michael Reese Hospital.)

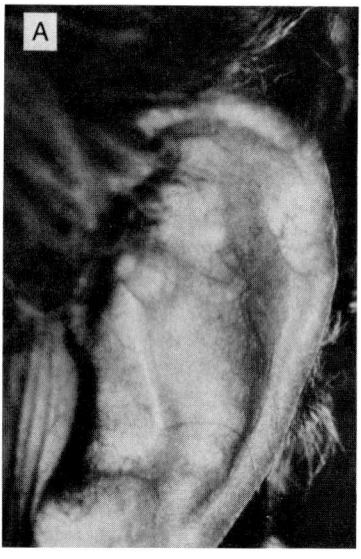

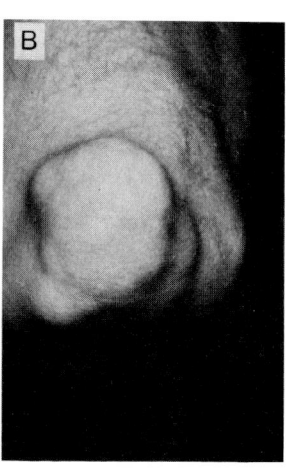

FIG. 104–5. *A,* Tophus in helix of ear. *B,* Olecranon bursa.

and prepatellar bursa often with a sandy or gritty sensation, ulnar surface of the forearm, and Achilles tendon. Deposits may produce irregular and often grotesque tumescences of the hands or feet with joint destruction and crippling. The "gouty" shoe is cut to accommodate such enlarged joints. The tense, shiny, thin skin overlying the tophus may ulcerate and extrude white, chalky material composed of myriads of needle-shaped (acicular) MSU crystals (Fig. 104–6). Ulcerated tophi rarely become secondarily infected. Bony ankylosis is also unusual, but certain patients may develop extensive ankylosis of multiple joints for unknown reasons—so-called *ankylosing gouty arthritis.*[52a]

As tophi and, possibly, renal disease advance, acute attacks recur less frequently and are milder; late in the illness they may disappear entirely or may be superimposed on indolently inflamed joints. The process of tophaceous deposition advances insidiously, the patient often noting progressive stiffness and aching of affected joints. Tophi or a secondary degenerative process may limit joint mobility by involvement of the joint and adjacent structures.

FIG. 104–6. Ulcerated tophi. (Courtesy Dr. Ira Melnicoff, Lutheran General Hospital.)

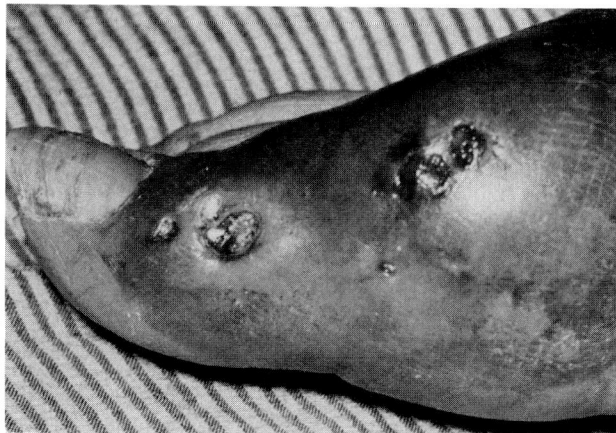

Unusual sites for tophaceous deposits include the aorta and myocardium, prepuce, corpora cavernosa, tarsal plate, cornea and sclerae, vocal cords, epiglottis, and tongue.[53-55] Likewise, the axial skeleton does not escape urate crystal deposition, which may mimic a tumor or protruded disc.[56] Tophaceous involvement of the sacroiliac joint (see Fig. 104–10) and osteonecrosis of the femoral head have been reported as manifestations of gout.[57,58] MSU crystals have been identified in avascular bone, although no cases of avascular necrosis of the femoral head were found in a systematic study of 138 gouty patients.[59]

Before the availability of uricosuric drugs, 50 to 70% of the gouty population developed visible tophi and permanent joint changes.[60,61] The incidence of tophi declined to less than 35% with the introduction of uricosuric agents.[62] A further decline in the past 20 years is probably attributable to the use of allopurinol. At the Mayo Clinic, the prevalence of tophi decreased from 11% in 1959 to 3% in 1972 without any appreciable change in the prevalence of acute gout.[63] Current figures are probably even lower.

PREVALENCE AND INCIDENCE RATES

The prevalence of gout varies in different populations worldwide, but it is similar in Europe (0.3%) and North America (0.27%).[64,65] A prevalence of 0.2% was found in Framingham, MA, among 5127 subjects (2283 men and 2844 women, aged 30 and 59 years, respectively, mean age, 44 years).[24] Fourteen years later, the prevalence had increased to 1.5% (mean age, 58 years); 2.8% in men, and 0.4% in women. Among 4663 Parisian men age 20 to 40 years, the prevalence was 1.1% in men 35 to 39 years and 2% in men 40 to 44 years.[66] The prevalence of gout is much higher among the islanders of the Mariana Islands and the Maori of New Zealand.[67,68] The prevalence of gout in the latter is 10.3% in men and 4.3% in women. The prevalence of gout is directly related to the serum urate levels[24] (Table 104–1).

Primary gout is predominantly a disease of men, with a peak incidence in the fourth to sixth decade.[29,69] Only 3 to 7% of cases occur in women, most of whom are postmenopausal.[70-72] Higher percentages of women have been recorded in series that included cases of gout complicating renal disease or diuretic therapy.[30a,48] It is uncommon before the third decade. In the Framingham study, the cumulative incidence rate in men appeared to be approaching a plateau at a mean age of 58 years, although only one third with urate levels of 8 mg/dl or more had developed gout.[24] A few patients with persistently normal serum urate levels developed clinical gout, although this was not proven by crystal identification.

DIAGNOSIS OF GOUTY ARTHRITIS

The diagnosis of gout should be established on firm criteria to ensure that expensive and potentially toxic medications are not prescribed. Available data do not support therapeutic intervention for patients with asymptomatic hyperuricemia. A definitive diagnosis of gout is made by the finding of intracellular MSU crystals in synovial fluid leukocytes (Fig. 104–7) (see Chapter 5). In a study conducted by the American Rheumatism Association subcommittee on diagnostic and therapeutic criteria, 84.4% of patients with gouty arthritis had demonstrable intracellular MSU crystals in acutely inflamed joints, a finding absolutely specific for gout.[35] This specificity, however, should not lead the physician to overlook the occasional patient with synovial fluid MSU crystals and another type of joint disease such as septic arthritis or pseudogout.

Extracellular MSU crystals have been described in the synovial fluid of approximately 70% of gouty patients when they were asymptomatic.[73] Only one of 19 asymptomatic, hyperuricemic controls had syn-

Table 104–1. Prevalence of Gouty Arthritis in Relation to Serum Uric Acid Level (Admitted at a Mean Age of 44 and Followed for 14 Years)

Serum Uric Acid Level (mg/dl)	Men			Women		
	Total No. Examined	Gouty Arthritis Developed in		Total No. Examined	Gouty Arthritis Developed in	
		No.	(%)		No.	(%)
6	1281	8	0.6	2665	2	0.08
6–6.9	790	15	1.9	151	5	3.30
7–7.9	162	27	16.7	23	4	17.40
8–8.9	40	10	25.0	4	0	0
9+	10	9	90.0	1	0	0
Total	2283	69	2.8	2844	11	0.4

(From Hall, A.P., et al.[24])

FIG. 104-7. Polymorphonuclear leukocyte containing a phagocytized monosodium urate monohydrate crystal.

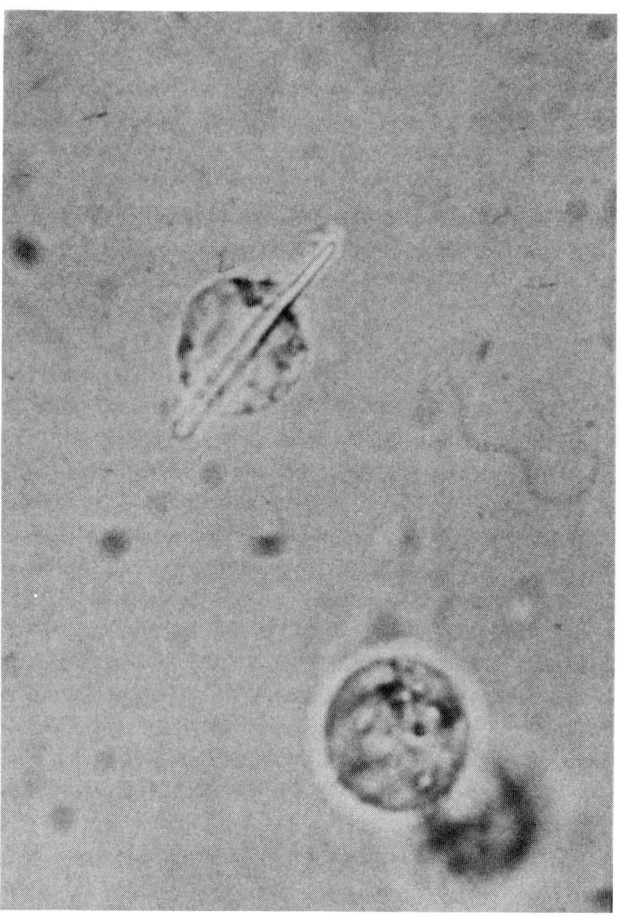

ovial fluid MSU crystals, whereas two of nine patients with renal failure and no history of synovitis had extracellular urate crystals. In another study of 31 subjects with asymptomatic hyperuricemia, MSU crystals were found in only one subject after joint lavage.[74] No crystals were found in the six patients with renal failure. Thus, extracellular MSU crystals in synovial fluid are common during intercritical gout, but this finding does not carry the specificity of intracellular urate crystals for establishing a diagnosis of gout.

The finding of urate crystals in tophi is nearly as specific as intracellular crystals in establishing a diagnosis of gouty arthritis; however, proven tophi are less sensitive, being found in less than 10% of patients with gout. In the absence of specific crystal identification, the following combination of findings are useful in diagnosing gout: (1) a classic history of monoarticular acute arthritis followed by an intercritical period free of symptoms, (2) rapid resolution of synovitis after colchicine therapy, and (3) hyperuri-

cemia.[35] Criteria for improvement as a result of colchicine therapy have been established, namely major subsidence of objective joint inflammatory changes within 48 hours and no recrudescence of inflammatory joint manifestations within 7 days.[75] Arthralgias or synovitis alone in a hyperuricemic patient is not sufficient to establish the diagnosis. Pseudogout (calcium pyrophosphate dihydrate [CPPD] crystal deposits) or basic calcium phosphate (BCP) crystal-induced inflammation are the most difficult diseases to differentiate; acute attacks caused by these crystals may also respond to colchicine therapy, especially if it is given intravenously.[76]

ROENTGENOGRAPHIC FINDINGS

The major value of radiographic examination is to exclude other types of arthritis and to detect tophaceous deposits in bone in patients with established gout. Sharply "punched-out," round or oval defects situated in the marginal areas of the joint and surrounded by a sclerotic border suggest gout (Fig. 104-8). *Bony tophaceous lesions almost always antedate subcutaneous tophi* and many be seen in joints that have never been clinically inflamed.[47] In about 40% of patients with gouty erosions in bone, an elevated margin extends outward into the soft tissue covering the tophaceous nodule.[77] This "overhanging margin" of bone may relate to bone resorption beneath the enlarging tophus with periosteal apposition of the involved cortex and helps to distinguish this radiologic feature from the "pocketed" erosions seen in RA. The "overhanging margin" is particularly common in patients with concomitant diffuse idiopathic skeletal hyperostosis (DISH). Bony erosions occur relatively late in the disease, and many patients with repeated gouty attacks show neither bone nor soft-tissue lesions.

Bony erosions caused by deposits of MSU crystals are related to both the duration and severity of the disease. In patients with advanced chronic tophaceous gout, joint destruction may be extensive. Bony ankylosis with obliteration of the joint space has been observed but is rare except in the interphalangeal joints of the hands and feet and in intercarpal regions.[78] Rather, the presence of a relatively normal joint space in an articulation with extensive erosions is an important radiologic characteristic of gout.

Deposition of tophi in soft tissue results in asymmetric nodular swelling that is particularly frequent in the feet, hands, ankles, elbows, and knees.[79] Soft-tissue prominence around the dorsum of the foot and calcaneus are also characteristic. Calcification of a tophus is unusual (Fig. 104-9).[80]

FIG. 104–8. Radiographic features of gout. Marginal erosions with sclerotic borders, osseous cysts, and ovehanging margins are seen. (From Dieppe, P.A., et al. (Eds): Gout. *In* Slide Atlas of Rheumatology. London, Gower Medical Publishing Ltd., 1985.)

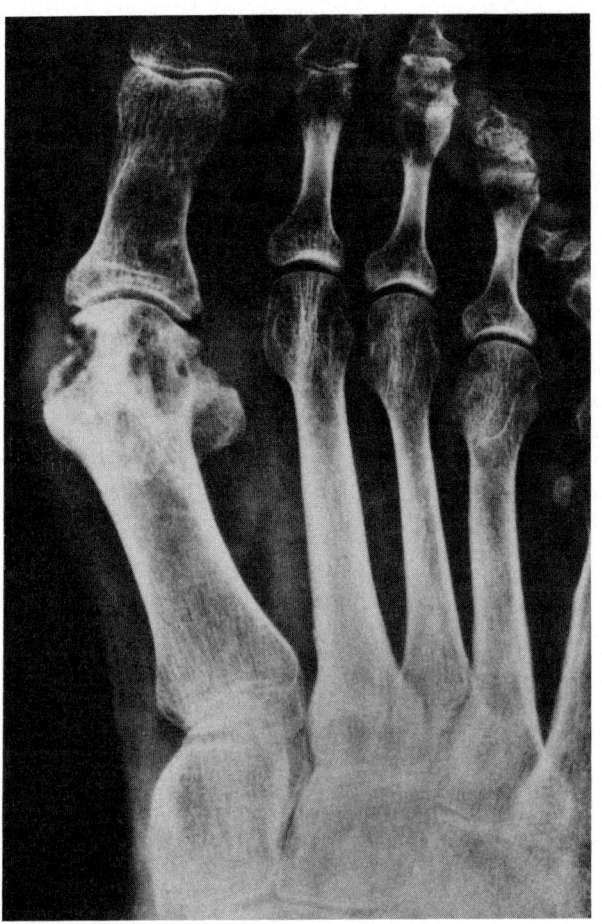

Dodds and Steinbach[81] found that 10 of 31 patients with gout had meniscal calcification of the type usually associated with CPPD crystal deposits. In another study, calcification of one or more menisci was found in only 2 of 43 patients (5%) with gout, roughly the incidence of chondrocalcinosis observed in elderly populations.[82] Because of the high incidence of gout in patients with pseudogout (5%) and vice versa, the presence of calcification in a patient with gout suggests coexistent CPPD crystal deposition.

Periarticular osteopenia can occur but is much less common in gout than in RA. As MSU crystals stimulate synovial cells to secrete PGE_2, which can mobilize calcium from bone, subchondral osteopenia in gout may be related to active synovitis.[83,84]

Subchondral lesions are occasionally observed near the sacroiliac joints in patients with chronic tophaceous gout (Fig. 104–10). Sclerotic "punched-out" lesions were found in the sacroiliac joints of 7 of 95 gouty patients.[85] In 6 of these patients, tophaceous deposits were also present in the extremities, and MSU crystals were documented in the sacroiliac lesions in two cases at autopsy. In a prospective radiologic survey of 143 gouty patients, 24 individuals with tophi had sacroiliac lesions, including sclerosis and irregularity of joint margins, focal osteoporosis, and cysts with sclerotic rims.[86]

Uric acid stones are radiolucent and appear radiologically as a "filling defect." Cysteine, xanthine, and 2,8-dihydroxyadenine stones are also radiolucent, but most radiolucent stones are composed of uric acid. Uric acid stones or gravel may be white or pink ("brick dust") as a result of absorption of a pigment that has still not been identified. Patients with *brick dust urine*

FIG. 104–9. Calcified soft tissue prominence over the dorsum of the foot and destruction of the talocalcaneous joint in a 63-year-old man with polyarticular tophaceous gout. (Courtesy Dr. David Tartof, Michael Reese Hospital.)

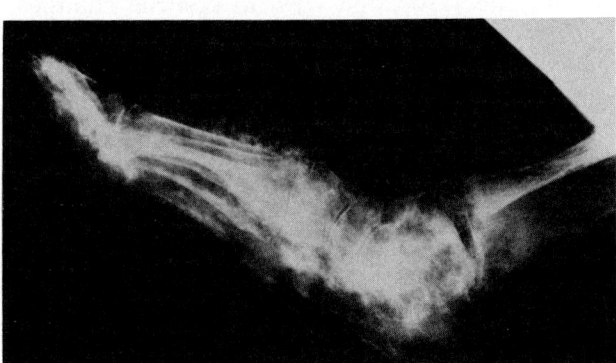

FIG. 104–10. Sacroiliac joint showing scalloped erosions and adjacent bony sclerosis in chronic tophaceous gout. (Courtesy Dr. Nancy Brown, Michael Reese Hospital.)

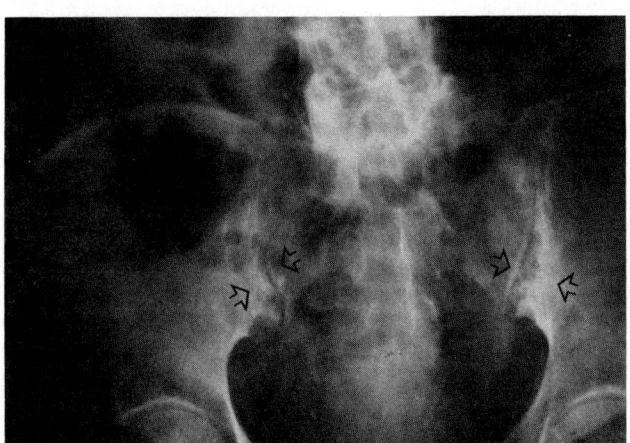

may present with what they believe to be hematuria. Radiopaque stones also occur in gouty subjects and are composed largely of calcium oxalate. These stones often contain a small amount of uric acid, which possibly serves as a nidus for the deposition of calcium oxalate by epitaxial overgrowth (vide infra).

HEREDITY

The familial nature of gout has long been recognized. English observers have reported a familial incidence of 38 to 81%, while in series reported from the United States, familial incidence has ranged from 6 to 18%.[87,88] Among hyperuricemic relatives of gouty patients, the incidence of gout averaged 20%.[89] In family members of gouty probands, asymptomatic hyperuricemia ranges from 25 to 27% in most series.[90,91]

From the available data, the serum urate concentration is controlled by multiple genes. A study of Blackfeet and Pima Indians showed a strong hereditary determinance of serum urate levels that appeared to be polygenic.[92] Transmission patterns suggested that some genes were autosomal dominant, others possibly X-linked. Other studies have also favored a multifactorial inheritance in which frequency histograms have shown a prevalence of high values without evidence of bimodality.[16,24] Studies of more restricted populations (i.e., racial selection, geographic isolation, families of gouty probands), however, have shown a bimodal distribution of serum urate values supporting a single-dominant gene hypothesis.[64,93–95] Polygenic control becomes increasingly prominent when the population studied is genetically heterogeneous.

PATHOLOGIC FEATURES

Monosodium urate crystals deposit in cartilage, epiphyseal bone, periarticular structures, and the kidney. Because they are water soluble, nonaqueous fixatives are necessary for their preservation in histologic sections. Urate deposits produce local necrosis, and unless the tissue is avascular, a foreign body reaction ensues with proliferation of fibrous tissues. The tophus consists of a multicentric deposit of urate crystals and intercrystalline matrix together with a foreign body reaction.[96] In some patients, very small, needle-shaped MSU crystals may be clustered radially in a spherulite form resembling beach balls. These may be seen in the synovial fluid[97] or synovium.[98] Affected joints can develop cartilaginous degeneration, synovial proliferation, destruction of subchondral bone, proliferation of marginal bone, and rarely, ankylosis (Fig. 104–11).[52a,99] No joint is exempt, although those of the lower extremities are more commonly involved. The significance of the tophaceous matrix rich in proteoglycans is uncertain.[100,101]

KIDNEY DISEASE

Apart from arthritis, renal disease is the most frequent complication of hyperuricemia.[102–104] Hyperuricemia may affect the kidney through (1) the deposition of MSU crystals in the renal interstitium, referred to as *urate nephropathy*; (2) the deposition of uric acid crystals in the collecting tubules, referred to as *uric acid nephropathy*; and (3) formation of *uric acid stone*. The distinction between the first two entities is often unclear, and the term "gouty kidney" has been used for both. Uric acid nephropathy is uncommon in the absence of malignant disease or enzymatic defects, leading to the overproduction and overexcretion of uric acid. Urate nephropathy is more common in patients with gout unassociated with the overproduction of uric acid. In addition to these direct effects of hyperuricemia, other causes of renal dysfunction such as hypertension and lead nephropathy are also prevalent in the gouty population.

Ordinarily, urate nephropathy is only slowly progressive and does not materially reduce life expectancy.[23a,105,106] The incidence of proteinuria varies from 15 to 20%.[107,108] Hypertension is as common as proteinuria.[103] It is not entirely clear whether hypertension is a result of hyperuricemia and urate nephropathy or whether it is a cause of renal dysfunction observed in gouty patients.[109] Uncontrolled hypertension is held responsible for a significant amount of the renal dysfunction observed in gouty patients.[108] Other studies also support this concept.[23a,110]

The only distinctive histologic feature of urate nephropathy is the presence of urate crystals and a surrounding giant cell reaction (Fig. 104–12). These crystals may be associated with interstitial changes, vascular changes, or both.[95] That some of the vascular changes can be related to concomitant hypertension emphasizes the difficulty of attributing pathologic changes to a single origin. In a review of the renal histology in 191 gouty patients at postmortem evaluation, only 3 showed neither urate crystals nor pyelonephritic or vascular changes.[103] These features were present in variable proportions and severity. A strong correlation existed between the clinical severity of gout and the severity of the renal lesions, both in patients with predominantly pyelonephritic changes

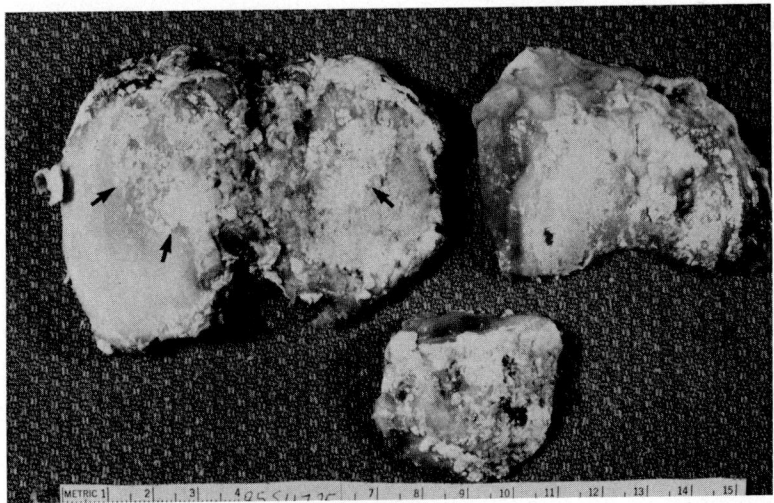

FIG. 104–11. Encrusted urate deposits on eroded articular cartilage of the tibial plateau (arrows), and fragments of the femoral condyle. (Courtesy Dr. Mitchell Krieger, Michael Reese Hospital.)

FIG. 104–12. *A,* Urate deposit in the medulla of the kidney fixed in alcohol (hematoxylin and eosin stain × 100). *B,* Same deposit stained with methenamine silver (× 375). (Courtesy Dr. Wellington Jao, Michael Reese Hospital.)

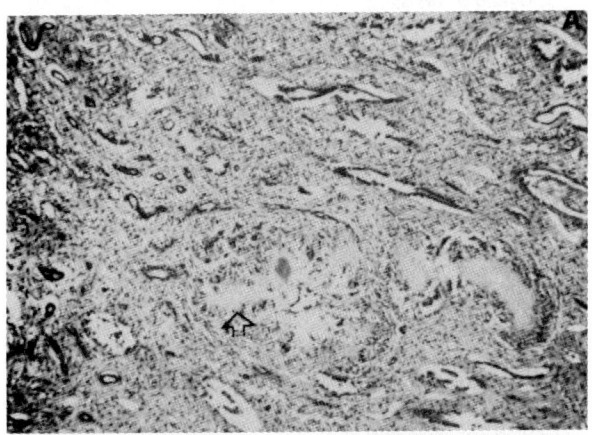

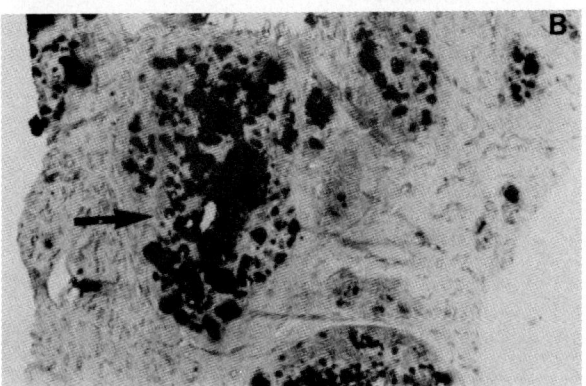

and in those whose kidneys showed predominantly vascular changes. Such vascular lesions included arterial and arteriolar sclerosis, and in 11 instances the findings were of malignant hypertension. Kidneys from 30 patients revealed both well-developed vascular changes and pyelonephritis with extensive structural alterations and urate crystal deposits.

A few notable exceptions from the correlated severity of clinical symptoms and renal disease were found. Some patients with severe tophaceous gout showed only minimal clinical evidence of renal insufficiency; conversely, other patients with severe renal disease had only minimal articular disease. In the latter, renal disease may have been the cause of premature death. The extreme degree of this phenomenon may be represented by the few reports of "gouty nephrosis" occurring without clinical evidence of gout.[111–113] In the rare patients purported to have this syndrome, however, no serum urate levels had been obtained during life.

A number of mechanisms have been proposed to explain the various pathologic findings reported in urate nephropathy. The renal lesions may stem from deposition of uric acid in collecting tubules with resultant obstruction, atrophy of the more proximal tubules, and secondary necrosis and fibrosis.[114] The associated interstitial inflammatory process has been attributed to complicating pyelonephritis.[115] Other studies have shown that tubular damage is an early structural abnormality associated with an interstitial reaction; this finding suggests a relationship between the interstitial and tubular changes.[116,117] The epithelial cells of the loop of Henle show early atrophy and occasional dilatation associated with brown pigment degeneration.[116] The interstitial reaction is maximal in the region near the loop of Henle, and the changes in the epithelial cells precede the interstitial reaction.

In kidneys without tophi, this reaction usually spares the medulla and the juxtamedullary cortex. Thus, the changes labeled as "chronic pyelonephritis" may not be of bacterial origin but rather an inflammatory reaction to urate crystals.[116] Gonick et al.[116] described a distinctive glomerulosclerosis in urate nephropathy, with uniform fibrillar thickening of glomerular capillary basement membranes different from that of nephrosclerosis or diabetic glomerulosclerosis. Heptinstall[118] does not believe that this lesion is distinctive.

A long-term study of a large population of patients with gout found that the onset of hypertension correlated with a reduction in glomerular filtration rate.[110] Nephrosclerosis associated with hypertension was postulated as the most common cause of renal damage. Excessive lead stores associated with a decreased creatinine clearance was found in gouty patients in a Veterans Administration Hospital, suggesting lead nephropathy as an unrecognized cause of renal dysfunction in gout.[119]

In the past, various authors have reported significant impairment of renal function in patients with gout, ranging from 10 to 40%.[102,103,120] In the experience of Talbott and Terplan,[103] renal failure was the eventual cause of death in 18 to 25% of their patients. More recent evaluations have de-emphasized a causal relation between hyperuricemia, gout, and renal disease.[23a,110] The incidence of renal disease is probably no higher than that of subjects of comparable age with similar degrees of hypertension, obesity, and primary renal disease.

PATHOGENESIS OF HYPERURICEMIA IN PRIMARY GOUT

Hyperuricemia, the prerequisite for gout, may result from an excessive rate of uric acid production, a decrease in its renal excretion, or a combination of both. *Primary hyperuricemia* refers to elevated serum urate levels found in the absence of a predisposing disorder or drug. *Secondary hyperuricemia* refers to elevated urate levels developing in the presence of such disorders or drugs. Further subdivision within these major categories is based on the identification of whether uric acid is overproduced or underexcreted (Table 104–2).

Uricolysis in men is due to the action of intestinal flora on uric acid entering the gastrointestinal tract in enteric secretions.[121,122] Gastrointestinal excretion is increased from the normal one third of excreted urate to about 50% in nearly all hyperuricemic subjects and may become the chief route of urate disposal in pa-

Table 104–2. Causes of Hyperuricemia in Man

Increased Purine Biosynthesis or Urate Production
  Inherited enzymatic defects
    Hypoxanthine-guanine phosphoribosyltransferase deficiency
    Phosphoribosylpyrophosphate synthetase overactivity
    Glucose-6-phosphatase deficiency
  Clinical disorders leading to purine overproduction
    Myeloproliferative disorders
    Lymphoproliferative disorders
    Polycythemia vera
    Malignant diseases
    Hemolytic disorders
    Psoriasis
    Obesity
    Tissue hypoxia
    Glycogenosis III, V, VII
  Drugs or dietary habits
    Ethanol
    Diet rich in purines
    Pancreatic extract
    Fructose
    Nicotinic acid
    Ethylamino-1,3,4-thiadiazole
    4-Amino-5-imidazole carboxamide riboside
    Vitamin B_{12} (patients with pernicious anemia)
    Cytotoxic drugs
    Warfarin

Decreased Renal Clearance of Urate
  Clinical disorders
    Chronic renal failure
    Lead nephropathy
    Polycystic kidney disease
    Hypertension
    Dehydration
    Salt restriction
    Starvation
    Diabetic ketoacidosis
    Lactic acidosis
    Obesity
    Hyperparathyroidism
    Hypothyroidism
    Diabetes insipidus
    Sarcoidosis
    Toxemia of pregnancy
    Bartter's syndrome
    Chronic beryllium disease
    Down's syndrome
  Drugs or dietary habits
    Ethanol
    Diuretics
    Low doses of salicylates
    Ethambutal
    Pyrazinamide
    Laxative abuse (alkalosis)
    Levodopa
    Methoxyflurane

tients with reduced renal function.[123] Impaired uricolysis is never a cause of hyperuricemia in man.

PRODUCTION OF URIC ACID

Chemical Balance

In theory, the rate of purine synthesis may be calculated as the difference between purine intake and excretion in the steady state. However, because the urinary excretion of uric acid represents a variable fraction of the total purine turnover and there are no convenient methods for the measurement of extrarenal disposal of urate, only gross estimates of purine production rates are possible by quantitation of urinary uric acid. Through severe dietary restriction of purines, *urinary uric acid becomes a minimal estimate of purine production.* Values in normal men on a purine-restricted diet range from 264 mg/day to 588 mg/day (mean, 425 ± 81 mg).[124]

In men with primary gout, urinary uric acid excretion ranges from <150 to ≥2400 mg/day. Lower values are found in patients with overt renal damage.

In some series, 21 to 28% of gouty patients excreted quantities of uric acid exceeding the mean +2 SD,[91,124] but the more general experience is that no more than 5 to 15% of patients with primary gout fall into this group. Decreased extrarenal disposal of urate has been excluded as a cause of uric acid overexcretion by the normal urinary recoveries of injected, isotopically labeled uric acid.[124] *Overexcretion of uric acid is therefore evidence of excessive synthesis of purines de novo. Conversely, however, a normal urinary uric acid excretion does not preclude purine overproduction because gastrointestinal disposal of urate may be increased.*

When isotopic uric acid is given intravenously and the isotope concentration in urinary uric acid is determined serially over several days, the size of the miscible pool of uric acid and its turnover rate can be estimated. In 25 normal men, the miscible pool averaged 1200 mg (range, 866 to 1587 mg), and the turnover rate averaged 696 mg/day (range, 513 to 1108 mg).[124-126] In five normal women, the pool ranged from 541 to 687 mg. In nontophaceous gout, the pool is enlarged to 2000 to 4000 mg,[121,127,128] while in patients with tophi the pool may enlarge to from 18,000 to 31,000 mg.[129] The miscible pool often represents only a small fraction of the total body urate in gouty subjects because only the outer layers of tophi are readily exchangeable with urate in solution. The turnover rate is uniformly increased in patients who overexcrete uric acid.[123,124,128] In patients having normal uric acid excretion and lacking visible tophi, turnover rates overlap with control values.[125]

Incorporation of Labeled Precursors Into Uric Acid

Purines are synthesized de novo from low-molecular-weight precursors including glycine, carbon dioxide, aspartic acid, formate, and glutamate (Fig. 104–13). The rate of urate production can be estimated by measuring the rate of incorporation of isotopically labeled precursors into urinary uric acid. When labeled glycine was fed to normal men, the isotopic enrichment of urinary uric acid reached a maximum on the second or third day and declined thereafter.[130,131] The pattern of incorporation was abnormal in gouty patients.[124,130–132] In overexcretors particularly, the peak enrichment values were higher, occurred earlier, and were followed by a more rapid decline because of increased urate synthesis. Marked overincorporation of precursor glycine into urinary uric acid occurred in all overexcretor subjects, and significant increased incorporation was found in many patients with normal excretion (Fig. 104–14). Glycine incorporation rates in subjects with primary gout showed urate production rates ranging from normal to four- or fivefold higher. "Correction" for large tophaceous deposits and poor renal function was accomplished by injecting urate labeled with a different isotope and determining the fraction that failed to appear in the urine.[124] Two of five gouty subjects whose uncorrected (^{14}C) glycine incorporation into uric acid was normal then showed excessive incorporation.

CONTROL OF DE NOVO PURINE BIOSYNTHESIS

Studies performed in vivo as well as in vitro with isolated enzymes and cells grown in tissue culture have documented an important role for phosphoribosylpyrophosphate (PRPP) and purine ribonucleo-

FIG. 104–13.   Precursors of purine ring.

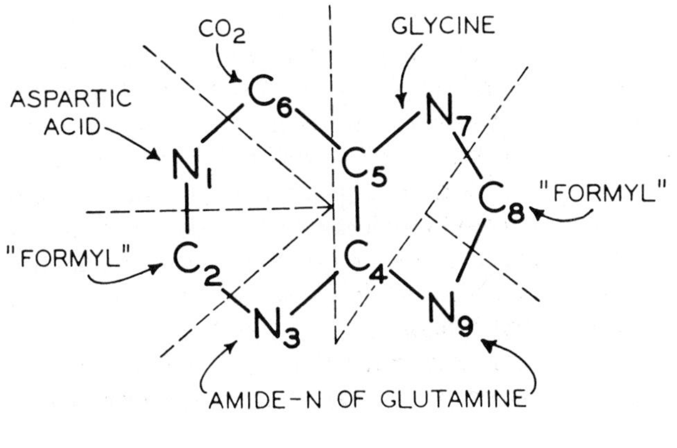

FIG. 104–14. Summary of ¹⁴C-glycine incorporation values in control and gouty subjects. (From Wyngaarden, J.B., and Kelley, W.N.[114]) PRPP = phosphoribosylpyrophosphate; PRT = hypoxanthine-guanine phosphoribosyltransferase.

FIG. 104–15. Pathway of purine biosynthesis showing the regulatory site of PRPP and nucleotides. AMP = adenosine monophosphate; GMP = guanosine monophosphate; IMP = inosine 5′-monophosphate; PRA = phosphoribosylamine; PRPP = phosphoribosylpyrophosphate.

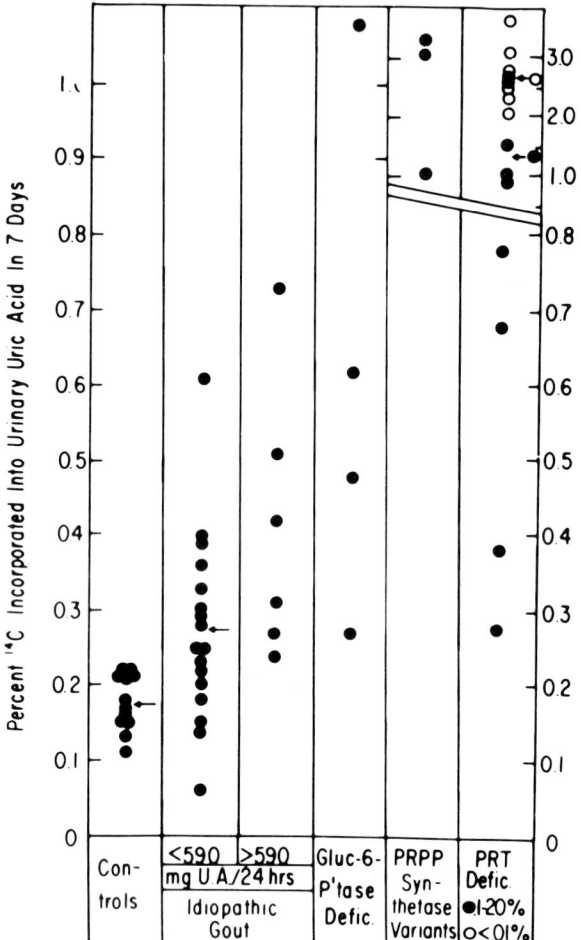

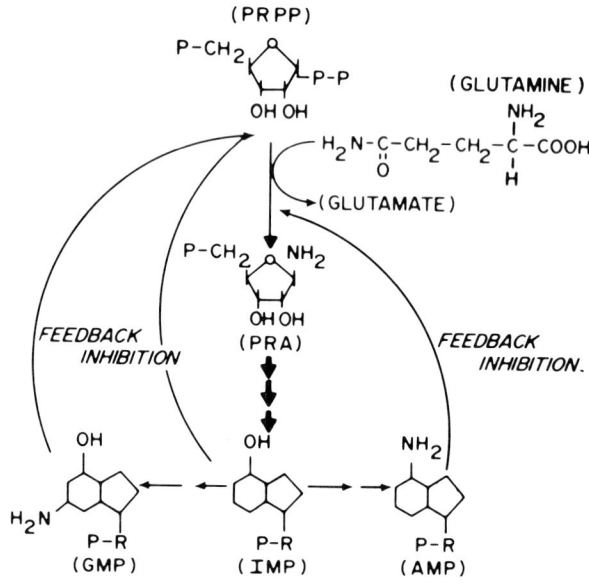

tides in the control of de novo purine biosynthesis.[133] Figure 104–15 illustrates some of the important steps in the purine biosynthetic pathway and indicates a common site at which PRPP and purine ribonucleotides regulate purine biosynthesis. This site is the first reaction unique to the pathway leading to the formation of inosinic acid, a reaction catalyzed by the enzyme *amidophosphoribosyltransferase*. PRPP and glutamic acid are substrates for this enzyme, and the purine ribonucleotide products inhibit catalytic activity through an allosteric feedback mechanism. Amidophosphoribosyltransferase activity and the rate of purine biosynthesis are regulated by the availability of the substrate PRPP and the concentration of the ribonucleotide inhibitors.

The mechanisms controlling the activity of amidophosphoribosyltransferase have been extensively studied.[134–137] The apparent Km (Michaelis constant) of human amidophosphoribosyltransferase for PRPP is approximately 0.5 mM, a value 10 to 100 times greater than the intracellular concentration of PRPP. It is unlikely that amidophosphoribosyltransferase is saturated with this substrate in vivo. Consequently, any change in PRPP concentration could lead to a corresponding change in the rate of purine biosynthesis.

Purine ribonucleotides inhibit the catalytic activity of human amidophosphoribosyltransferase (see Fig. 104–15). The molecular features of this inhibitory process have also been clarified.[134,135] The enzyme displays molecular heterogeneity, existing in a small active form of 133,000 daltons and in a large, inactive form of 270,000 daltons[135] (Fig. 104–16). The small form is converted to the large form by incubation of the enzyme with purine ribonucleotide, and the large form is converted to the small form by incubation with PRPP. Experiments in an animal model confirmed that interconversion between the small and large forms of amidophosporibosyltransferase actually occurs in vivo when the intracellular concentrations of PRPP and purine ribonucleotides are altered.[136]

FIG. 104–16. Schematic illustrating the control of human amidophosphoribosyltransferase. PRPP = phosphoribosylpyrophosphate.

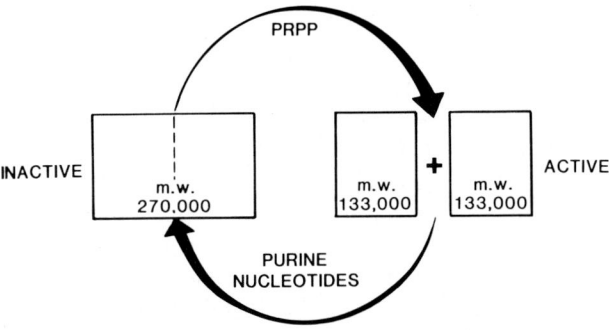

ENZYMATIC ABNORMALITIES LEADING TO PURINE OVERPRODUCTION IN MAN

A small minority of patients with primary gout (10% or less) show an increased rate of de novo purine biosynthesis. The florid overproducer of uric acid can be detected by quantifying the 24-hour urinary uric acid excretion. Up to 600 mg/day while on a purine-free diet is considered within the normal range for adults.[138,139] Because placing patients on a purine-restricted diet seldom is practical, collection of urine is often made when the patient is following his usual diet. Here, a value in excess of 1000 mg/day is clearly abnormal, while values between 800 and 1000 mg/day are borderline. The striking diurnal variation in the excretion of uric acid precludes the use of uric acid to creatinine ratios determined on spot-urine samples in assessing overproduction.[140] It is necessary therefore, in most gouty patients, to measure the 24-hour uric acid excretion. The much more sensitive and technically demanding isotopic incorporation techniques previously outlined are required to detect less pronounced urate overproduction.

A specific enzymatic defect has been identified in only a small percentage of patients who overproduce uric acid. These enzymatic abnormalities fall into two groups on the basis of the regulatory mechanisms previously discussed: (1) defects leading to an increased concentration or availability of PRPP and (2) defects leading to a decrease in the intracellular pool of purine nucleotides.

INCREASE IN PHOSPHORIBOSYLPYROPHOSPHATE

For each enzymatic alteration illustrated in Figure 104–17, it has been proposed that the concentration

FIG. 104–17. Enzymatic defects that may result in increased phosphoribosylpyrophosphate. NADP = nicotinamide-adenine dinucleotide phosphate; NADPH = reduced nicotinamide-adenine dinucleotide phosphate.

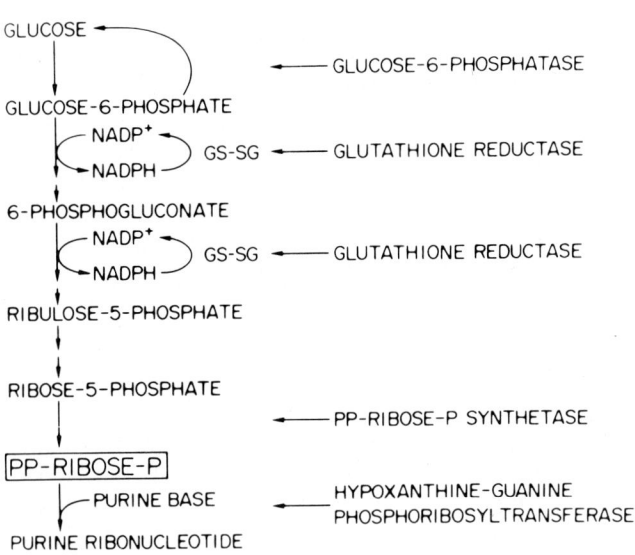

or availablity of PRPP is increased. This mechanism, however, has been established only in the case of the hypoxanthine-guanine phosphoribosyltransferase (HGPRTase) and PRPP synthetase mutants. With the exception of the glutathione reductase variants, each mutant has been associated with an increased rate of purine biosynthesis. *Glutathione reductase* generates nicotinamide-adenine dinucleotide phosphate (NADP), the cofactor in the first two steps of the pentose pathway. While theoretically, increased activity of this enzyme could result in excess synthesis of pentose phosphate compounds including PRPP and hence uric acid, an Israeli study failed to find either abnormal glutathione reductase activity or altered electrophoretic mobility in hemolysates of 52 gouty patients.[141]

Expansion of the PRPP pool in *glucose-6-phosphatase deficiency* (glycogen storage disease, type I) can occur by increasing the available substrate for the pentose phosphate pathway, because glucose-6-phosphatase is required for the hydrolysis of glucose-6-phosphate. A deficiency of this enzyme causes the intracellular accumulation of glucose-6-phosphate, a substrate for the pentose pathway,[142] and glucose-6-phosphatase deficiency could increase PRPP production by an additional mechanism. Hypoglycemia depletes the nucleotide pool in the liver of these patients. Depletion of purine nucleotides, such as adenosine diphosphate (ADP), in the liver of experimental animals may decrease the inhibition of PRPP synthetase.[136]

In patients with glucose-6-phosphatase deficiency (glycogen storage disease, type I), hyperuricemia appears in early infancy.[142a] Whereas gouty arthritis may develop by the end of the first decade, chronic tophaceous gout and gouty nephropathy become major problems only in the adult.

In cultured skin fibroblasts from two gouty patients, both ribose-5-phosphate and PRPP were increased, resulting in increased de novo purine biosynthesis.[143] The mechanisms responsible for the increase in ribose-5-phosphate and accelerated rate of purine biosynthesis are unknown. Increased activity of PRPP synthetase is, of course, associated with increased production of PRPP (vide infra).

Hypoxanthine-Guanine Phosphoribosyltransferase Deficiency

HGPRTase deficiency leads to an accumulation of PRPP because less of this substrate is consumed. The reaction catalyzed by this enzyme is shown in Figure 104–18. The substrates for HGPRTase include PRPP and either hypoxanthine or guanine; its products include inosine 5'-monophosphate (IMP), guanosine monophosphate (GMP), and inorganic pyrophosphate. HGPRTase deficiency results in decreased use of both PRPP and hypoxanthine; PRPP accumulation then provides more substrate for amidophosphoribosyltransferase, the first committed enzymatic step in the series of reactions leading to de novo purine

FIG. 104–18. Pathways showing purine ribonucleotide catabolism, salvage of purine bases, and oxidation to uric acid. GMP = guanosine monophosphate; HPRT = hypoxanthine-guanine phosphoribosyltransferase; IMP = inosine 5'-monophosphate; PNP = purine nucleoside phosphorylase; XO = xanthine oxidase.

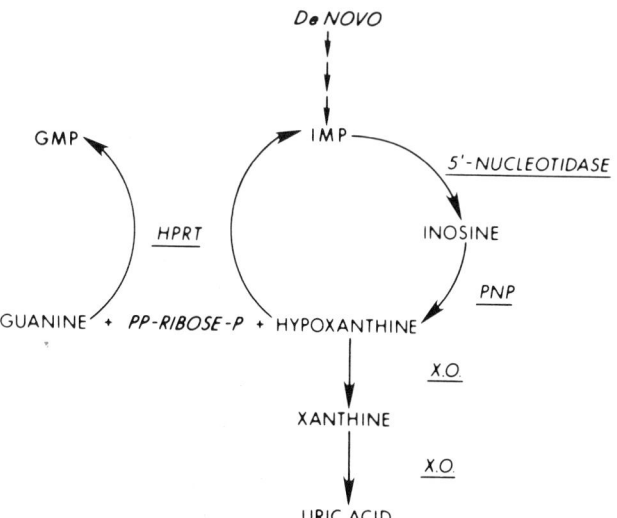

synthesis. The excess hypoxanthine is oxidized by xanthine oxidase to uric acid.

Purine nucleoside phosphorylase deficiency also leads to purine overproduction, probably as a result of decreased use of PRPP in the salvage pathway.[144] *Hypouricemia*, however, is the biochemical marker for this disorder because hypoxanthine, the substrate for xanthine oxidase, is not formed.

HGPRTase deficiency is an X-linked disorder due to a spectrum of enzyme activity in unrelated mutant hemizygous males ranging from undetectable levels to about 50% of normal.[145] Using immunochemical techniques, cell extracts from most patients have shown no demonstrable HGPRTase cross-reactive material. In others, the reduced catalytic activity is due to a decreased affinity for substrate or an increased sensitivity to inhibition by reaction products. Specific amino acid substitutions have been found in some of these mutant enzymes at sites predicted to affect either catalytic function or intracellular concentration of the enzyme.[146] Confirmation of single amino acid substitutions has been obtained by direct study of isolated DNA.[147] Using selective restriction enzymes and radiolabeled cDNA probes, a single nucleotide change in the codon for an amino acid was identified in one mutant.[148] This approach may prove useful in the antenatal diagnosis of HGPRTase deficiency.

The deficiency of this enzyme is expressed as two clinical phenotypes.[145,149] The *Lesch-Nyhan syndrome* occurs in young boys with a complete deficiency of enzyme catalytic activity. In addition to hyperuricemia, hyperuricosuria, and a tendency to form uric acid calculi, these patients also develop a central nervous system disorder, with mental retardation, spasticity, choreoathetosis, and compulsive self-mutilation (Fig. 104–19).[150] Although the basal ganglia are normally rich in HGPRTase activity, the neurologic sequelae are unrelated to hyperuricemia but rather to the dopaminergic pathway from the substantia nigra to the putamen and caudate nucleus.[151] In patients with only a *partial deficiency* of HGPRTase, the major manifestations are gouty arthritis beginning in the second or third decade and uric acid kidney stones related to the excessive uric acid excretion.[145] Neurologic findings are minimal or absent.

Increased Phosphoribosylpyrophosphate Synthetase Activity

PRPP synthetase catalyzes the synthesis of the purine regulatory substrate PRPP from adenosine triphosphate (ATP) and ribose-5-phosphate (Fig. 104–20).[152] Superactivity of PRPP synthetase, also an X-linked disorder, is characterized by marked over-

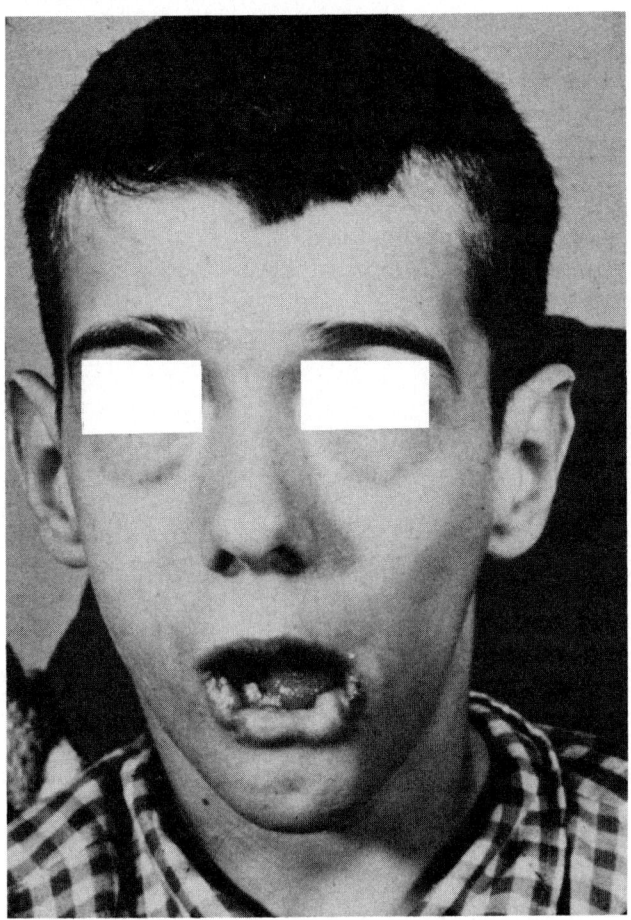

FIG. 104–19. Lesch-Nyhan syndrome. Note the mutilation of the lower lip. (Courtesy of Dr. Michael Becker, University of Chicago.)

FIG. 104–20. Control of phosphoribosylpyrophosphate synthetase activity by substrates and feedback inhibition. ADP = adenosine diphosphate; AMP = adenosine monophosphate; ATP = adenosine triphosphate; 2,3 DPG = diphosphoglycerate.

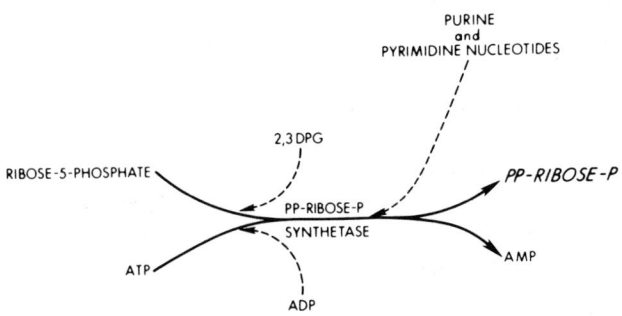

production of purines with hyperuricemia and hyperuricosuria.[153] Gouty arthritis and renal calculi occur at an early age. The excessive purine nucleotide production and uric acid excretion result from an increased concentration and rate of generation of PRPP. Considerable heterogeneity has been identified in the underlying kinetic defects. Abnormalities include both catalytic defects (increased maximal reaction velocity)[154,155] and regulatory defects with a diminished response to purine nucleotide inhibition.[156] Also, defects in substrate binding with increased affinity for ribose-5-phosphate[143] and combined catalytic and regulatory defects have been described.[157] The most common abnormality is an isolated catalytic defect due to increased maximal velocity of the enzymatic reaction. Neurologic impairment and sensorineural deafness have been described in three families with defective PRPP synthetase;[157-159] however, the data are insufficient to ascribe the neurologic abnormalities to the excessive enzyme activity.

DECREASES IN PURINE RIBONUCLEOTIDES

Theoretically, a deficiency of HGPRTase, a salvage pathway enzyme, could result in a decreased rate of synthesis of both IMP and GMP. However, quantitation of purine nucleotides in cell extracts deficient in HGPRTase has not documented a reduction.[160] By contrast, the hepatic content of purine nucleotides (ATP) does decrease in association with hypoglycemia or after glucagon administration in patients with glucose-6-phosphatase deficiency.[142] Studies in normal subjects and in animal models using fructose administration have provided insight into the pathogenesis of hyperuricemia in glucose-6-phosphatase deficiency and other conditions in which net ATP degradation results in elevation of uric acid and other oxypurines (Fig. 104–21).

The hepatic content of purine nucleotides is reduced because of increased catabolism of adenine nucleotides after fructose feeding, and this leads to increased purine synthesis de novo as well as direct conversion to uric acid from hypoxanthine. This is associated with an increased concentration of PRPP and a shift of amidophosphoribosyltransferase from the inactive to the active form.[136,161] Thus, disorders such as glucose-6-phosphatase deficiency, which also leads to intracellular nucleotide depletion, may also increase purine biosynthesis through decreased allosteric effects on amidophosphoribosyltransferase activity. Other conditions possibly associated with accelerated adenine nucleotide catabolism include sta-

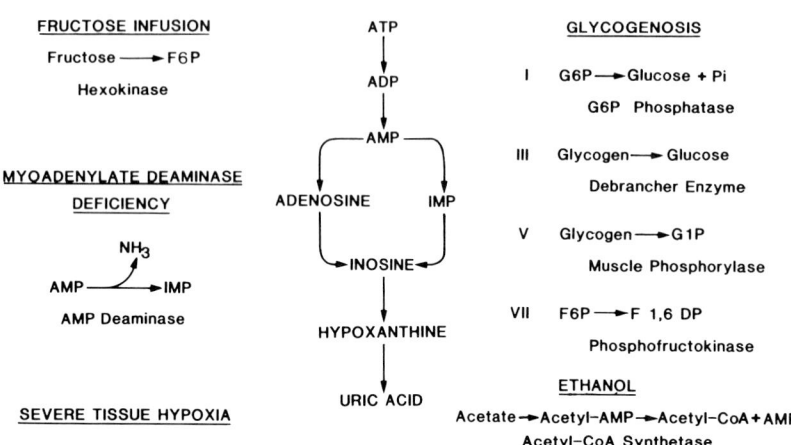

NUCLEOTIDE CATABOLISM

FIG. 104–21. Disorders proposed to result in accelerated adenine nucleotide catabolism. ADP = adenosine diphosphate; AMP = adenosine monophosphate; ATP = adenosine triphosphate; F6P = fructose-6-phosphate; F 1,6DP = fructose-1,6-diphosphate; G6P = glucose-6-phosphate; G1P = glucose-1-phosphate; IMP = inosine 5'-monophosphate.

tus epilepticus, myocardial infarction, and respiratory failure.[162,163] An elevated uric acid in such patients is thought to indicate a poor prognosis. This mechanism is also proposed for "myogenic" hyperuricemia of the glycogenosis type III (debrancher deficiency), type V (muscle phosphorylase deficiency), and type VII (muscle phosphofructokinase deficiency).[163a] The increased synthesis of uric acid during excessive alcohol consumption is also thought to be due, in part, to accelerated degradation of adenine nucleotides.[164]

EXCRETION OF URIC ACID

In normal man, approximately two thirds of uric acid produced daily is excreted by the kidney, one third is eliminated by the gastrointestinal tract and less than 1% is excreted in sweat.[122,165,166,167] In gouty patients, decreased renal clearance commonly leads to hyperuricemia despite increased gastrointestinal urate excretion. It is clear that extrarenal disposal of uric acid is *not* responsible for hyperuricemia.

CONTROL OF RENAL URIC ACID EXCRETION BY THE KIDNEY

Glomerular filtration and bidirectional urate transport including both tubular secretion and reabsorption are the essential physiologic functions that subserve the renal handling of uric acid. The discovery and relative contribution of each component has been used to define the various models proposed to explain the renal handling of uric acid and the final concentration of excreted urate. An early view held that uric acid was completely filtrable at the glomerulus and that all but 5 to 10% was reabsorbed in the tubule.[168]

A three-component system was next proposed on the basis of evidence for tubular secretion of uric acid in human and animal studies.[169–171] A four-component model was proposed later. This model includes glomerular filtration, proximal tubular reabsorption, tubular secretion, and finally, postsecretory reabsorption (Fig. 104–22).[172,173]

It is often assumed that urate is freely filtrable at

FIG. 104–22. Four-component model illustrating bidirectional urate transport by the kidney. Tubular secretion and reabsorption are shown as a percentage of filtered urate.

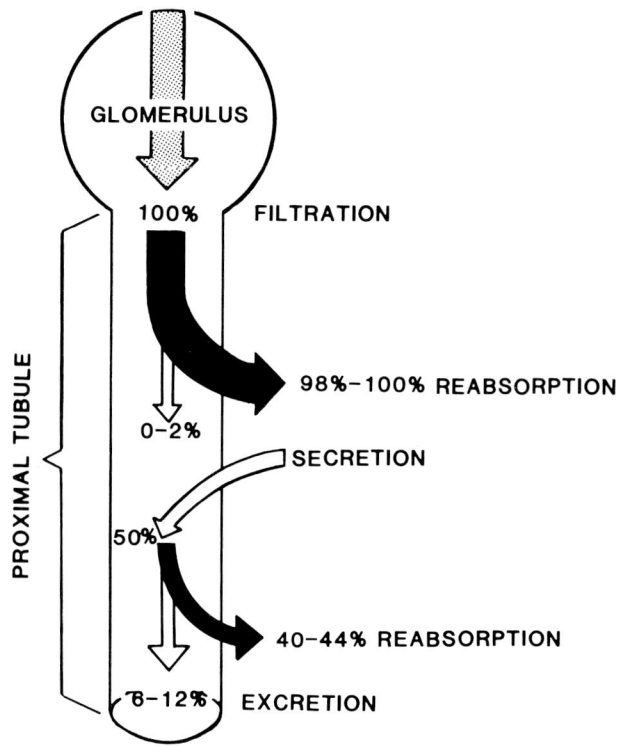

the glomerulus, and studies have yielded conflicting data with regard to urate binding to serum proteins. Whereas earlier studies focused on urate binding capacity of α_1-α_2-globulin found to be deficient in two gouty kindreds,[174] a specific urate-binding globulin could not be confirmed by others.[175] The evidence for extensive binding of urate to plasma proteins arose from in vitro studies conducted at low temperature, but urate binding becomes insignificant as the temperature approaches the physiologic range.[175–177] The current consensus is that in vivo binding of urate is very small and of no significance in the renal clearance of uric acid.[178,179]

Comparison of renal clearance of uric acid with that of inulin or creatinine (fractional excretion) gives ratios of 0.07:0.1 in normal subjects,[107] indicating that at least 90% of the filtered urate is reabsorbed by the tubules. Available animal studies suggest that the major site of such reabsorption is in the proximal tubule,[180–183] facilitated by active transport. In support of an active transport mechanism, the concentration of urinary uric acid may be only one tenth that of the plasma level during water diuresis and inhibition of urate secretion with pyrazinamide,[184] showing that reabsorption occurs against a concentration gradient. Because urate excretion is not influenced by changes in urinary pH, nonionic diffusion is not considered important.[185] The small transepithelial potential differences in the proximal tubule are unlikely to account for this phenomenon by passive forces alone.[186]

The mechanism of tubular secretion was first proposed to explain the paradoxic response of the kidney to salicylate and probenecid.[170] In low dosage, either drug decreases uric acid excretion, whereas high doses produce uricosuria. Inhibition of renal tubular secretion of urate was postulated at low drug doses, and inhibition of tubular reabsorption at higher doses.[187] Earlier, tubular secretion had been demonstrated in a healthy young man with hypouricemia, a human Dalmatian, whose urate clearance exceeded his inulin clearance by 46%.[169] Uric acid secretion was shown to occur in normal subjects after urate loading, mannitol diuresis, and large doses of probenecid.[188] Similar studies in patients with moderately reduced glomerular filtration rates (40 to 80 ml/min) produced urate clearances up to 23% above the glomerular filtration rate.[188] In virtually all animal studies using micropuncture techniques, the proximal nephron has been identified as a major site of tubular secretion,[186,189,190] facilitated by an active transport process. In a study in man, the proximal, but not the distal, nephron transported urate from plasma to tubular fluid.[191] Urate secretion in man is probably mediated by pathways common to other organic acids that in-

hibit urate excretion.[192] These include salicylates, acetoacetate, lactate and β-hydroxybutyrate, branched-chain ketoacids, and pyrazinoic acid.

Pyrazinamide virtually abolishes urate excretion in man.[193] Using stop-flow methods in the Dalmatian dog, this effect has been shown to be due to suppression of tubular secretion of urate.[194] This effect also formed the basis for the "pyrazinamide suppression test,"[195] which is no longer considered to be a valid tool for distinguishing between the relative contribution of nonreabsorbed and secreted urate to urinary uric acid excretion due to the existence of a postsecretory reabsorptive site.[172,173]

Pyrazinamide administration abolishes the uricosuria of Wilson's disease and Hodgkin's disease[196,197] and the uricosuric response to probenecid[198] or benzbromarone[173] as well as intravenous furosemide or volume expansion.[199,200] To accommodate these observations and the known effects of pyrazinamide and various uricosuric agents, a model has been proposed that includes extensive postsecretory reabsorption of secreted urate at a site either co-extensive with or distal to the secretory site.[172,173,200a] In support of this functional four-component model, hypouricemic subjects have been described with enhanced fractional excretion of urate, a normal response to pyrazinamide, and a reduced uricosuric response to benzbromarone or probenecid.[201–203] These data are interpreted as indicating an isolated defect in postsecretory reabsorption of uric acid. Further documentation and the relative flux of uric acid throughout the proposed four-component transport model will require additional study beyond in vivo pharmacologic manipulation.

DECREASED URIC ACID CLEARANCE

The concept that hyperuricemia in primary gout is due to an abnormality in the renal excretion of uric acid was first proposed by Garrod in 1876.[5] He noted that "gout would thus appear, at least partly, to depend on a loss of power . . . in the uric acid excretion function of the kidney." A reduction of uric acid clearance may contribute to hyperuricemia in 90% of patients with primary gout. Over a wide range of filtered urate loads, most gouty subjects have a lower urate clearance to glomerular filtration rate (filtration fraction) than nongouty subjects.[126] Simkin[204] has shown that the gouty individual excretes 41% less uric acid than normal subjects for any given plasma concentration of urate. Patients with primary hyperuricemia also have a greater increment in plasma urate in response to exogenous purines, which is also attributed to decreased urate clearances.[205] Gouty subjects require urate levels 2 to 3 mg/dl higher than nongouty subjects in order to achieve equivalent uric acid excretion rates.[204,204a]

Either reduced filtration of uric acid, enhanced reabsorption, or decreased secretion could lead to a decreased urate clearance in primary gout. The filtered load of urate could be decreased as a result of increased urate binding to plasma proteins. This defect has been proposed in the hyperuricemic Maori of New Zealand,[206] and in a few gouty subjects, but requires confirmation.

Both increased reabsorption and decreased secretion of uric acid have been suggested as accounting for the lower urate clearances observed in patients with gout. Although no compelling evidence fully excludes enhanced tubular reabsorption of uric acid as a cause, it has not received serious consideration in the past. Rather, diminished renal urate secretion per nephron has been postulated as a basis for hyperuricemia in primary gout not associated with urate overproduction.[207] The maximum uricosuric response induced by benzbromarone, which selectively inhibits postsecretory reabsorption, has been equated with the minimum secretory rate.[173] Using this measure, hyperuricemic patients with normal urate production have a significantly lower secretory rate compared to either patients with urate overproduction or normal subjects.

METABOLIC DEFECT IN IDIOPATHIC GOUT

Many gouty subjects exhibit both increased production and decreased renal clearance of uric acid. Glucose-6-phosphatase deficiency[142,151] and alcohol consumption[164] are examples in which both hyperlacticacidemia decreases urate secretion, and accelerated purine nucleotide catabolism enhances de novo purine biosynthesis. The concurrence of both pathogenic mechanisms leading to hyperuricemia is also found in idiopathic gout, albeit the precise metabolic defects are still unknown.[208]

HYPERURICEMIA AND GOUT ASSOCIATED WITH OTHER DISORDERS

HEMATOLOGIC DISORDERS

The mechanisms predisposing to secondary hyperuricemia and gout mirror the defects seen in primary gout, albeit the altered metabolism is brought into focus by an associated disease process or drug. In a series of patients with leukemia, myeloid metaplasia, polycythemia vera, and multiple myeloma, increased endogenous nucleotide catabolism resulted in hyperuricemia in 66% of 113 men and 69% of 73 women.[209] Gouty arthritis was noted in 10 patients (5.3%), an incidence similar to the 3.7% and 4.5% of gouty arthritis reported in other series.[28,71] In myeloid metaplasia, the incidence of gout, often complicated by tophaceous deposits, may be as high as 27%.

Mean urate excretion was 634 mg/24 hours in a group of 27 patients with gout complicating hematologic disorders, as compared to a mean value of 497 mg/24 hours in a control group.[71] In all of these conditions associated with increased marrow activity, the miscible pool is enlarged and the turnover of uric acid is increased.[128,210] The pattern of incorporation of labeled precursors into urinary purines and uric acid reflects early labeling within the first 2 days, suggesting rapid turnover of newly synthesized nucleotides, and secondary peaks at 1 to 2 weeks, suggesting the rapid turnover of myeloid and erythroid cells.[211]

Hyperuricemia is also common in secondary polycythemias,[212,213,213a] hemoglobinopathies,[214,215] pernicious anemia, especially after vitamin B_{12} therapy,[32] other chronic hemolytic states,[216,217] and occasionally, disseminated carcinomas characterized by rapid cell turnover.[218] In homozygous sickle cell disease, hyperuricemia ranges from 26 to 39%, principally in patients in the third decade with reduced renal secretory capacity.[215] The elevated urinary uric acid excretion seen at younger ages with normal or increased fractional excretion of uric acid, the excess labeled precursor incorporation into urinary uric acid, and the enlarged miscible pools all suggest excessive production of uric acid in this population.[219,220] Gouty arthritis is unusual, probably due to the shortened life span.[221]

DIURETIC DRUGS

Diuretic drug therapy represents one of the most important causes of secondary hyperuricemia. A study of hyperuricemic men admitted to a Veterans Administration Hospital implicated diuretics in 20%.[222] Fifty percent of new cases of gout in Framingham, MA, developed in subjects taking either thiazides or ethacrynic acid.[24] Surveillance of the Framingham population 26 years later showed that 20% of men and 25% of women reported taking antihypertensive medications,[223] and serum urate values were 0.8 mg/dl higher in these individuals. Other series report increments in urate values of 1.3 mg/dl and 1.8 mg/dl with chronic thiazide administration.[23,223a]

Enhanced tubular reabsorption of urate as a result of extracellular volume depletion appears to be of prime importance in urate retention because urate excretion remains at control values when volume depletion is prevented with intravenous saline.[199,224] In addition, furosemide and diazoxide can induce hyperlacticacidemia sufficient to suppress tubular secretion of urate. Neither mechanism appears to represent a direct effect on bidirectional urate transport. Spironolactone may decrease the renal clearance of uric acid but has no consistent effect on urate values.[225] The atypical presentation of tophaceous gout in elderly women with primary nodal osteoarthritis receiving chronic diuretic therapy has been discussed earlier.

ETHANOL

Epidemiologic studies show a strong correlation between serum urate levels and habitual alcohol intake[226,227] and intravenous infusion of ethanol results in hyperuricemia.[228] Gouty patients may consume more alcohol than a nongouty population.[226,227,229] Pathophysiologic mechanisms are as discussed earlier, and involve both increased urate production, and hyperlacticacidemia suppression of renal urate excretion.[228] Reduced nicotinamide-adenine dinucleotide (NADH) is generated in the metabolism of ethanol to acetaldehyde and acetate, resulting in excess conversion of pyurate to lactate. The increased adenine nucleotide catabolism in liver occurs after ethanol ingestion, which may account for elevated urate production, increased uric acid turnover, and increased oxipurine excretion.[164]

OTHER DRUGS

Besides diuretics and ethanol, a number of other drugs produce hyperuricemia. Low concentrations of salicylate in tubular urine (ingestion of approximately 2.0 g/day or less) suppress tubular secretion of urate, whereas high concentrations of free salicylate suppressed reabsorption as well as secretion; the net effect was uricosuria.[187] The antituberculous agents pyrazinamide[230] and ethambutol[231] decrease the renal clearance of uric acid. Nicotinic acid[232] operates through this mechanism but may also stimulate de novo purine biosynthesis, a mechanism also suggested for warfarin-induced hyperuricemia.[233]

BODY WEIGHT

Epidemiologic studies document a strong positive correlation between body weight and serum urate concentration, a relationship that is both complex and multifactorial.[234–240] In a study of 73,000 obese women, the crude relative risk for gout was 2.56, and women who were 85% above desirable body weight had gout 1.56 times more frequently than women less than 10% over ideal body weight.[241] In the Framingham study, the correlation between uric acid levels and weight was particularly marked in the age group 35 to 44 years, with lower correlations seen in older age groups.[242] In another study, 52% of gouty patients were more than 20% over ideal body weight.[42] That 85% of these patients were hypertensive, and 48% had abnormal glucose tolerance tests and hyperlipidemia points out the multiplicity of factors involved in obesity and its metabolic complications. An elevated ponderal index and decreased fractional excretion of uric acid have also been reported among hyperuricemic Maori men.[243] Obesity has a number of effects on urate metabolism including decreased clearance and increased production;[208] weight reduction is associated with a modest lowering of serum urate concentration.[238]

HYPERLIPIDEMIA

The relationship between hypertriglyceridemia and hyperuricemia is well established.[238,244,245] As many as 80% of individuals wih hypertriglyceridemia have hyperuricemia. From 50 to 75% of gouty patients have hypertriglyceridemia. The complexity of this relationship is evident, however, by the number of confounding variables observed in this population including both obesity and excessive alcohol intake. In one study of 40 gouty subjects, a correlation was found between the ponderal index and serum triglycerides, but the fasting triglyceride values were not significantly higher than those of obese controls.[246] The 17 gouty subjects in this study who drank excessive alcohol had higher triglyceride values than abstemious gouty patients. Another study reported a 1.6-fold increase in the frequency of hypertriglyceridemia independent of alcohol intake in a group of obese gouty patients whose hyperuricemia was normalized with either allopurinol or probenecid.[247] Hyperlipoproteinemia was seen in 56% of 108 gouty Japanese men and appeared to be independent of both alcohol intake and obesity.[248] Finally, no change was found in levels of serum urate or in uric acid excretion when triglycerides were acutely elevated in three gouty subjects receiving intravenous lipid.[249]

HYPERTENSION AND ATHEROSCLEROSIS

Hyperuricemia has been reported in 22 of 38% of untreated hypertensive patients and increases to 47 to 67% when therapy and renal disease are included.[250–252] The prevalence of gout in the hypertensive population is between 2 and 12%. Although the prevalence of hyperuricemia in the general population increases with increasing blood pressure, no consistent relationships emerge. In the Tecumseh, Michigan, study[253] no correlation was found between urate concentrations and age, sex, anthropometric data, or levels of blood pressure. Likewise, only 1% of blood pressure variation could be accounted for by serum urate values in the Israeli ischemic heart study of 10,000 men aged 40 years or older.[254] In patients with classic gout, conversely, 25 to 50% have hypertension that is unrelated to the duration of gout and is more common in the obese patient.[28,102,255]

Causal factors relating hyperuricemia and hypertension are unclear. Renal urate clearances, dependent on tubular secretory and post-secretory reabsorption rates, are reported to be inappropriately low relative to glomerular filtration rates in both adult and childhood essential hypertension.[250,251,256] This process may be regulated in part by renal blood flow. One study documented reduced renal blood flow and increased renal vascular resistance and total peripheral resistance in subjects with essential hypertension and hyperuricemia.[109] Glomerular filtration rates, cardiac output, and intravascular volume were unaffected. The authors suggest that hyperuricemia in patients with essential hypertension reflects early nephrosclerosis. The importance of this relationship should not be overlooked in the management of gout, because untreated hypertension may contribute greatly to renal morbidity.

Since the early description of excess hyperuricemia in a group of young patients with coronary heart disease, the question of hyperuricemia as an independent risk factor for atherosclerosis has been a subject of controversy.[257] Although additional reports have noted the relationship of hyperuricemia and atherosclerosis,[258,259] no clear association was found in the Tecumseh study when adjustments were made for age, sex, and relative weight.[253] Serum urate values were not significantly different in the coronary heart disease group from the mean value of the entire population. Using multivariate analysis of risk factors at the 13th biennial evaluation of the original Framingham cohort, serum urate values did not add independently to the prediction of coronary heart disease.[223] Among the Polynesians, hypertension, diabetes mellitus, and atherosclerosis are correlates of obesity rather than of hyperuricemia.[68] In hyperuricemic patients, risk factors such as obesity, hypertension, and hypertriglyceridemia appear to contribute to the observed association between elevated urate values and artherosclerosis.

CHRONIC RENAL INSUFFICIENCY

Hyperuricemia is common in uremic patients, whereas gouty arthritis is unusual, occurring in 1% or fewer patients. Among 882 patients with chronic renal insufficiency, Sarre and Mertz[260] found only two cases in which gouty arthritis was a complication. In another study, 17 cases were reported among 1600 patients with chronic renal disease of long duration.[261] Extremely high serum urate values are unusual in chronic renal disease, owing in part to an increase in the fractional excretion of uric acid. Tubular secretory capacity is preserved as glomerular filtration rate falls, and at glomerular filtration rates below 10 ml/min, tubular reabsorptive capacity for uric acid is reduced.[262] Increased extrarenal disposal of uric acid assumes a major role in homeostasis as renal function deteriorates.[263] The rarity of gout associated with uremia has been attributed to a shortened life span and a decreased ability to respond to an inflammatory stimulus.[264]

Recurrent attacks of acute arthritis or periarthritis may occur in patients with chronic renal failure treated with long-term hemodialysis. Although the clinical features of the acute inflammatory episodes and associated hyperuricemia have suggested gouty arthritis,[265] tissue and synovial fluid examination may show BCP (apatite)[266] and calcium oxalate crystals[267] in addition to MSU crystals.

LEAD INTOXICATION

An increased incidence of gout is found in chronic lead nephropathy and polycystic kidney disease.[268] In saturnine gout, the "moonshine malady," reduced renal clearance is the primary mechanism of hyperuricemia.[269] In Australia, the source of lead exposure has been leaded paint,[270] while in the Southeastern United States, the primary source has been illicit alcohol or "moonshine," which is contaminated during distillation or storage.[269,271,271a] A report questioning the significance of the association between moonshine ingestion and decreased urate clearance and gout has appeared.[42] No relationship was found between the reduced glomerular filtration rates and the amount of lead excreted following calcium EDTA (calcium edetate) infusion. Also, of 19 nongouty patients with a history of moonshine ingestion, 42% were found to have excess lead stores. Factors other than lead nephropathy such as obesity, alcohol consumption, and hypertension may contribute to the decreased urate clearance seen in this group of gouty subjects.

Isolated reports of familial nephropathy characterized by an interstitial nephritis, hyperuricemia, and gout may represent a distinct entity.[272–274] The features of this syndrome are variable but include a predominance of females, precocious gout and renal insufficiency, and an autosomal dominant pattern of inheritance.

STARVATION

Total caloric restriction results in hyperuricemia attributable to both reduced renal urate clearance and urate overproduction.[275,276] Urate retention is correlated best with ketosis, especially the serum concentrations of β-hydroxybutyrate and acetoacetate.[277] Carbohydrate, protein, or purine refeeding causes a prompt increase in urinary uric acid excretion and a return of serum urate to control values.[229] Ketosis persists when a fat diet succeeds a fast. Attacks of gout may occur during periods of starvation but are unusual except in patients with a history of prior gout.

HYPERPARATHYROIDISM

The incidence of hyperuricemia in hyperparathyroidism is high.[278,279] In most studies however, hypertension, obesity, and renal disease have obscured the significance of elevated serum urate levels.[279,280] Infusion of parathyroid hormone in 14 volunteers did not alter the renal excretion of uric acid.[281] In large series of patients with primary hyperparathyroidism, the incidence of "gouty" arthritis is reportedly between 3 and 9%[278,282] but synovial fluid examination to differentiate MSU crystals from the CPPD crystals of pseudogout was not performed in any of these earlier studies.

PSORIASIS AND SARCOIDOSIS

The relationship between psoriasis and hyperuricemia, postulated to result from an increase in epidermal cell turnover, is not clear. The occurrence of hyperuricemia in various series of patients with psoriasis ranges from no increase to 50%.[283,284] These dis-parate prevalence rates may reflect individual differences in bidirectional urate transport.[285] The pattern of labeled glycine incorporation into urinary uric acid has been interpreted as indicating increased nucleic acid turnover in psoriatic lesions.[283] The association of sarcoidosis, psoriasis, and gout has been regarded by some authors as a syndrome but as a chance occurrence by others.[286–287]

Hyperuricemia has also been reported in patients with Down's syndrome,[288] cystinuria,[289] primary oxaluria,[290] Paget's disease of bone,[291] and Bartter's syndrome.[292] Attendant episodes of gouty arthritis have been noted in Paget's disease and Bartter's syndrome, and uric acid nephrolithiasis has been described in cystinuria. Reduced renal urate clearance has been proposed for Bartter's syndrome, Down's syndrome, and hyperoxaluria.

UROLITHIASIS AND GOUT

Uric acid accounts for 5 to 10% of all renal stones in the United States and Europe[293,294] and 75% of renal stones in Israel.[295] The overall prevalence of uric acid stones in the adult United States population is estimated to be 0.01%.[296] In a series of 1258 patients with primary gout, the prevalence of renal lithiasis was 22% and climbed to 42% in 59 patients with secondary gout.[297] This figure remained remarkably stable 14 years later, when the primary gouty population increased to 2038; 23% gave a history of renal calculi.[298] Over 80% of calculi in these gouty patients were composed of uric acid. A central nidus of uric acid only, calcium oxalate, or calcium phosphate comprised the remaining stones. Renal stones antedated gouty arthritis in 40% of subjects with primary gout and occurred more frequently than arthritis before the fourth decade. When the prevalence of urolithiasis was related to serum urate in Framingham, 12.7% of male subjects with urate values between 7 and 7.9 mg/dl, and 40% of subjects with urate values greater than 9 mg/dl gave a history of renal stones[24] (Table 104–1). The risk of urolithiasis was shown to increase from 0.1%/year in normouricemic controls and 0.3%/year in asymptomatic hyperuricemic subjects, to 0.9%/year in patients with established gout.[23a] About one third of nongouty hyperuricemic patients who developed uric acid stones gave a family history of gout.[297]

From studies of gouty individuals, higher prevalence rates of uric acid urolithiasis are associated with increased uric acid excretion. In gouty patients excreting more uric acid than 1100 mg/day, the prevalence was 50%, or 4.5-fold greater, than in patients excreting less than 300 mg/day.[297] In addition to primary overproduction of uric acid, a number of other clinical situations may result in hyperuricosuria. These include inherited enzymatic defects and hematologic disorders that lead to accelerated purine biosynthesis, diets high in purine content,[205] and the administration of uricosuric drugs, which cause only a transient increase in uric acid excretion. The increase in uric acid excretion seen in patients ingesting large amounts of dietary purines may be associated with the development of calcium oxalate stones.[299] Low urine volume may be a predisposing factor to the development of uric acid calculi in patients with ileostomies or colostomies[300] as well as people living in hot arid climinates.[295] The maximum solubility of free uric acid is approximately 100 mg/L.[301]

Because the hydrogen ion concentration in urine is a critical determinant of uric acid solubility, the excretion of a persistently acid urine is another predisposing factor to the development of uric acid stones. For example, at pH 5.0, the solubility limit of uric acid is 15 mg/dl, but if urine pH is increased to 7.0, the solubility limit is raised to 200 mg/dl.[302] Because the biologically significant pKa of uric acid is 5.75, at a pH of 7.0, 95% of uric acid is present as the soluble urate salt. The finding of a low urinary pH is well documented in patients with uric acid calculi.[297,298,303] Also, patients with primary gout generally excrete an unusually acid urine.

The low urinary pH in patients with uric acid calculi has been interpreted by some as a defect in ammonium excretion,[304,305] and by others as an increase in titrable acidity.[306] At the present time, these conflicting results cannot be reconciled, because other variables may be important in assessing ammonium and titrable acid excretion. A reduced capacity for ammonium excretion is associated with aging,[306] a reduced nephron mass,[307] and diets high in protein and purines, which also increase titrable acidity.[303,308] These factors must be controlled in future studies of low urinary pH in patients with uric acid stones. A deficiency of renal glutaminase activity resulting in reduced glutamine use for ammonium production by the kidney was proposed,[309] but renal glutaminase was normal in gouty subjects by direct assay.[310]

A final factor to consider in the pathogenesis of uric acid stones and calcium oxalate stones in patients with idiopathic hyperuricosuria are substances that may affect both uric acid solubility and crystal growth. Regarding uric acid solubility, limited data suggest the presence of a nondialyzable mucoprotein in urine that retards uric acid precipitation.[311] There was no difference, however, in the amount of this substance in urine from patients with urolithiasis and healthy controls. Heterogeneous nucleation of calcium oxalate

crystals can occur either on monosodium urate or uric acid seed crystals in patients with hyperuricosuria.[312] In addition, a glycoprotein containing γ-carboxyl glutamic acid isolated from kidney and urine can inhibit calcium oxalate crystal growth.[313] The available data leave the exact mechanisms of crystal growth in doubt, but deserve further study.

HYPOURICEMIA

It is difficult to arrive at a precise value below which the serum concentration of urate is abnormally low. The problem arises because of the different methods used to determine urate values, and the non-Gaussian distribution of these values in the population. A conservative estimate of a serum urate concentration of 2 mg/dl or less was found in 0.8% of hospitalized patients and 1.0% of the residents of Tecumseh, Michigan.[16,314,315] Hypouricemia may result from diminished uric acid production, excess uric acid excretion, or a combinaiton of both mechanisms. No pathologic consequence of hypouricemia is recognized, and no therapy is required. Rather, the clinical significance of hypouricemia is determined by the underlying condition that causes this abnormal laboratory result. The congenital enzyme deficiencies of xanthine oxidase and purine nucleoside phosphorylase result in hypouricemia.

Xanthinuria is an autosomal recessive disorder characterized by the virtual absence of xanthine oxidase activity, hypouricemia and hypouricaciduria, elevated oxypurine excretion with a preponderance of xanthine, and recurrent xanthine stones.[316] Patients with arthritis and myopathy have also been reported. Treatment with allopurinol results in an acquired decrease in xanthine oxidase activity and elevation of urinary oxipurine excretion. (See Chapter 105.) *Purine nucleoside phosphorylase* deficiency is associated with T-cell dysfunction and an immunodeficiency state. Decreased activity of PRPP synthetase has been described in a mentally retarded male infant.[159]

Hypouricemia due to enhanced renal clearance of uric acid may be a biochemical feature of various diseases including Wilson's disease and Fanconi's syndrome, lymphomas, and carcinomas,[317] especially small cell carcinoma of the lung associated with inappropriate secretion of antidiuretic hormone.[318] Severe liver disease may cause hypouricemia, perhaps due to decreased purine biosynthesis.

A large list of medications in addition to uricosuric drugs may reduce serum urate concentrations. In a series of over 6000 consecutive urate measurements, the most frequently encountered agents included aspirin, x-ray contrast media, and glyceryl-guaiacholate.[314] Enhanced fractional excretions of uric acid and lowering of serum urate values is a common metabolic consequence of total parenteral nutrition, most likely related to the glycine content of the infusion solution.[33]

Finally, hypouricemia has been noted in several healthy adults with an isolated defect in the bidirectional tubular transport of uric acid.[169,201–203] Isolated defects that result in hypouricemia include diminished reabsorption of filtered urate, a defect in postsecretory reabsorption, and a defect characterized by urate clearances in excess of glomerular filtration rates (inulin clearance) due to deficient reabsorption of uric acid throughout the nephron. Hypouricemia detected during routine laboratory testing may be the initial clue leading to the proper diagnosis of one of these conditions.

REFERENCES

1. Hippocrates. The Genuine Works of Hippocrates. Vols. 1 and 2. Translated from the Greek with a preliminary discourse and annotations by Francis Adams. New York, Wood, 1886.
2. McCarty, D.J.: A historical note: Leeuwenhoek's description of crystals from a gouty tophus. Arthritis Rheum., 13:414–418, 1970.
3. Scheele, K.W.: Examen chemicum calculi urinarii. Opuscula, 2:73, 1776.
4. Wollaston, W.H.: On gouty and urinary concretions. Philos. Trans. R. Soc., Lond., 87:386–415, 1797.
5. Garrod, A.B.: Treatise on Gout and Rheumatic Gout (Rheumatoid Arthritis). 3rd Ed. London, Longmans, Green, 1876.
6. Fischer, E.: Untersuchungen in der Puringruppe. Berlin, Springer, 1907.
7. McCarty, D.J., and Hollander, J.L.: Identification of urate crystals in gouty synovial fluid. Ann. Intern. Med., 54:452–460, 1961.
8. Seegmiller, J.E., Howell, R.R., and Malwista, S.E.: The inflammatory reaction to sodium urate: Its possible relationship to the genesis of acute gouty arthritis. JAMA, 180:469–475, 1962.
9. Faires, J.S., and McCarty, D.J.: Acute arthritis in man and dog after intrasynovial injection of sodium urate crystals. Lancet, 2:682–684, 1962.
10. Seegmiller, J.E., and Howell, R.R.: The old and new concepts of acute gouty arthritis. Arthritis Rheum., 5:616–623, 1962.
11. Gutman, A.B., and Yu, T-F.: Benemid(p-di-n-propylsulfamyl)-benzoic acid) as uricosuric agent in chronic gouty arthritis. Trans. Assoc. Am. Physicians, 64:279–288, 1951.
12. Talbot, J.H., Bishop, C., Norcross, B.M., and Lockie, L.M.: The clinical and metabolic effects of Benemid in patients with gout. Trans. Assoc. Am. Physicians, 64:372, 1951.
13. Rundles, R.W., et al.: Effects of a xanthine oxidase inhibitor on thiopurine metabolism, hyperuricemia and gout. Trans. Assoc. Am. Physicians, 26:126–140, 1963.
14. Allen, D.J., Milosovich, G., and Mattock, A.M.: Inhibition of monosodium urate crystal growth. Arthritis Rheum., 8:1123–1133, 1965.
15. Emmerson, B.J., and Sandilands, P.: The normal range of plasma urate levels. Aust. Ann. Med., 12:46–52, 1963.
16. Mikkelsen, W.M., Dodge, H.J., and Valkenburg, H.: The distribution of serum uric acid values in a population unselected as to gout or hyperuricemia. Tecumseh, Michigan, 1959–1960. Am. J. Med., 39:242–251, 1965.
17. Crowley, L.V., and Alton, F.D.: Automated analysis of uric acid. Am. J. Clin. Pathol., 49:285–288, 1968.
18. Harkness, R.A., and Nicol, A.D.: Plasma uric acid levels in children. Arch. Dis. Child., 44:773–778, 1969.
19. Munan, L., Kelley, A., and Petitclerc, C.: Serum urate levels between ages 10 and 14: Changes in sex trends. J. Lab Clin. Med., 90:990–996, 1977.
20. Wolfson, W.Q., et al.: The transport and excretion of uric acid in man. V. A sex difference in urate metabolism. J. Clin. Endocrinol. Metab., 9:749–767, 1949.
21. Anton, F.M., et al.: Sex differences in uric acid metabolism in adults. Evidence for a lack of influence of Estradiol 17 (E_2) on the renal handling of urate. Metabolism, 35:343–348, 1986.
22. Campion, E.W., Glynn, R.J., and DeLabry, L.O.: Asymptomatic hyperuricemia. Risks and consequences in the normative aging study. Am. J. Med., 82:421–426, 1987.
23. Langford, H.G., et al.: Is thiazide-produced uric acid elevation harmful? Analysis of data from the hypertension detection and follow-up program. Arch. Intern. Med., 147:645–649, 1987.
23a. Fessel, J.W.: Renal outcomes of gout and hyperuricemia. Am. J. Med., 67:74–82, 1979.
24. Hall, A.P., Barry, P.E., Dawber, T.R., and McNamara, P.M.: Epidemiology of gout and hyperuricemia: A long term population study. Am. J. Med., 42:27–37, 1967.
25. Bergstrom, G., et al.: Prevalence of rheumatoid arthritis, osteoarthritis, chondrocalcinosis and gouty arthritis at age 79. J. Rheumatol., 13:527–534, 1986.
26. Copeman, W.S.C.: A short history of the gout. Berkley and Los Angeles, University of California Press, 1964.
27. Delbarre, F., Braun, S., and St. George-Chaumet, F.: La goutte: Problemes cliniques, biologiques et therapeutiques. Sem. Hop. Paris, 43:623–633, 1967.
28. Grahame, P., and Scott, J.T.: Clinical survey of 354 patients with gout. Ann. Rheum. Dis., 29:461–468, 1970.
29. Harth, M., and Robinson, C.E.G.: Gouty arthritis in a D.V.A. Hospital: A retrospective study. Med. Serv. J. Canada, 18:671–674, 1962.
30. Salzman, R.T., Howell, D.S., and Ricca, L.R.: Aberrancy in clinical hallmarks of gouty arthritis: Brief clinical report. Arthritis Rheum., 8:998–1001, 1965.
30a. Meyers, O.L., and Monteagudo, F.S.E.: Gout in females. An analysis of 92 patients. Clin. Exp. Rheumatol., 3:105–109, 1985.
31. Kernodle, G.W., and Allen, N.B.: Acute gout presenting in the manubriosternal joint. Arthritis Rheum., 29:570–572, 1986.
32. Sears, W.G.: The occurrence of gout during the treatment of pernicious anemia. Lancet, 1:24, 1933.
33. Derus, C.L., Levinson, D.J., Bowman, B., and Bengoa, J.M.: Altered fractional excretion of uric acid during total parenteral nutrition. J. Rheumatol., 114:978–981, 1987.
33a. Rodnan, G.P.: The pathogenesis of aldermanic gout: Procatarctic role of fluctuation in serum urate concentrations in gouty arthritis provoked by feast and alcohol. Clin. Res., 28:359A, 1980.
34. Linton, R.R., and Talbot, J.H.: The surgical treatment of tophaceous gout. Ann. Surg., 117:161–182, 1943.

35. Wallace, S.L., et al.: Preliminary criteria for the classification of the acute arthritis of primary gout. Arthritis Rheum., 20:895–900, 1977.

36. Gutman, A.B.: Gout and gouty arthritis. In Textbook of Medicine. Edited by P.B. Beeson and W. McDermott. Philadelphia, W.B. Saunders, 1958.

37. Raddatz, D.A., Mahowald, M.L., and Bilka, P.J.: Acute polyarticular gout. Ann. Rheum. Dis., 42:117–122, 1983.

38. Hadler, N.M., Franck, W.A., Bress, N.M., and Robinson, D.R.: Acute polyarticular gout. Am. J. Med., 56:715–719, 1974.

39. McCarty, D.J.: Crystal-induced inflammation: Syndromes of gout and pseudogout. Geriatrics, 18:467–478, 1963.

40. Ginsberg, M.H., Genant, H.K., Yu, T-F., and McCarty, D.J.: Rheumatoid nodulosis: An unusual variant of rheumatoid disease. Arthritis Rheum., 18:49–58, 1975.

41. Kozin, F., and McCarty, D.J.: Rheumatoid factors in the serum of gouty patients. Arthritis Rheum., 20:1559–1560, 1977.

42. Reynold, P.P., Knapp, M.J., Baraf, H.S.B., and Holmes, E.W.: Moonshine and lead. Relationship to the pathogenesis and hyperuricemia in gout. Arthritis Rheum., 26:1057–1064, 1983.

43. Agudelo, C.A., Turner, R.A., Panetti, M., and Pisko, E.: Does hyperuricemia protect from rheumatoid inflammation. Arthritis Rheum., 27:443–448, 1984.

44. Hench, P.S.: Diagnosis of gout and gouty arthritis. J. Lab. Clin. Med., 22:48–55, 1936.

45. Gutman, A.B.: The past four decades of progress in the knowledge of gout with an assessment of the present status. Arthritis Rheum., 16:431–445, 1973.

46. Nishioka, N., and Mikanagi, K.: Clinical features of 4,000 gouty subjects in Japan. Adv. Exp. Med. Biol., 122A:47–54, 1980.

47. Nakayama, D.A., et al.: Tophaceous gout: A clinical and radiographic assessment. Arthritis Rheum., 27:468–471, 1984.

48. Macfarlane, D.G., and Dieppe, P.A.: Diuretic-induced gout in elderly women. Br. J. Rheumatol., 24:155–157, 1985.

49. Doherty, M., and Dieppe, P.A.: Crystal deposition disease in the elderly. Clin. Rheum. Dis., 12:97–116, 1986.

50. Yu, T-F.: Secondary gout associated with myeloproliferative disease. Arthritis Rheum., 8:765–771, 1965.

51. Smythe, C.M., and Cutchin, J.H.: Primary juvenile gout. Am. J. Med., 32:799–804, 1962.

52. Wood, M.H., et al.: The Lesch-Nyhan syndrome: Report of three cases. Aust. N.Z. Med. J., 1:57–64, 1972.

52a.Ludwig, A.P., Bennett, G.A., and Bauer, W.: A rare manifestation of gout: Widespread ankylosis simulating rheumatoid arthritis. Ann. Intern. Med., 11:1248–1276, 1938.

53. Lichtenstein, L., Scott, H.W., and Levin, M.H.: Pathologic changes in gout; survey of 11 necropsied cases. Am. J. Pathol., 32:871–895, 1956.

54. Martinez-Cordero, E., Barreira-Mercado, E., and Katona, G.: Eye tophi deposition in gout. J. Rheumatol., 13:471–473, 1986.

55. Stark, T.W., and Hirokawa, R.H.: Gout and its manifestations in the head and neck. Otolaryngol. Clin. North Am., 15:659–664, 1982.

56. Varga, J., Giampaola, C., and Goldenberg, D.L.: Tophaceous gout of the spine in a patient with no peripheral tophi: Case report and review of the literature. Arthritis Rheum., 28:1312–1315, 1985.

57. McCallum, D.E., Mathews, R.S., and O'Neil, M.T.: Aseptic necrosis of the femoral head. Associated diseases and evaluation of treatment. South. Med. J., 63:241–253, 1970.

58. Hunder, G.G., Worthington, J.W., and Bickel, W.H.: Avascular necrosis of the femoral head in a patient with gout. JAMA, 203:101–103, 1968.

59. Stockman, A., Darlington, L.G., and Scott, J.T.: Frequency of chondrocalcinosis in the knees and avascular necrosis of the femoral head in gout: A controlled study. Ann. Rheum. Dis., 39:7–11, 1980.

60. Bauer, W., and Klemperer, F.: Gout. In Diseases of Metabolism. 2nd Ed. Edited by G. Duncan. Philadelphia, W.B. Saunders, 1947.

61. Bartels, E.C., and Matossian, G.S.: Gout: Six-year follow up on probenecid (Benemid) therapy. Arthritis Rheum., 2:193–202, 1959.

62. Yu, T-F.: Milestones in the treatment of gout. Am. J. Med., 56:676–685, 1974.

63. O'Duffy, J.D., Hunder, G.G., and Kelly, P.J.: Decreasing prevalence of tophaceous gout. Mayo Clin. Proc., 50:227–228, 1975.

64. Lawrence, J.S.: Heritable disorders of connective tissue. Proc. R. Soc. Med., 53:522–526, 1960.

65. Wyngaarden, J.B.: Gout. In The Metabolic Basis of Inherited Diseases. Edited by J.B. Stanbury, D.S. Fredrickson, and J.B. Wyngaarden. New York, McGraw-Hill, 1960.

66. Zalokar, J., Lellouch, J., and Claude, J.R.: Goutte et uricemia dans une population de 4663 hommes jeumes actifs. Sem. Hop. Paris, 14:664–670, 1981.

67. Lennane, G.A.Q., Rose, B.S., and Isdale, I.C.: Gout in the Maori. Ann. Rheum. Dis., 19:120–125, 1960.

68. Prior, I.A.M., Rose, B.S., Harvey, H.P., and Davidson, F.: Hyperuricemia, gout and diabetic abnormality in Polynesian people. Lancet, 1:333–338, 1966.

69. Turner, R.E., Frank, M.J., VanAusdal, D., and Bollet, A.J.: Some aspects of the epidemiology of gout: Sex and race incidence. Arch. Intern. Med., 106:400–406, 1960.

70. Bartels, E.C.: Gout as a complication of Surgery. Surg. Clin. North Am., 38:845–848, 1957.

71. Gutman, A.B., and Yu, T-F.: Secondary gout. (Abstract.) Ann. Intern. Med., 56:675, 1962.

72. Hoffman, W.S.: Some unsolved problems of gout. Med. Clin. North Am., 43:595–606, 1959.

73. Rouault, T., Caldwell, D.S., and Holmes, E.W.: Aspiration of the asymptomatic metatarsophalangeal joint in gout patients and hyperuricemic controls. Arthritis Rheum., 25:209–212, 1982.

74. Weinberger, A., et al.: Frequency of intra-articular monosodium urate (MSU) crystals in asymptomatic hyperuricemic subjects. Adv. Exp. Med. Biol., 195A:431–434, 1986.

75. Wallace, S.L., Bernstein, D., and Diamond, H.: Diagnostic value of colchicine therapeutic trial. JAMA, 199:525–528, 1967.

76. Spilberg, I., McLain, D., Simchowitz, L., and Berney, S.: Colchicine and pseudogout. Arthritis Rheum., 23:1062–1063, 1980.

77. Martel, W.: The overhanging margin of bone: A roentgenologic manifestation of gout. Radiology, 91:755–756, 1968.

78. Good, A.E., and Rapp, R.: Bony ankylosis. A rare manifestation of gout. J. Rheumatol., 5:335–337, 1978.

79. Vyhnanek, L., Lavicka, J., and Blahos, J.: Roentgenological findings in gout. Radiol. Clin., 29:256–264, 1960.

80. Talbott, J.H.: Gout. 3rd Ed. New York, Grune & Stratton, 1967.

81. Dodds, W.J., and Steinbach, H.L.: Gout associated with calcification of cartilage. N. Engl. J. Med., 275:745–749, 1966.

82. Good, A.E., and Rapp, R.: Chondrocalcinosis of the knee with gout and rheumatoid arthritis. N. Engl. J. Med., 277:286–290, 1967.

83. Hasselbacher, P., et al.: Stimulation of synovial fibroblasts by calcium oxalate and monosodium urate monohydrate. A

mechanism of connective tissue degradation in oxalosis and gout. J. Lab. Clin. Med., *100*:977–985, 1982.

84. Robinson, D.R., Tashjian, A.H., Jr., and Levine, L.: Prostaglandin induced bone resorption by rheumatoid synovia. (Abstract.) Clin. Res., *23*:443A, 1975.

85. Malawista, S.E., Seegmiller, J.E., Hathaway, B.E., and Sokoloff, L.: Sacroiliac gout. JAMA, *194*:954–956, 1965.

86. Alarcon-Segovia, D.A., Cetina, J.A., and Diaz-Jouanen, E.: Sacroiliac joints in primary gout: Clinical and roentgenographic study of 143 patients. AJR, *118*:438–443, 1973.

87. Cohen, H.: Gout and other metabolic disorders producing joint disease. *In* Textbook of the Rheumatic Diseases. Edited by W.S.C. Copeman. Edinburgh, Livingstone, 1955.

88. Neel, J.V.: The clinical detection of the genetic carriers of inherited disease. Medicine, *26*:115–153, 1947.

89. Smyth, C.J.: Hereditary factors in gout: A review of recent literature. Metabolism, *6*:218–229, 1957.

90. Smyth, C.J., Cotterman, C.W., and Freyberg, R.H.: The genetics of gout and hyperuricemia—An analysis of nineteen families. J. Clin. Invest., *27*:749–759, 1948.

91. Hauge, M., and Harvald, B.: Heredity in gout and hyperuricemia. Acta Med. Scand., *152*:247–257, 1955.

92. O'Brien, W.M., Burch, T.A., and Bunim, J.J.: Genetics of hyperuricemia in Blackfeet and Pima Indians. Ann. Rheum. Dis., *25*:117–119, 1966.

93. Cobb, S.: Hyperuricemia in executives. *In* The Epidemiology of Chronic Rheumatism. Vol. 1. Edited by J.H. Kellgren, M.R. Jeffrey, and J. Ball. Philadelphia, F.A. Davis, 1963.

93a. Laskarzewski, P.M., et al.: Familial hyper- and hypouricemias in random and hyperlipidemic recall cohorts. The Princeton school district family study. Metabolism, *32*:230–243, 1983.

94. Decker, J.L., Jane, J.J., Jr., and Reynolds, W.E.: Hyperuricemia in a male Filipino population. Arthritis Rheum., *5*:144–155, 1962.

95. Burch, T.A., O'Brien, W.M., Need, R., and Kurland, L.T.: Hyperuricemia and gout in the Mariana Islands. Ann. Rheum. Dis., *25*:114–119, 1966.

96. Sokoloff, L.: The pathology of gout. Symposium on Gout. Metabolism, *6*:230–243, 1957.

97. Fiechtner, J.J., and Simkin, P.A.: Urate spherulites in gouty synovia. JAMA, *245*:1533–1536, 1981.

98. Weinberger, A., et al.: Spherulite crystals in synovial tissue of a patient with recurrent monoarthritis. Clin. Exp. Rheumatol., *2*:63–65, 1984.

99. Catto, M.: Pathology of gout. Scot. Med. J., *18*(Suppl):232–238, 1973.

100. Hartung, E.F.: Symposium on gout: Historical considerations. Metabolism, *6*:196–208, 1957.

101. Perricone, E., and Brandt, K.D.: Enhancement of urate solubility by connective tissue. I. Effect of proteoglycan aggregates and buffer cation. Arthritis Rheum., *21*:453–460, 1978.

102. Barlow, K.A., and Beilin, L.J.: Renal disease in primary gout. Q. J. Med., *37*:79–96, 1968.

103. Talbott, J.H., and Terplan, K.L.: The kidney in gout. Medicine, *39*:405–468, 1960.

104. Wyngaarden, J.B.: The role of the kidney in the pathogenesis and treatment of gout. Arthritis Rheum., *1*:191–203, 1958.

105. Talbott, J.H., and Lilienfeld, A.: Longevity in gout. Geriatrics, *14*:409–420, 1959.

106. Reif, M.C., Constantiner, A., and Levitt, M.F.: Chronic gouty nephropathy: A vanishing syndrome? N. Engl. J. Med., *304*:535–536, 1981.

107. Gutman, A.B., and Yu, T-F.: Renal function in gout: With a commentary on the renal regulation of urate excretion, and

the role of the kidney in the pathogenesis of gout. Am. J. Med., *23*:600–622, 1957.

108. Yu, T-F., and Berger, L.: Renal disease in primary gout: A study of 253 gout patients with proteinuria. Semin. Arthritis Rheum., *4*:293–305, 1975.

109. Messerli, F.H., et al.: Serum uric acid in essential hypertension: An indicator of renal vascular involvement. Ann. Intern. Med., *93*:817–821, 1980.

110. Berger, L., and Yu, T-F.: Renal function in gout. IV. An analysis of 524 gouty subjects including long-term follow-up studies. Am. J. Med., *59*:605–613, 1975.

111. Brown, J., and Mallory, G.K.: Renal changes in gout. N. Engl. J. Med., *243*:325–329, 1950.

112. Ebstein, W.: Die Natur und Behandlung der Gicht. Wiesbaden, West Germany, Bergmanni, 1906.

113. Talbott, J.H.: Gout. 2nd Ed. New York, Grune & Stratton, 1964.

114. Wyngaarden, J.B., and Kelley, W.N.: Gout and Hyperuricemia. New York, Grune & Stratton, 1976.

115. Fineberg, S.K., and Altschul, A.: The nephropathy of gout. Ann. Intern. Med., *4*:1182–1194, 1956.

116. Gonick, H.G., and Rubini, M.E., Gleason, I.O., and Sommers, S.C.: The renal lesion in gout. Ann. Intern. Med., *62*:667–674, 1965.

117. Greenbaum, D., Ross, J.H., and Steinberg, V.L.: Renal biopsy in gout. Br. Med. J., *1*:1502–1504, 1961.

118. Heptinstall, R.H.: Diabetes mellitus and gout. *In* Pathology of the Kidney. 2nd Ed. Boston, Little, Brown, 1974.

119. Batuman, V., et al.: The role of lead in gout nephropathy. N. Engl. J. Med., *304*:520–523, 1981.

120. Schnitker, M.A., and Richter, A.B.: Nephritis in gout. Am. J. Med. Sci., *192*:241–252, 1936.

121. Sorensen, L.B.: Degradation of uric acid in man. Metabolism, *8*:687–703, 1959.

122. Wyngaarden, J.B., and Stetten, D.W., Jr.: Uricolysis in normal man. J. Biol. Chem., *203*:9–21, 1953.

123. Sorensen, L.B.: The pathogenesis of gout. Arch. Intern. Med., *109*:379–390, 1962.

124. Seegmiller, J.E., Grayzel, A.I., Laster, L., and Little, L.: Uric acid production in gout. J. Clin. Invest., *40*:1304–1314, 1961.

125. Scott, J.T., et al.: Studies of uric acid pool size and turnover rate. Ann. Rheum. Dis., *28*:366–373, 1969.

126. Wyngaarden, J.B.: Gout. Adv. Metab. Disord., *2*:1–78, 1965.

127. Benedict, J.D., Forsham, P.H., and Stetten, D.W., Jr.: The metabolism of uric acid in the normal and gouty human studied with the aid of isotopic uric acid. J. Biol. Chem., *181*:183–193, 1949.

128. Bishop, C., Garner, W., and Talbott, J.H.: Pool size, turnover rate, and rapidity of equilibration of injected isotopic uric acid in normal and pathological subjects. J. Clin. Invest., *30*:879–888, 1951.

129. Benedict, J.D., et al.: The effect of salicylates and adrenocorticotropic hormone upon the miscible pool of uric acid in gout. J. Clin. Invest., *29*:1104–1111, 1950.

130. Benedict, J.D., Roche, M., Yu, T-F., and Bien, E.J.: Incorporation of glycine nitrogen into uric acid in normal and gouty man. Metabolism, *1*:3–12, 1952.

131. Wyngaarden, J.B.: Overproduction of uric acid as the cause of hyperuricemia in primary gout. J. Clin. Invest., *36*:1508–1515, 1957.

132. Benedict, J.D., et al.: A further study of the utilization of dietary glycine nitrogen for uric acid synthesis in gout. J. Clin. Invest., *32*:775–777, 1953.

133. Holmes, E.W.: Regulation of purine biosynthesis de novo. *In*

Uric Acid: Handbook of Experimental Pharmacology. Vol. 51. Edited by W.N. Kelley an I.M. Weiner. New York, Springer-Verlag, 1978.

134. Holmes, E.W., et al.: Human glutamine phosphoribosylpyrophosphate amidotransferase: Kinetic and regulatory properties. J. Biol. Chem., 248:144–150, 1973.

135. Holmes, E.W., Wyngaarden, J.B., and Kelley, W.N.: Human glutamine phosphoribosylpyrophosphate amidotransferase: Two molecular forms interconvertible by purine ribonucleotides and phosphoribosylpyrophosphate. J. Biol. Chem., 248:6035–6040, 1973.

136. Itakura, M., Sabina, R.L., Heald, P.W., and Holmes, E.W.: Basis for the control of purine biosynthesis by purine ribonucleotides. J. Clin. Invest., 67:994–1002, 1981.

137. Wood, A.W., and Seegmiller, J.E.: Properties of 5-phosphoribosyl-1-pyrophosphate amidotransferase from human lymphoblasts. J. Biol. Chem., 248:138–143, 1973.

138. Coe, F.L., Moran, E., and Kavalich, A.G.: The contribution of dietary purine over-consumption to hyperuricosuria in calcium oxalate stone formers. J. Chronic Dis., 29:793–800, 1976.

139. Seegmiller, J.E., Grayzel, A.D., and Howell, R.R.: The renal excretion of uric acid in gout. J. Clin. Invest., 41:1094–1098, 1962.

140. Wortmann, R.L., and Fox, I.H.: Limited value of uric acid to creatinine ratios in estimating uric acid excretion. Ann. Intern. Med., 93:822–825, 1980.

141. Wasserzug, O., Szeinberg, A., and Sperling, O.: Altered physical properties of glutathione reductase in G-6PD deficiency. (Abstract.) Hum. Hered., 27:220, 1977.

142. Green, H.L., et al.: ATP depletion, a possible role in the pathogenesis of hyperuricemia in glycogen storage disease, Type I. J. Clin. Invest., 62:321–328, 1978.

142a. Howell, R.R., and Williams, J.C.: The glycogen storage diseases. In The Metabolic Basis of Inherited Diseases. 5th Ed. Edited by J.B. Stanbury et al. New York, McGraw-Hill, 1983.

143. Becker, M.A.: Patterns of phosphoribosylpyrophosphate and ribose-5-phosphate concentration and generation in fibroblasts from patients with gout and purine overproduction. J. Clin. Invest., 57:308–313, 1976.

144. Cohen, A., et al.: Abnormal purine metabolism and purine overproduction in a patient deficient in purine nucleoside phosphorylase. N. Engl. J. Med., 295:1449–1454, 1976.

145. Kelley, W.N., and Wyngaarden, J.B.: Clinical syndromes associated with hypoxanthine-guanine phosphoribosyltransferase deficiency. In The Metabolic Basis of Inherited Diseases. 5th Ed. Edited by J.B. Stanbury et al. New York, McGraw-Hill, 1983.

146. Wilson, J.M., and Kelley, W.N.: Molecular basis of hypoxanthineguanine phosphoribosyltransferase deficiency in a patient with the Lesch-Nyhan syndrome. J. Clin. Invest., 71:1331–1335, 1983.

147. Wilson, J.M., Young, A.B., and Kelley, W.N.: Hypoxanthine-guanine phosphoribosyltransferase deficiency. The molecular basis of the clinical syndromes. N. Engl. J. Med., 309:900–910, 1983.

148. Wilson, J.M., et al.: Human hypoxanthine guanine phosphoribosyltransferase. Detection of a mutant allele by restriction endonuclease analysis. J. Clin. Invest., 72:767–772, 1983.

149. Kelley, W.N., et al.: Hypoxanthine-guanine phosphoribosyltransferase deficiency in gout. Ann. Intern. Med., 70:155–206, 1969.

150. Christie, R., et al.: Lesch-Nyhan disease. Clinical experience with nineteen patients. Dev. Med. Child Neurol., 24:293–306, 1982.

151. Lloyd, K.G., et al.: Biochemical evidence of dysfunction of brain neurotransmitters in the Lesch-Nyhan syndrome. N. Engl. J. Med., 305:1106–1111, 1981.

152. Kornberg, A., Lieberman, I., and Simms, E.S.: Enzymatic synthesis and properties of 5-phosphoribosylpyrophosphate. J. Biol. Chem., 215:389–402, 1955.

153. Becker, M.A.: Abnormalities of PRPP metabolism leading to an overproduction of uric acid. In Uric Acid: Handbook of Experimental Pharmacology. Vol. 51. Edited by W.N. Kelley and I.M. Weiner. New York, Springer-Verlag, 1978.

154. Akaoka, I., et al.: A gouty family with increased phosphoribosylpyrophosphate synthetase activity: Case reports, family studies, and kinetic studies of the abnormal enzyme. J. Rheumatol., 8:563–574, 1981.

155. Becker, M.A., Losman, M.J., Itkin, P., and Simkin, P.A.: Gout with superactive phosphoribosylpyrophosphate due to increased enzyme catalytic rate. J. Lab. Clin. Med., 99:485–511, 1982.

156. Sperling, O., Persky-Brosh, S., Boer, P., and deVries, A.: Human erythrocyte phosphoribosylpyrophosphate synthetase mutationally altered in regulatory properties. Biochem. Med., 7:389–395, 1973.

157. Simmonds, H.A., Webster, D.R., Wilson, J., and Lingham, S.: An x-linked syndrome characterized by hyperuricemia, deafness, and neurodevelopmental abnormalities. Lancet, 2:68–70, 1982.

158. Becker, M.A., et al.: Variant human phosphoribosylpyrophosphate synthetase altered in regulatory and catalytic function. J. Clin. Invest., 65:100–120, 1980.

159. Becker, M.A., et al.: Phosphoribosylpyrophosphate synthetase superactivity. A study of five patients with catalytic defects in the enzyme. Arthritis Rheum., 29:880–888, 1986.

160. Becker, M.A.: Regulation of purine nucleotide synthesis: Effects of inosine on normal and hypoxanthine-guanine phosphoribosyltransferase deficient fibroblasts. Biochim. Biophys. Acta, 435:132–144, 1976.

161. Ravio, K.O., et al.: Stimulation of human purine synthesis de novo by fructose infusion. Metabolism, 24:861–869, 1975.

162. Woolliscroft, J.O., Colfer, H., and Fox, I.H.: Hyperuricemia in acute illness: A poor prognostic sign. Am. J. Med., 72:58–62, 1982.

163. Woolliscroft, J.O., and Fox, I.H.: Increased body fluid purine levels during hypotensive events: Evidence for ATP degradation. Am. J. Med., 81:472–478, 1986.

163a. Mineo, I., et al.: Myogenic hyperuricemia. A common pathophysiologic feature of glycogenosis types III, V, ad VII. N. Engl. J. Med., 317:75–80, 1987.

164. Faller, J., and Fox, I.H.: Ethanol-induced hyperuricemia. Evidence for increased urate production by activation of adenine nucleotide turnover. N. Engl. J. Med., 307:1598–1602, 1982.

165. Buzard, J., Bishop, C., and Talbott, J.H.: The fate of uric acid in the normal and gouty human being. J. Chronic Dis., 2:42–49, 1955.

166. Sorensen, L.B.: The elimination of uric acid in man studied by means of ^{14}C-labelled uric acid. Scand. J. Clin. Lab. Invest., 12:(Suppl):1–214, 1960.

167. Skupp, S., and Ayvazian, J.H.: Oxidation of 7-methylguanine by human xanthine oxidase. J. Lab. Clin. Med., 73:909–916, 1969.

168. Berliner, R.W., Hilton, J.G., Yu, T-F, and Kennedy, T.J., Jr.: The renal mechanism of urate excretion in man. J. Clin. Invest., 29:396–401, 1950.

169. Praetorius, E., and Kirk, J.E.: Hypouricemia: With evidence

for tubular elimination of uric acid. J. Lab. Clin. Med., 35:865–868, 1950.

170. Gutman, A.B., and Yu, T-F.: A three component system for regulation of renal excretion of uric acid in man. Trans. Assoc. Am. Physicians, 74:353–365, 1961.

171. Bordley, J., III, and Richards, A.N.: Quantitative studies of the composition of glomerular urine. VIII. The concentration of uric acid in glomerular urine of snakes and frogs, determined by an ultramicroadaptation of Folin's method. J. Biol. Chem., 101:193–221, 1933.

172. Diamond, H.S., and Paolino, J.S.: Evidence for a post-secretory reabsorptive site for uric acid in man. J. Clin. Invest., 52:1491–1499, 1973.

173. Levinson, D.J., and Sorensen, L.B.: Renal handling of uric acid in normal and gouty subjects: Evidence for a 4-component system. Ann. Rheum. Dis., 39:173–179, 1980.

174. Alvsaker, J.O.: Genetic studies in primary gout: Investigations on the plasma levels of the urate binding α_1-α_2-globulin in individuals from two gouty kindreds. J. Clin. Invest., 47:1254–1261, 1968.

175. Klinenberg, J.R., and Kippen, I.: The binding of urate to plasma proteins determined by means of equilibrium dialysis. J. Lab. Clin. Med., 75:503–510, 1970.

176. Kovarsky, J., Holmes, E.W., and Kelley, W.N.: Absence of significant urate binding to human serum proteins. J. Lab. Clin. Med., 93:85–91, 1979.

177. Sheikh, M.I., and Moller, J.F.: Binding of urate to proteins of human and rabbit plasma. Biochim. Biophys. Acta, 158:456–458, 1968.

178. Kelton, J.G., et al.: A method for monitoring dialysis patients and a tool for assessing binding to serum proteins in vivo. Ann. Intern. Med., 89:67–70, 1978.

179. Holmes, E.W., and Blondet, P.: Urate binding to serum albumin: Lack of influence on renal clearance of uric acid. Arthritis Rheum., 22:737–739, 1979.

180. Abramson, R.G., and Levitt, M.F.: Micropuncture study of uric acid transport in rat kidney. Am. J. Physiol., 228:1597–1605, 1975.

181. Greger, R., Lang, F., and Deetjen, P.: Handling of uric acid by the rat kidney. II. Microperfusion studies on bidirectional transport of uric acid in the proximal tubule. Pfluegers Arch., 335:257–265, 1972.

182. Greger, R., Lang, F., and Deetjen, P.: Handling of uric acid by the rat kidney: I. Microanalysis of uric acid in proximal tubular fluid. Pfluegers Arch., 324:279–287, 1971.

183. Roch-Ramel, F., and Weiner, I.M.: Excretion of urate by the kidneys of Cebus monkeys: A micropuncture study. Am. J. Physiol., 224:1369–1374, 1973.

184. Fanelli, G.M., Jr., and Weiner, I.M.: Pyrazinoate excretion in the Chimpanzee: Relation to urate disposition and the action of uricosuric drugs. J. Clin. Invest., 52:1946–1957, 1973.

185. Steele, T.H., Manuel, M.A., and Boner, G.: Diuretics, urate excretion, and sodium reabsorption: Effect of acetazolamide and urinary alkalinization. Nephron, 14:48–61, 1975.

186. Weiner, I.M., and Fanelli, G.M., Jr.: Renal urate excretion in animal models. Nephron, 14:33–47, 1975.

187. Yu, T-F., and Gutman, A.B.: Study of the paradoxical effects of salicylate in low, intermediate and high dosage on the renal mechanism for excretion of urate in man. J. Clin. Invest., 38:1298–1315, 1959.

188. Gutman, A.B., Yu, T-F., and Berger, L.: Tubular secretion of urate in man. J. Clin. Invest., 38:1778–1781, 1959.

189. Kessler, R.H., Hierholzer, K., and Gurd, R.S.: Localization of

urate transport in the nephron of mongrel and dalmatian dog kidney. Am. J. Physiol., 197:601–603, 1959.

190. Mudge, G.H., McAlary, B., and Berndt, W.O.: Renal transport of uric acid in the guinea pig. Am. J. Physiol., 214:875–879, 1968.

191. Podevin, R., et al.: Etude chez l'homme de la cinatique d'apparition dans l'urine de l'acide urique 2^{14}C. Nephron, 5:134–140, 1968.

192. Weiner, I.M., and Mudge, G.H.: Renal tubular mechanisms for excretion of organic acids and bases. Am. J. Med., 36:743–762, 1964.

193. Yu, T-F., et al.: Effect of pyrazinamide and pyrazinoic acid on urate clearance and other discrete renal functions. Proc. Soc. Exp. Biol. Med., 96:264–267, 1957.

194. Yu, T-F., Berger L., and Gutman, A.B.: Suppression of tubular secretion of urate by pyrazinamide in the dog. Proc. Soc. Exp. Biol. Med., 107:905–908, 1961.

195. Steele, T.H., and Rieselbach, R.E.: The renal mechanism for urate homeostasis in normal man. Am. J. Med., 43:868–875, 1967.

196. Wilson, D.M., and Goldstein, N.P.: Renal urate excretion in patients with Wilson's disease. Kidney Int., 4:331–336, 1973.

197. Bennett, J.S., Bond, J., Singer, I., and Gottlieb, A.J.: Hypouricemia in Hodgkin's disease. Ann. Intern. Med., 76:751–756, 1972.

198. Meisel, A.D., and Diamond, H.S.: Inhibition of probenecid uricosuria by pyrazinamide and para-aminohippurate. Am. J. Physiol., 232:F222–F226, 1977.

199. Steele, T.H., and Oppenheimer, S.: Factors affecting urate excretion following diuretic administration in man. Am. J. Med., 47:564–574, 1969.

200. Manuel, M.A., and Steele, T.H.: Pyrazinamide suppression of the uricosuric response to sodium chloride infusion. J. Lab. Clin. Med., 83:417–427, 1974.

200a. Puig, G.J.: Renal handling of uric acid in normal subjects by means of the pyrazinamide and probenecid tests. Nephron, 35:183–186, 1983.

201. Sorensen, L.B., and Levinson, D.J.: Isolated defect in post-secretory reaborption of uric acid. Ann. Rheum. Dis., 39:180–183, 1980.

202. Smetana, S.S., and Bar-Khayim, Y.: Hypouricemia due to renal tubular defect. A study with the Probenecid-Pyrazinamide test. Arch. Intern. Med., 145:1200–1203, 1985.

203. Tofukm, Y., Kuroda, M., and Takeda, R.: Hypouricemia due to renal urate wasting. Nephron, 30:39–44, 1982.

204. Simkin, P.A.: Urate excretion in normal and gouty men. Adv. Exp. Med. Biol., 76B:41–45, 1977.

204a. Levinson, D.J., Decker, D.E., and Sorensen, L.B.: Renal handling of uric acid in man. Ann. Clin. Lab. Sci., 12:73–77, 1982.

205. Zollner, N., and Griebsch, A.: Diet and gout. Adv. Exp. Med. Biol., 41B:435–442, 1974.

206. Campion, D.W., et al.: Does increased free serum urate concentration cause gout? (Abstract.) Clin. Res., 23:261A, 1975.

207. Rieselbach, R.E., Sorensen, L.B., Shelp, W.D., and Steele, T.H.: Diminished renal urate secretion per nephron as a basis for primary gout. Ann. Intern. Med., 73:359–366, 1970.

208. Emmerson, B.T.: Alteration of urate metabolism by weight reduction. Aust. N.Z. J. Med., 3:410–412, 1973.

209. Lynch, E.C.: Uric acid metabolism in proliferative diseases of the marrow. Arch. Intern. Med., 109:639–653, 1962.

210. Laster, L., and Muller, A.F.: Uric acid production in a case of myeloid metaplasia associated with gouty arthritis studied with N^{15}-labelled glycine. Am. J. Med., 15:857–861, 1953.

211. Wyngaarden, J.B., Seegmiller, J.E., Laster, L., and Blair, A.E.:

Utilization of hypoxanthine, adenine and 4-amino-5-imidazolecarboxamide for uric acid synthesis in man. Metabolism, 8:455–464, 1959.

212. Somerville, J.: Gout in cyanotic congenital heart disease. Br. Heart J., 23:31–34, 1961.

213. Martinez-Lavin, M., et al.: Coexistent gout and hypertrophic osteoarthropathy in patients with cyanotic heart disease. J. Rheumatol., 11:832–834, 1984.

213a. Ross, E.A., et al.: Renal function and urate metabolism in late survivors with cyanotic congenital heart disease. Circulation, 73:396–400, 1986.

214. Gold, M.S., Williams, J.C., Spivak, M., and Grann, V.: Sickle cell anemia and hyperuricemia. JAMA, 206:1572–1573, 1968.

215. Diamond, H.S., et al.: Hyperuricosuria and increased tubular secretion of urate in sickle cell disease. Am. J. Med., 59:796–802, 1975.

216. March, H.W., Schlyen, S.M., and Schwartz, S.E.: Mediterranean hemopathic syndromes (Cooley's anemia) in adults: Study of a family with unusual complications. Am. J. Med., 13:46–57, 1952.

217. Paik, C.H., Alavi, I., Dunea, G., and Weiner, L.: Thalassemia and gouty arthritis. JAMA, 213:296–297, 1970.

218. Ultmann, J.: Hyperuricemia in disseminated neoplastic disease other than lymphomas or leukemias. Cancer, 15:122–129, 1962.

219. Diamond, H.S., Meisel, A.D., and Holden, D.: The natural history of urate overproduction in sickle cell anemia. Ann. Intern. Med., 90:752–757, 1979.

220. Ball, G.V., and Sorensen, L.B.: The pathogenesis of hyperuricemia and gout in sickle cell anemia. Arthritis Rheum., 13:846–848, 1970.

221. Espinoza, L.R., Spillberg, I., and Osterland, C.K.: Joint manifestations of sickle cell disease. Medicine, 53:295–305, 1974.

222. Paulus, H.E., et al.: Clinical significance of hyperuricemia in routinely screened hospitalized men. JAMA, 211:277–281, 1970.

223. Brand, F.N., et al.: Hyperuricemia as a risk factor of coronary heart disease: The Framingham Study. Am. J. Epidemiol., 121:11–18, 1985.

223a. Bryant, M.J., et al.: Hyperuricemia induced by administration of chlorthalidone and other sulfonamide diuretics. Am. J. Med., 33:408–420, 1962.

224. Steele, T.H.: Evidence for altered renal urate reabsorption during changes in volume of the extracellular fluid. J. Lab. Clin. Med., 74:288–299, 1969.

225. Roos, J.C., Boer, P., Peuker, K.H., and Dorhout Mees, E.J.: Changes in intrarenal uric acid handling during chronic Spironolactone treatment in patients with essential hypertension. Nephron, 32:209–213, 1982.

226. Evans, J.G., Prior, I.A.M., and Harvey, H.P.B.: Relation of serum uric acid to body bulk, haemoglobin, and alcohol intake in two South Pacific Polynesian populations. Ann. Rheum. Dis., 27:319–324, 1968.

227. Saker, B.M., Tofler, O.B., Burvill, M.J., and Reilly, K.A.: Alcohol consumption and gout. Med. J. Aust., 1:1213–1216, 1967.

228. Lieber, C.S., Jones, D.P., Lasowsky, M.S., and Davidson, C.S.: Inerrelation of uric acid and ethanol metabolism in man. J. Clin. Invest., 41:1863–1870, 1962.

229. MacLachlan, M.J., and Rodnan, G.P.: Effects of food, fast and alcohol on serum uric acid and acute attacks of gout. Am. J. Med., 42:38–57, 1967.

230. Weiner, I.M., and Tinker, J.P.: Pharmacology of pyrazinamide: Metabolic and renal function studies related to the mechanism of drug-induced urate retention. J. Pharmacol. Exp. Ther., 180:411–434, 1972.

231. Postlethwaite, A.E., Bartel, A.G., and Kelley, W.N.: Hyperuricemia due to ethambutol. N. Engl. J. Med., 286:761–763, 1972.

232. Gershon, S.L., and Fox, I.H.: Pharmacologic effects of nicotinic acid on human purine metabolism. J. Lab. Clin. Med., 84:179–186, 1974.

233. Menon, R.K., et al.: Warfarin administration increases uric acid concentration in plasma. Clin. Chem., 32:1557–1559, 1986.

234. Brauer, G.W., and Prior, I.A.M.: A prospective study of gout in New Zealand Maoris. Ann. Rheum. Dis., 37:466–472, 1978.

235. Fessel, W.J., and Bar, G.D.: Uric acid, lean body weight and creatinine interactions. Results from regression analysis of 78 variables. Semin. Arthritis Rheum., 7:115–121, 1977.

236. Fessel, W.J., Siegelaub, A.B., and Johnson, E.S.: Correlates and consequences of asymptomatic hyperuricemia. Arch. Intern. Med., 132:44–54, 1973.

237. Glynn, R.J., Campion, E.W., and Silbert, J.E.: Trends in serum uric acid levels 1961–1980. Arthritis Rheum., 26:87–93, 1983.

238. Scott, J.T.: Obesity and hyperuricaemia. Clin. Rheum. Dis., 3:25–35, 1977.

239. Sturge, R.A., et al.: Serum uric acid in England and Scotland. Ann. Rheum. Dis., 36:420–427, 1977.

240. Seidell, J.C., et al.: Overweight and chronic illness—A retrospective cohort study with a follow-up of 6–17 years, in men and women of initially 20–50 years of age. J. Chronic Dis., 39:585–593, 1986.

241. Bray, G.A.: Complications of obesity. Ann. Intern. Med., 103:1052–1062, 1985.

242. Kannel, W.B., and Gordon, T.: Physiological and medical concomitant of obesity: The Framingham Study. In Obesity in America. Edited by G.A. Bray. Maryland, National Institutes of Health, DHEW No. (NIH) 79–359, 1979.

243. Gibson, T., et al.: Hyperuricemia, gout and kidney function in New Zealand Maori Men. Br. J. Rheumatol., 23:276–282, 1984.

244. Barlow, K.A.: Hyperlipidemia in primary gout. Metabolism, 17:289–299, 1968.

245. Berkowitz, D.: Blood lipid and uric acid interrelationships. JAMA, 190:856–858, 1964.

246. Gibson, T.J., and Grahame, R.: Gout, hypertriglyceridemia, and alcohol consumption. Ann. Rheum. Dis., 3:109–110, 1974.

247. Naito, H.K., and Mackenzie, A.H.: Secondary hypertriglyceridemia and hyperlipoproteinemia in patients with primary asymptomatic gout. Clin. Chem., 25:371–375, 1979.

248. Jiao, S., Kameda, K., Matsuzawa, Y., and Tarui, S.: Hyperlipoproteinemia in primary gout: Hyperlipoproteinemic phenotype and influence of alcohol intake and obesity in Japan. Ann. Rheum. Dis., 45:308–313, 1986.

249. Fox, I.H., et al.: Hyperuricemia and hypertriglyceridemia: Metabolic basis for the association. Metabolism, 34:741–746, 1985.

250. Cannon, P.J., et al.: Hyperuricemia in primary and renal hypertension. N. Engl. J. Med., 275:457–464, 1966.

251. Breckenridge, A.: Hypertension and hyperuricemia. Lancet, 1:15–18, 1966.

252. Dollery, C.T., Duncan, H., and Schumer, B.: Hyperuricemia related to treatment of hypertension. Br. Med. J., 2:832–835, 1960.

253. Myers, A.R., Epstein, F.H., Dodge, H.J., and Mikkelson, W.M.: The relationship of serum uric acid to risk factors in coronary heart disease. Am. J. Med., 45:520–528, 1968.

254. Kahn, H.A., et al.: The incidence of hypertension and associated factors: The Israel ischemic heart disease study. Am. Heart J., 84:171–182, 1972.

255. Rapado, A.: Relationship between gout and arterial hypertension. Adv. Exp. Med. Biol., 41B:451–459, 1974.

256. Prebis, J.W., Gruskin, A.B., Polinsky, M.S., and Baluarte, H.J.: Uric acid in childhood essential hypertension. J. Pediatr., 98:702–707, 1981.

257. Gertler, M., Garn, S.M., and Levine, S.A.: Serum uric acid in relation to age and physique in health and in coronary artery disease. Ann. Intern. Med., 34:1421–1431, 1931.

258. Dreyfuss, F.: The role of hyperuricemia in coronary heart disease. Chest, 38:332–334, 1960.

259. Hansen, O.E.: Hyperuricemia, gout and atherosclerosis. Am. Heart J., 72:570–572, 1966.

260. Sarre, H., and Mertz, D.P.: Sekundare Gicht bei Neirenin-suffizenz. Klin. Wochenschr., 43:1134–1140, 1965.

261. Richet, G., Mignon, F., and Ardaillou, R.: Goutte secondaire de nephropathies chroniques. Presse Med., 73:633–638, 1965.

262. Steele, T.H., and Rieselbach, R.E.: The contribution of residual nephrons within the chronically diseased kidney to urate homeostasis in man. Am. J. Med., 43:876–886, 1967.

263. Sorensen, L.B., and Levinson, D.J.: Origin and extrarenal elimination of uric acid in man. Nephron, 14:7–20, 1975.

264. Buchanan, W.W., Klinenberg, J.R., and Seegmiller, J.E.: The inflammatory response to injected microcrystalline monosodium urate in normal, hyperuricemic, gouty and uremic subjects. Arthritis Rheum., 8:361–367, 1965.

265. Caner, J.E.Z., and Decker, J.L.: Recurrent acute (?gouty) arthritis in chronic renal failure treated with periodic hemodialysis. Am. J. Med., 36:571–582, 1964.

266. McCarty, D.J., Jr.: The inflammatory reaction to microcrystalline sodium urate. Arthritis Rheum., 8:726–735, 1965.

267. Reginato, A.J., et al.: Arthropathy and cutaneous calcinosis in hemodialysis oxalosis. Arthritis Rheum., 29:1387–1396, 1986.

268. Newcombe, D.S.: Gouty arthritis and polycystic kidney disease. Ann. Intern. Med., 79:605, 1973.

269. Ball, G.V., and Sorensen, L.B.: Pathogenesis of hyperuricemia in saturnine gout. N. Engl. J. Med., 280:1199–1202, 1969.

270. Emmerson, B.T.: Chronic lead neuropathy: The diagnostic use of calcium EDTA and the association with gout. Aust. Ann. Med., 12:310–324, 1963.

271. Ball, G.V., and Moran, J.M.: Chronic lead ingestion and gout. South. Med. J., 61:21–24, 1968.

271a. Halla, J.T., and Ball, G.V.: Saturnine gout. A review of 42 patients. Semin. Arthritis Rheum., 11:307–314, 1982.

272. Simmonds, H.A., et al.: Familial gout and renal failure in young women. Clin. Nephrol., 14:176–182, 1980.

273. Massari, P.U., et al.: Familial hyperuricemia and renal disease. Arch. Intern. Med., 140:680–684, 1980.

274. Leumann, E.P., and Wegmann, W.: Familial nephropathy with hyperuricemia and gout. Nephron, 34:51–57, 1983.

275. Cristofori, F.C., and Duncan, G.G.: Uric acid excretion in obese subjects during periods of total fasting. Metabolism, 13:303–311, 1964.

276. Drenick, E.J., Swendseid, M.E., Blahd, W.H., and Tuttle, S.G.: Prolonged starvation as treatment for severe obesity. JAMA, 187:100–105, 1964.

277. Goldfinger, S., Klinenberg, J.R., and Seegmiller, J.E.: Renal retention of uric acid induced by infusion of beta-hydroxy-butyrate and acetoacetate. N. Engl. J. Med., 272:351–355, 1965.

278. Mallette, L.E., Bilezikian, J.P., Heath, D.A., and Aurback, G.D.: Primary hyperparathyroidism: Clinical and biochemical features. Medicine, 53:127–145, 1974.

279. Scott, J.T., Dixon, A. St. J., and Bywaters, E.G.L.: Association of hyperuricemia and gout with hyperparathyroidism. Br. Med. J., 1:1070–1073, 1964.

280. Castrillo, J.M., Diaz-Curiel, M., and Rapado, A.: Hyperuricemia in primary hyperparathyroidism: Incidence and evolution after surgery. Adv. Exp. Med. Biol., 165A:151–157, 1984.

281. Shelp, W.D., Steele, T.H., and Rieselbach, R.E.: Comparison of urinary phosphate, urate and magnesium excretion following parathyroid hormone administration to normal man. Metabolism, 18:63–70, 1969.

282. Dent, C.E.: Some problems of hyperparathyroidism. Br. Med. J., 2:1419, 1495, 1962.

283. Eisen, A.Z., and Seegmiller, J.E.: Uric acid metabolism in psoriasis. J. Clin. Invest., 40:1486–1494, 1961.

284. Lambert, J.R., and Wright, V.: Serum uric acid levels in psoriatic arthritis. Ann. Rheum. Dis., 36:264–267, 1977.

285. Puig, T.G., et al.: Uric acid metabolism in psoriasis. Adv. Exp. Med. Biol., 195A:411–416, 1986.

286. Bunim, J.J., Kimberg, D.V., Thomas, L.B., and Scott, J.: The syndrome of sarcoidosis, psoriasis, and gout. Ann. Intern. Med., 57:1018–1040, 1962.

287. Zimmer, J.G., and Demis, D.J.: Associations between gout, psoriasis, and sarcoidosis: With consideration of their pathologic significance. Ann. Intern. Med., 64:786–796, 1966.

288. Pant, S.S., Maser, H.W., and Krane, S.M.: Hyperuricemia in Down's syndrome. J. Clin. Endocrinol. Metab., 28:472–478, 1968.

289. Meloni, C.R., and Canary, J.J.: Cystinuria with hyperuricemia. JAMA, 200:257–259, 1967.

290. Aponte, G.E., and Fetter, T.R.: Familial idiopathic oxalate nephrocalcinosis. Am. J. Clin. Pathol., 24:1363–1373, 1954.

291. Altman, R.D., and Collins, B.: Musculoskeletal manifestations of Paget's disease of bone. Arthritis Rheum., 23:1121–1127, 1980.

292. Meyer, W.J., III, Gill, J.R., Jr., and Bartter, F.C.: Gout as a complication of Bartter's syndrome: A possible role for alkalosis in the decreased clearance of uric acid. Ann. Intern. Med., 83:56–59, 1975.

293. Herring, L.C.: Observations on the analysis of ten thousand calculi. J. Urol., 88:545–562, 1962.

294. Prien, E.L.: Crystallographic analysis of urinary calculi: A 23-year survey study. J. Urol., 89:917–924, 1963.

295. Atsmon, A., DeVries, A., and Frank, M.: Uric Acid Lithiasis. Amsterdam, Elsevier, 1963.

296. Boyce, W.H., Gavey, F.K., and Strawcutter, H.E.: Incidence of urinary calculi among patients in general hospitals, 1948 to 1952. JAMA, 161:1437–1444, 1956.

297. Yu, T-F., Gutman, A.B.: Uric acid nephrolithiasis in gout: Predisposing factors. Ann. Intern. Med., 67:1133–1148, 1967.

298. Yu, T-F.: Urolithiasis in hyperuricemia and gout. J. Urol., 126:424–430, 1981.

299. Coe, F.L., and Kavalach, A.G.: Hypercalciuria and hyperuricosuria in patients with calcium nephrolithiasis. N. Engl. J. Med., 291:1344–1350, 1974.

300. Clarke, A.M., and McKenzie, R.G.: Ileostomy and the risk of urinary uric acid stones. Lancet, 2:395–397, 1969.

301. Peters, J.P., and Van Slyke, D.D.: Quantitative clinical chemistry. Vol. 1. 2nd Ed. Baltimore, Williams & Wilkins, 1946.

302. Klinenberg, J.R., Goldfinger, S.F, and Seegmiller, J.E.: The effectiveness of the xanthine oxidase inhibitor allopurinol in the treatment of gout. Ann. Intern. Med., 62:639–647, 1965.

303. Plante, G.E., Durivage, J., and Lemieux, G.: Renal excretion of hydrogen in primary gout. Metabolism, *17*:377–385, 1968.

304. Henneman, P.H., Wallach, S., and Dempsey, E.F.: The metabolic defect responsible for uric acid stone formation. J. Clin. Invest., *41*:537–542, 1962.

305. Gutman, A.B., and Yu, T-F.: Urinary ammonium excretion in primary gout. J. Clin. Invest., *44*:1474–1481, 1965.

306. Brazel, U.S., Sperling, O., Frank, M., and De Vries, A.: Renal ammonium excretion and urinary pH in idiopathic uric acid lithiasis. J. Urol., *92*:1–5, 1964.

307. Wrong, O., and Davis, H.E.F.: The excretion of uric acid in renal disease. Q. J. Med., *28*:259–313, 1959.

308. Falls, W.F., Jr.: Comparison of urinary acidification and ammonium excretion in normal and gouty subjects. Metabolism, *21*:433–445, 1972.

309. Gutman, A.B., and Yu, T-F.: An abnormality of glutamine metabolism in primary gout. Am. J. Med., *35*:820–831, 1963.

310. Pollak, V.E., and Mattenheimer, H.: Glutaminase activity in the kidney in gout. J. Lab. Clin. Med., *66*:564–570, 1965.

311. Sperling, O., De Vries, A., and Kedem, O.: Studies on the etiology of uric acid lithiasis. IV. Urinary non-dialyzable substances in idiopathic uric acid lithiasis. J. Urol., *94*:286–292, 1965.

312. Coe, F.L., Lawton, R.L., Goldstein, R.B., and Tembe, V.: Sodium urate accelerates precipitation of calcium oxalate in vitro. Proc. Soc. Exp. Biol. Med., *149*:926–929, 1975.

313. Nakagawa, Y., Abram, V., and Coe, F.L.: Isolation of calcium oxalate crystal growth inhibitor from rat kidney and urine. Am. J. Physiol., *247*:F765–F772, 1984.

314. Ramsdell, M.C., and Kelley, W.N.: The clinical significance of hypouricemia. Ann. Intern. Med., *78*:239–242, 1973.

315. Van Peenen, H.J.: Causes of hypouricemia. Ann. Intern. Med., *78*:977–978, 1973.

316. Holmes, E.W., and Wyngaarden, J.B.: Hereditary xanthinuria. *In* The Metabolic Basis of Inherited Diseases. 5th Ed. Edited by J.B. Stanbury et al. New York, McGraw-Hill, 1983.

317. Dwosh, I.L., Roncari, D.A.K., Marliss, E, and Fox, I.H.: Hypouricemia in disease. A study of different mechanisms. J. Lab. Clin. Med., *90*:153–161, 1977.

318. Schichiri, M., et al.: Renal handling of urate in the syndrome of inappropriate secretion of antidiuretic hormone. Arch. Intern. Med., *145*:2045–2047, 1985.

105

MANAGEMENT OF HYPERURICEMIA

ROBERT L. WORTMANN

Hyperuricemia is a common clinical state with many possible causes. Progress in the understanding of purine metabolism, knowledge of the potential consequences of this condition, and the availability of excellent therapeutic measures have rendered hyperuricemia one of the most rationally manageable conditions in medicine. Because of these factors, the treatment of hyperuricemia should be safe, effective, and satisfying for both patient and physician.

GENERAL PRINCIPLES

Hyperuricemia refers to an elevated serum urate concentration. This laboratory finding is present in 2% of adult males in the United States,[1] and 17% in France.[2] The incidence of hyperuricemia was 13.2% in a large series of hospitalized adult male patients.[3] Hyperuricemia does not represent a specific disease, nor is it an indication for therapy. Rather, the finding of hyperuricemia is an indication to determine its origin, and a decision to treat this condition is based on the cause and the consequences in each hyperuricemic patient. Rational management requires that the physician answer the following questions: (1) Is the individual truly hyperuricemic? (2) What is the cause of the hyperuricemia? (3) Should the serum urate concentration be lowered?

DEFINITION OF HYPERURICEMIA
(see also Chapter 104)

Hyperuricemia is defined as a serum urate concentration greater than 7.0 mg/dl measured by the specific uricase method. The physicochemical saturation of urate in plasma occurs at this concentration, and in epidemiologic studies of healthy adults not selected for gout or hyperuricemia, 95% of the individuals had serum urate concentrations below this value.[4] The method used for urate determination is important because obsolete nonspecific colorimetric methods are still used and may detect reducing substances other than urate and may provide artificially high values, when compared to those obtained by the specific uricase method.* It is therefore important to know the method employed so that laboratory results may be interpreted properly.

Because the decision to treat hyperuricemia is usually a commitment to therapy for life, it is essential to document that the hyperuricemia is real and sustained. Certainly, the decision should not be based solely on the result of one test. Serum urate concentrations vary with age and sex, fluctuate throughout the day in some individuals, and may be subject to seasonal variation. Other factors, such as recent weight loss, heavy physical exertion, or renal functional impairment, may alter the serum urate concentration. The ingestion of many substances, such as alcohol, diuretics, or salicylates in doses under 2 g/day, may cause hyperuricemia.

WORKUP OF HYPERURICEMIA

Although the finding of hyperuricemia is not necessarily an indication for treatment, one must deter-

---

*Automated specific enzymatic methods are now used in most modern hospital clinical chemistry laboratories.

mine the cause. Hyperuricemia may be easily explained and judged clinically insignificant, or it may reflect a serious medical problem. Knowledge of the cause helps one to decide whether and how the condition should be treated. Fortunately, the cause can be easily determined in 70% of patients by means of medical history and physical examination alone.[3]

Traditionally, hyperuricemia has been classified as either primary or secondary. Primary hyperuricemia refers to an elevated serum urate concentration, the cause of which is not understood; or if the cause is known, as for example, hypoxanthine-guanine phosphoribosyltransferase deficiency, hyperuricemia is its first manifestation. Secondary hyperuricemias are those ascribed to some other disorder or therapy in which the basic defect is understood. A more practical classification of hyperuricemia is based on the underlying pathophysiologic features. As reviewed in Chapter 104, hyperuricemia results from urate overproduction, from decreased uric acid excretion, or from a combination of these two mechanisms.

A 24-hour urinary uric acid measurement can be obtained to determine whether hyperuricemia in a given patient is the consequence of overproduction or of decreased excretion.[5] On a purine-free diet, normal men excrete 164 to 588 mg uric acid/day.[6] Hyperuricemic individuals who excrete more than 600 mg uric acid/day while on a purine-free diet are hyperuricemic because of purine overproduction, and those excreting less than 600 mg are most often hyperuricemic because of inadequate excretion. If the assessment is performed while the patient is on a regular diet, then a value of 800 mg/24 hours can be used.

Interpretation of 24-hour urine uric acid excretion requires attention to three factors. First, the foregoing values were determined in subjects with normal renal function. Because impaired renal function decreases the amount of urate filtered in the glomeruli, less uric acid appears in the urine. Consequently, a 24-hour urinary uric acid value of under 600 mg, or under 800 mg with regular diet, does not necessarily rule out urate overproduction in a patient with renal failure. On the other hand, elevated values in the presence of renal failure are strong evidence of purine overproduction. Second, it is essential to know the method employed by the laboratory to measure the uric acid in urine. The normal values given previously are for the specific uricase method. Colorimetric methods are even less specific in urine than they are in serum because drugs and chromogens normally found in urine often cause spuriously high values. These normal chromogens are increased in patients with renal failure. Third, one must ascertain that the patient is not taking a uricosuric agent at the time of urine collection. Corticosteroids, ascorbic acid, salicylates in doses greater than 2 g/24 hours, and other agents (Table 105–1) promote urate excretion and interfere with the interpretation of results.

It is useful to know whether the hyperuricemia is due to overproduction or to decreased excretion because it narrows the list of conditions that may have caused the hyperuricemia (Table 105–2). If such a factor or disease is identified, the hyperuricemia should be considered secondary, and initial attempts at management should be directed to treating or eliminating the primary cause. In addition, knowing whether hyperuricemia is due to overproduction or to decreased excretion may help in the choice of drug, if one is indicated.

TREATMENT

Today, there is hardly any indication that specific urate-lowering drugs should be used to treat asymptomatic hyperuricemia. If the serum urate concentration can be lowered by treating an underlying disease or by removing a causal factor, however, such steps should be taken. Exactly when hyperuricemia should be treated in symptomatic patients remains the subject of much debate. Clearly, antihyperuricemic therapy is indicated in patients who suffer from frequent attacks of acute gouty arthritis or tophi. The use of specific urate-lowering drugs to treat hyperuricemia in patients who have had only a single episode of gouty arthritis is controversial.

Treatment with antihyperuricemic medicines is costly, inconvenient, and potentially toxic. Moreover, because these drugs are prescribed for life, they should not be used without definite indication. The decision to treat should be based on the needs of each

Table 105–1. Drugs with Uricosuric Activity

Acetohexamide	Estrogens
Adrenocorticotropic hormone (ACTH) and glucocorticoids	Glyceryl guaiacolate
Allopurinol	Glycopyrrolate
Ascorbic acid	Halofenate
Azauridine	Meclofenamate
Benzbromarone	Phenylbutazone
Calcitonin	Probenecid
Chlorprothixene	Salicylates
Citrate	Sulfinpyrazone
Dicumarol	Roentgenogram contrast agents
Diflunisal	Zoxazolamine

Table 105–2. Classification of Hyperuricemia (see also Table 104–1)

	Primary causes	Secondary causes

Overproduction
(24-hour urinary uric acid concentration greater than 600 mg on purine-restricted diet; 800 mg on unrestricted diet)
	Idiopathic
	Hypoxanthine-guanine phosphoribosyltransferase deficiency
	Increased phosphoribosylpyrophosphate synthetase activity
		Hemolytic process
		Myeloproliferative disease
		Lymphoproliferative disorder
		Psoriasis
		Paget's disease
		Exercise
		Glucose-6-phosphatase deficiency
		Artifactual
		    Nonspecific method to measure uric acid
		    Patient taking uricosuric agent

Underexcretion
(24-hour urinary uric acid concentration less than 600 mg on purine-restricted diet; 800 mg on unrestricted diet)
	Idiopathic	Renal insufficiency
		Hypertension
		Acidosis
		Drug ingestion
		    Salicylates (<2 g/24 hr)
		    Diuretics
		    Alcohol
		    Levodopa
		    Phenylbutazone (<200 mg/24 hr)
		    Ethambutol
		    Pyrazinamide
		    Nicotinic acid
		Sarcoidosis
		Lead intoxication
		Berylliosis

patient, with the potential benefit-to-risk ratio weighed individually.*

COMPLICATIONS OF ASYMPTOMATIC HYPERURICEMIA

Hyperuricemia can lead to gouty arthritis and renal disorders and has been considered by some authors to be a risk factor for coronary artery disease. Because of the fear of these consequences, for many years specific urate-lowering drugs were prescribed for the treatment of asymptomatic hyperuricemic individuals. Obviously, if evidence existed that maintaining serum urate concentrations within normal limits prevented renal failure or heart disease, there would be no debate over the treatment of this condition. Little data exist concerning the benefits of treating asymptomatic hyperuricema, however, and such treatment is no longer recommended, except in rare circumstances. The rationale for this position is provided by considering the complications of hyperuricemia that could develop if therapy is withheld.

*Editor's note. A mistake made in the treatment of a chronic disease is a chronic mistake.

GOUT

The risk of gouty arthritis rises both with increasing severity of hyperuricemia and with age.[1,7,8] In most cases, gout develops only after 20 or more years of sustained hyperuricemia. Although certain individuals may be at high risk for developing gouty arthritis, treatment of asymptomatic hyperuricemia simply to prevent the first episode of acute gouty arthritis is not indicated. No evidence indicates that structural kidney damage occurs before the first attack of gouty arthritis,[9,10] nor are tophi identifiable prior to that occurrence. Moreover, first attacks of gout are easily treated. It is best to withhold antihyperuricemic therapy until arthritis becomes manifest and the diagnosis is confirmed; this form of therapy is long term, and the drugs used are potentially toxic. The cost of the medication and the generally poor compliance in the treatment of asymptomatic problems both reinforce this position.

RENAL DISEASE

Chronic renal disease is an important potential consequence of hyperuricemia. Progressive renal failure, a major cause of death in patients with gout, accounts for 6.6 to 25% of the overall mortality.[11,12] An important question is whether asymptomatic hyperuricemia adversely affects renal function over time.

Hyperuricemia can affect the kidneys in three ways (see Chapter 104): (1) urate nephropathy, e.g., deposition of sodium urate crystals in the medullary interstitium and pyramids associated with a giant-cell inflammatory response; (2) nephrolithiasis; and (3) uric acid nephropathy, a reversible form of acute renal failure caused by the precipitation of uric acid crystals in the tubules, collecting ducts, pelvis, and ureters, and obstructing the flow of urine.

Urate nephropathy leading to renal failure is difficult to document and is rarely encountered today.[13] Concern about this manifestation does not warrant treatment of asymptomatic hyperuricemia. Urate nephropathy is a late event in the natural history of gout and has not been reported in the absence of previous gouty arthritis.[14-16] No evidence suggests that renal function is compromised at the time of the first gouty attack.[9,10]

The risk of renal failure from hyperuricemia alone is low. One study of 113 patients with asymptomatic hyperuricemia and of 193 normouricemic control subjects followed for 8 years found that azotemia, defined as a serum creatinine greater than 1.6 mg/100 ml in males and 1.3 mg/100 ml in females, occurred in 1.8 and 2.1%, respectively.[17] Thus, azotemia attributable to hyperuricemia alone is infrequent, mild, and probably of little clinical significance.

No evidence indicates that treatment of asymptomatic hyperuricemia alters the progression of renal disease. A study of 116 patients, followed for 2.5 or more years, compared the effects of allopurinol versus placebo therapy in nongouty patients matched for serum urate concentration, mean creatinine clearance, blood pressure, and size. No statistically significant differences were found among the groups, and it was concluded that normalization of the plasma urate did not alter renal function.[18]

Even in patients with gout, strong evidence indicates that hyperuricemia alone is rarely damaging to renal function.[19] Long-term followup of renal clearance in 149 gouty patients suggested that various, independently coexisting diseases with associated nephropathy have the most significant impact on renal function, with aging itself a second important factor.[20] Studies of renal hemodynamics in 624 gouty patients confirmed that hyperuricemia alone did not adversely affect renal function. Associated cardiovascular disease, especially hypertension, independently occurring intrinsic renal disease, and aging did correlate with decreased renal function, however. Reduced inulin clearance was attributed to hyperuricemia only

in patients with extensive tophaceous deposits, and even in this group, renal dysfuction was greater in patients with associated hypertensive vascular disease.[21]

The relationship between hyperuricemia and nephrolithiasis is complex.[22] Renal stones are 1000 times more prevalent in patients with primary gout than in the general population, but uric acid nephrolithiasis occurs in patients without manifestations of gout, only 20% of whom are hyperuricemic.[23,24] Moreover, some nongouty patients with calcium oxalate stones also have hyperuricosuria.[25-27]

In gouty patients, the risk of nephrolithiasis is related to the magnitude of the urinary uric acid excretion and, to a lesser degree, to the extent of serum urate elevation.[28] Such data are not available for individuals with asymptomatic hyperuricemia, but the risk of nephrolithiasis in such patients was assessed in one study. The rate of stone formation was 2.8 times higher in asymptomatic hyperuricemic individuals than in normouricemic control subjects; 1 stone per 295 asymptomatic hyperuricemic patients per year, as opposed to 1 stone per 825 control subjects per year.[17] This risk is sufficiently low to justify withholding therapy until the occurrence of the first stone.

Acute uric acid nephropathy is rare and occurs almost exclusively in patients receiving chemotherapy for hematologic malignancies. It is of little or no concern in the context of asymptomatic hyperuricemia, and its treatment is discussed later in this chapter.

CARDIOVASCULAR DISEASE

Whether hyperuricemia is an independent risk factor for atherosclerotic cardiovascular disease is unknown. Hyperuricemic individuals, with or without gout, have a high incidence of hypertension and coronary artery disease. In the Framingham study, patients with gout had twice the risk of coronary artery disease compared to normal subjects,[29] but the risk was not increased for hyperuricemic individuals without gouty arthritis. No correlation was observed between hyperuricemia and coronary artery disease in the Tecumseh Community Health study.[30] A Finnish health examination survey showed that hyperuricemia was associated with more advanced heart disease, but was not an independent cause of cardiovascular disease.[31] Attempts to relate hyperuricemia and heart disease have been complicated by the frequent coexistence of obesity and hypertension. One study demonstrated that the hypertension and atherosclerosis observed in gouty and hyperuricemic individuals were not simply the consequence of obesity.[32]

Therefore, hyperuricemia itself cannot be labeled a direct risk factor for cardiovascular disease, and it is best considered an indicator. In patients with essential hypertension, hyperuricemia most likely reflects early renal vascular involvement (nephrosclerosis),[33] and persistence of hyperuricemia following myocardial infarction is a sign of a poor prognosis.[34] No evidence indicates that lowering the serum urate concentration in either an asymptomatic hyperuricemic person or a patient with gout prevents cardiac disease.

In conclusion, little indication exists to screen asymptomatic individuals for hyperuricemia, and such screening is not recommended.[35] If hyperuricemia is encountered, however, its cause should be determined. The available data suggest that (1) renal function is not adversely affected by elevated serum urate concentrations; (2) renal disease accompanying hyperuricemia is often related to poorly controlled hypertension; (3) correction of hyperuricemia has no apparent effect on renal function; and (4) hyperuricemia is not a true risk factor for coronary artery disease. For these reasons and because of the inconvenience, cost, and potential toxicity of antihyperuricemic drugs, it is reasonable not to treat, but merely to observe, patients with asymptomatic hyperuricemia, regardless of the serum urate level. Correction of causal factors, if the condition is secondary, and control of associated problems such as obesity, hypercholesterolemia, diabetes, and particularly hypertension are definitely indicated.

SYMPTOMATIC HYPERURICEMIA

GOUT

The most common indication for lowering the serum urate concentration is articular gout. Because treatment is costly, lifelong, and potentially toxic, and because the differential diagnosis of acute monoarticular arthritis is extensive, accurate diagnosis must precede therapy. The finding of negatively birefringent crystals in polymorphonuclear leukocytes in synovial fluid or in subcutaneous tophi by compensated polarized light microscopy is definitive. The triad of acute monoarticular arthritis, hyperuricemia, and a dramatic response to colchicine is presumptive evidence of gouty arthritis in the absence of crystal identification. Criteria defining a colchicine ''response'' have been established as major subsidence of objective joint inflammatory changes within 48 hours of colchicine therapy and no recrudescence of inflam-

matory joint manifestations within 7 days.[36] Nevertheless, one should perform joint aspiration to search for crystals whenever possible until the diagnosis is proved.

Much debate exists concerning the appropriate moment to begin antihyperuricemic therapy in the course of gout. All authors agree that hyperuricemia should be treated in patients with recurrent attacks of gout, tophi, classic radiographic changes (bone tophi), or gout combined with nephrolithiasis. Some maintain that the first attack of acute gouty arthritis is sufficient indication to initiate therapy. Others argue that first attacks are easily, inexpensively, and effectively treated, and these physicians postpone urate-lowering therapy. Some individuals experience only a single gouty episode and may not have another for up to 42 years (mean 11.4 years).[37] In the Framingham study, 25% of the patients with acute gouty arthritis had only a single attack in 12 years of observation.[1]

A gouty patient should be educated about the disease and the logic and risks of therapy. Weight control is recommended for obese patients, and meticulous attention should be given to blood pressure control. A 24-hour urinary uric acid measurement helps determine the cause of the hyperuricemia and aids in selecting the most appropriate urate-lowering agent.[5,38,39] This measurement also influences the decision of whether to start antihyperuricemic therapy after a first gouty attack because the prevalence of renal stones in gouty subjects correlates with the amount of urinary uric acid. One study reported that 35% of patients excreting 700 to 900 mg uric acid/24 hours had nephrolithiasis; 50% of patients excreting more than 1100 mg/24 hours had renal stones.[28]

If urate-lowering therapy is withheld from the patient with gout, a definite risk of destruction to bone and cartilage exists from the sustained hyperuricemia. All patients with gout have deposits of monosodium urate in their tissues. If hyperuricemia is not controlled, these deposits enlarge and are radiographically evident before subcutaneous tophi are found. In a study of patients with intercritical gout, 42% without subcutaneous tophi had radiographic changes characteristic of bony tophi.[40] One could not predict from the frequency of acute attacks, the history of therapy, or the serum urate levels at the time of evaluation which patient would show bony changes. Thus, if urate-lowering therapy is withheld from patients with gout, radiography assessment is useful in defining the severity of the disease and in providing useful information concerning the advisability of treatment.[41]

Before giving specific antihyperuricemic agents, the

following criteria apply: (1) all signs of acute inflammation should be absent; (2) the patient should be counseled regarding factors capable of precipitating an acute attack and its prevention; (3) treatment with prophylactic colchicine should be started; (4) the patient should be advised that additional episodes of gouty arthritis are possible; and (5) he should be provided with anti-inflammatory medication with instructions concerning dosage, should such an episode occur.

The goal of antihyperuricemic therapy is the reduction of the total body urate pool. The serum urate concentration, which reflects this pool, is lowered with either a uricosuric agent or a xanthine oxidase inhibitor. Because any sudden increase or decrease in the serum urate concentration can prolong or trigger an acute attack, such therapy should be withheld until all signs of inflammation have resolved completely. Low doses of colchicine, 0.6 mg 1 to 3 times/day, are successful in preventing acute gouty attacks.[42,43] Prophylactic colchicine is most effective if started at least a week before the first dose of the urate-lowering agent is given and if continued until the serum urate concentration has been under control and the patient has been free of acute gouty attacks for a year. The use of prophylactic colchicine is generally well-tolerated and safe. Only an occasional patient will experience gastrointestinal side effects at these dosages. Neuromuscular toxicity may occur, but is rare. This manifests as a subacute myopathy with associated axonal neuropathy and elevated serum creatine kinase levels, usually occurs in individuals with renal insufficiency, and is reversible within 3 to 4 weeks after the drug is discontinued.[44]

Antihyperuricemic therapy, regardless of the agent employed, should be entirely successful, but it can succeed only if the dosage is adequate. Dosage is adequate when it is sufficient to maintain the serum urate concentration below 5.0 mg/dl. Extracellular fluid is saturated with urate at a concentration of approximately 6.4 mg/dl, and if the serum urate concentration remains above this level, tissue deposition of urate crystals will continue. A reduction of the serum urate concentration from 9.5 to 8.0 mg/dl, for example, will not reduce the total body urate pool, but will only retard the rate at which it increases.

NEPHROLITHIASIS

Medical prophylaxis of either uric acid or calcium stones in hyperuricemic patients is effective. Both types of stones occur in association with hyperuricosuria. The chemical composition of the stone should be identified whenever possible. Regardless of the nature of the calculi, patients should dilute their urine by ingesting fluid sufficient to produce a daily urine volume greater than 2 L. Alkalinization of the urine with sodium bicarbonate or acetazolamide may be justified for patients with uric acid stones because this process increases the solubility of uric acid. At pH 5.0, urine is saturated at a uric acid concentration of 15 mg/dl; at pH 7.0, saturation occurs with 200 mg/dl.[10]

Specific treatment of uric acid calculi is achieved by reducing urinary uric acid concentration with allopurinol, an inhibitor of xanthine oxidase. Allopurinol is also useful in reducing the recurrence of calcium oxalate stones in gouty subjects and in nongouty individuals with hyperuricemia or hyperuricosuria because uric acid may nucleate calcium stones.[45,46] Potassium citrate (30 to 80 mEq/day orally in divided doses) has been used successfully and can provide an alternative to allopurinol therapy for patients with uric acid stones alone or coexistent with calcium stones.[47]

URIC ACID NEPHROPATHY

This reversible form of acute renal failure is a result of the precipitation of uric acid in renal tubules and collecting ducts resulting in obstruction. Uric acid nephropathy may follow sudden urate overproduction with marked hyperuricosuria, dehydration, and acidosis. Autopsy studies have demonstrated intraluminal uric acid precipitates accompanied by dilated proximal tubules and normal glomeruli.[48] Work in animals suggests that the primary early pathogenetic events include obstruction of the collecting ducts by un-ionized uric acid and obstruction of the distal renal vasculature.[49,50] This form of acute renal failure develops most often in patients undergoing an aggressive or "blastic" phase of leukemia or lymphoma prior to or during cytotoxic therapy,[51,52] but it has also been observed in patients with disseminated adenocarcinoma,[53] after vigorous exercise with heat stress,[54] and following epileptic seizures.[55]

Uric acid nephropathy is important because it is often preventable and because immediate, appropriate therapy reduces the mortality rates associated with this condition from 47% to practically nil.[52] In addition to hyperuricemia, ranging from 12 to 80 mg/dl,[56,57] and oliguria, the distinctive clinical finding is probably the urinary uric acid concentration. In most forms of acute renal failure with decreased urine output, uric acid excretion is normal or reduced,[58] and the ratio of uric acid to creatinine is less than 1.0. A ratio of uric acid to creatinine greater than 1 in a random urine sample or in a 24-hour specimen may be diagnostic of uric acid nephropathy.[59]

Factors that favor uric acid precipitation should be reversed, and uric acid production should be blocked. Vigorous hydration by the intravenous route and furosemide administration are used to promote urine flow to 100 ml/hour or more. Acetazolamide, 240 to 500 mg every 6 to 8 hours, and sodium bicarbonate, 89 mEq/L, given intravenously, maximize the likelihood of achieving an alkaline urine.[60] It is important to monitor the patient's urine frequently to ensure that the pH remains above 7.0 and to watch for signs of circulatory overload.

In addition, antihyperuricemia therapy is administered to reduce the amount of urate that reaches the kidney. Allopurinol, which inhibits the production of urate and thereby decreases the concentration of urinary uric acid, is given in a single dose of 8 mg/kg. If renal insufficiency persists, subsequent daily doses should be reduced to 100 to 200 mg because oxipurinol, the active metabolite of allopurinol, is retained in this setting[61] (see the section on allopurinol in this chapter). Limited experience with urate oxidase, the enzyme that degrades uric acid to allantoin, has been reported.[62] Despite these measures, dialysis may be required. Hemodialysis should be employed because it is 10 to 20 times more effective than peritoneal dialysis in removing uric acid.[57]

THERAPEUTIC TECHNIQUES

DIET

Dietary considerations now play a minor role in the treatment of hyperuricemia, despite a fascinating history and abundant literature on the subject.[63] Strict restriction of purine intake reduces the mean serum urate concentration by only 1.0 mg/dl and urinary uric acid excretion by 200 to 400 mg/day.[64] Fortunately, modern therapeutic agents render attention to dietary purines rarely necessary.

Dietary counseling is important, however, and it should address the use of alcohol and associated medical problems such as obesity, hyperlipidemia, diabetes, or hypertension. Heavy alcohol consumption should be discouraged. An episode of excessive alcohol ingestion can cause temporary hyperlacticacidemia, elevate the serum urate concentration, and provoke an attack of gouty arthritis.[65] Long-term alcohol use increases uric acid production, hyperuricemia, and hyperuricosuria.[66,67]

URICOSURIC AGENTS

Candidates for uricosuric agents are gouty patients who meet all the following criteria: (1) hyperuricemia attributable to decreased uric acid excretion (less than 800 mg uric acid/24-hour urine specimen while the patient is on a regular diet; or less than 600 mg on a purine-restricted diet); (2) age under 60 years; (3) satisfactory renal function (a creatinine clearance greater than 80 ml/min is ideal, but it should be at least 50 ml/min); and (4) no history of nephrolithiasis.

Uricosuric agents reduce the serum urate concentration by enhancing the renal excretion of uric acid. This process occurs by the partial inhibition of proximal tubular reabsorption of filtered and secreted urate from the luminal side of the tubule at a site distal to the point of uric acid secretion.[68–71] If employed at a dosage sufficient to maintain the serum urate concentration at around 5.0 mg/100 ml, which is well below the level at which urate is saturated in extracellular fluid, these agents not only prevent urate deposition, but also allow dissolution of existing tophi.[72]

During the initial treatment period, the patient has a negative urate balance, and urinary uric acid excretion is elevated above pretreatment levels. Once the excess urate has been mobilized and excreted, urinary uric acid values return to original levels. At this point, the patient excretes uric acid at the pretreatment rate, but at a lower serum urate concentration.[73] Early in the course of treatment, before a steady state is reestablished, however, the risk of developing renal calculi is as high as 9%.[72]

Uricosuric agents may be effective in 70 to 80% of patients. In addition to drug intolerance, failure to control a serum urate concentration can be attributed to poor compliance, concomitant salicylate ingestion, or impaired renal function. Salicylates block the uricosuric effects of these agents, possibly by inhibiting urate secretion.[73a] These agents lose effectiveness as the creatinine clearance falls, and they are completely ineffective when glomerular filtration reaches 30 ml/min.[74,75]

Figure 105–1 illustrates the chemical structures of the three uricosuric agents discussed in the following paragraphs.

Probenecid

The "era of hypouricemic therapy" began in 1949 with the introduction of probenecid and the observations that sustained use of this agent controlled hyperuricemia, could mobilize tophi, and was well tolerated.[72,76,77] Probenecid is readily absorbed in the gastrointestinal tract. Its half-life ranges from 6 to 12

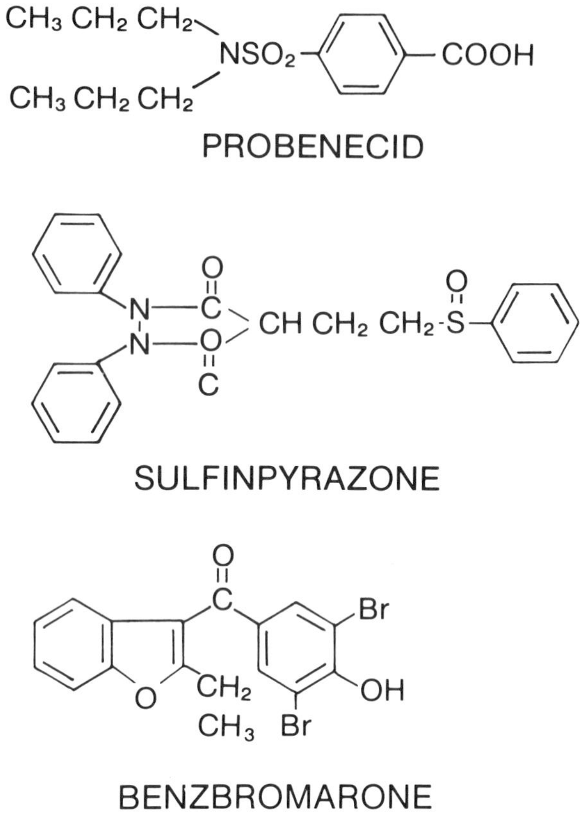

FIG. 105–1. Structures of uricosuric agents effective in the treatment of hyperuricemia.

PROBENECID

SULFINPYRAZONE

BENZBROMARONE

hours, is dose dependent,[78] and is prolonged by allopurinol.[79] This drug is extensively bound to plasma proteins, is largely confined to extracellular fluid, and is rapidly metabolized, with less than 5% of the administered dose recoverable in the urine in 24 hours.[72,79,80] Probenecid increases the half-life of penicillin, ampicillin, dapsone, acetazolamide, indomethacin, and sulfinpyrazone by decreasing renal excretion, of rifampin by impairing hepatic uptake, and of heparin by retarding its metabolism.[81]

Therapy is begun at 250 mg twice a day and is increased as necessary up to 3.0 g/day. A dose of 1 g/day is appropriate for about 50% of patients.[72,75] Because the half-life is 6 to 12 hours, probenecid should be taken in two to three evenly spaced doses.

The potential complications of probenecid most likely to occur early in the course of therapy include precipitation of acute gouty arthritis and nephrolithiasis. Gouty arthritis is prevented by the use of prophylactic colchicine. Nephrolithiasis is prevented by starting therapy at low doses and by increasing the dose at a rate of 0.5 g every 1 to 2 weeks, by liberally ingesting fluids, and possibly by alkalinizing the urine. Hypersensitivity, skin rash, and gastrointes-

tinal complaints are the major side effects. Serious toxicity is rare, but hepatic necrosis[82] and the nephrotic syndrome have been reported.[83,84]

Sulfinpyrazone

This analogue of a uricosuric metabolite of phenylbutazone possesses no anti-inflammatory activity and is a potent uricosuric agent. It is well absorbed through the gastrointestinal tract, with peak serum levels observed within an hour. The half-life of this agent is 1 to 3 hours.[85,86] Sulfinpyrazone is 98% bound to plasma proteins and is largely distributed in extracellular fluids. Although 20 to 45% of this drug is excreted unchanged in the urine the majority is excreted as the parahydroxyl metabolite, which is also uricosuric.[85,87] In addition to the uricosuric properties, sulfinpyrazone has antiplatelet activity, mediated by thromboxane synthesis inhibition, rather than by its urate-lowering effect.[88]

Sulfinpyrazone therapy is initiated at a dose of 50 mg twice a day. The usual maintenance level is 300 to 400 mg/day in 3 or 4 divided doses, but 800 mg/day may be required for satisfactory results.

Sulfinpyrazone has side effects similar to those of probenecid, and the drug is generally well tolerated. Bone marrow suppression can occur, but is rare.[89,90] Because of the rapid absorption and extreme potency of this drug, renal calculi are potentially more common early in the course of its use than with probenecid.

Benzbromarone

Benzbromarone is a halogenated uricosuric agent currently available outside the United States. This agent is debrominated in the liver and is excreted free or in the conjugated form primarily in the bile. Although a weak inhibitor of xanthine oxidase activity in vitro, the drug acts in vivo by inhibiting the tubular reabsorption of uric acid.[91–93]

Benzbromarone is effective and is well tolerated at daily doses of 25 to 120 mg.[91,94] This agent has been effective in patients with serum creatinine concentrations greater than 2.0 mg/dl and therefore may be useful for patients with renal insufficiency.[95]

INHIBITORS OF URIC ACID SYNTHESIS

Another approach for controlling the patient's serum urate concentration is the use of agents that decrease uric acid formation. Such agents are effective in the treatment of all types of hyperuricemia but are specifically indicated for the following: (1) patients with gout and: (a) evidence of urate overproduction

(24-hour urinary uric acid greater than 800 mg on a general diet; 600 mg on a purine-restricted diet); (b) nephrolithiasis; (c) renal insufficiency (creatinine clearance less than 80 ml/min); (d) tophaceous deposits; (e) age over 60 years; or (f) inability to take uricosuric agents because of ineffectiveness or intolerance; (2) patients with nephrolithiasis of any type and urinary uric acid excretion greater than 600 mg/24 hours; (3) patients with renal calculi composed of 2,8-dihydroxy-adenine; and (4) patients with, or at risk for, acute uric acid nephropathy.

The most widely used compound in this group is allopurinol, which inhibits xanthine oxidase. Oxipurinol, the major metabolite of allopurinol, is available outside the United States. Although useful in some patients who are sensitive to allopurinol,[96,97] the clinical utility of this drug is limited by its poor absorption from the gastrointestinal tract.[98] Thiopurinol, which probably inhibits de novo purine synthesis,[99] has had limited clinical use.

Allopurinol

This analogue of hypoxanthine originally synthesized to be an antitumor agent is a potent competitive inhibitor of xanthine oxidase.[100] It is also a substrate for the enzyme.[101] Oxypurinol, an analogue of xanthine, is the major metabolite of allopurinol and also effectively inhibits xanthine oxidase[102,103] (Fig. 105–2).

FIG. 105–2. Xanthine oxidase catalyzes the conversion of hypoxanthine to xanthine, of xanthine to uric acid, and of allopurinol to oxypurinol. Note the structural similarity of hypoxanthine to allopurinol and of xanthine to oxypurinol.

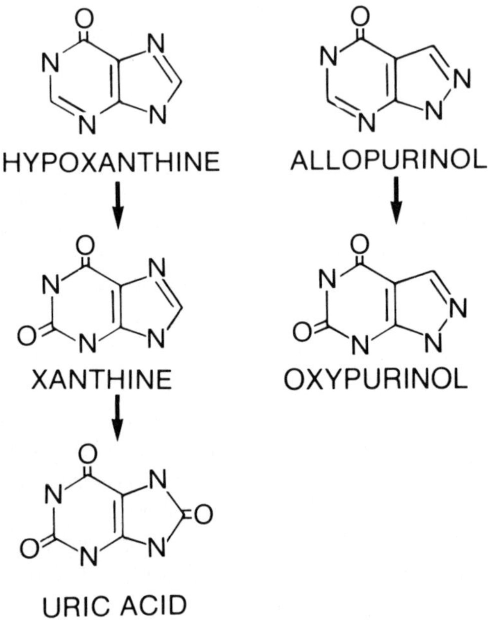

HYPOXANTHINE ALLOPURINOL

XANTHINE OXYPURINOL

URIC ACID

Allopurinol is completely absorbed from the gastrointestinal tract and has a half-life of 3 hours or less. Most oxypurinol formed is excreted unchanged in the urine and has a half-life of 14 to 28 hours.[104,105] Oxypurinol excretion is enhanced by uricosuric agents and is reduced by renal insufficiency.[106,107]

By inhibiting xanthine oxidase, these compounds block the conversion of hypoxanthine to xanthine and of xanthine to uric acid. The administration of allopurinol leads to decreases in serum urate concentration and in the urinary excretion of uric acid in the first 24 hours, and a maximum reduction occurs within 4 days to 2 weeks.[108,109] This change is accompanied by increased quantities of the oxypurines,* hypoxanthine and xanthine, which are the more readily excreted uric acid precursors in serum and urine.[110] Total purine excretion declines by 10 to 60% of pretreatment levels when allopurinol is taken.[98,109,110] This decline results from increased salvage of hypoxanthine to inosine 5'-monophosphate and from the concomitant reduction in the rate of de novo purine biosynthesis, the metabolic consequences of allopurinol conversion to allopurinol ribonucleotides[111–113] (Fig. 105–3). Allopurinol is also a potent inhibitor of de novo pyrimidine biosynthesis,[114] but the significance of this observation is uncertain.

Between 100 and 800 mg/day allopurinol is required to control the serum urate concentration adequately, and the dose for a specific patient depends on the severity of the tophaceous disease and on renal function. The average effective dose for most individuals is 300 mg/day.[115] The failure of a 400-mg dose to produce an adequate antihyperuricemic effect is rare and should cause one to question the patient's compliance. Allopurinol is effective in patients with renal insufficiency,[61] but the dose should be reduced because of the prolonged half-life of oxypurinol.[107] Therapy may be initiated at a low dose and may gradually be increased to minimize precipitation of acute gouty attacks or to find the lowest effective dose, but this regimen is not necessary for most patients. Because of the long half-life of oxypurinol, allopurinol need be taken only once a day.[116]

Allopurinol is clinically effective. Resolution of tophi is generally obvious, the frequency of gouty attacks is reduced, and the patient's functional status improves when the serum urate concentration has been controlled for 6 to 12 months. Although the incidence of recurrent gouty arthritis is low in patients who discontinue allopurinol therapy after 2 years despite the return of their serum urate concentrations

---

*Uric acid itself is the most "oxy" purine, but the term is usually meant to include only its "oxy" precursors.

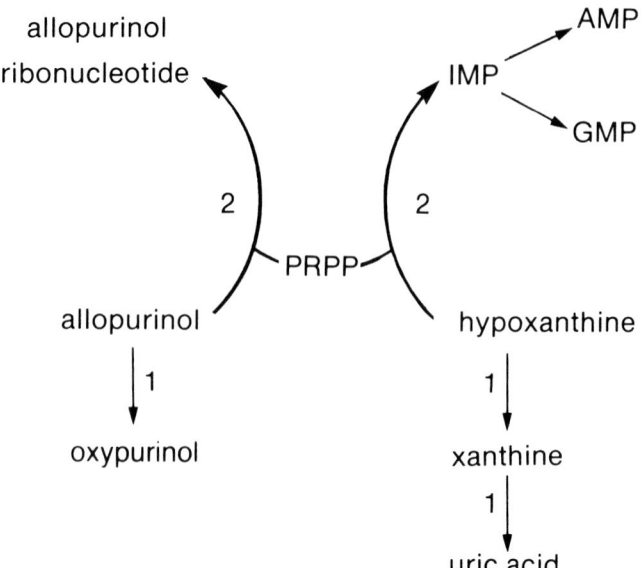

FIG. 105–3. Abbreviated scheme of allopurinol and hypoxanthine metabolism. The inhibition of xanthine oxidase (enzyme 1) by allopurinol and oxypurinol lowers uric acid formation by blocking the conversion of hypoxanthine to xanthine and xanthine to uric acid. Xanthine oxidase inhibition also results in the accumulation of hypoxanthine and allopurinol, which are converted to their respective ribonucleotide monophosphates by the action of hypoxanthine-guanine phosphoribosyltransferase (HGPRTase, enzyme 2). The formation of these ribonucleotides further decreases uric acid production by diminishing de novo purine biosynthesis by three mechanisms: (1) inhibition of amidophosphoribosyltransferase activity by allopurinol ribonucleotide; (2) inhibition of both amidophosphoribosyltransferase and phosphopyrophosphate (PRPP) synthetase activity by inosine 5'-monophosphate (IMP), adenosine 5'-monophosphate (AMP), and guanosine 5'-monophosphate (GMP); and (3) depletion of phosphoribosylpyrophosphate. PRPP is not only a substrate for HGPRTase, but also is an essential and rate-limiting substrate for de novo purine synthesis.

to pretreatment levels,[117] patients should continue to take the antihyperuricemic agent indefinitely once treatment is initiated.

Side effects, serious complications, and toxicity of allopurinol are unusual. Prophylactic colchicine is 85% effective in preventing episodes of acute arthritis that might be triggered by a sudden fall in serum urate concentration induced by allpurinol.[43] Because of the increased concentrations of oxypurines in the urine, xanthine renal calculi are possible. This complication is rare and has been demonstrated only five times, in patients with Lesch-Nyhan syndrome,[118–120] lymphosarcoma,[121] and Burkitt's lymphoma.[122] Microcrystalline deposits of oxypurinol, as well as of hypoxanthine and xanthine, have been demonstrated in muscle biopsy specimens from gouty patients taking allopurinol.[123] No clinical sequelae are known to result from that deposition, however.

The overall incidence of side effects from allopurinol is 5 to 20%, but only half the affected patients consider these effects sufficient to warrant discontinuing the medication.[79,124] The most frequent side effects include skin rash, gastrointestinal distress, diarrhea, and headache.[109,125] The most common rash is a maculopapular erythema, but exfoliative dermatitis and toxic epidermal necrolysis have been reported.[126,127] A mild rash is not a contraindication for further use of allopurinol. The drug should be stopped, but it may be reinstituted once the rash has cleared. Desensitization with low doses may be required in some individuals.[128,129]

More serious adverse effects include alopecia, fever, lymphadenopathy, bone marrow suppression,[130] hepatic toxicity,[131] interstitial nephritis,[132] renal failure, hypersensitivity vasculitis, and death.[133,134]

Some data also suggest that allopurinol may cause or may worsen existing cataracts.[135,136] Serious toxicity is fortunately rare, but it is most often seen in patients with renal insufficiency or in those taking thiazide diuretics.[107,133] Unfortunately, the majority of serious reactions and deaths have occurred in patients whose medical problems did not require allopurinol in the first place.[137]

Potentially important drug interactions must be considered when allopurinol is prescribed. Because 6-mercaptopurine and azathioprine are inactivated by xanthine oxidase, allopurinol prolongs the half-life of these agents and thus potentiates their therapeutic and toxic effects.[138] Cyclophosphamide toxicity may be enhanced,[139] and a threefold increase in the incidence of ampicillin- and amoxicillin-related skin rashes has been reported in patients taking allopurinol.[140,141] On the other hand, allopurinol can reduce the toxicity of 5-fluorouracil.[142]

Allopurinol and a uricosuric agent may be used simultaneously in the rare patient whose hyperuricemia cannot be controlled by a single medication.[143] Although uricosuric agents increase the urinary excretion of oxypurinol,[106] this effect is balanced because allopurinol increases the half-life of probenecid by inhibiting microsomal drug-metabolizing enzymes.[79] Clinically, the drugs can be used in combination without modifying the dosage schedule of either agent. The addition of a uricosuric drug to a therapeutic program including allopurinol usually increases the patient's urinary uric acid excretion and further lowers the serum urate concentration.[109]

The use of allopurinol in acute uric acid nephropathy and in the hyperuricemic individual with nephrolithiasis has been discussed in previous sections.

One additional indication for the use of this agent is in the treatment of 2,8-dihydroxyadenine kidney stones. Individuals with this condition have a homozygous deficiency of adenine phosphoribosyltransferase,[144] an enzyme that catalzyes the conversion of adenine to adenosine 5'-monophosphate. In the absence of this activity, adenine is converted by xanthine oxidase to the insoluble 2,8-dihydroxyadenine, which is excreted in the urine. Reports of 2,8-dihydroxyadenine stones are rare, most likely because of the chemical similarity between this compound and uric acid. X-ray powder diffraction analysis is necessary for correct identification. Stones of this type, however, may be more common than previously thought because the prevalence of the heterozygous state for this enzyme deficiency in the general population may be as high as 1%.[145]

REFERENCES

1. Hall, A.P., et al.: Epidemiology of gout and hyperuricemia: a long term population study. Am. J. Med., 42:27–37, 1967.
2. Zalokar, J., et al.: Serum uric acid in 23,923 men and gout in a subsample of 4,257 men in France. J. Chronic Dis., 25:305–312, 1972.
3. Paulus, H.E., et al.: Clinical significance of hyperuricemia in routinely screened hospitalized men. JAMA, 211:277–281, 1970.
4. Mikkelsen, W.M., Dodge, H.J., and Valkenburg, H.: The distribution of serum uric acid values in a population unselected as to gout or hyperuricemia: Tecumseh, Michigan, 1959–1960. Am. J. Med., 39:242–251, 1965.
5. Wortmann, R.L., and Fox, I.H.: Limited value of uric acid to creatinine ratios in estimating uric acid excretion. Ann. Intern. Med., 93:822–825, 1980.
6. Seegmiller, J.E., et al.: Uric acid production in gout. J. Clin. Invest., 40:1,304–1,314, 1961.
7. O'Sullivan, J.B.: The incidence of gout and related uric acid levels in Sudbury, Massachusetts. *In* Population Studies in the Rheumatic Diseases. Edited by P. Bennett and P. Wood. New York, Excerpta Medica, 1968, pp. 371–376.
8. Campion, E.W., Glynn, R.J., and DeLabry, L.O.: Asymptomatic hyperuricemia. Risks and consequences in the normative aging study. Am. J. Med., 82:421–426, 1987.
9. Emmerson, B.T.: The clinical differentiation of lead gout from primary gout. Arthritis Rheum., 11:623–634, 1968.
10. Klinenberg, J.R., Gonick, H.C., and Dornfield, L.: Renal function abnormalities in patients with asymptomatic hyperuricemia. Arthritis Rheum., 18 (Suppl.):725–730, 1975.
11. Talbott, J.H., and Terplan, K.L.: The kidney in gout. Medicine, 39:405–467, 1960.
12. Yu, T.-F., and Talbott, J.H.: Changing trends of mortality in gout. Semin. Arthritis Rheum., 10:1–9, 1980.
13. Beck, L.H.: Requiem for gouty nephropathy. Kidney Int., 30:280–287, 1986.
14. Brown, J., and Mallory, G.K.: Renal changes in gout. N. Engl. J. Med., 243:325–329, 1950.
15. Mayne, J.G.: Pathological study of renal lesions found in 27 patients with gout. Ann. Rheum. Dis., 15:61–62, 1965.
16. Sokoloff, L.: The pathology of gout. Metabolism, 6:230–243, 1957.
17. Fessel, W.J.: Renal outcomes of gout and hyperuricemia. Am. J. Med., 67:74–82, 1979.
18. Rosenfeld, J.B.: Effect of long-term allopurinol administration on GFR in normotensive and hypertensive subjects. Adv. Exp. Biol. Med., 41B:581–596, 1974.
19. Burger, L., and Yu, T.-F.: Renal function in gout. IV. An analysis of 524 gouty subjects including long-term follow-up studies. Am. J. Med., 59:605–613, 1975.
20. Yu, T.-F., et al.: Renal function in gout. V. Factors influencing the renal hemodynamics. Am. J. Med., 67:766–771, 1979.
21. Yu, T.-F., and Berger, L.: Impaired renal function in gout: its association with hypertensive vascular disease and intrinsic renal disease. Am. J. Med., 72:95–100, 1982.
22. Yu, T.-F.: Urolithiasis in hyperuricemia and gout. J. Urol., 126:424–430, 1981.
23. Armstrong, W.A., and Greene, L.F.: Uric acid calculi with particular reference to determinations of uric acid content of blood. J. Urol., 70:545–547, 1953.
24. Talbott, J.H.: Gout. New York, Grune and Stratton, 1957, p. 205.
25. Pak, C.Y.C., et al.: Mechanism for calcium urolithiasis among patients with hyperuricosuria. Supersaturation of urine with respect to monosodium urate. J. Clin. Invest., 59:426–431, 1977.
26. Coe, F.L.: Hyperuricosuric calcium oxalate nephrolithiasis. Kidney Int., 13:418–426, 1978.
27. Ettinger, B., et al.: Randomized trial of allopurinol in the prevention of calcium oxalate calculi. N. Engl. J. Med., 315:1386–1389, 1986.
28. Yu, T.-F., and Gutman, A.B.: Uric acid nephrolithiasis in gout. Predisposing factors. Ann. Intern. Med., 67:1,133–1,148, 1967.
29. Hall, A.P.: Correlations among hyperuricemia, hypercholesterolemia, coronary disease and hypertension. Arthritis Rheum., 8:846–851, 1965.
30. Meyers, A.R., et al.: The relationship of serum uric acid to risk factors in coronary heart disease. Am. J. Med., 45:520–528, 1968.
31. Reunanen, A., et al.: Hyperuricemia as a risk factor for cardiovascular mortality. Acta Med. Scand., 668 (Suppl.):49–59, 1982.
32. Fessel, W.J.: High uric acid as an indicator of cardiovascular disease: independence from obesity. Am. J. Med., 68:401–404, 1980.
33. Messerli, F.H., et al.: Serum uric acid in essential hypertension: an indicator of renal vascular involvement. Ann. Intern. Med., 93:817–821, 1980.
34. Woolliscroft, J.O., Colfer, H., and Fox, I.H.: Hyperuricemia in acute illness: a poor prognostic sign. Am. J. Med., 72:58–62, 1982.
35. Cebul, R.D., and Beck, J.R.: Biochemical profiles. Applications in ambulatory screening and preadmission testing of adults. Ann. Intern. Med., 106:403–413, 1987.
36. Wallace, S.L., Berstein, D., and Diamond, H.: Diagnostic value of colchicine therapeutic trial. JAMA, 199:525–528, 1967.
37. Hench, P.S.: The diagnosis of gout and gouty arthritis. J. Lab. Clin. Med., 22:48–55, 1936.
38. Wyngaarden, J.B., and Kelley, W.N.: Gout and Hyperuricemia. New York, Grune and Stratton, 1976, pp. 284–289.
39. Boss, G.R., and Seegmiller, J.E.: Hyperuricemia and gout: classification, complications and management. N. Engl. J. Med., 300:1,459–1,468, 1979.

40. Nakayama, D.A., et al.: Tophaceous gout: a clinical and radiographic assessment. Arthritis Rheum., 27:468–471, 1984.
41. Barthelemy, C.R., et al.: Gouty arthritis: a prospective radiographic evaluation of sixty patients. Skeletal Radiol., 11:1–8, 1984.
42. Cohen, A.: Gout. Am. J. Med. Sci., 192:448–493, 1936.
43. Yu, T.-F.: The efficacy of colchicine prophylaxis in articular gout—a reappraisal after 20 years. Arthritis Rheum., 12:256–264, 1982.
44. Kungl, R.W., et al.: Colchicine myopathy and neuropathy. N. Engl. J. Med., 316:1,562–1,568, 1987.
45. Coe, F.L.: Treated and untreated recurrent calcium nephrolithiasis in patients with idiopathic hypercalciuria, hyperuricosuria, or no metabolic disorder. Ann. Intern. Med., 87:404–410, 1977.
46. Pak, C.Y.C., et al.: Is selective therapy of recurrent nephrolithiasis possible? Am. J. Med., 71:615–622, 1981.
47. Pak, C.Y.C., Sakhaee, K., and Fuller, C.: Successful management of uric acid nephrolithiasis with potassium citrate. Kidney Int., 30:422–428, 1986.
48. Seegmiller, J.E., and Frazier, P.D.: Biochemical considerations of the renal damage of gout. Ann. Rheum. Dis., 25:668–672, 1966.
49. Conger, J.D., et al.: A micropuncture study of the early phase of acute urate nephropathy. J. Clin. Invest., 58:681–689, 1976.
50. Stavric, B., Johnson, W.J., and Grice, H.C.: Uric acid nephropathy: an experimental model. Proc. Soc. Exp. Biol. Med., 130:512–519, 1969.
51. Frei, E., et al.: Renal complications of neoplastic disease. J. Chronic Dis., 16:757–776, 1963.
52. Rieselbach, R.E., et al.: Uric acid excretion and renal function in the acute hyperuricemia of leukemia. Am. J. Med., 37:872–884, 1964.
53. Crittenden, D.R., and Ackerman, G.I.: Hyperuricemic acute renal failure in disseminated carcinoma. Arch. Intern. Med., 137:97–99, 1977.
54. Knochel, J.P., Dotin, L.N., and Hamburger, R.J.: Heat stress, exercise, and muscle injury: effects on urate metabolism and renal function. Ann. Intern. Med., 81:321–328, 1974.
55. Warren, D.J., Leitch, A.G., and Leggett, R.J.E.: Hyperuricemic acute renal failure after epileptic seizures. Lancet, 2:385–387, 1975.
56. Deger, G.E., and Wagoner, R.D.: Peritoneal dialysis in acute uric acid nephropathy. Mayo Clin. Proc., 47:189–192, 1972.
57. Kjellstrand, C.M., et al.: Hyperuricemic acute renal failure. Arch. Intern. Med., 133:349–359, 1974.
58. Steele, T.H., and Rieselbach, R.E.: The contribution of residual nephrons within the chronically diseased kidney to urate homeostasis in man. Am. J. Med., 43:876–886, 1967.
59. Kelton, J., Klley, W.N., and Holmes, E.W.: A rapid method for the diagnosis of acute uric acid nephropathy. Arch. Intern. Med., 138:612–615, 1978.
60. Kelley, W.N., et al.: Acetazolamide in phenobarbital intoxication. Arch. Intern. Med., 117:64–69, 1966.
61. Simmonds, H.A., Cameron, J.S., Morris, G.S., and Davies, P.M.: Allopurinol in renal failure and the tumor lysis syndrome. Clin. Chim. Acta, 160:189–195, 1986.
62. Jankovic, M., et al.: Urate-oxidase as hypouricemic agent in a case of acute tumor lysis syndrome. Am. J. Pediat. Hematol. Oncol., 7:202–204, 1985.
63. Talbott, J.H.: Solid and liquid nourishment in gout: selected historical excerpts, largely empiric or fashionable and current scientific(?) concepts in the management of gout and gouty arthritis. Semin. Arthritis Rheum., 11:288–306, 1981.
64. Gutman, A.B., and Yu, T.-F.: Gout, a derangement of purine metabolism. Adv. Intern. Med., 5:227–302, 1952.
65. Lieber, C.S., et al.: Interrelations of uric acid and ethanol metabolism in man. J. Clin. Invest., 41:1,863–1,870, 1962.
66. MacLachlan, M.J., and Rodnan, G.P.: Effect of food, fast, and alcohol on serum uric acid and acute attacks of gout. Am. J. Med., 42:38–57, 1967.
67. Faller, J., and Fox, I.H.: Ethanol-induced hyperuricemia: evidence for increased urate production and activation of adenine nucleotide turnover. N. Engl. J. Med., 307:1,598–1,602, 1982.
68. Steele, T.H., and Boner, G.: Origins of the uricosuric response. J. Clin. Invest., 52:1,368–1,375, 1973.
69. Fanelli, G.M., Jr.: Uricosuric agents. Arthritis Rheum., 18(Suppl.):853–858, 1975.
70. Meisel, A.D., and Diamond, H.S.: Inhibition of probenecid uricosuria by pyrazinamide and para-aminohippurate. Am. J. Physiol., 232:F222–F226, 1977.
71. Levinson, D.J., and Sorensen, L.B.: Renal handling of uric acid in normal and gouty subjects: evidence for a 4-component system. Ann. Rheum. Dis., 39:173–179, 1979.
72. Gutman, A.B., and Yu, T.-F.: Protracted uricosuric therapy in tophaceous gout. Lancet, 2:1,258–1,260, 1957.
73. Gutman, A.B., and Yu, T.-F.: Benemid (p-[di-n-propylsulfamyl] benzoic acid) as uricosuric agent in chronic gouty arthritis. Trans. Assoc. Am. Physicians, 64:279–287, 1951.
73a.Hansten, P.D.: Drug Interactions. 4th Ed. Philadelphia, Lea & Febiger, 1979, p. 255.
74. Wyngaarden, J.B.: Metabolic and clinical aspects of gout. Am. J. Med., 22:819–824, 1957.
75. Yu, T.-F.: Milestones in the treatment of gout. Am. J. Med., 56:676–685, 1974.
76. Gutman, A.B: Uric acid metabolism and gout: combined staff clinic. Am. J. Med., 9:799–817, 1950.
77. Talbott, J.H., Bishop, C., and Norcross, M.: The clinical and metabolic effects of Benemid in patients with gout. Trans. Assoc. Am. Physicians, 64:372–377, 1951.
78. Dayton, P.G., et al.: The physiological disposition of probenecid, including renal clearance in man, studied by an improved method for its estimation in biological material. J. Pharmacol. Exp. Ther., 140:278–286, 1963.
79. Tjandramaga, T.B., et al.: Observations on the disposition of probenecid on patients receiving allopurinol. Pharmacology, 8:259–272, 1972.
80. Dayton, P.G., et al.: Studies of the fate of metabolites and analogs of probenecid: the significance of metabolic sites, especially lack of ring hydroxylation. Drug Metab. Dispos., 1:742–751, 1973.
81. Wyngaarden, J.B., and Kelley, W.N.: Gout and Hyperuricemia. New York, Grune and Stratton, 1976, pp. 430–438.
82. Reynolds, E.S., et al.: Fatal massive necrosis of the liver as a manifestation of hypersensitivity to probenecid. N. Engl. J. Med., 256:592–596, 1957.
83. Ferris, T.F., Morgan, W.S., and Levitin, H.: Nephrotic syndrome caused by probenecid. N. Engl. J. Med., 256:592–596, 1957.
84. Hertz, P., Yager, H., and Richardson, J.A.: Probenecid induced nephrotic syndrome. Arch. Pathol., 94:241–243, 1972.
85. Burns, J.J., et al.: A potent new uricosuric agent, the sulfoxide metabolite of the phenylbutazone analogue. G-25671. J. Pharmacol. Exp. Ther., 119:418–426, 1957.
86. Dayton, P.G., et al.: Metabolism of sulfinpyrazone (Anturane) and other thio analogues of phenylbutazone in man. J. Pharmacol. Exp. Ther., 132:287–290, 1961.
87. Gutman, A.B., et al.: A study of the inverse relationship be-

tween pK$_a$ and rate of renal excretion of phenylbutazone analogs in man and dog. Am. J. Med., 29:1,017–1,033, 1960.

88. Ali, M., and McDonald, W.D.: Effects of sulfinpyrazone on platelet prostaglandin synthesis and platelet release of serotonin. J. Lab. Clin. Med., 89:868–875, 1977.

89. Persellin, R.H., and Schmid, F.R.: The use of sulfinpyrazone in the treatment of gout reduces serum uric acid levels and diminishes severity of arthritis attacks, with freedom from significant toxicity. JAMA, 175:971–975, 1961.

90. Emmerson, B.T.: A comparison of uricosuric agents in gout, with special reference to sulfinpyrazone. Med. J. Aust., 1:839–844, 1963.

91. deGery, A., et al.: Treatment of gout and hyperuricemia by benzbromarone, ethyl-2 (dibromo-3,5-hydrox-4-benzoyl)-3 benzofuran. Adv. Exp. Med. Biol., 41B:683–689, 1974.

92. Jain, A.K., et al.: Effect of single oral doses of benzbromarone on serum and urinary uric acid. Arthritis Rheum., 17:149–157, 1974.

93. Sinclar, D.S., and Fox, I.H.: The pharmacology of hypouricemic effect of benzbromarone. J. Rheumatol., 2:437–445, 1975.

94. Masbernard, A., and Giudicelli, C.P.: Ten year's experience with benzbromarone in the management of gout and hyperuricemia. S. Afr. Med. J., 59:701–706, 1981.

95. Zollner, N., Griebsch, A., and Fink, J.K.: Uber die Wirkung von Benzbromarone auf den Serumharnsaurespiegel und die Harnsaureausscheidung des Gichtkranken. Dtsch. Med. Wochenschr., 95:2,405–2,411, 1970.

96. Rundles, R.W.: Metabolic effects of allpurinol and alloxanthine. Ann. Rheum. Dis., 25:615–620, 1966.

97. Lockard, O., Jr., et al.: Allergic reaction to allopurinol with cross-reactivity to oxypurinol. Ann. Intern. Med., 85:333–335, 1976.

98. Delbarre, F., et al.: Treatment of gout with allopurinol: a study of 106 cases. Ann. Rheum. Dis., 25:627–633, 1966.

99. Auscher, C., et al.: Allopurinol and thiopurinol: effect in vivo on urinary oxypurine excretion and rate of synthesis of their ribonucleotides in different enzymatic deficiencies. Adv. Exp. Med. Biol., 41B:657–662, 1974.

100. Rundles, R.W.: The development of allopurinol. Arch. Int. Med., 145:1492–1503, 1985.

101. Feigelson, P., Davidson, J.K., and Robins, P.K.: Pyrazolo-pyrimidines as inhibitors and substrates of xanthine oxidase. J. Biol. Chem., 226:993–1,000, 1957.

102. Rundles, R.W., et al.: Drugs and uric acid in man. Annu. Rev. Pharmacol., 9:345–362, 1969.

103. Massey, V., Komai, H., and Palmer, G.: On the mechanism of inactivation of xanthine oxidase by allopurinol and other pyrazolo(3,4-d)pyrimidines. J. Biol. Chem., 245:2,837–2,844, 1970.

104. Elion, G.B., et al.: Metabolic studies of allopurinol, an inhibitor of xanthine oxidase. Biochem. Pharmacol., 15:863–880, 1966.

105. Hande, K., Reed, E., and Chabner, B.: Allopurinol kinetics. Clin. Pharmacol. Ther., 23:598–605, 1978.

106. Elion, G.B., et al.: Renal clearance of oxypurinol, the chief metabolite of allopurinol. Am. J. Med., 45:69–77, 1968.

107. Hande, K.R., Noone, R.M., and Stone, W.J.: Severe allopurinol toxicity. Description and guidelines for prevention in patients with renal insufficiency. Am. J. Med., 76:47–56, 1984.

108. Wyngaarden, J.B., Rundles, R.W., and Metz, E.N.: Allopurinol in the treatment of gout. Ann. Intern. Med., 62:842–847, 1965.

109. Rundles, R.W., Metz, E.N., and Silberman, H.R.: Allopurinol in the treatment of gout. Ann. Intern. Med., 64:229–258, 1966.

110. Klinenberg, J.R., Goldfinger, S.E., and Seegmiller, J.E.: The effectiveness of the xanthine oxidase inhibitor allopurinol in the treatment of gout. Ann. Intern. Med., 62:639–647, 1965.

111. Kelley, W.N., et al.: An enzymatic basis for variation in response to allopurinol: hypoxanthine-guanine phosphoribosyltransferase deficiency. N. Engl. J. Med., 278:287–293, 1968.

112. Fox, I.H., Wyngaarden, J.B., and Kelley, W.N.: Depletion of erythrocyte phosphoribosylpyrophosphate in man: a newly observed effect of allopurinol. N. Engl. J. Med., 283:1,177–1,182, 1970.

113. Edwards, N.L., et al.: Enhanced purine salvage during allopurinol therapy: an important pharmacologic property in humans. J. Lab. Clin. Med., 98:673–683, 1981.

114. Kelley, W.N., and Beardmore, T.D.: Allopurinol: alteration in pyrimidine metabolism in man. Science, 169:388–390, 1970.

115. Yu, T.-F.: The effect of allopurinol in primary and secondary gout. Arthritis Rheum., 8:905–906, 1965.

116. Brewis, I., Ellis, R.M., and Scott, J.T.: Single daily dose of allopurinol. Ann. Rheum. Dis., 34:256–259, 1975.

117. Loebl, W.Y., and Scott, J.T.: Withdrawal of allopurinol in patients with gout. Ann. Rheum. Dis., 33:304–307, 1974.

118. Sorenson, L., and Seegmiller, J.E.: Seminars on the Lesch-Nyhan syndrome: management and treatment, discussion. Fed. Proc., 27:1,097–1,104, 1968.

119. Greene, M.L., Fujimoto, W.Y., and Seegmiller, J.E.: Urinary xanthine stones—a rare complication of allopurinol therapy. N. Engl. J. Med., 280:426–427, 1969.

120. Kranen, S., Keough, D., Gordon, R.B., and Emmerson, B.T.: Xanthine-containing calculi during allopurinol therapy. J. Urol., 133:658–659, 1985.

121. Band, P.R., Silverberg, D.S., and Henderson, J.F.: Xanthine nephropathy in a patient with lymphosarcoma treated with allopurinol. N. Engl. J. Med., 283:354–357, 1970.

122. Albin, A., et al.: Nephropathy, xanthinuria, and orotic aciduria complicating Burkitt's lymphoma treated with chemotherapy and allopurinol. Metabolism, 21:771–778, 1972.

123. Watts, R.W.E., et al.: Microscopic studies on skeletal muscle in gout patients treated with allopurinol. Q. J. Med., 40:1–14, 1971.

124. McInnes, G.T., Lawson, D.H., and Jick, H.: Acute adverse reactions attributed to allopurinol in hospitalized patients. Ann. Rheum. Dis., 40:245–249, 1981.

125. Yu, T.-F., and Gutman, A.B.: Effect of allopurinol (4-hydroxypyrazolo-(3,4-d) pyrimidine) on serum and urinary uric acid in primary gout. Am. J. Med., 37:885–898, 1964.

126. Lang, P.G.: Severe hypersensitivity reactions to allopurinol. South. Med. J., 72:1,361–1,368. 1979.

127. Stratigos, J.D., Bartsokas, S.K., and Capetanakis, J.: Further experience of toxic epidermal necrolysis incriminating allopurinol, pyrazoline, and derivatives. Br. J. Dermatol., 86:564–567, 1972.

128. Fam, A.G., Paton, T.W., and Chaiton, A.: Reinstitution of allopurinol therapy for gouty arthritis after cutaneous reactions. Can. Med. Assoc. J., 123:128–129, 1980.

129. Webster, E., and Panush, R.S.: Allopurinol hypersensitivity in a patient with severe, chronic, tophaceous gout. Arthritis Rheum., 28:707–709, 1985.

130. Greenberg,M.S., and Zambrano, S.S.: Aplastic agranulocytosis after allopurinol therapy. Arthritis Rheum., 15:413–416, 1972.

131. Al-Kawas, F.H., et al.: Allopurinol hepatotoxicity: report of

two cases and review of the literature. Ann. Intern. Med., *95*:588–590, 1981.

132. Gelbart, D.R., Weinstein, A.B., and Fajardo, L.F.: Allopurinol-induced interstitial nephritis. Ann. Intern. Med., *86*:196–198, 1977.

133. Young, J.L., Jr., Boswell, R.B., and Nies, A.S.: Severe allopurinol hypersensitivity: association with thiazides and prior renal compromise. Arch. Intern. Med., *134*:553–558, 1974.

134. Lupton, G.P., and Odon, R.B.: The allopurinol hypersensitivity syndrome. J. Am. Acad. Dermatol., *1*:365–379, 1979.

135. Fraunfelder, F.T., et al.: Cataracts associated with allopurinol therapy. Am. J. Ophthalmol., *94*:137–140, 1982.

136. Lerman, S., Megaw J.M., and Gardner, K.: Allopurinol therapy and cataractogenesis in humans. Am. J. Ophthalmol., *94*:141–146, 1982.

137. Singer, J.Z., and Wallace, S.L.: The allopurinol hypersensitivity syndrome. Unnecessary morbidity and mortality. Arthritis Rheum., *29*:82–87, 1986.

138. Elion, G.B., et al.: Potentiation by inhibition of drug degradation: 6-substituted purines and xanthine oxidase. Biochem. Pharmacol., *12*:85–93, 1963.

139. Boston Collaborative Drug Surveillance Program: Allopurinol and cytotoxic drugs: interactions in relation to bone marrow depression. JAMA, *227*:1,036–1,040, 1974.

140. Boston Collaborative Drug Surveillance Program: Excess of ampicillin rashes associated with allopurinol or hyperuricemia. N. Engl. J. Med., *286*:505–507, 1972.

141. Jick, H., and Porter, J.B.: Potentiation of ampicillin skin reactions by allopurinol or hyperuricemia. J. Clin. Pharmacol., *21*:456–458, 1981.

142. Howell, S.B., et al.: Modulation of 5-fluorouracil toxicity by allopurinol in man. Cancer, *48*:1,281–1,289, 1981.

143. Kelley, W.N.: Pharmacologic approach to the maintenance of urate homeostasis. Nephron, *14*:99–115, 1975.

144. Gault, M.H., et al.: Urolithiasis due to 2,8-dihydroxyadenine in an adult. N. Engl. J. Med., *305*:1,570–1,572, 1981.

145. Fox, I.H., et al.: Partial deficiency of adenine phosphoribosyltransferase in man. Medicine, *56*:515–526, 1977.

PATHOGENESIS AND TREATMENT OF CRYSTAL-INDUCED INFLAMMATION

106

ROBERT A. TERKELTAUB, MARK H. GINSBERG,
and DANIEL J. McCARTY

Information pertaining to the cellular and molecular mechanisms of the inflammatory host response to several microcrystals characteristic of human rheumatic diseases and its treatment is considered in this chapter. A summary of crystals definitely identified in human joints appears in Table 5–7. Most but not all of these have been associated with joint inflammation.

HISTORICAL ASPECTS

Though acute gouty arthritis has been recogized for centuries as one of the most severe and painful forms of acute inflammation occurring in humans, it was not until 1961 that the constant presence of microcrystalline monosodium urate monohydrate (MSU) in gouty joint fluid was established.[1] Needle-shaped MSU crystals can often be seen under ordinary light microscopy, but compensated polarized light microscopy is much more sensitive and specific. The inventor of the microscope, Anton van Leeuwenhoek, born in 1632 was the first to describe these crystals, having obtained them from a draining tophus. Van Leeuwenhoek was unaware of their chemical composition because uric (lithic) acid was not discovered until 1776 by Scheele. Garrod used polarized light microscopic inspection of fresh tissue sections, cut by hand with a razor blade, to identify urate crystals; he wrote in 1876 that ". . . in the constancy of such deposition

lies the clue that has long been wanting; the occurrence of the deposit is at once pathognomonic and separates gout from every other disease which at first sight may appear allied to it."

Phagocytosis of MSU crystals by both polymorphonuclear and mononuclear cells was described in recently erupted human skin tophi by the Viennese dermatologist Gustav Riehl in 1897, a phenomenon rediscovered later in gouty joint fluid (Fig. 106–1).

At the turn of the century, Swiss investigators Wilhelm His, Jr. and Max Freudweiler, working in Germany, reported an inflammatory response to injected synthetic MSU and other crystals in man and in several other species. Subcutaneous injections of crystals (into Dr. Freudweiler) produced inflammation initially and later developed into tophi that were histologically indistinguishable from those seen in natural gout.

An acute inflammatory response associated with crystal phagocytosis after injection of synthetic urate crystals and control crystals composed of other substances into normal human and canine joints was described in 1962,[2] and a similar response to crystals injected into the joints of gouty patients was found the same year.[3] The terms crystal deposition disease and crystal-induced inflammation were coined; the latter was characterized as dose-related, completely reversible, and nonspecific with reference to both host species and chemical composition of the crystals, e.g., inflammation in human and canine joints after injection of microcrystalline adrenocorticosteroid esters

1691

FIG. 106–1. Natural monosodium urate crystals in a polymorphonuclear leukocyte (polarized light × 1250). The lysosomes have been stained supravitally with neutral red.

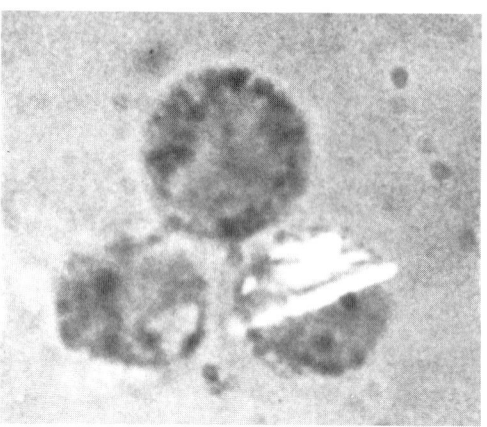

was postulated as responsible for the "poststeroid injection flare" sometimes observed after the therapeutic use of such preparations.[4]

RECENT DISCOVERIES

Dicalcium phosphate dihydrate crystals, CaHPO$_4$· 2H$_2$O, have been found in patients with arthritis.[5] These relatively soluble orthophosphate crystals (brushite) were originally found in cadaver cartilage.[6] Dicalcium phosphate dihydrate appeared as punctate desposits in multiple cartilages of 2.3% and calcium pyrophosphate dihydrate (CPPD) deposits were found in 3.2% of the 215 cadavers studied. With a single exception, these substances were mutually exclusive.

Gaucher and colleagues identified dicalcium phosphate dihydrate in cartilage removed surgically from a patient with radiologic chondrocalcinosis and destructive arthropathy.[5] These crystals appeared pyramidal by scanning electron microscopy (Fig. 106–2). Utsinger identified this substance by roentgenographic diffraction of crystals obtained from one patient with acute arthritis and two patients with chronic arthritis.[7] All three were men, and two of them had radiographic chondrocalcinosis. Dicalcium phosphate dihydrate crystals were identified only in two instances, and they coexisted with CPPD crystals in one synovial fluid; CPPD was found once. It is not yet resolved whether dicalcium phosphate dihydrate crystal deposition disease and crystal-induced inflammation are true entities.

The term apatite deposition disease was suggested by Dieppe and colleagues in 1976,[8] but as indicated

FIG. 106–2. *A,* Dicalcium phosphate dihydrate crystal from cartilage (scanning electron microscope × 1,900). *B,* Calcium pyrophosphate dihydrate from cartilage (scanning electron microscope × 10,000). (Courtesy of Dr. Gilbert Faure.)

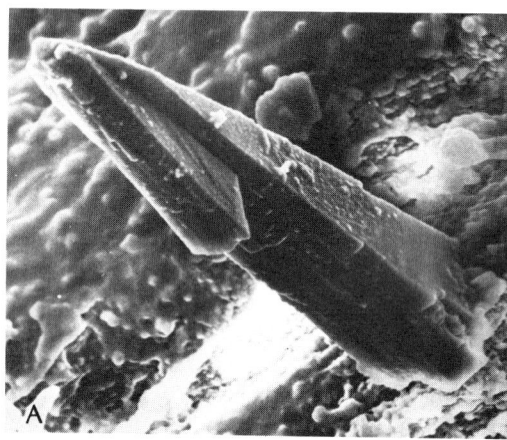

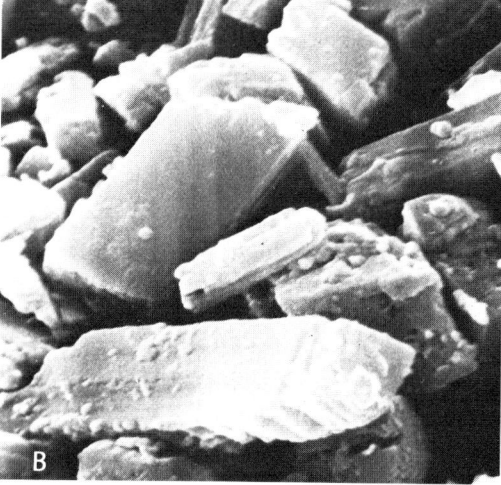

previously, the more precise term basic calcium phosphate (BCP) crystal deposition disease seems appropriate to describe their associated clinical syndromes (Chapter 108).

A single case of cystinosis with intermittent pain involving large and small joints was reported as "cystinosis with crystal-induced synovitis and arthropathy."[9] Crystals were found in bone marrow macrophages and histiocytes. Such crystals have been found in polymorphonuclear leukocytes of peripheral blood in this disease. Whether cystine crystals induced clinically significant inflammation remains questionable. The reported case had radiologic evidence of epiphysitis in two joints. No crystals were found in joint tissue or inside joint fluid leukocytes.

Tyrosine crystals have been found within cells in the destructive corneal lesions in children with tyrosinosis, and crystals, presumably tyrosine, formed within corneal epithelial cells, have been found in tyrosine-fed rats.[10] Moreover, some species of tyrosine crystals are membranolytic.[11] Charcot-Leyden crystals, some of which were intracellular, have been found in inflammatory joint fluids in association with eosinophilia (see Chapters 5 and 109).[12]

The inclusion of a variety of synovial lipids among entities provoking crystal-induced inflammation has been controversial. Nonbirefringent crystals of cholesterol are sometimes found in joint fluids, particularly in effusions of long duration in both degenerative and inflammatory joint diseases.[13,14] Similar crystals can be found in joint effusions experimentally induced in hyperlipidemic rabbits by a local Arthus reaction.[15] It is not clear whether inflammation is a direct consequence of the presence of intra-articular cholesterol crystals in vivo. Cholesterol crystals obtained commercially have activated complement through the alternative pathway,[16,17] and their injection into animal tissues has caused inflammation associated with phagocytosis.[18] However, cholesterol crystals have not been found within polymorphonuclear leukocytes in human joint effusions. Endotoxin contamination, or the presence of cholesterol oxidation products in commercial preparations not found in vivo, may invalidate any extrapolation of these experimental data to human arthritis. A possible relationship of cholesterol crystals to acute arthritis in familial type II hyperlipoproteinemia remains enigmatic, particularly as neutrophils from such patients may be more highly activated by soluble agonists in vitro than are normal neutrophils.[19] Additional clinical studies and experimental work with better-characterized crystals are needed.

Positively birefringent lipid spherulites are an occasional finding in a variety of synovial fluids (Chapter 5). Larger numbers of such extracellular and intracellular spherulites have been noted in a small number of patients with otherwise unexplained acute monoarthritis.[20,21] Trauma with resultant hemarthrosis might explain the acute joint manifestations in these patients and the possible derivation of the lipid spherulites from erythrocyte membranes.[22]

Calcium oxalate and aluminum phosphate crystals have both been described in patients undergoing long-term hemodialysis, and the consequences of deposition of these crystals are under investigation. Manifestations of oxalosis-associated arthropathy include podagra, olecranon bursitis, tenosynovitis, and calcified deposits in skin.[23,29] A symmetric polyarthritis of small joints of the hand associated with periarticular, dermal, and vascular calcification can occur.[24] Chondrocalcinosis may be an associated fea-

ture.[24] Crystallographic analysis of cartilage has not yet been carried out in these patients. It has been suggested that calcium oxalate monohydrate is the predominant synovial fluid form of oxalate associated with arthropathy.[24]

IDENTIFICATION OF CRYSTALS

Techniques useful in routine clinical practice and in experimental work are discussed in Chapters 5, 107, and 108.

SOURCES OF CRYSTALS

The following discussion focuses on the problems associated with the nucleation and growth of crystals in joint tissues.

MONOSODIUM URATE MONOHYDRATE (MSU)

In most instances, urate crystallizes as a monosodium salt from oversaturated joint fluids. MSU crystals found in joint fluid at the time of the acute attack may derive from rupture of preformed synovial deposits or may have precipitated de novo (Fig. 106–3). The recognition of urate spherulites and ultramicroscopic MSU crystals is discussed in Chapter 5. Acute attacks of gout in patients studied in a clinical research center correlated with the rate of change of serum uric acid content (either more or less) rather than with a sustained high or sustained low level.[25] Rodnan found that acute gout precipitated by an oral purine load, especially when ethanol was ingested, occurred 18 to 80 hours afterward, when serum urate levels were falling rapidly to prefeast levels.[26] This delay may account for the clinical finding of the occasional acute gouty patient with a normal serum urate level. Treatment with allopurinol commonly produces this abrupt decline in urate levels and acute attack of gout. Acute gouty attacks are also accompanied by a uric acid diuresis (see Chapter 104).

Arthroscopically, the earliest urate crystal deposits are apparently in the synovium, rather than in cartilage; they appear as white furuncles with an erythematous base. Investigators have found tophi in synovial membrane at the time of the first gouty attack.[27] Urate crystals are commonly found in asymptomatic metatarsophalangeal and knee joints that have not been involved in an acute attack of gout despite typical MSU crystal-associated gout in other

FIG. 106–3. Autoinjection of monosodium urate (MSU) crystals (a) from preformed tophus in synovium into adjacent joint space. Autoinjection of calcium pyrophosphate dihydrate (CPPD) crystals (b) from preformed cartilaginous deposit into adjacent joint space, as a result of crystal shedding. Both concepts are still hypothetic and have only indirect supportive evidence. See text for details.

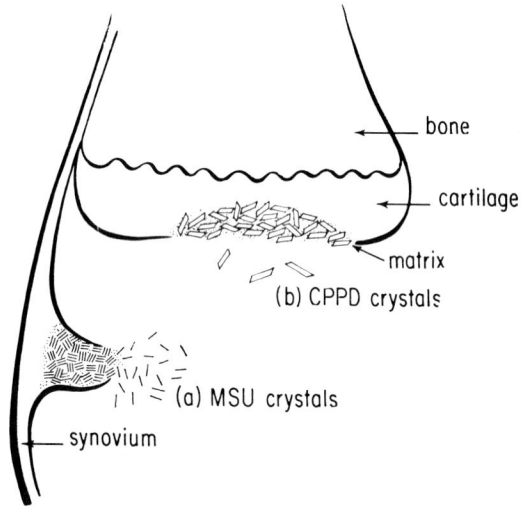

joints.[28–30] In addition, patients with asymptomatic hyperuricemia may have MSU crystals in metatarsophalangeal joint fluid.[31] These findings that confirm that gout, like CPPD crystal deposition, can exist in a lanthanic (asymptomatic) state, are discussed later.

Simkin has convincingly shown that the rate of diffusion of urate molecules from synovial space to plasma is only half that of water.[32] He envisions that the urate level in a small effusion in a dependent joint, such as the great toe, would equilibrate with plasma urate during the day. As the effusion resorbs during recumbency, a localized increase in urate level should occur. This phenomenon could account for those few patients who develop MSU crystals and acute gout in the absence of hyperuricemia, as well as for the usual nocturnal onset of symptoms in a dependent joint, but it cannot explain why only some hyperuricemic individuals develop clinical gout.

The decreased solubility of sodium urate at the lower temperatures of peripheral structures such as the toes and ears has been suggested as a reason why MSU crystals deposit in these areas.[33–35]

The finding by Katz of threefold elevations of serum uronic acid levels in patients with articular gout but not in patients with hyperuricemia or other inflammatory diseases provides a clue to the possible specificity of MSU crystal deposition.[36] The normalization of these elevated levels by the usual therapeutic doses of colchicine lends further credence to this finding and suggests that the prophylactic mechanism of colchicine may be different from that operating in the treatment of established acute gouty arthritis.[37] Katz was prompted to measure serum uronic acid levels, an index of serum glycosaminoglycans (GAGs), because he and Schubert had earlier found that cartilage proteoglycans enhanced urate solubility.[38] These researchers speculated that enzymes degrading proteoglycans might lead to local sodium urate crystallization. The elevated serum uronic acid levels in gout were thought to represent accelerated connective tissue turnover. The time- and dose-related suppression to normal levels of serum uronic acid by colchicine, but not by probenecid or allopurinol, suggests a presumed, as yet undefined, metabolic abnormality specific for gouty expression and unrelated to hyperuricemia.[37] The observations that hemiplegia appears to have a sparing effect on the development of tophi and acute gout on the paretic side,[38] and that tophi and acute gout occur in interphalangeal joints at the location of Heberden's nodes,[39] direct further emphasis to the potential importance of connective-tissue turnover.

The increased urate solubility in proteoglycans is due to their aggregation by hyaluronic acid.[40] The original results of Katz and Schubert were probably caused by the potassium used to precipitate the proteoglycan, rather than by the proteoglycan itself, because potassium urate is more soluble than sodium urate.

The fundamental mechanism of MSU crystal formation in joint and other tissues remains unclear. The lack of tophi in gout secondary to the hyperuricemia of renal disease is well documented, but unexplained.[41,42] The role of plasma protein binding to uric acid in maintaining its solubility was postulated to be a factor by Alvsaker,[43] who found a partial deficiency of a uric acid–binding α-globulin in a kindred with gout.[44a] Albumin has been demonstrated to slow monosodium urate crystallization from supersaturated uric acid solutions by some groups, but this activity has been variable and not universally reproducible.[44b] A number of other studies have concluded that uric acid binding to plasma proteins is generally weak and reversible and that plasma proteins have minimal effects on the distribution of uric acid in equilibrium dialysis.[45] Thus, this issue remains unresolved. The suggestion that lactate production by leukocytes in gouty joint fluid lowers the pH and causes further urate crystal formation has received support from in vitro studies showing that lowering of pH enhances nucleation by the formation of protonated solid phases.[46,47]

However, the solubility of *sodium* urate, as opposed to that of uric acid, actually increases as pH decreases from 7.4 to 5.8.[48] Actual measurements of both pH and buffering capacity in gouty joints, however, failed to demonstrate significant acidosis;[49] *pH changes, therefore, are unlikely to significantly influence MSU crystal formation*, and certainly not as strongly as the temperature effects already referenced.

Another series of studies examined the onset of MSU crystal nucleation by lengthy incubation of soluble sodium urate solutions.[35,50–52] The appearance of crystals was observed microscopically; the critical-threshold MSU concentration increased as the ratio of sodium to uric acid increased. Unfortunately, the physical instability of uric acid over time was ignored.

Although these data may indicate critical supersaturation levels, they give no information about the kinetics of crystal formation. The possible participation of a calcium urate phase was suggested by the finding that calcium affected MSU nucleation only when the solutions were also supersaturated with calcium urate.[50] Lead, at 1000 μg/L, effectively nucleated MSU from normal saline solution containing 10 mg/dl urate.[52] Because such high levels are found only in acute lead poisoning, it remains unlikely that lead acts as a nucleating agent, even in saturnine gout. The possible regulation of MSU crystal formation by substances in joint fluid has also been explored.[44b] Interestingly, joint fluid supernatants from gouty joints enhance nucleation, those from osteoarthritic joints have less activity, and rheumatoid joint fluids have almost none.[51] However, the possible participation of ultramicrocrystals in the gouty fluids as "seeds" was not definitely excluded in this study.

CALCIUM PYROPHOSPHATE DIHYDRATE

The initial site of CPPD crystal formation is probably articular cartilage. Precipitation de novo in synovial fluid or synovium has not been ruled out, and CPPD crystals are frequently found in these sites. In addition, CPPD crystal deposits are occasionally found in extra-articular tendons, ligaments, and bursae.[53] In hyaline cartilage, such crystals often lie in a granular matrix,[5,54,55] which stains more densely than surrounding cartilage with periodic acid-Schiff (PAS), alcian blue, colloidal iron, and ruthenium red.[56] These features suggest the presence of abnormal proteoglycan.

The generation of inorganic pyrophosphate (PPi) from cartilage and the nucleation and growth of CPPD crystals from solution and from gels are discussed in Chapter 107.

Assuming that the CPPD crystals lying in their cartilaginous mold of peculiar proteoglycan are in thermodynamic equilibrium with Ca^{++} and $P_2O_7^{-4}$, the ions from which they were formed, conditions that either lower ionized calcium or reduce Ca^{++} and $P_2O_7^{-4}$ should increase the solubility of these crystals and should free them from their mold. This still hypothetic phenomenon has been called *crystal shedding*.[57] The marked effect of even small changes in ionized calcium level on crystal solubility in vitro,[58] the onset of acute pseudogout after lavage of joints with solubilizers of CPPD crystals such as EDTA or Mg^{++}-containing buffers,[57] and the clinical correlation of acute arthritis with falling serum calcium concentrations[59,60] all support this hypothesis (Fig. 106–3). Joint fluid PPi levels are often higher than plasma levels.[61,62] Fluid PPi levels are lower during acute attack, owing to a more rapid clearance into the blood.[63,64] Thus, once an acute attack begins, the fall in ambient PPi may further increase crystal solubility and shedding.

Other postulated mechanisms for the autoinjection of CPPD crystals, which is presumed to precede acute pseudogout, are summarized in Table 106–1. Mechanical disruption of cartilage accompanying subchondral microfracture was implicated in an acute attack developing for the first time in a knee joint with acute neuropathic changes,[65] and trauma is a common antecedent of acute pseudogout. "Enzymatic stripmining" of crystals from preformed cartilaginous deposits was proposed to explain the occurrence of CPPD and MSU crystals in an osteoarthritic joint with superimposed acute pyogenic arthritis.[66] Many reports of this phenomenon have since appeared and are reviewed in Chapter 5. Presumably, any significant intrasynovial discharge of inflammatory proteases might digest the components of the "mold" and might thereby release crystals into the joint space. CPPD crystals were readily released from cartilage by synovial cell collagenase, for example.[67] Thus, the *mere presence of these or MSU crystals in joint fluid must be interpreted cautiously because they might be a result, as well as a cause, of joint inflammation.*

Finally, the reported association of silent CPPD crystal deposition and hypothyroidism with the onset of acute pseudogout after thyroid hormone therapy suggests that metabolically induced changes in cartilage matrix may also release crystals.[68]

BASIC CALCIUM PHOSPHATES

These ultramicrocrystals generally occur as aggregates, appearing as microspheroidal "snowballs" by

Table 106–1.   Proposed Mechanisms of Autoinjection of Calcium Pyrophosphate Dihydrate (CPPD) Crystals from Cartilage to Vascular Joint Tissue Space

Trigger	Hypothetic Mechanism	Clinical Circumstances of Acute Attack
Fall in synovial fluid (Ca^{++}) or inorganic pyrophosphate level	Partial dissolution crystal shedding	Postoperatively or during acute medical illness
Mechanic disruption of cartilage architecture	Microfractures of subchondral bone	Trauma
Increased activity of enzymes degrading cartilage matrix	Crystal shedding as a result of removal of matrix by "enzymatic strip-mining"	Pseudogout superimposed on another type of arthritis; i.e., pyogenic infection, acute gout, or osteoarthritis
Hypothyroidism with treatment	Altered cartilaginous "mold" with crystal shedding	Joint symptoms after thyroid hormone replacement

scanning electron microscopy. Hydroxyapatite, partially substituted with carbonate, and octacalcium phosphate or tricalcium phosphate have been identified in BCP aggregates in synovial fluid and in subcutaneous calcification from a patient with dermatomyositis.[69] The aggregates may appear purple with Wright's stain.[70] These crystals and clinical syndromes associated with them, are discussed in detail in Chapters 107 and 108.

Importantly, BCP crystals, like MSU and CPPD crystals, lie within a connective tissue matrix, the composition of which is poorly understood. They seem intimately associated with particulate collagens.[69] These crystals may gain access to joints or tendon spaces by rupture of preformed deposits,[70,71] or they may provoke extra-articular inflammation.[70–72]

CORTICOSTEROID ESTER

Synovitis occurs after some but not all injections,[4,73] probably because of the anti-inflammatory effect of that portion of the dose that is in solution. The appearance of these crystals varies with the type of ester, with the batch, and with storage conditions.[79]

MECHANISMS OF CRYSTAL-INDUCED INFLAMMATION

Gout was the first inflammatory crystal deposition disease to be defined and studied in detail and will serve as a paradigm for the following discussion. Acuteness, severity, and extension into periarticular soft tissues are the hallmarks of the articular inflammation in a gouty paroxysm. These features reflect the ability of MSU crystals to activate a remarkable number of humoral and cellular inflammatory mediator systems, some of which are depicted in Figure 106–4. The other crystals found in arthritis have been

less thoroughly studied, but they probably share many of the described reactivities of MSU.

COMPLEMENT ACTIVATION

Urate crystals activate the classic complement pathway in vitro.[75,76] Urate crystals can bind and induce cleavage of purified macromolecular C1 in the absence of immunoglobulin.[76,77] In addition, classic pathway activation is amplified by IgG[78] and C-reactive protein.[79] Alternative pathway activation also occurs in vitro at higher crystal concentrations[17,80] when classic pathway activation is inhibited.[81] Direct cleavage of C5 to C5a and C5b is also effected via a stable C5 convertase formed on the crystal surface.[82] Evidence from a number of laboratories supports the occurrence of complement activation in a substantial proportion of human gouty synovial fluids.[83–85] Though the amount of complement in normal joint fluid is low, C5a and C5a-des-arg are known to exert chemotactic effects at low concentrations (Chapter 25).

Despite the potential role of complement peptides in gouty synovitis, the degree of urate crystal-induced inflammation has been reduced only minimally, at most, by complement depletion in animal studies.[86–88] The results of such studies may reflect the use of urate crystals heated to 200° C to destroy endogenous pyrogen, as heating is known to reduce the complement-activating ability of MSU.[75,83,89] However, such results also reinforce the inherent redundancy of the inflammatory reactions to MSU crystals.

COAGULATION SYSTEM

Urate crystals activate Hageman factor (HF) and the contact system of coagulation in vitro, resulting in generation of kallikrein, bradykinin, plasmin, and other inflammatory mediators.[90] Joint fluids in both spontaneous acute gout and in synthetic urate crystal-

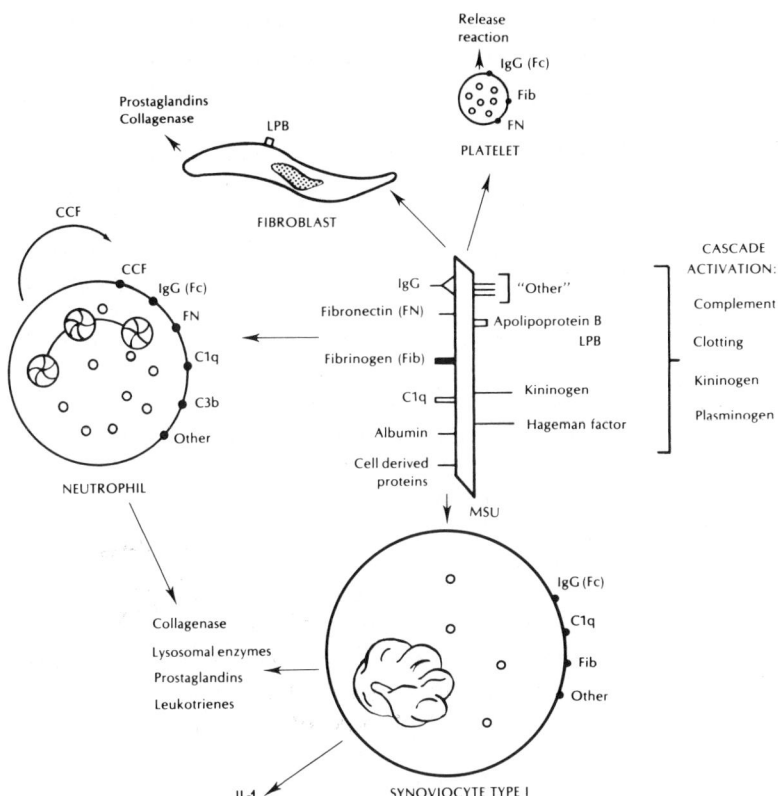

FIG. 106–4. Schematic representation of interaction of monosodium urate (MSU) crystals with various cells and molecules. See text for details of how these interactions may lead to acute gout and to chronic destructive (tophaceous) gout.

induced inflammation contain substantial amounts of kinins.[91,92] However, acute gout does occur in humans with HF deficiency,[93,94] and an acute inflammatory response to injected urate crystals is seen in chicks, which lack HF.[95] Thus, the contact system also does not appear necessary for acute gouty inflammation.

INFLAMMATORY CELL-DERIVED MEDIATORS

A central role for neutrophils and their products in gouty inflammation is supported by several lines of evidence. First, striking accumulation of these cells is present in both the joint fluid and synovial membrane in spontaneous and experimentally induced acute gout, in which these cells are seen both to phagocytose crystals actively and to be degranulated in the microvasculature in areas remote from crystals.[96,97] Second, experimental urate crystal-induced synovitis is diminished when neutrophils are depleted by cytotoxic drugs or antineutrophil antiserum.[98,99] The central role of neutrophils, and other inflammatory cells, in the pathogenesis of gouty inflammation is particularly emphasized by the efficacy of agents that modify neutrophil function in therapy of acute gout, e.g., colchicine.

Neutrophils exposed to urate crystals release acid

lysosomal proteases;[100] oxygen-derived free radicals;[101,102a] and lipoxygenase-derived products of arachidonic acid, including leukotriene B$_4$ (LTB$_4$) and hydroxyeicosatetraenoic acids.[103,104] They also release neutral proteases, including collagenase.[102] In addition, crystal phagocytosis is associated with secretion of a chemotactic, low-molecular-weight glycoprotein[105] termed crystal-induced chemotactic factor (CCF).[106] Injection of purified CCF induced a marked polymorphonuclear response in rabbit joints without altering vascular permeability.[107] LTB$_4$ and a CCF-like molecule have been identified in human gouty synovial fluids.[103,108]

Cells other than neutrophils also appear to be involved in the pathogenesis of gouty inflammation. First, acute gout has been described in the absence of neutrophils in human synovial fluid.[109] Second, urate crystals stimulate the release of vasoactive prostaglandins from synovial fibroblasts in vitro,[110] and phagocytosis of urate crystals by synoviocytes is an early event in experimental urate crystal-induced inflammation in canine joints.[111] Third, although outnumbered by neutrophils during the initial phase of gouty inflammation, synovial fluid mononuclear phagocytes become proportionately greater with time and are often seen to ingest urate crystals.[96,112] Urate crystals stimulate these cells to release prostaglandin E$_2$ (PGE$_2$), lysosomal enzymes,[113] and tumor necrosis factor-alpha in vitro. MSU crystals stimulate the production and release of interleukin-1 (IL-1) from mononuclear phagocytes in vitro.[114] Monocyte IL-1 release in response to MSU crystals does not appear to require phagocytosis and is not abrogated by colchicine.[114] In addition to mediating the fever, the peripheral blood leukocytosis, and the increased erythrocyte sedimentation rate (ESR) often associated with acute gout, IL-1 probably is involved in the initiation of acute gouty arthritis by stimulating leukocyte-endothelial interaction, and the intra-articular influx and activation of neutrophils.[115,116]

The participation of synovial mast cells, platelets, or both in acute gout is possible theoretically; platelets are among the earliest cells to mediate inflammatory responses (Chapter 24), and their interaction with urate crystals in vitro is described below. Mast cells are appreciated to reside in synovia, and stimulation of these cells in vitro by C3a, C5a, and IL-1 results in the release of a variety of inflammatory mediators, including histamine (Chapter 22). In experimental urate crystal-induced inflammation, early articular swelling has been diminished by antihistamines.[117]

MSU-MEMBRANE INTERACTION

Perturbation of plasma membranes and model liposomes by urate crystals results in membrane lysis.[100,118] In addition, nonlytic platelet serotonin secretion, the extracellular release from neutrophils of superoxide anion, and secretion of lysosomal proteases are associated with membrane perturbation by MSU crystals.[101,119–121] Critical factors mediating these events appear to include the crystal structure of MSU, substances coating the crystal surface, and membrane cholesterol and glycoproteins. First, Mandel and others have shown that negatively charged oxygen atoms prominent on the urate crystal surface impart a net negative surface charge.[112] However, atomic components with a partial positive charge are also exposed on the crystal surface.[122] Thus, urate crystals could associate with the plasma membrane by (1) hydrogen bonding, with crystals acting as hydrogen acceptors in interactions with positively charged phospholipid polar head groups, and acting as hydrogen donors in interactions with membrane glycoproteins;[100] and (2) formation of electrostatic bonds with polar membrane structures. Support for the latter hypothesis has been recently provided by the demonstration that MSU crystals interact with both positively and negatively charged electron spin resonance membrane probes.[123,124] The importance of membrane cholesterol has been elucidated by Weissmann; membranes and

liposomes not bearing cholesterol are not lysed by MSU crystals.[100] The role of native crystal structure is emphasized by the effects of heating urate crystals >200° C. Monosodium urate crystals are composed of parallel stacks of purine rings interspersed with sodium ions that bond to the oxygen atoms of the urate anions.[122] Water molecules of crystallization form hydrogen bonds with purines and lie in channels between the rings. Heating the urate crystal alters its structure by removing these water molecules.[125] Heated crystals appear less phlogistic when injected into rat foot pads in vitro[126] as well as less potent as stimulators of human neutrophils in vitro.[127] Alteration of the crystal lattice by heating is the likely reason for the diminution in the capacity of heated urate crystals to activate complement.[75,83,89]

Wallingford and McCarty demonstrated that coating the urate crystal surface with serum or with the hydrogen acceptor polyvinylpyridine N oxide inhibited urate-induced membranolysis,[118] thus pointing to a potential mechanism whereby gouty inflammation could be regulated in vivo by changes in the composition of absorbed molecules. Jaques and Ginsberg discovered that the adhesive platelet membrane glycoproteins Gp IIb/IIIa bind to urate crystals; this finding directed attention to the importance of crystal interaction with adhesive membrane glycoproteins, because proteolyic removal of these glycoproteins from the platelet surface, or direction of antibodies against these glycoproteins, suppressed urate-induced platelet serotonin secretion.[128] Because clustering of membrane proteins, such as might be induced by multivalent ligands, is a stimulus for secretion,[129] it can be hypothesized that urate crystals stimulate cells by binding to membrane proteins, leading to their clustering in the plane of the membrane (Fig. 106–5). Because a membrane protein bound to the surface of a rigid crystal is probably immobile, such clustering events probably occur at the junction between crystal-contacted and noncontacted plasma membrane, where freely diffusing membrane proteins could enter and be immobilized by binding to the crystal. Clustering could also be modulated by crystal-bound proteins; e.g., exposed Fc of IgG, or steric hindrance because of large hydrophobic proteins bound to the crystal surface such as apolipoprotein B (discussed below).

Phagocytosis of urate crystals by neutrophils is followed by rapid dissolution of the phagolysosomal membrane.[130–132] Internal release of lysosomal contents follows, and is associated with, cellular swelling and death (the so-called suicide sac hypothesis) (Fig. 106–6). The protein-coated crystals are probably stripped of surface proteins by enzymatic digestion

FIG. 106–5. Hypothetical mechanism of initial stimulation of inflammatory cells (e.g., human platelet) by urate crystals via clustering of plasma membrane urate crystal-binding glycoproteins. *A*, Platelet-membrane GPIIb/IIIa is initially homogeneously distributed in the membrane. GPIIb/IIIa, in close proximity to the rigid crystal surface, binds to it thereby immobilizing the glycoprotein in the plane of the membrane. *B*, Continued lateral diffusion of the unbound GPIIb/IIIa brings it to the junction zone where it becomes immobilized by binding to the crystal surface.

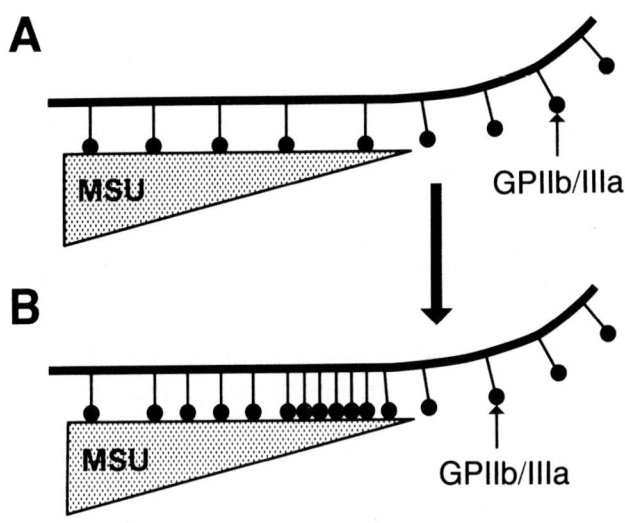

within phagolysosomes. Because the protein coat of urate crystals inhibits membrane injury, its removal would allow phagolysosome membrane lysis to proceed. Cell death following phagocytosis of other membranolytic crystals (silicon dioxide) appears to depend on an influx of extracellular calcium into the damaged cell and may not require phagolysosomal lysis under certain conditions.[133]

INITIATION, PROPAGATION, AND TERMINATION OF ACUTE GOUT

MSU crystals liberated from synovial microtophi or precipitated de novo are believed to activate these humoral and cellular mediator cascades in vivo (Fig. 106–4). Thus, early vasodilation, enhanced vascular permeability, and pain in gouty arthritis are likely mediated by vasoactive prostaglandins, kinins (which also potentiate prostaglandin synthesis via release of membrane arachidonate), complement peptides, and histamine. The role of prostaglandins as mediators of pain in gout is underlined by the strikingly complete suppression of tenderness (out of proportion to its effects on swelling, local heat, and volume of local effusion) in synovitis induced by MSU crystals in normal human volunteers pretreated with aspirin.[139] Evidence that prostaglandins and other arachidonic acid metabolites modify MSU crystal-induced inflammation also includes the finding that dietary enrichment with PGE_1 (known to inhibit certain neutrophil responses), fish oil or primrose oil (which provide alternative substrates to arachidonate for oxidative metabolism) are associated with suppression of inflammation in rats after injection of MSU crystals into subcutaneous air pouches.[135]

Pain signals may theoretically mediate inflammation in acute gout via the release from nociceptive afferent sensory nerve fibers of the undecapeptide neurotransmitter, *substance P.* Substance P is found in high concentrations in distal endings of sensory nerves in joints and has been shown to modulate the severity of adjuvant-induced arthritis in rats.[136] Its proinflammatory functions[137] include (1) potent vasodilatation and increased capillary permeability, (2) stimulation of histamine release from mast cells, (3) chemotaxis of monocytes, and (4) stimulation of PGE_2 and collagenase release from synoviocytes (possibly related to partial sequence homology shared by sub-

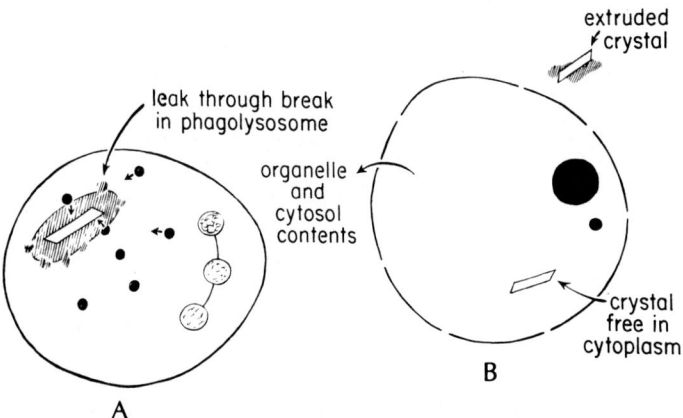

FIG. 106–6. *A*, Breaks occur in the phagosome and allow lysosomal materials to escape into the cytoplasm, producing autolysis and cell death. *B*, Monosodium urate crystal lies in the cytoplasm, and the cell membrane leaks potassium, lactic dehydrogenase, and other cytosol contents into the ambient medium. The crystal, now extracellular and with adherent parts of the dead cell, may again be phagocytosed by a fresh leukocyte.

stance P and interleukin-1).[138] Substance P increased foot pad swelling in rats injected with MSU crystals.[139]

Although neutrophils appear to be the usual effector arm of acute gouty inflammation, other cells and humoral mediators likely trigger neutrophil ingress into joints. Neutrophils are virtually absent in normal joint fluid. Neutrophil infiltration followed both the elevation in intra-articular pressure and crystal phagocytosis by synoviocytes in experimental MSU crystal-induced synovitis in canine joints.[111,140] The release of neutrophil-derived mediators (e.g., CCF, LTB₄, lysosomal proteases) in response to contact with intra-articular crystals and fluid-phase mediators (e.g., LTB₄, C5ₐ, kallikrein, IL-1) is believed to establish a cycle of further neutrophil ingress, neutrophil activation, and amplification of inflammation.

The mechanism whereby gouty attacks terminate (often without specific therapy) is likely multifactorial. Crystal sequestration may be a direct consequence of removal by phagocytic cells. Urate catabolism by myeloperoxidase[141] is too slow to effect any meaningful crystal removal. Furthermore, MSU crystal solubility could be modulated by increased local temperature because of tissue hyperemia; however, factors other than MSU crystal dissolution or catabolism must play a role in terminating attacks, as free MSU crystals are often found in synovial fluid for many weeks after subsidence of an acute gouty paroxysm. Clearly, anti-inflammatory pathways may balance the effects of released mediators. Such pathways might include inactivation of mediators (e.g., cleavage of bradykinin, C3a, and C5a by carboxypeptidases); ω-oxidation of LTB₄; tachyphylaxis to chemotaxins and IL-1 (which promotes both down-regulation of neutrophil extravasation in inflammatory lesions in vivo and inhibition of neutrophil phagocytosis in vitro[106,116,142]); induction by IL-1 of ACTH release with subsequent adrenal steroidogenesis (resulting in suppression of both IL-1 production and IL-1-mediated tissue responses); a shift in arachidonic acid metabolism (e.g., enhanced prostacyclin synthesis).

Changes in the adsorbed proteins during the evolution of a gouty paroxysm could also modulate the crystals' inflammatory potential. For example, binding of neutrophil lysosomal enzymes to MSU crystals[143] that may displace IgG from the crystal surface[121] renders MSU crystals less able to stimulate neutrophils in vitro.[144] Other mechanisms whereby molecules adsorbed to MSU crystal surfaces might determine the crystal's inflammatory potential are discussed below.

REGULATION OF INFLAMMATORY POTENTIAL OF MSU

The lack of direct correlation between the amount of urate crystal deposition and the severity of acute gouty inflammatory reactions is well accepted.[28–31,145] For example, large quantities of crystals ("joint milk") may be aspirated from joints that show little or no sign of inflammation. In other patients, few crystals might be detected despite full-blown acute gouty arthritis. A striking absence of inflammation about subcutaneous deposits of urate crystals is the rule, and some patients with chronic tophaceous gout give no history of acute attacks.[146] A multitude of factors, including host responsiveness as well as variable crystal structure and protein adsorption by crystals, could account for such observations.

HOST FACTORS

Host factors that may mediate MSU crystal-induced inflammation include renal failure and rheumatoid arthritis (RA). Patients with chronic renal insufficiency have diminished inflammatory responses to the subcutaneous injection of MSU crystals,[147] and it has been suggested that gouty attacks are less severe and less frequent in such individuals.[42,148] The high incidence of gouty arthritis in association with lead nephropathy seems paradoxic.

The coexistence of RA and gout is much rarer than expected statistically,[149,150] perhaps reflecting many factors, including the hypouricemic and anti-inflammatory effects of many agents employed continuously in RA. In addition, IgM rheumatoid factor binds to IgG-coated MSU crystals and suppresses their ability to stimulate neutrophils in vitro.[150]

Polymeric hyaluronic acid inhibits both neutrophil chemotactic mobility and phagocytosis of MSU crystals in a dose-dependent manner[151] and may thus regulate crystal inflammation. A fall in hyaluronate concentration as a result of development of an effusion, for example following trauma, might dilute its inhibitory effect on crystal-cell interactions and render the crystals more inflammatory. Uric acid in solution suppresses protein adsorption by neutrophil plasma membranes and could result in increased crystal-induced membranolysis.[152] Crystal size may be another important variable. Smaller crystals are phagocytized more avidly by human neutrophils and provoke higher leukocyte counts and phagocytic indices when injected into animal joints;[153] however, no correlation exists between crystal size and structure and severity of MSU-induced inflammation.[154]

PROTEIN ADSORPTION BY MSU CRYSTALS

Much attention has focused on the possibility that molecules adsorbed to crystal surfaces could be the critical determinant of their inflammatory potential. Isolated human IgG bound with high affinity to MSU,[155] and the binding was oriented so that the Fc part of the adsorbed molecule was exposed and functionally available.[156] High-resolution two-dimensional gel electrophoresis of the proteins adsorbed to MSU crystals exposed to plasma identified more than 30 crystal-associated polypeptides.[77] As expected from current knowledge of the MSU crystal surface structure already discussed, both anionic and cationic proteins bind to urate crystals.[77] Proteins more abundant in the crystal pellet than in starting plasma in vitro included $C1_q$, fibronectin, fibrinogen, and kininogen (Fig. 106–4).[77] Apolipoprotein B was also well represented in the eluate of MSU crystals exposed to plasma.[157] In contrast, the relative concentrations of a number of polypeptides, abundant in starting plasma (including albumin and IgG), were not increased in the crystal pellet.[77]

Urate crystals are capable of stimulating inflammatory cells in the absence of serum or plasma;[87,101,102,121] however, the presence of adsorbed purified IgG to urate crystals resulted in enhanced crystal-induced platelet secretion, increased superoxide generation, and augmented lysosomal enzyme release from neutrophils.[101,121,158] Though coating of urate crystals with IgG alone enhanced cellular stimulation, adsorption of whole plasma or serum to the crystal surface markedly inhibited membranolysis,[118] platelet secretion,[159] and neutrophil oxidative and secretory responses to urate crystals.[101,157] Using selective protein depletion and reconstitution, apolipoprotein B–bearing lipoproteins (LDL, IDL, VLDL) were identified as the major inhibitory species in plasma for MSU crystal-induced stimulation of human neutrophils and platelets.[157] LDL inhibited cellular responses to MSU, and certain other particulates, by binding to the crystal surfaces, thereby physically inhibiting particle-cell interaction and phagocytosis.[159] Apolipoprotein B is both necessary and sufficient for this activity of LDL.[160] Apolipoprotein B is normally excluded from uninflamed joints on the basis of size (Chapter 11). Thus, ingress of lipoproteins into the joint space during urate crystal-induced synovitis is a potential factor contributing to termination of acute gout.

Apolipoprotein B can be detected on urate crystals obtained from tophi.[127] Further clinical and animal studies are required to clarify the role, if any, of apolipoprotein B in the regulation of gouty arthritis. Thus far, LDL-coated MSU crystals have appeared to be as inflammatory as naked crystals when injected into rat tissues.[161,162] Certain glycosaminoglycans (GAGs) including hyaluronate, heparan sulfate, and heparin

not only block LDL-MSU crystal binding but also can elute bound LDL from crystals.[103] These effects are reduced by digestion of GAGs. The effects of GAGs on LDL binding to MSU may help explain not only the negative results using LDL-coated crystals in animal studies but also why acute gouty inflammation may proceed even when substantial intrasynovial concentrations of LDL are reached.

THE GOUT PARADIGM AND INFLAMMATION CAUSED BY OTHER CRYSTALS

The range in intensity of acute synovitis associated with intra-articular crystals other than MSU is broad. Similarly, the pathogenesis of inflammation induced by other microcrystals appears complex. For example, acute pseudogout is associated with neutrophil leukocytosis in synovial fluid and with intracellular crystals. CPPD crystals activate complement[81] and trigger release of CCF from neutrophils[106] but are relatively poor inducers of IL-1 release from macrophages.[115]

Negativity of crystal surface charge and surface irregularity appear to be important determinants of the inflammatory potential of crystals, that is, the crystal surfaces of more inflammatory membranolytic crystals (MSU, CPPD, the α-quartz form of silicon dioxide) are irregular and possess a high density of charged groups, whereas the surfaces of nonhemolytic noninflammatory crystals (e.g., diamond dust and the stishovite and anatase forms of silicon dioxide) are smooth.[122] Brushite and hydroxyapatite crystals present a lesser partial negatively charged surface atomic array than the more membranolytic CPPD crystals,[122] which may explain why these crystals are less frequently associated with acute inflammation.

BCP crystals have a remarkable tendency to form aggregates, the larger of which ("too big to swallow") may escape endocytosis. However, hydroxyapatite and other basic calcium phosphates stimulate leukocytes in vitro,[70] are phlogistic when injected into animals,[8] and are sometimes associated with severe acute articular and periarticular inflammation in humans.[8,70–72] They are also associated with widespread articular inflammation in ank/ank mice.[164,165] Thus, other factors that account for the remarkable lack of acute articular inflammation and leukocytosis generally associated with the presence of intra-articular BCP crystals in humans (Chapter 108) require an explanation. The low complement-activating potential, relative to MSU, of BCP crystals[81] and the diminished ability of BCP to stimulate human monocyte/macrophage IL-1 release in vitro[115] may partly explain this apparent impotency. Adsorbed molecules may mediate the inflammatory potential of BCP crystals as already demonstrated for MSU. α 2-HS glycoprotein, a serum protein produced by the liver that localizes to mineralizing bone, has been identified as a major specific inhibitor of neutrophil responses to basic calcium phosphate crystals in vitro.[166]

EXPERIMENTAL MODELS

Animal models of crystal-induced inflammation have used dog,[98,153,167] bird,[95] and rabbit joints;[86,107] rat paws;[126] and rat pleural spaces[8] (these are reviewed in detail in reference 168). More recently, a rodent subcutaneous air pouch, lined by cells histologically similar to synoviocytes, created by repeated injection of sterile air has been used.[162,169–172] However, such artificial "joints" do not contain hyaluronate-rich fluid. In addition, it has not been established that MSU crystal-induced inflammation in this tissue space is neutrophil dependent. Indomethacin treatment failed to suppress MSU crystal-induced neutrophil influx in this model system.[171]

A novel, natural animal model of crystal-induced inflammation is the progressive ankylosis disorder of ank/ank mice, characterized by the presence of basic calcium phosphate crystals in joint fluids, chronic inflammation, and joint fusion.[164,165]

Experimental crystal-induced inflammation has been successfully used for testing for drug effectiveness in humans,[134,174] and the effectiveness of pretreatment with colchicine, phenylbutazone, aspirin, or corticosteroids has been proven consistently.[160] The intradermal injection of MSU crystals in humans reproducibly provoked a transient, self-limiting local response with a systemic response detected by leukocytosis and a rise in serum amyloid A protein, the level of which peaks while the intradermal lesion is resolving.[174]

Although model systems of crystal-induced inflammation have been useful in the dissection of some critical features of the host response to crystals, the precise mode of action of drugs effective in the treatment of acute crystal synovitis in everyday clinical practice is still not known. The model systems in man and in animals have been used for this purpose only in a preliminary way. Even if further experimental work is done on the mechanism of action of anti-inflammatory drugs, the experimental models using synthetic crystals remain, at best, mere analogues of their natural counterparts.

TREATMENT OF CRYSTAL-INDUCED INFLAMMATION

The aims of therapy in gout are to alleviate pain, which is often excruciating, and to restore the inflamed joint to useful function. After protection of the joint by splinting and after administration of analgesics, a choice of effective drugs is at hand. The rationale for use of individual drugs is discussed below. Thorough aspiration of the joint, often possible at the time of diagnostic arthrocentesis to obtain fluid for crystal identification, may also be followed by local injection of microcrystalline adrenocorticosteroid esters. Such therapy is ideal in a single large joint; inflammation subsides predictably within 12 hours of treatment regardless of the prior duration of the acute attack.

COLCHICINE

This ancient drug is provided in 0.5 or 0.6 mg tablets or in vials (Lilly) containing 1 mg colchicine.

Although largely eclipsed by nonsteroidal anti-inflammatory drugs (NSAIDs) colchicine remains a useful primary therapeutic agent, especially when small joints are involved or with polyarticular inflammation. Importantly, colchicine can also be used in low doses (0.5 to 0.6 mg bid) as an adjunct to NSAIDs for therapy of severe attacks or for prophylaxis. As a primary treatment for acute gout, colchicine is most effective when administered in the first 24 hours after onset. The drug can be given orally, 0.5 mg every hour until relief or side effects occur. About 10 tablets are generally required.* Diarrhea is almost always produced; associated electrolyte imbalances in the elderly may be severe. Signs and symptoms of inflammation subside in 12 to 24 hours and pain is gone in over 90% of patients in 24 to 48 hours.[175]

Colchicine often cannot be given orally in persons with postoperative acute gout. The intravenous route must be used in these instances; 1 mg, diluted in 20 ml of normal saline, given as a single dose is adequate for most attacks. A total intravenous dose of greater than 2 mg and repeated intravenous administration time beyond 24 hours for one attack of gout are inadvisable.[176a]

The use of intravenous colchicine under any circumstances has been questioned.[176b] Two deaths occurring in a 4-year period in a teaching hospital were

---

*Editor's note. I know of one patient (unpublished data) who died of colchicine intoxication after receiving only 6 mg orally. I doubt whether any patient should be treated for any acute crystal problem with oral colchicine.

thought to represent 2% of patients treated with intravenous colchicine. One patient has renal insufficiency and the other was 91 years old; each had received the drug both orally and intravenously. *It is clear that this potent drug has been used in a cavalier fashion by many physicians in the mistaken belief that it is nearly completely safe.* In our experience, intravenous colchicine is relatively safe if certain guidelines are followed (Table 106–2).

Care is necessary to avoid extravasation because of the irritating properties of the drug. Gastrointestinal effects are prevented completely, and the anti-inflammatory effects are more rapid, becoming noticeable in 6 to 8 hours and affording complete relief in 24 hours. Particular caution is necessary as *potentially fatal marrow suppression or neuromyopathy may occur even with low doses of intravenous colchicine in patients with renal insufficiency.*[177]

Elderly patients, those individuals with significant renal, hepatic, and cardiac dysfunction, persons with hematologic malignant disease receiving chemotherapy, and those with severe infection have an elevated risk of colchicine toxicity. Contraindications are listed in Table 106–3. The effectiveness of colchicine in acute pseudogout is discussed below.

Prophylactic Use. Acute gouty attacks are effectively prevented by small daily doses of colchicine. Doses of 0.5 to 1.8 mg daily are given; the average patient requires about 1 mg. Such doses either completely prevented attacks or greatly reduced their frequency in 93% of a large series of gouty patients during many years of followup.[178] Only 4% had gastrointestinal tox-

Table 106–2. Suggested Guidelines for Colchicine Therapy*

Intravenous*
  One (1) mg diluted to 20 ml with 0.9% NaCl and administered slowly over not less than 10 minutes. (Do *not* use 5% glucose in water.) This dose may be repeated once within 24 hours in patients with good urinary output and *creatinine* clearance $\left(\dfrac{1}{\text{serum creatinine}} \times 100\right)$ >50 ml/min and who have not been taking the drug orally on a continuous daily regimen.
  Baseline peripheral blood total and differential leukocyte and platelet counts should be obtained.

Oral
  One to 3 tablets* (0.5 to 1.8 mg) may be given daily, beginning 24 hours after the last intravenous dose has been given.
  Peripheral blood total and differential leukocyte and platelet counts should be obtained 4 to 6 days after the last intravenous dose; stop therapy if significant leukopenia and/or thrombocytopenia has developed and monitor abnormality with serial counts obtained every 2 to 3 days.

*Colchicine is supplied in 0.432, 0.5, and 0.6 mg tablets and in 2 ml brown glass ampules containing 1 mg. Do not use if solution is cloudy. Roberts et al.[176b] recommend that the intravenous preparation be monitored by the hospital pharmacy.

Table 106–3. Contraindications to Use of Intravenous Colchicine

Absolute
- Pre-existing depressed bone marrow function
- Creatinine clearance <10 ml/min
- Anuria or severe oliguria
- Liver disease with bilirubin and/or alkaline phosphatase greater than twice the upper range of normal
- Severe sepsis with bacteremia

Relative
- Immediate prior use of oral colchicine, either therapeutically or in daily prophylactic doses
- Presence of borderline hepatic or renal function, localized infection
- Advanced age

Table 106–4. Toxic Manifestations of Colchicine

Intravenous
- Bone marrow depression producing peripheral thrombocytopenia and neutropenia—nadir of values about 3 to 6 days after drug is given; recovery in absence of additional drug in 4 to 6 days
- Cellulitis or thrombophlebitis at injection site
- Alopecia
- Gastrointestinal—abdominal pain, nausea, vomiting, diarrhea (rare)
- Peripheral neuritis
- Myopathy—weakness and elevated serum creatine kinase
- Shock—delayed, and associated with oliguria, hematuria, weakness, paralysis, delirium, convulsions, and (often) death

Oral
- Gastrointestinal—cramps, diarrhea (most common)
- Neuropathy ⎫
- Myopathy ⎬ uncommon
- Alopecia ⎭
- Bone marrow depression ⎫
- Shock ⎬ rare

icity, and many of these patients had underlying intestinal disease. Renal failure or concomitant cytotoxic drug treatment may predispose to more serious toxicity, including myopathy and neuropathy.[179,179a] Acute and chronic toxic manifestations of colchicine therapy are listed in Table 106–4. The mechanism of prophylaxis may be different from the effects of colchicine in primary treatment, as discussed already in connection with the elevated serum uronic acid levels in gouty arthritis.

Acute attacks may be heralded by "twinges" in the target joint. If attacks are relatively infrequent (<3/year), the patient not on daily prophylactic doses can often abort an attack by taking 1 mg of colchicine at the first symptom and 0.5 mg every 2 hours thereafter.

Diagnostic Use. The history of the diagnostic use of therapeutic trials is one of abandonment as better tests are developed. The colchicine therapeutic trial is no exception. Wallace and colleagues treated 58 patients with acute gout and 62 patients with other types of arthritis using rigidly defined criteria for clinical response;[180] 44 of 58 (75%) gouty patients and 3 of 62 (5%) control subjects showed major improvement. Colchicine had a weak general anti-inflammatory action in suppressing inflammation in rodent skin induced by staphylococcal toxin, and so it is not surprising that false positive trials occur. Patients with sarcoid arthritis, calcific tendinitis (apatite),[72] and pseudogout[181,182] sometimes show dramatic response to colchicine treatment.

Metabolism. A radioimmunoassay with a sensitivity of 0.05 ng colchicine showed measurable plasma levels in 5 of 7 patients given a single 2-mg dose intravenously 24 hours earlier.[183] Mean plasma half-life was 58 ± 20 minutes; zero time plasma concentration was 2.9 ± 1.5 μg/dl. Although maximal urinary excretion occurred 2 hours after drug administration, colchicine was found in the urine up to 10 days later. No breakdown products were noted despite published in vitro evidence of microsomal degradation.[184]

Colchicine has been measured in human serum, urine, and peripheral blood neutrophils after the intravenous administration of usual therapeutic doses.[185,186] The highest plasma concentration (zero time extrapolation of decay curve) was 7×10^{-7} M. Drug concentration in peripheral blood leukocytes was much greater, ranging from 1 to 2×10^{-5} M; at 72 hours, leukocyte colchicine levels approximated 5×10^{-6} M, and detectable drug levels were still found in cells isolated from the blood 10 days later. The increased concentration in leukocytes is probably related to their content of labile microtubules (tubulin), each dimer subunit of which specifically binds one molecule of colchicine.[187] Absorption after a single oral dose of 1 mg was variable; peak concentrations an order of magnitude lower than when the drug was given intravenously (0.3 ± 0.17 μg/dl) were reached in 0.5 to 2 hours. Interestingly, vinblastine also binds to tubulin dimers, produces metaphase arrest, and is effective in the treatment of gouty arthritis.

Mechanism of Action. Parameters of neutrophilic function suppressed by colchicine include random motility, adherence, chemotaxis, chemotactic factor (CCF and leukotriene B_4) release,[104,106] lysosomal discharge, and perhaps, lysosomal fusion with phagosomes.[188,189]

Two schools of thought on the mode of action of this drug exist. Malawista favors the concept that the anti-inflammatory and antimitotic effects of colchicine share a common mechanism.[190] The stabilization of labile microtubules normally needed for leukocyte motility may decrease chemotaxis, inhibit phagocytosis, lessen adhesiveness, and suppress leukocyte chemotactic factor release. Inhibition of the mitotic

spindle, which is largely tubulin, arrests mitosis in metaphase.

Wallace has pointed out certain paradoxes not explicable by this unitary theory.[175] Trimethylcolchicinic acid (TMCA), an experimental analogue of colchicine not now available, is as effective in treating acute gout as is colchicine itself, although it has no effect on microtubules and is not metabolized to colchicine in humans.[191] Comparison of the ability of various colchicine analogues to suppress polymorphonuclear leukocytic motility in vitro showed the same order of effectiveness as their clinical potency in treating gout.[191] On the other hand, lumicolchicine, which does not block mitosis, is also ineffective in the treatment of gout.[192] Colchicine binds to other proteins in living cells besides microtubules, especially membrane proteins, which might be tubulin-like attachment points for microtubules.[193] Moreover, colchicine is effective in preventing attacks of familial Mediterranean fever, but not in their treatment.[194]

On the cellular level, colchicine probably acts by inhibiting leukocyte-derived chemotactic factors because potent effects were seen in vitro with concentrations as low as 10^{-9} M.[195] Detectable effects on phagocytosis and lysosomal enzyme release in vitro in the same experiments required much larger levels of the drug.[195,196] Treatment of patients with acute gout with colchicine, 1.8 mg/day (3 tablets) orally for 1 week, was associated with partial, but significant, suppression of yeast phagocytosis by leukocytes ex vivo relative to both the baseline indices in patients and leukocytes from normal control subjects.[189]

NONSTEROIDAL ANTI-INFLAMMATORY AGENTS

Phenylbutazone, which is as effective orally as colchicine is intravenously, has long been employed for acute gout; 400 to 600 mg are given in divided doses. About 600 mg are given in the first 24 hours, followed by 100 mg, 3 to 4 times daily, for about a week. Nearly all attacks of acute gout can be controlled with this agent. Because fluid retention, hypertension, gastritis, and marrow toxicity are common, this drug has fallen into disuse. Indomethacin, 200 to 400 mg in the first 24 hours and 100 mg daily in divided doses over the next 4 to 5 days, is as effective as phenylbutazone. Like phenylbutazone, it interferes with CPPD crystal or starch granule phagocytosis; release of CCF is inhibited indirectly.[197] Naproxen, 750 mg as a single dose followed by smaller maintenance doses (250 mg tid), is also as effective as phenylbutazone in acute gout.[198] Other NSAIDs also provide effective therapy for acute gout.[200,201]

Patients receiving the large doses of NSAIDs needed to control acute gout are often dehydrated, elderly, or debilitated. The induction of hyporeninemic hypoaldesteronism with life-threatening hyperkalemia is a significant risk in such patients because their renal perfusion depends on vasodilatory prostaglandins. This risk probably exceeds that of intravenous colchicine.

Azopropazone, an NSAID related to phenylbutazone and possessing similar uricosuric effects at a dose of 0.6 to 1.2 g/24 hours, has successfully controlled acute gout, recurrent gout, and hyperuricemia in preliminary trials in Europe.[200,201] The frequency of renal and gastrointestinal side effects necessitates further evaluation of this drug for long-term use.[201,202a]

Adrenocorticotropic hormone and corticosteroids may be effective in severe cases of acute polyarticular gout, when administration of other agents is contraindicated. Corticosteroid administration may reduce pain, but inflammation can continue at a subdued level.

PSEUDOGOUT

Supportive measures are useful, as outlined previously. Thorough aspiration of a large joint often effectively controls acute inflammation even without local corticosteroid injection, presumably because of removal of sufficient crystals to control what is a dose-related response. Concomitant use of local corticosteroid ester crystals is virtually 100% effective in control of acute pseudogout in a single large joint, although a postinjection flare secondary to this use has been implicated as precipitating acute pseudogout.[202b] This effect may be due to the enzymatic "strip-mining" mechanism already discussed.

NSAIDs are effective in doses previously outlined for the treatment of acute gout. Colchicine effectiveness is less predictable when the drug is given orally, perhaps because of its less consistent suppressive effect on the release of the cell-derived chemotactic factor shown in vitro.[196] Intravenous colchicine (1 mg) more predictably controls acute pseudogout,[182] probably because it produces much higher blood levels, as outlined previously. The frequence of acute attacks of pseudogout can be diminished by the use of small daily prophylactic doses of colchicine as utilized for gout.[203,204]

REFERENCES

1. McCarty, D.J., and Hollander, J.L.: Identification of urate crystals in gouty synovial fluid. Ann. Intern. Med., 4:452–460, 1961.
2. Faires, J.S., and McCarty, D.J.: Acute arthritis in man and dog after intrasynovial injection of sodium urate crystals. Lancet, 2:682–685, 1962.
3. Seegmiller, J.E., Howell, R.R., and Malawista, S.E.: The inflammatory reaction to sodium urate. JAMA, 180:469–476, 1962.
4. McCarty, D.J., and Hogan, J.M.: Inflammatory reaction after intrasynovial injection of microcrystalline adrenocorticosteroid esters. Arthritis Rheum., (7)4:259–267, 1964.
5. Gaucher, A., et al.: Identification des cristaux observes dan les arthropathies destructrices de la chondrocalcinose. Rev. Rheum. Mal. Osteoartic., 44:407–414, 1977.
6. McCarty, D.J., et al.: Studies on pathological calcifications in human cartilage. I. Prevalence and types of crystal deposits in the menisci of two hundred and fifteen cadavera. J. Bone Joint Surg., 48:309–325, 1966.
7. Utsinger, P.D.: Abstract 448. In Proceedings of the Fourteenth International Congress of Rheumatology. San Francisco, 1977.
8. Dieppe, P.A., et al.: Apatite deposition disease. Lancet, 1:266–270, 1976.
9. Stepan, J., Petrova, S., and Pozderka, V.: Cystinosis with crystal-induced synovitis and arthropathy. Z. Rheumatol., 35:347–355, 1976.
10. Gibson, I.K., Burns, R.P., and Wolfe-Lande, J.D.: Crystals in corneal epithelial lesions of tyrosine fed rats. Invest. Ophthalmol., 14:937–941, 1975.
11. Goldsmith, L.A.: Hemolysis and lysosomal activation by solid state tyrosine. Biochem. Biophys. Res. Commun., 64:558–565, 1975.
12. Dougados, M., et al.: Charcot-Leyden crystals in synovial fluid. Arthritis Rheum., 26:1416, 1983.
13. Ettlinger, R.E., and Hunder, G.C.: Synovial effusions containing cholesterol crystals. Mayo Clin. Proc., 54:366–374, 1979.
14. Fam, A.G., et al.: Cholesterol crystals in osteoarthritic joint effusions. J. Rheumatol., 8:273–280, 1981.
15. Valente, A.J., and Walton, K.W.: Studies on increased vascular permeability in the pathogenesis of lesions of connective tissue diseases: 1. Experimental hyperlipidemia and immune arthropathy. Ann. Rheum. Dis., 37:490–499, 1978.
16. Hasselbacher, P.: Activation of the alternative pathway of complement by microcrystalline cholesterol. Atherosclerosis, 37:239–245, 1980.
17. Doherty, M., Whicher, J.T., and Dieppe, P.A.: Activation of the alternative pathway of complement by monosodium urate monohydrate crystals and other inflammatory particles. Ann. Rheum. Dis., 42:285–291, 1983.
18. Pritzker, K.P.H., et al.: Experimental crystal arthropathy. J. Rheumatol., 8:281–290, 1981.
19. Ludwig, P.W., Hunninghake, D.B., and Hoidal, J.R.: Increased leucocyte oxidative metabolism in hyperlipoproteinemia. Lancet, 1:348–350, 1982.
20. Reginato, A.J., Schumacher, H.R., Allan, D.A., and Rabinowitz, J.L.: Acute monoarthritis associated with lipid liquid crystals. Ann. Rheum. Dis., 44:537–543, 1985.
21. Trostle, D.C., Schumacher, H.R., Medsger, T.A., Jr., and Kapoor, W.N.: Lipid microspherule-associated acute monoarticular arthritis. Arthritis Rheum., 29:1166–1169, 1986.
22. Choi, S.J., Schumacher, H.R., Jr., and Clayburne, G.: Exper-

imental haemarthrosis produces mild inflammation associated with intracellular Maltese crosses. Ann. Rheum. Dis., 45:1025–1028, 1986.

23. Hoffman, G.S., et al.: Calcium oxalate microcrystalline-associated arthritis in end-stage renal disease. Ann. Intern. Med., 97:36–42, 1982.

24. Reginato, A.J., et al.: Arthropathy and cutaneous calcinosis in hemodialysis oxalosis. Arthritis Rheum., 29:1387–1396, 1986.

25. Maclachlan, M.J., and Rodnan, G.P.: Effects of food, fast and alcohol on serum uric acid and acute attacks of gout. Am. J. Med., 42:38–57, 1967.

26. Rodnan, G.P.: The pathogenesis of aldermanic gout: Procatartic role of fluctuation in serum urate cocentrations in gouty arthritis provoked by feast and alcohol. Arthritis Rheum., 23:737, 1980.

27. Schumacher, H.R.: Pathogenesis of crystal-induced synovitis. Clin. Rheum. Dis., 3:105–131, 1977.

28. Weinberger, A., Schumacher, H.R., and Agudelo, C.A.: Urate crystals in asymptomatic metatarsophalangeal joints. Ann. Intern. Med., 56:56–57, 1979.

29. Gordon, T.P., Bertouch, J.V., Walsh, B.R., and Brooks, P.M.: Monosodium urate crystals in asymptomatic knee joints. J. Rheumatol., 9:967–969, 1982.

30. Bomalaski, J.A., Lluberas, G., and Schumacher, H.R., Jr.: Monosodium urate crystals in the knee joints of patients with asymptomatic nontophaceous gout. Arthritis Rheum., 39:1480–1484, 1986.

31. Roualt, T., Caldwell, D.S., and Holmes, D.W.: Aspiration of the asymptomatic metatarsophalangeal joint in gout patients and hyperuricemic controls. Arthritis Rheum., 25:209–212, 1982.

32. Simkin, P.A.: The pathogenesis of podagra. Ann. Intern. Med., 86:230–233, 1977.

33. Loeb, J.N.: The influence of temperature on the solubility of monosodium urate. Arthritis Rheum., 15:189–192, 1972.

34. Kippen, I., et al.: Factors affecting urate solubility in vitro. Ann. Rheum. Dis., 33:313–317, 1974.

35. Wilcox, W.R., and Khalaf, A.A.: Nucleation of monosodium urate crystals. Ann. Rheum. Dis., 34:332–339, 1975.

36. Katz, W.A.: Deposition of urate crystals in gout. Arthritis Rheum., 18:751–756, 1975.

37. Katz, W.A.: Abstract 137. *In* Proceedings of the Fourteenth International Rheumatology Congress. Edited by International League Against Rheumatism. San Francisco, 1977.

38. Katz, W.A., and Schubert, M.: The interaction of monosodium urate with connective tissue components. J. Clin. Invest., 49:783–789, 1970.

38a. Simkin, P.A., Campbell, P.M., and Larson, E.B.: Gout in Heberden's nodes. Arthritis Rheum., 26:94–97, 1983.

39. Glynn, J.J., and Clayton, M.L.: Sparing effect of hemiplegia on tophaceous gout. Ann. Rheum. Dis., 35:534–535, 1976.

40. Perricone, E., and Brandt, K.: Enhancement of urate solubility by connective tissue. Arthritis Rheum., 21:453–460, 1978.

41. Emmerson, B.T., Stride, P.J., and Williams, G.: The clinical differentiation of primary gout from primary renal disease in patients with both gout and renal disease. Adv. Exp. Med. Biol., 122A:9–13, 1980.

42. Sorensen, J.B.: Gout secondary to chronic renal disease: Studies on urate metabolism. Ann. Rheum. Dis., 39:424–430, 1980.

43. Aakesson, I., and Alvsaker, J.O.: The urate-binding alpha$_{1-2}$ globulin. Isolation and characterization of the protein from human plasma. Eur. J. Clin. Invest., 1:281–287, 1971.

44. Alvsaker, J.O.: Genetic studies in primary gout: Investigations on the plasma levels of the urate-binding α_1-α_2-globulin in individuals from two gouty kindred. J. Clin. Invest., 47:1254–1261, 1968.

44a. Burt, H.M., and Dutt, Y.C.: Growth of monosodium urate monohydrate crystals: Effect of cartilage and synovial fluid components on in vitro growth rates. Ann. Rheum. Dis., 45:858–864, 1986.

45. Hardwell, T.R., Manley, G., Braven, J., and Whitaker, M.: The binding of urate to plasma proteins determined by four different techniques. Clin. Chim. Acta, 133:75–83, 1983.

46. Lam-Erwin, C.Y., Nancollas, G.H., and Ko, S.J.: The kinetics of formation and dissolution of uric acid crystals. Invest. Urol., 15:473–481, 1978.

47. Lam-Erwin, C.Y., and Nancollas, G.H.: The crystallization and dissolution of sodium urate. J. Crystal Growth, 53:214–223, 1981.

48. Klinenberg, J.R., et al.: Urate deposition disease. Ann. Intern. Med., 78:99–111, 1973.

49. Spilberg, I., Tanphaichitr, K., and Kantor, P.: Synovial fluid pH in acute gouty arthritis. Arthritis Rheum., 20:142, 1977.

50. Tak, H.K., and Wilcox, W.R.: Crystallization of monosodium urate and calcium urate at 37° C. J. Coll. Int. Sci., 77:195–201, 1980.

51. Tak, H.K., Cooper, S.M., and Wilcox, W.R.: Studies on the nucleation of monosodium urate at 37° C. Arthritis Rheum., 23:574–580, 1980.

52. Tak, H.K., Wilcox, W.R., and Cooper, S.M.: The effect of lead upon urate nucleation. Arthritis Rheum., 24:1291–1295, 1981.

53. Gerster, J.C., Lagier, R., and Boivin, G.: Olecranon bursitis related to calcium pyrophosphate dihydrate crystal deposition disease: Clinical and pathologic study. Arthritis Rheum., 25:989–996, 1982.

54. Bjelle, A.: Morphological study of articular cartilage of pyrophosphate arthropathy. Ann. Rheum. Dis., 31:449–456, 1972.

55. Reginato, A.S., Schumacher, H.R., and Martinez, V.A.: The articular cartilage in familial chondrocalcinosis: Light and electron microscopic study. Arthritis Rheum., 17:977–992, 1974.

56. Schumacher, H.R.: Ultrastructural findings in chondrocalcinosis and pseudogout. Arthritis Rheum., 19:413–425, 1976.

57. Bennett, R.M., Lehr, J.R., and McCarty, D.J.: Crystal shedding and acute pseudogout: an hypothesis based on a therapeutic failure. Arthritis Rheum., 19:93–97, 1976.

58. Bennett, R.M., Lehr, J.R., and McCarty, D.J.: Factors affecting the solubility of calcium pyrophosphate dihydrate crystals. J. Clin. Invest., 56:571–579, 1975.

59. Bilezikan, J.P., et al.: Pseudogout after parathyroidectomy. Lancet, 1:445–446, 1973.

60. O'Duffy, J.D.: Clinical studies of acute pseudogout attacks: Common on prevalence, predisposition and treatment. Arthritis Rheum., 19:349–352, 1976.

61. McCarty, D.: Crystals, joints and consternation. Ann. Rheum. Dis., 42:243–253, 1983.

62. Coswell, A., et al.: Pathogenesis of chondrocalcinosis and pseudogout. Metabolism of inorganic pyrophosphate and production of calcium pyrophosphate dihydrate crystals. Ann. Rheum. Dis., 42 (Suppl.):27–37, 1983.

63. Silcox, D.C., and McCarty, D.J.: Elevated inorganic pyrophosphate concentrations in synovial fluid in osteoarthritis and pseudogout. J. Lab. Clin. Med., 83:518–531, 1974.

64. Camerlain, M., et al.: Inorganic pyrophosphate pool size and turnover rate in arthritic joints. J. Clin. Invest., 55:373–381, 1975.

65. Bennett, R.M., Mall, J.C., and McCarty, D.J.: Pseudogout in

acute neuropathic arthropathy. A clue to pathogenesis? Ann. Rheum. Dis., 33:563–567, 1974.

66. Smith, R.J., and Phelps, P.: Septic arthritis, gout, pseudogout and osteoarthritis in the knee of a patient with multiple myeloma. Arthritis Rheum., 15:89–96, 1972.

67. Halverson, P.B., Cheung, H.S., and McCarty, D.J.: Enzymatic release of microspheroids containing hydroxyapatite crystals from synovium and of calcium pyrophosphate dihydrate crystals from cartilage. Ann. Rheum. Dis., 41:527–531, 1982.

68. Dorwart, B.B., and Schumacher, H.R.: Joint effusion chondrocalcinosis and other rheumatic manifestations in hypothyroidism. Am. J. Med., 59:780–789, 1975.

69. McCarty, D.J., Lehr, J.R., and Halverson, P.B.: Crystal population in human synovial fluid: Identification of apatite, octacalcium phosphate and beta tricalcium phosphate. Arthritis Rheum., 16:1220–1224, 1983.

70. Schumacher, H.R., et al.: Arthritis associated with apatite crystals. Ann. Intern. Med., 87:411–416, 1977.

71. McCarty, D.J., and Gatter, R.A: Recurrent acute inflammation associated with focal apatite crystal deposition. Arthritis Rheum., 9:804–819, 1966.

72. Thompson, G.R., et al.: Calcific tendinitis and soft tissue calcification resembling gout. JAMA, 203:464–472, 1968.

73. McCarty, D.J.: Treatment of rheumatoid joint inflammation with triamcinolone hexacetonide. Arthritis Rheum., 15:157–173, 1972.

74. Kahn, C.B., Hollander, J.L., and Schumacher, H.R.: Corticosteroid crystals in synovial fluid. JAMA, 211:807–809, 1970.

75. Naff, G.B., and Byers, P.H.: Complement as a mediator of inflammation in gouty arthritis. 1. Studies on the reaction between human serum complement and sodium urate crystals. J. Lab. Clin. Med., 81:747–760, 1973.

76. Giclas, P.C., Ginsberg, M.H., and Cooper, N.R.: Immunoglobulin G independent activation of the classical complement pathway by monosodium urate crystals. J. Clin. Invest., 63:759–765, 1979.

77. Terkeltaub, R., Tenner, A.J., Kozin, F., and Ginsberg, M.H.: Plasma protein binding by monosodium urate crystals. Analysis by two-dimensional gel electrophoresis. Arthritis Rheum., 26:775–783, 1983.

78. Hasselbacher, P.: Immunoelectrophoretic assay for synovial fluid C3 with correction for synovial fluid globulin. Arthritis Rheum., 22:243–250, 1979.

79. Russell, I.J., et al.: Effects of IgG and C-reactive protein on complement depletion by monosodium urate crystals. J. Rheumatol., 10:425–433, 1983.

80. Fields, T.R., et al.: Activation of the alternate pathway of complement by monosodium urate crystals. Clin. Immunol. Immunopathol., 26:249–257, 1983.

81. Hasselbacher, P.: C3 activation by monosodium urate monohydrate and other crystalline material. Arthritis Rheum., 22:571–578, 1979.

82. Russell, I.J., Mansen, C., Kolb, L.M., and Kolb, W.P.: Activation of the fifth component of human complement (C5) induced by monosodium urate crystals: C5 convertase assembly on the crystal surface. Clin. Immunol. Immunopathol., 24:239–250, 1982.

83. Hasselbacher, P.: C3 activation by monosodium urate monohydrate is enhanced by surface IgG. Arthritis Rheum., 11:620–625, 1979.

84. Kim, H.J., McCarty, D.J., Kozin, F., and Koethe, S.: Clinical significance of synovial fluid total hemolytic complement activity. J. Rheumatol., 7:143–152, 1980.

85. Moxley, G., and Ruddy, S.: Elevated C3 anaphylatoxin levels in synovial fluids from patients with rheumatoid synovitis. Arthritis Rheum., 28:1089–1095, 1985.

86. Spilberg, I., and Osterland, C.K.: Anti-inflammatory effect of the trypsin-kallikrein inhibitor in acute arthritis induced by urate crystals in rabbits. J. Lab. Clin. Med., 76:472–479, 1970.

87. Phelps, P., and McCarty, D.J.: Crystal-induced arthritis. Postgrad. Med., 45:87–93, 1969.

88. Webster, M.E., et al.: Urate crystal-induced inflammation in the rat: Evidence for the combined actions of kinins, histamine and components of complement. Immunol. Commun., 1:185–198, 1973.

89. Byers, P.H., et al.: Complement as a mediator of inflammation of acute gouty arthritis. II. Biological activities generated from complement and sodium urate crystals. J. Lab. Clin. Med., 81:761–769, 1973.

90. Ginsberg, M.H., Jaques, B., Cochrane, C.G., and Griffin, J.H.: Urate crystal-dependent cleavage of Hageman factor in human plasma and synovial fluid. J. Lab. Clin. Med., 95:497–506, 1980.

91. Kellermeyer, R.W., and Breckenridge, R.T.: The inflammatory process in acute gouty arthritis. II. The presence of Hageman factor and plasma thromboplastin antecedent in synovial fluid. J. Lab. Clin. Med., 67:455–460, 1966.

92. Melmon, K.L., Webster, M.E., Goldfinger, S.E., and Seegmiller, J.E.: The presence of a kinin in inflammatory synovial effusion from arthritides of varying etiologies. Arthritis Rheum., 10:13–20, 1967.

93. Green, D., Arsever, C.L., Grumet, K.A., and Ratnoff, O.D.: Classic gout in Hageman factor (factor XII) deficiency. Arch. Intern. Med., 142:1556–1557, 1982.

94. Londino, A.V., and Luparello, F.J.: Factor II deficiency in a man with gout and angioimmunoblastic lymphadenopathy. Arch. Intern. Med., 133:1497–1498, 1984.

95. Spilberg, I.: Urate crystal arthritis in animals lacking Hageman factor. Arthritis Rheum., 17:143–148, 1974.

96. McCarty, D.J.: Phagocytosis of urate crystals in gouty synovial fluid. Am. J. Med. Sci., 243:288–295, 1962.

97. Agudelo, C., and Schumacher, H.: The synovitis of acute gouty arthritis. A light and electron microscopic study. Hum. Pathol., 4:265–269, 1973.

98. Phelps, P., and McCarty, D.J.: Crytal-induced inflammation in canine joints. II. Importance of polymorphonuclear leukocytes. J. Exp. Med., 124(1):150, 1966.

99. Chang, Y.H., and Gralla, E.J.: Suppression of urate crystal-induced canine joint inflammation by heterologous anti-polymorphonuclear leukocyte serum. Arthritis Rheum., 11:145–150, 1968.

100. Weissmann, G., and Rita, G.A.: Molecular basis of gouty inflammation: Interaction of monosodium urate crystals with lysosomes and liposomes. Nature [New Biol.], 240:167–172, 1972.

101. Abramson, S., Hoffstein, S.T., and Weissmann, G.: Superoxide anion generated by human neutrophils exposed to monosodium urate. Arthritis Rheum., 15:174–180, 1982.

102a. Simchowitz, L., Atkinson, J.P., and Spilberg, I.: Stimulation of the respiratory burst in human neutrophils by crystal phagocytosis. Arthritis Rheum., 25:181–188, 1982.

102b. Cheung, H.S., Bohon, S., and Kozin, F.: Kinetics of collagenase and neutral protease release by neutrophils exposed to microcrystalline sodium urate. Con. Tiss. Res., 11:79–85, 1983.

103. Rae, A.A., Davidson, E.M., and Smith, M.J.H.: Leukotriene B4, an inflammatory mediator in gout. Lancet, 2:1122–1123, 1982.

104. Serhan, C.N., et al.: Formation of leukotrienes and hydroxy acids by human neutrophils and platelets exposed to monosodium urate. Prostaglandins, 17:563–581, 1984.

105. Phelps, P.: Polymorphonuclear leukocyte motility in vitro. III. Possible release of a chemotactic substance after phagocytosis of urate crystals by polymorphonuclear leukocytes. Arthritis Rheum., 12:197–203, 1969.

106. Spilberg, I., and Mandell, B.: Crystal-induced chemotactic factor. In Advances in Inflammation Research. Edited by G. Weissmann. New York, Raven Press, 1982.

107. Spilberg, I., Rosenberg, D., and Mandell, B.: Induction of arthritis by purified cell-derived chemotactic factor. J. Clin. Invest., 59:582–585, 1977.

108. Phelps, P., Andrews, R., and Rosenbloom, J.: Demonstration of chemotactic factor in human gout. J. Rheumatol., 8:889–894, 1981.

109. Ortel, R.W., and Newcombe, D.S.: Acute gouty arthritis and response to colchicine in the virtual absence of synovial fluid leukocytes. N. Engl. J. Med., 190:1363–1364, 1974.

110. Wigley, F.M., Fine, I.T., and Newcombe, D.S.: The role of the human synovial fibroblast in monosodium urate crystal-induced synovitis. J. Rheumatol., 10:602–611, 1983.

111. Schumacher, H.R., Phelps, P., and Agudelo, C.A.: Urate crystal-induced inflammation in dog joints: Sequence of synovial changes. J. Rheumatol., 1:102–113, 1974.

112. Schumacher, H.R.: Pathogenesis of crystal-induced synovitis. Clin. Rheum. Dis., 3:105–131, 1977.

113. McMillan, R.M., Hasselbacher, P., Hahn, J.L., and Harris, E.D.: Interactions of murine macrophages with monosodium urate crystals: Stimulation of lysosomal enzyme release and prostaglandin synthesis. J. Rheumatol., 8:555–562, 1981.

114. Duff, G.W., Atkins, E., and Malawista, S.E.: The fever of gout: Urate crystals activate endogenous pyrogen production from human and rabbit mononuclear phagocytes. Trans. Assoc. Am. Physicians, 96:234–245, 1983.

115. Malawista, S.E., et al.: Crystal-induced endogenous pyrogen production. A further look at gouty inflammation. Arthritis Rheum., 28:1039–1046, 1985.

116. Cybulsky, M.I., Colditz, I.G., and Movat, H.Z.: The role of interleukin-1 in neutrophil leukocyte emigration induced by endotoxin. Am. J. Pathol., 124:367–372, 1986.

117. Webster, M.E., et al.: Urate crystal-induced inflammation in the rat: Evidence of the combined actions of kinins, histamine and components of complement. Immunol. Commun., 1:185–198, 1972.

118. Wallingford, W.R., and McCarty, D.J.: Differential membranolytic effects of microcrystalline sodium urate and calcium pyrophosphate dihydrate. J. Exp. Med., 133:100–112, 1971.

119. Ginsberg, M.H., and Kozin, F.: Mechanisms of cellular interaction with monosodium urate crystals. Arthritis Rheum., 21:896–903, 1978.

120. Ginsberg, M.H., et al.: Mechanisms of platelet response to monosodium urate crystals. Am. J. Pathol., 94:549–568, 1979.

121. Kozin, F., Ginsberg, M.H., and Skosey, J.: Polymorphonuclear leukocyte responses to monosodium urate crystals: Modification by adsorbed serum protein. J. Rheumatol., 6:519–528, 1979.

122. Mandel, N.S.: The structural basis of crystal-induced membranolysis. Arthritis Rheum., 19:439–455, 1976.

123. Herring, F.G., Lam, E., and Burt, H.M.: A spin label study of the membranolytic effects of crystalline monosodium urate monohydrate. J. Rheumatol., 13:623–630, 1986.

124. Burt, H.M., et al.: Membranolytic effects of monosodium urate monohydrate: Influence of grinding. J. Rheumatol., 13:778–783, 1986.

125. Mandel, N.S.: Structural changes in sodium urate crystals on heating. Arthritis Rheum., 23:772–776, 1980.

126. Dieppe, P., et al.: Changes in monosodium urate crystals on heating or grinding. Arthritis Rheum., 24:975–976, 1981.

127. Terkeltaub, R.: Unpublished data.

128. Jaques, B.C., and Ginsberg, M.H.: The role of cell surface proteins in platelet stimulation by monosodium urate crystals. Arthritis Rheum., 25:508–521, 1982.

129. Henson, P.M., Ginsberg, M.H., and Morrison, D.C.: Mechanisms of mediator release from inflammatory cells. In Cell Surface Reviews, Vol. V. Edited by G. Poste and G.L. Nicholson. New York, Elsevier, 1978.

130. Schumacher, H.R., and Phelps, P.: Sequential changes in human polymorphonuclear leukocytes after urate crystal phagocytosis. Arthritis Rheum., 14:513–526, 1971.

131. Weissmann, G., Zurier, R.B., Speiler, P.J., and Goldstein, I.M.: Mechanisms of lysosomal enzyme release from leukocytes exposed to immune complexes and other particles. J. Exp. Med., 134:149–165, 1971.

132. Hoffstein, S., and Weissmann, G.: Mechanisms of lysosomal enzyme release from leukocytes. IV. Interaction of monosodium urate crystals with dogfish and human leukocytes. Arthritis Rheum., 18:153–165, 1975.

133. Kane, A.B., et al.: Dissociation of intracellular lysosomal rupture from the cell death caused by silica. J. Cell. Biol., 87:643–651, 1980.

134. Steele, A.D., and McCarty, D.J.: An experimental model of acute inflammation in man. Arthritis Rheum., 9:430–442, 1966.

135. Tate, G., Mandell, B.F., Schumacher, H.R., and Zurier, R.B.: Suppression of experimental urate crystal inflammation by prostaglandin E_1 (PGE_1) and dietary manipulation. Arthritis Rheum., 29(Suppl.):S36, 1986.

136. Levine, J.D., et al.: Intraneuronal substance P contributes to the severity of experimental arthritis. Science, 116:547–549, 1984.

137. Iverson, L.I.: Possible role of neuropeptides in the pathophysiology of rheumatoid arthritis. J. Rheumatol., 12:399–400, 1985.

138. Lotz, M., Carson, D., and Vaughan, J.H.: Substance P activation of rheumatoid synoviocytes: Neural pathway in pathogenesis of arthritis. Science, 235:893–895, 1987.

139. Denko, C.W., and Gabriel, P.: Effects of peptide hormones in urate crystal inflammation. J. Rheumatol., 12:971–975, 1985.

140. McCarty, D.J., Phelps, P., and Pyensen, J.: Crystal-induced inflammation in canine joints. I. An experimental model with quantification of the host response. J. Exp. Med., 124:99–114, 1966.

141. Howell, R.R., and Seegmiller, J.E.: Uricolysis by human leukocytes. Nature, 196:482–483, 1962.

142. Colditz, I.G., and Movat, H.Z.: Desensitization of acute inflammatory lesions to chemotaxins and endotoxin. J. Immunol., 133:2163–2168, 1984.

143. Ginsberg, M.H., et al.: Adsorption of polymorphonuclear leukocyte lysosomal enzymes to monosodium urate crystal. Arthritis Rheum., 20:1538–1542, 1977.

144. Rosen, M.S., Baker, D.G., Schumacher, H.R., Jr., and Cherian, P.V.: Products of polymorphonuclear cell injury inhibit IgG enhancement of monosodium urate-induced superoxide production. Arthritis Rheum., 29:1473–1479, 1986.

145. Arnold, W.J., and Simmons, R.A.: Clinical variability of the gouty diathesis. Adv. Exp. Med. Biol., 122A:33–46, 1980.

146. Hollingworth, P., Scott, J.T., and Burry, H.C.: Nonarticular gout: Hyperuricemia and tophus formation without gouty arthritis. Arthritis Rheum., 26:98–101, 1983.

147. Buchanan, W.W., Klinenberg, J.R., and Seegmiller, J.E.: The inflammatory response to injected microcrystalline monosodium urate in normal, hyperuricemic, gouty and uremic subjects. Arthritis Rheum., 8:361–367, 1965.

148. Emmerson, B.T., Stride, P.J., and Williams, G.: The clinical differentiaton of primary gout from primary renal disease in patients with both gout and renal disease. Adv. Exp. Med. Biol., 122A:9–13, 1980.

149. Wallace, D.J., et al.: Coexistent gout and rheumatoid arthritis. Case report and literature review. Arthritis Rheum., 22:81–86, 1979.

150. Gordon, T.P., Ahern, M.J., Reid, C., and Roberts-Thomson, P.J.: Studies on the interaction of rheumatoid factor with monosodium urate crystals and case report of coexistent tophaceous gout and rheumatoid arthritis. Ann. Rheum. Dis., 44:384–389, 1985.

151. Brandt, K.D.: The effect of synovial hyaluronate on the ingestion of monosodium urate crystals by leukocytes. Clin. Chim. Acta, 55:307–315, 1974.

152. Malawista, S.E., Van Blaricom, G.V., Cretella, S.B., and Schwartz, M.L.: The phlogistic potential of urate in solution: studies of the phagocytic process in human leukocytes. Arthritis Rheum., 22:728–736, 1979.

153. Schumacher, H.R., et al.: Comparison of sodium urate and calcium pyrophosphate crystal phagocytosis by polymorphonuclear leukocytes. Effects of crystal size and other factors. Arthritis Rheum., 18(Suppl.):783–792, 1975.

154. Antommattei, O., Schumacher, H.R., Reginato, A.J., and Clayburne, G.: Prospective study of morphology and phagocytosis of synovial fluid monosodium urate crystals in gouty arthritis. J. Rheumatol., 11:741–744, 1984.

155. Kozin, F., and McCarty, D.J.: Protein binding to monosodium urate monohydrate, calcium pyrophosphate and silicon dioxide crystals. I. Physical characteristics. J. Lab. Clin. Med., 89:314–325, 1977.

156. Kozin, F., and McCarty, D.J.: Molecular orientation of immunoglobulin G adsorbed to microcrystalline monosodium urate monohydrate. J. Lab. Clin. Med., 95:49–58, 1980.

157. Terkeltaub R., et al.: Lipoproteins containing apoprotein B are a major regulator of neutrophil responses to monosodium urate crystals. J. Clin. Invest., 73:1719–1730, 1984.

158. Kozin, F., et al.: Protein binding to monosodium urate crystals and its effect on platelet degranulation. Adv. Exp. Med. Biol., 76B:201–207, 1976.

159. Terkeltaub, R., Smeltzer, D., Curtiss, L.K., and Ginsberg, M.H.: Low density lipoprotein inhibits the physical interaction of phlogistic crystals and inflammatory cells. Arthritis Rheum., 29:363–370, 1986.

160. Terkeltaub, R., Martin, J., Curtiss, L.K., and Ginsberg, M.H.: Apolipoprotein B mediates the capacity of low density lipoprotein to suppress neutrophil stimulation by particulates. J. Biol. Chem., 261:15662–15667, 1986.

161. Gordon, T.P., Clifton, P., James, M.J., and Roberts-Thompson, P.J.: Lack of correlation between in vitro and in vivo effects of low density lipoprotein on the inflammatory activity of monosodium urate crystals. Ann. Rheum. Dis., 45:673–676, 1986.

162. Hutton, C.W., Hornby, J., and Dieppe, P.A.: Effects of low density lipoprotein and high density lipoprotein on monosodium urate crystal-induced inflammation (Abstract). Br. J. Rheumatol., 25:100, 1986.

163. Terkeltaub, R., Martin, J., Curtiss, L., and Ginsberg, M.: Gouty inflammation: Glycosaminoglycans regulate low density lipoprotein binding to urate crystals (Abstract). Arthritis Rheum. (in press).

164. Hakim, F.T., et al.: Hereditary joint disorder in progressive ankylosis (ank/ank) mice. I. Association of calcium hydroxyapatite deposition with inflammatory arthropathy. Arthritis Rheum., 27:1411–1420, 1984.

165. Hakim, F.T., Brown, K.S., and Oppenheim, J.J.: Hereditary joint disorder in progressive ankylosis (ank/ank) mice. II. Effect of high-dose hydrocortisone treatment on inflammation and intraarticular calcium hydroxyapatite deposits. Arthritis Rheum., 29:114–123, 1986.

166. Terkeltaub, R., and Santoro, D.: Alpha 2-HS glycoprotein is a major regulator of neutrophil stimulation by hydroxyapatite crystals (Abstract). Clin. Res. (in press).

167. McCarty, D.J., Phelps, P., and Pyenson, P.: Crystal induced inflammation in canine joints. I. An experimental model with quantification of the host response. J. Exp. Med., 124:99–114, 1966.

168. McCarty, D.J.: Pathogenesis and treatment of crystal-induced inflammation. In Arthritis and Allied Conditions, 10th ed. Edited by D.J. McCarty. Philadelphia, Lea & Febiger, 1983.

169. Edwards, J.C., Sedgwick, A.D., and Willoughby, D.A.: The formation of a structure with the features of synovial lining by subcutaneous injection of air: An in vivo tissue culture system. J. Pathol., 134:147–156, 1981.

170. Sin, Y.M., Sedgwick, A.D., Chea, E.P., and Willoughby, D.A.: Mast cells in newly formed lining tissue during acute inflammation: A six day air pouch model in the mouse. Ann. Rheum. Dis., 45:873–877, 1986.

171. Gordon, T.P., Kowasko, I.C., James, M., and Roberts-Thomson, P.J.: Monosodium urate crystal-induced prostaglandin synthesis in the rat subcutaneous air pouch. Clin. Exp. Rheumatol., 3:291–295, 1985.

172. Sin, Y.M., Sedgwick, A.D., Moore, A., and Willoughby, D.A.: Studies on the clearance of calcium pyrophosphate crystals from facsimile synovium. Ann. Rheum. Dis., 43:487–492, 1984.

173. Malawista, S.E., and Seegmiller, J.E.: The effect of pretreatment with colchicine on the inflammatory response to microcrystalline urate. Ann. Intern. Med., 62:648–657, 1965.

174. Hutton, C.W., et al.: Systemic response to local urate crystal induced inflammation in man: A possible model to study the acute phase response. Ann. Rheum. Dis., 44:533–536, 1985.

175. Wallace, S.L.: The treatment of the acute attack of gout. Clin. Rheum. Dis., 3:133–143, 1977.

176a. AMA Department of Drugs: Drugs used in gout. In AMA Drug Evaluations, 4th ed. Chicago, American Medical Association, pp. 109–119, 1980.

176b. Roberts, W.M., Liang, M.H., and Stern, S.H.: Colchicine in acute gout. JAMA, 257:1920–1921, 1987.

177. Bennett, W.M., et al.: Drug prescribing in renal failure: Dosing guidelines for adults. Am. J. Kidney Dis., 3:155–193, 1983.

178. Yu, T.F., and Gutman, A.B.: Efficiency of colchicine prophylaxis in gout. Ann. Intern. Med., 55:179–192, 1961.

179. Neuss, M.N.: Long-term colchicine administration leading to colchicine toxicity and death. Arthritis Rheum., 29:448–449, 1986.

180. Wallace, S.L., Bernstein, D., and Diamond, H.: Diagnostic value of the colchicine therapeutic trial. JAMA, 199:525–528, 1967.

181. Meed S.D., and Spilberg, I.: Successful use of colchicine in

acute polyarticular pseudogout. J. Rheumatol., *8*:689–691, 1981.

182. Spilberg, I., et al.: Colchicine and pseudogout. Arthritis Rheum., *23*:1062–1063, 1980.

183. Ertel, N.H., Mittler, J.C., and Akgun, S.: Radioimmunoassay for colchicine in plasma and urine. Science, *193*:233–239, 1976.

184. Wallace, S.L., and Ertel, N.H.: Plasma levels of colchicine after oral administration of a single dose. Metabolism, *11*:749–753, 1973.

185. Wallace, S.L., Omokoku, B., and Ertel, N.H.: Colchicine plasma levels—Implications as to pharmacology and mechanisms of action. Am. J. Med., *48*:443–448, 1970.

186. Ertel, N.H., and Wallace, S.L.: Measurement of colchicine in urine and peripheral leukocytes. Clin. Res., *19*:348–357, 1971.

187. Borisy, G.G., and Taylor, E.W.: The mechanism of action of colchicine. J. Cell Biol., *34*:525–548, 1967.

188. Pesante, E.L., and Axline, S.G.: Colchicine effects on lysosomal enzyme induction and intracellular degradation in the cultivated macrophage. J. Exp. Med., *141*:1030–1046, 1976.

189. Dallaverde, F., Fan, P.T., and Chang, Y.H.: Mechanism of action of colchicine. V. Neutrophil adherence and phagocytosis in patients with acute gout treated with colchicine. J. Pharmacol. Exp. Ther., *223*:197–202, 1982.

190. Malawista, S.E.: The action of colchicine in acute gouty arthritis. Arthritis Rheum., *18*:835–846, 1975.

191. Wallace, S.L.: Colchicine analogs in the treatment of acute gout. Arthritis Rheum., *2*:389–396, 1959.

192. Malawista, S.E., Chang, Y.H., and Wilson, L.: Lumicolchicine-lack of anti-inflammatory effect. Arthritis Rheum., *15*:641–643, 1972.

193. Stodler, J., and Franke, W.: Colchicine binding of proteins in chromatin and membranes. Nature,*237*:237–238, 1972.

194. Erlich, G.E.: Colchicine for Familial Mediterranean fever. N. Engl. J. Med., *288*:798, 1973.

195. Phelps, P.: Polymorphonuclear leukocyte motility in vitro. IV. Colchicine inhibition of chemotactic activity formation after phagocytosis of urate crystals. Arthritis Rheum., *131*:1–9, 1970.

196. Andrews, K., and Phelps, P.: Release of lysosomal enzymes from polymorphonuclear leukocytes after phagocytosis of monosodium urate and calcium pyrophosphate dihydrate crystals: Effects of colchicine and indomethacin. Arthritis Rheum., *14*:368, 1971.

197. Spilberg, I., et al.: A mechanism of action for non-steroid anti-inflammatory agents in calcium pyrophosphate dihydrate (CPPD) crystal induced arthritis. Agents Actions, *7*:153–160, 1977.

198. Struge, R.A., et al.: Multicentre trial of naproxen and phenylbutazone in acute gout. Ann. Rheum. Dis., *36*:80–82, 1977.

199. Chang, Y.H.: Studies on phagocytosis. II. The effect of non-steroidal anti-inflammatory drugs on phagocytosis and on urate crystal induced canine joint inflammation. J. Pharmacol. Exp. Ther., *182*:235–244, 1972.

200. Dieppe, P.A., Doherty, M., Whicher, J.T., and Walters, G.: The treatment of gout with azopropazone: Clinical and experimental studies. Eur. J. Rheumatol. Inflamm., *4*:392–399, 1981.

201. Gibson, T., et al.: Azopropazone—A treatment for hyperuricemia and gout. Br. J. Rheumatol., *23*:44–51, 1984.

202a. Sipola, R., Skrifurors, B., and Tornroth, T.: Reversible non-oliguric impairment of renal function during azopropazone treatment. Scand. J. Rheumatol., *15*:23–26, 1986.

202b. Masuda, I., and Ishikawa, K.: Clinical features of pseudogout attack—A survey of 50 cases (submitted for publication).

203. Bowles, C., et al.: Colchicine prevents recurrent pseudogout: Multicenter trial (Abstract). Arthritis Rheum., *29*:538, 1986.

204. Alvarellos, A., and Spilberg, I.: Colchicine prophylaxis in pseudogout. J. Rheumatol., *13*:804–805, 1986.

CALCIUM PYROPHOSPHATE CRYSTAL DEPOSITION DISEASE; PSEUDOGOUT; ARTICULAR CHONDROCALCINOSIS

107

LAWRENCE M. RYAN and DANIEL J. McCARTY

Microscopic examination of wet preparations of synovial fluid under compensated polarized light has provided a rapid, specific, and sensitive method for identification of crystals in gout, which might be called monosodium urate (MSU) crystal deposition disease.[1] Both monoclinic (unit cell with one obtuse and two right angles) and triclinic (unit cell with three obtuse angles) MSU crystals are seen, and "twinning" or pairing of crystals is observed frequently. Digestion with purified uricase has established the specific chemical composition of these crystals. See Chapters 5 and 108 for a discussion of various techniques of crystal identification.

Application of these methods to examination of synovial fluids led to the discovery of nonurate crystals in patients with a gout-like syndrome termed pseudogout.[2] These biaxial crystals were identified as calcium pyrophosphate dihydrate ($Ca_2P_2O_7 \cdot 2H_2O$, or CPPD)[3] (Fig. 107–1A). These crystals also exhibited monoclinic and triclinic dimorphism and frequently showed twinning. Polariscopically, they had a weakly positive birefringence and inclined extinction. Some crystals were isotropic under polarized light (nonrefractile). Urate crystals, on the other hand, were negatively birefringent under compensated polarized light and showed axial extinction. Fluid removed from acutely inflamed joints of patients with pseudogout invariably showed phagocytosed CPPD crystals (Fig. 107–1B).

Both MSU and CPPD crystals with morphologic features identical to natural crystals were synthe-sized.[4-6] Injection of such crystals into normal human and canine joints was followed by an acute inflammatory response. The phrase *crystal-induced synovitis* was coined to describe the tissue reaction provoked by either type of crystal,[7] and the responsible mechanisms are discussed in Chapter 106.

NOMENCLATURE

We initially termed the syndrome associated with CPPD deposition *pseudogout* because of the obvious parallel with true (urate) gout.[2] Many patients with symptomatic arthritis, however, do not have acute attacks, so this term should be reserved for the acute episodes associated with CPPD crystals. The term *chondrocalcinosis* was coined by Zitnan and Sitaj, based on the characteristic radiologic features.[8] Because subsequent analysis of cartilage calcifications showed at least three distinct mineral phases, this term is too broad and nonspecific, although it may suffice to indicate radiologic cartilage calcifications when crystal identification is lacking. *Pyrophosphate arthropathy* was coined in 1969 by H.L.F. Currey and is widely used in the United Kingdom.[9] No reason appears to justify blaming pyrophosphate for the arthropathy. Indeed, recent studies indicate that the calcium component of the crystal is responsible for profound biologic effects (see Chapter 108). It appears most prudent to use the specific term *CPPD crystal deposition disease* unless some good reason can be found to abandon it.

FIG. 107–1. *A,* Weakly birefringent monoclinic and triclinic calcium pyrophosphate dihydrate (CPPD) microcrystals in synovial fluid removed from a chronically symptomatic knee (polarized light × 1250). *B,* Phagocytosed crystal (arrow) in a polymorphonuclear leukocyte (phase contrast × 1250). *C,* Anteroposterior roentgenogram of the knee showing typical punctate and linear deposits of CPPD in the menisci and articular cartilage.

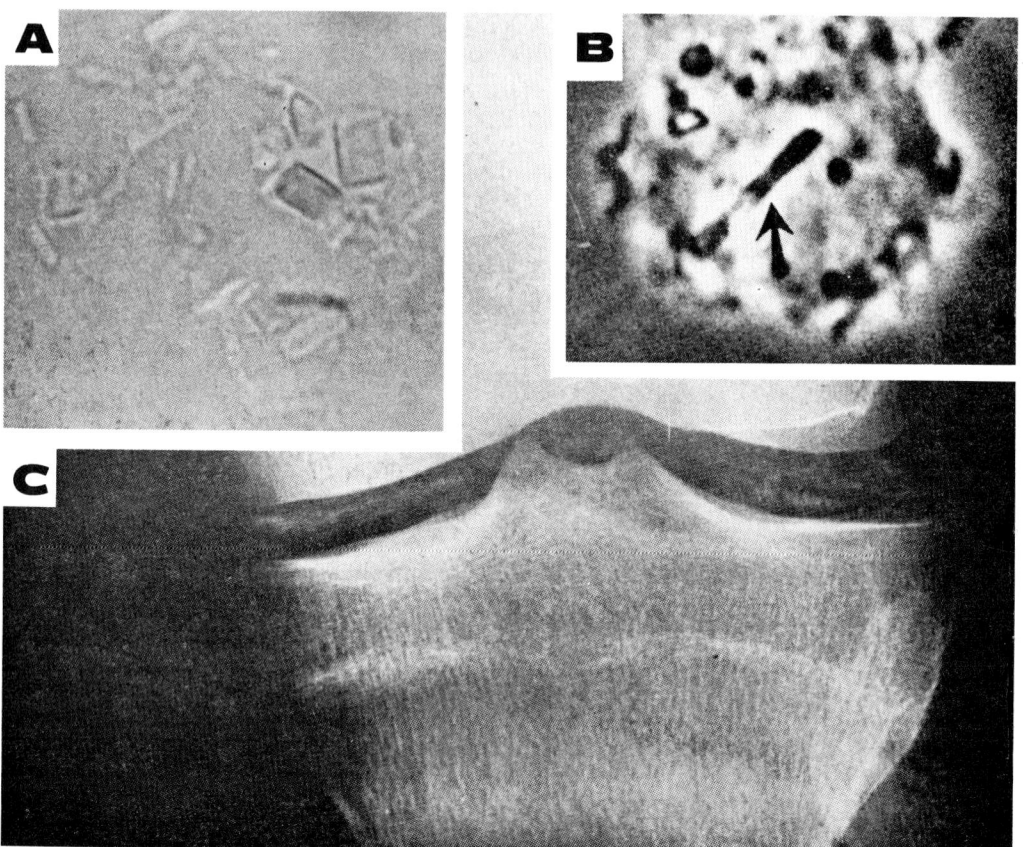

EARLY REPORTS

Initially, seven patients were studied, using the presence of microcrystalline CPPD as a common denominator (see Fig. 107–1A). The radiographic appearance of calcification of fibroarticular and hyaline articular cartilage was noted (see Fig. 107–1C). Analysis of such deposits showed CPPD crystals identical to those seen in joint fluid.

In addition to pseudogout attacks and a chronic degenerative arthropathy, other findings in this initial group of patients were confirmed by subsequent separate reports. For example, a destructive arthropathy resembling Charcot joints, radiologic lesions resembling osteochondromas, hemorrhagic joint fluids, prominent subchondral cysts, and urate crystals associated with gouty arthritis were all documented at least once in our initial series. When the clinical and roentgenographic findings in this group were analyzed, a review of the literature revealed a similarity

to chondrocalcinosis polyarticularis (familiaris), as described in 1958 by Zitnan and Sitaj.[8] These workers used the characteristic roentgenographic appearance as the unifying diagnostic feature. They pointed out that the menisci of the knee were most commonly involved (see Fig. 107–1C). These authors later reported 27 cases, 21 from 5 Hungarian families living in a single village in Slovakia.[10]

Perhaps the first report of CPPD deposition was made in 1903 by Bennett.[11] He described autopsy findings in an elderly man of mineral deposits in cartilages of the hips, shoulders, sternoclavicular joints, and temporomandibular joints. Chemical analysis indicated a substantial calcium and carbonate content, but no urates by the murexide test. The individual crystals were described as smaller than urate crystals and rhomboidal in shape under an ordinary light microscope.

Two types of meniscal calcification were differentiated on gross and microscopic pathologic grounds in 1927 by the Viennese surgeon Mandl.[12] A "primary" type predominated in the elderly and involved all four menisci with diffuse focal deposits of calcium salts; meniscal surfaces were smooth; the disorder occurred without antecedent trauma and was frequently asymptomatic. Microscopically, punctate deposits of granular calcific material and a striking hypocellularity of the involved cartilage were noted. A "secondary" type, found in a younger age group, involved a localized deposit in a single meniscus and usually followed trauma. The cartilage surface over the deposit was roughened, and the condition was symptomatic, frequently requiring meniscectomy.

A case reported in 1926 contained the first roentgenogram showing the characteristic pattern of "primary" calcification; the author correlated this pattern with the pathologic findings.[13] Calcifications were found in the menisci, hyaline articular cartilage, ligaments, and joint capsule. A metabolic disorder leading to arthritis deformans (osteoarthritis) was postulated. In 1929, Tobler systematically examined 400 menisci from 100 necropsies of cadavers ranging in age from several days to 86 years.[14] He found degenerative changes in 75% and calcification in 25% of menisci.

In their classic monograph on the effect of aging in the knee, Bennett, Waine, and Bauer described small deposits of "granular material" in semilunar cartilages showing interstitial matrix altered by degenerative changes.[15] Marked calcifications of the "primary" type were found in the lateral meniscus of a 90-year-old man; the medial meniscus, similarly involved, had been almost completely destroyed. Thus, 3 of 63 cadavers studied showed "primary" calcification (4.1%). None in their series had had symptomatic arthritis during life.

PREVALENCE

A summary of reported anatomic and radiologic studies of the prevalence of knee joint calcification is given in Table 107–1. The study of elderly Jewish subjects by Ellman and Levin, using high-resolution film, is of particular interest.[16] Fully 27.6% of their ambulatory volunteers showed calcific deposits. Assuming that all were CPPD deposits, this finding implicated age as a factor in the expression of the condition. These findings have been confirmed by a report using standard radiograms of the knee in 108 women over 80 years of age.[17] Meniscal calcification was found in 16% of the 55 women aged 80 to 89 and in 30% of 53 women aged 89 to 99; 22 of 25 with chondrocalcinosis had deposits in other joints as well. A radiographic

survey of patients admitted to a geriatric unit disclosed a 44% prevalence of chondrocalcinosis in patients over 84 years of age, when films of the hands and wrist, pelvis, and knees were examined.[18] The prevalence was 15% in patients between 65 and 74 years of age and 36% in those between 75 and 84 years.

X-ray diffraction powder patterns were obtained from at least one tissue deposit or from crystals harvested from synovial fluid in 51 of our first 80 cases; all were CPPD. A study of over 800 menisci from 215 anatomic cadavers was undertaken, using the CPPD crystal as a "marker."[19] At least one tiny deposit was seen in the type-M roentgenogram of 22% of excised menisci; most were too small to permit dissection, much less identification. Seven sets of menisci (3.2% of cadavers) showed linear and punctate deposits of CPPD; five sets (2.3% of cadavers) showed multiple punctate deposits of dicalcium phosphate dihydrate ($CaHPO_4 \cdot 2H_2O$, or DCPD); three single menisci (1.4% of cadavers) showed solitary deposits of "hydroxyapatite." Studies now suggest the term *basic calcium phosphate* (BCP) instead of hydroxyapatite (see Chapter 108). Four cadavers in this series had sodium urate deposits in the menisci.

Two reports have identified DCPD crystals in cartilage and in synovial fluid.[20,21] The crystals in synovial fluid were both free and intraleukocytic, so they too might be inflammatory. Apatite-like crystals in joint fluids,[22] and in joint fluid leukocytes, also occur.[23] At times, synovial fluids contain both BCP and CPPD crystals, leading to the term *mixed crystal deposition disease*.[24,25] CPPD crystals were also seen in joint fluids in 6 of 15 patients with Milwaukee shoulder–knee syndrome (see Chapter 108),[26] which is characterized by the presence of synovial BCP crystals.

A survey of a large number of pathologic nonarticular calcifications using crystallographic techniques showed no CPPD crystals and thus established their relative specificity for articular tissue.[28] Identification of crystals in aortic plaques, costal cartilages, pancreas, and pineal glands obtained from pseudogout patients at necropsy showed only "apatite." Periarticular deposits of crystallographically proved CPPD, however, have been reported in tendons, dura mater, ligamenta flava, and the olecranon bursa, as well as in isolated "tophi."[27]

JOINT FLUID FINDINGS

Nearly all fluids aspirated from inflamed joints showed phagocytosed CPPD microcrystals (Fig. 107–1B). Unlike urate crystals, they were often within

Table 107–1. Prevalence of Calcific Deposits in Knee Joints[27]

Anatomic Studies† (Authors)	Cadavers (No.)		Positive for Calcium Pyrophosphate Dihydrate (%)
Bennett et al.	63		4.1*
McCarty et al.	215		3.2
Lagier and Baud	320		6.8
Mitrovic et al.	108		18.5

Radiologic Studies (Authors)†	Subjects (No.)	Average Age (Year)	Positive for Calcific Deposits (%)
Bocher et al.	455	80	7.0
Cabanel et al.	200	—	6.5
Zinn et al.	131	65	4.6
Schmied et al.	52	66 (diabetic)	5.8
	45	61 (control)	2.2
Ellman and Levin	58	83	27.6
Mezard et al.	299	65	12.5
Glimet et al.	50	73	14
DeLauche et al.	62	85	32
Memin et al.	108	88	23
Wilkins et al.	100	79	34

*Crystals not identified specifically.
†See reference 27 for references to all studies.

phagolysosomes.[2] CPPD crystals are much more difficult to see by polarized light microscopy than are MSU crystals, and we routinely use phase-contrast in addition to polarized light at thousandfold magnification for crystal identification. Even using these sensitive techniques, ultramicrocrystals cannot be detected.[29,30] The number of crystals bears some relation to the acuteness of inflammation because pellets from joint fluid taken during acute attacks contained much more pyrophosphate on chemical analysis than did pellets from noninflamed joints.[27] Exceptions occur, however. Some fluids from inflamed joints have few CPPD crystals, and some fluids from noninflamed joints are milky on gross inspection because of the large number of crystals present. This same phenomenon has been noted in true gout. The mean leukocyte concentration in acute attacks is exactly the same as in urate gout, about 20,000/mm³, with over 90% polymorphonuclear (PMN) cells. The addition of acetic acid is more likely to yield a "good" mucin clot in pseudogout than in gout.[31] As already noted, the fluid in pseudogout may be tinged with blood, especially early in the acute episode.[27] In at least one case, such fluid was associated with subchondral bony fractures.[32]

DIAGNOSTIC CRITERIA

A diagnostic classification, based on the premise that CPPD crystals are the specific feature of the disease,[7] has been modified to include radiographic clues suggested by Resnick[33] and Martel[34] (Table 107–2). A case is considered "definite" if CPPD crystals are demonstrated in tissues or synovial fluid by definitive means or if crystals compatible with CPPD are demonstrated by compensated polarized light microscopy and typical calcifications are seen on roentgenograms. If only one of these criteria is found, a "probable" diagnosis is made. The clinical findings or the radiologic clues given in Table 107–2 should alert the clinician to the possible presence of underlying CPPD crystal deposition disease.

CLINICAL FEATURES

In our present series of over 600 "definite" and "probable" cases, men predominate in a ratio of 1.5:1. A similar sex ratio was recorded at the Mayo Clinic.[35] Female predominance has been reported in other surveys of patients with symptomatic CPPD deposition.[36,37] Our patients' ages averaged 72 years at the time of diagnosis. The average age at the time of diagnosis was lower in the Czechoslovakian and Chilean series because these studies included familial and asymptomatic cases detected radiographically. The absence of the putative associated diseases, such as hyperparathyroidism, hemochromatosis, and urate gout, in the familial cases is noteworthy.

The various patterns of arthritis encountered clinically are summarized graphically in Figure 107–2. We

Table 107–2. Revised Diagnostic Criteria for Calcium Pyrophosphate Dihydrate Crystal Deposition Disease (Pseudogout)

Criteria
    I. Demonstration of CPPD crystals, obtained by biopsy, necropsy, or aspirated synovial fluid, by definitive means; e.g., characteristic "fingerprint" by x-ray diffraction powder pattern or by chemical analysis.
    II. A. Identification of monoclinic or triclinic crystals showing a weakly positive, or a lack of, birefringence by compensated polarized light microscopy.
       B. Presence of typical calcifications on roentgenograms.*
    III. A. Acute arthritis, especially of knees or other large joints, with or without concomitant hyperuricemia.
       B. Chronic arthritis, especially of knees, hips, wrists, carpus, elbow, shoulder, and metacarpophalangeal joints, particularly if accompanied by acute exacerbations; the chronic arthritis shows the following features helpful in differentiating it from osteoarthritis:[33]
         1. Uncommon site for primary osteoarthritis; e.g., wrist, metacarpophalangeal joints, elbow, or shoulder.
         2. Radiographic appearance; e.g., radiocarpal or patellofemoral joint space narrowing, especially if isolated (patella "wrapped around" the femur†); femoral cortical erosion superior to the patella on the lateral view of the knee.
         3. Subchondral cyst formation.
         4. Severe progressive degeneration, with subchondral bony collapse (microfractures), and fragmentation, with formation of intra-articular radiodense bodies.
         5. Variable and inconstant osteophyte formation.
         6. Tendon calcifications, especially of Achilles, triceps, and obturator tendons.
         7. Involvement of the axial skeleton with subchondral cysts of apophyseal and sacroiliac joints, multiple levels of disc calcification and vacuum phenomenon, and sacroiliac vacuum phenomenon.

Categories
    A. Definite—criteria I or II(A) and (B) must be fulfilled.
    B. Probable—criteria IIA or IIB must be fulfilled.
    C. Possible—criteria IIIA or B should alert the clinician to the possibility of underlying CPPD deposition.

CPPD = calcium pyrophosphate dihydrate (CPPD); DCPD = dicalcium phosphate dihydrate.
*Heavy punctate and linear calcifications in fibrocartilages, articular (hyaline) cartilages, and joint capsules, especially if bilaterally symmetric; faint or atypical calcifications may be due to DCPD (CaHPO$_4$·2H$_2$O) deposits or to vascular calcifications; both are also often bilaterally symmetric.
†Also described as a feature of the arthritis of hyperparathyroidism.

FIG. 107–2. Diagrammatic representation of various clinical presentations of joint disease associated with calcium pyrophosphate dihydrate crystal deposition. (From McCarty, D.: The Heberden Oration, 1982. Crystals, joints, and consternation. Ann. Rheum. Dis., *42*:243–253, 1983.)

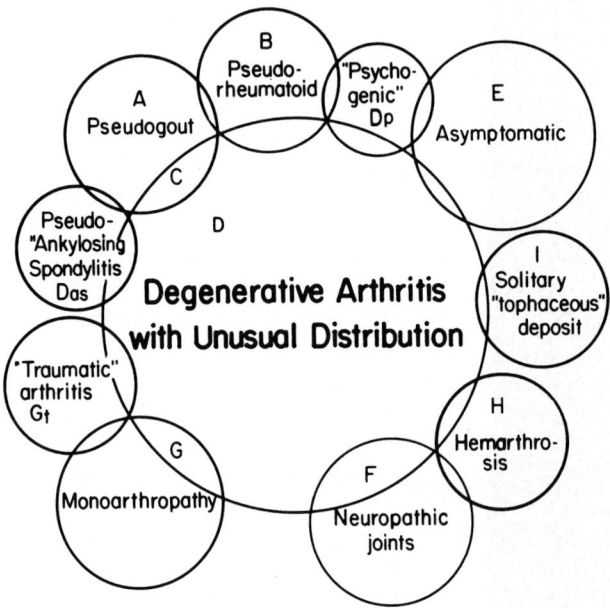

regard CPPD deposition as a great mimic because it often superficially resembles not only gout, but also rheumatoid arthritis (RA), osteoarthritis, and other types of joint disease.[9,38]

TYPE A—PSEUDOGOUT

The pseudogout pattern is marked by acute or subacute arthritic attacks lasting approximately 1 day to 4 weeks. These episodes are self-limited and generally involve only one or a few appendicular joints. Such attacks can be as severe as those of true gout, but they usually take longer to reach peak intensity and are less painful and disabling than gouty episodes. Inflammation may begin in a single "mother" joint with spread to involve other nearby "daughter" joints, the so-called cluster attack of the crystal deposition diseases. Mild "petite" attacks also occur, as in urate gout, and these may often outnumber full-blown attacks. Such attacks produce local effusions, joint stiffness, and warmth of the overlying skin, but they are not painful. Leukocytosis is noted in the synovial fluid. Injection of CPPD crystals into the joints of volunteers confirms that response is dose related and that pain is the last symptom to appear and the first to disappear (see Chapter 106).

Provocation of acute episodes by a surgical procedure or by medical illness is common in both gout and pseudogout. One study reported that the percentage of patients with either disease who had at least a single episode after operation was virtually identical: 8.3% of 168 gouty patients and 9.4% of 106 patients with pseudogout.[38] Parathyroidectomy is particularly likely to precipitate acute arthritis.[35,39] Similarly, severe medical illness, particularly vascular occlusion such as stroke or myocardial infarction, provoked attacks in 20.3% of 167 gouty subjects, as opposed to 24% of 104 patients with pseudogout. Trauma may provoke acute arthritis in patients with either gout or pseudogout. Because both types of crystals are often found in the same subject and because either may cause self-limited attacks under identical clinical circumstances and may respond similarly to treatment, joint aspiration and specific crystal identification are essential for precise differential diagnosis.

The knee joint is to pseudogout as the bunion joint is to gout, and it is the site of over half of all acute attacks. At least 11 crystal-proved instances of first metatarsophalangeal joint involvement, *pseudopodagra,* are known to us.

Although not nearly as predictably effective as in urate gout, oral colchicine may provide dramatic relief in pseudogout. The release of a chemotactic factor by PMN leukocytes after phagocytosis of either MSU or CPPD crystals[40] (see Chapter 106) is inhibited by colchicine in concentrations easily reached in serum by the usual therapeutic doses. The inhibition of urate crystal–induced release was more predictable than the inhibition induced by CPPD crystals, which provides in vitro results parallel to the clinical experience in patients. Spilberg and associates found that colchicine, 1 to 2 mg, given intravenously predictably controls acute attacks of pseudogout[41] (see Chapter 106).

Approximately 20% of patients with CPPD deposits have hyperuricemia, and about 5% have MSU crystal deposits as well. About 25% of our series of patients show this gout-like, type A pattern. Men predominate. As in gout, the patients are usually completely asymptomatic between attacks. Radiographic evidence of CPPD deposits is found in most patients with this pattern of disease (Figs. 107–3A and B, and 107–4 to 107–6).

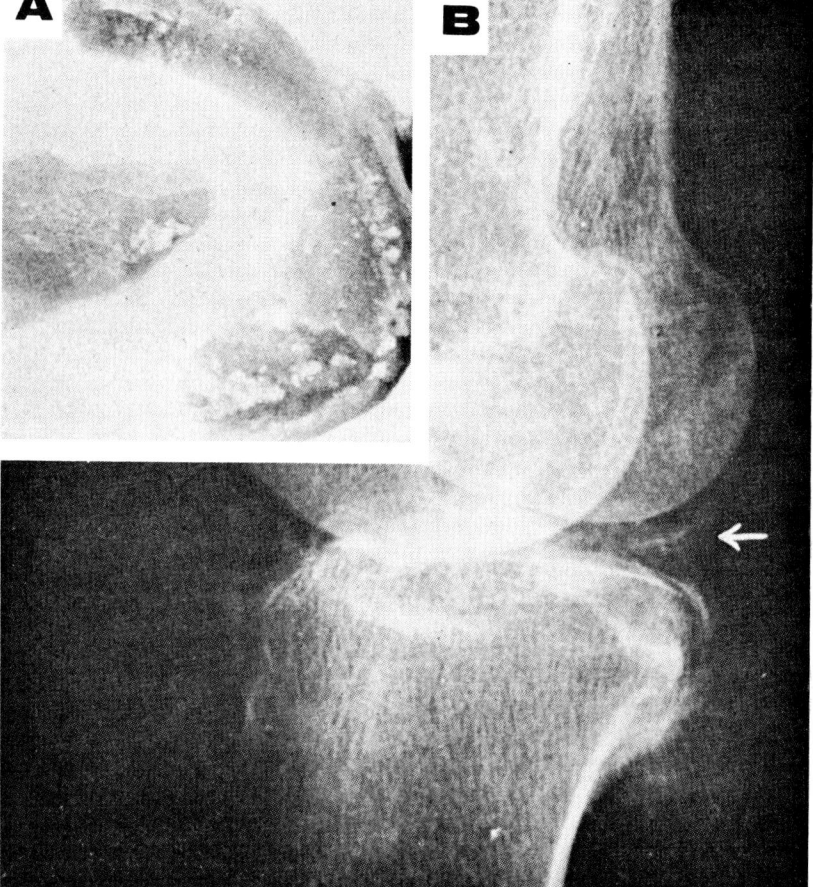

FIG. 107–3. *A,* Meniscus excised at necropsy showing punctate and linear aggregates of calcium pyrophosphate dihydrate microcrystals; a wedge of articular cartilage from the tibial plateau shows similar deposits. *B,* Lateral roentgenogram of the knee showing the typical Y-shaped appearance of meniscal calcification (arrow).

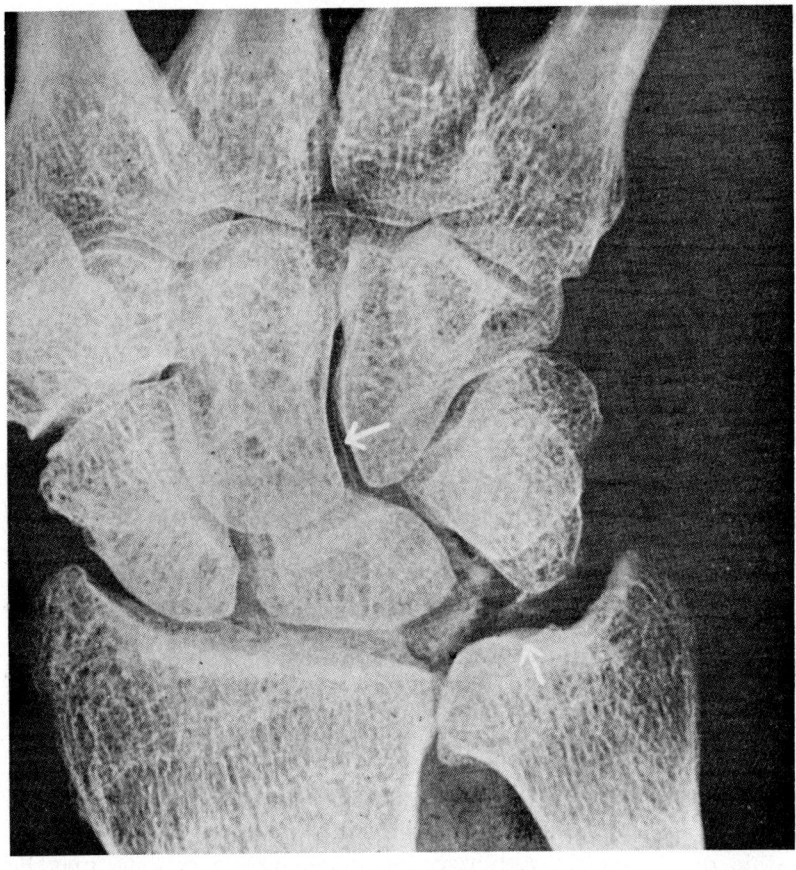

FIG. 107–4. Anteroposterior roentgenogram of the wrist showing calcification of the fibrocartilaginous articular disc and a fine line of calcification parallel to the radiodensity of the underlying bone, indicative of articular cartilage calcification (arrow).

TYPE B—PSEUDORHEUMATOID ARTHRITIS

Approximately 5% of patients have multiple joint involvement with subacute attacks lasting 4 weeks to

several months. Nonspecific symptoms of inflammation, such as morning stiffness and fatigue, are common; signs such as synovial thickening, localized pitting edema, limitation of joint motion due to inflammation or to flexion contractures, and elevated erythrocyte sedimentation rates are found. Such patients are often thought to have RA.[42] In addition,

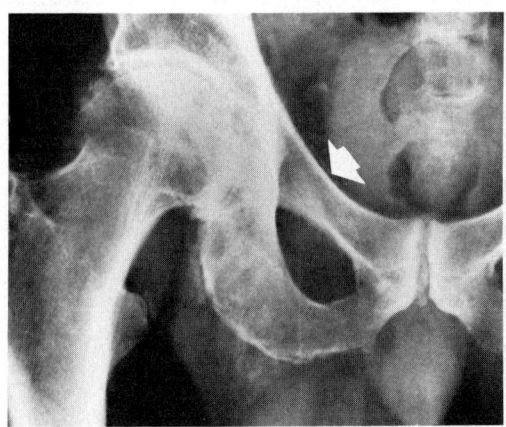

FIG. 107–5. Calcific deposits in the symphysis pubis, the hyaline cartilage, and the acetabular labrum of the hip, the origin of the adductor tendons on the ischium and lesser trochanter, and Cooper's ligament (arrow). (Courtesy Harry K. Genant, M.D.)

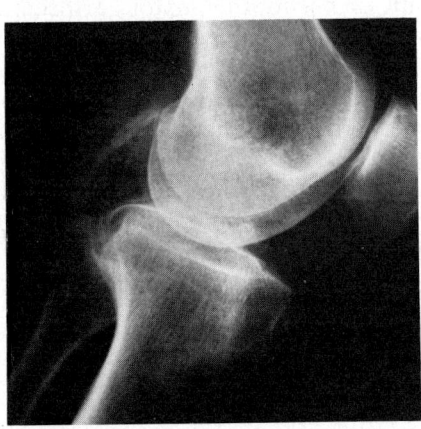

FIG. 107–6. Capsular calcification is prominent; deposits are also visible in the hyaline articular cartilage of the knee and in the proximal tibiofibular joints.

because about 10% of patients with CPPD-related arthritis have positive tests for rheumatoid factor (RF),[38] albeit usually in low titer, the opportunities for confusion abound. The presence of high titers of RF and typical radiographic erosions favor a diagnosis of "true" RA.[43] Interestingly, urate gout may also present with polyarticular involvement, RFs in 10% of cases, and symptoms mimicking those of RA.[43a]

CPPD deposits have been described both histologically[44] and radiographically[45] in patients with presumably bona fide RA. By chance alone, at least 1% of patients with CPPD joint deposits would be expected to have RA. This figure agrees with the finding of six cases of true RA in our series. A lower incidence (3%) of joint cartilage calcification in RA subjects was found in one study as compared to controls (14%), but the high incidence in the latter group, whose average age was 64.8 years, is more than is usually observed in an asymptomatic population.[46] This disparity may be due to the use as controls of patients presenting to the emergency unit with knee pain.[46] Conversely, we have studied over 600 cases of crystal-proved urate gout and only 1 showed a coincidence with RA. This patient had rheumatoid nodules and RF, hyperuricemia, and an ear tophus; the articular disease was unequivocally RA. The apparent negative association of urate gout and RA probably does not hold for CPPD deposits and RA.

The type-B pattern is intended to apply only to patients: (1) whose joints are inflamed "out of phase" with one another, as in gout, rather than "in phase," as in RA; (2) who form osteophytes; (3) who have CPPD crystals in joint fluid leukocytes; and (4) who do not have typical radiographic erosive disease. When RA and CPPD crystal deposition coexist, the typical radiographic appearance of the former is said to be atypical for RA.[46] Asymmetric disease, retained bone density, prominent osteophytes, well-corticated cysts, and paucity of erosions were found in 7 of 10 patients thought to have both diseases. It seems probable that those 7 patients actually had the *pseudorheumatoid* pattern of CPPD crystal deposition.

A variant of pseudorheumatoid arthritis (type B) can cause confusion clinically. The patient, usually elderly, when first seen, has multiple acutely inflamed joints, marked leukocytosis, fever of 102 to 104° F, and mental confusion or disorientation.[47] Systemic sepsis is suspected by the attending physicians, and antibiotics have usually been prescribed despite negative cultures. The entire clinical picture reverses with appropriate therapy.

TYPES C AND D—PSEUDO-OSTEOARTHRITIS

Approximately half of our patients have progressive degeneration of multiple joints (Figs. 107–7 to

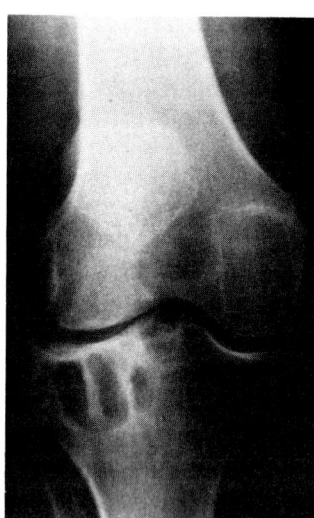

FIG. 107–7. Subchondral bone cyst under the lateral tibial plateau in a patient with generalized calcium pyrophosphate dihydrate deposition.

107–10). Women predominate. The knees are most commonly affected, followed by the wrists, metacarpophalangeal joints, hips, spine, shoulder, elbows, and ankles. Involvement is generally bilaterally symmetric, although the degenerative process may be much further advanced on one side, especially in joints that have been subjected to fracture or trauma. Flexion contractures of the involved joints are common. CPPD crystal deposition should be suspected in patients with bilateral varus deformities, unilateral valgus deformity, or flexion contractures of the knees, especially if accompanied by osteophytes and flexion contractures of other joints not usually affected by

FIG. 107–8. Calcifications in the insertion of the Achilles tendon and of the plantar fascia are seen in this lateral roentgenogram of the heel. Such deposits are particularly prominent in patients with hyperparathyroidism. (Courtesy Harry K. Genant, M.D.)

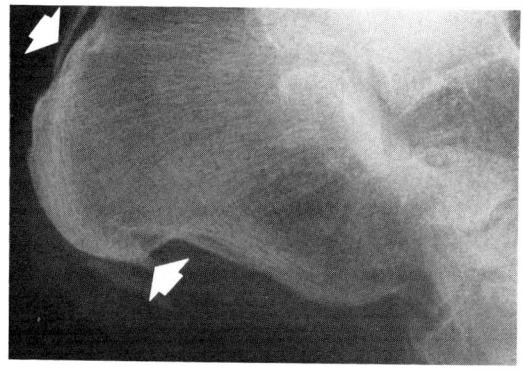

FIG. 107–9. Lateral roentgenograms of the knee showing peculiar erosion of the femoral cortex superior to the patella (arrow). Note the patella "wrapped around" the femur. (Courtesy Harry K. Genant, M.D.)

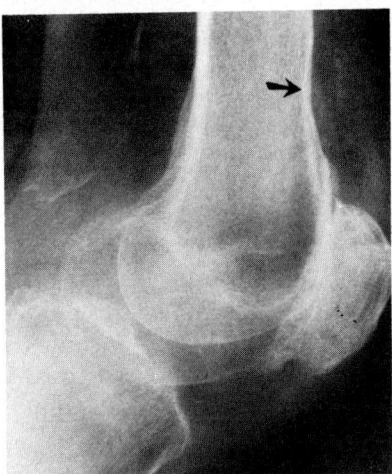

primary osteoarthritis, such as the wrists, elbows, shoulders, and metacarpophalangeal joints.

About 25% of the total series, or about half of those with types C and D disease, have a history of episodic, superimposed acute attacks and have been classified as type C. Those without an apparent inflammatory component have been classified as type D.

Characteristic CPPD deposits may or may not be visible on radiographs of involved joints. CPPD crystals are often found in radiographically negative joints, especially those with extensive degenerative change. Serial radiographic studies by Zitnan and Sitaj contain examples of joints with obvious CPPD deposits at an early phase of the disease that may be difficult to discern when severe degeneration has su-

FIG. 107–10. Anteroposterior roentgenogram of the shoulder showing neurotrophic joint appearance with extensive cystic bone lesions and powdered bony fragments in the synovial recesses inferiorly.

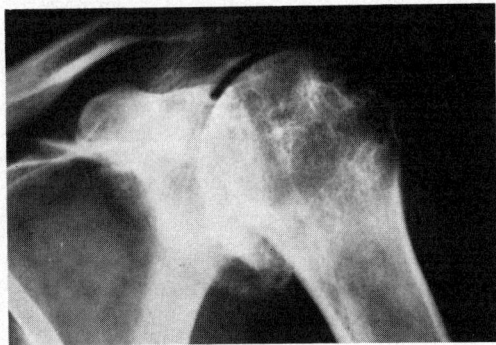

pervened.[48] Fine-detail roentgenograms are helpful in the detection of small or faint deposits.[49]

Martel and co-workers,[50] as well as Hamilton and his colleagues,[51] have described squaring of bone ends, subchondral cystic changes, and hooklike osteophytes, especially in the metacarpophalangeal joints. Atkins and associates compared the radiographic features of metacarpophalangeal degeneration in sporadic CPPD crystal deposition disease with that associated with hemochromatosis; they found more severe changes in a greater proportion of patients with hemochromatosis.[52]

Resnick and his colleagues have studied patients with CPPD deposition using age- and sex-matched control subjects. Useful diagnostic clues have been incorporated into the criteria outlined in Table 107–3. Axial skeleton involvement is frequent and is characterized by annular calcification, multiple levels of disc degeneration with vacuum phenomenon and subchondral erosions, and vacuum phenomenon of the sacroiliac joints.[33,34]

The pattern of joint degeneration in types C and D (e.g., wrists, metacarpophalangeal joints, elbow, and shoulder) is clearly different from that of primary osteoarthritis (e.g., proximal and distal interphalangeal and first carpometacarpal joints). The knee is commonly affected in both conditions. Concomitant Heberden's and Bouchard's nodes,[53] as well as other stigmata of primary osteoarthritis, often coexist with the pattern of joint involvement peculiar to CPPD crystal deposition, probably a chance association of two common conditions in elderly persons.

TYPE E—LANTHANIC (ASYMPTOMATIC) CALCIUM PYROPHOSPHATE DIHYDRATE CRYSTAL DEPOSITION

Type E CPPD crystal deposition may be the most common of all. Most joints with CPPD deposits plainly visible on roentgenograms are not symptomatic, even in patients with acute or chronic symptoms in other joints. Wrist complaints and genu varus deformities, but not acute joint inflammation, were more common in patients with CPPD deposits than in control subjects from the same population.[16]

TYPE F—PSEUDONEUROPATHIC JOINTS

One of the patients in our original report had a Charcot-like arthropathy of a knee in the absence of neurologic abnormality.[2] Subsequently, three of four cases of "neuropathic" arthritis of the knees associated with polyarticular CPPD deposition had mild tabes dorsalis; the fourth case also had late latent syphilis, but no neurologic abnormality.[54] One of these patients later developed an acute Charcot joint with hemorrhagic joint fluid and acute pseudogout.[32] Other reports of destructive arthropathy similar to neurotrophic arthropathy in patients with CPPD deposits and normal neurologic examinations underscore this association.[55-58] Severe degeneration of the neuropathic type has even been reported in the temporomandibular joints.[59]

Charcot knee joints develop in only 5 to 10% of patients with tabes dorsalis.[60] Because our three cases were seen consecutively and because CPPD deposition affects about 5% of the adult population (see Table 107–1), the two conditions might be expected to co-exist by chance alone in only 1 of 20 tabetics with Charcot joints. Thus, it was postulated that neurotrophic joints actually develop in the 5% of tabetic patients who have underlying CPPD crystal deposition.[54] That CPPD crystals alone can be associated with a destructive arthropathy, without the help of a neurologic deficit, reinforces this hypothesis (see Fig. 107–10).

OTHER PATTERNS OF CRYSTAL DEPOSITION

Multiple other patterns of disease have been described.[9] Stiffening of the spine that mimics ankylosing or diffuse idiopathic skeletal hyperostosis has been observed, particularly in familial CPPD deposition.[10,58] True bony ankylosis was observed in the Chilean series of familial cases, and none of the affected individuals were HLA-B27 positive.[61] Predominant symptoms of meningeal irritation[62] or radiculopathy have been reported and may be related to involvement of spinal joints or to CPPD deposits in the ligamentum flavum. A syndrome of acute neck pain ascribed to CPPD or BCP deposits is associated with tomographic appearance of calcification surrounding the odontoid process. This has been termed the "crowned dens" syndrome.[63] Monoarticular inflammation or degeneration may occur in CPPD secondary to trauma or attendant operations. This presentation is particularly common in the knee, years after meniscectomy,[63a] after operations to remove osteochondral fragments in osteochondritis dissecans,[64] or in disc fibrocartilage after lumbar surgical procedures.[65,66]

The frequent finding (8%) of polymyalgia rheumatica in a series from the United Kingdom suggests that CPPD deposition may mimic the proximal stiff-ness, pain, and elevated erythrocyte sedimentation rate of polymyalgia rheumatica.[35] Rarely, a localized, progressively destructive, solitary, "tophaceous" mass of CPPD crystals occurs in synovial tissue with chondroid metaplasia (Fig. 107–11). Seven cases have been reported, six in humans,[67-71] and one in the paw of a 12-year-old golden retriever.[72]

It is clear from the long-term observations of the natural history of CPPD joint deposition in familial cases by Zitnan and Sitaj that a given patient may show one pattern of arthritis early in the course of the disease and a different pattern later; many type-A patients may eventually have pattern C, D, or F, for example.[48]

Systemic findings during an acute attack are frequent but not invariable.[2] These include a fever of 99 to 103° F, leukocytosis of 12 to 15,000/mm³ with a "left shift," and an elevated erythrocyte sedimentation rate and serum acute-phase reactants.

FIG. 107–11. Lateral roentgenogram showing calcification in index finger pulp, demonstrated to consist of calcium pyrophosphate dihydrate crystal deposits in an area of chondroid metaplasia. (Reprinted from Arthritis and Rheumatism by permission.)

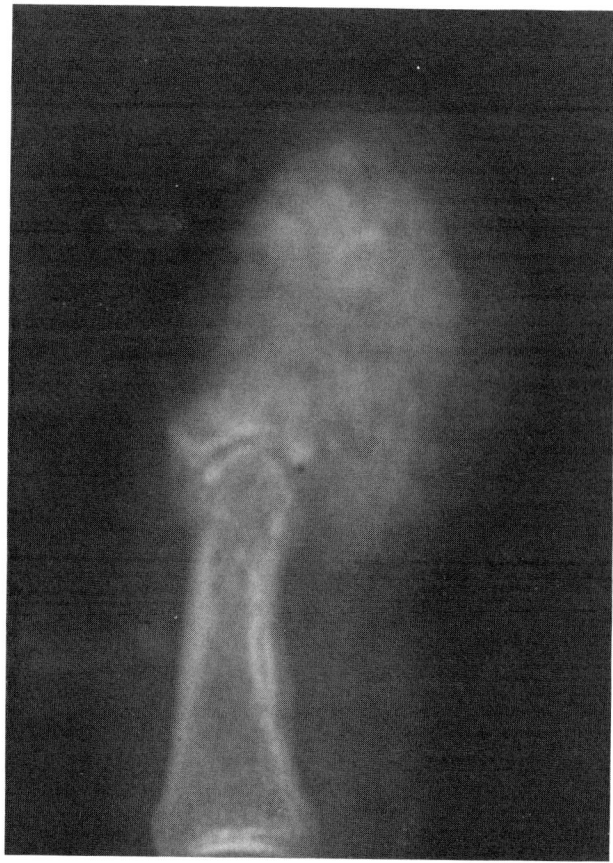

Table 107–3.   Etiologic Classification of Calcium Pyrophosphate Dihydrate Crystal Deposition Disease

I. Hereditary (see Table 107–4)
II. Sporadic (idiopathic)
III. Associated with metabolic disease (see Table 107–5)
IV. Associated with trauma or surgical procedures

CALCIUM PYROPHOSPHATE DIHYDRATE DEPOSITS IN ANIMALS

In addition to the previously mentioned dog, CPPD crystals have been identified in the cartilages of a barbary ape[73] and in elderly rhesus monkeys.[74,75] Calcifications in old rabbits have also been found, but were composed of apatite rather than of CPPD.[76]

ETIOLOGIC CLASSIFICATION

A tentative classification is given in Table 107–3. The genetic aberrations responsible for each of the nine largest reported series of *hereditary* cases probably differ.[27] Table 107–4 lists the evidence. Most families show disease transmission as an autosomal dominant trait. The Hungarian group has an HLA association, no male-to-male transmission, and symptomatic heterozygotes. Five of the other series showed male-to-male transmission of disease, indicating autosomal inheritance. Because nearly half the offspring of a heterozygote in all series developed radiographic evidence of CPPD crystal deposition, penetrance is nearly complete. "Associated" metabolic conditions, such as hyperparathyroidism, were rare in any of these kindreds. Phenotypic manifestations of the disease were severe in some kindreds and mild in others. The Hungarian homozygotes had severe disease, and the heterozygotes developed milder disease.[77]

The so-called *sporadic* or idiopathic cases deserve comment. Generally, no systematic search for the condition had been conducted among blood relatives, and none of the putative metabolic disease associations had been found. We examined 1 or more relatives clinically and radiologically in 12 of the first 18 cases and found 3 examples of familial disease. Such a study is difficult in the United States in view of the extreme mobility of our citizens and the widespread psychologic resistance to submit to study because of possible discovery of abnormality. In Spain, a study of 46 apparently "sporadic" cases revealed a familial incidence in 5 (11%).[78] This finding could represent a coincidence of sporadic cases in aged subjects. Another survey in Spain noted a 28% prevalence of familial CPPD deposition, in which at least one other blood relative had evidence of CPPD deposits.[78] It is likely that a thorough study of "sporadic cases" would result in reclassification of many as either hereditary or as associated with metabolic disease.

ASSOCIATED DISEASES

A number of metabolic diseases and physiologic stresses, such as aging and trauma, have been associated with CPPD deposition. Only aging and surgery have been statistically proved to occur with increased frequency in patients with CPPD deposition. Nonetheless, strong circumstantial evidence suggests that many of these associations are "true," and the converse has often been proved; that is, that radiographically evident chondrocalcinosis occurs more frequently in patients with several of these conditions, notably gout,[79] hemochromatosis,[80] and hyperparathyroidism,[81] than in age- and sex-matched control populations. Even when associations seem significant, however, a cause-and-effect relationship should not be inferred. If it is assumed that the putative associations are real, an immediate generalization is that all the metabolic diseases listed in Table 107–5 affect connective tissue metabolism in some way.

Table 107–4.   Characteristics of Hereditary Calcium Pyrophosphate Dihydrate Crystal Deposition Disease[27]

Series†	Type	Male-to-Male Transmission	Associations		
			Arthritis	Onset	HLA Antigens
Slovakian (Hungarian gene)		No	Severe	Early	Yes
Chilean (Spanish gene)	Autosomal dominant	Yes	Severe	Early	No
French	Autosomal dominant	Yes	Severe	Early	No
Japanese	Autosomal dominant	Yes	Severe	Early	NA*
Swedish	Autosomal dominant	Yes	Severe	Early	No
Dutch	Autosomal dominant	Yes	Mild	Early	No
Mexican-American	Autosomal dominant	Yes	Mild	Early	No
French-Canadian	Autosomal dominant	?	Mild	Early	No
Spanish	Autosomal dominant		Mild	Late	NA*

*NA = Not available.
†See reference 27 for references to all studies.

Table 107–5. Conditions Probably Associated With Calcium Pyrophosphate Dihydrate Crystal Deposition Disease*

Hyperparathyroidism
Familial hypocalciuric hypercalcemia
Hemochromatosis
Hemosiderosis
Hypophosphatasia
Hypomagnesemia
Hypothyroidism
Gout
Neuropathic joints
Aging
Amyloidosis
Trauma, including surgery

*Degenerative arthritis, included in our initial list, was deleted because it is probably an integral part of the basic disease process.

Analysis of our first seven cases and a review of the literature suggested that a number of metabolic and degenerative diseases are more prevalent than might be expected by chance.[2] Reported associations between CPPD deposition and other diseases must be interpreted with caution. Because CPPD deposits occur in about 5% of the adult population, they are associated with nearly all diseases on the basis of chance alone. Pragmatically, the clinician is well advised to keep the diseases listed in Table 107–5 in mind when confronted with a case of CPPD crystal deposition disease. Unsuspected hyperparathyroidism, hypothyroidism, and other metabolic abnormalities have been found repeatedly when appropriate laboratory studies were performed in such patients. Conversely, when arthritis supervenes in a patient with one of these metabolic conditions, the possibility of CPPD deposition disease should be considered in the differential diagnosis.

HYPERPARATHYROIDISM

Numerous reports of CPPD crystal deposition in patients with hyperparathyroidism have appeared,[81–84] and most series of patients with CPPD deposition show an incidence of 2 to 15%.[57,85,86] Conversely, 20 to 30% of patients with hyperparathyroidism have radiologic chondrocalcinosis.[81,87] Hyperparathyroid patients with CPPD deposits are older than those without such deposits. In most surgically treated cases, parathyroid adenoma rather than hyperplasia is found. Following parathyroidectomy, acute attacks of pseudogout are common.[35,39] During long-term postoperative followup study, the calcific deposits persist despite normalization of the serum calcium level.[88–90] An important effect of persistent hypercalcemia on the development of CPPD crystal deposits is reinforced by the reported associations of

joint symptoms and radiologic chondrocalcinosis suggestive of CPPD crystal deposits in persons with a benign lifelong condition called hypocalciuric hypercalcemia.[91,92] A better rheumatologic analysis of such patients is needed.

Elevated parathyroid hormone levels were found in 10 of 26 patents with CPPD deposition, only 4 of whom were hypercalcemic.[93] This finding has been confirmed, but its significance was obscured by the discovery of elevated parathyroid hormone levels in control patients with osteoarthritis of weight-bearing joints.[94] Nearly 75% of both groups had elevated levels of parathyroid hormone. One case of hypercalcemia was found in each group, but 2 additional patients with CPPD deposits had already undergone parathyroidectomy. Serum calcium levels showed a positive correlation with parathyroid hormone levels in both groups, rather than the expected inverse correlation, suggesting glandular autonomy. This relationship was not confirmed in a subsequent study using a different antibody in the parathyroid hormone assay.[95] Knee joint degeneration, as graded radiologically, correlated with the level of parathyroid hormone, and a positive correlation was seen between calcium levels and bone density, as quantified by radiodensitometry in both groups.[94] Normocalcemic hyperparathyroidism has been reported in patients with CPPD crystal deposition.[96]

Although the situation is far from clear, it appears that hyperparathyroidism may correlate with degenerative arthritis, rather than with the more obvious CPPD deposition. A well-known action of low doses of parathyroid hormone is to increase bone density; some patients with primary hyperparathyroidism may even have osteosclerosis.[82,97] It is possible that increased bone density, secondary to chronic, sustained, low-grade hyperparathyroidism, predisposes patients to osteoarthritis by the mechanism of subchondral microfractures of dense, less-compliant bone, as proposed by Pugh and colleagues.[98] Patients with primary osteoarthritis of the hip have increased bone density.[99]

HEMOCHROMATOSIS

The original report of arthritis in patients with hemochromatosis noted one example of articular cartilage calcification.[100] Many subsequent reports have documented this association.[27] Nearly half the patients with hemochromatosis have arthritis, and half of these have radiologic chondrocalcinosis.[101,102] Again, these are the older patients in the series.[102,103] CPPD deposition and related joint complaints are often present in patients with asymptomatic hemochromatosis. Involvement of metacarpophalangeal joints is more common in patients with hemochromatosis than in those with idiopathic chondrocalcinosis,[52] but the appearance of "squared off" bone ends, joint-space narrowing, and subchondral cysts in these joints was identical to that described by Martel and colleagues in patients with idiopathic chondrocalcinosis.[50] Adamson et al. pointed out more prevalent narrowing of the metacarpophalangeal joints, especially those in the fourth and fifth digits, peculiar hook-like osteophytes on the radial aspect of the metacarpal heads, and less prevalent scapholunate separation in CPPD crystal deposition.[103a] Appropriate treatment of the iron overload did not prevent the development of new calcifications over a 10-year period.[80] Radiologic evidence of CPPD crystal deposition increased from 7 to 13 of the 18 patients followed.

That the iron itself may be directly related to the calcific deposits is suggested by reports of CPPD deposition in patients with transfusion hemosiderosis.[27] Moreover, patients with hemophilia arthritis and chondrocalcinosis have been recorded.[104,105]

Just how tissue iron predisposes to CPPD crystal deposits is unclear. Ferrous, but not ferric, ions inhibited some inorganic pyrophosphatases[106]; ferric ions promoted CPPD crystal growth in vitro at lower inorganic pyrophosphate concentrations.[107] Synovial hemosiderosis slowed the metabolic clearance of radiolabeled CPPD crystals from rabbit joints by about 50%.[108] Finally, normocalcemic hyperparathyroidism may occur in 50% of patients with hemochromatosis.[109] Whether any of these mechanisms relate to the association of local tissue iron overload with CPPD crystals, however, is still conjectural.

OTHER DISORDERS

O'Duffy reported a patient with *hypophosphatasia* and CPPD deposits,[110] and subsequently several others have been described.[111,112] Inorganic pyrophosphate is a natural substrate of alkaline phosphatase,[113] and as urinary and plasma inorganic pyrophosphate levels are elevated in hypophosphatasia,[114,115] it is not surprising that hypophosphatasia may be associated with CPPD crystal deposition. Attempts at replacing alkaline phosphatase by infusing plasma from patients with Paget's disease of bone into a patient with infantile hypophosphatasia had no appreciable effect on the urinary excretion of inorganic pyrophosphate but may have improved the bony abnormalities.[116]

Hypomagnesemia associated with CPPD crystal deposition was first reported in 1974[94]; at least ten cases

have been recognized since (Table 107–6).[95,117–124a] This association makes sense teleologically, because magnesium increases the solubility of CPPD crystals[4] and is also an important cofactor for alkaline phosphatase[125] as well as for many inorganic pyrophosphatases.[106] In most reported instances, the defect appeared to be a failure of renal conservation of magnesium. In one case, magnesium replacement therapy decreased radiologic calcification.[119] A controlled study of oral magnesium therapy in patients with CPPD crystal deposits showed statistically significant beneficial effects.[126] CPPD deposition has also been reported in *Bartter's syndrome*,[123,124] perhaps secondary to the associated hypomagnesemia. Abnormalities in urinary or serum magnesium, however, are not present in most patients with CPPD crystal deposition.[94]

Hypothyroidism is associated with asymptomatic CPPD deposits, with frequent onset of joint inflammation after treatment with thyroid hormone.[127] One survey reported that 11% of 105 consecutive patients with CPPD deposition were hypothyroid.[128]

Periarticular and intra-articular *amyloid* deposits have been noted in association with CPPD deposition since the first report in 1976.[129] Four of five elderly patients with amyloid arthropathy, most of whom had carpal tunnel syndrome and pitting edema of the hands, had chondrocalcinosis.[130] Subsequent histologic studies have shown frequent amyloid deposits in cartilage and synovium, often in close proximity to the CPPD crystals.[27] Because most such patients are elderly, this association may represent the chance concurrence of two age-related processes. Amyloid is known to bind pyrophosphate analogues,[131] as well as calcium, however, and local sequestration could favor CPPD crystal formation. Amyloid has also been recently described in osteoarthritic cartilage[132,133] and has been reported in joints of senescent mice.[134]

Hyperuricemia, often accompanying mild azotemia, hypertension, or diuretic use, is common in the elderly population. The co-existence of pseudogout and *urate gout* varies from 2 to 8% in most reported series[27]; 5% of our series had both CPPD and MSU crystals. If the prevalence of MSU crystal deposition were 2% of the adult male population, as it might be,[19] then this association could be one of chance. Although 32% of a series of 31 gouty patients had radiologically evident chondrocalcinosis,[108] only 5% of another series of 43 gouty patients showed such deposits, a percentage no greater than in control subjects.[45] In carefully controlled prospective studies, the prevalence of chondrocalcinosis in patients with gout was 8 of 138; in age-matched normal control patients and in asymptomatic hyperuricemic patients, the prevalence was 0

Table 107–6. Cases of Hypomagnesemia Associated With CPPD Crystal Deposition

Author	No. of Cases	Age	Sex	Cause
McCarty et al.[94]	1	40	M	Unknown
Ellman et al.[95]	3	—	—	Renal wasting in one
Milazzo et al.[117]	1	40	F	Familial renal wasting
Rapado et al.[118]	1	38	M	Renal wasting
Runeburg et al.[119]	1	16	M	Renal wasting
Resnick and Rausch[120]	2	30	M	Renal wasting
		46	M	Renal wasting
Ishikawa;[121] Ishikawa et al.[124a]	5	35	M	Polycystic kidney
		43	F	Mild azotemia
		47	M	Mild azotemia
		55	M	Mild azotemia
		53	F	
Mayoux-Benhamou et al.[122]	2	—	—	Renal wasting
Bauer et al.[123]	2	36	M	Bartter's syndrome
		40	F	Bartter's syndrome
Goulon et al.[124]	2	41	F	Bartter's syndrome
		49	M	Bartter's syndrome

*These four are siblings who had severe destructive arthropathy and symptomatic arthritis associated with CPPD crystals with onset in the second and third decades of life.

of 142 and 1 of 84, respectively.[79,135] These results imply an association of CPPD with gout but not with hyperuricemia.

Diabetes mellitus, as defined by glucose intolerance, is common in the elderly. Controlled studies have not supported an association of CPPD deposition with diabetes.[60,136] A 26.5% incidence of diabetes in 49 patients with chondrocalcinosis was lower than that found (32.6%) in 46 control patients. If insulin requirement is used as a definition of diabetes, then the problem of small numbers in both patients and control groups supervenes.[94]

Ankylosing hyperostosis has been noted in serial studies of hereditary cases of CPPD deposition in Slovakia.[48] It appeared in one third of 18 Japanese patients,[137] and it was found in a number of hereditary cases studied in the Netherlands.[138] Conversely, CPPD deposits were found in 6% of 34 patients with ankylosing hyperostosis.

The association of chondrocalcinosis with acromegaly is probably fortuitous, despite the high plasma inorganic pyrophosphate levels in this disease.[139] The incidence of Paget's disease of bone is not increased in patients with CPPD deposits.[140] Definite crystal identification is still lacking in patients reported with Wilson's disease. The calcification in some patients with ochronosis appears to be CPPD.[27]

The routine examination of a newly diagnosed patient with CPPD deposition should include determinations of the following: serum calcium, magnesium, phosphorus, alkaline phosphatase, ferritin, iron and total iron-binding capacity, and thyroid-stimulating hormone, with further metabolic study if abnormalities are found.

TRAUMA/SURGERY

Mounting evidence links CPPD deposition with antecedent joint trauma or surgical procedures. In 1942, Weaver discussed monarticular calcific deposition following trauma.[141] Arthroscopic findings in such joints have been described.[142] Radiographic chondrocalcinosis has been recognized in hypermobile joints,[143] unstable joints,[144] and neuropathic joints.[54] The most compelling evidence was presented by Linden and Nilsson[64] and Doherty et al.[63] In the former study, 25 of 42 knees previously treated operatively for osteochondritis dissecans of the femoral condyle developed chondrocalcinosis in the operated, but not the contralateral, knee. A control group of meniscectomy patients developed chondrocalcinosis in 14 of 41 operated knees. In the latter study of postmeniscectomy patients, knee radiographs were obtained a mean of 25 years after operation; at that time, 20% of operated, but only 4% of contralateral, knees showed chondrocalcinosis.[63]

ROENTGENOGRAPHIC FEATURES

Heavy CPPD crystal deposits in fibrocartilaginous structures, hyaline (articular) cartilage, ligaments, and joint capsules have a characteristic appearance that is diagnostically helpful. Punctate and linear radiodensities are most frequently seen in the fibrocartilaginous menisci of the knee and usually involve both menisci of both knees (see Figs. 107–1C and 107–3B). Other fibrocartilaginous structures often calcified in this miliary fashion are the articular discs of the distal radioulnar joint (see Fig. 107–4), the symphysis pubis (see Fig. 107–5), the glenoid and acetabular labra, and the anulus fibrosus of the intervertebral discs. The articular discs of the sternoclavicular joints are often involved, but those of the temporomandibular joint are usually spared.

Calcification of the hyaline articular cartilage is common; the deposits in the midzonal layer appear as a radiopaque line paralleling the density of the underlying bone (see Figs. 107–3B and 107–4). The larger joints show these deposits most frequently, although they have been observed in nearly every diarthrodial joint. Calcifications of articular capsules or synovium, especially of the elbow, shoulder, hip, and knee, are frequent; the deposits appear as a broader, more diffuse, faintly opaque line (see Fig. 107–6).

Calcification of bursae, tendons, and ligaments also occurs in CPPD deposition disease. This calcification may represent BCP crystal deposition in some patients, but crystal-proved CPPD deposits have been reported in all the aforementioned sites. Synovial deposits may be so large as to mimic synovial chondromatosis,[145] and ligamentous or tendinous deposits may produce local compressive symptoms, such as carpal tunnel syndrome[146] or myelopathy, as already outlined.

Subchondral bone cysts are common and can attain a large size. Histologic examination of the walls of the lesion shown in Figure 107–7 confirmed that it was only a bone cyst. How such lesions are related to CPPD deposition disease is unknown, but they occur frequently enough to be a diagnostic clue.[33]

A number of distinct regional radiographic abnormalities may suggest CPPD deposition. A peculiar erosion of the femoral cortex superior to the patella has been reported.[147,148] This lesion appears to correlate with osteoarthritis of the patellofemoral compartment (see Fig. 107–9). Carpal instability reported in association with CPPD deposits resembles that of RA.[149] A particular propensity for radiocarpal involvement has been observed. Navicular-lunate dissociation is thought to result from degeneration of the ligamentous structures. Axial involvement has been described.[34] In the lumbar spine, multiple levels of anulus fibrosus calcification, vacuum disc phenomena, and disc narrowing are emphasized. A syndrome of acute neck pain associated with calcifications surrounding the odontoid process, the "crowned dens syndrome," has been described.[63] It has occurred in patients who have either BCP or CPPD crystal deposition in peripheral joints. Sacroiliac joint abnormalities include subchondral erosions, reactive sclerosis, and bilateral vacuum phenomena. Axial

involvement is particularly prominent in uremic patients with secondary hyperparathyroidism.[149a]

Features that may accompany CPPD crystal deposition include joint degeneration, tibial stress fractures, and avascular necrosis of the medial or lateral femoral condyle. Degenerative changes in joints not commonly involved in primary osteoarthritis, such as the metacarpophalangeal, radiocarpal, elbow, and shoulder joints may suggest underlying CPPD crystal deposition even in the absence of radiographic chondrocalcinosis. Subchondral cysts, bone and cartilage fragmentation, and variable osteophyte formation are characteristic (see Fig. 107–10). The best serial studies are those of the Hungarian familial cases.[48] CPPD deposits first appeared in radiographically normal cartilage, and degeneration inevitably followed. Tibial stress fractures were reported in five elderly patients with CPPD deposition and severe degenerative knee disease.[150] Because their knees were usually painful before the fractures, the source of increased pain was not readily apparent. Interestingly, 4 of 14 patients with osteonecrosis of the medial femoral condyle had CPPD knee deposits,[151] an association subsequently confirmed.[152]

An arthritic patient may be screened for CPPD deposition with four suitably exposed roentgenograms: (1 and 2) an anteroposterior view of each knee; (3) an anteroposterior view of the pelvis; and (4) a posteroanterior view of the wrists. If nothing diagnostic is seen on these films, a more extensive survey is unlikely to be helpful.

The chemical composition of the crystal deposits may be inferred with confidence from typical roentgenograms. Caution must be exercised when the calcifications are faint or atypical, however, because of the possibility of DCPD, BCP, or calcium oxalate crystal deposits or vascular calcifications, all of which are symmetric.[19]

PATHOLOGIC FEATURES

The joints of three cases at necropsy and seven anatomic cadavers were extensively examined.[19] The distribution of calcification generally paralleled that seen on radiogram. Joint capsules, especially in the hip and shoulder, and the hyaline articular cartilages, were often affected, but the heaviest deposits were in fibrocartilaginous structures. The menisci of the knee were involved in all cases (see Fig. 107–4A). Heavy deposits were often noted in tendons and in intra-articular ligaments, such as the cruciate ligaments in the knee. Microscopically, the deposits were composed of various-sized microcrystalline aggregates of CPPD (Fig. 107–12). Their diameters varied from 15 μm to 0.6 cm; the larger ones appeared grossly as white chalky deposits. It was difficult on gross inspection to distinguish these deposits (see Fig. 107-3A) from the white chalky lesions of true gout. These lesions were distributed diffusely in fibrocartilage, mainly in the midzonal or superficial areas of hyaline cartilage (Fig. 107-13).

The smallest, and presumably the earliest, crystals appeared at the lacunar margin of chondrocytes. When adjacent chondrocytes were damaged, pericellular matrix vesicles were often seen. Increased glycogen islands and rough endoplasmic reticulum were observed in the chondrocytes.[153] The surrounding matrix may appear normal or granular. Collagen fibril fragmentation in uncalcified areas of CPPD cartilage has been described in familial cases.[154] Larger superficial deposits occur in degenerative cartilages, usually at sites of surface ulcerations and fissuring and often associated with chondrocyte "cloning."

Ishikawa has shown convincing evidence of abnormal proteoglycan deposition within chondrocytes in the immediate vicinity of early CPPD crystal deposits (Fig. 107-14A and B). These "red cells," stained with safranin-0, were not seen if the tissue was first exposed to either papain or chondroitinase ABC, which confirms their proteoglycan nature. "Red cells" were a constant feature of evolving, but not of "mature," CPPD crystal deposits in fibrocartilage, hyaline cartilage, and synovium showing chondroid metaplasia.[154a] They were seen in tissue from both sporadic and familial cases. Ishikawa also found the following: (1) absence of normal safranin-0 staining in the matrix

in areas of early crystal deposition; (2) "packing" of the proteoglycan-denuded collagen fibers in these same areas; (3) hypertrophy and mitotic activity of the red cells (Fig. 107-14A and B); (4) the appearance of CPPD crystals in empty chondrocyte lacunae; and (5) "mature" deposits were ringed with dense, proteoglycan-free collagen, as shown in Figure 107-14C, but the crystals were coated with a thin film of proteoglycan. No collagen or cells could be identified within these crystal masses by light or electron microscopy. The surrounding matrix now contained normal-appearing cells and stained normally.

Ishikawa speculated that the cell-associated proteoglycan may indicate faulty release from the chondrocytes after synthesis, or that it may enter these cells by endocytosis. His findings deserve further exploration and, if confirmed, must be taken into account in any scheme of the pathogenesis of CPPD crystal deposition.

In three patients, superficial amyloid deposits were adjacent to CPPD crystals.[132] Isolated descriptions of CPPD crystals within chondrocytes have been reported,[155-157] indicating that chondrocytes may phagocytose crystals with attendant biologic consequences (see Chapter 108).

In no case has a cause-and-effect relationship been established between crystal deposits and morphologic changes.

Synovial biopsy material obtained with the Polley-Bickel needle showed inflammatory and reparative changes consistent with the clinical state of the joint at the time of biopsy. Early in an acute attack, the

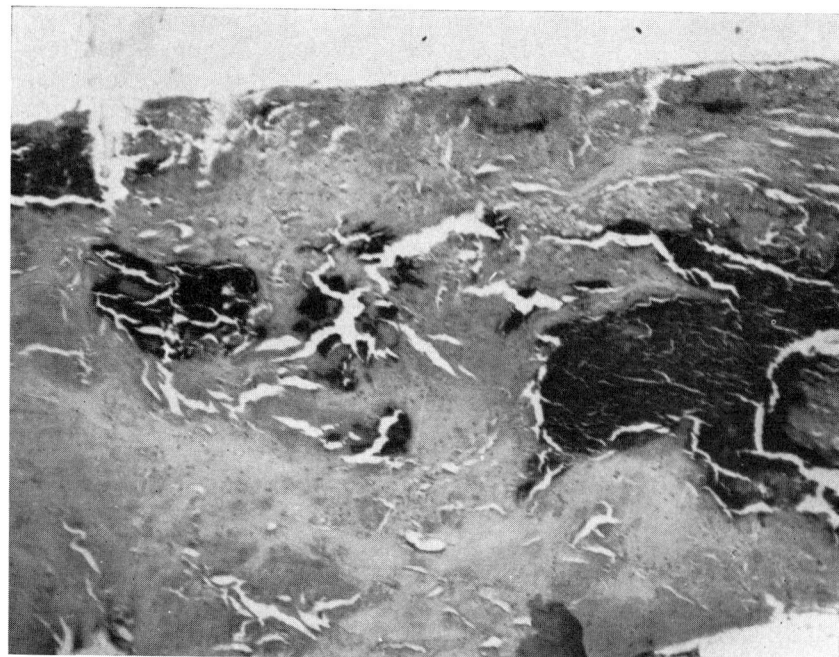

FIG. 107-12. Photomicrograph of a section through the meniscus shown in Figure 107-4A; various-sized aggregates of calcified material are distributed throughout (hematoxylin and eosin stain, ×26).

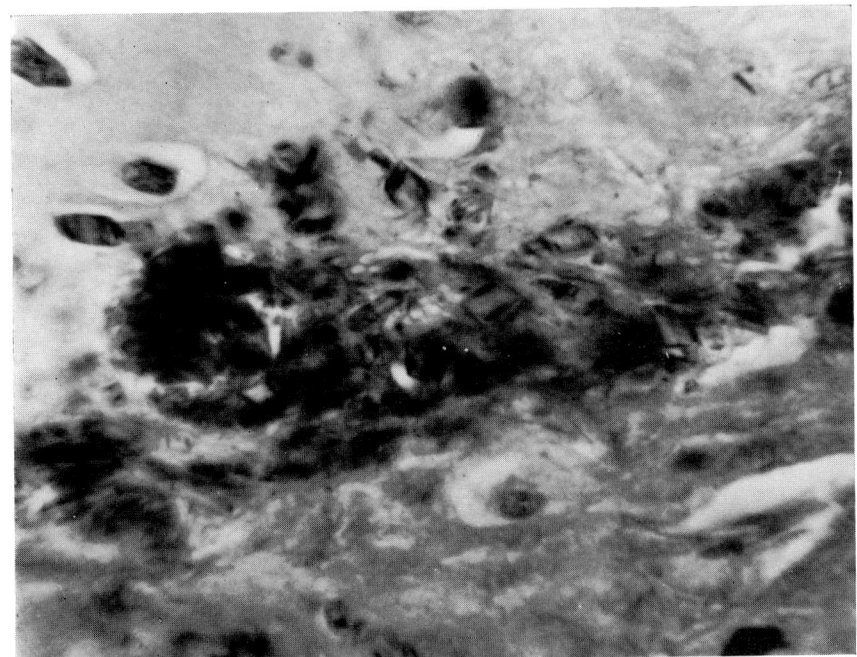

FIG. 107–13. Photomicrograph of the smallest deposits found shows them surrounding the lacunae of the chondrocytes. This process begins in the midzonal layer of articular cartilage, more diffusely in fibrocartilage. Individual crystals of calcium pyrophosphate dihydrate are visible in this section (alazarin red, ×800; linear magnification ×3).

edematous synovium was infiltrated with PMN leukocytes; later, mononuclear infiltration and fibroblastic proliferation were seen. Synovial proliferation and infiltration with chronic inflammatory cells in chronically symptomatic joints can resemble rheumatoid pannus. Crystals have been identified in the superficial synovium under polarized light and by electron microscopy.[156a] In patients with pseudo-osteoarthritis undergoing knee replacement, synovial deposits were focal and concentrated in avascular areas.[157]

PATHOGENESIS

The cause of CPPD crystal deposition is unknown. Conceptually, formation of CPPD crystals in cartilage may result from elevated levels of either calcium or inorganic pyrophosphate (PPi), from changes in the matrix that promote crystal formation, or from combinations of these factors (Fig. 107–15). Because CPPD crystal deposition is a clinically heterogeneous disorder, different factors probably predominate in individual cases, much as hyperuricemia preceding MSU crystal deposition may have different causes.

Bjelle favors the hypothesis that matrix changes antedate and predispose persons to CPPD crystal formation. In studies of Swedish patients with familial CPPD deposition, he found weakly staining midzonal matrix with decreased collagen content, some fragmentation of collagen fibers, and an abnormal hexosamine profile.[154] The proportions of keratan sulfate and chondroitin-6-sulfate were increased, and those of chondroitin-4-sulfate were decreased. A decrease in mucin-like oligosaccharides was found. Because these changes were independent of the amount of crystal deposits and because morphologically abnormal crystal-free areas in midzonal cartilage were seen by electron microscopy, Bjelle postulated a primary role of a matrix abnormality in promoting CPPD mineral phase.

The ionic composition of matrix may also affect CPPD crystal formation. Ferrous ions inhibit some pyrophosphatases[106]; ferric ions lower the formation product for CPPD crystals in vitro[107] and slowed the intracellular degradation of CPPD crystals injected into rabbit joints.[108] Hypomagnesemia, both primary and secondary to Bartter's syndrome, has also been associated with chondrocalcinosis. Magnesium is a cofactor for many pyrophosphatases and increases the solubility of CPPD crystals.[4] Therefore, its deficiency may decrease hydrolysis of PPi and may slow crystal dissolution. Profound hypomagnesemia induced by dietary magnesium deprivation did not change the rate of CPPD crystal clearance from rabbit joints, however.[158] Elevations of inorganic phosphate have promoted CPPD crystal nucleation and growth in vitro and may act similarly in vivo.[159] The effect of inorganic phosphate in aqueous solution on CPPD crystal formation is most prominent in the 0.01 to 1.0 mM range.[160] That such an aberration may exist is suggested by the finding of elevated levels of inorganic phosphate in synovial fluid in pseudogout.[161]

Studies of crystal formation in gels provide indirect

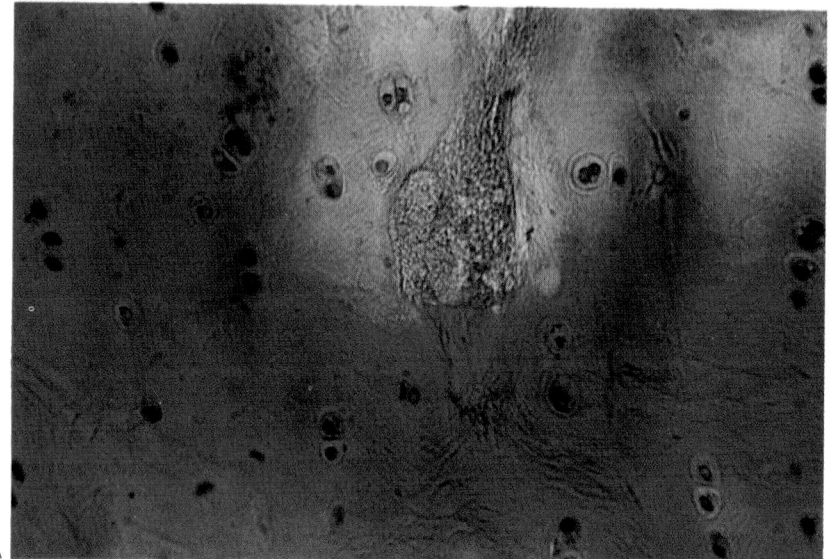

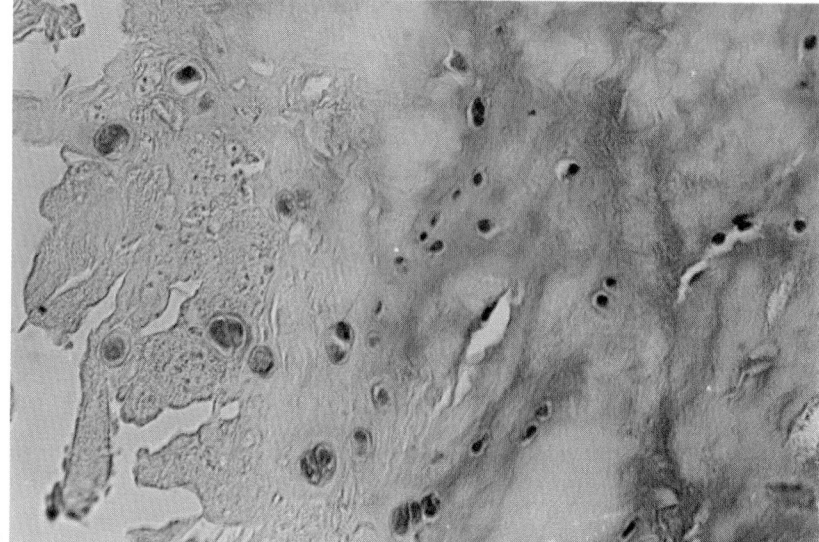

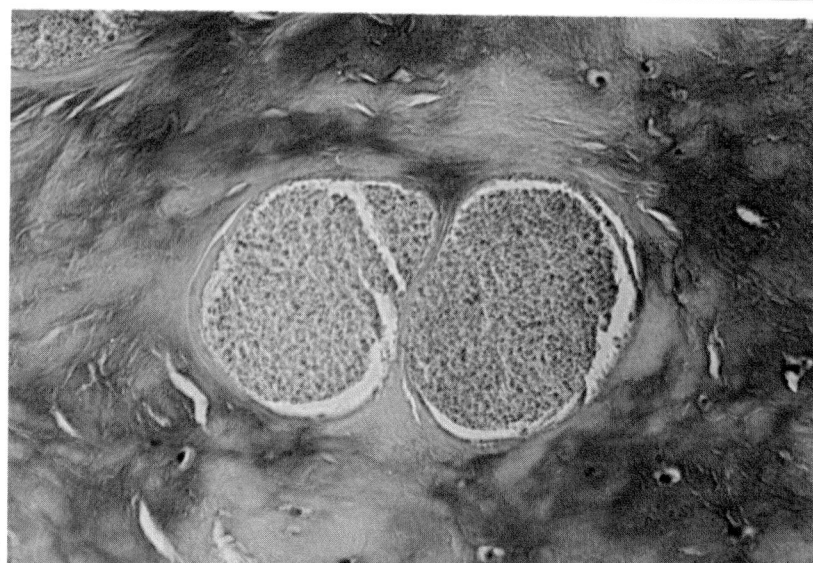

FIG. 107–14. *A,* Transitional zone articular cartilage from a 63-year-old man with sporadic calcium pyrophosphate dihydrate (CPPD) crystal deposition showing a small crystal deposit. The chondrocytes about the deposit have a characteristic loss of dark nuclear staining. Instead, they appear red because of their proteoglycan content. The matrix about the crystal deposit has lost its proteoglycan (safranin-O-fast green–iron hematoxylin ×370). *B,* Fibrocartilaginous meniscus from a 73-year-old woman with sporadic CPPD crystal deposition showing normal-appearing cartilage on the right. The area on the left, showing fibrillation and no matrix proteoglycan, contains the crystals. Again, the chondrocytes stain red and are hypertrophic, with some mitotic activity (same stains as *A,* ×370). *C,* Mature deposits in the same tissue showing crystal masses encapsulated by dense proteoglycan-free collagen. The crystals are coated with proteoglycan, but neither cells nor collagen exists among them. The surrounding matrix and chondrocytes now stain normally (same stains as *A,* ×370). (Courtesy Koichiro Ishikawa, M.D.)

FIG. 107–15. CPPD crystal deposition theoretically may result from abnormalities of matrix, calcium metabolism, or PPi metabolism. Possibilities are shown in the shaded areas of these Venn diagrams.

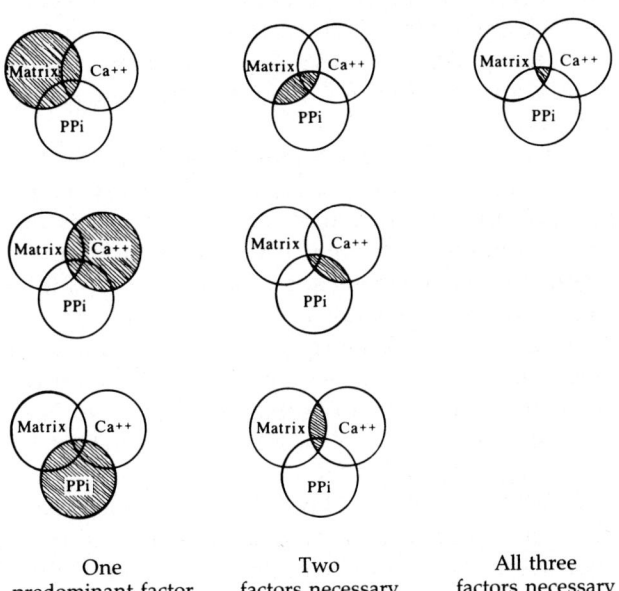

| One predominant factor | Two factors necessary | All three factors necessary |

evidence that organic matrix components may play a role as nucleating agents in CPPD crystal formation. In aqueous solutions, CPPD crystal synthesis occurs at acid pH or at high ionic concentrations.[5,158,160] In model collagen gels, however, crystals are formed at neutral pH[162] and at PPi concentrations between 2 and 20 μM.[163] Formation of amorphous calcium pyrophosphate and orthorhombic calcium pyrophosphate tetrahydrate preceded formation of monoclinic and triclinic CPPD crystals identical to those observed in vivo.[164] These studies seem particularly relevant because cartilage is a gel. The modulatory effect of other organic matrix components, such as proteoglycans, on CPPD crystal formation has not been studied systematically.

No systematic study has been made of cartilage interstitial fluid calcium in patients with CPPD deposition. Clearly, some of these patients have hyperparathyroidism, usually due to adenoma, with associated hypercalcemia. CPPD deposition has also been noted in patients with familial hypocalciuric hypercalcemia,[91,92] further supporting a role for calcium in promoting CPPD deposition.

PPi is produced by most biosynthetic reactions in macromolecular synthesis.[114] The ubiquitous pyrophosphatases, hydrolyzing PPi in inorganic orthophosphate, drive these reactions in the direction of synthesis, but the intracellular enzymatic hydrolysis of PPi does not go to completion, and detectable amounts are measurable in cells, including fibroblasts and chondrocytes.[165]

The amount of PPi produced in the body is immense. It has been calculated that 30 g are made daily in the human liver as a by-product of the synthesis of albumin alone.[114] Only a small amount of that synthesized appears in the urine (approximately 10 to 100 μmol daily), where it acts as a powerful inhibitor of crystal nucleation and growth. The turnover rate of plasma PPi in dogs is only about 2 minutes, which further complicates the interpretation of plasma values. Neither the source nor the fate of plasma PPi is known.

Much PPi is absorbed to bone mineral,[166,167] where it is thought to act as a regulator of mineralization. In addition to its effect on crystal precipitation, it retards the conversion of amorphous calcium phosphate into crystalline hydroxyapatite, inhibits crystal aggregation, and slows the dissolution rate of hydroxyapatite crystals. The diphosphonates, which have P-C-P bonds, instead of P-O-P bonds, are nonhydrolyzable analogues of PPi. These compounds have similar biologic effects and are used experimentally as therapeutic agents in various diseases of mineral metabolism and, coupled with tin and ^{99m}Tc, as bone-scanning agents.[114]

Studies of PPi metabolism were stimulated by recognition of this substance as a constituent of the crystal deposits. Because urinary levels are much easier to quantify than those in plasma, these were measured earliest and were found to be normal.[168,168a] Blood levels of PPi were later measured; serum contained two to three times the concentration of plasma.[169] This increase resulted from the release of PPi by platelets during clotting. Plasma levels were higher in venous blood than in arterial blood, increased with systemic exercise, and spuriously elevated by application of a venous tourniquet before phlebotomy.[170,171] Plasma concentrations in sporadic cases of CPPD deposition were similar to those in osteoarthritic or normal control subjects.[168,171,172] In patients with hypophosphatasia, a disease associated with CPPD deposition, both urinary and plasma levels of PPi were elevated,[115,173] presumably as a result of decreased hydrolysis.

Abnormal local metabolism of PPi was suggested by reports of elevated levels in synovial fluids from patients with CPPD crystal deposition, although elevations were also observed in synovial fluids from patients with gout, osteoarthritis, and even RA. The highest joint fluid levels were found in the most severely degenerated joints, as judged radiographically.[161] PPi levels were lower during acute attacks and rose as the episode subsided,[161] probably because of increased synovial blood flow during acute attacks with more rapid equilibration with plasma PPi. The elevated synovial fluid levels could not be explained by dissolution of crystals in the fluid. The gradient between synovial fluid and plasma implied a local origin of PPi.[161,172] The site of the synovial fluid production was expected to be cartilage, based on the histologic observation that the smallest and presumably the earliest crystals are seen adjacent to chondrocytes. Subsequent studies indicated that articular hyaline and fibrocartilages in organ culture liberated PPi into the ambient media, whereas synovium, subchondral bone, and nonarticular (elastic) cartilages did not.[174,175] Liberation of PPi correlated directly with uronic acid secretion in one study[175] but not in another.[176] Extrapolation of the amount produced by incubated slices to the amount of cartilage in a whole knee joint yielded figures for local production of the same order of magnitude as estimated from in vivo kinetic experiments.[174,177] Thus, cartilage is the most likely source of locally elevated concentrations of PPi in CPPD deposition.

Augmented PPi generation was found in the presence of adenosine triphosphate (ATP) by extracts of cartilages from patients with CPPD deposition, as compared with generation in extracts of osteoarthritic or normal cartilages.[178] ATP was enzymatically hydrolyzed to adenosine monophosphate and PPi by ATP pyrophosphohydrolase. A similar activity had been described in calcifying sheep cartilage.[179] Subsequent reports have verified the presence of this enzyme in matrix vesicle fractions of epiphyseal cartilage,[180,181] where it may play a role in calcium pyrophosphate precipitation.[182,183] We have characterized this activity as a chondrocyte nucleoside triphosphate pyrophosphohydrolase with broad substrate reactivity and as an ectoenzyme.[184] The cell surface location of this enzyme has been confirmed by Howell et al.[185] and Caswell and Russell.[186]

Because CPPD crystals appear to form extracellularly adjacent to chondrocytes and because PPi does not passively cross cell membranes,[187] the external position of this enzyme might allow the generation of PPi at the site of crystal formation in the presence of suitable substrate. Levels of nucleoside triphosphate pyrophosphohydrolase activity were higher in the synovial fluid of patients with CPPD deposition and osteoarthritis than in fluids from patients with RA or gout.[188] Enzyme activity correlated directly with the concentration of PPi in synovial fluid. In addition to elevated nucleoside triphosphate pyrophosphohydrolase activity in detergent extracts of cartilages with CPPD deposition, Tenenbaum et al. also described higher levels of 5'nucleotidase activity and

lower levels of alkaline phosphatase and PPiase activity than in osteoarthritic cartilages.[178] All these aberrations would favor the accumulation of PPi in the ectoenzyme system shown in Figure 107–16. A naturally occurring substrate for nucleoside triphosphate pyrophosphohydrolase in cartilage has not yet been conclusively demonstrated, but preliminary studies found concentrations of ATP in synovial fluid as high as 1 μM.[189]

Lust et al. found intracellular PPi levels twice those of control subjects in cultured skin fibroblasts and in lymphoblasts obtained from affected members of a French kindred with familial CPPD deposition.[165,190] A generalized metabolic abnormality phenotypically expressed only in chondrocytes was postulated. The PPi total and releasable content of platelets in 5 patients with sporadic or familial CPPD deposition was similar to that of 17 control subjects,[191] but a significant positive correlation was found between platelet PPi content and the age of the donor.

PPi levels in cultured skin fibroblasts from patients with both sporadic and familial CPPD crystal deposition were significantly elevated compared to those from normal persons or subjects with osteoarthritis.[192] Activity of ectonucleoside triphosphate pyrophosphohydrolase was elevated in fibroblasts from sporadic, but not familial, CPPD crystal deposition.[192] Lastly, intracellular PPi levels and ectonucleoside triphosphate pyrophosphohydrolase activity were positively correlated in fibroblasts from each of the groups studied.

Although these biochemical changes cannot yet be directly related to the pathogenesis of CPPD crystal deposition, they represent the earliest biochemical correlates of this metabolic arthropathy.

FIG. 107–16. Postulated enzymatic cascade of inorganic pyrophosphate (PPi) production from nucleotide triphosphate (NTP). Elevated NTP pyrophosphohydrolase and 5'nucleotidase activities and decreased inorganic pyrophosphatase activity in chondrocalcinosic cartilages all favor PPi accumulation. 5'NTase = 5'nucleotidase; PPiase = inorganic pyrophosphatase; Pi = inorganic phosphate; N = nucleotide; NMP = nucleotide monophosphate.

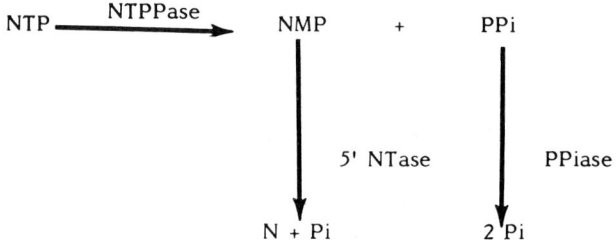

FIG. 107–17. Prevention of crystal formation or dissolution of CPPD crystals would have little effect on cartilage degeneration except in schema number 3 or if an amplification loop exists.
*amplification loop.[63a]

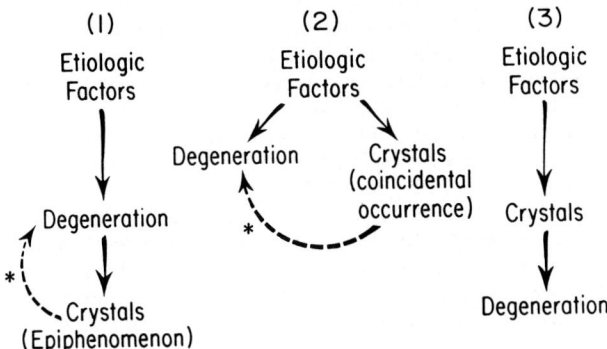

THERAPY

Acute attacks of pseudogout are readily treated by a number of methods, including (1) thorough aspiration of the joint to remove crystals; (2) administration of nonsteroidal anti-inflammatory drugs, such as indomethacin; (3) joint immobilization; and (4) local injection of microcrystalline corticosteroid esters. Intravenous colchicine works as well in pseudogout as it does in gout.[41] The prophylactic effectiveness of oral colchicine in patients who have recurrent attacks has been demonstrated.[193,194]

No known way exists to halt the progressive deposition of crystals or to remove those already deposited. Correction of associated metabolic disorders such as hyperparathyroidism, myxedema, and hemochromatosis has not resulted in the disappearance of radiographic cartilage calcification. New calcifications have developed in some such patients.[80] Attempts at lavage of affected joints with magnesium chloride were unsuccessful in removing significant amounts of crystal, but acute attacks were precipitated.[195] Several examples of spontaneous disappearance of calcific deposits have been reported. Wrist calcification disappeared in one case after immobilization and subsequent development of reflex sympathetic dystrophy.[196] The increased blood flow may have increased the clearance of pyrophosphate from the wrist. Another case associated with familial hypomagnesemia showed radiologic evidence of decreased meniscal calcification 2 years after institution of magnesium treatment.[119] In a double-blinded, placebo-controlled trial of magnesium carbonate treatment for sporadic CPPD crystal deposition, radiographic calcification did not change over 6 months, although symptoms improved significantly.[120]

Treatment of the frequently associated degenerative disease is the same as for osteoarthritis. Intraarticular injection with ^{90}Y was reported to ameliorate pain and stiffness and decrease the size of effusion in knee joints over a 6-month period.[197] Joint deformity and radiographic changes were not better than in the contralateral, uninjected knee, however.

Even if effective treatment were available, two problems would remain. First, no biochemical marker identifies those patients who will develop crystal deposition. We must await radiographic evidence of cartilage calcification or identification of crystals in joint fluids, both of which probably signal longstanding disease. Therapeutic interventions at this stage may be much less effective. Second, although treatment of the crystal deposition would probably ameliorate or would prevent acute pseudogout attacks, it might have no effect on the much more significant degenerative joint disease. Figure 107–17 illustrates three potential pathogenetic sequences relating degenerative disease to crystal deposition. Only in sequence 3, which is analogous to the pathogenesis of tophaceous gout, would removal or prevention of crystal formation affect cartilage degeneration. Dieppe has postulated that the biologic phenomena induced by crystals may act as an amplification loop, as shown by the hatched lines in sequences 1 and 2, which envision crystal formation as an epiphenomenon or as a coincidental phenomenon, respectively.[63a] If an amplification loop exists, then prevention of crystal formation or crystal removal would also have a salutary effect. Perhaps each of the paradigms shown here actually occurs in patients with CPPD crystal deposition, with varying sequences in different patients. Because the clinical importance of CPPD crystals will rise as the population ages, these therapeutic considerations are of more than theoretic interest.

REFERENCES

1. McCarty, D.J., and Hollander, J.L.: Identification of urate crystals in gouty synovial fluid. Ann. Intern. Med., 54:452–460, 1961.
2. McCarty, D.J., Kohn, N.N., and Faires, J.S.: The significance of calcium phosphate crystals in the synovial fluid of arthritis patients: The "pseudogout syndrome." I. Clinical aspects. Ann. Intern. Med., 56:711–737, 1962.
3. Kohn, N.N., et al.: The significance of calcium phosphate crystals in the synovial fluid of arthritis patients: The "pseudogout syndrome." II. Identification of crystals. Ann. Intern. Med., 56:738–745, 1962.
4. Bennett, R.M., Lehr, J.R., and McCarty, D.J.: Factors affecting the solubility of calcium pyrophosphate dihydrate crystals. J. Clin. Invest., 56:1571–1579, 1975.
5. Brown, E.H., et al.: Preparation and characterization of some

calcium pyrophosphates. J. Agr. Food Chem., *11*:214–222, 1963.

6. McCarty, D.J., and Faires, J.S.: A comparison of the duration of local anti-inflammatory effect of several adrenocorticosteroid esters: A bioassay technique. Curr. Ther. Res., *5*:284–290, 1963.

7. McCarty, D.J.: Crystal-induced inflammation: Syndromes of gout and pseudogout. Geriatrics, *18*:467–478, 1963.

8. Zitnan, D., and Sitaj, S.: Mnohopocentna familiarna kalcifikacin articularnych chrupiek. Bratisl. Lek. Listy, *38*:217–228, 1958.

9. McCarty, D.J.: The Heberden Oration, 1982. Crystals, joints, and consternation. Ann. Rheum. Dis., *42*:243–253, 1983.

10. Zitnan, D., and Sitaj, S.: Chondrocalcinosis articularis. Section I. Clinical and radiological study. Ann. Rheum. Dis., *22*:142–169, 1963.

11. Bennett, E.H.: Abnormal deposits in joints. Dublin J. Med. Sci., *65*:161–163, 1903.

12. Mandl, F.: Zur pathologie und therapie der Zwischenknorpilerkrankungen des Kniegelenks. Arch. Klin. Chir., *146*:149–214, 1927.

13. Werwath, K.: Abnormal depositions of calcium within the knee joints, an addition to the question of primary "meniscopathy." Acta Radiol., *37*:169–171, 1926.

14. Tobler, T.H.: The normal and pathological histology of the meniscus of the knee joint. Schweiz Med. Wochenschr., *59*:10–21, 1929.

15. Bennett, G.A., Waine, H., and Bauer, W.: Changes in the Knee Joint at Various Ages. New York, Commonwealth Fund, 1942.

16. Ellman, M.H., and Levin, B.: Chondrocalcinosis in elderly persons. Arthritis Rheum., *18*:43–47, 1975.

17. Memin, Y., Monville, C., and Ryckewaert, A.: La chondrocalcinose articulaire apres 80 ans. Rev. Rheum. Mal. Osteoartic., *45*:77–82, 1978.

18. Wilkins, E., et al.: Osteoarthritis and articular chondrocalcinosis in the elderly. Ann. Rheum. Dis., *42*:280–284, 1983.

19. McCarty, D.J., et al.: Studies on pathological calcifications in human cartilage. I. Prevalence and types of crystal deposits in the menisci of two hundred fifteen cadavera. J. Bone Joint Surg., *48A*:308–325, 1966.

20. Gaucher, A., et al.: Identification des cristaux observes dans les arthropathies destructives de la chondrocalcinose. Rev. Rheum. Mal. Osteoartic., *44*:407–414, 1977.

21. Utsinger, P.D.: Abstract 448. *In* Proceedings of the Fourteenth International Congress of Rheumatology, San Francisco, June, 1977.

22. Dieppe, P.A., et al.: Apatite deposition disease. Lancet, *1*:266–270, 1976.

23. Schumacher, H.R., et al.: Arthritis associated with apatite crystals. Ann. Intern. Med., *87*:411–416, 1977.

24. Dieppe, P.A., et al.: Mixed crystal deposition disease and osteoarthritis. Br. Med. J., *1*:150–151, 1978.

25. Doyle, D.V., et al.: Mixed crystal deposition in an osteoarthritic joint. J. Pathol., *123*:1–4, 1977.

26. Halverson, P.B., et al.: Milwaukee shoulder syndrome: Report of eleven additional cases with concomitant involvement of the knee in seven instances. Semin. Arthritis Rheum., *14*:36–44, 1984.

27. Ryan, L., and McCarty, D.: Calcium pyrophosphate crystal deposition disease; pseudogout; articular chondrocalcinosis. *In* Arthritis and Allied Conditions. 10th Ed. Edited by D.J. McCarty. Philadelphia, Lea & Febiger, 1985.

28. Gatter, R.A., and McCarty, D.J.: Pathological tissue calcification in man. Arch. Pathol., *84*:346–353, 1967.

29. Bjelle, A., Crocker, P., and Willoughby, D.: Ultra-microcrystals in pyrophosphate arthropathy. Acta Med. Scand., *207*:89–92, 1980.

30. Parel, H., Reginato, A., and Schumacher, H.R.: Alizarin red S staining as a screening test to detect calcium compounds in synovial fluid. Arthritis Rheum., *26*:191–200, 1983.

31. Cohen, A.S., Brandt, K.D., and Krey, P.R.: Synovial fluid. *In* Laboratory Diagnostic Procedures in the Rheumatic Diseases. 2nd Ed. Edited by A.S. Cohen. Boston, Little, Brown, 1975.

32. Bennett, R.M., Mall, J.C., and McCarty, D.J.: Pseudogout in acute neuropathic arthropathy: A clue to pathogenesis. Arthritis Rheum. Dis., *33*:563–567, 1974.

33. Resnick, D., et al.: Clinical, radiographic and pathologic abnormalities in calcium pyrophosphate dihydrate deposition disease (CPPD) pseudogout. Diagn. Radiol., *122*:1–15, 1977.

34. Martel, W., et al.: Further observations on the arthropathy of calcium pyrophosphate crystal deposition disease. Radiology, *141*:1–15, 1981.

35. O'Duffy, J.D.: Clinical studies of acute pseudogout attacks. Arthritis Rheum., *19*(Suppl.):349–353, 1976.

36. Dieppe, P.A., et al.: Pyrophosphate arthropathy: A clinical and radiological study of 105 cases. Ann. Rheum. Dis., *41*:371–376, 1982.

37. Fam, A.G., et al.: Clinical and roentgenographic aspects of pseudogout: A study of 50 cases and review. Can. Med. Assoc. J., *124*:545–550, 1981.

38. McCarty, D.J.: Diagnostic mimicry in arthritis: Patterns of joint involvement associated with calcium pyrophosphate dihydrate crystal deposits. Bull. Rheum. Dis., *25*:804–809, 1975.

39. Bilezikian, J.P., et al.: Pseudogout after parathyroidectomy. Lancet, *1*:445–449, 1973.

40. Phelps, P.: Polymorphonuclear leukocyte motility in vitro. IV. Colchicine inhibition of chemotactic activity formation after phagocytosis of urate crystals. Arthritis Rheum., *13*:1–9, 1970.

41. Spilberg, I., et al.: Colchicine and pseudogout. Arthritis Rheum., *23*:1062–1063, 1980.

42. Moskowitz, R.W., et al.: Chronic synovitis as a manifestation of calcium crystal deposition disease. Arthritis Rheum., *14*:109–116, 1971.

43. Resnick, D., et al.: Rheumatoid arthritis and pseudorheumatoid arthritis in calcium pyrophosphate dihydrate crystal deposition disease. Radiology, *140*:615–621, 1981.

43a. Wallace, S.L., et al.: Preliminary criteria for the classification of the acute arthritis of primary gout. Arthritis Rheum., *20*:895–900, 1977.

44. Bywaters, E.G.L.: Calcium pyrophosphate deposits in synovial membrane. Ann. Rheum. Dis., *31*:219–220, 1972.

45. Good, A.E., and Rapp, R.: Chondrocalcinosis of the knee with gout and rheumatoid arthritis. N. Engl. J. Med., *277*:286–290, 1967.

46. Doherty, M., Dieppe, P., and Watt, I.: Low incidence of calcium pyrophosphate dihydrate crystal deposition in rheumatoid arthritis, with modification of radiographic features in coexistent disease. Arthritis Rheum., *27*:1002–1009, 1984.

47. Bong, D., and Bennett, R.: Pseudogout mimicking systemic disease. JAMA, *246*:1438–1440, 1981.

48. Zitnan, D., and Sitaj, S.: Natural course of articular chondrocalcinosis. Arthritis Rheum., *19*(Suppl.):363–390, 1976.

49. Genant, H.K.: Roentgenographic aspects of calcium pyrophosphate dihydrate crystal deposition disease (pseudogout). Arthritis Rheum., *19*:307–328, 1976.

50. Martel, W., et al.: A roentgenologically distinctive arthropathy

in some patients with pseudogout syndrome. AJR, *109*:587–605, 1970.

51. Hamilton, E.B.D., et al.: The arthropathy of idiopathic haemochromatosis. Q.J. Med., *37*:171–182, 1968.

52. Atkins, C.J., et al.: Chondrocalcinosis and arthropathy: Studies in haemochromatosis and in idiopathic chondrocalcinosis. Q.J. Med., *39*:71–79, 1970.

53. Bourqui, M., et al.: Pyrophosphate arthropathy in the carpal and metacarpophalangeal joints. Ann. Rheum. Dis., *42*:626–630, 1983.

54. Jacobelli, S.G., et al.: Calcium pyrophosphate dihydrate crystal deposition in neuropathic joints: Four cases of polyarticular involvement. Ann. Intern. Med., *79*:340–347, 1973.

55. Gerster, J.C., Vischer, T.L., and Fallet, G.H.: Destructive arthropathy in generalized osteoarthritis with articular chondrocalcinosis. J. Rheumatol., *2*:265–269, 1975.

56. Hamilton, E.B.D., and Richards, A.J.: Destructive arthropathy in chondrocalcinosis articularis. Ann. Rheum. Dis., *33*:196–203, 1974.

57. Menkes, C.J., Simon, F., and Chourki, M.: Les arthropathies destructrices de la chondrocalcinose. Rev. Rhum. Mal. Osteoartic., *40*:115–123, 1973.

58. Reginato, A.J., et al.: Polyarticular and familial chondrocalcinosis. Arthritis Rheum., *13*:197–213, 1970.

59. Pritzker, K.P.H., et al.: Pseudotumor of temporomandibular joint: Destructive calcium pyrophosphate dihydrate arthropathy. J. Rheumatol., *3*:70–81, 1976.

60. Rodnan, G.P.: Arthritis with hematologic disorders, storage diseases and dysproteinemias. *In* Arthritis and Allied Conditions. 8th Ed. Edited by J.L. Hollander and D.J. McCarty. Philadelphia, Lea & Febiger, 1972.

61. Reginato, A.J., et al.: HLA antigens in chondrocalcinosis and ankylosing chondrocalcinosis. Arthritis Rheum., *22*:928–932, 1979.

62. LeGoff, P., Penunec, Y., and Youinou, P.: Signes cervicaux aigus pseudomeninge, relateurs de la chondrocalcinose articulaire. Sem. Hop. Paris, *56*:1515–1518, 1980.

63. Bouvet, J., et al.: Acute neck pain due to calcifications surrounding the odontoid process: The crowned dens syndrome. Arthritis Rheum., *28*:1417–1420, 1985.

63a. Doherty, M., Watt, I., and Dieppe, P.A.: Localised chondrocalcinosis in post-meniscectomy knees. Lancet, *1*:1207–1210, 1982.

64. Linden, B., and Nilsson, B.E.: Chondrocalcinosis following osteochondritis dissecans in the femur condyle. Clin. Orthop., *130*:223–227, 1978.

65. Andres, T.L., and Trainer, T.D.: Intervertebral chondrocalcinosis: A coincidental finding possibly related to previous surgery. Arch. Pathol. Lab. Med., *104*:269–271, 1980.

66. Ellman, M.H., et al.: Calcium pyrophosphate dihydrate deposition in lumbar disc fibrocartilage. J. Rheumatol., *8*:955–958, 1981.

67. DeVos, R.A., et al.: Calcium pyrophosphate dihydrate of the temporomandibular joint. Oral Surg., *51*:497–502, 1980.

68. Leisen, J.C., et al.: The tophus in calcium pyrophosphate deposition disease. JAMA, *244*:1711–1712, 1980.

69. Ling, D., Murphy, W.A., and Kyriakos, M.: Tophaceous pseudogout. Radiology, *138*:162–165, 1982.

70. Schumacher, H.R., et al.: Tumor-like soft tissue swelling of the distal phalanx due to calcium pyro-phosphate dihydrate crystal deposition. Arthritis Rheum., *27*:1428–1432, 1984.

71. Hensley, C., and Lin, J.: Massive intrasynovial deposition of calcium pyrophosphate in the elbow. J. Bone Joint Surg., *66A*:133–136, 1984.

72. Gibson, J.P., and Roenijk, W.J.: Pseudogout in a dog. J. Am. Vet. Med. Assoc., *161*:912–915, 1972.

73. Renlund, R.C., et al.: Calcium pyrophosphate dihydrate crystal deposition disease with concurrent diffuse idiopathic skeletal hyperostosis in Barbary ape. Arthritis Rheum., *26*:682–683, 1983.

74. Renlund, R., Prityker, K., Cheng, P., and Kessler, M.: Rhesus monkeys (Macaca mulatta) as a model for calcium pyrophosphate dihydrate crystal deposition disease. J. Med. Primatol., *15*:11–16, 1986.

75. Roberts, E., et al.: Calcium pyrophosphate deposition in nonhuman primates. Vet. Pathol., *21*:592–596, 1984.

76. Yosipovitch, Z., and Glimscher, M.J.: Chondrocalcinosis in adult rabbits. Metab. Bone Dis. Relat. Res., *7*:503–504, 1971.

77. Nyulassy, S., et al.: HL-A system in articular chondrocalcinosis. Arthritis Rheum., *19*(Suppl.):391–393, 1976.

78. Fernandez Dapica, M., and Gomez-Reino, J.: Familial chondrocalcinosis in the Spanish population. J. Rheum., *13*:631–633, 1986.

79. Hollingworth, P., Williams, P.L., and Scott, J.T.: Frequency of chondrocalcinosis of the knees in asymptomatic hyperuricemia and rheumatoid arthritis: A controlled study. Ann. Rheum. Dis., *41*:344–346, 1982.

80. Hamilton, E.B.D., et al.: The natural history of arthritis in idiopathic haemochromatosis: Progression of the clinical and radiological features over ten years. Q.J. Med., *50*:321–329, 1981.

81. Rynes, R.I., and Merzig, E.G.: Calcium pyrophosphate crystal deposition disease and hyperparathyroidism: A controlled prospective study. J. Rheumatol., *5*:460–468, 1978.

82. Aitken, R.E., Kerr, J.L., and Lloyd, H.M.: Primary hyperparathyroidism with osteosclerosis with calcification in articular cartilage. Am. J. Med., *37*:813–820, 1964.

83. Bywaters, E.G.L., Dixon, A. St. J., and Scott, J.T.: Joint lesions of hyperparathyroidism. Ann. Rheum. Dis., *22*:171–187, 1963.

84. Zvaifler, N.J., Reefe, W.E., and Black, R.L.: Articular manifestations in primary hyperparathyroidism. Arthritis Rheum., *5*:237–249, 1962.

85. Currey, H.L.F., et al.: Significance of radiological calcification of joint cartilage. Ann. Rheum. Dis., *25*:295–306, 1966.

86. Skinner, M., and Cohen, A.S.: Calcium pyrophosphate dihydrate crystal deposition disease. Arch. Intern. Med., *123*:636–644, 1969.

87. Dodds, W.J., and Steinbach, L.: Primary hyperparathyroidism and articular cartilage calcification. AJR, *104*:884–892, 1968.

88. Glass, J.S., and Grahame, R.: Chondrocalcinosis after parathyroidectomy. Ann. Rheum. Dis., *35*:521–525, 1976.

89. Harris, J., et al.: Ankylosing hyperostosis. Ann. Rheum. Dis., *33*:210–215, 1974.

90. Pritchard, M.H., and Jessop, J.D.: Chondrocalcinosis in primary hyperparathyroidism. Ann. Rheum. Dis., *36*:146–151, 1977.

91. Marx, S.J.: The hypocalciuric or benign variant of familial hypercalcemia: Clinical and biochemical features in fifteen kindreds. Medicine, *60*:397–412, 1981.

92. Marx, S.J., et al.: An association between neonatal severe primary hyperparathyroidism and familial hypocalciuric hypercalcemia in three kindreds. N. Engl. J. Med., *306*:257–263, 1982.

93. Phelps, P., and Hawker, C.D.: Serum parathyroid hormone levels in patients with calcium pyrophosphate crystals deposition disease (chondrocalcinosis, pseudogout). Arthritis Rheum., *16*:590–596, 1973.

94. McCarty, D.J., et al.: Diseases associated with calcium py-

rophosphate dihydrate crystal deposition: A controlled study. Am. J. Med., 56:704–714, 1974.

95. Ellman, M.H., Brown, N.L., and Porat, A.P.: Laboratory investigations in pseudogout patients and controls. J. Rheumatol., 7:77–81, 1980.

96. Pawlotsky, Y., et al.: Hyperparathormonemie normocalcemique et chondrocalcinose articulaire. Rev. J. Rheumatisme, 48:799–806, 1981.

97. Connor, T.B., et al.: Generalized osteosclerosis in primary hyperparathyroidism. Trans. Am. Clin. Climatol. Assoc., 85:185–196, 1976.

98. Pugh, J., Rose, R., and Radin, E.: Elastic and viscoelastic properties of trabecular bone: Dependence on structure. J. Biomech., 6:475–485, 1973.

99. Foss, M.V.L., and Byers, P.D.: Bone density in osteoarthritis of the hip and fracture of the upper end of the femur. Ann. Rheum. Dis., 31:259–264, 1972.

100. Schumacher, H.R.: Hemochromatosis and arthritis. Arthritis Rheum., 7:41–50, 1964.

101. Dorfmann, H., et al.: Les arthropathies des hemochromatoses: Resultats d'une enquete prospective portant sur 54 malades. Sem. Hop. Paris, 45:416–523, 1969.

102. Dymock, I.W., et al.: Arthopathy of hemochromatosis. Ann. Rheum. Dis., 29:469–476, 1970.

103. Hamilton, E.B.D.: Diseases associated with CPPD deposition disease. Arthritis Rheum., 19(Suppl.):353–357, 1976.

103a. Adamson, T.C., et al.: Hand and wrist arthropathies of hemochromatosis and calcium pyrophosphate deposition disease: Distinct radiographic features. Radiology, 146:377–381, 1983.

104. Jensen, P.S., and Putnam, C.E.: Chondrocalcinosis and haemophilia. Clin. Radiol., 28:401–405, 1977.

105. Leonello, P.P., Cleland, L.G., and Norman, J.E.: Acute pseudogout and chondrocalcinosis in a man with mild hemophilia. J. Rheumatol., 8:841–844, 1981.

106. McCarty, D.J., and Pepe, P.F.: Erythrocyte neutral inorganic pyrophosphatase in pseudogout. J. Lab. Clin. Med., 79:277–284, 1972.

107. Hearn, P.R., Russell, R.G.G., and Elliott, J.C.: Formation product of calcium pyrophosphate crystals in vitro and the effect of iron salts. Clin. Sci. Mol. Med., 54:29–33, 1978.

108. McCarty, D.J., Palmer, D.W., and Garancis, J.C.: Clearance of calcium pyrophosphate dihydrate crystals in vivo. III. Effects of synovial hemosiderosis. Arthritis Rheum., 24:706–710, 1981.

109. Pawlotsky, Y., et al.: Histomorphometrie osseuse et manifestations osteo-articulares de l'hemochromatose idiopathique. Rev. Rheum., 46:91–99, 1979.

110. O'Duffy, J.D.: Hypophosphatasia associated with calcium pyrophosphate dihydrate deposits in cartilage. Arthritis Rheum., 13:381–388, 1970.

111. Earde, A.W., Swannell, A.J., and Williamson, N.R.: Pyrophosphate arthropathy in hypophosphatasia. Ann. Rheum. Dis., 40:164–170, 1981.

112. Whyte, M.P., Murphy, W.A., and Fallon, M.D.: Adult hypophosphatasia with chondrocalcinosis and arthropathy: Variable penetrance of hypophosphatemia in a large Oklahoma kindred. Am. J. Med., 72:631–641, 1982.

113. Russell, R.G.G.: Pyrophosphate metabolism and pseudogout. Lancet, 2:461–476, 1976.

114. Russell, R.G.G.: Metabolism of inorganic pyrophosphate (PPi). Arthritis Rheum., 19(Suppl.):463–478, 1976.

115. Russell, R.G.G., et al.: Inorganic pyrophosphate in plasma in normal persons and in patients with hypophosphatasia, os-

teogenesis imperfecta and other disorders of bone. J. Clin. Invest., 50:961–969, 1971.

116. Whyte, M.P., et al.: Infantile hypophosphatasia: Enzyme replacement therapy by intravenous infusion of alkaline phosphatase-rich plasma from patients with Paget's bone disease. J. Pediatr., 101:379–386, 1982.

117. Milazzo, S.C., et al.: Calcium pyrophosphate dihydrate deposition disease and familial hypomagnesemia. J. Rheumatol., 8:767–771, 1981.

118. Rapado, A., et al.: Condrocalcinosis de hypomagnesemia: Un nuevo sindrome. Rev. Esp. Rheum. Enferm. Osteoartic., 3:283–291, 1976.

119. Runeberg, L., et al.: Hypomagnesemia due to renal disease of unknown etiology. Am. J. Med., 59:873–881, 1975.

120. Resnick, D., and Rausch, J.: Hypomagnesemia with chondrocalcinosis. J. Can. Assoc. Radiol., 35:214–216, 1984.

121. Ishikawa, K.: Personal communication.

122. Mayoux-Benhamou, M., et al.: Articular chondrocalcinosis and hypomagnesemia of renal origins. Apropos of two cases. Rev. Rhum. Mal. Osteoartic., 52:545–548, 1985.

123. Bauer, F., Glasson, M., Valloton, M., and Courvoisier, B.: Syndrome de Bartter, Articular chondrocalcinosis in a case. Chondrocalcinose et hypomagnesemie. Schweiz. Med. Wochenschr., 109:1251–1256, 1979.

124. Goulon, M., Raphael, J.C., and deRohan, P.: Syndrome de Bartter et chondrocalcinose. Nouv. Presse Med., 9:1291–1295, 1980.

124a. Matsubara, S., Ishikawa, K., and Kambara, T.: Calcium pyrophosphate dihydrate crystal deposition disease associated with hypomagnesemia. Submitted for publication.

125. McCarty, D.J., et al.: Inorganic pyrophosphate concentrations in the synovial fluid of arthritis patients. J. Lab. Clin. Med., 78:216–229, 1971.

126. Doherty, M., and Dieppe, P.A.: Double blind, placebo controlled trial of magnesium carbonate in chronic pyrophosphate arthropathy. (Abstract.) Ann. Rheum. Dis., 42(Suppl.):106–107, 1983.

127. Dorwart, B.B., and Schumacher, H.R.: Joint effusions, chondrocalcinosis and other rheumatic manifestations in hypothyroidism. Am. J. Med., 59:780–789, 1975.

128. Alexander, G.M., et al.: Pyrophosphate arthropathy: A study of metabolic associations and laboratory data. Ann. Rheum. Dis., 41:377–381, 1982.

129. Kaplinski, N., Biran, D., and Frankl, O.: Pseudogout and amyloidosis. Harefuah, 91:59, 1976.

130. Ryan, L.M., Liang, G., and Kozin, F.: Amyloid arthropathy: Possible association with chondrocalcinosis. J. Rheumatol., 9:273–278, 1982.

131. Yood, R.A., et al.: Soft tissue uptake of bone seeking radionuclide in amyloidosis. J. Rheumatol., 8:760–766, 1981.

132. Egan, M.S., et al.: The association of amyloid deposits and osteoarthritis. Arthritis Rheum., 25:204–208, 1982.

133. Ladefoged, C.: Amyloid in osteoarthritic hip joints: A pathoanatomical and histological investigation of femoral head cartilage. Acta Orthop. Scand., 53:581–586, 1982.

134. Shimizu, K., et al.: Amyloid deposition in the articular structures of AKR senescent mice. Arthritis Rheum., 24:1540–1543, 1981.

135. Stockman, A., Darlington, L.G., and Scott, J.T.: Frequency of chondrocalcinosis of the knees and avascular necrosis of the femoral heads in gout: A controlled study. Ann. Rheum. Dis., 39:7–11, 1980.

136. Schmied, P., et al.: Etude radiologique sur la frequence de

l'association entre la chondrocalcinose articulaire et le diabete. Schweiz. Med. Wochenschr., *101*:272–274, 1971.

137. Okazaki, T., et al.: Pseudogout: Clinical observations and chemical analyses of deposits. Arthritis Rheum., *19*:293–305, 1976.

138. VanderKorst, J.K., Geerards, J., and Driessens, F.C.M.: A hereditary type of idiopathic articular chondrocalcinosis. Am. J. Med., *56*:307–314, 1974.

139. Silcox, D.C., and McCarty, D.J.: Measurement of inorganic pyrophosphate in biological fluids, elevated levels in some patients with osteoarthritis, pseudogout, acromegaly and uremia. J. Clin. Invest., *52*:1863–1870.

140. Radi, J., Epiney, J., and Reiner, M.: Chondrocalcinose et maladie osseuse de Paget. Rev. Rhum. Mal. Osteoartic., *37*:385–388, 1970.

141. Weaver, J.B.: Calcification and ossification of the menisci. J. Bone Joint Surg., *24*:873–882, 1942.

142. Altman, R.D.: Arthroscopic findings of the knee in patients with pseudogout. Arthritis Rheum., *19*:286–292, 1976.

143. Bird, H.A., Tribe, C.R., and Bacon, P.A.: Joint hypermobility leading to osteoarthrosis and chondrocalcinosis. Ann. Rheum. Dis., *37*:203–211, 1978.

144. Settas, L., Doherty, M., and Dieppe, P.: Localized chondrocalcinosis in unstable joints. Br. Med. J., *285*:175–176, 1982.

145. Ellman, M., Krieger, M.I., and Brown, N.: Pseudogout mimicking synovial chondromatosis. J. Bone Joint Surg., *57A*:863–865, 1975.

146. Gerster, J.C., et al.: Carpal tunnel syndrome in chondrocalcinosis of the wrist. Arthritis Rheum., *23*:926–931, 1980.

147. Ahlgren, P.: Chondrocalcinois og knogleusurer. Nord. Med., *73*:309–313, 1965.

148. Lagier, R.: Case report: Rare femoral erosions and osteoarthritis of the knee associated with chondrocalcinosis. A histological study of this cortical remodeling. Virchows Arch. [A], *364*:215–223, 1974.

149. Resnick, D., and Niwyama, G.: Carpal instability in rheumatoid arthritis and calcium pyrophosphate deposition disease. Ann. Rheum. Dis., *36*:311–318, 1977.

149a. Frederick, N., et al.: Chondrocalcinosis in primary and in renal hyperparathyroidism. Kidney Int. (in press).

150. Ross, D.J., et al.: Tibial stress fracture in pyrophosphate arthropathy. J. Bone Joint Surg., *65B*:474–477, 1983.

151. Houpt, J.B., and Sinclair, D.S.: Spontaneous osteonecrosis of the medial femoral condyle. (Abstract.) J. Rheumatol., *1*(Suppl.):117, 1974.

152. Watt, I., and Dieppe, P.: Medial femoral condyle necrosis and chondrocalcinosis: A causal relationship. Br. J. Radiol., *56*:7–22, 1983.

153. Ali, S.Y., et al.: Ultrastructural studies of pyrophosphate crystal deposition in articular cartilage. Ann. Rheum. Dis., *42*(Suppl.):97–98, 1983.

154. Bjelle, A.: Cartilage matrix in hereditary pyrophosphate arthropathy. J. Rheumatol., *8*:959–964, 1981.

154a. Ishikawa, K.: Chondrocytes that accumulate proteoglycans and inorganic pyrophosphate in the pathogenesis of chondrocalcinosis. Arthritis Rheum., *28*:118–119, 1985.

155. Boivin, G., and Lagier, R.: An ultrastructural study of articular chondrocalcinosis in cases of knee osteoarthritis. Virchows Arch. [A], *400*:13–29, 1983.

156. Mitrovic, D.: Pathology of articular deposition of calcium salts and their relationship to osteoarthritis. Ann. Rheum. Dis., *42*(Suppl.):19–26, 1983.

156a. Schumacher, H.R.: The synovitis of pseudogout: electron microscopic observations. Arthritis Rheum., *11*:426–435, 1968.

157. Schumacher, H.R.: Articular cartilage in the degenerative arthropathy of hemochromatosis. Arthritis Rheum., *25*:1460–1468, 1982.

158. McCarty, D.J., Palmer, D.W., and James, C.: Clearance of calcium pyrophosphate dihydrate crystals in vivo. II. Studies using triclinic crystals doubly labeled with ^{45}Ca and ^{85}Sr. Arthritis Rheum., *22*:1122–1131, 1979.

159. Hearn, P.R., Guilland-Cumming, D.F., and Russell, R.G.G.: Effect of orthophosphate and other factors on the crystal growth of calcium pyrophosphate. Ann. Rheum. Dis., *42*(Suppl.):101, 1983.

160. Cheng, P.T., and Pritzker, K.: Pyrophosphate, phosphate ion interaction: Effects on calcium pyrophosphate and calcium hydroxyapatite crystal formation in aqueous solution. J. Rheumatol., *10*:769–777, 1983.

161. Silcox, D.C., and McCarty, D.J.: Elevated inorganic pyrophosphate concentrations in synovial fluid in osteoarthritis and pseudogout. J. Lab. Clin. Med., *83*:518–531, 1974.

162. Pritzker, K.P.H., et al.: Calcium pyrophosphate dihydrate crystal formation in model hydrogels. J. Rheumatol., *5*:469–473, 1978.

163. Mandel, N.S., and Mandel, G.S.: Nucleation and growth of CPPD crystals and related species in vitro. *In* Calcium in Biological Systems. Edited by R.P. Rubin, G. Weiss, and J.W. Putner. New York, Plenum, 1985.

164. Mandel, N., Mandel, G., Carroll, D., and Halverson, P.: Calcium pyrophosphate crystal deposition. An in vitro study using a gelatin matrix model. Arthritis Rheum., *27*:789–796, 1984.

165. Lust, G., et al.: Increased pyrophosphate in fibroblasts and lymphoblasts from patients with hereditary diffuse articular chondrocalcinosis. Science, *214*:809–810, 1981.

166. Jung, A., Bisaz, S., and Fleisch, H.: The binding of pyrophosphate and two diphosphonates by hydroxyapatite crystals. Calc. Tiss. Res., *11*:269–280, 1973.

167. McGaughey, C.: Binding of polyphosphates and phosphonates to hydroxyapatite, subsequent hydrolysis, phosphate exchange and effects on demineralization, mineralization, and microcrystal aggregation. Caries Res., *17*:229–241, 1983.

168. Russell, R.G.G., Bisaz, S., and Fleisch, H.: Inorganic pyrophosphate in plasma, urine and synovial fluid of patients with pyrophosphate arthropathy (chondrocalcinosis or pseudogout). Lancet, *2*:899–902, 1970.

168a. Pflug, M., McCarty, D.J., and Kawahara, F.: Basal urinary pyrophosphate excretion in pseudogout. Arthritis Rheum., *12*:228–231, 1969.

169. Silcox, D.C., Jacobelli, S.G., and McCarty, D.J.: The identification of inorganic pyrophosphate in human platelets and its release on stimulation with thrombin. J. Clin. Invest., *52*:1595–1600, 1973.

170. Ryan, L.M., Kozin, F., and McCarty, D.J.: Quantification of human plasma inorganic pyrophosphatase. II. Biologic variables. Arthritis Rheum., *22*:892–895, 1979.

171. Ryan, L.M., Kozin, F., and McCarty, D.J.: Quantification of human plasma inorganic pyrophosphate. I. Normal values in osteoarthritis and calcium pyrophosphate dihydrate crystal deposition disease. Arthritis Rheum., *22*:886–891, 1979.

172. Altman, R.D., et al.: Articular chondrocalcinosis: Microanalysis of pyrophosphate (PPi) in synovial fluid and plasma. Arthritis Rheum., *16*:171–178, 1973.

173. Sorensen, S.A., Flodgaard, H., and Sorensen, E.: Serum alkaline phosphatase, serum pyrophosphatase, phosphoreylethanolamine, and inorganic pyrophosphate in plasma and

urine: A genetic and clinical study of hypophosphatasia. Monogr. Hum. Genet., 10:66–69, 1978.

174. Howell, D.S., et al.: Extrusion of pyrophosphate into extracellular media by osteoarthritic cartilage incubates. J. Clin. Invest., 56:1473–1480, 1975.

175. Ryan, L.M., Cheung, H.S., and McCarty, D.J.: Release of pyrophosphate by normal mammalian articular hyaline and fibrocartilage in organ culture. Arthritis Rheum., 24:1522–1527, 1981.

176. Pieter, A., et al.: Inorganic pyrophosphate release by rabbit articular chondrocytes in vitro. Arthritis Rheum., 29:1485–1492, 1986.

177. Camerlain, M., et al.: Inorganic pyrophosphate pool size and turnover rate in arthritic joints. J. Clin. Invest., 55:1373–1381, 1975.

178. Tenenbaum, J., et al.: Comparison of phosphohydrolase activities from articular cartilage in calcium pyrophosphate deposition disease and primary osteoarthritis. Arthritis Rheum., 24:492–500, 1981.

179. Cartier, P., and Picard, J.: La mineralisation du cartilage ossifiable. III. Le mechanisme de la reaction atpasique du cartilage. Bull. Soc. Chim. Biol., 37:1159–1168, 1955.

180. Hsu, H.: Purification and partial characterization of ATP pyrophosphohydrolase from fetal bovine epiphyseal cartilage. J. Biol. Chem., 258:3463–3468, 1983.

181. Siegel, S.A., Hummel, C.F., and McCarty, R.P.: The role of nucleoside triphosphate pyrophosphohydrolase in in vitro nucleoside triphosphate-dependent matrix vesicle calcification. J. Biol. Chem., 258:8601–8607, 1983.

182. Hsu, H., and Anderson, H.: The deposition of calcium pyrophosphate and phosphate by matrix vesicles isolated from fetal bovine epiphyseal cartilage. Calcif. Tiss. Int., 36:615–621, 1984.

183. Hsu, H., and Anderson, H.: The deposition of calcium pyrophosphate by NTP pyrophosphohydrolase of matrix vesicles from fetal bovine epiphyseal cartilage. Int. J. Biochem., 18:1141–1146, 1986.

184. Ryan, L.M., et al.: Cartilage nucleoside triphosphate (NTP) pyrophosphohydrolase. I. Identification as an ectoenzyme. Arthritis Rheum., 27:913–918, 1984.

185. Howell, D., et al.: NTP pyrophosphohydrolase in human chondrocalcinotic and osteoarthritic cartilage. II. Further studies on histologic and subcellular distribution. Arthritis Rheum., 27:193–199, 1984.

186. Caswell, A., and Russell, R.: Identification of ecto-nucleoside triphosphate pyrophosphatase in human articular chondrocytes in monolayer culture. Biochim. et Biophys. Acta, 847:40–47, 1985.

187. Felix, R., and Fleisch, H.: The effect of pyrophosphate and diphosphonates on calcium transport in red cells. Experientia, 33:1003–1005, 1977.

188. Rachow, J., and Ryan, L.: Adenosine triphosphate pyrophosphohydrolase and neutral inorganic pyrophosphatase in pathologic joint fluids. Arthritis Rheum., 28:1283–1288, 1985.

189. Ryan, L., Rachow, J., and McCarty, D.: Synovial fluid ATP: A possible substrate for generation of inorganic pyrophosphate in calcium pyrophosphate dihydrate (CPPD) crystal deposition disease. Arthritis Rheum., S131, 1987.

190. Lust, G., et al.: Evidence of a generalized metabolic defect in patients with hereditary chondrocalcinosis. Arthritis Rheum., 24:1517–1521, 1981.

191. Ryan, L.M., Lynch, M.P., and McCarty, D.J.: Inorganic pyrophosphate levels in blood platelets from normal donors and patients with calcium pyrophosphate dihydrate crystal deposition disease. Arthritis Rheum., 26:564–566, 1983.

192. Ryan, L., et al.: Pyrophosphohydrolase activity and inorganic pyrophosphate content of cultured human skin fibroblasts. J. Clin. Invest., 77:1689–1693, 1986.

193. Bowles, C., et al.: Colchicine prevents recurrent pseudogout: Multicenter trial. Arthritis Rheum., 29:S38, 1986.

194. Alvarellos, A., and Spilberg, I.: Colchicine prophylaxis in pseudogout. J. Rheumatol., 13:804–805, 1986.

195. Bennett, R.M., Lehr, J.R., and McCarty, D.J.: Crystal shedding and acute pseudogout: A hypothesis based on a therapeutic failure. Arthritis Rheum., 19:93–97, 1976.

196. Fam, A.G., and Stein, G.: Disappearance of chondrocalcinosis following reflex sympathetic dystrophy. Arthritis Rheum., 24:747–749, 1981.

197. Doherty, M., and Dieppe, P.A.: Effect of intra-articular yttrium-90 on chronic pyrophosphate arthropathy of the knee. Lancet, 1:1243–1246, 1981.

BASIC CALCIUM PHOSPHATE (APATITE, OCTACALCIUM PHOSPHATE, TRICALCIUM PHOSPHATE) CRYSTAL DEPOSITION DISEASES

108

PAUL B. HALVERSON and DANIEL J. McCARTY

There are hundreds of reports of pathologic calcium phosphate mineral phase deposition in various human tissues. These reports are largely descriptive, and most present no clear pattern of disease. Basic calcium phosphate (BCP) crystals, formerly termed hydroxyapatite (HA), have long been associated with periarticular diseases such as calcific periarthritis and tendonitis.[1-5] Recently, BCP crystals have been found in synovial fluid by scanning electron microscopy (SEM) or transmission electron microscopy (TEM).[6,7]

CRYSTAL IDENTIFICATION

The study of BCP crystal–associated arthritis has been relatively difficult because of the lack of a simple, reliable diagnostic test (see also Chapter 5). Heterogeneity of crystal species in periarticular shoulder joint calcifications was first established by Faure et al., who directly measured the interplanar spacings of individual apatite crystals using high-resolution transmission electron microscopy.[8] These crystals were largely carbonate-substituted, and other non-apatite calcium phosphates were found. Intensive study of a subcutaneous calcification from a patient with scleroderma showed amorphous and poorly crystallized calcium phosphate in nodular aggregates with internodular apatite crystals.[9] Fourier transform infrared (FTIR) analysis of shoulder joint fluid crystals, of rabbit synovium calcified by calciphylaxis, and of subcutaneous calcifications from a girl with der-matomyositis showed that each contained partially carbonate-substituted HA, octacalcium phosphate (OCP), and particulate collagens (Table 108–1).[10] Samples from one patient had tricalcium phosphate (TCP) (whitlockite) instead of OCP. BCP is therefore used here to designate these crystal mixtures. Perhaps "BCP crystal deposition disease" is the most appropriate term for the associated clinical syndromes.

Radiography. Radiography of BCP crystal deposits has shown rounded or fluffy calcifications that vary in size from a few millimeters to several centimeters. They may occur either as solitary nodules or as multiple deposits. Although radiography is a useful diagnostic tool, it is both relatively insensitive and nonspecific in the diagnosis of BCP crystal arthropathies.[11] Asymptomatic periarticular calcific deposits are frequently observed as incidental findings.

Synovial Fluid. Phase-contrast polarized light microscopy, invaluable for the detection of the larger monosodium urate monohydrate and calcium pyrophosphate dihydrate crystals, provides little help with BCP crystals, because their size is below the limits of resolution of optical microscopy. Although these crystals tend to aggregate, their orientation within an aggregate is usually random, and they are not birefringent.[3] Rarely, birefringence is noted because thousands of ultramicroscopic crystals are oriented along the same axis.[13] Individual needle- or plate-shaped crystals are usually less than 0.1 μm long (Fig. 108–1). BCP crystal aggregates may be visible by light microscopy as shiny laminated "coins" (see Fig.

Table 108–1. Chemical Formulas and Molar Ratios of Calcium (Ca) to Phosphorus (P) of Calcium-Containing Crystals Found in Human Synovial Fluid, Cartilage, or Synovium

Crystal	Formula	Ca/P
BCP		
Hydroxyapatite (HA)	$Ca_5(PO_4)_3OH2H_2O$	1.67
Octacalcium phosphate (OCP)	$Ca_8H_2(PO_4)_65H_2O$	1.33
Tricalcium phosphate (TCP) (whitlockite)	$Ca_3(PO_4)_2$	1.5
OTHER		
Dicalcium phosphate dihydrate (brushite)	$CaHPO_42H_2O$	1.0
Calcium pyrophosphate dihydrate	$Ca_2P_2O_72H_2O$	1.0
Calcium oxalate	$CaC_2O_4H_2O$	∞

5–5B).[3,13–15] Alizarin red S staining of synovial fluid pellets has been suggested as a screening technique for BCP crystals.[16] The method is sensitive to 0.005 µg of HA standard/ml, but it is not specific for calcium phosphates and may provide many false positive results.[17]

A technique for semiquantitation of BCP in synovial fluid utilizing the binding of (^{14}C) ethane-1-hydroxy-1, 1-diphosphonate (EHDP) to BCP crystals has proved useful as a screening test.[18] The protocol for this method, sensitive to about 2 µg HA standard/ml, is shown in Table 108–2. Positive and negative controls are included routinely, and a detergent is added to release intracellular crystals if many cells are present. Diphosphonate binding in synovial fluid correlated strongly with the radiographic grade of osteoarthritis present (Fig. 108–2).[18,19] Synovial fluid pellets that bound EHDP were examined routinely by SEM. Microspheroidal aggregates approximately 1 to 19 µm in diameter were generally found (Fig. 108–3A).

These aggregates were then further characterized by x-ray energy dispersive analysis.[20] The spectrum is analyzed for calcium and phosphorus, and the relative molar amounts of each element are calculated using an on-line computer (Fig. 108–3B). Schumacher has suggested routine use of TEM,[21] which, while not quantitative, has the advantage of better definition of crystal morphology and location (e.g., in cells).

X-ray diffraction of BCP mineral by the powder method is relatively insensitive. Such small, poorly crystallized material yields broad diffraction minima that cannot differentiate between closely related calcium phosphate compounds. Electron diffraction, high-resolution TEM, and FTIR spectrophotometry are useful research tools, but are not practical for everyday clinical use.

Direct chemical analysis for calcium and phospho-

FIG. 108–1. Aggregate of needle-shaped crystals within a synovial fibrocyte. No limiting membrane can be identified ($\times$43,800). (From Garancis, J.C., et al.[13])

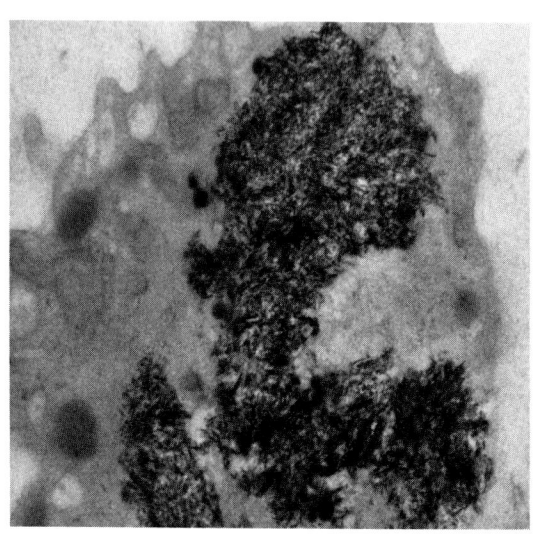

Table 108–2. Protocol for (^{14}C) Diphosphonate (EHDP) Binding

1. Collect 1–10 ml joint fluid in plastic tube containing 250 µl heparin and 1 mg hyaluronidase (300–800 units/mg). Incubate 30 min at room temperature. Transfer to plastic centrifuge tube with pipette. Record volume transferred.
2. Centrifuge 27,000 $\times$ g/20 min. Discard supernatant; resuspend in same volume of 0.1M tris Cl buffer pH 8.0.
3. Store at $-20°$ or proceed with assay.
4. Thaw and centrifuge 27,000 $\times$ g/20 min, resuspend in 0.5 ml tris Cl containing trypsin (180–220 units/ml), incubate 37° $\times$ 30 min. This step permits scanning EM and x-ray energy dispersive analysis to be performed on the pellet.
5. Centrifuge at 37,000 $\times$ g/20 min, discard supernatant, and resuspend in 1 ml of 20-mM phosphate buffer in normal saline containing 2 $\times$ 10^{-3}µCi (^{14}C) EHDP.
6. Rotate tube in roller drum $\times$ 2 hr, remove two 100-µl aliquots before and after centrifugation at 37,000 $\times$ g/20 min.
7. Count (^{14}C) in liquid scintillation spectrophotometer.
8. Calculate % binding of radionuclide. This can be related to a standard curve relating binding to various concentrations of a hydroxyapatite standard to express results in µg/ml.

$$100 - \frac{\text{initial CPM} - \text{postcentrifuge CPM}}{\text{initial CPM}} \times 100 = \% \text{ bound}$$

FIG. 108–2. Fluids that bound (^{14}C) EHDP generally were obtained from joints with advanced degenerative changes (radiologic grades 4 and 5). □ = internal derangement of knee; ● = osteoarthritis; ✦ = osteoarthritis with few CPPD crystals in fluid; × = inflammatory arthritis with WBC concentration >3,000 mm³; ⊗ = inflammatory arthritis with WBC concentration <3,000 mm³; ○ = miscellaneous arthritis. Positive results are shown in duplicate. (From Halverson, P.B., and McCarty, D.J.[18])

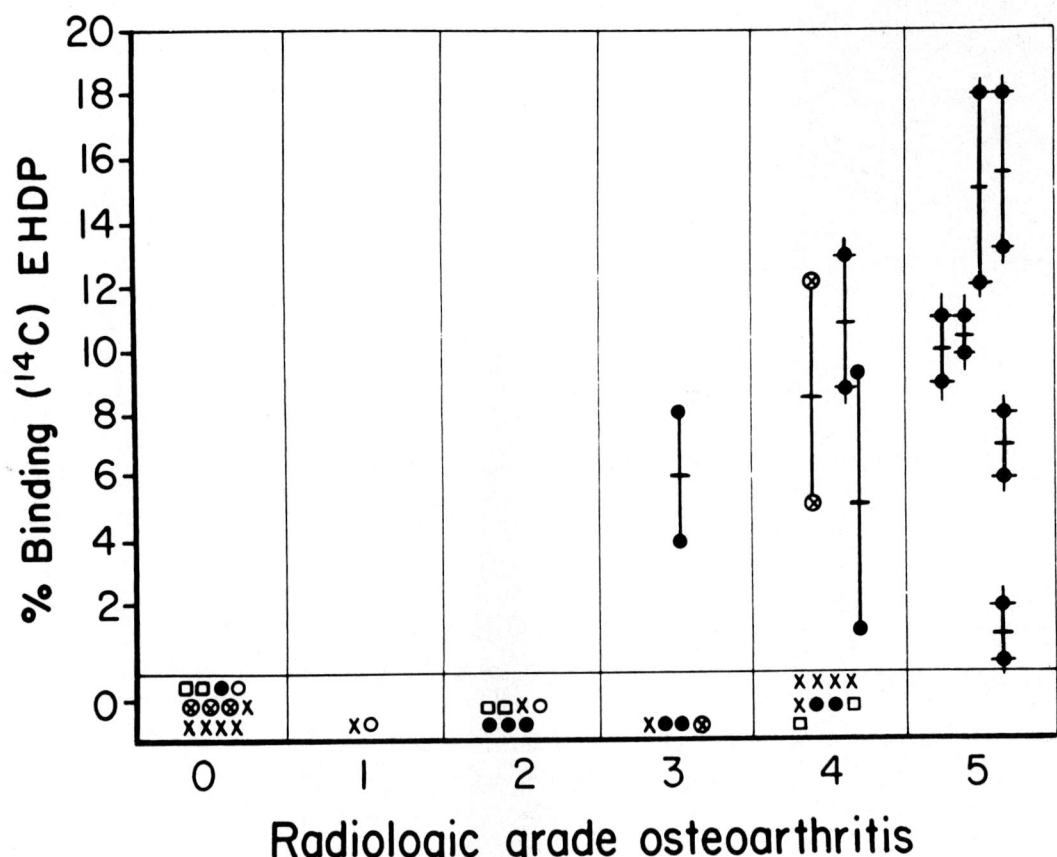

rus of several pellets from joint fluid that bound (^{14}C) EHDP showed levels of 12 to 45 μg BCP mineral per ml.[20]

DISEASES

Several articular and periarticular conditions associated with BCP crystals have been described (Table 108–3). Calcific tendonitis and calcific bursitis are discussed in Chapters 87 and 97, and calcinosis in Chapter 73. Calcific periarthritis has long been recognized, but acute and chronic synovitis associated with intraarticular BCP crystal deposition are more recent discoveries. The so-called secondary BCP arthropathies are known to predispose to articular and/or periarticular BCP crystal deposition (Table 108–3).

ROTATOR CUFF CALCIFICATIONS

In the shoulder, the location of rotator cuff calcifications has been related to etiopathogenesis, natural history, and prognosis.[33] Sarkar and Uhthoff found that calcifications at the tidemark of the rotator cuff insertion into the greater tuberosity of the humerus represented degenerative enthesopathy with *secondary calcifications*. These and the secondary calcification of the torn ends of a rotator cuff are irreversible.[69] On the other hand, *"primary" calcification* in the rotator cuff, approximately 1.5 cm away from the tidemark in "Codman's critical area,"[15] occurred in metaplastic fibrocartilage. These deposits were associated with matrix vesicles and with crystal phagocytosis by macrophages and giant cells. The natural history of such deposits is resorption. Scalloping of the fluffy radiodense deposits on roentgenograms represents the

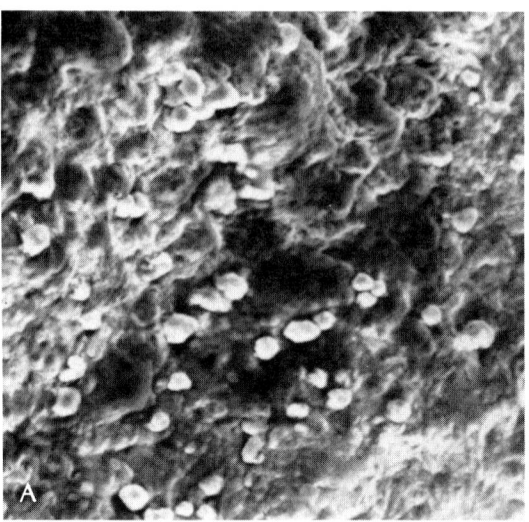

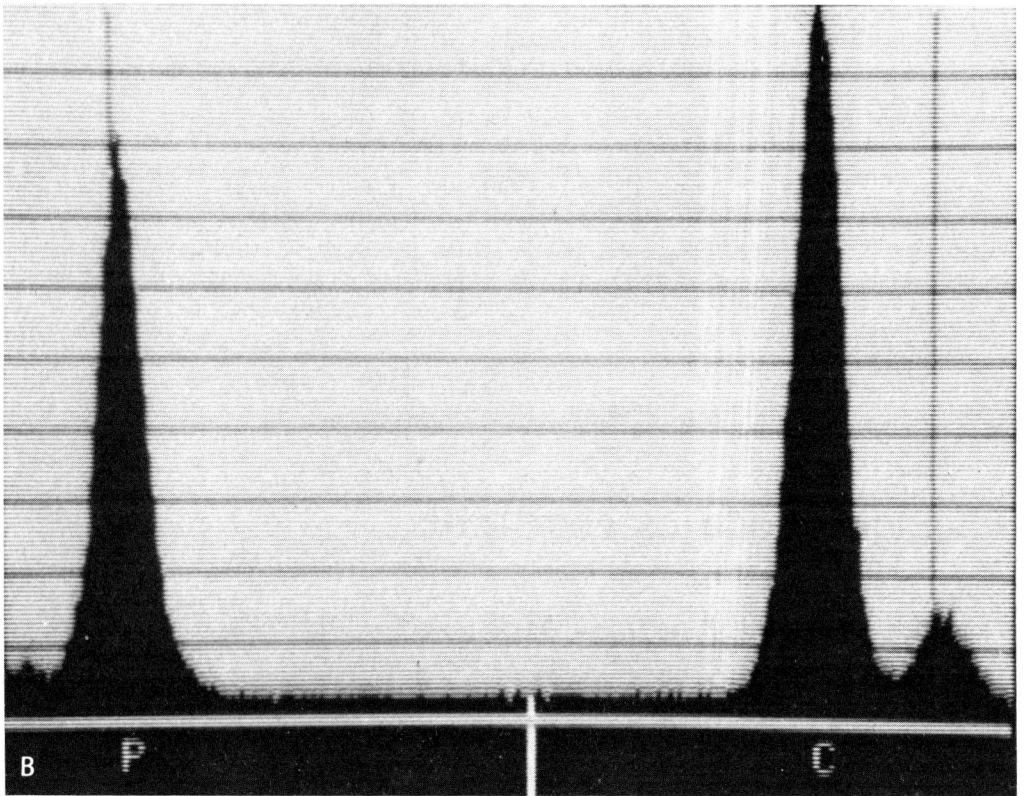

FIG. 108–3. *A,* Scanning electron micrograph of synovial fluid sediment showing typical microspheroidal crystal aggregates (×525). (From Halverson, P.B., et al.[20]) *B,* Spectrograph from x ray energy dispersive analysis showing peaks for phosphorus and calcium.

radiologic correlate of cellular resorption of mineral.[32] Others have not found chondroid metaplasia or matrix vesicles in calcific tenosynovitis, but found instead psammoma bodies and calcification within necrotic cells.[70]

Ali has presented electron microscopic evidence for pericellular matrix vesicles in normal articular cartilage, which he regards as a latent growth plate.[71] Vesicles were present at all levels of the cartilage, but were most numerous near the tidemark adjoining the subchondral bone. Microcrystals within mineral nod-

ules (0.6 μm in diameter) were noted in various stages of formation. Both vesicles and mineral were greatly increased in osteoarthritic cartilage; quantitatively, this increase was reflected by a marked increase (up to 30-fold) in alkaline phosphatase activity in osteoarthritic cartilage. Ali hypothesized that such abnormal mineralization may confer deleterious biomechanical properties to cartilage, and if shed into the synovial fluid may initiate attacks of joint inflammation. Further studies have shown three distinct types of calcification in osteoarthritic cartilage.[71,72] In addition to

Table 108–3. Basic Calcium Phosphate (BCP)
Crystal–Associated Joint Disease

Calcific Periarthritis
    Unifocal[4,15,22,23]
    Multifocal[2,3,15,24]
    Familial[24–30]
Calcific Tendonitis and Bursitis[5,15,22,23,31–33]
Intra-articular BCP Arthropathies
    Acute (gout-like) attacks[7,34–36]
    Milwaukee shoulder/knee syndrome[11,37–41]
        (Apatite-associated destructive arthritis; cuff tear arthropathy)
    Erosive polyarticular disease[42]
    Mixed crystal deposition disease (BCP + CPPD)[11,18,43,44]
Secondary BCP Crystal Arthropathies/Periarthropathies *
    Chronic renal failure†[35,45–49]
    "Collagen" diseases (calcinosis)[14,50,51]
    Sequel to severe neurologic injury[52–54]
    Post local corticosteroid injection[55,56]
    Other (see also Table 87–4)[57–60]
Tumoral Calcinosis
    Hyperphosphatemic[61–63]
    Nonhyperphosphatemic[64]

*Mineral deposits may also occur in fibrous tissues remote from joints in these conditions.
†Calcium oxalate[65,66] or aluminum salts[67] also may occur in joints in renal failure. Whitlockite ($Ca_3(PO_4)_2$) may deposit in lungs.[68]

the mineral nodules just discussed, dense cuboidal-shaped crystals resembling whitlockite morphologically, but with a molar Ca/P of 1.72, were found in pericellular matrix around the surface chondrocytes. Fine needle-shaped crystal clusters were observed on the cartilage surface in the acellular amorphous zone (lamina splendens). These clusters had a molar Ca/P of 1.7 and resembled the crystals found in synovial fluid. Matrix vesicles and crystals were seen in rabbit fibrocartilage that had formed from autologous grafts of synovial tissue implanted into defects produced surgically in hyaline cartilage, but not in sham-operated joints.[73]

A systematic study of articular cartilage from 28 patients with advanced osteoarthritis showed superficial HA-type needle-shaped crystals in 56%; calcified deposits were found in 36% in deeper repair-type fibrocartilage, and calcium pyrophosphate deposition (CPPD) crystals were seen in 11% of cases.[44] Overall, 75% of the cartilages had microcrystalline deposits of some kind.

Synovium from the same joints all showed a patchy lining cell hyperplasia and giant cells, whether or not calcific deposits were present in the area.[44] Calcific deposits were present in 70% of the specimens. All were of the HA type, but four specimens also showed CPPD deposits. The pathologic prevalence of 70 to 75% synovial calcification is in accord with a radiologic survey of osteoarthritic knee joints, wherein 72% showed periarticular or intra-articular calcification.[74]

CALCIFIC PERIARTHRITIS

Periarticular calcifications are found most commonly around the shoulder, but have been described near many other joints. Calcific scapulohumeral periarthritis was first described in 1870.[23] Roentgenographic demonstration of periarticular shoulder calcifications was first accomplished in 1907,[22] and a classic review of 329 cases of peritendinitis calcarea was presented in 1938.[23] An excellent study disclosed calcium deposits in one or both shoulders of 138 of 5,061 employees of a life insurance company.[75] More than 70% of patients were under age 40 and many remained asymptomatic, although serial study showed that large deposits usually caused acute painful inflammation eventually. Spontaneous resorption of some deposits, especially the smaller ones, occurred. Nearly half of these subjects had bilateral deposits.

Most cases of acute calcific periarthritis consist of a single attack in a single joint, frequently with localized warmth, erythema, swelling, and pain lasting up to a few weeks. The roentgenographic finding of periarticular calcification is useful as a confirmatory diagnostic aid (see Fig. 97–9).

Recurrent attacks of calcific periarthritis occurring at multiple sites suggest a more generalized condition rather than a chance localized process with resultant calcification.[2,3,15,24] Several reports describe familial occurrences of calcific arthritis and periarthritis.[24–30]

Episodic attacks of calcific periarthritis have been treated successfully with a variety of nonsteroidal anti-inflammatory drugs (NSAIDs) and colchicine.[5] Needle aspiration of the paste-like calcific deposits with or without irrigation may be helpful.[3,15,75] Mechanical disruption and dispersion of the deposits may speed their removal by phagocytosis as outlined by Sarkar and Uhthoff.[33,76] Surgical removal of large calcific deposits usually provides permanent symptomatic relief.[75] Codman considered this procedure to be essential for symptomatic relief.[15]

BCP CRYSTAL–RELATED ARTHRITIS

BCP is now recognized as another class of crystals that may be found within joints. Schumacher and associates have described both acute and chronic forms of arthritis.[7] Acute attacks of arthritis in relatively young persons occurred with extreme pain, swelling, and erythema closely resembling gout. Crystals resembling BCP were found by transmission electron microscopy in synovial fluid pellets with significantly elevated synovial fluid leukocyte counts and normal joint roentgenograms. The phlogistic potential of BCP crystals was also demonstrated by injection into rabbit joints. Persons with chronic degenerative arthropathy and three patients with erosive arthritis were also described.[42] Recurrent episodes of pain and swelling were associated with gradual erosion and destructive changes in metacarpophalangeal, proximal interphalangeal, and wrist joints. One of the three patients had chronic renal failure. Although all had radiographic evidence of periarticular calcific deposits, no synovial fluid was obtained; therefore, it remains unclear whether intrasynovial crystals were present.

In 1976, Dieppe et al. reported that synovial fluid from five patients with clinical evidence of osteoarthritis contained 0.15- to 0.8-μm crystals, which by x-ray energy dispersive analysis were compatible with apatite.[6] Other reports have established that crystals of the apatite family are found in approximately 30 to 60% of synovial fluid from patients with knee joint osteoarthritis.[19,77,78] Leukocyte levels in synovial fluid from osteoarthritic joints were no different if crystals were also present.[77] BCP and CPPD crystals are found more frequently together than either crystal alone.[19] A study of fluid from a series of patients with osteoarthritis of the knee suggested that BCP crystals correlated with greater joint deterioration, whereas CPPD crystals correlated with patient age.[19] BCP and CPPD crystals have also been found together in soft tissues in association with carpal tunnel syndrome.[79]

MILWAUKEE SHOULDER/KNEE SYNDROME

We have studied 30 cases of a peculiar arthropathy, which we named Milwaukee shoulder syndrome.[38] Robert Adams of Dublin was probably the first to describe this entity as rheumatic arthritis of the shoulder.[80] Salient clinical, radiographic, and synovial fluid findings are listed in Table 108–4.

Clinical Features. The primary findings include female predominance (80%), greater involvement of the dominant arm, glenohumeral joint degeneration, and gross loss of the rotator cuff. Others have described similar patients under a variety of descriptive terms, and a summary of all studies is shown in Table 108–5. The average age of our patients was 72.5 years with an age range of 53 to 90. Average duration of symptoms, when ascertainable, was 3.8 years, but the range was variable (1 to 10 years). The exact date of onset could not be determined in some cases. This syndrome appeared to evolve slowly over a span of years in most patients, with the exception of one

Table 108–4. Features of Milwaukee Shoulder/Knee Syndrome

Clinical Features
Elderly, female predominance
Dominant shoulder usually affected but often bilateral
Symptoms variable—asymptomatic to severe pain at rest; mostly painful after use and at night. Glenohumeral joint stiffness or instability

Roentgenographic Features
Glenohumeral joint degeneration
Soft tissue calcifications
Upward subluxation of the humeral head

Synovial Fluid
Low leukocyte counts
Basic calcium phosphate crystal aggregates
Particulate collagens
Elevated collagenase and neutral protease activities in some fluids.

woman in whom it occurred in less than 1 year. She had suffered a traumatic rotator cuff tear from a motor vehicle accident. A surgical repair was attempted but broke down when the shoulder became infected. After resolution of sepsis, a large, noninflammatory effusion that associated with chronic pain ensued. Symptoms also varied. Three patients with bilateral shoulder involvement had asymptomatic disease on the nondominant side. Most persons experienced mild to moderate pain, especially after use, but one patient had severe pain even at rest. Other symptoms included limitation of motion, stiffness, and pain at night. Examination showed reduced active range of motion in all affected shoulders, sometimes associated with pronounced joint instability. Crepitation and pain were often noted when the humerus was grated passively against the glenoid. Unusual features may include acromioclavicular joint cyst and acromial stress fracture.[81,82]

Aspiration of the affected shoulder joints routinely yielded 3 to 40 ml of synovial fluid that was frequently blood-tinged. Occasionally, hydrops of the shoulder yielding 130 ml or more of synovial fluid was encountered (Fig. 108–4). In two instances, hydrops was associated with joint rupture and dissection of fluid onto the anterior chest wall.

Associated Factors. Several factors that may predispose to the development of this syndrome have been identified.[83] Trauma or overuse was observed in 9 of our 30 cases. Four patients had fallen on an outstretched hand, and one was involved in a motor vehicle accident. Two men had "traumatic" professions (jackhammer operation and professional wrestling) and two other men had experienced recurrent shoulder dislocations.[84] Two patients with paraparesis used their shoulders as weight-bearing joints while crutch-walking and later using wheelchairs (im-

Table 108–5. Summary of Reports Describing 72 Patients with Severe Shoulder Degeneration

Study	No.	M:F	(%F)	Mean Age	(Range)	Bilateral	(%)	Knee
Dieppe et al.[37]	11	1:10	(91)	76.7	(69–83)	9	(82)	6
Neer et al.[39]	26	6:20	(77)	69	(50–87)	16	(62)	?
Weiss et al.[41]	4	0:4	(100)	75.3	(73–86)	2	(50)	1
Neuman et al.[40]	1	0:1		75		0		
Halverson et al.[11,83]	30	6:24	(80)	72.5	(53–90)	19	(63)	16
Totals	72	13:59	(82)	72.1	(50–90)	46	(64)	

pingement arthropathy).[85] Another had a dysplastic left shoulder from birth.

Eight patients were found to have BCP and CPPD crystals simultaneously, so-called mixed crystal deposition disease.[11,18,43,44] All but one of these also had symptomatic knee involvement. The significance of these two crystals' simultaneous occurrence is uncertain, but it is intriguing that certain joints are capable of generating multiple crystal species.

Three patients had severe neurologic disorders (syringomyelia in one and cervical radiculopathies in two). Thus, the shoulder disease was partially attributable to denervation resulting in neuropathic joints.

One patient had chronic renal failure requiring hemodialysis. The remaining one third of patients, all of them women, had no identifiable contributing factor.

Milwaukee shoulder/knee syndrome may represent the final common pathway of several conditions, although other factors must also be involved because these conditions do not always progress to severe joint destruction.

Neer et al. have described the clinical and pathologic findings in 26 patients encountered over an 8-year period with "cuff-tear arthropathy" for whom they attempted surgical correction by total replacement arthroplasty.[39] Nearly as many cases were encountered where surgery was not performed during the same period. The symptoms in this group of persons were nearly identical to those described by our patients. On examination, most patients had swollen shoulders caused by synovial fluid accumulation. The fluid was often blood-streaked, and five patients had periarticular ecchymoses. The tendon of the long head of the biceps was either ruptured or dislocated in 21 patients, with visible retraction or dislocation of the muscle belly. The incongruity of the glenohumeral joint surfaces resulted in an even greater limitation of motion than usually seen with tears of the rotator cuff per se. The syndrome of apatite-associated destructive arthritis, described by Dieppe,[37] also seems identical. Other affected joints included six knees, six hips, two elbows, and two ankles. Radiographic and synovial fluid findings, including the presence of "apatite" crystals, were remarkably similar to those described here. The similarity of findings in the 72 cases so far reported is striking (Table 108–5).

Roentgenographic Features. Roentgenographic study showed glenohumeral joint degeneration in 49 of 55 shoulders examined in our series of 30 cases. Soft-tissue calcifications were present in 55% of shoulders. Upward subluxation of the humeral head or arthrographic evidence of rotator cuff defects was evident in 46 of 55 shoulders in our series (Figs. 108–5 and 108–6). The distance from the superior rim of the humeral head to the acromion, measured on routine roentgenograms with the patient erect, was reduced to 2 mm or less in all but three patients in the series of Neer et al.[39] Erosion of the coracoid process, of the undersurface of the anterior third of the acromion, and of the acromioclavicular joint was common (Figs. 108–7, 108–8); in many instances a rounding off of the greater tuberosity occurred with loss of the sulcus demarcating the anatomic neck. Erosions, subchondral cysts, and roughening of the bony cortex over the greater tuberosity at the site of the insertion of the rotator cuff were also noted frequently.

Arthrograms or bursagrams were performed in all the patients studied by Neer et al.[39] Each showed a grossly defective rotator cuff with communication between the glenohumeral and acromioclavicular joints in 10 instances. Arthrograms of the contralateral shoulder were performed in 11 of the 26 patients, and all showed a complete tear of the rotator cuff, although only 5 had typical radiographic changes in the glenohumeral joint. Pseudarthrosis formation between the humeral head and the acromion and clavicle was common (see Fig. 108–7). Bony destruction of the humeral head was also common, whereas osteophyte formation was usually modest.[38,39] An area of collapse of the proximal aspect of the humeral articular surface was present in all patients in the latter series, and was a requirement for the diagnosis of cuff tear arthropathy. We agree with Neer that these changes are not those of osteoarthritis of the shoulder.

Synovial Fluid Features. Synovial fluid leukocyte counts were usually less than 1000 per mm³ (76 of 78 fluids). The fluids were assayed for BCP crystals by (^{14}C) diphosphonate binding as described previously; 73 of 78 fluids showed significant binding. CPPD crys-

FIG. 108–4. Photograph of a 62-year-old woman with grotesque swelling of the right shoulder. Inserts show two crystal masses found in a wet preparation of fresh joint fluid. Note the erythrocytes for size comparison (phase contrast ×1,000). (From McCarty, D.J., et al.[38])

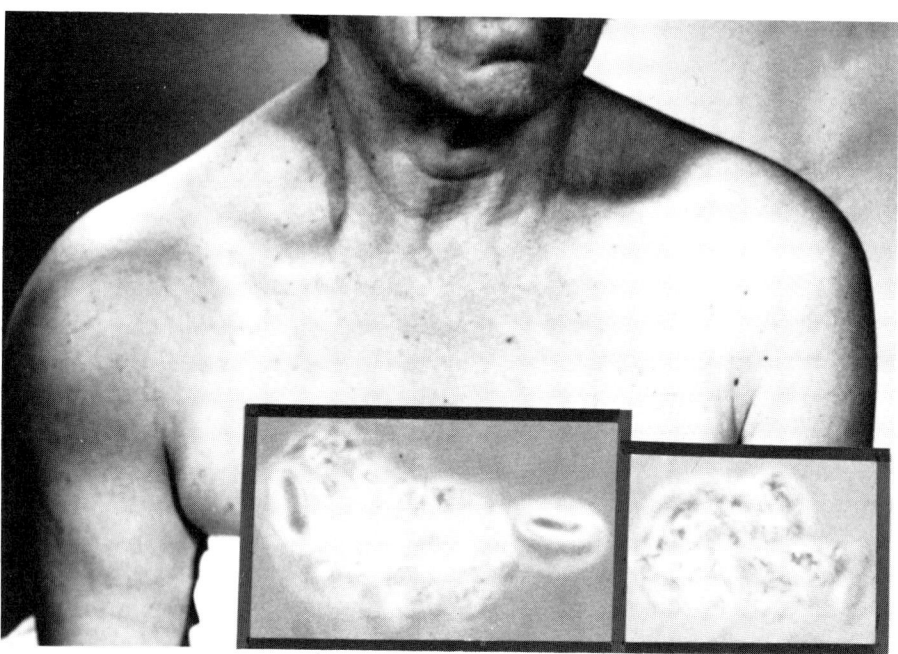

FIG. 108–5. Anteroposterior roentgenogram of the right shoulder showing soft tissue calcifications *(arrow)* and superior subluxation and sclerosis of the humeral head.

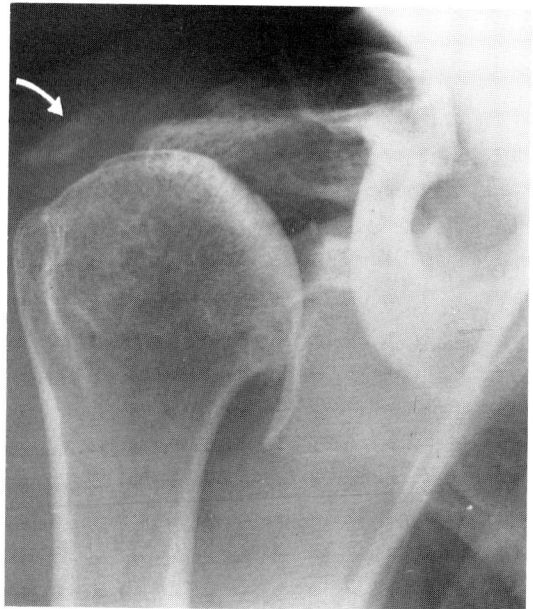

tals were also seen in eight fluids. Crystal concentrations estimated serially in fluids from two shoulders were remarkably constant for nearly a year, suggesting that they were under homeostatic control. Scanning electron microscopy detected microspheroidal aggregates in 33 of 46 fluids that bound (^{14}C) diphosphonate. The molar Ca/P of these aggregates ranged from 1.4 to 1.7 by x-ray energy dispersive analysis.[11]

Collagenase activity was found in at least one synovial fluid assay from half our patients. Although the total protein concentration in these fluids was 3 to 4 g/dl, most was albumin. Low levels of α_2-macroglobulin (a natural inhibitor of collagenase) and α_1-antitrypsin were found. Synovial fluids also demonstrated type I, II, and III particulate collagens and elevated neutral protease activities.[20] FTIR analyses also showed collagen as a constant feature in these joint fluid pellets.[10]

Knee Involvement. In our series of 30 patients with shoulder disease, 16 had symptomatic knee involvement. Lateral tibiofemoral compartment narrowing occurring in 14 of 36 patients (39%) (Figs. 108–9 and 108–10) such as is seen in CPPD disease (see Chapter 107) exceeded medial compartment narrowing in 11 of 36 patients (31%). This differed significantly from 56 patients (62 evaluable knees) with symptomatic osteoarthritis of the knee without shoulder involve-

FIG. 108–6. Anteroposterior roentgenogram of an asymptomatic left shoulder in a patient whose dominant right shoulder was severely involved. Calcifications are present in the rotator cuff, and cystic changes are noted at the site of insertion of the rotator cuff on the greater tuberosity of the humerus. An arthrogram showing complete rupture of the rotator cuff. This appearance is characteristic before bony collapse of the articulating surface of the humeral head occurs.

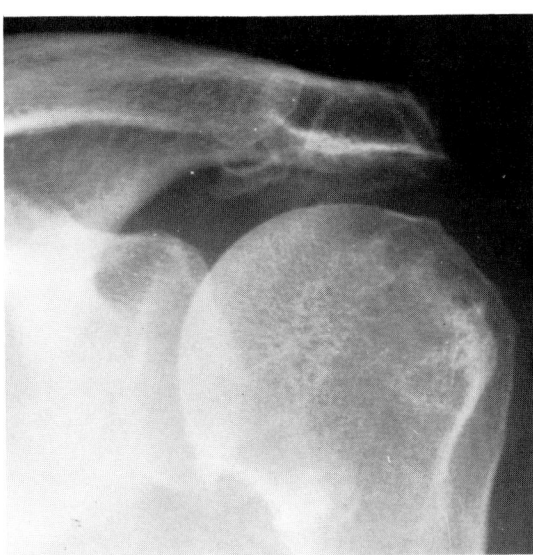

FIG. 108–7. Anteroposterior roentgenogram of the right shoulder in a patient showing more advanced changes. Superior displacement of the humeral head has resulted in a pseudoarticulation with the acromion. Sclerosis, cystic changes, and irregularity of the humeral head are also present. (From McCarty, D.J., et al.[38])

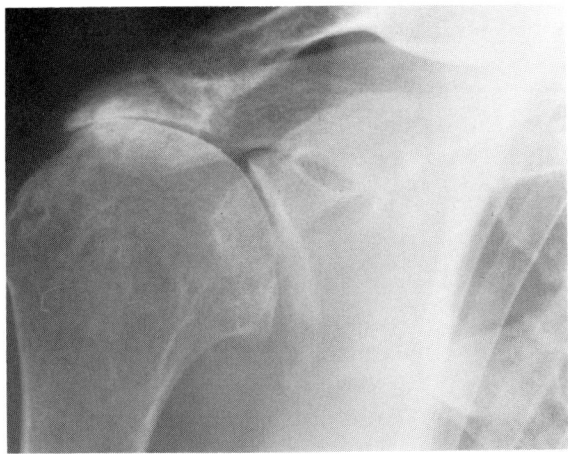

FIG. 108–8. Anteroposterior roentgenogram of the right shoulder of another patient showing superior displacement of the humeral head and pseudoarticulations with the clavicle, acromion, and coracoid process. The humeral head is partly collapsed with eburnation only in its inferomedial articulating surface. Note the absence of osteophytes.

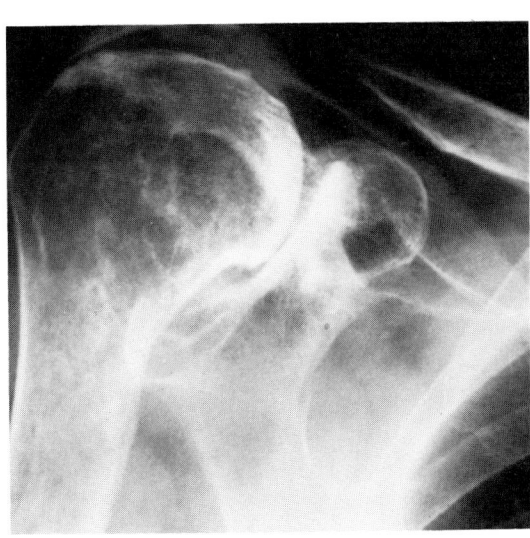

ment (p <0.01).[83] CPPD crystal deposition was detected either in synovial fluid or by radiographs in seven. One patient each had osteochondromatosis and lateral femoral condylar osteonecrosis, both of which have also been associated with CPPD deposition. The patients with the syndrome of "apatite-associated destructive arthritis" also showed primarily hip and lateral compartment knee involvement.[37] Thus, the pattern of knee joint degeneration in patients with shoulder joint disease appears to differ from that of ordinary osteoarthritis of the knee.

Other Joint Involvement. Two of our patients had severe degenerative arthritis of the hips, but because they already had prostheses there was no fluid to study. Whether a similar process was involved in pathogenesis is unclear. We have also studied a man with bilateral elbow joint degeneration and synovial fluid findings consistent with those of Milwaukee shoulder. As already discussed, the erosive arthropathy of wrists and small hand joints associated with periarticular calcific deposits described by Schumacher et al.[42] may share some of these features, although again, no fluid could be obtained for analysis.

Pathology. Synovial biopsies obtained at the time of operation from the shoulders of four patients demonstrated increased numbers of villi, focal synovial lining cell hyperplasia, a few giant cells, fibrin, and BCP crystal deposits (Fig. 108–11) (Table 108–6).[86] Electron microscopy showed crystals being engulfed

FIG. 108–9. Standing anteroposterior roentgenogram of the knees from a patient with Milwaukee shoulder syndrome showing lateral tibiofemoral compartment narrowing and incongruity with subchondral bony sclerosis, but minimal osteophyte formation.

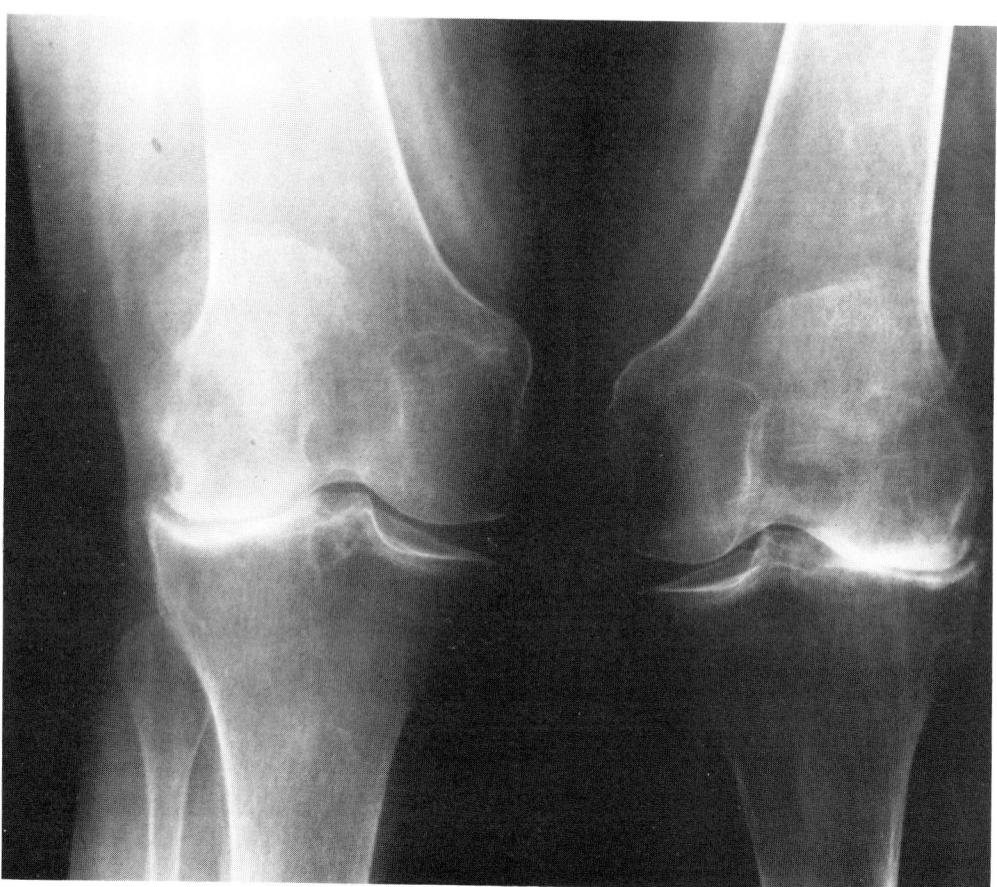

by synovial lining cells and histiocytes (Figs. 108–12, 108–13). Calcific deposits in synovial microvilli appeared to have access to the joint space through areas denuded of synovial lining cells (Fig. 108–14).

In the series of Neer et al., a large, complete cuff tear was found in each patient at operation.[39] The humeral head could be dislocated passively in 14 instances and was fixed in a dislocated position in the remaining 12 shoulders. The supraspinatus tendon was completely ruptured in all patients, and the infraspinatus tendon in all but one instance. The teres minor and subscapularis tendons were usually involved, but some vestiges remained in all patients. The tendon of the long head of the biceps was ruptured, dislocated, or frayed in 18, 3, and 5 patients, respectively. The subdeltoid bursa was thickened, forming a large loose pouch around the head of the biceps, and contained variable amounts of often sanguineous synovial fluid. The articular cartilage was pebble-like and the collapsed articular surface, the major point of contact with the acromion, was ebur-

nated and denuded of cartilage with small marginal osteophytes. The remainder of the humeral head was covered with degenerated cartilage and fibrous tissue. The subchondral bone could be indented easily with a finger. The anterior acromial epiphysis had failed to fuse in three patients, which may have contributed to subacromial impingement.

Histologically, the atrophic articular cartilage of the humeral head was covered to a variable degree with a fibrous membrane (pannus). In these areas, the adjacent bone was osteoporotic and hypervascularized with attempts at repair at points of bony collapse. At points of contact between the humeral head and scapula, the cartilage was completely denuded and the bone was sclerotic. Fragments of articular cartilage were found in the subsynovium. These fragments resembled those found in neuropathic joints, albeit less extensive.

Neer et al. point out that in glenohumeral osteoarthritis, the entire humeral head is sclerotic without large areas of cartilage atrophy and osteoporosis, and

FIG. 108–10. Lateral roentgenogram of the right knee of another patient showing isolated patellofemoral osteoarthritis (patella "wrapped around" the femur), femoral cortical defect, and chondrocalcinosis of the femoral articular cartilage. Osteochondromata can be seen in the posterior joint recess.

Table 108–6. Microscopic Features of Synovial Membrane in Milwaukee Shoulder/Knee Syndrome

Villous hyperplasia
Focal synovial lining cell hyperplasia
BCP crystal deposition (extracellular, intracellular)*
Fibrin deposition
Giant cells
Fibrosis
Vascular congestion
No inflammatory cells

*The only specific feature.

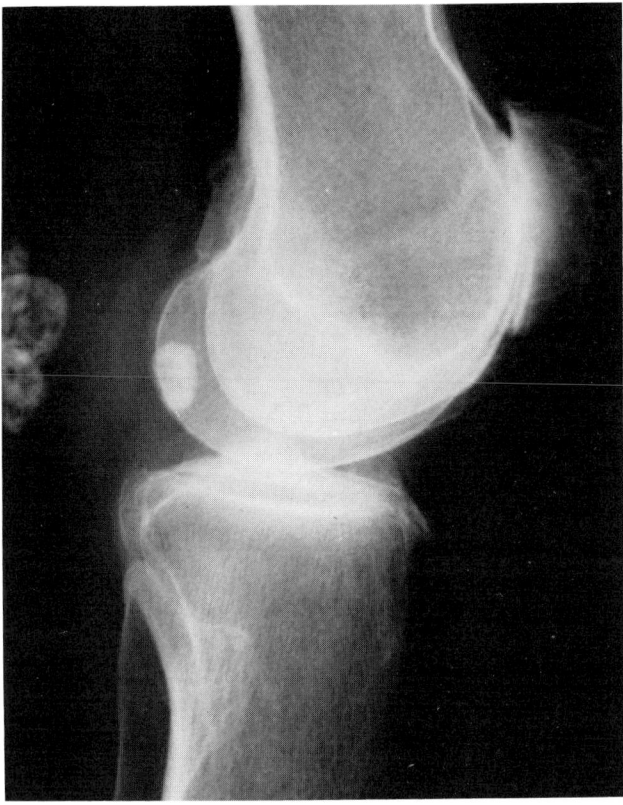

that it is enlarged by marginal osteophytes without bone atrophy and collapse.[39] The rotator cuff is nearly always intact.[87]

Pathogenesis. A hypothesis was formulated to link the synovial fluid findings to the genesis of this syndrome[20] (Fig. 108–15). BCP crystals, particulate collagens, and low leukocyte counts were associated with activated collagenase and neutral protease activities. Electron microscopy showed crystal aggregates enmeshed in synovial collagenous tissue and within synovial fixed macrophage-like cells. Werb and Reynolds demonstrated that particulates, such as latex beads, added to rabbit synovial cells in culture are phagocytized and stimulate increased secretion of proteases, including collagenase.[88] This increased secretion continued relentlessly until the ingested particles were biodegraded, at which time it returned to baseline. Collagen also stimulated collagenase release from cultured human skin fibroblasts,[89] and synovial fluid "wear" particles released neutral proteases from cultured synovial cells.[90]

We postulated that activated proteases synthesized and released after endocytosis of BCP crystals and particulate collagens might be instrumental (1) in causing the joint destruction and (2) in releasing additional crystals and particulate collagens into the joint space. Such enzymatic "strip-mining" had been envisioned previously for sodium urate and CPPD crystal release (see Chapter 107).

This hypothesis was tested by adding natural or synthetic BCP, CPPD, and other crystals to cultured human or canine synovial cells.[91] Neutral protease and collagenase secretion was augmented in a dose-related fashion approximately five to eight times over control cultures incubated without crystals. Chondrocytes in primary culture behaved similarly.[92] Because crystals have been described within human chondrocytes,[93,94] it is possible that autolysis of cartilage may occur without first the shedding of crystals into synovial fluid. Moreover, partially purified mammalian collagenase released BCP crystal microspheroidal aggregates from calcified synovial tissue in vitro.[95] The mean diameter and size ranges of the

FIG. 108–11. Light micrograph of synovium showing many villi and focal synovial cell hyperplasia. In cross section, the branching villi appear as free bodies. Some villi are partially covered with or contain fibrin in various stages of organization (×110).

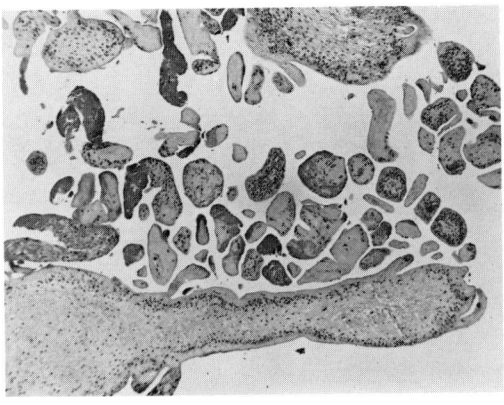

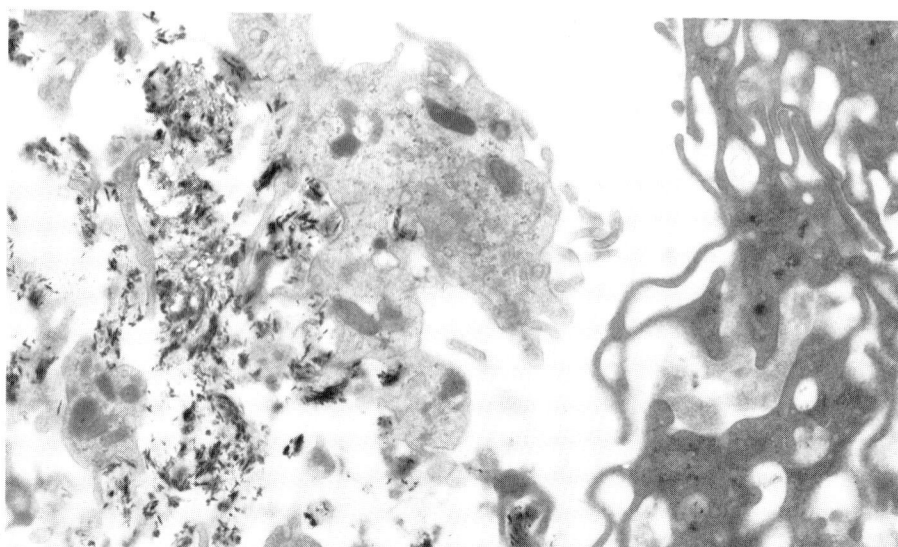

FIG. 108–12. Electron micrograph demonstrating hyperplastic synovial cells engulfing crystals, fibrin, and amorphous material. Extensive cytoplasmic processes form complex interdigitations with processes on adjacent cells ($\times$14,300).

released aggregates were virtually identical to those observed in synovial fluids obtained from the same patient. Fluid obtained several weeks after synovectomy of the affected shoulder in this patient showed no mineral by (^{14}C) EHDP binding and greatly reduced protease activities.[20] Although degenerating articular cartilage can form mineral as discussed previously, there is little doubt about the synovial origin of the crystals in this patient, who had synovial chondromatosis (chondrometaplasia of subsynovial fibroblasts).[13]

In addition to the stimulation of relentless enzyme secretion, BCP or CPPD crystal endocytosis was associated with a massive genesis of prostaglandins, especially PGE$_2$.[91,92] All PGE$_2$ release occurred in the first few hours after crystals were added to the cells.[96] Both PGE$_2$ release and collagenase release have been found after exposure of macrophages or synovial cells to sodium urate crystals and have been related to the hard tissue destruction in gout, as discussed in detail in Chapter 106. CPPD crystal–stimulated prostaglandin and protease release may account for the destruc-

FIG. 108–13. Electron micrograph of a hyperplastic synovial cell. Crystals within phagolysosomes are bounded by distinct limiting membranes. Many extracellular crystals are also present ($\times$26,400).

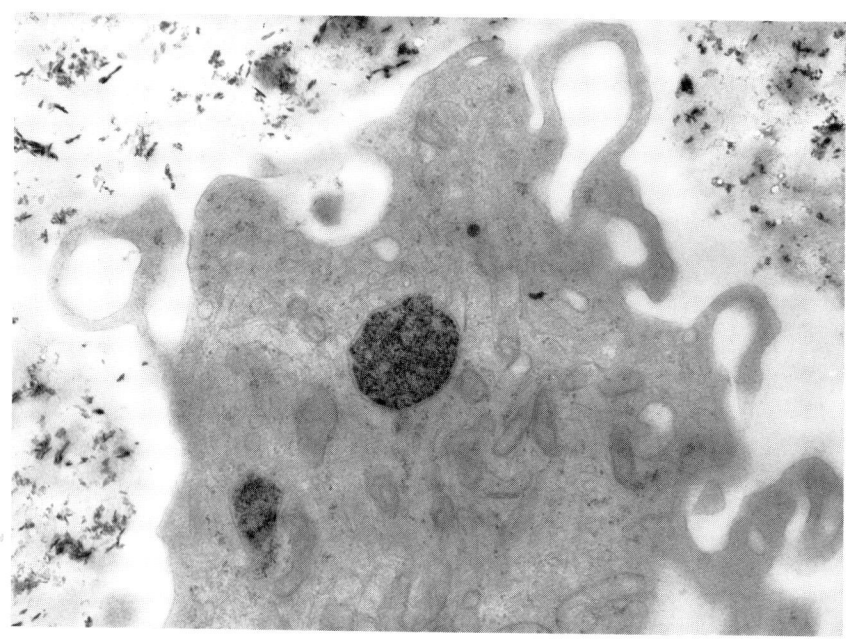

FIG. 108–14. Electron micrograph showing a small villus in cross section. Synovial lining cells are absent. Crystal microaggregates are seen dispersed among collagen fibers, lying free on the surface and in the synovial space. Several fibrocytes are present ($\times$6,400). (From Garancis, J.C., et al.[13])

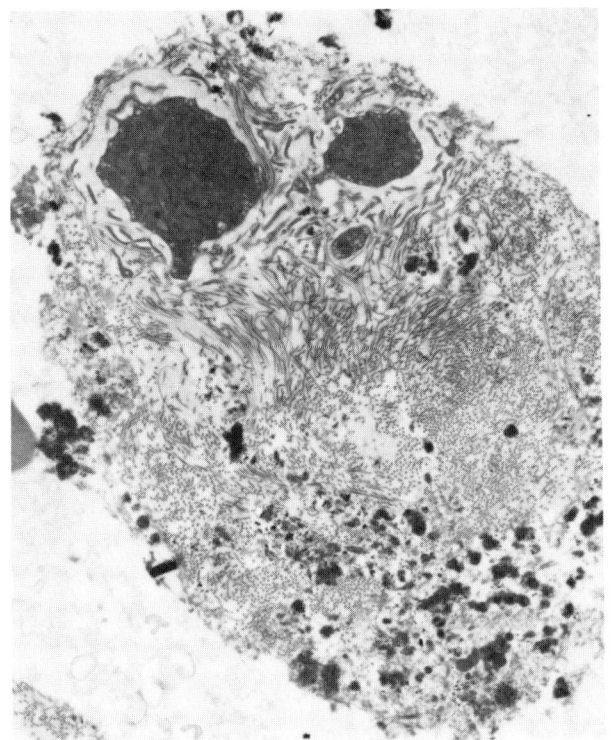

FIG. 108–15. Hypothetical schema relating the various features of Milwaukee shoulder/knee syndrome.

PATHOGENESIS OF MILWAUKEE SHOULDER/KNEE SYNDROME

Associated factors

Mechanical (overuse, trauma)
CPPD deposition
Denervation
Dialysis

BCP Crystals ← → "Degeneration"
& Particulate Collagen   Cartilege, Bone, Capsule
                              & Rotator Cuff

"Strip" mining

Endocytosis by   Collagenase
Synoviocytes   →   Neutral Protease
                         Prostaglandin E2
                         Interleukin I

Dissolution — → Mitogenesis — → Synoviocyte hyperplasia

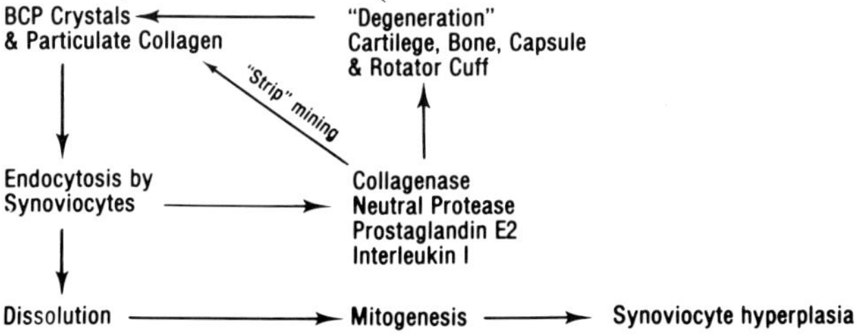

tive arthropathies associated with these crystals. PGE_2 was found in joint fluid from our patients[20] and was isolated from the periarticular calcium phosphate deposits from a patient with phalangeal osteolysis.[97] Alternatively, interleukin 1–like activity has been detected in crystal-containing synovial fluids and may stimulate chondrocytes to autolytic activity.[98] In another study, endogenous pyrogen production by mononuclear cells did not increase after exposure to BCP crystals.[99]

This hypothesis is consistent with the concept of "crystal traffic" derived from studies of the fate of radiolabeled CPPD or BCP crystals injected intrasynovially. One half of a dose of CPPD crystals was cleared from human joints in 30 to 90 days and from rabbit joints in 16 to 20 days.[100,101] Clearance rates were inversely proportional to crystal size. Injected crystals were phagocytized by synovial cells where virtually all dissolution appeared to take place. This phenomenon was evidenced by localization of all nuclide in synovial tissue, the finding of all crystals inside cells by electron microscopy, the lack of effect on clearance rate of extracellular magnesium depletion by dietary deprivation, the failure of joint lavage to remove significant radionuclide, and reduction of clearance rate by 65% in the presence of synovial cell hemosiderosis induced by injection of autologous blood.[102] Both CPPD crystals and hemosiderin were shown in the same cells by transmission electron microscopy and x-ray energy dispersive analysis. ^{85}Sr-labeled BCP crystals were cleared from rabbit joints with a half-life of about 6 days, about three times faster than for CPPD crystals.[103]

The focal cell hyperplasia found in the four synovial membranes we examined[86] was described by Doyle as a constant feature of synovial membranes containing calcium crystals.[104] This finding might be related to their mitogenic properties. BCP, CPPD, calcium urate, calcium diphosphonate, and calcium carbonate, but not crystals or particulates not containing calcium (such as sodium urate, diamond, silicon dioxide, or latex beads), were capable of substituting for serum growth factors in certain cell systems.[105] Crystals must undergo endocytosis by cells for mitogenesis to occur.[106] Dissolution of crystals follows phagocytosis and is also necessary for mitogenesis.[107,108] Calcium-containing crystals appear to act as a "competence" factor, because they can substitute for growth factors found in serum (platelet-derived growth factor, PDGF); like PDGF, calcium-containing crystals require a progression factor, such as somatomedin C, for full expression of mitogenic potency.[109,110] Similar intracellular biochemical events in cultured fibroblasts were observed in the presence of either PDGF or BCP crystals, although the appearance of certain proteins is delayed by 3 hours with the latter stimulus.[111] (^{45}Ca) BCP crystals added to cultured synovial cells, skin fibroblasts, or peripheral blood monocytes were phagocytized and degraded, probably by the ATPase-driven lysosomal proton pump.[112,113] Weak bases, such as chloroquine or NH_4^+, inhibited BCP crystal solubilization by all three cell types in a dose-dependent fashion.[108] Calcium crystal–induced mitogenesis was also reduced in a parallel dose-dependent fashion by these inhibitors, but mitosis stimulated by serum was unaffected.[108] Also, collagenase production by fibroblasts was not affected by inhibitors of crystal dissolution.[114] These data are consistent with the concept that intracellular crystal dissolution is associated with a rise in intracellular calcium, a known stimulus to cell division.

In contrast to these ideas, Neer et al. favor a pathogenesis based on disuse osteoporosis and mechanical instability.[39] The greater severity of the clinical symptoms, radiologic evidence of destruction, the greater joint fluid levels of crystals and enzymes in the shoulder on the dominant side, and the frequent history of increased joint use or trauma support a pathogenetic role of joint movement. But the finding of destructive arthropathies of the knee and possibly other joints in the same patients suggests that this may be a more generalized arthropathy. We agree that biomechanical factors probably play a role in the pathogenetic scheme outlined in Figure 108–15.

Treatment. The treatment of Milwaukee shoulder syndrome is generally unsatisfactory. A conservative approach including prescription of NSAIDs, repeated shoulder aspirations, and decreased shoulder use has sometimes controlled symptoms satisfactorily. Implantation of a subacromial spacer that depresses the humeral head into the glenoid fossa has been performed in two patients and resulted initially in improved motion and decreased pain. The spacer was later noted to have migrated in one of these patients. Several patients have successfully had semiconstrained total shoulder joint arthroplasty. Neer et al. suggest a resurfacing total shoulder joint replacement using a nonconstrained prosthesis with rotator cuff reconstruction when the full syndrome is present.[39] They admit that this procedure is difficult and that treatment goals must be limited. They envision three problems: (1) massive rotator cuff loss with instability, (2) painful incongruity of the glenohumeral joint, and (3) painful subacromial impingement. Treatment of the condition at the stage of "precollapse" of the humeral head (radiologic normal bony contour) is by anterior acromioplasty and repair of the rotator cuff. If collapse has occurred, they favor arthroplasty, often using

oversized, still experimental glenoid components for greater stability. Despite residual problems, all but one patient thought that arthroplasty was helpful. Radical acromionectomy had been performed in five patients by other surgeons and had increased the disability in all.

At the time of clinical diagnosis of our patients, advanced destructive changes were usually present, and in three shoulders these changes were asymptomatic. Thus, there is no way to identify persons at risk for this condition. Novel attempts to control the disease with inhibitors of calcification or collagenase inhibitors should probably be directed at the generally less involved nondominant shoulder in patients with established disease on the dominant side.

SECONDARY BCP ARTHROPATHIES

Several disease states, including chronic renal failure, the "collagen" diseases, and neurologic injury, have been associated with calcifications that may occur in almost any tissue. In these conditions, BCP crystals have been found in periarticular soft tissues, in bursae, and within joints and are often associated with rheumatic symptoms. For a more complete listing of conditions associated with calcinosis, see Table 73–4.

Soft-tissue calcifications involving the fibrous tissue in skin or muscle occur in the "collagen" diseases. Rare cases of intra-articular calcification, one with a chalky joint effusion, have been reported in scleroderma.[14,51] Another patient with an "overlap" collagen-vascular disease developed periarticular calcifications in multiple sites.[50]

Heterotopic ossification mimicking arthritis has been described following neurologic catastrophes.[52,53] Such ossification tends to occur in periarticular tissues. The mechanisms are unknown. In some cases of heterotopic ossification, low synovial fluid leukocyte counts and high protein concentrations have been found.[54]

Several miscellaneous causes of BCP crystal deposition have been described. An unusual patient had Laennec's cirrhosis, hypertrophic osteoarthropathy, and synovial calcifications in the knees, which may have been related to vitamin D intoxication.[58] A patient with "draft dodger's knee" developed calcifications around the knee many years after self-injection of olive oil.[57]

The intra-articular injection of triamcinolone hexacetonide has been associated with the formation of periarticular calcifications along the injection tract, which may become apparent months after the injection.[55,56] Such calcifications may gradually be resorbed over a period of months to years.

Tumoral Calcinosis. This condition, consisting of massive, expanding calcific deposits in or near one or more large joints, is rare in North America and Europe, but nonhyperphosphatemic cases are relatively common in Africa.[64] Phosphate deprivation constitutes definitive therapy for hyperphosphatemic cases, which are often familial.[61–63]

Arthropathy in Chronic Renal Failure. Uremia may predispose to several forms of arthritis or periarthritis. A portion of these may be associated with BCP crystals. Caner and Decker first described periarthritis occurring in hemodialysis patients.[46] Metastatic soft-tissue calcifications occur frequently in uremic patients with high calcium/phosphorus products.[47] This phenomenon has been described as a form of calciphylaxis in humans.[1] Several authors have suggested that recurrences of this form of calcific periarthritis could be prevented by control of serum phosphorus levels.[46,48,49]

One study of 28 patients undergoing long-term dialysis described articular symptoms in 57%.[115] Many were thought to have periarthritis or peritendinitis, but 38% had an erosive arthropathy. In the small joints of the hands, erosive arthropathy has been ascribed to secondary hyperparathyroidism.[116] Erosive disease has also been observed in axial joints and large joints, especially the shoulder.[117,118] "Erosive azotemic arthropathy" describes a subset of patients with erosive changes in large and small joints, "noninflammatory" synovial fluids, and renal osteodystrophy.[119] Histologic analysis of material found in bone cysts has shown amyloid composed of β_2-microglobulin.[129] Cases with carpal tunnel syndrome have consistently demonstrated this type of amyloid as well.[121] Amyloid has been detected in synovium, tenosynovium, capsule, and extra-articular locations as well.[122]

Crystal-induced arthritis appears to be common in uremia (Table 108–7). Hyperuricemia predisposes to acute gout, although attacks are less common than might be expected. BCP crystals are likely to form in or around joints and in other tissues in the milieu of excess phosphorus or calcium. CPPD crystal deposition has been associated with hyperparathyroidism.[123] Calcium oxalate has been found in the synovial

Table 108–7. Substances Deposited in Uremia

Monosodium urate monohydrate
Calcium pyrophosphate dihydrate
Basic calcium phosphates
Calcium oxalate
Aluminum phosphate
Amyloid (β_2-microglobulin)

fluid from patients on chronic hemodialysis, especially in those receiving ascorbic acid supplementation.[65,66,124] Finally, aluminum phosphate has been demonstrated in the synovium of patients taking aluminum compounds by mouth to bind intestinal phosphate.[67,125]

Synovial fluid leukocyte counts are generally not increased, although Good et al. found leukocytosis in two of three inflamed shoulders.[35] Intra-articular BCP crystals were found in two of these. BCP crystals have been found in an elbow joint without leukocytosis.[45]

Animal Models of BCP Crystal Deposition. Spontaneous periarticular calcinosis has been reported in dogs,[126,127] and may be familial.[127] Reginato et al. successfully calcified articular cartilage of synovium with vitamin D administration to rabbits.[128] These deposits were composed of BCP crystals identical to those found in the synovial fluid of patients.[10]

Treatment. The identification of the calcium-binding amino acid GLA (gamma carboxyglutamic acid) in pathologic soft-tissue calcification[129,130] provides a rationale for the use of warfarin therapy of these disorders. Synthesis of GLA-containing proteins, such as prothrombin, is vitamin K–dependent. Reports of success, however,[131] must be viewed in the light of the natural tendency for spontaneous resorption of at least some of these deposits. Probenecid has been used successfully to treat patients with calcinosis, but the same caveat applies in the absence of suitable controls.[132]

UNANSWERED QUESTIONS

Many questions about BCP crystal arthropathies and periarthropathies remain to be answered. Such crystals have been described in the synovial fluid of patients with advanced rheumatoid arthritis.[133] Whether BCP crystals participate in the inflammation of rheumatoid arthritis and other diseases or merely represent an epiphenomenon is unknown. Dieppe and Watt have suggested that crystal deposition is not the primary event but occurs secondarily as an opportunistic event in damaged joints.[134] Crystal deposition may then modify the arthropathy and contribute further to joint deterioration.

Perhaps the greatest mystery are the mechanisms of pathologic calcification. Codman considered the formation of periarticular calcific deposits in the shoulder to be the result of necrosis,[15] but Uhthoff et al. were unable to detect histologic evidence of necrosis.[33] They hypothesized that hypoxia induces the tendon to transform into fibrocartilage. BCP crystals then form in matrix vesicles generated by metaplastic chondrocytes, subsequently coalescing into larger deposits.[76] These data suggest that vascular invasion and resorption of the calcific deposits follow, leaving a reconstituted vascularized tendon.

Anderson has presented a unified concept of pathologic calcification encompassing both metastatic and dystrophic forms. Matrix vesicles or mitochondria may serve as repositories for calcium and, upon exposure to sufficient phosphate, mineralization begins.[135] The mechanism responsible for most pathologic calcifications that occur in the absence of hypercalcemia or hyperphosphatemia is unclear. Microcrystalline needles have been found in myelin bodies within degenerating fibrocytes in aging human[136] and rat[137] aortas. These crystals were presumed to originate in these cells, but the presence of calcifications on elastin or collagen fibers suggested that the crystals could have formed extracellularly with subsequent phagocytosis.

REFERENCES

1. Gipstein, R.M. et al.: Calciphylaxis in man. A syndrome of tissue necrosis and vascular calcification in 11 patients with chronic renal failure. Arch. Intern. Med., *136*:1273–1280, 1976.
2. Pinals, R.S., and Short, C.L.: Calcific periarthritis involving multiple sites. Arthritis Rheum., *9*:566–574, 1966.
3. McCarty, D.J., and Gatter, R.A.: Recurrent acute inflammation associated with focal apatite crystal deposition. Arthritis Rheum., *9*:804–819, 1966.
4. Swannell, A.J., Underwood, F.A., and Dixon, A.S.: Periarticular calcific deposits mimicking acute arthritis. Ann. Rheum. Dis., *29*:380–385, 1970.
5. Thompson, G.R., et al.: Calcific tendonitis and soft tissue calcification resembling gout. JAMA, *203*:464–472, 1968.
6. Dieppe, P.A., et al.: Apatite deposition disease. Lancet, *1*:266–269, 1976.
7. Schumacher, H.R., et al.: Arthritis associated with apatite crystals. Ann. Intern. Med., *87*:411–416, 1977.
8. Faure, G., et al.: Apatites in heterotopic calcifications. Scan. Electron Microsc., *4*:1624–1634, 1982.
9. Daculsi, G., Faure, G., and Kerebel, B.: Electron microscopy and microanalysis of a subcutaneous heterotopic calcification. Calcif. Tissue Int., *35*:723–727, 1983.
10. McCarty, D.J., Lehr, J.R., and Halverson, P.B.: Crystal populations in human synovial fluid. Identification of apatite, octacalcium phosphate, tricalcium phosphate. Arthritis Rheum., *26*:247–251, 1983.
11. Halverson, P.B., et al.: The Milwaukee shoulder syndrome: Eleven additional cases with involvement of the knee in seven. Semin. Arthritis Rheum., *14*:36–44, 1984.
12. Schumacher, H.R., Rothfuss, S., Bertken, R., and Linder, J.: Unusual laminated birefringent arrays of apatite crystals in inflammatory arthritis. Arthritis Rheum., *30*:S106, 1987.
13. Garancis, J.C., et al.: Milwaukee shoulder: Association of microspheroids containing hydroxyapatite crystals, active collagenase and neutral protease with rotator cuff defects. III. Morphologic and biochemical studies of an excised synovium showing chondromatosis. Arthritis Rheum., *24*:484–491, 1981.
14. Brandt, K.D., and Krey, P.R.: Chalky joint effusion. The result of massive synovial deposition of calcium apatite in progressive systemic sclerosis. Arthritis Rheum., *20*:792–796, 1977.
15. Codman, E.A.: The shoulder. Boston, Thomas Todd, 1934.
16. Paul, H., Reginato, A.J., and Schumacher, H.R.: Alizarin red S staining as a screening test to detect calcium compounds in synovial fluid. Arthritis Rheum., *26*:191–200, 1983.
17. Bardin, T., et al.: Alizarin red staining of synovial fluid (SF). Similar results in osteoarthritis (OA) and rheumatoid arthritis (RA). Arthritis Rheum., *28*:S53, 1985.
18. Halverson, P.B., and McCarty, D.J.: Identification of hydroxyapatite crystals in synovial fluid. Arthritis Rheum., *22*:389–395, 1979.
19. Halverson, P.B., and McCarty, D.J.: Patterns of radiographic abnormalities associated with basic calcium phosphate and calcium pyrophosphate dihydrate crystal deposition in the knee. Ann. Rheum. Dis., *45*:603–605, 1986.
20. Halverson, P.B., et al.: Milwaukee shoulder: Association of microspheroids containing hydroxyapatite crystals, active collagenase and neutral protease with rotator cuff defects. II. Synovial fluid studies. Arthritis Rheum., *24*:474–483, 1981.
21. Cherian, P.V., and Schumacher, H.R.: Diagnostic potential of rapid electron microscopic analysis of joint effusions. Arthritis Rheum., *25*:98–100, 1982.
22. Painter, C.F.: Subdeltoid bursitis. Boston Med. Surg. J., *156*:345–349, 1907.
23. Sandstrom, C.: Peritendinitis calcarea: A common disease of middle life; its diagnosis, pathology and treatment. Am. J. Roentgenol., *40*:1–21, 1938.
24. Zaphiropoulos, G., and Graham, R.: Recurrent calcific periarthritis involving multiple sites. Proc. R. Soc. Med., *66*:351–352, 1973.
25. Amor, B., et al.: Hydroxyapatite rheumatism and HLA markers. J. Rheumatol., *3*:101–104, 1977.
26. Cannon, R.B., and Schmid, F.R.: Calcific periarthritis involving multiple sites in identical twins. Arthritis Rheum., *16*:393–395, 1973.
27. Sharp, J.: Heredo-familial vascular and articular calcifications. Ann. Rheum. Dis., *13*:15–16, 1950.
28. Marcos, J.C., et al.: Idiopahic familial chondrocalcinosis due to apatite crystal deposition. Am. J. Med., *71*:557–564, 1981.
29. Hajiroussou, V.J., and Webley, M.: Familial calcific periarthritis. Ann. Rheum. Dis., *42*:469–470, 1983.
30. Doherty, M., Dieppe, P.A.: Multiple microcrystal deposition within a family. Ann. Rheum. Dis., *44*:544–548, 1985.
31. Faure, G., and Daculsi, G.: Calcified tendinitis: A review. Ann. Rheum. Dis., *42*:50–53, 1983.
32. McKendry, R.J.R., et al.: Calcifying tendinitis of the shoulder: Prognostic value of clinical, histologic and radiologic features in 57 surgically treated cases. J. Rheumatol., *9*:75–80, 1982.
33. Uhthoff, H.K., Sarkar, K., and Maynard, J.A.: Calcifying tendonitis. Clin. Orthop. Rel. Res., *118*:164–168, 1976.
34. Fam, A.G., et al.: Apatite-associated arthropathy: A clinical study of 14 cases and of 2 patients with calcific bursitis. J. Rheumatol., *6*:461–471, 1979.
35. Good, A.E., et al.: The dialysis shoulder. Arthritis Rheum., *25*:S34, 1982.
36. Gerster J.C., and Lagier, R.: Acute synovitis with intra-articular apatite deposits in an osteoarthritic metacarpophalangeal joint. Ann. Rheum. Dis., *44*:207–210, 1985.
37. Dieppe, P.A., et al.: Apatite associated destructive arthritis. Br. J. Rheumatol., *23*:84–91, 1984.
38. McCarty, D.J., et al.: Milwaukee shoulder: Association of microspheroids containing hydroxyapatite crystals, active col-

lagenase and neutral protease with rotator cuff defects. I. Clinical aspects. Arthritis Rheum., 24:464–473, 1981.

39. Neer, C.S., Craig, E.V., and Fukuda, H.: Cuff tear arthropathy. J. Bone Joint Surg., 69A:1232–1244, 1983.

40. Newman, J.H., et al.: Milwaukee shoulder syndrome: A new crystal induced arthritis syndrome associated with hydroxyapatite crystals—A case report. Del. Med. J., 55:167–169, 1983.

41. Weiss, J.J., Good, A., and Schumacher, H.R.: Four cases of "Milwaukee Shoulder" with a description of clinical presentation and long-term treatment. J. Am. Geriatr. Soc., 33:202–205, 1985.

42. Schumacher, H.R., et al.: Erosive arthritis associated with apatite crystal deposition. Arthritis Rheum., 24:31–37, 1981.

43. Dieppe, P.A., et al.: Mixed crystal deposition disease and osteoarthritis. Br. Med. J., 1:150, 1978.

44. Doyle, D.V., et al.: Mixed crystal deposition in an osteoarthritic joint. J. Pathol., 123:1–5, 1977.

45. Yano, E., Takeuchi, A., and Yoshioka, M.: Hydroxyapatite associated arthritis in a patient undergoing chronic hemodialysis. Int. J. Tissue React., 7:527–534, 1985.

46. Caner, J.E.Z., and Decker, J.L.: Recurrent acute (?gouty) arthritis in chronic renal failure treated with periodic hemodialysis. Am. J. Med., 36:571–582, 1964.

47. Kuzela, D.C., et al.: Soft tissue calcification in chronic dialysis patients. Am. J. Pathol., 86:403–424, 1977.

48. Mirahmadi, K.S., Coburn, J.W., and Bluestone, R.: Calcific periarthritis and hemodialysis. JAMA, 223:548–549, 1973.

49. Moskowitz, R.W., et al.: Crystal induced inflammation associated with chronic renal failure treated with periodic hemodialysis. Am. J. Med., 47:450–460, 1969.

50. Reginato, A.J., and Schumacher, H.R.: Synovial calcification in a patient with collagen-vascular disease: Light and electron microscopic studies. J. Rheumatol., 4:261–271, 1977.

51. Resnick, D., et al.: Intra-articular calcification in scleroderma. Radiology, 124:685–688, 1977.

52. Goldberg, M.A., and Schumacher, H.R.: Heterotopic ossifications mimicking acute arthritis after neurologic catastrophes. Arch. Intern. Med., 137:619–621, 1977.

53. Rosin, A.J.: Ectopic calcification around joints of paralysed limbs in hemiplegia, diffuse brain damage and other neurological diseases. Ann. Rheum. Dis., 34:499–505, 1975.

54. Yue, C.C., Regier, A., and Kushner, I.: The arthritis of heterotopic ossification shows elevated synovial protein concentration without synovial leukocytosis. Clin. Res., 31:808A, 1983.

55. Jalava, S., et al.: Periarticular calcification after intra-articular triamcinolone hexacetonide. Scand. J. Rheumatol., 9:190–192, 1980.

56. McCarty, D.J.: Treatment of rheumatoid joint inflammation with triamcinolone hexacetonide. Arthritis Rheum., 15:118–129, 1972.

57. Hood, R.W., and Insall, J.: Draft dodger's knee: Unusual pattern of calcification in the knee secondary to olive oil injection. A case report. Orthopedics, 4:1241–1244, 1981.

58. Kieff, E.D., and McCarty, D.J.: Hypertrophic osteoarthropathy with arthritis and synovial calcification in a patient with alcoholic cirrhosis. Arthritis Rheum., 12:261–271, 1969.

59. DiGiovanna, J.J., Helfgott, R.K., Gerber, L.H., and Peck, G.L.: Extraspinal tendon and ligament calcification associated with long term therapy with etretinate. N. Engl. J. Med., 315:1177–1182, 1986.

60. Butler, R.C., Dieppe, P.A., and Keat, A.C.S.: Calcinosis of joints and periarticular tissues associated with vitamin D intoxication. Ann. Rheum. Dis., 44:494–498, 1985.

61. Kirk, T.S., and Simon, M.A.: Tumoral calcinosis: Report of a case with successful medical management. J. Bone Joint Surg., 63A:1167–1169, 1981.

62. Lufkin, E.G., Kumar, R., and Heath, H.: Hyperphosphatemic tumoral calcinosis: Effects of phosphate depletion on vitamin D metabolism, and of acute hypocalcemia on parathyroid hormone secretion and action. J. Clin. Endocrinol. Metab., 56:1319–1322, 1983.

63. Prince, M.J., et al.: Hyperphosphatemic tumoral calcinosis. Association with elevation of serum 1,25 dihydroxycholecalciferol concentrations. Ann. Intern. Med., 96:586–591, 1982.

64. McKee, P.H., Liomba, N.G., and Hutt, M.S.R.: Tumoral calcinosis: A pathological study of fifty-six cases. Br. J. Dermatol., 107:669–674, 1982.

65. Hoffman, G., et al.: Calcium oxalate microcrystalline associated arthritis in end stage renal disease. Ann. Intern. Med., 97:36–42, 1982.

66. Reginato, A., et al.: Arthropathy and cutaneous calcinosis in hemodialysis oxalosis. Arthritis Rheum., 29:1387–1396, 1986.

67. Netter, P., et al.: Inflammatory effect of aluminum phosphate. Ann. Rheum. Dis., 42:114, 1983.

68. Conger, J.D., et al.: Pulmonary calcification in chronic dialysis patients. Clinical and pathologic studies. Ann. Intern. Med., 83:330–336, 1975.

69. Sarkar, K., and Uhthoff, H.K.: Rotator cuff tendinopathies with calcification. In Calcium in Biological Systems. Edited by R.P. Rubin, G. Weiss, and J.W. Putney. New York, Plenum, 1984.

70. Gravanis, M.G., and Gaffney, E.F.: Idiopathic calcifying tenosynovitis. Histopathologic features and possible pathogenesis. Am. J. Surg. Pathol., 7:359–361, 1983.

71. Ali, S.Y.: New knowledge of osteoarthritis. J. Clin. Pathol., 31:191–199, 1978.

72. Ali, S.Y., and Griffiths, S.: New types of calcium phosphate crystals in arthritis cartilage. Semin. Arthritis Rheum., 11:124–126, 1981.

73. Stein, H., Bab, I.A., and Sela, J.: The occurrence of hydroxyapatite crystals in extracellular matrix vesicles after surgical manipulation of the rabbit knee joint. Cell Tissue Res., 214:449–454, 1981.

74. Huskisson, E.C., et al.: Another look at osteoarthritis. Ann. Rheum. Dis., 38:423–428, 1979.

75. Bosworth, B.M.: Calcium deposits in the shoulder and subacromial bursitis. JAMA, 116:2477–2482, 1941.

76. Sarkar, K., and Uhthoff, H.K.: Ultrastructural localization of calcium in calcifying tendonitis. Arch. Pathol. Lab. Med., 102:266–269, 1978.

77. Dieppe, P.A., et al.: Synovial fluid crystal.. Q. J. Med., 192:533–553, 1979.

78. Gibilisco, P.A., Schumacher, H.R., Hollander, J.L., and Soper, K.A.: Synovial fluid crystals in osteoarthritis. Arthritis Rheum., 28:511–515, 1985.

79. Lagier, R., Boivin, G., and Gerster, J.C.: Carpal tunnel syndrome associated with mixed calcium pyrophosphate dihydrate and apatite crystal deposition in tendon synovial sheath. Arthritis Rheum., 27:1190–1195, 1984.

80. Adams, R.: Treatise on Rheumatic Gout. Dublin, John Churchill and Sons, 1873, pp. 91–161.

81. Craig, E.V.: The acromioclavicular joint cyst. Clin. Orthop. Rel. Res., 202:189–192, 1986.

82. Dennis, D.A., Ferlic, D.C., and Clayton, M.D.: Acromial stress fracture associated with cuff-tear arthropathy. J. Bone Joint Surg., 68A:937–940, 1986.

83. Halverson, P.B., Cheung, H.S., and McCarty, D.J.: Milwau-

kee shoulder syndrome (MSS): Description of predisposing factors. Arthritis Rheum., *30*:S131, 1987.

84. Samilson, R.L., and Prieto, V.: Dislocation arthropathy of the shoulder. J. Bone Joint Surg., *65A*:456–460, 1983.

85. Bagley, J.D., Cochran, T.P., and Sledge, C.B.: The weight-bearing shoulder—the impingement syndrome in paraplegics. J. Bone Joint Surg., *69A*:676–678, 1987.

86. Halverson, P.B., Garancis, J.C., and McCarty, D.J.: Histopathologic and ultrastructural studies of Milwaukee shoulder syndrome—a basic calcium phosphate crystal arthropathy. Ann. Rheum. Dis., *43*:734–741, 1984.

87. Neer, C.S.: Replacement arthroplasty in glenohumeral osteoarthritis. J. Bone Joint Surg., *56A*:1–13, 1974.

88. Werb, Z., and Reynolds, J.J.: Stimulation by endocytosis of the secretion of collagenase and neutral protease from rabbit synovial fibroblasts. J. Exp. Med., *140*:1482–1497, 1974.

89. Biswas, C., and Dayer, J.: Stimulation of collagenase production by collagen in mammalian cell cultures. Cell, *18*:1035–1041, 1979.

90. Evans, C.H., Mears, D.C., and Cosgrove, J.R.: Release of neutral proteinase from mononuclear phagocytes and synovial cells in response to cartilaginous wear particles in vitro. Biochim. Biophys. Acta, *677*:287–294, 1981.

91. Cheung, H.S., et al.: Release of collagenase, neutral protease and prostaglandins from cultured synovial cells by hydroxyapatite and calcium pyrophosphate dihydrate. Arthritis Rheum., *24*:1338–1344, 1981.

92. Cheung, H.S., Halverson, P.B., and McCarty, D.J.: Phagocytosis of hydroxyapatite or calcium pyrophosphate dihydrate crystals by rabbit articular chondrocytes stimulates release of collagenase, neutral protease and prostaglandins E_2 and $F_{2\alpha}$. Proc. Soc. Exp. Biol. Med., *173*:181–189, 1983.

93. Boivin, G., and Lagier, R.: An ultrastructural study of articular chondrocalcinosis in cases of knee osteoarthritis. Virchows Arch. (A), *400*:13–19, 1983.

94. Mitrovic, D.R.: Pathology of articular deposition of calcium salts and their relationship to osteoarthritis. Ann. Rheum. Dis., *42*:519–526, 1983.

95. Halverson, P.B., Cheung, H.S., and McCarty, D.J.: Enzymatic release of microspheroids containing hydroxyapatite crystals from synovium and of calcium pyrophosphate dihydrate crystals from cartilage. Ann. Rheum. Dis., *41*:527–531, 1982.

96. McCarty, D.J., and Cheung, H.S.: Prostaglandin (PG)E_2 generation by cultured synovial fibroblasts exposed to microcrystals containing calcium. Ann. Rheum. Dis., *44*:316–320, 1985.

97. Caniggia, A., et al.: Prostaglandin (PGE$_2$): A possible mechanism for bone destruction in calcinosis circumscripta. Calcif. Tissue Res., *25*:53–57, 1978.

98. Dieppe, P.A., Alwan, W., and Swan, A.: Synovial fluids (SF) in osteoarthritis (OA). Arthritis Rheum., *30*:S130, 1987.

99. Malawista, S.E., et al.: Crystal-induced endogeneous pyrogen production: A further look at gouty inflammation. Arthritis Rheum., *28*:1039–1046, 1985.

100. McCarty, D.J., Palmer, D.W., and Halverson, P.B.: Clearance of calcium pyrophosphate dihydrate (CPPD) crystals in vivo. I. Studies using ^{169}Yb labelled triclinic crystals. Arthritis Rheum., *22*:718–727, 1979.

101. McCarty, D.J., Palmer, D.W., and James, C.: Clearance of calcium pyrophosphate dihydrate (CPPD) crystals in vivo II. Studies using triclinic crystals doubly labelled with ^{45}Ca and ^{85}Sr. Arthritis Rheum., *22*:1122–1131, 1979.

102. McCarty, D.J., Palmer, D.W., and Garancis, J.C.: Clearance of calcium pyrophosphate dihydrate crystals in vivo. III. Ef-

fects of synovial hemosiderosis. Arthritis Rheum., *24*:706–710, 1981.

103. Palmer, D.W., and McCarty, D.J.: Clearance of ^{85}Sr labelled calcium phosphate (CP) crystals from normal rabbit joints. Arthritis Rheum., *27*:427–432, 1984.

104. Doyle, D.V.: Tissue calcification and inflammation in osteoarthritis. J. Pathol., *136*:199–216, 1982.

105. Cheung, H.S., Story, M.T., and McCarty, D.J.: Mitogenic effects of hydroxyapatite and calcium pyrophosphate on cultured mammalian cells. Arthritis Rheum., *27*:668–674, 1984.

106. Borkowf, A., Cheung, H.S., and McCarty, D.J.: Endocytosis is required for the mitogenic effect of basic calcium phosphate crystals in fibroblasts. Calcif. Tissue Int., *40*:173–176, 1987.

107. Owens, J.L., Cheung, H.S., and McCarty, D.J.: Endocytosis precedes dissolution of basic calcium phosphate crystals by murine macrophages. Calcif. Tissue Int., *38*:170–174, 1986.

108. Cheung, H.S., and McCarty, D.J.: Mitogenesis induced by calcium containing crystals: Role of intracellular dissolution. Exp. Cell Res., *157*:63–70, 1985.

109. Cheung, H.S., Van Wyk, J.J., Russell, W.E., and McCarty, D.J.: Mitogenic activity of hydroxyapatite: Requirement for somatomedin C. J. Cell Physiol., *128*:143–148, 1986.

110. Cheung, H.S., and McCarty, D.J.: Biological effects of calcium containing crystals on synoviocytes. *In* Calcium in Biological Systems. Edited by R.P. Rubin, G. Weiss, and J.W. Putney. New York, Plenum, 1984, pp. 719–724.

111. Borkowf, A., Cheung, H.S., and McCarty, D.J.: Effects of basic calcium phosphate crystals on specific protein synthesis in fibroblasts. Arthritis Rheum., *29*:S103, 1986.

112. Evans, R.W., Cheung, H.S., and McCarty, D.J.: Cultured canine synovial cells solubilize ^{45}Ca labeled HA crystals. Arthritis Rheum., *27*:829–832, 1984.

113. Evans, R.W., Cheung, H.S., and McCarty, D.J.: Cultured human monocytes and fibroblasts solubilize hydroxyapatite crystals. Calcif. Tissue Int., *36*:668–673, 1984.

114. Borkowf, A., and Cheung, H.S.: Basic calcium phosphate crystals stimulate mitogenesis and collagenase production by different mechanisms. Arthritis Rheum., *30*:S133, 1987.

115. Brown, E.A., Arnold, I.R., and Gower, P.E.: Dialysis arthropathy: Complication of long term treatment with hemodialysis. Br. Med. J., *292*:163–166, 1986.

116. Resnick, D.L.: Erosive arthritis of the hand and wrist in hyperparathyroidism. Radiology, *110*:263–269, 1974.

117. Kuntz, D., et al.: Destructive spondyloarthropathy in hemodialyzed patients: A new syndrome. Arthritis Rheum., *27*:369–375, 1984.

118. Goldstein, S., et al.: Chronic arthropathy in long-term hemodialysis. Am. J. Med., *78*:82–86, 1985.

119. Rubin, L.A., et al.: Erosive azotemic arthropathy. Arthritis Rheum., *27*:1086–1094, 1984.

120. Huaux, J., et al.: Erosive azotemic osteoarthropathy: Possible role of amyloidosis. Arthritis Rheum., *28*:1075–1076, 1985.

121. Bardin, T., et al.: Synovial amyloidosis in patients undergoing long-term hemodialysis. Arthritis Rheum., *28*:1052–1058, 1985.

122. Bardin, T., et al.: Hemodialysis-associated amyloidosis and beta-2 microglobulin. Am. J. Med., *83*:419–424, 1987.

123. Rynes, R., and Merzig, E.: Calcium pyrophosphate crystal deposition disease and hyperparathyroidism: A controlled prospective study. J. Rheumatol., *5*:460–468, 1978.

124. Worcester, E., Nakagawa, Y., Bushinsky, D., and Coe, F.: Evidence that serum calcium oxalate supersaturation is a consequence of oxalate retention in patients with chronic renal failure. J. Clin. Invest., *77*:1888–1896, 1986.

125. Netter P., et al.: Aluminum in joint tissues of chronic renal failure patients treated with regular hemodialysis and aluminum compounds. J. Rheumatol., *11*:66–70, 1984.

126. Ellison, G.W., and Norrdin, R.W.: Multicentric periarticular calcinosis in a pup. J. Am. Vet. Med. Assoc., *177*:542–546, 1980.

127. Woodard, J.C., et al.: Calcium phosphate deposition disease in Great Danes. Vet. Pathol., *19*:464–485, 1982.

128. Reginato, A.J., Schumacher, H.R., and Brighton, C.T.: Experimental hydroxyapatite synovial and articular cartilage calcification: Light and electron microscopic studies. Arthritis Rheum., *25*:1239–1249, 1982.

129. Lian, J.B., et al.: Gamma-carboxyglutamate excretion and calcinosis in juvenile dermatomyositis. Arthritis Rheum., *25*:1094–1100, 1982.

130. Lian, J.B., et al.: The presence of γ-carboxyglutamic acid in the proteins associated with ectopic calcification. Biochem. Biophys. Res. Commun., *73*:349–355, 1976.

131. Berger, R.G., and Hadler, N.M.: Treatment of calcinosis universalis secondary to dermatomyositis or scleroderma with low dose warfarin. Arthritis Rheum., *26*:S11, 1983.

132. Skuterud, E., Sydnes, A.O., and Haavik, T.K.: Calcinosis in dermatomyositis treated with probenecid. Scand. J. Rheumatol., *10*:92–94, 1981.

133. Reginato, A.J., Paul, H., and Schumacher, H.R.: Hydroxyapatite (HOA) crystals in rheumatoid arthritis (RA) synovial fluid. Clin. Res., *30*:662A, 1982.

134. Dieppe, P., and Watt, I.: Crystal deposition in osteoarthritis: An opportunistic event. Clin. Rheum. Dis., *11*:367–392, 1985.

135. Anderson, H.C.: Calcific diseases—a concept. Arch. Pathol. Lab. Med., *107*:341–348, 1983.

136. Kim, K.M., and Huang, S.N.: Ultrastructural study of calcification of human aortic valve. Lab. Invest., *25*:357–366, 1971.

137. Morgan, A.J.: Mineralized deposits in the thoracic aorta of aged rats: Ultrastructural and electron probe x-ray microanalysis study. J. Gerontol., *15*:563–573, 1980.

CALCIUM OXALATE AND OTHER CRYSTALS OR PARTICLES ASSOCIATED WITH ARTHRITIS

109

ANTONIO J. REGINATO

Besides monosodium urate monohydrate (MSU), calcium pyrophosphate dihydrate (CPPD), and other calcium phosphates, other crystals have been found in synovial fluid of arthritic patients (Table 109–1). Sufficient information is available to describe the clinical manifestations associated with calcium oxalate,[1-8] cholesterol,[9-19] lipid liquid crystals,[20-24] cryoglobulin crystals,[25-35] Charcot-Leyden crystals,[36-39] and synthetic corticosteroid crystals[40] (see also Chapter 5). Other crystals such as cystine,[41,42] hypoxanthine,[43-45] and aluminum phosphate[46,47] in synovial fluid, synovium, muscle, or bone have been described only in single case reports. Other endogenous compounds such as hemoglobin,[48,49] hematoidin,[50] myoglobin,[51] porphyrins,[52] tyrosine,[53,54] and a variety of proteins such as amyloid,[55] α-1 antitrypsin,[56] adenosinetriphosphatase,[57] and other less well identified proteins secreted by different tumors or leukemia cells,[58-60] as well as drugs,[61-63] can also crystallize in various body fluids and tissues.

Conceivably, some of these crystals could play a role in the pathophysiology of the clinical manifestations associated with hemoglobinopathies, porphyria cutanea tarda, or drug toxicity, but this remains speculative.

Exogenous particles described in association with foreign-body synovitis also often have a crystalline structure.[64-68] Sea urchin spines, for example, are formed from calcium carbonate crystals,[65] and talcum powder consists of magnesium silicate crystals, or starch granules.[67] Also, other foreign bodies such as plant thorns or polyethylene and polymethylmethac-

Table 109–1. Crystals and Birefringent Particles Uncommonly Found in Joint, Muscle, or Bone

Calcium oxalate
Cholesterol
Lipid liquid crystals
Other crystalline lipids
Corticosteroid esters crystals
Cystine
Xanthine
Hypoxanthine
Cryoglobulins
Charcot-Leyden (lysophospholipase) crystals
Aluminum
Foreign bodies
  Plant thorns
  Sea urchin spines (calcium carbonate)
  Polyethylene polymer
  Methylmethacrylate polymer

rylate polymer particles have a paracrystalline or crystalline structure.[65,68]

CALCIUM OXALATE CRYSTAL DEPOSITION

The articular manifestations of both primary oxalosis and secondary oxalosis occurring in uremic patients managed with long-term hemodialysis have been confused with those of gout and pseudogout.[1,3-5] Such patients may present a variety of articular manifestations (Fig. 109–1) as well as life-threatening organ involvement, which includes devastating peripheral vascular insufficiency with gangrene,[69-72]

FIG. 109–1. Clinical manifestations of oxalosis. A = acute.

CLINICAL SYNDROMES ASSOCIATED WITH OXALOSIS

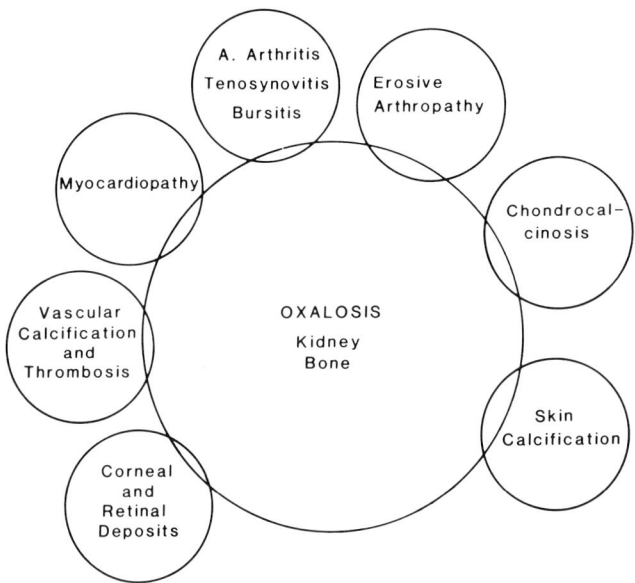

cardiomyopathy,[73–77] complete heart block,[74,75,77] peripheral neuropathy,[78] and aplastic anemia.[79,80]

ACQUIRED OXALOSIS

Oxalic acid is the metabolic end product of glycine, serine, other amino acids, and ascorbic acid.[81] Large amounts are also found in certain foods such as spinach and rhubarb. Oxalate is readily absorbed after ingestion. It is removed from the body almost entirely by glomerular filtration and secretion in the proximal tubule. Hyperoxalemia, hyperoxaluria, oxalate kidney stones, and crystalline tissue deposits may be the result of several contributing factors that may affect oxalate metabolism[81–83] (Table 109–2). Excessive oxa-

Table 109–2. Types of Oxalosis

Primary or Familial
Type I: Glycolic aciduria
Type II: Glyceric aciduria
Acquired
Diet rich in oxalate, e.g., rhubarb
Increased ingestion of oxalate precursors, e.g., ascorbic acid, ethyleneglycol
Increased absorption, e.g., small bowel resection or bypass, inflammatory bowel disease
Increased production, e.g., deficiency thiamine or pyridoxine
Decreased renal excretion; uremia
Dystrophic: retinal damage

late in the diet or increased absorption in patients with chronic inflammatory bowel disease, bowel resection, or intestinal bypass can lead to hyperoxalemia.[84] Methoxyflurane, ethyleneglycol, ascorbic acid, and xylitol are metabolized to oxalate.[81,85]

Thiamine and pyridoxine deficiencies may inhibit glyoxylate metabolism, increasing oxalate production.[82,83] Aspergillus niger can synthesize oxalic acid, which may crystallize in affected tissues and in aspergillomas.[86] Chronic renal failure can lead to serum oxalate levels 4 to 8 times greater than normal.[87] Serum levels parallel creatinine, becoming saturated when levels of the latter reach 8 to 9 mg/dl.[87] (Primary oxalosis is discussed later.)

The formation of calcium oxalate crystals in biologic fluids and tissues results when the limits of solubility are exceeded.[87] In the urine, the degree of saturation of calcium oxalate expressed in terms of the ionic concentration of calcium and oxalic acid is the most important single factor in the formation of oxalate stones.[88] Similar mechanisms may operate in serum and other tissues.[87] Some tissues, such as kidney, myocardium, and retina, and aspergillus infections produce oxalic acid, so that local acid concentration may exceed those of serum.[86,89–91] This may account for calcium oxalate crystal formation in aspergillosis and in dystrophic retinal damage.[86,90]

PRIMARY OXALOSIS

Primary oxalosis is a rare, recessive disorder characterized by excretion of excessive amounts of oxalate in the urine.[1,81,82,92–99] Two types of enzymatic defects have been recognized.

In type 1 (glycolic aciduria), excessive amounts of glyoxylic and glycolic acids are found in the urine. The increased oxalate and glycolic acid synthesis is the result of a blockage of glyoxylate alternate pathways (Fig. 109–2). Two enzyme deficiencies have been identified:[82,83,100] (1) *α-ketoglutarate glyoxylate carboligase*, which incorporates glyoxylate into α-hydroxy-β-keto adipate,[83] and (2) a peroxisomal liver enzyme, *alanine glyoxylate amino transferase*.[100] The latter defect can be diagnosed on liver tissue obtained through a needle biopsy. Assays of this enzyme activity may be useful in determining the prognosis and severity of the disease.[100]

Type-2 oxalosis (glyceric aciduria) is the result of a defect in hydroxypyruvate metabolism (see Fig. 109–2). Decreased activity of D glyceric acid dehydrogenase has been found in leukocytes of patients with this type of oxalosis.[83] Excessive hydroxypyruvate resulting from D glyceric dehydrogenase defi-

FIG. 109–2. Glyoxylate and oxalate metabolism. (From Ernest, D.L.: Enteric hyperoxaluria. Adv. Intern. Med., *24*:407, 1979.) LDH = Lactic dehydrogenase; NAD = Nicotinamide adenine dinucleotide; NADH = Reduced nicotinamide adenine dinucleotide.

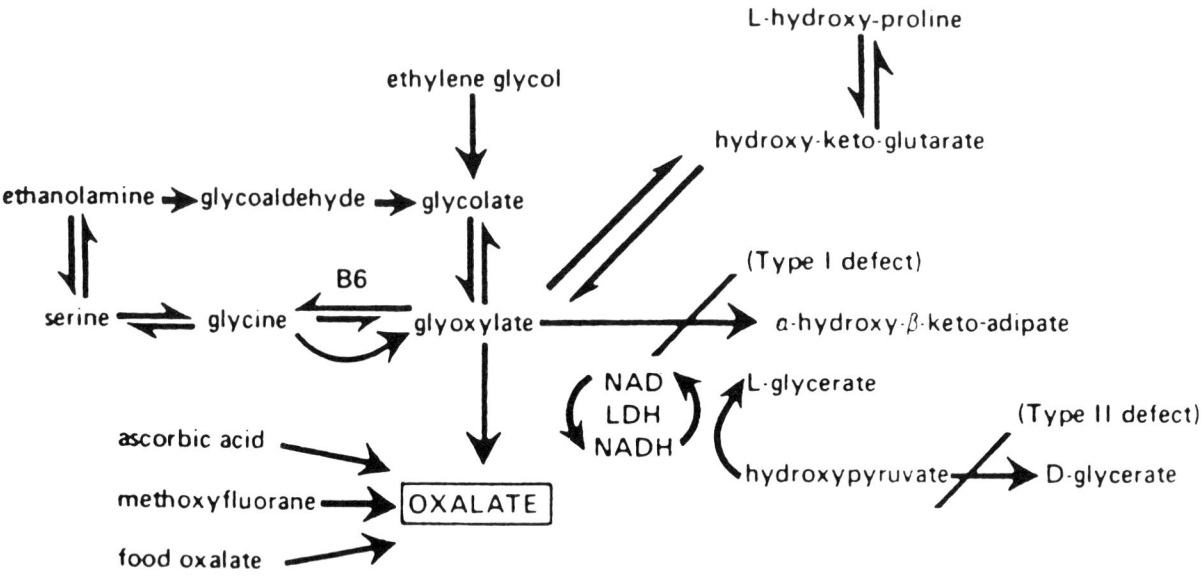

ciency is reduced to L glycerate with a parallel increase in the oxidation of glyoxylate to oxalate in a coupled reaction catalyzed by lactic acid dehydrogenase.[83]

Oxalosis symptoms begin during early childhood with nephrolithiasis and nephrocalcinosis, leading to renal failure and death before age 20.[94,95] Renal insufficiency is associated with rapid, progressive calcium oxalate crystal deposits in kidney, myocardium, skin, bone, and blood vessels. Oxalate crystals have been described in articular tissues at autopsies.[101] Over the past 50 years, tenosynovitis[102] and both acute and chronic arthritis have been described in these patients, but identification of crystals in synovial fluid or tissue has only rarely been possible.[3,93,98] As more patients with primary oxalosis are being managed with long-term hemodialysis, oxalate crystal deposition may become more important as a cause of morbidity.[99] Oxalate crystals have been identified in articular tissues of two patients with primary oxalosis, both older than 30 years at the time of diagnosis and both managed with long-term hemodialysis.[3,6] One presented with severe hand arthropathy with bony erosions and cysts and with large subcutaneous calcium oxalate crystalline deposits around his phalanges and olecranon mimicking tophaceous gout[3] (Fig. 109–3A and B).

ROENTGENOLOGIC MANIFESTATIONS

The roentgenologic appearance of primary and secondary oxalosis is similar, characteristically involving the hands and feet, with skin, vascular, periarticular, and intra-articular calcifications (Figs. 109–4 and 109–5).[103,104] Rosette-like areas of bony sclerosis in hands and feet, metaphyseal sclerotic bands, pathologic fractures, and pseudarthrosis[103–105] may be seen alone or in combination with the bony changes of renal osteodystrophy.[105–107] Chondrocalcinosis of larger joints and periarticular calcified masses has been described (Figs. 109–5 and 109–6).

PATHOLOGIC STUDIES

Synovium

Most synovium has been obtained during chronic synovitis and has shown mild synovial cell hyperplasia with hyperemia and pleomorphic calcium oxalate crystals lying in a mildly fibrotic interstitium with scarce mononuclear cells and a few giant cells[4,5] (Fig. 109–7A). Clumps of closely packed crystals with intensely and weakly positive birefringence may be seen in the subsynovium without an inflammatory reaction (Fig. 109–7B).

Cartilage, Meniscus, and Bone

Few studies of articular cartilage in oxalosis have been performed.[2,4] Kinnet and Bullough[2] described erosion of articular cartilage by chronically inflamed synovium containing oxalate crystals, and Hoffman et al.[4] found oxalate crystals in a large cystic area of a meniscus of a patient with hemodialysis oxalosis.

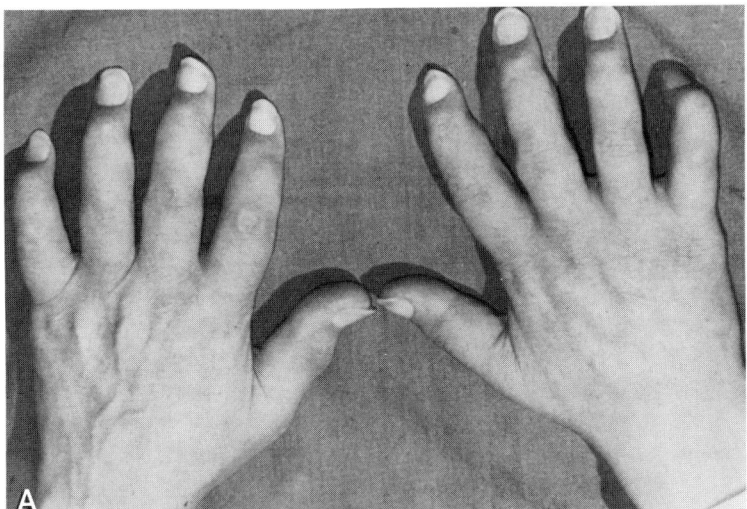

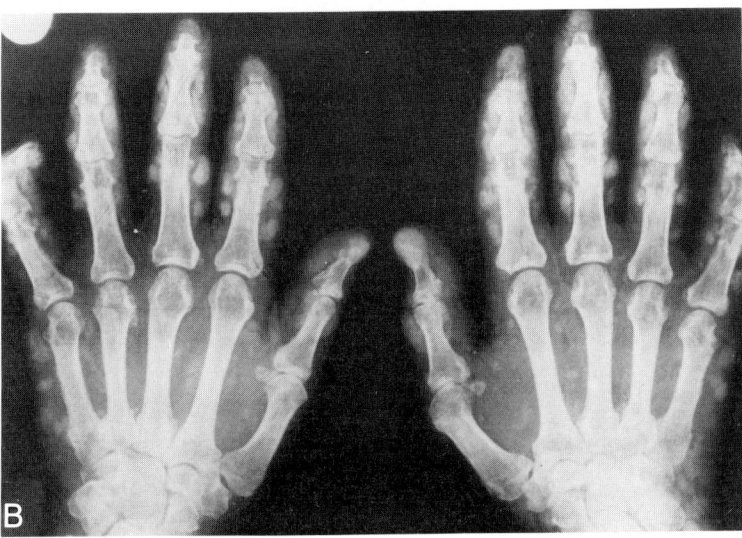

FIG. 109–3. *A,* Hands of a patient with primary oxalosis mimicking gout or rheumatoid arthritis. *B,* Radiographs of the same hands, showing periarticular calcific deposits, bony erosions, and resorption of distal phalanges. (From Schmidt, K.L., et al.: Arthropathies bei primarer Oxalose-Krystallsynovitis oder Osteopathie. Dtsch. Med. Wochenschr., *106*:19, 1981.)

Cartilage and bone obtained from a first metatarsophalangeal joint did not reveal any crystals although the synovium and capsule contained many.[5] However, bone histology in most patients with oxalosis shows oxalate crystal deposits surrounded by giant cells and bone marrow fibrosis. These deposits correlate with radiologic areas of subperiosteal resorption, endosteal erosion, pseudofractures, or localized osteosclerosis due to deposits of radiopaque calcium oxalate crystals in the bone marrow.[105,106]

CRYSTALLOGRAPHIC FEATURES

Calcium oxalate crystals deposit in bone,[1,2,92,93,101,105–112] tendon,[102] articular cartilage,[2,4,101,108] menisci,[4] and synovium.[1,2,4,5] These sites are probably the source of crystals found in joint fluid.[4,5] Two types of oxalate crystals have been identified: (1) characteristic dipyramidal crystals formed by calcium oxalate

dihydrate (weddellite) (see Fig. 109–7C) and (2) polymorphic crystals composed of calcium oxalate monohydrate (whewellite). The latter appear as irregular squares, chunks, short rods, stretched ovals, dumb-bells, and even microspherules.[4,5] Sizes range from 5 to 30 μm. Some calcium oxalate crystals show strongly positive birefringence, but most exhibit a weakly positive birefringence or none at all.* Most of them stain with alizarin red S on fresh preparations,[113,114] and those in tissue deposits can also be recognized with Pizzolato's stain,[115–117] a modification of the von Kossa stain. Under transmission electron microscopy, they are electron dense with sharp margins and a foamy structure similar to that of CPPD crystals.[4,5] Both x-ray diffraction analysis and scanning electron microscopy have been helpful in determining which of the two types of oxalate crystal is

---

Editor's note. Those crystals showing no birefingence are too small and thin to retard sufficient light waves (see Chapter 5).

FIG. 109–4. Miliary skin deposits in a patient with hemodialysis oxalosis. (From Reginato, A.J., et al.[5])

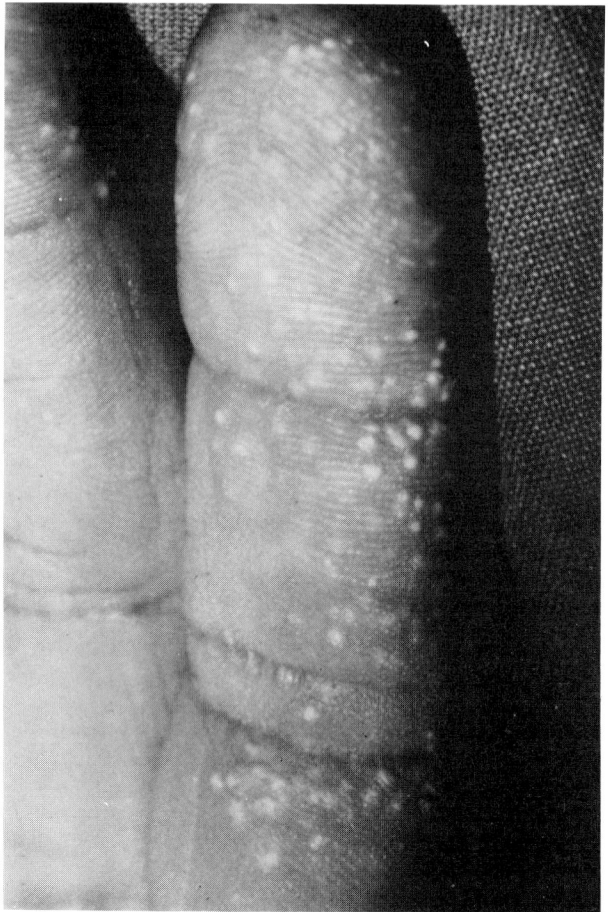

FIG. 109–5. Radiograph of a patient with hemodialysis oxalosis, showing skin, vascular, periarticular calcifications, and chondrocalcinosis. (From Reginato, A.J., et al.[5])

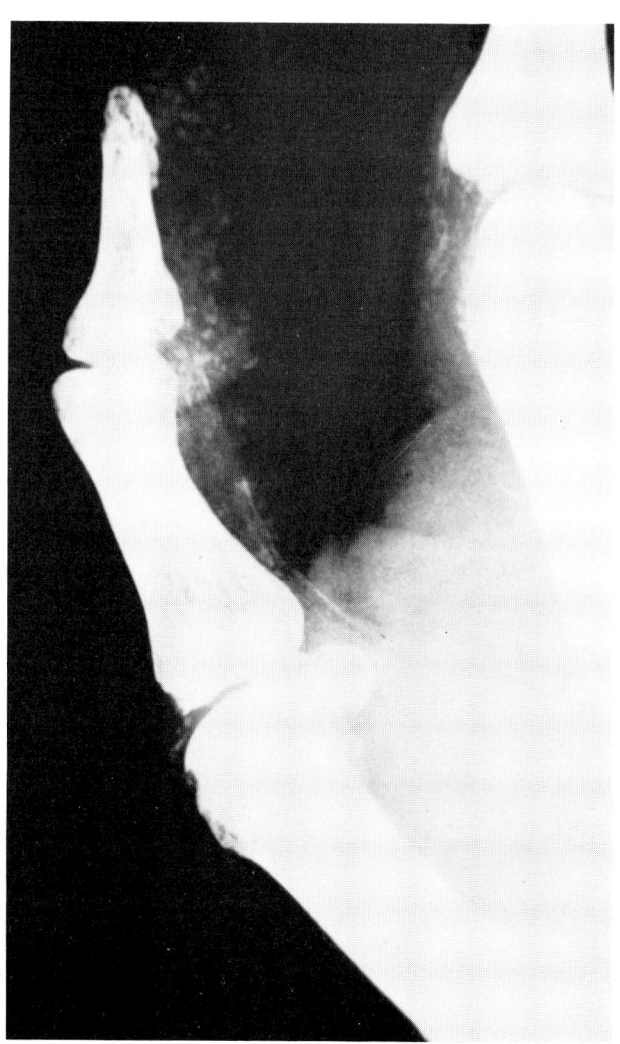

present and to correlate crystallographic structure with optical morphology.[118,119] (Fig. 109–8A to C). Due to their polymorphism and variable strength of birefringence, calcium oxalate crystals can easily be confused with CPPD crystals or even with apatite microspherules when synovial fluid is examined only by ordinary or compensated polarized light.[4,5] The phlogistic potency of calcium oxalate crystals is similar to that of MSU crystals or calcium phosphate crystals as assessed by injections of synthetic preparations into dog knees[120] or rat paws.[121] Crystalline calcium oxalate also stimulates synovial cells to synthesize and release latent collagenase and prostaglandins.[122] It seems possible that activation of synovial cells, fibroblasts, and osteoclasts by calcium oxalate crystals might play a role in inducing bone erosions, cysts, and even pathologic fractures like those seen in patients with bone and articular oxalosis.[4,5,105,106,122]

BIOCHEMICAL FEATURES

Serum oxalate levels have been measured in two of the three reports of articular oxalosis complicating long-term dialysis.[5,7] The levels ranged from 168 ± 36 mg/L, about eight times higher than normal. Synovial fluid oxalate levels in these patients were considerably higher than those found in fluid of patients with rheumatoid arthritis (RA), osteoarthritis or pseudogout.[4] Some patients had mild hypercalcemia and an increased calcium/phosphorous ratio due to secondary hyperparathyroidism and/or vitamin D administration.[5] Most patients with end-stage renal disease had a low serum calcium level, although a few were hypercalcemic.[105,106]

Hypercalcemia could be a contributory factor in pre-

FIG. 109–6. Knee radiograph of a patient with acquired oxalosis due to renal failure managed with chronic peritoneal dialysis and also to large calcified masses and arterial calcifications. (From Schumacher, J.R., Reginato, A.J., and Pullman, S.: Synovial fluid oxalate deposition complicating rheumatoid arthritis with amyloidosis and renal failure: Demonstration of intra-cellular oxalate crystals. J. Rheumatol., *14*:361, 1987.)

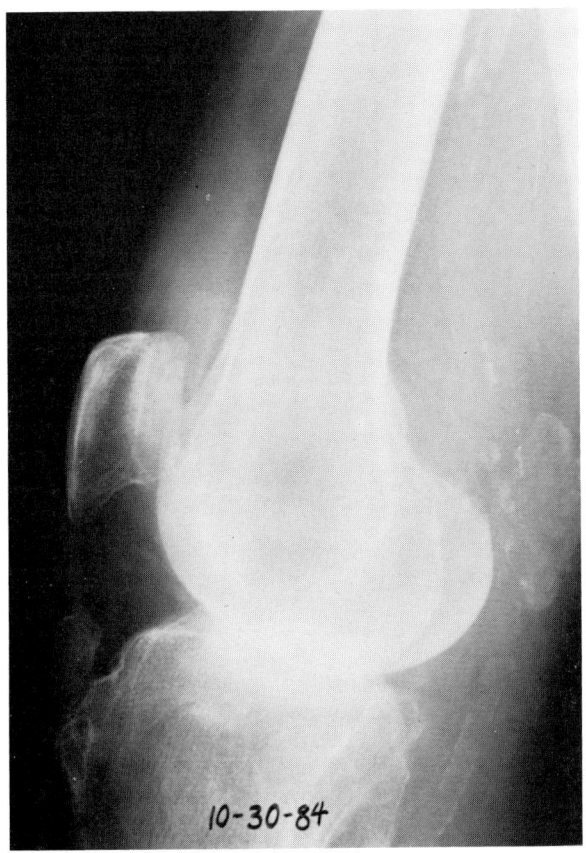

10-30-84

cipitating calcium oxalate crystals in tissues, but parathyroidectomy, performed in a few patients with bone oxalosis and end-stage renal disease, was ineffective in correcting the elevated serum calcium or in decreasing crystal deposits.[106] Another possible explanation for the hypercalcemia seen in these patients is increased osteoclastic bone resorption at the site of oxalate deposits in bone.[105,106]

Oxalate is removed by both hemodialysis and peritoneal dialysis, but neither procedure induces a negative balance that would result in effective removal of oxalate from tissues of patients with either primary oxalosis or end-stage renal disease.[123–129] Autopsy series show that renal and bone oxalosis occur in about 90% of patients with end-stage renal disease managed with long-term hemodialysis.[130–131] Because articular tissues have not been included in most of these stud-

ies, the frequency of articular oxalosis is unknown.[130,131] Several reports of articular oxalosis have implicated ascorbic acid administration in aggravating oxalate deposition.[4,5,7] In some dialysis protocols, ascorbic acid is added to dialysis solutions to neutralize chloramine and prevent hemolysis.[132] Because oxalate is a metabolic end product of ascorbic acid, large amounts given to patients receiving dialysis may result in higher serum oxalate levels and increased crystal deposition in tissues.[85,129,132,133] Most patients with articular oxalosis have received 500 to 1000 mg of ascorbic acid after each dialysis.[4,5,7]

CLINICAL MANIFESTATIONS

Symmetric proximal interphalangeal and metacarpophalangeal joints, acute arthritis, with or without flexor tenosynovitis, miliary calcific deposits of digits, and digital vascular calcification are the most characteristic clinical presentation[4,5] (see Figs. 109–3A to 109–5). Acute or chronic effusions of larger joints such as knees, elbows, or ankles may develop[4,5,7] (see Fig. 109–6). Podagra, Achilles tenosynovitis, and bursitis has been observed in single patients.[5] In most patients, the initial acute synovitis follows a chronic course, responding poorly to colchicine, nonsteroidal anti-inflammatory drugs (NSAIDs), intra-articular injections of corticosteroids, or even increased frequency of dialysis.[4,5] Synovial fluid from acute and chronic effusions has been clear or bloody with normal viscosity.[4,5,7] Leukocyte counts have been low, ranging from 150 to 2100 cells/μL with 60 to 90% of polymorphonuclear (PMN) cells in some samples.[4,5] In others, a predominance of large mononuclear cells was observed.[4,5] Abundant clumps of crystals are usually seen, most of which are extracellular (see Fig. 109–7C), but intracellular crystals were found in fluid from two patients.[5,7]*

MANAGEMENT

There is no effective therapy for either primary or secondary oxalosis.[134] Therapeutic methods that have been tried unsuccessfully for primary oxalosis include a low-oxalate diet[134]; allopurinol,[134] pyridoxine,[134–136] orthophosphate, and magnesium administration; combined hepatic and renal transplantation; and aggressive hemodialysis.[82,83,134–137]

*Editor's note. I have studied a drop of fluid from an interphalangeal joint from a dialysis patient that contained many intracellular oxalate crystals.

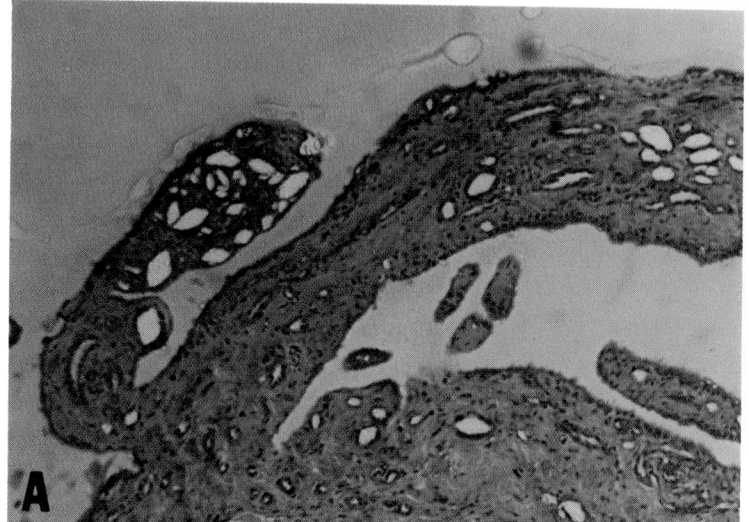

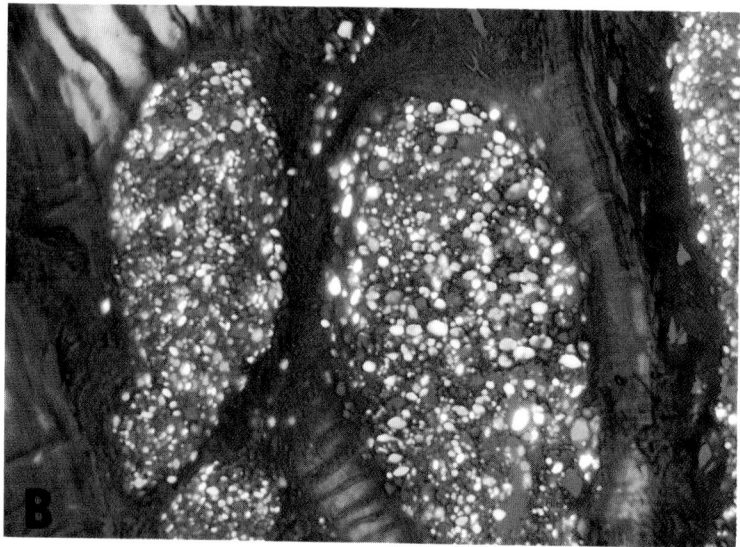

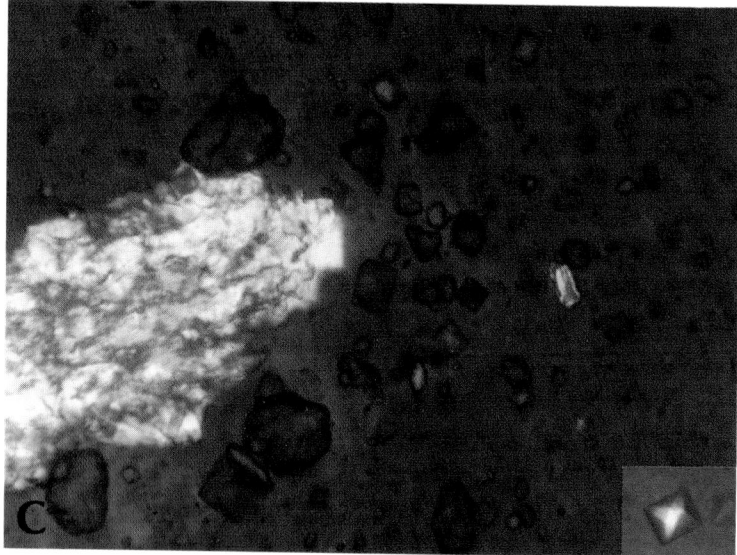

FIG. 109–7. *A,* Isolated calcium oxalate crystals in the superficial synovium (hematoxylin and eosin stain × 180). *B,* Large clumps of birefringent crystals lying between collagen fibers. Compensated light microscopy (× 180). *C,* Calcium oxalate crystals in synovial fluid. Pseudotophaceous deposits surrounded by abundant polymorphic and a few dipyramidal crystals showing no birefringence and weakly or intensely positive birefringence (insert). Compensated polarized (× 400). (From Reginato, A.J., et al.[5])

FIG. 109–8. Scanning electron micrographs. *A*, Rod-shaped and, *B*, hexagonal-shaped crystals of calcium oxalate monohydrate in synovial fluid (×4000). *C*, Energy dispersive analysis, showing calcium but no phosphorus. (From Reginato, A.J., et al.[5])

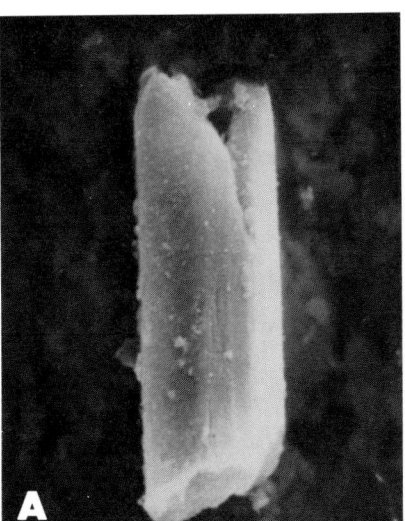
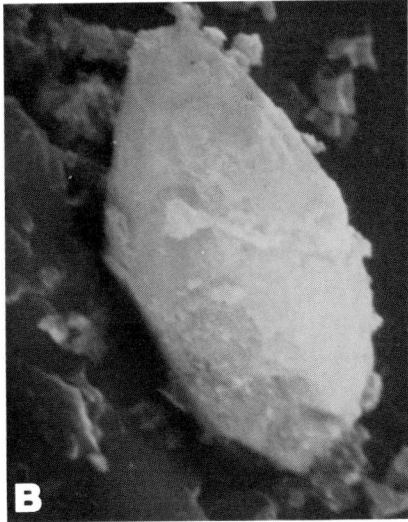
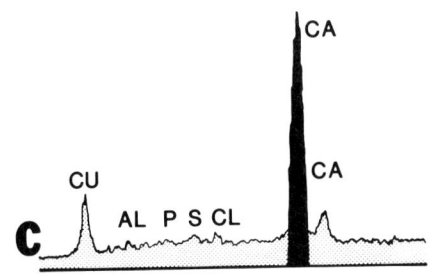

SYNDROMES ASSOCIATED WITH CHOLESTEROL CRYSTALS AND OTHER CRYSTALLINE LIPIDS

CHOLESTEROL CRYSTALS

Although cholesterol crystals are occasionally identified in rheumatoid joint fluid[9–14] or bursal effusions,[16,19] their possible contribution to either inflammation or joint deterioration is unclear.[138,139] Cholesterol crystals have also been observed (rarely) in synovial fluids from patients with osteoarthritis,[140] chronic tophaceous gout,[141–144] ankylosing spondylitis,[9] and even systemic lupus erythematosus.[143] These crystals also have been found in pleural[145,146] or pericardial effusions of patients with RA[147] as well as effusions due to tuberculosis or a tumor.[148] Cholesterol crystals have been seen in rheumatoid nodules,[149,150] tophi,[141,143] unicameral bone cysts,[151] and even as isolated granulomas or "cholesterol tophi" in the skin.[152] They have been demonstrated in bone granulomatosis (Erdhein Chester disease)[153] and in the kidneys of patients with nephrotic syndrome.[154] The few studies performed on synovial fluid of patients with arthritis associated with hyperlipoproteinemias have failed to show cholesterol or other crystalline lipids.[155–157] Synovium from two such patients has not shown crystalline lipid deposits either,[18,158] but in one of these, MSU deposits were found,[18] and in the other, apatite-like crystals were found inside synovial cells.[158] Xanthomas often develop in the Achilles ten-

dons and extensor tendon sheaths of the hands of patients with familial hypercholesterolemia.[159,160] Increased tendon size can produce pain and interfere with function, but tenosynovitis and tendon rupture occur rarely.[159] The syndrome of multiple cholesterol emboli may present a constellation of systemic manifestations mimicking necrotizing vasculitis[161,162] (see Chapter 75).

CRYSTALLOGRAPHIC FEATURES

Synovial fluid containing cholesterol crystals often has a golden-honey or yellow-brown color.[139] Cholesterol crystals in synovial fluid are extracellular but are often associated with intra- and extracellular birefringent "Maltese crosses" (Fig. 109–9A and B). Cholesterol crystals show two morphologic forms:[163] (1) highly birefringent, large, flat, rectangular plates with one or more notched corners, ranging from 8 to 100 μm (Fig. 109–10) and (2) rod or needle-shaped, strongly negative birefringent crystals ranging from 2 to 30 μm long (see Fig. 109–10, insert). Needle-shaped crystals are much more difficult to recognize and may be confused with MSU.[163] (See also Chapter 5.)

Under transmission electron microscopy, cholesterol crystals are electron dense and retain their platelike morphology before beam damage occurs. Under scanning electron microscopy, they appear as notched plates covered by synovial exudate.[140] X-ray diffraction analysis of joint fluid crystals showed that both

FIG. 109–9. Lipid liquid crystals. *A,* Single, large, double-positive birefringent microspherule. *B,* Extracellular small microspherules. *C,* Abundant intracellular small microspherules. Compensated polarized light (×200). (With permission of Ann. Rheum. Dis. From Reginato, A.J., et al.[21])

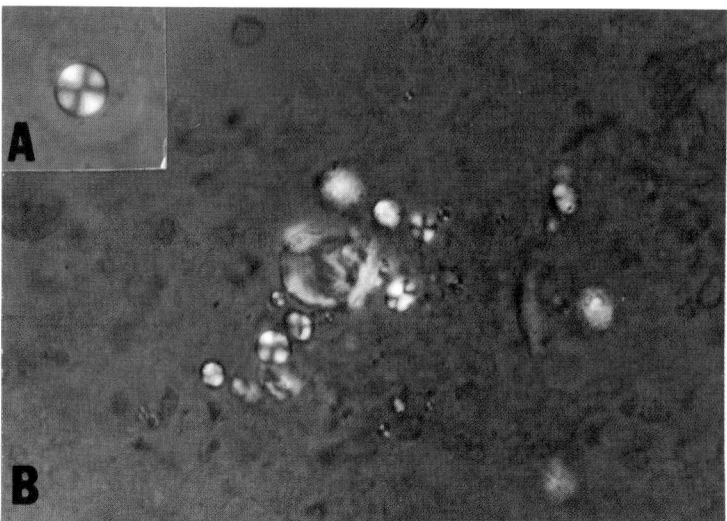

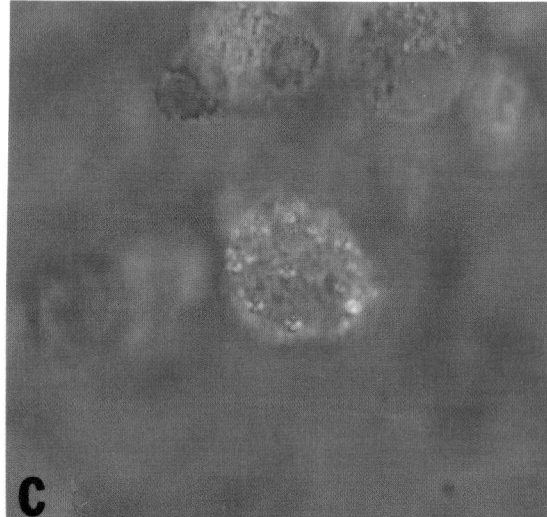

the needle and plate-like forms were anhydrous cholesterol,[163] but in studies of cholesterol crystals in bile, the plate-like crystals were identified as cholesterol monohydrate and the needle-shaped crystals as anhydrous cholesterol.[164] Small amounts of proteins and phospholipids may be entrapped in these crystals.[163]

Many factors are probably involved in the formation of cholesterol crystals in inflamed tissues including increased cholesterol synthesis,[138] in situ bleeding, lipid release from damaged cell membranes and organelles,[139] and abnormal intracellular transport of lipids due to chronic inflammation and/or infec-

tion.[139,165,166] The capability of synthetic cholesterol crystals to induce moderate acute and chronic inflammation in skin, subcutaneous tissue, and knee joint of rabbits have been demonstrated in studies performed by Bland et al.,[11] Denko and Petricevic,[167] and Pritzker et al.[168]* Although cholesterol crystals may

---

*Editor's note. I have never seen cholesterol crystals inside phagocytes, as occurs with MSU, CPPD, or basic calcium phosphate crystals. As pyrogen contamination was not ruled out or similarity of crystal structure with that of natural cholesterol crystals was not shown in any of these studies, extrapolation to human disease states remains speculative.

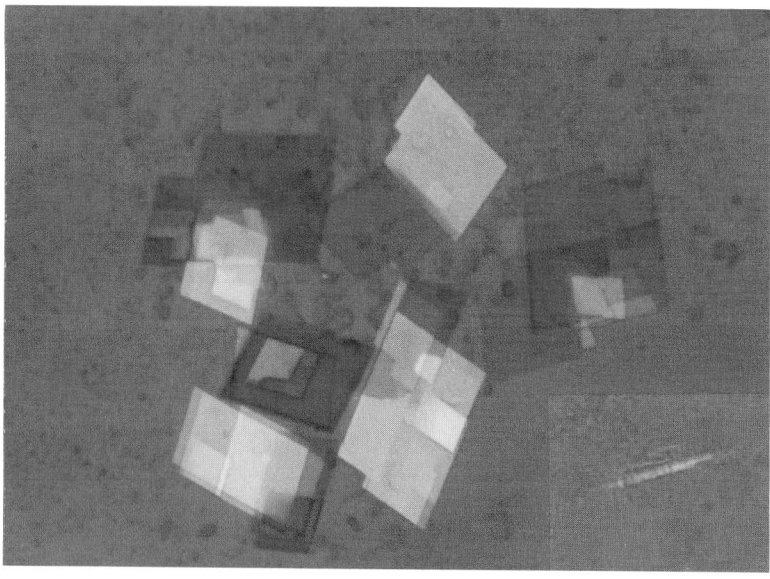

FIG. 109–10. Characteristic highly birefringent plate-like cholesterol crystals and a needle-like cholesterol crystal (insert). Compensated polarized light (×200).

activate serum complement,[169] which might potentiate inflammation and aggravate joint destruction in RA and even osteoarthritis, there is no clinical evidence to support this concept.[140]

LIPID LIQUID CRYSTALS

As already noted, birefringent Maltese crosses occasionally have been found in synovial or bursal fluids of patients with RA.[170] These structures are usually associated with increased synovial fluid lipid content and with cholesterol crystals and have been called "fluid spherocrystals,"[171] liposomes,[172] smetic mesophases,[173–175] or lipid liquid crystals.[173,176] They were found in the synovial fluid of 11 patients with otherwise unexplained acute monoarthritis,[20–22,24] in 7 patients with acute olecranon bursitis,[24] and in 1 patient with chronic unexplained symmetric polyarthritis[23] (see Fig. 109–9A to C).

Lipid liquid crystals represent states of matter having characteristics of both liquid and solids.[171,173–175] They have some degree of order in their molecular arrangement but also some degree of fluidity. Molecules that form liquid crystals are longer than they are wide, and have a polar or aromatic ring on the molecule.[173] The long shape and polar interactions permit molecular alignment in partially ordered *smetic* or *layered* arrays, similar to that of liposomes and in contrast to *nematic* arrays, in which the molecules are aligned side by side but not in mandatory layers.[173]

A liquid crystalline ordering of molecules has been described in both normal and pathologic biologic systems, e.g., normal cell membranes and organelles, myelin, bile, serum lipoproteins,[173] atherosclerotic plaques,[173,176] adrenal glands,[173] nephrotic kidneys,[171] and lipid storage diseases.[173–175] Inclusions with similar ultrastructure can be seen in muscles, myocardium, lung, and nerve as a result of toxicity with different medications such as amiodarone,[61] chloroquine, hydroxychloroquine,[177] and with some psychotherapeutic agents such as thioridazine and amitriptyline.[62] These inclusions are formed by phospholipids or by polar molecules of the drugs themselves, which can also be arranged as liquid crystals.[61,62,175]

CRYSTALLOGRAPHIC FEATURES

Under compensated polarized light, these microspherules have an intense double-positive birefringence (see Fig. 109–9A to C). Sizes range from 2 to 8 μm. Larger, irregularly birefringent plates (see Fig. 109–9B) probably represent transitional forms preceding the formation of cholesterol crystals.[173,176] In atherosclerotic plaques and in bile, these liquid lipid microspherules precede the formation of cholesterol crystals.[176] They are commonly seen inside cells, stain with Sudan black B, and are dissolved completely in 1:1 alcohol-ether.[21] Smaller microspherules may appear to be anisotropic (not birefringent). These positively birefringent Maltese crosses must be differentiated from the negatively birefringent MSU microspherules ("beachballs") rarely seen in patients with gout and from talcum powder crystals that may contaminate synovial fluids when gloves are used during arthrocentesis.[67] The latter are magnesium silicate or starch granules and show a positive birefringence, but their outlines are more irregular than MSU and lipid liquid crystal microspherules.

CLINICAL FEATURES

Acute Arthritis

All patients described have experienced the acute onset of monoarticular synovitis as often seen in other crystal-associated arthritis.[20–22,24] The knee is most commonly involved, although wrist involvement was noted in one instance.[21] Synovial fluid is inflammatory, with white cell counts ranging from 10,000 to 45,000/μL with 75 to 90% neutrophils. About 10 to 20% of these contain doubly birefringent microspherules (see Fig. 109–9A to C). Arthritis in all patients subsided completely within a week after NSAIDs were given. Synovium has been obtained in only two patients with acute synovitis;[22,24] mild inflammatory changes with rare lymphocytic, mononuclear, or PMN cell infiltrates were seen in both cases and in one specimen, intracellular birefringent microspherules were seen inside mononuclear cells.[23] Because both the clinical presentation and the subsequent course were similar to those seen in patients with gout or pseudogout, it was suggested that these crystals might induce inflammation as has been proposed for solid crystals.[21]

Synthetic lipid liquid crystals injected into rabbit knees induced either acute or subacute synovitis.[178] The origin of these microspherules in articular tissues is unknown. In the few cases reported, associated diseases included sarcoidosis and alcoholic cirrhosis in one patient each, while two other patients had recent joint trauma and hemarthrosis. Injection of autologous blood into rabbit knee joint was associated with formation of Maltese crosses.[179–181] Similar spherules seen in human joints may be formed by lipids derived from breakdown of membranes of platelets, erythrocytes, leukocytes, and even from serum lipids.[182]

Acute Bursitis

In one study, 7 of 18 bursal fluid samples contained positive birefringent microspherules.[24] One patient had gout, another had RA, while the remaining six had "traumatic" bursitis. Bursal fluid was inflammatory in all but the patient with gout.

Chronic Arthritis

The presence of lipid birefringent microspherules with chronic polyarthritis has been reported in one patient with otherwise unexplained symmetric polyarthritis resembling RA.[23]

Fabry's Disease

Fabry's disease, a sex-linked disorder affecting only males, is due to deposition of glycolipids in blood vessels, nerve, synovium, and kidney. Because of its unusual skin lesions, the disease is also known as angiokeratoma corporis universalis. Arthralgia and arthritis, usually exacerbated by warm weather, have been observed in patients with Fabry's disease.[98] Synovium and other tissues examined in these patients have shown glycolipidic inclusions with features of lipid liquid crystals.[183,184]

Other Crystalline Lipids

Other crystalline lipids, thought to be fatty acids, have been described in skin fat necrosis of newborns.[185] Identical structures have been observed in synovial fluid of patients with osteoarthritis associated with large bone cysts in hemarthrosis, and in synovial fluid examined several days after arthrocentesis.[186] Such crystals may have either a strongly positive or negative birefringence and may present with needle, plate, or rod shapes. Some may form clumps or rosettes. The rod- and needle-shaped crystals can be confused with CPPD or MSU crystals.

CRYOGLOBULIN CRYSTALS

Paraproteins and cryoglobulins can crystallize within plasma cells of patients with multiple myeloma[187,188] (Fig. 109–11). These crystals are usually seen in areas of tumor in the bone marrow and, more rarely, in plasma cell infiltrates in different organs.[189–193] Similar crystals can be seen independent of plasma cells in the renal glomeruli,[27,188,189] tubules,[189] lungs,[31] skin,[28] liver,[27,28] spleen, lymph nodes,[28] adrenals,[28] testis,[28] and cornea.[34,190–193] These deposits can be associated with variable degrees of organ failure.[27]

They may also occur in coronary and renal arteries and induce thrombosis and infarction.[27] Similar crystalline deposits have been observed in patients with essential cryoglobulinemia with purpuric and necrotic skin lesions[30] and in synovial fluid and synovium in association with arthritis.[25,26]

CRYSTALLOGRAPHIC FEATURES

Crystalline paraproteins are not associated with any particular type of heavy or light chains.[27,29,30] Their composition has been studied with trypsin digestion and immunofluorescent techniques.[33]

Paraprotein crystals are characterized by their large size, ranging from 3 to ≥60 μm, and their polymorphic shapes, which may vary with the cooling process used.[27,29,33,194,195] They usually appear as hexagonal, diamond-shaped, or polygonal crystals, but they may resemble squares, rectangles, rhomboids, or needles.[25,27,33,35] They may show either a strongly positive or a strongly negative birefringence. They stain with Giemsa and hematoxylin and eosin but not with Congo red or stains for lipids.[188] Under transmission electron microscopy they are electron dense, with sharply demarcated borders and a homogenous structure; they stain with osmium and uranyl acetate.[190,192,195]

CLINICAL FEATURES

Episodic joint pain followed by an erosive, chronic, symmetric polyarthritis involving joints of the hands, feet, and one ankle have been observed in one patient with cryoprecipitable immunoglobulin G (IgG) in his serum and cryoglobulin crystals in joint fluid and synovium.[25] Synovial fluid was inflammatory with a white cell count of 30,000/μL with 90% neutrophils and abundant large rectangular and rhomboid cryoglobulin crystals. Synovium revealed a chronic inflammatory reaction and a few giant cells surrounding crystal deposits. These crystals were identical to those obtained from the serum cryoprecipitates. This patient also had crystalline corneal deposits. The arthritis failed to improve with administration of several NSAIDs, penicillamine, and plasmapheresis but was better controlled with cyclophosphamide. Similar improvement of eye symptoms, with dissolution of corneal crystalline deposits, has been observed in a few patients with multiple myeloma managed with chemotherapy.[190] Another patient with erosive polyarthritis and crystallizable monoclonal cryoglobulin also has been reported.[26] Two patients with multiple

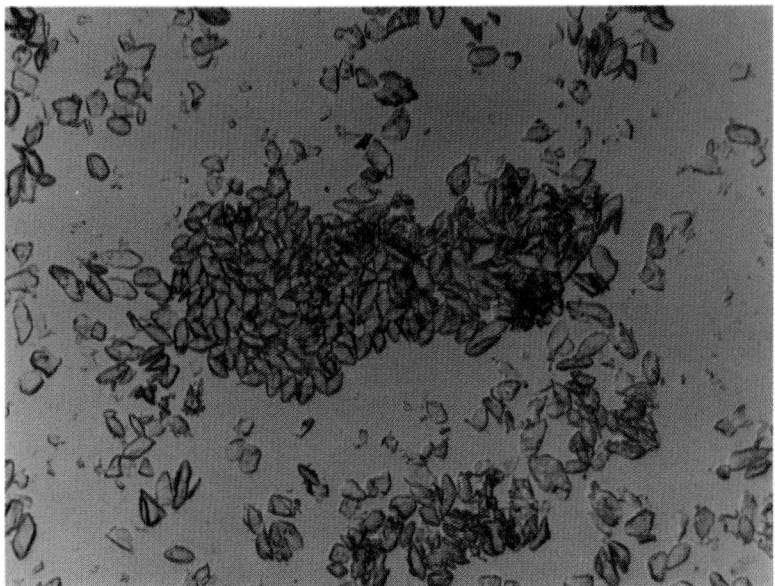

FIG. 109–11. Cryoglobulin crystals. Polygonal positive birefringent crystals of serum cryoprecipitate of a patient with multiple myeloma. Compensated polarized light (×200).

myeloma and corneal paraprotein crystalline deposits presented with foot arthritis, including podagra.[190] Arthritis associated with cryoglobulinemia but without paraprotein crystals in synovial fluid has also been reported.[196–198]

CYSTINOSIS

Cystinosis is an autosomal recessive inborn error of metabolism characterized by excessive accumulation of cystine in reticuloendothelial cells of liver, spleen, lymph nodes, and bone marrow.[199] The basic defect is an impairment of normal carrier-mediated transport of cystine across the lysosomal membrane.[200] Three different types have been described.[201] The most severe type is the infantile (nephrogenic), a milder type is seen in adolescents, and the most benign type is seen in adults. The form is characterized for polydipsia, polyuria, crystalline deposits in renal tubule and glomeruli, Fanconi's syndrome, and progressive renal failure. These patients also present with conjunctivitis, retinopathy, and vitamin D-resistant rickets.[199]

CRYSTALLOGRAPHIC FEATURES

Cystine crystals have a characteristic hexahedral shape with a weak-to-intense birefringence.[41,201] Typical crystals are rarely seen in tissue deposits, where they appear polymorphic, assuming square, rectangular, lozenge, and even acicular (needle-like) shapes.[41,201] Under transmission electron microscopy,

they are surrounded by osmiophilic dense bodies and almost always appear within lysosomes inside cells.[201] Histochemical studies showed crystals surrounded by membrane-bound structures staining positively for alkaline phosphatase and binding ferritin.[202] These intracellular crystals may form in situ rather than by phagocytosis of preformed crystals.[203,204]

CLINICAL FEATURES

Patients with the infantile type of cystinosis present with vitamin D-resistant rickets, that is, with growth retardation, pseudofractures, and bone pain.[199] Hypothyroidism has accompanied cystine deposits in the thyroid gland.[203,204] Symptomatic crystal deposits in bone were described in a single patient and correlated with localized focal demineralization.[42] In another patient, cystinosis of bone was associated with acute knee synovitis, wrist synovitis, and polyarthralgias of larger joints,[41] but no cystine crystals were found in his synovial fluid. Radiographs revealed coarse bone trabeculation with diffuse demineralization and flattening of one of the metacarpal heads with punctiform periarticular calcific deposits.

XANTHINE CRYSTALS

Xanthinuria is an uncommon hereditary disorder of purine metabolism resulting from a deficiency of the enzyme xanthine oxidase.[205] It is characterized by hypouricemia, decreased uric acid excretion in the urine, and the presence of xanthinuria, hypoxanthinuria, and xanthine kidney stones. Hypoxanthine and xanthine crystals have been identified in the muscle of three patients with xanthinuria and tender muscles.[43–45,206] Muscle pain was crampy and increased by walking. Another patient presented with acute arthritis mimicking gout; unfortunately no synovial fluid was obtained.[207] Xanthine, hypoxanthine, and oxipurinol crystals also have been identified in kidney stones and muscles of a patient with Lesch-Nyhan syndrome treated with allopurinol.[208] Similar deposits were found in kidneys of a patient with lymphosarcoma managed with aggressive chemotherapy and allopurinol.[209] Deposits of xanthine, hypoxanthine, and oxipurinol crystals have been found in skeletal muscle in absence of muscle pain or weakness of 10 patients with gout treated with allopurinol.[63]

CRYSTALLOGRAPHIC FEATURES

Xanthine crystals are plate-like or rhomboidal in shape, measure up to 2.5 μm, and are strongly birefringent. Hypoxanthine crystals are more polymorphic, although they may also appear as large plates or rhomboidal crystals. They range in size from 9.5 and 50 μm and show strong negative birefringence. Exact identification of these crystals requires electron or x-ray diffraction analysis.[206]

CHARCOT-LEYDEN CRYSTALS

The formation of protein crystals within cytoplasm of human cells is infrequent,[210,211] but Charcot-Leyden crystals represent an example of this phenomenon. They are formed in the cytoplasm of disrupted eosinophils and are found in the sputum of asthmatic patients,[210] the tissue of patients with hypereosinophilia,[39,219,211] eosinophilic disease processes such as eosinophilic bone granuloma,[212] hypereosinophilic syndrome,[39] the stool of patients with parasitic infections,[210] granulocytic leukemia,[210] and the synovial fluid of patients with eosinophilic synovitis.[36–38,213] Circulating Charcot-Leyden crystals have been observed in one patient with hypereosinophilic syndrome and crystalline deposits in thrombosed vessels and in the renal glomeruli.[39]

CRYSTALLOGRAPHIC FEATURES

Charcot-Leyden crystals are bipyramidal hexagonal-shaped crystals formed by a lysophospholipase or phospholipase B[214–216] (Fig. 109–12). Crystal sizes

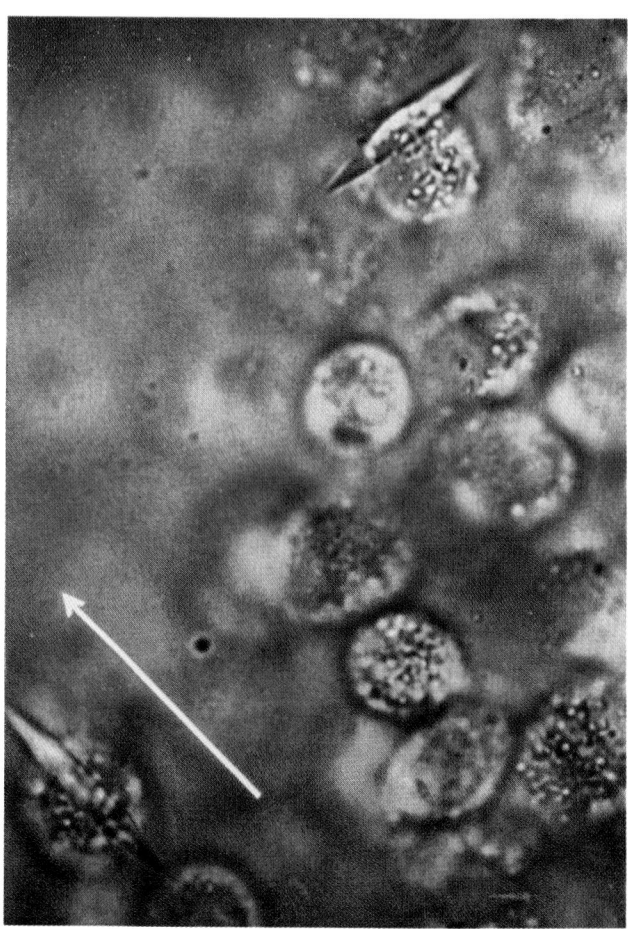

FIG. 109–12. Charcot-Leyden crystals in synovial fluid of a patient with eosinophilic synovitis. Compensated polarized light (×350). Arrow indicates compensator axis. (Courtesy Dr. H. Menard.)

range from 17 to 25 μm. With hematoxylin and eosin stain, they appear fairly eosinophilic; with Giemsa stain, they appear light purple or pink.[217] By transmission electron microscopy, these crystals are made of uniform, finely granular electron-dense material with a fine fibrillar pattern.[218,219] They may have a weakly positive birefringence,[36] but others have observed them to have a negative birefringence[212] or a very weak birefringence.[220]

CLINICAL FEATURES

Eosinophilic synovitis associated with Charcot-Leyden crystals on wet synovial fluid preparations has been recently documented in seven patients with a history of allergic reactions and dermatographism.[36–38] These patients developed painless monoarthritis after minor trauma without concurrent allergic symptoms. Joint swelling was seen in the knee of seven patients and in the first metatarsophalangeal joint of another patient. Each episode subsided within 1 to 2 weeks without therapy; three patients had recurrent episodes. Synovial fluid was mildly inflammatory, with leukocyte counts of $10,850 \pm 3,665/\mu L$ and up to 46% eosinophils. Charcot-Leyden crystals were seen inside cells on wet preparations. The in vitro formation of these crystals was facilitated by slight pressure on the coverslip and by overnight incubation at 4° C. It has been suggested that Charcot-Leyden crystals may be repository of human lysophospholipase by generating lysophospholipids and therefore possess a biologic function more significant than being solely a hallmark of an eosinophilic inflammatory process.[38,221]

ALUMINUM

In hemodialyzed patients, aluminum intoxication has been associated with a mineralization defect of bone matrix, resulting in osteomalacia, bone pain, and fractures.[47] Transmission electron microscopy and x-ray elemental microdispersive analysis have shown amorphous deposits of aluminum phosphate in mitochondria of bone cells and extracellular hexagonal crystals measuring 200 to 1000 Å at the mineralization front.[47] Aluminum levels in synovial fluid, synovium, and articular cartilage of patients undergoing chronic dialysis are higher than normal.[46] A high proportion of dialysis patients may also have amyloid and iron deposits in the synovium, as well as secondary hyperparathyroidism.[222,223] It has been difficult to separate such conditions from possible articular manifestations associated with intra-articular aluminum deposition.[222,223] Intra-articular injections of crystalline and amorphous aluminum phosphate in rabbits induced acute and chronic synovitis,[224,225] but these results cannot be extrapolated directly to humans.

FOREIGN-BODY SYNOVITIS

The introduction of hard penetrating particles into joints, tendon sheaths, and periarticular soft tissues, by causing infection or sterile inflammatory foreign-body reaction, can induce monoarticular synovitis, tenosynovitis, or cellulitis.[226] Those materials most commonly described with foreign-body synovitis include different vegetable particles such as plant thorns[65,226] and wood splinters,[227] which easily break inside the joint cavity (Table 109–3). Less often, sea

Table 109–3. Particles Associated With Foreign-Body Synovitis

Vegetal
Plant thorns
Date and sentinel plants
Blackthorn bushes
Roses, yuccas, hawthorns
Mesquites, bougainvilles
Ulex europeus (Tojo)
Wood splinters

Marine
Sea urchin spines
Crab spines
Fish bone

Minerals
Stone, gravel, silica
Brick fragments

Metals
Vitalium
Stainless steel
Lead

Miscellaneous
Silicone
Glass
Fiberglass
Polyethylene
Methylmethacrylate
Plastic
Rubber

urchin spines,[64,65] fish bone fragments,[65] crab spine,[228] stones, gravel, and brick fragments,[229] plastic,[230] rubber,[229] fiberglass,[231] and glass[229] can also be introduced into joints. Similar chronic granulomatous reaction of synovium can be induced by wear particles from articular implants such as metals,[232] silicones,[233] polyethylene,[68,234] and methylmethacrylate.[68,234] Bullet fragments, when lodged inside major joints, may induce mild synovitis and cause systemic manifestations of lead toxicity.[235] High-pressure injection injury of fingers with paint or grease guns usually induces a delayed necrotizing dactylitis, which requires immediate emergency surgical drainage and debridement.[236]

CLINICAL FEATURES

Clinical presentation of foreign-body synovitis is characterized by the sudden onset of pain at the site of the injury. Acute synovitis usually appears several days after the injury. Inflammation at the site of the penetrating injury may subside completely or become chronic with a steady or relapsing clinical course.[64,65,226] Frequently, the initial injury is forgotten by the patient or overlooked by the examiner. Joints most commonly involved are those of the hands and knees. Joint involvement is characterized by a variable degree of periarticular tender swelling and synovial thickening of small joints (Fig. 109–13), while larger joints may have large and persistent joint effusions. Fever, myalgias, lymph node enlargement, and synovitis of other noninjured joints have been observed in patients with sea urchin synovitis and subcutaneous silicone implants used for facial, breast, and small joint reconstruction.[64,65,237,238] In patients with high-pressure injection injury, the only initial clinical finding may be a painless puncture wound in the finger tip. After a few hours, however, signs of rapidly necrotizing dactylitis become apparent.[236]

Diving and other marine recreational activities, farming, and gardening are well-recognized risk factors.[65] Intravenous drug abuse also may be a possible risk factor.[65,239,240] Foreign-body synovitis must be differentiated from other conditions associated with acute, recurrent, or chronic monoarticular synovitis such as infectious arthritis,[239] gout, pseudogout and monoarticular juvenile RA,[239] or different causes of dactylitis.[65] These conditions include typical and atypical mycobacterial infections (tuberculous dactylitis or spina ventosa), erysipeloid, seal finger, sarcoidosis, psoriasis, tophaceous gout, and giant cell tumor of finger flexor tendon sheaths.

FIG. 109–13. Dactylitis of index finger and proximal interphalangeal joint synovitis due to plant thorn. (Courtesy Dr. J.L. Ferreiro.)

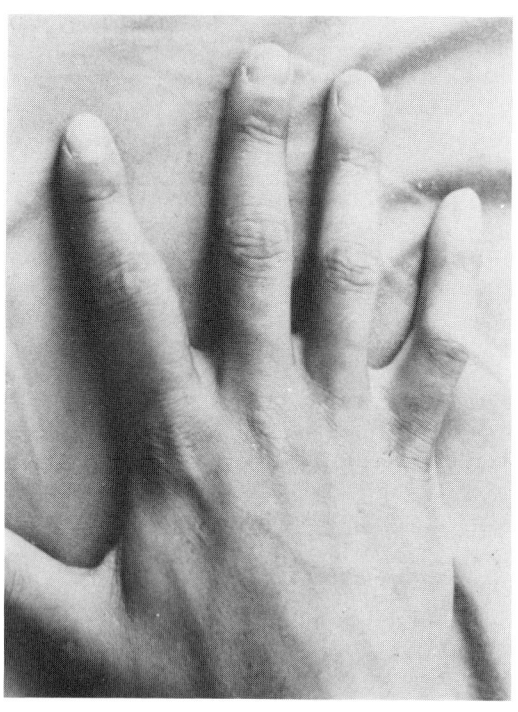

LABORATORY FINDINGS

White blood cell count and erythrocyte sedimentation rate are usually normal.[65] Synovial fluid can be cloudy or bloody; in those patients with detritic synovitis resulting from loose joint prostheses, it may be brownish and contain abundant debris.[232] Synovial fluid leukocyte counts range from 10,000 to 60,000/μL, with predominance of neutrophils.[239] Low-grade chronic infection is commonly seen in detritic synovitis associated with loose prostheses.[68,232,234] Fresh preparation of synovial fluid may reveal birefringent fragments of plant thorns, polyethylene, or polymethylmethacrylate,[65,68] or nonbirefringent particles such as needle-shape fiberglass and metallic particles.[231,232] Metallic particles appear as black rods or dots.[232]

RADIOGRAPHIC FEATURES

Radiographs are useful to detect radiodense particles of metals, fish bones, and sea urchin spines, but wood, plastic, and plant thorn particles are usually missed. Radiographs may reveal soft-tissue swelling[65,239] only, when obtained early. In patients with a chronic or relapsing course, however, periarticular demineralization, areas of localized osteolysis, osteosclerosis, and periosteal new bone formation can be seen[65] (Fig. 109–14). These changes may mimic those of osteomyelitis or primary bone tumors.[241] Ultrasonography[242] and computed tomography (CT)[243] may be helpful in detecting small pieces of nonmetallic, wood, or plastic foreign bodies.

PATHOLOGIC FEATURES

Excisional biopsy and bacteriologic studies of synovium, synovial fluid, and periarticular tissues are usually required for diagnosis and successful management of those with a chronic or relapsing course.[65,229,241] Synovium usually reveals synovial cell proliferation and diffuse infiltrates of lymphocytes and plasma cells with focal collections of PMN cells.[65,209,243,244] Giant cell formation in synovium is usually striking in those patients in whom foreign bodies are found inside the joint,[209,244] but it can be minimal or absent in patients in whom foreign particles are located in periarticular tissues or skin[239] (Fig. 109–15). Granulomas identical to those seen in sarcoidosis have been found in association with sea urchin synovitis.[65,245] Polarized light microscopy is useful in detecting birefringent fragments of plant thorn,

FIG. 109–14. Plant thorn synovitis with localized area of osteolysis, osteosclerosis, and periosteal new bone formation. (Courtesy Dr. J.L. Ferreiro.)

FIG. 109–15. Foreign-body synovitis. Characteristic plant thorn fragment surrounded by mononuclear and giant cells. Hematoxylin and eosin stain × 150. (Courtesy Dr. J.L. Ferreiro.)

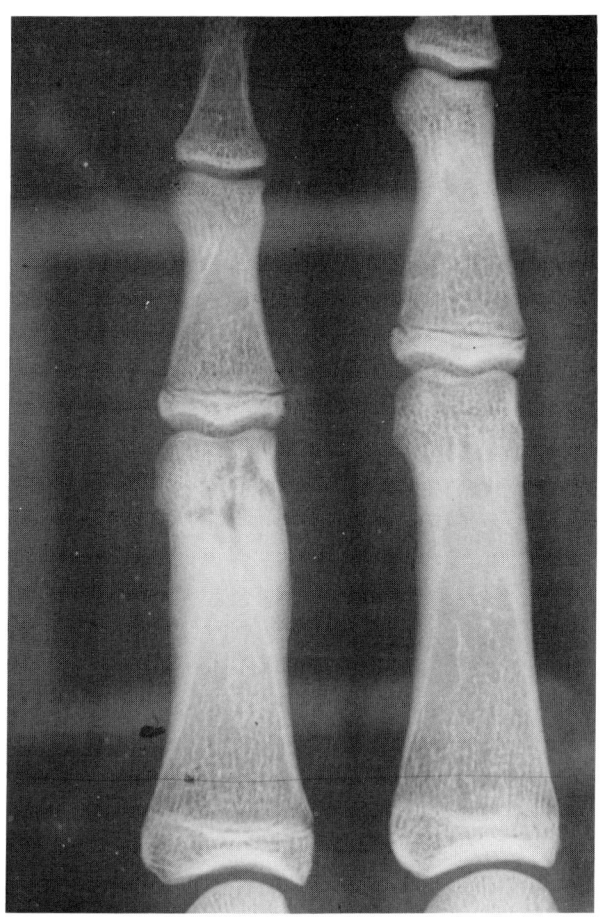

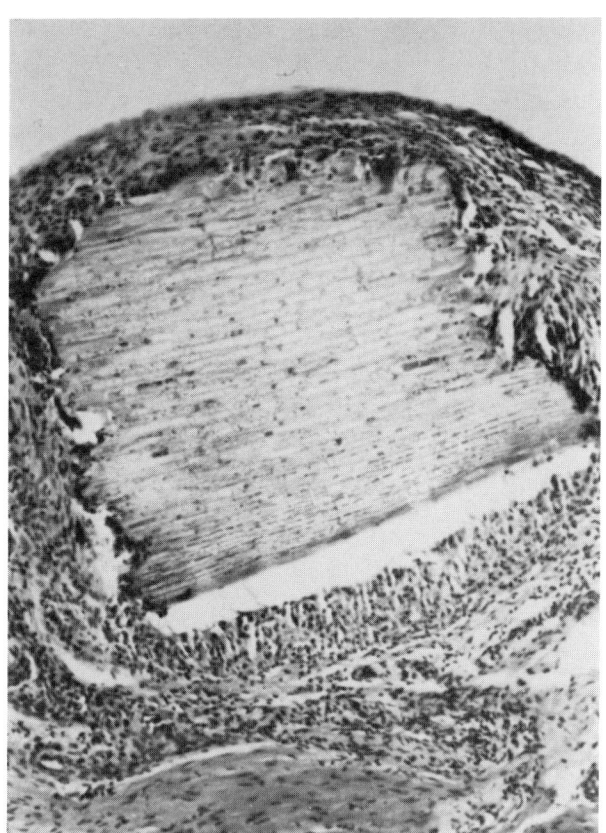

polyethylene, polymethylmethacrylate, and sea urchin spines (calcium carbonate crystals).[65] Elemental dispersive microprobe analysis may allow exact identification of metal particles, silica, silicon, and fiberglass.[231]

MECHANISM OF INFLAMMATION

Mechanisms mediating foreign-body synovitis are not well understood, but several have been postulated: associated low-grade infection, presence of toxins, alkaloid, mitogens, or other proteins on the surface of foreign bodies, as well as crystalline or paracrystalline structures with a negative surface charge.[230] Few experimental studies of foreign-body effects on synovium and skin of animals and humans have been performed.[230,246] In one study, minimal acute inflammation was induced by the injection of sterilized ground plant thorns or sea urchin spines

into rabbit knees and the rat skin air pouch model of synovium,[246] but 1 to 4 weeks later, both synovium and skin showed prominent chronic inflammation with lymphocytes, plasma cells, and giant cells. Dieppe injected plant thorns into rat paws and human forearm skin, and correlated the intensity of the inflammatory reaction with the surface charge of the thorns.[230]

MANAGEMENT

In about one third of patients with foreign-body synovitis due to exogenous particles, the inflammatory changes subside spontaneously. The remaining patients with a chronic or relapsing course usually require an excisional biopsy with synovectomy and articular lavage.[226,239,244] Occasionally, recurrent joint swelling with periosteal new bone formation can be seen after removal of the foreign body and synovectomy.[65]

REFERENCES

1. Chisholm, G.D., and Heard, B.E.: Oxalosis. Br. J. Surg., *50*:78–92, 1962.
2. Kinnett, J.G., and Bullough, P.G.: Identification of calcium oxalate deposits in bone by electron diffraction. Arch. Pathol. Lab. Med., *100*:656, 1976.
3. Schmidt, K.L., Leber, H.W., and Schutterle, G.: Arthropathies bei primarer Oxalose-Kristallsynovitis oder Osteopathie? Dtsch. Med. Wochenschr., *106*:19–22, 1981.
4. Hoffman, G.S., et al.: Calcium oxalate micro-crystalline-associated arthritis in end stage renal disease. Ann. Intern. Med., *97*:36–42, 1982.
5. Reginato, A.J., et al.: Arthropathy and cutaneous calcinosis in hemodialysis oxalosis. Arthritis Rheum., *29*:1387–1396, 1986.
6. Benhamou, C.L., et al.: Arthropathie microcristalline a oxalate de calcium au cours d'une oxalose primitive. Rev. Rhum. Med. Osteoartic., *52*:267–270, 1985.
7. Schumacher, H.R., Reginato, A.J., and Pullman, S.: Synovial fluid oxalate deposition complicating rheumatoid arthritis with amyloidosis and renal failure: Demonstration of intracellular oxalate crystals. J. Rheumatol., *14*:361–366, 1987.
8. Eade, A.W.T., Swannell, A.J., and Williamson, N.: Pyrophosphate arthropathy in hypophosphatasia. Ann. Rheum. Dis., *40*:164–170, 1981.
9. Ettlinger, E., and Hunder, G.G.: Synovial effusions containing cholesterol crystals. Report of 12 patients and review. Mayo Clin. Proc., *54*:366–374, 1979.
10. Griffin, P.E., and Bole, G.G.: Cholesterol-containing synovial effusions and cholesterosis of the synovial membrane. Univ. Mich. Med. Cent. J., *35*:170–176, 1969.
11. Bland, J.H., Gierthy, J.F., and Suhre, E.D.: Cholesterol in connective tissue of joints. Scand. J. Rheumatol., *3*:199–203, 1974.
12. Meyers, O.L., and Watermeyer, G.S.: Cholesterol-rich synovial effusions. S. Afr. Med. J., *50*:973–975, 1976.
13. Zuckner, J., Uddin, J., Gantner, G.E., and Dorner, R.W.: Cholesterol crystals in synovial fluid. Ann. Intern. Med., *60*:436–446, 1964.
14. Fam, A.G., et al.: Cholesterol associated synovitis: A clinicopathologic study of 8 cases. Ann. R. Coll. Phys. Surg. Can., *12*:94–103, 1979.
15. Bernal, L., Staphl, E., and Becerra, F.: Hyperlipidemic erosive arthritis. (Abstract.) Arthritis Rheum., *25*:4, 1982.
16. Taccari, E., and Teodori, S.: Rheumatoid chyliform bursitis: Pathogenic role of rheumatoid nodules. Arthritis Rheum., *27*:221–226, 1984.
17. Taccari, E., Teodori, S., and Manelli, H.: Les epanchements chyliformes de la polyarthritte chronique evolutive. Etude cytochimiques et ultrastructurales des cellules spumeuses. Rev. Rhum Mal. Osteoartic., *48*:555–562, 1981.
18. Zoppini, A., Teodori, S., and Taccari, E.: Valeur de la biopsie synoviale dans le diagnostic de arthropathies associees aux hyperlipoproteinemies. Rev. Rhum. Mal. Osteoartic., *47*:111–115, 1980.
19. Goldin, D.S., Stangler, D.A., and Canoso, J.J.: Rheumatoid subcutaneous bursitis. J. Rheumatol., *8*:974–978, 1981.
20. Weinstein, J.: Synovial fluid leukocytosis associated with intracellular lipid inclusions. Arch. Intern. Med., *140*:560–561, 1980.
21. Reginato, A.J., Schumacher, H.R., Allan, D.A., and Rabinowitz, J.: Acute monoarthritis associated with lipid liquid crystals. Ann. Rheum. Dis., *44*:537–643, 1985.
22. Trostle, D.C., Schumacher, H.R., Medsger, T.A., and Kapoor, W.N.: Microspherule associated acute monoarticular arthritis. Arthritis Rheum., *29*:1166–1168, 1986.
23. Schlesinger, P.A., Stillman, M.T., and Peterson, L.: Polyarthritis with birefringent lipid within synovial fluid macrophages: Case report and ultrastructural study. Arthritis Rheum., *25*:1365–1368, 1982.
24. Paul-Moya, H., and Abadi, I.: Monoartritis aguda y bursitis olecraneana asociada a liposomas. Artritis por cristales liquidos? (Abstract.) Libro de abstracts IX Congreso Panamericano de Reumatologia, November 1986, Buenos Aires, Argentina.
25. Langlands, D.R., et al.: Arthritis associated with crystallizing cryoprecipitable IG paraprotein. Am. J. Med., *68*:461–465, 1980.
26. Rosembaum, L.H., et al.: Cryo-crystalline arthropathy: Polyarthritis associated with unsuspected crystallizing monoclonal cryoimmunoglobulin. Presented at the meeting of the American Rheumatism Association, San Antonio, TX, June 1983.
27. Dornan, T.L., et al.: Widespread crystallization of paraprotein in myelomatosis. Q. J. Med., *222*:659–667, 1985.
28. Mullen, B., and Chalvardjian, A.: Crystalline tissue deposits in a case of multiple myeloma. Arch. Pathol. Lab. Med., *105*:94–97, 1981.
29. Grossman, J., et al.: Crystalglobulinemia. Ann. Intern. Med., *77*:395–400, 1972.
30. Berliner, S., et al.: Small skin blood vessels occlusions by cryoglobulins aggregates in ulcerative lesions in IgM-IgG cryoglobulinemia. J. Cutan. Pathol., *9*:96–103, 1982.
31. Chejfec, G., Natarelli, J., and Gould, V.E.: Myeloma lung. A previously unreported complication of multiple myeloma. Hum. Pathol., *14*:558–561, 1983.
32. Sikl, H.: A case of diffuse plasmocytosis with deposition of protein crystal in the kidney. J. Pathol. Bacteriol., *61*:149–164, 1949.
33. Mills, L.E., et al.: Crystallocryoglobulinemia resulting from human monoclonal antibodies to albumin. Ann. Intern. Med., *99*:601–604, 1983.
34. Rodrigues, M.M., et al.: Posterior corneal crystalline deposits in benign monoclonal gammopathy: A clinicopathologic case report. Arch. Ophthalmol., *98*:124–128, 1979.
35. Lutkitsch, O., Gebhardt, K.P., and Kovary, P.T.: Follicular hyperkeratosis and cryocrystalglobulinemia syndrome. Arch. Dermatol., *121*:795–798, 1985.
36. Menard, H.A., de Medicis, R., Lussier, A., and Brown, J.: Charcot-Leyden crystals in synovial fluid. (Letter.) Arthritis Rheum., *24*:1591–1593, 1981.
37. Dougados, M., Benhamod, L., and Amor, B.: Charcot-Leyden crystals in synovial fluid. Arthritis Rheum., *26*:1416, 1983.
38. Brown, J.P., Rola-Pleszcynski, M., and Menard, H.A.: Eosinophilic synovitis: Clinical observations on a newly recognized subset of patients with dermatographism. Arthritis Rheum., *29*:1147–1151, 1986.
39. Honsoon, P., Burton, T.J., and Van der Bel-Kahn, J.M.: Circulating Charcot-Leyden crystals in hypereosinophilic syndrome. Am. J. Clin. Pathol., *75*:236–242, 1981.
40. Kahn, C.B., Hollander, J.L., and Schumacher, H.R.: Corticosteroid crystals in synovial fluid. JAMA, *221*:807–809, 1970.
41. Stephan, J., Pitrova, S., and Pazderka, V.: Cystinosis with crystal-induced synovitis and arthropathy. Z. Rheumatol., *35*:347–355, 1976.
42. Antoci, B., and Gherlinzoni, G.: Cystinosis of bone. Ital. J. Orthop. Traumatol., *1*:81–97, 1975.
43. Berman, L., and Salomon, L.: Xanthine gout, crystal depo-

sition in skeletal muscle in a case of xanthinuria. Rheumatologie, 5:253–256, 1975.

44. Isaacs, A., Heffron, I.H., and Berman, L.: Xanthine, hypoxanthine and muscle pain: Histochemical and biochemical observations. S. Afr. Med. J., 49:1035–1038, 1975.

45. Chalmers, R.A., Watts, R.W.E., Bitenski, L., and Chayen, J.: Microsopic studies on crystals in skeletal muscle in two cases of xanthinuria. J. Pathol., 99:45–65, 1969.

46. Netter, P., et al.: Aluminum in the joint tissues of chronic renal failure patients treated with regular hemodialysis and aluminum compounds. J. Rheumatol., 11:66–70, 1984.

47. Plachot, J., et al.: Bone ultrastructure and x-rays microanalysis of aluminum-intoxicated hemodialyzed patients. Kidney Internat., 25:796–803, 1984

48. Ager, J.A.M., and Lehman, H.: Intra-erythrocytic hemoglobin crystals. J. Clin. Pathol., 10:336–340, 1957.

49. Bessis, M., Normarski, G., Thiery, J.P., and Breton-Gorius, J.: Etudes sur la falciformation des globules rougess au microscope polarizant et au microscope electronique. II. L'interiur du globule: Comparison avec les cristaux intra-globulaires. Rev. Hemat., 13:249–260, 1958.

50. Zahaopoulos, P., Wong, J.Y., and Keagy, N.: Hematoidin crystals in cervicovaginal smears. Report of two cases. Acta Cytol., 29:1029–1034, 1985.

51. Sussuki, T., Sugawara, Y., Sdatoh, Y., and Shikama, K.: Human oxymyoglobin: Isolation and characterization. J. Chromatogr., 195:227–280, 1980.

52. Waldo, E.D., and Tobias, H.: Needle-like cytoplasmic inclusions in the liver in porphyria cutanea tarda. Arch. Pathol., 96:368–371, 1973.

53. Thomas, K., and Hut, M.S.R.: Tyrosine crystals in salivary gland tumor. J. Clin. Pathol., 96:368–371, 1983.

54. Campbell, W.G., Priest, R.E., and Weathers, D.R.: Characterization of two types of crystalloids in pleomorphic adenomas of minor salivary glands. A light microscopic, electron microscopic, and histochemical study. Am. J. Pathol., 118:194–202, 1985.

55. Tischler, A.S., and Compagno, J.: Crystal-like deposits of amyloid in pancreatic islet cell tumors. Arch. Pathol. Lab. Med., 103:247–251, 1979.

56. Ordonez, N.G., Manning, J.T., and Mackay, B.: Crystals and alpha 1-antitrypsin-reactive globoid inclusions in an islet cell tumor of the pancreas. Ultrastruct. Pathol., 8:319–338, 1985.

57. Machinami, R., and Kikuchi, F.: Adenosine triphosphatase activity of crystalline inclusions in alveolar soft part sarcoma. An ultrahistochemical study of a case. Pathol. Res. Pract., 181:357–361, 1986.

58. Nesland, J.M., Langholm, R., and Marton, P.F.: Hexagonal crystals in the bone marrow in patients with myeloproliferative disease and preleukemia. Scand. J. Hematol., 32:552–558, 1984.

59. Staven, P., and Bjorneklett, A.: A light green crystal in May-Grunwald and Giemsa-stained bone marrow macrophages in patients with myeloid leukemia. Scand. J. Haematol., 18:67–72, 1977.

60. Nagano, T., and Ohtsuki, I.: Reinvestigation of the fine structure of Reinke's crystals in human testicular interstitial cell. J. Cell. Biol., 51:148–161, 1971.

61. Adams, P.C., et al.: Amiodarone pulmonary toxicity: Clinical and subclinical features. Quart. J. Med., 229:440–441, 1986.

62. Lullman, H., Lullman-Rauch, R., and Wasserman, O.: Drug induced phospholipidoses. CRC Crit. Rev. Toxicol., 4:185–218, 1975.

63. Watts, R.W.E., et al.: Microscopic studies on skeletal muscle

64. Cracchiolo, A., and Goldberg, L.: Local and systemic reactions to puncture injuries by the sea urchin spine and the date palm thorn. Arthritis Rheum., 20:1206–1212, 1977.

65. Ferreiro Seoane, J.L., Reginato, A.J., O'Connor, C.R., and Alvarez, B.: Foreign body synovitis, clinical and pathologic studies. Panamerican Congress of Rheumatology Abstract N, Buenos Aires, Argentina, November 1986.

66. Hollander, J.L.: Self-induced arthritis by intra-articular injection of talc. Unpublished observation.

67. Henderson, W.J., et al.: Identification of talc on surgeons gloves and in tissue from starch granulomas. Br. J. Surg., 62:941–944, 1975.

68. Crugnola, A., Schiller, A., and Radin, E.: Polymeric debris in synovium after total joint replacement. Histological identification. J. Bone Joint Surg., 59A:860–862, 1977.

69. Blackburn, W.E., et al.: Severe vascular complications in oxalosis after bilateral nephrectomy. Ann. Intern. Med., 82:44–46, 1975.

70. Dennis, A.J., et al.: Nitroglycerin as a remedy for peripheral vascular insufficiency associated with oxalosis. Ann. Intern. Med., 92:799–800, 1985.

71. Greer, K.E., Cooper, P.H., Campbell, F., Westervelt, F.B.: Primary oxalosis with livedo reticularis. Arch. Dermatol., 116:213–214, 1980.

72. Arbus, G.S., and Sniderman, S.: Oxalosis with peripheral gangrene. Arch. Pathol., 97:107–110, 1974.

73. Lewis, R.D., Lowenstam, H.A., and Rossman, G.R.: Oxalate nephrosis and crystalline myocarditis. Case report with postmortem and crystallographic studies. Arch. Pathol. Lab. Med., 98:149–155, 1974.

74. Tonkin, A.M., et al.: Primary oxalosis with myocardial involvement and heart block. Med. J. Aust., 1:873–874, 1976.

75. West, R.R., Salyer, W.R., and Hutchins, G.M.: Adult onset primary oxalosis with complete heart block. Johns Hopkins Med. J., 133:195–200, 1973.

76. O'Callahan, J.W., et al.: Rapid progression of oxalosis-induced cardiomyopathy despite adequate hemodialysis. Miner. Electrolyte Metab., 10:48–51, 1984.

77. Coltart, D.J., and Hudson, R.E.B.: Primary oxalosis of the heart: A cause of heart block. Br. Heart J., 33:315–317, 1971.

78. Moorhead, P.J., Cooper, D.J., and Timperley, W.R.: Progressive peripheral neuropathy in a patient with primary hyperoxaluria. Br. Med. J., 2:312–313, 1975.

79. McKenna, R.W., and Dehner, L.P.: Oxalosis: An unusual cause of myelophthisis in childhood. Am. J. Clin. Pathol., 66:991–997, 1976.

80. Hricik, D.E., and Hussain, R.: Pancytopenia and hepatosplenomegaly in oxalosis. Arch. Intern. Med., 144:167–168, 1984.

81. Hodgkinson, A., and Zarembski, P.M.: Oxalic acid metabolism in man: A review. Calcif. Tiss. Res., 2:115–132, 1968.

82. Williams, H.E., and Smith, L.H.: Disorders of oxalate metabolism. Am. J. Med., 45:715–735, 1968.

83. Williams, H.E., and Smith, L.H.: Primary hyperoxaluria. In The Metabolic Basis of Inherited Disease. Edited by J.B. Stanbury, J.B. Wyngarden, and D.S. Frederickson. New York, McGraw-Hill, 1983.

84. Earnest, D.L.: Enteric hyperoxaluria. Adv. Intern. Med., 24:407–427, 1979.

85. Pru, C., Eaton, J.R., and Kjellstrand, C.: Vitamin C intoxication and hyperoxalemia in chronic hemodialysis patients. Nephron, 39:112–116, 1985.

in gout patients treated with allopurinol. Quart. J. Med., 157:1–14, 1971.

86. Nime, F.A., and Hutchins, G.M.: Oxalosis caused by Aspergillus infection. Johns Hopkins Med. J., *133*:183–184, 1973.

87. Worcester, E.M., Nakagawa, Y., Bushinsky, D.A., and Coe, F.L.: Evidence that serum calcium oxalate supersaturation is a consequence of oxalate retention in patients with chronic renal failure. J. Clin. Invest., *77*:1888–1896, 1986.

88. Weber, D.V., et al.: Urinary saturation measurements in calcium nephrolithiasis. Ann. Intern. Med., *90*:180–184, 1979.

89. Hautman, R.A., et al.: Intrarenal distribution of oxalic acid, calcium, sodium, and potassium in man. Eur. J. Clin. Invest., *10*:173–176, 1980.

90. Cogan, D.G., et al.: Calcium oxalate and calcium phosphate crystals in detached retinas. Arch. Ophthalmol., *60*:366–371, 1958.

91. Albert, D.M., et al.: Flecked retina secondary to oxalate crystals from methoxyflurane anesthesia: Clinical and experimental studies. Trans. Am. Acad. Ophthalmol., *79*:817–826, 1975.

92. Dunn, H.G.: Oxalosis. Am. J. Dis. Child., *90*:58–80, 1955.

93. Hockaday, T.D.R., Clayton, J.E., Frederick, E.W., and Smith, L.H.: Primary hyperoxaluria. Medicine, *43*:315–345, 1964.

94. Daniels, R.A., Michels, R., Aisen, P., and Goldstein, G.: Familial hyperoxaluria. Report of a family review of the literature. Am. J. Med., *29*:820–831, 1960.

95. Boquist, L., Lindovist, B., Ostberg, Y., and Steen, L.: Primary oxalosis. Am. J. Med., *54*:673–681, 1973.

96. Burke, E.C., et al.: Oxalosis. Pediatrics, *15*:383–391, 1955.

97. Hall, E.G., Scowen, E.F., and Watts, R.W.E.: Clinical manifestations of primary oxaluria. Arch. Dis. Child., *35*:108–112, 1960.

98. Aponte, G.E., and Fetter, T.R.: Familial idiopathic oxalate nephrocalcinosis. Am. J. Clin. Pathol., *24*:1363–1373, 1954.

99 Morris, M.C., et al.: Oxalosis in infancy. Arch. Dis. Child., *57*:224–228, 1982.

100. Danpure, C.J., Jennings, P.R., and Watts, R.W.E.: Enzymological diagnosis of primary hyperoxaluria by measurement of hepatic alanine: Glyoxylate aminotransferase activity. Lancet, *1*:289–293, 1987.

101. Scowen, E.F., Stansfeld, A.G., and Watts, R.W.E.: Oxalosis and primary oxaluria. J. Pathol. Bacteriol., *77*:195–205, 1959.

102. Cohen, H., and Reid, J.B.: Tenosynovitis crepitans associated with oxaluria. Liverpool Med. Chirurg. J., *43*:193–199, 1935.

103. Nartijn, A., and Thijn, C.J.P.: Radiologic findings in primary oxaluria. Skeletal Radiol., *8*:21–24, 1982.

104. Halifa, G., Dossans, B., Gagnadoux, M.F., and Sauvegrain, J.: Aspect radiologiques de l'oxalose. J. Radiol., *60*:45–49, 1979.

105. Milgram, J.W.: Chronic renal failure. Recurrent secondary hyperparathyroidism. Multiple metaphyseal infractions, and secondary oxalosis. Bull. Hosp. Joint Dis., *35*:118–144, 1974.

106. Gherardi, G., et al.: Bone oxalosis and renal osteodystrophy. Arch. Pathol. Lab. Med., *104*:105–111, 1980.

107. Sherrard, D.J., Baylink, D.J., Wergedal, J.E., and Malone, N.A.: Quantitative histologic studies on the pathogenesis of uremic bone disease. J. Clin. Endocrinol. Metab., *39*:119–135, 1974.

108. Mathews, M., et al.: Bone biopsy to diagnose hyperoxaluria in patients with renal failure. Ann. Intern. Med., *90*:777–779, 1979.

109. Breed, A., et al.: Oxalosis induced bone disease. A complication of transplantation and prolonged survival in primary hyperoxaluria. Report of a case. J. Bone Joint Surg., *63*:310–316, 1981.

110. Milgran, J.W., and Salyer, W.R.: Secondary oxalosis of bone

in chronic renal failure. A histopathological study of three cases. J. Bone Joint. Surg., *56*:387–395, 1974.

111. Jahn, H., Frank, R.M., Voegel, J.C., and Shohn, D.: Scanning electron microscopy and x-ray diffraction studies of human bone oxalosis. Calcif. Tiss. Int., *30*:109–121, 1980.

112. Davis, J.S., Klinberg, W.G., and Stowell, R.E.: Nephrolithiasis with calcium oxalate crystals in kidney and bones. J. Pediatr., *36*:323–324, 1950.

113. Paul, H., Reginato, A.J., and Shumacher, H.R.: Alizarin red S stain as screening test to detect calcium compounds in synovial fluid. Arthritis Rheum., *26*:191–201, 1983.

114. Prioa, A.D., and Brinn, N.T.: Identification of calcium oxalate crystals using alizarin red S stain. Arch. Pathol. Lab. Med., *109*:186–190, 1985.

115. Chaplin, A.J.: Histopathologic occurrence and characterization of calcium oxalate. A review. J. Clin. Pathol., *30*:800–811, 1977.

116. Pizzolato, P.: Mercurous nitrate as a histochemical reagent for calcium phosphate in bone pathological calcification and for calcium oxalate. Histochem. J., *3*:463–469, 1971.

117. Pizzolato, P.: Histochemical recognition of calcium oxalate. J. Histochem. Cytochem., *12*:333–336, 1969.

118. Khan, S.R., Finlayson, B., and Hackett, R.: Scanning electron microscopy of calcium oxalate crystal formation in experimental nephrolithiasis. Lab. Invest., *41*:504–510, 1979.

119. Siew, S.: Investigation of crystallosis of the kidney by means of polarization, scanning transmission and high voltage electron microscopy. Isr. J. Med. Sci., *15*:698–710, 1979.

120. Faires, J.S., and McCarty, D.J., Jr.: Acute synovitis in normal joints of man and dog produced by injections of microcrystalline sodium urate, calcium oxalate and corticosteroid esters. (Abstract.) Arthritis Rheum., *5*:95, 1962.

121. Denko, C.W., and Whitehouse, M.W.: Experimental inflammation induced by naturally occuring microcrystalline calcium salts. J. Rheumatol., *3*:54–62, 1976.

122. Hasselbacher, P.: Stimulation of synovial fibroblasts by calcium oxalate and monosodium urate monohydrate. A mechanism of connective tissue degradation in oxalosis and gout. J. Lab. Clin. Med., *100*:977–981, 1982.

123. Balcke, P., et al.: Secondary oxalosis in chronic renal insufficiency. (Letter.) N. Engl. J. Med., *303*:944, 1980.

124. Op de Hock, C.T., et al.: Oxalosis in chronic renal failure. Proc. Eur. Dial. Transplant Assoc., *17*:730–735, 1980.

125. Zarembski, P.M., Hodgekinson, A., and Parson, F.M.: Elevation of the concentration of plasma oxalic acid in renal failure. Nature, *212*:511–512, 1966.

126. Ramsay, A.G., and Reed, R.G.: Oxalate removal by hemodialysis stage renal disease. Am. J. Kidney Dis., *4*:123–127, 1984.

127. Giboa, N., Largent, J.A., and Urizar, E.H.: Primary oxalosis presenting as anuric renal failure in infancy: Diagnosis by x-ray diffraction of kidney tissue. J. Pediatr., *103*:88–90, 1983.

128. Borland, W.W., Payton, C.D., Simpson, K., and Macdougall, A.I.: Serum oxalate in chronic renal failure. Nephron, *45*:119–121, 1987.

129. Balcke, P., et al.: Ascorbic acid aggravates secondary hyperoxalemia in patients on chronic hemodialysis. Ann. Intern. Med., *10*:344–345, 1984.

130. Fayemi, A.O., Ali, M., and Braun, E.V.: Oxalosis in hemodialysis patients: A pathologic study of 80 cases. Arch. Pathol. Lab. Med., *103*:58–62, 1977.

131. Salyer, W.R., and Keren, D.: Oxalosis as a complication of chronic renal failure. Kidney Int., *4*:61–67, 1973.

132. Sullivan, J.P., and Eisenstein, A.B.: Ascorbic acid depletion during hemodialysis. JAMA, *226*:1697–1699, 1972.

133. Ott, S.W., Andress, D.L., and Sherrard, D.J.: Bone oxalate in long term hemodialysis patients who ingested high doses of vitamin C. Am. J. Kidney Dis., *113*:450–454, 1986.

134. Scheimman, J.L.: The management of primary hyperoxaluria. The Kidney, *17*:13–17, 1984.

135. Watts, R.W.E., et al.: Primary hyperoxaluria (type I) attempted treatment with combined hepatic and renal transplantation. Q. J. Med., *57*:697–703, 1986.

136. Watts, R.W.E.: Studies of some possible biochemical treatments of primary hyperoxaluria. Q. J. Med., *48*:259–271, 1979.

137. Will, E.J., Bijvoet, O.L.M.: Primary oxalosis: Clinical and biochemical response to high dose pyridoxine therapy. Metabolism, *28*:542–548, 1979.

138. Newcombe, S.S., and Cohen, A.S.: Chylous synovial effusion in rheumatoid arthritis. Am. J. Med., *38*:156–164, 1965.

139. Wise, C.M., White, R.E., and Agudelo, C.: Synovial fluid lipid abnormalities in various disease states; review and classification. Semin. Arthritis Rheum., *16*:222–230, 1987.

140. Fam, A.G., Pritzker, K.P.H., Cheng, P.T., and Little, H.A.: Cholesterol crystals in osteoarthritic effusions. J. Rheumatol., *8*:273–280, 1981.

141. Chauffard, A., and Wolf, M.: Structure et evolution des tophus goutteux. Presse Med., *31*:1013–1015, 1923.

142. Sokoloff, L.: The pathology of gout. Metabolism, *6*:230–243, 1957.

143. Rodriquez, M.A., et al.: Multiple microcrystal deposition disease in a patient with systemic lupus erythematosus. Ann. Rheum. Dis., *43*:498–502, 1984.

144. Reginato, A.J., and Schumacher, H.R.: Cholesterol crystals in synovial fluid of chronic tophaceous gout. Unpublished observation.

145. Shiong, S.L., and Trimble, B.: Rheumatoid arthritis with bloody and cholesterol pleural effusion. Arch. Pathol. Lab. Med., *109*:769–771, 1985.

146. Dodson, W.N., and Hollingsworth, J.W.: Pleural effusion in rheumatoid arthritis. N. Engl. J. Med., *275*:1337–1342, 1966.

147. Nye, W.H.R., Terry, R., and Rosenbaun, D.L.: Observations on cholesterol effusions in rheumatoid arthritis and in idiopathic cholesterol pericarditis. (Abstract.) Arthritis Rheum., *9*:528, 1966.

148. Hillerdal, G.: Chyliform (cholesterol) pleural effusion. Chest, *88*:426–428, 1985.

149. Nixon, R.K., and Durham, R.H.: Lipoid nodules in chronic rheumatoid arthritis. Arthritis Rheum., *2*:27–29, 1959.

150. Weber, F.P.: A syndrome of rheumatoid arthritis combined with multiple xanthomatous connective tissue infiltrations. Ann. Rheum. Dis., *4*:3–10, 1944.

151. Gordon, S.L., Denton, J.R., McCann, P.D., and Parisien, M.V.: Unicameral bone cyst of the talus. Clin. Orthop., *215*:200–205, 1987.

152. Fam, A.G., Sugai, M., Gertner, E.M., and Lewis, A.: Cholesterol tophus. Arthritis Rheum., *26*:1525–1528, 1983.

153. Dalinka, M.K., Turner, M.L., Thompson, J.J., and Lee, R.E.: Lipid granulomatosis of the ribs: Focal Erdheim-Chester disease. Radiology, *142*:297–299, 1982.

154. Nast, C.C., and Cohen, A.H.: Renal cholesterol granulomas: Identification and morphological pattern of development. Histopathology, *9*:1195–1204, 1985.

155. Kieffer, D., et al.: Manifestations articulaires ou cours des dyslipedemies. A propos de deux observations personelles. Rev. Rhum. Mal. Osteoartic., *48*:569–573, 1981.

156. Mathon, G., et al.: Articular manifestations of familial hypercholesterolaemia. Ann. Rheum. Dis., *44*:599–602, 1985.

157. Rooney, P.J., et al.: Transient polyarthritis with familial hyperbetalipoproteinaemia. Q. J. Med., *67*:249–254, 1978.

158. Delbarre, F., Laoussadi, S., Kahan, A., and Aubony, G.: Le rhumatisme des thesaurismoses a lipides. Atteinte articulaire au cours de hyperdyslipidemie de type II. Presence de microcristaux dans les mitochondries des synoviocytes. C.R. Acad. Sci. Paris, *288*:181–184, 1979.

159. Shapiro, J.R., et al.: Achilles tendinitis and tenosynovitis. A diagnostic manifestation of familial Type II hyperlipoproteinemia in children. Am. J. Dis. Child., *128*:486–490, 1974.

160. Kruth, H.S.: Lipid deposition in human tendon xanthoma. Am. J. Pathol., *121*:311–315, 1985.

161. Smith, M.C., Chose, M.K., and Henry, A.R.: The clinical spectrum of renal cholesterol embolization. Am. J. Med., *11*:174–180, 1981.

162. Young, D.K., Burton, M.F., and Herman, J.: Multiple cholesterol emboli simulating systemic necrotizing vasculitis. J. Rheumatol., *13*:423–426, 1986.

163. Nye, W.H.R., Terry, R., and Rosenbaum, D.L.: Two forms of crystalline lipid in "cholesterol" effusions. Am. J. Clin. Pathol., *49*:718–728, 1968.

164. Sutor, D.J., and Gaston, P.J.: Anhydrous cholesterol: A new crystalline form in gallstones. Gut, *13*:64–65, 1972.

165. Fabricant, C.G., Krock, L., and Gillespe, J.H.: Virus-induced cholesterol crystals. Science, *181*:566–567, 1973.

166. Boucek, R.J., and Noble, N.L.: Biochemical studies on cholesterol in an in vivo cultivated connective tissue. Circulation Res., *5*:27–33, 1957.

167. Denko, C.W., Petricevic, M.: Modification of cholesterol induced inflammation. Agents Actions, *10*:353–357, 1980.

168. Pritzker, K.P.H., Fam, A.G., Omar, S.A., and Gertbein, S.D.: Experimental cholesterol crystal arthropathy. J. Rheumatol., *8*:281–290, 1981.

169. Hasselbacher, P., and Hahn, J.L.: Activation of the alternative pathway of complement by microcrystalline cholesterol. Arteriosclerosis, *37*:239–245, 1980.

170. Wild, J.H., and Zvaifler, N.J.: An office technique for identifying crystals in synovial fluid. Am. Fam. Physician, *12*:72–81, 1975.

171. Zimmer, J.G., Dewey, R., Waterhouse, C., and Terry, R.: The origin and nature of anisotropic urinary lipids in the nephrotic syndrome. Ann. Intern. Med., *54*:205–214, 1961.

172. Bangham, A.D.: Development of the liposome concept. *In* Liposomes in Biological Systems. Edited by G. Gregoriadis and A.C. Allison. New York, Wiley, 1980.

173. Small, D.M.: Liquid crystals in living and dying systems. J. Colloid. Interface Sci., *58*:581–602, 1977.

174. Ferguson, J.L.: Liquid crystals. Sci. Am., *211*:77–85, 1964.

175. Brown, G.H.: Structure and properties of the liquid crystalline state of matter. J. Colloid. Interface. Sci., *58*:534–538, 1977.

176. Small, D.M., and Shipley, G.G.: Physical chemical basis of lipid deposition in atherosclerosis. Science, *175*:222–229, 1974.

177. Ratliff, N.B., et al.: Diagnosis of chloroquine cardiomyopathy by endomyocardial biopsy. N. Engl. J. Med., *316*:191–193, 1977.

178. Choi, S.J., Schumacher, H.R., Clayburne, G., and Rothfuss, M.S.: Liposome-induced synovitis in rabbits. Arthritis Rheum., *29*:889–896, 1986.

179. Chadially, F.N.: Myelin Figures and Myelinoid Bodies, Ultrastructural Pathology of the Cell. Edited by F.N. Ghadially. Boston, Butterworth, 1975.

180. Roy, S., and Ghadially, F.N.: Pathology of experimental hemoarthrosis. Ann. Rheum. Dis., *26*:402–415, 1966.

181. Choi, S.J., et al.: Experimental haemarthrosis produces mild inflammation associated with intracellular Maltese crosses. Ann. Rheum. Dis., *45*:1025–1028, 1986.

182. Baldassare, J.J., et al.: Reconstitution of platelet proteins into phospholipid vesicles. Functional proteoliposomes. J. Clin. Invest., *75*:35–39, 1985.

183. Sheth, K.J., and Bernhard, G.C.: The arthropathy of Fabry's disease. Arthritis Rheum., *22*:781–783, 1979.

184. Delbarre, F., et al.: Le rhumatisme des thesuriamoses a lipides. Arthropathies au cours de la carence en alpha-galactosidase A (maladie de Fabry). Etude ultrastructurale de la membrane synoviale avec mise en evidences de micro-cristaux dans les mitrochondries des synoviocytes. C.R. Acad. Sci. Paris, *288*:579–582, 1979.

185. Black, M.M.: Panniculitis. J. Cutan. Pathol., *12*:366–380, 1985.

186. Reginato, A.J., et al.: Unusual birefringent crystals in synovial fluid of patients with osteoarthritis and subchondral bone cysts and in hemarthrosis. (Abstract.) Arthritis Rheum., *29*:S15, 1986.

187. Jennette, J.C., Wilkman, A.S., and Benson, J.D.: IgD myeloma with intracytoplasmic crystalline inclusions. Am. J. Clin. Pathol., *75*:231–235, 1981.

188. Neuman, V.: Multiple plasma cell myeloma with crystalline deposits in the tumor cells and in the kidneys. J. Pathol. Bacteriol., *61*:165–169, 1949.

189. Engle, R.L., and Wallis, L.A.: Multiple myeloma and the adult Fanconi syndrome. Report of a case with crystal-like deposits in the tumor cells and in the epithelial cells of the kidney. Am. J. Med., *34*:125–133, 1963.

190. Klintworth, C.K., Brodehoeft, S.J., and Reed, J.W.: Analysis of corneal crystalline deposits in multiple myeloma. Am. J. Ophthalmol., *86*:303–313, 1978.

191. Aronson, S.B., and Shaw, R.: Corneal crystals in multiple myeloma. Arch. Ophthalmol., *61*:541–546, 1959.

192. Cherry, P.M.H., et al.: Corneal and conjunctival deposits in monoclonal gammopathy. Can. J. Ophthalmol., *18*:142–143, 1983.

193. Hoisen, H., Ringvold, A., and Kildahl-Anderson, O.: Corneal crystalline deposits in multiple myeloma. A case report. Acta Ophthalmol., *61*:493–500, 1963.

194. Dotten, D.A., et al.: Cryocrystalglobulinemia. Can. Med. Assoc. J., *114*:909–912, 1976.

195. Stoebner, P., et al.: Ultrastructural study of human IgG–IgM crystalcryoglobulins. Am. J. Clin. Pathol., *71*:404–410, 1979.

196. An, H.S., Namey, T.C., Kim, K.: Essential cryoglobulinemia with intense and persistent synovitis of the knee. Clin. Orthop. Rel. Res., *215*:173–178, 1987.

197. Weinberger, A., Berlinger, S., and Pinkhas, J.: Articular manifestations of essential cryoglobulinemia. Semin. Arthritis Rheum., *10*:224–230, 1981.

198. Weinberger, A., Berlinger, S., and Pinkhas, J.: Spine manifestations in essential cryoglobulinemia. Rheumatol. Rehabil., *21*:127–133, 1982.

199. Chneider, J.A., Shulman, J.D., and Seegmiller, J.E.: Cystinosis. *In* The Metabolic Basis of Inherited Diseases. 5th Ed. Edited by J.B. Stanbury. New York, McGraw-Hill, 1983.

200. Gahl, W.A., et al.: Defective cystine exodus from isolated lysosome-rich fractions of cystinotic leucocytes. J. Biol. Chem., *257*:9570–9575, 1982.

201. Lietman, P.S., et al.: Adult cystinosis. A benign disorder. Am. J. Med., *40*:511–540, 1966.

202. Korn, D.: Demonstration of cystine crystals in peripheral white blood cells in a patient with cystinosis. N. Engl. J. Med., *262*:545–548, 1960.

203. Koizumi, F., et al.: Cystinosis with marked atrophy of the kidney and thyroid. Histological and ultrastructural studies in an autopsy case. Acta Pathol. Jpn., *35*:145–150, 1985.

204. Chan, A.M., et al.: Hypothyroidism in cystinosis: A clinical, endocrinologic, and histologic study involving sixteen patients with cystinosis. Am. J. Med., *48*:678–693, 1970.

205. Felicitas, A., et al.: Hereditary xanthinuria. Evidence for enhanced hypoxanthine salvage. J. Clin. Invest., *79*:847–852, 1987.

206. Chalmers, R.A., et al.: Crystalline deposits in striped muscle in xanthinuria. Nature, *221*:170–175, 1969.

207. Delbarre, F., et al.: Acces de goutte chez un xanthinurique. Nouv. Presse Med., *2*:2465–2466, 1973.

208. Greene, M.L., Fujimoto, W.Y., and Seegmiller, J.E.: Urinary xanthine stones. A rare complication of allopurinol therapy. N. Engl. J. Med., *280*:426–428, 1969.

209. Band, P.R., et al.: Xanthine nephropathy in a patient with lymphosarcoma treated with allopurinol. N. Engl. J. Med., *283*:354–360, 1970.

210. Thompson, J.H., and Paddock, F.K.: The significance of Charcot-Leyden crystals. N. Engl. J. Med., *223*:936–939, 1940.

211. Ayres, W.W., and Starkey, N.M.: Studies on Charcot-Leyden crystals. Blood, *5*:254–266, 1950.

212. Ayres, W.W., and Siliphant, W.M.: Charcot-Leyden crystals in eosinophilic granuloma of bone. Am. J. Clin. Pathol., *30*:323–327, 1958.

213. Amor, B., Benhamou, C.L., Dougados, M., and Grant, A.: Arthrites a eosinophiles et revue generale de la signification de l'eosinophilie articulaire. Rev. Rhum. Mal. Osteoartic., *50*:659–664, 1983.

214. Weller, P.F., Bach, D., and Austen, K.F.: Human eosinophil lysophospholipase: The sole protein component of Charcot-Leyden crystals. J. Immunol., *128*:1346–1349, 1982.

215. Weller, P.F., Goetzl, E.J., and Austen, K.F.: Identification of human eosinophil lysophospholipase as the constituent of Charcot-Leyden crystals. Proc. Natl. Acad. Sci.-U.S.A., *77*:7440–7448, 1980.

216. Acherman, S.J., Loegerine, D.A., and Gleich, G.J.: The human eosinophil Charcot-Leyden crystal protein: Characteristics and measurements by radioimmunoassay. J. Immunol., *125*:218–222, 1980.

217. Dawes, C.J., and Williams, W.L.: Histochemical studies of Charcot-Leyden crystals. Anat. Rec., *116*:53–71, 1953.

218. El-Hashimi, W.: Charcot-Leyden crystals. Formation from primate and lack of formation from non-primate eosinophils. Am. J. Pathol., *65*:311–325, 1971.

219. Welsh, R.A.: The genesis of the Charcot-Leyden crystal in the eosinophilic leukocyte of man. Am. J. Pathol., *35*:1091–1103, 1959.

220. Reginato, A.J.: Unpublished observation.

221. Samter, M.: Charcot-Leyden crystals: A study of the conditions necessary for their formation. Allergy, *18*:221–230, 1947.

222. Benhamou, C.L., et al.: Arthropathies des membres chez les insuffisants renaux dialyses. Presse Med., *16*:119–122, 1987.

223. Cary, N.R.B., et al.: Dialysis arthropathy: amyloid or iron? Br. Med. J., *293*:1392–1394, 1986.

224. Netter, P., et al.: Inflammatory effect of aluminum phosphate. Ann. Rheum. Dis., *42*:114, 1983.

225. Royer, D., et al.: Inflammatory effect of aluminum phosphate on rat paws. Pathol. Biol., *30*:211–215, 1982.

226. Kelly, J.J.: Blackthorn inflammation. J. Bone Joint. Surg., *48B*:474–478, 1966.

227. Solomon, S.D.: Splinter-induced synovitis. Arthritis Rheum., *21*:279, 1978.

228. Viegas, S.F.: Atypical causes of hand pain. Am. Fam. Physician, *35*:167–172, 1977.

229. Goodnough, C.P., and Frymore, J.W.: Synovitis secondary to non-metallic foreign bodies. J. Trauma, *15*:960–969, 1975.

230. Dieppe, P.: Miscellaneous crystals and particles. *In* Crystals and Joint Disease. Edited by P. Calvert. London, Chapman and Hall, 1983.

231. Cleland, I.G., Vernon-Roberts, B., and Smith, K.: Fibre-glass induced synovitis. Ann. Rheum. Dis., *43*:530–534, 1984.

232. Kitridou, R.C., Schumacher, H.R., Sbarbaro, J.L., and Hollander, J.L.: Recurrent hemarthrosis after prosthetic knee arthroplasty: Identification of metal particles in the synovial fluid. Arthritis Rheum., *12*:520–523, 1969.

233. Rosenthal, D.F., Rosenberg, A.E., Schiller, A.L., and Smith, R.J.: Destructive arthritis due to silicone: A foreign body reaction. Radiology, *149*:69–72, 1983.

234. Kaufman, R.L., Tong, I., and Beardmore, T.D.: Prosthetic synovitis: Clinical and histologic characteristics. J. Rheumatol., *12*:1066–1074, 1985.

235. Windler, E.C., Smith, R.B., Bryan, W.J., and Woods, G.W.: Lead intoxication and traumatic arthritis of hip secondary to retained bullet fragments. A case report. J. Bone Joint Surg., *60A*:254–255, 1978.

236. Conolly, W.B.: Color atlas of hand conditions. High pressure injection injury. 1st Ed. Chicago, Year Book Medical Publishers, 1980.

237. Christie, A.J., Weinberger, K.A., and Dietrich, M.: Silicone lymphadenopathy and synovitis. Complications of silicone elastomer finger joint prosthesis. JAMA, *237*:1463–1464, 1977.

238. Kumagai, Y., Shiokawa, Y., Medsger, T.A., and Rodnan, G.P.: Clinical spectrum of connective tissue disease after cosmetic surgery. Observation on eighteen patients and a review of the Japanese literature. Arthritis Rheum., *27*:1–12, 1984.

239. O'Connor, C.R., Reginato, A.J., and DeLong, W.: Foreign body reaction simulating acute septic arthritis. (Submitted to J. Rheumatol. for publication.)

240. Kiburz, D.: Intra-articular drug abuse. J. Bone Joint Surg., *66A*:1469–1470, 1984.

241. Maylahn, D.J.: Thorn-induced "tumors" of bone. J. Bone Joint Surg., *34A*:386–389, 1952.

242. Little, C.L., et al.: The ultrasonic detection of soft tissue foreign bodies. Invest. Radiol., *21*:275–277, 1986.

243. Bauer, A.R., and Yutani, D.: Computed tomography localization of wooden foreign bodies in children's extremities. Arch. Surg., *118*:1084–1086, 1983.

244. Sugarman, M., et al.: Plant thorn synovitis. Arthritis Rheum., *20*:1125–1128, 1977.

245. Kinmont, P.D.C.: Sea urchin sarcoidal granulomas. Br. J. Dermatol., *77*:336–343, 1965.

246. Reginato, A.J., Ferreiro, S.J.L., Clayburne, G., and Sieck, M.: Experimentally induced foreign body synovitis. Light and transmission electron microscopic studies. Panamerican Congress of Rheumatology. Buenos Aires, Argentina, November 1986.

METABOLIC DISEASES OF MUSCLE

110

ROBERT L. WORTMANN

A wide variety of conditions can be classified as metabolic diseases of muscle. These have in common an underlying abnormality in muscle glycogen, lipid, or adenosine triphosphate (ATP) metabolism. The study of metabolic muscle disease is relatively new. Myophosphorylase deficiency, the first described metabolic myopathy, was predicted in 1951[1] and the biochemical defect identified in 1959.[2,3] Subsequently, additional defects of glycogen metabolism and disorders of lipid and purine metabolism in muscle have been recognized. Other metabolic diseases of muscle assuredly await discovery. Clinically, these conditions must be considered in the differential diagnosis of individuals with proximal muscle weakness, myoglobinuria, or exercise intolerance as a result of fatigue, myalgias, or cramps. The evaluation of such patients requires an awareness of potential diagnoses, an understanding of energetics in normal muscle, and an acceptance that much remains to be learned about this general area before successful therapies will be available.

SKELETAL MUSCLE FIBERS

Skeletal muscle contains multinucleated cells called *fibers* (Fig. 110–1), functionally grouped in *motor units*. A motor unit is composed of all the fibers innervated by an individual *motor neuron*. The fibers within each motor unit have common histochemical and electrophysiologic properties and can be classified based on those characteristics (Table 110–1). Type 1 (red) fibers respond to stimulation slowly but are relatively resistant to fatigue. They are rich in lipids, mitochondria, and oxidative enzymes. In contrast, type 2B (white) fibers respond to stimulation briskly, with greater force, but fatigue rapidly. Their glycogen content and myophosphorylase activity are greater. The properties of type 2A fibers share some properties with each of the other types and respond to stimulation in an intermediate fashion. Individual human muscles are composed of mixtures of all fiber types.

CONTRACTION AND RELAXATION

Muscular activity can be initiated by electric, chemical, and mechanical stimulation to produce an *action potential* transmitted along the cell membrane. An action potential moves down the motor neuron to the *presynaptic nerve terminal*, where depolarization causes the release of acetylcholine, which diffuses to the postsynaptic membrane on a muscle cell and binds to specific receptors. Such binding causes conformational changes, opening channels permeable to sodium and potassium. As a consequence, sodium moves into the cell and potassium moves out, depolarizing the muscle fiber and generating a signal called an *end plate potential*. As the wave of depolarization spreads, the resting state of the membrane is restored and maintained, in part by an active sodium-potassium exchanger (Na-K-dependent ATPase). The wave of depolarization spreads from the membrane to the interior of the muscle fiber through the system

FIG. 110–1. Structure of a skeletal muscle fiber. Each muscle fiber is a multinucleated cell composed of fibrils that contain filaments of contractile proteins surrounded by a plasma membrane, the sarcolemma. Communication between the plasma membrane and fibrils is provided by the T system of tubules that runs along the border of the sarcomeres and connects to the sarcoplasmic reticulum that invests the fibrils. The varying refractile indices of the filaments give skeletal muscle its characteristic cross striated appearance by electron microscopy. The functional contractile unit of the muscle cell is the sarcomere and is defined as the area between two Z lines. The A band is composed of the thick filaments (myosin) and the M line is due to bulges in the centers of the thick filaments. At rest, the I band is the area occupied by thin filaments (troponin, tropomyosin, and actin) not overlapped by myosin. With contraction, cross bridges are formed between thick and thin filaments, Z lines move toward the M line, and the I bands become smaller.

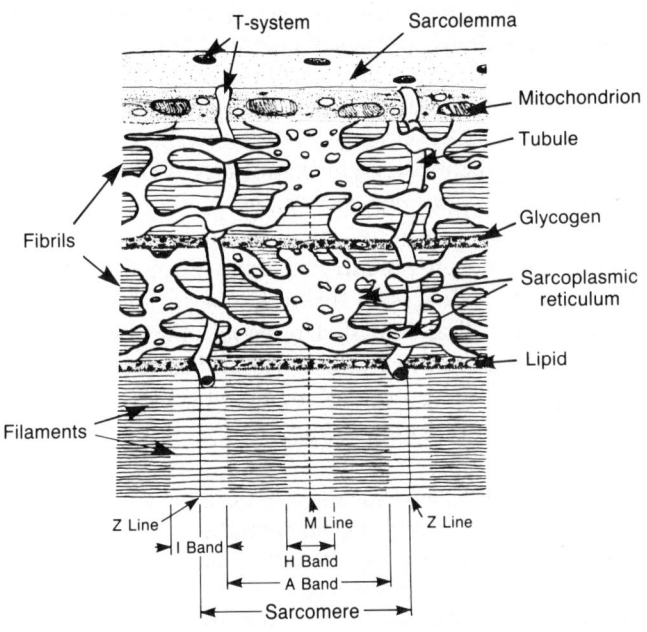

of T tubules, connecting the cell surface with the sarcoplasmic reticulum (Fig. 110–1). When the signal reaches the sarcoplasmic reticulum, calcium is released from the lateral sacs to diffuse among the fibrils, initiating *contraction*.

Contraction in muscle occurs as a consequence of a magnesium-dependent actomyosin ATPase. The activity of that enzyme results in the formation of *cross bridges between actin and myosin* and the *sliding of filaments*. At rest, actomyosin ATPase is inhibited and there are no cross bridges between the thick filaments (myosin) and thin filaments (troponin, tropomyosin, and actin). Troponin, along with tropomyosin, a protein that connects troponin to actin, inhibits the interaction of actin and myosin. As calcium concentra-

tions around myofibrils increase, calcium binds to troponin causing conformational changes that release the inhibition of the enzyme. With the hydrolysis of ATP, actin-containing filaments bridge with and slide along myosin, shortening the fiber.

Muscle fiber relaxation is also the result of an active process. Shortly after calcium is released, it is pumped back into the sarcoplasmic reticulum by a calcium-dependent ATPase. Once the concentration of calcium around the fibrils is lowered, calcium is displaced from troponin and the interaction between actin and myosin stops, cross-links are broken, and fiber lengthening occurs.

ENERGY METABOLISM IN SKELETAL MUSCLE

Energy necessary for muscle contraction is provided by the *hydrolysis of ATP*. Intracellular concentrations of ATP are maintained by the action of enzymes such as creatine phosphokinase (CPK), adenylate cyclase, and myoadenylate deaminase. The energy needed to replenish ATP when it is consumed during muscle contraction is provided by the *intermediary metabolism of carbohydrate and lipid* by the pathways of glycolysis, the Krebs (tricarboxylic acid) cycle, β-oxidation, and oxidative phosphorylation.

The immediate source of energy for skeletal muscle during work is found in preformed organic compounds containing high-energy phosphate such as ATP and creatine phosphate. At rest, the terminal phosphate of ATP is transferred to creatine, forming creatine phosphate and adenosine diphosphate (ADP) in a reaction catalyzed by CPK. Creatine phosphate thus acts as a reservoir of high-energy phosphate immediately available to reform ATP, and CPK acts to buffer cytoplasmic changes in ATP concentration.[4] CPK and its products, creatine and creatine phosphate, also play a significant role in the transport of energy from mitochondria to myofibrils. This latter action is referred to as the *creatine-creatine phosphate shuttle* (Fig. 110–2).[5,6]

During rest and less strenuous exercise, the activity of CPK renders the concentration of ATP within cells constant at the expense of creatine phosphate. When metabolic requirements such as those that occur during prolonged contraction and muscle fatigue exceed the capacity of oxidative phosphorylation to regenerate ATP, creatine phosphate is used to replenish ATP. When approximately 50% of the creatine phosphate has been converted to creatine, ATP levels begin to fall and inosine monophosphate (IMP) accumulates. ATP is hydrolyzed to ADP and then to AMP

Table 110–1. Properties of Muscle Fiber Types

Fiber Type Designation	1	2A	2B
	Red	Red	White
	SO	FOG	FG
	S	FR	FF
Motor unit properties			
Twitch speed	Slow	Intermediate	Fast
Tetanic force	Small	Large	Largest
Fatigue resistance	Highest	High	Low
Histochemical properties			
ATPase (pH 4.4)	High	Low	Low
ATPase (pH 10.6)	Low	High	High
Glycogen	Low	High	High
Lipid	High	Variable	Low
Myophosphorylase	Low	High	High
NADH dehydrogenase	High	Intermediate	Low

by adenylate kinase, and the AMP is converted to IMP by myoadenylate deaminase. During recovery from exercise, IMP is converted back to AMP by a two-step process. The conversion of AMP to IMP and back to AMP has been called the *purine nucleotide cycle* (Fig. 110–3).[9,10] The reactions of the purine nucleotide cycle (1) reduce AMP levels, which are inhibitory to ATP generating reactions; (2) generate ammonia, which stimulates glycolysis; and (3) release fumarate, an intermediate of the Krebs cycle and promoter of oxidative phosphorylation.[11–14]

The majority of cellular energy is produced in mitochondria by degradation of metabolites through the pathways of the Krebs cycle and respiratory (cytochrome) chain. Products of the aerobic degradation of carbohydrate (pyruvate) and fatty acids enter the Krebs cycle, generating reducing equivalents. The respiratory chain, a series of enzymes and coenzymes that function as hydrogen carriers, transfers reducing equivalents to molecular oxygen (Fig. 110–4 and Table 110–2). The large amount of free energy released is captured and conserved in the form of ATP by a process called *oxidative phosphorylation.*

Carbohydrates provide a major source of energy for cells. Glucose enters muscle fibers from the bloodstream and is degraded through a series of reactions to pyruvate (Fig. 110–5). Under aerobic conditions, pyruvate enters the Krebs cycle and is metabolized by that cycle and by oxidative phosphorylation to carbon dioxide and water. In the process, large amounts

FIG. 110–2. Scheme of the creatine-creatine phosphate shuttle. CPK is located on the inner mitochondrial membrane, on myofibrils, and in the cytoplasm. It provides a buffer mechanism for maintaining homeostatic concentrations of intracellular adenine nucleotides and plays an important role in energy transfer within the cell after ATP is produced in mitochondria. CPK also buffers ADP and inorganic phosphate levels. The cytosolic ADP concentration is an important metabolic regulator of mitochondrial respiration, and inorganic phosphate is a regulator of glycolysis.[7,8] Cr = creatinine; CrP = creatine phosphate; CPK = creatine phosphokinase; t = adenine nucleotide translocase.

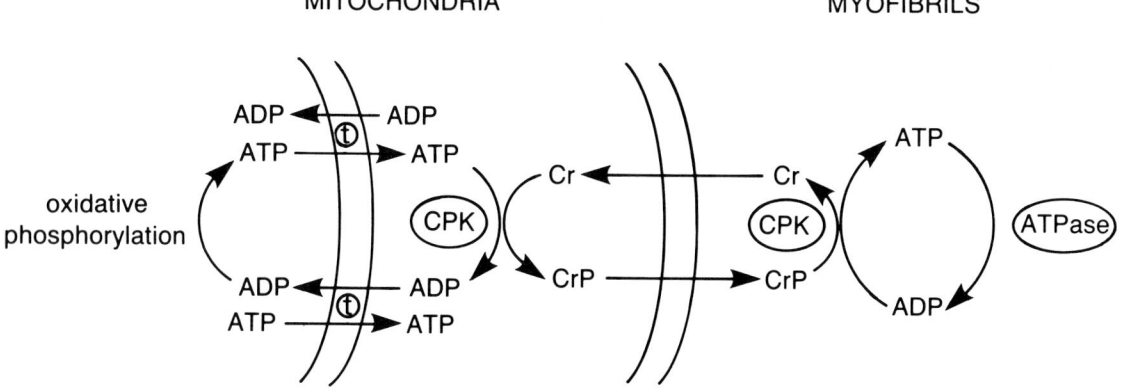

FIG. 110–3. The purine nucleotide cycle. When muscle contraction is sufficient to exceed the buffering capacity of creatine phosphate and deplete ATP, ADP and AMP are formed by the activity of adenylate kinase. Under these conditions, glycolysis becomes the major route for regeneration of ATP, and the enzymes of the purine nucleotide cycle play a critical regulatory role. The conversion of AMP to IMP by myoadenylate deaminase causes ammonia release and changes in nucleotide concentrations that stimulate glycolysis.[11–13] IMP accumulates until muscle activity decreases and recovery occurs. Oxidative conditions are restored and AMP is regenerated by a two-step process with the liberation of fumarate, an intermediate in the Krebs cycle. The higher concentrations of fumarate drive the Krebs cycle, causing efficient resynthesis of ATP by oxidative phosphorylation.[14,15b] 1 = myoadenylate deaminase; 2 = adenylsuccinate synthetase; 3 = adenylsuccinate lyase; 4 = adenylate kinase; SAMP = adenylsuccinate; NH_3 = ammonia; IMP = inosine monophosphate.

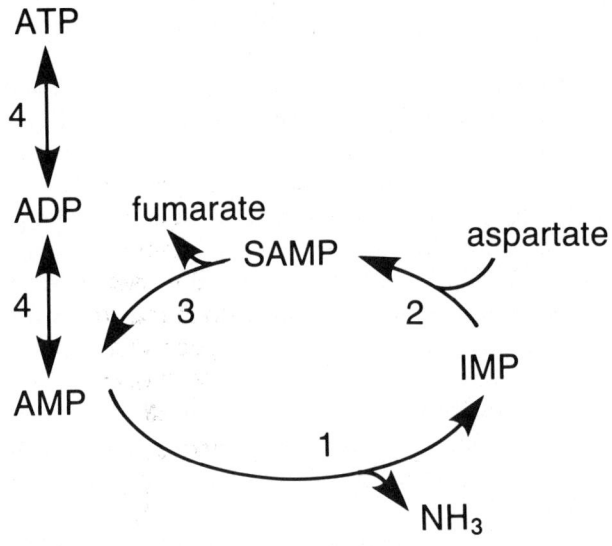

FIG. 110–4. Scheme of respiratory chain-linked oxidative phosphorylation. The respiratory chain takes reducing units from NADH and succinate derived from the Krebs cycle and passes them through a sequence of enzymes and coenzymes to molecular oxygen. In the process, the energy released is transferred to ATP by the action of ATP synthetase. I, II, III, and IV = respiratory chain complexes with enzymatic activity; cytochrome Q is also called ubiquinone.

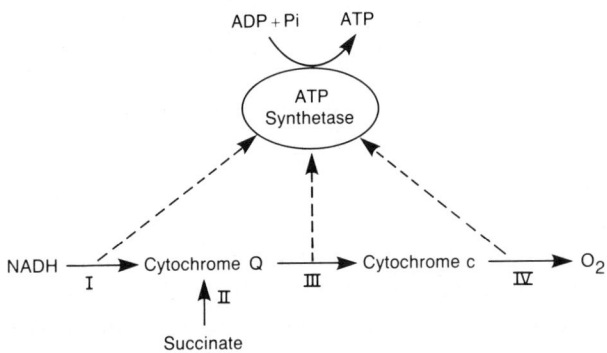

glucose unit from glycogen) compared to aerobic metabolism.

Lipids in the form of fatty acids (FAs) constitute the major substrates for energy production for muscles at rest, during contraction, and during recovery. Long-chain fatty acids move through the bloodstream from adipose tissues bound to albumin. These, plus smaller fatty acids, move across endothelial cells and into muscle cells, where they are available for energy production storage, or synthesis into membrane components. Each of these processes requires activation of the fatty acids to acyl-CoA derivatives. The resulting activated fatty acids can undergo oxidation following carnitine-mediated transport into mitochondria catalyzed by carnitine palmitoyltransferase (CPT) activities (Fig. 110–6) or esterification leading to the formation of cytosolic triglyceride droplets that provide a depot of lipid for future use. Once in the mitochondria, fatty acyl-CoA units are converted to acetyl-CoA by the process of β-oxidation, and acetyl-CoA is processed through the Krebs cycle. Although intracellular concentrations of free fatty acids play a role in determining the overall rate of fatty acid oxidation, the predominant regulating factor is the rate of ADP formation in working muscle.

of energy are liberated to form ATP. The metabolism of one molecule of glucose by aerobic glycolysis yields a net gain of 38 molecules of ATP.

However, during exercise of short duration and high intensity, the major source of energy is glycogen, not glucose.[15a] Glycogen, a branched homopolymer of glucose, is the major storage form of carbohydrate in the body and is distributed evenly between slow- and fast-twitch muscle fibers at rest.[16] Although glycogen products can enter the aerobic pathways described above, they can also be metabolized anaerobically. In *anaerobic glycolysis*, pyruvate does not enter the Krebs cycle, but is converted to lactate instead. This process produces smaller quantities of ATP (2 ATP per molecule of glucose or 3 ATP per

DISORDERS OF GLYCOGEN METABOLISM

The discovery in 1959 of myophosphorylase deficiency in muscle was the first report of a biochemical abnormality in an inherited myopathy.[2,3] This obser-

Table 110–2. Composition of Respiratory Chain Complexes

Complex (activity)		Major Components
I	(NADH dehydrogenase)	Flavin mononucleotide (FMN) Iron-sulfur
II	(Succinate dehydrogenase)	Flavin adenine dinucleotide (FAD) Cytochrome b Iron-sulfur
III	(Cytochrome Q dehydrogenase)	Cytochrome b Cytochrome c_1 Iron-sulfur Q-binding protein Antimycin A-binding protein
IV	(Cytochrome oxidase)	Cytochrome a Cytochrome a_3 Heme a Copper

vation occurred 8 years after McArdle had deduced that "a gross failure of the breakdown in muscle of glycogen to lactic acid" was responsible for lifelong exercise intolerance in a 30-year-old man.[1] Subsequently, additional inborn errors of glycogen metabolism associated with muscle symptoms have been reported (Table 110–3), and undoubtedly more remain to be described. Individuals with a glycogen storage disease are well at rest and perform mild exercise without difficulty, because free fatty acids are the major source of energy under those conditions. The enzymatic block that interferes with the use of carbohydrate to generate ATP causes problems only when exercise reaches a level that produces anaerobic conditions. The inability to replenish depleted high-energy phosphate stores then results in pain, contracture, and muscle necrosis.

DEFECTS OF GLYCOGENOLYSIS

Myophosphorylase Deficiency (McArdle's Disease)

The cardinal clinical manifestation of myophosphorylase deficiency is *exercise intolerance* associated with pain, fatigue, stiffness, or weakness. The degree of exercise intolerance varies among affected individuals. Symptoms can follow activities of high intensity and short duration or those that require less intense effort for longer intervals, but always resolve with rest. In fact, at rest affected individuals function well, provided they adjust their activities to a level below their individual threshold for symptoms. When they exceed their exercise tolerance, they become symptomatic. In addition to stiffness and weakness, painful muscle cramps are sometimes associated with muscle necrosis, myoglobinuria, and potentially reversible renal failure.[17] Some individuals experience a "second wind" phenomenon; if they stop their activities at the onset of myalgia or stiffness and rest briefly, they can

then resume exercising with increased tolerance.[18] This ability to tolerate gradually increasing workloads is probably due to the combination of increased blood flow in exercising muscles and mobilization of fatty acids.[19,20]

Although the onset of symptoms is usually noted in childhood, symptoms are often overlooked and recognized only in retrospect. For unknown reasons, severe cramps and myoglobinuria are rare before adolescence. The late development of significant symptoms accounts for the rarity of the diagnosis before age 10. Another possible reason is the clinical heterogeneity of the disease. Some individuals only complain of being tired and having poor stamina, but others develop progressive muscle weakness that tends to be proximal and may initially be misdiagnosed as polymyositis.[21] Rarely, symptoms develop so insidiously that the diagnosis is not made until after age 75.[22]

Elevated levels of serum CPK are a common finding in myophosphorylase deficiency, helping to distinguish it from the other significant metabolic myopathy that causes myoglobinuria, namely CPT deficiency. Electromyographic (EMG) studies are usually normal unless myoglobinuria is present, although nonspecific abnormalities including increased insertional activity and an increased number of polyphasic potentials, as well as evidence of muscular irritability with fibrillations and positive waves (changes that can also be seen in inflammatory muscle disease), have been reported. The cramps that follow voluntary activity or ischemic exercise are electrically silent.[1]

A useful, but nonspecific, tool used to study individuals suspected of being myophosphorylase deficient is the forearm ischemic exercise test (Table 110–4). This test exploits the abnormal biochemistry that results in the absence of myophosphorylase ac-

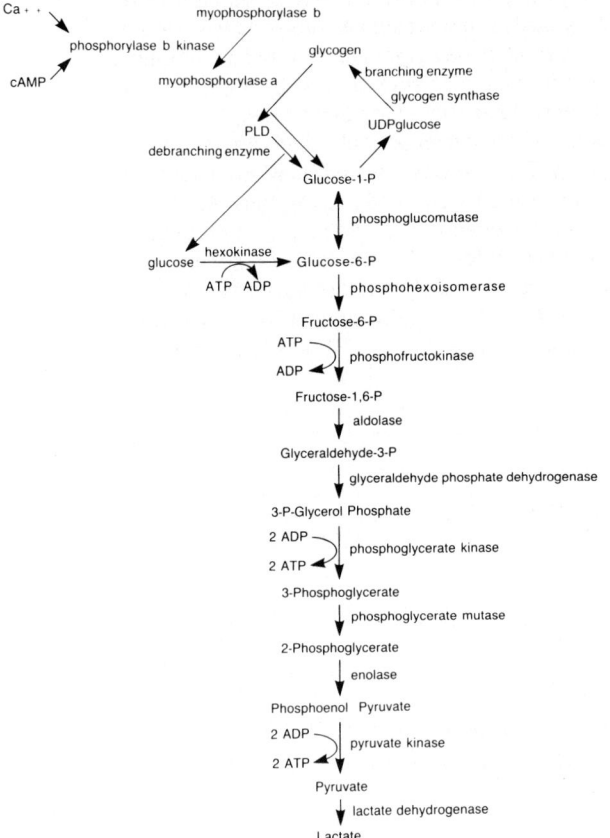

FIG. 110–5. Pathways for glycogen metabolism and glycolysis. Aided by insulin, glucose moves across the sarcoplasmal membrane into the cell, where it is immediately phosphorylated by the activity of hexokinase. The resulting glucose-6-phosphate is then converted to glucose-1-phosphate by phosphoglucomutase and then to UDPglucose by UDPglucose pyrophosphorylase. Glycogen synthesis then proceeds by a combination of reactions catalyzed by glycogen synthase, transferring glucose molecules from UDPglucose to a pre-existing polymeric chain of other glucose molecules, which are linked by α-1,4-glucosidic bonds in a linear fashion, and branching enzyme, which results in the formation of new outer side chains by forming α-1,6-glucosyl bonds.

Glycogen remains in the cell in reserve until metabolic demands lead to the activation of myophosphorylase (glycogen phosphorylase), degrading glycogen to glucose-1-phosphate, which can enter the glycolytic pathway, and degrading phosphorylase limit dextran (PLD). Myophosphorylase exists in active (phosphorylase a) and inactive (phosphorylase b) forms. Conversion of the inactive to the active form is regulated by the enzyme phosphorylase b kinase, which is stimulated either by calcium release from the sarcoplasmic reticulum after electric stimulation or by activity of cAMP-dependent protein kinase, which in turn is activated by β-adrenergic agonists such as epinephrine or glucagon.

Active phosphorylase can degrade only about 35% of a glycogen molecule to glucose-1-phosphate. In the process, it leaves PLDs, containing terminal α-1,6-glucosidically bound glucose units each covered by three α-1,4-glucosidically bound units. Further degradation of PLD requires the action of debranching enzyme (amylo-1,6-glucosidase), which rearranges the exposed 1,4-linked units to sites where they are accessible to myophosphorylase action and hydrolyzes the 1,6-linked units as well.

The glucose-1-phosphate formed is then available for entry into the glycolytic pathway. Under anaerobic conditions it is converted in ten steps to lactate. For each glucose unit entering the pathway, one ATP molecule is hydrolyzed but four ATP molecules are generated and two lactate molecules result. Under aerobic conditions, the end product of glycolysis is pyruvate. Pyruvate molecules can enter the Krebs cycle and proceed through oxidative phosphorylation. Rate limiting steps in glycolysis are those catalyzed by phosphofructokinase, glyceraldehyde phosphate dehydrogenase and phosphoglycerate kinase.

FIG. 110–6. Scheme of fatty acid metabolism in mitochondria. Short- and medium-chain fatty acids cross the mitochondrial membrane by diffusion but the process for long-chain fatty acids is more complex requiring four steps. First, the long-chain fatty acids must be activated, a reaction catalyzed by ACS in the outer mitochondrial membrane. The acyl-CoA products formed are substrate for the second step, the formation of acylcarnitine by the action of CPT I. L-carnitine is ubiquitous and has the primary function of transfering long-chain fatty acids across the inner mitochondrial membrane. Next, acylcarnitine is transported across the inner mitochondrial membrane by ACT. Finally, the long-chain acylcarnitine is converted to the corresponding acyl-CoA structure by CPT II, which is located on the matrix side of the inner mitochondrial membrane. Once in the mitochondrial matrix, the fatty acids are converted to acetyl-CoA by a repetitive process called β-oxidation. The β-oxidation process nets 5 molecules of ATP for each acetyl-CoA molecule generated, and each acetyl-CoA molecule formed is available for combustion through the Krebs cycle. Accordingly, the degradation of 1 molecule of palmityl-CoA requires seven β-oxidation cycles, yields 8 acetyl-CoA molecules, and produces 131 molecules of ATP. FA = fatty acid; ACS = acyl-CoA synthetase; CPT I = carnitine palmitoyltransferase 1; ACT = acylcarnitine translocase; CPT II = carnitine palmitolytransferase 2.

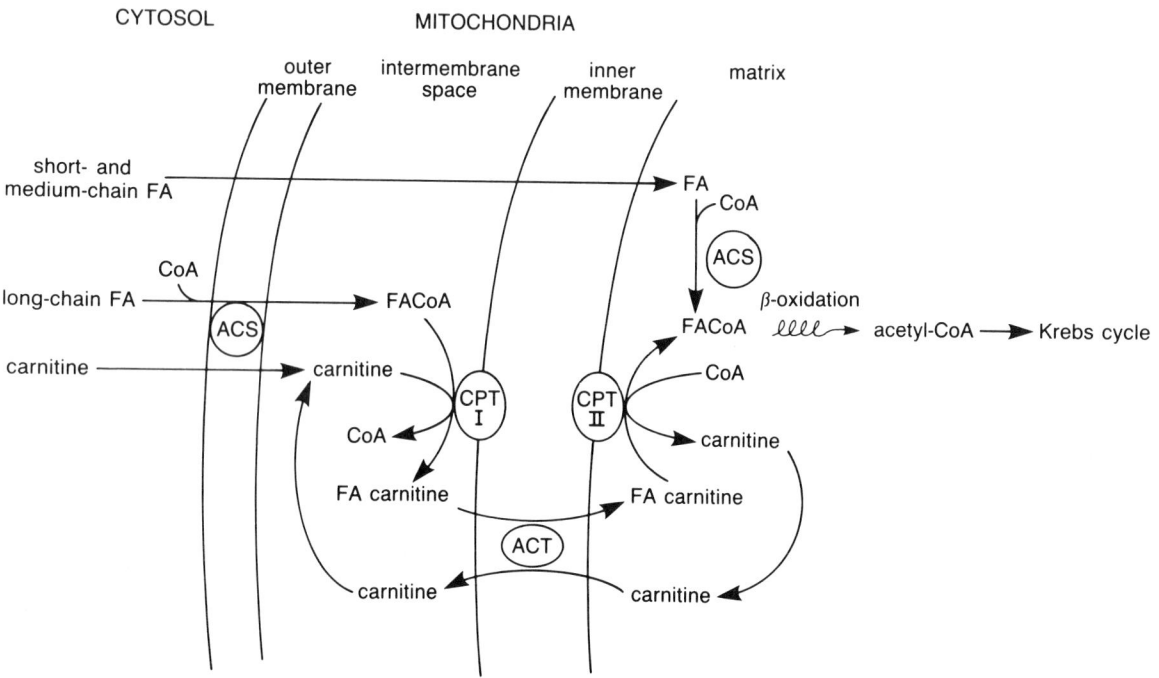

Table 110–3. Inborn Errors of Glycogen Metabolism That Affect Muscle

Enzyme Deficiency	Eponym	Symptoms
Acid maltase	Pompe's disease	Proximal weakness
Brancher enzyme	Andersen's disease	Hypotonia, weakness
Debrancher enzyme	Cori-Forbes' disease	Proximal weakness
Phosphorylase b kinase	—	Exercise intolerance, cramps, myoglobinuria
Myophosphorylase	McArdle's disease	Exercise intolerance, cramps, myoglobinuria
Phosphofructokinase	Tarui's disease	Exercise intolerance, cramps, myoglobinuria
Phosphoglycerate kinase	—	Exercise intolerance, myoglobinuria
Phosphoglycerate mutase	—	Exercise intolerance, myoglobinuria
Lactate dehydrogenase	—	Exercise intolerance, cramps, myoglobinuria

Table 110–4. Protocol for Forearm Ischemic Exercise Testing

1. A blood sample for analysis of baseline lactate and ammonia concentrations is drawn through an indwelling needle in an antecubital vein preferably without use of a tourniquet.

2. A sphygmomanometer cuff is placed on the upper arm and inflated to, and maintained at, a level at least 20 mm Hg above systolic pressure while the subject squeezes a tennis ball, or like object, vigorously at a rate of one squeeze every 2 seconds for 90 seconds.

3. After 90 seconds, the cuff is deflated and additional venous samples are obtained 1, 3, 5, and 10 minutes thereafter.

In normal individuals, lactate and ammonia concentrations increase at least threefold from baseline values. The major reason for a false positive result is insufficient work by the subject while exercising.[24] More work is required to increase ammonia levels than lactate levels.[25] When an abnormal result is obtained, the putative diagnosis should always be confirmed by muscle biopsy.

tivity. Normal muscle generates lactate from the degradation of glycogen when it exercises intensely under ischemic or anaerobic conditions (Fig. 110–5). This pathway is blocked when myophosphorylase activity is absent, and consequently no lactate is released into the circulation under anaerobic conditions. In addition, ammonia, inosine, and hypoxanthine concentrations increase significantly compared to normals, providing evidence of excessive purine nucleotide breakdown.[23] Similarly, other defects in the glycogenolytic and glycolytic pathways can interfere with lactate production during ischemic exercise and provide similar results.

In normal individuals, venous lactate levels increase three to sixfold shortly after ischemic exercise; in myophosphorylase-deficient individuals, levels do not change (Table 110–5).[1] The test can be painful if performed correctly. Some normal individuals cannot exercise more than a minute under ischemic conditions and find they are unable to fully flex or extend their fingers. The pain completely clears and full function is regained immediately after restoring the circulation. Painful persistent cramping, contracture, and even myoglobinuria can occur in an individual

with McArdle's disease. The major limitation of the test is that some individuals cannot or will not exercise with enough intensity to raise lactate concentrations above baseline, and thus given false positive results.[24,25] Thus, if lactate concentrations do rise after ischemic exercise, myophosphorylase deficiency is excluded but if lactate levels do not rise after ischemic exercise, the diagnosis is still a possibility.

The definitive diagnosis is made by analysis of muscle tissue. Classic changes observed with light microscopy include thick deposits of glycogen at the periphery and thinner, linear deposits within cells (Fig. 110–7). The amount of variation is wide and in milder cases deposits may not be obvious, even with periodic acid-Schiff (PAS) staining. The deposition is readily appreciated using the electron microscope (Fig. 110–8). Specific histochemical staining for myophosphorylase activity secures the diagnosis.[26,27] False positives can only be seen in patients with low residual activity[28,29] or when there are regenerating fibers after rhabdomyolysis. Regenerating fibers and immature muscle cells express a different isoenzyme.

Other Defects in Glycogen Metabolism

Deficiencies of *brancher and debrancher enzymes* have been reported but are rare. *Brancher enzyme* deficiency causes fatal hepatic failure in childhood, which can be associated with hypotonia and contracture[30,31] or exercise intolerance and cardiopathy.[32] It is characterized histologically by deposition of an abnormal PAS-positive polysaccharide.[33] Deficiency of *debrancher enzyme* results in phosphorylase limit dextran (PLD) accumulation and deposition in muscle, liver, and blood cells. This deficiency can cause hepatomegaly, fasting hypoglycemia, and failure to thrive in childhood, however, the first recognized manifestation of the disease may be slowly progressive muscle weakness sometimes associated with distal muscle wasting, beginning after age 20.[34,35] These individuals have elevated CPK levels and fail to generate lactate after forearm ischemic exercise. More recently, deficiency of muscle phosphorylase b kinase has been described.[36]

Table 110–5. Results of Forearm Ischemic Exercise Testing

Sample	Normal		Myophosphorylase Deficiency		Myoadenylate Deaminase Deficiency	
	Lactate*	NH₃*	Lactate	NH₃	Lactate	NH₃
Baseline	0.8	15	0.9	20	1.2	26
1 minute	5.9	106	0.8	94	3.8	26
3 minute	3.8	91	0.9	82	2.4	29
5 minute	2.0	45	0.9	40	1.6	230
10 minute	1.2	30	0.9	25	1.4	27

*Lactate in mEq/L; NH₃ (ammonia) in μmole/L.

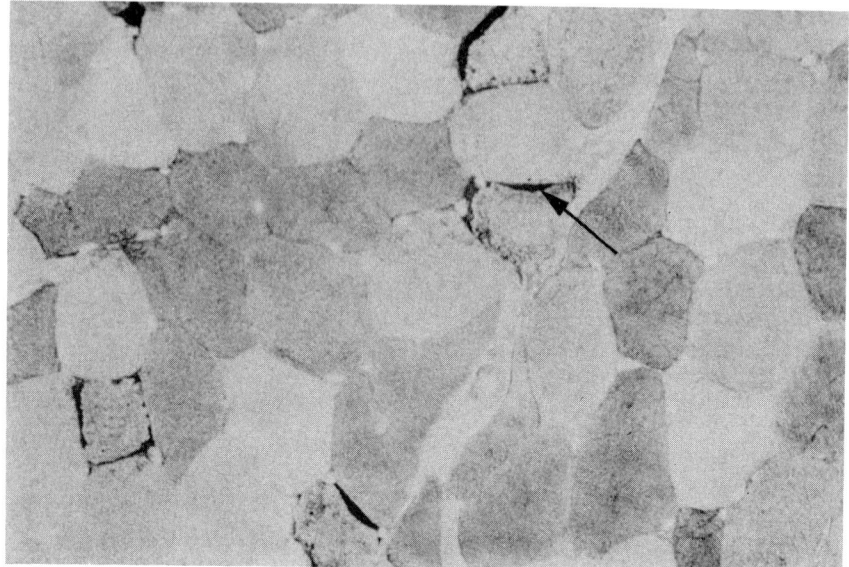

FIG. 110–7. Muscle biopsy specimen from a patient with myophosphorylase deficiency. The PAS-positive material (arrow) seen at the periphery of the cells and as lines within the cells, is excess glycogen.

This can cause a myopathy in childhood[37] or mimic McArdle's disease in adulthood.[38]

DEFECTS IN GLYCOLYSIS

Phosphofructokinase Deficiency (Tauri's Disease)

The clinical manifestations of *phosphofructokinase* (PFK) *deficiency* can be identical to McArdle's disease.[39–41a] Almost all patients are diagnosed as adults but in retrospect report having had problems with either exercise intolerance or cramps in their youth. PFK-deficient individuals differ from myophosphorylase deficient individuals in that the "second wind" phenomenon may be less common and exercise intolerance is likely to be associated with nausea and vomiting. About one third develop myoglobinuria

and most have elevated serum CPK levels at rest. EMG is either normal or provides nonspecific results, suggesting myopathy or inflammation. Predictably, these patients' venous lactate levels fail to increase after forearm ischemic exercise, and the test can initiate a prolonged contracture. Histochemical analysis of muscle tissue is needed to confirm the diagnosis.[42] In addition to increased glycogen deposition and decreased PFK activity, deficient muscle also contains an abnormal polysaccharide similar to that seen in brancher enzyme deficiency.[42a]

PFK deficiency can also cause hemolytic anemia.[40] This may be seen with or without myopathy, depending on the genetic defect. Isoenzymes of PFK vary in subunit composition. Generally, the muscle enzyme is composed of M subunits, and the eryth-

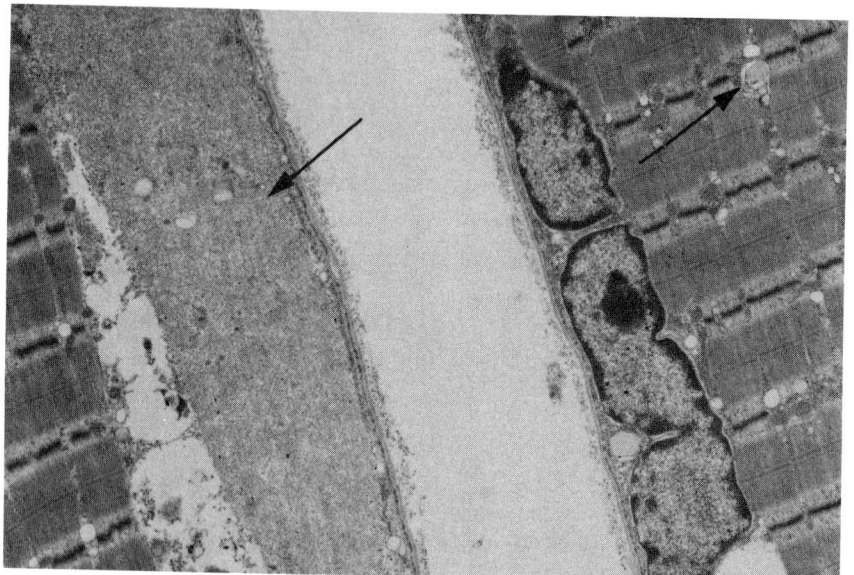

FIG. 110–8. Electron micrograph demonstrating increased glycogen deposition beneath the sarcolemma and between filaments (arrows). These changes could be seen in all glycogen storage diseases.

rocyte enzyme contains M and L subunits.[41a] Defects in the L subunit cause only hemolysis, but defects involving M subunits can affect both muscle and red cells. Much heterogeneity exists. The hemolysis associated with myopathic disease may be subclinical, causing only an increased reticulocyte count, or severe, causing jaundice and gallstones. Hyperuricemia and gout are common in these individuals, perhaps because of the high levels of purines released with hemolysis and during exercise.[23,43]

Other Defects in Glycolysis

Deficiencies of phosphoglycerate kinase,[43a] phosphoglycerate mutase,[44] and lactate dehydrogenase (LDH)[45] have been described in individuals whose problems began during adolescence or later and included exercise-induced myoglobinuria. These genetic defects all cause a failure of lactate release after ischemic exercise and require histochemical studies for diagnosis.

ACID MALTASE DEFICIENCY

Acid maltase is an enzyme, found in lysosomes, that catalyzes the release of glucose from maltose, oligosaccharides, and glycogen. Its precise role in cellular metabolism is not known. Deficiency of this enzyme is transmitted by autosomal recessive inheritance and produces three clinical syndromes that differ in age of presentation, organ involvement, and prognosis.[46] The *infantile* form causes symptoms of muscle weakness, hypotonia, and congestive heart failure that begin shortly after birth and progress to death within the first two years of life.[47,48] This form is characterized by massive glycogen deposits in cardiac, hepatic, neural, and muscular tissues. The second variety presents in *early childhood* with muscle weakness that is more proximal than distal and may affect respiratory muscles.[49,50] It tends not to involve the heart or liver and progresses slowly. Death, usually a result of respiratory failure, occurs before age 30.

The *adult* form causes few problems prior to age 20 and typically manifests as muscle weakness beginning in the third or fourth decade.[51] Although diaphragmatic involvement and respiratory failure dominate the clinical picture in about a third of cases,[52,53] most develop a slowly progressive myopathy that is easily confused with polymyositis or limb-girdle muscular dystrophy.[54] The weakness tends to occur in proximal muscles and the torso. Individual muscles or even parts of muscles can be affected, but craniobulbar muscles are spared. CPK is usually elevated but can be normal or only slightly increased. EMG is always abnormal, though variably. The characteristic changes include an unusually intense electrical irritability in response to movement of the needle electrode and myotonic discharges in the absence of clinical myotonia.[46] In some individuals, however, the changes are indistinguishable from those observed in some cases of polymyositis. Acid maltase–deficient subjects have no block in anaerobic glycolysis or nonlysosomal glycogenolysis because venous lactate concentrations increase normally after forearm ischemic exercise. This difference readily distinguishes them from individuals with other recognized forms of glycogen storage disease.

Acid maltase deficiency causes a vacuolar myopathy.[55,56] The vacuoles have a high glycogen content and stain for acid phosphatase. Small foci of acid phosphatase activity may also be found in muscle fibers that do not contain vacuoles. Glycogen is readily seen in involved muscle by electron microscopy, but the excess glycogen is not confined just to vacuolar structures. It is unclear why this nonlysosomal glycogen collects and why it is not degraded by cytosolic enzymes, nor is it clear what causes the muscular symptoms, because the pathways of glycogen and glucose metabolism for energy production are intact. The clinical heterogeneity is also not understood.

Biochemical studies are necessary to prove the diagnosis. Although characteristic EMG changes in the presence of typical vacuolar changes on biopsy from a patient with weakness involving respiratory muscles are strongly suggestive, they are not specific. Furthermore, these abnormalities tend to be less widespread and less striking in many adult cases. Assay of acid maltase in muscle, lymphocytes, cultured fibroblasts, or urine can be used to confirm the diagnosis.[57–59]

DISORDERS OF LIPID METABOLISM

Free fatty acids are the major source of energy while fasting, at rest, and exercising at low intensity and for long duration. Abnormalities involving the processing of long-chain fatty acids for energy lead to lipid storage myopathies, conditions in which the predominant pathologic alteration is the accumulation of abnormal amounts of lipid droplets between myofibrils (Fig. 110–6). Carnitine deficiency is the classic example of such a myopathy. CPT deficiency is the other major biochemical defect in the utilization of fatty acids for energy that causes human disease.

CARNITINE DEFICIENCY STATES

L-carnitine is essential for the transfer of long-chain fatty acids across the inner mitochondrial membrane and helps regulate CoA/acyl-CoA ratios in mitochondria.[60] Sources of carnitine include the diet, with red meat and dairy products containing large quantities, and de novo synthesis from lysine and methionine in liver, brain, and kidney. Carnitine is transported from the blood by an active saturable process into muscle, which contains 98% of the body stores. The major route of elimination from the body is in the urine.

In 1973, Engel and Angelini reported the first recognized case of muscle carnitine deficiency in an individual with lipid storage myopathy.[61] One year later, Karpati reported another form of carnitine deficiency, a systemic variety.[62] Carnitine deficiencies are now classified as either *primary* or *secondary*. Primary deficiencies have a genetic basis and can be further divided between *myopathic* and *systemic* forms. Secondary deficiencies are those that result from other disorders or that result from genetic defects in other pathways of intermediary metabolism.

Primary Carnitine Deficiencies

The syndrome of myopathic carnitine deficiency is characterized by progressive muscle weakness that, with some exceptions, begins in childhood.[63–65] The weakness is of the limb-girdle variety, but facial and pharyngeal muscle involvement is observed. Less common features are exertional myalgias, myoglobinuria, and cardiomyopathy. Half or more of patients have high CPK levels, and most have myopathic changes (polyphasic motor unit potentials of small amplitude and short duration) on EMG. Serum carnitine concentrations are usually normal, a finding consistent with the evidence indicating that a defect in carnitine transport into muscle cells underlies this form of the disease.[61–66] The only histologic abnormality in muscle is the nonspecific finding of increased lipid (Fig. 110–9). Similar changes can occur with ischemia and obesity. The diagnosis is made by biochemical analysis of muscle tissue.[67]

The first reported patient with systemic carnitine deficiency was an 11-year-old boy with progressive muscle weakness and a history of recurrent attacks that resembled Reye's syndrome.[62] The attacks began with vomiting and were followed by coma, hepatomegaly, liver function abnormalities, and hypoglycemia. Onset of this form is almost always in early childhood, with the attacks preceding the onset of muscle weakness in the majority of cases. The weakness is more proximal than distal and can affect cervical musculature, resulting in loss of head control.[68,69]

Cardiac muscle involvement, manifested by congestive heart failure, can occur.[70] Carnitine concentrations are reduced in skeletal muscle, heart, liver, and serum. A renal leak in carnitine is at least partially responsible for the deficiency in some patients, but the mechanism in other patients is unknown.[71]

Secondary Carnitine Deficiencies

Carnitine deficiency can be secondary to genetic defects in other reactions in intermediary metabolism or to other disorders. Attacks resembling Reye's syndrome occur in *acyl-CoA dehydrogenase deficiency* states,[72] and exercise intolerance occurs with defects in oxidative phosphorylation (see Mitochondrial Myopathies, below). The histologic features of lipid storage myopathy are present in these inborn errors of metabolism. Other disorders in which carnitine deficiency has been observed include renal failure requiring chronic hemodialysis (but not chronic peritoneal dialysis),[73–75] end-stage cirrhosis with cachexia,[76] valproic acid therapy for seizure disorders,[77] myxedema, adrenal insufficiency, hypopituitarism,[78,79] and pregnancy.[80]

Therapy

In theory, treatment of all types of carnitine deficiency should be effective with L-carnitine supplementation of the diet. In reality, however, the response to that therapy is variable. Attempts at treatment must include a diet rich in carbohydrates and medium-chain fatty acids and avoidance of fasting. During acute attacks, therapy should be designed to prevent hypoglycemia and to correct any electrolyte and acid-base imbalances that develop. Dietary supplementation with L-carnitine has sometimes been successful in improving each form of deficiency.[81–84] The dose for children is 100 mg/kg per day[85]; adults require 2 to 4 g in divided doses. Preparations containing the D-isomer of carnitine should not be used because it is not effective and can actually cause muscle weakness.[86,87] Some patients benefit from steroid therapy[88,89] or propranolol.[90]

CARNITINE PALMITOYLTRANSFERASE DEFICIENCY

DiMauro and Melis-DiMauro in 1973 first reported a deficiency of *carnitine palmitoyltransferase* in two brothers with recurrent myoglobinuria.[91] It is transmitted by autosomal recessive inheritance.[92] The clinical syndrome associated with CPT deficiency invariably includes attacks of exertional myalgias and muscular weakness associated with myoglobinuria.

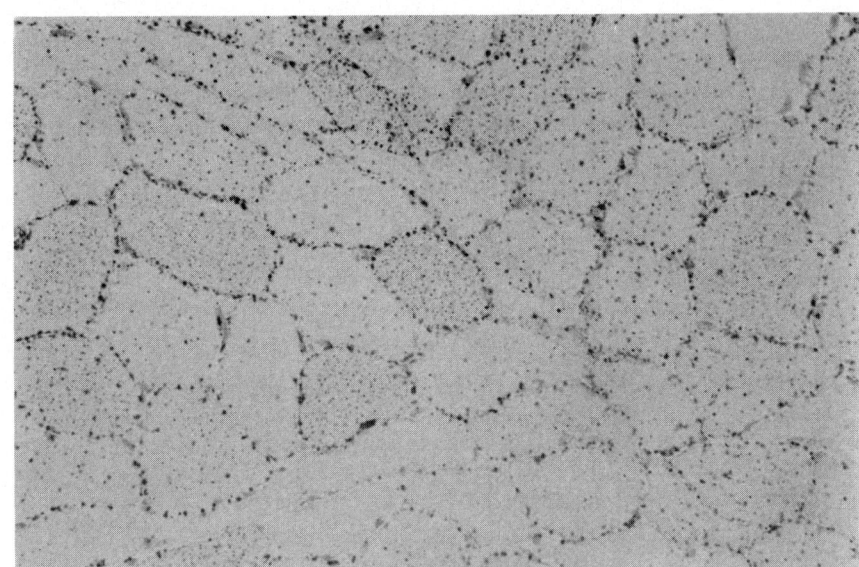

FIG. 110–9. Muscle tissue stained with oil red O. Lipid droplets of varying size are deposited between myofibrils. Large collections appear as vacuoles. The increased staining is typical of lipid storage myopathy, but by itself is a nonspecific finding.

CPT is necessary for transport of long-chain fatty acids into mitochondria for energy production. Because long-chain fatty acids provide the major source of cellular energy during prolonged exercise and in the fasting state, it is not surprising that attacks usually develop with prolonged exercise and fasting. Cold exposure and infection may also be important contributing and precipitating factors.[93] An episode of rhabdomyolysis culminating in respiratory failure followed initiation of ibuprofen therapy in one patient.[94] Mild attacks may be experienced in childhood, but severe attacks usually do not occur until the teenage years or later. About 25% of individuals develop renal failure with episodes of myoglobinuria,[95] but this is reversible. Respiratory failure may result during severe attacks.[94,96] Between attacks, CPT-deficient individuals feel and function well and have no abnormalities on physical examination.

The clinical picture of CPT differs in several ways from that of the glycogen storage diseases that also cause myoglobinuria. First, CPT-deficient patients do not experience severe cramping, and fixed proximal muscle weakness is rare. CPK is usually normal, except during episodes of rhabdomyolysis, or with prolonged fasting, and the increase in serum lactate concentration after forearm ischemic exercise is normal. Electrophysiologic studies and muscle tissue are entirely normal between attacks. Lipid accumulation is rarely observed in CPT-deficient muscle, and the diagnosis is made by measuring CPT activity in muscle.[97] Based on the known biochemistry, it could be predicted that CPT deficiency and carnitine deficiency would cause similar abnormalities, but this is not the case. Why the clinical and histologic features of these diseases differ is not understood.

Management consists of education. Avoidance of both prolonged strenuous exercise and fasting will prevent most attacks. Infection may not be preventable, but the need for adequate rest during an infection must be emphasized. Myoglobinuria constitutes a medical emergency. Interestingly, the development of renal failure does not correlate well with the amount of myoglobin in the urine. Treatment consists of hydration and use of an osmotic diuretic, such as mannitol, to force excretion of a dilute urine.[98,99] Alkalinizing the urine may also be prudent, but its efficacy has not been clearly established.

MITOCHONDRIAL MYOPATHIES

Mitochondrial myopathy is a term applied to cases of muscle disease in which the major morphologic abnormalities are alterations in the number, size, and structure of mitochondria. These changes are nonspecific and are associated with widely varying clinical syndromes. Perhaps it is more meaningful to consider mitochondrial myopathies to be disorders in muscle energetics caused by a defect in mitochondrial function that may be associated with structural changes. Defects in transport of pyruvate, fatty acids, and ketones into mitochondria as well as defects in the processing of these chemicals for energy to regenerate ATP are included in this category. Carnitine and CPT deficiency should be considered mitochondrial myopathies because of the biochemical defects, but they are not usually included under that classification because there are no associated changes in mitochondrial structure.

The most typical morphologic change in these diseases is the "ragged-red" fiber,[100] a distorted-appearing fiber that contains large peripheral and intermyofibrillar aggregates of abnormal mitochondria (Fig. 110–10). These appear as red deposits with the modified Gomori trichrome stain. An occasional ragged-red fiber is not diagnostic of a mitochondrial myopathy, but presence of these fibers does indicate the possibility of one of those diseases. On the other hand, many diseases that result from mitochondrial defects do not manifest this change. Additional changes, such as increased amounts of lipid or glycogen, intramitochondrial inclusions, or changes in mitochondrial size and/or shape, can be seen at the ultrastructural level.[101,102]

Mitochondrial myopathies recognized to date are associated with a variety of clinical manifestations. Many cause multisystem problems with involvement of the central nervous system, heart, and skeletal muscle.[101–103] Others cause problems primarily affecting muscle, with manifestations such as exercise intolerance,[104–107] muscle weakness that may have limb-girdle[108] or facioscapulohumeral distributions,[109] or extraocular muscle dysfunction with or without bulbar and limb muscle involvement.[110,111] Hypermetabolism,[112] salt craving,[113] and peripheral neuropathy[114] are reported in other cases, further indicating extreme heterogeneity.[115] Although some of these diseases affect infants, many cause symptoms in childhood that are recognized as the result of a disease only retrospectively, after the diagnosis is made later in life (Table 110–6).

To date, at least 25 different biochemical defects have been described in individuals with mitochondrial myopathies.[116] These defects can occur in nutrient transport into mitochondria, in the utilization of substrates such as pyruvate and fatty acids, in β-oxidation and the respiratory chain, or in energy conservation. There is little correlation between the biochemical defect, morphologic changes, and clinical picture. Precisely how these defects cause muscle fatigue and weakness is still not well understood.[120]

DISORDERED PURINE METABOLISM

Myoadenylate Deaminase Deficiency

Myoadenylate deaminase (MADA), a distinct isoenzyme of adenylate deaminase found only in skeletal muscle, catalyzes the irreversible deamination of AMP to IMP and plays an important role in the purine nucleotide cycle (Fig. 110–3).[121,122] In 1978, Fishbein reported the first cases of MADA deficiency.[123] The majority of MADA-deficient individuals complain of exercise intolerance as a result of fatigue and postexertional cramps and myalgias.[123–125] The diagnosis has been made at ages ranging from 7 to over 70 years, but individuals usually report that their symptoms began years earlier and gradually became more severe. A certain level of activity is required before symptoms develop in most MADA-deficient individuals. With increasing age, less activity is needed to bring on symptoms and more time is required for recovery.

MADA deficiency is probably the most common genetic cause of metabolic myopathy recognized at this time. Approximately 2% of large series of muscle biopsy specimens have been shown to be deficient in this enzyme.[123–125] The deficiency state has been described in association with many other disorders, including periodic paralysis, influenza-like illness, Kugelberg-Welander syndrome, amyotrophic lateral

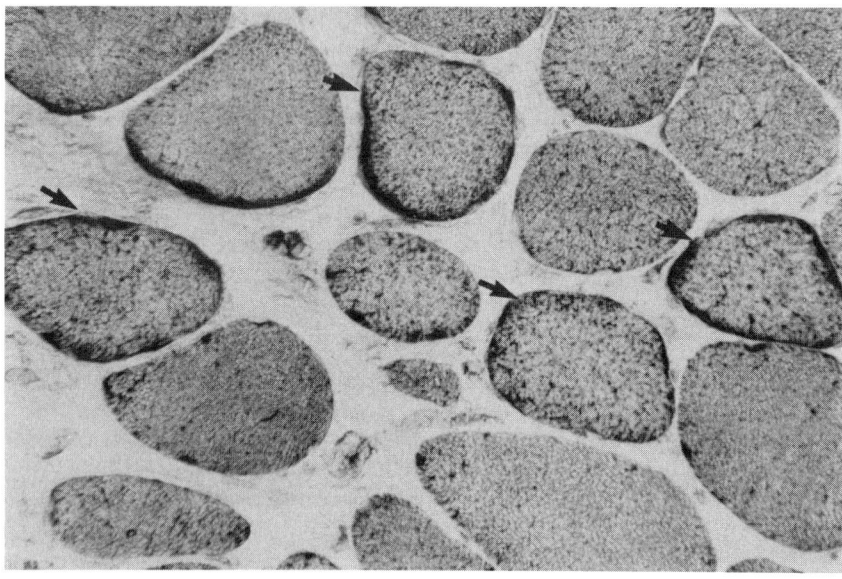

FIG. 110–10. Typical appearing ragged-red fiber is strongly suggestive, but not diagnostic, of a mitochondrial myopathy.

Table 110–6. Examples of Mitochondrial Myopathies Diagnosed in Adults

Deficiency	Age	Symptoms
Enzyme of β-oxidation[117]	33	Exercise intolerance, progressive weakness
NADH-CoQ reductase[116]	20–49	Exercise intolerance, progressive weakness
CoQ-cytochrome bc₁ reductase[102]	40, 43	Exercise intolerance, oculoskeletal myopathy
Cytochrome b[104]	38	Exercise intolerance, lacticacidemia
Cytochrome bc₁[118]	20	Exercise intolerance
Mitochondrial ATPase[119]	37	Nonprogressive weakness

sclerosis, spinal muscular atrophy, facial and limb-girdle myopathies, polymyositis, dermatomyositis, systemic lupus erythematosus, systemic sclerosis, diabetes, hyperthyroidism, and gout.[124–128] However, no associated neurologic, rheumatic, or metabolic disorder can be identified in half the individuals.[129] It is possible that MADA deficiency can occur in a primary form, inherited in an autosomal recessive pattern, and in a secondary form, caused by nonspecific muscle damage from a variety of neuomuscular disorders.

The precise relationship between MADA deficiency and muscular symptoms is unknown. The low exercise tolerance of these individuals is accompanied by rapid depletion of ATP in skeletal muscle, and the time required to replenish ATP to normal concentrations is prolonged compared to normals.[130] The response to forearm ischemic exercise is also abnormal in MADA deficiency (Table 110–5). Although the expected rise in venous lactate occurs, a corresponding change in ammonia concentration is not present. In addition, generation of the purine nucleotide degradation products adenosine, inosine, and hypoxanthine is diminished with exercise.[25,131,132]

Serum enzymes such as the CPK and aldolase are usually normal in MADA deficiency. Results of EMG are also normal or nonspecific. The measurement of venous lactate and ammonia concentrations following forearm ischemic exercise is effective for screening for MADA deficiency. However, submaximal exercise performance because of weakness, pain, or poor effort can be responsible for false positive results.[25] Consequently, failure to generate ammonia after exercise does not indicate MADA deficiency unless an adequate effort is documented. An abnormal result from forearm ischemic exercise testing should be followed by a muscle biopsy to confirm the putative enzyme deficiency. The structure of muscle tissue is usually normal. Histochemical techniques are useful in establishing the deficiency state.[133]

ENDOCRINE MYOPATHIES

A variety of endocrine diseases can cause symptoms of neuromuscular dysfunction. These include disorders of either hyperfunction or hypofunction of the adrenal, parathyroid, pituitary, and thyroid glands. A major mechanism responsible for the symptoms involves electrolyte imbalance.[134] This should not be surprising because muscle contraction requires transmembrane shifts in sodium, potassium, and calcium; inorganic phosphate is critical to the maintenance of high-energy compounds; and magnesium is an essential cofactor for ATPase activity. Thus, any hormonal change (or disease, drug, or other factor) that raises or lowers the concentrations of these ions can cause myopathic symptoms by altering surface membrane excitability, excitation-contraction coupling, or actin-myosin bridging. Endocrine disorders also cause skeletal muscle dysfunction through the effects of hormones on protein and carbohydrate metabolism.[135] The rheumatic aspects and myopathic syndromes of endocrinopathies are discussed in Chapter 113.

CLINICAL EVALUATION

The evaluation of patients with suspected metabolic muscle disease begins with a careful history and a thorough physical examination. Myopathies typically cause weakness, exercise intolerance as a result of fatigue, and postexertional myalgias, cramps, and stiffness. The weakness develops insidiously and is therefore ignored until it becomes truly limiting. The actual onset of the symptoms is often difficult to determine even in retrospect. Everyone experiences cramps, stiffness, and pain after certain exercise. Thus, the patient may deny the significance of his problems and others, including physicians, may disregard the patient's complaints for many years. Distinguishing between "normal" and "abnormal" exercise intolerance can truly be difficult.

The problem of diagnosing a metabolic muscle disease is confounded because at rest, patients are often completely asymptomatic and have no abnormal physical findings. The most significant complaints are severe, prolonged cramps and red wine–colored urine indicating myoglobinuria. Although these findings can hardly be ignored, special attention and questioning are required to determine the significance of the less dramatic symptoms. *The weakness of a metabolic myopathy is proximal and symmetrically distributed.* Initial complaints include difficulty climbing stairs or reaching a top shelf. Physical examination may be entirely normal and at most may show only weakness of a limb-girdle distribution. The prime importance of the physical examination in a neuromuscular disease may be to rule out evidence of a "neuro" component.

Measurement of muscle enzymes and electrodiagnostic studies follow if the patient's complaints are suspicious for myopathy or severe enough to alter his life-style. Increased levels of CPK, aldolase, serum glutamic-oxaloacetic transaminase (SGOT), serum glutamic-pyruvic transaminase (SGPT), and lactic dehydrogenase (LDH) may be observed in the blood of patients with muscle disease. Of these, the CPK is the most sensitive. However, when considering metabolic diseases of muscle, the presence of an elevated CPK is variable. Levels are usually increased in patients with glycogen storage diseases but are usually normal with the other diseases such as CPT or MADA deficiency. An isolated elevation of the CPK should be interpreted with caution. In normal individuals, spurious elevations can result from blunt trauma, intramuscular injection, aerobic exercise, EMG, muscle biopsy, and the use of medications such as morphine and barbiturates, which retard the excretion of the enzyme in the urine.[136,137] The patient's race and sex must also be considered in the interpretation of CPK levels. CPK values are significantly higher in healthy asymptomatic blacks than in whites or Hispanics and in males compared to females.[138] CPK levels are always raised in patients who have rhabdomyolysis. The MB isoenzyme fraction, which is usually considered as derived from cardiac muscle, may be increased under these conditions because regenerating skeletal muscle also produces this form.

Nerve conduction studies are entirely normal in metabolic myopathies. Finding normal nerve conduction in a patient with symptoms of muscle dysfunction defines the process as a myopathy by exclusion. EMG may also provide normal results in these individuals. Exceptions are in deficiencies of acid maltase, debrancher enzyme, and carnitine. But even in those conditions, the findings of abnormal motor unit potential and fibrillations are variable and nondiagnostic. The electromyogram, however, may be useful in clearly demonstrating myopathic changes and indicating preferential sites for muscle biopsy on the opposite side of the body.

Measurement of venous lactate and ammonia before and after forearm ischemic exercise provides a useful tool for ruling out MADA deficiency and all myopathic forms of glycogen storage disease except acid maltase deficiency. Individuals with MADA deficiency produce little ammonia compared to normal amounts of lactate under these conditions, whereas patients with the glycogenic and glycolytic defects produce the opposite result (Tables 110–4 and 110–5). Valid results from the forearm ischemic exercise test require an appropriate exercise effort on the part of the individual as false positive results can result from poor subject performance.[24,25,139] A positive result must be confirmed by tissue analysis.

A muscle biopsy provides the most important diagnostic information in the evaluation of a patient with a metabolic muscle disease. It is, however, the final step in the clinical evaluation and should not be performed until a preliminary diagnosis has been made. Selection of the muscle for biopsy is important. A clinically weak muscle that has not been traumatized (by intramuscular injection, EMG needle, or previous biopsy) is ideal. If weakness is not obvious, the biopsy site may be guided by EMG abnormalities on the opposite side of the body. Severely involved muscle, as seen acutely in rhabdomyolysis, should be avoided. The tissue can be severely distorted and the biochemical features of regenerating muscle can provide confusing information.

Routine histology can be helpful primarily in ruling out other conditions that can cause symptoms of muscle dysfunction such as inflammatory muscle disease and muscular dystrophies. *Histochemical studies* can provide the important information. The increased glycogen storage of disorders of glycogen metabolism can be detected with PAS staining (Fig. 110–7). Increased lipid accumulation, indicative of lipid storage myopathy, can be identified with Sudan or oil red O stains (Fig. 110–9). The Gomori modified trichrome stain reveals changes in mitochondria and the ragged-red fiber (Fig. 110–10). Acid phosphatase stains will demonstrate increased lysosomal enzyme activity indicative of acid maltase deficiency. Abnormal staining with NADH dehydrogenase, and other oxidative enzyme stains, suggests mitochondrial defects. Specific enzyme defects can be diagnosed with stains for myophosphorylase, phosphofructokinase, LDH, cytochrome oxidase, and MADA (Fig. 110–11). Carnitine concentration and CPT activity can be determined on muscle homogenate by radiochemical techniques.

Ultrastructural analysis by electron microscopy is clearly more sensitive than light microscopy in identifying glycogen (Fig. 110–8) and lipid deposition and reveals morphologic changes in mitochondria, mem-

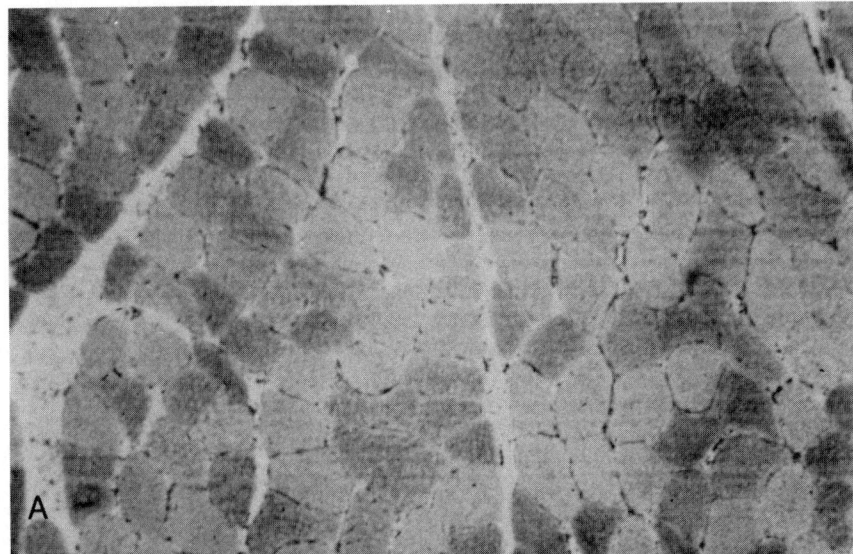

FIG. 110–11. *A,* Muscle stained for myoadenylate deaminase activity with normal results. *B,* Muscle from an individual with myoadenylate deaminase deficiency stained by the same method as the tissue in *A.*

branes, and sarcoplasmic reticulum. This technique will play an increased role in the evaluation of metabolic muscle diseases.

In the future, the evaluation of patients with symptoms of muscle dysfunction will include *^{31}P magnetic resonance spectroscopy.*[140,141] Presently this technique is used primarily for research purposes. Magnetic resonance spectroscopy can be used to measure tissue contents of ATP, creatine phosphate, and inorganic phosphate. This technique can be used to follow the shifts in these metabolites during exercise and to determine the pH of the tissue studied. It is noninvasive and harmless. Magnetic resonance spectroscopy has been applied to patients with McArdle's disease[142] and phosphofructokinase deficiency,[143] confirming the predicted rapid decreases in creatine phosphate and lack of pH change during ischemic exercise. At least

4 different patterns of metabolic change have been identified in muscle of patients with mitochondrial myopathies.[144,145] Additional studies with this technique will help elucidate normal patterns of muscle metabolism, detect altered states in various diseases and provide a valuable tool in following the effects of therapies.[146,147]

REFERENCES

1. McArdle, B.: Myopathy due to a defect in muscle glycogen breakdown. Clin. Sci., 24:13–36, 1951.
2. Mommaerts, W.F.H.M., et al.: A functional disorder of muscle associated with the absence of phosphorylase. Proc. Natl. Acad. Sci. USA, 45:791–797, 1959.
3. Schmid, R., Robbins, P.W., and Traut, R.R.: Glycogen syn-

thesis in muscle lacking phosphorylase. Proc. Natl. Acad. Sci. USA, 45:1236–1240, 1959.

4. Williamson, J.R.: Mitochondrial function in the heart. Ann. Rev. Physiol., 41:485–506, 1979.

5. Bessman, S.P., and Geiger, P.J.: Transport of energy in muscle: The phosphorylcreatine shuttle. Science, 211:448–452, 1981.

6. Erickson-Viitanen, S., Geiger, P., Yang, W.C.T., and Bessman, S.P.: The creatine-creatine phosphate shuttle for energy transport-compartmentation of creatine phosphokinase in muscle. Adv. Exp. Med. Biol., 151:115–125, 1982.

7. Moreadith, R.W., and Jacobus, W.E.: Creatine kinase of heart mitochondria. Functional coupling of ADP transfer to the adenine nucleotide translocase. J. Biol. Chem., 257:899–905, 1982.

8. Kushmerick, M.J.: Patterns in mammalian muscle energetics. J. Exp. Biol., 115:165–177, 1985.

9. Lowenstein, J.M.: Ammonia production in muscle and other tissues: The purine nucleotide cycle. Physiol. Rev., 52:382–414, 1972.

10. Meyer, R.A., and Terjung, R.L.: AMP deamination and IMP reamination in working skeletal muscle. Am. J. Physiol., 239 (Cell Physiol. 8):C32–C38, 1980.

11. Atkinson, D.E.: The energy charge of the adenylate pool as a regulatory parameter. Interaction with feedback modifiers. Biochemistry, 7:4030–4034, 1968.

12. Wy, T-F.L., and Davis, E.J.: Regulation of glycolytic flux in an energetically controlled cell-free system: The effects of adenine nucleotide ratios, inorganic phosphate, pH, and citrate. Arch. Biochem. Biophys., 209:85–99, 1981.

13. Aragon, J.J., Tornheim, K., and Lowenstein, J.M.: On a possible role of IMP in the regulation of phosphorylase activity in skeletal muscle. FEBS Lett, 117 (Suppl.):K56–K64, 1980.

14. Aragon, J.J., and Lowenstein, J.M.: The purine nucleotide cycle. Comparisons of the levels of citric acid intermediates with the operation of the purine nucleotide cycle in rat skeletal muscle during exercise and recovery from exercise. Eur. J. Biochem., 110:371–377, 1980.

15a. Bergstrom, J., and Hultman, E.: A study of the glycogen metabolism during exercise in man. Scand. J. Clin. Lab. Invest., 19:218–228, 1967.

15b. Goodman, M.N., and Lowenstein, J.M.: The purine nucleotide cycle. Studies of ammonia production by skeletal muscle in situ and in perfused preparations. J. Biol. Chem., 252:5054–5060, 1977.

16. Essen, B., and Henriksson, J.: Glycogen content of individual muscle fibers in man. Acta Physiol. Scand., 90:645–647, 1974.

17. DiMauro, S., and Bresolin, N.: Phosphorylase deficiency. In Myology. Edited by A.G. Engel and B.Q. Banker. New York, McGraw-Hill Book Company, 1986.

18. Pearson, C.M., Rimer, D.G., and Mommaerts, W.F.H.M.: A metabolic myopathy due to absence of muscle phosphorylase. Am. J. Med., 30:502–517, 1961.

19. Porte, D., et al.: Cardiovascular and metabolic response to exercise in a patient with McArdle's disease. N. Engl. J. Med., 275:406–412, 1966.

20. Pernow, B.B., Havel, R.J., and Jennings, D.B.: The second wind phenomenon in McArdle's syndrome. Acta Med. Scand., 472(Suppl.):294–307, 967.

21. Mastaglia, G.C., McCollum, J.P.K., Larson, P.F., and Hudgson, P.: Steroid myopathy complicating McArdle's disease. J. Neurol. Neurosurg. Psychiatry, 33:111–120, 1970.

22. Pourmand, R., Sanders, D.B., and Corwin, H.M.: Late-onset McArdle's disease with unusual electromyographic findings. Arch. Neurol., 40:374–377, 1983.

23. Mineo, I., et al.: Myogenic hyperuricemia. A common pathophysiologic feature of glycogenosis types III, V, and VII. N. Engl. J. Med., 317:75–80, 1987.

24. Munstat, T.L.: A standardized forearm ischemic exercise test. Neurology, 20:1171–1178, 1970.

25. Valen, P.A., et al.: Myoadenylate deaminase deficiency and forearm ischemic exercise testing. Arthritis Rheum., 30:661–668, 1987.

26. Takeuchi, K.T., and Kuriaki, H.: Histochemical detection of phosphorylase in animal tissues. J. Histochem. Cytochem., 3:153–160, 1955.

27. Engel, W.K., Eyerman, E.L., and Williams, H.E.: Late-onset type of skeletal muscle phosphorylase deficiency. A new familial variety with completely and partially affected subjects. N. Engl. J. Med., 268:135–137, 1963.

28. Mitsumoto, H.: McArdle's disease: Phosphorylase activity in regenerating muscle fibers. Neurology, 29:258–262, 1979.

29. DiMauro, S., Arnold, S., Miranda, A.F., and Rowland, L.P.: McArdle's disease: The mystery of reappearing phosphorylase activity in muscle culture: A fetal isoenzyme. Ann. Neurol., 3:60–66, 1978.

30. Fernandes, J., and Huijing, F.: Branching enzyme-deficiency glycogenosis: Studies in therapy. Arch. Dis. Child., 43:347–352, 1968.

31. Zellweger, H., et al.: Glycogenosis IV. A new cause of infantile hypotonia. J. Pediatr., 80:842–844, 1972.

32. Sernella, S., et al.: Severe cardiopathy in branching enzyme deficiency. J. Pediatr., 111:51–56, 1987.

33. Rowland, L.P., Araki, S., and Carmel, P.: Contracture in McArdle's disease. Stability of adenosine triphosphate during contracture in phosphorylase-deficient human muscle. Arch. Neurol., 13:541–544, 1965.

34. Brunberg, J.A., McCormick, W.F., and Schochet, S.S.: Type III glycogenosis. An adult with diffuse weakness and muscle wasting. Arch. Neurol., 25:171–178, 1971.

35. Garancis, J.C., Panares, R.P., Good, T.A., and Kuzma, J.F.: Type III glycogenosis. A biochemical and electron microscopic study. Lab. Invest., 22:468–477, 1970.

36. Lederer, B., Van de Werve, G., De Barsy, T., and Hers, H.G.: The autosomal form of phosphorylase kinase deficiency in man: Reduced activity of the muscle enzyme. Biochem. Biophys. Res. Commun., 92:169–174, 1980.

37. Ohtani, Y., et al.: Infantile glycogen storage myopathy in a girl with phosphorylase kinase deficiency. Neurology, 32:833–838, 1982.

38. Abarbanel, J.M., et al.: Adult muscle phosphorylase "b" kinase deficiency. Neurology, 36:560–562, 1986.

39. Tarui, S., et al.: Phosphofructokinase deficiency in skeletal muscle. A new type of glycogenosis. Biochem. Biophys. Res. Commun., 19:517–523, 1965.

40. Layzer, R.B., Rowland, L.P., and Ranney, H.M.: Muscle phosphofructokinase deficiency. Arch. Neurol., 17:512–523, 1967.

41. Tobin, W.E., et al.: Muscle phosphofructokinase deficiency. Arch. Neurol., 28:128–130, 1973.

41a. Rowland, L.P., DiMauro, S., and Layzer, R.B.: Phosphofructokinase deficiency. In Myology. Edited by A.G. Engel and B.Q. Banker. New York, McGraw-Hill Book Company, 1986.

42. Bonilla, E., and Schotland, D.L.: Histochemical diagnosis of muscle phosphofructokinase deficiency. Arch. Neurol., 22:6–12, 1970.

42a. Danon, M.J., et al.: Late-onset muscle phosphofructokinase (PFK) deficiency. Neurology, 35(Suppl.):207, 1985.

43. Kono, N., et al.: Increased plasma uric acid after exercise in muscle phosphofructokinase deficiency. Neurology, 36:106–108, 1986.

43a. DiMauro, S., Dalakas, M., and Miranda, A.F.: Phosphoglycerate kinase (PGK) deficiency: Another cause of recurrent myoglobinuria. Ann. Neurol., 13:11–19, 1983.

44. DiMauro, S., et al.: Muscle phosphoglycerate mutase deficiency. Neurology, 32:584–591, 1982.

45. Kanno, T., et al.: Hereditary deficiency of lactate dehydrogenase M-subunit. Clin. Chim. Acta, 108:267–276, 1980.

46. Engel, A.G., Gomez, M.R., Seybold, M.E., and Lambert, E.H.: The spectrum and diagnosis of acid maltase deficiency. Neurology, 23:95–106, 1973.

47. Hers, H.G.: Alpha-glucosidase deficiency in generalized glycogen-storage disease (Pompe's disease). Biochem. J., 86:11–16, 1963.

48. Hogan, G.R., et al.: Pompe's disease. Neurology, 19:894–900, 1969.

49. Martin, J.J., et al.: Acid maltase deficiency (type II glycogenosis): Morphological and biochemical study of a childhood phenotype. J. Neurol. Sci., 30:155–166, 1976.

50. Nakagawa, M., et al.: Muscle type acid maltase deficiency: An intermediate case between childhood type and adult type. Clin. Neurol. (Tokyo), 22:54–57, 1982.

51. Hudgson, P., et al.: Adult myopathy from glycogen storage disease due to acid maltase deficiency. Brain, 91:435–462, 1968.

52. Rosenow, E.C., and Engel, A.G.: Acid maltase deficiency in adults presenting as respiratory failure. Am. J. Med., 64:485–491, 1978.

53. Keunen, R.W.M., Lambregts, P.C.L.A., Op de Coul, A.A.W., and Joosten, E.M.G.: Respiratory failure as initial symptom of acid maltase deficiency. J. Neurol. Neurosurg. Psychiatry, 47:549–552, 1984.

54. Engel, A.G.: Acid maltase deficiency in adults: Studies in four cases of a syndrome which may mimic muscular dystrophy or other myopathies. Brain, 93:599–616, 1970.

55. Engel, A.G., and Dale, A.J.D.: Autophagic glycogenosis of late onset with mitochondrial abnormalities: Light and electron microscopic observations. Mayo Clin. Proc., 43:233–279, 1968.

56. Hudgson, P., and Fulthorpe, J.J.: The pathology of type II skeletal muscle glycogenosis: A light and electron-microscopic study. J. Pathol., 116:139–147, 1975.

57. Taniguchi, N., et al.: Alpha-glucosidase activity in human leucocytes: Choice of lymphocytes for the diagnosis of Pompe's disease and the carrier state. Clin. Chim. Acta, 89:293–299, 1978.

58. Schram, A.W., et al.: Use of immobilized antibodies in investigating acid alpha-gluocosidase in urine in relation to Pompe's disease. Biochim. Biophys. Acta, 567:370–383, 1979.

59. Loonen, M.C.B., et al.: Identification of heterozygotes for glycogenosis 2 (acid maltase deficiency). Clin. Genet., 19:55–63, 1981.

60. Bremer, J.: Carnitine-metabolism and functions. Physiol. Rev., 63:1420–1480, 1983.

61. Engel, A.G., and Angelini, C.: Carnitine deficiency of skeletal muscle associated with lipid storage myopathy: A new syndrome. Science, 179:899–902, 1973.

62. Karpati, G., et al.: The syndrome of systemic carnitine deficiency: Clinical, morphologic, biochemical and pathophysiologic features. Neurology, 25:16–24, 1975.

63. Markesbery, W.R., et al.: Muscle carnitine deficiency: Association with lipid myopathy, vacuolar neuropathy, and vacuolated leukocytes. Arch. Neurol., 31:320–324, 1974.

64. Carrier, H.N., and Berthillier, G.: Carnitine levels in normal children and adults and in patients with diseased muscle. Muscle Nerve, 3:326–334, 1980.

65. Rebouche, C.J., and Paulson, D.J.: Carnitine metabolism and function in humans. Annu. Rev. Nutr., 6:41–66, 1986.

66. Rebouche, C.J., and Engel, A.G.: Kinetic compartmental analysis of carnitine metabolism in the human carnitine deficiency syndromes: Evidence for alterations in tissue carnitine transport. J. Clin. Invest., 73:857–867, 1984.

67. McGarry, J.D., and Foster, D.W.: An improved and simplified radioisotope assay for the determination of free and esterified carnitine. J. Lipid Res., 17:277–281, 1976.

68. Bradley, W.G., Tomlinson, B.E., and Hardy, M.: Further studies of mitochondrial and lipid storage myopathies. J. Neurol. Sci., 35:201–210, 1978.

69. Chapoy, P.F., et al.: Systemic carnitine deficiency: A treatable inherited lipid-storage disease presenting as Reye's syndrome. N. Engl. J. Med., 303:1389–1394, 1980.

70. Tripp, M.E., et al.: Systemic carnitine deficiency presenting as familial endocardial fibroelastosis. N. Engl. J. Med., 305:385–390, 1981.

71. Rebouche, C.J., and Engel, A.G.: Carnitine transport in cultured muscle cells and skin fibroblasts from patients with primary systemic carnitine deficiency. In Vitro, 18:495–500, 1982.

72. Engel, A.G.: Carnitine deficiency syndromes and lipid storage myopathies. In Myology. Edited by A.G. Engel and B.Q. Banker. New York, McGraw-Hill Book Company, 1986.

73. Bohmer, T., Bergrem, H., and Eiklid, K.: Carnitine deficiency induced during intermittent haemodialysis for renal failure. Lancet, 1:126–128, 1978.

74. Savica, V., et al.: Plasma and muscle carnitine levels in haemodialysis patients with morphological-ultrastructural examination of muscle samples. Nephron, 35:232–236, 1983.

75. Moorthy, A.V., Rosenblum, M., Rajaram, R., and Shug, A.L.: A comparison of plasma and muscle carnitine levels in patients on peritoneal or hemodialysis for chronic renal failure. Am. J. Nephrol., 3:205–208, 1983.

76. Rudman, D., Sewell, C.W., and Ansley, J.D.: Deficiency of carnitine in cachectic cirrhotic patients. J. Clin. Invest., 60:716–723, 1977.

77. Laub, M.C., Paetzke-Brunner, I., and Jaeger, G.: Serum carnitine during valproic acid therapy. Epilepsia, 27:559–562, 1986.

78. Maebashi, M., et al.: Urinary excretion of carnitine in patients with hyperthyroidism and hypothyroidism: Augmentation by thyroid hormone. Metabolism, 26:351–356, 1977.

79. Maebashi, M., et al.: Urinary excretion of carnitine and serum concentrations of carnitine and lipids in patients with hypofunctional endocrine diseases: Involvement of adrenocorticoid and thyroid hormones in ACTH-induced augmentation of carnitine and lipid metabolism. Metabolism, 26:357–361, 1977.

80. Cederblad, G., Fahraeus, L., and Lindgren, K.: Plasma carnitine and renal-carnitine clearance during pregnancy. Am. J. Clin. Nutr., 44:379–383, 1986.

81. Angelini, C., Lucke, S., and Cantarutti, F.: Carnitine deficiency of skeletal muscle: Report of a treated case. Neurology, 26:633–637, 1976.

82. Prockop, L.D., Engel, W.K., and Shug, A.L.: Nearly fatal muscle carnitine deficiency with full recovery after replacement therapy. Neurology, 33:1629–1631, 1983.

83. Rocchi, L., et al.: Effects of carnitine administration in patients

with chronic renal failure undergoing periodic dialysis, evaluated by computerized electromyography. Drugs Exp. Clin. Res., *12*:707–711, 1986.

84. Carroll, J.E., et al.: Carnitine "deficiency": Lack of response to carnitine therapy. Neurology, *30*:618–626, 1980.

85. Strumpf, D.A., Parker, W.D., and Angelini, C.: Carnitine deficiency, organic acidemias, and Reye's syndrome. Neurology, *35*:1041–1045, 1985.

86. Bazzato, G., et al.: Myasthenia-like syndrome after D,L- but not L-carnitine. Lancet, *1*:1209, 1981.

87. Keith, R.E.: Symptoms of carnitinelike deficiency in a trained runner taking DL-carnitine supplements. JAMA, *255*:1137, 1986.

88. Engel, A.G., and Siekert, R.G.: Lipid storage myopathy responsive to prednisone. Arch. Neurol., *27*:174–181, 1972.

89. VanDyke, D.H., Griggs, K.R.C., Markesbery, W., and DiMauro, S.: Hereditary carnitine deficiency of muscle. Neurology, *25*:154–159, 1975.

90. Issacs, H., et al.: Weakness associated with the pathological presence of lipid in skeletal muscle: A detailed study of a patient with carnitine deficiency. J. Neurol. Neurosurg. Psychiatry, *39*:1114–1123, 1976.

91. DiMauro, S., and Melis-DiMauro, P.: Muscle carnitine palmitoyltransferase deficiency and myoglobinuria. Science, *182*:929–931, 1973.

92. Angelini, C., et al.: Carnitine palmitoyltransferase deficiency: Clinical variability, carrier detection, and autosomal recessive inheritance. Neurology, *31*:883–886, 1981.

93. Brownell, A.K.W., Severson, D.L., Thompson, C.D., and Fletcher, T.: Cold induced rhabdomyolysis in carnitine palmitoyltransferase deficiency. Can. J. Neurol. Sci., *6*:367–369, 1979.

94. Ross, N.S., and Hoppel, C.L.: Partial muscle carnitine palmitoyltransferase-A deficiency. Rhabdomyolysis associated with transiently decreased muscle carnitine content after ibuprofen therapy. JAMA, *257*:62–65, 1987.

95. DiMauro, S., and Papadimitriou, A.: Carnitine palmitoyltransferase deficiency. *In* Myology. Edited by A.G. Engel and B.Q. Banker. New York, McGraw-Hill Book Company, 1986.

96. DiDonato, S., et al.: Heterogeneity of carnitine-palmitoyltransferase deficiency. J. Neurol. Sci., *50*:207–215, 1981.

97. Zierz, S., and Engel, A.G.: Regulatory properties of a mutant carnitine palmitoyltransferase in human skeletal muscle. Eur. J. Biochem., *149*:207–214, 1985.

98. Gabow, P.A., Kaehny, W.D., and Kelleher, S.P.: The spectrum of rhabdomyolysis. Medicine, *61*:141–152, 1982.

99. Rowland, L.P.: Myoglobinuria, 1984. Can. J. Neurol. Sci., *11*:1–13, 1984.

100. Olson, W., Engel, W.K., Walsh, G.O., and Einaugler, R.: Oculocraniosomatic neuromuscular disease with "ragged-red" fibers: Histochemical and ultrastructural changes in limb muscles of a group of patients with idiopathic progressive external ophthalmoplegia. Arch. Neurol., *26*:193–211, 1972.

101. Carpenter, S., and Karpati, G.: Pathology of Skeletal Muscle. 1st ed. New York, Churchill Livingstone, 1984.

102. Karpati, G., et al.: The Kearns-Shy syndrome. A multisystem disease with mitochondrial abnormality demonstrated in skeletal muscle and skin. J. Neurol. Sci., *19*:133–151, 1973.

103. Ringel, S.P., Wilson, W.B., and Barden, M.T.: Extraocular muscle biopsy in chronic progressive external ophthalmoplegia. Ann. Neurol., *6*:326–339, 1979.

104. Morgan-Hughes, J.A., et al.: A mitochondrial myopathy characterized by a deficiency in reducible cytochrome b. Brain, *100*:617–640, 1977.

105. Morgan-Hughes, J.A., et al.: A mitochondrial myopathy with a deficiency of respiratory chain NADH Co-Q reductase activity. J. Neurol. Sci., *43*:27–46, 1979.

106. Land, J.N., Morgan-Hughes, J.A., and Clark, J.B.: Mitochondrial myopathy—Biochemical studies revealing a deficiency of NADH-cytochrome b reductase activity. J. Neurol. Sci., *50*:1–13, 1981.

107. Reichmann, H., et al.: Mitochondrial myopathy due to complex III deficiency with normal reducible cytochrome b concentration. Arch Neurol., *43*:957–961, 1986.

108. Salmon, M.A., Esiri, M.N., and Ruderman, M.B.: Myopathic disorder associated with mitochondrial abnormalities, hyperglycaemia and hyperketonaemia. Lancet, *2*:290–293, 1971.

109. Mechler, F., Fawcett, P.R.W., Mastaglia, F.L., and Hudgson, P.: Mitochondrial myopathy: A study of clinically affected and asymptomatic members of a six-generation family. J. Neurol. Sci., *50*:191–200, 1981.

110. Morgan-Hughes, J.A., and Mair, W.G.P.: Atypical muscle mitochondria in oculoskeletal myopathy. Brain, *96*:215–224, 1973.

111. Mechler, F., et al.: Mitochondrial myopathies. A clinico-pathological study of cases with and without extra-ocular muscle involvement. Aust. N.Z. J. Med., *16*:185–192, 1986.

112. DiMauro, S., et al.: Luft's disease: Further biochemical and ultrastructural studies of skeletal muscle in the second case. J. Neurol. Sci., *27*:217–232, 1976.

113. Spiro, A.J., Prineas, J.W., and Moore, C.L.: A new mitochondrial myopathy in a patient with salt-craving. Arch. Neurol., *22*:259–269, 1970.

114. Yiannikas, C., McLeod, J.G., Pollard, J.D., and Baverstock, J.: Peripheral neuropathy associated with mitochondrial myopathy. Ann. Neurol., *20*:249–257, 1986.

115. Berenberg, R.A., et al.: Lumping and splitting: "Ophthalmoplegia-plus" or Kearns-Sayre syndrome? Ann. Neurol., *1*:37–54, 1977.

116. Morgan-Hughes, J.A.: The mitochondrial myopathies. *In* Myology. Edited by A.G. Engel and B.Q. Banker. New York, McGraw-Hill Book Company, 1986.

117. Willner, J.H., et al.: Muscle carnitine deficiency. Genetic heterogeneity. J. Neurol. Sci., *41*:235–246, 1979.

118. Hayes, D.J., et al.: A new mitochondrial myopathy: Biochemical studies revealing a deficiency in the cytochrome-bc_1 complex (complex III) of the respiratory chain. Brain, *107*:1165–1177, 1984.

119. Schotland, D.L., et al.: Neuromuscular disorder associated with a defect in mitochondrial energy supply. Arch. Neurol., *33*:475–479, 1976.

120. Wilke, D.R.: Shortage of chemical fuel as a cause of fatigue: Studies by nuclear magnetic resonance and bicycle ergometry. *In* Human Muscle Fatigue: Physiological Mechanisms, Ciba Foundation Symposium 82. Edited by R. Porter and J. Whelan. London, Pitman Medical, 1981.

121. Lowenstein, J.M., and Goodman, M.N.: The purine nucleotide cycle in muscle. Fed. Proc., *37*:2308–2312, 1978.

122. Sugden, P.H., and Newsholme, E.A.: The effects of ammonium, inorganic phosphate and potassium ions on the activity of phosphofructokinase from muscle and nervous tissue of vertebrates and invertebrates. Biochem. J., *150*:113–122, 1975.

123. Fishbein, W.N., Armbrustmacher, V.W., and Griffen, J.L.: Myoadenylate deaminase deficiency: A new disease of muscle. Science, *200*:545–548, 1978.

124. Shumate, J.B., et al.: Myoadenylate deaminase deficiency. Muscle Nerve, *2*:213–216, 1981.

125. Kar, N.C., and Pearson, C.M.: Muscle adenylate deaminase deficiency. Arch. Neurol., 38:279–281, 1981.
126. DiMauro, S., et al.: Myoadenylate deaminase deficiency: Muscle biopsy and muscle culture in a patient with gout. J. Neurol. Sci., 47:191–202, 1980.
127. Mercelis, R., et al.: Myoadenylate deaminase deficiency in a patient with facial and limb girdle myopathy. J. Neurol., 225:157–166, 1981.
128. Gertler, P.A., and Jacobs, R.P.: Myoadenylate deaminase deficiency in a patient with progressive systemic sclerosis. Arthritis Rheum., 27:586–590, 1984.
129. Fishbein, W.N.: Myoadenylate deaminase deficiency: Inherited and acquired forms. Biochem. Med., 33:158–169, 1985.
130. Sabina, R.L., et al.: Disruption of the purine nucleotide cycle: A potential explanation for muscle dysfunction in myoadenylate deaminase deficiency. J. Clin. Invest., 66:1419–1423, 1980.
131. Patterson, V.H., Kaiser, K.K., and Brooke, M.H.: Exercising muscle does not produce hypoxanthine in adenylate deaminase deficiency. Neurology, 33:784–786, 1983.
132. Sinkeler, S.P.T., et al.: Ischaemic exercise test in myoadenylate deaminase deficiency and McArdle's disease: Measurement of plasma adenosine, inosine and hypoxanthine. Clin. Sci., 70:399–401, 1986.
133. Fishbein, W.N., Griffen, J.L., and Armbrustmacher, V.M.: Stain for skeletal muscle adenylate deaminase: An effective tetrazolium stain for frozen biopsy specimens. Arch. Pathol. Lab. Med., 104:482–486, 1980.
134. Knochel, J.P.: Neuromuscular manifestations of electrolyte disorders. Am. J. Med., 72:521–535, 1982.
135. Goldberg, A.L., Tischler, M., DeMartino, G., and Griffith, G.: Hormonal regulation of protein degradation and synthesis in skeletal muscle. Fed. Proc., 39:31–36, 1980.
136. Kagen, L.J.: Approach to the patient with myopathy. Bull. Rheum. Dis., 33:1–8, 1983.
137. Elin, R.J., et al.: Quantification of acute phase reactants after muscle biopsy. J. Lab. Clin. Med., 100:566–573, 1982.
138. Black, H.R., Quallich, H., and Gareleck, C.B.: Racial differences in serum creatine kinase levels. Am. J. Med., 81:479–487, 1986.
139. Sinkeler, S.P.T., et al.: The relation between blood lactate and ammonia in ischemic handgrip exercise. Muscle Nerve, 8:523–527, 1985.
140. Chance, B., et al.: Mitochondrial regulation of phosphocreatine/inorganic phosphate ratios in exercising human muscle: A gated ^{31}P NMR study. Proc. Natl. Acad. Sci. USA, 78:6714–6718, 1981.
141. Edwards, R.H.T., et al.: Clinical use of nuclear magnetic resonance in the investigation of myopathy. Lancet, 1:725–731, 1982.
142. Ross, B.D., et al.: Examination of a case of suspected McArdle's syndrome by ^{31}P nuclear magnetic resonance. N. Engl. J. Med., 304:1338–1342, 1981.
143. Chance, B., et al.: ^{31}P NMR studies of control of mitochondrial function in phosphofructokinase-deficient human skeletal muscle. Proc. Natl. Acad. Sci. USA, 79:7714–7718, 1982.
144. Ross, B.D., and Radda, G.K.: Application of ^{31}P NMR to inborn errors of muscle metabolism. Biochem. Soc. Trans., 11:627–630, 1983.
145. Radda, G.K., et al.: ^{31}P NMR examination of two patients with NADH-CoQ reductase deficiency. Nature, 295:608–609, 1982.
146. Taylor, D.J., et al.: Examination of the energetics of aging skeletal muscle using nuclear magnetic resonance. Gerontology, 30:2–7, 1984.
147. Argov, Z., et al.: Treatment of mitochondrial myopathy due to complex III deficiency with vitamins K_3 and C: A ^{31}P-NMR follow-up study. Ann. Neurol., 19:598–602, 1986.

OCHRONOSIS, HEMOCHROMATOSIS, AND WILSON'S DISEASE

111

H. RALPH SCHUMACHER, JR.

ALKAPTONURIA AND OCHRONOSIS

Alkaptonuria is a hereditary disorder characterized by homogentisic acid in the urine, which, when oxidized, imparts a brownish black color to the urine. The term "alkaptonuria," denoting an avidity for oxygen in alkaline solution, was coined by Boedeker in 1859 and is derived from fusion of an Arabic word meaning "alkali" and a Greek word (kaptein), meaning "to suck up avidly." When the freshly passed urine is alkalinized, polymerization of homogentisic acid is accelerated, and the urine turns black. Ochronosis denotes a bluish black pigmentation of connective tissue in patients with alkaptonuria, usually apparent clinically in the cartilage of the ear, in the skin, and in the sclera. This term was originated by Virchow in 1866, who described the microscopic appearance of this pigmentation as "ochre" or dark yellow.

Alkaptonuria itself is a symptomless condition. Clinical signs and symptoms develop when pigment is deposited in cartilage and other connective tissues (ochronosis). The relationship between alkaptonuria and ochronosis was first recognized in 1902 by Albrecht. Table 111–1 lists factors in the diagnosis of these and related conditions.

HISTORY

The earliest clinical observation, that of a boy who passed dark urine, was made by Scribonius in 1584. Boedeker, in 1859, was the first to isolate homogen-

tisic acid from the urine of a patient with alkaptonuria. Wolkow and Bauman in 1891 established the chemical structure of this compound as 2,5-dihydroxyphenylacetic acid and named it homogentisic acid. LaDu and his collaborators in 1958 demonstrated the absence of the enzyme homogentisic acid oxidase in the liver of a patient with alkaptonuria, ochronotic spondylosis, and peripheral arthropathy.[1]

NATURE OF THE BIOCHEMICAL LESION

Alkaptonuria is the result of a defect in the metabolic pathway for the aromatic amino acid tyrosine. Normally, the benzene ring of homogentisic acid is broken by the enzyme homogentisic acid oxidase, and maleylacetoacetic acid is formed. LaDu, et al. assayed liver homogenates from ochronotic patients and control subjects and demonstrated that the pattern of enzyme activities of the alkaptonuric liver was essentially the same as in the control liver, except with respect to homogentisic acid oxidase activity, which was completely missing in the alkaptonuric patient.[1] Of interest is the presence of the enzyme maleylacetoacetic acid isomerase in the alkaptonuric liver despite the apparent absence of the substrate maleylacetoacetic acid, which could be derived only from the metabolism of homogentisic acid. The presence of this enzyme in the absence of its substrate demonstrates that the genetic mechanism that controls the synthesis of this enzyme is not regulated by the substrate.

1798

Table 111–1. Diagnostic Features of Alkaptonuria, Ochronosis, Ochronotic Spondylitis, and Peripheral Arthropathy

Alkaptonuria
  Urine turns black:
    On alkalinization
    On standing
    When tested for sugar by Benedict's reagent; in addition, yellow-orange precipitate forms
  Positive family history

Ochronosis
  Pigmentation of cartilage and skin:
    Pinna of ear, eardrum, and cerumen
    Sclera
    Skin over malar area, nose, axilla, groin
  Prostatic calculi

Ochronotic spondylosis
  Calcification and ossification of intervertebral discs
  Disproportionately little osteophytosis
  Sacroiliac joints not fused and no "bamboo" spine
  Loss of lumbar lordosis
  Spine rigid and stooped, knees flexed, stance typical

Ochronotic peripheral arthropathy
  Knees, shoulders, and hips most commonly affected
  Synovial fluid contains small amounts of homogentisic acid and is noninflammatory, except with occasional calcium pyrophosphate crystal–associated inflammation
  Brittle cartilage fragments and pigmented "chards" in the synovium
  Osteochondral joint bodies common
  Small joints of hands and feet usually not affected

GENETIC FACTORS

Alkaptonuria is felt to be transmitted by a single recessive autosomal gene. The occasional occurrence of this disorder in successive generations of certain families may be the result of consanguineous marriages in which homozygotes mate with heterozygotes. The present concept of the mode of transmission of alkaptonuria, originally advanced by Garrod, and challenged at times, has been substantiated by several careful family studies in which complete pedigrees were available.[2] One family had HLA-B27 in 8 of 10 members with alkaptonuria.[3]

LABORATORY ASPECTS OF ALKAPTONURIA

The freshly passed urine of an alkaptonuric patient is of normal color and does not darken at once unless it is alkaline or contains less than a normal concentration of vitamin C or other reducing agents. On standing, it may turn brownish black as the homogentisic acid becomes oxidized. If Benedict's reagent is used in testing the urine for sugar, the yellowish orange precipitate that is formed because homogen-

tisic acid reduces the copper can be misinterpreted as indicating glucosuria. The color of the supernatant solution in these cases is always brownish black, which is diagnostic for alkaptonuria.

With the use of copper-reduction tablets (Clinitest), a black supernatant may also be seen in patients with malignant melanoma and after intravenous urography with sodium diatrizoate (Hypaque) and other x-ray contrast media.[4] Specific glucose oxidase tapes (Clinistix) may not detect urine glucose in diabetics with ochronosis because of interference with the peroxidase-indicator chromagen reaction by homogentisic acid.[5] Spuriously increased serum and urinary uric acid determinations have been described in ochronosis when colorimetric methods were used, but values were normal by the uricase spectrophotometric technique.[5] Homogentisic acid in the urine may also falsely elevate creatinine levels when measured by Jaffé's reaction.

DIAGNOSTIC TESTS FOR ALKAPTONURIA

Several presumptive, nonspecific tests for alkaptonuria are available. These tests are color reactions based on the reducing properties of homogentisic acid. Thus, in the Briggs tests, molybdate is reduced and a deep blue color is obtained. When a drop of urine is placed on photographic paper, a black spot indicates reduction of silver. When sodium hydroxide is added to the freshly passed urine, homogentisic acid is rapidly oxidized, and the urine properly darkens. A specific enzymatic method for quantitative determination of homogentisic acid in urine and blood has been developed.[6] Thin-layer chromatography can also be used.

PATHOLOGIC FEATURES OF OCHRONOSIS

The lesions of ochronosis result from the intercellular or intracellular deposition of pigment in many organs or structures. The exact chemical composition of the pigment has not yet been defined, although it is believed to be a polymer derived from homogentisic acid. Benzoquinoneacetic acid may be an intermediate compound that, when bound to connective tissue, may participate in a polymerization process leading to the final pigment formation.[7] Homogentisic acid is concentrated preferentially by connective tissue, but this process is reversible until after polymerization.[7] Homogentisic acid has been shown to inhibit hydroxylysine formation in vitro.[8] The predilection of ochronosis for cartilage that contains hydroxylysine-rich collagen may be in part related to this. The typical pathologic findings have been reviewed comprehensively.[9] Granules of insoluble, melanin-like pigment are usually found in the skin and subcutis, the cartilage of joints, the intervertebral discs, including the anulus fibrosus as well as the nucleus pulposus, the tracheal cartilages, the epithelial cells of the renal tubules, and the islets of the pancreas. Pigment granules impregnate the walls of large and medium-sized arteries and arterioles, including the aorta and the pulmonary, coronary, and renal arteries.

CLINICAL PICTURE OF OCHRONOSIS

Patients with alkaptonuria who live to the fourth decade almost invariably develop ochronosis. The cartilage of the ear, especially the concha and anthelix, is frequently involved and takes on a slate blue discoloration while becoming irregularly thickened and inflexible. When the pinna is transilluminated, the opaque pigmented area stands out prominently. The cerumen in the external canal is often black, and the periphery of the tympanic membrane is grayish black. Many patients with long-standing ochronosis have impaired hearing. Pigmentation of the sclera is usually localized to a small area midway between the limbus of the cornea and the inner or outer canthus. The skin over the malar areas, nose, axilla, and groin is often pigmented.

Deposition of pigment in the intervertebral discs and articular cartilages of the large joints leads to spondylosis and peripheral arthropathy.

Loud cardiac murmurs, mostly systolic, have been noted in about 15 to 20% of patients with ochronosis.[10] Pigment deposits in the mitral and aortic valves may be associated with deformity of the leaflets or cusps. Clinically significant aortic stenosis has been successfully treated by aortic valve replacement.[11]

Prostatic calculi occur in a large proportion of men with ochronosis and are readily palpable on rectal examination. Dysuria and frequency of urination may be present, and a prostatic operation may be necessary. Calculi may be passed spontaneously or removed surgically. These calculi have a characteristic black color and contain ochronotic pigment and calcium phosphate salts.

OCHRONOTIC SPONDYLOSIS

The majority of patients with ochronosis past the age of 30 develop spondylosis. Symptoms usually consist of stiffness and discomfort in the lower back. In about 10 to 15% of patients with ochronosis, the onset of spondylosis occurs with herniation of a nucleus pulposus.[10] In such instances, the symptoms and signs are indistinguishable from those in typical cases of herniated disc without alkaptonuria. The earliest site of spondylosis is the lumbar spine; years later, the dorsal and finally the cervical spine become involved. Stiffness of the lower back slowly progresses to rigidity and obliteration of normal lumbar lordosis. In many cases, lumbar kyphosis develops. Symptoms may be minimal despite prominent roentgenographic changes.

The earliest change apparent in roentgenograms of the spine consists of a wafer of calcification, and actual ossification, in the intervertebral disc of the lumbar spine (Fig. 111–1). Crystallographic study has shown the calcium in these discs to be hydroxyapatite.[12] Radiographic evidence of calcified intervertebral discs in adults is characteristic of ochronosis, but it is not diagnostic because similar changes can also be seen in pseudogout, in hemochromatosis, in chronic respiratory paralytic poliomyelitis, in spinal fusion of any origin, and occasionally in other disorders or without detectable associated disease. Secondary narrowing of the intervertebral spaces occurs. Osteophytes are usually small. Splits in disc material appear to account for radiolucencies in the discs that have been termed "vacuum discs."[13] In contrast to ankylosing spondylitis, the sacroiliac joints in ochronotic spondylosis are

FIG. 111–1. Roentgenogram of the lumbar spine of a 55-year-old man with ochronotic spondylosis. Note the calcification of intervertebral discs. The osteophytes are of only moderate size.

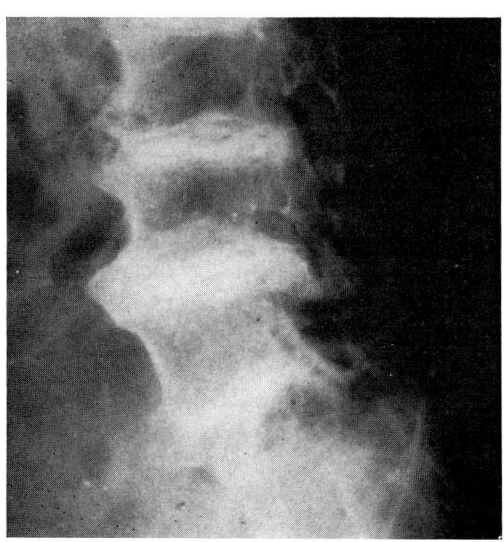

not fused, although they may show degenerative changes, the interfacetal articulations retain a normal radiographic appearance, and annular ossification with a "bamboo" pattern does not appear. The marked narrowing of multiple intervertebral spaces results in a loss of several inches in height. The spinal deformity and forward stoop cause the patient to stand with knees flexed and on a broad base. This posture imparts to the patient with ochronotic spondylosis a stance and gait similar to that of a patient with ankylosing spondylitis (Fig. 111–2).

OCHRONOTIC PERIPHERAL ARTHROPATHY

A degenerative arthritis of the peripheral joints also occurs, although it is less frequent and develops later than spondylosis. The joints most commonly affected are the knees, shoulders, and hips, in descending

FIG. 111–2. Typical posture and stance of a patient with ochronotic spondylosis: forward stoop, loss of lumbar lordosis, flexed hips and knees, wide-based stance. This 40-year-old man lost 6 inches in height.

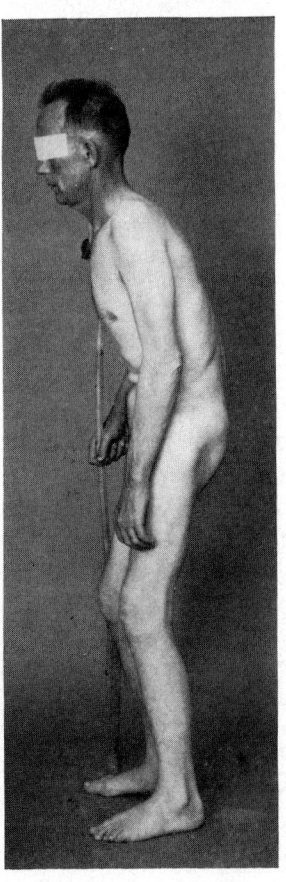

order of frequency. The knees are involved in the majority of cases of peripheral arthritis. Pain, stiffness, crepitation, flexion contractures, and limitation of motion are the most common features. In the peripheral joints, symptoms often antedate any visible roentgenographic changes. Effusion occurs in about half these cases. Synovial fluid is generally clear, viscous, and yellow, without darkening on exposure to alkali. Although homogentisic acid can be demonstrated, its concentration is much lower than in the urine. Occasionally, black specks of ochronotic cartilage are seen floating in the fluid.[14,15] Leukocyte counts in a large series by Huttl ranged from 112 to 700/mm³ with predominantly mononuclear cells.[16] Occasional cells have dark inclusions that appear to be phagocytized cartilage containing ochronotic pigment (Fig. 111–3). Synovial effusions or membrane can contain calcium pyrophosphate crystals without inflammation,[15,17–19] or the patient may have typical acute episodes of pseudogout with increased synovial fluid leukocyte counts.[20]

Pigmentation of the articular cartilage occurs initially in the deeper layers, with relative sparing of the surface. It is seen predominantly in the matrix of the tangential zone, but also in chondrocytes. Necrosis of chondrocytes occurs. Pigment appears by electron microscopy to be associated with the surface of collagen fibers in cartilage, but not in synovium.[18,21] The pigmented articular cartilage is brittle; minute fragments are broken off and are displaced into the synovial tissue (Fig. 111–4). In this location, they sometimes evoke a foreign-body reaction and new formation of bone tissue called osteochondral bodies (Fig. 111–5).[22] These bodies may be several centimeters in diameter and are readily palpable in and

FIG. 111–3. Synovial fluid mononuclear cells in ochronotic arthropathy. The dark cytoplasmic inclusions appear to be phagocytized pigmented debris (Giemsa stain × 1250). (Courtesy of S. Huttl and Acta Rheum. Baln. Pistiniana.)

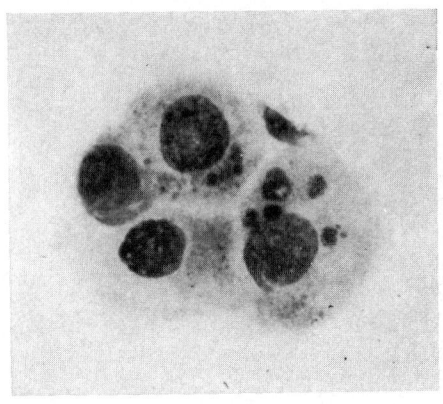

FIG. 111–4. Synovial tissue in ochronotic arthropathy. Minute fragments of darkly pigmented cartilage lie within the superficial portion of the tissue. The sharp edges of the "shards" are characteristic. A foreign-body cell reaction is present at the margins of a few and is accompanied by mild synovial fibrosis. Associated infiltration of lymphocytes and plasma cells may also be present (hematoxylin and eosin stain ×90).

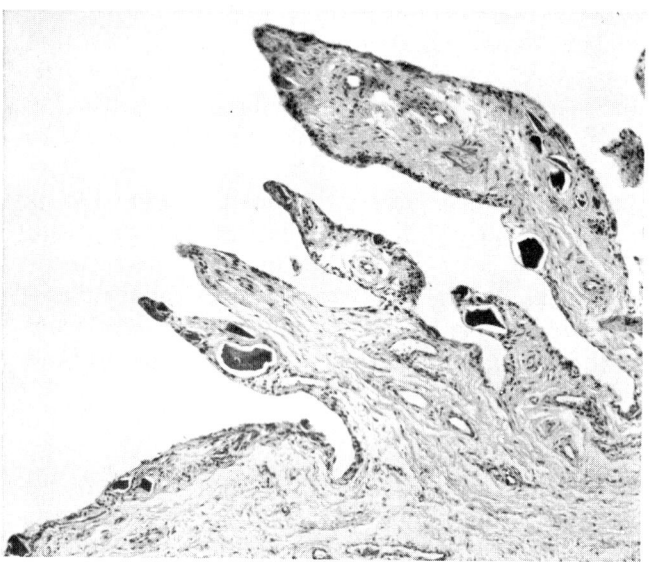

around the knee joint. They are often not tender and may be freely movable. Surgical removal may be necessary when the bodies interfere with motion.

The radiographic appearance of the large peripheral joints in ochronotic arthritis, virtually indistinguishable from that of primary osteoarthritis, demonstrates

FIG. 111–5. Synovial tissue in ochronotic arthropathy. Numerous pigmented deposits are present. A polypoid nodule has formed in the central portion as an osteochondroid reaction of the displaced cartilage fragments.

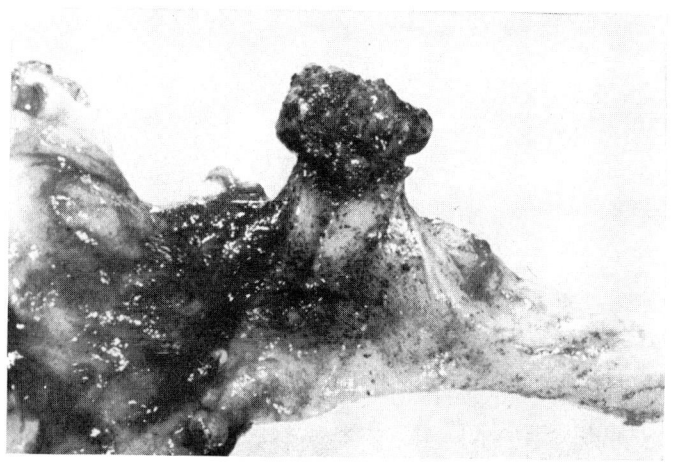

narrowing of the joint space, small marginal osteophytes, and eburnation. Rarely the diagnosis is first suggested at knee arthroscopy or surgery when the black pigmentation is encountered unexpectedly.[23] Protrusio acetabuli may be seen.[18] Ossification or calcification of the ligaments and tendons near the joints may be present.[24] Rupture of deeply pigmented ochronotic Achilles tendons has been reported.

In contrast to rheumatoid arthritis (RA) and osteoarthritis, the small joints of the hands and feet are rarely affected in ochronosis.

EXPERIMENTAL AND NONALKAPTONURIC PRODUCTION OF OCHRONOSIS

Rats fed with 8% L-tyrosine for 18 to 24 months develop pigment deposition in joint capsules and cartilages and a degenerative arthritis similar to that of spontaneous human alkaptonuria.[25] The cartilage pigment is melanin-like and includes phenolic bodies as in homogentisic acid or its metabolite benzoquinoneacetic acid.

A grossly bluish black connective tissue pigmentation associated with degenerative arthritis has also been described following prolonged administration of quinacrine in the absence of alkaptonuria. Ochronosis-like skin pigmentation attributed to enormous elastotic fibers has occurred in some blacks using hydroquinone bleaching creams.[26] Application of phenol dressings has been reported to produce ochronosis with alkaptonuria and arthropathy. Cartilage pigmentation does not occur in metastatic malignant melanoma.

TREATMENT

It is not yet feasible to compensate for the enzymatic deficiency of homogentisic acid oxidase. Attempts have been made to treat patients with a diet low in phenylalanine and tyrosine that is, unfortunately, unpalatable. Urinary excretion of homogentisic acid can be decreased, but clinical change was minimal in patients with advanced joint disease. Initiation of this diet at an early age before massive ochronosis develops has not been tried. Reduced protein intake can also decrease urine homogentisic acid levels, but this regimen is impractical for routine treatment. Although high doses of ascorbic acid do not decrease total urine homogentisic acid levels, they have been reported to reduce binding to connective tissue in experimental alkaptonuria of rats.[27] Long-term use of ascorbic acid has not been useful in limited trials in human ochronosis.

Symptomatic measures are of most practical value. Analgesics, braces, a program limiting joint overuse, and weight reduction have all provided some help. Adrenal corticosteroids, x irradiation, tyrosinase, insulin, various vitamins, and phenylbutazone are among the measures tried without benefit. Corrective orthopedic procedures have been helpful in several patients.[28]

HEMOCHROMATOSIS

Hemochromatosis is a chronic disease first recognized by Trousseau in 1865 and characterized pathologically by excessive iron deposition and fibrosis in many organs and tissues with ultimate functional impairment in untreated patients. This disorder occurs in a clinically detectable form in at least 1 in 7000 people in various populations of European origin. Clinical disease occurs five times more often in men than in women. Frequent clinical manifestations are hepatomegaly and cirrhosis, skin pigmentation, mostly from increased melanin, diabetes, other endocrine dysfunction, and heart failure.[29,30] Sicca syndrome has been reported, possibly adding to confusion with other rheumatic diseases.[31] Arthropathy occurs in 20 to 40% of patients. Hemochromatosis is often idiopathic, with a definite increased familial incidence first recognized by Sheldon in 1935.[30] It is inherited as an autosomal recessive trait. That patients have an increased frequency of HLA-A3 and HLA-B14 antigens suggests a hemochromatosis locus tightly linked to the HLA region on chromosome 6.[32] Because HLA haplotypes linked to the hemochromatosis alleles differ from family to family, HLA typing is best used after an index case has been identified in a family. Hemochromatosis can also be a late result of alcoholic cirrhosis or occasionally of multiple transfusions, refractory anemia, and long-term excessive oral iron ingestion. In all instances, iron absorption is excessive. Significant overload occurs only after many years, so the onset of symptoms is most common between 40 and 60 years. A form of hemochromatosis occurring before age 30 is often associated with hypogonadism and cardiac involvement. This is not obviously familial but may be associated with arthropathy as occurs in older patients.[33] Tables 111–2 and 111–3 list diagnostic features of hemochromatosis and its related arthropathy.

Table 111–2. Diagnostic Features of Hemochromatosis

Cirrhosis with iron deposition, predominantly in parenchymal cells
Iron deposition in other organs causing cardiomyopathy, diabetes, or other endocrine deficiencies
Increased skin pigmentation, largely by melanin
Elevated serum iron concentration and saturated iron-binding capacity

Table 111–3. Diagnostic Features of Arthropathy of Hemochromatosis

Degenerative arthropathy
Prominent involvement of metacarpophalangeal and proximal and distal interphalangeal joints, hips, and knees.
Chondrocalcinosis
Iron deposition in synovial lining cells

PATHOLOGIC FEATURES AND PATHOGENESIS

Iron as hemosiderin can be identified histologically in all the symptomatically affected tissues, as well as elsewhere. The largest iron deposits are in the liver, and diagnosis is most frequently established by liver biopsy. Large amounts of hemosiderin are seen in parenchymal cells in the liver and in other organs. Iron confined to reticuloendothelial tissues is termed hemosiderosis and does not produce the clinical picture seen in hemochromatosis. Although suspected, the iron has not been proved to be the cause of the tissue damage. Organ fibrosis, as in hemochromatosis, has not yet been produced by experimental iron overload alone. Iron may act in an additive fashion with nutritional deficiencies, alcohol, or other, still unidentified, hereditary factors.

DIAGNOSIS

The most important simple diagnostic laboratory test is the determination of serum iron concentration and the percentage of saturation of iron-binding capacity. Both values are elevated in hemochromatosis, but they can also be elevated in hemolytic anemia and other situations. Greater than 50% saturation of iron-binding capacity should raise consideration of hemochromatosis. Serum ferritin concentrations are often elevated, but may be normal in precirrhotic disease.[34] Magnetic resonance imaging showing reduced signal intensity can suggest liver iron overload.[35] Liver biopsy is needed to determine the extent of tissue iron deposition and the degree of tissue damage. One case of hemochromatosis with associated hypoxanthine-guanine phosphoribosyltransferase deficiency has been recorded where serum-iron concentrations and transferrin saturation were normal.[36]

OSTEOPENIA

Diffuse demineralization of bone can be seen, but its frequency and relationship to the hemochromatosis are difficult to ascertain. A diffuse osteopenia of the hands, without the periarticular demineralization as seen in RA, is most common. The mechanism for osteopenia is not known. Delbarre, who studied this topic extensively, postulated an androgen deficiency secondary to hemochromatosis.[37] Serum calcium, phosphorus, and alkaline phosphatase levels are normal. Biopsy specimens have shown osteoporosis rather than osteomalacia. Experimental acute iron overload can produce iron deposits in osteoblasts and trabeculae with decreased osteoblast numbers and activity.[38] More study of human hemochromatotic bone is needed. Because osteopenia is also seen in alcoholic cirrhosis, a direct relation to the defect in iron metabolism is not established.

DEGENERATIVE ARTHROPATHY AND CHONDROCALCINOSIS

An arthropathy associated with hemochromatosis was first described in 1964,[39] and since then more than 300 cases have been reported.[40-44] The most frequent joint involvement is degenerative, occurring in 20 to 50% of patients with hemochromatosis.[42] The age of onset varies from 20 to 70, but it is most common in the sixth decade. The onset of arthropathy is usually close in time to the onset of other symptoms of hemochromatosis, but joint symptoms and findings may antedate other clinical manifestations of hemochromatosis and may thus be the first clue to diagnosis.[41,45] Joint symptoms occasionally are first noted many years later, even after completion of phlebotomy therapy.

Hands, knees, and hips are most frequently involved, although other joints including the feet can be affected. Characteristic hand findings are a firm, only mildly tender, enlargement of the metacarpophalangeal and the proximal and distal interphalangeal joints. The second and third metacarpophalangeal joints are most often affected (Fig. 111-6). These joints are stiff and have limited motion, but no increased warmth or erythema. Ulnar deviation is not seen. Involvement is generally symmetric. Pain, when present, is accentuated on use. Morning stiffness usually lasts less than half an hour. This arthropathy is gradually progressive. Acute inflammation has occasionally been described, and whether it is always due to associated chondrocalcinosis and crystal-induced synovitis is not certain. Test results for rheumatoid factor are typically negative. Sedimentation rates are only occasionally elevated. Serum uric acid levels are generally normal and occasionally low.[36]

Roentgenograms often show the characteristic involvement of the metacarpophalangeal, proximal, and distal interphalangeal joints. Narrowing of the joint space, subchondral cysts, joint-space irregularity, subchondral sclerosis, and moderate bony proliferation with frequent hook-like osteophytes are seen[39,46] (Fig. 111-7). In 30 to 60% of those with arthropathy, especially older patients, chondrocalcinosis is also seen. Roentgenograms of other joints show changes similar to those in the hands and are often indistinguishable from degenerative arthritis and idiopathic chondrocalcinosis. Involvement of metacarpophalangeal joints 4 and 5 is rare in idiopathic chondrocalcinosis and is most suggestive of underlying hemochromatosis.

Synovial fluid is usually noninflammatory, with low leukocyte counts and predominantly mononuclear cells, adequate viscosity, and a pale yellow color. Iron measurements on synovial fluid are comparable to serum levels.[43] Synovial tissue shows a striking deposition of iron, mostly in the synovial lining cells, but also in some deeper cells. On hematoxylin and eosin staining, golden brown hemosiderin granules are seen. The iron can also be stained blue by Prussian blue (Fig. 111-8). By electron microscopy, the iron is principally seen in type B or synthetic lining cells (Fig. 111-9).[47] This distribution of synovial iron differs from that in hemarthrosis, RA, and other diseases in which iron is presumably derived from gross or microscopic bleeding into the joint. In these conditions, the iron is mostly found in deeper cells and macrophages. In addition to the iron, most synovial membranes in hemochromatosis show only mild lining-cell proliferation, fibrosis, and scattered chronic inflammatory cells. Biopsies of synovium during bouts of acute inflammation have not been reported.

Chondrocalcinosis with hemochromatosis, although usually associated with degenerative arthropathy, can also be an isolated joint finding.[45] Calcification is most commonly detected in menisci and articular cartilages at the knee, but it can also be seen at the wrists, fingers, elbows, shoulders, hips, ankles, toes, symphysis pubis, intervertebral discs, and the periarticular soft tissues and bursae.

Iron staining of cartilage has also been noted, but this characteristic is seen in chondrocytes and at the line of ossification, not at the crystal deposits.[47,48] Similarly, x ray diffraction and chemical studies have shown no iron at the sites of cartilage calcification.[42,48] Periarticular and bursal calcifications have not been studied to determine the type of calcium salt. Crystals

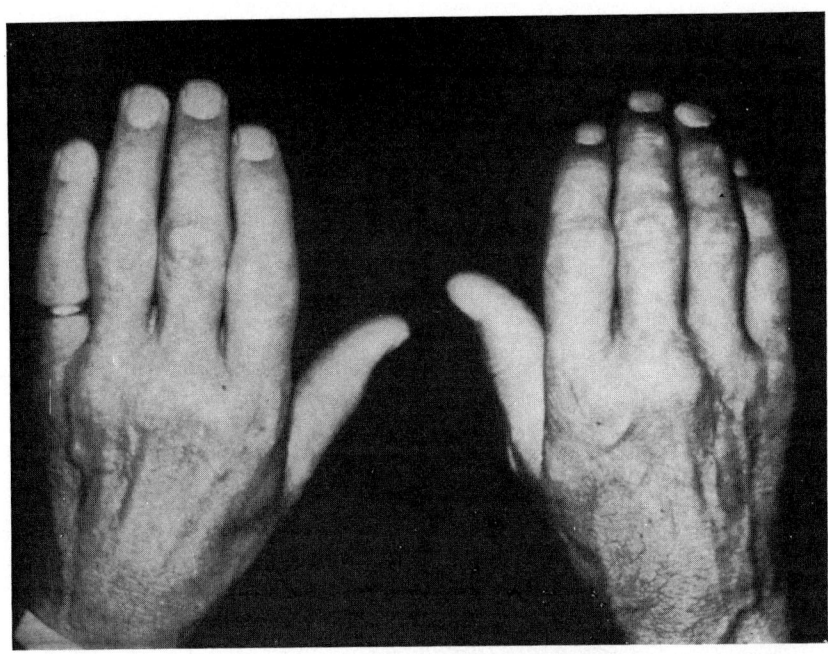

FIG. 111–6. Photograph of the hands of a 45-year-old man with hemochromatosis. Note the knobby enlargement at the metacarpophalangeal, proximal interphalangeal, and distal interphalangeal joints. He is unable to extend these joints fully.

resembling hydroxyapatite have been identified in hemochromatotic synovium and cartilage by electron microscopy.[47,48] Even when no calcification is radiographically visible, cartilage calcium pyrophosphate crystals or apatite are often identifiable by light and electron microscopy.[48]

POSSIBLE MECHANISMS FOR ARTHROPATHY

It is attractive to speculate that the iron directly or indirectly causes the osteoarthropathy, but such has

not been demonstrated. Arthropathy has only occasionally been reported in patients with transfusion siderosis[49,50]; this finding suggests that factors other than iron deposition are required. Patients with spherocytosis appear to develop iron overload only when they are also heterozygous for the hemochromatosis gene.[51] Many patients with iron-loading anemias do not survive long enough to develop tissue damage. Aseptic necrosis and osteopenia, but no other arthropathy, have been reported so far in Bantu siderosis. Kashin-Beck disease, an endemic growth disturbance and premature generalized degenerative

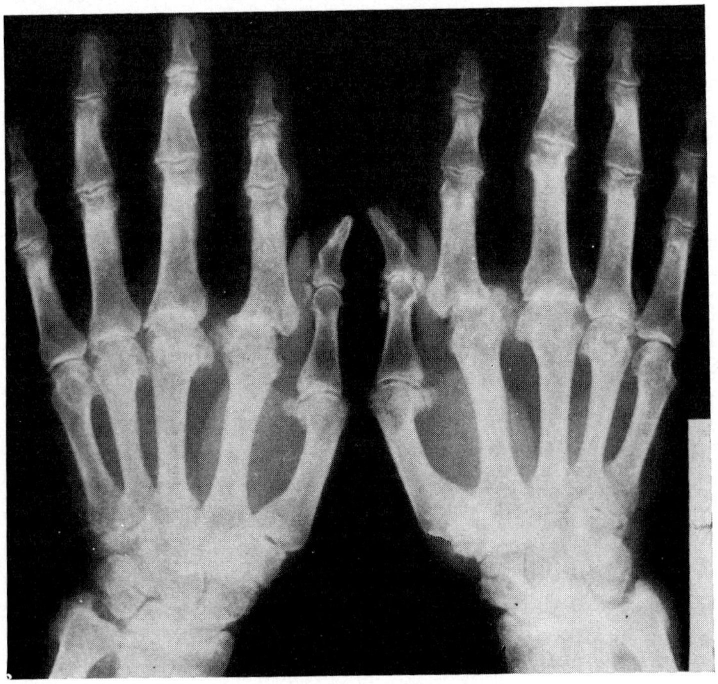

FIG. 111–7. Roentgenogram of hands showing involvement of the metacarpophalangeal and the proximal and distal interphalangeal joints, with characteristic joint-space narrowing, cystic subchondral lesions, joint-space irregularity, subluxation, some osteophytosis, and areas of bony sclerosis. Multiple periarticular calcifications are also present in the interphalangeal joint of the left thumb, and probable chondrocalcinosis is seen at the right ulnocarpal joint. Osteopenia is minimal in these hands.

FIG. 111–8. Synovium in hemochromatosis with dark Prussian blue–stained iron granules in the synovial lining cells (×400).

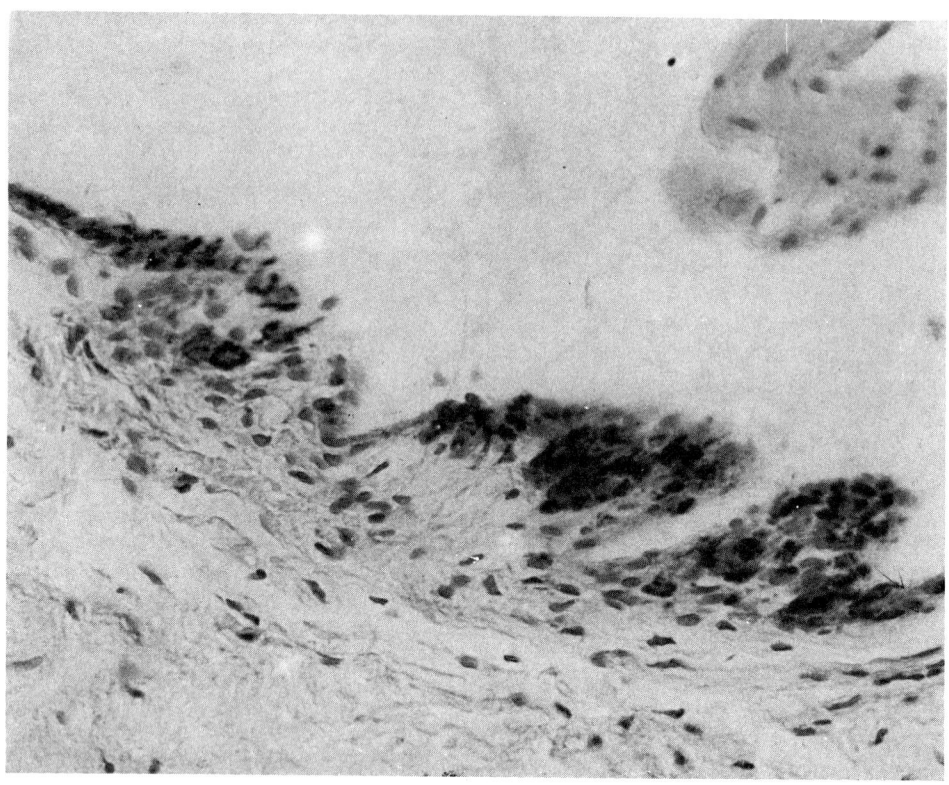

arthritis seen in Russia and Manchuria, has been attributed by Hiyeda to a high iron content in drinking water.[52] Hiyeda administered iron to vigorously exercised rabbits and believed that this regimen accelerated cartilage deterioration. That experimental iron loading of rabbits produced cartilage degeneration only when initiated early in life suggests the importance of early initiation of the toxic effect of iron.[53] Localized predominately in synthetic-type cells in cartilage or synovium, iron might cause joint damage by altering the protein polysaccharide or collagen produced by such cells. Iron can injure chondrocytes or other cells by lipid peroxidation of membranes. Ferric ion can irreversibly oxidize ascorbic acid and can impair hydroxylation of proline and thus allow deficient collagen formation.[53] Iron might produce damage by binding to connective tissue protein polysaccharides as it does in vitro in the Hale stain for protein polysaccharide. Some iron is present in lysosomes, and it could increase the release of lysosomal enzymes.

Iron in vitro inhibits pyrophosphatase and might in this manner help to allow the deposition of the calcium pyrophosphate of chondrocalcinosis.[54] Experimental synovial siderosis also inhibited clearance of calcium pyrophosphate crystals from rabbit joints.[55]

The primary site of joint damage is not established. The cartilage is most suspect in this degenerative process, but subchondral bone or synovial involvement may also be important because cartilage depends on both these areas for nutrition. No correlation has been found between the presence of advanced liver disease, generalized osteopenia, diabetes, or other endrocrine disease and the arthropathy. Classic RA has been reported to coexist in several cases, so the arthropathy is not an iron-altered rheumatoid disease.

TREATMENT

Present therapy of hemochromatosis is directed at prompt removal of the excess iron by phlebotomy, and this approach appears to reverse cardiac failure, to improve liver function, and to ameliorate diabetes. Improvement depends largely on the amount of existing tissue damage. Calcium pyrophosphate dihydrate crystal deposition is not reversed by such therapy. Prevention certainly would be preferable, so serum iron concentrations of relatives should be checked, and prophylactic phlebotomy should be

FIG. 111–9. Electron micrograph of electron-dense iron deposits in Type B synovial lining cells (B) in hemochromatosis. Type B cells are primarily synthetic in function and have profuse rough endoplasmic reticulum (ER). The type A cells (A) often have prominent filopodia and vacuoles and are believed to be more active in phagocytosis. Here they contain no identifiable iron (×13,000).

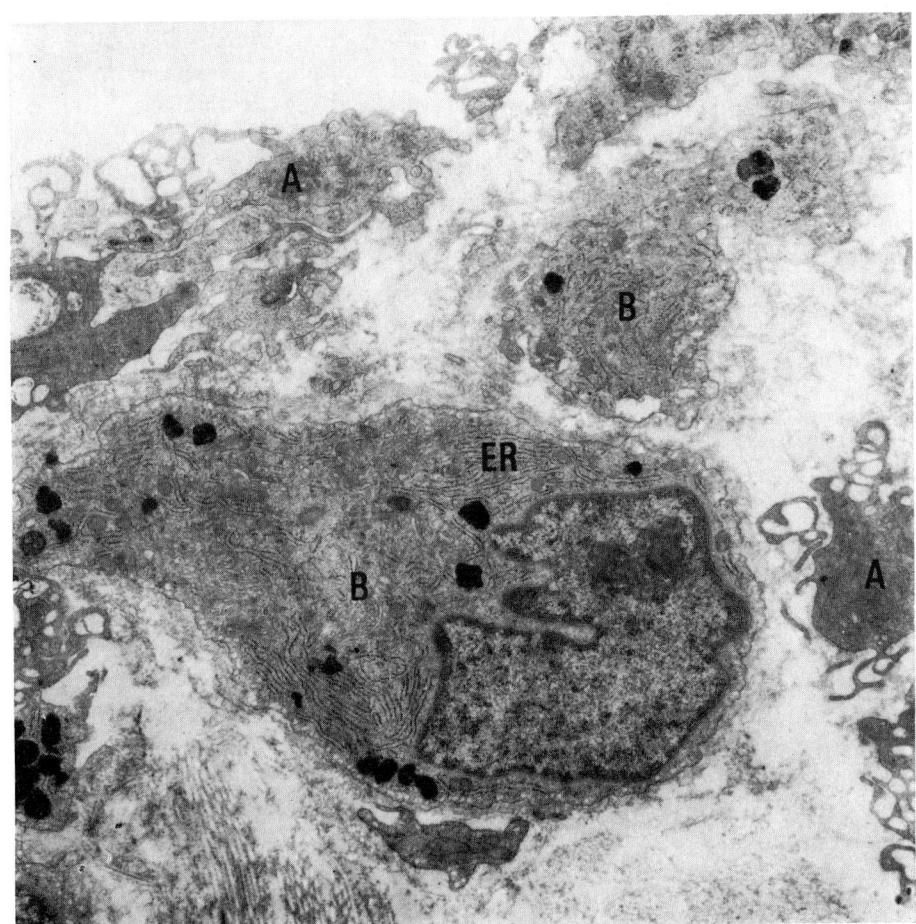

considered. Phlebotomy of 500 ml per week, until the development of mild iron deficiency anemia or demonstrable depletion of liver iron, is usual. Maintenance phlebotomy every 2 to 3 months is usually needed. Alcohol and excessive vitamin C ingestion can increase iron absorption and should be avoided.[56] Supportive treatment of the diabetes, liver disease, and heart failure is pursued as needed. Phlebotomy has not had any beneficial effect on the arthritis; arthritis and chondrocalcinosis may progress[42] and clinical arthritis has even developed after therapeutic phlebotomy. Irreversible connective tissue and joint change may well become established long before arthritis can be clinically or radiographically detected. Iron is easily demonstrable in the synovium of asymptomatic patients. Treatment of the arthritis is symptomatic; analgesics, nonsteroidal anti-inflammatory drugs, and systematic range-of-motion exercises are

most helpful. Prosthetic hip and knee arthroplasties have been successfully performed in patients with advanced disease, although further breakdown after 18 months has occurred in a knee after prosthetic arthroplasty.

WILSON'S DISEASE

Hepatolenticular degeneration (Wilson's disease), described by Wilson in 1912,[57] is an uncommon familial disease characterized by a ring of golden brown pigment at the corneal margin, known as the Kayser-Fleischer ring, sometimes visible only on slit-lamp examination, basal ganglion degeneration, and cirrhosis. The condition is inherited as an autosomal recessive trait. Symptoms may first appear between the ages of 4 and 50. Neurologic symptoms are usually earliest and include tremor, rigidity, dysarthria, incoordination, or personality change. Many patients also develop renal tubular disease manifested by aminoaciduria, proteinuria, glucosuria, renal stones, phosphaturia, defective urine acidification, or uricosuria. Uricosuria often results in low serum uric acid levels. Hemolytic anemia can occur. Untreated disease is invariably fatal.[58]

Characteristic disorders of copper metabolism are present.[59] Copper concentrations are increased in liver, brain, and other tissues; urine copper excretion is increased; and the serum copper-binding protein, ceruloplasmin, as well as total serum copper are almost always decreased. Measurement of the hepatic copper concentration appears to be the most reliable test. Although the basic underlying defect is not known, increased absorption of copper can be demonstrated. Copper may cause the tissue damage. Mobilization of copper from the body seems to produce an improvement in many patients. Although seen in at least 95% of patients, Kayser-Fleischer rings are not entirely specific and may be seen in other diseases.[60] Table 111–4 lists osseous and articular changes in Wilson's disease.

OSTEOPENIA

Radiographic evidence of demineralization of bone has long been recognized as part of Wilson's disease and is described in 25 to 50% of patients.[61,62] Osteopenia is seen at all ages and usually is asymptomatic. Occasional patients have pathologic fractures. Others have definite rickets,[63] or osteomalacia that can be attributed to the renal tubular disease.

ARTHROPATHY

Boudin, et al. first described articular alterations in Wilson's disease in 1957.[64] Joint changes are rare in childhood, but are seen in up to 50% of adults. Most patients studied have been 20 to 40 years old. Articular involvement ranges from premature osteoarthritis with pronounced symptoms to asymptomatic radio-

Table 111–4. Bone and Joint Changes in Wilson's Disease

Bone demineralization
Occasionally, rickets or osteomalacia attributable to renal tubular disease
Premature degenerative arthritis with prominent subchondral bone fragmentation
Prominent involvement of wrists, knees, and, less often, other joints
Periarticular calcifications and bone fragments

graphic findings.[61,62,65–69] Scattered subchondral bone fragmentations, cortical irregularity, and sclerosis at the margin of wrist, hand, elbow, shoulder, hip, and knee joints are seen (Fig. 111–10). The cartilage space is also often narrowed. Early age of onset and prominent involvement of wrists suggest a difference from the usual osteoarthritis. Tiny periarticular cysts,[62] vertebral wedging and marginal irregularity,[69] osteochondritis dissecans, and chondromalacia patellae[65] have been seen in several patients and may be related to Wilson's disease. Periarticular calcifications are common; many such calcifications occur in ligaments, tendons, and capsule insertions. Other calcifications seem to represent bone fragments. There is occasional radiographic evidence of chondrocalcinosis.[65,66,69] The cause of the chondrocalcinosis has not been well studied. Although copper could be identified in some cartilages by elemental analysis, calcium crystals were not found in one recent light and electron microscopic study.[68] Joint effusions are usually small, with clear, viscous fluid and 200 to 300 cells/mm³, predominantly mononuclear cells.[65,67] Synovial fluid copper and ceruloplasmin levels have not been studied. Only mild lining-cell hyperplasia and small numbers of chronic inflammatory cells have been noted on synovial biopsies.[67]

No correlation has been found between the severity of the disease, spasticity and tremors, osteopenia, liver or renal disease and the arthropathy. The primary defect may occur in the cartilage or subchondral bone, but no histologic or chemical studies of these tissues have been conducted. Although the joint involvement in Wilson's disease is generally milder, an analogy can be made with that of hemochromatosis. In both diseases, the metal excess is a possible mechanism for direct or indirect production of the arthropathy. Short-term experimental copper loading has not produced arthropathy. McCarty and Pepe have shown in vitro inhibition of inorganic cytosolic pyrophosphatase by cupric as well as by ferrous ions and have suggested this inhibition as a possible mechanism for deposition of calcium pyrophosphate producing chondrocalcinosis in Wilson's disease and hemochromatosis.[54]

TREATMENT

Penicillamine, 1 to 4 g/day orally, is the most successful chelating agent for mobilizing copper from the tissue and has produced definite clinical improvement in mental and neurologic changes in many patients. Treatment must be continued for life. Low-copper diets and potassium sulfide may also be used to de-

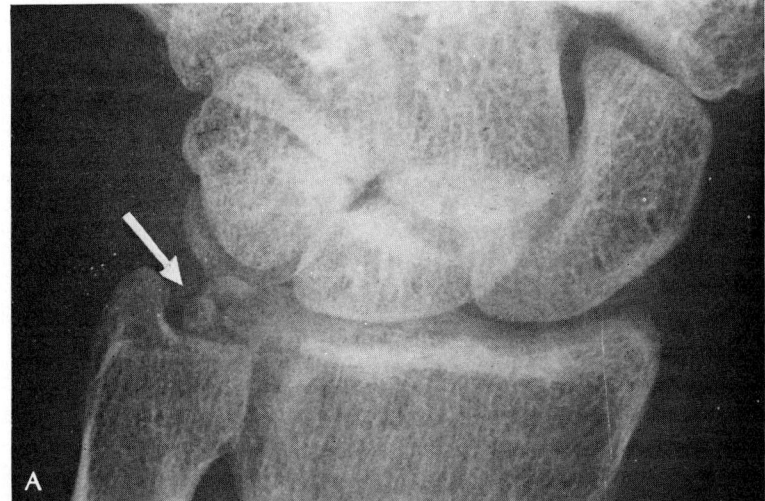

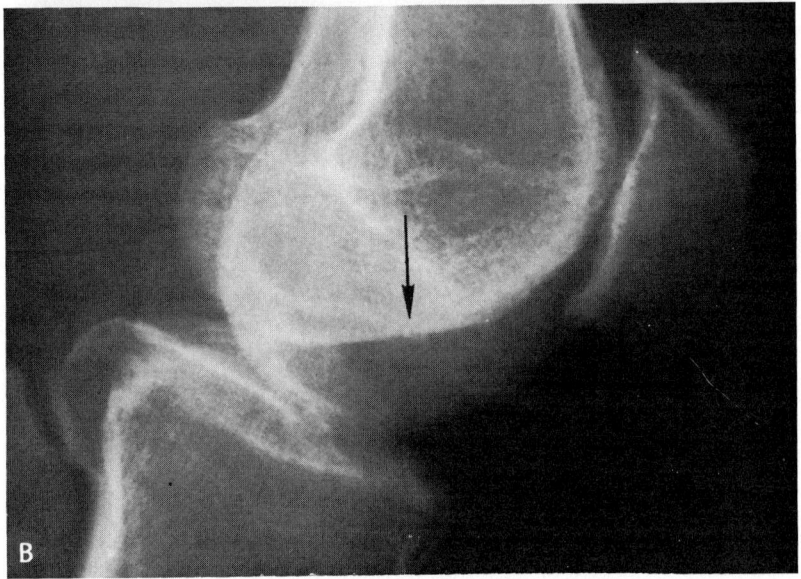

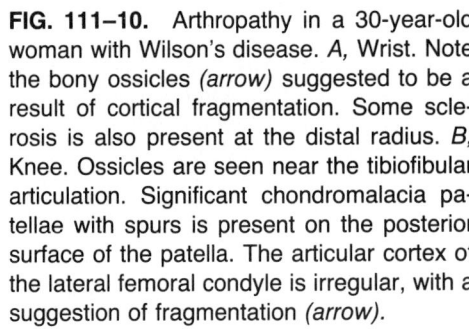

FIG. 111–10. Arthropathy in a 30-year-old woman with Wilson's disease. *A*, Wrist. Note the bony ossicles *(arrow)* suggested to be a result of cortical fragmentation. Some sclerosis is also present at the distal radius. *B*, Knee. Ossicles are seen near the tibiofibular articulation. Significant chondromalacia patellae with spurs is present on the posterior surface of the patella. The articular cortex of the lateral femoral condyle is irregular, with a suggestion of fragmentation *(arrow)*.

crease copper absorption. Symptomatic disease may be preventable by early D-penicillamine treatment of asymptomatic persons with biochemical abnormalities only.[70] Occasional patients treated with penicillamine still develop arthropathy. Whether early and long-term treatment will decrease the bone and joint disease is not yet known. Occasionally, penicillamine appears to cause polymyositis or lupus-like syndromes. Acute polyarthritis complicated penicillamine therapy in five patients with Wilson's disease.[66] There is some controversy about the safety of penicillamine in pregnancy.[71,72] Recent reports suggest that zinc[73] or trientine, a newer chelating agent,[72] may be considered as an alternative therapy in patients who cannot tolerate penicillamine.

REFERENCES

1. LaDu, B.N., et al.: The nature of the defect in tyrosine metabolism in alcaptonuria. J. Biol. Chem., *230*:251–260, 1958.

2. Knox, W.E.: Sir Archibald Garrod's inborn errors of metabolism. II. Alkaptonuria. Am. J. Hum. Genet., *10*:95–124, 1958.

3. Gaucher, A., et al.: HLA antigens and alkaptonuria. J. Rheumatol., *3*(Suppl.):97–100, 1977.

4. Lee, S., and Schoen, I.: Black copper reduction reaction simulating alkaptonuria—occurrence after intravenous urography. N. Engl. J. Med., *275*:266–267, 1966.

5. Kelley, W.M., et al.: Significant laboratory artifacts in alkaptonuria. Arthritis Rheum., *12*:673, 1969.

6. Seegmiller, J.E., et al.: An enzymatic spectrophotometric method for the determination of homogentisic acid in plasma and urine. J. Biol. Chem., *236*:774–777, 1961.

7. Zannoni, V.G., Malawista, S.E., and LaDu, B.N.: Studies on ochronosis. II. Studies on benzoquinoneacetic acid, a probable intermediate in the connective tissue pigmentation of alcaptonuria. Arthritis Rheum., *5*:547–556, 1962.

8. Murray, J.C., Lindberg, K.A., and Pinnell, S.R.: In vitro inhibition of chick embryo lysyl hydroxylase by homogentisic acid. J. Clin. Invest., *59*:1071–1079, 1977.

9. Lichenstein, L., and Kaplan, L.: Hereditary ochronosis: Pathologic changes observed in 2 necropsied cases. Am. J. Pathol., *30*:99–125, 1954.

10. O'Brien, W.M., LaDu, B.N., and Bunim, J.J.: Biochemistry, pathologic and clinical aspects of alcaptonuria, ochronosis and ochronotic arthropathy. Am. J. Med., 34:813–838, 1963.
11. Levine, H.D., et al.: Aortic valve replacement for ochronosis of the aortic valve. Chest, 74:466–467, 1978.
12. Bywaters, E.G.L., Dorling, J., and Sutor, J.: Ochronosis densification. (Abstract) Arthritis Rheum. Dis., 29:563, 1970.
13. Deeb, Z., and Frayha, R.: Multiple vacuum disks, an early sign of ochronosis: Radiologic findings in 2 biopsies. J. Rheumatol., 3:82–87, 1976.
14. Hunter, T., Gordon, D.A., and Ogryzlo, M.A.: The ground pepper sign of synovial fluid: A new diagnostic feature of ochronosis. J. Rheumatol., 1:45–53, 1974.
15. Reginato, A.J., Schumacher, H.R., and Martinez, V.A.: Ochronotic arthropathy with calcium pyrophosphate crystal deposition. Arthritis Rheum., 16:705–714, 1973.
16. Huttl, S.: Synovial effusion. A nosographic and diagnostic study. Part I. Acta Rheum. Baln. Pistiniana, 5:1–100, 1970.
17. Lagier, R.: The concept of osteoarthritic remodeling as illustrated by ochronotic arthropathy of the hip: An anatomico-radiological approach. Virchows Arch. (Pathol. Anat.), 385:293–308, 1981.
18. Schumacher, H.R., and Holdsworth, D.E.: Ochronotic arthropathy. 1. Clinicopathologic studies. Semin. Arthritis Rheum., 6:207–246, 1977.
19. McClure, J., Smith, P.S., and Gramp, A.A.: Calcium pyrophosphate dihydrate (CPPD) deposition in ochronotic arthropathy. J. Clin. Pathol., 36:894–902, 1983.
20. Rynes, R.J., Sosman, J.L., and Holdsworth, D.E.: Pseudogout in ochronosis: Report of a case. Arthritis Rheum., 18:21–25, 1975.
21. Mohr, W., Wessinghage, D., and Lendschaw, E.: Die Ultrastruktur von Hyalinem Knorpel und Gelenkkapsel-gewebe bei der alkaptonurischen Ochronose. Z. Rheumatol., 39:55–73, 1980.
22. O'Brien, W.M., Banfield, W.G., and Sokoloff, L.: Studies on the pathogenesis of ochronotic arthropathy. Arthritis Rheum., 4:137–152, 1961.
23. Lurie, D.P., and Musil, D.: Knee arthropathy in ochronosis: Diagnosis by arthroscopy with ultrastructural features. J. Rheumatol., 11:101–103, 1984.
24. MacKenzie, C.R., Major, P., and Hunter, T.: Tendon involvement in a case of ochronosis. J. Rheumatol., 9:634–636, 1982.
25. Blivaiss, B.B., Rosenberg, E.F., Katuzov, H., and Stoner, R.: Experimental ochronosis: Induction in rats by long-term feeding of L-tyrosine. A.M.A. Arch. Pathol., 82:45–53, 1966.
26. Horshaw, R.A., Zimmerman, K.G., and Menter, A.: Ochronosis-like pigmentation from hydroquinone bleaching creams in American Blacks. Arch. Dermatol., 121:105–108, 1985.
27. Lustberg, T.J., Schulman, J.D., and Seegmiller, J.E.: Decreased binding of ^{14}C-homogentisic acid induced by ascorbic acid in connective tissue of rats with experimental alcaptonuria. Nature, 222:770–771, 1970.
28. Detenbeck, L.C., Young, H.H., and Underdahl, L.O.: Ochronotic arthropathy. Arch. Surg., 110:215–219, 1970.
29. Finch, S.C., and Finch, C.A.: Idiopathic hemochromatosis: An iron storage disease. Medicine, 34:381–430, 1955.
30. Sheldon, J.H.: Haemochromatosis. London, Oxford University Press, 1935.
31. Blandford, R.L., et al.: Sicca syndrome associated with idiopathic hemochromatosis. Br. Med. J., 1:1323, 1979.
32. Cartwright, G.E., Edwards, C.Q., and Kravitz, K.: Hereditary hemochromatosis: Phenotypic expression of the disease. N. Engl. J. Med., 301:175–179, 1979.
33. Goldschmidt, H., et al.: Idiopathic hemochromatosis presenting as arthropathy and amenorrhea in a young woman. Am. J. Med., 82:1057–1059, 1987.
34. Wands, J.R., et al.: Normal serum ferritin concentrations in precirrhotic hemochromatosis. N. Engl. J. Med., 294:302–305, 1976.
35. Murphy, F.B., and Bernardino, M.E.: MR imaging of focal hemochromatosis. J. Comput. Assist. Tomogr., 10:1044–1046, 1986.
36. Rosner, I.A., et al.: Arthropathy, hypouricemia, and normal serum iron studies in hereditary hemochromatosis. Am. J. Med., 70:870–874, 1981.
37. Delbarre, F.: L'Ostéoporose des hémochromatoses. Sem. Hop. Paris, 36:3279–3294, 1960.
38. deVernejoul, M.C., et al.: Effects of iron overload on bone remodelling on pigs. Am. J. Pathol., 116:377–383, 1984.
39. Schumacher, H.R.: Hemochromatosis and arthritis. Arthritis Rheum., 7:41–50, 1964.
40. Delbarre, F.: Les manifestations ostéo-articulaires de l'hémochromatose. Presse Med., 72:2973–2978, 1964.
41. Dymock, I.W., et al.: Arthropathy of hemochromatosis. Ann. Rheum. Dis., 29:469–476, 1970.
42. Hamilton, E.B., et al.: The natural history of arthritis in idiopathic hemochromatosis: Progression of the clinical and radiological features over 10 years. Q.J. Med., 50:321–329, 1981.
43. Kra, S.J., Hollingsworth, J.W., and Finch, S.C.: Arthritis with synovial iron deposition in a patient with hemochromatosis. N. Engl. J. Med., 272:1268–1271, 1965.
44. Mitrovic, D., et al.: Etude histologique et histoclinique des lésion articulaires de la chondrocalcinose survenant au cous d'une hémochromatose. Arch. Anat. Pathol., 14:264–270, 1966.
45. Gordon, D.A., Clarke, P.V., and Ogryzlo, M.A.: The chondrocalcific arthropathy of iron overload. Arch. Intern. Med., 134:21–28, 1974.
46. Adamson, T.C., et al.: Hand and wrist arthropathies of hemochromatosis and calcium pyrophosphate deposition disease: Distinct radiographic features. Radiology, 147:377–381, 1983.
47. Schumacher, H.R.: Ultrastructural characteristics of the synovial membrane in idiopathic hemochromatosis. Ann. Rheum. Dis., 31:465–473, 1972.
48. Schumacher, H.R.: Articular cartilage in the degenerative arthropathy of hemochromatosis. Arthritis Rheum., 25:1460–1468, 1982.
49. Abbott, D.F., and Gresham, D.F.: Arthropathy in transfusional hemosiderosis. Br. Med. J., 1:418–419, 1972.
50. Sella, E.J., and Goodman, A.H.: Arthropathy secondary to transfusion hemochromatosis. J. Bone Joint Surg., 55A:1077–1081, 1973.
51. Mohler, D.N., and Wheby, M.S.: Case report: Hemochromatosis heterozygotes may have significant iron overload when they also have hereditary spherocytosis. Am. J. Med. Sci., 292:320–324, 1986.
52. Hiyeda, K.: On cause of endemic diseases prevailing in Manchoukuo (Kaschin-Beck's disease, so called Kokasan disease endemic goiter). Trans. Soc. Pathol. Jpn., 29:325–331, 1939.
53. Brighton, C.T., Bigley, E.C., and Smolenski, B.I.: Iron induced arthritis in immature rabbits. Arthritis Rheum., 13:849–857, 1970.
54. McCarty, D.J., and Pepe, P.F.: Erythrocyte neutral inorganic pyrophosphatase in pseudogout. J. Lab. Clin. Med., 79:277–284, 1972.
55. McCarty, D.J., Palmer, D.W., and Garancis, J.C.: Clearance of calcium pyrophosphate dihydrate crystals in vivo. III. Effects of synovial hemosiderosis. Arthritis Rheum., 24:706–710, 1981.
56. Cohen, A., Cohen, I.J., and Schwartz, E.: Scurvy and altered

iron stores in thalassemia major. N. Engl. J. Med., *304*:158–160, 1981.

57. Wilson, S.A.K.: Progressive lenticular degeneration: A familial nervous disease associated with cirrhosis of the liver. Brain, *34*:295–509, 1912.

58. Dobyns, W.B., Goldstein, N.P., and Gordon, H.: Clinical spectrum of Wilson's disease. Mayo Clin. Proc., *54*:35–42, 1979.

59. Perman, J.A., et al.: Laboratory measurements of copper metabolism in the differentiation of chronic active hepatitis and Wilson disease in children. J. Pediatr., *94*:564–568, 1979.

60. Weinberg, L.M., Brasitus, T.A., and Leskowitch, J.H.: Fluctuating Kayser-Fleischer-like rings in a jaundiced patient. Arch. Intern. Med., *142*:246–247, 1981.

61. Finby, N., and Bearn, A.G.: Roentgenographic abnormalities of the skeletal system in Wilson's disease (hepatolenticular degeneration). Am. J. Roentgenol., *79*:603–611, 1958.

62. Mindelzun, R., et al.: Skeletal changes in Wilson's disease: A radiological study. Radiology, *94*:127–132, 1970.

63. Cavallino, R., and Grossman, H.: Wilson's disease presenting with rickets. Radiology, *90*:493–494, 1968.

64. Boudin, G., et al.: Relapsing meningeal tuberculosis, cisternal blocking with symptoms similar to lethargic encephalitis (somnolence, ptosis, extrapyramidal syndromes). Bull. Soc. Med. Hop. Paris, *73*:559–561, 1957.

65. Feller, E., and Schumacher, H.R.: Osteoarticular changes in Wilson's disease. Arthritis Rheum., *15*:259–266, 1972.

66. Golding, D.N., and Walshe, J.M.: Arthropathy of Wilson's disease: Study of clinical and radiological features in 32 patients. Ann. Rheum. Dis., *36*:99–111, 1977.

67. Kaklamanis, P., and Spengos, M.: Osteoarticular change and synovial biopsy findings in Wilson's disease. Ann. Rheum. Dis., *32*:422–427, 1973.

68. Menerey, K., et al.: The arthropathy of Wilson's disease. J. Rheum., *15*:331–337, 1988.

69. Zakraoui, L., et al.: Les atteintes articulaires au cours de la maladie de Wilson. Rev. Rhum., *53*:345–348, 1986.

70. Sternlieb, I., and Scheinberg, I.H.: Prevention of Wilson's disease in asymptomatic patients. N. Engl. J. Med., *278*:352–359, 1968.

71. Endres, W.: D-Penicillamine in pregnancy—to ban or not to ban. Klin. Wochenschr., *59*:535–537, 1981.

72. Walshe, J.M.: The management of pregnancy in Wilson's disease treated with trientine. Q. J. Med., *58*:81–87, 1986.

73. Brewer, G.J., et al.: Treatment of Wilson's disease with oral zinc. Clin. Res., *29*:578A, 1981.

OSTEOPENIC BONE DISEASES

112

BEVRA H. HAHN

Diseases of bone constitute a major cause of pain and disability, especially in individuals over the age of 50. Many disorders can reduce bone mass until bone is inadequate to withstand the stresses of everyday life. Disability results from fractures, from increasing dorsal kyphosis, and from bone pain. The physiologic and histologic features of normal bone, methods of assessing bone mass, and methods of preventing and treating the most common metabolic bone diseases resulting in osteopenia are the subjects of this chapter.

PHYSIOLOGY OF NORMAL BONE

Bone has two major functions in humans: it provides a means of support, locomotion, and protection, and it serves as a reservoir of ions necessary to multiple body functions including calcium, phosphorus, magnesium, sodium, and carbonate metabolism. As with other body tissues, continual turnover and remodeling occur; during this process, rates of formation and rates of resorption are normally in equilibrium. The essential role of bone in maintaining normal ion and buffer concentrations in the extracellular fluid takes precedence over the supportive role when formation and resorption rates become uncoupled.

Bone is composed of connective tissue that becomes mineralized. Collagen, accounting for approximately 70% of the dry weight of bone, is its major component. Mucopolysaccharides, including chondroitin sulfate, keratan sulfate, and sialic acid, are also pres-

ent, as are recently discovered proteins including osteocalcin (gla-protein, a calcium-binding protein) and several glycoprotein growth factors that signal cells to proliferate. Bone collagen contains two α chains and one β chain; a mature collagen molecule consists of a left-hand helix coiled around another axis, which has a right-hand twist (see Chapter 12). Tropocollagen is formed by three such coils; its molecules stack together in rods. Mineralization begins in the spaces between rods. The mineral phase is composed predominantly of hydroxyapatite crystals.

During fetal life and early childhood, bones are formed from cartilaginous growth plates, which form the epiphysis and metaphysis of long bones and most of the mass of short bones such as vertebrae. The cortex of long bones derives from a perichondral area of new bone deposition. Until puberty, bone formation exceeds bone resorption. Bone growth is regulated by mechanical stimuli such as physical activity and weight bearing, which help to shape bone, and by the stimulus of several hormone systems including growth hormone and somatomedins. In adults, bone modeling has stopped, as has bone growth, and changes in bone are called *remodeling*.

The two major forms of mature mineralized bone are compact cortical bone, which forms the largest portion of long bones of the appendicular skeleton, and transverse interwoven trabecular bone, which forms the majority of bone in vertebral bodies and the flat bones of the skull and pelvis. Compact cortical bone is laid down around the haversian systems in ellipses or circles; the structure is more archlike in

1812

trabecular bone. The mechanical relationship of these types of bone and the direction in which they are laid down can be as important in determining skeletal strength as the total quantity of mineralized bone. Consider, for example, the high fracture rate in patients with Paget's disease, in whom the quantity of bone may be large in a given area, but in which structure is mechanically weak.

In both cortical and trabecular bone, the process of remodeling is continuous. Remodeling occurs from three "envelope" areas: from the haversian envelope, as shown in Figure 112–1; from the periosteal envelope; and from the endosteal envelope. The haversian envelope occurs within the structure of cortical bone and consists of tunneling canals in which bone is initially resorbed and then reformed.

The endosteal envelope covers the inner surface of the cortex and the trabecular bone surface, and separates bone from bone marrow. During adult life, the endosteal surface has a higher rate of resorption than formation; the bone marrow cavity consequently expands at the expense of the thickness of cortical and trabecular bone. Frost suggested the concept of bone modeling units, called basic multicellular units (Fig. 112–2). He suggested that two types of such units exist—one in which resorption is the major activity, and one in which bone formation is the major activity. These units occur on each skeletal envelope. In each basic multicellular unit, the following sequence of events occurs: (1) the unit is activated; (2) osteoclasts appear and begin to resorb bone, a process that takes on the average 2 weeks; (3) osteoblasts then synthesize osteoid, a process that takes approximately 6 weeks; and (4) mineralization of the new bone occurs. This entire process requires 2 to 6 months. In health, a steady state exists between rates of bone formation and resorption in the basic multicellular units. A number of factors can upset this balance, however, in-cluding change in the "birth rate" of new multicellular units, an uncoupling of rates of resorption and formation in multiple units, and failure to mineralize the osteoid that has been formed.

Adults have a wider variation in birth rates of basic multicellular units in the haversian and endosteal envelopes than in the periosteal envelope; loss of trabecular and cortical bone on the endosteal surface and loss of intracortical bone are more common than losses of subperiosteal bone. In cortical bone, remodeling caused by basic multicellular units occurs predominantly in the haversian system; in trabecular bone, remodeling occurs predominantly in Howship's lacunae. In most metabolic bone diseases in adults, the rate of remodeling determines whether total formation remains in equilibrium with resorption or whether bone is lost as the rates are uncoupled. The mechanisms by which these rates are controlled are largely unknown; several interesting reviews of this subject are available.[1-3]

Within the basic multicellular units, the origin of functional cells is clearly different. Osteoblasts are probably derived from precursor cells closely related to fibroblasts. They not only synthesize osteoid, but can produce matrix vesicles, which may be necessary for the initiation of mineralization. Osteoclasts, closely related to macrophages, are probably derived from bone marrow or from circulating monocytes that become functionally activated in haversian canals or Howship's lacunae. The osteocyte is a sessile bone cell—a mature osteoblast no longer capable of synthesizing either collagen or the ground substance of osteoid.

HORMONAL INFLUENCES

The movement of calcium and phosphorus ions in and out of the mineral phase of bone is under the

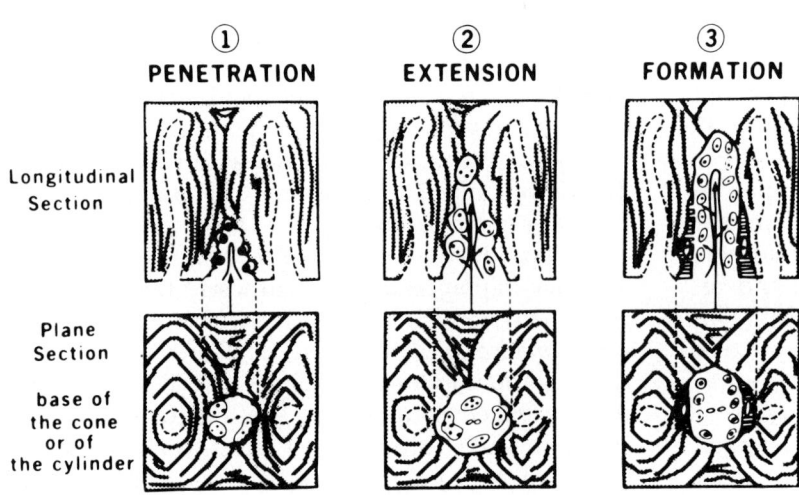

① **PENETRATION**   ② **EXTENSION**   ③ **FORMATION**

Longitudinal Section

Plane Section

base of the cone or of the cylinder

FIG. 112–1. A model of the sequential events in the formation of a new Haversian system in cortical bone (from Rasmussen, H., and Bordier, P.: The Physiological and Cellular Basis of Metabolic Bone Disease. Baltimore, Williams & Wilkins, 1974).

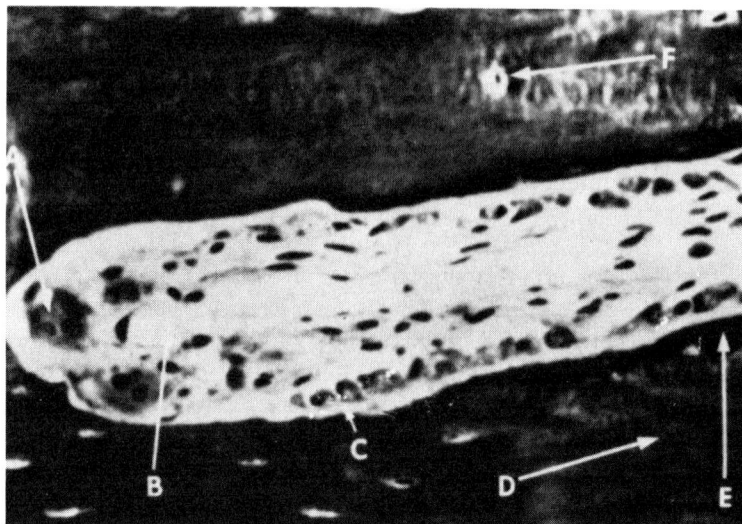

FIG. 112–2. A basic multicellular unit of bone; longitudinal section through an evolving Haversian system. At the front, the osteoclasts (A) are drilling a tunnel through the bone (D) from right to left, to make a temporary space filled by blood vessels and loose connective tissue (B). Further behind, the osteoblasts (C) lined up along the osteoid seam (E) are refilling the tunnel (from Parfitt, A.M.: Mineral Electrolyte Metab., 3:277, 1980; reprinted with permission of the publisher).

control of three major hormones: parathyroid hormone, the active metabolites of vitamin D, and calcitonin. Parathyroid hormone maintains the level of ionized calcium in the extracellular fluid by stimulating bone resorption, increasing resorption of calcium in the kidney tubules, and increasing intestinal calcium absorption by stimulating metabolism of vitamin D into its most active form, 1,25(OH)$_2$D. Parathyroid hormone is also capable of directly decreasing the synthesis of bone collagen. Vitamin D is formed in the skin from the conversion of 7-dehydrocholesterol to vitamin D$_3$ (cholecalciferol).[4] Cholecalciferol is hydroxylated to 25 OH D (calcifediol) in the liver and is further hydroxylated to 1,25(OH)$_2$D (calcitriol) in the kidney. Calcitriol is a potent stimulant of intestinal absorption of calcium and phosphorus. When this process is operating normally, calcitriol promotes bone growth and bone formation by providing adequate levels of mineral. When dietary intake of minerals is low, however, calcitriol is capable of directly resorbing calcium and phosphate from the skeleton. Calcitonin inhibits the resorption of calcium from bone, and thus reduces the concentrations of serum calcium. With age, the concentration of parathyroid hormone rises and the concentrations of 1,25(OH)$_2$D and calcitonin fall.

Several other hormones also influence bone, although their role is less clearly understood than that of the previously described hormones. Thyroid hormone is necessary for normal bone growth and remodeling, and excessive levels of thyroxin can stimulate bone resorption and a rapid birth rate of basic multicellular units. Sex hormones including estrogens, androgens, and progestins also affect bone. It has been thought for years that the decline in estrogen levels associated with menopause accounts for rapid loss of bone at that time. The effect of estrogen on bone may be indirect, mediated by lymphocytes or monocytes. However, recent data have suggested that osteoblast-like cells have receptors for estrogen, so there may be direct effects as well. As discussed in detail later, adrenal glucocorticoids also play an important role in skeletal remodeling. Pharmacologic levels decrease the intestinal absorption of calcium, the conversion of precursor cells to osteoblasts, and the formation of osteoid by osteoblasts. Physiologic levels are probably important in maintaining normal bone formation and resorption rates. Through its effects on somatomedins, growth hormone stimulates collagen synthesis and cell replication in adult bone, as well as growth in children. Insulin stimulates osteoblasts to synthesize collagen.

In addition to the hormones discussed, several others exert control over bone cell activation, acting as either paracrine or endocrine factors. Molecules that cause activation of bone resorption include interleukin-1 (IL-1), tumor necrosis factor (TNF-α and TNF-β), and prostaglandins (PG), especially of the E series. IL-1 is released by activated monocytes/macrophages as well as synovial lining cells and a few other cell types. It can probably cause bone resorption both locally and systemically. IL-1 release can be stimulated directly by antigens, T-cell products, and by TNF-α. IL-1 release from monocytes is accompanied by increased production of prostaglandin E$_2$, which causes feedback inhibition of IL-1 synthesis.[5] Evidence suggests that 1,25(OH)$_2$D can influence bone metabolism via regulation of IL-1 release. TNF-α is a product of activated monocytes/macrophages; TNF-β is released from activated lymphocytes. Both activate bone resorption locally through their effects on osteoblasts.

Each of these polypeptides, IL-1 and TNF, can also

act as mitogens for osteoblasts, thus promoting bone formation. For example, IL-1 reduces DNA synthesis by osteoblasts in vitro, unless prostaglandins are inhibited, in which case mitogenesis is increased.[5] Several other polypeptides act as growth factors for bone cells. These include somatomedins, especially insulinlike growth factor 1 (IGF-1); granulocyte-monocyte colony stimulating factor (GM-CSF); and platelet-derived growth factor. Polypeptides produced by bone cells also act as growth factors, such as bone morphogenetic protein and bone-derived growth factors I and II. Recent reviews treat the subject of hormones affecting bone resorption and formation in greater detail.[5-7] Mechanical stimulation of bone, probably modulated by the generation of small electrical currents, also enhances bone formation.

All these hormones have effects on both osteoblasts and osteoclasts, with the exception of calcitonin, which is a selective inhibitor of osteoclasts. The net results of interaction of these various hormones, mechanical stresses, and the components of the basic multicellular units at all three remodeling envelopes is that bone is in a constant dynamic equilibrium. In fact, bone turnover rates in children can be as high as 20% per year; in adults, those rates fall to 3 to 5% annually. To maintain normal bone, an adequate quantity of tropocollagen must be formed and arranged in the correct configuration to permit mineralization. Furthermore, adequate mineral must be available and mineralization must be mechanically sound to maintain normal tensile strength. When any one of these factors or any combination of them becomes abnormal, metabolic bone disease results.

HISTOLOGIC FEATURES

The morphologic results of the interaction of these multiple factors can be seen histomorphometrically, using the technique of examining stained, undecalcified bone biopsy sections, usually obtained from the iliac crest. A model of sequential events in a basic multicellular unit and the resultant histologic picture is shown in Figure 112–2. Osteoclasts, which can be clearly identified in this figure, form a "cutting cone," that is, a tunnel through cortical bone. Behind the osteoclasts are blood vessels and connective tissue, and farther behind is a line of osteoblasts forming osteoid, which appears as the dark area in Figure 112–2.

In the series of color plates in Figure 112–3 osteoid stains bright orange-pink and mineralized bone stains blue-black with the von Kossa stain. The osteoblasts and osteoclasts can be differentiated by their morphologic features. From similar bone biopsies, one can measure the quantity of osteoid per unit of bone, the width of the osteoid seam (a wide seam suggests lack of mineralization and osteomalacia), the quantity of trabecular bone, and the number of osteoclasts and resorbing surfaces or cavities. All these factors give a picture of the dynamic turnover of bone at the time of biopsy.

The *rate* of bone formation can be estimated more accurately by the technique of double tetracycline labeling developed by Frost. Before biopsy, two short courses of tetracycline are administered 7 to 14 days apart. Tetracycline forms fluorescent bands (Fig. 112–3G) after deposition at the mineralization front of bone. The distance between those fluorescent bands divided by the time interval between the midpoints of tetracycline administration is called the mean mineral apposition rate and is a measure of osteoblast function, rates of bone formation, and mineralization. Detailed discussions of bone histomorphometry are available elsewhere.[8,9]

METHODS OF MEASURING BONE MASS

Measurements of bone mass have presented difficulties with regard to sensitivity, accuracy, reproducibility, and general applicability to all parts of the skeleton. (Some areas of the skeleton with a high content of trabecular bone are more metabolically active than others.) Simple radiographic techniques have generally been unsatisfactory. Osteopenia in routine roentgenograms of any bone is defined as loss of trabeculae, and thinning of cortices. Because these changes are not apparent on standard roentgenograms until 30 to 50% of bone mass is lost, this technique is obviously unsuitable for the detection of early accelerated bone loss and for the measurement of increments in bone mass as systemic diseases are controlled or as other therapeutic interventions affecting bone are introduced.

Several simple radiographic techniques have been tried in the hope of providing greater sensitivity at a low cost. The techniques include metacarpal cortical width, Singh index, and comparison of bone density to an aluminum standard simultaneously irradiated (radiogrammetry). The thickness of several metacarpal bones from the endosteal to the periosteal surface of the cortex at a fixed distance from either the distal or proximal end of the bone can be used as a sequential measure of bone mass.[10] Although this technique is precise, it is insensitive. When my colleagues and I have used it in 12 to 18 month studies, during

FIG. 112–3.   Histologic specimen of bone obtained from iliac crest biopsies. Sections are undemineralized and are stained with the von Kossa stain. Mineralized bone stains blue-black; undemineralized osteoid stains pink-orange. *A,* Normal bone histologic specimen from a core biopsy of the iliac crest (× 10). *B,* Osteomalacia; note the large quantities of orange-staining undemineralized osteoid (arrows) laid down along all areas of previously mineralized bone (blue) (× 10). *C,* Low-turnover osteoporosis; note the small total quantities of mineralized bone. The absence of areas of osteoid formation and of resorption indicates a low rate of turnover (× 10). *D,* High-turnover osteoporosis; note the large area of resorption of a bone trabecula (arrows) and formation of osteoid (pink). This patient has osteoporosis with a high rate of turnover (× 100).

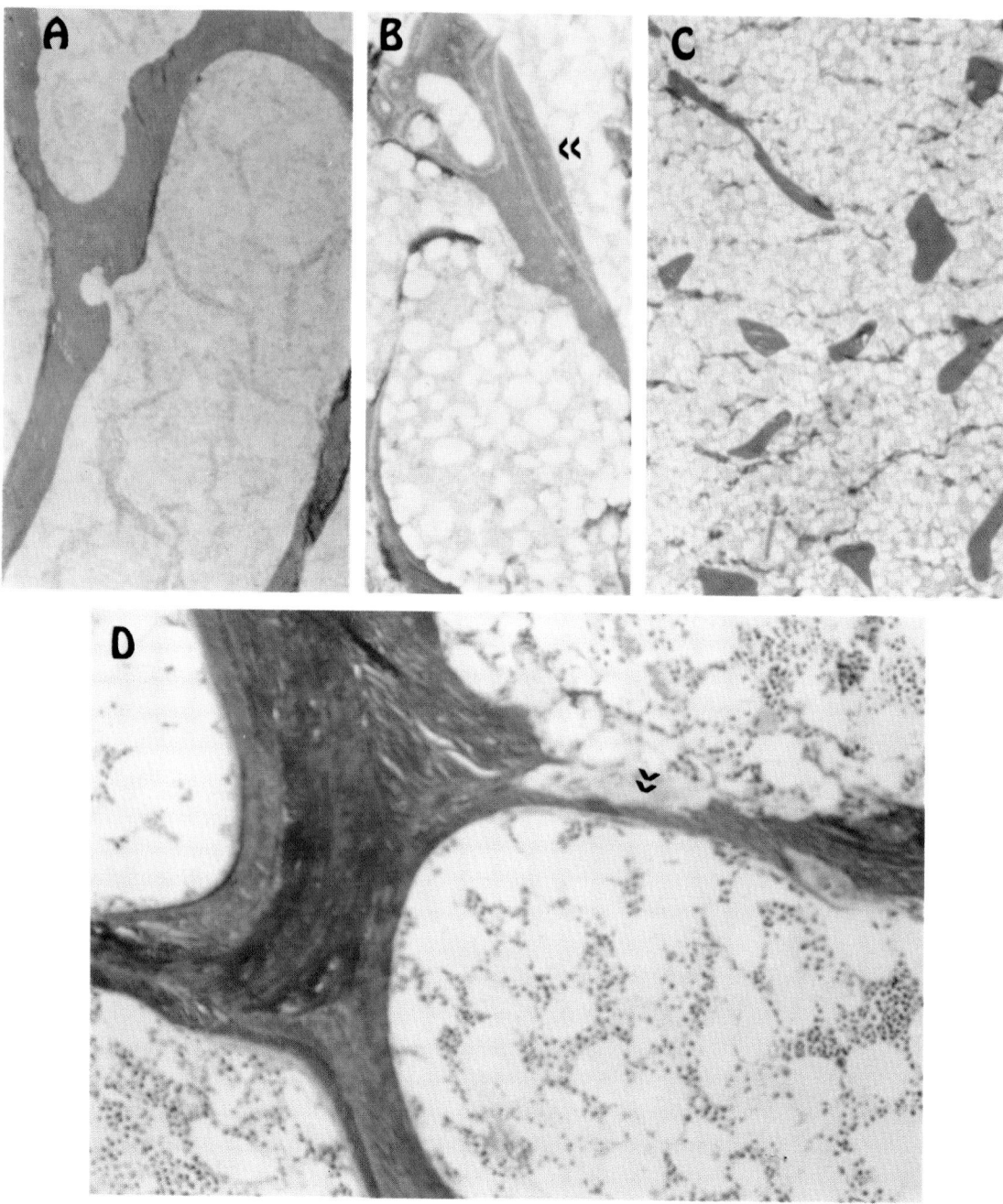

FIG. 112-3 Continued. *E,* Osteitis fibrosa of hyperparathyroidism. A line of osteoclasts has resorbed a large area along a trabecula. The space is being replaced by fibrous tissue. At the leading edge of resorption osteoid is being laid down (×400). *F,* Glucocorticoid-induced osteopenia. Osteoclasts have been activated and have resorbed part of the cortical bone at the endosteal surface (arrows). In contrast to *E,* however, no osteoid is forming (×100). *G,* Bone biopsy viewed under ultraviolet light after tetracycline labeling; tetracycline deposits at the mineralizing front of new bone. This patient received 3 days of tetracycline therapy twice, with a 2-week interval between doses. The distance between the two fluorescent bands of tetracycline is a measure of the rate of bone formation; the label of the bone indicates osteoid has been formed and mineralized (illustrations kindly provided by Steven Teitelbaum, M.D., Professor of Pathology, Washington University/Jewish Hospital of St. Louis).

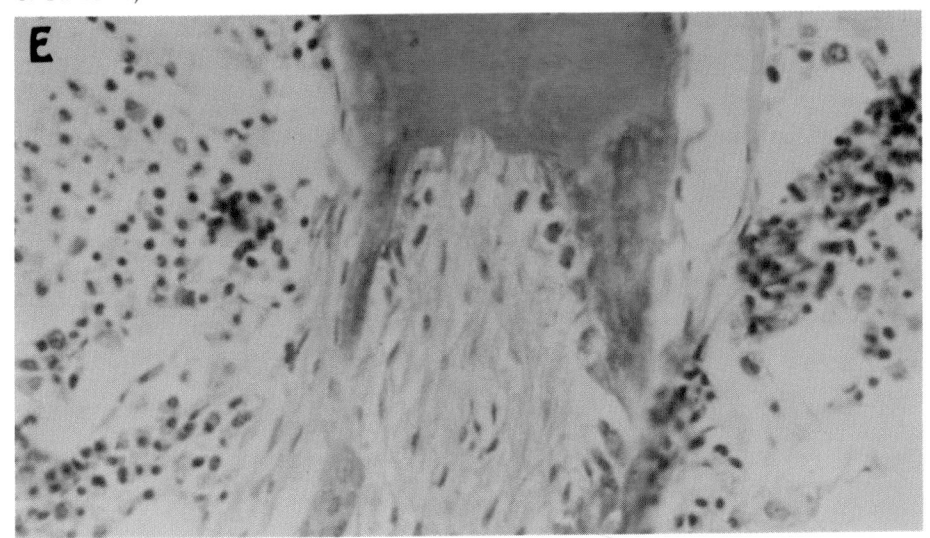

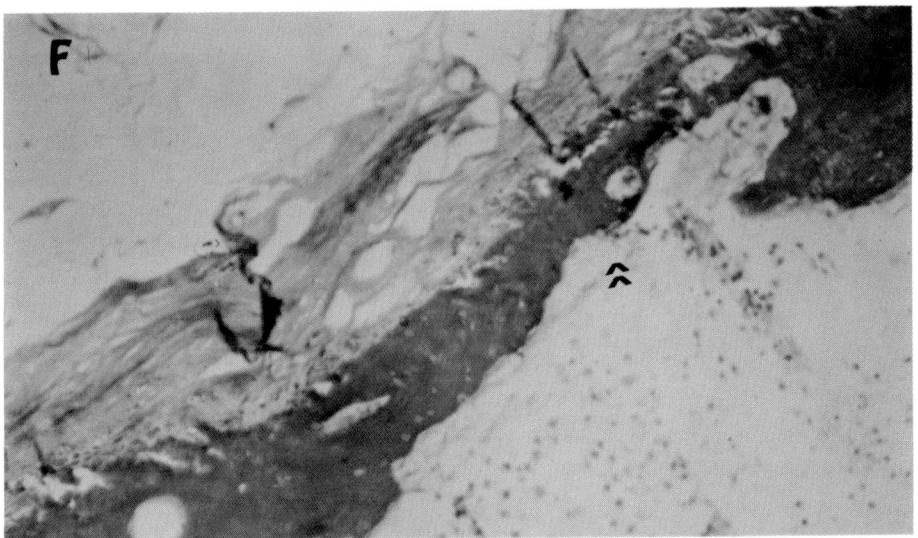

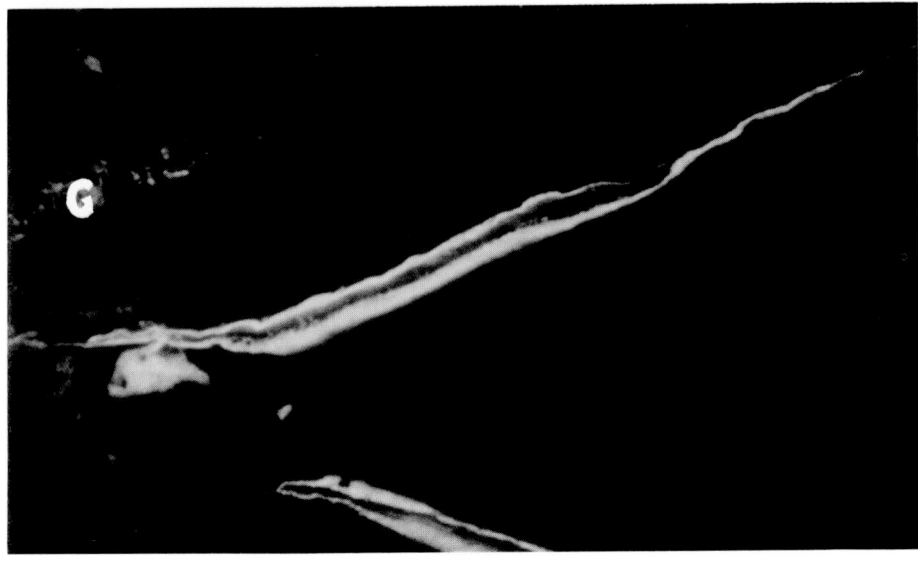

Table 112–1. Methods of Measuring Bone Mass

Technique	Advantages	Disadvantages
Measurement of the cortical width of selected long bones, usually several metacarpals	Simple; inexpensive; accurate for cortical mass; precise in longitudinal studies	Inability to detect loss of trabecular mass or intracortical bone loss; poor correlation with vertebral mass
Singh index, to grade trabecular pattern of the femoral neck	Simple; inexpensive	Better correlation with hip fractures than with vertebral or appendicular bone fractures
Radiogrammetry (density of bone compared to the density of aluminum standard)	Potential viewing of several bones on one film: bone size and shape and cortical mass measurable simultaneously; accurate correlation with single photon absorption of appendicular bone and with total body calcium by neutron activation	Precision lessened by uneven film background and large amount of soft tissue; technique largely replaced by single photon absorptiometry; not good for assessing vertebrae
Single-photon absorptiometry	Inexpensive; low radiation dose; accurate correlation of readings at midradius (diaphyseal mass) or at midmetacarpal with weight of that bone, weight of total skeleton, and total body calcium	Poor correlation with mass of vertebrae ($r = .6$); repositioning of arm is a source of error; precision is better at diaphysis than at metaphysis; single low-energy beam not allowing correction for differences in surrounding soft tissues
Dual photon absorptiometry	Second high-energy beam's penetration of soft tissue allows measurement of vertebral mass; correlation with vertebral fractures in osteoporosis more accurate than that of any foregoing techniques; can be used to measure mass of femoral neck	Repositioning a problem in longitudinal studies; arthritic spurs a possible source of error in vertebrae
Computed tomography of vertebrae	Definition of anatomy of vertebrae and separate measurements of cortical and trabecular bone; good correlation with vertebral fractures	Expensive; soft tissue variation around vertebrae and fat in bone marrow a source of error; scanner drifting with time
Neutron activation of restricted area, such as the hand, or of the whole body	Detection of small changes in regional or total body calcium (1–2%) over time	High radiation dose; expensive; time-consuming; unclear correlations with loss of bone mass at specific sites
Histomorphometry, to stain undecalcified iliac crest biopsy specimens	Clearer picture of dynamics of bone metabolism than static measures of bone mass	Poor correlations with vertebral fractures; better for assessing activity of bone formation and resorption than for quantitating mass

which time bone mass in the appendicular skeleton was shown to change by single photon osteodensitometry; the metacarpal width did not change. I have also found the Singh index disappointing as a measure of change in bone mass because of its insensitivity, although the measurement is easily reproducible. Radiogrammetry has been largely supplanted by the newer technique of photon absorption osteodensitometry and computed tomography (CT) scanning.

In *photon absorption osteodensitometry*, γ rays are directed through a selected portion of bone, and a scanning detector measures the degree of interference provided by the minerals contained in bone (Fig. 112–4).[11,12] This interference correlates directly with bone density and can be converted by computer to a number representing the grams of mineral content per square centimeter of bone scanned. Initially, osteodensitometry was performed using a single low-energy photon beam, which has limited scanning capacity in terms of the thickness of bone and soft tissue it can penetrate. It was applied to readily accessible peripheral bones of the appendicular skeleton; however, patterns of bone loss in the appendicular and axial skeletons ae often dissimilar. Reproducibility is a problem because the peripheral bone must be scanned at exactly the same position at each followup visit. Under optimal conditions, the variability of the test is approximately 3% at the midradius and 5% at the distal radius. Recently, there has been interest in single photon studies of density of the calcaneus, as a site of trabecular bone roughly comparable to vertebrae.

In the past few years, *dual photon absorptiometry* has come into use.[12] Because two photon sources are available, the density of large amounts of soft tissue can be penetrated and vertebral mass can be measured.

FIG. 112–4.   Single photon absorptiometry. The patient sits beside this absorptiometer, and his other arm or hand is placed above the γ beam and is surrounded with a water-filled cuff. The collimated detector can scan a selected area of the radius or the metacarpal bones.

FIG. 112–5.   Image of a vertebra analyzed by computerized axial tomography. The patient lies on a plastic board containing tubes (phantoms) filled with varying quantities of phosphates, and scanning is performed. The density of cortical or trabecular portions of vertebrae can be calculated by comparison to density of the phantoms.

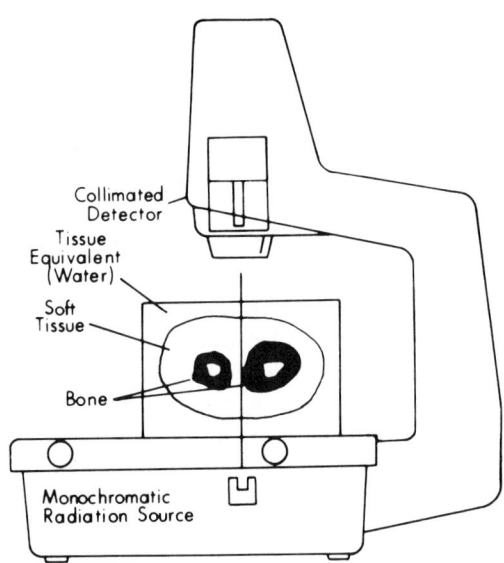

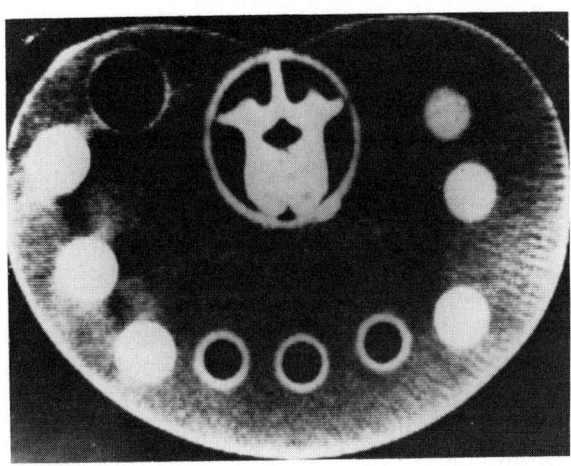

Currently available machines can scan lumbar vertebrae L1-L5 and their computers can delete the density readings in the soft-tissue areas occupied by intervertebral discs; an average reading for the density of the lumbar vertebrae results. The advantage of this apparatus is that it directly measures the density of bones with high trabecular content, such as vertebrae. Because vertebral crush fractures and hip fractures are the major disabling consequences of most forms of osteopenia, direct measurement of these areas is desirable. The disadvantages are that the technique is more cumbersome than measurement of the mass of radius or metacarpal bone, it is more expensive, and the level of radiation exposure is higher.

Quantitative CT scanning of selected vertebrae has been used at some centers to measure quantities of trabecular and cortical bone in the vertebrae.[13] Defined areas of target vertebrae can be selected for scanning, and the density of bone can be calculated by a computer by comparing energy absorption to that of phantoms containing varying quantities of phosphates (Fig. 112–5). The advantages of the technique are its ability to define the anatomic structures of the vertebrae and to obtain separate measurements of trabecular and cortical bone; the correlation of low density with increased risk of vertebral fracture is highly significant. The technique is time-consuming and expensive. Differences in the quantities of soft tissue surrounding vertebrae from one subject to another are a significant source of error, and the scanner drifts with time.

Neutron activation either of restricted areas of the body, such as the hand, or of the total body are available at a small number of centers.[14] Using this technique, the body is bombarded with photons that activate neutrons in the molecules of several different substances, including calcium, to produce ⁴⁶Ca. The emission of neutrons as the isotope decays can be measured by a detector and correlates accurately with the total amount of calcium present in the area bombarded. In population studies in the United States, whole-body neutron activation has been used most frequently to estimate changes in total body calcium as diseases progress, or as therapeutic regimens are introduced. The technique is sensitive enough to detect a 1 to 2% change in total-body calcium content. It is assumed that the change in calcium reflects mineralization of bone, but it is unclear how changes in whole-body calcium content relate to changes in specific areas of the skeleton. The technique requires a high dose of radiation and is expensive.

Histomorphometry can be used to assess total bone volume as well as to quantitate rates of formation and total resorptive surfaces.[8,9] Bone biopsies are obtained from the iliac crest with a .5-cm trocar after tetracycline labeling, and the specimens are stained without prior decalcification using a modified Masson trichrome stain. Fluorescence of the tetracycline label is studied with an ultraviolet microscope. Studies from some centers have *not* shown a strong correlation between total bone volume on biopsy and the number of vertebral compression fractures, the midradius bone density by single photon absorptiometry, or the metacarpal cortical width.[15] In contrast, studies by others have shown significant correlations between total bone volume on biopsy and autopsy diagnosis of osteoporosis.[16] Fractional trabecular bone volume is defined as the fraction of a volume of whole trabecular bone tissue, including marrow, occupied by trabecular bone, both mineralized and unmineralized. It does correlate with the weight of iliac bone, but not to a high degree; it also correlates well with the vertebral bone volume. Overall, reduced values for trabecular bone volume have been found in patients with osteoporosis, hyperthyroidism, and secondary hyperparathyroidism from renal disease or glucocorticoids. Nevertheless, the measurements of bone mass by photon absorptiometry or CT scanning are probably more sensitive than those by histomorphometry with regard to loss of bone mass over time; bone biopsy does provide a better understanding of the dynamics of that bone loss. For a detailed review of histomorphometry the reader is referred to other articles.[8,9]

DIAGNOSIS AND DIFFERENTIAL DIAGNOSIS OF OSTEOPENIA

Several different signs and symptoms should alert the physician to the possible diagnosis of osteopenia. These signs and symptoms include bone fractures after minor trauma or in the absence of trauma, loss of height, increasing dorsal kyphosis, and bone pain. In addition, some patients with osteomalacia or hyperparathyroidism have muscle symptoms, including stiffness and weakness, that can be confused with inflammatory myopathies. Some patients have no symptoms, but the diagnosis is suspected because of osteopenia seen on roentgenograms obtained for another reason.

The differential diagnosis of generalized osteopenia in adults is shown in Table 112–2. The disorders include osteoporosis, corticosteroid-induced osteopenia, osteomalacia, osteitis fibrosa, and other diseases such as hyperthyroidism, diffuse malignancies involving bone, and osteogenesis imperfecta tarda.

A complete evaluation of osteopenia should consist of medical history and physical examination; routine roentgenograms of affected portions of the skeleton; more sensitive measures of bone mass if available (see the preceding discussion of evaluation of bone mass); several measurements of fasting serum calcium, phosphorus, and alkaline phosphatase levels; meas-

urement of the serum parathyroid hormone level; measurement of the serum 25 OH D level; measurement of 24-hour urine calcium excretion: and iliac crest bone biopsy, if available.

Once the radiologic diagnosis of osteopenia is established and a diffuse malignant osteolytic process such as multiple myeloma has been excluded, one must establish the basis of the metabolic bone disorder. A good starting point is measurement of fasting serum calcium, phosphorus, and fractionated alkaline phosphatase levels. These determinations should be performed on fasting serum because postprandial rises in serum calcium and phosphorus can obscure mild abnormalities in basal levels. Most currently available parathyroid hormone assays can readily detect the marked increase in serum levels occurring in primary hyperparathyroidism and renal osteodystrophy, but these tests are less likely to detect the usual minor elevations found in states of mild secondary hyperparathyroidism, such as vitamin D deficiency and glucocorticoid-induced osteopenia. An elevated serum parathyroid value, in combination with other confirmatory data, is useful in establishing a diagnosis. Serum for parathyroid hormone determinations should also be drawn in the fasting state to increase the likelihood of detecting a minimally elevated basal level. Serum 25 OH D measurements provide a sensitive means of assessing vitamin D status. The normal ranges for a center in the midwestern United States was 10 to 25 ng/ml in the winter and 15 to 40 ng/ml in the summer. Values at or below normal limits indicate a deficiency state and warrant further evaluation for intestinal malabsorption, drug-induced osteomalacia, and other disorders. The 25 OH D assays are now available at an increasing number of medical centers and commercial laboratories. Malabsorption syndromes are best defined by determining 72-hour fecal fat excretion and D-xylose absorption.

Determination of 24-hour urinary calcium excretion is a simple and useful, albeit indirect, means of detecting abnormalities in calcium metabolism. With the patient on a 600- to 800-mg calcium diet for several weeks (the average American diet provides that amount), calcium urinary excretion should be between 100 and 200 mg/24 hours. Values below 100 mg on several determinations suggest intestinal calcium malabsorption with a decreased filtered calcium load or a secondary parathyroid hormone elevation, that promotes renal tubular calcium retention *unless* the patient is taking thiazide drugs, which usually decrease urine calcium excretion to 50 to 60% of basal values. An elevated urine calcium excretion and hyperchloremic acidosis would suggest acquired distal

Table 112–2. Differential Diagnosis of Generalized Osteopenia in Adults

Disorder	Possible Causes, Types, and Characteristics

Osteoporosis (parallel loss of mineral and matrix)	Aging
	    genetic, sex, race, and dietary predisposition (osteopenia or senile osteoporosis); fractures after minor trauma, especially of hip; senile osteoporosis tends to occur after age 70
	Postmenopausal
	    spontaneous fractures before age 70—usually of vertebrae, ribs, or radius
	Idiopathic
	Immobilization or reduced physical activity
	Premature menopause

Glucocorticoid-induced osteopenia	Iatrogenic Adrenal glucocorticoid overproduction

Osteomalacia (inadequate mineralization)	Vitamin D deficiency
	    inadequate intake and reduced sunlight exposure; drug-induced catabolism of vitamin D; intestinal malabsorption
	Phosphate-wasting syndromes
	    acquired renal tubular defects with isolated phosphate loss; combined tubular defects (Fanconi syndrome); renal tubular acidosis; antacid abuse

Osteitis fibrosa (parathyroid hormone-induced increase in mineral and matrix resorption)	Primary hyperparathyroidism Secondary hyperparathyroidism vitamin D deficiency states; decrease in intestinal calcium absorption with age; reduced renal mass
Other forms of osteopenia	Hyperthyroidism Osteogenesis imperfecta Malignant tumors replacing bone

renal tubular acidosis. This diagnosis can be confirmed by recording urine pH values for 2 to 3 consecutive days and by failure of urine pH to fall below 5.3 following NH_4Cl loading in the form of 0.1 mg/kg body weight in four divided doses. Other useful tests include determination of urinary hydroxyproline to detect states of increased bone turnover such as osteomalacia, a fasting 4-hour tubular reabsorption of phosphate test to detect renal phosphate wasting in hyperparathyroidism or renal tubular phosphate "leak" syndromes, and measurement of urinary free cortisol in suspected cases of excessive endogenous glucocorticoid production.

The utility of iliac crest bone biopsy to diagnose osteomalacia and low or high bone turnover has already been discussed.

OSTEOPOROSIS

The term osteoporosis refers to the parallel loss of both mineral and matrix that renders residual quantities of mineralized bone inadequate to withstand minor trauma without fracture. The term is confusing because it has been used to refer to the physiologic loss of bone that occurs with aging, as well as to the syndromes of accelerated or early bone loss that occur with inactivity, in menopausal or early postmenopausal women, and in men in late middle age. Thus, the terms "idiopathic osteoporosis," "postmenopausal osteoporosis," "involutional osteoporosis," "senile osteoporosis," "disuse osteoporosis," and "osteopenia" are all in use, with some confusion as to their exact meanings. I agree with the view, expressed by Riggs et al.,[17] that parallel loss of cortical and trabecular bone is physiologic and after many decades results in enough loss of mineralized bone to predispose a person to fractures. This phenomenon should be referred to as osteopenia or as senile or involutional osteoporosis. In contrast, a subset of women lose bone mass rapidly after menopause, often with a disproportionate loss of trabecular bone, and have a high rate of vertebral fractures in the early postmenopausal period. This disease is properly termed postmenopausal osteoporosis. The term osteopenia can refer to individuals with roentgenographic bone loss, and osteoporosis to individuals with bone fractures.

INCIDENCE

Data regarding the rate of bone loss as individuals age have been obtained from weighing bones at autopsy, from the various radiographic techniques discussed earlier, and from histomorphometry. Rates of bone loss vary with age, depending on the particular bone measured and the sex of the individual.

Males have a greater bone mass than females. In both sexes, after age 40 to 50, bone mass is lost from appendicular bone at an average annual rate of .5%. In women during the decade following menopause, however, that rate increases to approximately 1% per year, leveling off to the slower rate after age 60 to 65. Parallel to this accelerated postmenopausal appendicular bone loss is an increase in the negative calcium balance that occurs after age 40 and almost doubles

after menopause.[18] The patterns of bone loss from the midradius in women and in men are shown in Figure 112–6A and B. Loss of bone from the axial skeleton may occur in a different pattern and at a different rate from loss in the appendicular skeleton.[17,19] In vertebrae, bone loss may begin as early as 20 years of age, and it proceeds steadily at a high rate in women, approximately 7% per decade, and at a much slower rate in men, under 2% per decade (Fig. 112–6C and D). Total loss of bone mass in normal women and men over a lifetime, as estimated by the studies of Riggs and colleagues[17,19] is shown in Table 112–3. If

FIG. 112–6. Loss of bone mass with advancing age as determined by single and dual photon absorptiometry. *A*, Loss of bone mass from the midradius in normal United States women. Loss begins at age 35 to 40, accelerates around the time of menopause, and slows in rate after age 65. The center line represents the mean density for normal women; the shaded area encloses two standard deviations; dots are the bone mass in women who have osteoporosis and have had one or more vertebral fractures. *B*, Loss of bone mass from the midradius in normal United States men. The rate of loss is lower than in women. *C*, Loss of bone mass from lumbar vertebrae in normal United States women. The pattern is different from the pattern in the midradius. Bone mass begins to fall at age 20 and declines at a rapid rate unchanged by menopause. Dots represent bone mineral content in normal women. *D*, Loss of bone mass from lumbar vertebrae in normal United States men. The rate is much slower than in women. Dots represent values for normal men (from Riggs, B.L., et al.,[17] with permission of the publishers).

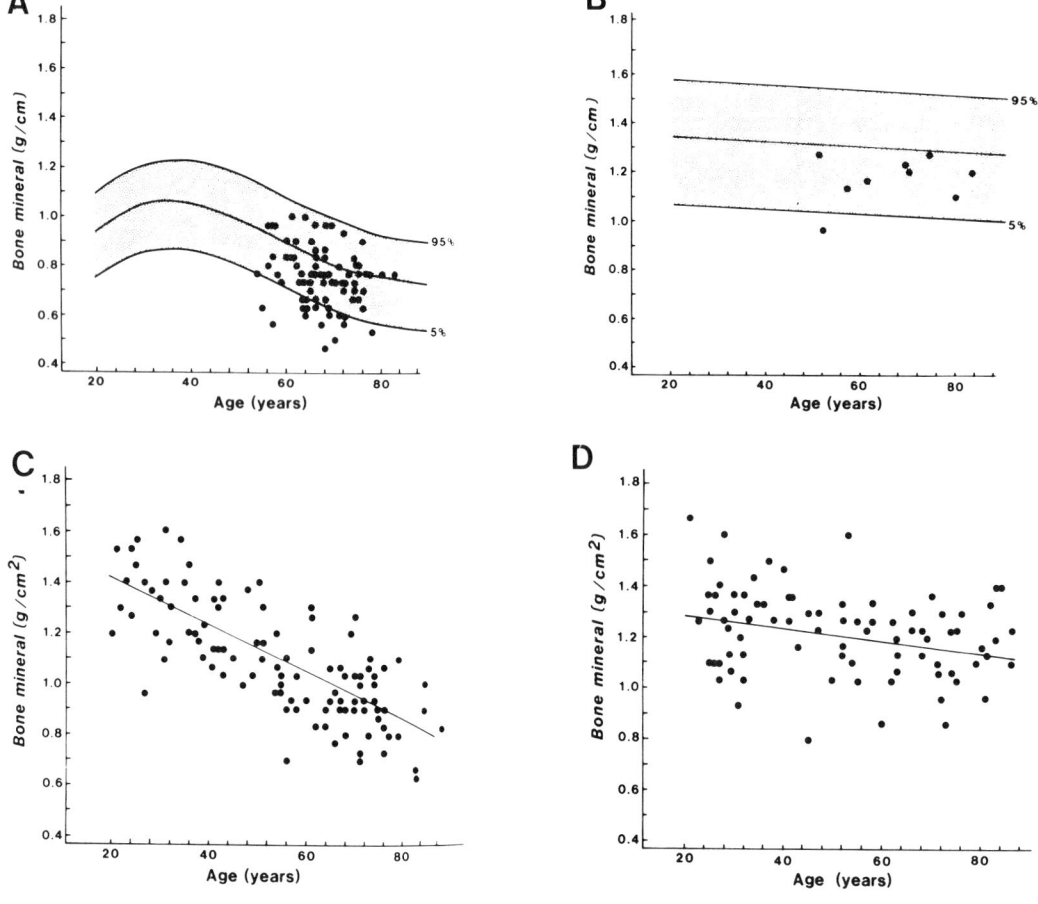

Table 112–3. Loss of Bone Mass in Normal Individuals

Location	Total Loss in Women	Total Loss in Men
	(%)	(%)
Lumbar vertebrae	42–47	13
Midradius	30	5
Distal radius	39	11
Neck of femur	58	36
Intertrochanteric area of femur	53	35

bone loss occurs at different rates in different areas of the skeleton, it is difficult to interpret changes in density or histologic features at a single location as measurements of the impact of a therapeutic intervention.

The incidence of vertebral, hip, and distal radial fractures undoubtedly increases with age. Hip fractures in the elderly are associated with a mortality rate of 12 to 20% in 6 months,[20] and costs of short- and long-term care for these problems constitute a major expenditure in our society.

PATHOGENESIS

Although bone turnover rates decrease progressively with age, bone formation is decreased to a slightly greater degree than is resorption, possibly because resorption rates increase. The result is a gradual net loss of bone. A variety of hypotheses regarding the nature of this pattern have been suggested, including relative osteoblast failure, calcium and vitamin D deficiencies related to dietary changes, decreased efficiency of intestinal calcium absorption and renal calcium retention, and imbalances between the various hormones that influence bone turnover. Certainly, physiologic osteopenia has many etiologic factors and different phenotypic expressions in different individuals. For example, some women with apparent postmenopausal osteopenia actually have osteomalacia on bone biopsy;[21] biopsies showing osteoporosis can contain a spectrum of changes from virtually inactive bone remodeling to high turnover.[15]

Diminished absorption of calcium by the intestine is a physiologic consequence of aging, although the reasons are unknown.[22] In some women, this malabsorption becomes severe enough to add a component of hyperparathyroidism to their osteoporosis. Estrogen loss after menopause probably enhances bone resorption; androgenic hormones and some progestins, levels of which also decline with time, may have positive effects on bone mass. Premature menopause, occurring before the age of 45, is associated with rapid bone loss in some women.[23] Early meno-

pause may be caused by the use of cytotoxic drugs in young women. Diminution in physical activity, in sunlight exposure, and in dietary intake of calcium and vitamin D probably play important roles in the osteopenia of aging.

Race and genetic factors are important in predisposing individuals to symptomatic osteoporosis.[24] Blacks have greater bone mass than whites, who in turn have greater bone mass than Orientals. Certain populations have a high incidence of osteoporosis, including Eskimos and Scandinavians.[25] Identical twins have a higher concordance for loss of bone mass than do dizygotic twins. Body build may also be important. Individuals who are "small boned" have low bone mass; osteoporosis is positively correlated with thinness and is negatively correlated with obesity.[26] Total immobilization results in severe bone loss, as much as 20% over 4 months.[27] Health habits other than nutrition and exercise also play a role in predisposing individuals to osteoporosis. Evidence suggests that alcohol ingestion, smoking, and coffee drinking all have deleterious effects on bone mass.[3,28] Many medications, including prostaglandin inhibitors, glucocorticoids, and methotrexate, reduce rates of bone turnover and may reduce mass. The factors that predispose persons to parallel loss of bone, mineral, and matrix are listed in Table 112–4.

DIAGNOSIS

The clinical diagnosis of idiopathic, postmenopausal, or involutional osteoporosis is essentially one of

Table 112–4. Factors Causing Bone Loss and Contributing to Idiopathic or Postmenopausal Osteoporosis

General	Specific
Aging	reduced intestinal absorption of calcium; change in hormone balance; senescence of bone multicellular units
Genetics	race; small body build; other
Sex	female (less bone mass and lost at higher rate)
Premature menopause	menopause before age 45
Menopause	declining levels of estrogen, androgens, progestogens
Drugs	glucocorticoids; prostaglandin inhibitors; methotrexate
Immobilization	—
Adverse health habits	little physical activity; low dietary intake of calcium; low dietary intake of vitamin D; little sunlight exposure; cigarette smoking; alcohol abuse; coffee drinking

exclusion. A middle-aged or elderly individual complains of loss of height, increasing dorsal kyphosis, or back pain. Fractures may have occurred. In general, patients with hip fractures are a different subset from patients with vertebral and wrist fractures. Radiologic osteopenia, measured either by routine roentgenograms or by one of the more sensitive radiographic techniques discussed previously, is evident. Serum studies show normal levels of calcium, phosphate, alkaline phosphatase, parathyroid hormone, and 25 OH D. Urine calcium may be low (<100 mg/24 hours) but is usually normal. Other causes of metabolic bone disease should be ruled out, including hyperthyroidism, malignancies, hypercortisolism, and alcoholism. Malabsorption, diminished renal function, renal tubular acidosis, or any other factors that might cause osteomalacia or secondary hyperparathyroidism should be excluded.

Initial evaluation should include the tests reviewed above. If special radiographic techniques to measure bone mass are available, baseline studies should be obtained. Similarly, if histomorphometry of bone is available, an iliac crest biopsy can be useful in ruling out an element of osteomalacia or osteitis fibrosa and in establishing the rate of bone turnover, because both high- and low-turnover forms occur, and such information may influence therapy.

PREVENTION

Because it is difficult to restore clinically significant quantities of bone once that mass is lost in individuals with osteopenia, it is appealing to construct programs that aim to prevent osteopenia or osteoporosis, rather than to treat symptomatic disease. To this end, a number of studies have evaluated the benefits of physical exercise and of dietary and hormonal supplementation in middle-aged, perimenopausal women. Osteoporosis is a heterogeneous disorder, and measurements of bone mass in a single site or in biopsies at a particular time, or calculations of total body calcium cannot be considered equivalent to studies of fracture rate. Therefore, studies that actually measure incidence of fractures determine whether an intervention is efficacious, provided all other variables are well controlled. Detailed discussions of prevention strategies are available elsewhere.[3,29,30]

Heavy exercise in adolescence leads to a measurable increase in bone mass, and 3 hours a week of the President's Council on Physical Fitness exercises for perimenopausal women increases total body calcium.[31,32] No firm data show that stimulation of bone formation by longitudinal compression of bone or by exercise against gravity translates into lower fracture rates, however.[27] Thus, moderate exercise programs remain a logical, but unproven, prevention strategy.

Certain nutritional modifications, on the other hand, may have positive effects on bone mass. Positive calcium balance correlates directly with increasing calcium intake. The average intake of calcium in the North American diet is 500 to 700 mg daily. To maintain positive calcium balance, most men and premenopausal white females require 1000 mg of elemental calcium a day; postmenopausal women require 1500 mg daily.[18,29,33] Therefore, supplements of 500 to 1000 mg elemental calcium daily may be desirable for many individuals at high risk for osteoporosis. An 8-ounce glass of milk contains approximately 300 mg calcium; calcium carbonate tablets contain about 40% calcium. Some studies have shown that supplementation with calcium alone reduces the rate of bone loss in postmenopausal women,[33,34] and one study showed significantly lower hip fracture rates in a Yugoslavian population with a high calcium intake than in another Yugoslavian group with a low calcium intake.[35] However, in more recent work, calcium supplementation of perimenopausal or postmenopausal women did *not* prevent loss of bone mass in either the appendicular or the axial skeleton (Fig. 112–7).[36,37] A high intake of calcium in childhood and adolescence probably increases total bone mass, but supplementing the intake later may not be effective. It is clear that addition of estrogen in the 5 years after menopause is much more effective in maintaining bone mass than is addition of calcium alone.[30,34,36,37]

Calcium supplementation is generally safe—hypercalcemia occurred in 1% of a population treated with calcium supplements; 1000 mg supplemental calcium increased urinary calcium by only 70 mg/24 hours. Whether such supplementation is effective, however, is controversial.

Strong evidence indicates that estrogens, and probably low doses of some progestins and androgens, also prevent or slow the rate of bone loss from both appendicular and axial skeleton in perimenopausal women.[36–38] In individuals who have premature menopause (before age 45), estrogen replacement clearly slows bone loss, is effective for at least 8 to 10 years, and cannot be discontinued without rapid bone loss.[23,38,39] Most authorities recommend that all women with premature menopause be treated with estrogen replacement, in cyclic form, at least .625 mg of conjugated estrogens 25 days out of 30, unless a specific contraindication exists. Alternatively, estrogens can be administered percutaneously, also in a cyclic regimen.[40]

Stabilization of bone mass, without much actual

FIG. 112–7. These data illustrate: (1) the increased effectiveness of estrogen compared to calcium alone in preserving bone mass in women within 3 years of menopause; (2) different rates of bone loss in different areas of the skeleton; and (3) use of multiple different methods to measure bone mass. Numbers in parentheses are the number of women entered into each treatment group. *Open circles* represent women who were not treated; *open squares* represent women treated with 1000 to 1500 mg of oyster shell calcium daily; *open diamonds* represent women treated with conjugated estrogen, .3 mg daily 25 days out of 30 (with a progestogen added from day 16 through 25) plus 1000 to 1500 mg of calcium daily. Bone mass was well maintained in all skeletal areas studied only in the groups that received estrogen; bone mass declined, especially in the spine, in the group receiving calcium alone. Bone loss was most marked in the lumbar spine compared to the radius or metacarpal bones. Metacarpal mass was measured as combined cortical thickness, radial mass as bone density by single photon absorptiometry, and spinal mass by quantitative CT scanning (reproduced from Ettinger, B., et al.;[36] with permission of the author and the publisher).

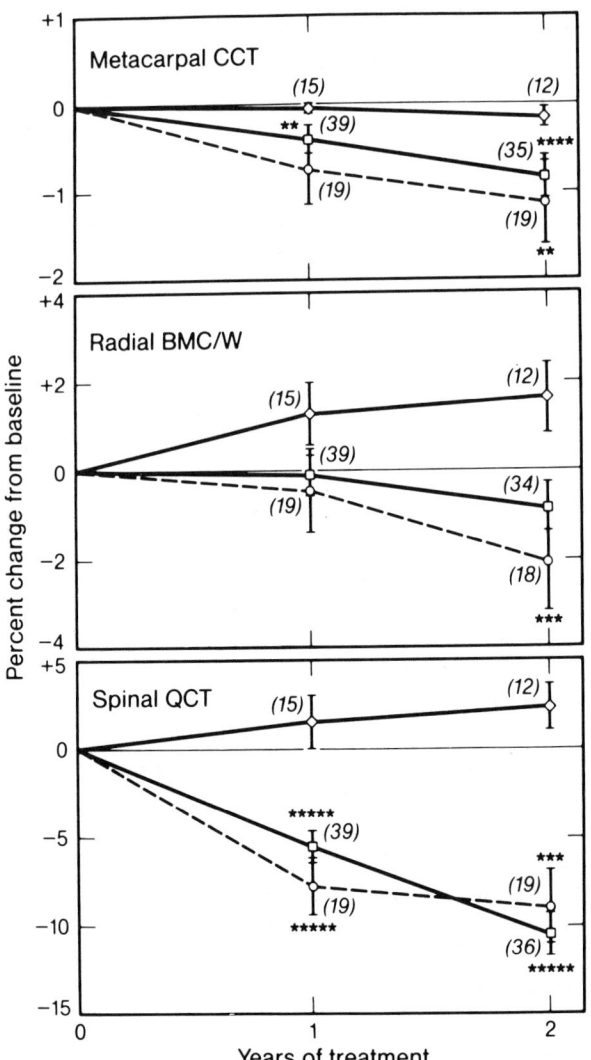

increase, can be achieved by administration of estrogen to women after a natural menopause, especially in those who are within 3 to 5 years of cessation of menses. Such replacement therapy is associated with a significantly reduced incidence of hip fractures.[41] The recent studies of Ettinger et al.[36] and of Riis et al.[37] showed that administration of estrogen for 2 years to women within 3 years of menopause maintained stable bone mass in the radius and the spine, whereas treatment with 1000 to 2000 mg of calcium carbonate daily, or no treatment, did not (Fig. 112–7). In the Ettinger study, the dose of estrogen used was .3 mg/day of conjugated estrogen orally, with 1000 mg of calcium carbonate; this was given cyclically 25 days of 30, with a progestogen added from day 16 to 25. In the Riis study, estrogen was administered percutaneously as 3 mg daily of 17 β-estradiol plus 2000 mg of calcium carbonate 24 of 28 days; some patients received progesterone on days 13 to 24. Therefore, cyclic administration of estrogen balanced by progesterone, which is considered to be the safest method of administering estrogen to postmenopausal women, is effective in maintaining bone mass for at least a few years if initiated shortly after menopause begins. Daily administration of estrogen is associated with increased risks for endometrial hyperplasia and carcinoma,[42] hypertension, migraine headaches, and hypercoagulable states. The risk of malignancy is *not* increased if administration of estrogen is cyclic and progestogens are also used. The use of transcutaneous estradiol may decrease the incidence of undesirable side effects of estrogen, which depend on increased synthesis of certain polypeptides by the liver, such as renin precursors.[40]

In summary, cyclic estrogen therapy should be considered for postmenopausal women who are thought to be at risk for osteoporosis, if there are no contraindications to its use. Data have been obtained primarily in whites, and risk factors have been identified in that group. If physicians and patients are to embark on such preventive therapy, it would be useful to have a method of measuring bone mass in areas of the skeleton at risk for fracture, such as the vertebrae and the hips. Dual photon absorptiometry probably serves this need best, although many followup measurements are necessary to confirm changes (or lack of change) in bone mass, given a decline of 2 to 10% in lumbar mass over 2 years in untreated women, and a variation in the dual photon measurements of 3 to 5%. The utility of such measurements is controversial,[43] but some experts find them helpful, and the measurements may help assess whether an intervention is having the desired effect of stabilizing bone mass. Increased bone formation is indicated by increasing serum levels of osteocalcin (gla-protein), which is produced only by activated osteoblasts.

If estrogen is to be used for prevention of osteoporosis in high risk subjects, .625 mg conjugated estrogen, or .3 mg accompanied by 1000 mg of calcium daily, is a minimal adequate dose to maintain vertebral mass. Transdermal estradiol, 100-µg patches, can probably be substituted.[40] The data suggest that the higher the dose of estrogens, the greater the positive effect on bone mass. For example, a minimal daily oral dose of 15 µg of estradiol were required to maintain bone mass; 25 µg or more were required to increase mass. The cyclic administration of estrogen, 25 days out of 30, is recommended. Progesterone, 10 mg daily during days 16 to 25, can be added to minimize endometrial stimulation. At a recent National Institutes of Health Consensus Conference on Osteoporosis, the Advisory Panel recommended that cyclic estrogen therapy be considered in all women within 5 years of natural menopause.

Androgens and some progestogens have effects similar to estrogens in maintaining bone mass in postmenopausal women.[44] Androgens may be useful in men with osteoporosis; estrogens are preferable in women.

Hypogonadism in men is associated with osteoporosis[45,46] whether as a result of idiopathic testosterone deficiency, hyperprolactinemia, anorexia nervosa, Klinefelter's syndrome, or idiopathic hypogonadotrophic states. Administration of androgens increases mass in the maturing skeleton of these individuals, and may be effective when administered to adults.

Prevention strategies are summarized in Table 112–5.

THERAPY

Therapy of symptomatic osteoporosis can be frustrating to both patient and physician because of the uncertainty that any interventions will increase bone mass enough to reduce pain and fractures. As discussed earlier, a high intake of calcium in childhood and adolescence probably increases total bone mass, but supplementing the intake later may not be effective. It is clear that addition of estrogen in the 5 years after menopause is much more effective in maintaining bone mass than is addition of calcium alone.

Calcium has many effects on bone. It is required for mineralization, and a positive calcium balance may help maintain bone mass, as discussed previously. That calcium also suppresses bone turnover may mean that it slows remodeling processes in which the bone-forming unit resorbs more net bone than it produces. Riggs and colleagues initially reported that recurrence of vertebral fractures can be diminished by approximately 50% if postmenopausal osteoporotic women are treated with calcium carbonate (1500 to 2500 mg daily) for more than a year.[47] This benefit was seen with or without pharmacologic doses of vitamin D. In more recent work, this benefit has not been seen, and the use of calcium as a sole agent to treat symptomatic osteoporosis is questionable.

Vitamin D and its metabolites are advocated by some authorities as therapy for osteoporosis, to ensure maximal absorption of dietary calcium and to maintain positive calcium balance. Several recent studies, however, have failed to demonstrate a reduction in fracture rates or an increase in bone mass accompanying vitamin D therapy for osteoporosis.[47] Hypercalciuria, defined as a urine calcium level >300 mg/24 hour, and hypercalcemia are complications of vitamin D therapy occurring in approximately 25% of patients, especially with 25 OH D and 1,25(OH)$_2$D regimens. Currently, I use supraphysiologic doses of vitamin D or its metabolites only in osteoporotic individuals who have urine calcium levels <100 mg/24 hour. For most patients, vitamin D supplementation of 400 to 800 IU/day may be adequate.

Estrogens act primarily as suppressors of bone resorption and thus reduce the rate of remodeling. I have already discussed the evidence that they reduce loss of bone mass and the hip-fracture rate in postmenopausal women.

In the studies of Recker and colleagues,[34] the combination of calcium and estrogen maintained bone mass in symptomatic postmenopausal women better than did calcium alone. In the studies of Riggs et al.,[47] the combination resulted in vertebral-fracture rates significantly lower than those in women receiving calcium alone. Studies showing maintenance of bone mass in asymptomatic postmenopausal women have been reviewed previously. Administration of estrogens to women with fractures who are within 3 to 8 years of menopause is probably effective in reducing fracture rates. Whether this intervention is useful in older women who are more than a decade past menopause is debatable. Some authorities have presented data supporting efficacy in that group; others have reported that estrogens are not efficacious in that setting. Patients with symptomatic osteoporosis who are treated with estrogen should receive cyclic therapy with conjugated estrogens orally or with transcutaneous estradiol. The regimens are the same as those recommended for prevention of osteoporosis, as discussed in the section, "Prevention."

Sodium fluoride may be chosen to treat sympto-

Table 112–5. Prevention of Osteoporosis

Approach	Specifics
Identification of subjects at high risk	Small, white women; positive family history; low calcium intake
Prescription of a regular program of physical activity	3 hour/week exercise against gravity; 1–1.5 miles walking daily (suggested regimen)
Ensuring adequate calcium intake	1000 mg/day elemental calcium in men and premenopausal women; 1500 mg/day in postmenopausal women
Ensuring adequate vitamin D intake	400 IU/day
Estrogen replacement therapy in women with premature menopause (before age 45)	cyclic estrogen therapy—choices are conjugated estrogens .625 mg a day orally, or conjugated estrogens .3 mg a day plus calcium 1000 mg a day orally, or 100 μg transcutaneous estradiol; each should be given 25 days out of 30; consider administration of a progestogen from days 16–25
Estrogen replacement therapy in all women at risk beginning within 5 years of menopause	Cyclic estrogen therapy—choices are conjugated estrogens .625 mg a day orally, or conjugated estrogens .3 mg a day plus calcium 1000 mg a day orally, or 100 μg transcutaneous estradiol; each should be given 25 days out of 30; consider administration of a progestogen from days 16–25

matic osteoporosis in patients who are not candidates for estrogen or who fail to improve on estrogen. Sodium fluoride is the only medication currently available that stimulates formation of osteoid, even in areas that do not contain bone-remodeling units. The danger that the osteoid will not mineralize properly is real, however, so osteomalacia can be induced by fluoride treatment if the dose is high or if inadequate quantities of mineral are available. Therefore, calcium and vitamin D should be given with fluoride (see Table 112–6 for recommended regimens). In addition to stimulating bone formation, fluoride incorporated into the hydroxyapatite crystal increases the density of bone. Whether that denser bone is stronger, rather than more brittle, is a point of debate. Therapy of more than one year's duration with fluoride, vitamin D, and calcium has been associated with reduced fracture rates.[47] Common undesirable side effects of fluoride therapy include dyspepsia, nausea, diarrhea, anorexia, peptic ulcer, rheumatic symptoms (especially plantar fasciitis), and acne; these side effects occur in 34 to 40% of patients. Fractures of long bones have been reported in fluoride-treated patients, but issues of whether optimal doses of fluoride were used, and whether adequate amounts of minerals and vitamin D were supplied, can be raised in interpreting these reports.

In the study by Riggs et al.,[47] the combination of calcium, fluoride, vitamin D, and estrogen was more

Table 112–6. Treatment of Symptomatic Osteoporosis

1. Measure serum and urine calcium levels
2. If urine calcium <120 mg/24 hours
   A. Give: calcium, 1,000 mg/daily
         vitamin D 50,000 U, 2 to 3 times/week*
         or 25 OH D 20 μg/day
   B. Monitor urine and serum calcium every 3 to 4 months
3. If urine calcium >120 mg/24 hour
       Give: calcium, 1,000 mg/day
         vitamin D 400 IU/day
4. If patient is within 10 years of menopause
       Add: cyclic estrogen therapy as recommended in Table 112–5
5. If patient is a man, or if patient is more than 10 years postmenopausal
       Add: sodium fluoride 25 mg twice a day with meals
         calcium 1,000–1,500 mg daily
         vitamin D 400–800 IU daily if urine calcium >120 mg/24 hr
         50,000 units 1 to 3 times weekly if urine calcium <120 mg/24 hr or 25 OH D, 20 μg/day
6. If new fractures occur after 1 year of treatment with regimen 4 or 5, combine the regimens

Note: If iliac crest bone histomorphometry is available, biopsy may be useful to determine whether regimen 4 or 5 is a more desirable initial intervention.

If dual photon osteodensitometry is available, assessment of vertebral and hip mass before and at 6 to 12 month intervals after institution of therapy is useful to determine efficacy.

*See text for discussion of incidence of undesirable side effects.

effective than any two or three of the agents in reducing vertebral-fracture rates in osteoporotic women.

Other, less frequently used therapeutic regimens include calcitonin, thiazide, parathyroid hormone, anabolic hormones, and diphosphanates. Their use as single therapeutic agents for osteoporosis is controversial, and the reader is referred to review articles for more information.[30,48–50] Each of these agents may be useful in combination therapy.

Frost proposed an approach to therapy of osteoporosis in which one cycle of therapy activates bone remodeling units; the next cycle inactivates the remodeling units before a large quantity of bone is resorbed; and in the third cycle, no therapy is given, so osteoblasts are free to form bone.[1] The sequence is then repeated. Activators of bone-remodeling units might include parathyroid hormone, growth hormone, thyroxine, or regional electrical stimulation. Suppressors could include diphosphanates, calcitonin, estrogen, and calcium. A related idea has been offered by Whyte et al.,[15] who select therapy according to histologic features. If the patient has low bone turnover with little osteoid and little uptake of tetracycline, one might stimulate osteoid formation with fluoride, in addition to calcium and vitamin D. If the patient has a high rate of bone turnover with multiple areas of osteoid and many resorption sites, remodeling should be suppressed with calcium or estrogen, biopsy should be repeated in 6 to 9 months, and fluoride should be prescribed only if bone turnover has been reduced.

In summary, several available therapeutic approaches to symptomatic osteoporosis, although officially considered experimental, probably reduce fracture rates (Table 112–6). Of these, calcium supplementation, which is of questionable benefit, is associated with negligible side effects. Estrogen therapy, if administered cyclically, may also be relatively safe. How aggressive the physician should be with these and other therapies depends on the degree of disability of the patient and the presence of concomitant disorders.

GLUCOCORTICOID-INDUCED OSTEOPENIA

Glucocorticoid-induced osteopenia is an important subset of osteoporosis.

DEFINITION

The bone loss associated with glucocorticoid therapy may be defined as another state in which the rate of bone resorption exceeds the rate of bone formation. The uncoupling of formation and resorption caused by supraphysiologic glucocorticoid levels has two mechanisms: reduction of formation and increase of resorption. As in many other metabolic bone diseases, especially hyperparathyroid states, bone with a large surface area available for endosteal osteoclastic resorption is lost at a faster rate than compact cortical bone. Therefore, bones with high trabecular content, such as vertebrae and ribs, are at a high risk of fracture—a fact recognized for decades in both spontaneous and iatrogenic Cushing's syndrome (Fig. 112–8).[51–56,56a] Bones of the appendicular skeleton also fracture at a high rate in individuals with rheumatic diseases who are treated on a long-term basis with glucocorticoids (Table 112–7).[57]

Based on the more rapid loss of metabolically active trabecular bone than of compact cortical bone in glucocorticoid osteopenia, a technique for identifying the disease in a population of individuals treated with glucocorticoids was developed.[58,59] As shown in Figure 112–9, the metaphyseal site of the distal human radius has a higher proportion of trabecular bone than the diaphyseal midradius.[60] In addition, endosteal resorption of cortical bone is more easily measured at metaphyseal than at diaphyseal sites of long bones. Therefore, if a single photon is passed through both diaphyseal and metaphyseal sites of the radius, one can detect differential loss of bone in these two areas. As shown in Figure 112–10, our studies have confirmed this theory; individuals receiving daily glucocorticoid therapy on a long-term basis had significantly more loss of metaphyseal mass than of diaphyseal mass, whereas individuals with rheumatoid arthritis (RA) who had never received glucocorticoids had a similar loss of metaphyseal and diaphyseal mass.[52,59] Similar results were reported in patients with asthma receiving long-term glucocorticoid therapy.[58] The simplest way to express these data is as the ratio of diaphyseal mass to metaphyseal mass (DM/MM). This ratio is constant after puberty and is the same in males and females and in blacks and whites. It does not have to be adjusted for age, sex, or race, as do separate measures of diaphyseal and metaphyseal mass. As discussed previously, the technique of single photon osteodensitometry has its problems, and measurements of appendicular bone mineral content do not correlate as well with vertebral mass as with long bone mass, but the technique is rapid, inexpensive, and useful in screening populations.

Most individuals with rheumatic diseases who receive chronic glucocorticoid therapy develop elevated DM/MM ratios because they lose metaphyseal mass

FIG. 112–8. Roentgenograms of patients with glucocorticoid-induced osteopenia. *A*, Multiple vertebral compression fractures in a middle-aged woman with rheumatoid arthritis treated for several years with 10 to 15 mg prednisone daily. Note the anterior wedging of thoracic vertebrae (T12) in contrast to the central collapse of lumbar vertebrae (L1–L5). Similar radiographic findings occur in idiopathic or postmenopausal or senile osteoporosis. *B*, Lumbar spine and pelvis in a 24-year-old man treated for 10 years with prednisone to suppress glomerulonephritis. Note the mottled appearance of bone in the lumbar vertebrae and ilia indicating bone loss and the failure of the epiphyses of the ilia to close (arrows) (courtesy of Richard H. Gold, M.D., Professor of Radiology, University of California, Los Angeles).

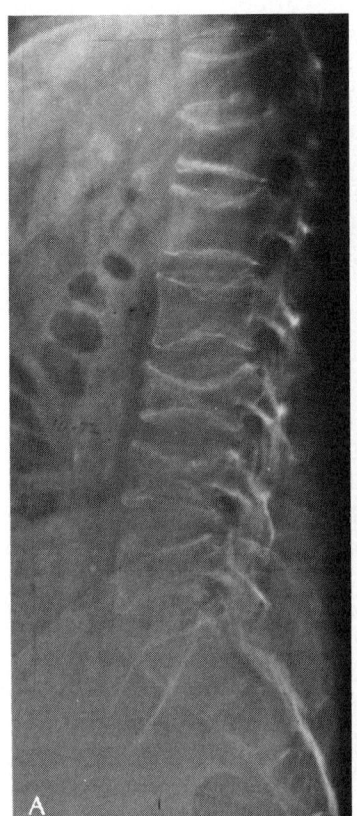
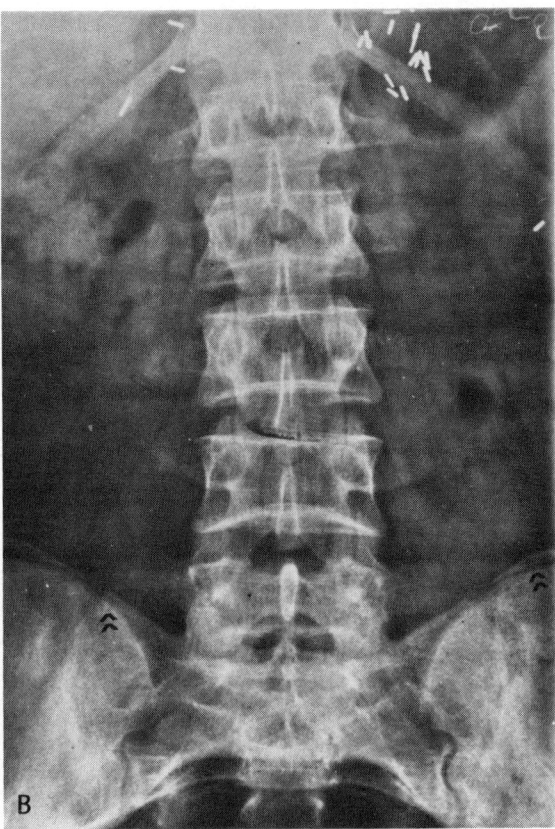

at a faster rate than diaphyseal mass. Although patients with primary hyperparathyroidism have a similar pattern of loss (Fig. 112–10), glucocorticoid osteopenia can be distinguished easily from primary hyperparathyroidism by the presence of normal serum calcium levels, and from other types of secondary hyperparathyroidism by the absence of renal failure, intestinal malabsorption, and hepatic dysfunction.

Although measures of DM/MM ratios have been a useful screening test for us, the technique is not widely available to the practicing physician, who must rely on other techniques to confirm the suspicion that bone mass is declining at a worrisome rate.

The histologic features of iliac crest bone biopsies can be helpful in understanding glucocorticoid osteopenia (see Fig. 112–3).[61,62] Formation rates are usually low, and numbers of resorption sites are increased.

Table 112–7. Incidence of Fractures in Rheumatic Disease Patients Receiving Long-Term Glucocorticoid Therapy

	Fractures		
	Vertebral (%)	Extravertebral (%)	All (%)
Patients never receiving systemic glucocorticoid therapy	5–8	6	9
Patients receiving long-term glucocorticoid therapy	12–18	19	30

FIG. 112–9. Sketch of the human radius. The midportion of the radius (diaphyseal mass—DM) contains predominantly compact cortical bone. The distal end (metaphyseal mass—MM) contains a high proportion of trabecular bone.

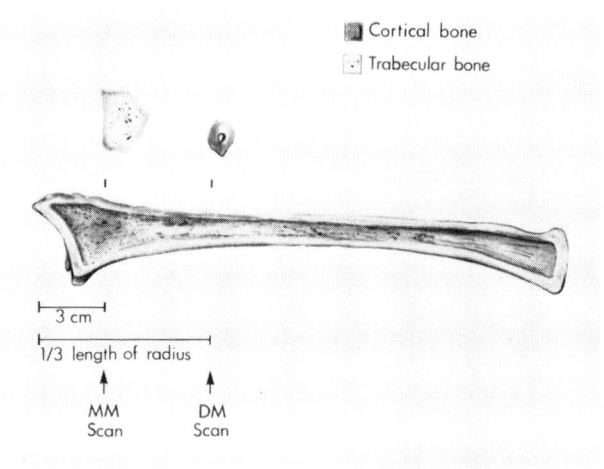

Trabecular bone volume is usually low. Sometimes the biopsy shows increased formation or little resorption. None of the histomorphometric findings are specific for glucocorticoid osteopenia.

INCIDENCE

Bone fractures of both the axial and the appendicular skeleton in patients receiving glucocorticoid therapy remain a major clinical problem. Such fractures occur in highest frequency in older individuals; therefore, glucocorticoid osteopenia is usually an insult added to bone loss resulting from age, the postmenopausal state, RA, or inactivity. We have seen vertebral fractures as early as 3 months after the institution of glucocorticoid therapy in older individuals.

The incidence of glucocorticoid osteopenia is not clear because of variations in definition and in populations studied. In studies in which bone mass was measured by direct weight of bones at autopsy or by calculation of trabecular bone volume from iliac crest biopsies, 85 to 90% of patients treated with glucocorticoids had significantly less bone mass than age-, sex-, and race-matched normal individuals.[5,6,9] In a cross-sectional study of 161 patients with rheumatic disease treated for more than 6 weeks with various doses of daily or alternate-day prednisone,[57] the incidence of glucocorticoid osteopenia, defined as a greater loss of metaphyseal mass than of diaphyseal mass on single photon absorptiometry of the radius, correlated directly with the cumulative dose of pred-

nisone (Tables 112–7, 112–8, and 112–9). More than 80% of individuals who had received >30 g of prednisone had glucocorticoid osteopenia. Most individuals receiving glucocorticoid therapy on a long-term basis will lose bone to the extent that their risk of fracture is increased.

Fracture rates in individuals with rheumatic diseases, with or without glucocorticoid therapy, depend on the population studied. For example, 60% of adults in one series had sustained vertebral or rib fractures,[16] and 18% in our study had vertebral collapse.[57] In our group of rheumatic disease patients receiving chronic glucocorticoid therapy, the incidence of all fractures is shown in Table 112–7.

In summary, the data suggest that patients with rheumatic diseases have a twofold to threefold increase in incidence of axial or appendicular bone fractures if they are receiving glucocorticoid therapy on a long-term basis (Table 112–7).

RISK FACTORS

Elderly individuals, especially white women, are the group at highest risk for disabling fractures after the institution of glucocorticoids.[57,58] This risk is not surprising, because white postmenopausal women are also the highest-risk group for fractures related to idiopathic osteoporosis. Children, with their rapidly growing bones, are also at high risk.[63] Factors that may alter this risk include sex, age, race, body build, type of rheumatic disease, duration of disease, glucocorticoid dose, duration of therapy, concomitant therapies, level of activity, nutritional status (especially vitamin D and calcium intake) and amount of exposure to sunlight.

Table 112–9 summarizes the factors that increase the risk of elevated DM/MM ratio and the risk of fractures.[57] An increasing cumulative glucocorticoid dose gave the strongest positive correlation with rising ratio of diaphyseal to metaphyseal mass (see Table 112–8). Daily prednisone dose and duration of therapy did not correlate with this rising ratio, but both are obviously related to total cumulative doses. Moreover, others have shown that bone mass at the metaphyseal site of the radius falls rapidly with prednisone use, with approximately a 4% loss after 6 months and a 30% loss after 100 months.[64] Therefore, the duration of glucocorticoid therapy probably correlates inversely with bone mass. With regard to daily dose, my colleagues and I could show no direct effect beyond its relationship to total cumulative dose. Some have suggested that a low daily dose level of glucocorticoids at which most individuals do not malabsorb

FIG. 112–10. Differential loss of bone mass from the diaphyseal (DM) and metaphyseal (MM) areas of the radius in different disease states. Bone mass is expressed as the percentage of decrease from age- and sex-matched normal individuals living in the same geographic area. In individuals receiving long-term glucocorticoid therapy, more MM is lost than DM; this pattern of bone loss is similar to that seen in primary hyperparathyroidism. RA = Rheumatoid arthritis; numbers in parentheses are the number of patients in each diagnostic group.

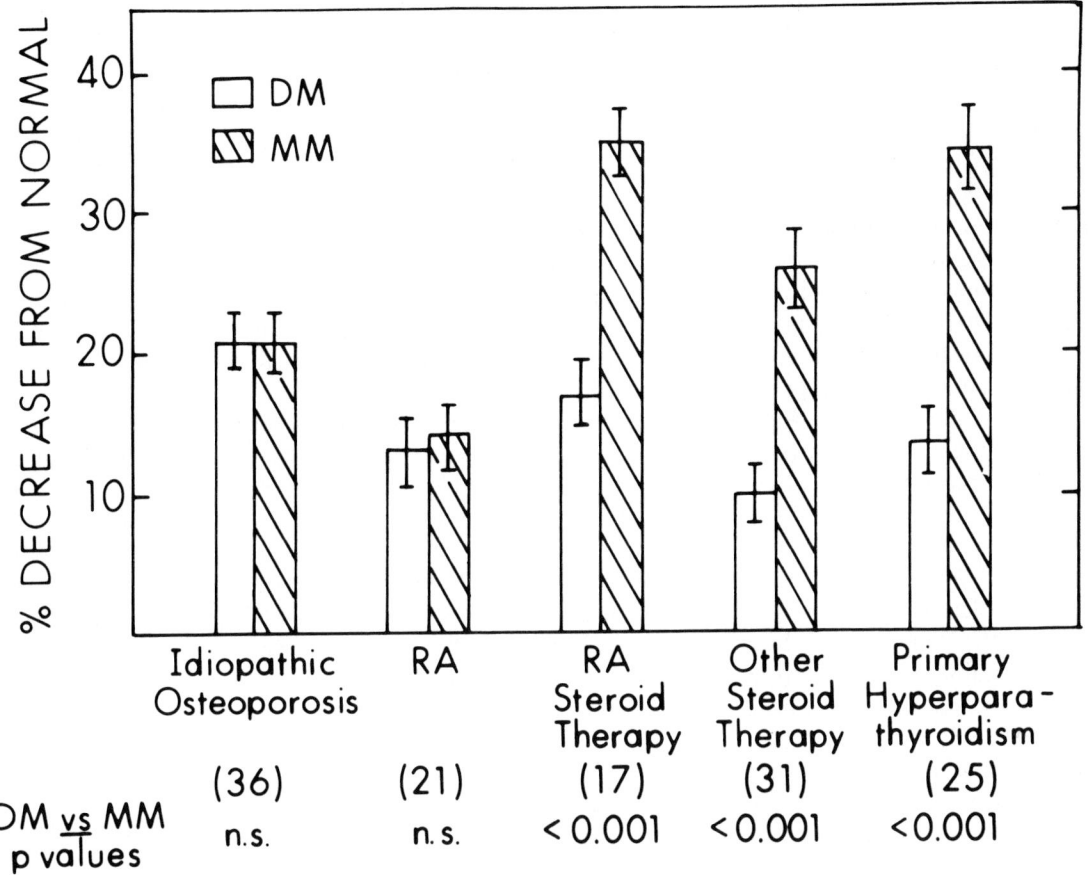

Table 112–8.   Daily and Cumulative Effect of Glucocorticoid Doses on Diaphyseal-to-Metaphyseal Mass (DM/MM) Ratios and Fractures

	Elevated DM/MM (%)	p*	Fractures (%)	p*
Daily Dose (mg)				
≤5	11/32 (34)		6/29 (32)	
6–20	42/105 (40)	NS	18/58 (31)	NS
>20	8/24 (33)		4/16 (25)	
Total Dose (g)				
<10	18/77 (23)		10/45 (22)	
10–30	25/61 (40)	<.002	10/33 (33)	<.03
>30	18/23 (78)		8/15 (53)	

*Probability by multiple regression analysis. Data are based on a cross-sectional survey of 161 patients with various rheumatic diseases attending clinics at Washington University in St. Louis and receiving long-term glucocorticoid therapy. Radiographs were available in 93; the median age was 50 years, the mean prednisone dose was 15.6 mg per day, and the mean duration of therapy was 48 months.[57]

Table 112–9. Risk Factors for Development of Glucocorticoid-Induced Osteopenia

Definite	Probable	Unlikely
High total cumulative dose of glucocorticoids	Increasing duration of glucocorticoid therapy	Type of rheumatic disease (when corrected for age of susceptible population)
Increasing age; individuals >50 years old (men or women) at higher risk	High daily doses of glucocorticoids Age <15 years	
Postmenopausal state	Small body size White race Female sex (before menopause or age 50)	Sex (after age of 50 years)

calcium may be safe for bones. Klein et al.[65] reported that prednisone doses <10 mg daily do not cause calcium malabsorption in healthy persons, but the level required to reduce synthesis of osteoid has not been determined. Furthermore, abnormally low intestinal uptake of calcium has been found in several patients with rheumatic disease taking only 5 mg prednisone daily. An overall fracture rate of 26% occurred in 29 patients receiving ≤5 mg prednisone daily—a rate similar to that of patients taking higher doses.[57] It is my opinion that *no dose of exogenous glucocorticoids is safe in terms of bone loss;* however, it is logical that the lower daily doses are safer. Our data also show that *alternate-day glucocorticoid regimens cause bone loss similar to that of daily regimens,*[66] again suggesting that the total cumulative dose may be a more powerful risk factor than the daily dose. Others have reported less calcium malabsorption in humans on alternate-day therapy than on daily therapy,[65] and better bone growth in animals.[67]

The second strongest risk factor correlating positively with increasing ratios of diaphyseal to metaphyseal mass and fracture rates was increasing age. Individuals over age 50 had a significantly higher incidence of fractures than did younger individuals;[57] these findings were similar to those reported by others.[58] Postmenopausal women, including those with premature menopause, had a significantly higher fracture rate than did premenopausal women. Before age 50, the fracture rate was much lower in men than in women, but thereafter the rates were essentially the same in both sexes.

Individuals of small body size may be at greater risk for development of glucocorticoid osteopenia. We showed a significant negative correlation between increasing body surface area (presteroid) and abnormal bone mass; however, we could not demonstrate a difference in fracture rates.

Interestingly, no correlations were noted between type of rheumatic disease and either DM/MM ratio or fracture rates when data were corrected for age. Clinically, we suspect that older individuals with polymyalgia rheumatica are at high risk for glucocorticoid-

related fractures, individuals with RA are at moderate risk, and those with systemic lupus erythematosus are at lower risk. Data reported by my associates support these perceptions and show a closer relationship to age than to disease process.[57] This finding is surprising because patients with RA who never received glucocorticoids had significantly lower bone mass than age-, sex-, and race-matched healthy control subjects.[59]

We were not able to show significant differences in the prevalence of glucocorticoid osteopenia in DM/ MM or fracture rates when we compared black individuals to white, but our numbers were relatively small, and we did not have enough Oriental and Hispanic individuals in our study group to make any conclusions regarding race or ethnicity as a risk factor.

Factors likely to increase risk of fractures in patients with rheumatic diseases treated with glucocorticoids are listed in Table 112–10.

MECHANISMS OF GLUCOCORTICOID OSTEOPENIA

Several reviews of the pathogenesis of glucocorticoid-induced osteopenia have appeared.[52,64,68] The effects resulting in loss of bone are summarized in Table 112–10.

Glucocorticoids undoubtedly inhibit bone formation in vitro and in vivo.[16,54,69–74] In children and young animals, glucocorticoids suppress growth hormone.[74]

Table 112–10. Mechanisms by Which Glucocorticoids Cause Bone Loss

Suppression of Bone Formation
  Reduced conversion of precursor cells to osteoblasts
  Reduced synthesis of osteoid by osteoblasts

Enhancement of Bone Resorption
  Reduced intestinal absorption of calcium
  Stimulation of parathyroid hormone, which activates osteoclasts in spite of direct suppression of osteoclast function by glucocorticoids

Net result: rate of resorption > rate of formation

Proliferation of epiphyseal cartilage is retarded and complete cessation of longitudinal growth can result (Fig. 112–7). Osteoblasts in culture reduce their synthesis of collagen if glucocorticoids are added to the media.[73] Collagen and noncollagen protein synthesis declines in cultures of fetal rat bone treated with glucocorticoids for more than 72 hours, and precursor cells do not differentiate into osteoblasts.[69] Decreased bone formation has been found in bone biopsies from humans treated with cortisone or related compounds.[71,72]

The mechanism by which glucocorticoids increase bone resorption is complicated. Many investigators have observed increased numbers of osteoclast-resorbing surfaces in bone biopsies from patients receiving glucocorticoids.[16,72] In culture systems, however, glucocorticoids directly inhibit osteoclast activity.[68,75] Furthermore, short-term administration of these hormones to rats can decrease bone resorption.[76] In humans receiving chronic glucocorticoid treatment, the indirect effect of those hormones on parathyroid hormone levels predominates. Glucocorticoids decrease the intestinal absorption of calcium and phosphate,[62,65,77] sometimes as early as 7 days after the institution of glucocorticoid therapy. Malabsorption of calcium stimulates the secretion of parathyroid hormone, and osteoclasts are then activated.[78] In animals, parathyroidectomy abolishes this osteoclastic response to glucocorticoids.[54]

Some studies have shown that levels of circulating parathyroid hormone are higher in patients or animals treated with glucocorticoids compared to those not receiving glucocorticoid therapy.[62] Other studies have not confirmed that finding.[61,65] In any case, the sensitivity of bone cells to the effects of parathyroid hormone is increased by glucocorticoids. The result is a state of secondary hyperparathyroidism in which the effects of hyperparathyroidism predominate over inhibitory effects on osteoclasts, and osteoclastic resorption of bone is increased. These effects are probably greatest in osseous areas with a large surface for osteoclasts to attack, such as trabecular bone and the endosteal surfaces of cortical bone at the metaphyses of long bones.

Investigators have debated possible alterations in vitamin D metabolism during glucocorticoid therapy. Serum levels of $1,25(OH)_2D$ were decreased in glucocorticoid-treated children in one study,[79] and their low levels correlated with decreased bone mass. In another study,[65] serum levels of 25 OH D correlated inversely with the daily prednisone dose. In studies in adults, my colleagues and I have not detected any differences in the circulating levels of 25 OH D or $1,25(OH)_2D$.

In summary, the bone loss of glucocorticoid osteopenia is caused by direct suppression of bone formation and increased bone resorption from functional hyperparathyroidism. The results are negative calcium balance[16] and a loss of bone mass that contributes to an increased risk of both vertebral and extravertebral fractures, especially when associated with senile, idiopathic, or disease-related osteoporosis in adults, or in rapidly modeling bones in children.

DIAGNOSIS

As discussed previously, no inexpensive, simple techniques are widely available to confirm a specific diagnosis of glucocorticoid-induced osteopenia. The clinician can only suspect its presence in most individuals who have received daily or alternate-day doses of glucocorticoids for several months. If routine roentgenograms, especially of vertebrae, show osteopenia, the patient is probably at high risk for fracture. Simple screening tests should be done to rule out other conditions, including hyperparathyroidism, hyperthyroidism, osteomalacia, and malignancies in bone. Generally, a complete blood count, creatinine determination, electrolyte measurement, liver function tests, and determination of serum levels of calcium, phosphorus, and alkaline phosphatase should suffice. Serum levels of calcium and phosphate are almost always normal in untreated glucocorticoid osteopenia. Alkaline phosphatase is usually normal, but may be mildly elevated.

TREATMENT

The best therapy for glucocorticoid-induced osteopenia is *complete withdrawal of the glucocorticoids*. I have observed exuberant new bone formation in iliac crest bone biopsies obtained from patients with rheumatic disease 3 to 6 months after discontinuation of prednisone therapy. Unfortunately, in patients with chronic allergic or inflammatory conditions, it is often undesirable to discontinue glucocorticoids, so other strategies are used, always with the goal of administering the smallest possible dose of this agent.

Two additional strategies might be employed. First, a glucocorticoid less toxic to bone might be formulated. Comparisons of the different types of glucocorticoid currently available in the United States have been made. At equivalent anti-inflammatory doses, they all have similar effects on calcium balance.[64] One molecule currently designated deflazacort (formerly oxazacort) in which an oxazoline ring has been added to the prednisolone molecule has been developed in Europe.[80] In short-term studies in healthy volunteers and longer-term studies in patients with RA, less calcium wasting was seen with deflazacort than with equivalent doses of prednisone or betamethasone.[64,80,81] Whether this drug will become available in the United States, whether its calcium-sparing effects persist after several months, and whether fracture rates will be diminished remain to be seen.

For the present, only the second strategy, that is, one designed to counteract the adverse effects of glucocorticoids on bone, is practical (Table 112–11).

As noted in the discussion of idiopathic osteoporosis, there is controversy regarding whether calcium supplementation alone can diminish the rate of bone loss in postmenopausal women. Patients with rheumatic diseases who were receiving long-term glucocorticoid therapy and had elevated DM/MM ratios and intestinal malabsorption of calcium were randomized into two groups.[61] The first received $1,25(OH)_2D$ and 500 mg calcium, as carbonate, daily; the second group received 500 mg calcium, as carbonate, alone. During the subsequent 18 months, most individuals in the calcium-alone group did *not* show a decline of diaphyseal or metaphyseal mass, and the appearance of their iliac crest biopsies did not change; most continued to show increased resorption surfaces. These data suggested that calcium supplementation might be useful to maintain bone mass, at least in the appendicular skeleton.

The use of vitamin D or its metabolites to prevent or to treat glucocorticoid osteopenia is somewhat controversial because of the risk of hypercalciuria and hypercalcemia. Treatment with vitamin D, 25 OH D, or $1,25(OH)_2D$, can partially overcome the intestinal malabsorption of calcium induced by glucocorticoids.[49,52,61,62] The treatment is usually associated with an increase in urinary calcium excretion, so regular monitoring of serum and urine calcium levels is required. Patients with past or present evidence of nephrolithiasis should probably be excluded from such therapy.

Our studies in rheumatic disease patients with elevated DM/MM ratios while receiving glucocorticoids demonstrated a significant increase of 8 to 15% in metaphyseal bone mass after 12 months of therapy with vitamin D (50,000 units 3 times a week)[52] or 25 OH D (20 to 40 µg daily).[62] In the patients receiving 25 OH D, we found increased intestinal absorption of calcium, reduced serum parathyroid hormone levels, and reduced resorption surfaces and osteoclast numbers on iliac crest biopsies. Bone formation rates, judged by tetracycline labeling, were unchanged or increased. In contrast, an 18-month trial of $1,25(OH)_2D$ resulted in improved calcium absorption and reduced parathyroid hormone levels, but metaphyseal mass did not increase. Although resorption surfaces were significantly diminished in iliac crest biopsies, so was the quantity of osteoblastic osteoid.[61] In all of these studies, the numbers of patients were inadequate to detect a difference in fracture rates.

In summary, *I recommend addition of vitamin D to the therapeutic regimen of any patient with rheumatic disease receiving chronic glucocorticoid therapy, if the 24-hour urinary excretion of calcium is <120 mg, which suggests intestinal malabsorption of calcium.* The vitamin D preparation of choice is 25 OH D, because it is eliminated

---

Table 112–11. Strategies to Minimize Adverse Effects of Glucocorticoid-Induced Osteopenia

1. Maintain glucocorticoid dose at lowest level possible to control disease
2. Encourage regular exercise (against gravity) when possible to stimulate bone formation
3. Identify high-risk patients and consider prophylactic therapy as follows:
   a. Allow glucocorticoid dose to stabilize and hypercalciuric effect of glucocorticoids to diminish (approximately 4–12 weeks)
   b. Measure serum calcium, phosphate, alk phosphatase, and 24-hour urine calcium levels

Serum studies normal Urine calcium >120 mg/24 hour	Serum studies normal Urine calcium <120 mg/24 hour No history of nephrolithiasis	Serum studies abnormal
Add calcium—500 mg if <50 years old, 1000 mg if >50 years old	Add calcium—500 mg if <50 years old; 1000 mg if >50 years old	Evaluate for additional cause of bone disease
Monitor serum and urine calcium levels every 6 months	Add 25 OH D, 20 mcg daily or vitamin D, 50,000 units 3 times/week	
	Monitor serum and urine Ca	

4. In patients who develop bone fractures after 12–18 months of the foregoing therapy:
   Consider adding fluoride, estrogens, or calcitonin; histologic bone study is helpful at this point; estrogen or calcitonin might be useful (or 25 OH D if it has not been added) when resorption is occurring at a high rate; fluoride may be useful in patients with little bone formation

Note: All the regimens listed under 3 and 4 must be considered experimental because none have been proved to reduce fracture rates in glucocorticoid-induced osteopenia.

more quickly than vitamin D. Rapid elimination is desirable if hypercalciuria or hypercalcemia occur. Vitamin D, however, is cheaper and more widely available, and it is effective. The use of 1,25(OH)$_2$D is probably undesirable.

Other investigators could *not* show an increase in bone mass in patients with hematologic and rheumatic diseases treated from the onset of prednisone therapy for 6 months with vitamin D, calcium phosphate and sodium fluoride.[82] Studies have not been done to determine if treatment with either calcium alone or calcium and vitamin D or its metabolites reduces fracture rates in patients with glucocorticoid-induced osteopenia.

For patents who begin or continue to experience bone fractures after 6 to 12 months of therapy with calcium with or without vitamin D, other experimental approaches must be considered. The addition of sodium fluoride should increase bone formation rates; the addition of estrogens or calcitonin might decrease resorption rates. (The use of these therapies is discussed in the section of this chapter on idiopathic osteoporosis.) In this situation, I find bone biopsy helpful. If the biopsy shows a large amount of osteoid, indicating a surprisingly high formation rate, I am reluctant to institute fluoride. If histology suggests active resorption of bone, then estrogen or calcitonin might be indicated. Baylink[49] reported that combination therapy with sodium fluoride, calcium, and vitamin D, with addition of hydrochlorthiazide if hypercalciuria occurs, is effective in increasing trabecular bone mass in patients receiving prednisone therapy.

Hypercalcemia and hypercalciuria must be sought at regular intervals in patients receiving vitamin D or its metabolites. We do not permit the patient's 24-hour urine calcium excretion to exceed 350 mg; no one knows at what level of urinary calcium the risk of nephrolithiasis increases, so our choice is arbitrary.

In conclusion, glucocorticoid-induced osteopenia is a major problem in terms of high incidence and high association with disability. Although the mechanisms and risk factors are understood and some potential therapies have been studied, none have been shown to lower fracture rates. The need for further investigation is clear.

OSTEOMALACIA

Osteomalacia is a pathologic loss of mineralized bone caused by reduction of calcium phosphate levels to below that required for normal mineralization of bone matrix. As a result, the ratio of bone mineral to matrix is reduced, undecalcified matrix (osteoid) accumulates, and bone strength declines. The most common causes of osteomalacia beginning after early childhood are reduced vitamin D absorption due to biliary, proximal small-bowel mucosal, or ileal disease; increased vitamin D catabolism as a result of drug-induced increases in liver oxidase enzymes; and acquired renal tubular defects with renal phosphate wasting. This third group includes acquired renal tubular phosphate leaks (adult-onset vitamin D-resistant rickets"), Fanconi syndrome, and renal tubular acidosis of the variety seen with the chronic dysproteinemias associated with Sjögren's syndrome, systemic lupus erythematosus, monoclonal gammopathies, and heavy metal poisoning. Additionally, an occasional patient with peptic ulcer disease develops phosphate depletion because of magnesium-alumina gel antacid abuse; large amounts of these substances convert dietary phosphate to insoluble complexes in the intestine.

CLINICAL AND DIAGNOSTIC FEATURES

Clinically, patients with osteomalacia have many of the symptoms commonly associated with the rheumatic diseases, including generalized aching and fatigability, proximal myopathy, periarticular tenderness, and sensory polyneuropathy.[2,83,84] When osteomalacia is treated, these symptoms all remit rapidly. Radiographs may show only mild generalized demineralization, or they may be more diagnostic and reveal multiple old rib fractures with poor callus formation, or pathognomonic pseudofractures, termed Looser's zones (Fig. 112–11). The presence of nephrocalcinosis suggests renal tubular acidosis.

Characteristic of vitamin D deficiency osteomalacia are a low-normal to decreased calcium level, hypophosphatemia, an elevated bone alkaline phosphatase level, a mild parathyroid hormone elevation, and decreased 25 OH D levels. In the renal phosphate leak syndromes, levels of serum calcium and 25 OH D are normal, but serum phosphate levels are low. A mild hyperchloremic acidosis is compatible with severe vitamin D deficiency and secondary hyperparathyroidism leading to proximal tubular bicarbonate wasting. Marked hyperchloremic hypokalemic acidosis suggests renal tubular acidosis, a diagnosis that can be confirmed by inadequate urine acidification after an ammonium chloride load. Vitamin D deficiency decreases urine calcium excretion, sometimes to undetectable levels. In the renal phosphate leak syndromes, urine calcium excretion is generally normal or, in renal tubular acidosis, elevated. In both

FIG. 112–11. Roentgenogram of the pelvis and hips of a patient with osteomalacia. Note the generalized osteopenia and symmetric pseudofractures in both femoral necks (arrows) (courtesy of Richard H. Gold, M.D., Professor of Radiology, University of California, Los Angeles).

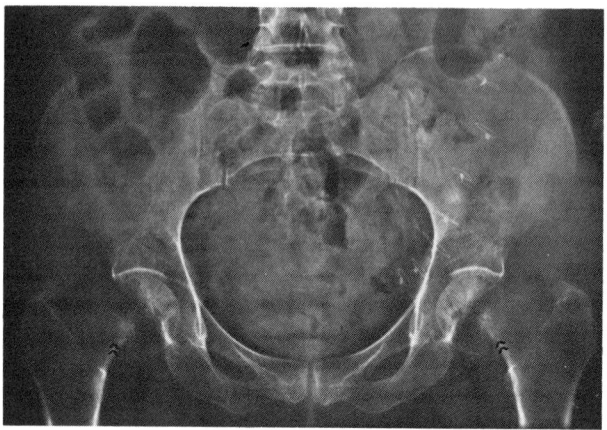

varieties of osteomalacia, tubular reabsorption of phosphate is appropriately low for the level of serum phosphate. Bone biopsy in patients with vitamin D deficiency shows changes of both osteomalacia and osteitis fibrosa. In pure phosphate deficiency, osteomalacia predominates.

The differential diagnosis of osteomalacia caused by vitamin D deficiency includes severe dietary deprivation, which is rare, intestinal fat malabsorption syndromes, and drug-induced acceleration of hepatic vitamin D catabolism. The diagnosis of dietary deficiency can be established by a careful history, and the patient can be treated with vitamin D (or its metabolites), 50,000 IU three times weekly, in addition to calcium supplementation until serum chemistries and urinary calcium excretion return to normal. At that point, an adequate diet with a 400-IU supplement of vitamin D daily is sufficient. Intestinal fat malabsorption may be readily apparent by the patient's medical history, but it is more often occult, as in smoldering ileitis with deficient bile salt reabsorption and consequent deficient solubilization of ingested fats. An adequate evaluation should include appropriate radiologic studies, quantitation of intestinal fat absorption, assessment of mucosal function by D-xylose uptake, and jejunal biopsy, if indicated. Proper treatment involves both control of the primary intestinal disorder and replenishment of body vitamin D and mineral stores. Depending on the severity of the malabsorption syndrome and the degree of vitamin D depletion, one should administer vitamin D, 50,000 IU three to seven times/week and calcium, 1000 mg/ day. In patients with unusually severe malabsorption, even higher doses may be required.

Therapeutic response can be assessed by following levels of serum calcium, phosphorus, alkaline phosphatase, and 25 OH D as well as 24-hour urine calcium excretion. A period of several months or longer may be required before these parameters return to normal. At that point, doses of vitamin D and calcium can be reduced to maintain normal serum and urine calcium levels. In these disorders especially, it is essential to monitor patients' serum and urine calcium levels frequently because improved intestinal absorption following treatment of the primary disease can lead to vitamin D intoxication if the dose is not adjusted promptly.

In the renal tubular phosphate leak syndromes, therapy is directed toward reversing the acidosis, if present, compensating for renal phosphate wasting, and maintaining normal calcium absorption with supplemental vitamin D. In the case of an isolated tubular phosphate leak, one should prescribe vitamin D, 50,000 IU three times weekly, and phosphate, 1.8 to 2.4 g/day in two to four divided doses. In patients with Fanconi syndrome, it is important to correct the acidosis with bicarbonate or Shol's solution because the acidosis itself impairs bone mineral content. The effect of acidosis appears to be the result of removal of buffering anions and calcium from bone, with resultant renal calcium and phosphate loss. In pure renal tubular acidosis, alkali therapy and calcium supplementation, in addition to vitamin D, is usually sufficient. It is essential to supplement with calcium and vitamin D in renal tubular acidosis because alkali therapy alone may well precipitate tetany in a severely osteomalacic patient. When healing has occurred, vitamin D supplementation should be discontinued; relapse does not usually occur if the acidosis is controlled.

The active metabolites of vitamin D (25 OH D_3 or 1,25(OH)$_2$D) may be substituted for vitamin D in the treatment of osteomalacia. Both metabolites have a shorter half-life than vitamin D; therefore, toxicity can be treated more quickly. Because 1,25(OH)$_2$D is the "final" metabolite, however, it may not be associated with feedback control; hypercalciuria and hypercalcemia are more frequent with 1,25(OH)$_2$D than with vitamin D supplementation. For a more detailed discussion of osteomalacia and its treatment, the reader is referred to recent reviews.[2,83,84,85]

DRUG-INDUCED OSTEOMALACIA

The primary basis of this recently recognized disorder appears to be drug induction of hepatic microsomal oxidase enzymes that accelerate the conversion of vitamin D and its active metabolites to polar, inactive compounds that are rapidly excreted.[86] The anticonvulsant drugs, particularly phenobarbital and phenytoin, have been most commonly implicated. All long-acting barbiturates, many sedatives, and a variety of drugs used in rheumatic disease, such as diazepam and phenylbutazone, are potent hepatic oxidase inducers that could possibly reduce the levels of vitamin D metabolites. The disorder is most severe in patients with high drug doses, marginal vitamin D intake, and reduced exposure to sunlight. Serum calcium and phosphate levels may be within the normal range in all but the most severe cases; however, serum 25 OH D levels and urinary calcium excretion are uniformly reduced in patients with clinically significant disease.

Needle biopsy of iliac crest bone is useful to confirm a doubtful diagnosis. It is essential to have a high index of suspicion of this disorder. The diagnosis may be obvious in a patient who experiences seizures and has been treated with anticonvulsants for a long time; it may be less apparent in an elderly patient with marginal dietary intake who is confined indoors and who has received barbiturate sedatives or phenylbutazone on a long-term basis. Treatment consists of repleting body vitamin D stores with 25,000 to 100,000 IU/week until serum and urine calcium as well as serum 25 OH D levels are normal; then one must compensate for the increased hepatic catabolism by supplementing with vitamin D, 1000 to 2000 IU/day.

OSTEITIS FIBROSA

Osteitis fibrosa is a histologic diagnosis based on the findings of increased osteoclast numbers and resorption sites with ultimate replacement of bone by fibrous tissue. The sole basis of these changes is increased secretion of parathyroid hormone, either as a primary process or as a secondary response to a prolonged hypocalcemic stimulus, such as calcium malabsorption as a result of vitamin D deficiency or decreased intestinal calcium absorption in the aged.

PRIMARY HYPERPARATHYROIDISM

The initial manifestations of primary hyperparathyroidism occasionally include generalized osteopenia with vertebral compression or long-bone fractures. Associated clinical findings are a history of weakness and easy fatigability, weight loss, muscular aches and proximal muscle weakness, arthralgias,

morning stiffness, or pseudogout, as well as the more classic symptoms of epigastric pain and renal colic.[87] Hypertension and proximal myopathy may be observed on physical examination; band keratopathy is an infrequent finding. Radiologic clues include subperiosteal bone resorption, especially in the phalanges (Fig. 112–12A), occasional brown tumors ap-

FIG. 112–12. Roentgenograms of patients with hyperparathyroidism. *A,* Hand film from a middle-aged woman with long-standing primary hyperparathyroidism. Note erosions and resorption of digital tufts, subperiosteal resorption of shafts of the proximal and middle phalanges, and bony erosions at the second and fifth metacarpophalangeal joints. *B,* Bilateral erosive changes in the sacroiliac joints in a young man with severe secondary hyperparathyroidism resulting from chronic renal failure. The right femoral head has been replaced because of ischemic necrosis (courtesy of Richard H. Gold, M.D., Professor of Radiology, University of California, Los Angeles).

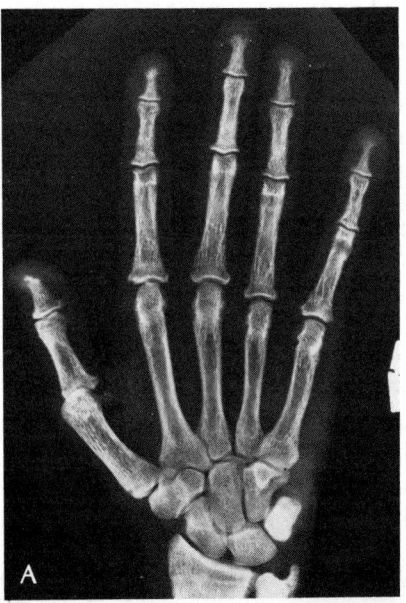

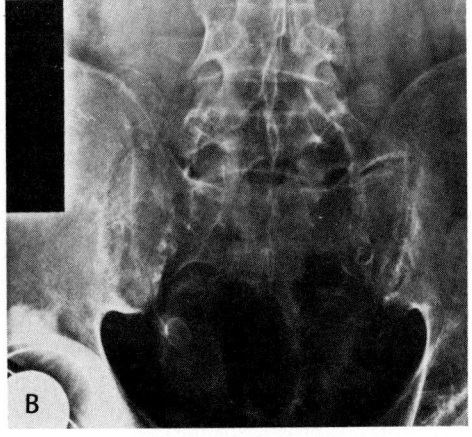

pearing as smooth, sharply demarcated, cyst-like lesions in any part of the skeleton, and renal calculi. Subperiosteal resorption is the most consistent radiologic finding. Occasionally, erosive and sclerotic changes in the sacroiliac joints mimic ankylosing spondylitis (Fig. 112–12B).

The diagnosis can be readily established by demonstrating a consistently elevated serum calcium level, a reduced serum phosphate level, and an elevated parathyroid hormone level. The tubular reabsorption of phosphorus is inappropriately low for the level of serum phosphate. In patients with significant bone disease, the bone fraction of serum alkaline phosphatase is likely to be elevated. Hyperuricemia is frequently observed. Whereas urinary calcium excretion may be normal or even low in patients with mild primary hyperparathyroidism because of the renal calcium-retaining effects of parathyroid hormone, patients with significant bone disease usually have an elevated urinary calcium excretion because of the increased filtered load.

The only curative treatment of osteopenia caused by primary hyperparathyroidism is parathyroidectomy, following which some return of bone mass is noted.[87] In patients who are not operative candidates, serum and urine calcium levels may be reduced by the administration of phosphorus. The resultant elevation of urinary phosphate excretion increases the risk of calcium-phosphate stone formation, however, and the increased calcium × phosphate product makes metastatic soft-tissue calcification more likely.

Ectopic tumor production of parathyroid hormone accounts for about 15% of cases of hypercalcemic (autonomous) hyperparathyroidism in adults, but because of the rapid progression of the underlying malignant process, osteopenia is rarely observed. Approximately 90% of parathyroid hormone–producing tumors occur in the lung, kidney, or urogenital tract; therefore, a normal chest roentgenogram and intravenous urogram adequately exclude this diagnosis unless definite clinical signs of malignant disease are present elsewhere.

SECONDARY HYPERPARATHYROIDISM

Hyperparathyroidism may be secondary to disorders that decrease intestinal calcium absorption. The most common of these are vitamin D deficiency states and the idiopathic reduction in intestinal calcium absorption seen occasionally in older individuals. In cases of vitamin D deficiency, fatigability and myopathic symptoms are common. Diagnostic findings include low-normal to mildly reduced serum calcium levels, reduced serum phosphate levels, a mild parathyroid hormone elevation, and much-reduced urinary calcium excretion. Treatment consists of restoring intestinal calcium absorption to normal (see the sections on osteoporosis and osteomalacia in this chapter). Although severe secondary hyperparathyroidism is common in chronic renal disease, the radiologic bone picture is generally mixed and can include osteomalacia, osteitis fibrosa, osteoporosis, and even patchy osteosclerosis. The osteitis fibrosa component responds to therapy with $1,25(OH)_2D$ or $1\ \alpha\text{-OH}\ D$, which is metabolized to $1,25(OH)_2D$, and most patients with bone pain and myopathy benefit. The response of the osteomalacic component to this treatment is variable, however. At least some of the osteomalacia in patients undergoing renal dialysis is due to aluminum toxicity rather than to a deficiency of vitamin D.[88]

In summary, the management of the bone disease associated with renal failure and dialysis is complex and beyond the scope of this chapter; the reader is referred to detailed reviews of the subject.[88,89]

HYPERTHYROIDISM (HIGH-TURNOVER OSTEOPOROSIS)

The bone disease of hyperthyroidism is high-turnover osteoporosis. Patients may have bone pain and fractures, in addition to other features of hyperthyroidism. Although the disease is usually endogenous, severe osteoporosis can probably be caused by the exogenous administration of thyroid hormones after decades of treatment, possibly in association with postmenopausal osteoporosis.[90] Radiographs usually show diffuse osteopenia; occasionally, abnormal striations of cortical bone are seen. Biochemical parameters usually include slight elevations in serum calcium levels and elevated serum levels of alkaline phosphatase. Urinary studies often show high levels of calcium and hydroxyproline.

The mechanism of this disease is probably direct stimulation of bone resorption by excessive levels of thyroid hormone. This process reduces the levels of serum parathyroid hormone and thereby causes renal retention of phosphate and mild elevations of serum phosphate. Both low parathyroid hormone levels and high serum phosphate levels lead to reduced activity of renal 1-α-hydroxylase[91] with a subsequent decrease in serum levels of $1,25(OH)_2D$ and an increase of $24,25(OH)_2D$. In spite of low $1,25(OH)_2D$ levels, bone biopsies rarely show osteomalacia. Typical findings include a high rate of bone turnover, characterized by an increase of osteoclasts and osteoclastic surfaces and increased osteoid formation surfaces, involving cortical as well as trabecular bone; mineralization is normal.[90,91] Increased porosity of cortical bone is typical.

The treatment of this disorder is correction of the hyperthyroid state.

OSTEOGENESIS IMPERFECTA

Occasionally, an adult with multiple fractures, especially in the long bones of the legs, and radiographic osteopenia, actually has osteogenesis imperfecta (see Chapters 12 and 85). This group of disorders is characterized by a genetically determined inability to form quantitatively or qualitatively normal collagen; most defects are probably in type I collagen. To date, different mutations in the gene for type I procollagen have been identified in several variants of type I, II, III, and IV osteogenesis imperfecta: all result in formation of unstable collagen helices.[92] Most patients develop bone fractures in childhood. One prenatal form is lethal. Some of these individuals are deaf or have blue sclerae, but others have only osseous manifestations. If the disease begins in childhood, bones may grow abnormally. Extremities are short, legs are bowed, and saber shins occur. Pectus excavatum or carinatum can appear, as well as a dome-shaped forehead and lateral widening of the skull. Some individuals have lax joints, are easily bruised, or have small, misshapen, discolored teeth. Fractures usually diminish in frequency at puberty, but they often increase around the time of menopause in women and at a similar age in men.

If none of the phenotypic characteristics of osteogenesis imperfecta are present except for fragile bones, the diagnosis can be difficult. A positive family history and a history of multiple fractures in childhood are helpful in establishing the diagnosis. Radiographs show thinning of cortical and trabecular areas of bones indistinguishable from that seen in other osteopenias. Platybasia of the skull and bone islands in the cranium also suggest osteogenesis imperfecta. Bone biopsy shows diminished quantities of osteoid with replacement by a blue-staining material. Therapy with sodium fluoride or with sex hormones has been advocated, but it is not clear whether any interventions reduce fracture rates. For a discussion of the different types of this disorder, the reader is referred to a recent review[92] and to Chapters 12 and 85.

REFERENCES

1. Frost, H.M.: The pathomechanics of osteoporosis. Clin. Orthop., 200:198–225, 1985.
2. Goldring, S.R., and Krane, S.M.: Metabolic bone disease: Osteoporosis and osteomalacia. D.M., 27:1–103, 1981.
3. Raisz, L.G.: Osteoporosis. J. Am. Geriatr. Soc., 30:127–138, 1982.
4. Mawer, E.B., Blackhouse, J., and Holman, C.: The distribution and storage of vitamin D and its metabolites in man. Clin. Sci., 43:413–420, 1972.
5. Canalis, E.: Interleukin-1 has independent effects on deoxyribonucleic acid and collagen synthesis in cultures of rat calvariae. Endocrinology, 118:74–81, 1986.
6. Canalis, E., and Centrella, M.: Isolation of a nontransforming bone-derived growth factor from medium conditioned by fetal rat calvariae. Endocrinology, 118:2002–2008, 1986.
7. Raisz, L.G., and Kream, B.E.: Regulation of bone formation. N. Engl. J. Med., 309:83–89, 1983.
8. Melson, F. and Mosekilde, L.: The role of bone biopsy in the diagnosis of metabolic bone disease. Orthop. Clin. North Am., 12:571–602, 1981.
9. Meunier, P.J., and Bressot, C.: Endocrine influence on bone cells and bone remodeling evaluated by clinical histomorphometry. *In* The Endocrinology of Calcium Metabolism. Edited by J.A. Parson. New York, Raven Press, 1982.
10. Meema, H.E., and Meema, S.: Radiogrammetry in non-invasive measurements of bone mass and their clinical application. *In* Noninvasive Bone Measurements of Bone Mass and their Clinical Application. Edited by S.H. Cohn. Boca Raton, CRC Press, 1981.
11. Colbert, C., and Bachtell, R.S.: Radiographic absorptiometry (photodensitometry). *In* Noninvasive Bone Measurements of Bone Mass and their Clinical Application. Edited by S.H. Cohn. Boca Raton, CRC Press, 1981.
12. Mazess, R.B.: Photon absorptiometry. *In* Noninvasive Bone Measurements of Bone Mass and their Clinical Application. Edited by S.H. Cohn. Boca Raton, CRC Press, 1981.
13. Firooznia, H., et al.: Rate of spinal trabecular bone loss in normal perimenopausal women: CT measurement. Radiology, 161:735–738, 1986.
14. Cohn, S.H.: Total body neutron activation. *In* Noninvasive Bone Measurements of Bone Mass and their Clinical Application. Edited by S.H. Cohn. Boca Raton, CRC Press, 1981.
15. Whyte, M.P., et al.: Postmenopausal osteoporosis. A heterogeneous disorder as assessed by histomorphometric analysis of iliac crest bone from untreated patients. Am. J. Med., 72:193–201, 1982.
16. Nordin, B.E.C., et al.: The effects of sex steroid and corticosteroid hormones on bone. J. Steroid Biochem., 15:171–174, 1981.
17. Riggs, B.L., et al.: Differential changes in bone mineral density of the appendicular and axial skeleton with aging: Relationship to spinal osteoporosis. J. Clin. Invest., 67:328–335, 1981.
18. Heaney, R.P., Recker, R.R., and Saville, P.D.: Menopausal changes in calcium balance performance. J. Lab. Clin. Med., 92:953–963, 1978.
19. Riggs, B.L., et al.: Changes in the bone mineral density of the proximal femur and spine with aging: Difference between the postmenopausal and senile osteoporosis syndromes. J. Clin. Invest., 70:716–723, 1982.
20. Jensen, J.S., and Tondevold, E.: Mortality after hip fractures. Acta Orthop. Scand., 50:161–167, 1979.
21. Johnson, K.A., et al.: Osteoid tissue in normal and osteoporotic individuals. J. Clin. Endocrinol. Metab., 33:745–751, 1971.

22. Avioli, L.V., McDonald, J.E., and Lee, S.W.: The influence of age on the intestinal absorption of ^{47}calcium in women and its relation to ^{47}Ca absorption in postmenopausal osteoporosis. J. Clin. Invest., 44:1960–1967, 1965.

23. Aitken, J.M., et al.: Osteoporosis after oophorectomy for non-malignant disease in premenopausal women. Br. Med. J., 2:325–328, 1973.

24. Smith, D.M., et al.: Genetic factors in determining bone mass. J. Clin. Invest., 52:2800–2808, 1973.

25. Mazess, R.B., and Mather, W.E.: Bone mineral content in Canadian Eskimos. Hum. Biol., 47:45–63, 1975.

26. Dalen, N., Hallberg, D., and Lamke, B.: Bone mass in obese subjects. Acta Med. Scand., 197:353–355, 1975.

27. Hartman, D.A., et al.: Attempts to prevent disuse osteoporosis by treatment with calcitonin, longitudinal compression, and supplementary calcium and phosphate. J. Clin. Endocrinol. Metab., 36:845–858, 1973.

28. Spencer, H., et al.: Chronic alcoholism: Frequently overlooked cause of osteoporosis in men. Am. J. Med., 80:393–397, 1986.

29. Heaney, R.P.: Management of osteoporosis: Nutritional considerations. Clin. Invest. Med., 5:185–187, 1982.

30. Recker, R.R.: Continuous treatment of osteoporosis: Current status. In Symposium of the Osteoporoses. Edited by H.M. Frost. Orthop. Clin. North Am., 12:611–627, 1981.

31. Aloia, J.F., et al.: Prevention of involutional bone loss by exercise. Ann. Intern. Med., 89:356–358, 1978.

32. President's Council on Physical Fitness: Adult Physical Fitness: A Program for Men and Women. Washington, D.C., United States Government Printing Office, 1965.

33. Heaney, R.P., Recker, R.R., and Saville, P.D.: Calcium balance and calcium requirements in middle-aged women. Am. J. Clin. Nutr., 30:1603–1611, 1977.

34. Recker, R.R., Saville, P.D., and Heaney, R.P.: Effect of estrogens and calcium carbonate on bone loss in postmenopausal women. Ann. Intern. Med., 87:649–655, 1977.

35. Matkovic, V., et al.: Fracture rates in two regions of Yugoslavia. Am. J. Clin. Nutr., 32:540–549, 1979.

36. Ettinger, B., Genant, H.K., and Cann, C.E.: Postmenopausal bone loss is prevented by treatment with low-dosage estrogen with calcium. Ann. Intern. Med., 106:40–45, 1987.

37. Riis, B., Thomsen, K., and Christiansen, C.: Does calcium supplementation prevent postmenopausal bone loss? A double-blind, controlled clinical study. N. Engl. J. Med., 316:173–177, 1987.

38. Lindsay, R., Hart, D.M., and Baird, C.: Prevention of spinal osteoporosis in oophorectemized women. Lancet, 2:1151–1157, 1980.

39. Aitken, J.M., Hart, D.M., and Lindsay, R.: Estrogen replacement therapy for prevention of osteoporosis after oophorectomy. Br. Med. J., 2:515–518, 1973.

40. Chetkowski, R.J., et al.: Biologic effects of transdermal estradiol. N. Engl. J. Med., 314:1615–1620, 1986.

41. Paganini-Hill, A., et al.: Menopausal estrogen therapy and hip fractures. Ann. Intern. Med., 95:28–31, 1981.

42. Antunes, C.M.F., et al.: Endometrial cancer and estrogen use. N. Engl. J. Med., 300:9–13, 1979.

43. Cummings, S.R., et al.: Should perimenopausal women be screened for osteoporosis? Ann. Intern. Med., 104:817–823, 1986.

44. Chesnut, C.H., et al.: Effect of metandrostendone on postmenopausal bone wasting as assessed by changes in total bone mineral mass. Metabolism, 26:267–277, 1977.

45. Finkelstein, J.S., et al.: Osteoporosis in men with idiopathic

46. Seeman, E., et al.: Risk factors for spinal osteoporosis in men. Am. J. Med., 75:977–983, 1983.

47. Riggs, B.L., et al.: Effect of the fluoride calcium regimen on vertebral fracture occurrence in postmenopausal osteoporosis: Comparison with conventional therapy. N. Engl. J. Med., 306:446–450, 1982.

48. Fatourechi, V., Health, H. 3rd: Salmon calcitonin in the treatment of postmenopausal osteoporosis. Ann. Intern. Med., 107:923–925, 1987.

49. Baylink, D.J.: Glucocorticoid-induced osteoporosis. N. Engl. J. Med., 309:306–308, 1983.

50. Frost, H.M.: Clinical management of the symptomatic osteoporotic patient. In Symposium of the Osteoporoses. Edited by H.M. Frost. Orthop. Clin. North Am., 12:671–681, 1981.

51. Curtiss, P.H., Clark, W.S., and Herndon, C.H.: Vertebral fractures resulting from prolonged cortisone and corticotrophin therapy. JAMA, 156:467–470, 1954.

52. Hahn, T.J., and Hahn, B.H.: Osteopenia in patients with rheumatic diseases: Principles of diagnosis and therapy. Semin. Arthritis Rheum., 6:230–253, 1976.

53. Howland, W.J., Pugh, D.G., and Sprague, R.G.: Roentgenologic changes of the skeletal system in Cushing's syndrome. Radiology, 71:69–78, 1958.

54. Jee, W.S.S., et al.: Corticosteroid and bone. Am. J. Anat., 129:477–480, 1970.

55. Soffer, L.J., Iannaccone, A., and Gabrilove, J.L.: Cushing's syndrome: A study of 50 patients. Am. J. Med., 30:129–138, 1961.

56. Sussman, C.B.: The roentgenologic appearance of the bones in Cushing's syndrome. Radiology, 39:288–292, 1942.

56a.Seeman, E., et al.: Differential effects of endocrine dysfunction on the axial and appendicular skeleton. J. Clin. Invest., 69:1302–1308, 1982.

57. Dykman, T.R., et al.: Evaluation of factors associated with glucocorticoid-induced osteopenia in patients with rheumatic diseases. Arthritis Rheum., 28:361–368, 1985.

58. Adinoff, A.D., and Hollister, J.R.: Steroid-induced fractures and bone loss in patients with asthma. N. Engl. J. Med., 309:265–268, 1983.

59. Hahn, T.J., Boisseau, V.C., and Avioli, L.V.: Effect of chronic corticosteroid administration on diaphyseal and metaphyseal bone mass. J. Clin. Endocrinol. Metab., 39:274–282, 1974.

60. Schlenker, R.A., and von Seggen, W.W.: The distribution of cortical and trabecular bone mass along the lengths of the radius and ulna and the implications for in vivo bone mass measurements. Calcif. Tissue Res., 20:41–52, 1976.

61. Dykman, T.R., et al.: Effect of oral 1,25-dihydroxyvitamin D and calcium on glucocorticoid-induced osteopenia in patients with rheumatic diseases. Arthritis Rheum., 27:1336–1343, 1984.

62. Hahn, T.J., et al.: Altered mineral metabolism in glucocorticoid-induced osteopenia: Effect of 25-hydroxyvitamin D administration. J. Clin. Invest., 64:655–665, 1979.

63. Bradley, B.W., and Ansell, B.M.: Fractures in Still's disease. Ann. Rheum. Dis., 19:135–142, 1960.

64. Caniggia, A., et al.: Pathophysiology of the adverse effects of glucoactive corticosteroids on calcium metabolism in man. J. Steroid Biochem., 15:153–161, 1981.

65. Klein, R.G., et al.: Intestinal calcium absorption in exogenous hypercortisonism—Role of 25-hydroxyvitamin D and corticosteroid dose. J. Clin. Invest., 60:253–259, 1977.

66. Gluck, O.S., et al.: Bone loss in adults receiving alternate day

glucocorticoid therapy. A comparison with daily therapy. Arthritis Rheum., 24:892–898, 1981.

67. Sheagren, J.N., et al.: Effect on bone growth of daily versus alternate-day corticosteroid administration: An experimental study. J. Lab. Clin. Med., 89:120–130, 1977.

68. Raisz, L.G.: Effect of corticosteroids on calcium metabolism. Prog. Biochem. Pharmacol., 17:212–219, 1980.

69. Dietrich, J.W., et al.: Effects of glucocorticoids on fetal rat bone collagen synthesis in vitro. Endocrinology, 104:715–721, 1979.

70. Follis, R.H.: Effect of cortisone on growing bones of the rat. Proc. Soc. Exp. Biol. Med., 76:722–724, 1954.

71. Frost, H.M., and Villanueva, A.R.: Human osteoblastic activity. III. The effect of cortisone on lamellar osteoblastic activity. Henry Ford Hosp. Med. J., 9:97–100, 1961.

72. Jowsey, J., and Riggs, B.L.: Bone formation in hypercortisonism. Acta Endocrinol., 63:21–31, 1970.

73. Peck, W.A., Brandt, J., and Miller, T.: Hydrocortisone-induced inhibition of protein synthesis and uridine incorporation in isolated bone cells in vitro. Proc. Natl. Acad. Sci. U.S.A., 57:1599–1602, 1967.

74. Baxter, J.D.: Mechanisms of glucocorticoid inhibition of growth. Kidney Int., 14:330–333, 1978.

75. Raisz, L.G., et al.: Effects of glucocorticoids on bone resorption in tissue culture. Endocrinology, 90:961–967, 1972.

76. Yasumura, S.: Effects of adrenal steroids on resorption in rats. Am. J. Physiol., 230:90–93, 1976.

77. Collins, E.J., Garret, E.R., and Johnston, R.L.: Effects of adrenal steroids on radio-calcium metabolism in dogs. Metabolism, 11:716–726, 1962.

78. Fucik, R.F., Kukreja, S.C., and Hargis, G.K.: Effect of glucocorticoids on function of the parathyroid glands in man. J. Clin. Endocrinol. Metab., 40:152–155, 1975.

79. Chesney, R.W., et al.: Reduction of serum 1,25 dihydroxyvitamin D in children receiving glucocorticoids. Lancet, 2:1123–1125, 1978.

80. Caniggia, A., et al.: Effects of a new glucocorticoid, oxazacort, on some variables connected with bone metabolism in man: A comparison with prednisone. Int. J. Clin. Pharmacol. Biopharm., 15:126–134, 1977.

81. Hahn, T.J., et al.: Comparison of subacute effects of oxazacort and prednisone on mineral metabolism in man. Calcif. Tissue Int., 31:109–115, 1980.

82. Rickers, H., et al.: Corticosteroid-induced osteopenia and vitamin D metabolism: Effect of vitamin D_2, calcium, phosphate and sodium fluoride administration. Clin. Endocrinol (Oxf)., 16:409–415, 1982.

83. Frame, B.: Osteomalacia. In Internal Medicine. Edited by J.H. Stein. Boston, Little, Brown and Co., 1983.

84. Krane, S.M., and Holick, M.F.: Rickets and osteomalacia. In Harrison's Principles of Internal Medicine. Edited by E. Braunwald, et al. New York, McGraw-Hill Book Company, 1987.

85. Singer, F.: Osteomalacia. In Textbook of Rheumatology. 2nd Ed. Edited by W.N. Kelley, et al.: Philadelphia, W.B. Saunders Co., 1985, pp. 1662–1670.

86. Hahn, T.J.: Drug-induced disorders of vitamin D and mineral metabolism. J. Clin. Endocrinol Metab., 9:107–129, 1980.

87. Potts, J.T., Jr.: Diseases of the parathyroid gland and other hyper- and hypocalcemic disorders. In Harrison's Principles of Internal Medicine. Edited by E. Braunwald, et al. New York, McGraw-Hill Book Company, 1987.

88. Drucke, T.: Dialysis osteomalacia and aluminum intoxication. Nephron, 26:207–210, 1980.

89. Avioli, L.V.: Renal osteodystrophy. In The Kidney. Edited by B. Brenner and F.C. Rector, Jr. Philadelphia, W.B. Saunders, 1976.

90. Fallon, M.D., et al.: Exogenous hyperthyroidism with osteoporosis. Arch. Intern. Med., 143:442–444, 1983.

91. Jastrup, B., et al.: Serum levels of vitamin D metabolites and bone remodeling in hyperthyroidism. Metabolism, 31:126–132, 1982.

92. Prockop, D.J., and Kivrikko, K.I.: Heritable diseases of collagen. N. Engl. J. Med., 311:376–380, 1984.

113

RHEUMATIC ASPECTS OF ENDOCRINOPATHIES

MARY E. CRONIN

Hormonal excess or deprivation can lead to a variety of syndromes with musculoskeletal manifestations. Their recognition is important because they are often treatable. Awareness of these features can suggest the appropriate diagnosis. Such states of altered hormonal balance, including pregnancy, have shed light on the pathogenesis of some rheumatic disorders and promise new insights into their treatment. These relationships are described here.

The role of the neuroendocrine system in immunity is a relatively new area of research, but it is now well recognized that the neuroendocrine system has direct and indirect regulatory functions affecting the immune system. A number of hormones and neuropeptides can modulate lymphocyte function, probably by specific receptors. These peptides include adrenocorticotropic hormone (ACTH), growth hormone, insulin, acetylcholine, endorphins, enkephalins, prolactin, vasoactive intestinal peptide (VIP), and substance P. The intracellular level of cyclic nucleotides can be affected by hormones and neurotransmitters, thus effecting activation or suppression of immune cells.[1,2] Lymphoid cells themselves may produce ACTH, thyroid-stimulating hormone (TSH), and endorphin-like substances that could also act as immune messengers.[3] The study of the clinical implications of these systems to rheumatic diseases is just beginning but merits close attention.[4]

ACROMEGALY

Pituitary adenomas may produce excessive quantities of growth hormone, the anabolic effects of which can lead to significant changes in connective tissues. Such tumors usually occur in older persons, in whom epiphyseal closure has already taken place, and *acromegaly* results. Excessive growth hormone production before puberty results in *gigantism*. Although many anabolic influences derive from the direct action of this hormone, stimulation of chondroitin sulfate and collagen synthesis by articular chondrocytes are due to a hepatically derived serum factor called somatomedin induced by growth hormone.[5] Somatomedin is one of a family of insulin-like growth promoting factors. Somatomedin C is the best known of these and corresponds to insulin-like growth factor I (IGF-I); IGF-II corresponds to somatomedin A. These and other substances that stimulate cellular proliferation are discussed in Chapter 14.[6]

Growth hormone itself stimulates the proliferation of soft tissues including bursae, joint capsules, synovium, cartilage (Fig. 113–1), and bone. Soft-tissue changes include coarse, thickened digits; bursal thickening caused by noninflammatory fibrous hyperplasia, particularly of the prepatellar, olecranon, and subacromial bursae; and joint capsular hypertrophy and laxity permitting hypermobility. Synovial thickening, villous and usually noninflammatory, is due to increased adipose and fibrous tissue rather than to synoviocyte hyperplasia. An abnormally thickened heel pad can be found in 35% of acromegalic patients.[7]

Most endochondral tissues are not as susceptible to growth hormone in adults as they are in the prepubertal state, but some cartilage remains responsive, as in the mandibular condyle, in which the jaw may

FIG. 113–1. Midsagittal section through the distal toe of a 50-year-old acromegalic man; irregular hypertrophy and hyperplasia of the cartilage, and bony overgrowth at the joint margins with sparse, thickened trabeculae has occurred. (Courtesy of R.T. McCluskey, M.D., Department of Pathology, Massachusetts General Hospital, Boston.)

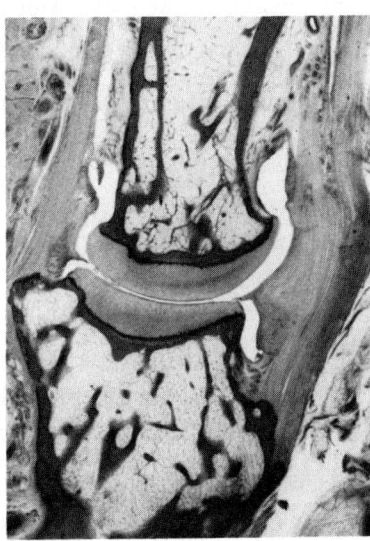

Table 113–1.   Rheumatic Manifestations of Acromegaly

Tissue overgrowth	Bursal hyperplasia
	Capsular thickening
	Synovial proliferation and edema
	Cartilage hyperplasia
	Bony proliferation
Arthropathy	Hypermobility of joints
	Cartilage degeneration
	Bony remodeling with osteophytosis and periosteal reaction
	Intermittent (crystal-induced?) synovitis
Muscle abnormalities	Increased muscle mass
	Proximal weakness, fatigue, myalgias, cramps
Neuropathy	Palpable peripheral nerves
	Peripheral neuropathy
	Carpal tunnel syndrome
Others	Back pain and hypermobility
	Kyphosis
	Raynaud's phenomenon

actually lengthen, and in the costochondral junctions, in which fusiform enlargement may take place leading to a beading pattern and rib lengthening.[8] This process results in an increased anteroposterior diameter of the chest. Cartilaginous overgrowth may even occur in the larynx, interfering with speech and, rarely, with respiratory function. Bony thickening results in a thickened calvarium, an enlarged mandible, and *hyperostosis frontalis interna*. Another characteristic finding is widening of the distal ungual tufts, seen in 67% of patients.[9] This can lead to an appearance of the hands similar to that of clubbing. The sesamoid bones are enlarged in approximately half these patients, and even the stapedial footplate of the ear may be affected, causing auditory symptoms.

The rheumatologic manifestations of acromegaly listed in Table 113–1 are found frequently if sought by careful medical history, physical examination, and laboratory testing. Their presence correlates more with the duration of disease than with absolute levels of growth hormone. Rheumatic complaints, however, may arise early in the disease and can be the presenting manifestation. With the exception of soft-tissue thickening, carpal tunnel symptoms, and paresthesias, many of these rheumatologic consequences of prolonged exposure to growth hormone may not remit with ablative pituitary therapy, but earlier recognition and treatment of this endocrine disorder may change this pessimistic view.[10]

ARTHROPATHY

The usual manifestations of acromegalic arthropathy resemble those of osteoarthritis, with cartilaginous thickening and hypermobility as important distinguishing features. Involvement of large and small peripheral joints may occur in as many as 75% of patients. The arthropathy may consist of a noninflammatory proliferation of articular and periarticular structures, with osteophytosis and degenerative changes of the articular cartilage. The arthropathy has been divided into an early form consisting of hypermobility, recurrent effusions, and widened joint spaces, and an advanced form with bony hypertrophy, loss of motion, and deformities.[11] Human necropsy studies and animal experimentation using exogenous growth hormone to produce polyarticular lesions have shed light on the pathogenesis of these changes.[12] The cartilaginous matrix, although massively thickened in acromegaly, is laid down in a random manner, and degenerative changes arise in the middle and basal layers, leading to friability, fissuring, and ulceration. Joint hypermobility caused by capsular hypertrophy and redundancy accelerate this degenerative process.

Such osteoarthritis-like changes may be monoarticular or polyarticular, and can affect the knees, shoulders, hips, or hands; the elbows and ankles are involved less frequently. Some patients develop intermittent painful episodes lasting weeks or months. The exact mechanism responsible for these episodes and the possible role of crystals remain to be determined. Less commonly, patients complain initially of joint pain and morning stiffness. This presentation, together with the elevated erythrocyte sedimentation rate seen in some patients,[11] can cause confusion with rheumatoid arthritis (RA).

Physical examination often reveals many of the characteristics of osteoarthritis, but the pronounced degree of joint crepitation, attributed to cartilaginous thickening and joint hypermobility, help to differentiate acromegalic arthropathy from primary osteoarthritis. Palpable dorsal phalangeal ridging just distal to the proximal interphalangeal joints may also be useful diagnostically. Thickened synovium and periarticular tissues may have a swollen appearance, but effusions are relatively rare, and when present are noninflammatory, contain no crystals, and have low leukocyte counts just as in osteoarthritis.

The radiographic features of acromegaly include widened cartilage spaces, enlarged bones with periosteal remodeling and increased density along the shaft, marginal osteophyte formation, and calcified tendinous and capsular insertions.[11,12] The cartilage space in the bones can be easily quantitated by measuring the second metacarpophalangeal joint space on an anteroposterior radiogram. The normal space in men is less than 3 mm and in women is less than 2 mm. Approximately one third of acromegalic individuals have increased joint spaces.[9] Exostoses at the sites of ligamentous attachments produce a "squared-off" appearance at the bone ends. Although thickening of the trabeculae at the epiphyses occurs, their simultaneous widening may lead to an osteoporotic appearance while the diaphyses remain dense; this is especially common at the metacarpal and metatarsal heads (Fig. 113–2). The humeral and femoral heads may develop a mushroom configuration along with

FIG. 113–2. Radiograph of an acromegalic foot showing widened joint spaces, periosteal proliferation, dense diaphyses with pipe-stem configuration, and thickened and widely spaced trabeculae giving a porotic appearance of the metatarsal heads. (From Kellgren, J.H., et al.[11])

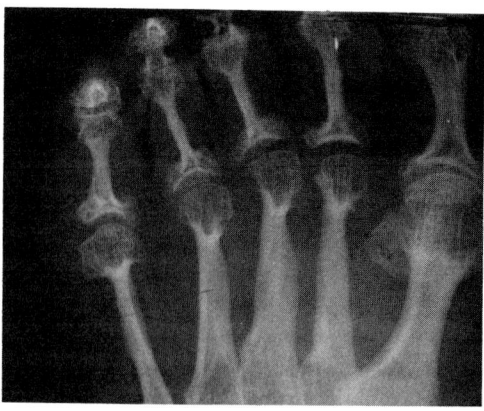

joint-space widening. Hypertrophic spurring with flaring of the femoral and tibial condyles may be found in knee films.

Troublesome symptoms can be treated with nonsteroidal anti-inflammatory agents and other conservative measures, as in osteoarthritis (see Chapter 103). Although intra-articular corticosteroids are reported to be ineffective, no controlled studies are available. Advanced degenerative changes may be treated surgically; a preoperative corticosteroid may be required in a previously treated acromegalic patient with pituitary insufficiency.

MYOPATHY

Up to 50% of acromegalic patients with long-standing disease develop a proximal myopathy. Growth hormone preferentially increases proximal muscle mass in experimental animals but the muscle is functionally inefficient. Muscle biopsies from patients with acromegaly have shown both hypertrophic and atrophic changes occurring separately or concurrently. Type I fiber hypertrophy, perhaps secondary to peripheral neuropathy, and type IIa and type IIb muscle fiber atrophy predominate. The atrophy is not that of disuse, which primarily affects type I fibers. Disease duration, but not growth hormone levels, correlated with biopsy findings.[13] Ultrastructurally, glycogen and lipofuscin deposits, coiled membranous bodies (probably phospholipid),[14] and pleomorphic mitochondria with abnormal cristae and vacuolization has been found, consistent with the known influence on glycogen uptake in skeletal muscle by growth hormone and its stimulation of ribonucleic acid (RNA) turnover. But a causal relationship between the mitochondrial disruption and the decreased muscle strength noted clinically has not been established.

Proximal weakness and decreased exercise tolerance are the usual complaints, followed by myalgias, cramps, and muscle twitching. The muscles may feel flabby, with weakness out of proportion to muscle mass.

The serum creatine kinase and aldolase levels, although usually normal, may be increased as a reflection of patchy necrosis. The electromyogram is abnormal in most acromegalic patients with myopathy, even those without demonstrable weakness, but the findings of low-amplitude, short-duration, and polyphasic potentials are nonspecific myopathic findings.

Return of normal strength after pituitary ablative therapy is gradual and may be incomplete even after 2 years.[15]

NEUROPATHY

As noted in Table 113–1, several forms of neuropathy are associated with acromegaly. These neuropathies do not correlate with increased growth hormone levels, may be independent of carpal tunnel syndrome, and may occur without concomitant diabetes mellitus. Their pathogenesis is varied and consists of the following: (1) possible metabolic effects on the neuron directly or indirectly related to growth hormone; (2) compression of the spinal cord secondary to bony (foramen magnum, vertebral body) and paraspinal connective tissue overgrowth; and (3) ischemic neuropathy secondary to proliferation of endoneural and perineural tissues. Vague paresthesias involving several peripheral nerves may be the earliest symptoms and these resolve after treatment. Five of eleven acromegalic patients had palpable enlargement of the ulnar or popliteal nerves with paresthesias, decreased or absent deep tendon reflexes, distal wasting, and even footdrop.[16] Decreased vibratory and position sense has also been described. Microscopic studies of peripheral nerves revealed a decrease in both myelinated and unmyelinated fibers, with segmental demyelination and remyelination and occasional axonal degeneration. The supporting neural tissues were increased, with significant proliferation, particularly in the hypertrophic form.[16]

CARPAL TUNNEL SYNDROME

Typical carpal tunnel syndrome, usually bilateral, develops in as many as 50% of patients with acromegaly.[12] Although encroachment on the carpal tunnel by enlarging bone and soft tissue is a major part of the pathogenesis of this disorder, local swelling and hypertrophy of the median nerve itself may also contribute. Edema has been observed beneath the transverse carpal ligament at operation. The disappearance of this soft-tissue swelling after pituitary therapy can account for the rapid improvement in symptoms after surgery but the return to normal of nerve conduction velocities is more prolonged.

BACK PAIN

Nearly half of acromegalic patients complain of back pain during the course of their disease. Although most symptoms are in the lumbosacral spine, cervical and thoracic involvement may also occur. In spite of severe pain and sometimes advanced radiographic changes, such patients may show hypermobility of the spine. This striking finding may be a key in distinguishing between this and other spinal disorders and is presumably due to the enlarged intervertebral discs, which retain their resiliency and turgor.[12] Such mobility may accelerate spinal degeneration and osteophyte formation. Radiographically, disc spaces are normal or increased, and occasionally calcified. Hypertrophic spurring develops at the anterior vertebral margin. Posteriorly, the exaggeration of the normal concavity of the vertebral body is probably caused by remodeling or pressure from paraspinal tissues. Kyphosis is frequently observed, possibly secondary to the barrel-chest deformity related to rib elongation.

RAYNAUD'S PHENOMENON

Raynaud's phenomenon occurred in 14 of 25 acromegalic patients in one series.[11] Although the exact mechanism is uncertain, thickening of the blood vessel walls may contribute to its development.

GIGANTISM

The accelerated endochondral ossification and lengthening of tubular bone occurring in prepubertal patients with a pituitary adenoma is termed gigantism. The disorder is rare and the true incidence of rheumatic manifestations is not known; the arthropathy, myopathy, and hypertrophic neuropathy noted in acromegaly may also occur in gigantism. The incidence of carpal tunnel syndrome may be less frequent. Bony and soft tissue growth occur in tandem, and thus the carpal tunnel may not be compromised.

HYPOTHYROIDISM

In primary hypothyroidism, hyaluronic acid and other mucoproteins deposit in many organs and tissues. Many of the numerous rheumatic syndromes associated with this disorder are probably secondary to such deposits in connective tissues and basement membranes (Table 113–2). The stimulus for the synthesis of the excess hyaluronic acid could be thyroid-stimulating hormone.[17] If this hypothesis is correct, it would account for the apparent paucity of musculoskeletal syndromes in secondary hypothyroidism, in which concentrations of thyroid-stimulating hormone are low. Other reasons for the infrequency of rheumatologic problems in secondary hypothyroidism include its rarity and its association with other endo-

Table 113–2. Rheumatic Manifestations of Thyroid Disorders

Hypothyroidism	Peripheral neuropathy—carpal tunnel syndrome
	Arthropathy—noninflammatory viscous effusions, chondrocalcinosis (calcium pyrophosphate crystals), Charcot-like joint destruction, hyperuricemia and gout, flexor tenosynovitis, epiphyseal dysplasia
	Myopathy—aches, pain, stiffness, cramping, weakness, myoedema, hypertrophy
Hyperthyroidism	Thyroid acropachy—clubbing, periosteal proliferation, soft tissue swelling, pretibial myxedema, exophthalmos, LATS (long-acting thyroid stimulator)
	Periarthritic osteoporosis
	Myopathy—atrophy, exophthalmic ophthalmoplegia, myasthenia gravis, periodic paralysis
Autoimmune (Hashimoto's) thyroiditis	Fibrositis syndrome
	Chest-wall pains
	Association with connective tissue diseases

crine deficiencies, which might mask musculoskeletal symptoms.

NEUROPATHY

Neurologic features, although frequent in myxedema, are easily overlooked. Hypothyroid patients have few spontaneous complaints, and the neurologic examination is difficult to perform, owing to the patient's inability to cooperate. Several authors have emphasized the generalized nature of the *peripheral neuropathy*.[18–20] Originally believed to be caused by nerve compression by mucinous deposits, it is now thought to be due to a neuronal metabolic dysfunction secondary to the hypothyroid state. Segmental demyelination of nerve fibers has been detected with a proliferation of Schwann cells, together with mucinous infiltration of the endoneurium and perineurium. The neuropathy is primarily sensory; slowed sensory conductive velocities have been found in the ulnar, median, and posterior tibial nerves. Abnormalities of conduction in the motor fibers have been found also although the reported frequency is variable.

All 25 patients with myxedema in one series complained of paresthesias, and 60% had diminished peripheral sensation. Sensory loss primarily involved pain and light touch; decreased vibratory sensation was less common. One of the best recognized neurologic complications of hypothyroidism is *carpal tunnel syndrome*. Approximately 10% of all patients with carpal tunnel syndrome have myxedema.[21] Conversely, median nerve compression can be documented in from 5 to 80% of those with hypothyroidism.[17,18] Symptoms of carpal tunnel syndrome can occur before clinical hypothyroidism is apparent. This association is important because treatment by thyroid

replacement is followed by complete relief of the neuropathy, thus avoiding surgery.

In addition to the effects of hypothyroidism on peripheral nerves, the cerebral cortex, cerebellum, and cranial nerves may also be involved. In hypothyroid patients, the cerebral spinal fluid protein concentration averages 115% above normal, with γ-globulin levels over 3 times normal.[18,20] With rare exceptions, all neurologic manifestations of hypothyroidism disappear completely after treatment.

ARTHROPATHY

The initial studies of Bland and Frymoyer,[17] and the subsequent clinical pathologic study by Dorwart and Schumacher,[22] have defined a joint disorder distinctive for myxedema whose characteristic features are listed in Table 113–2. Joint involvement usually develops concurrently with the onset of hypothyroidism, but occasionally antedates the development of clinical myxedema. Approximately one third of hypothyroid patients have symptomatic synovial effusions. Inflammation is neither common nor severe, with minimal pain and tenderness and only slight warmth and erythema. The arthritis is usually bilateral, most often affecting the knees; the ankles, metacarpophalangeal joints, and small joints of the hands and feet are less frequently involved. Periarticular tissues appear thickened, and the increased intra-articular fluid is reflected in a sluggish "bulge" sign. This finding, caused by hyperviscosity, is secondary to an increased concentration of synovial fluid hyaluronic acid.[22] The synovial fluid otherwise is generally noninflammatory, with a leukocyte count less than 1000/mm³.

Radiographs are characteristically normal except for signs of effusions. A single case of a patient with hypothyroidism presenting with an erosive arthropathy of the fingers and responsive to therapy with thyroxine has been reported.[23]

In addition, although Frymoyer and Bland excluded patients with hyaline cartilage calcification from their series, they did comment that radiographs in three cases showed destructive lesions of the tibial plateau and what appeared to be pathologic compression fractures.[21] Because a Charcot-like destructive arthropathy has been associated with chondrocalcinosis (see Chapter 107), these three patients may have had associated calcium pyrophosphate dihydrate (CPPD) crystal deposition. Dorwart and Schumacher found chondrocalcinosis of the knee in 7 of 12 myxedematous patients; 9 patients had knee effusions, with calcium pyrophosphate crystals demonstrable in 6.[22] Conversely, an increased incidence of hypothyroidism (10.5%) was found in a study of 105 patients with chondrocalcinosis.[24] Both intraleukocytic and extracellular calcium pyrophosphate and sodium urate crystals were noted, but *without* an associated inflammatory response.

The frequent failure of patients with myxedema to manifest intense inflammatory joint effusions in response to either sodium urate or calcium pyrophosphate crystals is of interest. Two findings may provide the explanation. First, neutrophil functions are reduced in hypothyroidism, an abnormality corrected after treatment with thyroxine.[25] Second, the high intrinsic viscosity and elevated concentration of hyaluronic acid in synovial fluid impedes the chemotactic movement of leukocytes and diminishes the rate of crystal endocytosis.[26] After treatment with thyroid hormone, several patients developed typical crystal-induced inflammatory joint attacks, in contrast to the resolution of noncrystal-related joint pain and effusions.

Asymptomatic hyperuricemia often occurs in hypothyroid men, but not women.[27] The increased incidence of clinical myxedema in patients with gout is small but significant.[28] The contributions of obesity and the influence of thyroid hormone on renal urate excretion remain unclear, and as a result, the association of gout and hypothyroidism remains controversial.

Wrist flexor tenosynovitis associated with hypothyroidism[22] was reported not to respond to thyroid therapy, but to subside promptly after injections of corticosteroid into the tendon sheaths. Although biopsies were not performed, hyaluronate deposition was believed to be responsible for the thickened, tender, and boggy palmar sheaths.

Ligamentous laxity occurs in approximately one third of patients with myxedema. The synovial effusions with edematous, lax joint capsules, ligaments, and tendons resemble the changes seen in an animal model of hypothyroidism thought to be due to increased concentrations of hyaluronate in the involved tissues. Myxedematous joint disease has been described only in primary hypothyroidism, in which levels of thyroid-stimulating hormone are increased. This hormone may increase synovial synthesis of hyaluronate, which may result in the changes described.[29]

Both the congenital and the acquired forms of hypothyroidism in children can delay epiphyseal closure and can retard maturation and ossification. This phenomenon, most often seen in the femoral head, may cause slipped capital femoral epiphysis. Helpful diagnostic features in such children include hip pain, limping, and an elevated serum creatine kinase level.[30]

MYOPATHY

Myopathic features may accompany many different endocrinopathies, but numerically their occurrence in hypothyroidism is probably the most important. Besides the slow movement and the delayed muscle contraction and relaxation classically seen in hypothyroidism, about half these patients complain of *weakness* and *muscle cramps, aches* and *pains,* or *stiffness.*[31] Muscle hypertrophy occurs in about 12% of patients. Pain and stiffness may be present during rest and are exacerbated on exposure to cold, thus resembling primary fibrositis. Such muscular symptoms may be the presenting complaints in many patients without overt clinical hypothyroidism. Like the neuropathy and arthropathy, myopathy can antedate the diagnosis of hypothyroidism by several months. The various muscle symptoms of hypothyroidism probably constitute a continuous spectrum, beginning with aches and pains and progressing to muscle cramping, proximal weakness, and even hypertrophy in association with severe, long-standing hypothyroidism. A case of rhabdomyolysis with hypothyroidism has been reported.[32]

On physical examination, weakness usually is not severe. The proximal muscles are principally affected. Muscle contraction and relaxation are slowed, owing more often to muscle disease than to altered nerve conduction or to defective neuromuscular transmission. Direct percussion of the muscle with a reflex hammer leads to an interesting sign, termed the "mounding phenomenon" or *myoedema.* This transient focal ridging seen in response to striking or pinching the muscle persists for several seconds and can also be present in patients with hypoalbuminemia. Muscles are usually of normal bulk; atrophy is rare in hypothyroidism. Generalized hypertrophy of muscles, when observed in infants and children, is called the *Kocher-Debre-Semelaigne syndrome,* and in adults, *Hoffman's syndrome.* This unusual finding, producing an athletic or "Herculean" appearance, disappears with therapy. Percussion of these hypertrophic muscles produces prolonged contractions resembling myotonia, although electromyographic studies have shown these muscle responses to be electrically silent.

The activities of most "muscle" enzymes are increased in the serum of patients with hypothyroidism.[33] Creatine kinase has been best studied and its concentrations correlate well with the severity of hypothyroidism. The exact contribution of the cardiac muscle isoenzyme to the serum creatine kinase level in hypothyroidism remains to be resolved. The creatine kinase level returns to normal within 2 months after restoration of the euthyroid state. In the few studies of patients with hypopituitarism and secondary hypothyroidism, myopathy was not a clinical feature, and serum creatine kinase levels were normal suggesting a role of thyroid-stimulating hormone in the pathogenesis of hypothyroid myopathy.

Electromyographic changes are independent of muscle bulk. Approximately half the patients demonstrate increased needle insertional activity and hyperirritability. An equal number manifest polyphasic motor unit action potentials. Frequently, chains of repetitive discharges are observed after reflex motion. These changes are nonspecific indicators of a myopathy and not pathognomonic of hypothyroid muscle disease.

Although biopsies may be normal, light microscopy reveals evidence of muscle degeneration in many patients as well as areas of focal necrosis, regeneration, and basophilia with vacuolization of fibers. Fiber size varies, and the sarcolemmal nuclei are numerous, enlarged, and centrally positioned. Mucoprotein deposits, widespread in multiple organs in hypothyroidism, are found in the muscles of one third of patients. Histochemical staining has demonstrated a decrease in type II fibers proportional to the severity of the hypothyroidism. This lower percentage of type II fibers correlates with the severity of the disease and with the elevation of creatine kinase levels. With treatment, the ratios of the fiber types return to normal.[34]

Although most cases of connective tissue disease have occurred in patients with autoimmune thyroiditis, a case of hypothyroidism secondary to panhypopituitarism with Raynaud's phenomenon has been reported; all symptoms resolved after thyroid hormone replacement.[35]

HYPERTHYROIDISM

THYROID ACROPACHY

This extraordinary rheumatic manifestation of hyperthyroidism usually follows treatment for thyrotoxicosis.[36] Thyroid acropachy, or thickening of small parts, occurs in approximately 1% of patients with past or present thyroid disease and usually develops approximately 1 year after either thyroidectomy or radioablation. The fingers and toes become *clubbed,* and patients develop *periostitis* of the digits and distal extremities with swelling of soft tissues. Usually, these patients also have *exophthalmos* and *pretibial myxedema.* These features, in addition to the presence in the serum of long-acting thyroid stimulator (LATS), help to differentiate thyroid acropachy from other causes of hypertrophic osteoarthropathy. When this syndrome appears, patients are often clinically hypothyroid. Signs of inflammation are not prominent, although the syndrome is *painful,* especially on palpation over the periosteal new bone. Partial improvement, with incomplete resolution of pains in the extremities and digits and subsidence of the periosteal new bone proliferation, occurs in some patients after treatment with thyroid hormone or prednisone (see also Chapter 86).

Immune factors appear to participate in the pathogenesis of Graves' disease and possibly in its extrathyroidal manifestations, including acropachy.[37] Patients with Graves' disease have circulating thyroid-stimulating immunoglobulins, considered to be antibodies to the thyroid-stimulating hormone receptor on thyroid cell membranes. The presence of other thyroid autoantibodies suggests a close relationship between Graves' disease and Hashimoto's thyroiditis. Evidence indicates cell-mediated immunity in both diseases, with the finding of T-lymphocytes sensitized to a thyroid antigen.[37] It has been postulated that local interferon production induces Ia-like antigens on the surface of thyroid cells with a subsequent immune response to the tissue adjacent to the Ia molecule.[38] Additional evidence linking these disorders includes the development of acropachy in both, their occurrence in the same families, and their histopathologic coexistence within the same thyroid gland. The significant excess of the histocompatibility antigens HLA-B8 and HLA-DR3 in patients with Graves' disease is evidence of a genetic association. The exact role of organ-specific autoantibodies or sensitized leukocytes in the production of either of these thyroid disorders or of the acropachy remains unclear.

Another rheumatic association of uncertain pathogenesis is periarthritis of the shoulder, which is said to coexist with hyperthyroidism and to respond to restoration of the euthyroid state.[39] Marked osteoporosis, with subsequent fractures, is also frequently seen in thyrotoxicosis and is due to bone resorption stimulated by thyroid hormone, possibly by osteoclast activating factor (OAF), or interleukin-1, with subsequent elevation of serum calcium and phosphorus levels. Both parathyroid hormone and 1,25 dihydroxyvitamin D_3 concentrations are decreased.[40] This osteoporosis is also reversible when the thyroid disorder is treated.

THYROTOXIC MYOPATHY

Clinical evidence of weakness can be found in almost all thyrotoxic patients.[31] The myopathy of thyrotoxicosis can be mild, characterized by weakness, fatigability, and minimal atrophy, or it can be extreme, characterized by proximal wasting and severe weakness, resembling polymyositis. Unlike polymyositis, acute inflammatory changes are not evident, and laryngeal and pharyngeal muscles are usually not involved. Atrophy and infiltration by fat cells and lymphocytes occur. "Muscle" enzymes are generally not increased in the serum, although creatinuria is present. Electromyographic abnormalities include short-duration motor unit potentials and an increased percentage of polyphasic potentials. Full recovery of muscle strength occurs as patients become euthyroid. There is controversy over the possible beneficial effect of β blockade on thyrotoxic myopathy.[41]

Three other forms of myopathy are less common. *Exophthalmic ophthalmoplegia* usually parallels the severity of exophthalmos. Associated findings include swelling of the eyelid and conjunctiva and sometimes of the optic nerve head. A second form is the coexistence of Graves' disease in 5% of patients with *myasthenia gravis*. The association of these disorders has a distinct female sex preponderance. Patients respond to prostigmine, but improvement is incomplete, owing to the thyrotoxicosis. *Thyrotoxic periodic paralysis* is the third of the rarer forms of skeletal muscle involvement in thyrotoxicosis. It is similar to the periodic paralysis of primary hypokalemia. This syndrome has the cardinal features of flaccid paralysis of the extremities, with absent reflexes and diminished electrical excitability. Precipitating factors are thought to be exercise, a high carbohydrate intake, and the administration of insulin or epinephrine. This disor-

der is rare in whites and is more common in Oriental males. Serum potassium concentrations are usually low, and the administration of potassium salts can prevent or abort attacks. Restoration of the euthyroid state leads to resolution of the paralytic attacks.

AUTOIMMUNE (HASHIMOTO'S) THYROIDITIS

Early in the course of autoimmune thyroiditis, as the thyroid gland gradually enlarges, most patients are euthyroid and some are hyperthyroid. But with progressive lymphocytic infiltration, fibrosis, and obliteration of thyroid follicles nearly half of these patients develop hypothyroidism. This common cause of diffuse goiter, with a female predilection, is frequently associated with musculoskeletal symptoms. The most common rheumatic syndrome resembles *fibrositis*; patients complain of stiffness of the joints and muscles, exacerbated by cold or dampness and worse on arising in the morning or after any period of immobility. This syndrome resembles that seen in hypothyroidism and can be present in autoimmune thyroiditis even in the absence of thyroid deficiency.[2] Another rheumatic symptom is *unusual chest-wall pains* of intermittent nature. Described in 12% of patients with Hashimoto's disease, these thoracic and shoulder-girdle pains, lasting for several minutes to hours, are relieved by changes of position or by mild exercises.[42] Half the patients with Hashimoto's disease have an *elevated erythrocyte sedimentation rate*, with or without rheumatic symptoms.

Most patients with Hashimoto's disease have high serum titers of *thyroid antibodies*, both to thyroglobulin and to microsomal antigens. Cellular immunity may also be important in the pathogenesis of the disease.[37] Biologic false-positive tests for syphilis, rheumatoid factors, and antinuclear antibodies are also common. Hashimoto's disease coexists with other autoimmune disorders, especially pernicious anemia and hemolytic anemia, and possibly with RA, systemic lupus erythematosus (SLE), and Sjögren's syndrome.[42–45] These disorders appear in family members of patients with autoimmune thyroiditis too often to be coincidental.

The frequency of thyroid disease in patients with rheumatic disorders has also been examined. Although patients with connective tissue diseases, notably systemic lupus erythematosus and RA, have a high incidence of antibodies to thyroid antigens, the majority are euthyroid and do not have detectable goiters. A prospective study showed frequent thyroid function test abnormalities, including elevated thyroid-stimulating hormone, in patients with SLE without clinically evident thyroid disease. The most common abnormalities were consistent with incipient or true hypothyroidism. Mild to moderate hypothyroidism may be missed because of the similarity of some of its symptoms with those of SLE.[46] Despite this and other uncontrolled series, the coexistence of either hyperthyroidism or hypothyroidism with RA, polymyositis, scleroderma, or systemic lupus erythematosus may be coincidental and deserves further investigation. Two other situations associated with thyroid disorders are known: (1) the administration of antithyroid drugs may be followed by syndromes resembling either RA or systemic lupus erythematosus, especially in children[47]; and (2) falsely low values of serum thyroxine can be seen in patients treated either with salicylates or with corticosteroid hormones.

PARATHYROID DISORDERS

A number of rheumatic findings are associated with parathyroid hormone excess (Table 113–3). A more detailed discussion of the osseous consequences of increased levels of this hormone, including osteitis fibrosa cystica, may be found in Chapter 112.

The resorptive effects of parathyroid hormone on bone may lead to the characteristic *subperiosteal erosive* radiographic appearance, particularly at the radial aspect of the middle phalanges, the medial aspect of the proximal femur or tibia, and the inferior aspect of the distal third of the clavicle. *Erosions* may also occur in juxta-articular sites, especially at the interphalangeal, metacarpophalangeal, carpal, and acromioclavicular joints. These lesions can be found in the absence of subperiosteal resorption, can be symmetric, and can be associated with morning stiffness, thus mimicking RA. Several features distinguish parathy-

roid disorders: (1) the erosions may have a shaggy appearance; (2) they often occur at the distal interphalangeal joints and spare the proximal interphalangeal joints; (3) joint-space narrowing in association with these erosions is uncommon because parathyroid hormone does not directly induce inflammatory synovitis or cartilage dissolution; and (4) concurrent articular calcification is common.

Parathyroid hormone increases collagenase activity,[48] which may account for the *laxity of capsular and ligamentous structures* seen in this disorder. *Tendon ruptures and avulsions* have been reported.[49] *Vertebral subluxation* occurs, especially in the cervical spine; *dorsal kyphosis* is present, with anterior bowing of the sternum; the lumbar spine is *hypermobile*. Additional changes include *sacroiliac erosions* and *intervertebral disc calcifications*. The laxity leads to joint abuse, which contributes to the back pain, disc protrusion, and degenerative joint changes seen in hyperparathyroidism.

Chondrocalcinosis has been reported in 18 to 25% of patients with hyperparathyroidism[50,51] (see also Chapter 108). Calcium pyrophosphate dihydrate (CPPD) crystal deposition may cause attacks of pseudogout, which can precede the recognition of parathyroid hormone excess and may thus be an initial manifestation of this disease. *Pseudogout* attacks may flare within 2 to 3 days of parathyroidectomy, or they may occur later, often coincident with the postoperative nadir of the serum calcium level.[52] Once chondrocalcinosis is present, it usually persists in spite of parathyroidectomy, and the frequency of episodes of pseudogout continues unabated or even increases. Bywaters and co-workers have described subchondral cyst formation with subsequent destructive joint changes in 15 of 19 patients with hyperparathyroidism.[53] More than half their patients had chondrocalcinosis. Because similar joint changes with severe destruction and the development of Charcot-like joints have been de-

Table 113–3. Rheumatic Manifestations of Parathyroid Disorders

Hyperparathyroidism	Osteitis fibrosa cystica
	Subperiosteal resorption
	Bony erosions
	Joint laxity
	Tendon avulsions/ruptures
	Back abnormalities
	Degenerative arthritis
	Chondrocalcinosis and pseudogout
	Charcot-like joints
	Hyperuricemia and gout
	Ectopic calcifications
	Neuromyopathy
Hypoparathyroidism and pseudohypoparathyroidism	Subcutaneous calcifications; myopathy
	Paraspinal ligament calcifications (spondylitis without sacroiliitis)

scribed in association with chondrocalcinosis per se, the relative contribution of CPPD crystals and parathyroid hormone to this type of arthropathy remains to be elucidated. The presence of severe osteoarthritis should prompt a search for CPPD crystals, and if these are found, for the metabolic diseases associated with them, including hyperparathyroidism.

The persistently elevated serum calcium levels in primary hyperparathyroidism may result in nephrocalcinosis and a nephropathy characterized by an impaired tubular-concentrating mechanism. Some hyperparathyroid patients have a decreased uric acid clearance, which may exlain the finding of hyperuricemia. The incidence of actual gouty attacks in hyperparathyroidism varies from 3 to 45%.[27] Because hyperuricemia and gout do not seem to occur without underlying renal changes, they may persist after parathyroidectomy. Elevated levels of parathyroid hormone were found in about 70% of patients with CPPD crystal deposits and in age- and sex-matched control subjects with osteoarthritis of the knee.[54] Chemical hyperparathyroidism occurred in patients in both groups. Serum levels of parathyroid hormone correlated directly with serum calcium levels, female patients having the most severe osteoarthritis, and with bone density. These findings have not been confirmed.

In secondary hyperparathyroidism, as well as in other disorders in which metastatic calcifications are found, deposits of amorphous and crystalline basic calcium phosphate salts may occur in periarticular or articular tissues. Their presence can induce a local inflammatory reaction with pain and swelling (see also Chapter 109). Treatment consists of prophylaxis with aluminum hydroxide gels and the use of anti-inflammatory agents or intra-articular corticosteroids during acute episodes.

Fatigue, generalized weakness, and other neuromuscular complaints occur in the majority of patients with primary or secondary hyperparathyroidism. Weakness is usually in the *proximal muscles,* often only in the lower extremities. This symptom is most commonly secondary to a *peripheral neuropathic process.*[55,56] Other neurologic findings include abnormalities of the cranial nerves, long-tract signs, and decreased vibratory sensation. Muscle enzyme levels are not elevated, and nerve conduction velocities are reported normal despite other electromyographic findings suggesting a neuropathic process. Muscle biopsy reveals neurogenic atrophy of both fiber types, with type II atrophy predominating.[56] Parathyroidectomy usually rapidly reverses these abnormalities. Other causes of neuromuscular symptoms in hyperparathyroid patients are a polymyositis-like myopathy[57] and an

ischemic myopathy caused by intravascular calcifications[58] that occurs in the seondary hyperparathyroidism associated with uremia.

Hypoparathyroidism. In addition to the bony features of hypoparathyroidism, pseudohypoparathyroidism, and pseudopseudohypoparathyroidism, *subcutaneous* and *ectopic calcifications* may be seen. *Spondylitis without sacroiliitis,* wih extensive paraspinal calcifications in hypoparathyroidism and pseudohypoparathyroidism, has been reported.[59] *Myopathy,* in association with elevated serum levels of creatine kinase and normal muscle biopsy has also been seen in hypoparathyroidism.[60]

DIABETES MELLITUS

The musculoskeletal complications of diabetes mellitus, both articular and periarticular, are listed in Table 113–4. Some of these, such as destructive arthropathy, reflex sympathetic dystrophy, carpal tunnel syndrome, interosseous muscle wasting, and proximal weakness, may be primarily the result of neuropathic changes. Ischemic vascular disease may also contribute to their genesis. Complications that appear to be related to a proliferation of fibrous tissue include the increased incidence of capsulitis of the shoulder, Dupuytren's contractures and flexor tenosynovitis in adults, and flexion contractures in juvenile-onset diabetics. The collagen from skin and tendon samples of young diabetics is stiff and stabilized, similar to samples from normal control subjects 50 to 65 years older. Possible reasons for the excessive fibrosis and accelerated aging of collagen is discussed in Chapter 94.

The association between diabetes and hyperuricemia or gout remains controversial. Joslin, et al. reported only one case of gout in 1500 diabetic patients,[62] and studies of patients with hyperuricemia compared with age- and weight-matched controls showed no difference in results of glucose tolerance tests. Nonobese, type II, diabetic patients have no greater incidence of gout than the normal population. Similarly, there is a consensus that there is no increase in the incidence of diabetes in gout.[27] Less clearly defined is the putative association with ankylosing hyperostosis.[63] Controlled studies have failed to support an association of diabetes mellitus (see Chapter 108) with CPPD crystal deposition.

NEUROPATHY

Diabetic neuropathy may take several forms: (1) a peripheral symmetric sensory or sensorimotor loss;

Table 113–4. Rheumatic Manifestations of Diabetes Mellitus

Neuropathy	Distal sensory and sensorimotor disorders
	Mononeuropathy multiplex
	Diabetic amyotrophy
	Radiculopathy
	Autonomic neuropathy
Neuroarthropathy	Osteolysis
	Osteoporosis
	Charcot joint
	Coexistent osteomyelitis
	Periarthritis of the shoulder (adhesive capsulitis)
Other Associations	Hyperuricemia and gout?
	Ankylosing hyperostosis
	Flexion contractures (Dupuytren's contractures, limited joint mobility)
	Tenosynovitis

(2) a mononeuropathy multiplex with an increased frequency of cranial nerve involvement; (3) a neuropathy resulting in proximal muscle weakness, termed diabetic amyotrophy; (4) a radiculopathy leading to lancinating pains in a dermatomal distribution; (5) an autonomic neuropathy; and (6) carpal tunnel syndrome. With *peripheral neuropathic* involvement, patients frequently have a stocking-glove distribution of sensory loss, with decreased vibratory and position sense and decreased or absent deep-tendon reflexes. Wasting of the interosseous muscles of the hands and feet may give a claw-hand or hammer-toe appearance.

Mononeuropathies most commonly affect the third and sixth cranial nerves, and occasionally the fourth and seventh as well. Mononeuropathy involving the motor supply of the proximal hip and leg muscles, and less often of the upper extremities, occurs more in men, often in those with only mild diabetes. This so-called *diabetic amyotrophy* is usually bilateral but asymmetric. Muscle biopsy shows a predominance of type I fibers, with type II atrophy and no evidence of significant necrosis or inflammation. Muscle enzyme levels are normal, and the electromyogram shows some fibrillation potentials. The weakness may spontaneously remit. Evidence also indicates that control of hyperglycemia contributes to recovery.[64] *Diabetic radiculopathy* may occur secondary to infarction of a nerve root, with resultant lancinating pains. These pains are sometimes confused with the symptoms of a herniated disc. When proprioceptive loss and ataxia accompany this shooting pain, it is called "diabetic pseudotabes."

Involvement of the *autonomic nervous system* results in orthostatic hypotension, impotence, dyshidrosis, and diarrhea. Autonomic dysfunction may be related to the unilateral or bilateral reflex dystrophy and to the apparently increased shoulder pain seen in diabetes. *Periarthritis (adhesive capsulitis) of the shoulder,*

often bilateral, was found in 11% of a large group of diabetic patients.[65] Conversely, in another study, approximately 25% of patients with periarthritis were diabetic.[66] This entity occurs more commonly in women on the nondominant side of the body and produces aching with limitation of shoulder motion. Calcific bursitis and tendinitis may be present. The natural course of the disorder varies, but spontaneous remissions may occur. Physical therapy, anti-inflammatory drugs, and local corticosteroid injections are helpful. Although 5 to 17% of patients with carpal tunnel syndrome have diabetes, systematic, controlled observations have not demonstrated a significant association.[67]

ARTHROPATHY

As a consequence of sensory neuropathy, severe arthropathy with Charcot-like changes develops in approximately 0.1% of long-standing diabetes.[68] The tarsometatarsal and metatarsophalangeal joints are by far the most common sites of involvement, but changes may rarely affect joints above the ankle. A combination of microfragmentation from trauma, ischemia from small blood vessel disease, and superimposed infection can contribute to the clinical and radiographic changes of neuroarthropathy. All patients with diabetic neuroarthropathy have peripheral neuropathy. In advanced disease, the longitudinal arch of the foot collapses, leading to an unstable gait and a "rocker-sole" appearance. Ulcerations and plantar callosites occur over hypoesthetic pressure points. Osteolysis of bone can develop, with periosteal reaction and remodeling, whittling of the metatarsal bones, cupping deformities, and telescoping of the phalanges.[68] Fractures may be the initial lesion in a Charcot joint or may simply contribute to more extensive joint damage. In all involved joints, the discrepancy between pain, which is minimal or absent, and the destructive radiographic appearance, which is severe, is striking. The mainstay of therapy is rest of the involved area, attention to care of the feet including proper shoes, treatment of concomitant osteomyelitis, and amputaiton if required (see Chapter 81).

A group of disorders of more obscure pathogenesis has in common excessive proliferation of fibroblastic tissue. *Fibrous palmar nodules* with subsequent Dupuytren's contractures have been reported in as many as 21% of diabetic patients; diabetes was found in 10% of those with Dupuytren's contractures (see Chapter 94).[69] Diabetes has also been described in 10 to 30% of all adult cases of trigger finger or flexor tenosynovitis.[70] In addition, reports exist of interphalangeal flexion deformities (cheiroarthropathy or limited joint mobility), initially described in insulin-dependent, juvenile-onset diabetic patients.[71] Noninsulin-dependent adult-onset diabetics have deformities as severe as juvenile-onset diabetics.[72,73] This progressive stiffness has been seen only in the hands and is not related to Dupuytren's contractures or flexor tenosynovitis. The stiffness and limited mobility appear to be related to a thick, tight, waxy skin. A simple screening test for limited joint mobility consists of asking the patient to place both hands on a table palm down with fingers fanned. The entire palmar surface of the fingers makes contact in normal persons.[71] Rosenbloom et al. showed that, in patients who had had diabetes for an average of 16 years, the presence of stiff joints increased the risk of retinal and renal complications from 25 to 83%.[74] The clinical signs and the presence of microvascular disease are reminiscent of scleroderma, but nailfold capillaroscopy is normal.[75]

Type B insulin-resistant diabetes mellitus secondary to insulin receptor antibodies[76] has been associated with multiple rheumatic complaints suggestive of systemic lupus erythematosus, Sjögren's syndrome, or progressive systemic sclerosis.[77,78] Fourteen such patients developed features of an autoimmune disease; 8 of the 14 met the American Rheumatic Association criteria for systemic lupus erythematosus, and 4 developed glomerulonephritis histologically consistent with lupus nephritis.[79] Whenever a patient has extremely insulin-resistant diabetes mellitus and features of a systemic rheumatic disease, the possibility of circulating antibodies to insulin receptors should be considered.

CORTICOSTEROID ADMINISTRATION

Corticosteroid excess due to adrenal hyperproduction or secondary to exogenous administration can profoundly affect the musculoskeletal system. Generalized osteoporosis, osteonecrosis* of the humeral and femoral heads, and pathologic fractures are consequences in bone. Changes in the vertebral column can cause severe pain, kyphosis, and loss of height. In children, growth is retarded, and, if not corrected, results in permanently short stature. A noninflammatory proximal myopathy may progress from the pelvic to the shoulder girdle and, ultimately, to the distal musculature. Serum muscle enzyme levels are usually normal in states of corticosteroid excess, but urinary creatine excretion is increased.[80] Following correction of hypercortisolism, creatinuria subsides. This dissociation between serum and urine laboratory tests may help to differentiate corticosteroid-related from inflammatory myopathies. The electromyogram in corticosteroid myopathy has yielded confusing results and is not helpful diagnostically. Muscle biopsy reveals a type II atrophy without inflammatory change. Although some recovery of muscle strength occurs within days after reduction of corticosteroid dose, complete resolution usually takes 1 to 4 months.

Adrenal insufficiency after corticosteroid withdrawal may be associated with constitutional symptoms of weakness, fatigue and lassitude, and arthralgias. Addison's disease is generally associated with weakness, but flexion contractures caused by progressive stiffening of the pelvic girdle and thigh muscles can occur. This painful condition, also seen in patients with hypopituitarism, responds to therapy with corticosteroids but not mineralocorticoids.[81]

CARCINOID ARTHROPATHY

Distinctive rheumatologic findings occur in at least 10% of carcinoid patients. Arthralgias of the wrists and hands, constant stiffness and pain on movement, and marked intensification of pain after a sustained grip are characteristic complaints. Because the arthralgias can be rapidly reversed with parachlorophenylalanine, which blocks serotonin synthesis, serotonin is believed to be responsible for these symptoms. Bradykinin and histamine may also be involved. One may detect juxta-articular demineralization and erosions at the metacarpophalangeal joints and at the proximal and distal interphalangeal joints, with subchondral cystic changes.[82]

Editor's note. Paradoxically, osteonecrosis in natural Cushing's disease or syndrome is exceedingly uncommon although the other bony changes noted with exogenous corticosteroid use are frequent. The reason for this is a conundrum.

ECTOPIC HORMONAL SYNDROMES

Tumor cells can synthesize polypeptide hormones, such as adrenocorticotropic hormone, growth hormone, thyroid-stimulating hormone, and parathyroid hormone, with structural and functional characteristics similar or identical to those of normal hormones.[83] Because the bony, myopathic, and neuropathic changes associated with endocrinopathies require prolonged hormonal exposure, these syndromes are not seen with ectopic hormone production by malignant tissues. Several cases of *hypertrophic pulmonary osteoarthropathy* have been reported in patients with *acromegalic* physical features and increases in growth hormone or similar substances that resolved when the tumor was removed, suggesting a possible relationship.[84] The periosteal proliferation seen in this osteoarthropathy may resemble the periosteal remodeling of acromegaly, but further clarification is needed to determine whether any humeral substance mediates this syndrome.

PREGNANCY

The symptoms of RA frequently remit during pregnancy. Since Hench's description in 1938 of the beneficial action of pregnancy,[85] improvement has been reported in numerous other rheumatic disorders as well (Table 113–5).[86] Many of these reports have dealt with a few patients or even a single patient, however, and with rare exception, the observations have been retrospective and anecdotal.

Table 113–5. Disorders Reported to be Ameliorated by Pregnancy

Rheumatoid arthritis	Sarcoidosis
Ankylosing spondylitis	Polymyositis
Psoriatic arthropathy (and psoriasis)	Raynaud's phenomenon
	Gout (possibly)
Behçet's syndrome	Cutaneous anaphylaxis
Fibrositis	Angioneurotic edema
Intermittent hydrarthrosis	Bronchial asthma
Periodic diseases	Hay fever
Erythema nodosum	Migraine headache

Experimental Animal Diseases

Experimental vasculitis (dogs)	Carrageenan inflammation (rats)
Adjuvant arthritis (rats)	Allergic thyroiditis (guinea pigs)

Disorders with Variable Course

Systemic lupus erythematosus	Inflammatory bowel diseases
Scleroderma	Necrotizing cutaneous vasculitis
Myasthenia gravis	

The most complete data have been accumulated on the course of RA during gestation and in the postpartum period.[87] As shown in Figure 113–3, improvement of disease was not noted in all these 296 pregnancies. Only 219 (74%) had some degree of subsidence of arthritis activity during gestation. Fifty percent of patients with RA had some degree of subsidence of disease activity during the first trimester of pregnancy. Thereafter, an additional 24% experienced relief of symptoms throughout the second and third trimesters, some even waiting until the last month of gestation for improvement. In 26% of published cases, patients failed to note an amelioration of arthritis. Some even had more severe symptoms; still others experienced the onset of their disease during pregnancy.

After delivery, the symptoms of RA recurred in more than 90% of patients, although complete data are not available. Information has been published on the postpartum experience of only 128 patients (Fig. 113–4).[87] All had an exacerbation following parturition; 64% noted a return of symptoms by the eighth week after delivery. Thirty-six percent had no joint inflammation until more than 8 weeks postpartum. These data indicate that the benefits of pregnancy are temporary, lasting an average of 6 weeks after delivery. The return of symptoms can be abrupt or insidious and is not related to the resumption of menstruation or to the termination of lactation. A careful quantitation of disease activity has not been performed, but it is generally stated that postpartum RA is at least as severe as prior to gestation.

FIG. 113–3. Time of onset of symptomatic improvement in rheumatoid arthritis activity during 296 pregnancies. A total of 50% improved during the first trimester, and an additional 24% improved throughout the remainder of gestation. (From Neely, N.T., and Persellin, R.H.[87])

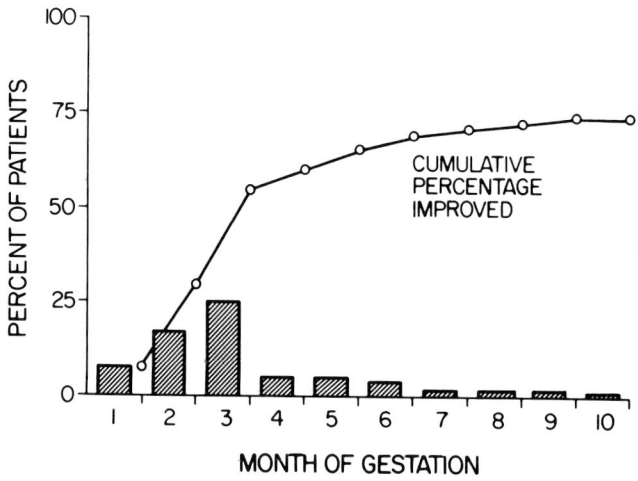

FIG. 113–4. Recurrence of rheumatoid arthritis symptoms in each 2-week period post partum in 128 patients. The cumulative percentage is also presented. (From Neely, N.T., and Persellin, R.H.[87])

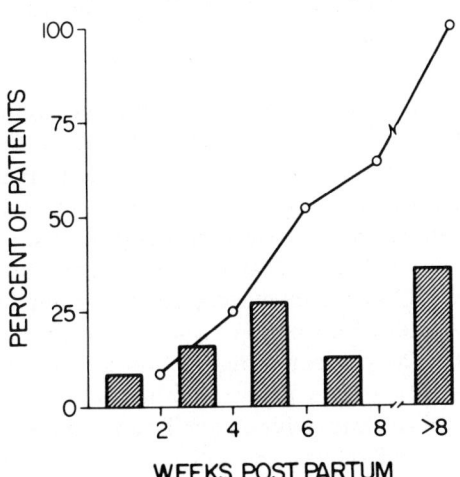

There are few studies of the effect of rheumatoid arthritis on fertility or on the fetus. One retrospective study found that the fertility rate of patients with rheumatoid arthritis was normal although the rate of spontaneous abortion was slightly higher.[88]

Another disorder in which a considerable clinical experience during pregnancy has been accumulated is systemic lupus erythematosus.[86] Most authors have noted a high spontaneous abortion rate in pregnancies occurring before the onset of their first recognizable manifestation of this disease, as well as in pregnancies after the onset of clinical disease. Spontaneous abortions may be related to antiphospholipid antibodies, particularly antibodies to cardiolipin.[89] The possibility of heart block in offspring of mothers with systemic lupus erythematosus is now well known[90] and is related to anti-Ro (SSA) antibody.[91] Mothers of babies born with complete heart block should be monitored for signs of lupus because the diagnosis may not be known before delivery. One mother did not develop the disease until 16 years after the birth of the first of three children with congenital heart block.[92]

Less certain is the relationship between disease activity and pregnancy, including the progression of renal or other organ dysfunction. As with RA, exacerbations of systemic lupus have been documented frequently in the postpartum period. Less frequent exacerbations, usually of minor consequence, have been noted in more recent studies. Renal function deterioration is not frequent and usually reversible.[93] These results may be due to more aggressive therapy

and/or differences in the definition of a lupus flare. It can be difficult to differentiate changes caused only by pregnancy from true disease exacerbation. Serum hemolytic complement levels may be helpful, because these are usually high in normal pregnancies. Because of these uncertainties, a number of investigators have suggested that pregnancies be delayed in these patients until their disease has been inactive for 6 months or more prior to conception.[94] The same risks during pregnancy have been reported in patients with mixed connective tissue disease[95] (see also Chapters 67 and 71).

FACTOR RESPONSIBLE FOR AMELIORATION

The factor responsible for improvement of rheumatoid arthritis during pregnancy is not yet known. The increased susceptibility of pregnant women to certain infectious diseases and the specific suppression of normal immune responses during pregnancy might be relevant. During gestation, women are believed to suffer increased morbidity and mortality from certain infectious agents, chiefly viruses and fungi.[96] The virulence of these intracellular microorganisms may be related to impaired cell-mediated immunity. Skin-graft rejection is delayed and in vitro T-lymphocyte responses are depressed, effects believed to be mediated by the serum or plasma of pregnancy.[97] The ameliorating substance may be responsible for all the clinical alterations associated with gestation.

Because the concentration of blood cortisol increases during pregnancy, it has been related to the suppression of rheumatoid activity.[98] Subsequent studies have shown, however, that the increased corticosteroid concentrations alone were not fully responsible for the observed improvement.[86] Measurement of plasma cortisol levels did not correlate with disease activity during pregnancy. Plasma cortisol levels fall to normal by 48 hours after delivery, and yet RA remains suppressed post partum for more than 6 weeks in 50% of patients. The hormone is mostly transcortin-bound during gestation and is therefore not biologically active. Thus, despite the original enthusiasm for cortisol, other factors responsible for improvement during gestation have bene sought.

A variety of other products of pregnancy, including placental extracts, umbilical cord serum, and blood or urine fractions, have been used to treat RA without reproducible improvement. The concentrations of many plasma proteins are increased during gestation, including: (1) the carrier proteins, such as transcortin, thyroxin-binding globulin, testosterone-binding globulin, estrogen-binding globulin, transferrin, and ceruloplasmin; (2) the coagulation proteins, including fibrinogen and factors VII, VIII, and IX; (3) plasminogen; (4) α_2-macroglobulin; (5) C-reactive protein and other so-called "acute phase" proteins; and (6) the pregnancy-associated plasma proteins.[99]

Of these proteins, studies on the biologic activities of the pregnancy zone protein (PZP) have been the most promising. This glycoprotein is found at low concentrations in the serum of women who are not pregnant and increases during gestation in most individuals.[100] Following delivery, the level falls at a slower rate than the other pregnancy-associated plasma proteins. The timing of changes in the concentration of plasma pregnancy zone protein paralleled both the remissions and the postpartum exacerbations of RA. Additionally, approximately 25% of women have only minimal elevations of this protein in their plasma during gestation; this finding may explain the failure of this percentage of patients to experience clinical improvements.[96] This substance affects a variety of in vitro parameters of inflammation and acts on the membranes of isolated organelles, polymorphonuclear leukocytes, and lymphocytes as well.[96] Unlike previous observations using corticosteroid hormones, pregnancy zone protein is effective in vitro in physiologic concentrations.

The dramatic changes in the metabolism of the sex hormones during pregnancy are well known. Estrogens reduce the metabolic activity of neutrophils, alter delayed skin-test reactivity in experimental animals, and suppress the development and severity of adjuvant arthritis in rats. Progesterone has also been shown in vitro to suppress leukocyte functions. Most of these effects have resulted from large, nonphysiologic amounts of these sex hormones, however.[97] Despite original enthusiasm, the beneficial effects of sex hormones on patients with RA have not been substantiated by clinical trials, but carefully controlled studies have not been performed. Because estrogenic hormones are known to induce a vaiety of serum protein changes similar to those in pregnancy, their effect on serum concentrations of pregnancy zone protein has been studied. Significant increases in this protein were observed during the administration of either combinations of estrogen and progesterone or of estrogen alone. Serum concentrations of pregnancy zone protein induced by exogenous sex hormone administration reached only one tenth the levels usually found during pregnancy,[96] however, and this factor may account for the failure of estrogens to produce the clinical response observed during gestation. Thus, sex hormones, corticosteroids, and pregnancy zone protein, the plasma constituents increased during pregnancy, have been demonstrated in vitro and in some animal models to possess anti-inflammatory activity.

SEX HORMONES IN AUTOIMMUNE DISORDERS

Many autoimmune diseases are more common in women than in men. In systemic lupus erythematosus (SLE), the best example, the female to male ratio can be as high as 15:1. The ratio does vary with age. In premenarcheal or postmenopausal women, the ratio falls to 2:1. This change in ratio suggests hormonal influence. Oral contraceptive agents either may exacerbate latent SLE or may induce the formation of antibodies to nuclear antigens. In a series of eight patients with antinuclear antibodies believed secondary to oral contraceptive use, all had rheumatic complaints of arthralgias, myalgias, and morning stiffness, and two had synovitis.[101] A subsequent prospective study by the same investigators confirmed the development of autoantibodies in response to these agents, but other investigators were unable to find either rheumatic symptoms or autoantibodies in large groups of women using oral contraceptives.[102] Studies using the newer low-dose estrogen contraceptives in SLE have not been done. These preparations may be a safe, effective alternative for contraception in women with SLE.

In addition to the exacerbating effects of estrogens, it is postulated that androgens play a protective role in autoimmune disease. Indeed, there is a higher incidence of SLE in patients with Klinefelter's syndrome. Treatment of these patients with testosterone may have a therapeutic effect on their autoimmune disease as well.[103]

The effects of sex steroid hormones on autoimmune disease have been studied in murine lupus models. Androgens suppressed murine lupus, and estrogens accelerated the disease. Estrogen receptor-like binding has been found in mouse thymus tissue, and estrogens may inhibit the clearance of immune complexes; these findings reflect the probable influence of sex hormones on the immune system by means of thymus epithelium and the reticuloendothelial system. Thymic hormones are also influenced by sex hormones. T cells, however, appear to be the primary target for hormones. Hormonal manipulation has a profound effect on T cells, with effects on B cells probably orchestrated through the T cells.[104] Additionally, that androgens have preserved interleukin-2 activity in some mice with lupus suggests a relationship between interleukin-2 and sex hormones.[104]

Metabolism of estrogens and androgens in patients with lupus has been investigated. Patients with SLE showed an elevation of 16 hydroxylated metabolites with increased estrogenic activity. First-degree relatives of these patients also had higher levels of 16 hydroxylated metabolites; a genetic predisposition to altered estrogen metabolism is implied.[105]

The results of these and other studies suggest an important role for hormonal modulation of the immune system in autoimmune disorders, in particular systemic lupus erythematosus, and may lead to novel therapeutic techniques (see Chapter 38).

REFERENCES

1. Ahlquist, J.: Hormonal influences on immunologic and related phenomena. Psychoneuroimmunology. Edited by R. Ader. New York, Academic Press, 355–403, 1981.
2. Hadden, J.W.: Cyclic nucleotides and related mechanisms in immune regulation. A minireview. *In* Immunoregulation. Edited by N. Fabris, E. Garaci, J. Hadden, and N.A. Mitchison. New York, Plenum Press, 1983.
3. Smith, E.M., et al.: Human lymphocyte production of immunoreactive thyrotropin. Proc. Natl. Acad. Sci. USA., *80*:6010–6013, 1983.
4. Levine, J.D., Moskowitz, M.A., and Basbaum, A.I.: The contribution of neurogenic inflammation in experimental arthritis. J. Immunol., *135*:843s, 1985.
5. Sledge, C.: Growth hormone and articular cartilage. Fed. Proc., *32*:1503–1505, 1973.
6. Van Wyk, J.J., et al.: Role of somatomedin in cellular proliferation. *In* The Biology of Normal Human Growth. Edited by M. Ritzen, et al. New York, Raven Press, 1980.
7. Steinbach, H.L., and Russell, W.: Measurement of the heel-pad as an aid to diagnosis of acromegaly. Radiology, *82*:418–423, 1964.
8. Waine, H., Bennett, G.A., and Bauer, W.: Joint disease associated with acromegaly. Am. J. Med. Sci., *209*:671–687, 1945.
9. Anton, H.C.: Hand measurements in acromegaly. Clin. Radiol., *23*:445–450, 1972.
10. Lacks, S., and Jacobs, R.P.: Acromegalic arthropathy: A reversible rheumatic disease. J. Rheumatol., *13*:634–636, 1986.
11. Kellgren, J.H., Ball, J., and Tutton, G.K.: The articular and other limb changes in acromegaly. Q. J. Med., *21*:405–424, 1952.
12. Bluestone, R., et al.: Acromegalic arthropathy. Ann. Rheum. Dis., *30*:243–258, 1971.
13. Nagulesparen, M., et al.: Muscle changes in acromegaly. Br. Med. J., *2*:914–915, 1976.
14. Revel, J.P., Ito, S., and Fawcett, D.W.: Electron micrographs of phsopholipids simulating intercellular membranes. J. Biophys. Biocytol., *4*:495–498, 1958.
15. Pickett, J.B.E., III, et al.: Neuromuscular complications of acromegaly. Neurology, *25*:638–645, 1975.
16. Low, P.A., et al: Peripheral neuropathy in acromegaly. Brain, *97*:139–152, 1974.
17. Bland, J.H., and Frymoyer, J.W.: Rheumatic syndromes of myxedema. N. Engl. J. Med., *282*:1171–1174, 1970.
18. Nickel, S.N., et al.: Myxedema neuropathy and myopathy: A clinical and pathologic study. Neurology, *11*:125–137, 1961.
19. Rao, S.N., et al.: Neuromuscular status in hypothyroidism. Acta Neurol. Scand., *61*:167–177, 1980.
20. Swanson, J.W., Kelly, J.D., and McConahey, W.M.: Neurologic aspects of thyroid dysfunction. Mayo Clin. Proc., *56*:504–512, 1981.
21. Frymoyer, J.W., and Bland, J.: Carpel-tunnel syndrome in patients with myxedematous arthropathy. J. Bone Joint Surg., *55A*:78–82, 1973.
22. Dorwart, B.B., and Schumacher, H.R.: Joint effusions, chondrocalcinosis and other rheumatic manifestations in hypothyroidism. A clinicopathologic study. Am. J. Med., *59*:780–790, 1975.
23. Gerster, J.C., Quadri, P., and Saudan, Y.: Hypothyroidism presenting as destructive arthropathy of the fingers. Postgrad. Med. J., *61*:157–159, 1985.
24. Dieppe, P.A., et al.: Pyrophosphate arthropathy: A clinical and radiological study of 105 cases. Ann. Rheum. Dis., *41*:371–376, 1982.
25. Farid, N.R., et al.: Polymorphonuclear leukocyte function in hypothyroidism. Horm. Res., *7*:247–253, 1976.
26. Brandt, K.D.: The effect of synovial hyaluronate on the ingestion of monosodium urate crystals by leukocytes. Clin. Chim. Acta, *55*:307–315, 1974.
27. Newcombe, D.S.: Endocrinopathies and uric acid metabolism. Semin. Arthritis Rheum., *2*:281–300, 1973.
28. Durward, W.F.: Gout and hypothyroidism in males. Arthritis Rheum., *19*:123, 1976.
29. Newcombe, D.S., Ortel, R.W., and Levey, G.S.: Activation of synovial membrane adenylate cyclase by thyroid stimulating hormone. Biochem. Biophys. Res. Commun., *48*:201–214, 1972.
30. Hirano, T., et al.: Association of primary hypothyroidism and slipped capital femoral epiphysis. J. Pediatr., *93*:262–264, 1978.
31. Ramsey, I.D.: Thyroid Disease and Muscle Dysfunction. London. Whitefriars Press, 1974.
32. Halverson, P.B., et al.: Rhabdomyolysis and renal failure in hypothyroidism. Ann. Intern. Med., *91*:57–58, 1979.
33. Griffiths, P.D.: Serum enzymes in diseases of the thyroid gland. J. Clin. Pathol., *18*:660–663, 1965.
34. McKeran, R.O., et al.: Muscle fibre type changes in hypothyroid myopathy. J. Clin. Pathol., *28*:659–663, 1975.
35. Shagan, B.P., and Friedman, S.A.: Raynaud's phenomenon and thyroid deficiency. Arch. Intern. Med., *140*:831–832, 1980.
36. Gimlette, T.M.D.: Thyroid acropachy. Lancet, *1*:22–24, 1960.
37. Volpé, R.: The role of autoimmunity in hypoendocrine and hyperendocrine function: With special emphasis on autoimmune thyroid disease. Ann. Intern. Med., *87*:86–99, 1977.
38. Londei, M., et al.: Epithelial cells expressing aberrant MHC class II determinants can present antigen to cloned human T cells. Nature, *312*:639–641, 1984.
39. Gorman, C.A.: Unusual manifestations of Graves' disease. Mayo Clin. Proc., *47*:926–933, 1972.
40. Auwerx, J., and Bouillon, R.: Mineral and bone metabolism in thyroid disease: A review. Q. J. Med., *60*:737–752, 1986.
41. Miller, J.L., Ismail, F., Waligora, J.K., and Gevers, W.: Modulating influence of D,L-propranolol on triiodothyronine-induced skeletal muscle protein degradation. Endocrinology, *117*:869–871, 1985.
42. Becker, K.L., Ferguson, R.H., and McConahey, W.M.: The connective tissue diseases and symptoms associated with Hashimoto's thyroiditis. N. Engl. J. Med., *268*:277–280, 1963.
43. Gordon, M.B., et al.: Thyroid disease in progressive systemic sclerosis: Increased frequency of glandular fibrosis and hypothyroidism. Ann. Intern. Med., *95*:431–435, 1981.

44. Oren, M.E., and Cohen, M.S.: Immune thrombocytopenia, Red cell aplasia, lupus and hyperthyroidism. South. Med. J., 71:1577–1578, 1978.
45. Withrington, R.H., and Seifert, M.H.: Hypothyroidism associated with mixed connective tissue disease and its response to steroid therapy. Ann. Rheum. Dis., 40:315–316, 1981.
46. Miller, F.W., Moore, G.F., Weintraub, B.D., and Steinberg, A.D.: Prevalence of thyroid disease and thyroid function test abnormalities in patients with systemic lupus erythematosus. Arthritis Rheum., 30:1124–1131, 1987.
47. Cassorla, F.G., et al.: Vasculitis, pulmonary cavitation and anemia during antithyroid drug therapy. Am. J. Dis. Child., 137:118–122, 1983.
48. Stern, B.D., et al.: Studies of collagen degradation during bone resorption in tissue culture. Proc. Soc. Exp. Biol. Med., 119:577–583, 1965.
49. Preston, E.T.: Avulsion of both quadriceps tendons in hyperparathyroidism. JAMA, 221:406–407, 1972.
50. Hamilton, E.B.D.: Diseases associated with CPPD deposition disease. Arthritis Rheum., 19:353–357, 1976.
51. Pritchard, M.H., and Jessop, J.D.: Chondrocalcinosis in primary hyperparathyroidism: Influence of age, metabolic bone disease and parathyroidectomy. Ann. Rheum. Dis., 36:146–151, 1977.
52. Bilezikian, J.P., et al.: Pseudogout after parathyroidectomy. Lancet, 1:445–446, 1973.
53. Bywaters, E.G.L., Dixon, A. St. J, and Scott, J.T.: Joint lesions of hyperparathyroidism. Ann. Rheum. Dis., 22:171–184, 1963.
54. McCarty, D.J., et al.: Diseases associated with calcium pyrophosphate dihydrate crystal deposition: A controlled study. Am. J. Med., 56:704–714, 1974.
55. Mallette, L.E., Patten, B.M., and Engel, W.K.: Neuromuscular disease in secondary hyperparathyroidism. Ann. Intern. Med., 82:474–483, 1975.
56. Patten, B.M., et al.: Neuromuscular disease in primary hyperparathyroidism. Ann. Intern. Med., 80:182–193, 1974.
57. Frame, B., et al.: Myopathy in primary hyperparathyroidism: Observations in three patients. Ann. Intern. Med., 68:1023–1027, 1968.
58. Richardson, J.A., et al.: Ischemic ulcerations of skin and necrosis of muscle in azotemic hyperparathyroidism. Ann. Intern. Med., 77:129–138, 1969.
59. Chaykin, L.B., Frame, B., and Sigler, J.W.: Spondylitis: A clue to hypoparathyroidism. Ann. Intern. Med., 70:995–1000, 1969.
60. Kruse, K., et al.: Hypocalcemic myopathy in idiopathic hypoparathyroidism. Eur. J. Pediatr., 138:280–282, 1982.
61. Hamlin, C.R., Kohn, R.R., and Luschin, J.H.: Apparent accelerated aging of human collagen in diabetes mellitus. Diabetes, 24:902–904, 1975.
62. Treatment of Diabetes Mellitus. 9th Ed. Edited by E.P. Joslin, H.F. Root, P. White, and A. Marble. Philadelphia, Lea & Febiger, 1952.
63. Julkunen, H., Heinonen, O.P., Pyrörälä, K.: Hyperostosis of the spine in an adult population: Its relation to hyperglycaemia and obesity. Ann. Rheum. Dis., 30:605–612, 1971.
64. Locke, S., Lawrence, D.G., and Legg, M.A.: Diabetic amyotrophy. Am. J. Med., 34:775–785, 1963.
65. Bridgeman, J.E.: Periarthritis of the shoulder and diabetes mellitus. Ann. Rheum. Dis., 31:69–71, 1972.
66. Lequesne, M., et al.: Increased association of diabetes mellitus with capsulitis of the shoulder and shoulder hand syndrome. Scand. J. Rheumatol., 6:53–56, 1977.
67. Pastan, R.S., and Cohen, A.S.: The rheumatologic manifes-

tations of diabetes mellitus. Med. Clin. North Am., 62:829–839, 1978.
68. Sinha, S., Munichoodappa, C.S., and Kozak, G.P.: Neuropathy (Charcot joints) in diabetes mellitus. Medicine, 51:191–210, 1972.
69. Viljanto, J.A.: Dupuytren's contracture—a review. Semin. Arthritis Rheum., 3:155–176, 1973.
70. Strom, L.: Trigger finger in diabetes. J. Med. Soc. N.J., 74:951–954, 1977.
71. Grgic, A., et al.: Joint contracture—common manifestation of childhood diabetes mellitus. J. Pediatr., 88:584–588, 1976.
72. Campbell, R.R., Hawkins, S.J., Maddison, P.J., and Reckless, J.P.D.: Limited joint mobility in diabetes mellitus. Ann. Rheum. Dis., 44:93–97, 1985.
73. Fitzcharles, M.A., et al.: Limitation of joint mobility (cheiroarthropathy) in adult noninsulin-dependent diabetic patients. Ann. Rheum. Dis., 43:251–254, 1984.
74. Rosenbloom, A.L., et al.: Limited joint mobility in childhood diabetes mellitus indicates increased risk for microvascular disease. N. Engl. J. Med., 305:191–194, 1981.
75. Trapp, R.G., Soler, N.G., and Spencer-Green, G.: Nailfold capillaroscopy in type I diabetes with vasculopathy and limited joint mobility. J. Rheumatol., 13:917–920, 1986.
76. Kahn, C.R., et al.: The syndromes of insulin resistance and acanthosis nigrans. N. Engl. J. Med., 294:739–745, 1976.
77. Hardin, J.G., and Siegal, A.M.: A connective tissue disease complicated by insulin resistance due to receptor antibodies: Report of a case with high titer nuclear ribonucleoprotein antibodies. Arthritis Rheum., 25:458–463, 1982.
78. Weinstein, P.S., et al.: Insulin resistance due to receptor antibodies: A complication of progressive systemic sclerosis. Arthritis Rheum., 23:101–105, 1980.
79. Tsokos, G.C., et al.: Lupus nephritis and other autoimmune features in patients with diabetes mellitus due to autoantibody to insulin receptors. Ann. Intern. Med., 102:176–181, 1985.
80. Askari, A., Vignos, P.J., and Moskowitz, R.W.: Steroid myopathy in connective tissue disease. Am. J. Med., 61:485–492, 1976.
81. Ebinger, G., Six, R., Bruyland, M., and Somers, G.: Flexion contractures: A forgotten symptom in Addison's disease and hypopituitarism. Lancet, 2:858, 1986.
82. Plonk, J.W., and Feldman, J.M.: Carcinoid arthropathy. Arch. Intern. Med., 134:651–654, 1974.
83. Odell, W.D., and Wolfsen, A.R.: Humoral syndromes associated with cancer. Annu. Rev. Med., 29:379–406, 1978.
84. DuPont, B., et al.: Plasma growth hormone and hypertrophic osteoarthropathy in carcinoma of the bronchus. Acta Med. Scand., 188:25–30, 1970.
85. Hench, P.S.: The ameliorating effect of pregnancy on chronic atrophic (infectious rheumatoid) arthritis, fibrositis and intermittent hydrarthrosis. Mayo Clin. Proc., 13:161–167, 1938.
86. Cecere, F.A., and Persellin, R.H.: The interaction of pregnancy and the rheumatic diseases. Clin. Rheum. Dis., 2:747–768, 1981.
87. Neely, N.T., and Persellin, R.H.: Activity of rheumatoid arthritis during pregnancy. Tex. Med., 73:59–63, 1977.
88. Kaplan, D.: Fetal wastage in patients with rheumatoid arthritis. J. Rheumatol., 13:875–877, 1986.
89. Lockshin, M.D., et al.: Antibody to cardiolipin as a predictor of fetal distress or death in pregnant patients with systemic lupus erythematosus. N. Engl. J. Med., 313:152–156, 1985.
90. Chameides, L., et al.: Association of maternal systemic lupus erythematosus with congenital complete heart block. N. Engl. J. Med., 297:1204–1207, 1977.

91. Ramsey-Goldman, R., et al.: Anti-SSA antibodies and fetal outcome in maternal systemic lupus erythematosus. Arthritis Rheum., *29*:1269–1273, 1986.

92. Kasinath, S.B., and Katz, A.I.: Delayed maternal lupus after delivery of offspring with congenital heart block. Arch. Intern. Med., *142*:2317, 1982.

93. Fine, L.G., et al.: Systemic lupus erythematosus in pregnancy. Ann. Intern. Med., *94*:667–677, 1981.

94. Hayslett, J.P.: Effect of pregnancy in patients with SLE. Am. J. Kidney Dis., *2*:223–228, 1982.

95. Kaufman, R.L., and Kitridou, R.C.: Pregnancy in mixed connective tissue disease: Comparison with systemic lupus erythematosus. J. Rheumatol., *9*:549–555, 1982.

96. Persellin, R.H.: Inhibitors of inflammatory and immune responses in pregnancy serum. Clin. Rheum. Dis., *7*:769–780, 1981.

97. Schiff, R.I., Mercier, D., and Buckley, R.H.: Inability of gestational hormones to account for the inhibitory effects of pregnancy plasmas on lymphocyte responses in vitro. Cell. Immunol., *20*:69–80, 1975.

98. Hench, P.S.: Potential reversibility of rheumatoid arthritis. Mayo Clin. Proc., *24*:167–178, 1949.

99. Lin, T.M., Halbert, S.P., and Spellacy, W.N.: Measurement of pregnancy-associated plasma proteins during human gestation. J. Clin. Invest., *54*:576–582, 1974.

100. Von Schoultz, B.: A quantitative study of the pregnancy zone protein in the sera of pregnant and puerperal women. Am. J. Obstet. Gynecol., *119*:792–797, 1974.

101. Bole, G.G., Friedlander, M.H., and Smith, G.K.: Rheumatic symptoms and serological abnormalities induced by oral contraceptives. Lancet, *1*:323–326, 1969.

102. Tarzy, B.J., et al.: Rheumatic disease, abnormal serology and oral contraceptives. Lancet, *2*:501–502, 1972.

103. Bizzaro, A., et al.: Influence of testosterone therapy on clinical and immunological features of autoimmune diseases associated with Klinefelter's syndrome. J. Clin. Endocrinol. Metab., *64*:32–36, 1987.

104. Ansar Ahmed, S., Penhale, W.J., and Talal, N.: Sex hormones, immune responses, and autoimmune diseases. Mechanisms of sex hormone action. Am. J. Pathol., *12*:531–551, 1985.

105. Lahita, R.G., et al.: Abnormal estrogen and androgen metabolism in the human with systemic lupus erythematosus. Am. J. Kidney Dis., *2*:206–211, 1982.

section **XI**

INFECTIOUS
ARTHRITIS

PRINCIPLES OF DIAGNOSIS AND TREATMENT OF BONE AND JOINT INFECTIONS

114

FRANK R. SCHMID

Bone and joint infections are curable if antimicrobial drugs active against the invading microorganisms are given early and promptly, and if retained necrotic material is drained. A rational therapeutic program based on these principles is outlined in Table 114–1. Its use will anticipate problems that can compromise the outcome. When the infection is eradicated before irreversible tissue damage has occurred, complete restoration of function can be expected.

PATHOGENESIS OF BONE AND JOINT INFECTIONS

SEPTIC ARTHRITIS, BURSITIS, AND TENDINITIS

Except in rare cases of direct penetration by instrumentation or trauma,[1,2] invasion of the joint cavity by microorganisms occurs through the blood and usually reflects the culmination of a series of successive failures of the host's systemic defense mechanisms. A primary focus of infection is first established at a portal of entry, usually remote from the joint. Microorganisms escaping from this site enter the circulation, where they must resist serum bactericidal activity,[3] as well as elude an active reticuloendothelial system in sufficient numbers and for an adequate time to allow colonization of synovial tissue or juxta-articular bone. Finally, the joint cavity itself must be penetrated from this periarticular location to permit the full-blown expression of acute septic arthritis. In normal circumstances, therefore, the joint is a privileged sanctuary. For each example of overt sepsis, countless instances of failure to infect must occur, considering the low incidence of infectious arthritis in comparison with the much higher incidence of systemic infectious diseases and bacteremia.[4]

Thus, the likelihood of infectious arthritis is greater if host resistance is impaired by prior disease[5-8] or by treatment with drugs that interfere with defense mechanisms, such as corticosteroids or immunosuppressive agents.[9-11] Although sepsis may develop in normal joints, particularly with gonococcal and staphylococcal infections, previous damage by trauma or by another arthritic disease predisposes a joint to infection.[9,12-15] The characteristic monoarticular presentation of septic arthritis suggests that local factors, even within an apparently "normal" joint, favor its colonization over that of other joints equally exposed to the same blood-borne agent.

As microorganisms penetrate the joint cavity, a rapid series of events occurs. Although studies of the inflammatory process in septic arthritis are sparse,[16] the process is similar to that produced by other phlogistic stimuli. The synovial microvasculature dilates, subsynovial tissue becomes edematous, and the volume of synovial fluid increases dramatically with a rise in intra-articular pressure.[17,18] Microvascular injury may cause intravascular thrombosis and ischemia, leading to microabscess formation and, in adjacent bone, ischemia and foci of avascular necrosis.[19] Concentrations of macromolecules, such as immunoglobulins and complement proteins in joint

1863

Table 114–1. Guidelines for Management of a Patient with Infectious Arthritis

INITIAL EVALUATION
Objective: Develop support for diagnosis of infectious arthritis
1. Historical and physical data
—Primary site of infection
—Septicemia: fever, chills, skin rash, polyarthralgia, other metastatic sites of infection
—Host defense impairment
—Pre-existing joint damage
2. Initial joint fluid examination
—Joint fluid analysis: order of priority if amount of joint fluid is limited; smear and culture (or antigen detection); microscopy of wet-mount preparation; glucose measurement; cell count
3. Joint visualizaiton
—Radiographs of affected and contralateral joint
—Radioisotope joint scan, especially for deep-seated joints

INITIAL THERAPEUTIC DECISION
Objective: Selection of antibiotic for the most probable infecting microorganism
1. Identification of suspected microorganism
—Clinical clues: age, geography, environment, primary site of infection
—Bacteriologic smear of joint fluid
2. Selection of antibiotic(s)
—Route for administration: intravenous or intramuscular, usually
—Dosage
3. Joint immobilization and support, analgesia

REAPPRAISAL: 24–72 HOURS
Objective: Reassessment of initial antibiotic choice and decision concerning joint drainage
1. Confirmation of antibiotic choice
—Culture report and sensitivity of invading microorganism to antibiotic drugs
—Review of dosage requirements: bacterial assay of synovial fluid if adequacy of drug levels in doubt
2. Institution of joint drainage
—Needle aspiration and lavage
—Arthrotomy: reserved initially for such special circumstances as infancy, some deep-seated joint infections, or grossly contaminated wounds
3. Monitoring treatment response
—Clinical parameters: systemic findings and primary site of infection
—Infected joint(s): appearance and size; synovial fluid appearance, volume, glucose, white blood cell count, antigen assay if possible, culture

REAPPRAISAL: 5–8 DAYS
Objective: Assessment of efficacy of joint drainage and antibiotic treatment
1. Assessment of frequency and type of joint drainage
—Review clinical and laboratory data from monitoring system
—Criteria for arthrotomy/arthroscopy: microorganism, treatment response, radiographic changes
2. Problems associated with antibiotic usage
—Inability to detect an invading microorganism
—Hypersensitivity to initial drug choice
—Decision for duration and dosage: microorganism, treatment response
—Postinfectious synovitis
3. Passive or active range-of-motion exercises

REAPPRAISAL: 2–8 WEEKS
Objective: Planning out-patient care
1. Choice of drug for oral use: dosage and duration
2. Joint function
—Sequential monitoring system to maximal improvement
—Radiologic comparison with initial films
—Joint use and weight-bearing

REAPPRAISAL: 3–6 MONTHS OR LONGER
Objective: Planning corrective surgical procedure or supportive measures for patients with incomplete restoration of joint function or structure
1. Joint function and structure
—Evaluation of residual inflammation, motion, and structural integrity of joint
—Radiologic comparison with previous films
—Criteria for surgical reconstruction

fluid, approach those in plasma.[20] Because hematogenous dissemination usually occurs at least several days after the infection has become established at a primary site, lymphocyte activation and antibody production against the microorganisms ordinarily will have begun. Thus, immune complexes can form between the antibody and the microorganism or its antigenic fragments, some of which may have become fixed within the cartilage matrix; this both favors its destruction and acts as a reservoir to prolong the inflammation of the entire joint.[21] These complexes can induce such complement-mediated events in the joint as histamine release, chemotaxis, and phagocytosis.[18,22] Bacterial products alone, even in the absence of antibody, can trigger complement activation through the alternate pathway.[23]

A major difference between a closed-space infection, such as septic arthritis, and one dispersed throughout the fibrillar scaffolding of connective tissue, such as cellulitis, is the slower rate of exchange of its contents with the surrounding vascular and lymphatic spaces. Solutes in synovial fluid must diffuse across the synovial lining, often tamponaded by increased pressure,[24] in contrast to the rapid access of molecules in interstitial tissues to and from nearby capillary networks. Diffusion of solutes between joint fluid and blood, although slowed, finally reaches equilibrium, but only after several hours.[25] Thus, the diminished effectiveness of antibiotics against bacteria in a closed-space infection is not because of suboptimal local concentrations of the drug. Rather, the slowed diffusion from the joint of metabolic by-products of the infection retards bacterial cell growth.[26-31] *Bacteria remain dormant under these conditions and survive in the presence of otherwise bactericidal drug concentrations.* For this reason, the time-honored principle of relief of pressure by drainage of pus is a critical component of an effective therapeutic program.

Other synovial tissues, such as bursae and tendon sheaths, share the same pathogenetic mechanism for infection as described for the joint synovium, except direct penetration of microorganisms from the skin might be a more common means of infection of superficial sacs, such as the olecranon and prepatellar bursae.[32,33]

Structures at risk for injury by the infectious process are those lying within the confines of the synovial-lined capsule or sheath, although surrounding soft tissues outside this space are sometimes invaded in rare instances of rupture or sinus formation. Damage to the synovium and capsule of a bursa is reversible, but tendons within synovial sheaths are vulnerable to the effects of the inflammatory process and lose a significant degree of function. Even more vulnerable

is articular cartilage. Chondrolysis is readily demonstrated in the presence of pus,[16,24,34-36] and destroyed hyaline cartilage cannot be totally or effectively replaced. These anatomic considerations influence the need for drainage, which is obviously even more critical for joints and tendons than for bursae.

OSTEOMYELITIS

Bone becomes infected from the blood or from a site of contiguous infection. Hematogenous osteomyelitis most often involves rapidly growing bone, characteristically the metaphysis of long bones in children.[37,38] In adults, the vertebrae are more commonly involved.[39] Osteomyelitis from an adjacent area of infection may result from trauma, open wounds, compound fractures, or an operative infection.[39,40] In recent years, problems relative to infection of joint prostheses have been of great importance.[41]

The acquisition and spread of such infections are tied closely to differences in the microvascular anatomic structures of growing and of mature bone[39] (Fig. 114–1). Between the age of 1 year and puberty, osteomyelitis usually starts in the metaphyseal sinusoidal vein. This site is favored because the afferent loop of the metaphyseal capillary lacks phagocytic lining cells and the efferent loops are frequently multiple, with a broad diameter in which blood flow becomes slow and more turbulent. Furthermore, the capillary loops adjacent to the epiphyseal growth plate are nonanastomotic, so necrosis can result from obstruction caused by microbial emboli and vascular thrombosis.[16] The metaphyseal infection does not cross the epiphyseal growth plate in children, but spreads laterally, perforating the cortex and lifting the loose periosteum to cause a subperiosteal abscess (route 4, Fig. 114–1). In some joints, such as the hip and shoulder, the synovial reflection reaches beyond the epiphyseal growth plate, so infection penetrates directly into the joint through cortical bone (route 1, Fig. 114–1). In the infant less than a year old, capillaries perforate the growth plate, and the infection may thereby spread into the epiphysis and, by further extension, into the joint, with destruction of the epiphyseal growth center (route 3, Fig. 114–1). An analogous situation can occur in the adult.[42] After resorption of the growth cartilage, anastomoses form between the metaphyseal and the epiphyseal blood vessels and allow the spread of infection from the epiphyseal portion of bone to the joint cavity (route 2, Fig. 114–1).

Once microorganisms have colonized the perivascular bone, edema, cellular infiltration, and accu-

FIG. 114–1. Schematic representation of the vascular supply to the bone and joint in the infant, the child, and the adult. Blood-borne microbial emboli reach the metaphysis where conditions favor their lodgment. The bone abscess that forms can spread in several directions, depending on the age of the patient. In children older than 1 year, the epiphyseal growth plate blocks extension of the infection, so the abscess penetrates laterally to the subperiosteum (route 4) or to the joint, in the case of the shoulder, in which the synovial reflection extends beyond the epiphysis to the metaphysis (route 1). In the infant, small capillaries cross the epiphyseal growth plate and thus permit extension of the infection to the epiphysis and subsequently to the joint (route 3). In the adult, osteomyelitis can spread by the anastomotic metaphyseal-epiphyseal vessels to the subperiosteum and then to the joint (route 2). (Adapted from Waldvogel, F.A., Medoff, G., and Schwartz, M.[39] and from Atcheson, S.G. and Ward, J.R.[42])

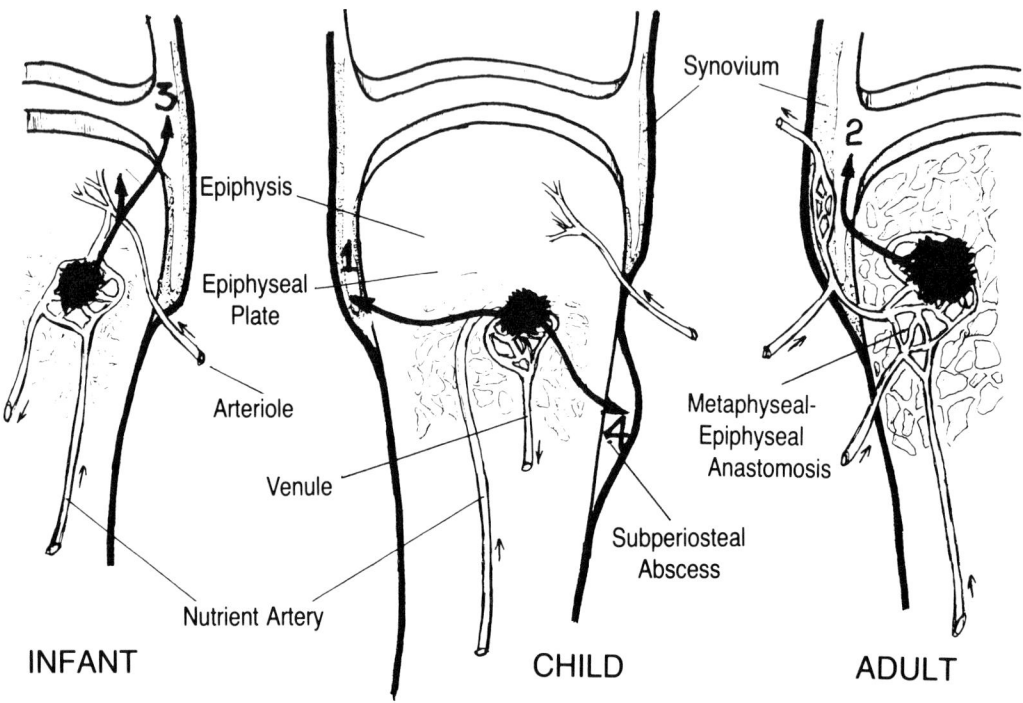

mulation of products of inflammation develop in much the same manner as in septic arthritis and contribute to the necrotic breakdown of bone trabeculae and loss of matrix and mineral. The part played by vascular obstruction is even more important in bone infection. Large segments of bone devoid of blood supply can separate to form sequestra. In cross section, the infected bone shows a core of necrosis with fibrin deposits and massive polymorphonuclear cell infiltration surrounded by an area with granulation tissue containing lymphocytes and plasma cells, and finally an outer layer of fibrous tissue in which new bone is formed. When the infection ruptures beneath the periosteum, more common in children than in adults, the periosteum overgrows to form an involucrum. Cortical destruction can predispose such a patient to fractures.[39]

The vertebral body is the most common site of hematogenous osteomyelitis in the adult. This infection spreads readily along the adjacent ligaments by means of freely anastomosing venous channels, thus commonly involving two adjacent vertebral bodies. The disc between each vertebra loses its vascular supply early in life, but it can be infected by direct extension from the vertebral abscess. The infection can also extend centrally into the spinal canal under the dura mater, with resulting spinal cord compression, or externally to paraspinal soft tissues. In the cervical region, osteomyelitis can cause a retropharyngeal abscess or mediastinitis; in the thoracic spine, mediastinitis, empyema, or pericarditis; and in the lumbar spine, peritonitis or an abscess beneath the diaphragm or along fascial planes of the iliopsoas muscle.

An infection established in any soft tissue or viscus may spread directly to adjacent bone. The source may be exogenous, as in sepsis introduced into a postsurgical or post-traumatic wound, or it may be an already infected neighboring tissue, such as a nasal sinus, tooth, or abdominal organ. The propensity for bone to become infected in these instances appears to be enhanced by concomitant arterial disease. In diabetic feet or in the extremities of patients with rheumatoid vasculitis, an infection in necrotic tissue may involve the underlying bone.[39]

MICROORGANISMS RESPONSIBLE FOR BONE AND JOINT INFECTIONS

Almost any microorganism can cause infectious arthritis, but most infections are caused by a few common agents (Table 114–2). In children who have a high incidence of pyogenic arthritis,[43] Staphylococcus aureus and other cocci are often found, but Haemophilus influenzae is most frequent in the younger child,[37,44,45] probably as a result of an immature immune system. In those under age 2, the absence of antibody has been linked to vulnerability to H. influenzae. Even gonococcal arthritis, although rare, occurs in children.[46] In adults, gonococci and staphylococci now cause the majority of joint infections.[5,8,47-52]

Gram-positive cocci are also the most frequent invaders of bone in hematogenous osteomyelitis (Table 114–2). Gram-negative bacilli are next, but Neisseria species are rare. In some settings, as in osteomyelitis in heroin addicts, infection with Pseudomonas aeruginosa or Serratia species stands out,[53] in patients with sickle cell disease, Salmonella species are prominent;[39,54,54a] and in the neonate, group B streptococci.[55] Although fungi and mycobacteria are only occasionally the cause of musculoskeletal infections (see Chapter 117), they have a propensity to localize in bone. Diagnosis is especially difficult unless the bone lesion can be aspirated and the material from the lesion cultured. These microorganisms should always be considered whenever routine cultures are sterile. Occasionally, infection may be caused by several microorganisms, as, for example, septic arthritis of the hip after perforation of an abdominal organ,[2] or osteomyelitis from a contiguous infection. Both aerobic and anaerobic bacteria may be present in a polymicrobial infection.[56,57]

The microorganisms that usually infect bone and joint tissues are not the most common causes of clinical septicemia. Gram-negative bacilli, other than Haemophilus species, are common causes of septicemia, but they invade osseous or synovial tissue usually only when the tissue has suffered previous damage,[5,58] or when the host has become immunocompromised. Thus, the staphylococcus and other cocci may thus have a special affinity for bone and synovial structures.

MICROORGANISMS ASSOCIATED WITH STERILE JOINT INFLAMMATION

Hematogenous infections of bones and joints almost always occur after the host has had sufficient time to mount an immune response. As part of that response, committed lymphocytes and plasma cells respond to the various products made by the infecting microbial agents or to portions of its structure.[59,60] Immune complexes that form between these antigens and specific antibody or human cells that are cytolytic for antibody-coated or other target tissues can induce inflammation even in the absence of viable microorganisms. Furthermore, host tissues that cross-react with microbial antigens may also participate in this response. Thus, a pathogenic spectrum varying, on the one hand, from an inflammatory process gener-

Table 114–2.   Estimate of the Incidence of Microorganisms Commonly Responsible for Acute Pyogenic Arthritis and Osteomyelitis

Microorganism	Septic Arthritis		Hematogenous Osteomyelitis	
	Adults (%)	Children* (%)	Adults (%)	Children* (%)
Gram-positive cocci				
Staphylococcus aureus	35	27	65	75
Streptococcus pyogenes, S. pneumoniae, viridans-group streptococci	10	16	10	15
Gram-negative cocci				
Neisseria gonorrhoeae and meningitidis	50	8	—	—
Haeomophilus influenzae†	<1	40	—	5
Gram-negative bacilli				
Escherichia coli, Salmonella sp., *Pseudomonas,* etc.	5	9	20	5
Mycobacteria, fungi	<1	<1	<5	<1

*Data of Fink, C.W., and Nelson, J.D.[37]

†H. influenzae are actually coccobacilli, but are listed under "cocci" because they are frequently mistaken on smears for cocci.

ated mainly by virulence factors of the actively metabolizing microbe, to sterile inflammation generated by the host's immune system, on the other hand, may account to varying degrees for the signs of inflammation seen in different patients infected by the same agent or seen at various times during the course of the disease in a single patient[18] (Fig. 114–2).

IMMUNE-MEDIATED FORMS OF ARTHRITIS

Well-known examples of inflammation associated with immune complexes are found in patients with the disseminated gonococcal syndrome[61] (see Chapter 116), with hepatitis[62] and rubella[63] virus infections (see Chapter 118), and most recently, with Lyme disease[64] (see Chapter 119). In each instance, viable bacteria, viruses, and spirochetes have been cultured from the inflamed joint, and immune complexes have been detected in the plasma or joint fluid. When both are present at the same time, the relative contribution of either to the inflammation cannot be determined. When cultures of synovial fluid or tissue are sterile, the cause of the inflammation may be attributed to the host's immune response. Yet even in such patients, special culture techniques may be necessary to uncover the presence of a viable agent. For example, spirochetes were recovered from the skin and joints of patients with Lyme disease only after a long search,[65] and rubella virus was "rescued" from the peripheral blood lymphocytes of an arthritic patient who had received live rubella vaccine 2 years earlier.[66] A unique illustration of the combination of both infectious and noninfectious inflammation in the same patient may be the development of sterile, so-called *sympathetic* effusions in a bursa or joint adjacent to a primary site of septic arthritis or osteomyelitis. No explanation is known for these effusions, but it is assumed that inflammatory mediators are transported from the infected region to the nearby sac to cause the inflammation. The implications of such observations for antibiotic therapy are discussed later in the section of this chapter on postinfectious synovitis.

A few observations have been made about the immune response in osteomyelitis. Antibodies to a staphylococcal cell-wall constituent, teichoic acid, have been found mainly in the serum of patients with bone infections.[67] Rheumatoid factors develop, but less commonly in staphylococcal osteomyelitis than in staphylococcal endocarditis.[68] The possible relevance of these serologic findings to the pathogenesis of the bone disease is not known.

REACTIVE ARTHRITIS

The pathogenesis of sterile inflammation in the joints of patients with infectious diseases at extra-articular sites is even more elusive. Examples are streptococcal pharyngitis in patients with rheumatic fever (see Chapter 77), enteritis resulting from Salmonella, Shigella, or Yersinia species, urethritis resulting from Mycoplasma agents in patients with Reiter's syndrome (see Chapter 60), or bowel lesions related to parasitic infestations,[69] and to bacterial residues in patients with Whipple's disease (see Chapter 62). The type of immune or other response that induces the arthritis in these cases is not known. Pathogenetic immune complexes either have not been found or, if found, do not correlate with the disease process. In some cases, success attends eradication of the triggering infecting agent by administration of appropriate drugs, although most often this approach fails to control the arthritis.

CLINICAL PRESENTATIONS

Infectious arthritis may become manifest in a variety of ways, both typical and atypical.

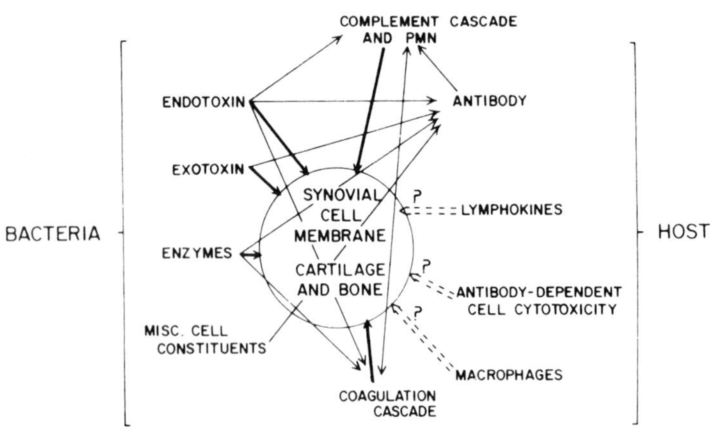

FIG. 114–2. Interaction of bacterial and host factors in the inflammatory process of septic arthritis. A thick arrow indicates a final and direct pathway of tissue damage; a thin arrow represents the interaction of one component with another leading to induction of synovial inflammation; and an interrupted arrow signifies a possible, but insufficiently documented, host effect. PMN = Polymorphonuclear leukocytes. (From Tesar, J.T., and Dietz, F.[18])

TYPICAL PRESENTATION

Pyogenic arthritis affecting single or, less commonly, two or more joints is usually of acute onset.[5,8,37] A migratory polyarthritis may precede this phase, especially in gonococcal and meningococcal arthritis.[70–73] Large joints, such as the knee and hip, are involved most often, but articular structures of any size or location, including the sacroiliac and spinal joints, may be affected. The infected joint is typically warm, painful, and distended with fluid. Because bacterial entry into a joint is most often hematogenous, the patient may have fever with chills.[50] Signs and symptoms of a primary infection should be sought. Careful examination may reveal pneumonia as a source of pneumococci or a carbuncle as a source of staphylococci. A history of urethritis, pharyngitis, or prostatitis suggesting gonococcal infections might be obtained. In staphylococcal or streptococcal joint disease, and less often in gram-negative bacillary arthritides, a primary site of infection may not be found, however.[5]

ATYPICAL PRESENTATIONS

Unfortunately, septic arthritis may present in an atypical fashion. In a joint damaged by prior disease, superimposed infection may not be obvious because the new process may become "lost" among other painful, chronically swollen joints.[9,14,56] Careful questioning usually reveals that the infected joint has become more symptomatic than it was before, however. Elderly patients, or those under treatment with immunosuppressive or corticosteroid drugs, are more vulnerable to superimposed infection and may show less evidence of inflammation than other patients. Some locations may be overlooked, such as a popliteal cyst,[74] the sternoclavicular or sternomanubrial joints,[53,75] or the hip joints.[76] Infected superficial bursae such as the prepatellar and olecranon bursae are sometimes mistaken for the adjacent knee and elbow joints, respectively.[32,33,77]

Infection of the deeply situated axial joints of the body, such as the hip, shoulder, pubic, and sacroiliac joints, can present major difficulties in diagnosis and treatment because evidence of inflammation may be masked, or, if present, may be ascribed to noninfectious causes until the process is far advanced.[76,78–81] This situation is of particular concern in the evaluation of acute shoulder pain. Delay in diagnosis may result in severe joint destruction and loss of motion.[78]

JOINT INFECTIONS IN CHILDREN

Septic arthritis most often resulting from Staphylococcus aureus, group B streptococci and gram-negative bacilli, in neonates 1 to 28 days of age may induce signs and symptoms of septicemia, such as lethargy, fever, tachycardia, and hypotension. Decreased spontaneous movement of the involved extremity, even in the absence of pain and swelling, helps to locate the infection. Multiple joints may be involved. Although bacteria can gain access into the joint directly by lodging in subsynovial vessels, more commonly they do so from a region of adjacent osteomyelitis (see route 3, Fig. 114–1). Predisposing factors are a low birth weight and perinatal complications that necessitate instrumentation, such as fetal monitoring or exchange transfusions.[37,55]

In older children, the clinical appearance of septic arthritis more closely parallels that observed in adults.

Diagnostic problems are magnified in children, especially those with an infection of the hip. This joint is affected more often than any other except the knee, particularly in children below the age of 6 months.[43] Unless treatment is started promptly, irreversible destruction can occur within days.[82–84] Distension of the joint can rapidly deprive the femoral head of its blood supply, and purulent fluids destroy cartilage and bone. Hematogenous dissemination of microorganisms from a primary portal of entry to the joint or adjacent bone is usual, and prior joint disease or associated illness predisposes the child to infection in the hip, just as in other joints.[85] Direct penetration may occur as a complication of femoral venipuncture,[86] or it may result from infection extending from an abdominal abscess into the retroperitoneal space near the iliopsoas muscle.[2]

Symptoms of sepsis in the hip include pain in the groin, lateral upper thigh, or buttocks. Referred pain along the obturator nerve to the knee is common.[87] The thigh is usually held in flexion, adduction, and internal rotation, and pain permits only a few degrees of motion. In adults, external signs of inflammation are rare, but in children, the massive increase in the volume of joint fluid may distend the capsule, obliterating the inguinal crease and causing generalized edema of the thigh. Marked tenderness may be elicited by local pressure.

INFECTIONS OF BONE

Hematogenous osteomyelitis commonly affects rapidly growing bones in children, frequently the metaphysis of the tibia or the femur. In a large series, more than 80% of the cases were found in children below age 10, and almost 60% below age 5.[37] In recent years, the prevalence of bone infections in adults has increased, especially in the vertebral bodies.[39]

Most patients have fever, with or without chills, constitutional symptoms such as weight loss and fatigue, and symptoms referable to the local site of bony involvement. Thus, osteomyelitis of the long bones of the lower extremity may be associated with local pain, sometimes accompanied by swelling and erythema, a limp, or in a young child, refusal to walk. Vertebral osteomyelitis may be associated with back pain and local tenderness, spasm of paraspinal or psoas muscles, and limitation of motion. Pelvic osteomyelitis may cause abdominal pain or pain referred to the hip or lower extremities.[88] Findings in patients with spinal or pelvic osteomyelitis may be so subtle that infection in these regions should be considered in any individual who only has systemic signs of inflammation, such as a fever of unknown origin.[89] In such patients, a positive blood culture increases the likelihood of deep-seated osteomyelitis. Sepsis of the sacroiliac joint should be considered in the differential diagnosis of low-back or hip pain, particularly when unilateral sacroiliac disease is noted on a radiograph or scintiphotograph.[90,91]

INFECTED JOINT PROSTHESES

Infection following a joint implant is a serious complication. Rates of infection initially were greater than 10%, but with extensive experience, they have dropped to only a few percent in most large centers.[41] Although most infections occur during the early postoperative months (40% in the first 3 months and another 45% within 1 year[92]), some appear several years later.[93]

In the postoperative period, systemic signs such as fever may be falsely attributed to other complications such as pneumonia or a urinary tract infection. Persistent joint pain may be the only finding that suggests the real cause of the problem. Its character helps to distinguish mechanical loosening of the prosthesis from infection. With infection, pain is generally dull, is present also at night, is described as deep gnawing or throbbing, and may diminish after the use of antibiotics. Pain with loosening is related to motion or weight-bearing, and may be accentuated by sharp movement.[92] If purulent material drains from the wound, and if the infection does not respond to antibiotics, a deep infection around the prosthesis rather than a superficial wound infection should be considered, and exploration of the operative site may be

required. Staphylococcus aureus or S. epidermidis are the most common causes of an infected joint prosthesis; gram-negative bacilli and anaerobic and other bacteria are less common.[41,57,94,95] Anaerobic organisms have fastidious growth requirements, and their presence must be looked for carefully by appropriate culture techniques when the routine cultures are sterile and the index of suspicion for infection is high.[41]

DIAGNOSTIC STUDIES

DIFFERENTIAL DIAGNOSIS OF SEPTIC ARTHRITIS

Other acute arthritic disorders, such as gout, pseudogout, palindromic rheumatism, rheumatic fever, trauma, and the oligoarticular syndromes associated with the spondyloarthropathies or with juvenile rheumatoid arthritis (RA), may be confused with infectious arthritis. Constitutional symptoms, such as high fever or chills and marked leukocytosis, are uncommon in these conditions. Even when a noninfectious form of arthritis is actually present, an added infectious process must be excluded by bacteriologic examination of synovial fluid. An unusual but distressing example of superimposed infection occurs in crystal-induced synovitis, in which the previous deposition of urate or calcium pyrophosphate crystals in the joint predisposes the patient to sepsis,[12,13,15,96] or more likely, tissue breakdown by septic inflammation releases pre-existing crystal deposits into the joint space, a phenomenon aptly termed "enzymatic strip mining"[15,97] (see Chapter 107). Patients with RA have a high incidence of joint infection, usually as a result of staphylococci.[9,14] Therefore, suspicion of sepsis should be heightened whenever a primary site of infection or evidence of septicemia is recognized in any arthritic patient.

DIFFERENTIAL DIAGNOSIS OF BONE INFECTION

Infections of the vertebral body, disc, or sacroiliac joint may be overlooked because symptoms and signs can mimic other conditions, such as post-traumatic thinning of a disc, congenital absence of a disc, osteochondritis of a disc, metastatic carcinoma, Paget's disease, or Charcot arthropathy.[39] Ankylosing spondylitis or the spondyloarthropathy associated with Reiter's disease, psoriasis, or bowel disease may present problems in the differential diagnosis of sacroiliac joint disease; these conditions usually affect both sacroiliac joints, however, whereas infection is almost always unilateral.[79] Correct diagnosis may require identification or exclusion of an infecting microorganism by aspiration under fluoroscopic control or rarely by surgical exploration.[98,99]

GENERAL STUDIES

A complete medical history and physical examination are essential, with special attention to the portals of entry for infection: skin, nasal passages, including sinuses and the middle ear, lungs, rectum, urethra, and pelvis.

Initial studies in a patient with acute septic arthritis or hematogenous osteomyelitis may reveal leukocytosis with an increased percentage of immature leukocytes, but the absence of leukocytosis does not rule out sepsis, particularly in a debilitated individual. Anemia is not likely to be present early, unless an underlying disease antedates the infectious process. The erythrocyte sedimentation rate and other acute-phase reactants, such as C-reactive protein and the serum precursor of amyloid protein AA (SAA),[100] are elevated both in infectious arthritis and in noninfectious inflammatory states. That elevated C-reactive protein levels failed to identify infection in patients with systemic lupus erythematosus dashed a hope raised by an earlier study.[101,102] The form of α_1-acid glycoprotein that reacts with concanavalin A can be measured in the serum and may offer real promise in deciding whether an infection has occurred, however. Lupus patients who became infected had significantly higher values for this acute-phase reactant than did noninfected lupus patients.[103] Serum calcium, phosphorus, and alkaline phosphatase levels are usually normal in osteomyelitis. At least two blood cultures for aerobic and anaerobic organisms should be taken within the first several hours in every suspected case of pyogenic arthritis or osteomyelitis. A single positive blood culture may be difficult to interpret because of possible contamination during collection. Two blood cultures containing the same organism virtually rule out contamination. Cultures should also be made of any exudate or secretion at a suspected portal of entry.

RADIOLOGIC EXAMINATION

Several weeks are usually needed before cartilaginous or bony abnormalities can be detected in previously normal bone or joints. In septic arthritis, rarefaction of subchondral bone develops first, followed

FIG. 114–3. *A,* Ankle joint of a 36-year-old man 3 weeks after it was injected for pain. *Pseudomonas aeruginosa* grew from the culture of synovial fluid. The joint space is normal and the white line of the articular cortical margin is normal. *B,* Same ankle joint 5 weeks later. The white line of the articular margin *(open arrows)* is destroyed on both sides of the joint. Underlying bone trabeculae are bare and irregularly destroyed, causing the fuzzy appearance of the bone margins. (From Hendrix, R.W., and Fisher, M.R.[104])

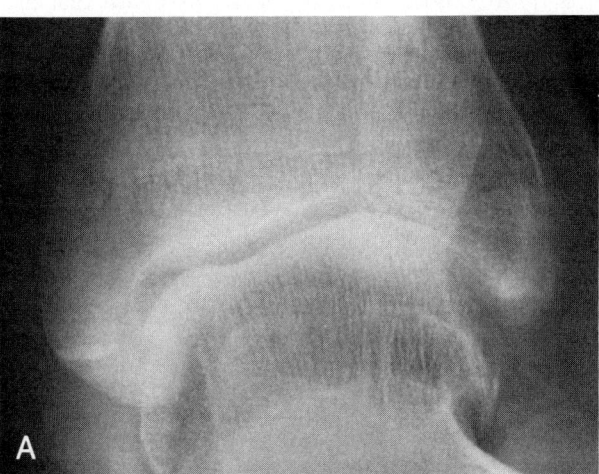
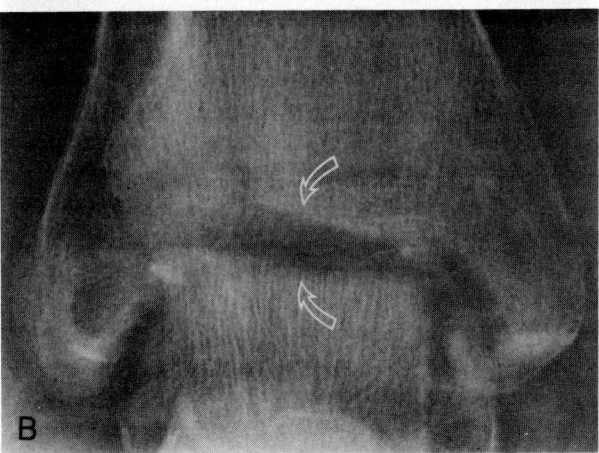

by erosion of juxta-articular bone and narrowing of the joint space[104] resulting from destruction of articular cartilage (Fig. 114–3). When superimposed on a diseased joint, changes caused by infection may be indistinguishable from those already present. The decalcification resulting from infection is particularly troublesome in children, in whom skeletal immaturity already makes significant bony structures radiolucent.

In osteomyelitis, bone is destroyed locally, but this change does not become visible for 2 to 3 weeks when 30 to 50% of bone mineral has been removed. New bone also forms, but about a month is required for the deposition of mineral to be sufficient to be detected. Thus, areas of lysis and increased bone density appear at about the same time radiographically, although soft-tissue swelling and periosteal elevation may be seen earlier. For the same reason, radiologic evidence of healing of osteomyelitis also lags behind clinical improvement and actual bone reconstruction.[39]

Within a few weeks of the onset of vertebral disc or bone infection, thinning of the involved disc and destruction of vertebral bone may occur. Tomograms may more clearly outline lesions that are obscure on standard films (Fig. 114–4). Lesions may heal by fusion. Most infections of the sacroiliac joint are unilateral, in contradistinction to bilateral involvement by the sterile spondylitic syndromes.

In deep-seated joints, such as the hip, soft-tissue changes resulting from joint-space distension may be helpful in diagnosis. The *obturator sign*, a widening and curving of the border of the obturator internus tendon adjacent to the capsule of the hip joint, may be helpful if positive. A radiolucent *air sign* is an unusual finding in lesions produced by some gas-forming microorganisms. This sign was noted in the disc space of a patient with vertebral osteomyelitis and in joints of patients with septic arthritis resulting from Clostridium perfringens,[105,106] Streptococcus milleri, anaerobic bacteria, and gram-negative bacilli.[107]

Although evidence of sepsis may not be evident, films taken early document the extent of prior damage and permit an estimate of the degree to which function might ultimately be restored. Comparison with

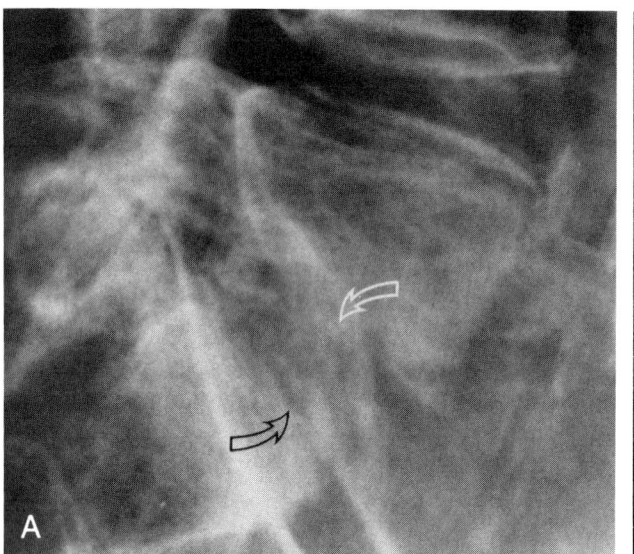

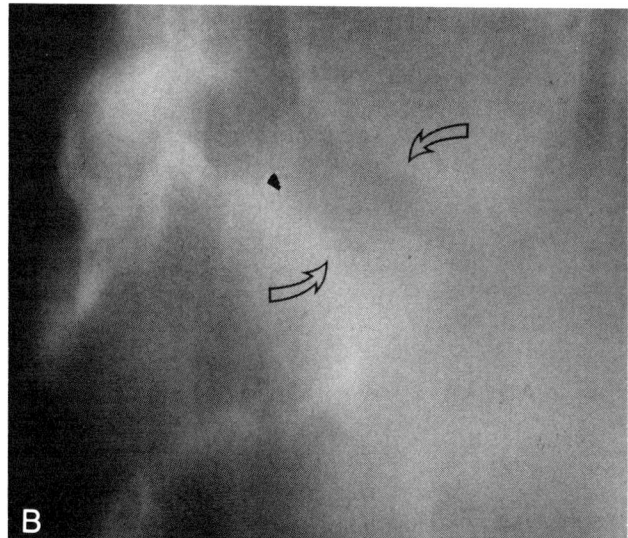

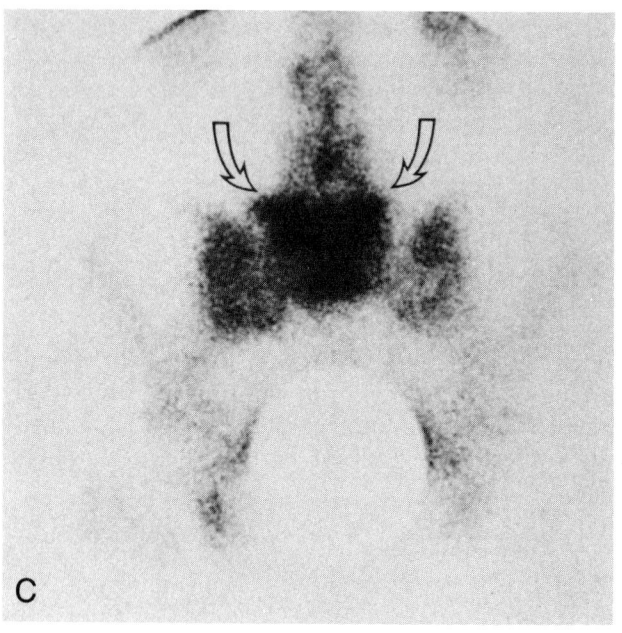

FIG. 114–4. *A,* The vertebral end-plates at L5-S1 of a 58-year-old woman are indistinct *(open arrows)* because of destruction by a disc space-vertebral infection by Staphylococcus aureus. *B,* A conventional tomogram demonstrates this indistinctness more clearly *(open arrows)*. *C,* The ^{99m}Tc-disphosphonate bone scintigram shows increased activity at the L5-S1 level *(open arrows)*. The greater sacroiliac activity in the left compared to the right is a result of patient rotation; the left sacroiliac joint is closer to the crystal detector of the gamma camera. (From Hendrix, R.W., and Fisher, M.R.[104])

radiographs of the contralateral bone and joint may reveal subtle changes in the involved side. Sequential films are helpful to monitor treatment (see Table 114–1).

ARTHROGRAPHY

In addition to determining placement of structures within the joint, arthrograms may reveal capsular or ligamentous damage. The contrast material does not exacerbate the infectious process, nor does it interfere with antibiotic treatment. Rupture of the rotator cuff, with or without superior subluxation of the humeral head,[78] and delineation of the position and integrity of the femoral head, especially in children,[108–110] are often detectable by arthrography. Synovial fluid obtained should be examined for microorganisms by staining and culture before the contrast dye is injected.

COMPUTED TOMOGRAPHY (CT) SCANNING

This procedure is most valuable when the anatomic structures are complex, as in the spine, or when the involved areas are surrounded by bone; it is less valuable in examining peripheral joints and the neck (see Chapter 81).[111] Osteomyelitis in a long bone increases the density of medullary tissues, presumably because of vascular congestion and edema, even before bone destruction becomes apparent. Later, just as on standard radiographs and conventional tomograms, CT scanning can be used to document bone destruction, cavitation, and sequestration.[112] In the spine, this technique permits identification of a soft-tissue abscess.[104] Swelling and effusion can be recognized in a deep-seated area such as the sacroiliac joint.[113]

MAGNETIC RESONANCE IMAGING (MRI)

Magnetic resonance imaging (MRI) can demonstrate, in superb anatomic detail, soft-tissue structures of the musculoskeletal system with striking differentiation between muscles, fibrous structures, and blood vessels. These structures on the CT scan have an almost indistinguishable appearance.[104] Articular cartilage and, in children, growth cartilage can be depicted. In the knee, the fibrous cartilage of the meniscus is seen as a very low intensity structure distinctly different from the articular cartilage. The increased anatomic visualization afforded by MRI can

be compared to the findings on standard radiographs and CT scans in the case of an infected hip joint (Fig. 114–5) and in the case of osteomyelitis of the spine in a child (Fig. 114–6).

RADIOISOTOPE SCANNING TECHNIQUES

^{99m}Technetium (^{99m}Tc) diphosphonate and ^{67}gallium (^{67}Ga) citrate scintigraphy may detect the presence of infection at an early stage; these techniques are particularly useful in examining deep joints such as the hip, shoulder, and spine.[104,114] Positive results by either isotope are not specific for infection because other inflammatory or even degenerative joint diseases can create the same image.[115] Specificity for bone and joint infection, however, may be enhanced by giving more weight to a positive ^{67}Ga citrate scintigram than to a positive ^{99m}Tc scintigram,[116] for osteomyelitis, one may perform a three-phase study, consisting of the radionuclide angiogram, the immediate postinjection "blood pool" image, and the 2- to 3-hour delayed image, to distinguish bone infection from soft-tissue infection and from noninfectious skeletal disease.[117] Using these techniques, the pathologic process can be localized to a joint rather than to overlying tissue, as in cellulitis. This feature has been particularly useful in evaluating disease in the sacroiliac joint.[90,114]

In acute osteomyelitis, ^{99m}Tc-diphosphonate often fails to demonstrate a high-uptake lesion in the neonate, in contrast to the expected greater yield of abnormal images in the slightly older infant or child.[118] Even in older children, however, fulminant osteomyelitis may escape detection. Instead, a focal decrease in nuclide accumulation occurs, considered to be a result of thrombosis in the microcirculation[16] or of intraosseous pressure on the nutrient artery.[119]

Radionuclide studies should always be interpreted together with findings revealed by the standard radiograph because the detailed anatomic information provided by the radiograph often complements the functional information provided by scintigraphy.

RADIOLOGY OF AN INFECTED JOINT PROSTHESIS

Several weeks or months may elapse before conventional radiographs indicate changes compatible with infection in an endoprosthesis. These changes include the formation of a radiolucent zone at the bone-cement interface, scalloping of the cortical margin, a periosteal reaction resembling lamination, and

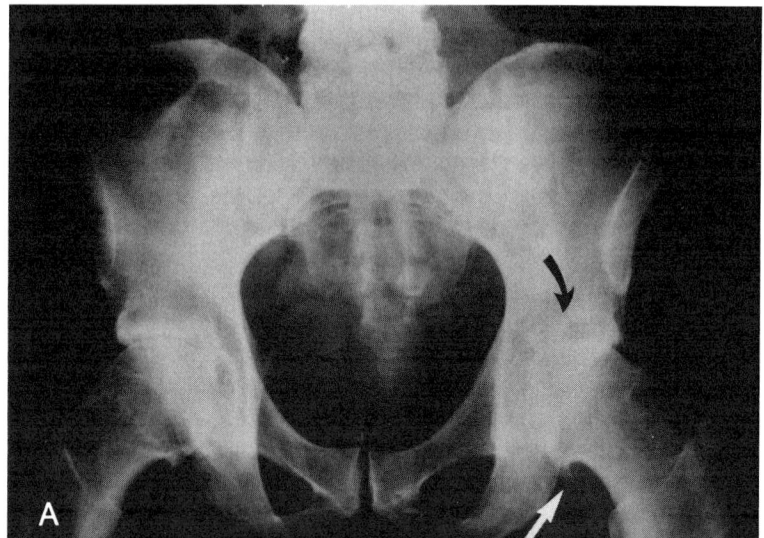

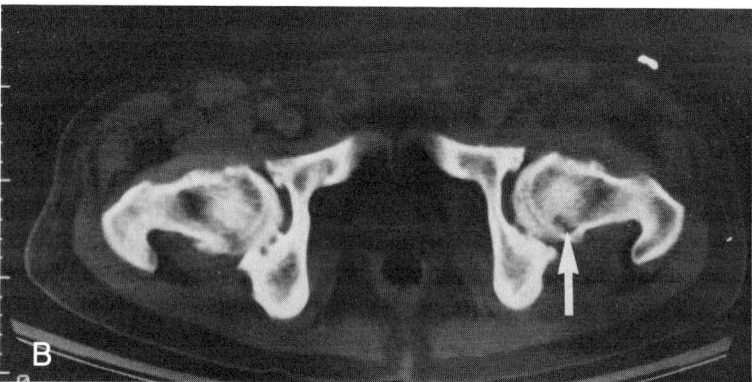

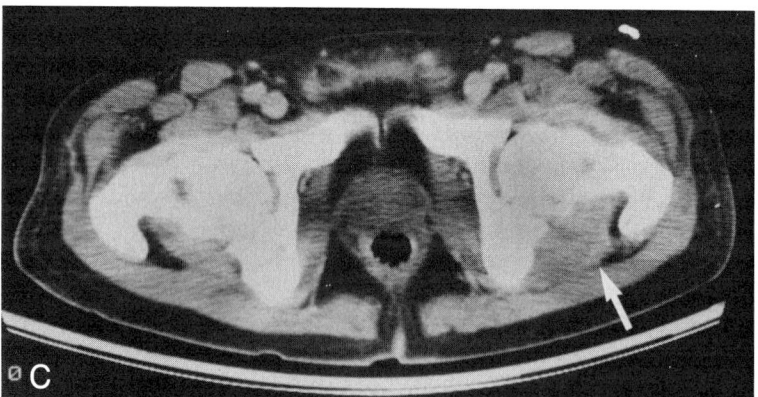

FIG. 114–5. Infectious arthritis of the left hip in a 53-year-old drug-addicted patient. *A,* In the conventional radiograph, narrowing of the joint space is greater on the left than the right, with associated evidence of prior osteoarthritis *(straight arrow showing osteophytes).* The ill-defined left acetabular margin *(curved arrow)* is suspicious for infection. *B,* In the CT scan at the level of the hip joints with a bone window setting, minimal differences exist between the bone density and joint space of the left and right hip, except for a vague area *(arrow)* of decreased bone density along the posterior aspect of the left femoral head; *C,* in the CT scan with a soft-tissue window setting, there is enlargement of the surrounding musculature *(arrow).*

regions of increased bone density and radiolucency typical of osteomyelitis (Fig. 114–7). Early and minor alterations are not recognizable without a comparison with previous films. Arthrograms are not helpful for the diagnosis of infection itself, but they can demonstrate the extent and location of soft tissue involvement, such as a sinus tract. If a sinus tract has perforated to the exterior, a sinogram can be done. Subtraction technique is essential to verify details when radiopaque cement is present. ^{99m}Tc-diphos-

phonate uptake may fail to distinguish mechanical loosening from infection; as mentioned earlier, imaging by ^{67}Ga citrate may be more specific for infection.[120]

JOINT FLUID EXAMINATION

Aspiration and examination of joint fluid are mandatory whenever infection is considered. These procedures must be done immediately and must not be deferred.

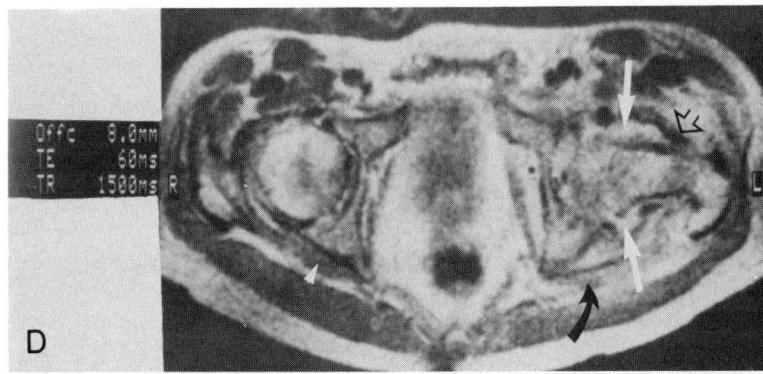

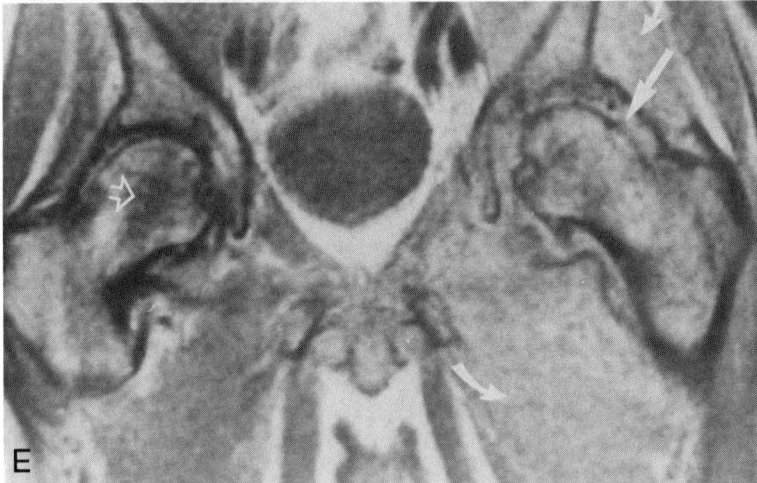

FIG. 11–5. (Continued) *D*, A transverse MRI at a similar level shows an abnormal collection of material *(closed straight arrows)* within the left hip joint displacing the joint capsule *(open arrow)* outward. The signal intensity within the surrounding musculature *(curved arrow)* is increased on the left compared to the opposite normal side *(arrowhead)*. The left femoral head and neck have a nonhomogeneous signal intensity. *E*, In a coronal MRI through the hip joints, the abnormal collection within the joint *(closed arrow)* and the enlarged adjacent musculature with an increased intensity *(curved arrows)* are shown. The low-intensity line on the right femoral neck is the site of normal trabecular thickening *(open arrow)*. (From Hendrix, R.W., and Fisher, M.R.[104])

Arthrocentesis requires strict asepsis (see Chapter 39). Inadvertent introduction of infection from skin, blood, or a para-articular focus into a joint cavity represents a hazard of joint aspiration. For this reason, a careful examination of the area is required to define anatomically the exact site of infection. The needle should be introduced into the joint through uninvolved subcutaneous tissue.

An arthrocentesis tray should contain sterile culture tubes. If indicated, joint fluid should be inoculated into these tubes as well as into tubes for chemical determinations and tubes with heparin or ethylene diamine tetracetate anticoagulant for cell examination. These culture samples should be taken directly to a laboratory by the physician. Lacking such tubes, the syringe into which the joint fluid was aspirated can be refitted with a new capped, sterile needle and carried to the laboratory where its contents can be distributed, first for smears and cultures and then for other studies. The synovial fluid should still be warm when inoculated into appropriate bacteriologic media. Some even recommend bedside inoculation of the fluid onto media when infection with fastidious microorganisms, such as the gonococcus, are anticipated. If only one or two drops of synovial fluid can

be obtained, they should be cultured, and any remaining fluid should be smeared onto a slide for Gram's staining. Rank order priority for studies on joint fluid are given in Table 114–1.

SYNOVIAL OR BONE BIOPSY

Tissue may be required to confirm a diagnosis of sepsis in patients whose synovial fluid has not yielded a positive culture. In some cases, this procedure may prove helpful because the density of bacteria may be greater in tissue,[121] and in other cases, such as in tuberculous and fungal infections,[122] because microbial growth, even on appropriate culture media, is slow and thus may delay diagnosis and appropriate treatment. Tissue can be obtained by a blind synovial biopsy or under direct vision at arthroscopy or arthrotomy. Bone biopsy can be performed either with a needle or surgically. The fresh tissue specimen should be transported to the laboratory in a sterile container or in a sterile sponge moistened with saline solution. In addition to the appropriate bacteriologic studies, a portion of the tissue should be fixed and submitted for histologic examination.

FIG. 114–6. Osteomyelitis of the spine in a child. *A*, A sagittal MRI through the lumbosacral region demonstrates decreased signal intensity of the involved L5 and S1 vertebral bodies and disc. Note disc space narrowing *(closed straight arrow)* compared to the high intensity of normal disc material *(open arrow)*. The extension into the epidural space is well visualized *(curved arrow)*. *B*, The same view by CT demonstrates irregularity of the L5-S1 end-plates *(arrows)* and loss of disc height. The degree of bone involvement and extension into the spinal canal is not as well delineated as with MRI. (From Hendrix, R.W., and Fisher, M.R.[104])

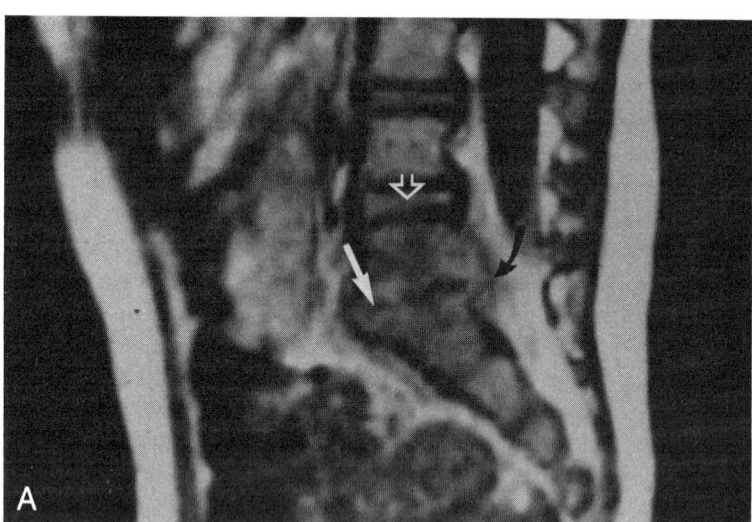
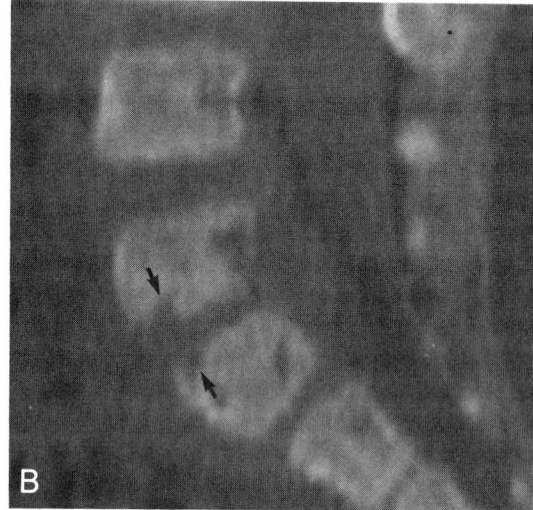

BACTERIOLOGIC STUDIES

Blood agar should be used routinely for culturing all synovial fluid or tissue specimens, with chocolate agar used in addition when Neisseria gonorrhoeae or Haemophilus infection is suspected. The medium designed by Thayer and Martin is suitable for gonococcal isolation, but it contains vancomycin and colistin methanesulfonate because it was designed to isolate gonococci from the mixed flora of the female genital tract.[123] Therefore, many other bacteria such as Haemophilus species do not grow on Thayer-Martin media. Media of higher ionic strength have been advocated to culture gonococcal protoplasts. In one patient with gonococcal arthritis, standard cultures were negative, but growth occurred on such hypertonic media.[124] Haemophilus species can easily be isolated on peptic digest of blood agar, which is prepared from commercially available products. Placement of about 1 ml synovial fluid in thioglycolate broth allows recovery of many anaerobic and aerobic bacteria. Many microaerophilic bacteria actually grow more rapidly after primary inoculation in thioglycolate broth than on solid media.

Isolation of strict anaerobes may require special anaerobic techniques. Fungal media, such as Sabouraud agar, should be inoculated in most instances. If fungal media are not inoculated, fungi may be recovered from the blood agar plates after incubation for as long as 2 weeks at room temperature. Drying of ordinary blood agar plates can be retarded by sealing the plate with paraffin tape. Culture of Mycobacterium species is best done with at least two kinds of media, an egg-glycerol-potato medium, suh as A.T.S. medium, and a synthetic medium, such as Middlebrook 7H10 agar. If a large volume of synovial fluid is available, it should be concentrated by centrifugation before inoculating mycobacterial cultures. Because of improvements in culture media, one no longer needs to use guinea pig inoculation as a means of recovering M. tuberculosis; results in the guinea pig are rarely positive when mycobacterial cultures are negative.[125] Furthermore, atypical Mycobacterium species, which also infect joints, are nonpathogenic for guinea pigs (see also Chapter 117).

After inoculation of joint fluid into all appropriate media, smears are prepared on glass slides, which are air dried, and Gram's stain, Wright's stain, and appropriate stains for acid-fast and fungal organisms are applied. Examination of such slides provides the necessary information to begin treatment.

Certain additional studies of joint fluid are regularly performed (Table 114–3). The total leukocyte count can be determined manually or with an automated cell counter *using physiologic saline solution as a diluent.* The acid diluents used for blood leukocyte counts

FIG. 114–7. Infected total hip replacement resulting from Staphylococcus aureus 18 months after insertion shows well-defined cement-metal *(open arrow)* and bone-cement *(closed arrows)* lucent zones. (From Hendrix, R.W., and Fisher, M.R.[104])

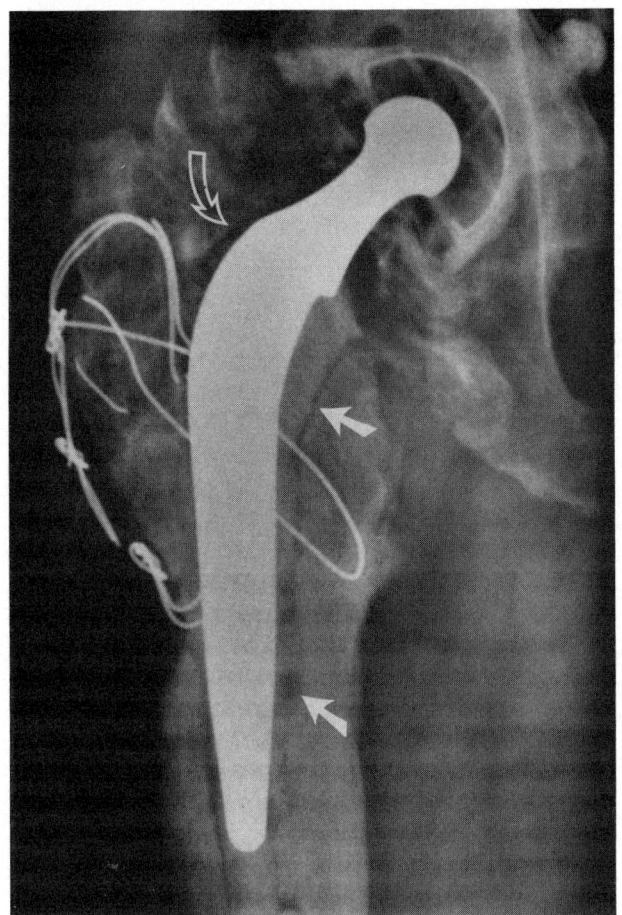

coagulate the hyaluronate of synovial fluid and trap leukocytes, so counts are falsely low. Although fluids in septic arthritis often appear grossly purulent and have elevated cell counts, predominantly of polymorphonuclear leukocytes, high white blood cell counts containing many polymorphonuclear cells can appear in noninfected fluids obtained from some patients with acute gout, pseudogout, or RA.[126] Therefore, microbiologic stains and cultures provide the only absolute confirmation of sepsis.

The fasting synovial fluid glucose value is usually reduced to less than half the blood glucose value obtained simultaneously.[52] Reductions of this magnitude are unusual in inflammatory joint fluids of nonseptic origin, in infectious arthritis resulting from viruses, and in gonococcal arthritis. Determinations should be made only on specimens obtained 6 or more hours after eating or after termination of glucose infusions

to allow equilibration of glucose between blood and synovial fluid. Reduction of glucose concentration in fluid from joints infected with gonococci is often less dramatic than in infections with other microorganisms.[71]

The synovial fluid lactate level is higher in patients with bacterial arthritis than in those with noninfectious inflammatory states, such as RA. Lactate values are often just barely elevated, however, in gonococcal arthritis and in partially treated cases of infectious arthritis resulting from other bacteria.[26,127–129] Lactate, along with other metabolites, such as succinic acid,[26] may be measured by gas-liquid chromatography, which detects end products of bacterial and host-tissue metabolism, but the method is laborious. A simpler and quicker technique makes use of the enzymatic oxidation of lactate to pyruvate.[128,130] Although the measurement of lactate levels may provide useful information in the diagnosis of joint sepsis, its limitations in patients with gonococcal and, probably, viral disease and in partially treated patients with bacterial sepsis make this test no more informative than the ratio of synovial fluid to serum glucose levels.

Inflammation from any cause increases the vascular permeability of the fenestrated synovial capillaries and augments the influx of serum proteins with a larger proportion of macromolecules, such as the complement proteins. In infectious arthritis, the level of these proteins in synovial fluid does not approach that found in serum because they are consumed intra-articularly in the inflammatory process. Complement proteins of both the classic and the alternate pathways are involved. Therefore, the ratio of C3 to total protein concentration of joint fluid is lower than the ratio of C3 to total serum protein.[131] A similar reduction is well recognized in RA, but not in other inflammatory arthritides, such as gout, pseudogout, and seronegative spondyloarthropathy. Thus, decreased joint fluid complement levels are of interest in understanding the pathogenesis of sepsis, but they have a minor role in its diagnosis (see Chapter 5).

ANTIGEN DETECTION

Countercurrent immunoelectrophoresis has been used to identify soluble bacterial antigens in various body fluids.[132,133] The method has been particularly helpful to detect the antigens of microorganisms such as the pneumococcus, meningococcus, and Haemophilus influenzae, and of viruses such as hepatitis B. Results, available within several hours, provide a quantitative measurement of the amount of antigen within body fluids. In studies of cerebrospinal and

Table 114–3. Synovial Fluid Findings in Acute Pyogenic Arthritis (see also Chapter 5)

Joint Fluid Examination	Noninflammatory Fluids	Inflammatory Fluids Noninfectious	Inflammatory Fluids Infectious
Color	Colorless, pale yellow	Yellow	Yellow
Turbidity	Clear, slightly turbid	Turbid	Turbid, purulent
Viscosity	Not reduced	Reduced	Reduced
Mucin clot	Tight clot	Friable	Friable
Cell count (per mm³)	200 to 1000	3000 to >10,000	10,000 to >100,000
Predominant cell type	Mononuclear	PMN*	PMN*
Synovial fluid/blood glucose ratio	0.8–1.0	0.5–0.8	<0.5
Lactic acid	Same as plasma	Higher than plasma	Often very high
Gram's stain for organism	None	None	Positive†
Culture	Negative	Negative	Positive†

*PMN = polymorphonuclear leukocyte
†In some cases, especially in gonococcal infection, no organisms may be demonstrated.

pleural fluids, the quantity of antigen has borne a direct relation to the severity of the infection and to prognosis.[134]

A reliable test for the diagnosis of active gonococcal disease, using antigens such as pili from the bacterial wall for the detection of specific antibody, is not yet at hand,[135,136] nor have tests for gonococcal antigens in body fluids been developed.

MISCELLANEOUS TESTS

Assays using limulus amebocyte lysate to detect endotoxin in body fluids have not been able to distinguish septic arthritis, not even that owing to gram-negative organisms, from noninfectious inflammatory arthritis.[137]

Teichoic acid antibodies to staphylococci have been found in the serum of many patients with osteomyelitis, but only infrequently in the serum of patients with septic arthritis resulting from this organism.[67] The value of this test as a diagnostic procedure seems marginal because staphylococci can be readily cultured from infected fluids and tissues. When the culture is negative or when material for culture is unavailable, the detection of such antibodies may complement the information obtained from the clinical, radiologic, and scanning examinations.

The nitroblue-tetrazolium (NBT) reduction test is useless in confirming the presence of infection in joint fluids. The test depends on the conversion of a soluble, colorless compound into an insoluble, blue granule on phagocytosis by polymorphonuclear or other phagocytic cells. Synovial fluid polymorphonuclear cells usually show a positive reaction, whether they come from infected or noninfected joints. The study of peripheral blood polymorphonuclear cells also does not discriminate between infectious and noninfectious inflammation.[138]

ANTIBIOTIC TREATMENT

IMMEDIATE MANAGEMENT

Antibiotics should be given in cases of clear-cut or strongly suspected bone and joint infections, even before an exact identification of the infecting microorganism is made. When the microorganism has been identified and its sensitivity to antimicrobial drugs has been assayed, the choice and dose of antibiotic can be reconsidered. If no microorganism is recovered from the bone or joint, further decisions about drug treatment will depend on the use of other, albeit nonspecific, laboratory tests and on the clinical course.

Antibiotic treatment for septic arthritis should begin within the first few hours after the patient's admission to the hospital. A preliminary estimate of the type of infecting microorganism can be made on the basis of the findings noted on the Gram's-stained smear of synovial fluid, which may show gram-positive cocci, gram-negative cocci or coccobacilli, gram-negative bacilli, or no microorganisms.

If no organism is detected in an otherwise healthy young or middle-aged adult, I treat with penicillin G intravenously (Table 114–4), which is adequate for most infections caused by pneumococci, gonococci, penicillin G–susceptible staphylococci, and several less-common bacteria. Gonococcal arthritis in the adult is frequently accompanied by a negative Gram's-stained smear, despite clinically convincing evidence of infection.[70–73] Improvement, often in 4 to 7 days of treatment with large amounts of penicillin G alone, may be dramatic and may suggest the probable cause of the disease. If penicillinase-producing gonococci are present in a community, however, a third-generation cephalosporin such as ceftriaxone should be used. These new strains are appearing more frequently and retain their invasiveness despite a tendency for gonococci associated with arthritis to

Table 114–4. Antibiotic Selection Based on Patient's Age and Gram's-Stain Findings

Age (Years)	Gram-Negative Bacilli	Gram-Negative Cocci	Gram-Positive Cocci	No Organism Seen
<½	Aminoglycoside (*Enterobacteriaceae* or *Pseudomonas aeruginosa*)*	Penicillin G OR extended-spectrum cephalosporin (*Neisseria gonorrhoeae*)	Penicillinase-resistant penicillin OR vancomycin (staphylococci or streptococci)	Penicillinase-resistant penicillin AND aminoglycoside (staphylococci, group B streptococci, or coliforms)
½ to 2–4	Extended-spectrum cephalosporin (*Haemophilus influenzae*)	As above	As above	Extended-spectrum cephalosporin (*Haemophilus influenzae* or streptococci)
2–4 to 14	Aminoglycoside (*Enterobacteriaceae* or *Pseudomonas aeruginosa*)	As above	As above	Penicillinase-resistant penicillin OR vancomycin (staphylococci or streptococci)
15 to 59	As above	As above	As above	Penicillin G OR extended-spectrum cephalosporin (*Neisseria gonorrhoeae*)
>60	Extended-spectrum cephalosporin (*Enterobacteriaceae* or *Pseudomonas aeruginosa*)	As above	As above	Extended-spectrum cephalosporin AND vancomycin (staphylococci, coliforms)

*Presumed identity of pathogenetic microorganism in parentheses. If other microorganisms are suspected, consult appropriate sources for alternative antibiotic selection.

be sensitive to penicillin.[139] In an ill or elderly patient, particularly with reduced renal function, in whom gram-negative bacillary infection is suspected, I use a third-generation cephalosporin or a monobactam. Initial treatment in the newborn in whom infection owing to staphylococci, group B streptococci, or coliform organisms might occur should be a penicillinase-resistant penicillin or vancomycin plus an aminoglycoside.[37] Beyond the neonatal period and until 4 to 5 years of age when β-lactamase–positive strains of Haemophilus influenzae are a common cause of septic arthritis, chloramphenicol has been recommended,[140] but cefuroxime may be as effective without the bone marrow toxicity associated with chloramphenicol.[37] If β-lactamase–negative microorganisms are found later on culture, ampicillin can be substituted.[140]

Initial antibiotic treatment for acute hematogenous osteomyelitis is usually a penicillinase-resistant penicillin. If gram-negative sepsis is suspected, an aminoglycoside is added. In nonhematogenous osteomyelitis, which may be a result of a polymicrobic infection, dual antibiotic therapy is appropriate, as in the case of gram-negative sepsis.

During the acute phase of the illness, antibiotics should be given parenterally. If the drug is administered intravenously, the daily dose should be divided into fractions, and a fractional dose should be given every 6 to 8 hours over a span of 30 to 60 minutes into a constant infusion. This "piggyback" technique is preferred to continual delivery of the drug by intravenous infusion, to avoid loss owing to interruption of flow that might result from subcutaneous infiltration or blockage of the needle or tubing.

When a specific bacterium is seen on the Gram's-stained smear, one may attempt a closer approximation to definitive antibiotic therapy. Types and doses of drugs currently recommended for several different kinds of infection are listed in Table 114–4. Infections caused by gram-negative bacilli such as Escherichia coli and Pseudomonas require a more aggressive approach, usually with two antibiotics.

Suggestions for antibiotic therapy given here provide only general guidelines. Such information quickly becomes outdated as more effective drugs are discovered or changing patterns of drug resistance emerge in some strains of bacteria. For these reasons, the therapist must have access to current knowledge concerning antibiotics. Knowledge of drug toxicity is also essential. The dosage of antibiotic must be appropriately reduced in a patient with diminished renal function. Blood levels of antibiotic determined by the tube-dilution technique provide the necessary information.

TRANSPORT OF ANTIBIOTICS INTO SYNOVIAL FLUID

Antibiotics diffuse readily from the circulation into infected and uninfected inflamed joints.[25,141–147] Early studies of synovial fluid concentrations of penicillin showed inadequate amounts of this drug in the joint, but the dose was much lower than currently recommended. Effective synovial fluid concentrations of a number of common antibiotics were measured in a study of 75 paired samples of synovial fluid and blood obtained from 29 adult patients with a presumptive diagnosis of infectious arthritis.[146] Parenteral administration of penicillin G, phenoxymethyl penicillin (penicillin V), nafcillin, cloxacillin, cephaloridine, tetracycline, erythromycin, and lincomycin in conventional doses produced bactericidal fluid concentrations within the joint (Fig. 114–8). Similar results have been reported in infants and children for ampicillin, methicillin, penicillin G, and cephalothin.[144] Knowledge of such effective concentrations in infected joints obviates the need for direct instillation of antibiotics into the joint space and thus reduces the risk of introducing a new infectious agent, as well as the risk or producing a "chemical synovitis" from local irritation by excessively high local concentrations of some drugs.[47,142]

Protein binding of the antibiotic and the degree of the inflammatory response influence the rate of diffusion of serum constituents into the joint. When the diffusion of nafcillin, which is strongly bound to serum protein, was compared to another penicillin analogue, ampicillin, which shows little protein binding, comparable, effective joint fluid levels of both

drugs were found at 4 hours, although the rate of entry of ampicillin was initially more rapid than that of nafcillin (Fig. 114–9). Thus, protein binding does not impair the entry into the joint or the efficacy of an antibiotic administered extra-articularly.[25] *The general rule in the use of antibiotics in infectious arthritis is that most drugs reach therapeutic levels in the synovial fluid if adequate amounts are given systemically.*

Amphotericin B may be an exception to this rule because data on this drug are sparse and contradictory.[148–150] Information on newly marketed antibiotics may also be unavailable. Therefore, until such data are provided, it is recommended that adequate transport of these drugs be documented by studies in each patient in which they are used. If diffusion of the drug is inadequate, local instillation into the joint might be done once or twice a day, or another antibiotic known to enter the joint more readily can be substituted. Finally, aminoglycoside effectiveness decreases by an order of magnitude at pH 6.5. Thus, effective removal of purulent exudate, which correlates with low pH, is especially important when this antibiotic is used.[97]

TRANSPORT OF ANTIBIOTICS INTO BONE

Although measurement of antibiotics in bone poses more difficulties than in synovial fluid,[151] most studies

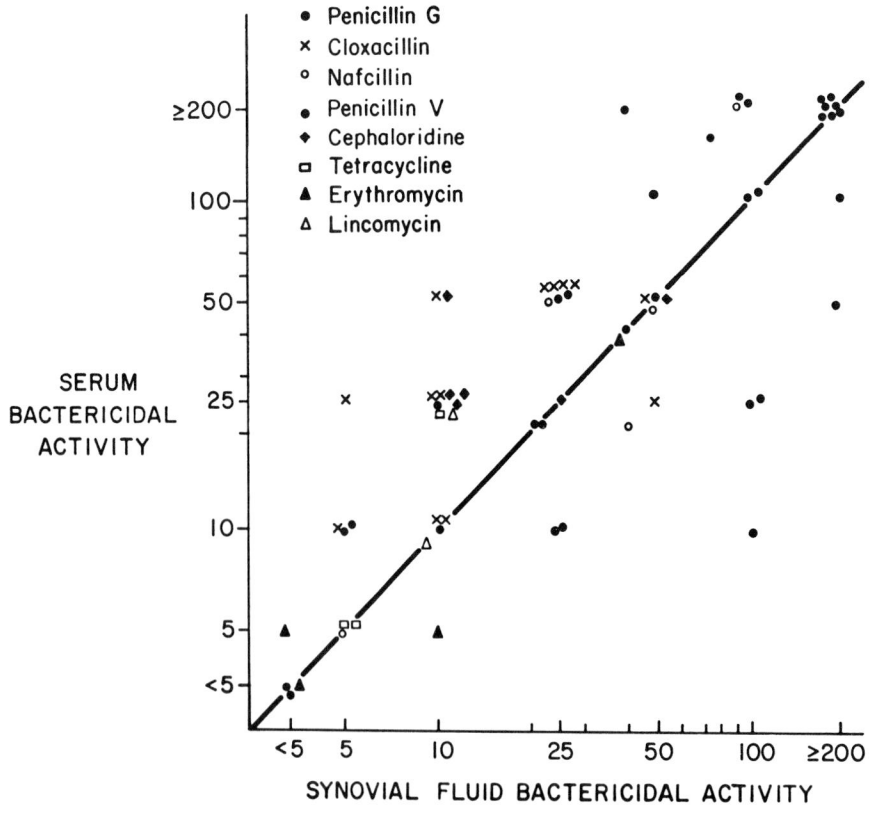

FIG. 114–8. Comparison of the bactericidal activity of 75 paired specimens of serum and synovial fluid obtained from 29 patients during systemic antibiotic therapy. Points on the diagonal line indicate pairs with equal activity. Bactericidal activity is expressed as the reciprocal of the maximum dilution showing this activity. (From Parker, R.H., and Schmid, F.R.[146])

FIG. 114–9. Comparison of serum and synovial fluid concentrations of ampicillin and nafcillin in 6 patients receiving a single dose of each drug, 500 mg intramuscularly, in a cross-over study. (From Parker, R.H., Birbara, C., and Schmid, F.R.[25])

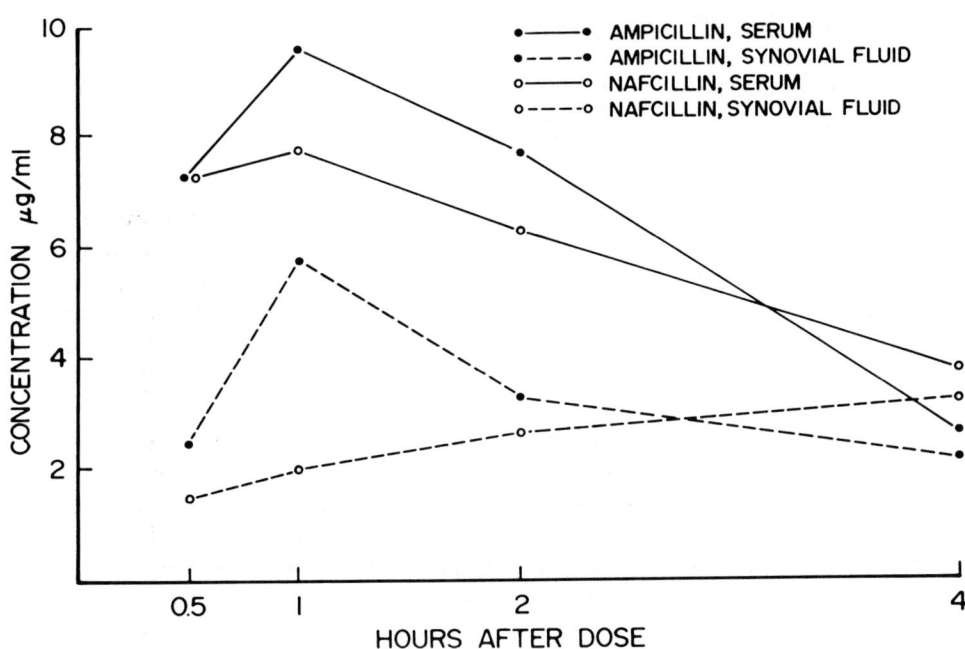

indicate that, as in synovial fluid, adequate concentrations of antibiotics are reached when bactericidal doses have been administered systemically. Problems in interpreting drug levels in bone are the use of normal, uninfected bone for the assay, usually from uninfected patients undergoing elective operations, the variations in porosity of cancellous and cortical bone, destruction of the test antibiotic by the heat generated by the pulverization process used to grind the bone, and contamination of the specimen by plasma not removed in the washing process. Therefore, only approximate drug levels can be measured. These levels are usually far below those obtained in plasma, yet they are often greater than the concentration needed to achieve bacterial inhibition and killing. Some data are available on most penicillins, cephalosporins, erythromycin, lincomycin, and clindamycin, but few data are available on aminoglycosides.[152]

DEFINITIVE MANAGEMENT OF INFECTIOUS ARTHRITIS

As soon as the exact identity of the microorganism and its susceptibility to antibiotics are known, definitive therapy can be planned. Details of such management are provided in Chapters 115 through 119. Either the initial antibiotic is continued at the same

or modified dose, or a more appropriate antibiotic is selected. Proof that the intravenous antibiotic is actually entering the joint in bactericidal concentrations should be obtained by determining antibacterial activity in paired samples of synovial fluid and serum. A simple tube-dilution technique can be performed in most clinical bacteriologic laboratories, using either the bacterium isolated from the patient or a bacterial species with identical antibiotic susceptibility.[146] Test results indicate the limiting dilution of serum and synovial fluid that still retains bacteriostatic or bactericidal activity. A margin of bactericidal effect ten or more times that found in undiluted synovial fluid provides sufficient antibiotic for antimicrobial action. One should rely on a regimen that produces bactericidal, not just bacteriostatic, activity. If this end has not been achieved, the dose of antibiotic should be increased until adequate bactericidal activity is reached, or else another antibiotic should be substituted. An excellent correlation exists between this simple tube-dilution test and the more quantitative agar-diffusion technique.[146]

Parenteral antibiotic administration should be maintained until clinical signs of active synovitis and inflammatory changes in the joint fluid begin to revert toward normal.[153] Synovial fluid should be recultured repeatedly during the initial stages of therapy to demonstrate sterility. If prolonged use of an antibiotic is anticipated, intravenous administration can be attempted with the placement of a subcutaneous reservoir that feeds into a large central vein, such as the subclavian vein. An external pump can be attached to deliver a constant amount of the antibiotic through a needle inserted into the reservoir. Use of this type of device allows treatment for a protracted infection to be carried out at home. When one is certain that the infection is controlled, the antibiotic may be given orally. The oral route is unreliable in early treatment because patients with sepsis often have nausea, vomiting, and other gastrointestinal disturbances. Sterility and a progressive decline in total joint fluid leukocyte concentration are signs of a good prognosis; conversely, continued bacterial growth and a steady or rising leukocyte level suggest the need to reassess the treatment regimen.

Infections caused by the gonococcus and certain other coccal organisms, such as the pneumococcus and the streptococcus, generally respond rapidly to appropriate antibiotic management. In patients with such infections, the duration of therapy might be expected to be brief, perhaps 2 weeks or less. Infections caused by staphylococci and gram-negative bacteria respond more slowly to treatment.[5,44,58] A satisfactory explanation for these differences is not available. Local factors may play a role, but a change in the drug sensitivity of the microorganisms present within the joint fluid is not likely to be a factor. In most cases, the strain of organism infecting the joint remains constant and is not replaced by another drug-resistant, variety unless a contaminating strain is carried into the joint inadvertently during arthrocentesis. This finding contrasts with the changing bacterial flora noted during the treatment of "open" infections in bone in which a sinus tract has formed, or during the open drainage and suction sometimes carried out after arthrotomy. In addition, staphylococci do not usually show spontaneous mutation in their patterns of drug sensitivity. Thus, a strain of Staphylococcus aureus sensitive to penicillin G at the outset remains sensitive to this drug during treatment.

DEFINITIVE MANAGEMENT OF OSTEOMYELITIS

In patients with osteomyelitis, plasma bactericidal levels of antibiotics are an indication of the adequacy of the drug dose. If this information is correlated with the sensitivity of the microorganism obtained either from blood or an aspirate of the bone lesion, an informed decision can be made. How long to continue drug therapy is contingent on an evaluation of the

clinical response, which, although less quantitative than the assessment of synovitis and joint fluid changes, provides useful evidence of the effects of treatment.

SERUM SICKNESS ARTHRITIS FROM ANTIMICROBIAL AGENTS

Serum sickness is a well-known but unusual complication of drug therapy. Almost any antibiotic, acting as a hapten, can induce this reaction. When symptoms of fever, rash, and flare of arthritis develop during the course of treatment of infectious arthritis, one must distinguish between a relapse of the primary joint disease and the onset of the polyarthritis of serum sickness.

Careful examination of the bacterial status of the inflamed joint is mandatory and, if necessary, one must use an unrelated drug. In the interval between stopping the original drug and giving the new antibiotic, the joint fluid should be tested for the presence of microorganisms by smear and culture, along with cell count and glucose level. Pending the results of these tests, antibiotic treatment can be administered with a drug to which the patient is not known to be sensitive.

POSTINFECTIOUS SYNOVITIS

Tissue injury in septic arthritis is caused directly by toxic factors produced by viable microorganisms and indirectly by the host's response to microbial antigens. The killing of microorganisms by the action of antibiotics does not remove microbial products. Such materials may persist within the joint for prolonged periods, either in loculated areas or possibly embedded in articular cartilage. The retention of these substances may thereby contribute to persistence of the inflammatory response.

Such postinfectious synovitis leads to confusion about the adequacy of antibiotic treatment. Because viable microorganisms may still be present in tissues even after synovial fluid cultures have become sterile, antibiotics are usually not discontinued. Instead, a nonsteroidal anti-inflammatory drug is added, but only after several days or more of antibiotic drug treatment. If the combination of antibiotic and anti-inflammatory therapy controls the inflammatory process, both drugs can be continued until all signs of active disease have disappeared. It is not advisable to initiate nonspecific anti-inflammatory drug use earlier because such drugs are also antipyretic; the patient's initial response to the antibiotic alone provides reassurance that the infection is coming under control. A rapid response, particularly in the case of a gonococcal infection, provides added weight for the diagnosis, especially in bacteriologically unproved cases.

ANTIBIOTIC PROPHYLAXIS FOR PATIENTS WITH JOINT PROSTHESES

Infection is the most feared complication of total joint replacement, and removal of the prosthesis is often necessary to eradicate the septic process successfully. Thus, during the perioperative period, ways to avoid infection are emphasized. Attention is also directed to the prevention of a late infection, particularly in situations that might favor bacteremia.

PERIOPERATIVE PROPHYLAXIS

In addition to the use of scrupulously sterile technique, special operative clothing, avoidance of unnecessary personnel or traffic in the operating room, and sometimes, laminar air-flow systems at the operating table, almost all patients undergoing total joint replacement receive antibiotics (usually antistaphylococcal agents such as oxacillin or vancomycin) prior to and during the procedure and for a number of days postoperatively.[41,154-156] The rationale for the use of systemic antibiotics is that, despite precautions, most wounds may become contaminated during the course of a long operation. In most centers, the rate of infection has dropped as surgical experience has grown and as the operative time has been shortened. Transient bacteremia with hematogenous seeding of microorganisms is also a possibility. For this reason, any known focus of infection elsewhere in the body is treated aggressively prior to the operation.

Antibiotic-impregnated cement has also been used; the idea is that a drug reservoir can be maintained at the operative site from which an antibiotic, such as gentamicin, can diffuse throughout the wound.[157] Evidence for its added value to an otherwise exemplary surgical program is not clear; some are concerned that the antibiotic might weaken the mechanical properties of the cement.

PROPHYLAXIS AGAINST LATE BACTEREMIA

A few well-placed prostheses become infected months after operation, most likely by hematogenous seeding of bacteria to the implant area.[41,158] For this reason, antibiotics have been used prophylactically in circumstances in which bacteremia is known to occur. A recommended regimen after oropharyngeal, bronchial, gastrointestinal, and urologic procedures is listed in Table 114-5.[41]

DRAINAGE OF INFECTED BONE AND JOINTS

DRAINAGE OF SYNOVIAL FLUID

Except for infants with septic arthritis of the hip, who require open surgical drainage as soon as the diagnosis is made,[85,159,160] drainage can be accomplished by needle aspiration in almost all cases of uncomplicated infectious arthritis. Patients with a prosthetic joint infection or an infection secondary to prior trauma or surgery may require early surgical drainage. All possible fluid and debris are removed on a regular basis, sometimes daily, or even more frequently if needed. Because some material always remains in the joint and may be compartmentalized by fibrinous adhesions, some clinicians suggest lavage of the joint cavity with sterile physiologic saline or Ringer's solution.[161] At each aspiration, the volume, cell count, culture, and, at appropriate intervals, the fasting glucose or lactate levels should be determined (see Table 114-1).

In the deep-seated joint of the older child or adult, the decision whether to perform open surgical drainage or needle drainage poses a problem because of the difficulty associated with repeated aspiration. If sepsis is recognized early, and if the organism recovered from the joint is sensitive to antibiotics, particularly if it is a gonococcus or another nonstaphylococcal coccus, then needle drainage is still preferred because it prevents the conversion of a closed-space infection into an open wound. If recognition of sepsis is delayed, however, or if sepsis is a result of "difficult" organisms, such as staphylococci or gram-negative bacilli, or if the infected joint is the result of extension of infection from a periarticular site, such as a contiguous bone or soft tissue, then open drainage may be needed.[162,163] Open drainage is indicated if needle aspiration fails to decompress the joint adequately.

SURGICAL DRAINAGE

Except for the foregoing circumstances, surgical drainage is withheld unless one sees little or no clin-

Table 114–5.   Prophylactic Antibiotic Schedules Suggested for Adults with a Joint Prosthesis*

| Procedure | Antibiotic Schedule | |
	Parenteral	Oral
Oropharyngeal	Procaine penicillin G 1.2 × 10⁶ units 30 to 60 min. prior to procedure; then penicillin V 500 mg p.o. 6 hourly × 8 doses If allergic to penicillin, clindamycin 600 mg IM/IV, then 300 mg p.o. according to the same schedule as penicillin	Penicillin V 2.0 g p.o. 30 to 60 min. prior to procedure, then 500 mg p.o. 6 hourly × 8 doses If allergic to penicillin, clindamycin 450 p.o., then 300 mg p.o. according to the same schedule as penicillin
Genitourinary and gastrointestinal	Procaine penicillin G 2.4 × 10⁶ units IM OR ampicillin 1.0 g IM/IV PLUS gentamicin 1.0 mg/kg IM/IV (not to exceed 80 mg)—ALL 8 hourly × 3 doses commencing 30 to 60 min. prior to procedure	Probenecid 1.0 g p.o. 90 min. prior to procedure PLUS ampicillin 3.5 g p.o. 60 min. prior to procedure, then 1.0 g p.o. 6 hourly × 8 doses PLUS gentamicin 2.0 mg/kg IM 60 min. prior to procedure, then 1.5 mg/kg IM 12 hourly × 3 doses
Surgery on infected or contaminated tissue (variable depending on anticipated pathogen. Information is provided for *Staphylococcus aureus*)	Nafcillin 2.0 g IV 30 to 60 min. prior to procedure; then dicloxacillin 500 mg p.o. 6 hourly × 8 doses OR cefazolin 1.0 g IM/IV, then cephradine 500 mg p.o. OR clindamycin 600 mg IM/IV, then 300 mg p.o. according to the same schedule as nafcillin/dicloxacillin	Dicloxacillin 1.0 g p.o. 30 to 60 min. prior to procedure, then 500 mg p.o. 6 hourly × 8 doses OR cephradine 2.0 g p.o., then 500 mg p.o. OR clindamycin 450 mg p.o., then 300 mg p.o. according to the same schedule as dicloxacillin

*Modified from Brause, B.D.[41]

ical or laboratory evidence of improvement during the first 4 to 7 days of treatment. This time interval is arbitrary. I would still continue to treat a slowly responding gonococcal infection by needle aspiration for another 4 to 7 days. On the other hand, infections owing to staphylococci or to gram-negative bacilli, unrelenting synovitis present a week after treatment is begun call for arthrotomy or arthroscopy. No adequately controlled study to support this opinion is available, although almost all large series in which this question is examined have failed to demonstrate an advantage of initial open drainage over deferred open drainage (Fig. 114–10).[161,164,165]

ARTHROSCOPY

This technique offers the prospect of inspecting the joint cavity and the opportunity to lavage its contents and to remove fibrotic or necrotic tissue, some of which might be further examined by culture and histologic study for evidence of persisting infection.[166,167] Morbidity is much lower with arthroscopy than with open drainage. The procedure can be repeated at a later stage if further local debridement is required. Its limitations need to be recognized, however, because current models of arthroscopes are used only for the knee and for a few other large joints, such as the shoulder or ankle. Moreover, when adjacent osteomyelitis is extensive, open drainage and debridement may still be needed.

DEBRIDEMENT IN OTEOMYELITIS

For hematogenous osteomyelitis, the prognosis for recovery of function is good with suitable antibiotic therapy. Little or no disability is apt to result, even with spontaneous vertebral fusion, and surgical debridement is not necessary. A diagnostic aspiration of exudate from the body of the vertebra or from the disc space can be done, if necessary, to identify the microorganism and its drug sensitivities. If an abscess

FIG. 114–10. The outcome of joint function in 242 joints that received needle aspiration and in 125 that received either arthrotomy or arthroscopy. (From Broy, S.B., and Schmid, F.R.[161])

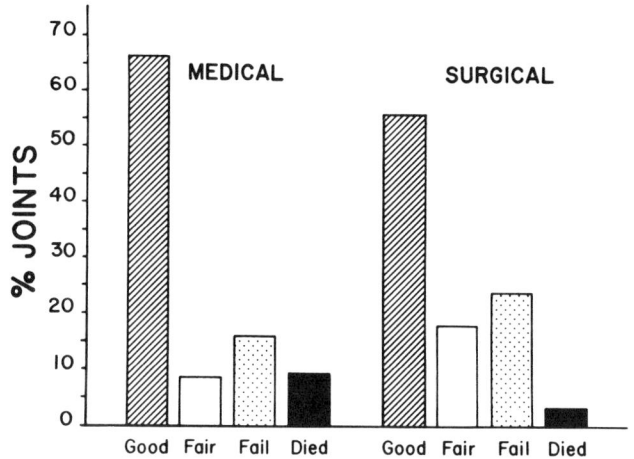

OUTCOME BY METHOD OF DRAINAGE

or spinal cord compression develops, however, surgical drainage and debridement of the infected area are indicated.

DEBRIDEMENT OF AN INFECTED JOINT PROSTHESIS

If an infection occurs during the immediate postoperative period after insertion of the prosthesis, surgical drainage of an infected hematoma and antibiotic therapy can frequently eradicate the infectious process and salvage a functional arthroplasty. With an established infection, however, the prosthetic device and associated acrylic bone cement almost always must be removed. Three surgical approaches are then possible: (1) immediate reconstruction during the same surgical procedure—a one-stage exchange arthroplasty; (2) delayed reconstruction at a future date—a two-stage arthroplasty; and (3) if the bone stock is insufficient, a new approach with debridement followed by a bone grafting procedure in 6 months and a reconstructive arthroplasty 12 to 18 months after debridement—a three-stage arthroplasty. The one-stage procedure with gentamicin-impregnated cement may provide short-term success, but long-term results are less favorable. The two-stage procedure, however, can usually be successfully performed 3 months after resection arthroplasty for infections from which streptococci other than enterococci, methicillin-susceptible staphylococci, and gram-positive bacilli were isolated. For all other agents, reconstruction should be delayed for 12 months. These guidelines are suggested for an infection in the hip but can be extrapolated to other sites as well.[168]

GENERAL SUPPORTIVE MEASURES

The affected joint must be kept at rest during the acute phases of the illness. A splint helps to reduce pain and, by immobilization, to control inflammation. A posterior resting splint of the leg or arm is usually sufficient. In an experimental model of infectious arthritis in the rabbit, use of continuous passive motion (CPM) for the infected joint was associated with less articular cartilage damage.[169] Therefore, the use of a CPM device in a patient with sepsis of the knee might prove effective in much the same way such a device improves function in the patient who receives a total knee replacement. Patients in the acute phase of infectious spondylitis should be treated by bed rest. If

a danger of subluxation exists, the spine should be immobilized in a plaster shell or brace.

As the inflammatory process subsides, one should attempt to restore range of motion and to increase muscle strength gradually. Passive exercises, followed by graded active exercises, are begun with the assistance of a physical therapist. Weight-bearing should be deferred until signs of acute inflammation have disappeared.

In addition to treatment of the joint, efforts are needed to control the primary infection that led to the arthritis, to supply fluids and nutrition, and to control pain. Anti-inflammatory drugs, including aspirin, should be withheld for several days or longer until the response of the joint to the antibiotic can be correctly assessed. Codeine or propoxyphene, which have no anti-inflammatory properties, can be used to control pain.

ONGOING EVALUATION OF THE TREATMENT PROGRAM

Clinical and laboratory studies are used to monitor the outcome of infectious arthritis.

ACUTE STAGE OF INFECTIOUS ARTHRITIS

The response of the infection to treatment is assessed by changes in tenderness, heat, swelling, and range of motion of the affected joint. The frequency of aspiration is reduced as the volume and the inflammatory character of the fluid decrease. If one is uncertain whether effective bactericidal levels have been achieved because of a change in the type, dose, or route of administration of an antibiotic drug, a tube-dilution assay of paired serum and synovial fluid should be performed. If joint fluid is no longer obtainable, assay of antibiotic concentrations of blood alone provides an acceptable approximation of the drug concentration in the joint. The results of this continuous monitoring should be charted chronologically, so the effectiveness of the treatment program can be accurately determined.

Antibiotic therapy is ordinarily continued for about a week after all systemic or local findings of inflammation have subsided. In staphylococcal and in some gram-negative bacillary infections, which respond more slowly, this period is extended to several weeks. The patient should be observed for another few weeks after cessation of antibiotic therapy for any sign of relapse. If the infection is slow to improve or if it worsens during any phase of the treatment period, one must review all aspects of the program. The following questions should be asked: Was the joint fluid rendered sterile? Were bactericidal levels of antibiotic in the joint fluid achieved? Was needle aspiration successful in decompressing the joint? Answers to these questions dictate the appropriate change in the type or the dosage of antibiotic administered or in the method of drainage. Consultation from the outset with an infectious-disease specialist and with an orthopedic surgeon is invaluable in planning a co-ordinated approach.

ILLUSTRATIVE CASE

A patient with septic arthritis illustrates the value of continued monitoring of the repsonse to treatment (Fig. 114–11). Gram-positive cocci, subsequently proved to be Staphylococcus aureus, were identified in the smear of fluid obtained from the knee. Penicillin G was given intravenously. On the second day of treatment, bactericidal levels of antibiotic against the staphylococcus recovered from the joint were present, but the patient developed an intense allergic response that required the substitution of lincomycin. Again, suitable bactericidal drug concentrations were achieved. As the patient improved, smaller amounts of fluid were obtained by needle aspiration from the

joint. For the balance of the treatment schedule, erythromycin was given. Initially by the intravenous route and later orally, bactericidal levels of drug were noted. After the patient's discharge from the hospital after 29 days, oral medication was continued for another 2 weeks. Although this patient had developed septic arthritis in a joint already damaged by RA, prompt diagnosis and therapy prevented further loss of joint function.

LATE OUTCOMES OF INFECTIOUS ARTHRITIS

Any septic joint untreated or inadequately treated for more than 1 or 2 weeks may develop some of the pathologic changes of a chronic infection. These manifestations include damage to cartilage and bone, increased fibrosis, and ultimately, destruction of the normal joint mechanism.[159] Fortunately, the number of such complications has decreased since the introduction of antibiotic therapy. In one large clinic, the number of cases of bacterial arthritis decreased approximately by half from 1952 to 1957, when compared to two periods extending, respectively, from 1939 to 1945 and from 1946 to 1951. This reduction occurred in the number of patients with chronic, rather than acute, disease.[43]

In patients with chronic disease, a major effort

FIG. 114–11. Response of a 56-year-old white male patient with septic arthritis to antibiotic treatment. Comparable bactericidal drug levels were achieved in the joint fluid and blood for each drug. I.V. = intravenously; I.M. = intramuscularly.

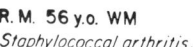

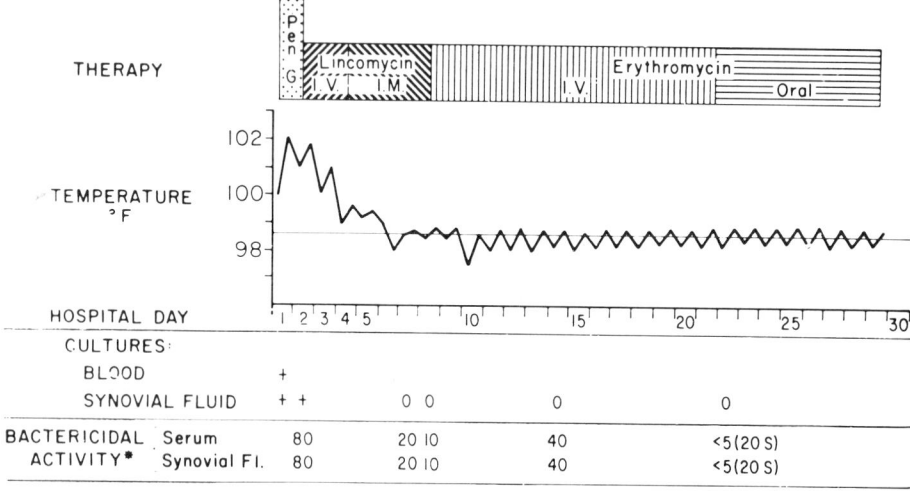

should be directed toward analysis of the factor(s) responsible for the failure of the therapeutic regimen. The bacterial status of the joint should be reevaluated by a synovial fluid culture obtained several days after withdrawal of all antibiotics and again a week or two later if active synovitis persists.

Open arthrotomy or arthroscopy may be required for adequate drainage and excision of necrotic bone and soft tissue, including sinuses.[162,164,166] Tissue should be obtained for culture as well as for histologic examination. Culture of synovial tissue may be positive when the synovial fluid is sterile. Care must be taken to inoculate a wide range of culture media to facilitate the recovery of fungi or mycobacteria, agents that may have eluded earlier detection. Moreover, during inspection of the joint, a nonradiopaque foreign body, such as a plant thorn, that had allowed the inflammatory process to persist may be found and removed.

Antibiotics, such as the penicillins and cephalosporins, that inhibit bacterial cell-wall synthesis may induce the formation of cell-wall-free bacteria or protoplasts. Little evidence suggests that these crippled bacteria are pathogenic.[49,54,124] In one case familiar to me, such forms of bacteria, as well as native bacterial forms of Staphylococcus aureus, were cultured from the necrotic remnants of a patient's patella after several months of continuous penicillin therapy. In the postoperative period, this patient was treated successfully with erythromycin because this drug influences bacterial metabolism by means other than the inhibition of cell-wall synthesis.

The prognosis for the complete recovery of function in a previously normal joint infected with antibiotic-sensitive bacteria is generally excellent when treatment is begun within a few days of the onset of infection. Delayed diagnosis is directly related to a poorer outcome. The prognosis may be difficult to judge at the outset.[37] In one study, the predictability of good results was not completely ascertained until many months later.[159] Thus, long-term observation is necessary to determine the end result.

RECONSTRUCTION OF DAMAGED JOINTS

If a joint has been damaged, reconstructive procedures may be considered, but the operation should be deferred until all evidence of infection has been absent for several months. Arthroplasty or fusion of a joint may be indicated.[170,171] Prosthetic replacement to restore normal joint function is now widely accepted.[172–174] Guidelines for this procedure generally follow those that were given previously for the insertion of a new prosthesis into the site of a prior infected joint prosthesis.[168] The possibility of re-exacerbating a dormant infection, however, must always be considered, particularly in patients with tuberculosis. Nevertheless, prosthetic replacement of a damaged hip, knee, and other joint has been undertaken with satisfactory results.

LATE OUTCOMES OF OSTEOMYELITIS

The therapeutic program for patients with osteomyelitis needs closer monitoring than that for patients with septic arthritis. Clinical findings at the site of the bone infection and serial radiologic and scintiphotographic examinations are used to determine whether the infection has been eradicated. In hematogenous osteomyelitis of a long bone or a vertebra, antibiotics are given orally for several weeks after initial intravenous use; in chronic osteomyelitis, most often when secondary to continuous infection, long-term oral therapy has been successful.[40] Surgical treatment of osteomyelitis is largely empiric and is based on concepts that have gained wide acceptance, some with and others without scientific documentation. Included are drainage of infected areas, excision of necrotic bone, and removal of sequestra and foreign material, such as cement and prostheses.[40]

The likelihood of only partial eradication of the infection is greater in osteomyelitis than in septic arthritis. Reactivation has been recognized many years after the implantation of the original infection. The late outcome of acute hematogenous osteomyelitis in children between 1947 and 1976 was failure to cure or recurrence in almost 20% of cases, most often in the first year. Half of these patients had more than a single recurrence. With the more effective use of antibiotics, especially in those over age 16, the failure rates were lower.[175] Treatment of a recurrence requires extended antibiotic administration, usually for months.[176] For staphylococcal osteomyelitis, a penicillinase-resistant penicillin can be given orally or, in some cases, intravenously by a pump mechanism that delivers the antibiotic into a subcutaneously implanted reservoir. At the same time, the involved bone needs to be evaluated by the surgeon for possible osteotomy to remove residual necrotic materials. Persistent treatment almost always eradicates the infection.

REFERENCES

1. Chusid, M.J., Jacobs, W.M., and Sty, J.R.: Pseudomonas arthritis following puncture wounds of the foot. J. Pediatr., 94:429–431, 1979.

2. Smith, W.S., and Ward, R.M.: Septic arthritis of the hip complicating perforation of abdominal organs. JAMA, 195:1148–1150, 1966.

3. Schoolnick, G.K., Ochs, H.O., and Buchanan, T.M.: Immunoglobulin class responsible for gonococcal bactericidal activity of normal human sera. J. Immunol., 122:1771–1779, 1979.

4. Cluff, L.E., et al.: Staphylococcal bacteremia and altered host resistance. Ann. Intern. Med., 69:859–873, 1968.

5. Goldenberg, D.L., and Cohen, A.S.: Acute infectious arthritis: a review of patients with nongonococcal joint infections (with emphasis on therapy and prognosis). Am. J. Med., 60:369–377, 1976.

6. Mathews, M., et al.: Septic arthritis in hemodialyzed patients. Nephron, 25:87–91, 1980.

7. Petersen, B.H., et al.: Neisseria meningitidis and Neisseria gonorrhoeae bacteremia associated with C6, C7, or C8 deficiency. Ann. Intern. Med., 90:917–920, 1979.

8. Willkens, R.F., Healey, L.A., and Decker, J.L.: Acute infectious arthritis in the aged and chronically ill. Arch. Intern. Med., 106:354–364, 1960.

9. Kellgren, J.H., et al.: Suppurative arthritis complicating rheumatoid arthritis. Br. Med. J., 1:1193–1200, 1958.

10. Mills, L.C., et al.: Septic arthritis as a complication of orally given steroid therapy. JAMA, 164:1310–1314, 1957.

11. Vincenti, F.: Septic arthritis following renal transplantation. Nephron, 30:253–256, 1982.

12. Heinicke, M.: Crystal arthropathy as a complication of septic arthritis. J. Rheumatol., 8:529–531, 1981.

13. McConville, J.H., et al.: Septic and crystalline joint disease: a simultaneous occurrence. JAMA, 231:841–842, 1975.

14. Mitchell, W.S., et al.: Septic arthritis in patients with rheumatoid disease: a still undiagnosed complication. J. Rheumatol., 3:124–133, 1976.

15. Smith, J.R., and Phelps, P.: Septic arthritis, gout, pseudogout and osteoarthritis in the knee of a patient with multiple myeloma. Arthritis Rheum., 15:89–96, 1972.

16. Mahowald, M.L.: Animal models of infectious arthritis. Clin. Rheum. Dis., 12:403–421, 1986.

17. Reginato, A.J., et al.: Synovitis in secondary syphilis: clinical, light, and electronmicroscopic studies. Arthritis Rheum., 22:170–176, 1979.

18. Tesar, J.T., and Dietz, F.: Mechanisms of inflammation in infectious arthritis. Clin. Rheum. Dis., 4:51–61, 1978.

19. Mahowald, M.L., et al.: Experimental septic arthritis in rabbits with antigen induced arthritis following intra-articular injection of *Staphylococcal aureus*. J. Infect. Dis., 154:273–282, 1986.

20. Kushner, I., and Somerville, J.A.: Permeability of human synovial membrane to plasma proteins: relationship to molecular size and inflammation. Arthritis Rheum., 14:560–570, 1971.

21. Bobechko, W.P., and Mandell, L.: Immunology of cartilage in septic arthritis. Clin. Orthop. Res., 108:84–89, 1975.

22. Hadler, N.M.: Phlogistic properties of microbial debris. Semin. Arthritis Rheum., 8:1–16, 1978.

23. Ward, P.A., et al.: Generation by bacterial proteinases of leukotactic factors from human serum and human C3 and C5. J. Immunol., 111:1003–1006, 1973.

24. Phemister, D.B.: The effect of pressure on articular surfaces in pyogenic and tuberculous arthritides and its bearing on treatment. Ann. Surg., 80:481–500, 1924.

25. Parker, R.H., Birbara, C., and Schmid, F.R.: Passage of nafcillin and ampicillin into synovial fluid. *In* Staphylococci and Staphylococcal Diseases. Edited by J. Jeljaszewicz. Stuttgart, New York, Gustav Fischer Verlag. pp. 1151–1123, 1976.

26. Borenstein, D.G., Gibbs, C.A., and Jacobs, R.P.: Gas-liquid chromatographic analysis of synovial fluid: succinic acid and lactic acid as markers for septic arthritis. Arthritis Rheum., 25:947–953, 1982.

27. Eagle, H.: Experimental approach to the problem of treatment failure with penicillin. I. Group A streptococcal infection in mice. Am. J. Med., 13:389–399, 1952.

28. Harris, E.D., Jr., and Krane, S.M.: Collagenases. N. Engl. J. Med., 291:605–609, 1974.

29. McCarty, D.J., Jr., Phelps, P., and Pyenson, J.: Crystal-induced inflammation in canine joints. I. An experimental model with quantification of the host response. J. Exp. Med., 124:99–114, 1966.

30. Steere, A.C., et al.: Elevated levels of collagenase and prostaglandin E_2 from synovium associated with erosion of cartilage and bone in a patient with chronic Lyme arthritis. Arthritis Rheum., 23:591–599, 1980.

31. Yaron, M., et al.: Stimulation of prostaglandin E production by bacterial endotoxins in cultured human synovial fibroblasts. Arthritis Rheum., 23:921–925, 1980.

32. Canoso, J.J., and Sheckman, P.R.: Septic subcutaneous bursitis: report of sixteen cases. J. Rheumatol., 6:96–102, 1979.

33. Ho, G., Jr., and Tice, A.D.: Comparison of nonseptic and septic bursitis: further observations on the treatment of septic bursitis. Arch. Intern. Med., 139:1269–1273, 1979.

34. Curtiss, P.H., and Klein, L.: Destruction of articular cartilage in septic arthritis. J. Bone Joint Surg., 45A:797–806, 1963.

35. Roy, S., and Bhawan, J.: Ultrastructure of articular cartilage in pyogenic arthritis. Arch. Pathol., 99:44–47, 1975.

36. Ziff, M., Gribetz, H.J., and LoSpalluto, J.: Effect of leukocyte and synovial membrane extracts on cartilage mucoprotein. J. Clin. Invest., 39:405–412, 1960.

37. Fink, C.W., and Nelson, J.D.: Septic arthritis and osteomyelitis in children. Clin. Rheum. Dis., 12:423–435, 1986.

38. Peterson, S.: Acute haematogenous osteomyelitis and septic arthritis in childhood: a 10 year review and follow-up. Acta Orthop. Scand., 51:451–457, 1980.

39. Waldvogel, F.A., Medoff, G., and Schwartz, M.N.: Osteomyelitis: a review of clinical features, therapeutic considerations and unusual aspects. N. Engl. J. Med., 282:198–206, 260–266, 316–322, 1970.

40. Waldvogel, F.A., and Vasey, H.: Osteomyelitis: the past decade. N. Engl. J. Med., 303:360–370, 1980.

41. Brause, B.D.: Infection associated with prosthetic joints. Clin. Rheum. Dis., 12:523–536, 1986.

42. Atcheson, S.G., and Ward, J.R.: Acute hematogenous osteomyelitis progressing to septic synovitis and eventual pyarthrosis: the vascular pathway. Arthritis Rheum., 21:968–971, 1978.

43. Newman, J.H.: Review of septic arthritis throughout the antibiotic era. Ann. Rheum. Dis., 35:198–205, 1976.

44. Borrela, L., et al.: Septic arthritis in childhood. J. Pediatr., 62:742–747, 1963.

45. Nelson, J.D.: The bacterial etiology and antibiotic management of septic arthritis in infants and children. Pediatrics, 50:437–440, 1972.

46. Fink, C.W.: Gonococcal arthritis in children. JAMA, 194:237–238, 1965.

47. Argen, R.J., Wilson, C.H., Jr., and Wood, P.: Suppurative arthritis: clinical features of 42 cases. Arch. Intern. Med., 117:661–666, 1966.

48. Chartier, Y., Martin, W.J., and Kelly, P.J.: Bacterial arthritis: Experiences in the treatment of 77 patients. Ann. Intern. Med., 50:1462–1474, 1959.

49. Garcia-Kutzbach, A., et al.: Identification of Neisseria gon-

orrhoeae in synovial membrane by electron microscopy. J. Infect. Dis., 130:183–186, 1974.

50. Rosenthal, J., Bole, G.G., and Robinson, W.D.: Acute non-gonococcal infectious arthritis. Arthritis Rheum., 23:889–897, 1980.

51. Sharp, J.T., et al.: Infectious arthritis. Arch. Intern. Med., 139:1125–1130, 1979.

52. Ward, J., Cohen, A.S., and Bauer, W.: The diagnosis and therapy of acute suppurative arthritis. Arthritis Rheum., 3:522–535, 1960.

53. Roca, R.P., and Yoshikawa, T.T.: Primary skeletal infections in heroin users: clinical characterization, diagnosis and therapy. Clin. Orthop., 144:238–248, 1979.

54. Palmer, D.W., and Ellman, M.H.: Septic arthritis and Reiter's syndrome in sickle cell disorders: case reports and implications for management. South. Med. J., 69:902–904, 1976.

54a.Ebong, W.W.: Septic arthritis in patients with sickle-cell disease. Br. J. Rheum., 26:99–102, 1987.

55. Memon, I.A., et al.: Group B streptococcal osteomyelitis and septic arthritis: its occurrence in infants less than two months old. Am. J. Dis. Child., 133:921–923, 1979.

56. Dodd, M.J.: Pyogenic arthritis due to Bacteroides complicating rheumatoid arthritis. Ann. Rheum. Dis., 41:248–249, 1982.

57. Fitzgerald, R.H., Jr.: Anaerobic septic arthritis. Clin. Orthop., 164:141–148, 1982.

58. Goldenberg, D.L., et al.: Acute arthritis caused by gram negative bacilli: a clinical characterization. Medicine, 53:197–208, 1974.

59. Goldings, F.A., and Jericho, J.: Lyme disease. Clin. Rheum. Dis., 12:343–367, 1986.

60. Aaskov, J.G., Fraser, J.R.E., and Dalglish, D.A.: Specific and non-specific immunological changes in epidemic polyarthritis patients. Aust. J. Exp. Biol. Med. Sci., 59:599–608, 1981.

61. Manicourt, D.H., and Orloff, S.: Gonococcal arthritis-dermatitis syndrome: study of serum and synovial fluid immune complex levels. Arthritis Rheum., 25:574–578, 1982.

62. Dienstag, J.L., et al.: Circulating immune complexes in non-A, non-B hepatitis. Lancet, 1:1265–1267, 1979.

63. Chantler, J.K., Tingle, A.J., and Petty, R.E.: Persistent rubella virus infection associated with chronic arthritis in children. N. Engl. J. Med., 313:1117–1123, 1985.

64. Hardin, J.A., Steere, A.C., and Malawista, S.E.: Immune complexes and the evolution of Lyme arthritis: dissemination and localization of abnormal C1q-binding activity. N. Engl. J. Med., 301:1358–1363, 1979.

65. Steere, A.C. et al.: The spirochetal etiology of Lyme disease. N. Engl. J. Med., 308:733–740, 1983.

66. Chantler, J.K., Ford, D.K., and Tingle, A.J.: Rubella-associated arthritis: rescue of rubella virus from peripheral blood lymphocytes two years postvaccination. Infect. Immun., 32:1274–1280, 1981.

67. Tuazon, C.U.: Teichoic acid antibodies in osteomyelitis and septic arthritis caused by Staphylococcus aureus. J. Bone Joint Surg., 64A:762–765, 1982.

68. Williams, R.C., Jr., and Kunkel, H.G.: Rheumatoid factor, complement and conglutinin aberrations in patients with subacute bacterial endocarditis. J. Clin. Invest., 41:666–675, 1962.

69. Bocanegra, T.S., et al.: Reactive arthritis induced by parasitic infestation. Ann. Intern. Med., 94:207–209, 1981.

70. Brandt, K.D., Cathcart, E.S., and Cohen, A.S.: Gonococcal arthritis: clinical features correlated with blood, synovial fluid, and genitourinary cultures. Arthritis Rheum., 17:503–510, 1974.

71. Garcia-Kutzbach, A., Dismuke, S.E., and Masi, A.T.: Gono-coccal arthritis: clinical features and results of penicillin therapy. J. Rheumatol., 1:210–221, 1974.

72. Keefer, C.S., and Spink, W.W.: Gonococcic arthritis: pathogenesis, mechanism of recovery and treatment. JAMA 109:1448–1453, 1937.

73. Keiser, H., Ruben, F.L., and Wolinsky, E.: Clinical forms of gonococcal arthritis. N. Engl. J. Med., 279:234–240, 1968.

74. Richards, A.J.: Ruptured popliteal cyst and pyogenic arthritis. Br. Med. J., 282:1120–1121, 1981.

75. Nitsche, J.F.: Septic sternoclavicular arthritis with Pasteurella multocida and Streptococcus sanguis. Arthritis Rheum., 25:467–469, 1982.

76. Kelly, P.J., Martin, W.J., and Coventry, M.B.: Bacterial arthritis of the hip in the adult. J. Bone Joint Surg., 47A:1005–1018, 1965.

77. Ho, G., Jr., and Mikolich, D.J.: Bacterial infection of the superficial subcutaneous bursae. Clin. Rheum. Dis., 12:437–457, 1986.

78. Gelberman, R.H., et al.: Pyogenic arthritis of the shoulder in adults. J. Bone Joint Surg., 62A:550–553, 1980.

79. Gordon, G., and Kabins, S.A.: Pyogenic sacroiliitis. Am. J. Med., 69:50–56, 1980.

80. Schaad, U.B., McCracken, G.H., and Nelson, J.D.: Pyogenic arthritis of the sacroiliac joint in pediatric patients. Pediatrics, 66:375–379, 1980.

81. Sequeira, W., et al.: Pyogenic infections of the pubic symphysis. Ann. Intern. Med., 96:604–606, 1982.

82. Fielding, J.W., and Lieber, W.A.: Septic dislocation of hip joint in infancy: follow-up of fifteen years. N.Y. State J. Med., 61:3916–3917, 1961.

83. Lunseth, P.A., and Heiple, K.G.: Prognosis in septic arthritis of the hip in children. Clin. Orthop., 139:81–85, 1979.

84. Stetson, J.W., DePonte, R.J., and Southwick, W.O.: Acute septic arthritis of the hip in children. Clin. Orthop., 56:105–116, 1968.

85. Morrey, B.F., Bianco, A.J., and Rhodes, K.H.: Suppurative arthritis of the hip in children. J. Bone Joint Surg., 58A:388–392, 1976.

86. Asnes, R.S., and Arendar, G.M.: Septic arthritis of the hip: a complication of femoral venipuncture. Pediatrics, 38:837–841, 1966.

87. Flatman, J.G.: Hip disease with referred pain to the knee. JAMA, 234:967–968, 1975.

88. Morrey, B.F., Bianco, A.J., and Rhodes, K.H.: Hematogenous osteomyelitis at uncommon sites in children. Mayo Clin. Proc., 53:707–713, 1978.

89. Bernard, T.N., Jr., and Haddad, R.J.: Fever of undetermined etiology masks vertebral osteomyelitis. Orthop. Rev., 9:63–71, 1982.

90. Coy, J.T., III, et al.: Pyogenic arthritis of the sacro-iliac joint: long-term follow-up. J. Bone Joint Surg., 58A:845–849, 1976.

91. Delbarre, F., et al.: Pyogenic infection of the sacro-iliac joint: report of thirteen cases. J. Bone Joint Surg., 57A:819–825, 1975.

92. Gristina, A.G., and Kolkin, J.: Total joint replacement and sepsis. J. Bone Joint Surg., 65A:128–134, 1983.

93. Inman, R.D., et al.: Clinical and microbiological features of prosthetic joint infection. Am. J. Med., 77:47–53, 1984.

94. Booth, J.E., et al.: Infection of prosthetic arthroplasty by Mycobacterium fortuitum: two case reports. J. Bone Joint Surg., 61A:300–302, 1979.

95. Prince, A., and Neu, H.C.: Microbiology of infections of the prosthetic joint. Orthop. Rev., 8:91–96, 1979.

96. Hamilton, M.E., et al.: Simultaneous gout and pyarthrosis. Arch. Intern. Med., 140:917–919, 1980.

97. McCarty, D.J.: Joint sepsis: a chance for cure: (Editorial.) JAMA, *247*:835, 1982.

98. Miskew, D.B., Block, R.A., and Witt, P.F.: Aspiration of infected sacro-iliac joints. J. Bone Joint Surg., *61A*:1071–1072, 1979.

99. Hendrix, R.W., Lin, P.P., and Kane, W.J.: Simplified aspiration or injection technique for the sacroiliac joint. J. Bone Joint Surg., *64A*:1249–1252, 1982.

100. Scheinberg, M.A., and Benson, M.D.: SAA amyloid protein levels in amyloid-prone chronic inflammatory disorders: lack of association with amyloid disease. J. Rheumatol., *7*:724–726, 1980.

101. Honig, S., Gorevic, P., and Weissmann, G.: CRP in SLE patients: an aid in diagnosing superimposed infections. Arthritis Rheum., *20*:121, 1977.

102. Zein, N., Ganuza, C., and Kushner, I.: Significance of serum C-reactive protein elevations in patients with systematic lupus erythematosus. Arthritis Rheum., *21*:605, 1978.

103. Mackiewicz, A., et al.: Marcinkowska-Pieta, R., Ballou S., Mackiewicz, S., and Kushner, I.: Microheterogeneity of alpha₁-acid glycoprotein in the detection of intercurrent infection in systemic lupus erythematosus. Arthritis Rheum., *30*:513–518, 1987.

104. Hendrix, R.W., and Fisher, M.R.: Imaging of septic arthritis. Clin. Rheum. Dis., *12*:459–487, 1986.

105. Pate, D., and Katz, A.: Clostridia discitis: a case report. Arthritis Rheum., *22*:1039–1040, 1979.

106. Schiller, M., et al.: Clostridium perfringens septic arthritis. Report of a case and review of the literature. Clin. Orthop., *139*:92–96, 1979.

107. Lever, A.M.L., Owen, T., and Forsey, J.: Pneumoarthropathy in septic arthritis caused by Streptococcus milleri. Br. Med. J., *285*:24, 1982.

108. Crawford, A.H., and Carothers, T.S.: Hip arthrography in the skeletally immature. Clin. Orthop., *162*:54–60, 1982.

109. Glassberg, G.B., and Ozonoff, M.B.: Arthrographic findings in septic arthritis of the hip in infants. Radiology, *128*:151–155, 1978.

110. Schwartz, A.M., and Goldberg, M.J.: Medial adductor approach to arthrography of the hip in children. Radiology, *132*:483, 1979.

111. Rosenthal, D.I., Mankin, H.J., and Bauman, R.A.: Musculoskeletal applications for computed tomography. Bull. Rheum. Dis., *33*:1–4, 1983.

112. Azouz, E.M.: Computed tomography in bone and joint infections. J. Can. Assoc. Radiol., *32*:102–106, 1981.

113. Morgan, G.J., Jr.: Early diagnosis of septic arthritis of the sacroiliac joint by use of computed tomography. J. Rheumatol., *8*:979–982, 1981.

114. Majd, M., and Frankel, R.S.: Radionuclide imaging in skeletal inflammatory and ischemic disease in children. AJR, *126*:832–841. 1976.

115. Coleman, R.E.: Imaging with Tc-99m MDP and Ga-67 citrate in patients with rheumatoid arthritis and suspected septic arthritis. J. Nucl. Med., *23*:479–482, 1982.

116. Lisbona, R., and Rosenthall, L.: Observations on the sequential use of ⁹⁹ᵐTc-phosphate complex and ⁶⁷Ga imaging in osteomyelitis, cellulitis, and septic arthritis. Radiology, *123*:123–129, 1977.

117. Maurer, A.H.: Utility of three-phase skeletal scintigraphy in suspected osteomyelitis. J. Nucl. Med., *22*:941–949, 1981.

118. Ash, J.M., and Gilday, D.L.: The futility of bone scanning in neonatal osteomyelitis. J. Nucl. Med., *21*:417–420, 1980.

119. Murray, I.P.C.: Photopenia in skeletal scintigraphy of suspected bone and joint infection. Clin. Nucl. Med., *7*:13–20, 1982.

120. LaManna, M.M., et al.: An assessment of technetium and gallium scanning in the patient with painful total joint arthroplasty. Orthopedics, *6*:580–582, 1983.

121. Wofsy, D.: Culture-negative septic arthritis and bacterial endocarditis: diagnosis by synovial biopsy. Arthritis Rheum., *23*:605–607, 1980.

122. Enarson, D.A., et al.: Bone and joint tuberculosis: a continuing problem. Can. Med. Assoc. J., *120*:139–145, 1979.

123. Thayer, J.D., and Martin, J.E.: Improved medium selective for cultivation of N. gonorrhoeae and N. meningitidis. Public Health Rep., *81*:559–562, 1966.

124. Holmes, K.K., et al.: Recovery of Neisseria gonorrhoeae from "sterile" synovial fluid in gonococcal arthritis. N. Engl. J. Med., *284*:318–320, 1971.

125. Klein, S.J., Craggs, E., and Konwaler, B.E.: Guinea pig inoculation versus culture for isolation of M. tuberculosis. Am. Rev. Respir. Dis., *87*:451, 1963.

126. Ropes, M.W., and Bauer, W.: Synovial Fluid Changes in Joint Disease. Cambridge, Harvard University Press, 1953.

127. Brook, I., et al.: Synovial fluid lactic acid: a diagnostic aid in septic arthritis. Arthritis Rheum., *21*:774–779, 1978.

128. Mossman, S.S.: Synovial fluid lactic acid in septic arthritis. N.Z. Med. J., *93*:115–117, 1981.

129. Riordan, T.: Synovial fluid lactic acid measurement in the diagnosis and management of septic arthritis. J. Clin. Pathol., *35*:390–394, 1982.

130. Behn, A.R., Matthews, J.A., and Phillips, I.: Lactate UV-system: a rapid method for diagnosis of septic arthritis. Ann. Rheum. Dis., *40*:489–492, 1981.

131. Bunch, T.W., et al.: Synovial fluid complement determination as a diagnostic aid in inflammatory joint diseases. Mayo Clin. Proc., *49*:715–720, 1974.

132. Dorff, G.J., Ziokowski, J.S., and Rytel, M.W.: Detection by counterimmunoelectrophoresis of pneumococcal antigen in synovial fluid from septic arthritis. Arthritis Rheum., *18*:613–615, 1975.

133. Merritt, K., et al.: Counter immunoelectrophoresis in the diagnosis of septic arthritis caused by Haemophilus influenzae. J. Bone Joint Surg., *58A*:414–415, 1976.

134. Rytel, M.W.: Rapid diagnostic methods in infectious diseases. Adv. Intern. Med., *20*:37–60, 1975.

135. Reimann, K., Lind, I., and Andersen, K.E.: An indirect haemagglutination test for demonstration of gonococcal antibodies using gonococcal pili as antigen. II. Serological investigation of patients attending a dermatovenereological outpatient clinic in Copenhagen. Acta Pathol. Microbiol. Scand., *88*:155–162, 1980.

136. Salit, I.E., Blake, M., and Gotschlich, E.C.: Intra-strain heterogeneity of gonococcal pili is related to opacity colony variance. J. Exp. Med., *151*:716–725, 1980.

137. Spagna, V.A., and Prior, R.B.: The limulus amebocyte lysate assay. Am. Fam. Physician, *22*:125–128, 1980.

138. Steigbigel, R.T., Johnson, P.K., and Remington, J.S.: The nitroblue tetrazolium reduction test versus conventional hematology in the diagnosis of bacterial infection. N. Engl. J. Med., *290*:235–238, 1974.

139. Rinaldi, R.Z., Harrison, W.O., and Fan, P.T.: Penicillin-resistant gonococcal arthritis: a report of four cases. Ann. Intern. Med., *97*:43–45, 1982.

140. Chang, M.J., Contron, G., and Rodriguez, W.J.: Ampicillin-resistant Hemophilus influenzae type B septic arthritis in children. Clin. Pediatr., *20*:139–141, 1981.

141. Drutz, D.J., et al.: The penetration of penicillin and other antimicrobials into joint fluid: three case reports with a reappraisal of the literature. J. Bone Joint Surg., 49A:1415–1421, 1967.

142. Hirsch, H.L., Feffer, H.L., and O'Neil, C.B.: A study of the diffusion of penicillin across the serous membranes of joint cavities. J. Lab. Clin. Med., 31:535–543, 1946.

143. Latif, R., et al.: Pharmacokinetic and clinical evaluation of moxalactam in infants and children. Rev. Pharmacol. Ther., 3:222–231, 1981.

144. Nelson, J.D.: Antibiotic concentrations in septic joint effusions. N. Engl. J. Med., 284:349–353, 1971.

145. Pancoast, S.J., and Neu, H.C.: Antibiotic levels in human bone and synovial fluid used in the evaluation of antimicrobial therapy of joint and skeletal infections. Orthop. Rev., 9:49–61, 1980.

146. Parker, R.H., and Schmid, F.R.: Antibacterial activity of synovial fluid during therapy of septic arthritis. Arthritis Rheum., 14:96–104, 1971.

147. Sattar, M.A.: The penetration of metronidazole into synovial fluid. Postgrad. Med. J., 58:20–24, 1982.

148. Murray, H.W., Fialk, M.A., and Roberts, R.B.: Candida arthritis: a manifestation of disseminated candidiasis. Am. J. Med., 60:587–595, 1976.

149. Noyes, F.R., McCabe, J.D., and Fekety, F.R., Jr.: Acute Candida arthritis: report of a case and use of amphotericin B. J. Bone Joint Surg., 55A:169–176, 1973.

150. Poplack, D.G., and Jacobs, S.A.: Candida arthritis treated with amphotericin B. J. Pediatr., 87:989–990, 1975.

151. Quinlan, W.R., Hall, B.B., and Fitzgerald, R.H., Jr.: Fluid spaces in normal and osteomyelitic canine bone. J. Lab. Clin. Med., 102:78–87, 1983.

152. Smith, B.R., et al.: Bone penetration of antibiotics. Orthopedics, 6:187–193, 1983.

153. Ho, G., Jr.: Therapy for septic arthritis. JAMA, 247:797–800, 1982.

154. Carlsson, A.S., Lidgren, L., and Lindberg, H.: Prophylactic antibiotics against early and late deep infection after total hip replacement. Acta Orthop. Scand., 48:405–410, 1977.

155. Hill, C., et al.: Prophylactic cefazolin versus placebo in total hip replacement. Lancet, 1:795–797, 1981.

156. Hirschmann, J.V., and Inui, T.S.: Antimicrobial prophylaxis: a critique of recent trials. Rev. Infect. Dis., 2:1–23, 1980.

157. Wahlig, H., et al.: The release of gentamicin from polymethylmethacrylate beads. J. Bone Joint Surg., 60B:270–275, 1978.

158. D'Ambrosia, R.D., Shoji, H., and Heater, R.: Secondarily infected total joint replacements by hematogenous spread. J. Bone Joint Surg., 58A:450–453, 1976.

159. Howard, J.B., Highgenboten, C.L., and Nelson, J.D.: Resid-

ual effects of septic arthritis in infancy and childhood. JAMA, 236:932–935, 1976.

160. Samilson, R.L., Bersani, F.A., and Watkins, M.B.: Acute suppurative arthritis in infants and children. The importance of early diagnosis and surgical drainage. Pediatrics, 21:798–803, 1958.

161. Broy, S.B., and Schmid, F.R.: A comparison of medical drainage (needle aspiration) and surgical drainage (arthrotomy or arthroscopy) in the initial treatment of infected joints. Clin. Rheum. Dis., 12:501–522, 1986.

162. Ballard, A., et al.: Functional treatment of pyogenic arthritis of the adult knee. J. Bone Joint Surg., 57A:1119–1123, 1975.

163. Kawashima, M., et al.: The treatment of pyogenic bone and joint infections by closed irrigation-suction. Clin. Orthop., 148:240–244, 1980.

164. Goldenberg, D.L., et al.: Treatment of septic arthritis: comparison of needle aspiration and surgery as initial modes of joint drainage. Arthritis Rheum., 18:83–90, 1975.

165. Mielants, H.: Long-term functional results of the non-surgical treatment of common bacterial infections of joints. Scand. J. Rheumatol., 11:101–105, 1982.

166. Jarrett, M.P., et al.: The role of arthroscopy in the treatment of septic arthritis. Arthritis Rheum., 24:737–739, 1981.

167. Broy, S.B., Stulberg, S.D., and Schmid, F.R.: The role of arthroscopy in the diagnosis and management of the septic joint. Clin. Rheum. Dis., 12:489–500, 1986.

168. Fitzgerald, R.H., Jr.: Problems associated with the infected total hip arthroplasty. Clin. Rheum. Dis., 12:537–554, 1986.

169. Salter, R.B.: The protective effect of continuous passive motion on living articular cartilage in acute septic arthritis: an experimental investigation in the rabbit. Clin. Orthop., 159:223–247, 1981.

170. Price, C.T.: Thompson arthrodesis of the hip in children. J. Bone Joint Surg., 62A:1118–1123, 1980.

171. Tuli, S.M.: Excision arthroplasty for tuberculous and pyogenic arthritis of the hip. J. Bone Joint Surg., 63B:29–32, 1981.

172. Jupiter, J.B., et al.: Total hip arthroplasty in the treatment of adult hips with current or quiescent sepsis. J. Bone Joint Surg., 63A:194–200, 1981.

173. McLaughlin, R.E., and Allen, J.R.: Total hip replacement in the previously infected hip. South. Med. J., 70:573–575, 1977.

174. Salvati, E.A.: Total hip replacement in current or recent sepsis. Orthop. Rev., 9:97–102, 1980.

175. Gillespie, W.J.: The management of acute haematogenous osteomyelitis in the antibiotic era: a study of the outcome. J. Bone Joint Surg., 63B:126–131, 1981.

176. Black, J., Hunt, T.L., Godley, P.H., and Matthew, E.: Oral antimicrobial therapy for adults with osteomyelitis or septic arthritis. J. Infect. Dis., 155:968–972, 1987.

115

BACTERIAL ARTHRITIS

GEORGE HO, JR.

The general principles of septic arthritis are discussed in Chapter 114. Characteristics of the host and the microorganisms and the clinical setting in which bacterial arthritis occurs are the subjects of this chapter.

BACTERIAL ARTHRITIS IN CHILDREN*

The largest American experience on septic arthritis in children comes from Dallas. Fink and Nelson[1] reviewed a series of 591 cases collected over 30 years and concluded that there probably has not been a significant increase in the incidence of septic arthritis between 1955 and 1984. The proportion of cases wherein a specific pathogen was identified has remained fairly constant at an overall average of 66%. Table 115–1 summarizes the data from the Dallas series along with four other recent series, bringing the total number of patients available for analysis to 865. The percentages of cases with bacteriologic confirmation varied from 64 to 100%, which in part reflected the nonuniform inclusion criteria used by the different authors. Overall, 611 of 865 children with septic arthritis (71%) had an identified bacterial etiology.

Cultures of the synovial fluid were positive in only 70 to 97% of the cases of septic arthritis with bacteriologic confirmation (Table 115–1). When antibiotic

*Editor's note. It is very important to remember that septic arthritis in children can be secondary to contiguous acute osteomyelitis (metaphysis). Bony tenderness next to a swollen joint is an important clue to this situation.

treatment had been instituted prior to joint aspiration, the yield of positive synovial fluid culture dropped to 36%.[4] Similarly, the likelihood of identifying microorganisms on the Gram-stained smear of the synovial fluid was higher in those who had not received antibiotic therapy (54%) than in those who had (19%).[4] Approximately one third of all Gram-stained smears of infected synovial fluid in children were positive for bacteria.[1]

Blood cultures were positive in 33 to 46% of children with septic arthritis, and may be the only clue in identifying the responsible pathogen. The importance of obtaining blood cultures as well as cultures of other extra-articular sites of infection cannot be overemphasized because positive results enhance the yield of bacteriologic confirmation and aid in the specific antimicrobial drug therapy.

The age of the child is a very important determinant of the susceptibility of the host to a specific pathogen. The environment in which the infection is acquired, whether community-acquired or nosocomial, is another factor that has an influence on the most likely causative microorganism. The most common bacteria in childhood septic arthritis are Hemophilus influenzae and Staphylococcus aureus. In those centers whose experience includes a large number of patients who are 2 years of age and younger, Hemophilus influenzae has been the most common pathogen.[1,2,5] Although this predominance of H. influenzae as a cause of joint infection in children between 6 months and 2 years of age is well recognized (Table 115–1),

Table 115–1. Septic Arthritis in Children

	Fink and Nelson	Sequeira et al.	Wilson and DiPaola	Speiser et al.	Welkon et al.
Year published	1986	1985	1986	1985	1986
Reference no.	1	2	3	4	5
Study years	30 (1955–84)	10 (1972–81)	10 (1972–81)	10 (1974–83)	10 (1975–85)
Study location	Dallas, TX	Chicago, IL	Glasgow, Scotland	St. Louis, MO	Philadelphia, PA
Total no. of cases	591	32	61	86	95
No. of cases with bacteriologic confirmation	390	32	56	72	61
% of total no. of cases	66	100	92	84	64
I. Among those with bacterial etiology (%)					
Positive gram stain of synovial fluid	33	—	—	19–54*	—
Positive synovial fluid culture	79	97	71–80†	36–70*	84
Positive blood culture	33	—	41	46	46
II. Site of Infection (%)					
Knee	40	37	29	30	49
Hip	23	27	40	29	27
Ankle	13	15	22	17	17
Sum of above	76	79	91	76	93
Polyarticular	7	—	5	7	8
III. Microbiology (%)					
Staphylococcus aureus	17	25	44	37	13
Hemophilus influenzae	25	37	16	17	29
Others	25	38	32	29	22
Culture negative	33	—	8	16	36
Patients <2 years old	51	55	26	49	69

*The lower percentages reflect results in patients receiving antibiotics; the higher values are from patients not yet treated with antibiotics.
†71% positive for specimens obtained at arthrotomy and 80% positive for aspirated samples.

a trend toward fewer cases has been observed in Saint Louis.[4]

Among children over 5 years old, and in neonates or infants of less than 6 months Staphylococcus aureus is the major pathogen. The bacteria causing septic arthritis in the neonatal and early infancy periods can be further subdivided according to where the infection was acquired.[6] Pathogens in community-acquired joint infections include group B streptococcus (52%), staphylococcus (25%), gonococcus (17%) and gram-negative bacilli (5%). In sharp contrast, the relative frequencies of the hospital-acquired pathogens are staphylococcus (62%), Candida (17%), gram-negative enteric bacilli (13%), and streptococcus and Hemophilus influenzae (4% each). Whether these data derived from a review of the medical literature are representative of any or all regions is uncertain. The need to determine the local pattern of bacterial causes of septic arthritis is of utmost importance, since the selection of the initial antimicrobial drugs may depend solely on this information. Knowledge about the antibiotic sensitivities of the local bacterial isolates is also crucial. For example, in the Dallas study 18% of the H. influenzae are β-lactamase-positive and resistant to ampicillin.[1] Similarly, there are regions in the United States, namely metropolitan Detroit, where methicillin-resistant Staphylococcus aureus is quite prevalent.[7] Neisseria gonorrhoeae remains a possible cause of septic arthritis in the adolescent and in the young infant, especially when the disease is polyarticular. Gonococcal joint disease in children is polyarticular in 50% of cases, whereas all the other common bacteria cause monoarticular disease (93%) rather than polyarticular (7%).[1]

Joint infections in children favor the large joints of the lower extremities. In a review of infections in 1023 joints, 39% affected the knee, 26% the hip, and 13% the ankle.[1] These three joint sites accounted for 79% of the joint infections in 948 patients. The figures from other recent studies (Table 115–1) confirm this general distribution of joint involvement, although in some series, hip infections were more common than infections of the knee.[3]

THERAPY

The age-dependent vulnerability to a specific pathogen, the circumstances under which the joint infection is acquired, the knowledge of the regional trends in the bacterial causes of septic arthritis, and the local antibiotic susceptibility patterns, in addition to the fact that approximately 30% of the cases of presumed bacterial arthritis in children were not bacteriologically confirmed, must all be taken into account in the drug treatment of childhood bacterial arthritis. The principle of choosing the most efficacious and specific, the least toxic, and the least expensive drug should be followed. A positive Gram-stained smear of the synovial fluid and the results of the laboratory investigation on extra-articular sites of infection (i.e., cerebral spinal fluid, sputum and urine) are used to determine the most appropriate antibiotic treatment prior to culture confirmation. When the Gram-stained smear shows no microorganisms, the initial, empirically chosen antimicrobial agent(s) should be broad-spectrum with optimal activity against the most likely pathogens. For example, in the neonate with hospital-acquired bacterial arthritis, the antibiotic regimen must be directed at S. aureus as well as the gram-negative enteric bacilli. Thus, the use of a penicillinase-resistant penicillin along with an aminoglycoside is appropriate while culture results are pending. On the other hand, empiric treatment of community-acquired infection should be directed against group B streptococcus, staphylococcus, and gonococcus. In children between 6 months and 5 years of age, if Hemophilus influenzae is suspected but Staphylococcus aureus cannot be ruled out, initial treatment should be chloramphenicol and a penicillinase-resistant penicillin[8] or cefuroxime alone.[4] In the older child (over 5 years old) and the adolescent, the initial antibiotic treatment is directed at S. aureus for monoarticular joint disease. Vancomycin should be chosen over a penicillinase-resistant penicillin or a cephalosporin as the initial antistaphylococcal drug in areas where the prevalence of methicillin resistance is high. Polyarticular disease in a sexually active adolescent deserves treatment directed at Neisseria gonorrhoeae.

The duration of antibiotic therapy and the mode of joint drainage have not been rigorously studied in a controlled, prospective fashion. Recommendations on the duration of antibiotic treatment vary between 2 to 4 weeks for uncomplicated bacterial arthritis caused by less virulent pathogens and 4 to 6 weeks for joint sepsis caused by S. aureus or gram-negative bacilli and for joint infections complicated by osteomyelitis. The length of hospitalization may be reduced by the use of home intravenous therapy[9,10] or the substitution of oral antibiotic treatment[11] in carefully controlled situations. The obvious advantages are the return of the child to the home environment, the decreased likelihood of nosocomial infections, and the reduction of the cost of prolonged hospitalization.

General agreement regarding the drainage of an infected joint in the child includes the prompt surgical decompression of hip infections and the need for open drainage when repeated needle aspirations show the persistence of infection or when they cannot be carried out satisfactorily because of technical difficulty. The morbidity associated with arthrotomy must be weighed against the benefit gained by initial open drainage. One recent study clearly showed that joint infection of sites other than the hip had an excellent chance of responding to nonoperative treatment when there was minimal delay in diagnosis and treatment.[12]

The outcome of treated bacterial arthritis in childhood is a function of the patient's age, the joint infected, the infecting microorganism, and the promptness of diagnosis and treatment. Overall, about 25% of children with bacterial arthritis had some degree of residual abnormality on long-term followup.[13,14] Infants, especially those with infected hips, have poorer results.[3] Hip infection in general has a less favorable outcome than that of the knee and ankle.[13,14] Of the two most common causes of childhood septic arthritis, Staphylococcus aureus is more likely to lead to residual impairment than Hemophilus influenzae,[4] although this finding is not invariable.[14] Finally, delay in diagnosis and treatment is certainly detrimental to the outcome of treatment.[12]

BACTERIAL ARTHRITIS IN THE ELDERLY

In 1900 barely 4% of the total American population, or 3 million people, were 65 years and older. Today 12% of the population in the United States, or 28 million people, are 65 or older. By the year 2000, 35 million Americans will be 65 and over.[15] Although the incidence of septic arthritis in adults has not changed significantly over the last several decades,[16] a British study spanning a 30-year period showed that the percentage of those older than 60 had increased from 19% between 1954 and 1963 to 45% in the following decade of 1964 to 1973.[17] These observations suggest that the number of cases of acute bacterial arthritis will increase proportionally to the growth of the population, but a larger percentage will come from the geriatic population. An analysis of 402 adults with septic arthritis reported from 1960 to 1986 found that 163 (41%) were more than 60 years old.[18]

Systemic factors impairing the ability of the host to combat infections are numerous. The more prevalent illnesses among adults with septic arthritis are diabetes mellitus, cirrhosis, chronic renal failure, rheumatoid arthritis (RA), and neoplastic disease.[19] Two other major risk factors for infectious complications are associated with the management of these chronic illnesses. One is the employment of invasive diagnostic procedures and surgical interventions, and the other is the iatrogenic lowering of the host's resistance by the use of immunosuppressive drugs. Even in the absence of overt systemic illness, the aging process itself may lead to the decline of the immune function and an increased susceptibility to infectious diseases.[20]

Table 115–2 summarizes the data from 4 retrospective studies examining nongonococcal bacterial arthritis in the elderly.[21–24] The mean age of the 68 patients was 69.6 years. The prevalence of an underlying joint disease ranged from 23 to 71% with a mean rate of 57%. Osteoarthritis and RA were the most common underlying joint diseases, but gout, systemic lupus erythematosus, and hemophiliac arthropathy were also noted. Many patients had a history of trauma to the joint, which subsequently became infected.* The infection most often affected the knee joint. The next most frequent sites were the hip, shoulder, and wrist.

Finding the presence of monosodium urate or calcium pyrophosphate dihydrate crystals in highly inflammatory joint fluids does not preclude the coexistence of a septic

---

*Editor's note. Trauma may rupture synovial capillaries. If a patient has coincident bacteremia, this may result in inoculation of the joint from the blood.

process. The simultaneous occurrence of septic arthritis and crystal-induced arthritis appears to be a problem unique to the geriatric population (see Septic Arthritis Associated With Crystalline Arthritis later in the chapter).

The rate of finding the microorganism on Gram-stained smears of the synovial fluid is estimated to be 75% for staphylococcal and 50% for gram-negative bacillary infections.[19] The microbiology of acute bacterial joint infection in the elderly is not different from that of nongonococcal septic arthritis in all adults. Staphylococcus aureus was the predominant microorganism responsible for 43 to 64% of the cases of septic arthritis in the elderly (Table 115–2). Other less common gram-positive coccal causes included the various species of streptococci, pneumococcus, and Staphylococcus epidermidis, in that order. Neisseria gonorrhoeae is a much less frequent cause of arthritis in the elderly, but the clinical features are quite similar to those in the young person with gonococcal arthritis (see Chapter 116).[25,26]

Gram-negative bacilli have emerged as a significant cause of septic arthritis in the last 2 decades[27] because of the increased incidence of bacteremia caused by gram-negative bacillary organisms in general[28] and because of the predilection of septic arthritis in intravenous drug-abusers caused by Pseudomonas aeruginosa[29] and Serratia marcescens.[30] The latter situation is much less likely in the geriatric population than in young adults. The percentages of the elderly with septic arthritis caused by gram-negative bacilli were 14%, 18%, and 35% in three series (Table 115–2). Combining these figures, the overall rate is 24%, in excellent agreement with the 23% figure reported from the Boston University Medcal Center experience of 97 adults between 1965 to 1982.[19]

THERAPY

Treatment of septic arthritis in these four series of elderly patients was examined retrospectively. The

---

Table 115–2. Septic Arthritis in the Elderly

	Cooper and Cawley[21] (1986)	McGuire and Kauffman[22] (1985)	Ho and Su[23] (1982)	Willkens et al.[24] (1960)
Study period	1973–82	1973–83	1975–80	1954–59
No. of patients	21	23	11	13
Mean age (yr)	73.8	67.1	66.7	69.9
Age range (yr)	60–85	60–87	60–78	60–82
Underlying joint disease	71%	65%	55%	23%
Knee infections	48%	43%	55%	54%
Next most frequent site	Hip (38%)	Wrist (17%)	Shoulder (27%)	Shoulder (38%)
Staphylococcus aureus	43%	52%	64%	62%
Gram-negative bacilli	14%	35%	18%	—
In-hospital mortality	33%	22%	9%	—
Poor functional outcome	52%	—	40%	46%

approach taken did not differ significantly in principle from the current recommendations on antibiotic treatment[31] and drainage[32] of an infected joint. The outcome of treatment of septic arthritis in the elderly was generally disappointing with mortality ranging from 9 to 33% and an overall mortality of 24% (Table 115-2). Such high mortality was not due solely to the infectious disease that affected the joint. Nosocomial pseudomonas infection contributed significantly in one series.[22] Other age-related chronic diseases could have contributed to the demise of some of these patients, although the contribution of pre-existing conditions was difficult to assess. Among the survivors, the functional outcome was poor in approximately half the patients (Table 115-2). These results compare unfavorably with the mortality (9%) and morbidity (34%) of adult nongonococcal septic arthritis in general.[33] Factors portending a poor outcome included delay in diagnosis, underlying joint disease, especially RA with polyarticular infection,[33] gram-negative bacillary septic arthritis, involvement of the hip joint, and serious chronic debilitating illnesses and their associated treatments.

SEPTIC ARTHRITIS COMPLICATING RHEUMATOID ARTHRITIS

Bacterial infection of a joint already affected by RA is "dangerous, not only to limb but to life."[34] That a joint previously damaged by RA is prone to bacterial invasion has been recognized since the 1958 report of Kellgren and associates[35] and by other researchers.[36-44] Impairments of normal host defenses in RA include decreased chemotaxis[45] and phagocytosis[46] of neutrophils. The therapeutic use of corticosteroid and/or cytotoxic drugs, and other defects, such as the depressed hemolytic complement levels and decreased bacteriolytic activity of synovial fluid, may play a role.[47] Which factor is most responsible for the susceptibility to joint infection is unclear, but septic arthritis in a patient with RA can have catastrophic results, especially when the diagnosis is delayed.

Typically, the patient is older with longstanding seropositive, erosive disease and significant functional impairment and debilitation (Table 115-3). Nearly half of the patients (45%) were receiving systemic corticosteroid therapy. Thus, the clinical expression of joint infection may be blunted. The onset may be insidious rather than abrupt, and the usual signs of fever and toxicity may be absent (Table 115-3). Only 56% of cases had peripheral blood leukocytosis. Increased pain in one or more joints may easily be mistaken for a flare-up of the rheumatoid disease, the

diagnosis of bacterial joint infection is delayed, and the patient is treated at a more advanced stage of the infection.

Table 115-3 also shows the relative frequencies of the various bacteria found in infections of the rheumatoid joint. Gram-positive cocci cause 89% of the infections, and Staphylococcus aureus is the major pathogen. Gram-negative bacilli are responsible for the remaining cases, with Enterobacteriaceae accounting for most of them. Polymicrobial infection occurred in one of 116 cases, an infection of an Austin-Moore hip prosthesis caused by two enteric bacilli, Escherichia coli and Proteus mirabilis.[37] The spectrum of bacterial etiologies continues to broaden with reports of cases caused by uncommon and opportunistic pathogens, including Plesiomonas shigelloides,[48] Pasteurella multocida,[49] Kingella kingae,[50] Listeria monocytogenes,[51] Micrococcus luteus,[52] Bacteroides melaninogenicus,[53] and Bacteroides fragilis.[53] Polyarticular infections occurred in 25% of cases. Some microorganisms may have a predilection to cause disease in multiple joints, for example, Bacteroides fragilis,[54-56] pneumococcus,[57] and group G streptococcus.[58] On the other hand, rheumatoid damage in multiple joints may predispose to the localization of infection in more than one joint. Large joints, especially the knee, are the most commonly affected. Unusual sites include the temporomandibular joint[59] and the cricoarytenoid joint.[60]

THERAPY

Treatment of septic arthritis superimposed on RA adheres to the principles of therapy for acute bacterial arthritis in general. Systemic antibiotic administration and adequate drainage of the purulent synovial fluid are both necessary. Whether the infected rheumatoid joint is better served by immediate open surgical drainage and debridement[39] is debatable. Open drainage, however, may be indicated since the diagnosis of infection is often delayed and rheumatoid joints are often difficult to aspirate completely because of adhesions and debris (rice bodies). The deleterious effect of delayed diagnosis on outcome is well illustrated by a study showing that patients with full recovery had an average delay of 6.6 days between onset of symptoms to diagnosis compared with those with a poor outcome where the average delay was 18.0 days.[44]

The mortality of 25% in patients with RA complicated by acute septic arthritis (Table 115-3) is much higher than the rate of 9% in adults with nongonococcal septic arthritis.[33] Such high mortality is due in

Table 115–3.   Bacterial Arthritis in Rheumatoid Arthritis Patients*

No. of patients	116
Patient characteristics	
Mean age in years (range)	56 (27–82)
Mean duration of RA in years (range)	14 (1–55)
Systemic corticosteroid therapy	45% (51/113)
Clinical features	
Fever	76% (62/82)
Leukocytosis >10,000 cells/mm³	56% (43/77)
Polyarticular infection	25% (22/89)
Microbiology of 109 bacterial isolates†	
Grám-positive cocci	89% (97/109)
Staphylococcus aureus	77%
Staphylococcus epidermidis	2%
Hemolytic streptococcus	7%
Streptococcus pneumoniae	3%
Gram-negative bacilli	11% (12/109)
Escherichia coli	6%
Proteus mirabilis	1%
Morganella morganii	1%
Salmonella sp.	1%
Pseudomonas aeruginosa	1%
Hemophilus influenzae	1%
Fusobacterium necrophorum	1%
Outcome	
Deaths	25% (29/116)
Range of mortality rates	0–88%
Survivors with fair to good outcome	50% (25/50)
Survivors with poor outcome	50% (25/50)

*Analysis of 89 cases taken from reference nos. 36 to 44 published between 1966 and 1986 plus 27 cases from 1958 to 1964 reviewed in reference no. 36.
†See text for other bacteria responsible for septic arthritis in rheumatoid patients.

part to the extremely poor outcome of rheumatoid patients with polyarticular septic arthritis (mortality of 56%).[33] Half of surviving patients recovered the preinfection level of function, and the other half experienced further loss of function. Thus, septic arthritis is a serious complication of RA that requires early diagnosis and treatment.

BONE AND JOINT INFECTIONS ASSOCIATED WITH INTRAVENOUS DRUG ABUSE

Parenteral abuse of drugs is associated with many infectious complications. These include viral infections such as hepatitis B and human immunodeficiency virus infection, bacterial infections such as skin abscesses or endocarditis, and fungal infections such as candidemia. Bacterial infections of the skeletal system include osteomyelitis and septic arthritis. The pathogenesis is believed to be by the hematogenous dissemination of bacteria injected into the bloodstream with the illicit drug. Staphylococcus aureus comes from the patient himself because of the high carrier rate of S. aureus in the nose and throat and on the skin of parenteral drug abusers.[61] Contamination of dirty needles and syringes shared by addicts serves as a reservoir for Pseudomonas aeruginosa.[62] The predilection for such infections to involve the bones of the vertebral column and the fibrocartilaginous joints of the pelvis and the sternum is well recognized but poorly understood.[29,63]

Combining the 1976–1979 Cook County Hospital experience[29] with the 1969–1978 Harbor–UCLA Medical Center series[63] and review of 101 cases,[63] 158 cases were analyzed for the relative frequencies of the different sites of skeletal infection in intravenous drug abusers. Most common was the vertebral column (49%) in the order of lumbar, cervical, and thoracic.[63] The least common sites were the large peripheral diarthrodial joints (17%). The fibrocartilaginous articulations of the pelvis and the sternum were involved in 33% of cases, including the sacroiliac joint (9 to 20%),[64] the symphysis pubis (3 to 9%),[65] the ischium (3 to 9%),[63] the sternoclavicular joint (6 to 10%),[66] and the other sternoarticulations (8%). The latter included sternocostal[66] and sternomanubrial joints.[67]

The bacteriology of skeletal infections in intravenous drug abusers reflected primarily pathogens contaminating the blood. In the review by Roca and Yoshikawa,[63] 78% of the infections were caused by Pseudomonas aeruginosa, 11% were due to gram-positive cocci including staphylococci and streptococci, and the remainder were due to the Klebsiella (3%), Enterobacter (4%), and Serratia (5%) group of gram-negative microorganisms. The prevalence of the different bacterial pathogens varied from region to region. The changing trends over time are illustrated by a report from Detroit, comparing their experience of 1966 to 1977 with that of 1981 to 1982.[7] An increased incidence of bacterial arthritis, an increased number of drug addicts among their patients with septic arthritis, a decreased number of cases caused by Pseudomonas, and an increased number of cases resulting from methicillin-resistant Staphylococcus aureus were found.

Intravenous drug abusers with bacterial bone and joint infections are generally young and, except for drug addiction, healthy. This contrasts to the non-addicted adults with nongonococcal septic arthritis, who are older and often have underlying joint and/or systemic diseases (see earlier section, Bacterial Arthritis in the Elderly).[63] Infections affecting the axial skeleton in addicts caused by gram-negative bacilli have a more insidious clinical presentation with less toxicity[29] and longer duration of symptoms[63] than an acute staphylococcal infection of a knee. Similarly, the physical findings in patients with axial skeleton involvement are less obvious than in those with a peripheral joint infection. Bone scintigraphy is useful in localizing skeletal infections when plain radiographs are unrevealing. Once the site of suspected infection is localized, the bacterial cause should be sought aggressively. Aspiration of synovial fluid, needle biopsy or aspiration under fluoroscopic guidance, or open biopsy and culture of the affected bone or joint tissues may be needed.

THERAPY

Antimicrobial treatment is directed at the isolated bacteria according to the in-vitro antibiotic sensitivities. Against Pseudomonas, the combination of an aminoglycoside and an antipseudomonal penicillin is generally recommended. The duration of antibiotic treatment is usually prolonged, varying from 4 to 6 weeks. Surgical decompression, drainage, or debridement are necessary in patients with epidural or paravertebral abscess complicating vertebral infection, with osteomyelitis and/or retrosternal abscess accompanying sternoarticular disease, with abscess or se-

questrum in periarticular osteomyelitis of the sacroiliac joint or the symphysis pubis, or with hip infection or infection of another peripheral joint that fails to respond to repeated needle aspirations and adequate systemic antibiotic therapy. The immediate outcome of treatment of these skeletal infections in drug addicts is generally favorable, but long-term followup results in this population are rarely available.

BACTERIAL INFECTION OF PROSTHETIC JOINTS

Bacterial infection occurring in a prosthetic joint is an extremely grave and costly complication of total joint replacement (TJR). Besides the expense of prolonged hospitalization for antibiotic treatment and surgery to eradicate the infection, there is the agony of the return of symptoms and loss of function, the cost of further surgery to salvage the failed implant, and the risk of uncontrolled infection resulting in the loss of limb or life. However, millions worldwide have benefited from TJR for advanced osteoarthritis or rheumatoid arthritis of the hip and knee joints. In 1985, 111,000 total hip replacements and 73,000 total knee replacements were done in the United States (excluding federal hospitals),[68] compared with the 80,000 (hip) and 40,000 (knee) performed in 1976.[69] Since the need for these operations is greatest in people over 60 years old,[70] as the aging population in the United States is enlarging,[15] such increases are not surprising. The number of people needing prosthetic joint surgery will clearly continue to rise.

Under optimal conditions, the overall infection rate of TJR is probably close to 1%,[71,72] which is below the 2% for total hip replacement and 4% for total knee replacement cited in a 1983 review.[73] The experience with total replacement of the shoulder, elbow, or ankle is limited in both number and duration of followup. Reported infection rates appear high, for example, 6% for total elbow replacement at one center[72] to 9% at another.[74] Such figures are similar to the high infection rates for hip or knee prostheses when they were first performed.[73]

There are two ways to classify prosthetic joint infections: (1) by the route of bacterial invasion, that is, direct introduction at the time of surgery versus hematogenous seeding from an extra-articular site, and (2) by the time of occurrence of infection after implantation of the prosthesis, that is, early or acute (usually within 12 weeks), delayed or subacute (up to 12 months), and late (greater than 1 year). Neither classification is totally satisfactory. For the former, accurate categorization is difficult because the source of the bacteria is often obscure. In the latter classification, the subdivisions are criticized as being artificial and arbitrary. Early infections are mostly related to postoperative wound infection and respond to prompt aggressive treatment; retention of the original prosthesis is more likely. Late infections usually result from hematogenous dissemination of bacteria and are more common in rheumatoid arthritis patients.[75,76] The relative frequencies are 36 to 50% for early, 23 to 45% for delayed, and 15 to 27% for late infections.[73,76–78] Hematogenous seeding has been responsible for 20 to 40% of all cases of prosthetic joint infection.[79] While the orthopedic surgeon usually evaluates and treats the patient with early infectious complications associated with TJR, the internist is more apt to see the patient with late infection after years of being asymptomatic. Thus, awareness of the clinical, laboratory, therapeutic, and prognostic aspects of bacterial infection in total joint replacement is essential.

Certain patients are at greater risk of prosthetic joint infection. The many factors predisposing to infection include impairment in host defense, surgical technique and duration of operation, and material and design of the prosthesis. Rheumatoid arthritis carries a higher risk of prosthetic joint infection, especially the late hematogenous type.[72,75,76] Revision arthroplasty is technically more difficult than primary joint replacement and often prolongs the operation. Increased operative time contributes to the increased infection rate in joints that have undergone previous surgery.[72,80] Changing from a posterior to a posterolateral surgical approach in total elbow replacement was thought to have lowered the rate of infection from 6 to 2.5%.[72] The less constrained design of joint prostheses, allowing for the natural multiaxial movement of the knee, may have reduced the incidence of both septic and aseptic failures.[72]

Pain most commonly (95%) heralds an infection in a joint prosthesis. Fever (43%), swelling (38%), and drainage through the skin (32%) occur less commonly among these patients.[79] Presentation may be acute and fulminant or it may be quite indolent, with the gradual onset of pain in a previously painless prosthesis. The virulence of the causative bacteria influences the acuteness and the severity of the clinical presentation. The possibility of infection must always be entertained when a prosthetic joint becomes painful, when there are signs of local inflammation or drainage, or when there is progressive radiographic evidence of loosening of the prosthesis.

Aspiration of joint fluid for the isolation of the bacterial pathogen is the most specific means of establishing the diagnosis. The Gram-stained smear of the joint aspirate is positive for microorganisms in approximately 30% of cases.[79] Estimates of culture-negative joint aspirates vary between 2 to 15%[79] and 7 to 15%,[73] and the diagnosis of prosthetic joint infection in these cases is made at the time of surgery when periprosthetic specimens are examined bacteriologically and histologically.

Prosthetic joint infection may be caused by aerobic gram-positive cocci (75 to 80%), aerobic gram-negative rods (10 to 20%), and anaerobic microorganisms (5 to 10%).[78,79] Staphylococci account for 75 to 90% of the gram-positive coccal infections. Staphylococcus epidermidis may be twice as common as Staphylococcus aureus in prosthetic joint infections,[79] in contrast with septic arthritis in natural joints, in which S. aureus predominates and Staphylococcus epidermidis is an extremely uncommon pathogen. The presence of a foreign body may play a permissive role in infections caused by the less virulent microorganisms.[81] The other gram-positive cocci found in infected prosthetic joints are the various streptococci including groups A, B, G, D (enterococci)[58,82,83] as well as Streptococcus pneumoniae.[84] Among the gram-negative bacilli, Escherichia coli, Proteus mirabilis, and Pseudomonas aeruginosa are the major culprits.[85] The less common gram-negative pathogens include Enterobacter aerogenes, Pasteurella multocida, Moraxella, Klebsiella, Salmonella, and Serratia.[75,77,85,86] Anaerobic bacteria, accounting for 5 to 10% of infections, include Peptococcus species, Peptostreptococcus species, Clostridium perfringens, and Bacteroides fragilis.[82,87] Other rare causes are corynebacteria (aerobic diphtheroides), Propionibacterium acnes (anaerobic diphtheroides),[74] Hemophilus influenzae,[72] Listeria monocytogenes,[77] Aeromonas hydrophila,[75] Pseudomonas pyocyanea,[76] and Mycoplasma hominis.[88] Infections caused by mixed microorganisms, or polymicrobial disease, range from 6%[82] to 25%,[72] and these are usually early infections.

THERAPY

Antibiotics directed at the isolated pathogen(s) and surgical debridement or removal of the infected prosthesis are essential steps in management. The best chance for retention of the prosthesis is in the patient with early, postoperative infection that is diagnosed and treated promptly. The Mayo Clinic experience with 61 infected total knee prostheses from 1970 to 1981 resulted in retention of the prosthesis by early debridement for acute infection in 6, arthrodesis in 35 (success rate of 83%), early reimplantation in 13 (38% success rate), and resection arthroplasty in 5, and amputation in 2.[89] At the Hospital for Special Surgery, a two-stage revision arthroplasty protocol with 6 weeks of parenteral antibiotic therapy guided by quantitative in-vitro sensitivity testing before reimplantation[90] had a 100% success rate for 40 infected total knee prostheses and 93% success rate for 80 infected total hip prostheses after 2 years of followup.[79]

One-stage revision for infected total hip prostheses with[91,92] or without[93] antibiotic-impregnated cement had success rates of 90 to 91% and 86%, respectively. The success of the latter approach may lie in the utilization of an antibiotic regimen consisting of three agents followed by prolonged oral treatment.[93] A review on antibiotic-impregnated cement concluded that it is "not known whether the combination of systemically delivered antibiotics and antibiotic-impregnated cement might be superior to either used separately" in the management of infected total hip prostheses.[94] Excision arthroplasty or Girdlestone's pseudarthrosis is an alternative treatment for infected total hip prostheses if reimplantation is not feasible, but poor functional outcome is to be expected.[95] A final option in the treatment of an infected total joint replacement may be chronic suppressive antibiotic therapy in very selected patients: (1) the retained prosthesis must not be loose; (2) the pathogen has to be of low virulence and/or exquisitely sensitive to the oral antibiotic agent used; and (3) the patient must be able to tolerate the long-term antibiotic program. Even with these rigid criteria, the success rate is only 50%.[79]

A recent survey of 1112 total joint replacements, with an average followup of 6 years, found an overall incidence of 0.27% for late hematogenous infections or an annual incidence of only 0.04%.[76] But, no matter how small the risk of hematogenous infection may be, antibiotic prophylaxis against the transient bacteremia associated with certain diagnostic and/or therapeutic procedures may be warranted to avoid the disastrous consequences of an infected total joint replacement. This is especially applicable to high-risk patients, such as those with rheumatoid arthritis or others who are predisposed to bacterial infections. *An appropriate prophylactic regimen parallels the recommendations for patients with prosthetic cardiac valves.*[96]

SEPTIC ARTHRITIS ASSOCIATED WITH CRYSTALLINE ARTHRITIS

The simultaneous occurrence of septic arthritis and crystalline arthritis is relatively uncommon, but undiagnosed infection in the presence of acute gout or pseudogout may result in delayed treatment and poor outcome. On the other hand, inappropriate treatment for joint sepsis in acute arthritis caused by crystalline disease without infection can lead to serious side effects associated with antibiotic administration.[97] Coexistent septic arthritis and crystalline arthritis is often a disease of the elderly. The mean age in the 31 reported cases was 73 years with a median of 75 years, and ranged from 42 to 94 years.[98–100] In the 10 cases of coincident septic arthritis and gout, 6 had more than one affected joint. In the 17 cases of septic arthritis and pseudogout, the disease was monoarticular in all. Two of the four cases of septic arthritis coincident with both gout and pseudogout had polyarticular involvement. Overall, the knee was the most commonly affected joint.

Of these 31 patents 29 had bacterial causes; Mycobacterium marinum[101] and Candida albicans[102] were responsible for one case each. Mixed bacterial infection was present in only one case (caused by Pasteurella multocida and Pseudomonas aeruginosa).[103] Gram-positive and gram-negative organisms were isolated in 16 and 14 patients, respectively. Staphylococcus, streptococcus, and pneumococcus caused the gram-positive infections, whereas the spectrum of gram-negative microorganisms included bacilli (e.g., Escherichia coli, Serratia marcescens, and Pseudomonas aeruginosa), coccobacilli (e.g., Hemophilus influenzae and Pasteurella multocida), and cocci (e.g., Neisseria meningitidis and N. gonorrhoeae).

Experimental evidence suggests that the presence of infection promotes crystal "shedding" and precipitates acute crystalline arthritis superimposed on sepsis.[100] On the other hand, a joint previously damaged by crystalline arthritis may be more susceptible to infection during bacteremia. Thus, the coexistence of septic arthritis and acute crystalline arthritis may be more than a mere coincidence. Synovial fluid analysis of highly inflammatory or purulent-appearing joint fluid should include examination for crystals and microbiologic studies to ensure that neither condition is overlooked.*

SEPTIC ARTHRITIS OF THE FIBROCARTILAGINOUS JOINTS IN THE AXIAL SKELETON

The sternomanubrial joint and the symphysis pubis are midline fibrocartilaginous joints of the axial skel-

---

Editor's note. This situation is a genuine clinical problem. I know of a patient with gout who eventually suffered bilateral leg amputations from uncontrolled staphylococcal sepsis in both feet. The attending rheumatologist, finding urate crystals in joint aspirate, treated only with anti-inflammatory drugs until septic shock ensued.

eton that lack a synovial membrane. Various disease states, including many rheumatic diseases, can affect these two sites.[104,105] Primary bacterial infection is a rare cause of inflammation in these joints. Staphylococcus aureus infections of the sternomanubrial joint have been reported in a 38-year-old man with systemic lupus erythematosus,[106] a 20-year-old heroin user,[67] and a 42-year-old healthy man,[107] and Pseudomonas pseudomallei was cultured from the sternomanubrial joint of a 49-year-old Vietnam veteran.[108]

Bacterial infections of the symphysis pubis occur in children, in elderly debilitated patients, and in parenteral drug abusers.[109] Staphylococcus aureus is the major pathogen in children, whereas Pseudomonas aeruginosa is most common in adults. In the elderly, infection of the symphysis pubis is often related to diseases of the genitourinary system and their associated treatment. The susceptibility of intravenous drug abusers to bone and joint infections, with a propensity to affect the fibrocartilaginous articulations of the axial skeleton, has already been discussed. The clinical features of pyogenic osteitis pubis, or septic arthritis of the symphysis pubis, in drug addicts have been reviewed with an emphasis on the difficulty of diagnosis because of the poorly localized pain, the potentially misleading physical finding of hip disease, and the often normal radiographs.[65] Bone scintigraphy is useful to confirm inflammation of the symphysis pubis. Attempts to establish a bacterial etiology should include open biopsy of the joint and/or adjacent bone.

The sternoclavicular and sacroiliac joints are paired fibrocartilaginous joints of the axial skeleton that are synovial-lined. They are also affected by a variety of diseases[110,111] including bacterial infections where unilateral involvement is the rule. Predispositions to sternoclavicular joint infection include previous damage by an underlying arthritis and contamination of the venous bloodstream through venous channels, for example,. a subclavian catheter, hemodialysis, and intravenous drug abuse.[112] The diagnosis of a shoulder joint problem is often mistakenly made because the pain is diffuse and the motion of the shoulder is limited. Skillful physical examination and bone scintigraphy are useful to pinpoint the sternoclavicular joint. Tomograms may be necessary to visualize the destructive effects of infection. Microorganisms may be isolated from aspirated joint fluid, but surgical exploration may be necessary to obtain an adequate specimen for culture.

Infections of the sternoclavicular joint have been caused by Staphylococcus aureus, Streptococcus pneumoniae, other streptococci, Pseudomonas, Salmonella, Brucella, Escherichia coli, Hemophilus influenzae, Bacteroides species, Neisseria meningitidis, and Neisseria gonorrhoeae.[110] And infections caused by Streptococcus milleri,[112,113] group B streptococcus,[114] Serratia marcescens,[115] Acinetobacter anitratus,[66] and one case of polymicrobial infection caused by Streptococcus sanguis and Pasteurella multocida[116] have been reported.

Infection of the sacroiliac joint is an uncommon cause of sacroiliitis.[64,117–119] It is usually seen in young adults who present with acute or subacute pain in the buttock, hip, or flank associated with inability to bear weight because of pain. Mistaken diagnosis of intrinsic hip, back, intra-abdominal, or retroperitoneal disease and delayed therapy may accompany unfamiliarity with this entity and misleading physical findings. Pressure over the joint or any maneuver that distracts or compresses the joint[111] reproduces the pain. Blood cultures are positive in about one third of the cases.[64,120] The affected joint is best aspirated under fluoroscopy[121] or computed tomography (CT) guidance.[117]

The bacteriology of pyogenic sacroiliitis reflects the primary site of infection that seeds the joint through bacteremia. Staphylococcus aureus is the most frequently isolated pathogen in both children[122] and adults,[118–120] skin infections being the most common primary source. Tonsillitis, dental manipulation, and an infected tooth impaction were responsible for pyogenic sacroiliitis resulting from group A,[118] group B,[64] and group G[123] streptococcus, respectively. Urinary tract infections were associated with Escherichia coli and enterococcus sacroiliitis,[119] upper respiratory tract infection with Branhamella catarrhalis,[64] enteritis with Salmonella schwarzengrund,[118] and cervical carcinoma with group B streptococcus.[64] Intravenous drug abuse has led to sacroiliitis from Pseudomonas aeruginosa, Serratia marcescens, Staphylococcus aureus, and Enterobacter aerogenes.[64,124] Fusobacterium necrophorum,[125] Clostridium septicum, and Peptostreptococcus[126] are anaerobic microorganisms that have been found in sacroiliac joint infection. Brucellar sacroiliitis is discussed later under Microorganisms Acquired From Animals.

Rapid improvement follows early diagnosis and appropriate antibiotic treatment, but antibiotic treatment of bacterial infections affecting the fibrocartilaginous joints must often be prolonged because osteomyelitis of the adjacent bone is frequently present. Surgical exploration and drainage is indicated when a juxta-articular abscess is present or when sequestrectomy is necessary.[66,105,106,118,119]

OTHER PREDISPOSITIONS TO SEPTIC ARTHRITIS

Two uncommon underlying joint diseases that may provide fertile soil for superimposed septic arthritis are hemophiliac arthropathy and Charcot (neuropathic) joints. Staphylococcus aureus has caused infection of the "target" joint of hemophiliacs where recurrent intra-articular bleedings have previously occurred.[127] Traumatic hemarthrosis in elderly patients with osteoarthritis can become secondarily infected by S. aureus.[128] Charcot joints caused by tabes dorsalis, syringomyelia, or congenital insensitivity to pain have been sites of bacterial infection. Gram-positive cocci have caused this infectious complication in the knee,[129,130] shoulder,[130,131] and ankle.[132]

Other specific examples of increased host susceptibility to bacterial infections of bone and joint are illustrated by patients with chronic renal failure,[133,134] renal transplant,[135] and sickle cell anemia.[136,137] A report from a renal unit detailed the varied presentations and the difficulties in diagnosis and management of serious bone and joint infections among their patients.[134] Extradural abscesses in the lumbar region and diskitis with vertebral osteomyelitis and paravertebral abscess of the thoracic spine were commonly caused by Staphylococcus aureus. Infections of the sternoclavicular joint, and the large peripheral joints and long bones by Staphylococcus aureus, Pseudomonas, Serratia, and Proteus species are reminiscent of the skeletal infections seen in intravenous drug abusers (see Bone and Joint Infections Associated With Intravenouse Drug Abuse). Bomalaski et al. reviewed the spectrum of infectious arthritis among renal transplant patients.[135] In addition to Staphylococcus aureus and the more common gram-negative bacilli, other causes included Nocardia asteroides, Cryptococcus neoformans, Mycobacterium tuberculosis, M. chelonei, M. fortuitum, M. kansasii, M. scrofulaceum. M. gordonae, and cytomegalovirus. Immunosuppression against transplant rejection leaves the patient vulnerable to opportunistic infections, including septic arthritis.

Bacterial infections are a major cause of morbidity and mortality among patients with sickle cell anemia.[138] These patients and those with related hemoglobinopathies are at increased risk of bacterial meningitis, pneumococcal bactermia, and Salmonella osteomyelitis.[138] The musculoskeletal manifestations of sickle cell disease are protean and result from different pathogenetic mechanisms ranging from ischemic necrosis of the bone to synovitis, hemarthrosis, and secondary gout.[139] Bone and joint infections are relatively uncommon. The predilection of Salmonella species to cause osteomyelitis, and Streptococcus pneumoniae to cause septic arthritis are noteworthy.[136,137] The differentiation of ischemic bone infarcts from multifocal bacterial osteomyelitis is often difficult, and the exclusion of a bacterial cause of in-

flammatory joint fluid must be made.[139] Epidemiologic factors within a geographic region impact on the frequency of infection as well as the bacterial etiology.

Profound suppression of normal immunity is acquired through infection by the human immunodeficiency virus (HIV). Opportunistic infections abound among patients with the acquired immune deficiency syndrome (AIDS). Many are incurable and lead to death. Cases of septic arthritis caused by fungi, for example, Sporothrix schenckii,[140] and Cryptococcus neoformans[141] have been reported in AIDS patients.

POLYARTICULAR SEPTIC ARTHRITIS

Acute bacterial arthritis is most often monoarticular. Polyarticular infection, or multijoint (more than one joint) involvement, occurs in 5 to 8% of pediatric cases (see Table 115–1) and in 10 to 19% of nongonococcal adult cases.[33,142] Polyarticular infection is a function of the bacteria as well as the host.[33] Bacteria that have a predilection for polyarticular involvement are Neisseria gonorrhoeae,[19] Streptococcus pneumoniae, group G streptococcus, and Hemophilus influenzae.[33] But the most common microorganism recovered in cases of multijoint septic arthritis is Staphylococcus aureus. Prior disease in multiple joints predisposes to polyarticular septic arthritis. Patients with septic joints superimposed on RA have an 18[33] to 35%[143] rate of polyarticular involvement. Of the cases reviewed in Table 115–3, 25% had polyarticular septic arthritis. Septic arthritis superimposed on gout had a polyarticular pattern in 60% of the cases compared with only monoarticular infections among the patients with concomitant pseudogout. The importance of polyarticular septic arthritis is at least twofold. First, knowledge of its relative frequency may avoid misdiagnosis or delay in diagnosis. Second, its poor outcome (23% mortality) is primarily due to the subgroup of patients with RA who had 56% mortality.[33]

POLYMICROBIAL SEPTIC ARTHRITIS

Polymicrobial septic arthritis (two or more bacterial species) is rare in a natural joint unless penetrating trauma occurred or recent surgery was performed. Combinations of gram-positive, gram-negative, mixed gram-positive and gram-negative, aerobic, and anaerobic microorganisms have all been encountered.[144,145] Most instances of polymicrobic infection involve two different microorganisms, but cases with three or four microbes have been reported.[144,145] In one review,[144] hip infections were most common among the 12 adults, many resulting from a communication of a retroperitoneal or pelvic abscess directly with the hip. In prosthetic joint infections, 6 to 25% of the cases were polymicrobic,[72,82] and early postoperative wound infections accounted for most of these infections.

PATHOGENS CAUSING BACTERIAL ARTHRITIS

ANAEROBIC BACTERIA

Anaerobic bacteria are probably responsible for less than 1% of all cases of acute hematogenous septic arthritis affecting natural joints. Finegold's review included data from the preantibiotic era,[146] and found that over one third of 180 anaerobic joint infections were caused by Fusobacterium necrophorum. Anaerobic cocci, Bacteroides fragilis, and other Fusobacterium, Bacteroides, and Clostridium species accounted for most of the other cases of anaerobic bacterial arthritis.

Anaerobes are found more frequently (5 to 10%) in infected joint prostheses.[78,79] The Mayo Clinic experience noted two different clinical settings where anaerobic bacteria caused joint infection[147]; most cases occurred after joint surgery, 53% after reconstructive surgery, and 28% after trauma. In these postoperative infections, anaerobic cocci, for example, Peptococcus and Peptostreptococcus species, were the major pathogens. But Bacteroides fragilis was the most frequent cause of a second type of infection (19%), occurring in patients with chronic illnesses such as inflammatory bowel disease, rheumatoid arthritis, psoriatic arthritis, and chronic osteomyelitis. The anaerobic bacteria seeding the joints by the bloodstream arose from intra-abdominal sources or decubitus ulcers. Another route of infection was the extension of chronic osteomyelitis into the adjacent joint. This latter group of patients with nonsurgery-related anaerobic septic arthritis had 50% mortality, and the poor outcome was attributed to their debilitated antecedent condition.

GRAM-POSITIVE COCCI

The gram-positive cocci of the Micrococcaceae and Streptococcaceae families are responsible for the great majority of all cases of nongonococcal bacterial arthritis.[148-152] Staphylococcus species, predominantly Staphylococcus aureus and occasionally coagulase-negative staphylococci, and rarely Micrococcus species,[52] represent the Micrococcaceae family. The Strep-

tococcaceae family includes the various species of hemolytic streptococci, the different groups of viridans streptococci including the pneumococcus, and Aerococcus species. These gram-positive cocci account for 50 to 90% of all cases of nongonococcal septic arthritis.

Staphylococci are the major cause of septic arthritis among the gram-positive cocci. In the elderly, Staphylococcus aureus causes 43 to 64% of all cases (see Table 115–2). In rheumatoid arthritis patients, 77% of joint infections are caused by S. aureus (see Table 115–3). In prosthetic joint infections, 75 to 90% of the gram-positive microorganisms are staphylococci, albeit S. epidermidis may be more common than S. aureus. In the neonate, staphylococci are responsible for 25% of the community-acquired joint infections and 62% of the nosocomial cases of septic arthritis. Overall, 13 to 44% of all cases of childhood septic arthritis are due to S. aureus (see Table 115–1), a low estimate because many cases are not bacteriologically confirmed (about 30%), and Hemophilus influenzae is another predominant pathogen among young children.

Staphylococcus aureus may cause *septic diskitis* (Fig. 115–1). CT and/or radionuclide scintigraphy are often positive early in the course of the condition when plain films are negative. Needle aspiration of the disc under fluoroscopic guidance using an image intensifier, or direct surgical tissue biopsy should be done to obtain a precise diagnosis.

The microbiologic, clinical, therapeutic, and preventive aspects of diseases caused by Staphylococcus aureus have been reviewed recently.[153] Special therapeutic consideration against methicillin-resistant staphylococci includes the empiric use of vancomycin in areas where resistant microorganisms are prevalent[7] while culture and antibiotic-sensitivity results are pending. Vancomycin resistance has been reported in coagulase-negative staphylococci isolated from the peritoneal fluid of a diabetic patient receiving continuous ambulatory peritoneal dialysis.[154] A promising class of antimicrobial agents, the fluoroquinolones, are active in vitro against methicillin-resistant S. aureus, as well as multiply antibiotic-resistant gram-negative bacilli and β-lactamase-producing Neisseria gonorrhoeae.[155] Use of the fluoroquinolones might be considered in patients with serious infections caused by methicillin-resistant staphylococci when vancomycin cannot be used, or when β-lactams or aminoglycosides are contraindicated.[156]

Streptococcal septic arthritis accounts for 15 to 30% of all nongonococcal causes of bacterial arthritis and is second only to the staphylococci. Most are due to Streptococcus pyogenes (group A). Joint infections caused by group B (S. agalactiae) and group G strep-

FIG. 115–1. Septic infection of the spine due to staphylococci. *A,* Conventional lateral radiograph demonstrates mild disc-space narrowing and dissolution of the vertebral end plate. The extensive destruction of the cancellous bone may only be detected tomographically, as shown in lateral *(B)* and anteroposterior *(C)* projections.

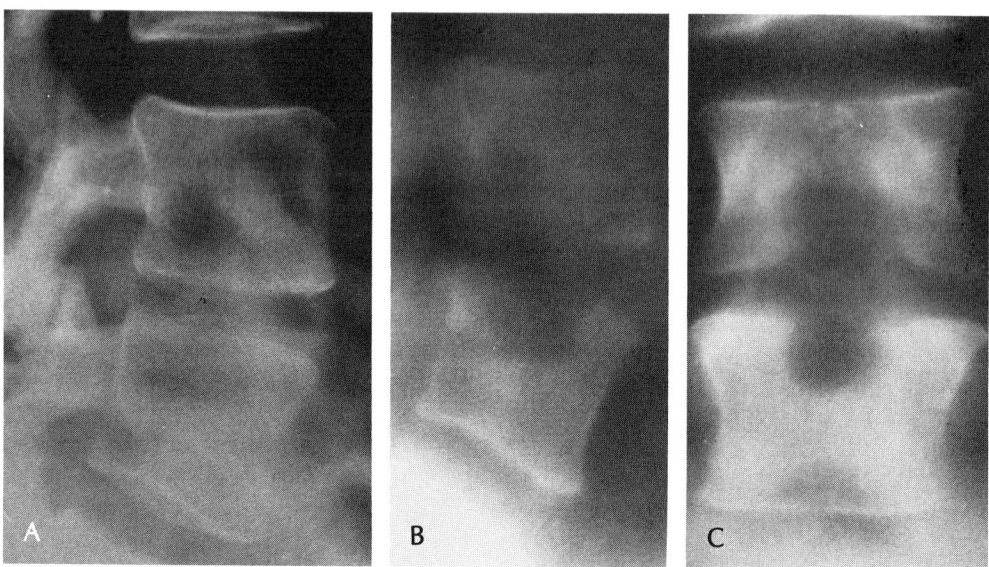

tococci have been further elucidated. Diabetes mellitus is a major predisposition to group B streptococcal septic arthritis.[83,157] Among adults with group B streptococcal joint infection, 20% have polyarticular disease,[33,158] and involvement of the joints of the axial skeleton[157] and prosthetic joints[83] is common. The disease can be aggressive, leading to functional loss and significant morbidity and mortality.[83,157] Group B streptococcus is also a major pathogen of community-acquired septic arthritis in neonates.[6]

Serious group G streptococcal infection occurs in patients with neoplastic disease, alcoholism, and diabetes mellitus.[159] Septic arthritis caused by group G streptococcus was often polyarticular (25% of 36 cases).[58] More than one-third of the patients had underlying rheumatoid disease, and over one fourth of the infections affected a prosthetic joint. Polymicrobial infection, frequently associated with Staphylococcus aureus, probably indicates the skin as the common portal of entry.[58,159] Prepatellar bursitis caused by group G streptococcus was noted in 8% of 38 cases.[58]

Streptococcus pneumoniae has remained an uncommon cause of joint infection. Predispositions include alcoholism, hypogammaglobulinemia,[160] underlying joint disease such as RA,[57] gout,[161] and joint prostheses.[84] Often, the primary pneumococcal infection is meningitis, pneumonia, or rarely endocarditis, with secondary bacteremic seeding of the joint, but one or more joints may be the primary and only site(s)

of infection.[160] Polyarticular pneumococcal infection is common[33] possibly reflecting impairments in host defense such as decreased serum chemotactic factors[162] or rheumatoid disease.[57]

Septic arthritis caused by group C streptococcus is rare. Reported cases include a 13-year-old boy with a neuropathic ankle joint[132] and three adults,[163–165] including one with polyarticular infection in conjunction with gouty arthritis[164] and another patient, a 42-year-old horse trainer, with a septic knee who may have acquired the infection from a horse.[165] Group D enterococcus is another rare cause of septic arthritis. Zwillich et al. reported two adults, one with a knee infection and another with rheumatoid arthritis and enterococcal infection in a hip prosthesis.[166] The first patient required an above-knee amputation because of recurrence and osteomyelitis, and the second underwent a Girdlestone excision arthroplasty. Unlike other streptococcal joint infections where penicillin is the drug of choice, enterococcal disease requires a combined regimen of ampicillin and gentamicin similar to that used in enterococcal endocarditis.[166] A woman with septic arthritis of a hip caused by Aerococcus viridans responded to treatment with penicillin and open drainage.[167] This microorganism is similar to other viridans streptococci, but may be confused with enterococcus. Other viridans streptococci that have caused septic arthritis include Streptococcus sanguis,[116] S. milleri,[113] ad S. anginosus-constellatus.[112]

GRAM-POSITIVE BACILLI

Gram-positive bacillary septic arthritis is extremely rare. Listeria monocytogenes most commonly causes meningitis and bacteremia in hosts who are compromised by hematologic or lymphoproliferative malignancy, renal transplantation or other nonmalignant disease requiring corticosteroid therapy, or alcoholism.[168] Septic arthritis caused by L. monocytogenes has been reported in patients with long-standing rheumatoid disease[51,169] or gout.[170] Other gram-positive bacilli include Corynebacterium pyogenes, seen in a septic knee of a 70-year-old man with advanced osteoarthritis,[171] Bacillus cereus, cultured from the knee fluid of a 24-year-old Marine after diagnostic arthrography,[172] and Bacillus species, isolated from the metatarsophalangeal joint of the great toe of a 27-year-old woman following repair of a flexor tendon injury complicated by a wound infection.[173]

GRAM-NEGATIVE COCCI AND COCCOBACILLI

The two most important gram-negative cocci that infect joints are Neisseria gonorrhoeae and Neisseria meningitidis. The former is the subject of Chapter 116 and the latter is discussed below. Other members of the family Neisseriaceae that have caused joint infection include Branhamella, Moraxella, and Kingella species. Branhamella catarrhalis was implicated in pyogenic sacroiliitis in a 15-year-old girl with an upper respiratory tract infection[64] and septic arthritis of the hip in a 23-year-old Navajo man.[174]

Joint infections caused by Moraxella or Kingella species are uncommon and usually have an indolent course because of the low pathogenicity of these bacteria.[175] Morphologic resemblance to Hemophilus influenzae and Neisseria gonorrhoeae has been noted.[175,176] Young children (under 4 years) appear especially vulnerable.[175-179] Kingella kingae septic arthritis has been reported in a 49-year-old alcoholic,[180] a 51-year-old woman with rheumatoid arthritis and Felty's syndrome,[50] and a 76-year-old man with chronic lung disease.[181]

Neisseria Meningitidis

Arthritis is estimated to complicate 2 to 10% of all cases of meningococcal disease.[182] The articular manifestations of meningococcal infection have been divided arbitrarily into three types based on the clinical features of the systemic illness.[183] Most common is *joint involvement accompanying acute meningococcal disease.* Among 15,387 cases of acute meningococcal infection, 1075 (7%) had this type of arthritis, monoarticular in 56% and polyarticular in 44%. Its onset either coincided with the acute systemic illness or was delayed from 1 to 12 days after the appearance of the acute meningococcal disease. Often the patient has responded to antibiotic treatment when the joint problem appears, which had led to speculation on pathogenetic mechanisms other than direct bacterial invasion of the synovium. Evidence supporting an immunologic pathogenesis includes immune complex formation and complement activation but is not conclusive.[184] The presence of Neisseria meningitidis in the synovial fluid documented by culture and/or by Gram-stain proves the direct seeding by the bloodstream, but joint fluid cultures have been positive in only 21% of the cases studied (47/222).[183]

The other two types of joint involvement are much less common, and include the *arthritis of chronic meningococcemia* and *primary meningococcal arthritis.* Rather than distinct and separate clinical entities, these represent segments within the spectrum of meningococcal joint disease. Synovial fluid cultures are rarely positive in chronic meningococcemia but are often positive (80 to 90%) in primary meningococcal arthritis. Blood cultures are, by definition, positive in chronic meningococcemia, and are positive in approximately 40% of the cases of primary meningococcal arthritis. Primary meningococcal arthritis is more often monoarticular (66%) than polyarticular (33%) and almost invariably affects the large joints, especially the knee.[183] A rash can be seen in all three types of articular involvement and requires differentiation from other acute arthritis-dermatitis syndromes, the most common of which is disseminated gonococcal infection (DGI). Helpful differential points are the number of skin lesions and their location and appearance. Skin lesions are more numerous in meningococcemia than in gonococcemia.[185] The lesions associated with meningococcemia are generalized and maculopapular or petechial in nature, whereas the skin manifestations of gonococcemia are located distally and usually consist of petechial lesions that evolve into pustules on an erythematous base.[186] Tenosynovitis is a prominent feature of gonococcal joint disease, seen in upward of two thirds of all cases, but it also occurs in some cases of meningococcal arthritis.[186-188] A survey from Seattle notes the increasing importance of Neisseria meningitidis relative to Neisseria gonorrhoeae as the cause of the acute arthritis-dermatitis syndrome.[185]

Hemophilus Influenzae

Hemophilus influenzae is an aerobic, pleomorphic, gram-negative coccobacillus. Of the typeable strains, type B is the major pathogen in humans. In adults, it is an important cause of pneumonia, meningitis, epiglottitis, and acute sinusitis.[189] Less commonly, it infects the diarthrodial joint. H. influenzae is the etiologic agent in less than 1% of all bacterial causes of septic arthritis in adults.[151] In children, the spectrum of disease caused by H. influenzae includes bacteremia, meningitis, pneumonia, epiglottitis, arthritis, cellulitis, osteomyelitis, and pericarditis.[190] Septic arthritis accounts for about 8% of all H. influenzae infections in children.[190] Among the bacterial causes of septic arthritis in children, H. influenzae is a major pathogen that rivals Staphylococcus aureus (see Bacterial Arthritis in Children).

Peak vulnerability to Hemophilus influenzae arthritis is between the ages of 6 months and 2 years old. Children under 3 months and over 5 years old are much less likely to experience H. influenzae joint infection. The disease in children is usually monoarticular and affects predominantly the large joints of the lower extremity.[1] Joint infection often follows an upper respiratory tract infection and/or otitis media and results from the hematogenous dissemination of the bacteria.[190,191] Hemophilus influenzae arthritis in children is associated with concurrent meningitis (8 to 30%) and osteomyelitis (12 to 22%).[190,191]

The adult disease has some different clinical features in addition to its rarity. Systemic or local predisposition to infection was present in two thirds of 25 cases.[192] The infection was monoarticular in 12 (48%) polyarticular in 6 (24%), and accompanied by tenosynovitis and/or bursitis in 7 (28%). Six additional cases have been reported since 1983,[193-195] and five of the six had a systemic predisposition to infection.[193,195] Four had polyarticular infection,[194,195] one had septic olecranon bursitis without joint involvement,[193] and the other had an infected hip prosthesis.[195] Thus, Hemophilus influenzae arthritis in an adult can mimic the polyarthritis and tenosynovitis of gonococcal infection, resemble septic olecranon bursitis most commonly caused by Staphylococcus aureus,[196] or involve a prosthetic joint. Although ampicillin is the drug of choice against *sensitive* Hemophilus influenzae, the initial antibiotic agent directed at suspected H. influenzae infection should be chloramphenicol or cefuroxime because of possible ampicillin resistance.

GRAM-NEGATIVE BACILLI

Gram-negative bacilli account for 7 to 26%[27,197] of adult nongonococcal cases of septic arthritis. Ruth-berg and Ho[198] noted that 17% of 412 cases of septic arthritis in adults between 1934 and 1980 had been caused by these microorganisms. Analysis of the data from three periods (pre-1960, 1960s, and 1970s) showed a steady increase in the frequency of gram-negative bacillary arthritis of 6%, 14%, and 27% respectively. This trend could reflect the progressively increasing frequency of gram-negative bacteremia in general.[28] Among the elderly with septic arthritis, 24% of cases are due to gram-negative bacilli (see Table 115–2). Among rheumatoid patients, the percentage is 11%. Intravenous drug abusers are especially prone to bone and joint infections from Pseudomonas,[29,199] Serratia,[30,124] and Staphylococcus. Gram-negative bacilli are responsible for less than 10% of joint infections among children over 2 years of age,[197] but those under 2 years old are more susceptible to gram-negative bacillary joint infection (28%)[197] and these are also more prevalent in nosocomial than in community-acquired infections among neonates.[6] Of prosthetic joint infections, 10 to 20% are due to aerobic gram-negative rods.

Two series of cases highlight the major features of the two ends of the spectrum of gram-negative bacillary joint infections.[27,200] Host factors determine many of the clinical features including the microbiology, the site of the joint infection, and the outcome of treatment. The series of 13 patients from Boston University[27] is characteristic of the older patient population (mean age 56 years) with serious underlying systemic diseases and pre-existing joint disease who had Escherichia coli or Proteus mirabilis septic arthritis seeded hematogenously from the urinary tract or the biliary tract. Less commonly, Serratia marcescens, Pseudomonas aeruginosa, and Salmonella species caused the infections. The patients were often receiving antibiotic and/or corticosteroid medications, and the monoarticular infection most commonly affected the knee. Many failed to respond to medical treatment and required subsequent surgical debridement. The mortality was high and the cure rate low. In contrast, the series of 21 patients from UCLA[200] is representative of the younger patient population (mean age 29 years) whose primary predisposition was intravenous drug abuse. Otherwise healthy, many had infections localized to the sternal articulations caused by Pseudomonas aeruginosa. Escherichia coli and Proteus mirabilis were less commonly encountered, and single cases were due to Enterobacter aerogenes, E. liquefaciens, Klebsiella pneumoniae, Eikenella corrodens, Acinetobacter anitratus, and Bacteroides fragilis. Despite the frequent occurrence of juxta-articular osteomyelitis and/or periarticular abscess requiring surgery, the cure rate was 90% and the mortality only 5%.

Among the members of the Enterobacteriaceae family, Escherichia coli and Proteus mirabilis are the most frequent causative agents of septic arthritis followed by Klebsiella, Enterobacter, Serratia, and Morganella species. Salmonella species,[201,202] Arizona hinshawii,[203] Yersinia enterocolitica,[204,205] and Campylobacter fetus[206] have been isolated from synovial fluids, but reactive arthritis following gastrointestinal infection by Salmonella, Yersinia, Shigella flexneri, or Campylobacter jejuni is a more common problem associated with these pathogens (see Chapter 60).[207,208]

Pseudomonas aeruginosa is a member of the Pseudomonadaceae family and is an important cause of gram-negative septic arthritis in chronically debilitated older patients with serious systemic illnesses as well as younger parenteral drug abusers (see Bone and Joint Infections Associated With Intravenous Drug Abuse). In addition to an aminoglycoside, usually gentamicin, an antipseudomonal semisynthetic penicillin is often used for its prolonged treatment of up to 4 to 6 weeks.[31] A case of P. aeruginosa infection of the knee in a 73-year-old diabetic woman failed to respond to gentamicin and azlocillin. Treatment with a third-generation cephalosporin, ceftazidime, intravenously and intra-articularly was then successful.[209] The direct instillation of antibiotics into infected joints has not been studied extensively because most parenterally administered antibiotic agents penetrate into the synovial fluid without difficulty.[210,211]

The spectrum of gram-negative bacillary septic arthritis is constantly expanding with reports of a new isolation. Examples of such occurrences include joint infections caused by Capnocytophaga ochracea,[212] Plesiomonas shigelloides,[48] and Aeromonas hydrophila.[75,213,214]

MICROORGANISMS ACQUIRED FROM ANIMALS

Pasteurella Multocida

This small, aerobic, facultatively anaerobic, gram-negative coccobacillus is found in the normal oral flora of many domestic and wild animals.[215] Human infections can result from casual contact with cats or dogs or more commonly from their bites and scratches. Of 446 cases of human infection by Pasteurella multocida, 48% affected the skin, 14% the oral and respiratory tract, 13% the cardiovascular system, 13% the skeletal and articular system, followed by the central nervous system (5%), the gastrointestinal tract (4%), the genitourinary tract (2%), and the eye (1%).[215] The bone and joint infections separate into three distinct categories: osteomyelitis, septic arthritis with osteomyelitis, and septic arthritis alone.[216] Osteomyelitis results as the soft-tissue wound infection extends to the adjacent bone or by direct inoculation of P. multocida into the periosteum by a bite. Common sites of osteomyelitis are the forearm, leg, hand, and wrist. Almost all the cases of septic arthritis with osteomyelitis affect the small joints and bones of the hand after cat bites. Few patients had any underlying systemic illness predisposing to bacterial infection.

In sharp contrast, septic arthritis caused by P. multocida without osteomyelitis rarely occurs in the host who is not immunocompromised or in a joint not previously damaged. Chronic RA requiring corticosteroid treatment is the most common pre-existing illness and is also the most common underlying joint disease. Here the hematogenous route of bacterial dissemination rather than local extension or direct penetration is important. This route is suggested by the presence of bacteremia and polyarticular infection.[86,217] The infection is usually monoarticular and affects the knee joint most commonly. Almost a third of the reported cases have involved total knee replacements.[216] This observation may merely reflect the increased susceptibility to infection of a patient with long-standing RA. However, P. multocida infection of bilateral knee prostheses in a patient with osteoarthritis has been reported.[86] Joint infection with P. multocida has been reported in association with Staphylococcus aureus in a prosthetic knee,[218] with Streptococcus sanguis in a sternoclavicular joint,[116] and with Pseudomonas aeruginosa in a patient with bilateral knee prostheses.[86]

Penicillin is the agent of choice for treatment of Pasteurella multocida septic arthritis. Drainage of the infected joint is necessary. In the cases of infected knee prostheses, some were able to retain the artificial joint,[217,219] but others required its eventual removal.[86,218]

Rat-bite Fever

Another infectious disease that affects the articular system is transmitted by the bite of rodents. Two microorganisms, Streptobacillus moniliformis, a pleomorphic gram-negative rod, and Spirillum minus, a spirochete, can cause rat-bite fever. Both are normal flora in the oropharynx of many rodents. Streptobacillary infection presents with fever, a morbilliform or petechial rash, and polyarticular pain 2 to 10 days after a rodent bite. Rarely, Streptobacillus moniliformis has been isolated from the joint fluid.[220,221] Spirillum minus causes a febrile illness after an incubation period of over 10 days. Joint symptoms are rare, but regional adenopathy draining the site of the bite is common. Treatment of rat-bite fever is with penicillin for both causative agents.

Brucellosis

Brucellosis has a worldwide distribution, and the pathogenic species differ depending on the geographic location. The four species that cause human disease are Brucella melitensis, B. abortus, B. suis, and B. canis. The clinical manifestations and the severity of disease vary according to the responsible species and the host.[222,223] Human hosts acquire the disease from infected animals. Ingestion of raw milk or dairy products made from unpasteurized milk, inhalation of aerosolized bacteria, or contact with the contaminated animal through broken skin or conjunctiva are the known routes of acquiring the infection. The spectrum of organ system involvement by brucellosis has been reviewed by Young.[222] Examples of ingestion-acquired, laboratory-acquired, and abattoir-acquired disease are well illustrated. A comprehensive review of 304 cases of human infection by B. melitensis from Lima, Peru found joint involvement in a third (33.8%) of the patients.[223] Sacroiliitis (46.6%), peripheral arthritis (38.8%), or the combination of sacroiliitis and arthritis (7.8%) accounted for 93.2% of the musculoskeletal involvement and tended to occur in young patients with acute infection. Spondylitis (6.8%) was most common in the lumbosacral region and tended to affect older patients with more chronic infection. The pathogenesis of the latter is believed to be infection beginning at the disc space with contiguous involvement of the adjacent vertebral body and eventual vertebral osteomyelitis. Paraspinal abscess formation can complicate vertebral brucellosis and may be the cause of resistance to antibiotic treatment until the abscess is found and drained.[224] Sacroiliitis is usually unilateral and nondestructive and responds to antibiotic treatment. The peripheral arthritis also responds to antibiotic treatment, but remits spontaneously at times, raising the possibility of a reactive form of brucellar arthritis.[223] Recovery of the microorganism from the sacroiliac joint, sternoclavicular joint, or other peripheral joints is uncommon but well-documented.[222,223,225,226]

In the United States, Brucella melitensis infections are uncommon relative to B. abortus and B. suis. Brucella canis has been responsible for at least two cases of septic arthritis in children.[222,227] A popular antibiotic regimen against brucellosis consists of tetracycline plus streptomycin, but trimethoprim-sulfamethoxazole, rifampin, and the third-generation cephalosporins have all been used with some success.[222,227,228]

SPIROCHETES

Spirillum minus is a rare cause of rat-bite fever in the United States. Lyme arthritis, first described by Steere and Malawista is now known to be caused by Borrelia burgdorferi and is the subject of Chapter 119. Another spirochete, Treponema pallidum, is responsible for syphilitic joint disease.[229] Arthritis as a result of primary or secondary syphilis is rare. In tertiary syphilis, arthritis can result from gummata deposited in the juxta-articular tissue, cartilage, or bone. Large, usually painless, effusions with little evidence of limitation of motion are the characteristics of gummatous arthritis. Syphilitic spondylitis is an osteitis caused by the invasion of bone and periosteum by Treponema pallidum. Charcot's joint secondary to lues is a complication of tabes dorsalis and primarily involves the weight-bearing articulations (see Chapter 81).

Congenital syphilis has been associated with several musculoskeletal syndromes. *Parrot's pseudoparalysis* is an osteochondritis affecting the epiphysis and articular cartilage of the humerus or the tibia of neonates and infants within the first 3 months of life. *Clutton's joint* is a late sequela of congenital syphilis

Table 115–4. Summary of Principles for Diagnosis and Management of Septic Arthritis Caused by Bacteria[236]

1. Suspect septic arthritis in a patient: (a) with debilitating disease, especially neoplastic or hepatic disease; (b) who is taking corticosteroids or immunosuppressive agents; (c) who has infection elsewhere, even if receiving antibiotics; or (d) who has pre-existing joint damage from another type of arthritis.

2. Diagnose septic arthritis by synovial fluid smear and culture, or by counterimmunoelectrophoresis for bacterial antigens. High fluid concentrations of lactate and other organic acids, especially succinate, fluid glucose levels 40 mg/dl or more below plasma glucose levels (after fasting), and poor mucin clot suggest bacterial sepsis. Fluid leukocyte concentrations are usually high; polymorphonuclear leukocytes predominate (>90%).

3. Splint affected joint initially, give analgesic, and mobilize joint as inflammation subsides with antibiotic treatment.

4. Treat with parenteral antibiotics after obtaining synovial fluid and blood cultures but before obtaining the results; time is important. A direct correlation exists between the duration of symptoms before treatment and the time needed to sterilize joint fluid once treatment is begun.[23] Prescribe empiric antibiotic regimen using clinical clues as to the probable causative agent. Do not inject antibiotics into the joint because they are irritants and may confuse the clinical picture. Aminoglycoside effectiveness decreases by an order of magnitude at pH 6.5; synovial fluid pH correlates with local leukocyte concentration.[237] Hence, drainage of exudate is particularly important.

5. Decompress joint by daily needle drainage, which gives better results than open drainage, except in infections of long duration and in deeply situated joints, where needle drainage is technically difficult.

6. Follow daily joint fluid leukocyte count and cultures for prognosis. Serial fall in leukocyte count and sterile fluid correlate with a good outcome.[23]

Table 115–5. Antibiotic Therapy Regimens for Bacterial Arthritis*

Microorganism	Antibiotic of Choice	Alternative Drugs
Enterobacteriaceae	A third-generation cephalosporin (cefotaxime, ceftizoxime, or ceftriaxone)	Imipenem Aztreonam Ampicillin An aminoglycoside (not alone)
Pseudomonas aeruginosa	Ticarcillin or other antipseudomonal penicillin plus an aminoglycoside	An aminoglycoside plus ceftazidime, imipenem, or aztreonam
Hemophilus influenzae	Ampicillin	Cefuroxime A third-generation cephalosporin Chloramphenicol
Neisseria gonorrhoeae	Penicillin G	Ceftriaxone Erythromycin
Streptococcus	Penicillin G	Cefazolin Vancomycin Clindamycin
Enterococcus	Penicillin or ampicillin plus gentamicin	Vancomycin plus an aminoglycoside
Staphylococcus aureus	Nafcillin	Cefazolin Vancomycin Clindamycin
Methicillin-resistant staphylococcus	Vancomycin	

*Table prepared with the assistance of John M. Boyce, M.D., and Antone A. Medeiros, M.D. of the Division of Infectious Diseases at the Miriam Hospital.

manifested by chronic hydrarthrosis of one or both knees in children between 6 and 16 years old.

MYCOPLASMA

Mycoplasmas as agents of human disease have been reviewed by Cassell and Cole.[230] Septic arthritis has resulted from infection by Mycoplasma hominis, M. pneumoniae, and Ureaplasma urealyticum. Some patients with hypogammaglobulinemia develop polyarthritis resembling rheumatoid disease, and from their joint fluids, mycoplasmas and ureaplasmas have been cultured.[231,232] Mycoplasma joint disease is responsive to antibiotic treatment; tetracycline or erythromycin are used most frequently. Prosthetic joint infection with Mycoplasma hominis has been reported in a patient with RA[88] and treated successfully with ciprofloxacin.

NOCARDIA

Nocardia are aerobic, gram-positive, partially acid-fast bacteria that form branching filaments. Nocardia asteroides and N. brasiliensis are the major pathogens causing human disease. Septic arthritis from either organism is rare. The reported cases are usually in compromised hosts receiving corticosteroids or other immunosuppressive drugs.[233–235] Trimethoprim and sulfamethoxazole appear to be the antibiotic combination of choice. Treatment duration is usually prolonged, from months to a year.

THERAPY

Suggested antimicrobial therapy has been discussed in the sections dealing with specific organisms. The principles for diagnosis and management are summarized in Table 115–4. Draining with repeated needle aspiration must produce repeated success in relieving local pus accumulation. Serial fall in total leukocyte count and sterility of aspirate are good omens and correlate with a good outcome.[23]

A summary of recommended antimicrobials and alternative drugs is provided in Table 115–5 for the most common organisms causing bacterial arthritis. Drug dosages and duration of treatment must be determined for each case.

REFERENCES

1. Fink, C.W., and Nelson, J.D.: Septic arthritis and osteomyelitis in children. Clin. Rheum. Dis., 12:423–435, 1986.
2. Sequeira, W., Swedler, W.I., and Skosey, J.L.: Septic arthritis in childhood. Ann. Emerg. Med., 14:1185–1187, 1985.
3. Wilson, N.I.L., and Di Paola, M.: Acute septic arthritis in infancy and childhood: 10 years' experience. J. Bone Joint Surg., 68B:584–587, 1986.

4. Speiser, J.C., et al.: Changing trends in pediatric septic arthritis. Semin. Arthritis Rheum., 15:132–138, 1985.

5. Welkon, C.J., Long, S.S., Fisher, M.C., and Alburger, P.D.: Pyogenic arthritis in infants and children: A review of 95 cases. Pediatr. Infect. Dis., 5:669–676, 1986.

6. Dan, M.: Septic arthritis in young infants: Clinical and microbiologic correlations and therapeutic implications. Rev. Infect. Dis., 6:147–155, 1984.

7. Ang-Fonte, G.Z., Rozboril, M.B., and Thompson, G.R.: Changes in nongonococcal septic arthritis: Drug abuse and methicillin-resistant Staphylococcus aureus. Arthritis Rheum., 28:210–213, 1985.

8. Scoles, P.V., and Aronoff, S.C.: Antimicrobial therapy of childhood skeletal infections. J. Bone Joint Surg., 66A:1487–1492, 1984.

9. Poretz, D.M., et al.: Intravenous antibiotic therapy in an outpatient setting. JAMA, 248:336–339, 1982.

10. Rehm, S.J., and Weinstein, A.J.: Home intravenous antibiotic therapy: A team approach. Ann. Intern. Med., 99:388–392, 1983.

11. Tetzlaff, T.R., McCracken, G.H., Jr., and Nelson, J.D.: Oral antibiotic therapy for skeletal infections of children. II. Therapy of osteomyelitis and suppurative arthritis. J. Pediatr., 92:485–490, 1978.

12. Herndon, W.A., Knauer, S., Sullivan, J.A., and Gross, R.H.: Management of septic arthritis in children. J. Pediatr. Orthop., 6:576–578, 1986.

13. Gillspie, R.: Septic arthritis in childhood. Clin. Orthop., 96:152–159, 1973.

14. Howard, J.B., Highgenboten, C.L., and Nelson, J.D.: Residual effects of septic arthritis in infancy and childhood. JAMA, 236:932–935, 1976.

15. U.S. Senate Special Committee on Aging: Size and growth of the older population. In Aging America. Trends and Projections. 1985–86 Edition. U.S. Govt. Printing Office, 1986.

16. Kelly, P.J.: Bacterial arthritis in the adult. Orthop. Clin. North Am., 6:973–981, 1975.

17. Newman, J.H.: Review of septic arthritis throughout the antibiotic era. Ann. Rheum. Dis., 35:198–205, 1976.

18. Ho, G., Jr., et al.: Rheumatologic disorders in the elderly. In Contemporary Geriatric Medicine. Vol. III. Edited by S.R. Gambert. New York, Plenum Medical Publishers (in press).

19. Goldenberg, D.L., and Reed, J.I.: Bacterial arthritis. N. Engl. J. Med., 312:764–771, 1985.

20. Schneider, E.L.: Infectious diseases in the elderly. Ann. Intern. Med., 98:395–400, 1983.

21. Cooper, C., and Cawley, M.I.D.: Bacterial arthritis in the elderly. Gerontology, 32:222–227, 1986.

22. McGuire, N.M., and Kauffman, C.A.: Septic arthritis in the elderly. J. Am. Geriatr. Soc., 33:170–174, 1985.

23. Ho, G., Jr., and Su, E.Y.: Therapy of septic arthritis. JAMA, 247:797–800, 1982.

24. Willkens R.F., Healey, L.A., and Decker, J.L.: Acute infectious arthritis in the aged and chronically ill. Arch. Intern. Med., 106:354–364, 1960.

25. Geelhoed-Duyvestijn, P.H.L.M., et al.: Disseminated gonococcal infection in the elderly patients. Arch. Intern. Med., 146:1739–1740, 1986.

26. Straus, S.E., Vest, J.V., and Glew, R.H.: Gonococcal arthritis in the elderly. South. Med. J., 71:214–215, 1978.

27. Goldenberg, D.L., Brandt, K.D., Cathcart, E.S., and Cohen, A.S.: Acute arthritis caused by gram-negative bacilli: A clinical characterization. Medicine (Baltimore), 53:197–208, 1974.

28. Kreger, B.E., Craven, D.E., Carling, P.C., and McCabe, W.R.: Gram-negative bacteremia. III. Reassessment of etiology, epidemiology and ecology in 612 patients. Am. J. Med., 68:332–343, 1980.

29. Miskew, D.B., Lorenz, M.A., Pearson, R.L., and Pankovich, A.M.: Pseudomonas aeruginosa bone and joint infection in drug abusers. J. Bone Joint Surg., 65A:829–832, 1983.

30. Donovan, T.L., Chapman, M.W., Harrington, K.D., and Nagel, D.A.: Serratia arthritis: Report of seven cases. J. Bone Joint Surg., 58A:1009–1011, 1976.

31. Schmid, F.R.: Routine drug treatment of septic arthritis. Clin. Rheum. Dis., 10:293–311, 1984.

32. Broy, S.B., and Schmid, F.R.: A comparison of medical drainage and surgical drainage in the initial treatment of infected joints. Clin. Rheum. Dis., 12:501–522, 1986.

33. Epstein, J.H., Zimmermann, B., and Ho, G., Jr.: Polyarticular septic arthritis. J. Rheumatol., 13:1105–1107, 1986.

34. Septic arthritis in rheumatoid disease. Leading article. Br. Med. J., 2:1089–1090, 1976.

35. Kellgren, J.H., Ball, J., Fairbrother, R.W., and Barnes, K.L.: Suppurative arthritis complicating rheumatoid arthritis. Br. Med. J., 1:1193–1200, 1958.

36. Rimoin, D.L., and Wennberg, J.E.: Acute septic arthritis complicating chronic rheumatoid arthritis. JAMA, 196:617–621, 1966.

37. Karten, I.: Septic arthritis complicating rheumatoid arthritis. Ann. Intern. Med., 70:1147–1158, 1969.

38. Myers, A.R., Miller, L.M., and Pinals, R.S.: Pyarthrosis complicating rheumatoid arthritis. Lancet, 2:714–716, 1969.

39. Gristina, A.G., Rovere, G.D., and Shoji, H.: Spontaneous septic arthritis complicating rheumatoid arthritis. J. Bone Joint Surg., 56A:1180–1184, 1974.

40. Resnick, D.: Pyarthrosis complicating rheumatoid arthritis. Radiology, 114:581–586, 1975.

41. Mitchell, W.S., Brooks, P.M., Stevenson, R.D., and Buchanan, W.W.: Septic arthritis in patients with rheumatoid disease: A still underdiagnosed complication. J. Rheumatol., 3:124–133, 1976.

42. Gelman, M.I., and Ward, J.R.: Septic arthritis: A complication of rheumatoid arthritis. Radiology, 122:17–23, 1977.

43. Kraft, S.M., Panush, R.S., and Longley, S.: Unrecognized staphylococcal pyarthrosis with rheumatoid arthritis. Semin. Arthritis Rheum., 14:196–210, 1985.

44. Blackborn, W.D., Jr., Dunn, T.L., and Alarcon, G.S.: infection versus disease activity in rheumatoid arthritis: Eight years' experience. South. Med. J., 79:1238–1241, 1986.

45. Mowat, A.G., and Baum, J.: Chemotaxis of polymorphonuclear leukocytes from patients with rheumatoid arthritis. J. Clin. Invest., 50:2541–2549, 1971.

46. Turner, R.A., Shumacher, H.R., and Myers, A.R.: Phagocytic function of polymorphonuclear leukocytes in rheumatic diseases. J. Clin. Invest., 52:1632–1635, 1973.

47. Pruzanski, W., Leers, W.D., and Wardlaw, A.C.: Bacteriolytic and bactericidal activity of sera and synovial fluids in rheumatoid arthritis and in osteoarthritis. Arthritis Rheum., 17:207–218, 1974.

48. Gordon, D.L., Philpot, C.R., and McGuire, C.: Plesiomonas shigelloides septic arthritis complicating rheumatoid arthritis. Aust. N.Z. J. Med., 13:275–276, 1983.

49. Barth, W.F., Healey, L.A., and Decker, J.L.: Septic arthritis due to Pasteurella multocida complicating rheumatoid arthritis. Arthritis Rheum., 11:394–399, 1968.

50. Lewis, D.A., and Settas, L.: Kingella kingae causing septic arthritis in Felty's syndrome. Postgrad. Med. J., 59:525–526, 1983.

51. Wilson, A.P.R., Prouse, P.J., and Gumpel, J.M.: Listeria monocytogenes septic arthritis following intra-articular yttrium-90 therapy. Ann. Rheum. Dis., 43:518–519, 1984.

52. Wharton, M., Rice, J.R., McCallum, R., and Gallis, H.A.: Septic arthritis due to Micrococcus luteus. (Letter.) J. Rheumatol., 13:659–660, 1986.

53. Dodd, M.J., Griffiths, I.D., and Freeman, R.: Pyogenic arthritis due to bacteroides complicating rheumatoid arthritis. Ann. Rheum. Dis., 41:248–249, 1982.

54. Dawes, P.T., and Hothersall, T.E.: Septic polyarthritis due to Bacteroides fragilis in a patient with rheumatoid arthritis. Clin. Rheumatol., 3:381–383, 1984.

55. Schorn, D., and Pretorius, J.A.: Septic polyarthritis due to Bacteroides fragilis in a patient with rheumatoid arthritis. S. Afr. Med. J., 62:213–214, 1982.

56. Ryden, A.-C., Schwan, A., and Agell, B.-O.: A case of septic arthritis in multiple joints due to Bacteroides fragilis in a patient with rheumatoid arthritis. Acta Orthop. Scand., 49:98–101, 1978.

57. Good, A.E., Gayes, J.M., Kauffman, C.A., and Archer, G.L.: Multiple pneumococcal pyarthrosis complicating rheumatoid arthritis. South. Med. J., 71:502–504, 1978.

58. Gaunt, P.N., and Seal, D.V.: Group G streptococcal infection of joints and joint prostheses. J. Infect., 13:115–123, 1986.

59. Trimble, L.D., Schoenaers, J.A.H., and Stoelinga, P.J.W.: Acute suppurative arthritis of the temporomandibular joint in a patient with rheumatoid arthritis. J. Maxillofac. Surg., 11:92–95, 1983.

60. Berger, A.J., and Calcaterra, V.E.: Septic cricoarytenoid arthritis. Otolaryngol. Head Neck Surg., 91:211–213, 1983.

61. Tuazon, C.U., and Sheagren, J.N.: Increased rate of carriage of Staphylococcus aureus among narcotic addicts. J. Infect. Dis., 129:725–727, 1974.

62. Rajashekaraiah. K.R., Rice, T.W., and Kallick, C.A.: Recovery of Pseudomonas aeruginosa from syringes of drug addicts with endocarditis. J. Infect. Dis., 144:482, 1981.

63. Roca, R.P., and Yoshikawa, T.T.: Primary skeletal infections in heroin users: A clinical characterization, diagnosis and therapy. Clin. Orthop., 144:238–248, 1979.

64. Gordon, G., and Kabins, S.A.: Pyogenic sacroiliitis. Am. J. Med., 69:50–56, 1980.

65. Magarian, G.J., and Reuler, J.B.: Septic arthritis and osteomyelitis of the symphysis pubis (osteitis pubis) from intravenous drug use. West. J. Med., 142:691–694, 1985.

66. Bayer, A.S., Chow, A.W., Louie, J.S., and Guze, L.B.: Sternoarticular pyoarthrosis due to gram-negative bacilli. Arch. Intern. Med., 137:1036–1040, 1977.

67. Lopez-Longo, F.J., et al.: Primary septic arthritis of the manubriosternal joint in a heroin user. Clin. Orthop., 202:230–231, 1986.

68. Detailed Diagnoses and Procedures for Patients Discharged from Short-Stay Hospitals, United States, 1985. Series 13, No. 90. Washington, DC, Department of Health and Human Services. National Center for Health Statistics, 1987.

69. Hori, R.Y., Lewis, J.L., Zimmerman, J.R., and Compere, C.L.: The number of total joint replacements in the United States. Clin. Orthop., 132:46–52, 1978.

70. Melton, L.J., III, Stauffer, R.N., Chao, E.Y.S., and Ilstrup, D.M.: Rates of total hip arthroplasty: A population-based study. N. Engl. J. Med., 307:1242–1245, 1982.

71. Total hip joint replacement in the United States. (Consensus Conferences.) JAMA, 248:1817–1821, 1982.

72. Poss, R., et al.: Factors influencing the incidence and outcome of infection following total joint arthroplasty. Clin. Orthop., 182:117–126, 1984.

73. Gristina, A.G., and Kolkin, J.: Total joint replacement and sepsis. J. Bone Joint Surg., 65A:128–134, 1983.

74. Morrey, B.F., and Bryan, R.S.: Infection after total elbow arthroplasty. J. Bone Joint Surg., 65A:330–338, 1983.

75. Stinchfield, F.E., et al.: Late hematogenous infection of total joint replacement. J. Bone Joint Surg., 62A:1345–1350, 1980.

76. Ainscow, D.A.P., and Denham, R.A.: The risk of haematogenous infection in total joint replacements. J. Bone Joint Surg., 66B:580–582, 1984.

77. Grogan, T.J., Dorey, F., Rollins, J., and Amstutz, H.C.: Deep sepsis following total knee arthroplasty. J. Bone Joint Surg., 68A:226–234, 1986.

78. Hunter, G., and Dandy, D.: The natural history of the patient with an infected total hip replacement. J. Bone Joint Surg., 59B:293–297, 1977.

79. Brause, B.D.: Infections associated with prosthetic joints. Clin. Rheum. Dis., 12:523–536, 1986.

80. Hofammann, D.Y., Keeling, J.W., and Meyer, R.D.: Total hip arthroplasty: Comparison of infection rates in a VA and a University hospital. South Med. J., 79:1252–1255, 1986.

81. Gristina, A.G., Costerton, J.W., Hobgood, C.D., and Webb, L.X.: Bacterial adhesion, biomaterials, the foreign body effect, and infection from natural ecosystems to infections in man: A brief review. Contemp. Orthop., 14:27–35, 1987.

82. Inman, R.D., et al.: Clinical and microbial features of prosthetic joint infection. Am. J. Med., 77:47–53, 1984.

83. Small, C.B., et al.: Group B streptococcal arthritis in adults. Am. J. Med., 76:367–375, 1984.

84. Mallory, T.H.: Sepsis in total hip replacement following pneumococcal pneumonia. J. Bone Joint Surg., 55A:1753–1754, 1973.

85. Prince, A., and Neu, H.C.: Microbiology of infections of the prosthetic joint. Orthop. Rev., 8:91–96, 1979.

86. Orton, D.W., and Fulcher, W.H.: Pasteurella multocida: Bilateral septic joint prostheses from a distant cat bite. Ann. Emerg. Med., 13:1065–1067, 1984.

87. Eftekhar, N.S.: Wound infection complicating total hip joint arthroplasty. Orthop. Rev., 8:49–64, 1979.

88. Sneller, M., Wellborne, F., Barile, M.F., and Plotz, P.: Prosthetic joint infection with Mycoplasma hominis. (Letter.) J. Infect. Dis., 153:174–175, 1986.

89. Rand, J.A., Bryan, R.S., Morrey, B.F., and Westholm, F.: Management of infected total knee arthroplasty. Clin. Orthop., 205:75–85, 1986.

90. Insall, J.N., Thompson, F.M., and Brause, B.D.: Two-stage reimplantation for the salvage of infected total knee arthroplasty. J. Bone Joint Surg., 65A:1087–1098, 1983.

91. Buchholz, H.W., et al.: Management of deep infection of total hip replacement. J. Bone Joint Surg., 63B:342–353, 1981.

92. Wroblewski, B.M.: One-stage revision of infected cemented total hip arthroplasty. Clin. Orthop., 211:103–107, 1986.

93. Turner, R.H., Miley, G.D., and Fremont-Smith, P.: Septic total hip replacement and revision arthroplasty. In Revision Total Hip Arthroplasty. Edited by R.H. Turner and A.D. Schiller. New York, Grune & Stratton, 1982.

94. Trippel, S.B.: Antibiotic-impregnated cement in total joint arthroplasty. J. Bone Joint Surg., 68A:1297–1302, 1986.

95. McElwaine, J.P., and Colville, J.: Excision arthroplasty for infected total hip replacements. J. Bone Joint Surg., 66B:168–171, 1984.

96. Shulman, S.T., et al.: Prevention of bacterial endocarditis. Circulation, 70:1123A–1127A, 1984.

97. Radcliffe, K., Pattrick, M., and Doherty, M.: Complications resulting from misdiagnosing pseudogout as sepsis. Br. Med. J., 293:440–441, 1986.

98. Baer, P.A., Tenebaum, J., Fam, A.G., and Little, H.: Coexistent septic and crystal arthritis. Report of four cases and literature review. J. Rheumatol., 13:604–607, 1986.

99. Brancos, M.A., et al.: Septic arthritis and pseudogout. (Letter.) J. Rheumatol., 12:1021–1022, 1985.

100. Gordon, T.P., Reid, C., Rozenbilds, M.A.M., and Ahern, M.: Crystal shedding in septic arthritis: Case reports and in vivo evidence in an animal model. Aust. N.Z. J. Med., 16:336–340, 1986.

101. Zyskowski, L.P., Silverfield, J.C., and O'Duffy, J.D.: Pseudogout masking other arthritides. J. Rheumatol., 10:449–453, 1983.

102. Ide, A., Jacobelli, S., and Zenteno, G.: Candida arthritis associated with positive birefringent crystals without chondrocalcinosis. (Letter.) J. Rheumatol., 4:327–328, 1977.

103. Heinicke, M., Gomez-Reino, J.J., and Gorevic, P.D.: Crystal arthropathy as a complication of septic arthritis. J. Rheumatol., 8:529–531, 1981.

104. Parker, V.S., Malhotra, C.M., Ho, G., Jr., and Kaplan, S.R.: Radiographic appearance of the sternomanubrial joint in arthritis and related conditions. Radiology, 153:343–347, 1984.

105. Sequeira, W.: Diseases of the pubic symphysis. Semin. Arthritis Rheum., 16:11–21, 1986.

106. Gruber, B.L., Kaufman, L.D., and Gorevic, P.D.: Septic arthritis involving the manubriosternal joint. J. Rheumatol., 12:803–804, 1985.

107. Glushakow, A.S., Carlson, D., and DePalma, A.F.: Pyarthrosis of the manubriosternal joint. Clin. Orthop., 114:214–215, 1976.

108. Borgmeier, P.J., and Kalovidouris, A.E.: Septic arthritis of the sternomanubrial joint due to Pseudomonas pseudomallei. Arthritis Rheum., 23:1057–1059, 1980.

109. Sequeira, W., et al.: Pyogenic infections of the pubic symphysis. Ann. Intern. Med., 96:604–606, 1982.

110. Yood, R.A., and Goldenberg, D.L.: Sternoclavicular joint arthritis. Arthritis Rheum., 23:232–239, 1980.

111. Bellamy, N., Park, W., and Rooney, P.J.: What do we know about the sacroiliac joint? Semin. Arthritis Rheum., 12:282–313, 1983.

112. Hynd, R.F., Klofkorn, R.W., and Wong, J.K.: Streptococcus anginosus-constellatus infection of the sternoclavicular joint. J. Rheumatol., 11:713–715, 1984.

113. Seviour, P.W., and Dieppe, P.A.: Sternoclavicular joint infection as a cause of chest pain. Br. Med. J., 288:133–134, 1984.

114. Tabatabai, M.F., Sapico, F.L., Canawati, H.N., and Harley, H.A.J.: Sternoclavicular joint infection with group B streptococcus. (Letter.) J. Rheumatol., 13:466, 1986.

115. Watanakunakorn, C.: Serratia marcescens osteomyelitis of the clavicle and sternoclavicular arthritis complicating infected indwelling subclavian vein catheter. Am. J. Med., 80:753–754, 1986.

116. Nitsche, J.F., Vaughan, J.H., Williams, G., and Curd, J.G.: Septic sternoclavicular arthritis with Pasteurella multocida and Streptococcus sanguis. Arthritis Rheum., 25:467–469, 1982.

117. Kerr, R.: Pyogenic sacroiliitis. Orthopedics, 8:1030–1034, 1985.

118. Shanahan, M.D.G., and Ackroyd, C.E.: Pyogenic infection of the sacroiliac joint. J. Bone Joint Surg., 67B:605–608, 1985.

119. Delbarre, F., et al.: Pyogenic infection of the sacro-iliac joint. J. Bone Joint Surg., 57A:819–825, 1975.

120. Iczkovitz, J.M., Leek, J.C., and Robbins, D.L.: Pyogenic sacroiliitis. J. Rheumatol., 8:157–160, 1981.

121. Miskew, D.B., Block, R.A., and Witt, P.F.: Aspiration of infected sacroiliac joints. J. Bone Joint Surg., 61A:1071–1072, 1979.

122. Schaad, U.B., McCracken, G.H., and Nelson, J.D.: Pyogenic arthritis of the sacroiliac joint in pediatric patients. Pediatrics, 66:375–379, 1980.

123. Quevedo, S.F., Mikolich, D.J., Humbyrd, D.E., and Fisher, A.E.: Pyogenic sacroiliitis caused by group G streptococcus. (Letter.) Arthritis Rheum., 30:115, 1987.

124. Ross, G.N., Baraff, L.J., and Quismorio, F.P.: Serratia arthritis in heroin users. J. Bone Joint Surg., 57A:1158–1160, 1975.

125. Ziment, I., Davis, A., and Finegold, S.M.: Joint infection by anaerobic bacteria. Arthritis Rheum., 12:627–635, 1969.

126. Longoria, R.R., and Carpenter, J.L.: Anaerobic pyogenic sacroiliitis. South. Med. J., 76:649–651, 1983.

127. Scott, J.P., Maurer, H.S., and Dias, L.: Septic arthritis in two teenaged hemophiliacs. J. Pediatr., 107:748–751, 1985.

128. Helliwell, M.: Staphylococcus aureus infection complicating haemarthroses in elderly patients. Clin. Rheumatol., 4:90–92, 1985.

129. Martin, J.R., Root, H.S., Kim, S.O., and Johnson, L.G.: Staphylococcus suppurative arthritis occurring in neuropathic knee joints. Arthritis Rheum., 8:389–402, 1965.

130. Rubinow, A., Spark, E.C., and Canoso, J.J.: Septic arthritis in a charcot joint. Clin. Orthop., 147:203–206, 1980.

131. Goodman, M.A., and Swartz, W.: Infection in a charcot joint. J. Bone Joint Surg., 67A:642–643, 1985.

132. Ascuitto, R., Drennan, J., and Fitzgerald, V.: Group C streptococcal arthritis an osteomyelitis in an adolescent with a hereditary sensory neuropathy. Pediatr. Infect. Dis., 4:553–554, 1985.

133. Mathews, M., Shen, F.H., Lindner, A., and Sherrard, D.J.: Septic arthritis in hemodialyzed patients. Nephron, 25:87–91 1980.

134. Spencer, J.D.: Bone and joint infection in a renal unit. J. Bone Joint Surg., 68B:489–493, 1986.

135. Bomalaski, J.S., Williamson, P.K., and Goldstein, C.S.: Infectious arthritis in renal transplant patients. Arthritis Rheum., 29:227–232, 1986.

136. Mallouh, A., and Talab, Y.: Bone and joint infection in patients with sickle cell disease. J. Pediatr. Orthop., 5:158–162, 1985.

137. Syrogiannopoulos, G.A., McCracken, G.H., and Nelson, J.D.: Osteoarticular infections in children with sickle cell disease. Pediatrics, 78:1019–1096, 1986.

138. Barrett-Connor, E.: Bacterial infection and sickle cell anemia. Medicine, 50:97–112, 1971.

139. Espinoza, L.R., Spilberg, I., and Osterland, C.K.: Joint manifestations of sickle cell disease. Medicine, 53:295–305, 1974.

140. Lipstein-Kresch, E., et al.: Disseminated Sporothrix schenckii infection with arthritis in a patient with acquired immunodeficiency syndrome. J. Rheumatol., 12:805–808, 1985.

141. Ricciardi, D.D., et al.: Cryptococcal arthritis in a patient with acquired immune deficiency syndrome. Case report and review of the literature. J. Rheumatol., 13:455–458, 1986.

142. Smith, J.W.: Infectious arthritis. In Principles and Practice of Infectious Diseases. Edited by G.L. Mandell, R.G. Douglas, Jr., and J.E. Bennett. 2nd Ed. New York, John Wiley & Sons, 1985, Chapter 83.

143. Wolski, K.P.: Staphylococcal and other Gram-positive coccal arthritides. Clin. Rheum. Dis., 4:181–196, 1978.

144. Esposito, A.L., and Gleckman, R.A.: Acute polymicrobic sep-

tic arthritis in adult: Case report and literature review. Am. J. Med. Sci., 267:251–254, 1974.

145. Petty, B.G., Sowa, D.T., and Charache, P.: Polymicrobial polyarticular septic arthritis. JAMA, 249:2069–2072, 1983.

146. Finegold, S.M.: Anaerobic Bacteria in Human Disease. New York, Academic Press, 1977, pp. 443–454.

147. Fitzgerald, R.H., Jr., Rosenblatt, J.E., Tenney, J.H., and Bourgault, A.: Anaerobic septic arthritis. Clin. Orthop., 164:141–148, 1982.

148. Goldenberg, D.L., and Cohen, A.S.: Acute infectious arthritis. A review of patients with nongonococcal joint infections (with emphasis on therapy and prognosis). Am. J. Med., 60:369–377, 1976.

149. Rosenthal, J., Bole, G.G., and Robinson, W.D.: Acute nongonococcal infectious arthritis. Evaluation of risk factors, therapy, and outcome. Arthritis Rheum., 23:889–897, 1980.

150. Manshady, B.M., Thompson, G.R., and Weiss, J.J.: Septic arthritis in a general hospital 1966–1977. J. Rheumatol., 7:523–530, 1980.

151. Sharp, J.T., Lidksy, M.D., Duffy, J., and Duncan, M.W.: Infectious arthritis. Arch. Intern. Med., 139:1125–1130, 1979.

152. Cooper, C., and Cawley, M.I.D.: Bacterial arthritis in an English health district: A 10 year review. Ann. Rheum. Dis., 45:458–463, 1986.

153. Sheagren, J.N.: Staphylococcus aureus. The persistent pathogen. N. Engl. J. Med., 310:1368–1373, 1437–1442, 1984.

154. Schwalbe, R.S., Stapleton, J.T., and Gilligan, P.H.: Emergence of vancomycin resistance in coagulase-negative staphylococci. N. Engl. J. Med., 316:927–931, 1987.

155. Wolfson, J.S., and Hooper, D.C.: The fluoroquinolones: Structures, mechanisms of action and resistance, and spectra of activity in vitro. Antimicrob. Agents Chemother., 28:581–586, 1985.

156. Hooper, D.C., and Wolfson, J.S.: The fluoroquinolones: Pharmacology, clinical uses, and toxicities in humans. Antimicrob. Agents Chemother., 28:716–721, 1985.

157. Pischel, K.D., Weisman, M.H., and Cone, R.O.: Unique features of Group B streptococcal arthritis in adults. Arch. Intern. Med., 145:97–102, 1985.

158. Laster, A.J., and Michels, M.L.: Group B streptococcal arthritis in adults. Am. J. Med., 76:910–915, 1984.

159. Vartian, C., Lerner, P.I., Shlaes, D.M., and Gopalakrishna, K.V.: Infections due to Lancefield group G streptococci. Medicine, 64:75–88, 1985.

160. Kauffman, C.A., Watanakunakorn, C., and Phair, J.P.: Pneumococcal arthritis. J. Rheumatol., 3:409–419, 1976.

161. Edwards, G.S., Jr., and Russell, I.J.: Pneumococcal arthritis complicating gout. J. Rheumatol., 7:907–910, 1980.

162. Andersen, B.R., Mayer, M.E., Geiseler, P.J., and Niebel, J.R.: Multi-joint pneumococcal pyarthrosis in a patient with a chemotactic defect. Arthritis Rheum., 26:1160–1162, 1983.

163. Mitnick, H., Mitnick, J.S., Rafii, M., and Wetherbee, R.: Septic arthritis secondary to Group C streptococcus. (Letter.) J. Rheumatol., 9:974–976, 1982.

164. Hamilton, M.E., Parris, T.M., Gibson, R.S., and Davis, J.S.: Simultaneous gout and pyarthrosis. Arch. Intern. Med., 140:917–919, 1980.

165. Gorman, P.W., and Collins, D.N.: Group C streptococcal arthritis, a case report of equine transmission. Orthopedics, 10:615–616, 1987.

166. Zwillich, S.H., Hamory, B.H., and Walker, S.E.: Enterococcus: An unusual cause of septic arthritis. Arthritis Rheum., 27:591–595, 1984.

167. Taylor, P.W., and Trueblood, M.C.: Septic arthritis due to Aerococcus viridans. J. Rheumatol., 12:1004–1005, 1985.

168. Nieman, R.E., and Lorber, B.: Listeriosis in adults: A changing pattern. Rev. Infect. Dis., 2:207–227, 1980.

169. Newman, J.H., Waycott, S., and Cooney, L.M., Jr.: Arthritis due to Listeria monocytogenes. Arthritis Rheum., 22:1139–1140, 1979.

170. Breckenridge, R.L., Jr., Buck, L., Tooley, E., and Douglas, G.W.: Listeria monocytogenes septic arthritis. Am. J. Clin. Pathol., 73:140–141, 1980.

171. Norenberg, D.D., Bigley, D.V., Virata, R.L., and Liang, G.C.: Corynebacterium pyogenes septic arthritis with plasma cell synovial infiltrate and monoclonal gammopathy. Arch. Intern. Med., 138:810–811, 1978.

172. Robinson, S.C.: Bacillus cereus septic arthritis following arthrography. Clin. Orthop., 145:237–238, 1979.

173. Morrison, V.A., and Chia, J.K.S.: Septic arthritis due to Bacillus. South Med. J., 79:522–523, 1986.

174. Craig, D.B., and Wehrle, P.A.: Branhamella catarrhalis septic arthritis. J. Rheumatol., 10:985–986, 1983.

175. Patel, N.J., Moore, T.L., Weiss, T.D., and Zuckner, J.: Kingella kingae infectious arthritis: Case report and review of literature of Kingella and Moraxella infections. Arthritis Rheum., 26:557–559, 1983.

176. Feigin, R.D., San Joaquin, V., and Middelkamp, J.N.: Septic arthritis due to Moraxella osloensis. J. Pediatr., 75:116–117, 1969.

177. Redfield, D.C., Overturf, G.D., Ewing, N., and Powars, D.: Bacteria, arthritis, and skin lesions due to Kingella kingae. Arch. Dis. Child., 55:411, 1980.

178. Gay, R.M., Lane, T.W., and Keller, D.C.: Septic arthritis caused by Kingella kingae. J. Clin. Microbiol., 17:168–169, 1983.

179. Powel, J.M., and Bass, J.W.: Septic arthritis caused by Kingella kingae. Am. J. Dis. Child., 137:974–976, 1983.

180. Vincent, J., Podewell, C., Frankin, G.W., and Korn, J.H.: Septic arthritis due to Kingella (Moraxella) kingii. J. Rheumatol., 8:501–503, 1981.

181. Salminen, I., Von Essen, R., Koota, K., and Nissinen, A.: A pitfall in purulent arthritis brought out in Kingella kingae infection of the knee. Ann. Rheum. Dis., 43:656–657, 1984.

182. Pinals, R.S., and Ropes, M.W.: Meningococcal arthritis. Arthritis Rheum., 7:241–258, 1964.

183. Schaad, U.B.: Arthritis in disease due to Neisseria meningitidis. Rev. Infect. Dis., 2:880–888, 1980.

184. Greenwood, B.M., Mohammed, I., and Whittle, H.C.: Immune complexes and the pathogenesis of meningococcal arthritis. Clin. Exp. Immunol., 59:513–519, 1985.

185. Rompalo, A.M., et al.: The acute arthritis-dermatitis syndrome. Arch. Intern. Med., 147:281–283, 1987.

186. Rosen, M.S., Myers, A.R., and Dickey, B.: Meningococcemia presenting as septic arthritis, pericarditis, and tenosynovitis. Arthritis Rheum., 28:576–578, 1985.

187. Kidd, B.L., Hart, H.H., and Grigor, R.R.: Clinical features of meningococcal arthritis: A report of four cases. Ann. Rheum. Dis., 44:790–792, 1985.

188. Pollet, S.M., and Leek, J.C.: Tenosynovitis in meningococcemia. (Letter.) Arthritis Rheum., 30:232–233, 1987.

189. Hirschmann, J.V., and Everett, E.D.: Haemophilus influenzae infections in adults: Report of nine cases and a review of the literature. Medicine (Baltimore), 58:80–94, 1979.

190. Dajani, A.S., Asmar, B.I., and Thirumoorthi, M.C.: Systemic Hemophilus influenzae disease: An overview. J. Pediatr., 94:355–364, 1979.

191. Rotbart, H.A., and Glode, M.P.: Haemophilus infuenzae type b septic arthritis in children: Report of 23 cases. Pediatrics, 75:254–259, 1985.

192. Ho, G., Jr., Gadbaw, J.J., Jr., and Glickstein, S.L.: Hemophilus influenzae septic arthritis in adults. Semin. Arthritis Rheum., 12:314–321, 1983.

193. Knisely, G.K., Gibson, G.R., and Reichman, R.C.: Hemophilus influenzae bursitis and meningitis in an adult. Arch. Intern. Med., 143:1465–1466, 1983.

194. Cohen, M.A., Levy, I.M., and Habermann, E.T.: Multiple joint sepsis by Hemophilus influenza in an adult. Clin. Orthop., 209:198–201, 1986.

195. Borenstein, D.G., and Simon, G.L.: Hemophilus influenzae septic arthritis in adults. A report of four cases and a review of the literature. Medicine (Baltimore), 65:191–201, 1986.

196. Ho, G., Jr., Tice, A.D., and Kaplan, S.R.: Septic bursitis in the prepatellar and olecranon bursae. Ann. Intern. Med., 89:21–27, 1978.

197. Goldenberg, D.L., and Cohen, A.S.: Arthritis due to Gram-negative bacilli. Clin. Rheum. Dis., 4:197–210, 1978.

198. Ruthberg, A.D., and Ho, G., Jr.: Nongonococcal bacterial arthritis. In Orthopedic Infections. Edited by R.L. Marier and R.D. D'Ambrosia. Thorofare, NJ, Slack, Inc. (in press).

199. Gifford, D.B., Patzakis, M., Ivler, D., and Swezey, R.L.: Septic arthritis due to Pseudomonas in heroin addicts. J. Bone Joint Surg., 57A:631–635, 1975.

200. Bayer, A.S., et al.: Gram-negative bacillary septic arthritis: Clinical, radiographic, therapeutic, and prognostic features. Semin. Arthritis Rheum., 7:123–132, 1977.

201. David, J.R., and Black, R.L.: Salmonella arthritis. Medicine, 39:385–403, 1960.

202. Brodie, T.D., and Ehresmann, G.R.: Salmonella dublin arthritis: An initial case presentation. J. Rheumatol., 10:144–146, 1983.

203. Quismorio, F.P., Jr., et al.: Septic arthritis due to Arizona hinshawii. J. Rheumatol., 10:147–150, 1983.

204. Spira, T.J., and Kabins, S.A.: Yersinia enterocolitica septicemia with septic arthritis. Arch. Intern. Med., 136:1305–1308, 1976.

205. Taylor, B.G., Zafarzai, M.Z., Humphreys, D.W., and Manfredi, F.: Nodular pulmonary infiltrates and septic arthritis associated with Yersinia enterocolitica bacteremia. Am. Rev. Resp. Dis., 116:525–529, 1977.

206. Kilo, C., Hagemann, P.O., and Marzi, J.: Septic arthritis and bacteremia due to Vibrio fetus. Am. J. Med., 38:962–971, 1965.

207. Aho, K., Leirisalo-Repo, M., and Repo, H.: Reactive arthritis. Clin. Rheum. Dis., 11:25–40, 1985.

208. Ford, D.K.: Reactive arthritis: A viewpoint rather than a review. Clin. Rheum. Dis., 12:389–401, 1986.

209. Walton, K., Hilton, R.C., and Sen, R.A.: Pseudomonas arthritis treated with parenteral and intra-articular ceftazidime. Ann. Rheum. Dis., 44:499–500, 1985.

210. Nelson, J.D.: Antibiotic concentrations in septic joint effusions. N. Engl. J. Med., 284:349–353, 1971.

211. Pancoast, S.J., and Neu, H.C.: Antibiotic levels in human bone and synovial fluid. Orthop. Rev., 9:49–61, 1980.

212. Winn, R.E., Chase, W.F., Lauderdale, P.W., and McCleskey, F.K.: Septic arthritis involving Capnocytophaga ochracea. J. Clin. Microbiol., 19:538–540, 1984.

213. Dean, H.M., and Post, R.M.: Fatal infection with Aeromonas hydrophila in a patient with acute myelogenous leukemia. Ann. Intern. Med., 66:1177–1179, 1967.

214. Chmel, H., and Armstrong, D.: Acute arthritis caused by Aeromonas hydrophila: Clinical and therapeutic aspects. Arthritis Rheum., 19:169–172, 1976.

215. Weber, D.J., Wolfson, J.S., Swartz, M.N., and Hooper, D.C.: Pasteurella multocida infections. Report of 34 cases and review of the literature. Medicine (Baltimore), 63:133–154, 1984.

216. Ewing, R., et al.: Articular and skeletal infections caused by Pasteurella multocida. South. Med. J., 73:1349–1352, 1980.

217. Mellors, J.W., and Schoen, R.T.: Pasteurella multocida septic arthritis. Conn. Med., 48:221–223, 1984.

218. Sugarman, M., Quismorio, F.P., and Patzakis, M.J.: Joint infection by Pasteurella multocida. Lancet, 2:1267, 1975.

219. Griffin, A.J., and Barber, H.M.: Joint infection by Pasteurella multocida. Lancet, 1:1347–1348, 1975.

220. Mandel, D.R.: Streptobacillary fever. An unusual cause of infectious arthritis. Cleve. Clin. Q., 52:203–205, 1985.

221. Anderson, D., and Marrie, T.J.: Septic arthritis due to Streptobacillus moniliformis. (Letter.) Arthritis Rheum., 30:229–230, 1987.

222. Young, E.J.: Human brucellosis. Rev. Infect. Dis., 5:821–842, 1983.

223. Gotuzzo, E., et al.: Articular involvement in human brucellosis: A retrospective analysis of 304 cases. Semin. Arthritis Rheum., 12:245–255, 1982.

224. Ariza, J., et al.: Brucellar spondylitis: A detailed analysis based on current findings. Rev. Infect. Dis., 7:656–664, 1985.

225. Porat, S., and Shapiro, M.: Brucella arthritis of the sacro-iliac joint. Infection, 12:205–207, 1984.

226. Baranda, M.M., et al.: Sternoclavicular septic arthritis as first manifestation of brucellosis. (Letter.) Br. J. Rheumatol., 25:322, 1986.

227. Tosi, M.F., and Nelson, T.J.: Brucella canis infection in a 17-month-old child successfully treated with moxalactam. J. Pediatr., 101:725–727, 1982.

228. Gomez-Reino, F.J., Mateo, I., Fuertes, A., and Gomez-Reino, J.J.: Brucellar arthritis in children and its successful treatment with trimethoprim-sulphamethoxazole. Ann. Rheum. Dis., 45:256–258, 1986.

229. Clark, G.M.: Syphilitic joint disease. In Arthritis and Allied Conditions. 8th Ed. Edited by J.L Hollander and D.J. McCarty, Jr. Philadelphia, Lea & Febiger, 1972, pp. 1255–1259.

230. Cassell, G.H., and Cole, B.C.: Mycoplasma as agents of human disease. N. Engl. J. Med., 304:80–89, 1981.

231. Taylor-Robinson, D., Gumpel, J.M., Hill, A., and Swannell, A.J.: Isolation of Mycoplasma pneumoniae from synovial fluid of a hypogammaglobulinemic patient in a survey of patients with inflammatory polyarthritis. Ann. Rheum. Dis., 37:180–182, 1978.

232. Vogler, L.B., et al.: Ureaplasma urealyticum polyarthritis in agammaglobulinemia. Pediatr. Infect. Dis., 4:687–691, 1985.

233. Boudoulas, O., and Camisa, C.: Nocardia asteroides infection with dissemination to skin and joints. Arch. Derm., 121:898–900, 1985.

234. Cons, F., Trevino, A., and Lavalle, C.: Septic arthritis due to Nocardia brasiliensis. (Letter.) J. Rheumatol., 12:1019–1021, 1985.

235. Rao, K.V., O'Brien, T.J., and Andersen, R.C.: Septic arthritis due to Nocardia asteroides after successful kidney transplantation. Arthritis Rheum., 24:99–101, 1981.

236. McCarty, D.J.: Joint sepsis: A chance for cure. (Editorial.) JAMA, 247:835, 1982.

237. Ward, T.T., and Steigbigel, R.T.: Acidosis of synovial fluid correlated with synovial fluid leukocytosis. Am. J. Med., 64:933–936, 1978.

116

GONOCOCCAL ARTHRITIS

DON L. GOLDENBERG

In 1879 Neisser described the characteristic gram-negative diplococcus, Neisseria gonorrhoeae, and soon thereafter gonococcal arthritis was reported.[1,2] During the past 20 years the structural and immunologic features of N. gonorrhoeae have been studied extensively, helping to further our understanding of host-microbial interactions in disseminated gonococcal infection (DGI).[3-5] The clinical and laboratory characteristics of DGI have been described and contrasted with other types of bacterial arthritis.[3,6-12] This chapter reviews the microbiologic, serologic, clinical, and therapeutic manifestations of DGI and discusses the possibility that certain of these clinical manifestations may not require the existence of viable organisms.

NEISSERIA GONORRHOEAE

Neisseria gonorrhoeae is a gram-negative diplococcus identified in the laboratory by its growth characteristics and its sugar-fermentation patterns. The Gram-stained smear of body secretions reveals the characteristic kidney-bean–shaped pair of organisms, although Hemophilus as well as other Neisseria species may have a similar appearance. The nutritional requirements of N. gonorrhoeae are fastidious, and these bacteria require special care for optimal growth. Genitourinary, anal, and throat secretions should be plated on antibiotic-impregnated media, such as Thayer-Martin or modified New York City plates, to inhibit the growth of other bacteria. All other body fluids should be immediately plated on chocolate agar, prepared by heating red blood cells, and then placed in an atmosphere of increased carbon dioxide tension. Even when optimal culture techniques are followed, the recovery of the organism from body fluids has been disappointing. Growth of the organisms in standard broth cultures can be delayed, and blood or joint fluid should be repeatedly checked for bacterial growth for up to 7 days. The cell wall of N. gonorrhoeae is a complex structure, which consists of an outer capsule, pili, or protein filaments; an outer membrane that contains protein, lipopolysaccharide, and peptidoglycan; and an inner cytoplasmic membrane. Several of these components have identifiable structural or serologic characteristics that vary among specific gonococcal strains. For example, three outer membrane proteins have been identified, including protein I, which provides a means for serotyping gonococci, and protein II, responsible for colonial opacity.

At least 60 different pili serologic types have been characterized. These pili are important in cell adherence and help to determine gonococcal strain virulence.[2,13] The pili can change their individual antigenicity. The lipopolysaccharide of the outer membrane contains a hydrophobic component, lipid A, and is also characterized serologically into major antigenic determinants, based on variations in carbohydrate structure. One or more of these cell-wall determinants may be important in the virulence of a specific strain.[3-5] For example, the nutritional requirements of strains producing DGI are different from those of strains producing uncomplicated local gonococcal infections.[4] Nearly two thirds of DGI-producing strains possess a nutritional requirement for arginine, hypoxanthine, and uracil, as compared with only 8% of strains from cases of uncomplicated gonorrhea.[3] DGI-producing strains also possess unique principal outer membrane proteins and are resistant to the bactericidal activity of normal human sera, in contrast to many localized strains,[3,14] particularly those that cause severe pelvic inflammatory disease in women. Despite this serum resistance, the DGI-producing strains are still uniquely sensitive to antibiotics.[15] Laboratory growth characteristics also distinguish the strains that cause disseminated infections. For example, piliated phenotypes, easily identified on the basis of the growth characteristics of their morphologic colonies, are isolated in primary culture and are probably responsible for DGI.[13] Transparent colonies are also more common in gonococcal isolates from sites such as the blood or joint, whereas opaque colonies are more often isolated from local sites.[3,5]

INCIDENCE

Gonococcal arthritis is currently the most common form of bacterial arthritis reported by United States urban medical centers.[6] There are about 4 million cases of gonorrhea reported each year in the United States and about 2.5 cases of DGI per 100,000 population.

Most patients with DGI are young and healthy and have no host-defense impairment that might predispose them to bacteremia. Although gonococcal arthritis was more common in men than in women prior to the development of antibiotics, in the past 25 years more women than men developed DGI.[3,7-12] The interval from the onset of sexual exposure or genitourinary tract symptoms to DGI varies from a day to many weeks. Patients with DGI do not usually complain of genitourinary symptoms such as pelvic inflammatory disease or prostatitis.

The absence of local symptoms and the female predominance of DGI may be due to failure of a mucosal inflammatory response to block the organism's entrance into the circulation. For example, women are prone to develop DGI during the menses or early in pregnancy. N. gonorrhoeae can change its colonial phenotype during menses from opaque to transparent. Thus, the characteristics of the host's mucosa and the adherence traits of the organism, such as the presence of pili, which promotes attachment, are important in the initial gonococcal infection.

The major independent host-defense factor that predisposes individuals to DGI is complement-component deficiency. Patients with congenital complement-component deficiencies, especially those with terminal C5-C8 deficiencies, develop recurrent DGI as well as other recurrent neisserial infections.[16] I have also noted C3 and C4 deficiency in my patients with DGI.[3]

Some of the foregoing interrelated host-microbial factors determine whether a strain of N. gonorrhoeae will cause a local infection or whether it will disseminate. Tissue penetration and circulatory invasion seem to depend on specific cell-wall properties that can be altered by genetic mutations.[17,18] Perhaps the most important factor in dissemination, as well as in the clinical manifestations of DGI, is the ability of the various gonococcal strains to resist the bactericidal activity of normal human serum.[3] This activity depends on a natural antibody, which is directed against gonococcal lipopolysaccharide, and an uncharacterized unique interaction of gonococci with complement. DGI-producing strains may also effectively bind naturally occurring "blocking antibodies," with a resulting inability of bactericidal antibodies and complement to kill the organism.

CLINICAL MANIFESTATIONS

Most patients with DGI first experience either migratory or additive polyarthralgias (Table 116–1). Fever, chills, and other constitutional symptoms are common; however, genitourinary symptoms are unusual. Only 5 of our 37 patients with positive genitourinary cultures had genitourinary symptoms.[3] Only 1 of 5 patients with positive pharyngeal cultures and none of 10 patients with positive rectal cultures had local symptoms. Tenosynovitis is present in two thirds of patients with DGI. The tenosynovitis usually involves multiple joints and is especially common over the wrists, fingers, ankles, and toes. Polyarthritis or monoarthritis was present in 42% of our patients

Table 116–1. Initial Symptoms and Signs in 49 Patients With Disseminated Gonococcal Infection*

	(%)
Polyarthralgias	70
Tenosynovitis	67
Dermatitis	67
Fever	63
Arthritis†	42
Monoarthritis	32
Polyarthritis	10

*Patients seen from 1975 to 1982 with positive blood or synovial fluid culture or clinical symptoms typical of this infection and positive local cultures.
†Documented with synovial fluid aspiration.
(Data from O'Brien, Goldenberg, and Rice.[3])

Table 116–2.   Clinical and Laboratory Characteristics of Patients With Disseminated Gonococcal Infection With Tenosynovitis and Dermatitis and With Suppurative Arthritis*

	Tenosynovitis and Dermatitis		Suppurative Arthritis	
Number of patients	30		19	
Duration of symptoms prior to hospitalization (median number of days)	4		4	
Tenosynovitis	26	(87%)	4	(21%)
Dermatitis	27	(90%)	8	(42%)
Positive blood culture	13	(43%)	0	
Positive joint fluid culture	0		9	(47%)
Number of patients with a twofold or greater rise in bactericidal antibody activity	3/18	(17%)	9/13	(69%)
Number of gonococcal strains resistant to all 10 normal sera	18/24	(75%)	9/19	(47%)

*Patients seen at Boston University Medical Center from 1975 to 1982.
(Data from O'Brien, Goldenberg, and Rice.[3])

with DGI. Although the knees, wrists, and ankles are usually affected, hip, spinal, and temporomandibular joint involvement may occur. In fact, any joint may be affected. When joint effusions can be aspirated, the synovial fluid is usually purulent, with a mean leukocyte count of 50,000 cells/mm³. Occasionally, a small joint effusion that is relatively acellular is present for a few days.

Dermatitis occurs in two-thirds of patients with DGI (Tables 116–1, 116–2).[3,7,12] Skin lesions are usually multiple and are most often found on the extremities or on the trunk, but rarely on the face, palms, or soles (Fig. 116–1). These lesions are often painless, and patients may be unaware of their existence, although some skin lesions are painful. The most common skin lesions are hemorrhagic macules or papules, but pustules, vesicles, bullae, erythema nodosum, or erythema multiforme have also been described. New skin lesions may develop during the initial 24 to 48 hours of antibiotic therapy.

Most patients are febrile, although the average temperature is usually only moderately elevated. A modest peripheral blood leukocytosis is common. Transiently elevated liver function studies have been described, probably representing subclinical hepatitis during bacteremia.[3,8] Additionally, a perihepatitis, termed the Fitz-Hugh–Curtis syndrome, may occur in women secondary to adhesions between the surfaces of the liver and the peritoneum as a result of intraperitoneal spread of infection. Gonococcal meningitis and endocarditis are rarely reported in the antibiotic era. A presumed immune-mediated glomerulonephritis secondary to DGI has been reported.[19]

Some investigators have proposed that DGI progresses sequentially from a bacteremic phase, characterized by chills, tenosynovitis, and skin lesions, to a joint-localized phase manifested by purulent arthritis.[7,8] The diagnostic utility of such a classification is suspect, however, because of the significant clinical

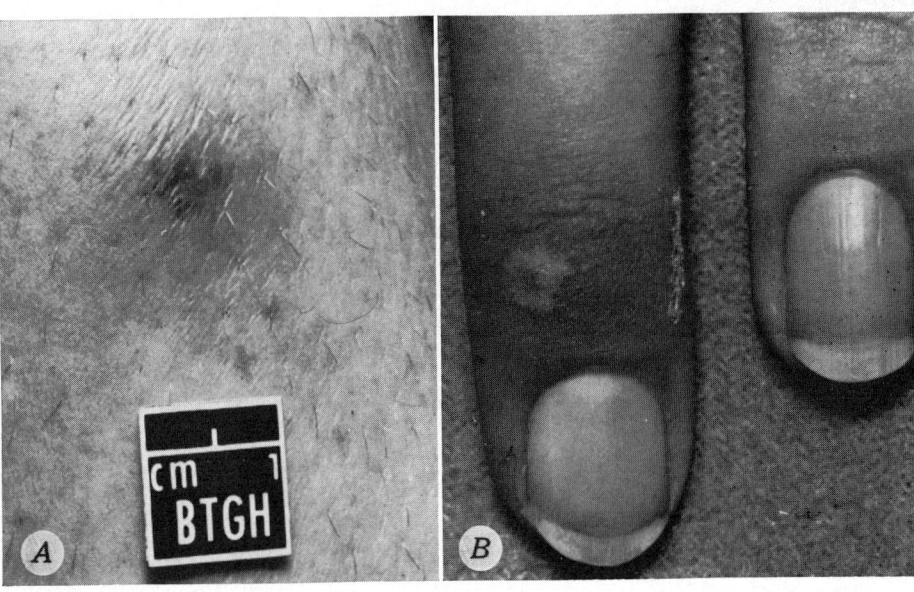

FIG. 116–1.   Skin lesions characteristic of septicemia due to Neisseria gonorrhoeae, N. Meningitidis, Streptobacillus moniliformis, and Hemophilus influenzae. A, Hemorrhagic spot 5 to 6 mm in diameter on the upper arm; the gray area 1 to 2 mm in diameter in the center indicates necrosis. B, Pustulovesicular lesion on the finger of the same patient; the necrotic center is evident as a dark gray area.

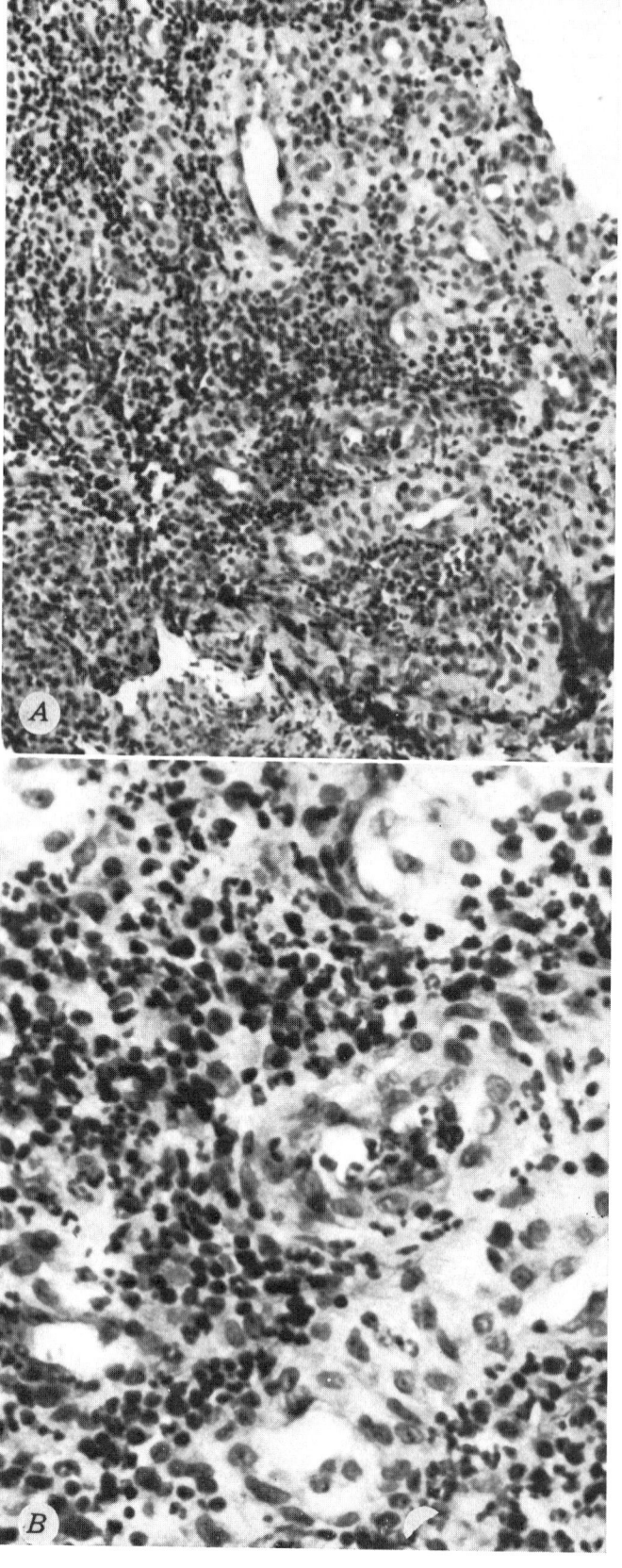

FIG. 116–2. A 38-year-old man had abrupt onset of pain and swelling in the distal interphalangeal (DIP) joint of the left third finger. One day later, he developed pain and swelling in the right wrist and the dorsum of the right hand, and 2 days later, he had swelling and pain in the right ankle. Ten days after onset, examination confirmed involvement of these areas. No skin lesions or urethral discharge were present. On the eleventh day of illness, the left ankle became swollen and painful. Blood cultures were sterile, and synovial fluid cultures from the right wrist and the left ankle on the fifteenth day of illness showed no growth. Serum uric acid levels, antistreptolysin O titer, and electrocardiograph findings were normal. LE cell preparations and latex fixation for anti-IgG were negative. Nineteen days after onset, the left third DIP and the right wrist joint remained inflamed; the other joints were clear. Fever was present. Diagnostic biopsy was advised by the consultant on the twenty-first day of illness. Tissue from the wrist joint grew Neisseria gonorrhoeae. A section of biopsy tissue stained with hematoxylin and eosin is shown in A (×185) and in B (×460). The biopsy shows proliferation of new tissue including prominent neovascularization. Synovial lining cells are not seen on the surface of the section (A, right) and are infrequently present throughout the ttissue. The inflammatory infiltrate consists of a mixture of cell types. Collections of polymorphonuclear leukocytes are scattered through the section, along with mononuclear cells and lymphocytes. In some areas not shown, plasma cells are prominent.

FIG. 116–3. Roentgenograms of the patient whose biopsy specimen is shown in Figure 116–2. *A* was obtained on the eleventh day of illness, 10 days after the onset of pain and swelling in the right wrist; the film is normal. *B* was taken on the nineteenth day of illness; one sees demineralization of the carpal and metacarpal bone along the carpometacarpal articulations, with a loss of clearly defined trabecular bone markings and a loss of articular cartilage in the same area. *C* was obtained 11 weeks after the onset of arthritis; remineralization has occurred. Joint-space narrowing is present along the carpometacarpal row, the intercarpal articulations, and the radiocarpal joints.

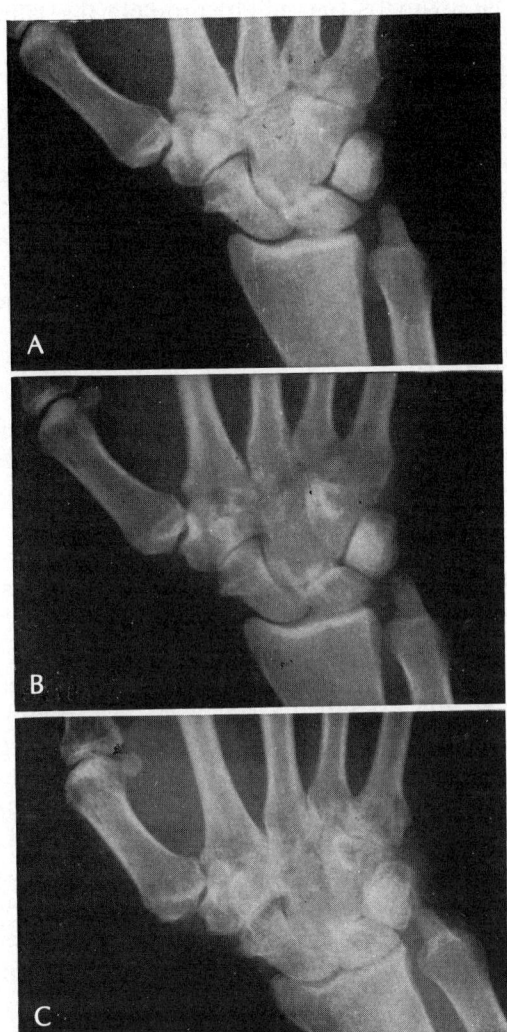

overlap and the inconsistent temporal sequence of the articular manifestations.[3,9,10] I find that most patients initially have either a predominantly joint-localized disease or tenosynovitis and dermatitis (Table 116–2, Figs. 116–2 and 116–3). No difference is noted in the duration of symptoms prior to the diagnosis of DGI in patients with suppurative arthritis and in those with tenosynovitis. These initial clinical manifesta-

tions may be determined by certain microbiologic and serologic features of the strain of N. gonorrhoeae.[4] For example, the strains of N. gonorrhoeae isolated from patients with purulent arthritis are generally phenotypically different from those isolated from patients with dermatitis and tenosynovitis (see Table 116–2). Seventy-five percent of the N. gonorrhoeae isolates from patients with tenosynovitis and dermatitis were resistant to the bactericidal activity of normal human sera, whereas only 47% of strains isolated from patients with suppurative arthritis were resistant. Sixty-nine percent of patients with suppurative arthritis, but only 17% of patients with tenosynovitis and dermatitis, developed a significant rise in bactericidal antibody activity, as measured in their serum during the acute illness and in convalescence.

PATHOGENESIS

Suppurative arthritis caused by N. gonorrhoeae is generally considered secondary to bacteremic spread of the organisms to the synovium, with replication of bacteria and the subsequent release of proteolytic enzymes from synovial lining cells and of polymorphonuclear leukocytes (Table 116–3). Eventually, cartilage is destroyed. This process is the same as in most other types of bacterial arthritis. Gonococcal bacteremia is more likely to cause arthritis or tenosynovitis than infection with pneumococci or other common bacteria. Microscopically, the synovial membrane initially reveals lining-cell hyperplasia and infiltration by polymorphonuclear leukocytes (see Fig. 116–2). Gram-stained smears of the synovial fluid or synovial membrane are sometimes initially positive. If a second synovial membrane specimen is obtained 5 to 7 days after treatment, most of the acute infiltrate will have subsided, but chronic inflammatory cells will be prominent. Synovial fluid and synovial membrane Gram-stained smears and cultures will no longer show N. gonorrhoeae. Rarely, a chronic synovitis persists despite appropriate antibiotic therapy.[20] This sterile synovitis may be responsible for persistent pain and joint effusions despite eradication of the acute infection, a phenomenon termed "postinfectious" arthritis.

Although the synovial membrane and fluid characteristics of acute gonococcal arthritis are generally similar to those of arthritis caused by other bacteria, DGI rarely destroys cartilage or bone. Even in the preantibiotic era, untreated gonococcal arthritis rarely caused permanent joint destruction.[1] I have also seen patients with DGI undergo complete resolution of arthritis and tenosynovitis without antibiotic treatment.

Table 116–3. Pathogenesis of Clinical Manifestations of Disseminated Gonococcal Infection

Mechanism	Evidence
Bacteremic seeding of synovium	Recovery of Neisseria gonorrhoeae from synovial fluid
Development of "postinfectious" or "reactive" arthritis	Negative synovial fluid cultures; laboratory models of cell-wall-induced arthritis
Immune mediation	Circulating immune complexes; antibody, complement deposits in skin lesions; clinical resemblance to serum sickness

Clinical and laboratory evidence indicates that the arthralgias, tenosynovitis, dermatitis, and the "sterile" arthritis associated with DGI may be due to immune-mediated mechanisms or hypersensitivity (Table 116–3). The initial presentation of DGI often resembles that of serum sickness, with tenosynovitis and migratory polyarthralgias that are usually transient and often disappear without antimicrobial therapy. Similar musculoskeletal symptoms are common in immune-complex-related infections such as hepatitis, but they are absent in non-neisserial bacterial arthritis. Furthermore, N. gonorrhoeae is recovered from fewer than 50% of purulent synovial effusions, in contrast with nongonococcal bacterial arthritis.[6] Positive blood cultures are found in fewer than one third of patients with DGI, and positive blood and synovial fluid cultures are mutually exclusive (see Table 116–2). Investigators have attributed the frequent absence of positive blood and synovial fluid cultures to the fastidious growth requirements of N. gonorrhoeae, yet the organisms are easily recovered from the genitourinary tract or other local sites in most cases of DGI. Therefore, some investigators have questioned the role of immune-mediated phenomena or hypersensitivity in the synovitis and dermatitis associated with DGI. Gonococcal urethritis might initiate a "reactive," sterile arthritis. Scandinavian investigators have reported that an aseptic arthritis, clinically similar to Reiter's syndrome, occurs commonly following gonococcal urethritis.[21] Nonviable bacterial antigenic components could also cause a persistent yet sterile synovitis. In some patients with DGI, purulent synovitis does not occur, and circulating or deposited immune complexes may be more important.[20]

The dermatitis associated with DGI is almost always sterile, and the cause of the skin lesions does not seem to be secondary to embolic spread of viable organisms.[22–24] Erythema nodosum, erythema multiforme, and vasculitis, which have all been reported in DGI, suggest immune-mediated or hypersensitivity reactions. Although viable N. gonorrhoeae are rarely recovered from these skin lesions, immunofluorescent evidence exists of gonococcal cell-wall components, gonococcal antibody, and complement.[23,24] Circulat-

ing immune complexes have also been detected in patients with DGI.[25,26] These complexes are especially prominent early in the clinical course and could cause a sterile synovitis that might promote the later entrance of bacteria into the joint.[25]

Higher levels and frequency of immune complexes, determined by the Raji cell immunofluorescent assay or the C1q polyethylene glycol binding assay, were detected in the synovial fluid when compared to the serum.[27] The synovial fluid immune complexes more often contained IgM, whereas the serum immune complexes were predominantly IgG, suggesting primary immune complex formation within the synovial cavity.

My colleagues and I have investigated the role of nonviable bacterial components in DGI using an experimental model of gonococcal arthritis in rabbits.[28] Intra-articular injections of N. gonorrhoeae caused an acute arthritis within 24 hours, and at 7 to 10 days, a chronic synovitis developed. Histologically, the changes were identical to those following the intra-articular injection of gram-positive cocci and Escherichia coli into rabbits' knees. N. gonorrhoeae could not be recovered from the infected joint even 48 hours after injection, however, whereas the gram-positive cocci and the Escherichia coli were persistently recovered for days to weeks following their injection. Intra-articular injections of nonviable Neisseria gonorrhoeae or gonococcal lipopolysaccharide isolated from the cell wall of Neisseria gonorrhoeae also caused an initially acute and then chronic, persistent synovitis.[29] A lipopolysaccharide concentration as low as 5 µg (10^{-6} g dry weight) caused arthritis, whereas much larger concentrations of another gonococcal antigenic component, the outer membrane protein, did not cause synovitis. Therefore, clinical and laboratory evidence indicates that, in some circumstances, the synovitis, tenosynovitis, and dermatitis associated with DGI may not require viable N. gonorrhoeae.

DIAGNOSIS

The diagnosis of DGI should be suspected in any young, sexually active patient who has acute arthritis

Table 116–4.   Differential Diagnosis of Disseminated Gonococcal Infection

Clinical Diagnosis	Patient	Musculoskeletal Manifestations	Dermatitis	Genitourinary Manifestations	Blood Tests	Therapy
Disseminated gono-coccal infection	Young, healthy, more often women	Tenosynovitis (70%); migratory polyar-thralgias (70%); monoarthritis, joint fluid culture positive (<25%)	Common (70%), but culture positive in only 80%	Symptoms in <25%, but positive cul-tures in 80%	Positive cultures in 10 to 30%	Antibiotics (complete and rapid re-sponse)
Non-neisserial bacte-rial arthritis	Often immunocom-promised	Monoarthritis with positive joint fluid culture	None	None, unless urinary tract infection is source of bacter-emia	Positive cultures in 50 to 70%	Antibiotics, drainage
Hepatitis	Exposed to hepatitis	Tenosynovitis, polyar-thritis	Rash, usually urti-carial	None	Abnormal liver func-tion tests; HB$_s$Ag	Salicylates or other nonsteroidal anti-inflammatory drugs
Reiter's syndrome	Young, healthy, more often men, with re-cent history of ure-thritis, dysentery	Asymmetric arthritis, sacroiliitis	Keratodermia, circin-ate balanitis	Nongonococcal urethritis	HLA-B27 positive or (+)	Nonsteroidal anti-in-flammatory drugs
Acute rheumatic fever	Children, young adults	Migratory arthritis	Erythema margina-tum; subcuta-neous nodules	None	Serologic evidence of recent streptococcal throat infection	Salicylates
Bacterial endocarditis	Any age	Arthralgias, myalgias, arthritis	Emboli, macules	None	Positive blood culture	Antibiotics
Juvenile rheumatoid arthritis	Children, young adults	Mono- or polyarthritis	Evanescent rash	None	Possibly, striking leu-kocytosis	Salicylates, other nonsteroidal anti-inflammatory drugs
Lyme disease	Children, young adults; appropriate geo-graphic exposure	Mono-or oligoarthritis	Circular, enlarging lesion 2 weeks before arthritis	None	Antibody to spirochete	Initially antibiotics; later, salicylates, nonsteroidal anti-inflammatory drugs, and anti-biotics

and dermatitis. Although tenosynovitis can occur with other types of arthritis, the presence of teno-synovitis or arthritis in association with a skin rash is sufficient clinical grounds for a presumptive diagnosis of DGI. Most patients are febrile, demonstrate pe-ripheral blood leukocytosis, and have an elevated erythrocyte sedimentation rate. These nonspecific findings are not always present, however. If synovial fluid can be aspirated, the leukocyte count is generally 30,000 to 100,000 cell/mm^3, although the range is wider than in the joint effusions of nongonococcal bacterial arthritis, and some fluids are relatively acel-lular. A Gram-stained smear of concentrated synovial fluid is positive in fewer than 25% of purulent joint effusions, in contrast with other forms of bacterial arthritis.[6] In most recent series, the genitourinary cul-tures provided the best yield of Neisseria gonor-rhoeae, whereas blood and skin cultures were rarely positive (Table 116–4).[5,9–12] The urethra should be swabbed to obtain a specimen for culture because most men do not have a urethral discharge. In women, a specimen should be obtained directly from the cervix. Rectal and pharyngeal cultures should be obtained, particularly the latter because pharyngeal gonorrhea may lead to disseminated infection. In-vestigators are currently using specific polyclonal and monoclonal antisera in attempts to identify gonococ-cal antigens in sterile joint fluid and blood in patients with DGI. Tests for immunologic detection of gono-coccal antigens in cervical specimens are already com-mercially available.

When Gram-stained smears or cultures of the syn-ovial fluid or blood are negative, a therapeutic re-sponse to penicillin or other appropriate antibiotic is so rapidly effective that it may be an important di-agnostic clue to DGI. Therefore, it is common to ini-tiate antibiotic therapy in patients with suspected DGI while awaiting the identification of the organisms in the culture specimen. Most patients become afebrile and their clinical manifestations subside within 48 to 72 hours. Some other forms of bacterial arthritis or viral arthritis have initial features similar to those of DGI. Meningococcal arthritis is the most difficult bac-terial arthritis to differentiate from DGI, and the mus-culoskeletal manifestations of the disorders are vir-tually identical.[30] A chronic purulent monoarthritis may occur in chronic meningococcemia.[30] As in DGI, evidence suggests toxic or immunologic mechanisms because depressed serum complement and deposi-tion of IgG, IgM, complement, and meningococcal antigen have been identified in the synovial membrane and the synovial fluid, and the synovial fluid is usually sterile.

Non-neisserial bacterial arthritides share many clinical features distinct from those of DGI.[6] Gram-positive coccal arthritis or arthritis caused by gram-negative bacilli often occurs in the extremely young or in the elderly, it almost always causes monoarthritis, and it often occurs in compromised hosts. These disorders are not associated with tenosynovitis or dermatitis, and they do not usually respond quickly to treatment; repeated needle aspirations or surgical drainage, as well as prolonged parenteral antibiotics, are often required (Table 116-4). Even with optimal treatment, permanent joint destruction is common.

Other major differential diagnostic considerations include hepatitis, Reiter's syndrome, acute rheumatic fever, bacterial endocarditis, other bacteremias, and other connective tissue diseases (Table 116-4). Polyarthritis, tenosynovitis, and a skin rash are common in hepatitis; the rash and arthritis generally occur in the anicteric phase. The skin rash is usually urticarial, and the synovial fluid leukocyte count is usually lower than in DGI. The most helpful diagnostic features are elevated hepatocellular enzymes and the identification of hepatitis surface antigen (HB$_s$Ag) in the blood, with negative blood and synovial fluid cultures. Reiter's syndrome may also cause arthritis, tenosynovitis, and urethritis. In classic Reiter's syndrome, the urethritis is not due to Neisseria gonorrhoeae, but rather is nongonococcal. Other helpful clinical features include the presence of conjunctivitis, characteristic mucocutaneous lesions, circinate balanitis, and keratoderma blennorrhagicum. Clinical and radiologic evidence of sacroiliitis and the presence of HLA-B27 on lymphocytes are also characteristic of Reiter's syndrome. Acute rheumatic fever may cause polyarthritis in young adults without carditis, chorea, or subcutaneous nodules. Some investigators have termed this disorder poststreptococcal arthritis rather than acute rheumatic fever. If a skin rash is present, it usually is transient (erythema marginatum). The diagnosis relies on evidence of a recent streptococcal throat infection, confirmed by culture or by serologic testing of blood, and a rapid response to salicylates or other anti-inflammatory agents.

Many bacteremias or other systemic infections can cause musculoskeletal and dermatologic manifestations that mimic DGI. Bacterial endocarditis is especially important to differentiate from DGI. Purulent arthritis is not common in bacterial endocarditis unless hematogenous spread to the synovium occurs, such as occasionally seen in endocarditis caused by Staphylococcus aureus. Myalgias, arthralgias, tendinitis, and back pain are common musculoskeletal manifestations associated with bacterial endocarditis, particularly subacute disease already present for several weeks. Viral diseases including measles and rubella, as well as various arboviral infections not commonly seen in the United States, can also cause skin lesions and arthritis. Rarely, infections caused by herpesviruses are accompanied by a skin rash and arthralgias.

Lyme disease, caused by a spirochete, is also associated with a skin rash, but the rash is a characteristic enlarging annular lesion (erythema chronicum migrans) and antedates the onset of the arthritis by a few weeks (see Chapter 104). Another disease caused by spirochetes, secondary syphilis, also may cause arthritis and a skin rash.

Patients with rheumatoid arthritis (RA), systemic lupus erythematosus, or other connective tissue diseases may have initial manifestations similar to those of DGI. Adult-onset juvenile RA is especially confusing, in view of the fever, skin rash, polyarthralgias, and leukocytosis. In addition, patients with underlying connective tissue disease may develop superimposed gonococcal arthritis or other forms of infectious arthritis. Therefore, septic arthritis must always be considered in patients who have an acute exacerbation of an existing joint inflammation.[6]

THERAPY

The principles of therapy of DGI are similar to those of other forms of infectious arthritis, with some notable exceptions. As mentioned, antibiotic therapy is usually so successful that patients are dramatically better within a few days. Patients who predominantly have arthralgias, fever, and dermatitis are often asymptomatic following 24 to 48 hours of antibiotics. These patients do not usually require more than a single needle aspiration of an inflamed joint for diagnostic purposes. Patients with large, purulent joint effusions, however, often require repeated needle aspirations of the joint and longer antimicrobial treatment, such as 7 to 10 days of parenteral antibiotics. In the experience of my colleagues and myself, the average duration of hospitalization of patients with dermatitis and arthralgias was 4 days, whereas the duration of hospitalization in patients with purulent gonococcal arthritis was 8 days.[3] Other investigators also have determined that a large, purulent joint effusion is the single most important determinant of the length of hospitalization in patients with DGI.[31] The response to treatment of patients with DGI and with purulent effusions is more complete and is faster than that of patients with nongonococcal bacterial arthritis.

However, even in patients with gonococcccal arthritis of the hip, joint drainage is not generally a problem, and only twice in the last 10 years have our patients with gonococcal arthritis required surgical drainage for a recurrent effusion. This finding is in contrast with patients with nongonococcal bacterial arthritis, in whom drainage by needle aspiration is sometimes inadequate, and who often require open drainage, especially when effusions involve the hip or shoulders.[6]

Until recently, the choice of antibiotic in patients with DGI was not difficult because DGI-producing strains were rarely resistant to penicillin. In fact, DGI-producing strains isolated from patients in the United States have been more sensitive to penicillin than strains isolated from patients with local infections.[3] The mean inhibitory concentration to penicillin of DGI-producing strains was 0.0527 µg/ml, as compared to a mean inhibitory concentration of 0.14 µg/ml of strains causing pelvic inflammatory disease and isolated during the same period.[3] None of these DGI-producing strains were penicillinase producing; however, some penicillinase-producing strains causing DGI have been reported,[32] and DGI caused by penicillinase-producing strains is becoming more common in the Far East.

The resistance of certain strains to antibiotics is due to selective mutations that may be promoted by the host-microbial environment. Thus, homosexual males may be infected with organisms that are resistant to the hydrophobic surroundings present in the rectum, and this resistance may also be accompanied by resistance to certain antimicrobial agents. If penicillinase-producing strains become a more common cause of DGI, the choice of antibiotics as well as the utility of a diagnostic trial of antibiotics in DGI will not be nearly as successful. Spectinomycin or some of the newer cephalosporins have been effective in eradicating the penicillin-resistant organisms thus far associated with DGI.[32] At this time, in most patients with DGI, penicillin is the antibiotic of choice. However, in areas where penicillinase-producing strains predominate, initial antibiotic therapy should include a third-generation cephalosporin. Cultures of local and disseminated sites must be checked for multiple antibiotic-resistant strains, because some penicillinase-producing strains are also chromosomally mediated resistant to penicillin, tetracycline, and cefoxitin sodium.

Various treatment regimens have been recommended, and essentially all of them are successful. Large doses of parenteral antibiotics, such as 10 million U penicillin G administered daily for 7 to 10 days, have been recommended by some, but 1.2 million U penicillin intramuscularly or 2 g erythromycin orally have been administered by others (Table 116–5).[31,33] At present, no single antibiotic regimen is felt to be superior to others. I generally hospitalize patients with DGI and begin parenteral therapy with 2 to 4 million U penicillin intravenously daily. If the patient responds dramatically or if no large joint effusions are present, I discharge the patient after a few days of parenteral antibiotics and complete a 7-day course of antibiotics with oral drugs. Patients who have significant joint effusions or who are more resistant to therapy receive parenteral antibiotics for 7 days in the hospital or until all signs of joint inflammation have subsided.

In conclusion, DGI has become the most common cause of septic arthritis and is a leading cause of acute arthritis necessitating hospitalization. DGI occurs most often in young, healthy women and generally causes initial polyarthralgias, tenosynovitis, and dermatitis. In contrast with other types of bacterial arthritis, purulent joint effusions are present in fewer than half these patients, and Neisseria gonorrhoeae can be recovered from only half the effusions. Other sites of dissemination such as the skin and blood cultures are also usually sterile; therefore, the diagnosis is usually made by a typical clinical picture and by positive genitourinary, pharyngeal, or rectal cultures.

Treatment consists of antibiotic administration and, if necessary, joint drainage with needle aspirations. Response to treatment is rapid, and permanent joint destruction is rare. Antibiotic-resistant strains have only recently been recovered from patients with DGI, and unless these strains become more prevalent, a

Table 116–5. Treatment of Disseminated Gonococcal Infection*

Patients with arthralgias and tenosynovitis
   24 to 48 hours of moderate-dose penicillin IM or IV, followed by 5 to 7 days of oral ampicillin or other antibiotic
   Outpatient management possible, although with an initial 24 to 48 hours of hospitalization

Patients with large effusions
   Hospitalization until signs of sepsis and joint inflammation have disappeared
   Large doses of penicillin (4 to 10 million U/day) IM or IV for 7 to 10 days
   Joint drainage with repeated needle aspirations until purulent effusions fail to reaccumulate

Patients allergic to penicillin
   Same as above, but with spectinomycin, erythromycin, or tetracyclines

Patients possibly infected with a penicillinase-producing strain
   Same as above, but with spectinomycin or one of the newer cephalosporins and a determination of the sensitivity of the organism

*Always repeat cultures in 3 to 5 days to determine cure.
IM = Intramuscularly; IV = intravenously.

rapid therapeutic response to penicillin can be used for diagnostic purposes.

The clinical features of DGI that resemble serum sickness and the frequency of negative blood, skin, and joint fluid cultures support the theory that certain of the manifestations of DGI may not require the presence of viable Neisseria gonorrhoeae, but rather may relate to toxic or immune-mediated inflammation. The relationship of these mechanisms with certain host and microbial characteristics will require further elucidation.

REFERENCES

1. Wehrbein, H.L.: Gonococcus arthritis—a study of 610 cases. Surg. Gynecol. Obstet., 49:105–113, 1929.
2. Keefer, C.S., and Spink, W.W.: Gonococcic arthritis: Pathogenesis, mechanism of recovery and treatment. JAMA, 109:1448–1453, 1937.
3. O'Brien, J.P., Goldenberg, D.L., and Rice, P.A.: Disseminated gonococcal infection: A prospective analysis of 49 patients and a review of the pathophysiology and immune mechanisms. Medicine, 62:395–406, 1983.
4. Rice, P.A., and Goldenberg, D.L.: Clinical manifestations of disseminated infection caused by Nesseria gonorrhoeae are linked to differences in bactericidal reactivity of infecting strains. Ann. Intern. Med., 95:175–178, 1981.
5. Britigan, B.E., Cohen, M.S., and Sparling, P.F.L.: Gonococcal infections: A model of molecular pathogenesis. N. Engl. J. Med., 312:1683–1694, 1985.
6. Goldenberg, D.L., and Reed, J.I.: Bacterial arthritis. N. Engl. J. Med., 312:764–771, 1985.
7. Keiser, H., Ruben, F.L., Wolinsky, E., and Kushner, I.: Clinical forms of gonococcal arthritis. N. Engl. J. Med., 279:234–240, 1968.
8. Holmes, K.K., Counts, G.W., and Beaty, H.N.: Disseminated gonococcal infection. Ann. Intern. Med., 74:979–993, 1971.
9. Brandt, K.D., Cathcart, E.S., and Cohen, A.S.: Gonococcal arthritis: Clinical features correlated with blood, synovial fluid and genito-urinary cultures. Arthritis Rheum., 17:503–512, 1974.
10. Brogadir, S.P., Schimmer, B.M., and Myers, A.R.: Spectrum of the gonococcal arthritis-dermatitis syndrome. Semin. Arthritis Rheum., 8:177–183, 1979.
11. Gelfand, S.C., Masi, A.T., and Garcia-Kutzbach, A.: Spectrum of gonococcal arthritis. J. Rheumatol., 2:83–90, 1979.
12. Masi, A.T., and Eisenstein, B.I.: Disseminated gonococcal infection and gonococcal arthritis. Semin. Arthritis Rheum., 10:173–198, 1981.
13. Salit, I.E., Blake, M., and Gotschlich, E.C.: Intra-strain heterogeneity of gonococcal pili is related to opacity colony variance. J. Exp. Med., 151:716–725, 1980.
14. Cannon, J.G., Buchanan, T.M., and Sparling, P.F.: Confirmation of association of protein I serotype of Neisseria gonor-rhoeae with aiblity to cause disseminated infection. Infect. Immun., 40:816–819, 1983.
15. Wiesner, P.J., Handsfield, H.H., and Holmes, K.K.: Low antibiotic resistance of gonococci causing disseminated infection. N. Engl. J. Med., 288:1221–1222, 1973.
16. Petersen, B.H., Lee, T.J., Snyderman, R., and Brooks, G.F.: Neisseria meningitidis and Neisseria gonorrhoeae bacteremia associated with C6, C7, or C8 deficiency. Ann. Intern. Med., 90:917–920, 1979.
17. Heckels, J.E.: Structural comparison of N. gonorrhoeae outer membrane proteins. J. Bacteriol., 145:736–742, 1981.
18. Segal, E., et al.: Role of chromosomal rearrangement in N. gonorrhoeae pilus phase variation. Cell, 40:293–300, 1985.
19. Ebright, J.R., and Komorowski, R.: Gonococcal endocarditis associated with immune complex glomerulonephritis. Am. J. Med., 68:793–796, 1980.
20. Goldenberg, D.L.: "Post-infectious" arthritis: A new look at an old concept with particular attention to disseminated gonococcal infection. Am. J. Med., 74:925–928, 1983.
21. Rosenthal, L., Olhagen, B., and Elk, S.: Aseptic arthritis after gonorrhoeae. Ann. Rheum. Dis., 39:141–146, 1980.
22. Barr, J., and Danielson, D.: Septic gonococcal dermatitis. Br. J. Med., 1:482–485, 1971.
23. Scherer, R., and Braun-Falco, O.: Alternative pathway complement activation: A possible mechanism inducing skin lesions in benign gonococcal sepsis. Br. J. Dermatol., 95:303–309, 1976.
24. Shapiro, L., Teisch, J.A., and Brownstein, M.H.: Dermatohistopathology of chronic gonococcal sepsis. Arch. Dermatol., 107:403–406, 1973.
25. Manicourt, D.H., and Orloff, S.: Gonococcal arthritis-dermatitis syndrome. Arthritis Rheum., 25:574–578, 1982.
26. Walker, L.C., et al.: Circulating immune complexes in disseminated gonorrheal infection. Ann. Intern. Med., 89:28–33, 1978.
27. Shiel, W.C., et al.: Immune complexes in synovial fluid and serum from patients with disseminated gonococcal infection: evidence for local immune complex formation within the joint. Ann. Rheum. Dis., 45:816–820, 1986.
28. Goldenberg, D.L., Chisholm, P.L., and Rice, P.A.: Experimental models of bacterial arthritis: A microbiologic and histopathologic characterization of the arthritis after the intra-articular injection of Neisseria gonorrhoeae, Staphylococcus aureus, group A streptococci and Escherichia coli. J. Rheumatol., 10:1–7, 1983.
29. Goldenberg, D.L., Reed, J.I., and Rice, P.A.: Arthritis in rabbits induced by killed Neisseria gonorrhoeae and gonococcal lipopolysaccharide. J. Rheumatol., 11:3–8, 1984.
30. Fam, A.G., Tenebaum, J., and Stein, J.L.: Clinical forms of meningococcal arthritis: A study of five cases. J. Rheumatol., 6:567–573, 1979.
31. Handsfield, H.H., Wiesner, P.J., and Holmes, K.K.: Treatment of the gonococcal arthritis-dermatitis syndromes. Ann. Intern. Med., 84:661–667, 1976.
32. Rinaldi, R.Z., Harrison, W.O., and Fan, P.T.: Penicillin-resistant gonococcal arthritis. Ann. Intern. Med., 97:43–45, 1982.
33. Thompson, S.E., et al.: Gonococcal tenosynovitis-dermatitis and septic arthritis: Intravenous penicillin vs. oral erythromycin. JAMA, 244:1101–1102, 1980.

ARTHRITIS DUE TO MYCOBACTERIA, FUNGI, AND PARASITES

117

RONALD P. MESSNER

MYCOBACTERIA

Tuberculous, mycotic, and parasitic infections are relatively rare causes of arthritis. They are important because they are potentially curable. Proper diagnosis requires awareness of their clinical presentations together with identification of the organism in synovial fluid or tissue. Certain immunologic tests are helpful but do not replace the need to examine material directly from the involved joints. Constitutional symptoms and radiographic evidence of extra-articular involvement are often absent. These infections should be sought in the evaluation of patients with chronic monoarticular arthritis and should be considered in various other situations, including spondylitis, tendonitis, and erythema nodosum (Table 117–1).

TUBERCULOSIS

The incidence of new cases of tuberculosis of all types has decreased dramatically in the United States in the last 40 years. In 1932 there were 77 new cases per 100,000 population, and in 1984 only 9.4 per 100,000. The incidence is highest in congested cities. Tuberculosis affects nonwhites six times more frequently than whites, and males twice as often as females. Immigrants from developing countries, elderly nursing home patients, and hemodialysis patients appear to be at increased risk. Approximately 15% of cases involve extrapulmonary sites,[1] and 1 to 3% of patients have bone and/or joint tuberculosis.[2,3] The rarity of bone and joint tuberculosis has lowered the index of suspicion in the medical community, often resulting in unfortunate delays in diagnosis.[4] There is evidence that the number of newly reported cases

Table 117–1. Typical Clinical Presentations of Arthritis Due to Tuberculosis or Mycoses

Tuberculosis	Spondylitis; monoarticular disease of large weight-bearing joints.
Atypical tuberculosis	Tendonitis in hand or wrist.
Leprosy	Polyarthritis with erythema nodosum leprosum; destruction of small bones and joints of hands and feet; neuropathic wrists or ankles.
Coccidioidomycosis	Polyarthritis with erythema nodosum; monoarticular arthritis of knee.
Blastomycosis	Monoarticular arthritis of large weight-bearing joints associated with lung and skin involvement; spondylitis.
Cryptococcosis	Monoarticular arthritis secondary to osseous infection; spondylitis.
Histoplasmosis	Polyarthritis with erythema nodosum.
Sporotrichosis	Monoarticular arthritis of knee, wrist, or hand; polyarthritis with disseminated skin lesions.
Candidiasis	Monoarticular arthritis of the knee in patient with serious concurrent illness.
Actinomycosis	Spondylitis.

of extrapulmonary tuberculosis remained constant throughout the last decade.[5] On a global scale, there are an estimated 10 million new cases of all types of tuberculosis per year, and one half of the world's population has been infected with this organism.[6]

In the nonimmune host, primary tuberculosis begins in the lungs. It is characterized by rapid multiplication of tubercle bacilli and dissemination by way of blood and lymph to all parts of the body. The disease usually resolves coincident with development of delayed hypersensitivity and cellular immunity. In a few patients, it progresses and may result in disseminated tuberculosis or progressive disease limited to one or two organ systems. In contrast, tuberculosis in the immune person is characterized by a vigorous tissue response with local necrosis but relative containment of the infection. Dissemination does not occur unless a bronchus or blood vessel is eroded. Tuberculosis of bone can develop in three ways: by hematogenous spread, by lymphatic spread from chronic pleural, renal, or lymph node foci, or by reactivation of latent infection at sites seeded in the primary illness.[7] Involvement of joints may be direct by the hematogenous route or may occur secondary to osseous infection. Articular tuberculosis is often a combination of osteomyelitis and arthritis.[2] The inflammatory reaction in the synovium is followed by formation of granulation tissue, effusion, and production of a pannus. Cartilage destruction begins in the periphery of the joint and proceeds slowly compared with pyogenic infections. Ultimately, the process results in severe destruction of bone, cold abscesses, and sinus tract formation.

Fifty percent of cases of skeletal tuberculosis occur in the spine. The next most common sites are large weight-bearing joints. The hip and knee are each affected in about 15% of cases and the ankle or wrist in 5 to 10% of cases. Skeletal infection often occurs in the absence of active or even inactive pulmonary disease. The incidence of coexistent active pulmonary infection varies from 10 to 50% in various series.[7–9] Evidence of previous infection has been found in up to 40% of patients and other extrapulmonary disease in about 20% of patients. Multiple skeletal lesions are more common in children but occur in only 5 to 15% of all patients.

Tuberculosis of the Spine. In developing countries, spinal tuberculosis (Pott's disease) is seen primarily in children and young adults. In the United States and Europe, cases in which the patients are in the first decade of life have almost disappeared, and most patients are over 40. Typically, the infection starts in the margins of the vertebral bodies and invades the disc space early. The disc space narrows, destruction

of bone leads to vertebral collapse with kyphosis or gibbous deformity, and a cold paraspinous abscess forms. The midthoracic to upper lumbar area is usually affected.[7,10] Skip areas with radiographically normal vertebrae in-between occur in about 10% of patients. Paraspinous abscesses are common (50 to 96%) and may dissect for long distances up or down the spine or out along the ribs to point in the neck, groin, chest wall, or sternum.[7,10] The most common symptom is back pain.[11] Muscle spasm, local tenderness, kyphosis, and referred pain from root compression complete the typical clinical picture. Neurologic symptoms caused by cord compression (Pott's paraplegia) occur in 10 to 25% of patients with spinal tuberculosis.[8,12] Kyphosis, which is more common in paraplegic patients, is associated with destructive vertebral lesions in the thoracic area more often than in the lumbar area. Altered sensation is present below the level of the lesion. Lower motor neuron weakness caused by coexistent root compression is sometimes observed.[12] Cerebral spinal fluid examination reveals a partial or complete block and increased protein with normal cell count and sugar.

Another complication of spinal tuberculosis is a mycotic aneurysm of the aorta, usually created when a paraspinous abscess penetrates the vessel wall. The resulting hematoma walls off to form a false aneurysm. Penetration of the abscess into the arterial blood may lead to secondary hematogenous spread and miliary disease.[13] Other notable frequent sites of tuberculosis of the axial skeleton are the sacroiliac joints and the ribs. Rib lesions are often associated with a local soft-tissue mass and pain. They generally occur in patients with other skeletal involvement, particularly in the spine. Sacroiliac joint involvement, usually unilateral, occurs in about 7% of patients with skeletal tuberculosis.

Tuberculosis of Peripheral Joints. Articular tuberculosis presents as chronic monoarticular disease in approximately 85% of patients. Though it may occur at any age, as with spinal tuberculosis it is now rare in patients in the first decade of life in developed countries. The peak incidence is in the fourth and fifth decades. The incidence in males and nonwhites is twice that in females and whites. In the hip, tubercle bacilli may localize in the synovium, acetabulum, or proximal femur. Bony destruction is seen most commonly in the acetabulum. The femoral neck and capital and trochanteric epiphyses are also frequent sites of involvement. Symptoms include mild to moderate pain in the groin, knee, or thigh, and limitation of motion. A limp is the most common presenting complaint in children. Atrophy of the gluteal muscles and tenderness in the groin are often present. At rest, the hip is held in flexion and abduction. Later severe destruction of the femoral neck and acetabulum occurs with formation of a cold abscess and sinus tract, which usually points to the outer thigh.

In the knee, pain is the first symptom of tuberculosis in 70% of patients. It is insidious in onset and may persist for years before the patient seeks medical attention. About 20% of patients describe swelling, and 10% have stiffness as the initial complaint.[14] Localized heat and muscular wasting are usually present on examination. A limp, synovial swelling, and limitation of motion are common. Although pure synovial infection does occur, most patients have involvement of both synovium and bone.[14] Symptoms in other joints are similar to those described in the hip and knee: chronic low-grade pain, swelling, and stiffness with slowly progressive loss of function and eventual abscess formation. Tuberculosis involving tendons in the hand and wrist may cause a carpal tunnel syndrome.[15] Infection of the trochanteric bursa has also been reported. A rare patient with tuberculosis may present with acute polyarticular arthritis, a high swinging fever, and evidence of active disease in the chest or lymph nodes (Poncet's disease). In these patients, joints are normal radiographically, and articular symptoms resolve several weeks after initiation of antituberculous drugs.[16]

Radiographic Signs. There are no pathognomonic roentgenographic signs of skeletal tuberculosis. In general, tuberculosis causes destruction of bone without stimulating much reactive new bone formation. Destructive osseous lesions adjacent to joints[7] are often oval with clear margins and no periosteal reaction (Fig. 117–1). As they expand and erode the cortex, some periosteal reaction occurs. Sequestra formation is rare. When the joint itself is involved, local osteopenia and soft-tissue swelling are early signs. Later small subchondral erosions appear at the margins of the joint (Fig. 117–2). The cartilage space tends to be preserved until extensive destruction of adjacent cortical bone has occurred (Fig. 117–3). With advanced disease, total destruction of the joint can occur. Destruction is not accompanied by osteophyte formation, but the shadow of a cold abscess may be seen.

In the spine, the classic picture is narrowing of the disc space with vertebral collapse and a paraspinous abscess. Scalloping of the anterior vertebral surface is common.[10] Occasional infection of the central portion of the vertebrae may cause extensive bone destruction without disc space invasion. In about 10% of patients productive or sclerotic changes, which are difficult to see radiographically, may occur in infected vertebrae.

FIG. 117–1.   Tuberculosis of the knee and femur in a child.

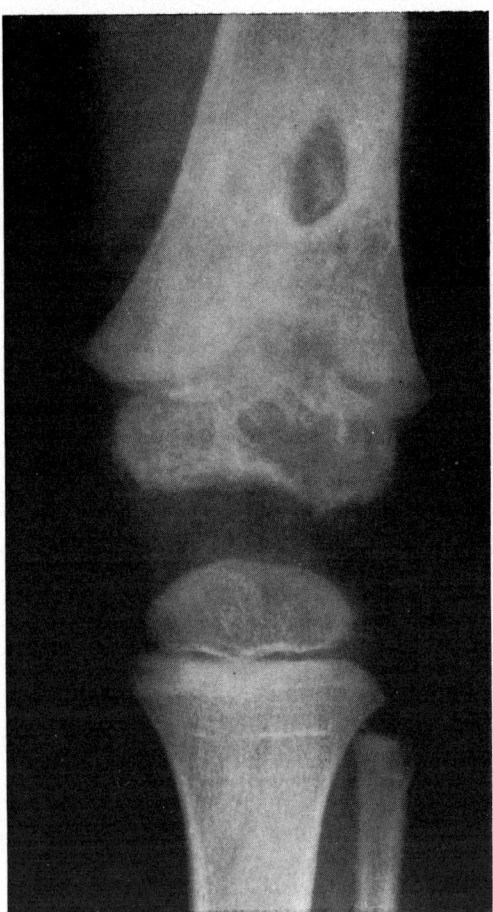

Computerized tomographic scanning is helpful in determining the extent of the involvement.[11]

Diagnostic Tests. Diagnosis of tuberculous arthritis requires an index of suspicion and a willingness to obtain material for histologic examination and culture. The quickest and most reliable method of diagnosis is biopsy. A positive diagnosis can be made by either histology or culture of synovial tissue in over 90% of specimens. Synovial fluid culture is positive in approximately 80% of cases and smear in 20% of cases.[17,18] Synovial fluid protein is always elevated, whereas 60% of patients have fluid with low glucose levels. The synovial white blood cell count varies widely but is usually between 10,000 and 20,000/mm^3. Polymorphonuclear leukocytes may account for 90% of the total white cell count. In the case of spinal disease, material for culture is best obtained with a needle biopsy guided by fluoroscopy or computed tomography (CT). The Mantoux test with stabilized purified protein derivative (PPD-S) is positive in most cases of skeletal tuberculosis. In advanced disease or

FIG. 117–2. Tuberculosis of the knee in an adult. (Courtesy of Donald Resnick, M.D.)

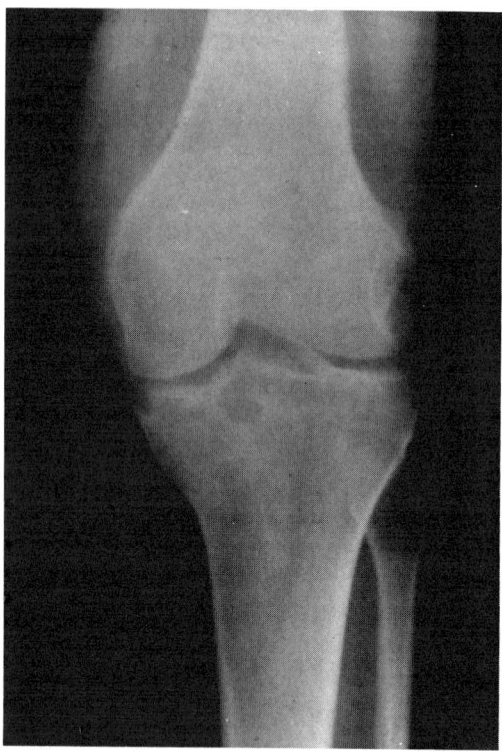

FIG. 117–3. Advanced tuberculosis of the knee. (Courtesy of Donald Resnick, M.D.)

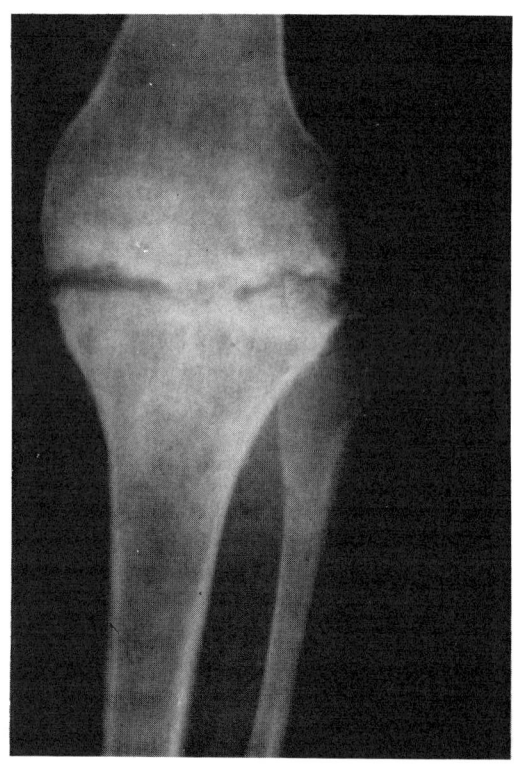

old age, anergy may be present. Anergy may be nonspecific or it may be specific for PPD-S.

Treatment. The keystone of treatment of skeletal tuberculosis is the use of combinations of chemotherapeutic agents. Because skeletal infection is rare compared with pulmonary involvement, the bulk of information on therapy comes from experience with pulmonary disease. The recommended initial combination is isoniazid (5 mg/kg, up to 300 mg orally daily) and rifampin (10 mg/kg, up to 600 mg orally daily) and pyrazinamide (15 to 30 mg/kg, up to 2 g daily). Pyrazinamide should be discontinued after 2 months. Ethambutol, 15 mg/kg daily, should be added until drug sensitivity is confirmed if the patient has emigrated from an area with a known high level of initial drug resistance or has a history of previous antituberculosis chemotherapy.[19] The optimum duration of treatment of skeletal tuberculosis has not been defined. Short-course therapy using isoniazid and rifampin for 9 months has proved equal or superior to other regimens in initial treatment of pulmonary disease. It is suggested that this form of treatment is also adequate for extrapulmonary disease, but the response to treatment must be evaluated in each case. The major contraindication to the combined use of isoniazid and rifampin is the presence of active liver disease. If alternative drug combinations are used, treatment must be continued for 18 to 24 months.

The role of surgery is more controversial, but some general guidelines can be drawn. In articular disease with absent or minimal bone involvement, drug therapy alone is effective. If bone involvement is extensive, debridement of the foci of bone infection may hasten healing. Synovectomy with curettage may be important in children with hip disease. When destruction is extensive in weight-bearing joints, arthrodesis has been the procedure of choice. In developing countries where sitting cross-legged and squatting are important, Girdlestone excision arthroplasty has been used effectively for hip disease.[20] Total hip replacement may be successful if the active infection is controlled.[21]

A series of reports from around the world on spinal tuberculosis indicate that chemotherapy is as successful alone as when combined with surgery.[9,11,22] Immobilization offers no benefit, and debridement procedures are indicated only when material for culture cannot be obtained by needle biopsy. Even in Pott's paraplegia, surgery may not be needed unless there is severe neurologic dysfunction when the patient is first seen or unless progressive neurologic deterioration occurs on adequate chemotherapy.[11,23]

Atypical Tuberculosis. Atypical mycobacteria are ubiquitous, generally saprophytic organisms that have low pathogenicity for man.[24] Surveys with skin tests have shown that up to 48% of healthy young adults have developed delayed hypersensitivity to various members of this group. In addition to producing pulmonary disease resembling typical tuberculosis, these mycobacteria can infect joints, tendons, and bursae. Patients with arthritis rarely have active pulmonary disease. Approximately 50% of patients with articular disease have involvement of tendon sheaths or joints in the hand and wrist, while 20% have infection of the knee.[25-27] Infection of the hip, elbow, ankle, and prepatellar and olecranon bursae, as well as periarticular tissue simulating arthritis, have also been described. Several patients with flexor tendonitis at the wrist have had carpal tunnel syndrome. Polyarticular disease has occurred in about 15% of patients. A history of prior trauma or operation has been obtained in 45% of patients, and 36% have had prior intra-articular injection of corticosteroids. About one quarter of these patients have an underlying illness, most commonly another form of arthritis, such as degenerative joint disease, rheumatoid arthritis, or systemic lupus. The group I photochromogens Mycobacterium kansasii and M. marinum are the most frequent offenders, followed by the group III nonphotochromogen M. intracellularis.

Skin testing with PPDs prepared from atypical mycobacteria correlates well with culture results in children. In adults, cross-reactivity between various PPDs can lead to confusion. Microscopic examination of synovial fluid or biopsy material may reveal granuloma and acid-fast bacilli, but definitive diagnosis of the type of infection requires culture. Although data are not as plentiful on atypical infections, it appears that the yield of positive cultures from biopsies and synovial fluid will be similar to that obtained with M. tuberculosis. Treatment should be based on in-vitro sensitivity testing because these organisms are often resistant to the standard antituberculosis drug regimen. A combination of four or five drugs and/or synovectomy may be necessary.

LEPROSY

Joint involvement was noted as a prominent symptom of leprosy in the Chinese medical writings of the *Nei Ching* in 600 BC.[28] The "stiff joints" described by these ancient physicians may occur in several ways. The indolent course of leprosy is punctuated by reactions. In *lepromatous leprosy*, these reactions take the form of erythema nodosum leprosum, in which inflamed subcutaneous nodules develop in crops. This condition may be accompanied by fever and arthralgia, by pitting edema of the hands from the metacarpal joints to the midforearm, or by a frank polyarthritis that involves knees, ankles, and small joints of the hands.[29] Synovial biopsy reveals an acute inflammatory reaction.[30] In most patients, lepra organisms are not detected in the synovium, and the synovial fluid is a transudate.[31] It has been postulated that this form of arthritis has an immunologic basis. However, group III fluid, which contains lepra cells with ingested organisms and high synovial fluid complement values, has been found, suggesting that the synovitis in some patients is due to infection.[32] Reactions in *tuberculoid* or *borderline leprosy* may also be accompanied by joint symptoms that on occasion may simulate rheumatoid arthritis. Another form of arthritis occurs secondary to bone disease. *Direct infection of bone* occurs most commonly in the distal ends of the phalanges. During a reaction, subchondral bone may collapse and cause destruction of the adjacent joint.[30,33]

The most common joint deformities in leprosy occur secondary to disease in the peripheral nerves. Neurotrophic changes lead to absorption of bones, especially in the distal ends of the metatarsals. Sensory loss and repeated trauma are responsible for degenerative changes and aseptic necrosis of bone. These changes, accompanied by infection in soft tissue and bone, are responsible for loss of terminal digits and severe deformities of the hands and feet.[33] The claw hand that occurs secondary to nerve damage can further compound the disability. Finally, true neuropathic joints with complete disorganization of the weight-bearing surfaces and supporting bone may occur. Charcot joints are most frequently seen at the wrist and ankle. In addition to arthritis, a necrotizing vasculitis, the Lucio phenomenon, may occur in the lower legs.[29]

One of the puzzling aspects of leprosy is why some patients develop the lepromatous form of diffuse involvement with anergy and large numbers of bacilli present in macrophages, whereas others develop the tuberculoid form of more localized disease with well-organized, lymphocyte-rich granulomas containing few viable organisms. The T-lymphocytes in lepromatous lesions belong primarily to the CD8-positive suppressor subset, whereas those in the tuberculoid lesions are predominantly CD4-positive helper cells.[34,35] It has been postulated that the predominance of suppressor cells in the lepromatous form reduces the production of lymphokines, which are critical to effective macrophage killing of the organisms. In the lepromatous form, serum antibodies to a unique phenolic glycolipid of Mycobacterium leprae are high, and delayed hypersensitivity is negligible. This situation is reversed in the tuberculoid form, while borderline leprosy covers the gradient in between.

The diagnosis of leprosy rests on demonstration of acid-fast bacilli in skin smears and histologic evidence of lepra organisms, with involvement of peripheral nerves on skin biopsy. From a clinical standpoint, the cardinal sign is anesthesia of the skin. Typically, thermal and tactile senses are lost before the ability to sense pain and pressure. The ulnar and peroneal nerves frequently are involved early.

Treatment of leprosy requires a coordinated effort that includes attention to the social needs of the patient as well as specialized drug therapy and physical measures to protect the skin and joints and to reduce contractures. In response to the increasing incidence of primary and secondary dapsone resistance, the World Health Organization now recommends the use of three drugs in combination for patients with multibacillary disease: dapsone, rifampin, and clofazimine. Dapsone and rifampin are recommended for those with paucibacillary disease.[35] In the United States, patients with leprosy are entitled to treatment by the US Public Health Service.

FUNGI

COCCIDIOIDOMYCOSIS

Coccidioidomycosis is caused by a fungus found in the soil throughout the lower Sonoran life zone. This zone includes the semiarid areas of southern California, Arizona, and New Mexico as well as western Texas and northern Mexico. It is characterized by hot summers, moderately wet winters, and infrequent freezes. The fungus multiplies in the soil after the winter rains, resulting in a higher incidence of disease in the summer months. Primary infection occurs 1 to 3 weeks after inhalation of spores. Clinical signs, which are usually self-limited, include fever, malaise, cough, chest pain, and erythema nodosum. A chronic pulmonary infection closely resembling tuberculosis occurs in about 2% of patients, whereas 0.2% develop widely disseminated disease. Dissemination is more common in black and Filipino males. Patients with collagen vascular diseases or lymphomas who are taking corticosteroids may be at greater risk, and acquired immune deficiency syndrome (AIDS) patients appear to be particularly susceptible.[36,37]

Arthritis occurs in both the benign primary illness and the chronic disseminated form. In primary disease, it is usually associated with erythema nodosum and clears without residual deformity. In chronic disseminated disease, arthritis may occur alone or secondary to bone infection. Bayer and Guze have reviewed 57 cases of coccidioidal arthritis.[38] The most common presentation was a chronic monoarticular arthritis of the knee. The mean age was 36 years, and males outnumbered females by 4 to 1. Patients were otherwise in good health. Only one patient had a major underlying illness. A history of antecedent arthritis or joint injury was rare and only 6 patients (10%) had evidence of coccidioidal infection in extra-articular sites. If the organisms seeded directly to synovium, symptoms of an indolent synovitis with effusion, stiffness, and mild pain dominated the early course. If infection began in adjacent bone with later penetration into the joint, the early signs were pain and loss of motion without effusion. In either case, untreated synovial infection gradually progressed to villous hypertrophy and pannus formation, which often led to bony erosive changes later in the course. The indolent nature of this process is reflected in the long interval from onset of symptoms to diagnosis, a mean of 4.5 years. Its destructive nature is clear; 11 of 26 (42%) of patients whose initial radiographic examination was available showed destructive changes and/or adjacent osteomyelitis at diagnosis. The knee was involved in 39 (70%) of cases, and the wrist, hand, and the ankle were the next most commonly affected sites.

Infection of bone occurs in 10 to 20% of patients with disseminated disease. Sites most often involved are the ends of the long bones, the skull, vertebrae, and ribs. Metacarpals, metatarsals, the tibial tubercle, the malleoli, and the acromial process also appear to be favorite sites of localization. Approximately 60% of patients have involvement of a single site, while 15 to 20% have infection in three or more sites. Multiple bone lesions are associated with rapid dissemination and a poor prognosis. In the more indolent forms of disseminated disease, solitary bone lesions are common. The course of these solitary lesions is one of slow destruction of bone that may progress to involve adjacent joints.

Most joint infections are diagnosed by culture or histologic examination of synovial tissue. Fewer than 5% of synovial fluid cultures have been positive. In purulent material, the characteristic spherules are best seen after digestion with 20% potassium hydroxide. Coccidioides immitis can be cultured on Sabouraud's agar. It is important to notify the bacteriology laboratory if coccidioidomycosis is suspected because the spore-forming mycelial cultures are highly infectious.

Although most patients with disseminated coccidioidomycosis are anergic, 80% of those with coccidioidal arthritis have a positive skin test to coccidioidin. Serologic tests may also be helpful. The tube precipitation test is useful for detecting early primary disease. It is positive within 1 to 3 weeks of infection in 80% of cases, reverts to negative after 6 months, but becomes positive again with relapse or reinfection. In disseminated disease, complement fixation (CF) and immunodiffusion tests are usually positive. Ninety percent of patients with coccidioidal arthritis have positive CF tests. Circulating immune complexes containing coccidioidin antigen have been found in most patients with active disease. It has been suggested that these complexes or free anticoccidioidin antibodies may play a role in the depressed T-lymphocyte responses that may accompany progressive disease.[39]

If the diagnosis is made prior to bone involvement, the development of villonodular synovitis, or pannus formation, treatment with amphotericin B alone may be effective. If any of these events have occurred, drug treatment should be combined with surgery. Intra-articular amphotericin B has been used with success for a few patients.[40] Ketoconazole, a broad-spectrum fungistatic agent with relatively low toxicity, can be given orally and requires gastric acid for absorption. About 80% of patients with osteoarticular disease have shown a good initial response. Unfortunately, 40% have relapsed while still taking the drug or after it has been discontinued.[41,42] It should thus be considered second choice to amphotericin B.

BLASTOMYCOSIS

In the continental United States, blastomycosis occurs primarily in the Ohio and Mississippi river valleys and Middle Atlantic States. Peak incidence is in the 20- to 50-year age group. The organism exists in the soil, apparently in geographically restricted microfoci.[43] Males are affected 10 times more often than females, presumably owing to their greater exposure through outdoor activities.[44] There is only one documented case of human-to-human transmission. Despite the unique susceptibility of dogs to infection, dog-to-human transmission has been documented in only one instance of a bite from an infected animal. Infection, which begins in the lungs after inhalation of spores, may produce a variety of results ranging from an asymptomatic or acute self-limited illness to acutely or insidiously progressive disease. Extrapulmonary infection spreads from the lungs by lymphatic or hematogenous routes. Skin and bone are the most frequent sites. Skeletal involvement occurs in one half

of patients, and approximately 5% will present with joint pain.[45,46]

Articular blastomycosis usually presents as an acute monoarticular synovitis in a patient who is systemically ill with pulmonary and multifocal extrapulmonary disease. Fully 90% of these patients have active lung infections, and 70% have cutaneous abscesses. The knee is the most frequently involved joint, followed by the ankle and elbow. In approximately 70% of patients, joint infection results from hematogenous seeding to synovium; in 30% it is a consequence of extension of an underlying osteomyelitis. Osseous blastomycosis is most common in the vertebrae, ribs, tibia, tarsus, and skull, although involvement of almost every site in bone has been reported. Direct extension into the joint is most often seen at the knee. Spinal infection is associated with destruction of disc spaces, erosion of anterior vertebral bodies, proximal rib development of paraspinal soft tissue, and dissection of the infection beneath the anterior longitudinal ligament. Vertebral infection usually occurs in the thoracic and/or lumbar areas, but is rare in the cervical spine.

Blastomyces dermatitidis organisms are usually seen on potassium hydroxide–treated smears of synovial fluid, sputum, or material from abscesses. Cytologic analysis may reveal the organisms when routine smears are negative.[46] Definitive diagnosis is made on culture. An immunodiffusion test using the A and B antigens of the yeast phase of the organism is specific for B. dermatitidis and has a sensitivity of 80%. The drug of choice for treatment of blastomycotic arthritis is amphotericin B. Ketoconazole is an effective alternative in patients with mild to moderate disease.[47] Although the role of operative treatment has not been fully defined, debridement of devitalized bone or synovium may benefit patients who fail to respond to antifungal drugs.

CRYPTOCOCCOSIS

Infection with Cryptococcus neoformans begins in the lungs with inhalation of spores and spreads to other organs, especially the central nervous system. Predisposing factors for susceptibility to this disease include lymphoma, Hodgkin's disease, diabetes mellitus, sarcoidosis, and corticosteroid treatment.[48,49] The organism is widely distributed in nature. The most dangerous source of infection appears to be pigeon droppings. Bone infection occurs in only about 10% of patients and follows a slowly progressive course.[50] Radiologic changes consist of lytic lesions with sharply scalloped margins and little reaction in adjacent bone or periosteum. These lesions may be found in the metaphyses of long bones, in the flat bones or vertebrae, the ribs, tarsal bones, or carpal bones. Vertebral infection resulting in paraspinal abscess formation can mimic tuberculosis. Only a few detailed reports of cryptococcal arthritis exist in the literature.[51,52] One half involved the knee and three quarters were monoarticular. About three quarters of these patients had an identifiable underlying illness. The synovial fluid of some patients was grossly purulent, whereas others had a relatively low white blood cell count of about 2000 cells/mm[3].

Serologic tests for antibody to cryptococcal antigens are positive in fewer than 50% of proved cases. Cryptococcal antigens in sera or synovial fluid have been detected by agglutination of latex particles coated with rabbit anticryptococcal antibody. Rheumatoid factors can react with rabbit IgG and give a false-positive test. Amphotericin B given in combination with 5-fluorocytosine is the recommended treatment. Although debridement of joints may also be advisable, the data are insufficient to conclude whether medical or combined medical-surgical treatment is more effective.

HISTOPLASMOSIS

Histoplasma capsulatum grows in mycelial form in soil, where it produces spores that infect humans when inhaled. It thrives in ground contaminated with chicken, bird, or bat excreta. The highest incidence of positive histoplasmin skin tests occurs in persons from states adjacent to the confluence of the Mississippi and Ohio rivers. In this area, 60 to 90% of young men are positive. Fortunately, both primary infection and reinfection are usually benign, self-limited diseases. Symptoms range from a transient pneumonitis to more generalized disease characterized by fever, malaise, chest pain, dyspnea, and weight loss. An acute polyarthritis may occur alone or in association with erythema nodosum, and polyarthritis or an additive polyarthralgia may be the presenting symptom of primary histoplasmosis.[53-55] Both types of joint involvement clear without residual deformity.

Progressive disease occurs in only 5% of infected persons. The most common form is a localized pulmonary infection in middle-aged white men. Disseminated histoplasmosis occurs in fewer than 0.1% of infections, usually in older or immune-compromised persons. Its manifestations are protean, and prognosis is poor. In the chronic form of disease, arthritis is truly an unusual clinical problem. Chronic infection of the knee (both unilateral and bilateral) and of the

wrist have been reported.[51] The diagnosis depends on demonstration of Histoplasma capsulatum in histologic sections or culture of involved tissues. Immunologic tests play a minor role in diagnosis. In sensitized persons, the histoplasmin skin test may induce antibodies that will influence serologic tests drawn more than a few days after the skin test. The complement fixation test is positive in 50% of patients with disseminated disease and may also be positive in other fungal diseases. While useful in a few very ill patients, these tests must be interpreted with caution.[56]

SPOROTRICHOSIS

Sporotrichosis is a rare cause of chronic granulomatous arthritis. The organism is a ubiquitous fungus that lives on plants or in the soil. Infection with this organism is usually limited to the skin, where it begins as a painful red nodule at the site of a scratch or a thorn prick. Cutaneous sporotrichosis may spread proximally by the lymphatics to form multiple necrotic secondary satellite lesions, or it may penetrate directly into adjacent tissues. Only a small percentage of people exposed to the fungus develop the systemic form of infection.

Systemic sporotrichosis occurs primarily in men 40 years of age or older. It has been associated with outdoor occupations or hobbies, alcohol abuse, and diseases or drugs that compromise the immune system.[57,58] In many patients, however, it develops without a history of predisposing factors. Two forms of the disease have been described, unifocal and multifocal.[59] Unifocal systemic sporotrichosis most commonly affects the lungs as cavitary disease of the upper lobes closely resembling tuberculosis. The other common presentation is as a chronic monoarthritis or oligoarthritis. Morning stiffness and fever are absent, but synovial thickening and effusions are found in the involved joints. A history of transient improvement with intra-articular steroids but poor response to oral steroids or aspirin may be obtained. The knee is most often involved, followed in decreasing frequency by the wrist, small joints of the hand, ankle, and elbow. Tenosynovitis may occur in the hand or wrist.[60]

Multifocal systemic sporotrichosis typically involves the skin, joints, and bones. These patients are more likely to have a compromised immune system than those who develop unifocal disease. Skin lesions differ from those in cutaneous sporotrichosis. Dusty red nodules up to several centimeters in diameter develop randomly anyplace on the body except the palms and soles. The lesions eventually ulcerate and may heal while new ones appear. The skin around joints, on the face, and on the scalp is most often involved.[61] Skin lesions usually precede joint symptoms. In this form of the disease, the arthritis is polyarticular in about two thirds of patients. As in the unifocal form, tendonitis may be present, and fistulas may develop after surgical procedures on the joints if proper antifungal therapy is not given. Infection of bones spares the vertebrae, ribs, and jaw, but involves long bones near the joints. Joint infection is rarely related to extension of osseous infection. Pulmonary involvement occurs in fewer than 20% of patients with multifocal disease. It differs from unifocal lung disease in that nodules are smaller and do not cavitate. Central nervous system involvement is rare.

Diagnosis of sporotrichosis arthritis rests on culture of Sporothrix schenckii from joint fluid or synovial tissue. Both have yielded positive results, but the percentage of positives appears to be higher with cultures of tissue. The best yield occurs with culture of both tissue and fluid. The organisms are difficult to see in tissue sections. The sedimentation rate is elevated, but peripheral white blood cell counts are normal. Joint fluid shows the pattern of low-grade inflammation with cell counts of 8,000 to 20,000/mm^3, a fair to good mucin clot, and decreased glucose concentration.[60,61] Two serologic tests are available for diagnosis. The latex slide test is preferred because it has fewer false positive reactions and comparable sensitivity (94%) with the tube agglutination test. Titers of 1:4 or greater are presumptive evidence of active disease. Soft-tissue swelling, osteoporosis, decreased joint space, and erosions similar to those occurring in rheumatoid arthritis may be seen radiographically.

Treatment consists of amphotericin B alone or in combination with surgical debridement of infected joints.[60] In a patient unable to tolerate amphotericin B, iodide therapy plus surgical debridement may be a reasonable alternative. Ketoconazole does not appear effective in this disease.[62] Results of treatment of unifocal disease are usually excellent. The main cause of poor results is a long delay between onset of disease and diagnosis. The outcome of multifocal sporotrichosis is less certain. In one report, 11 deaths occurred in 37 patients with this form of disease.[61]

CANDIDAL ARTHRITIS

Arthritis caused by Candida species has been reported with increasing frequency in the past several years. An underlying illness or direct predisposing cause has been present in all patients. Two thirds of the adults were hospitalized with a serious illness, such as cancer, renal failure, sepsis, or a connective tissue disease. Most were receiving antibiotics, chemotherapy, or immunosuppressive treatment and often had indwelling intravenous catheters.[63,64] The remainder of the adults were ambulatory. In these instances, predisposing causes included osteoarthritis with repeated corticosteroid injections, recent joint surgery, and previous joint infection. A similar pattern is seen with candidal osteomyelitis.[65] Heroin addiction has also been noted as a predisposing cause. A distinctive syndrome of follicular and nodular lesions of the scalp, beard, and pubis with ocular infection or osteoarticular lesions of the intervertebral discs, knee, or chondrocostal junctions has been noted in this group of individuals.[66] Ninety percent of children with candidal arthritis have been less than 1 year old. All have had a serious underlying illness, and most were critically ill from other causes at the time the arthritis was diagnosed. As in adults, antibiotics, immunosuppression, and catheters were frequently implicated as predisposing causes. Candidal arthritis may occur in as many as 2% of infants receiving hyperalimentation.[67] Only one case has been reported in association with chronic mucocutaneous candidiasis.

In both adults and children, the knee is involved in 75% of cases. The hip and shoulder are the next most frequently involved joints. Small joint involvement is rare. Multiple joint infections occur about twice as often in infants as in adults (35 vs. 15%), and coexistent osteomyelitis is more common in infants. Infection seeds from the blood to the synovium and may follow fungal septicemia by intervals of 2 to 12 weeks. Symptoms include pain, tenderness, synovial thickening, and effusion, but red hot joints are infrequent. Isolated candidal arthritis following direct injection of organisms into the joint by trauma or arthrocentesis follows a more indolent course. It is not associated with systemic symptoms and is usually caused by less virulent strains of Candida species.[68]

The synovial fluid contains a mean of 38,000 leukocytes/mm^3 with 80% polymorphonuclear leukocytes, but lower counts may be found in patients with leukemia.[64] Synovial fluid glucose levels have been low in 70% of reported cases. Culture of synovial fluid is a highly reliable method for identifying Candida species. Gram stain is not reliable, however, being negative in 80% of culture-positive samples. Candida albicans is the most frequent offender followed by C. tropicalis. Serologic tests for serum antibodies to C. albicans antigens may show a rising titer with dissemination of infection, but these tests do not clearly differentiate heavy colonization of systemic disease.

The relatively small number of reported cases makes it difficult to draw firm conclusions regarding optimum treatment. Amphotericin B alone has resulted in eradication of the infection in about 60% of cases in which it has been used. The failure rate appears to be somewhat less if it is combined with surgical operation or 5-fluorocytosine. The latter drug alone is not a good choice. A few reports on the successful use of ketoconazole have appeared.[69] Overall, 60% of adults and 40% of infants have recovered with normal joint function. Twenty percent of patients in both groups have died of Candida sepsis or of the underlying disease. The remainder have survived with significant disability resulting from destruction of the joint.

ACTINOMYCOSIS

Actinomycosis is caused by an anaerobic bacterialike obligate parasite, Actinomyces israelii, which is a normal resident of the human mouth. Infection occurs through the gastrointestinal tract, particularly after dental procedures or injury to the mouth and jaw. It may also follow aspiration into an atelectatic portion of the lung. Abscesses form in the neck, jaw, lung, or abdomen. Bone involvement is frequent in the jaw and spine, and is usually secondary to abscesses in adjacent tissues. Infection of the spine typically involves several vertebrae, but not the intervening discs. Adjacent pedicles, transverse processes, and the heads of contiguous ribs may be eroded. In the vertebrae, channels of infection surrounded by sclerotic bone cause a "honeycomb" or "soap bubble" radiographic appearance. Long, dense, longitudinal spurs and sclerotic changes in the lateral portions of the vertebrae are sometimes seen when infection spreads from the abdomen to the spine by way of the psoas muscle. Dense trabeculae and sclerosis make vertebral collapse uncommon.[70] Any level of the spine may be affected. Symptoms vary from mild local pain to severe restriction of motion, radicular pain, or weakness. Extension of the infection into the spinal canal may result in meningitis. Diagnosis is made by identification of sulfur granules on Gram's stain of pus from the abscesses and is confirmed by growth of the organism in anaerobic culture. Blood cultures are rarely positive. No serologic test is currently available for actinomycosis. Treatment with tetracycline has been successful, but penicillin is the drug of choice.

MYCETOMA (MADUROMYCOSIS, MADURA FOOT)

Mycetoma is an indolent tumor-like infection found in tropical and semitropical climates. It is caused by a variety of actinomycetes or fungi that gain entrance through the skin. Allescheria boydii is the most common cause in North America, whereas Nocardia brasiliensis is the usual cause in Central and South America. Mycetoma commonly involves the foot, where it invades subcutaneous tissue, bone, and ligaments.[71] In long-standing cases, swelling, sinus formation, and clubbing with pronounced deformity may occur. A similar process may involve the hand. Systemic symptoms and regional lymphadenopathy are uncommon. Effective treatment requires accurate identification of the infecting organism, prolonged high-dose administration of the appropriate antimicrobial agent, and surgical debridement. Prognosis depends to some extent on the causative organism and is better with actinomycotic than with true fungal mycetoma. In some cases, amputation may be necessary.

PARASITES

Parasitic infections may cause arthritis by direct invasion of the joints or through secondary immune mechanisms. They may also involve periarticular tissues and produce nonarticular or soft-tissue rheumatic syndromes (Table 117–2). These mechanisms are not mutually exclusive. Joint involvement is relatively rare in these diseases but a very large number of people in developing countries are involved. For example, 600 million people are estimated to have schistosomiasis or filariasis. Thus even a low incidence of arthritis may result in significant morbidity in these populations.

FILARIASIS

The lymphatic-dwelling filarial parasite Wuchereria bancrofti is transmitted by mosquitoes and is found

Table 117–2. Typical Rheumatologic Syndromes Associated With Parasites

Filariasis	Chylous effusion of the knee
	Monoarthritis or oligoarthritis of large joints
Trichinosis	Myositis
Cisticercosis	Myalgia, skin and muscle nodules
Echinococcosis	Bone cysts
Schistosomiasis	Low back, thigh, knee, and heel pain
Giardiasis	Seronegative arthritis of knees, ankles, and feet

in tropic and subtropic areas. The adult worms live in the lymphatics where they cause first reversible and then irreversible damage to lymph flow, resulting in brawny edema and elephantiasis. An acute inflammatory arthritis of the knee may occur associated with fever and inguinal lymphadenopathy. The initial episode typically lasts only 7 to 10 days but recurrent, less inflammatory effusions may follow. The synovial fluid in these cases is chylous and devoid of parasites. Lymphangiographic studies suggest the presence of a fistula between the abnormal lymphatics and the synovial space.[72] In other instances an acute or chronic monoarthritis or oligoarthritis of large joints, usually involving the knee, occurs with a nonchylous effusion and few if any constitutional symptoms. In these persons the sedimentation rate is often normal, and the rheumatoid factor is usually negative. Resolution of the arthritis with treatment of the underlying filariasis provides the most convincing evidence for a causal relationship between the arthritis and the helminthic infection.[73]

Infection with the guinea worm Dracunculus medinensis can involve the joints by several mechanisms. The adult female worm, which infects millions of people on the Indian subcontinent and in West Africa, migrates into the subcutaneous tissues usually of the lower leg, ankle, or foot where it emerges from the base of a cutaneous ulcer to discharge its larvae. A septic arthritis may occur secondary to bacterial infection of periarticular ulcers. In other cases a mild synovitis occurs in joints adjacent to deep-seated worms. The most dramatic form of arthritis occurs when the worm enters the synovial space and discharges its larvae. An intense inflammation results, probably from the toxic effects of the uterine secretions. The synovial fluid is exudative and the diagnosis can be confirmed by the finding of the larvae in the fluid. Surgical removal of the worm and irrigation of the joint cavity results in prompt relief of symptoms.[74] Other filaria may cause arthritis through direct invasion of the joint. In both *loa loa* and *onchocerciasis*, microfilaria have been found in the synovial fluid of patients with inflammatory arthritis of the knee. In the latter disease a symmetric polyarthritis, possibly caused by deposition of immune complexes, has also been described.

TRICHINOSIS

Trichinella spiralis is a tissue-dwelling round worm that is transmitted directly from host to host by eating contaminated meat. The adult worm causes few if any symptoms in the intestine, but systemic invasion by the larvae, which occurs about 2 weeks after infection, typically results in myositis, with myalgia, weakness and swelling associated with fever, periorbital edema, and headache. Muscle enzymes are elevated in the serum but the erythrocyte sedimentation rate is usually normal. Frequent involvement of the extraocular muscles and eosinophilia help to distinguish trichinosis from polymyositis. A definitive diagnosis can be made with serologic testing.

SCHISTOSOMIASIS

Schistosomes are blood flukes that parasitize the venous channels of the human host. They are endemic in Africa, Asia, South America, and the Caribbean islands. Infection is usually acquired in childhood. Like other helminths, schistosomes do not multiply in man. They do, however, produce eggs that release enzymes to facilitate their exit from the body. The immune response to the eggs and their products results in granuloma formation and subsequent disruption of the function of the tissues in which they lie. Arthritis, when it occurs, usually presents as low-back, thigh, knee, or heel pain. In one series of 124 patients with joint complaints, radiographs of the sacroiliac joints and heels were each abnormal in 40% of the cases.[75] None of the patients had morning stiffness or symptoms in the hands. Tests for rheumatoid factors were negative. In 3 of 11 biopsies of the knee, ova were identified in the synovium; but the other biopsies showed chronic synovitis with lymphocytic plasma cell infiltrates and no ova or adult worms. Thus, the majority of patients appear to have a reactive type of arthritis resembling Reiter's syndrome.

CESTODE INFECTION

Infection with the pork tapeworm Taenia solium may cause fever, eosinophilia, and myalgia during the invasive phase. Later in the disease, cysticerci are frequently found in subcutaneous tissue or muscle, where they form painless nodules. Actual joint involvement is extremely rare. In echinococcosis the embryos are freed from the eggs in the intestine and enter the bloodstream, where they are usually filtered out in the capillary beds of the liver or lung. Occasionally they may lodge in bone, where the formation of the bladder-like cyst results in an enlarging mass that may cause chronic bone pain or spontaneous fracture. Rarely the cyst may involve a joint.[76]

OTHER HELMINTHIC INFECTIONS

Reactive arthritis or "parasitic rheumatism" has been described with Strongyloides stercoralis, Taenia saginata, and Toxocara canis infections.[77] Patients have presented with symmetric polyarthritis, asymmetric oligoarthritis, and also muscle pain and stiffness reminiscent of polymyalgia rheumatica. Most, but not all, have had eosinophilia. The sedimentation rate is usually elevated and the rheumatoid factor is often negative. In all reported cases the joint symptoms have resolved with treatment of the underlying infection. Examination of synovial biopsies or synovial fluid has failed to reveal the organism, but not all patients with this syndrome have had a definitive search for the organisms in the joints. Immune complexes were found in serum and synovial fluid in two patients, and in one case immunoglobulin and complement deposits were found in the synovium. These cases may represent a reactive arthritis or immune complex–mediated disease, but the present data are insufficient to determine the pathologic mechanism with certainty.

PROTOZOAN INFECTION

A seronegative arthritis involving primarily the knees, ankles, and feet may occur in children infected with Giardia lamblia.[78] In some children the arthritis is associated with fever, abdominal pain, diarrhea, and headache, while in a few it is the only symptom. More than one course of treatment with metronidazole may be needed to eliminate the parasite and thus alleviate the joint symptoms. This syndrome is also thought to represent a reactive arthritis.

REFERENCES

1. Glassworth, J., Robins, A.B., and Snider, D.E.J.: Tuberculosis in the 1980's. N. Engl. J. Med., 302:1441–1450, 1980.
2. Davidson, P.T., and Horowitz, I.: Skeletal tuberculosis. Am. J. Med., 48:77–84, 1970.
3. Enarsen, D.A., et al.: Bone and joint tuberculosis: A continuing problem. Can. Med. Assoc. J., 120:139–145, 1979.
4. Evanchick, C.C., Davis, D.E., and Harrington, T.M.: Tuberculosis of peripheral joints: An often missed diagnosis. J. Rheumatol., 13:187–189, 1986.
5. Alvarez, S., and McCabe, W.R.: Extrapulmonary tuberculosis revisited: A review of experience at Boston City and other hospitals. Medicine, 63:25–55, 1984.
6. Ellner, J.J.: Immune dysregulation in human tuberculosis. J. Lab. Clin. Med., 108:142–149, 1986.
7. Nathanson, L., and Cohen, W.: A statistical and roentgen analysis of two hundred cases of bone and joint tuberculosis. Radiology, 36:550–567, 1941.
8. LaFond, E.M.: Analysis of adult skeletal tuberculosis. J. Bone Joint Surg., 40:346–364, 1958.
9. Fancourt, G.J., et al.: Bone tuberculosis: Results and experience in Leicestershire. Br. J. Dis. Chest, 80:265–272, 1986.
10. Bailey, H.L., et al.: Tuberculosis of the spine in children: Operative findings and results in one hundred consecutive patients. J. Bone Joint Surg., 54:1633–1657, 1972.
11. Gorse, G.J., et al.: Tuberculous spondylitis: A report of 6 cases and a review of the literature. Medicine, 62:178–193, 1983.
12. Ginsburg, S., et al.: The neurological complications of tuberculous spondylitis. Arch. Neurol., 16:265–276, 1967.
13. Felson, R., et al.: Mycotic tuberculous aneurysm of the thoracic aorta. J.A.M.A., 237:1104–1108, 1977.
14. Key, L.A.: Tuberculosis of the knee joint in adults. Br. Med. J., 1:408, 1940.
15. Kofkorn, R.W., and Steigerwald, F.C.: Carpal tunnel syndrome as the initial manifestation of tuberculosis. Am. J. Med., 60:583–586, 1976.
16. Allen, S.C.: A case in favor of Poncet's disease. Br. Med. J., 283:952, 1981.
17. Berney, S., Goldstein, M., and Bishko, F.: Clinical and diagnostic features of tuberculous arthritis. Am. J. Med., 53:36–42, 1972.
18. Wallace, R., and Cohen, A.S.: Tuberculous arthritis: A report of two cases with review of biopsy and synovial fluid findings. Am. J. Med., 61:277–282, 1976.
19. American Thoracic Society: Treatment of tuberculosis and tuberculosis infection in children and adults. Am. Rev. Respir. Dis., 134:355–363, 1986.
20. Tulis, M., and Mukherjee, S.K.: Excision arthroplasty for tuberculosis and pyogenic arthritis of the hip. J. Bone Joint Surg., 63B:29–32, 1981.
21. Jupiter, J.B., et al.: Total hip arthroplasty in the treatment of adult hips with current or quiescent sepsis. J. Bone Joint Surg., 63A:194–200, 1981.
22. Martini, M., Adjrad, A., and Boudjemaa, A.: Tuberculous osteomyelitis: A review of 125 cases. Int. Orthop., 10:201–207, 1986.
23. Pattisson, P.R.M.: Pott's paraplegia: An account of the treatment of 89 consecutive patients. Paraplegia, 24:77–91, 1986.
24. Woods, G.L., and Washington, J.A.: Mycobacteria other than *Mycobacterium tuberculosis*: Review of microbiological and clinical aspects. Rev. Infect. Dis., 9:275–294, 1987.
25. Hoffman, G.S., et al.: Septic arthritis associated with Mycobacterium avium: A case report and literature review. J. Rheumatol., 5:199–209, 1978.
26. Sutker, W.L., Laukford, L.L., and Thompsett, R.: Granulomatous synovitis: The role of atypical mycobacteria. Rev. Infect. Dis., 1:729–735, 1979.
27. Travis, W.E., et al.: The histopathologic spectrum in *Mycobacterium marinum* infection. Arch. Pathol. Lab. Med., 109:1109–1113, 1985.
28. Cochrane, R.G., and Davey, T.F.: Leprosy in Theory and Practice. Baltimore, Williams & Wilkins, 1964, p. 3.
29. Chavez-Legaspi, M., Gomez-Vazquez, A., and Garcia-DeLa Torre, I.: Study of rheumatoid manifestations and serologic abnormalities in patients with lepromatous leprosy. J. Rheumatol., 12:738–741, 1985.
30. Karat, A.B.A., et al.: An exudative arthritis in leprosy–rheumatoid arthritis-like syndrome in association with erythema nodosum leprosum. Br. Med. J., 3:770–772, 1967.
31. Modi, T.H., and Lele, R.D.: Acute joint manifestations in leprosy. J. Assoc. Physicians India, 17:247–254, 1969.
32. Louie, J.S., and Glovsky, M.: Complement determinations in

the synovial fluid and serum of a patient with erythema nodosum leprosum. Int. J. Lepr., *43*:252–255, 1975.

33. Paterson, D.E., and Job, C.K.: Leprosy in Theory and Practice. Baltimore, Williams & Wilkins, 1964, p. 425.

34. Van Vorris, W.C., et al.: Cutaneous infiltrates in leprosy. N. Engl. J. Med., *307*:1593–1597, 1982.

35. Shepard, C.C.: Leprosy today. N. Engl. J. Med., *307*:1640–1641, 1982.

36. Johnson, W.M., and Gall, E.P.: Fatal coccidiomycosis in collagen vascular diseases. J. Rheumatol., *10*:79–84, 1983.

37. Bronnimann, D.A., et al.: Coccidiomycosis in the acquired immunodeficiency syndrome. Ann. Int. Med., *106*:372–379, 1987.

38. Bayer, A.S., and Guze, L.B.: Fungal arthritis II. Coccidioidal synovitis: Clinical, diagnostic, therapeutic and prognostic considerations. Semin. Arthritis Rheum., *8*:200–211, 1979.

39. Yoshinoza, S., Cox, R.A., and Pope, R.M.: Circulating immune complexes in coccidioidomycosis. J. Clin. Invest., *66*:655–663, 1980.

40. Bried, J.M., and Galgiani, J.N.: *Coccidioides immitis* infection in bones and joints. Clin. Orthop. Rel. Res., *211*:235–243, 1985.

41. Catanzaro, A., et al.: Treatment of coccidiodomycosis with ketoconazole: An evaluation utilizing a new scoring system. Am. J. Med., *74*:64–69, 1983.

42. Stevens, D.A., et al.: Experience with ketoconazole in three major manifestations of progressive coccidioidomycosis. Am. J. Med., *74*:58–63, 1983.

43. Klein, B.S., et al.: Isolation of *Blastomyces dermatitidis* in soil associated with a large outbreak of blastomycosis in Wisconsin. N. Engl. J. Med., *314*:529–534, 1986.

44. Tenebaum, J.J., Greenspan, J., and Kerkering, T.M.: Blastomycosis. CRC Crit. Rev. Microbiol., *9*:139–163, 1982.

45. Cooperative Study of the Veterans Administration: Blastomycosis: A review of 198 collected cases in Veterans Administration hospitals. Am. Rev. Respir. Dis., *89*:659–672, 1964.

46. George, A.L., Hays, J.T., and Graham, B.S.: Blastomycosis presenting as monoarticular arthritis: The role of synovial fluid cytology. Arthritis Rheum., *28*:516–521, 1985.

47. National Institute of Allergy and Infectious Disease Mycoses Study Group: Treatment of blastomycosis and histoplasmosis with ketoconazole: Results of a prospective randomized clinical trial. Ann. Intern. Med., *103*:861–872, 1985.

48. Lewis, J.L., and Rabinovich, S.: Wide spectrum of cryptococcal infections. Am. J. Med., *53*:315–322, 1972.

49. Prefect, R.F., Durack, D.T., and Gallis, H.A.: Cryptococcemia. Medicine, *62*:98–109, 1983.

50. Collins, V.P.: Bone involvement in cryptococcosis (torulosis). Am. J. Roentgenol., *63*:102, 1950.

51. Bayer, A.S., et al.: Fungal arthritis. V. Cryptococcal and histoplasmal arthritis. Semin. Arthritis Rheum., *9*:218–227, 1980.

52. Ricciardi, D.D., et al.: Cryptococcal arthritis in a patient with acquired immune deficiency syndrome: Case report and review of the literature. J. Rheumatol., *13*:455–458, 1986.

53. Wheat, L.J., et al.: A large urban outbreak of histoplasmosis: Clinical features. Ann. Intern. Med., *94*:331–337, 1981.

54. Thornberry, D.R., et al.: Histoplasmosis presenting with joint pain and hilar adenopathy. Arthritis Rheum., *25*:1396–1402, 1982.

55. Rosenthal, J., et al.: Rheumatic manifestations of histoplasmosis in a recent Indianapolis epidemic. Arthritis Rheum., *26*:1065–1070, 1983.

56. Dratz, D.J., and Graybill, J.R.: Infectious disease. *In* Basic and Clinical Immunology. Edited by D.P. Stites, J.D. Stobo, and J.V. Wells. Norwalk, CT, Appleton and Lange, 1987, pp. 534–581.

57. Gullberg, R.M., et al.: Sporotrichosis: Recurrent cutaneous, articular and central nervous system infection in a renal transplant recipient. Rev. Infect. Dis., *9*:369–375, 1987.

58. Lipstein-Kresch, E., et al.: Disseminated *Sporothrix schenckii* infection with arthritis in a patient with acquired immune deficiency syndrome. J. Rheumatol., *12*:805–808, 1985.

59. Wilson, D.E., et al.: Clinical features of extracutaneous sporotrichosis. Medicine, *46*:265–279, 1967.

60. Bayer, A.S., Scott, V.J., and Guze, L.B.: Fungal arthritis III. Sporotrichal arthritis. Semin. Arthritis Rheum., *9*:66–74, 1979.

61. Lynch, P.J., Voorhees, J.J., and Harrell, E.R.: Systemic sporotrichosis. Ann. Intern. Med., *73*:23–30, 1970.

62. Dismukes, W.E., et al.: Treatment of systemic mycosis with ketoconazole: Emphasis on toxicity and clinical response in 52 patients. Ann. Intern. Med., *98*:13–20, 1983.

63. Bayer, A.S., and Guze, L.B.: Fungal arthritis. Part I. Candida arthritis. Semin. Arthritis Rheum., *3*:142–150, 1978.

64. Fainstein, V., et al.: Septic arthritis due to Candida species in patients with cancer: Report of 5 cases and review of literature. Rev. Infect. Dis., *4*:78–85, 1982.

65. Gathe, J.C., Jr., et al.: Candida osteomyelitis: Report of five cases and review of the literature. Am. J. Med., *82*:927–937, 1987.

66. Dupont, B., and Drouket, E.: Cutaneous, ocular, and osteoarticular candidiasis in heroin addicts: New clinical and therapeutic aspects in 38 patients. J. Infect. Dis., *152*:577–591, 1985.

67. Yousefzadeh, D.K., and Jackson, J.H.: Neonatal and infantile candidal arthritis with or without osteomyelitis: A clinical and radiographic review of 21 cases. Skeletal Radiol., *5*:77–90, 1980.

68. Katzenstein, D.: Isolated Candida arthritis: Report of a case and definition of a distinct clinical syndrome. Arthritis Rheum., *28*:1421–1424, 1985.

69. Duquesnoy, B., et al.: Ketoconazole for treatment of Candida arthritis. J. Rheumatol., *11*:105–107, 1984.

70. Crank, R.N., Sundaram, M., and Shields, J.B.: Case report 197. Skeletal Radiol., *8*:164–167, 1982.

71. Mariat, F., Destembes, P., and Segretain, G.: The mycetomas: Clinical features, pathology and epidemiology. Contrib. Microbiol. Immunol., *4*:1–39, 1977.

72. Das, G.C., and Sen, S.B.: Chylous arthritis. Br. Med. J., *2*:27–29, 1968.

73. Salfield, S.: Filarial arthritis in the Sepik district of Papua New Guinea. Med. J. Aust., *1*:264–267, 1975.

74. Sivaramappa, M., et al.: Acute guinea worm synovitis of the knee joint. J. Bone Joint Surg., *51A*:1324–1330, 1969.

75. Bassiouni, M., and Kamel, M.: Bilharzial arthropathy. Ann. Rheum. Dis., *43*:806–809, 1984.

76. Naaseh, G.A.: Hydatid disease in bone and joint. J. Trop. Med. Hyg., *79*:243–244, 1975.

77. Bocanegra, T.S., et al.: Reactive arthritis induced by parasitic infestation. Ann. Intern. Med., *94*:207–209, 1981.

78. Woo, P., and Panayi, G.: Reactive arthritis due to infection with *Giardia lamblia*. J. Rheumatol., *11*:79, 1984.

118

VIRAL ARTHRITIS

ALLEN C. STEERE

Arthritis may be associated with a number of viral infections (Table 118–1). Since the last edition of this textbook, rubella virus has been further implicated as a cause of chronic arthritis, and parvovirus has been shown to be the cause of erythema infectiosum. Although each agent causes particular syndromes, several generalizations can be made.

Many viral arthritides begin with the nonspecific symptoms often observed with viral infections: malaise and fatigue, chills and fever, headache, stiff neck, sore throat, or nausea and vomiting (Table 118–2). There is often a rash, usually macular or papular, but mild temperature elevation and regional lymphadenopathy may be the only nonarticular physical findings.

No single pattern of joint involvement is characteristic (Table 118–3); in hepatitis B alone, the arthritis may be symmetric, asymmetric, migratory, or additive and may affect one or many joints. Periarticular structures (tendons and bursae) may also become inflamed. Morning stiffness is usually mentioned only in affected joints. On examination, joints may be red, hot, and swollen, or arthralgia may be the only sign of involvement.

Routine laboratory tests usually show few, if any, abnormalities (Table 118–4). Some patients may be mildly anemic or may have a few atypical lymphocytes. Tests are usually negative for rheumatoid factor and for antinuclear antibodies. Elevated erythrocyte sedimentation rates (ESR) are the most commonly observed abnormality. Cryoprecipitates and depressed serum complement levels have been found in the serum of patients with hepatitis B. Synovial fluid analyses reflect varying degrees of inflammation, but the findings are nonspecific (Table 118–5). The usual finding, 15,000 to 25,000 cells/mm³ with predominantly polymorphonuclear leukocytes, is also typical for rheumatoid arthritis (RA). However, biopsies generally show less intense signs of synovial inflammation than in RA.

Little is known about how viruses induce arthritis. In hepatitis B, the evidence suggests an immune-com-

Table 118–1. Viral Infections and Arthritis

I. VIRAL INFECTIONS OFTEN ASSOCIATED WITH ARTHRITIS
   Hepatitis B
   Rubella (including vaccine-induced)
   Parvovirus (erythema infectiosum)
   Group A arboviruses
      Epidemic polyarthritis of Australia (Ross River virus)
      Chikungunya
      O'nyong-nyong
      Sindbis
      Mayaro
   Mumps
   Smallpox (including vaccinia)

II. VIRAL INFECTIONS ASSOCIATED WITH ARTHRITIS IN A FEW PATIENTS
   Adenovirus type 7
   Herpes viruses
      Varicella-zoster
      Herpes simplex type 1
      Infectious mononucleosis (Epstein-Barr virus)
      Cytomegalovirus
   Enteroviruses
      Coxsackie viruses
      ECHO viruses

Table 118–2. Viral Arthritis: Associated Findings

Disease	Symptoms	Skin Lesions	Other Signs
I. VIRAL INFECTIONS OFTEN ASSOCIATED WITH ARTHRITIS			
Hepatitis B	Sore throat; nausea, vomiting; myalgias; chills; malaise	Urticarial; macular; papular; petechial	Lymphadenopathy; low-grade fever
Rubella	Coryza; cough; sore throat; headache; myalgia; malaise; fatigue	Morbilliform	Lymphadenopathy; low-grade fever
Rubella vaccine (HPV-77 DK12)	Coryza; cough; sore throat	Morbilliform (often absent)	Lymphadenopathy; low-grade fever; myeloradiculitis
Parvovirus (erythema infectiosum)	Headache; coryza; ocular and abdominal pain	Three stages: red cheeks; maculopapular rash; recurrent lesions	
Epidemic polyarthritis of Australia	Headache; rhinorrhea; sore throat; nausea, vomiting	Maculopapular; vesicular; petechial (minor)	Lymphadenopathy; low-grade fever
Chikungunya	Headache and backache; myalgia; malaise; cough; sore throat; mild gastrointestinal complaints	Maculopapular (faint, confluent); petechial (minor)	Conjunctivitis; high fever; lymphadenopathy
O'nyong-nyong	Headache and backache; eye pain; myalgia; cough; coryza; gastrointestinal complaints	Morbilliform; maculopapular	Lymphadenitis; low-grade fever; conjunctivitis
Mumps	Chills; headache; stiff neck; sore throat; vomiting; myalgias		Fever; parotitis; orchitis; pancreatitis
Smallpox	Headache; myalgia; abdominal pain; vomiting	Vesicular	Fever
II. VIRAL INFECTIONS ASSOCIATED WITH ARTHRITIS IN A FEW PATIENTS			
Adenovirus type 7	Sore throat	Maculopapular	Low-grade fever; pericarditis; meningitis
Varicella-zoster	Malaise	Vesicular	Fever
Herpes simplex type 1		Vesicular	
Infectious mononucleosis	Headache; malaise; sore throat	Maculopapular	Lymphadenopathy; sore throat
Cytomegalovirus			Fever
Coxsackie viruses	Sore throat; pleuritis pain	Maculopapular	Fever; myopericarditis
ECHO viruses	Fever; headache; vomiting; sore throat; diarrhea	Macular	Fever; meningitis

plex–mediated pathogenesis. In rubella, recovery of the virus from the synovial fluid of multiple patients suggests that it may replicate in synovium. Varicella, herpes simplex type 1, cytomegalovirus and ECHO virus type 11 have been isolated from joint fluid in only one patient each.

Because many findings are nonspecific, how does one recognize or suspect viral arthritis? Information about exposures can be helpful: a history of drug abuse for hepatitis B, or recent immunization for rubella, or of recent exposure to an endemic area and seasonal onset for arboviruses or enteroviruses. The most characteristic feature of the known viral arthritides, however, is their usual short duration. If inflammatory arthritis disappears in 1 or 2 weeks and if the patient has no preceding drug exposures (e.g., penicillin therapy), one thinks of viral arthritis. Indeed, the short duration of arthritis without deforming changes is the biggest difference between known types of viral arthritis and established RA.

However, observations in recent years have blurred this distinction. Hepatitis B arthritis may last for months, and a vasculitis indistinguishable from polyarteritis nodosa may occur. It now appears that both rubella virus and human parvovirus may occasionally cause chronic arthritis and that rubella, mumps, and coxsackie viruses may be associated with a condition similar to Still's disease. These reports lend credence to the hypothesis that infectious agents may play a role in a number of chronic rheumatic diseases.

VIRAL INFECTIONS OFTEN ASSOCIATED WITH ARTHRITIS

HEPATITIS B

Although Robert Graves, in 1843, described eight patients who had transient arthritis followed by jaun-

Table 118–3. Viral Arthritis: Musculoskeletal System

Disease	Percentage with Arthritis	Type of Involvement	Duration, Days
I. VIRAL INFECTIONS OFTEN ASSOCIATED WITH ARTHRITIS			
Hepatitis B	10–30%	Symmetric or sometimes asymmetric, migratory, or additive; small, sometimes large joints; tendinitis; bursitis	14 (7–180)
Rubella	15–35% of adult women; uncommon in men, children	Symmetric; knees, wrists; PIPs; carpal tunnel syndrome; tendinitis	5–30
Rubella vaccine (HPV-77 DK12)	1–10% of children; more common in women	Symmetric (PIPs) or monoarticular (knees); carpal tunnel syndrome	7–21; recurrences common
Parvovirus (erythema infectiosum)	70% of adults; 5% of children	Wrists, knees	5–9
Epidemic polyarthritis of Australia	Majority of adults	Symmetric or sometimes asymmetric or additive; small, sometimes large joints; tendinitis; periarticular swelling	14–21; sometimes months
Chikungunya	Majority	Large (especially knees), sometimes small joints; swelling rare	5–7; may recur for months
O'nyong-nyong	Majority	Large, sometimes small joints; no swelling	~5
Mumps	0.4%	Migratory; large and small joints; tenosynovitis	14 (2–90)
Smallpox	0.25–0.5%	Elbow, other large joints	up to 60
II. VIRAL INFECTIONS ASSOCIATED WITH ARTHRITIS IN A FEW PATIENTS			
Adenovirus type 7	5 patients	Large and small joints	7–35; recurrences possible
Varicella-zoster	8 patients	Knee, other large joints	7
Herpes simplex type 1	3 patients	Knee, other large joints	21 (14–120)
Infectious mononucleosis	4 patients	Large and small joints	68 (7–126)
Cytomegalovirus	1 patient	Knee	7
Coxsackie viruses	9 patients	Large and small joints	unknown
ECHO viruses	3 patients	Large and small joints	9–84

dice, arthritis associated with liver disease received little attention until the discovery of HB$_s$Ag over a century later. The arthritis typically affects many joints symmetrically, precedes the onset of frank hepatitis, and is often associated with a diffuse urticarial, macular, papular, or petechial rash. Both skin and joint lesions usually disappear when the liver disease becomes apparent. Although hepatitis A has rarely been associated with extrahepatic features, two patients have been reported who developed relapsing hepatitis A complicated by arthritis in both cases and cutaneous vasculitis in one.[1] There is still no direct evidence that non-A, non-B hepatitis is associated with arthritis.

Pathogenesis. Several observations suggest that circulating immune complexes may play a pathogenetic role in the arthritis and urticaria associated with hepatitis B infection. The complexes appear in the prehepatic period when HB$_s$Ag is in excess and when joints and skin are likely to be clinically active (Fig. 118–1). They contain HB$_s$Ag and anti-HB, other immunoglobulins, and complement components.[2] Their IgG subtypes are primarily 1 and 3, the ones that bind complement,[2] and concomitant serum complement levels, particularly C4 and CH$_{50}$, may be depressed.[3,4] Immune complexes containing HB$_s$Ag, IgM, and C3 have been found in affected dermal vessels.[5] With the development of antibody excess, the complexes disappear, and the arthritis and rash resolve. This sequence is similar to that in experimental "one-shot" serum sickness.[6] The circulating immune complexes may become localized in the synovium or dermal vessels where they elicit an inflammatory response.

Alternatively, hepatitis B virus may invade the synovium directly and replicate there. Particles consistent with HB$_s$Ag, including particles apparently budding from the cell membrane, have been seen in synovial lining cells.[7] Because normal cell structures may re-

Table 118–4. Viral Arthritis: Laboratory Findings in Blood

Disease	Hct	WBC	ESR	RF	ANA	C3	C4	Cryoglobulins	Specific Serology
I. VIRAL INFECTIONS OFTEN ASSOCIATED WITH ARTHRITIS									
Hepatitis B	↔ ↓*	↔ ↑; rel 1' cytosis†; atypical lymphs‡	↔ ↑	Negative	Negative	↓ ↔	↓ ↔	Often positive	Yes
Rubella		↔ ↑	↔ ↑	Often positive					Yes
Rubella vaccine (HPV-77 DK12)			↔ ↑	Rarely positive	Rarely positive	↔ ↓			Yes
Parvovirus (erythema infectiosum)		↔; rel 1' cytosis	↔ ↑	Rarely positive	Negative				Yes
Epidemic polyarthritis of Australia		↔ ↓; rel 1' cytosis; atypical lymphs	↔ ↑	Usually negative	Negative	↔ (1 patient)	↔		Yes
Chikungunya	↔	↔ ↑ ↓	↔ ↑						Yes
O'nyong-nyong		↔ ↓; rel 1' cytosis							Yes
Mumps	↔	↔ ↑	↔ ↑	Rarely positive					Yes
II. VIRAL INFECTIONS ASSOCIATED WITH ARTHRITIS IN A FEW PATIENTS									
Adenovirus type 7			↔ ↑	Negative	Negative	↓	↓		Yes
Varicella-zoster			↔ ↑	Negative	Negative			Negative	Yes
Infectious mononucleosis			↔ ↑	Negative	Usually negative	↑ ↔	↑ ↔	Usually negative	Yes

*↔ normal, ↓ decreased, ↑ increased
†Relative lymphocytosis
‡Atypical lymphocytes

semble viral particles ultrastructurally, however, this finding is not definitive.

Epidemiology. The reported frequency of joint manifestations in patients with hepatitis B infection is variable, but is generally between 10 and 30%.[8,9] Most studies report an age range from the first through the sixth decades (mean, third decade) with males and females affected equally.[3,8,10–12]

Clinical Characteristics. The arthritis typically begins with symmetric involvement of many joints.[8,10,13,14] In some patients, however, the pattern of involvement may be asymmetric,[15] migratory,[16,17] or additive.[8] The small joints of the fingers, particularly the proximal interphalangeal joints, but also the metacarpophalangeal and the distal interphalangeal joints, are most commonly affected, followed by the knee, shoulder, ankle, elbow, and wrist (Fig. 118–2). These joints may be markedly tender and sometimes swollen, red, and hot, or objective signs of inflammation may be absent. Some patients have localized tender areas over the joint, and others have tendinitis.[16,18] Two patients have been reported with subcutaneous nodules on the extensor surfaces of the forearm.[15,16] The histology of the nodule in one was indistinguishable from that seen in RA.[16] The arthritis lasts from several days to 6 months, but usually only for a few weeks.[3,10,16]

The arthritis is often accompanied by a rash that is most commonly urticarial, but may be macular, papular, or petechial.[3,8,10,12,18] All three types of rash may coexist in one patient.[18] In a review of 96 patients, one-half of those with arthritis had an urticarial rash that was often pruritic.[10] The Koebner phenomenon may be noted with respect to urticaria. In another report of 18 patients, 6 had an urticarial eruption and 2 had maculopapular eruptions.[3] The rash is usually on the lower extremities, but it may also involve the upper extremities, trunk, and face.[8] Angioneurotic edema of the soles may occur.[3] Like the arthritis, the rash lasts from days to weeks.[8]

Patients may experience malaise, sore throat, anorexia, nausea and vomiting, fever and chills, and myalgias.[8,10,17] Fever,[8,16] if present, is low-grade (100 to 102° F). Regional adenopathy may be present.[8,16] These symptoms appear 1 day to 12 weeks before the arthritis.[8]

The joint manifestations usually subside before liver involvement becomes apparent.[10,12] Serum glutamic-oxaloacetic transaminase (SGOT) levels may be elevated while the arthritis is still present; alternatively, some patients never develop abnormal SGOT levels.[8]

Laboratory Findings. When the arthritis is present, HB$_s$Ag is usually recoverable from blood, although it

Table 118–5. Viral Arthritis: Findings in Synovial Fluid or Synovium

Disease	Synovial Fluid				Synovium
	WBC × 10⁻³/mm³	Predominant Cell Type	Total Protein (g/dl)	Virus Cultured	
I. VIRAL INFECTIONS OFTEN ASSOCIATED WITH ARTHRITIS					
Hepatitis B	25 (0.5–90)	PMN or mononuclear cells	4 (2.5–6)	No (HB$_s$Ag detectable)	Limited mononuclear infiltrate
Rubella	30 (15–60) (5 patients)	Mononuclear cells or PMN	2–3.8	Yes	Synovial hyperplasia (2 patients), with ↑ vascularity, mononuclear infiltrate (1 patient)
Epidemic polyarthritis of Australia	10 (1.5–13.8)	Mononuclear cells		No	
Mumps		PMN (1 patient)		No	
Smallpox	Pus	PMN		No (Elementary bodies seen)	
Vaccinia	44 (1 patient)	PMN (1 patient)		Yes	
II. VIRAL INFECTIONS ASSOCIATED WITH ARTHRITIS IN A FEW PATIENTS					
Adenovirus type 7	3–25 (4 patients)	PMN or mononuclear cells		No	
Varicella-zoster	~4 (4 patients)	Mononuclear cells		Yes	
Herpes simplex type 1	~10 (2 patients)	Mononuclear cells		Yes	
Infectious mononucleosis	40 (3 patients)	PMN		No	
Cytomegalovirus	37 (1 patient)	PMN		Yes	
Coxsackie viruses	7–46 (4 patients)	PMN		No	
ECHO viruses	2.2–32 (2 patients)	PMN and large mononuclear cells		Yes	

may be necessary to test multiple samples before one obtains a positive result.[8] HB$_s$Ag has been detected in synovial fluid as well as in serum.[8,16,19] As the arthritis improves, HB$_s$Ag usually disappears, and the test for anti-HB becomes positive (see Fig. 118–1). Patients rarely have a positive test for HB$_s$Ag and anti-HB in the serum at the same time.[8]

Cryoprecipitates have been detected in the serum of some patients when the arthritis is present. These precipitates derive from large, circulating immune complexes that may contain HB$_s$Ag, anti-HB, immunoglobulins M, G, and A, and the complement components, C1q, C3, C4, and C5.[2] In addition, putative Dane particles have been seen in the precipitates by electron microscopy.[20]

Complement components may be consumed most quickly when the arthritis is first present (see Fig. 118–1). At such times, C4 and CH$_{50}$ levels are often markedly depressed, C3 levels are low-normal to de-

pressed, and C1q levels are variable.[3,4] Higher concentrations of HB$_s$Ag have been associated with lower levels of C4 and C1q. However, low complement levels are not found in all patients. In one study, only 13 of 29 patients had C3 levels below 120 mg/dl, and only 8 had C4 levels below 20 mg/dl.[8] The complement system apparently may be activated by both the classic and alternative pathways.[2]

In most patients, the hematocrit and the total white cell count are normal; sometimes a relative lymphocytosis and a few atypical lymphocytes are present.[3] However, hematocrits as low as 31% and total white cell counts as high as 21,500 cells/mm³ have been noted.[8] The presence of microscopic hematuria and red-cell casts[8] may lead to chronic glomerulonephritis.

The synovial fluid was first thought to be mostly noninflammatory, with a predominance of lymphocytes,[16,18] although counts as high as 5,600 WBC/mm³ with 56% polymorphs had been recorded. Subse-

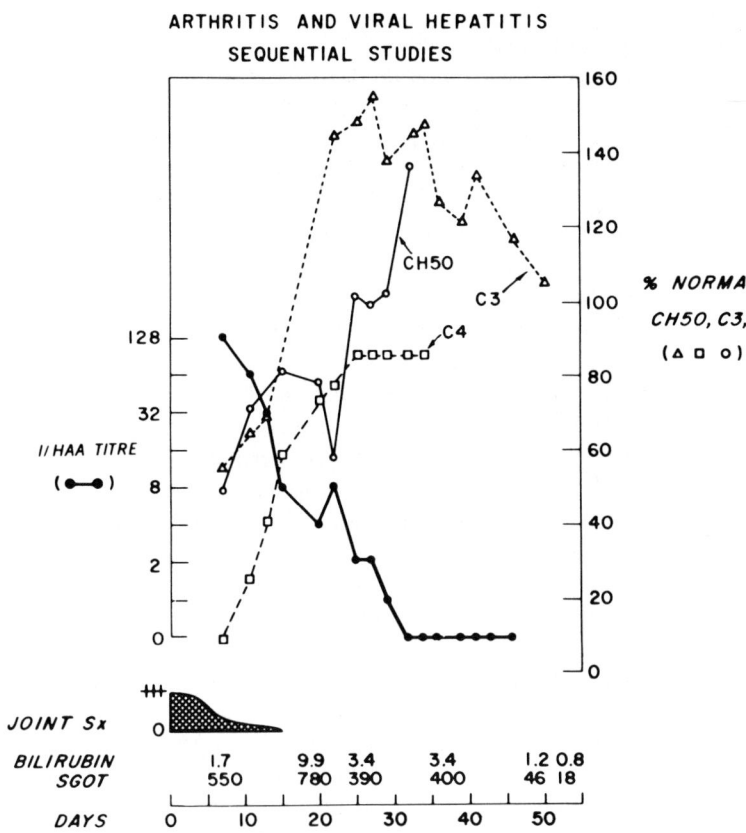

ARTHRITIS AND VIRAL HEPATITIS
SEQUENTIAL STUDIES

FIG. 118–1. Changes in CH_{50}, C3, and C4 serum concentrations and HB_sAg titers are seen during the course of HB_sAg-associated arthritis followed by hepatitis. HB_sAg is present, and complement components are depressed when the joints are active. With the development of antibody excess (not shown), the arthritis resolves and the hepatitis becomes apparent. (From Alpert, E., Schur, P.H., and Isselbacher, K.J.: Sequential changes of serum complement in HAA related arthritis. N. Engl. J. Med., 287:103, 1972.)

quent observations, however, have shown that white cell counts may be highly variable. In fluid from six patients, white counts ranged from 465 to 90,000 cells/mm^3 (mean 24,172), and most were polymorphonuclear leukocytes.[8] The joint fluid total protein and glucose also varied a great deal: protein 2.6 to 6.1 g/dl (mean 4.2) and glucose 62 to 260 mg/dl (mean 114).[8] Joint fluid C3 levels were not low when adjusted for total protein, but CH_{50} was markedly reduced in a fluid with a positive HB_sAg titer.[16]

Synovial biopsies in two patients showed only limited inflammatory changes.[7] Synovial lining cells were one to five layers thick, some vessels were congested, and occasional scattered lymphocytes were seen. HB_sAg was demonstrated throughout the synovium by direct immunofluorescence, and possible viral particles were observed by electron microscopy in synovial lining cells, blood vessels, and other deep synovial structures.

Treatment. The duration of the arthritis and rash is usually brief regardless of therapy. The rash, which may be quite pruritic, responds poorly to antihistamines or to epinephrine.[8] Some patients have noted dramatic relief of the arthritis with salicylates.[8]

RUBELLA

Arthritis as a complication of rubella was mentioned in Sir William Osler's textbook, *Principles and*

Practice of Medicine, in 1906, and joint symptoms have been noted since in many rubella outbreaks.[21–23] Rubella arthritis typically occurs in women,[23,24] while the rash is present, or occurs a few days later, often involving the fingers, wrists, and knees symmetrically. Its duration is usually brief.

Pathogenesis. The mechanism by which rubella virus induces arthritis is uncertain. The virus has been isolated from the synovial fluid of affected patients on many occasions,[25–28] suggesting that the organism may invade and replicate in synovium. Alternatively, the observed sequence of viral isolation from the pharynx or blood, followed by the appearance of the rash and arthritis and the detection of circulating antibody, is compatible with an immune complex–associated arthritis.[23] However, tests for circulating immune complexes and complement levels have generally been normal.[29,30]

Epidemiology. Joint involvement occurs in about one third to one sixth of women with rubella.[23,31] It is much less common in adult men or in children. In an outbreak in Great Britain in 1953, 16 of 50 patients (32%) developed joint symptoms. All 16 were adults, and 15 were women.[32]

Clinical Characteristics. Patients often have the characteristic morbilliform rash of rubella, posterior cervical lymphadenopathy, low-grade fever, malaise, and fatigue. The onset of arthritis associated with ru-

FIG. 118–2. Frequency of joints involved is seen in three viral arthritides. Small joints of the fingers, then knees, are most often affected in hepatitis B[2,4,12,17,18] and rubella.[24,33,43,49,53] Ankles, toes, fingers, and knees are affected most often in epidemic polyarthritis of Australia.[72]

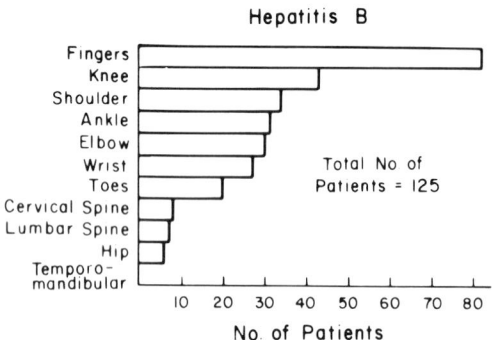

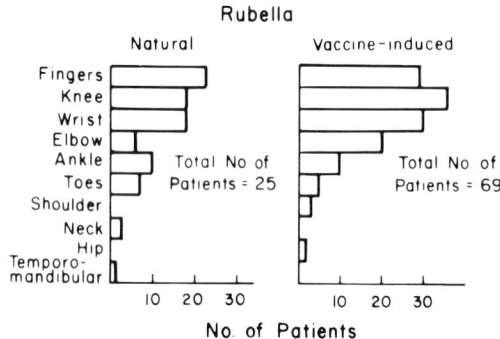

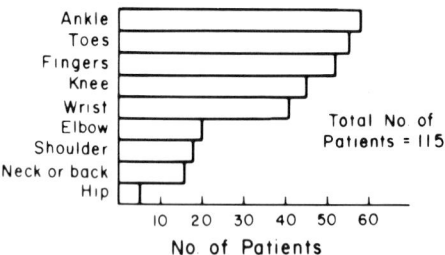

bella is usually sudden, commonly affecting the fingers, knees, and wrists symmetrically (see Fig. 118–2). Pain on motion and stiffness are often the only symptoms of inflammation. Some patients may also develop carpal tunnel syndrome[33] or tenosynovitis.[34] The arthritis occurs from 6 days before to 6 days after the rash, but usually a few days after its onset.[34] The arthritis may occasionally occur without the rash. The joint symptoms usually do not last longer than 1 month,[21,33–35] but some patients have had persistent

joint involvement for more than 1 year.[36] Aspirin may provide partial relief.[33,37]

Laboratory Findings. Blood counts in most patients are normal; a few patients have mild leukocytosis or an elevated ESR. In two series, most patients had a positive test for rheumatoid factor;[21,35] in two others, only a few patients did.[24,33] Joint effusions, if present, are usually small (e.g., 20 ml). In fluids aspirated from five patients, synovial fluid white cell counts ranged from 14,600 to 60,000.[27,34,38] Four patients had predominantly mononuclear cells with no polymorphonuclear leukocytes; the other had 95% polymorphonuclear leukocytes. Rubella antigen was demonstrated in mononuclear cells by immunofluorescence.[27] The total protein content ranged from 1.9 to 3.8 g/dl. One synovial biopsy showed a nonspecific inflammatory reaction with synovial cell hyperplasia, increased vascularity, a predominantly mononuclear cell infiltrate, and a fibrinopurulent exudate;[24] another showed only mild hyperplasia of synovial lining cells.[27] Rubella virus has been cultured from the synovial fluid of one infant[28] and three adults[27] with acute naturally acquired disease.

Chronic Arthritis. Recent articles report the isolation of rubella virus from the synovial fluid or lymphoreticular cells of patients with chronic arthritides.[25,26,39] In some patients, rubella antigen was seen in synovium and synovial fluid mononuclear cells by immunofluorescence, and particles resembling the electron-dense cores of rubella virus were found in synovium by electron microscopy.[26] In another study, the joint fluid mononuclear cells of a patient with unexplained knee arthritis underwent blast transformation when exposed to rubella antigens, but peripheral blood mononuclear cells did not.[25] Rubella virus was subsequently isolated from his joint fluid. More recently, rubella virus was isolated from the lymphoreticular cells of one of five children with Still's disease, two of two with polyarticular juvenile rheumatoid arthritis (JRA), two of six with pauciarticular JRA, and two of six with seronegative spondyloarthritis, but none of 16 control subjects.[39] These reports suggest that rubella virus may occasionally cause chronic rheumatic disease syndromes, such as RA, JRA, or Still's disease. Alternatively, the virus may simply be present in synovium as an epiphenomenon and may not be the inciting agent.

RUBELLA ARTHRITIS (VACCINE-INDUCED)

Because of teratogenic effects of rubella virus on the fetus, rubella vaccines were developed. In 1969, three live attenuated vaccines (HPV-77 DK12, HPV-77 DE5, and Cendehill) became available. It soon became apparent that all three strains, but particularly HPV-77 DK12, could induce arthritis in both children and adults similar to that caused by natural rubella. HPV-77 DK12 has been withdrawn from the market.

Pathogenesis. As with natural rubella, the mechanism of vaccine-induced rubella arthritis is uncertain. The virus has been cultured from synovial fluid following vaccination in four reported cases (3 or 4 months after the onset of symptoms in three patients).[37,40] Because of these isolates, it has been postulated that the organism may invade and replicate in synovium. Alternately, three patients with vaccine-induced rubella arthritis had putative circulating immune complexes, determined by the C1q-binding assay.[38] In other reports, complement levels (B1c and CH_{50}), with one exception,[29] were normal.[41,42]

Epidemiology. Each rubella vaccine, including the newer RA 27/3, has been associated with joint involvement in 5 to 10% of those receiving it.[43-47] These attack rates are somewhat lower than has been found with HPV-77 DK12 vaccine.[41,42,48,49] As in natural rubella, the frequency of this complication is greatest in women: 43% of women and 39% of postpubescent, adolescent girls given the HPV-77 DE5 vaccine developed arthralgias or arthritis, whereas only 3% of children given the same vaccine developed these complications.[23,37,50,51]

In several studies, the mean rubella titers were not significantly different in those who developed arthritis compared to those who did not.[24] In addition, the titers were not significantly different in those with only one attack of arthritis compared to those with recurrent attacks.[41] Arthritis rarely accompanied vaccination if the individual was previously immune due to natural infection.[42]

Clinical Characteristics. The joint symptoms following rubella vaccination are similar to those associated with the natural infection, except that isolated knee involvement and carpal tunnel syndrome are apparently more common (see Fig. 118–2). Of 40 children with arthritis following vaccination with HPV-77 DK12, 50% had predominantly knee complaints, 33% had symptoms that suggested carpal tunnel syndrome, and only 17% had polyarthritis.[42] Pain and stiffness (often mild) are the usual findings in affected joints; swelling, heat, and redness are unusual.[41]

The arthritis usually occurs 2 to 4 weeks after vaccination (range 8 to 55 days); arthralgias typically last a few days and arthritis 1 to 3 weeks (range 1 to 46 days).[41,42,48-50,52] However, a third to a tenth of those with knee involvement after HPV-77 DK12 vaccination had recurrent attacks for as long as 3 years,[23,41,49]

and three patients had them for as long as 5 years.[53] Recurrent attacks, usually affecting the same joint, typically last 1 to 5 days with longer intervening periods of complete remission (range 2 weeks to 1 year). Patients tend to have fewer attacks the longer the time from vaccination, but the frequency in an individual patient is unpredictable. One patient experienced synovial hypertrophy in the intercondylar notch 5 years after onset,[53] but permanent joint damage was not reported.[41,49] Recently, six women were reported who continued to have chronic or recurrent arthralgia or arthritis for 2 to 7 years after vaccination. In 5% of these patients, chronic rubella viremia was detected in peripheral blood mononuclear cells for up to 6 years after vaccination.[54]

As in the natural infection, patients with vaccine-induced arthritis sometimes have the characteristic rash, coryza, cough, sore throat, posterior cervical lymphadenopathy, or low-grade fever.[42,49] However, a rash is less common than in the natural infection; in one study, only 8 of 40 patients developed a rash.[48]

Two distinct neuropathic syndromes have been noted after rubella immunization. One type is characterized by numbness and tingling in the hands and sharp, shooting pains in the arms,[52] and the other by pain mostly in the back of the legs.[55] These children sometimes assume the so-called catcher's crouch position, particularly in the morning. In one study of 13 children, 11 had slowing of nerve conduction,[55] a finding also recorded by others.[35]

As in natural rubella, aspirin therapy often provides some symptomatic relief.[42]

Laboratory Findings. Although blood counts are usually normal, white cell counts as high as 11,600 cells/mm³ and sedimentation rates as high as 46 mm/hour (Westergren) have been seen.[41,48] Tests for rheumatoid factor and for antinuclear antibodies are rarely positive,[42,49] immunoglobulin levels are usually normal,[40] and complement components (B1c and CH_{50}), except in one instance,[29] have also been normal.[40,41]

PARVOVIRUS (ERYTHEMA INFECTIOSUM)

Erythema infectiosum, "fifth disease," a mild exanthematous illness usually of childhood, was first described by Tshamer in 1886 as a variant of rubella and by Escherich in 1896 as a separate entity. It is distinguished by a characteristic recurrent rash. Joint involvement occurs primarily in adults and affects both large and small joints. In 1983, the illness was linked serologically to human parvovirus infection.[56-58]

The disease occurs in localized epidemics, often

during the winter, and usually affects children of school age. It is presumably spread from person to person. The incubation period is approximately 4 to 14 days.[59]

Clinical Characteristics. The illness is defined by a characteristic three-stage rash. The first stage consists of a bright red rash on the face, the so-called slapped cheek appearance. Discrete macules may also appear on the forehead, chin, and neck. The rash is warm to the touch and sometimes pruritic. The second stage begins within 1 to 4 days when a lace-like eruption spreads to the extensor surface of the arms and legs and to the buttocks. This stage lasts a few days to several weeks. In the third stage, the lesions may recur for as long as 10 months. Trauma, sunlight, changes in temperature, and emotional stress have been thought to activate the lesions.[60]

Although many patients have no other signs or symptoms, some experience headache, sore eyes, mild coryza, slight sore throat, gastroenteritis, abdominal pain, irritability, depression, or malaise and fatigue. A few patients may have low-grade fever or posterior cervical lymphadenopathy.[59,60]

With two exceptions,[61,62] early reports of erythema infectiosum do not mention joint involvement.[60] However, in an outbreak of 364 cases in 1966,[59] 44 of 57 adults (77%) noted joint pain compared to 24 of the 307 children (8%). Sixty-eight percent of those with joint pain also had joint swelling. The arthritis was confined to large joints, usually the wrists or knees.

In 1983, an outbreak of erythema infectiosum in Scotland was linked serologically to human parvovirus infection.[56,57] Arthritis occurred primarily in adult females, and one quarter of those with joint involvement had neither rash nor viral prodromata. In contrast to previous descriptions, most of the patients had symmetric polyarthritis, commonly affecting the small joints of the hands, wrists, and knees. Joint involvement usually resolved within several weeks but sometimes persisted for months. Subsequently, of 153 patients attending an "early synovitis" clinic in Bath, England, 19 were found to have serologic evidence of recent parvovirus infection.[58] Joint involvement usually improved somewhat within 2 weeks, but in 17 patients, symptoms persisted for more than 2 months, and in 3 patients for more than 4 years. One patient with evidence of recent parvovirus infection had arthritis and cutaneous vasculitis.[63]

The epidemiology and clinical characteristics of parvovirus arthropathy are similar to those of rubella arthritis. However, erythema infectiosum differs from rubella by the usual absence of fever and lymphad-

enopathy and by the longer duration of the rash. If there is confusion, the two illnesses can now be separated serologically.

Laboratory Findings. Human-parvovirus-specific IgM, determined by capture assay, is present early in the illness and may persist for months.[64] Specific IgG appears during this period, but the diagnostic value of a single elevated IgG titer late in the illness is not yet clear. The virus has not been cultured yet from affected patients. Synovial biopsies, done in two cases, showed increased vascularity and stromal edema, but no significant inflammatory infiltrate.[58] Patients sometimes have an elevated ESR or an increased ^{125}I-C1q binding capacity, but most have a normal white blood cell count. Tests for rheumatoid factor and antinuclear antibodies are almost always negative. A distinct parvovirus, RA-1, has been cultured from the synovium of one patient with RA.[64a]

ARBOVIRUSES

Joint pain is a common manifestation of many illnesses caused by arboviruses, including dengue. In the following five entities, all caused by group A arboviruses (alphaviruses), joint pain is the predominant feature.

Epidemic Polyarthritis of Australia

Epidemic polyarthritis was first described by Nimmo in New South Wales, Australia, in 1928. Outbreaks have been reported subsequently in Australia, New Guinea, the Solomon islands, Fiji, American Samoa, and a number of South Pacific islands.[65] The illness, caused by a group A arbovirus (the Ross River virus) and transmitted by mosquitoes, usually affects small (and sometimes large) joints, is frequently associated with a diffuse maculopapular rash, and typically lasts for several weeks.

Pathogenesis. The mechanism by which the Ross River virus induces arthritis is unknown. There is no evidence of direct invasion and replication in synovium or for the presence of immune complexes. The virus has been recovered several times from blood samples of seronegative patients early in the illness.[66,67] Attempts to isolate the virus from synovial fluid specimens have been unsuccessful.[68] Unlike classic immune-complex-mediated serum sickness, circulating antibody has always been present when patients are symptomatic rather than appearing as symptoms subside,[69] and levels of complement components (C3 and C4) have been normal in serum and synovial fluid.[70] In one study, patients with epidemic polyarthritis had an increased frequency of the B-cell alloantigen, DR 7.[71]

Epidemiology. Epidemic polyarthritis primarily affects adults of either sex.[66,69,72] Children may show seroconversion against Ross River virus, but they are usually asymptomatic.[69] The illness occurs primarily from December through May (the equivalent of summer and fall in the northern hemisphere).[68,69,72,73] Attack rates in the affected areas may be quite high. During 1979 and 1980, major epidemics of Ross River virus infection occurred in several South Pacific islands; these outbreaks sometimes involved 40 to 50% of the local population.[65] The number of asymptomatic cases may also be high.[74]

The causative agent, the Ross River virus, was first recovered from mosquitoes, Aëdes vigilex, in 1959[75] and has been isolated subsequently from other Aëdes species and from Culex and Mansonia mosquitoes.[65,76] The incubation period from the bite to the onset of symptoms is thought to be 2 to 15 days.[68,77] Person-to-person transmission has not been noted.[68,72,77]

Clinical Characteristics. The arthritis, which may begin gradually or suddenly, typically affects two or more joints and may be symmetric, asymmetric, or additive.[72,78–80] The ankle and small joints of the toes and fingers are involved most often, followed by knees and wrists (see Fig. 118–2). Although the affected joints are frequently stiff, tender, and painful to move, swelling is rare, and redness and heat are not reported.[80] In addition to arthritis, symptoms that patients may experience include periarticular swelling, tendinitis, and pronounced localized tenderness over one part of a joint capsule or ligament.[78,80] Joint symptoms often persist longer than other manifestations of the illness, typically for 2 to 3 weeks, but sometimes for months.[68,69,72,78] Roentgenograms of affected joints show no abnormality, and no patients have had permanent joint damage.

A fine, nonconfluent, maculopapular rash often accompanies the arthritis,[68,72,78,80] but may precede it by as much as 11 days or follow it by as much as 15 days.[69] The rash may become vesicular, and a few petechiae are sometimes noted. The lesions often begin on the trunk, but in many patients spread quickly to cover the entire body, including the scalp, palms, and soles (lesions on the palms and soles are usually macular).[68,69,78] In a few patients, dark red macules have been noted on the hard and soft palates. The rash, which may be painless or slightly pruritic, typically lasts about 1 week (range 1 to 18 days) and usually fades without desquamation.[68,72,78] It may occur without arthritis, and vice versa.[69]

Constitutional symptoms are often mild. However, some patients experience headache, rhinorrhea, sore throat, nausea and vomiting, myalgia in the legs, malaise, and marked lethargy, particularly at the beginning of the illness.[68,69] Paresthesias with numbness and tingling or soreness of the fingers and toes may be the most distressing symptoms.[69,72,78,80] Temperatures are usually normal or mildly elevated (101° F). Regional or generalized lymphadenopathy may be present, and nodes are sometimes tender.

Aspirin and other analgesic drugs may give partial but not dramatic relief.[71,72]

Laboratory Findings. Complement fixation, hemagglutination inhibition, and neutralization tests are available for serodiagnosis.[79] The white cell count and ESR are usually normal.[69,80] A few patients have had mild leukopenia, relative lymphocytosis, and a few atypical lymphocytes.[72] In joint fluid from eight patients, white cell counts ranged from 1,500 to 13,800 cells/mm^3 and consisted primarily of monocytes, in which Ross River virus antigen was detected by specific immunofluorescence.[81] In one patient, tests for rheumatoid factor and antinuclear antibodies in serum and synovial fluid were negative, and complement levels (C3 and C4) were normal.[70]

Chikungunya

A large epidemic of a "dengue-like illness" called chikungunya, "that which bends up," was first described in southern Tanganyika (now Tanzania) in 1952.[82–84] Epidemics of the same illness have been recognized subsequently in wide areas of Africa, southern India, southeastern Asia, and the Philippine Islands.[65,85–88] American servicemen were affected during the Vietnam war.[89] The illness, caused by a group A arbovirus (the chikungunya virus) and transmitted by mosquitoes, is characterized by high fever, severe joint pains, and a maculopapular rash. It usually lasts 5 to 7 days, but residual joint pain may recur for months or years in some patients.

Epidemiology. Arthritis occurs more often in adults than in children,[83,85,86] and there is no sex predilection. Attack rates during epidemics, which affect primarily rural populations, may be high. During the first outbreak described, 60 to 80% of the inhabitants of affected villages acquired the infection within 2 to 3 weeks.[83] The onset is seasonal, from April through August, during and shortly after periods of unusually heavy rainfall.[86,89]

The virus is usually transmitted by mosquitoes of the species Aëdes aegypti,[82,84] although it has also been isolated from A. africanus and A. furcifer.[65,90] The incubation period from the bite to the onset of symptoms is thought to be 3 to 12 days.[83]

Clinical Characteristics. The illness usually begins abruptly with the onset of high fever and severe, generalized joint pains often associated with prolonged morning stiffness.[83,84,86,91] In some patients, only large joints are involved, particularly the knees.[83] Joint swelling is rare; only 6 of 115 patients experienced it in one epidemic.[83] The arthritis usually lasts from 5 to 7 days, but joint pain and swelling may recur intermittently for more than a year, often in different joints.[83,91,92] The severity and duration of the joint pain are the primary clinical features distinguishing chikungunya from dengue.[83,87]

The rash is usually a faint, confluent, macular, or maculopapular eruption occurring on the trunk, extremities, or over the entire body,[88,89] and is indistinguishable from the nonhemorrhagic rash of dengue. A few scattered petechiae are sometimes found.[89] Although the rash may precede arthritis, it more often occurs 4 to 5 days after joint symptoms and lasts 2 to 5 days.[83] The rash may also occur without arthritis, and vice versa.

High fever (up to 105° F) is characteristic; it usually lasts for several days, but may be biphasic as in dengue.[83,86,89] Headache, myalgia, backache, and malaise are common. Eye suffusion and conjunctivitis, retroorbital pain, mild gastrointestinal complaints (vomiting, diarrhea, or constipation), cough, and sore throat occur less often. One patient was described as having paresthesias on the dorsal surface of the arms.[86] Regional lymphadenopathy, particularly of the cervical nodes, is common, and a few patients may have generalized lymphadenopathy and splenomegaly. Mild hemorrhagic phenomena (e.g., a positive tourniquet test, a low normal platelet count, and epistaxis) have been noted in some patients.[87]

Analgesics ranging from aspirin to morphine have been used for relief from the severe joint pain. Chloroquine phosphate treatment has been tried in patients with chronic chikungunya arthritis.[93]

Laboratory Findings. Chikungunya virus has been recovered on numerous occasions from blood specimens of affected patients as long as 3 days after the onset of symptoms.[84-86,89] Complement fixation, hemagglutination inhibition, and neutralization tests are available for serodiagnosis.[88] In most instances, the hematocrit is normal, but mild leukopenia or leukocytosis is sometimes found.[83,87,89] The ESR is sometimes elevated as high as 40 mm/hour.[89] In one study, 2 of 20 patients had positive tests for rheumatoid factor.[91] There have been no reports of synovial fluid analyses.

O'nyong-nyong

A large outbreak of a disease similar to chikungunya, called o'nyong-nyong, was first recognized in northern Uganda in 1959.[94-97] During the subsequent 2 years, the illness was estimated to have affected about two million inhabitants of Uganda, Kenya, Tanzania, and the Sudan.[96] O'nyong-nyong, caused by a group A arbovirus and transmitted by mosquitoes, is characterized by generalized joint pains, a morbilliform rash, and lymphadenitis. It usually lasts about 5 days, but joint symptoms sometimes persist longer.

Although persons of any age and either sex may be affected, those 10 to 39 years of age are affected most, females more often than males.[95] Attack rates may be high, as many as 78% of the inhabitants of certain villages.[95] Subclinical infections occur in a ratio of 1:6 to overt infections.[97]

The o'nyong-nyong virus has been recovered from both Anopheles funestes and A. gambiae mosquitoes.[95] The incubation period from the bite to the onset of symptoms is thought to be at least 8 days.[95]

Clinical Characteristics. Onset is sudden with associated fever, rigor, and generalized symmetric joint pain.[95] The knees, elbows, wrists, fingers, and ankles are most frequently involved. The pain in affected joints may range from excruciating to vague weakness and stiffness; swelling, redness, and heat have not been reported. The illness usually lasts about 5 days, but the joint pain may persist longer.

The rash, which is sometimes quite pruritic, is morbilliform, macular, or maculopapular, and cannot be distinguished from that of measles.[95] It generally starts on the face and may descend over the neck, the arms, or the entire body. Punctate erythema of the soft palate is also common. The rash typically erupts on the fourth day of the illness, but may appear at the first sign of symptoms or as long as 7 days later. It lasts approximately 4 to 7 days and then fades without desquamation. About 60 to 70% of individuals with arthritis also have the rash.

Headache, ranging from moderate to severe, is almost universal.[95] Eye pain and suffusion, throbbing postorbital pain, backache, particularly in the lumbar region, dry cough, coryza, colicky abdominal pain, and constipation or diarrhea are also common. About two thirds of patients have moderate fever (101° F), but high fever is unusual. Lymphadenitis, particularly of the posterior cervical nodes, may be striking and is the principal clinical finding that permits differentiation of this entity from chikungunya.

Laboratory Findings. O'nyong-nyong virus, which is similar to the virus that causes chikungunya, has been isolated from the blood of only a few patients.[96] Complement fixation, hemagglutination inhibition, and neutralization tests are available for serodiagnosis.[96,97]

The white cell count is usually normal, but some

patients have had neutropenia and a relative lymphocytosis.[95]

Sindbis

Sindbis, a group A arbovirus first isolated from Culex and Mansonia mosquitoes in 1952,[98] has been reported in Europe, Africa, Asia, Australia, and the Philippines.[65] Its basic maintenance cycle involves mainly Culex mosquitoes and wild birds.[65] Although clinical descriptions of the illness are few, it is typically characterized by joint pains, rash, headache, myalgias, and lethargy.[99,100] Arthritis begins suddenly and usually involves small (but sometimes large) joints. Swelling is common, and tendinitis is sometimes present. The rash, which may appear as long as 15 days after the onset of arthritis, is maculopapular, pruritic, and nonconfluent. Vesicles may form on the hands and feet. Red blotches or small ulcers may appear in the pharynx. Headache, stiff neck, periocular pain, myalgias, paresthesias, low-grade fever, and lethargy may accompany the illness. Symptoms usually last 10 to 15 days, but joint involvement has been noted for as long as 10 weeks.

Mayaro

Mayaro, a mosquito-transmitted group A arbovirus, is found in Trinidad, Surinam, Brazil, Colombia, and Bolivia.[65] Forest-dwelling mosquitoes of the genus Haemagogus are believed to be the principal vector.[101] The most frequent manifestations of the illness are fever, maculopapular rash, and polyarthralgias; about 20% of the patients develop joint swelling.[101] Associated signs and symptoms include headache, eye pain, myalgia, nausea and vomiting, diarrhea, and lymphadenopathy. The arthritis may persist for more than 2 months.

MUMPS

Arthritis as a rare complication of mumps was first mentioned by Rettier in 1850. In the Paris mumps epidemic of 1923 to 1924, it was estimated that 6 of 1334 patients (0.44%) developed arthritis.

This complication occurs most commonly in men, but may affect either sex at any age.[102] The arthritis, which is often migratory, usually involves large joints, but may also affect small ones. Monarticular involvement, fleeting arthralgias, and tenosynovitis have also been described.[102–107] Affected joints may become red, hot, and swollen, or tenderness and pain on motion may be the only signs of inflammation. Although arthritis may precede parotitis by several days, joint symptoms most commonly follow it by 1 to 2 weeks; they usually last only a few weeks but may linger for months.[103,108] Roentgenograms of affected joints show no signs of permanent damage. The clinical features of mumps arthritis have been reviewed.[109]

Nonspecific findings may include chills and fever (to 106° F), headache, stiff neck, sore throat, vomiting, and myalgia.[103,105,106] Although patients with mumps arthritis usually experience parotitis, a few cases without parotitis have been recognized by serologic criteria.[108,110] One of these patients had a clinical picture suggestive of adult Still's disease.[108]

Patients often show a leukocytosis (up to 21,000 white cells/mm³) and an elevated ESR (up to 100 mm/hour).[103,105,106] Several patients have had positive tests for rheumatoid factor.[102,111] Synovial fluid, reported only once, contained many neutrophils; no cell count was given.[102]

Salicylates are completely ineffective, but both phenylbutazone and corticosteroids have been reported to be beneficial.[102,110]

SMALLPOX (AND VACCINIA)

Smallpox, now thought to be extinct, caused arthritis in about 0.25 to 0.5% of patients[112] and usually affected children. The elbow joints were most commonly involved, followed by the wrists, ankles, and knees. In some instances, the arthritis resulted from direct extension of the virus from the metaphysis of bone (osteomyelitis variolosa) to the articular surface. Complete recovery usually occurred within a few months.

Arthritis may also occur as a complication of vaccinia immunization.[113] One such patient developed pain, heat, and swelling of a knee 10 days after vaccination. The joint fluid contained 44,000 white cells/mm³ with 79% polymorphonuclear leukocytes; vaccinia virus was recovered from the fluid. The arthritis resolved completely in 9 days.

VIRAL INFECTIONS ASSOCIATED WITH ARTHRITIS IN A FEW PATIENTS

ADENOVIRUS TYPE 7

Arthritis related to adenovirus type 7 was first reported in 1974;[114] four additional cases have been noted subsequently.[115,116] Illness begins with pharyngitis and low-grade fever. Within a few days, symmetric arthralgias of large and small joints, myalgias, and a diffuse maculopapular rash develop, and some large joints may become swollen. The arthritis lasts approximately 1 to 5 weeks, although recurrent attacks are noted in some patients.[115] In addition to arthritis, one patient had aseptic meningitis,[114] and another had pericarditis.[115] An immunodeficient patient with chronic, rheumatoid-like polyarthritis was reported to have persistent adenovirus type 1 infection in synovial tissue.[117] Aspirin has been used for symptomatic relief.

The ESR is usually elevated during attacks. Tests for rheumatoid factor and antinuclear antibodies are negative. Joint fluid white cell counts range from 3,300 to 24,800 cells/mm³, and either polymorphonuclear leukocytes or monocytes may predominate. In one patient, synovial biopsy showed inflammatory synovitis, but attempts to recover the virus from joint fluid were unsuccessful.[114] Complement fixation, hemagglutination inhibition, and neutralization tests are available for serodiagnosis.

HERPES VIRUSES

All the herpes viruses—varicella-zoster, herpes simplex, Epstein-Barr, and cytomegalovirus—are rare causes of arthritis.

Varicella-Zoster

Arthritis is an unusual complication of chickenpox.[118–123] The joint involvement, which typically begins 1 to 5 days after the onset of the rash, most commonly affects the knee, followed by other large joints. In one child, several metatarsophalangeal joints were involved.[122] Some affected joints may become hot and swollen. Complete resolution usually occurs within a week.[124]

The ESR may be elevated, but tests for rheumatoid factor, antinuclear antibodies, and cryoglobulins are negative. The joint fluid in three patients had 3,600 to 6,000 white cells/mm³, with predominantly mononuclear cells.[119,120,123] In one instance, 90% of the cells were shown to be monocytes.[120] Varicella virus was grown from one knee effusion.[121] Aspirin has been used for treatment.

Arthritis associated with herpes zoster was reported in 1979[125] and again in 1983.[126] One patient experienced involvement of the knees; the other, of a hip. In one instance, varicella antigen was demonstrated in the cytoplasm of joint fluid macrophages by indirect immunofluorescence, but the virus was not recovered from synovial fluid.[125]

Herpes Simplex Type 1

Four patients have had monoarticular arthritis in either a knee or an ankle associated with diffuse ve-sicular rash due to herpes simplex type 1.[127,128] Only one patient had known immunologic impairment. In two cases, the virus was recovered from synovial fluid; in both instances, the joint fluid white cell counts were 10,000 cells/mm³ with predominantly mononuclear cells.[128,129] Joint involvement lasted 1 week to 4 months.

Infectious Mononucleosis

Although arthralgias occur in approximately 2% of patients with infectious mononucleosis,[130] frank arthritis is rare.[131] Several case reports, however, suggest that this complication occurs more often than previously thought.[132–134] Perhaps the wider availability of serologic tests for Epstein-Barr virus (EBV) has allowed better documentation of unusual cases.

Of the four well-documented cases in the literature, two patients had monoarticular or oligoarticular involvement of large joints.[131,132] The other two experienced symmetric polyarthritis.[133,134] The duration of joint involvement ranged from 8 days to 4½ months. Sedimentation rates ranged from 10 to 110 mm/hour, and joint fluid leukocyte counts ranged from 18,900 to 80,000 cells/mm³. Antinuclear antibodies were found in low titer in one subject;[134] tests for rheumatoid factor were negative in all four. Three of the four patients lacked heterophil antibody production, but they were diagnosed by a rise in specific EBV antibody titers. In a serologic survey of nine patients with the acute onset of seronegative polyarthritis, four had either acute or continuing active infection with EBV.[135] They did not show other signs and symptoms often associated with infectious mononucleosis.

The pathogenesis of arthritis associated with infectious mononucleosis is not known. Both viral replication within synovium and precipitation of immune complexes have been postulated. However, EBV is known to replicate only within B lymphocytes, and although one patient had cryoglobulins,[134] another lacked abnormal ¹²⁵I-C1q binding activity.[133]

Cytomegalovirus

The only patient reported with arthritis associated with cytomegalovirus developed hip pain, knee pain and swelling, fever, and urinary retention 3 months following renal transplantation.[127] Cytomegalovirus was isolated from the synovial fluid. More recently, the virus has also been recovered from the joint fluid of a patient who had classic seropositive RA for 17 years, but who had not been taking corticosteroids or immunosuppressive agents.[136] The meaning of this isolate is unknown.

ENTEROVIRUSES

There are only a few case reports of arthritis induced by either coxsackie or ECHO viruses.[137–140] However, enteroviruses may cause arthritis more commonly than these few case reports might indicate because documentation of these infections is often difficult. There is no single serologic test for enteroviruses; each one must be sought individually.

Coxsackie Viruses

Nine patients are known to have had acute febrile polyarthritis associated with rising or elevated antibody titers against various coxsackie viruses, generally B_2 and B_4.[138,139] In addition to fever and arthritis, symptoms in these patients included rash, sore throat, and pleuritic pain. Three of them also had myopericarditis. Joint fluid white cell counts ranged from 7,000 to 46,000 cells/mm³ with predominantly neutrophils. One of these patients, a 15-year-old boy, had prolonged polyarthritis suggestive of Still's disease.[139]

ECHO Viruses Types 6, 9, and 11

Only three patients have been reported with arthritis associated with an ECHO virus infection (types 6, 9, and 11).[137,140,141] Two of the patients had polyarthritis of large and small joints, one for 9 days and the other for 3 months. The remaining patient experienced monoarthritis of a knee for 2 days. Associated symptoms included fever, myalgias, rash, diarrhea, sore throat, or meningismus. For one patient, the synovial fluid showed 2,250 leukocytes/mm³,[137] and in another, 32,300 leukocytes/mm³.[141] ECHO virus type 11 was isolated from the joint fluid of one patient.[141]

REFERENCES

1. Inman, R.D., et al.: Arthritis, vasculitis, and cryoglobulinemia associated with relapsing hepatitis A infection. Ann. Intern. Med., 105:700–703, 1986.
2. Wands, J.R., et al.: The pathogenesis of arthritis associated with acute hepatitis-B surface antigen-positive hepatitis. J. Clin. Invest., 55:930–936, 1975.
3. Alpert, E., Isselbacher, K.J., and Schur, P.H.: The pathogenesis of arthritis associated with viral hepatitis. N. Engl. J. Med., 285:185–189, 1971.
4. Alpert, E., Schur, P.H., and Isselbacher, K.J.: Sequential changes of serum complement in HAA related arthritis. N. Engl. J. Med., 287:103, 1972.
5. Dienstag, J.L., et al.: Urticaria associated with acute viral hepatitis type B: Studies of pathogenesis. Ann. Intern. Med., 89:34–40, 1978.
6. Dixon, F.J., et al.: Pathogenesis of serum sickness. Arch. Pathol., 65:18–28, 1958.
7. Schumacher, H.R., and Gall, E.P.: Arthritis in acute hepatitis and chronic active hepatitis. Am. J. Med., 57:655–664, 1974.
8. Duffy, J., et al.: Polyarthritis, polyarteritis, and hepatitis B. Medicine, 55:19–37, 1976.
9. Koff, R.S., and Galambos, J.: Viral hepatitis. In Diseases of the Liver. Edited by L. Schiff. Philadelphia, J.B. Lippincott Co., 1987, pp. 457–581.
10. Alarcon, G.S., and Townes, A.S.: Arthritis in viral hepatitis: Report of two cases and review of the literature. Johns Hopkins Med. J., 132:1–15, 1973.
11. Segool, R.A., Lejtenyi, C., and Jaussig, L.M.: Articular and cutaneous prodromal manifestations of viral hepatitis. J. Pediatr., 87:709–712, 1975.
12. Shumaker, J.B., et al.: Arthritis and rash. Arch. Intern. Med., 133:438–485, 1974.
13. Inman, R.D.: Rheumatic manifestations of hepatitis B infection. Semin. Arthritis Rheum., 11:406–420, 1982.
14. Reference omitted.
15. Wenzel, R.P., et al.: Arthritis and viral hepatitis. Arch. Intern. Med., 130:770–771, 1972.
16. McCarty, D.J., and Ormiste, V.: Arthritis and HB Ag-positive hepatitis. Arch. Intern. Med., 132:264–268, 1973.
17. Onion, S.K., Crumpacker, C.S., and Gilliland, B.C.: Arthritis of hepatitis associated with Australia antigen. Ann. Intern. Med., 75:29–33, 1971.
18. Fernandez, R., and McCarty, D.J.: The arthritis of viral hepatitis. Ann. Intern. Med., 74:207–211, 1971.
19. McKenna, P.J., et al.: Hepatitis and arthritis with hepatitis-associated antigen in serum and synovial fluid. Lancet, 2:214–215, 1971.
20. Farivar, M., et al.: Cryoprotein complexes and peripheral neuropathy in a patient with chronic active hepatitis. Gastroenterology, 71:490–493, 1976.
21. Johnson, R.E., and Hall, A.P.: Rubella arthritis. Report of cases studied by latex tests. N. Engl. J. Med., 258:743–745, 1958.
22. Lee, P.R., et al.: Rubella arthritis. A study of twenty cases. California Med., 93:125–128, 1960.
23. Lerman, S.J., et al.: Immunologic response, virus excretion, and joint reactions with rubella vaccine. Ann. Intern. Med., 74:67–72, 1971.
24. Yanez, J.E., et al.: Rubella arthritis. Ann. Intern. Med., 64:772–777, 1966.
25. Ford, D.K., et al.: Synovial mononuclear cell responses to rubella antigen in rheumatoid arthritis and unexplained persistent knee arthritis. J. Rheumatol., 9:420–423, 1982.
26. Grahame, R., et al.: Chronic arthritis associated with the presence of intrasynovial rubella virus. Ann. Rheum. Dis., 42:2–13, 1983.
27. Fraser, J.R.E., et al.: Rubella arthritis in adults. Isolation of virus, cytology and other aspects of the synovial reaction. Clin. Exp. Rheumatol., 1:287–293, 1983.
28. Hildebrandt, H.M., and Maasab, H.F.: Rubella synovitis in a one-year-old-patient. N. Engl. J. Med., 274:1428–1429, 1966.
29. Panush, R.S.: Serum hypocomplementemia with rubella arthritis. Case report. Milit. Med., 140:117–120, 1975.
30. Singh, V.K., Tingle, A.J., and Schulzer, M.: Rubella-associated arthritis. II. Relationship between circulating immune complex levels and joint manifestations. Ann. Rheum. Dis., 45:115–119, 1986.
31. Geiger, J.C.: Epidemic of German measles in a city adjacent to an army cantonment. J.A.M.A., 70:1818, 1918.
32. Loudon, I.S.L.: Polyarthritis in rubella. Br. Med. J., 1:1388, 1953.

33. Kantor, T.G., and Tanner, M.: Rubella arthritis and rheumatoid arthritis. Arthritis Rheum., 5:378–383, 1962.
34. Chambers, R.J., and Bywaters, E.G.L.: Rubella synovitis. Ann. Rheum. Dis., 22:263–267, 1963.
35. Kilroy, A.W., et al.: Two syndromes following rubella immunization. Clinical observations and epidemiological studies. J.A.M.A., 214:2287–2292, 1970.
36. Tingle, A.J., et al.: Rubella-associated arthritis. I. Comparative study of joint manifestations associated with natural rubella infection and RA 27/3 rubella immunization. Ann. Rheum. Dis., 45:110–114, 1986.
37. Weibel, R.E., et al.: Rubella vaccination in adult females. N. Engl. J. Med., 280:682–685, 1969.
38. Vergani, D., et al.: Joint symptoms, immune complexes, and rubella (letter). Lancet, 2:321, 1980.
39. Chantler, J.K., Tingle, A.J., and Petty, R.E.: Persistent rubella infection associated with chronic arthritis in children. N. Engl. J. Med., 313:1117–1123, 1985.
40. Ogra, P.L., and Herd, J.K.: Arthritis associated with induced rubella infection. J. Immunol., 107:810–813, 1971.
41. Spruance, S.L., et al.: Recurrent joint symptoms in children vaccinated with HPV-77 DK12 rubella vaccine. J. Pediatr., 80:413–417, 1972.
42. Thompson, G.R., Ferreyra, A., and Brackett, R.G.: Acute arthritis complicating rubella vaccination. Arthritis Rheum., 14:19–26, 1971.
43. Farquhar, J.D., and Curretjer, J.E.: Clinical experience with Cendehill rubella vaccine in mature women. Am. J. Dis. Child., 118:266–268, 1969.
44. Gold, J.A., Prinzie, A., and McKee, J.: Adult women vaccinated with rubella vaccine. Am. J. Dis. Child., 118:264–265, 1969.
45. Horstmann, D.M., Liebhaber, H., and Kohorn, E.I.: Postpartum vaccination of rubella-susceptible women. Lancet, 2:1003–1006, 1970.
46. Plotkin, S.A., Farquhar, J.D., and Ogra, P.L.: Immunologic properties of RA27/3 rubella virus vaccine. J.A.M.A., 225:585–590, 1973.
47. Rogers, K.D., et al.: Clinical response to immunization with Cendehill strain rubella vaccine. Pediatrics, 47:7–14, 1971.
48. Spruance, S.L., and Smith, C.B.: Joint complications associated with derivatives of HPV-77 rubella vaccine. Am. J. Dis. Child., 122:105–111, 1971.
49. Thompson, G.R., et al.: Intermittent arthritis following rubella vaccination. Am. J. Dis. Child., 125:526–530, 1973.
50. Austin, S.M., et al.: Joint reactions in children vaccinated against rubella. Am. J. Epidemiol., 95:53–58, 1972.
51. Grand, M.G., et al.: Clinical reactions following rubella vaccination. J.A.M.A., 220:1569–1572, 1972.
52. Cooper, L.Z., et al.: Transient arthritis after rubella vaccination. Am. J. Dis. Child., 118:218–225, 1969.
53. Spruance, S.L., et al.: Chronic arthropathy associated with rubella vaccination. Arthritis Rheum., 20:741–747, 1977.
54. Tingle, A.J., et al.: Postpartum rubella immunization: Association with the development of prolonged arthritis, neurological sequelae, and chronic rubella viremia. J. Infect. Dis., 152:606–612, 1985.
55. Gilmartin, Jr., R.C., Jabbour, J.T., and Duenas, D.A.: Rubella vaccine myeloradiculoneuritis. J. Pediatr., 80:406–412, 1972.
56. Anderson, M.J., et al.: Human parvovirus, the cause of erythema infectiosum (Fifth disease) (letter). Lancet, 1:1378, 1983.
57. Reid, D.M., et al.: Human parvovirus-associated arthritis: A clinical and laboratory description. Lancet, 1:422–425, 1985.
58. White, D.J., et al.: Human parvovirus arthropathy. Lancet, 1:419–421, 1985.
59. Ager, E.A., Chin, T.D.Y., and Poland, J.D.: Epidemic erythema infectiosum. N. Engl. J. Med., 275:1326–1331, 1966.
60. Auriemma, P.R.: Erythema infectiosum: Report on a familial outbreak. Am. J. Public Health, 44:1450–1454, 1954.
61. Lawton, A.L., and Smith, R.E.: Erythema infectiosum. Arch. Intern. Med., 47:28–41, 1941.
62. Shaw, H.L.K.: Erythema infectiosum. Am. J. Med. Sci., 129:16–22, 1905.
63. Li-Loong, T.C., et al.: Human serum parvovirus associated vasculitis. Postgrad. Med. J., 62:493–494, 1986.
64. Anderson, M.J., et al.: The development and use of an antibody capture radioimmunoassay for specific IgM to a human parvovirus-like agent. J. Hyg. (Lond.), 88:309–324, 1982.
64a.Simpson, R.W., et al.: Association of parvoviruses with rheumatoid arthritis in humans. Science, 223:1425–1428, 1984.
65. Tesh, R.B.: Arthritides caused by mosquito-borne viruses. Ann. Rev. Med., 33:31–40, 1982.
66. Doherty, R.L., Carley, J.G., and Best, J.C.: Isolation of Ross River virus from man. Med. J. Aust., 1:1083–1084, 1972.
67. Aaskov, J.G., et al.: Isolation of Ross River virus from epidemic polyarthritis patients in Australia. Aust. J. Exp. Biol. Med. Sci., 63:587–597, 1985.
68. Anderson, S.G., and French, E.L.: An epidemic exanthem associated with polyarthritis in the Murray Valley, 1956. Med. J. Aust., 2:113–117, 1957.
69. Clarke, A.J., Marshall, I.D., and Gard, G.: Annually recurrent epidemic polyarthritis and Ross River virus activity in a coastal area of New South Wales. Am. J. Trop. Med. Hyg., 22:543–550, 1973.
70. Clarris, B.J., et al.: Epidemic polyarthritis: A cytological, virological, and immunochemical study. Aust. N.Z. J. Med., 5:450–457, 1975.
71. Fraser, J.R.E., et al.: Possible genetic determinants in epidemic polyarthritis caused by Ross River virus infection. Aust. N.Z. J. Med., 10:597–603, 1980.
72. Seglenieks, Z., and Moore, B.W.: Epidemic polyarthritis in South Australia: Report of an outbreak in 1971. Med. J. Aust., 2:552–556, 1974.
73. Doherty, R.L., et al.: Epidemic polyarthritis. Occurrence in Eastern Australia 1959–1970. Med. J. Aust., 1:5–8, 1971.
74. Doherty, R.L., et al.: Studies of arthropod-borne virus infections in Queensland. V. Survey of antibodies to group A arboviruses in man and other animals. Aust. J. Exp. Biol. Med. Sci., 44:365–377, 1966.
75. Doherty, R.L., et al.: The isolation of a third group A arbovirus in Australia, with preliminary observations on its relationship to epidemic polyarthritis. Aust. J. Sci., 26:183–189, 1963.
76. Gard, G., Marshall, I.D., and Woodroofe, G.M.: Annually recurrent epidemic polyarthritis and Ross River virus activity in a coastal area of New South Wales. II. Mosquitoes, viruses, and wildlife. Am. J. Trop. Med. Hyg., 22:551–559, 1973.
77. Fuller, C.O., and Warner, P.: Some epidemiological and laboratory observations on an epidemic rash and polyarthritis occurring in the upper Murray region of South Australia. Med. J. Aust., 2:117–120, 1957.
78. Dowling, P.G.: Epidemic polyarthritis. Med. J. Aust., 1:245–246, 1946.
79. Shope, R.E., and Anderson, S.G.: The virus etiology of epidemic exanthem and polyarthritis. Med. J. Aust., 1:156–158, 1960.
80. Sibree, E.W.: Acute polyarthritis in Queensland. Med. J. Aust., 2:565–567, 1944.

81. Fraser, J.R.E., et al.: Cytology of synovial effusions in epidemic polyarthritis. Aust. N.Z. J. Med., *11*:168–173, 1981.

82. Lumsden, W.H.R.: An epidemic of virus disease in southern province, Tanganyika territory, in 1952–53. II. General description and epidemiology. Trans. R. Soc. Trop. Med. Hyg., *49*:33–57, 1955.

83. Robinson, M.C.: An epidemic of virus disease in southern province, Tanganyika territory, in 1952–53. I. Clinical features. Trans. R. Soc. Trop. Med. Hyg., *49*:28–32, 1955.

84. Ross, R.W.: The Newala epidemic. III. The virus: Isolation, pathogenic properties and relationship to the epidemic. J. Hyg., *54*:177–191, 1956.

85. Moore, D.L., et al.: Arthropod-borne viral infections of man in Nigeria, 1964–1970. Ann. Trop. Med. Parasitol., *69*:49–64, 1975.

86. Moore, D.L., et al.: An epidemic of chikungunya fever in Ibadan, Nigeria, 1969. Ann. Trop. Med. Parasitol., *68*:59–68, 1974.

87. Nimmannitya, S., et al.: Dengue and chikungunya virus infection in man in Thailand, 1962–1964. I. Observations on hospitalized patients with hemorrhagic fever. Am. J. Trop. Med. Hyg., *18*:954–972, 1969.

88. Tesh, R.B., et al.: The distribution and prevalence of group A arbovirus neutralizing antibodies among human populations in southeast Asia and the Pacific Islands. Am. J. Trop. Med. Hyg., *24*:664–675, 1975.

89. Deller, J.J., and Russell, P.K.: Chikungunya disease. Am. J. Trop. Med. Hyg., *17*:107–111, 1968.

90. Weinbren, M.P., Haddow, A.J., and Williams, M.C.: The occurrence of chikungunya virus in Uganda. Trans. R. Soc. Trop. Med. Hyg., *52*:253–262, 1958.

91. Kennedy, A.C., Fleming, J., and Solomon, L.: Chikungunya viral arthropathy: A clinical description. J. Rheumatol., *7*:231–236, 1980.

92. Brighton, S.W., and Simson, I.W.: A destructive arthropathy following chikungunya virus arthritis—A possible association. Clin. Rheumatol., *3*:253–258, 1984.

93. Brighton, S.W.: Chloroquine phosphate treatment of chronic chikungunya arthritis. S. Afr. Med. J., *66*:217–218, 1984.

94. Haddow, A.J., Davies, C.W., and Walker, A.J.: O'nyong-nyong fever: An epidemic virus disease in East Africa. I. Introduction. Trans. R. Soc. Trop. Med. Hyg., *54*:517–522, 1960.

95. Shore, H.: O'nyong-nyong fever: An epidemic virus disease in East Africa. III. Some clinical and epidemiological observations in the northern province of Uganda. Trans. R. Soc. Trop. Med. Hyg., *55*:361–373, 1961.

96. Williams, M.C., Woodhall, J.P., and Gillett, J.D.: O'nyong-nyong fever: An epidemic virus disease in East Africa. VII. Virus isolations in man and serological studies up to July 1961. Trans. R. Soc. Trop. Med. Hyg., *59*:186–197, 1965.

97. Williams, M.C., Woodhall, J.P., and Portersfield, J.S.: O'nyong-nyong fever: An epidemic virus disease in East Africa. V. Human antibody studies by plaque inhibition and other serological tests. Trans. R. Soc. Trop. Med. Hyg., *56*:166–172, 1962.

98. Taylor, R.M., et al.: Sindbis virus: A newly recognized arthropod-transmitted virus. Am. J. Trop. Med. Hyg., *4*:844–862, 1955.

99. Malherbe, H., Strickland-Cholmley, M., and Jackson, A.L.: Sindbis virus infection in man. Report of a case with recovery of virus from skin lesions. S. Afr. Med. J., *37*:547–552, 1963.

100. McIntosh, M., et al.: Illness caused by Sindbis and west Nile viruses in South Africa. S. Afr. Med. J., *38*:291–294, 1964.

101. Pinheiro, F.P., et al.: An outbreak of Mayaro virus disease in Belterra, Brazil. Am. J. Trop. Med. Hyg., *30*:674–681, 1981.

102. Appelbaum, E., et al.: Mumps arthritis. Arch. Intern. Med., *90*:217–223, 1952.

103. Caranasos, G.J., and Felker, J.R.: Mumps arthritis. Arch. Intern. Med., *119*:394–398, 1967.

104. Filpi, R.G., and Houts, R.L.: Mumps arthritis. J.A.M.A., *205*:216–217, 1968.

105. Ghosh, S.K., and Reddy, T.A.: Arthralgia and myalgia in mumps. Rheumatol. Rehab., *12*:97–99, 1973.

106. Gold, H.E., Boxerbaum, B., and Leslie, Jr., H.J.: Mumps arthritis. Am. J. Dis. Child., *116*:547–548, 1968.

107. Lass, R., and Shephard, E.: Mumps arthritis. Br. Med. J., *2*:1613–1614, 1961.

108. Gordon, S.C., and Lauter, C.B.: Mumps arthritis: Unusual presentation as adult Still's disease. Ann. Intern. Med., *97*:45–47, 1982.

109. Gordon, S.C., and Lauter, C.B.: Mumps arthritis: A review of the literature. Rev. Infect. Dis., *6*:338–344, 1984.

110. Solem, J.H.: Mumps arthritis without parotitis. Scand. J. Infect. Dis., *3*:173–175, 1971.

111. Tracey, J.P., and Riggenbach, R.D.: Mumps arthritis associated with positive latex fixation reaction. South. Med. J., *63*:1122–1123, 1970.

112. Cockshott, P., and MacGregor, M.: Osteomyelitis variolosa. Q. J. Med., *27*:369–387, 1958.

113. Silby, H.M., et al.: Acute monoarticular arthritis after vaccination. Ann. Intern. Med., *62*:347–350, 1965.

114. Panush, R.S.: Adenovirus arthritis. Arthritis Rheum., *17*:534–536, 1974.

115. Rahal, J.J., Millian, S.J., and Noriega, E.R.: Coxsackie and adenovirus infection. J.A.M.A., *235*:2496–2501, 1976.

116. Utsinger, P.D.: Immunologic study of arthritis associated with adenovirus infection (abstract). Arthritis Rheum., *20*:138, 1977.

117. Fraser, K.J., et al.: A persistent adenovirus type 1 infection in synovial tissue from an immunodeficient patient with chronic, rheumatoid-like polyarthritis. Arthritis Rheum., *28*:455–458, 1985.

118. Friedman, A., and Naveh, Y.: Polyarthritis associated with chickenpox. Am. J. Dis. Child., *122*:179–180, 1971.

119. Mulhern, L.M., Friday, G.A., and Perri, J.A.: Arthritis complicating varicella infection. Pediatrics, *48*:827–829, 1971.

120. Pascual-Gomez, E.: Identification of large mononuclear cells in varicella arthritis (letter). Arthritis Rheum., *23*:519, 1980.

121. Priest, J.R., et al.: Varicella arthritis documented by isolation of virus from joint fluid. J. Pediatr., *93*:990–992, 1978.

122. Shuper, A., et al.: Varicella arthritis in a child. Arch. Dis. Child., *55*:568–569, 1980.

123. Ward, J.R., and Bishop, B.: Varicella arthritis. J.A.M.A., *212*:1954–1955, 1970.

124. Gibson, N.F., IV, and Ogden, W.S.: Varicella arthritis. South. Med. J., *79*:1028–1030, 1986.

125. Cunningham, A.L., et al.: A study of synovial fluid and cytology in arthritis associated with herpes zoster. Aust. N.Z. J. Med., *9*:440–443, 1979.

126. Devereaux, M.D., and Hazelton, R.A.: Acute monoarticular arthritis in association with herpes zoster (letter). Arthritis Rheum., *26*:236, 1983.

127. Friedman, H.M., et al.: Acute monoarticular arthritis caused by herpes simplex virus and cytomegalovirus. Am. J. Med., *69*:241–247, 1980.

128. Shelley, W.B.: Herpetic arthritis associated with disseminate

herpes simplex in a wrestler. Br. J. Dermatol., *103*:209–212, 1980.

129. Remafedi, G., and Muldoon, R.L.: Acute monoarticular arthritis caused by herpes simplex type I. Pediatrics, *72*:882–883, 1983.

130. Schooley, R.T., and Dolin, R.: Epstein-Barr virus (infectious mononucleosis). *In* Principles and Practice of Infectious Diseases. 2nd Ed. Edited by G.L. Mandell, R.G. Douglas, Jr., and J.E. Bennett. New York, John Wiley & Sons, Inc., 1985, pp. 971–982.

131. Adebonojo, F.O.: Monoarticular arthritis: An unusual manifestation of infectious mononucleosis. Clin. Pediatr., *11*:549–550, 1972.

132. Pollak, S., Enat, R., and Barzilai, D.: Monoarthritis with heterophile-negative infectious mononucleosis: Case of an older patient. Arch. Intern. Med., *142*:1109–1111, 1980.

133. Sigal, L.H., Steere, A.C., and Niederman, J.C.: Symmetric polyarthritis associated with heterophile-negative infectious mononucleosis. Arthritis Rheum., *26*:553–556, 1983.

134. Urman, J.D., and Bobrove, A.M.: Acute polyarthritis and infectious mononucleosis. West. J. Med., *136*:151–153, 1982.

135. Ray, C.G., et al.: Acute polyarthritis associated with active Epstein-Barr virus infection. J.A.M.A., *248*:2990–2993, 1982.

136. Hamerman, D., Gresser, I., and Smith, C.: Isolation of cytomegalovirus from synovial cells of a patient with rheumatoid arthritis. J. Rheumatol., *9*:658–664, 1982.

137. Blotzer, J.W., and Myers, A.R.: Echovirus-associated polyarthritis. Arthritis Rheum., *21*:978–981, 1978.

138. Hurst, N.P., et al.: Coxsackie B infection and arthritis. Br. Med. J., *286*:605, 1983.

139. Rahal, J.J., Millian, S.J., and Noriega, E.R.: Coxsackie and adenovirus infection. J.A.M.A., *235*:2496–2501, 1976.

140. Sanford, J.P., and Sulkin, S.E.: The clinical spectrum of ECHO-virus infection. N. Engl. J. Med., *261*:1113–1121, 1959.

141. Kujala, G., and Newman, J.H.: Isolation of ECHO virus type 11 from synovial fluid in acute monocytic arthritis. Arthritis Rheum., *28*:98–99, 1985.

119

LYME DISEASE

STEPHEN E. MALAWISTA

Lyme disease is a tick-borne, immune-mediated inflammatory disorder caused by a newly recognized spirochete, Borrelia burgdorferi. Its clinical hallmark is an early expanding skin lesion, erythema chronicum migrans (ECM), which may be followed weeks to months later by neurologic, cardiac, or joint abnormalities. Symptoms may refer to any one of these four systems alone or in combination. All stages of Lyme disease may respond to antibiotics, but treatment of early disease is the most successful. Foci of Lyme disease are widely distributed within the United States and Europe.

HISTORY

Lyme *arthritis* was first recognized in November, 1975 because of unusual geographic clustering of children with inflammatory arthropathy in the region of Lyme, Connecticut.[1] Its early elucidation—natural history,[1-6] immunopathogenesis,[7-11] epidemiology,[12-15] pathology,[2,4,11] and therapy[16-19]—was carried out primarily at Yale University by Steere, Malawista, and their colleagues. It soon became clear that this was a multisystem disorder (Lyme *disease*[2-6]) occurring at any age and in both sexes and often preceded by a characteristic expanding skin lesion, erythema chronicum migrans (ECM, Afzelius, 1909[20]). In Europe, ECM had been associated with the bite of the sheep tick, Ixodes ricinus,[21] and with tick-borne meningopolyneuritis (Garin-Bujadoux, 1922,[22] Bannwarth, 1941 and 1944[23]). These syndromes are now often subsumed under the name Lyme disease. In the Lyme region, a closely related deer tick, Ixodes dammini (a member of the so-called I. ricinus complex), was implicated as the principal disease vector on epidemiologic grounds.[12-15]

In 1982, Burgdorfer and associates[24] isolated the spirochete that bears his name from Ixodes dammini collected on Shelter Island, New York, and linked it serologically to patients with Lyme disease. Within months this organism had been cultured from blood, skin, and cerebrospinal fluid of patients, and specific IgM and IgG antibody responses to it had been delineated.[25,26] Because it is infectious in origin but inflammatory or "rheumatic" in expression, Lyme disease, beyond its intrinsic interest as a new nosologic entity, presents a unique human model for an infectious etiology of rheumatic disease.[27]

PATHOGENESIS

In morphology, physiology, and DNA nucleotide composition, the spirochetes found in ticks and patients resemble Borrelia rather than Leptospira or Treponema, the other two spirochetes pathogenic for humans, and isolates in the United States and Europe appear so far to belong to a single species: Borrelia burgdorferi (Fig. 119–1)[28]; there is, however, antigenic variation.[29] This organism is also responsible for some cases of an early skin lesion, benign lymphocytoma,[30] and for a late one, acrodermatitis chronica atrophicans,[30,31] both seen primarily in Europe.

1955

FIG. 119–1. Scanning electron micrograph of Borrelia burgdorferi isolated from the spinal fluid of a patient with meningoencephalitis[25] whose Lyme disease had begun 2½ months earlier with erythema chronicum migrans. (bar = 0.5 μm). (From Johnson, R.C., Hyde, F.W., and Rumpel, C.M.: Taxonomy of the Lyme disease spirochetes. Yale J. Biol. Med., 57:529–537, 1984.)

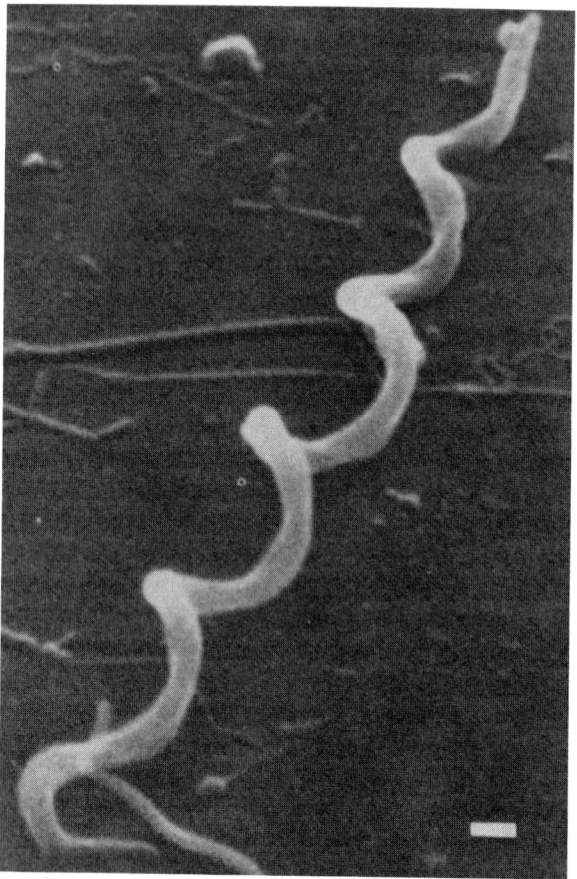

Recovery of B. burgdorferi is straightforward from the tick but generally difficult from patients, perhaps in part because of a relative paucity of organisms in most specimens of human tissues and fluids. An exception is its isolation from ECM biopsy specimens in improved media; for example, 6 of 14 in one study[32]; 9 of 13 in another.[31] Nevertheless, rare positive cultures are reported at all stages of the illness—from blood (early),[25,26] secondary annular lesions,[31] meningitic cerebrospinal fluid,[25] joint fluid,[33] and even from an acrodermatitis chronica atrophicans that had been present for over 10 years.[31] Spirochetes have been identified by silver stain or by immunofluorescence in some histologic sections of ECM,[34] and rarely of secondary annular lesions,[35] synovium,[36] brain,[37] eye,[38] heart,[39] spleen, kidney, and bone marrow.[40] From these data, combined with clinical and epi-

demiologic features of Lyme disease, the following pathogenetic sequence is likely. B. burgdorferi is transmitted to the skin of the host by the tick vector. After an incubation period of 3 to 32 days,[6] the organism migrates outward in the skin (causing ECM), spreads in lymph (causing regional adenopathy), or disseminates in blood to organs (e.g., central nervous system and presumably liver and spleen) or other skin sites (causing secondary annular lesions). Maternal-fetal transmission can occur.[40] Although organisms are hard to find in later stages of Lyme disease, it is likely that persistent live spirochetes are driving the illness throughout its course. Evidence for this interpretation includes the responsiveness of many patients to antibiotics, the rare sightings of spirochetes in affected tissues and fluids, the antigen-specific proliferation of lymphocytes from these fluids,[41,42] and an expansion of the antibody response to additonal spirochetal antigens over time.[43]

Lyme disease is associated with characteristic immune abnormalities.[7–10] At disease onset (ECM), almost all patients have evidence of circulating immune complexes.[9,10] At that time, the findings of elevated serum IgM levels and cryoglobulins containing IgM predict subsequent nervous system, heart, or joint involvement[7,8] (i.e., *early humoral findings have prognostic significance*). Serial determinations of serum IgM are often the single most helpful laboratory indicator of disease activity. These abnormalities tend to persist during neurologic or cardiac involvement. Later in the illness, when arthritis is present, serum IgM levels are more often normal. By then, immune complexes are usually lacking in serum but are present uniformly in joint fluid,[10] where their titers correlate positively with the local concentrations of polymorphonuclear leukocytes.[44] Mononuclear cells from peripheral blood increase their antigen-specific proliferative response as the disease progresses, but the greatest reactivity to antigen is seen in cells in fluid from inflamed joints.[41] On biopsy one sees a proliferative synovium, often replete with lymphocytes and plasma cells[2] that presumably are capable of producing immunoglobulin locally. Thus, an initially disseminated, immune-mediated, inflammatory disorder becomes localized and propagated in the joints of some patients. (Inflammatory mediators are noted below in the section entitled Arthritis.) Patients with arthritis or with another late manifestation, acrodermatitis chronica atrophicans, appear to have an increased frequency of the B-cell alloantigen, DR2.[4,45]

EPIDEMIOLOGY

Lyme disease is widespread. In the United States there are three distinct foci: the Northeast from Massachusetts to Maryland, the Midwest in Wisconsin and Minnesota, and the West in California, southern Oregon, and western Nevada.[14,46] However, the illness has also been reported in over half the states, as well as throughout Europe and in Australia.[46,47] The earliest known U.S. cases occurred on Cape Cod in 1962 and in Lyme, Connecticut in 1965[14]; cases now number in the thousands. Disease can occur at any age and in either sex.[15] Onset of illness is generally between May 1 and November 30, the peak, in June and July.[6]

The primary vectors of Lyme disease are tiny hard ticks of the Ixodes ricinus complex; major foci of disease correspond to the distribution of I. dammini (Northeast and Midwest),[14,46] I. pacificus (West),[14,46] and I. ricinus (Europe).[46,47] However, Australia has Lyme disease but lacks the I. ricinus complex,[48] and other vectors, including the lone star tick, Amblyomma americanum, are likely in some areas of the United States.[49,50] Biting insects are possible secondary vectors.[51]

In one U.S. study, 31% of 314 patients recalled a tick bite at the skin site where ECM developed days to weeks later.[6] The six ticks that were saved were invariably nymphal I. dammini, whose peak questing period is May through July; the nymphal stage seems to be the stage primarily responsible for transmission of disease.[52] Preferred hosts for I. dammini nymphs are white-footed mice, and for adults, white-tailed deer, in whose fur they may survive the winter.[13,52,53] The prevalence of B. burgdorferi in nymphal I. dammini ranges from about 20% to over 60%[24,25,50] (compare with I. pacificus: 0.9–2%[54]). The organism has been isolated, or specific antibody found, in blood and tissues of a wide variety of large and small animals, including domestic dogs (which can develop arthritis) and birds.[55–59] Indiscriminate feeding on a variety of animals by immature I. dammini may favor the spread of infection.

CLINICAL CHARACTERISTICS

Lyme disease is conveniently divided into three clinical stages, but with the understanding that the stages may overlap, and that most patients do not exhibit all of them (in fact, seroconversion can occur in asymptomatic individuals[60,61]). The illness usually begins with ECM and associated symptoms (*stage 1*), sometimes followed weeks to months later by neurologic or cardiac abnormalities (*stage 2*), and weeks to years later by arthritis (*stage 3*). Chronic neurologic and skin involvement may also occur years after onset.

EARLY MANIFESTATIONS

Erythema chronicum migrans (ECM), the unique clinical marker for Lyme disease, begins as a red macule or papule at the site where the tick vector, usually long gone, had engorged.[2,6] As the area of redness expands to 15 cm or so (range, 3 to 68 cm), there is usually partial central clearing (Fig. 119–2). The outer borders are red, generally flat, and without scaling. The centers are occasionally red and indurated, even vesicular or necrotic. Variations may occur—multiple rings, for example. The thigh, groin, and axilla are particularly common sites. The lesion is warm to touch but not often sore, and easily missed if out of sight. Routine histology is nonspecific: a heavy dermal infiltrate of mononuclear cells, without epidermal change except at the site of the tick bite.

Within days of onset of ECM, about half of U.S. patients develop multiple annular secondary lesions (Fig. 119–2; Table 119—1). They resemble ECM itself, but are generally smaller, migrate less, and lack indurated centers; they are not associated with previous tick bites. Individual lesions may come and go, and their borders sometimes merge. Other occasional skin lesions are noted in Table 119–1. In addition, benign lymphocytoma cutis has been reported in Europe.[30] ECM and secondary lesions fade in 3 to 4 weeks (range, 1 day to 14 months). They may recur.

Skin involvement is often accompanied by flulike symptoms—malaise and fatigue, headache, fever and chills, myalgia and arthralgia (Table 119–2).[2,6] Some patients have evidence of meningeal irritation or mild encephalopathy—for example, episodic attacks of excruciating headache and neck pain, stiffness, or pressure—but typically lasting only for hours at this stage of the illness, and without spinal fluid pleocytosis or objective neurologic deficit.[3] Except for fatigue and lethargy, which are often constant, the early signs and symptoms are typically intermittent and changing. For example, a patient may have meningitic attacks for several days, a few days of improvement, and then the onset of migratory musculoskeletal pain. This last may involve joints (generally without swelling), tendons, bursa, muscle, and bone. The pain tends to affect only one or two sites at a time and to last a few hours to several days in a given location. The various associated symptoms may occur several days before ECM (or without it) and last for months (especially fatigue and lethargy) after the skin lesions have disappeared.

In Europe, untreated ECM more commonly has a prolonged course, and it is less commonly associated with multiple annular lesions, pronounced general

FIG. 119–2. Dermatologic manifestations of Lyme disease. *A,* Erythema chronicum migrans (ECM). An early lesion is seen 4 days after detection. *B,* In a 10-day lesion of ECM, the red outer ring has expanded and central clearing is beginning. *C,* Eight days after onset of ECM, similar secondary lesions have appeared, and several of their borders have merged. (From Steere, A.C., et al.: The early clinical manifestations of Lyme disease. Ann. Intern. Med., *99*:76–82, 1983.)

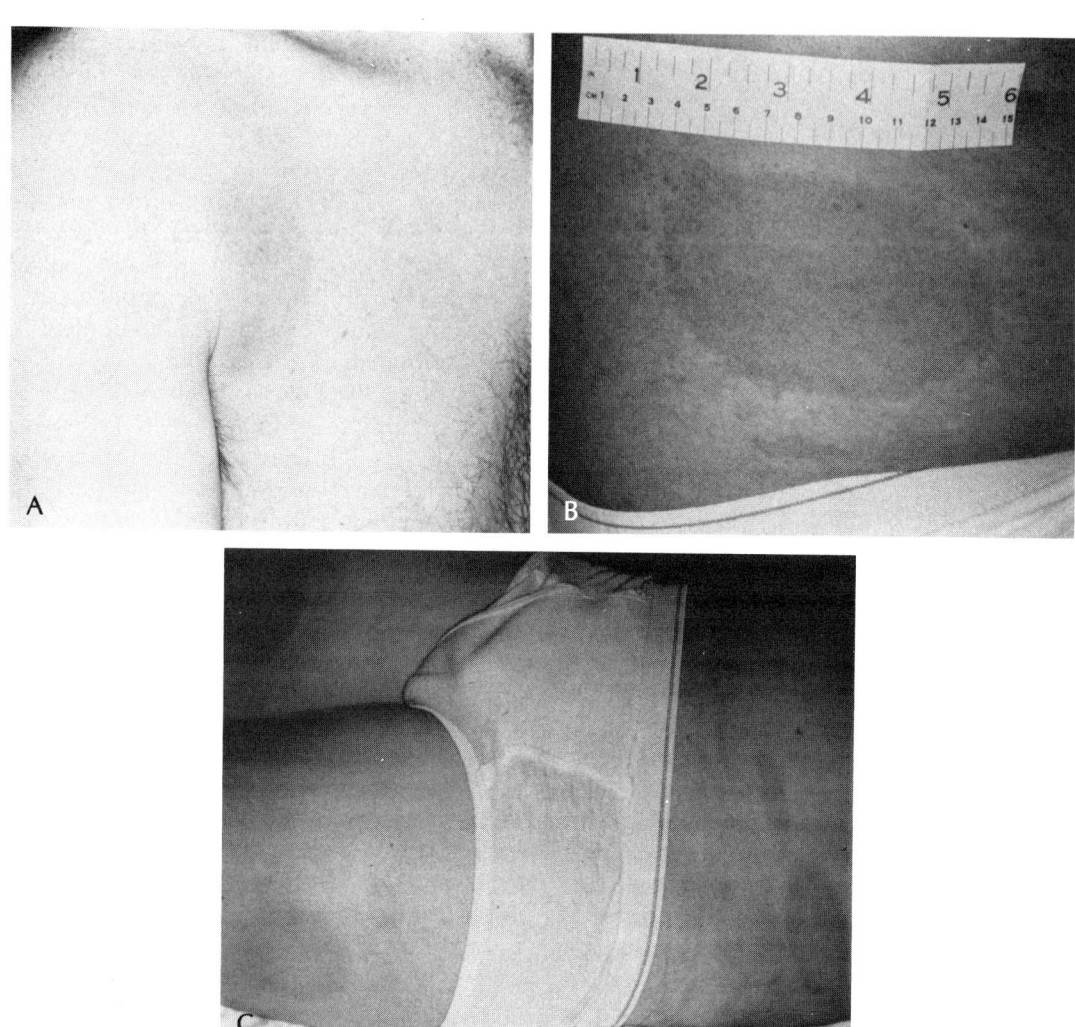

symptoms, laboratory abnormalities, or subsequent arthritis.[62]

LATER MANIFESTATIONS

Neurologic Involvement. Within several weeks to months of the onset of illness, about 15% of patients develop frank neurologic abnormalities including meningitis, encephalitis, chorea, cranial neuritis (including bilateral facial palsy), motor and sensory radiculoneuritis, or mononeuritis multiplex, in various combinations.[3,63] The usual pattern is fluctuating meningoencephalitis with superimposed cranial nerve (particularly facial) palsy and peripheral radiculoneuropathy (Fig. 119–3), but Bell's palsy may occur *alone*. By now, patients with meningitic symptoms have a lymphocytic pleocytosis (about 100 cells/mm³) in cerebrospinal fluid and sometimes diffuse slowing on electroencephalogram. However, the neck is rarely stiff except on extreme flexion; Kernig and Brudzinski signs are absent. Neurologic abnormalities typically last for months but usually resolve completely (late neurologic complications are noted below).

Cardiac Involvement. Within weeks to months of onset, about 8% of patients develop cardiac involve-

Table 119–1. Early Signs of Lyme Disease*

Signs	No. of Patients N = 314	(%)
Erythema chronicum migrans†	314	(100)
Multiple annular lesions	150	(48)
Lymphadenopathy		
Regional	128	(41)
Generalized	63	(20)
Pain on neck flexion	52	(17)
Malar rash	41	(13)
Erythematous throat	38	(12)
Conjunctivitis	35	(11)
Right upper quadrant tenderness	24	(8)
Splenomegaly	18	(6)
Hepatomegaly	16	(5)
Muscle tenderness	12	(4)
Periorbital edema	10	(3)
Evanescent skin lesions	8	(3)
Abdominal tenderness	6	(2)
Testicular swelling	2	(1)

*From Steere, A.C., et al.: The early clinical manifestations of Lyme disease. Ann. Intern. Med., *99*:79, 1983.
†Erythema chronicum migrans was required for inclusion in this study.

Table 119–2. Early Symptoms of Lyme Disease

Symptoms	No. of Patients N = 314	(%)
Malaise, fatigue, and lethargy	251	(80)
Headache	200	(64)
Fever and chills	185	(59)
Stiff neck	151	(48)
Arthalgias	150	(48)
Myalgias	135	(43)
Backache	81	(26)
Anorexia	73	(23)
Sore throat	53	(17)
Nausea	53	(17)
Dysesthesia	35	(11)
Vomiting	32	(10)
Abdominal pain	24	(8)
Photophobia	19	(6)
Hand stiffness	16	(5)
Dizziness	15	(5)
Cough	15	(5)
Chest pain	12	(4)
Ear pain	12	(4)
Diarrhea	6	(2)

(From Steere, A.C., et al.: The early clinical manifestations of Lyme disease. Ann. Intern. Med., *99*:79, 1983.)

ment.[5] The most common abnormality is fluctuating degrees of atrioventricular block (first degree, Wenckebach, or complete heart block). Some patients have evidence of more diffuse cardiac involvement including electrocardiographic changes compatible with acute myopericarditis, radionuclide evidence of mild left ventricular dysfunction, or, rarely, cardiomegaly.[5] Gallium-positive myocarditis[64] and, in one fatal case,

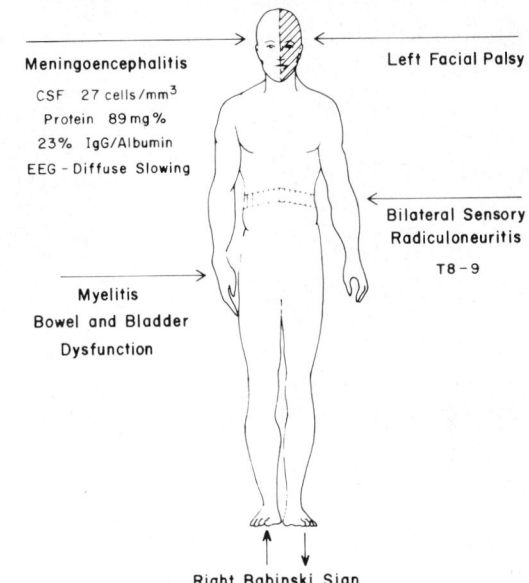

FIG. 119–3. Neurologic abnormalities of Lyme disease that occurred in a 58-year-old man. Three weeks after the onset of erythema chronicum migrans, the patient developed meningoencephalitis, left facial palsy, and bilateral sensory radiculoneuritis. Although long-tract signs are unusual in Lyme disease, this patient had bowel and bladder dysfunction and a right Babinski sign suggestive of myelitis.

spirochete-positive pancarditis[39] are reported. No patients have had significant heart murmurs (compare with acute rheumatic fever).[5] Cardiac involvement is usually brief (3 days to 6 weeks), but it may recur.

Arthritis. From weeks to as long as 2 years after the onset of illness, about 60% of patients develop frank arthritis,[2,4,11] usually characterized by intermittent attacks of asymmetric joint swelling and pain primarily in large joints, especially the knee, one or two joints at a time. Affected knees are commonly more swollen than painful, often hot, rarely red. Baker's cysts may form and rupture early. However, both large and small joints may be affected, and a few patients have had symmetric polyarthritis. Attacks of arthritis, which generally last from weeks to months, typically recur for several years. Fatigue is common with active joint involvement, but fever or other system symptoms at this stage are unusual. Joint fluid white cell counts vary from 500 to 110,000 cells/mm³ with an average of about 25,000 cells/mm³, mostly polymorphonuclear leukocytes.[2] Total protein ranges from 3 to 8 g/dl. C3 and C4 levels are generally greater than one third, and glucose levels usually greater than two thirds, that of serum. Tests for rheumatoid factor and antinuclear antibody are negative.

In about 10% of patients with arthritis, involvement

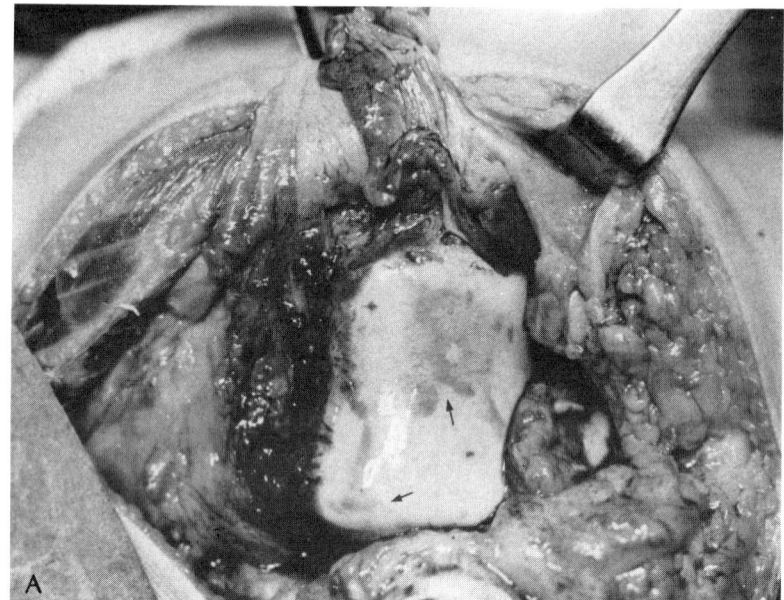

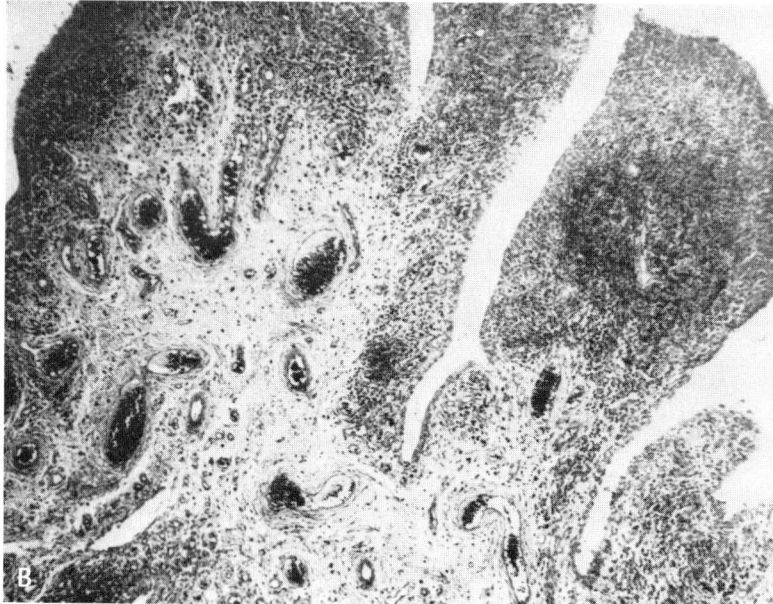

FIG. 119–4. *A*, The knee of a patient with Lyme disease at the time of synovectomy. The patient had typical erythema chronicum migrans in June, 1974 followed by intermittent migratory polyarthritis. Two years later, he developed persistent swelling of the right knee. After 7 months, he underwent a synovectomy. The articular surface of the femur can be seen; the arrows indicate what was the advancing border of pannus, now stripped away from the underlying eroded cartilage. *B*, Tissue structure of affected synovium. Individual polypoid stalks show central edema and vascular proliferation. Surrounding this central core is a rim of predominantly mononuclear cells. In one area an aggregate resembling a lymphoid follicle is seen. (From Steere, A.C., et al.: Erythema chronicum migrans and Lyme arthritis: The enlarging clinical spectrum. Ann. Intern. Med., *86*:693, 1977.)

in large joints may become chronic, with pannus formation and erosion of cartilage and bone (Fig. 119–4*A*).[4,11] Synovial biopsies may mimic those of rheumatoid arthritis (RA) with surface deposits of fibrin, villous hypertrophy, vascular proliferation, and a heavy infiltration of mononuclear cells (Fig. 119–4*B*).[2,4,11] In addition, there may be an obliterative endarteritis and (rarely) demonstrable spirochetes.[36] Borrelia burgdorferi are potent stimulators of mononuclear phagocytes to produce interleukin-1, found in synovial fluids.[65] In one patient with chronic Lyme arthritis, synovium grown in tissue culture produced large amounts of collagenase and prostaglandin E$_2$.[11] Thus, in Lyme disease the joint fluid cell counts, the

immune reactants (except for rheumatoid factor), the synovial histology, the amounts of synovial enzymes released, and the resulting destruction of cartilage and bone may be similar to those in RA.[66]

Other late findings (years after onset of illness) associated with this infection include a chronic skin lesion—acrodermatitis chronica atrophicans[30,31]—well known in Europe but still rare in the United States. Violaceous infiltrated plaques or nodules, especially on extensor surfaces, eventually become atrophic. There may be underlying joint changes. Late chronic neurologic disease includes transverse myelitis, demyelinating lesions of the central nervous system, psychiatric illness, or recurrent episodes of severe fatigue.[67,68] "Progressive Borrelia encephalomyelitis"[69] is currently recognized more frequently in Europe than in the United States.

LABORATORY TESTS

Determination of specific antibody titers is currently the most helpful diagnostic test for Lyme disease. Culture of B. burgdorferi from patients permits definitive diagnosis, but is rarely successful except from skin.[25,31,32] Similarly, spirochetes are not often seen by direct examination of blood, plasma, plasma pellets, or skin transudate specimens of ECM,[25] and special tissue staining techniques[34-36] are low-yield and not readily available.

In serum, specific IgM antibody titers against B. burgdorferi usually reach a peak between the third and sixth week after the onset of disease; specific IgG antibody titers rise more slowly and are generally highest months later when arthritis is present (Fig. 119–5).[25,70] To date, *no one with established Lyme arthritis has failed to have an elevated titer of specific IgG antibody.* This finding makes antibody titers against B. burgdorferi particularly useful in differentiating Lyme disease from other rheumatic syndromes, especially when ECM is missed, forgotten, or absent. This antibody cross-reacts with other spirochetes, including Treponema pallidum, but patients with Lyme disease do not have positive tests for VDRL.[6,70]

The most common nonspecific laboratory abnormalities, particularly early in the illness, are a high erythrocyte sedimentation rate (ESR), an elevated serum IgM level, or an increased serum glutamic oxaloacetic transaminase (SGOT) level (Table 119–3).[2,7] The enzyme levels generally return to normal within several weeks. Patients may be mildly anemic early in the illness and occasionally have elevated white cell counts with shifts to the left in the differential count. A few patients have had microscopic hematuria, sometimes with mild proteinuria (dipstick); values for creatinine and blood urea nitrogen have been normal. Throughout the illness, serum C3 and C4 levels are generally normal or elevated. Tests for rheumatoid factor or antinuclear antibodies are usually negative.

DIFFERENTIAL DIAGNOSIS

Erythema chronicum migrans is the unique herald lesion of Lyme disease (Fig. 119–2); little else can be confused with it in its classic form. However, some patients are not aware of having had erythema chronicum migrans, and in others, its appearance is not characteristic. Secondary lesions might suggest erythema multiforme, but blistering, mucosal lesions and involvement of the palms and soles are not features of Lyme disease. Malar rash may suggest systemic lupus erythematosus (SLE), an urticarial rash, hepatitis B infection, or serum sickness. Evanescent blotches and circles may resemble erythema marginatum, but blotches and circles of Lyme disease do not expand.

Early flulike symptoms may be misleading, especially when erythema chronicum migrans is absent or missed or is not the first manifestation. Severe headache and stiff neck may resemble aseptic meningitis; abdominal symptoms, hepatitis; and generalized tender lymphadenopathy and splenomegaly, infectious mononucleosis. As in the last infection, profound fatigue in Lyme disease may be a major and persistent complaint.

In later stages Lyme disease may mimic other immune-mediated disorders. Like rheumatic fever, Lyme disease may be associated with sore throat followed by migratory polyarthritis and carditis, but without evidence of valvular involvement or of a preceding streptococcal infection. Migratory pain in tendons and joints may also suggest disseminated gonococcal disease. An isolated facial weakness may mimic other causes of Bell's palsy. Late neurologic involvement may suggest multiple sclerosis (transverse myelitis), Guillain-Barré syndrome (symmetric peripheral neuropathy), primary psychosis, or brain tumor. In adults with Lyme arthritis the large knee effusions can resemble those in Reiter's syndrome, and the occasional symmetric polyarthritis can resemble that of RA. In children, the attacks of arthritis, although generally shorter, may be identical to those seen in the oligoarticular form of juvenile rheumatoid arthritis (JRA), but without iridocyclitis.

TREATMENT

STAGE 1

If patients are treated early with antibiotics, erythema chronicum migrans and its associated symptoms resolve in days, and subsequent major sequelae (myocarditis, meningoencephalitis, or recurrent arthritis) usually do not occur.[17] Prompt treatment is therefore important, even though such patients may be susceptible to reinfection.[71] For adults, therapy in order of preference includes oral tetracycline, 250 mg four times a day, phenoxymethyl penicillin, 500 mg four times a day, or erythromycin, 250 mg four times

FIG. 119–5. Antibody titers against Borrelia burgdorferi in serum samples from 135 patients with different clinical manifestations of Lyme disease, from 40 control patients with infectious mononucleosis or inflammatory arthritis, and from 40 normal control subjects, determined by indirect immunofluorescence. The heavy bar shows the geometric mean titer for each group; the shaded areas indicate the range of titers generally observed in control subjects. Note that all patients with Lyme arthritis have elevated IgG antibody titers. (From Steere, A.C., et al.: The spirochetal etiology of Lyme disease. N. Engl. J. Med., *308*:733–740, 1983.)

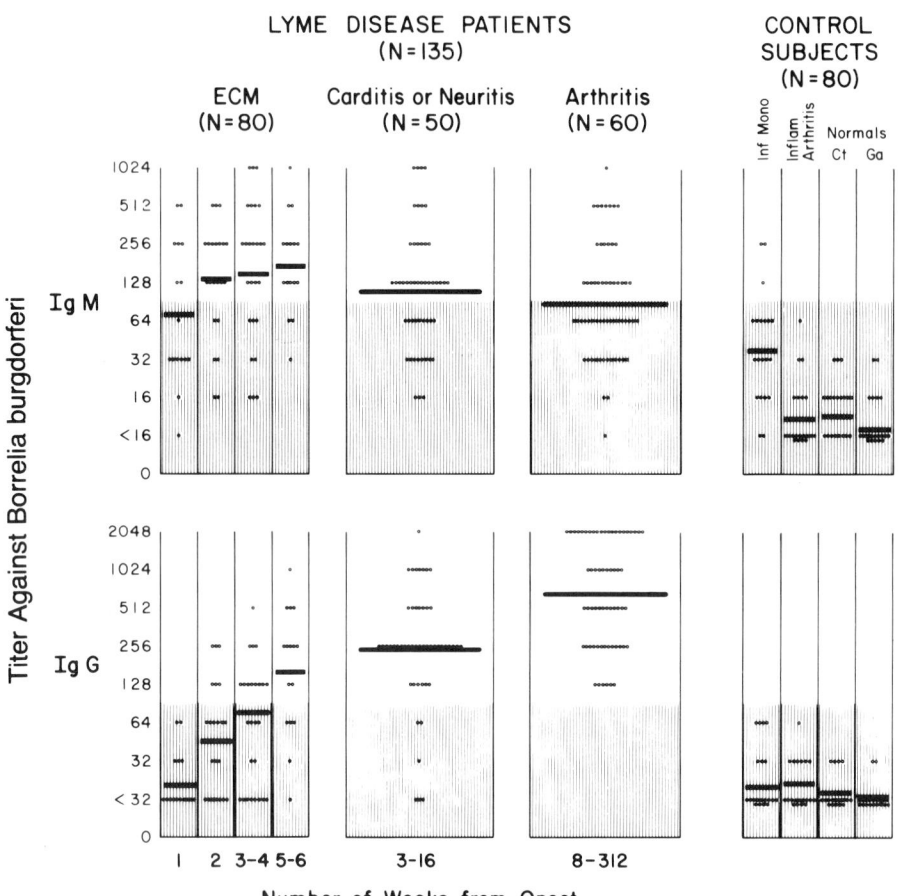

a day, each for 10 to 20 days depending on the response.[17] In children, phenoxymethyl penicillin, 50 mg/kg/day (not less than 1 g or more than 2 g per day), is given in divided doses for the same period, or, in cases of penicillin allergy, erythromycin, 30 mg/kg/day, in divided doses for 15 or 20 days. Although adverse outcomes of pregnancy have not been directly ascribable to maternal B. burgdorferi infection, that potential provides additional impetus for early treatment with penicillin or erythromycin for Lyme disease occurring during pregnancy.[40,72]

About 10% of patients experience a Jarisch-Herxheimer-like reaction (higher fever, redder rash, or greater pain) during the first 24 hours of therapy.[17] Whichever drug is given, nearly half of patients have brief (hours to days) recurrent episodes of headache or pain in joints, tendons, bursae, or muscles, often with lethargy, which may continue for extended periods.[17] Such symptoms may represent undergraded antigen rather than persistent live spirochetes.

STAGE 2

For meningitis and cranial or peripheral neuropathies, intravenous penicillin G, 20 million U a day in six divided doses for 10 days is effective therapy.[18] Headache, stiff neck, and radicular pain usually begin to subside by the second day of therapy and disappear by 7 to 10 days; motor deficits frequently require 7 to 8 weeks for complete recovery. Although not studied systematically, carditis also responds rapidly (in days)

Table 119–3. Laboratory Findings in Early Lyme Disease

Laboratory Test	No. of Patients with Abnormal Values		Median (Range) of Abnormal Values
	N = 314	(%)	
Hematology			
Hematocrit	37	(12)	35 (36–31)
Leukocytes >10 cells × 10³/mm³	24	(8)	12 (11–18)
ESR >20 mm/hour	166	(53)	35 (21–68)
Immunoglobulins			
IgM >250 mg/dl	104	(33)	310 (252–930)
IgG >1500 mg/dl	10	(3)	1580 (1520–1760)
IgA >400 mg/dl	12	(4)	440 (410–580)
Liver Function			
SGOT >35 U/ml	59	(19)	71 (36–251)
SGPT >32 U/ml*	47	(15)	125 (42–491)
LDH >600 U/ml*	49	(16)	775 (608–1080)
Renal Function			
Microscopic hematuria (red cells/hpf)	18	(6)	15 (10–25)

*Tested only in the 55 patients with abnormal SGOT; CPK was normal in all these patients.
(From Steere, A.C., et al.: The early clinical manifestations of Lyme disease. Ann. Intern. Med., *99*:80, 1983.)

to this regimen. Prednisone, 40 to 60 mg a day in divided doses, may be added when a strong anti-inflammatory effect is important (e.g., persistent complete heart block or deteriorating cardiac function).[5] For patients with allergy to penicillin, tetracycline, 500 mg four times a day for 30 days (an alternative recommended for tertiary syphilis) is reasonable but unevaluated.

STAGE 3

For established Lyme arthritis, even with unremitting involvement, parenteral penicillin is curative in some patients.[19] During treatment, the affected joint should be at rest, and accumulated fluid should be removed by needle aspirations. In a double-blinded placebo-controlled trial, 7 of 20 patients given intramuscular benzathine penicillin, 2.4 million U weekly for 3 weeks, were cured (mean followup 33 months), versus none of 20 control patients.[19] This regimen provides low serum levels of penicillin for about 6 weeks. The high-dose intravenous regimen of penicillin G (above), which yields much higher serum levels over its 10-day course, cured 11 of 20 patients, including 2 in whom benzathine penicillin had failed.[19] Optimal therapy for this problem and for the later neurologic complications of Lyme disease is not yet clear. In difficult cases current thinking favors longer periods of the highest tolerated oral doses of penicillin (with probenecid) or tetracyclines, or longer intravenous regimens of penicillin. Experience with parenteral ceftriaxone is limited at present.[73] Synovectomy may be useful for treatment failures. The infiltrative lesions of acrodermatitis chronica atrophicans are usually cured by 3 weeks of oral phenoxymethyl penicillin, 2 to 3 g daily in divided doses.[74]

REFERENCES

1. Steere, A.C., et al.: Lyme arthritis: an epidemic of oligoarticular arthritis in children and adults in three Connecticut communities. Arthritis Rheum., 20:7–17, 1977.
2. Steere, A.C., et al.: Erythema chronicum migrans and Lyme arthritis: The enlarging clinical spectrum. Ann. Intern. Med., 86:685–698, 1977.
3. Reik, L., et al.: Neurologic abnormalities of Lyme disease. Medicine, 58:281–294, 1979.
4. Steere, A.C., et al.: Chronic Lyme arthritis: Clinical and immunogenetic differentiation from rheumatoid arthritis. Ann. Intern. Med., 90:286–291, 1979.
5. Steere, A.C., et al.: Lyme carditis: Cardiac abnormalities of Lyme disease. Ann. Intern. Med., 93:8–16, 1980.
6. Steere, A.C., et al.: The early clinical manifestations of Lyme disease. Ann. Intern. Med., 99:76–82, 1983.
7. Steere, A.C., Hardin, J.A., and Malawista, S.E.: Erythema chronicum migrans and Lyme arthritis. Cryoimmunoglobulins and clinical activity of skin and joints. Science, 196:1121–1122, 1977.
8. Steere, A.C., et al.: Lyme arthritis: Correlation of serum and cryoglobulin IgM with activity and serum IgG wth remission. Arthritis Rheum., 2:471–483, 1979.
9. Hardin, J.A., et al.: Circulating immune complexes in Lyme arthritis: Detection of the ¹²⁵I-C1q binding, C1q solid phase and Raji cell assays. J. Clin. Invest., 63:468–477, 1979.
10. Hardin, J.A., Steere, A.C., and Malawista, S.E.: Immune complexes and the evolution of Lyme arthritis: Dissemination and localization of abnormal C1q binding activity. N. Engl. J. Med., 301:1358–1363, 1979.
11. Steere, A.C., et al.: Elevated levels of collagenase and pros-

taglandin E$_2$ from synovium associated with erosion of cartilage and bone in a patient with chronic Lyme arthritis. Arthritis Rheum., 23:591–599, 1980.

12. Steere, A.C., Broderick, T.E., and Malawista, S.E.: Erythema chronicum migrans and Lyme arthritis: Epidemiologic evidence for a tick vector. Am. J. Epidemiol., *108*:312–321, 1978.

13. Wallis, R.C., Brown, S.E., Kloter, K.O., and Main, A.J., Jr.: Erythema chronicum migrans and Lyme arthritis: Field study of ticks. Am. J. Epidemiol., *108*:322–327, 1978.

14. Steere, A.C., and Malawista, S.E.: Cases of Lyme disease in the United States: Locations correlated with distribution of Ixodes dammini. Ann. Intern. Med., *91*:730–733, 1979.

15. Steere, A.C., and Malawista, S.E.: The epidemiology of Lyme disease. *In* Current Topics in Rheumatology: Epidemiology of the Rheumatic Diseases. Proceedings of the Fourth International Conference. Edited by R.C. Lawrence and L.E. Schulman. New York, Gower Medical Publishing Limited, 1983, pp. 33–42.

16. Steere, A.C., et al.: Antibiotic therapy in Lyme disease. Ann. Intern., Med., *93*:1–8, 1980.

17. Steere, A.C., et al.: Treatment of the early manifestations of Lyme disease. Ann. Intern. Med., *99*:22–26, 1983.

18. Steere, A.C., Pachner, A.R., and Malawista, S.E.: Neurologic abnormalities of Lyme disease: Successful treatment with high-dose intravenous penicillin. Ann. Intern. Med., *99*:767–772, 1983.

19. Steere, A.C., et al.: Successful parenteral antibiotic therapy of established Lyme arthritis. N. Engl. J. Med., *312*:869–874, 1985.

20. Afzelius, A.: Verhandlungen der Dermatologischen Gesellschaft zu Stockholm on October 29, 1909. Arch. Dermatol. Syph., *101*:404, 1910.

21. Thone, A.W.: Ixodes ricinus and erythema chronicum migrans (Afzelius). Dermatologica, *136*:57–60, 1968.

22. Garin-Bujadoux, C.: Paralysie par les tiques. J. Med. Lyon, *71*:765–767, 1922.

23. Bannwarth, A.: Zur Klinik und Pathogenese der "chronischen lymphozytaren Meningitis." Arch. Psychiat. Nervenkr., *117*:161–185, 1944.

24. Burgdorfer, W., et al.: Lyme disease—A tick-borne spirochetosis? Science, *216*:1317–1319, 1982.

25. Steere, A.C., et al.: The spirochetal etiology of Lyme disease. N. Engl. J. Med., *308*:733–740, 1983.

26. Benach, J.L., et al.: Spirochetes isolated from the blood of two patients with Lyme disease. N. Engl. J. Med., *308*:740–742, 1983.

27. Malawista, S.E., Steere, A.C., and Hardin, J.A.: Lyme disease: A unique human model for an infectious etiology of rheumatic disease. Yale J. Biol. Med., *57*:473–477, 1984.

28. Johnson, R.C., et al.: *Borrelia burgdorferi* sp. nov.: Etiologic agent of Lyme disease. Int. J. Syst. Bacteriol., *34*:496–497, 1984.

29. Barbour, A.G., Heiland, R.A., and Howe, T.R.: Heterogeneity of major proteins in Lyme disease Borrelia: A molecular analysis of North American and European isolates. J. Infect. Dis., *152*:478–484, 1985.

30. Weber, K., Schierz, G., Wilske, B., and Preac-Mursic, V.: European erythema migrans disease and related disorders. Yale J. Biol. Med., *57*:463–471, 1984.

31. Asbrink, E., and Hovmark, A.: Successful cultivation of spirochetes from skin lesions of patients with erythema chronicum migrans Afzelius and acrodermatitis chronica atrophicans. Acta Pathol. Microbiol. Immunol. Scand. [B], *93*:161–163, 1985.

32. Berger, B.W., Kaplan, M.H., Rothenberg, I.R., and Barbour, A.G.: Isolation and characterization of the Lyme disease spirochete from the skin of patients with erythema chronicum migrans. J. Am. Acad. Dermatol., *3*:444–449, 1985.

33. Snydman, D.R., et al.: *Borrelia burgdorferi* in joint fluid in chronic Lyme arthritis. Ann. Intern. Med., *104*:798–800, 1986.

34. Berger, B.W., Clemmensen, O.J., and Ackerman, A.B.: Lyme disease is a spirochetosis: A review of the disease and evidence for its cause. Am. J. Dermatopathol., *5*:111–124, 1983.

35. Berger, B.W.: Erythema chronicum migrans of Lyme disease. Arch. Dermatol., *120*:1017–1021, 1984.

36. Johnston, Y.E., et al.: Lyme arthritis: Spirochetes found in synovial microangiopathic lesions. Am. J. Pathol., *118*:26–34, 1985.

37. MacDonald, A.B.: Borrelia in the brains of patients dying with dementia (letter). J.A.M.A., *256*:2195–2196, 1986.

38. Steere, A.C., Duray, P.H., Kauffman, D.J., and Wormser, G.P.: Unilateral blindness caused by infection with the Lyme disease spirochete, *Borrelia burgdorferi*. Ann. Intern. Med., *103*:382–384, 1985.

39. Marcus, L.C., et al.: Fatal pancarditis in a patient with coexistent Lyme disease and babesiosis. Demonstration of spirochetes in the myocardium. Ann. Intern. Med., *103*:374–376, 1985.

40. Schlesinger, P.A., Duray, P.H., Burke, B.A., and Steere, A.C.: Maternal-fetal transmission of the Lyme disease spirochete, *Borrelia burgdorferi*. Ann. Intern. Med., *103*:67–68, 1985.

41. Sigal, L., Steere, A.C., Freeman, D.H., and Dwyer, J.M.: Proliferative responses of mononuclear cells in Lyme disease. Arthritis Rheum., *29*:761–769, 1986.

42. Pachner, A.R., Steere, A.C., Sigal, L.H., and Johnson, C.J.: Antigen-specific proliferation of CSF lymphocytes in Lyme disease. Neurology, *35*:1642–1644, 1985.

43. Craft, J.E., Fischer, D.K., Shimamoto, G.T., and Steere, A.C.: Antigens of *Borrelia burgdorferi* recognized during Lyme disease: Appearance of a new immunoglobulin M response and expansion of the immunoglobulin G response late in the illness. J. Clin. Invest., *78*:934–939, 1986.

44. Hardin, J.A., Steere, A.C., and Malawista, S.E.: The pathogenesis of arthritis in Lyme disease: Humoral immune responses and the role of intra-articular immune complexes. Yale J. Biol. Med., *57*:589–593, 1984.

45. Kristoferistch, W., et al.: HLA-DR in Lyme borreliosis (letter). Lancet, 2(8501):278, 1986.

46. Schmid, G.P.: The global distribution of Lyme disease. Rev. Infect. Dis., *7*:41–50, 1985.

47. Stanek, G., Flamm, H., Barbour, A.G., and Burgdorfer, W. (Eds.): Lyme Borreliosis: Proceedings of the Second International Symposium on Lyme Disease and Related Disorders, Vienna 1985. Gustav Vischer Verlag, Stuttgart and New York, 1987.

48. Fraser, J.R.E.: Lyme disease challenges Australian clinicians. The implications of Australia's first reported case of Lyme arthritis. Med. J. Aust., *1*:101–102, 1982.

49. Schulze, T.L., et al.: *Amblyomma americanum:* A potential vector of Lyme disease in New Jersey. Science, *224*:601–603, 1984.

50. Magnarelli, L.A., et al.: Spirochetes in ticks and antibodies to *Borrelia burgdorferi* in white-tailed deer from Connecticut, New York State, and North Carolina. J. Wildl. Dis., *22*:178–188, 1986.

51. Magnarelli, L.A., Anderson, J.F., and Barbour, A.G.: The etiologic agent of Lyme disease in deer flies, horse flies, and mosquitoes. J. Infect. Dis., *154*:355–358, 1986.

52. Spielman, A., Wilson, M.L., Levine, J.F., and Piesman, J.: Ecology of *Ixodes dammini*-borne human babesiosis and Lyme disease. Annu. Rev. Entomol., *30*:439–460, 1985.

53. First International Symposium on Lyme Disease. Edited by A.C. Steere, et al. Yale J. Biol. Med., *57*:445–713, 1984.

54. Burgdorfer, W., et al.: The western black-legged tick, *Ixodes pacificus:* A vector of *Borrelia burgdorferi.* Am. J. Trop. Med. Hyg., *34:*925–930, 1985.

55. Bosler, E.M., et al.: Natural distribution of the *Ixodes dammini* spirochetes. Science, *220:*321–322, 1983.

56. Magnarelli, L.A., Anderson, J.F., Burgdorfer, W., and Chappell, W.A.: Parasitism by *Ixodes dammini* (Acari: Ixodidae) and antibodies to spirochetes in mammals at Lyme disease foci of Connecticut, U.S.A. J. Med. Entomol., *21:*52–57, 1984.

57. Anderson, J.F., Johnson, R.C., Magnarelli, L.A., and Hyde, F.W.: Identification of endemic foci of Lyme disease: Isolation of *Borrelia burgdorferi* from feral rodents and ticks *(Dermacentor variabilis).* J. Clin. Microbiol., *22*(1):36–38, 1985.

58. Kornblatt, A.N., Urband, P.H., and Steere, A.C.: Arthritis caused by *Borrelia burgdorferi* in dogs. J. Am. Vet. Med. Assoc., *186:*960–964, 1985.

59. Anderson, J.F., Johnson, R.C., Magnarelli, L.A., and Hyde, F.W.: Inolvement of birds in the epidemiology of the Lyme disease agent *Borrelia burgdorferi.* Infect. Immun., *51:*394–396, 1986.

60. Hanrahan, J.P., et al.: Incidence and cumulative frequency of endemic Lyme disease in a community. J. Infect. Dis., *150:*489–496, 1984.

61. Steere, A.C., et al.: Longitudinal assessment of the clinical and epidemiological features of Lyme disease in a defined population. J. Infect. Dis., *154:*295–300, 1986.

62. Åsbrink, E., and Olsson, I.: Clinical manifestations of erythema chronicum migrans Afzelius in 161 patients. A comparison with Lyme disease. Acta Derm. Venereol. (Stockh.), *65:*43–52, 1985.

63. Pachner, A.R., and Steere, A.C.: The triad of neurologic manifestations of Lyme disease: Meningitis, cranial neuritis, and radiculoneuritis. Neurology, *35:*47–53, 1985.

64. Alpert, L.I., Welch, P., and Fisher, N.: Gallium-positive Lyme disease myocarditis. Clin. Nucl. Med., *10:*617, 1985.

65. Habicht, G.S., et al.: Spirochetes induce human and murine interleukin-1 production. J. Immunol., *134:*3147–3154, 1985.

66. Zvaifler, N.J.: Etiology and pathogenesis of rheumatoid arthritis. *In* Arthritis and Allied Conditions. 11th Ed. Edited by D.J. McCarty. Philadelphia, Lea & Febiger, 1988.

67. Reik, L. Jr., Smith, L., Khan, A., and Nelson, W.: Demyelinating encephalopathy in Lyme disease. Neurology, *35:*267–269, 1985.

68. Pachner, A.R.: Spirochetal diseases of the CNS. Neurol. Clin., *4:*207–222, 1986.

69. Ackermann, R., Gollmer, E., and Rehse-Kupper, B.: Progressive Borrelien-Enzephalomyelitis. Chronische Manifestation der Erythema-chronicum-migrans-Krankheit am Nervenstem. Dtsch. Med. Wochenschr., *26:*1039–1042, 1985.

70. Craft, J.E., Grodzicki, R.L., and Steere, A.C.: The antibody response in Lyme disease: Evaluation of diagnostic tests. J. Infect. Dis., *149:*789–795, 1984.

71. Shrestha, M., Grodzicki, R.L., and Steere, A.C.: Diagnosing early Lyme disease. Am. J. Med., *78:*235–240, 1985.

72. Markowitz, L.E., et al.: Lyme disease during pregnancy. J.A.M.A., *255:*3394–3396, 1986.

73. Dattwyler, R.J., Halperin, J.J., Pass, H., and Luft, B.: Ceftriaxone—Effective treatment in refractory Lyme disease. J. Infect. Dis. *155:*1322–1325, 1987.

74. Åsbrink, E., Hovmark, A., and Hederstedt, B.: Serological studies of erythema chronicum migrans Afzelius and acrodermatitis chronica atrophicans with indirect immunofluorescence and enzyme-linked immunosorbent assay. Acta Derm. Venereol. (Stockh.), *65:*509–514, 1985.

EXTRA-ARTICULAR RHEUMATOID ARTHRITIS

PAUL A. BACON

The extra-articular features of rheumatoid arthritis (RA) are of major importance to rheumatologists. These are not just clinical curiosities to intrigue collectors, nor should they be seen simply as complications of arthritis. They are an important and integral part of the rheumatoid disease process, and are also common, occurring in the majority of RA patients.[1-3] It is unfortunate that the name rheumatoid arthritis concentrates on the articular features of a disease that both clinically and pathologically is a systemic disease from the onset. The designation "rheumatoid disease" would be more accurate.

It is essential for the rheumatologist to learn about systemic rheumatoid disease in order to cope with the disease in the whole patient, as well as to consider illness arising during the long course of RA as a possible manifestation of the disease before it is dismissed as an unrelated intercurrent event. It is the essential chronicity of RA that emphasizes the importance of the systemic manifestations. Clinically apparent lesions may be infrequent at any one time but probably only represent the tip of an iceberg of low-grade inapparent disease. This may be detectable only on special testing but may contribute to the widespread general malaise characteristic of RA. The incidence of the lesions of systemic RA is cumulative over the course of the chronic disease and the severity of individual

lesions when fully developed can be of major importance and even life threatening.

It must be emphasized that RA has a definite influence on mortality, although this is easily missed by the casual observer since it is measured in years rather than in minutes. The application of actuarial statistics has made this apparent and stressed its importance.[4] Thus there may be a loss of life expectancy of as much as 18 years for a middle-aged man developing rheumatoid disease, especially if it is classic seropositive disease. Indeed the vast majority of systemic extra-articular RA complications occur in the group of patients with classic RA, in accord with other evidence that this is a discrete disease entity,[5] separate from the other less well defined diseases previously grouped under the broad umbrella of RA. Rheumatoid arthritis patients die by slow degrees, often with multiple problems that make it difficult to ascribe the exact final cause of death. There is good evidence, however, that systemic RA is a major factor contributing directly to the mortality of RA and indirectly by adding to the inability to deal with other events such as drug problems and infections.[6]

CLASSIFICATION

A precise classification of the extra-articular features of RA will remain difficult until the underlying etio-

---

Due to unforeseen circumstances the manuscript for this chapter was delayed, preventing us from placing the material in its proper sequence.

The Publisher and Author regret any inconvenience this situation may cause the reader.

pathogenesis has been established in detail. Nevertheless, it is useful to the clinician to have a file system for use, even if not perfect, rather than a lengthy undigested list. A personal classification system is proposed here (Table 44–1).

Systemic Rheumatoid Disease

Systemic rheumatoid disease, the first group listed in Table 44–1 contains those features that appear to be an integral part of the rheumatoid disease process. This implies that they can occur in any patient with the rheumatoid diathesis. The factors that lead to their localization remain elusive, equally so for the common feature of synovitis as for the less frequent nodule or vasculitis. This remains an important area for research in the future.

Rheumatoid serositis occurs most obviously as synovitis in joints, although synovitis in tendon sheaths is also a major feature. Serositis occurring in the pleural or pericardial membranes is much less common as an overt clinical feature, but clinically inapparent involvement is not rare. The immunopathologic features of such serositis has many similarities to that of rheumatoid synovitis, including inflammatory cell infiltrates suggesting a local immune response, together with local rheumatoid factor (RF) production. The feature that these two membranes have in common with the synovial membrane is of course that of movement, suggesting that local trauma (perhaps microbleeding) could have an important role. The rarity of peritoneal or arachnoid involvement in systemic rheumatoid disease would support this concept.

Subcutaneous nodules also typically occur at sites of local pressure or trauma, while internal nodules occur especially at sites of movement such as tendon sheaths or pericardium. Vasculitic lesions at the surface again frequently relate to sites of pressure, such as the nail edge,[7] or to internal flow pressure changes, such as sites of branching.[8] These observations all accord with the idea that physiologic and anatomic features, especially those relating to movement and trauma, may be of the utmost importance in determining the sites of disease involvement in an individual patient even when the underlying disease process appears to be clearly mediated by immunologic features. In this respect RA may not differ from the chronic inflammatory disease induced by infections, such as tuberculosis.

There are several reasons why the systemic rheumatoid features of serositis, vasculitis, and nodules should be regarded as essential features of rheumatoid arthritis and not as complications. The first is the timing of the lesions. All these features are often thought of as late manifestations of RA and indeed their incidence is cumulative during chronic arthritis. More important is the fact that they can occur at the time of diagnosis[9] or even before the development of chronic polyarthritis, which is the way RA is defined at present. In this respect they may be thought of as analogous to palindromic rheumatoid arthritis in which transient synovitis can in some, but not all, cases progress to chronic RA. The identification of a specific trigger or even a genetic marker might allow us to define those cases of rheumatoid serositis that do not progress to established RA, a concept already accepted for rheumatoid nodules.

The second point is that complications of arthritis may be expected when the disease is most severely active, as well as accumulating with time. Serositis can occur with very active early disease of explosive onset but may also occur in late RA, as can nodules. Vasculitis in RA appears to have a greater likelihood of occurring in the presence of inactive synovitis than when the synovitis has flared up.[10,11] Finally there is the question of the etiopathogenesis. Certainly there are different serologic markers, with possible pathogenetic relevance, for rheumatoid vasculitis and rheumatoid synovitis. The most obvious is the nature of the rheumatoid factors themselves, which are classically IgM in synovitis, whereas IgG RF is particularly elevated in vasculitis.[12] This speaks strongly against the idea of vasculitis being simply due to the overflow of some pathogenetic factor or factors, such as immune complexes, from the inflamed joint.[13]

Table 44–1. Classification of Extra-articular Features of RA

I. *Essential systemic rheumatoid disease*
    Serositis
    Vasculitis
    Granulomata (nodules)

II. *Features related to chronic immune stimulation*
    Anemia
    Lymphadenopathy
    (? Felty's syndrome)

III. *Associated syndromes occurring in RA*
    (These syndromes also occur in other connective tissue disease or in isolation.)
    Sicca syndrome
    Fibrosing alveolitis

IV. *Complications of RA*
    Amyloidosis
    Osteopenia

V. *Drug-induced complications*
    Drug-induced problems form both a separate group of clinical importance *and* may contribute to classes II, III, or IV.

Features Relating to Chronic Immune Inflammation

The second group of extra-articular features includes those that are not specific to rheumatoid arthritis but that do result directly from the ongoing systemic inflammatory process. This implies that these factors are more or less universal and that their severity reflects the activity of the rheumatoid inflammatory process. The latter is easily measured only in terms of synovial joint inflammation. Extensive evidence does exist that the activity of the arthritis does broadly correlate with the anemia of RA. Less attention has been directed to the correlation with other factors such as lymphadenopathy, but the same association appears to apply.

Associated Syndromes

The relationship of features such as the sicca syndrome and fibrosing alveolitis to rheumatoid arthritis is intriguing and problematic. They may present as an apparent part of the rheumatoid disease process but they also occur as part of other connective tissue diseases or as a lone disease, so they are better regarded as associated syndromes separate from either of the above two groups. Their pathogenesis may relate in part to the chronic immune inflammatory stimulation occurring in RA (for example, the contribution of circulating immune complexes to fibrosing alveolitis), but they are neither universal features nor do they appear to reflect current synovial activity. The intriguing possibilities that they represent either a general genetic predisposition to autoimmune disease or, since they both represent the site of interaction with external antigens, a response to an exogenous trigger factor common to many autoimmune diseases remain pure speculation at present.

Complications of RA

Complications of RA arise as a direct result of the rheumatoid disease process and therefore become progressively more common with increasing disease duration. Despite this they are not universal, nor do they obviously relate to disease activity. The prime example is amyloidosis, which clearly occurs as a result of the rheumatoid inflammatory process stimulating chronic high levels of serum amyloid A (SAA), the building block of AA amyloid.[14] However, not all patients with RA or all those with elevated SAA develop clinical amyloidosis even if followed for a long period. Clearly other, as yet undefined, factors are involved in the pathogenesis of amyloidosis. These may be entirely unrelated to RA. It is interesting that the incidence of AA amyloid complicating the chronic infectious process of leprosy is similar to the approximately 6% incidence of amyloidosis observed in chronic rheumatoid arthritis.[15]

Drug-Induced Complications

The relationship of drugs to rheumatoid extra-articular features cannot be ignored because it is both an important clinical problem and also presents conceptual difficulties. Drug-associated problems deserve inclusion here because apparently drug-induced lesions such as gastritis or nephropathy appear to have a considerably higher frequency in rheumatoid arthritis patients than they do when a comparable drug intake is seen in other groups without systemic disease, for instance, osteoarthritis patients taking nonsteroidal drugs. This suggests a contribution from both the rheumatoid disease and from the drug. These features can occur at any stage of the disease or any type of drug prescription but are not universal nor do they reflect disease activity. They may in part relate to the generalized effect of the chronic inflammatory state and can certainly contribute to such features as anemia. They may also appear to relate to the direct complications of RA. For instance, the incidence of infection in RA appears increased in longstanding disease, in those with amyloidosis, and in those taking certain drugs. This emphasizes the multifactorial nature of systemic features occurring in chronic rheumatoid arthritis.

Specific organ involvement in RA is discussed in detail later in the light of this classification to see how far current knowledge allows these disease manifestations of RA to be fitted into the above scheme.

RHEUMATOID NODULES

Nodules are the most characteristic feature of rheumatoid arthritis but are not unique to the disease. Lesions of similar pathologic character are seen in granuloma annulare, although the clinical picture is different.[16] An identical clinical and histologic picture may be seen rarely in people, usually males, with no evidence of arthritis or other disease.[17-22] Such nodulosis is thought to be a part of the rheumatoid spectrum, likened by Bywaters to the Cheshire cat.[23] Occasionally a progression to recognizable arthritis occurs, confirming this viewpoint.

Nodules are seen in approximately 30 to 40% of white patients with classic rheumatoid arthritis, all of whom have seropositive disease. The incidence of nodules varies in an unexplained way with both race and geography. For example, nodules are an exceptional rarity in Asian patients with RA seen in the Indian subcontinent[24] and the same is true in some parts of Africa.[25,26]

Clinically, nodules may be classified as superficial or deep. The prime site for surface nodules is at the elbow, where they occur either over the trochanter or in relation to the subcutaneous border of the ulnar extending into the forearm. Initially the latter may appear fixed to the periosteum but as they enlarge they may appear more mobile. At the elbow they may develop in the wall of the trochanteric bursa, and it has been suggested that nodules characteristically arise in relation to a bursa.[27,28] Nodules may be single or multiple and vary from a few millimeters to 2 centimeters or more in size. They are usually painless but may be unsightly and interfere with function. The elbow and the forearm are important pressure points when patients sit with elbows on the arm of a chair or use their arms to push themselves upright. The majority of superficial nodules similarly occur at pressure points. The sacrum is another typical site for a rheumatoid nodule, which in a bed or chairbound person may ulcerate through leading to a chronic sinus disorder.[29,30] In some cases a sacral pressure sore is the first sign of a previous nodule.[31] Occasionally multiple nodules appear at pressure sites, including the spine, the scalp, the heels, and the sacrum. Such multiple nodules usually occur in generally ill patients with severe long-standing RA, but not necessarily with active synovitis at the time. A single or few nodules is far more common and can occur at any stage of RA from early to late disease, even developing before synovitis on occasions. They are often persistent but in some cases may soften, diminish in size, or even disappear. In other cases they may develop at a time when the patient otherwise feels well.

Tendon sheath nodules are also common. They may be visible at some sites, particularly in the tendon sheaths around the ankle where they may be seen both anteriorly and posteriorly in the Achilles tendon. Flexor tension sheath nodules in the palm of the hand are also common. They are more easily appreciated by palpation than by inspection. At this site they may impede tendon movement through the tendon sheaths causing triggering of the fingers. Tendon sheaths are sites of movement, so local pressure or trauma may again be a determining factor.

Intracutaneous nodules are seen more rarely, manifesting as multiple small nodules close to the surface. They particularly affect the fingers and again may relate to pressure or local trauma. They can be seen at other sites including the soft tissues of the buttocks. This variety of nodules is often linked to vasculitis[9] both because crops of them can occur when there are vascular lesions elsewhere and because the surface of such intracutaneous nodules may show small infarcted areas. The initial appearance of such lesions may be accompanied by sharp pain. Such nodules often last a few weeks only before disappearing completely, although crops of nodules may be recurrent. Occasionally the surface may break down, leading to ulceration. Unlike other nodules, the small intracutaneous variety often respond to aggressive antirheumatic or immunosuppressive therapy. The suggestion that all rheumatoid nodules are related to local vasculitis is an old one,[32,33] but has not been confirmed by recent evidence.[34]

The eye may also become involved by a lesion pathologically similar to a nodule in the condition known as scleromalacia.[35] There is characteristic discoloration of the white sclera occurring laterally or superiorly to the iris. Rarely this can progress to perforation of the eye, known as scleromalacia perforans,[36] with leakage of orbital contents. This usually occurs in patients with aggressive vasculitis. In the more chronic stages scleromalacia appears to be associated with thinning of the sclera, but accurate measurement using ultrasonography has suggested that this is more apparent than real.[37]

Deep nodules occur in internal organs, particularly at sites of movement. This includes the pleural and pericardial surfaces and the parenchymal tissue of the lung or heart. Like surface nodules, these granuloma are asymptomatic unless they interfere with function, so their exact incidence is unknown. Isolated examples have been reported of clinically important complications arising from nodules in the aorta,[38] kidney,[39] and retroperitoneum.[40] Postmortem studies suggest that they may not be as rare as often believed. For the heart, for example, quoted figures range from 3 to 20%,[33,41,42] but average about 10%.[43]

It is interesting that rheumatoid nodules have very rarely been described within the joint[43a] although this is a prime site of the movement and minor trauma that is thought to contribute to the location of nodules elsewhere. It is possible that high intra-articular pressure or direct trauma actually prevents the development of an organized granuloma recognizable as a nodule. Another possibility is that the rice bodies[44] frequently found in rheumatoid joints represent the development of a nodule determined by the physical characteristics of the joint. Certainly they contain fibrinoid, fibronectin, and inflammatory cells although they lack the organized layer of epithelioid cells seen in classic nodules.[45]

RHEUMATOID VASCULITIS

Vasculitis as a specific complication of rheumatoid arthritis was first described by Sokoloff and colleagues in 6 out of 57 muscle biopsies.[46] The previous clinical recognition of vascular involvement in RA was ascribed to coexisting polyarteritis nodosa.[47] However, 50 years earlier the pathologic features were described at necropsy in a patient who previously had evidence of peripheral neuropathy.[32] Bywaters was the first to describe the focal ischemic digital lesions, particularly of the fingernail edges, initially observed in a patient who also developed gangrene and severe internal organ involvement.[48]

The clinical lesions of vasculitis remain the rarest manifestation of rheumatoid diseases with an incidence of less than 1 per 100,000 population.[10] That figure was based on my personal series, which used a strict definition of classic features and/or pathologic confirmation of necrotizing arteritis.[49] Nail edge lesions alone are more common (Fig. 44–1). The incidence of vascular lesions at postmortem examination has been as high as 25%.[50] In support of this, a significant incidence of immune complex deposits in vessel walls has been noted in biopsies from uninvolved skin in RA.[51,52] Rheumatoid vasculitis occurs equally in both sexes. It is often found in long-standing severe disease but can occur early on. In rare cases it occurs as the first symptom of the disease and is therefore not just a complication of rheumatoid arthritis.[53] It may have been more prevalent in the early steroid era of the 1950s[54] but has not disappeared.[10]

Clinical features of systemic rheumatoid vasculitis show a wider spectrum than the classic descriptions of mononeuritis or peripheral gangrene would sug-gest.[49,55–60] Cutaneous manifestations are the most frequent, but peripheral gangrene (Fig. 44–2), the most definitive cutaneous manifestation, is relatively uncommon.[10,49,59] Nail edge lesions, a variety of rashes, and skin ulcers are much more common. The latter usually develop suddenly as deep punched-out ulcers at sites unusual for venous ulceration, such as the dorsum of the foot or the upper calf (Fig. 44–3). They are often complicated by secondary infection. Leg ulcers are not uncommon in chronic RA in the absence of clinical signs of vasculitis.[61,62] These are usually more chronic and sited around the ankle but are not always distinguishable from vasculitis ulcers. Rheumatoid nodules are present in the majority of cases,[49] although some series have noted a far lower incidence,[60] supporting the idea that nodules and vasculitis do not share the same pathogenetic mechanisms in RA.

Systemic features of vasculitis are very common, so that unexplained weight loss in severe RA should raise a high index of suspicion for vasculitis. Hepatosplenomegaly may be seen in one fifth of patients, but neutropenia is rare despite the known association of Felty's syndrome with vasculitis.[63,64] Mononeuritis multiplex, usually with an abrupt onset of motor neuropathy, is very characteristic of rheumatoid vasculitis,[65–67] but was seen in less than half of my and my colleagues' patients. This was supported by a recent literature review,[60] although other recent series have continued to find a high incidence[68,69] perhaps owing to different selection methods. Central nervous system involvement can occur,[70] but may be easily missed particularly in the elderly.[71]

Eye manifestations are seen in one fifth of patients, usually as symptomatic scleritis. The association of severe scleritis with rheumatoid vasculitis is well described,[72] and conversely a significant increase in mortality in RA patients with severe persistent episcleritis has been documented.[73,74] The complication of scler-

FIG. 44–1.   *A*, Prominent nail fold arterioles. *B.* Nail edge infarction. *C*, Volar finger pump brown spot. All these patients had RA.

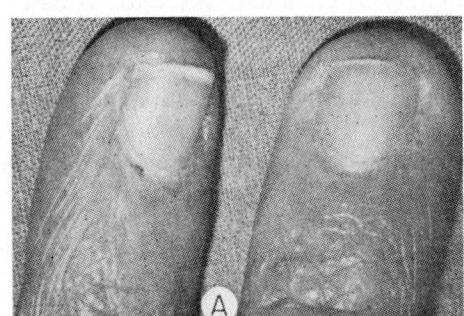
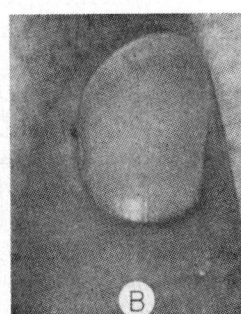
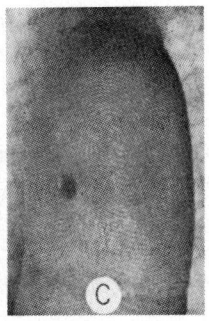

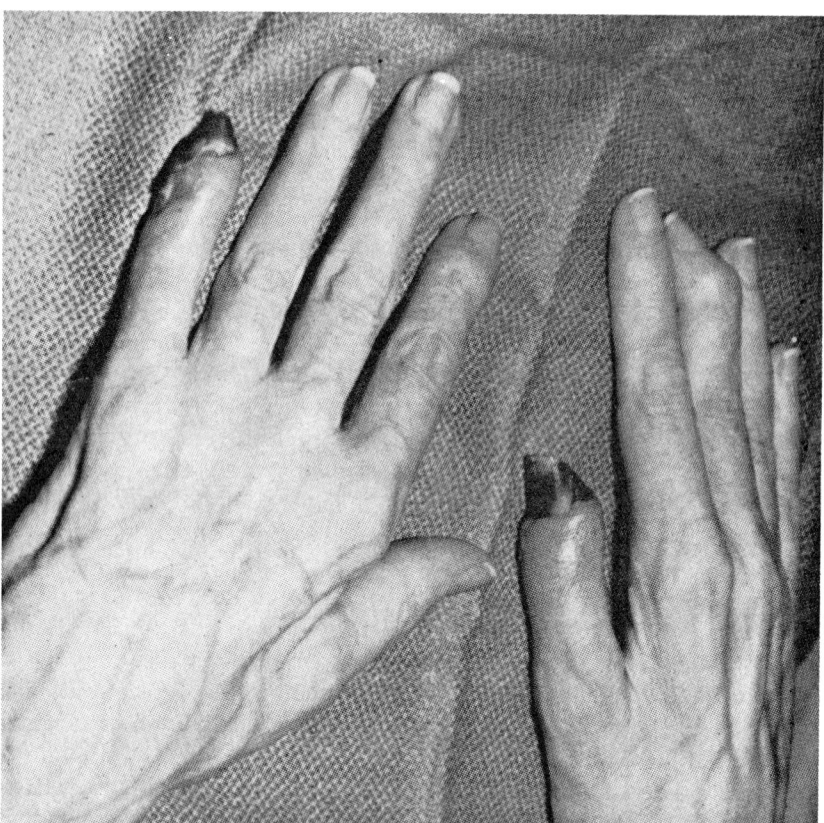

FIG. 44–2. Gangrenous fingertips of the same patient as in Figure 44–1. The necrotic fingers showed their first cyanosis five weeks earlier.

omalacia perforans is rare. Corneal involvement producing corneal melting is another serious but rare complication.[75]

Heart and lung involvement both occurred in approximately one third of our series. The most common pulmonary problem is alveolitis often of abrupt onset and sometimes transient. Acute pleurisy is also seen. Clinically overt pericarditis is the most common cardiac manifestation, but arrhythmias are also quite frequent. Aortic regurgitation developed acutely in a small number of patients[76] in relation to aortic root dilatation or valve rupture, requiring urgent surgery in some cases. Both heart block[77] and myocardial infarction[78] have been reported as fatal complications of rheumatoid vasculitis. The diagnosis has been established in life by endomyocardial biopsy with subsequent good response to therapy.[78a]

Renal involvement, a major feature of most forms of necrotizing vasculitis, was present in only one fifth of our rheumatoid vasculitis patients and only one fourth of these developed chronic renal failure.[10] A significant association between abnormal urinary sediment and subsequent mortality in systemic rheumatoid vasculitis has been noted.[69] Major gastrointestinal involvement is an uncommon but serious manifestation that may present as an acute abdomen and carries a high mortality.[55]

Rheumatoid vasculitis is an episodic relapsing phenomenon but the flares of activity seem to bear little relationship to the activity of the synovitis. In the small number of cases in which vasculitis occurs within the first year of RA, all manifestations including synovitis, nodule formation, and vasculitis appear to progress at the same time, but aggressive therapy that halts the vasculitis may have little effect on the joint disease. Early onset of vasculitis in RA is associated with a poor outcome.[80] In the majority of cases, particularly in long-standing disease, vasculitis develops when the arthritis is relatively quiescent.[49] This divergence between joint and vascular inflammation has been noted by others.[69] The clinical manifestations of vasculitis seen in relapse are not necessarily the same as those of previous episodes. The serious systemic involvement in rheumatoid vasculitis is associated with a significant morbidity together with a definite mortality.[10,49,61,66–69] The high recurrence rate correlates with the accumulative mortality and varies from 30 to 50% over 5 years.[49,61,69] The progressive cumulative mortality in our series related largely to active vasculitis with its 50% recurrence rate, rather than to other complications. Mortality was highest in those with other histologic evidence of necrotizing vasculitis or those with neuropathy. Patients with cutaneous small vessel vasculitis had a lower mortality,

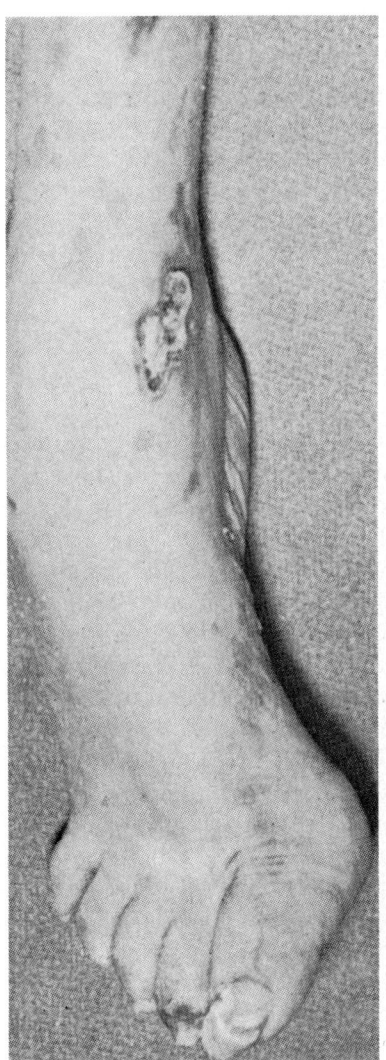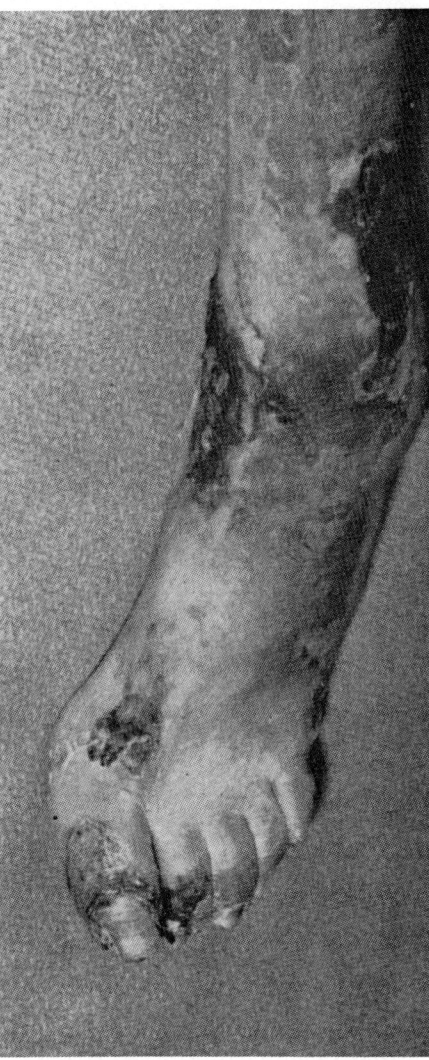

FIG. 44–3. The feet of a 69-year-old woman who had had RA for 10 years and had been treated with large amounts of steroids. She had high titers of rheumatoid factor, abundant joint erosion visible radiographically, and biopsy-demonstrated active and healed arteritis with arterial wall necrosis. The ankle inversion of bilateral foot drop, extensive necrotic skin ulceration about the left ankle, and multiple cyanotic or gangrenous toe tips are all features of rheumatoid arteritis.

but deaths still occurred largely because of cardiac involvement. The presence of leukocytoclastic vasculitis in a skin biopsy does not rule out the existence of more serious necrotizing vasculitis elsewhere. A rectal biopsy may be a useful prognostic indicator, since it reveals positive necrotizing vasculitis particularly in patients with a high instance of systemic features, neuropathy, and a higher mortality.[81] The decreased survival of patients with systemic rheumatoid vasculitis, compared with the general population or to definite RA, has been confirmed in a careful epidemiologic analysis.[69]

Pathologic studies show a wide spectrum of vascular involvement in rheumatoid vasculitis. The acute lesions in small muscle arteries may be identical to those in polyarteritis nodosa, and are characterized by fibrinoid necrosis of the intima together with a cellular infiltrate of lymphocytes plus occasional polymorphonuclear leukocytes in the outer coats. Occasionally a less acute picture is seen with few inflammatory cells and more marked intimal proliferation, reminiscent of a healing scar. Progression from the acute to a subacute stage has been seen in sural nerve biopsies[82] and in rectal biopsies.[81] The chronic obliterative endarteritis described in the occlusive digital lesions of Bywaters[83] presumably represents a previous necrotizing arthritis in that site as well. A leukocytoclastic vasculitis (LV) may also be seen in small arterioles through to venules and can coexist with the necrotizing arteritis.[10,49] LV is classically described in the skin but is occasionally seen in other tissues. The coexistence of abnormal urinary sediment with cutaneous leukocytoclastic vasculitis suggests that transient small vessel involvement can also occur in the kidney, where necrotizing arteritis is relatively rare. The immunopathogenesis of rheumatoid vasculitis is not fully elucidated but there are well-established associations with serologic abnormalities. Classically, IgM factors are present in the majority of, though not all, cases. Clinical features correlate more strongly in serial studies with IgG rheumatoid factor levels,[12,84,85] which are present in higher levels in serum than in synovial fluid.[86] Immune complexes containing IgG rheumatoid factor have complement-activating properties[13] and may be relevant in rheumatoid vasculitis pathogenesis. Other autoantibodies including antinuclear antibodies[87] and an unidentified precipitin to rabbit thymus extract[88] are also reported in higher incidence in rheumatoid vasculitis than in uncomplicated RA. There is extensive evidence for circulating immune complexes but these are not always distinguishable between rheumatoid vasculitis and uncomplicated synovitis. However, both cryoglobulins[89] and hypocomplementemia[12,90] are common in vasculitis, whereas elevated complement levels are usually seen in uncomplicated rheumatoid synovitis. Assessment of disease activity is difficult in rheumatoid vasculitis. The acute-phase proteins more commonly indicate active synovitis and leukocytosis is rare, in contrast to polyarteritis nodosa. Recent studies suggest that plasma levels of factor VIII–related antigen, which is present in platelets and endothelial cells, may reflect significant vascular damage,[91] but further experience is required.

Treatment of rheumatoid vasculitis requires aggressive therapy in view of the significant mortality. Oral steroids may have contributed to the increased reports of vasculitis in the 1960s and 1970s.[54,57,58] A decision to institute or increase steroids had a significant association with decreased survival in a recent analysis.[69] Pulse methylprednisolone alone offers little benefit and may be associated with an increase in sepsis. Cyclophosphamide has made a major difference in the treatment of rheumatoid vasculitis, as with other systemic necrotizing vasculitides.[12,89,92] An intermittent bolus regimen of cyclophosphamide plus steroid appears rapidly effective and well tolerated in rheumatoid vasculitis patients, and demonstrates several advantages over continuous oral regimens.[93] An oral intermittent cyclophosphamide and steroid regimen can be used in less acutely ill patients and appears to be a suitable maintenance regimen.[94] I favor increasing the interval between doses rather than altering the dose of each bolus. Maintenance treatment may be necessary for several years with the aim of preventing the relapses typical of this disease.

THE HEART

Cardiac involvement fits most easily, but still not completely, into the concept that organ involvement in RA consists of serositis, nodules, and vasculitis, together with some complications. The serositis is ob-

viously restricted to the pericardium, but granulomata are found at pericardial, endocardial, and myocardial locations. Active vasculitis is exceptionally rare. It is not clear how far nonspecific myocarditis can be ascribed to scarring following healed specific rheumatoid disease, or to other RA-related events such as alternative immune mechanisms or amyloid deposition, or whether it has to be ascribed to nonrheumatologic events, especially atherosclerosis.

Pericarditis

Involvement of the pericardium in the rheumatoid disease process is both common, being the most frequent cardiologic manifestation of RA, and well recognized. It was first well-documented in necropsy studies by Charcot in 1881,[95] when he was examining the then current dogma that cardiac involvement in arthritis meant rheumatic fever rather than rheumatoid arthritis. Many descriptions of it since have expanded the understanding of the clinical picture and the extent of rheumatoid pericarditis.

The incidence of pericardial involvement depends on the diagnostic criteria used. Symptomatic pericarditis occurs in approximately 1% of hospitalized RA patients, but the incidence increases to 10% in the face of careful, repeated examination.[96] Use of sensitive echocardiographic screening increases the incidence of detection to about one third of all RA patients,[97] while in those selected for seropositive nodular disease it may be as high as 50%.[98] This high incidence correlates with the postmortem findings of pericardial fluid or pericardial scarring in RA patients.[42,99,100] Pericarditis may occur at any time during RA and one careful longitudinal study using clinical detection methods has suggested an annual incidence of 0.34% in females and 0.44% in males.[101] These figures emphasize the male predominance, although it is not as great as for pleurisy. Even over a 20-year period this would give a much lower overall prevalence of pericarditis than the 30% noted in one large review,[96] which most likely reflects patient selection, since this study was based on hospitalized patients at a special referral center, representing severe disease.

The discrepancy between the echocardiographic or postmortem figures and the clinical incidence emphasizes how a small collection of pericardial fluid frequently may be asymptomatic. Symptomatic pericarditis can develop at any stage of rheumatoid disease but is most common early on and is occasionally the presenting feature. It usually occurs when RA is very active and there are often nonspecific systemic features in addition.[43,76] Laboratory tests confirm the presence of active disease and virtually all patients have seropositive results, many showing IgG as well as IgM rheumatoid factors. Examination of the pericardial fluid reveals the presence of rheumatoid factors, together with immune complexes and evidence of complement consumption.[102] The high cell count may contain both polymorphonuclear leukocytes and mononuclear cells and is often heavily blood-stained.[103] The pericardial fluid is characterized by particularly low glucose levels, relating to the high cell count.[104] Cholesterol content is often high, particularly in chronic effusions, and cholesterol crystals are occasionally seen.[43,105] Histologic examination of the pericardium reveals nonspecific inflammatory changes with features of both acute and chronic inflammation.[43] There are similarities to the synovial reaction in RA.[106] Proliferation of serosal lining cells is seen with an intense underlying infiltrate of inflammatory cells, including lymphocytes and plasma cells. Patches of fibrinoid necrosis may be seen at the pericardial surface, with an underlying layer of palisadic histiocytes or epithelioid cells surrounded by chronic inflammation. These have the appearance of an opened-out rheumatoid nodule.[107] Distinct granulomas or nodules may also be seen dotted on the pericardial surface.[43] As well as the increased fluid effusion, the striking feature in RA is the pronounced inflammatory thickening of both pericardial layers,[43] leading to the typical "bread and butter" pericarditis seen in both acute cases and in those with the complication of chronic constriction.

The outcome of rheumatoid pericarditis is favorable in the majority of cases, although the low-grade postmortem findings in approximately 40% of cases shows that complete healing does not occur. Recurrences are not uncommon, being seen in as many as 15% of cases.[96] The serious complications are tamponade and constriction, both of which are rare. The dramatic nature of their occurrence tends to lead to overreporting with exaggeration of their frequency.

Tamponade is certainly rare. The salient features have been described by Iveson and colleagues,[43,108] who were able to collect only 19 cases from the literature in the 20 years since the first description of it. Tamponade usually occurred in patients with established severe arthritis who had preceding evidence of pericardial involvement for several weeks, but occasionally the tamponade occurred abruptly. Exertional dyspnea or ankle edema were the usual presenting features, but ascites or radiographically detected cardiomegaly have also been recorded. Considerable delay has been noted in making the diagnosis in some cases, perhaps reflecting its rarity. Delay is serious, since treatment of such an effusion requires urgent pericardiocentesis. Steroids have been injected locally into the pericardial space after aspiration with reported benefit,[102,109] but most physicians advocate pericardectomy, particularly if repeated attempts to aspirate fluid are necessary or are unsuccessful.[43,108]

Constrictive pericarditis is less rare than tamponade with more than twice as many cases reported, but is still uncommon.[43] Thould[110] has estimated the prevalence of pericardial constriction as 0.64% for men and 0.06% for women, again emphasizing a significant male predominance. In the past constrictive pericarditis was widely regarded as a result of tuberculosis, but with the decline in that disease RA has been increasingly recognized as an important if uncommon cause. It again usually occurs in patients with severe seropositive RA who have twice the incidence of subcutaneous nodules seen in uncomplicated disease. The majority of patients have clinical evidence of preceding pericarditis, and constriction, which is less dramatic in its presentation than tamponade, may develop very insidiously over a prolonged period. Because of this, a high index of suspicion is required to differentiate constrictive pericarditis from congestive cardiac failure. The diagnosis can be confirmed by intracardiac pressure recordings at cardiac catheterization, or angiography may confirm the presence of pericardial thickening. In difficult cases computed tomography (CT) scanning can provide the best differentiation between pericardial thickening and inflamed pericardial fluid.[111] There is a 75% incidence of associated pleural effusion in patients with tamponade or constriction.

Constrictive pericarditis is a serious complication that is frequently fatal; early surgery is therefore indicated.[43] Delays may contribute to mortality, particularly if overaggressive attempts to control intractable edema produce electrolyte imbalances. Surgery removes only the outer layers of the pericardium, leaving the visceral pericardium intact. This can cause persistent symptoms and relapses and additional immunosuppressive therapy is usually required. Direct involvement of the underlying myocardium by the inflamed visceral pericardium may also contribute to postoperative morbidity and occasional mortality. In contrast, uncomplicated pericarditis usually responds to steroids alone or in combination with cytotoxic drugs. Interestingly, use of second-line drugs such as gold or penicillamine to control the underlying joint disease appears to have no effect in preventing the progression of pericarditis to constriction.[112]

Endocarditis

The aortic valve is the one most commonly affected by a wide variety of immune connective tissue diseases. Regurgitation is the predominant problem, and stenosis is rare.[76] In rheumatoid arthritis the most common lesion is a nonspecific valvulitis, reported in up to 20% of cases at necropsy.[43] Despite this, symptoms or signs of aortic valve dysfunction during life are rare in RA, but regurgitation requiring surgery is reported.[76,113-116] Nonspecific valvulitis consists of diffuse thickening and fibrosis. Specific nodules within the cusps are detected in 3 to 5% of necropsy cases.[42,117] They are usually associated with rheumatoid nodules both at the surface and at other deep sites including the mitral valve. Histologic examination may show the presence of nonspecific granulomatous thickening of the cusps, perhaps analogous to the opened-out nodule appearance of the pericardium, as well as discrete nodules.[117] Nodules can cause perforation of the cusp, usually presenting clinically as acute valve incompetence that requires emergency surgery.[113,117] We have personal experience of 11 such patients over a 10-year period.[76] In common with other reports, other extra-articular features of RA were frequent, including other valve lesions, pleurisy, and cutaneous vasculitis in half the patients. This stresses the widespread systemic nature of such rheumatoid disease. Although rare, this can be a serious complication; three patients have died, and four have had successful valve replacements. Infective endocarditis is surprisingly a very rare complication of rheumatoid valve disease, despite concurrent steroid medication and apparent predisposition to infection in RA.

Rheumatoid granulomata can involve all four heart valves.[118] After the aortic, the mitral valve is the most common site of involvement, being described at between 1% and 6% of autopsy studies.[117] The echocardiographic demonstration of severe slowing of mitral valve movement has a similar incidence[98] but the clinicopathologic significance of this is uncertain. Mitral or tricuspid valve involvement sufficiently severe to produce symptoms is limited to occasional case reports. Mitral valve granulomata have been found in a surgical specimen only once.[119]

Myocarditis

Clinically significant myocardial disease is rare in rheumatoid arthritis, unlike other connective tissue diseases such as scleroderma, but fatal necrotizing myocarditis,[79] diffuse myocardial disease,[117,120] and complicating hypertrophic cardiomyopathy[121] have been reported. Assessment of its importance is complicated by the sedentary life enforced on many severe arthritics. Autopsy studies suggest that a nonspecific

focal myocarditis occurs in as many as 15% of patients.[42] This is more common than the more diagnostic finding of rheumatoid nodules seen in the myocardium in less than 5% of patients.[33,99] Focal myocardial fibrosis may also be seen.[122] Antibodies apparently specific for heart and skeletal muscle have been described in RA,[123] but the role of immune mechanisms in rheumatoid myocarditis is unknown. Scarring from previous arteritis could also contribute to the picture.

Coronary arteritis diagnosed during life is limited to single case reports.[124,125] Our review of 90 patients with systemic rheumatoid vasculitis[10] showed evidence of myocardial infarction in five patients but only one had proven coronary arteritis at autopsy. Diagnosis during life has been confirmed by endomyocardial biopsy and may be important in determining the need for aggressive therapy.[78a] Autopsy studies suggest a very different incidence, with changes consistent with small vessel vasculitis in up to 20% of cases.[42,117] Early aggressive therapy with cyclophosphamide and steroids may produce significant improvement in coronary arteritis as in other forms of vasculitis, so a high incidence of suspicion is warranted.

Arrhythmias may occur in rheumatoid arthritis when the sensitive, specialized myocardial fibers making up the conduction system are injured by direct mechanical obstruction from rheumatoid granuloma, by infarction, by vasculitis, or by spread of inflammation affecting the nearby pericardium. This last occurs particularly with the sinoatrial node, which lies close to the pericardium. The most easily recognized abnormality is complete heart block[126] but this is rare, involving approximately only 0.1% even of hospitalized patients.[127] His bundle studies suggest that the block is distal to the atrioventricular node.[128] Most patients have long-standing erosive nodular RA with other extra-articular manifestations including vasculitis. Despite this, nodal vasculitis has not yet been described although pressure from a rheumatoid nodule has been detailed.[129] Minor degrees of heart block frequently predate the complete heart block, but the effect of drugs in preventing the progression of such disease is not established. Pacemakers are being used successfully, when the post-operative prognosis will depend on the presence of other cardiac lesions.

Amyloidosis is another potential cause of myocardial dysfunction in RA, but clinically significant cardiac amyloid deposition appears to be almost restricted to primary or AL amyloidosis. In our series of 47 cases of amyloidosis associated with RA[130] some evidence of cardiac involvement was a common finding at autopsy. However, no patients developed symptoms of restrictive cardiomyopathy or arrhythmias that were well documented in the AL amyloidosis patients, although one case has been described.[131] A higher incidence of clinical cardiac involvement in AA amyloidosis secondary to all causes has been noted.[132]

The rarity of clinically detected rheumatoid processes or complications involving the heart contrasts with the twofold increase in mortality related to cardiac disease in RA compared with the general population.[133] The major contribution to this is ischemic heart disease, but the mechanism of action is unclear. It is possible that it represents previous immune-mediated vascular damage to the coronary arteries, perhaps aggravated by steroids, as has been documented for systemic lupus erythematosus (SLE).

THE LUNG

There has been extensive discussion on whether certain types of pulmonary disease are specifically associated with rheumatoid arthritis or whether such disorders occur concurrently by chance.[134,135] Pulmonary nodules are easy to accept as a specific rheumatoid manifestation, and the histologic and immunologic features of pleurisy strongly support the same contention. With diffuse pulmonary involvement the question is not so easily solved despite three large radiographic surveys.[134,136,137] The first, published in 1955, found a wide range of pulmonary disorders in patients with rheumatoid arthritis, some of which were specific to RA, whereas others were related to chronic immune stimulation predisposing, for instance, to lung infections. In this case therapy, especially steroids, might also play a part. Other disorders might represent chance associations. Two subsequent surveys failed to show differences in the incidence of interstitial lung disease between RA patients and control populations. Detailed epidemiologic studies with large numbers of case histories and carefully specified diagnostic criteria would be needed to provide definitive answers. If an association is specific but uncommon then large numbers of patients with RA must be studied. The association may be more easily detected by analyzing a group of patients with a less common disorder for the frequency of RA. One such analysis of 220 patients with cryptogenic fibrosing alveolitis[138] revealed that 16% had rheumatoid arthritis compared with the expected prevalence of less than 4% in a middle-aged population. The use of screening methods more sensitive than chest radiography, such as pulmonary function studies, also suggests a considerably higher incidence of abnormalities of diffusion capacity,[139–142a] or obstructive lung disease in RA.[140,143,144] Cigarette smoking may make some contribution to this but the impairment still exceeds that in smoking control subjects.[140,143,145]

Pleurisy

Inflammation of the serous lining of the lung in association with inflammation of synovial membranes has been recognized for many years.[137,146,147] As with pericardial inflammation, this classically occurs even in patients with seropositive and often nodular rheumatoid arthritis, with an increased incidence in males.[137,148] The overall incidence in a hospital-based population is approximately 1%. It is lower in the milder form of disease seen in population-based surveys but many of the latter would not meet either the stricter New York criteria for RA nor the updated American Rheumatism Association (ARA) criteria. One outpatient survey[149] found an annual incidence of pleural effusion in 0.3% of females and 1.54% of males, indicating a very striking male preponderance. Pleural effusion may occur at any time during the course of rheumatoid disease, so the 20-year prevalence would be approximately 20% of RA patients, a figure similar to the incidence of effusions or old pleural adhesions found in postmortem studies. The effusions are frequently asymptomatic, and routine detailed examination and chest x-ray studies are necessary to detect them.[150,151] The latency of such rheumatoid pleural effusions is often overlooked.[152] Symptomatic pleurisy usually occurs early in the disease. It may be one of the presenting manifestations,[153] together with weight loss, severe malaise, and even fever suggesting an infective or neoplastic basis.

Examination of pleural fluid shows a low glucose level and low levels of complement components despite a high total protein content.[152,153a] Rheumatoid factor titers may be higher than the corresponding serum.[154] The cytologic findings show a high cell count with degenerate phagocytic cells, often predominantly lymphocytes.[135] Eosinophils have been reported.[155] More typical are macrophages with cytoplasmic inclusions of IgM (ragocytes),[156,157] together with occasional multinucleate giant cells that may show the appearance of comet cells.[158] These have a tail of cytoplasm streaming away from the rounded head containing up to 12 nuclei. Such comet cells, together with a massive deposit of a morphous proteinaceous debris, are sufficiently typical of RA to confirm the diagnosis.[159] The debris consists largely of fragments of immunoglobulin, indicating an active local immune reaction. Biopsy of the pleural membrane is often nonspecific[160] but necessary to exclude diseases such as tuberculosis and neoplastic disease. Less commonly the pleural fluid may show a picture of acute and chronic inflammation similar to that seen in rheumatoid pericarditis and reminiscent of rheumatoid synovitis. There is a dense lymphocytic infiltrate in which plasma cells are seen, suggesting that local formation of immune complexes contributes to the low complement levels found in the fluid.[135] Biopsy may also reveal typical rheumatoid granulomata,[161–163] and the appearance of an opened-out rheumatoid nodule as described in the pericardium can also be seen. Inspection of the pleural surface on fiberoptic examination or at thoracotomy may reveal multiple small white nodules reminiscent of tuberculomata studding the pleural surface.

Resolution of pleurisy usually occurs as the rheumatoid disease improves spontaneously or with antirheumatic drugs. A diagnostic pleural fluid biopsy is normally the only procedure necessary. Rarely the inflamed pleural membrane may become significantly thickened, sufficient to interfere with lung expansion to the extent of necessitating pleurectomy. Pleural adhesions frequently form during resolution and may even calcify, presenting diagnostic problems on chest x-ray study. Occasionally large effusions may be very persistent, necessitating drainage. Such procedures are not without hazard and empyema has been reported in a few cases.[164]

Rheumatoid Nodules

Pulmonary granulomata associated with rheumatoid arthritis are well recognized although considerably less frequent than pleurisy.[151] They are more common in the upper rather than the lower lobes and may be solitary or multiple.[165–167] They can occur at any stage of the disease and again have been described as a presenting feature of RA or even antedating it by many years.[167–169] Nodules may persist unchanged over medical followup for years or may resolve spontaneously. Cavitation is described,[170] in which hemoptysis may occur or even superinfection. Nodules may occur successively in one or both lungs.

When rounded shadows are seen in the chest x-ray study of a patient with established RA, the diagnosis may be suspected. When the nodules precede arthritis they have usually been excised on a proper suspicion of bronchial carcinoma.[170a] The development of techniques such as needle or transbronchial biopsy may allow histologic material to be obtained without resorting to thoracotomy.[135] The serum rheumatoid factor has been reported negative when pulmonary nodules preceded joint symptoms, and is therefore of no value in diagnosis in such cases.[168]

Caplan's Syndrome

The presence of intrapulmonary nodules in coal miners with rheumatoid arthritis was first reported by Caplan in 1953.[171] This suggested that the development of the rheumatoid lesion was associated in some way with a modified tissue response to coal dust. Similar lesions have since been described in workers with RA exposed to other inorganic dusts such as silica[172,173] and asbestos.[174] Interestingly, an association between smaller rounded pulmonary lesions and the presence of circulating rheumatoid factor has since been reported in coal miners without any evidence of arthritis.[175,176] The pulmonary lesions in Caplan's syndrome are usually multiple rather than single and may be considerably larger than the usual pulmonary rheumatic nodules (Fig. 44–4). Some patients develop widespread progressive pulmonary fibrosis in association with inorganic dust disease. The antinuclear antibodies that are frequently seen may develop early and may persist as documented in longitudinal studies, suggesting that they may contribute to the development of more florid lesions rather than simply being a consequence of them.[135]

Fibrosing Alveolitis

This condition may be seen as an idiopathic syndrome but it can also occur in rheumatoid arthritis. The first recognition of fibrosing alveolitis in RA led to the term "rheumatoid disease" being coined.[47] Early series[177] using analysis of chest x-ray studies failed to find an increased incidence of interstitial pulmonary disease in RA compared with control subjects. From the chest physician's viewpoint, however, a substantial proportion of patients with interstitial fibrosis have RA or another type of arthritis. Rheumatoid factors and antinuclear antibodies are common even in those patients without joint involvement.[135,178–181] A more recent series of 309 patients[151] has suggested an incidence of pulmonary fibrosis in RA of 11.3%. The pattern of diffuse reticulonodular fibrosis had a frequency of 4.5%, considerably higher than matched control subjects. In addition, a number of surveys[139,140,142] have shown altered pulmonary function, with reduction of vital capacity and of transfer factor in the presence of a normal chest radiograph. This suggests a higher incidence of inapparent disease than either chest x-ray studies or clinical

FIG. 44–4. *A* and *B,* Two examples of rheumatoid pneumoconiosis in the classic form. (Courtesy of Dr. A. Caplan.)

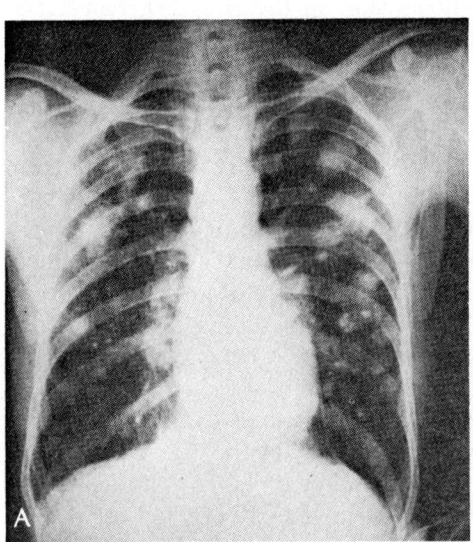
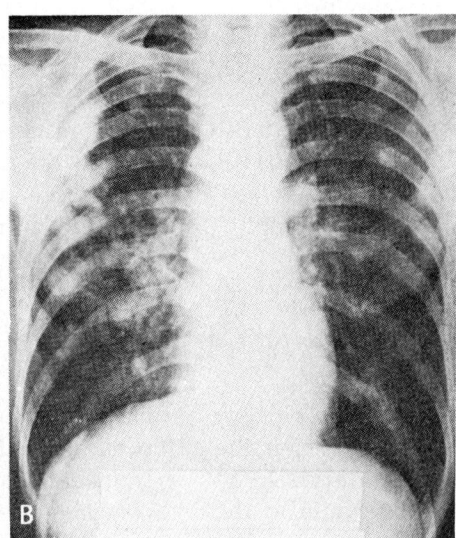

symptoms has indicated. Impaired pulmonary function appears to relate to RA in being associated with disease severity and the presence of extra-articular disease.[145] The same series also noted an association with smoking and with gold therapy. Another survey suggested the D-penicillamine could protect against the development of airways disease.[182] As with most other extra-articular rheumatoid disease a male preponderance is found. Fibrosing alveolitis is not a late complication of RA since in the majority of cases the two conditions develop together within a few years.[135] Joint disease usually precedes lung involvement but rarely the lungs are involved first with an interval of up to 5 years before joint disease becomes apparent.

The clinical features of fibrosing alveolitis in rheumatoid patients do not differ from those with the idiopathic syndrome although exertional dyspnea may be a less prominent feature in patients with restricted mobility. Crepitations are invariable and finger clubbing is common. Chest radiographs usually show extensive shadowing, frequently including the upper zones. Interestingly, associated pleural effusions are uncommon.

There is a significantly increased risk of death from respiratory disease in RA,[183] and fibrosing alveolitis developing in rheumatoid disease carries a serious prognosis with a 5-year mortality of approximately 50% of cases. This survival rate is similar to that seen in idiopathic fibrosing alveolitis.[133] Steroids are often advocated for therapy but reports of the response are conflicting.[135] A useful response occurs in only a mi-

nority of patients and complete remission is very rare. In other cases steroids appear to induce more rapid deterioration.[184] It is not clear whether corticosteroids may slow the rate of disease progression and thus prolong survival in cases not actually showing improvement. A similar variable response to immunosuppressive agents such as azathioprine and cyclophosphamide has also been reported. Penicillamine may slow disease progression in some cases.[185]

Pathologic findings show an infiltration of lymphocytes and plasma cells in alveolar spaces in the acute stages of disease. Desquamative interstitial pneumonia has occasionally been seen. In more chronic disease widespread interstitial fibrosis with lung destruction is found with only scanty inflammatory elements. Changes in pulmonary hypertension may be seen, and rarely pulmonary vasculitis is documented on lung biopsy.[186] Digital vasculitis has been noted in patients with fibrosing alveolitis, adding to the serologic evidence that circulating immune complexes may relate to the pathogenesis of the pulmonary involvement. Despite the extensive pathologic findings that may be documented on lung biopsy there is little overall correlation between histology and the clinical or x-ray picture.[187]

Obliterative Bronchiolitis

Obliterative bronchiolitis is a rare pulmonary manifestation that is most commonly linked with rheumatoid arthritis.[188-191] It often first manifests as breathlessness of abrupt onset that may suggest pulmonary embolism. The chest x-ray picture shows only slight hyperinflation. Pulmonary function tests show an obstructive pattern of small airways disease. Only scanty crepitations are heard at the bases of the lungs, sometimes accompanied by a dry cough, but there is little evidence of inflammatory bronchitis and most patients are nonsmokers. The syndrome may be rapidly fatal and examination of the lungs confirms widespread small airways obstruction without emphysema or alveolar wall fibrosis.

MINOR OR INFREQUENT ORGAN INVOLVEMENT

Involvement of almost every organ or system in the body has been reported in rheumatoid arthritis. Even when not a major feature, these contribute to the overall morbidity of rheumatoid disease. Subclinical lesions may be far more common than clinically apparent disease indicates, although autopsy data suggesting this have to be viewed with some caution since they may represent only terminal events. The precise relationship of many organ or system manifestations to true systemic rheumatoid disease is unclear. Certainly complications of disease such as amyloidosis and iatrogenic disease, related to antirheumatic drugs, make a significant contribution.

Renal Disease

Depression of renal function in patients with rheumatoid arthritis has been noted with considerable regularity in series reported from different countries and at different times.[192-196] The impairment of function is often mild and appears clinically insignificant. Nevertheless, renal-related deaths have been reported as making a significant contribution to the increased mortality of TA.[4,195,197]

The causes of altered renal function in RA may be multiple. Certainly amyloidosis, vasculitis, and drugs can all affect the kidney. In addition a correlation has been noted between depressed renal function and the duration or severity of rheumatoid arthritis, the presence of nodules, the presence of arthritis elsewhere, and with rheumatoid factor positivity.[196] These observations have led to the suggestion that renal disease might be an intrinsic part of the rheumatoid disease process but the evidence for this is still imprecise.

Amyloid deposits in the kidney occur in the majority of patients who develop AA (secondary) amyloidosis as a complication of rheumatoid arthritis. Renal involvement makes a significant contribution to the mortality of amyloidosis patients[15] (see discussion of amyloidosis later in the chapter). Nevertheless, the probability of amyloidosis involvement is only about 5% of even severe RA patients with 20 years of disease.[15] This does not account for the total pool of depressed renal function seen in RA, which is reported to affect twice that number of patients or even more. Vasculitis affects the kidneys in RA surprisingly infrequently (see previous section, Rheumatoid Arthritis). The glomerulus is a very vascular site that is known to be the site of immune complex deposits in other autoimmune diseases. Additionally the necrotizing vasculitis of RA is histologically identical to that of polyarteritis nodosa, in which renal involvement is both frequent and clinically very important. In RA, however, despite the suggestions from early autopsy studies,[146] biopsy studies have consistently failed to show evidence for renal vasculitis,[195,199,200] except in rare cases.[201] This may in part be due to the patchy nature of vascular involvement in RA, where skip lesions are common, and a recent autopsy study has again suggested a high instance of renal vasculitis in severe RA.[49] Clinically it is rare to observe severe renal failure in patients even with extensive rheumatoid vasculitis.[10] Minor and often transient alteration of glomerular function may be seen more commonly if patients are closely monitored, together with transient hematuria indicating local inflammation. This would be consistent with the autopsy findings but suggests that the vascular inflammation observed is not causing significant tissue damage.

Three classes of drugs used in rheumatoid arthritis may affect the kidney and may make a substantial contribution to renal impairment in RA. Analgesic nephropathy was the first disease to be widely recognized but is becoming less significant now. It appeared as an apparently new disease entity in the 1950s, initially in Europe.[202] In the next 2 decades the association between analgesic abuse and both interstitial nephritis and capillary necrosis was recognized worldwide. Analgesic nephropathy was seen as a major cause of chronic renal failure in some countries such as Australia,[203] but with wide regional variation. The geographic distribution of this entity shows some correlation with the rate of analgesic consumption.[203] The subsequent fall in acetaminophen (paracetamol) use has certainly been associated with a fall in the incidence of clinically recognizable analgesic nephropathy. The pathologic lesion may be attributed either to direct tubular damage[204] or to interference with the capillary blood flow.[205] The earlier evidence emphasized phenacetin as the chief culprit. However, phenacetin was a common constituent of many widely used analgesic compound preparations. Acetaminophen is the main metabolite of phenacetin but there is little evidence that acetaminophen alone is nephrotoxic in humans. Aspirin is a major constituent of many of the commonly abused analgesic mixtures and in high dosage can produce capillary necrosis in rats.[206] Nevertheless most clinical studies have emphasized the importance of analgesic mixtures in the pathogenesis. Experimentally, renal capillary necrosis in rats again occurs with aspirin mixtures and is seen particularly when the animals are dehydrated. Analgesic nephropathy is important to diagnosis since the cessation of analgesic abuse often leads to stabilization or even improvement in renal function. It is typically seen more commonly in women with a long history of high doses of analgesic consumption, most often bought as over-the-counter medicine rather than as prescriptions for arthritis. However, large-series studies of analgesic nephropathy patients have included between 10% and 30% of patients with RA.[203] Patients often have minor evidence of psychiatric disturbance such as depression or alcohol abuse. They usually are diagnosed with symptoms related to chronic renal failure, but a few patients present acutely with renal colic or hematuria relating to shedding of renal papillae. Acute renal failure may follow an episode of dehydration associated with intercurrent illness or major surgery.

The nonsteroidal anti-inflammatory drugs (NSAIDs) currently available are all potent inhibitors of cyclo-oxygenase, an important enzyme in the metabolic pathway producing prostaglandins from arachidonic acid. In the kidney, inhibition of this pathway leads to loss of the ability to compensate for ischemic stress by increasing the production of the vasodilatory prostaglandins PGE_2 and PG_{12}, so as to maximize cortical blood flow. This may be of no consequence under normal circumstances but becomes important in at-risk patients, including those in specific disease groups such as SLE as well as those with pre-existing renal failure, congestive cardiac failure, diminished extracellular fluid volume caused by diuretics, or the elderly. The extent to which this causes clinical problems is still unclear. Aspirin was initially associated with the analgesic nephropathy syndrome, particularly when used in analgesic compound mixtures. More recently NSAIDs have been associated with interstitial nephritis, with or without proteinuria[207] and subsequently with acute renal failure.[208] The belief that this only occurs in patients with associated risk factors is challenged by the finding of a uniform improvement in renal function (creatinine clearance) in a group of RA patients who had their nonsteroidal drug discontinued after admission to the hospital.[209] The findings of this small group need to be repeated and the relationship of the RA to nonsteroidal therapy requires clearer definition. The disease process, if any, in such cases has not been studied. Renal biopsy obtained in patients presenting with both acute and chronic renal failure associated with NSAIDs has shown interstitial nephritis that may progress to fibrosis.[210] The mechanisms whereby NSAIDs might cause interstitial nephritis are currently unknown but it is noteworthy that interstitial nephritis has been described both in Sjögren's syndrome and as the most common cause of disease in RA patients presenting with uremia,[196,211] as well as being frequently seen in analgesic nephropathy. The contribution of rheumatoid disease alone or in association with drugs to this lesion will certainly be the subject of future studies.

The slow-acting antirheumatic drugs, gold and D-penicillamine have also been associated with renal disease but of a different sort.[212] Chrysotherapy is associated with the development of proteinuria in 2 to 10% of patients but in only 1 to 2% is it sufficiently severe to cause nephrotic syndrome. D-Penicillamine has been associated with significant proteinuria in up to one third of patients and the nephrotic syndrome is correspondingly more common, being seen in as many as 5% or even 10% of patients in some series. With gold, proteinuria may occur at any time during therapy, but with D-penicillamine the maximum concentration is in the second 6 months of therapy. The degree of proteinuria may be highly variable with either drug. Proteinuria may persist or even increase for the first 1 or 2 months after discontinuing therapy before gradually decreasing. It may take up to 2 years to resolve completely. Renal function is often normal but may be moderately impaired, and occasionally severe reduction has been observed.[213,214] The pathologic findings revealed on biopsy in both cases is classically an immune complex glomerular nephritis similar to the early stages of idiopathic membranous glomerular nephritis. Light microscopy reveals normal glomeruli or mild mesangial cell proliferation, but epimembranous spikes may be revealed when thick secretions are examined. On immunofluorescence granular deposits of immunoglobulin, especially IgG, and complement (C3) are seen. Electron microscopy shows characteristic subepithelial electron-dense deposits with loss of epithelial foot processes. Some patients show only mild mesangial cell proliferation. The finding of immune complex deposits in the kidney in chronic autoimmune disease indicates that the rheumatoid disease process might contribute to this lesion. It is suggested as being much more common in RA than in, for example, Wilson's disease patients treated with D-penicillamine. The mechanism is probably associated with the accumulation of drug in the proximal and distal tubules. This can lead to interstitial fibrosis and to damage to the brush border of the renal tubular epithelial cells, causing the release of the autoantigen RTE. This induces the formation of small soluble immune complexes that localize in the subepithelial space, leading to membranous glomerular nephritis. The mechanism is thus similar to the experimental lesions induced in rats following the injection of autologous kidney immune complex.[215] The lack of severe renal dysfunction or of inflammatory changes associated with this immune complex deposition in the kidneys is intriguing. It has been noted in SLE that the presence of rheumatoid factor is associated with less severe renal disease.

Similar proteinuria or even nephrotic syndrome is reported occasionally in RA patients not taking gold or penicillamine.[216–219] The early suggestion of a true rheumatoid glomerulitis with glomerular hypercellularity reported at autopsy to be common in RA, has not been confirmed by renal biopsies.[220,221] Thus these case reports probably represent the chance association of two unrelated disorders.

Gastrointestinal Involvement

Nonsteroidal anti-inflammatory drugs, with their known ulcerogenic potential, are administered to virtually all patients with rheumatoid arthritis. This makes any estimation of the prevalence of peptic ulcer relating to rheumatoid disease itself extremely difficult. Endoscopy studies have suggested that gastric erosions are both more common than clinical symptoms suggest and may have an increased incidence in RA.[222] Nevertheless, drug-induced upper gastrointestinal lesions remain the chief clinical concern. The entire gastrointestinal tract may be affected by diffuse rheumatoid vasculitis. Again personal experience with gastric and rectal biopsy suggests that this occurs considerably more often than is usually suspected. Clinically overt gastrointestinal lesions of vasculitis are a serious complication with a high mortality (see previous section, Rheumatoid Vasculitis). They usually present as an abdominal emergency, particularly perforation, but occasionally massive bleeding is seen.[49] In a similar way amyloid deposits may be shown at autopsy to involve the entire intestine, and the rectal mucosa is a good site for blind biopsy to establish the diagnosis.[223] Yet like vasculitis, gastrointestinal symptoms relating to this amyloid deposition are uncommon (see later section, Amyloidosis). In-

volvement of the small intestine in the rheumatoid disease process has been suggested by the findings of altered mucosal permeability, but again this may well relate to the administration of nonsteroidal drugs.[224] Ultrastructural changes have been described in rectal mucosal cells,[225] including increased iron deposition in siderosomes and more pronounced cytoplasmic filaments, abnormalities that have already been well described in synovial tissue, but the significance of these observations is not yet clear.

Neuromuscular Manifestations

Neuromuscular manifestations add considerably to the burden of chronic rheumatic disease and make a major difference in the functional capacity of RA patients. Patients with prominent joint pain may not specifically complain of additional symptoms such as weakness or paresthesia, which would suggest neuropathy. The evaluation of the contribution of neuromuscular features in a patient with actively inflamed or deformed joints represents a time-consuming and difficult task for the physician, but it is important since recognition of such features leads to institution of different therapies.

Neurologic lesions can be protean[70] and several classification schemes of neurologic lesions seen in RA have been devised.[226] The simplest approach is to consider the entrapment neuropathies, diffuse peripheral sensory neuropathy, and the more dramatic mononeuritis multiplex. The entrapment neuropathies are related to pressure caused by inflammation or edema at a point where the nerve is restricted by nondistensible structures. In rheumatoid arthritis inflammation may be primarily in tendon sheaths or in the joint itself and the sites of compression are usually juxta-articular. Relief of inflammation by the use of rest, local splinting, local steroid injection, or adequate systemic therapy is often successful. Less commonly, surgical intervention is required and is often dramatically successful.

The carpal tunnel syndrome, causing compression of the median nerve, is by far the most common entrapment neuropathy found in RA.[227] Conversely, RA is the most common cause of all cases of median nerve compression.[228] These symptoms may occur at any time and indeed have been recognized as the presenting manifestation of RA.[227] Carpal tunnel compression is particularly common in early disease in which electromyographic (EMG) studies suggest that as many as two thirds of patients may have some evidence of median nerve compression. The clinical symptoms are insidious and the early changes are largely sensory. The ulnar nerve can also be affected at the wrist, but more commonly is involved at the elbow. The radial or posterior interosseous nerve is less often involved at the elbow as it passes anterior to the lateral epicondyle.[229] The nerve compression causes loss of finger extension with preserved wrist extension, which must be distinguished from an extensor tendon rupture. In the lower limb, anterior tibial nerve palsy with footdrop can be associated with popliteal space compression. External compression of the nerve as it rounds the fibular head caused by splints or braces can also occur. The posterior tibial nerve can be compressed in the tarsal tunnel beneath the flexor retinaculum distal to the medial malleolus.[230,231] Again this relates to the flexor tendon sheaths. A clinical syndrome of burning pain with paresthesias has to be distinguished from true joint pain, which may be difficult in the absence of a clear history.

Cervical myelopathy may be considered a form of pressure neuropathy that occurs from narrowing of the cervical canal caused by either atlantoaxial dislocation or subluxation at lower levels of the cervical spine. Radiographic evidence of atlantoaxial subluxation is seen in about 20% of RA patients if a lateral view in full flexion is taken.[232,233] Fortunately this is rarely associated with evidence of cervical myelopathy, perhaps owing to the generous width of the cervical canal at this level (Fig. 44–5A). Forward luxation of the upper cervical vertebrae below this level is seen less commonly in RA but may have a more serious prognosis, relating to the narrower confines of the spinal canal here (see Fig. 44–5B).

Cervical cord compression is most likely to develop in patients in whom it is most difficult to detect, that is, in those with long-standing, seropositive, erosive, deforming RA.[234,235] Localized cervical pain may occur, often with radiation up to the occiput owing to the involvement of the posterior occipital nerve. Pain in the cervical spine may be entirely absent and the patient may present with upper motor neuron signs such as weakness or unexplained "giving way" of the legs. The classic clinical signs such as a positive Babinski reflex and increased deep tendon reflexes are more difficult to elicit in the presence of joint deformities. Careful sensory examination is most important, particularly because sensory changes are frequently presenting problems.[236] The findings can range from a barely detectable abnormality to a full-blown tetraplegia. The rare cases of sudden death relate not just to direct cord compression but also to acute ischemia from vertebral artery thrombosis.[237,238] This is again due to involvement in the deformed cervical spine. Trauma is dangerous to these patients, particularly

any form of whiplash injury while traveling. Special care must be taken with neck manipulation for surgical procedures, especially during endotracheal intubation and anesthesia induction. Conservative management is often possible,[239] with patient instruction and the use of a collar to immobilize the neck in midposition. A rigid Philadelphia or halo collar may be required to control pain or in the presence of acute neurologic symptoms. A variety of surgical procedures have been tried with some success[240]; nevertheless, they should be reserved for severe cases with definite neurologic signs.[241] Remarkable spontaneous improvement has been observed occasionally in patients considered unfit for surgical procedures.

Central nervous system involvement is largely remarkable by its absence in RA, perhaps surprisingly in view of the widespread nature of this disorder. Rheumatoid granulomata impinging on the central nervous system are the subject of scattered case reports. These involve principally the dura mater in the cranium,[242–245] but the choroid plexus has rarely been the site of similar granulomata at postmortem examination.[246,247] Extradural rheumatoid nodules can involve the spinal canal and produce nerve root compression,[248,249] or even spinal cord compression.[250] The neural tissue may be directly involved in rheumatoid vasculitis. Such complications are well described[70] but the significance of an apparent cerebrovascular accident may not always be appreciated in the context of rheumatoid disease, leading to an underestimate of its frequency. Finally mental confusion, with or without other central neurologic signs, has been described in elderly women withdrawn from corticosteroids, which was responsive to the readministration of these drugs.[251,252] It is unclear whether this relates directly to cerebral vascular inflammation.

Muscle weakness and wasting are a prominent feature of rheumatoid arthritis. The weakness may cause as much functional disability as does joint pain. The wasting is most marked in connection with acutely inflamed joints, but weakness and muscle stiffness may be generalized. Despite this there is little evidence for muscle inflammation in RA. The concurrence of true polymyositis with rheumatoid arthritis is exceptionally rare and may simply be a coincidence of two diseases.[253,254] Significant elevations of muscle enzyme levels are not observed although elevated serum creatine/creatinine ratios are increased, consistent with diminished muscle mass.[255] Electromyographic studies may show evidence of either "myositis" or "myopathy" but the findings relate poorly to clinically observed weakness and wasting, or to synovial disease activity.[256] Muscle biopsy may show

FIG. 44–5. *A,* Flexion films of the upper cervical spine with the odontoid process of C2 outlined by arrows. The dislocation measured 7 mm. The patient, a 59-year-old woman, had had seropositive RA with nodules for 17 years. She had severe deformities with finger extensor tendon destruction. She had had posterior cervical pain, but neither symptoms nor findings of neural compression. *B,* Mild subluxation of C4 on C5 in long-standing RA. This less-common change can be, but here was not, accompanied by findings of spinal cord compression. (Courtesy of Dr. John Bland.)

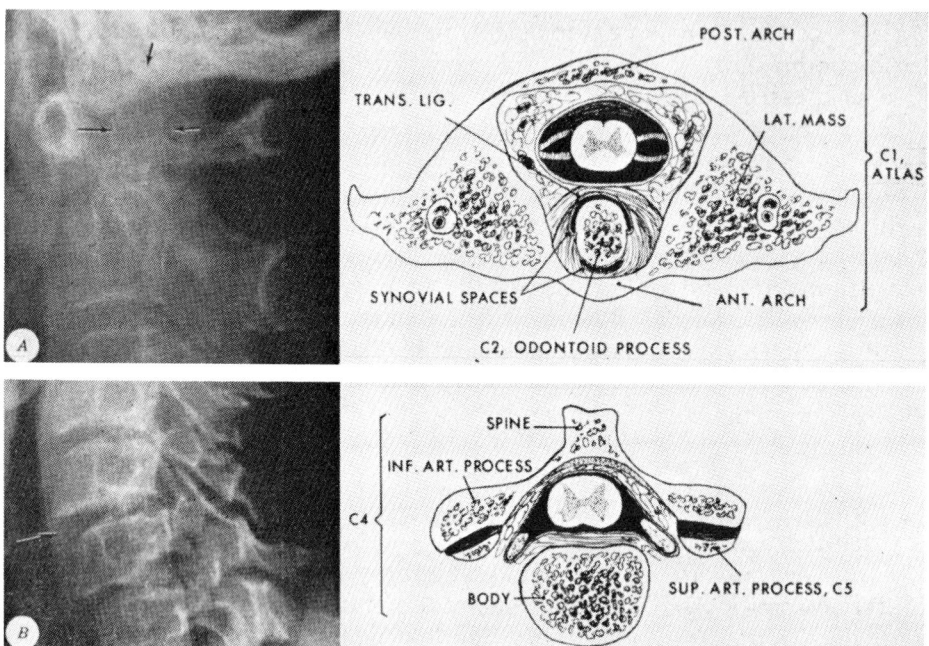

the presence of "lymphorhages," that is, small aggregates of lymphocytes between muscle fibers. These do not appear to be associated with any inflammatory process or muscle fiber destruction and are not specific to RA.[257,258] Steroids can induce myopathy and may be an added cause of weakness in RA patients thus treated. Another antirheumatic drug, D-penicillamine may rarely induce myasthenia gravis.[259] It is important to recognize the cause of this additional weakness, since it responds well to withdrawal of the D-penicillamine, although supportive therapy may be needed for a brief period.

Bone Disease

Osteopenia, or thinning of the bone visible on x-ray study, is recognized to occur not just in juxta-articular bone but may be widespread, particularly in long-standing rheumatoid arthritis. A fracture following minimal trauma may be the last straw that permanently immobilizes a disabled patient. Osteoporosis is the chief contributing factor, which in RA may relate to immobility and the use of steroids, in addition to well-recognized postmenopausal osteoporosis in women. Other factors may contribute to osteopenia. Vitamin D deficiency can occur particularly in immobilized elderly patients who do not get out into the sunlight and subsist on a poor diet.[260] A contribution by the rheumatoid disease itself stimulating increased osteoclastic activity in the bone was described by several authors over 80 years age.[261] Recent sophisticated measurements of bone mineral content using photonabsorptiometry in serial studies have also suggested that rheumatoid disease activity as well as steroid use contribute to the observed bone loss.[262]

Ocular Manifestations

Ocular manifestations have been traditionally related to two portions of the eye, the sclera and the anterior uveal tract. However, it has become apparent that anterior uveitis is no more common in RA than in the general population despite its involvement in other granulomatous diseases such as sarcoidosis or chronic infection. Indeed nongranulomatous anterior uveitis, a typical feature of both ankylosing spondylitis and juvenile chronic arthritis, helps to distinguish these diseases from RA, as discussed in detail elsewhere.[263,264] Corneal and conjunctival manifestations of the sicca syndrome are the most common ophthalmologic features of RA, and many of the drugs used in RA may also affect the eye.[265] Disease of the sclera is rare but characteristic.

Drug-related disorders include gold deposition in the cornea, corneal and retinal changes related to antimalarial agents, and posterior subcapsular cataracts caused by corticosteroids. Episcleritis appears over the anterior sclera, most frequently close to the limbus. It may be localized or diffuse and typically appears as a raised lesion a few millimeters in diameter surrounded by intense hyperemia of the deeper vessels.[72] It may appear a darker purple compared with the bright red of conjunctival hyperemia. Discomfort is common but pain is not. The lesions may be transient but can persist for weeks or months despite the use of topical steroids. They may involve one or both eyes and are sometimes multiple. They seem to be more prevalent in women and are common in patients with rheumatoid arteritis. Indeed followup of patients with severe and persistent episcleritis has shown a considerable mortality caused by associated vasculitic lesions elsewhere.[73,74]

Scleritis is a rarer and potentially serious problem.[265] It may manifest as a painful inflammatory condition with widespread necrosis known as necrotizing nodular sclerosis (Fig. 44–6). The specificity of this lesion is established by its histopathologic features, which are typical of an acellular rheumatoid nodule.[35] More commonly an indolent and very slowly progressive asymptomatic nodular destruction of the sclera occurs.[73] This is known as scleromalacia perforans, although actual perforation is fortunately very rare. Lesions are most common superiorly in the sclera of the anterior eye, with associated hyperemia. As the condition progresses the sclera may become thinned and transparent leaving slate-blue scars. Despite the appearance, ultrasound studies have suggested that actual thinning is less common than was previously thought.[266]

Less well recognized ocular complications of rheumatoid disease include Brown's syndrome, with diplopia on upward inward gaze, caused by tenovaginitis of the superior oblique tendon.[267] The melting cornea syndrome also appears to have an increased frequency in rheumatoid arthritis.[75]

Laryngeal and Ear Manifestations

Laryngeal symptoms are ascribed to typical rheumatoid synovitis in the cricoarytenoid joints, which has been well documented by careful autopsy dissection.[268,269] Clinical manifestations are rare although detailed assessment of patients with generalized rheumatoid disease suggests that some findings may

FIG. 44–6. *A,* Medial sclera showing vascularity overlying nodular scleritis in a 52-year-old woman with 18 years of seropositive RA. Subcutaneous nodules had first appeared 5 years before, and scleromalacia perforans had developed in the opposite eye 2 years earlier. (Courtesy of Dr. Vernon Wong.) *B,* This patient was 67 years old; RA had been apparent since about age 35. The darkening of the lateral sclera had the distinctly bluish hue of choroidal pigmentation, seen because of scleral thinning from previous scleritis. The destruction had occurred in 3 episodes over a year's time, the last ending a year earlier. (Courtesy of Dr. Werner Barth.)

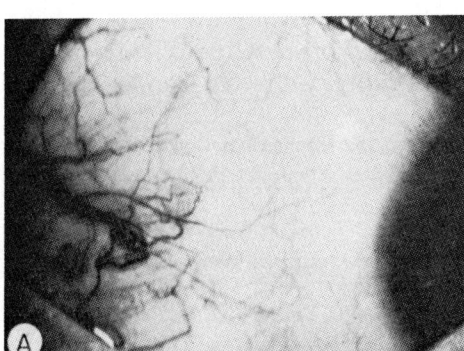
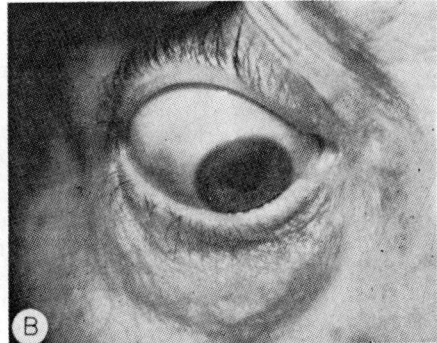

be present in up to 25% of patients.[270] Pain, dysphagia, and hoarseness are common. Occasionally stridor may be seen or dyspnea on exertion. These symptoms may develop acutely or persist over extending periods. Dyspnea and stridor may be absent simply because arthritis limits exertion, but the number of patients without voice change is remarkable. Indirect laryngoscopy may show acute redness and swelling over the involved joints with immobilized cricoarytenoid joints and the vocal cords adducted to the midline. If this is symmetric the airway may be reduced to a significant degree.[271] Attempts to move the arytenoid cartilage induce pain. Superimposed respiratory infection can put the patient at substantial risk because of laryngeal and vocal cord edema that may require emergency tracheotomy. Local steroid infiltration may be helpful after control of infection, if it is necessary. Surgical intervention is rarely required.

NONSPECIFIC FEATURES AND COMPLICATIONS OF RHEUMATOID ARTHRITIS

Nonspecific malaise is a common feature during a flare-up of joint activity, particularly in the early stages of rheumatoid arthritis. It contributes to the notable functional loss seen in early disease, which actually improves in the majority of cases as the patient comes to terms with chronic disease. The continual feeling of being unwell, without having much to show for it early on, disturbs a number of patients. Indeed the impact of the disease on the emotional life of the patient can be devastating and makes a major contribution to the quality of the sufferer's life. Significant depression is a common feature in rheumatoid arthritis whatever the premorbid personality, particularly in the first year or two of disease. With the progress of time, most patients learn to cope with their disease either by coming to terms with it or less satisfactorily by apparently denying its effects.[272] The cheerful way with which patients cope with the long-term problems of advanced disease evokes the admiration of rheumatologists.

The malaise is not all psychologic, and weight loss may be apparent, again particularly in the early stages of disease. In later disease, imobility may promote obesity. Weight loss can be a sign of serious extra-articular systemic RA at any stage and is particularly prominent when there is active arteritis. Indeed, severe unexplained weight loss in a patient with rheumatoid arthritis should lead to suspicion of vasculitis.[49] Fever can also occur, particularly when other extra-articular features are present. It is usually a low-grade fever and night sweats can be a problem. High fever is uncommon and again should suggest arteritis. Infections of all sorts, especially pulmonary and urinary tract infections, have been suggested in the past to be increased in RA, but the evidence for this has not been well controlled except in patients with Felty's syndrome. It is important to avoid increasing the risk of infection by the unnecessary use of steroids or immunosuppressive drugs. However, in a debilitated patient with long-standing arthritis complicated by vasculitis and perhaps amyloidosis, it is difficult to assess whether the disease or the therapy contributes most to a terminal infection.

Anemia

Moderate normochromic normocytic anemia almost invariably occurs with rheumatoid arthritis and is certainly the most common extra-articular disease manifestation. The degree of anemia is related to disease activity and recedes as the disease is brought under control. The pathophysiologic mechanisms causing anemia in RA have been the subject of numerous investigations over the years[273] and the association is clearly multifactorial (Table 44–2). In spite of the many facts that have emerged, the central mechanism for the anemia of chronic RA is still not established.

A tendency to hyperchromia and microcytosis exists in some patients, particularly women. Chronic blood loss from the gastrointestinal tract, related to salicylate use and to a lesser extent to the newer nonsteroidal drugs, does occur regularly but does not appear to be the major causative factor.[274] In the majority of patients, anemia is not the iron deficiency type. Serum iron is frequently depressed, as is the saturation of transferrin, but the total transferrin-binding capacity is also depressed compared with the increase expected in true iron deficiency. This relates to the role of transferrin as a negative acute-phase reactant. By contrast, serum ferritin levels may be increased in RA, as part of the acute-phase reaction, compared with the depressed levels seen in true iron

Table 44–2. Pathophysiologic Mechanisms Contributing to the Anemia of RA

Iron deficiency
Iron withholding
Impaired production and response to erythropoietin
Ineffective erythropoiesis
Immune suppression of CFUe
Shortened red blood cell survival

deficiency.[275,276] Assessment of the iron stores in the bone marrow gives the most clear-cut evidence of iron status, but this invasive procedure is not usually required. It was previously suggested that giving oral iron supplements until the hemoglobin concentration stopped rising was the simplest clinical way of assessing how much the anemia was related to iron deficiency.[277] More recent evidence suggests that iron may be harmful in RA by contributing to iron overload in the synovial tissues and promoting free radical–induced inflammation.[278]

Iron withholding in the bone marrow seems to be the chief mechanism of anemia in RA, which occurs in the presence of increased total body iron stores.[279] Massive iron deposits are seen in the inflamed synovium,[280] presumably relating to local microbleeding, but they also occur in other tissues, particularly lymphoid tissues.[281] The iron is laid down in the form of hemosiderin, which is unavailable for marrow uptake. However, when an iron-chelating agent such as deferoxamine is given to RA patients, iron excretion is greater than normal. In the normal state, the iron used in hematopoiesis is derived primarily from the breakdown of effete erythrocytes but the release of this iron may be diminished in RA. Intravenously administered iron is cleared more rapidly from the plasma than normal but is not used for hematopoiesis. Such a study suggests that the major defect rests in an increased uptake and diminished release of iron from a site where it is unavailable for erythropoiesis. The avidity of this iron withholding is directly related to disease activity. Acute suppression of disease by steroids or adrenocorticotropic hormone (ACTH) is followed by rapid iron utilization in hematopoiesis, together with elevation of serum iron levels in the absence of iron supplements, later followed by a rising hemoglobin concentration.[282]

A number of other mechanisms may contribute to the anemia of rheumatoid arthritis. Ineffective erythropoiesis has been described.[283,284] Erythropoietin levels, although increased in RA, are not raised appropriately for the degree of anemia present and the response to erythropoietin appears to be depressed in RA.[285] Recent evidence has also suggested a direct effect of the disordered immune response in the anemia of RA, similar to the mechanisms described in Felty's syndrome (see later section). In the case of anemia, rheumatoid plasma to a small extent and rheumatoid peripheral T lymphocytes to a large extent inhibited the formation of human bone marrow erythroid colony-forming units.[286] Red cell life span is shortened to some degree in most patients with active RA. Although the normal bone marrow should be easily able to compensate for this shortened life

cycle, this is clearly not true of the depressed bone marrow in RA. Expanded plasma volume with secondary hemodilution may also play a small role in patients with active disease, depressed serum albumin, and a degree of splenomegaly.

Lymphadenopathy

Lymph node enlargement is common in rheumatoid arthritis, being seen in 50 to 75% of patients.[287,288] The exact incidence depends on the definition of lymphadenopathy. Special soft tissue radiography or lymph angiograms reveal that deep as well as superficial nodes are enlarged. The prevalence is higher in men, and nodal enlargement is more common in rheumatoid-factor-positive patients with active joint disease. A relationship between local synovitis and lymphadenopathy in the nodes draining the involved limb has recently been demonstrated.[289] Lymph node enlargement may be sufficiently marked to suggest neoplasia. Biopsy shows significant follicular hyperplasia extending uniformly throughout all the node.[290] This uniformity helps to distinguish a rheumatoid lesion from a low-grade lymphoma, which the marked cellularity may suggest. Cytologic studies of lymph node aspirate may reveal active centriblast cells without malignant features.[291] Their presence correlates with markers of T-cell activation in the peripheral blood.

Significant lymphadenopathy in RA thus correlates with clinical markers of disease severity, duration, and male sex. It is also associated with depressed lymphocyte reactivity and alterations of CD4:CD8 subset ratios, abnormalities similar to those seen in Felty's syndrome. It is tempting to speculate that these changes may be a predisposing factor to the increased incidence of lymphoma now well documented to occur in RA, again particularly in male patients with severe prolonged disease.[292]

Felty's Syndrome

In 1924 Felty described 5 patients with deforming arthritis who had developed splenomegaly and leukopenia.[293] This triad, together with a few other common symptom accompaniments, is often thought to represent a specific syndrome.[294] An alternative viewpoint is to regard it as the aggregation of multiple nonspecific features of RA, representing the end of the spectrum of severe extra-articular rheumatoid disease. The syndrome includes features already discussed, such as anemia and lymphadenopathy. The splenomegaly may be regarded simply as a part of the latter symptom. Weight loss, fever, and infection are all common but nonspecific features of this syndrome. Vasculitic lesions are also often seen, underlining the relationship of Felty's syndrome to systemic rheumatoid disease. In contrast to this extra-articular activity, synovitis is often quiescent in patients with Felty's syndrome. The etiopathogenesis of the syndrome also appears to be multifactorial, supporting the idea that it is a nonspecific collection of symptoms rather than a true syndrome. It is often seen in patients with long-standing and severely deforming RA, particularly white patients; it almost never occurs in blacks.[295] The suggestion of a genetic element is reinforced by the very high frequency of HLA-DR4 antigen observed in Felty's syndrome patients, an unusually high proportion of them being homozygous for HLA-DR4.[296] An extended sibship with Felty's syndrome showing a common haplotype including HLA-DR4 has also been reported.[297]

Felty's original description included weight loss and pigmentation of exposed surfaces in addition to the classic triad of symptoms. A number of features have been added since and some modification made to the triad.[294] Felty's syndrome patients were described at a time when the classification of inflammatory polyarthritis was much less complete than currently. However, the syndrome is now seen only in those patients who would fit rigid definitions of RA, are seropositive, and have a high proportion of positive antinuclear antibodies.[298] The leukopenia that Felty described is characteristically a neutropenia seen in the absence of other causes, such as drug-induced suppression of the bone marrow. The neutrophil count may range from a mild depression to an apparent total absence of these cells in the peripheral blood. Some depression of circulating lymphocyte numbers is often seen but may not be pronounced. Monocytes and eosinophils are not reduced; rarely a relative eosinophilia is seen. The platelet count is normal or somewhat reduced, in contrast to the thrombocythemia seen in active rheumatoid synovitis.[299] Leukopenia is accompanied by anemia that is severe even by the standards of rheumatoid arthritis. It is hypochromic but in addition the red blood cell destruction may be accelerated. The administration of chromium-labeled red cells shows increased spleen and liver uptake in such cases, in which the anemia may be alleviated by splenectomy.[300] Isotope labeling studies have also shown increased platelet destruction in the spleen in some cases. An additional factor is the dilutional anemia commonly observed in the presence of marked splenomegaly.

The presence of recurrent infections has been stressed by some authors and may be the feature bringing the patient to a physician's attention. However, infections are not as common as the depressed neutrophil count might suggest. Studies have shown that the rate of infection is not related to the level of the circulating white cells.[301] Neutrophil incompetence may be more important in the infection than actual neutrophil numbers, and recent studies have documented a depressed ability to release reactive oxygen species in response to phagocytic events.[302] This important neutrophil function, essential to bacterial killing, can be depressed in normal polymorphonuclear leukocytes incubated with plasma from Felty's syndrome,[302a] an activity that correlated with the content of circulating immune complexes and binding of IgG to polymorphonuclear leukocytes. An increase in neutrophil count and in the ability to generate superoxide has been observed in Felty's syndrome following chrysotherapy.[303]

The spleen ranges from barely palpable to a large size. It is occasionally massive and tender, probably related to splenic infarcts, but is usually detected on routine examination. Hypersplenism may contribute to Felty's syndrome but is not essential. Splenic enlargement is not detected in up to one third of patients with neutropenia and RA who otherwise have features typical of Felty's syndrome.[294] Certainly splenomegaly is not specific to the Felty's syndrome end of the rheumatoid disease spectrum, since a palpable spleen is common in RA in the absence of leukopenia.[304] Splenomegaly appears to relate to the diffuse lymphoid hyperplasia seen in rheumatoid arthritis. It is interesting that liver disease, even with portal hypertension, may occur in Felty's syndrome. An apparently typical noncirrhotic condition with increased liver fibrosis has been termed nodular regenerative hyperplasia of the liver.[305] This again has been rarely seen in RA patients without Felty's syndrome, and when it has occurred it has been generally ascribed to active vasculitis rather than to neutropenia or the effects of splenic-induced portal hypertension. Other manifestations of vasculitis are quite frequently seen in Felty's syndrome patients including episcleritis, peripheral neuropathy, and pericarditis. One characteristic feature is chronic leg ulcers particularly seen in long-standing cases.[301] These again may be vasculitic in origin and regional biopsies have shown arteritis with fibrinoid necrosis and low-grade inflammation occluding small blood vessels.[306] Leg ulcers are common in rheumatoid vasculitis but are also seen in patients with chronic RA without any overt evidence of vasculitis. Even here the occasional dramatic response to cytotoxic drugs suggests a vasculitic basis. Other ulcers may start as minor local trauma, particularly in steroid-thin skin, or at the site of breakdown of a rheumatoid nodule. However, after all known causes have been considered, there remains a group of elderly patients with deforming rheumatoid arthritis and chronic leg ulcers. In one study of such patients, 6 of 8 patients had either splenomegaly or leukopenia.[307] The relationship of the pigmentation originally noted by Felty to leg ulceration and chronic ischemic disease of the leg is a matter of speculation.

The etiopathogenesis of neutropenia in Felty's syndrome is still not fully elucidated. Studies of the mechanisms of leukopenia have revealed a number of abnormalities, but no one of them clearly explains the pathogenesis of the entire syndrome. Increased neutrophil destruction caused by hypersplenism is frequently invoked as a mechanism, but there is surprisingly little direct evidence to support this. The occurrence of neutropenia without splenomegaly has already been noted. The response to splenectomy is variable but does not support more than a contributing role of the spleen to the disease.[308–311] The white cell count usually rises initially but does not show the overshoot commonly seen after splenectomy in other conditions. Neutropenia tends to recur with increasing frequency the longer the followup of splenectomy patients and this can only be infrequently related to the development of an accessory spleen. Antibodies to the surface of white cells have been described,[312,313] as well as antinuclear factors specific for granulocyte nuclei.[314,315] Neutrophils appear to have increased immunoglobulin on their surface that may return to normal following splenectomy.[313] Nevertheless, the relationship between such antibodies and neutropenia is very tenuous. Recent studies showed that the polymorphonuclear leukocyte binding reactivity of immunoglobulins seen in the serum of Felty's syndrome patients was related to the binding of immune complexes and not to the presence of antineutrophil antibodies.[316] The granulocytes may also show large inclusions suspected to be ingested immune complexes,[317] and neutropenia appears to correlate better with levels of circulating complexes.[298] The relevance of these complexes was stressed by the experimental injection of Felty's syndrome serum into normal mice, which produced neutropenia in contrast to the neutrophilia following injection of normal human serum.[318] The infusion of Felty's syndrome plasma into a normal human subject can also cause transient leukopenia.[319] More importantly, autologous presplenectomy plasma from a patient with Felty's syndrome reinfused after splenectomy may cause the return of defective release of granulocytes following an injection of etiocholanolone.[320] This points more to an abnormality at the level of the bone mar-

row. A factor that can stimulate the in-vitro growth of marrow cells is diminished in the urine and serum of patients with Felty's syndrome.[321,322] The suppression of granulocyte-colony-forming activity of normal bone marrow cells has been observed in T cells from Felty's syndrome patients but not from those in nonneutropenic RA or drug-induced neutropenia.[323–325] These interesting studies by Abdou suggest that several different mechanisms are at work in different Felty's syndrome patients.[323] A role for an alternative lymphocyte population is suggested by the recent description of neutropenia in rheumatoid arthritis associated with large granular lymphocytosis.[326] One recent series found such lymphocytosis in one fourth of their patients with Felty's syndrome.[327] The abnormal lymphocytes are similar to the cells seen in large granular T-cell leukemia but do not have the T-cell receptor β- and γ-chain rearrangements seen in that condition.[327] The cells also resemble natural killer cells although they may not bear all the markers for this lineage and many are CD8-positive. An autoimmune neutropenia associated with T-cell γ-chain lymphocytosis occurring in patients without rheumatoid arthritis also shows the presence of such large granular cells.[328] Finally, the role of margination should not be forgotten. About one half of intravascular granulocytes are adherent to the vascular endothelium. This marginated pool is increased in virtually all patients with Felty's syndrome and may be the major cause of neutropenia in some.[299] Certainly the presence of an elevated white cell count in the synovial fluid when there is a joint effusion in Felty's syndrome, or the presence of suppurating leg ulcers, points to the existence of this marginated pool even in patients with a significantly reduced circulating neutrophil count.

The therapy of Felty's syndrome is a matter of controversy. The results of splenectomy are difficult to assess because of the tendency to report favorable results, although some longer term followup study has been reported.[310,311] Splenectomy is usually limited to patients with recurrent infection but is associated with an increased risk. Perioperative infection is not infrequent in Felty's syndrome and the disappearance of recurrent infection is by no means assured.[301,310] The effect of splenectomy on ulcers is irregular and the procedure does not have any recognized effects on the associated polyarthritis. It is rarely justified by the low-grade hemolytic anemia seen in the disease. Two features that do often improve are weight loss and severe malaise. Corticosteroids have been advocated but at tolerable doses do not alleviate leukopenia. High doses do elevate the white cell count, but relapse is usually when the dose is lowered again. Steroids may also contribute to the risk of infection. Steroids combined with cytotoxic drugs to suppress the underlying disease process may be more rational, particularly in those cases related to lymphocyte-mediated suppression of bone marrow function.[329] Personal experience has suggested that intermittent-bolus cyclophosphamide administration plus a corticosteroid can be effective without the increased risk in infection seen with daily dosing. The use of low-dose oral methotrexate has also been advocated for Felty's syndrome patients.[330] Chrysotherapy has long found favor with some physicians although special attention needs to be paid to monitoring. Support for this approach comes from the recent observations that neutrophil function as well as neutrophil numbers improve following chrysotherapy.[303]

Amyloidosis

Secondary or AA-associated amyloidosis remains the most common type of amyloidosis in the United Kingdom and Europe, although American reports suggest that, in hospital practice at least, primary or AL amyloidosis is more frequent.[132] Of the amyloidosis secondary to systemic disease, rheumatoid arthritis is now the major contributor since the demise of widespread tuberculosis. The incidence of amyloidosis in RA may be between 5 and 10%.[15] Personal observation showed a cumulative incidence of 6% by the 20-year assessment of 100 patients followed from the onset of rheumatoid arthritis. Other authors have suggested an incidence as high as 15%,[331] but the study was a small one. A large detailed study in Finland again suggested that the incidence was approximately 5%.[332] The importance of amyloidosis in RA is that in the majority of cases the disease is progressive, but there is wide variation and a small group of patients has apparently nonprogressive disease.[332] In the progressive cases amyloidosis leads to progressive organ dysfunction and makes a significant contribution to the increased mortality of RA.

Clinically, amyloidosis in rheumatoid arthritis presents most commonly as renal involvement.[130] Proteinuria on routine testing is the most frequent presentation but up to one fourth of patients may develop nephrotic syndrome. Insidious development of chronic renal failure is also not uncommon. Other features of amyloidosis lead to the diagnosis much less rarely. Gastrointestinal disturbance is described but is uncommon in amyloidosis secondary to rheumatoid arthritis. It presents as intermittent diarrhea often alternating with obstinate constipation. Organ-

omegaly, a frequent finding in AL amyloidosis, is remarkably uncommon in rheumatoid amyloidosis. This applies to cardiomegaly as well as hepatosplenomegaly, and clinically significant cardiac involvement is not a feature of reactive amyloidosis. However, the renal deposition is a major contributor to the mortality of this condition.[15]

Pathologic features show remarkably widespread deposition of AA amyloid fibrils, in contrast to the clinical findings. The gastrointestinal tract is frequently involved from the stomach through to the rectum, explaining why rectal biopsy is the best site for a blind biopsy.[223] Amyloid deposits are usually present in liver, spleen, and pancreas, the adrenal and thyroid glands, and the heart, as well as being present in subcutaneous fat. However, it is the consistent and extensive glomerular amyloid deposition that is the most important feature. The pathogenesis has become more explicable since the finding that the fibrils of AA amyloidosis are derived from a serum precursor SAA, which acts like an acute-phase protein. The finding of persistently elevated SAA levels after other acute-phase proteins had been depressed to the normal range by antirheumatic therapy[333] may explain amyloid deposition in some apparently quiescent cases of chronic rheumatoid arthritis. The presence of SAA as the building block of amyloid does not explain the incidence of amyloidosis, since SAA is elevated in all RA patients with active inflammation. Other factors relating to the removal of SAA or perhaps the degradation of AA fibrils are clearly important. These may be genetically determined.

Treatment of amyloidosis in rheumatoid arthritis remains unsatisfactory. Aggressive suppression of the disease with second-line drugs or, better, with cytotoxic therapy has been successful in some cases.[334] Chlorambucil has been advocated for amyloidosis associated with Still's disease,[335] but whether this is better than other agents more frequently used in RA such as cyclophosphamide or azathioprine has not been tested. Preservation of renal function by attention to hypertension, to nephrotoxic drugs, and to infection or obstruction, together with good conservative management of chronic renal failure improves the quality of life. It also ensures better results for those patients entering dialysis and transplant programs that have been successfully applied to systemic amyloidosis.[130]

REFERENCES

1. Gordon, D.A., Stein, J.L., and Broder, I.: The extra-articular features of rheumatoid arthritis. A systematic analysis of 127 cases. Am. J. Med., 54:445–452, 1973.

2. Williams, R.C.: Rheumatoid Arthritis as a Systemic Disease. Philadelphia, W.B. Saunders, 1974.

3. Dieppe, P.A., et al.: Rheumatological Medicine. Edinburgh, Churchill Livingstone, 1985.

4. Symmons, D.P.M.: Mortality in RA. Br. J. Rheum., 27 (Suppl 1):44–54, 1988.

5. Mitchell, D.M., and Fries, J.S.: An analysis of the American Rheumatism Association criteria for rheumatoid arthritis. J. Arthritis Rheum., 25:481–487, 1982.

6. Rasker, J.J., and Cosh, J.A.: Cause and age at death in a prospective study of 100 patients with rheumatoid arthritis. Ann. Rheum. Dis., 40:115–120, 1981.

7. Edwards, J.C.W.: Relationship between pressure and digital vasculitis in rheumatoid disease. Ann. Rheum. Dis., 39:138–140, 1980.

8. Kniker, W.T., and Cochrane, C.G.: The localisation of circulating immune complexes in experimental serum sickness: the role of vasoactive amines and hydrodynamic forces. J. Exp. Med., 127:119–135, 1968.

9. Ansell, B.M., and Loewi, G.: Rheumatoid arthritis—general features. Clin. Rheum. Dis., 3:385–401, 1977.

10. Bacon, P.A., and Scott, D.G.I.: La Vascularite Rhumatoide. In Polyarthrite Rhumatoide. Edited by J. Sany. Paris, Medecine-Sciences, Flammarion, 1987.

11. Vollertsen, R.S., et al.: Rheumatoid vasculitis: survival and associated risk factors. Medicine (Baltimore), 65:365–375, 1986.

12. Scott, D.G.I., et al.: IgG rheumatoid factor, complement and immune complexes in rheumatoid synovitis and vasculitis: comparative and serial studies during cytotoxic therapy. Clin. Exp. Immunol., 43:54–63, 1981.

13. Elson, C.J., et al.: Complement activating properties of complexes containing rheumatoid factor in synovial fluids and sera from patients with rheumatoid arthritis. Clin. Exp. Immunol., 59:285–292, 1985.

14. Natvig, J.B., and Anders, R.J.: Characterization of four different immunochemical classes of amyloid fibril proteins. Clin. Rheum. Dis., 3:589–601, 1977.

15. Tribe, C.R., and Mackenzie, J.C.: Amyloidosis. In The Kidney and Rheumatic Disease. Edited by P. Bacon and N.M. Hadler. Butterworths International Medical Reviews: Rheumatology, 1:297–322, 1982.

16. Collins, D.M.: The subcutaneous nodule of rheumatoid arthritis. J. Path. Bact., 45:97–117, 1937.

17. Askari, A., Moscowitz, R.W., and Goldberg, V.M.: Subcutaneous rheumatoid nodules and serum rheumatoid factor without arthritis. JAMA, 229:319–320, 1974.

18. Causey, J.Q.: Isolated subcutaneous rheumatic-like nodules in an adult. South Med. J., 65:633–634, 1972.

19. Gander, O.P., and Caplan, H.I.: Rheumatoid disease without joint involvement. JAMA, 288:339, 1974.

20. Ginsberg, M.H., et al.: Rheumatoid nodulosis, an unusual variant of rheumatoid disease. Arthritis Rheum., 18:49–58, 1975.

21. Wisnieski, J.J., and Askari, A.D.: Rheumatoid nodulosis. A relatively benign rheumatoid variant. Arch. Intern. Med., 141:615–619, 1981.

22. Moore, C.P., and Willkens, R.F.: The subcutaneous nodule: its significance in the diagnosis of rheumatic disease. Semin. Arthritis Rheum., 7:63–79, 1977.

23. Bywaters, E.G.L.: Vasculitis in rheumatoid arthritis. In Nonarticular Forms of Rheumatoid Arthritis. Edited by T.E.W. Feltkamp. Proc. IV ISRA Symposium. Stafleu's Scientific Publications, Leyden, 82–84, 1976.

24. Sattar, M.A., and Sughayer, A.A.: A clinical profile of rheumatoid arthritis in Kuwait. J. Kuwait Med. Assoc., 20:21–28, 1986.

25. Moolenburgh, J.D., Valkenburg, H.A., and Fourie, P.B.: A population study on rheumatoid arthritis in Lesotho, southern Africa. Ann. Rheum. Dis., 45:691–695, 1986.

26. Reference deleted.

27. Aherne, M.J., et al.: Immunohistochemical findings in rheumatoid nodules. Virchows Arch. (Pathol. Anat.), 407:191–202, 1985.

28. Reference deleted.

29. Bywaters, E.G.L., and Scott, J.T.: The natural history of vascular lesions in rheumatoid arthritis. Ann. Rheum. Dis., 12:114–121, 1953.

30. Shapiro, R.F., Resnick, D., and Castles, J.: Fistulization of rheumatoid joints. Ann. Rheum. Dis., 34:489–498, 1975.

31. Laine, V.A.I., and Vainio, K.J.: Ulceration of the skin in rheumatoid arthritis. Acta. Rheum. Scand., 1:113–118, 1955.

32. Bannatyne, G.A.: Rheumatoid Arthritis. Bristol, John Wright, 1898.

33. Sokoloff, L., McCluskey, R.T., and Bunim, J.J.: Vascularity of the early nodule of rheumatoid arthritis. A.M.A. Arch. Pathol., 55:475–495, 1953.

34. Rasker, J.J., and Kuipers, F.C.: Are rheumatoid nodules caused by vasculitis? A study of 13 early cases. Ann. Rheum. Dis., 42:384–388, 1983.

35. Ferry, A.P.: The histopathology of rheumatoid episcleral nodules: an extraarticular manifestation of rheumatoid arthritis. Arch. Ophthalmol., 82:77–78, 1969.

36. Jayson, M.I.V., and Jones, D.E.P.: Scleritis and rheumatoid arthritis. Ann. Rheum. Dis., 30:343–347, 1971.

37. Rooney, P.J., et al.: Thin sclera: a clinical illusion. Ann. Rheum. Dis., 34:464–465, 1975.

38. Shearn, D.L.: Aneurysm of the sinus of valsalva secondary to rheumatoid nodulosis. Arthritis Rheum., 24:978, 1981.

39. Ziegler, P., and Albukerk, J.: Rheumatoid granuloma of kidney. Urology, 12:84–86, 1978.

40. Adelson, G.L, Saypo, D.C., and Walker, A.N.: Ureteral stenosis secondary to retroperitoneal rheumatoid nodules. J. Urol., 127:124–125, 1982.

41. Goehrs, H.R., Baggenstoss, A.H., and Slocumb, C.H.: Cardiac lesions in rheumatoid arthritis. Arthritis Rheum., 3:298–308, 1960.

42. Lebowitz, W.B.: The heart in rheumatoid disease. Geriatrics, 21:194–198, 1966.

43. Iveson, J.M.I., and Pomerance, A.: Cardiac involvement in rheumatic disease. Clin. Rheum. Dis., 3:467–500, 1977.

44. Chamberlain, M.A.: Intra-articular rheumatoid nodules of the knee. J. Bone Joint Surg., 53b:507–509, 1971.

45. Popert, A.J., et al.: Frequency of occurrence, mode of development, and significance of rice bodies in rheumatic joints. Ann. Rheum. Dis., 41:109–117, 1982.

46. Sokoloff, L., Wilens, S.L., and Bunim, J.J.: Arteritis of striated muscle in rheumatoid arthritis. Am. J. Pathol., 27:157–173, 1951.

47. Ellman, P., and Ball, R.E.: Rheumatoid disease with joint and pulmonary manifestations. Br. Med. J., 2:816–820, 1948.

48. Bywaters, E.G.L.: Peripheral vascular obstruction in rheumatoid arthritis and its relationship to other vascular lesions. Ann. Rheum. Dis., 16:84–103, 1957.

49. Scott, D.G.I., Bacon, P.A., and Tribe, C.R.: Systemic rheumatoid vasculitis: a clinical and laboratory study of 50 cases. Medicine (Baltimore), 60:288–297, 1981.

50. Cruickshank, B.: The arteritis of rheumatoid arthritis. Ann. Rheum. Dis., 13:136–145, 1954.

51. Westedt, M.L., et al.: Rheumatoid arthritis. The clinical significance of histo-immunopathological abnormalities in normal skin. J. Rheumatol., *11*:448–453, 1984.
52. Fitzgerald, O.M., et al.: Direct immunofluorescence of normal skin in rheumatoid arthritis. Br. J. Rheumatol., *24*:340–345, 1985.
53. Kinsey, S., Scott, D.G.I., and Bacon, P.A.: Systemic vasculitis as the presenting feature of rheumatoid arthritis. Br. J. Rheumatol., *25*:455, 1986.
54. Hart, F.D.: Rheumatoid arthritis: extra-articular manifestations. Br. Med. J., *3*:131–136, 1969.
55. Adler, R.H., Norcross, B.M., and Lockie, L.M.: Arteritis and infarction of intestine in rheumatoid arthritis. JAMA, *180*:922–926, 1962.
56. Epstein, W.V., and Engleman, E.P.: The relation of the rheumatoid factor content of serum to clinical neurovascular manifestations of rheumatoid arthritis. Arthritis Rheum., *2*:250–258, 1959.
57. Johnson, R.L., et al.: Steroid therapy and vascular lesions in rheumatoid arthritis. Arthritis Rheum., *2*:224–249, 1959.
58. Kemper, J.W., Baggenstoss, A.H., and Slocumb, C.H.: The relationship of therapy with cortisone to the incidence of vascular lesions in rheumatoid arthritis. Ann. Intern. Med., *46*:831–851, 1957.
59. Mongan, E., et al.: A study of the relation of seronegative and seropositive rheumatoid arthritis to each other and to necrotizing vasculitis. Am. J. Med., *47*:23–25, 1969.
60. Schneider, H.A., et al.: Rheumatoid vasculitis: experience with 13 patients and review of the literature. Semin. Arthr. Rheum. *14*(4):280–286, 1985.
61. Wilkinson, M., and Kirk, J.: Leg ulcers complicating rheumatoid arthritis. Scot. Med. J., *10*:175–182, 1965.
62. Nishikawa, J.A.: Are leg ulcers in rheumatoid arthritis due to vasculitis? Eur. J. Rheum. Inflam., *6*:288–290, 1983.
63. Bennett, R.M.: Haematological changes in rheumatoid disease. Clin. Rheum. Dis., *3*:443–465, 1977.
64. Weisman, M., and Zvaifler, N.J.: Cryoimmunoglobulinaemia in Felty's syndrome. Arthritis Rheum., *19*:103–110, 1976.
65. Schmid, R.F., et al.: Arteritis in rheumatoid arthritis. Am. J. Med., *30*:56–83, 1961.
66. Ferguson, R.H., and Slocumb, C.H.: Peripheral neuropathy in rheumatoid arthritis. Bull. Rheum. Dis., *11*:251, 1961.
67. Pallis, C.A., and Scott, J.T.: Peripheral neuropathy in rheumatoid arthritis. Br. Med. J., *1*:1141–1147, 1965.
68. Gierson, A.J., Sturfelt, G., and Truedsson, L.: Clinical and serological features of severe vasculitis in rheumatoid arthritis—prognostic implications. Ann. Rheum. Dis., *46*:727–733, 1987.
69. Vollertsen, R.S., et al.: Rheumatoid vasculitis: survival and associated risk factors. Medicine (Baltimore), *65*:365–375, 1986.
70. Kim, R.C., and Collins, G.H.: The neuropathology of rheumatoid disease. Hum. Pathol., *12*(1):5–15, 1981.
71. Ramos, M., and Mandylbur, T.I.: Cerebral vasculitis in rheumatoid arthritis. J. Arch. Neurol., *32*:271–275, 1975.
72. Lyne, A.J., and Pitkeathley, D.A.: Episcleritis and scleritis; assocation with connective tissue disease. Arch. Ophthalmol., *80*:171–176, 1968.
73. Jayson, M.I.V., and Jones, D.E.P.: Scleritis and rheumatoid arthritis. Ann. Rheum. Dis., *30*:343–347, 1971.
74. Foster, S., Forsot, S.L., and Wilson, L.A.: Mortality rate in rheumatoid arthritis patients developing necrotising scleritis or peripheral ulcerative keratitis. Ophthalmology, *91*:1253–1263, 1984.

75. Scharf, Y., et al.: Marginal melting of cornea in rheumatoid arthritis. Ann. Ophthalmol., *16*(10):924–926, 1984.
76. Scott, D.G.I., and Bacon, P.A.: Cardiac involvement in immunological diseases. Clin. Immunol. Allergy, *1*:537–575, 1987.
77. Wilsher, M., et al.: Complete heart block and bowel infarction secondary to rheumatoid disease. Ann. Rheum. Dis., *44*:425–428, 1985.
78. Morris, P.B., et al.: Rheumatoid arthritis and coronary arteritis. Am. J. Cardiol., *57*:689–695, 1986.
78a.Slack, J.D., and Waller, B.: Acute congestive heart failure due to the arteritis of rheumatoid arthritis: early diagnosis by endomyocardial biopsy: a case report. Angiology, *37*:477–482, 1986.
79. Bevans, M., et al.: The systemic lesions of malignant rheumatoid arthritis. Am. J. Med., *16*:298–304, 1954.
80. Lakhanpal, S., Conn, D.L., and Lie, J.T.: Clinical and prognostic significance of vasculitis as an early manifestation of connective tissue disease syndromes. Ann. Intern. Med., *101*:743–748, 1984.
81. Tribe, C.R., Scott, D.G.I., and Bacon, P.A.: The place of rectal biopsy in the diagnosis of systemic vasculitis. J. Clin. Pathol., *34*:843–850, 1981.
82. Conn, D.L., McDuffie, F.C., and Dyke, P.J.: Immunopathological study of sural nerves in rheumatoid arthritis. Arthritis Rheum., *15*:135–143, 1972.
83. Bywaters, E.G.L., and Scott, J.T.: The natural history of vascular lesions in rheumatoid arthritis. J. Chronic Dis., *16*:905–914, 1963.
84. Theophilopolous, A.N., et al.: IgG rheumatoid factor and low molecular weight IgM: an association with vasculitis. Arthritis Rheum., *17*:272–284, 1974.
85. Pope, R.M., and McDuffy, S.J.: IgG rheumatoid factor: relationship to seropositive rheumatoid arthritis and absence in seronegative disorders. Arthritis Rheum., *22*:988–998, 1979.
86. Elson, C.J., et al.: A new IgG rheumatoid factor assay and its use to analyse rheumatoid factor activity with human IgG isotopes. Rheumatol. Intern., *5*:175–179, 1985.
87. Venables, P.J.W., Erhardt, C.C., and Maini, R.N.: Antibodies to extractable nuclear antigens in rheumatoid arthritis: relationship to vasculitis and circulating immune complexes. Clin. Exp. Immunol., *39*:146–153, 1980.
88. Scott, D.G.I., et al.: Precipitating antibodies to nuclear antigens in systemic vasculitis. Clin. Exp. Immunol., *56*:601–606, 1984.
89. Weisman, M.H., and Zvaifler, N.J.: Vasculitis in connective tissue diseases. Clin. Rheum. Dis., *6*:351–372, 1980.
90. Franco, A.E., and Schur, P.H.: Hypocomplementemia in rheumatoid arthritis. Arthritis Rheum., *14*:231–238, 1971.
91. Woolf, A.D., et al.: Factor VIII related antigen in the assessment of vasculitis. Ann. Rheum. Dis., *46*:441–447, 1987.
92. Abel, T., et al.: Rheumatoid vasculitis: effect of cyclophosphamide on the clinical course and levels of circulating immune complexes. Ann. Intern. Med., *93*:407–413, 1980.
93. Scott, D.G.I., and Bacon, P.A.: Intravenous cyclophosphamide plus methylprednisolone treatment in systemic rheumatoid vasculitis. Am. J. Med., *76*:377–384, 1984.
94. Bacon, P.A.: Vasculitis—clinical aspects and therapy. *In* Biology of Vascular Disease, Acta. Med. Scand., Symposium Series 3 (Suppl 1) *715*:157–163, 1987.
95. Charcot, J.M.: Clinical lectures on senile and chronic diseases. Translated by Tuke, W.S. London, The New Sydenham Society, *95*:172–175, 1881.
96. Kirk, J., and Cosh, J.: The pericarditis of rheumatoid arthritis. Q. J. Med., *152*:397–423, 1969.

97. Nomeir, A.M., Turner, R., and Watts, E.: Cardiac involvement in rheumatoid arthritis. Ann. Intern. Med., 79:800–806, 1973.

98. Bacon, P.A., and Gibson, D.G.: Cardiac involvement in rheumatoid arthritis. Ann. Rheum. Dis., 33:20–24, 1974.

99. Cathcart, E.S., and Spodick, D.H.: Rheumatoid heart disease—a study of the incidence and nature of cardiac lesions in rheumatoid arthritis. N. Engl. J. Med., 266:959–964, 1962.

100. Bonfiglio, T., and Atwater, E.C.: Heart disease in patients with seropositive rheumatoid arthritis—a controlled autopsy study and review. Arch. Intern. Med., 124:714–719, 1969.

101. Jurik, A.G., and Graudal, H.: Pericarditis in rheumatoid arthritis. A clinical and radiological study. Rheumatol. Int., 6:37–42, 1986.

102. Richards, A.J., et al.: Rheumatoid pericarditis: comparison of immunologic characteristics of pericardial fluid, synovial fluid and serum. J. Rheumatol., 3:275–282, 1976.

103. Thomas, P., and Hare, J.: A case of rheumatoid arthritis and haemopericardium. Rheum. Rehab., 13:32–36, 1974.

104. Latham, B.A.: Pericarditis associated with rheumatoid arthritis. Ann. Rheum. Dis., 25(3):235–241, 1966.

105. Michet, C.J., and Hunder, G.G.: Pericarditis. In The Heart and Rheumatic Disease. Edited by B.M. Ansell and P.A. Simkin. Cornwall, Butterworths International Medical Reviews: Rheumatology, 2:1–26, 1984.

106. Bywaters, E.G.L.: The relation between heart and joint disease including 'rheumatoid heart disease' and chronic post-rheumatic arthritis (Type Jaccoud). Br. Heart J., 12:101–131, 1950.

107. Champion, G.D., Robertson, M.R., and Robinson, R.G.: Rheumatoid pleurisy and pericarditis. Ann. Rheum. Dis., 21:521–530, 1968.

108. Thadani, U., Iveson, J.M.I., and Wright, V.: Cardiac tamponade, constrictive pericarditis and pericardial resection in rheumatoid arthritis. Medicine (Baltimore), 54:261–270, 1975.

109. Scharf, J., et al.: Pericardial tamponade in juvenile rheumatoid arthritis. Arthritis Rheum., 19:760–762, 1976.

110. Thould, A.K.: Constrictive pericarditis in rheumatoid arthritis. Ann. Rheum. Dis., 45:89–94, 1986.

111. Isner, J.M., et al.: Computed tomography in the diagnosis of pericardial heart disease. Ann. Intern Med., 97:473–479, 1982.

112. Franco, A.E., Levine, H.D., and Hall, A.P.: Rheumatoid pericarditis: report of 17 cases diagnosed clinically. Ann. Intern. Med., 77:837–844, 1972.

113. Liew, M., et al.: Successful valve replacement for aortic incompetence in rheumatoid arthritis with vasculitis. Ann. Rheum. Dis., 38:483–484, 1979.

114. Newman, J.H., and Cooney, L.M., Jr.: Cardiac abnormalities associated with rheumatoid arthritis: aortic insufficiency requiring valve replacement. J. Rheumatol., 7:375–378, 1980.

115. Iveson, J.M.I., et al.: Aortic valve incompetence and replacement in rheumatoid arthritis. Ann. Rheum. Dis., 34:312–320, 1975.

116. Leak, A.M., Millar-Craig, M.W., and Ansell, B.M.: Aortic regurgitation in seropositive juvenile arthritis. Ann. Rheum. Dis., 40:229–234, 1981.

117. Cosh, J.A., and Lever, J.V.: The aortic valve. In The Heart and Rheumatic Disease. Edited by B.M. Ansell and P.A. Simkin. Cornwall, Butterworths International Medical Reviews: Rheumatology, 2:83–119, 1984.

117a. Cruikshank, B.: Heart lesions in rheumatoid disease. J. Pathol. Bacter., 76:223–240, 1958.

118. Roberts, W.C., et al.: Cardiovascular lesions in rheumatoid arthritis. Arch. Intern. Med., 122:141–146, 1968.

119. Good, A.E., et al.: Cardiac necrobiotic (rheumatoid?) granu-

120. Lebowitz, W.B.: The heart in rheumatoid arthritis (rheumatoid disease)—a clinical and pathological study of 62 cases. Arch. Intern. Med., 58:102–123, 1963.

121. Voncina, D., Rozman, B., and Cijan, A.: Felty's and Sjogren's syndromes and hypertrophic obstructive cardiomyopathy (case report). Zeitschrift fur Rheumatologie, 43:97–99, 1984.

122. Schwartz, S.: Rheumatoid carditis. JAMA, 201:556–558, 1967.

123. Kaplan, M.H., and Rakita, L.: Myocardial disease. In Immunological Diseases. Edited by M. Samter. Boston, Little Brown, 1971, p. 1378.

124. van Albada-Kuipers, G.A., et al.: Coronary arteritis complicating rheumatoid arthritis. Ann. Rheum. Dis., 45:963–965, 1986.

125. Morris, P.B., et al.: Rheumatoid arthritis and coronary arteritis. Am. J. Cardiol., 57:689–690, 1986.

126. Chausse, J.D., Blanchot, P., and Warin, J.: Atrioventricular block in rheumatoid arthritis. Rev. Rheum., 43:177–183, 1976.

127. Ahern, M., Lever, J.V., and Cosh, J.: Complete heart block in rheumatoid arthritis. Ann. Rheum. Dis., 42:113–115, 1983.

128. Gelso, A., Sanderson, J.M., and Carson, P.: Rheumatoid pericardial effusion with heart block treated by pericardectomy and implantation of permanent pacemaker. Br. Heart J., 39:113–115, 1977.

129. Davies, M.J.: Disorders of the conduction system. In The Kidney and Rheumatic Disease. Edited by P. Bacon and N.M. Hadler. Butterworths International Medical Reviews: Rheumatology, 2:65–82, 1984.

130. Browning, M.J., et al.: Ten years' experience of an amyloid clinic—a clinicopathological survey. Q. J. Med., 54:213–227, 1985.

131. Thery, C., Lekieffre, J., and Grosselin, B.: Le bloc auriculoventriculaire de la polyarthrite rhumatoide. Etude histologique due systeme de His-Tawara. Archives des Maladies du Coeur, 10:1181–1191, 1974.

132. Brandt, K., Cathcart, E.S., and Cohen, A.S.: Amyloid in an arthritis clinic. Am. J. Med., 44:955, 1968.

133. Prior, P., et al.: Cause of death in rheumatoid arthritis. Br. J. Rheumatol., 23:92–99, 1984.

134. Aronoff, A., Bywaters, E.G.L., and Fearnley, G.R.: Lung lesions in rheumatoid arthritis. Br. Med. J., 2:228–232, 1955.

135. Turner-Warwick, M., and Courtenay Evans, R.: Pulmonary manifestations. Clin. Rheum. Dis., 3(3):549–564, 1977.

136. Talbott, J.A., and Calkins, E.: Pulmonary involvement in rheumatoid arthritis. JAMA, 189:911, 1964.

137. Walker, W.C., and Wright, V.: Rheumatoid pleuritis. Ann. Rheum. Dis., 26:467, 1967.

138. Turner-Warwick, M., Burrows, B., and Johnson, A.: Cryptogenic fibrosing alveolitis: response to corticosteroid treatment and its effect on survival. Thorax, 35:593–599, 1980.

139. Popper, M.S., Bagdonoff, M.L., and Hughes, R.L.: Interstitial rheumatoid lung disease. Chest, 62:243, 1972.

140. Davidson, C., Brooks, A.G.F., and Bacon, P.A.: Lung function in rheumatoid arthritis. Ann. Rheum. Dis., 33:4, 1974.

141. Laitinen, O., et al.: Pulmonary involvement—patients with rheumatoid arthritis. Scand. J. Resp. Dis., 56:297, 1975.

141a. Hills, E.A., and Geary, M.: Membrane diffusing capacity and pulmonary capillary volume in rheumatoid disease. Thorax, 35:851–855, 1980.

142. Whorwell, P.J., Wojtulewski, J.A., and Lacey, B.W.: Respiratory function in rheumatoid arthritis. Br. Med. J., 2(5964):175, 1975.

142a.Oxholm, P., et al.: Pulmonary function in patients with rheumatoid arthritis. Scand. J. Rheumatol., *11*:109–112, 1982.

143. Collins, R.L., et al.: Obstructive pulmonary disease in rheumatoid arthritis. Arthritis Rheum., *19*:623–628, 1976.

144. Geddes, D.M., Webley, M., and Emerson, P.A.: Airways obstruction in rheumatoid arthritis. Ann. Rheum. Dis., *38*:222–225, 1979.

145. Gordon, D., et al.: Pulmonary involvement in RA. J. Rheumatol., *10*:395–440, 1983.

146. Baggenstoss, A.H., and Rosenberg, E.F.: Visceral lesions associated with chronic infectious (rheumatoid) arthritis. Arch. Path., *35*:503, 1943.

147. Sinclair, R.J.G., and Cruickshank, B.: A clinical and pathological study of sixteen cases of rheumatoid arthritis with extensive visceral involvement ('rheumatoid disease'). Q. J. Med., *25*:313–332, 1956.

148. Emerson, P.A.: Pleural effusion complicating rheumatoid arthritis. Br. Med. J., *i*:428, 1956.

149. Jurik, A.G., and Graudal, H.: Pleurisy in rheumatoid arthritis. Scand. J. Rheumatol., *12*:75–80, 1983.

150. Sievers, K., et al.: Studies of rheumatoid pulmonary disease; a comparison of roentgenological findings among patients with high rheumatoid factor titres and with completely negative reactions. Acta Tuberc. Scand., *45*:21–34, 1964.

151. Jurik, A.G., Davidsen, D., and Grandal, H.: Prevalence of pulmonary involvement in rheumatoid arthritis and its relationship to some characteristics of the patients. A radiological and clinical study. Scand. J. Rheumatol., *11*:217–224, 1982.

152. Delcambre, B., et al.: Rheumatoid pleurisy. Rev. Rheum., *47*:621–629, 1980.

153. Pauli, G., et al.: Pleural effusion as the presenting feature of RA. Poumom Coeur, *37*:213–217, 1981.

153a.Bankhurst, A.D., and Rowe, T.: Rheumatoid pleural effusions: the case for a primary glucose transport defect. J. Rheumatol., *7*:110–111, 1980.

154. Rothwell, R.S., and Davis, P.: Relationship between serum ferritin, anaemia, and disease activity in acute and chronic rheumatoid arthritis. Rheumatol. Int., *1*:65–67, 1981.

155. Portner, M.M., and Gracie, W.A., Jr.: Rheumatoid lung disease with cavity nodules, pneumothorax and eosinophilia. N. Engl. J. Med., *275*:697, 1968.

156. Berger, H.W., and Sekler, S.G.: Pleural and pericardial effusions in rheumatoid disease. Ann. Intern. Med., *64*:1291, 1960.

157. Carmichael, D.S., and Golding, D.N.: Rheumatoid pleural effusion with 'RA' cells in the pleural fluid. Br. Med. J., *ii*:814, 1967.

158. Boddington, M.M.L., and Spriggs, A.I.: Cytodiagnosis of rheumatoid pleural effusions. J. Clin. Pathol., *24*:95–106, 1971.

159. Engel, U., Aru, A., and Francis, D.: Rheumatoid pleurisy. Specificity of cytological findings. Acta Pathol. Microbiol. Immunol. Scand. (A), *94*:53–56, 1986.

160. Brennan, S.R., and Daly, J.J.: Large pleural effusions in rheumatoid arthritis. Br. J. Dis. Chest, *73*:133–140, 1979.

161. Heller, P., Kellow, W.F., and Chomet, B.: Needle biopsy of the parietal pleura. N. Engl. J. Med., *225*:684, 1956.

162. Portner, M.M., and Gracie, W.A., Jr.: Rheumatoid lung disease with cavity nodules, pneumothorax and eosinophilia. N. Engl. J. Med., *275*:697, 1968.

163. Campbell, G.D., and Ferrington, E.: Rheumatoid pleuritis with effusion. Chest, *53*:521, 1968.

164. Dieppe, P.A.: Empyema in rheumatoid arthritis. Ann. Rheum. Dis., *34*:181–185, 1975.

165. Gruenwald, P.: Visceral lesions in a case of rheumatoid arthritis. Arch. Pathol., *46*:59, 1948.

166. Scadding, J.G.: The lung in rheumatoid arthritis. Proc. R. Soc. Med., *62*:227, 1969.

167. Eraut, O.D., Egans, J., and Caplin, M.: Pulmonary necrobiotic rheumatoid nodules without rheumatoid arthritis. Br. J. Dis. Chest, *72*:301–306, 1978.

168. Hull, S., and Matthews, J.A.: Pulmonary necrobiotic nodules as a presenting feature of rheumatoid arthritis. Ann. Rheum. Dis., *41*:15–20, 1982.

169. Johnson, T.S., et al.: Endobronchial necrobiotic nodules antedating rheumatoid arthritis. Chest, *82*:199–200, 1982.

170. Panettiere, F., Chandler, B.F., and Libcke, J.H.: Pulmonary cavitation in rheumatoid disease. Am. Rev. Respir. Dis., *97*:89, 1968.

170a.Beumer, H.M., and Van Belle, C.J.: Pulmonary nodules in rheumatoid arthritis. Respiration, *29*:556, 1972.

171. Caplan, A.: Certain unusual radiological appearances in the chest of coal-miners suffering from rheumatoid arthritis. Thorax, *8*:29, 1953.

172. Hayes, D.S., and Posner, E.: A case of Caplan's syndrome in a roof tile maker. Tubercle, *41*:143, 1960.

173. Klockars, M.: Silica exposure and rheumatoid arthritis: a follow up study of granite workers 1940–81. Br. Med. J., *294*:997–1000, 1987.

174. Telleson, W.G.: Rheumatoid pneumoconiosis (Caplan's syndrome) in an asbestos worker. Thorax, *16*:372, 1961.

175. Caplan, A., Payne, R.B., and Withey, J.L.: A broader concept of Caplan's syndrome related to rheumatoid factors. Thorax, *17*:205, 1962.

176. Lindars, D.C., and Davies, D.: Rheumatoid pneumoconiosis. A study in colliery populations in the East Midlands coalfields. Thorax, *22*:525, 1967.

177. Stack, B.H.R., and Grant, I.W.B.: Rheumatoid interstitial lung disease. B. J. Dis. Chest, *59*:202, 1965.

178. Thomasi, T.B., Jr., Fudenberg, H.H., and Finby, N.: Possible relationship of rheumatoid factors and pulmonary disease. Am. J. Med., *33*:243–248, 1962.

179. Turner-Warwick, M., and Doniach, D.: Autoantibody studies in interstitial pulmonary fibrosis. Br. Med. J., *1*:886–891, 1965.

180. Pearsall, H.R., et al.: Disseminated pulmonary infiltrates associated with protein abnormalities. II. Pulmonary findings in patients with an elevated serum rheumatoid factor titre. Bull. Mason Clin., *21*:151–155, 1967.

181. Crystal, R.G., et al.: Idiopathic pulmonary fibrosis; clinical, histologic, radiographic, physiologic, scintigraphic, cytologic and biochemical aspects. Ann. Intern. Med., *85*:769–788, 1976.

182. Wolfe, F., et al.: Upper and lower airway disease in penicillamine treated patients with rheumatoid arthritis. J. Rheumatol., *10*:406–410, 1983.

183. Symmons, D.P.M., et al.: Factors influencing mortality in rheumatoid arthritis. J. Chron. Dis., *39*(2):137–145, 1986.

184. Dixon, A. St J., and Ball, J.: Honeycomb lung and chronic rheumatoid arthritis. A case report. Ann. Rheum. Dis., *16*:241, 1957.

185. Goodman, M., Knight, R.K., and Turner-Warwick, M.: Pilot study of penicillamine therapy in steroid failure patients with interstitial lung disease. *In* Modulation of Autoimmunity and Disease. Edited by R.N. Maini and H. Berry. New York, Praeger. Clinical Pharmacology and Therapeutics Series, *1*:41–299, 1981.

186. Wade, G.: Pulmonary hypertension in rheumatic heart disease. *In* The Heart and Rheumatic Disease. Edited by B.M.

Ansell and P.A. Simkin. Butterworths International Medical Reviews: Rheumatology, 2:151–185, 1984.

187. Yousem, S.A., Colby, T.V., and Carrington, C.B.: Lung biopsy in rheumatoid arthritis. Am. Rev. Respir. Dis., 131(5):770–777, 1985.

188. Geddes, D., Brewerton, D.A., and Turner-Warwick, M.: Obliterating airways in rheumatoid arthritis. Q. J. Med., 46:427–444, 1977.

189. Cooney, T.P.: Interrelationship of chronic eosinophilic pneumonia, bronchiolitis obliterans, and rheumatoid disease: a hypothesis. J. Clin. Pathol., 34:129–137, 1981.

190. Herzog, C.A., Miller, R.R., and Hoidal, J.R.: Bronchiolitis and rheumatoid arthritis. Am. Rev. Respir. Dis., 124:636–639, 1981.

191. Jansen, H.M., et al.: Progressive obliterative bronchiolitis in a patient with rheumatoid arthritis. Eur. J. Respir. Dis., 121(suppl.):43–52, 1982.

192. Sorenson, A.W-S.: The Waaler-Rose test in patients suffering from rheumatoid arthritis in relation to 24 hour endogenous creatinine clearance. Acta Rheum. Scand., 7:304, 1961.

193. Allander, E., et al.: Renal function in rheumatoid arthritis. Acta Rheum. Scand., 9:116, 1963.

194. Bulger, R.J., Healey, L.A., and Polinsky, P.: Renal abnormalities in rheumatoid arthritis. Ann. Rheum. Dis., 27:339, 1968.

195. Burry, H.C.: Reduced glomerular function in rheumatoid arthritis. Ann. Rheum. Dis., 31:65, 1972.

196. Whaley, K., and Webb, J.: Liver and kidney disease in rheumatoid arthritis. Clin. Rheum. Dis., 3(3):527–547, 1977.

197. Mutru, O., et al.: Ten year mortality and causes of death in patients with rheumatoid arthritis. Br. J. Med., 290:1797–1799, 1985.

198. Wegelius, O., et al.: Follow up study of amyloidosis secondary to rheumatic disease. In Amyloid and Amyloidosis. Edited by G.G. Glenner, P.P. e Costa, and A.F. de Freitas. Amsterdam, Excerpta Medica, 1980, pp. 183–190.

199. Pollack, V.E., et al.: The kidney in rheumatoid arthritis; study by renal biopsy. Arthritis Rheum., 5:1, 1962.

200. Camp, A.V., et al.: A study of renal disease in rheumatoid arthritis. Ann. Rheum. Dis., 32:278–279, 1973.

201. Mulhallawy, M.N.E., and Sabour, M.S.: Renal lesions in rheumatoid arthritis. Lancet, 2:852, 1959.

202. Lindvall, N.: Renal papillary necrosis. Acta Radiologica (Suppl.), 192:1–153, 1960.

203. Cove-Smith, R.: Analgesic nephropathy: pathogenesis, clinical features and association with rheumatoid arthritis. In The Kidney and Rheumatic Disease. Edited by P. Bacon and N.M. Hadler. Butterworths International Medical Reviews: Rheumatology, 1:228–245, 1982.

204. Burry, A.F.: The evolution of analgesic nephropathy. Nephron., 5:185–201, 1965.

205. Nanra, R.S., Chirawong, P., and Kincaid-Smith, P.: Medullary ischaemia in experimental analgesic nephropathy: the pathogenesis of renal papillary necrosis. Aust. NZ J. Med., 3:580–586, 1973.

206. Molland, E.A.: Experimental renal papillary necrosis. Kidney Int., 13:5–14, 1978.

207. Blackshear, J.I., et al.: Renal complications of non-steroidal anti-inflammatory drugs: identification and monitoring of those at risk. Semin. Arthritis Rheum., 14:163–175, 1985.

208. Walshe, J.J., and Venuto, R.C.: Acute oliguric renal failure induced by indomethacin; possible mechanism. Ann. Intern. Med., 91:47–49, 1979.

209. Unsworth, J., et al.: Renal impairment associated with non-steroidal anti-inflammatory drugs. Ann. Rheum. Dis., 46:233–236, 1987.

210. Adams, D.H., et al.: Non-steroidal anti-inflammatory drugs and renal failure. Lancet, 1:57–59, 1986.

211. Webb, J., et al.: Studies of renal function in Sjogren's syndrome and rheumatoid arthritis. Rheuma, 3:263, 1975.

212. Hall, C.L.: Gold and D-penicillamine induced disease. In Kidney and Rheumatic Disease. Edited by P. Bacon and N.M. Haldler. Butterworths International Medical Reviews: Rheumatology, 1:246–266, 1982.

213. Bacon, P.A., et al.: Penicillamine nephropathy in rheumatoid arthritis. Q. J. Med., 45:661–684, 1976.

214. Samuels, B., et al.: Membranous nephropathy in patients with rheumatoid arthritis: relationship to gold therapy. Medicine, 57:319–327, 1977.

215. Haymann, W., et al.: Production of nephrotic syndrome in rats by rat kidney suspension and Freund's adjuvant. Proc. Soc. Exp. Biol. Med., 100:660–664, 1959.

216. Davis, J.A., et al.: Glomerulonephritis in rheumatoid arthritis. Arthritis Rheum., 22:1018–1023, 1979.

217. Skrifvars, B.: Immunofluorescence study of renal biopsies in chronic rheumatoid arthritis. Scand. J. Rheumatol., 8:234–240, 1979.

218. Helin, H., et al.: Mild mesangial glomerulopathy—a frequent finding in rheumatoid arthritis patients with hematuria or proteinuria. Nephron, 42:224–230, 1986.

219. Higuchi, A., Suzuki, Y., and Okada, T.: Membranous glomerulonephritis in rheumatoid arthritis unassociated with gold or penicillamine treatment. Ann. Rheum. Dis., 46:488–490, 1987.

220. Pollak, V.E., et al.: The kidney in rheumatoid arthritis, studied by renal biopsy. Arthritis Rheum., 5:1–8, 1962.

221. Sellars, L., et al.: Renal biopsy appearance in rheumatoid disease. Clin. Nephrol., 20:114–120, 1983.

222. Willoughby, J.M.T., et al.: Smoking and peptic ulcer in rheumatoid arthritis. Clin. Exp. Rheumatol., 4:31–35, 1986.

223. Tribe, C.R., Bacon, P.A., and Mackenzi, J.C.: The accuracy of rectal biopsy in the diagnosis of systemic amyloidosis; pathological correlations. Amyloidosis E.A.R.S. Proc. First Eur. Amyloidosis Res. Symp., Bristol and Bath: 183–186, 1981.

224. Bjarnason, I.: Intestinal permeability and inflammation in rheumatoid arthritis: effects of non-steroidal anti-inflammatory drugs. Lancet, 2:1171–1174, 1984.

225. Struthers, G.R., et al.: Ultrastructural changes in the rectal mucosa of patients with rheumatoid arthritis. Ann. Rheum. Dis., 44:625–630, 1985.

226. Pallis, C.A., and Scott, J.T.: Peripheral neuropathy in rheumatoid arthritis. Br. Med. J., 1:1141–1147, 1965.

227. Chamberlain, M.A., and Bruckner, F.E.: Rheumatoid neuropathy: clinial and electrophysiological features. Ann. Rheum. Dis., 29:609–616, 1970.

228. Yamaguchi, D.M., Lipscomb, P.R., and Soule, E.H.: Carpal tunnel syndrome. Minn. Med., 48:22–33, 1965.

229. Fernandes, L., Goodwill, C.J., and Srivatsa, S.R.: Synovial rupture of rheumatoid elbow causing radial nerve compression. Br. Med. J., 2:17–18, 1979.

230. Grabois, M., Puentes, J., and Lidksy, M.: Tarsal tunnel syndrome in rheumatoid arthritis. Arch. Phys. Med. Rehabil., 62:401–403, 1981.

231. Lloyd, K., and Agarwa, A.: Tarsal-tunnel syndrome, a presenting feature of rheumatoid arthritis. Br. Med. J., 3:32, 1970.

232. Winfield, J., et al.: A prospective study of the radiological changes in the cervical spine in early rheumatoid disease. Ann. Rheum. Dis., 40:109–114, 1981.

233. Reference deleted.

234. Conlon, P.W., et al.: Rheumatoid arthritis of the cervical spine: an analysis of 33 cases. Ann. Rheum. Dis., 25:120–126, 1966.

235. Matthews, J.A.: Atlanto-axial subluxation in rheumatoid arthritis. Ann. Rheum. Dis., 28:260–266, 1969.

236. Marks, J.S., and Sharp, J.: Rheumatoid cervical myelopathy. Q. J. Med., 50:307–319, 1981.

237. Martel, W., and Abell, M.R.: Fatal atlanto-axial subluxation in rheumatoid arthritis. Arthritis Rheum., 6:224–231, 1963.

238. Webb, F.W.S., Hickman, J.A., and Brew, D. St. J.: Death from vertebral artery thrombosis in rheumatoid arthritis. Br. Med. J., 2:537–538, 1968.

239. Smith, P.H., Benn, R.T., and Sharp, J.: Natural history of rheumatoid cervical luxations. Ann. Rheum. Dis., 31:431–439, 1972.

240. Santavirta, S., et al.: Evaluation of patients with rheumatoid cervical spine. Scand. J. Rheumatol., 16:9–16, 1987.

241. Crellin, R.Q., MacCabe, J.J., and Hamilton, E.B.D.: Severe subluxation of the cervical spine in rheumatoid arthritis. J. Bone Joint Surg., 52B:244–251, 1970.

242. Ellman, P., Cudkowicz, L., and Elwood, J.S.: Widespread serous membrane involvement by rheumatoid nodules. J. Clin. Pathol., 7:239–244, 1954.

243. Markenson, J.A., et al.: Rheumatoid meningitis: a localized immune process. Ann. Intern. Med., 90:786–790, 1979.

244. Schachenmayr, W., and Friede, R.L.: Dural involvement in rheumatoid arthritis. Acta Neuropathol., 42:65–66, 1978.

245. Spurlock, R.G., and Richman, A.V.: Rheumatoid meningitis. A case report and review of the literature. Arch. Pathol. Lab. Med., 107:129–131, 1983.

246. Kim, R.C.: Rheumatoid disease with encephalopathy. Ann. Neurol., 7:86–91, 1980.

247. Kim, R.C., Collins, G.H., and Parisi, J.E.: Rheumatoid nodule formation within the choroid plexus. Report of a second case. Arch. Pathol. Lab. Med., 106:83–84, 1982.

248. Linquist, P.R., and McDonnell, D.E.: Rheumatoid cyst causing extradural compression: a case report. J. Bone Joint Surg., 52A:1235–1240, 1970.

249. Friedman, H.: Intraspinal rheumatoid nodule causing nerve root compression: case report. J Neurosurg., 32:689–691, 1970.

250. Hauge, T., et al.: Treatment of rheumatoid pachymeningitis involving the entire thoracic region. Scand. J. Rheumatol., 7:209–211, 1978.

251. Gupta, V.P., and Ehrlich, G.E. Organic brain syndrome in rheumatoid arthritis following steroid withdrawal. Arthritis Rheum., 19:1333–1338, 1976.

252. Skowronski, T., and Gatter, R.A.: Cerebral vasculitis associated with rheumatoid disease—a case report. J. Rheumatol., 1:473–475, 1974.

253. Adams, R.D.: Diseases of Muscle; A study in Pathology. 3rd Ed. New York, Harper & Row, 1975.

254. Reza, J.M., and Verity, M.A.: Neuromuscular manifestations of rheumatoid arthritis: a clinical and histomorphological analysis. Clin Rheum. Dis., 3(3):565–588, 1977.

255. Wegelius, O., Pasternack, A., and Kuhlback, B.: Muscular involvement in rheumatoid arthritis. Acta Rheumatol. Scand., 15:257–261, 1969.

256. Morgora, A., Wolf, E., and Gonen, B.: Electrodiagnostic investigation of the neuromuscular lesions in rheumatoid arthritis. Acta Rheumatol. Scand., 16:280–292, 1970.

257. Haslock, D.I., Wright,V., and Harriman, D.G.F.: Neuromuscular disorders in rheumatoid arthritis: a motorpoint muscle biopsy study. Q. J. Med., 39:335–358, 1970.

258. Kaplan, H., and Brooke, M.H.: Histochemical study of muscle in rheumatic disease. Arthritis Rheum., 14:168, 1971.

259. Bucknall, R.C., et al.: Myasthenia gravis associated with penicillamine treatment for rheumatoid arthritis. Br. Med. J., 1:600–602, 1975.

260. Maddison, P.J., and Bacon, P.A.: Vitamin D deficiency, spontaneous fractures, and osteopenia in rheumatoid arthritis. Br. Med. J., 4:433–435, 1974.

261. Kennedy, A.C., and Lindsay, R.: Bone involvement in rheumatoid arthritis. Clin. Rheum. Dis., 3:403–420, 1977.

262. Reid, D.M., et al.: Corticosteroids and bone mass in asthma: comparison with rheumatoid arthritis and polymyalgia rheumatica. Br. Med. J., 293:1463–1466, 1986.

263. Van Metre, T.D., et al.: The relationship between non-granulomatous uveitis and arthritis. J. Allergy, 36:158–174, 1965.

264. Kimura, S.J., et al.: Uveitis and joint diseases; clinical findings in 191 cases. Arch. Ophthalmol., 77:309–316, 1967.

265. Hazleman, B.L., and Watson, P.G.: Ocular complications of rheumatoid arthritis. Clin. Rheum. Dis., 3:501–526, 1977.

266. Rooney, P.J., et al.: Thin sclera: a clinical illusion. Ann. Rheum. Dis., 34:464–465, 1975.

267. Killian, P.J., McLain, B., and Lawless, O.J.: Brown's syndrome; an unusual manifestation of rheumatoid arthritis. Arthritis Rheum., 20:1080–1084, 1977.

268. Bridger, M.W., Jahn, A.F., and van Nostrand, A.W.: Laryngeal rheumatoid arthritis. Laryngoscope, 90:296–303, 1980.

269. Bienenstock, H.,. Ehrlich, G.E,., and Freyberg, R.H.: Rheumatoid arthritis of the cricoarytenoid joint: a clinicopathologic study. Arthritis Rheum., 6:48–63, 1963.

270. Lofgren, R.H., and Montogmery, W.W.: Incidence of laryngeal involvement in rheumatoid arthritis. N. Engl. J. Med., 267:193–195, 1962.

271. Polisar, I.A., et al.: Bilateral midline fixation of crico-arytenoid joints as a serious medical emergency. JAMA, 172:901–906, 1960.

272. Viney, L.L., and Westbrook, M.T.: Coping with chronic illness. J. Chronic. Dis., 37:489–502, 1985.

273. Mowat, A.G.: Hematological abnormalities in rheumatoid arthritis. Semin. Arthritis Rheum.,. 2:195–216, 1972.

274. Barager, F.D., and Duthie, J.J.R.: Importance of aspirin as a cause of anemia and peptic ulcer in rheumatoid arthritis. Br. Med. J., 1:1106–1108, 1960.

275. Bentley, D.P., and Williams, P.: Serum ferritin concentation as an index of storage iron in rheumatoid arthritis. J. Clin. Pathol., 27:786–788, 1974.

276. Hansen, T.M., and Hansen, N.E.: Serum ferritin as an indicator of iron responsive anemia in patients with rheumatoid arthritis. Ann. Rheum. Dis., 45:596–602, 1986.

277. Reference deleted.

278. Blake, D.R., et al.: The importance of iron in rheumatoid disease: an hypothesis. Lancet, 2:1142–1144, 1981.

279. Bentley, D.P.: Anemia and chronic disease. Clin. Haematol., 11:465–479, 1982.

280. Muirden, K.D.: The anaemia of rheumatoid arthritis: the significance of iron deposits in the synovial membrane. Aust. Ann. Med., 2:97–104, 1970.

281. Muirden, K.D.: Lymph node in iron in rheumatoid arthritis; histology, ultrastructure and chemical concentration. Ann. Rheum. Dis., 29:81–88, 1970.

282. Mowat, A.G., Hothersall, T.E., and Aitchison, W.R.C.: Nature of anaemia in rheumatoid arthritis. XI. Changes in iron metabolism induced by the administration of corticotrophin. Ann. Rheum. Dis., 28:303–309, 1969.

283. Dinant, H.J., and de Maat, C.G.: Erythropoiesis and mean

red-cell lifespan in normal subjects and in patients with the anaemia of active rheumatoid arthritis. Br. J. Haematol., 39:437–444, 1978.

284. Cavill, I., and Bentley, D.P.: Erythropoiesis in the anaemia of rheumatoid arthritis. Br. J. Haematol., 50:583–590, 1982.

285. Baer, A.N., et al.: Blunted erythropoietin response in rheumatoid arthritis. Br. J. Haematol., 66:559–564, 1987.

286. Sugimoto, M., et al.: Immunological aspects of the anemia of rheumatoid arthritis. Am. J. Hematol., 25:1–11, 1987.

287. Short, C.L., Bauer, W., and Reynolds, W.E.: Rheumatoid Arthritis. Cambridge, MA, Harvard University Press, 1957.

288. Robertson, M.D.J., et al.: Rheumatoid lymphadenopathy. Ann. Rheum. Dis., 27:253–260, 1968.

289. Symmons, D.P.M., Salmon, M., and Bacon, P.A.: The significance of lymphadenopathy in rheumatoid arthritis. Q. J. Med., 65:873–874, 1987.

290. Nosanchuk, J.S., and Schnitzer, B.: Follicular hyperplasia in lymph nodes from patients with rheumatoid arthritis; a clinicopathologic study. Cancer, 24:343–354, 1969.

291. Symmons, D.P.M., Salmon, M., and Bacon, P.A.: A study of lymph node lymphocytes in rheumatoid arthritis. Adv. Exp. Med. Biol., 186:1027, 1985.

292. Symmons, D.P.M.: Neoplasms of the immune system in rheumatoid arthritis. Am. J. Med., 78:22, 1985.

293. Felty, A.R.: Chronic arthritis in the adult, associated with splenomegaly and leukopenia; a report of five cases of an unusual clinical syndrome. Bull. Johns Hopkins Hosp., 35:16–20, 1924.

294. Spivak, J.L.: Felty's syndrome: an analytical review. Johns Hopkins Med. J., 141:156–162, 1977.

295. Termini, T.E., Biundo, J.J., Jr., and Ziff, M.: The rarity of Felty's syndrome. Ann. Rheum. Dis., 41:486–489, 1982.

296. Klouda, P.T., et al.: Felty's syndrome and HLA-DR antigens. Tissue Antigens, 27:112–114, 1986.

297. Runge, L.A., et al.:The inheritance of Felty's syndrome in a family with several affected members. J. Rheumatol., 13:39–42, 1986.

298. Bucknall, R.C., et al.: Neutropenia in rheumatoid arthritis: studies on possible contributing factors. Ann. Rheum. Dis., 41:242–247, 1982.

299. Bennettt, R.M.: Haematological changes in rheumatoid disease. Clin. Rheum. Dis., 3:433–465, 1977.

300. Hume, R., et al.: Anemia of Felty's syndrome. Ann. Rheum. Dis., 23:267–271, 1964.

301. Ruderman, M., Miller, L.M., and Pinals, R.S.: Clinical and serological observations on 27 patients wth Felty's syndrome. Arthritis Rheum., 11:377–384, 1968.

302. Davis, P., et al.: Depressed superoxide radical generation by neutrophils from patients with rheumatoid arthritis and neutropenia: correlation with neutrophil reactive IgG. Ann. Rheum. Dis., 46:51–54, 1987.

302a. Friman, C., et al.: Suppression of superoxide generation by normal polymorphonuclear leukocytes preincubated in plasma from patients with Felty's syndrome. Scand. J. Rheumatol., 16:113–120, 1987.

303. Bertouch, J.V., Johnston, C., and Davis, P.: Reversal of depressed neutrophil superoxide production in Felty's syndrome after gold therapy. J. Rheumatol., 14:52–54, 1987.

304. Isomaki, H., Koivisto, O., and Kivinity, K.: Splenomegaly in rheumatoid arthritis. Acta Rheumatol. Scand., 17:23–26, 1971.

305. Blendis, L.M., et al.: Nodular regenerative hyperplasia of the liver in Felty's syndrome. Q. J. Med., 43:25–32, 1974.

306. Laine, V.A.I., and Vainio, K.J.: Ulceration of the skin in rheumatoid arthritis. Acta Rheumatol. Scand., 1:113–118, 1955.

307. Wilkens, R.F., and Decker, J.L.: Rheumatoid arthritis with serological evidence of systemic lupus erythematosus. Arthritis Rheum., 6:720–735, 1973.

308. Laszlo, J., et al.: Splenectomy for Felty's syndrome. Clinicopathological study of 27 patients. Arch. Intern. Med., 138:597–602, 1978.

309. Logue, G.L., Huang, A.T., and Shimm, D.S.: Failure of splenectomy in Felty's syndrome. The role of antibodies supporting granulocyte lysis by lymphocytes. N. Engl. J. Med., 304:380–383, 1981.

310. Moore, R.A., et al.: Felty's syndrome: long term follow-up after splenectomy. Ann. Intern. Med., 75:381–385, 1971.

311. Thorne, C., and Urowitz, M.B.: Long-term outcome in Felty's syndrome. Ann. Rheum. Dis., 41:486–489, 1982.

312. Rosenthal, R.D., et al.: White cell antibodies and the aetiology of Felty's syndrome. Q. J. Med., 43:187–203, 1974.

313. Logue, G.: Felty's syndrome: granulocyte-bound immunoglobulin G and splenectomy. Ann. Intern. Med., 85:437–442, 1976.

314. Wilk, A., and Munthe, E.: Complement-fixing granulocyte-specific antinuclear factors in neutropenic cases of rheumatoid arthritis. Immunology, 26:1127–1134, 1974.

315. Rosenberg, J.N., et al.: Eosinophil-specific and other granulocyte-specific antinuclear antibodies in juvenile chronic polyarthritis and adult rheumatoid arthritis. Ann. Rheum. Dis., 34:350–353, 1975.

316. Breedveld, F.C., et al.: Felty syndrome: autoimmune neutropenia or immune-complex-mediated disease? Rheumatol. Int., 5:253–258, 1985.

317. Hurd, E.R., LoSpalluto, J., and Ziff, M.: The role of immune complexes in the production of the neutropenia of Felty's syndrome. J. Rheumatol., I (Suppl.):105, 1974.

318. Breedveld, F.C., et al.: Immune complexes and the pathogenesis of neutropenia in Felty's syndrome. Ann. Rheum. Dis., 45:696–702, 1986.

319. Calabresi, P., Edwards, E.A., and Schilling, R.F.: Fluorescent antiglobulin studies in leukopenic and related disorders. J. Clin. Invest., 38:2091–2100, 1959.

320. Kimball, H.R., et al.: Marrow granulocyte reserves in the rheumatic diseases. Arthritis Rheum., 16:345–352, 1973.

321. Duckham, D.J., et al.: Retardation of colony growth of in vitro bone marrow culture using sera from patients with Felty's syndrome, disseminated lupus erythematosus (SLE), rheumatoid arthritis, and other disease states. Arthritis Rheum., 18:323–333, 1975.

322. Gupta, R., Robinson, W.A., and Albrecht, D.: Granulopoietic activity in Felty's syndrome. Ann. Rheum. Dis., 34:156–161, 1975.

323. Abdou, N.I., et al.: Suppressor cell-mediated neutropenia in Felty's syndrome. J. Clin. Invest., 61:738–743, 1978.

324. Reference deleted.

325. Reference deleted.

326. Barton, J.C., et al.: Rheumatoid arthritis associated with expanded populations of granular lymphocytes. Ann. Intern. Med., 104:314–323, 1986.

327. Freimark, B., et al.: Comparison of T cell receptor gene rearrangements in patients with large granular T cell leukemia and Felty's syndrome. J. Immunol., 138:1724–1729, 1987.

328. McCullough, J., Clay, M.E., and Thompson, H.W.: Alloimmune and autoimmune cytopenia. Bailliere's Clinical Immunology and Allergy. 1, No2:303–326, 1987.

329. Wiesner, K.G., et al.: Immunosuppressive therapy in Felty's syndrome. N. Engl. J. Med., 296:1172, 1977.

330. Allen, L.S., and Groff, G.: Treatment of Felty's syndrome with

low dose oral methotrexate. Arthritis Rheum., *29*:902–905, 1986.

331. Lender, M., and Wolf, E.: Incidence of amyloidosis in rheumatoid arthritis. Scand. J. Rheumatol., *1*:109–112, 1972.

332. Wegelius, O., et al.: Follow up study of amyloidosis secondary to rheumatic disease. *In* Amyloid and Amyloidosis. Edited by G.G. Glenner, P.P. e Costa, and A.F. de Freitas. Amsterdam, Excerpta Medica, 1980, pp. 183–190.

333. Grindulis, K.A., et al.: Serum amyloid A protein during the treatment of rheumatoid arthritis with second-line drugs. Br. J. Rheum., *24*:158–163, 1985.

334. Bacon, P.A., et al.: Treatment regimes for AA amyloidosis. Amyloidosis E.A.R.S. Proc. First Eur. Amyloidosis Res. Symp., Bristol and Bath: 131–135, 1981.

335. Schnitzer, T.J., and Ansell, B.M.: Amyloidosis in juvenile chronic polyarthritis. Arthritis Rheum., *20*:245–252, 1977.

index

Page numbers in *italics* indicate illustrations; page numbers followed by "t" indicate tables.

1999